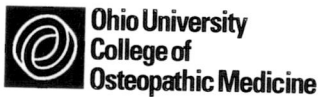

Principles of Geriatric Medicine and Gerontology

FIFTH EDITION

Principles of Geriatric Medicine and Gerontology

Editors

WILLIAM R. HAZZARD, M.D.

Professor of Medicine
University of Washington School of Medicine
Director, Geriatrics and Extended Care
VA Puget Sound Health Care System, Seattle, Washington

JOHN P. BLASS, M.D., PH.D.

Winifred Masteron Burke Professor of Neurology, Neuroscience, and Medicine
Director, Dementia Research Service
Weill Medical College of Cornell University
Burke Medical Research Institute, White Plains, New York

JEFFREY B. HALTER, M.D.

Professor of Internal Medicine
Director, Geriatrics Center and Chief, Division of Geriatric Medicine
Senior Research Scientist, Institute of Gerontology
University of Michigan
Research Scientist, GRECC, VA Ann Arbor Healthcare System, Ann Arbor, Michigan

JOSEPH G. OUSLANDER, M.D.

Professor of Medicine and Nursing
Director, Division of Geriatric Medicine and Gerontology
Chief Medical Officer, Wesley Woods Center of Emory University
Research Scientist, Birmingham/Atlanta VA GRECC, Atlanta, Georgia

MARY E. TINETTI, M.D.

Gladys Phillips Crofoot Professor of Medicine, Epidemiology, and Public Health
Director, Program on Aging, Yale University School of Medicine
New Haven, Connecticut

McGRAW-HILL

Professional

New York   Chicago   San Francisco   Lisbon   London   Madrid
Mexico City   Milan   New Delhi   San Juan   Seoul   Singapore   Sydney   Toronto

1234567890   KGPKGP   09876543

ISBN: 0-07-140216-0

This book was set in Times Roman by The GTS Companies/York, PA Campus
The editors were James Shanahan, Kathleen McCullough, and Karen G. Edmonson.
The production supervisor was Richard Ruzycka.
The cover designer was Janice Bielawa.
The indexer was Kathi Unger.
Quebecor World Kingsport was printer and binder.

This book is printed on acid-free paper.

Library of Congress Cataloging-in-Publication Data

CONTENTS

COLLEGE OF OSTEOPATHIC MEDICINE
LEARNING CENTER

PART I
PRINCIPLES OF GERONTOLOGY

PART II
PRINCIPLES OF GERIATRIC CARE

SECTION A   ASSESSMENT

SECTION D SURGICAL MANAGEMENT

PART III
ORGAN SYSTEMS AND DISEASES

SECTION A CARDIOLOGY

SECTION B RESPIRATORY SYSTEM

SECTION H   INFECTIOUS DISEASES AND IMMUNOLOGY

PART IV

CROSS CUTTING DOMAINS

SECTION A   NUTRITION

PART V

NEUROPSYCHIATRY

PART VI

GERIATRIC SYNDROMES

      Color plates appear between pages 788 and 789

Itamar B. Abrass, M.D. [124]
Professor and Chief, Division on Geriatrics
University of Washington School of Medicine
Harborview Medical Center
Seattle, Washington

Joseph V. Agostini, M.D. [117]
Robert Wood Johnson Clinical Scholar
Yale University School of Medicine
Department of Internal Medicine-Geriatrics
New Haven, Connecticut

Neil B. Alexander, M.D. [71]
Associate Professor of Medicine
Division of Geriatric Medicine
University of Michigan
Ann Arbor, Michigan

George S. Alexopoulos, M.D. [112]
Professor of Psychiatry
Weill Medical College of Cornell University
Cornell Institute of Geriatric Psychiatry
White Plains, New York

Richard M. Allman, M.D. [122]
Professor of Medicine
University of Alabama-Birmingham
Director, Birmingham/Atlanta VA GRECC
Birmingham, Alabama

Sonia Ancoli-Israel, Ph.D. [119]
Professor of Psychiatry
University of California, San Diego
Department of Psychiatry
San Diego, California

Toni C. Antonucci, Ph.D. [22]
Professor of Psychology
Program Director, Institute for Social Research
University of Michigan
Ann Arbor, Michigan

William J. Apfeldorf, M.D., Ph.D. [112]
Assistant Professor of Psychiatry
Weill Medical College of Cornell University
Cornell Institute of Geriatric Psychiatry
White Plains, New York

William B. Applegate, M.D., M.P.H. [40]
Dean, Wake Forest University School of Medicine
Senior Vice President
Wake Forest University Health Sciences
Winston-Salem, North Carolina

James A. Ashton-Miller, Ph.D. [71]
Senior Distinguished Research Scientist
Department of Mechanical Engineering
University of Michigan
Ann Arbor, Michigan

James L. Bailey, M.D. [45]
Professor of Medicine
Emory University School of Medicine
Renal Division
Atlanta, Georgia

Arthur K. Balin, M.D., Ph.D., F.A.C.P. [59]
Clinical Senior Investigator
Lankenau Institute for Medical Research
Jefferson Health System
Media, Pennsylvania

Steven Barczi, M.D. [93]

Assistant Professor of Medicine
University of Wisconsin-Madison
Associate Director, Clinical/GRECC
Madison, Wisconsin

Daniel R. Bensimhon [35]

Fellow, Division of Cardiology
Duke University Medical Center
Durham, North Carolina

Richard W. Besdine, M.D. [120]

Professor of Medicine
Brown Medical School
Director, Division of Geriatrics
Providence, Rhode Island

Adil E. Bharucha, M.D. [51]

Assistant Professor of Medicine
Mayo Medical School
Gastroenterology Research Unit
Rochester, Minnesota

Rex Biedenbender, M.D. [89]

Assistant Professor of Medicine
Glennan Center for Geriatrics and Gerontology
Eastern Virginia Medical School
Norfolk, Virginia

Marc R. Blackman, M.D. [20]

Clinical Director and Chief
Laboratory of Clinical Investigation
National Center for Complementary and Alternative Medicine
Bethesda, Maryland

John P. Blass, M.D., Ph.D. [107]

Winifred Masteron Burke Professor of Neurology, Neuroscience
and Medicine
Director, Dementia Research Service
Weill Medical College of Cornell University
White Plains, New York

Deborah T. Blumenthal, M.D. [58]

Assistant Professor of Neurology
Director, Division of Neuro-oncology
Huntsman Cancer Institute
Salt Lake City, Utah

Sidney S. Braman, M.D., F.C.C.P. [42]

Professor of Medicine
Brown Medical School
Director, Pulmonary, Critical Care, and Sleep Medicine
Providence, Rhode Island

Julie A. Braun, J.D., L.L.M. [27]

Attorney at Law
Law Office of J. A. Braun
Chicago, Illinois

Wendy Weinstock Brown, M.D., M.P.H. [46]

Professor of Internal Medicine
St. Louis University School of Medicine
Director, Clinical Nephrology
St. Louis, Missouri

Ferdinando S. Buonanno, M.D. [106]

Assistant Professor of Neurology
Harvard Medical School
Massachusetts General Hospital
Boston, Massachussetts

James R. Burke, M.D., Ph.D. [109]

Associate Professor of Medicine
Division of Neurology
Duke University Medical Center
Durham, North Carolina

Robert N. Butler, M.D. [98]

President and CEO, International Longevity Center
Professor of Geriatrics and Adult Development
Mt. Sinai Medical Center
New York, New York

Michael Camilleri, M.D. [51]

Professor of Medicine and Physiology
Mayo Medical School
Consultant, Division of Gastroenterology and Hepatology
Rochester, Minnesota

Elizabeth A. Capezuti, R.N., Ph.D. [27]

Associate Professor and Independence Foundation
Wesley Woods Chair in Gerontologic Nursing
Nell Hodgson Woodruff School of Nursing
Emory University
Atlanta, Georgia

Richard K. Capling, D.O. [46]

Fellow in Nephrology
St. Louis University School of Medicine
St. Louis, Missouri

Donald O. Castell, M.D. [50]

Professor of Medicine
Director, Esophageal Disorders Program
Medical University of South Carolina
Charleston, South Carolina

Marc F. Catalano, M.D. [57]

Associate Professor of Medicine
Medical College of Wisconsin
Milwaukee, Wisconsin

Jane A. Cauley, Dr.P.H. [99]

Associate Professor
Department of Epidemiology
University of Pittsburgh
Pittsburgh, Pennsylvania

Alan Chait, M.D. [34]

Professor of Medicine
Head, Division of Metabolism, Endocrinology, and Nutrition
University of Washington School of Medicine
Seattle, Wisconsin

Mary Y. Chang, Ph.D. [34]

Acting Assistant Professor
University of Washington School of Medicine
Seattle, Washington

Gurkamal S. Chatta, M.D. [60],[61]

Associate Professor of Medicine
Division of Hematology/Oncology
University of Pittsburgh
UPMC Cancer Pavilion
Pittsburgh, Pennsylvania

Joshua Chodosh, M.D., M.S.H.S. [25]

Assistant Professor of Medicine
Division of Geriatrics
UCLA School of Medicine
VA Greater Los Angeles Health System
Department of Research and Development
Los Angeles, California

Brenna Cholerton, Ph.D. [105]

Senior Fellow
VA Puget Sound Health Care System
Tacoma, Washington

Giovanni Cizza, M.D., Ph.D. [20]

Clinical Neuroendocrinology Branch
National Institute of Mental Health
National Institutes of Health
Bethesda, Maryland

Harvey Jay Cohen, M.D. [53]

Professor of Medicine
Duke University Medical Center
Director, Aging Center
Chief, Division of Geriatrics
Durham, North Carolina

Mairav Cohen-Zion, M.S. [119]

University of California, San Diego
Joint Doctoral Program in Clinical Psychology
Veterans Affairs Healthcare System
San Diego, California

Eric A. Coleman, M.D., M.P.H. [13]

Associate Professor of Medicine
University of Colorado Health Sciences Center
Hartford/Jahnigen Geriatric Center for Excellence
Denver, Colorado

Leo M. Cooney, M.D. [79]

Humana Foundation Professor of Geriatric Medicine
Chief, Section of Geriatric Medicine
Yale University School of Medicine
New Haven, Connecticut

Suzanne Craft, Ph.D. [105]

Adjunct Professor of Psychiatry
University of Washington School of Medicine
Seattle, Washington

Jeffrey L. Cummings, M.D. [9]

Professor of Neurology
UCLA School of Medicine
Los Angeles, California

Toni M. Cutson, M.D. [24]

Associate Clinical Professor
Department of Medicine/Geriatrics
Duke University Medical Center
Durham, North Carolina

Osvaldo Delbono, M.D., Ph.D. [70]

Associate Professor of Medicine and Physiology/Pharmacology
Wake Forest University School of Medicine
Winston-Salem, North Carolina

Mauro Di Bari, M.D., Ph.D. [40]

Department of Critical Care Medicine and Surgery
Unit of Gerontology and Geriatrics
Azienda Ospedaliera Careggi
Florence, Italy

Margaret A. Drickamer, M.D. [10]

Associate Professor of Medicine
Yale University School of Medicine
New Haven, Connecticut

Catherine E. DuBeau, M.D. [101]

Assistant Professor of Medicine
Harvard Medical School
Gerontology Division, Beth Israel Deaconess Medical Center
Urban Medical Group
Jamaica Plain, Massachusetts

Gustave Duque, M.D. [75]

Assistant Professor of Medicine
Division of Geriatric Medicine
McGill University
Montreal, Quebec
Canada

E. Wesley Ely, M.D., M.P.H. [15]

Associate Professor of Medicine
Division on Allergy, Pulmonary and Critical Care Medicine
Center for Health Services Research of Vanderbilt University
Nashville, Tennessee

Paul L. Enright, M.D. [41]

Research Associate Professor of Medicine
University of Arizona
Tucson, Arizona

William B. Ershler, M.D. [63]

Director, Institute for Advanced Studies in Aging and
Geriatric Medicine
Washington, DC

Viktor E. Eysselein, M.D. [57]

Professor of Medicine
Chief of Gastroenterology
UCLA School of Medicine
Torrance, California

Monsignor Charles J. Fahey [28]

Professor Emeritus
Fordham University
Loretto Institute for the Frail Elderly
Bronx, New York

Stanley Fahn, M.D. [108]

Professor of Neurology
Director, Center for Parkinson's Disease and Other Movement
Disorders
Columbia University College of Physicians and Surgeons
New York, New York

David Felson, M.D. [74]

Professor of Medicine & Public Health
Chief, Section of Clinical Epidemiology
Boston University School of Medicine
Boston, Massachusetts

Bruce A. Ferrell, M.D. [25]

Associate Professor of Medicine
Division of Geriatrics
UCLA School of Medicine
Los Angeles, California

James Ferrendelli, M.D. [111]

Kraft W. Eidman Professor and Chairman
Department of Neurology
University of Texas-Houston Medical School
Houston, Texas

Luigi Ferrucci, M.D., Ph.D. [4]

Coordinator of the Laboratory of Clinical Epidemiology
Chief of the Geriatric Section, INRCA Geriatric Department
Italian National Institute on Aging
Florence, Italy

Ellen Flaherty, R.N., Ph.D.(C), G.N.P. [21]

Project Director, GITT Resource Center
New York University
The Steinhardt School of Education
Division of Nursing
New York, New York

Liana Fraenkel, M.D., M.P.H. [74]

Assistant Professor of Medicine
Yale University School of Medicine
Chief, Section of Rheumatology
New Haven, Connecticut

Linda P. Fried, M.D., M.P.H. [116]

Professor of Medicine, Epidemiology and Health Policy
Director, Center on Aging and Health
Deputy Director for Clinical Epidemiology and Health Services
Research
Johns Hopkins Medical Institutions
Baltimore, Maryland

Terry Fulmer, Ph.D., R.N., F.A.A.N. [21]

Interim Division Head & Professor of Nursing
New York University
The Steinhardt School of Education
New York, New York

Curt D. Furberg, M.D., Ph.D. [40]

Professor of Public Health Sciences
Wake Forest University School of Medicine
Winston-Salem, North Carolina

Elizabeth Gardner, Ph.D. [3]

Assistant Professor
Department of Bioscience and Biotechnology
Drexel University
Philadelphia, Pennsylvania

Andrew W. Gardner, Ph.D. [39]
Professor, Department of Health and Sport Sciences
University of Oklahoma
Norman, Oklahoma

Thomas A. Glass, Ph.D. [5]
Assistant Professor
Johns Hopkins Bloomberg School of Public Health
Department of Epidemiology
Baltimore, Maryland

Andrew P. Goldberg, M.D. [68]
Professor, Division of Gerontology
University of Maryland School of Medicine
Director, GRECC
Baltimore VA Maryland Healthcare System
Baltimore, Maryland

Stefan Gravenstein, M.D., M.P.H. [89]
Professor of Medicine
Glennan Center for Geriatrics and Gerontology
Eastern Virginia Medical School
Norfolk, Virginia

Tomas L. Griebling, M.D. [100]
Assistant Professor of Urology
Assistant Scientist–Center on Aging
University of Kansas
Kansas City, Kansas

David A. Gruenewald, M.D. [65]
Associate Professor of Medicine
University of Washington School of Medicine
VA Puget Sound Healthcare System
Seattle, Washington

Jack M. Guralnik, M.D., Ph.D. [4]
Chief, Epidemiology and Demography Office
Laboratory of Epidemiology, Demography and Biometry
National Institute on Aging
Bethesda, Maryland

Jerry H. Gurwitz, M.D. [19]
The Dr. John Meyers Professor of Primary Care Medicine
University of Massachusetts Medical School
Executive Director, Meyers Primary Care Institute
Worcester, Massachusetts

Karen E. Hall, M.D., Ph.D. [48]
Assistant Professor of Internal Medicine
University of Michigan Healthcare System
Ann Arbor VA Medical Center
Ann Arbor, Michigan

Jeffrey B. Halter, M.D. [67]
Professor of Internal Medicine
Director, Geriatrics Center and Chief, Division of
Geriatric Medicine
Senior Research Scientist, Institute of Gerontology
University of Michigan
Research Scientist, GRECC, VA Ann Arbor Healthcare System
Ann Arbor, Michigan

Danielle Harari, M.B.B.S. [52]
Clinical Senior Lecturer in Elderly Medicine
King's College London
Consultant Physician, St. Thomas' Hospital
London, England

Tamara B. Harris, M.D., M.S. [91]
Chief, Geriatrics Epidemiology Section
Laboratory of Epidemiology, Demography and Biometry
National Institute on Aging
Bethesda, Maryland

Sima Hassani, D.O. [66]
West Los Angeles VA Medical Center
UCLA School of Medicine
Los Angeles, California

William R. Hazzard, M.D. [6],[34],[97]
Professor of Medicine
University of Washington School of Medicine
Director, Geriatrics and Extended Care
VA Puget Sound Health Care System
Seattle, Washington

Beth A. Hellerstedt, M.D. [55]
Fellow, Division of Hematology and Oncology
University of Michigan Medical Center
Ann Arbor, Michigan

Jerome M. Hershman, M.D. [66]
Professor of Medicine
UCLA School of Medicine
West Los Angeles VA Medical Center
Los Angeles, California

Kevin P. High, M.D. [82]
Associate Professor of Medicine
Section on Infectious Diseases
Wake Forest University School of Medicine
Winston-Salem, North Carolina

Amine Hila, M.D. [50]
Research Fellow
Medical University of South Carolina
Division of Gastroenterology and Hepatology
Charleston, South Carolina

John H. Hodges, D.P.M. [80]

Instructor
Department of Orthopaedic Surgery
Wake Forest University School of Medicine
Winston-Salem, North Carolina

Helen Hoenig, M.D. [24]

Assistant Professor of Medicine
Duke University Medical Center
Chief, Physical Medicine and Rehabilitation Service
Durham VA Medical Center
Durham, North Carolina

Kathryn Hyer, Dr.P.A. [21]

Director, Training Academy on Aging
FPECA
University of South Florida
Tampa, Florida

Sharon K. Inouye, M.D. [117]

Associate Professor of Medicine
Yale University School of Medicine
New Haven, Connecticut

Bryan D. James, M.Bioethics [29]

University of Pennsylvania
Ralston-Penn Center
Philadelphia, Pennsylvania

Cheryl A. Jay, M.D. [86]

Associate Clinical Professor
Department of Neurology
University of California, San Francisco
San Francisco, California

Larry E. Johnson, M.D. [90]

Medical Director, Extended Care Unit
Central Arkansas Veteran's Healthcare System
North Little Rock VA Hospital
North Little Rock, Arkansas

Theodore M. Johnson, II, M.D., M.P.H. [123]

Manager, Geriatrics and Extended Care Service Line
Atlanta VA Medical Center
Atlanta Site Director, Birmingham/Atlanta GRECC
Decatur, Georgia

Barry D. Jordan, M.D., M.P.H. [110]

Director, Head Injury Service
The Burke Rehabilitation Hospital
White Plains, New York

Amy C. Justice, M.D., Ph.D. [87]

Associate Professor
University of Pittsburgh School of Medicine
VA Pittsburgh Healthcare System
Pittsburgh, Pennsylvania

Balu Kalayam, M.D. [115]

Associate Professor of Clinical Psychiatry
Weill Medical College of Cornell University
The New York Presbyterian Hospital–Westchester Division
White Plains, New York

Lillian Kao, M.D. [32]

Assistant Professor, Surgery
University of Texas, Health Sciences Center at Houston
Houston, Texas

Jason H. T. Karlawish, M.D. [29]

Assistant Professor of Medicine
University of Pennsylvania
Ralston-Penn Center
Philadelphia, Pennsylvania

Paul R. Katz, M.D. [17]

Professor of Medicine
University of Rochester Medical School
Monroe Community Hospital
Rochester, New York

Leslie I. Katzel, M.D., Ph.D. [68]

Associate Professor, Division of Gerontology
University of Maryland
Associate Director, GRECC
Baltimore VA Medical Center
Baltimore, Maryland

Rose Anne Kenny, M.D., F.R.C.P.I. [121]

Professor of Cardiovascular Research
University of Newcastle-Upon-Tyne
Institute for Ageing and Health
Newcastle-Upon-Tyne,
United Kingdom

Howard L. Kim, M.D. [111]

Department of Neurology
University of Texas-Houston Medical School
Houston, Texas

Gretchen G. Kimmick, M.D. [54]

Assistant Professor of Medicine
Section on Hematology/Oncology
Wake Forest University School of Medicine
Winston-Salem, North Carolina

Abby C. King, Ph.D. [23]
Associate Professor of Health Research and Policy and Medicine
Stanford University School of Medicine
Palo Alto, California

Mary B. King, M.D. [118]
Assistant Professor of Clinical Medicine
University of Connecticut School of Medicine
Hartford Hospital Geriatric Program
Hartford, Connecticut

Marvin M. Kirsh, M.D. [30]
Professor of Surgery
University of Michigan School of Medicine
Director, Cardiothoracic Surgery
Ann Arbor, Michigan

J. Phillip Kistler, M.D. [106]
Professor of Neurology
Harvard Medical School
Director, Stroke Service
Boston, Massachusetts

Mary Ann Knovich, M.D. [64]
Fellow, Section on Hematology and Oncology
Wake Forest University School of Medicine
Wintston-Salem, North Carolina

Wendy M. Kohrt, Ph.D. [72]
Professor of Medicine
Division of Geriatric Medicine
University of Colorado Health Sciences Center
Denver, Colorado

Anand Kumar, M.D. [114]
Professor of Psychiatry
UCLA Neuropsychiatric Institute and Hospital
Los Angeles, California

Mark S. Lachs, M.D., M.P.H. [125]
Co-Director, Division of Geriatric Medicine and Gerontology
Weill Medical College of Cornell University
New York, New York

Edward G. Lakatta, M.D. [33]
Director, Laboratory of Cardiovascular Science
Gerontology Research Center
Intramural Research Program
National Institute on Aging
Baltimore, Maryland

Eric B. Larson, M.D., M.P.H. [11]
Professor of Medicine and Medical Director
University of Washington Medical Center
Seattle, Washington

Bruce Leff, M.D. [18]
Associate Professor of Medicine
Johns Hopkins University School of Medicine
Johns Hopkins Geriatric Center
Baltimore, Maryland

Cari R. Levy, M.D. [15]
Fellow, Division of Geriatrics
University of Colorado Health Sciences Center
Denver, Colorado

Myrna I. Lewis, Ph.D. [98]
International Longevity Center
New York, New York

David A. Lipschitz, M.D., M.P.H. [60],[61]
Professor and Chair
Donald W. Reynolds Department of Geriatrics
University of Arkansas for Medical Sciences
Little Rock, Arkansas

Mark B. Loeb, M.D., M.Sc. [82]
Associate Professor
Departments of Pathology and Molecular Medicine
Clinical Epidemiology and Biostatistics
Hamilton, Ontario
Canada

Richard F. Loeser, M.D. [70]
Associate Professor of Medicine
Rush Medical College
Rush-Presbyterian-St. Luke's Medical Center
Chicago, Illinois

Karl Lorenz, M.D., M.S.H.S. [26]
Clinical Instructor in Medicine
UCLA School of Medicine
General Medicine Staff and Consultant
VA Greater Los Angeles Healthcare System
Los Angeles, California

Kenneth W. Lyles, M.D. [69]
Professor of Medicine
Duke University Medical Center
Clinical Director, GRECC
Durham VA Medical Center
Durham, North Carolina

Joanne Lynn, M.D. [26]
Director, RAND Center to Improve Care of the Dying
Arlington, Virginia

George L. Maddox, Ph.D. [5]
Professor Emeritus of Medical Sociology
Duke University Medical Center
Center for Aging
Durham, North Carolina

Edward R. Marcantonio, M.D., S.M. [16]
Assistant Professor of Medicine
Harvard Medical School
Director of Quality and Outcomes Research
Hebrew Rehabilitation Center for Aged
Boston, Massachusetts

Thomas J. Marrie, M.D. [83]
Professor and Chair
Department of Medicine
University of Alberta
Edmonton, Alberta
Canada

Alvin M. Matsumoto, M.D. [65]
Professor of Medicine
University of Washington School of Medicine
VA Puget Sound Health Care System
Seattle, WA

Karen A. Matthews, Ph.D. [99]
Professor, Department of Psychiatry
University of Pittsburgh
Department of Psychology
Pittsburgh, Pennsylvania

Mark P. Mattson, Ph.D. [104]
Gerontology Research Center
National Institute on Aging
Baltimore, Maryland

Melissa Matulis, M.D. [64]
Fellow, Section on Hematology and Oncology
Wake Forest University School of Medicine
Wintston-Salem, North Carolina

Annette Medina-Walpole, M.D. [17]
Assistant Professor of Medicine
University of Rochester Medical School
Monroe Community Hospital
Rochester, New York

Stephen W. Meldon, M.D. [14]
Assistant Professor of Emergency Medicine
Case Western Reserve University
MetroHealth Medical Center
Cleveland, Ohio

Esteban Mezey, M.D. [49]
Professor of Medicine
Johns Hopkins University School of Medicine
Division of Gastroenterology
Baltimore, Maryland

Myron Miller, M.D. [47]
Professor of Medicine
Johns Hopkins University School of Medicine
Sinai Hospital of Baltimore
Baltimore, Maryland

Richard A. Miller, M.D., Ph.D. [1]
Professor of Pathology
Associate Director, Geriatrics Center
Senior Research Scientist, Institute of Gerontology
University of Michigan
Ann Arbor, Michigan

John H. Mills, Ph.D. [96]
Professor and Vice Chairman
Department of Otolaryngology-Head and Neck Surgery
Medical University of South Carolina
Charleston, South Carolina

Nadeem Mirza, M.D. [113]
Clinical Fellow
Geriatric Psychiatry Branch
National Institute of Mental Health
Bethesda, Maryland

John E. Morley, M.D., B.Ch. [102]
Dammert Professor of Gerontology
Director, Division of Geriatric Medicine
St. Louis University Health Sciences Center
St. Louis, Missouri

Donna M. Murasko, Ph.D. [3]
Office of the Dean
College of Arts and Sciences
Drexel University
Philadelphia, Pennsylvania

Hyman B. Muss, M.D. [54]
Professor of Medicine
Director, Hematology/Oncology
University of Vermont
Fletcher Allen Health Care
Burlington, Vermont

Aman Nanda, M.D. [120]
Assistant Professor of Medicine
Brown Medical School
Division of Geriatrics
Providence, Rhode Island

Lindsay E. Nicolle, M.D. [85]
Professor of Medicine
University of Manitoba, Health Sciences Center
Winnipeg, Mannitoba
Canada

Kenneth S. O'Rourke, M.D. [77],[81]
Associate Professor of Medicine
Head, Section on Rheumatology
Wake Forest University School of Medicine
Winston-Salem, North Carolina

Mark B. Orringer, M.D. [30]
John Alexander Distinguished Professor of Thoracic Surgery
University of Michigan School of Medicine
Head, Section of Thoracic Surgery
Ann Arbor, Michigan

Joseph G. Ouslander, M.D. [123]
Professor of Medicine and Nursing
Director, Division of Geriatric Medicine and Gerontology
Chief Medical Officer, Wesley Woods Center of
Emory University
Investugator, Birmingham, Atlanta VA Grecc, Atlanta, Georgia

John Owen, M.D. [64]
Professor of Internal Medicine
Section on Hematology and Oncology
Wake Forest University School of Medicine
Wintston-Salem, North Carolina

Marco M. Pahor, M.D. [40]
Professor of Internal Medicine
Director, J. Paul Sticht Center on Aging
Wake Forest University School of Medicine
Winston-Salem, North Caolina

Alireza Pakkar, M.D. [9]
UCLA School of Medicine
Los Angeles, California

Robert M. Palmer, M.D., M.P.H. [14]
Associate Professor of Medicine
Ohio State University
The Cleveland Clinic Foundation
Cleveland, Ohio

Miguel A. Paniagua, M.D. [6]
Senior Fellow/Acting Instructor
University of Washington School of Medicine
Harborview Medical Center
Seattle, Washington

Michael C. Perry, M.D. [56]
Professor of Internal Medicine
Director, Division of Hematology and Medical Oncology
University of Missouri
Ellis Fischel Cancer Center
Columbia, Missouri

Eric Peterson, M.D. [35]
Associate Professor of Medicine
Division of Cardiology
Duke University Medical Center
Durham, North Carolina

Elizabeth A. Phelan, M.D., M.S. [6]
Acting Assistant Professor of Medicine
University of Washington School of Medicine
Harborview Medical Center
Seattle, Washington

Kenneth J. Pienta, M.D. [55]
Professor of Internal Medicine and Urology
Director, Urologic Oncology Program
University of Michigan
Ann Arbor, Michigan

Jerome B. Posner, M.D. [58]
Evelyn Frew American Cancer Society Clinical Research Professor
George C. Cotzias Chair of Neuro-oncology
Memorial Sloan-Kettering Cancer Center
New York, New York

Bayard L. Powell, M.D. [62]
Professor of Internal Medicine
Head, Section on Hematology and Oncology
Wake Forest University School of Medicine
Winston-Salem, North Carolina

Karen M. Prestwood, M.D. [75]
Assistant Professor of Medicine
University of Connecticut School of Medicine
Center on Aging
Farmington, Connecitut

Bruce M. Psaty, M.D., Ph.D. [40]
Professor of Medicine
University of Washington
Cardiovascular Health Research Unit
Seattle, Washington

Peter V. Rabins, M.D. [113]

Professor of Psychiatry
Department of Psychiatry and Behavioral Sciences
Johns Hopkins University School of Medicine
Baltimore, Maryland

Shobita Rajagopalan, M.D. [84]

Associate Professor of Medicine
Division of Infectious Diseases
Charles R. Drew University of Medicine and Sciences
King-Drew Medical Center
Los Angeles, California

Vikram Jala Reddy, M.D. [38]

Department of Medicine
Mullenburg Hospital
Robert Wood Johnson Medical School
New Brunswick, New Jersey

Mark Reger, Ph.D. [105]

Senior Fellow
University of Washington School of Medicine
Seattle, Washington

Sonya Reicher, M.D. [57]

Resident in Internal Medicine
Harbor-UCLA Medical Center
Torrance, California

David B. Reuben, M.D. [8]

Professor of Medicine
Chief, Geriatric Medicine & Gerontology
UCLA School of Medicine
Los Angeles, California

Michael W. Rich, M.D. [37]

Associate Professor of Medicine
Cardiovascular Division
Washington University School of Medicine
St. Louis, Missouri

JoAnne Robbins, Ph.D. [93]

Associate Professor of Medicine
University of Wisconsin-Madison
Associate Director of Research/GRECC
Madison, Wisconsin

Paula A. Rochon, M.D., M.P.H. [19]

Associate Professor of Medicine and Public Health Sciences
University of Toronto
Scientist, Institute for Clinical Evaluative Sciences
Toronto, Ontario
Canada

Eugenio R. Rocksmith, M.D. [110]

Head Injury Service
The Burke Rehabilitation Hospital
White Plains, New York

G. Alec Rooke, M.D., Ph.D. [31]

Professor of Anesthesiology
University of Washington School of Medicine
VA Puget Sound Health Care System
Seattle, Washington

Linda A. Russell, M.D. [76]

Assistant Professor of Medicine
Weill-Cornell Medical College
The Hospital for Special Surgery
New York, New York

Sanjeev Saksena, M.D., F.A.C.C. [38]

Arrhythmia and Pacemaker Service
Cardiovascular Institute
Atlantic Health System (East)
Warren, New Jersey

Jeff M. Sands, M.D. [45]

Professor of Medicine and Physiology
Emory University School of Medicine
Renal Division
Atlanta, Georgia

John Santinga, M.D. [36]

Associate Professor of Internal Medicine
Divisions of Geriatric Medicine and Cardiology
University of Michigan
Ann Arbor, Michigan

Kenneth Schmader, M.D. [88]

Associate Professor of Medicine
Division of Geriatrics
Duke University Medical Center
Durham, North Carolina

Richard Schulz, Ph.D. [22]

Professor of Psychiatry
Director, University Center for Social and Urban Research
The University of Pittsburgh
Pittsburgh, Pennsylvania

Robert S. Schwartz, M.D. [72]

Professor of Medicine
Division Head, Geriatric Medicine
University of Colorado Health Sciences Center
Denver, Colorado

Marie-Florence Shadlen, M.D. [11]
Assistant Professor of Medicine
University of Washington School of Medicine
Seattle, Washington

Nasir Shahab, M.D. [56]
Assistant Professor of Clinical Medicine
University of Missouri-Columbia
Ellis Fishel Cancer Center
Columbia, Missouri

Jonathan A. Ship, D.M.D. [94]
Professor, Department of Oral Medicine
New York University College of Dentistry
Director, Bluestone Center for Clinical Research
New York, New York

Shahid Sial, M.D. [57]
Assistant Professor of Medicine
Director of Endoscopy, Division of Gastroenterology
UCLA School of Medicine
Torrance, California

Mika Sinanan, M.D., Ph.D. [32]
Associate Professor of Surgery
University of Washington School of Medicine
Seattle, Washington

John D. Sorkin, M.D., Ph.D. [39]
Department of Medicine, Division of Gerontology
University of Maryland, GRECC
VA Medical Center
Baltimore, Maryland

Stephanie Studenski, M.D., M.P.H. [73]
Professor of Medicine
University of Pittsburgh
Division of Geriatric Medicine
Pittsburgh, Pennsylvania

Dennis H. Sullivan, M.D. [90]
Associate Professor of Medicine and Geriatrics
Vice Chairman, Donald W. Reynolds Department of Geriatrics
University of Arkansas for Medical Sciences
Little Rock, Arkansas

Trey Sunderland, M.D. [113]
Chief, Geriatric Psychiatry Branch
National Institute of Mental Health
Bethesda, Maryland

George E. Taffet, M.D. [33]
Associate Professor of Medicine
Chief, Section of Geriatrics and Cardiovascular Sciences
Baylor College of Medicine
Houston, Texas

Syed Tariq, M.D. [102]
Fellow, Geriatric Medicine
St. Louis University Health Sciences Center
St. Louis, Missouri

Robert D. Teasdall, M.D. [80]
Associate Professor
Department of Orthopaedic Surgery
Wake Forest University School of Medicine
Winston-Salem, North Carolina

J. Lisa Tenover, M.D., Ph.D. [103]
Associate Professor of Medicine
Emory University School of Medicine
Chief of Medicine
Wesley Woods Center of Emory University
Atlanta, Georgia

Victor J. Thannickal, M.D. [43]
Assistant Professor of Internal Medicine
Division of Pulmonary and Critical Care Medicine
University of Michigan, School of Medicine
Ann Arbor, Michigan

Mary E. Tinetti, M.D. [7]
Gladys Phillips Crofoot/Professor of Medicine, Epidemiology, and Public Health
Director, Program on Aging, Yale University School of Medicine
New Haven, Connecticut

Galen B. Toews, M.D. [43]
Professor of Internal Medicine
Chief, Division of Pulmonary and Critical Care Medicine
University of Michigan School of Medicine
Ann Arbor, Michigan

M. A. Topcuoglu, M.D. [106]
Fellow, Neurology Service
Massachusetts General Hospital
Boston, Massachusetts

Jack I. Twersky, M.D. [88]
Assistant Clinical Professor of Medicine
Division of Geriatrics
Duke University Medical Center
Durham, North Carolina

Peter Vaitkevicius, M.D. [30]

Assistant Professor of Geriatrics and Cardiology
University of Michigan School of Medicine
VA Ann Arbor Health Care System
Ann Arbor, Michigan

Philip A. Vedovatti, M.D. [32]

Clinical Assistant Professor of Medicine
University of Washington School of Medicine
Medicine Consult Service
Seattle, Washington

Subir Vij, M.D., M.P.H. [89]

Assistant Professor of Medicine
Glennan Center for Geriatrics and Gerontology
Eastern Virginia Medical School
Norfolk, Virginia

Jeffrey I. Wallace, M.D., M.P.H. [92]

Associate Professor of Medicine
Division of Gerontology and Geriatric Medicine
University of Colorado Health Sciences Center
Denver, Colorado

Jeremy D. Walston, M.D. [116]

Associate Professor of Medicine
Johns Hopkins University School of Medicine
Johns Hopkins Asthma and Allergy Center
Baltimore, Maryland

Louise C. Walter, M.D. [12]

Assistant Professor of Medicine
University of California, San Francisco
Staff Physician, San Francisco VA Medical Center
San Francisco, California

Eugenia Wang, M.D. [2]

Professor, Department of Biochemistry and Molecular Biology
University of Louisville
Louisville, Kentucky

Gale R. Watson, Med, C.L.V.T. [95]

Research Health Scientist
Rehabilitation Research and Development Center on Vision Loss
and Aging
Atlanta VA Medical Center
Decatur, Georgia

Andrew D. Weinberg, M.D., F.A.C.P. [27]

Associate Professor of Medicine
Emory University School of Medicine
Medical Director for Long-Term Care
Wesley Woods Center for Emory University
Atlanta, Georgia

Aviva D. Wertkin, B.S. [20]

Laboratory of Clinical Investigation
National Center for Complementary and Alternative
Medicine
National Institutes of Health
Bethesda, Maryland

Jocelyn Wiggins, B.M., B.Ch., M.R.C.P. [44]

Lecturer, Division of Geriatric Medicine
University of Michigan School of Medicine
Ann Arbor, Michigan

Sara Wilcox, Ph.D. [23]

Assistant Professor
University of South Carolina
Department of Exercise Science
Columbia, South Carolina

Thomas T. Yoshikawa, M.D. [84]

Professor and Chair
Department of Medicine
King/Drew Medical Center
Los Angeles, California

Raymond Yung, M.D. [78]

Assistant Professor of Internal Medicine
Division of Geriatric Medicine
University of Michigan
Ann Arbor, Michigan

Mark Yurkofsky, M.D., C.M.D. [16]

Clinical Instructor in Medicine
Harvard Medical School
Director, Extended Care Facilities Program
Harvard Vanguard Medical Associates
Boston, Massachusetts

PREFACE

Five years have passed since the publication of the fourth edition of the *Principles of Geriatric Medicine and Gerontology*. In the interval, we have entered a new millennium, the human genome has been mapped, and the scourge of human immunodeficiency virus (HIV)-related illness has become less terrifying.

In the same interval, baby boomers have become another five years older. The leading edge of the boomer generation has begun to anticipate both the glowing prospect of a life of fulfillment and unfettered freedom in retirement, while also nervously wondering whether retirement will be affordable. They are also concerned about when the physical and psychological challenges of old age will begin to encroach upon that freedom.

During those same five years, the complementary fields of geriatric medicine and gerontology, which are the dual foci of this volume, have continued to mature in parallel with the progressive aging of the population. Advances continue apace on genetic and subcellular aspects of aging at the one extreme and continued extension of functional independence and average longevity at the other. To reflect this progress, while facilitating mastery of the various domains of geriatric medicine, the fifth edition has been extensively reorganized. The opening section on the "Principles of Gerontology" is substantially truncated, to just 6 chapters, highlighting areas with broad, cross-cutting implications for the practice of geriatric medicine. Conversely, chapters dealing with the aging-related (gerontologic) aspects of the physiology of the various organ systems are grouped together with chapters focused on the disorders of those systems in elderly patients (e.g., the chapters on "Circulatory Function" [33] and "Atherosclerosis" [34] are included in the section on "Cardiology"). In addition several of the sections focused upon problems of specific organ systems are expanded (e.g., the section on "Oncology and Hematology" now has 12 chapters, one dealing with general principles and the other 11 dealing with specific forms of malignancy and hematological disease). This mirrors the inclusion of a substantial number of chapters (12) covering neurospsychiatry that began with the second edition, in recognition of the central position of these issues and

diseases in geriatric care. In addition, the major section on the "Principles of Geriatric Care," comprising 26 chapters, is updated to address both patient-focused and systems issues. A major outcome of the redesign of the fifth edition is the addition and clustering of chapters on other areas of major concern to geriatricians, namely nutrition; sensory function; and gender, sex, and sexuality. The volume closes with 10 chapters that highlight the progress made over the past 5 years in understanding and managing geriatric syndromes, the health conditions that perhaps best define the field of geriatrics and that often constitute the primary focus of the medical care of the frail elderly patient. All in all, 125 chapters in the fifth edition strive to encompass a vast and growing field.

The physical constraint posed by attempting to provide comprehensive coverage of an expanding field within a constant page limit proved a challenge to the authors and editors of the fifth edition. Of substantial help in this regard, and in keeping with trends in medical communication, we instructed authors to select a limited number of key references to landmark studies and critical reviews that will readily provide entry to the primary and secondary medical literature for the reader eager to pursue a topic in depth.

Thus, as with the first four editions, the fifth edition attempts to provide a comprehensive array of chapters that are all relevant to the care of the oldest, frailest, and most vulnerable patients. Again, it is designed according to the organizing assumption that such patients will be cared for by virtually all practicing physicians and that trained and certified geriatricians will comprise but a small fraction of that physician workforce. Encouragingly, that philosophy appears to be increasingly embraced by virtually all sectors of the American medical profession, acknowledging the special role of geriatricians as teachers, researchers, organizational leaders, and physicians to a limited number of perhaps the most frail, complex, and challenging patients. Accordingly, the curricula of medical students, residents, and fellows from a broad array of disciplines (with the sole exception of pediatrics, perhaps) are being enriched in gerontologic and geriatric content and experience, a new generation of teachers and leaders with focused expertise in this arena are rising through the ranks of the academic disciplines and professional societies, and aging research is growing rapidly in both quality and quantity. But none too soon. The age wave keeps approaching, and unless we prevail in providing that first-quality expertise, our health care system may yet be inundated by a tsunami of unmet need and demand.

The editors are indebted to the authors of the chapters and the McGraw-Hill's James Shanahan, who shepherded this edition to publication with deft organizing skill. We also acknowledge those who have supported our editorial efforts from our academic offices. These include Anna Marie Ciresi at Yale University School of Medicine, Ann Pine and Judy Seeger at the University of Michigan, Susan Ratliff at Emory University, and Carol Montanaro at Burke Medical Research Institute. And we all pay special tribute to Nancy Woolard at the J. Paul Sticht Center on Aging at Wake Forest University School of Medicine. As with the last three editions, Nancy has served as senior editorial assistant and final common pathway for assembly of the fifth edition of the *Principles of Geriatric Medicine and Gerontology*.

Willliam R. Hazzard, M.D.

Principles of
Geriatric Medicine
and Gerontology

PART I

PRINCIPLES OF GERONTOLOGY

The Biology of Aging and Longevity

RICHARD A. MILLER

Aging is a process that converts healthy adults into frail ones with diminished reserves in most physiologic systems and an exponentially increasing vulnerability to most diseases and to death. Aging is a mystery, in the sense that cancer, heredity, development, and infection were once mysteries, and cognition still is: a process so poorly understood that we cannot yet be sure how to go about seeking an explanation. The impact of aging on health and well-being dwarfs that of any single category of illness, because aging is itself the principal risk factor for most important diseases of late life. For this reason, the ability to modify the aging rate in humans to the degree that is now routine in mice and some other animals would be of greater benefit than the entire abolition of cancer, cardiovascular diseases, and diabetes (see Fig. 1-1).

This chapter provides a brief overview of what is now known, or suspected, about the basic biological processes of aging: what aging is, what aging does, why aging occurs at all (from an evolutionary perspective), and what biochemical processes seem likely to contribute to age-associated decline. The chapter finishes with an annotated selection of some promising research areas in basic gerontology. Readers interested in deeper and broader introductions can turn to several monographs and review collections listed at the end of the chapter.

MATTERS OF TERMINOLOGY AND RECOMMENDED DEFINITIONS

Although laypersons and physicians alike can tell young people apart from old people, and although researchers generate hundreds of papers each year describing the effects of age at ever finer levels of cellular and molecular detail, the fundamental processes that control the rate at which people age and that can explain how aging leads to the diseases of aging are still essentially unknown. Experimental work over the last 30 years has, however, ruled out theories of aging that once seemed promising, while providing new support for several others. Before we delve into

these results, however, it may be helpful to focus first on a set of working definitions.

The definition that began this chapter—aging as a process that converts healthy adults into frail ones with diminished reserves in most physiologic systems and an exponentially increasing vulnerability to diseases and death—was proposed to help focus attention on uniform, broadly based, deteriorative changes as the fundamental concern for experimental gerontology. Some authorities have argued that aging should be viewed as an extension of the normal developmental process that turns fertilized eggs into reproductively mature adults. This idea seems seriously flawed: although there may well be senescent processes that begin in early life or that depend upon embryogenic and maturational processes, there is no good reason to suspect that the mechanisms that convert zygotes into adults will closely resemble those that turn adults into 90-year-olds. In fact, the two processes differ in a fundamental way: the steps of development are strongly regulated by darwinian selection, while in contrast, the degenerative changes of aging reflect the cumulative damage permitted by the absence of strong selective pressures at advanced ages. The steps that convert steel and glass into new automobiles are very different from those that produce used cars from new ones.

A second set of confusions arises from borrowed terminology, the use of common terms to describe more than one biological phenomenon. Thus the term *senescence* has been used to describe annual leaf abscission from deciduous plants, the removal of erythrocytes from circulation, and the conversion of proliferative cell cultures to differentiated, nondividing progeny, as well as the effects of aging on whole animals. While it is possible that important insights into organismal aging can be gained from the study of such models (see the discussion of clonal senescence below in the "Four Hot Topics" section), it is important to avoid the tempting assumption that study of senescence in these senses will necessarily prove relevant to the study of senescent change in intact, multicellular organisms. The same caveat can be applied to the analysis of various forms of programmed (apoptotic) cell death, whose analysis is

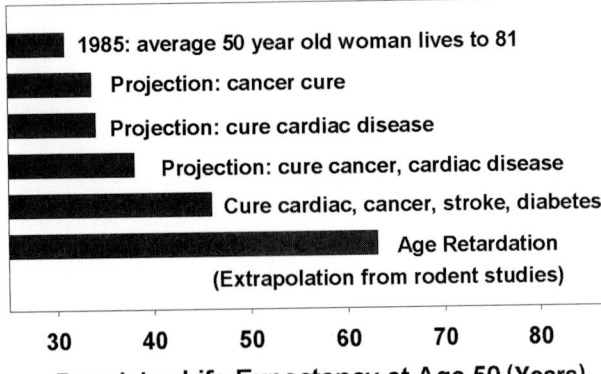

Remaining Life Expectancy at Age 50 (Years)

Figure 1-1 Theoretical remaining life expectancy of a 50-year-old white woman in the United States under a variety of demographic assumptions. The *top bar* shows remaining life expectancy with disease-specific mortality rates that prevailed in 1985. The four middle bars show projected life expectancy under the assumption that mortality risks for the indicated diseases were in fact zero. Data from Olshansky SJ et al: *Science* 250:634, 1990. The *bottom line* shows projected longevity if it were possible to retard human aging to the same degree that is obtained in the typical study of caloric restriction in rats or mice. Figure reprinted with permission from Miller RA: *Milbank Q* 2002 (in press).

neither more nor less likely to reveal important insights into aging than investigation of other major biological processes with less-suggestive names.

A less-tractable set of confusions arises from our inability to measure aging directly, as it occurs, in any single individual. We can measure a huge variety of age-sensitive outcomes, including gray hair, skin wrinkles, collagen cross-linking, maximum work output and endurance, number of hepatomas, and antibody responses, in individual subjects, but each of these, and probably all other indirect indices of aging, are also influenced by genetic and environmental factors besides aging per se. It is tempting to argue from this perspective that there is no single process worth calling aging, because no two people age in exactly the same way, and to argue that gerontologists are merely studying the effects of a variety of diseases that afflict some, but not all, old people. We have not, however, abandoned the idea of a unified process of embryogenesis simply because newborns differ from one another. One 70-year-old person may be hard of hearing, another vulnerable to influenza, and a third no longer able to climb five flights of stairs, but it is rare to find a 20-year-old with any of these problems, and rare to find a 90-year-old who has avoided all of them. It is also unlikely to be merely coincidental that a spectrum of disabilities, including declines in cardiovascular reserve, neurosensory function, immune response, and increased incidence of neoplastic and degenerative diseases, affects old mice, old horses, and old dogs in patterns recognizably similar to those seen in aging humans.

The relationship between aging and disease can be seen as a special case of the question of interindividual differences just discussed. The details of how aging contributes to, and alters, various diseases will be addressed in most of the other chapters in this text. Here, however, we confront the more general issue: which age-dependent changes can be considered a part of "normal" aging, and which are aspects of disease? The matter is not merely semantic: researchers who wish to measure the effects of normal aging on some end point (immune function, perhaps, or speed in the 100 meter dash) typically try to compare disease-free young and old subjects to avoid the objection that any differences seen might not be a result of aging per se but instead be a result of diseases present in a proportion of the elderly subject pool. This makes excellent sense: a group of 80-year-olds of whom 10% are cardiac patients and another 10% suffer from Alzheimer's disease is unlikely to produce a good average time in the 100 yard dash. On the other hand, classification of an 80-year-old as "disease-free" is itself problematic. An 80-year-old who has osteoporosis but no broken bones, prostatic hypertrophy but no malignancy, or coronary atherosclerosis but no angina may be classified disease-free by some conventions and for some purposes, but it is clear that the dividing line, wherever it is drawn, will be arbitrary from the perspective of basic biology. If one does locate a group of 80-year-olds that meet a rigorous set of exclusion criteria, is it reasonable to allow this highly atypical group to represent the "typical" aged human?

One way to deal with this chronic debate is to acknowledge that while it may not be possible to decide whether a specific condition (loss of visual acuity, or atheromatous change, etc.) represents an effect of aging with variable expression in different individuals, or is, instead, a disease that accompanies aging in some but not all people, it is in practice often possible to discern an effect of aging despite the confounding effects of age-related disease. It is important to realize that while the effects of aging may not become obvious until the last quarter of life, the process by which aging produces 70-year-olds acts throughout adult life. Changes that occur progressively and (almost) universally throughout the middle half of life are likely to be reflections of aging rather than of illness. It is difficult to study aging by studies of elderly people, in whom aging effects are confounded by latent or apparent disease and by the effects of selective prior mortality. The proper study of the biogerontologist is the middle-aged.

TWO FUNDAMENTAL OBSERVATIONS

A discussion of the mechanisms of aging should start from two observations that are so obvious that they typically go unstated, their implications ignored. The first is that old mice, old dogs, old horses, and old people all resemble one another. The second is that old people are older than old horses, dogs, or mice: it takes longer to produce an old human than it does to produce an old dog, with the same collection of tooth problems, diminished muscle strength and cardiovascular endurance, impaired protective immunity, cataracts, and benign and potentially lethal neoplastic lesions. These two generalities, so commonplace that they are familiar to children, nonetheless constitute the central "core" observations that will need to be explained by any comprehensive molecular model of the aging process.

Aged mice, dogs, and humans share a common loss of physiologic reserve in most cellular and physiologic systems, which, in turn, leads to an exponentially increasing vulnerability to most forms of life-threatening illnesses. The details, particularly of the final failure mode, can differ from species to species, and indeed from strain to strain: some rodents are more susceptible than others to kidney degeneration, and some are more susceptible to lymphomas, while no rodent seems at risk for the atherosclerosis and Alzheimer's disease that often lead to death in humans. Yet in each mammalian species, aging brings easily recognizable changes in phenotype, some biochemical, some physiologic: alterations in hair coloration; loss of immune function; decline in cardiovascular capabilities; alterations in collagen and crystallin structure; increases in pigment deposition; changes in protein synthesis and degradation rates; impaired balance, strength, coordination, and memory; and declining reproductive performance among many others. The challenge is to explain why all these deleterious changes occur in rough synchrony within each species, but over time-scales that differ as much as 30-fold among the species of mammals. The eye lens, thymic tissue, and skeletal muscle of a young adult mouse look very similar, histologically, to the corresponding sections of a young adult human, and yet all three will start to fail, in the rodent, within 2 to 3 years, for reasons that are at present entirely inexplicable at the molecular and cellular levels. There is no physical law that prevents a rodent or dog from owning teeth and hearts that last 60 years, as they do in humans; the basis for these differences in synchronized longevity are fundamentally understood in evolutionary terms, but not yet in molecular terms.

EVOLUTIONARY INSIGHTS INTO THE AGING PROCESS

Unlike the biochemists and cell physiologists, the evolutionary biologists have, over the last 35 years, produced a convincing picture of the way in which evolutionary pressures lead to the development of aging, a picture that explains how longevity is distributed across species and makes predictions that can be (and have been) tested in laboratory and field situations. The modern evolutionary theory of aging, based on ideas of Medawar and Haldane, fully stated by G. Williams in 1957, and then developed quantitatively by Charlesworth and his colleagues, has already had a substantial influence on thinking about aging, and is just beginning to exert a salutary effect on selection of experimental models.

Why do we age? The naive intuition that aging evolves in order to remove old individuals and thus prevent them from competing with their offspring is now known not to have any merit: there is no evolutionary advantage in ceasing to produce offspring at an age when others of the same species, lacking the gene(s) that induce senescence, are still reproductively active. Aging is not "programmed" in the genes, in the same sense that developmental processes are programmed. Instead, the modern model begins from the observation that individuals would have a substantial probability of dying even in the absence of any effect of aging. In the absence of aging, the mortality rate would be unrelated to chronologic age, and the survival curve

would resemble the familiar exponential decay curve of radioisotopes. Thus members of a nonaging population are in no sense immortal, even though they do not exhibit the characteristic age-related exponential increase in mortality risk. In a hypothetical nonaging population, in which half the individuals die each year as a consequence of predation, starvation, infection, or other ill fortune, the fraction of individuals surviving to the fifth year will be small; and those surviving to 15 years vanishingly so.

In this nonaging population, there would be very little selection pressure against genes whose harmful effects are "late" relative to ages at which most individuals are likely already to have died. In addition, there would be strong pressure in favor of genes that were beneficial early in life, even if these genes carried with them harmful effects later in the life span. In a species in which half the individuals die each year, for example, a mutant gene that prevents some degenerative disease that only affects 10-year-old members of the species will have no chance of fixation, because there will be few, if any, 10-year-old individuals in the population. On the contrary, genes that increase the fitness of 1-year-olds and 2-year-olds would be highly favored, even if as a side effect they lead to lethal diseases in 5- and 10-year-olds, because they have a good chance of "saving" some lucky recipients and little chance of doing any harm by killing a 10-year-old (because 10-year-olds are very rare). Both these pressures favor the evolution of genetic alleles whose negative effects are postponed until late in life; that is, genes that cause aging, as a side effect.

Thus evolutionary considerations predict that nearly all species (or more precisely, species in which the germ line cells can be distinguished from somatic tissues) will evolve an aging phenotype, in which the risk of mortality increases with time as a consequence of (1) selective pressures for genes whose beneficial early effects more than compensate for any injurious late life effects, and (2) a lack of selection pressure against genes whose effects, though entirely negative, are delayed until very late in life. It is not hard to suggest plausible examples. A gene that leads to calcium deposition, for example, may promote the rapid development of the bones needed to support independent locomotion, and yet predispose to arterial calcification in later life. A gene that promotes rapid cell division in embryogenesis may also render an animal vulnerable, in later life, to rapid growth of neoplastic tissue.

Why do we age at the rate we do? The power of selective pressures on genes that have distinct effects on reproductive fitness in young and old individuals depends greatly on the details of the ecologic niche of the species in question. Animals subjected to high predation pressures as adults, for example, evolve genomes that favor rapid production of large litters. Diminished predation pressure (e.g., as a consequence of size, fierceness, habitat, speed or the ability to fly), or lifestyles that require intensive protection or education of juveniles by adults, diminish the pressures for rapid reproduction, and thus increase the reproductive value of the later stages of adult life. A subpopulation of a species that finds itself isolated in a new habitat relatively free of predators, for example, will feel weaker selective pressures for rapid reproduction; conversely, genes that lead to disabilities at more advanced ages are now for the first time themselves subjected to darwinian pressures as more individuals reach the ages in question. Thus the species may, given sufficient population size, time, and genetic heterogeneity, evolve into a new species or subspecies with postponed physiologic senescence and a longer life span; that is, a species that ages more slowly than did the ancestral population.

Laboratory and field work has illustrated these principles in action. Several groups have found evidence for genes in fruit flies that accelerate reproduction (and are hence usually highly favored) but that also accelerate the aging process. Artificial selection for flies that could produce eggs late in life creates, over many generations, a population that produces fewer offspring early in life, and thus would have lowered darwinian fitness under natural conditions, but which lives longer than did the flies in the initial starting population. Biochemical studies of these flies and their shorter-lived relatives may produce some insights into the aging process in flies, and offer clues about the controls of aging in mammals.

It is not yet clear whether similar breeding schemes will work in mammals; this will depend in part on whether a given species retains allelic differences that could contribute to increased longevity even at the expense of impaired reproductive fitness. Austad's work, however, suggests that such polymorphisms are likely to have been retained by natural mammalian populations. Austad compared survival and reproduction in two groups of closely related opossums, one population of which has lived on an island unconnected to the mainland for 4500 years, and thus been subject to greatly diminished levels of predation pressure, that is, with less selection for extremely rapid reproduction. In good agreement with the evolutionary ideas, the island population was found to age more slowly, as measured both by longevity and alterations in collagen biochemistry, and to devote a diminished amount of effort to early reproduction (see Fig. 1-2). This study shows that selective pressures can lead fairly quickly to changes in the frequency of genes that alter aging rate in mammals. Studies of the genetic and physiologic differences between these two closely related groups of opossums, or between populations of mice selectively bred for differences in reproductive scheduling, could provide important insights into the control of the aging rate.

Analyses of the distribution of longevity among species have also generated support for predictions of the evolutionary model. Among mammals, for example, bats are remarkably long-lived as compared to nonflying mammals of similar mass; gliding mammals also tend to have longer maximum life spans than closely related nongliding species. It is worth noting that this relationship between life span and reduced predation pressure is not the trivial result of decreased death by predation per se, but rather an evolved, intrinsic change, induced by differences in selective pressures but demonstrable in predator-free environments. The exceptional longevity of birds, turtles, and porcupines also reflects their relative invulnerability to predation, and the accompanying advantages of genetic alleles that prolong survival, and therefore reproductive competence, for extended periods of time, even at the cost of an initial rapid burst of reproduction. Biochemists and

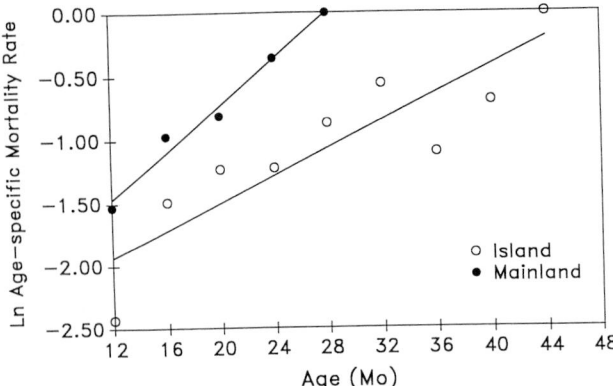

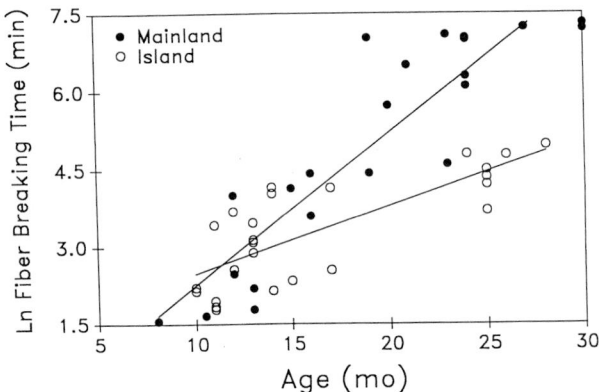

Figure 1-2 Differential aging in two closely related populations of opossums. *Top panel:* Gompertz analysis shows lower aging rate in island opossums. *Bottom panel:* Island opossums show a slower rate of collagen cross-linking as measured by tail tendon break time. From Austad J: Zool. London 229:695, 1993.

cell physiologists have been lamentably slow to exploit these insights from comparative biology. Birds that live 5 to 10 times longer than comparably sized mammals have apparently evolved protective mechanisms, for example, antioxidant pathways and controls on oncogene expression, that account for their resistance to age-related pathology and dysfunction, and which might well be worth careful molecular analysis.

Comparative biogerontology, that is, the analysis of the distribution of aging patterns across species, supports an important conclusion: the generation of a long-lived species from shorter-lived ancestors occurs quite frequently in the evolutionary radiation. In addition to the aforementioned bats, birds, turtles, and porcupines, the evolutionary record contains a wealth of other examples, including elephants, whales, hyenas, hippopotami, and naked mole rats among the more photogenic. Nature seems to have no difficulty decelerating life history transitions, and aging along with them, when this provides a way to use a low hazard ecologic niche effectively. It is difficult to see how such a commonplace evolutionary event could arise, over and over again in separate lineages, if aging rate were indeed regulated by a very large number of system-specific genetic switches—some regulating the rate of immune aging, others timing the effects of aging on bone, still others with influence on the pace of aging in teeth, vascular endothelia, oncogenesis, the eye lens, the skin, and so forth. Furthermore, genetic alleles that ensured 50 years of protective immunity would be of little use (and thus have little selective advantage) in a creature whose other systems began to show critical failures after a single decade. The frequency with which evolutionary process give rise to coordinated deceleration of so many forms of age-related dysfunction provides support for the hypothesis that the timing of life history trajectories, including aging, may be tunable by changes in a rather small number of genetic loci or physiologic pathways.

FOUR KEY DISCOVERIES IN MODERN BIOGERONTOLOGY

Much of the current excitement in biogerontology reflects a recent consilience of research agendas pursued separately, sometimes for 50 years or more, that have only now begun to converge into a prototheory of the connections between aging and development at the cellular level. This coalescence of ideas can be presented in the context of four key discoveries: (1) the extension of life span in rodents by caloric restriction; (2) stress-resistance as a unifying feature of long-lived mutant worm strains; (3) single-gene mutants that extend mouse longevity by alterations in hormone levels and growth trajectories; and (4) the role of insulin and insulin-like signals in modulating aging rates in widely separated species of animals.

Caloric Restriction

The oldest of these four key discoveries is that reduction of caloric intake to a level approximately 60 percent of that which a mouse or rat would consume voluntarily leads to an increase, typically 40 percent, in both mean and maximal longevity (see Fig. 1-3). Many different regimens for

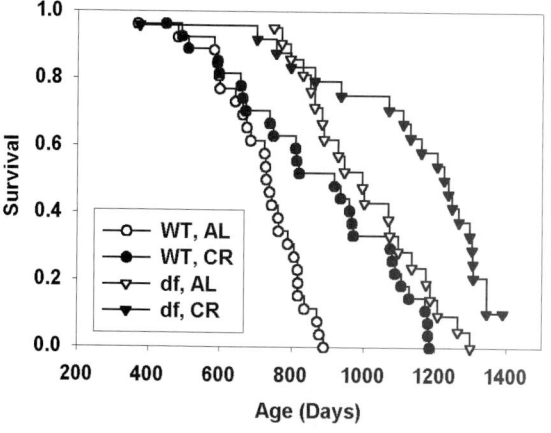

Figure 1-3   Survival curves for genetically normal (wild-type [WT]) or Ames dwarf (df) mice on caloric-restricted diet (CR) or on unrestricted ad libitum (AL) food intake. Each symbol represents a mouse dying at the indicated age. The dwarf mice live longer than the WT mice on either diet, and the CR diet extends the life span of mice of either genotype. Data from Bartke et al: *Nature* 414:412, 2001.

caloric restriction (CR) seem to work about equally well (e.g., smaller daily portions or every-other-day feeding) as long as the total calorie intake is reduced to approximately 60 percent of the ad libitum intake and as long as protein, vitamins, and micronutrients are provided in amounts adequate to prevent malnutrition. CR imposed at the time of weaning has the largest effect, but substantial effects both on longevity and on physiologic measures of aging can also be seen in rodents placed on a low-calorie diet in midlife. The CR regimen is severe enough to delay or prevent sexual maturation in rats, and is thus unlikely to resemble dietary conditions encountered by free-living wild rodent populations, for which delayed sexual competence would lead to extinction. CR-treated rodents are not only long-lived, but just as importantly they display a deceleration of the effects of aging on a wide range of age-dependent changes, including patterns of gene expression; alterations in cell function in proliferative and nonproliferative cell types; modifications in acellular tissues such as lens and connective tissues; and changes in the responsiveness of multicellular organs including brain, immune system, and endocrine networks. CR rodents remain active and vigorous even when very old; CR rats permitted access to a running wheel will typically clock more than 2 km per day even at ages at which controls have long since died (see Fig. 1-4). This slowing down of multiple facets of the aging process leads to diminished mortality risks for most diseases, including autoimmune, neoplastic, and degenerative illnesses. The ability of the CR diet to retard such a wide range of age-related changes is one of the strongest arguments that aging itself can be regarded as a unitary process whose timing may be regulated by a very small number of physiologic control systems.

It is still uncertain whether the CR effect will be seen in long-lived animals, including humans and nonhuman primates. Three major studies, using rhesus and squirrel monkeys, are underway to determine whether caloric restriction will retard aging and disease, and increase life span, if initiated in young or in middle-aged primates. Preliminary data show that the CR protocol increases life span of monkeys that were, at the outset of the study, already obese and showing early signs of adult-onset diabetes; but whether similar effects will be observed in monkeys not suffering from these particular late-life maladies remains to be determined. Because many of these animals are likely to live 30 or more years, definitive results will be long in coming. It is important, though not surprising, that the restricted monkeys are much lighter and leaner than controls, and differ from control animals in biochemical and physiologic tests that reflect obesity and hypertension. Data using outcomes that are age-dependent but less strongly associated with adiposity, such as age-dependent changes in muscle, immune, or cognitive function, are just now beginning to emerge from these ambitious studies.

The degree of CR needed to achieve an antiaging effect is far too severe to be a practical preventive regimen for more than a tiny fraction of the human population. Thus work to define the biochemical mechanism by which CR alters age-dependent physiologic decline is likely to provide the best clues to clinically useful preventative strategies. One line of inquiry starts with the set of known, dramatic changes

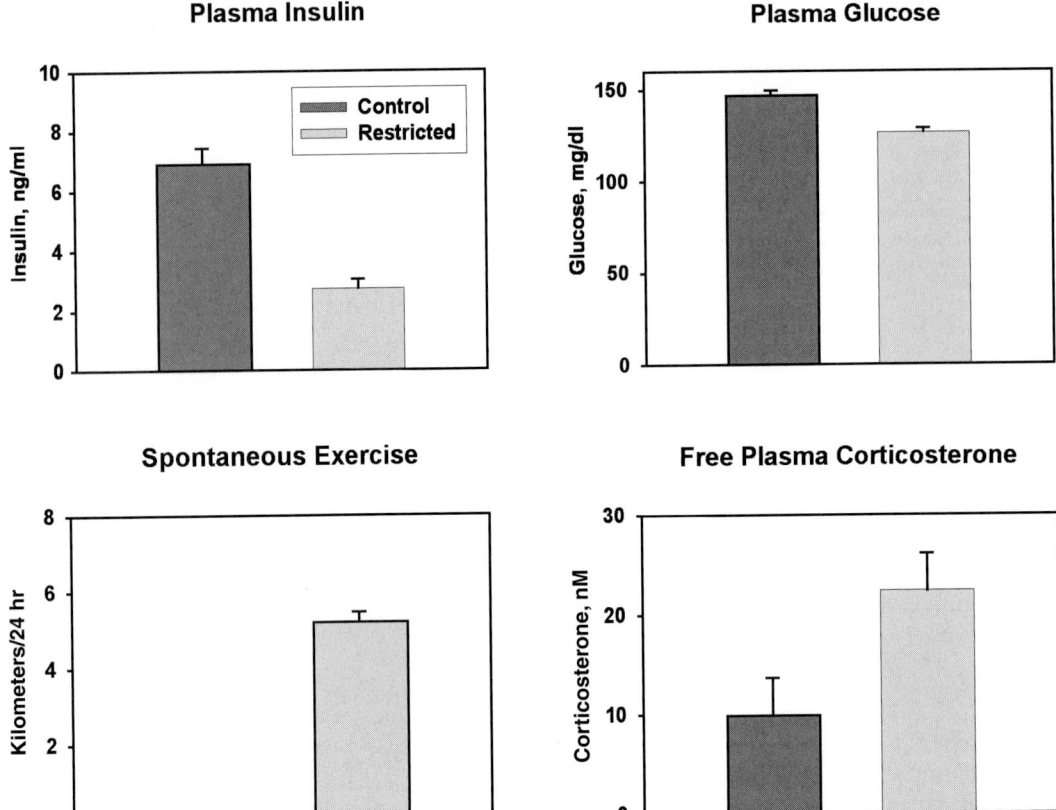

Figure 1-4 Physiologic effects of caloric restriction in rats: changes within the first 8 to 10 months. Panels show, *clockwise from upper left*, plasma insulin concentrations at 0800 hours, mean 24-hour plasma glucose concentrations, spontaneous running wheel exercise as kilometers run per day, and mean 24-hour free plasma corticosterone levels in 9- to 13-month-old F344 male rats on a calorie-restricted diet (60 percent of control food intake) from 6 weeks of age. Each bar shows means and standard errors. These findings are examples of dramatic alterations induced relatively early after imposition of the CR protocol, which do not reflect merely a delayed development of traits seen in normal aged rats. Insulin and glucose data from Masoro et al: *J Gerontol Biol Sci* 47:B202, 1992. Exercise data from McCarter et al; *Aging Clin Exp Res* 9:73, 1997. Corticosterone data from Sabatino et al: *J Gerontol Biol Sci* 46:B171, 1991.

induced by the CR protocol, and attempts to determine whether one or more of these changes can by themselves produce the same effects on aging and longevity. CR rodents exhibit several provocative effects that do not represent merely a postponement of normal aging changes, and thus are plausible candidates for primary mediators of CR. These include declines in serum glucose and insulin levels, mild increases in free serum glucocorticoid levels, a drop of about 0.5° to 1° in basal body temperature, and an increase in cellular protection against oxidant-mediated damage (see Figure 1-4). Each of these effects could, in principle, lead to major changes in a wide range of proliferative and nonproliferative cell and tissue types. Attempts to mimic some of these CR effects, either pharmacologically or by the genetic manipulation of experimental mice, will help to clarify the causal connections among these changes and their relationship to aging and disease. There is also some evidence that other dietary manipulations, such as reductions of the available levels of the amino acid methionine, also extend rodent life span; analysis of the physiologic consequences of these diets may help to suggest which alterations in hormonal milieu and cellular biochemistry are key mediators of the CR effect, and which merely incidental.

Mutant Flies and Worms

The great advantage of the famous invertebrates (the fruit fly *Drosophila melanogaster* and the soil nematode *Caenorhabditis elegans*) for aging studies comes from their exceptional tractability for genetic manipulation, while their great disadvantage comes from the disparities between their physiology and that of people. Their relevance to human aging rests on two sources: their value in testing general ideas about aging and longevity, and the hope—already realized in many other areas of developmental genetics—that genetic loci that regulate the timing of life history changes in these species may have homologs with similar functions in mammals.

Studies of nematode worms were the first to illustrate the important principle that mutations in single genes can radically lengthen life span (Fig. 1-5), by as much as two- to fourfold in certain cases. This observation by itself provides strong evidence against models of aging in which longevity is regulated by scores or hundreds of genetic loci, each controlling independently some aspect of the aging process. It is of course still possible—indeed, likely—that many components of the aging process, and many varieties of late-life disease, are influenced by numerous polymorphic

Survival Curves of Mutant Worm Strains

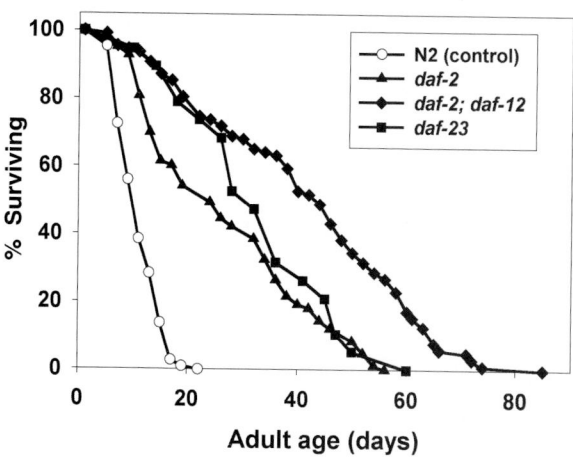

Figure 1-5   Survival curves for normal and mutant strains of the nematode worm *C. elegans*. Strain N2 is the normal control strain; 50 percent of the worms die by age 10 days, and all are dead by day 24. Single-gene mutant strains *daf-2(e1370)* and *daf-23* have about threefold longer mean and maximal life spans. The double-mutant *daf-2(e1370); daf-12(m20)* is still longer-lived, with mean and maximal life span about fourfold greater than the normal control from which the mutants were derived. Data provided by Pam Larsen; see Larsen et al: *Genetics* 139:1567, 1995 for additional details.

genes. The existence of long-lived single-gene mutants, however, suggests that the timing of these coordinated late-life changes can be altered synchronously, and thus that they are likely to be linked to a small number of fundamental timing mechanisms.

The analysis of long-lived mutant worms has produced two surprising and important results. The first of these is that nearly all of the life span extending mutations in these worms share a common physiologic basis: they produce resistance to cellular damage produced by ultraviolet light, oxidizing agents, and overheating (Fig. 1-6). It is thus tempting to speculate that a generalized resistance to such injuries might contribute to longevity, and information about how resistance to these diverse calamities might be conveyed by a single-gene mutation could provide useful clues to human pathophysiology. The "heat shock" genes that are induced by a similarly wide range of stresses in human as well as worm and fly cells are among the most attractive candidates for such a link, and indeed worms genetically engineered to express higher levels of certain heat shock proteins show extended longevity.

The second surprising finding is that normal, nonmutant worms possess at least one gene (*daf16*) that would lead to prolonged life span were it not that *daf16* is, in normal worms, turned off in adult life. The mutant genes that lead to life span prolongation in these animals do so by failing to turn off *daf16* and thus allowing continued expression of *daf16* in adult life to increase longevity. Head-to-head competition experiments show that neither long-lived mutants nor short-lived controls have a selective advantage when food supplies are steady and ample, but that the long-lived mutant stocks are at a disadvantage when confronted with fluctuating environments in which food supply is

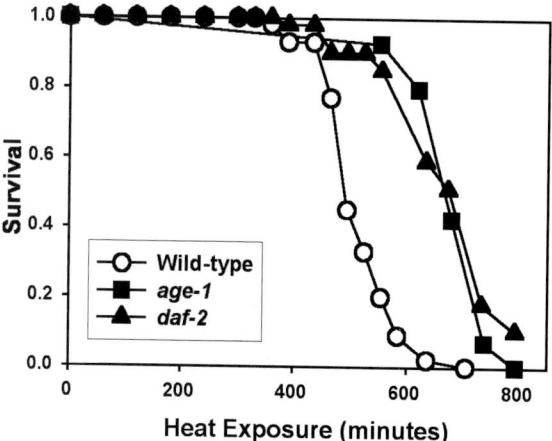

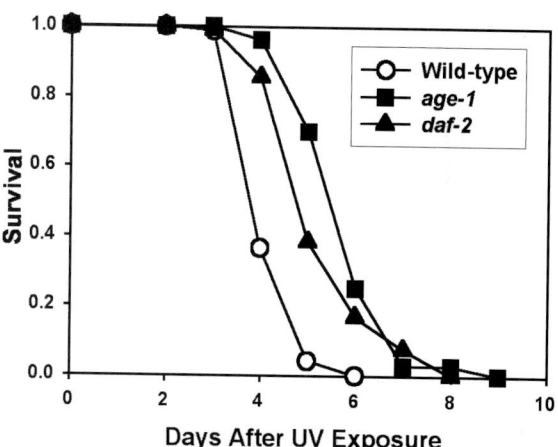

Figure 1-6   Long-lived mutant strains of worms are also more resistant than controls to UV-induced damage and to thermal stress. *Top panel* shows survival of normal (wild-type) worms and two different strains of long-lived mutants (*age1* and *daf2*) at elevated temperatures. *Bottom panel* shows survival of these three strains after exposure to ultraviolet light (UV). Data provided by Shin Murakami and Thomas Johnson. See Johnson et al: *J Gerontol Biol Sci* 51:B392, 1996.

periodically short. Thus, turning off the *daf16* gene in adult life is a good move for worms whose natural environment, in a soil in which rotting vegetation is discontinuous, calls for boom-or-bust spurts of reproduction, even though continuous expression of *daf16* would slow the aging process and increase maximal longevity.

Is the *daf16* story a worm-specific curiosity or an important clue to regulation of aging rate throughout the animal kingdom? *C. elegans* has an unusual life history strategy, similar in some ways to mammalian hibernation, that involves the ability to enter a "dauer larva" stage well-suited to surviving long periods of food shortage or low moisture, and then to resume normal development when food and water once again become available; this process is regulated by *daf16*. Some have speculated that the ability of caloric restriction to extend rodent life span may represent a similar adaptation to resource scarcity, and the idea that the caloric restriction phenomenon involves activation of

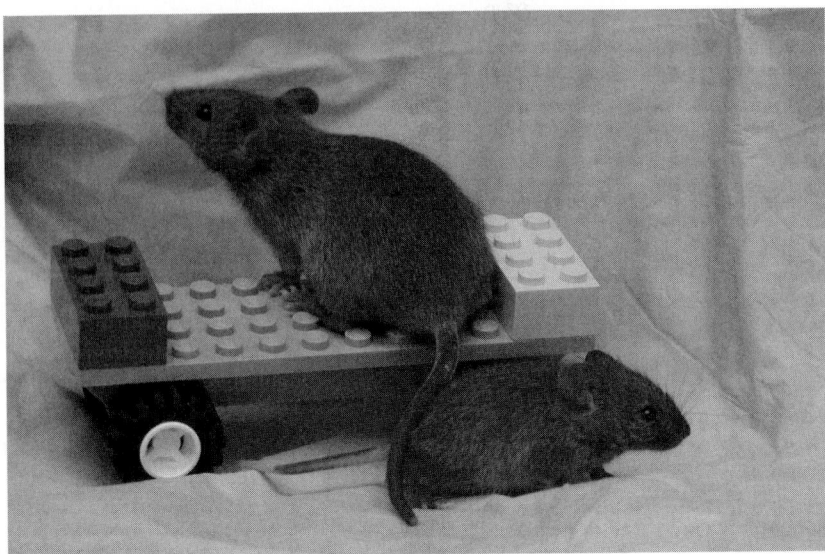

Figure 1-7   Young adult mouse of the Snell dwarf stock (*on the ground*) and a normal size, nonmutant, littermate control (*on the vehicle*).

genetic pathways similar to those that mediate the life span-extension pathways in worms is an interesting, although unproven, idea. Work is now in progress to clarify what the daf16 protein does, what cell types it is expressed in, and what role, if any, homologous genes (members of the forkhead family of transcription factors) play in modulating mammalian responses to food abundance and mammalian aging.

Genetic analysis of aging in the fruit fly *Drosophila melanogaster* has lagged slightly behind analysis of *C. elegans*, but there are now reports of at least four mutations that extend life span in flies, with a large number of additional unpublished examples, and in the next few years this organism will begin to provide insights into the molecular control of aging and suggest new ideas for parallel analysis of mammalian models.

Mutant Mice with Altered Hormone Patterns and Growth Trajectories

The 1996 discovery by Andrzej Bartke and his colleagues that mice carrying the Ames dwarf mutation lived approximately 50 percent longer than normal mice provided the first evidence that longevity in mammals can be substantially extended by single genetic changes, as it can in worms and flies. This finding, like the evidence on caloric restriction, strongly supports the idea that multiple aspects of aging can be coordinately controlled by shared timing mechanisms. The Ames dwarf mutation, a mutation at the Prop1 gene on chromosome 11, acts in embryogenesis to block development of certain cells of the anterior pituitary. As a result, Ames dwarf mice are defective in production of growth hormone (GH) and its mediator insulin-like growth factor 1 (IGF-1), defective in production of thyroid-stimulating hormone (TSH) and its mediators the thyroxines T3 and T4, and defective in production of the lactation hormone prolactin. The deficiencies of IGF-1 and T4 lead to postnatal growth retardation, and as young adults these

mice (Fig. 1-7) are only approximately one-third the size of controls with normal forms of the Prop1 product. Mice carrying the Snell dwarf mutation show an essentially identical set of hormonal deficiencies, and these mice, too, live at least 40 percent longer than nonmutant control mice. The mutations appear to slow aging per se, rather than merely a specific class of lethal illness, because Snell dwarf mice not only live longer but also show slower progression of age-related changes in T cells, joints, and skin. Although there are similarities between dwarf and CR rodents, including small body size, some shared alterations in hormone levels, and variable declines in body temperature, the dwarf mutations do not merely recapitulate the CR syndrome. For one thing, dwarf mice do not show the exceptional leanness typical of CR animals. In addition, the effects of the CR diet and the dwarf mutations are at least additive, and dwarf mice placed on the CR regime are substantially longer lived than either normally fed dwarf mice or CR-treated mice of normal genotype (see Figure 1-3).

Dwarf mice differ from normal mice in many respects; a study comparing gene expression patterns in the liver of young dwarf and normal mice has shown statistically significant differences in at least 72 genes, or approximately 3 percent of the genes examined. It seems likely that defects in the GH and IGF-1 pathway account for at least some of the effects on aging, because two other mutant mouse lines, those with mutations in the GH receptor or in the growth hormone-releasing hormone receptor gene, also show extended longevity without major alterations in the prolactin and thyroid specific pathways. It will be of great interest to learn whether any or all four of these dwarfing mutations increase the stress resistance of cells or tissues of the affected mice. There may prove to be multiple genetic pathways that regulate both body size and ultimate life expectancy in rodents: mouse stocks selected for small body size and slow early life growth rates do live longer than mice selected for rapid early growth, but do not differ from controls in IGF-1 levels, at least when these are measured in young adults. These mutant mice provide valuable tools for further analysis of the pathways linking hormone

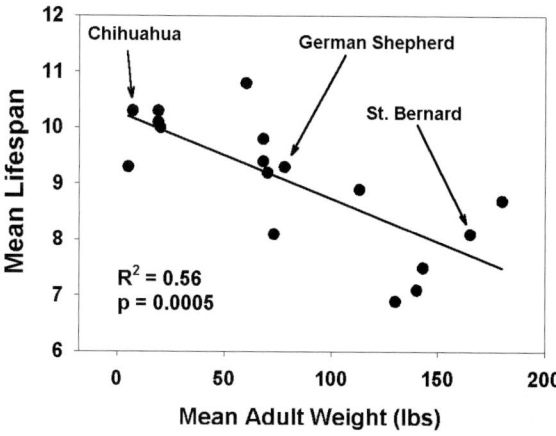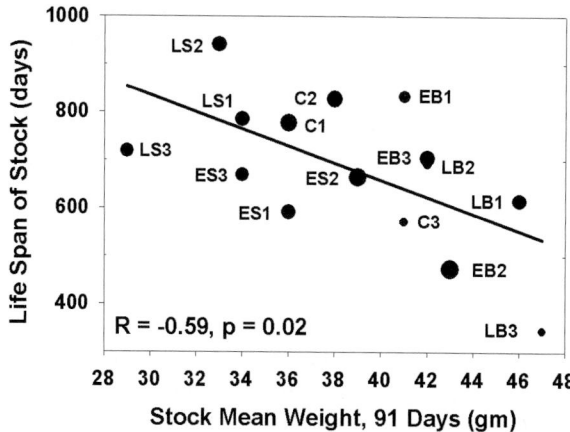

Figure 1-8 Big dogs and big mice die young. *Left panel:* Each data point represents a breed of dog; three of these are indicated by named arrows. The points show approximations of mean life span and mean adult weight recalculated from data presented in Li et al: *J Gerontol Biol Sci* 51:B403, 1996. The regression line fitted by least squares is also shown. The regression coefficient is highly significant, with 56 percent of the variation in breed life span "explained" by interbreed variation in adult weight. *Right panel:* Each point shows a stock of mice from an experiment in which mice were selectively bred for more than 15 generations for differences in growth rate during the first 2 months of life. The size of the symbol is proportional to the number of mice tested for each of the 15 stocks. The regression line illustrates the significant association of small body size (at 91 days) with life expectancy. Data from Miller RA, Chrisp C, Atchley W: *J Gerontol Biol Sci* 55A:B455, 2000.

levels, growth trajectories, the rate of aging, and vulnerability to late life illnesses.

Insulin-like Hormones, Fuel Abundance, and Aging

The studies of caloric restriction, mutant worms and flies, and long-lived mutant mice have led to a recognition of a common theme: the potential importance of insulin-like signals in regulation of longevity in widely separated species of animals. In worms, the levels of the antiaging molecule *daf16* are controlled by a pathway that senses food availability and requires action of a receptor, encoded by the *daf2* gene, that closely resembles the human receptors for insulin and IGF-I. Working with flies, two research groups have found mutations of the insulin receptor that lead to dramatic increases in life span. Four mouse mutations that interfere with production of IGF-1 all lead to extended longevity. Small breeds of dogs and small strains of mice are also long-lived as compared to larger stocks (Figure 1-8), and in the two cases examined to date, the small size of the long-lived dog breeds has been found to reflect lower levels of IGF-1 as compared to closely related but larger breeds of dogs. Even in the yeast *Saccharomyces cerevisiae,* cell life span and resistance to oxidation stress are controlled by a protein kinase whose homologs are required for response to insulin in mammals and which mediates the level of *daf16* in worms. In terms of evolutionary distance (i.e., time since their derivation from a common ancestor), worms, flies, and yeast are as distant from one another as each is distant from dogs, mice, and humans. The involvement of insulin and IGF-1 signals in regulation of longevity in all of these species thus suggests that this relationship may be very deeply rooted in evolutionary history. Even in the earliest eucaryotes, pathways may have evolved that sense food abundance and translate this information into

decisions about life history, committing resources to immediate reproduction in times of abundance but delaying developmental transitions and instead increasing cellular stress resistance under conditions of scarcity. Such a pathway could in principle have been co-opted, in mammals, as an important timer of developmental pace, and might now play a key role in allocating resources alternately towards rapid growth or towards producing stress-resistant cells and tissues that trade reproductive speed for endurance.

It is clear that the relationship of insulin and IGF-1 to aging and disease in humans is too complex to be captured by such a simple paradigm. Insulin and its actions play well-known roles in many late life diseases, and there is little likelihood that simple abrogation of insulin pathways will enhance human health. Similarly, there is some evidence that pharmacologic elevation of IGF-1 levels may have some benefits in a subset of elderly people, although there is still uncertainty about the ratio of risks to benefits for such an intervention. Further work in mice is needed to establish whether or not alterations of IGF-1 or other insulin-like signals at early stages of the life span might serve to diminish disease risks at older ages, and do so without unacceptable side effects.

FOUR HOT TOPICS IN CONTEMPORARY BIOGERONTOLOGY

Clonal "Senescence" and Telomere Biology

The famous observation of Hayflick that human diploid fibroblasts cease to grow in culture after a limited number of population doublings sparked a line of experimentation that continues to yield important insights into the molecular control of cell growth, differentiation, and neoplastic transformation. Human fibroblasts placed in tissue culture will continue to divide until approximately 50 cell doublings have occurred, after which the remaining cells can survive indefinitely in a healthy but nondividing state. This clonal senescence model seemed to a generation of biogerontologists the most attractive approach to the genetics and cell biology of aging, and a coherent model of the alterations in gene expression that lead to and maintain the growth-impaired state of the late passage cells is emerging from ongoing studies. In vitro growth limitations are seen not only in fibroblasts, but in a wide range of other cell types in both humans and other mammals.

The challenge of showing that this in vitro system can deliver important clues about the biology of aging, that is, the process that converts healthy young adults into old people, has remained a serious hurdle. The most obvious possibility is that some of the diseases and disabilities of the elderly might represent a loss, with age, in proliferative capacities of one or more cell types. There is some evidence, for example, that vascular endothelial cells in regions of the arterial tree especially prone to atherosclerosis may have progressed through more cell divisions than endothelial cells in atheroma-resistant areas of the vasculature. Whether these differences contribute to the pathophysiology of atherosclerosis, or are a secondary consequence of the disease, is still an open issue. Research into the pathologic consequences, if any, of clonal senescence has been hindered by a paucity of evidence that tissues of elderly individuals actually contain cells that have reached the limits of their growth potential. Tests using an isoform of the enzyme β-galactosidase that seems to be synthesized only by late passage cells suggested that this marker enzyme is produced by a small proportion of the fibroblasts in the skin of old, but not young, individuals. This finding, however, has proven difficult to replicate, and there are no corresponding data for other markers or other cell types or other tissues, and no evidence yet that the presence of these cells causes alterations of tissue function. The dramatic changes induced by aging in cells that do not divide in postnatal life, such as neurons, as well as in extracellular structures such as teeth and cartilage, have also posed a clear challenge to the idea that blocks to cell division are a key timer of aging in mammals.

Studies of the role of telomere length in clonal senescence have now buttressed the claims that replicative senescence of the sort shown by late passage human fibroblasts is an important element in tumor biology while simultaneously weakening the case for this system as a model for aging in whole animals. The enzymes that replicate DNA in mammalian chromosomes cannot replicate DNA at the very ends of the chromosomes, called the telomeres. A separate enzyme, telomerase, is responsible for replication of telomeric DNA in dividing cells. Many human cell types, including fibroblasts, do not express telomerase, and for these cells each individual cell division leads to a slight decline in the length of the DNA at the telomeric end of each chromosome. There is now strong evidence that the gradual loss of telomere length over the course of 50 to 100 mitotic divisions leads, through unknown mechanisms, to a switching off of genes required for passage through the cell cycle. Restoration of functional telomerase to a growing culture of fibroblasts prevents the progressive shortening of telomeres and prevents the block to cell replication typically seen at the "Hayflick limit" of 50 to 70 in vitro doublings. The observation that telomerase is spontaneously turned back on, and telomere diminution prevented or reversed, in approximately 90 percent of clinically significant human cancers, has led to the important idea that the telomere clock evolved, in humans, to guard against unbridled proliferation of early neoplastic clones.

Such a mechanism cannot be responsible for the effects of aging in mice or rats. For one thing, rodents, like most mammals that have been studied, have much longer telomeres than humans. If the 70 years of human life span are just sufficient to produce perceptible shortening of the 6 to 10 kilobases of human telomeres, it is hard to see how the 2 to 3 years of rodent life span could have much impact on the 20 to 100 kilobases of telomeric deoxyribonucleic acid (DNA) with which rats and mice are endowed. Furthermore, genetic manipulations have produced lines of mice whose telomeres are indeed at the same, short, length seen in proliferating cell types in elderly humans, and while these mice show specific abnormalities (skin ulceration, infertility, frequently lethal gastrointestinal lesions, and increased frequencies of certain forms of neoplasia), they do not resemble normal aged mice in most respects.

Thus it now seems increasingly unlikely that replicative senescence plays a major role in aging, at least in those many aspects of the aging process that are similar in rodents and humans. It remains a possibility that clonal senescence could contribute to some aspects of aging that are seen only in humans, or whose regulation is fundamentally different in long-lived versus short-lived species. Evidence that clonal senescence did indeed contribute to some aspects of aging in humans, other than as a defense against tumors, would be an important contribution to biogerontology.

Gene Mapping

There is ample evidence, reviewed in other chapters of this volume, that genetic polymorphisms can modify the risk of specific diseases; genes that increase the risk of Alzheimer's disease, atherosclerosis, or type 2 diabetes, for example, will have a substantial impact on life expectancy and provide key clues to the pathogenesis of specific syndromes. There is substantially less evidence, however, for the possible effects of genetic polymorphisms that might, in principle, alter the rate of aging and hence influence the pace of a wide range of late-life processes including multiple diseases.

One approach has been to search for genetic alleles whose frequency is higher in extremely old individuals (centenarians, or at least those well into their nineties) than in matched population samples. The logic of this approach comes from the argument that to obtain centenarian status one needs to have some resistance, presumably at least partly genetic, to multiple forms of disease, including the most common cardiovascular, renal, endocrine, and cognitive illnesses. If this is correct, then those specific alleles that promote exceptional longevity should be somewhat more common among the very old than among matched samples of middle-aged people, very few of whom will ever achieve centenarian status. This program can be pursued through surveys of candidate genes, that is, genes thought on theoretical grounds to be of particular importance in the aging process, or else through a systematic genome scan experiment involving arbitrarily selected marker genes, scattered throughout the genome, that might be linked to genes that actually influence aging.

Both candidate and genome scan approaches present practical difficulties. It is difficult to identify and recruit the hundreds of centenarians (or near-centenarians) needed to provide adequate statistical power for such mapping calculations. Obtaining an appropriately matched reference population of middle-aged people is also difficult, because population shifts and varying ethnic composition of successive age cohorts can modify the frequency of individual genetic alleles and thereby produce differences in gene frequencies between age groups that are unrelated to health effects. Lastly, both approaches are likely to come across genetic loci whose over-representation in the centenarian group reflects an effect on specific, common illnesses; alleles that increase the risk of Alzheimer's disease or type 2 diabetes or heart attacks, for example, are unlikely to be very common among the exceptionally old. Distinguishing hypothetical antiaging genes from those that simply alter risks of specific common diseases may eventually prove to depend on assessment of the extent to which such genes modify age-dependent traits that do not themselves pose a risk to survival. At this point, the literature contains well over a dozen studies showing overrepresentation of candidate genes in specific populations of centenarians, with only modest success at replication in independent populations. There is also a single report of a locus, on human chromosome 4, whose overrepresentation among the very old was documented by a genome scan.

Three groups have used genome scanning approaches to try to identify mouse loci that predict life span, and each has reported from two to six such loci; whether such mapping data will prove to be replicable in other stocks of mice, and whether these loci will be shown to influence a wide range of age-sensitive traits is yet to be examined. There is some evidence, from these studies and from comparable studies of longevity genes in fruit flies, that the effects of some of the loci may be sex-specific, that is, apparent only in males, or only in females, but not in both, and that some of the loci may have effects that vary depending on inheritance at other, unlinked, genes (Fig. 1-9). Such effects would, if generally true, greatly complicate attempts to detect human genes with effects on the aging process.

Werner's Syndrome and Other Alleged Progerias

Patients who inherit two copies of the null allele at the WRN locus on human chromosome 8 develop Werner's syndrome, characterized by growth retardation in the teenage years, cataracts, premature graying of the hair, and a set of characteristic skin and facial abnormalities. By their thirties these patients typically have developed osteoporosis, diabetes, and atherosclerosis; they also show an

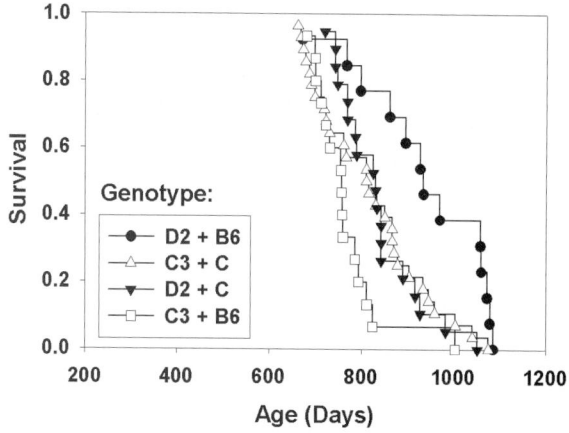

Figure 1-9 Interaction effects between genes that influence longevity in mice. In this experiment genetic alleles linked to the chromosome 10 locus D10Mit15 and the chromosome 16 locus D16Mit182 were found to predict life span in male mice of a segregating stock. Each symbol shows a mouse dying at the indicated age. The longest-lived mice, shown by the *filled circles,* inherit the D2 allele at D10Mit15 and the B6 allele at D16Mit182. Neither of these alleles is associated with extended life span except when in combination with the other, and indeed mice that inherit the B6 allele at D16Mit182 but not the D2 allele at D10Mit15 (*open squares*) are particularly short-lived. Interaction effects of this kind would greatly complicate analysis of the genetics of longevity and aging in humans. Unpublished data of Miller RA et al.

unusually high risk for mesenchymal tumors, although they show no risk of the more common epithelial and endothelial neoplasias.

Because many of these features also appear as a consequence of normal aging, some have been tempted to consider Werner's syndrome a form of accelerated or premature aging. This is an unfortunate oversimplification: there are many features of normal aging that are not seen in Werner's patients, and many features of Werner's syndrome that are not seen in normal old individuals. Werner's syndrome patients, for example, do not show signs of Alzheimer's disease or other amyloidoses, hypertension, immune failure, or nonmesenchymal cancers, which are so typical of normal aging, but they do show subcutaneous calcifications, altered fat distribution, vocal changes, flat feet, malleolar ulcerations, high levels of urinary hyaluronic acid, and a number of other idiosyncrasies not seen commonly in elderly individuals. Nonetheless, the cooccurrence of so many age-associated changes as a consequence of a change at a single genetic locus suggests that these signs of aging may be connected to one another at some fundamental level.

The cloning of the WRN gene and the discovery that it encoded a protein likely to play a role in DNA repair, together with the earlier observation that cultured cells from Werner's syndrome patients were unusually prone to develop mutations in culture, have drawn new attention to the old idea that accumulation of mutations in somatic cells could play a role in multiple facets of normal aging. Mice in which the product of the WRN gene has been eliminated have not, so far, shown any signs of premature aging or shortened life span, perhaps because the role played by

WRN in human cells is subsumed in rodents by another enzyme.

George Martin has coined the term "segmental progeroid syndrome" to cover illnesses, such as Werner's, Down's, and Hutchinson–Gilford syndromes and many other inborn errors of metabolism, in which patients show a variety of changes reminiscent of changes typically seen in elderly subjects; by symptom count, Down's syndrome (trisomy 21) shows the strongest resemblance to normal aging in Martin's catalog. It is possible that further studies of the WRN locus may reveal other mutations that are less severe than those which lead to full-blown Werner's syndrome and yet which lead to altered risks of important diseases of later life. In any case, investigation of the cell biology and molecular details by which mutations of the WRN locus contribute to so many forms of pathology may provide key clues to the basis for the coordinated appearance of these changes as a part of normal aging.

Transgenic Models to Test Specific Mechanistic Theories of Aging

The development of experimental methods that can add extra copies, or remove copies, of specific genes from lines of laboratory mice has made it possible to develop new strains of animals useful for testing specific molecular ideas about aging and its relationship to late life diseases. A comprehensive review of this bustling area is beyond the scope of this chapter, although a review article is included in the list of citations for those who wish to pursue the topic further. A representative sampling of the ongoing work includes:

- Production of mice with unusually high levels of enzymes that remove free radicals and other potentially toxic byproducts of oxidative metabolism, to test the idea that free radical damage to proteins, lipids, or nucleic acids contributes to multiple aspects of aging.
- Production of mice with unusually high levels of proteins that regulate heat production by alteration of mitochondrial ion fluxes, to see if uncoupling fuel usage from adenosine triphosphate (ATP) generation might mimic some of the benefits of calorically restricted diets.
- Development of mice with alterations in insulin receptor levels, altered glucocorticoid levels, or altered levels of growth hormone responsiveness to see if these endocrine system changes might delay aging by mimicking the hormonal changes seen in long-lived mutant and in calorically restricted rodents.
- Studies of mice with altered rates of DNA methylation or improvements in DNA repair enzymes, to test the idea that systematic changes in gene sequence or genetic expression patterns are a key element in normal aging.
- Development of multiple lines of mice in which some aspect of aging is deliberately accelerated, for example by curtailing telomere length or crippling antioxidant defenses, to see which aspects of aging are correspondingly hastened. Interpretation of such efforts, however, is fraught with peril, because there are many ways to impair health by interference with developmental and homeostatic pathways, and it is difficult to distinguish these from alterations in aging per se.

FOUR CHALLENGES FOR FUTURE RESEARCH

This final section touches briefly on four areas of biogerontology that are likely to repay future investment, topics that are not yet areas of intense activity but which deserve to be, chosen, respectively, from the molecular, organismic, ecologic, and medical branches of gerontologic research.

The first area is that of control of protein synthesis rates. Over the last 30 years, many studies have established that both the rate of synthesis and the rate of degradation of most proteins is much slower in tissues of old rodents and humans than in younger subjects. The cause of this slowdown is unknown; it is not even known yet whether the decline in synthesis rate is the cause of, or rather the result of, the alteration in degradation rate. What is clear, however, is that this fundamental change in cell biology leads to increases in the mean lifetime of individual protein molecules, and that as a consequence, individual proteins are substantially more likely to be converted, by covalent modification or by intramolecular rearrangement, to forms not typically present in cells from younger individuals. It is easy to speculate that such changes in protein conformation caused by this increase in "dwell time" could contribute to the accumulation of damaged cells seen in Parkinson's, Alzheimer's, and other late-life forms of neurodegeneration. They might also contribute to the autoimmune reactions implicated in atherosclerosis and other vascular abnormalities, and might impair cellular activation and homeostasis in a range of key cells and tissues.

The second neglected problem is that of validating biomarkers of aging, that is, of finding age-sensitive traits that can distinguish among middle-aged individuals those whose systems have been relatively altered, or proven relatively resistant, to the aging process. In a sense, studying the rate of aging without a set of validated biomarkers is akin to trying to study the causes and cures of hypertension without a way to measure blood pressure, or to study fever without a thermometer. To qualify as a biomarker of aging, a measurement would need to show consistent and statistically significant correlations with age-dependent changes in multiple cells and tissues, among individuals of the same chronologic age; ultimately, such a test or set of tests would also need to be useful predictors of life span and the pace of functional decline. Tests that can be conducted cheaply and without any harm to the subject would be required for use of these tests in human epidemiology. By these criteria, there are at present no useful validated biomarkers of aging available for either rodents or humans. Developing evidence for biomarkers would require coordinated studies of large populations by a team of biochemists, physiologists, and statistical epidemiologists, but the outcome of such an effort would be an invaluable addition to the research infrastructure for studies of aging.

The third area nominated for special mention is that of comparative biology. The best that can be accomplished by caloric restriction or by genetic manipulations within a given species of mammal is an increase in life span of

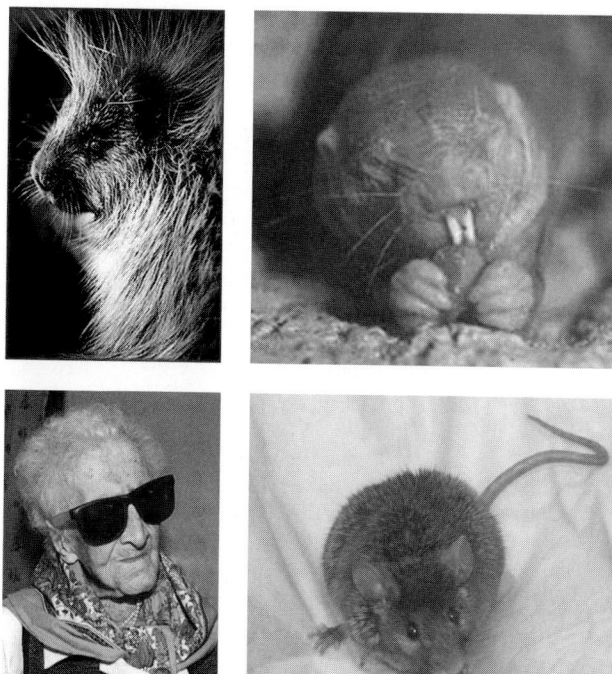

Figure 1-10   Longevity extremes, within and across species. The *top two panels* present the contenders for the honor of longest-lived species of rodent. At *upper left* is a porcupine; some species of porcupines are reported to live 27 years. At *upper right* is a naked mole rat; although the same size as a common laboratory mouse, 85 percent of naked mole rats live at least 20 years (T. O'Connor, personal communication), and the maximal longevity is probably close to 30 years. The longest lived primate, Mme. J. Calment (*lower left*), died at the age of 122 years in 1997. The *lower right panel* shows a mouse, bred in the laboratory from wild-trapped grandparents, who died at the age of 1450 days; so far as is known, this is the maximum extent of mouse longevity in the absence of caloric restriction and gene deletion.

approximately 40 percent. By contrast, natural selection has created species of mammals whose maximal longevity differs by a factor of about 30-fold (comparing mice or voles to humans), and even within a given order of mammals (the primates, for example) species-specific maximum life span may vary as much as 10-fold (Fig. 1-10). This wealth of similarly constructed animals with such varying powers of endurance provides a corresponding wealth of scientific opportunity. Comparative analysis of the repair processes, feedback controls, growth regulators, and metabolic allocations between sister species with major differences in life span are very likely to furnish us with new insights into the basic biology of aging and the factors that link development, aging, and the timing of late-life diseases.

The fourth item on this list of desiderata is the nearly empty field of gerontologic pathology. At first glance, such a term may seem an unnecessary redundancy, like American baseball or theoretical philosophy: surely most research pathologists concern themselves with diseases that largely afflict the elderly? Most investigation into the pathophysiology of late-life diseases, however, is directed at the study of factors that distinguish among diseases: Why does this patient develop the mural lesions of atherosclerosis? Why does this patient develop Alzheimer's disease, while others succumb instead to hypertension or cataracts or diabetes or emphysema? It is time to focus some research attention on the factors that synchronize each of these forms of illness, that postpone them for six decades in humans but for only a few years or a few decades in other species. The most important, still hypothetical, contribution to be made by biogerontologists to the medical enterprise will be to learn enough about the mechanisms that postpone so many human illnesses for so many decades of good health in the majority of young and middle-aged adults so that we can start to turn these insights into practical forms of preventive intervention.

ACKNOWLEDGMENTS

Unpublished data from my own laboratory were collected with the support of NIA grants AG08808, AG13283, and AG13711, and AG11687. I appreciate the willingness of several colleagues, mentioned in the figure legends, to share their own data with me for inclusion in this chapter.

REFERENCES

Austad SN: *Why We Age: What Science is Discovering about the Body's Journey Through Life.* New York, John Wiley & Sons, 1997.

Brown-Borg HM et al: Dwarf mice and the ageing process. *Nature* 384:33, 1996.

Campisi J: Aging and cancer: The double-edged sword of replicative senescence. *J Am Geriatr Soc* 45:482, 1997.

Finch CE: *Longevity, Senescence, and the Genome.* Chicago, University of Chicago Press, 1990.

Kapahi P et al: Positive correlation between mammalian life span and cellular resistance to stress. *Free Radic Biol Med* 26:495, 1999.

Masoro EJ (ed): *Handbook of Physiology.* Section 11, Aging. New York, Oxford University Press, 1995.

Miller RA: When will the biology of aging become useful? Future landmarks in biomedical gerontology. *J Am Geriatr Soc* 45:1258, 1997.

Miller RA: Kleemeier award lecture: Are there genes for aging? *J Gerontol Biol Sci* 54A:B297, 1999.

Miller RA: Genetics of increased longevity and retarded aging in mice. In: Masoro EJ, Austad SN (eds): *Handbook of the Biology of Aging.* San Diego, CA, Academic Press, 2001 p 369.

Morgan WW et al: Application of exogenously regulatable promoter systems to transgenic models for the study of aging. *J Gerontol A Biol Sci Med Sci* 54:B30, 1999.

Olshansky SJ et al: Demography. Prospects for human longevity. *Science* 291:1491, 2001.

Weindruch R: Caloric restriction and aging. *Sci Am* (January) 274:46, 1996.

Genetics of Age-Dependent Human Diseases

EUGENIA WANG

This chapter focuses on understanding how and why age-dependent diseases emerge and how our genetic makeup sets the course from birth to frailty and diseases 60, 80, or 90 years later. Genes never act in isolation but always interact with the environment; how this interaction determines the path leading to the emergence of disease toward the end of a long life is a challenge to every investigator who dares to ask the question. Understanding the genetics of human diseases in this century largely means understanding age-dependent diseases such as cancer, cardiovascular disorders, neurodegeneration, type 2 diabetes, osteoarthritis, osteoporosis, macular degeneration, and so on. The first step in studying the genetics of age-dependent human disease is identifying the genes and environmental factors that deprive elderly people of a healthy life span. Identification of these genes and factors will pave the way to success in treating, reducing, or delaying disease and achieving a maximal healthy life span with dignity, independence, and disease-free normal aging in the last decades of life.

This chapter presents a synopsis of topics dealing with the cell and molecular biology of aging. It should serve as a point of reference for questions such as What is aging? What genetic factors determine the aging process? What genes endow a normal aging process or extremely successful aging? What genes dictate the development of age-dependent diseases? Unified answers to all these questions are not yet available, nor is a utopian world of remaining forever young—free from aging and age-dependent diseases. This chapter considers the genetics of aging with a view ranging from genes to cells to tissues to organs, a vertical view of how genes function in totality in an organism, and how they exert their impact on developing frailties and diseases in the elderly population.

SINGLE GENE VERSUS COMPLEX GENES, REDUCTIONIST VERSUS COMPLEX TRAIT ANALYSIS

Signal Transduction and Complexity in Cellular Functions

One of the most subtle paradigm shifts in the last decade involves our understanding of the complexity of the genetic makeup of living organisms. Embedded in this shift is an awakening appreciation that the success or failure of every physiologic function depends on the orchestrated operation of hundreds of genes in concerted action. A single functional modality such as eating is actually a complex action requiring the coordinated functions of motor neurons and chewing and swallowing jaw muscles, which at the cellular level is controlled by a signal transduction network coordinated in a way to activate the neurons to send signals to the muscles to perform the repetitive actions of chewing and swallowing. Furthermore, products of hundreds of genes are involved in creating the microenvironment of the oral cavity that facilitates these repetitive actions; for example, a common debility of elderly people, dry mouth syndrome, results from the failure of salivary gland cells to secrete the appropriate amount of fluid to maintain a moist environment for chewing and swallowing. What genes and cells are involved in the signals for muscle contractility for chewing and swallowing and for the secretion of fluid into the oral cavity by the salivary glands? The same players perform these actions but with different functional manifestations, as the musicians in an orchestra stay the same although the concert pieces they play change.

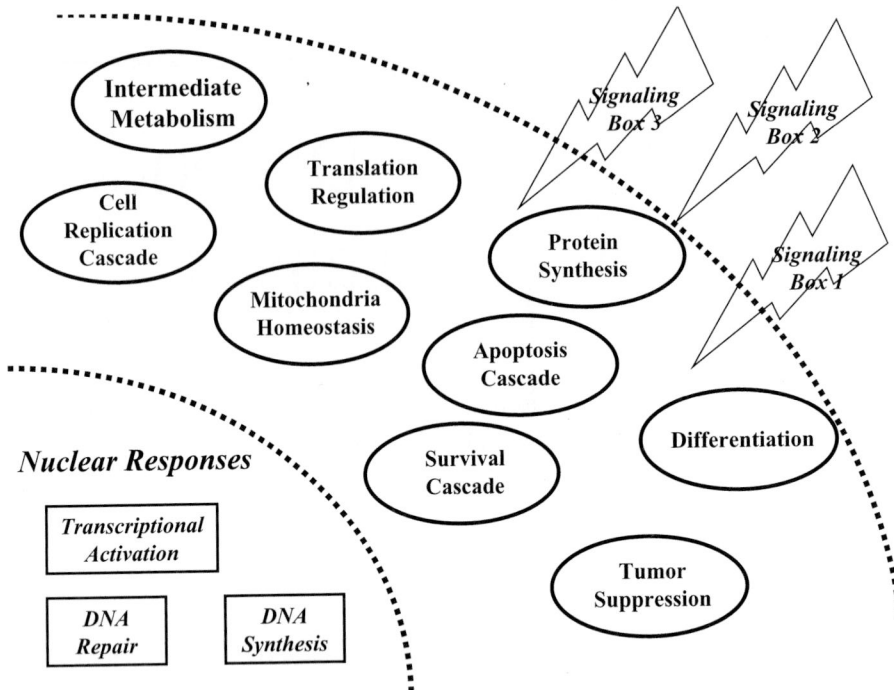

Figure 2-1   Diagram of signal transduction pathways showing signals generated from the extracellular environment binding to their corresponding receptors (lightning) on the cell membrane, cytoplasmic response boxes (ovals), and nuclear response boxes.

Thousands of molecular players are involved in signal transduction pathways. A glance at a few of them reveals several facts: (1) cellular actions are never controlled by single genes; (2) key gene products may serve as "master" switches; (3) "boxes" of molecular actions allow complex signals to be carried in a compartmentalized fashion; and (4) a mismatch of boxes of molecular actions may allow cross-talk among different components of the network (Figure 2-1). The processing of signals in a muscle cell for the repetitive action of chewing is carried out by the activity of certain selected boxes of gene products while other boxes in this complex network remain silent.

As each cell type has a designated function, a particular chain of molecular boxes may be focused on performing continuous actions to support the essential activity of the cells in their tissue. Cell functions can be classified into three categories: (1) specialized cell functions such as cardiomyocyte contraction, neuronal transmission, and the defensive actions of B or T cells, which are vital to survival and can be performed without being constantly prompted by new signals; (2) temporal cell action such as muscle cells contracting when they are called on; and (3) ad hoc cell actions such as those needed for repair or regeneration. Each of these actions requires different sets of signal processing. The sensory network responsible for efficient processing of cell action involves a surveillance system that constantly monitors the operational status of each cell to ensure that it serves properly as a building block, contributing to the critical mass for optimal functioning of the host tissue.

It is important to realize that for every molecular action to be executed, precise spatial and temporal factors are involved. A misfired gene activation is as deleterious as a missing gene activation. We know little of how, in a three-dimensional intracellular environment, the hierarchic order of gene activations is arranged spatially and temporally. Many genes are found to be important because their molecular product regulates a specific reaction; for example, the gene for MAP kinase kinase, an enzyme that can phosphorylate the downstream MAP kinase, serves as the master gene for several key signal pathways (Figure 2-2) Even as well known as this gene and its product are, we know little of when, where, and how enzymatic action actually takes place when the proper signal is sent to a cell. Nevertheless, the importance of MAP kinase in supporting our continual survival is illustrated by the recent interest in anthrax. In inhalation anthrax, a bacterial protein enters human lung epithelial cells and cleaves MAP kinase into fragments, causing death by depriving the cells of this essential enzyme.

The Reductionist Approach and Age-Dependent Diseases

The success of some biomedical advances in the last century has left us with the biased and misleading notion that disease can be cured by the eradication of a single culprit. Transferring this concept to the study of the genetics of aging, some researchers are driven by a fervent desire to identify a single genetic defect that serves to explain everything associated with the changes seen in aging. This zeal for identifying single genetic defects was fostered by successes in molecular biology in the 1980s and early 1990s involving a series of pivotal discoveries of how genetic action

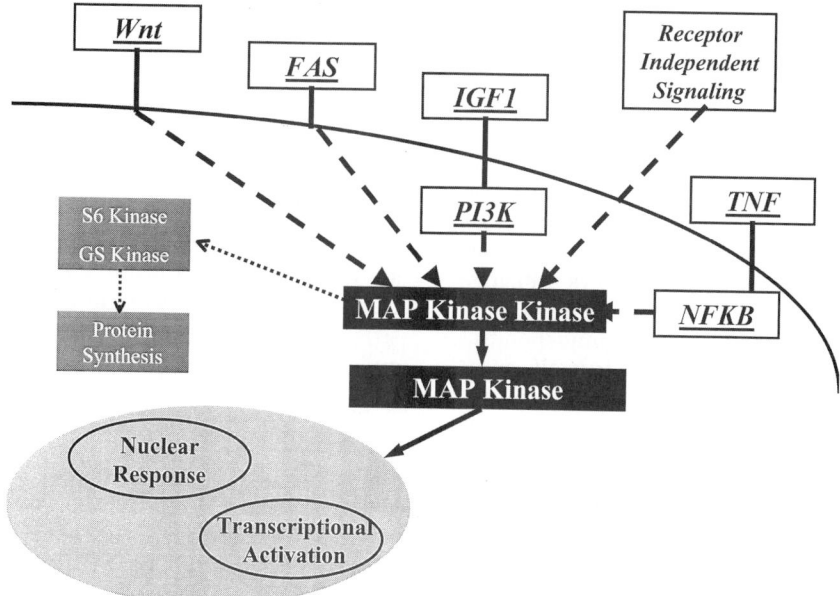

Figure 2-2 Diagram of the PI3 kinase/MAP kinase pathway.

takes place in a cell. Therefore, subconsciously we hope to investigate the genetics of aging or age-dependent diseases, such as cardiovascular problems, neurodegeneration, type 2 diabetes, cancer, osteoporosis, and so on, with the goal of identifying a single mutation of a crucial gene or a group of homologous genes that can explain all the diseases associated with the elderly population.

For every success in deleting or adding a gene action, by either transfection-associated introduction in cell cultures or transgenic methods, there are probably 100 more experiments in which overexpressing or repressing a single gene action exerted no observable effect on the organism. The negative results of such experiments are not due simply to technical failure but rather to the fact that complexity is involved; thus the deletion or addition of a single gene may be able to exert an effect in a test tube, or even in a single cultured cell, but fail to produce the expected results in a complex system where gene actions are manifested by an entire assembly of genes and cells in a three-dimensional cell milieu. Of course, timing, or temporal order, adds to this scenario yet another dimension of complexity, making the understanding of gene actions even more challenging.

The advent of high-throughput DNA sequencing has allowed us to map most of the entire human genome. This revolutionary giant step, while affording invaluable insights into the details of the genetic map, does not provide an operational manual explaining how genes are segregated into functional units or how, where, or when each gene functions when it is expressed. Nevertheless, it does offer tools for studying how changes in a single nucleotide, that is, single nucleotide polymorphisms (SnPs), may serve as the missing element in the sequence of events leading to the evolution of a special type of age-dependent disease. Identifying a defective gene may provide the first step in the investigation of a complex genetic process involving multiple gene actions. One example is the success in identifying

longevity assurance genes (LAGs) in *Caenorhabditis elegans* as described below.

Genetics of Life Span Determination and Signal Transduction Pathways

Do LAGs determine the life span of each species? Emerging pictures from the genetic study of animal models such as *C. elegans* and *Drosophila* provide a resounding yes in answer to this question.

The first identification of a gene essential in regulating the life span of a living organism may be the discovery of *age1* (*daf23*) in the nematode *C. elegans*; it was found that mutation of this gene extends the worm's life span to twice that of its normal counterparts. The sequence of *daf23* shares homology with the genetic sequence of PI3 kinase in mammalian cells. This finding, coupled with the discovery of *daf2*, which initiates this pathway, and its homology with the insulin growth factor 1 (IGF1) receptor, presented the fact that the life span of a worm can be controlled in part by the IGF pathway.

This successful research on worms has been paralleled by work done with two other model systems, yeast and fruit flies, where LAGs have also been discovered. Their links to basic cellular functions such as signal transduction pathways and chromosomal structural integrity provide yet another exciting insight: Mutation in key genes serves as the fundamental basis for the determination of life span. However, it is important to bear in mind that mutation in worms causing life span extension involves a *loss* of function. It is as if reducing the expenditure of energy leads to a gain in life span. This then leads to the question of whether one can manipulate the rate of cellular intermediary metabolism, conserving overall energy use in order to extend overall life span.

The discovery of a retrograde connection between mitochondria and the nucleus (i.e., that mitochondria can send signals to either activate or silence nuclear transcription) provides an entirely different outlook on mitochondrial function. Mitochondria, which act as the cellular powerhouse, have their own genetic machinery. The mitochondrial genome in general has been thought of as controlling mitochondrial function in the generation of adenosine triphosphate (ATP), and therefore mutations in mitochondrial genes have been expected to work primarily in determining the functionality of the mitochondria. This retrograde type of communication between mitochondria and other cellular compartments may prove to be the missing link, explaining how survival genes such as *bcl2* and killing genes such as caspases, although located in or associated with mitochondria, can send signals to the nucleus to execute anti- or pro-apoptotic transcription programs. How the control of intermediate metabolism is related to life span extension, mitochondrial function, and ATP production, and further to retrograde mitochondrial function, remains to be investigated. It is important to realize that the genetic determination of life span may involve hundreds of interacting genes. The pieces of this genetic jigsaw puzzle are just starting to be put together.

Caloric Restriction and Age-Dependent Diseases

Perhaps the most noted manipulation of maximal life span is the effect of dietary restriction observed in rodents. Restriction of caloric intake can extend life in several strains of mice and rats, to two more years in most cases. This restriction, in general, works best when caloric intake is controlled very soon after birth. Although life span extension has been observed for a long time, the genetic mechanism determining this phenotype remains elusive. Two clues as to how caloric restriction extends life span have emerged: similar regimens of dietary restriction can also extend life span in fruit flies; and growth hormone–deprived dwarf Ames mice, which also have an extended life span, can further increase their life span with caloric restriction. These findings suggest that with the wealth of genetic mutant stock available and the knowledge obtained so far from the *Drosophila* model system, the mechanisms controlling the gain in life span obtained with caloric restriction may provide further insights to the genetics determining life span in other species, possibly even humans. The Ames mice provide a further indication that life span can be controlled by growth hormone regulation.

What remains the central issue in studying genetic mechanisms extending life span is whether mutations in worms or flies, or dietary restrictions in rodents, merely delay the progression of death-causing diseases. What do the worms or flies die of at the end of their life span? Do the mutations simply delay death by delaying the activation of death-causing genes? Death in elderly mice generally results from cancer, most frequently lymphoma. It has been shown that dietary-restricted animals have a delayed onset of tumors compared with age-matched controls. Therefore, it seems that dietary-restricted animals may have "younger"

physiologic phenotypes similar to those of their younger counterparts. This suggests the possibility of genetic mechanisms working to delay death; according to the hypothesis that life span extension can be achieved by avoiding death, LAGs may prove to be "death delaying genes" (DDGs). This hypothesis can be tested in worms and fruit flies, where the life span is relatively short and where an abundant stock of mutant strains are available. However, a major handicap is that the causes of death in worms and flies simply are not known. As a result, we do not know definitively whether LAGs are indeed equal to DDGs, how dietary restriction extends life span, or how mutations in worms and flies ultimately extend life span at the organismic level.

Multihit Theory of Age-Dependent Diseases

By definition, a major factor in the etiology of age-dependent diseases is the time required for disease to become manifest. Some individuals experience the onset of disease in their fifties, whereas in others it may be delayed until their eighties or nineties. This observation suggests that the symptomatic presentation of a clinically defined disease is the result of an accumulation of abnormal gene functions. One example of an age-dependent disease is breast cancer, which shows a steep increase in incidence in white women after 70 years of age. In postmenopausal women, the ductal epithelial cells, having fulfilled their designated function (the secretion of milk for breast feeding) usually undergo a cell suicide program, committing to apoptosis in order to be eliminated from breast tissues; this cellular process for eliminating unwanted cells is the chief operation occurring in involuted breast tissue.

Both the rate and extent of regression during involution vary among women. Often involution is not seen uniformly throughout breast tissue, resulting in a patchy or localized distribution and leaving residual ductal and lobular structures that are refractile to the involution process and persist into older age. These persistent tissues in an otherwise regressed organ may be a focal time bomb leading to breast cancer.

During involution, the ductal, lobular, or stromal cells are not sloughed off in sheets, as occurs in the endometrium during menstruation; rather, individual dying cells are scattered throughout the involuting tissues. This cell loss may be controlled by programmed cell death (i.e., a deliberate action to eliminate unwanted cells), as seen in other tissues. The benefit of cell death is most notable during development; for example, programmed cell death occurs in the development of the gut and nervous system and in remodeling of the limb buds, cartilage, and bones. Interference with the timing or frequency of this suicide program can turn a beneficial effect into deleterious consequences, as suggested here for breast cancer oncogenesis.

What factors contribute to this defect in the involution process? The contrast between North American and European populations and Asian, especially Japanese, populations is that breast cancer incidence decreases with age in the latter but increases in the former. A similar contrast is also seen between American Indian women living

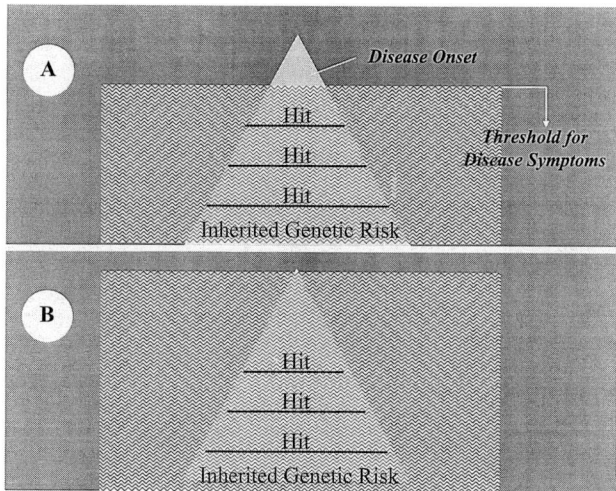

Figure 2-3 Diagram of the "iceberg" multihit model of the development of age-dependent diseases. (A) Accumulation of hits emerging above the threshold level, producing disease symptoms. (B) Asymptomatic accumulation of hits below the threshold level of disease presentation.

in New Mexico and their white neighbors; American Indian women, known for their low breast cancer risk, usually experience involution much earlier and exhibit an early shift to low-density parenchymal patterns. This early activation of involution may indicate a substantial loss of epithelial functional elements, leading to a more complete involution process. Although other variables such as diet and lifestyle may contribute to this epidemiologic difference, a set of genetic factors may also exist that influence the scope of the involution process. Incomplete involution may be affected by inherent genetic factors, permitting resilient cells to remain and form an initial "seed" for tumor development.

The scenario described for breast cancer development may pertain to other age-dependent diseases; that is, the genetic abnormality may start out as a seed. The germination of this genetic seed may occur only when a specialized cell function such as apoptosis is called into action. With time, germinated seeds grow in number, and with further insults, uncontrolled seed growth leads to symptomatic manifestation of disease. This "iceberg-like" hidden accumulation of functional defects stemming from an inherited flaw in the genetic makeup, along with environmental risks, contributes to the ultimate causes of age-dependent diseases, as shown in Figure 2-3. Obviously, familial age-dependent diseases involve genes having a high degree of polymorphism, and those who inherit "bad" alleles are likely to exhibit an earlier onset of disease, such as *APOE4* in persons with familial Alzheimer's disease and *BRCA 1* and *BRCA 2* in breast cancer patients.

ORDER OF GENE FUNCTIONS DURING AGING

Timing of the Functional Genomic State

A complex organism such as a human being requires genes to function in different stages: (1) developmental growth, (2) puberty and maturation, (3) adult maintenance, and (4) postreproductive sustenance (Fig. 2-4). Gene functions required for the first stage are those needed to generate cell mass that can be differentiated to form specialized organs and tissues (e.g., heart, brain, muscle). Gene functions required for the second stage are largely involved in maturation, specifically sexual maturation for reproduction; once sexual maturity is achieved, a stable program for this stage is controlled by genes involved in adulthood maintenance. Finally, the last program, postreproductive sustenance, known as the aging process, is largely controlled by yet a fourth program of gene expression.

Each of these four programs is regulated by a set of genes whose primary functions may operate in promoting or repressing cell growth. For example, during embryonic development, the need to create cell mass in a short period of time requires the intense effort of genes that function in cell cycle traverse. Soon after birth, these genes are silenced, to be expressed later only on occasions requiring cell growth such as wound healing and tissue regeneration. Obviously, the control of timing for this stage is a key factor in maintaining the overall balance of gene actions. Embryonic-like, pro–cell growth gene expression in an adult tissue can have a devastating effect, with the potential consequence of neoplastic growth leading to cancer. Therefore, correct timing of the actions of a specific set of genes in a given tissue is absolutely essential to maintaining a healthy genomic state. We know little of how this timing is governed and even less about how a defect in timing contributes to irregular physiologic functioning of each organ, and over time to the development of age-dependent diseases. Resetting the timing device for the regulation of gene expression could be a key to better health for elderly individuals.

The Yin-yang Mechanism and "Good" and "Bad" Genes

In general, for any given cellular event, genes functioning in groups can be categorized as pro or con in their actions. For example, pro- and anti-apoptotic genes are involved in controlling the molecular events that regulate programmed cell death, or apoptosis, a cell suicide process integrated into all tissues to dispose of excess, unwanted, infected, or damaged cells (Fig. 2-5). Proapoptotic genes act largely to activate a killing program that results in cell suicide; antiapoptotic genes act largely to counteract this killing action biochemically and are therefore known as survival factors. These two groups of genes, the proapoptotic represented mainly by caspases and the antiapoptotic known best by the *bcl2* gene family, work in a yin-yang balancing act to control whether a tissue in a given microenvironment needs to undergo the apoptotic or the survival program. Functional manifestations of each group of genes are largely controlled by an interwoven network of signal transduction pathways; cross-talk among them can eventually determine whether a cell lives or dies (Figures 2-1, 2-2, and 2-5).

We often erroneously consider genes "good" or "bad" according to their functional action. For example, we might categorize genes encoding caspases as bad genes because

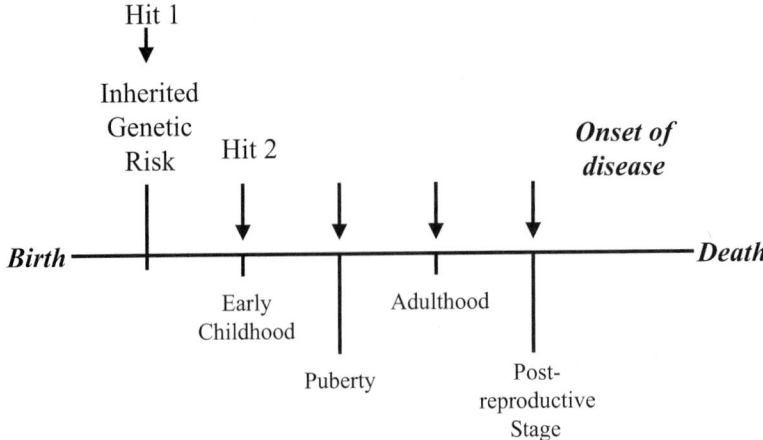

Figure 2-4 Multihit model of the etiology of age-dependent diseases in chronologic order over the entire life span.

their killing action causes the loss of neurons, possibly contributing to neurodegeneration seen in elderly people. However, a lack of caspase gene action in breast ductal epithelial cells or endometrial epithelium in postmenopausal women may be the genetic seed leading to breast or endometrial cancer in these patients. Furthermore, during embryonic development, caspase gene action is essential for tissue sculpturing to attain precise anatomic size and shape. By program design, during development the goal is first to produce extra cells; then, once the tissue is formed, the extra cells are eliminated by the apoptotic program. Caspase-3 knockout transgenic mice die during embryonic development because their brains develop twice as fast as those of normal control mice because of a failure to eliminate the excess neurons that are produced.

Thus, this genetic balance between two counteracting groups of gene actions in space and time is part of the ultimate beauty Mother Nature has endowed us with. As discussed above, age-dependent diseases often result from an accumulation of multiple hits; inheriting a defective expression in terms of the timing or location of caspase or

bcl2 genes may be one of the hits contributing to the heritability of familial early-onset age-dependent diseases such as breast cancer and Alzheimer's disease. A great effort is under way at many large pharmaceutical companies to develop pharmacogenomic drugs to correct the actions of caspase and *bcl2* genes. Success in this area may result in progress in combating cancer and neurodegenerative diseases in the elderly population.

Master Genes and Compensatory Gene Functions

Identification of the "concertmaster" of the genetic orchestra may be critical, as the heavy burden of the success or failure of the symphony lies on this player's shoulders. A concertmaster generally is a relatively permanent fixture, while a conductor can be a guest. Thus, in transducing a cellular event, the conductor may initiate the signal triggering activation of the event, whereas the concertmaster is the key to carrying out the tasks. As indicated in

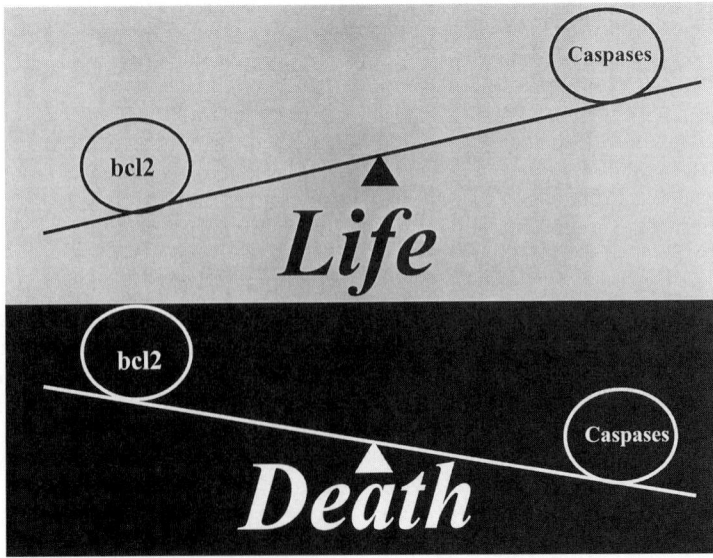

Figure 2-5 The seesaw effect of killer gene actions, represented by caspases, and survival gene actions, represented by *bcl2*. The upper panel shows the balance tilting toward life, and the lower shows the balance tilting toward death.

Figures 2-1 and 2-2, the PI3 kinase and MAP kinase pathways are so named because PI3 kinase and MAP kinase are the molecules that act as concertmasters for their respective pathways. These two pathways are not isolated in a cell, but rather function in a coordinated action, with constant cross-talk to ensure that multiple parallel cellular actions can be carried out simultaneously.

Signal transduction pathways can also be viewed as complex but organized cellular highways, with master genes situated at the major "hubs". These highways can be traversed from the nucleus to the plasma membrane, or vice versa. There may be one- or two-way traffic overall, but essential to the design is an alternate route to the destination. Thus, in a signal transduction pathway, nature provides many alternate routes to reduce the burden on one route compared to another or, more importantly, compensatory functions so that if one route is damaged, normal function can be carried out via other detours while the main route is being repaired. We would have been evolutionarily doomed to extinction if such compensatory gene actions did not exist. In other words, redundant, parallel, or compensatory biochemical networks are the rule of the game in the design of our genetic makeup.

Obviously, age-dependent diseases may result from heritable genetic defects in master genes and/or in the inefficiency several compensatory biochemical networks. It is not hard to visualize that clogging of either the PI3 kinase or the MAP kinase pathway (or both) will adversely affect the functional health of a cell. The excessive burden at each or both sites can slow down traffic and cause the entire system to be jammed, resulting in reduced efficiency and eventually in total system failure. Genetic defects, in terms of the optimal functioning of these two genes, are likely essential risk factors leading to age-dependent diseases.

Trade-off Between Gene Actions

Evolutionary biogerontologists often debate the theory of a "trade-off" between reproduction and longevity. Because (in this view) the primary goal of an organism's life is procreation, the genetic mechanisms for reproduction to ensure the survival of the species are the best-crafted designs of nature. Such mechanisms for enhanced reproduction may actually have a negative impact on longevity but would still be favored from the evolutionary viewpoint. However, this trade-off between reproduction and longevity does not necessarily apply. The emerging picture of the genetics of *C. elegans,* for example, shows that there may be no trade-off between fertility and longevity. In other words, compared to their shorter-lived counterparts, long-lived worms have an equal ability to produce progeny.

Genetically, the most difficult, yet most fascinating, task is identifying the timing of each gene expression. In other words, a gene or a group of genes may be functionally manifested at a precise time during the physiologic history of the organism. A "right" gene expressed at the "wrong" time may be devastating to the organism's overall need at the time. Such a mistake would be similar to an orchestra member playing the right music during the wrong movement,

leading to chaotic disharmony. The sharp rise in breast cancer among professional women may be due simply to delayed pregnancy. In a perimenopausal woman, the breast tissues are undergoing an involutional process, and the key ductal epithelial cells are programmed to commit apoptotic suicide. At this juncture, a pregnancy produces entirely different signals, stimulating the same cells not to die but to live and replicate so that they can grow into the critical mass required to perform the milk-producing function. These opposing demands, being scheduled to die but called on to live, place conflicting demands on a system designed to be shut down at a certain time. These cells receiving confused signals may be the very event that leads to breast cancer two decades later. Therefore, although there may be arguments as to whether evolutionarily there is a trade-off between fertility and longevity, there is certainly a trade-off between late pregnancy and risk for breast cancer in American women.

Gain or Loss of Gene Action

Most of the mutations studied as possible determinants of the life span of *C. elegans* indicate that longevity is extended by the loss of function of the specific genes involved. This notion of a survival-oriented loss of gene action is contrary to the unconscious assumption that death-causing frailty in elderly people is caused by the loss of normal gene functions, suggesting that a "cure" should involve restoring these lost functions. Work on *C. elegans* reveals that a loss of function, rather than a gain of function, may be the key to a healthy life span. Genetically, this loss of function operates like a dimmer switch for a light bulb; it is not intended to shut down the action but to maintain it at a reduced level. The remarkable discovery that the IGF1 receptor in *C. elegans* LAGs is also involved in *Drosophila* longevity suggests that the dimming effect of IGF1 in longevity extension may be a general rule for life span determination across species.

Here, we take at face value the notion that genetic control of a long life equals control of delaying death. If indeed this is the case, does the loss of gene functions seen in worms and flies occur in mammals, and even in humans? The answer to these questions may be both yes and no because the majority of the cell mass in *C. elegans* and *Drosophila* is "postmitotic," like our muscles, neurons, and cardiomyocytes, which do not replicate throughout our adult life. The findings of longevity related to the model systems of worms and flies are good, powerful models for these postmitotic cells in mammalian systems. What then represents a model for the mitotic cells in the human body, such as colonic epithelium, where scheduled cell replication is essential to the renewal of intestinal crypts? Here, gains of tumor suppressor gene function may be more essential to keep cell replication in balance, in order to avoid excessive cell proliferation and colon cancer formation.

However, the fact that growth factor knockout dwarf mice show a long-life phenotype suggests that a loss of function may be a positive factor for life span extension in mammals also, just as in lower organisms such as nematodes and flies. Moreover, the fact that long-lived caloric-restricted animals experience a delayed onset of cancer may mean that the issue is not whether or not to replicate but rather that the function of the IGF1/PI3 kinase signaling pathway in different cell types may be entirely different. In a postmitotic cell, it may direct proper signaling for neuronal axonal transport (or cardiomyocyte or muscle contraction), whereas in mitotic cells the same signaling pathway operates to drive replication, requiring additional tumor suppressor genes to keep cell cycle traverse in balance. "Overdrive" of IGF1/PI3 kinase signaling in either postmitotic or mitotic cells could lead to various abnormalities, either degenerated neurons or neoplastic colon epithelial cells. Therefore, the loss of function in a key gene may ensure the preservation of metabolic function, with gains of other gene functions, such as controlling tumor suppressors, as a complementary compensatory balance.

Key Genes, Vital Organs, and Age-Dependent Diseases

At the time of death, not all organs are at the end of their functional life span. In general, mortality results from a failure of one or a few vital organs. What genetic factors help avoid cardiomyocyte or neuronal failure, which can lead to death or denervation or to malfunctioning of bone and muscle cells, which can lead to reduced activities of daily living (ADL) indices? Are there common threads that are under genetic control in diverse organs? The answer may be yes because every cell in our body has similar networks of complex signal transduction pathways. The functional operation of this cellular network may differ among the various cell types. Key genes regulating the hubs of the highway network are essential to ensure the success of the signaling events required for each cell. Inherited defects in these key genes may lay a foundation for an iceberg-like buildup of leading to age-dependent diseases.

GENETICS, COMORBIDITY, AND EARLY ONSET OF AGING

Genes and Comorbidity

The concept of comorbidity may be the first lesson to be learned by every student combating age-dependent diseases. Here, the most elementary rule is appreciation that the same genetic defects, in principle, exist in all tissue systems but may not be manifested everywhere in the same fashion. Nevertheless, functional manifestations of these defects can occur in different cell types, with the same mechanism of iceberg buildup but with a different topographic appearance. For example, neurons and cardiomyocytes are the most long-lived cell types in our body, becoming postmitotic immediately after birth and remaining in this nonproliferating state throughout life. The prosurvival or antiapoptotic genes must operate in perfect pitch to allow neurons and cardiomyocytes to live as long as possible. Genes defective in the ability to maintain this lifelong survival program may be the nucleus of events leading to death in either type of cell. For example, shared cellular dysfunction resulting in apoptotic loss of both neurons and cardiomyocytes, caused by the same inherited gene defects, could be a determinant of vascular dementia.

Genes, Early-Onset Aging, and Familial Alzheimer's Disease

It is easy to understand why increased numbers of inherited genetic defects may be the prime reason for the early onset of an age-dependent disease simply because the starting point for the buildup is already high. Inherited defective genes contributing to age-dependent diseases cannot be totally functionless; if they were, the manifestation of their genetic defects would occur early in life or might even be lethal to the embryo. An epidemiologic geneticist studying Alzheimer's disease (AD) in general prefers to work with many families with early-onset forms of the disease because early onset is likely probably genetically transmitted and thus would be useful in the quest for the genetic culprits behind age-dependent diseases. Therefore it is not surprising that the first genes to be identified as being associated with AD were of the familial and early-onset type.

The identification of *APOE* as a gene involved in AD opened the door to mechanistic investigation of this complex neurodegenerative debility. Other genes associated with the development of AD have also been discovered. Nevertheless, the best linkage study on *APOE* provides at most only a 12 percent linkage frequency. In other words, *APOE* and other identified AD genes may contribute to only a small fraction of cases of AD. What genetic mechanisms are involved in *sporadic* AD? Do individuals with this condition carry no heritable genetic defects? Is their disease evolution caused entirely by stochastic environmental insults, and if so, which gene functions are compromised thereby? We shall address these issues in the section on genes and environmental factors.

GENETICS OF NORMAL AGING AND AGE-DEPENDENT DISEASES

A Continuum of Normal and Diseased Aging Processes

Biogerontologists often debate which genetic mechanisms determine the normal aging process and which cause diseases. The truth of the matter is that normal and disease-associated aging are on a continuum, with the ultimate symptomatic presentation of disease as the endpoint.

How does a normal aging process reach the threshold of a disease state? A goal of increasing the functional life span of elderly individuals is to retard the process leading to this threshold. Identifying genes contributing to aging may then simplify the search for genes that make individuals vulnerable to crossing this threshold.

Normal Versus Diseased Aging as Seen by Bone and Muscle Aging, Osteoporosis, and Osteoarthritis

The dream of a "fountain of youth" is for every senior citizen to have the vigor and strength of youth. Can we reverse the degeneration in aging muscles by providing young muscle to rejuvenate them? The answer is no; when muscles of young mice are grafted onto the muscle of old mice, they die. However, if we graft in the opposite direction, old muscle into young hosts, the muscle lives. These results indicate that the old muscle environment is hostile to the survival of young muscle. Therefore, the foremost need here is to understand the genes that render the old muscle environment hostile to new muscle survival; similar reasoning may pertain to the old bone environment as well.

One simple explanation of why old muscle is a hostile host for new muscle survival may be depletion of growth factors from the microenvironment in old muscle tissues. As discussed above, nature has engineered a program for living or dying for every cell. A cell's survival depends on the continual presence of antideath factors, that is, antiapoptotic genes. If the tissue environment is deprived of these gene products, the cells are automatically channeled toward the death route. In old muscle, the age-dependent decrease in the abundance of growth factors may simply represent the lack of a safety net for muscle cell survival. Consequently, the death of muscle cells occurs to a degree that produces a loss of muscle mass and unavoidable age-dependent muscle weakness.

Similarly, age-dependent dysregulation of gene functions in pro- and antiapoptotic death may also apply to bone aging. Bone health status is largely dependent on the constant replication of osteoblasts to supply new cells to the tissue and on constant apoptotic suicide of osteoclasts to dispose of old cells. The balance between these two cell behaviors, generating new cells and disposing of old cells, is a genetic wonder occurring for most of our adult life. Moreover, it is not hard to envision that tilting the balance of expression of pro- versus antiapoptotic genes can easily trigger more loss than gain, a prelude to bone degeneration. When the balance tilts strongly in favor of significant loss, the degree of bone degeneration approaches the threshold of the onset of osteoporosis.

Genes, Determination of Tissue-Specific Abundance of Survival Factors, and Normal Versus Diseased Aging Processes

If deprivation of growth factors is one of the genetic principles governing bone and muscle degeneration, why are the effects of this deprivation localized to these two tissues? Do other tissues suffer the same deprivation without experiencing disease phenotypes? The answer is that we do not know. Although estrogen withdrawal is well known to occur in postmenopausal women, there has never been a systematic study revealing specific age-dependent loss of growth factors in each type of tissue. We do not know the comprehensive profiles of all the growth factors in every body tissue, much less how much of each kind of growth factor is needed and where. Systematic studies on the temporal and spatial expression of growth factors will provide the first clues regarding the type, the amount, and the site of growth factors needed for the optimal healthy functioning of each tissue. Mutation in essential genes regulating these processes could exacerbate the damage, speeding up the process and changing the threshold of disease onset during the normal aging process.

Genes and Tissue-Specific Aging Processes

Do all our tissues respond similarly to a synchronized aging process or do they differ qualitatively and quantitatively en route to age-dependent disease states? One answer is that death is in general caused by the failure of one or two vital organs, although other organs may remain perfectly functional. Nevertheless, analytical answers to questions about the genetic mechanisms determining the differential aging processes of organs may not emerge until new technology allows us to examine in vivo the operational efficiency of each organ during life. Currently, it is almost impossible to identify the genes that determine tissue-specific aging processes and thereby tissue-specific vulnerability to age-dependent disease.

DNA Polymorphism, Individual Variations in Aging Processes, and Age-Dependent Diseases

The general message emerging from the previous discussion is that for each tissue to function optimally, gene actions determining cell survival must be balanced. These gene products, strategically located either extracellularly as growth factors or their respective receptors, or intracellularly as biochemical members of signal transduction pathways, are generated by the many base-pair sequences defining each gene's function and level of expression. Except for a few identified mutation changes, we know little of how changes in these DNA sequences govern the qualitative and quantitative manifestation of each gene's function. Just as we know little about how inheritable traits determine our facial features, we know even less about the magnitude of gene expression needed for the process determining cell survival. Therefore, interpersonal variation in the aging process or in the preferential vulnerability of one's vital organs to aging or age-dependent diseases may depend largely on the totality of DNA polymorphisms that determine our genetic individuality.

GENES AND ENVIRONMENT

Obviously, a healthy life span is achievable only when "bad" genetic and environmental factors are eliminated. However, in making a therapeutic attempt to eliminate these two groups of factors, it should be remembered that they do not work in isolation but are integrated. For the functional operation of every gene, there are four possibilities: (1) good gene and good environment, (2) good gene and bad environment, (3) bad gene and good environment, and (4) bad gene and bad environment. Although we are seeking a perfect world of good genes and good environment, a more practical approach may be to study what constitutes a bad environment to avoid damage to our good genes. In this section, we summarize how environmental factors can damage our genetic makeup and accumulate over time, leading to the development of age-dependent diseases.

Programmed Versus Stochastic, and Development Versus Aging

Discussions of aging mechanisms often focus on whether the aging process is programmed or stochastic. The popular analogy between an aging individual and an old car equates human organs to mechanical parts, which deteriorate over time. Thus, the aging process can be seen as a collection of many stochastic events, with death occurring when the accumulated stochastic insults cause vital organs to cease to function. In reality, the programmed theory and stochastic hypothesis are both likely correct. The regulation of gene expression, constituting the operating manual for every cell, is programmed, whereas insults to this regulation from environmental factors may be stochastic.

In order to understand how stochastic insults can occur intracellularly to induce dysfunction of the genetic program, we need to understand how the program of gene expression is first installed and organized during development. All the base pairs inherited from our parents and defined for a particular gene are organized according to a simple principle with two separate functional domains: coding and noncoding regions, with the latter located proximal to the beginning (the 5' end) or the tail (the 3' end) of the former. In general, the base-pair sequence in coding regions defines the genetic code for the gene product, the protein, whereas 5' and 3' ends define the regulatory mechanism for the gene action—"switching the light bulb on or off."

A precisely controlled program for gene expression is present very early in development. For example, there is a highly organized program supporting cell replication because there is a need to generate a critical mass for the formation of each tissue. Along with the requirement to produce optimal tissue mass, there is a parallel program of differentiation to achieve the specialized function of each cell type. The concerted efforts of gene expression can be seen as a continuum with different patterns of gene expression (embryonic-specific versus adult-specific) and another group for transition between these two stages (Figure 2-6). Many genes share considerable sequence homology but are expressed at different stages of an organism's life. These genes are considered isoforms of each other, with most of their functions shared but specialized for different physiologic needs. Thus, during development and maturation, there is a constant shift from embryonic to adult isoforms and therefore a change from embryonic to adult gene expression.

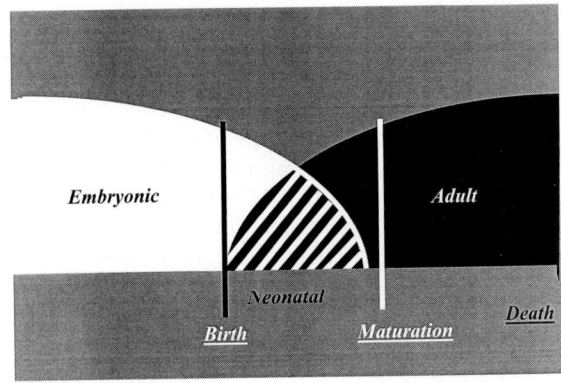

Figure 2-6 Diagram of the programmed shift from the expression of embryonic genes to the expression of their adult counterparts.

Promoters, Silencers, Enhancer Regulation of Transcription, and Age-dependent Diseases

The postdevelopmental profile of gene expression must be maintained throughout adult life. Practically, how can this program be sustained with a surveillance program to ensure perfect coordination? The answer lies in the exquisite regulation of gene expression at three different levels: (1) transcriptional decisions, whether or not a gene is activated by transcribing its genetic code to messenger RNA (mRNA); (2) translational operations to produce the protein prescribed by the transcribed mRNA; and (3) posttranslational biochemical modifications of the protein. Thus, the coordination of this operation is under an intricate checks-and-balances system, involving many layers of players in order to provide failure-proof molecular governing of our 3-billion-base-pair genome.

Operationally, it is essential to realize that regulation at these three levels is not simple. Rather, there are pro- and antimolecular forces for every gene action, and the balance between these forces controls the level of each gene action. In this regard, the regulation of gene action can be compared to the electrical control provided by numerous switch boxes in a house. The brightness of any light bulb in a particular room is controlled first by the main switch panel with its fuses and then by the switches in an individual room, which may function as a dimming rheostat. Molecularly, the intensity of each gene's expression resembles the shining of a light bulb resulting from the totality of all functional units—switch boxes with fuses, electric cables and wires, individual room switches, and finally light bulbs.

En route to maturation, a specific program is gradually activated in all cells to ensure that development-specific gene expressions are deactivated. For example, the task of creating neuronal cell mass needed during development is no longer required in an adult, and the expressions of certain genes necessary for cell replication are thus permanently shut down by a program of transcriptional repression. However, the action of some genes, such as those required for protein synthesis, may be needed in different degrees in different cell types; replicating cells may require high levels of expression, whereas quiescent cells need a reduced level. The intensity of expression of these genes can be modified by a "dimmer" switch providing for the different needs of different cell types. Therefore, promoter, enhancer, silencer, and repressor sequences are embedded in our genetic makeup and function together to define a precise level of expression for each gene in a particular environment.

This analogy involving light bulbs and switches presents a scenario for describing age-dependent disease. With age, deterioration of a system may make electrical conductance less efficient and thus result in the failure of individual operational units. For example, transcriptional activation of dormant gene expression for the cell cycle in neurons may be detrimental to the health of the neural system because some of these gene expressions are shared by cell replication and apoptotic death. In either case, replication or death, neurons lose their destined mission, which is to maintain the steady, nonproliferating state needed for neuronal transmission. Therefore, dysregulation of the intensity of the expression of cell cycle genes may contribute to the development of age-dependent diseases. In permanently nonmitotic cells such as neurons and cardiomyocytes, neither replication nor death is operationally optimal, and for mitosis-capable cells, excessive expression of genes involved in the cell cycle may set the stage for neoplastic growth. Therefore, the ultimate goal of genetics in preserving health in old age is to ensure that all the molecular light bulbs function with balanced efficiency as long as possible.

Genomic Stability, Methylation and Acetylation, DNA Repair, and Environmental Insults

Most genes expressed during embryonic development are not needed in adult life; vice versa, many adult gene expressions are kept silent during embryonic development. The embryonic and adult forms are sometimes sister genes whose genetic code sequences may be similar but not identical.

These minor sequence differences may represent the exact decision point for the functional divergence between the two sister genes. The shift from embryonic to adult gene expression occurs during the neonatal and postnatal periods, at the juncture where the task of creating tissue critical mass is completed and assumption of the total functional status of a given tissue commences with full intensity. For some genes this shift is an abrupt process, whereas for others it is drawn out. In some tissues this shift will be revisited during adult life. For example, in liver regeneration, wound healing, and breast feeding, the cells involved may revert to the embryonic state to meet the sudden requirement for critical mass building and then shift back to adult gene expression once the need is met.

Engineering of the embryonic-to-adult shift requires programmed control of gene expression similar to an electric switch box, with the special molecular design to qualitatively and/or quantitatively activate each gene. As described above, many sequence elements determine the on, off, or dimmer status of each encoded gene's expression. However, turning genes on or off involves the binding of

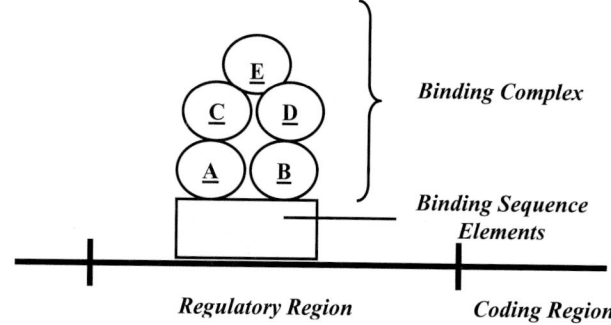

Figure 2-7 Diagram of the biochemical interaction between a binding complex and binding elements located in the 5′ regulatory region proximal to the coding region of a gene.

regulatory proteins in elaborate complexes that precisely dictate the level of gene expression (Figure 2-7). The binding of the nucleotide sequence base with the protein complex resembles the fit of a hand in a glove, requiring an exact three-dimensional topographic and biochemical match; if the glove is tightened with a rubber band, it will not fit the hand (nor, analogously, can genes be expressed). What molecular design permits these genetic gloves to fit just right? This process is mostly accomplished by two pairs of reciprocal biochemical actions: methylation and demethylation, and acetylation and deacetylation.

In general, genes to be expressed must be demethylated or acetylated, with the opposite biochemical states silencing other genes. Systematic regulation by methylation and acetylation may be nature's answer to activating or silencing gene expression. Thus, the shift from embryonic to adult gene expression can be arranged through the strategic methylation of a given embryonic gene and the simultaneous demethylation of its sister adult gene. These coupled biochemical reactions can also occur with acetylation but in the opposite direction, with acetylation turning the gene on and deacetylation turning it off (Figure 2-8).

Competitors for binding sites on the same protein often form complexes and function in opposite ways. For example, c-myc, a well-known oncogene, and MAD4, a tumor suppressor gene, both bind to a protein called MAX, forming a heterodimer which can then bind to a genetic sequence element CACGTG, known as an E-box. When the MAD4/MAX heterodimer binds to the E-box, acetylation occurs, allowing all 200 or so E-box–binding genes to be expressed; however, MAD4/MAX binding induces deacetylation, with subsequent silencing of the same genes. Needless to say, c-myc and MAD4 are two genes whose expression may be dominant factors in this biochemical scenario. The methylated state of these two genes may in turn affect their own expression and therefore produce a downstream acetylation state in E-box gene expressions. Therefore, avoiding tumor development requires that these two key proteins be in the proper biochemical state, with c-myc methylated and MAD4 demethylated.

Ideally, in any given adult tissue, chromosomal structural architecture should be arranged to allow a balance of methylation and demethylation, and likewise for acetylation and deacetylation, preventing embryonic genes from

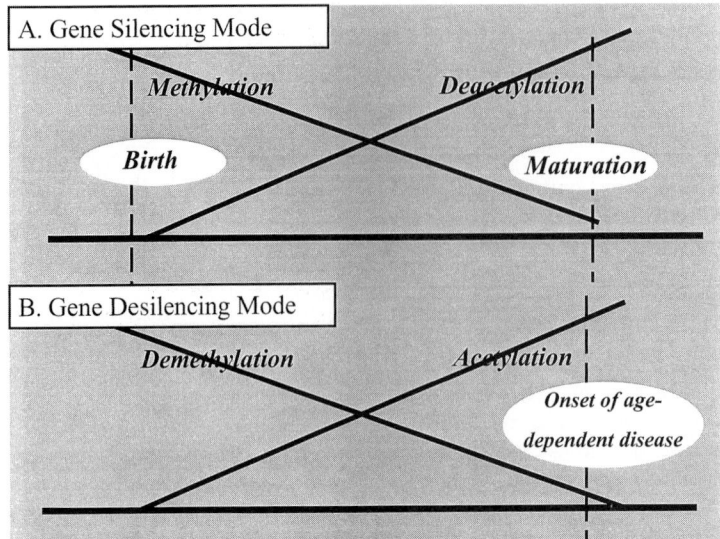

Figure 2-8 Diagram of biochemical actions on embryonic gene expression, programmed for the mode of gene silencing (A) or desilencing (B) of embryonic gene expression at the onset of age-dependent diseases.

being expressed and allowing adult genes to be expressed instead. In reality, this is a troublesome program, with many challenging tasks for the surveillance of damage and the structural repair of DNA. Chromosomal structures are constantly under bombardment from environmental insults such as free radicals, ultraviolet (UV) light, and so on. Accumulating excessive insults such as these can overwhelm the DNA repair system, resulting in irreversible damage. Therefore, somatic mutation or genomic instability is probably the most important contributing factor in the multihit theory of age-dependent diseases; our heritable traits for maintaining genomic stability may be essential in determining the early or late onset of disease.

Gene Doses, Oxidative Damage and Stress, and the Theory of Age-Dependent Diseases

Each of us inherits from our parents two copies of all genes except those on the sex chromosomes. As described above, the expression of each of these copies can be modulated by on, off, or dimmer functions. Therefore, genetic determination of the individual variance for a given gene can be qualitatively and quantitatively defined by the gene dose effect, ranging from zero to maximal capacity. For example, a person who inherits DNA repair genes in a maximal dose may be able to tolerate nicotine-induced damage to lung epithelial cells better than genetically disadvantaged individuals who inherit a lower dose. This may explain why in some cases cohorts with the same smoking habits experience widely different onsets of lung cancer.

Genes and environment are constantly interacting in every cell, the overriding principle being that when balance is lost, a disruption in cellular function may occur. Therefore, the decision points for the hits leading to the development of age-dependent diseases are probably determined by the qualitative and quantitative gene doses we

have inherited, which are integrated with the qualitative and quantitative environmental insults we are subjected to. Future research in individualized medicine, based on assaying our genomic heritable makeup, may reveal our total qualitative and quantitative genetic traits. Until then, the best strategy is to minimize the environmental insults and keep our genes always on the winning side in the battle with oxidative damage and stress.

Caloric Restriction and the Multihit Theory of Age-Dependent Diseases

The challenging lesson to be learned in combating any age-dependent disease is acceptance that there may never be a "cure" but rather many therapeutic interventions to delay a disease and restrict its damage. This delaying strategy may be the way to extend a healthy functional life span as long as possible. (For details on life span extension by caloric restriction, the reader should refer to Chapter 1.) Caloric-restricted animals usually manifest a delayed onset of cancer compared to counterparts fed ad libitum. The food restriction may in itself affect the speed of developing the hits leading to age-dependent diseases (Figure 2-4).

Dietary restriction may work at the molecular level to slow down metabolic rates that are too fast for cells to handle homeostatically, resulting in chromosome structural reorganization and in turn favoring dysregulation of the methylation and acetylation balance. This dysregulation may then cause a shift from the adult to the embryonic form of gene expression in a reversal of normal development. For some long-lived cells such as neurons and cardiomyocytes, reversion to the embryonic form would be detrimental and could lead to intolerable cell proliferation, disrupting the permanency of axonal transport or cardiac synchrony. For other cells such as liver and peripheral lymphocytes, such a reversion might cause hyperproliferation, a prelude to neoplastic growth. Therefore, instituting a program of dietary restriction and thus reducing intermediate metabolism may be the very intervention needed to maintain the molecular balancing act in methylation and acetylation biochemical programs.

We do not know specifically which genes are targeted by caloric restriction. Furthermore, all successful experiments on caloric restriction have been performed with genetically inbred laboratory-kept animals. It is hard to know whether results derived from such controlled-environment experiments with laboratory rats and mice are applicable to genetically diverse populations. Moreover, even from birth, we are not fed a constant diet like the food designed for laboratory rats and mice. Nevertheless, future investigations identifying which genes are directly or indirectly affected by caloric restriction, and determining how they work, may provide genetic clues to the use of nutritional modification to modulate the speed at which hits develop and later lead to age-dependent diseases.

DNA POLYMORPHISM, PREMATURE AGING, AND EXTREME LONGEVITY

In the previous section, we described enzymatic actions such as methylation and acetylation serving as switches controlling gene transcription. Environmental or genetic factors causing dysregulation of methylation or acetylation may produce consequential deregulated gene expression, thereby contributing multihits leading to the development of age-dependent diseases. The question then arises, What if the genes themselves become defective as a result of environmental insults? What do the cells do then? The answers can be found in the intricate assembly of a cadre of DNA repair enzymes whose primary mission is to localize the site of damage requiring repair.

Single Nucleotide Polymorphism and the Genetics of Aging

Single nucleotide polymorphisms are nucleotide based differences between two individuals in any given segment of the genomic sequence. There may be millions of SnPs scattered throughout our 3 billion base pairs. So far, we do not understand the mechanisms dictating the origination of SnPs in our genome, but they can occur anywhere along the chromosomes. If these SnPs are located in strategic sites, either in the coding region of a gene or in regulatory regions such as promoter regions, they may contribute to heritable defects.

The search for SnPs and their chromosomal locations can be a long, drawn-out process requiring large amounts of time and effort. In general, this kind of project starts with a population or cohort easily identified by phenotype. With the aid of quantitative trait lineage (QTL) analysis, the specific disease phenotype can be eventually mapped to a chromosomal location. This represents the beginning of a effort to perform finer mapping of the workable segments approachable by high-speed sequencing in order to identify the specific gene(s) bearing the SnP. Needless to say, once the entire human genome is decoded and mapped out, this laborious effort of sequencing will be reduced, and we may know just which genes serve as candidate segments bearing disease-associated SnPs.

Because SnPs exist and are known to be associated with the evolution of disease (e.g., *BRCA 1* represents an increased risk for breast cancer), we cannot ignore the possibility that the genetic factors linked with multihits leading to age-dependent diseases may be dependent on the frequency and locations of SnPs in our genome. It is reasonable to expect that there are many bad SnPs whose existence may not be lethal to an individual but may contribute to suboptimal functioning of our molecular machinery. Ultimately, the enormous challenge of identifying individual personalized SnPs may be the answer to mapping out the specific risks inherited from our parents.

Microsatellite Polymorphism and the Genetics of Age-Dependent Diseases

In addition to SnPs, another class of significant heritable traits determining our genetic makeup consists of microsatellites in our DNA; repetitive sequences of nucleotide base pairs in different configurations. For example, the best-known types are dinucleotide repeats such as CGCGCGCG . . . , called CpG islands, and trinucleotide repeats such as CAGCAGCAG. . . . The length of these repeats varies among individuals; short tandem repeats (STRs) are polymorphic and hereditary, but microsatellites can expand to greater lengths during the prezygotic stage, when the set of paternal chromosomes tries to match with the set of maternal chromosomes. In order to establish identical repeat numbers in progenitor cells, the shorter of the two parental sets is extended to match the longer set in order and length. Thus the expansion of microsatellite length generally occurs during the first stage of embryo formation, at the precise moment when sperm and oocyte fuse and two sets of chromosomes merge.

Both CpG islands and CAG repeats are well-known genetic structural elements defined as STRs of nucleotide sequences in strings of two (dinucleotides) or three (trinucleotides). STRs can vary in length and are found in coding regions (e.g., the CAG repeats within the Huntington's protein) in the 5′ or 3′ untranslated regions (e.g., the CTG repeats of myotonic dystrophy [103]), and in proximal noncoding regions (e.g., the CpG island [106–109] or the CA repeat associated with familial colon cancer). The length of microsatellite regions is intimately associated with the etiology of some age-dependent diseases. For example, the number of trinucleotide repeats, in general, determines the age of onset of Huntington's disease, whereas the length of dinucleotide repeats such as the CpG island is often associated with colon cancer development. It is not entirely clear what the optimal length of trinucleotide repeats such as CAG should be; longer CAG repeats, exceeding 200 units, are associated with an earlier onset of Huntington's disease. However, emerging results show that if the CAG repeat is located in the androgen receptor gene, CAG island segments shorter than eight repeats constitute a high risk for the early onset of prostate cancer. Thus, "good" or "bad" lengths of microsatellite repeats are in general determined by the specific genes where they occur rather than by the repeat size itself. Future fine mapping of our entire genome may reveal the optimal length for each of these microsatellite regions.

The Huntington's disease contig is a region known for gene richness; that is, a large number of genes have been discovered in this region. So far, besides the *HD* gene, others include α-adducin, *IT11*, and a G-protein-coupled receptor kinase. The fact that this region contains a high frequency of CpG islands, together with the trinucleotide (CAG) repeats found within the *HD* gene, makes the region most interesting in the study of mechanisms leading to human genetic diseases. This region is suggested to be a "hotbed" of genetic instability caused by mutation and expansion. Genomic instability is often found in these nucleotide repeat regions or microsatellites and usually results in expansion of the length of the repeats. As described above, although expansion of the length of repeats is thought to occur in germ line cells in the prezygotic stage, increasing evidence shows that somatic expansion also occurs and may contribute to the nonhereditary instability associated with some diseases.

Genetic diseases linked to trinucleotide repeats involve a repeated sequence becoming expanded beyond a critical length and thus poised for further uncontrolled expansion during DNA replication. This unregulated expansion may cause the silencing of transcription, message instability, or the formation of breakage points leading to segments of chromosome loss. Early, restricted expansion of a specific locus renders it an unstable "premutation"; but once subsequent large-scale expansion occurs, the fragile locus becomes a problematic "full mutation" site. The CAG repeats of Huntington's disease occur within the coding region, resulting in long stretches of glutamine within the huntingtin protein and a gain of function involved in enhanced promoter binding, possibly via transglutaminase, which is currently hypothesized to be a possible cause of Huntington's disease. CpG islands, described above, are a kind of dinucleotide repeat frequently found to be expanded in cancers; for example, the $(CA)_n(GT)_n$ repeats are well known to be associated with hereditary nonpolyposis colorectal cancer. The CpG island is thought to be involved in DNA methylation (and therefore transcriptional silencing).

Although the expansion of either tri- or dinucleotide repeats is thought to occur during oogenesis or spermatogenesis, it can also occur postzygotically. It may even take place during DNA replication with each round of cell division, in cells engaged constantly in replication, as a sort of inverse reflection of telomere shortening. For cell lines that are permanently growth-arrested after birth, such as neurons, cardiomyocytes, and myotubes, the expansion of a repetitive sequence may occur in a late stage of life when signals holding cells in a growth-arrested state are no longer effective, producing subsequent defective control of the expansion. The expansion of di- or trinucleotide repeats may occur as a reversion to meiosis during oogenesis or spermatogenesis; if the expansion occurs at sites proximal to key cell proliferation or death suppressor genes, the result may be deleterious to the proper regulation of their expression, leading either to hyperproliferation in the case of neoplastic growth or to death of selective neurons in the case of neurodegeneration. The final determination of whether repeats such as CAG and CpG islands have deleterious effects genetically and contribute to the multihits needed for the development of age-dependent diseases may depend on (1) the proximity of a key regulatory gene, (2) the inherited length and frequency of the repeats, and (3) the environmental insults imposed on the genomic instability of these genetic hotbeds.

DNA Repair and Premature Aging

Somatic mutation refers to the occurrence of an SnP or a change in the length of microsatellite repeats in adult non–germ line cells. These mutations usually are the result of environmental insults, such as UV or oxidative stress damage, which can cause the loss of a nucleotide or a change in the identity of a nucleotide base. When such losses or changes occur, a complex molecular repair machinery is called into play to repair the damage. Surveillance for DNA damage is associated with the transcriptional machinery involved in reading the genetic information. When DNA damage is encountered during transcription, transcription pauses and DNA repair takes over. Among the repair proteins associated with RNA polymerase II are helicases and endonucleases, which first melt the DNA duplex in the damaged region and then excise the damaged strand of DNA. The resulting gap is repaired by DNA polymerase delta, and the nick in the DNA strand is sealed. The newly repaired DNA can then be successfully transcribed, restoring the genome to a healthier state.

As noted above, DNA helicases associated with the transcriptional machinery play an essential role in repairing damage to DNA bases that can affect the readout of genetic information. Interestingly, premature aging is caused by mutations in another DNA helicase whose exact function within the cell is still unknown. This helicase is encoded by the gene responsible for Werner's syndrome. Mutations in this gene cause multiple disease phenotypes, such as early development of cancer, cardiovascular disorders, and a host of other clinical abnormalities. Werner's syndrome helicase appears to recognize DNA structures found at replication and transcription forks, and it has been proposed that this helicase may function to resolve aberrant DNA structures formed at these locations. The defect repair in this case may be related to higher-order levels of DNA structure beyond the sequence of bases within the DNA.

Transcriptional Infidelity and Neurodegeneration

Errors in the readout of genetic information that occur with aging are not limited to changes in DNA structure, either through base changes or DNA modification. Errors introduced during transcription may have important roles in age-dependent neurodegenerative diseases. These mistakes are introduced by RNA polymerase II during the transcription of GAGAG repeat sequences of neuronal mRNAs. The mRNAs affected include those encoding the beta amyloid precursor protein (betaAPP) and ubiquitin B. This phenomenon, known as molecular misreading, causes frameshift mutations in neuronal mRNAs. These mRNAs in turn encode proteins that contain additional amino acids at their carboxyl termini relative to their normal counterparts. These extended proteins are found in pathologic lesions associated with Alzheimer's disease, such as neurofibrillary tangles, neuritic plaques, and neurophil threads, suggesting that they may have a role in disease etiology.

At the present time the extent to which molecular misreading contributes to other age-related diseases is unclear. GAGAG repeats are thought to occur quite frequently in random sequences, indicating that there are likely many other mRNAs that may be targets for molecular misreading. In addition, it is not known whether this phenomenon is restricted to neuronal cells or if it is more widespread throughout the body.

The potential for errors in the readout of genetic information extends beyond the transcriptional machinery to the translational apparatus. In fact, one of the early theories of aging, the error catastrophe theory, was based in part on the idea that errors occurring during translation create abnormal proteins, which can then affect the fidelity of other processes such as DNA replication and repair, transcription, and translation, creating a positive feedback loop of errors leading to a catastrophic decline in cellular function. Thus the hundreds of genes involved in various aspects of the protein synthetic machinery are targets for mutational events that may affect translational fidelity and contribute to age-related diseases.

Finally, as noted above, ubiquitin B mRNA is a target of molecular misreading, indicating that defects in protein degradation may have a role in the development of age-related diseases. With all these potential sources of errors increasing with aging, one would predict that an efficient means of eliminating affected proteins would be necessary. And yet, just the opposite is true. All these factors may therefore contribute to the genetic basis of age-dependent diseases.

Repair Versus Suicide, and Age–Dependent Disease

In the case of genomic damage beyond repair, a signal activates the suicide program, apoptosis, to eliminate the cells involved. Interestingly, the first proteins found to be substrates for apoptosis-associated killers, caspases, are all involved in the DNA repair mechanism. Therefore, it is not hard to conceive that the molecular decision for a particular cell to live or die is strategically targeted to genes that function in the DNA repair process, the best known of which is polyadenosine diphosphate ribose polymerase. The best way to guarantee the functional status of each tissue is to dispose of cells that are damaged beyond repair in order to ensure the functioning of the majority of healthy cells unencumbered by the presence of damaged cells.

An imperfect apoptotic process may occur largely because of defects in the decision for life or death. The defective forms of the p53 gene provide an example of this. In general, p53 has dual functions, tumor suppression and apoptosis activation; it can act either to inhibit cell proliferation, restraining cells from improper replication that leads to neoplastic growth, or to activate the apoptosis program when damage beyond repair occurs, such as that associated with UV exposure. Thus the p53 gene is a master gene whose function is vital to our well-being. Failed p53 function usually means a failure in both tumor suppressor and apoptosis programs, resulting in an uncontrolled proliferation of cells with DNA damage beyond repair. It is no wonder that mutations associated with the p53 gene were among the early genes identified in the search for the mechanism of early onset of widespread age-dependent heritable cancers.

DNA Repair, Centenarians, and Extreme Longevity

The notion of a perfect environment, void of every insult to our genetic makeup, is not realistic. For example, sunlight is the very source of our existence on the planet; on the other hand, too much sunlight results in excess UV exposure, which produces the DNA damage described above. Thus an indispensable resource also constitutes a risk for cancer in photosensitive individuals. Facial basal cell carcinoma associated with prolonged sunlight exposure, which is found especially in individuals of Scandinavian ancestry, is usually genetically determined. In this context, a continuous battle between genetic damage and repair may be occurring over our entire life span. As repeatedly discussed in this chapter, winning or losing this battle determines how long we can last before we exhaust the repair reservoir of our genetic makeup. On an individual basis, it is obvious that those who inherit a larger reservoir have a better reserve to combat this "gene versus environment" warfare. Integrated into this equation, emerging knowledge of good environmental factors such as caloric restriction will help to reduce the rate at which our genetic reservoir is exhausted.

As described earlier, DNA polymerase is a key determinant of life or death. It is no wonder that the life spans of different species are correlated with the abundance of this gene product; long-lived animals have more abundant DNA polymerase than species with a shorter life span. In human populations, extremely long-lived individuals such as centenarians and nonagenarians survive or escape age-dependent diseases. What explains their long-lived phenotype at the genetic level? How can these extremely long-lived individuals delay or override the hits contributing to the development of age-dependent diseases such as cancer, neurodegeneration, and cardiovascular disorders? The answer may lie in the genetic robustness of their DNA repair systems. Subjected to the same environmental impacts, extremely long-lived individuals may be privileged to have efficient repair systems.

Human Longevity Assurance Genes and the Genetics of Aging

It is possible that long-lived individuals may indeed possess genes whose functions can restrict diseases to a temporary course without complications. These genes might counteract age-dependent processes and therefore count as DDGs, or in the opposite sense, human longevity genes. There may be countless examples of such genes, such as perhaps anti–mercury toxin genes and anti–biological hazard genes protecting against air or water pollution. It is therefore essential to identify and investigate whether such genes indeed figure in our hereditary endowment. Ultimately, the search for the genes determining extreme human longevity will merge with the search for genes functioning as anticancer, anti–cardiovascular failure, anti–neurodegenerative debility, antiosteoporosis, antiarthritis, and so on. Of course, the ultimate prize will be the identification of "golden genes" that counteract all these disorders.

HUMAN GENOME MAPPING, THE BIOTECHNOLOGY REVOLUTION, AND SUCCESSFUL AGING

We are poised to take giant leaps beyond the information age and into the postgenome era, fortified to embark on a future world of personalized medicine based on the genetics of our individual aging processes. This section introduces recent cutting-edge enabling technology and examines how it might be applied in investigating the genetics of aging and age-dependent diseases.

Human Genome Mapping, Chip Technology, and Biosignatures for Individualized Aging Processes

Sequencing of the human genome has become the centerpiece of a biological revolution. Eventually, mapping the entire sequenced 3 billion base pairs will allow us to determine the physical locations of all the genes that in totality determine the makeup of our entire being. The human genome is composed of about 30,000 genes, and with the increasing complexity of our environment, it is hard to understand how the integration of our genes and our surroundings creates a disease-predisposed state. Perhaps an individual's "genetic signature" can provide a means to prevent and treat diseases in an individual manner, creating individualized medicine for prognostic, diagnostic, and therapeutic purposes.

Parallel to the human genome sequencing effort is another enormous technologic breakthrough in which DNA or mRNA chip platforms are used to decipher the genomic status associated with physiologic processes as well as with disease stages. Biochip technology, otherwise known as high-throughput gene screening, gene discovery, or microarray technology, is a rapidly developing field of biomedical research in which molecular medicine is combined with state-of-the-art computer and engineering science. A biochip is a platform containing multiple samples of genetic or gene message information, perhaps hundreds or thousands of gene fragments or mRNAs; the simultaneous analysis of dozens or hundreds of these biochips covers a significant fraction of our 30,000 genes at a glance.

The success of DNA chip technology will allow the development of pioneering research products that can be used in geriatric medicine in areas such as (1) genetic or gene expression profiling of risk factors involved in the development of disorders such as cancer, cardiovascular disease, and neurodegenerative disease; (2) molecular assessment of disease-prone genes to identify environmental risk factors; (3) gene-based diagnoses; and (4) clinical evaluation with advanced diagnostic technologies.

Genome Mapping of Model Animal Systems, and Age-Dependent Diseases of Humans

The biochip approach may facilitate determining and triaging health care customized to individual needs and may also speed up the development of new drugs. The idea that gene sequences are largely conserved between species provides biologists with an immediate lead to the molecular identity and candidate putative functions of each novel gene as it is identified. A simple search in the GeneBank for genes sharing entire or fragmentary sequences can provide a step toward understanding the possible connection between the involvement of a gene in a cellular function and how it may be related to the determination of life span across species. Thus, the discovery of genes that determine life span in genetic model systems such as yeast, *C. elegans, Drosophila,* and mice may provide clues leading to the discovery of homologous human genes that may functionally determine an individual's life span.

Artificial Intelligence and the Genetics of Aging and Age-Dependent Diseases

Computerized artificial intelligence expert systems for recognizing patterns, such as handwriting on personal checks and addresses on envelopes, or detecting written language differences, have been under development for decades. Using the same science of pattern recognition to recognize changes in multiple gene expressions is a fast-developing field in the discipline of bioinformatics. Advances in this direction will expand from the presently popular single-gene analysis approach to investigating 10 to 100 or more gene differences simultaneously. Such an approach is necessary in analyzing the volume of data generated by multiple biochips and addressing how a halffold or onefold difference in about 50 genes can create a molecular pattern leading to the development of cancer or cardiovascular debility in an individual elderly patient.

Computerized expert systems can be expanded beyond genes to address how changes in patterns of clinical, cognitive, and epidemiologic risk factor analyses differ among individuals. This linkage between genetic and clinical, cognitive, and epidemiologic data recognized by expert systems may support the design of new research programs and generate new questions, for example, how to take care of each elderly patient as an individual in a cost-effective manner. Identifying unique genes and their expressions associated with healthy human longevity, as well as the technology of biochip production, may open up new areas of research in preparation for twenty-first century biomedical progress.

From Genomic Studies to Health Care Delivery

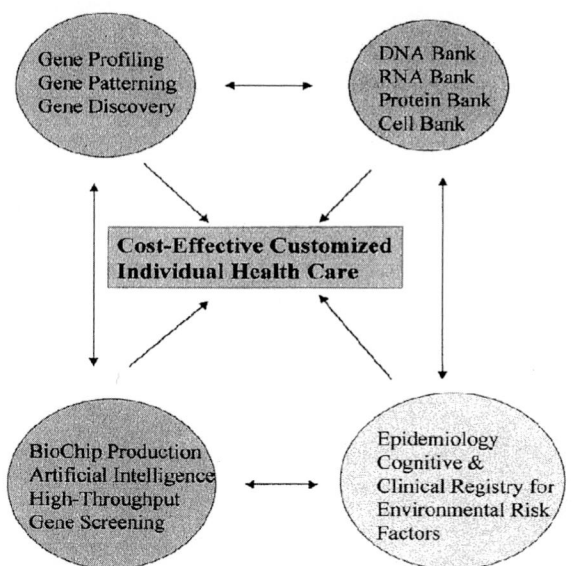

Figure 2-9 Diagram showing how genomic studies could potentially contribute to improved health care delivery.

CONCLUSIONS

The most powerful gain from understanding the genes that determine normal aging and age-dependent disease processes is likely to be the ability to link genetic information with epidemiologic risk factors and cognitive functional assessment in one continuous approach to analyzing mechanisms controlling the dynamics of life span determination from genes to environmental and behavioral factors (Fig. 2-9). The success of this linkage may provide high-tech genomic approaches along with low-tech corrections of problems related to life-long preventive medicine, education, and behavioral and pharmacogenomic therapeutic treatment, with the ultimate goal of creating a new total medicine for geriatric care directed toward achieving a healthy, functional life span.

ACKNOWLEDGMENTS

The author is deeply indebted to Alan N. Bloch and Steve R. Ellis for discussions shared and comments offered during the preparation of this chapter. I am also grateful for the laborious proofreading efforts of Alan N. Bloch and for graphics work by Angel Wang.

Eugenia Wang's research program in the biology of aging has been supported by a MERIT award from the National Institute on Aging of the National Institutes of Health, as well as by a grant from the Defense Advance Research Project Agency (DARPA) of the US Department of Defense.

REFERENCES

Amuthan G et al: Mitochondria-to-nucleus stress signaling induces phenotypic changes, tumor progression, and cell invasion. *EMBO J* 20(8):1910, 2001.

Bartke A et al: Genes that prolong life: Relationships of growth hormone and growth to aging and life span. *J Gerontol* 56A(8):B340, 2001.

Carlson BM, Faulkner JA: Muscle transplantation between young and old rats: Age of host determines recovery. *Am J Physiol* 256(6 pt 1):C1262, 1989.

Cheung VG et al: Making and reading microarrays. *Nat Genet Suppl* 21:15, 1999.

Dorman JB et al: The *age-1* and *daf-2* genes function in a common pathway to control the lifespan of *Caenorhabditis elegans*. *Genetics* 141:1399, 1995.

Finch CE, Tanzi R: Genetics of aging. *Science* 278:407, 1997.

Franke TF et al: P13K: Downstream action blocks apoptosis. *Cell* 88:435, 1997.

Hamilton ML et al: Does oxidative damage to DNA increase with age? *Proc Natl Acad Sci U SA* 28;98(18):10469, 2001.

Henson DE, Tarone RE: On the possible role of involution in the natural history of breast cancer. *Cancer* 71(6):2154, 1993.

International Human Genome Consortium: The 24 volumes of the Human Book of Life (October 2000 edition). *Nature* 409:860, 2001.

Kimura KD et al: *daf-2*, An insulin receptor-like gene that regulates longevity and diapause in *Caenorhabditis elegans*. *Science* 277:942, 1997.

Kinney BA et al: Evidence that Ames dwarf mice age differently from their normal siblings in behavioral and learning and memory parameters. *Hormones Behav* 39:277, 2001.

Mochizuki A et al: The evolution of genomic imprinting. *Genetics* 144:1283, 1996.

Morris JZ et al: A phosphatidylinositol-3-OH kinase family member regulating longevity and diapause in *Caenorhabditis elegans*. *Nature* 382:536, 1996.

Olshansky SJ et al: In search of Methuselah: Estimating the upper limits to human longevity. *Science* 250(4981):634, 1990.

Tatar M et al: A mutant *Drosophila* insulin receptor homolog that extends life-span and impairs neuroendocrine function. *Science* 6;292(5514):107, comment on 41-3, 2001.

van Leeuwen FW et al: Molecular misreading: A new type of transcript mutation expressed during aging. *Neurobiol Aging* 21(6):879, comment on 893-2, discussion on 903-4, 2000.

Warren ST: The expanding world of trinucleotide repeats. *Science* 271:1374, 1996.

CHAPTER 3

Immunology of Aging

DONNA M. MURASKO • ELIZABETH M. GARDNER

The maintenance of an effective immune system is essential in conferring protection against infection, cancer, and autoimmune diseases. Although aging is accompanied by a decline in the effectiveness of immune function, a causal relationship between decreased immunity and increased rates of infection, cancer, and autoimmune disease in the elderly population has not been established because of confounding factors that include environment, genetics, nutrition, and age-related diseases. Even if age-associated changes in immune functions are not solely responsible for the increased morbidity and mortality among the elderly population with this group of diseases, an altered immune system undoubtedly influences those increased rates significantly. Therefore, it is important for those who care for the elderly person to understand age-associated changes in immune function. To more fully appreciate the alterations in immune response that occur in specific alterations that occur during immunosenescence, an overview of normal immune function is provided below.

OVERVIEW OF THE IMMUNE SYSTEM

Cells of the Immune System

Lymphocytes, monocytes, and granulocytes are the major cell types that constitute the immune system (Table 3-1). Multipotent stem cells in the bone marrow give rise to cells of the lymphoid lineage (T cells, B cells, and natural killer [NK] cells) and to the myeloid lineage (monocytes/macrophages, neutrophils, eosinophils, and basophils). The primary lymphoid organs—thymus and bone marrow—are the sites of T- and B-cell maturation, respectively. Lymphocytes migrate from the bone marrow or thymus to the secondary lymphoid organs (lymph nodes, spleen, and mucosal-associated lymphoid tissue), which are the sites of maximal interaction of immune cells with antigens, such as microbial pathogens and allergens. Cells of the immune system communicate with each other through the release and uptake of soluble factors called cytokines (Fig. 3-1). Cytokines have autocrine and paracrine effects that modulate interactions among cells of the immune system and between the immune system and other organs. The immune system recognizes and responds to

"nonself" and "altered self" antigens through two major effector arms: cell-mediated immunity and humoral immunity. T cells are the primary mediator of cell-mediated immunity, whereas B cells play the comparable role in humoral immunity. Both arms are amplified by cytokines and by the involvement of phagocytic cells (e.g., macrophages and neutrophils) and NK cells.

T Cells

T cells constitute approximately 70 percent of the lymphoid pool in blood. T-cell precursors from the bone marrow migrate to the thymus, where they undergo maturation. In the thymus, genes responsible for encoding the T-cell receptor (TCR) are rearranged so that each mature T cell has a unique receptor that is specific for an antigenic determinant (also called an epitope). The result is an extensive array of T cells specific for a vast range of antigens. The TCR, however, does not interact with soluble antigens. Antigenic molecules must be processed into small peptides and presented to a T cell by another cell (antigen-presenting cell [APC]) in the context of molecules on the surface of the APC. These molecules are coded within the major histocompatibility complex (MHC). In addition, the TCR of all T cells is associated with another surface marker, CD3 (Table 3-2). CD3 is a complex of five distinct polypeptide chains. The association of TCR with CD3 is required for T-cell function. The TCR has antigen specificity but requires CD3 to transmit activation signals intracellularly. Other surface molecules, such as CD28 (Table 3-3), that are not associated with the TCR are costimulatory molecules that are also involved in signal transduction in T cells. This complex system allows for specificity and, importantly, for control of T-cell reactivity.

Mature T cells can be subdivided into two subpopulations: T helper cells (Th) and cytotoxic T lymphocytes (CTLs). Th cells, which are characterized by expression of the CD4 surface marker, are capable of stimulating proliferation and differentiation of both CTLs and B cells. CD4+ cells recognize antigen in the context of MHC class II molecules. Th cells accomplish their functions in part through the secretion of substances called cytokines. Because many of the cytokines are produced by one white blood cell and induce activity in another white blood cell,

Table 3-1   Cells of the Immune System in Blood

	Leukocytes, %	Function
Lymphocytes	20–40	
T cells	60–75*	Cell-mediated immunity
B cells	10–20*	Humoral immunity
Natural killer cells	10–15*	Cytotoxicity
Monocytes	1–5	Phagocytosis Antigen presentation
Granulocytes		
Neutrophils	50–70	Phagocytosis
Eosinophils	1–2	Phagocytosis; defense against parasites
Basophils	<1	Nonphagocytic; allergic reactions through release of actives substances

*Percent of total lymphocytes in blood.

they have been called interleukins (ILs) (Table 3-4). The pattern of cytokine secretion by Th cells determines the clinical manifestations of the immune response.

Analyses of Th cell clones have defined several subgroups of Th cells, which are distinguished by their cytokine profile. Th1 cells secrete IL-2 and interferon-γ (IFN-γ) and are the major mediators of cytotoxic and inflammatory reactions. Th2 cells secrete IL-4, IL-5, IL-6, and IL-10 and function mainly to stimulate B cells to proliferate and differentiate. Although most immune responses are neither exclusively Th1 nor Th2, the balance of Th1 and Th2 cytokine production shifts a response toward one reaction or the other. For example, high levels of IFN-γ downregulate the production of Th2 cytokines; an inflammatory response is the dominant clinical manifestation. In contrast, high concentrations of IL-4 result in low levels of IFN-γ and predominantly an antibody response. Th cells that secrete both Th1 and Th2 cytokines are designated Th0 cells.

Mature T cells that have not yet encountered antigens are considered naïve. After antigen-induced clonal proliferation and differentiation, some T cells become long-lived memory cells. Naïve cells can be distinguished from memory cells by their expression of various isoforms of CD45, activation requirements, and cytokine production. Naïve T cells are characterized by the expression of CD45RA. CD45RA+ cells have stringent activation requirements, proliferate preferentially to mitogens, and secrete primarily IL-2 in response to stimulation. After activation

of T cells, CD45RA is replaced by CD45RO. Cells that express CD45RO are considered memory T cells. These cells have upregulated costimulatory and adhesion molecules and have TCR with increased avidity for antigen, making CD45RO+ cells well suited for recall responses to antigen. Unlike naïve T cells, which secrete IL-2, memory T cells secrete a wide range of cytokines, including IL-3, IL-4, IL-10, IFN-γ, and high levels of IL-2, on stimulation and thus allow for varied clinical manifestations of the immune response.

CTLs play a very important role in clearing "altered self" cells, such as tumor cells, and cells infected with intracellular pathogens (e.g., viruses). CTLs are characterized by the expression of the CD8 surface marker and the ability to bind via their TCRs to cells that express antigen in the context of MHC class I molecules. In addition, cytokines produced by Th cells (e.g., IL-2) are needed for maximal proliferation and differentiation of CTLs. Once activated, CTLs can bind to target cells and can induce a target cell to undergo apoptosis (programmed cell death) through the secretion of perforin and serine proteases.

B Cells

B cells, which constitute 15 to 25 percent of lymphocytes in peripheral blood, originate and mature in the bone marrow. B cells, like T cells, express an antigen-specific surface receptor. The B-cell receptor (BCR) is composed of a surface immunoglobulin (sIg) with antigen specificity and a signal transduction complex of CD79a (Igα) and CD79b (Igβ). During B-cell maturation, immunoglobulin genes of individual cells are rearranged to produce a unique BCR. After rearrangements, mature naïve B cells express IgM alone or coexpress IgM and IgD. However, once B cells are exposed to antigen, they further differentiate into effector cells (antibody-producing plasma cells) or cells capable of recall responses to specific antigens (memory B cells). The sIg expressed on mature B cells after exposure to antigen may be IgM, IgG, IgE, or IgA. The switching of immunoglobulin class that occurs after exposure to antigen is dependent on cytokine signals (e.g., IL-4, IL-5, IFN-γ) from Th cells. Mature B cells also express other surface markers that participate in signal transduction, such as CD19, CD21, CD40, and B7 (CD 80) (see Table 3-3). Although no unique surface markers distinguish memory B cells from naïve B cells, memory B cells express high-affinity sIg obtained through the process of antibody affinity maturation. This process occurs in the germinal center of the lymph node by means of antigen-driven somatic hypermutation of sIg. The result is selection of B-cell clones with increasing affinity for specific antigens. Both naïve B cells and memory B cells can differentiate into plasma cells, which can secrete up to 2000 molecules of antibody per second. These antibodies are the effector arm of the humoral response, binding to a bacteria, virus, or allergen.

Phagocytes

Phagocytes (neutrophils and mononuclear phagocytes) bind to foreign substances (e.g., microbial pathogens and

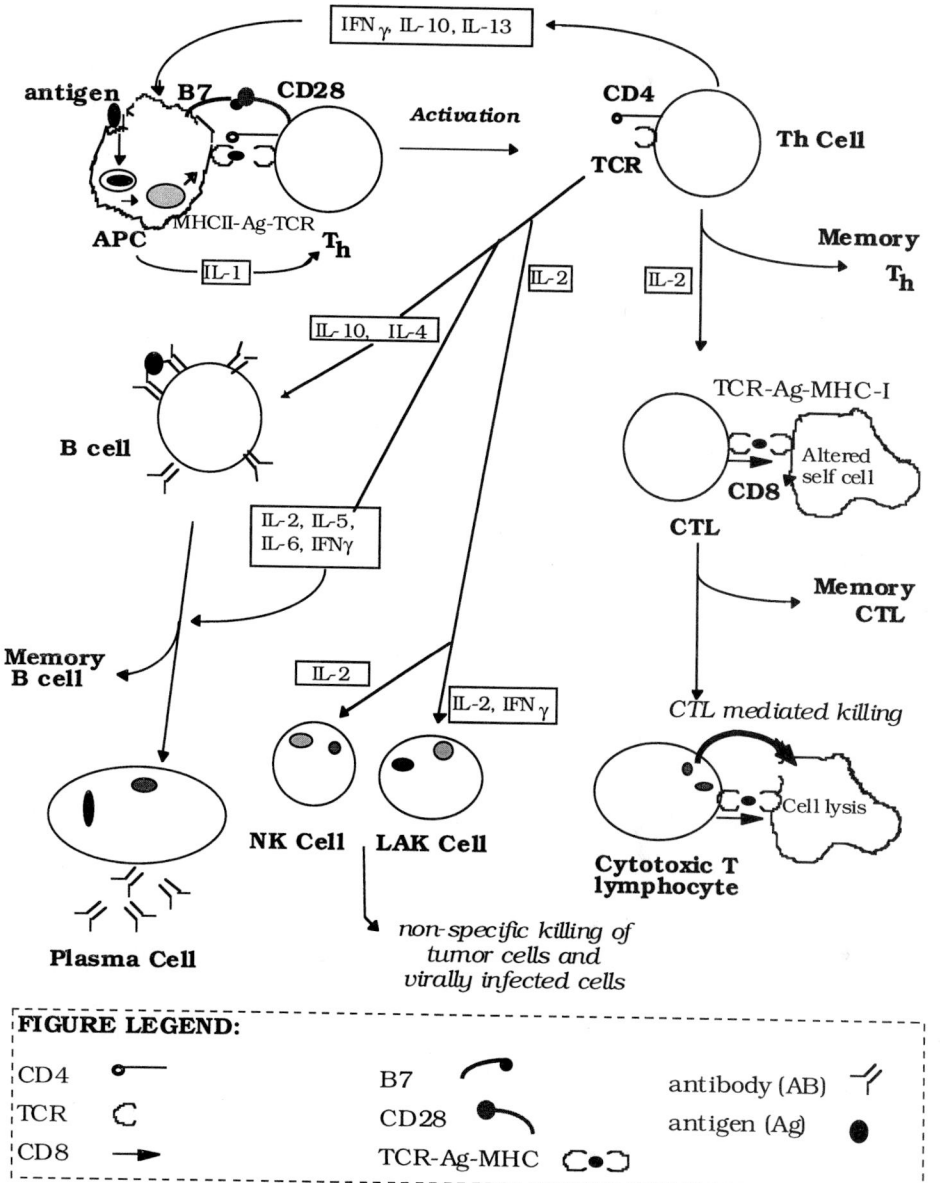

Figure 3-1 Interactions among cells of the immune system.

environmental pollutants) and then internalize and degrade them. Mononuclear phagocytes circulate in blood as monocytes or reside as macrophages in specific organs, such as Kupffer's cells in the liver, alveolar macrophages in the lung, microglia in the brain, and sinus macrophages in the spleen. These cells play an essential role in the first line of defense against invading substances. They are also key players in the inflammatory response to tissue injury, in which a series of chemical mediators allow for extravasation of leukocytes from capillaries to the site of injury. At the site of injury, phagocytes engulf foreign material and secrete substances, such as IL-1, IL-6, and tumor necrosis factor-alpha (TNF-α), which are responsible for many of the local and systemic effects of inflammation.

In addition to serving as scavengers, a subset of these phagocytes—macrophages—act as APCs. They process the internalized substances into immunogenic peptides

Table 3-2   Surface Markers of Lymphocytes

Lymphocytes	Surface Markers
T Cells	
T helper	CD3, CD4
Cytotoxic T	CD3, CD8
T naive	CD3, CD4 or CD8, CD45RA
T memory	CD3, CD4 or CD8, CD45RO
B cells	
Immature	CD19
Mature	CD19, CD21, CD79a and b
Natural killer cells	CD56, CD16

Table 3-3 Common Surface Markers Used to Identify Leukocytes

	Common Synonym	Primary Expression	Function
CD2*	Sheep red blood cell receptor	T cells, NK cells	Adhesion, activation
CD3	Pan-T-cell marker	T cells	Signal transduction; associated with TCR
CD4		Th cells	Adhesion: binds MHC class II; signal transduction
CD8		CTL	Adhesion: binds MHC class I; signal transduction
CD16	FcγRIII	NK, macrophages, granulocytes	Receptor for Fc of Ig; ADCC[†]
CD19	B4	B cells	Activation
CD21	B2, CR2	B cells	Activation, receptor for C3d[‡]
CD25	IL-2 receptor α chain, TAC	Activated T cells and B cells	Cell growth
CD28		T cells	Interacts with costimulatory molecule B7 on antigen-presenting cells
CD40		B cells, macrophages, dendritic cells	Activation
CD45 　CD45RA 　CD45RO 　CD45RB	Common leukocyte antigen	Leukocytes Naïve T cells Memory T cells B cells	Signal transduction
CD56	Leu 19	NK cells, T cells	Adhesion
CD79a	Igα	B cells	Associated with B-cell antigen receptor
CD79b	Igβ	B cells	
CD80	B7-1	Macrophages, activated B cells	Costimulator for T-cell activation; binds CD28 on T cells

CTL, cytotoxic T lymphocyte; Ig, immunoglobulin; IL, interleukin; MHC, major histocompatibility complex; NK, natural killer cells; TAC, T cell actuation antigen; TCR, T-cell receptor; Th, T-helper cells.
*CD antigens: cell membrance molecules that are used to identify populations of leukocytes. These molecules are detected by using monoclonal antibodies. Because molecules have many antigenic determinants, two monoclonal antibodies may react with the same molecule, but with different antigenic determinants. Monoclonal antibodies that react with the same molecule are grouped together, and the grouping is termed a cluster of differentiation (CD).
[†] Antibody-dependent cell-mediated cytotoxicity.
[‡]Complement factor.

and present those peptides in the context of the MHC to T cells. APCs include macrophages, Langerhans' cells, follicular dendritic cells, interdigitating cells, and B cells. The presentation of antigenic peptides (epitopes) by APCs to T cells is one form of communication between the non-specific (i.e., phagocytic) and the specific (i.e., T-cell) responses of the host to foreign substances. APCs secrete IL-1, which promotes maturation and clonal proliferation of lymphocytes; IL-6, which promotes terminal maturation of B cells into plasma cells; and IL-12, which induces IFN-γ and, along with IL-2 secreted by T cells, induces differentiation of CTL.

Although macrophages and other APCs act as initiators of the specific immune responses of T cells, they also function as effectors of T-cell-mediated activities. As was stated above, cytokines produced by Th cells, induce a wide range of macrophage functions, including phagocytosis, enzymatic degradation, cytokine secretion, and cytotoxicity. In addition, IFN-γ and IL-4 can enhance MHC class II expression and thus further enhance antigen presentation to T cells. In fact, many of the clinical manifestations of cell-mediated immunity are a result of the activation of macrophages by T-cell–produced cytokines.

Table 3-4 Cytokines Important in the Immune Response

	Produced by	Interacts with	Primary Effect on Traget
IL-1	Monocytes, macrophages, B cells, dendritic cells	T cells B cells NK cells	Activation Maturation Increased activity
IL-2	Th1 cells	Th and CTL NK and CTL	Induction of proliferation Increased activity
IL-3	Th1 and Th2 cells, NK cells	Hematopoietic cells	Growth and differentiation
IL-4	Th2 cells, mast cells	T cells B cells B cells and macrophages	Switch from IgG to IgE Proliferation Increased MHC class II
IL-5	Th2 cells	B cells Eosinophils	Proliferation; switch to IgA Growth and differentiation
IL-6	Monocytes, macrophages, Th2 cells	B cells Plasma cells	Differentiation Increased antibody secretion
IL-8	Macrophages	Neutrophils	Enhanced chemotaxis
IL-10	Th1 cells	Macrophages Th1 cells	Suppressed cytokine production
IL-12	Macrophages, B cells	T cells, NK cells	Stimulate proliferation Increased IFN-γ production
IFN-α	Leukocytes	Wide range of cells NK	Increased MHC class I Increased activity
IFN-γ	Th1 cells, CTL, NK	Wide range of cells Macrophages B cells	Increased MHC classes I and II Increased phagocytosis Switch to IgG2a
TNF-α	Macrophages	Macrophages and neutrophils	Induction of cytokines Increased phagocytosis
TNF-β	Th, CTL	Macrophages and neutrophils	Induction of cytokines Increased phagocytosis

CTL, cytotoxic T lymphocytes; IFN, interforon; Iq, immunoglobulin; MHC, major histocompatibility complex; NK, natural killer cells; Th, T-helper cells.

Natural Killer Cells

NK cells are lymphocytes that were originally called null cells because they have neither the pan-T-cell marker CD3 nor the surface immunoglobulin of B cells. Morphologically, they are large granular lymphocytes (LGLs). NK cells constitute up to 15 percent of circulating lymphocytes. They are characterized by the expression of the membrane-associated molecules CD56, CD57, and CD16 (see Table 3-2). NK cells are also part of the first line of host defenses, because they can recognize and kill tumor cells and virally infected cells without prior sensitization. Although NK cells can function without interacting with other cells, cytokines, such as IL-2, IL-12, and IFN-γ or IFN-α, can enhance NK activity. NK cells can effect target cell death directly through the secretion of perforin and serine proteases

(e.g., granzyme B). They also can act through their receptors for the constant region of immunoglobulin (FcR [Fc receptor]) to effect antibody-dependent cellular cytotoxicity (ADCC). In ADCC, cells without antigen-specific receptors (i.e., NK cells and macrophages) are directed to kill specific targets through the binding of antibody to the target cell and the localization of the cytotoxic effector cell to the target cell through the binding of the antibody by the FcR of the effector cell. NK cells secrete IFN-γ and TNF-α.

Immune Response

The immune response consists of cells that respond to stimuli through nonspecific or specific interactions. Nonspecific responses provide the initial interaction directed against foreign substances and include phagocytosis by macrophages and neutrophils and cytotoxicity by NK cells. Specific immunity, also known as the adaptive immune response, allow for the recognition of specific pathogens or altered self antigens (e.g., tumor cells) and the development of memory so that successive exposures to the same foreign substance result in increasingly improved responses that ultimately culminate in the ability to prevent the symptoms induced by that foreign substance (e.g., an infectious disease). The primary cells of the adaptive immune response are B cells.

T and B cells mediate their actions through the secretion of cytokines and antibodies and through interactions among cells via constitutively expressed and newly induced surface adhesion molecules (see Fig. 3-1). Briefly, an APC takes up a foreign substance, degrades it, and presents it in the context of MHC class II to a Th cell. The Th cell having a TCR specific for the presented epitope binds to the peptide-loading MHC class II molecules of the APC. Other surface molecules participate in maintaining the T cell–APC interaction and transmitting activation signals that induce T cells to enter the cell cycle.

While the TCR itself is unable to induce signal transduction, the CD3 complex, along with CD4 and CD45, mediates a series of phosphorylation and dephosphorylation events that lead to the activation of many genes important in clonal proliferation and the secretion of cytokines (Fig. 3-2). Major participants in this scheme include the tyrosine kinases (e.g., lck and ZAP 70) and the mitogen-activated protein (MAP) kinases. Activation of these kinases results in an increase in protein kinase C (PKC) activity and an increase in the Ca^{2+} concentration in the cytoplasm of a T cell. The scheme continues through the activation of nuclear transcription factors (e.g., c-Fos/c-Jun, AP-1 [activation protein-1], NF-AT [nuclear factor-activated T cell], and NF-kB [(nuclear factor-kappa B)]) that are necessary for cell proliferation and for specific T-cell function. To illustrate, the AP-1 complex consists of deoxyribonucleic acid (DNA)-binding proteins from the Fos and Jun protein families. AP-1 induction is essential for transcription of NF-AT, which, in turn, is essential to the transcription of the IL-2 gene. IL-2, previously called T-cell growth factor, is essential for T-cell proliferation. Interaction of other costimulatory molecules, such as B7 on the APC with CD28 on the T cell, supports sustained production of IL-2 and stabilization of IL-2 messenger ribonucleic acid (mRNA). IL-2 functions in an autocrine and paracrine manner, causing proliferation and differentiation of Th cells. In a similar manner, the genes responsible for the production of the other Th cytokines are subsequently activated. The cytokines of the Th cells direct the immune response to a cell-mediated immunity response characterized by inflammation and cytotoxicity or to humoral immunity.

Humoral Immunity

The interaction of B cells with antigen, with subsequent activation and differentiation, is key to the generation of antibodies, which are the effectors of the humoral response. B cells are stimulated to differentiate into plasma cells which produce large amounts of antibody specific for the inducing antigen. Antibody can eliminate antigen through a number of mechanisms, including promoting phagocytosis by macrophages or neutrophils (opsonization), or through immune complex activation of complement. Antibody also can prevent the interaction of a foreign substance with its cellular receptor by binding the relevant epitope on the substance. This type of interaction (often referred to as neutralization) can prevent the action of a toxin or infection by a virus. Humoral responses are particularly effective at clearing extracellular pathogens and their products.

B cells can be induced to proliferate and differentiate into plasma cells by both T-cell–dependent and T-cell–independent mechanisms. T-cell–dependent mechanisms require Th cells to induce B-cell proliferation and differentiation. The activation signals from T cells include cytokines (e.g., IL-4, IL-5, and IFN-γ), as well as interactions between surface molecules. One such interaction is between CD40 on a B cell and CD40 ligand (CD40L) on a T cell, which results in a highly potent activation signal for the B cell. This interaction also increases the production of IL-2 and other cytokines by the T cell and thus sustains the activation signals being transmitted to the B cell.

B cells also can differentiate with minimal help from Th cells through T-cell–independent mechanisms. These responses occur when B cells encounter repetitive polymeric structures such as bacterial lipopolysaccharides, pneumococcal polysaccharides, and staphylococcal protein A, which are capable of cross-linking the B-cell surface immunoglobulin receptor. Unlike T-cell–dependent B-cell responses, T-cell–independent responses do not induce long-lasting memory for the antigen and result primarily in the production of IgM as a result of the lack of Th cytokines required for immunoglobulin class switching.

Cell-Mediated Immunity

The classic example of a cell-mediated immune response is the delayed-type hypersensitivity reaction (DTH). Histologic examination of the site of DTH reveals that the infiltrating cells are primarily lymphocytes and mononuclear phagocytes. Initiated by a sequence of events that use APCs to present antigen in the context of MHC class II to CD4+ cells, the DTH response is an example of a Th response mediated primarily through Th1-type cytokines. IL-2 and IFN-γ not only activate the T cells in the area but recruit and enhance the activity of the mononuclear cells, which subsequently secrete their own cytokines (e.g., IL-1, IL-6, TNF-α) and various enzymes (e.g., lysozyme and esterase). This enhanced macrophage reactivity results in an amplified inflammatory response which is clinically observable about 7 days after primary exposure or 2 to 3 days after secondary exposure.

In addition to the DTH response, a cell-mediated response may be manifest by CTL reacting to altered self cells (e.g., virally infected cells and tumor cells) or nonself cells (e.g., allogeneic transplants). Although CD8+ cells can be activated independently by their TCR recognizing an antigenic epitope in the context of MHC class I on APC or the target cells, they have maximal activity when CD4+ T cells also are involved in the reaction. This interaction relies

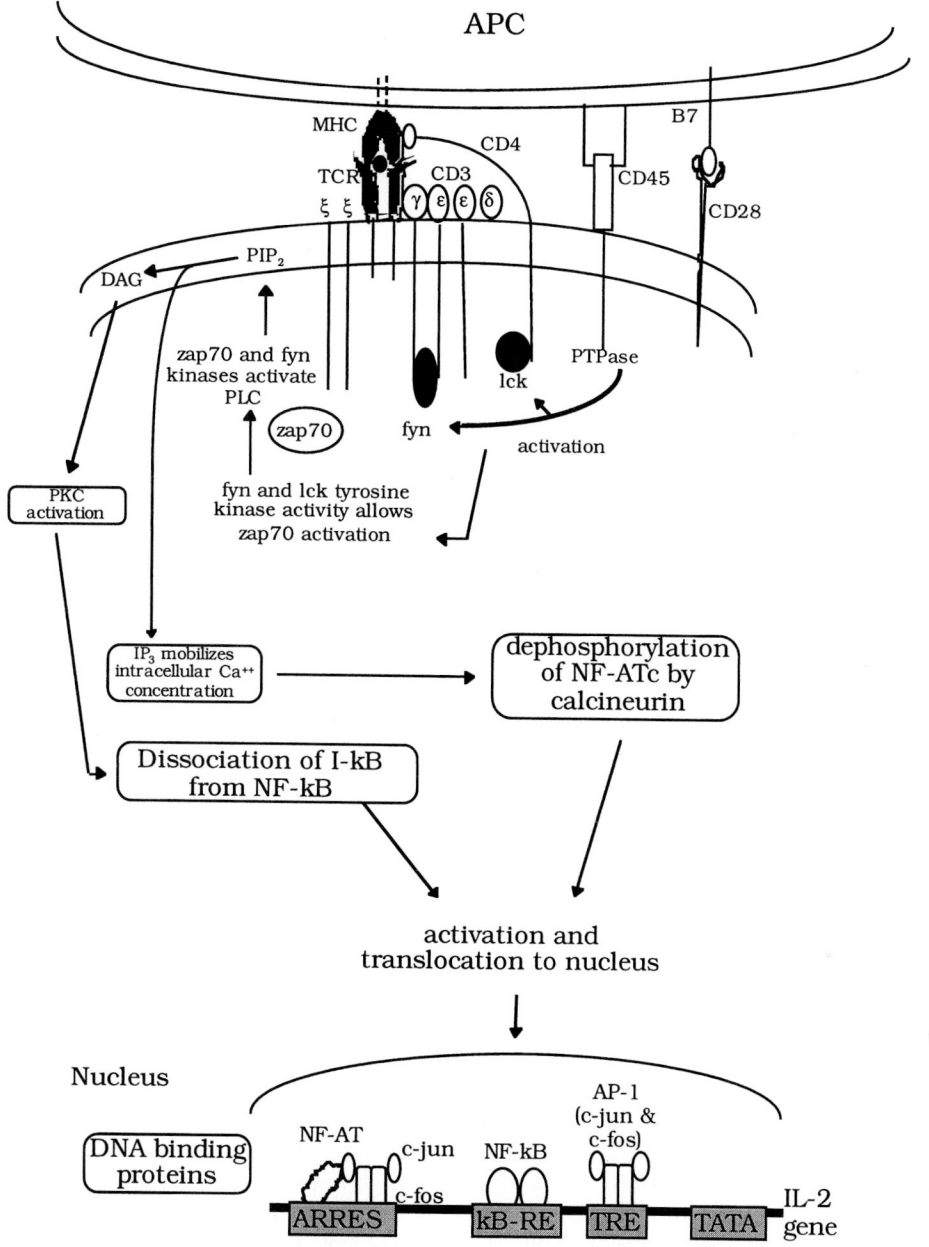

Figure 3-2 Molecular mechanism of T-cell activation.

on the release by CD4+ cells of cytokines, such as IL-2 and IFN-γ, that maximally activate the CTL. Although it is possible to observe reactions that depend primarily on Th cells and macrophages or on CTL, most cell-mediated immune responses demonstrate both CTL activity and the enhanced activities of macrophages mediated by the cytokines produced by Th cells.

Although cytotoxicity by CTL is mediated through an interaction of the TCR of the CTL with the antigenic epitope in the context of MHC class I on the target cell, not all cell-mediated cytotoxicity occurs through this mechanism. While NK cells and activated macrophages can discriminate tumor cells or virally infected cells from normal cells and can directly kill those cells, the recognition elements of these cells have not been precisely defined. The cytotoxic activities of NK cells and macrophages can

be enhanced by the cytokines released by Th cells during a specific immune interaction. In addition, NK cells and macrophages can function through a mechanism involving antibody (ADCC). Through this mechanism, the humoral and cell-mediated arms of the system interact with each other, resulting in maximal effectiveness of the immune system against the foreign substance.

AGE-RELATED CHANGES IN IMMUNE FUNCTION

The finely tuned orchestration of the immune response is dependent on regulation at many levels. Although disruption at one level may still allow for adequate responses,

Table 3-5   Summary of Age-Related Changes in Immune Function

Cell Type	Parameter	Age-Related Changes
T cells	Thymus	Involution after puberty
	Circulating number or percent	Declines or no change
	Memory phenotype	Increases
	DTH	Declines
	Cytotoxicity	Declines
	Proliferative response	Declines
	Cytokine production	
	IL-2	Declines
	IL-4	Increases or no change*
	IL-6	Increases or no change*
	IL-10	Decreases or no change*
	IFN-γ	Increases, decreases, or no change*
B cells	Circulating number or percent	No change
	Antibody production to specific antigens	Declines
	Autoantibody production	Increases
NK cells	Circulating number or percent	Increases
	Basal or induced activity	No change
LAK cells	Induced activity	Declines
Accessory Cells	Circulating number or percent	No change
	Phagocytosis	Declines or no change
	Cytokine production	Declines*

DTH, delayed-typed hypersensitivity; IFN, interferom; IL, interleukin; LAK, lympiuvine-actuated killer; NK, natural killer.
*Data are limited and inconclusive.

alteration of key regulators or dysfunction of several regulatory steps may abrogate a response or may manifest as a suboptimal immune response or an inappropriate response, such as autoreactivity. Aging is accompanied by many modifications of immune reactivity, with the most significant changes being observed in the T-cell compartment. Peripheral blood mononuclear cells (PBMCs) demonstrate decreased reactivity to both antigens and nonspecific stimuli. Antibody responses to vaccination and infection are decreased, while levels of autoreactive antibodies are increased. Table 3-5 summarizes the major changes seen in the immune response in the elderly subject. While the majority of immunosenescence research has been descriptive, an impressive effort has been made in recent years to understand the mechanisms of the age-related decline in immune function. The following subsections highlight the major age-associated changes in the immune system.

T Cells

As was outlined above, T cells play a central role in orchestrating the overall immune system as well as functioning as direct effectors of immune reactivity. It is therefore not surprising that the most pronounced effects of age on the immune system are manifested in the T-cell population. One of the first identified age-associated functional changes

in immune response was decreased DTH responses. It has been reported that 40 percent of individuals older than age 70 years demonstrate decreased reactivity to a skin test panel, regardless of their overall health status. Although DTH responses can be designed to assess the ability to respond to a new antigen (e.g., dinitrochlorobenzene) or a recall antigen (e.g., streptokinase/streptodornase), it is difficult to quantitate changes in reactivity accurately and even more difficult to address the mechanism of age-associated declines. A decreased DTH response can result from changes in the initial activation of T cells, a shift in cytokine production by the activated cells, or altered reactivity by macrophages. In addition, age-associated alterations in the physical and chemical properties of the skin have been implicated as nonimmune mechanisms responsible for this decrease in DTH reactivity. Therefore, much of the information regarding age-associated changes in T-cell response has been obtained from in vitro evaluations.

Multiple age-associated changes have been observed in vitro, including decreased proliferative responses, modified activation signals, and altered cytokine production profiles. Because it has been postulated that the cumulative defects seen in the T-cell compartment contribute significantly to all the immune dysregulation that occurs with advancing age, these changes merit close attention by health care professionals. The material below summarizes the changes in T-cell function seen with increasing age and attempts to evaluate the contribution of each particular change to the overall immune dysregulation that has been observed.

T-Cell Proliferative Responses

Although many events are required before T cell proliferation, assessment of lymphocyte proliferation often has been used as an indicator of the cell-mediated immune potential of an individual. Therefore, many studies have utilized the proliferative response to assess age-associated changes in T-cell response.

A decreased ability of PBMCs to proliferate in response to T-cell stimuli is among the most consistent age-associated alterations of the immune system. Polyclonal stimuli used to demonstrate this decreased proliferative response have included mitogens such as phytohemagglutinin (PHA) and concanavalin A (conA), antibodies to T cell surface markers (e.g., anti-CD3 and anti-CD28), and superantigens such as toxic shock syndrome toxin (TSST). In addition, age-associated decreases have been observed in response to specific antigens after immunization. These antigens include influenza vaccine, tetanus toxoid, and purified protein derivative (PPD) of *Mycobacterium tuberculosis*. Figure 3-3 shows representative data from such studies. Although a significant age-associated decrease in lymphoproliferation (usually a ≥50 percent decline) is observed in most studies that compare the mean response of healthy young adults (18 to 40 years old) with the mean response of healthy elderly adults (≥65 years old), this decrease is not observed in all studies. Many factors can contribute to this discrepancy among studies.

The general health of the subjects can have a major influence on immune responsiveness. Most studies exclude subjects who have had cancer or autoimmune diseases or who are taking medications that are known to alter the immune response (e.g., steroids). However, within the populations studied, there is great variation in overall health. As is shown in Fig. 3-4, the response of three populations of elderly subjects who meet these criteria demonstrated very different proliferative responses to influenza vaccine after immunization. Elderly persons living in the community who exercised regularly demonstrated the greatest increase in response from preimmunization to postimmunization and included the largest proportion of subjects showing an increased response after immunization. Subjects who also lived in the community, but did not exercise, demonstrated a smaller increase from preimmunization to postimmunization, although the difference between this group and the group that exercised is not significant. Subjects residing in a nursing home and requiring assistance for the performance of daily activities showed the lowest rate of response to immunization. Because the age of the three groups was fairly comparable (72, 69, and 76 years, respectively), other diseases and overall health appear to contribute significantly to the lymphoproliferative results.

In an effort to minimize the potentially confounding effect of age-associated diseases, investigators have established the Senieur Protocol, a set of stringent criteria for the inclusion of elderly subjects in studies evaluating the direct effects of aging on particular functions. Although

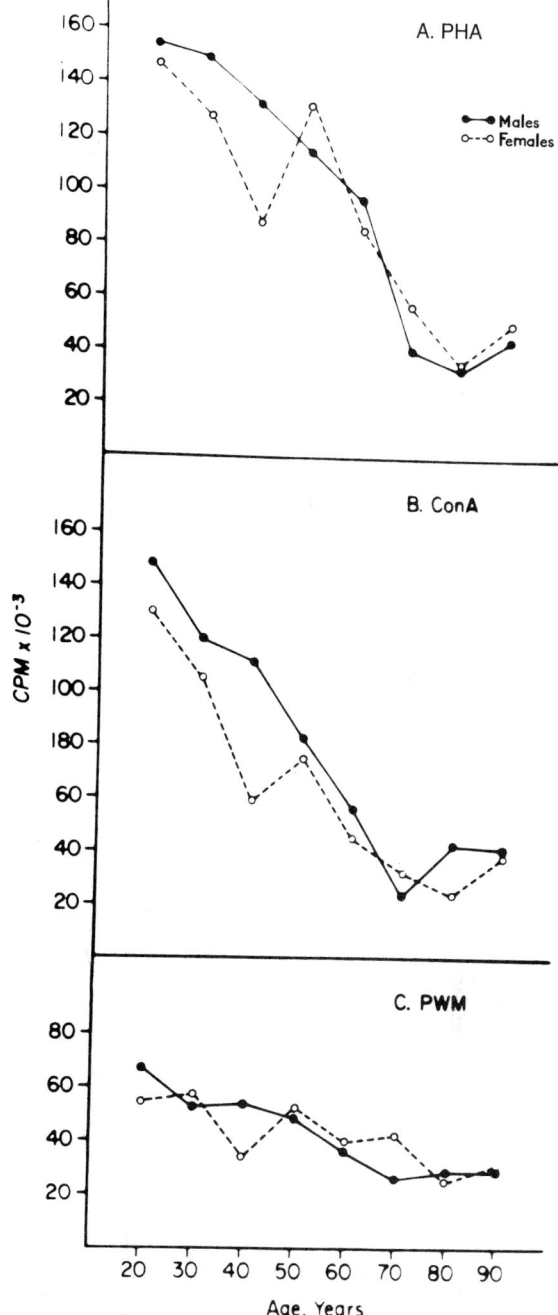

Figure 3-3 Proliferative response of PBMCs to mitogenic stimuli. Shown are mean values of response to the T-cell mitogen (PHA) (panel A), the T-cell mitogen concanavalin A (conA) (panel B), and the T-cell–dependent B-cell mitogen pokeweed mitogen (PWM) (panel C). Each point represents the mean of 10 to 15 individuals for a total of 20 to 30 individuals at each decile. Reproduced with permission from Murasko DM et al: Decline in mitogen-induced proliferation of lymphocytes with increasing age. *Clin Exp Immunol* 70:440, 1987.

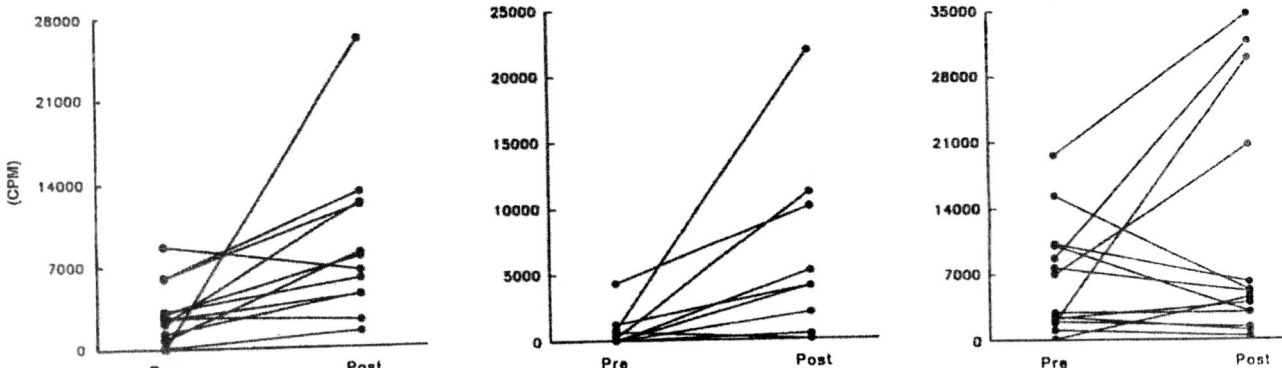

Figure 3-4   Proliferative response to influenza vaccine before and after immunization. PBMCs were obtained from individuals immediately before immunization with influenza vaccine and 4 weeks later. Cells were cultured for 5 days in the presence of vaccine, and net proliferation (cpm of ^{3}H-thymidine – cpm of ^{3}H-thymidine with media) was calculated. The connected points are results from the same individual. Panel A represents individuals (mean age, 72 years) who regularly exercise; panel B represents individuals (mean age, 69 years) living in the community but recruited from the medical clinic; and panel C represents nursing home individuals (mean age, 76 years). Note that most subjects in panel A and panel B demonstrate an increased response from preimmunization to postimmunization, while only a limited number in panel C show an increase. The mean responses of the subjects in both panel A and panel B are significantly increased from preimmunization to postimmunization, and postimmunization responses of both groups are significantly higher than those of subjects in panel C ($P < .05$, student t test) (unpublished results).

such stringent criteria are necessary to control for the effects of age-associated diseases, it must be recognized that elderly persons who meet these criteria represent a group of exceptional individuals. Studies employing such criteria may therefore underestimate the magnitude of immunosenescence observed in the general population. If the goal is to determine the direct effects of age on immune function, studies employing the most stringent health criteria should be utilized as the benchmarks. However, if the purpose is to define age-associated alterations in immune function so that strategies for more effective immunizations or cancer immunotherapies for the elderly can be developed, the results from a study population that reflects the general elderly population should be the standard. The results summarized in this chapter primarily reflect studies of the general population, because many of these studies have used less-stringent definitions of the "healthy elderly person."

Studies that employ the more-stringent health criteria, however, also demonstrate conflicting results. While most still observe decreased proliferative responses to polyclonal stimuli, some do not reveal age-associated alteration in proliferation. Therefore, heterogeneity of the immune response in the elderly person is not limited to individuals with overt differences in health or level of daily activities. Using the same individuals included in Fig. 3-3, the heterogeneity of responses seen among elderly persons living independently in apartments in one retirement community is considerable (Fig. 3-5). Specifically, some elderly persons have responses comparable to those of the young, some have responses greatly reduced relative to those of the young, but the majority demonstrate a 30 to 50 percent decrease in response. As a result of this heterogeneity, it is possible to observe results that are skewed toward either high or low responses in a random sampling of small numbers of individuals. Therefore, while all reports regarding the immune response must be considered, a discrepancy among studies can reflect a sampling error. Despite the

discrepancies, however, the overwhelming proportion of studies, including several that examined more than 100 subjects, have clearly demonstrated that there is an age-related decrease in the ability of T lymphocytes to proliferate in response to various stimuli.

Thymus

The thymus is the site of T-cell maturation. This organ demonstrates the first age-associated changes by beginning to involute at the time of puberty, with a concomitant decrease in thymic hormones. This age-associated involution of the thymus has been suggested repeatedly to be a major contributor to the functional decline of T-cell immunity with age. Although thymic involution certainly accounts for some of the age-related changes in the T-lymphocyte pool, this process cannot be the primary mediator of the decline, because less than 10 percent of thymic function remains intact at age 25 years, while T-cell proliferative responses demonstrate little decline for the majority of individuals until 65 to 70 years of age.

Changes in T-Cell Phenotypes

Numerous studies over the last three decades have examined whether phenotypic changes in the T-cell compartment accompany human aging. Although it is generally accepted that normal healthy aging is accompanied by a slight decrease in circulating lymphocytes, there is considerable controversy regarding which cells demonstrate that decline. Some studies indicate a decline in the number of total T cells (CD3+ cells), while others find decreases in only CD4+ or CD8+ cells. Some reports indicate changes in absolute numbers of cells but not in percentages, while others report differences in percentages but not in absolute numbers; some reports indicate differences in absolute numbers as well as in percentages. In one of the largest of

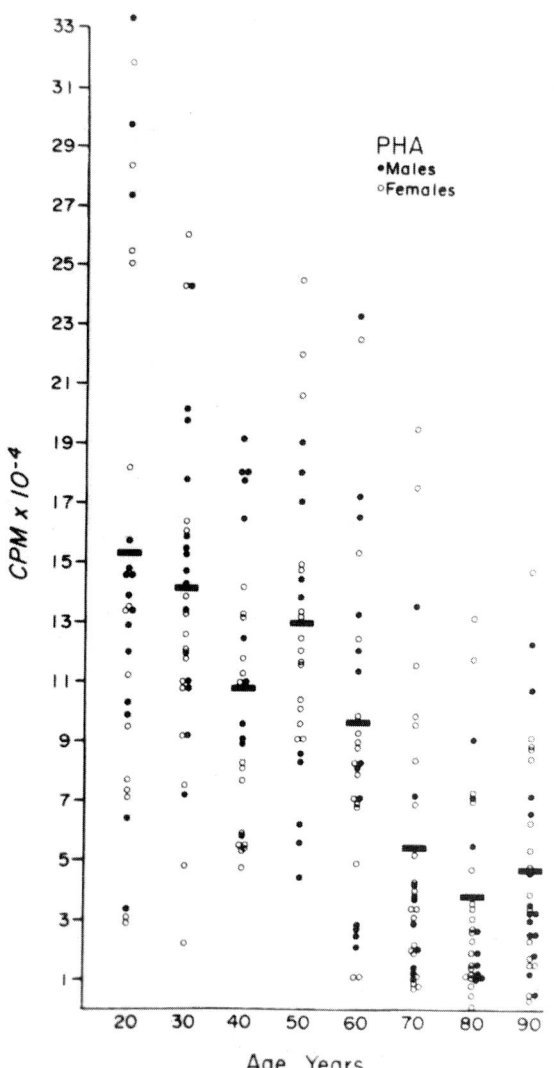

Figure 3-5 Heterogeneity of the proliferative response in elderly individuals. Individuals included in Fig. 3-3 are now represented as individual responses. Only the response to PHA (Fig. 3-3[A]) is indicated.

these studies, the relationship between T-cell phenotype and lymphoproliferation was evaluated in 149 healthy elderly persons and 101 young controls. The conclusion of this study, as well as that of another large study, was that the small decline in CD3+, CD4+, or CD8+ cells in the elderly persons was not correlated with the age-associated decline in mitogen-induced lymphoproliferation. Thus, while small changes in CD3+, CD4+, or CD8+ T-cell subsets occur, the relevance of these changes to the age-associated decline in T-cell responses is questionable.

In contrast, an age-associated shift from naïve (CD45RA+) T cells to memory (CD45RO+) T cells of both the CD4+ and the CD8+ subsets is observed consistently in humans. Investigators have theorized that this shift is caused by an increasing pool of memory cells after years of antigenic stimulation, with a concomitant decreased introduction of new naïve cells into the periphery by the involuted thymus. Some reports have argued that the increased ratio of memory to naïve T cells accounts for many

of the functional changes seen in the T-cell compartment with aging. Importantly, the percentage of naïve CD4+ cells is directly related to the ability of lymphocytes to proliferate in response to stimulation with mitogens (e.g., PHA or anti-CD3 antibody). While an increased population of memory T cells, which do not proliferate as well to mitogens as do naïve T cells, can explain much of the age-related decrease in mitogen-induced proliferative responses, the increased percentage of memory cells does not explain the decline in secondary responses of T cells to recall antigens. A few studies suggest that there is an intrinsic defect specific to the memory cells of elderly subjects that results in decreased responses to recall antigens. However, other studies argue for the presence of a generalized T-cell defect present in both CD45RA+ and CD45RO+ cells that leads to decreased proliferative responses to both mitogen and recall antigens.

While the percentages of CD4+ and CD8+ cells in peripheral blood do not reflect the lymphoproliferative response of PBMCs to mitogenic stimuli, there is an age-associated shift in the percentage of these cells that survive after activation in vitro. It has been demonstrated repeatedly that upon mitogenic stimulation, CD8+ cells are preferentially expanded in young humans. This expansion of CD8+ cells after in vitro culture with mitogens does not occur in the elderly. Thus, while young persons and elderly individuals may initially have comparable numbers of CD4+ and CD8+ cells, the proportion of CD8+ cells that respond after in vitro stimulation is decreased in the elderly.

The mechanism for this decreased response of CD8+ cells may be related to another phenotypic alteration seen with aging. A number of reports have demonstrated an age-related decline in CD28+ T cells, with the largest decline observed in CD28 expression on CD8+ cells. As was mentioned earlier, the binding of the costimulatory molecule CD28 on T cells by B7 (CD80) on APC is critical for transducing activation signals to the T cell. If binding of CD28 does not occur, T cells can become anergic rather than activated. It is not known whether the age-related decrease in CD28 expression results in a greater number of anergic responses. However, this is an attractive explanation for the age-related decrease in the number of CD8+ cells in culture after in vitro activation.

The CD8+/CD28− population can maintain its cytotoxic activity. It has been suggested that the CD8+/CD28− population may represent a subset of memory CD8+ cells that cannot proliferate because of the loss of CD28 but are still available for antigen-specific killing. Interestingly, the largest expansion of CD8+/CD28− cells has been observed in centenarians. Whether the accumulation of these cells in the oldest old represents an age-associated defect or a compensatory mechanism that contributes to successful aging remains to be seen.

Alterations in T-Cell Cytokine Production

Murine studies have suggested that aging is accompanied by a shift in cytokine production such that a predominating Th1 cytokine profile (IL-2, IFN-γ) is replaced by a Th2 cytokine profile (IL-4, IL-5, IL-10). Attempts to apply this

Table 3-6 Age-Associated Changes in Cytokine Production*

Category	Cytokine	Stimulus	Number of Studies Demonstrating		
			Decrease	No Change	Increase
Th1	IL-2	Mitogen	10	5	
		Antigen	1	2	1
	IFN-γ	Mitogen	2	4	2
		Antigen	3	2	
	IL-12	Mitogen		2	
Th2	IL-4	Mitogen	1	3	1
	IL-10	Mitogen		2	
		Antigen		2	
Proinflammatory	IL-1	Mitogen	2	2	1
		Antigen			1
	IL-6	Mitogen		2	1
		Antigen		1	
	TNF-α	Mitogen	1	1	1
		Antigen			1

IFN, interferon; IL, interleukin; Th, T helper cell; TNF, tumor necrosis factor.
*Restricted to human data.

paradigm of a switch from Th1 to Th2 with aging in humans have provided more controversy than answers (Table 3-6). The most consistent age-related change in cytokine production by human PBMCs after stimulation with mitogens or anti-CD3 antibody is decreased production of IL-2. Approximately 60 percent of studies that assessed IL-2 production after mitogen stimulation observed a decrease; the remaining studies reported no change in IL-2 production with age. When assessed concomitantly, decreased production of IL-2 was reflected in decreased levels of IL-2 mRNA. Whether this decrease in IL-2 reflects a smaller number of T cells producing IL-2 or a lower production of IL-2 per cell is unclear.

The addition of IL-2 to PBMC cultures from elderly people increases proliferative responses in most cases. However, it does not restore lymphoproliferation to the level achieved by PBMCs of young subjects. Interestingly, responses of individuals (rather than the mean response of the population) show that the addition of exogenous IL-2 increased the level of response to the level of the young in only about 30 percent of elderly subjects. The PBMCs of the remaining elderly subjects demonstrated little or no response to the IL-2.

These results could be explained by a defect in the expression of the IL-2 receptor (IL-2R). Similar to the results of assessment of IL-2, approximately 80 percent of studies have observed decreased IL-2R expression after mitogenic stimulation. The kinetics of the induction of IL-2R expression may explain the inconsistent results. Induction of early expression of IL-2R on PBMCs of elderly subjects is decreased, while later expression is equivalent to that of PBMCs from young controls. However, when PBMCs from elderly individuals were selected for "normal" expression of IL-2R in one study, exogenous IL-2 was still unable to restore the proliferative response to the level of young subjects. Because the affinity of the IL-2R binding was not ascertained in this study, alteration in IL-2R may still be responsible for the decreased proliferative response of T cells from aged subjects.

Another Th1 cytokine—IFN-γ—has been reported to increase, decrease, or remain unchanged with age. These inconsistencies may be a result of the experimental stimulus and/or the phenotype of the responding cells. IFN-γ is produced by both CD4+ and CD8+ cells, as well as by NK cells. Furthermore, the level of IFN-γ production by T cells may depend on the stimulus used for induction. For example, 8 of 14 studies using mitogenic stimuli showed comparable or even increased IFN-γ production by PBMCs of the elderly, while 3 of 5 studies that used specific antigens showed an age-related decrease in IFN-γ. These findings suggest that under the appropriate conditions, the elderly may be capable of producing IFN-γ at levels comparable to those of the young. However, because few studies have assessed isolated T cells, no statement can be made at this time regarding a possibly decreased ability of T cells of elderly persons to produce Th1 cytokines.

Information regarding Th2 cytokine production by PBMCs of the elderly is more limited. In studies in which lymphoproliferation was decreased in the elderly, IL-4 and IL-10 production by PHA-induced PBMCs from young and elderly subjects was comparable. In one study, no age-related difference was observed in proliferative responses of PBMCs after stimulation with PHA, anti-CD3, or anti-CD2 and anti-CD28 together, but IL-4 production by PBMCs of elderly subjects was increased compared with that of young subjects. Although these studies suggest that IL-4 production has the potential for dysregulation in the elderly, the current results are insufficient to conclude that such dysregulation plays a role in the altered T-cell response seen with increasing age.

Increased IL-4 without a change in lymphoproliferation argues against a Th1-to-Th2 cytokine shift as the explanation for the age-related decrease in lymphoproliferation in humans. Investigations of another Th2 cytokine, IL-10, results in a similar conclusion. Stimulation of PBMC with two superantigens demonstrated no age-associated change (TSST) or increased (staphylococcal enterotoxin B [SEB]) IL-10, while stimulation with PHA resulted in either no change or an age-associated decrease in IL-10. There may be antigen-specific alterations in IL-10 production. For example, PBMCs from influenza-vaccinated elderly individuals produce less IL-10 after restimulation in culture with influenza than do PBMCs from vaccinated young controls.

A cytokine that has received more attention in humans with regard to aging is IL-6. IL-6 is produced by monocytes, macrophages, endothelial cells, and, to a more limited extent, T cells. Although IL-6 is involved in T-cell activation, B-cell differentiation, and antibody secretion, it plays a major role in inflammatory responses. While one study reported an age-associated increase in IL-6 levels of healthy individuals, three of four additional studies found no age difference of IL-6 levels. Similar variability was observed after in vitro stimulation of PBMCs with mitogen or antigen, with four of six studies finding no age change.

The variability in IL-6 may be a result of a number of factors. First, although all the subjects were reported to be healthy, none of them were screened specifically for inflammatory diseases (e.g., arthritis), which are known to be associated with higher levels of IL-6. Second, in several of the studies the IL-6 level was very low and, furthermore, was not detectable in many subjects. It is therefore quite possible that the higher levels of IL-6 observed in elderly people reflect the increased incidence of inflammatory conditions rather than a general age-associated increase in the production of IL-6.

Alterations in CTL Activity

Assessing CTL activity of humans is technically difficult because of the requirement for extended in vitro culture to expand the specific CTL to detectable levels and for strict matching of the MHC class I antigens of the target cells and the responding T cells of the subject. Although limited in number, these studies generally have observed decreased CTL activity in elderly subjects as compared with young subjects. This decreased CTL response has been seen in responses to influenza vaccine, tetanus toxoid, and allogeneic cells. An interesting observation made by one group is that the CTL response of elderly subjects is not tightly restricted by MHC class I. For example, after immunization with influenza A/Texas, young subjects who possess human leukocyte antigen (HLA)-A2 and -A4 can kill only target cells that express HLA-A2 or HLA-A4 infected with influenza A/Texas. In contrast, some elderly subjects who also possess HLA-A2 and HLA-A4 can kill influenza-infected target cells that express HLA-A2, -A4, or -A6. While this is a provocative finding, it has not been observed in other studies which also investigated the requirement for matched

MHC class I antigen expression on both target cells and CTL.

In summary, current studies suggest that there is an age-associated decrease in CTL activity. Whether this reflects a smaller number of CTLs specific for the antigenic determinant or decreased function of each CTL through impaired binding to the target cells or altered lytic mechanisms has not been explored directly in humans. However, there is some indication from studies in mice using tetramer technology to identify antigen specific CD8+ cells that a decrease in the number of antigen-specific cells is at least one component of this decrease.

B Cells

A number of age-associated changes in the B-cell compartment have been observed, including (1) decreased antibody production to vaccination or infection; (2) altered immunoglobulin classes and subclasses such that circulating levels of IgG and/or IgA are increased; (3) decreased affinity of antibodies; (4) dysregulation of the antiidiotype network; and (5) increases in autoantibodies. Although the mechanisms of these alterations have not been established, they do not appear to be due to age-associated changes in B-cell numbers. The majority of studies show no age-related alteration in the proportion of B cells in peripheral blood, although one group of investigators consistently demonstrated decreased proportions of CD19+ cells (pan-B-cell marker) among the elderly population.

An age-associated decrease in humoral response was recognized more than 50 years ago. At that time, it was reported that the titer of serum antibodies to foreign erythrocytes decreased with increasing age. Subsequent studies extended this observation of decreased antibody response to "naturally exposed" antigens (e.g., foreign erythrocytes) and to antigens introduced via immunization. Several investigators have attempted to increase the responses of the elderly person to vaccination administration by booster immunization 1 month after primary immunization with influenza. Although the mean response of the elderly cohort was higher after the second, as compared with the first, immunization, 75 percent of subjects who had not achieved a positive response (hemagglutination antibody [HA] titer ≥40) after the first immunization still did not reach this level after the second immunization. It is possible that when primary immunization occurs early in life (e.g., tetanus, measles/mumps/rubella), the secondary response is maintained throughout life. However, when the primary immunization occurs late in life (age 65 years or after), the secondary response also may demonstrate an age-associated decline.

Even when the level of antibody production by the elderly person is comparable to that of young individuals, the antibodies often do not neutralize antigen as effectively as do those from the young. Several reports from experimental systems including influenza and pneumococcal vaccination have shown that antibodies from vaccinated elderly individuals do not protect as well as do those from the young even when the actual titers of antibodies are equivalent. These alterations in the neutralizing capability of antibodies in the elderly may be due to multiple factors. Evidence exists for decreased affinity maturation of the antibody in the germinal centers of lymph nodes as a result of a decreased level of B7 expression on the surface of B cells that interact with CD28 on T cells. A few reports suggest that reduced binding of CD40 on B cells by costimulatory CD40L on T cells is responsible for the decreased activation response observed in aged subjects. A decreased interaction between T cells and B cells could result in less cytokine production by Th cells and subsequently impaired stimulation of B cells. Equally suggestive data indicate that rather than lower cytokine production by Th cells, an altered cytokine profile by Th cells results in inappropriate isotype switching by the B cell for the specific antigen.

In addition to quantitative and qualitative changes in antibody production to foreign antigens, there is a parallel rise in autoantibodies. Several studies show an inverse relation between the titers of autoantibodies and the titers of antibodies to foreign antigens, such as antitetanus antibodies and antierythrocyte antibodies (anti-A or anti-B antibodies). A causal relation between the increase in autoantibodies and the decrease in antibodies to foreign antigens, however, has not been established. It has been reported that up to 20 percent of individuals older than age 65 years have detectable levels of antibodies to DNA, thyroglobulin, or other autoantigens in their sera. In spite of the high incidence of autoantibodies in the elderly population, the presence of autoantibodies seldom is associated with the symptoms of autoimmune disease.

When sensitive techniques have been used, as many as 50 percent of individuals older than age 65 years have been reported to demonstrate a monoclonal gammopathy. Although the antigenic reactivity of these immunoglobulins is unknown in most cases, some have been shown to be reactive with autoantigens. While there is an increased incidence of monoclonal B-cell neoplasms in the elderly population, many of these monoclonal gammopathies occur without any apparent disease.

It is unclear whether the age-associated changes in antibody responses reflect primary B-cell defects or defects in Th cells that result in decreased B-cell function. As a result of the extensive communication between B cells and T cells during the generation of antibody responses to most antigens, it is possible that the majority of changes with age in the B-cell compartment can be attributed to alterations in the T-cell compartment. Although there currently is no treatment to effectively increase either T-cell or B-cell responses, knowledge of the mechanism of the decrease in antibody production will be important when such specific therapies become available.

Natural Killer Cells

NK cells play an important role in the control of viral infections and the eradication of tumor cells. Because the elderly population is disproportionately affected by both cancer and viral infections, a number of investigators have evaluated age-related changes in NK cells. The proportion of NK cells in the circulating lymphocyte pool, as assessed by the NK markers CD16 and/or CD56, appear to be increased in the elderly population. However, in spite of this increase, a review of 31 studies of comparable design indicated that basal NK function, as measured by antitumor cytotoxicity, remains relatively intact with age. In addition, enhancement of NK activity by IL-2, IL-12, and IFN-γ and IFN-α is comparable in young subjects and elderly subjects in regard to level, kinetics, and dose responses. The relationship between the increased percentage of NK cells with age and the lack of a resultant increase in function has not been elucidated.

Phagocytes

The number of studies evaluating neutrophil, monocyte, and macrophage function in the elderly population is limited. The few reports investigating neutrophil function have yielded conflicting data regarding age-related changes and have little information on the mechanisms of functional changes of neutrophil with age. However, there have been some consistent observations. Neutrophil and monocyte/macrophage numbers remain constant throughout life. Phagocytic capacity and bactericidal mechanisms, particularly those initiated by contact with opsonized yeast or bacteria, appear to be decreased in both healthy and debilitated elderly persons. While the significance of this age-related decreased on phagocytosis by granulocytes is unclear, it is possible that decreased phagocytosis by macrophages may result in decreased antigen presentation activity and thus contribute to the observed decrease in T-cell reactivity.

While monocytic APC numbers in peripheral blood remain unchanged with age, a greater number of dendritic cells (DCs), which are highly efficient APCs, were isolated from the blood of elderly subjects than from the blood of young subjects. Thus, aging may be accompanied by increased compartmentalization of DC to the blood, with decreased migration to peripheral organs. This hypothesis is supported by previous studies in mice and humans showing age-related decreases in the DC population of the skin. This decreased migration of DC is not likely to be a result of changes in the surface molecules that normally mediate homing and migration, because no such differences were found between DCs from young and elderly individuals.

Other studies indicate that there may be abnormalities in APC function with age. Using allogeneic T cells of young subjects, monocytes from elderly subjects supported a lower proliferative response to a nonspecific stimulus (PHA) than did monocytes from young controls. This decreased activity could not be explained by altered cytokine production or cell adhesion molecule expression, because the monocytes from young and old subjects showed similar production of cytokines (IL-1, IL-6, tumor necrosis factor), expression of cell adhesion molecules (intercellular cell adhesion molecule [ICAM]-1 and leukocyte factor antigen [LFA]-3), and MHC class II.

Although the cytokines produced by macrophages and other accessory cells may have a major impact on immune responses, the effect of aging on these cytokines has received little attention. Dysregulation of the balance between IL-1 and TNF-α and their antagonists results in pathologic plasma concentrations of either the cytokines (e.g., in sepsis and cachexia) or the antagonists (e.g., in afebrile infections and inadequate immune responses). The six studies assessing IL-1 and the four studies assessing TNF-α showed the pattern observed frequently in cytokine evaluation in the elderly: a fairly even distribution of results among studies showing an age-associated decrease, an increase, or no change. One study assessing the ability of monocytes isolated from healthy elderly and young subjects to produce granulocyte colony-stimulating factor (G-CSF), granulocyte-macrophage colony-stimulating factor (GM-CSF), TNF-α, and IL-8 after stimulation with lipopolysaccharide observed significantly lower production of all these cytokines by monocytes from elderly subjects, as compared with monocytes from young controls. In contrast, another study using the same stimulus demonstrated an age-related increase in IL-1 but no change in TNF-α production. A study of 122 healthy elderly persons and 100 young adults demonstrated age-related increases in plasma concentrations of IL-1 and TNF-α antagonists, with no detectable IL-1 or TNF-α in either cohort. The age-related increase in plasma concentrations of IL-1 antagonists was inversely correlated with IL-2 production by PHA-stimulated PBMCs from the same individuals. These data suggest that the age-related increase in IL-1 antagonist production may contribute to the age-related decrease in T-cell function. This conclusion is consistent with results of studies using PBMCs from young subjects that demonstrated that the addition of IL-1 antagonists to PBMC cultures inhibits proliferation and IL-2 production.

Although it is apparent that more studies are required before definitive statements can be made regarding the effect of age on proinflammatory cytokine production, the studies cited above seem to indicate that the interplay between age-related alterations in cytokines and their antagonists may contribute to the immune dysregulation observed in the elderly. Because the number of studies is low, it is also difficult to reach a definitive conclusion regarding age-associated changes in monocytes/macrophages and neutrophil function. Further studies are needed to definitively establish whether age-associated changes occur in (1) activities of these cells as the first line of defense (e.g., phagocytic activity and the production of cytokines); (2) the ability of these cells to act as APCs; and (3) the ability of these cells to be activated by T-cell cytokines.

GENERAL MECHANISMS OF IMMUNOSENESCENCE

Alterations in Activation Signals

The most dramatic age-related changes in immune function occur when the experimental stimulus requires interaction with the TCR complex. Experimental systems using stimuli that bypass the receptor (such as phorbol esters with ionomycin) indicate that age-related alterations in lymphoproliferation can be partially, if not totally, overcome. For this

reason, early signal transduction events have been studied to identify the mechanisms responsible for immunosenescence. However, limited studies have addressed each potential site of age-related alteration in humans.

Figure 3-6 illustrates the sites of reported age-related alterations in signal transduction. There is no significant or consistent age-related alteration in TCR–CD3 receptor complex number or affinity. The lipid composition of lymphocyte membranes from elderly donors was found to contain an increased ratio of cholesterol to phospholipids. This change was associated with increased membrane viscosity and decreased lymphoproliferative responses. However, the exact role of this alteration in lipid composition in the age-related decline in immune function has not been explored.

Many other postreceptor signal transduction events show age-related changes. The actin polymerization of the cytoskeleton that accompanies receptor-mediated responses in immune cells from young donors is absent in cells from elderly individuals. Age-related alterations in cytoskeleton function could diminish further signal transduction by destabilizing receptor interactions through their cytoplasmic tails.

Normal signal transduction across the membrane requires the interaction of several stimuli with appropriate receptors to induce a series of phosphorylation and dephosphorylation events that increase Ca^{2+} mobilization and PKC activity, ultimately resulting in activation of transcription factors and gene transcription. There is an age-related decline in cytoplasmic Ca^{2+} concentration and PKC activity in both T and B lymphocytes after stimulation through the membrane. Because PMA (PKC activator) and ionomycin (increases Ca^{2+} flux) only partially rescue the age-related decline in lymphocyte function, alterations in other downstream events may play a significant role in the diminished responses observed with increasing age.

There is a decline with age in nuclear transcription factors (AP-1, NF-AT, and NF-kB) and thus decreased expression of genes whose transcription depends on AP-1, NF-AT, and NF-kB activity. The age-related decline in AP-1 and NF-AT activity appears to be caused by a selective decrease in c-Fos protein, which is necessary for full AP-1 activity and thus for NF-AT expression. The mechanism for the age-related decline in c-Fos mRNA and protein levels may be in the proximal signal transduction steps. For example, aberrant phosphorylization–dephosphorylization by the MAP kinase family of serine/threonine kinases has been implicated as the mechanism of this decrease in some studies.

Age-related alterations also have been demonstrated in another nuclear transcription factor: NF-kB. In a resting cell, NF-kB is found in the cytoplasm bound to an inhibitor, IkB. Degradation of IkB results in translocation of NF-kB to the nucleus, in instances where NF-kB is active. There is decreased activity of NF-kB in activated T cells from elderly donors relative to young donors. This age-related decrease in NF-kB activity was not a result of differences in constitutive levels of NF-kB available for activation or to alteration in the subunit composition of NF-kB. A role for an age-related alteration in IkB degradation has been proposed. In summary, no single age-sensitive step in the signal transduction pathway has been delineated, but several

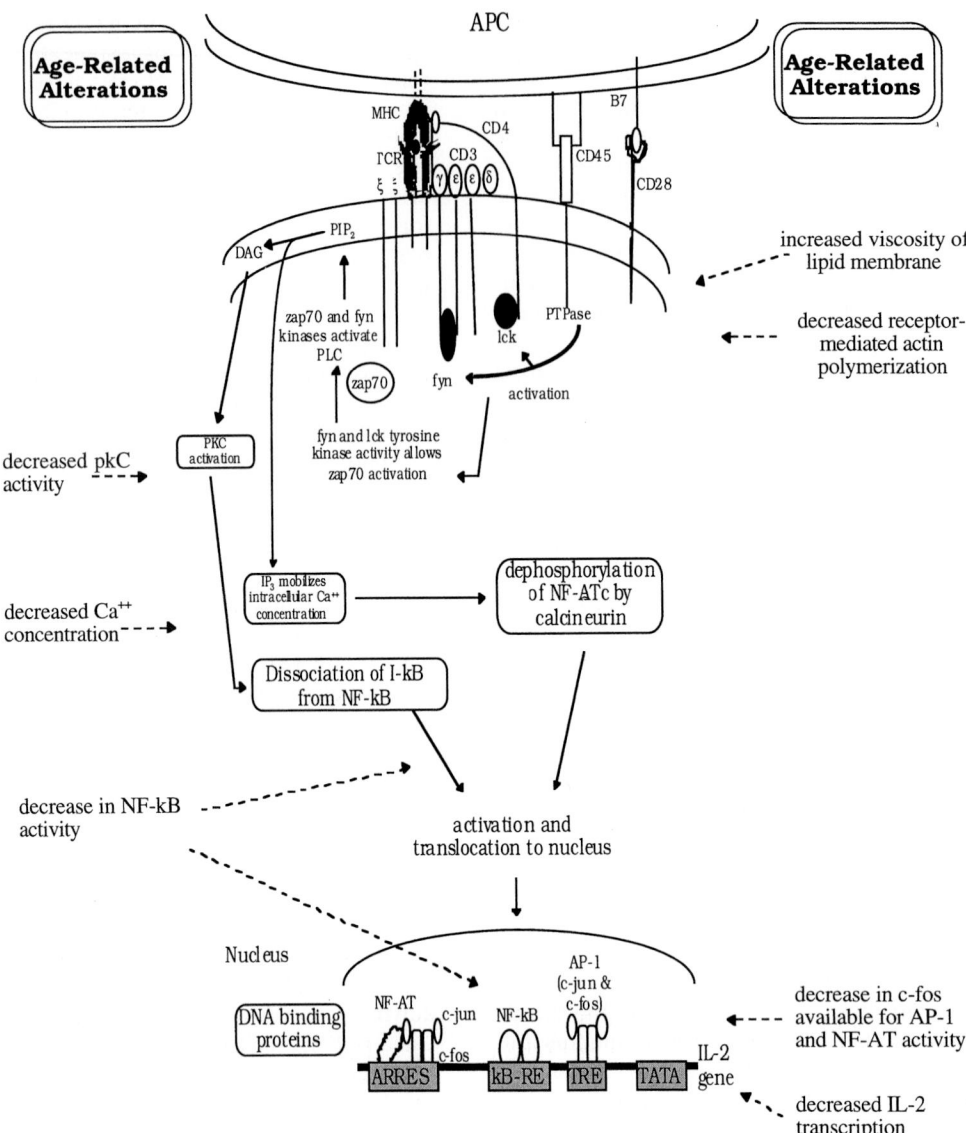

Figure 3-6 Age-associated changes in T-cell activation.

age-related alterations appear to contribute to the abnormal activation of lymphocytes in the elderly.

Alterations in Cellular Life Span

Although antigen stimulation of T cells results in activation and clonal proliferation of the responding T cells, this antigen-induced activation ultimately leads to greater than 95 percent death of antigen-specific T cells by a mechanism called apoptosis, programmed cell death, or activation-induced cell death (AICD). The process is necessary to maintain normal homeostasis and regulate the immune response so that it does not become pathologic, as in toxic shock syndrome. Apoptosis is induced by ligand binding of the transmembrane receptor CD95 (Fas). CD95 is expressed on many cells, including T cells. Activation of T cells induces increased expression of CD95 and new expression of the ligand for CD95. Interactions

between Fas (CD95) and Fas ligand trigger AICD. Alterations in apoptosis have been suggested as a theoretical mechanism to explain both age-related decreases in cell-mediated immunity and increases in autoimmunity. It has been hypothesized that decreased expression of CD95 on cells results in the accumulation of dysfunctional senescent cells and self-reactive cells.

However, limited studies that have addressed age-associated alterations in apoptosis in lymphocytes of humans report that aging is associated with a higher percentage of cells undergoing apoptosis after activation. Both CD4+ and CD8+ T cells of elderly subjects increase expression of both Fas and Fas L and demonstrate more apoptosis after exposure to anti-Fas antibody. A similar increase in apoptosis occurs after treatment with TNF-α. While the percentage of lymphocytes undergoing apoptosis is higher in memory (CD45RO+) as compared to naïve (CD45RA+) cells of both young and elderly, memory and naïve subsets of both CD4+ and CD8+ T cells of elderly subjects exhibit a higher percentage of apoptotic cells as compared to cells of young subjects. None of the studies, however, correlate the level of immune response (e.g., as assessed by proliferation) with the extent of apoptosis. The relationship between alterations in apoptosis in human lymphocytes and immunosenescence remains an area for further investigation.

CLINICAL IMPLICATIONS OF ALTERED IMMUNE RESPONSE IN THE ELDERLY POPULATION

Three issues are critical in bringing research on the mechanisms of the age-related decline in immunity from "bench to bedside" to help with the prevention and treatment of age-associated illnesses, such as infection, malignancy, and autoimmunity.

First, it is important to recognize the characteristics of the subject population participating in any given study. Conclusions drawn from research involving nursing home-dwelling elderly persons may not be applicable to healthy, ambulatory elderly people and vice versa. Frail elderly persons (e.g., nursing home residents) generally exhibit substantially decreased immune function, whereas the decline in the immune status of independently living elderly persons is more subtle. Thus, application of the results from a particular study should carefully consider the characteristics of both the study population and the individual elderly patient.

Second, it is critical to understand that even within defined subpopulations of the elderly there is considerable heterogeneity of the immune response. This heterogeneity is evident both in baseline responses and in responses to efforts to augment those responses. For example, the mean immune response of a population of elderly individuals to various stimuli is consistently decreased compared to that of the young. However, the level of response of some elderly individuals is so profoundly affected that their response is negligible, while the immune response of others is similar to the response of young individuals. While all the factors responsible for this heterogeneity have not been established, general health status is one factor. Genetic differences may represent a major component of this heterogeneity, a factor that cannot be controlled or even identified at this time. However, the magnitude of age-related changes in immune function may be exacerbated by factors such as poverty, environmental pollutants, nutritional status, depression, mental illness, smoking, medications, alcohol and/or drug abuse, comorbid diseases, and genetics. The geriatric team must consider the impact of these factors on each older individual, while keeping in mind the general high risk of decreased immune function among the elderly. Thus, efforts to increase immune function (e.g., nutritional supplements and booster vaccines) may not be effective in all geriatric patients even though published reports demonstrate significant increases in average immune function. Such reports only provide a starting point from which to evaluate the immune function of an individual geriatric patient.

Third, the implications of immunosenescence for clinical outcomes are not fully understood. Although increased rates of infection, malignancy, and autoimmunity are associated with the dysregulated immune response characteristic of the elderly person, the changes in the immune response have not been causally related to the increased incidence of disease. However, there is little doubt that the interplay between immunosenescence and other age-related physiologic changes does appear to make the elderly person susceptible to increased morbidity and mortality from infection, autoimmunity, and cancer.

Elderly individuals who demonstrate low lymphoproliferation in response to mitogens (<20 percent of the mean response of the young) exhibit a higher rate of mortality over 2 years as compared with elderly persons with higher lymphoproliferative response (≥50 percent of the mean response of the young). No association was found between level of lymphoproliferative response and increased incidence of infection or cancer; instead, a similar distribution of causes of mortality was observed among all the subjects. In contrast, one study observed that a decreased overall immune response was associated with an increased rate of infection. Although this literature is not yet definitive, the results suggest that general immune responsiveness may be an indicator of overall health status. Advances expected in the next decade should permit clinicians to assess individual age-related changes in immune response with specificity and accuracy and should lead to new therapeutic interventions targeted precisely at strengthening specific attributes of the immune system without fear of disrupting or dysregulating others.

ACKNOWLEDGMENTS

We would like to thank Ms. Christine Kinsinger for her excellent administrative support. This effort was supported by NIH AG18641.

REFERENCES

Bruce IN et al: Age-related changes in non-receptor dependent generation of reactive oxygen species from phagocytes of healthy adults. *Mech Ageing Dev* 94:135, 1997.

Butcher S et al: Ageing and the neutrophil: no appetite for killing? *Immunology* 100:411, 2000.

Fagnoni FF et al: Expansion of cytotoxic CD8 CD28 T cells in healthy ageing people, including centenarians. *Immunology* 88:501, 1996.

Fietta A et al: Influence of aging on some specific and nonspecific mechanisms of the host defense system in 146 healthy subjects. *Gerontology* 40:237, 1994.

Fulop T: Signal transduction changes in granulocytes and lymphocytes with ageing. *Immunol Lett* 40:259, 1994.

Gardner EM, Murasko DM: Age-related changes in type 1 and type 2 cytokine production in humans. Biogerontology 3:271, 2002.

Gross PA et al: The efficacy of influenza vaccine in elderly persons: A meta-analysis and review of the literature. *Ann Intern Med* 123:518, 1995.

Gupta S: Molecular and biochemical pathways of apoptosis in lymphocytes from aged humans. *Vaccine* 18:1596, 2000.

Hallgren HM et al: Changes with age in CD4+ memory and naïve T lymphocyte proliferative responses to both mitogen and recall antigens in healthy humans. *Aging Immunol Infect Dis* 5:109, 1994.

Kutza J et al: Basal natural killer cell activity of young versus elderly humans. *J Gerontol Biol Sci* 50A:B110, 1995.

LeMaoult J et al: Effect of age on humoral immunity, selection of the B-cell repertoire and B-cell development. *Immunol Rev* 160:115, 1997.

Miller RA: The aging immune system: Primer and prospectus. *Science* 273:70, 1996.

Mountz JD et al: Cell death and longevity: Implications of Fas-mediated apoptosis in T-cell senescence. *Immunol Rev* 160:19, 1997.

Murasko DM, et al: Role of humoral and cell-mediated immunity in protection from influenza disease after immunization of healthy elderly. *Exp Gerontol* 37:427, 2001.

Paganelli R et al: Humoral immunity in aging. *Aging Clin Exp Res* 6:143, 1994.

Pawelec G et al: The T cell in the aging individual. *Mech Ageing Dev* 93:35, 1997.

Steger MM et al: Morphologically and functionally intact dendritic cells can be derived from the peripheral blood of aged individuals. *Clin Exp Immunol* 105:544, 1996.

Whisler RL et al: Impaired induction of c-fos/c-jun genes and of transcriptional regulatory proteins binding distinct c-fos/c-jun promoter elements in activated human T cells during aging. *Cell Immunol* 175:41, 1997.

Demography and Epidemiology

JACK M. GURALNIK • LUIGI FERRUCCI

Over the past century there have been truly remarkable changes in the numbers and characteristics of older persons throughout the world. The growth of the older population has resulted from a general increase in the overall population size but has been particularly affected by major declines in several of the leading causes of mortality. The increased survival of older persons has also been accompanied by declining birth rates; so the proportion of the population aged 65 years and older has increased dramatically and will continue to increase for the next 50 years. These demographic transformations have an effect on society that reverberates well beyond the increased medical care needs associated with an older population.

As more people live to advanced old age, it is important to gain a greater understanding of more than just the individual diseases that affect them. It is critical to appreciate the global picture of older persons who may have multiple chronic conditions, decrements in functional abilities, and social and psychological problems that may have an impact on many facets of their health and quality of life. In contrast to the previous stereotype, older people become more heterogeneous, not more alike, as they age, and understanding this process is one of the key challenges of geriatric medicine. Adding to the clinical perspective on single patients or small samples of patients, geriatric epidemiology has provided a useful tool with which to approach these challenges by studying representative populations of older persons. Going beyond the demographic focus of counting and projecting the number of older people in the population, epidemiology has made additional contributions to our understanding of the health status and functional trajectory of the older population. In the past two decades, epidemiologic researchers either have utilized previously initiated cohort studies that include persons who have aged during the study or have begun new cohorts focusing on older people. These epidemiologic studies have assessed the distribution and determinants of specific diseases and have evaluated issues of relevance to an aging population, such as quality of life, geriatric syndromes, comorbidity, functional status, and end-of-life issues. Many of the chapters in this book refer to epidemiologic research on specific diseases and conditions. This chapter focuses on the more general or "geriatric" outcomes, particularly disability, that

have also been the subject of much epidemiologic investigation.

The chapter begins by documenting the rapid growth and impressive increases in the number of older persons in the United States and other countries. It then examines improvements in survival and life expectancy. Selected demographic characteristics are then considered, including living situation and labor force participation across many developed countries. The second section, on mortality, depicts current causes of death in the older population in the United States and considers the change in death rates with increasing age. Data on overall and disease-specific changes in mortality rates from 1950 through 1999 show the dramatic changes in these rates. The third section addresses chronic disease in the older population by using data from national surveys on self-reporting of chronic conditions, ambulatory medical visits, and hospital discharges. Data are then presented for two conditions, cancer and dementia, as examples of conditions where the use of only mortality data would provide an incomplete picture. The fourth section presents epidemiologic data on disability in older persons. This section describes the prevalence of disability, its causes and consequences, individual transitions in functional status, population changes in disability prevalence, and measurement issues. Finally, the chapter provides a description of important behavioral risk factors for chronic disease, injury, and disability and the prevalence rates of these risk factors in the older population.

DEMOGRAPHICS

One-hundred-fifty years of aging in America are summarized in Table 4-1, beginning with 1900 and including projections through 2050. This table demonstrates how the older population has grown, as well as how the oldest segment of the older population has grown even more rapidly. In 1900 only 4.1 percent of the 76 million persons in the United States were aged 65 years and older, and among those in this age group only 3.2 percent were aged 85 years and older. By 1950 more than 8 percent of the total population was aged 65 years and older, and by 2000 this percentage had increased to 12.6 percent. The US Census Bureau

Table 4-1   Actual and Projected Growth of the Older US Population, 1900–2050 (Millions)

Year	Total Population (All Ages)	65 Years and Older		85 Years and Older	
		Number	Percent of Total Population	Number	Percent of 65 Years and Older Population
1900	76.1	3.1	4.1	0.1	3.2
1950	152.3	12.3	8.2	0.6	4.9
2000	276.1	34.9	12.6	4.4	12.6
2050	403.7	82.0	20.3	19.4	23.7

SOURCE: Population Division, US Census Bureau, Washington, DC 20233.

creates several alternative mortality scenarios when developing population projections, and according to their middle mortality assumption, there will be 82 million persons aged 65 years and older in the United States in 2050. If mortality declines faster than projected under this assumption, the number of older people will be even higher. In 2050 one in five Americans will be aged 65 years or older. The growth of the 85 and older population, termed by some the oldest old, will be even more dramatic. By 2050, when the current baby boom generation will be in this age group, it is projected that 19 million persons, representing nearly a quarter of all persons aged 65 years and older, will be 85 years and older. There will be more than 4 times as many people in the 85 years and older age group as there are now, and almost 200 times as many as there were in 1900. Thus, the numbers of older people are rising dramatically, the proportion of the total population aged 65 years and older is increasing, and the older population itself is getting older, with increasing proportions in the 85 years and older subgroup.

Population aging is taking place throughout the world. Figure 4-1 presents data on the current and projected percentage of the population aged 65 years and older for six regions of the world. Change in the proportion of a population that is elderly depends on changes both in the survival of older persons and in the birthrate. Improved survival at older ages and a low birthrate have resulted in European countries having the oldest populations in the world. In fact, of the world's 25 countries with the oldest populations, 24 are in eastern or western Europe. The country with the oldest population is Italy, where 18.1 percent of the population was 65 years and older in 2000. The only non-European country on the list of the oldest 25 populations is Japan, which has the fourth oldest population in the world, with 17.0 percent aged 65 years and older. Europe will continue to have the oldest populations in the world in the twenty-first century, with almost one in four Europeans projected to be aged 65 years or older by 2030. The current percentage aged 65 years and older in Latin America, the Caribbean, Asia, the Near East, and North Africa is low, ranging from about 4 percent to 6 percent. However, growth of the older population will be rapid in these countries, and it is projected that in 2030 the proportion of the population in this age range will double. Sub-Saharan Africa has few older persons, and it is expected that the percentage of older people in the general population will not grow substantially in the future.

Populations have aged at different speeds and during different time periods throughout the world. Figure 4-2 shows the number of years it took, or is projected to take,

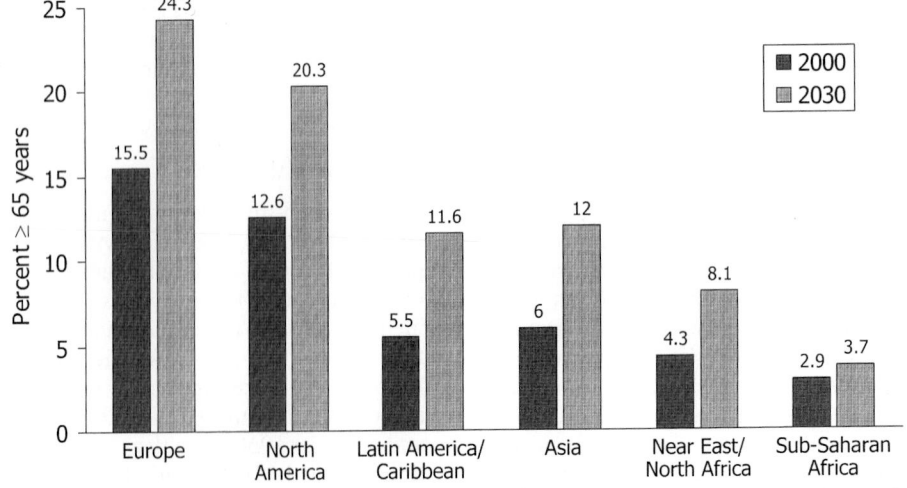

Figure 4-1   Percentage of population aged 65 years and older, 2000 and projected for 2030. Reprinted with permission from Kinsella K, Velkoff VA: *An Aging World: 2001.* US Census Bureau, Series P95/01–1. Washington, DC, US Government Printing Office, 2001.

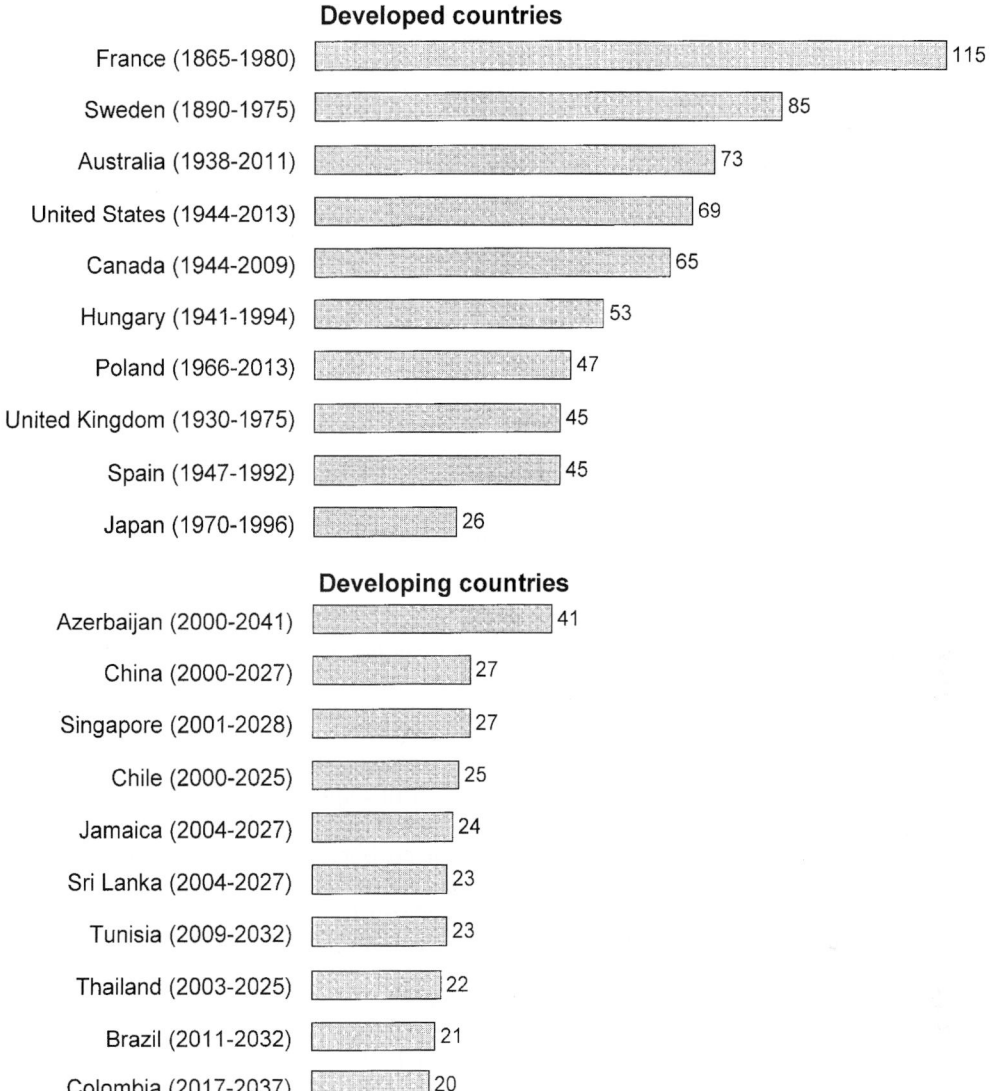

Figure 4-2   Speed of aging: number of years and time period in which percent of population aged 65 and over doubled or will double from 7 percent to 14 percent. Reprinted with permission from Kinsella K, Velkoff VA: *An Aging World: 2001*. US Census Bureau, Series P95/01–1. Washington, DC, US Government Printing Office, 2001.

for specific countries to progress from having 7 percent of the population aged 65 years and older to having 14 percent of the population in this age range. The United States is expected to reach 14 percent in 2013 and will have taken 69 years to make the transition. Sweden and the United Kingdom reached the 14 percent level in 1975, with Sweden taking 85 years to go from 7 percent to 14 percent and the United Kingdom taking about half that time. Japan has already reached the 14 percent mark and took only 26 years to do so. A particularly clear message about the speed of aging in developing countries is presented in Figure 4-2. Although the developing countries shown will generally not reach the 14 percent mark until the third decade of this century, they will have spent less than 27 years making the transition. The rapid aging of these countries will certainly have a large societal impact, with less ability to adapt than in countries that have aged more slowly.

There has always been a fascination with extreme longevity, but the demographics of very long life have been

formally studied only in recent years. Previous claims for the world record for longevity were often unsubstantiated, and pockets of the world where claims were made for general high longevity usually turned out to be no different than other parts of the world. However, recent data from places like Sardinia, Italy, have identified areas of increased longevity that have been meticulously validated. Better age documentation has made it possible to be more confident about the numbers of centenarians and changes in these numbers. It has been estimated that the number of centenarians in western Europe has doubled every decade since 1950, and estimates for the United States also show a doubling between 1980 and 1990 and again from 1990 to 2000, when the total number of centenarians rose from 28,000 to 68,000. These numbers are probably inflated, but there has still been an impressive rise in the number of centenarians. However, future increases will be spectacular, with a projected 1 million centenarians in the United States in 2050. In 1990, 78 percent of US centenarians were non-Hispanic

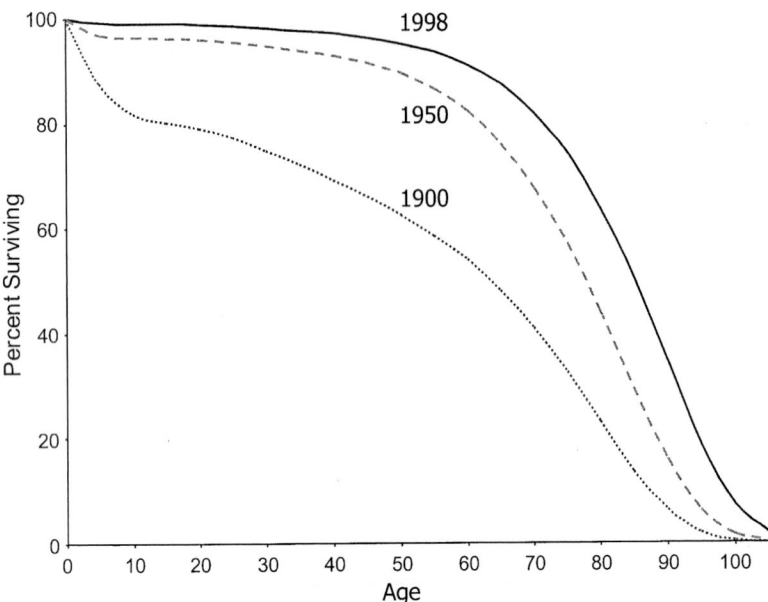

Figure 4-3   Survival curves for US population. Reprinted with permission from Anderson RN: *United States life tables, 1998*. National Vital Statistics Reports, vol. 48, no. 18. Hyattsville, MD, National Center for Health Statistics, 2001.

whites, but centenarians in the future are expected to be much more ethnically diverse.

Better survival at all ages has had a major impact on the size and age distribution of the older population. Figure 4-3 depicts survival curves for the total US population over the course of the twentieth century. In 1900 there was substantial mortality in infancy and early childhood, with the survival curve in midlife being somewhat steeper than at the end of the century. By 1950 a large proportion of early-life mortality had been removed, although survival in this age range was still improving by the end of the century. By 1998 a large proportion of persons were living to age 60 years, and only at age 70 years did the survival curve start to fall rapidly. The change observed in the shape of survival curves has been termed the rectangularization of survival, and it has been proposed that at some point in time full rectangularization will be reached, with no further increases in life expectancy. When this will occur is not yet clear, and the US Census Bureau and Social Security Administration are projecting continued increases in survival for at least the next 50 years.

Life expectancy at age *x* is defined as the average number of years remaining to be lived by a member of a survivorship group who is exactly age *x*. Most life expectancy estimates use current life tables, meaning that they use the age-specific mortality experience of the current population. With this approach, life expectancy at birth gives an estimate of the average length of life of a cohort of children who are born now and then experience today's age-specific mortality rates as they proceed through life. This is an artificial construct, but it provides a way to represent the overall mortality experience of a current population and allows us to compare this experience across countries and over time. If mortality rates continue to decline, as is expected, the average child born today will live considerably longer than the estimate shown on a current life table. Given these caveats, it is nonetheless useful to examine changes in life expectancy over the last century and life expectancy at specific ages. Life expectancy at birth was only 47.3 years in 1900 and rose to 68.2 years by 1950, affected to a large extent by improvements in infant and child mortality. Life expectancy continued to rise through the second half of the twentieth century, driven mainly by increases in survival in middle and old age. Table 4-2 shows life expectancy at birth and at ages 65, 75, and 85 years for the year 2000. At all ages females have a higher life expectancy than males,

Table 4-2   Life Expectancy in 2000 (Years)

	Male			Female		
Age	All	White	Black	All	White	Black
At birth	74.1	74.8	68.3	79.5	80.0	75.0
65 years	16.3	16.3	14.6	19.2	19.2	17.5
75 years	10.2	10.1	9.4	12.1	12.1	11.2
85 years	5.6	5.5	5.8	6.7	6.6	6.5

SOURCE: Minino AM, Smith BL: Deaths: Preliminary data for 2000. National Vital Statistics Reports, vol 49, no 12. Hyattsville, MD, National Center for Health Statistics, 2001.

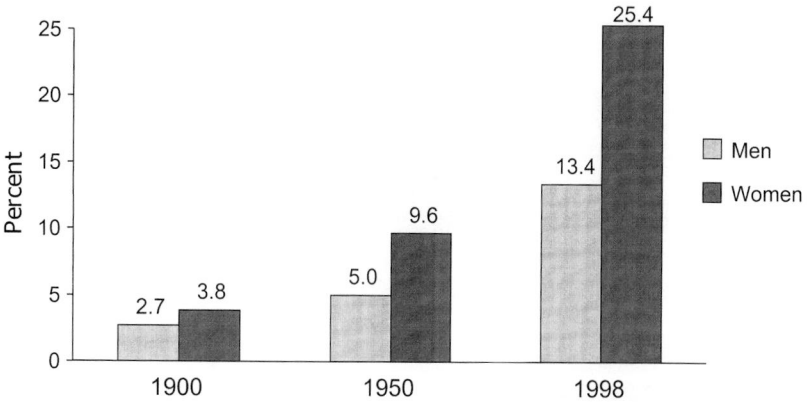

Figure 4-4 Probability of 50-year-old living to 90, 1900 to 1998. Computed from US life tables in Anderson RN: *United States life tables, 1998*. National Vital Statistics Reports, vol. 48, no. 18. Hyattsville, MD, National Center for Health Statistics, 2001.

with the differential at birth being 5.4 years. The gender differential for blacks (6.7 years) is greater than for whites (5.2 years). Blacks have a lower life expectancy than whites through age 75 years and then have a similar life expectancy at age 85 years. The observations of importance to geriatric medicine in these estimates are that the average 75-year-old man will live about 10 more years and the average 75-year-old woman will live 12 more years. At age 85, the average person will still live another 5 to 6 years.

The estimates shown in Table 4-2 do not include Hispanics. Although the National Center for Health Statistics does publish data on Hispanic mortality rates, these data come with warnings of problems associated with their accuracy. The denominator for Hispanic rates comes from the US Census, where Hispanic ethnicity is self-reported. At the time of death, Hispanic ethnicity is reported by the person completing the death certificate, and there is likely a large amount of underreporting. It is also known that a not insignificant number of Hispanic persons return to their native countries to spend the last years of their lives, and so their deaths are not enumerated as deaths in the United States. Thus, there is substantial underascertainment of the numerator for Hispanic death rate calculations, leading to an underestimation of the true rates.

The improvements in survival over the last century are relevant to the field of geriatric medicine, as the decline in

mortality rates throughout life has resulted in a population with a large proportion of individuals who will survive to advanced old age. This point is made compellingly by the data shown in Figure 4-4. This figure was generated using data from 1900, 1950, and 1998 life tables and illustrates the proportion of 50-year-old men and women who can expect to live to age 90 years or older. Only about 3 percent to 4 percent of 50-year-olds could expect to live to this age in 1900. By 1950 this proportion had hardly risen at all in men but had gone up to 10 percent in women. The large decreases in old-age mortality in the second half of the century led to large changes by 1998, when 13 percent of 50-year-old men and more than 25 percent of 50-year-old women could expect to reach the age of 90 years. All these estimates are derived from current life tables; so if mortality continues to decline, these percentages will be even higher in the current cohort of 50-year-olds. The consequence of these changes is that an unprecedented proportion of the current middle-aged population will live to very old age.

Further demographic characteristics relevant to the social environment in which older persons find themselves living are shown in Figures 4-5 and 4-6. In Figure 4-5, the elderly ratio, defined as the number of persons aged 65 years and older divided by the number of persons aged 20 to 64 years, multiplied by 100, is shown for the total population and racial and ethnic subgroups in 1990 and

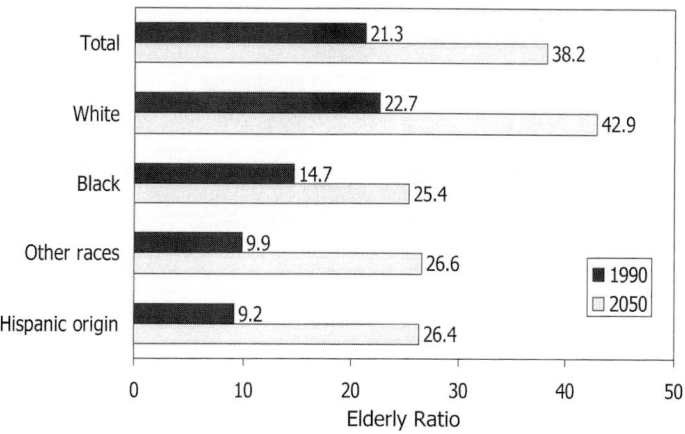

Figure 4–5 Elderly ratio: number of persons aged 65 years and over divided by number of persons aged 20 to 64, times 100. Reprinted with permission from US Census Bureau: *65+ in the United States*. Current Population Reports, Special Studies, P23–190. Washington, DC, US Government Printing Office, 1996.

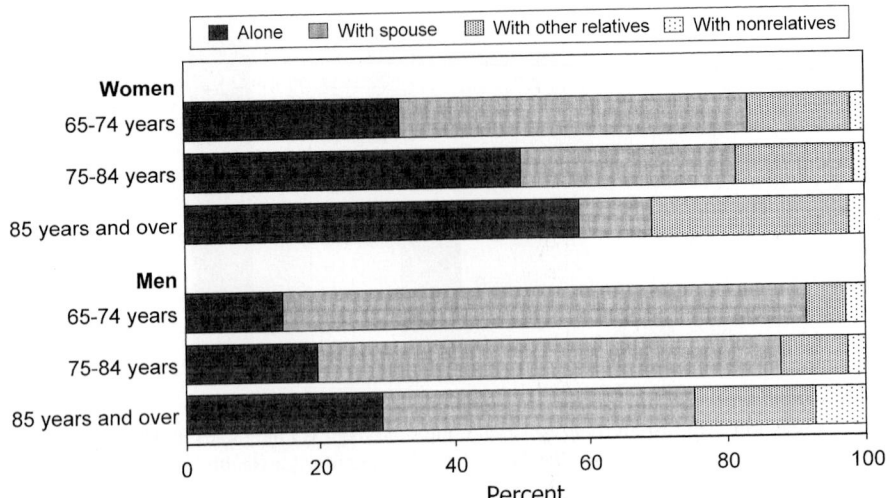

Figure 4-6 Living arrangements of community-dwelling persons 65 years and over United States, 1997. Reprinted with permission from Kramarow E, Lentzner H et al: *Health, United States, 1999.* Health and Aging Chartbook. Hyattsville, MD, National Center for Health Statistics, 1999.

projected to 2050. With the faster growth of the older population and the less rapid increase in the younger population, this ratio will rise dramatically in the future. Currently there are about 21 older people for every 100 persons aged 20 to 64 years. By 2050 there will be 38 older people for

every 100 persons in the younger age group, the group who will be called on to care for older parents and grandparents and whose Social Security payments will be used to provide for retirees. Now and in the future the elderly ratio is highest in whites. Blacks currently have a higher

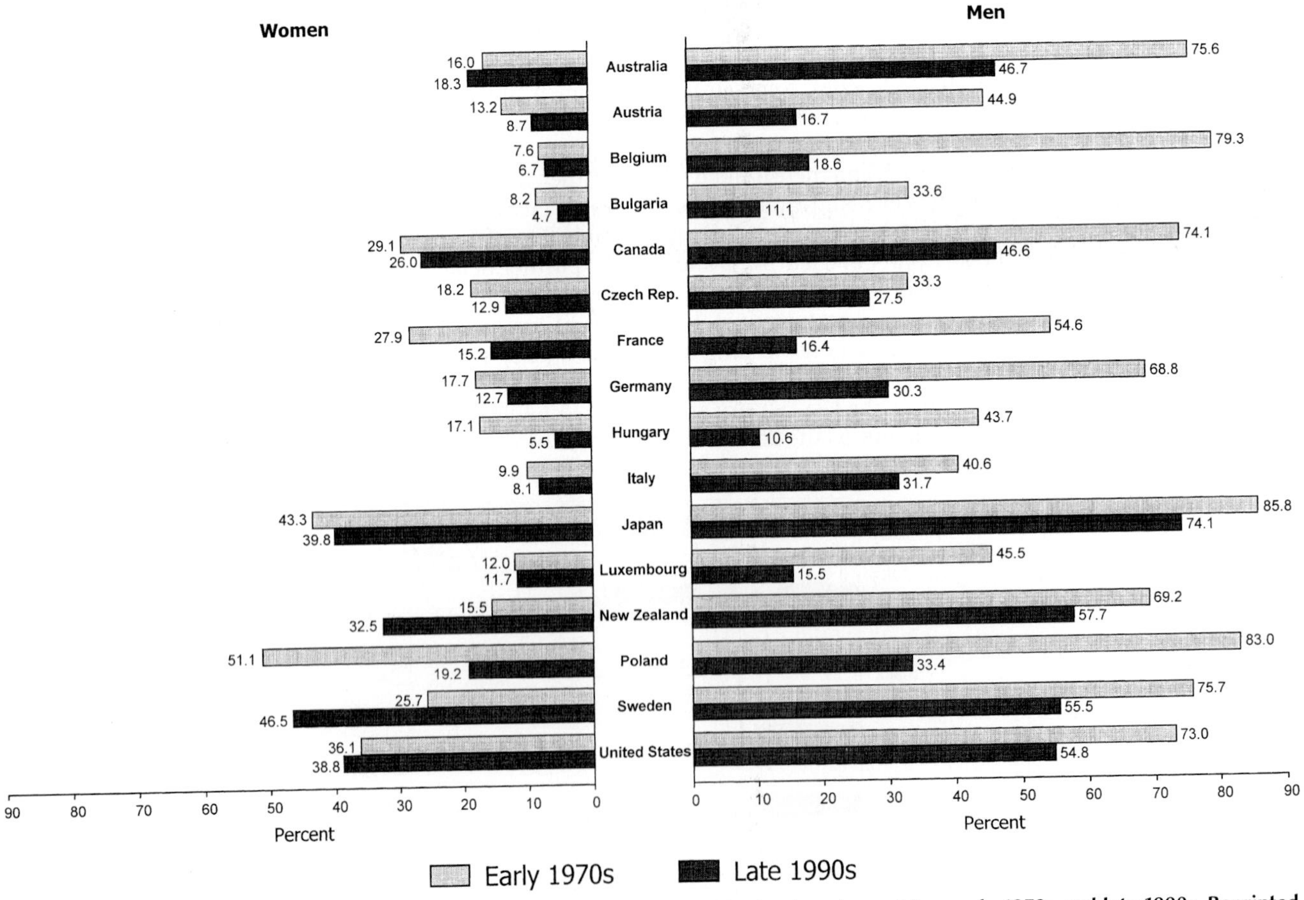

Women

Country	Early 1970s	Late 1990s
Australia	16.0	18.3
Austria	13.2	8.7
Belgium	7.6	6.7
Bulgaria	8.2	4.7
Canada	29.1	26.0
Czech Rep.	18.2	12.9
France	27.9	15.2
Germany	17.7	12.7
Hungary	17.1	5.5
Italy	9.9	8.1
Japan	43.3	39.8
Luxembourg	12.0	11.7
New Zealand	15.5	32.5
Poland	51.1	19.2
Sweden	25.7	46.5
United States	36.1	38.8

Men

Country	Early 1970s	Late 1990s
Australia	75.6	46.7
Austria	44.9	16.7
Belgium	79.3	18.6
Bulgaria	33.6	11.1
Canada	74.1	46.6
Czech Rep.	33.3	27.5
France	54.6	16.4
Germany	68.8	30.3
Hungary	43.7	10.6
Italy	40.6	31.7
Japan	85.8	74.1
Luxembourg	45.5	15.5
New Zealand	69.2	57.7
Poland	83.0	33.4
Sweden	75.7	55.5
United States	73.0	54.8

☐ Early 1970s   ■ Late 1990s

Figure 4-7 Labor force participation rates for men and women aged 60–64 in developed countries, early 1970s and late 1990s. Reprinted with permission from Kinsella K, Velkoff VA: *An Aging World: 2001.* US Census Bureau, Series P95/01–1. Washington, DC, US Government Printing Office, 2001.

ratio than Hispanics, but by 2050 there will be about 26 elderly blacks, Hispanics, and persons of other races for every 100 people aged 20 to 64 years.

Living situation is determined by health, financial factors, and widowhood and varies considerably by gender and age, as seen in Figure 4-6. Among community-living persons in the United States, women are much more likely to live alone, with about 60 percent of women aged 85 years and older living alone. A large proportion of men live with their spouses. Women are more likely to outlive their husbands not only because they live longer but also because they tend to marry older men. Very modest percentages of older persons live with other relatives, and a very small proportion live with nonrelatives.

In recent years, the percentage of older people who work and the average age of retirement have fallen throughout the developed countries. In Figure 4-7 the percentage of persons working is shown for the early 1970s and the late 1990s for the 60 to 64-year age group, the group that was traditionally preretirement. Overall, women work less than men, but in a few countries, including the United States, the percentage of women working rose during this time. In many countries, there have been extremely large declines in the percentage of men in this age group who work. For example, the percentage of men 60 to 64 years old who were employed declined over this 25-year period from 76 percent to 47 percent in Australia, from 79 percent to 19 percent in Belgium, from 55 percent to 16 percent in France, and from 69 percent to 30 percent in Germany. An increase in societal wealth has been the main driving force for decreased workforce participation, but other factors include obsolescence

of the skills of older workers, pressure for older workers to leave their jobs to make room for younger workers in countries with high unemployment, and the growth of financial incentives for early retirement. The percentage of persons in the 65 years and older age group who work has also declined. For example, in the United States the percentage of men in this age group who work dropped from 24.8 percent in the early 1970s to 16.9 percent in the late 1990s. The corresponding percentages for men in Germany were 16.0 percent and 4.5 percent, in France 10.7 percent and 2.3 percent, and in Japan 54.5 percent and 35.5 percent. With earlier retirement and longer life expectancy, the number of years people live after retirement has increased greatly. The Organization for Economic Cooperation and Development (OECD) has estimated that in 1960 men in developed countries could expect to spend 46 years in the labor force and a little more than 1 year in retirement. By 1995 years in the labor force had decreased to 37, whereas years in retirement had increased to 12.

MORTALITY

The increasingly greater life expectancy of the population has been driven in part by reduced mortality at older ages. It is instructive to review the US vital statistics data on causes of death in the older population, changes in these rates with increasing age, and trends in overall and disease-specific mortality over time. Table 4-3 lists the leading causes of death in the population age 65 years and older employing the newly instituted ICD-10 classification system, which

Table 4-3 Leading Causes of Death in Persons 65 Years and Older in 2000

Cause of Death	Number of Deaths	Death Rate (per 100,000 Population)	Percent of All Deaths in Persons 65 Years and older
Heart disease	595,440	1,712.2	33.0
Malignant neoplasms	392,082	1,127.4	21.7
Cerebrovascular disease	146,725	421.9	8.1
Chronic lower respiratory tract disease	107,888	310.2	6.0
Influenza and pneumonia	60,261	173.3	3.3
Diabetes mellitus	52,102	149.8	2.9
Alzheimer's disease	48,492	139.4	2.7
Nephritis, nephrotic syndrome and nephrosis	31,588	90.8	1.7
Motor vehicle accidents	7,165	20.6	0.4
All other accidents	24,167	69.5	1.3
Septicemia	25,143	72.3	1.4
All other causes (residual)	314,134	903.3	17.4
Total	1,805,187	5,190.8	100.0

SOURCE: Minino AM, Smith BL: Deaths: Preliminary data for 2000. National Vital Statistics Reports, vol 49, no 12. Hyattsville, MD, National Center for Health Statistics, 2001.

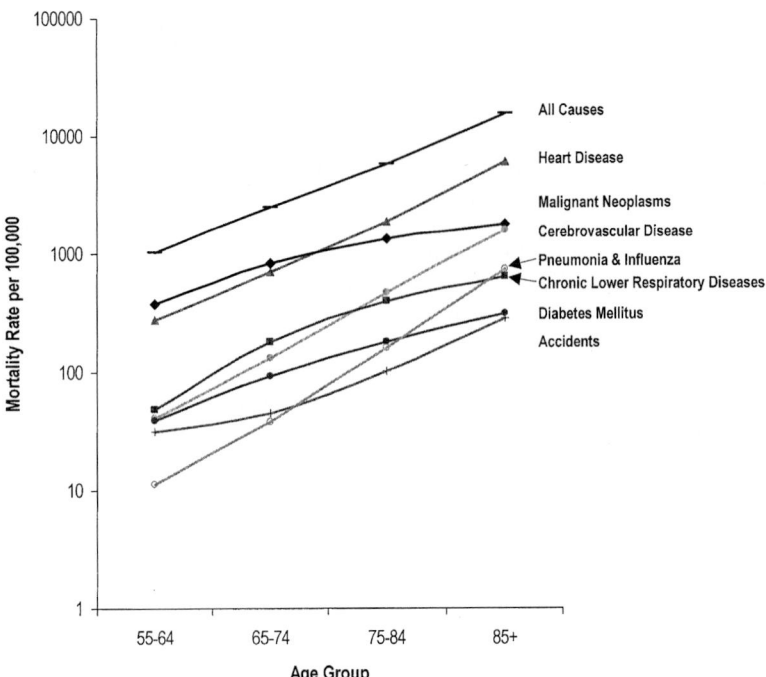

Figure 4-8 Age-specific death rates for leading cause of death in the older population, United States, 1999. Reprinted with permission from Hoyert DL, Arias E et al: *Deaths: Final data for 1999.* National Vital Statistics Reports, vol. 49, no. 8. Hyattsville, MD, National Center for Health Statistics, 2001.

was first used for national data in 1999. As in younger individuals, heart disease is by far the most common cause of death, followed by cancer. The five leading causes of death—heart disease, cancer, stroke, chronic lower respiratory tract disease, and influenza and pneumonia account for 72.1 percent of all deaths. Alzheimer's disease, which in the past was rarely assigned as the underlying cause of death and was not on the list of leading causes of death, is now listed as the seventh leading cause, responsible for 2.7 percent of deaths. This is still likely a gross underestimation, and the contribution of Alzheimer's disease in the future will probably grow substantially. It is well recognized that assigning a single underlying cause of death is fraught

with problems when an individual dies in advanced old age and has multiple chronic conditions. What is surprising is that despite this difficulty the distribution of causes of death in the United States remains quite stable from year to year.

Age-specific mortality rates for selected leading causes of death are depicted in Figure 4-8. On this logarithmic scale a straight-line increase indicates an exponential increase in mortality rate with age. Exponential increases, which are remarkably parallel, are present for all causes of death—heart disease, cerebrovascular disease, and pneumonia and influenza. The mortality rates for cancer and lower respiratory tract disease do not maintain as steep a

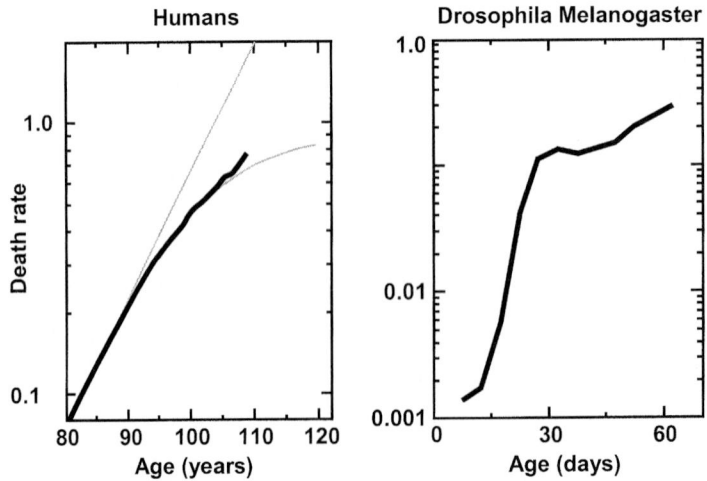

Figure 4-9 Death rates at advanced old age in women and from age 0 to 60 days for a genetically homogeneous line of *Drosophila melanogaster*. Human estimates come from data aggregated from 14 countries for which data were available over the period from 1950 to 1990 for ages 80 to 109, and to 1997 for ages 110 and over. Data on *Drosophila* are from 6333 flies reared under usual laboratory conditions. Reprinted with permission from Vaupel JW, Carey JR et al: Biodemographic trajectories of longevity. *Science* 280:855, 1998.

rise with increasing age, perhaps because the people who contribute substantially to these categories are smokers, who die at younger ages and are less represented in the oldest segment of the population. Diabetes mortality rates also do not show an exponential increase with advancing age, again because diabetic patients may die disproportionately at younger ages. The one condition in this figure for which the mortality rate slope becomes steeper with advancing age is accidents. Although motor vehicle accidents are an issue of real concern in older persons, it is important to note, as shown in Table 4-3, that there are 3½ times as many deaths from other types of accidents as from motor vehicle accidents.

The graph of the exponential rise in mortality with increasing age, which has been described for many species, has been termed the Gompertz curve. It has been difficult to evaluate whether the exponential increase is maintained to the very end of life, as the numbers of extremely old individuals available for study have traditionally been quite small. Recently, larger populations of very old humans and other species have been evaluated to examine whether the Gompertz curve continues to describe mortality rates at advanced old age. Figure 4-9 shows death rates for humans and fruit flies at the extremes of old age, and in both these examples the Gompertz function, which is represented as a straight line in the human example, is not consistent with the data. The conclusion from these studies and from studies on a variety of other species is that the force of mortality declines somewhat in individuals who survive to very old age, although the causes of this phenomenon remain unclear.

The first half of the twentieth century saw large declines in mortality in infants and children, but in the second half of the century there were unprecedented declines in mortality in the older segment of the population. In the total population, mortality rates between 1950 and 1999 fell by 36.6 percent in males and 39.8 percent in females (Figure 4-10). What was notable during the latter half of the century was that this magnitude of decline was also seen in men and women in the 65- to 74- and 75- to 84-year-old

age groups. Even for people 85 years and older there was a mortality rate decline that exceeded 20 percent.

Mortality change over this time period is further explored in Table 4-4, which lists 1950 and 1999 death rates and percentage changes in these rates for heart disease, stroke and cancer, diseases that account for nearly two-thirds of deaths in older adults. For the total population, heart disease mortality declined more than 50 percent, and stroke mortality dropped more than 65 percent, a truly remarkable decline in these diseases that reflects major advances in both prevention and treatment as well as a secular trend that is not fully understood. For both these diseases, the declines in the 65- to 74- and 75- to 85-year old age groups kept pace with or exceeded the percentage decline seen for the total population. In persons aged 85 years and older, heart disease mortality declined by more than 30 percent, with stroke mortality dropping by more than 50 percent in men and more than 40 percent in women, impressive declines in this very old segment of the population. Unfortunately, the declines in mortality seen for heart disease and stroke were not seen for cancer. In women, the overall population showed a slight decline in cancer mortality, but the older population had a modest rise in rates. Cancer mortality rates in men rose more than 30 percent in those older than age 65 years, a larger increase than that seen for the total male population. Heavy cigarette smoking in the cohort of men who were in the older age groups at the end of the last century was probably a major contributing factor to this increase in cancer rates.

DISEASE STATUS

Although there is much useful information to be gained by observing the diseases responsible for mortality, a full picture of disease status in the older population cannot be obtained by looking only at diseases that cause death. A number of ascertainment approaches that work well to characterize morbidity in the general population are used here to give an overview of important diseases prevalent

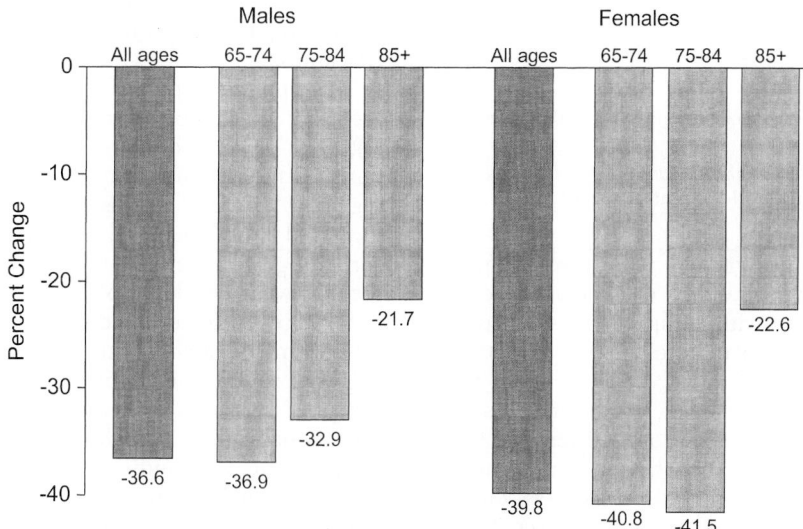

Figure 4–10   Percent change in mortality rates, United States, 1950 to 1999, for all ages (age-adjusted using year 2000 standard population) and for older age groups. Calculated from data in *Health, United States, 2001, with urban and rural health chartbook*. Hyattsville, MD, National Center for Health Statistics, 2001.

Table 4-4 Age-Adjusted and Age-Specific Mortality, United States, 1950 and 1999

Disease*	1950	1999	Percent Change
Diseases of the heart			
Males			
All ages	697.0	328.1	−52.9
65–74	2292.3	961.6	−58.1
75–84	4825.0	2308.9	−52.1
85+	9659.8	6313.3	−34.6
Females			
All ages	484.7	220.9	−54.4
65–74	1419.3	503.2	−64.5
75–84	3872.0	1562.5	−59.6
85+	8796.1	5913.8	−32.8
Cerebrovascular disease			
Males			
All ages	186.4	62.4	−66.5
65–74	589.6	149.0	−74.7
75–84	1543.6	494.5	−68.0
85+	3048.6	1455.5	−52.3
Females			
All ages	175.8	60.5	−65.6
65–74	522.1	118.5	−77.3
75–84	1462.2	458.2	−68.7
85+	2949.4	1670.6	−43.4
Malignant neoplasms			
Males			
All ages	208.1	251.6	20.9
65–74	791.5	1031.2	30.3
75–84	1332.6	1746.2	31.0
85+	1668.3	2619.2	57.0
Females			
All ages	182.3	169.9	−6.8
65–74	612.3	676.6	10.5
75–84	1007.7	1068.1	6.0
85+	1299.7	1449.1	11.5

*Data for "all ages" are age-adjusted using the US 2000 standard population.

SOURCE: *Health, United States, 2001, with urban and rural health chartbook.* Hyattsville, MD, National Center for Health Statistics, 2001.

in older persons. This overview is not meant to provide a comprehensive epidemiology of all medical conditions that often develop with aging but to show data that allow for a comparison of rates across the major conditions.

When a medical history is obtained, a clinician begins to construct a profile of disease status from self-reporting by the patient. In extending this approach to surveys of large, representative samples of older persons, it has been found that self-reporting works quite well for most diseases. Table 4-5 lists the 10 most commonly reported chronic conditions among people aged 65 years and older in the United States. The most commonly reported condition is arthritis

Table 4-5 Most Commonly Reported Chronic Conditions per 1000 Persons 65 Years or Older in 1996

Condition	Male	Female
Arthritis	411.2	534.5
Hypertension	298.0	410.8
Heart disease	311.3	238.0
Hearing impairment	386.8	243.2
Cataracts	140.1	194.3
Deformity or orthopedic impairment	156.5	158.4
Chronic sinusitis	109.6	122.5
Diabetes	121.8	84.3
Tinnitus	117.4	66.1
Visual impairment	103.8	70.0

SOURCE: Adams PF, Hendershot GE et al: Current estimates from the National Health Interview Survey, 1996. National Center for Health Statistics. *Vital Health Stat 10*(200), 1999.

and it, like most of the conditions on the list, has a large impact on overall health and quality of life but does not appear on the list of the most common conditions causing death. In fact, only heart disease and diabetes are among the most commonly reported chronic conditions and are also on the list of the 10 most common causes of death. There are some differences in the prevalence rates of chronic conditions according to race and ethnicity. For example, in persons aged 70 years and older, diabetes is more common in non-Hispanic black and Hispanic persons than in non-Hispanic whites. Non-Hispanic blacks have $1\frac{1}{2}$ times as much hypertension as non-Hispanic whites. Non-Hispanic white men report more heart disease than Hispanic whites or non-Hispanic blacks, whereas non-Hispanic black women report more stroke than non-Hispanic whites or Hispanics.

An important aspect of disease status that distinguishes the older population from the younger population is the high rate of the cooccurrence of multiple chronic conditions, termed comorbidity. Because the risk of developing most diseases increases progressively with age, the increased prevalence and severity of comorbidity is not surprising. However, several lines of research suggest that the observed prevalence of comorbidity is higher than the prevalence expected based on the rates of individual diseases, implying a clustering of diseases in certain individuals. The concept of comorbidity is a useful one in considering the burden of disease in older people. However, the operationalization of a definition for comorbidity depends on the number of conditions being ascertained and the intensity of the diagnostic effort to identify prevalent diseases. The longer the list of conditions and the harder one works to find prevalent diseases, the greater the prevalence of comorbidity. In a national survey that used self-reporting of 9 common conditions, comorbidity was present in almost

Table 4-6 Ambulatory Medical Visits, Reasons for Visit*, and Drug Prescriptions According to Age Group, and Hospital Discharges by Age Group, United States, 1999

Age Group	Average Number of Visits per Person per Year	Percent of Visits for Acute Problems	Percent of Visits for Chronic Problems (Routine or Flare-up)	Percent of Visits with 4+ Drugs Prescribed or Continued	Number of Hospital Discharges per 1000 Population
<15	1.9	50.8	16.9	5.3	40.8
15–24	1.6	39.7	26.9	3.0	74.2
25–44	2.3	36.7	32.7	5.6	86.6
45–64	3.4	31.7	44.4	15.0	116.9
65–74	5.2	26.9	48.6	21.6	270.6
75+	6.8	27.2	51.4	24.6	481.6

*This table does not account for pre- or postsurgery/injury follow-up, nonillness care, or unknown reason for visit.

Source: Cherry DK, Burt CW et al: National Ambulatory Medical Care Survey: 1999 summary. Advance Data From Vital and Health Statistics, no. 322. Hyattsville, MD, National Center for Health Statistics, 2001. Popovic JR: 1999 National Hospital Discharge Survey: Annual summary with detailed diagnoses and procedure data. National Center for Health Statistics. *Vital Health Stat 13* (151), 2001.

50 percent of persons aged 60 years and older. Among those aged 80 years and older, 70 percent of women and 53 percent of men had comorbidity. Although comorbidity is a characteristic of older patients that is dealt with regularly by clinicians, there has been a limited amount of research on the classification of specific patterns of comorbidity and on the impact of comorbidity. In particular, certain combinations of conditions seem to occur at a higher rate than would be expected by chance alone, and certain pairs of conditions may have a synergistic effect on functional loss.

Data on physician visits and hospitalizations can also provide insight into the disease status of older people. Data from the National Ambulatory Medical Care Survey reveal that the three most common reasons for physician office visits are essential hypertension, acute upper respiratory tract infections, and arthropathies and related disorders. However, these three conditions account for only about 10 percent of office visits, with a wide range of problems accounting for the remainder. Table 4-6 shows data on medical visits and hospitalizations in 1999 for the full age spectrum. With increasing age the number of physician visits increases steadily, and persons aged 75 years and older make, on average, nearly seven visits per person per year. The proportion of each age group's visits that are for acute problems and for chronic problems are shown separately, and there is a clear trend in both, with acute problems decreasing steadily with increasing age and chronic problems rising with age and accounting for more than half of office visits in persons aged 75 years and older. The percentage of office visits at which four or more drugs are prescribed or continued also rises steeply with age, and more than one-fifth of visits in persons aged 65 years and older involve patients taking this many drugs. Finally, the table lists overall rates of hospital discharge, which go up dramatically with increasing age. For every 1000 persons aged 65 to 74 years there are 271 hospital discharges in a year, and for every 1000 persons aged 75 years and older there are 482 hospital discharges in a year.

The actual causes of hospitalization in persons aged 65 years and older are represented in Table 4-7, which uses data from the National Hospital Discharge Survey. Heart disease is the most important cause of hospitalization by far, with congestive heart failure a slightly more common cause of hospitalization than other manifestations of heart disease. Other diseases that are frequent causes of death in older adults (pneumonia, cancer, and stroke) are also common reasons for hospitalization, but so are diseases not as strongly associated with mortality, including fractures,

Table 4-7 The Ten Leading Causes of Hospitalization in Persons Aged 65 and Older, First Listed Diagnosis, United States, 1999

	Discharge Rate per 10,000 Population
1. Heart disease	843.7
Acute myocardial infarction	148.6
Coronary atherosclerosis	189.2
Cardiac dysrhythmias	143.5
Congestive heart failure	221.1
2. Pneumonia	236.5
3. Malignant neoplasms	212.8
4. Cerebrovascular disease	205.5
5. Fractures, all sites	155.2
Fractures, neck of femur	85.2
6. Chronic bronchitis	107.8
7. Osteoarthrosis and allied disorders	88.6
8. Volume depletion	72.2
9. Septicemia	70.5
10. Psychoses	62.0

Source: Popovic JR: 1999 National Hospital Discharge Survey: Annual summary with detailed diagnoses and procedure data. National Center for Health Statistics. *Vital Health Stat 13* (151), 2001.

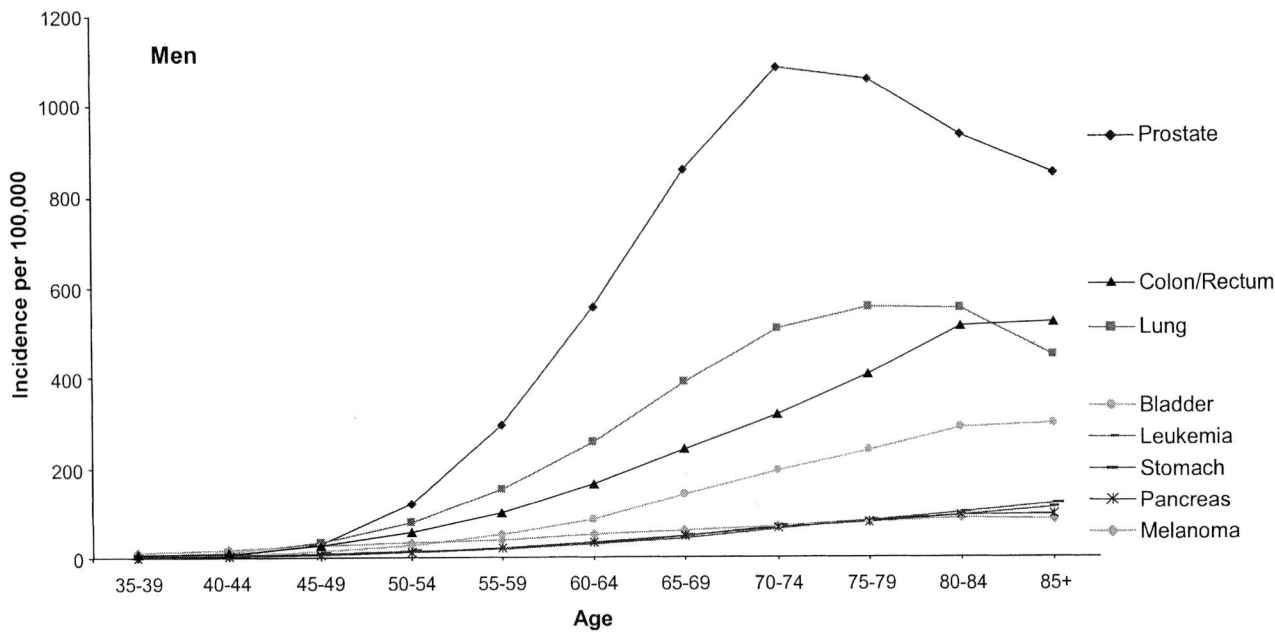

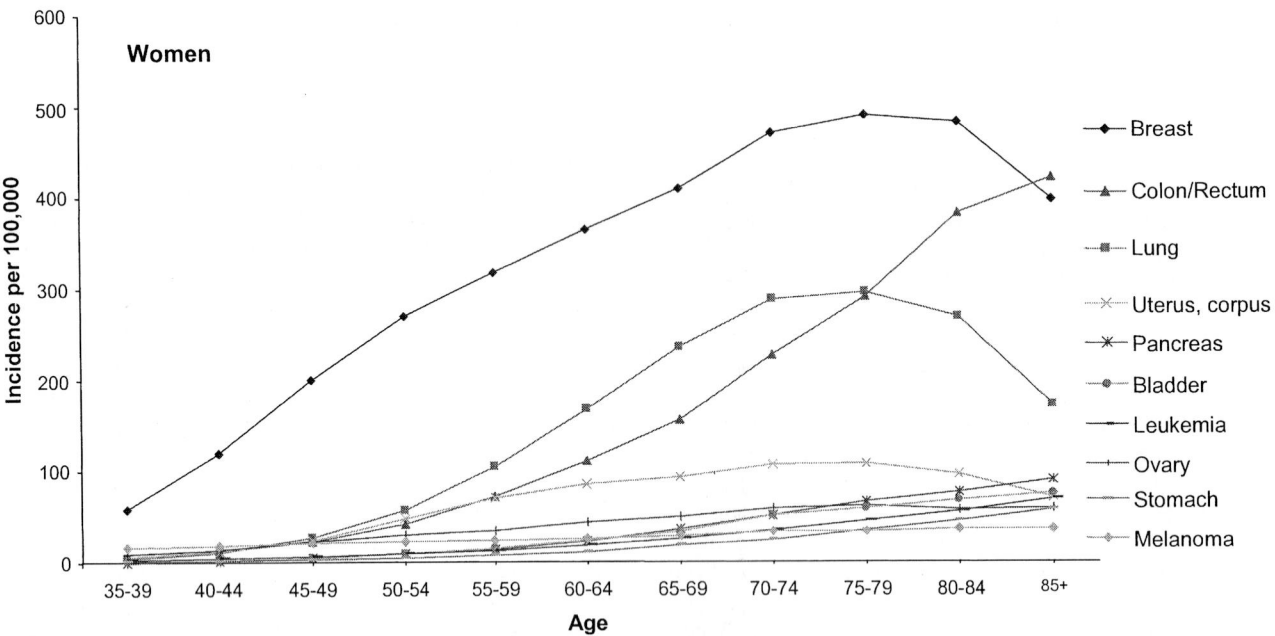

Figure 4-11 Incidence rates of specific cancers in men (top) and women (bottom) by age. Reprinted with permission from SEER cancer statistics review, 1973–1998. Surveillance, Epidemiology and End Results Program, National Cancer Institute. seer.cancer.gov/Publications/

chronic bronchitis, osteoarthritis, and psychosis. The presence of volume depletion and septicemia on this list of the leading causes of hospitalization reflects the fact that a portion of the older population is frail and at high risk for these kinds of illnesses.

Cancer mortality rates do not always reflect the incidence rates of newly diagnosed cancers. The latter data are available from the Surveillance, Epidemiology and End Results (SEER) survey of the National Cancer Institute and

other cancer registries. Figure 4-11 depicts the age-specific incidence of the most common cancers that affect men and women. The highest incidence rates in men are seen for prostate, lung, colon and rectum, and bladder cancers, and in women for breast, colon and rectum, lung, and uterine cancers. The incidence of most of these cancers rises steadily with increasing age, but several, including prostate, breast, and lung cancers, begin to drop in incidence at the oldest ages.

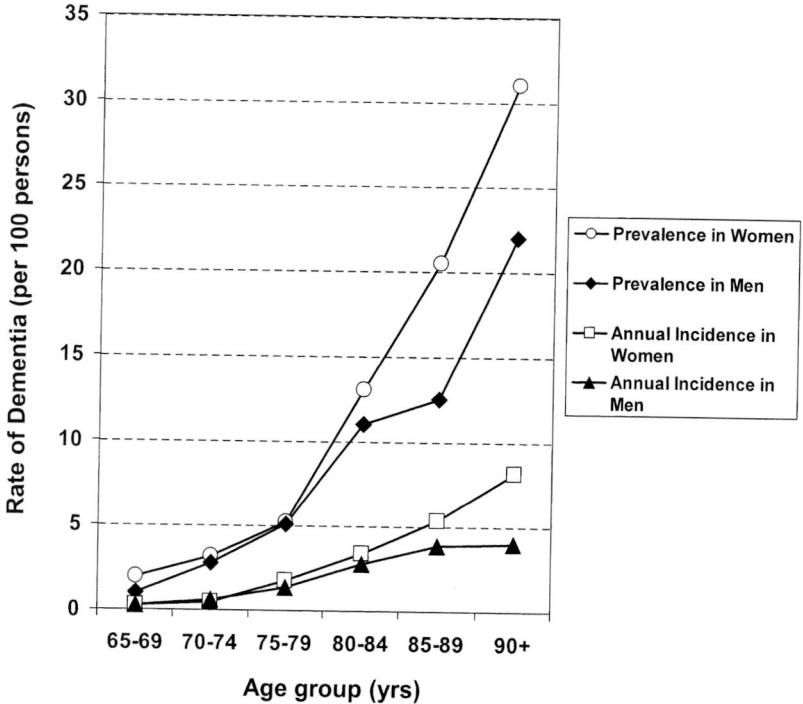

Figure 4-12   Age- and gender-specific prevalence and annual incidence of dementia in persons aged 65 and older. Data from pooled analyses of 11 studies carried out in 8 European countries (prevalence) and in 8 studies in 7 countries (incidence). Adapted with permission from Lobo A, Launer LJ et al: Prevalence of dementia and major subtypes in Europe: A collaborative study of population-based cohorts. *Neurology* 54(suppl 5):S4, 2000. Fratiglioni L, Launer LJ et al: Incidence of dementia and major subtypes in Europe: A collaborative study of population-based cohorts. *Neurology* 54(suppl 5):S10, 2000.

Dementia is a condition of aging for which prevalence and incidence rates cannot be validly obtained from either national survey data or registries. Because of the complexities of diagnosing dementia, data on the occurrence of the condition must rely on well-designed epidemiologic studies in local geographic areas. A network of dementia studies in Europe used comparable diagnostic techniques, which allowed for the aggregation of data on both prevalence and incidence (Figure 4-12). These pooled results show that both incidence and prevalence increase with age, with a steep rise in prevalence after age 80 years, when the prevalence in women becomes somewhat higher than in men. The incidence data show a clear rise in women to age 90 years and older, but some leveling off in men after age 85 years. The incidence rates are about 15 percent to 30 percent of the prevalence rates. In a condition such as dementia, which cannot be cured, this relationship between incidence and prevalence indicates that mortality occurs about 3 to 5 years after diagnosis. An even larger collection of studies on dementia incidence from around the world supported an exponential increase in dementia with age and demonstrated that rates tend to be lower in East Asia than in Europe and the United States.

DISABILITY

A hallmark of geriatrics is emphasis on the functional ability of older patients, and this subject is discussed from a clinical point of view in several chapters in this book. This approach recognizes that although individual diseases are

important and that our system of modern medicine is oriented toward the diagnosis and treatment of specific diseases, the consequences of single and multiple diseases can be understood best by evaluating the functional status of the patient. A large body of epidemiologic work undertaken over the past two decades has treated disability as a condition that can be studied in much as if it were a well-defined chronic disease by using epidemiologic tools to assess prevalence, incidence, and a wide range of risk factors. This work has led to a greater understanding of the occurrence, determinants, and consequences of disability in the older population and has provided insights into strategies for the prevention of disability.

Measures of disability were originally developed for use in the clinical setting and were aimed at quantifying the impact of severe medical conditions such as stroke on physical and mental functioning, obtaining standard information on the rate and degree of recovery from these conditions, and assessing work ability and the need for formal and informal care. These assessment tools were gradually applied in clinical research and population-based studies, and almost all research studies in older populations now assess disability status. Federal data collection efforts did not include very old populations as recently as 20 years ago, but these surveys now have no upper age limit and include various instruments to assess disability. This type of assessment is illustrated in Figure 4-13, which is based on data from the National Health Interview Survey. Data are shown for both difficulty in performing and inability to perform three different kinds of tasks. Physical activity is a general term that describes a set of tasks that have come to be classified as

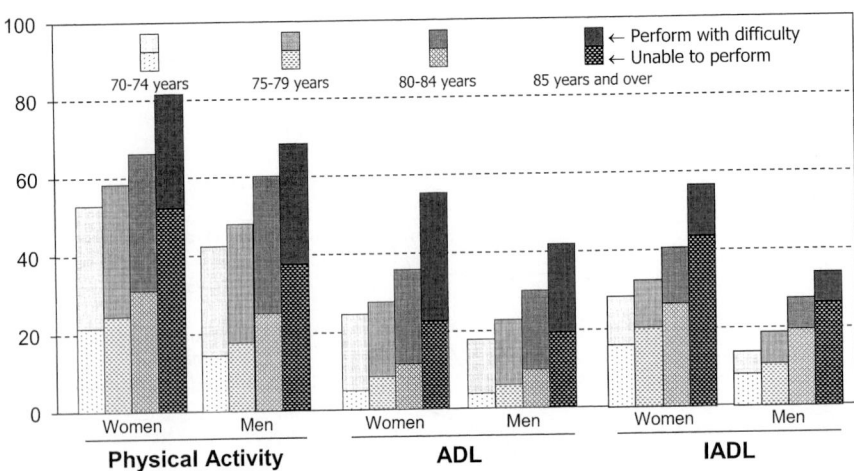

Figure 4–13 Difficulty and inability to perform physical activity, activities of daily living (ADL), and instrumental activities of daily living (IADL), United States, 1994 National Health Interview Survey, Second Supplement on Aging. Physical activities include walking for a 1/4 mile; walking up 10 steps without resting; standing or being on one's feet for 2 hours; sitting for 2 hours; stooping, crouching, or kneeling; reaching up over one's head; reaching out (as if to shake someone's hand); using one's fingers to grasp or handle; lifting or carrying something as heavy as 10 lb. ADLs include bathing or showering; dressing; eating; getting in and out of bed or chairs; walking; going outside; using the toilet. IADLs include preparing one's own meals; shopping for groceries and personal items; managing money; using the telephone; doing heavy housework, like scrubbing floors or washing windows; doing light housework. Reprinted with permission from Kramarow E et al: *Health, United States, 1999*. Health and Aging Chartbook. Hyattsville, MD, National Center for Health Statistics, 1999.

functional limitations rather than disabilities. These are the kinds of actions that are the building blocks of activities of daily living (ADL) and include tasks such as walking, standing, reaching, and grasping. ADLs are basic self-care tasks. Instrumental ADL (IADL) are tasks that are physically and cognitively somewhat more complicated and difficult than self-care tasks and are necessary for independent living in the community. ADL and IADL are measures of disability and reflect how an individual's limitations interact with the demands of the environment. The prevalence rates in Figure 4-13 indicate difficulty in doing or inability to do one or more of the tasks in each of three categories. For each category there is a consistent pattern of increasing prevalence with increasing age and greater disability in women than in men.

Disability has been assessed with a wide variety of instruments, and even when instruments contain the same items, they may differ in how they assess specific aspects of performing the task or the severity of limitation in performing the task. For example, it is always debatable whether it is better to ask people whether they actually perform a specific task or whether they should be asked to judge whether they could perform the task even if they have not done it for long time. The former approach gives more concrete information, but respondents could be classified as disabled simply because they have chosen not to do a task that they are perfectly capable of performing. The latter approach allows for classification of people regardless of whether or not they have actually done the task recently but is limited because respondents who have not done the task are required

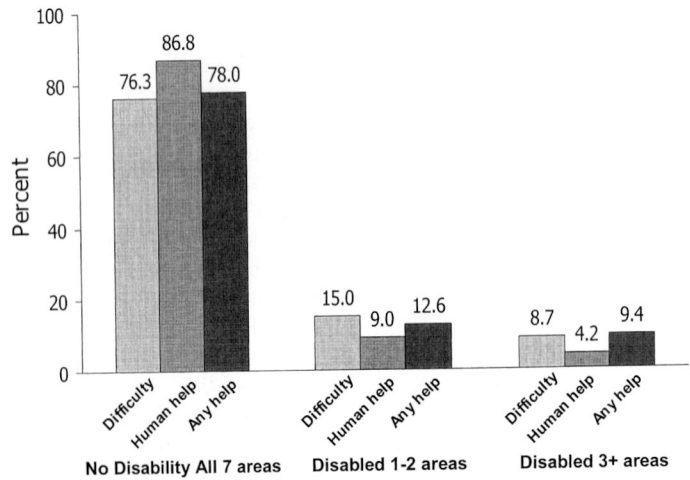

Figure 4–14 Disability estimates using three different measurements methods. Reprinted with permission from Jette AM: How measurement techniques influence estimates of disability in older populations. *Soc Sci Med* 38:937, 1994.

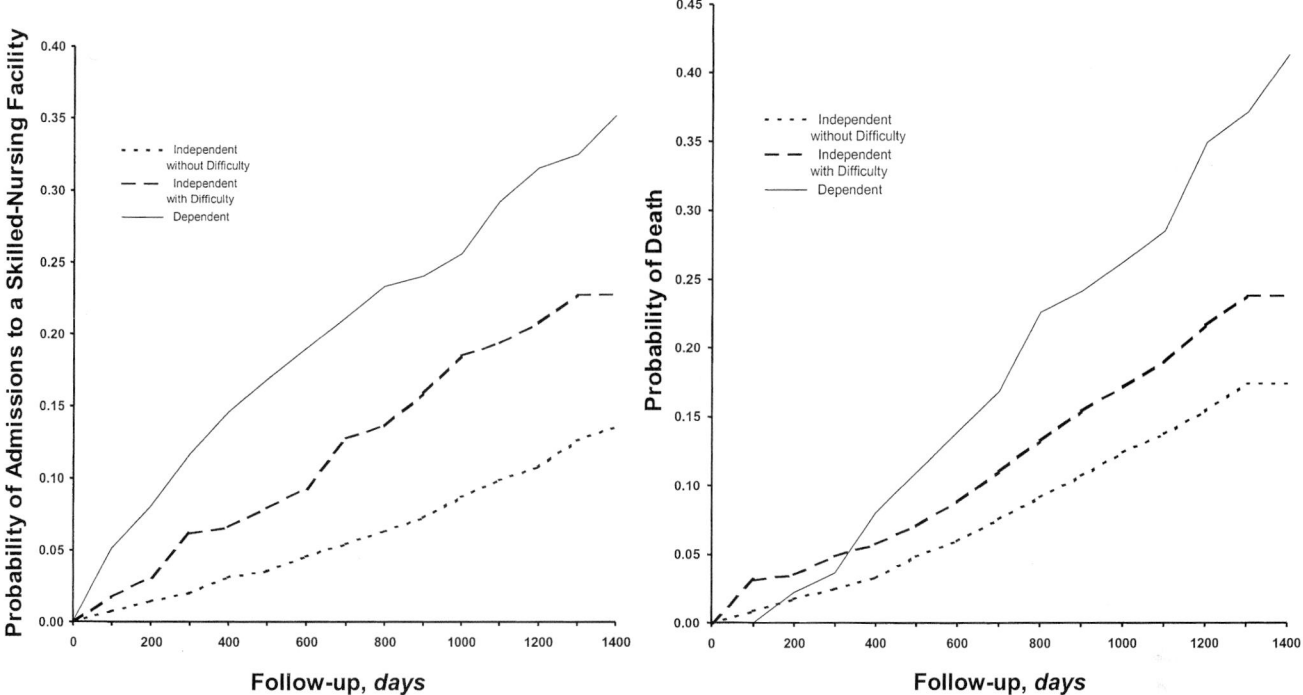

Figure 4-15 Cumulative probability of admission to a skilled-nursing facility (left) and death (right) for three basic activities of daily living groups. Reprinted with permission from Gill TM, Robison JT et al: Difficulty and dependence: Two components of the disability continuum among community-living older persons. *Ann Intern Med* 128:96, 1998.

to speculate as to their ability. For this and other issues in disability assessment, there is no single best way to perform an assessment, and there is therefore no single instrument that is ideal. The lack of standardization that results from the use of multiple competing instruments makes it difficult to compare rates of disability across studies. The differences in prevalence rates that different methods of assessment yield are demonstrated in the methodologic study of ADL disability shown in Figure 4-14. Disability classified as having any difficulty or being unable to perform a task had a higher prevalence than disability classified as requiring human assistance or being unable to perform. Disability classified as requiring human help or help from an assistive device had a higher prevalence rate than disability requiring human help only and was similar in prevalence to the classification using difficulty. This study found that for individual ADL the assessments that relied on difficulty produced estimates of disability 1.2 to 5.0 times greater than assessments that used human assistance as the criterion for disability. Thus, in evaluating research that reports on disability rates, it is critical to examine the way questions are asked and how responses are used to determine the presence of disability.

Disability status has been demonstrated in epidemiologic studies to be one of the most potent of all health status indicators in predicting adverse outcomes. This is probably because disability measures are able to capture the impact of the presence and severity of multiple pathologies, including physical, cognitive, and psychological conditions, as well as the potential synergistic effects of these conditions on overall health status. The powerful prognostic power of disability presence is illustrated in Figure 4-15, which

considers a hierarchy of disability statuses that are defined as independent in ADL, independent but reporting some difficulty with ADL, and dependent on personal assistance for ADL. For these three groups, there were different cumulative probabilities over a 4-year follow-up period of the two outcomes shown here—admission to a nursing home and mortality. These results support the discussion in the previous paragraph that different disability criteria can identify population subgroups with different prognoses. They also support the validity of disability measurement, with level of disability being highly predictive of two important outcomes.

The higher prevalence rate of disability in women shown in Figure 4-13 has been repeatedly demonstrated in many studies and is consistent across a variety of measures and in studies using both self-reporting and objective assessments. Indeed, the fact that women live longer than men in spite of their worse health and higher rate of disability at all ages is one of the most interesting paradoxes in the epidemiology of aging. Another valuable measure of disability that has received increasing attention is mobility disability and is usually evaluated using questions related to walking and climbing stairs. Figure 4-16a shows that mobility disability, defined as the inability to walk $\frac{1}{2}$ mile or climb stairs, increases with age and has a higher prevalence in women than in men at all ages after 65 years. The dynamics of this difference in prevalence are highly instructive. Prevalence is a snapshot at a single point in time and is a function of the flow into and out of the condition being assessed. In the case of mobility disability, women have a higher incidence (new occurrence) of disability (Figure 4-16b) and are less likely to exit from the disabled state than

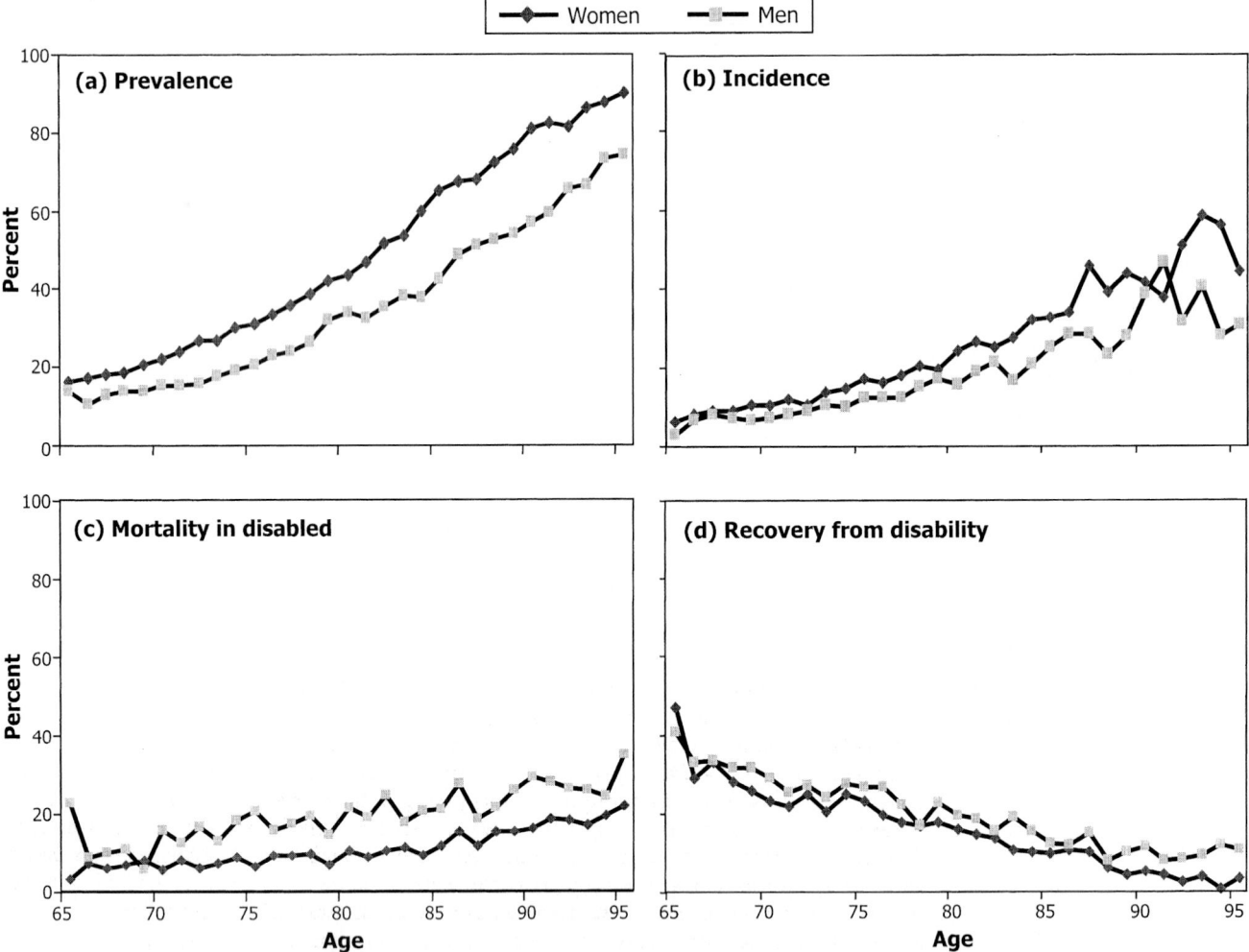

Figure 4-16 Women's and men's prevalence of mobility disability (a), 1-year incidence among nondisabled persons (b), and 1-year mortality (c) and recovery (d) among disabled persons, by age. Established Populations for the Epidemiologic Study of the Elderly. Reprinted with permission from Leveille SG, Penninx BW et al: Sex differences in the prevalence of mobility disability in old age: The dynamics of incidence, recovery, and mortality. *J Gerontol Soc Sci* 55:S41, 2000.

men because they have lower mortality than men when they are disabled (Figure 4-16c) and because they are less likely to recover from disability than men (Figure 4-16d). Thus, the prevention of disability and better treatment of women who have become disabled are likely to have a beneficial effect in lowering the disability rates of women to the level of those of men. Reduction in mortality in disabled men would also contribute to reducing gender differences in disability prevalence.

In addition to gender, a wide array of risk factors for disability has been found in longitudinal studies in older populations. Although the disability definitions were not consistent across these studies, the relative risk of disability for many risk factors was found to be consistent across different definitions, providing strong support for the importance of these risk factors. The most commonly and consistently reported risk factors for disability are listed in Table 4-8, which comes from a review of 78 community-based longitudinal studies that assessed factors related to decline in functional status in older persons. Risk factors are divided into two sections: behavioral factors and

individual characteristics, and specific chronic conditions. There is a great deal of interdependence between these risk factors. Behavioral risk factors such as physical inactivity and smoking can promote the development of a variety of diseases, which can then go on to cause disability. It is becoming evident that these behavioral risk factors may also have direct effects of their own. For example, physical inactivity may be a risk factor for the onset of specific diseases, and it also may have a direct negative impact on muscle, bone, and the central and peripheral nervous systems. These changes can move an individual closer to the physiologic and functional threshold beyond which functioning is impaired to the point that disability occurs.

The role that cognitive impairment plays in physical disability has been generally underappreciated in epidemiologic studies. For clinicians attending to severely disabled persons in nursing homes, however, it is evident that dementia itself prevents these individuals from being independent. Figure 4-17, based on data from population-based studies in Tuscany, Italy, shows estimates of the numbers of men and women with ADL disability in 1999 according to

Table 4-8   Risk Factors for Functional Status Decline

Behavioral risk factors and individual characteristics

Low physical activity

Smoking

High and low body mass index, weight loss

Heavy and no alcohol consumption

Increased age

Lower socioeconomic status (income, education)

High medication use

Poor self-rated health

Reduced social contacts

Chronic conditions

Cardiovascular disease
   Hypertension
   Coronary heart disease
   Myocardial infarction
   Angina pectoris
   Congestive heart failure
   Stroke
   Intermittent claudication

Osteoarthritis

Hip fracture

Diabetes

Chronic obstructive pulmonary disease

Cancer

Visual impairment

Depression

Cognitive impairment

Comorbidity

SOURCE: Stuck et al: Risk factors for functional status decline in community-living elderly people: A systematic literature review. *Soc Sci Med* 48:445, 1999.

age. It also separates these people into those with and without dementia. There is an overall increase in the number of disabled persons through the mid-eighties in men and through the late eighties in women, with a drop-off in the numbers after that because of the decline in the total number of persons in the population at these advanced ages. The obvious gap in these otherwise smooth curves is a result of the low birthrate during and just after World War I, which translated into a smaller population 80 years later. In both men and women, most ADL disability before age 75 years is not associated with dementia. From age 75 to 90 years about half of ADL disability is accompanied by dementia, and after age 90 years the majority of persons with ADL disability have dementia. It should be noted that these data do not prove that dementia is what caused the disability in these individuals. Serious physical impairments and diseases cooccur with dementia, and it may not be possible to always understand just what the cause of disability is. Nevertheless, it is impressive that such a large proportion of disabled persons have dementia, and it is clear that cognitive functioning must be considered when developing interventions to prevent or treat disability.

Longitudinal epidemiologic studies have revealed much about the dynamics of disability onset and progression. Figure 4-18 demonstrates incidence of and recovery from disability, the dynamic process whereby people become severely disabled, and the feasibility of assessing functional limitations that precede the onset of disability. In effect, disability is a product of the disease or diseases from which an individual suffers, sedentary lifestyle or disuse, and physiologic declines that may be the result of aging or pathologic processes that are not specific diseases but result from factors such as inflammation or endocrine changes. As these predisposing conditions change, they have an impact on the initiation of disability and on changes in the status of already established disability.

It has been found that, contrary to previous belief, a substantial proportion of individuals who are disabled report improvement on subsequent assessments. Figure 4-18 shows data for men and women from a US national database that demonstrates change in disability state over a 6-year period. Four hierarchic disability levels at baseline are considered, and at follow-up, participants are classified into one of these states or as institutionalized, dead, or missing. For example, of the 1932 men who were non-disabled in 1984, 48.5 percent remained nondisabled in 1990, 3.6 percent had moderate ADL disability, and 1.8 percent had severe ADL disability. The validity of the hierarchy is supported by the gradient of institutionalization and mortality risk seen in both men and women. The 6-year mortality according to the four baseline disability states ranges from 27 percent to 69 percent in men and from 14 percent to 52 percent in women. Institutionalization rates according to baseline disability status range from 2 percent to 6 percent in men and from 3 percent to 6 percent in women. For individuals with any level of disability at baseline, more than 10 percent have less disability 6 years later (shaded area in Figure 4-18). Even in those with moderate or severe ADL disability, a small percentage have no disability 6 years later. Other studies have observed improvement in disability status over shorter intervals, usually ranging from 1 to 2 years, and in these studies an even larger proportion of disabled persons report no or less disability at follow-up. This improvement in function could result from inaccurate self-reporting of disability over time (unreliability of instrument), a true change in disability status, or both. There is some evidence that both these explanations play a role, but there is consistent evidence that there is a certain amount of real improvement in disability. Both community-based studies and studies on persons hospitalized after an acute event have evaluated factors that predict recovery from disability. Age less than 85 years, good cognitive function, remaining physically mobile, absence of depression, and good social support have all been associated with a greater probability of recovery.

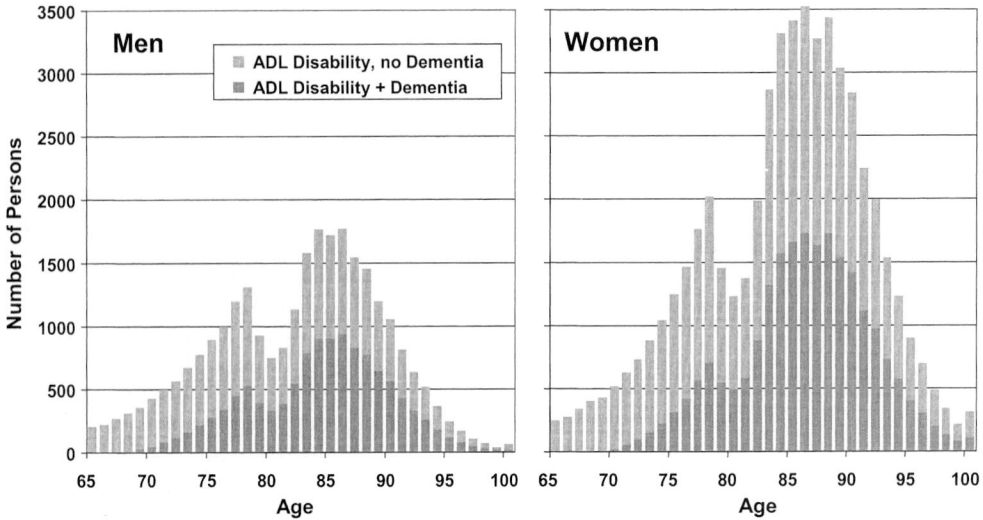

Figure 4-17 Estimated number of men and women with activities of daily living disability (need for help of another person) with and without an additional diagnosis of dementia according to age, Tuscany, Italy, 1999. The figure was obtained by applying estimates from three large population-based epidemiologic studies in the Tuscany population, the Italian Longitudinal Study on Aging, JCARE Dicomano, and InCHIANTI. The original analyses and population estimates are from Istituto Nazionale di Statistica: National Statistical Institute of Italy, 1999.

In understanding the dynamics of disability progression it is useful to consider the pace at which disability develops. The terms "progressive disability" and "catastrophic disability" have been used, indicating a slow downhill course and a very rapid decline, respectively. Progressive disability results from one or more ongoing chronic conditions and causes disability over months or years, whereas catastrophic disability can occur in moments as a result of a stroke or a hip fracture. The prevalence of both progressive and catastrophic severe ADL disability, defined as needing help with three or more ADL, increases with increasing age, although progressive disability rises faster than catastrophic disability. Among those with severe ADL disability, the proportion that has catastrophic ADL disability is much higher at the young old ages, and the proportion that has progressive ADL disability is much higher at the oldest ages

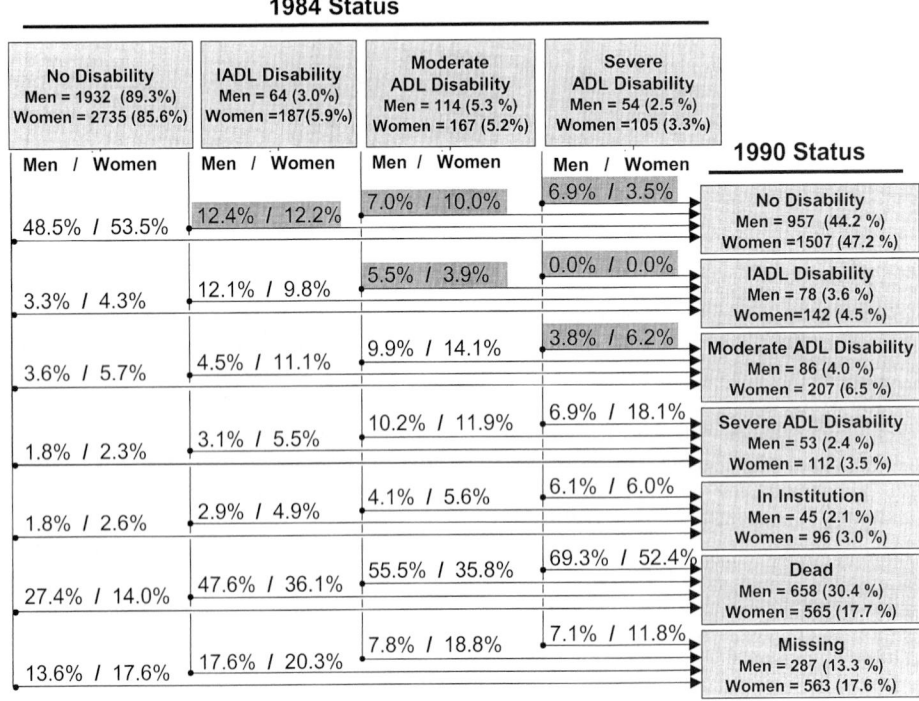

Figure 4-18 Six-year disability transition rates for initially community-dwelling men and women aged 70 to 79. Transition rates are for men and women. Shaded areas represent improvement. Adapted with permission from Mor V et al: Functional transitions among the elderly: Patterns, predictors, and related hospital use. *Am J Public Health* 84(8):1274, 1994.

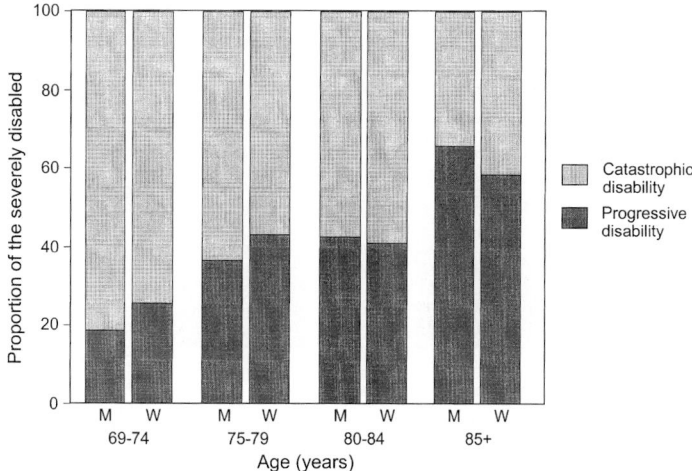

Figure 4-19   Proportion of population needing help with three or more activities of daily living (ADL) who have catastrophic disability (no ADL disability in preceding year) and progressive disability (need for help with one or two ADL in previous year), by age and gender. Reprinted with permission from Ferrucci L et al: Progressive versus catastrophic disability: A longitudinal view of the disablement process. *J Gerontol Med Sci* 51:M123, 1996.

(Figure 4-19). A similar age pattern has been found for on-set of severe mobility disability (inability to walk across a room), where it has been demonstrated that progressive disability is much more common in people who have three or more chronic conditions.

The dynamics of disability can also be approached by studying the pathologic changes that precede its onset. Most disability results from disease, and different theoretical pathways have been proposed to describe the changes that occur as a person proceeds from disease to disability. The theoretical pathway that has received substantial empirical support in aging research is that proposed by Nagi and endorsed by the Institute of Medicine. In this pathway, two intermediate steps, impairment and functional limitation, follow disease and lead to disability (see Verbrugge and Jette, 1994). Impairment describes the dysfunction and structural abnormalities in specific body systems that result from pathology. Functional limitation describes restrictions in basic physical and mental actions that result from impairments. Functional limitations are the basic building blocks of functioning, and the interaction of these components of functioning with the environmental demands faced by an individual determine whether that person is disabled. Conventional study of the consequences of disease describes the physiologic organ impairments that result from specific conditions. More recent work in aging has gone on to describe further steps in the pathway. The impacts of impairments such as poor balance, muscle weakness, and visual deficits on functional limitations and disability have been demonstrated. Furthermore, the relationship between functional limitations, such as reduced gait speed, and subsequent disability also supports the pathway.

Objective measures of physical performance have received increasing attention as assessments that can measure functioning in a standardized manner in both the research and clinical settings. These measures can be used to represent impairments, functional limitations, or actual disability, but most are indicators of functional limitations. A short, standardized battery of performance tests was administered to a large number of participants in the Established Populations for the Epidemiologic Study of the Elderly (EPESE). This battery, which included gait speed, time required to rise from a chair and sit down five times, and hierarchic measures of balance, was used to create a summary score of lower extremity performance that ranged from 0 to 12 (see Guralnik et al, 1995). This measure has been found to predict mortality, the need for nursing home admission, and health care utilization in the overall older population. Furthermore, in a population that had no disability at the time the performance battery was administered, the score was found to be highly predictive of who developed ADL and mobility disability 1 and 4 years later (Figure 4-20). These findings have been replicated in other populations and with other, similar performance measures and indicate that there is a state of preclinical disability, expressed as impairments and functional limitations, that indicates a high risk of proceeding to full-blown disability. This finding also provides a way of identifying high-risk older persons for whom preventive interventions may be highly effective.

Because disability status is a good way of representing overall health status in older persons with complex patterns of disease, and because disability also has direct implications for the long-term care needs of an older person, there has been much interest in evaluating disability trends over time. Although a number of national surveys now assess disability, uniform disability assessment done over time has been available only since the mid-1980s in just a few studies with nationally representative samples. Although these studies use different assessment instruments, a convincing decline in age- and gender-specific rates of disability was observed from the mid-1980s through the 1990s. The National Long Term Care Survey has similar assessments of ADL and IADL disability available from 1982 through 1999, and recent findings indicate that the decline in disability observed for the first 12 years of the study continued and

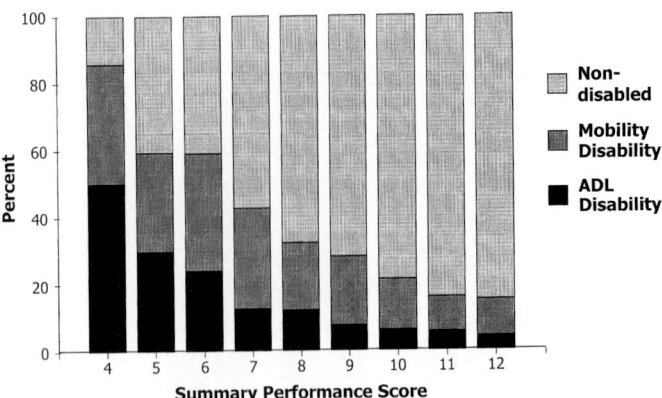

Figure 4-20 Disability status at four years according to baseline summary performance score in persons age 71 and older with no disability at baseline. Reprinted with permission from Guralnik JM, Ferrucci L et al: Lower extremity function in persons over the age of 70 years as a predictor of subsequent disability. *N Engl J Med* 332:556, 1995.

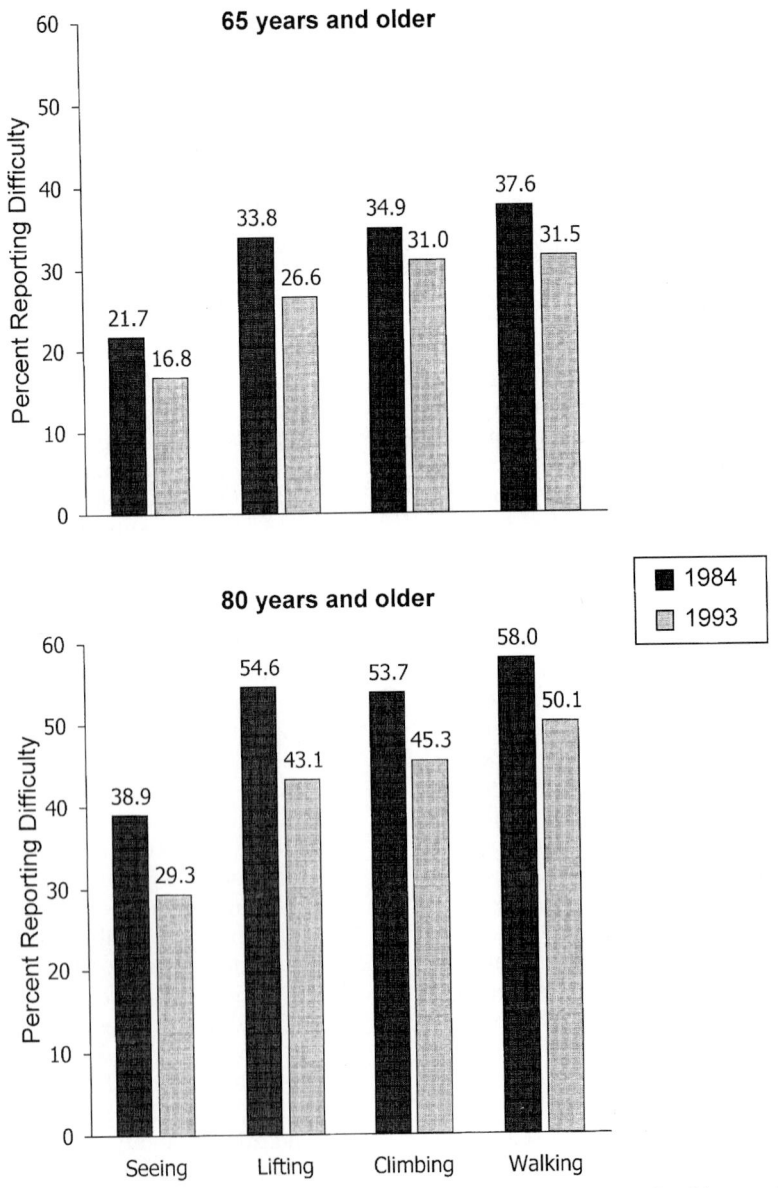

Figure 4-21 Prevalence of functional limitations, United States, 1984 and 1993. Adapted with permission from Freedman VA, Martin LG: Understanding trends in functional limitations among older Americans. *Am J Public Health* 88:1457, 1998.

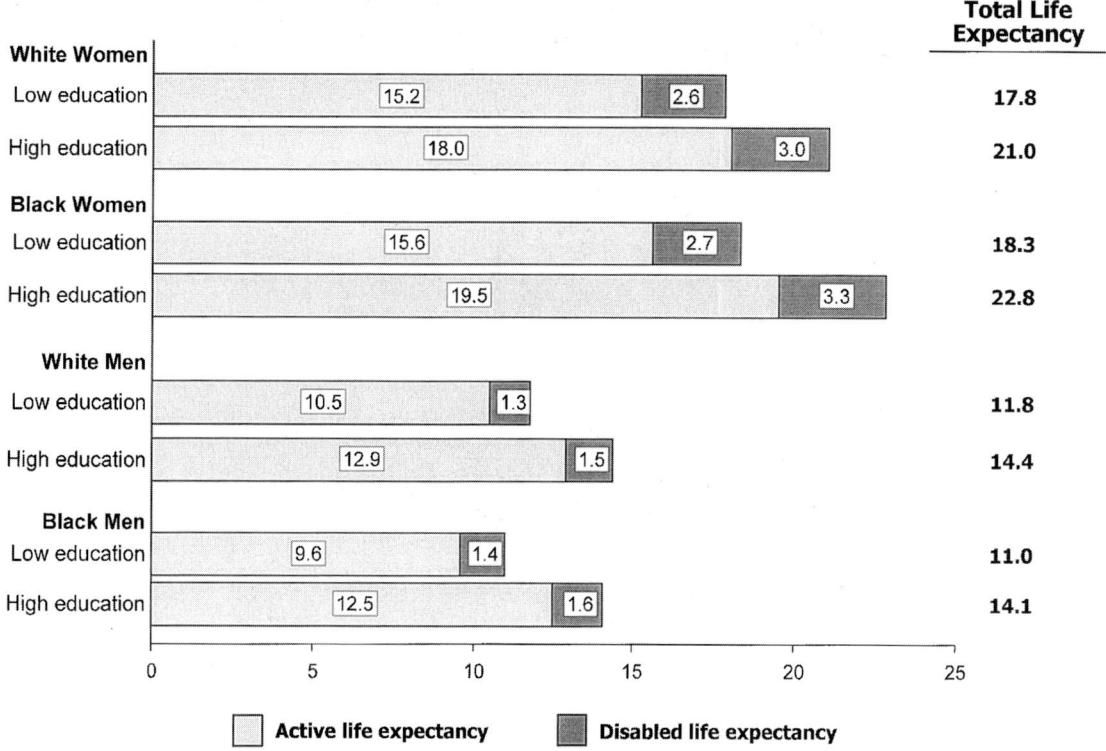

Figure 4-22   Total life expectancy, active (nondisabled) life expectance, and disabled life expectancy at age 65 according to gender, race, and educational status. Lower education defined as less than 12 years of school, and higher education as 12 or more years of school. Adapted with permission from Guralnik JM, Land KC et al: Educational status and active life expectancy in older blacks and whites. *N Engl J Med* 329:110, 1993.

actually accelerated from 1994 through 1999 (see Manton and Gu, 2001). In another study that utilized reports of functional limitations, including lifting and carrying 10 lb, climbing stairs, walking 1/4 mi, and seeing words in a newspaper, changes in prevalence were evaluated between 1984 and 1993. Declines were seen in the inability to perform all four of these tasks in the 65 years and older population and as well as the 80 years and older population (Figure 4-21). Functional limitations, assessing more basic tasks than disability, are an excellent way to follow trends over time because they are influenced less by changing roles that can affect disability assessment (more men cooking in more recent surveys and more women managing money). The observed declines in disability and functional limitations can be attributed to a number of factors. Educational status is strongly associated with disability, and it has been estimated that anywhere from 25 percent to 75 percent of the observed functional declines are related to a higher educational level in more recent cohorts. Other factors proposed as explanations for the decline in disability include reductions in the prevalence of several chronic diseases, changes in nutrition and public health at the time when these cohorts were young, and improved health promotion and medical therapy.

There is an interplay among time of disability onset, duration of disability, and time of death that determines the number of years that older individuals live in the disability-free state, termed active life expectancy, and the number of years spent in the disabled state. Life table approaches have been used to calculate active and disabled life

expectancy, utilizing data from population-based longitudinal studies on transitions from the nondisabled state to disability and death and from the disabled state to nondisability and death. Using this approach may provide insight into the mechanisms and risk factors that affect the quality of aging and suggest potential targets for intervention. In Figure 4-22 an example is shown using data from the EPESE study on the impact of race and educational status on total, active, and disabled life expectancy. This demonstrates that low education (less than 12 years) is associated with shorter total life expectancy and shorter active life expectancy in both black and white women and men but that, comparing persons with the same educational status, there are only small differences between blacks and whites. Alternative methods have been developed to estimate active life expectancy that utilize mortality data and prevalence of disability, which is easier to obtain in a national survey than 1-year transition probabilities. As more data become available to estimate both active and disabled life expectancy, we will gain more insight into the prospects for a compression of morbidity, which is the reduction in disabled life expectancy that results from compressing chronic disease and disability into a smaller number of years between disease and/or disability onset and mortality (see Fries, 1980).

BEHAVIORAL RISK FACTORS

An important role for epidemiology is to elucidate risk factors for disease, injury, and disability, and many risk factors

Table 4-9 Behavioral Risk Factors in Middle-Aged and Older Persons, United States, 1997–2000.

	Percent in Each Age Group			
	35–44	45–54	55–64	65+
Current smoker	28.2	24.3	20.4	11.1
Last blood pressure check				
Never checked	0.2	0.1	0.0	0.1
Past 6 mo	68.9	74.7	79.7	87.2
6 mo to 1 y	15.5	14.3	11.4	7.9
1–2 y	7.9	5.9	3.7	2.4
2–5 y	3.7	2.6	2.3	1.0
5+ y ago	2.8	2.4	1.9	1.2
Any physical activity, past month	74.9	73.3	70.0	65.3
Fruit and vegetable consumption				
Never or <1 time/day	3.8	3.2	2.2	1.5
1–2 times/day	38.0	33.6	28.2	21.1
3–4 times/day	37.6	40.8	42.6	44.8
5+ times/day	19.8	21.8	26.9	31.7
Overweight				
Body mass index $\geq$27.8 (men) $\geq$27.3 (women)	31.7	38.2	39.8	31.4
5+ drinks on one or more occasions, past month	28.3	20.8	15.3	7.4
Influenza immunization, past 12 mo	20.5	28.2	40.8	67.4
Pneumonia immunization, ever	6.4	9.9	18.7	54.9
Teeth cleaned, past year	69.1	73.5	72.6	73.1
Use of seatbelts				
Always	69.5	70.9	70.3	74.4
Nearly always	13.9	14.2	13.4	12.1
Sometimes	7.5	7.5	7.4	5.3
Seldom	3.5	3.2	3.1	2.5
Never	3.8	3.5	3.5	3.2
Smoke detector in home	97.1	96.1	94.9	93.5
Among persons with smoke detectors, smoke detector tested, past year	82.7	81.6	82.7	82.7

	Percent in Each Age Group			
	40–49	50–59	60–64	65+
Mammogram, ever	80.1	88.5	88.8	84.3
Among women who had a mammogram, last mammogram				
Past year	58.0	70.8	71.5	65.4
1–2 y	22.6	15.2	13.9	18.2
2–3 y	7.3	4.1	3.8	5.2
3–5 y	5.6	3.8	3.0	3.8
5+ y ago	5.7	4.5	5.5	7.2
Sigmoidoscopy/colonoscopy, ever	15.7	33.0	45.4	51.5

SOURCE: Behavioral Risk Factor Surveillance System, Centers for Disease Control and Prevention. ww.cdc.gov/nccdphp/brfss.

have been shown to have a large impact in older persons. Although certain risk factors that are potent predictors of major diseases in middle age may have less or no impact at old age, most behavioral risk factors continue to be important throughout old age. Cigarette smoking, for example, continues to predict mortality even in smokers who have survived past age 65 years, and stopping smoking even in old age is associated with better outcomes. The Centers for Disease Control and Prevention perform national surveys on a wide range of behavioral risk factors and include the older population in these assessments. Table 4-9 demonstrates the prevalence of risk factors and protective factors across four age groups, from 35 to 44 years through 65 years and older. For almost all these health practices older persons have similar or somewhat better rates than younger individuals.

These results are compatible with findings that adherence to physicians' recommendations and medication schedules is better in older than in younger persons. Thus, this is a population that faces increasing risk of disease and disability with increasing age but one that cares about its health, has a positive risk factor profile, and is willing to comply with interventions to prevent or improve adverse health outcomes. Applying what has been learned in epidemiologic studies on older populations so that effective prevention and treatment strategies will be available to older persons is a continuing challenge for the field.

REFERENCES

Ettinger WH et al: Long-term physical functioning in persons with knee osteoarthritis from NHANES I: Effects of comorbid medical conditions. *J Clin Epidemiol* 47:809, 1994.

Ferrucci L et al: Hospital diagnoses, Medicare charges, and nursing home admissions in the year when older persons become severely disabled. *JAMA* 277:728, 1997.

Fried LP, Guralnik JM: Disability in older adults: Evidence regarding significance, etiology, and risk. *J Am Geriatr Soc* 45:92, 1997.

Fries JF: Aging, natural death, and the compression of morbidity. *N Engl J Med* 303:130, 1980.

Gill TM et al: Predictors of recovery in activities of daily living among disabled older persons living in the community. *J Gen Intern Med* 12:757, 1997.

Guralnik JM: Assessing the impact of comorbidity in the older population. *Ann Epidemiol* 6:376, 1996.

Guralnik JM et al: Disability as a public health outcome in the aging population. *Ann Rev Public Health* 17:25, 1996.

Kramarow E et al: *Health and Aging Chartbook, Health, United States, 1999.* Hyattsville, MD, National Center for Health Statistics, 1999. http://www.cdc.gov/nchs/data/hus/hus99.pdf.

Manton KG, Gu X: Changes in the prevalence of chronic disability in the United States black and nonblack population above age 65 from 1982 to 1999. *Proc Natl Acad Sci* 98:6354, 2001.

Stuck AE et al: Risk factors for functional status decline in community-living elderly people: A systematic literature review. *Soc Sci Med* 48:445, 1999.

Verbrugge LM, Jette AM: The disablement process. *Soc Sci Med* 38:1, 1994.

Psychosocial Aspects of Aging

THOMAS A. GLASS • GEORGE L. MADDOX

Decades of research and scholarship have reinforced the need to study aging as a synergistic product of biological, behavioral, and social factors. Each of these domains is complex and, to a degree not yet determined, modifiable. This chapter summarizes the role of psychosocial factors in aging processes and outcomes as that role is currently understood. Special emphasis is placed on those factors that appear to play a role in the modifiability of aging, and that are therefore appropriate targets for intervention at the societal, organizational, and individual levels.

The study of aging requires the collaboration of biological scientists, clinicians, and epidemiologists, as well as behavioral and social scientists. A fundamental commitment to the intellectual interdependence of these disciplines remains deep and persistent within the professional identity of gerontology. At the same time, we have just begun to create languages and methods necessary to allow the full potential of this multilevel collaboration to be realized. This chapter illustrates ways in which the connections and synergies between psychosocial and biological factors can be better understood. Toward these ends, two propositions guide the development of this chapter:

1. The observed heterogeneity of aging processes and outcomes can be explained only by examination of contextual factors external to the individual. Social science has contributed to an understanding of how many of the common health problems associated with later life have their roots in social phenomenon. The mechanisms that underlie these associations are just now beginning to be understood. This chapter is structured within an analytic framework that specifies three levels of social context: the macro-social (societal) level, the messo-social (organizational) level, and the micro-social (individual) level. Each level plays an integral part in shaping the patterns observed in aging populations both within and across societies.

2. The importance of psychosocial factors in human aging, both directly and as regulators of biological processes, is increasingly recognized. Researchers are increasingly emphasizing the complex manner in which psychosocial processes regulate and interact with biological processes in ways that might create additional opportunities for intervention. As researchers move toward the development and testing of intervention models, the real promise of psychosocial factors can begin to be seen.

AGING DEPENDS ON SOCIAL CONTEXT

As normally practiced and taught, scientific research places considerable emphasis on succinct empirically derived generalizations about the phenomena under study and, consequently, tends to be reductionistic. Every statistical mean has a companion estimate of dispersion (variance) and shape (normality). However, in most of science, our eye is drawn toward measures of location (the mean), while dispersion around the mean is often ignored or de-emphasized. While variance is comprised partly of nuisance factors such as measurement error, the systematic variance seen in late life is undoubtedly of crucial importance. This heterogeneity, seen among all higher animals, must be explained, in part, by psychosocial factors external to the individual. As an organizing principle, the discussion relies on a distinction between three levels of analysis commonly differentiated in social scientific discussions. These levels are described in Fig. 5-1. The figure is not intended as a causal model per se, but rather as a depiction of the separate but interconnected layers of causal influence that allow for a clearer explication of the role of social context in aging. The field of social gerontology focuses on understanding the role of these factors and how they are related within and across levels to the processes and outcomes of aging. The three levels are the *macro-social level* (society-wide structures and processes), the *messo-social level* (related to the social organization and dynamics of formal and informal institutions), and the *micro-social level* (related to the interaction that occurs at the level of interpersonal communication). It is assumed that each of these levels is important but analytically independent layers of causal influence; analogous to biomedical research when shifting between the level of the organism, the cell and molecular levels of analysis.

Psychosocial Factors at the Macro–Social Level

The macro-social level refers to broad systems of social structure as reflected in social policy, systems of

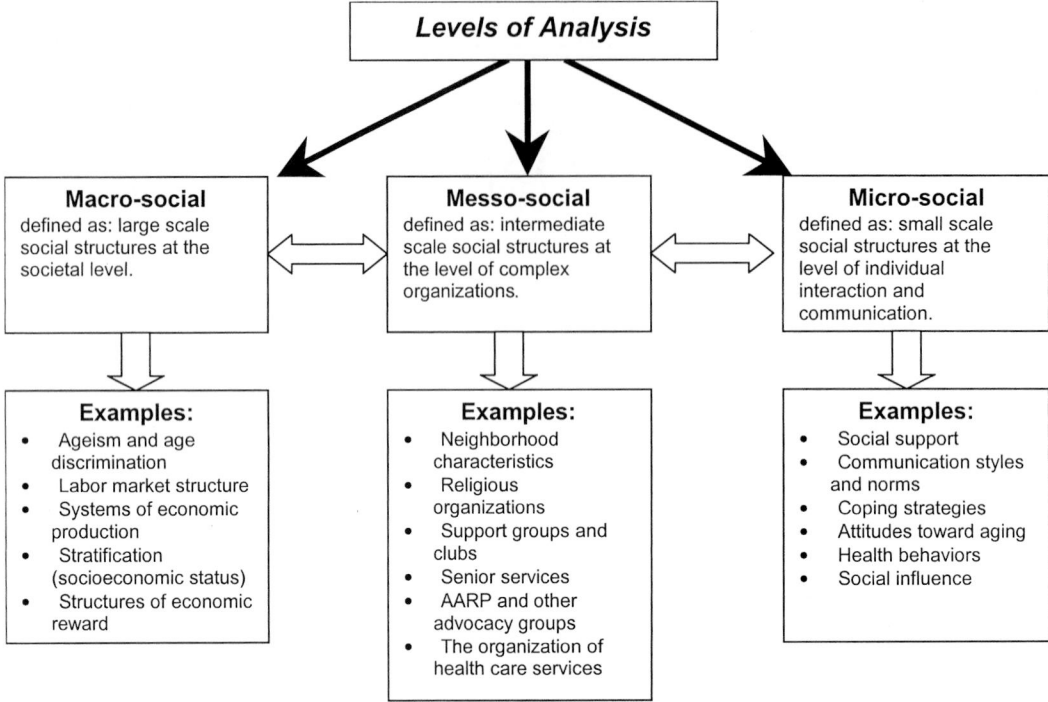

Figure 5-1 Levels of analysis in social gerontology.

stratification, politics, and various features of economic structure (such as labor markets). These societal-level effects can be illustrated in at least two ways. One effect is seen in the distinction between societies that are *more* or *less* developed. The other effect focuses on the implications of socioeconomic differentiation in resource distribution within a society, an occurrence known as stratification.

Differential Resource Allocation Across Societies

Demographic data show clearly that survival to old age as an average expectation at birth is a recent achievement. Beginning in the mid-1800s spectacular advances in life expectancy at all ages, as well as for older persons, began to occur. The twentieth century saw a doubling of life expectancy for many nations, including the United States, from approximately 47 years in 1900 to the 77.1 years by the century's end. Even at age 65 years, age-specific expected years of life remaining rose from 13 to 16 years in just the period between 1970 and 1998 for US males (see Chap. 4).

These achievements, however, cannot be taken for granted. In a few developing nations, average life expectancy continues to be about the same as it was in the United States at the turn of the century. Estimated life expectancy for all less-developed nations in the 1990s was 56 years, and for Africa, it was 49.7 years. Average life expectancy at birth in the year 2020 is now estimated to be 70.6 years for less-developed countries and 78.7 years for more-developed countries.

Changes in the former Soviet Union illustrate the effect of macro-social change particularly well. In the period between 1987 and 1994, male life expectancy at birth plummeted 7.3 years as a result of significant changes that

occurred as a result of political and economic changes. Differences in life expectancy are substantially greater among lesser-developed nations than they are in the developing world, owing to the consequences of a variety of factors that occur at the societal level that have implications across the entire life course of individuals.

Social Stratification

Differential availability of resources occurs within, as well as among, societies. Within a given society, material and social resources are inevitably distributed unequally. The rationale for inequalities can be found in societal values and preferences. All societies generate systems of differential rewards of goods, status, honor, and power. The magnitude of inequality has been convincingly linked to higher mortality rates in both cross-national data as well as within the United States. The process by which resources become differentially distributed is referred to as *social stratification*. In any society, to be at the top of the system of stratification means more than the prospects of having access to material and social rewards such as prestigious occupation, higher pay, and a maximum degrees of self-determination. These rewards, in turn, affect patterns of morbidity and mortality in a favorable direction and increase the prospects of perceived well-being in later life. Social status continues, given such correlates, to be one of the most powerful predictors or health and well-being in epidemiological research.

The impact of social stratification can be seen in differential outcomes in late life. Growing old poor, uneducated, and without access to resources is clearly not the same as growing old rich, educated, and well connected. In a series of papers, House and colleagues show that the effects of socioeconomic status accumulate throughout the life course, culminating in substantial differences in health and functioning in late life. In an analysis of the 1985 National Health Interview Survey, this group showed that the effects of both age and socioeconomic status on health are substantial and that their effects are interactive rather than additive. A more recent replication showed that these findings to be robust in longitudinal analyses. In this latter study, the socioeconomic status (SES) gradient in health outcomes was explained substantially by differential exposure to a number of psychosocial risk factors including smoking, social isolation, and both acute and chronic stressful life circumstances. These findings strengthen the view that socioeconomic factors at the macro-social level create fundamentally different outcomes in an aging population predominately through the regulation of important exposures throughout adulthood.

The relationship between the distribution of social resources and differential outcomes of aging was demonstrated with special effectiveness in a Canadian study by Wilkins and Adams. In this study, the authors develop the concepts of *health expectancy* (i.e., disability-free life expectancy at birth) and *quality-adjusted life expectancy* (i.e., a weighted measure to indicate the probability of capacity for self-care in a noninstitutional setting) and apply these to the experience of Canada. These concepts make an important distinction between survival in the biological sense and living personally and socially satisfying lives. This research illustrates the diversity of aging outcomes in relation to both individual and neighborhood-level measures of socioeconomic status. The nearly 5-year average differentials in life expectancy at birth between those with lowest versus highest income is overshadowed by the even larger income-related differentials in quality-adjusted life expectancy (7.7 years) and disability-free life expectancy (11 years). Life expectancy at birth is 9.1 years greater for those residing in middle-class neighborhoods as compared to those who reside in poor neighborhoods. The same differential is 10.8 years for quality-adjusted life expectancy and 13.3 years for disability-free years.

In sum, whether one survives into later life and whether one ages well are substantially affected by external macro-social factors. The operation of these factors is illustrated through the structures that govern food availability and distribution, the allocation of roles and statuses, and related social policy regarding the perceived differential worth of individuals.

Psychosocial Factors at the Messo-Social Level

The *messo-social* level represents an intermediate layer of causal influences occurring between large scale structural and psychological factors. Messo-social effects result from the dynamics of complex organizations that are both formal (schools, work places, religious organizations, labor unions) and informal (neighborhood associations, fraternal groups, interest and support groups). Societies are natural experiments in the effects of alternative organizational arrangements for providing and maintaining income in

adulthood, delivering health care, and structuring living environments. The social roles traditionally allocated to women and the effects of this allocation on economic security in later life illustrate this point particularly well. In a comparative analysis of the incomes of older women and men in both the United States and Sweden, O'Rand documents the inferior economic outcomes for older women as compared with older men in both societies, and explains why this outcome is observed. The explanation reflects similar institutional arrangements in both societies regarding family responsibility, careers within the workplace, and pension policies. In both societies, although more so in the United States than in Sweden, women have continued to have more extensive responsibilities than men for child rearing. These responsibilities, in turn, affect entry into and continuation in the work force, influence career advancement and related income, and determine the probability of working in industries likely to provide additional private pensions in retirement. Consequently, women in both societies tend to have lower average incomes in retirement than men. Gender in a society, then, has social connotations for economic security as well as for survival. Social roles related to gender become proxies for shared understandings about social obligations, which have consequences for careers and the resources available in the postretirement years.

The Social Organization of Health Care

The effects of psychosocial factors at the messo-social level are well illustrated by examining the effects of how health care is organized. Health services research shows that older adults do not conform to stereotypes about high health care use and poor health status in general. In fact, a minority of older adults have a disabling chronic illness, and only a relatively small proportion of them have high rates of health care use (occurring mostly in the last year of life). Elevated rates of disability and health care costs among a subset of the older population reflects age-related biological decrements as well as the unintended effects of public policy that ensures that chronic and particularly terminal illnesses will be treated in the high-technology environments of hospitals. It is increasingly clear that systems of care in the United States are not optimal for the treatment of chronic illnesses that disproportionately effect seniors. The mismatch between a medical and hospital system designed primarily to deal with acute disease and the need for more community-based health care options capable of serving an aging population is increasingly noted. In societies whose populations are aging, these policy decisions ensure that large concentrations of older adults in high-cost medical settings will achieve very high social visibility, particularly if the treatment involves public expenditure. Consequently, a society's institutional arrangements determine where older adults are treated, what kind of care they receive, and who pays for that care. These factors, in turn, contribute significantly to the public discourse on rights and generational equity.

The landmark 1965 Medicare and Medicaid legislation in the United States led, indirectly, to the creation of a new component of the health care industry—the nursing home.

This industry came to dominate thinking about long-term care to the degree that long-term care traditionally has been equated with nursing home care. Contemporary discussions of long-term care, however, tend to emphasize alternatives to institutionalization and to stress home- and community-based care. Assisted-living arrangements that integrate housing with assistance in activities of daily living have proved to be particularly attractive. While national policy on long-term care continues to be ambivalent, public policy discussions are including a broader range of options for financing and location of services than ever before. Canada and a number of countries in Western Europe, which include long-term care as a basic component of their national health-financing schemes, have relatively high rates of disabled older adults in a variety of non-institutionalized settings. The United States has tended, until recently, to concentrate on nursing homes for impaired older adults, rather than a continuum of sheltered housing environments or community-based care. Evidence suggests that forces are now shifting and alternative models are emerging. These alternative structures are likely to illustrate further the effects of psychosocial factors at the messo-social level.

Neighborhood Characteristics

Interest in the role of psychosocial factors in aging has followed a larger trend within epidemiology to begin to study characteristics of places, rather than just characteristics of people, in order to describe their impact on health in late life. This is not, however, a new idea. Much of the recent epidemiologic work on neighborhoods and aging owes a substantial debt to the seminal work of Lawton and Nahemow who developed a model of person–environment fit; that is, the matching of personal capabilities and preferences with the demands and opportunities of different milieus. Lawton and Nahemow argued that environments that were either too challenging or not sufficiently stimulating could provoke dysfunctional responses equally, leading to deterioration of capacity. This model is the origin of the now popular "use-it-or-lose-it" idea. This model was recently extended in a review article on neighborhood influences on aging by Glass and Balfour. This work has begun to show that various features of the way neighborhoods are organized and structured has potentially substantial impact on the capacity of older adults to remain living in the community. To the extent this is the case, it is increasingly clear that population aging will require rethinking current models of gentrification and suburban sprawl if the needs of older adults are to be taken into account in the design of residential living spaces. A variety of factors, such as noise, graffiti, the availability of stores and services, and socioeconomic factors, have been linked to a range of outcomes, including mortality, disability, cognitive function, and institutionalization. There appear to be fairly clear answers to the question of what kind of neighborhoods older persons prefer. These types of neighborhoods, however, are disappearing rapidly from many cities. Consideration of the design of neighborhoods and the built environment remains on the horizon as key policy objectives for the next several decades.

Psychosocial Factors at the Micro-Social Level

Micro-social factors may be defined as resources and processes operating at the level of interpersonal interaction and communication. This category of influences is illustrated by patterns of variation in health and well-being observed in the various milieus recognizable in everyday life. In the remainder of this section, the variables that have received the most attention are reviewed briefly with emphasis on those factors that have shown promise as potential targets of intervention.

Self-efficacy and Sense of Control

One consistent theme that emerges from a review of the literature on psychosocial factors in aging is the importance of perceived control over circumstances. Several landmark studies have demonstrated the health-related benefits of both *mastery* (perceived control over the outcome of circumstances) and *self-efficacy* (beliefs about one's ability to successfully accomplish tasks or meet goals). Both concepts are grounded in a social cognition framework whereby an individual's perceptions of control over events is partially a function of the feedback they receive from the social environment. This contrasts with a strictly psychological view of self-efficacy as a purely psychological trait or a component of personality. This is good news because it suggests that alterations in the messages that older persons receive from the social world can have important and salutary impacts on their health and well-being. Self-efficacy beliefs have been perhaps the strongest and most consistent predictors of a variety of indicators of successful aging including cognitive and physical function.

Social Networks and Support

The most commonly studied aspect of social context is social integration, although this term has been used rather broadly and without adequate clarity about the differentiation among related concepts such as social networks, social support, and more recently, social engagement. Social networks refer to the structural features of an individual's social ties and relationships. These characteristics include the size, density, and proximity of the network of friends and acquaintances an individual possess. Social networks are the conduits that allow for the potential exchange of resources such as assistance, information, and material goods among persons. The resources that can flow across these conduits are referred to as social supports. Four distinct types of social support can be defined including *instrumental support* (aid and assistance of a practical and tangible nature), *emotional support* (expressions of affection, belonging, and support of an intangible nature), *informational support* (knowledge and resources that allow for access to and understanding of other resources), and *financial support* (which can include the promise of financial aid).

A solid body of research documents the salutary effects of social networks and social support. Social networks are associated with lower mortality risk in more than a dozen prospective population-based studies. The magnitude of this association is equal to other well-known risk factors such as cigarette smoking. Social network characteristics also predict survival after the onset of illness. One interesting facet of the association between social networks and well-being in late life is that ties with friends and relatives that are more distant (meaning not immediate family or friends) appear to be more important than ties with immediate family. The Duke Longitudinal Studies of Aging, for example, found that frequency of contact with secondary networks (social groups and more distant friends) but not primary groups predicted who would age successfully. In the Established Populations for Epidemiologic Studies of the Elderly (E.P.E.S.E.), ties with friends and relatives (but not children or a confidant) were associated with both the onset of and recovery from physical disability.

While social networks are strong predictors of long-term outcomes such as mortality, the quality and quantity of available social support appears to be more closely associated with shorter-term outcomes such as illness recovery. For example, the lack of emotional support measured before myocardial infarction was found to be associated with an increased mortality in both men and women after myocardial infarction, controlling for disease severity, comorbidity, smoking, and sociodemographic factors. Other studies show that social support protects against the risk of several diseases, although the link between social support and disease onset is clearly weaker than for other outcomes. In a review of 51 studies that examined the link between social support and cardiovascular disease, Anderson and colleagues conclude that the evidence for the view that those without social support have worse recovery and adaptation after myocardial infarction is convincing. In this review, they suggest several mechanisms appear to underlie this association, including improved motivation for recovery, optimal adherence to medical regimens, and the prevention of depression. As yet, few attempts have been made to translate these insights into intervention strategies.

Stress and Stressful Life Events

Another area that has received considerable attention is life stress. Chronic life strains have been repeatedly observed to be significant predictors of late-life depression. The stress of bereavement has been closely studied as a risk factor for both mortality and depression. The literature remains equivocal on the question of whether old age leaves persons more vulnerable to the effects of stress. Some work suggests that the aging body is more susceptible to the deleterious influences of stressful events, while other literature points to the "steeling" influence of repeated stressors. Given the potential to intervene in the stress process, through both environmental change and pharmacologic intervention, the need to study this association more carefully is urgent.

Social Engagement

Little doubt remains that physical activity and fitness are health promoting. What is beginning to be clear is that social and productive activities (or social engagement) is also related to physical and cognitive health. Social engagement can be defined as the performance of meaningful social roles. As such, social engagement provides not only opportunities for physical and social activity, but also acts as a scaffolding for the maintenance of a coherent sense of identity in the face of the age-related changes that accrue with advancing age. The continuity in social engagement is recognized as a core aspect of successful aging, in part because it appears to play an especially vital role in the health of older persons. Social engagement is predictive of a variety of health outcomes including mortality, cognitive function, and disability.

An additional aspect of social engagement that confers particular benefits is religious participation. As with other forms of social engagement, the mechanisms underlying this association are known to be complex. Religious participation also illustrates ways in which micro-social factors (social support and purpose in life) interact with organizational and neighborhood factors (the organization of religious organizations and their location and role within society). While it has been observed that religious participation may not be an ideal area for intervention for ethical reasons, it would be useful to understand how and why religious involvement has such robust health benefits in late life.

Biological Mechanisms: How Do Social Factors Get Into the Body?

A major contribution of social gerontology has been to document the important contribution of psychosocial variables to the etiology of diseases of the aged. To suggest the importance of psychosocial factors is not to diminish the importance of physiologic processes, but rather to acknowledge that physiologic processes alone are inadequate to explain the social patterning of disease states. A more complex understanding of disease causation must attend to the synergistic influences of social, ecologic, and physiologic processes. This has led to a search for multilevel models that recognize the interdigitation and mutually reinforcing aspects of the biopsychosocial matrix. From this perspective, the important scientific question is not whether psychosocial factors or physiologic factors are more important, but how do psychosocial factors influence biologic and physiologic functions. Answers to this question can suggest strategies for individual and societal intervention.

Mounting evidence suggests that various psychosocial factors modify basic biological parameters such as blood lipids, heart rate, blood pressure, and immune responsiveness. Research on the biological penetrants of psychosocial factors has focused attention on the neurohormonal systems that regulate cardiovascular parameters. For example, a review by Uchino argues that social support has robust influences on the cardiovascular, endocrine, and immune systems. Interventions to improve outcomes in patients with myocardial infarction and stroke are now under way that seek to increase social support.

Recent work has established the link between environmental stress and well-being in late life. Extending earlier work on stress and adaptation, McEwen and Stellar introduced the concept of allostatic load, defined as the cumulative strain on the body produced by repeated physiologic

response across multiple systems in response to life experiences. Seeman and colleagues developed measures of
allostatic load based on levels of physiologic activity across
a range of regulatory systems pertinent to disease risk.
Those measures were associated with poorer cognitive and
physical function and predicted larger decrements in cognitive and physical functioning among participants of the
MacArthur Studies of Successful Aging. That group later
showed that allostatic load was associated with 7-year survival and (marginally) with incident cardiovascular disease
events, independent of standard sociodemographic characteristics and baseline health status. Measures of allostatic
load (particularly urinary cortisol excretion) also predict
memory function. The study of environmental stress and
the resulting allostatic load shows considerable promise,
although it is not clear whether biomarkers of stress are attributable to environmental or more endogenous stressors
such as depression or attribution.

THE MODIFIABILITY OF AGING PROCESSES AND THE CASE FOR INTERVENTION

This chapter has emphasized the social patterning of variation in human aging across and within societies. These
patterns in late-life outcomes are the result of a synergistic
interaction of internal biological factors and characteristics of the social environment at the macro-, messo-, and
micro-social levels. Biology identifies not just what may be
necessary for survival, but our biological inheritance makes
possible a range of developmental scenarios over the life-
course that are shaped by characteristics of the social milieu. Following this general theme, the discussion moves
to the question of the modifiability of aging processes as
suggested by the arguments above. The basic structure of
the argument is maintained by pointing to intervention approaches at the same three levels of analysis.

Intervention at the Macro-Social Level: The Importance of Public Policy

At the macro-social level, intervention in the form of public policy to modify institutional arrangements for income
and access to health care has been an area of demonstrable success over the past two decades in the United States.
The effect of income maintenance policy in later adulthood
is a particularly successful story, although recent evidence
suggests that important concerns remain. Social Security
legislation and improved private pensions in the United
States have reduced the rate of poverty among older adults
by half in less than two decades, from 25 percent to less than
12 percent. The reduction is sufficient to produce a rate of
poverty among older adults that is substantially less than
that of children. This fact has caused concern about generational equity. There is no obvious answer to questions
about generational equity, although it is equally clear that
the benefits of aging policy have not benefited all groups
to the same degree (particularly women and minorities).
While the official rate of poverty dropped to its lowest point
in the 1990s, subgroups of older adults (e.g., single women,

minority populations) continue to have very high rates of
poverty. In addition, the replacement rate for earned income provided by Social Security in the United States is
the lowest observed among major industrial nations.

Intervention at the Messo-Social Level: Implications for Geriatrics

The above arguments about the importance of psychosocial
factors in human aging have important practical implications for geriatricians and, more generally, for the organization of health care services. Geriatricians can expect successive cohorts of older persons to differ, reflecting a life-time
of differential exposure to environments and behaviors.
This heterogeneity argues further for caution against
stereotypic images of older persons, their expectations,
and their capacities. Another implication of this for health
care providers is the urgent need to view aging in a multidisciplinary context. Long-term care is a good illustration.
In their comparative study of long-term care in three
Canadian provinces, Kane and Kane noted the persistent
tension between two competing perspectives on long-term
care. One perspective is that the disabling impairments of
later life are the domain of medicine and hospitals, with
social intervention playing a minor role. The competing
perspective is that geriatric care is essentially a social process best pursued in a community setting with collaborative
participation by physicians, nurses, social workers, therapists, and even policy practitioners. The attractiveness of
these alternative viewpoints is very much dependent on sociocultural values and how the preferences related to these
values are embedded in the training of professional caregivers and the expectations of laypersons. The Kanes argue
persuasively that geriatric care is most efficiently and effectively pursued when care is conceived of as a social process
with medical aspects, and not the other way around.

In the United States, the care of older adults has generally been based in institutional settings such as hospitals
and nursing homes. Geriatrics as a specialized field has
maintained a high degree of commitment to the need to
take social factors into consideration. However, the full
realization of the promise of geriatric medicine and the appropriate models of care have been slow to develop. There
are signs that this is changing. The penetration of managed care and for-profit medicine, along with rising consumer demand for alternatives, have led to increasing rates
of experimentation in the organization of care. A variety of
alternatives to institutionalized models for long-term care
have also emerged. Home hospital models and preventive
home-visitation have begun to demonstrate effectiveness.

Many societies in Europe and Asia are pursuing noninstitutionalized socially oriented approaches more vigorously. For example, the United Kingdom and Sweden both
have hospital-based geriatricians, but also have integrated
social and medical services, and a broad range of housing
strategies (other than nursing homes) for dependent older
persons. Geriatric care in Britain and Sweden is unambigu-
ously the primary responsibility of the public sector. In
contrast, the United States, has continued to insist that the
private sector can solve the technical and fiscal problems

that will follow population aging. This has continued to be the case even as public investment in geriatric care has escalated in the past several decades. Certainly there is little evidence of political consensus about a national health service or a national health insurance system, or the systematic integration of health and social services. Evidence points to a growing preference for private market-based solutions for the care of older persons.

Even though relatively high-cost nursing homes have not uniformly ensured quality care, community-based care has not fully emerged as more than a theoretically cost-effective alternative to institutionalization because no acceptable alternative to a fragmented health and welfare system has been identified. Consequently, long-term care remains the last great risk of life that has remained inadequately insured even for most middle- and upper-income individuals. Even in the 1990s, half of the expenditures for long-term care were paid for privately. The majority of LTC is still provided by family in the home. While the baby boom generation is likely to retire "economically rich," it is likely also to be "socially poor" in terms of family resources to meet long-term care needs. Moreover, the need for sound policy interventions to address the long-term care needs of the baby boom generation will grow substantially in the coming decades.

Intervention at the Micro-Social Level: The Case for Psychosocial Intervention

The beneficial effects of a variety of individual-level interventions on the quality of life in later adulthood have been suggested and sometimes effectively demonstrated (for a systematic review, see Glass). Included among the successful models of psychosocial intervention that have thus far been shown to be effective in older populations are programs to modify health behaviors including smoking cessation and diet modification (see also Chap. 23). The benefits of aerobic exercise on cardiovascular efficiency and mood in older populations has been repeatedly demonstrated (see Chap. 72). However, the literature on exercise in older adults highlights the importance of thinking broadly about psychosocial issues in intervention research. Many of the exercise studies attempted thus far illustrate how difficult it can be to recruit and retain older adults in health promotion programs and how complex issues of adherence can be in this population.

Intervention research at the individual level has also sought to target several cognitive mechanisms discussed above. Studies such as Advanced Cognitive Training for Independent and Vital Elderly (ACTIVE) are currently under way to determine whether cognitive functioning can be restored through retraining. In a seminal example of a successful intervention on a psychosocial variable, Rodin and colleagues conducted a study to determine whether encouraging personal responsibility and reinforcing self-efficacy can alter the trajectories of well-being in nursing home residents. In this study, members of a treatment group were compared to control subjects after a simple intervention in which subjects were given a houseplant to care for and were told that they would be asked to take more

responsibility for themselves and their daily activities. Intervention subjects were observed to have longer survival, better mood, and less illness. One implication of this study is that some portion of the deterioration of capacity seen in institutional settings may be a function of how those settings induce a sense of disengagement from self-care responsibility and thereby undermine self-efficacy. A second implication is that if level of self-efficacy (and by extension dependency) is manipulable, then the construction of appropriately stimulating milieus should be a core feature of the design not only of nursing homes, but also community-living, neighborhoods, and rehabilitation facilities.

CONCLUSION

As adequate food, water, and sanitation are increasingly available worldwide, there is every reason to expect that life expectancy at birth and age-specific life expectancy in adults will continue to increase in all societies, and this is what one now observes worldwide. This achievement, sometimes referred to as the "first revolution in health," ensures the necessity in every society of a "second" revolution as populations age and chronic disease replaces acute disease as the primary mission of public health. This second revolution in health must focus on behavioral and environmental issues, which are central to the understanding of, and in the response to, age-related chronic impairments, disabilities, and handicaps.

The demonstrated potential for change indicates a realistic basis for optimism without, however, identifying the feasible and reasonable limits of change in aging processes. We therefore do not know the limits of desirable change even when change is feasible. In any case, what is feasible is a scientific question; what is desirable is an ethical and political question. Whether we should expect to delay the onset of morbidity and to what degree we should expect to delay it are clearly debatable. The issue will continue to be debated, particularly in the absence of definitive evidence. What will be increasingly needed is research that attempts to bridge the gaps that currently exist between basic science and intervention, between biological and social processes, and between the study of social factors at multiple levels and social policies that affect them.

REFERENCES

Anderson D et al: Social support, social networks and coronary artery disease rehabilitation: A review. *Can J Card* 12:739, 1996.

Anderson NB: Levels of analysis in health science. A framework for integrating sociobehavioral and biomedical research. *Ann N Y Acad Sci* 840:563, 1998.

Berkman LF, Glass TA: Social integration, social networks, social support, and health, in Berkman LF, Kawachi I (eds): *Social epidemiology.* New York, Oxford University Press, 2000, p 137.

Berkman LF et al: Emotional support and survival after myocardial infarction: A prospective, population-based study of the elderly. *Ann Intern Med* 117:1003, 1992.

Binstock RH, George LK: *Handbook of Aging and the Social Sciences* (5th ed.). San Diego, Academic Press, 2001, p 513.

Crystal S: Economic status of the elderly, in Binstock RH et al. (eds): *Handbook of Aging and the Social Sciences (4thed.).* San Diego, Academic Press, 1996, p 531.

Dannefer D: What's in a name? An account of the neglect of variability in the study of aging, in Birren JE, Bengston VL (eds): *Emergent Theories of Aging.* New York, Springer Publishing Co., 1988, p 356.

Ferraro KF: *Gerontology: Perspectives and Issues (2nded.).* New York, Springer Publishing Co., 1997.

Glass TA, Balfour JL: Neighborhood effects on the health of the elderly, in Kawachi I, Berkman LF (eds): *Neighborhoods and Health.* New York, Oxford University Press, in press.

Glass TA: Psychosocial interventions, in Berkman LF, Kawachi I (eds): *Social Epidemiology.* New York, Oxford University Press, 2000, p 267.

Hemingway H, Marmot M: Evidence-based cardiology: Psychosocial factors in the aetiology and prognosis of coronary heart disease. Systematic review of prospective cohort studies. *BMJ* 318:1460, 1999.

House JS et al: Age, socioeconomic status, and health. *Milbank Q* 86:383, 1990.

House JS et al: The social stratification of aging and health. *J Health Soc Behav* 35:213, 1994.

House JS et al: Social relationships and health. *Science* 241:540, 1988.

Kane R, Kane R: *A Will and a Way: What the United States Can Learn from Canada about Caring for the Elderly.* New York, Columbia University Press, 1985.

Lawton MP, Nahemow L: Ecology and the aging process, in Eisdorger C, Lawton MP (eds): *The Psychology of Adult Development and Aging.* Washington, DC, American Psychological Association, 1973, p. 464.

Lawton MP: *Environment and Aging.* Monterey, CA, Brooks/Cole, 1980.

Levin JS et al: Religion and spirituality in medicine: Research and education. *JAMA* 278:792, 1997.

Maddox GL: Aging differently. *Gerontologist* 27:557, 1987.

McEwen BS, Stellar E: Stress and the individual. Mechanisms leading to disease. *Arch Intern Med* 153:2093, 1993.

Mendes de Leon CF et al: Social networks and disability transitions across eight intervals of yearly data in the New Haven E.P.E.S.E. *J Gerontol B Psychol Sci Soc Sci* 54B:S162, 1999.

Mendes de Leon CF, Glass TA: Personal resources and social support as factors in ethnic disparities in aging health, in (eds): *Ethnic Disparities and Aging Health.* National Academies of Science Press, in press, p.

O'Rand AM: Convergence, institutionalization and bifurcation: Gender and the pension acquisition process, in Maddox G, Lawton MP (eds): *Varieties in Aging: Annual Review of Gerontology and Geriatrics.* New York, Springer, 1988, p. 132.

Palmore E: *Social Patterns in Normal Aging: Findings from the Duke Longitudinal Study.* Durham, NC, Duke University Press, 1981.

Pillemer K et al: *Social Integration in the Second Half of Life.* Baltimore, Johns Hopkins University Press, 2000, p 318.

Rodin J, Langer EJ: Long-term effects of a control-relevant intervention with the institutionalized aged. *J Pers Soc Psychol* 35:897, 1977.

Rodin J: Aging and health: Effects of the sense of control. *Science* 233:1271, 1986.

Rosow I: *Social Integration of the Aged.* New York, The Free Press, 1967.

Ryff CD, Marshall VW: *The Self and Society in Aging Processes.* New York, 1999.

Schulz R et al: *Intervention Research with Older People.* New York, Springer Publishing Co., 1998, p 18.

Seeman T et al: Self-efficacy beliefs and change in cognitive performance: MacArthur studies of successful aging. *Psychol Aging* 11:538, 1996.

Seeman TE et al: Allostatic load as a marker of cumulative biological risk: MacArthur studies of successful aging. *Proc Natl Acad Sci U S A* 98:4770, 2001.

Seeman TE et al: Price of adaptation—Allostatic load and its health consequences. MacArthur studies of successful aging. *Arch Intern Med* 157:2259, 1997.

Smedley B, Syme L: *Promoting Health: Intervention Strategies from the Social and Behavioral Sciences.* Washington DC, National Academy Press, 2001.

Stuck AE et al: Home visits to prevent nursing home admission and functional decline in elderly people: Systematic review and meta-regression analysis. *JAMA* 287:1022, 2002.

Taylor SE et al: Health psychology: What is an unhealthy environment and how does it get under the skin? *Ann Rev Psychol* 48:411, 1997.

Uchino BN et al: The relationship between social support and physiological processes: A review with emphasis on underlying mechanisms and implications for health. *Psychol Bull* 119:488, 1996.

Wilkins R, Adams O: *Healthfulness of Life: A Unified View of Mortality, Institutionalization and Non-institutionalized Disability Research.* Montreal, Canada, Institute for Research in Public Policy, 1978.

Yi KM: Psychosocial factors in geriatric care. *J Am Geriatr Soc* 40:976, 1992.

Preventive Gerontology: Strategies for Optimizing Health Across the Life Span

ELIZABETH A. PHELAN • MIGUEL A. PANIAGUA • WILLIAM R. HAZZARD

In developed societies, the success of disease prevention strategies over the last century, coupled with more effective treatments for many diseases, has resulted in a decline in mortality caused by acute disease. However, this decline in mortality is associated with a rise in chronic illness and attendant morbidity in the form of chronic disability in old age. The sheer magnitude of the elderly population of the near future will place critical demands on existing health care delivery systems. Consequently, continued independent functioning of the elderly population is a major challenge to public health. The ability to perform activities of daily living is essential for ensuring independent living. Thus, preventive gerontology—the study of individual and population health strategies across the life span aimed at maximizing both the quality and quantity of human longevity—must now aim not just to retard chronic disease but also to prevent functional decline.

Aging is a lifelong process in which early- and mid-life events and behaviors can have an important influence on the health and functioning of individuals as they age. Development of chronic disease, functional decline, and loss of independence are not inevitable consequences of aging. Health and function in late life can be seen to a great degree as under one's own personal control. Disability is associated with chronic conditions that are potentially preventable, and changes in behavior and lifestyle will reduce risk factors that lead to many chronic conditions. This is true throughout life, and has been shown to apply even for persons of advanced age.

What should the primary care provider advise his/her young adult and middle-aged patients about how to maintain optimal health and function into their later years? Health promotion efforts at the level of the individual should ideally be established early in life and maintained throughout life. Chronic disease, an avoidable outcome intermediate in the pathway to functional decline or death (see Fig. 6-1), is unlikely to have a single cause but rather, to

be the result of the interactions of multiple factors. Efforts to prevent such disease require a comprehensive approach that focuses primarily on behavioral modification.

Individuals who pursue a healthy lifestyle have a lower risk of developing a chronic disease. A healthy lifestyle can be conceptualized as one that involves avoidance of health damaging behaviors along with the adoption of a proactive approach to one's health. This chapter first examines those behaviors that should be avoided and then turns to those behaviors that should be adopted if one is to maximize the time spent in a state of independent functioning.

AVOIDANCE OF HEALTH-DAMAGING BEHAVIORS

Achieving and maintaining health and function in advanced years can be aided by a commitment to a lifestyle that involves avoidance of smoking and other behaviors that adversely affect health. Large cohort studies, including the Multiple Risk Factor Intervention Trial (MRFIT) and the Chicago Heart Association Detection Project in Industry (CHA) showed that nonsmokers with favorable levels of cholesterol and blood pressure and no history of diabetes, myocardial infarction, or electrocardiogram (ECG) abnormalities have far lower risk of coronary heart disease and greater longevity. Similarly, the Nurses Health Study found that middle-aged women who did not smoke, drank alcohol in moderate amounts, were not overweight, consumed a healthy diet, and exercised at least 30 minutes daily had an 83 percent reduction in their risk of coronary events as compared with all the other women, and that each factor independently and significantly predicted risk, even after adjustment for age, family history, presence or absence of diagnosed hypertension or diagnosed high cholesterol, and menopausal status. The online

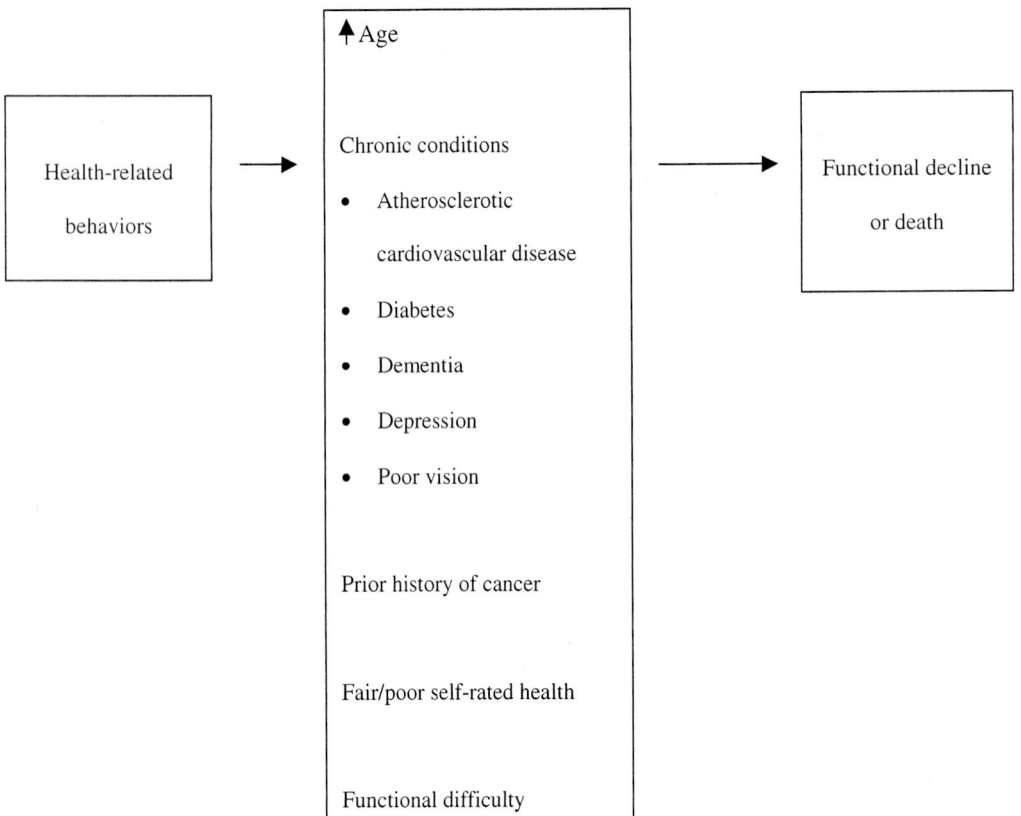

Figure 6-1   Conceptual model of how health behaviors impact the combined outcome of functional decline or death.

publication of *Healthy People 2010* (http://www.health.gov/healthypeople/BeHealthy/) contains links to reliable information about behavioral risk factors that lead to chronic disease and disability for individuals at every age. At http://www.healthfinder.gov/, information on these topics is organized by age, race, ethnicity, and gender, and for parents, caregivers, and health professionals.

Tobacco Use

Tobacco use is clearly the largest single preventable cause of illness and premature deaths in the United States. Illnesses related to tobacco use (coronary artery disease [CAD]; cancers of the lung, larynx, oral cavity, esophagus, pancreas, and urinary bladder; stroke; chronic obstructive pulmonary disease) account for one of every five deaths in the United States. Evidence from the National Health and Nutrition Examination Survey (NHANES) indicates that tobacco use predicts shorter survival time for middle-aged (45 to 54 years of age) and older (65 to 74 years of age) men. Although studies of prevalent cases have suggested that tobacco use either has no effect or is protective against Alzheimer's disease, prospective data investigating incident cases found that, quite to the contrary, tobacco use is associated with an increased risk of dementia, including that attributable to Alzheimer's disease. Tobacco use can also multiply the risk associated with other carcinogenic agents; for example, heavy alcohol consumption, associated with esophageal cancer, carries an even greater risk

when combined with cigarette smoking. In addition, the relative risk of developing lung cancer is at least additive in those who also have a history of exposure to certain occupational agents such as arsenic, asbestos, chromium, nickel, and vinyl chloride.

It is increasingly evident that exposure to environmental tobacco smoke may also be a risk factor for lung cancer in lifelong nonsmokers. The adverse health effects of environmental tobacco smoke are far reaching—in one case study, the attributable risk of death for second-hand smoke was similar to that of melanoma and motor vehicle collisions. Remarkably, tobacco use is a voluntary activity and therefore the diseases, disabilities, and deaths attributable to its use are all clearly preventable.

Tobacco dependence should be viewed as a chronic condition requiring ongoing assessment and repeated intervention. However, effective treatments are available that can lead to long-term, and in some cases, permanent, abstinence. Studies show that individuals at any age can benefit from quitting the tobacco habit. Benefits include reduction in the risk of CAD, cancers, stroke, and even hearing loss, along with improved pulmonary function, arterial circulation, and pulmonary perfusion.

Studies have found that not all health care providers routinely inquire about their patients' tobacco habits or advise patients who use tobacco to quit. Data indicate that, if physicians advise patients not to use tobacco, as many as 25 percent of patients will quit or reduce the amount they use. Thus, providers should ask all patients at each clinic visit about tobacco use and advise all tobacco users about the importance of quitting, emphasizing factors that have been found to contribute most to successful attempts to quit: health concerns (symptoms); a desire to set an example for children; the expense of the habit; odor of breath, home, and clothing; and loss of taste for food. Providers should then assess a patient's willingness to attempt to quit. Patients who are unwilling to attempt to quit should be provided with a brief intervention designed to increase their motivation to quit. Patients who are willing to quit should be provided with treatments that have been identified as effective. First-line pharmacotherapies that increase long-term smoking abstinence rates include bupropion and nicotine (gum, inhaler, nasal spray, or patch). Second-line therapies include clonidine and nortriptyline. Additional information about these therapies, as well as descriptions of brief clinical interventions for patients willing and unwilling to make a quit attempt, can be found in the June 2000 guideline, "Treating tobacco use and dependence," available at http://www.ahrq.gov/clinic.

Substance Abuse

The harmful health effects of substance abuse are well documented. Studies show that individuals at any age can benefit from quitting these habits, and effective, brief interventions are available. Providers might consider participating in continuing education programs to hone screening and counseling skills.

Alcohol

Epidemiologic studies support a survival benefit associated with moderate alcohol consumption (1 to 2 ounces daily), primarily through reduction of cardiovascular risk, perhaps through elevation of high-density lipoprotein (HDL) cholesterol. Additionally, both epidemiologic and experimental studies suggest a protective effect against the development of cardiovascular disease with moderate consumption of red wine. The exact mechanism of the protective effect remains to be established, although it has been attributed to the properties of tannins or phenolic compounds, as well as alcohol content. Weaker associations with moderate alcohol consumption include a protective effect against bone loss in older women, Alzheimer's disease, intermittent lower-extremity claudication, ischemic stroke, and prevention of hearing loss.

However, alcohol is clearly a two-edged sword as it relates to health. Consumption of alcohol beyond a moderate level can induce adverse effects on every organ system, including increased risk of hypertension; breast, esophageal, liver, and head and neck cancer; cirrhosis; gastrointestinal bleeding; pancreatitis; cardiomyopathy; seizures; cerebellar degeneration; peripheral neuropathy; cognitive dysfunction; insomnia; depression; and suicide. Counseling about problem drinking following a few screening questions has been identified as a high-impact, cost-effective service that is nevertheless currently delivered to less than 50 percent of the adult population (see "Priorities among recommended clinical preventive services" at http://www.prevent.org, under the "Publication" link). Screening can be accomplished by taking a careful history of alcohol use or by using a standardized screening questionnaire. All adults should be counseled on the health risks associated with excess alcohol consumption, as well as the risk of injury after drinking alcohol (e.g., motor vehicle crashes or other equipment-related injury). Nondependent heavy drinkers, as well as those with alcoholism (a chronic illness involving a state of dependency), should be counseled about the benefits of decreasing alcohol intake. Brief counseling by primary care providers can result in a significant reduction in alcohol use. Dependent drinkers should be referred to formal alcohol treatment programs and considered for a trial of naltrexone, an opioid antagonist that reduces the pleasurable effects of alcohol and may reduce relapse to heavy drinking.

Illicit Drugs

Injection drug use continues to be a major risk factor for acquisition of human immunodeficiency virus (HIV), hepatitis B virus (HBV), and hepatitis C virus (HCV). Injection drug users typically initiate injection drug use during late adolescence (before age 21 years); however, a sizable subgroup begins injecting during early and late adulthood.

Noninjection drug use (crack smokers, methamphetamine, intranasal heroin or cocaine, etc.) contributes to development of gastroduodenal ulcers, chest pain, and myocardial infarction, and to an increased risk of death. In survival analyses, individuals identified as both drug users and drug-dependent were more likely to die and to have a younger median age at death. As might be expected, higher levels of drug involvement also were associated with increased age-adjusted mortality.

Prescription Drug Misuse

Prescription drug misuse is poorly described in the medical literature. Misuse of prescription medications may be related to insomnia, chronic pain, depression, or anxiety. The potential misuse of benzodiazepines is well recognized and has led to prescribing recommendations that suggest only short-term use and use only for intended indications. Amphetamine-like stimulants have abuse potential, but addiction to these drugs is seldom documented. Other medications that are often misused are sedative-hypnotics, opioid analgesics, and barbiturates. Chronic use of such agents may lead to physical dependency and the development of withdrawal symptoms with attempts to discontinue use. Treatment may require detoxification followed by rehabilitation.

The Task Force on Community Preventive Services, an independent, nonfederal, multidisciplinary group charged with reviewing and assessing the quality of available evidence on the effectiveness and cost-effectiveness of essential community preventive health services, will be publishing their reviews in an online document entitled, The Guide to Community Preventive Services. Proposed topics coordinate with *Healthy People 2000/2010* objectives and address actual causes of death, as described by McGinnis et al. in their 1993 *JAMA* article, as well as prevalent risk behaviors. The list of topics selected for initial review includes addictive drugs. As topic reviews are completed, they will be available at http://www.thecommunityguide.org, by following the "Topics" link and then clicking on the topic of interest listed on the left navigation bar.

Injury

Head Trauma and Risk for Alzheimer's Disease

A number of case-control studies indicate that, in addition to maximizing one's years of education and minimizing exposure to neurotoxins, avoidance of significant head trauma (that which results in loss of consciousness or seeking of medical attention) may lower the risk of eventual development of Alzheimer's disease. It therefore stands to reason that with implementation of cranioprotective measures during early life, such as wearing helmets during high-risk activities and avoidance of high-risk behaviors that may put one at risk for head trauma, the risk of eventual cognitive decline may be reduced.

Ultraviolet Light and Risk for Skin Cancers and Cataracts

Increased risk of melanoma and nonmelanoma skin cancers, as well as cataracts, is associated with exposure to ultraviolet B (UVB, or 280 to 320 nanometer) rays. More than five sunburns has been found to double the risk of melanoma, irrespective of the timing in life. Avoiding peak exposures, wearing protective clothing, and using sunscreen with a sun protection factor (SPF) of at least 15, indicating protection against UVB, along with a star rating for ultraviolet A (UVA, or 320 to 400 nanometer rays) protection of 3 to 4, might reduce the risk of melanoma and other skin cancers. Wearing sunglasses that afford UVB protection along with hats with brims can reduce the risk of cataracts by lowering eye exposure to UVB light. Thus, patients should be advised to change behaviors that may increase the risk of skin cancer and cataracts. However, the United States Preventive Services Task Force (USPSTF), in its third edition of the *Guide to Clinical Preventive Services* (available at http://www.ahrq.gov/clinic/prevenix.htm), concluded that there is insufficient evidence to recommend for or against a periodic skin examination by clinicians.

Excessive Noise and Risk for Hearing Loss

Noise-induced hearing loss ranks second only to presbycusis as a leading cause of sensorineural hearing loss, and the interaction between the two makes hearing loss a major source of social isolation and disability in the elderly. The noise-induced element is a well-described disability that is unarguably preventable. Such an insult can occur at any age and can affect one's life for years thereafter. Importantly, progression of cell death at the level of the cochlear cilia can be halted with avoidance of the offending recreational or occupational noise and using hearing protection, such as earplugs. Patients who have been exposed to excessive noise should be screened for hearing loss. When hearing loss is suspected, a thorough history, physical examination, and audiometry should be performed. If these examinations disclose evidence of hearing loss, referral for full audiologic evaluation is recommended.

Sleep Deprivation and Motor Vehicle Crash Fatalities

Impaired driving continues to be a considerable cause of morbidity and mortality in this country. In 1998, alcohol was involved in 38 percent of all fatal motor vehicle collisions. Sleep deprivation is evolving as another significant risk factor for fatal motor vehicle accidents, and may be as dangerous as driving under the influence of alcohol (and the combination of the two all too commonly lethal). Both medical (i.e., obstructive sleep apnea) and environmental (i.e., nightshift-requiring occupations) factors contribute to daytime sleepiness, putting drivers at risk, and in some studies, causing 16 to 20 percent of vehicle accidents. Patients, families, and employers need to be educated about the dangers of this phenomenon, and how to best prevent its potentially devastating consequences.

Obesity

In American adults, obesity is defined as a body mass index (BMI) of 30 kg/m^2 or more, while overweight is a BMI of 25 to 30 kg/m^2. Despite public health messages that focus on reducing fat intake and increasing energy expenditure, the incidence of obesity in America is increasing. There is strong evidence that obesity is associated with increased cardiovascular risk as well as a higher incidence of hypertension, dyslipidemia, and diabetes (all associated with insulin resistance and "the metabolic syndrome"). Obesity is one of the leading factors associated with functional limitations, including such disabling conditions as osteoarthritis and stroke, as well as premature death. Moreover, those who are obese may suffer from social stigmatization, discrimination, and low self-esteem. Excess body weight or weight gain, particularly from ages 25 to 50 years, contributes to the development of chronic conditions (cardiovascular disease, diabetes mellitus, hypertension, and osteoarthritis) in later years.

Efforts to maintain a healthy weight should start early in life and continue throughout adulthood, as this is likely to be more successful than efforts to lose substantial amounts of weight and to maintain weight loss after obesity has developed. Adults who are trying to maintain a healthy weight after weight loss are advised to get even more physical activity than the 30 minutes per day (described below) that is currently recommended. Weight management leading to a slow, steady weight loss is more beneficial than a pattern of weight cycling, which may actually contribute to an elevated risk of mortality. The basal metabolic rate decreases with age, in parallel with the decline in lean body mass, that begins as early as the third decade, and body fat increases proportionally. Thus, in order to most readily achieve normalization of body weight and body composition, an energy-sufficient (but not excessive) diet should be combined with exercise to permit maintenance of basal metabolic rate. Obese individuals who are trying to lose a substantial amount of weight should seek the guidance of a health care provider.

TAKING A PROACTIVE APPROACH TO PERSONAL HEALTH AND WELL-BEING

Achieving and maintaining health and function in advanced years—successful preventive gerontology—is rooted in a personal commitment to a lifestyle that promotes proper nutrition, physical fitness, social connections, and use of preventive health care. Whereas the advice and encouragement of the health care provider can facilitate preventive gerontology, it is the acceptance by the individual of primary responsibility in managing his or her health and behavior that is central to the concept.

Nutrition

A healthful diet can contribute to an increase in life expectancy and better health. Healthy diets show the potential to lower blood pressure and blood cholesterol. Optimal diets are also associated with lower risk of chronic diseases, notably coronary artery disease, diabetes, obesity, and some forms of cancer. A diet with adequate calcium and vitamin D reduces the risk of osteoporosis, which is a major cause of fractures and concomitant disability and threatened independence, especially in postmenopausal women. NHANES III data show potentially important decreases with age in median protein and zinc intakes, as well as intakes of calcium, vitamin E, and other nutrients. Subclinical nutrient deficiencies can adversely affect health and physical functioning. Longitudinal studies show that caloric intake and, as expected, macronutrient (fat, protein, and carbohydrate) intake decrease with age.

The traditional Mediterranean diet, dominated by consumption of olive oil, vegetables, and fruits, meets the criteria for a healthy diet. Direct evidence in support of this diet has become available. Antioxidants represent a common element in these foods and an antioxidant mechanism is a plausible explanation for the benefits. The fifth edition of *Nutrition and Your Health: Dietary Guidelines for Americans*, available online at http://www.health.gov/dietaryguidelines/, can serve as a reference for providers in counseling adults about healthful eating patterns.

Physical Activity

Physical activity and physical fitness can help prevent or delay the onset of chronic illnesses such as coronary artery disease, type 2 diabetes, osteoporosis, and obesity, protect against the development of functional decline, improve mood, reduce stress, and increase active life expectancy, as well as total life expectancy. Physical activities that improve endurance, strength, and flexibility will delay impairments in mobility and may preserve the ability to perform tasks of daily living. Regular, moderate-intensity physical activity increases muscle mass and oxidative capacity, improves immune function, increases antioxidant defense against oxygen free radicals, and reduces oxidative stress. The current recommendation that every American exercise at least 30 minutes on most, and preferably all days derives from evidence that even moderate physical activity is associated

with a substantial drop in all-cause mortality. The cumulative, lifetime activity pattern may be the most influential factor in terms of providing protection from most diseases, especially those with a long developmental period, as well as mediating secondary disease complications associated with coronary artery disease, diabetes, and hypertension.

However, despite an enormous amount of information about the positive effects of exercise in preventing disease and increasing life expectancy, the majority of adults do not engage in regular, sufficient physical activity. For example, only 15 percent of the US adult population met the 30 minutes per day goal in 1997, and 40 percent of adults engaged in no leisure-time physical activity. Women are less likely than men to report regular leisure time physical activity; the lowest levels typically are among women of Hispanic or African American descent. Furthermore, aging appears to be associated with a rise in the prevalence of inactivity, especially among women, such that by age 75 years, one in three men and one in two women engage in *no* regular physical activity. Societal changes over the past 50 years, including increased dependence on cars for transportation, the advent of television and computers, and rise in number of desk jobs, have virtually engineered physical activity out of the daily routines of many Americans. Many mid-life and older adults are unaware of the benefits of physical activity. Thus, encouraging and prescribing physical activity for adults of all ages is imperative, and this can be viewed as a central tenet of preventive gerontology. Regular participation in activities of moderate intensity (such as walking, climbing stairs, biking, yard work), which increase caloric expenditure and maintain muscle strength, should be recommended. It is especially activity of moderate intensity that appears to allow health benefits to accrue. Building such activity into one's daily routine (e.g., taking the stairs rather than an elevator) is recommended as the most practical and efficacious way to achieve the goal of 30 minutes of exercise each day.

What factors determine regular participation in physical activity? Several psychological and environmental factors determine physical activity behavior throughout the life span. Self-efficacy, or confidence in one's ability to perform a particular behavior (in this case, regular exercise), is strongly associated with both adoption of and adherence to physical activity among adolescents, young adults, and older adults. Strategies suggested by Bandura to enhance self-efficacy, such as assessing readiness for exercise using a behavior change philosophy, using motivational interviewing techniques, weekly action planning and feedback, collaborative problem-solving, and addressing barriers to exercise may all enhance self-efficacy for exercise. These techniques can be learned and implemented by health care providers. Affective disorders such as depression and anxiety are inversely associated with physical activity participation at any age. Thus, evaluation for the presence of these conditions and institution of treatment may be necessary before adoption of an exercise program can occur. Social influences on physical activity appear to be strong throughout the life span. Peer reinforcement is particularly important in youth, while social support from spouses and friends is correlated with vigorous activity in younger and older adult populations. Finally, environmental factors—particularly safety and accessibility—influence activity participation across the age span. These latter factors are increasingly becoming a focus of community intervention efforts.

Social Connections

Ongoing involvement in a social network permits social contact (integration), the provision of social support, and the opportunity for social influence, and is associated with positive health outcomes and self-assessed well-being. Through opportunities for social engagement, such as attending social functions, getting together with friends and family, and going to church, meaningful social roles are defined and reinforced, creating a sense of belonging and identity that is made possible by the network context. Measures of social integration or "connectedness" are powerful predictors of mortality, likely because ties give meaning to an individual's life by enabling and obligating him/her to be fully involved in his/her community and thereby to feel attached to it.

In turn, there are several pathways most proximate to health by which social networks are thought to influence health: (1) a health behavioral pathway; (2) a psychological pathway; and (3) a physiologic pathway. Regarding the health behavioral pathway, social ties influence the likelihood that certain behaviors will be adopted and that behavior will change. *Social influence* refers to the way members of a social network obtain normative guidance about health-relevant behaviors (physical activity, smoking, etc.). For example, several studies show that marriage and friendship ties promote a healthier diet, more regular exercise, less smoking and drinking, and more cancer screening. Spouse pairs demonstrate a concordance in their level of exercise, smoking, and drinking. However, studies also show that family and friends carry the potential for encouraging detrimental health behaviors; for example, the presence of a smoker in one's social network is associated with greater relapse in efforts to quit. Adherence and nonadherence to medical treatments have each been linked to the presence of more social ties. Thus, the evidence indicates that ties can serve as role models of appropriate or undesirable behavior. Evidence also suggests that social network size is inversely related to risk-related behaviors. Data from Alameda County show a gradient between increasing social disconnection and the prevalence of both health damaging behaviors and mortality.

Psychological pathways are another mechanism by which social networks influence health. Evidence suggests that ongoing participation in one's social network is essential for the maintenance of self-efficacy beliefs throughout life. For example, studies have observed the indirect influence of social support through enhanced self-efficacy in smoking cessation and exercise. In addition, it is generally accepted that social ties have a salutary effect on mental health and psychological well-being, regardless of whether an individual is under stress. Integration in a social network may also directly produce positive psychological states, such as a sense of self-worth, purpose, and belonging. These positive states, in turn, may benefit mental health as a result of direct modulation of the neuroendocrine response to stress, and may increase the likelihood of social support, protecting against psychological distress (depression and anxiety).

Physiologic pathways are the third mechanism by which social networks influence health. The basic premise is that human physiologic homeostasis is influenced by the social environment. Social relationships may influence health via alteration in immune response, by effects on the hypothalamic-pituitary-adrenal axis, or by cardiovascular reactivity. For example, a low number of contacts with acquaintances is associated with high resting plasma levels of epinephrine, and people with low social support have higher levels of urinary norepinephrine, regardless of their level of stress. Studies of medical students show that those who were lonely had lower levels of natural killer cell activity.

Cognitive Activity

Continuing cognitive activity helps maintain cognitive function. Crossword puzzles and reading are two examples of activities that can help maintain cognitive skills. Higher levels of education (and cognitive ability, for which education could be a marker) are associated with less age-related loss in cognitive function.

Health Care

A primary purpose of health care in an aging society is to help each individual set and achieve personal health-related goals, that is, goals that will enhance active life expectancy and quality of life. Adults should be instructed to seek medical attention early for bothersome symptoms. They should receive education about self-management of chronic conditions, including the importance of long-term adherence to medications (e.g., for treatment of hypertension or dyslipoproteinemia) prescribed to treat such conditions. Finally, they should be advised to participate fully in the periodic preventive screening and health care activities described below (see also Chap. 12). Providers should be aware that although *Healthy People 2000* had a stated goal of screening 80 percent of Americans for lifestyle risk factors just discussed (i.e., tobacco, alcohol, and drug use, diet, and exercise), only 56 percent of Americans have actually been screened. Thus, in addition to the interventions described below, the routine work of health care providers should include regular counseling about health behavior change to prevent disease and making referrals to health care system and community resources as indicated.

Blood Pressure Evaluations

A recent study supported by the National Heart, Lung, and Blood Institute indicates that middle-aged Americans face a 90 percent chance of developing high blood pressure at some time during the rest of their lives. All patients should be counseled that the development of high blood pressure is not an inevitability; however, they should be educated about the role of abstaining from smoking, following a healthy eating plan that includes low sodium intake, maintaining a healthy weight, being physically active, and consuming alcohol in moderation in the prevention of hypertension altogether.

The Framingham study showed that men aged 45 to 64 years with blood pressures above 160/95 have two to three times the coronary artery disease rate of those with pressures under 140/90. Among those with systolic pressures above 160, strokes were three times as frequent as among those with systolic pressures under 140. Other studies (e.g., Systolic Hypertension in the Elderly Person [SHEP]) have demonstrated the efficacy of blood pressure lowering in reducing the complications of hypertension. Thus, treating high blood pressure with lifestyle modification and medication will reduce the risk of CAD and stroke.

Lipid Evaluations

Premature heart disease is unequivocally associated with elevated blood cholesterol levels. Data from the Framingham study indicate that for a 1 percent rise in cholesterol there is a 2 percent rise in CAD, while for a 1 percent rise in HDL cholesterol there is a 2 percent fall in risk of CAD. Strategies to increase HDL levels while lowering low-density lipoprotein (LDL) cholesterol to the total cholesterol:HDL cholesterol ratio of 3.5 or less are recommended. The third edition of the USPSTF's *Guide to Clinical Preventive Services* (available at http://www.ahrq.gov/clinic/prevenix.htm) recommends that all adults (men beginning at age 35 years and women beginning at age 45 years) be screened routinely for lipid disorders to determine whether their cholesterol levels increase their risk for heart disease. Younger adults should be screened for lipid disorders if they have other risk factors for heart disease, especially a family history of premature heart disease. Providers should counsel all patients about lifestyle changes (reducing saturated fat in the diet, exercising, and losing weight) that can improve their lipid levels. Individuals at highest risk may require medication to control their lipid abnormalities.

Diabetes Screening and Prevention

Diabetes is an important risk factor for CAD. Diabetics tend to have more severe atherosclerosis, two to three times as many myocardial infarctions, and twice as many strokes as nondiabetics of the same age. This is especially germane for women, in whom diabetes appears to nullify their relative (5- to 10-year) protection from CAD conferred by their gender. In other words, a woman with diabetes is at equal risk of CAD at any given age as a man with diabetes. Current interventions for the prevention of type 2 diabetes mellitus are targeted toward modifying lifestyle risk factors, such as reducing obesity and promoting physical activity. Awareness of risk factors for developing type 2 diabetes (i.e., strong family history of diabetes, age, obesity, physical inactivity, and having a personal history of gestational diabetes or being an offspring of a woman who had gestational diabetes) is important to permit screening, early detection, and treatment in high-risk populations.

Recent evidence suggests that weight reduction (via caloric restriction and increased physical activity) can reduce the risk of developing type 2 diabetes in overweight adults. This strategy appears to be more effective than pharmacologic intervention (with metformin) in reducing insulin resistance (58 percent reduction in incidence of diabetes with lifestyle modification versus 31 percent with metformin, each compared to placebo). Other lines of evidence (chiefly from clinical trials of statins that have included diabetics) underscore the importance and efficacy of CAD risk reduction in diabetics, in whom the risk of CAD events in the absence of clinical CAD is equivalent to that of nondiabetics with CAD. This has led to a more ambitious goal for LDL cholesterol reduction in diabetics in the 2001 Adult Treatment Panel III (ATP III) National Cholesterol Education Program (NCEP), to 100 mg/dL or less, the same as in nondiabetics with CAD or other atherosclerotic vascular disease. The NCEP report can be viewed at http://www.nhlbi.nih.gov/guidelines/cholesterol/index.htm.

Cancer Screening

Cancers and cancer deaths can be prevented both by limiting exposure to known carcinogens and through early detection and treatment before a cancer has spread. Available screening procedures for colon and cervical cancer, if more widely applied to asymptomatic persons, would likely prevent many deaths from these diseases. For example, The Minnesota Colon Cancer Control Study showed that annual fecal occult-blood testing reduced mortality by 33 percent. A large body of observational studies suggests that early detection through periodic Papanicolaou (Pap) testing lowers mortality from cervical cancer by 20 to 60 percent. Mammographic screening for breast cancer remains controversial, given the risks (e.g., low sensitivity and specificity of mammography; false-positive results that generate additional testing and result in anxiety; overdiagnosis and unnecessary treatments) and costs associated with periodic (every 1 to 2 years beginning at age 40 years) screening. Debate continues over whether a survival benefit is derived from mass screening for breast cancer. Clinicians and women should discuss individual risk factors and personal preferences to determine when to have a first mammogram and how often to have them thereafter. Screening for early detection of prostate cancer also remains controversial, especially beyond age 70 years (see also Chap. 55).

Immunizations for Pneumococcal Pneumonia and Influenza

Both pneumococcal pneumonia and influenza can lead to hospitalization and disability. Vaccinations should be administered to any adult with a chronic condition regardless of age and universally for those over 65, annually for influenza and once for pneumococcus.

Aspirin for Primary Prevention of Myocardial Infarction

There is compelling evidence that aspirin decreases the incidence of coronary artery disease in middle-aged and older adults who are at increased risk (i.e., a 5-year risk of

3 percent or more) but who have never had a myocardial infarction or a cerebrovascular accident (CVA). Combined data from five clinical trials show that aspirin therapy lowers the risk of CAD by 28 percent. However, there is no reduction in the risk of CVA with aspirin; the risk of having a hemorrhagic CVA is actually slightly increased. There is also an increased risk of gastrointestinal bleeding with aspirin. Thus, the risk may outweigh the benefits for those who are at average or low risk for CAD. A risk calculator can be found at http://hin.nhlbi.nih.gov/atpiii/calculator.asp.

CONCLUSION

Adoption and maintenance of a healthy lifestyle should be emphasized from childhood through older adulthood. Sound health habits not only help people survive longer but postpone the onset of disability and compress functional loss into fewer years at the end of life. Among the most important self-care behaviors are those that involve adequate nutrition, avoidance of tobacco use, and regular physical activity. As the population ages, the potential for strain on health care systems will increase, because the greatest use of health services has tended to occur during the last years of life. Thus, in the present health care environment, health promotion is an important focus for providers who care for individuals of any age.

REFERENCES

Alessio HM, Blasi ER: Physical activity as a natural antioxidant booster and its effect on a healthy life span. *Res Q Exerc Sport* 68(4):292, 1997.

Armstrong BK, Kricker A. The epidemiology of UV induced skin cancer. *J Photochem Photobiol B* 63:8, 2001.

Barrett-Connor E, Kritz-Silverstein D: Gender differences in cognitive function with age: The Rancho Bernardo study. *J Am Geriatr Soc* 47:159, 1999.

Berkman LF, Kawachi I: *Social Epidemiology*. New York, Oxford University Press, 2000.

Brownson RC et al: *Chronic Disease Epidemiology and Control*, 2nd ed. Washington, DC, American Public Health Association, 1998.

DiPietro L: Physical activity in aging: Changes in patterns and their relationship to health and function. *J Gerontol A Biol Sci Med Sci* 56(Spec No 2):13, 2001.

Fleming MF et al: Brief physician advice for problem alcohol drinkers. A randomized controlled trial in community-based primary care practices. *JAMA* 277:1039, 1997.

Graves AB et al: The association between head trauma and Alzheimer's disease. *Am J Epidemiol* 131:491, 1990.

Horne JA, Reyner LA: Sleep related vehicle accidents. *BMJ* 310:565, 1995.

Knowler WC et al: Reduction in the incidence of type 2 diabetes with lifestyle intervention or metformin. *N Engl J Med* 346(6):393, 2002.

Laux G, Puryear DA: Benzodiazepines—Misuse, abuse and dependency. *Am Fam Physician* 30:139, 1984.

Neumark YD et al: "Drug dependence" and death: Survival analysis of the Baltimore ECA sample from 1981 to 1995. *Subst Use Misuse* 35:313, 2000.

Olsen O, Gotzsche PC: Screening for breast cancer with mammography (Cochrane Review). *Cochrane Database Syst Rev* 4, 2001.

Ott A et al: Smoking and risk of dementia and Alzheimer's disease in a population-based cohort study: The Rotterdam Study. *Lancet* 351:1840, 1998.

Popelka MM et al. Moderate alcohol consumption and hearing loss: A protective effect. *J Am Geriatr Soc* 48:1273, 2000.

Rabinowitz PM: Noise-induced hearing loss. *Am Fam Physician* 61:2749, 2759, 2000.

Rollnick S et al: *Health Behavior Change: A Guide for Practitioners*. Philadelphia, Churchill Livingstone, 1999.

Stamler J et al. Low risk-factor profile and long-term cardiovascular and noncardiovascular mortality and life expectancy: findings for 5 large cohorts of young adult and middle-aged men and women. *JAMA* 282:2012, 1999.

Taylor HR et al: Effect of ultraviolet radiation on cataract formation. *N Engl J Med* 319:1429, 1988.

Tinsley JA, Watkins DD: Over-the-counter stimulants: Abuse and addiction. *Mayo Clin Proc* 73:977, 1998.

Wakimoto P, Block G: Dietary intake, dietary patterns, and changes with age: An epidemiological perspective. *J Gerontol A Biol Sci Med Sci* 56(Spec No 2):65, 2001.

Wollin SD, Jones PJ: Alcohol, red wine and cardiovascular disease. *J Nutr* 131:1401, 2001.

Woodward A, Laugesen M: How many deaths are caused by second hand cigarette smoke? *Tob Control* 10:383, 2001.

PRINCIPLES OF GERIATRIC CARE

Approach to Clinical Care of the Older Patient

MARY E. TINETTI

CLINICAL DECISION MAKING

Clinical decision making, including diagnosis, treatment, and outcomes, differs between younger and older adult patients. The primary goal of medical care in younger adult patients usually is diagnosis of the disease causing the presenting symptoms, signs, and/or laboratory abnormalities. Treatment is targeted toward the pathophysiologic mechanisms deemed responsible for the disease. Relevant clinical outcomes are determined by the specific diseases and include cure if the disease is acute, and control or modification if the disease is chronic.

The conventional disease-specific approach is not optimal in older patients for several reasons. First, the average 75-year-old suffers from 3.5 chronic diseases. With multiple coexisting chronic diseases, there is a less consistent relationship between pathology and disease or between disease and clinical manifestations. One disease may obscure or change the pathology, manifestations, or accuracy of laboratory evaluation of coexisting diseases. Treatment of one disease may increase the severity of another. With multiple coexisting diseases it becomes difficult, and often impossible, to assess the severity or manifestations of individual diseases and to ascribe health and/or functional status to specific disease processes.

Second, many distressing symptoms or impairments among older persons, such as pain, dizziness, fatigue, sleep problems, sensory impairments, and gait disorders cannot be ascribed to a single disease; instead, they result from the accumulated effect of physical, psychological, social, environmental, and other factors. A clinical focus solely on diagnosing and treating discrete diseases may lead to expensive diagnostic testing with inconclusive results, to unnecessary, or even harmful, interventions, or, conversely, to ignoring potentially remediable symptoms. While clinicians may be reluctant to treat symptoms in younger and middle-aged patients without a specific diagnosis, treatment focused on improving symptoms in multiply ill and impaired older patients is often appropriate, because comfort and function are primary goals of health care in this population.

Third, older patients vary in the importance they place on potential health outcomes. When asked, older persons are able to prioritize among the often competing goals of increased survival, comfort, cognitive function, and physical function. Optimal clinical decision making in the care of older patients includes the articulation of patient preferences or goals of care; the identification of the diseases, impairments, and non–disease-specific factors affecting the attainment of these preferences and goals; and the selection of treatment options based on the modifiable impediments to individual patient goals. In contrast to the increased emphasis on disease management, which aims to reduce interindividual variability in treatment and monitoring among younger and middle-aged patients, optimal care of older patients is highly variable and individualized. The multiplicity of impairments and diseases; the contribution of psychological, social, and environmental factors to health conditions; the enhanced likelihood of harm as well as benefit from many interventions; and the interindividual variability in patient preference all combine to make clinical decision making in the care of older persons very complex.

Clinical decision making is further complicated in older patients because other persons, including the spouse, adult children, other relatives, and significant others, are often actively involved, particularly when cognitive impairment is present. Involvement of family and friends is helpful and often crucial, since they may provide additional sources of information, facilitate adherence to treatment recommendations, and offer both emotional and instrumental support. Conflicts may arise, however, when goals of the patient and family differ. Striking a balance between patient confidentiality and family involvement, between independence and support, and between patient and family goals is a constant challenge. When based on an understanding of these factors, however, the clinical care of older persons is both effective and immensely gratifying.

PRESENTATION

At least three factors affect clinical presentation in older persons: underreporting of symptoms and impairments, changes in the patterns of presentation of individual illnesses, and an altered spectrum of health conditions. Contrary to a popular perception of older persons as complainers, they tend, if anything, to underreport significant symptoms. One reason for underreporting is that both older persons and their clinicians often dismiss treatable symptoms and impairments as age-related changes for which nothing can be done. Denial, resulting from fear of economic, social, or functional consequences, is suggested as another reason for underreporting health conditions. Cognitive impairment and depressive symptoms may further limit the ability or desire of some older persons to report symptoms and health conditions. This tendency to underreport means that clinicians must actively inquire about symptoms and concerns.

Altered presentation is a second characteristic of illness in older persons. While both acute and chronic illnesses may, and often do, present with "classic" signs and symptoms, age-related changes and coexisting conditions may combine to obscure these classic presentations in older persons. Symptoms or signs of one condition may exacerbate or mask those of another condition, complicating clinical evaluation. For example, arthritis, if it limits physical activity, may mask the presence of severe cardiovascular disease. Manifestations of clinically important disease may be attenuated in older persons, particularly those who are frail. Chest pain may be absent in older persons presenting with myocardial infarction, as may shortness of breath in persons with congestive heart failure. Another common phenomenon is that symptoms in one organ system may reflect disease in another system. Pneumonia may present as confusion or anorexia; a urinary tract infection may present as an unsteady gait or a fall. A corollary of these altered presentations is that signs and symptoms are often nonspecific. That is, while suggesting that the older persons is experiencing an acute illness or an exacerbation of a chronic condition, the signs and symptoms may offer limited help in determining what the illness or condition might be. These altered presentations mean that the clinician must be particularly diligent in ascertaining all symptoms and signs. She must rely on combinations of findings from the history, physical examination, and ancillary testing to determine the diagnosis, or, as is often the case, to identify the treatable contributors to the illness or health condition.

Third, the spectrum of health conditions in older persons differs from younger patients. Important clinical entities include not only acute and chronic diseases but also geriatric syndromes as well as cognitive and physical disabilities. Geriatric syndromes are health conditions common in older persons that result from the accumulated effect of multiple predisposing factors and that may be precipitated by an acute insult. Examples, described in Chaps. 116 to 125, include delirium, falls, and incontinence. Geriatric syndromes and disabilities are relevant both because they may be the presenting manifestation of another underlying illness and because they are treatable causes of morbidity in their own right.

EVALUATION

Interindividual variability in preferences and goals of care, multiple coexisting illnesses and diseases, altered presentations, underreporting, and a broader spectrum of health conditions all combine to make clinical evaluation particularly challenging in older persons. A clinical evaluation grounded in a clear understanding of these issues can, however, be effective. These factors dictate changes in the conventional clinical encounter in both the content and method of ascertainment for both the history and physical examination. It is important to bear in mind that, contrary to the conventional history and physical that is aimed at identifying the presence of discrete diseases, the aim of the clinical encounter in older patients is to identify the impairments, diseases, and other factors impeding the attainment of individual patient preferences and goals.

History/Interview

The setting and sources of information may need to be adapted to the specific impairments of some older persons. Impairments in hearing, visual acuity, and cognition, each prevalent among older persons, mandate a quiet, well-lit, and unhurried setting—not easily obtained in today's health care environment—in order to obtain thorough and accurate information. Multiple encounters may be required to complete the history and to gather the necessary information. While the patient remains the key informant, the history often needs to be supplemented by information obtained from the family, friends, and other care providers, particularly if the older person has cognitive impairment.

As clinical decision making should occur within the context of individual preferences and goals, ascertainment of these preferences should occur early in the clinical encounter. Older persons rarely volunteer their preferences. Active solicitation of priorities and preferences, therefore, needs to be an integral part of the patient and family interview. While the articulation of specific goals necessitates the identification of underlying diseases, impairments, health conditions, and other factors, the elicitation of priorities among general, often competing goals, including longevity, comfort/symptom relief, cognitive functioning, and physical functioning should drive all subsequent evaluation and management decisions.

The altered, often attenuated, presentation of diseases, the coexistence of multiple processes and the underreporting of symptoms and conditions in older patients mandate a reordering of the importance of various components of the history. The chief complaint, the cornerstone of history-taking in younger patients, has decreased relevance in older persons. Indeed, overreliance on the chief complaint leads to the oft cited, though inaccurate, comment that older persons are "vague or poor historians." Older patients are not necessarily poor historians. Rather, they may be accurately reporting the often vague, nonspecific manner in which their illnesses present.

The review of systems takes on greater importance in older persons and is often the vehicle by which treatable health conditions are revealed. Complementary to the conventional review of systems, physicians should perform a review of syndromes, targeting modifiable multifactorial geriatric syndromes common in older persons including sleep problems, incontinence, pain, dizziness, falls, depressive symptoms, fatigue, anorexia, and weight loss. As noted earlier, these syndromes are both relevant targets of intervention themselves as well as clues to the existence of other acute and chronic illnesses. Difficulty, degree of dependence, and change in ability in both self-care or basic activities of daily living (ADL—eating, dressing, grooming, bathing, walking, and transferring) and instrumental activities of daily living (IADL—taking medication, handling finances, using transportation, preparing meals, housekeeping, communicating outside the home, and shopping) are integral components of the history in older persons constituting the inventory of functional status, as are frequency of participation in social and higher level physical activities. These functional activities often are the primary outcomes targeted in the treatment of older patients. Furthermore, changes in the frequency or difficulty in participating in these activities often herald the onset of a new, or worsening of an existing, illness.

The clinical history of older persons should also include assessments of cognitive function, affect and mood (depressive symptoms), social supports, and economic and environmental factors because problems in these domains are prevalent in older persons, contribute to a wide range of health conditions, and are often modifiable. All patients should undergo quick screens of cognition, such as three-item recall, and affect, such as the two-question depressive screen (In the past month, have you been sad, blue, or down in the dumps? Have you lost interest in most things or been unable to enjoy them?). More formal, systematic assessments in these areas should be undertaken if there is any question of cognitive impairment or depression.

Physical Examination

The physical examination in older persons differs from younger persons in content and purpose. The purpose of the physical examination in younger persons is primarily to diagnose specific diseases. The physical examination in older persons, however, serves also to identify treatable impairments such as muscle weakness, gait instability, or sensory impairments, and to directly observe the performance of key functional tasks.

While the technique of physical examination in an older person is often the same as in younger persons, direct observation and functional testing play particularly important roles in older persons. Observing the older patient as he/she walks down the hall, gets on and off the exam table or in and out of bed, and arises from a chair and gets dressed and undressed is a valuable and time-efficient way to ascertain relevant information concerning muscle strength, joint range of motion, and gait stability as well as difficulty with daily functional tasks. Similarly, buttoning and unbuttoning a shirt or blouse, taking shoes on and off, and writing a sentence are simple tests of fine-motor coordination, manual dexterity, and motor planning. Reading a prescription bottle or a magazine provides information on visual acuity. Observing a patient's ability to follow multiple step commands such as during finger-to-nose testing provides valuable information on cognitive, as well as neurologic, functioning. Information on nutritional status can be inferred from observations of the face (e.g., temporal wasting) and hands (e.g., interossei atrophy). Recent weight loss can be judged from clothing that is too large, especially at the collar and waist.

In considering interpretation of physical examination findings, it is important to bear in mind that the coexistence of multiple diseases and the occurrence of non–disease-specific physical impairments in older persons compromise the sensitivity and specificity and, consequently the predictive value of the physical examination in older persons. Abnormal findings may be linked to any of several diseases. Rales, for example, may result from any congestive heart failure, interstitial fibrosis, or pneumonia, each common and often coexistent in older persons. A decreased neck range of motion may result from arthritis or be a secondary manifestation of voluntarily limiting neck turning because of dizziness caused by vestibular dysfunction. Conversely, the coexistence of multiple diseases may attenuate the physical findings of one or another disease process, such as when the sensitivity of the physical findings of congestive heart failure are compromised by the coexistence of chronic obstructive pulmonary disease.

Physical findings may also have important clinical and functional consequence, even when not linked to any specific disease. Peripheral neuropathy, manifested as decreased vibratory or position sense, for example, may be caused by any number of diseases, including diabetes mellitus, alcohol effect, or vitamin B_{12} deficiency, or may occur in the absence of any clinically detectable disease process. Regardless of whether an underlying disease is causative, peripheral neuropathy is an important physical finding in its own right because it leads to gait unsteadiness and a predisposition to falling.

While the content of the physical examination will be much the same for older, as for younger patients, given time constraints, high-yield, relevant, but not as yet traditional, examination items should substitute for low-yield items. Low-yield items are those that have low specificity in older persons or that do not provide useful information concerning diagnosis, prognosis, or treatment. Examples include the Weber and Rinne tests, undilated eye examinations, Papanicolaou (Pap) smear after age 65 years if previous results were normal, and routine testing of patellar reflexes because of the wide variation in "normal range." Conversely, high-yield items that should become part of the standard physical examination of older persons are defined as findings common in older persons that provide useful diagnostic or prognostic information or suggest the presence of a modifiable condition associated with morbidity.

The functional tests described above are one example of high-yield items that should be part of the standard examination. Postural blood pressure, gait examination, inspection of ear canal for cerumen, hearing, visual acuity, and foot examination are other such examples.

Laboratory and Ancillary Tests

As for the physical examination, the coexistence of diseases and age-related changes may affect the sensitivity, specificity, predictive value, and interpretability of laboratory, imaging, and other ancillary tests. In addition, age-referenced normal values and ranges have been developed for many laboratory tests. Issues related to diagnostic testing in older persons are discussed further in Chaps. 11 and 12.

MANAGEMENT

Treatment decisions should be predicated on attaining feasible patient goals, particularly as treatment of one condition may worsen another and as many treatments adversely effect comfort and functioning. The increased chance of harm as well as benefit of most interventions in older persons dictate that a delineation of risks, benefits, and tradeoffs should constitute an initial step in management. Furthermore, the coexistence of multiple conditions and the contribution of multiple factors to individual conditions require a prioritization of possible interventions to maximize adherence and benefit and minimize harm and burden.

Medication prescribing offers a particular challenge. There are an ever expanding list of medications available for treating chronic diseases and nondisease specific symptoms. Prescribing decisions need to be made within the context of patient preference and with an appreciation of total medication burden not solely the benefit and harm of each individual medication for an individual disease. The cost of medications is another significant medication-related issue in many older patients. Issues related to medication use in older patients are discussed in Chap. 19.

Because many health conditions in older persons result from the accumulated effect of psychological, social, and environmental, as well as purely medical, factors, a multicomponent, integrated treatment plan represents the most effective strategy. The use of nonpharmacologic interventions is one of the most effective ways to minimize medication use. For many health conditions, including diabetes mellitus, arthritis, congestive heart failure, depression, pain, and sleep disorders, treatment should include a combination of pharmacologic, rehabilitative, psychosocial, and environmental interventions. Exercise and physical activity are proven interventions for each of these conditions. Counseling and cognitive behavior therapy are important treatment components for depression, pain, and sleep disorders. Interdisciplinary teams, as discussed in Chap. 21 are essential to the successful implementation of these multicomponent interventions.

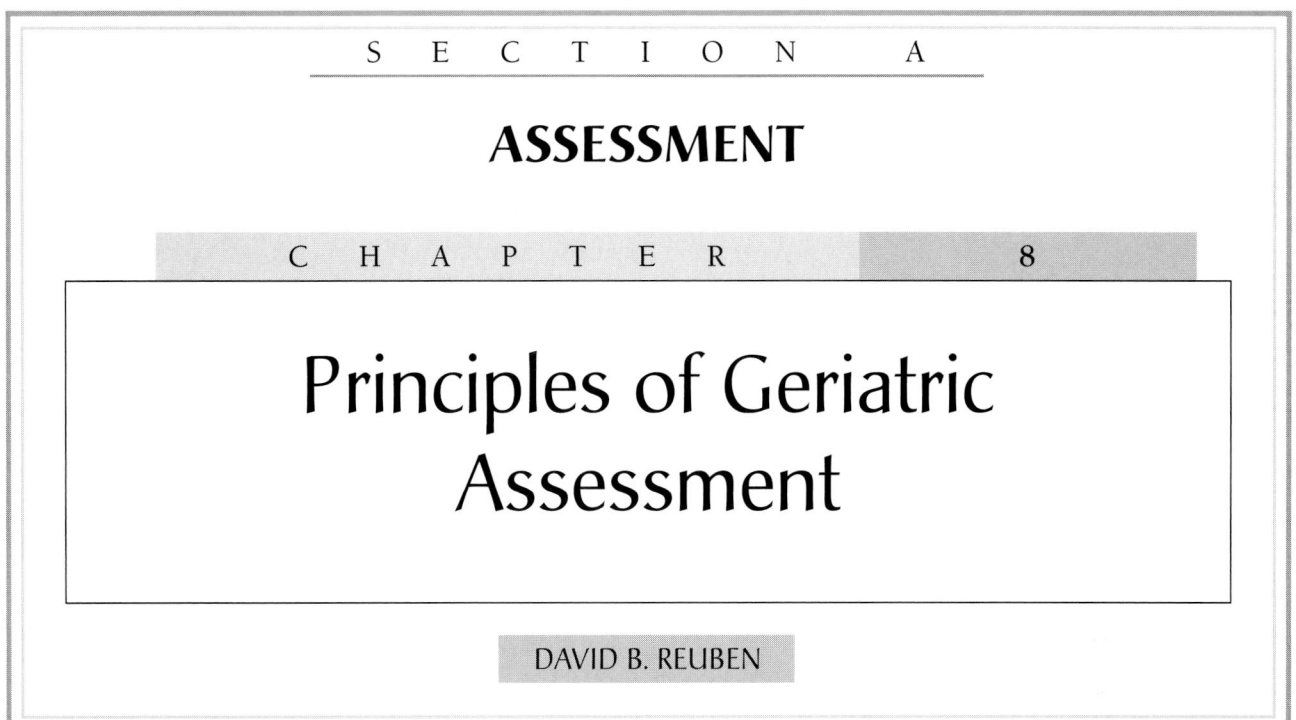

S E C T I O N   A

ASSESSMENT

C H A P T E R   8

Principles of Geriatric Assessment

DAVID B. REUBEN

Geriatric assessment is a broad term used to describe the health evaluation of the older patient, which emphasizes an approach different from that of the standard medical evaluation. This approach recognizes that the health status of older persons is dependent upon influences beyond the manifestations of their medical conditions. Among these are social, psychological and mental health, and environmental factors. Geriatric assessment also places high value upon functional status, both as a dimension to be evaluated and as an outcome to be improved or maintained.

Although in the strictest sense geriatric assessment is a diagnostic process, many use the term to include both evaluation and management. Moreover, geriatric assessment is sometimes used to refer to evaluation by the individual clinician and at other times is used to refer to a more intensive interdisciplinary process, comprehensive geriatric assessment (CGA). The terminology is further clouded because the latter process has evolved since its inception with respect to sites where the assessment is provided, the participating health professionals, the nature of the assessment, and the amount of follow-up and management that is included. Accordingly, any discussion of geriatric assessment must be precise in its description of the process of interest. This chapter is divided into these components: (1) geriatric assessment by the individual clinician, with an emphasis on the outpatient setting; (2) a strategic approach to geriatric assessment for the practicing clinician; (3) comprehensive geriatric assessment and evidence for its effectiveness; and (4) lessons learned from geriatric assessment that have been applied to health care delivery of older persons.

GERIATRIC ASSESSMENT BY THE INDIVIDUAL CLINICIAN

Geriatric assessment (Fig. 8-1) by the individual clinician extends beyond the traditional medical evaluation of older persons' health to include assessment of cognitive, affective, functional, social, economic, environmental, and spiritual status, as well as a discussion of patient preferences regarding advance directives. Assessment instruments can be used to guide these evaluations but do not substitute for clinical skills and judgment, including the skill of eliciting important items from the patient's history and physical examination. Information obtained from assessment instruments can direct the clinician's attention to issues that are particularly relevant to an individual patient. Systematic assessment of the multiple domains noted above ensures that the evaluation is comprehensive. Some clinicians may prefer to rely on less-formal questions to probe into potential problems. (Examples of potential open-ended questions are provided later in this chapter.)

Geriatric assessment differs according to the setting where the patient is being evaluated. In the hospital setting, the initial assessment is usually directed at the acute medical problem that precipitated the hospitalization. As the patient begins to recover and plans are initiated for discharge, other components (e.g., social support, environment) assume increasing importance in the assessment. The inpatient setting can be problematic for geriatric assessment because of the rapidly changing status of several key dimensions. For example, a patient may temporarily

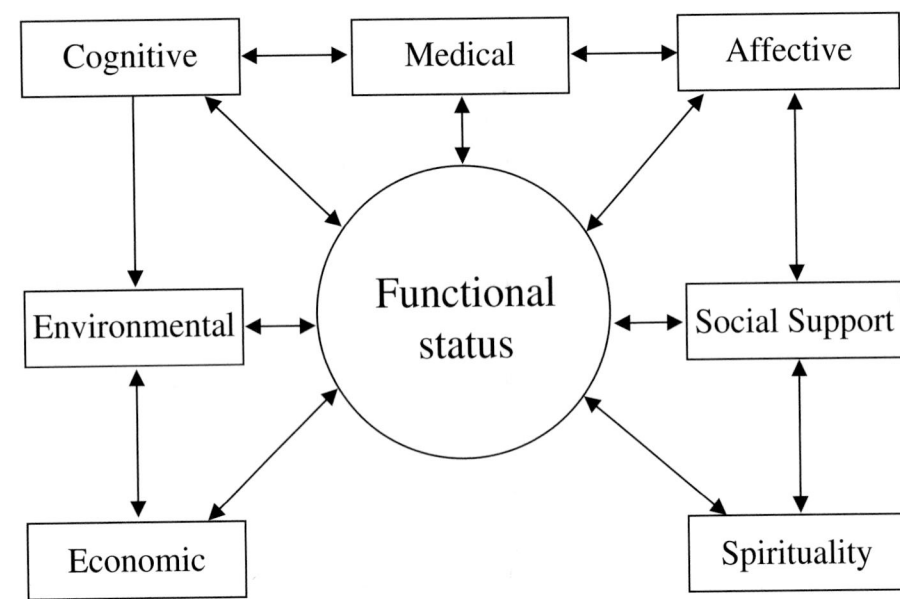

Figure 8-1 Interacting dimensions of geriatric assessment.

become "dependent" on all measures of functional status when acutely ill and gradually improve prior to discharge. Because patients may overestimate their functional status based on their previous level of functioning, direct observational methods (e.g., by nurses or physical therapists) may provided a more accurate assessment. The patient's full potential to participate in rehabilitation may not be known until near the time of discharge.

Nursing home geriatric assessment requires that closer attention be directed to selected aspects of assessment such as nutritional status and self care activities. Other components such as functional status at the instrumental activities of daily living level are less relevant in this setting. Geriatric assessment conducted in the patient's home provides an opportunity for an entirely different type of assessment; environmental factors can be directly assessed while other aspects of the traditional examination (e.g., the gynecologic examination) are much more difficult.

Because the primary site of most clinicians' practices is the office setting, assessment techniques are described primarily for this setting. When appropriate, differing or particularly important information about assessment in other settings is added.

Components of the Geriatric Assessment

In addition to the standard medical history and physical examination, the clinician should systematically search for specific conditions that are common among older persons and that might have considerable impact on function. In the course of the traditional medical evaluation, these problems may go unnoticed because older patients fail to report them spontaneously. For example, they may not recognize that falling is a treatable medical problem. They also may be embarrassed to mention problems with maintaining urinary continence or with sexual function. Finally, they may believe that these symptoms, such as hearing loss, are normal aspects of aging that cannot be helped.

Visual Impairment

Although many older persons seek eye care directly from optometrists, opticians, and ophthalmologists, the high rates of vision disorders and impairment and the brevity of the screening process justifies screening. Each of the four major eye diseases (cataract, age-related macular degeneration, diabetic retinopathy, and glaucoma) increases in prevalence with age. Moreover, presbyopia is virtually universal and the vast majority of older persons require eyeglasses.

The standard method of screening for problems with visual acuity is the Snellen eye chart, which requires the patient to stand 20 feet from the chart and read letters, using corrective lenses. Patients fail the screen if they are unable to read all the letters on the 20/40 line with their eyeglasses (best corrected vision).

Several interviewer and self-administered instruments to detect functional problems caused by visual impairment have been developed, including the "Activities of Daily Vision Scale" and the VF-14. These are primarily used in research settings, but may hold some promise as screening instruments in the future.

Hearing Impairment

Hearing impairment is among the most common medical conditions reported by older persons, affecting approximately one-third of those 65 years of age or older. Hearing impairment is associated with reduced cognitive, emotional, social, and physical function in older persons and the use of amplification devices has led to improved functional status and quality of life of older persons.

Screening for hearing loss can be accomplished by several methods (Table 8-1). The most accurate of these is the Welch Allyn AudioScope 3 (Welch Allyn, Inc., Skaneateles Falls, NY), a hand-held otoscope with a built-in audiometer. The AudioScope 3 can be set at a several different levels of intensity, but should be set at 40 dB to evaluate hearing in older persons. A pretone at 60 dB is delivered and then four tones (500, 1000, 2000, and 4000 Hz) at 40 dB are

Table 8-1 Simple Tests of Hearing Loss

Question/Test	Time to Administer	Comments
Audioscope	1–2 minutes	Sensitivity 87–90%, specificity 70–90%
Whisper test	1 minute	Sensitivity 80–100%, specificity 82–89%
Hearing handicap	2 minutes	Sensitivity 48–63%, specificity 75–86% at cutpoint >8

Inventory for the elderly NHANES* battery
  Age >70 = 1
  Male sex = 1
  ≤12th grade education = 1
  previously saw doctor about trouble
    hearing = 1
  without hearing aid, cannot hear
    whisper across the room = 1
  without hearing aid, cannot hear
    normal voice across the room = 2
	<2 minutes	Sensitivity 80%, specificity 80% at cutpoint of >3

*National Health and Nutrition Examination Survey

delivered. Patients fail the screen if they are unable to hear either the 1000- or 2000-Hz frequency in both ears or both the 1000- and 2000-Hz frequencies in one ear, indicating the need for formal audiometric testing.

An alternative is the whispered voice test, which is administered by whispering three to six random words (numbers, words, or letters) at a set distance (6, 8, 12, or 24 inches) from the person's ear and then asking the patient to repeat the words. The examiner should be behind the person to prevent speech reading and the opposite ear should be covered or occluded during the examination. Patients fail the screen if they are unable to repeat half of the whispered words correctly.

Similar to vision screening, a self-administered test of emotional and social problems associated with impaired hearing, the Hearing Handicap Inventory for the Elderly–Screening Version (HHIE-S) was developed. Although this questionnaire is brief and easy to administer, its accuracy when compared to audiometry is less than the audiometer. Another screening instrument that uses sociodemographic information coupled with three simple questions (Table 8-1) about hearing loss has high accuracy in identifying older persons with hearing loss.

Malnutrition/Weight Loss

Malnutrition is a global term that encompasses many different nutritional problems that are associated with diverse health consequences. Both extremes of body weight place older people at risk for subsequent functional impairment, morbidity, and mortality. Among community-dwelling older persons, the most common nutritional disorder is obesity. In addition, a small percentage of community-dwelling older persons have energy or protein energy undernutrition, which places them at higher risk for death and functional decline. Protein energy undernutrition is defined by the presence of clinical (physical signs such as wasting, low body mass index) *and* biochemical (albumin or other protein) evidence of insufficient

intake. Although the importance of low serum albumin and low cholesterol as prognostic factors for mortality in community-dwelling, hospitalized, and institutionalized older persons has been demonstrated, these tests may reflect inflammation rather than malnutrition.

Several methods of nutritional screening can be applied in office settings. On their initial visit, patients should be asked about weight loss within the previous 6 months. All patients should be weighed at every office visit. Height should also be measured on the initial visit to allow calculation of body mass index (weight in kg/[height in meters]^2). Several self-administered nutritional questionnaires are available, most notably the Nutrition Screening Initiative's 10-item checklist and the Mini-Nutritional Assessment. Although the validity of these instruments has been questioned, they are being increasingly used in community-based screening programs.

In hospital settings, when nutritional needs are great, energy and protein intake should be monitored closely. Intake can be measured through formal calorie counts. Laboratory monitoring may also be useful. Although serum albumin levels can drop acutely during inflammatory states, physiologic stress, and in response to trauma or surgical conditions, this protein has a long half-life (approximately 18 days). Accordingly, obtaining serum albumin level at the time of hospital admission provides an idea of the patient's baseline nutritional status. Prealbumin, which has a much shorter half-life (approximately 2 days) may be a better means of monitoring response to nutritional treatment. Serum cholesterol may also be valuable in monitoring hospitalized patients as falling values have been associated with increased morbidity and mortality.

Urinary Incontinence

Urinary incontinence is common, especially among older women, and is underrecognized. Women may be embarrassed to raise the issue; they also may regard it as a normal aspect of aging.

Table 8–2   Simple Tests of Lower Extremities: Strength, Balance, Gait, and Fall Risk

Question/Test	Time to Administer	Comments
Timed up and go	<1 minute	Sensitivity 88%, specificity 94% compared to geriatrician's evaluation using cutpoint >15 seconds

Office-based maneuvers
  Observed gait
  Resistance to nudge
  Tandem/semitandem stand
  Rising from chair
  360° turn
	2–3 minutes	Some are part of Performance-Oriented Assessment of Mobility

Functional reach	2 minutes	Adjusted odds ratios for >2 falls within 6 months
		  8.1 if unable to reach
		  4.0 if reach ≤6″
		  2.0 if reach ≥6″ but <10″

Incontinence can be screened for by asking two questions: (1) "In the last year, have you ever lost your urine and gotten wet?" and if so, (2) "Have you lost urine on at least six separate days?" In a recent study, those who answered positive to both questions had high rates (79 percent for women and 76 percent for men) of urinary incontinence as determined by a clinician's evaluation (see Chap. 123).

Balance and Gait Impairments and Falling

The risk of falling can be assessed (Table 8-2) by testing balance, gait, and lower extremity strength (see Chap. 118). Moreover, the assessment of these components may also help identify methods to improve the patient's function beyond simply reducing the risk of falling.

Clinicians should ask their older persons specifically about falls, which should be included in the review of systems at each visit. The report of any fall should prompt subsequent questions by the clinician to determine the circumstances of the fall. Patients with recurrent falls or falls with any injury should receive a more detailed evaluation, including assessment of gait and balance, orthostatic blood pressure readings, vision testing, and reviewing medications that may contribute to the risk of falling (see chap. 118). Balance and gait disorders are best assessed by observing patients walking and performing balance maneuvers. Once the clinician is trained to assess gait, this evaluation can be performed while the patient is entering or leaving the examining room.

Several simple tests of balance and mobility can also be performed quickly in the office setting, including the ability to maintain a side-by-side, semitandem, and full-tandem stance for 10 seconds; resistance to a nudge; and stability during a 360-degree turn. Quadriceps strength can be briefly assessed by observing an older person arising from a hard armless chair without the use of his or her hands. The timed "up and go" test is a timed measure of the patients ability to rise arm chair, walk 3 meters (10 feet), turn, walk back, and sit down again; those who take longer than 20 seconds to complete the test merit further evaluation. The Performance-Oriented Assessment of Mobility is a standardized battery that measures gait and balance; it has been widely used in research and in some clinical settings, but may take too long to administer to be practical in most office settings. The ability to stretch as measured by functional reach, a test of balance, can predict subsequent recurrent falls.

Polypharmacy

Because older persons often receive care from multiple providers and because they may fill prescriptions at several pharmacies, each patient should be instructed to bring in all current medications—both prescription and nonprescription medications,—to each visit. Office personnel can check these against the medication list in the medical record and discrepancies can be brought to the clinician's attention at the time of the patient encounter. Several drug interaction programs are commercially available to check for potential drug–drug interactions. With the introduction of personal digital assistants and drug software programs, clinicians can easily assess the potential for drug–drug interactions at the time of prescribing any new medication. The use of four or more prescription and nonprescription medications should trigger a review and consideration of continued need for each medication given the increased risk of adverse drug effect with increasing number of medications.

Cognitive Assessment

Because the prevalence of Alzheimer's disease, other dementias, and cognitive impairment, rises considerably with advancing age, the yield of screening for cognitive impairment increases with age. The most commonly used screen is the Mini-Mental State Examination, a 30-item interviewer-administered assessment of several dimensions of cognitive function. However, it is too long for most practitioners to routinely incorporate into their clinical practices. Several shorter screens (Table 8-3) have also been validated including recall of three items at 1 minute, the clock drawing test, and the Mini-Cog test, which

Table 8-3 Predictive Value of Brief Screening Questions for Cognitive Impairment

Test	Test Result	Likelihood Ratio
Orientation		
Day	Abnormal	6.3
	Normal	0.5
Month	Abnormal	16
	Normal	0.4
Year	Abnormal	37
	Normal	0.5
Forward digit-span	≤4 digits	7.1
	5 digits	2.0
	6 digits	0.8
	7 digits	0.1
Recall of 3 items	Recalls <2	3.1
	Recalls 2	0.5
	Recalls all 3	0.06
Clock drawing	Abnormal	24
	Almost normal	0.8
	Normal	0.2
Mini-Cog	Abnormal	14.1
	Normal	0.01
Time and Change	Abnormal	3.0
	Normal	0.2

SOURCE: Adapted from Siu AL (1991).

combines three-item recall and clock drawing. The Time-and-Change test, which employs clock recognition and counting change, is another valid screening test. The clock drawing components of these tests evaluate executive function (which includes higher cognitive processing) and appear to be less influenced by educational level or culture than some other cognitive assessments. Although normal results on these tests vastly reduce the probability of dementia and abnormal results increase the likelihood that the patient has dementia, these tests are neither diagnostic for dementia nor do normal results exclude the possibility of this disorder. Patients who have abnormal findings on a cognitive screening test should receive more in-depth evaluation of memory, language, visual–spatial, and executive function.

Among hospitalized patients, mental status should be assessed at the time of hospital admission and then periodically because older persons are especially prone to develop delirium during the hospital stay. Abnormal findings on the mental status examination in hospitalized patients must be interpreted in the context of change from baseline and the clinical situation. The Confusion Assessment Method provides a guide to interpreting such changes.

Affective Assessment

Although major depression is no more common among the elderly than among the younger population, symptoms of depression and other affective disorders are common and cause considerable morbidity. A simple inquiry such as "Do you often feel sad or depressed?" can be used as a screen. This single question, however, tends to be overly sensitive and may be better used in tandem with a second screen such as the Geriatric Depression Scale, which has 5-, 15-, and 30-item versions. A variety of other screens for depression are available and each has its advantages and disadvantages.

Assessment of Function

Measurement of functional status is an essential component of the assessment of older persons. The patient's ability to function can be viewed as a summary measure of the overall impact of health conditions in the context of his or her environment and social support system. Moreover, in older persons, the ability to function consistent with their personal lifestyle desires should be an important consideration in all care planning. Therefore, changes in functional status should prompt further diagnostic evaluation and intervention. An early indicator of impending functional disability is self-perceived difficulty with performing functional tasks. Measurement of functional status is also valuable in monitoring response to treatment and may provide prognostic information that will help plan for long-term care.

Functional status can be assessed at three levels: basic activities of daily living (BADLs), instrumental or intermediate activities of daily living (IADLs), and advanced activities of daily living (AADLs). Basic activities of daily living refer to self-care tasks such as bathing, dressing, toileting, continence, grooming, feeding, and transferring. Instrumental activities of daily living refer to the ability to maintain an independent household such as shopping for groceries, driving or using public transportation, using the telephone, meal preparation, housework, home repair, laundry, taking medications, and handling finances, whereas AADLs refer to the ability to fulfill societal, community, and family roles as well as participate in recreational or occupational tasks. These advanced activities vary considerably from individual to individual but may be valuable in monitoring functional status prior to the development of disability.

Scales that measure functional status at each of these levels have been developed and validated. Questions that ask about specific BADL and IADL functions have also been incorporated into a variety of more generic health-related quality-of-life instruments (e.g., the Medical Outcomes Study Short-form 36 and its shorter version, the SF-12). Some AADLs (e.g., exercise and leisure time physical activity) can be also be ascertained by using standardized instruments, but open-ended questions about how older persons spend their days might provide a better assessment of function in healthier older persons.

Over the past decade, there has been emerging interest in assessment of physical functioning by directly observing the performance of functional tasks (see also Chap. 73). Instruments have been developed for use in ambulatory, nursing home, and hospital settings, and predictive validity has been demonstrated for many. To date, these instruments are rarely incorporated into clinical practice, but some demonstration projects are in place that are attempting to use performance-based instruments in practice, much like vital signs, to monitor patients. Some recent studies demonstrate that combining self-reported functional with performance-based measures can provide more refined prognostic information than either method alone.

Assessment of Social Support

The composition of the older patient's social support structure can be assessed by asking a few questions about it when obtaining the social history. The quality of these relationships should also be determined. For very frail older persons, the availability of assistance from family and friends is frequently the determining factor of whether a functionally dependent older person remains at home or is institutionalized. If dependency is noted during functional assessment, the clinician should inquire as to who provides help for specific BADL and IADL functions and whether these persons are paid or voluntary help. Even in healthier older persons, it is often valuable to raise the question of who would be available to help if the patient becomes ill. Early identification of problems with social support may prompt planning to develop resources should the necessity arise.

Economic Assessment

Although some clinicians feel uncomfortable in assessing the economic status of their patients, insurance status is routinely collected by office staff. The patient's income can also be assessed and eligibility for state or local benefits (e.g., In Home Supportive Services through Medicaid) to provide services for the functionally impaired can be determined. For the frail and functionally impaired, physicians may need to begin discussions of planning to mobilize savings and other resources to provide personal attendant care.

Environmental Assessment

Environmental assessment encompasses two dimensions, the safety of the home environment and the adequacy of the patient's access to needed personal and medical services. Particularly among frail individuals and those with mobility and balance problems, the home environment should be assessed for safety. Although most physicians do not personally conduct environmental assessments, the National Safety Council has developed a home safety checklist that patients and their families can complete. For those receiving home health services, in-home safety inspections can be performed, including recommendations for installation of adaptive devices such as shower bars and raised toilet seats.

Older persons who begin to develop IADL dependencies should be evaluated for the geographic proximity of necessary services such as grocery shopping and banking, their need for use of such services, and their ability to use these services in their current living situations.

Spirituality

Spirituality, whether affiliated with a formal religious denomination or nonreligious intangible elements, has increasingly been recognized as an important influence on health. Recent data indicate that frequent attendance of religious services is associated with lower health care utilization and mortality rates. Formal instruments assessing spirituality have been developed but are not yet widely used in clinical practice. Simply asking older persons whether religion or spirituality is important to them may provide insights that may facilitate their care. Especially in hospital settings, involvement of pastoral care may be valuable in supporting the patient and in framing medical decisions in the context of the patient's personal belief system.

Advance Directives

Discussions of advance directives are important for all patients and should be initiated early on to discuss the patients' goals and preferences for care should they become unable to speak for themselves because of progressive cognitive impairment or acute illness. A particularly important time to discuss such preferences is prior to surgery because of the possibility of surgical complications or postoperative delirium, which may preclude discussions following the procedure. The durable power of attorney for health care, which asks the patient to designate a surrogate to make medical decisions if the patient loses decision-making capacity, is often less emotionally laden than specifying treatments that the patient may or may not want. Such discussions should be revisited any time there are significant changes in a patient's medical condition and a better understanding about prognosis becomes available. Patients often revise their thoughts about the benefits of treatment. Cultural differences regarding preferences for advance directives and end-of-life care should be recognized and respected.

A Strategic Approach to Geriatric Assessment

The practice of medicine in office settings is in a state of transition from a previous era of medicine when physicians practiced more like individual artisans to an approach in which physicians function as members of a health care team. Much of the germane information of the medical history can be obtained from old records, other professional or nonprofessional staff, or by self-report from patients or family members completing forms, rather than from direct physician interview. Although many physicians and patients lament such changes, this efficiency allows the physician to spend more time following up on issues raised by the available information, conducting the physical examination, discussing treatment, and providing health education.

One effort adopted by many clinical practices has been the use of previsit questionnaires that can be completed by the patient or proxy before the clinical encounter. These questionnaires typically gather information on past medical history, medications, preventive measures, and functional status, including information on who helps when the patient is functionally dependent. As a result, they can markedly reduce the time needed to conduct an initial assessment and can ensure a consistent level of

Table 8-4 Multidimensional Screening Instruments

Problem	Screening Measure	Screening Package Characteristics		
		Positive Screen	Positive Predictive Value	Negative Predictive Value
Vision	Two parts: Ask: "Do you have difficulty driving, or watching television, or reading, or doing any of your daily actvites because of your eyesight?" If yes, then: Test each eye with Snellen chart while patient wears corrective lenses (if applicable).	Yes to question and inability to read greater than 20/40 on Snellen chart.	0.75	0.89
Hearing	Use audiometer set at 40 dB. Test hearing using 1000 and 2000 Hz.	Inability to hear 1000 or 2000 Hz in both ears or either of these frequencies in one ear.	0.75	0.91
Leg mobility	Time the patient after asking: "Rise from the chair. Walk 20 feet briskly, turn, walk back to the chair and sit down."	Unable to complete task in 15 seconds.	0.91	0.92
Urinary incontinence	Two parts: Ask: "In the last year, have you ever lost your urine and gotten wet?" If yes, then ask: "Have you lost urine on at least 6 separate days?"	Yes to both questions.	0.86	0.96
Nutrition/weight loss	Two parts: Ask: "Have you lost 10 lbs. over the past 6 months without trying to do so?" Weigh the patient.	Yes to the question or weight <100 lb.	0.62	0.92
Memory	Three-item recall.	Unable to remember all three items after 1 minute.	0.60	0.92
Depression	Ask: "Do you often feel sad or depressed?"	Yes to the question.	0.71	0.90
Physical disability	Six questions: "Are you able to . . . : ". . . do strenuous activities such as fast walking or bicycling?" ". . . do heavy work around the house such as washing windows, walls, or floors?" ". . . go shopping for groceries or clothes?" ". . . get to places out of walking distance?" ". . . bathe, either a sponge bath, tub bath, or shower?" ". . . dress, such as putting on a shirt, buttoning and zipping, or putting on shoes?"	No to any of the questions.	0.88	0.77

SOURCE: Adapted from Moore AA and Siu AS (1996).

Table 8–5   Multidimensional Case-Finding Instruments Used, with References and Average Performance Time

Problem	Instrument (Reference)	Average Time to Perform (min)($n = 37$)	Cost Per Case Receiving a New Diagnosis or Treatment
Cognitive impairment	Mini-Mental State Examination	9.2	$68
Depression	Geriatric Depression Scale	5.1	$17
Gait instability	Performance-Oriented Assessment of Mobility	2.5	$15
Malnutrition	Mid-arm circumference using gender-specific criteria	1.0	$15
Recent weight loss	Review of weights in chart	0.275	$8
Hearing impairment	Whisper test	0.55	<$1
Vision impairment	Hand-held Snellen chart	2.1	$10
Urinary incontinence	Specific question	0.275	<$1
Sexual problem	Questions regarding general function and specific problems	0.825	$14

Source: Adapted from Miller et al. (1995).

comprehensiveness for every patient. By including validated screening instruments, they can also be used to case-find individuals with common geriatric syndromes.

A second method of streamlining the office visit is to delegate the administration of screening instruments for many of the important geriatric problems to trained office staff. Thus, the clinician may spend a short period of time reviewing the results of these screens and then decide which dimensions, if any, need greater evaluation. Several groups (Table 8-4) have demonstrated the feasibility and yield of using office staff to administer case-finding and screening instruments that assess many of the dimensions described above. This approach can dramatically improve the practitioner's efficiency and increase the number of new and treatable problems detected in their older patients. However, using office-based staff to screen or case-find has cost implications. Office staff must be properly trained to administer these instruments, which can be quite time-consuming. One published method takes approximately 22 minutes to administer and another takes an estimated 10 minutes to administer. This time must be taken from other office tasks and the cost of screening may be considerable (Table 8-5). Clinicians must also be able to effectively act on this information to improve clinical outcomes. Nevertheless, as physicians become increasingly pressured to increase their productivity, such methods may be the only way to feasibly ensure that older patients' diverse health needs are addressed comprehensively.

Table 8-6 shows a strategy that optimizes the clinician's time by employing the most efficient methods to obtain assessment information. The initial step provides the clinician with basic information that can quickly be processed and followed with more extensive data gathering, when appropriate. Such a strategy begins with the pre-visit questionnaire and then is supplemented by information obtained by office staff. These two data sources are reviewed by the clinician and additional information is obtained from the patient and family at the time of the visit.

COMPREHENSIVE GERIATRIC ASSESSMENT

Comprehensive geriatric assessment is based on the premise that a systematic evaluation of frail older persons by a team of health professionals may uncover treatable health problems and lead to better health outcomes. Early randomized clinical trials provided convincing evidence that such programs conducted in hospital-based and rehabilitation units, which typically required several weeks of treatment, could lead to better survival rates, improved functional status, and more desirable placement (e.g., home rather than nursing home) following discharge from the hospital. Conceptually, comprehensive geriatric assessment is a three-step process: (1) screening or targeting of appropriate patients, (2) assessment and development of recommendations, and (3) implementation of recommendations, including physician and patient adherence with recommendations. Each of these steps is essential if the process is to be successful at achieving health and functional benefits.

Within this broad conceptualization, CGA has been implemented using many different models in various health care settings (Table 8-7). Because of changes in length of hospital stays, an increasing number of CGA programs are relying on postdischarge and community-based assessment. Furthermore, most of the early programs focused on restorative or rehabilitative goals (tertiary prevention), whereas many newer programs are aimed at primary and secondary prevention.

Table 8-6   Strategy for Efficient Office-based Assessment

Aspect Being Assessed	Method and Depth of Assessment*				
	Previsit Questionnaire	Office Staff Administered	Clinician Routine	Clinician as needed	Referral† as needed
Past medical history	D		R		
Geriatric syndromes/ health conditions					
Visual impairment	B	B	R		Ophthalmologist or optometrist
Hearing impairment	B	B (if needed)	R		Audiologist
Urinary incontinence	B		R	D(office urodynamics)	Geriatrician, urologist, or gynecologist
Malnutrition	D		R		Dietitian or social worker
Sexual dysfunction	B		R		Urologist or geriatrician
Polypharmacy	B		R		Pharmacist or geriatrician
Dental Problems	B		R		Dentist
Gait, balance, falls	B		B	D	Physical therapist
Affective problems	D		R	D	Psychiatrist
Cognitive problems		B	R	D	Geriatrician, psychiatrist, or neurologist
Functional disability	D		R	D	Physical or occupational therapist social worker
Environmental problems	D		R		Home health
Preventive services	D		R		

*B, brief screen (e.g., less than 2 minutes); D, detailed evaluation (usually 5 minutes or more); R, review of collected information
† Examples of referrals to specific health professional or comprehensive geriatric assessment might be used.

The purpose of the first step, targeting, is to distinguish elderly patients who are appropriate and will benefit from CGA, from those who are either too sick or are too well to benefit. To date, no easily administered targeting criteria have been demonstrated and validated to readily identify patients who are likely to benefit from CGA in different settings. Specific strategies used by CGA programs to identify older persons who are most appropriate for CGA have included chronological age, functional disability, physical illness, geriatric conditions, psychosocial conditions, and previous or predicted high health care utilization. All of these criteria have randomized clinical trial support for their effectiveness in identifying older persons likely to benefit from CGA. However, the definitions of these criteria and the interventions that have followed have varied from study to study.

Most CGA programs exclude patients who are unlikely to benefit because of terminal illness, severe dementia,

Table 8-7   Spectrum of CGA-like Interventions

	Most Intensive	← →	Least Intensive
Setting	CGA, GEM, and rehabilitation units	CGA consultation inpatient or outpatient	Community-based and in-home outreach programs
Targeting	Most restrictive		Least restrictive
Process	Large team, extensive evaluations		Screening and referral
Cost	Very expensive		Relatively inexpensive

CGA, comprehensive geriatric assessment; GEM, geriatric evaluation and management.

complete functional dependence and inevitable nursing home placement. Exclusionary criteria have also included identifying older persons who are "too healthy" to benefit.

The second step of CGA, the assessment process itself, continues to be highly variable across programs. The types of health care professionals included in the assessment team, the content of information collected, and the types and intensity of services provided have differed in studies of the effectiveness of CGA. In many settings, the CGA process relies on a core team consisting of a physician, nurse, and social worker and, when appropriate, draws upon an extended team of various combinations of physical and occupational therapists, nutritionists, pharmacists, psychiatrists, psychologists, dentists, audiologists, podiatrists, and opticians. Although these professionals are usually on staff in hospital settings and are available in the community, access to and reimbursement for these services have limited the effectiveness of the CGA process. Frequently, the composition of the team is determined by local expertise and availability of resources rather than programmatic needs. Increasingly, CGA programs are moving towards a "virtual team" concept in which members are included as needed, assessments are conducted at different locations on different days, and conferencing is completed via telephone or electronically.

Traditionally, the various components of the evaluation are completed by different members of the team. There is considerable variability in which professional conducts the assessments. For example, the medical assessment of older persons may be conducted by a physician, nurse practitioner, or physician's assistant. The core team may conduct only brief initial assessments or screens for some dimensions. These may be subsequently augmented with more in-depth evaluations by additional professionals. For example, a dietitian may be needed to assess dietary intake and provide recommendations; an audiologist may need to conduct a more extensive assessment of hearing loss and evaluate an older person for a hearing aid.

Components of Comprehensive Geriatric Assessment

The key elements of the process of care rendered by CGA teams can be divided into six steps: (1) data gathering; (2) discussion among the team; (3) development of a treatment plan; (4) implementation of the treatment plan; (5) monitoring response to the treatment plan; and (6) revising the treatment plan.

Data Gathering

In early studies of CGA, the data-gathering process simply identified the members of the team and mentioned that each conducted an evaluation. Such descriptions are problematic because of the variability of evaluations among health professionals. A formal training process can reduce this variability, but a popular approach is to standardize the assessment. Standardized assessments can either use

instruments developed specifically for clinical purposes or assemble standard instruments that have previously been studied for validity and reliability. The advantage of the former is that teams can customize the information being gathered to best suit the clinical needs of the program. The advantage of the latter is that patients in the program can be compared to patients in other programs. Frequently, however, these instruments were developed for purposes other than to guide clinical decision-making and may provide information that is not very helpful in the care of patients.

Discussion Among Team

Following initial data gathering, the team meets to discuss the patient's geriatric needs. Although any member of the team could theoretically lead the conference, the leadership is usually determined by local culture. Each conference typically begins with short discipline-specific presentations followed by interactive discussions among professionals. Sometimes additional information will need to be obtained before final recommendations can be made. The team then identifies problems that need action and might be responsive to treatment.

Development of Treatment Plan

Based upon this discussion, the team develops an initial treatment plan and goals for the patient. If the number of recommendations resulting from CGA is large, it is necessary to prioritize recommendations. CGA teams should advise primary care physicians and patients to focus on the major recommendations, those that are most likely to produce the desired outcomes. The urgency of recommendations must also be determined. Although some recommendations may need to be implemented immediately to confer short-term benefit such as stopping a medication that may be the cause of delirium, many more may be better implemented once the patient is stable.

At the time of the assessment, a plan for implementation of each recommendation must be developed. It needs to be determined who will assume responsibility for initiation and completion of the recommendation. Similarly, the team must establish a plan for monitoring the patient's progress as treatment is being delivered.

Implementation of the Treatment Plan

Because of the problem of poor adherence to CGA recommendations, the issue of implementation is particularly critical to the success of CGA consultation programs. Among inpatient CGA models, poor implementation rates may explain some negative trials of hospital consultation models of CGA. Failure to implement recommendations is usually attributable to three problems: (1) poor receptivity among primary care physicians whose patients have been assessed using consultative models; (2) inadequate resources to implement recommendations; and (3) poor continuity or follow-through on recommendations after hospital discharge. In ambulatory settings, patient adherence to recommendations emanating from CGA looms as an even larger obstacle to implementation. Patients may simply choose not to return to see the CGA team (in continuity of care models) or ignore recommendations in a consultative model.

A variety of options for implementation are available ranging from direct implementation of recommendations by the team to merely advising physicians and patients by a note in the chart or verbally. In consultative models of CGA in some ambulatory settings, patients have been provided with direct advice and instructions on how to approach their physicians to discuss CGA recommendations (patient empowerment). This method, coupled with direct communication to primary care physicians, has resulted in high implementation rates of CGA recommendations. Other approaches to improve adherence by primary care physicians have been by direct telephone contact, letters, faxes, and e-mail.

Monitoring

To ensure that recommendations are implemented and to follow a patient's progress through the treatment plan, patients must be monitored directly by the CGA team or by the primary care physician. If the team is to monitor the patient, key issues are how frequently and for how long this monitoring should occur. The more intensively and the longer patients are followed, the more resource intensive the consultation becomes. In some models (described below), the CGA team may temporarily assume primary care for several months before returning the patient to the primary care physician for ongoing care.

Revising the Treatment Plan

By monitoring the patient, CGA teams can continually assess the patients progress toward meeting the goals established by the team. If progress is not proceeding according to expectations, the team may need to reevaluate the patient and resume the team discussion. Treatment recommendations and implementation plans may need to be revised. Any modification will require additional monitoring. The frequency and extensiveness of reevaluations and additional discussions are important influences on the cost of CGA consultation. The more extensive this continued reevaluation becomes, the more expensive the consultation becomes.

Effectiveness of CGA

In virtually all studies of CGA, the process itself has resulted in improved detection and documentation of geriatric problems. However, such identification of problems has not always led to improved outcomes. A 1993 meta-analysis of five models of CGA (geriatric evaluation and management units, inpatient geriatrics consultation services, home assessment services, home assessment services for patients who had recently been discharged, and outpatient assessment services) summarized the evidence to date on traditional models of CGA.

Geriatric Evaluation and Management Units

The most consistent findings of the meta-analysis indicated that the hospital or rehabilitation unit model of CGA had the strongest and most consistent benefits on mortality, living at home, and functional status. However, the geriatric evaluation and management unit may no longer confer the same benefits in the current environment. A recently completed multisite randomized clinical trial within the US Department of Veterans Affairs demonstrated little benefit of such units when compared to usual care, which may have improved considerably since the early 1980s.

Inpatient Consultation

Both the meta-analysis and a subsequent large negative randomized clinical trial of inpatient geriatric assessment consultation, have suggested little benefit from this model of comprehensive geriatric assessment and it has largely been abandoned.

Posthospital Discharge Assessment and Management

Similarly, posthospitalization CGA conducted in the home was ineffective in the meta-analysis in reducing mortality, functional decline, or readmission rates. Although a subsequent randomized clinical trial confirmed these negative findings, a nursing-led program of comprehensive discharge planning and home follow-up has been more effective. Key elements included use of targeting criteria to identify appropriate patients, a program of comprehensive discharge planning (including multidimensional assessment) and home follow-up with advanced practice nurses who visited the patients at least every other day during the hospitalization and at least twice during the 4 weeks following discharge. These visits were supplemented by telephone calls. In a randomized clinical trial, this intervention was associated with reduced hospital readmissions and costs.

Outpatient Consultation

The meta-analysis did not demonstrate any benefit from outpatient CGA consultation. A subsequent randomized clinical trial was also negative. More recently, a model that combines CGA with an adherence intervention has been developed and tested. This program provided outpatient comprehensive geriatric assessment for community-dwelling older persons with functional disability, urinary incontinence, falls, or depressive symptoms. The assessment was then linked to an adherence intervention that was designed to empower the patient to take action and educate the physician. In a randomized clinical trial, this strategy was associated with less functional decline, less fatigue, and better social functioning and was cost-effective when compared with many commonly used treatments.

In-home Assessment

In the 1993 meta-analysis, home assessment programs, all of which were implemented and tested in Europe, demonstrated survival benefit at 36 months. Subsequently, a model of geriatric preventive services for unselected community-dwelling older persons used a geriatric nurse practitioner to provide periodic in-home assessments that were subsequently discussed with a multidisciplinary team. This intervention delayed functional decline and reduced nursing home placement in a randomized clinical trial. In a replication study, however, the benefit was confined to persons who were at low risk for nursing home admission.

LESSONS LEARNED FROM GERIATRIC ASSESSMENT

Despite unresolved issues regarding the effectiveness of CGA, the principles of comprehensive geriatric assessment have been incorporated into a number of programs that have been demonstrated to be effective. Several new models of outpatient care for older persons modify the basic structure of care. These models adopt various components of CGA including targeting, assessment, and interventions.

Geriatric evaluation and continuity management is a direct outgrowth of comprehensive geriatric assessment. These programs differ from CGA in that they become the source of ongoing primary care usually by interdisciplinary teams in geriatrics clinics. Randomized trials have indicated that this ongoing care has resulted in better perceived health, life satisfaction, affective health status, and quality of health and social care. One study demonstrated a significant benefit of geriatric evaluation and management (GEM) on instrumental activity of daily living functional status at 2 years. However, a recently completed trial of GEM within the Department of Veterans Affairs demonstrated no effect on most outcomes. Another type of continuity GEM assumes primary care of older persons who are at high risk for high health care utilization for an average of 6 months and then returns patients to the care of their primary care physicians. When evaluated in a randomized clinical trial, this approach reduced the risk of functional decline and reduced the likelihood of depression at a modest cost ($1250 per person). Randomized trials of collaborative practice models using physicians, nurses, and case assistants, and physicians, nurses, and social workers for targeted patients have demonstrated reduced 2-year mortality and fewer hospitalizations, respectively.

In summary, geriatric assessment continues to evolve beyond simply spending more time evaluating older persons. As assessment techniques become better standardized and validated, more efficient yet comprehensive approaches are possible. To date, implementation of such strategies has not occurred on a widespread basis. Cost, logistical, and training issues are still important barriers. The research agenda still must include testing whether these more efficient strategies can lead to better health outcomes.

Comprehensive geriatric assessment has also changed considerably as medicine has become increasingly cost conscious. Though effective, the long-stay units can no longer be sustained and the emphasis must shift to extending the effective components and principles into less expensive settings and programs. Although several examples of such successful progeny have already been developed and tested, undoubtedly, additional generations of CGA-like interventions will be forthcoming.

REFERENCES

Boorson S et al: The Mini-Cog: A cognitive "vital signs" measure for dementia screening in multi-lingual elderly. *Int J Geriatr Psychiatry* 15:1021, 2000.

Boult C et al: A randomized clinical trial of outpatient geriatric evaluation and management. *J Am Geriatr Soc* 49:351, 2001.

Cohen HJ et al: A controlled trial of inpatient and outpatient geriatric evaluation and management. *N Engl J Med* 346:905, 2002.

Gill TM et al: Difficulty and dependence: Two components of the disabled among community-living older persons. *Ann Intern Med* 128(2):96, 1998.

Halter JB, Reuben DB: Indicators of function in the geriatric population, in Finch CE, Vaupel JW, Kinsella K (eds): *Cells and Surveys: Should Biological Measures be Included in Social Science Research?* Washington, DC, National Academy Press, 2000, p 159.

Hays JC et al: The spiritual history scale in four dimensions (SHS-4): Validity and reliability. *Gerontologist* 41:239, 2001.

Hoyl MT et al: Development and testing of a five-item version of the Geriatrics Depression Scale. *J Am Geriatr Soc* 47:873, 1999.

Inouye SK et al: The time and change test: A simple screening test for dementia. *J Geron Med Sci* 53A:M281, 1998.

Inouye SK et al: Clarifying confusion: The confusion assessment method. A new method for detection of delirium. *Ann Intern Med* 113:941, 1990.

Mangione CM et al: Development of the "Activities of Daily Vision Scale": A measure of visual functional status. *Med Care* 30:1111, 1992.

Miller DK et al: Efficiency of geriatric case-finding in a private practitioner's office. *J Am Geriatr Soc* 43:533, 1995.

Moore AA, Siu AL: Screening for common problems in ambulatory elderly: Clinical confirmation of a screening instrument. *Am J Med* 100:438, 1996.

Mulrow CD, Lichtenstein MJ: Screening for hearing Impairment in the elderly. *J Gen Intern Med* 6:249, 1991.

Naylor MD et al: Comprehensive discharge planning and home follow-up of hospitalized elders: A randomized clinical trial. *JAMA* 281(7):613, 1999.

Reuben DB: Organizational interventions to improve health outcomes of older persons. *Med Care* 2002; 40:416–428.

Reuben DB et al: Nutrition screening in older persons. *J Am Geriatr Soc* 43:415, 1995.

Siu AL: Screening for dementia and investigating its causes. *Ann Intern Med* 115:122, 1991.

Steinberg EP et al: The VF-14: An index of functional impairment in patients with cataract. *Arch Opthalmol* 112:630, 1994.

Stuck AE et al: Comprehensive geriatric assessment: A meta-analysis of controlled trials. *Lancet* 342:1032, 1993.

Tinetti ME: Performance-oriented assessment of mobility problems in elderly patients. *J Am Geriatr Soc* 34:119, 1986.

Tombaugh TN, McIntyre NJ: The Mini-Mental State Examination: A comprehensive review. *J Am Geriatr Soc* 40:922, 1992.

Mental Status and Neurologic Examination in the Elderly

ALIREZA PAKKAR   •   JEFFREY L. CUMMINGS

In normal aging, changes in cognitive and neurologic functions are expected. To distinguish overt neurologic dysfunction from the neurologic concomitants of normal aging, the clinician must conduct a comprehensive mental status and neurologic examination. When establishing a neurologic diagnosis, the clinical history (i.e., history of the present illness, past medical history, social habits, occupational experience, family illness and disorders) generates a differential diagnosis that is further explored by pertinent observations documented on the mental status and neurologic examinations. Mental status assessment should evaluate cognition, emotion, and behavior. The neurologic examination provides data to develop diagnostic hypotheses formulated on the basis of the mental status examination. These clinical hypotheses determine the necessary laboratory, imaging, or specialized assessments. This chapter outlines the components of the mental status and neurologic examinations and the relevant assessment of the elderly.

MENTAL STATUS EXAMINATION

The elements of a comprehensive mental status examination include observational, neuropsychiatric, and cognitive assessments. Although each of these elements is presented separately, they are interrelated and collectively characterize the neurobehavioral function of the patient.

Observational Assessment

Observation of a patient's level of arousal or alertness, appearance, emotion, behavior, movements, and speech provides insight into their mental status.

Arousal/Alertness

An accurate assessment of a patient's mental status and neurologic function must first document the patient's alertness or level of arousal. Altered levels of consciousness can directly impact the patient's cognitive performance on

mental status testing and influence the examiner's interpretation of the test results. Furthermore, impaired consciousness (e.g. coma, stupor) may be indicative of a medical or neurologic condition requiring immediate medical intervention (e.g., cardiopulmonary intervention, neurosurgical evaluation).

Abnormal patterns of arousal include hypo-aroused or hyper-aroused states. Decreasing levels of arousal include lethargy, obtundation, stupor, and coma. The lethargic patient is drowsy or fatigued and falls asleep if not stimulated. Obtundation refers to a state of moderately reduced alertness with diminished ability to consistently engage the environment. The stuporous patient requires vigorous stimulation to be aroused. Coma, which represents the end of the continuum of hypo-arousal states, is a state of unresponsiveness to the external environment. In the elderly, hypo-arousal states can be associated with systemic infection, meningoencephalitis, increased intracranial pressure, toxic-metabolic insults, traumatic brain injury, or cerebrovascular disease. Coma requires either bilateral hemispheric dysfunction or brainstem dysfunction. Hyper-arousal is characterized by anxiety, autonomic hyperactivity (tachycardia, tachypnea, hyperthermia), tremor or exaggerated startle response. In the elderly, hyper-arousal states are most often encountered in toxic-metabolic disorders including withdrawal from alcohol, opiates, or sedative-hypnotic agents. Some patients may experience both periods of hypo- and hyper-arousal.

Appearance

Assessment of a patient's physical appearance should acknowledge body size and type, apparent age, posture, facial expressions, eye contact, hygiene, dress, and general activity level. A disheveled appearance may indicate dementia, delirium, frontal lobe dysfunction or schizophrenia. Wearing excessive makeup or flamboyant grooming or attire in an old individual should raise the suspicion of a manic episode. Patients with unilateral neglect may fail to dress, groom, or bathe one side of their body. Patients with

Parkinson disease may display a flexed posture, whereas patients with progressive supranuclear palsy have an extended posture. The overall appearance of an individual should also provide information regarding their general health status. The cachectic patient may harbor a systemic illness (e.g., cancer), or have anorexia or depression.

Emotional State

Traditionally, *mood* and *affect* have been used to describe one's emotional state. Some authors use affect to describe several entities, including feeling tone associated with mental representations of external reality and the outward and transient display of emotion, while mood refers to the patient's constant and internal emotional state or summation of affects. To help resolve this inconsistency, some authors have abandoned the use of mood and affect in mental status examination. Instead, they favor the use of *objective component of emotion* to describe the way in which emotion is expressed through facial grimaces, vocal tone, and body movements, and *subjective component of emotion* to describe patient's report of what he or she feels internally: "I feel sad, happy, apprehensive, cynical," and so on.

The predominant emotional state helps to categorize the behavioral diagnosis. Depression is the most frequent mood disturbance and can occur in a variety of neurologic disorders (Table 9-1). Euphoria or full-blown mania occurs less often than depression in the course of neurologic illness. Euphoria is most common with frontal lobe dysfunction (trauma, frontotemporal degenerations, infections) and with secondary mania. Table 9-1 lists the neurologic disorders associated with maniform symptoms. Anxiety occurs in a variety of neuropsychiatric conditions including anxiety disorders, metabolic encephalopathies (e.g., hyperthyroidism, anoxia), toxic disorders (e.g., lidocaine toxicity), and degenerative diseases (e.g., Alzheimer's disease, Parkinson's disease).

Objective and subjective emotional components may be incongruent in certain psychiatric disorders (e.g., schizophrenia and schizotypal personality disorder), in developmental disorders (e.g., velocardiofacial syndrome), and in neurologic conditions such as pseudobulbar palsy.

Range and intensity of the observable component of emotion should be noted. Constriction or flatness is observed in apathetic states; for example, in the context of negative symptoms of schizophrenia, severe melancholic depression, autism spectrum, or in demented patients with apathy. Increased intensity, on the other hand, is seen in mood disorders such as bipolar illness, and in cluster B personality disorders such as borderline personality.

Lability is a disorder of emotional regulation. Patients with marked lability are irritable and shift rapidly among anger, depression and euphoria. The emotional outbursts are usually short-lived. Labile mood is seen in mood disorders such as bipolar illness and in certain personality disorders such as borderline personality. It also may occur in frontotemporal dementia.

Behavior

Behavioral observations can reveal important information regarding the mental status and neurologic function of the patient. A variety of personality alterations can be encountered with focal brain lesions (Table 9-2).

Table 9-1 Neurologic Conditions Associated with Mood Disorders

Depression
Stroke
Alzheimer's disease
Dementia with Lewy bodies
Parkinson's disease
Epilepsy
Multiple sclerosis
Huntington's disease
Wilson disease
Idiopathic basal ganglia calcification
Vascular dementia
Corticobasal degeneration
Mania
Huntington's disease
Wilson's disease
Idiopathic basal ganglia calcification
Stroke
Trauma
Multiple sclerosis
General paresis
Viral encephalitis
Postencephalitic syndromes
Frontotemporal dementia
Thalamotomy

Table 9-2 Personality and Behavioral Alterations Associated with Focal Brain Lesions

Focal Lesions	Personality Alteration
Orbitofrontal	Irritability, impulsiveness, "pseudopsychopathic"
Medial frontal	Apathy, loss of motivation and initiative
Right hemisphere (childhood)	Schizoid
Right hemisphere (adult)	Alexithymia
Left hemisphere (Wernicke area)	Suspiciousness, anger
Bilateral temporal lobe	Placidity (component of the Kluver-Bucy syndrome)
Ventromedial hypothalamus	Rage

Orbitofrontal dysfunction may be characterized by impulsiveness or undue familiarity with the examiner, lack of judgment or lack of social anxiety, and antisocial behavior. Individuals with dorsolateral frontal lobe dysfunction may be inattentive and distractible. Apathy (lack of motivation, energy, emotional reciprocity, social isolation) may be caused by medial frontal dysfunction. Psychomotor retardation (i.e., slowed central processing and movement) may be indicative of vascular dementia, subcortical neurologic disorders, medial frontal syndromes, or depression.

Speech

Observation of spontaneous speech is the first step in formal language testing and can be assessed during history taking as well as in the course of the mental status examination. The examiner first observes whether speech is absent or present. Mutism may be encountered in several neurologic conditions such as akinetic mutism, vegetative state, locked-in syndrome, catatonic unresponsiveness, or large left hemispheric lesions. Akinetic mutism is characterized by absent speech in the setting of alert-appearing immobility. The patient's eyes are open, and the individual may follow environmental events. The patient exhibits regular sleep–wake cycles but may be completely inert or display brief movements or postural adjustments spontaneously or in response to vigorous stimulation. Akinetic mutism may be seen with large frontal lobe injuries, bilateral cingulate gyrus damage, or midbrain pathology. Akinetic mutism should be distinguished from a vegetative state where the patient exhibits sleep–wake cycles with open eyes. A vegetative state can occur after severe brain injury. Locked-in syndrome occurs with bilateral pontine lesions, rendering the patient mute and paralyzed. Intellectual function, however, is not impaired and the patients can communicate by eye movements or eye blinks.

Spontaneous speech is characterized by its rate, rhythm, volume, response latency, and inflection. Accelerated speech may be encountered in mania, disinhibited orbitofrontal syndromes or festinating parkinsonian conditions, whereas a reduced rate of speech output can occur as a component of psychomotor retardation or nonfluent aphasias. Response latencies may be prolonged or the patient may impulsively interrupt the examiner, anticipating the question. Perturbed speech prosody (loss of melody or inflection) can be encountered in brain disorders affecting the right hemisphere or the basal ganglia. Empty speech with hesitations or circumlocutions can be exhibited in patients with word-finding difficulties. Word-finding impairment may occur in aphasias, metabolic encephalopathies, physical exhaustion, sleep deprivation, anxiety, depression, or dorsolateral frontal lobe damage in the absence of an anomia. Empty speech is a characteristic feature of fluent aphasia.

Movements

Observation of patient's movements may provide evidence of parkinsonism, chorea, myoclonus, or tics.

Neuropsychiatric Assessment

The neuropsychiatric interview of the patient includes the evaluation of thought form, thought content, and insight. The new onset of disturbances in any of these domains in the elderly is unusual in the absence of a brain disease. Their emergence should trigger the search for a neurologic condition.

Thought Form

Formal thought disorders such as tangentiality, circumstantiality, loose associations, illogicality, derailment, and thought blocking are less common than delusions as a manifestation of psychosis in neurologic diseases. Thought disorders have been observed in the psychoses accompanying epilepsy, Huntington's disease, and idiopathic basal ganglia calcification.

Perseveration and incoherence are disorders of the form of thought that are common in neuropsychiatric conditions. Perseveration refers to the inappropriate continuation of an act or thought after conclusion of its proper context. Intrusions are a special case of perseveration with late recurrences of words or thoughts from an earlier context. Perseverations and intrusions are seen in aphasias and dementing illnesses. Incoherence refers to the absence of logical association between words or ideas. It is observed in extreme cases of psychotic verbigeration, delirium, advanced cortical dementias such as Alzheimer's disease, and the jargon output of fluent aphasia.

Thought Content

Several types of disorders of thought content occur in neurologic diseases. Delusions are the most common manifestation of psychosis in neurologic disorders and are characterized by false beliefs based on incorrect inference about external reality. Common types of delusions encountered involve being followed or spied on, theft of personal property, spousal infidelity, or the presence of unwelcome strangers in one's home. Theme-specific delusions such as the Capgras syndrome (the belief that someone has been replaced by an identical-appearing impostor) may also be observed in neurologic illnesses. Delusions are common in Alzheimer's disease and dementia with Lewy bodies, and may occur in vascular dementia, frontotemporal dementia, Huntington's disease and a wide variety of other neurologic disorders.

Hallucinations occur in many neurologic disorders. Hallucinations are sensory perceptions that occur without stimulation of the relevant sensory organ. Hallucinations and delusions occur together in psychosis; hallucinations are nondelusional when the patient recognizes the sensory experience to be unreal. Hallucinations may involve any sensory modality (visual, auditory, tactile, gustatory, olfactory) and hallucinations may be formed (e.g., visual hallucinations of people or things) or unformed (flashing lights or colors). Hallucinations occur with ocular and structural brain disorders as well as epilepsy, narcolepsy, and migraine. Visual hallucinations are prominent in dementia with Lewy bodies.

Insight

Patients with neuropsychiatric disease may display limited insight and be unaware of their medical conditions or limitations in function. Accordingly, assessment of a patient's insight into the severity of their illness can yield useful diagnostic information. For example, Alzheimer's disease patients have impaired insight into their memory and cognitive difficulties, whereas patients with vascular dementia often exhibit more appropriate concern regarding their cognitive dysfunction. Lesions of the parietal lobe of the right hemisphere are associated with unawareness, neglect, or denial of the abnormalities of the contralateral hemibody.

Cognitive Assessment

The assessment of cognitive function should be conducted methodically and should assess comprehensively the major domains of neuropsychological function (attention, memory, language, visuospatial skills, executive ability). The patient's age, handedness, educational level, and sociocultural background may all influence cognitive function and should be determined prior to initiating or interpreting the evaluation.

Attention

Two tests are useful in assessing attention: digit span and continuous performance tests. In the digit span forward test, the patient is asked to repeat increasingly long series of numbers. The examiner says the numbers at a rate of one per second. A normal forward digit span is seven digits; fewer than five is abnormal. Concentration is evaluated by a continuous performance test. In the "A" test, the clinician says a series of random letters at a rate of one per second. The patient is asked to raise their hand each time the letter "A" is said. Distractible patients fail to detect one or more of the "As." Confusional states are characterized by impaired attention.

Memory

Learning, recall, recognition, and memory for remote information are assessed in the course of mental status examination. Asking the patient to remember three words and then asking him or her to recall the words 3 minutes later can help assess learning, recall, and recognition. Patients having difficulty with recall are given clues (e.g., the category of items to which the word belongs or a list of words containing the target) to distinguish between storage and retrieval deficits. Prompting and clues will not aide patients with storage deficits (e.g., amnesia); patients with intact storage but poor recall (e.g. retrieval-deficit syndrome) are aided by clues. Hippocampal–thalamic circuit lesions produce amnesia; impairment of frontal–basal ganglia circuitry causes a retrieval-deficit syndrome.

Information is gathered on the patient's remote memory function while taking a history of the patient's illness, inquiring about the patient's life events (marriage, births of children, etc.), and asking about important historical events. The temporal profile of remote memory may be diagnostically important. Amnestic syndromes feature normal, nonmemory cognitive functions, a period of retrograde amnesia following the onset of the disorder, variable periods of anterograde amnesia, and intact remote memory beyond the period of the retrograde amnesia.

Language

Language assessment includes evaluation of spontaneous speech, comprehension, repetition, naming, reading, and writing.

The two types of aphasic disturbances are referred to as fluent or nonfluent. Fluent aphasias are characterized by normal or excessive amounts of speech, preserved phrase length, intact speech melody, and a paucity of information. Phonemic paraphasias, substitution of one phoneme for another; semantic paraphasias, the replacement of one word with another; or neologistic paraphasias, the construction of new words, may occur. Wernicke, transcortical sensory, conduction, and anomic aphasias are fluent aphasic syndromes. Nonfluent aphasias feature reduced verbal output, short or one-word replies, agrammatism, poor speech initiation, reduced speech prosody, and dysarthria. There are few paraphasias. Broca, transcortical motor, global, and mixed transcortical aphasias are nonfluent aphasic disorders.

Primary progressive aphasia is a disorder seen in patients with asymmetric frontotemporal degeneration that involves primarily the left side of the brain. There are two major subtypes: a nonfluent aphasia and a fluent aphasia. Progressive nonfluent aphasia involves primarily unilateral left frontal, left frontoparietal, or left frontotemporal degeneration and is characterized by agrammatism, paraphasias, and anomia. Bilateral temporal lobe atrophy and hypoperfusion with more pronounced involvement of the left anterior temporal lobe may cause semantic dementia that is characterized by progressive loss of knowledge about objects, people, facts, and words, that is often accompanied by visual agnosia.

Language comprehension is tested by asking the patient to follow increasingly complex linguistic constructions. The easiest commands are one-step orders such as "stand up" and "turn around," "open your mouth," and "stick out your tongue." Asking the patient to point to room objects or body parts is the next level of comprehension difficulty. Finally, more complex questions, such as "If a lion is killed by a tiger, which animal is dead?," are asked. Impaired comprehension usually implies dysfunction of parietotemporal regions of the left hemisphere. Comprehension is abnormal in most fluent and global aphasic syndromes. In the elderly, it is important to establish that hearing is intact before testing comprehension. Failure to comprehend commands may reflect the inability to hear as opposed to impaired comprehension.

Repetition is assessed by asking the patient to repeat increasingly long phrases or sentences. Omissions and paraphasic substitutions may disrupt accurate repetition. Repetition is impaired in Wernicke, Broca, conductive and global aphasia.

Naming tests involve asking the patient to name objects, parts of objects, and colors. Errors include paraphasias, circumlocutory responses, and simply making no response. Anomia occurs in aphasias, dementias, and deliria. Adequate vision and object recognition must be ensured before errors are ascribed to naming deficits.

When assessing reading, the patient's ability to read aloud and to comprehend what is read must both be tested. Adequate vision must be ensured before failures are ascribed to an alexia. Most aphasias have concomitant alexias; in alexia with agraphia and alexia without agraphia, reading abnormalities occur without aphasic disturbances.

Mechanical or aphasic abnormalities may cause agraphia. Micrographia is a characteristic aspect of parkinsonism in which the script becomes progressively smaller as the patient writes a sentence or extended series of numbers or letters, and mechanical agraphias occur in patients with limb paresis, limb apraxia, or movement disorders such as tremor and chorea. Aphasic agraphias accompany aphasic syndromes and errors similar to those noted in verbal output are present in written form. In Gerstmann syndrome (agraphia, acalculia, right–left disorientation, finger agnosia), alexia with agraphia, and disconnection agraphia (occurring with injury of the corpus callosum), agraphia occurs without aphasia. Agraphia also occurs in dementia and delirium.

Word List Generation

Word list generation involves asking the patient to think of as many members of a specific category as possible within 1 minute. Patients may be asked to name as many animal names as possible within 1 minute. Normal individuals can name approximately 18 animals within 1 minute. Word list generation deficits occur with anomia, frontal-subcortical systems dysfunction, and psychomotor retardation. It is a highly sensitive test but lacks specificity.

Visuospatial Skills

There are a number of visuospatial abilities including spatial attention, perception, construction, visuospatial problem solving, and visuospatial memory. Constructional tasks are most widely used to assess visuospatial ability. In the clock drawing test, the patient is asked to draw a clock and draw in the clock hands to indicate a specific time. Patients with executive dysfunction may draw a clock face that is too small to contain the required numbers (poor planning), whereas patients with unilateral neglect will ignore half of the clock face.

Tests of copying involve having the patient reproduce figures such as a circle, intersecting circle and triangle, overlapping pentagons, cube, or more complex figures. Abnormalities include failures to reproduce the shapes accurately, perseveration on individual elements, drawing over the stimulus figure, or unilateral neglect. Drawing disturbances are common with many types of neurologic conditions including focal brain damage, degenerative disorders, and toxic and metabolic encephalopathies.

Calculation

In assessing calculation skills, patients are asked to add or multiply one or two digits mentally or to execute more demanding problems with pencil and paper. Calculation abilities are related to education and occupation. Acalculias occur in aphasic syndromes, visuospatial disorders leading to incorrect alignment of columns of numbers, and primary anarithmetias. Anarithmetias are produced by damage to the posterior left hemisphere.

Executive Function

Executive function is assessed by asking the patient to perform tasks mediated by frontal–subcortical systems. Frontal–subcortical systems are complex neural circuits that include the frontal cortex, striatum, globus pallidus/substantia nigra, thalamic nuclei, and connecting white matter tracts. Executive function is mediated by the frontal–subcortical circuit originating in the dorsolateral prefrontal cortex. Patients with dorsolateral prefrontal–subcortical systems dysfunction manifest perseveration; motor programming abnormalities; reduced word list generation (left dorsolateral dysfunction); reduced nonverbal fluency (right dorsolateral dysfunction); poor set shifting; abnormal recall with intact recognition memory; loss of abstraction abilities; poor judgment; and impaired mental control. These abnormalities are common following head trauma, in frontal lobe degenerations, with frontal lobe neoplasms, in chronic multiple sclerosis, with Huntington's disease and other basal ganglia disorders, following multiple subcortical infarctions, and in some brain infections such as syphilis.

Digit span in reverse is a test of mental control and complex attention, as well as executive dysfunction. It entails saying increasingly long series of numbers and asking the patient to say them backwards. A normal digit span in reverse is five digits; fewer than three is abnormal.

Abstraction

Similarities, differences, idioms, and proverbs are used to assess abstracting capacity. These tests are not culture fair and abstraction abilities are influenced by culture and education. Abstraction abnormalities are a nonspecific indicator of cerebral dysfunction. Patients with frontal lobe disorders have disproportionately severe abstracting disturbances.

Judgment

Assessing judgment assists in exploring the patient's interpersonal and social insight. Judgment is impaired in many neurologic conditions. Damage to orbitofrontal subcortical circuit (e.g., in frontotemporal dementia, trauma or focal syndromes) produces marked alterations in social judgment.

NEUROLOGIC EXAMINATION

The neurologic examination includes assessment of cranial nerve function, strength, coordination, sensation, muscle stretch reflexes, pathologic/primitive reflexes, and neurovascular status. Examination of head and neck may provide additional important information.

Cranial Nerve Examination

Cranial Nerve I

Olfaction is tested by asking the patient to identify a variety of odors. In normal aging, loss of olfaction may be a nonspecific or clinically insignificant finding.

Cranial Nerve II

Examination of the optic nerve includes visual inspection of the nerve head, testing of visual acuity, and mapping of the visual fields. In aging, visual acuity may be impaired and this is typically associated with glaucoma, cataracts, or refractive error. Unilateral visual field deficits can also be associated with glaucoma. Abrupt changes in visual fields or acuity should alert the clinician to potential cerebrovascular or retinovascular disease. Homonymous field deficits reflect disruption of the postchiasmatic geniculocalcarine radiations.

Cranial Nerves III, IV, and VI

The oculomotor, trochlear, and abducens nerves mediate ocular motility, pupillary responses, and eyelid position. In aging, ocular motility may be reduced. Normal elderly can exhibit restricted convergence and limitation of conjugate upward gaze. Other nonspecific concomitants of normal aging include the evolution of small sluggishly reactive pupils, loss of Bell phenomenon (upward eye deviation on eye closure) and the inability to dissociate ocular movements from head movements. The clinician should be concerned when an elderly patient exhibits new onset diplopia, pupillary asymmetry, or extraocular movement disorders that are not typical of normal aging.

Cranial Nerve V

The trigeminal nerve innervates the muscles of mastication and mediates facial and corneal sensation. Tumors of the middle fossa and in the cerebellopontine angle may compress the fifth cranial nerve and produce a cranial nerve syndrome with decreased corneal reflex and sensory loss on the ipsilateral face.

Cranial Nerve VII

The facial nerve supplies the facial musculature, lacrimal and salivary glands, stapedius, muscles of the middle ear, and taste fibers of the anterior tongue.

Cranial Nerve VIII

Hearing and balance are mediated by the eighth cranial nerve. Deafness results from auditory nerve damage. Vestibular lesions produce nystagmus and vertigo. Vestibular nystagmus is horizontal or combined horizontal–rotatory and is typically accompanied by vertigo and nausea, whereas lesions disrupting vestibular connections in the central nervous system can produce nystagmus in any direction and are usually not associated with vertiginous or nauseous sensations. Decreased hearing for high pitched

Table 9-3   Differential Diagnosis of Vertigo

Peripheral etiology
  Vestibular neuronitis
  Labyrinthitis
  Benign positional vertigo
  Ménière's syndrome
  Labyrinthine imbalance
  Posttraumatic vertigo
  Peulymphatic fistula

Central etiology
  Brainstem ischemia
  Multiple sclerosis
  Basilar artery migraine
  Posterior fossa tumors

sounds and lack of perception of background noise are common concomitants of aging and should not be considered a pathologic finding. However, progressive hearing loss, associated with tinnitus and vertigo should prompt further medical evaluation. The complaint of dizziness in the elderly is not uncommon; however, the examiner must determine whether the dizzy patient is experiencing lightheadedness or true vertigo. If true vertigo is present, then the clinician should further discern whether it is peripheral (vestibular) or central (brainstem) in origin (Table 9-3). Causes of vertigo associated with vestibular disease include benign positional vertigo, Ménière's syndrome and trauma.

Cranial Nerves IX and X

The ninth and tenth cranial nerves control pharyngeal and laryngeal function, taste, and the gag reflex. Hoarseness, aphonia, and dysphagia occur with vagus nerve lesions. In normal aging, the gag reflex can be reduced and, when accompanied by a decrease in the cough reflex, can result in difficulty handling bronchial secretions.

Cranial Nerve XI

The spinal accessory nerve innervates the upper half of the trapezius and the sternocleidomastoid muscle. In the normal elderly, frank weakness of the trapezius or sternocleidomastoid muscle is not a typical finding and, if present, should be investigated further. A delayed shrug may be an indication of a mild ipsilateral hemiparesis.

Cranial Nerve XII

The hypoglossal nerve innervates the tongue. Tongue weakness is common in pseudobulbar palsy and motor neuron disease.

Motor System Examination

Muscle bulk, strength, tone, and coordination are assessed as part of the motor system examination. Muscle bulk is examined by visual inspection and palpation. Muscle wasting may occur with disuse; muscle, nerve, or spinal disease; and in generalized weight loss secondary to malnutrition, systemic illness, or advanced brain diseases. Muscular wasting without associated weakness can be encountered in normal aging. The interossei and calf muscles are the muscle groups that are most commonly involved.

Strength is graded as 0 (no evidence of muscle contraction), 1 (muscle contraction without movement of the limb), 2 (limb movement after gravity eliminated), 3 (limb movement against gravity), 4 (limb movement against partial resistance), or 5 (normal strength). Distal weakness is most indicative of peripheral neuropathies, whereas proximal weakness is more consistent with primary muscle disease. Hemipareses occur with lesions of the pyramidal system. In aging, mild generalized weakness may occur; however, focal weakness is indicative of a neuropathologic process.

Muscle tone may be increased or decreased in neurologic disorders. Muscle tone is decreased in muscle and peripheral nerve disease, with cerebellar disorders, early in the course of many choreiform disorders, and acutely following an upper motor neuron lesion. Increased muscle tone (rigidity) is encountered in spasticity with pyramidal tract lesions and plastic rigidity with extrapyramidal disorders. Cogwheel rigidity results from the occurrence of tremor that is palpated when manipulating the limbs. "Gegenhalten" refers to the active resistance to movement encountered in advanced brain diseases.

Coordination may be disrupted by many types of motor and sensory abnormalities and is dependent on intact cerebellar function. Tests of coordination include rapid alternating movements, fine finger movements, finger-to-nose movements, heel-knee-shin maneuvers, and rebound check tests. During aging, there is an overall decrease in speed of coordinated movements that is of no pathologic consequence. In addition, mild appendicular dysmetria and/or slowed rapid rhythmic alternating movements may be encountered. However, gross abnormalities in cerebellar function are not anticipated and should be evaluated thoroughly.

Adventitious movements should be assessed during the motor reexamination. There are four general classes of movement disorders. These include parkinsonism, dystonia, hyperkineses (chorea, myoclonus, tics), and tremor.

Gate and posture depend on motor and sensory function. In normal aging, changes in gait and posture are expected. As an individual ages, posture becomes more flexed. Older patients without evident neurologic disease may exhibit a slightly slowed and unsteady gait. When assessing gait in the elderly, it is important to recognize gait abnormalities that may be secondary to joint pain and arthritic conditions. Table 9-4 lists the causes of gait disturbance in the elderly.

Sensory Examination

Primary modalities, including light touch and temperature, and cortical sensory modalities, including joint position sense, two-point discrimination, graphesthesia, and stereognosis, are tested to assess sensory function. A variety

Table 9-4 Etiologies of Gait Disturbances in the Elderly

Parkinson's disease
White matter ischemic injury
Normal pressure hydrocephalus
Cervical spondylosis
Lumbar spondylosis
Cerebellar disease
Peripheral neuropathy
Myelopathy
Hemiparesis
Myopathy
Vestibulopathy
Impaired vision
Arthritis of lower extremities
Hip replacement surgery
Foot disease

of sensory changes can occur in normal aging. Nearly invariably, elderly individuals will experience decreased vibratory sensation at the toes bilaterally; diminished vibratory sensation should be considered abnormal if it extends to the knees. Causes of pathologic decreased vibratory sensation include peripheral neuropathies, tabes dorsalis, vitamin B_{12} deficiency, and myelopathies. Mild impairment of light touch, pain, and vibration can occur in uncomplicated aging, but more severe abnormalities are indicative of pathologic sensory loss. Unilateral sensory loss occurs with lesions of primary sensory cortex or its projections.

Muscle Stretch Reflexes

Decreased muscle stretch reflexes are found in muscle, peripheral nerve, and nerve root disorders, while increased reflexes occur with upper motor neuron lesions. Lateralized hyperactive reflexes in conjunction with spasticity and the Babinski sign are indicative of a contralateral lesion of the pyramidal system. In aging, deep tendon reflexes tend to become hypoactive. Ankle reflexes may be absent in normal aging, but knee reflexes persist. Absent or diminished reflexes may be encountered in advanced cervical and lumbar spondylosis if nerve roots are compromised.

Pathologic and Primitive Reflexes

Babinski sign is dorsiflexion of the great toe with plantar stimulation. It is produced by upper motor neuron lesions.

The grasp reflex (involuntary gripping of objects in or near the patient's hand) occurs in patients with advanced brain disease and with lesions restricted to the medial frontal lobes.

The sucking reflex (sucking movements of the lips, tongue, and jaw elicited by stimulation of the lips) occurs in patients with frontal lobe and diffuse brain dysfunction.

The palmomental reflex (ipsilateral contraction of the mentalis muscle in response to stroking of the thenar eminence of the hand) can be seen in normal aged individuals and may be regarded as pathologic when it is unilateral or when it does not fatigue with repeated palmar stimulation.

Neurovascular Assessment

Examination of vascular system, including auscultation for cranial and carotid bruits and assessment of blood pressure, complements the neurologic exam.

CONCLUSION

Several neurologic disorders (e.g., stroke, Parkinson's disease, Alzheimer's disease, and other dementias) preferentially afflict the elderly. Comprehensive mental status and neurologic examination should document changes in neurologic function (i.e., memory/cognition, behavior/personality, cranial nerves, motor function, and sensory perception) that are associated with pathologic conditions that affect the nervous system, and distinguish them from the functional changes associated with normal aging.

Limited memory and cognitive function changes occur as one ages. Subtle changes in memory that do not interfere with normal functioning in society and that do not impair activities of daily living occur in normal aging or age-related cognitive decline (age-associated memory impairment). More significant declines in memory and cognitive function can be encountered in dementia and delirium.

Altered cognitive function in the setting of a clear sensorium is consistent with dementia secondary to a neurodegenerative process or medical illness. The primary dementias (e.g., Alzheimer's disease, frontotemporal dementias, dementia with Lewy bodies) are characterized by a specific constellation of signs and symptoms. In Alzheimer disease the individual typically exhibits limited insight into their cognitive deficits that involve memory, language, and visuospatial skills. Patients with frontotemporal dementias present with a predominance of features consistent with frontal and/or temporal degeneration. These individuals exhibit early changes in behavior and personality, such as social inappropriateness, disinhibition, apathy, perseveration, and oral/dietary changes. Other accompanying features may include language/speech impairment, executive dysfunction, and preserved posterior functions (e.g., visuospatial ability, calculations). In dementia with Lewy bodies, patients may exhibit fluctuating cognition, recurrent well-formed and detailed visual hallucinations, and extrapyramidal signs consistent with parkinsonism. Dementia can occur as a consequence of other neurological and medical illnesses such as cerebrovascular disease,

vitamin B_{12} deficiency, hypothyroidism, Parkinson's disease, and meningoencephalitis.

If someone first develops symptoms of a personality disorder (e.g., antisocial symptoms in a person with no such history) late in life, consideration should be given to a general medical or neurologic condition such as Huntington's disease, neurodegenerative disorders (e.g., frontotemporal dementia, Alzheimer disease, Parkinson's disease), traumatic brain injury, stroke, a substance-induced condition, or another psychiatric disorder (such as mania). However, some personality disorders (e.g., antisocial and borderline personality disorders) may become less evident or remit with age. Disorders such as obsessive-compulsive or schizotypal personality are less likely to improve.

A functional decline in some aspects of cranial nerve function (e.g., vision, hearing, vestibular function, taste, and smell) can be anticipated in normal aging and should be distinguished from pathological conditions afflicting the nervous system. Similarly, older individuals experience decreased mobility as they age. Subtle changes in gait, posture, coordination, and strength are expected concomitants of aging. However, more profound changes that significantly alter mobility and/or present as focal weakness or impaired coordination should alert the clinician to the possibility of a neuropathologic disorder. Common neurologic causes of gait disturbance in the elderly include Parkinson's disease, cervical and lumbar spondylosis, and cerebrovascular disease.

Alterations in sensory perception can be indicative of neuropsychiatric dysfunction in the aged. Subtle deficits in vibration and other primary sensory modalities may be encountered in normal aging. However, marked deficits in sensory function are suggestive of neurologic disease involving either the peripheral or central nervous system and require further diagnostic testing.

In conclusion, neurologic concomitants of normal aging include subtle declines in cognitive function, mildly impaired motor function, and altered sensory perceptions. Exaggerated impairments in cognitive, behavioral, motor, and sensory function may be encountered in pathologic conditions that afflict the elderly. A comprehensive mental status and neurologic examination is the foundation for identifying neuropathologic conditions that necessitate further laboratory and imaging investigation.

ACKNOWLEDGMENTS

This project was supported by a National Institute on Aging (NIA) Alzheimer's Disease Center grant (AG 16570), an Alzheimer's Disease Research Center of California grant, and the Sidell-Kagan Foundation.

REFERENCES

Adams RD, Victor M: *Principles of Neurology*, 4th ed. New York, McGraw-Hill, 1989.

Bolla KI et al: Memory complaints in older adults. Fact or Fiction? *Arch Neurol* 48:61, 1991.

Borclay L: *Clinical Geriatric Neurology.* Philadelphia, Lea & Febiger, 1993.

Critchley M: Neurologic changes in the aged. *J Chronic Dis* 3:459, 1956.

Cummings JL et al: Organic personality disorder in dementia syndrome: An inventory approach. *J Neuropsychiatry Clin Neurosci* 2:261, 1990.

Cummings JL, Victoroff JI: Noncognitive neuropsychiatric syndromes in Alzheimer's disease. *Neuropsychiatry Neuropsychol Behav Neurol* 3:140, 1990.

Cummings JL: *Clinical Neuropsychiatry.* New York, Grune and Stratton, 1985.

Cutting J: *The Right Cerebral Hemisphere and Psychiatric Disorders.* New York, Oxford Medical, 1990.

Damasio H, Damasio AR: *Lesion Analysis in Neuropsychology.* New York, Oxford University Press, 1989.

Edwards-Lee T: The temporal variant of frontotemporal dementia. *Brain* 120:1027, 1997.

Fossati A: Latent class analysis of DSM-IV schizotypal personality disorder criteria in psychiatric patients. *Schizophr Bull* 27(1):59, 2001.

Galasko D et al: Neurological findings in Alzheimer's disease and normal aging. *Arch Neurol* 47:625, 1990.

Hilty D: The psychotic patient, primary care. *Clin Office Pract* 26(2):327, 1999.

Jenkyn LR et al: Neurologic signs in senescence. *Arch Neurol* 42:1154, 1985.

Kiernan RJ et al: The neurobehavioral cognitive status examination: A brief but differentiated approach to cognitive assessment. *Ann Intern Med* 107:481, 1987.

Kokmean E et al: Neurological manifestations of aging. *J Gerontol* 32:411, 1977.

Laplane D et al: Obsessive-compulsive and other behavioural changes with bilateral basal ganglia lesions. *Brain* 112:699, 1989.

Locke S: Neurological concomitants of aging. *Geriatrics* 19:722, 1964.

Manley MRS: *Kaplan & Sadock's Comprehensive Textbook of Psychiatry,* 7th ed. CD-ROM, chapter 7.1.

Martin RL: Late-life psychiatric diagnosis in DSM-IV. *Psychiatr Clin North Am* 20(1):12, 1997.

Mesulam MM: Slowly progressive aphasia without generalised dementia. *Ann Neurol* 11:592, 19828

Miller BL et al: Hypersexuality or altered sexual preference following brain injury. *J Neurol Neurosurg Psychiatry* 49:867, 1986.

Neary D et al: Frontotemporal lobar degeneration, a consensus on clinical diagnostic criteria. *Neurology* 51(6):1546, 1998.

O'Leary K: Borderline personality disorder neuropsychological testing results. *Psychiatr Clin North Am* 23(1):41, 2000.

Plum F, Posner JB: *The Diagnosis of Stupor and Coma,* 3rd ed. Philadelphia, FA Davis, 1980.

Quattrocolo G et al. Autosomal dominant late-onset leukoencephalopathy. Clinical report of a new Italian Family. *Eur Neurol* 37:53, 1997.

Rauch S, Savage C: Neuropsychiatry of the basal ganglia, neuroimaging and neuropsychology of the striatum, bridging basic science and clinical practice. *Psychiatr Clin North Am* 20(4):741, 1997.

Robinson RG, Starkstein SE: Current research in affective disorders following stroke. *J Neuropsychiatry Clin Neurosci* 2:1, 1990.

Rosen H et al: Frontotemporal dementia. *Neurol Clin* 18(4): 2000.

Shukla S et al: Mania following head trauma. *Am J Psychiatry* 144:93, 1987.

Skre H: Neurological signs in a normal population. *Acta Neurol Scand* 48:575, 1972.

Snowden JS et al: Semantic dementia: A form of circumscribed cerebral atrophy. *Behav Neurol* 2:167, 1989.

Starkstein SE et al: Mania after brain injury: Neuroradiological and metabolic findings. *Ann Neurol* 27:652, 1990.

Strub RL, Black FW: *The Mental Status Examination in Neurology,* 2nd ed. Philadelphia, FA Davis, 1985.

Sultzer DL, Cummings JL: Drug-induced mania—Causative agents, clinical characteristics and management. *Med Toxic Adverse Drug Exp* 4: 127, 1989.

Tinetti ME: Performance-oriented assessment of mobility problems in elderly patients. *J Am Geriatr Soc* 34:119, 1986.

Torgersen S: "True" schizotypal personality disorder: A study of co-twins and relatives of schizophrenic probands. *Am J Psychiatry* 150(11):1661, 1993.

Tweedy J et al: Significance of cortical disinhibition signs. *Neurology* 32:169, 1982.

Wragg RE, Jeste DV: Overview of depression and psychosis in Alzheimer's disease. *Am J Psychiatry* 146:577, 1989.

Assessment of Decisional Capacity and Competency

MARGARET A. DRICKAMER

The medical profession has been charged with the seemingly conflicting responsibilities of respecting patients' autonomy while protecting from harm those patients who are incapable of protecting themselves. Assessing a patient's ability to make decisions is a role with which all clinicians should be familiar. Although certain situations may call for specialized assessment, generalists, internists, subspecialists, and geriatricians should be familiar with the principles and process sufficiently well to handle most situations. This chapter explains some of the ethical underpinnings to these responsibilities, highlights the strengths and weaknesses of approaches to assessing decisional capacity, and describes the types of situations in which the clinician may play a role.

Autonomy is defined as self-determination. Respect for individual autonomy is understood to be an elemental principle of our society. Nonetheless, all of us face limitations on how much we can truly determine our fates. Limitations of resources and opportunity, societal and legal prohibitions, and the limits imposed by the rights of others not to have *their* autonomy infringed upon are examples of such limitations. There are also limitations on who qualifies as an autonomous "self." The full right to self-determination is generally recognized to apply only to adults who are "of sound mind."

Paternalism is defined as limiting an individual's autonomy in order either to prevent that individual from doing harm to himself or herself or to prevent the person from missing a substantial benefit. The circumstances under which paternalism is acceptable are not defined by the action the individual may wish to undertake, or by the probable untoward consequences of an action, but rather by the individual's ability to make decisions. In other words, the clinician's desire to protect an individual from doing himself or herself harm does not justify paternalism; an individual cannot be prevented from doing things that may cause him or her harm (overeating, Bungee jumping, etc.). Intervention can only be justified if it is judged that an individual lacks the capacity to make decisions. In that case, responsibility for protecting the person from the possible harm of a decision rests on the clinician.

The interplay between these concepts becomes apparent when the person is no longer felt to be "of sound mind." This chapter will focus on those individuals who have cognitive impairment or a clouded sensorium (fixed lesions, dementia or delirium). The competence of individuals with psychiatric illness will not be addressed. When patients are cognitively impaired, clinicians have an obligation both to respect their rights and to protect their persons. These dual obligations often require a complex balancing act.

WHAT IS BEING DECIDED?

For an individual to be competent, in the broadest sense of the word, means that the individual is well qualified to do whatever task he or she is doing. In this context, competence is viewed as a legal term. Competence refers to a judge's ruling as to whether an individual has been deemed capable of making his or her own decisions. An individual adjudicated to be incompetent must have a guardian appointed to make the decisions for the area (or areas) in which the person has been found to be incompetent. Although guidelines vary somewhat from state to state, it is generally accepted that a ruling of incompetence cannot be made solely on the basis of a medical diagnosis, age, level of education, or personal eccentricity. A judgment of competence or incompetence is based on an assessment of the individual's decisional capacity and demonstrated ability or inability to carry out a plan.

Assessment of decisional capacity is made by a professional based on the patient's ability to make decisions. There are three necessary elements to making a capable decision. First, the individual must be able to understand the information being considered sufficiently well enough to make a decision. That information must have been presented in an understandable way and every effort must have been made to ensure that barriers such as hearing impairment and language difference do not constitute the sole reasons that the person is unable to understand the information. Second, the individual must have the conceptual ability to understanding the consequences of the decision that he or she is making. Finally, the person must be able to communicate the decision.

Two secondary considerations are sometimes used in judging an individual's decisional capacity. The considerations are consistency and rationality. The inconsistency of an individual's decision with past decisions made by that person provides an important clue to possible underlying cognitive or psychiatric problems that require exploration. In and of itself, however, inconsistency does not negate the person's right to make decisions.

Judging the rationality of a decision can be difficult. Even if it is felt—and even if most of society would feel—that an individual's decision is irrational, that does not negate the person's right to self-determination. Society has a great respect for individuality and one's right to express that individuality in a wide variety of ways. Nonetheless, the ability of an individual to give a rationale for their decision is sometimes used as secondary evidence of decisional capacity. That is to say, if the person is capable of explaining the basis for making the decision, be it religious belief, personal values, or some other rationale, the person's ability to explain provides assurance that the decision is not being made in the context of decreased cognitive capacity or a psychiatric illness that would need further investigation before the decision could be accepted.

Legal Aspects

In protecting an individual who is unable to make decisions, an application to the local probate court requesting that the individual be adjudicated to be incompetent may be needed. Although specifics of probate statutes vary from state to state, most follow the general pattern articulated in the Uniform Probate Code. Once an individual has been adjudicated incompetent, another person is appointed to represent his or her interests. This person is referred to as a guardian, conservator, or legal surrogate. The term conservator is used in this chapter. Although there are movements toward "limited conservatorship" that limits the powers of the conservator to decision making in specific areas where a person has been shown to be incapable, generally there are two broad categories of conservatorship that are commonly used, those of finance and of person. Conservatorship of finance is a fairly self-evident term. Conservatorship of person grants a more global responsibility for assuring that the individual is kept safe and that decisions are made either as substituted judgment or on the basis of the individual's best interests (see Chap. 29). These decisions may involve, for example, medical care, where a person will live, and what help the person will receive to maintain himself or herself. The person may retain the ability to make a will, referred to as testamentary competence, even when he or she has been adjudicated as incompetent of person and finance.

It should be emphasized that not all incapacitated individuals need to be conserved. There are no statistics available to say how many incapacitated individuals receive informal care management from relatives and never require

probate action. These individuals likely represent the majority of cases. Probate adjudication of a conservator may not be needed if financial management has been allocated to a family member by a power of attorney prior to the individual becoming incapacitated, and if there is a general agreement among concerned and interested parties that decisions should be made by a specific individual. Probate can be avoided if family members and other interested parties agree on the need for specific actions. If the individual involved has granted someone a durable power of attorney for health affairs (see Chap. 29), there may not be a need for court action. Involvement of the court is unnecessary even when interested parties disagree, provided they are willing to respect the individual's appointment of surrogate decision makers.

Even when the court has been asked to take action, 75 to 85 percent of the time the court appoints a family member as conservator. The ability of these individuals to act as an appropriate surrogate varies considerably. One advantage of having a court-appointed conservator is that the probate court has some oversight responsibilities for the management of the individual's affairs. This oversight by a judge may prove beneficial if the conservator is not scrupulous about managing a capacitated individual's funds. A judge who does not choose a family member as conservator may appoint an individual from the community, an attorney, a social worker, or an agency to fill that role.

Practical Aspects

Although courts tend to see the ability to make decisions as an all-or-nothing phenomenon, a person's ability to make decisions often falls somewhere on a continuum ranging from complete capability to incapacity. Furthermore, not only ability, but also circumstances, influence the need for intervention. For instance, a person's ability to capably manage financial affairs will be influenced by the size and complexity of the finances requiring management. If the need for complex medical decision-making does not arise, then the ability of an individual to make those types of decisions is not questioned. If the individual is in a situation where others are managing household affairs and looking out for the person's needs, then the person's ability to care for himself or herself may not be examined. It is only when a problem arises that the individual's ability to make these types of decisions becomes an issue. Also, as mentioned above, even if the patient is incapable and others need to make decisions, this can often be handled without court participation.

PROCESS OF DETERMINING CAPABILITY

The individual's inability to make decisions is determined in two different ways. Specific testing can measure dysfunction while observing the person's decision-making process can demonstrate his or her inability to complete the decision-making task capably. To understand and apply both of these methods, one needs to understand the cognitive processes involved in decisional capacity. These processes can be understood both as discrete neuropsychiatric functions and as contributors to the holistic process of making decisions.

The brain functions that contribute to decision-making are centered in the cortex and frontal lobes. Cortical, parietal and temporal lobe functions involved in decision-making include immediate memory and language. Cortical function includes immediate memory, which is defined as the ability to remember rehearsed or consolidated materials for 30 seconds to 30 minutes, for example, first repeating three objects and then recalling them in 5 minutes. Immediate memory is clearly important in the individual's ability to participate in a discussion around a specific decision. Cortical language abilities are those that affect comprehension and the ability to produce the intended words when expressing one's thoughts in both spoken and written communication. The ability to understand language is highly correlated with an individual's ability to comprehend the information needed to make a decision. Problems with expressive language ability from cortical lesions can lead to statements by the individual that misrepresent his or her thoughts such as through the misuse of words, word substitutions, or paraphrasic errors. Ability to understand and manipulate numbers may also come in to play.

Frontal lobe functions involved in the process of making capable decisions include the abilities to concentrate, express oneself, use abstract reasoning, initiate actions, solve problems, monitor one's behavior, and use judgment. The frontal lobe is responsible for filtering out both internal and external stimuli that interfere with the individual's ability to concentrate and to understand instructions or explanations. Frontal lobe dysfunction can lead to inattention that interferes with the ability to complete necessary tasks appropriately. The intrusion of internal stimuli can lead to inappropriate and impulsive behaviors that can interfere with the individual's functioning and decision making.

Traditional Mental Status Tools

Tools commonly used for the assessment of cognition in patients, such as the Mini-Mental State Examination (MMSE) or the Executive Interview (EXIT) exam, test specific cognitive functions (memory, language, praxis, concentration, etc.) or the integration of these functions into simple processes (three-step command, story telling). Reviewing performance on individual items and extrapolating to predict how performance will affect the processes necessary for decision making may help the clinician to evaluate a patient. No single cutoff score on any of these tests will divide those capable of making a decision from those not capable. This is particularly true since different types of decisions require different skills. These tests also do not look at the patient's function. On the other hand, a score may signal a level of such diminished cognitive abilities that it is highly unlikely that person with that score will be capable of making decisions. Knowledge of how the cognitive functions tested may influence the individual's ability to make decisions is important. These tests may also serve as important

triggers to further investigation of the individual's decisional capacity.

The Folstein MMSE is representative of tests for cortical function that have been shown to have some correlation with an individual's ability to make decisions. The MMSE tests skills that may affect a person' ability to make decisions, including immediate memory, word finding; understanding simple verbal and written material, ability to integrate that understanding into a simple action, and the ability to express basic ideas in writing. MMSE scores of less than 10 are diagnostic of impairment so severe as to preclude the ability to make decisions.

Testing of frontal lobe or executive functioning is less commonly done, but is of great importance. The EXIT examination and clock drawing are the two most commonly used measures by clinicians. The EXIT 25 has been shown to have the best correlation with subjective measures of competency of available neuropsychological tests. An overall score of 15 on the EXIT exam (higher being less capable) indicates very significant impairment. Functions that may be most reflective of problems with decisional capacity include poor insight, impulsivity, poor self-monitoring and impaired ability to plan and follow through on the plan. Although individual items on these tests do not correlate directly with each of these functions, observing the individual as he or she does the test with these functions in mind can clarify areas of deficits. For example, when the individual makes an obvious error, does he or she realize it and go back and correct the mistake? Is the person able to plan how to draw the face of a clock? If the person draws a clock face that is too small, does he or she notice this and correct it? Does the concrete stimulus of the numbers interfere with the abstraction of how the hands indicate time? Similar observations can be made while watching an individual take the EXIT examination. Does the person plan out how to approach a problem such as telling a story? Can the person correct errors in sequencing? Does the person let internal over-learned stimuli interfere with his or her ability to hear and repeat?

Test results can be deceptive. Individuals may have frontal lobe dysfunction sufficient to impair their capacity for making decisions yet score very well on the MMSE. There are more complex neuropsychological tests that can be done to test the same areas of function in more detail. These tests are not practical in the clinical setting. The clinician should thus refer the patient to a neuropsychologist if there is any question of the nature or severity of neuropsychological deficits.

Tests of Decisional Capacity

There are tests that are specifically designed to assess an individual's capacity for making medical decisions. These tests may use hypothetical vignettes to demonstrate whether the individual is capable of the three elements of decision-making: understanding the vignette (usually written at a sixth-grade level), being able to reason with the material, and then being capable of verbalizing an opinion. An example of such a test is the Capacity to Consent to

Treatment Instrument (CCTI). The CCTI consists of a series of case vignettes that the individual must read and then consider two different treatment options. The Hopkins Competency Assessment Test consists of a short essay that describes informed consent and durable power of attorney and a series of questions to assess the individual's comprehension of the material. The MacArthur Competence Assessment Tool-Treatment (MacCAT-T) is an example of a structured interview that allows the clinician to test the individual's ability to make a specific decision. The first two tests deal with theory or theoretical situations and can be used prior to the need for a decision. The MacCAT-T focuses on an individual's ability to make a specific decision at the time of the testing.

Specific Decisions

It is not always possible to make a definitive and enduring diagnosis of decisional incapacity. It is important to bear in mind that decisional incapacity is task specific and may be time-limited. Although one is legally adjudicated incompetent or competent in two broad categories, the ability of an individual to make decisions or at least to participate in decisions needs to be thought of in much more flexible terms. In the following sections, incapacity in matters of person (medical decisions and ability for self-care), finance, wills, advance directives, and research are discussed.

Medical Decisions

Because patients have the right to refuse medical interventions and the right to be informed before consenting to medical treatments, their ability to make these decisions has been widely discussed. The need to make a medical decision often prompts the first assessment of decisional capacity, often at a time when clinicians face pressure to make speedy judgments. For the patient facing these types of decisions, the neuropsychological functions of memory, language, and reasoning are the most crucial. Memory and language are both cortical and frontal in nature.

Although tests can help to measure the patient's ability to make medical decisions, observing the patient's ability to handle the information given is more valuable, and more important, than administering any test. Among tests, the EXIT examination has been shown to have the highest correlation (specificity and sensitivity) for testing medical decisional capacity when compared to expert assessment. Sometimes a formal structure or score is necessary, in which case the MacCAT-T provides a good framework from which to work. The interviewer is asked to stop and rate the individual's abilities in the following six steps of the process: (1) appreciation of the disorder; (2) understanding of the treatment and risks or discomforts; (3) appreciation of the treatment benefits; (4) understanding of alternate treatments; (5) reasoning; and (6) expressing a choice. Documentation of a formal score for any test is not necessary in most cases when a patient faces medical decisions. A thoughtful interview with the patient and a written description of the areas in which the patient is unable to function is usually sufficient for this purpose.

Problems of Self-Care

Circumstances may at times require formal testing. Testing may be necessary when a patient is demonstrating an inability to care for himself or herself or to accept the help needed to remain safely in his or her present environment. Issues of cognitive impairment versus denial may be hard to sort through without formal testing. A person's tendency to be "eccentric" is not always easily distinguishable from dangerous behaviors stemming from increasing cognitive impairment. Gross impairment of cortical functioning, especially short-term memory, can pose problems for day-to-day function. The impact of frontal lobe dysfunction is more evident. The inability to plan, initiate action, monitor ones behavior, and self-correct are essential to being able to care for oneself. A combination of findings on frontal lobe testing and demonstrated inability to care for oneself is usually sufficient evidence for action.

Problems of Finances

There are times when an individual remains able to make medical decisions and decisions related to self-care but can no longer handle finances. When bills are going unpaid or gross mistakes made in handling money, then someone else will need to take over financial management. Specific tests of the ability to calculate, to understand a checkbook, to monitor bank accounts, for example, can be administered by an occupational therapist or a neuropsychologist. A demonstrated problem with these areas, however, is sufficient to warrant supervision without formal testing. If the individual has enough insight to understand the problem and a reliable person is available to help, granting that person power of attorney for finances should suffice. If the incapacitated person is reluctant to relinquish control, or court monitoring is deemed advisable, then the family, the clinician, or other concerned party should seek a conservator of finance.

OTHER ISSUES OF DECISIONAL CAPACITY AND CONSENT

Wills and Testaments

The ability to make a Last Will and Testament is often believed to be retained even after the ability to handle finances and make decisions have been lost. An individual's ability to remember his or her estate plans and to express some logic behind these choices is usually sufficient evidence of capability. Despite the risk of exploitation of an impaired person, the courts usually are very liberal in allowing someone to change a will, even if cognitive problems exist.

Living Wills

In contrast, the ability to grant someone durable power of attorney for health affairs or to make a Living Will requires higher levels of cognitive function than does day-to-day decision making. Both of these areas deal with hypothetical situations that can often be hard even for cognitively intact individuals to understand fully. Scales such as the Hopkins Competency Assessment Test or the Capacity to Consent to Treatment Instrument may help to establish this ability, but these instruments are not practical in most clinical situations. The clinician should question the individual's ability to understand the process fully if he or she has demonstrated problems with memory or language or shown signs of frontal lobe dysfunction. On the other hand, as noted below, an individual may still portray wishes and desires even when very cognitively impaired.

Participation in Research

An individual's ability to consent to participate in research is also difficult to judge. The understanding of the risks and benefits of being in a research trial must be even greater than that for accepting or declining an established medical treatment. The risks and benefits are more theoretically based and therefore harder to make concrete to an individual who may be having difficulty with abstract thinking. This is an important time for dual decision making as outlined in the section below.

Temporary Loss of Decisional Capacity

Individuals may be transiently incapacitated for decision making or the likelihood of recovery of cognition may not be known, for example when the patient is delirious or has suffered a recent stroke. In such situations, the clinician should seek an interim solution. An informal surrogate, the person granted durable power of attorney for health affairs, or a temporary conservator can make decisions while the clinician clarifies the prognosis for decisional-capacity. The decisions needed during a time of uncertainty should fall on the side of aggressive protection of the individual's life or continued function until the person can make his or her wishes known or the permanence and extent of the impairment becomes clear.

Consent versus Assent

Even when an individual is no longer able to give informed consent to a procedure or a change in living situation, he or she may still participate in the decision-making process. Substituted judgment is the process that a surrogate, legal or otherwise, is supposed to apply as the basis on which a decision should be made. Substituted judgment enjoins one to take into account the patient's prior wishes and long-held beliefs as the basis for one's decision, "deciding as they would have decided." Assent refers to the impaired individual's willingness to cooperate with a plan of care. It is, in essence, a way of taking into consideration the individual's present desires when making a decision. Although it has been used primarily in the ethics and legal literature when looking at the role of adolescents in the process of medical decision-making, the principles apply to impaired adults as well. In cognitively impaired adults there is a continuum of incapacity, even among those who do not retain the full capacity to make decisions. An individual who is incapable of understanding the complexities of a situation or decision may retain high levels of understanding around specific aspects of the process and be able to express their opinions. Even very cognitively impaired patients can give indications of what brings them pleasure and what gives them pain, and clinicians should consider this information in the decision-making process.

Clinicians attempting to obtain consent for medical treatment or research protocols may wish to use a combination of surrogate consent and patient assent. This combination may be essential in situations in which the patient's ability to cooperate is needed in order to carry out the treatment or procedure. Even the courts are moving towards the recognition of the need for "limited conservatorship" that reflects that decisional capacity is not an all-or-nothing phenomenon. Decisional capacity is situation-dependent and can change with time.

REFERENCES

Grisso T, Appelbaum PS: *Assessing Competence to Consent to Treatment: A Guide for Physicians and Other Health Professionals.* 6th ed. New York, Oxford University Press, 1998 p 124.

Holzer JC et al: Cognitive functions in the informed consent evaluation process: A pilot study. *J Am Acad Psychiatry Law* 25:531, 1997.

Janofsky JS et al: The Hopkins Competency Assessment Test: A brief method for evaluating patients' capacity to give informed consent. *Hosp Commun Psychiatry* 43:132, 1992.

Marson DC: Loss of competency in Alzheimer's disease: Conceptual and psychometric approches. *Int J Law Psychiatry* 24:267, 2001.

Schindler BA et al: Competency and the frontal lobe: The impact of executive dysfunction on decisional capacity. *Psychosomatics* 36:400, 1995.

Wendler D, Prasad K: Core safeguards for clinical research with adults who are unable to consent. *Ann Intern Med* 135:514, 2001.

Diagnostic Tests

MARIE-FLORENCE SHADLEN • ERIC B. LARSON

APPROPRIATE USE OF NEW DIAGNOSTIC TECHNIQUES IN OLDER PERSONS

Sackett and colleagues have described eight guides for deciding the clinical usefulness of a diagnostic test (Table 11-1). This decision relies on the severity of the disease, the patient's prognosis, and the probability of treatment response as reported in study populations similar to the individual patient. Regardless of the reason, the overriding criterion for seeking diagnostic information is the usefulness of the given piece of data to the clinician who seeks it and to the patient who generates it. In this context, the clinician also assesses the value of new diagnostic technologies and incorporates these tests into practice.

The definition of normal can be particularly challenging in geriatrics. For example, imaging of brain atrophy with prominent sulci and ventricles was attributed to Alzheimer's disease until these signs were shown to be age-related changes. For both computed tomography (CT) and magnetic resonance imaging (MRI), there was also failure to appreciate that so-called periventricular lucencies—although similar to changes resulting from stroke—can be seen in persons with "normal" aging and thus do not constitute a criterion for diagnosing multiinfarct dementia.

The bulk of geriatric treatment is directed toward chronic diseases, palliation, and health promotion to optimize patient function, not the complete cure or prevention of disease. There are potentially limitless opportunities to apply diagnostic tests. The geriatric caregiver will need to seek increasingly good evidence of test utility, especially in the context of progressive escalation of test costs. The ultimate criterion for any clinical maneuver, including a diagnostic test, is whether a patient is better off for it. Although this may seem like a tall order for new tests, it is a notion that gains support in an age of limited health resources and managed care.

FEATURES OF DIAGNOSTIC TEST PERFORMANCE

MRI is more sensitive than CT for diagnosis of certain strokes. MRI is more accurate for visualizing lesions in the temporal lobes, posterior fossa, brainstem, and spinal cord. But do the high quality images warrant the 30 to 100 percent higher cost as compared to CT? With regard to routine clinical practice, there are instances where MRI neuroimaging is preferred, but there are many other circumstances where its marginal value is modest to nil as compared with CT.

A screening test should be highly sensitive because it is used to rule out a diagnosis. Screening with fecal occult-blood testing remains a controversial intervention because of its high false negative rate. The sensitivity of fecal occult blood testing for colon cancer has been reported to be 33 percent and false positives are common. Therefore, routine screening for fecal occult blood has a small but definite effect on colon cancer mortality. A confirmatory test should be highly specific because a positive diagnosis may lead to subsequent procedures or surgery with potential risks and costs. Because sensitivity and specificity of a test when properly established do not depend on the underlying disease probability, the values determined by other investigators can be applied in any clinical setting. This allows comparison to test results obtained on different patient groups.

Once the results of a test are known, its predictive value is the probability of interest. The predictive values of a test depend both on test accuracy and on the prevalence of disease in the particular clinical scenario. Figure 11-1 shows that predictive values can be calculated according to Bayes' theorem of probability. Bayes' theorem tells us how sensitivity, specificity, and probability of a disease give the predictive value of a positive or negative test. The positive predictive value tells us what proportion of patients who had positive test results had the disease (true positive/true positive + false positive). For instance, screening with fecal occult blood testing has been reported to have a positive predictive value of 2.2 percent, making it a costly screening strategy when the subsequent testing is taken into account. The negative predictive value tells us what proportion of patients who had negative test results did not have the disease (true negative/false negative + true negative).

A test that is very useful for diagnosing a disease in a patient with symptoms (higher pretest probability) may be nearly useless for screening an asymptomatic person (lower pretest probability). The more specific the diagnostic test, the better the positive predictive value, and the more confident the clinician will be that the positive test result

Table 11-1   Eight Guides for Deciding the Clinical Usefulness of a Diagnostic Test

1. Has there been an independent, "blind" comparison with a "gold standard" of diagnosis?
2. Has the diagnostic test been evaluated in a patient sample that included an appropriate spectrum of mild and severe, treated and untreated disease, plus individuals with different but commonly confused disorders?
3. Was the setting for this evaluation, as well as the filter through which study patients passed, adequately described?
4. Have the reproducibility of the test result (precision) and its interpretation (observer variation) been determined?
5. Has the term normal been defined sensibly as it applied to this test?
6. If the test is advocated as part of a cluster or sequence of tests, has its individual contribution to the overall validity of the cluster or sequence been determined?
7. Have the tactics for carrying out the test been described in sufficient detail to permit their exact replication?
8. Has the utility of the test been determined?

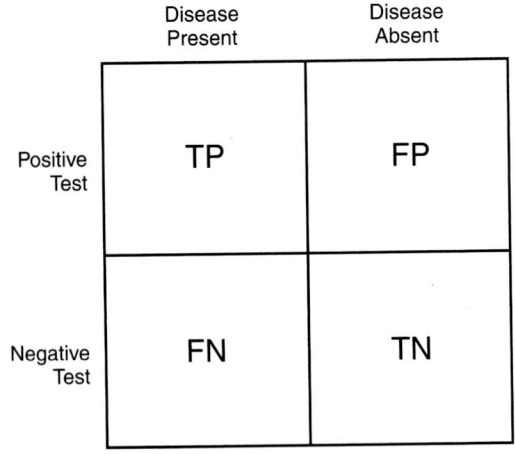

Figure 11-2   The relationship between a diagnostic test result and the occurrence of disease. There are two possibilities for the result to be correct (true positive and true negative) and two possibilities for the result to be incorrect (false positive and false negative).

The odds ratio measures the odds of having a positive test if the disease is present divided by the odds of having the positive test if the disease is absent. An odds ratio of 1 represents the point at which the odds of disease are the

indicates disease. Conversely, the more sensitive the test, the higher the negative predictive value, and the clinician can be more confident that a patient with a negative test result does not have the disease.

The higher the prevalence, or pretest probability of a disease, the higher the positive predictive value. When the test is applied to patients among whom the prevalence of a given disease is low, "positive" results may be largely false-positive results. The relationship of prevalence on positive predictive value for a test is shown in Figure 11-2 and Table 11-2.

LIKELIHOOD RATIOS

Summary test performance characteristics are the so-called likelihood ratio statistics. The main advantage of likelihood ratio statistics is that measures of test accuracy can be readily communicated with patients. Likelihood ratios of several independent diagnostic tests can also be multiplied to estimate their joint value. Like sensitivity and specificity, likelihood ratios are not influenced by the prevalence of the disease.

$$+PV = \frac{(Se)(P)}{(Se)(P) + (1 - Sp)(1 - P)}$$

where: Se = sensitivity;
Sp = specificity;
P = prevalence;
+PV = positive predictive value

Figure 11-1   Predictive value is calculated according to Bayes' theorem of probability.

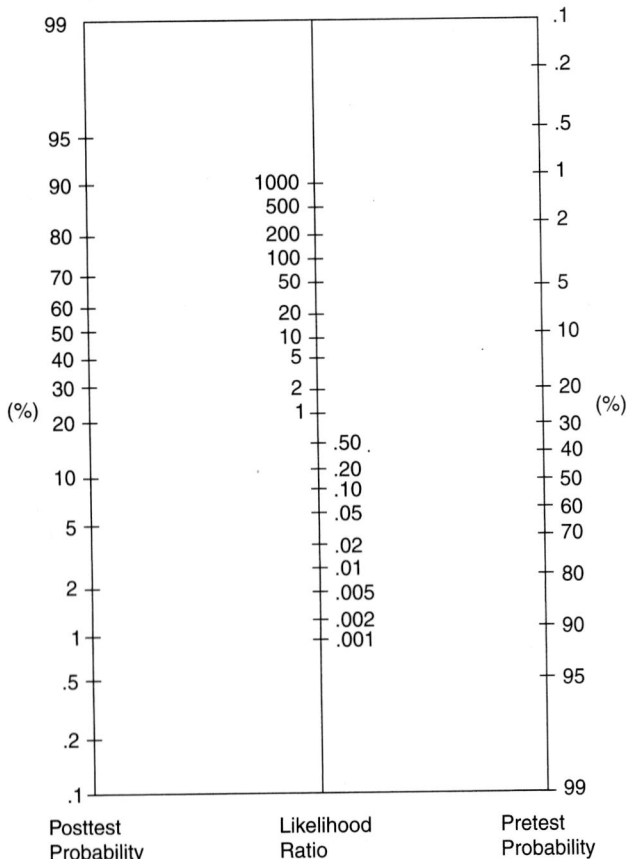

Figure 11-3   Nomogram for calculating post-test probabilities, given probabilities and likelihood ratios as reported by Fagan. To use the nomogram, find the pretest probability on the right hand scale and the likelihood ratio on the center scale. Connect these two points with a straight line, extending the line to intercept the left-hand scale. Read the post-test probability at this intercept.

same whether or not the test result is positive. A probability can be converted to odds by writing the probability to the left of the colon and the difference between 1 and the probability (1 − probability) to the right. For example, a probability of 0.75 (or 75 percent) becomes odds of 0.75:0.25, which, after dividing both sides by 0.25, becomes 3:1. To convert an odds ratio into a probability, the expression on the left of the colon is divided by the sum of the numbers on both sides of the denominator. For example, odds of 4:1 becomes a probability of $4/(4+1) = 4/5 = 0.80$ (or 80 percent).

The *likelihood ratio positive* (LR+) is the odds of disease among those in whom the test yielded positive results divided by the odds of disease in the entire population. The likelihood ratio is also defined as sensitivity/1 − specificity. The LR+, therefore, indicates how much the odds of disease was increased if the test result was positive. The likelihood ratio for a negative test (LR−) is the odds of having disease among those in whom the test yielded negative results divided by the odds of disease in the entire population. The LR−, therefore, shows how much the odds of disease was decreased if the test result was negative. The likelihood ratio can be summarized as the odds of disease

given a specific test value divided by the odds of disease in the general population.

The confidence interval on an odds ratio allows us to say (usually with 95% confidence) that the odds ratio is present not only in our sample but in the larger population from which the sample was obtained. Thus, if the 95% confidence interval around the observed odds ratio fails to extend beyond or overlap 1, one can conclude that the odds ratio is statistically significant with a p-value less than or equal to 0.05.

The posttest odds of disease equal the pretest odds multiplied by the likelihood ratio. Figure 11-3 shows that the conversion to odds, multiplication by the likelihood ratio, and conversion back to probability can also be accomplished by means of the nomogram.

The most effective tests will have high likelihood ratios for positive tests (greater than 10 or 20) and lower likelihood ratios for negative tests (less than 0.2). Such tests will have the greatest effect on posttest probability for a target disorder as compared to diagnostic tests with intermediate values of likelihood ratios. Likelihood ratios greater than 1 give posttest odds that are greater than pretest odds, whereas likelihood ratios less than 1 give posttest odds that

Table 11-2   Standard 2 × 2 Table Comparing the Test Results and the True Disease Status of the Subjects Tested

		TRUE DISEASE STATUS		
		DISEASED	NONDISEASED	TOTAL
Test result	Positive	a	b	a + b
	Negative	c	d	c + d
	Total	a + c	b + d	a + b + c + d

a = Subjects with a true-positive test result
b = Subjects with a false-positive test result
c = Subjects with a false-negative test result
d = Subjects with a true-negative test result
$a + b$ = All subjects with a positive test result
$c + d$ = All subjects with a negative test result
$a + c$ = All subjects with the disease
$b + d$ = All subjects without the disease

Formulas are as follows:
$a/(a + c)$ = Sensitivity
$d/(b + d)$ = Specificity
$b/(b + d)$ = False-positive error rate (alpha error rate, type I rate)
$c/(a + c)$ = False-negative error rate (beta error rate, type II rate)
$a/(a + b)$ = Positive predictive value
$d/(c + d)$ = Negative predictive value

$[a/(a + c)]/[b/(b + d)] = (a/b)/[(a + c)/(b + d)]$ = Likelihood ratio positive (LR+)
$[c/(a + c)]/[d/(b + d)] = (c/d)/[(a + c)/(b + d)]$ = Likelihood ratio negative (LR−)

$(a + c)/(a + b + c + d)$ = Prevalence

SOURCE: Reproduced with permission from Jekel et al. (1996).

are less than pretest odds. Likelihood ratios near 1 give posttest odds that are similar to pretest values. Likelihood ratios are often published in critical reviews or so-called meta-analyses of diagnostic test efficacy.

Another useful application of the odds method is in sequential testing where the posttest odds from the first test become the pretest odds for the next test, thereby avoiding the need to construct a series of 2×2 tables (Table 11-2). Note, however, that this use of Bayes' theorem rests on the assumption that the tests in the sequence are conditionally independent, that is, a particular result of one test is not associated with a particular result on the other.

ASSESSING THE VALIDITY OF SCREENING TESTS: INSTRUCTIVE EXAMPLES RELEVANT TO GERIATRIC PRACTICE

Apolipoprotein E Screening for Alzheimer's Disease

A 70-year-old woman has made an appointment to ask for your advice. She has no cognitive complaints. However, her brother has been diagnosed with Alzheimer's disease at the age of 75 years. She heard that a genetic test is now available to screen for susceptibility to this disease. She asks you if

screening certain members of her family for Alzheimer's disease might be warranted.

Fewer than 2 percent of Alzheimer's disease patients have an autosomal dominant pattern of disease transmission. By and large, familial early onset Alzheimer's disease cases are associated with the B-amyloid precursor protein gene (APP) on chromosome 21, the presenilin 1 gene on chromosome 14, or the presenilin 2 gene on chromosome 1. The apolipoprotein E epsilon 4 (apoE4) gene on chromosome 19 is a susceptibility gene that increases the risk of developing Alzheimer's disease and appears to reduce the age of onset. However, fewer than 25% of persons with sporadic, late-onset Alzheimer's disease have the apoE4 gene, and as many as 50% of people having at least one apoE4 allele never develop Alzheimer's disease. For the general population, the lifetime risk of Alzheimer's disease is 1 percent. The main risk factor for Alzheimer's disease is advanced age. A sibling, child, or parent of a person with late-onset, sporadic Alzheimer's disease is unlikely to develop the disease.

Several companies are offering the apolipoprotein E genotype polymerase chain reaction assay as a diagnostic test. How accurate is apoE genotyping for diagnosing Alzheimer's disease? The usefulness of a test rests on its comparison to the gold standard. Because the diagnosis of Alzheimer's disease is definitive only at autopsy, there is no antemortem gold standard with which to assess its diagnostic efficacy. A study of subjects in the Framingham cohort

First scenario: Evaluate the predictive value of APOE testing for diagnosis of Alzheimer's disease in a 70-year-old with 3 percent pretest probability.

	DX ALZHEIMER'S DISEASE		
	GOLD STANDARD ALZHEIMER'S DISEASE	GOLD STANDARD ALZHEIMER'S DISEASE-FREE	TOTAL
Positive	$a = 15$	$b = 242.5$	$a + b = 257.5$
Negative	$c = 15$	$d = 727.5$	$c + d = 742.5$
Total	$a + c = 30$	$b + d = 970$	$a + b + c + d$ $= 1000$

a = Number of individuals with AD who had 1 E4 allele.
b = Number of individuals without AD who had 1 E4 allele.
c = Number of individuals with AD who are negative for E4 allele.
d = Number of individuals without AD who are negative for E4 allele.
$a + c$ = Total number of positives.
$b + d$ = Total number of negatives.
$a/a + c$ = Sensitivity = 0.50
    $a = 15, c = 15; 15/(15 + 15) = 0.50$
$d/(b + d)$ = Specificity = 0.75
    $b = 242.5, d = 727.5; 727.5/(242.5 + 727.5) = 0.75$
$a/(a + b)$ = Predictive value of a positive test = 5.8%
    $a = 15, b = 242.5; 5/(15 + 242.5) = 0.058 = 5.8\%$
$d/(c + d)$ = Predictive value of a negative test = 98%
    $c = 15, d = 727.5; 727.5/(15 + 727.5) = 0.979 = 98\%$

Second scenario: Evaluate the predictive value of apoE testing for diagnosis of Alzheimer's disease in an 80-year-old with 20 percent pretest probability.

	DX ALZHEIMER'S DISEASE		
	GOLD STANDARD ALZHEIMER'S DISEASE	GOLD STANDARD ALZHEIMER'S DISEASE-FREE	TOTAL
Positive	$a = 100$	$b = 200$	$a + b = 300$
Negative	$c = 100$	$d = 600$	$c + d = 700$
Total	$a + c = 200$	$b + d = 800$	$a + b + c + d$ $= 1000$

a = Number of individuals with AD who had 1 E4 allele.
b = Number of individuals without AD who had 1 E4 allele.
c = Number of individuals with AD who are negative for E4 allele.
d = Number of individuals without AD who are negative for E4 allele.
$a + c$ = Total number of positives.
$b + d$ = Total number of negatives.
$a/a + c$ = Sensitivity = 0.50
     $a = 100, c = 100; 100/(100 + 100) = 0.50$
$d/(b + d)$ = Specificity = 0.75
     $b = 200, d = 600; 600/(600 + 200) = 0.75$
$a/(a + b)$ = Predictive value of a positive test = 33%
     $a = 100, b = 200; 100/(100 + 200) = 0.33$
$d/(c + d)$ = Predictive value of a negative test = 86%
     $c = 100, d = 600; 600/(100 + 600) = 0.857$

Third scenario: Evaluate the predictive value of apoE testing for diagnosis of Alzheimer's disease in an 90-year-old with 50 percent pretest probability.

	DX ALZHEIMER'S DISEASE		
	GOLD STANDARD ALZHEIMER'S DISEASE	GOLD STANDARD ALZHEIMER'S DISEASE-FREE	TOTAL
Positive	$a = 250$	$b = 125$	$a + b = 375$
Negative	$c = 250$	$d = 375$	$c + d = 625$
Total	$a + c = 500$	$b + d = 500$	$a + b + c + d$ $= 1000$

a = Number of individuals with AD who had 1 E4 allele.
b = Number of individuals without AD who had 1 E4 allele.
c = Number of individuals with AD who are negative for E4 allele.
d = Number of individuals without AD who are negative for E4 allele.
$a + c$ = Total number of positives.
$b + d$ = Total number of negatives.
$a/a + c$ = Sensitivity = 0.50
     $a = 250, c = 250; 250/(250 + 250) = 0.50$
$d/(b + d)$ = Specificity = 0.75
     $b = 125, d = 375; 125/(125 + 375) = 0.75$
$a/(a + b)$ = Predictive value of a positive test = 66%
     $a = 250, b = 125; 250/(250 + 125) = 0.66$
$d/(c + d)$ = Predictive value of a negative test = 60%
     $c = 250, d = 375; 375/(250 + 375) = 0.60$

by Myers et al. found apoE genotyping had a sensitivity of 49 percent, specificity of 81 percent, positive predictive value of 10 percent, and negative predictive value of 97 percent. A case-control study in Seattle by Kukull et al. reported the presence of one apoE4 allele had a sensitivity of 52 percent and specificity of 74 percent. Hence, only a small proportion of persons with the apoE4 allele are diagnosed with Alzheimer's disease. In comparison with genotyping, the study by Crum et al. reported that the Folstein Mini-Mental State Exam with a cutoff score of 24 points has a sensitivity of 87 percent and a specificity of 82 percent for the diagnosis of Alzheimer's disease. Thus while apoE genotyping remains a useful research tool for evaluating the interaction of risk factors and for identifying potential subgroups of patients with differential treatment responses, it is neither a sensitive nor specific diagnostic marker for Alzheimer's disease.

The relationship between the effect of prevalence on predictive value for a test with dichotomous results (presence or absence of one apoE4 allele) is demonstrated below. Calculate the predictive values of the presence of one apoE4 allele with the diagnosis of Alzheimer's disease in three scenarios: among persons ages 65 to 74 years (3 percent prevalence), persons ages 75 to 85 years (19 percent prevalence), and persons ages 85 years and older (47 percent prevalence). Assume sensitivity of 50 percent and specificity of 75 percent for the diagnosis of Alzheimer's disease.

These calculations indicate that the probability of a disease being present or absent after obtaining the results of a test is dependent on the best possible estimate of the probability of disease made before performance of the test. When the probability of Alzheimer's disease is relatively low as in an asymptomatic 70-year-old, even a positive test leaves a 94.2 percent probability that the disease is absent. When the pretest probability of Alzheimer's disease is moderately high as in an asymptomatic 90-year-old, even a negative test—that is the absence of the apoE4 allele—leaves a 40 percent probability that the patient has Alzheimer's disease.

The sensitivity, specificity and predictive value of apoE4 testing for Alzheimer's disease was evaluated by Saunders in a group of 57 patients with Alzheimer's disease and 10 patients with dementias from other causes. A positive test for one apoE4 allele was shown to have a sensitivity of 75 percent, a specificity of 100 percent, a positive predictive value of 100 percent, and a negative predictive value of 42 percent. Based on these data, one might assume that apoE genotyping was well suited for screening the general population because 100 percent of those with one apoE4 allele will have the diagnosis of Alzheimer's disease. For this study, the apoE4 test was applied to a group in which 85 percent of patients had neuropathologically confirmed Alzheimer's disease. Thus the pretest probability of Alzheimer's disease in the test group was 85%. The predictive value of a positive test depends on the prevalence of the disease in the group of individuals tested. Even among nonagenarians, the prevalence of Alzheimer's disease will be much lower than 85 percent. Consequently, the predictive value of a positive apoE4 as a screening test is well below 100 percent.

Serum Prostate-Specific Antigen

On a routine office visit a 70-year-old white male requests a test of his serum prostate-specific antigen (PSA) level for early detection of prostate cancer. His close friend died recently of metastatic prostate cancer. The patient has no family history of prostate cancer. He denies any symptoms of urinary frequency, incomplete emptying, dribbling, hematuria, or bony pains. His chart review shows that he had a normal PSA 3 years previously. His physical exam is unremarkable. The digital rectal exam reveals no evidence of a prostate nodule. Do you recommend PSA screening?

The patient's concern about occult prostate cancer is valid. It is a common disease with an annual incidence rate of 187.4 cases per 100,000 men. The median age at diagnosis of prostate cancer is 72 years. Prostate cancer often does not cause symptoms for many years and the mean lead time from increased PSA to clinical diagnosis of prostate cancer is estimated to be 7 years. On the other hand, the survival of men who have stage I prostate cancer is similar to that of their age-matched normal counterparts. To be a useful screening tool, the PSA test must not only improve survival but must also reduce the burdens associated with detection of prostate cancer that otherwise would not have been diagnosed within the patient's lifetime. The best estimates from the literature on the operating characteristics of PSA screening for prostate cancer show a sensitivity of 79 percent, specificity of 59 percent, positive predictive value of 40 percent and negative predictive value of 89 percent. Hence, a positive PSA (>4 ng/mL) leaves a 60 percent probability that an asymptomatic patient does not have prostate cancer. The PSA is a reliable confirmatory test. A positive PSA in the presence of clinically suspicious prostatic nodules increases the probability that cancer will be diagnosed at biopsy. Moreover, the PSA is useful for monitoring treatment response once prostate cancer is diagnosed.

Randomized studies to address mortality reductions in PSA and free prostate antigen screening are currently ongoing and results may not be available for a decade. These trials were not designed to test the efficiency of varying screening intervals or ages of starting and stopping PSA screening. The aggregate cost of follow-up biopsies resulting from one-time PSA screening for men older than age 50 years in the United States would be approximately $12 billion. In a computer-simulation model, annual screening of men ages 50 through 75 years with a cutoff of 4.0 ng/mL saved 0.16 person-years of life per man screened. If the interval were increased to biennial PSA screenings, there would be a 50 percent reduction in the number of false-positive PSA tests, while retaining 93 percent of years of life saved.

The American Cancer Society and the American Urological Association currently recommend annual screening in most men ages 50 to 70 years using digital rectal exams and PSA testing. Asian and Native American men are at lower risk, whereas African American men are at higher risk of prostate cancer. African American men have twice the mortality of white Americans from prostate cancer. Men of all races with history of a brother or father diagnosed with prostate cancer are also at higher risk of prostate cancer. In the higher risk groups, screening is recommended starting at age 40 years. Although some urologists suggest workup of PSA levels greater than 2.5 ng/mL in men at higher risk for prostate cancer, the performance of PSA at varying cutoffs in populations with higher pretest probabilities of prostate cancer has not been formally tested. Until there is further evidence to support the efficacy of routine PSA screening in low-risk groups, an individualized approach is recommended. For instance, it is reasonable to screen the 70-year-old white male presented in this section who had a normal PSA 3 years previously but who requests PSA screening for reassurance.

Bone Mineral Density Screening

A 75-year-old white female of Scandinavian ancestry volunteers for a free dual-energy x-ray absorptiometry (DXA) scan. The patient has no family history of fractures. She denies use of corticosteroids and has no history of hyperparathyroidism or hyperthyroidism. She does not smoke nor drink alcohol. The results of the DXA scan showed an average bone mineral density of 0.817 g/cm^2 of the lumbar spine (0.06 standard deviations below a 75-year-old mean) and 0.649 g/cm^2 of the left hip (1.13 standard deviations below a 75-year-old mean). She returns to your office with a report indicating that she has moderate osteopenia of the spine and severe osteopenia of the left hip. She is at moderate to relatively high risk for an osteoporosis-related fracture. She is wondering why you are not screening the bone mineral density for older women in your practice.

The patient's concern about the public health consequences of osteoporosis is valid (as detailed in Chap. 75). However, the assumption implicit in the patient's question is that offering DXA scan screening to older women will prevent the devastating consequences of osteoporosis.

A meta-analysis by Marshall et al. studied the usefulness of measurements of postmenopausal women's bone density for prediction of later fractures. The positive predictive value of a bone density measure 1 standard deviation below the age-adjusted mean was 58 percent among women with multiple risk factors for fracture (pretest probability 30 percent) as compared with a positive predictive value of 9 percent among women with low prevalence of fractures (pretest probability 3 percent). Thus, as many as 42 percent of women with bone density one standard deviation below the age-adjusted mean did not have fractures during the 1.8 to 24 years of follow up. The source of error is the large overlap in the bone densities of patients with fracture and in the bone densities of those without a fracture. Moreover, bone density tests such as the DXA scan do not take into account other factors that contribute to frailty.

Until there is evidence to support the cost-effectiveness of routine DXA scan screening, an individualized approach is recommended (in spite of the recent decision to reimburse such screening by Medicare). Bone density measurements should be recommended to patients receiving chronic glucocorticoid therapy or when measurement will help the patient decide whether to institute long-term treatment to prevent osteoporotic fractures. There is no evidence in support of monitoring response to antiresorptive agents with serial DXA scan measurements. Thus older patients should be instructed to have calcium intake of 1,000 to 1,500 mg/d and vitamin D of 400 to 600 IU/d and take the other measures outlined in Chap. 75 to minimize bone mineral loss and prevent fractures.

CLINICAL DECISION MAKING

Diagnostic tests are most useful when the pretest estimates of disease probability are intermediate, neither very high nor very low. Thus, the physician has most to gain from a test when the pretest estimate is most uncertain. When evaluating relative odds of disease, it is the relative change in probabilities that matters. That is, from 75 percent to 25 percent represents a relative reduction by threefold in disease likelihood. For instance, the relative risk of dying of breast cancer after screening mammography as compared with no screening has been estimated at 0.72 (95% confidence interval, 0.54 to 0.88) for women 60 to 69 years of age. This would represent a relative reduction by 1.39-fold likelihood of breast cancer mortality (1 divided by 0.72). Measurements of relative changes in probabilities of disease are more meaningful than absolute magnitudes of change.

Clinicians often lack confidence in their estimates of pretest probabilities. It is only after some reflection that skilled clinicians recognize their implicit assessment of odds of disease before ordering a test. Even crude estimates in disease prevalence are unlikely to distort the test interpretation. Assuming that the diagnostic test has good operational characteristics, diagnostic testing will result in reduced uncertainty. Even normal results are likely to increase certainty of likelihood of absence of disease.

PRINCIPLES OF DIAGNOSTIC TECHNOLOGY ASSESSMENT

In the wake of societal concerns about the high costs of diagnostic technologies, taxonomies of diagnostic efficacy have been developed. The most commonly cited taxonomy describes a hierarchy of five levels consisting of technologic capacity, diagnostic accuracy, diagnostic impact, therapeutic impact, and patient outcomes. Ideally, a new diagnostic technology will have clinical research and development describing its effect in all five levels. In fact, there are very few instances when we have evidence of a diagnostic technology favorably affecting patient outcomes.

Technologic capacity deals with the capacity for a diagnostic technique to measure a phenomenon with accuracy. In imaging, this capacity is measured by such variables as image quality and reliability. Diagnostic accuracy refers to the technology's ability to detect and classify pathology accurately. These properties are measured by the diagnostic test performance variables described earlier, including sensitivity, specificity, and true-positive and false-positive rates. Diagnostic impact refers to the accuracy and clinical value of a new technique compared to the alternative diagnostic test. This impact is typically measured according to the same properties used to measure diagnostic accuracy but, at this level, these properties are compared with some alternative and not simply described in isolation.

Therapeutic impact relates to the effect of diagnostic technology on patient care. Desirable effects would be to reduce risk and discomfort to patients, improve treatment selection by clinicians, and perhaps provide more reassurance to patients or clinicians. Finally, patient outcome refers to whether a diagnostic test leads to a longer life, relief of pain and suffering, or improved functional status. These outcomes are difficult to prove but are certainly important when one is considering widely used tests like screening tests. Nonetheless, it is certainly not unreasonable to expect that well-established diagnostic tests should have fairly good information on at least the first four levels of efficacy.

USE AND SELECTION OF NEW DIAGNOSTIC TESTS

Clinicians tend to develop practice patterns that "work" to solve problems for them and their patients. New diagnostic tests can be viewed as offering added efficiencies in solving clinical problems or in enhancing the quality of information available to the physician. The principles described in the preceding section should be helpful in deciding whether to use a new test, in whom, and how to interpret the results.

Health services research has demonstrated considerable variation among physicians in the use of diagnostic tests. In general, the variation in test ordering leads to widespread differences in the costs generated by those tests without any measurable difference in value to patients. This has led to increased efforts to establish practice standards or guidelines for common clinical problems. Such efforts occur at all levels, from local hospital or clinic practice guidelines, to specialty society standard settings, to efforts sanctioned by national governments to establish national guidelines. Both the United States and Canada have also charged ongoing task forces to describe those elements of the periodic health exam that have been demonstrated to be efficacious. These guidelines are formulated to assist physicians in using diagnostic tests effectively and were designed to help produce more standardized and cost-effective practice patterns.

New tests pose a particular challenge to practicing physicians, because most clinicians will not have experienced new tests in a training situation. The guides described in this chapter should be helpful to clinicians in determining the extent to which a test's value has been demonstrated and will thus likely be of value for patients. In addition, given the vastness of the medical literature, groups like the Clinical Efficacy Assessment Project of the American College of Physicians have commissioned clinical reviews of carefully peer-reviewed statements of clinical efficacy.

These guidelines help clinicians determine those clinical instances when a new test—for example, MRI of the brain and spine—will be valuable. The most useful reviews are likely to be those that use principles of clinical epidemiology and so-called rules of evidence to determine value rather than those which rely solely on expert opinion or the enthusiastic reports of a test's developer.

A study in 1985 found that internists left unanswered 70 percent of the questions that arose when seeing patients and almost never consulted the medical literature for the rest. Their reasons for failing to do so included lack of time, disorganization of their own journal collection, and a lack of knowledge about where to look for answers. Clinicians now increasingly rely on electronic searches of the medical literature in their offices, clinics, and homes. There are now compendia of diagnostic tests plus a continuing series of articles in *Annals of Internal Medicine* from the Clinical Efficacy Assessment Project of the American College of Physicians. To set up a Medline search, specify the appropriate medical subject headings for one or more clinical problems or areas that you want to keep abreast with and combine these with the subheadings for diagnostic tests with the terms: sensitivity, specificity, predictive value of tests or receiver operating characteristics (ROC) curves.

SCREENING TESTS

Decisions to screen for a disease initiated by a health care provider are based on a society's assessment of the burden of the disease, the diagnostic accuracy of the test, the consequences of false-positive and false-negative results, and the outcome of early detection of disease. The latter is particularly relevant in the practice of geriatric medicine where patients are frequently already close to their life expectancy. As reported by Goldberg and Chabin, most clinicians regard age 85 with an average remaining life expectancy of 5 years as a general cutoff range beyond which routine screening tests are unlikely to be warranted. The data on false-positive and false-negative rates for many screening tests have been obtained in younger populations which tend to have less physiologic heterogeneity and longer estimated remaining longevity. Table 11-3 shows the US Preventive Services Task Force (USPSTF) criteria for the periodic use of selected screening tests in older persons. As reported by Kerlikowske et al., the USPSTF recommends screening mammograms every 1 to 3 years until age 85 years in selected women, screening sigmoidoscopy every 5 years in selected older adults, and screening thyroid function studies in older women with unexplained symptoms. The USPSTF does not recommend screening for the following in asymptomatic persons older than 75 years of age: serum glucose, serum cholesterol, serum prostate specific antigen, the digital rectal exam, bone density testing, or electrocardiogram. These recommendations emphasize selective screening instead of routine periodic screening of all older persons at average risk of disease. These guidelines cannot only assist physicians in using diagnostic tests effectively, but can help produce more standardized and cost-effective practice patterns.

Table 11-3   U S Preventive Services Task Force (USTF) Criteria for Periodic Use of Selected Screening Tests in Older Adults

Test	Criteria	USTF Recommendations
Routine hematocrit	Institutionalized elderly persons	No
Routine urinalysis	Age >60 years	Yes
Routine cholesterol	>75 years old	NR
Routine thyroid testing	Women >60 years old	Yes
Routine fasting plasma glucose	Age >50 years	No
Prostate specific antigen	Men >65 years old	No
Routine electrolytes	Age >65 years	NR
Stool for occult blood	Age >65 years	NR
Routine electrocardiography	Age >65 years	No
Routine bone mineral analysis	Women >50 years	No
Routine mammography	Age 50–75 years or beyond: yearly	Yes
Routine cervical Cytologic screening	Age >65 years if no cytologic testing in previous 10 years;	Yes
	If previous screening with normal results.	No
Routine sigmoidoscopy	Age >65 years	NR
Routine colonoscopy	Age >65 years	NR

NR, no recommendation.

SOURCE: Adapted from Sox (1994) and Beers (1991).

REFERENCES

Beers MH et al: Screening recommendations for the elderly. *Am J Public Health* 81:1131, 1991.

Brunader R: Radiologic decision-making: Radiologic bone assessment in the evaluation of osteoporosis. *Am Fam Physician* 65(7):1357, 2002.

Carter HB et al: Recommended prostate-specific antigen testing intervals for detection of curable prostate cancer. *JAMA* 277:1456, 1997.

Carter HB et al: Prostate-specific antigen testing of older men. *J Natl Cancer Inst* 91(20):1733, 1999.

Crum RM et al: Population-based norms for the Mini-Mental State Examination by age and educational level (see comments). *JAMA* 269:2386, 1993.

Etzioni R: Overdiagnosis due to prostate-specific antigen screening: lessons from US prostate cancer incidence trends. *J Natl Cancer Inst* 94(13):981, 2002.

Etzioni RA et al: Serial prostate-specific antigen screening for prostate cancer: A computer model evaluates competing strategies. *J Urol* 162:741, 1999.

Evans DA et al: Prevalence of Alzheimer's disease in a community population of older persons: Higher than previously reported. *JAMA* 262:2551, 1989.

Fagan TJ: Nomogram for Bayes' theorem [letter]. *N Engl J Med* 293:257, 1975.

Farrer LA et al: Statement on use of apolipoprotein E testing for Alzheimer's disease. *JAMA* 274(20):1627, 1995.

Feussner JR, White LJ: The clinical efficacy assessment program of the American College of Physicians. *Ann N Y Acad Sci* 703:268, 1993.

Fleming C et al: A decision analysis of alternative treatment strategies for clinically localized prostate cancer. *JAMA* 269:2650, 1993.

Gann PH et al: A prospective evaluation of plasma prostate-specific antigen for detection of prostate cancer. *JAMA* 25: 273:289, 1995.

Goldberg TH, Chabin SI: Preventive medicine and screening in older adults. *J Am Geriatr Soc* 45:344, 1997.

Hugosson J et al: Would prostate cancer detected by screening with prostate-specific antigen develop into clinical cancer if left undiagnosed? A comparison of two population-based studies in Sweden. *BJU Int* 85(9):1078, 2000.

Jekel JF et al: *Epidemiology, Biostatistics and Preventive Medicine.* Philadelphia, WB Saunders, 1996.

Kerlikowske K et al: Efficacy of screening mammography: A meta-analysis. *JAMA* 273:149, 1995.

Kim DE, Berlowitz DR: The limited value of routine laboratory assessments in severely impaired nursing home residents. *JAMA* 272(18):1447, 1994.

Kukull WA et al. Apolipoprotein E in Alzheimer's disease risk and case detection: A case-control study. *J Clin Epidemiol* 49(10):1143, 1996.

Larson EB, McGee SR: Update in general internal medicine. *ACP J Club* September/October:A-12, 1995.

Mandel JS et al: Reducing mortality from colorectal cancer by screening for fecal occult blood [erratum *N Engl J Med* 329:672, 1993]. *N Engl J Med* 328:1365, 1993.

Marshall D et al: Meta-analysis of how well measures of bone mineral density predict occurrence of osteoporotic fractures. *BMJ* 312:1254, 1996.

McKibbon KA, Walker-Dilks CJ: How to harness MEDLINE for diagnostic problems. *ACP J Club* September/October:A-10, 1994.

Myers RH et al: Apolipoprotein E e4 association with dementia in a population-based study: The Framingham study. *Neurology* 46:673, 1996.

Panzer RJ et al. (eds): *Diagnostic Strategies in Common Medical Problems.* Philadelphia, American College of Physicians, 1992 p 1, 499.

Riegelman RK, Hirsh RP: *Studying a Study and Testing a Test,* 2nd ed. Riegelman Children's Trust, Toronto, 1989.

Ross KS et al: Comparative efficiency of prostate-specific antigen screening strategies for prostate cancer detection. *JAMA* 284(11):1399, 2000.

Sackett DL et al: *Clinical Epidemiology: A Basic Science for Clinical Medicine,* 2d ed. Boston, Little, Brown, 1991 p 3, 52.

Saunders AD et al: Specificity, sensitivity, and predictive value of apolipoprotein E genotyping for sporadic Alzheimer's disease. *Lancet* 348:90, 1996.

Selby JV et al: Effect of fecal occult blood testing on mortality from colorectal cancer. *Ann Intern Med* 118:1, 1993.

Selby JV et al: A case-control study of screening sigmoidoscopy and mortality from colorectal cancer. *N Engl J Med* 326:653, 1992.

Sox HC Jr: Preventive health services in adults. *N Engl J Med* 330:1589, 1994.

Williamson JW et al: Health science information management and continuing education of physicians. *Ann Intern Med* 110:151, 1989.

Principles of Screening in Older Adults

LOUISE C. WALTER

This chapter focuses on the topic of screening, specifically the issues that need to be considered when making a decision to screen an older person for cancer, because this decision highlights many of the special philosophical and practical challenges inherent in recommending preventive services to older persons. One obvious challenge to recommending cancer screening (and many other preventive services) to older adults is that few studies of preventive interventions have enrolled persons older than age 75 years. The absence of age-specific data requires clinicians to extrapolate data about the effectiveness of screening in younger persons and apply it to older persons. Furthermore, even if trials suggest that the effectiveness of screening is similar in younger and older populations, challenges remain about how to apply data from trials to an individual older person. Trials show the average effectiveness of an intervention, but they generally do not address individual patient characteristics, such as comorbid conditions or functional status, which may change the likelihood of receiving benefit or harm from screening. Given these challenges, the need to individualize screening decisions is especially important for older people, because individuals become increasingly unique in their particular combination of health, function, remaining life expectancy, and values with advancing age.

The important issues that need to be considered when making individualized screening decisions in elderly persons are not addressed by current guidelines that base their recommendations primarily on age. Although many screening guidelines that recommend upper age limits for stopping screening are now including caveats about screening an older person if he/she has a "reasonable life expectancy," current guidelines offer little guidance about how to estimate life expectancy or how patient preferences should factor into screening decisions. This chapter outlines a systematic framework for individualizing cancer screening decisions in older adults that includes consideration of an individual's life expectancy and his/her preferences regarding the potential benefits and harms of screening (Fig. 12-1). Like many medical decisions, informed screening decisions are best made by using quantitative estimates of life expectancy and screening outcomes to anchor decisions, tempered by qualitative consideration of how an older person values the potential benefits and harms of screening. While potential benefits of screening include increased survival, this should be balanced against the potential harms of screening, which encompass adverse effects on survival, comfort, function, and psychological well-being emanating from all procedures that result from screening.

GENERAL FRAMEWORK FOR MAKING INFORMED CANCER SCREENING DECISIONS

Estimate Life Expectancy

The first step in individualizing cancer screening recommendations is to estimate an older person's life expectancy, because life expectancy affects the likelihood of receiving benefit versus harm from screening. For example, finding an asymptomatic cancer in a person who will die of something else before the cancer would become symptomatic does not benefit the person and may cause considerable harm. The risk of such a scenario depends upon the life expectancy of the individual and the age-specific mortality rate of the particular cancer. With advancing age, the mortality rates of most cancers increase, yet overall life expectancy decreases. The need to weigh these two opposing factors when estimating the likelihood that a person will die of a screen-detectable cancer makes cancer screening decisions in older people complex.

In estimating life expectancy, it is useful to have a general idea of the distribution of life expectancies at various ages. For example, when estimating the life expectancy of an 80-year-old woman, it is useful to know that approximately 25 percent of 80-year-old women will live more than 13 years, 50 percent will live at least 8.6 years, and 25 percent will live less than 4.6 years. Figure 12-2 presents the upper, middle, and lower quartiles of life expectancy for the US population according to age and sex, and illustrates

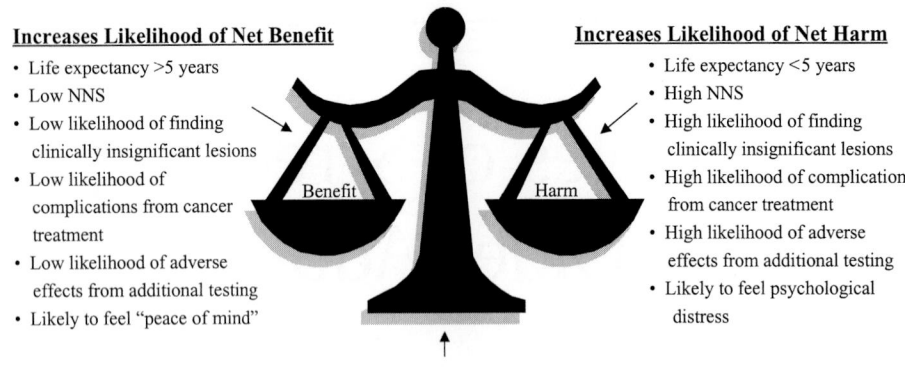

Figure 12-1   The benefits and harms that need to be weighed when making informed cancer screening decisions. Patient preferences act like a moveable fulcrum of a scale to shift the magnitude of the benefits or harms needed to tip the decision toward recommending the screening test (net benefit likely) or recommending against the screening test (net harm likely). NNS, number needed to screen to prevent one cancer-specific death.

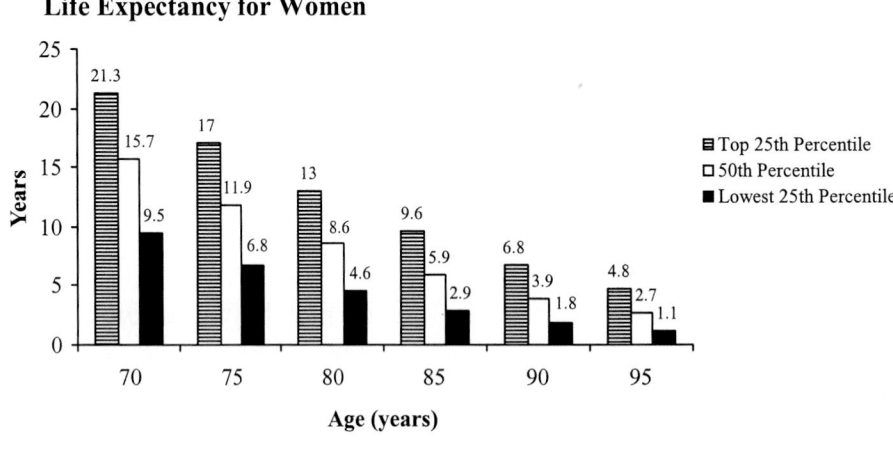

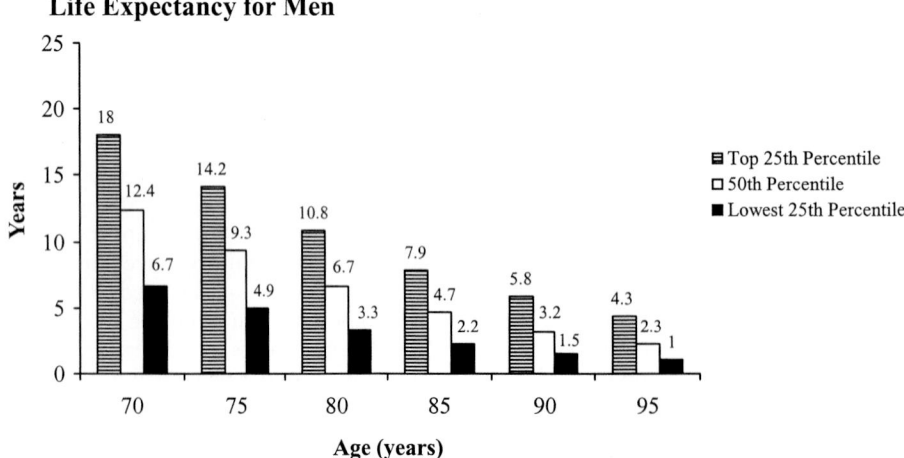

Figure 12-2   Upper, middle, and lower quartiles of life expectancy for women and men at selected ages. Data from the Life Tables of the United States, 1997. Adapted from Walter LC, Covinsky KE: Cancer screening in elderly patients: A framework for individualized decision making. *JAMA* 285:2750, 2001.

the substantial variability in life expectancy that exists at each age. Although it is impossible for clinicians to predict the exact life expectancy of an individual person, it is possible to make reasonable estimates of whether a person is likely to live substantially longer or shorter than an average person in his/her age cohort. Such estimates, while not perfect, would allow for better estimations of potential benefits and harms of screening than focusing on age alone.

There are many factors clinicians can use to estimate whether an older person is typical of someone at the middle of their age-sex cohort or is more like someone in the upper or lower quartiles. For example, the number and severity of comorbid conditions and functional impairments are much stronger predictors of mortality in older people than chronological age. Congestive heart failure, end-stage renal disease, oxygen-dependent chronic obstructive lung disease, severe dementia, or functional dependencies in several activities of daily living are examples of factors that would cause an elderly person to have a life expectancy substantially below the average for his/her age. The absence of significant comorbid conditions or presence of excellent functional status identifies older individuals who are likely to live longer than average.

Estimate Benefits of Cancer Screening

The next step is to consider the potential benefits of screening. Survival is generally the benefit described for cancer screening, because the impact of cancer screening on quality of life or functional decline has not been studied. There is good evidence that mammography, fecal occult blood testing (FOBT), and Papanicolaou (Pap) smears are effective in reducing cancer-specific mortality. However, the strength of the evidence that these tests are effective in older adults is limited by the small number of older patients included in screening trials. In addition, even screening tests likely to be effective in older populations may not provide survival benefit to individuals with short life expectancies, because the benefit from screening is not immediate. For example, in the randomized controlled trials of FOBT and mammography, the cancer-specific survival curves between the screened and unscreened groups do not separate significantly until at least 5 years after the start of screening. This period is likely even longer for persons older than 70 years of age because some evidence suggests that the length of time that a screen-detectable cancer remains clinically asymptomatic increases with advancing age for both breast and colorectal cancer. This suggests that older persons who have life expectancies of less than 5 years will not derive survival benefit from cancer screening.

For patients with estimated life expectancies greater than 5 years, it is important to have a general idea of the potential benefit of screening tests in absolute terms. The absolute benefit of a screening test can be conveyed by the absolute risk reduction (the absolute difference in proportions of persons with a given outcome from two treatments or actions), or more effectively by calculating the number needed to screen (NNS), which is the reciprocal of the absolute risk reduction. Considering older persons at average risk for developing cancer, the approximate NNS to prevent one cancer-specific death is listed in Table 12-1

for screening tests that have been shown effective in reducing cancer-specific mortality. All the numbers in Table 12-1 assume a 5-year delay between the onset of screening and survival benefit. The numbers are presented according to age and life expectancy because life expectancy defines the potential number of years available for screening. For example, 240 very healthy 80-year-old women would have to be screened with mammography during their remaining lifetime to prevent one death from breast cancer. Table 12-1 emphasizes the importance of considering life expectancy when making cancer screening decisions, as illustrated by the example that an 85-year-old woman in the upper quartile of life expectancy is more likely to benefit from screening than a 75-year-old woman in the lowest quartile.

Estimate Harms of Cancer Screening

The third step is to consider the potential harms of screening, as all screening tests pose direct and indirect harms. Harms that would be accepted to treat a symptomatic person with known disease are less acceptable when they are caused by screening tests, which benefit only a few individuals but expose all screened individuals to the harms. In addition, harms occur immediately, whereas it takes several years for a mortality benefit to occur after cancer screening. Therefore, as the likelihood of benefit declines with decreasing life expectancy, the balance between harms and benefits from screening will shift in the direction of net harm.

Individuals who are found not to have cancer after work-up of an abnormal screening result (false-positive result) clearly have experienced harm from screening, as they were subjected to physical and psychological distress from additional testing and procedures that would not have been necessary had they not been screened. However, what is often forgotten is that in older persons some of the greatest harms from screening occur by finding and treating cancers that would never have become clinically significant. The risk of identifying an inconsequential cancer increases with decreasing life expectancy as well as with the increasing likelihood that screening will detect certain neoplasms that are unlikely to progress to symptoms in older persons, such as ductal carcinoma in situ (DCIS). Fewer than 25 percent of DCIS lesions progress to invasive cancer within 5 to 10 years, yet because of the inability to distinguish which lesions will progress, many older women with DCIS will undergo surgery. Women who have surgery for DCIS that would never have become symptomatic in their lifetime have suffered serious harm from screening.

In addition to physical harms, the psychological distress caused by cancer screening should be considered. Potential psychological harms range from the emotional pain of a diagnosis of cancer in persons whose lives were not extended by screening, through the alarm of false-positive results to the stress of undergoing the screening test itself. Many older persons may have cognitive, physical, or sensory problems that make screening tests and further work-up particularly difficult, painful, or frightening. Considering factors that increase the likelihood of harm is vital to making appropriate screening decisions.

Table 12–1   Number Needed to Screen Over Remaining Lifetime to Prevent One Cancer-Specific Death for Women and Men at Selected Ages and Life Expectancy Quartiles

WOMEN

Screening Test	Age 70 Life Expectancy (yrs)			Age 75 Life Expectancy (yrs)			Age 80 Life Expectancy (yrs)			Age 85 Life Expectancy (yrs)			Age 90 Life Expectancy (yrs)		
	21.3	15.7	9.5	17	11.9	6.8	13	8.6	4.6	9.6	5.9	2.9	6.8	3.9	1.8
Mammography	142	242	642	176	330	1,361	240	533	—	417	2,131	—	1,066	—	—
Pap smear	934	1,521	4,070	1,177	2,113	8,342	1,694	3,764	—	2,946	15,056	—	7,528	—	—
Fecal occult blood	178	340	1,046	204	408	1,805	262	581	—	455	2,326	—	1,163	—	—

MEN

Screening Test	Age 70 Life Expectancy (yrs)			Age 75 Life Expectancy (yrs)			Age 80 Life Expectancy (yrs)			Age 85 Life Expectancy (yrs)			Age 90 Life Expectancy (yrs)		
	18	12.4	6.7	14.2	9.3	4.9	10.8	6.7	3.3	7.9	4.7	2.2	5.8	3.2	1.5
Fecal occult blood	177	380	1,877	207	525	—	277	945	—	554	—	—	2,008	—	—

Life expectancy quartiles correspond to upper, middle, and lower quartiles as presented in Fig.12-2. Persons with life expectancies less than 5 years are unlikely to derive any survival benefit from cancer screening, which is denoted by "—."

SOURCE: Adapted from Walter LC and Covinsky KE (JAMA, 2001).

Integrate Patient Values and Preferences

The final step is to assess how individuals value the potential harms and benefits of screening and to integrate their preferences into screening decisions. Because many cancer-screening decisions in older persons will not be answered solely by quantitative assessments of benefits and harms, talking to older persons about their values and preferences is especially important. The value placed on different health outcomes will vary among older people, as will preferences for screening. For example, some women undergoing screening mammography value "peace of mind" after a negative screening result, whereas women with dementia likely receive no such comfort. In considering the benefits versus harm of screening, clinicians must elicit how individual persons value the tradeoffs among longer survival, comfort, and functional status.

Clinicians should consider a person's usual approach to medical decision making to decide how to approach the discussion of screening. In some cases, clinicians will need to learn a person's values, apply them to the known benefits and harms of screening, and make a formal recommendation. For other people, the clinician will want to discuss the benefits and harms with the person and allow the person to apply his/her values to the outcomes and come to a decision together. For people with dementia, discussion about preferences should be held with an involved caregiver. However, it should be remembered that despite being unable to articulate consent, many persons with dementia can still effectively communicate refusal. If a person with dementia is likely to be frightened or agitated by a screening test, the caregiver and clinician should forgo the test. Also, there should be a general discussion prior to screening about the possible procedures and treatments that may be required after an abnormal screening result. Persons who would not want further workup or treatment of an abnormal result should not be screened.

APPLICATION OF SCREENING PRINCIPLES TO SPECIFIC CANCERS

Breast Cancer

Risk of Dying of Breast Cancer

For very healthy 75-year-old women who have life expectancies in the top twenty-fifth percentile, the lifetime risk of dying of breast cancer is approximately 2.8 percent. The risk of dying of breast cancer declines with decreasing life expectancy, such that unhealthy women older than age 75 years who have estimated life expectancies in the lowest twenty-fifth percentile for their age cohort have less than a 1 percent chance of dying of breast cancer.

Benefits of Breast Cancer Screening

Methods for screening for breast cancer are mammography and clinical breast exam. Mammography has the strongest evidence for screening efficacy based on pooled evidence from randomized controlled trials showing an overall relative risk reduction in breast cancer-related mortality of 27 percent for women between the ages of 50 and 69 years. There is little information regarding the absolute benefits of screening mammography in women older than age 70 years, so data from trials in younger people must be extrapolated to older people (Table 12-1).

Harms of Breast Cancer Screening

On average, 1 in 15 elderly women sent for a screening mammogram will have a false-positive result and 1 in 1000 women will have DCIS detected, which would otherwise not have been found without screening. Most DCIS lesions are unlikely to have an effect on the life expectancy of older women, yet many will undergo surgery once DCIS has been found by screening. Frail older women are at increased risk for experiencing harms from screening. One study of frail community-living women found that 17 percent experienced burden from screening mammography as a result of work-up refusals, false-positive results, or identification of clinically insignificant lesions. Women with multiple comorbid conditions are also likely to experience adverse effects from surgery, radiation, and chemotherapy.

Recommendations

Most guidelines recommend mammography alone or supplemented by clinical breast exam. The American Cancer Society (ACS) recommends yearly mammography and clinical breast exam for women starting at age 40 years. The US Preventive Services Task Force (USPSTF) recommends mammography every 12–33 months between ages 40 and 70 years. The American Geriatrics Society (AGS) recommends biennial screening mammography for healthy older women until age 85 years. The author recommends against screening for breast cancer if a woman has an estimated life expectancy of less than 5 years. For women who have a life expectancy between 5 and 10 years, the decision to screen is a close call, and patient preferences should play a major role in the decision to screen. For healthy older women who have a life expectancy greater than 10 years, biennial screening mammography, regardless of age, is a reasonable recommendation based on the data available.

Colorectal Cancer

Risk of Dying of Colorectal Cancer

For very healthy 75-year-olds who have life expectancies in the top twenty-fifth percentile, the lifetime risk of dying of colorectal cancer is approximately 3.5 percent for men and 3.3 percent for women. The risk of dying of colorectal cancer declines with decreasing life expectancy, such that men and women older than age 70 years with life expectancies in the lowest twenty-fifth percentile for their age cohort have less than a 1 percent chance of dying of colorectal cancer.

Benefits of Colorectal Cancer Screening

Methods for screening for colorectal cancer include FOBT, flexible sigmoidoscopy, and colonoscopy. Nonrehydrated fecal occult blood testing has the strongest evidence for screening efficacy based on two randomized controlled trials showing a relative risk reduction in colorectal cancer-related mortality of 15 to 18 percent for persons between the ages of 45 and 75 years. Table 12-1 lists estimates of absolute benefits of screening fecal occult blood testing according to life expectancy. Case-control studies show that sigmoidoscopy provides protection from distal colorectal cancer that lasts up to 10 years.

Harms of Colorectal Cancer Screening

Approximately 1 of 10 older adults who submit a screening nonrehydrated fecal occult blood testing will have a false-positive result. Colonoscopy is the standard work-up following a positive fecal occult blood testing and may have serious complications, such as perforation (1/1000), serious bleeding (3/1000), and cardiorespiratory events (5/1000). Complications may be higher if polypectomy is performed or if persons are in poor health. Discomfort from flexible sigmoidoscopy or colonoscopy may occur, and many older persons may experience substantial distress from the bowel preparation.

Recommendations

Most guidelines recommend annual screening fecal occult blood testing and/or flexible sigmoidoscopy every 5 years for average-risk persons starting at age 50 years. There is no evidence available to determine which screening method is preferable or when screening should stop. Colonoscopy every 10 years is also a screening strategy supported by the American Cancer Society. The author recommends against screening for colorectal cancer if a person has an estimated life expectancy of less than 5 years. For persons with life expectancies between 5 and 10 years, the decision to screen is a close call, and patient preferences should play a major role in the decision to screen. For healthy older people who have a life expectancy greater than 10 years, screening with fecal occult blood testing and/or flexible sigmoidoscopy, regardless of age, is reasonable recommendation based on available data.

Cervical Cancer

Risk of Dying of Cervical Cancer

For very healthy 75-year-old women who have life expectancies in the top twenty-fifth percentile and who have not been previously screened for cervical cancer, the lifetime risk of dying of cervical cancer is approximately 0.2 percent. The risk of dying of cervical cancer declines with decreasing life expectancy and is extremely low for older women who have had normal screening exams in the past.

Benefits of Cervical Cancer Screening

The principal method for screening for cervical cancer is through the use of cervical cytology. Since screening with Pap smears was initiated, population studies in the United States show a 20 to 60 percent decline in mortality rates from cervical cancer. Table 12-1 lists estimates of absolute benefits of screening Pap smears according to life expectancy. Decision models suggest that older women who have had repeated normal Pap smears during their reproductive years do not benefit from continued Pap testing beyond age 65 or 70 years. However, these models make variable recommendations about the number of normal Pap smears required prior to stopping screening.

Harms of Cervical Cancer Screening

For women older than age 70 years, the risk of a false-positive Pap smear result has not been studied, but for postmenopausal women with a normal Pap result in the previous 2 years, the positive predictive value of an abnormal cervical smear is less than 1 percent. Harms of false-positive results include needless patient concern and invasive procedures, such as colposcopy or biopsy. Discomfort and anxiety during Pap smears also occurs as does the identification and treatment of clinically unimportant cervical lesions.

Recommendations

The USPSTF recommends Pap smears at least every 3 years for all women who are or have been sexually active and who have a cervix. Pap testing may be discontinued after age 65 years in women who have had previous normal screening results. The American Cancer Society recommends annual Pap smears for all women who have reached age 18 years. Pap smears may be performed less frequently after three or more smears have been normal, but the ACS does not recommend an upper age limit. The American Geriatrics Society recommends Pap smears every 1 to 3 years until age 70 years, then stopping if tests have been normal. If previous results have been abnormal, then the American Geriatrics Society recommends continued testing every 1 to 3 years. Screening for cervical cancer is unnecessary if an elderly person has an estimated life expectancy of less than 5 years, has had previous normal screening results, or lacks a cervix. For average-risk elderly persons with life expectancies greater than 5 years, little data about benefits and harms exist to guide decision making. Therefore, the decision to screen is a close call and patient preferences should play a major role in the decision to screen.

Other Cancers

Although prostate-specific antigen (PSA) testing is frequently performed, no compelling evidence demonstrates that PSA testing reduces prostate cancer mortality and the harms of treating prostate cancer are substantial, including incontinence and impotence. The American Cancer Society

Table 13-1 Simple Rules for the Twenty-first–Century Health Care System

Current Approach	New Rule
Care is based primarily on visits.	Care is based on continuous healing relationships.
Professional autonomy drives variability.	Care is customized according to patient needs and values.
Professionals control care.	The patient is the source of control.
Information is a record.	Knowledge is shared and information flows freely.
Decision making is based on training and experience.	Decision making is evidence based.
Do no harm is an individual responsibility.	Safety is a system property.
Secrecy is necessary.	Transparency is necessary.
The system reacts to needs.	Needs are anticipated.
Cost reduction is sought.	Waste is continuously decreased.
Preference is given to professional roles over the system.	Cooperation among clinicians is a priority.

SOURCE: Reprinted with permission from *Crossing the Quality Chasm.* Copyright 2001 by the National Academy of Sciences. Courtesy of the National Academy Press, Washington, D.C.

the right amount of care, by the right practitioner, in the right location, at the right time.

To accomplish the objectives of this vision, the focus of the current system must shift from being "provider-centered" or "payment-centered" to "patient-centered." Table 13-1 provides 10 simple rules for how this shift could be accomplished. CMS has taken steps toward this goal by committing to put beneficiaries' needs ahead of all other concerned parties. However, additional system-wide actions are required to facilitate this change. In particular, professional and financial incentives need to be aligned to make it easy for practitioners to "do the right thing" when it comes to delivering high-quality geriatric care. For example, financial incentives need to be created to promote interdisciplinary collaboration that will lead toward the development and execution of common care plans that are respected across various health care settings, but also allow for individual refinements.

In addition, changes in the financial structure of the health care system need to be implemented. New systems need to be developed that better integrate the financing of acute and long-term care to facilitate more comprehensive health care for older adults. Risk adjustment techniques also need to be reengineered to provide more equitable reimbursement for the care of the sickest and frailest older adults. Irrespective of the current debates weighing the merits of managed care for older adults, capitated care undoubtedly will be a central feature of the health care system in the future. This capitation must be used to leverage the design of more rational care systems and reimbursement based on the entire episode of illness rather than the setting in which the care is being delivered.

Practitioners also need greater support from the health care system to better serve older patients. First, population-based care tools need to be employed. These should include evidence-based, computerized systems that prompt caregivers when preventive care (e.g., influenza vaccination and

mammography) is due. Second, specific structural changes (e.g., more time) and content modifications (e.g., simple algorithms to optimize care for common geriatric conditions) should be implemented. Third, risk identification protocols are needed to identify older adults at greatest risk for adverse health outcomes. Mechanisms need to be in place to ensure that (1) high-risk older patients receive active, ongoing, coordinated primary medical care, (2) the care management of older patients is centralized irrespective of the setting, and (3) evidence-based protocols are available for addressing common geriatric conditions. Finally, greater collaboration is needed between medical care providers and community service agencies to facilitate patients' access to complementary community programs that support their care plans (e.g., incontinence self-management programs, supervised physical activity programs, and layperson-led chronic illness self-management courses).

Older patients also need greater support in terms of managing their chronic conditions, improving the quality of their lives, and navigating the health care system. The goal is for older patients to feel confident in initiating care for new problems and to participate in the development of care plans for existing problems. This can be achieved by providing older patients with access to both peer and professional support that, among other things, will empower them to prepare specific questions for their medical encounters. By necessity, this system also should include assistance to informal caregivers, including specific training programs for the management of dementia, support groups, and respite programs.

Information technology (IT) also should play a prominent role in improving health care delivery for older adults. IT is essential for supporting ongoing communication between practitioners and institutions. With appropriate mechanisms to safeguard confidentiality, sharing clinical information across settings improves and reduces medical errors. Essential patient information that should be

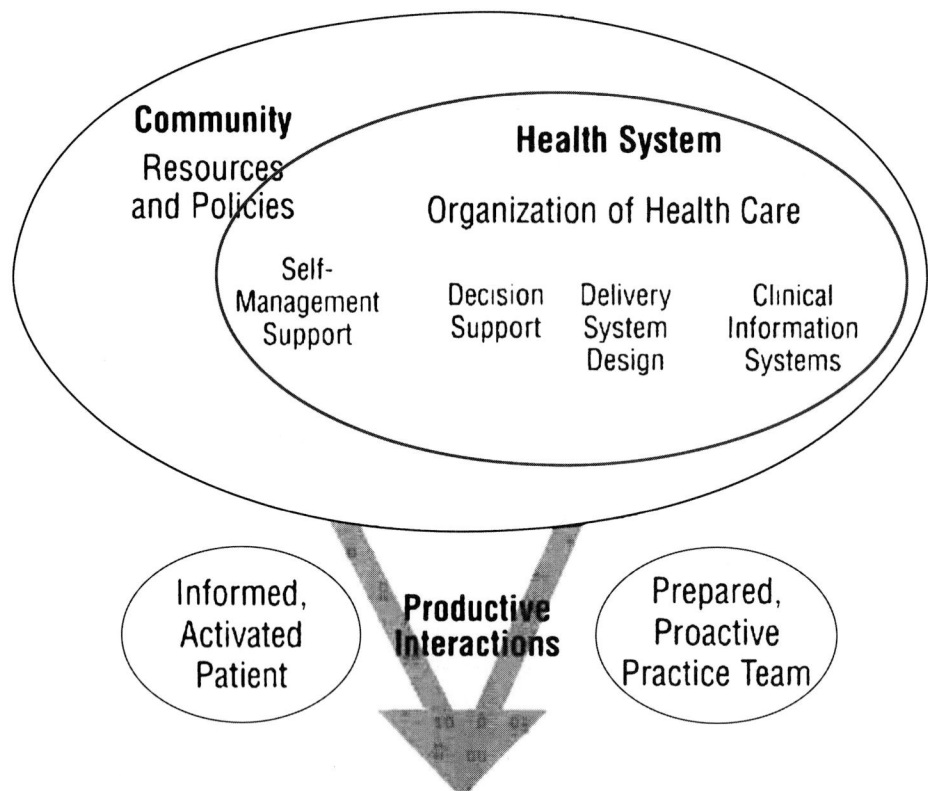

Functional and Clinical Outcomes

Figure 13-5   The chronic care model.

available to all relevant practitioners includes a current list of problems, the overall care goals tailored for the patient and specific goals for the particular setting, treatment preferences and advanced directives, an accurate medication regimen and a list of medication allergies, an assessment of baseline physical and cognitive function, and contact information for both professional and informal care providers. In keeping with the practice of population-based care, registries should be created to facilitate the identification and management of older persons with common geriatric conditions and ensure their adherence to protocols designed to promote health and reduce disability. In addition, the ability to run queries using this electronic clinical information would create opportunities for quality improvement strategies that allow for "real-time" corrective action.

Overall changes in the structure of the health delivery system also are necessary to improve the quality of geriatric care. The chronic care model (CCM) is an empirically derived model for system change that incorporates many of the ideas proposed in this proposed vision (Fig. 13-5). The CCM postulates that functional and clinical outcomes can be improved through more productive interactions between patients and practitioners, provided that coordinated changes occur in six areas of the health delivery system: (1) links to relevant community resources, including physical activity and peer support programs; (2) the organization of care, including changes at a systems level, with a commitment from leadership to improve clinical outcomes and rational incentives to provide better

care; (3) support for patients' self-management of chronic conditions; (4) decision-making support, including the use of evidence-based practice guidelines or protocols and the opportunity to collaborate with practitioners who possess complementary expertise; (5) delivery system design or redesign including changes in the way that care is organized and staffed, the manner in which follow-up care is arranged, and the roles that different practitioners play; and (6) clinical information systems, including programs that can provide timely and useful information at the point of care and systematize population-based care, such as disease registries. Improvements in these six areas should facilitate productive interactions between practitioners who are prepared and patients who are informed and actively engaged in their treatment.

Finally, the role of the clinical geriatrician needs to be enhanced so that she or he can more explicitly serve as a population-based health care specialist to older adults. Ideally, the geriatrician should design and champion new models of care, and support primary care and hospital-based physicians in managing the unique needs of their older patients. In the primary care arena, geriatricians could act as "roving specialists," bringing their expertise to the primary care setting, thereby reducing the potential for care fragmentation and miscommunication. In this scenario, older patients would simultaneously see their primary care physician and the geriatrician, who together would formulate a treatment plan, including a scheduled return visit. While the emphasis of these visits would be on the collaborative management of the patient, the arrangement would enable primary care physicians to gain one-on-one geriatric training that they could incorporate into the management of other older patients.

Geriatricians could play a similar role by bringing their expertise to less-traditional care settings, such as residential care communities, assisted-living communities, or large facilities that provide multiple levels of care. One benefit of this arrangement is that certain economies of scale can be created when the geriatrician is able to evaluate a significant number of residents. These savings can justify a more intense interdisciplinary team approach to care (e.g., a GNP, pharmacist, social worker, physical therapist) and specific programs (e.g., a falls prevention program, urinary incontinence self-management classes). In addition, as stated previously, providing care on-site enables practitioners to gain considerable insight into the functional capability of residents in their living environments. This knowledge can be particularly vital for developing realistic care plans. Finally, and perhaps most importantly, on-site care can result in the timely management of acute problems, thereby reducing transports to the emergency department and hospitalization admissions while improving the outcomes of care.

ACKNOWLEDGMENTS

Funding support was provided by Paul Beeson Faculty Scholars in Aging Research/American Federation for Aging Research and the National Institute on Aging Grant No. 1 K23 AG19652-01.

REFERENCES

Beck A et al: A randomized trial of group outpatient visits for chronically ill older HMO members: The Cooperative Health Care Clinic. *J Am Geriatr Soc* 45(5):543, 1997.

Bergman H et al: Care for Canada's frail elderly population: Fragmentation or integration? *CMAJ* 157:1116, 1997.

Boult C et al: Systems of care for older populations of the future. *J Am Geriatr Soc* 46(4):499, 1998.

Coleman E, Besdine R: Integrating quality assurance across sites of geriatric care, in Calkins E, Wagner E.H., Boult C, Pacala JT (eds): *New Ways to Care for Older People*. New York, Springer, 1999, p 185.

Coleman E et al: Reducing emergency visits in older adults with chronic illness: A randomized controlled trial of group visits. *Eff Clin Pract* 2:49, 2001.

Coleman E, on behalf of the HMO Care Management Workgroup: *Improving the Care of Older Adults with Common Geriatric Conditions*. Washington, DC, AAHP Foundation, 2002, p 1.

Fama T, Fox P: Efforts to improve primary care delivery to nursing home residents. *J Am Geriatr Soc* 45(5):627, 1997.

Institute of Medicine, Committee on Quality of Health Care in America (ed).: *Crossing the Quality Chasm: A New Health System of the 21st Century*. Washington, DC, National Academy Press, 2001.

Kramer AM et al: Effects of nurse staffing on hospital transfer quality measures for new admissions, in *Appropriateness of Minimum Nurse Staffing Ratios for Nursing Homes*. Baltimore, Health Care Financing Administration, 2000.

Leveille S et al: Preventing disability and managing chronic illness in frail older adults: A randomized trial of a community-based partnership with primary care. *J Am Geriatr Soc* 46(10):1191, 1998.

Lorig K et al: Evidence suggesting that a chronic disease self-management program can improve health status while reducing hospitalization. *Med Care* 37(1):5, 1999.

National Chronic Care Consortium: Self-Assessment for System Integration Tool (SASI). Bloomington MN, National Chronic Care Consortium, 1998.

National Health Information. Web-based senior care management program takes flight in California. *Senior Care Manager* 4(12):187, 2001.

Naylor M et al: Comprehensive discharge planning and home follow-up of hospitalized elders: A randomized clinical trial. *JAMA* 281(7):613, 1999.

Portner G et al: An Analysis of Rehabilitation Services "Flow" Patterns and Payments by Provider Setting for Medicare Beneficiaries. Washington, DC, Muse and Associates, 1996.

von Sternberg T: The role and responsibilities of the geriatrician in managed care: Opportunities and responsibilities. *J Am Geriatr Soc* 47(5):605, 1999.

Wagner EH: The promise and performance of HMOs in improving outcomes in older adults. *J Am Geriatr Soc* 44(10):1251, 1996.

Wagner EH et al: Organizing care for patients with chronic illness. *Milbank Q* 74(4):511, 1996.

Acute Care

ROBERT M. PALMER • STEPHEN W. MELDON

AGING AND HOSPITALIZATION

Patients 65 years of age and older comprise 13 percent of the American population, but they account for 40 percent of all discharges from non-federal acute hospitals and 48 percent of inpatient days of care. Compared with younger patients, older patients have longer and more frequent hospitalizations and their illness severity is greater. Among older patients, rates of hospitalization are more than twice as great for the age group 85 years and older as compared to the age group 65 to 74 years. Although admission of adults to hospitals has declined since the introduction of the prospective payment system, admission rates of elderly patients, and the age group 85 years and older in particular, continue to increase. A relatively small percentage of elderly patients account for a large percentage of hospital admissions. Only approximately 5 percent of elderly patients have consistently high rates of hospitalization, averaging one or more admissions annually.

Rates of in-hospital mortality are higher in the elderly population. In 1999, 78 percent of hospital deaths occurred in patients age 65 years and older. Prospective studies have identified predictors of mortality during or in the one to three years following hospitalization for acute medical illnesses. Predictors include demographic, medical, and functional measures. In one study, three measures of functional status—seven or more depressive symptoms on the shortened Geriatric Depression Scale, cognitive impairment indicated by a score less than 20 on the Mini-Mental State Examination, and physical impairment indicated by dependence at baseline in one or more instrumental activities of daily living (IADL)—were independent predictors of 2-year mortality in patients aged 70 years and older. Each of these measures added to the prognostic ability of commonly used indices of burden of illness. Among seriously ill patients age 80 years and older 2-year mortality is increased in those with weight loss, cognitive dysfunction, impaired functional status, high chronic disease class, and acute physiology score. The importance of functional measures as predictors of 1-year mortality was also demonstrated in a study of hospitalized patients with a mean age of 80 years. Independent risk factors for mortality included male sex, number of dependent activities of daily living (ADL) at discharge, congestive heart failure, cancer, creatinine level >3.0 mg/dL, and serum albumin <3.5 g/dL. Other studies of hospitalized elderly patients show that depressive symptoms present at hospital admission increase the risk of mortality subsequent to hospitalization. Patients with six or more symptoms of depression on the shortened Geriatric Depression Scale were more likely to die over the next 3 years as compared to patients with fewer than six depressive symptoms. Likewise, delirium prevalent at or incident to admission increases the risk of 1-year mortality even after adjustment for covariates known to be predictive of mortality. Together these studies imply that interventions designed to improve functional outcomes of hospitalization could improve the prognosis of patients in the years following their discharge.

Costs of hospitalization are higher in elderly patients compared to younger adults. The greatest expenditures are for patients in the age group 70 to 79 years, despite a longer average length of stay for patients in older age groups. Medicare expenditures in the last year of life decrease with age, especially among patients aged 85 years or older. This observation is attributable to less-aggressive medical care of the oldest patients, including fewer intensive care unit admissions, and less-frequent cardiac catheterization, hemodialysis, and ventilator support. However, with trends toward greater use of intensive resources for very old patients increasing in the United States, the costs of treating patients age 85 years and older is likely to grow, underscoring the importance of allocating resources based on prognostic indices and measures of functional status. Medicare expenditures are greater in the subset of patients who have repeated unplanned hospitalizations. Risk factors for repeated hospital admission among people age 70 years or older include older age; male sex; poor self-rated general health; availability of an informal caregiver; history of coronary artery disease; history of hospital admission during the previous year; six or more visits to physicians; or diabetes mellitus. The presence of these risk factors more than doubles the risk of hospital admission, when compared to low-risk patients, and is associated with a higher rate of mortality and higher hospital charges. Other sources of Medicare expenditures that occur more commonly in older hospitalized patients are transfers to skilled nursing facilities or to home care services. Again, functional status is a predictor of the use of these services.

Indeed, hospitalization of elderly patients typically focuses on the medical care of disease-specific and life-threatening illnesses, while less attention is generally given to functional outcomes such as physical and cognitive functioning. Although functional outcomes are not usually the focus of care in the hospital, they may be critical determinants of the quality of life, physical independence, cost of care, and prognosis among elderly patients. The patient's impairment in the performance of basic activities of daily living (BADL) and IADL and diagnoses of delirium or depression often go undiagnosed by physicians. A study of hospitalized elderly medical patients revealed that medical records contained no documentation of most individual BADL or IADL items. If functional outcomes are to be improved in hospitalized patients, their functional status will need to be better documented. Appropriate assessment of elderly patients should begin in the emergency department (ED) and continue in the acute care hospital.

EMERGENCY CARE OF ELDERLY PATIENTS

Older patients who present to the emergency department often have functional impairments and multiple comorbidities that leave them vulnerable to functional decline and a loss of physical independence. Elderly patients comprise an increasing proportion of emergency medical services users. The highest rate of ED use when analyzed by age group is by patients age 75 years and older. Elderly patients are more likely to present to an emergency department for serious medical illnesses, to arrive by ambulance, and to require hospital admission. One-third of older ED patients arrive by emergency medical services transport. The admission rate for elderly ED patients in one study was 46 percent, representing by extrapolation more than seven million hospital admissions.

Following an ED visit, older patients are at increased risk for adverse outcomes, including unplanned ED revisits, hospital admission, and functional decline (a loss of independent functioning in activities of daily living). Approximately one-fourth of elderly patients return to the emergency department within 90 days. Male gender, living alone, and functional problems are significantly associated with a repeat ED visit.

Emergency Department Challenges

The evaluation of elderly patients in the emergency department is challenging because of the busy and episodic nature of emergency care and the common occurrence of multiple medical problems, communication difficulties, and cognitive impairment among older patients. Elderly patients spend significantly more time in the emergency department, require more radiographic and laboratory evaluations, and have higher emergency department charges than do non-elderly patients. In surveys, practicing emergency physicians indicate that caring for elderly patients is more difficult and more time-consuming for most clinical complaints, including abdominal pain, altered mental status, dizziness, and trauma. They also report that the aging population has a major impact on ED flow and availability of hospital and intensive care unit beds. They are concerned about potential social and ethical issues common in older patients, including the costs of caring for elderly patients, access to care and lack of primary care providers, and elder abuse and neglect.

Pitfalls in Emergency Care of Older Patients

The physiologic changes associated with aging often interact with disease processes to alter the manifestations and presentations of common diseases. Common, life-threatening illnesses that often present atypically include acute myocardial infarction, serious infections such as pneumonia and urinary tract infections, and intra-abdominal emergencies. Functional decline is often worsened by acute illness that is initially evaluated in the emergency department. Table 14-1 summarizes the pitfalls of geriatric emergency care. Atypical presentations are not confined to medical diseases. Important psychosocial issues, such as elder abuse, alcoholism, and depression may also present atypically and be difficult to detect in the older age group. Drug prescribing in the ED is also a challenge. In one ED study, nearly one-third of older patients had a potential drug–drug interaction, with 7 percent of those interactions being considered a potentially major problem. This underscores the importance of obtaining a complete medication list and, perhaps, of using computerized programs or personal digital assistants to alert physicians to potential interactions (Table 14-1). A challenge to health professionals working in the ED is to identify elderly patients at increased risk of adverse health outcomes including death, admission to a long-term care institution, or functional decline. A self-reported screening tool, Identification of Seniors At Risk (ISAR), identifies older patients at increased risk of these adverse health outcomes (Table 14-2). The ISAR screen includes six self-report questions on functional dependence (baseline and acute), recent hospitalization,

Table 14-1   Geriatric Emergency Care Pitfalls

- Not recognizing atypical presentation of life-threatening disease
- Not recognizing the importance of acute functional decline as a marker of serious illness
- Not obtaining a thorough history from caregivers, emergency medical services, or nursing home personnel
- Not differentiating normal from abnormal laboratory values and vital signs
- Not considering adverse drug reactions, including increased side effects and drug–drug interactions
- Not considering psychosocial issues such as abuse, depression, or alcoholism

SOURCE: Adapted from Meldon SW: Our aging population and its impact on the practice of emergency medicine, in *Geriatric Emergency Report Monograph*. Atlanta, American Health Consultants, 2000, p 1.

Table 14-2 Identification of Seniors at Risk (ISAR): Screening Questions

1. Before the injury or illness that brought you to the emergency department, did you need someone to help you on a regular basis? (*yes*)
2. Since the illness or injury that brought you to the emergency department, have you needed more help than usual to take care of yourself? (*yes*)
3. Have you been hospitalized for one or more nights during the past 6 months (excluding a stay in the emergency department)? (*yes*)
4. In general do you see well? (*no*)
5. In general do you have serious problems with your memory? (*yes*)
6. Do you take more than two different medications every day? (*yes*)

The ISAR comprises six items. The number of high-risk responses (shown in parentheses) are summed to give a scoring range from 0 to 6.

SOURCE: Adapted from McCusker J et al: Prediction of hospital utilization among elderly patients during the six months after an emergency department visit. *Ann Emerg Med* 36:438, 2000. Used with permission.

Table 14-3 Principles of Geriatric Emergency Medicine

1. The patient's presentation is frequently complex.
2. Common diseases present atypically in this age group.
3. The confounding effects of comorbid diseases must be considered.
4. Polypharmacy is common and may be a factor in presentation, diagnosis, and management.
5. Recognition of the possibility for cognitive impairment is important.
6. Some diagnostic tests may have different normal values.
7. The likelihood of decreased functional reserve must be anticipated.
8. Social support systems may not be adequate, and patients may need to rely on caregivers.
9. A knowledge of baseline functional status is essential for evaluating new complaints.
10. Health problems must be evaluated for associated psychosocial adjustment.
11. The emergency department encounter is an opportunity to assess important conditions in the patient's personal life.

SOURCE: From Sanders AB et al: Principles of care and application of the emergency care model, in, Sanders AB (ed): *Emergency Care of the Elder Person*. St. Louis, Beverly Cracom Publications, 1996, p 59. Used with permission.

impaired memory and vision, and multiple medication use. An intervention that included use of the ISAR, a brief standardized nursing assessment in the ED, and notification of the primary care physician and home care providers and referrals as needed increased the rate of referral to primary care physicians and home care services. Functional decline was reduced by 40 percent at 4 months.

Principles of Geriatric Care in the Emergency Department

The traditional approach in the ED focuses on the medical history and physical examination to determine if an acute illness is life-threatening (for example, identifying an urgent disease process or injury that needs prompt attention). It further focuses on common conditions that may cause the patient's acute symptoms. While the traditional assessment model works well for the majority of ill adults and injured patients in the ED, it may not apply as well to elderly patients. Consequently, principles for evaluating elderly patients in the ED have been developed (Table 14-3).

Older patients often present with complex symptoms rather than a single chief complaint. The acute symptom may be vague or ambiguous (e.g., "weakness," "dizziness," "not feeling well") yet may signify serious medical conditions such as myocardial infarction, exacerbation of congestive heart failure, or sepsis. Recognizing atypical presentations of diseases in elderly patients may help to prevent delays or misdiagnoses and the associated increases in morbidity or mortality. In addition, comorbid diseases may have a major impact on the diagnosis made in the emergency department. For example, acute infection may cause exacerbation of chronic heart failure, thereby obscuring the diagnosis of an acute pneumonia. Polypharmacy is

common and might influence the presentation and management of a patient in the ED. For example, a patient with dementia might develop agitation and delirium after taking over-the-counter sleeping pills. Although cognitive impairment, most often caused by delirium or dementia, is common, it often goes unrecognized by emergency physicians. Cognitive impairment may alter the patient's presentation of acute illness, interfere with the effective evaluation of the patient in the emergency department, and impact the disposition of the patient from the ED. For example, patients with a relatively minor acute illness such as a cellulitis might be admitted to the hospital, whereas a cognitively normal patient could have been sent home. Acute illness or physiologic stresses impact organ system function, resulting in rapid deterioration and complications while the patient is in the emergency department. Functional and psychosocial issues become important factors in the patient's disposition. Social support systems, including the social support network, the capability of the primary caregiver at home, and the availability of transportation home and to subsequent medical follow-ups, need to be carefully assessed before vulnerable elderly patients are sent home from the ED. At least a brief assessment of the caregivers is needed to determine the risk of elder mistreatment or neglect at home. A change in baseline functional status may signify the occurrence of a more serious medical condition than might have been suspected. For example, a patient presenting to the ED with a fall and difficulty walking might have an evolving stroke or an early presentation of pneumonia. In addition, assessments of baseline functional status such as personal care needs and ADL independence are important when evaluating treatment and disposition decisions for older patients. In summary, the ED visit is often a sentinel event for an elderly patient. In addition to identifying significant medical problems the visit may reveal serious psychosocial and functional issues. This underscores the need for rapid detection of high risk patients, appropriate initial evaluation in the ED, and a coordinated effort to further evaluate and manage these issues following the patient's hospitalization or return to home.

FUNCTIONAL DECLINE: RECOGNIZING THE HAZARDS OF ACUTE ILLNESS AND HOSPITALIZATION

Approximately one-third of elderly patients admitted to the hospital for treatment of acute medical illness decline in their performance of one or more basic ADL. Approximately 40 percent of these patients lose independence in one or more IADL when compared to their pre-illness IADL 90 days after discharge. The loss of independent functioning is related to both elements of hospitalization and to characteristics of patients. Iatrogenic illness and forced immobility, altered sleep wake cycles, disorienting effects of the environment, sensory deprivation, and undernutrition are factors that place the frail elderly patient at risk for functional decline in hospital. Many patients enter the hospital with chronic diseases and pre-existing functional impairments that predispose them to functional decline. Increasing age, cognitive impairment at hospital admission, and lower pre-admission independence in instrumental activities of daily living increase the risk of functional decline in hospital. The presence of a pressure sore, functional dependence at admission, cognitive dysfunction and a low social activity level prior to admission are other predictors of functional decline in hospital. Depressive symptoms present at admission predict functional decline. Although a comprehensive geriatric assessment is an ideal method to detect patients at risk for functional decline, it is often time consuming and hence impractical to perform in the hectic setting of the acute care hospital. Table 14-4 offers a practical suggestion for "bedside" geriatric assessment during hospital rounds.

Iatrogenic Illness

Iatrogenic illness is any illness that results from a diagnostic procedure or therapeutic intervention that is not a natural consequence of the patient's disease. Older patients are predisposed to iatrogenic illness related to their diminishing homeostatic reserves, high level of comorbid illnesses, and polypharmacy, which increases the probability of adverse drug events. Generally, iatrogenesis is categorized as illness resulting from either medications, diagnostic and therapeutic procedures, nosocomial infections, or environmental hazards. Adverse hospital events can also occur from negligence or medical systems errors (e.g., dispensing the wrong medication). In a study of 15,000 hospitalized

patients in the United States, the incidence of adverse events was 5.3 percent among elderly patients as compared to 2.8 percent among non-elderly patients. The incidence of preventable adverse events was 1.6 percent among elderly patients. These preventable events were related to medical procedures (e.g., thoracentesis, cardiac catheterization), preventable adverse drug events and preventable falls. The higher rate of adverse events in this study was attributable to the greater burden of illness of elderly as compared to younger patients. Adverse drug events in hospitalized patients are associated with prolonged hospital stay, higher medical care costs, and an increase risk of death. Explicit criteria have been developed for determining potentially inappropriate medication use by elderly patients. A recent quality improvement study suggests that the incidence of inappropriate drug prescribing can be decreased through professional education, care pathways, and formulary changes. The study succeeded by advocating the avoidance of drugs with anticholinergic properties, the avoidance of psychotropic agents (particularly those with long elimination half-life), and the avoidance of meperidine for pain control.

Preventing Adverse Drug Events

Guidelines to prevent adverse drug events in elderly patients may include a variety of strategies. These strategies include reviewing all medications (over-the-counter as well as prescribed), assessing the patient's prior compliance with prescription medications, assuring consistency of drug prescribing of medications prior to and after hospitalization, and rational drug prescribing. Rational drug prescribing requires a knowledge of the pharmacology of drugs in relation to aging, the use of lower than usual doses when the geriatric dose in unknown, the avoidance of psychoactive drugs when alternatives such as behavioral or environmental alternatives are available, and the cautious monitoring of patients receiving two or more drugs that are inducers or inhibitors of phase I hepatic metabolism (cytochrome P450), or are highly protein bound.

Nosocomial Infections

Nosocomial infections caused by resistant microorganisms are a growing problem in hospitalized elderly patients (Table 14-5). In particular, methicillin-resistant staphylococcus aureus (MRSA) and vancomycin-resistant enterococcus (VRE) infections are common in hospitalized patients. The VRE infections are associated with prolonged hospitalization, intra-hospital transfer between floors, and use of broad spectrum anti-microbials, including third-generation cephalosporins and vancomycin. VRE are likely to be transmitted from patient to patient by the unwashed hands of health care workers or contaminated medical equipment and environmental surfaces. Nosocomial infections are potentially preventable. Infection and antibiotic control procedures including the restriction of vancomycin and better selection of empiric antibiotics are warranted. Hospital personnel should be educated about the risks of nosocomial infection and the need to wash hands and clean medical devices.

Table 14-4   Bedside Assessment of Functional Status

Functional Area	Bedside Assessment	Recommendations
Activities of daily living	• Review patient's baseline performance of ADL. • Review nurses' notes and observations about patient's ability to bathe, dress, toilet, and eat. • Review ADL status on rounds daily. • Ask about bowel and bladder function.	• Consult occupational therapy for more formal ADL assessment if ADL decline/impairment is present. • Prescribe assistive devices and aids to enable patient self-care.
Mobility/gait	• Observe patient sitting up in bed, dangling legs, transferring to chair or standing up. • Observe patient walking to bathroom and in hallway corridor ("walk rounds").	• Consult physical therapy if patient has mobility, transfer or gait impairments. • Avoid "bed rest" orders. • Avoid physical restraints. • Encourage patient to get out of bed. • Flex and extend patient's ankles and knees during bedside rounds.
Cognitive function	• Ascertain patient's baseline level of cognition from interviews with patient and family, and from a review of medical records and nurses' notes. • Screen for delirium each visit: change in alertness, inattention, fluctuating mental status, inappropriate behavior or thought processes. • Probe patient's cognition with questions that require attention and short-term memory: "How are you feeling today?" "How did the studies go this morning?" • Consider a screening instrument: Short Portable Mental Status Questionnaire, Mini-Mental State Examination, Clock Drawing Test, digit span.	• For patient with risk factors for delirium, "reality orientation": introduce yourself each visit, remind patient of day, reason for hospitalization, upcoming diagnostic studies and consultants, and plans for follow-up visit. • Optimize vision (corrective lenses, diffuse lighting in room) and hearing (aids, amplifying devices, face-to-face conversations with door of patient's room closed). • Encourage family visits and social interactions, or assign sitter for demented patients at risk of falls or therapy disruption.
Mood/affect	• Review medical history for depression or anxiety. • Assess patient's affect: observe for dysphoria, apathy, irritability, poor eye contact. • Ask, "Do you feel sad or depressed?" • Assess for symptoms of anxiety: impaired concentration, insomnia, fearfulness, tachycardia, restlessness. • Consider screening instrument: Geriatric Depression Scale.	• Offer reassurance and gentle touch. • Encourage visits from family (and pets if permitted). • Therapeutic activities; supportive counseling. • Anxiolytics or antidepressants if symptoms cannot be improved with behavioral approaches and supportive counseling.
Nutrition (undernutrition)	• Observe for clinical features suggesting protein-energy malnutrition: low body mass index, muscle wasting, generalized weakness. • Review laboratory parameters suggesting protein–energy malnutrition: low serum albumin (<3.5 g/dL), low serum cholesterol (<160 mg/dL), unexplained anemia. • Observe for evidence of poor wound healing (pressure ulcer), dehydration (poor skin turgor, postural hypotension). • Review laboratory parameters suggesting dehydration: electrolytes (serum sodium), ratio of blood urea nitrogen to serum creatinine.	• Assess nutritional status at admission (physical examination, laboratory tests). • Refer to Table 14-7. • Speech therapy consultation and modified barium swallow for patients with suspected oropharyngeal dysphagia.

Table 14-5   Factors Promoting and Potential Prevention of Nosocomial Infection

Infection	Factors Promoting	Prevention
Vancomycin-resistant enterocci (VRE)	Urethral catheterization; transmission from patient to patient by health care workers; contaminated medical equipment or surfaces (e.g., bed rails, blood pressure cuffs)	Infection and antibiotic control procedures; restriction of vancomycin use; improved selection of empiric antibiotic usage; hand and equipment washing; isolation of colonized patients; cleansing of the environment; limited bladder catheterization
Methicillin-resistant staphylococcal aureus (MRSA)	Intravenous and intra-arterial lines and devices; intra-institutional transmission of resistant bacteria; poor hand washing by health care workers; institutional transfer of colonized patients	Wash hands and equipment; shorten duration of central intravenous or intra-arterial lines; disinfect patient's skin (e.g., with chlorhexidine gluconate) prior to catheterization; use triple-lumen catheter impregnated with antimicrobal agents; remove lines promptly with suspected infection
Nosocomial pneumonias	Intensive care units colonized with resistant pathogens; colonization of the upper and gastrointestinal tracts; ventilator use; gastric aspiration; spread of pathogens by unwashed hands; fecal–oral spread of pathogens; cross-contamination from other patients.	Clean respiratory and medical equipment; wash hands between patients, maintain patient in semi-upright position; use proton pump inhibitors (preferred to histamine-2 antagonists)

Resistant urinary tract infections often follow prolonged indwelling urinary catheterization. The incidence of nosocomial urosepsis can be limited by avoiding persistent indwelling catheterization, choosing intermittent catheterization instead as needed, and by avoiding prophylactic anti-microbial therapies.

Nosocomial pneumonia is potentially preventable. Nosocomial pneumonia results from colonization of the upper respiratory and gastrointestinal tracts and occurs most often in ventilator dependent patients. Factors promoting nosocomial pneumonia include gastric aspiration, the spread of pathogens by the hands of medical and nursing personnel, fecal–oral spread of pathogens, and cross contamination from other patients. Prevention of nosocomial pneumonia includes the cleaning of respiratory equipment, hand washing between patient contacts and maintaining the patient in an upright position to minimize the risk of gastric aspiration.

Intravascular infections are associated with the use of central intravenous or intra-arterial lines. To minimize the risk of intravascular infection the patient's skin should be disinfected prior to catheterization, triple lumen catheters impregnated with antimicrobial agents should be used when a multilumen catheter is necessary, and the line should be removed when there is clinical evidence of infection from the catheter.

Cognitive Dysfunction

Impaired cognition, usually caused by dementia or delirium, is present in approximately one-third of hospitalized elderly patients admitted to general medical services.

Cognitive dysfunction is often attributable to delirium, dementia, or depression. Delirium is a major predictor of functional decline, prolonged length of stay, alternate-site placement following hospitalization, and mortality (see Chap. 117). Delirium is more common in elderly patients with baseline cognitive and sensory impairments, and dehydration. Medications, especially those with psychotropic properties (e.g., anticholinergic agents, antihistamines, opiates) are associated with delirium. Delirium can be precipitated by processes of medical care that are modifiable. In one study, the use of physical restraints, the addition of three or more new medications to the patient's initial regimen, undernutrition in hospital, and iatrogenic complications preceded the incidence of delirium in elderly patients.

To detect patients with baseline dementia or delirium on admission, a mental status examination should be performed and combined with an interview with family caregivers to determine the patient's baseline level of cognition. Progress notes from physicians, nurses and other health care professionals should be reviewed for evidence of possible delirium. For example, certain behaviors (agitation, restlessness, inappropriate verbalizations) are often suggestive of the diagnosis of delirium. The notation of a "change in mental status" generally implies the development of delirium. The diagnosis of delirium can be made confidently by applying standardized criteria such as the confusion assessment method.

Delirium in medically ill hospitalized elderly patients can be reduced by 40 percent with a multicomponent targeted risk factor intervention (see Chap. 117). The intervention is targeted at patients age 70 years and older who have one or more risk factors for delirium (cognitive impairment, sleep deprivation, immobility, dehydration, vision or hearing impairment). The interventions are implemented by an interdisciplinary team including a geriatric nurse specialist, trained volunteers and a volunteer coordinator, and geriatricians working closely with primary nurses. The interventions include daily visitors and reality orientation, therapeutic activities, early mobilization, visual protocols (visual aids), hearing protocols (e.g., amplifying devices), oral volume repletion and/or feeding assistance, and sleep enhancement (e.g., non-pharmacologic sleep protocol). An analysis of the multicomponent intervention concludes that it is a cost-effective option for patients at intermediate risk for delirium in hospital.

Depression and Anxiety

Mood disorders are found in 20 to 25 percent of hospitalized older patients, although clinical depression is often undetected or untreated by physicians. The patient's presentation of acute illness, the presence of cognitive impairment, and the presence of significant comorbid conditions may complicate the diagnosis of depression. For example, symptoms of depression (e.g., fatigue, weight loss) may be attributed to the acute illness or comorbid conditions (e.g., heart failure). An extensive and prolonged diagnostic work-up looking for medical causes of somatic symptoms may delay the diagnosis of depression and the delivery of effective therapies. Depression can be detected through a careful medical history of treatment for a mood disorder. Depressive symptoms can be elicited with the use of screening instruments such as the Geriatric Depression Scale. Patients with adjustment disorders caused by acute or chronic diseases may present with depressive symptoms that improve with treatment of their medical conditions. Major depression will require psychological and/or pharmacologic therapy. Although definitive clinical trials are lacking, an effort to detect and treat depression in the hospital is warranted given its adverse effects on clinical outcomes. Because response to antidepressant therapy is often delayed for several weeks, therapy begun in the hospital needs to be continued after the patent's discharge.

Anxiety is also common in hospitalized patients. Insomnia, depression, agitation, or delirium may accompany anxiety. Behavioral and environmental therapies, such as those described for the prevention of delirium, may also help alleviate anxiety. Anxiolytics (e.g., lorazepam) while useful for treatment of acute anxiety may worsen cognition or increase the risk of falls. Their use should be carefully monitored and the lowest effective dose used for the shortest time necessary in order to avoid adverse effects.

Immobility

Patients often become immobile during the course of an illness that results in admission to the hospital. Impaired homeostatic reserves, reduced muscle mass and strength, disuse atrophy, and the catabolic effects of severe disease predispose to a loss of independent ambulation. The immobility may be exacerbated by prolonged bed rest, leading to the loss of ability to transfer from bed to chair or to stand without assistance. Immobility is associated with postural hypotension, skin tears, pressure ulcers, and venous thromboses. Hypoxemia, constipation, reduced cardiac output, and bone demineralization may also occur with prolonged immobility.

Processes of care in the hospital further promote impaired mobility. The use of various tethers—intravenous and intraarterial lines, nasogastric tubes and other hardware, and physical restraints—limit the patient's free movement or ability to transfer from bed or to walk. Physical restraints are frequently used by physicians or nurses to prevent elderly patients from disrupting life-sustaining medical treatments or to prevent falls. However, reducing the use of physical restraint in hospitalized patients is a major focus of accrediting and regulatory agencies, including the Joint Commission on Accreditation of Healthcare Organizations (JCAHO) and the Health Care Financing Administration (Center for Medicare and Medicaid Services [CMS]). Clinical trials to reduce the use of restraints in the hospital have not been reported. However, a quality improvement program employing an interdisciplinary model of consultation has shown that a clinically important reduction of 20 percent or more in the rate of use of physical restraints is achievable in selected hospital units without increasing the incidence of patient falls or therapy disruptions. The program included a clinical nurse specialist consultation on patients deemed at risk of restraint or admitted to the hospital unit in restraint, a selection of "alternatives" to restraint (e.g., moving patients closer to the nurses station, reality orientation for cognitively impaired patients, sitters or companions), interdisciplinary team rounds twice weekly to review difficult management problems, ongoing recommendations to the nurses and physicians and feedback to the nurse and team.

Reducing the use of restraints is not easily achieved in the hospital setting. Despite an absence of supportive data, surveys suggest that clinicians believe in the efficacy of physical restraints to prevent disruption of therapy and to prevent falls, and they believe they are vulnerable to legal liability resulting from patient harm related to not using restraints. A reasonable approach to restraint use is to avoid them until alternative approaches have been implemented or determined not to be feasible and the underlying reason for the restraint is addressed. Table 14-6 describes alternatives to physical restraint usage.

To further reduce the adverse risks of immobility, the patient's physical activity should be fostered through environmental adaptations (e.g., handrails, grab bars in bathroom, uncluttered hallway corridors) and specific exercise orders. Range-of-motion, low-impact endurance, and low-intensity resistive exercises will help to maintain or improve muscle strength in the lower extremities and improve standing balance. In a clinical trial, a hospital exercise program combined with a 1-month home exercise program included 12 exercises for flexibility and strengthening and a walking regimen. The intervention was performed twice daily in hospital and following discharge and three times a week at home for 1 month. The exercise program was

Table 14-6   **Alternatives to Physical Restraint**

Restraint Risk: Disruption of Therapy
  Patient Assessment
    Is patient delirious or demented?
    Are there reversible causes of agitation or confusion?
      Polypharmacy: narcotics (e.g., meperedine), H_2 blockers, psychoactive drugs (e.g., benzodiazepines), anticholinergic
        agents.
      Delirium caused by infections, hypoxia, neurologic event.
      Physical discomfort: urinary retention, fecal impaction, musculoskeletal pain, limb ischemia.
  Interventions
    Treat underlying cause of delirium or agitation.
    Maximize communication with patient.
      Low, calm tone of voice.
      Assistive devices as appropriate: hearing aids, headphone amplifiers, eyeglasses, communication boards.
      Explain all actions and instructions in clear, simple terms.
    Orient and reassure patient.
    Introduce yourself each time you see patient.
    Maintain anxiety-reducing techniques: calm manner, gentle touch, pleasant demeanor.
    Involve family in bedside care of patient.
    Pharmacotherapy for agitated or psychotic patients.
    Discontinue treatment modalities no longer essential to patients care (e.g., IV lines)

Restraint Risk: Accidental Falls
  Patient Assessment
    Fall risk factors: ≥ 75 years, history of falls, impaired gait, orthostatic hypotension or dizziness, impaired cognition, sensory
      impairments, incontinence, psychoactive drug use.
    Observe patient transfer and gait: evidence of weakness, unsteadiness.
  Interventions
    Environmental considerations
      Assure safe environment: nonslip floors, diffuse overhead lighting, eliminate room and hallway clutter.
      Grab bars in bathrooms, handrails in rooms and hallway corridor.
      Bedside and bathroom call system.
      Low bed positions.
      Move patient to room near nurse's station.
      Nonskid footwear.
      Remove unneeded tethers: bladder catheters, intravenous lines.
    Exercises to increase lower extremity and hip muscle strength
      Physical therapy consultation.
      Low-intensity resistive and endurance exercises.
    Assisted ambulation in hallway.
    Active or passive range-of-motion exercises for immobile patients.
    Treat orthostatic hypotension: modify drug regimen (e.g., decrease doses of vasodilators, α-blockers), increase dietary salt,
      apply compression stockings, leg-pumps.

associated with better function in instrumental activities of daily living at 1 month following discharge.

Environmental adaptations may foster greater mobility. Hand rails in hallway corridors, grab bars in bathrooms, non-glare lighting and carpeting, or textured flooring may help foster the patient's independent functioning while reducing caregivers' concerns for patient safety. Activity orders should specify whether patients can be allowed out of bed without restriction or with assistance. Physical therapy consultation is warranted when patients have difficulty with transfers or have generalized weakness or gait impairment. Occupational therapy may help patients to improve performance of ADL that will enable them to return to independent living.

Undernutrition

Undernutrition, especially protein–energy malnutrition (PEM) and specific nutrient deficiencies are common in chronically ill patients who are hospitalized for treatment of acute exacerbations of chronic diseases. PEM is associated with functional dependency, chronic medical illnesses (e.g., congestive heart failure, chronic obstructive pulmonary disease), cognitive impairment, social isolation, poor dentition, reduced thirst perception, and limited access to food and fluids. PEM contributes to the excess risk of death from various chronic diseases, such as congestive heart failure. Nutritional needs of elderly patients are frequently unrecognized or unaddressed early in the patients' hospital course often resulting in delays in recovery from an acute illness or in the healing of wounds and pressure ulcers. Evidence of this was shown in a prospective study of non-terminally ill hospitalized elderly veterans: 20 percent of the patients had a nutrient intake less than 50 percent of their calculated maintenance energy requirements. Compared to patients whose nutrient intake was adequate, the low-nutrient patients at discharge had lower serum cholesterol and albumin levels, a higher rate of in-hospital mortality and 90-day mortality, and were more likely to become functionally dependent at hospital discharge. Patients were frequently ordered to have nothing by mouth and neither canned supplements nor nutritional supports were used effectively.

The diagnosis of malnutrition is based on clinical evaluation, anthropometric measurements, laboratory markers, and measures of food intake (see Chap. 92). In the hospital, the diagnosis of PEM can be suspected by obtaining a history of a patient's unintentional weight loss, by observing the patient for physical evidence of muscle atrophy, and by documenting low levels of serum proteins (e.g., serum albumin <3.5 g/dL). However, the evaluation of nutritional status is hampered by the interactions of sarcopenia (loss of muscle mass) with aging, the effects of chronic diseases (e.g., chronic lung and heart diseases, cancer) and the effects of inflammatory diseases on the measures of nutritional status (for example, serum transferrin, serum albumin). Nonetheless, PEM should be suspected in elderly patients who have a documented history of weight loss, low body weight, muscle atrophy, and generalized muscle weakness. Treatment for undernutrition should be started in the hospital and continued after the patient's discharge (Table 14-7).

A team approach is usually needed to assess and manage PEM. Although definitive trials of nutritional intervention for non-critically ill elderly patients are lacking, several studies suggest that nutritional supplements containing balanced mixtures of amino acids, fat, carbohydrate, vitamins, and minerals improve the prognosis of elderly patients with specific illnesses. In a systematic review, the strongest evidence for the effectiveness of nutritional supplementation exists for oral protein and energy requirements for treatment of hip fractures. While oral feedings are preferred to peripheral alimentation, a percutaneous endoscopic gastrostomy (PEG) tube is superior to a nasogastric tube in patients suffering strokes and could be considered for use in any patient whose nutritional status is compromised by severe dysphagia, PEM, or contraindications to oral feeding. However, a high short-term mortality in hospitalized patients who have advanced dementia has been observed in patients with PEG tubes. In one prospective study of hospitalized patients with advanced dementia, a 50 percent 6-month median mortality was observed and tube feeding was not associated with survival. There is no evidence that PEG tubes prevent aspiration pneumonia

or other infections. Consequently, in the absence of clinical trials, a PEG tube is best considered for treatment of patients with acute illnesses, whose prognosis for improvement is good but their ability to take food by mouth is predicted to be delayed for weeks to months. Calorie-dense, nutritious, and palatable food supplements or snacks are recommended for malnourished, dyspneic, and weak patients who may be unable to consume a standard meal. Patients at risk for aspiration pneumonia because of generalized weakness or oropharyngeal dysphagia should undergo formal evaluation of swallowing conducted by a speech therapist, usually followed by a modified barium swallow. Patients with dysphagia for liquids may benefit from a pureed diet or thickened liquids that enable them to swallow safely, and provide sufficient calories and hydration (Table 14-7).

GENERAL MEASURES

Hospitalization for treatment of an acute illness can be an emotionally stressful experience for elderly patients and their families. Removed from the familiar routines of home and the support of family members, the elderly patient may experience anxiety, disruption of sleep patterns, and loss of personal autonomy. To allay these effects of hospitalization, it is important to ensure the patients' personal comfort and safety and to respect their personal wishes for care. Privacy and quiet at night, visits from family members, and opportunities to socialize in hallway corridors or activity rooms may help to lessen the stressful experience of hospitalization. Attention to bowel and bladder function through a toileting schedule, and bedside commode or urinal for men, also helps make the hospital experience easier for patients. Fiber supplements or routine use of hyperosmolar laxatives (e.g., lactulose) may be needed to prevent fecal impaction in high risk patients such as those who are immobile or are taking opiates or drugs with anticholinergic properties. Assistive devices, including canes and walkers, should be made readily available to the patient. Prophylactic anticoagulation with either unfractionated heparin or low-molecular-weight heparin is warranted to prevent venous thrombosis in immobile patients and those with recent history of cancer, surgery, heart failure or a past history of deep vein thrombosis.

Advanced Directives

Upon admission, the patient's advanced directives, either a living will or a durable power of attorney for healthcare, should be reviewed and copies of them included in the medical record. In discussing advance directives with patients, physicians should also seek their wishes for end-of-life care, including cardiopulmonary resuscitation, intensive care, or nutritional support during acute or end-stage illness. Despite the importance of advanced directives, decisions are often made under emergent conditions, and it may be unclear what course of action to take for a patient facing critical illness. In these instances, frequent discussions with the patient and family to further identify the patients' personal values about health and their expectations of hospitalization will prove most useful.

Table 14-7 Nutritional Interventions: Clinical Recommendations

Route	Patient Characteristics	Nutritional Considerations
Oral	Alert, normal swallowing mechanics, or normally nourished or mildly malnourished.	Monitor hydration and calories: optimal levels determined by nutritional assessment Calorie-dense foods. Consider nutritional supplements between meals.
Intravenous fluids	Acutely ill, impaired swallowing, decreased oral fluid intake, dehydration. Ability to eat anticipated in <48 hours.	Glucose solutions with electrolytes. Sole source of nutrition limited to <48 hours.
Enteral	Oropharyngeal dysphagia, unsafe to eat (e.g., delirium), severely malnourished; capacity for oral feeding expected to return within days to 2 weeks; cyclic use needed to augment oral nutrition.	Nasoenteric tube feeding (continuous or intermittent) with lactose-free solutions; either balanced-protein or high protein solutions. Cyclic or continuous infusions. Nasogastric tube not recommended.
Peripheral parenteral nutrition	Oral and nasoenteric routes are temporarily (e.g., ≤2 weeks) contraindicated (e.g., small-bowel obstruction, acute pancreatitis).	Peripheral intravenous (large-bore catheter) infusion with isotonic glucose-electrolyte-lipid solution. Limited capacity to deliver high-calorie nutrition. Observe for hypertriglyceridemia.
Total parenteral nutrition	Severely malnourished; enteral route contraindicated (e.g., bowel obstruction, short bowel); hypermetabolic state (e.g., sepsis) while enteral route delivery is not sufficient.	Central intravenous (e.g., subclavian vein) catheter (large bore). Infusion of high-calorie, hypertonic and balanced infusions (protein, amino acid, carbohydrate) is achievable.
Percutaneous endoscopic gastrostomy	Severely malnourished; oropharyngeal dysphagia unlikely to resolve soon; oral feeding contraindicated (e.g., stroke); enteral nutrition required for 2 or more weeks or indefinitely.	Superior to nasoenteric tubes for administering medications (e.g., tablets). No evidence of benefit for severely demented patients.

INTERDISCIPLINARY DISCHARGE PLANNING

The interdisciplinary process of discharge planning serves to identify patients who will need nursing home placement or home care services; to estimate the patient's hospital length of stay; to educate the patient and family about the patient's diagnosis, prognosis, and choices for discharge location; and to review medications, home safety, and the promotion of self-care. The effectiveness of interdisciplinary discharge planning is well established by clinical trials. In a randomized clinical trial conducted at two hospitals, an advanced practice nurse (APN) provided comprehensive discharge planning and home follow-up in collaboration with the patient's attending physician. The APN conducted a geriatric assessment, coordinated the patient's discharge planning with the primary physician, and provided home visits and telephone follow-up after hospital discharge. By week 24 after the initial hospital discharge patients receiving the intervention were less likely to be readmitted to the hospital. Even when they were readmitted, the intervention patients spent fewer total days in hospital.

Interdisciplinary care also helps to clarify the discharge location that is appropriate for the patient. The process of

discharge planning is aided by an awareness of the patient's baseline functional status (i.e., prior to the acute illness), the expected length of hospital stay, and the degree of anticipated recovery of self-care in that time. The input of nurses, social workers, physical therapists and occupational therapist are especially valuable to physicians.

Most medically ill elderly patients are discharged from hospital to home, while others are transferred to transitional care sites (e.g., subacute units or skilled nursing facilities) or long-term care facilities. Patients able to perform daily activities independently usually return home with or without home care services. Skilled nursing care and home physical therapy often enable patients to return home for completion of their medical treatment and rehabilitation. An inpatient rehabilitation hospital is an option for patients with a categorical illness such as hip fracture or stroke and who have good rehabilitative potential and adequate home support. Increasingly, complex patients are discharged to subacute care units or to skilled nursing facilities for short-term rehabilitation or skilled nursing care until they are able to return to independent living. Patients lacking sufficient supports at home and who require only chronic disease management may be eligible for home

Table 14-8   The Acute Care of Elders Unit Intervention

The prepared environment

Modified to enhance independent functioning by patients.

Hallway corridor and patient rooms carpeted and clocks and calendars prominently placed in each room.

Carpeting patterns and wall coverings with visual contrast chosen to aid in patient orientation and way-finding.

Special beds with floor lighting added and additional lighting installed behind each patient's bed.

A large common space (activity room), created to encourage dining outside of rooms, socializing, and light exercise.

Multidimensional assessment linked to nonpharmacologic prescriptions

Nurse-initiated guidelines direct the primary nurse's assessment of the patient's functional status and suggest interventions to restore independent functioning or to prevent functional decline.

Nurse's assessment is routine part of the evaluation of all elderly patients admitted to the ACE unit.

The clinical nurse specialist reviews the functional status of each patient daily and discusses findings and recommendations daily with the interdisciplinary team.

Medical care review

Medical director reviews the patient's medical care to assure that standards of medical care are maintained on the unit.

Recommendations for changes in diagnostic or therapeutic interventions are made to the resident or attending physician.

Clinical guidelines describe the optimal choices of psychoactive drugs, alternatives to physical restraints, nutritional therapies, and pressure ulcer management.

Interdisciplinary team rounds and comprehensive discharge planning

All patients are reviewed daily at team rounds.

Team members are directly involved in the patient's care, enabling rounds to be brief and highly task oriented.

Team members review the patient's baseline functional status, daily functional status, and trajectory of expected cognitive and physical functioning by hospital discharge.

Length of stay is estimated and postdischarge plans are begun.

Transition of care extends hospital interventions to the outpatient setting.

Patients are assessed for signs of clinical instability on the day of planned hospital discharge.

Medicaid waiver programs, programs of all inclusive care of the elderly (PACE), or admission to a long-term care facility. Palliative care, either in the hospital or in the community, is an option for patients who have an illness that will be terminal, and hospice is recommended for patients who are terminally ill (life expectancy less than 6 months).

Patients should not be discharged from the hospital if they have evidence of clinical instability on the day preceding the planned discharge. While clinical trials to define "clinical stability" for hospital discharge are lacking, a retrospective Medicare review identified signs of clinical instability that are associated with a greater risk of mortality in the 30 days following discharge. These signs include a new finding of incontinence, chest pain, dyspnea, delirium, tachycardia or hypotension; a temperature >38.3°C (100.9°F); or a diastolic blood pressure >105 mmHg.

MULTICOMPONENT INTERVENTIONS TO IMPROVE CLINICAL OUTCOMES OF HOSPITALIZATION

Clinical trials of hospitalized elderly patients have focused on improving functional status, reducing nursing home admission or functional decline, reducing costs of care, decreasing length of stay, or reducing mortality. The interventions include consultative-based geriatrics, improved systems of care, and interdisciplinary discharge planning. Trials of geriatric consultation have proven generally disappointing. Greater successes have been reported with specialized units—inpatient geriatric evaluation and management (GEM) units, acute care of elders (ACE) units and, stroke units. The Hospital Elder Life Program (see Chap. 117) reduces the incidence of delirium and is a model of hospital care for all vulnerable elderly patients.

Geriatric Evaluation and Management Units

Inpatient and outpatient intervention teams at the Veteran Affairs Medical Centers have improved short-term and long-term clinical outcomes. Earlier studies had suggested that GEM units could improve moral and physical functioning among elderly veterans and decrease mortality. A recent multicenter randomized trial of hospitalized patients supports the effectiveness of the GEM intervention to improve some functional and mental health outcomes, although mortality was not reduced by the intervention. Frail hospitalized patients, whose medical condition had stabilized were assigned to either inpatient GEM or to usual hospital care. At discharge the patients were assigned outpatient follow-up in either the geriatric clinic or to usual outpatient care. Patients receiving the intervention in the hospital reported higher health-related quality of life, better performance of basic activities of daily living, and less bodily pain. However, after 1 year, only mental health was reportedly better in the patients attending the geriatric clinic. Over the 1-year period of the trial there were no significant differences in mortality, functional status or overall costs of inpatient and outpatient care.

Acute Care for Elders Units

Improvements in clinical outcomes have been found with ACE units. In one clinical trial, medically ill patients age 70 years or older were randomly assigned to either usual care on a general medical service or to the specially designed ACE unit. The ACE unit provided a standardized and structured intervention (Table 14-8). Compared to patients receiving usual care patients receiving the ACE intervention were less likely to lose independence in one or more basic ADL and more likely to regain independence in ADL. Fewer patients in the intervention group were discharged for the first time to institutional long term care. Mean hospital charges and length of stay were not increased by the intervention. A clinical trial of ACE in a community hospital demonstrated less impressive results on ADL outcomes but did show a decrease in the composite outcome of ADL decline from baseline or nursing home placement in patients receiving the ACE intervention compared to usual care. The process of care was significantly better and patient mobility determined by a performance based measure was better at hospital discharge in patients receiving the intervention.

Stroke Units

Stroke units vary in their description and process but meta-analyses suggest benefits on functional outcomes and reduced risks of nursing home transfers. Recent quality improvement programs are attempting to improve stroke outcomes by including the principles of geriatric assessment and interdisciplinary care to usual stroke management by neurologists. These and related studies support the importance of assessment and intervention of hospitalized elderly patients and the potential to improve the processes and outcomes of hospitalization for this vulnerable population.

REFERENCES

Agostini JV et al: Cognitive and other adverse effects of diphenhydramine use in hospitalized older patients. Arch Intern Med 161:2091, 2001.
Avenell A, Handoll HH: Nutritional supplementation for hip fracture aftercare in the elderly. Cochrane Database Syst Rev 1, 2002.
Bogardus ST et al: What does the medical record reveal about functional status? A comparison of medical records and interview data. J Gen Intern Med 16:728, 2001.
Cohen HJ et al: A controlled trial of inpatient and outpatient geriatric evaluation and management. N Engl J Med 346:905, 2002.
Counsell SR et al: Effects of a multicomponent intervention on functional outcomes and process of care in hospitalized older patients: a randomized controlled trial of acute care for elders (ACE) in a community hospital. J Am Geriatr Soc 48:1572, 2000.
Covinsky KE et al: Depressive symptoms and three year mortality in older hospitalized medical patients. Ann Intern Med 130:563, 1999.
Ferris D, Menyah DK: Reducing the use of inappropriate medications in the hospitalized elderly. Am J Health Syst Pharm 58:1588, 2001.
Inouye SK et al: Importance of functional measures in predicting mortality among older hospitalized patients. JAMA 279:1187, 1998.
Inouye SK et al: The hospital elder life program: A model of care to prevent cognitive and functional decline in older hospitalized patients. J Am Geriatr Soc 48:1697, 2000.
Levinsky NG et al: Influence of age on Medicare expenditures and medical care in the last year of life. JAMA 286:1349, 2001.
McCusker J et al: Delirium predicts 12-month mortality. Arch Intern Med 162:457, 2002.
McCusker J et al: Rapid emergency department intervention for older people reduces risk of functional decline: results of a multi-center randomized trial. J Am Geriatr Soc 49:1272, 2001.
Meier DE et al: High short-term mortality in hospitalized patients with advanced dementia: Lack of benefit of tube feeding. Arch Intern Med 161:594, 2001.
Mion LC et al: Outcomes following physical restraint reduction programs in two acute care hospitals. Jt Comm J Qual Improv 27:605, 2001.
Naylor MD et al: Comprehensive discharge planning and home follow-up of hospitalized elders. A randomized clinical trial. JAMA 281:613, 1999.
Popovic JR: 1999 National hospital discharge survey: Annual summary with detailed diagnosis and procedure data. National Center for Health Statistics. Vital Health Stat 13(151), 2001.
Siebens H et al: A randomized controlled trial of exercise to improve outcomes of acute hospitalization in older adults. J Am Geriatr Soc 48:1545, 2000.
Strange GR, Chen EH: Use of emergency departments by elder patients: A five-year study. Acad Emerg Med 5:1157, 1998.
Sullivan DH et al: Protein-energy undernutrition among elderly hospitalized patients: A prospective study. JAMA 281:2013, 1999.
Teno JM et al: Prediction of survival for older hospitalized patients: The HELP survival model. J Am Geriatr Soc 48:S16, 2000.
Thomas EJ, Brennan TA: Incidence and types of preventable adverse events in elderly patients: Population-based review of medical records. BMJ 320:741, 2000.
Walter LC et al: Development and validation of a prognostic index for one-year mortality in older adults after hospitalization. JAMA 285:2987, 2001.
Wu AW et al: Predicting functional status outcomes in hospitalized patients aged 80 years and older. J Am Geriatr Soc 48:S6, 2000.

Critical Care in the Elderly: Optimizing Outcomes for Older Patients Admitted to Intensive Care

CARI R. LEVY • E. WESLEY ELY

This chapter addresses some of the most commonly encountered medical and ethical dilemmas facing physicians when their elderly patients are admitted to an intensive care unit (ICU). Upon developing a potentially life-threatening condition, the possibility of an ICU admission mandates a reexamination of a patient's preferences for medical care. This reexamination is fueled by uncertainty about outcomes in this population, as well as by a fear that the treatments offered might be overly burdensome and pose undue risk in relation to the potential for benefit. To aid in these difficult decisions and in order to make evidence-based decisions, we must be knowledgeable about outcomes in this population.

The elderly are the most rapidly growing segment of the ICU population. Approximately two-thirds of all ICU beds are occupied by patients older than age 65 years, and the number of days spent in the ICU is seven times greater for patients older than age 75 years than it is for those patients younger than age 65 years. The landmark Study to Understand Prognosis and Preferences for Outcomes and Risks of Treatment (SUPPORT) was designed to help the medical community understand how care is provided to seriously ill patients. More than 9000 seriously ill adult patients were enrolled from five clinical sites. Data from the SUPPORT investigation indicated that age >70 years is associated with lower intensity of care (Fig. 15-1). Similarly, Nuckton and List demonstrated that physicians use age as a factor in the decision to admit an elderly patient to the ICU. Should age alone be used as a foundation for determining aggressiveness of care? If not, what evidence is there to help guide such decisions? This chapter reviews outcomes among the elderly after an ICU stay in an attempt to answer these and other relevant questions.

We are just beginning to understand the many ethical, medical and social factors that affect the decision to admit elderly patients to an ICU. It is likely, however, that the outcomes literature we report represents a highly selected group of elderly individuals. The information in the following sections will assist health care professionals as they make decisions about aggressiveness of care for critically ill elderly patients.

ICU MORTALITY AND ESTIMATING PROGNOSIS

The mortality rate of elderly patients admitted to the ICU ranges widely across studies (Table 15-1). Champion et al. reported ICU mortality of 8 percent among patients aged 65 to 74 years and 10 percent for those older than 74 years. Most investigators, however, report overall ICU mortality rates of 20 to 30 percent for patients over age 65 years. In-hospital mortality after leaving the ICU ranges from 16 to 50 percent, but rates most typically range from 30 to 50 percent. When elderly ICU patients require mechanical ventilation for support of dysfunctional lungs, mortality increases substantially. Although some studies report increased mortality among the elderly, other studies fail to demonstrate consistent evidence of uniformly poor survival, even in patients older than age 80 years. For example, in a retrospective analysis by Chelluri et. al., the mortality rate was 38 percent among patients older than age 85 years, a rate similar to those observed for cohorts younger than age 85.

Predicting which elderly patients will die in the ICU is difficult given the variability among individual patients. In

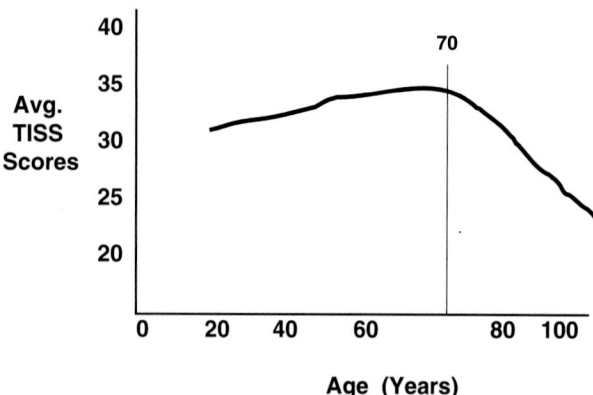

Figure 15-1 The relationship between patient age and the intensity of care delivered to patients enrolled in the SUPPORT trial is depicted as patient age (x axis) versus average Therapeutic Intervention Scoring System (TISS) on days 1 and 3 (y axis). TISS is a valid and reliable method of measuring resource use in cohorts of patients. The solid line represents the TISS scores after adjustment for severity of illness and functional status, and shows that intensity of care was lower for older patients even after these adjustments. Adapted with permission from Hamel MB et al.: Patient age and decisions to withhold life-sustaining treatments from seriously ill, hospitalized adults. *Ann Intern Med* 130:116, 1999.

the study by Lynn et al., at a time point of only 7 days before death, experienced physicians prospectively estimated that 50 percent of patients with congestive heart failure, chronic obstructive pulmonary disease, and cirrhosis would live for at least 6 months. For patients with acute respiratory failure and multiple organ dysfunction syndrome, the same physicians estimated that 20 percent of the patients would live for 6 months, when in actuality they lived for only 7 days. Whether or not age independently predicts increased mortality, two of three elderly patients do survive ICU admission and most return to productive lives. The challenge is to identify those elderly most likely to survive and to provide alternative management strategies for those unlikely to survive.

To provide physicians with prognostic information, several investigators have designed and validated prognostic models. Walter et al. used six independent risk factors, including gender, number of dependent activities of daily living (ADL), congestive heart failure, cancer, elevated creatinine, and low albumin to estimate the likelihood of 1-year mortality after hospitalization. As reported by Knaus et al., a mortality prediction model was also developed by the SUPPORT investigators to estimate survival of seriously ill hospitalized adults over a 180-day period. Predictor variables included diagnosis, age, number of days in the hospital before study entry, presence of cancer, neurologic function, and 11 physiologic measures on day 3 following study entry. The model was as accurate as physician estimates and accuracy improved when the model was combined with physician estimates of survival.

While prediction tools may assist physicians in avoiding serious errors in clinical judgment, they are difficult to apply at the bedside because caring for critically ill or dying patients is emotionally charged. Goals of care are likely to be influenced more by the preferences of patients, families, and physicians than by prognostic models. Even when physicians are provided with prognostic information on their seriously ill patients, as noted by Lynn et al., their behavior is not altered by such information.

FUNCTIONAL OUTCOMES AND QUALITY OF LIFE AFTER AN ICU STAY

As many as 1 in 3 elderly patients will be alive 1 year after an ICU stay. The majority of elderly survivors return to normal or near-normal function after discharge from the hospital. Although functional status and health-related quality of life (HRQOL) are often used interchangeably, elderly patients are more frequently satisfied with their lives in spite of chronic illness and functional impairment. It is important not to assume that patients with an impaired quality of life (QOL) want less-aggressive treatment. Elderly patients are more likely to consider burdens of treatment than younger adults, but as reported by Tsevat et al., they are also more likely to value living longer in suboptimal health versus living less time in excellent health.

Many of the studies on functional outcomes are limited by methodologic flaws and small sample size, but consistent findings across studies include some decline in function but return to prior living situation and preservation of perceived quality of life (Table 15-2). Chelluri et al. found that 100 percent of patients aged 65 to 74 years and 80 percent of those older than age 75 years had returned to their homes 1 year following their ICU stay. There was no change in perceived quality of life at 1 year, and 84 percent were independent in ADL as compared to 94 percent at baseline. Ninety percent of the survivors were independent in ADL prior to the hospitalization, and 84 percent of them remained independent at 1 year.

Predictors of poorer functional outcome include age >85 years, poor baseline function, the need for mechanical ventilation, and impairment of 2 or more organ systems during hospitalization. Longer length of stay and Acute Physiology and Chronic Health Education (APACHE II) scores do not consistently predict functional decline. Predictors of perceived quality of life include baseline QOL and illness severity.

Despite worse function, patients surviving an ICU stay frequently perceive their health as good or better than before their critical illness and superior to the health of their contemporaries. Furthermore, many elderly patients that have been in the ICU are willing to accept the high burden of ICU treatment again. When asked if they would be willing to be admitted to the ICU again, 71 to 90 percent of the elderly surveyed said they would if admission were indicated.

CARDIOPULMONARY RESUSCITATION OUTCOMES

The probability of surviving cardiopulmonary resuscitation (CPR) is frequently debated during the hospitalization of critically ill adults. Data on outcomes after in-hospital cardiopulmonary resuscitation is included in this chapter to

Table 15-1 Mortality of Elderly Patients Who Are Admitted to Intensive Care

Reference and Country	ICU	Age Range (years)	Elderly Patients (n)	ICU	In-hospital	Postdischarge
Champion et al. (1981) USA	MICU/CCU	65–74	624	8	14	33 (6–18 months)
		≥75	560	10	16	43 (6–18 months)
		≥70		—		
LeGall et al. (1982) France	Multi	≥70	40	—	—	69 (1 year)
Fedullo and Swinburne (1983) USA	MICU	70–79	61	26	41	—
		80–89	23	30	34	—
Nicolas et al. (1987) France	Med/Surg 7 hospitals	>65	191	37	—	—
Sage et al. (1987) USA	Med/Surg	>65	134	—	12	28 (18 months)
Chalfin and Carlon (1990) USA	Med/Surg (cancer hospital)	65–74	324	27	36	—
		≥75	163	17	30	—
Ridley et al. (1990) Scotland	MICU	65–74	102	29	—	38 (18–42 months)
		75–84	39	21	—	
		≥85	3	0	—	
Wu et al. (1990) USA	MICU	≥75	130	17	51	—
Mahul et al. (1991) France	Med/Surg 4 hospitals	>70	295	20–29 (4 hospitals)	—	49 (1 year)
Mayer-Oakes et al. (1991) USA	MICU, 3 hospitals	65–74	104	—	30	45 (6 months)
		≥75	153	—	38	49
Chelluri et al. (1992) USA	All adult	≥85	34	26	38	—
Heuser et al. (1992) USA	All adult, 78 hospitals	≥65	2208	—	8	—
Kass et al. (1992)	Med/Surg	≥85	105	30	—	64 (1 year)
Chelluri et al. (1993) USA	All adult (excluded cancer patients with "poor prognosis")	65–74	43	21	40	58 (1 year)
		≥75	54	31	39	63
Rockwood et al. (1993) Canada	Multi, 2 hospitals	>65	406	16	—	49 (1 year)
Cohen and Lambrinos (1995) USA	All beds for MV patients, 243 NY hospitals	70–74	5613	—	51	—
		75–79	5874	—	56	—
		80–84	4910	—	62	—
		85–89	3145	—	67	—
		90+	1812	—	75	—
Djaini and Ridley, 1997 England	ICU	>70	474	19	—	47 (1 year)
		70–74		12	—	—
		75–79		17	—	—
		80–84		26	—	—
		≥85		34	—	—

CCU, cardiac care unit; Med/Surg, medical/surgical ICU; Multi, multidisciplinary ICU; MV, mechanically ventilated; mo, months

Source: Nelson JE and Nierman DM (2001), with permission.

Table 15-2 Functional Outcomes and Quality of Life of the Elderly after Intensive Care

Reference and Country	ICU	Age Range (years)	Elderly Patients (n)	Measures/Follow-up Period	Results
Campion et al. (1981) USA	MICU/CCU	65–74 ≥75	624 560	Physical activity at 6–18 months vs. pre-ICU	In both elderly groups, no change in % home at f/u vs. baseline. Lifestyle with mild or more exertion: 65–74 years, 76% (baseline); 70% (f/u) ≥75 years, 68% (baseline); 50% (f/u) Sedentary lifestyle: 65–74 years, 11% (baseline); 26% (f/u) ≥75 years, (baseline); 43% (f/u)
LeGall et al. (1982) France	Med/Surg	≥50 ≥70	67 18	Functional status at 3 months pre-ICU, 1 year post-ICU	49% of survivors ≥50 years; no change at 1 year; 51% had worse function; functional outcome influenced by age + number of organ failures
McClean et al. (1985) Canada	Multi-RICU	≥75	14	Functional status, attitudes re: QOL and ICU, 12–24 months post-ICU	43% with activity level at f/u ≥ baseline 85% QOL worthwhile 77% would repeat ICU if indicated
Sage et al. (1987) USA	Med/Surg	>65	59	SIP-uniscale at 18 months post-ICU	90% self-rated as "acceptably" or "extremely" healthy Slightly (not significant) lower adjusted SIP and uniscale for ICU survivors vs. elderly controls
Zaren and Hedstrand (1987) Sweden	Med/Surg	≥65	199	Functional status at 1 year post-ICU vs. 3 years post-ICU	80% of patients independent at home vs. 90% at baseline Poor baseline function, ICU LOS ≥1 week, MV, predicted worse functional outcome
Zaren and Hedstrand (1989) Sweden	Med/Surg	≥65	350	Functional status at 1 year post-ICU vs. 3 years post-ICU	73% of patients' functional status at 1 year ≥ baseline MV but not ICU LOS associated with worse functional outcome
Mundt et al. (1989) USA	Med/Surg	≥70	262	Functional status in physical, psychological, and social domains at 6 months post-ICU	Most had worse functional status, but more contact with family 72% of previously working patients still working
Ridley and Wallace (1990) Scotland	Multi	≥60	40	PQOL, Katz's ADL, other functional capacity 1–3 years post-ICU	82% of patients had same or improved status; 7% deteriorated
Mahul et al. (1991) France	Med/Surg (4 hospitals)	≥70	106	Residence and functional status at 1 year post-ICU	88% at home, 70% independent at 1 year 80% functional status ≥ baseline No clinical parameters at ICU admission predicted functional outcome

(Continued)

Table 15–2 (*Continued*) Functional Outcomes and Quality of Life of the Elderly after Intensive Care

Reference and Country	ICU	Age Range (years)	Elderly Patients (n)	Measures/Follow-up Period	Results
Chelluri et al. (1992) USA	Med/Surg	≥85	21	Residence and level of activity, attitudes re: QOL and ICU	86% of patients from home; 43% independent 62% discharged to home, 5% to rehab hospital 8/10 QOL = good or fair; 9/10 would receive ICU care again
Mata et al. (1992) Spain	Med/Surg		155 33	Function and PQOL at ICU admission and 1 year post-ICU	50% worse function, 50% same or better function vs. baseline Lower function not mirrored by lower subjective perception of QOL 1-year QOL influenced by baseline QOL age, illness severity
Chelluri et al. (l993) USA	ICU	≥65	38	Kat's ADL, PQOL, CES-D at 1 year post-ICU	All 65–74-year-olds from home back at home at 1 year; 85% patients ≥75 years at home at 1 year 84% independent ADL at 1 year vs. 94% at baseline No decline in PQOL from baseline; no difference in PQOL compared to community elderly controls CES-D same as controls 71% willing to repeat ICU if indicated
Rockwood et al. (1993) Canada	Multi, 2 hospitals	>65	175	Health status, functional capacity, attitudes re: ICU at 1 year post-ICU	Majority independent in ADL Compared to control in community, same proportion perceived health as good to very good despite worse function. 70% satisfied with health status 54% had health status ≥ 5 years before ICU 66% had health status ≥ contemporaries
Konopad et al. (1995) Canada	Med/Surg	66–76 >75	46 175	Spitzer's QOL at ICU admission and 1 year post-ICU	Activity level and ADL worse for all age-groups Patients >75 years perceived health status as better 82% of 66–75-year-olds, 71% of patients >75 years home at 1 year

ADL, activities of daily living; CCU, cardiac care unit; CES-D, Center of Epidemiologic Studies—Depression Score; f/u, follow-up; LOS, length of stay; Med/Surg, medical/surgical ICU; Multi, multidisciplinary ICU; MV, mechanically ventilated; PQOL, perceived quality of life; QOL, quality of life; RICU, respiratory ICU; SIP, Sickness Impact Profile.
SOURCE: From Nelson JE and Nierman DM (2001), with permission.

Table 15-3 Survival Rates after In-Hospital Cardiac Arrest

Reference	Cardiac Rhythm	Number of Patients (n)	Survival to Hospital Discharge (%)	Age Influences Outcome Unfavorably	Comments
Gulati RS et al: CPR of old people. *Lancet*: 267, 1983	All	52	17	No	Of those alive at 1 month, none had neurologic injury or physical dependence
Bedell SE et al: Survival after CPR in the hospital. *N Engl J Med* 309:569, 1983	All VF	294	14 24	No	75% of survivors alive at 6 months
Taffet GI et al: In-hospital CPR. *JAMA* 260:2069, 1988	All VF	≥70 = 77 <70 = 322	0 0	Yes	
George AL et al: Pre-arrest morbidity and other correlates of survival after in-hospital CPR. *Am J Med* 87:28, 1989	All VF	140	24 36	Yes	No absolute predictor of mortality
Murphy DI et al: Outcomes of CPR in the elderly. *Ann Intern Med* 111:199, 1989	All VF	259 (≥70)	3 21	Yes	Un-witnessed arrest survival <1%
Peterson MW et al: Outcome of CPR in a medical intensive care unit. *Chest* 100:168, 1991				No	Poor outcome: hypotension, sepsis, elevated APACHE II
Rosenberg M et al: Results of CPR. *Arch Intern Med* 153:1370, 1993	All	>70 N = 178	22	No	Survival similar in age <50
Schneider AP et al: In-hospital CPR: A 30-year review. *J Am Board Fam Pract* 6:91, 1993		Meta-analysis	12		For age >90, 0% survived to discharge; community vs. teaching hospitals (19% vs. 14%)
Schwenzer KJ et al: Selective application of CPR improves survival rates. *Anesth Analg* 76:478, 1993	All	Age ≥70 and <80 N = 137	22	No	Age ≥70 less likely to receive CPR but when CPR was performed, survival = younger patients
Di Bari M et al: CPR of older, inhospital patients: Immediate efficacy and long-term outcome. *Crit Care Med* 28:2320, 2000	All	245 Mean age 70	33	No	At 2-year follow-up 60% still alive and survival curve similar in older and younger patients
Tresch DD et al: CPR in elderly patients hospitalized in the 1990s: A favorable outcome. *J Am Geriatr Soc* 42:137, 1994	All VF	50 28 Age ≥70	24 39	No	86% of survivors alive at 1 year; outcomes were similar to younger patients; 76% of arrests were witnessed; most were functionally active before admission; cardiac disease predicted success

prepare health care professionals for such conversations. Although some have described cardiopulmonary resuscitation in the elderly as "an exercise in futility," age alone is not the most significant determinant of survival in patients who receive CPR. Survival to hospital discharge after CPR in elderly patients ranges from 0 to 39 percent (Table 15-3). Some studies report very poor outcomes, whereas more recent studies demonstrate improved survival similar to that among patients younger than 65 years. If a patient survives the event that required CPR, then survival to discharge from the hospital is likely. Furthermore, many elderly patients remain highly functional after CPR especially if their primary illness is cardiac. As discussed below, data in this area are somewhat conflicting, and it is important to have a full understanding of the evidence both in support of and against CPR in elderly patients.

Two studies (Taffet et al. and Murphy et al.) reported very poor outcomes among hospitalized elderly who received CPR. These studies received much attention and led to pessimism regarding CPR. Taffet et al. found immediate survival of older (>70 years) patients was 31 percent versus 43 percent in the younger cohort, but none of the elderly patients survived to hospital discharge as compared to 16 percent of patients younger than age 70 years surviving to hospital discharge. Murphy et al. retrospectively analyzed the survival of 259 hospitalized elderly patients (≥70 years) who were resuscitated between 1977 and 1987. Only 6.5 percent of those resuscitated while hospitalized survived to hospital discharge. Half of these survivors required placement in a long-term care facility or a rehabilitation unit, and half of all survivors had significant functional or neurologic impairment. The conclusion from these two authors was that CPR is rarely beneficial to hospitalized elderly patients.

In contrast, recent studies demonstrate better outcomes among elderly patients, which are similar to those for younger patients. Bedell et al. found that 75 percent of CPR survivors were still alive 6 months after CPR. DiBari et al. reported 60 percent survival at 2 years among patients who received CPR in an ICU (n = 221) or on a general medical ward (n = 24). Patients older than 70 years of age had an immediate survival of 39.4%, and advancing age was not a predictor of immediate or long-term survival. Tresch et al. evaluated survival after resuscitations performed in the 1990s and noted no significant difference between those 70 years of age or older versus those younger than 70 years of age. There were no significant differences in functional status pre- and postarrest among patients surviving to hospital discharge. Survival at 1, 2, and 3 years in elderly versus younger survivors was also not greatly dissimilar (86% versus 80%, 76% versus 67%, and 71% versus 61%, respectively).

Age is not a consistent predictor of mortality in many studies. The two most consistent predictors of survival after CPR are "a witnessed arrest" and a cardiac rhythm of ventricular fibrillation or ventricular tachycardia versus asystole or pulseless electrical activity. Patients presenting with ventricular fibrillation or ventricular tachycardia have a survival rate up to seven times greater compared to those with asystole or pulseless electrical activity. Similarly, survival of in-hospital CPR doubles if the arrest is witnessed. Most investigators also concur that a diagnosis of metastatic cancer portends a poorer prognosis immediately after CPR. Other factors variably associated with increased mortality include respiratory failure, increased number of comorbidities, greater severity of illness, very advanced age (>89 years), poor functional status, sepsis, creatinine >2.0, albumin <3, hypotension, CPR lasting longer than 15 minutes, and a HCT <35 mg/dL.

MECHANICAL VENTILATION IN THE ELDERLY PATIENT

Clinicians have difficulty accurately predicting patient preferences for mechanical ventilation. As reported by Hamel et al., physician error rates in estimating patients' preferences for mechanical ventilation increase from 36 percent at ages younger than 50 years to 79 percent at ages greater than 80 years.

The probability of withholding mechanical ventilation increases with patient age (Fig. 15-2) yet the effect of age on outcomes after mechanical ventilation in the ICU is not clear. Many prior investigations of mechanical ventilation (MV) in the elderly are limited by their retrospective design and the absence of adjustment for severity of illness (Table 15-4). In a review of 21 published reports with data on mechanically ventilated elderly patients, the investigators' conclusions differ regarding the effect of age on outcome. One important limiting factor is the inability to know how many elderly patients choose to forego mechanical interactions even though they meet criteria for intubation and mechanical ventilation. Three recent cohort investigations have advanced the understanding of outcomes of older persons receiving mechanical ventilation.

The first report in this series, by Ely et al. (1999), was from a medical ICU and showed that intubated patients over 75 actually passed a daily screen of weaning at a faster rate than younger patients. This study also found that mechanically ventilated older persons (with respiratory failure of various etiologies not confined to acute lung injury) had

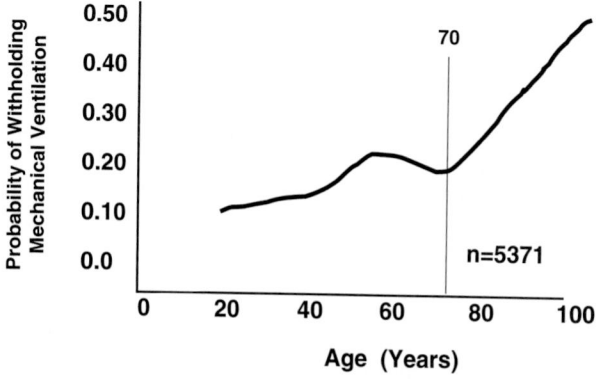

Figure 15-2 The relationship between patient age and the adjusted probability of a decision to withhold mechanical ventilation by study day 30 in the SUPPORT investigation. At age 70 to 79 years, relative risk 1.5 (1.2 to 1.9), and at age >80 years, relative risk 2.1 (1.6 to 2.7). Adapted with permission from Hamel MB et al: Patient age and decisions to withhold life-sustaining treatments from seriously ill, hospitalized adults. *Ann Intern Med* 130:116, 1999.

Table 15-4   Investigations Describing Outcomes after Mechanical Ventilation in Older Patients

Author/Year/ Reference	Elderly (N) and Definition		Design of Study	Inclusion Criteria	Hospital Mortality (%)	Multivariate Analysis	Severity Adjustment	Age Influences Outcome[†]
Nunn (1979)	15	>75	Prospective	ICU*	73	No	No	Yes
Campion (1981)	565	≥75	Retrospective	ICU/CCU	16	No	No	No
Fedullo (1983)	84	≥70	Retrospective	MICU only	39	No	No	No
Witek (1985)	51	>70	Prospective	ICU*	51	No	No	Yes
McLean (1985)	49	≥75	Prospective	ICU*	43	No	No	No
Elpern (1989)	95	≥60	Retrospective	ICU ≥3 days	66	No	No	Yes
Tran (1990)	92	>70	Retrospective	MICU only	46	No	No	Yes
O'Donnell,	17	>70	Retrospective	ICU*	59	No	No	No
Pesau (1992)	99	≥70	Retrospective	ICU	60	Yes	Yes	No
Gracey (1992)	496	>65	Retrospective	ICU	46	No	No	Yes
Chelluri (1992)	34	≥85	Retrospective	MICU only	38	No	No	No
Stauffer (1993)	118	>70	Retrospective	ICU	62	Yes	No	Yes
Swinburne and	282	≥80	Retrospective	ICU	69	No	No	No
Cohen (1993)	109	≥80	Retrospective	ICU ≥3 days	62	No	No	Yes
Papadakis et al.	138	≥70	Retrospective	ICU	76	Yes	Yes	Yes
(1995)	110	≥70	Retrospective	ICU	38	No	No	No
	21,342	≥70	Retrospective	ICU	59	No	No	Yes
Steiner (1997)	40	>65	Prospective	ICU/Stroke patients	32 at 2 mo	Yes	No	Yes
Kurek (1997)	3,256	≥70	Retrospective	Tracheostom	64	No	No	Yes
Zilberberg (1998)	31	>65	Prospective	MICU	74	Yes	Yes	Yes
Kurek (1998)	4,101	≥75	Retrospective	ICU	55	No	No	Yes
Ely (1999)	63	≥75	Prospective	MICU/CCU	39	Yes	Yes	No
Ely (2002)	173	≥70	Prospective	ARDS/ALI	50 at 28 days	Yes	Yes	Yes
Esteban (2002)	1038	≥70	Prospective	ICU	52	Yes	Yes	Yes

Ely EW, Evans GW, Haponik, EF. Mechanical ventilation in a cohort of elderly patients admitted to an intensive care unit. Annals of Internal Medicine. 131:1999,96–104.

*Investigations including only mechanically ventilated patients

[†]Indicates the predominant conclusion of the authors as to whether or not age is independently important

total days on the ventilator and survival rates that were comparable to their younger counterparts.

The second cohort from an international study of respiratory failure, reported by Esteban et al., demonstrated that 1038 patients 75 years of age and older spent a similar amount of time on the ventilator and in the hospital as compared to 4118 patients younger than 75 years of age (both P > 0.2). The older patients did have higher ICU mortality than did younger patients (38 percent versus 30 percent, respectively, P < 0.001) and higher in-hospital mortality (52 percent versus 37 percent, respectively, P < 0.001).

The third report, a recently published analysis by Ely et al. (*Semin Respir Crit Care Med*, 2001), of 902 patients from the ARDS (acute respiratory distress syndrome) network's acute lung injury investigations in the United States, was the largest prospectively collected cohort to date. Patients 70 years of age and older had 28-day and 180-day mortality rates that were nearly twice those of patients younger than 70 years of age, with steady reductions in survival age by decades (i.e., 50 to 59, 60 to 69, 70 to 79, ≥80 years of age). Even after adjusting for covariates, age was a strong predictor of mortality. Interestingly, older persons who did survive achieved initial recovery land-marks at the same rate as their younger counterparts (i.e., they passed conventional weaning criteria and were able to sustain spontaneous breathing without mechanical support), yet they were delayed in their further progression through convalescence and much more likely to be reconnected to the ventilator.

In summary, the duration of mechanical ventilation has been shown to be an independent predictor of mortality, even after adjusting for covariates such as severity of illness. Elderly patients have rates of initial physiologic recovery (i.e., ability to breathe spontaneously) comparable to their younger counterparts, but they have a delay in successful liberation from the ventilator and are reintubated more often.

COGNITIVE OUTCOMES AFTER AN ICU STAY

Delirium is an organic mental disorder characterized by the acute onset of altered level of consciousness, fluctuating course, and disturbance in orientation, memory, attention, thought, and behavior. Delirium has been described as the brain's form of "organ dysfunction." According to the National Research Council, "For many people in good physical condition who succumb to an acute illness, cognitive decline is the main threat to their ability to recover and enjoy their favorite activities; for those whose physical activities were already limited, cognitive decline is a major additional threat to quality of life." Delirium is frequently not recognized by clinicians, and when recognized, is often considered an inevitable outcome of critical illness.

Neurologic deficits may complicate the ICU course of patients with sepsis, ARDS, and other severe illness. Hopkins et al. demonstrated that cognitive impairment was present in 100 percent of ARDS patients at hospital discharge, and in 80 percent at 1 year. Similarly, in a general ICU population not restricted to ARDS, neuropsychological abnormalities were present in over 50 percent of survivors following mechanical ventilation at hospital discharge. Deficits included clinically relevant abnormalities in psychomotor speed, executive function, visuoconstruction abilities, memory, and verbal fluency at 6 months.

A significant percentage of individuals developing delirium in the hospital continue to demonstrate symptoms of delirium after discharge (Fig. 15-3). Survivors of ICU studied within 24 hours of leaving the hospital show that 1 in 2 patients were significantly impaired by Folstein Mini-Mental State Examination, 1 in 5 had some features of delirium, and 1 in 10 met full delirium criteria at the time of hospital discharge. Such patients demonstrate decreased cerebral activity and increased cognitive deterioration, and are more likely to develop dementia than patients without delirium.

Delirium in ICU patients is associated with increased overall cost and morbidity, including increased length of stay, the need for subsequent institutionalization, and higher mortality rates. Mechanically ventilated, delirious ICU patients take longer to wean from the ventilator, are more likely to develop nosocomial pneumonia, and have increased length of stay. However, most data on delirium

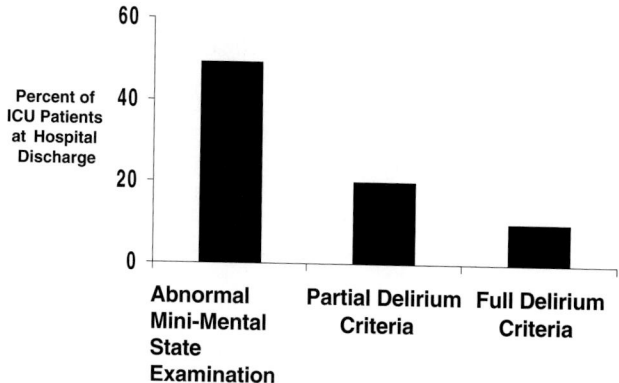

Figure 15-3 Rate of ongoing cognitive deficits and delirium at hospital discharge following mechanical ventilation. These data from survivors of ICU studied within 24 hours of leaving the hospital show that 1 in 2 patients were significantly impaired by Folstein Mini-Mental State Examination, 1 in 5 had partial delirium, and 1 in 10 met full delirium criteria at the time of hospital discharge. Adapted with permission from Ely EW et al. Delirium in mechanically ventilated patients: Validity and reliability of the confusion assessment method for the intensive care unit (CAM-ICU). *JAMA* 286(21):2703, 2001.

have been derived from non-ICU hospitalized patients, and few data exist concerning delirium in the ICU. This paucity of data has been attributed in part to a lack of validated instruments for assessing delirium in ventilated patients. In a recently published study, investigators validated a delirium assessment instrument called the Confusion Assessment Method for the ICU (CAM-ICU). The CAM-ICU is a 2-minute assessment instrument, which demonstrated a sensitivity of 93 to 100 percent, a specificity of 98 to 100 percent, and high interrater reliability (kappa = 0.96) in the detection of delirium, as compared to diagnosis by a psychiatrist. First in 48, and then in 96, consecutive mechanically ventilated patients, reported by Ely et al. (*JAMA,* 2001), delirium occurred in greater than 80 percent of patients in the ICU. In the subgroups expected to pose the greatest challenges for the CAM-ICU (i.e., those aged 65 years and older, those with suspected dementia, and those with the highest severity of illness), the instrument retained excellent sensitivity, specificity, and interrater reliability.

Cognitive Outcomes after CPR

In a meta-analysis by Schneider et al. of successful CPR (defined as discharge alive from the hospital) in 2994 patients, central nervous system impairment was noted in only 1.6 percent. In another literature review that included 19 studies, only 16 of 7324 (0.2 percent) remained in a vegetative state for up to 6 weeks until death, but up to 14 percent in some series were in a chronic vegetative state. Rogove et al. studied a total of 774 patients who were initially comatose after successful resuscitation from cardiac arrest. The analyses include both in- and out-of-hospital cardiac arrests. Mortality rate was 94 percent for the oldest group (>80 years of age) as compared to 68 percent for the youngest group (≤45 years of age) (p < .01). Recovery of good neurologic function was seen in 27 percent of the 774 patients. There was no statistically significant difference in neurologic recovery rates by age. Multivariate analysis showed that predictors of good neurologic outcome were a cardiac cause of arrest, short arrest time, short cardiopulmonary resuscitation time, and no history of diabetes mellitus. Importantly, increasing age was not an independent predictor of poor neurologic outcome on either univariate or multivariate analyses.

ADVANCE DIRECTIVES (SEE ALSO CHAP. 29)

Establishing goals of care consistent with patient wishes is the intent of executing an advance directive prior to an ICU admission. Elderly patients do want to discuss advance directives, and despite the importance of establishing preferences for care, the vast majority of patients report not having had a discussion with their physician about advance directives. Singer et al. suggest that while patients prefer to participate actively in determining their "code status," they are frequently asked during an acute illness when they feel poorly and often get confused by the precise treatment options and implications of such decisions. Therefore, the ICU may be the one of the most challenging places to initiate such discussions, and underscoring the importance of having such discussions in the outpatient setting or early in the course of an illness.

In the SUPPORT investigation, the presence of an advance directive did result in limited interventions at the end of life. In contrast, patients without an advance directive but for whom an order was written to limit resuscitation during their ICU stay had the longest length of stay, the most interventions and highest mortality. Most patients died in the ICU shortly after orders were written to limit resuscitative efforts.

The SUPPORT study demonstrated that less than 40 percent of patients recalled discussing prognosis or their preferences for life-sustaining treatments with their physician, and even when preferences were elicited for palliative care, only 29 percent of those who preferred palliative care felt their care reflected that preference. Only 47 percent of physicians knew that their patient did not want resuscitation, and 46 percent of do not resuscitate (DNR) orders were written within 2 days of death. In another investigation, when patients and physicians were presented with medical vignettes, 40 percent of physicians chose a level of care different from that requested by the patient. In fact, 10 percent of physicians would have done CPR on a patient with a DNR request. Interestingly, although this study was using hypothetical examples, the SUPPORT investigation revealed that CPR was performed on 11 percent of patients who had requested not to be resuscitated.

Fried et al. suggest that patients are able to incorporate probabilistic thinking into advance care planning and recommend focusing advance care discussions on potential outcomes and burdens of treatment, rather than on specific interventions. In this investigation, seriously ill patients were asked if they wanted to receive a given treatment depending on the burden of treatment and the outcome. Patients were willing to accept high treatment burdens if they would return to their current health status. However, if the outcome were severe functional or cognitive impairment, the majority of patients (74.4 percent and 88.8 percent, respectively) would decline treatment, even if the alternative were death.

Although there was initial enthusiasm about cost savings as a result of establishing advance directives, Emanuel suggested that substantial cost savings are unlikely to result. Thus, the merit of establishing advanced directives is to spare patients unwanted aggressive care rather than an effort to reduce medical expenditures.

LIMITING CARE AND FUTILITY (SEE ALSO CHAP. 26)

The probability of limiting life-sustaining treatment increases with advancing age (Fig. 15-4). Futility is often invoked as a justification for such limitation of care but futility is an inherently difficult term to define in medical care. Quantitative futility is an intervention where the estimate of success is less than or equal to 1 percent. Very few medical conditions are known to have a survival of less than 1 percent; hence, there is rarely an opportunity to apply the principle of quantitative futility when deciding whether or not to limit care. Qualitative futility is an intervention that merely preserves permanent unconsciousness or fails to end total dependence on intensive medical care. Again, it is difficult to know how long a patient will need intensive care and what interventions will or will not assist in liberating them from the need for ICU care. Given these definitions, it is not surprising that futile care has been described as uncommon in the ICU.

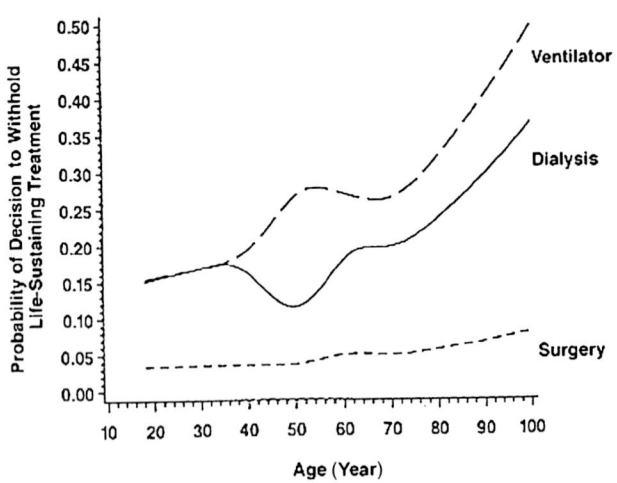

Figure 15-4 The relationship between patient age and the adjusted probability of a decision to withhold each life-sustaining treatment by study day 30. Results are calculated on the basis of Cox proportional hazard models, representing age as cubic spline functions, and are adjusted for sex, income, education, insurance, prognosis, comorbid conditions, baseline function, study site, and preferences for cardiopulmonary resuscitation and life-extending care. Adapted with permission from Hamel MB et al: Patient age and decisions to withhold life-sustaining treatments from seriously ill, hospitalized adults. *Ann Intern Med* 130:116,1999.

To aid in this complicated ethical dilemma, we refer the reader to the 1999 report of the Council on Ethical and Judicial Affairs of the American Medical Association (AMA). The AMA recommends a standardized "fair process" rather than a strict definition of futility. The process includes deliberation and resolution among all involved parties, securing alternatives in the case of irreconcilable differences, and a final step focused on providing closure when all alternatives have been considered. Physicians should base futility decisions on factors such as clinical efficacy of treatments, likelihood of mortality, and subsequent quality of life considerations rather than on chronologic age alone.

Although futility as a means of justifying the limitation of care can be onerous, as reported by Halvy et al., limitation of life support prior to death is common in the ICU setting. The circumstances of withdrawal vary widely from one institution to another and are unrelated to ICU, hospital type, mortality rate or admission rate. The active withdrawal of life-sustaining therapy occurs more often in patients without access to a private attending physician (29.9 percent versus 80.8 percent; $p < 0.001$) and death as a result of withholding life support occurs more frequently in community than in teaching hospitals (11.9 percent versus 3.8 percent, respectively, $p = 0.004$).

In a national survey, by Prendergast and Luce, of all American postgraduate training programs with significant clinical exposure to critical care medicine, including 6303 ICU-related deaths, active limitation of life support was common. Standard ICU care including failed cardiopulmonary resuscitation occurred in 26 percent (range, 4 to 79 percent); 24 percent (range, 0 to 83 percent) received standard ICU care without CPR; 14 percent (range, 0 to 67 percent) had life support withheld, and 36 percent (range, 0 to 79 percent) had life support actively withdrawn.

In the process of limiting therapy and transitioning to comfort care, health care professionals must continue to provide quality end-of-life care. Singer et al. sought to identify and describe elements of quality end-of-life care from patients' perspectives by using in-depth, open-ended, face-to-face interviews. This study showed that patients considered the following five domains of quality of end-of-life care to be the most important:

1. Receiving adequate pain and symptom management.
2. Avoiding inappropriate prolongation of death.
3. Achieving a sense of control.
4. Relieving burden.
5. Strengthening relationships with loved ones.

These domains are difficult to reconcile in the ICU because, traditionally, the ICU represents aggressive care. For example, adequate pain management may be sacrificed because consequent sedation may interfere with weaning from mechanical ventilation. How does one know when the prolongation of life is no longer appropriate? How can a patient with multiple IV lines and monitoring equipment achieve a sense of control? How can a patient expect to strengthen relationships with family when visitation is limited to several hours each day?

However, health care professionals must proceed in the face of prognostic uncertainty and seek to relieve suffering for all ICU patients. Palliative care must not be reserved for those "at the end of life." Holding to the principles of such care, specific domains of palliative care in the ICU might include:

1. Relief of pain.
2. Relief of dyspnea.
3. Relief of anxiety.
4. Regular communication between family and medical team.
5. Spiritual and psychological support for family and medical team.
6. Respect for patients' wishes regarding health care.

The elderly will continue to represent a large percentage of patients treated in the ICU. Several important conclusions can be drawn from this review of ICU care for the elderly. First, although an ICU admission may serve as a catalyst for discussions about preferences for care, such discussions would be better held in the outpatient setting when patients are able to fully consider their treatment options, seek a better understanding of the implications of their decisions, and, ultimately, articulate their choices regarding health care. All too often decisions about life-sustaining care fall to surrogates and clinicians who are frequently inaccurate in their assessment of the patient's preferences for care. Second, despite their older age, many scenarios result in outcomes that are acceptable and valued by elderly patients. Decisions about the aggressiveness of care must be carefully considered on a case-by-case basis. Finally, regardless of the degree to which a seriously ill patient desires aggressive care, health care providers must attend to all aspects of care and keep the patient free of pain, anxiety, and dyspnea while creating a supportive medical environment.

REFERENCES

1. Angus DC et al, for the committee on manpower for pulmonary and critical care societies (COMPACCS). Current and projected workforce requirements for care of the critically ill and patients with pulmonary disease: Can we meet the requirements of an aging population? *JAMA* 2000; 284:2762–2770.

2. Nuckton TJ, List ND: Age as a factor in critical care unit admissions. *Arch Intern Med* 1995; 155(10):1087–1092.

3. Hamel MB et al: Seriously ill hospitalized adults: do we spend less on older patients? *J Am Geriatr Soc* 1996; 44:1043–1048.

4. Nelson JE, Nierman DM. Special Concerns for the Very Old. In: Curtis JR, Rubenfeld GD, editors. Managing Death in the Intensive Care Unit: The Transition from Cure to Comfort. New York: *Oxford University Press*, 2001: 49–367.

5. Lynn J et al: Prognoses of seriously ill hospitalized patients on the days before death: implications for patient care and public policy. *New Horiz* 1997; 5:56–61.

6. Walter LC et al: Development and validation of a prognostic Index for 1-year mortality in older adults after hospitalization. *JAMA* 2001; 285(23):2987–2994.

7. Knaus WA et al: The SUPPORT prognostic model. Objective estimates of survival for seriously ill hospitalized adults. Study to

understand prognoses and preferences for outcomes and risks of treatments. *Ann Inter Med* 1995; 122(3):191–203.

8. Tsevat J et al: Health values of hospitalized patients 80 years and older. *JAMA* 1998; 279:371–375.
9. Tresch DD, Thakur RK: Cardiopulmonary resuscitation in the elderly. *Emergency Medicine Clinics of North America* 1998; 16:649–663.
10. Faber-Langendoen K: Resuscitation of patients with metastatic cancer. *Arch Intern Med* 1991; 151:235–239.
11. Vitelli CE et al: Cardiopulmonary resuscitation and the patient with cancer. *J Clin Oncol* 1991; 9:111–115.
12. Hamel MB et al: Patient age and decisions to withold life-sustaining treatments from seriously ill, hospitalized adults. *Ann Intern Med* 1999; 130:116–125.
13. Ely EW et al: Mechanical ventilation in a cohort of elderly patients admitted to an intensive care unit. *Ann Intern Med* 1999; 131:96–104.
14. Ely EW et al: Mechanical Ventilation in a Cohort of Elderly Patients Admitted to an Intensive Care Unit. *Ann Intern Med* 1999; 131:96–104.
15. Esteban A et al: Indications for, complications from, and outcome of mechanical ventilation: effect of age. *Am J Respir Crit Care Med* 2000; 161(A385).
16. Ely EW et al: Delirium in the intensive care unit: An under-recognized syndrome of organ dysfunction. *Seminars in Respiratory and Critical Care Medicine* 2001; 22:115–126.
17. Inouye SK et al: Delirium: a symptom of how hospital care is failing older persons and a window to improve quality of hospital care. *Am J Med* 1999;(106):565–573.
18. Hopkins RO et al: Neuropsychoogical sequelae and impaired health status in survivors of severe acute respiratory distress syndrome. *Am J Respir Crit Care Med* 1999; 160(1):50–56.
19. Ely EW et al: Delirium in mechanically ventilated patients –validity and reliability of the confusion assessment method for the intensive care unit (CAM-ICU). *JAMA* 2001; 286(21):2703–2710.
20. Schneider AP et al: In-hospital cardiopulmonary resuscitation: A 30-year review. *Journal of the American Board of Family Practice* 1993; 6:91–101.
21. Singer PA et al: Quality end-of-life-care: patients' perspectives. *JAMA* 1999; 281:163–168.
22. Teno J et al: Murphy D, Wenger NS et al. Decision-making and outcomes of prolonged ICU stays in seriously ill patients. *Journal of American Geriatrics Soc* 2000; 48:S70–S74.
23. Fried TR et al: Understanding the Treatment Preferences of Seriously Ill Patients. *NEJM* December 2002; 346(14):1061–1066.
24. Emanuel EJ: Cost saving at the end of life: what do the data show. *JAMA* 1996; 275:1907–1914.
25. Council on Ethical and Judicial Affairs AMA. Medical futility in end-of-life care: report of the council on ethical and judicial affairs. *JAMA* 1999; 281:937–941.
26. Halevy A et al: The low frequency of futility in an adult intensive care unit setting. *Arch Intern Med* 1996; 156:100–104.
27. Prendergast TJ et al: A national survey of end-of-life care for critically ill patients. *Am J Respir Crit Care Med* 1998; 158:1163–1167.
28. Kollef MH et al: The influence of access to a private attending physician on the withdrawal of life-sustaining therapies in the intensive care unit. *Crit Care Med* 1999; 27:2125–2132.

29. Nunn JF et al: Survival of patients ventilated in an intensive therapy unit. *Br Med J* 1979; 1(6177):1525–1527.
30. Campion EW et al: Medical intensive care for the elderly. A study of current use, costs, and outcomes. *JAMA* 1981; 246(18):2052–2056.
31. Fedullo AJ et al: Relationship of patient age to cost and survival in a medical ICU. *Crit Care Med* 1983; 11(3):155–159.
32. Witek TJ et al: Mechanically assisted ventilation in a community hospital:immediate outcome, hospital charges, and follow-up of patients. *Arch Intern Med* 1985; 145:235–239.
33. McLean RF et al: Outcome of respiratory intensive care for the elderly. *Crit Care Med* 1985; 13(8):625–629.
34. Elpern EH et al: Long-term outcomes for elderly survivors of prolonged ventilator assistance. *Chest* 1989; 96(5):1120–1124.
35. Tran DD et al: Age, chronic disease, sepsis, organ system failure, and mortality in a medical intensive care unit. *Crit Care Med* 1990; 18(5):474–479.
36. O'Donnell A et al: Outcome in patients requiring prolonged mechanical ventilation: Three year experience. *Chest* 100[2], 29S. 1991 (Abstr).
37. Pesau B et al: Influence of age on outcome of mechanically ventilated patients in an intensive care unit. *Crit Care Med* 1992; 20(4):489–492.
38. Gracey DR et al: Hospital and posthospital survival in patients mechanically ventilated for more than 29 days. *Chest* 1992; 101:211–214.
39. Chelluri L et al: Outcome of intensive care of the "oldest-old" critically ill patients. *Crit Care Med* 1992; 20(6):757–761.
40. Stauffer JL et al: Survival following mechanical ventilation for acute respiratory failure in adult men. *Chest* 1993; 104:1222–1229.
41. Swinburne AJ et al: Respiratory failure in the elderly. Analysis of outcome after treatment with mechanical ventilation. *Arch Intern Med* 1993; 153(14):1657–1662.
42. Cohen IL et al: Mechanical ventilation for the elderly patient in intensive care. Incremental changes and benefits. *JAMA* 1993; 269(8):1025–1029.
43. Papadakis MA et al: Prognosis of mechanically ventilated patients. *Western Journal of Medicine* 1993; 159(6):659–664.
44. Dardaine V et al: Outcome of elderly patients requiring ventilatory support in intensive care. *Aging* 1995; 7(4):221–227.
45. Cohen IL, Lambrinos J. Investigating the impact of age on outcome of mechanical ventilation using a population of 41,848 patients from a statewide database. *Chest* 1995; 107(6):1673–1680.
46. Steiner T et al: Prognosis of stroke patients requiring mechanical ventilation in a neurological critical care unit. *Stroke* 1997; 28(4):711–715.
47. Kurek CJ et al: Clinical and economic outcome of patients undergoing tracheostomy for prolonged mechanical ventilation in New York state during 1993: analysis of 6,353 cases under diagnosis-related group 483. *Crit Care Med* 1997; 25(6):983–988.
48. Zilberberg MD et al: Acute lung injury in the medical ICU. Comorbid conditions, age, etiology, and hospital outcome. *Am J Respir Crit Care Med* 1998; 157:1159–1164.
49. Kurek CJ et al: Clinical and economic outcome of mechanically ventilated patients in New York state during 1993. *Chest* 1998; 114:214–222.
50. Ely EW et al: Recovery rate and prognosis in older persons who develop acute lung injury and the acute respiratory distress syndrome. *Annals of Internal Medicine* 2002; 136:25–36.

Subacute Care

EDWARD R. MARCANTONIO • MARK YURKOFSKY

A recently aired radio advertisement states, "Nursing Homes: not just for the end of life anymore." While the number of elderly persons residing permanently in nursing homes has remained stable over the past several years, increasing numbers are admitted to nursing homes for short-term stays, usually for rehabilitation or continuing medical management after an acute hospitalization. Indeed, the past 10 years has seen the establishment of a whole new area of medicine, termed subacute care, postacute care, or transitional care, along with units that specialize in this care, both in free-standing skilled nursing facilities, and in hospital-based transitional care units. Subacute care has become an increasingly important component of the continuum of care for elderly persons, and care in this setting is frequently provided by geriatricians and geriatric nurse practitioners. In fact, subacute care has become one of the clinical niches of geriatric medicine.

This chapter discusses the fundamentals of subacute care from the perspective of clinicians actually delivering care in this setting. After defining subacute care and its providers, the chapter follows the timeline of subacute care, beginning at the hospital, to subacute admission, assessment, care planning, medical management, and discharge planning. The chapter also briefly touches upon the financial and medicolegal aspects of providing care in this setting and highlights aspects of medical management and decision making that may be unique in the subacute setting.

DEFINITION OF SUBACUTE CARE

There is some debate about the exact definition of subacute care. In fact, there is a great deal of variation in the settings, patients, and providers encompassed within subacute care. In this chapter, subacute care is defined as the management of discrete episodes of illness requiring medical management and/or functional rehabilitation within the skilled nursing facility. The intensity of the medical management is generally less than that provided on a general medical/surgical unit in an acute care hospital, but greater than what can be provided in the traditional nursing home setting, or at home. The level of functional rehabilitation provided is less intense than in a specialized rehabilitation hospital, but greater than that provided at home. Usually, but not always, subacute care provides a continuation of a treatment plan initiated in the hospital. The frequency of medical encounters, and the costs of care are also intermediate between the hospital and long-term care settings.

A major distinction between acute care and subacute care is a focus on function. This makes it an ideal setting for geriatricians. Acute care in hospitals is focused on diagnosis and targeted aggressive treatment of acute medical problems. Unfortunately, as a result of hospitalization, many elderly persons suffer nosocomial complications and functional decline that persist well after the acute problem is corrected. Innovative models have been developed to reduce the risk of delirium and functional decline in acute care hospitals; nonetheless, these problems remain rampant, particularly in frail individuals with underlying dementia or chronic medical illnesses. Add to this the continuing pressure to shorten length of stay, and many acutely hospitalized elderly persons are unable to return to their residences at discharge. Subacute care has filled the need for a place where these patients can receive ongoing medical and nursing care, in addition to skilled rehabilitation and discharge planning for eventual return to the community. Length of stay in subacute care varies widely, from less than 1 week up to 100 days (the Medicare limit), but the average is generally 1 to 3 weeks.

Subacute care plays a particularly important role in the managed care system for several reasons. First, the cost pressures engendered under managed care require treating patients in the least costly environment that meets their needs. Second, many managed care plans have per diem rates with acute care hospitals, leading to even more intense pressure for discharge than the traditional Medicare DRG (diagnosis-related group) system. Third, managed care plans are exempt from the "3-day" hospital rule (in traditional Medicare, patients must be hospitalized for at least 3 nights to qualify for a skilled nursing benefit), so that these patients can access their skilled nursing facility benefit with a shorter hospital stay, or even be directly admitted from the community (often via the doctor's office or emergency department). For all of these reasons, managed care plans tend to admit sicker patients to skilled nursing facilities (SNFs) for shorter lengths of stay, and managed care providers have been the leaders in developing expertise in subacute care. Foremost has been the establishment of teams of physicians and nurse practitioners who spend most or all of their professional lives delivering subacute care. These teams have developed protocols for facilitating hospital transfers, assessing patients, delivering sophisticated medical care, addressing acute medical problems, minimizing re-hospitalizations, providing case management, and proactive discharge planning. Each of these is discussed in greater detail later in this chapter. In general, fee-for-service systems have not developed as sophisticated programs for providing subacute care, although many of the managed care principles are eminently translatable.

SUBACUTE CARE PATIENTS

Compared to the usual nursing home population, subacute patients tend to be younger (average age in seventies rather than late eighties), more acutely ill, but less likely to have dementia or major chronic functional limitations. Most patients admitted for subacute care come directly from hospitals and are expected to return to their homes after a specific, planned treatment. However, a small but significant proportion of subacute patients (10 to 33 percent) never achieve their discharge goals and "convert" to long-stay nursing home patients. Another significant proportion of patients become medically unstable in the subacute setting and need to be rehospitalized (up to 25%). These figures depend on the acuity of illness and underlying frailty of the population, as well as on the quality of care provided at the facilities. Maximizing return to the community, and minimizing rehospitalizations and long-term care placements are worthy goals of subacute care. Typical subacute diagnoses include hip fracture, other fractures (upper extremity or vertebral), stroke, cardiac and pulmonary conditions, postoperative care, pressure and vascular ulcers, and pneumonia. Subacute patients may need intensive medical management, functional rehabilitation, or a combination of both.

SUBACUTE CARE PHYSICIANS

Delivering effective care to the subacute population requires a much greater physician presence than traditional long-term care. *SNFist* and *subacutist* are novel terms occasionally used to describe clinicians practicing primarily in this environment. Practicing as a long-term care and subacute care clinician requires a special set of skills. Physicians working in SNFs and subacute units are usually geriatricians or other clinicians with strong geriatric skills such as internists, osteopathic physicians, and family practitioners.

A number of clinical, administrative, and interpersonal skills are important for a physician to achieve success in the area of subacute care. To properly manage this challenging patient population, the nursing facility clinician must have *clinical expertise* in managing conditions that are a blend of office, hospital, and geriatric practice (see Table 16-1).

Administrative skills are also important for the subacute care practitioner. Nursing facilities have a relatively simple administrative structure. The administrator and director of nursing are the primary salaried personnel that run the facility. There is a facility medical director as well. Attending

Table 16-1   Areas of Clinical Expertise in Subacute Care

Geriatric syndromes including delirium, dementia, and urinary incontinence

Postoperative orthopedic and surgical patients

Skin breakdown issues

Pain and symptom control in the dying patient

Non-ICU hospital conditions such as congestive heart failure and infections

Medication administration and dosing in an elderly population

Wound care

Geriatric rehabilitation

physicians have the opportunity to work closely with these three individuals in a facility. Attending physicians, even if they are not the medical director, can make significant contributions to the quality of care of subacute patients (Table 16-2).

Interpersonal skills are the third key area for subacute care practitioners. The ability to form trusting collaborative relationships with patients and families quickly, is critical to effective care in nursing facilities. Patients currently entering nursing facilities are often critically ill, are more dependent than previously, fear loss of independence, have caregivers under great stress, and often have financial and housing pressures. They are often suspicious of nursing facilities and may not understand all of the medical issues. Table 16-3 summarizes the interpersonal skills needed in a subacute care provider.

ROLE OF ADVANCED PRACTICE CLINICIANS

Daily rounding by a clinician with round-the-clock phone availability is essential to providing effective subacute care. To provide this enhanced clinical coverage, physicians may collaborate with advanced practice clinicians (APCs) such

Table 16-2   Areas of Administrative Expertise in Subacute Care

Improving care transitions from hospital to subacute facility

Improving facility systems regarding ancillary supports (especially lab, x-ray, and pharmacy), training staff, documentation, and communication

Knowledge regarding OBRA regulations

Working effectively within the constraints of the reimbursement system for nursing facilities under Medicare and managed care

OBRA, Omnibus Budget Reconciliation Act of 1987.

Table 16-3   Interpersonal Skills Needed to Provide Effective Subacute Care

Understand and appreciate the nursing home culture

Be a skilled leader of the interdisciplinary team

Work well with families regarding discharge planning and end-of-life care

Teach staff within the facility

Interface effectively with hospital and outpatient clinicians

Be a good listener and a good communicator

Table 16-5   Key Aspects of the OBRA Regulations

The medical regimen must be comprehensive and part of an interdisciplinary care plan

A decline in the resident's physical, mental, and psychosocial well-being must be demonstrably unavoidable

Restraint use requires rigorous individual clinical assessment

The resident's drug regimen must be justifiable

OBRA, Omnibus Budget Reconciliation Act of 1987.

as nurse practitioners and physician's assistants. APCs play a major role in providing care in many subacute units. States and facilities vary regarding the scope of practice for APCs. In some locales, nurse practitioners practice as independent clinicians, while in others, direct physician supervision is required. Many facilities require written guidelines that describe the scope of practice of the APC as well as the manner by which physician supervision will be provided.

The physician working in a subacute care setting may find tremendous benefit from working with an APC. Many APCs have specialized areas of expertise that complement the skills and knowledge of the physician. Table 16-4 lists the roles and duties an APC can assume in a subacute unit.

A physician practicing with an APC has the opportunity to form a team that can improve the quality of care provided and can improve job satisfaction for both providers. As in other teams, excellent communication, trust, availability and support are essential.

The model of physician–APC collaboration in the subacute setting has many similarities to an inpatient hospital model. The APC may operate much like a first-year resident, managing day-to-day issues, identifying new issues, and requesting support from the physician when needed. By rounding together on a regular basis the MD–APC care team have the opportunity to assess patients together. Patients can be reassured seeing their care team together. There is no substitute for a bedside evaluation in assessing issues such as pain control, cognitive status, anxiety, and medical stability. APCs are able to participate in night and weekend on-call duties. It is essential that if an APC is

Table 16-4   Roles of Advanced Practice Clinicians in Subacute Care

Specialized areas of expertise including management of dementia, pressure ulcers, gynecology issues, congestive heart failure

Patient/family education regarding diabetes, home safety, medication administration, medication simplification

Training facility staff

Working out problems with nurses, nurses' aides, patient, and family

taking "first call" that there always be a physician available for consultative support.

It is preferable to have a model of on-call coverage that uses clinicians who not only know the patient but also the capabilities of the facility. When it is not possible to have a clinician who is a direct caregiver providing on-call coverage, effective signouts are important. Key clinical information can be transmitted by direct verbal communication or by written summaries that can be faxed or e-mailed to the covering clinician.

SUBACUTE CARE REGULATIONS

Subacute care units are licensed and regulated under the same regulations as nursing homes. In 1987, a set of regulations regarding patient care in nursing facilities was enacted in the Omnibus Budget Reconciliation Act (OBRA). These regulations laid out a number of principles that were used to standardize care in nursing facilities. In 1995 the nursing home certification and enforcement regulations took effect. Unless nursing facilities were found to comply with the standards laid out in OBRA, they would not be allowed to participate in the Medicare and Medicaid programs. Table 16-5 summarizes key aspects of the OBRA regulations. These principles provide a framework for providing appropriate clinical care. Physicians must work collaboratively with nursing facility staff to maintain compliance with OBRA regulations. It is particularly challenging managing a high turnover, higher acuity population under these regulations. Excellent assessment skills, complete and accurate documentation, and a well-functioning interdisciplinary team are necessary to meet regulatory requirements, and are also the cornerstone of good subacute care.

DEFINING QUALITY IN SUBACUTE CARE

Quality in subacute care goes beyond traditional medical process and outcome measures emphasized in hospitals. Perhaps most important is the quality and availability of the nursing staff. Because of the stress of managing high acuity patients in the nursing home setting, many subacute facilities are chronically understaffed, or experience high staff turnover, especially of licensed nurses and nursing aides. Significant use of "agency" personnel, with little knowledge of the facility or its patients, can have a major negative impact on quality. Additional issues that are of great importance in the subacute setting include the quality of the rehabilitation and palliative care services. Subacute facilities are also judged on their hotel services in addition to their medical services. Good food, pleasant ambiance, television, and clean rooms are all part of the reasonable expectations of patients and their families. Subjective measures, such as patient and family satisfaction, and the facility's reputation in the community, can be good overall measures of quality.

ADMITTING A SUBACUTE PATIENT: THE HOSPITAL PERSPECTIVE

The vast majority of subacute patients are transferred from acute care hospitals. The providers at the hospitals have a critical role in ensuring the success of the subacute stay. Often, hospital providers operate with little knowledge of the facilities to which they are sending their patients. A brief communication between the hospital and subacute clinicians can help to answer questions about appropriateness, timing of transfer, specific treatments, and overall goals of care. Unfortunately, this type of communication is more the exception than the rule. In general, if the acute care hospital providers have any questions or concerns about transfer of a patient, it is best to ask before acting.

The first question to be asked is who should be sent to subacute care, and who should not? Subacute facilities vary widely in terms of their capabilities, so there is no general answer. Hospital physicians often make the naïve assumption that the nurses "screening" patients for facilities have intimate knowledge of them and can make appropriate referrals. Often, these screeners work for large corporations that may have several facilities in a large urban area. The screeners focus more on "filling beds," and leave it up to the clinicians to determine appropriateness.

A few rules of thumb hold: in general, a patient requiring the ICU is *not* appropriate for subacute care. The rare exception is a stable ventilated patient who is being transferred from an ICU to a specialized pulmonary subacute facility. In addition to ICU care, few subacute facilities have sophisticated cardiac monitoring, so patients with active cardiac issues such as unstable angina, poorly controlled congestive heart failure, or arrhythmias requiring continuous monitoring are rarely good candidates for subacute care.

Nursing care in subacute facilities is much less intensive than in acute care hospitals. While hospitals rarely have more than 7 patients per nurse, subacute units may have 20 or more patients per nurse—in an 8-hour shift, that averages 20 minutes per patient. Therefore, a patient with hemodynamic instability, one receiving active intravenous cancer chemotherapy, or other situations requiring close nursing monitoring, may be poor candidates for subacute care. In general, patients with a relatively straightforward treatment plan for acute illness that has shown evidence of improvement, combined with established treatment of chronic illnesses and functional rehabilitation needs, are the most ideal for this setting.

On the opposite end of the spectrum is a patient who will likely be able to go home within a few days. For these patients, an additional facility transfer is probably not worthwhile or necessary, and runs the risk of introducing further discontinuity. In general, subacute stays substantially shorter than 1 week should be avoided, if possible, in favor of direct discharge to home.

Another issue is selecting the best facility for the patient. This is a complex issue that involves both clinical and psychosocial factors. Screeners and hospital case managers may be more focused on getting a bed quickly rather than finding the best facility for the patient. Facilities vary widely in their capabilities, and some have specialized programs in specific areas, such as orthopedics and stroke care. In general, knowledge of a proven track record of success handling a particular kind of patient is the best proof of the wisdom of transfer. In addition to these clinical issues, patients and family members may prefer a facility close to home, which can facilitate family visits and the like. These preferences should be honored if all else is equal. However, it should be explained to patients and family members that because only a short-term stay is anticipated, established medical care linkages and proven clinical excellence should outweigh geographic convenience to ensure the best possible outcome.

The optimal time for transfer can be defined as the point when the patient's needs can be met as well or better at the subacute facility as in the hospital. In practice, this is often hard to define, and discharge is often dictated by bed availability or "critical pathways" that predetermine length of stay. Ultimately, it is the physician's responsibility to determine whether the patient is clinically ready for transfer, and for ensuring adequate transfer of information with the patient to ensure continued implementation of the plan of care. It is better to keep the patient for an extra day in the hospital than to risk a rapid readmission for medical instability or poorly coordinated transfer.

When the time for transfer comes, it is crucial that the appropriate information accompany the patient. Table 16-6 describes the key information required by the SNF. In addition, the physicians at the hospital should review the discharge summary and other key transfer documents to ensure that there are no discrepancies—if so, these should be remedied.

Developing better systems whereby receiving facilities and sending hospitals coordinate the transitions of care is crucial to improving patient care and optimizing outcomes. One approach can be achieved through sharing information via computer systems. Clearly, this is easiest for onsite transitional care units. However, even free-standing subacute facilities can have dial-up or hard-wired computer links with sending hospitals. Only certain members of the subacute staff (particularly the physicians, who may also be on staff at the sending hospital) receive access to key elements of the patient's record, as well as the ability to e-mail hospital providers.

Understanding the limitations of subacute care facilities can help hospital providers better manage the transfer of care. First, consider the timing of transfer. Unfortunately, most patients arrive for admission to SNFs between 4 and 7 P.M. However, staffing at most SNFs is best on the day

Table 16-6 Key Data Needed for Transfer to a Subacute Unit

A list of clinical problems

Complete medication list matched with the clinical diagnosis

Summary of hospital course

Code status/advanced directives

Name of health care proxy/guardian

Wound-care instructions

Weight-bearing instructions

Recent significant laboratory test results

Key health care providers involved in care and how to contact them

Diet including consistency of food/liquids if swallowing is impaired

If on tube feeding, type of tube, rate/time of feeding, amount/time of water flushes

Recent focused physical exam findings

Goals for the subacute stay

Pending tests and how to follow up

Follow-up appointments

Clear anticoagulation orders with recent PT/INR results, INR goals

Indications for urinary catheter if present and when it can be removed

Last bowel movement

Family contacts with accurate names, phone numbers, and addresses

Type of intravenous access

INR, international normalized ratio; PT, prothrombin time.

(7 to 3) shift. Therefore, hospitals should attempt to transfer the patient as early as possible during the day, preferably before noon. Before sending the patient, hospital providers should ensure that all patient needs are met for the next several hours. Second, consider that most SNFs do not have onsite pharmacies and that it may take several hours for ordered medications to be delivered to the patient. Therefore, all medications, particularly pain medications that the patient will need over the next 4 to 6 hours, should be administered prior to transfer. Finally, SNFs may have difficulty inserting and maintaining intravenous access. Therefore, stable access should be ensured prior to transfer. If the patient will need more than 1 to 2 days of treatment, a more permanent "long-line" catheter is advisable.

One special case deserves mention: direct admissions from the community to subacute care. Because of Medicare's "3-day rule," direct admissions come only in managed care patients (who are exempt from this rule), or patients who have had a 3-day hospital admission in the previous 30 days. Direct admissions should be medically stable and should not require immediate diagnostic or therapeutic intervention. In these cases, it is crucial that appropriate information, including reason for admission, medical history, physical examination, medications, treatments, allergies, and the like, be transmitted from the emergency room or doctor's office. A direct dialog between the sending and receiving physician is often required. Only systems that can care for very high acuity subacute patients should consider direct admission.

ADMITTING A SUBACUTE PATIENT: THE FACILITY PERSPECTIVE

Those who work in a subacute environment need to understand the crucial role played by the first 24 hours postadmission. From a clinical outcome, patient satisfaction, and a risk-management perspective, the first day and night in the facility is key. Case 1 illustrates some of the perils of the hospital–subacute transfer.

Case 1: Transition of Care Issues in the First 24 hours

An 85-year-old male retired professor is admitted with a hip fracture, hypertension, and diabetes. Here are some common issues that arise that can impact outcomes in a subacute setting:

1. Family communication: The patient's daughter does not know if and when her father is going to the subacute facility and does not know how to get to the subacute facility.
2. Timing of admission: The patient is scheduled for a 2 P.M. arrival, but arrives at 6 P.M. because the hospital nurse had another sick patient and did not get the paperwork done. The patient left the hospital before dinner was served and arrived at the subacute facility after dinner was over.
3. Avoidable complications: His blood glucose was 40 mg/dL and he was lethargic by the time his dinner arrived.
4. Missing information:
   The weight-bearing status is not given on the hospital referral.
   The page 1 referral had a "titrate Coumadin to INR of 2.0" order but no dose and no INRs.
   The discharge summary did not arrive with the patient. The hospital was not aware that the patient took glaucoma drops and therefore these medications were not noted on the referral form.
5. Facility issues:
   Physical therapy had left by the time the patient arrived and nursing was not comfortable transferring the patient out of bed to the toilet.

Diapers were placed on the patient.

The room smelled because the patient was incontinent. Pain medicine was ordered but was not delivered until the next morning.

The daughter arrives, sees her father in diapers, in pain, more confused, and the nurses unsure about his medications, and wants to send the patient back to the hospital and says she is going to write a complaint letter to the Department of Public Health.

The issues that arise in Case 1 are not unusual. Patients arrive unexpectedly, and the information transmitted is inadequate and sometimes contradictory. Interagency referral forms may be done at different times than discharge summaries and can contain conflicting information.

Nursing home clinicians often manage new SNF admissions telephonically for the first 24 hours. Accurate, complete nursing assessments are important to the SNF clinician who is attempting to manage a patient he or she has never met over the phone. Nurses who work on subacute units need to work effectively with their offsite physician colleagues. An important aspect of this collaboration is judgment when to page the physician/APC and what information to have available. Nurses need to perform an appropriate assessment of the patient based on the clinical situation. In addition, it is important to have information on medications being given, as well as recent laboratory results.

A comprehensive history and physical examination is required within 72 hours of subacute admission. It is best practice if this can be performed within the first 24 hours. In addition to understanding the medical problems identified at the hospital, key issues for the subacute clinician to consider when admitting a new patient include understanding the goals for the SNF stay, making sure medications are appropriately dosed, and assessing pain, bowels, and cognition.

In addition to the history and physical by the physician–APC team, the newly admitted subacute patient must have a number of assessments performed by many disciplines. The physician or APC, as leader of the interdisciplinary team needs to be aware of key findings from these team members and integrate them into the initial treatment plan. Table 16-7 provides examples of the assessments that need to be done and the disciplines that do them.

In addition to the medical issues identified by the hospital, patients may arrive with unidentified issues, such as skin breakdown, constipation, pain, fall risk, urinary retention, and delirium, that may require immediate attention. The subacute clinician has to organize this information and prioritize issues that need immediate attention.

Nursing facilities do not have onsite pharmacies. Delivery of medications can take several hours. To help with this issue, facilities have drug "emergency boxes" that contain dozens of frequently used medications including intravenous antibiotics and a small selection of opioids. Familiarity with the contents of these boxes is important for the subacute care provider to practice effectively. At times, short-term substitutions must be made until the exact medication can be delivered. In addition, like hospitals, facilities have formularies. Medications may need to be changed to meet formulary requirements.

Table 16-7 Initial Assessment of the New Patients by Subacute Staff

Rehabilitation team	Screens by physical, occupational, therapy, and speech
Nursing	Skin, cognition, fall risk, pain, bowel/bladder, medication review
Dietary	Nutritional needs/diet
Kitchen	Food preferences
Social service	Psychosocial evaluation, end-of-life preferences
Case management	Discharge planning including equipment and home care
Administration	Valuables assessment

PATIENT/FAMILY/STAFF INTERACTIONS

In addition to being astute and thorough when assessing a new patient, the subacute clinician must be skilled at establishing trusting relationships with the patient and key family members as soon as possible after admission. Any time a patient changes setting and new caregivers assume care, there are opportunities and dangers. We have already identified that there may be inaccuracy, omissions, and ambiguity in transfer information. The initial hours after admission are an important window period in which the receiving clinicians can form a strong collaborative relationship with the patient and family.

Family members provide important clinical and functional information that may otherwise be unavailable. Speaking with family members may help to identify areas of concern related to past care and can point special issues on which to focus immediately on admission. The physician can establish him or herself as a patient advocate and a problem solver. By establishing an early, strong family connection, the subacute clinician is better able to identify and ultimately meet the goals of care, and overcome barriers to discharge.

PHYSICIAN'S ROLE IN REHABILITATION

In the subacute setting, an interdisciplinary team meeting plays a crucial role in formulating and assessing the plan of care. At the team meeting, key issues of function, medical condition, cognition, mood, and interactions between family, patient, and staff can be shared. The interdisciplinary team needs to gather and communicate information regarding medical condition, treatment and prognosis, rehabilitation potential and level of function, psychosocial needs, financial options, and family/patient teaching needs. Most internists, primary care physicians, family practitioners, and general practitioners do not receive formal training in rehabilitation. Many physicians working in nursing facilities do not take an active role in assessing the patient's rehabilitation needs, goals, and progress. It is clear that there is a vital role that a physician can play in this regard that benefits the facility and the patients, as well as the patients' families.

The physician understands the pathophysiology of disease processes better than any other member of the interdisciplinary care team. Therefore, the physician has a critical role to play in leading the team in identifying realistic functional goals for patients, understanding and explaining the impact of intercurrent medical illnesses on patient function, and communicating with patients, staff, and families regarding realistic goals and expected level of function. The physician does not need to know how best to identify weakness in a particular muscle group and what exercises to do to strengthen it, nor what the best assistive device will be for a patient. However, the physician does need to understand whether the goals of treatment outlined by the therapy team are realistic.

How to get the patient walking again is often the major challenge to face nursing facility staff. Generally, physical and occupational therapists are able to provide 1 to 3 hours of therapy per day in the subacute setting. It is essential that other members of the care team provide an environment that encourages patients to get out of bed and ambulate when the therapists are not working with the patient. Nurses and aides need to be taught by the therapists how best to transfer the patient, to observe any weight-bearing precautions, and to learn which assistive devices need to be used. Often schedules need to be set up to get the patient out of bed. The physician needs to oversee the care being provided. Identifying what is not working well and brainstorming with other members of the care team to identify solutions is an important role for the physician. There are a number of roles that the physician may be required to fill in the interdisciplinary team (see Table 16-8).

Clear communication between all members of the interdisciplinary team is essential. The physician, nurse practitioner, and physician assistant play an important goal in helping set realistic goals and making sure that each member of the care team is providing care that is geared towards achieving those goals. They also play a key role in communicating with family members.

Case 2 outlines the key role of physicians in communicating between providers and altering the plan of care to optimize patient outcomes.

Case 2: Importance of Communication in Subacute Care

A 78-year-old female with a left hip fracture repair and a history of mild dementia presents to the nursing facility for rehabilitation. The patient arrives with a non–weight-bearing status on her left leg. The physician sees the patient and finds she has poor memory and impaired judgment. She lives with her frail but independent husband in a home with eight stairs separating the bedroom and kitchen. The physician orders occupational and physical therapy evaluations.

On day 2 of the admission, the physician realizes that the patient's functional and cognitive deficits will likely prevent her from keeping weight off the operated leg. Furthermore, it is clear that very few 78-year-olds can ambulate safely on

Table 16-8 Physician's Roles in the Interdisciplinary Team

Provide medical expertise on prognosis

Determine realistic, achievable functional goals

Determine whether medical improvement is likely, resulting in improved function, or whether medical status has plateaued or will deteriorate with stable or reduced function

Adjust treatment based on input from team members (pain/bowel/anxiety, etc.)

Gather input from specialists and share with team members

Participate in brainstorming to identify solutions

Guide discussions around ethical issues

Determine when skilled care is not beneficial or needed

Facilitate family communication

Determine when discharge to another setting is appropriate

Provide constructive feedback

Assess/improve teamwork between rehabilitation/nurses/ nurses aides

one leg using a walker or crutches. In such situations, the end result is often that until the weight-bearing restriction is removed, which often takes 1 to 2 months, the patient will not be able to ambulate and will require a prolonged nursing home stay. This places the patient at high risk for needing permanent long-term care. The physician calls the operating surgeon and explains the dilemma. Upon further reflection, the surgeon states that the fracture was minimally displaced, the alignment was good, the repair was reasonably strong and the patient is only 105 pounds and advances her to a weight-bearing as tolerated status. The treatment plan for this patient has now changed dramatically. Achieving independence with transfers now becomes a realistic possibility. She may be able to negotiate stairs. The plan is now for a 1- to 2-week stay with discharge to a home setting with community supports and the family paying for extra assistance.

Patients with advanced dementia may have great difficulty learning new strategies or compensatory techniques. The physician plays a vital role in identifying patients who can benefit from therapy. In addition to dementia, patients with delirium, depression, pain, or other medical illnesses may have difficulty participating in and benefiting from a rehabilitation program. The physician must identify and treat the depression, pain, or congestive heart failure that is limiting participation in and benefit from the rehabilitation program.

It is often appropriate and necessary to teach nursing facility staff such as nurses' aides how best to feed, transfer, and ambulate patients. The goal is to provide for the patient's safety while maximizing their autonomy. There is a tension at times between getting things done quickly by helping the patient and having the same task be done more slowly but with the patient doing all the work. The patient may take 20 minutes to get dressed, needing periodic verbal cues from the nurses' aide during the process. If the nurses' aide did more of the work the job might be done in 10 minutes. The patient may even prefer to have the aide do more of the work. However, a cornerstone of care for the elderly patient is to encourage as much independence as possible.

PHYSICIAN'S ROLE IN FAMILY MEETINGS

Family meetings are an invaluable means of sharing information, reviewing goals, making decisions, and identifying action steps. Family meetings should generally take place after there has been an interdisciplinary team meeting without the family present. Complex information needs to be presented in an organized manner that allows time for questions, discussion, and identifying action steps. Ideally, all this needs to be done in less than 45 minutes, so that staff can resume other duties and patients and family members are not overwhelmed. Family meetings can include the patient, key family members, the physician/nurse practitioner/physician's assistant; case manager; social service; the rehabilitation team, including physical, occupational, and speech therapy; nursing; and even aides. Formulating an agenda and goals for the meeting ahead of time helps identify who needs to be present. Table 16-9 summarizes common goals for family meetings.

It is important that a staff member such as the physician, case manager, or social worker run the meeting. It is often very helpful for the senior clinician to provide a brief update regarding the medical issues and prognosis.

Knowing what different team members are going to recommend is essential for family meetings to go well. Major differences in the treatment plan between team members should be addressed before the family meeting. For example, the therapist may find the confused patient with a resolving pneumonia is not participating in rehabilitation.

However, the physician may be able to explain that the confusion is likely related to a delirium and may improve quickly as the pneumonia responds to antibiotics. Without the physician present to provide this input, the facility caregivers and family members may not have an accurate picture regarding disease progression, clinical improvement, and overall prognosis. Providing a clear, realistic picture of function and medical prognosis is also a critical part of the discharge planning process.

Several conditions are especially common among subacute patients. Key aspects of these conditions relevant to subacute care are discussed below. Other chapters in this text discuss these conditions in more detail.

MEDICAL MANAGEMENT IN THE SUBACUTE SETTING

Pain Management

It is well recognized that pain, especially in the elderly person, is often unrecognized and undertreated. Effective pain relief is an essential aspect of subacute care. Table 16-10 outlines some of the negative consequences of untreated pain.

Recognizing and relieving pain are critical skills for the subacute clinician. It is beyond the scope of this chapter to review the broad area of pain relief. However, opioid use in the subacute setting merits special mention.

Opioids play an important role in pain control. Whether for postoperative pain or end-stage cancer, a sound knowledge of principles of pain control and an understanding of nursing facility regulations regarding opioid use is essential. Opioids can be delivered in several different forms. Familiarity with the different routes of administration for opioids is an important aspect of providing pain management. Table 16-11 summarizes routes of administration.

Patients arriving from hospitals may have orders written for intravenous "push" narcotics. Nurses in nursing facilities do not generally give narcotics, or other

Table 16-9   Goals of Family Meetings

Information gathering regarding:
Previous function
Caregiver supports
Financial resources
Home environment
Goals of care
Decision making regarding:
End-of-life care
Rehabilitation goals that need to be attained
Discharge site, e.g., home, long-term care, assisted living
Setting a discharge date
Resolving areas of conflict:
Between family members
Between family and patient
Regarding facility services

Table 16-10   Impact of Pain in Subacute Patients

Decreased mobility
Incontinence
Constipation/impaction
Pressure ulcers
Delirium
Depression
Anxiety
Malnutrition
Pneumonia
Increased risk of needing long-term care
Family stress

Table 16-11 Routes of Opioid Administration

Oral tablets in both short- and long-acting form

Oral liquids

Sublingual liquids in concentrate form

Rectal suppositories

Transdermal patches

Subcutaneous injections

Subcutaneous infusions

Table 16-12 Key Issues Regarding Opioid Use in Subacute Care

Be specific regarding dosing/frequency when ordering opioids

Know the contents of the facility's "emergency box"

Prompt faxing/phoning reduces delays in getting opioids

Order a bowel program with opioids

Evaluate whether a sustained release product is needed with prn "rescue" doses

For new admissions, consider developing a system where it is known what the medications (including opioids) will be before the patients arrives and *preorder* them so there will not be delays

medications, in this manner. The clinician in the nursing facility needs to reorder these medications in a form that is appropriate for the facility.

The regulatory issues in nursing facilities can, at times, complicate and impair the provision of good pain control. Unlike the hospital setting, nursing facilities regulations require a prescription for each opioid order. The physician must either fax a prescription to the pharmacy or call the pharmacy to obtain an emergency 72-hour supply of the medication. In nursing facilities, exact doses and parameters for "as needed" indications are required, for instance: Percocet (5/325 mg) 1 tablet orally q4h prn for moderate hip pain (4 to 7 on pain scale) and 2 tablets orally q4h prn for severe hip pain (8 to 10 on pain scale).

Many patients, such as the one in this example, may experience a roller coaster effect when given prn doses of short acting pain medications. The result is many hours of discomfort with just a few hours of pain relief. Familiarity with and use of sustained-release oral opioids is an essential aspect to being able to provide successful pain control in the nursing facility. It should also be noted that most extended release medications should not be crushed. If the patient is not able to swallow the tablet, then an alternate dosing route needs to be considered, such as a transdermal patch.

Finally, a standing bowel program needs to be ordered along with the opioids. Orders for "milk of magnesia prn" or Colace are inadequate for most patients on opioids. Table 16-12 summarizes key points regarding opioid use in subacute care.

Urinary Incontinence and Catheters

Many patients arriving at subacute facilities have indwelling catheters or were incontinent at the hospital. Urinary catheters are most commonly used to monitor urine output when patients are first admitted to the hospital. Most patients arriving with catheters from the hospital can have them removed immediately. From both an infection control and a nursing home regulatory perspective, urinary catheters should be used in very limited situations. The two main ones are in the setting of urinary retention when intermittent catheterization is not practical and in the case of severe skin wounds when healing would be impaired by urine from an incontinent patient. Before committing a patient to permanent catheterization for urinary retention it is important to determine whether there is a

reversible cause for the retention, such as stool impaction or a medication side effect. Anticholinergic medications are particularly likely to inhibit proper bladder emptying.

The hospitalized patient with new incontinence often has an etiology that can be diagnosed and treated in the nursing facility, without sophisticated studies. It is important to determine the prehospitalization continence status and the etiology for the incontinence. Infections, medications (diuretics), delirium, immobility, fecal impaction, urinary retention, and deconditioning are common causes of incontinence that are readily treated. Nurses' aides, nurses, and therapists are very important to the clinician as a source of information regarding continence. An interdisciplinary meeting is an excellent way in which to obtain information on continence and to develop a plan to manage it. Table 16-13 summarizes some ways of rapidly assessing and managing incontinence in the nursing facility.

There are effective medications for urge incontinence. These medications come in long-acting forms and, unlike their predecessors, have much less in the way of anticholinergic side effects. The subacute setting can be used to monitor patients for urinary retention related to these medications.

Swallowing Issues

An appropriate diet and feeding plan can be crucial in the subacute setting. Hospitals may not always supply detailed information on food and beverage consistencies for patients at the time of admission to the nursing facility. Patients with strokes, impaired cognition, and other neuromuscular disorders require special types of diets because of dysphagia. The subacute clinician should be familiar with these diets. Solid foods can be ground or pureed to facilitate swallowing. Liquids can be thickened to nectar or honey thick consistencies to reduce aspiration risk. Contacting the sending hospital prior to feeding the patient may be necessary to determine the proper diet in a dysphagia patient.

Speech therapists are important members of the rehabilitation team in nursing facilities. Speech therapists have a dual role. They work on communication techniques and strategies and also screen for and evaluate swallowing

Table 16-13   Assessing and Managing Incontinence

Treat a diaper as a red flag: ask why it is on and if not needed make sure it stays off

Do a rectal exam: stool impaction is commonly overlooked and is very treatable

Consider a bedside commode if the patient is slow transferring and ambulating

Make sure there is not a problem with delays answering call lights; if there are delays, involve the director of nursing in formulating a solution

Avoid anticholinergics, especially in men, as they may cause urinary retention or confusion

Get a good history from the patient/family regarding prehospitalization continence

Consider obtaining a postvoid residual volume to rule out urinary retention

Review medications and lab work for causes of incontinence

difficulties. Speech therapists can assess whether food consistencies are appropriate and whether other interventions are needed such as elevation of the head of the bed, tucking the chin, or turning the head with swallowing.

Swallowing difficulties can develop in the setting of an acute or a chronic illness. Delirium and dementia contribute to swallowing problems, especially if an acute medical illness develops. Stroke, neuromuscular illnesses, anatomical abnormalities, and infections also may cause dysphagia. Coupled with swallowing problems is the fact that elderly patients entering nursing facilities often have poor dentition, ill-fitting dentures, or have lost their dentures.

The role of the speech therapist in reducing aspiration risk includes items listed in Table 16-14. Table 16-15

Table 16-14   Speech Therapist's Role in Aspiration Management

Screening new admissions for swallowing difficulties

Assessing swallowing capabilities

Recommending food and liquid consistency

Teaching the patient compensatory swallowing strategies, e.g., chin tuck

Deciding whether further diagnostic studies are needed, e.g., modified barium swallow

Training facility staff and family members proper techniques

Table 16-15   Physician's Role in Aspiration Management

Order appropriate food and fluid consistencies

Order aspiration precautions when appropriate

Coordinate the interdisciplinary team to ensure that the proper diet is provided at all times

Assess whether a feeding tube might be indicated

Identify reversible medical causes of dysphagia

summarizes the physician's role in helping to manage the patient with swallowing difficulties.

Falls

A significant challenge in managing patients in nursing facilities is the tension between safety and autonomy. Many patients in nursing facilities have cognitive impairment as well as a functional deficit that hinders transfers or ambulation. The physician plays a vital role in working with facility staff in identifying risk factors for falls and reducing those risks. Table 16-16 identifies some of the common causes of falls in a subacute setting.

If a patient does fall, a review of the above issues needs to be undertaken to determine why the fall occurred and to take corrective measures. The use of restraints, whether physical or chemical, to prevent activities or behaviors that increase the risk of falls needs to be carefully scrutinized. Physical restraints may result in injury or even death if improperly used or monitored. Chemical restraints have significant morbidity associated with them as well. Finding ways to manage problematic behaviors to decrease the risk of falls or to keep patients safer is challenging (Table 16-17).

The attending physician or facility medical director may be asked to review cases prior to admission where restraints

Table 16-16   Causes of Falls in Subacute Settings

Medication-related postural hypotension

Medication-related confusion

Pain

Poorly fitting footwear

Inadequate lighting

Delays in answering call lights

Incontinence causing a slip and fall

Lack of familiarity with environment

Environmental hazards such as oxygen tubing, bedside trays that roll when leaned on

New stroke or fracture causing weakness in a limb(s)

Subacute physicians and APCs are instrumental in helping nursing facilities succeed under PPS and managed care. The clinical expertise provided by these practitioners enables facilities to better evaluate the scope and severity of clinical conditions for each patient. Having enhanced clinical presence in the nursing facility can identify new illnesses sooner, thereby implementing less-costly interventions and avoiding complications. For example, identifying and treating pneumonia before the patient becomes delirious, dehydrated, and septic is certainly better for the patient and can lead to a reduced need for intravenous therapies, emergency room visits, and ambulance services. The result is a better financial outcome for the facility, as well as a better clinical outcome for the patient.

REIMBURSEMENT FOR PHYSICIANS

A nursing home practice has some distinct advantages over an office practice. For instance, a nursing home practice can have less overhead costs. A physician who only practices in skilled nursing facilities does not have to pay rent on a large office with multiple exam rooms, needs less nursing and administrative staff, and does not have to pay for as much equipment and other office supplies.

Physician billing in nursing facilities is currently based on eight codes organized into three categories. The first two categories are codes related to discharges and follow-up visits. The third category relates to the performance of a full history and physical on admission, for a yearly physical, or when a significant change in resident status takes place. All eight codes require face-to-face, hands-on patient contact. For any of the codes, a progress note must be written documenting the evaluation that was performed and the care provided, and reflect the complexity of the medical decision-making that took place. The billing code selected must be based on the documentation in the progress note. Nurse practitioners and physician's assistants can bill Medicare for the care they provide in nursing facilities. At present, the Medicare fee schedule is 85 percent of the physician payment for the same level of service code. Individual states and insurance carriers may not view coding similarly. It is suggested that physicians learn about coding guidelines in their specific geographic regions. The American Medical Directors Association is an excellent resource for obtaining up to date billing information (www.amda.com).

SUBACUTE CARE AS A SAFETY NET

Subacute care is becoming an increasingly important setting to provide medical and rehabilitative services, as well as end-of-life and palliative care. The interdisciplinary approach upon which subacute care is based should benefit patients and society from both quality of care and cost perspectives. Because of hospital pressures to discharge increasingly complex patients who are just getting over a critical illness, have just been started on new medications, and have symptoms that are continuing to evolve, the subacute site serves as a safety net in the continuum of care for older persons. A large cadre of physicians and APCs are needed who are able to practice effectively in this setting.

REFERENCES

Burl JB et al: Geriatric nurse practitioners in long-term care: Demonstration of effectiveness in managed care. *J Am Geriatr Soc* 46:506, 1998.

Burl JB, Campbell I: Impact of a paradigm change in the management of HMO patients admitted for subacute care. *Ann Long-term Care* 12:426, 1997.

Buxbaum R, Yurkofsky M: Wernicke's encephalopathy: The subacute setting as safety net. *Ann Long-term Care* 9:71, 2001.

Creditor MC: Hazards of hospitalization of the elderly. *Ann Intern Med* 118:219, 1993.

Friedman M et al: Post-acute and ongoing assessment of elders: Where to begin? In: Faulkner and Grey's Healthcare Information Center, New York, NY, *2000 Post-Acute Outcomes Sourcebook.*

Hutt E et al: Precipitants of emergency room visits and acute hospitalization in short-stay medicare nursing home residents. *J Am Geriatr Soc* 50:223, 2002.

Levenson S: Subacute care: Why nursing home practitioners should take notice. *Ann Long-term Care* 3:23, 1994.

Levenson S: The new OBRA enforcement rule: Implications for attending physicians and medical directors. *Ann Long-term Care* 9:214, 1995.

Marcantonio ER et al: Delirium symptoms in post-acute care: Prevalent, persistent, and associated with poor functional recovery. *J Am Geriatr Soc* 51:4–9, 2003.

Murley J: The role of the nurse practitioner in quality improvement in nursing homes. *Ann Long-term Care* 3:11, 1994.

Von Sternberg T et al: Post-hospital subacute care: An example of a managed care model. *J Am Geriatr Soc* 45:87, 1997.

Weinberg A: Risk Management in Long-term Care—A Quick Reference Guide. New York: Springer Publishing, 1998.

Nursing Home Care

ANNETTE MEDINA-WALPOLE • PAUL R. KATZ

Nursing homes have evolved from alms houses, common at the turn of the century, into highly regulated institutions for individuals with profound physical and mental disabilities. Although nursing homes have become an integral part of the United States health care system, in many respects they remain poorly understood. Expectations of nursing homes vary considerably from acute hospital systems to individual health care professionals, the lay public, policy makers, and regulatory bodies. Divergent expectations, when combined with ever increasing resource constraints and staff shortages, create a set of very unique and complex care issues. To fully understand these issues, this chapter examines the nursing home from a number of perspectives. These perspectives encompass population needs, government policy, reimbursement, and staffing patterns, as well as medical care and administrative issues, knowledge of which is key to quality care in the nursing home setting.

DEMOGRAPHICS AND ECONOMICS

Nursing home practitioners will readily attest that nursing homes have changed dramatically over the past decade. While still affording long-term care to severely disabled individuals, often with limited social supports, nursing homes also care for patients recovering from acute illness or injury, as well as those suffering from terminal illness (19 percent of all deaths occur in nursing homes). The scope of care has changed in response to the increasing heterogeneity of the nursing home resident population, and with it, provider responsibilities and challenges have changed.

The lifetime risk of nursing home placement for an individual 65 years of age and older is estimated at 43 percent, with a third of lifetime risk applicable to nursing home stays of 90 days or less. Whether this estimate changes dramatically in the years to come depends heavily on the manner in which long-term care services are financed. Currently, an increasing percentage of all nursing home admissions are "subacute" or rehabilitative in nature, with relatively short stays and eventual discharge back into the community. Of all nursing home admissions, short stayers (3 months or less) currently account for 25 percent of admissions, in contrast to 50 percent of admissions who will spend at least 1 year in the nursing home. One in five nursing home admissions will reside in the nursing home almost 5 years. In contrast to the more traditional longer-stay resident, the short-stay population is reimbursed primarily through Medicare and, to a lesser extent, other private long-term care insurance. A change in these funding streams would dramatically impact nursing home occupancy.

Interestingly, occupancy rates in nursing homes nationally have declined over the past several years and now stand at 88 percent. This decline is despite a rise in total nursing home admissions, reflecting the dynamic nature of this sector of the long-term care continuum. While many observers have attributed the decline in occupancy to the availability of other long-term care options such as assisted living, there are likely several other causal social and financial variables that have yet to be defined. Indeed, older populations cared for at different long-term care sites are not interchangeable, as evidenced by the fact that the availability and use of home care services for Medicare-eligible patients has not been found to reduce nursing home admissions. Declines in Medicare spending on home health care as part of the prospective payment system ($9.7 billion in 1999 versus $17.5 billion in 1997) may eventually force some individuals into nursing homes for lack of affordable home care options.

Needless to say, the average nursing home resident is characterized by significant impairments in physical and instrumental activities of daily living as illustrated in Table 17-1. Only 2.8 percent of nursing home residents are completely independent in their activities of daily living (ADL). Approximately 14 percent require assistance with one or two ADL and 83 percent require assistance with three or more ADL. Overall, the level of disability in the nursing home has increased over the past decade and exceeds that found in persons receiving home care. In addition to impairments of activities of daily living, 81 percent of nursing home residents are impaired in their ability to make daily decisions, two-thirds have orientation difficulties and/or memory problems, and more than half (54 percent) have either bowel or bladder incontinence. Hearing and visual impairment are found in 36 percent and 39 percent of residents, respectively. Dementia remains the most frequently occurring condition in the nursing home with estimates ranging from 50 to 70 percent. Behavioral

Table 17-1   Functional Disabilities in the Nursing Home

Function		% Affected
Dressing	Assistance Required	52.3
	Totally Dependent	35.9
Bathing	Assistance Required	49.5
	Totally Dependent	47.0
Eating	Assistance Required	41.2
	Totally Dependent	18.5
Transferring	Assistance Required	45.2
	Totally Dependent	28.4
Mobility	Assistance Required	36.5
	Totally Dependent	30.0
Toileting	Assistance Required	41.5
	Totally Dependent	38.3

problems, understandably, are also common, occurring in at least one-third of nursing home residents. Such behaviors include verbal and physical abuse, social inappropriateness, resistance to care, and/or wandering. Communication problems are noted in 60 percent of residents, while 44 percent have difficulty with being understood and with understanding others. Depression is diagnosed in 20 percent of nursing home residents.

Almost half of all nursing home residents are 85 years of age and older, with less than 9 percent younger than age 65 years. The risk of nursing home admission rises steeply with age: 19 percent of persons age 85 years and older reside in nursing homes versus 1 percent for those persons 65 to 74 years of age. The majority are women (72 percent), white (89 percent), and unmarried (60 percent widowed) with limited social supports. The percentage of black residents in nursing homes has increased in recent years (9 percent) approaching national population norms. In fact, black persons 65 to 74 years of age are more likely than whites to be admitted to a nursing home. Nonetheless, other nonwhite populations, such as Hispanics, Asians, and Native Americans, are under represented in nursing homes despite even higher disability rates. Older adults with developmental disabilities comprise another unique population that is requiring increasing nursing home care as their elderly parents die off. These individuals often require specialized care that many nursing homes have difficulty providing.

Although there is a significant chance of being admitted to a nursing home with increasing age, quantifying risk is complex. Age, male gender, low income, poor family supports (especially lack of spouse and children), and low social activity have been used as predictors of institutionalization. Cognitive and functional impairments have also predicted nursing home placement, often of a permanent nature. Interestingly, education and caregiver support delay the need for nursing home institutionalization for up to 1 year for patients with dementia. Not surprisingly, older adults with more-positive attitudes toward nursing homes are more likely to use skilled nursing facilities (SNF)

than are adults with less-favorable dispositions. Although nurses, physicians, and social workers tend to agree in their estimates of the probability of nursing home placement, mental and functional impairments are commonly underestimated and potentially impede the discharge process. Hospital discharge planners are often more focused on bed utilization/occupancy and may not focus in a comprehensive fashion on the long-term needs of medical patients. The range of long-term care services that are now available (i.e., SNF, home care, assisted living) further complicate placement decisions as the relative value and merits of one over the other have not been empirically tested. Interestingly, the use of formal (i.e., paid for) community services does not necessarily counter the risk of nursing home placement for patients with severe disabilities.

Currently there are 17,000 nursing homes with 1.8 million beds, 1.6 million residents, and 2.4 million discharges (i.e., to home, hospital, or secondary to death). Of these facilities, 65 percent are proprietary (for-profit) with voluntary nonprofit (25 percent) and government nursing homes (10 percent) accounting for the remainder. The average nursing home operates 107 beds, with a minority (8 percent) operating more than 200 beds. A little more than half of all nursing homes (56 percent) are part of a chain.

While occupancy rates in nursing homes have declined in recent years, this may be a short-lived phenomena. Assuming that the prevalence of chronic disease does not change dramatically as a result of new discoveries (e.g., a cure for Alzheimer's disease), it is estimated that between 4.3 and 5.3 million elderly will require nursing home care by the year 2030.

Nursing home expenditures currently total $90 billion and are projected to increase to $150 billion by 2007. Public expenditures comprise almost two-thirds of all nursing home spending. In 1998 Medicaid expenditures totaled $22.7 billion while Medicare outlays equaled $13.4 billion for nursing home care. Under the new prospective payment system (PPS) enacted as part of the balanced budget act of 1997, Medicare payments to skilled nursing facilities are no longer cost-based but predicated on functional needs and rehabilitative potential. While PPS has not conclusively limited access to skilled nursing care for Medicare beneficiaries, it has definitely forced nursing homes to be more diligent as regards to admission policies. Those patients in need of expensive services (i.e., IVs, ventilators, tube feedings) may be passed over for individuals receiving high reimbursement rates, such as those with strokes and joint replacements. Reimbursement limits or caps on certain rehabilitative therapies and/or equipment may also constrain specific types of admissions. Not unexpectedly, physical, occupational, and speech therapies are commonly prescribed in the nursing home, with half of all nursing home admissions receiving at least 90 minutes of these rehabilitation services in one recent study. While SNF rehabilitation offers quality care that costs much less than in acute care hospitals, eligibility requirements at times disenfranchise those truly in need. For example, eligibility for SNF care under part A Medicare mandates hospitalization within 30 days of the nursing home admission, which must be of a duration of at least 3 days. Restoration of lost function is a requirement for payment, and custodial care is not covered.

Nursing home residents today are clearly sicker and more disabled than nursing home residents in the past. Unfortunately, the number of nurses available to provide the necessary care remains suboptimal. Studies confirm the correlation between the provision of quality care and total nursing hours and the ratio of professional [i.e., registered nurses (RNs)] to nonprofessional nursing staff. A 1996 Institute of Medicine report recommended increasing nurse staffing levels to enhance the quality of nursing home care and has spurred Congress to debate the merits of mandatory minimum staffing ratios. Even if eventually mandated, the finances to achieve significantly higher staffing ratios remains elusive. Recruiting and retaining staff, particularly nursing assistants who comprise the bulk of the nursing home workforce, remains problematic. Turnover rates for all nursing personnel remain incredibly high (50 to 90 percent per year); likely a measure of low wages, intense public scrutiny, lack of peer respect, and overall job demands.

PHYSICIAN PRACTICE

The "typical" nursing home physician is a primary care internist or family physician who devotes 2 hours or less per week to nursing home care. Only one in five physicians seek out a nursing home practice, in large part because of perceptions of excessive regulations and paperwork, and limited reimbursement. In addition, historically there has been a paucity of credible role models for physicians-in-training who are involved in nursing home care and who might engender interest and involvement in long-term care issues.

Such limited involvement often precludes a full integration of the physician into the culture of the nursing facility and potentially impedes interdisciplinary communication and treatments. Surveys of nursing home physicians and nurses have highlighted a lack of trust and respect between professions which might be circumvented by more closed medical staffs. Closed staffs attract a limited number of more committed physicians to care for a facility's residents with evidence now suggesting that the closed staff model delivers a higher intensity and quality of care. While resident choice of physicians may be limited with closed medical staff models, this must be balanced against access and quality issues.

Medical care of nursing home residents, despite misconceptions to the contrary, offers practitioners unique challenges and demands exemplary clinical skills as well as sensitivity to a host of ethical, legal, and interdisciplinary issues. Medical interventions, whether they are curative, preventative, or palliative in nature, require an individualized approach that recognizes the complex interplay between resident, family, and staff needs. Care is further complicated by the spotty evidence available upon which to base treatment. The biopsychosocial complexities that accompany most decision making and care planning for nursing homes residents requires a team approach of health care professionals that relate to each other in a truly interdisciplinary fashion. A well-functioning team assures that medical interventions will be coordinated among all relevant disciplines in the nursing home and will be based on a shared knowledge of patient values and goals for care. The physician's role as a member of the health care team need not be compromised due to a lack of a constant physical presence in the facility. Success in the nursing home depends more on a physician's willingness to seek out and listen to the opinion of others, whatever their professional standing. Rather than feel threatened, the physician must make a concerted effort to understand each individual's role in the nursing home including the manner in which it is governed by state and federal regulations. This is especially important if the physician is to forge a successful, constructive relationship with the nursing home administrator, director of nursing, pharmacist consultant, and medical director.

In the context of the team, and through interventions with staff, residents, and families, physicians often serve as role models in the nursing home. Skill at communication, clear and concise documentation in the medical record, and an overriding respect for individual rights and dignity are cornerstones of nursing home practices. Table 17-2 highlights the role of physicians practicing in nursing

Table 17-2   Physician Responsibilities in the Nursing Home

1. Comprehensively assess each resident and, in concert with the care team, resident, and family, assist in care plan development and coordination of all aspects of medical care. (Tag 272, 279)
2. Periodically review the care plan and assure that the goals and objectives designed to meet the highest practicable well-being of each resident are rational and functionally relevant. (Tag 272, 279, F250, F309)
3. Implement specific treatments and services to enhance or maintain physical and psychosocial function, and to avoid accidents, if at all possible. (Tag F502–F512, F310, F311, F323, F324)
4. Physically attend to each resident in a manner consistent with established state and federal guidelines (visit every 30 days for the first 90 days following admission and at least every 60 days thereafter), while assuring that appropriate diagnostic tests are performed and followed up in a timely fashion. (Tag F387, F500–F512)
5. Respond in a timely and appropriate fashion to resident's change in function. (Tag F157)
6. Inform residents of their health status and optimize ability for self-determination whenever possible. (Tag F154, F151, F152)
7. Determine each resident's decision-making capacity while assisting in establishing advance directives. (Tag F151, F152)
8. Assure that resident's are free from unnecessary drugs by periodic review of drug regimens and consultant pharmacist recommendations. (Tag F329–F331, F428, F429)

homes and reflects accepted standards of care as well as specific regulations. These regulations encompass several domains, each of which corresponds to a regulatory code known as a tag number. These domains specifically address physician services, resident assessment function, resident rights, and quality of care.

While each nursing home resident must be seen by a physician, nurse practitioner, or physician assistant every 30 or 60 days, scheduling routine visitations (chart or bedside rounds) with the nursing staff is an effective way to share pertinent clinical information and ensure ongoing communication. The efficiency of physician care may be enhanced by scheduling several residents for evaluation per visit, as well as providing nurses with protocols that define routine, emergent, and urgent medical situations and provide guidelines for care in each instance. Scheduled/structured progress notes have been used in some nursing homes to ensure comprehensive and easily retrievable data collection that meets or exceeds all regulatory requirements. Figure 17-1 is an example of a nursing home medical progress note. While none of these approaches have been rigorously tested as regards to impact on care outcomes, they highlight the many opportunities to improve upon nursing home practice.

Nurse practitioners (NPs) and physician assistants (PAs) are increasingly becoming involved in nursing home care. Whether employed by the nursing facility directly or by a physician, they have taken on important functions in as much as 20 percent of nursing homes. Studies to date suggest that NPs and PAs who act in concert with the primary care physician, provide more intensive care to the nursing home resident, enhance satisfaction with care, and may decrease hospitalization rates while maintaining cost neutrality.

THE ACUTE/LONG-TERM CARE INTERFACE

The bidirectional transfer of patients between nursing home and hospital brings with it a host of clinical, research, and policy issues. Most nursing home admissions originate from acute care hospitals while acutely ill nursing home residents, often with serious infections, are frequently admitted to the hospital. Problems frequently encountered on transfer to the nursing home are outlined in Table 17-3, many of which reflect process issues that will require system wide solutions to resolve.

The increasing acuity and rapid turnover of patients transferred to nursing homes has put increasing stress on long-term care facilities where resources and trained staff are often in short supply. Conversely, many nursing home residents are transferred to the hospital inappropriately or with inadequate documentation. A recent study, based on a structured implicit review of medical records, noted

MEDICAL PROGRESS NOTE

Date:	30 day ____ 60 day ____
Active/Chronic/Past Medical Problems:	
Changes in Condition Since Last Medical Progress Note:	
Change in Function: □ Yes □ No Describe: Continence Bladder ____ Functional Status: ____ Continence Bowel ____ Falls (number of): ____	
Medication/Indication:	AIMS: __/__/__
Diet/Nutritional Status:	Weight: ____ Gain: ____ Loss: ____
Review of Systems HEENT ____ Chest ____ GI ____ GU ____ Lymphatic ____	Extremities ____ Joints ____ Neuro ____ Skin ____ Behavior ____

PE-General B/P ____ Pulse ____ Respiratory Rate ____		
Mental/Cognitive Status:		
	NP/PA/FELLOW	ATTENDING PHYSICIAN
HEENT		
Lymphatic		
Lungs		
Heart		
Abdomen		
Extremities		
Skin		
Neuro		
Laboratory Data:		
Assessment/Plan (Address 3 Or More Chronic Conditions) Colon		
Advance Directives:	Code Status:	

FORM COMPLETED BY:

Signature of PA/NP/Fellow ____ Please Print Name ____

I was present and personally participated in the key elements of this evaluation. I verified the essential points of today's visit.Upon review,I agree with the fellow's assessment and plan of care.

Signature of Physician ____ Please Print Name ____

ICP Reviewed: ____

Figure 17-1 Sample medical progress note. Developed at Monroe Community Hospital, Rochester, NY.

Table 17-3 Problems Encountered with Acute Care to Long-Term Care Transfers

1. Illegible or nonexistent transfer summary.
2. Omission of prescribed medications on transfer form.
3. Nonspecific rehabilitation instructions following orthopedic procedures.
4. Inconsistencies in transfer data.
5. Lack of information pertaining to recent procedures, labs, radiographs, and electrocardiograms.
6. Lack of documentation of advanced directives.
7. Lack of psychosocial information and related behavioral issues.

that 44 percent of emergency department transfers and 40 percent of hospital admissions from nursing homes were inappropriate (controlling for advance directives) and thus could have been adequately cared for at the SNF level of care. The factors underlying inappropriate transfers related to suboptimal evaluation and/or care of acute illness in the nursing home, the over- and misinterpretation of the patient's chief complaint, and/or lack of knowledge of available resources. Increased physician and nurse practitioner/physician assistant involvement in the nursing home, as well as the availability of special care units, may reduce transfers to the hospital.

SUBACUTE CARE

Nursing homes have responded to the increasing postacute needs of older persons and declining lengths of hospital stays with the development of subacute programs. While the types of subacute services and programs vary significantly from one locale to another (i.e., dialysis, orthopedic, ventilator, postoperative, rehabilitative, or wound care), they remain distinct from the standard nursing home services by integrating the features of acute medical, long-term care nursing, and rehabilitative cultures. The challenge in subacute care is that of accommodating to patients with varying degrees of disease severity, functional dependence, and comorbidities. In selected patient populations, subacute care in the nursing home may achieve equal or better outcomes when compared to acute hospitals. Definitions as to what constitutes subacute care, however, vary widely as do regulatory standards, thus making comparison studies difficult.

QUALITY OF CARE IN THE NURSING HOME

Quality care in nursing homes has been a subject of intense debate over the past several decades ultimately leading to extensive regulatory reform. The essence of the nursing home reform act of 1987 (OBRA 87) can be summarized in one of its overriding mandates: "to assure the highest practicable quality of life for each nursing home resident." To accomplish this goal, the federal government has

established training guidelines, minimum staffing requirements, and basic resident rights, as well as mandated periodic comprehensive assessments. This standardized assessment is known as the minimum data set (MDS) and focuses specifically on clinical issues relevant to quality care. The MDS quantifies real or potential problems in a host of clinical, psychosocial, and functional domains, thus forming the basis for all care planning. Resident assessment protocols (RAPs) further outline standard diagnostic and therapeutic approaches to specific problems (i.e., pressure ulcers, incontinence, delirium, depression) and are meant to be used by the care team in much the same way as practice guidelines. Figure 17-2 is an example of a Behavioral Symptoms RAP Key. A recent survey of physicians caring for nursing home residents revealed that only 11 percent the entire MDS, and 21 percent reported reviewing part of the MDS, for all of their patients. Furthermore, 19 percent of the sample failed to review the care plan for any of their patients, while 56 percent voiced negative or derogatory comments concerning the MDS.

Additional regulatory mandates have been introduced that require physicians to clearly document the need for medications, particularly psychoactive agents. Unnecessary drugs are defined as those that are given in excessive doses for excessive periods of time, without adequate monitoring or indications for use, or in the presence of adverse consequences that indicate the need for dose reduction or discontinuation. In addition to these generic instructions, specific types of drugs are banned (i.e., usage will warrant a citation from the state survey inspection team unless a clear rationale for use is documented in the chart) from use in the nursing home based upon criteria developed by a group of experts.

While it is difficult to dispute the goals of current nursing home regulations, their overall impact on care has been difficult to measure. In part, this stems from the survey process itself, which is under the direction of each state's own survey, licensing, and certification agency. Surveys occur at a minimum of every 15 months and are designed to monitor compliance with federal regulations. The survey process, however, has been criticized for its inconsistencies and its punitive and adversarial underpinnings, which are detailed in Table 17-4.

The current regulatory paradigm in the United States, according to many observers, is at the core of much of the controversy regarding effectiveness of the nursing home survey system. Regulations in the United States are "deterrent," based on the underlying premise that nursing facilities are "amoral calculators," willing to "break the rules" when and if necessary. The result is regulation that is formal, legalistic, punitive, and sanction oriented. Regulation that focuses on "compliance," however, views institutions as good, not evil, and generally emphasizes cooperation and respect, in a true quality improvement environment. A system that combines the features of both a compliance and deterrence regulatory system might well meet the needs of all concerned while allowing for maximum decision-making flexibility.

A relatively new initiative to enhance quality care in the nursing home involves the use of quality indicators (QIs). Quality indicators, shown in Table 17-5, are designed to

BEHAVIORAL SYMPTOMS RAP KEY (For MDS Version 2.0)

TRIGGER – REVISION	GUIDELINES

Review of behavior status suggested if one or more of following present

- Wandering*
  [E4aA = 1,2,3]

- Verbally abusive
  [E4bA = 1,2,3]

- Physically abusive
  [E4cA = 1,2,3]

- Socially inappropriate
  [E4dA = 1,2,3]

- Resists Care
  [E4eA = 1,2,3]

- Behavior improved
  [E5 = 1]

Review and describe behavioral symptom:

- Evaluating the seriousness and stability / change of behavioral symptoms. Review of intensity, duration, frequency and, if any, pattern of behaviors, their development over time, and their effect on resident and others **[E4aB, E4bB, E4cB, E4dB, E4eB, from record]**

Review potential causes that could be addressed or resolved:

- **Cognitive status problems.** Delirium [B5], Alzheimer's Disease **[I1q]** or other dementia **[I1u]**, Effects of stroke **[C4, C5, C6; G5, G6; I1r, I1t]**
- **Mood or relationship problems.** Sad or anxious mood **[E1]**, Unsettled relationships **[F2]**, Psychiatric diagnosis **[11dd, 11ee, 11ff, 11gg]**
- **Environmental conditions.** Departure from resident's normal routines prior to entering facility **[F3c]**, Staff responses, presence of stressful conditions of physically aggressive resident **[from record, interviews with staff, resident]**
- **Illness/conditions.** Onset of acute illness, worsening of chronic illness **[J5a,b]**, and other related problems, such as Constipation **[H2b]**, Diabetes **[I1a]**, CHF **[11f]**, Pneumonia **[I2e]**, Septicemia **[I2g]**, UTI **[I2j]** or other infection **[I2,I3]**, Fever **[J1h]**, Delusions **[J1e]**, Hallucinations **[J1i]**, Pain [J2], Fall with physical trauma to head **[J4a,b; I1cc]**
- **Communications deficits.** Difficulty making self understood **[C4]** or Understanding others **[C6]**
- **Sensory impairments.** Hearing problem **[C1]**, Visual problem **[D1]**, Visual Limitations **[D2]**
- **Treatment/management procedures.** Antipsychotics, antianxiety, antidepressants, hypnotics [O4a,b,c,d], Behavior management program **[P2]**, Trunk, limb or chair restraints **[P4c,d,e]**

* **Note** –This item also triggers on the Fall RAP

Figure 17-2 Example of behavioral symptoms RAP key. From long-term care facility resident assessment instrument (RAI) user's manual. Official replica edition, September 2000. RAP 9, behavioral symptoms, p. 6.

Table 17-4   Problems with Nursing Home Surveys

1. Lack of due process.
2. Disassociation between outcomes and processes, penalizing facilities for unpreventable events.
3. Failure of deficiencies to discriminate between trivial and important quality issues.
4. Subjectivity of surveyors allowing for significant regional variations in type and scope of deficiencies cited.
5. Inadequate quality improvement system for survey teams.
6. Inconsistent application of regulations.
7. Inappropriate punishment.

highlight extant or potential problems as a means to guide each facility's own QI program. Quality indicators may be compared between facilities that are similar in size and complexity as a way to benchmark standards. The debate continues, however, concerning the most appropriate risk adjustment methodology for QIs, which are meant to adjust for the case mix of a given facility. While each nursing home must conduct its own QI program representing all major disciplines, the design of such programs is not standardized. Nursing home-based quality improvement programs can, however, be invaluable in defining problems and designing interventions that improve resident care. Interestingly, although most older adults would choose assisted living over a nursing home if necessary, many are under the mistaken belief that both are under the same stringent regulatory mandates.

Table 17-5   Examples of Nursing Home Quality Indicators

Domain / Quality Indicator
Accidents
1. Incidence of new fractures
2. Prevalence of falls
Behavior/Emotional Patterns
3. Prevalence of behavioral symptoms affecting others
High risk
Low risk
4. Prevalence of symptoms of depression
5. Prevalence of symptoms of depression without antidepressant therapy
Clinical Management
6. Use of nine or more different medications
Cognitive Patterns
7. Incidence of cognitive impairment
Elimination/Incontinence
8. Prevalence of bladder or bowel incontinence
High risk
Low risk
9. Prevalence of occasional or frequent bladder or bowel incontinence without a toileting plan
10. Prevalence of indwelling catheter
11. Prevalence of fecal impaction
Infection Control
12. Prevalence of urinary tract infection
Nutrition/Eating
13. Prevalence of weight loss
14. Prevalence of tube feeding
15. Prevalence of dehydration
Physical Functioning
16. Prevalence of bedfast residents
17. Incidence of decline in late loss ADL
18. Incidence of decline in range of motion
Psychotropic Drug Use
19. Prevalence of antipsychotic use in the absence of psychotic or related conditions
High risk
Low risk
20. Prevalence of antianxiety/hypnotic use
21. Prevalence of hypnotic use more than two times in last week
Quality of Life
22. Prevalence of daily physical restraints
23. Prevalence of little or no activity
Skin Care
24. Prevalence of stage 1 to 4 pressure ulcers
High risk
Low risk

MEDICAL CARE ISSUES IN THE NURSING HOME

Caring for nursing home residents has become increasingly complex over the past several years, commensurate with an increasing level of medical acuity in an environment constrained by lack of adequate resources. Comprehensive, ongoing assessment within an interdisciplinary framework provides the practitioner the opportunity to address the basic geriatric principles of care, restore function, whenever possible, and always to enhance quality of life. Although the nursing home is likely the most challenging setting in which to practice geriatric medicine, the relationships developed between patients, families, physicians, and staff are among the most rewarding. Clinical challenges abound in the nursing home setting, in part, by the atypical or more subtle presentation of illness so characteristic of patients with such profound physical and psychological frailty and a high prevalence of cognitive impairment. Additionally, the medical decision making is complicated by intense regulatory oversight, limited access to technology, and dependence on nursing and other nonphysician staff for patient assessment.

The heterogeneity among nursing home residents is another factor that affects overall care and precludes a uniform approach for each resident. Success in this setting demands diligence on the part of the physician and a thoughtful, reasoned, often individualized approach to the medical and ethical problems frequently encountered. Medical problems encountered in the nursing home often require unique diagnostic and therapeutic strategies. Many are best managed using an interdisciplinary team approach to care. Relevant medical issues include infections such as nursing home-acquired pneumonia, falls, malnutrition, incontinence, behavioral disturbances, polypharmacy and prevention/screening.

MODELS OF INTERDISCIPLINARY TEAM APPROACH TO COMMON GERIATRIC SYNDROMES

Several interdisciplinary programs aimed at addressing common geriatric syndromes have been developed and described. Geriatrics is rooted in the interdisciplinary team approach to care and this model can be expanded to teams that specifically address behavior, falls, and incontinence, as examples. The successful implementation of interdisciplinary teams that include physicians often relates to the staffing organization of the facility. This can become an issue if the physician team is not physically in the building. Nursing home with closed medical staff limit provider privileges to those based at the facility, compared with open staffing, where community providers play a role in the care of the patients. Facilities with closed medical staffing are more likely to have providers on site daily, more rapid response time to patient care and administrative issues and greater provider participation in interdisciplinary teams. Although a closed medical staff environment may be ideal to the team approach, the team model can also be successful with providers that are available for team meetings on a weekly or bimonthly basis and are available by phone for interim discussions. Regardless of staffing patterns, physicians should play a key role and be fully integrated within interdisciplinary teams. Several interdisciplinary models that address specific geriatric syndromes and issues are described below.

Prevention and Cancer Screening in the Nursing Home

The issue of prevention and screening is an important, yet challenging, issue in the nursing home setting. It is difficult to generalize specific guidelines for such a mixed population of functional impairment, cognitive impairment and various comorbid illnesses. Certain areas of prevention, such as yearly influenza vaccination, tuberculosis screening, and monthly weight screening, are more easily incorporated as routine procedure, whereas decisions regarding screening for cancer really need to be made on a case-by-case basis. A framework that incorporates the risk of dying, the benefits and harms of cancer screening, and the values and preferences of the older adult has been described. This individualized approach is well suited to the nursing home where cancer screening may not be indicated given life expectancy and impairments in function and cognition.

Health maintenance screening is an essential aspect of nursing home care. Certain prevention issues are mandated at regular intervals such as tuberculosis testing, annual history and physical examination, dental and medical reviews. Others are recommendations for quality care and include functional assessment including gait and mental status examination; visual, auditory, and podiatry evaluations; and selected laboratory tests. Although there is scant evidence to support routine laboratory monitoring, nursing home experts do recommend focused disease-specific testing such as hemoglobin (Hgb) A1C in diabetics, chemistries to monitor renal function and calculate creatinine clearance, albumin for nutrition monitoring, and certain drug levels (e.g., digoxin, antiepileptics, warfarin). Because subclinical thyroid disease and vitamin B_{12} deficiency are common issues in the nursing home population, even among those younger than age 65 years with chronic medical illness, screening for these conditions should be performed. Other preventive measures include yearly influenza vaccine, pneumococcal vaccination following established guidelines, and tetanus booster every 10 years or primary tetanus vaccination for those never immunized. Progressive resistance exercise training is an effective means of counteracting muscle weakness and physical frailty in frail nursing home residents. Additionally, exercise strategies and nursing-based rehabilitation as facility-wide interventions can result in a reduction of ADL decline rates and maintenance of involvement in ADL activities.

Urinary Incontinence

Urinary incontinence affects approximately half of nursing home residents, is associated with significant morbidity and cost, and is a common reason for long-term care placement. Urinary incontinence is not a normal consequence of aging and its prevalence in the nursing home setting largely reflects the high degree of functional and cognitive impairment seen in long-term care residents. It may also reflect the acceptance by many staff and providers that urinary incontinence is "the norm" rather than "the exception" in most nursing home residents. Based on the Omnibus Budget Reconciliation Act (OBRA) regulations, in 1987, facilities should have an incontinence program in place. Additionally, 3 of the 24 quality indicators from the Health Care Financing Administration (HCFA) *State Operations Manual* are directly related to urinary incontinence. This is further reason for a comprehensive, facility-wide approach to this prevalent issue.

The etiology, pathophysiology, diagnosis, and pharmacologic and nonpharmacologic treatment of urinary incontinence are well documented, including guidelines from the American Medical Director's Association. Interdisciplinary and individualized approaches to manage urinary incontinence in the nursing home setting have proven successful. Most long-term care residents require caregiver-dependent behavioral interventions that can be effective in 25 to 40 percent of cases. These include prompted voiding and toileting schedules to maintain continence. Nighttime incontinence care in particular should be individualized to minimize sleep disruption. A team approach to urinary incontinence in long-term care residents that includes the involvement, education, and empowerment of certified nursing assistants as members of a urinary incontinence management team lead by advanced practice nurses has been described. Although there are many residents with potentially treatable incontinence, the cost of regimens requiring intense staff time remains prohibitive in many facilities.

Management of Behavioral Disturbances

Behavioral disturbances in dementia are a frequent occurrence and a challenge to clinicians and caregivers alike, particularly in the institutional setting. These behaviors include depression in approximately 40 percent, psychosis in 40 percent, and agitation in 60 percent of patients. Undiagnosed medical problems, including delirium, pain, and sleep disturbances, are often associated with behavioral disturbances. Providers and caregivers can often successfully identify and modify causative and exacerbating factors, and then work toward resolution with behavioral and, if needed, pharmacologic therapy. A multifaceted program to address behavioral issues in transitional care setting at a VA Medical Center was recently described. This "behavior management program" involved an interdisciplinary approach to the management of behavioral disturbances. The program includes the development of a behavior team and a comprehensive behavior observation record that assists caregivers and staff in identifying and monitoring target behaviors. Both nonpharmacologic and pharmacologic interventions play a role in reducing behavioral episodes, promoting education and staff camaraderie and creating a productive liaison between the transitional care unit (TCU) and the psychiatry service. The behavior team meets in

1-hour sessions every 2 weeks to discuss behaviors and management strategies for TCU residents with behavioral disturbances. The behavior observation record, a weekly observational tool, is used to track behaviors by staff, as well as the success or failure of various management approaches (both nonpharmacologic and pharmacologic). The team and staff carefully document any changes in behavior as well as the team discussion in the resident's medical record. Overall, this represents a successful model of the interdisciplinary team approach to the management of behavioral disturbances in long-term or transitional care residents. This model can be reproduced in facilities capable of incorporating the team approach, even if the medical provider or geriatric psychiatrist is only available on a biweekly or monthly basis for input.

A Consultation Service to Reduce Falls and a Falls Prevention Program

Falls and fall-related injuries are a major issue in nursing homes with serious clinical, social and economic implications. Approximately half of nursing home residents fall each year, representing twice the rate for community-dwelling older adults. Injuries range from minor soft-tissue abrasions and swelling to serious injuries with significant morbidity and hospitalization risk, such as fractures and subdural hematomas.

Several studies in community-dwelling elderly have documented a reduced incidence of falls with various interventions—exercise, balance, and a multifactorial risk reduction approach. Studies among nursing home residents have not been as fruitful. In an effort to target falls reduction in the nursing home setting, one randomized controlled trial involved a falls consultation service aimed at modifying behavioral and environmental factors in four domains: environmental and personal safety, wheelchairs, psychotropic drugs, and transferring and ambulation. The consult service aimed to modify and improve safety practices in each domain as well as encourage facility-wide interventions to improve staff safety behavior. The intervention facilities had 19 percent fewer recurrent fallers and 31 percent fewer injurious falls among study subjects, although the latter was not statistically significant. The program was most effective in those for whom the recommendations were followed and who had three or more falls in the prior year. In this group, the intervention residents had 50 percent fewer injurious falls than control residents. Examples of the most frequent recommendations by the consultation team include labeling wheelchairs and equipment; repairing and replacing furniture; using properly fitted shoes; adjusting and repairing wheelchair brakes; cleaning and lubricating moving parts; installing antitip rods and brake extensions; tapering and discontinuing benzodiazepines or changing to as-needed dosing; reducing antipsychotic medication doses and implementing a behavior management plan; increasing observation of residents; toileting and nourishing every 2 hours; and safety reminders and assistance with transfers. The biggest challenge to this model is the staff, resident, and facility compliance with the recommendations.

Because many nursing homes may not be able to reproduce a full-scale consultation intervention, alternative models exist. Although not formally tested, one such model incorporates an interdisciplinary fall prevention program in an attempt to identify residents at high risk of falls, emphasizing prevention and interventions to minimize falls and related injuries. This model, operationalized at a 566-bed academic nursing home, includes a fall risk assessment, shown in Fig. 17-3, which is completed upon admission, annually, and when changes in status occur that can place an individual at an increased risk for falls. Once an individual is identified as being at risk for falls, the interdisciplinary team reviews and changes the care plan to incorporate the status of conditions predisposing the resident to falling, specific fall prevention efforts, and the resident's response to the interventions. All facility direct care staff are required to be competent in the identification and prevention of falls. The fall prevention program is reviewed in a staff member's initial orientation and included as an annual mandatory educational session. The facility also collects data to record the program's effectiveness and to identify trends through the use of Minimum Data Set 2.0 and the resident incident reporting system.

ENSURING NUTRITION AND HYDRATION IN THE NURSING HOME SETTING

There is a high potential for nutritional deficits in nursing home residents both on admission and during their long-term course. Community-dwelling elders entering the nursing home may have had poor eating habits, insufficient funds for food, and an inability or lack of interest to prepare nutritionally balanced meals. It is therefore imperative that a nutritional assessment be performed upon admission and then at regular intervals thereafter. The American Medical Director's Association has new guidelines focused on altered nutritional status, dehydration, and fluid maintenance, which emphasize finding the underlying cause of the nutritional problem, the team approach to maintaining optimal nutrition and hydration, and the individual patient's eating preferences and desires. This process begins with an initial assessment that includes measurement of weight, calculation of body mass index, and evaluation of food preferences. Risk factors for nutritional impairment and dehydration should be identified and will warrant involvement from multiple disciplines. These risk factors include recent weight loss, cognitive impairment, dysphagia, inability to self-feed, medications (e.g., those that cause sedation, xerostomia), dietary restrictions, depression, acute infection, fluid loss (e.g., diarrhea, excessive sweating or urination, fever), comorbid illnesses and pressure sores. The final step is detecting, identifying and treating the cause of the weight loss, deterioration in nutrition, or inadequate intake. Weight loss that would warrant assessment is the loss of 5 percent in 1 month, 7.5 percent in 3 months, or 10 percent in 6 months. After ruling out dehydration as a cause, monitoring of caloric and fluid intake is warranted. If intake is greater than 75 percent, evaluation for increased caloric need should ensue (infection, hypermetabolic state,

Fall Risk Assessment

A fall is defined as a problem characterized by the failure to maintain an appropriate lying, sitting, or standing position resulting in an individual's abrupt, undesired relocation to the ground.

Directions: Complete the following upon admission, annually and when changes occur in resident status which could place him/her at increased risk for falls.	Date			Date			Date			Date		
	Yes	No	Unknown	Yes	No	Unknown	Yes	No	Unknown	Yes	No	Unknown
History of fall												
Coma ('If yes stop here)												
Unsteady gait, dizziness, imbalance, weakness												
Mental status: inability to understand or follow directions, impulsivity												
Combative												
Anxiety / Depression												
Sensory deficits												
Altered communications												
Cardiovascular Medications(check): ( )diuretic, ( ) beta blocker, ( ) digitallis prep, ( ) vasodilator												
CNS Medications: ( ) tranquilizers, ( ) psychotropics, ( ) hypnotic / analgesic sedative, ( ) antidepressant												
Pain												
Chronic illness exacerbation												
Acute illness												
Nocturia (altered bladder control)												
( ) Environmental changes: ( ) equipment attached												
Assistive Devices												
Other												
initials												

If any yes: review / revise care plan for fall reducation (Review-resdient assessment protocol #11)

Date:_____   Reviwed: _____

Figure 17-3 Fall risk assessment. Developed at Monroe Community, Hospital, Rochester, NY.

acute illness, wounds etc.). If intake is less than 75 percent, exploration of the environment and resident-specific causes of anorexia or inability to eat should be pursued. This includes an evaluation for depression, dementia, dysphagia, odynophagia, and medication review.

In many but not all residents, the cause of weight loss or malnutrition can be identified. An interdisciplinary approach is again key. The interventions to address weight loss could include facility-wide changes to enhance the dining experience of all residents and providing choices

about food and fluid preferences. These recommendations may be difficult to carry out given the staff constraints of many facilities. Although federal regulations mandate that facilities must provide each resident with sufficient fluids to maintain proper hydration and health, inadequate fluid intake and a high risk for dehydration occurs when staffing is inadequate and supervision poor.

The treatment of feeding disorders and poor nutrition also raises additional problems. For example, determining the risks and benefits of tube feedings for frail nursing home residents, particularly in those with dementia, must be predicated not only on underlying illness but also on the resident/family's value system, resources available in the nursing home, and staff acceptance of the intervention. Given that the evidence for and against enteral feeding in nursing home residents is controversial, the practitioner must continue to individualize therapy. There are alternatives to enteral nutrition for residents with decreasing intake or dysphagia. One option is spoon-feeding which can provide physical, environmental, and social stimulation.

PRESSURE ULCERS

Pressure ulcers have a prevalence of 2.4 to 23 percent in long-term care facilities and an incidence of new ulcers up to 12 percent over a 6-month period. Pressure ulcers are a critically important issue in nursing homes as the development of a pressure ulcer in a low-risk patient is considered a sentinel event. The American Medical Director's Association has published clinical practice guidelines on pressure ulcers, which specifically address nursing home-related issues. Implementation of a wound care program may be an efficient, cost-effective means of addressing and preventing pressure ulcers in nursing homes. Programs that use practice guidelines such as those developed by the Agency for Health Care Policy and Research have been shown to reduce the incidence and length of time to pressure ulcer development. Key to the establishment of a wound care program is a specially trained wound care nurse to organize and oversee the program. This may be a luxury at some nursing homes, but the creation of this position should be a high priority given the breadth of the problem of skin care. Prior to implementation of a wound care program, measurement of the facilities incidence and prevalence of ulcers and pressure ulcer management protocols should be established to set appropriate goals. A wound care team including representation from medicine, nursing, therapy, nutrition, and a wound care nurse should be developed and round regularly. Systems should be established for referrals, data collection, documentation, and orders. Program interventions might include risk assessment, skin assessment/protection, nutritional assessment, pressure, shear and friction reduction, activity/mobility, and education.

POLYPHARMACY AND MEDICATION PRESCRIPTION

Medication prescription in the older nursing home resident is complicated by several factors. Polypharmacy is widespread in long-term care facilities, with an average of eight medications prescribed per resident. In the setting of age-related changes in pharmacokinetics and pharmacodynamics, this high number of medications provides the scenario for drug–drug and drug–disease interactions when new medications are added. Criteria determining inappropriate medication use in nursing home residents have been suggested. Additionally, in July 1999, the HCFA developed surveyor guidelines, which include a list of drugs and drug–diagnosis combinations with potential for adverse

outcomes in persons older than 65 years of age. Based upon these guidelines, physicians and pharmacists are required to justify the use of these drugs with details of alternative regimens, ongoing monitoring for adverse side effects, and documentation of attempts to lower doses or discontinue medications. Nursing home residents are expected to be maintained on no more than nine medications if possible. Adherence to this rule may compromise the standard of medical care for some nursing homes. For example, a resident with several chronic illnesses (diabetes, hyperlipidemia, and hypertension) may require multiple medications to control their illnesses. If health maintenance is practiced, they may be on additional medications such as a multivitamin, calcium, and vitamin D. If a bowel regimen is added, the number of medications easily exceeds nine. The authors believe careful documentation and justification of each medication targeted to each illness is equally as important as the actual number of prescribed medications.

Renal function should be considered when prescribing medications to older adults, particularly in a nursing home environment. One study examined the adherence of renal dosing guidelines in long-term care facilities and found that 34 percent of prescriptions were considered inappropriate for the calculated creatinine clearance of long-term care residents. Improper medication dosing is associated with adverse drug reactions, drug toxicity, hospitalization, and mortality.

Appropriate medication prescription involves coordination with the facilities' pharmacists to review the appropriateness, dosage, and clinical indication for each medication prescribed on a regular basis. Ideally, the pharmacist and the medical providers will have a cohesive linkage and open communication to discuss the pharmacist's recommendations, as this can potentially lead to important cost savings and a decrease in adverse drug reactions. The medical director or facility can also institute policies to improve the overall prescription of medications in compliance with state and federal regulations. Examples include automatic stop dates for certain medications such as antibiotics or prn medications not used, and regularly scheduled laboratory assessment of drug levels and renal function, liver function, and complete blood count as determined based upon potential side effects.

INFECTIONS AND INFECTION CONTROL

The nursing home population has profound vulnerability to infections as a consequence of decrements in host defense mechanisms related to age and chronic illness and the closed institutional environment. The average incidence rate is about 1 to 2 infections per resident per year, and most commonly involve the respiratory tract, urinary tract, and skin/soft tissue. It is highly recommended that each nursing home have an infection control program or policy with an appointed infection control practitioner. The reality in many homes is that this position becomes another job of the director of nursing or a staff nurse, who lack the necessary time and experience. Written policies and procedures are essential and should follow federal state and regulatory agency requirements. Comprehensive infection control programs that include hand washing and environmental cleaning and disinfecting reduce infections among older adults residing in long-term care facilities. Components of an infection control program include surveillance of infections; detection and control of outbreaks; isolation and precaution system; antibiotic use monitoring and microbial resistance patterns; education; resident and employee health programs; and reporting disease to authorities.

Nursing home-acquired pneumonia has been a distinct clinical entity since its description in 1978, and has a higher mortality rate and hospital transfer rate than do other nursing home-acquired infections. Risk factors for pneumonia among nursing home residents include dependence in activities of daily living, age, bed-fast state, aspiration, dysphagia, feeding tubes, sedative-hypnotic drug use, cognitive impairment, and cardiac and pulmonary disease. Data on risk factors for pneumonia mortality specifically in nursing home residents is limited but includes, dependence in activities of daily living, hypothermia, infiltrate on chest radiograph, tachypnea, and comorbidity score. An eight-variable predictive model for 30-day mortality includes serum urea nitrogen, white blood cell count, absolute lymphocyte count <800/L, pulse, male sex, activities of daily living, body mass index, and deterioration in mood in past 90 days.

The pathogenesis of pneumonia in older adults is believed to result primarily from aspiration of organisms colonizing the oropharynx. Definitive bacteriologic diagnoses are not often pursued in the nursing home setting because of difficulty with specimen collection. Older studies document that the common pathogens are similar to those for community-acquired pneumonia and include *Streptococcus pneumoniae* (20 percent), *Haemophilus influenzae* (10 percent), *Staphylococcus aureus* (10 percent), aerobic gram-negative bacilli (30 percent), and normal flora (15 percent). Outbreaks from influenza A, influenza B, and respiratory syncytial virus have all been documented.

Diagnostic and therapeutic guidelines were recently recommended. The chest radiograph is believed by most to be the "gold standard" of diagnosis as clinical signs and symptoms may be atypical in the nursing home resident. A subtle change in functional or cognitive status or tachypnea can be the sole initial clinical finding, often detected by astute nursing staff. Sputum examination is not directly recommended. Prior studies of expectorated sputum do not reveal etiologic organisms in most cases, coupled with the difficulty of obtaining adequate specimens in older adults. Blood cultures may be helpful in identifying the etiologic organism if positive and white blood cell counts may aid in determining severity of infection. Serum chemistries may influence a provider's choice of antibiotics and allow calculation of creatinine clearance to appropriately dose antibiotics or antiviral agents.

The decision to hospitalize for pneumonia has received much attention in the literature. Many infections can and should be treated in the nursing home setting, as clinical outcomes may not be significantly different. Hospitalization decisions will be based on patient-related factors such as prior advanced directives or patient and family wishes regarding acute hospitalization, high-risk clinical indicators,

and clinical factors such as oxygen saturation, vital signs, acute cognitive decline, fluid intake, and uncontrolled co-morbid illness. Additionally, the nursing home environment will also dictate the level of care that can be provided to the patient with pneumonia based on the availability of RN coverage, frequency of vital sign assessment, parenteral hydration, and laboratory access.

Treatment of pneumonia in the nursing home is primarily on an empiric basis targeting *S. pneumoniae, H. influenzae, S. aureus,* and gram-negative rods. Various treatment regimens are acceptable, but the recent recommendations for empiric therapy are an antipneumococcal quinolone or a Beta- lactam and a newer macrolide for a total of 10 to 14 days.

Nursing homes must take a multifaceted approach to the prevention of pneumonia. This includes minimizing the incidence of aspiration; optimizing nutritional status; cautious use of sedative-hypnotic medications; ensuring regular dental care; establishing and enforcing a tuberculosis surveillance program for all staff and nursing home residents; and administration of the pneumococcal and influenza vaccination. The medical director can also play an active role in prevention by assuring updated infection control policies and procedures; by collaborating with the pharmacist and infection control practitioner to ensure appropriate antibiotic use; by assuring the availability and review of antibiograms; by issuing automatic stop orders for antibiotics; and by making dose adjustments for renal impairment. Implementation of standard protocols for the diagnosis and treatment of nursing home acquired pneumonia is also recommended.

PALLIATIVE CARE

Palliative care has become increasingly important in the nursing home, where one in five Americans will eventually die and where there is a substantial amount of physical and psychological suffering. While pain has been reported in over half of nursing home residents, a sizable percentage of residents with pain remain undertreated. Furthermore, advance directives, when they exist, often lack specificity to effectively guide care in the setting of an acute or chronic life-threatening illness. Hospice is commonly used in nursing homes and appears to be as effective as when it is provided for individuals residing in the community. The fact that nursing home residents have only an 11-day median survival time versus 19 days for community dwellers speaks to the need to initiate end-of-life care sooner rather than later. Increasing awareness of the need for more comprehensive and targeted palliative care services has resulted in innovative quality improvement initiatives in nursing homes as well as incorporation of palliative care issues into the Minimum Data Set.

ROLE OF THE MEDICAL DIRECTOR

To ensure compliance with Medicare and Medicaid regulations, all nursing homes must appoint a medical director. While the roles and responsibilities of medical directors have been clearly delineated by national organizations, the unique culture and needs of individual nursing facilities dictate how these responsibilities are operationalized. Ideally, the medical director functions as chief of the medical staff and oversees the development of all policies and procedures relevant to medical care delivery, directs a medical quality improvement program, and, when necessary, serves as a public spokesperson for the nursing home. Unlike the chief of staff at an acute hospital, however, the nursing home medical director must work closely with all disciplines, constantly cognizant of the unique interplay between laws, ethics, regulations, and the organization of medical care. Medical directors are most effective when they can work closely with the facility administrator and director of nursing to foster true interdisciplinary team care and ongoing staff education.

The relationship between the medical director and the medical staff is critical in ensuring that all quality standards set forth by the medical director are instituted. Expectations must be clearly communicated and outcomes to be measured agreed upon. Medical directors who provide both primary patient care and administrative support often serve as key role models for other practitioners.

Certification for medical directors is offered through the American Medical Director's Association following completion of a formal course. Further information regarding medical director responsibilities, certification requirements, and relevant policies and procedures can be found on the American Medical Director's Association's web site (www.AMDA.com).

REFERENCES

Beers MH: Explicit criteria for determining potentially inappropriate medication use by the elderly. An update. *Arch Intern Med* 157:1531, 1997.

Casarett DJ et al: Does hospice have a role in nursing home care at the end of life? *J Am Geriatr Soc* 49:1493, 2001.

Fenner SP: Developing and implementing a wound care program in long-term care. *JWOCN* 26:254, 1999.

Hughes TL, Medina-Walpole AM: Implementation of an interdisciplinary behavior management program. *J Am Geriatr Soc* 48:581, 2000.

Jogerst G et al: Physician use of and attitudes regarding the minimum data set. *JAMA* 2:4, 2001.

Katz PR et al: Medical practice with nursing home residents: Results from the national physician professional activities census. *J Am Geriatr Soc* 45(8):911, 1997.

Kayser-Jones J et al. Factors contributing to dehydration in nursing homes: Inadequate staffing and lack of professional supervision. *J Am Geriatr Soc* 47:1187, 1999.

Krauss NA, Altman BM: *Characteristics of Nursing Home Residents—1996.* AHCPR Pub. No. 99-0006. Rockville, MD, Agency for Health Care Policy and Research, 1998.

Makris AT et al: Effect of a comprehensive infection control program on the incidence of infections in long-term care facilities. *Am J Infect Control* 28:3, 2000.

Medina-Walpole AM, Katz PR: Nursing home-acquired pneumonia. *J Am Geriatr Soc* 47:1005, 1999.

Mehr DR et al: Predicting mortality in nursing home residents with lower respiratory tract infection. The Missouri LRI study. *JAMA* 286:2427, 2001.

Morris JN et al: Nursing rehabilitation and exercise strategies in the nursing home. *J Gerontol* 54A:M494, 1999.

Ouslander J et al: *Medical Care in the Nursing Home,* 2nd ed. New York, McGraw-Hill, 1999.

Papaioannou A et al: Assessment of adherence to renal dosing guidelines in long-term care facilities. *J Am Geriatr Soc* 48:1470, 2000.

Ray WA et al: A randomized trial of a consultation service to reduce falls in nursing homes. *JAMA* 278:557, 1997.

Saliba D et al: Appropriateness of the decision to transfer nursing facility residents to the hospital. *J Am Geriatr Soc* 48:154, 2000.

Walshe K: Regulating US nursing homes: Are we learning from experience? *Health Aff (Millwood)* 20:128, 2001.

Yoshikawa TT, Ouslander JG (eds): *Infection Control in Long-Term Care.* New York, Marcel Dekker, 2002.

Community-Based Long-Term Care and Home Care

BRUCE LEFF

An estimated seven million older Americans require long-term care of some kind, mostly as a result of chronic medical conditions and illnesses that render them functionally impaired. The vast majority of these people live in the community, and their numbers are sure to increase over the coming decades as the population ages. However, the issue of how best to care for and pay for the care of frail, noninstitutionalized older persons is one that poses significant challenges. Most older persons, given a choice, would prefer to remain in the community rather than enter an institution, if the need arises. Family caregivers, who provide the bulk of community-based long-term care, and whose ranks are thinning relative to the increasing number of older persons, may prefer to have their family member remain in the community, but are often left to their own devices to provide and/or pay for such care. Policymakers and governments struggle with issues of how to provide quality long-term care in the community within budgetary constraints.

Community-based long-term care in the United States is decentralized and includes family or paid caregivers caring for an older person at home; adult day care; skilled home health care services provided by home health agencies under the Medicare system; custodial services under the Medicaid system and some local governments; and various types of residential settings ranging from the spartan to the luxurious. The heterogeneity among these models and access to them is emblematic of the fact that there is no organized regional or national system for community-based long-term care.

This chapter discusses community-based long-term care and home care in the United States as these relate to the care of older persons, recognizing that a substantial portion of those receiving such services are younger disabled persons. Evidence related to community-based long-term care and other models of home care and house calls, the role of physicians in home care, policy issues, and a look toward the future of home care in the US medical system are discussed.

SEMANTICS

Home care, *community-based long-term care*, and *house calls* are used interchangeably in the literature and can refer to any of a number of health care services provided in the home. Mostly these terms refer to nursing, hygienic, or formal or informal social support services provided to older disabled persons in need of chronic care, with the explicit goal of maintaining them in the community. Such care is usually provided by a family caregiver or one or more members of an interdisciplinary healthcare team, the latter under the general prescription of a physician. Home care may also refer to postacute hospital care, geriatric assessment services, prevention health strategies, formal rehabilitation services, and high-technology programs. Often, these services overlap and it can be difficult to put a discrete label on a service intervention. For example, a physician-led community-based house calls program that provides geriatric assessment and continuing longitudinal care to older persons upon discharge from the acute hospital using an interdisciplinary team may be difficult to categorize discreetly. These semantic difficulties have engendered substantial challenges in combining studies for meta analytic purposes, at times to the detriment of the field. For the purposes of this chapter, the *house calls* refers specifically to physician house calls and models of home care that include a significant physician component; otherwise *home care* or *community-based long-term care* is used, with the understanding that there is substantial overlap between these categories.

CHALLENGES IN STUDYING HOME CARE

Home care, in its many forms, has been studied extensively in the last several decades. In fact, some argue that home care is one of the most studied of all health services interventions. This reflects, in some measure, the fierce beliefs of some that home care itself is a virtue that should not be discarded even in the absence or relative dearth of data supporting its use. However, it also reflects the fact that regardless of the model of home care or house calls that is examined, there are inherent difficulties in studying the interventions. In studies of community-based long-term care, these difficulties are especially complex and include the ability to allocate resources randomly, controlling for severity of illness or disability, significant subject attrition, concurrent changes in the health care system, and examination of varied outcome measures. Finally, there is a "black box" phenomenon. That is, home care interventions tend to be complex and multifaceted. Hence, it is difficult to understand the effect of individual components of an intervention or identify that part of an intervention responsible for its success or failure. In addition, it is often difficult to combine these studies for the purposes of meta analysis because they often differ with regard to the targeted population, the specific nature of the home care intervention, or the outcomes evaluated.

COMMUNITY-BASED LONG-TERM CARE

Community-based long-term care usually refers to the provision of personal care services or health care to persons in their homes with the goal of maintaining them in the community rather than moving them to an institutional setting such as a nursing home. By some estimates, for every person in a nursing home, there are as many as three persons in the community who are equally impaired or frail. The majority of community-based long-term care services, up to 80 percent by some estimates, are provided by informal caregivers. While home care and community-based long-term come under the rubric of the health care system, much of what it provides is in the social realm. Formal services cover a wide range. Some are provided under the Medicare home health benefit such as skilled nursing care, physical therapy, occupational therapy, social work, and a home health aide. Medicaid also provides services. These services vary by state with some mix of skilled and unskilled services provided, with an emphasis on the latter, providing ongoing supportive custodial services. Other formal services fall outside the Medicare home health benefit and include services such as meals on wheels, homemaker services, congregate meals, respite care, adult day care, adult protective services, and case management services. Area agencies on aging are an excellent source of information on the nature and availability of these services in one's own community.

Recently, there has been a wave of new programs at the state level that have introduced consumer-directed home-based services. In such models, the responsibility for key service decisions is shifted from professionals to care recipients. Home care recipients can choose to hire and pay their family member to provide community-based long-term care services with state funds. Early studies suggest that they may be less costly than professionally directed services and associated with improved client satisfaction and quality of life.

In the academic realm, community-based long-term care has been studied extensively. This research has been difficult and criticized for a number of reasons. Studies often lacked methodologic sophistication. Studies lumped together under the rubric of "home care" or "community-based long-term care" were, in fact, describing many different types of interventions, some social, others medical, and still others combining medical and social approaches. In addition, the studies targeted disparate populations of patients and examined a variety of outcome measures. Data will be presented related to community-based long-term care, adult day care, life care at home, and two integrated models of care, the Program of All-Inclusive Care for the Elderly (PACE), and social health maintenance organizations (SHMO). These models are aging-in-place models. Multilevel residential facilities, typically called continuing care retirement communities, are becoming increasingly popular with older persons. Other residential facilities include group and foster homes, sheltered housing, and assisted living facilities. Table 18-1 depicts the basic characteristics of these care models.

Studies of community-based long-term care have been reviewed in depth by Hedrick (1986) and her colleagues. The Channeling National Long-term Care Demonstration Project was a massive study, carried out in 10 states in the United States. It compared case management with and without an infusion of a broad array of purchased services. The trial served a very frail population. However, the intervention failed to lower hospital use or nursing home placement or to affect the function abilities of patients. There was no major effect on the provision of informal caregiving, and there was increased use of formal community services. The comprehensive assessment and follow-up did decrease unmet care needs, produced a transient improvement in life satisfaction, and appealed to caregivers. This important and essentially negative study set a pessimistic tone for home care research; that home care may be preferred by patients but difficult to justify on clinical grounds, especially in a time of budgetary constraints. However, in a recent landmark study by Shaughnessy, a national demonstration program with more than 150,000 patients studied in 54 home health agencies achieved a greater than (1989) 20% reduction in hospitalization and a 7.7% selective improvement in targeted clinical outcomes. The quasi-experimental intervention was the use of an outcomes-based quality improvement program.

In addition, meta-analysis of the effects of home care on mortality and nursing home placement by Hedrick (1989) demonstrated a small, beneficial effect of home care on mortality that fell short of statistical significance, and stronger evidence of a reduction in nursing home placement. Another meta-analysis by Hughes found a small to moderate positive impact of home care in reducing hospital days, ranging from 2.5 to 6 days per 180 days of follow up. A more recent meta analysis by Stuck (2002) of various types of home visit programs found that such programs are effective. Programs that provided more than 9 follow-up visits, when compared to those offering fewer follow-up visits, were associated with lower rates of admission to nursing home (relative risk 0.66); programs with multidimensional assessment, when compared to those without multidimensional assessment, were associated with better functional outcomes (relative risk 0.76); programs that focused on the

Table 18-1   Community-Based Long-Term Care Services Requiring a Change in Residence

	Usual Architecture	Funding	Services Provided in Addition to Room and Board	Comments
Continuing care retirement community	Community— bungalow, apartments, condominium	Private pay—most require substantial entry fee and monthly fee for rent and supportive services. Usually very expensive	Social, cultural, educational, recreational facilities	Allows for aging in place with transition from independent to assisted living to nursing home care
Group home	Single-family home	Private—costs shared by residents	Usually some assistance with activities of daily living	Licensed in most states
Foster home	Single-family home	State department of social services subsidy	Assistance with activities of daily living by sponsoring family or paid caregiver	Facilities licensed in some states
Assisted-living facility	Apartment-like building	Mostly private, some Medicaid programs subsidize in lieu of nursing home placement	Social supportive services	Licensed in some form by all states
Sheltered housing	Apartment-like building	Department of Housing and Urban Development (HUD) subsidy	Social work services	

young old (approximately 73 to 77 years old) rather than old old (approximately 80 to 82 years old) were associated with reduced mortality (relative risk 0.76).

Adult day care or senior centers provide social and medical programs for older persons in the community. Social programs focus on highly functional and independent older persons, while medically oriented adult day care focuses on a frailer population and in addition to social programs and activities, have a primary medical component. Adult day care is usually privately financed, although Medicaid provides some coverage for eligible persons. Adult day care has been studied formally. The Adult Day Health Care (ADHC) Evaluation Study had two components: a randomized controlled trial of ADHC compared with usual care in eight Veteran's Administration Medical Centers and a prospective cohort study comparing community-based ADHC with Veteran's Administration-based ADHC and usual care. In this well-designed and well-implemented study, there were no differences in health outcomes between groups and costs were generally higher in the intervention groups. One subgroup of patients, those with severe disabilities, had lower nursing home, clinic, home care, pharmacy, and laboratory costs. Patients with moderate and low levels of disability and few behavioral problems had significantly higher costs.

A life care at home care model is analogous to a continuing care retirement community (see Table 18-1), but

for the fact that the patient remains in the patient's own home, rather than moving to a retirement community setting. There are several variations of this model, but most charge an entrance and monthly fee that provides lifelong in-home skilled and unskilled care in the event that the participant develops an impairment in function, usually defined as an impairment in one ADL.

The Program of All-Inclusive Care for the Elderly (PACE), is an integrated health care system that provides all acute and long-term care services for approximately 8000 frail older persons at approximately 25 sites across the United States. The model, derived from the On Lok experience in San Francisco, uses a day health center model and provides primary care by an interdisciplinary team, specialty care by contract, and other services, including home care, transportation, durable medical equipment, acute hospital care, and nursing home care. PACE enrollees are required to be nursing home eligible and both Medicare and Medicaid eligible or, in some states, be willing to spend down to Medicaid eligibility. The PACE providers receive a combined, regionally adjusted Medicare and Medicaid capitation for each of its members and is responsible for all the health care needs of the PACE member. Because of the capitation model, PACE is free to spend monies outside standard Medicare rules and may, for example, provide skilled home care services to patients who would not meet Medicare standards for skilled service eligibility. The average

PACE enrollee is approximately 80 years of age with 7 to 8 medical conditions and 2.7 limitations in activities of daily living. In early studies, PACE appears to be a quality, cost-effective model. Congress has made PACE a legislated benefit, meaning that any healthcare organization meeting certain criteria can apply to open a PACE site.

SHMOs started in the middle 1980s. Like PACE, SHMOs attempt to deliver integrated acute and long-term care services, but serve the full range of Medicare beneficiaries, not just low-income, disabled seniors. The SHMO receives the Medicare capitation and provides usual Medicare benefits as well as limited long-term care services. Studies suggest that the first round SHMOs did not realize the true integration of medical and social services, nor did they achieve cost savings compared with the fee-for-service sector. A second round of SHMOs is currently underway that will attempt to better integrate care, implement more extensively geriatric principles of care, and focus on patients with chronic illnesses, as well as disability. Capitation rates have been adjusted to improve the economic feasibility of the model.

MODELS OF HOME CARE

Data related to specific home care models are reviewed: physician house calls/interdisciplinary home care, home geriatric assessment, postacute hospital disease-specific home-based case management strategies, and home hospital. In general, these models of home care, are notable for targeting specific at-risk populations and delivering a tailored home care intervention, often with some level of physician involvement.

Physician House Calls/Interdisciplinary Home Care

The literature describes several physician house calls programs. These programs are usually designed to provide longitudinal medical care to frail, usually older, patients for whom making an office visit is a hardship. Some of these programs are academic hospital-based programs, and in addition to providing a needed service to such patients, serve a significant medical educational function for medical students and resident trainees in geriatrics training and in fostering positive attitudes toward older persons. Others have been established in the private, fee-for-service sector. This market niche seems to be expanding, especially as physician reimbursement rates were increased under the Medicare system and physicians realized that practices devoted to home care substantially reduce the office-based component of overhead expenses.

Successful programs share several key organizational features. A functioning multidisciplinary team of physicians, nurses, home health aides, social workers, and therapists dedicated to the program is critical to success. The linchpin of many such programs is a patient or program coordinator whose function it is to orchestrate the function of

this team. Team meetings occur on a regularly scheduled, often weekly, basis to allow group discussion of active patients. These programs have been termed "interdisciplinary home care" to distinguish them from typical community-based long-term care programs, and the integration of medical and supportive services are the critical element in their success. Such programs have been able to demonstrate improvement in function, reduced costs, decreased medication use, improved satisfaction, better end-of-life care, and fewer nursing home admissions and outpatient visits.

Comprehensive Home Geriatric Assessment and Prevention Models

Comprehensive geriatric assessment (CGA) is a process of evaluation designed to identify patient problems in several spheres and to provide targeted interventions with the aim of improving clinical outcomes for patients. In theory, the home is an ideal environment in which to implement CGA because patients can be examined in the reality of their daily lives, allowing accurate assessment of medical, functional, psychological, and social issues. Results of these studies have varied, probably as a result of differences in the precise nature of various home CGA interventions, as well as differences in research design, targeted populations, and outcomes assessed. Meta-analysis by Stuck and colleagues (1993) found that home CGA had a favorable effect on mortality. One of the more interesting studies from this period by Stuck (1995) and colleagues, was of a home-based CGA that targeted patients older than age 75 years from voter registration roles and consisted of initial assessment by a nurse practitioner, review with a geriatrician, and every 3-month follow-up by the nurse practitioner to monitor implementation of the recommendations that came out of the initial CGA. Importantly, in complex situations, the study personnel contacted the patient's primary physician directly. Employing this strategy, 47 percent of recommendations were implemented. The intervention resulted in a higher level of physical function and decreased admission to nursing homes. A more recent systematic review by van Haastregt of a variety of home-based interventions included under the CGA rubric, suggested that although some studies demonstrated positive outcomes, the evidence was unclear that home CGA consistently improved specific outcomes related to physical or psychological function, falls, admissions to institutions, or mortality.

Postacute Hospital Disease-Specific Home-Based Case Management Strategies

The home has been used as the site of case management models focused on the care of specific medical conditions. The case management model includes identification of suitable patients, care planning, and intervention. The majority of studies have focused on patients with common costly conditions such as congestive heart failure. In a seminal randomized controlled study by Rich, study patients received intensive education by nurses regarding their illness, dietary assessment and instructions by a dietitian, discharge planning by a social worker, review and consolidation of medical regimen by a gerocardiologist, and intensive follow-up by nurses by phone and home visits, with continued physician involvement in the decision process. The intervention resulted in a significant reduction in the number of readmissions for heart failure and in the number of multiple readmissions. It remains unclear which element or combination of elements of this intervention was most important in producing these beneficial effects. Translating this and similarly positive studies into results at health systems levels has yet to be demonstrated.

Home Rehabilitation Care

Providing rehabilitation care following a stroke has several theoretical advantages. These include avoiding prolonged stays in inpatient rehabilitation settings, the ability to personalize the rehabilitation approach to maximize function, satisfying patient choice, and cost savings. Several randomized controlled trials have been performed in the United Kingdom and Australia. Consistently, these studies demonstrate that home-based rehabilitation following stroke is feasible, acceptable to patients and caregivers, and as effective as hospital-based rehabilitation. End points such as cost savings, functional advantages, and caregiver stress demonstrate more variability.

Home Hospital

Although the acute hospital represents the current paradigm of care for acutely ill patients, the hospital environment may not be ideal for older patients. Iatrogenic complications and functional decline are common among hospitalized older persons. Varied models of home hospital have been described. The most attractive from a geriatric viewpoint are those that substitute entirely for an inpatient admission. Other programs have been developed that facilitate early hospital discharge by providing services that many in the United States would consider standard post acute hospital discharge home care. Most home hospital studies have come from the United Kingdom and Australia, countries with national health insurance schemes. Although a recent review of the evidence on home hospital concluded that home hospital had no notable effects on patients' or caregivers' health and had mixed cost effects, this review may have suffered from inclusion of studies of models that were not truly home hospital models and selection of inappropriate outcomes. Randomized controlled trials of home hospital for older persons that have substituted entirely for an acute inpatient admission of medical illnesses have demonstrated comparable clinical outcomes, reduced length of stay, and striking reductions in important geriatric complications such as confusion, urinary and bowel complications. Home hospital is a model in evolution. A demonstration study of home hospital is currently

being conducted in the United States in the Medicare managed care and Veterans Administration settings. Results are expected from this study in 2003.

DISSEMINATING MODEL PROGRAMS OF HOME CARE

Although a number of home care models have been demonstrated to be effective, it has been difficult to translate favorable results in home care into practical home care models for the general public. This is a result of a number of factors: a relative dearth of physicians who wish to provide home care, a system of home care that requires medicalization of what are often social issues; few or no incentives in the health care system to provide such care; and the difficulties inherent in health care systems adapting models of home care to their own environment. The reasons for this difficulty in translating models of care into widespread reality are complex and have been discussed by Boult and colleagues.

THE ROLE OF THE PHYSICIAN IN HOME CARE

Despite the fact that much home care occurs in the absence of physicians, physicians nonetheless must play an important role in providing care in the home. The focus of the physicians role varies, to some extent, by the nature and circumstances of the patient, whether it be long-term care, postacute care home care, or acute care. In long-term care, the physician provides ongoing medical services, coordinates activities of the interdisciplinary team when skilled services are involved, and serves as an advocate for the patient, referring them to appropriate community services to foster continued independence. In postacute care and home rehabilitation care, the focus is on restoring function and completing the management of medical problems. The interdisciplinary care team provides much of the care in this setting. In acute home care, the physician is actively involved in management of acute illness. Physician home visits and close coordination of the interdisciplinary care team are crucial in this setting to assess and manage the patient.

PRACTICAL REGULATORY ISSUES RELATED TO THE PRACTICE OF HOME CARE MEDICINE

Medicare will pay for certain home care services and physicians who care for older persons should be familiar with the basic entry criteria for Medicare home health services. First, the patient must be homebound, defined loosely that the patient needs significant assistance to leave home or that it requires considerable effort. The patient need not be absolutely homebound to meet this requirement. Medicare, developed in the 1960s, was designed as an acute illness benefit, rather than insurance to help care for the long-term care of older persons with chronic conditions. As such, the Medicare home health benefits are linked to transitions from the acute care settings (i.e., hospital or skilled nursing facility) to what Medicare refers to as a "skilled need." A skilled need represents services that can be provided only by a skilled health care professional, for example, nursing services, physical therapy services, or speech therapy services. Skilled services fall into four categories: observation and assessment, teaching and training, therapy, and management and evaluation of a care plan. If the patient is homebound and requires skilled services of some type, then other services become available for the patient under the Medicare benefit as long as the skilled need persists. These additional services include home health aide services, occupational therapy, and social work services. Services must be intermittent for Medicare to reimburse. The rationale for this requirement is to prevent Medicare home health services from becoming a de facto long-term care benefit. Intermittent services cannot total more than 35 hours a week, nor can they usually occur on a daily basis. In addition, the skilled need must be reasonable and necessary. The Medicaid system for low-income persons also pays for home health care. Medicaid is a state administered program and eligibility and benefits vary by state. Medicaid commonly pays for custodial and personal care services for ongoing support of daily living needs. In addition, in certain states, Medicaid may pay for some skilled services.

The physician is responsible for certifying the plan of care by signing the Health Care Financing Administration (HCFA, now Center for Medicare and Medicaid Services [CMS]) Form 485. The physician should review the plan of care, services to be provided, and patient's medications. The patient will not receive care nor will the home health agency receive payment for its services until the physician has properly signed the document. In addition, physicians can bill Medicare part B services for certifying the plan of care as well as for providing care plan oversight (CPO), services provided in overseeing and coordinating the care of a home care patient. To bill for CPO, the physician must have been seen the patient in the previous 6 months and the physician must spend at least 30 minutes in a month on the patient in providing care plan oversight. Such plan oversight time includes time spent discussing the patient with interdisciplinary team members, coordinating care, talking with pharmacist. Time spent talking with family members may not be counted toward care plan oversight. Eligibility requirements for Medicare home health benefits, definitions of services, physician requirements, and billing issues have been reviewed in detail by Oldenquist and colleagues.

Recently, changes have been made in Medicare home health care in the areas of reimbursement at the level of the home health agencies. In the early and mid-1990s, home health care was the fastest growing component of the Medicare system. However, by 1997, this growth in home health care, marked regional variations in utilization, insufficient proof that such expenditures provided savings in other areas of the health care system, and the suspicion of fraud and abuse within the system provided the impetus for the Balanced Budget Amendment of 1997 (BBA). The BBA established a prospective payment system (PPS) for home health care services. Under PPS, Medicare home health agencies are paid prospectively in 60-day increments on the basis of assignment of a home health patient into a Home Health Related Group (HHRG). HHRGs are determined by using 18 items on the 89-item Outcome Assessment Information Set (OASIS). Although OASIS was developed as a tool to determine patient needs and to facilitate care plan development and quality improvement in home health, it is now a requirement for Medicare home health and must be completed at the start of care and then every 60 days that care is provided. Recent data on the ability of OASIS to enhance home health agency performance suggest strongly that outcome-based quality improvement using OASIS can produce significant patient benefits in reducing hospitalization and improving health status. Under PPS and other provisions of the BBA, many home health agencies failed and by early 2000, Medicare home health spending dropped by approximately 50 percent. The effects on beneficiaries are not yet known.

TECHNOLOGY AND TELEMEDICINE

In the last few years there has been considerable interest in technology and telemedicine as a means to expand the role of home care medicine in the US health care system. In the technology realm, certain devices once found only in the hospital are now relatively commonplace in the home. Such items include ultrasound, electrocardiography, infusion therapies, pulse oximetry, feeding pumps, ventilators, and hand-held blood analyzers, to name but a few. Telemedicine comes in various forms, including store-and-forward services that collect clinical data, store them, and forward them to be interpreted later; self-monitoring and testing telemedicine services that enable physicians to monitor physiologic measurements, test results, images, and sounds; and clinician interactive telemedicine services that are real time clinician patient encounters. A review of telemedicine services by the Agency for Healthcare Research and Quality identified several hundred telemedicine programs in the US. The review concluded that the use of telemedicine was small but growing, and demonstrated that the technology can work and can be used beneficially from clinical and economic standpoints and that further studies were necessary.

SUMMARY

Currently, the long-term care system in the United States is fragmented and decentralized. Home care in its various forms constitutes a significant part of that system and allows older persons to retain their independence. Studies suggest that community-based long-term care is effective. There are models of home care and house calls that are effective, although barriers exist to their widespread implementation. Technological developments will likely help home care to continue to develop. However, the influence of health care policy in the home care realm, especially payment policy, will be crucial to develop the proper incentives to ensure home care's proper place in the health care system.

REFERENCES

Benjamin AE: Consumer-directed services at home: a new model for persons with disabilities. *Health Affairs* 20:80, 2001.

Binstock RH, Cluff LE (eds): *Home Care Advances.* New York, Springer, 2000.

Boult C et al: Systems of care for older populations of the future. *J Am Geriatr Soc* 46:499, 1998.

Calkins E et al (eds): *New Ways to Care for Older People—Building Systems Based on Evidence.* New York, Springer, 1999.

Callahan JJ: Do we need a surgeon general's report on home and community based services? A personal and policy journey. *Gerontologist* 41:149, 2001.

Caplan GA et al: Hospital in the home: A randomized controlled trial. *Med J Aust* 170:156, 1999.

Hedrick SC et al: Meta-analysis of home care effects on mortality and nursing home placement. *Med Care* 27:1015, 1989.

Hedrick SC, Inui TS: The effectiveness and cost of home care: An information synthesis. *Health Serv Res* 20:851, 1986.

Hedrick SC et al: Summary and discussion of methods and results of the adult day health care evaluation study. *Med Care* 31:SS94, 1993.

Hersh WR, Wallace JA, Patterson PK, et al. Telemedicine for the Medicare Program. Evidence Report/Technology Assessment No. 24 (Prepared by Oregon Health Sciences University, Portland, OR under Contract No. 290-97-0018). AHRQ Publication No. 01-E012. Rockville (MD) Agency for Healthcare Research and Quality. July 2001.

Hughes SL et al: Impact of home care on hospital days: A meta analysis. *Health Serv Res* 32:415, 1997.

Leff B, Burton JR: The future history of home care and physician house calls in the United States. *J Gerontol A Biol Sci Med Sci* 56A:M603, 2001.

McCall N et al: Medicare home health before and after the BBA. *Health Aff (Millwood)* 20:189, 2001.

Oldenquist GW et al: Home care: What a physician needs to know. *Cleve Clin J Med* 68:433, 2001.

Rich MW, Beckham V, Wittenberg C, Leven CL, Freedland KE, Carney RM. A multidisciplinary intervention to prevent the readmission of elderly patients with congestive heart failure. *N Engl J Med.* 1995 Nov 2;333(18):1190–5. PMID: 7565975 [PubMed-indexed for MEDLINE]

Shaughnessy PW et al: *Improving Patient Outcomes of Home Health Care: Findings from Two Demonstration Trials of Outcome-Based Quality Improvement,* JAGS 50:1354–1364, 2002.

Soderstrom L et al: The health and cost effects of substituting home care for inpatient acute care: A review of the evidence. *CMAJ* 160:1151, 1999.

Steel K et al: A home care annotated bibliography. *J Am Geriatr Soc* 46:898, 1998.

Stuck AE et al: Comprehensive geriatric assessment: A meta-analysis of controlled trials. *Lancet* 342:1032, 1993.

Stuck AE et al: A trial of annual in-home comprehensive geriatric assessments for elderly people living in the community. *N Engl J Med* 333:1184, 1995.

Stuck AE et al: Home visits to prevent nursing home admissions and functional decline in elderly people. Systematic review and meta-regression analysis. *JAMA* 287:1022, 2002.

Tell EJ et al: Life care at home: A new model for financing and delivering long-term care. *Inquiry* 24:245, 1987.

van Haastregt JC et al: Effects of preventive home visits to elderly people living in the community: A systematic review. *BMJ* 320:754, 2000.

Weissert WG, Hedrick SC: Lessons learned from research on effects of community-based long-term care. *J Am Geriatr Soc* 42:348, 1994.

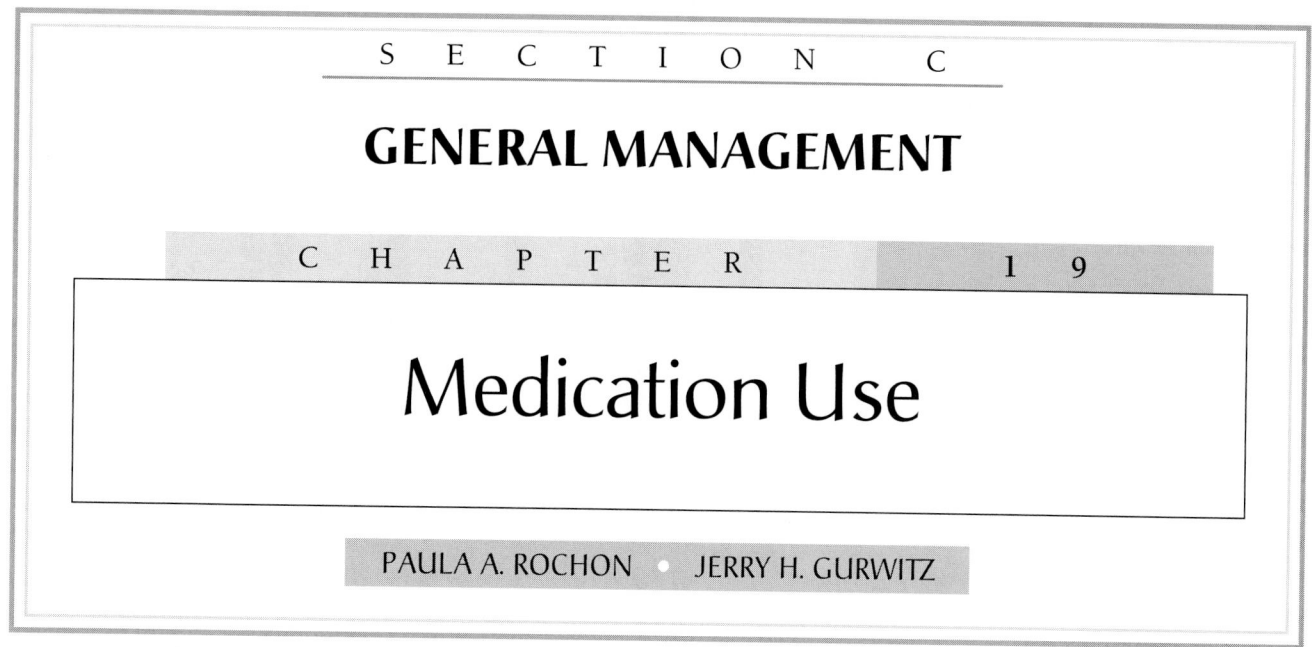

S E C T I O N   C

GENERAL MANAGEMENT

C H A P T E R   1 9

Medication Use

PAULA A. ROCHON • JERRY H. GURWITZ

Prescribing for older patients offers special challenges. Older people take about three times as many prescription medications as do younger people, mainly because of an increased prevalence of chronic medical conditions among the older patient population. Taking several drugs together substantially increases the risk of drug interactions and adverse events. Many medications need to be used with special caution because of age-related changes in pharmacokinetics (i.e., absorption, distribution, metabolism, and excretion) and pharmacodynamics. For some drugs, an increase in the volume of distribution (e.g., diazepam) or a reduction in drug clearance (e.g., lithium) may lead to higher plasma concentrations in older patients than it does in younger patients. Pharmacodynamic changes with aging may result in an increased sensitivity to the effects of certain drugs, such as opioids, for any given plasma concentration. The pharmacokinetic and pharmacodynamic changes with aging have been discussed extensively elsewhere.

While a physician can usually do little to alter the characteristics of individual older patients to affect the kinetics or dynamics of drugs, the decision whether to prescribe any drug, the choice of drug, and the manner in which it is to be used (e.g., dose and duration of therapy) are all factors that are under control of the prescriber. This chapter discusses ways to optimize prescribing of drug therapy for older adults.

EPIDEMIOLOGY OF DRUG THERAPY

Writing a prescription is the most frequently employed medical intervention. Yet, creating optimal drug regimens that meet the complex needs of older persons requires thought and careful planning. Avoidable adverse drug events are the most serious consequences of inappropriate drug prescribing. Advanced age, frailty, and increased drug utilization are all factors that contribute to an individual patient's risk for developing a drug-related problem. As many as 28 percent of hospital admissions for older patients result from drug-related problems. Up to 70 percent of these drug-related admissions are attributed to adverse drug reactions.

A random sample of 2590 noninstitutionalized older adults in the United States during the years 1998 and 1999 provides information on the use of prescription and over-the-counter medications in the community. This survey demonstrated that use of all medications (prescriptions, over-the-counter drugs, vitamins/minerals, and herbals/supplements) (Fig. 19-1) and the use of prescribed drug therapies (Fig. 19-2) increases dramatically with advancing age. The highest prevalence of medication use was among women aged 65 years and older. Among these women, 12 percent took 10 or more medications and 23 percent took at least 5 prescribed drug therapies. The widespread use of over-the-counter drug therapies identified in this survey indicates the importance of routinely inquiring about their use when evaluating a drug therapy regimen.

Herbal medicines are frequently used by older adults; physicians often do not question patients about such use. An estimated 14 percent of the US population takes an herbal medicine or supplement such as ginseng, ginkgo biloba extract, and glucosamine. In a survey of 1539 adults, 34 percent of whom were 50 years of age or older, almost 75 percent did not inform their physician that they were using unconventional treatments including herbal medicines. Herbal medicines may interact with prescribed drug therapies leading to adverse events, underscoring the

219

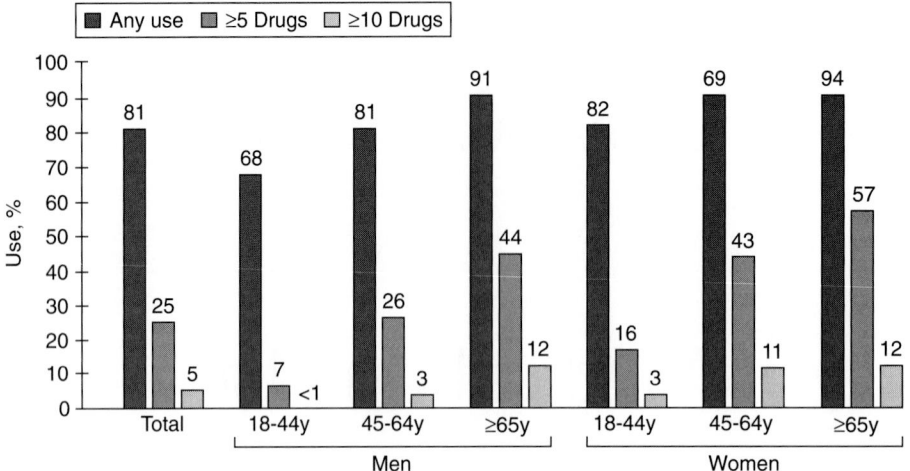

Figure 19-1 Use of medications during the preceding week, by sex and age. Adapted from Kaufman (2002).

importance of routinely questioning patients about their use of these unconventional therapies. Examples of herbal–drug therapy interactions include warfarin in combination with ginkgo biloba extract leading to an increased risk of bleeding and serotonin-reuptake inhibitors in combination with St. John's wort leading to serotonin syndrome in older adults.

MEASURING THE QUALITY OF DRUG PRESCRIBING IN OLDER PERSONS

Various criteria have been developed by expert panels in Canada and in the United States to assess the quality of medication use in elderly patient populations. The most widely used criteria employed for the assessment of inappropriate prescribing are based on the Beers criteria. These criteria were developed in 1991 by a consensus panel of experts in geriatric medicine, geriatric psychiatry, and pharmacology to evaluate inappropriate prescribing in nursing home residents. This expert group identified a list of medications considered inappropriate for older patients, either because they are ineffective or because they pose a high risk for adverse events. The list included

long-elimination half-life benzodiazepines (e.g., diazepam) and hypoglycemics (chlorpropamide), antidepressants with strong anticholinergic properties (e.g., amitriptyline) and ineffective dementia treatments (e.g., cyclandelate). The Beers criteria were revised in 1997 to make them more relevant to current prescribing issues and to generalize them beyond the nursing home setting.

Use of drug therapies considered inappropriate according to the Beers criteria has been identified as an ongoing problem among community-dwelling older adults. Using the subset of the 20 drug therapies that should be entirely avoided, 23.5 percent of community-dwelling older adults in the United States, as identified using the 1987 National Medical Expenditure Survey, were found to be taking one or more of the inappropriate medications. More recently, a panel of seven experts recategorized the 33 medications deemed inappropriate according to the Beers criteria into three groups: (1) drugs that should always be avoided (e.g., barbiturates, chlorpropamide); (2) drugs that are rarely appropriate (e.g., diazepam, propoxyphene); and (3) drugs with some indications, but that are often misused (e.g., oxybutynin, diphenhydramine). Using these three categories of inappropriate drug therapy, 2455 respondents to the 1996 Medical Expenditure Panel Survey were

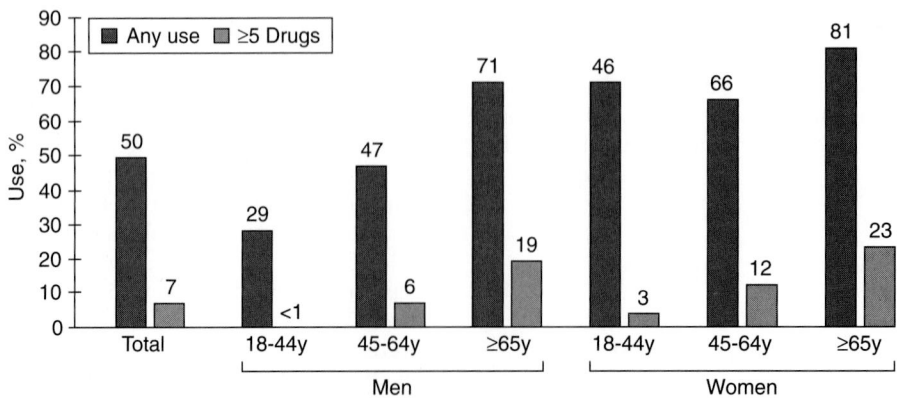

Figure 19-2 Use of prescription drugs during the preceding week, by sex and age. Adapted from Kaufman (2002).

evaluated; 20 percent were found to be using at least one of these potentially inappropriate drug therapies. Three percent used at least 1 of the 11 drug therapies that the panel determined should always be avoided by older adults.

The Health Care Financing Administration expert consensus panel drug utilization review criteria have also been used to evaluate inappropriate prescribing in community-dwelling older adults. These criteria target eight prescription drug classes (i.e., digoxin; calcium channel blockers; angiotensin-converting enzyme inhibitors; histamine-2 receptor antagonists nonsteroidal antiinflammatory drugs (NSAIDs); benzodiazepines; antipsychotics; and antidepressants) and focus on four types of prescribing problems: (1) use of an inappropriate dosage; (2) duplication of therapies; (3) potential for drug–drug interactions; and (4) inappropriate duration of therapy. Based on the criteria, almost 20 percent of 2508 community-dwelling older adults were found to be using one or more medications inappropriately. NSAIDs and benzodiazepines were the drug classes identified with the most frequent potential problems.

Unfortunately, the vast majority of medications that are commonly implicated in preventable adverse drug events are not identified by these widely used "bad drug" lists. Inappropriate prescribing is often more subtle, more pervasive, and often unrecognized. "Good drugs" prescribed in an inappropriate manner may be far more common and problematic. Very few drugs that cause difficulty for older adults are inherently bad. When drugs do cause problems, it is because they are prescribed, dosed, taken, combined with other medications, or monitored inappropriately. Our ability to assess the quality of medication use in older patients remains limited because of a lack of appropriate assessment methods.

Quality indicators were developed as a way for improving the appropriate use of medication by older adults. Knight and Avorn identified 12 quality indicators for appropriate medication use. Table 19-1 describes each of the 12 indicators and summarizes the rationale for its need. These indicators start with the need to document the indication for a new drug therapy, to educate patients on the benefits and risks associated with the use of a new therapy, the need to maintain current medication lists in patient medical records, the importance of documenting response to therapy and the need for a periodic review of drug therapies. In addition, these indicators specify seven drug therapies that either should not be prescribed for older adults (i.e., hypoglycemic agent chlorpropamide, drugs with strong anticholinergic properties, barbituates, and meperidine) or that warrant careful monitoring after they have been initiated (i.e., warfarin, diuretic, and angiotensin-converting enzyme inhibitor therapy).

PRESCRIBING CASCADES

Perhaps the most concerning aspect of suboptimal medication use in the elderly relates to the occurrence of prescribing cascades. A prescribing cascade begins when an adverse drug event is misinterpreted as a new medical condition. An additional drug therapy is prescribed, and the patient is placed at risk for the development of additional adverse drug events relating to this potentially unnecessary treatment (Fig. 19-3). Prescribing cascades and other risks associated with drug therapy are particularly important for older adults with multiple chronic diseases who are likely to be prescribed multiple drug therapies. Selected examples of prescribing cascades are described below.

Drug-Induced Parkinsonism

Among 95 new cases of Parkinson's disease from community-dwelling older adults referred to a geriatric medicine department in the United Kingdom, more than half were found to have drug-induced parkinsonism. Neuroleptic medications such as haloperidol, prochlorperazine, and thioridazine were among the major drug therapies implicated.

The association between neuroleptic drug exposure and subsequent treatment of parkinsonism was identified among 3512 adults aged 65 to 99 years who were enrolled in a Medicaid program and initiated on a drug therapy for the treatment of parkinsonian symptoms. Patients dispensed a neuroleptic therapy in the 90 days prior to the initiation of anti-Parkinson's therapy were more than five times more likely to begin anti-Parkinson's therapy relative to control patients who were not dispensed neuroleptic therapy. Furthermore, a dose-response relationship was demonstrated.

Neuroleptic therapy is widely used in older adults for the management of behavioral problems associated with dementia. Antidopaminergic-related adverse effects associated with these agents have long been recognized, including the development of extrapyramidal signs and symptoms. This drug-related symptom may be potentially misdiagnosed as a new medical condition (i.e., Parkinson's disease). Patients who are placed on antiparkinsonian therapy then become vulnerable to the adverse events associated with this new therapy, including hypotension and delirium. A better approach is to discontinue or reduce the dose of the neuroleptic therapy. If a neuroleptic is deemed essential, it is prudent to select a therapy with a more favorable adverse effect profile and to use this therapy at the lowest feasible dose. Even newer agents have adverse effects at higher doses.

Drug-induced parkinsonism has also been reported with other drug therapies, including metoclopramide. A case-control study of adults aged 65 years and older in the New Jersey Medicaid Program demonstrated that metoclopramide users were three times more likely to begin drug treatment for Parkinson's disease as compared with nonusers. Risk increased with increasing daily metoclopramide dose such that the odds ratio was 1.19 for up to 10 mg/d, 3.33 for 10 to 20 mg/d, and 5.25 for >20 mg/d. Thus, drug-induced parkinsonism may lead to the initiation of anti-Parkinson drug therapy. Such drug-induced symptoms in an older person can be misinterpreted as indicating the presence of a new disease or be attributed to the aging process rather than to the drug therapy. This misinterpretation is particularly likely when the symptoms are indistinguishable from an illness, such as Parkinson's disease that is seen in greater frequency in older persons.

Table 19-1   Quality Indicators for Appropriate Medication Use in Older Adults

Indicator Title	Description	Rationale
Indication	When prescribing a new drug, the therapy should have a clearly defined indication documented in the medical record.	The medication may have been prescribed for an indication that was unclear or transient.
Patient education	When prescribing a new drug, the patient or caregiver should be educated about the optimal use of the therapy and the anticipated adverse events.	Education may improve adherence, clinical outcomes, and alert patients or caregivers to potential adverse events.
Medication list	Medical records (outpatient or hospital) should contain a current medication list.	Allows identification and elimination of duplicate therapies, corrects drug interactions, and streamlines the drug regimen to improve adherence.
Response to therapy	Every new drug prescribed on an ongoing basis (e.g., for a chronic condition) should have documentation of response of therapy within 6 months.	Provides a rationale for continuation of the therapy if effective, or change or discontinuation if ineffective.
Periodic drug review	Annual drug regimen review.	Provides an opportunity to discontinue unnecessary therapy or to add needed drug therapies.
Monitoring warfarin therapy	When warfarin is prescribed, international normalized ratio (INR) should be evaluated within 4 days and at least every 6 weeks.	Older adults are at high risk for drug toxicity that can be identified earlier if there is close monitoring for agents with a narrow therapeutic range.
Monitoring diuretic therapy	When a thiazide or loop diuretic therapy is prescribed, electrolytes should be checked within 1 week after initiation and at least annually.	Risk of hypokalemia because of diuretic therapy.
Avoid use of chlorpropamide as a hypoglycemic agent	When prescribing an oral hypoglycemic agent, chlorpropamide should not be used.	This therapy has a prolonged half-life that can result in serious hypoglycemia and is more likely than other agents to cause the syndrome of inappropriate secretion of antidiuretic hormone.
Avoid drugs with strong anticholinergic properties	Do not prescribe drug therapies with a strong anticholinergic effect if alternative therapies are available.	These therapies are associated with adverse events such as confusion, urinary retention, constipation, and hypotension.
Avoid barbituates	If older adult does require the therapy for control of seizures, do not use barbiturates.	These therapies are potent central nervous system depressants, have a low therapeutic index, are highly addictive, cause drug interactions, and are associated with an increased risk for falls and hip fracture.
Avoid meperidine as an opioid analgesic	When analgesia is required, avoid use of meperidine.	This therapy is associated with an increased risk for delirium and may be associated with the development of seizures.
Monitor renal function and potassium in patients prescribed angiotensin-converting enzyme inhibitors	If angiotensin-converting enzyme inhibitor therapy is initiated, potassium and creatinine levels should be monitored with 1 week of initiation of therapy.	Monitoring may prevent the development of renal insufficiency and hyperkalemia.

SOURCE: Adapted from Knight EL and Avorn J (2001).

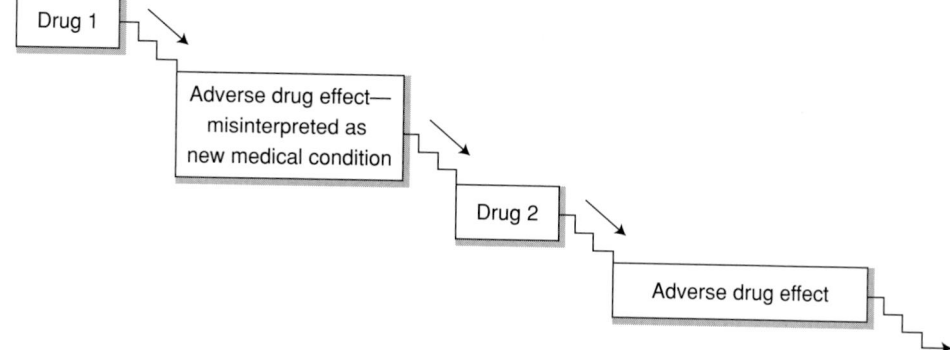

Figure 19-3 Prescribing cascade.

NSAID Therapy and Hypertension

The effects of NSAIDs in elevating blood pressure have been documented and are most apparent in patients with existing hypertension. The antiinflammatory properties of NSAIDs appear to result from their ability to inhibit cyclo-oxygenase, a critical enzyme in the biosynthesis prostaglandins. There is good evidence to suggest an important role of prostaglandins in the modulation of two major determinants of blood pressure, vasoconstriction of arteriolar smooth muscle and control of extracellular fluid volume.

In a case-control study of older patients in the New Jersey Medicaid Program, patients who were initiated on an antihypertensive medication were compared with a similar number of randomly selected control patients. The adjusted odds ratio for the initiation of antihypertensive therapy for recent NSAID users as compared to nonusers was 1.66. Given the widespread use of NSAID use by elderly persons and the complications associated with hypertension, this association could have important public health implications for the care of older patients. The challenge is for the clinician to recognize the association between NSAID use and blood pressure elevations, so that the initiation or intensification of antihypertensive therapy may be avoided. Because NSAID therapy is available as an over-the-counter preparation, it is important to obtain information on use of all therapies including prescribed medications and over-the-counter preparations.

Other prescribing cascade scenarios, such as the association between the use of hydrochlorothiazide therapy and the initiation of antigout therapy, have been identified. Many more potential prescribing cascades will become apparent as physicians carefully consider the relationship between the initiation of a new drug therapy, the adverse event profile of that therapy and the development of a new medical condition. The increased recognition of similar prescribing scenarios hopefully will reduce the occurrence of inappropriate prescribing decisions.

UNDER USE OF BENEFICIAL THERAPY

Prescribing strategies that seek to simply limit the overall number of drugs prescribed to older adults in the name of improving quality of care may be misdirected. For example, a patient with a myocardial infarction may be prescribed three essential drug therapies: a betablocker, an angiotensin-converting enzyme (ACE) inhibitor, and acetylsalicylic acid. If this patient has elevated lipid levels and diabetes, three or more additional medications may be required. Accordingly, many elderly persons may benefit from taking six or more essential medications. Underuse of beneficial drug therapy by older adults may be associated with increased morbidity, mortality, and reduced quality of life. This suggests a need for a more complex model for assessing the quality and appropriateness of prescribing for older persons than simply counting the number of different medications that a patient is receiving. This complex model should be directed toward assessing the potential benefit versus harm of the patient's total medication regimen.

For patients of advanced age with multiple medical problems, secondary prevention may not be given a high priority. Among patients 65 years of age or older who have a chronic condition, unrelated diseases often go untreated. For example, older adults with diabetes as indicated by insulin use, were significantly less likely to be dispensed estrogen replacement therapy (for osteoporosis prevention) relative to patients without this condition (2.4 percent relative to 5.9 percent, p < 0.001). Similarly patients with psychotic syndromes, as indicated by use of haloperidol, were significantly less likely to be dispensed arthritis therapy relative to patients without psychoses (18 percent relative to 27 percent, p < 0.001). While an understanding of the logic behind these decisions for individual patients remains uncertain, potential explanations for under treatment include "a belief that treatment of the patient's primary problem is enough; a judgment that the adverse effects of additional medications are too great and the benefits insufficient; or a patient's preference for taking fewer medicines." Selected examples of underprescribing of beneficial therapy are described below.

Example of Undertreatment: Hypertension

Despite the availability of guidelines to facilitate hypertension management, this condition is inadequately treated even when physicians are monitoring their patients in a clinic. For example, among 800 men with hypertension with a mean age of 65 years receiving care in Veterans Affairs outpatient clinics in New England, approximately 40 percent had a blood pressure of 160/90 mmHg despite an average of more than six hypertension-related visits in a year. At visits in which a diastolic blood pressure of <90 mmHg and a systolic blood pressure of >165 mmHg were recorded, increases in the antihypertensive regimen occurred only 22 percent of the time. The systolic hypertension in the elderly person (SHEP) study demonstrated that treating isolated systolic hypertension in people 60 years of age and older reduced the risk of stroke by 36 percent (p = .0003) and also reduced major cardiovascular events relative to the placebo condition.

Example of Underuse of Beneficial Therapy: Betablocker Therapy Postmyocardial Infarction

Studies demonstrate that older adults, including those at high-risk for poor outcomes, benefit from betablocker therapy postmyocardial infarction. The relation between betablocker use and subsequent mortality was evaluated among New Jersey Medicare recipients sustaining an acute myocardial infarction between 1987 and 1992. Among those dispensed betablocker therapy, mortality was decreased by 43 percent relative to nonrecipients of this agent (aRR = 0.57). In a sample of "ideal" betablocker therapy candidates in the Cooperative Cardiovascular Project's cohort of myocardial infarction survivors between 1994 and 1995, being discharged from hospital with a prescription for betablocker therapy was associated with a 14 percent mortality reduction.

Withholding betablocker therapy may be most harmful to seniors of advanced age and with potential contraindications to betablocker therapy. Among 201,752 seniors participating in the Cooperative Cardiovascular Project, patients at high-risk for betablocker related complications (i.e., patients with heart failure, pulmonary disease, and diabetes) obtained substantial mortality reduction when prescribed betablocker therapy relative to those who were not prescribed this treatment. For example, patients with congestive heart failure treated with betablocker therapy had a 40 percent mortality reduction relative to nonrecipients. Despite this knowledge, observational studies document continued underprescribing of betablocker therapy to seniors some 20 years after these agents were proven effective in randomized control trials (RCTs).

Example of Underuse of Beneficial Therapy: Osteoporosis

Osteoporosis is a common condition, particularly among older women. Guidelines are available for the management of the condition (see Chap. 75). To treat osteoporosis, it must first be diagnosed. Despite increasing attention, this condition continues to be underdiagnosed. The findings obtained from the National Osteoporosis Risk Assessment (NORA) study illustrate this problem. The NORA study is a longitudinal observational study of more than 200,000 postmenopausal women to evaluate the relationship between bone mineral density and the risk for fractures. Ambulatory, postmenopausal women with no previous diagnosis of osteoporosis and not on osteoporosis therapy (i.e., bisphosphonate, calcitonin, or raloxifene) were eligible. Of the patients evaluated 39.6 percent were classified as having osteopenia and 7.2 percent with osteoporosis. Among the individuals with follow-up information at 1 year, those

with osteopenia were almost twice as likely to develop a fracture relative to those with normal bone mineral density. Those older women with a diagnosis of osteoporosis were four times as likely to develop a fracture during the 1 year of follow-up relative to those with a normal bone mineral density. These findings suggest that undiagnosed low bone mineral density is very common in postmenopausal women and is associated with a high rate of fractures. Improved measures aimed at primary prevention in combination with better diagnosis could lead to better outcomes for older women.

Example of Underuse of Beneficial Therapy: Opioid Analgesia and Cancer Pain

Opioid analgesia reduces pain and improves quality of life for cancer patients. Underprescribing of analgesia for cancer pain means that older patients may suffer needless discomfort. Pain guidelines are available to assist physicians in managing pain associated with metastatic cancer. In a study of 1308 outpatients with metastatic cancer being followed by oncologists, 769 patients reported experiencing pain, which 62 percent described as being substantial. Furthermore, older patients were more likely than younger patients to report that their pain was not being adequately managed. Older persons may be at risk of undertreatment because of a reluctance to prescribe opioid analgesics to older cancer patients. If analgesics are prescribed, the dose may not be adequate to achieve pain control. Efforts to address underprescribing of beneficial therapy in the elderly population must focus on educating healthcare providers, improving the adherence to prescribed drug regimens by older patients, and reducing the financial barriers to access to essential medications.

Underuse of Beneficial Therapy: Warfarin in Atrial Fibrillation

Warfarin is recommended in evidence-based guidelines for stroke prevention for older adults with atrial fibrillation, but is often inappropriately prescribed to older adults in long-term care setting. Among 429 residents of long-term care facilities with atrial fibrillation, 42 percent were prescribed warfarin therapy. Of the 83 older adults who were classified as being "ideal" candidates for warfarin therapy (i.e., no known risk factors for hemorrhage), only half (53 percent) were prescribed this therapy. Furthermore, international normalized ratio (INR) readings were often found to be either below or above the therapeutic range. In fact, INR values were maintained in the therapeutic range only 51 percent of the time, placing patients at unnecessary risk for an adverse event, despite long-term care residents residing in a supervised setting.

A more systematic approach to decision making regarding the use of warfarin for stroke prevention in frail older persons would be welcome. An organized strategy would encourage more appropriate use of warfarin therapy and help to maintain patients receiving warfarin in the therapeutic range. More widespread use of specialized anticoagulation clinics in order to provide coordinated anticoagulation care may offer an option to improve the effectiveness and safety of warfarin therapy in this particularly high-risk group of patients.

SPECIAL CONSIDERATIONS REGARDING DRUG THERAPY IN THE LONG-TERM CARE SETTING

Long-term care residents include a disproportionate number of women, people of advanced age, and those with multiple medical problems, in particular dementia. Of all types of therapeutic interventions, medications are the most commonly used in the nursing home setting. The average US nursing home resident uses 6 different medications; more than 20 percent use 10 or more different drugs, placing this group at increased risk of adverse drug events.

Neuroleptic Therapy in the Long-term Care Setting

In long-term care facilities excess use of neuroleptic therapy for the management of behavioral problems is an area of concern. An Institute of Medicine report on improving the quality of care in nursing homes in the United States, determined that excessive use of neuroleptic therapy was evidence of poor quality of care.

Concern about overuse of neuroleptic therapy led to the introduction of guidelines and legislative action in the United States designed to reduce neuroleptic therapy use in long-term care. As a result of these US federal regulations implemented in 1990, the indication for treatment with a neuroleptic therapy now has to be documented, nonpharmacologic approaches must be tried first, and a record of gradual reduction of therapy has to be on file after 6 months of treatment. Following the institution of these federal guidelines, neuroleptic therapy in nursing homes decreased by 27 percent with no compensatory increase in use of other psychoactive medications.

Risk of Adverse Drug Events in the Long-term Care Setting

The occurrence of adverse drug events that may have been prevented is among the most serious concerns regarding suboptimal medication use in the nursing home setting. Few studies have systematically examined the incidence of adverse drug events in the nursing home population. A retrospective review of incident reports relating to adverse and unexpected events in an academically oriented, 700-bed, long-term care facility identified 50 reports of adverse drug reactions over a 1-year period. Skin rashes were the most frequently reported events, and antibiotics were the most commonly implicated medication category. The limited number of reports of drug-related events suggests that voluntary reporting systems in the nursing home setting lead to very-low reporting rates of only a very narrow spectrum of events.

In a study of all long-term care residents of 18 community-based nursing homes in Massachusetts over a 12-month observation period, drug-related incidents were detected by reports by nursing home staff and by periodic review of all nursing home resident records by trained nurse and pharmacist investigators. Incidents were classified by physician reviewers, according to whether they represented an adverse drug events, and if so, the severity (significant, serious, life-threatening, and fatal) and preventability of the event. During 28,839 nursing home resident-months of observation in the 18 participating nursing homes, 546 adverse drug events were identified (1.89 adverse drug events per 100 resident-months). Of all adverse drug events, 1 was fatal, 31 (6 percent) were life-threatening, 206 (38 percent) were serious, and 308 (56 percent) were significant. Overall, 50.5 percent of adverse drug events were judged preventable. Of the 238 fatal, life-threatening, or serious adverse drug events, 72 percent were considered preventable, compared with 34 percent of the 308 significant adverse drug events. Psychoactive drugs (i.e., antipsychotics, antidepressants, and sedatives/hypnotics) and anticoagulants were the most commonly implicated drug categories associated with the occurrence of preventable adverse drug events (Table 19-2). Confusion, oversedation, delirium, falls, and hemorrhagic events were the most commonly identified preventable adverse drug events (Table 19-3). Errors resulting in preventable adverse drug events occurred most often at the stages of ordering and monitoring. Transcription, dispensing, and administration errors were less commonly identified. Independent risk factors for experiencing a preventable adverse drug event included having a greater comorbidity burden and being on a higher number of medications. Extrapolating from the results of this research, 350,000 adverse drug events per year may occur among US nursing home residents and more than half may be preventable. There are almost 20,000 fatal or life-threatening adverse drug events per year, of which 80 percent may be preventable. Drug-related morbidity and mortality is an important area to target in efforts to both improve the quality of medical care for older persons and reduce the costs of healthcare for this population.

Failures in the design of systems of care often contribute to the occurrence of medical errors, as well as the injuries that result from some of those errors. Enhanced surveillance and reporting systems for adverse drug events occurring in the nursing home setting are required as are continued educational efforts relating to the optimal use of drug therapies in the frail elderly patient population. However, as Leape concluded in regard to the occurrence of serious medication errors in the hospital setting, "Preventive efforts that focus solely on the individual provider or which rely on inspection alone have limited impact. Analysis and the correction of underlying systems faults is much more likely to result in enduring changes and significant error reduction." Ordering and monitoring errors in the nursing home setting may be particularly amenable to prevention strategies that use systems-based approaches. The benefits of such an approach to error reduction in the hospital setting that uses computerized order entry have been reported; such a system could be designed to focus on ordering and monitoring issues in the nursing home. Successes in the hospital setting pave the way for similar efforts in the

Table 19-2   Frequency of Adverse Drug Events and Potential Adverse Drug Events by Drug Class*

Drug Class	Adverse Drug Events No. (%) (n = 546)	Preventable Adverse Drug Events No. (%) (n = 276)	Nonpreventable Adverse Drug Events No. (%) (n = 270)
Antipsychotics	125(23)	72(26)	53(20)
Antibiotics/antiinfectives	109(20)	13(5)	96(36)
Antidepressants	68(13)	50(18)	18(7)
Sedatives/hypnotics	68(13)	49(18)	19(7)
Anticoagulants	51 (9)	37(13)	14(5)
Antiseizure	47(9)	27(10)	20(7)
Cardiovascular	35(6)	25(9)	10(4)
Hypoglycemics	27(5)	14(5)	13(5)
Nonopioid analgesics	22(4)	13(5)	9(3)
Opioids	15(3)	7(3)	8(3)
Antiparkinsonians	12(2)	7(3)	5(2)
Gastrointestinal	11(2)	6(2)	5(2)

*Drugs in more than one category were associated with some events. Frequencies in each column sum to greater than the total number of events.
Adapted from Gurwitz (2000).

nursing home setting aimed at reducing drug-related injuries and disability and improving the quality of care provided to the frail elderly patient population.

DEFICIENCIES IN INFORMATION ABOUT DRUG THERAPY IN OLDER ADULTS

Selecting the right medication and the right dose to prescribe for an older person is difficult because so little evidence is available to guide choices. Decision-making often has to draw on information obtained from the experience of patients very different from those encountered in clinical practice, where patients often have several medical conditions and are taking more than one drug. The findings of clinical trials of treatments for conditions commonly affecting older people cannot directly be extrapolated to that age group, as older persons, particularly frail persons and those with multiple illnesses, have often been excluded from participation in such studies. There are several ways in which the quality and availability of information about the use of drugs in older persons might be improved. These include enhancing the inclusion of older persons in drug trials, and using observational studies and systematic reviews to provide information to guide clinical decision making.

Inclusion of Older Persons in Clinical Trials

More than two decades ago the United States Food and Drug Administration published Guidelines for the Study of Drugs Likely to be Used in the Elderly. The guideline was intended to encourage routine and thorough evaluation in elderly populations of the effects of new drugs being proposed for federal approval so that physicians would have sufficient information to use such drugs properly in their older patients. The guidelines state "there is no good basis for the exclusion of patients on the basis of advanced age alone, or because of the presence of any concomitant illness or medication, unless there is a reason to believe that the concomitant illness or medication will endanger the patient or lead to confusion in interpreting the results of the study." In short, drug trials should include subjects that reflect the group that would eventually be prescribed the therapy.

Despite these guidelines, older adults, continue to be underrepresented in clinical trials. For example, while almost 50 percent of older people report some form of arthritis, RCTs of NSAID therapy include few older people and hardly any older than age 85 years. National funding agencies, particularly the National Institutes of Health in the United States, have also developed guidelines to ensure that the trials they fund adequately represent women. These guidelines are very important for older adults because women outnumber men in the older age groups. While these guidelines have been received with enthusiasm, their impact on the inclusion of older women in clinical trials is less encouraging. For example, despite the fact that 80 percent of deaths caused by acute myocardial infarction occur in persons aged 65 years and older, older patients continue to be excluded from clinical trials. In a review of 214 randomized trials of treatments for acute myocardial infarction, 60 percent were found to exclude patients older than 75 years of age. Similarly, it was found that women represented, on average, less than a quarter of participants in trials evaluating the benefit of drug therapy for myocardial infarction. In a comparison of the inclusion of elderly

Table 19-3 Frequency of Adverse Drug Events by Type*

Type	Adverse Drug Events (n=546)	Preventable (n=276)
Neuropsychiatric	150(27)	83(30)
Falls	67(12)	55(20)
Gastrointestinal	65(12)	30(11)
Dermatologic/allergic	59(11)	7(3)
Hemorrhage	57(10)	40(14)
Extrapyramidal symptoms/tardive dyskinesia	52(6)	19(7)
Infection	34(6)	1 (0.4)
Metabolic/endocrine	27(5)	14(5)
Anorexia/weight loss	20(4)	14(5)
Ataxia/difficulty with gait	18(3)	9(3)
Cardiovascular	15(3)	10(4)
Electrolyte/fluid balance abnormality	9(2)	5(2)
Syncope/dizziness	8(1)	5(2)
Functional decline†	7(1)	6(2)
Respiratory	3(0.5)	3(1)
Anticholinergic‡	3(0.5)	2(0.7)
Renal	3(0.5)	1 (0.4)
Hematologic	2(0.4)	2(0.7)
Hepatic	1 (0.2)	1 (0.4)

*Adverse drug events could manifest as more than one type.

†Adverse drug event manifested only as decline in activities of daily living without any other more specific type of event. Other types of events may have been associated with functional decline.

‡Anticholinergic effects include dry mouth, dry eyes, urinary retention, and constipation.

Adapted from Gurwitz et al (2000).

persons and women in trials of acute coronary syndromes (myocardial infarction, unstable angina, or acute coronary syndromes) published between 1966 and 1990 relative to those published between 1991 and 2000, trials with explicit age-related exclusion criteria were noted to decrease from 58 percent to 40 percent in more recent years. The inclusion of older patients (i.e., 75 years of age and older) increased from 2 percent between 1966 and 1990 to 9 percent between 1991 and 2000. The inclusion of women in these trials increased from 20 percent from 1966 to 1990 to 25 percent in the more recent years. However, this number remains below the number of women presenting with myocardial infarction. These findings suggest that federal guidelines have not yet met their expectation.

Using Alternative Study Designs to Study Drug-Related Risks and Benefits

Using alternative study designs as a complement to clinical trials may help to improve the quality and availability of information about the use of drug therapy by older persons. RCTs have long been considered the gold standard for evaluating the efficacy of a drug therapy. Ethical concerns may prevent the inclusion of the very impaired and the very old in RCTs and it may be unrealistic to expect these studies to include adequate numbers of all relevant subgroups in the elderly population. In addition, there is mounting concern that such clinical trials are not the optimal way to evaluate adverse drug events in older adults. Drug trials are of relatively short duration. Drug-related problems that present months after initiating therapy may not be identified during the course of these relatively short trials. In general, drug trials focus on the efficacy of the therapy and give less emphasis to the potential risks associated with the use of the therapy. For example, in a survey of 192 randomized drug trials, the severity of clinical adverse events was adequately defined in fewer than 40 percent of the published trials. The amount of text devoted to the discussion of the adverse events was similar to that given to the listing of contributors name and affiliations, suggesting underreporting of adverse events. Furthermore, the older persons included in RCTs have fewer comorbid illnesses than their age-matched peers. Thus, RCT results may not reflect the benefits or adverse effects of medications in frailer older persons or persons with multiple chronic illnesses.

Well-designed observational studies provide a promising approach for evaluating the relative risk and benefit of new drugs among subgroups of older persons who were not represented in clinical trials. Observational data may detect rare adverse events that become of major public health importance when a drug therapy is taken by very large numbers of people. For example, a study of adults 60 years and older from the Tennessee Medicaid program found that patients currently dispensed an NSAID were almost five times more likely as those not dispensed an NSAID to die from a peptic ulcer or a gastrointestinal hemorrhage. This study made an important contribution to alerting health care providers to important risks associated with commonly used therapy.

Observational data may also provide information about the benefits of drug therapy at doses that were not evaluated in clinical trials. The major RCTs demonstrating the benefit of betablocker therapy postmyocardial infarction evaluated doses of betablocker therapy that are higher than those generally used in clinical practice. Using linked Ontario provincial databases, 10,991 myocardial infarction survivors were identified who were dispensed one of the evaluated betablocker therapies (i.e., atenolol, metoprolol, propranolol, or timolol). Almost 90 percent received a lower dose of a betablocker than have been evaluated in a clinical trial. Among 13,623 older myocardial infarction survivors in the province of Ontario, relative to those not dispensed betablocker therapy, the adjusted risk ratios for mortality were lower for all three doses (low, standard, or high) of betablocker therapy. In a study from the United States, myocardial infarction survivors dispensed betablocker therapy at doses less than half of that evaluated in clinical trials received substantial benefit from the therapy. These findings support the strategy of initiating betablocker therapy at low dose and titrating the dose as tolerated.

While there are many challenges in using observational data, careful attention to design and methodologic issues maximize the likelihood of obtaining high quality usable data. Inception cohorts using strict criteria ensure the identification of the populations at risk and the time of exposure. Risk-adjustment techniques enable the modeling of outcomes controlling for observed differences between exposed and unexposed groups. Despite their limitations, observational studies provide valuable information on the benefits and harms of medications when prescribed to actual patient in a real world setting.

Systematic Reviews to Guide Therapeutic Decision Making

A systematic review provides another important source of information. Systematic reviews can be a useful way to organize and synthesize the vast amount of information available from clinical trials, which, individually, may include relatively small numbers of older people. By combining the information from older individuals obtained from a series of trials, useful information can be retrieved. Standardized reporting of trial data by age would make such analyses easier. The high quality systematic reviews produced and maintained by the Cochrane Collaboration provide important information to improve the care of older adults with a specific medical condition. For example, in a systematic review of the evidence for pharmacotherapy for hypertension treatment in elderly persons, 15 hypertension trials involving 21,908 adults who were at least 60 years of age or older were evaluated. This review demonstrated that treating hypertension in elderly persons, at least the spectrum of elderly persons included in RCTs, reduces coronary heart disease and cerebrovascular morbidity and mortality. Systematic reviews can be used to summarize data and inform clinical decisions that clinicians have had to make empirically.

Better representation of older and frailer adults in clinical trials, the evaluation of the risks and benefits of drug therapy through the use of observational data, and the use of high-quality systematic reviews are examples of ways to improve the quality of information available to clinicians in making prescribing decisions for older patients. In the meantime, limitations on what is known about drug treatments for many common conditions in older persons suggest the need for special care in prescribing and extra caution in considering use of new products in older patients.

POLICY ISSUES RELATED TO DRUG THERAPY IN OLDER ADULTS

A prescription may be written but not filled, or filled and not taken regularly, because of financial considerations. The use of drug therapy has been shown to be directly related to coverage of drug costs. It is estimated that more than 40 percent of all Medicare enrollees in the United States have no coverage for outpatient drug expenditures. In the United States, cost has been identified as an important reason that patients did not take medication that was prescribed by their health care provider. Specifically, among older adults, cost was identified by 7.7 percent with no prescription coverage, 3 percent with partial coverage, and 2 percent with full coverage as being the factor responsible for older adults taking less than the prescribed amount of their drug therapy.

Enhanced drug coverage for elderly persons may encourage the use of beneficial treatments. Among two groups of Medicare patients with heart disease, statin use ranged from 4.1 percent in those without coverage to 27 percent in those with employer-sponsored drug coverage (p < .001). Significant differences were also seen for use of relatively inexpensive betablocker therapy (20.7 percent versus 36.1 percent; p = .003) and nitrates (20.4 percent versus 38.0 percent; p = .005). This study suggests that older adults without drug coverage are less likely to be dispensed inexpensive life-saving drug therapy relative to those with drug coverage. Whether this difference is caused by the differences in drug coverage or to differences in characteristics of persons with and without such coverage is not clear.

Limited Manufacturing of Low-Dose Formulations of Recommended Drug Therapy

Limited manufacturing of low-dose formulations of drug therapy may make it more difficult for patients to take their prescribed drug therapy. Low-dose therapy is often recommended for older adults. For example, there is considerable evidence supporting the efficacy and greater safety, of low doses of thiazide diuretic therapy in the treatment of hypertension in the older patient population. The Joint National Committee on Detection, Evaluation and Treatment of High Blood Pressure (JNC VI) guidelines and the *Canadian Guidelines for the Treatment of Uncomplicated Hypertension* suggest starting antihypertensive therapy at low doses in all patients. Specifically, these guidelines suggest that therapy be initiated with a 12.5 mg dose of a thiazide diuretic. Low doses of thiazide diuretics (e.g., 12.5 mg of hydrochlorothiazide) often produce as large an antihypertensive effect as larger doses, with a reduced risk of metabolic abnormalities. In fact, there is evidence that a dose of hydrochlorothiazide as low as 6.25 mg can be as efficacious in treating hypertension in many older patients, when combined with a low dose of another antihypertensive medication.

PRACTICAL APPROACH TO PRESCRIBING MEDICATIONS TO OLDER PERSONS

Review Current Drug Therapies

A periodic evaluation of the drug regimen that a patient is taking is an essential component of the medical care of an older person. Such a review may indicate the need for

Table 19-4 Practical Steps to Consider in Optimizing Drug Regimens for Older Adults

Review current drug therapy
Discontinue unnecessary therapy
Consider adverse drug events as a potential cause for any new symptom
Consider nonpharmacologic approaches
Substitute with safer alternatives
Reduce the dose

SOURCE: *Modified from Rochon PA, and Gurwitz JH (1995).

changes to prescribed drug therapy. These changes may include discontinuation of a therapy prescribed for an indication that no longer exists, substitution of a required therapy with a potentially safer agent, reduction in dosage of a drug that the patient still needs to take, or an increase in dose or even addition of a new medication (Table 19-4). The physician should ask the patient to bring to the visit all of the bottles of pills that they are using. For example, patients may not consider over-the-counter products, ointments, vitamins, ophthalmic preparations, or herbal medicines to be drug therapies. Patients need to be specifically told to bring these therapies to the visit. In addition, patients should be instructed to keep a complete, accurate, and up-to-date medication list including over-the-counter medications and herbal preparations. This list should be brought to every physician visit. A patient-generated list is particularly important as patients are prescribed medications from several physicians and receive their medications from several pharmacies. Although there are an increasing number of effective medications for preventing or controlling a range of illnesses and for alleviating many symptoms, several studies show that adherence decreases, and adverse medication effects increase, with the complexity of the medication regimen. The goal should thus be the simplest regimen that controls the patient's symptoms and illnesses, and optimizes disease prevention. A medication grid which displays each medication with dosage and frequency has been found effective at facilitating the reduction in medication complexity.

Discontinue Potentially Unnecessary Therapy

Physicians are often reluctant to stop medications, especially if they did not initiate the treatment and the patient seems to be tolerating the therapy. Sometimes, however, this exposes the patient only to the risks for an adverse event with limited or no therapeutic benefit. The use of chronic digoxin therapy among older adults with normal systolic function is one such example. Use of digoxin therapy by older adults is not without risk. Renal impairment that progresses over time or dehydration associated with a gastrointestinal or respiratory illness, or urinary tract infection, may predispose older adults to digoxin toxicity.

Often digoxin therapy has been prescribed for years for reasons that were not well documented. In a small study of 23 nursing home residents with normal sinus rhythm, normal ejection fraction and no clinical evidence of heart failure, digoxin was discontinued in 14 residents. One patient developed a decreased ejection fraction (from 60 to 50 percent) and digoxin therapy was restarted even though the patient remained clinically asymptomatic. At 2 months following the discontinuation of digoxin therapy, all patients with digoxin therapy discontinued remained clinically stable. These findings suggest that digoxin can be safely discontinued in selected nursing home residents. Other investigators, however, have found that discontinuation of digoxin therapy in patients with impaired systolic function can have a detrimental effect.

Physicians should carefully consider whether the development of a new medical condition could be linked to an existing drug therapy before adding a new drug therapy to the patient's drug regimen. For example, tricyclic antidepressants such as amitriptyline are used for a variety of indications in elderly patients, from depression to the relief of chronic pain. The tricyclic antidepressants tend to have especially strong anticholinergic properties with the potential for side effects including constipation. A patient started on a strongly anticholinergic antidepressant may develop constipation. As a result, laxative therapy may be prescribed. A better alternative may be to discontinue the anticholinergic therapy.

Consider Nonpharmacologic Approaches

Physicians should limit prescribing of a new drug therapy to situations in which benefits clearly out weigh risks and to use drug therapy only after potentially safer alternatives have been attempted. For example, NSAIDs may be extremely useful in treating patients with rheumatoid arthritis. However, the use of this medication to manage pain in older adults with osteoarthritis may be inappropriate because safer options are available. Epidemiologic and clinical studies have characterized the adverse consequences of NSAID use in older persons, particularly the association between NSAID use and gastrointestinal bleeds and renal impairment. Thus, alternative approaches should be considered before NSAIDs are prescribed for indications such as osteoarthritis. Possible nonpharmacologic approaches, such as gentle exercise and weight reduction, may be beneficial alternatives to treatment with NSAIDs. When pharmacologic therapy is required, a drug therapy with a less-adverse event profile, such as acetaminophen, should be used.

Hypertension is another example of a condition for which nonpharmacologic treatments may be beneficial. Drug therapy is beneficial in reducing the risk of stroke and coronary heart disease associated with hypertension in older adults. However, use of drug therapy is associated with the potential for drug-related adverse events and can be costly, particularly when the therapy is required long-term. Nonpharmacologic approaches are an attractive option. The benefit of dietary sodium reduction and weight loss in the treatment of hypertension was recently examined. Three months following the intervention, a withdrawal of hypertension therapy was attempted and patients were followed for the combined outcome measure (i.e., occurrence of high blood pressure, treatment with an antihypertensive medication, or the occurrence of a cardiovascular event). Among 585 obese older adults, participants assigned to reduced sodium intake, weight loss alone, or to reduced sodium intake and weight loss were significantly more likely to remain free of an outcome relative to those participants assigned to usual care without a lifestyle intervention. This trial indicates restricting sodium intake and weight reduction are beneficial nonpharmacologic therapies for hypertension management in older adults.

Often when drug therapy is deemed necessary for the patient, a safer alternative to the current regimen is available. For example, if a patient is taking a long elimination half-life benzodiazepine such as diazepam and continued therapy is required, a shorter half-life agent may reduce risks associated with drug accumulation with repeated dosing especially in the context of age-related pharmacokinetic changes. Longer-half life agents are more likely to produce central nervous system adverse events such as daytime somnolence, confusion, and impaired motor coordination. The evidence remains inconclusive as to whether long acting benzodiazepines are associated with an increased risk of hip fractures relative to shorter-acting preparations. A recent study suggests that the benzodiazepine dose is a more important risk factor for hip fracture than the elimination half-life. Given this information, a prudent approach would be to avoid using both long elimination half-life and high doses of benzodiazepine therapy in older adults.

Reduce the Dose

Many adverse drug events are dose-related. A classic example of dose-related adverse events comes from a study which explored the association between use of long-elimination half-life hypnotic-anxiolytics, neuroleptics, and tricyclic antidepressants and the development of hip fracture. Investigators documented a dose-related association for each class of drug. This study is one of many to illustrate dose-related adverse drug events. When prescribing drug therapies it is important to use the minimal dose required to obtain clinical benefit.

SUMMARY

Optimizing drug therapy means achieving the balance between overprescribing of inappropriate therapy and underprescribing of beneficial therapy. Particular attention should be given to using all drug therapies only when required and at the minimum effective dose. Beneficial therapy should be prescribed when indicated. Financial pressures need to be recognized and strategies developed to make sure that older adults have access to drug therapies when needed. Adverse drug events are common and system-level approaches need to be developed to minimize their impact.

REFERENCES

Avorn J et al: Use of psychoactive medication and the quality of care in rest homes: Findings and policy implications of a statewide study. N Engl J Med 227:320, 1989.

Bates DW et al: Effect of computerized physician order entry and a team intervention on prevention of serious medication errors. JAMA 280:1311, 1998.

Beers MH et al: Explicit criteria for determining inappropriate medication use in nursing home residents. Arch Intern Med 151:1825, 1991.

Berlowitz DR et al: Inadequate management of blood pressure in a hypertensive population. N Engl J Med 339:1957, 1998.

Eisenberg DM et al: Unconventional medicine in the United States: Prevalence, costs, and patterns of use. N Engl J Med 328:246, 1993.

Federman AD et al: Supplemental insurance and use of effective cardiovascular drugs among elderly medicare beneficiaries with coronary heart disease. JAMA 286:1732, 2001.

Griffin MR et al: Nonsteroidal anti-inflammatory drug use and increased risk for peptic ulcer disease in elderly persons. Ann Intern Med 114(4):257, 1991.

Gurwitz J et al: Incidence and preventability of adverse drug events in nursing homes. Am J Med 109:87, 2000.

Gurwitz JH et al: The exclusion of the elderly and women from clinical trials in acute myocardial infarction. JAMA 268:1417, 1992.

Gurwitz JH et al: Atrial fibrillation and stroke prevention with warfarin in the long-term care setting. Arch Intern Med 157:978, 1997.

Ioannidis JPA, Lau J: Completeness of safety reporting in randomized trials. JAMA 285(4):437, 2001.

Kaufman DW et al: Recent patterns of medication use in the ambulatory adult population of the United States: The Slone Survey. JAMA 287:337, 2002.

Knight EL, Avorn J: Quality indicators for appropriate medication use in vulnerable elders. Ann Intern Med 135:S703, 2001.

Krumholz HM et al: National use and effectiveness of beta-blockers for the treatment of elderly patients after acute myocardial infarction. National Cooperative Cardiovascular Project. JAMA 280:623, 1998.

Leape LL et al: Systems analysis of adverse drug events. ADA Study Group. JAMA 274:35, 1995.

Lee PY et al: Representation of elderly persons and women in published randomized trials of acute coronary syndromes. JAMA 286:708, 2001.

Mulrow C et al: Pharmacotherapy for hypertension in the elderly, in The Cochrane Library, edited by TC Collaboration. Cochrane Collaboration, 2002.

Ray WA et al: Psychotropic drug use and the risk of hip fracture. N Engl J Med 316(7):363, 1987.

Redelmeier DA et al: The treatment of unrelated disorders in patients with chronic medical diseases. N Engl J Med 338(21):1516, 1998.

Rochon PA et al: Age and gender-related use of low-dose drug therapy: The need to manufacture low-dose therapy and evaluate the minimum effective dose. J Am Geriatr Soc 47:954, 1999.

Rochon PA, Gurwitz JH: Drug therapy. Lancet 346:32, 1995.

Rochon PA, Gurwitz JH: Optimizing drug treatment for elderly people: The prescribing cascade. BMJ 315:1096, 1997.

Rochon PA et al: Rate of heart failure and 1-year survival for older people receiving low-dose beta-blocker therapy after myocardial infarction. Lancet 356:639, 2000.

Shorr RI et al: Changes in antipsychotic drug use in nursing homes during implementation of the OBRA-87 regulations. JAMA 271:358, 1994.

Siris ES et al: Identification and fracture outcomes of undiagnosed low bone mineral density in postmenopausal women. JAMA 286:2815, 2001.

Tamblyn R et al: Adverse events associated with prescription drug cost-sharing among poor and elderly persons. JAMA 285(4):421, 2001.

Whelton PK et al: Sodium reduction and weight loss in the treatment of hypertension in older persons: A randomized controlled trial of nonpharmacologic interventions in the elderly (TONE). JAMA 279:839, 1998.

Zhan C et al: Potentially inappropriate medication use in the community-dwelling elderly. JAMA 286:2823, 2001.

Complementary and Alternative Medicine in Aging

AVIVA D. WERTKIN • GIOVANNI CIZZA • MARC R. BLACKMAN

INTRODUCTION

Definition of Complementary and Alternative Medicine

Complementary and alternative medicine (CAM) modalities constitute a diverse group of consumer-driven medical and health care practices outside the realm of conventional medicine, which are yet to be validated using scientific methods. Considered as such, CAM practices are ever changing. Most CAM use is complementary, that is, as an adjunct to conventional practices, and only a minority is used as an alternative to mainstream medical care. A main tenet of CAM therapy is that it stimulates and strengthens the body's own natural defense systems to prevent and treat diseases. Thus, elderly as well as nonelderly individuals use CAM practices with the hope of improving wellness and for relief of symptoms attributable to chronic, "stressful," degenerative, or fatal conditions.

From a conceptual perspective, the panoply of CAM modalities can be divided into five major groupings: alternative medical systems, mind–body interventions, biologically based treatments, manipulative and body-based methods, and energy therapies (Table 20-1). The reasons for CAM use are multiple, but include dissatisfaction with conventional medicine because of its ineffectiveness in producing cures, cost, adverse effects, and depersonalization. CAM use also empowers the individual to take control over personal health decisions, and it focuses on the individual's values, spiritual and religious philosophy, and beliefs regarding the nature and origins of illness. The fragmentation of care by busy specialists, and provision by CAM therapists of "touch, talk, and time," as well as media reports of dramatic results, all contribute to the increasing interest in CAM therapies. Surveys indicate that those who use CAM tend more often to be women; to be of higher educational level and economic status; suffer from poorer health status (e.g., chronic anxiety, pain, back problems, urinary tract infections); possess a holistic orientation to health; and report having had a "transformational life experience."

Use and Misuse of CAM Modalities

In recent years, the use of CAM has steadily increased among adults of all ages. In the largest US study to date, nearly 29 percent of 30,801 respondents to a 1999 National Health Interview Survey reported using at least one CAM modality in the prior year. This prevalence of CAM usage is somewhat less than that reported in other surveys. According to Eisenberg's follow-up of his earlier national survey, the probability of an adult American visiting a CAM provider increased by 30 percent during the 1990s, to 46.3 percent in 1997, accounting for approximately $27 billion in out-of-pocket expenses. It was estimated that nearly 60 percent of CAM use was not disclosed to health care providers. The therapies of escalating usage included botanicals, massage, vitamins, self-help group, folk remedies, energy healing, and homeopathy. Alternative therapies were most frequently pursued for chronic conditions including back problems, anxiety, depression, and headaches.

To evaluate the predictors and patterns of CAM use among the elderly, Blue Shield Medicare conducted a 1-year mail-in survey of a population receiving Medicare coverage for acupuncture and chiropractic services. Among 728 responders, 41 percent reported use of one or more CAM practices. The most frequently used therapies were herbs (24 percent), chiropractic (20 percent), therapeutic massage (15 percent), and acupuncture (14 percent). Results from this survey may not reflect the entire aged population, because trends in alternative medicine have shown that while many people will pay out-of-pocket for these expenditures, insurance coverage of CAM increases the probability of its use. As with younger adults, elderly persons more likely to employ CAM modalities tend to be younger; female; white; better educated; report depression, anxiety, or arthritis; and are engaged in more disease prevention activities, such as exercise or frequent physician visits. Whereas 80 percent stated that they perceived benefits from using CAM in the Blue Shield Medicare survey, only 42 percent discussed the use of these therapies with their primary care physicians, consistent with reports in younger adults.

Table 20-1   CAM Domains

Alternative medical systems	Complete systems that evolved independent of and often prior to conventional medicine, e.g., traditional systems • Traditional Chinese medicine • Ayurveda • Native American medicine • Homeopathy • Naturopathy
Mind–body interventions	Application of techniques designed to facilitate the mind's ability to affect one's body symptoms and functions. • Meditation or guided imagery • Dance, music, and art therapy • Prayer • Biofeedback
Biologically based treatments	Natural and biologically based practices, interventions, and products • Herbal therapies • Dietary supplements • Special diets • Orthomolecular therapies
Manipulative and body-based methods	Modalities based upon manipulation and/or movement of the body • Chiropractic • Osteopathic manipulation • Therapeutic massage
Energy therapies	Focus on energy fields believed to originate within the body or from other sources • Biofields (internal), e.g., reiki, qi gong, therapeutic touch • Bioelectromagnetic based (external), e.g., electroacupuncture, magnetic fields

Ineffective communication between the mainstream provider and patient is likely to be multifactorial and influenced by the provider's knowledge and interest in CAM and the patient's fear of reproach.

In the US, CAM practices are widely available (Table 20-2), but are largely unregulated. Among CAM practices, only five (acupuncture, chiropractic, massage, naturopathy, and homeopathy) are licensed in multiple states, whereas several others (art therapy, traditional Chinese Medicine, reflexology) are licensed in only a few

Table 20-2   CAM Practitioners and their Utilization

- *Chiropractic:* 55,000 licensed, $8 billion estimated market for services
- *Massage:* 1 million, 150,000–200,000 certified. $6 billion market.
- *Acupuncture:* 5000–8000 licensed (1000 MD's) $0.5–1 billion
- *Homeopathy*– 3000 (500 MD's), $0.2 billion
- *Naturopathy* – 1000–3000 licensed; $0.2 billion.

SOURCE: (The state of healthcare in America—1998 Business & Health)

states, and still others (biofeedback, hypnosis) require only certification. Moreover, the scope of practice may vary from state to state (e.g., acupuncture). The American public spends more out-of-pocket for CAM practices than for all other healthcare needs. Most consumers believe that their health plans should pay for CAM treatments, and an increasing number of insurers and HMO's are now doing so.

Current Issues in the Use of CAM Modalities

Validating the efficacy, safety, and mechanisms of action of the broad spectrum of CAM practices poses unique scientific challenges and opportunities, as CAM products and practices are already in widespread use; product and practice standards are inconsistent; there is a dearth of credible scientific information; there are substantial market disincentives to research; most CAM practitioners lack research experience; and most scientists lack CAM training. Among the safety issues that need to be addressed are those relating to standardization for ensuring safety, efficacy, and quality control; regulation of herbal/botanical supplements; research methodology for safety and efficacy of CAM therapies and products; improved communication between physicians and consumers; more widespread CAM

Table 20-3 Safety Concerns Related to Four Herbal Products Commonly Used by Elderly Persons

Common Name	Indication	Adverse Effects	Drug Interactions
Ginkgo Biloba	Dementia	Usually mild but rare serious effects include bleeding and seizures.	Anticoagulants
Saw Palmetto	Benign prostatic hyperplasia	Constipation, diarrhea, decreased libido, headaches, hypertension, urine retention (all usually rare and mild)	None described
Echinacea	Respiratory infections	Allergic reactions, hepatitis, asthma, vertigo, anaphylaxis (rare)	Immunosuppressants
St. John's wort	Antidepressant	Nausea, allergic reactions, photosensitization (rare)	Anticoagulants, antiviral agents, oral contraceptives, SSRIs

SSRIs, selective serotonin reuptake inhibitors.

SOURCE: Adapted from Ernst E. *Ann Intern Med* 136:42, 2002.

training for mainstream providers; and reliable information for the public on rational use of CAM therapies. Despite the general lack of product and practice standardization and uncertain safety of some products, most consumers are satisfied, and few malpractice or wrongful injury lawsuits are filed.

As noted above, and contrary to popular belief, people aged 65 years or older do seem to use CAM as frequently as do younger populations, and the use is increasing. This finding underlies the importance of the scientific and clinical validation for the use of these treatments in more vulnerable groups, such as children, pregnant women, and the elderly. This chapter discusses CAM use for certain musculoskeletal, neurobiological, endocrine–metabolic, cardiovascular, and malignant diseases that commonly afflict the elderly population. Unfortunately, at this juncture, the nature of CAM is largely one of anecdotal and not scientifically evidence-based medicine. As such, it is a challenge to precisely summarize the beneficial application of these therapeutic interventions.

USE OF CAM MODALITIES FOR DISORDERS OF THE ELDERLY PATIENT

Musculoskeletal

Osteoarthritis

Osteoarthritis is one of the most common chronic diseases, affecting 49 percent of the elderly population. It is also one of the most common conditions for which elderly persons seek CAM treatments. Current pharmacologic treatments are useful in managing certain aspects of this disabling condition but do not halt cartilage degeneration or modify the natural course of the disease, and sometimes they are associated with serious side effects. CAM treatments for osteoarthritis are used as frequently as conventional therapies and account for a similar monetary cost. In one survey, nearly half (47 percent) of osteoarthritic patients aged 55 to 75 years reported using some form of CAM treatment,

principally massage therapy (57 percent), chiropractic care (21 percent), and various CAM medications (17 percent).

Glucosamine and chondroitin sulfate have both been publicized as potentially effective dietary supplements for treating chronic osteoarthritis. However, only a few small studies have been published in the scientific literature. The National Institutes of Health (NIH) is currently sponsoring a Phase III multicenter trial to assess the separate and combined effects of glucosamine and/or chondroitin-sulphate in the treatment of pain associated with osteoarthritis of the knee. Herbal preparations may have limited, but unproven, efficacy in reducing pain and improving mobility, including capsaicin cream and Phytodolor, which are thought to modulate the local release of substance P and to influence the cyclooxygenase and lipoxygenase pathways, respectively, similar to conventional nonsteroidal antiinflammatory treatments.

Dietary modifications that are sometimes suggested include increasing sulfur-containing foods such as eggs, asparagus, and onions. Sulfur is an important element necessary for repairing bone, cartilage, and connective tissue, as well as in promoting the absorption of calcium. In addition, it may be helpful for others to avoid what are considered the nightshade vegetables because they contain solanine, a substance that interferes with muscle enzymes and may contribute to discomfort. The nightshade vegetables include peppers, eggplant, tomato, and white potato.

Because pain can be influenced by one's expectations, any intervention, including CAM treatments, could be perceived as effective in reducing the pain and discomfort associated with osteoarthritis. Similarly, negative beliefs in reference to a medical procedure may often be associated with augmented pain perception and decreased tolerability. The specific mechanism(s) of the placebo and nocebo effects are yet to be elucidated. Social support and maintenance of close personal relationships are predictors of successful aging; and their lack is associated with worsening of symptoms of osteoarthritis.

Various stress-reducing techniques may be of benefit as adjunctive treatments for osteoarthritis. Music therapy has been used successfully for pain relief in elderly and disabled patients. Self-selected taped music, together with relaxation techniques, decreases chronic pain. There are no specific data on the effects of music therapy in elderly patients with osteoarthritis. Specific forms of exercise, such as yoga, tai chi, and qigong, have been used widely to treat various musculoskeletal abnormalities. Any of these gentle movements may be a useful alternative or adjunctive to traditional exercise programs for patients with limited mobility.

Small-scale studies suggest that acupuncture affords relief of pain and improves functional status in osteoarthritic patients. To further investigate this hypothesis, the NIH is sponsoring a randomized, controlled trial comparing the effects of traditional Chinese acupuncture, sham acupuncture, and conventional education/attention in patients with knee osteoarthritis.

Osteoporosis

Osteopenia, osteoporosis, and nontraumatic fractures of the spine, wrist, and hip increase in frequency with age in both women and men. Early recognition and treatment of risk factors for osteopenia may help reduce accelerated bone loss and fractures. Keeping physically active, including weight-bearing exercise such as walking is strongly encouraged. The more alternative exercises such as tai chi and yoga, which promote balance and strength, may also be supportive for reducing the number of falls and hip fractures.

Major depression is associated with accelerated osteoporosis, attributed in part to increased cortisol secretion. Given the high prevalence of depression in the elderly population, more research is needed to evaluate the effectiveness of various mind–body interventions in preventing or treating osteoporosis in this age group.

Soy and phytoestrogen products obtained from dietary or supplemental sources are often used as an alternative to conventional hormone therapy of osteoporosis in menopausal women, although data supporting their efficacy in preventing or treating established osteoporosis are lacking. In contrast, the benefits of proper daily consumption of calcium are well established. Good dietary sources of calcium are green leafy vegetables, dairy products, almonds, beans, and fortified whole grains. Calcium can only be assimilated if it is accompanied by sufficient amounts of endogenous or exogenous vitamin D and magnesium. Several studies suggest that added magnesium may improve bone mineral density, but further investigation of magnesium in relation to osteoporosis is needed. All of these vitamins and minerals are easily obtained in supplemental pill form, as are folic acid, pyridoxine, boron, and silica. The latter have all been promoted for their bone-strengthening or bone-maintaining activity, although these claims have not been substantiated by clinical trials. Dehydroepiandrosterone (DHEA), a widely used dietary supplement, is the most abundant adrenal steroid in humans. Circulating DHEA levels decline progressively with age. Small-scale trials of DHEA supplementation in older individuals have produced conflicting results regarding effects on bone density, and further studies are needed to determine its possible use in preventing or treating osteoporosis in elderly individuals.

Chronic Low Back Pain

Chronic low back pain is one of the conditions for which CAM treatments are most often sought. In one 10-week, randomized trial comparing the efficacy of therapeutic massage, traditional acupuncture, and self-care in patients with back pain, who were 20 to 70 years of age, subjects in the massage group experienced fewer severe symptoms and less medication use and restricted activity than did those in the self-care group. The effect on symptoms and medication use persisted after 1 year of treatment. Self-care educational material exerted little effect initially, but after 1 year it was as effective as massage. Traditional acupuncture was not effective in this trial. However, acupuncture has been helpful for alleviating back pain in other clinical trials. Chiropractic treatment remains on the fringes of mainstream medicine, but is progressing toward acceptance as its popularity increases. There is considerable evidence supporting the efficacy of spinal manipulation for low back pain; however, there is limited research pertaining specifically to its use in the elderly population. Side effects of spinal manipulation may include headaches, localized discomfort, or fatigue; these generally resolve within 48 hours. Serious complications from lumbar spine manipulation are estimated to be extremely rare. The extract white willow bark contains natural salicylic acid (like aspirin). Despite claims of its purported efficacy in treating headaches and low back pain, this has yet to be proved. Moreover, this biological agent may interfere with the absorption of iron and other minerals.

Neurobiological

Depression

Nutritional status can exert a significant impact on emotional well-being. Diets too low in complex carbohydrates can deplete serotonin levels and contribute to depression, whereas increased protein and essential fatty acid intake may increase alertness and uplift spirits. Equally as important is avoidance of excess alcohol, tobacco, processed sugars, and caffeine, all of which can contribute to irritability and depression. Identifying and controlling food allergies can be a significant factor in alleviating depressive symptoms.

Based on conflicting data from multiple clinical trials, controversy remains as to whether the botanical known as St. John's wort (Hypericum perforatum) is as effective as standard antidepressant medications in alleviating signs and symptoms of major depression, and with fewer side effects. A recent NIH multicenter study failed to demonstrate significant improvement in psychological outcome measures in patients with major depression of mild to moderate severity when taking either St. John's wort or a standardized antidepressant. Additional studies are being conducted to examine its potential use in patients with mild symptoms of depression, social phobia, and seasonal affective disorder. Side effects of St. John's wort include photosensitivity, gastrointestinal upset, fatigue, dizziness, headache, and dry mouth. Importantly, St. John's wort interacts with the hepatic P450 enzyme system that contributes to metabolism of many drugs, contributing to clinically significant, adverse botanical–drug interactions with various antiretroviral, oral contraceptive, anticoagulant, immunosuppressant, antidepressant, and chemotherapeutic medications.

S-adenosyl-methionine (SAM-e), a naturally occurring compound necessary for the brain to manufacture serotonin and dopamine, is marketed as an antidepressant. In one study of 195 patients, depressive symptoms lessened after taking 400 mg of SAM-e daily for 2 weeks.

Ginkgo biloba is another herb that may help alleviate some of the symptoms of depression. It has been speculated that use of extracts of ginkgo biloba leaves (EGb 761) might be particularly effective in older individuals with mild depression resulting from cognitive decline or poor quality of sleep. In addition to increasing blood flow to the brain, studies have shown an increase in the number of serotonin receptor sites after supplementation of ginkgo biloba. The latter effect, if validated, could prove to be of special benefit in the elderly population.

Kava kava is an herb that until recently was widely used to reduce the anxiety, stress, and restlessness that can accompany other symptoms of depression. It is claimed to be useful for promoting both physical and emotional relaxation and enhancing sleep. Some European studies have found that kava kava is just as effective as synthetic tranquilizers for reducing anxiety. Although kava kava was thought to be well tolerated, there are increasing reports of serious hepatotoxicity leading to death resulting from kava kava intake, and the product has been banned from use in a number of countries.

Supplementing 5-hydroxytryptophan (5-HTP) may be another beneficial method for relieving depression-related symptoms of anxiety and sleeplessness. Several studies have found that 5-HTP is as effective as tricyclic antidepressants, and more effective than the selective serotonin reuptake inhibitor (SSRI) Luvox. Advantages of this extract are said to be that it is equally as effective as antidepressant drugs, less expensive, and better tolerated. However, there may be safety issues related to the use of these compounds and their contaminants. In 1989, more than 1500 patients with eosinophilia-myalgia syndrome and approximately 40 deaths were reported in the United States among people ingesting tryptophan for various reasons, including sleep disorders and depressive symptoms.

Recent research has identified light therapy is a promising modality for the treatment of a specific type of depression, seasonal affective disorder (SAD). Light therapy uses a full-spectrum fluorescent light to boost both serotonin and melatonin levels when a person experiences insufficient exposure to natural sunlight. Some of the nonspecific, constitutional symptoms of SAD, such as lack of energy, depressed mood, nonspecific pain symptoms, and easy fatigability, are sometimes also observed in subjects suffering from vitamin D deficiency. Both conditions are exacerbated during the winter season, are more common at higher latitude, improve during summer, and are ameliorated by light therapy. It is therefore possible that some subjects diagnosed with SAD may indeed suffer from vitamin D deficiency. Therefore, before prescribing light therapy, it is important to rule out hypovitaminosis D. Aromatherapy is sometimes suggested to alleviate sadness. While there are several aromas from which to choose, Rosemary (*Rosmarinus officinalis*) is a scent containing cineol, which has been shown to be a central nervous system (CNS) stimulant.

Aerobic exercise is widely used as treatment for mild to moderate depression in older patients. In one 16-week study, 56 men and women with major depression, ages 50 to 77 years, were randomly assigned to a program of aerobic exercise (three 45-minute exercise sessions per week), antidepressants (sertraline HCl), or combined exercise and medication. At the end of the study, all groups exhibited clinically significant reductions in depressive scores. Patients receiving medications exhibited a faster initial response; however, by week 16, exercise was as effective as the study medication. Aerobic exercise may prove to be a practical and effective treatment for depression in some older persons.

Expressing emotions through journal writing is another activity that may help to sort out feelings and perhaps provide relief from ongoing unhappy thoughts. Additionally, recent research has delineated the health benefits of spirituality and prayer. For some people, writing could be used as a venue for prayer. It may also have particular benefits for someone dealing with a chronic or newly diagnosed illness.

Dementia

Alzheimer's disease and cerebrovascular insufficiency are the two most common causes of dementia in the elderly. Ginkgo biloba extract, EGb 761, is widely used to increase memory and cognitive ability. Despite the contradictory reports on the efficacy of EGb 761, there is some suggestive evidence that it may be beneficial for enhancing cognitive ability and daily living for patients with both vascular and Alzheimer's dementia. Adverse effects of ginkgo biloba are generally mild. However, there have been serious cases of associated bleeding and seizures. It is also recommended not to use ginkgo biloba in conjunction with anticoagulants because of its antiplatelet nature. The NIH is currently sponsoring a large, multicenter study to examine the efficacy and safety of EGb 761 in the treatment of dementia caused by Alzheimer's disease.

Melatonin secretion decreases with healthy aging, and falls to an even greater extent in patients with dementia. The potential antioxidant and antiamyloidogenic properties of melatonin are under investigation for their potential actions in dementia prevention or treatment. To date, however, there are no reports of controlled, double-blinded clinical studies of melatonin for the prevention or treatment of Alzheimer's disease or vascular dementia.

Vitamins A, C, and E, carotenoids, and selenium all slow the progression of Alzheimer's disease. Brain tissue from patients with Alzheimer's disease shows higher levels of oxidized proteins and lipid peroxidation products, which represent potential therapeutic targets for these antioxidants. Spinal fluid concentrations of vitamins C and E are reduced in patients with Alzheimer's disease, offering yet another rationale for supplementing with these vitamins. Whether the above-noted vitamins can retard brain aging in healthy people with no existing cognitive deficits is unknown. Several studies are underway to investigate whether vitamin E or donepezil may keep patients with mild cognitive impairment from developing Alzheimer's disease and whether reducing homocysteine levels with high-doses of folate/B$_6$/B$_{12}$ supplements can slow the rate of cognitive decline in people with Alzheimer's disease.

Parkinson's Disease

One alternative approach to treating Parkinson's disease is to supplement with glutathione. Brain levels of glutathione, an antioxidant that serves significant neuroprotective functions, are reduced in patients with Parkinson's disease. In one study, intravenous injection of glutathione slowed the progression of Parkinson's disease and reduced symptom severity. Nicotinamide adenine dinucleotide (NADH) and coenzyme Q10 have also been advocated to remedy the deficit in neuronal cell energy that is a component of Parkinson's disease. Coenzyme Q10 declines with age, but is more deficient in Parkinson's disease patients. It has been suggested that older individuals eat foods containing higher amounts of coenzyme Q10, such as mackerel, salmon, and sardines. Recent research confirms that the brains of patients with Parkinson's disease exhibit increased oxidative activity, so that the use of antioxidant vitamins may counteract deleterious free radical production and strengthen antioxidant defenses. Alpha-lipoic acid, an antioxidant itself, serves to regenerate vitamins C, E, and glutathione. Moreover, alpha-lipoic acid serves as a metal chelator, enhancing the excretion of potentially toxic metals, a possible beneficial effect considering the high amounts of metal found in the brain biopsies of Parkinson's patients. N-acetyl-cysteine and acetyl-L-carnitine, two other significant antioxidants, may also slow progression of the disease. Ginkgo biloba is also being evaluated for its possible role in treating this condition.

Traditional Chinese medicine teaches that age-related dementia results from a deficiency of qi, or vital energy, caused by a blockage in phlegm. Acupuncture has been used to treat dementia because of its supposed enhancement of qi and blood circulation. Current literature suggests that acupuncture may exert beneficial effects in patients with vascular dementia and Parkinson's disease.

The standard of care in managing patients with Parkinson's disease includes physical therapy to reduce disabilities from the associated symptoms. For many years, music therapy has been suggested to boost the social, emotional, and cognitive function of elderly individuals. Some studies have found that music therapy increases feelings of relaxation and reduces the anxiety and depression commonly experienced by elderly persons with dementia. Additional methods of relaxation, such as deep-breathing exercises may also be beneficial as adjuncts to conventional treatments. Relaxation techniques and music therapy can be useful tools to alleviate some of the emotional and psychological concerns of the elderly, which in turn could also help their memory retention skills.

Sleep Disorders

Clinically significant alterations in sleep quality and quantity are common in both healthy and unhealthy older persons. Epidemiologic studies suggest that nearly 40 percent of people age 65 years and older are dissatisfied with their sleep patterns. Recent studies suggest that abnormalities in slow wave sleep and/or rapid eye-movement (REM) sleep may contribute to significant endocrine–metabolic, immune, and psychological dysfunctions, and augment cardiovascular and neurovascular risk. Mainstream and CAM therapies that address the underlying pathophysiology of age-related sleep disruption remain to be identified.

Nutritional interventions may be among the safer approaches for promoting a relaxed and restful sleep state. A glass of warm milk is one of the oldest remedies used to induce feelings of sleepiness, which can be mildly effective as it contains tryptophan. In the brain, tryptophan is a precursor of serotonin and may therefore be helpful in depression-induced insomnia. Other foods that are rich in tryptophan include turkey, brown rice, peanuts, and bananas. Drinking a hot cup of decaffeinated tea can sometimes be soothing. There are several herbal teas, which are promoted for their relaxing and mild sedative effects. This list includes chamomile, passion flower, hops, and California poppy.

Valerian is a botanical product that is touted for its mildly sedative properties. Several small-scale double-blind studies suggest that valerian can exert a mild calming effect and enhance sleep, possibly by increasing slow-wave sleep. St. John's wort has also been reported to increase REM sleep latency. Melatonin, the main product of the pineal gland, is secreted cyclically at night, is thought to contribute to normal sleep–wake cyclicity, and naturally declines with age. In one 4-week study, melatonin administration was found to produce a significant decrease in fatigue and sleepiness scores, as well as sleep onset latency, as compared with placebo, in patients with delayed sleep-phase syndrome. Further research is needed to determine the efficacy, safety, and potential clinical use of these biological products for treating diverse sleep disorders in the elderly population.

Several studies have examined the sleep-enhancing effects of exercise. Much of the evidence points to aerobic exercise as a contributor to deepened sleep. Additional research is needed to evaluate the benefit of exercise related to late-life insomnia. Finally, music therapy, aromatherapy, or a hot bath may be helpful accompaniments for encouraging a calm and relaxed state in patients with anxiety related insomnia.

Endocrine—Metabolic

Menopause

Surveys by the North American Menopause Society suggest that CAM use during the menopause is perceived as a natural extension of interest in nutrition, exercise, and other behavioral, nonpharmacologic interventions to improve or maintain quality of life. More than 30 percent of menopausal women use acupuncture, natural or plant estrogens, and/or herbal supplements. Most studies of these interventions reveal a 20 percent response rate in the placebo groups. Given the uncertainty that exists in the minds of many women and their health care providers regarding hormone replacement therapy, it can be anticipated that the use of uninvestigated "natural" products and practices to manage menopausal symptoms and signs will continue to burgeon.

Several botanical and nutritional products that contain estrogen-like ingredients are being evaluated for their possible benefits in relieving certain menopausal symptoms. Among these, phytoestrogens are the most prominent. Phytoestrogens are classified into three groups: isoflavones (e.g., genistein, daidzein), which are plant sterols found in soy, garbanzo beans, and other legumes; lignans, which derive from the cell walls of plants, and are found in seed husks (e.g., flaxseed) used to make oils; and coumestans, found in red clover, sunflower seeds, and bean sprouts. Several studies suggest that soy and isoflavones may be helpful in short-term (<1 to 2 years) management of vasomotor symptoms. It is as yet uncertain whether initiating use of phytoestrogens later in life will also provide other health benefits or risks, such as developing osteoporosis, cardiovascular and/or neurovascular disease, memory, mood, and sleep disorders, endometrial and/or breast cancer. Whether the different groups of phytoestrogens exert characteristic positive and/or adverse effects is unknown, as is the extent to which they can act as agonists or antagonists of the estrogen receptor (alpha and/or beta). Thus, to date, information remains inconclusive on the use of phytoestrogens as an alternative to postmenopausal hormone therapy, and caution is needed in recommending these agents to women with hormone-dependent cancers.

Currently, there is a lengthy list of marketed dietary supplements that are claimed to relieve various menopausal symptoms. However, the majority of the claims have not been verified by means of rigorous clinical trials. The following herbs have shown some degree of benefit: black cohosh (Cimicifuga racemosa) is commonly used for menstrual disorders and related health problems. Research has been conducted on this herb for many years and has shown it to be useful for relieving sleep disorders, mood disturbances, and hot flashes; chaste tree berry (Vitex agnus-castus) is another popular herb that is used for menstrual irregularities and premenstrual syndrome. This extract is claimed to revitalize vaginal tissue and to relieve cyclical breast pain, but there is limited information regarding its value in treating menopausal symptoms; dong quai is a Chinese botanical advertised for its hormone-balancing action. Used alone, it does not appear to be useful in treating menopausal symptoms; however, in Chinese remedies it is usually dispensed in a formula combined with other herbs; whether St. John's wort beneficially influences mood changes that can accompany menopause is unknown; the German Commission E has approved lemon balm (Melissa officinalis) to help treat nervous disturbances. Balm has sedative, antispasmodic, antihormonal, and antiviral actions in animal models.

Relaxation techniques may be useful for some women to manage certain psychological and physical manifestations of the menopause. Finally, acupuncture may also be useful for relieving some of the unwanted menopausal symptoms.

Benign Prostatic Hyperplasia

Symptomatic benign prostatic hyperplasia (BPH) affects more than 40 percent of men older than 70 years of age.

During the past several years men have increasingly begun to self-treat this condition with the herbal compound Serenoa repens, known as saw palmetto, which has become the fifth leading medicinal herb consumed in the United States. In a recent meta-analysis, patients with moderate benign prostatic hypertrophy averaged 65 years of age and were studied for at least 3 months. Saw palmetto was found to be superior to placebo and to exhibit similar efficacy to the standard pharmacologic treatment. Few side effects were reported other than intermittent slight abdominal distress. However, the rigor of the experimental design of these trials has been questioned, and a large, multicenter, NIH-sponsored clinical trial is currently under way to assess the effect of saw palmetto extract in men with moderate to severe BPH.

Pygeum is an African tree bark powder that has been extensively studied for its potential benefits in relieving urinary problems. In a review of 18 clinical trials in men with BPH, pygeum extract improved overall urodynamic patterns while decreasing nocturnal urination. Side effects were mild and similar to those experienced in the placebo groups. Several trials have shown that the astringent nettle root can significantly increase urinary flow in men with BPH, with adverse effects consisting of mild gastrointestinal distress, sweating, and allergic skin reactions. Several European studies reported that eating pumpkin seeds or taking a supplemented extract alleviates symptoms associated with BPH. Pumpkin seeds contain phytosterols, carotenoids, and unsaturated fatty acids, which are all hypothesized to exert beneficial actions.

Diabetes Mellitus

In a recent survey among diabetics, 57 percent reported using one or more CAM modalities within the prior 12 months, and 35 percent described using a CAM treatment specifically for diabetes. The CAM practices most commonly used were prayer/spiritual practice, herbal remedies, commercial diets, and folk remedies. Because the incidence and prevalence of type II diabetes mellitus and its major public health impact continue to increase, there is an urgent need to generate rigorous data regarding the benefits, risks, and mechanisms of action of potentially useful CAM therapies that might be used in conjunction with weight reduction, exercise, and dietary modifications. Some preclinical and clinical data suggest that chromium administration may exert beneficial effects on glucose and insulin homeostasis in patients with type II diabetes, but a definitive, large-scale clinical trial is necessary to establish its possible value. Until then, chromium administration should not be recommended for this purpose.

Vitamin C, an important antioxidant, is thought to exert potentially beneficial effects on insulin sensitivity, glucose tolerance, and vascular endothelial function. Further studies are warranted to evaluate the possible clinical relevance and health benefits of these observations.

Vanadium is a compound found in tiny amounts in plants and animals. A recent, small-scale study found that when people with diabetes were given vanadium, they developed a modest increase in insulin sensitivity and decrease in insulin requirements.

Certain foods may contain substances that interfere with the gastrointestinal absorption of saccharides, thus exerting a preventive effect towards type II diabetes and may explain the low prevalence of diabetes observed in certain geographic areas in which these foods are consumed.

Acupuncture has been a means of providing relief in a number of chronic pain syndromes and has been able to alleviate symptoms in some people with diabetic neuropathy. Further laboratory and clinical research will be required to determine the validity of these claims.

Cardiovascular Disease

Coronary artery disease (CAD) affects more than 60 to 70 percent of the population older than age 65 years. The use of CAM modalities to help lower blood pressure and high cholesterol is increasing. It is generally recommended that a heart-healthy diet is one that limits sodium, saturated fat, and refined sugar, while encouraging intake of complex carbohydrates, fruits, and vegetables. In the Dietary Approach to Stop Hypertension (DASH) trial, approximately 70 percent of the participants following this diet significantly decreased both systolic and diastolic blood pressures. Dietary modifications such as a reduced consumption of saturated fatty acids and an increased intake of unsaturated fatty acids, accompanied by other lifestyle interventions such as exercise, are likely to decrease the incidence and prevalence of obesity, type II diabetes mellitus, and coronary heart disease.

Flavonoids and phytoestrogens can exert beneficial effects on cardiac risk factors in patients with existing coronary artery diseases. Flavonoids are present in fruits, vegetables, tea, wine, beer, and grains. The flavonoids in wine have been studied extensively, and in moderate consumption, they decrease platelet aggregation, low-density lipoprotein (LDL) oxidation, and coronary disease. Phytoestrogens and soy products consumed over time may improve lipoprotein profiles. In October 1999, based on a series of studies, the FDA concluded that a daily intake of 25 g of soy protein with a diet low in cholesterol and saturated fat may reduce the risk of coronary heart disease by lowering total cholesterol and LDL cholesterol levels. Epidemiologic evidence suggests that increased consumption of certain nuts, such as walnuts, reduces cholesterol levels. Multiple studies show that garlic taken in dietary form or by pill can reduce total and LDL cholesterol levels, although its effects on blood pressure remains uncertain. The known adverse effects of taking garlic supplements include unfavorable breath and body odor, flatulence, abdominal and esophageal pain, allergies, and bleeding. Whether long-term consumption of these products can influence the frequency of coronary heart disease or cardiovascular morbidity and mortality remains to be determined.

Various dietary supplements are claimed to be effective in the prevention and/or treatment of cardiovascular disease. Consumption of L-carnitine has been suggested as a means of reducing triglyceride and cholesterol levels in the blood, increasing oxygen uptake, and reducing heart damage from cardiac surgeries. Coenzyme Q10 may act to normalize blood pressure and reduce total cholesterol

as well as increase oxygenation of heart tissue and possibly prevent recurrences of heart attacks. In one study of middle-aged and elderly men, small doses of DHEA were associated with a 48 percent reduction in death from heart disease. Whether DHEA administration reduces the incidence, progression, or mortality of heart disease in elderly women or men is unknown.

Hawthorne is a botanical supplement containing flavonoids, catechins, triterpene saponins, amines, and oligomeric proanthocyanidins. This herb is thought to dilate coronary blood vessels and to lower blood pressure and cholesterol. Olive leaf extract contains several phytochemicals, which may also act as vasodilators, lowering blood pressure and preventing heart attacks. In a 3-month study conducted in hypertensive patients supplementing olive leaf extract, a significant reduction in blood pressure levels was observed, without adverse effects. Essential fatty acids are available via dietary and supplemental sources. Omega-3 fatty acids can be found in fresh deepwater fish and in certain oils such as flaxseed oil. Omega-6-linoleic acid is found in raw nuts, seeds, and some oils such as primrose oil. Recent research suggests that consumption of these fatty acids is essential for healthy fat metabolism and may also lower blood pressure, lower levels of triglycerides and LDL and increase those of high-density lipoproteins (HDL). Although vitamin C and E administration may lower blood pressure in hypertensive patients, these vitamins have not been shown to be beneficial for preventing and treating cardiovascular disease. The antioxidant nature of these vitamins may be helpful for strengthening the immune system and reducing the oxidative stress associated with heart failure.

Aerobic exercise for at least 30 minutes three times a week may promote weight loss and reduce the risk of developing hypertension. Insufficient sleep, common in the elderly population, is associated with increased blood pressure; whether improving the quality and quantity of sleep will beneficially affect hypertension is not known. Stress management techniques such as yoga may help control high blood pressure. Yoga is an example of a low-impact activity that tones the body, promotes tranquility, and focuses on breathing. Other relaxation techniques, such as music therapy combined with deep breathing have been demonstrated to reduce blood pressure in hypertensive patients.

Cancer

Increasing numbers of cancer patients now use one or more CAM treatments. In one recent survey, as many as 50 percent of breast cancer patients and 37 percent of prostate cancer patients use CAM modalities in the course of their treatments. In another study of older patients with breast, colorectal, prostate, or lung cancer, nearly 33 percent reported using CAM therapy, and these individuals, as in other reports, were more likely to be women and to have a higher level of education. The three most frequently used therapies were exercise, herbal therapy, and spiritual healing. Some CAM therapies aim to strengthen the body's natural defense mechanisms, whereas others are used to alleviate the side effects of mainstream treatments, such as chemotherapy.

Many cancer patients perceive CAM therapies as a means of providing self-control over their disease and its management, which in itself may enhance quality of life. Given the lack of standardization and quality control of many CAM biological products used to treat cancer, and the potential for adverse herb/botanical–drug interactions, there is a clear need for more research related to cancer and CAM.

Breast Cancer

Controversy remains regarding the role of diet as a possible risk factor for development of breast cancer, with recent reports of unusual geographic concentrations of this disease highlighting the need for more research regarding this issue. High fiber, low-fat diets, rich in fresh organic fruits and vegetables, whole grains, legumes, fish, and other protein sources have been recommended for the prevention and/or treatment of breast cancer, although their efficacy is unproved. Obesity (and the associated increased estrogenicity) in postmenopausal women is associated with increased risks of de novo breast cancer and recurrence after early stage disease. Consequently, weight control via dietary and exercise interventions may be useful. Excess alcohol consumption is also associated with an increased risk of breast cancer, and thus temperate use of alcohol is warranted.

Various CAM biological agents have been used in the management of patients with breast cancer. Mistletoe extract has been a major agent in cancer therapy in Germany for several decades. In a 30-year study of more than 35,000 patients with diverse, advanced solid tumors, including breast cancer, iscador, an extract of the mistletoe plant, was reported to lengthen survival time of cancer patients by approximately 40 percent. Although this botanical agent has been shown to exert immunostimulatory and cytotoxic activity in vitro, conclusive data as to its benefits in patients with breast or other cancers have yet to be obtained.

Melatonin has been evaluated for its possible use as a CAM treatment for breast cancer patients. Women with estrogen-receptor–positive breast cancer exhibit reduced melatonin production, and supplementing melatonin for its antiestrogen and anticancer effects has been proposed as an adjunct therapy. Future clinical trials are needed to clarify the potential value of this supplement.

Use of high doses of antioxidants such as coenzyme Q10 or vitamin C is a controversial therapeutic approach to patients receiving chemotherapy or radiation. Some data suggest that these dietary supplements may help to protect healthy cells from free radical scavengers, whereas other information suggests that they may safeguard cancer cells. Clearly, further research is needed to decipher the role of supplemental antioxidant vitamins as an intervention when combined with chemotherapy.

A variety of teas, including black and green teas, are claimed to contain different elements that promote good health. Green tea contains EGCG, a polyphenolic antioxidant believed to be accountable for the tea's anticancer effects. Ginger tea and candied ginger are frequently recommended to soothe nausea. However, the use of ginger for chemotherapy-induced nausea has not been clinically evaluated. Peppermint tea is another frequently suggested but unproved means of reducing nausea.

Astragalus is a Chinese medicinal root that has been widely used for its purported enhancement of immune system function. The benefit of astragalus for cancer patients is related to its apparent ability to increase energy and stamina, protect the immune system, and promote overall healing.

Medicinal mushrooms, such as shiitake and maitake mushrooms, have been used in traditional medicine settings for thousands of years and have recently become the focus of scientific investigation. This research has indicated a potential therapeutic value in enhancing immunity and generating antitumor activity; however, the mechanisms of these actions and proof of their efficacy and safety in clinical trials remain to be clarified.

The lifestyle changes and somatic symptoms associated with breast cancer and its treatment not infrequently elicit signs and symptoms of stress, mild to moderate depression, or a posttraumatic stress syndrome-like state. Psychosocial interventions, such as a support group or individual therapy, may be adjunctively beneficial in easing the devastation that can accompany coping with cancer. For example, studies conducted by Spiegel have included a mixture of psychological interventions, such as support expressive groups, imagery, or self-hypnosis for patients with metastatic breast cancer. While initial reports suggested increased survival time for the intervention participants, as compared with a control group, more recent studies have not duplicated this outcome. Even if behavioral and supportive interventions do not prolong survival, these mind–body techniques have therapeutic value in improving physical and mental well-being for patients with breast cancer. Similarly, regular exercise of moderate intensity that does not contribute to discomfort may also be helpful in elevating mood. Relaxation and stress-reducing activities, such as yoga, meditation, breathing exercises, biofeedback, hypnosis, music therapy, guided imagery, and prayer, can enhance quality of life and positively affect the course of breast cancer patients.

Acupuncture may serve as another useful means of CAM cancer treatment. Acupuncture studies have demonstrated an immune enhancing effect as well as an inhibitory effect on mammary cancer cells in mice. An NIH consensus conference concluded that acupuncture treatment is a safe and effective means for reducing acute chemotherapy-induced nausea and vomiting, especially in breast cancer patients. Current trials are examining the potential utility of acupuncture for management of chronic or anticipatory postchemotherapy nausea and vomiting, as well as the neurologic and physiologic mechanisms of action underlying acupuncture's apparent efficacy.

Prostate Cancer

Prostate cancer is the most commonly diagnosed cancer in men. While there are several potential conventional treatments, men may also prefer some CAM interventions to reduce discomfort, enhance quality of life, and, possibly, to increase longevity.

Prostate cancer in older men usually develops slowly. Older men with early stage prostate cancer are at a higher risk of death from heart disease than from prostate cancer.

Not surprisingly, they are often encouraged to eliminate foods from animal sources and high saturated fat that are thought to increase the risks of both diseases. Lycopene, a red-orange carotenoid antioxidant found in high levels in tomato-based foods, is recommended for prostate cancer patients. Diets high in tomato products, especially cooked tomato, are also associated with lower prostate cancer incidence.

Drinking a moderate amount of red wine or supplementing grape seed extract is potentially beneficial in protecting against prostate cancer. In one recent study, grape seed extract suppressed the growth of androgen-responsive prostate cancer cells while augmenting that of normal cells.

Until recently, one of the most promising CAM therapies for patients with prostate cancer was PC-SPES, a dietary supplement containing eight different Chinese herbs. Several small clinical trials reported substantial decreases in serum prostate-specific antigen (PSA) levels, decrease in pain, and improvement in quality of life in patients with advanced prostate cancer. Initially reported adverse effects included breast tenderness, decreased libido, blood clots, leg cramps, and diarrhea. However, in June 2002, the sole US distributor of PC-SPES officially terminated all operations because their product was found to contain undeclared prescription drug ingredients, including diethylstilbestrol, nonsteroidal antiinflammatory agents, and warfarin. While all US-based clinical trials have been discontinued, properly controlled preclinical studies will continue to assess the cellular and molecular mechanisms of action of this complex biological agent. This widely publicized experience highlights some of the problems and pitfalls inherent in the use of complex "natural" products.

Vitamin E (alpha-tocopherol) is a potent antioxidant that is sometimes suggested when considering vitamin supplements to fight cancer. Natural vitamin E prevents the oxidation of lipids, improves oxygen use, and enhances immunity. The mineral selenium is another powerful antioxidant that may enhance the absorption of vitamin E. Currently, the NIH is sponsoring a Phase III randomized controlled study to determine the efficacy of selenium and/or vitamin E in the prevention prostate cancer in 32,400 healthy men. This is the largest chemoprevention trial of prostate cancer ever conducted in the United States.

A common side effect of a radical prostatectomy is urinary incontinence. A behavioral approach to "reeducate" the pelvic floor is being evaluated as a possible adjunctive treatment of this vexing problem. Whether regular, moderate physical activities, such as walking, swimming, playing tennis or golf can improve quality of life or slow the progression of prostate cancer remains to be determined.

Lung Cancer

In addition to smoking, nutritional intake seems to be one of several significant risk factors contributing to lung cancer occurrence. In this regard, high intakes of fruits and vegetables, vitamin A carotenoids (found in yellow and orange vegetables), and flavonoids from apples and broccoli, are considered to be cancer protective, whereas consumption of excess amounts of red meat, dairy products, and saturated fats are thought to pose an increased risk for

developing lung cancer. In one study assessing the effects of selenium on skin cancer, fewer reports of lung cancer were noted in the group taking this supplement. The use of selenium is now being investigated as a potential CAM medicine for lung cancer.

Participation in support group programs, and learning relaxation and stress management techniques may help lung cancer patients cope with their illness, decrease physical and emotional distress, and enhance quality of life. Behavioral interventions have also been shown to help reduce nausea and vomiting associated with chemotherapy treatment. In a small study to assess a nonpharmacologic approach to assisting breathlessness, lung cancer patients, underwent breathing retraining, relaxation, and counseling. This approach appeared to be helpful in managing the symptom of breathlessness and its related discomforts.

Although dietary vitamin A intake is generally considered to be helpful for cancer patients, ingestion of this vitamin by people who smoke may be harmful. The mechanisms of this apparent adverse effect is unknown.

Small-scale clinical studies report mixed results regarding the use of shark cartilage in treating lung cancer. The NIH is currently sponsoring a Phase III multicenter study to investigate the effects of a specific shark cartilage extract, AE-941, in combination with chemotherapy and radiotherapy for patients with non–small-cell lung cancer.

Colon Cancer

To date, there is no widely used CAM treatment for colon cancer, although several foods have been reported or hypothesized to help prevent colon cancer and to increase the survival time once a diagnosis has been made. Based on a review of animal studies, almonds, peanuts, and black tea all contain components that may reduce the risk of developing colon cancer. The American Dietetic Association has advised that a fiber-rich diet is associated with a lower risk of colon cancer, although results from recent clinical trials suggest that increasing fiber intake does not protect against colon cancer. In one study, consumption of the carotenoid lutein, present in broccoli, spinach, carrots, tomatoes, and oranges, was beneficial in preventing colon cancer. One study demonstrated a protective effect on colon cancer of drinking large amounts of orange juice. Oranges are not only a major source of vitamin C but also contain flavonoids that may inhibit colon carcinogenesis.

Qigong is an ancient Chinese healing art that has recently been viewed as an effective tool for strengthening patient response to chemotherapy. Whether this and selected other mind–body techniques are beneficial as CAM treatments in cancer patients can only be answered by controlled clinical studies.

SAFETY OF CAM MODALITIES

There are several important concerns regarding the safety of CAM modalities in the elderly population. One area relates to the use of dietary supplements. Vitamin and herbal products are among the most popular CAM therapies in older persons, and, unfortunately, consumers often assume that the term "natural" means that a product is both safe and effective. In 1994, the US Congress passed The Dietary Supplement Health and Education Act (DSHEA) to classify dietary supplemental products. Under DSHEA, a dietary supplement is a product that contains an ingredient intended to supplement the diet and contains one or more of the following: a vitamin, mineral, herb or other botanical, amino acid, or any other dietary substance. Dietary supplements are used for oral intake as a concentrate, metabolite, extract, constituent, or in combination. The FDA is not empowered to evaluate or regulate dietary supplements, and industry is not required to prove that the advertised ingredients provide the health benefits or safety they claim. Multiple studies have found that dietary supplements often can contain little, none, or more of what the product labels claim, as well as contaminants or adulterants with unlisted products and prescription drugs.

This category of CAM therapy is also a potential cause for great public health concern in elderly people, because of the general lack of scientific research on these products, the easy access, and the tendency for the public to self-medicate without the supervision of a medical professional. The trend of "silent use" among patients can put physicians in a challenged position to optimally treat their patients and can put the individual at an increased risk for unintended, self-prescribed serious harm. Of the limited number of studies reported to date, it has become clear that that some vitamins and herbal products have the potential to cause serious adverse events and fatalities. There is also a dearth of information related to possible differences in the pharmacokinetics and pharmacodynamics of various CAM biological agents in the elderly population, so that proper dosage adjustments for these compounds are unknown. Coupled with the increased susceptibility of the elderly population to concomitant use of multiple medications, there is an increased risk for adverse herb–drug interactions in older persons. Without the knowledge of what these products contain in their entirety or the consequences of their use, consumers and providers must increase communication while continued research is conducted to provide accurate evaluations.

CONCLUSION

The escalating use of CAM modalities by the US public, including the elderly population, and the paucity of information supporting the safety, efficacy, and mechanisms of action of these diverse modalities, argue strongly for increasing the scope and rigor of CAM-related research. To address important public health needs in the elderly population, including those who are underserved, it would seem prudent to investigate the basic biology and potential clinical utility of selected CAM modalities that may allay or attenuate a variety of a life "stressors," including depression, cognitive decline, chronic pain, musculoskeletal frailty, and sleep disorders. Of particular note is that the aforementioned conditions are disproportionately more problematic in older persons than in younger persons, often coexist in the same individual, and account for substantial use of one or more CAM modalities. Moreover,

from a pathophysiologic perspective, each of these age-related stressors exhibits derangements in the interrelationships among endocrinologic, neurologic, and immunologic functions. Thus further research efforts might profitably be directed towards unraveling the interactions among these three important physiologic systems, particularly as they affect aged individuals.

Identifying an appropriate agenda for future CAM studies in the elderly population poses significant challenges. To select among the myriad CAM modalities that are currently being used by consumers, several considerations appear warranted, including the extent of use by aged persons; the public health importance of the diseases or conditions being treated; the quality and quantity of reported data, which allows for determination of whether to emphasize preclinical versus clinical studies; and the feasibility and cost of conducting the research. Integrating allopathic and CAM approaches in the design of the next generation of CAM studies represents another exciting yet daunting opportunity to advance the discipline of CAM in the twenty-first century.

REFERENCES

Abbasi F et al: Relationships between obesity, insulin resistance, and coronary heart disease risk. *J Am Coll Cardiol* 5:40, 2002.

ACOG practice bulletin: Clinical management guidelines for obstetrician-gynecologists. Use of botanicals for management of menopausal symptoms. *Obstet Gynecol* 97:Suppl (1), 2001.

Astin J et al: Complementary and alternative medicine use among elderly persons: One-year analysis of a Blue Shield medicare supplement. *J Gerontol A Biol Sci Med Sci* 55:M4, 2000.

Brown J et al: Nutrition during and after cancer treatment: A guide for informed choices by cancer survivors. *CA Cancer J Clin* 51:153, 2001.

Cherkin DC et al: A randomized trial comparing traditional Chinese medicine, medical acupuncture, therapeutic massage, and self-care education for chronic low back pain. *Arch Intern Med* 161:1081, 2001.

Cizza G et al: Depression: A major, unrecognized risk factor for osteoporosis? *Trends Endocrinol Metab* 12:198, 2001.

Davidson JRT: Effect of hypericum perforatum (St. John's wort) in major depressive disorder. *JAMA* 287:1807, 2002.

Dvorkin L, Song KY: Herbs for benign prostatic hyperplasia. *Ann Pharmacother* 36:1443, 2002.

Eisenberg DM et al: Trends in alternative medicine use in the United States, 1990–1997: Results of a follow-up national survey. *JAMA* 280:1569, 1998.

Ernst E: The risk-benefit profile of commonly used herbal therapies: Ginkgo, St. John's wort, ginseng, echinacea, saw palmetto, and kava. *Ann Intern Med* 136:42, 2002.

Gaytan R, Prisant LM: Oral nutritional supplements and heart disease: A review. *Am J Ther* 8:255, 2001.

Khosh F, Khosh M: Natural approach to hypertension. *Altern Med Rev* 6:590, 2001.

Kontush A et al: Influence of vitamin E and C supplementation on lipoprotein oxidation in patients with Alzheimer's disease. *Free Radic Biol Med* 31:345, 2001.

Mansky PJ: Mistletoe and cancer: Controversies and prospectives. *Semin Oncol* 29:589, 2002.

Murray M, Pizzorno J: *The Encyclopedia of Natural Medicine.* Roseville CA, Prima Health, 1998.

Nahin R, Straus S: Research into complementary and alternative medicine: Problems and pitfalls. *BMJ* 322:161, 2001.

Ni H et al: Utilization of complementary and alternative medicine by United States adults. *Med Care* 40:353, 2002.

Perlmutter D: New advances in Parkinson's disease. *Townsend Letter for Doctors & Patients* 216:52, 2001.

Ramsey SD et al: Use of alternative therapies by older adults with osteoarthritis. *Arthritis Care Res* 45:222, 2001.

Richardson MA et al: Complementary/alternative medicine use in comprehensive cancer center and the implications for oncology. *J Clin Oncol* 18:2505, 2000.

Spiegel D: Mind matters—Group therapy and survival in breast cancer. *N Engl J Med* 345:1767, 2001.

Warren MP et al: Use of alternative therapies in menopause. *Best Pract Res Clin Obstet Gynaecol* 16:411, 2002.

Writing Group for the Women's Health Initiative Investigators: Risks and benefits of estrogen plus progestin in healthy postmenopausal women: Principle results from the Women's Health Initiative randomized controlled trial. *JAMA* 288:321, 2002.

Yeh GY et al: Use of complementary and alternative medicine among persons with diabetes mellitus: Results of a national survey. *Am J Public Health* 92:1648, 2002.

Yesavage J: Relaxation and memory training in 39 elderly patients. *Am J Psychiatry* 141:778, 1984.

Team Care

ELLEN FLAHERTY • KATHRYN HYER • TERRY FULMER

Managing the complex syndromes experienced by frail older adults requires skills beyond the training of one discipline. Older adults are best cared for by a team of health professionals. Interdisciplinary team care improves functional status, perceived well-being, mental status, and depression scores. The cost-effectiveness of team care has been demonstrated by a reduction in patient readmission rates and numbers of physician office visits.

In 1993, the Pew Health Professions Commission predicted that health professionals would need 17 competencies to practice health care in 2005. Anticipating a shift toward population-based medicine, increasing use of technology and managed care, the competencies included an emphasis on primary care, participation in coordinated care, involvement of patients and families in decision making, and ensuring cost-effectiveness. While regulators and policy makers almost a decade later seem less enthralled with managed care, the forces driving managed care—increasing costs, concerns about cost-effectiveness, and a focus on prevention—have not slowed.

To be effective in managing the complex care of older adults, team knowledge and skills must emphasize multidimensional geriatric assessment, interdisciplinary team care planning, maximization of self-care and function, self-determination in the care plan, and improving quality of life. Future health professionals providing care to older individuals will be expected to apply the knowledge and skill in practice. Clinical care managers will need to evaluate providers on patient satisfaction, cost-effectiveness, productivity, and quality of care. Geriatric teams of the future will be expected to identify individuals at greatest risk of functional limitations and manage groups of older persons with similar problems in a cost-effective manner. In this context, the task for educators of future health professionals and practice-based managers becomes one of ensuring that providers are knowledgeable about the principles and practices of team care.

For almost a decade, the John A. Hartford Foundation of New York City has supported an effort to incorporate team training into graduate medical, nursing, and social work education. The program, Geriatric Interdisciplinary Team Training (GITT), has trained more than 1800 health care students and professionals across the country, and developed training materials to encourage the development of effective geriatric teams. Two important principles were realized in the development of curriculum and programs. Effective teams require a structure and an understanding of group process; skills that can be taught and should continue to evolve during professional development. However, teams must focus on the outcome of the team process, the creation of an interdisciplinary care plan or the management of the complex patient. While structure and process increase the efficiency of teams, assessing the team's effectiveness must be based on the outcome of the team meeting and the ability of the team to address or improve the patient's and family's needs.

According to the American Congress on Rehabilitation Medicine, a team is capable of achieving results with patients that individuals who constitute the team cannot achieve in isolation. Simply forming a team comprised of several disciplines does not, however, guarantee that the team will function well or that the outcome of the process will be the desired one. Effective teaming as an interdisciplinary group requires structure, the use of agendas, agreement upon ground rules and process, attention to issues of leadership, communication, and respect for one another's expertise.

COLLABORATION AND THE IMPORTANCE OF GERIATRIC INTERDISCIPLINARY TEAMS

Collaboration implies a process of shared planning, decision making, accountability, and responsibility in the care of the patient. In collaborative practice, providers work together. They demonstrate effective communication, trust, mutual respect, and understanding of others' skills. While skills and services may overlap, most skills and services are complementary and reinforce each other.

With advanced technology and the growth of community-based care, providers frequently provide home treatments or treatments in the nursing home that were previously delivered exclusively in the hospital setting. Monitoring older adults in these community settings requires well-honed communication skills, because providers need to understand and correctly implement complex plans of care. It is crucial to recognize when to alert other providers of change in status. It is also important to learn what information other team members require to make decisions about treatment.

With the advent of managed care, there is an emphasis on efficiency and appropriate use of resources. Skills in coordinating care and being responsive to older adults increases in importance. Physicians, nurses, social workers, and other providers must recognize when referrals to other providers are necessary and know what outcome to expect. Understanding the skills of other health providers is increasingly important for all patients, but is critical in the care of frail older adults.

PRINCIPLES OF SUCCESSFUL TEAMWORK

To provide the important benefits of team care to the client, team members must know their functions and how to interact to make the team effective. The essential elements of teamwork are coordination of services, shared responsibility, and communication. Effective teams must work across settings and have well-organized mechanisms to share information. Assessment of older adults is usually shared with one or more providers who administer geriatric assessment tests. Because the focus of the team is on the older person, providers must share information clearly and effectively. By focusing on the client, the team shares a common goal. Hence, effective teaming requires rules to govern the team and team member behavior, plans to make meetings run efficiently, clarity about the skills and boundaries for the roles and responsibilities of each team member, team communication skills, and mechanisms for managing team conflict.

TEAMS AND TEAM MEMBER RULES

Team rules, both for team governance and for member behavior, are needed in the early stages of team development. Table 21-1 provides an overview of the eight principles of successful team work. Not having these rules is a primary cause of team problems later on and can slow or stop

team development completely. Rules for team governance should include some or all of the following:

- Share a clear understanding by all members (and the larger organization within which it operates) about the overall purpose of the team and the goals for each meeting.
- Determine the composition of the team, including which disciplines are needed as members and the number of members (enough to get the job done; not so many that the work cannot get done). Allow the problem to define the composition of the team, not vice versa.
- Determine how often the team needs to meet and specify attendance requirements. (Is there a core team of doctor, nurse, and social worker? Are other disciplines asked to participate on cases that require their expertise?)
- Identify time, place, and duration of team meetings.
- Determine a system by which cases are to be presented and by whom. Identify how care plans and action will be carried out and documented. (Is one member chosen to write down the care plan or does this responsibility rotate?)
- Identify opportunities or requirements for team-building meetings and/or team training.
- Create mechanism for enforcing both governance and behavior rules through ongoing evaluation of the effectiveness of the meeting (if rules are made and not enforced, the team can quickly become ineffective and be a negative experience for everyone involved).

People are usually more willing to expend time and energy if there is a clear understanding of what is going to occur and why it is needed. The time spent with participants clarifying rules and getting a commitment for involvement will prevent team problems and support the development of an effective and efficient team.

While the above governance rules provide a structure for team interaction, behavior rules are also needed for each team. They can include some or all of the following:

- Ensure clear understanding by all team members of what an interdisciplinary team is and what members should bring to the group.
- Promote understanding and respect for others' expertise.

Table 21-1   Eight Principles of Successful Team Work

1. All team members share a common purpose and work together to establish explicitly stated patient care goals.
2. The patient and family are at the center of all team activities and are active team members.
3. The full scope of the professional capabilities of each team member is clearly understood by everyone on the team; professional roles are dynamic and are determined by the needs of the team, individual experience, and the knowledge and skills of team members.
4. All team members should contribute to team function through constructive individual behaviors, including rotating leadership.
5. There must be effective team communication across all work and care settings.
6. The team must have tools or strategies for the effective management of conflict.
7. The team should have explicit rules about participation and decision making.
8. The team must be adaptable, responding to new challenges and conditions as they develop over time.

Source: GITT Medicine Special Interest Group: Team Pocket Card. New York: GITT Resource Center, New York University; 1999.

- Recognize the implications of idioms by the professionals involved. Learn how to articulate information clearly to others. (Do client and patient mean the same thing in different professional groups?) Health care goals will come from different perspectives and from different disciplines.
- Share information and expertise openly.
- Identify and follow a decision process when roles overlap. Resist setting rigid boundaries on roles. Instead, promote effective ways of sharing responsibilities and tasks.
- Define acceptable behavior (willingness to work with other professionals to develop a care plan, active participation, respect for others' roles).

THE WELL-PLANNED MEETING

Teams with poorly planned and organized meetings become ineffective and inefficient. This cultivates negative attitudes towards teams, and leads to poor attendance and less than enthusiastic participation by the team members. Elements essential to the structure of an effective meeting include:

1. Agenda (what do we expect to accomplish?)
2. Estimated timeline for completing agenda (reasonable time frames).
3. Establishment of meeting roles. Members can and should rotate the following roles but every meeting should include:

- Leader (calls meeting to order, has agenda, sets expectations).
- Timekeeper (keeps group on task).
- Recorder (keeps track of agreements about the care plan and modifications, and is responsible for recording changes to care plan).

4. Summary of agreements (recorder reports agreements).
5. Evaluation/reflection on team process (both team process and outcome of the meeting are discussed).

SUGGESTED STRUCTURE FOR REGULAR HEALTH CARE TEAM MEETINGS

Creating a structure and format for health care team meetings standardizes the meeting process and assists in making teams more efficient and effective. By using a standard agenda, health care team members are more prepared for meetings and the flow of the meeting is predictable. Table 21-2 provides tips on how to facilitate a team meeting. Key elements are an agenda with time frames and a responsible party for each agenda item, a timekeeper to encourage the group to stay on track, and a recorder who captures the group decisions and delineates the responsible person for specified tasks. Evaluating meetings is important and improves the quality of the structure and process, especially if evaluation is a routine part of the regularly

Table 21-2 How to Facilitate a Team Meeting

The role of the facilitator is to:

1. Ensure goals and objectives of the meeting are clear to all members.
2. Observe and value the participation of each member.
3. Acknowledge both verbal and nonverbal communication, and address dysfunctional behaviors within the team.
4. Identify conflict, exploring thought processes that lead to differing conclusions.
5. Seek mutual understanding.
6. Assure shared decision making.
7. Suggest tools/techniques to enhance meeting flow, information gathering, decision making, and future planning.
8. Give constructive feedback.
9. Encourage team to evaluate its progress.

SOURCE: GITT Medicine Special Interest Group: Team Pocket Card. New York: GITT Resource Center, New York University; 1999.

scheduled meetings. The following format should work for most meetings.

1. Review meeting objectives to ensure that all members understand and are in agreement with the meeting objectives.
2. Review agenda and order of items. Add, reorder, or delete items as the group decides. Ensure that all team members agree with the agenda items.
3. Assign timekeeper, recorder, and leader roles. Confirm time intervals timekeeper will use to cue group.
4. Report follow-up from last meeting.
5. Discuss issues or patients as listed on the agenda.
6. Summarize action items from this meeting. Decide who will do what before the next meeting.
7. Decide what the objectives and agenda items will be for the next meeting.
8. Evaluate the meeting. Ask each member to evaluate the meeting. Evaluation can be written or verbal but the questions should focus on: What did the team do well that it should continue doing? What could the team do differently to improve the meeting?

SKILLS OF DIFFERENT PROFESSIONALS ON TEAMS

Team members from different disciplines bring a unique set of skills (Table 21-3), but those skills also overlap. Understanding the skills and education of various team members contributes to respect but also allows team members to refer elderly clients appropriately to other professionals. Because each profession trains its members in a culture that reflects a common language, professional behaviors, values, and beliefs, disagreement between professionals may occur because of different professional expectations and

Table 21-3   Team Members Overview

Discipline	Practice Roles/Skills	Education/Training	Licensure/Credentials
Nurse	Licensed vocational nurse (LVN)—basic nursing skills that are dictated by the facility; registered nurse (RN)—BA or higher and has increased scope of practice, including planning for optimal functioning, coordination of care, teaching, and direct and indirect patient care.	LVN—1 year of training; RN with associate degree—2 years of training, usually in a community college; BS, RN—4 years in college; MS, RN—2 years of postgraduate speciality study; PhD RN—3–4 years of postgraduate studies	LVN-exam required for licensing; CE requirements. RN—can be RN; BS, RN; APN; MS, GNP or other speciality RNs; PhD, RN: all must pass the national licensure exam and are required to have 20 hours of CEUs per year.
Nurse practitioner	Health assessment, health promotion skills, histories and physicals in outpatient settings; order, conduct, and interpret some lab and diagnostic tests; teaching and counseling.	Master's degree with a defined speciality area such as gerontology (GNP).	In addition to RN licensure, NP must pass a National Certification Exam in the appropriate speciality area (e.g., gerontology or family practice)
Physician	Treat diseases and injuries, provide preventive care, do routine checkups, prescribe drugs, and do some surgery.	Physicians complete medical school (4 years) plus 3 to 7 years of graduate medical education	State licensure required for doctor of medicine degree; exam required and possible exams required for speciality areas. CE requirements.
Geriatrician	Physician with special training in the diagnosis, treatment, and prevention of disorders in older people; recognizes aging as a normal process and not a disease state.	Complete a 1- to 3-year postgraduate fellowship training program in geriatric medicine or pass an exam. Certificate of Added Qualification (CAQ) in geriatrics.	Doctor of medicine state exam required as above.
Physician assistant (PA)	Practice medicine with the supervision of licensed physicians; exercise autonomy in medical decision making and provide a broad range of diagnostic and therapeutic services; practice is centered on patient care.	Specially designed 2-year PA program located at medical colleges and universities. Most have bachelor's degree and more than 4 years of health care experience before entering a PA program.	NCCPA certifying exam—the credentials PAC will be used if certified; PA will be used if not certified. This exam is given every fall (October) for first-time takers. Every 6 years a PA must take a recertification exam and this is given in the spring. Requires 100 hours of CEUs every 2 years.
Social Worker	Assessment of individual and family psychosocial functioning and provision of care to help enhance or restore capacities; this can include locating services or providing counseling.	There is a 4-year college degree (BSW); 2 years of graduate work (MSW), and doctoral degree (Ph.D.); 15 hours of continuing education is required every year.	State certification is required for clinical social workers. The LMSW (for masters level); LSW (BS level); SWA is a social work associate with a combination of education and experience. ACP—signifies licensure for independent clinical practice.

(Continued)

Table 21-3 (*Continued*) Team Members Overview

Discipline	Practice Roles/Skills	Education/Training	Licensure/Credentials
Psychologist	Assessment, treatment, and management of mental disorders; psychotherapy with individuals, groups, and families.	Graduate training consists of 5 years beyond undergraduate training; most course work includes gerontology and clinical experience.	Ph.D. or EdD or PsyD are degrees awarded. State licensure; the American Psychological Association has ethics codes, as do most states.
Psychiatrist	Medical doctors who treat patients' mental, emotional, and behavioral symptoms.	Medical school and residency specializing in psychiatry. Residency includes both general residency training and 2–3 years in area of specialization (e.g., geriatrics, pediatrics).	State exam to practice medicine; Board of Psychiatry and Neurology offers exam for diplomat in psychiatry, although not required for psychiatric practice in Texas.
Pharmacist	Devise and revise a patient's medication therapy to achieve the optimal regimen that suits the individual's medical and therapeutic needs; information resource for the patient and medical team.	Pharmacists can receive a baccalaureate (B.S.)- 5 year program; or doctorate degree (Pharm.D.). Annual CEUs required range from 10 to 15 hours.	State exam required-Texas uses the national exam (NABPLEX); given every quarter; RPh is the title for a registered pharmacist in Texas; board certifications in specialities available (pharmacotherapy, nuclear pharmacy, nutrition, psychiatric, and oncology in near future).
Occupational Therapist (OT)	One who utilizes therapeutic goal-directed activities to evaluate, prevent, or correct physical, mental, or emotional dysfunction or to maximize function in the life of the individual.	BS or MS in OT with a minimum of 6 months of field work; for OT assistant, an associate degree or OT assistant certificate is required with a minimum of 2 months' field work.	State exam required for the credential of OTR (occupational therapist registered). Exam also required for COTA (certified occupational therapy assistant). These exams are given at least 2 times/year.
Physical Therapist	The evaluation, examination, and utilization of exercises, rehabilitative procedures, massage, manipulations, and physical agents including, but not limited to, mechanical devices, heat, cold, air, light, water, electricity, and sound in the aid of diagnosis or treatment.	Four-year college degree in physical therapy is required to be eligible for the state exam; master's degree in physical therapy is available; 3 CEUs every 2 years are required.	PT is the credential that is used by licensed physical therapists and PTA is the credential for licensed physical therapist assistant. To use either of these titles, one must pass a state exam. CEUs are required for both; titles and licenses must be renewed biannually.
Chaplain	Provide visits and ministry to patients and family.	Master's degree in theology, plus a minimum of 1 year of clinical supervision. If fully certified, can work in some settings without being fully certified.	Certification is through the Chaplaincy Board of Certification—credentials for this are BCC; however, credentials are not normally used. Most chaplains are ordained ministers, but not all. CEUs required are 50 hours per year.

(*Continued*)

Table 21-3 *(Continued)* Team Members Overview

Discipline	Practice Roles/Skills	Education/Training	Licensure/Credentials
Dietitian	Evaluate the nutritional status of patients; work with family members and medical team to determine appropriate nutrition goals for patient.	BS degree in food and nutrition and experience are required to be eligible for exam; CEU's are required for both the LD (6 clock hours/year) and RD (67 clock hours every 5 years); Ms degree is available also.	RD is the credential for a registered dietitian in the state of Texas. For RD, must pass the national exam of the American Dietetic Association; LD is the credential for a licensed dietitian in the state of Texas; same exam is required but processing of paperwork/fees are different.

SOURCE: Adapted from Long DM, Wilson NL (eds): *Houston Geriatric Interdisciplinary Team Training Curriculum*. Houston, TX: Baylor College of Medicine's Huffington Center on Aging; 2001.

language. Most professionals do not recognize the training of others and learn what other professionals do only after being in professional practice. Although a range of individuals can be found as members of an interdisciplinary team in geriatrics, the core professional members are typically the physician, nurse, social worker, and pharmacist. The extended professional members of the team might include nonphysician providers (nurse practitioners, physician assistants), physical therapist, occupational therapist, speech pathologist, dietitian, and psychologist or psychiatrist. That the older client and the client's family are also important members of the team cannot be emphasized enough.

Knowledge about the preparation, expertise, and scope of practice affects individual team member performance, in that it can:

- Reduce tension that occurs around who is doing what;
- Help members accept role overlap as necessary and positive;
- Foster positive views toward the efforts of several disciplines; and
- Increase the ability to problem solve beyond a single discipline.

SPECIFIC ROLES/SKILLS OF TEAM MEMBERS

Table 21-3 provides an overview of the different practice roles/skills, education/training, and licensure/credentials of different professionals who commonly participate as members of interdisciplinary teams.

The Physician

The physician treats diseases and injuries, provides preventive care, performs routine checkups, prescribes drugs, and may perform surgery. A geriatrician is a physician with special training in the diagnosis, treatment, and prevention of disorders affecting older people. The geriatrician recognizes that aging is a normal process and not a disease state.

The GITT Medicine Special Interest Group has guidelines on the physician's role on an interdisciplinary team:

- Responsibilities to team members don't differ according to discipline. They involve cooperation, participation in the tasks at hand, and respect for the contributions of others.
- The physician should model these behaviors and teach them to students as well.
- The physician should serve as a mentor not only to physicians-in-training but also to students from all disciplines.
- The physician should ensure that medical issues are given the proper weight in the decision-making process. He or she can accomplish this by describing the relevant medical aspects of cases, so that they are fully understood by everyone participating in the development of the interdisciplinary care plan.

The Geriatric Nurse Practitioner

The GITT Nursing Special Interest Group defined the professional skills and interdisciplinary team skills of the nurse practitioner. Upon completion of a formal educational program, gerontological nurse practitioners are able to do the following:

- Elicit a comprehensive health history from the client and/or caregivers, including an evaluation of developmental maturation, physiologic/psychosocial/functional status, cultural orientation, perception of health, health-promoting behaviors, risk factors for illness, response to stressors, activities of daily living (instrumental and functional), service utilization, and support systems.
- Complete a comprehensive functional assessment, mental status assessment, and psychoemotional assessment.
- Perform a complete physical examination on the older adult, employing techniques of observation, inspection, palpation, auscultation, and percussion.

- Discriminate among normal findings, normal changes of aging, pathologic findings, and abnormal findings that require collaboration with a physician.
- Use pertinent screening tools to determine health status.
- Order and/or perform pertinent diagnostic tests.
- Analyze the data collected in collaboration with the health care team to determine health status and need for consultation with or referral to other agencies or resources.
- Formulate a problem list.
- Develop and implement, with the client, caregiver(s) and/or significant other(s), and health care team a plan of care to promote, maintain, and rehabilitate health.
- Evaluate the client's response to the health care provided and the effectiveness of the care with the client.
- Collaborate with other health professionals and agencies involved in the client's care.
- Modify the plan and intervention as needed.
- Record all pertinent data about the client, including the health history, functional assessment, physical examination, problems identified, interventions planned and/or provided, results of care, and plans for consultation or referral.
- Coordinate the services required to meet the client's need for primary health care and/or long-term care and monitor outcomes.
- Act as an advocate for the older adult to improve his or her health status.
- Provide for continuity of care over time and in a variety of settings.
- Provide patient/family-centered care.
- Participate in lifelong learning, peer review, and Continuous Quality Improvement (CQI).

The Social Worker

The role of the social worker on an interdisciplinary team includes, but is not limited to, the following:

1. Diagnosis/assessment: The goal of a bio-psycho-social assessment is to identify the strengths and limitations of the patient and family and to assist them in creating a treatment plan with clearly defined goals. It provides a holistic view of the patient/family. The social worker can identify barriers to medical compliance and assist others on the team in the management of an acute or chronic illness. The social worker can also help to assess whether the presenting medical problem is compounded by mental health problems. The social work assessment takes into consideration how well the patient (and the family or caregiver) is functioning in six areas:

    - Physical—a brief medical history, functional abilities, appearance, and observed behavior.
    - Psychological—affect, mood, outlook, attitude, personality characteristics, cognitive functioning, self-image.
    - Social—vocation, social roles, support networks, education, and financial status.
    - Cultural—values, general rules of behavior, definition of the "sick role," beliefs about the root causes of illness and prescribed treatments, communication patterns that encompass varied language and speech patterns, as well as bilingual issues.
    - Environmental—living conditions and home surroundings, with focus on safety and maintaining functional independence.
    - Spiritual—beliefs about people's roles and responsibilities, rules for living, belief system, diet, and acceptable medical treatments.

2. Care management: Also referred to as case management, this social work role includes problem identification (e.g., lack of financial resources, need for help with activities of daily living, or mental health intervention), as well as links to and coordination of community resources to facilitate the highest practical level of functioning for the patient and family. It requires knowledge of community resources and entitlements, and skills in matching patient/family with resources, linking resources, and serving as an interpreter and advocate for the patient/family.

3. Individual counseling: Psychosocial counseling includes treatment of mental health problems such as depression and anxiety through various techniques, including family therapy, relaxation, and stress management training for the patient and/or caregiver. This is intended to assist patients and families in adjusting to major life stressors and transitions such as illness, disability, institutionalization, and loss, as well as to empower the client. A patient's ability to adapt to an illness has a profound impact on quality of life, as well as on the patient's willingness/ability to comply with the prescribed treatment and is paramount to recovery, physical, and emotional healing, timely discharge from the hospital, risk management, and effective decision making. The social worker brings skills in listening, problem resolution, and negotiation, with attention to community and environmental factors.

4. Group work: Group psychotherapy and supportive psychoeducational groups are designed to help patients/families and/or caregivers cope with a specific illness, such as depression, Alzheimer's disease, cancer, or diabetes. The social worker brings skills in group development and facilitation.

5. Liaison: The social worker can also serve as a liaison between the patient/family and the professional community. This is particularly pertinent when the family lives out of the area and their input must be obtained via long-distance communication.

6. Advocacy: A social worker's training, including a working knowledge of ethics, confidentiality, advance directives, cultural/ethnic factors, and patient/family rights, serves to help teams face the challenge of balancing patient needs with the system demands. Often the most important service provided by a geriatric/gerontological social worker to patients is assistance negotiating an overwhelmingly bureaucratic system, such as Medicaid, Social Security disability, funeral arrangements, or dealing with insurance and hospital

paperwork, by acting on the patient's behalf, and/or teaching them to help themselves.

7. Community resource expertise: Knowledge of community resources and how to access them is an invaluable piece of the social work profession. This involves high-level skills in negotiation and bargaining in order to broker for appropriate resource allocation. A working knowledge of financial systems, including federal, state, and county programs is part of this expertise. Serving as a resource referral coordinator requires negotiation and collaboration to assist patients and families in setting priorities, care goals, and balancing issues.

The Patient, Family, and/or Caregivers

The patient's, family's, or caregiver's roles as team members can be described in terms of their contributions to the care planning process of the interdisciplinary team:

- Extent of commitment to problem management plan;
- Understanding of goals and components of treatment plan; and
- Self-determination and rights.

EFFECTIVE TEAM COMMUNICATION

Communication is the foundation for all team functioning. It requires that all team members cooperate to establish ongoing communication with each other, with the patient, and with the family for the sole purpose of developing an integrated care plan that addresses each aspect of the needed care.

Barriers to communication range from the lack of a shared language born of differences in core values and terminology used by different disciplines, to systems and organizational barriers. Moreover, in a busy health care organization, a major hurdle is finding the time for a team meeting and developing methods for effective team communication. In an organization where care is being provided in multiple locations and settings, informal communication often occurs in hallways and elevators, and by telephone, voice mail, and e-mail. The provision of effective coordinated care requires the team to have an effective mechanism for the exchange of information. At the simplest level, this requires the time, space, and regular opportunity for members to meet and discuss patient cases. An ideal system for interdisciplinary team communication includes:

- A well-designed record system.
- A regularly scheduled forum for members to discuss patient management issues.
- A regularly scheduled forum to discuss and evaluate team function and development, and to address related interpersonal issues.
- A mechanism for communicating with the external system (e.g., hospital administration) within which the team operates.

Effective communication also relies on listening, explaining perceptions, acknowledging, and discussing the differences and similarities in views, recommending appropriate treatment, and negotiating agreement. In our increasingly diverse workplaces, language and cultural barriers can exist among members of a team. These barriers can make it difficult for one member to understand the finer points in the meanings, intentions, and reactions of other team members. Our cultural heritage, our gender, our socioeconomic status, and our stage of life—all of these influence our use of language and our perception of others. Some degree of cultural competency must be in place for team members to effectively communicate with each other as well as with patients and family members. Additional barriers to effective communication and teamwork can include:

- Lack of a clearly stated, shared and measurable purpose.
- Lack of training in interdisciplinary collaboration.
- Role and leadership ambiguity.
- Team too large or too small.
- Team not composed of appropriate professionals.
- Lack of appropriate mechanisms for timely exchange of information.

Even among team members of similar cultural backgrounds, members need to recognize and value the different competencies and approaches of different disciplines. People do not need to think the same to be unified. The key to team success is to value the differences on the team and use such diversity to achieve the team's common purpose.

VALUING DIVERSITY

Values are a major source of conflicting and competing communication patterns among health professionals. The education and training of health care professionals vary according to different modes and methods of practice. For example, a patient who is being seen by a team may have a problem with depression. A pharmacist might see a patient with no drug therapy; a social worker might see a socially isolated patient; and a physician might see a patient with possible dementia. Furthermore, if members of an interdisciplinary team do not possess at least a basic understanding of each other's knowledge and values, then it is likely that misunderstandings will result. For example, most physicians equate quality of life with mental status or freedom from mental impairment, while many nurses relate quality of life to physical strength, seeing, hearing, and having someone who cares.

The following tips may be helpful for valuing diversity on a team:

- Reasonable people can—and do—differ with each other. No two people are the same. Diversity among team members enhances creativity.
- Learn as much as you can from others. Learning the various backgrounds, cultures, and professional values of others can enrich your own skills and abilities.
- Evaluate a new idea based on its merits. Avoid evaluating ideas based on who submitted them or how closely they mirror your own personal preferences.

- Avoid comments and remarks that draw negative attention to a person's unique characteristics. Humor is a key factor in a healthy team environment but should never be used at the expense of another's identity or self-esteem.

Don't ignore the differences among team members. The differences should be honored and utilized to advance the goals of the team. Decision making and conflict resolution are also components of the communication process that must be acknowledged by teams. The group process must integrate openness and confrontation, support and trust, cooperation and conflict, sound procedures for solving problems and getting things done, and good communication. Establishing a planned process for decision-making is essential. The process must also take resolution of conflicts into account, because conflict is inevitable.

TEAM CONFLICT

Conflict is a natural and unavoidable part of human affairs, especially in such groups as interdisciplinary health care teams that seek to grow and develop. The various health professionals on a team have underlying differences in their modes and methods of practice that affect their relationships with each other, as well as with their patients. Professionals may differ in their logic of geriatric clinical assessment, that is, how to define the problem.

This difference may be characterized by two different styles of practice. One, a "ruling-out problem" approach systematically eliminates possibilities until only one problem and a corresponding solution remain. The other, a "ruling-in problem" approach, relies on expanding the range of professional view to encompass an increasingly long list of potential factors. For example, physicians are trained in diagnostic techniques that narrow the range of options, relying heavily on such objective data as laboratory tests in the process. Social workers, on the other hand, are taught to go beyond the narrow presenting problems to view it within larger, encompassing psychosocial issues, such as income, family relationships, and environment. In addition to the diverse professional perspectives, team members also have different personalities that influence interactions among team members. Other factors that may lead to conflict in team care include scarce resources and organizational or professional change that threatens individuals or the overall program. Table 21-4 provides guidelines for using conflict to promote interdisciplinary problem solving.

The discussion of different points of view promotes growth and development which lead to improved outcomes. This sort of discussion often leads to conflict, a natural and unavoidable part of human affairs. Successful resolution of conflict requires the ability to communicate effectively as well as to confront issues, not people, focusing on the search for win–win solutions in which both sides achieve a benefit. Table 21-5 lists common approaches to negotiation and conflict resolution.

EMPHASIZING CARE GOALS AND INTERDISCIPLINARY CARE PLANNING

The concept of goals is essential on at least two levels within interdisciplinary geriatric care teams. Teams are generally organized to achieve specific programmatic goals. Health care teams work with patients, families, and others to achieve patient-specific goals. For an interdisciplinary team to function effectively, the team's purpose and goals should be understood clearly and agreed upon by all members. With the increasing cost consciousness in health care, the goals of teamwork and the products of interdisciplinary collaboration are of paramount importance. In managed care, the measurement of outcomes is an important and widely accepted way of demonstrating that adequate care is being provided. Goals established—whether long- or short-term—need to be feasible, because interdisciplinary teams function in a variety of settings (e.g., home care, inpatient), the team membership, types and intensity of services provided, and overall goals will vary. One step toward establishing goals is to have the team answer the question, "What do we want to achieve with this patient?"

INTERDISCIPLINARY CARE PLANNING

After programmatic goals are determined, team members next must agree on what they mean in reality. For example, if "improve patient outcome" is a goal used by a team, successful outcome will need to be defined case by case. The process of interdisciplinary team care planning is the means of achieving consensus on desired patient outcomes. One discipline might want to save the patient's life at all costs, while another discipline might want comfort and less aggressive medical care. For example, when a patient shows signs of confusion and an inability to care for herself, a doctor might want the patient hospitalized for her own safety, while a social worker might want to bring social services or health care into the home first. These choices can keep the team in a conflict mode without reaching a decision on the care plan unless the purpose and goals are clear and the patient or a surrogate is meaningfully involved in the decision about care.

An interdisciplinary team developing care plans and treatment goals for patients must be able to conceptualize patients broadly, incorporating all relevant information and knowing how different pieces of information relate. The ability of each discipline to add to the overall care plan will depend on each team member's understanding of the linkages between problems. A general treatment outcome goal of optimum health for the patient can be agreed upon easily by team members but the best means of obtaining that goal will be considered differently by the various disciplines represented on the team. Professionals will share their views of plan initiatives based on their professional knowledge or previous experience. This exchange will lead the group into areas that might not be considered if it weren't for the team expertise available. If the patient is having problems with fatigue, sleeping, and eating, one professional may believe depression needs to be considered and another team member will bring up overmedication as

Table 21-4   Using Conflict to Promote Interdisciplinary Problem Solving

Methods/Strategies	Power	Conclusion	Use/Don't Use
Coerce–Force One defensive; one offensive; emphasize differences; judge and accuse	Imbalance (real or perceived); attempt to retain imbalance	One yields or standoff	Emergency; unpopular issue, fixed resources, need decision/need support or long-term relationship
Withdraw–Avoid One defensive; one offensive; emphasize differences	Imbalance (real or perceived); attempt to retain imbalance or create new imbalance	One yields or standoff	Trivial issue; little power; nonrecurring problem; part of larger problem/serious issue; critical goals; recurring problem
Negotiate–Compromise Bargain; hoard information	Relatively equal; attempt to increase relative power	Different factions agree to accept decision; all win and lose	Mutually exclusive goals of moderate importance; balanced power; focused on roles/early in problem; need more information
Accommodate–Oblige Share *all* information, clarify *all* disagreements; equalize input	Relatively equal; attempt to further equalize power	Overt agreement; covert disagreement	When wrong; need social credits; goals not critical; to promote member responsibility/issue important to team and relationships
Collaborate–Integrate Openly present problems; use all power strategies; balance conflict and cooperation	Universal and unequal; members free to get more power; team controls power for decision making	Comprehensive solution and reevaluation	Critical needs and goals; ill-defined problem; need commitment/no time; no trust

SOURCE: Adapted from Drinka, Clark: *Health care teamwork: Interdisciplinary practice and teaching.* Westport, CT: Auburn House; 2000.

Table 21-5   Common Approaches to Negotiation and Conflict Resolution

1. Welcome conflict and use it as potential for change. Address data, facts, assumptions, and conclusions.
2. Clarify the nature of the problem as seen by all parties.
3. Try to identify areas of agreement. Focus on common interests, not positions.
4. Deal with one problem at a time, beginning with the easier issues.
5. Listen with understanding. Reflect and clarify when communicating.
6. Brainstorm.
7. Use objective criteria when possible.
8. Invent new solutions where all parties again.
9. Evaluate and review the problem-solving process after implementing the plan.

SOURCE: Adapted from Long D: Houston, TX: Huffington Center on Aging, Baylor College of Medicine; 1999.

a possible physical cause. Within a team, these ideas need to be shared for the overall benefit of the patient. Members must communicate these as their own professional opinions and all members need to respect the different kinds of expertise each brings to the group.

For all the great effort put into developing a care plan, a plan cannot work unless the team has a system for documenting it and indicating clearly who will be responsible for what and by when. This documentation should be completed before the end of the meeting and available to all team members to remind them of their responsibilities. In addition, there must be in place a system (formal and informal) for communicating and continuing with the next steps of the care plan between team meetings. This is most often done informally with the different disciplines talking with each other as needed.

CONCLUSION

Good interdisciplinary care teams can enhance management of the complex syndromes experienced by older adults. Good teams require team members with excellent clinical skills who are schooled in the knowledge and skills of teaming. Good teaming doesn't happen by accident but is a function of well developed team structure which includes rules to govern the team and team member behavior, plans to make meetings run efficiently, clarity about the skills and boundaries for the roles and responsibilities of each team member, team communication skills, and mechanisms for managing team conflict. Fulfilling these requirements can lead to care goals and care planning that emphasizes the particular needs of the older adult.

REFERENCES

American Congress on Rehabilitation Medicine, cited in Long DM, Wilson NL (eds). *Houston Geriatric Interdisciplinary Team Training Curriculum.* Houston, TX, Baylor College of Medicine, Huffington Center on Aging, 2001.

Cassel C et al (eds): *Mount Sinai Geriatric Interdisciplinary Team Training Resource Manual.* New York, Mount Sinai School of Medicine, 2000.

Clark P: Values in health care professional socialization: Implications for geriatric education in interdisciplinary teamwork. *Gerontologist* 37(4):441, 1997.

Clark PG: Quality of life, values, and teamwork in geriatric care: Do we communicate what we mean? *Gerontologist* 35:402, 1995.

Drinka T, Streim J: Case studies from purgatory: Maladaptive behavior within geriatric health care teams. *Gerontologist* 34(4):541, 1994.

Fisher K et al: *Tips for Teams: A Ready Reference for Solving Common Team Problems.* New York, McGraw-Hill, 1995.

Grant RW, Finocchio LJ: *California Primary Care Consortium Subcommittee on Interdisciplinary Collaborative Teams in Primary Care. A Model Curriculum and Resource Guide.* San Francisco, Pew Health Professions, 1995.

Harrington-Machkin DH: *Let's Meet: Team Meetings. The Team-Building Toolkit: Tips, Tactics, and Rules for Effective Workplace Teams.* New York, American Management Association, 1994 p 31.

Hyer K et al (eds): *The GITT Curriculum Guide.* New York, NYU GITT Resource Center, 2001.

Hyer K et al (eds): *The GITT Implementation Manual.* New York, NYU GITT Resource Center, 2001.

Long D, Wilson N (eds): *Houston Geriatric Interdisciplinary Team Training Curriculum.* Houston, TX, Baylor College of Medicine, Huffington Center on Aging, 2001.

Mezey M et al (eds): *Ethical Patient Care: A Casebook for Geriatric Health Care Teams.* Baltimore, Johns Hopkins, 2002.

Pew Health Professions Commission and California Primary Care Association: *Interdisciplinary Collaborative Teams in Primary Care: A Model Curriculum and Resource Guide.* San Francisco, Pew Health Professions Commission, 1995.

Qualls SH, Czirr R: Geriatric health teams: Classifying models of professional and team functioning. *Gerontologist* 28:372, 1988.

Siegler EL et al (eds): *Geriatric Interdisciplinary Team Training.* New York, Springer, 1998 p 3.

Walker P et al: Building community: Developing skills for interprofessional health professions education and relationship-centered care. NLN Appointed Interdisciplinary Health Education Panel. *J Allied Health* 27(3):173, 1998.

Woodcock M, Francis D: *Teambuilding Strategy.* VT, Gower Publishing, Brookfield, VT 1994.

Woods AM, Coutts L: Communication, in Long DM and Wilson, NL (ed): *Geriatric Interdisciplinary Team Training: A curriculum from the Huffington Center on Aging at Baylor College of Medicine.* 2001, p.76.

INTERNET RESOURCES

The Great Lakes GITT: http://www.gitt.cwru.edu.

The Huffington Center on Aging at Baylor College of Medicine: http://www.hcoa.org/hgitt/.

The Mount Sinai School of Medicine GITT: http://www.mssm.edu/geriatric.

The NYU GITT Resource Center: http://www.gitt.org.

The University of California at Los Angeles: http://www.geronet.med.ucla.edu.

The University of Colorado Health Sciences Center: http://www.uchsc.edu.

Families, Social Support, and Caregiving

TONI C. ANTONUCCI • RICHARD SCHULZ

This chapter focuses on social relations and considers two special aspects of social relations, families, and caregiving. To elucidate the general concept of *social relations,* we emphasize its life span and cumulative nature. We consider the various aspects of social relations including social networks, social support, and satisfaction with support. We note that the exchange of social support is common in most relationships and can consist of a range of exchanges from affection to sick care. There are different types of social networks that essentially describe the structure within which most support is exchanged. One of the most common social network structures is the family—mother, father, husband, wife, child, parent—which represents the most common exchange patterns, and is also the most common composition of caregiving dyads. Thus, understanding the nature of social relations provides important information about family and caregiving interactions.

SOCIAL RELATIONS

Social relations are widely recognized as an important aspect of health and patient care. While it has long been known that social relations influence psychological factors, their influence on physical and mental health has also become increasingly clear. Social relations can be assumed to contribute to the health and well-being of the elderly person through their influence on the caregiving relationship specifically, as well as through their potential to influence successful aging more generally. As the aging individual is faced with increasing physical and mental challenges, medicine can help, but only to a point. Social relations are important to the individual's ability to prepare for, cope with, and recover from many of the exigencies of life that are faced with increasing frequency as one ages. These include providing care to loved ones, as well as personally experiencing the challenges of age.

Relevant Terms and Definitions

The generalized term *social relations* is used to describe the broad array of factors and interpersonal interactions that characterize the social exchanges among people. Under this rubric, we consider three useful terms: social networks, social support, and sense of control. *Social networks* can best be understood in terms of the objective characteristics that describe the people with whom an individual maintains interpersonal relations, that is, their family and friends. Thus, one can describe one's social network members in terms of their age, gender, role relationship, years known, residential proximity, frequency of contact, and the like. Describing a social network reveals critical information about the people with whom an individual has a relationship, about those from whom one might expect to receive care and, at the same time, about those to whom one might be expected to, or feel obligated to, provide care. However, these objective characteristics of the social network reveal nothing about the nature, content, or quality of those relationships.

To describe the content of social relations we use the term *social support.* Social support refers to the actual exchange of support. Social support can be described as an interpersonal transaction involving one of three key elements: aid, affect, or affirmation. Aid refers to instrumental or tangible support such as lending money, helping with chores, or providing sick care. Affect refers to emotional support such as love, affection, and caring. Affirmation refers to agreement or acknowledgment of similarities or appropriateness of one's values or point of view. While the normal exchange of aid, affect, and affirmation have been described as social support, these exchanges are generally characterized by reciprocity and, therefore, are distinctly different from the detailed or explicit expectations of caregiving. However, since, as noted earlier, the people who provide caregiving are often the same people with whom social support was exchanged previously, awareness of the prior relationship can be critical. The transition from a reciprocal supportive relationship to a nonreciprocal caregiving one can be a traumatic one. The degree to which that transition is successful can set the tone for the entire late life experience. It is very likely that much about the caregiving relationship has a basis in the earlier exchange of social support.

Several characteristics of social support exchanges have been shown to be important. The first to consider is source of support, e.g. family, friend, neighbor. This issue clearly parallels the caregiving experience where, at least in this country, the two most common caregivers are spouse and children. Substantially different caregiver issues arise depending on whether the caregiver is a spouse or child. The psychological characteristics of the caregiving relationship, which include the satisfaction one feels with the support received, that is, its quality, content, or quantity; and even the perception that the support was provided, whether or not it actually was, are also important.

An emerging issue is the *sense of control* an individual feels in any particular situation. Of particular interest to the study of social relationships is how individuals cognitively represent information about people and social situations and then use that information to guide their behavior. Many factors are thought to influence how a person processes and represents information. Among the included factors are fundamental cognitive processes as well as such characteristics as memories of the past, perceptions of self, and attributions about others. Social cognition, generally, can be very helpful to understanding fundamental aspects of social relations. In this consideration of social relations, families, and caregiving, it is proposed that the degree to which social relations lead to, influence, or are influenced by a sense control, is especially relevant. This association is further explored below.

Theoretical Perspectives: Importance of the Life Course

It is now generally recognized that a life span perspective provides a critical underlying base to the study of social relations, and by extension caregiving. The most important social relations usually involve long-lasting, significant, close relationships such as those between parent and child, siblings, husband and wife. Interpersonal relationships are life span in nature either because they have existed over the life course or because they are built upon earlier relationships that influence the type, style, and content of later relationships. To understand how an individual experiences a relationship at any one in time, it is most useful to understand the history of that specific relationship as well as other relationships in the person's life. Thus, the study of a 50-year-old woman and her 70-year-old mother is best conceptualized as a relationship that has continued from when the 50-year-old was an infant through her early childhood, adolescence, young adulthood, into the current state of middle age. Similarly, her mother was at one time a 20-year-old mother and has loved and cared for her child throughout the subsequent 50 years. In the case of spousal caregiving, a wife may willingly care for her husband with advanced Alzheimer's disease as she remembers her husband's care of their child years earlier when she was

hospitalized with a major illness. The resultant mother–child or spousal relationship, as well as the nature of their caregiving relationship, is likely to be understood very differently depending on these lifetime-accumulated experiences. One could even argue that what might be perceived by others to be an onerous caregiving burden is easily and even happily undertaken because of a lifetime of positive, supportive experiences. Or, to the contrary, a contemporaneous, relatively simple caregiving task might be refused or resented because of a lifetime of disappointment or neglect. Several theories have been suggested as useful for conceptualizing this cumulative and life span aspect of social relations. A representative example is considered below.

The *convoy model* provides a framework within which to study social relationships because it uses a life span perspective as the fundamental basis upon which to conceptualize the longitudinal nature of social relations. The convoy can be thought of as a structural concept shaped by personal (age, gender, personality) and situational (role expectations, resources, demands) factors that influence the support relations experienced by the individual. People form the convoy and the convoy, under ideal conditions, provides a protective, secure base or cushion that allows the individual to learn about, cope with, and experience the world. These personal and situational factors and social relations, in turn, affect that individual's health and well-being, both contemporaneously and longitudinally. The protective base provided by convoy members leads to better mental health and less psychological distress because it allows the individual to optimally grow and develop, and to successfully meet the challenges of life. This protective base is both objective and subjective, providing the individual with practical help but also, and perhaps most importantly, a psychological basis upon which to view the world. This is critical because we know that subjective and perceived support can be far more effective than objective and actual support in effecting the health and well-being of the individual. This fact indicates that, in addition to the actual support or caregiving provided, it is also critically important to consider the individual's cognitive construction and interpretation of the situation in order to explain how and why social relations effect an individual's health and well-being.

Most unique and especially relevant to the caregiving situation is the conceptualization of the individual as part of a dynamic network that moves through time, space, and the life course surrounding, embracing, and supporting the individual through the multiple experiences of life. The individual changes, grows, and develops. The situation within which the individual exists changes. It may become more or less complex, involve more or less people. And the interaction between the individual and the situation changes in response to both the individual's changes and the situational changes, thus exactly describing the type of situation that can lead to a caregiving relationship. The convoy reflects this dynamic aspect of social relations. As the individual ages, people are added to the convoy, subtracted from the convoy and move in and out of the convoy in response to both internal and external events. Under optimal conditions, this dynamic aspect of the convoy allows it to meet and be responsive to the changing needs of the individual.

Hence, the convoy can provide critical structure for anticipating and understanding the caregiving situation.

Other recent theoretical work has focused on explaining how social support positively effects the health and well-being of the individual. The *support/efficacy model* suggests that it is not only the exchange of specific support that accomplishes these effects, but the cumulative expression by one or several individuals to another that communicates to the target person that he or she is an able, worthy, capable person. Assuming that the support recipient perceives the support provided as accurate and altruistically motivated, the support recipient will come to internalize this same belief communicated by the supportive other. Thus, with multiple and repeated exchanges of this type, the supported person accumulates a belief in his or her own ability that will enable that person to face and succeed in the multiple goals and challenges of life, that is, to cope with problems across the life span. Not all people receive support from those who surround them and not all support is positive. Thus, some people instead of being told that they are competent, capable, and worthy may be led to believe that they are incompetent, incapable, and unworthy. Just as the cumulative effect of positive exchanges can have a positive affect on an individual's health and well-being, so the opposite can have a devastating and cumulative negative effect of health and well-being. Some support networks can have a negative effect by supporting or encouraging behaviors detrimental to health and well-being. Drug buddies, drinking buddies, eating buddies, and buddies who discourage exercise are all examples of people who help or "support" behaviors that simply are not good for you. The potential for these influences are certainly evident within the caregiving relationship and serve to explain why caregiving experiences are so varied. It is the goal of the health care professional to help maximize the positive potential of the caregiving situation and, to the extent possible, minimize the negative. In some cases the role of the health care professional might be to encourage certain caregiving behaviors or certain caregiver relationships, but clearly in other cases the most important role of the geriatric professional might be to discourage certain caregiving behaviors or caregiver relationships.

Some consider social support a coping mechanism. It is argued that as people are confronted with stress, the receipt of social support from important close others is a critical and significant coping strategy. This might be a useful way to conceptualize caregiving. Others argue that social support is actually personality based. People with specific personality characteristics seek and benefit from different types of social relations including specific types of social support exchanges. Thus, family and caregiving interactions will be more or less successful depending on the personality characteristics of the family members and of both the caregiver and the care receiver. Still others suggest an interweaving of social relationships, emotional development, and life span experiences. The *socioemotional selectivity theory* suggests that at younger ages people are more likely to seek out and be advantaged by numerous exchanges and social contacts, whereas as they age people reduce the number of exchanges with which they engage to only those which are perceived as most close. Within

the family and caregiving context this might explain why interactions and care from a significant few seems to be so much more important to people than from a larger number of people to whom the individual-recipient feels less close.

Sociodemographic and Cultural Issues

There are both sociodemographic and cultural similarities and differences in social relations that effect the general exchange of support and caregiving. Most people report immediate family—mother, father, spouse, children, and siblings—as their closest relationships, but people differentiate their feelings of closeness among these relationships. While all these relationships can be important, it is clear that the closest relationships are the most important in most circumstances and that under most circumstances it is these close relationships to which people turn for support and later caregiving. At the same time, it should be recognized that while close relationships are pervasively important, there can be special circumstances under which a person generally not considered very close can have a significant effect on the individual. One example is that of a nonrelated caregiver who uses a special skill to take on a special task such as feeding or bathing. The friend of a family member who has experienced a similar illness or treatment is another example. Generally, however, as with people of all ages, the social networks of the elderly person consist mainly, although not exclusively, of close family and friends.

The Importance of Age, Gender, Race, and Culture

Age   While it is commonly believed that the size of social networks, that is, the number of people in one's network, and the exchange of social support decreases with age, this is an overly simplistic view. Studies using large representative samples indicate that there are relatively few changes in social relations over time, at least until extreme old age. While it may be true that the total number of social relations decreases with age, the number of close relationships sustained by people and the amount of emotional support are relatively stable over time. In fact, an especially interesting finding is that people become more positive and less negative about their social relations with age.

Examination of the stability of social relations across age has yielded relatively consistent findings across cultures. Data from a variety of countries indicate considerable stability in social relations until very late in life. There is no doubt, however, that as one reaches ages 80, 90, and 100 years old, there are significantly fewer people who have been close supporters who are still alive. At the same time, these relationships are so close and long lasting that they are not easily replaced. Data from several countries in Western Europe concerning social networks and support relationships of the elderly person indicate a great many similarities in both size and composition of social networks. Most people have networks which average three to seven members, with the closest members being spouse, children, other family members, and friends. Data available from Asian countries such as Japan and China support similar findings. These social network data have important implications for who is available to exchange support with or to provide care when an elderly person requires it.

An interesting question arises over the issue of frequency of interactions by age. While there seems to be a general decrease in the quantity of interactions with age, some data suggest that there is an increase. It may very well be that there is a general decline in contact frequency with age under normal conditions. With the onset of a crisis, however, there is a concomitant increase in network contact, especially among close relations, to meet the needs brought on by the crisis. The question of network size over time is important because people with larger networks get more help in times of illness and, more informal support at an early period in life leads to less decline in health at a later period. Thus, the simple question, does network size increase, decrease or remain the same with age, appears to have a complex answer. Available evidence suggests that network size remains the same except at advanced old age. It may be that rather than network size increasing in times of crises, the existing, although perhaps dormant, network is activated under certain specialized "crisis" conditions.

Gender Perhaps the most complex and controversial issue in the study of social relations is the study of gender differences. While men and women have social relations with the same people, that is, spouse, children, other family, and friends, the nature of these relationships is quite different. It has been assumed that women are benefited by their relationships because the social relations of women are more intimate, of higher quality, and of greater intensity. Although these facts are still assumed to be true, more recent research questions the benefits of these differences. While women's relationships do seem to be more intimate, this apparently translates to a much greater, more in-depth sharing of both problems and concerns. Although relationships have been thought to be of higher quality among women, mainly because of the expression of greater closeness with larger numbers of people, evidence suggests that, in fact, women have both more positive and more negative relationships with others, often the same people. Thus, women are more likely to feel strong, positive feelings of affection toward their spouse, children, family, and friends, but they are also more likely to report higher levels of conflict, disagreement, and frustration with these same relationships. With respect to the intensity of their relationships it has been shown that while men and women may both express concern about the problems and crises faced by their close relationships, women feel responsible for and try to help solve the problems of their network members, while men, although wishing their support network members well in the resolution of their problems, do not feel personally responsible for them. These perspectives have critical implications for social relations, especially caregiving relationships, where women tend to assume more responsibility and take more personally the needs of their loved ones. Health care professionals may need to take an active role in limiting or distributing the responsibilities that women might assume, while men may need help arranging the provision of care for their spouse.

The increasing labor participation among women might be thought to have important implications for their social relations and for caregiving. Women at midlife do not have fewer people in their networks. It appears that they maintain the same, if not more (adding on coworkers), relationships but have less time to spend with them. One might speculate about both the positive and negative implications of these changes. On the one hand, working women have less time to invest in other people's problems but on the other, they may also have less time to garner support from their network members. While these multiple roles may lead to more stress, they can also lead to more sources of satisfaction.

Interestingly, in light of the gender differences just described, there appears to be a protective effect from social relations for men but not women. For this reason, the association between social relationships and mortality may be gender-specific, but little is known about the nature of this specificity. In sum, while men and women have close social relations with the same people, the nature, content, and effect of these relationships differ by gender. This appears to also be true of the caregiving relationship.

Race, Ethnicity, and Culture Renewed attention has been given to recognizing the influence of race, ethnicity, and culture. With this recognition comes the crucial next step of understanding when there are racial, ethnic, and cultural universals in social relations and when there are unique differences. Some fundamental characteristics of social relationships appear to transcend group membership. Thus, for example, most support networks consist of close family members. However, different groups seem to have different customs and sometimes different characteristics, which influence support relationships as well as caregiving relationships. The following examples illustrate this point.

It has been noted that social relations, in particular social networks and social support, have served important adaptive strategies among ethnic minorities. For example, the role of family, friends, and the church as support providers is especially important among the African American community and has implications for caregiving. The literature on kin and nonkin as sources of help among African Americans indicates that both are crucial and major sources of informal aid. However, as with whites, marital status is also important. African Americans who are married most often turn to their spouse for caregiving. While this is also true for whites, the fact that African Americans are more likely than whites to be never married, separated, divorced, or widowed suggests that fewer African Americans will have this source of support and caregiving available to them. Nevertheless, in general among older people, age, rather than race, is more predictive of social network and caregiving characteristics. For example, differences between whites and blacks in frequency of contact and proportion of kin disappear among older people.

Other racial and ethnic groups also show distinctive patterns of social relations. Dense and supportive networks of the nuclear and extended family among Hispanics has been noted as critical in the lives of elderly Hispanics. Elderly Chinese immigrants in the United States report that children are their primary support providers followed by friends and family. At the same time, different customs in different countries affect the expectation and enactment of social relations and by extension caregiving in different ways. In the United States, the daughter is often the most significant support provider and caregiver for older parents. However, in Japan, daughters-in-law are more likely to provide support than are daughters because the traditional living arrangements in Japan require daughters-in-law to live with her husband in his parents' house. It is, nevertheless, important to remember that structure and culture do not always predict perception, expectation, and/or quality of support. Older people in Italy who often live with their children report less social integration and more loneliness than do older people in The Netherlands who often live alone. It may be that Italians expect more, perceive less, and, therefore, are more likely to downgrade the quality of the support they receive. These imply important distinctions of which we are often aware but about which we understand little. For example, people who are lonely or have more hostile interactions with others are much more likely to become ill, develop heart disease, cope less well with stress, and take longer to recover from health problems.

The Importance of Socioeconomic Status Social relations vary by socioeconomic status. People at lower socioeconomic status levels have smaller networks, which tend to be sex segregated and to consist mainly of family members. They exchange support with fewer people and are often, although not always, less satisfied with the support they do receive. Generally speaking, social relations are more strained among people with fewer resources, that is, those at the lower end of the socioeconomic status continuum, people with less education, income, or occupational status.

In some circumstances, it may be socioeconomic status rather than ethnicity that shapes social relations. Comparing the social networks of African Americans, Asian Americans, white Americans, and Hispanic Americans, far more similarities than differences were found once education (an indicator of socioeconomic status) was controlled. Increased education is likely associated with greater financial resources and increased independence, which may explain the decreased reliance on family. With limited resources all ethnic group elders turn to family, especially children, for support. But once more resources are available other family members and nonkin may also be called upon.

It is, however, difficult to generalize about socioeconomic status and social relations. Although education, a common measure of socioeconomic status, is positively related to support, another common indicator of socioeconomic status, family income, is completely unrelated. While relationships among people of lower socioeconomic status may be of less quality than those of higher socioeconomic status overall, no such socioeconomic status difference is evident in the appraisal of close relationships. In fact, low socioeconomic status men who have an adult child on whom they can rely are as healthy as high socioeconomic status men. One interpretation of this finding is that the key to the socioeconomic status–health link for low socioeconomic status men may be close family ties. These ties are associated with less loneliness, better self-care, better immunologic functioning and, consequently, better health.

Thus, it appears that rather than sweeping generalizations concerning social relations, caregiving, and socioeconomic status, greater specificity is required to understand the association across all ages, but especially among the elderly population. These sociodemographic variables should be of special interest to health care professionals because they provide important insights into how membership in these groups influence the social relations and caregiving experiences of individuals.

FAMILY CAREGIVING

Health care professionals need to be sensitive to the social relations and family history of each individual. Doing so will provide important insight when an individual faces a specific illness or when caregiving becomes necessary. Simply stated, because it is necessary to find ways to maximize positive aspects of support and caregiving and minimize the negative aspects, using knowledge about the family and social support history should be especially useful. The transition from social support exchanges to caregiving is a delicate one. We turn to a consideration of this transition and definition of caregiving next.

Definition

The provision of assistance and support by one family member or friend to another is a pervasive aspect of everyday human interactions. Providing help to a family member with a chronic illness or disability is not very different from the tasks and activities that characterize interactions among families and close friends without the presence of illness or disability. Thus, when a wife provides care to her husband with Alzheimer's disease by preparing his meals, it may be an activity she would normally do for an unimpaired husband. However, if a wife also assists her cognitively impaired husband with bathing and dressing, few would question whether or not caregiving is taking place. The difference is that providing assistance with bathing and dressing or assisting with complex medical routines clearly represents "extraordinary" care and exceeds the bounds of what is "normative" or "usual." Similarly, parents caring for a child with a chronic illness may need to assist with daily medical routines (e.g., insulin injections or chest physical therapy) that are time-consuming and difficult and are in addition to normal parenting responsibilities. Caregiving involves significant expenditure of time and energy, often for months or years, requiring the performance of tasks that may be physically demanding and unpleasant, and frequently disrupting other family and social roles of the caregiver.

Although caregivers may perform tasks similar to those carried out by paid health professionals, they perform these services for no compensation and do so either voluntarily or because they feel there are no other alternatives. Because the physical and mental health consequences of taking on this role are sometimes severe, and because caregivers represent an invaluable resource to the well-being of our population, research on caregiving has become a high priority among scholars in many disciplines as well as among policy makers.

Prevalence of Caregiving

Although the definition and boundaries of what is meant by the term caregiving often vary depending on the purpose for which such definitions are used, there is strong consensus that regardless of how caregiving is defined, its prevalence is high. A broadly inclusive approach might argue that a caregiver is needed for every person with health-related mobility and self-care limitations which makes it difficult to take care of personal needs, such as dressing, bathing, and moving around the home. Current estimates indicate that 4 percent of the noninstitutionalized US population younger than age 55 years meet these criteria. Beyond the age of 55 years, the proportion of persons with mobility and/or self-care limitations increases dramatically; fully half of the population falls into this category after age 85 years. If we assume that these individuals minimally require one caregiver, these estimates yield more than 15 million caregivers in the US. Indeed, these estimates are somewhat lower than in a 1997 national survey of caregivers by the National Alliance for Caregiving, which indicated that there were 22.4 million households that met broad criteria for the presence of a caregiver in the previous 12 months.

Who Provides Care and What Type of Care is Provided?

Caregivers to elderly individuals are generally differentiated by age and relationship to the care recipient. One large group consists of adult children, usually daughters or daughters-in-law, in their fifties and sixties; the second group of caregivers is comprised of spouses of care-recipients and is generally older and has a higher proportion of male caregivers than adult children caregivers.

The roles and functions of family caregivers vary by type and stage of illness and include both direct and indirect activities. Direct activities can include provision of *personal care assistance,* such as helping with bathing, grooming, dressing, or toileting; *health care assistance* such as catheter care, giving injections, or monitoring medications; and *checking and monitoring tasks,* such as continuous or periodic supervision, and telephone monitoring. Indirect tasks include *care management,* such as locating services, coordinating service use, monitoring services, or advocacy, and *households tasks,* such as cooking, cleaning, shopping, money management, and transportation of the family member to medical appointments or day care programs. The intensity at which some or all of these caregiving activities are performed varies widely, with some caregivers having only limited types of involvement for a few hours per week, while other caregivers might provide more than 40 hours a week of care and are on call 24 hours per day. Regardless of the intensity of the caregiving, it is clear that the caregiving relationship, because of the nature of the role relationships most often shared—that is, parent–child, spouse—is most often a continuation of a very long-term social relationship. Knowledge about interpersonal relationships and social support provides an important base upon which to build an understanding of the caregiving relationship.

Conceptual Approaches to the Study of Caregiving

The dominant conceptual model for caregiving assumes that the onset and progression of chronic illness and physical disability is stressful for both patient and caregiver and, as such, can be studied within the framework of traditional stress-coping models. Indeed, caregiving may be similar to being exposed to a severe, long-term, chronic stressor. Within this framework, objective stressors include measures of patient disability, cognitive impairment, and problem behaviors, as well as the type and intensity of caregiving provided. Key outcome variables for the caregiver include psychological distress and burden, often referred to as caregiver burden, psychological and physical morbidity, and patient outcomes, such as institutionalization and death.

There is a moderate relationship between level of patient disability and psychological distress of the caregiver. However, there is considerable variability in caregiver outcomes, which is thought to be mediated and/or moderated by a variety of factors including economic and social support resources available to the caregiver; a host of individual difference factors, such as gender and personality attributes (optimism, self-esteem, self-mastery); coping strategies used; and the quality of the relationship between caregiver and care recipient. Stress-coping models also include examination of secondary stressors, such as role conflict engendered by caregiving demands. Many additional theoretical perspectives borrowed from social and clinical psychology, sociology, and the health and biological sciences have also been applied to help understand specific aspects of the caregiving situation. Finally, a variety of physiologic mechanisms including the pituitary–adrenal axis, the sympathetic nervous system, and the immune system may modulate the stress–health relationship and contribute to the finding that caregiving is a risk factor for a number of adverse outcomes.

The wide range of caregiving effects include disruption of family routines, psychological distress, psychological and physical morbidity including mortality, financial hardship, and work-related problems. Feeling burdened or distressed by the demands of caregiving is the most frequently reported outcome associated with caregiving, although this is not a universal phenomenon, particularly among spousal caregivers. Psychiatric morbidities such as depression and anxiety are also common. Physical health effects such as increased susceptibility to illness have been more difficult to demonstrate, although they are likely to occur in high-demand situations among vulnerable (e.g., frail) caregivers. Possible mediators of illness effects are increased depression associated with caregiving and changes in health related behaviors such as sleeping and eating patterns and medical compliance. Positive effects of caregiving such as increased self-esteem, the satisfaction of knowing that one's relative is being properly cared for, as well as improved mental health have also been reported.

The demands and negative impacts of dementia caregiving are generally higher than nondementia caregiving. Dementia care is different from other types of family caregiving. Not only do dementia caregivers spend significantly more hours per week providing care than nondementia caregivers, they also report greater employment complications, caregiver strain, mental and physical health problems, reduced time for leisure and other family members, and family conflict. Factors that are likely to account for this greater level of strain include having to contend with behavioral problems of the care-recipient (e.g., wandering, aggressiveness), and the unpredictable nature and course of dementing illnesses.

Interventions for Caregivers

Given the complexity of the caregiving experience and the variability in caregiver resources, we should not be surprised to find that there is no silver bullet solution to alleviating caregiver distress. There is no single, easily implemented, and consistently effective method for eliminating the stresses of caregiving. There exists strong consensus that all caregivers are likely to benefit from enhanced knowledge about the disease, the caregiving role, and resources available to caregivers. Once the informational needs have been met, the caregiver may additionally benefit from the opportunity to access needed resources, training in general problem-solving skills, as well as training in more specific skills needed to manage patient behaviors or their own emotional response to caregiving. Recent intervention studies also suggest that there may be important synergies achieved by simultaneously treating the care recipient (e.g., giving medications or memory retraining) and the caregiver. The combination of an experimental cognitive enhancing drug for the patient and limited education and support for the caregiver resulted in a significant reduction in caregiver distress when compared to the group receiving a placebo.

The rich array of methods for delivering interventions to caregivers include traditional methods, such as individual in home and community group sessions, but also newer technologies involving enhanced telephone systems and microcomputers and web sites. As sophisticated communication technologies become more available to individuals, treatment delivery options will increase. Although new technology has the potential to overwhelm already-stressed caregivers, it can be effective if introduced in a graduated step-wise fashion.

Helping the Caregiver

Primary care physicians who care for community residing older adults may be in the best position to identify caregivers at risk. A number of instruments are currently available for identifying caregivers at risk for negative health outcomes (see, for example, Caregiver Self-Assessment Questionnaire of the American Medical Association) and they provide valuable guidance in alerting the health care provider as to what to look for.

Because older individuals may be at high risk for negative health outcomes, it is particularly important to carefully assess the circumstances of older individuals caring for their disabled spouse. Older married couples should be evaluated as a unit, in terms of their health status as well as the caregiving demands that exist in the home environment. To the extent that caregiving demands are high, opportunities for restorative activities are limited, and the individual is physically compromised, an intervention that reduces caregiving demands such as the provision of respite services may be needed. Under extreme circumstances it may be appropriate to permanently relieve a vulnerable older person from caregiving responsibilities by finding an alternative caregiver or even institutionalizing the care recipient.

Implications for the Health Professional

Although traditional conceptual models of caregiving are important, it is also useful to consider the health continuum which most people, but especially older people, experience. People experience a range of health statuses, from healthy with no chronic or acute illness, through to the experience of acute illnesses and/or the accumulation of chronic illnesses, to the final status of terminal illness. From this perspective, it is clear that one embarks on a health continuum which, for almost everyone, includes an element of caregiving. Health care providers can serve their patients by shepherding them through this experience, helping them to understand, anticipate, and prepare for each stage of the health continuum that both they and their loved one are likely to experience.

For the caregiver, one might think of the health continuum as involving parallel stages of caregiving, namely the early stages, the full-blown stages, and the advanced stages of caregiving. Health providers do not always see it as their role to engage the caregiver in a preparatory or planning process but it could be especially useful for their patients. Regardless of whether a disease has been diagnosed, it is advisable to help patients and their families anticipate and plan for the future. The philosophy of continuity of care facilitates this approach because, especially in the primary care setting, one is likely to continue to care for the same patients and their families over the course of a number of years. This continuity of care provides an excellent opportunity to introduce topics that are both personally targeted and generally useful. The health care provider can address the particular issues most relevant to the individual patient and family and thus begin to allow them to plan for potential health care needs, caregiver and otherwise, at a very early stage. Thus, a care provider who knows their patient is in a rural setting or a multistory dwelling can suggest that the patient and family begin to plan for a time when a rural setting or multistory home will both limit their independence and maximize the potential for harm, or at the very least, limit their access to care. There are some characteristics of the physical and social environment that are known to be better or worse for people as they age. The current cohort of older people are, in many ways, pioneering a productive, sometimes independent, sometimes dependent, but certainly extended, old age. Previous cohorts had less time to live and thus less need to plan for this time.

Those who work with older people know that it is often difficult to persuade an older person to actually engage in the kind of planning outlined above. Tactics that are likely to work are also best personally or individually based. Thus, if one knows there are children waiting to inherit the farm, it may be easier to convince the elder to move out of the family home. Or it may be persuasive to note that if a couple engages in a certain activity it will greatly facilitate the adjustment of the surviving spouse (assuming, of course, a positive spousal relationship). The health care provider who knows the patient's personal circumstance is likely to be able to make the most persuasive case for planning for future caregiving needs.

The next stage of the health continuum involves the onset of either acute or chronic illness. While acute illnesses are characterized by the relatively quick recovery one experiences, with age, acute illnesses often trigger an awareness of what the future might hold. Acute and chronic illnesses are usually accompanied by a need for caregiving. Both the caregiver and the care receiver begin to understand at a very personal level how illness will impact their daily lives. Many at this point choose to isolate and ignore, if not deny, the implications of this experience. Rather than have this initial, often neither life-threatening nor permanent, event serve as a wake-up call to what the future will bring, patients and their families often move from event to recovery and completely avoid the implications of this experience. Once again, the health care provider can be critically helpful in suggesting how one might begin to prepare for the future caregiving needs of both the care provider and the care receiver. One must be realistic at this point as well and attempt to identify whomever might be the most open to preparation and learning. Thus, in some cases the patient will simply refuse to consider a reasonable plan that will minimize the burden on the caregiver. This might include refusing follow-up care, rehabilitation services, or diet or exercise modifications. If the patient refuses to plan for the future, the health care provider would, nevertheless, do well to attempt to engage the family or other potential caregiver in a dialogue that would allow them to understand what the future might bring and consider various preparatory strategies that might prove beneficial.

And finally, all patients eventually reach a stage of advanced ill health. Of course, there is great variation in how long one experiences this stage and what the caregiving needs of the individual might be. This full-blown caregiving stage is also dynamic because the caregivers ability to meet the needs of the care receiver can change. The health care professional can help the primary caregiver be less burdened through a variety of steps, for example, by recommending a support group, suggesting respite care, and calling a family meeting for both educational and relief purposes. Once again, knowledge of the family that one acquires from patients over the long-term is helpful. Perhaps preserving the caregivers capability would be best achieved by hiring someone to help with cleaning or bathing, or perhaps it is most important that the caregiver be able to meet the demands of their employment so that the financial needs of the patient and family can be met, or perhaps simply preserving a 2-hour jog or visit with grandchildren once a week is a critical contributor to the caregiver's mental health and well-being. Similarly, it may be the health care provider's role to give the caregiver "permission" to maintain or develop these well-being links. Sometimes a health care provider can convince the caregiver to take these steps because it will, in fact, make them a better caregiver. Often the role of the health care professional is not over when the patient dies or is institutionalized. With institutionalization a caregiver might need guidance about how to continue giving care when their loved one is in this new setting. When the care recipient dies, the caregiver often feels a tremendous loss, a terrible void in their life. They might need help adjusting to their postcaregiving status. Praise and recognition of their caregiving role, the job they did as a caregiver, can often play an important part in helping the caregiver recover and readjust to life post-caregiving.

FUTURE OF FAMILIES, SOCIAL RELATIONS, AND CAREGIVING

A number of important interrelated demographic, health, and social trends are shaping families, social relations, and caregiving. First, families are becoming smaller with fewer children. This is changing the nature of their social relations. Future cohorts of elderly people will have smaller families and fewer children available to provide care. Second, the sustained increase in labor force participation by women is also changing the nature of family and social relations. Women have less time to maintain the types of social relations they maintained in the past and are less likely to have the energy to engage in the types of social interactions that may have characterized families in the past. A third trend involves the decrease in traditional families, that is, families with one father, one mother, one marriage, and only their biological children. For example, little is known about the effect multiple marriages and multiple divorces will have on family and social relations. If these trends weaken family ties, it may be that other nonkin social relations will become more important. Another unknown of the future is the mobility of families. It is not clear whether families will increase or decrease their mobility in the future and consequently increase or decrease their availability for family interactions, social interactions, and caregiving.

There will be a worldwide increase in the number of older individuals, and possibly increased numbers of disabled individuals with longer life expectancies because of medical interventions. A key question will be the extent to which increases in life expectancy are associated with increasing years of disability. Some early evidence suggests that future cohorts of elderly individuals will be healthier and more functional than current cohorts; thus, adding years to life may not necessarily increase the need for caregiving assistance. These healthy elderly people may be important sources of support for their family and friends. Alternatively, one can speculate that some types of medical interventions (e.g., drug therapies that enable Alzheimer's disease patients to spend more years at home) will extend the family caregiving career. In sum, families, social relations, and caregiving are experiencing extraordinary changes and challenges. The degree to which these challenges are successfully met will fundamentally influence the health and well-being of older people and their families.

REFERENCES

Ajrouch KJ et al: Social networks among blacks and whites: The interaction between race and age. *Journal of Gerontology: Social Sciences* 56:S112, 2001.

Antonucci TC, Jackson JS: Social support, interpersonal efficacy, and health, in Carstensen LI Edelstein BA (eds): *Handbook of clinical gerontology.* New York, Pergamon Press, 1987, p291.

Beach SR et al: Negative and positive health effects of caring for a disabled spouse: Longitudinal findings from the Caregiver Health Effects Study. *Psychol Aging* 15:259, 2000.

Biegel DE, Schulz R: Caregiving and caregiver interventions in aging and mental illness. *Family Rel* 48:345, 1999.

Carstensen LL et al: Taking time seriously: A theory of socioemotional selectivity. *American Psychologist* 54:165, 1999.

Due P et al: Social relations: Network support, and relational strain. *Social Science and Medicine* 48:661,1999.

Haidt J, Rodin J: Control and efficacy as interdisciplinary bridges, *Review of General Psychology* 3:317, 1999.

Haley WE et al: Appraisal, coping, and social support as mediators of well-being in black and white family caregivers of patients with Alzheimer's disease. *Consul Clin Psychol* 64:121, 1996.

Kiecolt-Glaser JK et al: Spousal caregivers of dementia victims: Longitudinal changes in immunity and health. *Psychosom Med* 53:345, 1991.

National Alliance for Caregiving and the American Association of Retired Persons: Family caregiving in the US. Findings from a national survey. Final Report. Bethesda, MD, National Alliance for Caregiving, 1997.

Ory MG et al: Prevalence and impact of caregiving: A detailed comparison between dementia and non-dementia caregivers. Dementia and non-dementia caregiving. *Gerontologist* 39:177, 1999.

Pearlin LI et al: The forms and mechanisms of stress proliferation: The case of AIDS caregivers. *J Health Social Behav* 38:223, 1997.

Pearlin LI et al: Caregiving and its social support, in Binstock RH, George LK (eds.): *Handbook of Aging and the Social Sciences,* 4th ed. New York, Academic Press, 1995 p 283.

Quittner AL et al: Chronic parenting stress: Moderating vs. mediating effects of social support. *J Pers Soc Psychol* 59:1266, 1990.

Schulz R (ed.): *Handbook of Dementia Caregiving.* New York, Springer, 2000.

Schulz R, Beach S: Caregiving as a risk factor for mortality. The caregiver health effects study. *JAMA* 282:2215, 1999.

Schulz R et al: Psychiatric and physical morbidity effects of Alzheimer's disease caregiving: Prevalence, correlates, and causes. *Gerontologist* 35:771, 1995.

Schulz R et al: Psychiatric and physical morbidity effect of caregiving. *J Gerontol* 45:P181, 1990.

Uchino BN et al: The relationship between social support and physiological processes: A review with emphasis on underlying mechanisms and implications for health. *Psychological Bulletin* 119:488, 1996.

US Bureau of the Census: *The Need for Personal Assistance with Everyday Activities: Recipients and Caregivers. Current Population Reports, Household Economic Studies* (Series P-70, No. 19). Washington, DC, Department of Commerce, 1990.

Vitaliano PP et al: Research on physiological and physical concomitants of caregiving: Where do we go from here? *Ann Behav Med* 19:117, 1997.

Walen HR, Lachman ME: Social support and strain from partner, family, and friends: Costs and benefits for men and women in adulthood. *Journal of Social and Personal Relationships* 17:5, 2000.

Wallsten SM et al: Disability and depressive symptoms in the elderly: The effects of instrumental support and its subjective appraisal. *International Journal of Aging and Human Development* 48:145, 1999.

Zarit SH et al: Subjective burden of husbands and wives of caregivers: A longitudinal study. *Gerontologist* 26:260, 1986.

Health Behaviors and Adherence

SARA WILCOX • ABBY C. KING

Healthful behaviors can prevent or control many chronic diseases and can reduce functional disabilities that tend to increase with age. Older adults who do not smoke, are normal weight, and are physically active (low-risk group) delay the onset of minimal disability by approximately 7 years relative to those who are smokers, overweight, and sedentary (high-risk group). This finding, called the "compression of morbidity," is shown in Fig. 23-1. Healthful behaviors also enhance the quality of life and well-being of older adults. Despite these benefits, clinicians and researchers are faced with a major challenge of promoting the adoption and maintenance of healthy lifestyles.

This chapter describes two commonly applied theoretical approaches to health behavior change and reviews the prevalence, determinants, and interventions targeted toward six major health behaviors as they relate to older adults. These behaviors include medication adherence, smoking, alcohol consumption, sleep, physical activity, and nutrition. Where appropriate, Healthy People 2010 goals for individual and health care provider behaviors are also presented. Finally, future directions in health behaviors, adherence research, and practice are discussed.

MODELS OF HEALTH BEHAVIOR CHANGE

Social learning/social cognitive theories and the transtheoretical model are two of the more widely cited approaches to describing how individuals adopt, change, and adhere to health behaviors. Both models have been applied to health behaviors in age groups spanning childhood through old age. These theories and others are described in more detail in Glanz and colleagues' text.

Social Learning/Social Cognitive Theories

Social learning/social cognitive theories view human behavior as the result of a reciprocal interaction among behavior, personal factors, and environmental influences (physical and social). These theories emphasize that people have the ability to change their behavior by setting short-term, intermediate, and long-term goals; monitoring their

progress toward reaching these goals; reinforcing their progress towards goals through rewards and incentives; using problem-solving skills to overcome obstacles; and altering their social and physical environments to support their behaviors. The theories emphasize the importance of observational learning of behaviors through role models. A core component of these theories is the idea that people are more likely to attempt a behavior if they believe the behavior will lead to a desired outcome (referred to as outcome expectations) and if they are confident that they will be able to successfully perform the behavior, even in the face of barriers (referred to as self-efficacy).

Health care providers can incorporate these behavioral principles into practice. For example, providers can help patients to set specific, realistic, and quantifiable behavioral goals; encourage patients to monitor their behavior and reward themselves when goals are met; encourage patients to seek support for their behavior change from family and friends; and recommend ways that patients can modify their physical environment to support behavior change. Also consistent with this theory, providers can emphasize the benefits of the behavior, can encourage patients to identify potential barriers to change and how they can overcome these barriers, and can directly provide reinforcement in the way of verbal encouragement to patients for making change.

Transtheoretical Model

The *transtheoretical model* proposes that individuals adopting or changing a behavior progress through a series of five stages. Those in the *precontemplation stage* have no intention to adopt or change a behavior. They may be unaware of the consequences of their behavior, may deny that they need to change a behavior, or may be unwilling to change, perhaps because they have had unsuccessful past attempts. Those in the *contemplation stage* are considering adopting or changing a behavior in the near future. These individuals are aware of the possible benefits of changing their behavior, but they are often equally aware of the barriers to change. Individuals in the *preparation stage* intend to take

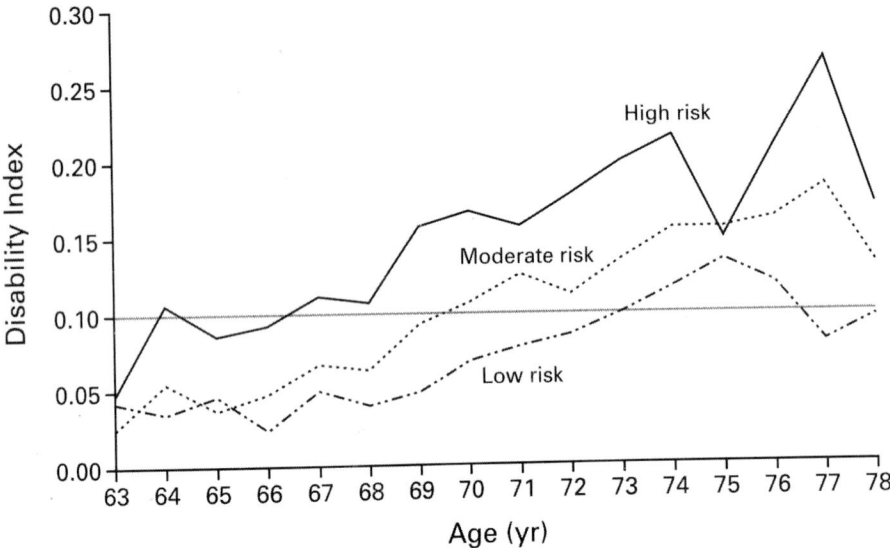

Figure 23-1 Disability index according to age at the time of the last survey and health risk in 1986. Average disability increased with age in all three risk groups, but the progression to a given level of disability was postponed by approximately seven years in the low-risk group as compared with the high-risk group. The horizontal line indicates a disability index of 0.1, which corresponds to minimal disability. From Vita AJ et al: Aging, health risks, and cumulative disability. *N Engl J Med* 338:1035, 1998. Copyright © 1998, Massachusetts Medical Society. All rights reserved. Reproduced with permission.

action to change their behavior in the immediate future, and they have generally taken initial steps toward change. Those in the *action stage* have actively made changes but have not yet maintained the behavior for a long period of time. Finally, individuals in the *maintenance stage* have been engaging in the desired behavior for a period of at least 6 months.

The transtheoretical model postulates that interventions are most successful when they are tailored to the individual's readiness for change. The model describes a number of cognitive and behavioral processes of change that help move individuals through the five stages. Finally, the transtheoretical model incorporates other dimensions of behavior change, including self-efficacy and the balance of pros versus cons of making change (decisional balance). The pros of making change tend to outweigh the cons of making change among individuals in later stages of behavior change.

Health care providers can apply the transtheoretical model to practice by first assessing their patient's readiness for change, and then by tailoring their intervention approach. For example, when working with a sedentary patient who states that she or he is not interested in beginning an exercise program, the provider's goal should be to encourage the patient to *consider* beginning an exercise program. This could be done by providing the patient with information about exercise, tying the patient's current health problem to his or her sedentary lifestyle, and asking the patient to consider the personal benefits of and barriers to exercise. Thus, the provider attempts to influence the patient's cognitions rather than actual behavior. In contrast, a patient who has already begun to make change can be provided with information on behavioral strategies to support and encourage further change, such as the importance of rewarding oneself, enlisting social support, and creating a supportive physical environment.

HEALTH BEHAVIORS AMONG OLDER ADULTS

Medication Adherence (See also Chapter 19, Medication Use)

Older adults are disproportionate users of both prescribed and over-the-counter medications, and polypharmacy becomes increasingly common with advanced age. It is estimated that between 25 and 59 percent of older adults make errors in the self-administration of prescribed medications. Not only do these errors contribute to poorer management of chronic conditions, but nonadherence to drug therapy is also a principal factor in hospitalizations among older adults.

There are several methods to measure medication adherence. Blood, serum, and urine samples can be used to detect the presence of medications, but these methods detect less than half of all drugs taken by older patients. Self-report measures include patient interviews, questionnaires, and self-monitoring diaries. Although self-report measures are simple and inexpensive, patients tend to overestimate their adherence. Self-monitoring logs may be more useful than patient interviews or questionnaires because they serve as both a record of adherence and a visual reminder for the patient. Conducting a pill count is another relatively inexpensive method of assessing adherence. One limitation of pill counts is that they only tell the number of pills missing over a specific period of time; they do not indicate whether the medication was taken properly (e.g., correct time of day) or at all (e.g., patient may have discarded pills to appear more compliant). Electronic medication monitoring devices, such as the Medication Event Monitoring System (MEMS), contain computer chips in the pill caps that record the time and date when the pill bottle was opened. Monitoring devices tend to be more accurate than

Table 23-1 Healthy People 2010 Goals for Health Behavior Counseling by Health Care Providers and Current Practices

Health Care Provider Goal	2010 Target Goal	Current Practice
Increase the proportion of patients who receive verbal counseling from *prescribers* on the appropriate use and potential risks of medications.	95	24
Increase the proportion of patients who receive verbal counseling from *pharmacists* on the appropriate use and potential risks of medications.	95	14
Increase the proportion of *internists* who counsel about smoking cessation.	85	50
Increase the proportion of *family physicians* who counsel about smoking cessation.	85	43
Increase the proportion of *dentists* who counsel about smoking cessation.	85	59
Increase the proportion of *primary care providers* who counsel about physical activity.	85	22
Increase the proportion of physician office visits made by patients with a diagnosis of cardiovascular disease, diabetes, or hyperlipidemia that include counseling or education related to diet and nutrition.	75	42

*All numbers represent percents. Data sources include NIH, NCI, CDC, NCHS, and FDA.

CDC, centers for Disease Control; FDA, Food and Drug Administration; NCHS, National Center for Health Statistics; NCI, National Cancer Institute; NIH, National Institutes of Health.

SOURCE: US Department of Health and Human Service: *Healthy People 2010: Understanding and Improving Health,* 2nd ed. Washington, DC, US Government Printing Office, 2000.

self-report measures. However, like pill counts, these devices do not confirm ingestion of a pill. These devices are generally cost-prohibitive in clinical settings, but are often used in research.

Medication adherence is a complex, multidetermined behavior. Factors associated with patient and provider, as well as factors associated with the medication itself, interact to influence adherence. There is no clear evidence that age is related to medication adherence; most studies show that age is *not* an important predictor. Characteristics that are positively associated with age, but that are not age-dependent, such as the number of medications prescribed and the complexity of the medication regimen, appear more important than age per se. In addition, having a greater number of physicians is associated with poorer medication adherence in older adults. An older adult's illness beliefs as well as their beliefs regarding medication effectiveness are important factors to consider in adherence. Misunderstandings regarding the purpose of the medication, its effects and side effects, and proper dosage contribute to lower adherence. Declines in cognitive ability and sensory abilities (e.g., vision and hearing), as well as lower literacy levels, are also associated with poorer medication adherence. The perceived cost of a medication to the individual can be a limiting factor: patients may decrease their dosage to make a medication last for a longer period of time or they may prioritize medications and forgo more expensive ones. Provider behaviors also influence medication adherence. Providers who clearly explain the purpose of a medication and how to take it, using both oral and written instructions, increase the likelihood of adherence. As shown in Table 23-1, a Healthy People 2010 goal is to increase to 95 percent the proportion of patients who receive verbal counseling from prescribers and pharmacists on the appropriate use and potential risks of medications. As of 1998, only 24 percent of prescribers and 14 percent of

pharmacists were providing this counseling. Patient–provider communication styles can also impact adherence. Patients are more likely to follow medication instructions when they have good rapport with their provider. Experiencing negative side effects is the most common medication-related factor associated with poor adherence. Other medication-related factors include difficulties with childproof containers, the use of a small font size in instructions, high cost, and medications that require more doses in a given day.

Several reviews of interventions to promote medication adherence have been reported in the past several years. These reviews have criticized the methodology of many of the intervention trials conducted to date, and have recommended that well-controlled randomized clinical trials be conducted. Interventions to increase patient's knowledge regarding medications have not generally been effective in increasing adherence rates. Forgetting to take pills is a greater barrier to adherence than is knowledge regarding the medication. Thus, automated telephone reminders, written medication schedules, and pill organizers are fairly inexpensive yet somewhat effective techniques to prompt pill taking. Prompting systems that use pictures in addition to words, such as showing a clock and pictures of the number of pills to be taken, can be even more effective, especially for lower literate adults. In one study, the actual pills in the correct number were glued to a reminder card to show the patient the actual pill and proper dose. Blister packs are also helpful for reminding patients to take pills, although many drugs are not available in this form, and the packaging generally increases cost. Self-medication programs involve educating hospitalized patients about their medications and giving the patient increasing responsibility for taking their own pills in the hospital. These programs have been associated with greater adherence and knowledge after discharge.

White Pills

Identifying your medicine
1. Name of doctor:
    Your doctor is Dr. Farley. You can call Dr. Farley at (603) 436-2200.

2. Name of medicine:
    The name of your medicine is White Pills.

3. Purpose of medicine:
    Your White Pills are for relief of symptoms from seasonal allergies.

How to take your medicine
4. Dose:
    Take two pills each time.

5. Time to take medicine:
    Take the White Pills four times each day. You should take your medicine at 8 a.m. in the morning, 12 noon, 4 p.m. in the afternoon, and 8 p.m. in the evening.

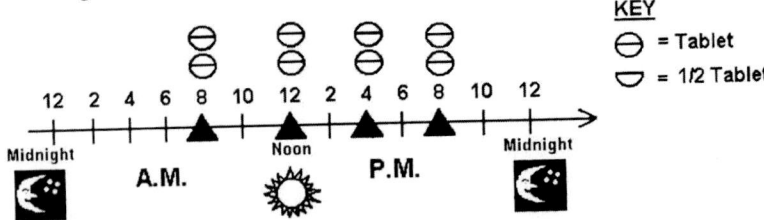

6. How long to take medicine:
    Take your White Pills for two weeks.

7. Warnings:
    Take with a full glass of water. If you miss a dose, take immediately upon remembering.

Possible side effects
8. Mild side effects:
    Continue to take your medicine even if you experience an increase in appetite or feel weak. Consult your doctor only if these symptoms persist.

9. Dangerous side effects:
    Stop taking the White Pills and call Dr. Farley if you experience heart palpitations or perspire excessively.

10. In case of emergency, use your telephone and dial 911.

Figure 23-2   An example of medication instructions that are organized by patient's medication schema. These instructions include a time line icon. From Morrow D, Leirer VO: Designing medication instructions for older adults, in Park DC et al. (eds): *Processing of Medical Information in Aging Patients. Cognitive and Human Factors Perspectives.* Mahwah, NJ: Lawrence Erlbaum, 1999, p 249. Copyright © 1999, Lawrence Erlbaum. Reproduced with permission.

Research in cognitive psychology underscores the importance of presenting medication instructions and reminders in ways that are consistent with a patient's medication schema. Schemas are knowledge structures in long-term memory that represent stereotypical situations. Both older and younger adults have a medication schema that organizes medication information in the following order: (1) general information about the medication, including its name and purpose; (2) how to take the medication, including dose and times; and (3) possible outcomes of the medication, such as side effects. Thus, information that is presented with general information about the medication first, then the steps needed to accomplish the task (in proper order) increases the likelihood that instructions will be remembered. In addition, memory for critical information declines with longer medication instructions. This memory limitation is likely a result of the amount of information that must be maintained in short-term memory. When critical instructions are given in simpler forms, they will be better consolidated into long-term memory. Consistent with this memory factor, Morrow and colleagues have shown that list instructions and the use of icons improve medication comprehension to a greater extent than paragraph and text-only instructions. Figure 23-2 shows an example of written medication instructions that use these principles. Medication adherence is further discussed in Chap. 19.

Smoking

Cigarette smoking is the leading cause of preventable morbidity and premature mortality in the United States. Among individuals aged 60 years and older, smoking is a major risk factor for 6 of the 14 leading causes of death, and is a complicating factor for 3 others. Although the United States has experienced a marked decrease in smoking rates since the 1960s, 23.5 percent of adults continue to smoke (1999 data). Smoking rates are slightly higher among men (25.5 percent) than women (23.1 percent); however, the decline in smoking rates over time has been less in women than men. Smoking rates are highest among American Indian/Alaskan Natives (40.8 percent) and lowest among Hispanics (18.1 percent) and Asian/Pacific Islanders (15.1 percent). Finally, smoking rates are higher among persons with lower levels of education and income. A Healthy People 2010 goal is to reduce to 12 percent or less the proportion of adults who smoke.

Despite the relatively low rate of smoking among older adults in the United States (10.6 percent) as compared to other age groups, smoking has great health costs for older adults who do smoke. Smoking exacerbates preexisting illnesses and conditions that are more prevalent among older than younger adults (e.g., cardiovascular disease, circulatory and vascular conditions, diabetes), leading to high health care utilization and poor quality of life. Smoking also interferes with the effectiveness of many medications prescribed to older adults. Moreover, unless smoking rates among younger populations significantly decline, smoking-related illnesses will be even more serious in upcoming years. For example, of those who are approaching older age (currently, 45 to 64 years of age), the rate of smoking remains elevated (23.3 percent). As this large group of smokers age, they will continue to accrue smoking-related diseases and disabilities unless smoking cessation rates increase.

Studies conducted over the past two decades clearly document that smoking cessation leads to immediate and long-term health benefits among all age groups, including older adults. Some of these health benefits include a reduced risk of heart disease, stroke, and mortality, and improvements in circulation and pulmonary function. Even older adults with preexisting diseases such as cardiovascular disease can significantly improve their chances of survival by quitting smoking, and they can experience reductions similar to those of younger adults.

Data from recent observational, prospective, and intervention trials have identified important age differences among smokers and have underscored the importance of age-tailored smoking cessation messages. In terms of demographic variables, older smokers tend to be less educated, have lower levels of income, and are more likely to be women than younger smokers. With the exception of longer smoking histories in older smokers, smoking habits and quitting histories do not vary dramatically by age. Smokers of all ages overwhelmingly prefer self-help over formal smoking cessation programs. Smokers entering formal programs tend to be more highly addicted to nicotine with a history of more quit attempts than smokers who quit on their own.

Age differences have also been reported in smoking-related attitudes. Older smokers minimize both the negative impacts of smoking on their health and the potential health benefits of smoking cessation to a greater extent than younger smokers. For example, close to half of older smokers do not believe that continued smoking will harm their health. Although older smokers cite similar motivations for wanting to quit smoking as do younger smokers (e.g., effects on current and future health and impact on others), older smokers rate these factors as significantly less important than their younger counterparts. In addition to these attitudes, older smokers have less confidence, or self-efficacy, in their ability to quit smoking than younger smokers. This finding could be related to older adults' longer smoking histories. Older adults are less likely to attempt quitting than are younger adults (35 percent of older adults versus 41 percent of all adults stopped smoking 1 day or longer in 1998; Healthy People 2010 goal is 75 percent). However, among those who do attempt to quit, older smokers are at least as successful as younger smokers.

Only a handful of randomized clinical trials of smoking cessation in older adults exist. These studies indicate that intervention success rates are similar in older and younger adults. Participants in an intensive 3-month program tailored specifically to older smokers had 1-year abstinence rates three times higher than control participants (28 to 38 percent versus 10 percent). In response to older adults' preference for self-help interventions, Rimer and Orleans developed a self-help guide, *Clear Horizons,* tailored specifically to the needs of older smokers. Older adults who were mailed the age-tailored guide reported significantly higher rates of abstinence (20 percent) than those who were mailed the age-general guide (15 percent) at the 12-month follow-up. Morgan and colleagues used a multifaceted age-tailored intervention that combined the "4 A's" protocol (Ask, Advise, Assist, and Arrange), the *Clear Horizons* guide, the transtheoretical model, and nicotine gum in a primary care setting. Patients in the age-tailored intervention had 6-month abstinence rates that were twice as high as in the control group (15.4 percent versus 8.2 percent, respectively) and were significantly more likely to discuss smoking-related issues with their physician. Orleans and colleagues combined the *Clear Horizons* guide with computer-generated tailored messages that were delivered by mail. Both quit attempts and abstinence rates in the intervention were higher than in the usual care condition at 6 months; differences in abstinence rates were not maintained at 12 months. A major challenge to smoking cessation interventions is promoting longer-term adherence. Ossip-Klein and colleagues found that self-help interventions produced comparable 3- and 6-month abstinence rates in older adults as in other populations. Gender differences were noted: men did better with smoking cessation mailings, whereas women did better with telephone counseling.

A Healthy People 2010 goal is to increase to at least 85 percent the proportion of internists, family physicians, and dentists who routinely advise smoking cessation and provide assistance and follow-up for their tobacco-using patients. Actual percentages, shown in Table 23-1, are substantially lower. Health care providers play a major role in

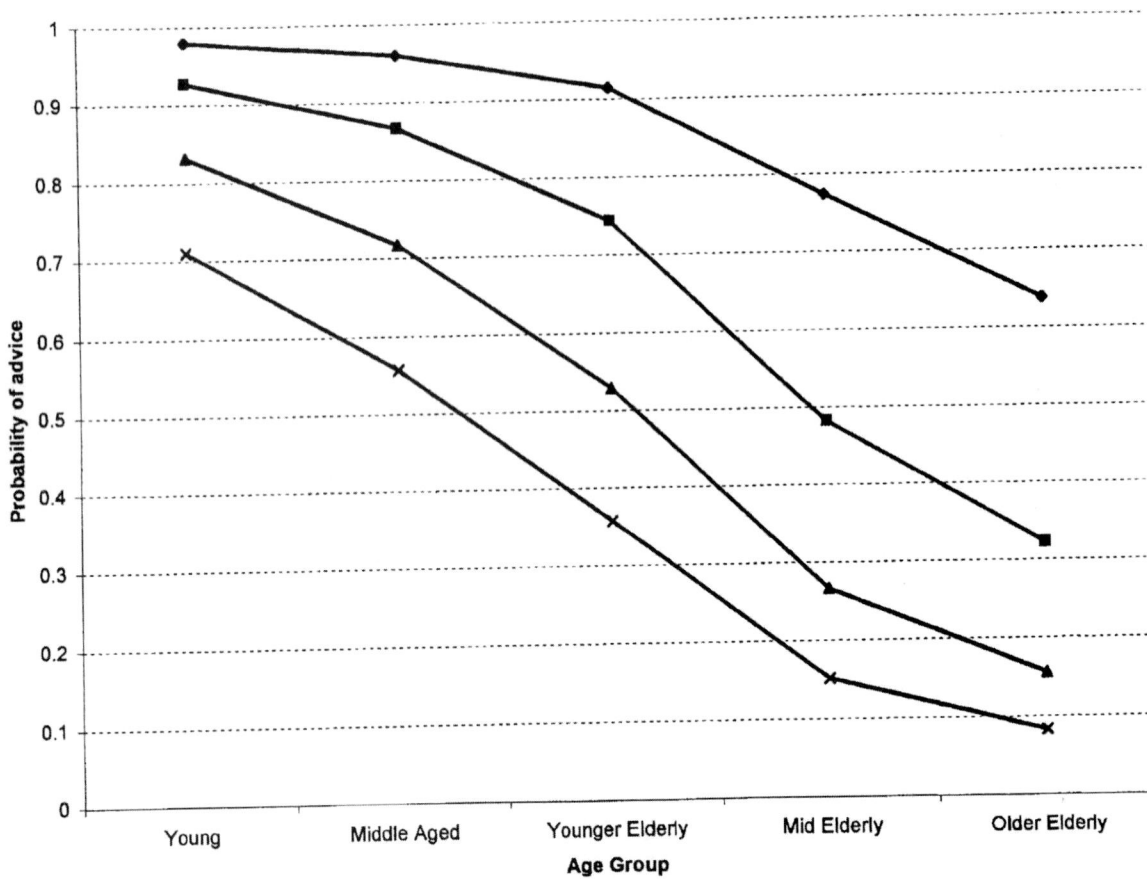

Figure 23-3 Probability of receiving advice about cessation of cigarette smoking as a function of patient age and medication condition: ♦, risk factors for coronary heart disease; ■, no medical problems; ▲, psychiatric illness; ×, terminal cancer. From Maguire CP et al: Do patient age and medical condition influence medical advice to stop smoking? *Age Ageing* 29:264, 2000. Copyright © 2000, British Geriatrics Society. Reproduced with permission.

facilitating quit attempts in their patients. Indeed, most tobacco users have contact with a physician each year, and a high percentage of users wish to quit. Unfortunately, studies in the United States and elsewhere show that older adults are significantly less likely to be counseled to quit smoking relative to other age groups. In a recent study, physicians were given vignettes in which the participants varied by age and health status, and they were asked whether they would advise the patient to quit smoking. Figure 23-3 shows that the probability of advice declined with patient age, regardless of patient health status. Interventions that target older adults should emphasize the detrimental health effects for the individual of continued smoking as well as the health benefits of cessation. In addition, confidence in one's ability to quit smoking is a consistent predictor of both intentions to quit and successful quit attempts. Physicians and other health professionals can assist in this process by recommending behavioral smoking cessation techniques, including helping the smoker to set a quit date, plan and prepare for triggers to smoking and ways to avoid them, find healthier ways to cope with stress (e.g., exercise, relaxation, recreational activities), set short-term goals, and enlist support from others. Table 23-2 shows an example of the "5 A's" protocol; these techniques are described in more detail in the recent U.S. Department of

Health and Human Services (USDHHS) publication. Finally, when counseling patients to quit smoking, it is important to remember that quitting smoking is an ongoing process that typically requires several quit attempts before cessation is achieved.

Alcohol Consumption

Alcohol consumption in older adults is one of the most difficult health behaviors to study, but it has important public health implications. Prevalence data regarding alcohol use in older persons are highly variable, most likely because of the different subpopulations studied, geographic variations in alcohol use, different time periods in which studies were conducted, differing criteria for alcohol consumption, and reporting biases on the part of the individual. Large, national studies estimate that approximately 60 percent of older adults have consumed at least 12 drinks sometime in their lifetime. When defined as drinking at least 12 drinks in a *single year* and at least 1 drink in the *past year*, more than half of elderly men (56 percent) and close to one-third of elderly women (31 percent) are current drinkers. Rates of alcohol use are lower and rates of lifetime abstinence are higher among older adults when compared to younger

Table 23-2   The "5 A's" for a Brief Smoking Cessation Intervention

5 As	Action	Strategies for Implementation
ASK about tobacco use. **ADVISE** to quit.	Query and document tobacco-use status for *every* patient at *every* clinic visit. In a *clear, strong,* and *personalized* manner, urge every tobacco user to quit.	Expand the vital signs to include tobacco use or use an alternative universal identification system. Advice should be: • *Clear*—"I think it is important for you to quit smoking now and I can help you." • *Strong*—"As your clinician, I need you to know that quitting smoking is the most important thing you can do to protect your health now and in the future." • *Personalized*—Tie tobacco use to current health/illness, and/or its social and economic costs, motivation level/readiness to quit, and/or the impact of tobacco use on others.
ASSESS willingness to make a quit attempt.	Ask every tobacco user if he or she is willing to make a quit attempt at this time (e.g., within the next 30 days).	Assess patient's willingness to quit: • If the patient is willing to make a quit attempt at this time, provide assistance (see ASSIST below) • If the patient will participate in an intensive treatment, deliver treatment or refer. • If the patient clearly states that he or she is unwilling to make a quit attempt at this time, provide a motivational intervention (see USDHHS publication).
ASSIST in quit attempt.	• Help the patient with a quit plan. • Provide practical counseling (problem solving/skills training). • Provide intratreatment social support. • Help patient obtain extratreatment social support. • Recommend approved pharmacotherapy. • Provide supplementary materials.	• Encourage patients to set quit date; tell family, friends, and coworkers; anticipate challenges; remove tobacco products from environment; prior to quitting, avoid smoking where one spends a lot of time. • Emphasize total abstinence; review past quit experiences; discuss challenges/triggers and how to overcome; have patients encourage others in household to also quit or not smoke in their presence. • Provide a supportive clinical environment while encouraging the patient in his or her quit attempt. "My office staff and I are available to assist you." • Help patient develop social support for his or her quit attempt in his or her environments outside of treatment. • *Sources:* federal agencies, nonprofits, or local/state health departments; *Type:* culturally, racially, educationally, and age appropriate.
ARRANGE follow-up.	Schedule follow-up contact, either in person or via telephone.	• *Timing*—Have first follow-up within 1 week of the quit date, and second follow-up within the first month. Schedule further follow-up contacts as indicated. • *Actions during follow-up contact*—Congratulate success. If tobacco use has occurred, review circumstances and elicit recommitment to total abstinence. Remind patient that a lapse can be used as a learning experience. Identify current and anticipated challenges. Assess pharmacotherapy use and problems. Consider use or referral to more intensive treatment.

SOURCE: Adapted from Fiore MC et al: *Treating Tobacco Use and Dependence. Clinical Practice Guideline.* Rockville, MD, US Department of Health and Human Services, Public Health Service, June 2000.

adults. Because longitudinal data are lacking, it is unclear whether alcohol consumption actually declines with age. Other explanations are also plausible. Premature mortality of the heaviest drinkers; the greater proportion of women, who tend to drink less than men at all ages and in old age; and cohort differences in drinking (a result of factors such as Prohibition and the Great Depression) could all account for lower current alcohol consumption among older adults. Although the risks of alcohol consumption are emphasized here, it is important to note that low to moderate alcohol consumption is associated with cardiovascular health benefits.

The proportion of heavy drinkers (generally defined as consuming more than two drinks per day) is relatively low in population samples of older adults (approximately 9 percent of men and 2 percent of women). Sixteen percent of men and 15 percent of women who were current drinkers in the National Health and Nutrition Examination Survey (NHANES) I were classified as heavy drinkers (more than two drinks a day for men and more than one drink a day for women). The prevalence of heavy drinking is reported to be even higher in several subpopulations of older adults. Among residents of retirement communities, as many as one in three men and one in five women are heavy drinkers. Rates are also higher among older patients assessed in primary care settings, emergency rooms, medical inpatient units, and psychiatric inpatient units.

The assessment and treatment of alcohol abuse or dependence in older adults is further explored in a recent report by the American Medical Association. Even low to moderate levels of alcohol consumption can have deleterious effects in some older adults because of physiologic changes that occur with age, the increased likelihood of drug–alcohol interactions, and the increased likelihood that alcohol will exacerbate preexisting medical conditions, as well as traumatic injuries related to falls and automobile accidents.

With increasing age, changes in body composition as well as pharmacodynamic and pharmacokinetic changes increase the magnitude of the effects of alcohol. Because alcohol is distributed through the body's water, and water volume decreases with age, the same amount of ingested ethanol leads to a greater blood alcohol concentration in an older person as compared to a younger person. In addition, even when blood alcohol concentrations are comparable, an older adult is more sensitive to the effects of alcohol than is a younger adult.

The disproportionate use of over-the-counter and prescription medications places older adults at increased risk for drug-alcohol interactions. It is estimated that alcohol interacts with at least half of the 100 most frequently prescribed medications. Depending on the drug, these interactions can have additive, synergistic, or inhibitory effects. Alcohol consumption is also contraindicated for a number of medical conditions that increase with age, including diabetes and hypertension. In addition, the potential for drug–alcohol interactions combined with the increased sensitivity to alcohol can lead to a number of serious complications in older adults, including impaired cognition, confusion, falls, bone fractures, and psychomotor impairment.

Despite its importance, alcohol consumption can be particularly difficult to assess as a result of both patient and health care provider biases and because existing screening measures tend to focus exclusively on alcohol abuse or dependence. Older adults, especially older women, are more reluctant to report alcohol use because of the stigma associated with alcohol. This is particularly true for cohorts who lived through Prohibition. Health professionals may not ask about alcohol use, often because they do not expect older adults to drink and/or have alcohol-related problems. A recent random survey found that physicians underestimated alcohol use disorders among older adults. Symptoms such as cognitive impairment, depression, malnutrition, falls, and incontinence may be interpreted as age- or medically related, when these symptoms could also be a result of alcohol misuse. Finally, professionals unfamiliar with pharmacokinetic and pharmacodynamic changes with age might underestimate the effects of even moderate amounts of alcohol (often defined as *up to* one drink per day in older adults) on their older patients. A final barrier to assessing alcohol consumption in older persons is that existing screening measures do not assess low to moderate alcohol consumption that may be negatively affecting the elder's health and/or functioning for reasons described earlier.

The majority of older individuals who are moderate or heavy drinkers do not seek professional help specifically for alcohol use. Nearly nine in ten older adults, however, visit their physician on a yearly basis, providing an opportunity for health care providers to assess alcohol consumption, make recommendations to alter consumption, and provide referrals as needed. A potentially effective way to assess alcohol use in a less-threatening and less-judgmental manner is to embed questions regarding consumption in more general dietary or health assessments. Individuals whose drinking may be impacting their health should be provided with education regarding the health impact of alcohol on older adults and direct information regarding their need to reduce or abstain from alcohol. If the patient is in agreement, including family or significant others in these changes could prove useful.

A number of studies demonstrate that alcohol counseling delivered in health care settings can reduce heavy drinking, but most of these studies have been relatively time intensive. In contrast, several studies show that relatively brief health care provider interventions can reduce high-risk alcohol use. Ockene and colleagues found that physicians and nurse practitioners who were trained in patient-centered counseling and who delivered a brief (5- to 10-minute) screening and intervention reduced alcohol consumption in the high-risk drinkers aged 21 to 70 years group (a reduction of 5.8 drinks per week versus a reduction of 3.4 drinks per week at 6 months). Project GOAL (Guiding Older Adult Lifestyles) found that physician counseling (two 10- to 15-minute counseling sessions) delivered to older patients ($\geq$65 years of age) who were problem drinkers led to significant reductions in alcohol use, binge drinking, and excessive drinking, as compared to the control group, at 3, 6, and 12 months postintervention. Interventions that target more moderate but nonetheless problematic drinking in older adults deserve further study. For example, one approach is to classify drinking as nonhazardous, hazardous, or harmful by using algorithms that considered alcohol quantity/frequency information and medical problems, medication use, and functional status. This broader conceptualization (e.g., beyond sheer level of alcohol consumption) is critical when working with older populations.

Sleep

More than one-third of community-dwelling adults aged 65 years and older report insomnia, and rates are even higher among institutionalized older adults and older adults with dementia. Insomnia is associated with emotional distress, a decreased sense of well-being, the use of sleep medications, and in some cases, an increased risk of disease and mortality. Furthermore, older adults disproportionately consume sedative-hypnotic and over-the-counter sleep medications, despite the age-specific documented risks and questionable benefits of these agents.

Difficulties in sleep initiation or onset, sleep maintenance, early morning awakenings, and daytime tiredness are all relatively common in older age. Older adults take more daytime naps than younger adults and they have poorer sleep efficiency percentages (total time asleep/time in bed × 100) because older individuals tend to remain in bed longer but sleep for shorter periods than younger adults. There are also age-related changes in sleep architecture such that older adults have less deep sleep (stages 3 and 4) and less rapid eye-movement (REM) sleep than younger adults. Their sleep tends to be more fragmented, shorter, and lighter.

Several recent epidemiologic studies provide useful information regarding correlates of sleep problems in older persons. Among older individuals, women consistently report more sleep impairments than men, including longer sleep onset latencies, more nighttime awakenings, more problems with early morning awakenings, and greater use of sedative-hypnotics. These findings are inconsistent with studies that used objective measurement of sleep (polysomnography) that have shown that men often have more fragmented sleep than women. Men also report more daytime naps, snoring, and, in some studies, daytime tiredness. Dissatisfaction with sleep is greater among white than African American older adults. Health problems, particularly angina, heart disease, arthritis, respiratory symptoms, nocturia, and functional limitations are all associated with sleep problems in older persons. The use of sedative-hypnotics, alcohol, caffeine, over-the-counter medications (particularly analgesics containing caffeine), and psychotropics, as well as physical inactivity, are also consistently associated with sleep problems. Psychosocial factors associated with sleep disturbances include depression, anxiety, and a lack of social support. When health and physical functioning variables are considered, age per se is often not associated with sleep complaints, indicating that insomnia is not age dependent.

Treating sleep disorders involves identifying and treating possible underlying causes. For example, treating depression, sleep apnea, periodic leg movements, or other disorders known to cause insomnia are likely to substantially reduce sleep impairments. Sleep difficulties, however, are often the result of a complex interaction of physical, psychosocial, and behavioral factors, necessitating broader biopsychosocial assessment and interventions. Unfortunately, the most common treatment for sleep disorders in older persons is the long-term use of sedative-hypnotics. Because of the problems associated with these drugs, including falls, confusion, and poor efficacy, nonpharmacologic treatments are of great importance. A number of empirically supported behavioral treatments for insomnia exist, including sleep hygiene, stimulus control therapy, sleep-restriction therapy, relaxation training, and cognitive-behavioral therapy.

Sleep hygiene involves educating individuals about behaviors that may interfere with sleep, with the goal of modifying these behaviors. For example, individuals are advised to avoid alcohol, tobacco, caffeine intake (from drugs and food), excess fluid intake in the evening, heavy evening meals, daytime napping, lack of daytime activities, irregular bed and wake times, and poor sleeping environments (e.g., too warm, loud, bright). Sleep hygiene is generally incorporated as part of formal behavioral treatments of insomnia. It is considered a necessary but not sufficient treatment for chronic insomnia.

Stimulus control therapy is based on behavioral principles that the bed is no longer a discriminative stimulus for sleep because it has become associated with sleep-incompatible behaviors such as watching television, worrying, and eating. Individuals are instructed to go to bed only when they are tired and not before their scheduled bedtime, to use the bed only for sleeping and sex, to leave the bedroom if they are awake for longer than 10 to 30 minutes (varies by study), and to return to bed when they are tired. Stimulus control therapy reduces sleep onset latency by as much as 60 percent. In addition, this form of treatment decreases time awake after sleep onset and increases total sleep time by as much as 1 hour. The requirement to get out of bed if a person is not sleeping may pose a challenge to treatment adherence. A modified form of stimulus control therapy, *countercontrol therapy,* is based on similar principles but eliminates the necessity of having to leave the bed when awake. Instead, participants are instructed to engage in a nonarousing activity, such as reading a dull book, until they become tired. Countercontrol therapy has received little empirical study in older adults.

Sleep restriction or *sleep compression therapy* is based on the idea that excessive time in bed perpetuates insomnia. Treatment involves setting a regular bedtime and wake time based on the total time the individual reports sleeping per night. For example, a person reporting 5 hours of actual sleep per night is instructed to set a bedtime and wake time that will allot only approximately 5 hours in bed. As individuals increase their sleep efficiency, the allotted time in bed is increased. Sleep restriction therapy significantly improves quality of sleep in older adults, and to a greater extent than relaxation training.

Relaxation training is a general term for a variety of activities that aim to achieve a state of relaxation, and it is perhaps the most frequently studied insomnia treatment. Common relaxation techniques include deep breathing,

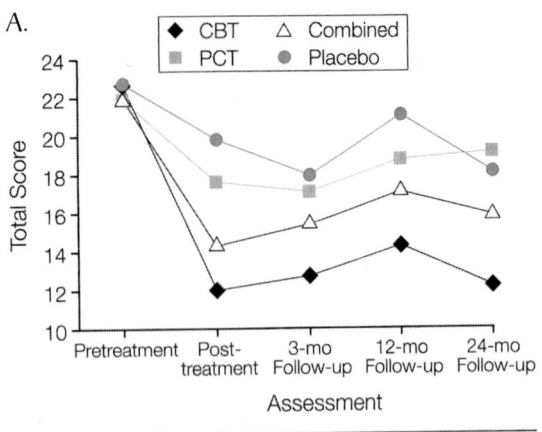

CBT indicates cognitive-behavior therapy; PCT, pharmacotherapy.

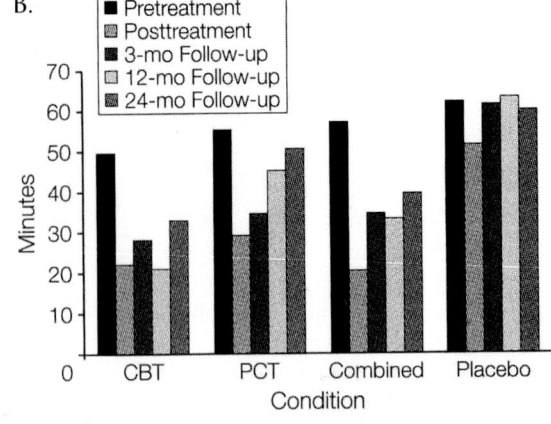

CBT indicates cognitive-behavior therapy; PCT, pharmacotherapy.

Figure 23-4 *A.* Pretreatment, posttreatment, and follow-up changes in total scores for the sleep impairment index (patient version). *B.* Changes in wake after sleep onset as measured by sleep diaries over assessment periods. From Morin CM et al: Behavioral and pharmacological therapies for late-life insomnia. A randomized controlled trial. *JAMA* 281:991, 1999. Copyright © 1999, American Medical Association. Reproduced with permission.

imagery, meditation, and progressive muscle relaxation. Several studies show that relaxation training improves sleep quality in older insomniacs to a greater extent than no treatment. However, relaxation training appears less effective than the other behavioral treatments described in this section. There is some evidence to suggest that relaxation training may be most useful for individuals reporting significant daytime impairment due to tiredness, as it may extend sleep. Relaxation training also leads to a reduction in sedative–hypnotic use in older insomniac women without further deterioration in sleep quality. It is hypothesized that the relaxation may serve as a buffer against sedative–hypnotic withdrawal. This hypothesis warrants further study, given the relatively high use of sedative–hypnotics in older individuals.

Finally, *cognitive–behavioral therapy (CBT)*, as applied specifically to insomnia, is based on the idea that insomnia is caused by the interactions among emotional, cognitive, and physiologic arousal factors; dysfunctional cognitions (e.g., worry over lack of sleep); maladaptive habits (e.g., irregular sleep and wake schedule); and the consequences of insomnia (e.g., fatigue or impaired activities of daily living). Cognitive–behavioral therapy uses a number of techniques aimed at altering the individual's thought patterns and behaviors in an attempt to create healthier cognitions, emotions, and behaviors conducive to restful sleep. Cognitive–behavioral therapy for insomnia has typically consisted of components of stimulus control, sleep restriction, sleep hygiene, and cognitive restructuring. In recent years, there has been a substantial increase in the number of randomized clinical trials of cognitive–behavioral therapy applied to older adults. These interventions have been delivered in group settings by both psychologists and nurses, and a recent study tested a self-help form of cognitive–behavioral therapy. Although results vary somewhat from study to study, overall findings indicate that cognitive–behavioral therapy results in long-term (up to 2 years),

clinically significant improvements on a wide range of sleep outcomes (both self-report and objective), and is more effective than other types of behavioral treatments. Furthermore, behavioral treatments can be successfully integrated into routine clinical practice, and patients with chronic insomnia and those using hypnotics respond equally well to cognitive–behavioral therapy relative to patients with less severe insomnia.

Morin and colleagues compared cognitive–behavioral therapy, pharmacotherapy (temazepam), or cognitive–behavioral therapy plus pharmacotherapy with placebo control in older adults with sleep-onset or maintenance insomnia. As shown in Fig. 23-4, cognitive–behavioral therapy-only and combined patients rated themselves as significantly more improved than did the placebo or pharmacotherapy-only patients at posttreatment, and patients treated with cognitive–behavioral therapy surpassed all groups at the follow-up periods (assessed for 24 months). Furthermore, older adults reported more satisfaction with the behavioral treatment, which is important for promoting long-term adherence to treatment.

Finally, two randomized controlled trials, one of moderately sleep-impaired older adults and the other of depressed older adults, have shown that physical activity can significantly improve sleep. King and colleagues (1997) found that after 16 weeks of regular, moderate-intensity exercise training, older participants with moderate sleep impairments reported significant improvements in global sleep scores, sleep quality, sleep onset latency, sleep duration, and sleep efficiency, relative to controls. Participants in the exercise group reduced their sleep onset latencies by about one-half and increased their total sleep time by almost 1 hour. Singh and colleagues' study of depressed older adults found that a regimen of progressive resistance training led to a similar magnitude of improvement in these sleep variables over a 10-week period. Sleep is discussed further in Chap. 119.

Physical Activity

The role of regular physical activity in promoting health and preventing disease and disability is well established and is reviewed in detail in the recent Surgeon General's Report on physical activity and health, and in a position stand specific to older adults by the American College of Sports Medicine. Regular physical activity lowers blood pressure and reduces the risk of coronary heart disease, colon cancer, breast cancer, type 2 diabetes mellitus, and osteoporosis. Physical activity is also beneficial for the ongoing management of chronic diseases. For example, both endurance and resistance training have been shown to relieve symptoms and improve the functioning of individuals with osteoarthritis, rheumatoid arthritis, heart failure, and chronic obstructive pulmonary disease. Furthermore, regular physical activity can reduce the risk of falls and increase one's ability to carry out activities of daily living by improving balance, gait, and strength. Finally, regular physical activity can improve psychological well-being and health-related quality of life by reducing depression and anxiety, improving sleep, and improving mobility. The health and psychological benefits of physical activity extend to older adults, and in some instances, may be especially relevant for this age group.

The most recent national recommendations from the Centers for Disease Control and Prevention and the American College of Sports Medicine indicate that "every US adult should accumulate 30 minutes or more of moderate-intensity physical activity on most, preferably all, days of the week." Walking at a brisk pace (3 to 4 miles per hour in healthy adults) is an example of a moderate-intensity activity. The current recommendations also emphasize the benefits of incorporating routine physical activity into one's daily life (e.g., walking up stairs rather than using the elevator). It is recommended that individuals with chronic diseases or chronic disease risk factors

and inactive men older than 40 years of age or inactive women older than 50 years of age who plan to begin a *vigorous* exercise regimen first consult their physician. Furthermore, previously inactive persons should gradually increase the intensity and duration of their physical activity over time so as to avoid overexertion or overuse problems. Finally, although these guidelines focus largely on endurance exercise, a regular program of strength and flexibility exercises is also recommended, particularly for older individuals.

Table 23-3 shows the Healthy People 2010 goals for physical activity. Despite the health benefits of regular physical activity, however, half of those aged 65 to 74 years and two-thirds of those aged 75 years and older report no leisure-time physical activity. Furthermore, only 7 to 10 percent of older adults participate in strength training, and 22 to 24 percent participate in stretching exercises.

Physical activity is generally measured with self-report questionnaires, diaries, or logs; interviewer-administered surveys; and objective monitors (accelerometers). Each method has strengths and weaknesses. Many self-report measures assess activities that are uncommon in the older persons, such as sports and vigorous physical activities, producing floor effects. Individuals may have difficulty accurately recalling low- and moderate-intensity activities that are more common. Several self-report questionnaires have been developed specifically for older adults. Self-report diaries, while providing useful information, tend to require a great deal of time and accuracy on the part of the individual. A number of clinical trials have shown that simple self-report logs are a valid measure of physical activity adherence. Objective monitors eliminate reliance on the self-report of the individual, but they may not capture patterns of activity over the course of the day, tend to be less reliable for activities other than walking and jogging, and tend to be expensive. Pedometers are a lower-cost (generally less than $20) objective monitor that can serve as

Table 23-3 Healthy People 2010 Physical Activity Targets and the Percent of Older Adults (65-74 and 75+ years) and Adults in General who Meet these Targets*

Physical Activity Behavioral Goal	2010 Target Goal	65–74 Years of Age	75+ Years of Age	All Adults 18+ Years of Age
Reduce the proportion of adults who engage in no leisure-time physical activity.	20	51	65	40
Increase the proportion of adults who engage in moderate physical activity for 30+ minutes per day, 5+ days per week.	30	16	12	15
Increase the proportion of adults who engage in vigorous physical activity 3+ days per week for 20+ minutes per occasion.	30	13	6	23
Increase the proportion of adults who perform physical activities that enhance and maintain muscular strength and endurance.	30	10	7	18
Increase the proportion of adults who perform physical activities that enhance and maintain flexibility.	43	24	22	30

*All numbers represent percents. Data sources include Centers for Disease Control and National Center for Health Statistics.

SOURCE: US Department of Health and Human Services: *Healthy People 2010: Understanding and Improving Health,* 2nd ed. Washington, DC, US Government Printing Office, 2000.

both a measure of physical activity (specifically, steps) and a motivational tool.

Correlates of physical activity can be generally grouped into three categories: personal characteristics, program or regimen-based factors, and environmental factors. *Personal characteristics* include demographic and health variables; knowledge, attitudes, and beliefs associated with physical activity; and psychological or behavioral attributes and skills that may enable or constrain regular physical activity. In terms of demographic variables, women, particularly ethnic minority women, those 85+ years of age, smokers, those who are overweight, those who live in rural areas, and those with low income and education levels have the highest rates of physical inactivity. Of particular relevance for older adults, individuals in poor physical condition and health are less active than their healthy counterparts. Illness has also been shown to be a strong predictor of poor adherence to physical activity programs in older age groups. Arthritic pain is a significant barrier to physical activity in older adults, although moderate physical activity is often indicated in the treatment of arthritis. In addition, fear of falling or suffering an exercise-related injury, such as a heart attack, are potent barriers to physical activity, especially for older women.

Positive attitudes toward physical activity and accurate knowledge and beliefs are necessary but insufficient factors in the adoption of physical activity. Knowledge of and beliefs in the health benefits of physical activity and exercise self-efficacy relate to both the adoption and maintenance of physical activity. Older adults, especially older women, may hold more negative attitudes and beliefs about physical activity. For example, believing that exercise will "wear out" the body, that physical declines occurring with increasing age are inevitable and irreversible, and that exercise is socially "inappropriate" in older persons have been cited as barriers unique to older individuals. Additionally, sedentary older adults, particularly those without physical limitations, may erroneously believe that they are active enough and may not be aware of the necessary intensity, frequency, and duration needed to accrue health benefits. Lack of time is the most frequently cited barrier to physical inactivity in adults in general, but this factor appears to be less important among older individuals. Enjoyment of the physical activity is also associated with higher levels of physical activity, and may be especially important for older adults.

Psychological factors negatively associated with the adoption and maintenance of physical activity include low levels of self-motivation and high levels of psychological distress, such as depression and anxiety. The potential for achieving health-related benefits through exercise is a stronger motivator for older adults than for younger adults. Potential mental health benefits through exercise equally motivate younger and older adults. Previous experience and success with physical activity have also been positively associated with exercise participation. Current cohorts of older women have had less exposure to exercise and sports at younger ages; consequently, they may be less likely to initiate an exercise regimen.

Program- or *regimen-based factors* include the structure, format, complexity, intensity, convenience, and financial and psychological costs associated with the activity. Older

adults prefer moderate-intensity activities over more vigorous activities. Physical activities that are convenient, inexpensive, and noncompetitive are preferred. For example, walking and gardening are cited most often by older adults as preferred physical activities. Approximately two-thirds of older women and men, regardless of current physical activity levels and race/ethnicity, prefer physical activities that can be undertaken outside of a formal class or group setting. Furthermore, adherence to supervised home-based programs is higher than adherence to class- or group-based programs. As shown in Fig. 23-5, participants (aged 50 to 65 years) assigned to telephone-supervised home-based (lower- or higher-intensity) as compared to group-based exercise had significantly higher adherence rates in the first year of the study. During the second year of the study, adherence was highest among those assigned to higher-intensity (e.g., walk/jogging) home-based exercise that required fewer sessions per week. Recently, King and colleagues (2000) reported that adherence to home-based exercise sessions (92 percent) was significantly higher than adherence to class-based sessions (65 to 68 percent) among adults aged 65 years and older participating in a 1-year randomized clinical trial.

Finally, *social* and *physical environmental factors* influence physical activity participation. Social support from friends, family, and health professionals is positively associated with physical activity participation. The importance of social support appears to be stronger in older women than men, yet many older women do not perceive that they receive support from their physician and family to be physically active. Physical environmental factors such as the travel distance required for exercise, aversive climate and weather, neighborhood safety, and availability of facilities for physical activity (e.g., parks, walking/jogging paths) could also impact physical activity, but they have received little systematic investigation.

Many of the determinants of physical activity described above can be modified with intervention. For example, misconceptions and lack of knowledge regarding the risks and benefits of exercise in old age, self-efficacy for exercise, social support, exercise program factors, and type of exercise engaged in are examples of determinants that could be targeted for change. Thorough reviews of physical activity interventions are included in two recent reviews by King and colleagues (1998, 2001). Briefly, interventions based on the principles of social learning/social cognitive theories (e.g., self-monitoring, goal setting, self-reward, problem solving, self-efficacy, improving attitudes and knowledge, social support) and the transtheoretical model (i.e., psychological readiness to change) have received the most support for increasing physical activity in adults in general and older adults in particular. Similar to smoking cessation, older adults who participate in physical activity interventions comply at rates similar to younger adults and derive similar benefits. Much less is known, however, about older individuals who currently have no intention of becoming more active. These individuals have the most to gain by increasing their level of physical activity. Correlate of home-based, moderate-intensity activities warrant further study given the potential public health importance of these types of activities.

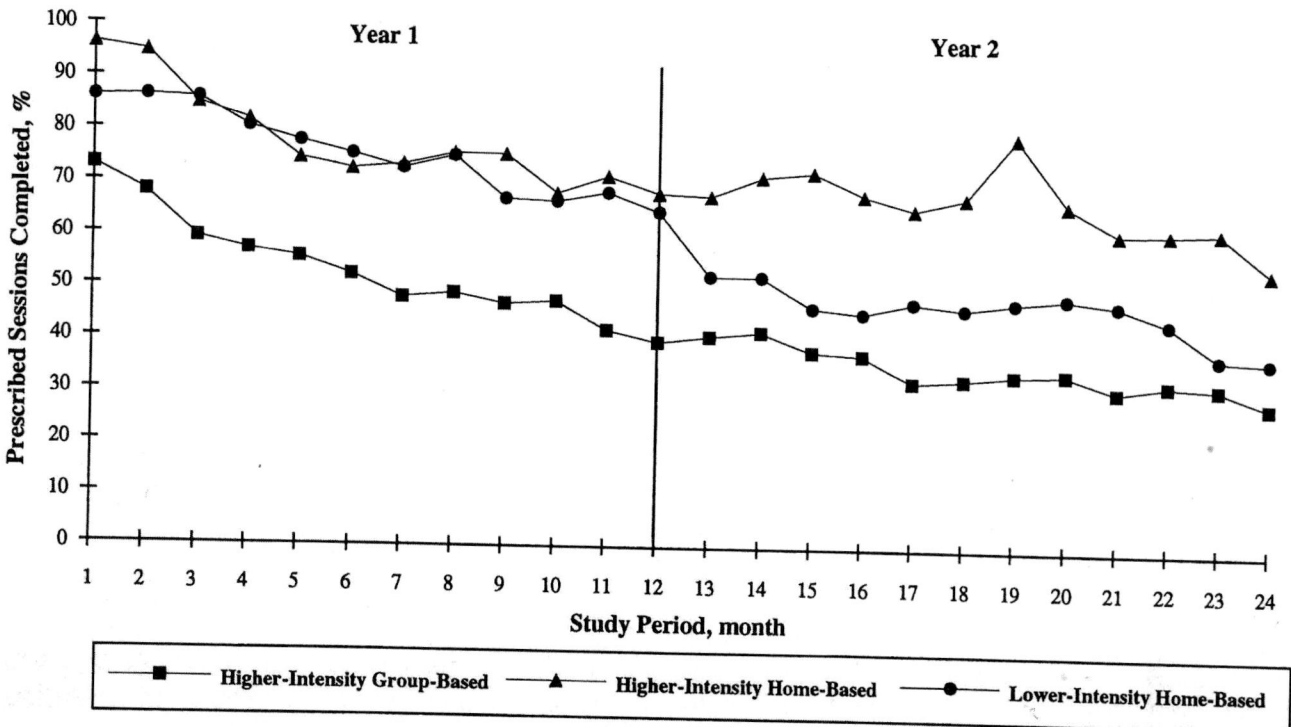

Figure 23-5 Monthly adherence rates (percentage of prescribed exercise sessions completed) across the 2-year period by exercise training condition assignment. Note: During year 1, group-based training condition differed from the other two conditions at P < .0005. During year 2, higher-intensity, home-based training condition differed from the other two conditions at P < .0029. From King AC et al: Long-term effects of varying intensities and formats of physical activity on participation rates, fitness, and lipoproteins in men and women aged 50 to 65 years. *Circulation* 91:2596, 1995. Copyright © 1995, American Heart Association. Reproduced with permission.

As with all of the health behaviors discussed in this chapter, physicians and other health professionals can play a major role in encouraging older adults to become more physically active. As shown in Table 23-1, a Healthy People 2010 goal is to increase to at least 85 percent the proportion of primary care providers who counsel their patients about physical activity. Unfortunately, rates of counseling are substantially lower, with estimates ranging from 15 to 34 percent. In the Physician-based Assessment and Counseling for Exercise (PACE) study, brief (3 to 5 minutes) physician counseling produced significant increases in walking at the 6-week follow-up relative to a control group. The recently completed Activity Counseling Trial (ACT; participants were 35 to 75 years of age) used a randomized design and had a substantially longer follow-up period than PACE. Both a less-intensive ("assistance") and more-intensive ("counseling") intervention increased cardiorespiratory fitness over 2 years relative to recommended care ("advise") in women, but the three interventions were equivalent at 2 years for men. At 2 years, men and women had increased their self-reported physical activity relative to baseline, but there were no significant differences by intervention group. The Physically Active for Life (PAL) project evaluated physician-delivered physical activity counseling for older adults. Although the intervention produced short-term increases in motivational readiness for physical activity in intervention, but not in control, patients, effects were not maintained at the 8-month follow-up. In addition, physical activity did not significantly change as a result of the intervention. A recent review

of physical activity interventions delivered in health care settings indicated that intervention effects were small but significant, and were larger in samples with a mean age of 50 years or greater versus younger than 50 years. Effects, however, were smaller at longer follow-up periods. Together, these results suggest that physical activity counseling from primary care physicians may produce gains in both fitness and physical activity, but more research is needed to understand how to sustain behavioral changes in older patients over longer periods of time. In light of the high regard in which older adults hold physicians and other health professionals, continued efforts to involve health professionals in supporting regular physical activity among older adults remains a critical goal.

Nutrition

Overweight and obesity are the most prevalent nutritional problems in the United States and other industrialized nations. (See Table 23-4 for definitions of overweight and obesity.) Excess weight is associated with cardiovascular disease, type 2 diabetes mellitus, hypertension, stroke, dyslipidemia, osteoarthritis, and some cancers. Results from NHANES III indicate that 67 percent of men aged 55 years and older (versus 60 percent of men aged 25 to 54 years) and 61 percent of women aged 55 years and older (versus 49 percent of women aged 25 to 54 years) are overweight or obese. There is some controversy regarding the importance of overweight in older adults. A

Table 23-4   Classification of Overweight and Obesity by Body Mass Index (BMI), Calculated as kg/m²

	Obesity Class	BMI
Underweight		<18.5
Normal		18.5–24.9
Overweight		25.0–29.9
Obesity	I	30.0–34.9
	II	35.0–39.9
Extreme obesity	III	≥40

SOURCE: Adapted from the NHLBI Expert Panel: Executive summary of the clinical guidelines on the identification, evaluation, and treatment of overweight and obesity in adults. *J Am Diet Assoc* 98:1178, 1998.

recent review of prospective studies in which both Body Mass Index (BMI) and mortality were assessed found that overweight was not associated with excess mortality risk in older persons, and obesity was a smaller risk factor in older adults relative to younger adults. The authors concluded that federal guidelines for normal weight may be overly restrictive for older persons. It is important, however, to consider other outcomes in addition to mortality. For example, a prospective analysis of the Nurses' Health Study found that weight gain was associated with decrements in quality of life (decreased physical function and vitality and increased bodily pain), whereas weight loss was associated with improvements in quality of life, regardless of age (<65 years and ≥65 years).

Nutritional deficiencies, while less prevalent than obesity in the general population of older adults, are also of concern and are more common in older persons who are isolated and economically deprived, and in frail older adults. For example, it is estimated that between 5 and 10 percent of free-living older adults and between 30 and 60 percent of hospitalized or institutionalized older adults in the United States experience malnutrition.

Risk factors for poor nutrition in older adults are multidimensional. Health factors that are associated with malnutrition include chronic diseases and conditions that interfere with the ability to chew, swallow, digest, and absorb food; poor oral health, including loose-fitting dentures, tooth loss, mouth sores, cavities, and decreased salivation; physical disabilities and frailty that interfere with shopping and meal preparation; sensory impairments that limit one's ability to taste and smell foods; alcohol use; and polypharmacy. Psychosocial factors associated with poor nutrition include social isolation, recent bereavement, depression and other mental illnesses, and cognitive impairments. Finally, socioeconomic factors, including poverty and low levels of education, put individuals at much greater risk of malnutrition. Older women, those who live alone, and those from ethnic minority groups experience the highest rates of poverty and are at greatest risk for malnutrition. With the exception of mental illness and alcohol use, each of these factors becomes more common with advanced age, resulting in an increased risk of malnutrition with increasing age.

Until recently, the dietary behaviors and specific nutritional needs of older adults received inadequate attention. For example, "51 years and above" is the oldest age category in the 1989 edition of the Recommended Dietary Allowances (RDAs). However, recent revisions to the Dietary Reference Intakes (DRIs) have extended the age range: DRIs for adults aged 51 to 70 years and older than 70 years are provided. In addition, a number of health and professional organizations, such as the American Dietetic Association, have issued age-specific recommendations for nutrition and health.

Despite the fact that older adults have higher rates of overweight and obesity than younger adults, older adults actually consume fewer calories than younger adults. This apparent contradiction is explained by the fact that energy requirements decline with age because of a reduction in lean body mass and increased sedentary lifestyles. Age-related reductions in caloric intake can make it difficult for older adults to meet recommended values for foods and nutrients and to ensure adequate diet diversity. Thus, physical activity also has an important role in nutrition: active older adults have greater energy requirements, which provides an opportunity to eat more food, ideally translating into more variety and improved nutritional quality. Another important but often overlooked area in geriatric nutrition is hydration. Dehydration is responsible for approximately 7 percent of hospitalizations in older age. In consideration of these issues, a modified food guide pyramid was developed at Tufts University for adults aged 70 years and older. The base of the pyramid was narrowed to reflect the reduced energy requirements of older adults. It also emphasizes nutrient-dense foods to maximize nutrients for a given level of calories (e.g., fortified foods, whole grains), the role of dietary supplements for some older adults, and the importance of fluid intake. Figure 23-6 shows this pyramid.

Data from NHANES III and other sources indicate that older adults' intakes of calories, calcium, dietary fiber, carbohydrates, and fruits and vegetables are below recommended levels, whereas dietary fat consumption is higher than recommended. Older ethnic minorities are at greater risk of malnutrition than are whites. Protein deficiency, while relatively uncommon in most individuals, is prevalent in some subgroups of older adults, including those who are homebound and those who live in poverty. Despite the fact that many older adults are not meeting nutritional recommendations, older adults are typically as or more adherent to dietary recommendations than younger adults, with some exceptions (e.g., calcium intake declines with age, especially in women). Table 23-5 shows the Healthy People 2010 goals and actual proportions for targeted areas.

Nutritional problems and adherence are generally assessed by a combination of self-report dietary measures, anthropometric measures (e.g., BMI), weight change history, and laboratory measures. Self-report methods of assessing diet within the time constraints of clinical settings are reviewed elsewhere (see recent reviews by Calfas et al. and Vellas et al.). The Nutrition Screening Initiative (NSI) was begun in 1990 and emphasized the identification, intervention, and treatment of nutritional problems in older adults by increasing consumer and professional

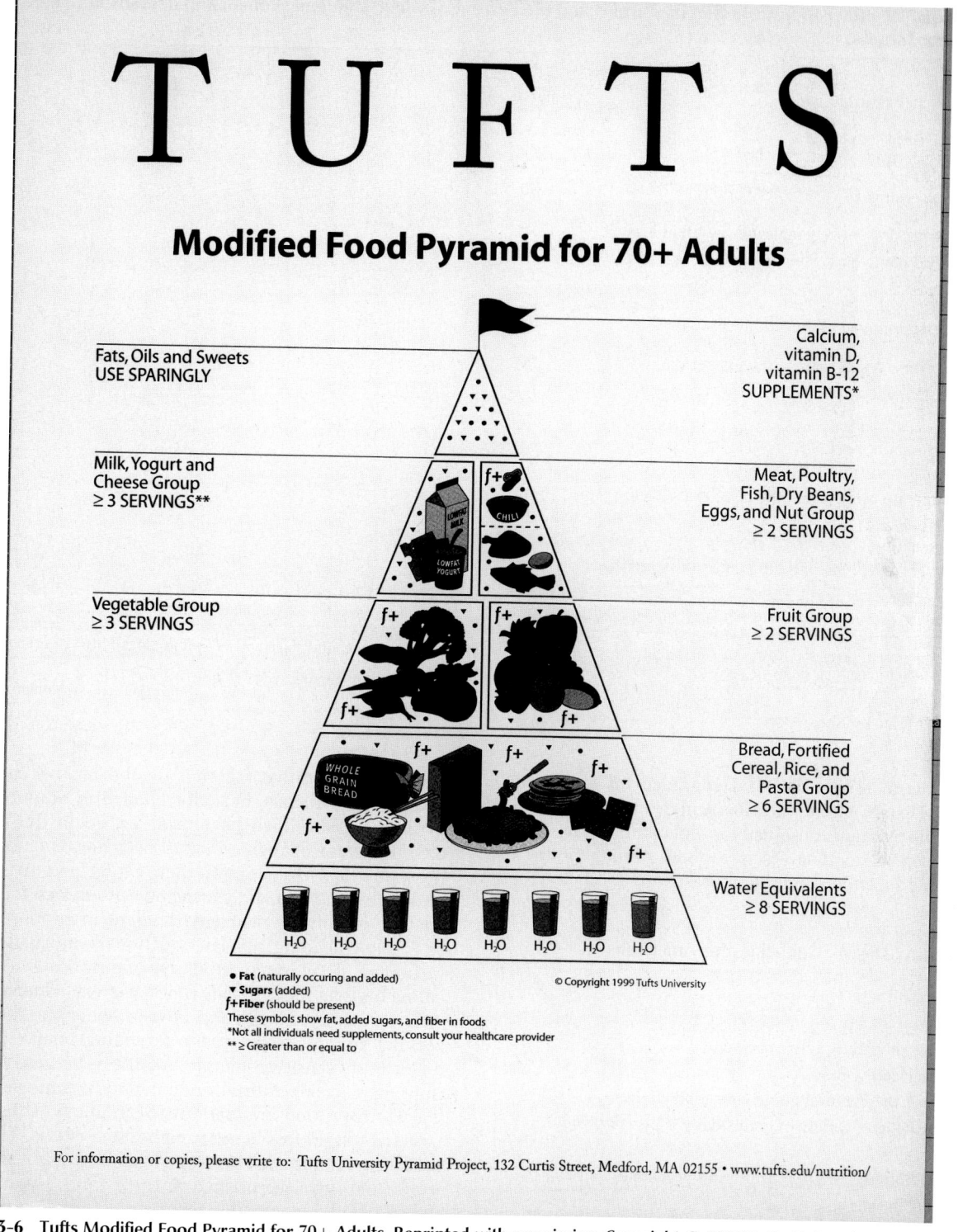

Figure 23-6 Tufts Modified Food Pyramid for 70+ Adults. Reprinted with permission. Copyright © 1999 Tufts University. Development of this pyramid is described in Russell RM et al: Modified food guide pyramid for people over seventy years of age. *J Nutr* 129:751, 1999.

awareness of the subject. Although not meant to be diagnostic, the NSI developed a brief, self-administered checklist that assesses older adults' risk of poor nutritional status (shown in Fig. 23-7). This screening measure is widely used. The NSI also outlined two levels of screening that can be used to further assess and diagnose malnutrition in those who score high on the screening checklist. These widely

disseminated materials provide a cost- and time-effective method for increasing awareness of nutritional factors among older adults.

Few dietary behavior interventions specific to older adults exist. Based on other age groups, components of an effective intervention include nutrition education and behavioral change skills training. Instructing older

Table 23–5 Healthy People 2010 Dietary Targets and the Percent of Older Men and Women and Persons in General who Meet these Targets*

Dietary Behavioral Goal	2010 Target Goal	Women, 60+ Years of Age	Men, 60+ Years of Age	All persons, 2+ Years of Age
Eat 2+ servings of fruit per day	75	35	39	28
Eat 3+ servings of vegetables per day	50	43	57	49
Eat 3+ servings of vegetables/day, with at least one-third being dark green or orange vegetables per day	50	13	11	8
Eat 6+ servings of grain products per day	50	28	54	51
Eat 6+ servings of grain products per day, with at least 3 being whole grains	50	6	12	7
Consume less than 10% of calories from saturated fat	75	47	42	36
Consume no more than 30% of calories from total fat	75	40	34	33
Consume less than 2400 mg of sodium per day	65	NR	NR	21
Meet dietary recommendations for calcium	75	27	35	46

*All values represent percents. Note: For calcium intake, current percentages reflect data from adults aged 50 years and older. NR = not reported. Data sources include USDA, CDC, and NCHS.

Source: From US Department of Health and Human Services: *Healthy People 2010: Understanding and Improving Health,* 2nd ed. Washington, DC, US Government Printing Office, 2000.

individuals to follow the US Department of Agriculture (USDA) Dietary Guidelines for Americans (Table 23-6), food guide pyramids designed for older adults (Fig. 23-6), and/or to read food labels is a good starting point for nutrition education. Techniques based on social learning

Table 23-6 Dietary Guidelines for Americans

Aim for Fitness...
- Aim for a healthy weight.
- Be physically active each day.

Build a Healthy Base...
- Let the Pyramid guide your food choices.
- Choose a variety of grains daily, especially whole grains.
- Choose a variety of fruits and vegetables daily.
- Keep food safe to eat.

Choose Sensibly...
- Choose a diet that is low in saturated fat and cholesterol, and moderate in total fat.
- Choose beverages and foods to moderate your intake of sugars.
- Choose and prepare foods with less salt.
- If you drink alcoholic beverages, do so in moderation.

Source: USDA: Nutrition and Your Health: Dietary Guidelines for Americans, 2000.

and social cognitive theories are the most widely used strategies for dietary behavior change in adults. Similar to the other health behaviors described in this chapter, techniques for changing dietary behaviors include assisting individuals to monitor their eating patterns; setting nutrition-related goals; increasing self-efficacy for dietary change; modifying their environment to support change (e.g., avoid keeping high fat, nutritionally unbalanced food in home); developing alternative coping skills to replace eating high-fat foods during times of stress; addressing barriers to dietary change and how to overcome them; and seeking support from others. Providing interventions in a culturally sensitive manner is critical, because food has important social, cultural, and religious meanings. The Dietary Intervention: Evaluation of Technology (DIET) study targeted weight loss in overweight older adults. This CBT-based intervention led to weight loss and improved glucose levels that were maintained at the 2- and 3-year follow-ups. Age-tailored nutrition newsletters and other mail- and telephone-mediated interventions also appear to improve both nutritional knowledge and selected dietary components in older adults. It is unclear how well these strategies apply to problems related to nutritional deficiencies. Assisting elders in using federal programs (e.g., home-delivered meals, food stamps) and treating underlying medical and psychological problems (e.g., dental problems, depression) are important in cases of malnutrition. Interventions with older adults are most likely to succeed when they combine traditional techniques described above with age-tailored

The Warning Signs of poor nutritional health are often overlooked. Use this checklist to find out if you or someone you know is at nutritional risk.

Read the statements below. Circle the number in the "yes" column for those that apply to you or someone you know. For each "yes" answer, score the number in the box. Total your nutritional score.

DETERMINE YOUR NUTRITIONAL HEALTH

	YES
I have an illness or condition that made me change the kind and/or amount of food I eat.	2
I eat fewer than 2 meals per day.	3
I eat few fruits or vegetables or milk products.	2
I have 3 or more drinks of beer, liquor or wine almost every day.	2
I have tooth or mouth problems that make it hard for me to eat.	2
I don't always have enough money to buy the food I need.	4
I eat alone most of the time.	1
I take 3 or more different prescribed or over-the-counter drugs a day.	1
Without wanting to, I have lost or gained 10 pounds in the last 6 months.	2
I am not always physically able to shop, cook and/or feed myself.	2
	TOTAL

Total Your Nutritional Score. If it's –

0-2 **Good!** Recheck your nutritional score in 6 months.

3-5 **You are at moderate nutritional risk.** See what can be done to improve your eating habits and lifestyle. Your office on aging, senior nutrition program, senior citizens center, or health department can help. Recheck your nutritional score in 3 months.

6 or more **You are at high nutritional risk.** Bring this checklist the next time you see your doctor, dietitian, or other qualified health or social service professional. Talk with them about any problems you may have. Ask for help to improve your nutritional health.

Remember that warning signs suggest risk, but do not represent a diagnosis of any condition. Turn the page to learn more about the Warnings Signs of poor nutritional health.

These materials are developed and distributed by the Nutrition Screening Initiative, a project of:

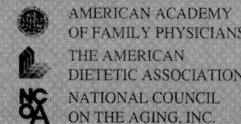

AMERICAN ACADEMY OF FAMILY PHYSICIANS
THE AMERICAN DIETETIC ASSOCIATION
NATIONAL COUNCIL ON THE AGING, INC.

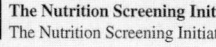

The Nutrition Screening Initiative • 1010 Wisconsin Avenue, NW • Suite 800 • Washington, DC 20007
The Nutrition Screening Initiative is funded in part by a grant from Ross Products Division of Abbott Laboratories.

Figure 23-7 *A.* Determine Your Nutritional Health Checklist. Reprinted with permission of the Nutrition Screening Initiative, a project of the American Academy of Family Physicians, the American Dietetic Association, and the National Council on the Aging, Inc., and funded in part by a grant from Ross Products Division, Abbott Laboratories Inc.

approaches (e.g., address how such factors as bereavement, social isolation, poverty, poor dentition, and illness and disability impact dietary behaviors and adherence).

A Healthy People 2010 goal is to increase to 75 percent the proportion of physicians who provide counseling or education related to diet and nutrition to patients with a diagnosis of cardiovascular disease, diabetes, or hyperlipidemia (see Table 23-1). Currently, only 42 percent of

physicians provide such counseling or education. Furthermore, among adults older than 65 years of age who attended general medical/gynecologic visits, only 23 percent received dietary counseling, indicating even lower rates for preventive counseling. Health care providers are well-positioned to provide nutrition counseling to their older patients, but many feel unprepared to provide this counseling. Interventions that have trained residents in dietary

The Nutrition Checklist is based on the Warning Signs described below. Use the word DETERMINE to remind you of the Warning Signs.

DISEASE

Any disease, illness, or chronic condition which causes you to change the way you eat, or makes it hard for you to eat, puts your nutritional health at risk. Four out of five adults have chronic diseases that are affected by diet. Confusion or memory loss that keeps getting worse is estimated to affect one out of five or more older adults. This can make it hard to remember what, when or if you've eaten. Feeling sad or depressed, which happens to about one in eight older adults, can cause big changes in appetite, digestion, energy level, weight, and well-being.

EATING POORLY

Eating too little and eating too much both lead to poor health. Eating the same foods day after day or not eating fruit, vegetables, and milk products daily will also cause poor nutritional health. One in five adults skip meals daily. Only 13% of adults eat the minimum amount of fruit and vegetables needed. One in four older adults drink too much alcohol. Many health problems become worse if you drink more than one or two alcoholic beverages per day.

TOOTH LOSS/MOUTH PAIN

A healthy mouth, teeth and gums are needed to eat. Missing, loose, or rotten teeth or dentures which don't fit well, or cause mouth sores, make it hard to eat.

ECONOMIC HARDSHIP

As many as 40% of older Americans have incomes of less than $6,000 per year. Having less -- or choosing to spend less -- than $25-30 per week for food makes it very hard to get the foods you need to stay healthy.

REDUCED SOCIAL CONTACT

One-third of all older people live alone. Being with people daily has a positive effect on morale, well-being, and eating.

MULTIPLE MEDICINES

Many older Americans must take medicines for health problems. Almost half of older Americans take multiple medicines daily. Growing old may change the way we respond to drugs. The more medicines you take, the greater the chance for side effects such as increased or decreased appetite, change in taste, constipation, weakness, drowsiness, diarrhea, nausea, and others. Vitamins or minerals, when taken in large doses, act like drugs and can cause harm. Alert your doctor to everything you take.

INVOLUNTARY WEIGHT LOSS/GAIN

Losing or gaining a lot of weight when you are not trying to do so is an important warning sign that must not be ignored. Being overweight or underweight also increases your chance of poor health.

NEEDS ASSISTANCE IN SELF CARE

Although most older people are able to eat, one of every five have trouble walking, shopping, buying and cooking food, especially as they get older.

ELDER YEARS ABOVE AGE 80

Most older people lead full and productive lives. But as age increases, risk of frailty and health problems increase. Checking your nutritional health regularly makes good sense.

 The Nutrition Screening Initiative • 1010 Wisconsin Avenue, NW • Suite 800 • Washington, DC 20007
The Nutrition Screening Initiative is funded in part by a grant from Ross Products Division of Abbott Laboratories.

Figure 23-7 *B. (Continued).*

counseling have improved provider self-efficacy for dietary counseling. When this training is combined with provider prompts (e.g., chart reminders, providing patient's blood cholesterol levels), health care providers are more likely to deliver dietary counseling. A recent review of dietary interventions delivered in health care settings (not older adult specific) indicated that these interventions produce small but significant improvements in dietary outcomes. Nutrition is further discussed in Chap. 90.

SUMMARY AND RECOMMENDATIONS

Improving the health and functioning of older adults is an ever-increasing health care priority. Promoting healthful behaviors has the potential for greatly reducing the personal and societal burden resulting from chronic diseases. Despite the importance of health promotion, far less is known about the most effective health intervention approaches for older adults. From what is known, components of effective interventions appear to be similar across age groups. Furthermore, as clearly demonstrated in the smoking cessation literature, the effectiveness of health promotion interventions can probably be enhanced by incorporating age-specific components into existing interventions. In all health behaviors reviewed in this chapter, the use of self-help and/or mail- or telephone-mediated interventions show significant improvements in target behaviors. These approaches are also preferred by most older adults. Further development of these cost-effective interventions, translation of these interventions from research to clinical and community practice, and age-tailoring of these interventions (where needed) are priorities. Another priority for future research is to examine subgroups of older adults who have received very little empirical study. Examples of these subgroups include ethnically diverse older adults, rural older adults, less-educated and impoverished older adults, the frail elderly, and those 85 years of age and older. Understanding the health practices and barriers to health practices in these subgroups is an essential first step in developing effective interventions. Finally, research is accumulating that health care providers can have a major impact on the health and well-being of adults of all ages. The challenges of limited time and financial constraints necessitate the development of brief yet reliable and valid assessment instruments and effective interventions. Most older adults hold their physicians in high regard, and the majority of older adults have visited their physicians within the last year, providing an important opportunity to assess the older adult's health behaviors and to intervene and/or refer when necessary.

ACKNOWLEDGMENTS

We wish to thank Brook Harmon for her assistance in preparing this chapter.

REFERENCES

American Medical Association: Alcoholism in the elderly. *JAMA* 275: 797, 1996.

ADA: Position of the American Dietetic Association: Nutrition, aging, and the continuum of care. *J Am Diet Assoc* 100:580, 2000.

Brownell KD, Cohen LR: Adherence to dietary regimens. 2: Components of effective interventions. *Behav Med* 20:155, 1995.

Calfas KJ et al: Practical nutrition assessment in primary care settings: a review. *Am J Prev Med* 18:289, 2000.

Dornelas EA et al: The DIET study: Long-term outcomes of a cognitive–behavioral weight-control intervention in independent-living elders. Dietary Intervention: Evaluation of Technology. *J Am Diet Assoc* 98:1276, 1998.

Edinger JD et al: Cognitive–behavioral therapy for treatment of chronic primary insomnia: A randomized controlled trial. *JAMA* 285:1856, 2001.

Fleming MF et al: Brief physician advice for alcohol problems in older adults: A randomized community-based trial. *J Fam Pract* 48:378, 1999.

Glanz K et al: *Health Behavior and Health Education. Theory, Research, and Practice.* San Francisco, CA: Jossey-Bass, 1997.

Heiat A et al: An evidence-based assessment of federal guidelines for overweight and obesity as they apply to elderly persons. *Arch Intern Med* 161:1194, 2001.

King AC et al: Moderate-intensity exercise and self-rated quality of sleep in older adults. A randomized controlled trial. *JAMA* 277:32, 1997.

King AC et al: Physical activity interventions targeting older adults. A critical review and recommendations. *Am J Prev Med* 15:316, 1998.

King AC et al: Comparative effects of two physical activity programs on measured and perceived physical functioning and other health-related quality of life outcomes in older adults. *J Gerontol* 55:M74, 2000.

King AC: Interventions to promote physical activity by older adults. *J Gerontol* 56A:36, 2001.

Lichstein KL, Morin CM: *Treatment of Late-Life Insomnia.* Thousand Oaks, CA: Sage, 2000.

McGee M, Jensen GL: Nutrition in the elderly. *J Clin Gastroenterol* 30:372, 2000.

Moore AA et al: Drinking habits among older persons: Findings from the NHANES I Epidemiologic Followup Study (1982–84). National Health and Nutrition Examination Survey. *J Am Geriatr Soc* 47:412, 1999.

Morgan GD et al: Reaching midlife and older smokers: Tailored interventions for routine medical care. *Prev Med* 25:346, 1996.

Must A et al: The disease burden associated with overweight and obesity. *JAMA* 282:1523, 1999.

Ockene JK et al: Brief physician- and nurse practitioner-delivered counseling for high-risk drinkers: Does it work? *Arch Intern Med* 159:2198, 1999.

Orleans CT et al: Computer-tailored intervention for older smokers using transdermal nicotine. *Tob Control* 9:153, 2000.

Ossip-Klein DJ et al: Self-help interventions for older smokers. *Tob Control* 6:188, 1997.

Rimer BK, Orleans CT: Tailoring smoking cessation for older adults. *Cancer* 74:2051, 1994.

Ryan AA: Medication compliance and older people: A review of the literature. *Int J Nurs Stud* 36:153, 1999.

Singh NA et al: A randomized controlled trial of the effect of exercise on sleep. *Sleep* 20:95, 1997.

The Writing Group for the Activity Counseling Trial Research Group: Effects of physical activity counseling in primary care: The Activity Counseling Trial: A randomized controlled trial. *JAMA* 286:677, 2001.

US Department of Health and Human Services: *Physical Activity and Health: A Report of the Surgeon General.* Atlanta, GA: National Center for Chronic Disease Prevention and Health Promotion, Centers for Disease Control and Prevention, US Department of Health and Human Services, 1996.

Vellas B et al: Nutrition assessment in the elderly. *Curr Opin Clin Nutr Metab Care* 4:5, 2001.

White JV: Risk factors for poor nutritional status. *Prim Care* 21:19, 1994.

Wilcox S et al: Nutrition and physical activity interventions to reduce cardiovascular disease risk in health care settings: A quantitative review with a focus on women. *Nutr Rev* 59:197, 2001.

Wilcox S et al: Physical activity patterns, assessment, and motivation in older adults, in Shephard RJ (ed): *Gender, Physical Activity, and Aging.* Boca Raton, FL, CRC Press, 2002, p 13.

Geriatric Rehabilitation

HELEN HOENIG • TONI M. CUTSON

HOW DISABILITY OCCURS

The goal of rehabilitation is to improve disability caused by physical and/or psychological pathology. To achieve this goal, rehabilitation makes use of a wide variety of therapeutic interventions. The essential goals and techniques used in rehabilitation do not differ for older versus younger persons. There are, however, important differences in rehabilitation approach and in outcomes related to age. Even among the subset of patients older than 65 years of age there may be important age-related differences in outcomes of care. For example, many rehabilitation patients older than 80 years of age are less independent at the time rehabilitation is discontinued than are patients between the ages of 65 and 80 years. The etiology of age-related differences in rehabilitation outcomes is unknown. One key difference, however, is that many older patients suffer from multiple conditions that may interact to exacerbate functional disability and that may affect response to some rehabilitation interventions. Young adults with disability primarily experience catastrophic disability, usually as a consequence of a single underlying cause. Many older adults, in contrast, acquire disability more slowly. Disability in older patients often is due to the interplay of multiple underlying causal factors. Even when the disability itself is due to a single catastrophic event like a stroke or a hip fracture, multiple comorbid conditions are common in the older patient. Older rehabilitation patients with multiple comorbid conditions tend to have longer lengths of stay and worse functional outcomes. An understanding of the disablement process, which tends to be much more complicated than in young adults, is critical to geriatric rehabilitation.

Disability is a complex behavior with social, economic, and biological causes (e.g., deconditioning, age-related changes, illness). Table 24-1 compares several common theoretical frameworks for the causation of disability.

The Initial Stages in the Development of Disability: Disease and Impairment

All of the models divide the disablement process into four basic stages. For many older people, the disablement process does not necessarily consist of four discrete steps but rather is an incremental process of gradual decline, in contrast to the more familiar catastrophic disability typical of stroke or hip fracture. However, the four steps provide a useful framework for understanding and treating disability. The first step of the process is "disease," the underlying pathology or disorder. The disease process causes dysfunction at the organ system level, that is, impairment, which is the second step in the disablement process. There is substantial empirical evidence in support of this disease–impairment relationship. For example, poorly controlled diabetes mellitus may result in end-organ damage such as retinopathy or neuropathy. Inflammation from rheumatoid arthritis causes pain and destruction of the joint space, while interrupting the inflammatory process slows joint destruction.

The Final Stages in the Development of Disability: Disability and Handicap

If organ system impairment is severe enough, or in the presence of other facilitating factors, it may manifest as a "disability." Disability refers to a limitation in the ability to perform an activity in a normal manner or a disturbance in the performance of daily tasks like dressing or bathing. The term *physical disability* often is used interchangeably with the term *functional limitation* to refer to this stage. The disablement process culminates in difficulty maintaining social role function, such as employment. This stage is referred to as a social disability or a handicap. Recent models for the disablement process attempt to use empowering terminology, referring to "activities" rather than "disability," and "participation" rather than "handicap." These various terms are used interchangeably in this chapter, depending on the context.

Substantial epidemiologic evidence supports a causal relationship between impairment and functional limitations or physical disability. Prospective studies show, for example, that slow gait speed precedes the development of frank disability. Many of the relationships between specific impairments and specific disabilities can be understood through simple physics. For example, patients who are unable to fully extend the hips, a common problem

Table 24-1 Comparison of Different Models for the Disablement Process

Source	Pathology	Organ System	Self-care Function	Social Role Function	Social and Physical Environment
World Health Organization, 1980*	Disease	Impairment	Disability	Handicap	
Institute of Medicine†	Disease	Impairment	Functional limitation	Social disability	Biopsychosocial risk factors
World Health Organization, 2000‡	Disease	Impairment	Activities	Participation	Personal and environmental contextual factors

SOURCE: Authors own work summarizing models for the disablement process from *International Classification of Impairments, Disabilities, and Handicaps: Manual of Classification Relating to Consequences of Disease.* Geneva, Switzerland, WHO, 1980; †Pope AM, Tarlov AR (eds): *Disability in America.* Washington, DC, National Academy Press, 1991, p 1; ‡http://www.worldhealth.org/.

in patients who have been at bed rest for any length of time may have difficulty maintaining balance or walking long distances. This difficulty results because hip flexion moves the trunk forward, moving the body's center of gravity in front of its base of support. People can compensate for decreased hip extension by flexing the knees so as to bring the body back over the base of support. As the quadriceps muscles rest when the knee is fully extended, during the stance phase of the gait cycle, however, lack of full knee extension causes the quadriceps to fatigue more rapidly, reducing endurance while walking. If the quadriceps muscles are weak, also a common occurrence after prolonged bed rest, standing with the knees flexed for more than a few seconds may be difficult. The legs may give way suddenly. A common compensatory strategy to help with this problem is use of a walker, which acts to broaden the patient's base of support allowing for full knee extension while accommodating the lack of hip extension.

Diseases differ both in prevalence and the degree of disability produced. On average, for example, stroke produces more disability than does arthritis, but stroke occurs much less often than does arthritis. The difference in their respective prevalences is the reason why, among men older than age 70 years, arthritis ranks as the number one cause of activity limitation, whereas cerebrovascular disease ranks as number seven.

Interactions Among Diseases, Impairments, and Disability

Diseases and impairments may interact with one another in a synergistic fashion, exacerbating the risk of disability beyond the additive effect of each condition in isolation. Among community dwelling older Americans, for example, the risk of mobility disability is 2 times higher among persons with heart disease alone, 4 times higher among persons with arthritis alone, and 14 times higher among persons with both heart disease and arthritis, when compared with persons with neither disease. This synergy occurs because any condition that affects the biomechanical integrity of the joints of the lower extremity, such as arthritis, use of a brace, or amputation, increases the work of walking. Merely having the knee immobilized by a brace can increase the work of walking by more than 20 percent as compared to walking without the knee immobilized. The degree to which joint impairment increases the work of walking depends on the number of joints affected and the degree to which normal joint function is impaired. Compensatory strategies include reducing gait speed because walking quickly requires more energy than walking slowly and taking advantage of strength reserves in other limbs through use of a cane or crutches. The natural walking pace of older persons with early osteoarthritis, for example, may be 10 percent slower than in older persons without osteoarthritis. When walking slowly is not an option, cardiac output must be increased to accommodate the increased work of walking, which can be problematic in the presence of significant heart or lung disease. This interaction accounts for the excess disability seen in people with both heart disease and arthritis. In addition to appreciating the potential for interactions among diseases, it is important to realize that the disablement process is not necessarily unidirectional. The presence of a disability or handicap may increase the risk of developing other diseases and impairments. Immobility due to a stroke or hip fracture, for example, may increase the risk of developing a pressure sore or aspiration pneumonia.

Contextual Factors Influence Disability

In addition to considering specific medical conditions, it is critical to consider the contribution of social and environmental factors to the disablement process. The disablement process can be modified by a number of factors. These are referred to as extrinsic and intrinsic modifiers or as contextual factors. The development of end-organ damage from diabetes provides a useful example. Exposure to nicotine in tobacco, an environmental influence, will exacerbate the effects of diabetes on the vascular system, resulting in development of end-organ damage more rapidly. The availability of a caregiver to help ensure that the patient uses insulin properly or follows a proper diet may favorably influence the progression of diabetes-related end-organ damage by ensuring better control of the diabetes.

Key contextual factors include social support, cognition, affect, finances, and environment. Social supports are critically important to disabled older patients staying in the community; failure of social supports may be one reason older patients require institutional placement. Coexisting depression or cognitive impairment can adversely affect functional outcomes in many diseases. Stroke patients, for example, who are depressed or cognitively impaired have poorer functional outcomes. Financial supports enable people to pay for personal assistance or equipment that in turn increases independence. While most insurance policies cover the more basic types of adaptive equipment, it may be difficult to obtain reimbursement for anything other than a standard wheelchair or commode. For example, few insurance policies cover motorized scooters. Similarly, the physical environment is a key factor influencing functional outcomes among people with physical impairments. The Americans with Disabilities Act was enacted with this in mind. If the environment is wheelchair accessible, someone who must use a wheelchair for mobility will be able to carry out activities in their home and outside their home. There are some excellent free resources available to consumers and businesses describing how to design environments, or to adapt existing structures, to maximize access for people with physical disabilities. Useful web sites include the web site for the American with Disabilities Act (ADA) at http://www.adata.org/, the Center for Design and Environmental Access at http://design6.ap.buffalo.edu/~idea/index.html, and The Center for Universal Design at http://www.design.ncsu.edu/cud/index.html.

Disability and handicap often are a result of complex interactions among physical and cognitive impairments, environmental influences, social, and psychological supports. The effects of contextual factors are particularly influential over time. For example, while high correlations between the amount of motor impairment and the amount of disability are seen after acute spinal cord injury, the correlations are lower among persons with chronic spinal cord injury. Self-perceptions can play an important role in how people interpret and cope with physical impairment. People with major mobility limitations may not perceive themselves as having a disability, whereas others with relatively minor physical limitations may report experiencing substantial disability.

EVALUATION

Goals of the Evaluation

An important consideration in rehabilitation treatment planning is whether or not rehabilitative treatment should be directed at the disability irrespective of the underlying disease process. Referring patients who report functional difficulty to rehabilitation without a medical evaluation might be appropriate if the outcomes of rehabilitation

treatment are the same irrespective of the underlying cause(s).

On the other hand, identifying the underlying disablement process is important if the effectiveness of rehabilitation interventions differs according to the causal disease(s). For example, exercise has been embraced enthusiastically by geriatric practitioners. Yet a recent systematic review shows that while exercise may result in improvement at the organ-system level (e.g., increased strength), these improvements generally have not resulted in improved functional skills. Those studies targeting persons with chronic arthritis, however, did show improvement in functional skills as well as strength. Thus, the underlying causal disease may influence response to a rehabilitative intervention like exercise. Several examples of various treatments for walking disability further illustrate the importance of establishing the underlying diagnosis.

If a tear of the medial meniscus causes difficulty walking, surgical intervention often is the most effective way to restore mobility. If difficulty walking is caused by mild to moderate osteoarthritis of the knee, an exercise intervention often will reduce pain and increase function. Much of the stability of the knee is because of the surrounding muscular and tendinous support. Resistance and flexibility exercises help to increase muscular support around the knee, normalize knee range of motion, and improve the biomechanical integrity of the arthritic knee joint, so long as the knee is not grossly unstable due to ligamentous injury or deformity. On the other hand, difficulty walking because of osteoarthritis of the hip often is treated most effectively by reducing the weight borne across the joint, for example, by use of a cane in the hand opposite to the affected hip. Strengthening exercises for the hip are relatively ineffective because the hip is a ball-and-socket joint and is unaffected by modest variations in muscle strength. Regular aerobic and resistive exercise may help prevent generalized deconditioning caused by inactivity from the painful hip, and may help prevent bursitis caused by impaired flexibility, but will do little for the pain and dysfunction from degeneration of the hip joint. As these examples illustrate, adequate assessment of the underlying cause(s) of the disability ensures the identification of the most effective treatment, targeted, as indicated, at the disease, impairment, or disability. Therefore, the goals of the evaluation of the rehabilitation patient include identifying the cause of the disability and the comorbidities (e.g., cardiac or pulmonary disease) that may have direct or indirect influence on patient function and rehabilitation effort.

The next section outlines the evaluation process that can be used to help individualize treatment according to the patient's unique disablement process.

Disability Oriented History and Physical Exam

Determining the causes of disability in a given patient begins by characterizing the disability. Fully characterizing the disability gives important clues to the underlying etiology and helps to identify the type of treatment that may be most effective. Identifying the time span over which the functional decline occurred and the patient's symptoms

Table 24-2 Physical Exam Maneuvers, the Organ Systems Tested by Those Maneuvers, and the Activities Potentially Affected by Poor Performance

Physical Task	Muscles and Joints Tested	Activities Affected
Clasp hands behind head	External rotation and abduction of the shoulder, elbow flexion	Dressing upper body, grooming, bathing, and housework
Clasp hands behind the back	Internal rotation of the shoulder	Dressing upper body, bathing, and housework
Place ankle on opposite knee	External rotation of the hip, hip flexion, and knee flexion	Walking, bathing, toileting, dressing lower body, stair climbing, and balance
Flex one knee to the chest while supine (the other leg should be able to stay flat)	Hip and knee extension in the extended leg and hip and knee flexion in the flexed leg	Balance and ambulation
Dorsiflex ankle to 90 degrees	Ankle strength and range of motion	Balance and ambulation
Put a heavy book on a shelf	Arm strength	Housework
Grasp a piece of paper and resist its removal	Pinch strength	Cooking, feeding self, grooming, housework
Rise and stand from sitting 3 to 5 times	Lower extremity strength (especially hip and knee)	Balance, ambulation, bathing, toileting
Rise on tip toes 5 to 10 times	Lower extremity strength (especially ankle strength)	Balance, stair climbing
Gentle nudge (5 to 10 pounds pressure) to the sternum	Ankle, hip, and trunk strength	Balance

SOURCE: Modified with permission from Twersky J, Hoenig H: Rehabilitation, in Salerno J (Ed): *Geriatric Review Syllabus: A Core Curriculum in Geriatric Medicine.* New York, American Geriatrics Society, 1999, p. 84.

when attempting to do the activity often give important clues to the cause of the disability. For example, rapid functional decline would lead to a suspicion of an acute process, for example a fracture or stroke, whereas an insidious process might be more characteristic of a chronic condition, such as arthritis. Asking about the symptoms the patient may experience when attempting to do the impaired activity is particularly useful because symptoms are relatively organ system specific. For example, shortness of breath with walking would point towards a cardiopulmonary problem, whereas unilateral leg pain would be more characteristic of a musculoskeletal disorder. The diagnostic work-up becomes much more manageable if causation is first narrowed down at the level of the organ-system impairment. For example, walking can be adversely affected by impairment in three major organ systems (neurologic, musculoskeletal, cardiopulmonary) as compared to more than 50 different diseases that can affect walking.

In addition to the patient's symptoms, physical exam maneuvers can be used to screen for the most likely causal impairments. Table 24-2 outlines some specific exam maneuvers (e.g., rising to stand without using the hands), the organ system tested by the maneuver (e.g., hip and knee strength), and the type of functional deficit that might be expected with impaired performance (e.g., difficulty climbing stairs, getting in and out of the bathtub). These

physical examination maneuvers can be used to screen for the causal impairments when evaluating a patient whose chief complaint is disability. The screening tests are designed to be rapid, but they are not as accurate as other, more time-consuming, exam maneuvers, so if a screening test is abnormal, then a more detailed examination should be carried out to confirm the causal impairment. For example, rising from a chair primarily tests hip and knee strength, but hip and knee contractures also could affect the ability to stand up from the seated position. If the screening test is abnormal (i.e., the patient is unable to stand up without using the arms to assist), manual muscle testing should be performed to confirm hip and/or knee weakness, and if these are normal, then hip and knee range of motion should be tested. It can be difficult to test strength and range of motion accurately in the typical physician's examining room, and relatively minor but functionally significant abnormalities can be missed. In some cases, referral to physical therapy may be needed to test strength and range of motion adequately. When examining the patient, special attention should paid to suspicious organ system(s) based on the patient's symptom(s) when performing the activity (e.g., unilateral leg pain with ambulation would lead to a focus on the musculoskeletal system for possible arthritic causes, whereas symmetric leg pain with ambulation would lead to concern for vascular claudication or pseudoclaudication from spinal stenosis and a focus on the vascular and neurological systems). Once the underlying impairments are identified, it is often fairly straightforward to identify the causal diseases.

Assessments of cognition, affect, social supports, financial situation, and environment are all components of a disability evaluation. Another element of the evaluation is ascertainment of the methods the patient has been using already to cope with the disability. How much personal assistance and what kinds of adaptive devices (e.g., cane, walker) are being used? Has the patient cut back on specific activities (e.g., no longer going shopping at the supermarket)? With a complete picture of the disablement process in hand, an appropriate treatment plan is developed.

MANAGEMENT

Differing rehabilitation interventions have their greatest impact at different levels of the disablement process. Exercise targets the impaired organ system (weak muscles), assistive devices target the disability (e.g., a bath tub bench for difficulty getting in and out of the bathtub), and removal of environmental barriers targets handicap. Personal contextual factors can be modified through patient and family education (e.g., vocational retraining), and by use of peer support groups. Multimodal interventions are particularly helpful in the geriatric population often is multifactorial in etiology. See Fig. 24-1 for an example of a multimodal rehabilitation treatment plan targeting the different levels of the disablement process.

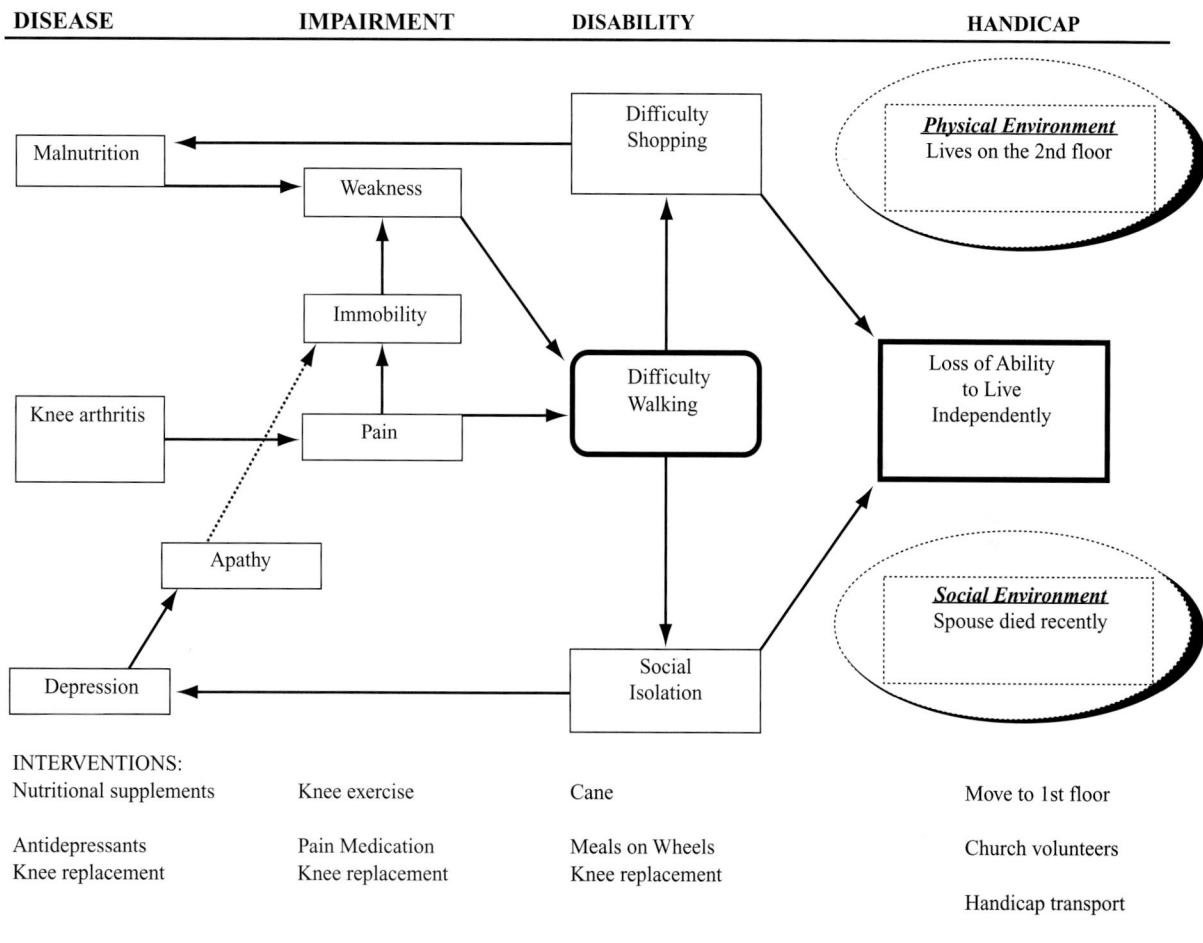

Figure 24-1 An example of a multicausal disability and multimodal treatment plan typical in the geriatric population. The column headings indicate the type of information listed below. For example, column one lists three diseases that are responsible for significant impairment in this person (malnutrition, arthritis, and depression). Treatment interventions are directed at all levels of the disablement process (diseases, impairments, disabilities, and handicaps), and these are detailed on the bottom three rows of the figure. In the disability column, walking is indicated as the key disability from which the patient's other problems stem. If the patient's mobility can be improved, many of his other problems would be ameliorated. In the handicap column, the key issue is the patient's ability to live independently (role functioning). Because of his social and environmental circumstances, the patient's difficulty walking is threatening to force him to move into a nursing home. However, nursing home placement may not be necessary if treatment of the patient's disease, impairment, and disability are undertaken, along with some environmental modifications (e.g., moving to the first floor). Knee replacement surgery would be considered if other interventions (exercise, pain medication, and cane) failed. Reprinted with permission from Hoenig H et al: Geriatric rehabilitation: State of the art. *J Am Geriatr Soc* 45:1371, 1997.

When to Use Rehabilitation to Treat Disability

Individuals who may benefit from rehabilitation referral include people with pre-existing functional limitations, those who have had a recent change in functional ability, and selected patients who are at risk for loss of function. Treatment choices often involve tradeoffs between improvements in quality of life and the potential risks of the intervention. Furthermore, priorities and preferences may differ among individuals. The decision to prescribe a motorized scooter for difficulty walking, for example, might depend upon the degree of limitation in ambulation, the potential activities that would be made available to the patient by use of a scooter, and the patient's willingness to engage in regular exercise to prevent deconditioning. A number of factors affect whether rehabilitation in general, or a specific intervention in particular, is appropriate for a given patient, irrespective of the type of disability or the underlying cause of the disability. Medical stability, cognition, patient motivation, and how long the patient has had the disability may affect the goals of rehabilitation or alter the specific interventions employed to treat the patient. Sometimes a meaningful assessment of rehabilitation potential cannot be determined until acute medical conditions, such as delirium or pneumonia, are resolved or improved. Sometimes the best approach will be concurrent medical and rehabilitative treatment, particularly in older persons where medical conditions (e.g., angina) and medical interventions (e.g., orthostatic hypotension from antihypertensives) can affect both the types of rehabilitative interventions that are used and functional outcomes. Consultation with a rehabilitation expert may be appropriate if the causal pathway is unclear and/or there is a question about the optimal treatment.

Table 24-3 lists a variety of factors that may affect use of rehabilitation and the specific ways they may affect use of rehabilitation. A variety of organizations have developed guidelines that include recommendations about use of rehabilitation for specific diseases. The National Guideline Clearinghouse provides a comprehensive database of guidelines published by the Agency for Healthcare Research and Quality, the American Medical Association, and others at http://www.guideline.gov/index.asp.

COMPONENTS OF REHABILITATION

The Organization of Rehabilitative Care

Settings for Care

There are a variety of settings in which rehabilitation can be provided. There are three levels of inpatient medical rehabilitation (rehabilitation units in an acute care or rehabilitation hospitals, high-level nursing home rehabilitation, and low-level nursing home rehabilitation). Detailed information concerning these levels can be requested through the CARF web site (http://www.carf.org), but generally speaking, rehabilitation is most intense in terms of the diversity of providers available to the patient and the amount of care provided in the acute rehabilitation or rehabilitation hospital, followed by a subacute rehabilitation

unit or a skilled nursing facility with a dedicated rehabilitation unit, followed by a nursing home that does not offer specialized rehabilitation services. Rehabilitation also can be provided in the outpatient or home settings. In addition to differences in the types of providers and the amount of rehabilitative treatment provided, other important care processes may differ by setting. For example, one study found that compliance with federal guidelines for stroke rehabilitation varied substantially across VA hospitals, and that better compliance with the guidelines predicted better 6-month outcomes for stroke patients. A meta-analysis of randomized trials of stroke rehabilitation showed that stroke patients had better outcomes when treated in specialized stroke units compared to standard medical treatment. Similarly, treatment in geriatric evaluation units is associated with improved functional outcomes as compared to usual care for frail, older inpatients. However, costs vary across rehabilitation settings and some third-party payers regulate the settings for which they will provide reimbursement. Important considerations in determining whether care in a rehabilitation hospital or geriatric evaluation unit is appropriate include the patient's prognosis, the duration of disability, the ability of the patient to learn, and how much daily therapy the patient can tolerate.

Rehabilitation Providers

There are many different types of rehabilitation providers. Training of rehabilitation providers may vary according to years of education (e.g., master's degree for a occupational therapist [OT] versus an associate's degree for a certified OT assistant), training in specific therapeutic techniques (e.g., speech and language pathologist versus OT), and licensure or certification (e.g., unlicensed OT aide versus certified OT assistant). There may be considerable overlap in the actual services rendered by the different types of providers. Although this overlap often is beneficial for the patient, helping to reinforce and generalize newly learned skills, it can cause some confusion for medical care providers new to a particular rehabilitation team. Table 24-4 outlines the most common targets of treatment by different types of rehabilitation providers and the modalities commonly used by those providers in their treatment.

Use of a multidisciplinary, comprehensive treatment team is a central tenant of rehabilitation, but evidence for its effectiveness is sparse. Coordinated multidisciplinary rehabilitation is one of the characteristics of successful stroke units. However, use of a single rehabilitation provider type is common, particularly for people with a unicausal disability and/or disabling conditions whose effects are limited to a single organ system, for example osteoarthritis or uncomplicated orthopedic surgery. Until further data are available, use of a multidisciplinary team is suggested for patients whose functional deficits are sufficiently severe to warrant inpatient rehabilitation, for patients with multiple functional deficits or multiple diseases interacting together to cause or exacerbate disability, and for patients in whom cognitive, psychological, social, environmental, and other factors seem to play a role in functional disability handicap.

Table 24-3   Factors that Might Affect Use of Rehabilitation

Factors that Might Alter Rehabilitation Interventions, Prognosis, and/or Goals	Potential Effect
Cognitive impairment	Goals may be more limited. Take advantage of skills the patient already has, use interventions that do not require carry-over.
Disability has been present for many years	Goals may be more limited and directed to compensatory strategies or treatment of deconditioning.
Motivation is limited	Goals need to be well defined and reached in measurable steps.
Patient had prior rehabilitation for the same problem	Rehabilitation may be limited unless new functional decline has occurred.
Terminal illness	Intervention is directed towards reducing caregiver burden and patient discomfort.
Severity of disability	Extremely mild disability may not require intervention. Extremely severe disability may have very limited potential for benefit.
Social and cultural circumstances	Absence of a caregiver, financial limitations, and cultural beliefs may preclude use of certain techniques or technologies.
Malnutrition	Unable to build muscle; rehabilitative interventions may be limited unless nutritional status is improved.
Delirium or altered level of consciousness	Unable to learn or cooperate; rehabilitation may not be appropriate until resolved.
Hemodynamic instability	May make it unsafe to carry out certain types of exercise; rehabilitation may not be appropriate until resolved.
Occult fracture, bony metastasis	Weight-bearing or resistance exercise could worsen fracture or cause fracture; rehabilitation interventions may be limited.
Acute infection (e.g., bladder infection, pneumonia)	May cause confusion and/or fatigue and/or hypotension; rehabilitation may not be appropriate until problem resolved.
Acute skin or joint infection	May cause fatigue, pain, and/or muscle splinting; rehabilitation may not be appropriate until resolved.
Acute inflammatory disease (e.g., certain rheumatologic and neuromuscular conditions)	Resistive exercise may impair recovery; rehabilitative interventions may be limited.
Acute orthopedic conditions	Joint instability may preclude use of certain exercises and functional goals may be limited.
Medications: psychotropics, β-blockers, anticholinergics, antihypertensives, anticoagulants	May alter ability to cooperate during rehabilitation, to carry out certain types of exercise, or reduce the effectiveness of treatment.

SOURCE: Modified with permission from Hoenig H, Odom C: Rehabilitation, in Mezey MD, Bottrell MM et al. (eds): *Encyclopedia of Elder Care: The Comprehensive Resource on Geriatric and Social Care.* New York: Springer, 2000, p. 559.

Process of Care: Rehabilitation Interventions

Rehabilitation providers use a variety of interventions to treat physical impairment and disability. These are divided into four major categories: (1) exercise; (2) adaptive techniques and technology; (3) physical modalities (e.g., heat, cold, ultrasound); and (4) orthotics (braces, splints) and prosthetics (artificial limbs). These are briefly summarized below and in Table 24-5, followed by an in-depth review of exercise and assistive technology.

Exercise is used for multiple purposes including to improve muscle function, to preserve or increase bone density, to reduce joint pain, to increase balance, and to enhance cardiovascular conditioning. Adaptive techniques and

Table 24-4   Types of Rehabilitation Providers and the Primary Aspect of the Disablement Process Targeted by Their Treatment and the Methods They Typically Use in Evaluation and Treatment

Discipline	Primary Target of Treatment	Primary Methods Used in Evaluation and Treatment
Physical therapist	Impairment, disability	• Assessment of joint range of motion and muscle strength • Assessment of gait and mobility • Exercise training to increase range of motion, strength, endurance, balance, coordination, and gait • Treatment with physical modalities (heat, cold, ultrasound, massage, electrical stimulation)
Occupational therapist	Disability, handicap, environmental contextual factors	• Evaluate self-care skills and other activities of daily living • Home safety evaluation • Self-care skills training; recommendations and training in use of assistive technology • Fabrication of splints and treatment of upper extremity deficits
Speech therapist	Impairment, disability	• Assessment of all aspects of communication • Assessment of swallowing disorders • Treatment of communication deficits • Recommendations for alterations of diet and positioning to treat dysphagia
Nurse	Disability, handicap, contextual factors	• Evaluation of self-care skills • Evaluation of family and home care factors • Self-care training • Patient and family education • Liaison with community
Social worker	Handicap, personal and environmental contextual factors	• Evaluation of family and home care factors • Assessment of psychosocial factors • Counseling • Liaison with the community
Dietician	Impairment	• Assess nutritional status • Alter diet to maximize nutrition
Recreation therapist	Disability, handicap	• Assess leisure skills and interests • Involve patients in recreational activities to maintain social roles

SOURCE: Reprinted with permission from Twersky J, Hoenig H: Rehabilitation, in Salerno J (ed): *Geriatric Review Syllabus: A Core Curriculum in Geriatric Medicine.* New York, American Geriatrics Society, 1999, p. 84.

technology are used to modify a task so that it can be performed despite physical impairment. Adaptive techniques and technology enable people with physical limitations to interact with the environment more favorably. Methods range from altering the way an activity is performed to altering the environment itself to using special equipment. Physical modalities use physical methods to apply the treatment, including ultrasound, diathermy, electrical stimulation, whirlpool, massage, and application of heat or cold. Data are limited on the efficacy of many physical modalities, although there is substantial anecdotal support for some modalities (e.g., heat for chronic musculoskeletal pain). Generally speaking, orthotic devices are externally applied devices used to support rather than replace an existing body structure, as would a prosthetic

device like an artificial limb. Examples of orthotics include shoe inserts, splints (e.g., for carpal tunnel syndrome) and straps (e.g., for lateral epicondylitis), and braces to support an unstable joint (e.g., an ankle–foot orthosis after a stroke).

Exercise

Exercise can be classified into five major types: resistance; aerobic (endurance); balance; flexibility; and functionally based. There are various exercise subclasses depending on the way in which the exercise is delivered (e.g., weight-bearing versus in a pool, isotonic versus isokinetic), the way in which the difficulty of the exercise is increased (e.g., progressive resistive exercise), and the frequency of

Table 24-5   Types of Rehabilitation Treatment Interventions, the Target(s) of the Treatment and Methods of Application

Intervention	Subtypes	Target of Treatment	How Applied
Exercise	1. Aerobic 2. Resistive 3. Flexibility 4. Balance 5. Functionally-based	1. Cardiopulmonary and musculoskeletal impairment 2. Musculoskeletal impairment 3. Musculoskeletal impairment 4. Vestibular and musculoskeletal impairment 5. Multiple organ systems	• Number of repetitions and frequency vary • Supervision may be needed • Special equipment may be used • Reimbursement may be limited to "therapeutic," in contrast to "maintenance," exercise • Physician prescription may be needed for reimbursement
Assistive technology	1. Mobility 2. Bathroom 3. Selfcare 4. Augmentative	1. Transfering and Walking 2. Toileting, bathing 3. Eating, dressing, housework 4. Hearing, vision	• Used during specific activities • Permanent or temporary use • Physician prescription may be needed for reimbursement
Physical modalities	1. Heat and cold 2. Whirlpool 3. Massage 4. TENS	1. Musculoskeletal impairment 2. Skin and subcutaneous tissue 3. Musculoskeletal/neurologic impairment 4. Musculoskeletal/neurologic impairment	• Supervision required for some modalities • Special equipment required for some modalities • Physician prescription may be needed for some modalities
Orthotics and prosthetics	1. Orthotics (casts, braces, splints, shoe inserts) 2. Prostheses	1. Musculoskeletal impairment 2. Musculoskeletal (artificial limb) or sensory (prosthetic eye) impairment	• Professional fitting may be needed; some types available over the counter • Worn some or all of the time

TENS, transcutaneous electrical neuromuscular stimulator.

exercise (e.g., 30 minutes per day, two to three times per week). Considerable research has been performed examining the merits of different types of exercises for specific conditions. Exercise is further described in Chap. 72.

Resistance Exercise   Resistance exercise or strength training has received considerable attention because of the age-related decline in muscle strength. Epidemiologic studies show a relationship between muscle strength and physical function in the older population. Leg weakness predicts decline in walking speed 2 years later. Slower gait speed, in turn, predicts the development of frank disability. Older adults are able to gain strength with resistance exercise. Thus, there is a logical chain of evidence in support of resistance exercise for the older population. However, a recent meta-analysis of randomized trials of exercise in the older population showed that improvements in organ system function gained with resistance exercise did not necessarily translate to improvements in self-care function. The greatest functional benefit from resistance exercise was found in the studies that focused on people with arthritic disorders. Thus, resistance exercise may be most useful for specific types of musculoskeletal disorders particularly amenable to benefit from increased muscle strength. Methods for performing resistive exercises are described in Chap. 72.

Aerobic (Endurance) Exercise (See also Chap. 72)
There is a substantial body of research on aerobic exercise in older persons. The majority of studies show that aerobic exercise is effective at improving aerobic capacity in older persons. In a meta-analysis of endurance exercise studies, maximum oxygen uptake in older people was significantly improved with aerobic exercise, although the magnitude of improvement was slightly less than in younger people, being inversely related to age. Systematic reviews of aerobic exercise for specific conditions have shown a variety beneficial effects as well, for example, increased pain-free walking distance in patients with intermittent claudication, reduced symptoms and improved survival in patients with coronary heart disease. However, while longitudinal studies consistently show that long-term physical activity is associated with postponement of disability in older adults, randomized trials of aerobic training do not always show similar benefits. The reason for this discrepancy is unknown. The effect size seen in randomized trials often is lower than that seen in epidemiologic studies. In addition, much of the physiologic benefit of aerobic exercise occurs via prevention or reduction in the severity of diseases whose end-organ effects cause disability (e.g., reducing the occurrence of stroke because of uncontrolled hypertension). Thus, it may take many years for the functional benefits from aerobic exercise to be apparent. Persons who are disabled

already may experience less benefit from aerobic exercise as they suffer already from the conditions that aerobic exercise helps prevent.

Balance Exercise Balance exercises deliberately stress both the musculoskeletal system and the vestibular system. "Habituation exercises" are a type of balance exercise used specifically to treat benign positional vertigo by having the patient repetitively assume the position causing the vertiginous sensation. Various types of exercise interventions, including exercises that focus specifically on balance, are effective in preventing falls among persons at risk for falls, particularly when used as a part of a multifaceted approach to treatment. The relative merits of one type of exercise versus another type in treatment of falls is an active area of investigation. Insufficient evidence is available at this point to make a definitive statement.

Flexibility Exercise Benefits attributed to stretching exercises include reduction in musculoskeletal injury, alleviation of muscles cramps, pain and stiffness, and improved balance. Most studies showing correlations between limited flexibility and certain types of musculoskeletal injury have been performed in adolescents and young adults. There is no reason to believe, however, that mechanism of injury caused by lack of flexibility differs in the older adult. A reduction in the sensation of stretching can occur within as little as 2 weeks of regular stretching exercise. This sensory adaptation may underlie the relief that stretching exercise provides for painful muscles. Limitations in hip and ankle range of motion appear to be common among older persons with a history of falls, but intervention studies for falls have not tested flexibility exercise in isolation of other types of exercise.

Limited data suggest that stretching exercise can improve flexibility in older persons. For example, exercise to enhance axial flexibility in patients with Parkinson disease increased measured axial rotation and functional reach. Interestingly, a comparison in older men of flexibility exercise alone with flexibility plus resistance exercise showed that range of motion increased in the group performing flexibility exercise alone, but did not increase in the group performing both flexibility and resistance exercise. It is likely that the resistance exercise itself acted to decrease flexibility, and this effect was only partially counteracted by the flexibility exercises. Notwithstanding the lack of specific studies of flexibility exercise in the geriatric population, diseases commonly occurring with advanced age such as stroke, arthritis, and parkinsonism can adversely affect flexibility. The general clinical belief is that age does not impair the utility of flexibility exercises.

Functionally Based Exercises Functionally based exercise takes advantage of normal activities to provide the exercise. This type of exercise may be particularly beneficial for certain populations, including some stroke patients and patients with cognitive impairment who may have difficulty comprehending and complying with exercise instructions. A variety of names have been applied to this type of exercise, and both occupational and recreational therapy may use functional activities as treatment.

Functionally based exercises incorporated into daily care routines appear to be effective. For example, a randomized trial in nursing home patients with dementia found use of physical assistance with daily care and disruptive behavior decreased with use of a graded system that sequentially required the patient to independently perform an increasing portion of their activities of daily living. However, while more independent, the study subjects took longer to complete self-care tasks, with a consequent increase in the amount of time nursing staff actually had to spend with the patient. This is an important avenue for further research.

Functional activities also may be used as a part of a novel treatment for stroke patients. In this form of treatment, sometimes termed massed activity, the patient performs a variety of exercises and activities for up to 8 hours per day. As a part of this treatment, the patient may have the unaffected arm constrained so that they are forced to use the affected arm during functional activities. Massed activity in conjunction with constraint therapy appears to have substantial efficacy for selected patients with acute or chronic stroke. This therapeutic approach may be effective for stroke-related language deficits, as well as for motor deficits.

Studies Comparing Differing Types of Exercise Data are sparse on the relative merits of one type of exercise versus another for the same condition, and results of the studies to date in the older population either show little or no difference according to type of exercise. A randomized trial comparing resistance exercise, aerobic exercise, and health education for knee osteoarthritis found both resistance and aerobic exercise more effective than health education alone, but they were not significantly different from one another. In another study, functionally based exercise with demented nursing home patients had essentially equivalent functional outcomes compared with a regimen of aerobic plus resistance exercise. A meta-analysis of falls exercise trials showed that the adjusted fall incidence ratio was 0.90 for general exercise treatment and 0.83 for balance exercise treatment.

Adaptive Techniques and Technology

Adaptive techniques and technology encompass a diverse group of interventions designed to enable people with physical limitations to continue to participate in a broad range of activities. Adaptive techniques are specific to the organ system affected and usually are taught by occupational therapists or experts in that particular type of physical limitation (e.g., blind rehabilitation specialists). Adaptive techniques may be taught as well by nursing personnel and through peer support groups such as those with the Arthritis Foundation.

Information on environmental modifications and assistive technology has been greatly facilitated by national legislative activity that has promoted the availability of substantial informational resources on the Internet for people with disabilities. The general concept of environmental modification to enhance access sometimes is termed universal design to highlight the overarching goal of enabling environmental access for the widest possible breadth of physical abilities. The ADA, enacted in 1990, speaks to enhancing access in public locations, including the workplace, public buildings, and transportation. Technical information on the ADA is available at www.adata.org. In addition, several federally funded centers provide information on universal design for the home, as well as in public buildings (see the Center for Design and Environmental Access at http://design6.ap.buffalo.edu/~idea/index.html and the Center for Universal Design at http://www.design.ncsu.edu/cud/index.html).

Assistive technology is an increasingly common way of coping with disability. The majority of assistive device users are older than 65 years of age, reflecting the greater proportion of the older population coping with disability as compared to younger adults. Approximately one in four older adults report using an assistive device; one-third of whom report using more than one assistive device. However, recent increases in use of most assistive devices far exceed the increase in size of the US population, even accounting for the aging of the US population. From 1980 to 1994, the age-adjusted use of leg braces increased by 52.1 percent, canes by 37.0 percent, walkers by 70.1 percent, and wheelchairs by 82.6 percent, while the size of the US population only increased by 19.1 percent. In part, the increased use of assistive technology is caused by remarkable improvements in the functionality and appearance of many devices, and availability of greater diversity and choice. For example, design options for wheelchairs now include lighter weight and motorized wheelchairs, and diverse seating options to accommodate the physical dimensions and sitting balance of the wheelchair user.

However, despite widespread use, research on assistive technology is relatively sparse, both in general and in the older persons in particular. In addition, federal oversight of assistive technology is limited. New technology is developed and disseminated by widely divergent sources. Thus, information on useful technology is not necessarily readily available to the consumer. Available data show that many disabled people lack potentially helpful devices, many of the devices that are provided are never used or are discarded soon after use, devices commonly are in disrepair or do not fit properly, and problems with device use are reported commonly. While some disuse may be due to improved health and/or personal preferences, the process by which assistive devices are acquired by older adults also appears to contribute to suboptimal use of assistive devices. Numerous problems exist with current methods for provision of assistive technology, including lack of funds to purchase the most suitable equipment, fraud, abuse by providers, and denial of needed equipment by third-party payers.

Increased use of professional assistance to fit and train people in correct use of assistive technology may be helpful. It is fairly common for older adults to obtain mobility aids without professional assistance. Wheelchair users who obtain their wheelchair without professional assistance are more likely to report problems with their wheelchair. For example, patients whose homes are not adapted for their wheelchair are less likely to use the wheelchair. A home visit to ensure mobility aids and bathroom devices fit the home and are used safely may improve device utilization and patient safety. Physical therapists can provide expert input regarding safety and fit of mobility aids, occupational therapists and/or nursing staff can provide expert input in to the safety and use of assistive devices used for various types of self-care. To address some of the problems with obtaining information on assistive technology, the Assistive Technology Act of 1998 helped establish centers on assistive technology in each state and it has facilitated availability of information for people. A state-by-state listing of assistive technology centers can be found at www.resna.org/taproject/index.html/at/statecontacts.html. Other useful web sites on assistive technology include http://www.abledata.com/, which provides a listing of more than 17,000 different assistive devices, http://www.wheelchairnet.org/, which is a web site specifically focused on wheelchairs, and http://www.resna.org/, which is the web site for the Rehabilitation Engineering and Assistive Technology Society of North America.

The geriatric practitioner needs to know how to detect aids that are in disrepair, that fit poorly, or that are used unsafely. Because they are the most commonly used assistive devices, mobility aids are discussed in some detail. Bathroom and self-care aids and computerized technology are also discussed.

Mobility Aids   Table 24-6 lists commonly used mobility aids with their typical purpose, design options, correct fit, contraindications to use, and potential problems. The cane is the most commonly used mobility aid because of its light weight and general versatility. Using a cane requires good hand and arm strength and it provides only minimal support. It is important that the handle of the cane allows for strong grip; an adapted handle (e.g., pistol grip) may increase the support gained from a cane. Most canes are adjustable either by cutting a wooden cane or by a ratchet in the stem of an aluminum cane. Most canes have a rubber tip to provide better grip on the floor that must be replaced when worn. Canes typically are used to reduce the weight borne across an arthritic joint, thereby reducing pain, or to assist with balance when the balance problem is caused by impaired sensation and/or mild leg weakness. A cane can transmit proprioceptive input to the hands and arms, which can be helpful to people with neuropathic problems or visual deficit. A cane should be used in the hand opposite to the affected leg and the handle of the cane should be at the level of the wrist with the arm fully extended. Canes are most useful when the gait problem is unilateral and/or mild.

Crutches should be used cautiously for older patients, as they require excellent arm and shoulder function. When used by someone lacking sufficient arm and shoulder strength, crutches can result in shoulder and neuropathic injuries. Moreover, correct crutch use requires learning a novel gait pattern, which can be challenging for someone who is acutely ill, delirious, or demented.

Table 24-6   Indications for Use of Commonly Prescribed Mobility Aids

Cane
- Uses: supports minimal (15–20%) of body weight
- Options: single point, quad-, and hemi-cane
- Fitting/use: to ulnar styloid with arm extended, use on side opposite affected limb
- Contraindications: arm weakness, moderate-severe gait or balance deficit
- Potential problems: inadequate support

Walker
- Uses: supports up to 30% of body weight; easy to learn how to use
- Options: 4 post; 2 wheel/2 post; 3 wheel; 4 wheel; 4 wheel with seat and hand brakes (Rollator); 4 wheel with safety bars and sling seat (Merry Walker); forearm supports
- Fitting/use: to ulnar styloid with arm extended, do not pull on walker to help with rising or seating
- Contraindications: environmental barriers (steps), severe arm weakness, severe gait deficit
- Potential problems: slows gait, hard to maneuver

Crutches
- Uses: supports full body weight
- Options: underarm, forearm
- Fitting: 2 inches under shoulder; do not lean armpit on crutch
- Contraindications: arm weakness, shoulder arthritis, cognitive impairment
- Potential problems: neuropathy, shoulder pain, difficult to learn to use properly

Wheelchair
- Uses: supports full body weight
- Options: manual or motorized; various accessories (cushions, armrests, legrests, headrests); lower to ground or one-sided drive (hemi-chair); racing wheelchair; handcycle
- Fitting: 1–1.5 inches around hips and under knees; footplates clear floor by 1–2 inches; armrest at elbow height; removable footplates and armrests are safer and more convenient
- Contraindications: unable to sit or able to walk to desired destinations safely
- Potential problems: deconditioning, contractures, pressure sores

SOURCE: Modified with permission from Hoenig H et al: Rapid assessment of rehabilitation options for functional disability. *Cleve Clin J Med* 67(5):361, 2000.

Walkers are commonly used. Walkers generally are used to treat bilateral gait problems or when greater support is needed than can be provided with a cane. Walkers may be used to decrease pain from spinal stenosis or osteoporosis as leaning forward on a walker can open up the spinal canal or offload some of the pressure on the painful vertebrae. The most commonly used type of walker is a two-wheel or front-wheel walker. A four-point, or pick-up, walker requires more arm strength to use than the front-wheel walker, it is more complicated to operate correctly, it offers little additional stability over a front-wheel walker, and it requires twice as much energy to use as a two-wheel walker. There are several types of four-wheel or rolling walkers, with various indications for use. A rolling walker can be helpful for patients with parkinsonism as it facilitates initiation of walking. In addition, patients with parkinsonism tend to fall backwards when they fall, a tendency that is counteracted by the tendency of the rolling walker to roll forward. A Rollator is a 4-wheel walker with brakes located on the handles (like a bicycle), a platform seat in the middle, and an optional basket on the front (for examples, see http://www.footsmart.com or http://www.nursingshop.com/). The Rollator is somewhat less stable than a standard two-wheel walker, requires good hand coordination to safely use the brakes, and is more expensive than a standard two- or four-wheel walker. However, the Rollator may be an excellent choice for patients whose primary gait deficit is poor endurance because of pain or shortness of breath, as such patients often have the balance and hand coordination to manipulate this type of walker and the seat allows for rest breaks whenever the patient might need it. Finally, a Merry Walker is a type of four-wheel walker that is sometimes used for patients with more severe balance and coordination deficits and who are at significant fall risk with a standard walker or even with a wheelchair. It has four wheels, a sling seat, and railing all around the patient so that they are protected from falling yet are able to propel themselves safely (for example see http://www.merrywalker.com). The Merry Walker is bulkier than other walkers and typically is most appropriate for a setting with wide doorways. Three-wheel walkers may offer greater maneuverability than four-wheel walkers, but they are used infrequently because they do not offer the seating advantages possible with a four-wheel walker and lack the stability of a two-wheel walker.

Wheelchairs usually are used for patients in whom bilateral leg weakness and/or motor incoordination are of sufficient severity that safe use of a walker is not possible, or for whom weightbearing is completely prohibited. The wheelchair used most commonly is a manual wheelchair with a sling seat that folds and has removable footrests and armrests. Wheelchairs should be inspected visually for wear and tear. When the sling seat wears, the bowing in the seat may reduce the ability to shift weight while seated and therefore increase risk of pressure sores as well as increasing discomfort. A seat cushion generally should be used with the wheelchair. Special air and gel cushions are available to reduce risk of pressure sores in patients with limited ability to shift their weight while seated. Specialized seating can be fabricated for patients with postural problems or deformity and can substantially improved comfort, independence, and safety with seated activities such as eating. While cost-savings may be achieved by use of nonremovable arm and foot rests, these increase the difficulty of transferring in and out of the chair. Fixed foot rests are a fall hazard. Elevating leg rests and reclining back rests are additional options that may help some patients. Lighter weight wheelchairs, while more expensive than standard manual wheelchairs, appear to have equal or better durability and may be easier to propel. Expert assessment is recommended for patients with a history of pressure sores, who are at risk of pressure sores (e.g., because of incontinence and inability to shift weight), who have postural problems, for whom a motorized mobility aid is being considered, or who will spend most of the day in the wheelchair.

One recent development is a "power-assisted" manual wheelchair that uses a small battery to assist with manual propulsion. It offers some of the advantages of a power wheelchair while maintaining the dimensions of a manual wheelchair. A review of this device can be found at http://www.wheelchairnet.org. However, like a power wheelchair, the power-assisted manual wheelchair is most suitable for use out of doors rather than in the small confines of the home because of slightly greater difficulty with maneuvering when compared to a standard manual wheelchair. Motorized wheelchairs and scooters are increasingly common. Motorized wheelchairs and scooters are most helpful for patients whose primary problem is with community mobility rather than in-home mobility. Even the most compact motorized wheelchair requires greater width and turning radius than a manual wheelchair, making them problematic for use in the home. The clinician and patient must trade-off the potential increased participation in activities that a motorized scooter or wheelchair might allow versus the potential for deconditioning that might occur with overdependence on such technology. One study showed that wheelchair users appear to choose the locations in which they use their wheelchairs based on needs, abilities, and environmental constraints.

Bathroom and Self-Care Aids Bathroom aids typically include raised seats for the tub, shower, and toilet, as well as grab bars and hand-held showers. It requires more effort to rise from a lower-level seat than from a higher-level seat, therefore a raised toilet seat or tub bench may be helpful to someone with weak legs or painful arthritic joints. Freestanding commodes are available with fairly high seats and the free-standing commodes can be placed directly over the toilet or used in a separate room.

Bars may allow patients to rise more safely by allowing the patient to compensate for weak legs with strength in their arms. Some raised toilet seats have bars attached to the seat itself as do most free-standing commodes. In addition, bars are available that attach easily to the back of the toilet. ADA regulations provide guidelines for grab bars. Newer grab bar technologies such as grab bars that can swing away, may be preferred by older adults. Bars can be attached to the side of the tub or to the wall. Special attachment techniques are available to attach bars to prefabricated tubs or showers. There are differences in the stability and sturdiness of various tub and shower chairs. It is important to ensure that the equipment provided will fit in the patient's bathroom and will enhance safety. A visit by a home health nurse and a physical and/or occupational therapist can help ensure bathroom equipment is optimal. Many people find a hand-held shower is helpful when using a tub bench or shower, and designs are available that can be attached to most faucets and showerheads. Helpful information on a variety of bathroom aids and their installation, and bathroom design, can be found at the web sites for the Center for Design and Environmental Access (http://design6.ap.buffalo.edu/~idea/index.html) and the Center for Universal Design (http://www.design.ncsu.edu/cud/index.html).

Higher seating may be helpful in other areas of the house. Lift chairs are chairs with an elevating seat. Similar to a standard recliner type chair, lift chairs have fairly soft seats that may increase the risk of a pressure sore for people with limited ability to shift their weight. In addition, while the seat rises slowly, adequate standing balance must be present or stand-by assistance available to ensure safe use. Hydraulic lifts can be helpful for patients who have extremely limited mobility. These lifts can be easily used even by quite frail caregivers.

Special utensils and dinnerware may be helpful for people with hand or arm weakness, deformity, or poor coordination. An occupational therapist can recommend the most useful type of eating equipment. For example, utensil handles can be enlarged for poor hand grip or weighted for tremor or lack of coordination. Nonskid mats (e.g., Dycem) may help people with poor coordination or suboptimal functional use of one upper extremity by preventing the plate from slipping during a meal. People with dysphagia may benefit from special feeding techniques (e.g., chin tucking, using a double swallow) and/or dietary modifications. Recommendations for special feeding techniques for dysphagia should be developed in conjunction with radiographic evaluation of the swallow and by a specialist in treatment of dysphagia. Experts who may be helpful in developing an individualized treatment plan for someone with dysphagia include a speech and language pathologist, nutritionist, and/or occupational therapist (see Chap. 93).

Electronic Devices, Including Environmental Control Units and Augmentative Communication Aids Electronic devices are available that allow for control of a switch by very limited movement, including eyeblinks, tongue movements, or finger movements. The switch, in turn, controls a variety of other devices, thus allowing a disabled person to perform tasks, such as turning on and off appliances or lights, and opening and closing doors. Software allows use of this technology with a speech synthesizer and a computer, enabling people with severe paralysis and aphasia to communicate. Computerization is allowing for greater functionality from devices as diverse as prosthetic limbs and hearing aids. The Internet alone can facilitate communication for people who are otherwise socially isolated. By using large screens, adapted keyboards, and/or specialized software, Internet access can be made available to the blind and deaf. State assistive technology centers (for a state-by-state listing see www.resna.org/taproject/index.html/at/statecontacts.html), the local telephone company, and other vendors can provide guidance in selection of devices. The Assistive Technology Provider Certification offered by Rehabilitation Engineering and Assistive Technology Society of North America (RESNA) includes training in such devices and it may be helpful to consult a certified assistive technology provider when considering expensive electronic technology. RESNA can be contacted at http://www.resna.org/.

SPECIFIC CONDITIONS TREATED WITH REHABILITATION

Arthritic and Related Musculoskeletal Conditions

At first glance, it makes sense to consider painful musculoskeletal conditions as a general group. However, there may be important differences in response to rehabilitation depending on the underlying pathophysiology of the musculoskeletal disorder. While exercise may be provided as a form of "prehabilitation" for someone with an acute musculoskeletal injury, the exercise usually consists of cautious range of motion and isometric exercise; weight-bearing and most resistance exercise would be contraindicated. On the other hand, there is good evidence for benefit from resistive exercise for osteoarthritis of the knee.

A recent systematic review of exercise for osteoarthritis jointly summarized studies of exercise for the hip and the knee, and found no significant benefit. From an anatomic point of view, exercise may be less effective for a deep ball-and-socket joint like the hip, than for a joint like the knee or shoulder where the muscles and tendons provide considerable support to the joint. Thus, a meta-analysis that jointly summarizes studies of exercise for hip arthritis with studies of exercise for knee arthritis might show no overall effect from exercise because the negative hip studies outweigh the positive knee studies rather than because exercise truly is ineffective for both hip and knee arthritis.

The first step in managing a painful joint should be to rule out acute pathology (e.g., swelling, ecchymosis), inflammatory disease (e.g., heat, erythema), and systemic illness (e.g., fever, weight loss) by pursuing appropriate radiologic and laboratory studies prior to referral to physical therapy (see Chap. 81). If acute pathology and systemic disease have been ruled out, exercise, assistive technology,

and orthotics reduce disability caused by diverse musculoskeletal disorders. The specific type of exercise and the most useful device or orthotic depends on the specific joints affected and the underlying pathology. The following provides a brief review of rehabilitative treatment of rotator cuff tendonitis, osteoarthritis of the hip and knee, and plantar fasciitis. Excellent texts are available that cover rehabilitation of musculoskeletal conditions in detail.

Symptomatic shoulder pathology is common in older persons, the most common diagnosis being rotator cuff tendonitis. Symptoms often persist over time despite treatment. Ultrasound can shorten the course of calcific rotator cuff tendonitis, although the time and financial costs of ultrasound merit trial of other approaches first. Corticosteroid injections may have a more rapid effect than physical therapy for relief of symptoms; differences between the two approaches often are negligible in 6 months or a year. Resistance exercise to strengthen the shoulder girdle combined with flexibility exercise may help prevent recurrent problems and relieve symptoms. While surgery may prevent progression of chronic rotator cuff tendonitis to a rotator cuff tear, there may be important differences in response to surgery between older and younger patients because of age-related changes in collagen. Shoulder surgery should be approached cautiously in the older patient, and only after failure of more conservative treatment.

Hip pain may be caused by osteoarthritis of the hip or inflammation of one of the bursa around the hip (most commonly the subtrochanteric bursa), or it may radiate from the low back. It is important to differentiate the etiology, as bursitis may respond to local corticosteroid injections, range-of-motion exercise, and/or eliminating precipitating factors. Patients with hip pain radiating from the back should be evaluated for neurologic abnormalities, and if present, referred to neurosurgery or orthopedic surgery. If indicated, acute medical causes of low back pain should be ruled out (e.g., metastatic disease), then a trial of conservative treatment is indicated and may include nonsteroidal medication, home-based exercise, physical therapy, or chiropractic treatment (see Chap. 79). The American College of Rheumatology offers guidelines for treatment of hip osteoarthritis. Improvement in gait may be seen by off-loading weight from the hip through use of a cane in the opposite hand. There are few data to support substantial benefit from exercise interventions for hip arthritis. Nonetheless, it makes good sense to carry out exercise to prevent deconditioning and maintain hip flexibility and strength. There is considerable anecdotal support for water-based exercises for arthritis patients. For patients with severe hip arthritis, hip replacement should be considered. (See Chap. 74 for further discussion of arthritis of the hip.)

In contrast to hip arthritis, mild to moderate knee arthritis often responds well to exercise. Exercise for knee arthritis usually includes resistance exercise to strengthen the quadriceps and flexibility exercise to the hamstrings, quadriceps, and iliotibial band. Simply walking daily can be helpful. However, in the presence of frank instability or severe deformity, surgery may be necessary. Bracing can be helpful with patellofemoral arthritis, but is less helpful with valgus or varus deformity. Like hip arthritis, use of a cane to off-load weight from a painful joint can provide symptomatic relief. (See Chap. 74 for further discussion of arthritis of the knee.)

Heel pain is a common type of foot pain. Painful heel conditions often improve with orthotics. Randomized trials comparing prefabricated to custom orthotics for plantar fasciitis showed equivalent or better results for prefabricated orthotics in terms of pain and the proportion of patients improving with the intervention. Long-term compliance, however, may be better with the custom orthotics. Stretching often is used in combination with orthotics. Steroid injections may provide short-term relief.

Stroke

Poststroke rehabilitation can be provided in a variety of locations, including a rehabilitation hospital, skilled nursing facility, in the patient's own home, or in outpatient facilities. There is good evidence that poststroke care in a designated stroke unit results in improved functional outcomes compared with rehabilitation in other settings. There is less benefit to be gained, however, among patients who have little functional disability or who are unable to participate fully in rehabilitation activities. The choice of rehabilitation setting should be guided by the patient's medical stability, physical endurance, amount of poststroke functional disability, and support available in the home. Most of neurologic recovery occurs in the first 3 to 6 months. Some improvement, however, can be seen for up to 2 years following the injury. There is increasing evidence that neural plasticity is important in the poststroke patient and can be taken advantage of to further improve functional outcomes. For example, massed activity involving intensive exercise for up to 8 hours per day appears to improve motor function in carefully selected patients, even many months after the original stroke. Current investigations are examining combinations of exercise plus pharmacologic treatment (e.g., sympathomimetics) to further enhance neural plasticity.

Motor loss can be disabling, but associated problems of sensory or perceptual loss, balance impairment, and neglect can be equally disabling, and may be less amenable to rehabilitation interventions. Unilateral neglect is a common problem with right hemispheric strokes. It is thought to negatively impact functional recovery and rehabilitation. While visual scanning and "tracking" are current methods of treatment, there are a number of interesting newer approaches to rehabilitation of neglect including L-dopa, eye patching, visual imagery, and videotape feedback. Comorbid conditions can affect outcomes after a stroke. Treatment of these comorbidities has an important role in stroke rehabilitation. For example, depression is associated with poor stroke outcomes. Treatment of depression may improve cognitive and motor function poststroke. Stroke patients with dysphagia are at risk for malnutrition, and early nutritional support can reduce poststroke mortality.

Cardiopulmonary and Peripheral Vascular Disease

Cardiac rehabilitation is used less frequently in older patients as compared to younger patients. While there are important age-related changes in cardiac function, and while future research may show that cardiac rehabilitation should be modified in specific ways for elderly patients, there are no known age-specific differences in rehabilitation strategies for older cardiac patients from those used for younger cardiac patients. Cardiac rehabilitation is quite safe and reduces symptoms and/or improves survival in diverse cardiac conditions, including ischemic heart disease, congestive heart failure, and postmyocardial infarction. Most cardiac rehabilitation programs use a combination of graded aerobic exercise, educational, and nutritional interventions. More strenuous exercise interventions may be needed for patients with minimal impairment to experience benefit. The educational and psychosocial components of cardiac rehabilitation help reduce disability by providing accurate information on risks related to various activities such as sexual activity.

Many people with cardiovascular disease also have pulmonary disease and/or peripheral vascular disease. Rehabilitation is helpful for both pulmonary conditions and cardiac conditions. Aerobic exercise (usually walking to exercise large muscles), inspiratory muscle resistance training, and education are the mainstays of pulmonary rehabilitation. A recent randomized trial showed that a comprehensive rehabilitation program significantly improved exercise tolerance and respiratory symptoms over patient education alone. Patients with claudication can benefit by daily walking for about 30 minutes, walking to the onset of pain and then resting briefly, and walking again to the onset of pain. A meta-analysis showing that walking exercise increased the distance walked prior to onset of pain by 179 percent, which compares quite favorably to pharmacologic treatment. Adequate treatment and rehabilitation of cardiopulmonary disease is important both because of the direct effects of cardiopulmonary impairment function limitations and because of the data suggesting that cardiac disease in combination with other conditions have multiplicative effects on disability.

Hip Fracture Rehabilitation

Many people have substantial decline in physical function after hip fracture. While randomized controlled trial data are lacking, several cohort studies have shown that high-intensity postoperative physical therapy (more than five visits per week) may prevent postoperative complications and promote better functional outcomes. A combination of early mobilization, comprehensive rehabilitation, and postdischarge continuity of care showed a 17 percent reduction in costs of care. Early mobilization may be facilitated by early surgical repair. Early surgery can be safely carried out in most hip fracture patients, although further study is needed to clarify which patients might benefit from delay and further medical work-up. Early mobilization may be difficult in patients with cognitive impairment in whom simplifying the rehabilitative approach can be helpful. For example, directions for partial weight bearing (e.g., "touch down weight bearing") can be difficult to comprehend. So long as there is adequate fracture stabilization, most hip fracture patients do well with "weight bearing as tolerated," and using a walker as needed. Discharge from the acute hospital usually occurs when patients are medically stable and able to transfer to a chair. Rehabilitation may be continued in a rehabilitation hospital, nursing home, or at home. The optimal duration and location of high intensity physical therapy after acute hip fracture needs further study. (See Chap. 76 for discussion of hip fracture).

Amputation

Amputation in older persons often occurs in the setting of severe peripheral vascular disease rather than traumatic injury. This means the rehabilitation of the older amputee often is more complicated than for the younger patient. Vascular disease is systemic and the adult who undergoes a lower extremity amputation has a 28 to 66 percent chance of requiring another amputation within 2 to 5 years. Successful prosthetic rehabilitation for the second amputation is dependent upon the person having completed successful prosthetic rehabilitation for the initial amputation. Because severe peripheral vascular disease often occurs in the patients with long-standing diabetes mellitus, and/or hypertension, and/or tobacco abuse, the effects of these comorbid diseases can affect the surgical care, postoperative medical care, and rehabilitation.

Premorbid functional limitations and comorbid conditions must be considered both preoperatively and postoperatively in the older adult, especially cardiac and pulmonary disease. Because the work of walking is substantially higher after an amputation, cardiac function should be optimized both during and after surgery, and rehabilitation may need to proceed more slowly in the face of significant cardiopulmonary disease. Efficiency of gait, which places less stress on the cardiopulmonary reserve, is dependent upon limb length (e.g., transtibial is more efficient than transfemoral). Therefore, every effort should be made to preserve limb length. However, the functional benefits of greater limb length must be weighed against the surgical risks to the patient if repeat surgery becomes necessary because of a poorly healing wound. Wound healing is more likely to preclude immediate postoperative weight bearing and to delay final fitting of the prosthesis in older patients as compared to treatment of younger amputees, so aggressive wound care is of great importance in the older amputee. In addition to wound healing, avoidance of knee or hip contracture and maintenance of joint mobility is essential for successful prosthetic rehabilitation. Patients at particular risk for joint contractures include those who are unable to tolerate immediate postoperative weight bearing or who are at bedrest or predominantly in a wheelchair. Phantom limb pain is experienced by 60 to 80 percent of adults undergoing a lower extremity amputation; approximately 10 percent of these individuals report severe pain that is disabling. There is conflicting evidence as to whether adequate pain control preoperatively and perioperatively reduces the incidence of severe phantom pain. However, it makes inherent sense that pain should be treated aggressively.

Prosthetic limbs continue to improve in design, comfort, and functionality; however, costs of the newer prosthetic limbs can be considerable and may not be covered by third party payers. Geriatric patients with lower extremity amputations benefit from light-weight, comfortable prostheses than are easy to don and doff. Newer technology with multiaxis feet and pneumatic/hydraulic knees may be appropriate for some individuals, but the usual lightweight prosthesis with hinge knee and SACH (solid ankle, cushion heel) foot suffices for many.

Parkinsonism

While it is unclear whether rehabilitative techniques have direct effects on the pathologic processes underlying parkinsonism, rehabilitation provides significant functional benefits. A number of studies show improvement in physical function with exercise, including resistance and flexibility exercise, and water-based exercise. The disability associated with Parkinson disease results from the direct effects of the disease, such as rigidity and bradykinesia, and from the subsequent indirect effects such as kyphosis, stiffness, knee contractures, or general deconditioning. Pharmacologic interventions may help ameliorate the direct effects of the disease, but rehabilitative interventions, such as exercise or assistive technology, are necessary to ameliorate the indirect effects. Investigators currently are examining whether novel exercise interventions such as partial body weight-supported treadmill training may result in greater improvement in physical function, and whether that improvement persists, compared to standard physical therapy exercise.

One contributing factor to the physical disability associated with Parkinson disease is a lack of internal cue production. Patients thus may rely on environmental or external cues for motor function. Therefore, visual (mirrors, tracking lines), auditory, tactile, or other sensory cues appear to be of benefit at the time an activity is undertaken. Sustained benefit from these cues may be limited.

A variety of assistive technologies may facilitate coping with the disabling effects of the bradykinesia and motor incoordination. For example, rolling walkers and motorized scooters may provide significant assistance in maintaining functional mobility.

Deconditioning and Sarcopenia

Decreases in activity levels, particularly bed rest, are associated with a variety of physiologic changes including loss of strength, loss of flexibility, and hemodynamic abnormalities (e.g., orthostatic hypotension). Prevention and treatment of deconditioning typically includes early mobilization during hospitalization as well as participation in exercise both during hospitalization and after discharge. There is good evidence for the benefit of early mobilization out of bed to chair. Evidence for efficacy of exercise among acutely ill older patients is just beginning to appear.

Sarcopenia refers to the decline in muscle strength and wasting sometimes seen with aging. Deconditioning is thought to play a role in sarcopenia. There is evidence, however, that sarcopenia is a complex condition resulting from the interaction of multiple factors both hormonal and environmental, leading to loss of muscle fibers. Research on deconditioning and sarcopenia is highly pertinent to geriatric rehabilitation. The major focus of current research is exercise of various types alone and in combination with other treatments such as hormonal and nutritional support. As reviewed in the section on exercise earlier in this chapter, there is good reason to believe that exercise can reverse impairment in muscle strength and function. The translation of gains in strength to improved function in frail elderly persons, however, remains elusive. As the complex physiologic abnormalities underlying sarcopenia become better understood, the efficacy of rehabilitation for this condition likely will be enhanced.

Falls

Rehabilitation interventions, along with other medical and nonmedical interventions, are commonly used to prevent falls. Rehabilitation interventions typically used in fall prevention programs are various types of exercise and environmental modification. While there is some evidence that reduction of fall hazards in the home can reduce fall rates, the effect of this intervention has been inconsistent across studies. Nonetheless, there is little to be lost by improving lighting and removing obvious fall hazards. A recent Cochrane Systematic Review of fall prevention trials and one preplanned meta-analysis concluded that exercise alone did not appear effective for protection against falls, but that exercise did appear effective if it was used as one of multiple interventions specifically targeting identified risk factors (see Chap. 118 for discussion of falls).

Pain

Pain is extremely common in the geriatric population given the prevalence of musculoskeletal problems and malignancies. In addition to pain medications and psychological interventions, rehabilitation specialists have much to offer the patient in pain. Many physical modalities are effective, including massage, pressure, vibration, heat, cold, exercise, and mobilization. For bed-bound patients, correct positioning and range-of-motion exercises may alleviate pain or discomfort. Positioning may involve the use of devices such as splints, foam blocks, or slings to achieve correct positioning and comfort. Rehabilitation efforts can help provide comfort for the patient with chronic pain, which can be disabling, or for the patient who is terminally ill.

CONCLUSION

One of the great difficulties in a review of geriatric rehabilitation is that older patients commonly have multiple comorbid conditions. Unfortunately, most rehabilitation research has focused on rehabilitation of a single condition (e.g., stroke), largely ignoring the role of comorbid conditions and without specifying the interventions being used. At the same time, most geriatric research has focused on functional outcomes from a specific rehabilitation intervention (e.g., resistive exercise) or from multifocal interventions (e.g., stay in a geriatric rehabilitation unit with treatment by a multidisciplinary team), but without discriminating the underlying conditions at all. While it is likely that the optimal outcomes would be obtained if rehabilitation treatment interventions were selected in light of the patient's comorbid conditions, definitive proof is lacking. At this point, the most prudent approach is to define the underlying disablement process as thoroughly as possible, and then target specific treatments to identified conditions.

REFERENCES

Asplund K et al: How do stroke units improve patient outcomes—A collaborative systematic review of the randomized trails. *Stroke* 28:2139, 1997.

Cohen HJ et al: Effect of geriatric evaluation and management units and clinics on survival, health related quality of life, and functional status: A VA cooperative trial. *N Engl J Med* (under review).

deGoede CJ et al: The effects of physical therapy in Parkinson's disease: A research synthesis. *Arch Phys Med Rehabil* 82(4):509, 2001.

Duncan PW et al: Adherence to post-stroke rehabilitation guidelines improves functional recovery. *Stroke* (in press).

Ettinger WH et al: A randomized trial comparing aerobic exercise and resistance exercise with a health education program in older adults with knee osteoarthritis—The Fitness Arthritis and Seniors Trial (FAST). *JAMA* 277(1):25, 1997.

Gillespie LD et al: Interventions for preventing falls in the elderly (Cochrane Review). The Cochrane Library, issue 1, 2002. Oxford: Update Software.

Grabois M et al (eds): *Physical Medicine and Rehabilitation—The Complete Approach.* Malden, MA, Blackwell Science, 2000.

Green JS, Crouse SF: The effects of endurance training on functional capacity in the elderly: A meta-analysis. *Med Sci Sports Exer* 27(6):920, 1995.

Hochberg MC et al: Guidelines for the medical management of osteoarthritis: Part I. Osteoarthritis of the hip. *Arthritis Rheum* 38:1535, 1995.

Hoenig H et al: Geriatric rehabilitation: State of the art. *J Am Geriatr Soc* 45:1371, 1997.

Hoenig H et al: Wheelchair users are not necessarily wheelchair bound. *J Am Geriatr Soc* (in press).

Jagger C et al: Patterns of onset of disability in activities of daily living with age. *J Am Geriatr Soc* 49:404, 2001.

Jolliffee JA et al: Exercise-based rehabilitation for coronary heart disease. *Cochrane Database Syst Rev* Issue 2, 2001.

Keysor JJ, Jette AM: Have we oversold the benefit of late life exercise? *J Gerontol A Biol Sci Med Sci* 56A(7):M412, 2001.

Krivickas LS: Training flexibility, in Dawson DM, Slovik DM (eds): *Exercise in Rehabilitation Medicine. Human Kinetics.* Champaign, IL, 1999.

Martin JE et al: Mechanical treatment of plantar fasciitis. A prospective study. *J Am Podiatr Med Assoc* 91(2):55, 2001.

Miltner WH et al: Effects of constraint-induced movement therapy on patients with chronic motor deficits after stroke: A replication. *Stroke* 30:586, 1999.

Morris JN et al: Nursing rehabilitation and exercise strategies in the nursing home. *J Gerontol A Biol Sci Med Sci* 54A:M494, 1999.

Morrison RS et al: The medical consultant's role in caring for patients with hip fracture. *Ann Intern Med* 128:1010, 1998.

Oakley A et al: Preventing falls and subsequent injury in older people. *Qual Health Care* 5(4):243, 1996.

Rogers JC et al: Improving morning care routines of nursing home residents with dementia. *J Am Geriatr Soc* 49:1049, 1999.

Russell JN et al: Trends and differential use of assistive technology devices: United States, 1994. *Adv Data* 292:1, 1997.

Siebens H et al: A randomized controlled trial of exercise to improve outcomes of acute hospitalization in older adults. *J Am Geriatr Soc* 48:1545, 2000.

van der Windt DA et al: Ultrasound therapy for musculoskeletal disorders: A systematic review. *Pain* 81:257, 1999.

van Baar ME et al: Effectiveness of exercise therapy in patients with osteoarthritis of the hip or knee. A systematic review of randomized clinical trials. *Arthritis Rheum* 42:1361, 1999.

C H A P T E R   2   5

Pain Management

BRUCE A. FERRELL   •   JOSHUA CHODOSH

DEFINITION

Pain is defined as an unpleasant sensory and emotional experience. It is derived from complex physiologic processes that include elements of neural sensation and nerve transmission integrated with central nervous system processing of memory, expectations, and emotions. Pain management is particularly challenged by the lack of objective biological markers. There are no measurements in blood, electroencephalographic, or other imaging devices that accurately reflect the intensity or character of pain experiences. The most accurate and reliable evidence for the existence and intensity of pain is the patient's description. Pain complaints are quite variable in description, character, and intensity. To better understand, predict, and treat pain, a variety of classification schemes have been used. Pain management is predicated in part upon its categorization as acute or chronic.

Acute Pain

Acute pain is often defined by its distinct onset, obvious cause, and short duration. Trauma, burns, infarction, and inflammation are examples of pathologic processes that can result in acute pain. Acute pain is often associated with autonomic nervous system signs including tachycardia, diaphoresis, or mild hypertension. The presence of acute pain often indicates an acute injury or acute disease; the intensity of acute pain often indicates the severity of injury or disease. Thus acute pain should trigger an urgent search for an underlying cause that might be life threatening or require immediate intervention.

Chronic Pain

The International Association for the Study of Pain has defined chronic pain as pain that lasts more than 3 months. Moreover, painful symptoms persisting beyond an expected time frame for healing are usually classified as chronic. Intensity of chronic pain is often out of proportion to the observed pathology and often associated with prolonged functional impairment, both physical and psychological. Autonomic signs are often absent due to desensitization from chronic stimuli. Underlying causes of chronic pain are often associated with chronic disease and are less curable.

Chronic pain is often more difficult to manage because the underlying cause is less remedial and many treatment strategies are either short-lived, difficult to maintain, or associated with long-term side effects. Chronic pain usually requires a multidimensional approach to treatment including use of both analgesic drug and nondrug strategies, with attention to sensory, emotional, and behavioral components of the pain experience.

In reality, the definition of chronic pain is not as simple as it seems, and it has led to considerable differences in research design and limited generalizability of many published studies. Some researchers have used arbitrary time frames to define chronic pain, such as pain that persists longer than 6 months. Although chronic pain has been defined as pain that persists beyond an expected time frame for healing, for many conditions, a time-framed definition is not very meaningful because healing may never be expected to occur. In other cases, chronic pain has been defined as persistent pain that is not amenable to "routine" pain control methods. In the final analysis, there are many differences in what may be regarded as chronic pain. Thus, the definition of chronic pain remains flexible and is often related to a specific diagnosis and case. In addition, a variety of successful new approaches to pain management have blurred the distinction between acute and chronic pain with respect to treatment decisions. Strategies such as fast acting oral medications and infusion therapy have become widespread in chronic as well as acute pain situations.

Unfortunately for many elderly persons, the term *chronic pain* has become a label associated with negative images and stereotypes often associated with long-standing psychiatric problems, futility in treatment, malingering, or drug-seeking behavior. For this reason, the term *persistent pain* is favored in the medical literature and may foster a more positive attitude by patients and clinicians for more active and vigilant intervention and management of these recalcitrant problems.

CLASSIFICATION BASED ON PATHOPHYSIOLOGY

The classification of pain by pathophysiologic mechanisms may help clinicians choose and target pain-management strategies more effectively. Treatments, when directed at specific pathophysiologic pain mechanisms, may be more effective. The American Geriatrics Society Panel on Persistent Pain identified four basic pathophysiologic pain mechanisms that have important implications for choosing pain management strategies (Table 25-1). Pain that results largely from stimulation of pain receptors is called nociceptive pain. Nociceptive pain may arise from tissue injury, inflammation, or mechanical deformation. Nociceptive pain may be visceral (related to the internal organs or viscera) or somatic (related to body walls and musculoskeletal system). Examples include trauma, burns, infection, mass lesions leading to tissue distortion, arthritis, myofascial pain syndromes, and ischemic disorders. Nociceptive mechanisms usually respond well to traditional approaches to pain management, including common analgesic medications and nondrug strategies for pain. Neuropathic pain results from pathophysiologic processes that arise in the peripheral or central nervous system. Examples include diabetic neuralgia, postherpetic neuralgia, poststroke "central" or "thalamic pain," and posttraumatic neuralgia (postamputation or "phantom limb" pain). In contrast to nociceptive pain, neuropathic pain syndromes often respond to nonconventional analgesic medications such as tricyclic antidepressants and anticonvulsant drugs. Mixed pain syndromes are often thought to have multiple or unknown pathophysiologic mechanisms. Treatment of these problems is more problematic and often unpredictable. Examples include recurrent headaches and some vasculitic syndromes. Finally, rare psychologically based pain syndromes may exist when psychological factors are judged to have a major role in the onset, severity, exacerbation, or maintenance of pain. Examples include somatoform disorders and conversion reactions. These patients may benefit from specific psychiatric intervention, but traditional pain strategies are probably not indicated. It is important to remember that the pathophysiologic basis of pain may be multifactorial for many diseases. Cancer, for instance, may cause pain from tumor distention and deformation of surrounding tissues, invasion of peripheral nerves, or chronic inflammation. Arthritis may cause pain from inflammation, joint distortion with associated strain on muscles and connective tissue, and microfracture from eroded cartilage or bone. Unfortunately for many diseases, the pathophysiologic basis of pain is only partially understood.

The approach to pain assessment and management is often different for older people as compared to younger persons. Older people often present with multiple medical problems and many potential sources of pain. Older persons more frequently experience adverse medication effects from common analgesic drugs. Alternative care settings such as nursing homes, assisted-living arrangements, and home care also present logistic challenges to providing good pain control. Each of these issues makes pain more difficult to manage in older persons.

Table 25-1   Pathophysiologic Classification of Pain

I. Nociceptive pain
   Trauma or burns
      Infection or inflammation
      Ischemia
      Mechanical deformity
      Distension
      Arthropathies (e.g., rheumatoid arthritis, osteoarthritis, gout, posttraumatic arthropathies, mechanical neck and back syndromes)
   Myalgia (e.g., myofascial pain syndromes)
   Nonarticular inflammatory disorders (e.g., polymyalgia rheumatica)
   Visceral pain (pain of internal organs and viscera)

II. Neuropathic pain
   Peripheral nervous system
      Postherpetic neuralgia
      Trigeminal neuralgia
      Painful diabetic polyneuropathy
      Post amputation (phantom limb) pain
   Central nervous system
      Poststroke pain ("central pain")
      Myelopathic/radiculopathic pain (e.g., multiple sclerosis, spinal stenosis, arachnoiditis, root sleeve fibrosis)
   Sympathetic nervous system
      Reflex sympathetic dystrophy
      Causalgia-like syndromes (complex regional pain syndromes)

III. Mixed or undetermined pathophysiology
   Chronic recurrent headaches (e.g., tension headaches, migraine headaches, mixed headaches)
   Vasculopathic pain syndromes (e.g., painful vasculitis)

IV. Psychologically based pain syndromes
   Somatization disorders
      Hysterical reactions (conversion)

Pain management has reached a high level of sophistication over the last 20 years. The success of specialized pain centers, multidisciplinary pain teams, and the development of technology (e.g., drug-delivery systems) have defined a variety of options for pain control. Several organizations have sponsored consensus panels and summarized available medical evidence to publish clinical practice guidelines on acute and postoperative pain, cancer pain, acute back pain, use of analgesic drugs, and, most recently, noncancer-related pain specifically for elderly people. Unfortunately, few randomized trials have been conducted to definitively evaluate pain management strategies specifically in older persons, particularly the oldest old. For the most part, information has been extrapolated from experience with younger patients and those with pain caused by cancer.

PATHOPHYSIOLOGY OF PAIN PERCEPTION

Pain is a universal experience. Except for the rare condition of hereditary polyneuropathy (a congenital anomaly associated with poorly developed spinal ganglia and almost total anesthesia to pain), all people experience pain associated with trauma or disease. As a teleologic explanation, pain probably serves a protective purpose that signals tissue injury or potential injury. Theories of pain as a simple sensation have long ago been abandoned. Pain is now recognized as a complex experience that includes sensory stimuli, but also includes emotional components. Pain cannot be understood without recognizing this dual nature of the pain experience.

Neuroanatomic and neurochemical connections in pain perception are extremely complex. Figure 25-1 provides a simplified illustration of the anatomic connections in simple pain perception. It is now known that many sensory receptors are capable of detecting pain if stimulated

appropriately. Painful stimuli are conducted primarily in two types of nerve fibers. Large myelinated fast conducting A-delta fibers convey phasic pain information that gives rise to location and intensity. Slower conducting nonmyelinated C fibers conduct tonic pain information that often gives rise to pain character descriptions such as "dull," "aching," or "burning." Sensory neurons are usually bipolar neurons whose cell bodies reside in the dorsal root ganglia and enter the spinal column through the dorsal roots where they synapse with interneurons in the ascending lateral and posterior spinothalamic tracts. These tracts relay sensory information to the brainstem and thalamus with projections to the cerebral cortex. There are also descending pain pathways in the spinal cord that transmit inhibitory pain information from the cortex, limbic system, thalamus, and midbrain to the spinal level. Activity in the descending pathway can actually inhibit pain at the spinal level. These anatomic findings may help explain the results of treatments such as transcutaneous nerve stimulation, acupuncture, tricyclic antidepressants, and placebo effects. It is now known that pain can also be transmitted via sympathetic nerves that accompany blood vessels and internal organs. In fact, local sympathetic nerve or ganglia blockade helps some neuropathic conditions that have subsequently been described specifically in the pain literature as sympathetically maintained pain (SMP) and reflex sympathetic dystrophy (RSD).

Identification of specific neurotransmitters in pain perception has also added to our knowledge of pain perception. Table 25-2 lists some of the neurotransmitters associated with pain perception. Their function in modulating pain is elaborate, complex, and often not entirely understood. Specific neurotransmitters may enhance or inhibit pain information. Serotonergic antidepressants, for example, may excite descending pathways that attenuate some pain perceptions at the spinal level. A large number of opioid mediators have been identified in three major classes including endorphins, enkephalins, and dynorphins. Five types of opioid receptors have also been identified in various areas of the brain, spinal cord, and ganglia. The complexity of this system probably accounts for the variable effects of many analgesic drugs that may include pain relief, narcosis, depression, central nervous system excitement, euphoria, hunger, and many other sensations. Unfortunately, little is known about the effect of aging on these complex neural functions.

Age-associated changes in pain sensation have been a topic of interest for many years. Elderly people have been observed to present with painless myocardial infarction, painless intraabdominal catastrophes, and other unusual manifestations of common illnesses. Whether these clinical observations represent age-related changes in pain perception remains controversial. Although changes in sensory organs, nerve conduction, and integrative function may occur, age-associated observations are difficult to differentiate from disease and environmental injuries. Studies using a variety of methodologies to induce pain and measure it in "normal" volunteers have shown mixed results. Some studies show an age-associated increase in pain threshold with respect to thermal skin sensitivity, whereas others demonstrate no difference. The change in

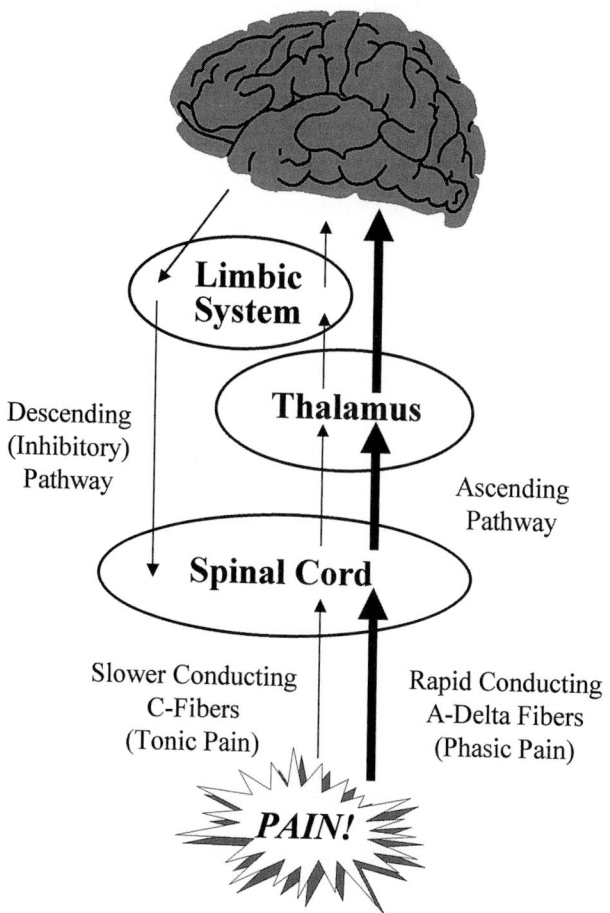

Figure 25-1 Simplified schematic of the major neural connections in the perception of pain.

pain threshold with respect to electric shock has been widely divergent across studies. The most elegant of studies recently measured differences in A-delta but not C fiber function associated with aging. Unfortunately, because of differences in methodologies and sampling, a formal meta-analysis of pain studies is not possible. The divergent results of these studies do not suggest any consensus about age-associated changes in pain threshold. Moreover, it is not clear that these induced stimuli are analogous to the sensation of pain mediated from a clinical disease or injury. In the final analysis, age-associated changes in pain perception are probably not clinically significant.

Table 25-2 Neurochemical Mediators Identified in Pain Perception

Sensory neurons
  Glutamate
  ATP (adenosine triphospate)
  Bradykinin
  5-HT (5-hydroxytryptophan)
  Histamine
  Arachinodonic acid metabolites
  Nitric oxide
  CGRP (calcitonin gene-related peptide)
  Mechanotransduction (mechanisms not clearly understood)

Ascending pathway (dorsal horn neurons)
  Glutamate
  Substance P
  Neurotensin
  Cholecystokinin
  Somatostatin

Descending pathway (midbrain and spinal cord)
  Serotonin
  Norepinephrine
  γ-Aminobutric acid (GABA)
  Glycine
  Acetylcholine

Assorted areas (brain, spinal cord, nerves, ganglia)
  Dopamine
  Neuropeptide Y
  N-methyl-D-aspartate (NMDA) receptors
  Opiate receptors
    Five types: mu, kappa, delta, gamma, sigma (mu, kappa, and delta receptor types most often associated with analgesia; all have multiple subtypes)
  Endogenous opioids (many compounds in three classes)
    Endorphins
    Enkephalins
    Dynorphins

EPIDEMIOLOGY OF PAIN IN ELDERLY PEOPLE

Pain is one of the most common complaints heard in physicians' offices. However, from population-based studies, a precise incidence and prevalence is not known. Epidemiology studies of pain in general populations have suffered from the lack of a standard definition for what might be regarded as "significant pain." Despite this limitation, a number of population-based studies suggest that pain-related problems are present in 25 to 50 percent of community-dwelling elders. For example, a random survey of 500 households in Ontario, Canada, identified a twofold increase in painful conditions in those older than age 60 years, as compared to those younger than age 60 years (25 percent versus 12.5 percent). In other studies, prevalence rates have ranged from 36 percent to 88 percent, depending on definitions used and sampling methods. A Louis Harris telephone survey found that 1 in 5 elderly Americans (18 percent) are taking analgesic medications regularly (several times a week or more) and that 63 percent of those had taken prescription pain relievers for more than 6 months.

Pain is also common in nursing home populations. In a random survey of patients in 10 community nursing homes in Los Angeles, 62 percent of those who could make their needs known had pain that affected their daily lives. Others who have studied the problem in nursing home settings have found 49 to 83 percent of nursing home residents have important pain problems.

The most common causes of pain in elderly people are probably related to musculoskeletal disorders. The Louis Harris survey found that elderly patients who took analgesics regularly were more likely to suffer from arthritis, joint disorders, and back pain, than any from other condition. Reports from a rural population based survey in Iowa suggested that the most prevalent pain in the preceding year was joint pain (66.3 percent) followed by nocturnal leg pain (56.4 percent), back pain (28.3 percent), and leg pain while walking (21.4 percent). In nursing homes, musculoskeletal problems were also found to be the most common complaints. From the random sample from 10 community-based nursing homes in Los Angeles, authors reported arthritis was the most likely cause in 70 percent of patients with pain, followed by old fracture sites (13 percent), neuropathy (10 percent) and malignancy (4 percent).

Elderly people are disproportionately affected by a number of specific painful medical problems. Osteoarthritis may affect 80 percent of those older than age 65 years and most have significant pain. Cancer is a source of severe pain in this age group, especially near the end of life. Herpes zoster, temporal arteritis, polymyalgia rheumatica, and atherosclerotic peripheral vascular disease are all more common in elderly people than in younger people.

The consequences of pain are also common in elderly people. Depression, decreased socialization, sleep disturbance, impaired ambulation, and increased health care use, and costs are associated with pain in elderly people. Although less-thoroughly explored, deconditioning, gait disturbances, slow rehabilitation, and polypharmacy are among the many conditions often made worse by the presence of pain. Most importantly, poor pain control is an important determinant of quality of life and quality of care, especially among those near the end of life and those in long-term care settings.

PRESENTATION OF PAIN

Older patients are often reticent to bring forth pain complaints. Thus, inquiry about pain should be a routine part of every new patient encounter with health care professionals and repeated at regular intervals. The care of older patients includes special problems in recognizing painful conditions. Multiple concurrent illnesses, underreporting of symptoms, and the presence of cognitive impairment may make pain recognition more difficult. With no objective biological markers for pain, clinicians must rely on patients' self-reports and, at times, other signs or symptoms. Elderly patients often use a variety of words to describe pain experiences. Many patients do not use the word "pain," but refer to the problem as hurting, aching, burning, or other descriptive terms. A decline in functional status, altered mental status, or recent depression may be the only presentation of an underlying painful condition.

EVALUATION OF PAIN IN ELDERLY PEOPLE

Any pain complaint that has an impact on physical function or quality of life should be recognized as a significant problem. Accurate pain assessment begins when clinicians believe patients and take their pain complaints seriously.

Initial evaluation begins with a thorough pain history. The history is important to establish a definitive diagnosis and a baseline description of the pain experience. Pain treatment is most successful when the underlying cause of pain is identified and treated definitively. An appreciation of the interplay between coexisting disease and a thorough review of past and present medication use are important aspects of pain evaluation. Although past medical and surgical history is important, care must be taken to avoid attributing acute pain to preexisting conditions. Successful evaluation is further challenged by the fact that chronic pain may fluctuate with time. Injuries due to trauma as well as acute inflammatory arthritis (e.g., gout or calcium pyrophosphate arthritis) can be easily overlooked in this setting. Only astute questioning and comprehensive evaluation will help avoid these pitfalls. Among those for whom the underlying cause is not remediable or only partially treatable, a multidisciplinary assessment and treatment strategy is often necessary.

A baseline description of pain is important to compare with treatment outcomes. Figure 25-2 provides a chart form that can be used to summarize the pain history and pain description. The pain description should include information about the pattern, duration, location, and character of the pain problem. Clinicians should probe for descriptions that may not include the word "pain" and use these descriptions in the initial assessment and during subsequent follow-up evaluations.

Pain intensity can be measured quantitatively using a variety of pain scales that have been validated in older patients. Figure 25-3 provides examples of some existing pain scales that are known to be useful. At least one investigation has shown that 80 percent of nursing home patients, including those with substantial cognitive impairment can provide meaningful information about pain intensity using these types of scales. Although several multidimensional pain scales are also available for the assessment of pain (e.g., McGill Pain Questionnaire and others), they are often laborious and difficult to administer in clinical settings. In general, pain measurement is more reliable when the clinician is asking about pain at the moment. Because of memory impairment and difficulty integrating pain experiences over time, the measurement of "average" pain over the last few weeks or months may be more problematic. In some cases, more accurate evaluation may require a pain record or diary with information gathered over several days or weeks.

Persons with moderate to severe cognitive impairment may present substantial challenges to pain assessment. Although it has often been assumed that those in deep coma do not experience pain, it is not clear that such brain damage necessarily results in complete anesthesia. Patients with "locked-in syndrome" (having intact perception and cognitive function, but not purposeful motor function, and no means of communication) may suffer severely. Health care providers must be aware of these situations and provide analgesia empirically, at least during procedures or for conditions known to be uncomfortable or painful. More often, the majority of those with severe cognitive impairment can and do make their needs known through simple yes and no answers communicated in a variety of ways. Those with profound aphasia can often provide accurate and reliable answers to yes and no questions when confronted by a sensitive and skilled interviewer. For these patients, it is important for health care providers to be creative in establishing communication methods for the purpose of pain assessment.

Behavioral cues in pain assessment have been a topic of interest for many years. Behaviors such as facial grimace, groaning, and guarding may provide clues for pain assessment in some patients. Table 25-3 lists some behaviors commonly associated with pain. It is important to remember, however, that some patients may demonstrate a lack of behavior when in pain. Some patients are observed to lie still, sleep, and withdraw from social or other activity that may be the only clue to a new or recurrent problem.

Finally, family and caregivers are often very helpful in the evaluation of pain. Among those with cognitive impairment, family or other caregivers may be the only source for qualitative information such as history, medication use, behavior, or actions that seem to reduce pain. Family and caregivers are, however, limited in their interpretation of events and behaviors. In fact, data suggest that when it comes to estimating pain intensity, proxies are not always accurate or reliable. Physicians and nurses have often been found to underestimate pain intensity and provide inadequate pain medication. In the final analysis, family and caregivers can be important sources for qualitative information, but they probably should not be relied on entirely for

GERIATRIC PAIN ASSESSMENT

Date:_____   Medical Record Number_____

Patient's Name_____

Problem List: Medications:

_____   _____
_____   _____
_____   _____
_____   _____
_____   _____

Pain Description:

Pattern: Constant   Intermittant
Duration:_____
Location:_____
Character:
Lancinating   Burning   Stinging Radiating
       Shooting   Tingling

Other Descriptors:

_____
_____
_____

Exacerbating Factors:

_____
_____

Relieving Factors:

_____
_____

Other Assessments or Comments:

_____
_____
_____

Most Likely Cause of Pain_____

Plans:_____
_____
_____
_____

Pain Intensity:
0 1 2 3 4 5 6 7 8 9 10
None   Moderate   Severe

Worst Pain in Last 24 hours:
0 1 2 3 4 5 6 7 8 9 10
None   Moderate   Severe

Mood:_____

Depression Screening Score: _____

Gait and Balance Score: _____
Impaired Activities:

_____
_____
_____

Sleep Quality: _____
Bowel Habits:_____

_____

Figure 25-2   Example of a medical record form that can be used to summarize the initial evaluation of pain.

quantitative assessment of pain intensity or distress, especially among patients able to communicate their own pain experiences.

A thorough evaluation of pain also includes a thorough physical examination. The physical examination should focus on the musculoskeletal and nervous system. It is important to palpate for trigger points, swelling, and inflammation. Trigger points that result from myofascial pain syndromes, tendinitis, muscle strain, or nerve irritation may benefit from specific treatment such as local injections or physical therapy. Neurologic examination should include a search for signs of sensory, motor, and autonomic deficits suggestive of neuropathic conditions and nerve injuries that may require specific treatments. Maneuvers that

reproduce pain, such as range of motion evaluation and straight leg raising can provide both diagnosis and assessment of functional status.

The evaluation of functional status is important as an outcome measure for pain management so that mobility and independence can be maximized. Functional assessment may include information from the history and physical examination as well as the use of several available self-report or performance-based functional assessment scales.

Psychosocial impairments related to pain should also be evaluated. Pain is often associated with depression, anxiety, and decreased socialization. When these complications occur, pain is more difficult to manage. Depression can be evaluated using one of several available screening tools.

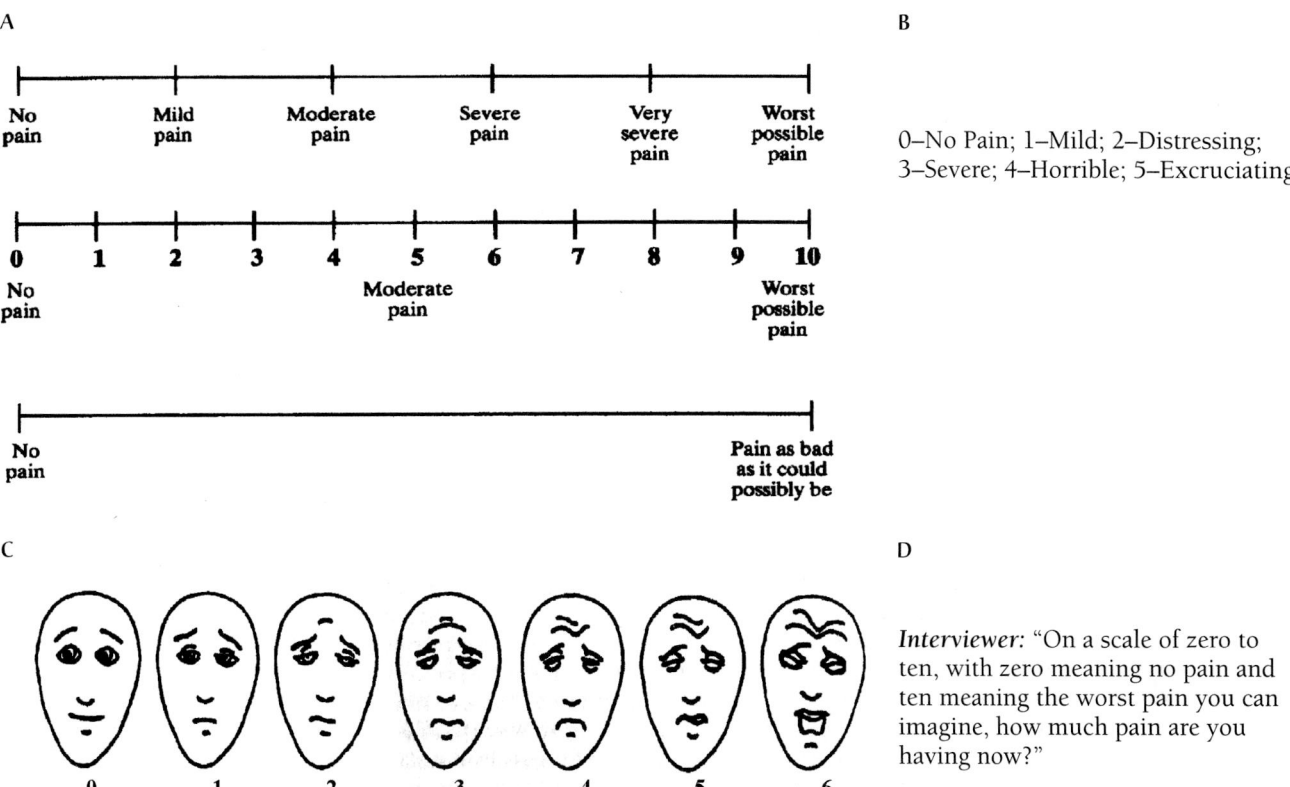

A

No pain | Mild pain | Moderate pain | Severe pain | Very severe pain | Worst possible pain

0   1   2   3   4   5   6   7   8   9   10
No pain   Moderate pain   Worst possible pain

No pain   Pain as bad as it could possibly be

B

0–No Pain; 1–Mild; 2–Distressing; 3–Severe; 4–Horrible; 5–Excruciating

C

0   1   2   3   4   5   6

D

Interviewer: "On a scale of zero to ten, with zero meaning no pain and ten meaning the worst pain you can imagine, how much pain are you having now?"

Figure 25-3   Examples of one-dimensional pain scales for quantifying pain at the moment. *(A)* Visual analog scales; *(B)* a word descriptor scale; *(C)* a graphic picture scale; *(D)* a verbal scale.

Clinicians should also inquire about fears and the meaning of pain. To some patients, pain may represent atonement for past transgressions or may mean they are approaching death. These emotional issues may make pain assessment and treatment more difficult. For most patients, healthy coping skills can be very helpful. An exploration of coping skills may include discussions about behavior and recognizing which behaviors are helpful and harmful to the overall pain management process. Finally, patients with pain often withdraw and become socially isolated. Recognition and intervention of this complication can help to improve mood disorders and quality of life for many of these patients.

PAIN MANAGEMENT

Most problems encountered in elderly people can be improved with careful use of medications and other effective nonpharmacologic strategies. Existing clinical practice guidelines suggest a combination of pharmacologic and nonpharmacologic techniques results in more effective pain control and less reliance on medications alone that have major adverse effects in this population. Elderly people with pain may benefit most from physicians, nurses, and restorative care personnel who use an interdisciplinary approach to this complex problem.

Elderly people should be given an expectation of pain relief, but it is unrealistic to suggest or sustain an expectation of complete relief for some patients with chronic pain. The goals, expectations, tradeoffs, and limitations of possible therapies need to be discussed openly. For patients anticipating surgery or a painful procedure, preoperative education and preparation cannot be overemphasized. A period of trial and error should be anticipated when new strategies are initiated and while titration of medication occurs. Review of medications, treatments, and adverse effects should be a regular process of care, and seemingly ineffective strategies should be discontinued.

Economic issues do play a role in current pain management and should enter into decision-making processes at some level. Economic considerations should be used to make balanced decisions after sound principles of assessment and treatment have been followed. Clinicians should be aware of economic barriers patients and their families may encounter, including lack of Medicare reimbursement for some strategies, limited formularies, delays in referrals in some managed care environments, delays from mail-order pharmacies, and limited availability of strong opioid analgesic medications in some pharmacies.

Finally, elderly people have been systematically excluded from many clinical trials. Of the nearly 4000 papers published each year on pain management, fewer that 1 percent involve elderly subjects. A report of 83 randomized trials of nonsteroidal antiinflammatory drugs (NSAIDs) that included nearly 10,000 subjects, found less than 3 percent of subjects were age 65 years or older and no subjects older than age 85 years were included. A dearth of information

Table 25-3 Behaviors Commonly Associated with Pain

Facial expressions
　Grimacing
　Tightly closed eyes
　Facial distortion

Verbalizations
　Grunting, chanting
　Groan, moaning
　Verbal abuse

Body movements
　Rigid body posture, guarding
　Figeting, restlessness
　Pacing, rocking, repetitive movements
　Restricted movement, gait changes

Changes in activity
　Refusing food, decreased appetite
　Increased sleep, change in sleep pattern
　Cessation of common routines

Changes in personal interactions
　Aggressive, combative, agitation, disruption
　Social withdrawal

Changes in mental status
　Increased confusion
　Crying, tears
　Depression, distress

is also available on commonly used nondrug strategies for pain management such as the use of heat, cold, massage, and many other physical modalities. Thus, much of what is known about what works and what doesn't work for the management of pain in older persons is largely derived from extrapolation of studies of younger patients and those with cancer. Most treatment principles remain largely based on clinical judgement tailored to individual patient situations.

Pharmacologic Therapies

Analgesic Drugs

The most common treatment strategy for pain management is the use of oral or injectable medications. Any patient who has pain that impairs functional status or quality of life is a candidate for pharmacologic therapy. All pharmacologic interventions carry a balance of benefits and burdens. Although analgesic drugs are safe and effective when used properly, elderly people are more likely to experience adverse drug reactions. For some classes of pain-relieving medications (opioids, for example), elderly patients have greater analgesic sensitivity. However, elderly people are a heterogeneous population; thus, optimum dosage and side effects are difficult to predict. Recommendations for age-adjusted dosing are not available for most analgesics. The adage "start low and go slow" is probably appropriate

for most drugs known to have high adverse effect profiles in the elderly. In reality, dosing for most patients requires careful titration, including frequent assessment and dosage adjustments for optimum pain relief, while monitoring and managing potential adverse effects.

Some analgesic combinations are known to produce synergistic effects. The combination of opioid analgesic drugs with acetaminophen or NSAIDs may produce a synergism for analgesia. This has been shown to be particularly effective in the treatment of bone pain related to metastatic cancer. It is recognized that there is a significant potential for problems with multiple drug use in older patients. However, the use of more than one agent to affect a therapeutic end point may be necessary to minimize dose-limiting adverse effects of a particular drug class. Combining smaller effective doses of differing classes may produce pain relief without as much risk of the adverse effects associated with higher doses of a single medication. Close monitoring is important when multiple medications are prescribed, particularly for patients with multiple concurrent medical problems. It is important to note that combinations of the same class (i.e., two or more opioids, or two or more NSAIDs) usually offer no advantage and often counteract each other's effect on serum-protein-binding sites or pain-receptor mechanisms. This results in no analgesic advantage, but substantial increased risk of adverse effects.

Route of Administration

The least-invasive route of drug administration should always be used. This is usually the oral route. A variety of other routes and drug delivery systems are available including subcutaneous, intravenous, transcutaneous, sublingual, and rectal. Many drugs are limited to only a few safe routes of administration, but new delivery systems are being created and studied each year. It is best to consult package inserts for the most accurate information on available routes of administration. The oral route is preferable because of its convenience and associated relatively steady blood levels. Drug effects are often seen in 30 minutes to 2 hours for most analgesics given orally, which may be a drawback in acute, rapidly fluctuating pain. Intravenous bolus provides the most rapid onset and shortest duration of action, which may be appropriate for acute pain and postoperative pain control. Subcutaneous and intramuscular injection, although commonly used, has disadvantages of wider fluctuations in absorption and rapid fall off of action compared to oral routes. Transcutaneous, rectal, and sublingual routes should probably be reserved for those with difficulty swallowing.

Timing of Administration

Timing of medications is also important. Fast-onset, short-acting analgesic drugs should be used for episodic pain. Medications for intermittent or episodic pain can usually be prescribed as needed. For continuous pain, medications should be provided around the clock. In these situations, a steady-state analgesic blood level is more effective in maintaining comfort. Long-acting or sustained-release preparations should only be used for continuous pain. Most patients with continuous pain also need fast-onset short-acting drugs for break-through pain. Break-through pain includes (1) end-of-dose failure as the result of decreased blood levels of analgesic with concomitant increase in pain prior to the next scheduled dose; (2) incident pain, usually caused by activity that can be anticipated and pretreated; and (3) spontaneous pain, common with neuropathic pain that is often fleeting and difficult to predict.

Most patients can cope better if medications are prescribed in an effort to support appropriate exercise, enjoyable activities, and uninterrupted sleep. Chronic pain is an exhausting experience. Deconditioning, inadequate sleep, and poor eating habits can arise from uncontrolled pain and make pain management more difficult. Clinical end points for pharmacologic interventions should not concentrate on reduced drug dose but rather focus on decreased pain, improved function and improved mood and sleep. With these goals in mind, clinicians can often simplify drug regimens. Patients and caregivers should have some flexibility in designing regimens for their particular needs and lifestyles.

Acetaminophen

Acetaminophen is most often the drug of choice for elderly persons with mild to moderate pain, especially that of osteoarthritis and other musculoskeletal problems. As an analgesic and antipyretic, acetaminophen appears to act in the central nervous system but remains classified separately from opioids or NSAID drugs. Despite the lack of antiinflammatory activity, recent studies suggest that acetaminophen is as effective as ibuprofen for chronic osteoarthritis of the knee. Acetaminophen may also have deleterious effects on renal function (over a long period of time) and may interfere with the concomitant administration of warfarin. Nonetheless, given in a dose of 650 to 1000 mg four times a day, it remains the safest analgesic medication, as compared to NSAIDs and other analgesic drugs, for most patients. It is important to remember that acetaminophen overdose can result in irreversible hepatic necrosis. Therefore, the maximum daily dose should never exceed 4000 mg per day.

Nonsteroidal Antiinflammatory Drugs

NSAIDs have analgesic activity both peripherally and centrally. NSAIDs are appropriate for short-term use in inflammatory arthritic conditions such as gout, calcium pyrophosphate arthropathy, acute flare-ups of rheumatoid arthritis, and other inflammatory rheumatic conditions. They have also been reported to relieve the pain of headache and other mild to moderate pain syndromes. These drugs can be used alone for mild to moderate pain or in combination with opioids for more severe pain. They have the advantage of being nonhabit forming. Individual drugs in this class vary widely with respect to antiinflammatory activity, potency, analgesic properties, metabolism, excretion, and adverse-effect profiles. Moreover, it has been observed that failure of response to one NSAID may not predict the response to another. A disadvantage of NSAIDs is that they all demonstrate a ceiling effect, that is, a level at which an increased dose results in no further increase in analgesia.

Although a large number of NSAIDs are now available, there is no evidence to support a particular compound as the NSAID of choice. Several NSAIDs are available over-the-counter without a prescription. Table 25-4 lists selected NSAIDs for pain management.

NSAIDs are potent inhibitors of prostaglandin synthesis that have effects on inflammation, pain receptors, and nerve conduction, and may have central effects as well. It is now known that there are two major NSAID-sensitive cyclooxygenase enzymes (COX-1 and COX-2) synthesized in a variety of organs. COX-1 is present in most organ systems and plays a role in normal organ function such as gastric mucosal blood flow and barrier function, renal blood flow, hepatic blood flow, and platelet aggregation. COX-2, normally present in lower concentrations, is an inducible enzyme in response to injury or inflammation. It is now known that selective inhibition of COX-2 gives rise to analgesic and antiinflammatory activity with potentially less toxicity compared to the non-selective inhibition of both enzymes (COX-1 and COX-2). These findings resulted in new NSAIDs reaching the market that may have less gastric toxicity as compared to older NSAID medications. In fact, clinical trials have found COX-2 inhibitors to be similarly effective to traditional NSAIDs in terms of peak pain relief, total pain relief, and in indices of joint inflammation in patients with arthritis. It is important to note that, like other NSAIDS, these drugs have limited effectiveness and potency for patients with moderate to severe pain problems. Even though in some studies the COX-2 agents have demonstrated a reduction in gastrointestinal erosions and dyspepsia as compared to other NSAIDs, the supporting safety data on serious peptic ulcer bleeding remains more controversial. Because these drugs do not effect platelet function, patients who need cardioprotective antiplatelet therapy should also receive aspirin or other antiplatelet drugs. However, a secondary analysis of one study suggested that concomitant antiplatelet therapy may negate some of the gastrointestinal (GI) protection afforded by COX-2 drugs. Thus, additional studies will be important to clarify limitations of these new agents and clinicians must stay alert to new findings as they come available.

High-dose NSAIDs for long periods of time should be avoided in elderly patients. Of major concern is the high incidence of adverse reactions in elderly patients, including GI bleeding, renal impairment and bleeding diathesis from platelet dysfunction. The concomitant use of misoprostol or proton pump inhibitors is partially successful at reducing the risk of significant GI bleeding associated with NSAID use. Also, the adverse-effect profiles of gastroprotective drugs in this population must be weighed against their limited benefits. These gastroprotective medications do nothing to prevent renal impairment or other adverse effects. For those with multiple medical problems, NSAIDs are associated with increased risk of drug–drug and drug–disease interactions. For example, NSAIDs may interact with antihypertensive therapy. Thus, the relative risks and benefits of NSAIDs must be weighed carefully against other available treatments for older patients with chronic pain problems. For some patients, chronic opioid therapy, low-dose or intermittent corticosteroid therapy, or many other nonopioid analgesic drug strategies may have

Table 25–4   Selected Nonsteroidal Antiinflammatory Drugs for Pain*

Drug	Maximum Dose	Description	Comments
Celecoxib (Celebrex)	200 mg bid	Selective COX-2 inhibition; pain and antiinflammatory activity similar to other NSAIDs	Less gastric toxicity; less platelet inhibition
Refocoxib (Vioxx)	50 mg q24h	Selective COX-2 inhibition; pain and antiinflammatory activity similar to other NSAIDs	Less gastric toxicity; less platelet inhibition
Valdecoxib (Bextra)	10 mg q24h	Similar to other COX-2 agents	Similar to other COX-2 agents
Relafen (Nabumetone)	2000 mg/24 h (q24h dosing)	Partially COX-2 selective; gastric toxicity may be less; occasionally requires q12h dosing	Avoid maximum dose for prolonged periods
Aspirin	4000 mg/24 h (q4–6h dosing)	Prototype NSAID	Salicylate levels may be helpful in monitoring
Salsalate (Disalcid)	3000 mg/24 h (q6–8h dosing)	Hydrolyzed in small intestine to aspirin	Elderly may require dose adjustment downward to avoid salicylate toxicity; salicylate levels may be helpful in monitoring
Ibuprofen (Motrin by prescription; Advil, Nuprin, and others otc[2])	2400 mg/24 h (q6–8h dosing)	Gastric, renal, and abnormal platelet function may be dose dependent; constipation, confusion, and headaches may be more common in older persons	Avoid high doses for prolonged periods of time
Diflunisal (Dolobid)	1000 mg/24 h maximum dose Loading = 1000 mg then 500 mg q12h or 750 mg then 250 mg q8h in small patients or frail elderly	Relatively good analgesic properties, but requires loading dose	Dose may need downward adjustment for small patients or frail elderly
Sulindac (Clinoril)	400 mg/24 h (q12h dosing)	Same as ibuprofen	Same as ibuprofen
Naproxen (Naprosyn by prescription; Aleve and others OTC)	1000 mg/24 h (q8–12h dosing)	Same as ibuprofen; may require a loading dose for better pain control	Same as ibuprofen
Choline magnesium trisalicylate (Trilisate)	5500 mg/24 h (q12h dosing)	Lower effect on platelet function	Salicylate levels may be helpful to avoid toxicity
Indomethacin (Indocin)	200 mg/24 h (q8–12h dosing)	Extremely high toxicity in frail elderly; should be reserved for acute inflammatory conditions (e.g., gout)	Keep dose to a minimum (25 mg q8h) and for short-term use only; avoid use for osteoarthritis or other noninflammatory problems
Ketorolac (Toradol)	IM: 120 mg/24 h (30–60 mg loading dose; followed by half the loading dose; 15–30 mg q6h limited to not more than 5 days) PO: 60 mg/24 h (q6h dosing limited to not more than 14 days)	Substantial gastrointestinal toxicity as well as renal and platelet dysfunction; relatively high postoperative complications have been documented	Duration of treatment limited because of high toxicity; reduce dose in half for those less than 50 kg or older than 65 years of age

COX, cyclooxygenase; OTC, over-the-counter or available without prescription; IM, intramuscular injection; PO, per os (orally or by mouth).

*A limited number of examples is provided. For comprehensive lists of other available NSAIDs and a host of brand names, clinicians should consult other sources.

fewer life-threatening risks as compared to long-term, high-dose NSAID use.

Opioid Analgesic Medications

Opioid analgesic medications act by blocking receptors in the central nervous system (brain and spinal cord), resulting in a decreased pain perception. Some of these drugs (including morphine) may act similarly to local anesthetics and now have widespread use in epidural anesthesia. Opioid drugs have no ceiling to their analgesic effects and have been shown to relieve all types of pain. Data from short-term studies indicate that elderly persons, as compared to younger persons, are more sensitive to the pain-relieving properties of these drugs. This has been shown for acute postoperative pain, as well as for chronic cancer pain. One study noted enhanced analgesia in elderly women even when morphine was administered by the epidural route. Advanced age is associated with a prolonged half-life and altered pharmacokinetics of opioid drugs. Thus, elderly persons may achieve pain relief from smaller doses of opiate drugs than typical doses used in younger persons. Table 25-5 lists some examples of opioid drugs for older patients.

Opioid drugs have the potential to cause respiratory depression, cognitive disturbances, constipation, and habituation in older persons. They are safe for older persons, however, when used correctly. Drowsiness, respiratory depression, and decline in performance-based measures of cognitive impairment should be anticipated when opioids are initiated and doses are escalated rapidly. Such changes occur in a dose dependent fashion and can be used to estimate dose escalations. If patients have unrelieved pain with little drowsiness or cognitive impairment, doses may be escalated more rapidly. Fortunately, tolerance to these adverse effects develops quickly (usually in just a few days) at which time, patients usually return to a fully alert status and baseline cognitive function. Until tolerance develops, patients should be instructed not to drive and to take precautions against falls or other accidents. But once tolerance to these effects has developed, patients can often return to normal activities including driving and other demanding tasks even in the presence of high doses. In fact, cancer patients are often observed to have improved physical function on opioid analgesics once pain is adequately relieved.

Constipation is a complication of opioid drugs for which older patients do not develop tolerance. Fortunately, opioid-associated constipation can be prevented and relieved. The management of constipation usually includes increasing fluid intake, maintaining mobility, and use of other cathartic strategies. Some patients find relief through previously used remedies like prune juice or other natural laxatives. Other patients may need more potent osmotic laxatives such as milk of magnesia, lactulose, or sorbitol. But for many patients, opioid-induced constipation may require potent stimulant laxatives such as senna or bisacodyl. It should be remembered that stimulants should not be used unless impactions have been removed and obstruction has been ruled out. Finally, some patients require regular enemas to ensure bowel evacuation during high-dose opioid administration for severe pain.

Nausea also occasionally complicates opioid therapy. Nausea from opioid medications may result from several mechanisms. Opioid drugs may stimulate chemoreceptors directly in the midbrain resulting in nausea and vomiting. They may also cause nausea related to gastric and/or colonic paresis. Opioids in high doses may stimulate vestibular activity and resultant nausea. Identification of the most likely mechanism may help plan an appropriate strategy for control of nausea. If vertiginous symptoms are present, an antihistamine antiemetic may be more appropriate. If gastroparesis is present, medications that increase gastric propulsion (e.g., metoclopramide) may be helpful. For those with nausea as a result of direct chemoreceptor triggers in the brain, traditional neuroleptic antiemetics such as prochlorperazine and chlorpromazine have been the mainstay of treatment for nausea in younger patients. Recent anecdotal reports suggest that low-dose haloperidol has a lower adverse effect profile than do other neuroleptic drugs. All of these agents have high adverse-effect profiles in elderly patients, including movement disorders, delirium, and anticholinergic effects. Some patients may develop tolerance to mild nausea after a few days. For more severe cases, clinicians should choose antiemetic medications with the least-adverse effects and continue to monitor patients frequently.

It is important for clinicians who prescribe opioid analgesics to understand issues of tolerance, dependency, and addiction. Tolerance is a pharmacologic phenomenon that occurs with many drugs. Tolerance is described as diminished effect of a drug that occurs over time, as the individual is constantly exposed to the drug. For opioid drugs, tolerance to adverse effects such as drowsiness and respiratory depression occur much faster than tolerance to analgesic properties of the drug. In fact, tolerance to analgesia is difficult to predict among individuals. Many previous reports that described tolerance among cancer patients resulting in the need for massive doses of morphine to achieve adequate analgesia were probably misinterpreted because those patients had rapidly advancing cancer and escalating pain symptoms. More recent studies of opioid-managed arthritis pain have noted that significant tolerance was infrequent. In fact, some patients have been noted to remain on stable doses of opioids for many years without demonstrating significant tolerance.

Dependency is also a pharmacologic phenomenon associated with many drugs including corticosteroids and beta-blockers. Dependency is present when patients experience uncomfortable adverse effects when the drug is withheld abruptly. The development of drug dependence requires constant exposure to the drug for some period of time. This is, however, difficult to predict. The minimum dose and time relationship between drug exposure and development of dependent withdrawal symptoms is not precisely known and it appears to vary with individual opioid compounds. Symptoms associated with opioid withdrawal may include anorexia, nausea, diaphoresis, tachycardia, mild hypertension, and mild fever. Worsening symptoms may include skin mottling, gooseflesh, and frank autonomic crisis. Fortunately, these symptoms can be ameliorated easily by tapering opioids over a few days. In fact, one rule of thumb is to cut the dose of opioid by 25 percent every

Table 25-5 Opioid Analgesic Medications for Pain*

Drug	Starting Dose (Oral)	Characteristics	Precautions
Morphine (Roxanol, MSIR)	30 mg (q4h dosing)	Intermediate half-life; older people are more sensitive than younger people to side effects	Titrate to comfort; continuous use for continuous pain; intermittent use for episodic pain; anticipate and prevent side effects
Codeine (plain codeine, Tylenol #3, other combinations with acetaminophen or NSAIDs)	30–60 mg (q4–6h dosing)	Acetaminophen or NSAIDs limit dose; constipation is a major issue	Begin bowel program early; do not exceed maximum dose for acetaminophen or NSAIDs
Hydrocodone (Vicoden, Lortab, others)	5–10 mg (q3–4h dosing)	Toxicity similar to morphine; acetaminophen or NSAID combinations limit maximum dose	Same as above
Oxycodone (Roxicodone, Oxy IR; or in combinations with acetaminophen or NSAIDs such as Percocet, Tylox, Percodan, others)	20–30 mg (q3–4h dosing)	Toxicity similar to morphine; acetaminophen or NSAID combinations limit maximum dose; oxycodone is available generically as a single agent	Same as above
Hydromorphone (Dilaudid)	4 mg (q3–4h dosing)	Half-life may be shorter than morphine; toxicity similar to morphine	Similar to morphine
Sustained-release morphine (MS Contin, Oramorph, Kadian)	MS Contin: 30–60 mg (q12h dosing) Oramorph: 30–60 mg (q12h dosing) Kadian: 30–60 mg (q24h dosing)	Morphine sulfate in a wax matrix tablet or sprinkles; MS Contin and Oramorph should not be broken or crushed; Kadian capsules can be opened and sprinkled on food	Titrate dose slowly because of drug accumulation; rarely requires more frequent dosing than q12h; immediate-release opioid analgesic necessary for breakthrough pain
Sustained-release oxycodone (Trilisate)	15–30 mg (q12h dosing)	Similar to sustained-release morphine	Similar to sustained-release morphine
Transdermal fentanyl (Duragesic)	25 μg patch (q72h dosing)	Reservoir for drug is in the skin, not in the patch; equivalent dose compared to other opioids is not very predictable (see package insert); effective activity may exceed 72 h in older patients	Titrate slowly using immediate-release analgesics for breakthrough pain; peak effect of first dose may take 18–24 h; not recommended for opioid naïve patients

*A limited number of examples is provided. For comprehensive lists of other available opioids, clinicians should consult other sources.

24 to 48 hours. In severe cases, clonidine given in titrated doses over a short time period will usually control serious autonomic signs. The physiologic effects of opioid withdrawal are usually not life-threatening when compared to serious withdrawal from alcohol, benzodiazepines, or barbiturates.

Addiction is a behavioral problem and is defined as a pattern of compulsive drug use characterized by a continued craving for an opioid and the need to use the opioid for effects other than pain relief. Addicted patients often have erratic behavior that can be seen in the clinical setting in the form of missed appointments, solicitation of prescriptions from multiple physicians, selling, buying, and procuring drugs on the street, and the use of medication by bizarre means such as dissolving tablets for intravenous self-administration. Table 25-6 lists common behaviors that are often associated with addiction. It is now clear that drug use alone is not the major factor in the development of addiction. Other medical, social, and economic factors play immense roles in addictive behavior. It is also important to not construe certain behaviors as necessarily addictive behaviors. Hoarding of medications, persistent or worsening pain

Table 25-6   Behaviors Often Associated with Addiction

Probable Addictive Behavior	Possible Addictive Behavior
• Intravenous use of oral preparations • Illicit drug use: heroin, crack, etc. • Self-inflicted injury for prescriptions • Sex for drugs • Criminal offenses	• Intoxication • Missed appointments • Early refill requests • Hoarding medications • Multiple physicians • Multiple pharmacies

complaints, frequent office visits, requests for dose escalations, and other behaviors associated with unrelieved pain is characterized by the term *pseudoaddiction*. Laws, regulations, and unintentional behavior by prescribing clinicians may require patients to hoard medication and seek other physicians for additional help. In fact, true addiction is rare among patients taking opioid analgesic medications for medical reasons. In one study of 12,000 hospital records, only 4 cases of addiction were documented. Among older people, the incidence of opioid addiction appears to be even less. Those older than age 60 years account for less than 1 percent of all patients admitted to methadone maintenance clinics. This is not meant to imply that opioid drugs can be used indiscriminately, only that fear of addiction and adverse effects do not justify failure to treat pain in elderly patients, especially those near the end of life.

Fear of addiction has been identified as a major barrier to pain management in elderly people. Unfortunately, fears by clinicians and patients have been overinfluenced by social pressures to reduce illegal drug use among younger people and those that take narcotics for emotional rather than medical reasons. Regulation of controlled substances by state and federal authorities, as well as scrutiny of physicians practices by state license boards, have intimidated many clinicians to not prescribe potent analgesic medications, even for those with severe pain near the end of life. It is feared that this issue may actually contribute to patients who seek suicide rather than endure inadequately managed pain. More recently, many organizations, such as the American Medical Association, the American College of Physicians, and the American Geriatrics Society have released position statements supporting the comfort and control of pain in patients near the end of life. These organizations emphasize that clinicians have an obligation to provide comfort, pain relief, and dignity for patients, even if such interventions may shorten life by a few hours or days.

Today, a variety of opioid analgesic drugs are available and they differ widely with respect to potency and adverse effect profiles. Table 25-5 lists some of the opioid analgesic drugs that are available. Because of special problems among elderly patients several opioid drugs deserve special mention. Propoxyphene is an opioid drug that is controversial because it has never been shown to be superior to aspirin or acetaminophen, yet it has the potential for dependency and renal impairment. Meperidine (Demerol) is a second-line opioid drug because it is metabolized to an active form that is prone to accumulation causing central nervous system (CNS) excitement and seizures. Because of low potency orally and erratic absorption from muscles, it should only be used intravenously for acute pain when morphine or other potent opioids are contraindicated. Pentazocine (Talwin) is a drug that has both agonist and antagonist opiate receptor activity and it is associated with a high incidence of delirium in elderly people. Butorphanol (Stadol) is a drug that should be used with caution in patients already taking opioid analgesic medications. Like pentazocine, butorphanol has mixed opiate receptor activity and can displace opioid analgesic compounds presently occupying pain receptors. This may result in immediate withdrawal symptoms including autonomic crisis. Methadone should also be used with caution in elderly people because of its long half-life that may be even more prolonged in elderly people. And, finally, transdermal fentanyl should not be used in opioid naïve patients, or in those who have not developed tolerance to the potential respiratory depressant side effects of this drug. Fentanyl is perhaps 50 times as potent as morphine and the dose is not as predictable as that of other opioid drugs (see package insert). It should heighten concern that the reservoir for this transdermal delivery system is the skin rather than the patch. The dermal reservoir results in a 72-hour half-life, which may be even longer in frail elderly persons. If patients become inadvertently overdosed, prompt removal of the patch will do little to abort drug delivery. The long half-life also requires slow titration and frequent rescue doses of immediate-release medications for breakthrough pain. Thus, transdermal fentanyl should be reserved for patients who cannot take medications by mouth and who are already accustomed to high-dose opioid drugs.

Other Nonopioid Medications for Pain

A variety of other medications not formally classified as analgesics have been found to be helpful in certain specific pain problems. The term *adjuvant analgesic drugs,* although frequently used, is a misnomer in that some of these nonopioid drugs may be the primary pain-relieving pharmacologic intervention in certain cases. Table 25-7 provides some examples of nonopioid drugs that may help certain kinds of pain. The largest body of available evidence relates to the use of these drugs for neuropathic pain, such as diabetic neuropathies, postherpetic neuralgia, and trigeminal neuralgia. Tricyclic antidepressants, anticonvulsants, and local anesthetics are the most frequently used nonopioid analgesics for neuropathic conditions. In general, these drugs have had limited success in pain syndromes that are not associated with neuropathic mechanisms. Most reports have found that these agents are only partially successful. Typically, approximately 50 to 70 percent of patients have a measurable response, and of those, most experience only partial relief. Thus, these drugs are often panaceas and are rarely totally successful as single agents. One exception may be trigeminal neuralgia where carbamazepine is probably the drug of choice. Usually these agents work better in combination with other traditional drug and nondrug strategies in an effort to improve pain and to keep other

Table 25-7 Nonopioid Medications for Pain*

Drug	Specific Indications	Precautions	Recommendations
Antidepressants (amytriptyline, desipramine, doxipin, imipramine, nortriptyline, others)	Neuropathic pain, major depression, sleep disturbance	Older people are more sensitive than younger people to side effects, especially anticholinergic effects; desipramine may be as effective as amytriptyline with a lower side-effect profile	Complete relief not often seen; more effective as adjunct to other pharmacologic and nonpharmacologic strategies for pain management; monitor closely for side effects; start low and increase slowly every 3–5 days
Anticonvulsants (clonazapam, carbamazepine)	Only for neuropathic pain; carbamazepine is probably the drug of choice for trigeminal neuralgia	Carbamazepine may cause leukopenia, thrombocytopenia, and, rarely, aplastic anemia; clonazepine side effects may be similar to other benzodiazapines in the elderly patient	Start low and increase slowly; check blood counts on carbamazepine
Gabapentin (also an anticonvulsant; Neurontin)	Neuropathic pain only	May prove to have less serious side effects than carbamazepine	Start with 100 mg and titrate up slowly tid dosing; monitor for idiosyncratic side effects such as ankle swelling and ataxia; effective dose anecdotally reported to be 100–800 mg q8h
Antiarrythmics (mexiletine or Mexitil)	Neuropathic pain only	Effective pain dose may be less than effective cardiac dose; common side effects include tremor, dizziness, paresthesias; rarely may cause blood dyscrasias and hepatic damage	Avoid use in patients with preexisting heart disease; start low and titrate slowly; monitor ECGs; q6–8h dosing
Local anesthetics (intravenous lidocaine)	Diagnostic test	Delirium common	May be useful predictor of response to mexiletine or other local anesthetics; should be used as a diagnostic test or in a monitored environment where emergency procedures are readily available to control seizures, cardiac arrest, or other complications
Tramadol (Ultram)	Acute and chronic pain	Partial opioid and serotonin agonist; more of a norepinephrine antagonist; may cause drowsiness, nausea, vomiting, and constipation	Has ceiling effect; dose >300 mg/24 h usually not tolerated because of nausea; q4–6h dosing
Muscle relaxants (blacofen, chlorzoxazone [Paraflex], cyclobenzaprine [Flexaril])	Skeletal muscle spasm	Sedation; anticholinergic effects; aburpt withdrawl of baclofen may cause CNS irritability	Mechanism of action not precisely known; monitor for sedation and anticholinergic effects; taper baclofen on discontinuation

(Continued)

Table 25-7 (*Continued*) Nonopioid Medications for Pain*

Drug	Specific Indications	Precautions	Recommendations
Substance P inhibitors (capsician) available OTC; for topical use only	Neuropathic and other chronic pain; inhibits reuptake of substance P from primary afferent sensory neuron synapses	Burning pain during depletion of substance P may be intolerable by as many as 30 percent of patients; may take 14 days for maximum response; avoid eye contamination	Start with small doses; can be partially removed with vegetable oil
NMDA inhibitors (Ketamine)	No indications outside of operating rooms at this time	Available only as intravenous anesthetic agent	Oral agents are not yet available

CNS, central nervous system; ECG, electrocardiogram; NMDA, N-methyl-D-asparte; OTC over-the-counter.

*A limited number of examples is provided. For comprehensive lists of other available medications for pain, clinicians should consult other sources.

drug doses to a minimum. Failure of response to one particular class of drugs does not necessarily predict failure with another class of agents. In general, nonopioid medications for neuropathic pain should be chosen according to the least-adverse-effect profile. Treatment should usually start with lower doses than recommended for younger patients and doses should be increased slowly based on known pharmacokinetics of individual drugs and appropriate knowledge of disease-specific treatment strategies. Unfortunately, most of the nonopioid medications for pain management have high adverse-effect profiles in elderly persons. Therefore, these medications often have to be monitored carefully.

Antidepressants have been the most widely used class of nonopioid medications for pain. The mechanism of action for these drugs is not entirely known, but probably has to do with interruption of norepinephrine and serotonin mediated mechanisms in the brain. With respect to neuropathic pain, the major effect of these drugs is not their mood-altering capacity, although this may also be helpful in those with depressive symptoms. More is probably known about tricyclic antidepressants than the other subclasses. A randomized placebo-controlled trial of amitriptyline, desipramine, and fluoxetine has indicated that desipramine may be as effective as amitriptyline, but fluoxetine was no better than placebo for the treatment of diabetic neuropathy. Thus, desipramine may be a better choice because it has a lower adverse-effect profile in elderly persons than amitriptyline. Other studies of the selective serotonin reuptake inhibitors (SSRIs), which may have lower side-effect profiles for elderly people, have had mixed reviews, and most are ineffective for pain management.

It has been known for many years that some medications with local anesthetic, antiepileptic, and antiarrhythmic activity may relieve the pain of trigeminal neuralgia (tic douloureux). Studies have shown that other compounds such as Dilantin, Tegretol, and valproic acid may also improve diabetic neuralgia symptoms and other neuropathic pains in some patients. The usefulness of these drugs has been limited by frequency and severity of adverse effects in elderly persons and the fact that most patients respond only partially, making the overall risk:benefit ratio rather large in this population. Indeed, these drugs are not simple analgesics and should not be used for the relief of trivial aches and pains. More recently, newer agents, such as gabapentin, that are reasonably effective for neuropathic pain and have substantially better side-effect profiles have been introduced. In fact, gabapentin may provide a good first choice for most elderly patients with neuropathic pain problems.

Several local anesthetics have also been shown to relieve neuropathic pain when administrated systemically in addition to their known local anesthetic effects. Intravenous lidocaine has been studied and found to sometimes predict the response to other anticonvulsant and systemically administered local anesthetics. Unfortunately, lidocaine is not effective orally and requires continuous IV infusion, which is often associated with delirium and other serious side effects. More recently, mexiletine (Mexitil; similar to lidocaine but active orally) has shown some activity against neuropathic pain of diabetic neuralgia. Although this drug also has a high risk:benefit ratio, some studies report response rates at one-third to one-half of the dose often recommended for cardiac arrhythmias.

Finally, chronic pain associated with osteoporosis has often been shown to improve with calcitonin. Most studies on the effects of calcitonin include anecdotal reports of significant improvement in pain symptoms that are encouraging.

Placebos

Placebos are unethical and there is no place for their use in clinical care. Placebos, in the form of inert oral medications, sham injections, or other fraudulent procedures are only justified in certain research designs where patients have given informed consent and understand that they may be receiving a placebo as a part of the research design. In research, placebos may be useful in identifying and measuring random or uncontrollable events that may confound results of some research designs. In clinical settings, a placebo effect might be observed under a variety

Table 25-8   Anesthetic and Neurosurgical Techniques for Pain Management

Procedure	Possible Indications
Continuous infusion opioids (morphine, hydromorphone, fentanyl)	Perioperative pain; rarely, severe cancer pain when all-oral route has failed
Epidural analgesia (intermittant local anesthetics or opioids, or continuous opioids)	Perioperative pain; rarely, severe cancer pain when oral route has failed
Nerve blocks	Mononeuropathies, postherpetic neuralgia, intercostal nerve pain (postthoracotomy or postherpetic neuralgia)
Intrathecal analgesia	Perioperative pain
Stellate ganglia blockade	Sympathetically mediated pain of the upper extremity
Lumbar sympathetic blockade	Smypathetically mediated pain of the lower extremity, peripheral vascular disease
Celiac plexus blockade	Severe pain from carcinoma of pancreas
Neuroablation (permanent nerve destruction)	Severe recalcitrant mononeuropathic pain
Cordotomy	Severe recalcitrant cancer pain
Neurostimulation (dorsal column or thalamic)	Severe recalcitrant focal pain

of clinical situations, but it is neither diagnostic of pain nor a reliable indicator of a therapeutic response. In fact, placebo effects are usually short-lived and most patients eventually learn the truth. The use of placebos in clinical practice often results in loss of patient trust for the entire health system, and causes greater suffering.

Anesthetic and Neurosurgical Approaches to Pain Management

A wide variety of anesthetic and neurosurgical approaches to pain are available and some require highly specialized skills. Table 25-8 lists some of these technical procedures. Although it is beyond the scope of this chapter to review many of these techniques, a few deserve mention.

Trigger-point injections have been used extensively for the treatment of myofascial pain syndromes. Myofascial pain with trigger points was first recognized more than 50 years ago. In a relatively high percentage of cases, trigger points may initiate a reflex mechanism that produces referred pain, tenderness, and muscle spasm. With local injection of the trigger point followed by stretching and reconditioning of the muscles, the myofascial pain syndrome usually subsides. More recently, similar results have been obtained by using ice massage or vapo-coolant spray applied topically followed by specific muscle stretching and physical therapy techniques. Nonetheless, trigger-point injection with dilute local anesthetics may be highly effective when combined with specific physical therapy for many myofascial pain syndromes.

Continuous opioid infusions are highly effective for providing steady-state analgesic drug levels. Continuous infusions can be maintained by continuous pump via intravenous, subcutaneous, intrathecal, and epidural routes.

Continuous infusions, either IV, subcutaneous, or epidural, are the method of choice for perioperative pain management in most hospitals. These methods are safe and effective for most frail elderly people, as compared to traditional perioperative analgesia using intermittent injections. At least one study of patient controlled analgesia in frail elderly men reported results similar to previous studies in younger patients, including overall less medication use, better pain management, and fewer adverse effects, including less confusion. These techniques have also found widespread use in severe chronic cancer pain, especially among those near the end of life. Whether these invasive high-tech strategies are appropriate for patients with other kinds of chronic pain remains controversial. These techniques are very expensive, but third-party payers, including Medicare, often reimburse for their use. Ethical issues have been raised about the application of high-tech strategies for patients who might be equally well managed by using oral medications that are not reimbursable. In general, these methods should be used only when oral medications become ineffective or the oral route of administration is no longer viable. More work needs to be done to justify these risky and expensive techniques that need to be carefully monitored in nursing homes, home care, and other low-tech long-term care settings.

Nonpharmacologic Strategies for Pain Management

Nonpharmacologic strategies, used alone or in combination with appropriate analgesic medications, should be an integral part of the care plan for most elderly patients with significant pain problems. Nonpharmacologic strategies for pain management encompass a broad range of treatments

Table 25-9   Nonpharmacologic Strategies for Pain Management

Treatment	Indications	Comments
Education	All patients and caregivers.	Content should include basic knowledge about pain (diagnosis, treatment, complications, and prognosis), other available treatment options, and information about over-the-counter medications and self-help strategies.
Exercise	All patients with stable chronic pain.	Can be tailored for individual patient needs and lifestyle. Moderate-intensity exercise should be maintained for 30 minutes or more three to four times a week and continued indefinitely.
Cognitive-behavioral therapy	Most patients with chronic pain and good cognitive function.	Should be conducted by a trained therapist.
Physical modalities (heat, cold, and massage)	Most patients with chronic pain. Avoid heat on acute injuries. Use caution against thermal injuries on patients with cognitive impairment.	A variety of techniques are available for application.
Physical or occupational therapy	Impaired range of motion, specific muscle weakness, or other physical impairments associated with acute or chronic pain.	Should be conducted by a trained therapist.
Chiropractic	Stable acute or chronic back pain.	Potential spinal cord or nerve root impingement should be ruled out prior to any spinal manipulation.
Acupuncture	Postoperative dental pain; data less convincing for headache, fibromyalgia, low-back pain, tennis elbow, and carpel tunnel syndrome.	Should be provided only by a qualified acupuncturist.
Transcutaneous electrical nerve stimulation (TENS)	Acute or chronic regional pain.	Should initially be applied and adjusted by an experienced professional.
Relaxation and distraction techniques	Patients with good attention.	Patients with cognitive impairment may not be good candidates.

and physical modalities. Table 25-9 lists some common nonpharmacologic strategies for pain management along with some comments about their use. Many of these strategies carry little risk for adverse effects. Although many of these interventions provide short-term relief, few have greater benefit than control groups in randomized trials for elderly patients. Nonetheless, nonpharmacologic interventions used in combination with appropriate drug regimens often improve overall pain management, enhancing therapeutic effects while allowing medication doses to be kept to a minimum to prevent adverse drug effects.

The importance of patient education cannot be overstated. Studies show that patient education programs alone significantly improve overall pain management. This is especially true of preoperative preparation for surgery or other painful procedures. Such programs often include content about the nature of pain, how to use pain diaries and pain assessment instruments, how to use medications appropriately, and how to use self-help nondrug strategies. Family caregiver education is also important for many patients. Whether conducted in groups or individually, it should be tailored for individual patient needs and level of understanding. Use of written materials and appropriate methods of reinforcement is important to the overall success of the program.

Physical exercise is important for most patients with pain. A program of exercise can be tailored to most patients needs and is extremely important for rehabilitation, and the maintenance of strength, flexibility, and endurance. Clinical trials of older patients with chronic musculoskeletal pain show that moderate levels of exercise (aerobic and resistance training) on a regular basis are effective in improving pain and functional status. Initial training for chronic pain patients usually requires 8 to 12 weeks of supervision by a professional with expertise in the needs of older people with musculoskeletal disorders. A training program can be tailored for the individual's needs, lifestyle, and preference, given the lack of evidence of one form of exercise being more effective than another. The intensity of exercise along with frequency and duration must be adjusted to avoid exacerbation of the underlying condition while gradually increasing, and later maintaining, overall conditioning. Creating a disciplined routine of regular exercise is important because improvement in symptoms may suggest otherwise. Continued encouragement and reinforcement is often required. Unless complications arise, the program of exercise should be maintained indefinitely to prevent deconditioning and deterioration.

Psychological strategies are also helpful for some patients with significant pain. Cognitive therapies are aimed at altering belief systems and attitudes about pain and suffering. They include various forms of distraction, relaxation, biofeedback, and hypnosis. Behavioral therapies are aimed at enhancing healthy behaviors and at discouraging abnormal behavior that is unpredictable and self-defeating. Cognitive therapy can be combined with behavioral approaches, and together they are known as cognitive-behavioral therapy. Cognitive-behavioral therapy in its purest form includes a structured approach to teaching coping skills that might be used alone or in combination with analgesic medications and other nondrug strategies for chronic pain control. Trained professionals can conduct effective programs with individual patients or in groups, and there is some evidence that the effect is enhanced with caregiver involvement. Although it may not be appropriate for those with significant cognitive impairment, there is evidence from randomized trials to support the use of cognitive-behavioral therapy for many patients with significant chronic pain.

Finally, many patients use a variety of alternative therapies with or without the knowledge or recommendation of their physician or other primary care provider. Alternative medicine approaches to chronic pain may include homeopathy, spiritual healing, or the growing market of nutriceuticals (vitamin, herbal, and natural remedies). Although there is little scientific evidence to support these strategies for pain control, it is important that health care providers not abandon patients or leave them with a sense of hopelessness in an effort to debunk health care quackery and fraud.

SPECIAL ISSUES

Improving the Quality of Chronic Pain Care for Vulnerable Older Patients

Health care systems have an obligation to improve the quality of pain management for older persons. Beyond epidemiology studies that suggest many older persons in hospitals and nursing homes suffer substantially, little is known about existing quality of medical care provided to frail older patients with chronic pain. There is often little consensus among clinicians regarding specific structures and processes that insure good pain management. Recently, regulators and survey organizations turned their attention to assessment of quality of care in pain management. The Joint Commission on Hospital Accreditation, state license boards, and other agencies are scrutinizing hospitals, nursing homes, and other facilities' care of pain problems. The American Geriatric Society's clinical practice recommendations on chronic and persistent pain management have raised attention and helped fuel the need for quality improvement in pain management. Finally, recent development and publication of valid indicators for measuring quality of care for elderly patients with chronic pain may finally provide substantial methods for defining and measuring quality of care for older persons with chronic pain. Table 25-10 lists recently published valid indicators for quality of care in elderly persons with chronic pain.

Care Settings

Nursing homes and home care settings may present some unique challenges to pain management. Initial assessment of acute and chronic pain is often difficult in these settings. Medical records are often inadequate. Consultants

Table 25-10   Validated Indicators of Quality of Care for Chronic Pain in Vulnerable Elderly Persons

- All vulnerable elderly people should be screened for chronic pain during the initial evaluation period.
- All vulnerable elderly people should be screened for chronic pain every 2 years.
- If a vulnerable elderly person has a newly reported chronic painful condition, then a targeted history and physical should be initiated within 1 month.
- If a vulnerable elderly person has been prescribed a nonsteroidal antiinflammatory drug (NSAID) for the treatment of chronic pain, then the medical record should indicate whether he or she has a history of peptic ulcer disease, and if a history is present, justification of NSAID use should be documented.
- If a patient with chronic pain is treated with opioids, then the patient should be offered a bowel regimen or the medical record should document the potential for constipation or explain why bowel treatment is not needed.
- If a vulnerable elderly person has a newly reported chronic painful condition, then treatment should be offered.
- If a vulnerable elderly person is treated for a chronic painful condition, then he or she should be assessed for a response within 6 months.

SOURCE: Chodosh J et al: Quality indicators for pain management in vulnerable elders. *Ann Intern Med* 135(8 Pt 2):731, 2001.

are often not available. These settings do not routinely provide diagnostic laboratories, x-rays or other procedures that are common in hospitals and clinics. Lack of convenient transportation can make frequent clinic visits impossible or fraught with iatrogenic complications such as missed medications, missed meals, and records that are unavailable or unshared. For some patients, short hospitalization may be required while a diagnosis is established, a plan of care is formulated, and severe pain is stable. It is important for clinicians who care for these patients to recognize the limitations of such settings and plan effective strategies to overcome some of the barriers to pain management.

Clinicians who care for patients in nursing homes and home care settings must help to establish a care plan that is reasonable given the limited resources and skills often available in these settings. Medication regimens should be simplified as much a possible. Long-acting medications should be used whenever possible to provide longer durations of comfort and fewer doses that nurses or other caregivers have to administer. Short-acting, fast-onset medications should also be available for pain associated with physical activities or other circumstances. Treatment should be simplified so that nighttime monitoring and sleep interruptions can be minimized. It is important to remember that patients in nursing homes and at home do not usually have pharmacies and other medical resources on a 24-hour basis. Contingency plans for pain management must be anticipated so that delays do not occur during medication changes or dosage adjustments. Institutional limits on use of heating pads for fear of thermal injuries, limits on visiting hours, or use of television or radios for distraction techniques should not be so rigid as to create barriers to pain relief for some patients in nursing homes.

Although it is often assumed that patients will be more comfortable at home, this is not always the case. Despite the willingness of some patients to sacrifice good pain management in order to be at home, the tradeoff can result in substantial suffering. In fact, being home bound often results in having limited access to medications and many nondrug strategies. For patients with severe pain, home care often places substantial demands on family caregivers who see loved ones in pain and don't know what to do.

Studies of elderly cancer patients and their informal caregivers suggest that caregivers often administer medication, deciding what to give and when to give it. Family members often miss work to provide transportation to and from distant facilities. Also, they are interrupted from sleep for medication doses and other treatments. At the same time, family members are often stressed by seeing themselves in the role of reducing suffering while controlling medications and preventing addiction. Intense demands on inexperienced family and friends can result in substantial stress and caregiver burnout. These issues may lead to patients being sent to local emergency rooms to solve health care access problems. This results in many iatrogenic complications from health care personnel who are unfamiliar with individual patient needs and primary goals of care. Clinicians who work in nursing homes and home care need to help develop appropriate structure and processes of care that insure delivery of quality pain management services, especially for those who are physically disabled and near the end of life.

REFERENCES

AGS Panel on Persistent Pain in Older Persons: The management of persistent pain in older persons. *J Am Geriatr Soc* 50:5205–24, 2002.

Arthritis Pain Management Panel: *Guidelines for the Management of Pain in Osteoarthritis, Rheumatoid Arthritis, and Juvenile Chronic Arthritis.* Glenview, IL, American Pain Society, 2002.

Ferrell BA: Pain, in Osterweil D et al. (eds): *Comprehensive Geriatric Assessment.* New York, McGraw-Hill, 2000, p 381.

Gibson SG, Helme RD: Age-related differences in pain perception and report. *Clin Geriatr Med* 17:433, 2001.

Gloth FM III: Pain management in older adults: Prevention and treatment. *J Am Geriatr Soc* 49:188, 2001.

MacLean CH: Quality indicators for the management of osteoarthritis in vulnerable elders. *Ann Intern Med* 135:711, 2001.

O'Grady M et al: Therapeutic and physical exercise prescription for older adults with joint disease: An evidence-based approach. *Rheum Dis Clin North Am* 26:617, 2000.

Pain and Policy Studies Group: Annual review of state pain policies 2000. University of Wisconsin, 2000. Available: http://www.medsch.wisc.edu/painpolicy.

C H A P T E R 2 6

Care of the Dying Patient

KARL LORENZ • JOANNE LYNN

DEFINITION AND HISTORY OF PALLIATIVE CARE

Although coming to the end of life often entails physical and existential suffering, it can also be a time of extraordinary insight for patients and families. Increased attention to the distinctive challenges of caring for persons with chronic, eventually fatal illness has led to a type of practice called *palliative care,* which is defined by the World Health Organization as, "the active total care of patients whose disease is not responsive to curative treatment. Control of pain, of other symptoms, and of psychological, social, and spiritual problems is paramount. The goal of palliative care is achievement of the best possible quality of life for patients and their families." In other words, physicians have a responsibility to help persons with life-limiting illness to live as well as possible. Geriatricians have a special obligation to excel in palliative care because elderly persons do not usually "graduate" to some other care provider before the end of life, so almost every geriatric patient lives out the end of life in our care.

In 1900, most Americans died of an unexpected, relatively quick disease process. However, advances in housing, sanitation, food production, and medical care have altered life expectancy. Most Americans born in the latter half of the twentieth century can expect to live beyond the age of 70 years and to die of complications of chronic diseases (Table 26-1). Although physicians may be prompted to consider palliation because the patient has an obviously terminal condition such as metastatic cancer, geriatricians must consider incorporating palliative principles into care across the full spectrum of conditions represented by chronic, eventually fatal illness. The field of palliative care initially developed in response to patients and families seeking an alternative to aggressive, costly, and unwanted life-sustaining medical treatments, and palliative care offers helpful approaches to clinicians in the care of all patients approaching the end of their lives.

Demographic trends contribute to the urgent need to address deficiencies in end-of-life care. In the United States, very large numbers of the baby boomers born just after World War II will begin turning 65 years old in 2011, and aged persons living with chronic illness will constitute an increasingly large proportion of the population.

Throughout the world, increasing longevity is translating into rapidly growing elderly populations. In addition, because much health care spending occurs near the end of life, growth in aged populations, as well as numbers of chronically ill persons, will create pressure on health care budgets and require new approaches to care in order to restrain health care costs in the chronically ill, elderly population.

PALLIATIVE CARE APPROACH TO THE PATIENT

Palliative medicine starts with recognition by the patient, family, and physician that the patient is in the last phase of his or her life. Trajectories of illness at the end of life vary by disease (Fig. 26-1). Some patients, mostly those with common cancers, often have a prolonged period of slow loss in function followed by an evident and steep decline in their functional status in their last 1 to 2 months. In contrast, patients with chronic organ system failures like congestive heart failure have more severe ongoing disability, with background decline that is punctuated by episodes of acute decompensation. Persons in a third category, "frailty," experience gradual, prolonged decline from a multitude of conditions, often including cognitive impairment. Predicting death within a few months for patients with malignancy is fairly reliable once their function begins to decline. Prognostication for those with congestive heart failure or dementia is much less precise (Fig. 26-2). Prediction of duration of life and course in those with frailty may be least precise, given the as yet incomplete characterization of this perhaps quintessential geriatric syndrome (Chap. 117). Because of these considerations and because attention to palliation addresses important patient needs (e.g., symptom relief, treatment planning), providers should implement a palliative approach concurrently with other types of treatment such as rehabilitation and secondary prevention.

Although addressing symptoms, family concerns, and emotional caring are part of good care in general, a palliative approach should be considered when disease, age, and frailty raise the concerns and challenges of the last phase of life, even though death may be months or years

Table 26-1   How Americans Die: A Century of Change

	1900	2000
Age at death:	46 years	78 years
Top causes:	Infection Accident Childbirth	Cardiovascular disease Cancer Organ-system failure
Disability:	Not much	2–4 years before death
Financing:	Private, modest	Public and substantial—83% in Medicare Approximately 50% of women die in Medicaid
Site of death:	Home	Hospital, nursing home

Trajectory of Dying for Lung Cancer or CHF

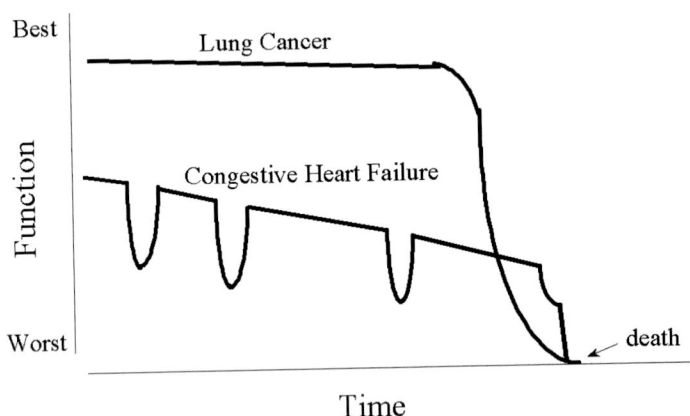

Figure 26-1   Trajectory of dying for lung cancer or congestive heart failure.

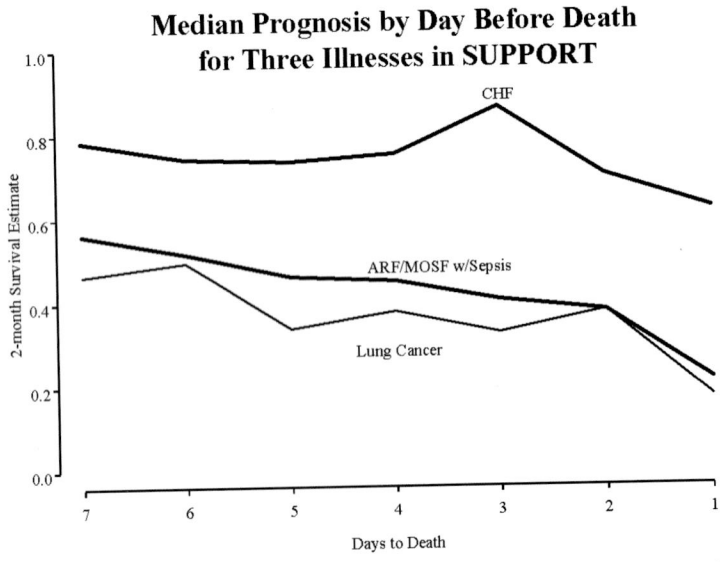

Figure 26-2   Median prognosis by day before death for three illnesses in SUPPORT (Study to Understand Prognosis and Preferences for Outcomes and Risks of Treatment).

Table 26-2   Hospice and the Medicare Hospice Benefit

Characteristics of the Hospice Approach	Characteristics of the Medicare Hospice Benefit
Nursing directed	Enrollment requires prognosis of 6 months or less
Home centered	Comprehensive (all services provided for typical rate of about $100 per day)
Holistic (includes explicit spiritual care and bereavement support)	Recertification required but no lifetime benefit limit
Family as unit of care	Permits hospice care in home, nursing home, and other residential settings
Focus on pain and symptom management and very basic medical care	Includes routine home, continuous home, respite, and inpatient levels of care

in coming. Although it does not identify all patients who could benefit from palliative approaches, one empirically helpful way to identify patients who might benefit from a palliative approach has been to ask the simple question "Would you be surprised if this patient died in the next year?" Providers' affirmation of the possibility of death signals that they should carefully consider palliative issues in the total plan of care. In contrast, to qualify for formal hospice care, Medicare specifically requires a 6-month prognosis, and this requirement has been translated into specific criteria. This high standard of prognostic precision is usually unobtainable until very late in the course of disease, particularly in the care of persons with noncancer conditions. Hence, hospice care is a more rigidly defined subset of palliative care, which has a coherent set of philosophical principles and practices without a specific timeline for their application in a particular case (Table 26-2).

FACILITATING END-OF-LIFE DECISIONS

Facilitating end-of-life decisions is a challenging aspect of providing good palliative care. Physicians often need to help patients and their families come to terms with the possibility of death, yet physicians, patients, and their families are often reluctant to engage this subject directly. After assessing what patients actually know, physicians must be sensitive to patients' varying desires for information. Some patients may demand full disclosure while other patients prefer not to be informed directly about their condition. Similarly, some patients may wish to discuss such issues privately while others desire to involve significant friends or family members. Moreover, coming to terms with these issues often requires time and multiple encounters and is always potentially subject to change. Hence, mapping the course of this complex and dynamic process in any given patient requires patience on the part of practitioners of palliative care.

Making allowance for patients' cultural preferences and by using everyday language, physicians should directly address medical conditions and prognosis. Such discussions can be highly emotional, and patients and families may

often forget important details following such discussions. Asking patients and families to repeat the most important information during such discussions is helpful, and allowing sufficient time for empathetic emotional communication is essential. Frequently asking patients and family members how they are feeling permits participants to reflect upon and find meaning in their emotions and thoughts. Expert physician communicators are noted for extensive listening, giving less technical information, and fully exploring psychosocial issues.

From the patient's perspective, coming to terms with dying is a developmental process, and "acceptance" is neither inevitable nor predictable. The physician's role is to facilitate that development in a culturally appropriate manner—throughout the chronology of illness to provide clear, accurate information, involve important persons, and avoid undesired outcomes. Palliative care requires more rather than less medical skill; in addition to a sophisticated knowledge of what is medically possible, palliative care requires a humanistic sensitivity to the patient that integrates these goals and values in specific treatment decisions. Because patients and families often lack the physician's technical medical knowledge, clinicians inevitably must elicit general guidance from patients and families and anchor treatment decisions in those values and assumptions (Table 26-3). Providing appropriate preference-guided care means constantly reassessing patients' and families' general goals, because they may change in unanticipated ways over the course of illness.

Disagreement about medical treatment can occur among providers, patients, and their families near the end of life. In the case of a competent patient, providers should provide care that is both consistent with the patient's best interests and respectful of the patient's autonomy. While ultimately respecting the patient, providers should be sensitive to family concerns in decision making, because family members must continue to live with the consequences of decisions made. On one hand, patients may make requests of providers that conflict with provider values or that are medically ineffective (e.g., chelation therapy for metastatic cancer). Physicians are not obligated to provide treatments when patient or family requests are medically ineffective.

Table 26-3 Helpful Questions in Eliciting Patient and Family Goals and Values

What are you expecting?

What do you most want to accomplish?

What is most important in your life right now?

What are you hoping for?

What do you hope to avoid?

What do you think will happen?

What are you afraid will happen?

What gives your life joy or meaning?

What would be left undone, if you were to die soon?

SOURCE: Emanuel LL et al: *Goals of Care. EPEC Participants Handbook.* EPEC Project [Module 7] Chicago, American Medical Association, 1999, pM7.

However, competent patients may also express seemingly irrational treatment preferences that differ from the choices providers would make for themselves. When the situation permits, simply deferring and revisiting decisions can be helpful. In addition, providers can explore the personal context (e.g., values, past experiences, emotions, psychosocial context) that lead patients to make such decisions. Through sensitively exploring the context underlying treatment decisions, physicians can understand how the patient is viewing the situation and therefore how a successful decision can be made (Table 26-4). Physicians should also be aware that the way treatments are presented (e.g., "framing effects") can have significant impacts on how patients perceive choices; one approach is to present treatment alternatives by using alternative framings of an issue (e.g., 50 percent of persons will live versus 50 percent of persons will die).

Conflict can also occur between families and physicians. Often, patients do not have clearly expressed wishes regarding treatment, even though they may have expressed

Table 26-4 Issues Important to Persons at the End of Life

Pain and symptom management

Communication about treatment decisions

Preparation for death

Achieving completion

Contributing to others

Being known as a whole person

SOURCES: Steinhauser KE et al: In search of a good death: Observations of patients, families, and providers. *Ann Internal Med* 132(10):825, 2000, and Steinhauser KE et al: Factors considered important at the end of life by patients, family, physicians, and other care providers. *JAMA* 284(19):2476, 2000.

general goals that help guide care. Families often seek information from sources other than the medical team, and they may have difficulty assimilating information because of denial, grieving, guilt, or other emotional conflict because of its sheer volume and complexity. Families may also be uncertain about the goals or outcomes of care, and dysfunctional relationships often noted in long histories of family dysfunction may be unmasked by stress (but potentially healed in the palliative care process). Conflicts may be rooted in basic disagreement over values among family members and between the family and healthcare providers (e.g., differences on the priority of the sanctity over quality of life). Serving these patients well requires that physicians provide empathetic listening to concerns, explore the decision-making dynamic and values underlying treatment choices, allow emotional expression and grieving, and patiently express genuine concern and commitment to promote the well-being and interests of the patient.

MEDICAL MANAGEMENT OF SPECIFIC SYMPTOMS

General Principles

Minimizing physical symptoms is a very important goal for most persons with chronic, eventually fatal illness. Unrelieved physical symptoms can promote psychological distress in both patients and caregivers. All physicians should be competent to palliate some common symptoms (e.g., pain), although the diseases and treatment settings that typify a physician's practice will affect the specific symptoms that a physician is called upon to treat. Although they are not population-based, surveys of community hospice providers and palliative medicine services give some insight into the rate of common symptoms at the end of life (Table 26-5). Conventional medical treatments have an important role in treating physical symptoms (e.g., anticancer therapies), but one also must minimize treatments that will not be effective in helping patients achieve desired goals and especially those that are likely to cause harm.

Symptom Management
Pain (See also Chap. 25)

Of all the symptoms common in end-of-life care, pain is one of the most feared and most prevalent. Attending to any other activity becomes impossible when a person is overwhelmed by pain. Pain may reflect distress as a result of physical, psychological, and spiritual factors. The prevalence and intensity of pain varies with the type of disease; although the majority of cancer patients experience serious pain, especially as their disease progresses, pain also commonly occurs in noncancer conditions, and pain is a frequent iatrogenic complication of medical treatments. Skilled practitioners should become familiar with a variety of pain syndromes that can occur in the course of illness at the end of life.

Table 26-5   Taxonomy of Physician–Patient Treatment Conflicts and Approaches

Source of Conflict	Approach
1. Bias toward present and near future harms or benefits	1. Clarify the future harm or benefit
2. Belief in personal invulnerability	2. Distinguish between patients who acknowledge but accept risk and patients who deny the possibility of untoward events (e.g., "It can't happen to me")
3. Fear of the medical experience	3. Help patients distinguish between a fear they wish to overcome and a deliberate choice with which they are truly comfortable
4. Unusual or rationally incompatible goals	4. Distinguish between an authentic but unusual request (e.g., religious refusal of blood transfusion) and a distorted decision based on a condition such as depression

SOURCE: Brock DW and Wartman SA (1990).

Pain varies temporally in an individual patient (i.e., with activity, emotional state, and treatment), and individual patient perceptions and reports of pain vary widely. Good care therefore requires regular assessment of pain intensity over time to understand the individual factors that exacerbate pain and promote pain relief (in certain contemporary circles, pain is called the "fifth vital sign"). In addition, because of individual variation in perception and expression, pain intensity should be evaluated with standard rating instruments, especially when multiple providers are involved in assessing and treating an individual patient. Monitoring these ratings at various times of day and over several days may improve evaluation of the patient's chronic pain burden and response to treatment.

The goal of treatment is not just pain relief, but also its prevention. Therefore, one should aim for continuous and efficacious medication treatment matched to the various mediators of chronic pain. In addition to evaluating psychological and spiritual factors that can contribute to pain perception, pain assessment should include a careful physical exam and identification of nociceptive and neuropathic components because these factors can be considered separately in terms of treatment. Evaluation of pain and other symptoms should include eliciting understanding of how the symptom impacts daily life. This is helpful in assessing pain severity and in evaluating the effectiveness of treatment.

Opioids can be administered orally and by a variety of mucosal routes, intravenously, or directly to the central nervous system (e.g., intraspinal). Limited only by side effects, opioids should be increased to whatever dose is necessary to relieve pain in the patient being managed according to the principles of palliative care. Patients usually accommodate after a few days to adverse opioid side effects of sedation and nausea while maintaining benefit in terms of pain relief. Other opioid side effects can include histamine-induced pruritus and myoclonus at high doses. The regular side effect of constipation should be anticipated and prevented by a concomitant bowel program of regular and aggressive laxatives whenever chronic opioids are initiated. The opioid class includes many drugs that are available as combinations with aspirin, acetaminophen, and other compounds, and the dosing of combination products is usually limited by the toxicity of the nonopioid components (Table 26-6).

When initiating pain treatment in institutionalized settings, physicians should be cognizant of barriers to the use of "as-needed" medication. An alternative approach is to prescribe opioids on a regular schedule and provide parameters (e.g., for excessive sedation or reduced respiratory frequency) for calling the physician to avoid withholding treatment. Expert opinion suggests that patients whose pain becomes severe while on opioids may benefit from total daily dose increases of 50 to 100 percent above baseline, and patients who develop mild to moderate pain may have their total daily dose increased 25 to 50 percent above baseline. These rates of increase apply even at large baseline doses.

When patients are taking large daily doses of short-acting opioids, it is helpful to convert to longer-acting agents, with short-acting drugs for management of breakthrough pain. Short-acting opioid doses may be escalated every 2 hours, and long-acting oral opioids are best increased daily with short-acting supplements to bridge any shortfall. Changing from short-acting to longer-acting drugs involves dose conversion when drugs have differing potencies. Physicians can consult a standard table of relative potencies when changing from one opiate to the other, but partial cross-tolerance may require reducing the total dose by up to 50 percent. Conversion must also make allowance for differences in the route of administration. The equally effective dose of oral morphine is generally about one-third of the IV or SQ dose (e.g., divide the oral dose by three when changing po to IV or SQ). Impaired renal and hepatic function should modify the timing and amount of dose escalation or lead to consideration of drugs with alternative metabolism (e.g., methadone in renal failure). In a pain emergency, or when permanent intravenous access facilitates, IV opioids can be given continuously with close monitoring and titrated to pain relief or sedation. Cognitively intact patients may effectively participate in their own treatment using patient-controlled analgesia (PCA).

Although opioids can be effective in treating all types of pain, other medications may be more specific, especially in treating neuropathic pain. Irritation, damage, or

Table 26-6 Common Symptoms in Colorado Community Hospice Patients

Symptom	Present (%)*	Severe, When Symptom Present(%)‡
Lack of energy	83	46
Pain	76	14
Lack of appetite	63	31
Feeling drowsy	61	21
Difficulty concentrating	60	31
Feeling sad	51	19
Shortness of breath	48	26
Agitation	48	17
Worrying	43	15
Cough	42	11
Nervousness	42	16
Constipation	39	18
Irritability	38	13
Swelling of arms or legs	36	24
Difficulty sleeping	35	11
Weight loss	35	15
Dry mouth	34	17
Difficulty swallowing	30	30
Changes in skin	26	34

N = 348

*Present: answer other than "do not have" or "do not know."

‡Severe: "severe" or "very severe."

SOURCE: Kutner JS et al. (2001).

destruction of the nerve itself results in pain that patients often characterize as sharp, lancinating, tingling, or burning. Antidepressant, anticonvulsant, and other medications have been found to be quite helpful in relieving these symptoms, sometimes even without the addition of narcotic analgesia. Adjuvant medications may make other analgesic medications much more effective. Anxiolytics decrease the amplification of specific pain sensations and allow the patient to perceive the presence of pain with less discomfort. Many clinicians prefer lorazepam for anxiolysis because of its equal efficacy when given by oral, intramuscular, or intravenous routes. However, many other anxiolytics are also commonly used, including other

benzodiazepines, buspirone, and major tranquilizers with sedative effects.

Patients may find other nondrug treatments of pain helpful, including splinting, local wound or injury treatment, biofeedback, or acupuncture. Although many nondrug and alternative treatments have not been rigorously studied, patients may benefit and physicians may endorse such efforts when they carry a low risk of harm. Physicians should be aware of toxicities and interactions of herbal preparations with conventional therapy. Certain drugs are contraindicated in treating chronic pain. These include meperidine, pentazocine, butorphanol, and nalbuphine. Meperidine is a relatively weak and short-acting analgesic compared with morphine, and causes accumulation of normeperidine, a toxic metabolite that can lead to seizures or delirium after a few doses. Pentazocine, butorphanol, and nalbuphine should generally be avoided because of their psychotomimetic effects and low maximal efficacy. In addition, partial agonists should be used with care because they block pain receptors from stronger medications, and thus combined use may cause withdrawal.

Depression

Depression is often entangled with the many other symptoms that patients experience at the end of life. For example, depression and pain are mutually reinforcing and must be considered together. In addition, the usual diagnostic criteria for depression do not account for the fact that reduced appetite, weight loss, fatigue, difficulty sleeping, declining activity, and diminishing social involvement are so common as to be the norm with advancing illness at the end of life. Finally, patients understandably experience grief in anticipation of their own death, and normal grieving and depression share many features. Because they are not actually an enduring component of normal dying, psychological criteria such as depressed mood, feelings of worthlessness or guilt, feelings of helplessness or hopelessness, or suicidal ideation are more helpful than vegetative symptoms in distinguishing depression from other conditions at the end of life. A time-limited trial of antidepressant treatment is often warranted.

A great number of drugs are available to treat depression, so the choice depends on the short-term prognosis, likely efficacy, and side effects. One important aspect of addressing depressive symptoms is providing empathetic emotional and spiritual support which can be highly therapeutic. Successfully addressing pain and other physical symptoms can also have a remarkable impact on affective symptoms. Methylphenidate, dextroamphetamine, and pemoline have rapid response time, which is an advantage when the patient's prognosis is very limited. Conventional antidepressants may be effective and should be considered when patients have longer life expectancy (i.e., several months) or when they may have particular efficacy for troubling symptoms (e.g., tricyclics for neuropathic pain). Treatment should consider the potential side effects of various strategies that can be harmful (e.g., appetite suppression) or helpful (e.g., sedative, anxiolytic), depending on the clinical situation (Table 26-7).

Dyspnea

Dyspnea, or difficulty breathing, is a common symptom with a multifactorial etiology. Both chronic and acute dyspnea may occur in the course of terminal illness. If a reversible or treatable lung condition is present, such as upper airway obstruction, pleural effusion, or bronchospasm, this should be addressed directly. When such a reversible etiology for dyspnea is not present, low doses of narcotics, especially morphine, are often effective, whether given orally or parenterally. Morphine often reduces "air hunger" by resetting the sensitivity of the brain to hypoxia or hypercarbia. Low doses of morphine, titrated to effect, are very unlikely to cause death by respiratory depression. Instead, a dose of morphine can usually be found that relieves the person's dyspnea and allows him or her to live more comfortably. Morphine risks being a lethal respiratory depressant only in high doses, and generally only in the opioid-naïve patient.

Carefully titrated anxiolytics such as the benzodiazepines may relieve dyspnea without respiratory depression. Oxygen can be of subjective assistance in relieving dyspnea in some patients and is commonly used. Increasing airflow to the patient's face by means of a portable fan may be effective. In addition, airway secretion management by means of anticholinergic drugs (e.g., hyoscyamine, atropine, scopolamine), and suctioning can be helpful.

Constipation

Constipation is a common symptom at the end of life that may be caused directly by diseases that affect the gastrointestinal tract or its innervation, associated with metabolic complications (e.g., hypercalcemia), or it may result from side effects of medications commonly used in palliative care (e.g., opioids). Plain radiography can help to distinguish bowel obstruction when patients present with obstipation, abdominal distention, and pain. In addition to general medical measures, specific treatments (e.g., surgery) may maintain bowel patency and alleviate symptoms in gastrointestinal malignancy, but they must be considered in light of the patient's longevity and goals of care.

Constipation should be anticipated and prevented when initiating chronic opioid therapy by adding stimulant laxatives to the pain regimen. Physical maneuvers (e.g., disimpaction and enemas) may be helpful in the initial treatment of constipation. Bulk laxatives and stool softeners are not useful in acute treatment and may not be as useful in preventing constipation, because many causes of constipation in palliative care are associated with decreased bowel motility. Stimulant laxatives, such as senna, cascara, and bisacodyl usually are more helpful as preventatives. Similarly, lubricants, such as mineral oil, or osmotically active laxatives, such as sorbitol or magnesium citrate, can be highly effective prophylactically or in treating constipation when obstruction is not present.

Anorexia and Weight Loss

Patients and families often are troubled by anorexia and weight loss. Families usually see providing food as part of basic human caring—and anorexia and weight loss may provoke anticipatory grief and guilt. Patients and families can be reassured that anorexia often accompanies the dying process. In addition, for the dying person, eating can become intrusive and uncomfortable. Artificial feeding by means of nasogastric tubes, gastrostomy tubes, or intravenous nutrition may lead only to more complications, discomfort, and earlier death. Meta-analysis of parenteral feeding studies in cancer patients found that increased calorie consumption leads to faster tumor growth and earlier death. Artificial feeding with dementia patients may yield more pneumonia and aspiration.

However, feeding and artificial feeding have so many layers of meaning to patients and families that physicians need to raise and discuss this issue thoughtfully when planning care. Physicians should attend to the entire gastrointestinal tract when evaluating a patient with anorexia and cachexia. Recognizing the risk, patients and families may be reassured and given permission to attempt feeding as tolerated when medical complications (e.g., aspiration) are not a paramount concern. A patient may benefit from a trial of appetite stimulants such as megestrol acetate which sometimes restores a sense of well being to the patient. Other interventions that may be tried include low-dose steroids and dronabinol.

Nausea and Vomiting

When nausea and vomiting occur in the dying patient, concomitant constipation should be a foremost consideration. Ileus without constipation is also common during the dying process, as the bowel becomes less active in peristalsis. Standard antiemetic medications, such as prochlorperazine and promethazine, can be helpful. Many palliative care specialists prefer haloperidol because this drug is an effective antiemetic without much sedation and counteracts some of the mood-altering effects of narcotics. Tetrahydrocannabinol may also be mildly efficacious. When partial or complete obstruction occurs, reducing the normal bowel secretions by use of the somatostatin synthetic analog octreotide has proven effective in avoiding nasogastric suctioning or even surgical intervention. A combination of efforts usually is successful in gaining comfort without incurring the risks and discomfort of surgery.

Other Symptoms

Hiccups are uncommon but can be a particularly difficult symptom to deal with in terminal care. While intramuscular chlorpromazine is commonly recommended for breaking the cycle of intractable hiccups, it often does not work well with dying patients. Stimulation of the vagus nerve by touching the posterior pharynx with a nasogastric tube may be stop hiccups for a few minutes or a few hours. Decompression of over inflated bowels is one possible specific remedy. Some patients may require anesthesia or transection of the phrenic nerve.

Dry mouth can be quite bothersome near the end of life. Cardiac failure and hypotension, mouth breathing with

Table 26-7 Antidepressants Used in Palliative Care*

Agent	Advantages	Disadvantages	Onset of Action	Starting Dose (mg)	Usual Daily Dose (mg)	Maximum Dosage (mg/d)	Side Effects	Schedule
Psychostimulants[†] Methylphenidate Dextroamphetamine	Act rapidly, are well tolerated in elderly and debilitated patients; are effective adjuvant analgesic agents; counter opioid-induced fatigue; improve appetite and energy; are effective in 70%	Cardiac decompensation can occur in elderly patients and patients with heart disease, can cause confusion in old or cognitively impaired patients; infrequently, tolerance may develop	<24 h <24 h	25–5 25	10–20 5/10	60–90 60–90	A mean of 11% of patients experience restlessness, dizziness, nightmares, insomnia, palpitations, arrhythmia, tremor, and dry mouth; psychosis is rare	8:00 am and 12:00 noon 8:00 am and 12:00 noon
Premoline		Premoline can cause hepatocellular injury and choreoathetosis; hepatic function must be monitored regularly; should be used with caution in patients with renal failure	1–2 d	18.75	37.5	150	Produces minimal cardiac stimulation	Twice daily
SSRIs Sertraline	Are safe and effective with few side effects; cause little orthostatic hypotension, urinary retention, and	Inhibit cytochrome P45026, causing interactions with other drugs	2–4 wk	125–25	50–1000	200	Nausea, gastrointestinal distress	Once daily
Fluoxetine Paroxetine	sedation; have no effect on cardiac conduction; are easy to tritate	Fluoxetine has a long half-life; not tolerated as well as paroxetine and sertraline		5–10 10	20–40 20–40	60 60		Once daily Once daily

330

Tricyclics	Therapeutic response		2–4 wk	10–25	25–100	150	Adverse effects	At bedtime
Amitriptyline‡	Therapeutic response often seen at low dose; are effective for treatment of neuropathic pain; can be given parenterally	Not tolerated as well as nortriptyline and desipramine	2–4 wk	10–25	25–100	150	Adverse effects occur in as many as 34% of patients with cancer; not well tolerated in terminally ill patients because of anticholinergic side effects (dry mouth, delirium, constipation)	At bedtime
Imipramine	or compounded for rectal administration; drug levels can be monitored	Not tolerated as well as nortriptyline and desipramine		10–25	25–100	150		At bedtime
Doxepin‡				10–25	25–100	150		At bedtime
Desipramine				10–25	25–100	150		At bedtime
Nortriptyline				10–25	25–75	125		At bedtime

*Numbers in parentheses are reference numbers. SSRI, selective serotonin reuptake inhibitor.

†Physician should first prescribe a low dose, then increase dose gradually every 1 to 2 days until a therapeutic response or side effects occur or until the maximum dosage is reached.

‡Can be used in patients who have difficulty sleeping.

SOURCE: Block SD: Assessing and managing depression in the terminally ill patient. ACP-ASIM End-of-Life Care Consensus Panel. American College of Physicians - American Society of Internal Medicine. Ann Intern Med 132(3):209, 2000.

excessive drying of oral tissues, dehydration, or inadequate oral hygiene may cause a sensation of dry mouth. Local hygiene and assiduous moisturizing are helpful. Intravenous fluid challenge is usually not necessary or desirable because of its intrusiveness and its risks of pulmonary edema with worsening dyspnea.

As a person's body fails, the brain's changes may be manifest as anxiety, depression, delirium, hallucinations, or even seizures. As noted earlier, anxiety and depression, whether associated with pain or not, can be relieved with anxiolytics and antidepressants. Delirium needs to be evaluated on an individual basis, because it may be the result of drug side effects, sepsis, hypoxia, or some other remediable process. Control of patients' psychotic symptoms with antipsychotic medications is appropriate and efficacious when they are disturbing. Haloperidol is usually the drug of choice. Seizures may arise anew, especially as the person nears death. Intramuscular lorazepam is usually the best drug to try first, with phenytoin or phenobarbital as alternatives for recurrent and prolonged seizures.

Keeping a dying person clean is a valued labor that must not be overlooked. Attention to basic hygiene prevents skin breakdown, promotes more interaction with family and friends, and simply enhances basic human dignity. The need for personal care increases during the dying process. Sphincter control is often lost, leading to incontinence of urine and stool. Medications to increase sphincter tone or decrease detrusor activity are not usually appropriate, nor is toilet training or prompting. Instead, diapers, frequent changes of clothing, and bathing are often more comfortable and dignified. This points to the need for adequate resources, because this is time-intensive labor.

Pressure ulcers are common in the dying, although they should not be. Incontinence, hypotension, blood chemistry alterations, tissue shear forces when the patient is moved, and prolonged rest in one position all lead to pressure ulcers. These predisposing factors are difficult to avoid in the dying, although assiduous nursing care and use of special mattresses can prevent most breakdown. When pressure ulcers do develop, aggressive curative interventions, such as skin and tissue flaps or vigorous débridement, are uncomfortable and usually fail. Instead, local dressing treatments to maintain hygiene and analgesic medications to treat pain usually serve patients best.

Fungating tumors also can cause considerable discomfort because of the need for aggressive hygienic measures and because of disfigurement. Localized radiation treatment may be of some value in selected patients, such as those in whom superficial bleeding is prominent. Local measures to improve cleanliness and decrease smell (using topical antibiotics and frequent dressing changes) are important.

Pruritus is bothersome to many terminally ill persons. Itching may be caused by excessive washing of the skin with resulting xerosis. Liver dysfunction and stasis of bile acids, drug reaction, and other metabolic derangements also cause pruritus. Symptomatic treatment with skin emollients or anesthetics, with antihistamines, or with sedatives is usually effective. Treatment of the underlying disorder is worth considering.

Bereavement

Patients and families usually start the mourning process at the time a life-threatening disease is recognized. This anticipatory grief is a healthy part of normal end-of-life adjustments. Denial, anger, bargaining, depression, and acceptance often occur during this period, although with widely varying sequences and emphases. Care providers do well not to suggest one type of grief reaction over another. They should be supportive of the pattern evidenced, promote adaptive behaviors, and monitor for prolonged dysfunctional reactions that might require counseling intervention.

After a patient's death, family members and friends usually have a profound sense of loss. Hallucinations of seeing or hearing the dying person can be a normal part of the grieving process for up to 3 months after the death. Overreaction to perceived helpfulness or slights is common during the grieving process. Spousal loss is especially difficult and is associated with increased morbidity and mortality in the survivor. Those grieving often have considerable work to do in getting their lives put back together in a functional way while also making sense of the loss. The Medicare hospice benefit specifies that bereavement support should continue for at least 1 year after the death of the patient. Providing some follow-up support and assessment would be in order for deaths outside of hospice. Contact allows assessment of the progress of normal grieving and provides access to more focused treatment for those who are having serious problems.

HOSPICE AND OTHER PALLIATIVE SERVICES

Our modern approach to care at the end of life began when Dr. Cicely Saunders demonstrated a better approach to end-of-life care. In 1967, Dr. Saunders founded the famous St. Christopher's Hospice in South London. In 1983, Congress enacted the Medicare hospice benefit in the United States leading to rapid hospice growth; in the last decade, annual hospice admissions have increased from approximately 200,000 to 700,000 persons. Hospice provides comprehensive, continuous care directed at achieving comfort and encompassing social, spiritual, and psychological needs at the end of life. Almost all hospice services are provided in patients' homes, although some hospice programs may also provide service in nursing homes and other residential settings. In addition, the hospice benefit provides coverage for services not available under fee-for-service Medicare, including outpatient prescription drugs, respite care, homemakers, and bereavement support (Table 26-2). The management of pain and other symptoms is a particular focus of hospice care. The importance of such services to dying patients and family members has been substantiated in surveys of providers, families, and patients.

Medicare is the primary payer for hospice in the United States, and Medicaid's, and often private insurers', hospice benefits are usually modeled after Medicare. Medicare patients with an expected prognosis of 6 months or less are eligible for hospice services, and patients must

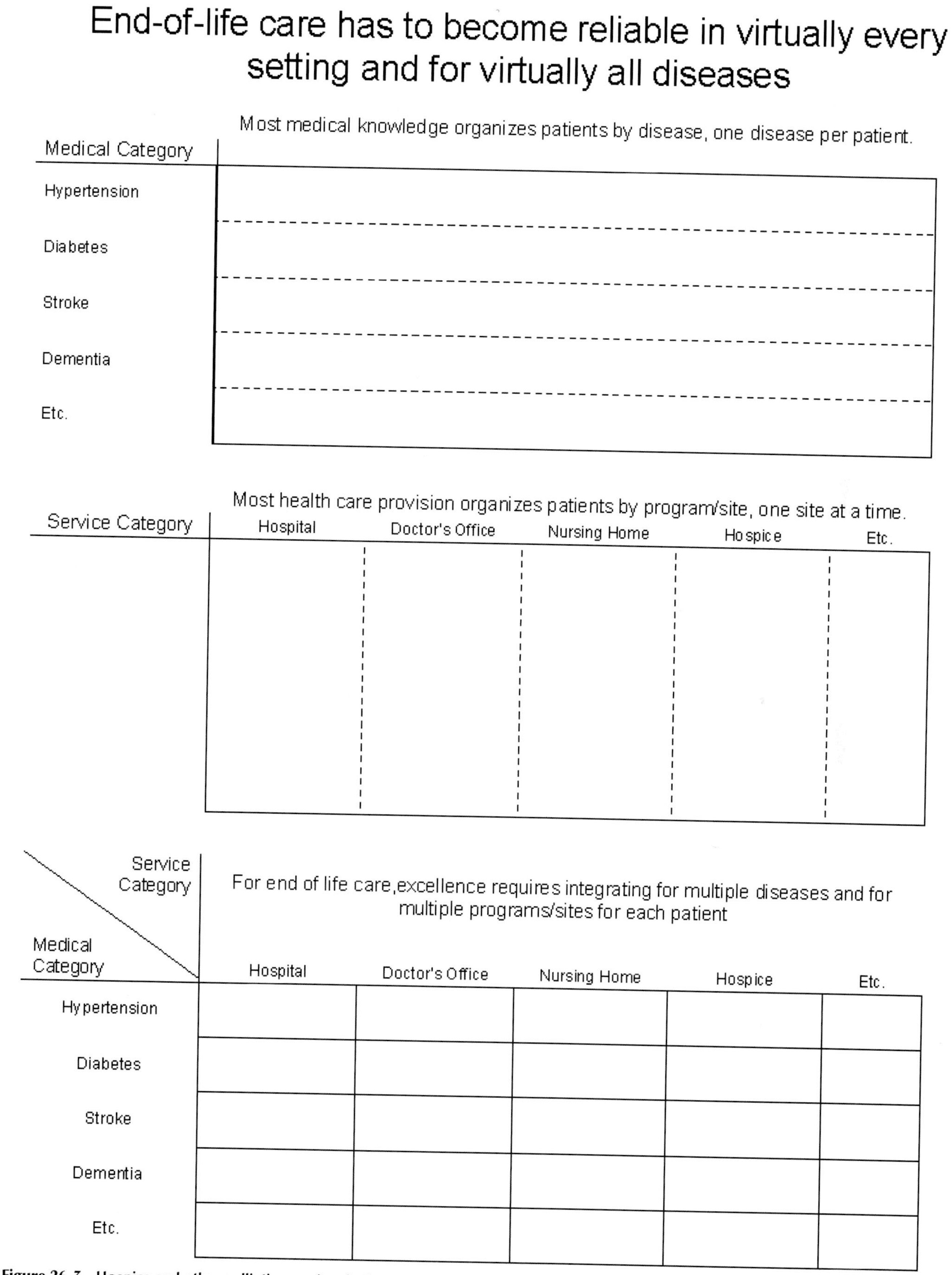

End-of-life care has to become reliable in virtually every setting and for virtually all diseases

Most medical knowledge organizes patients by disease, one disease per patient.

Medical Category
Hypertension
Diabetes
Stroke
Dementia
Etc.

Most health care provision organizes patients by program/site, one site at a time.

Service Category	Hospital	Doctor's Office	Nursing Home	Hospice	Etc.

For end of life care, excellence requires integrating for multiple diseases and for multiple programs/sites for each patient

Service Category / Medical Category	Hospital	Doctor's Office	Nursing Home	Hospice	Etc.
Hypertension					
Diabetes					
Stroke					
Dementia					
Etc.					

Figure 26-3   Hospice and other palliative services in the spectrum of end-of-life illness.

be recertified periodically based on their clinical condition. Hospice providers are paid a daily capitation rate for all services, although that rate varies with the intensity of service and includes all drugs, diagnostic and therapeutic treatment, equipment, and services related to the care of the terminal illness. Persons who elect hospice relinquish other Medicare coverage related to their terminal illness, although they retain Medicare coverage for unrelated conditions. An important implication is that any treatment for the terminal illness, for example, chemotherapy for end-stage cancer patients, must be reimbursed by the hospice out of its capitated payment.

The pioneering example of hospice has contributed importantly to subsequent efforts to improve the care of the dying. Patients and physicians often face a stark choice between curing and palliation when making a decision about enrolling in hospice, a decision that does not reflect the multiplicity of goals and treatments at the end of life. For example, patients may desire both symptom relief and longevity and their care system may make them give up access to anti-tumor therapy when entering hospice. Physicians and others have desired to eliminate the artificial distinction between curative and palliative care by offering comprehensive care such as that offered by hospice earlier in the care of serious illness.

In addition, the Study to Understand Prognoses and Preferences for Outcomes and Risks of Treatment (SUPPORT) and other research demonstrated serious deficiencies in the care of dying hospitalized patients. The realization that better hospital care was needed for the terminally ill has spurred the development of hospital-based palliative services. A growing number of hospitals currently have palliative care programs. In general, the organization and nomenclature of palliative services is in great flux. However, growing support for palliative care promises to eventually make palliative care available across all treatment settings, something that is badly needed and promises to benefit persons with life-limiting illness (Fig. 26-3).

REFERENCES

Brock DW, Wartman SA: When competent patients make irrational choices. *N Engl J Med* 322:1595, 1990.

Buckman R: *How to Break Bad News: A Guide for Health Care Professionals.* Baltimore, Johns Hopkins University Press, 1992.

Derek Doyle, Geoffrey W. Hanks and Neil MacDonald. Eds.: Oxford Textbook of Palliative Medicine. 2nd Edition. 1997. Oxford University Press.

Fox E et al: Evaluation of prognostic criteria for determining hospice eligibility in patients with advanced lung, heart, or liver disease. SUPPORT Investigators. Study to Understand Prognoses and Preferences for Outcomes and Risks of Treatments. *JAMA* 282(17):1638, 1999.

Goold SD et al: Conflicts regarding decisions to limit treatment: A differential diagnosis *JAMA* 283:909, 2000.

Kutner JS et al: Symptom burden at the end of life: Hospice providers' perceptions. *J Pain Symptom Manage* 21(6):473, 2001.

Lynn J: Perspectives on care at the close of life. Serving patients who may die soon and their families: the role of hospice and other services. *JAMA* 285(7):925, 2001.

Porter S, Knight C: *Assessment and Treatment of Pain in the Terminally Ill. American Academy of Hospice and Palliative Medicine UNIPAC Series.* Dubuque, IA, Kendall/Hunt Publishing, 1997.

Rosenfeld KE et al: End-of-life decision making: A qualitative study of elderly individuals. *J Gen Intern Med* 15(9):620, 2000.

Roter DL et al: Experts practice what they preach: A descriptive study of best and normative practices in end-of-life discussions. *Arch Intern Med* 160(22):3477, 2000.

Somogyi-Zalud E et al: Elderly persons' last six months of life: Findings from the Hospitalized Elderly Longitudinal Project. *J Am Geriatr Soc* 48(Suppl 5):S122, 2000.

The SUPPORT Investigators: A controlled trial to improve care for seriously ill hospitalized patients. Study to Understand Prognoses and Preferences for Outcomes and Risks of Treatments (SUPPORT). *JAMA* 274(20):1591, 1995.

Weissman D: *Fast Facts and Concepts #20: Opioid Dose Escalation.* September, 2000. End-of-Life Physician Education Resource Center. www.eperc.mcw.edu.

WHO: *Cancer Pain Relief and Palliative Care. Technical Support Series 804.* Geneva: World Health Organization, 1990.

Legal Issues

JULIE A. BRAUN • ELIZABETH A. CAPEZUTI • ANDREW D. WEINBERG

The legal issues in geriatrics derive from the principal relationship in health care—that between physician and patient—and the rights and obligations that flow from this relationship. The legal relationship between physician and patient is contractual and, like any other contract, requires agreement and commitment, one or more exchanges of valuable commodities, and a natural conclusion when the purposes of each party have been fulfilled.

PATIENT AUTONOMY AND SELF-DETERMINATION

The Doctrine of Informed Consent

The doctrine of informed consent imposes a duty on physicians to disclose material information to a patient so that the patient can make an informed decision regarding medical treatment. The doctrine, born from a strong, judicial deference to individual autonomy or self-determination, establishes boundaries for the physician–patient relationship and guides medical decision making. The judicial development of the informed consent doctrine has evolved from little more than disclosure by physicians of proposed treatment in the mid-twentieth century to present requirements that demand disclosure of various factors to satisfy the elements of informed consent as articulated by most courts. Today, all 50 states recognize, by statute or by court decision, an individual's right to self-determination. For a competent patient's consent to be valid, the decision must be made without any undue influence, coercion, or duress.

Informed Consent Document Constitutes a "Best Practice"

Medicare and Medicaid reimbursement rules and Joint Commission on Accreditation of Healthcare Organizations (JCAHO) certification standards all require documentation of informed consent in a patient's chart. Good patient care also demands full disclosure by the patient's physician prior to treatment of the risks, benefits, and alternatives. A general informed consent document constitutes a "best practice" by the geriatrician and by health care institutions serving older adults. A broadly drafted document should apply to all services provided, with the ability to append information specific to a particular procedure. Do not include exculpatory language, disclaimers, or waivers of liability or the right to sue in the general informed consent document as such language is not likely to have any binding effect on the patient, physician, or institution and it may inflame a jury or public opinion in the event of a lawsuit.

Standards of Disclosure: Physician-Based Standard and Reasonable Patient Standard

Two separate standards measure a physician's duty to disclose in informed consent actions. Most states rely upon a "reasonable physician" standard where a physician must disclose whatever information a reasonable, prudent health care professional would share with a patient under the circumstances. Expert testimony is required to prove this physician-based standard. A minority of states mandate disclosure under the "reasonable patient" standard where a physician must disclose information that a reasonable patient would need to make an informed choice. Expert testimony is not required under this standard. The two legal standards usually represent very similar information.

Informed Refusal

A patient's right to informed refusal is the logical correlative to the right to informed consent. Under most circumstances, a competent patient also can decline treatment that health care providers may believe to be in the patient's best interests. If a patient refuses treatment, it is the health care provider's responsibility to inform the patient of the risks inherent in this action. In addition, the provider should document the refusal and any discussion of potential outcomes because of the decision.

Factors to Disclose

The laws of the various states determine the nature and scope of information disclosed by the physician. For instance, the physician should explain the medical steps preceding diagnosis and describe the diagnosis. Such disclosure is so basic to the physician–patient relationship that few legal cases consider a physician's failure to discuss it. Depending on the jurisdiction, other information conveyed might include the intervention's nature and purpose; associated risks with the threshold of disclosure governed by probability and severity; outcome data for and practitioner success rates related to the treatment; results of inaction if the recommended treatment is declined; prognosis with treatment; treatment alternatives and their risks; and relating any conflict of interest. Notably, some state statutes mandate disclosure of specific risks. Iowa and Georgia, for example, require physicians to disclose the known risks of death, brain damage, quadriplegia, paraplegia, loss of organ function, and disfiguring scars.

Exceptions to Physician's Duty to Disclose

The four recognized exceptions to the informed consent doctrine involve a medical emergency, therapeutic privilege, waiver, and patient incompetence. In a medical emergency, a physician may dispense with informed consent and treat the patient in conformity with customary practice. Courts commonly interpret emergency circumstances broadly to allow treatment immediately and find consent implied or presumed. However, even when treatment is urgent, a competent and conscious patient generally can refuse any intervention.

Informed consent may not be required where, in the physician's opinion, full disclosure of diagnosis, prognosis, and treatment options would be medically harmful to the patient or fail to produce a rational decision. This is known as the *doctrine of therapeutic privilege*. The scope of this exception is unclear and seldom invoked to dismiss a case. Accordingly, it is prudent for a physician who wishes to rely on therapeutic privilege to document discussion with the patient as well as any indications that disclosure would be unwise.

Either by statute or by judicial ruling, a patient may voluntarily waive their right to be fully informed and give consent. Patients may waive the right to informed consent by advising their physician that they do not want to hear about the treatment and prefer to let the physician make all treatment decisions. As expected, physicians who prefer to involve patients in the medical decision-making process will attempt to override expressions of refusal to participate. In addition, the patient may choose to designate another person to make health care decisions. Both designating a family member and deferring to physician judgment are recognized as longstanding practices in medicine. However, like therapeutic privilege, the exception could be used to avoid the requirements of informed consent, so it is sensible to document communications refusing information and choosing another decision maker.

Finally, informed consent does not need to be obtained from an incompetent patient. However, in such instance, consent must be secured from someone with legal authority to act on the patient's behalf. Determination of competency and appropriate surrogate decision makers are significant components of geriatric medical practice.

Capacity/Competency: The Threshold Issue

The outcome of any discussion about informed consent and its validity hinges on an older person's competency, or actual capacity to make informed medical decisions. A competent patient's constitutionally based fundamental right to give or refuse consent applies to all treatment decisions, although refusal may lead to death. This principle applies to artificial nutrition and hydration, which the law does not distinguish from other invasive treatments. It applies to terminally ill and nonterminally ill individuals, even though a patient might want palliative care while refusing treatment that might prolong life.

The law requires different levels of capability in decision making, depending on the nature of the decision. The capacity required to make health care decisions is the subject of extensive legal commentary. In general, a patient possesses legal competence as long as he or she has attained the age of majority and has not been declared incompetent, incapacitated, or disabled by a court during a guardianship proceeding (described in a later section Guardianship). In some states, such as Illinois, the patient's physician has the duty to ascertain, to a reasonable degree of medical certainty, whether the patient has such clinical competence when the opportunity arises to obtain informed consent.

A history of decisions contrary to the person's well-being may be cause to question competency, but it does not conclusively resolve the issue. As a practical matter, an individual whose decision is challenged for refusing professional recommendations for treatment must have some recognition of the objective facts of his or her condition (e.g., physically obvious symptoms) and the reasonable results of refusing treatment in order to retain the right to make the health care decision.

The legal determination of decision-making capacity is illustrated by comparing the facts and outcomes of *Tennessee Department of Human Services v. Northern*, 563 S.W. 2d 197 (Tenn. App. 1978, *cert. denied*, S.Ct. 1978), and *Lane v. Candura*, 376 N.E.2d 1232 (Mass. App. 1978). Both cases involve diabetic elderly women with seriously deteriorated tissues on their feet who refuse amputation.

In *Tennessee Department of Human Services v. Northern*, a hospital secured a court order declaring an elderly patient, Mrs. Northern, mentally incapacitated and authorizing a guardian to consent to the recommended amputation. The judge who interviewed Mrs. Northern found that her train of thought wandered and her concept of time was distorted. Furthermore, the judge believed her decision to refuse amputation was irrational and unwise. The court opinion relates that Mrs. Northern "looked at her feet and refused to recognize the obvious fact that the flesh was dead, black, shriveled, rotting, and stinking." She "wants to live and keep her dead feet, too, and refuses to consider the impossibility of such a desire," although the eventuality of death was estimated at 90 to 95 percent. The court would have accepted and honored her decision, however unreasonable to others, if the evidence had showed a comprehension of the facts of her condition.

In contrast, consider *Lane v. Candura* in which the state was unable to obtain an order authorizing surgery for Mrs. Candura because she exhibited "a high degree of awareness and acuity [w]hen responding to questions concerning the proposed operation." She made it clear that she did not wish the amputation "even though that decision will in all likelihood lead shortly to her death." According to the court, an individual must be cognizant of the specific need for and purpose of the procedure, as well as the consequences of refusing treatment.

Physician-Assisted Suicide

State laws that prohibit assisting a suicide memorialize the state interest in preventing suicide. Distinguish this interest from Oregon's controversial state law allowing physician-assisted suicide for competent individuals who wish to refuse continued treatment because of pain or perceived poor quality of life and who wish to avoid a prolonged or painful death. The law remains unclear, however, as to whether such statutes are appropriate expressions of patient autonomy interests or, instead, represent unacceptable breaches of significant state interests in life and professional integrity.

Life-Sustaining Treatment

Geriatricians often face difficult decisions and conflict regarding starting, continuing, or stopping life-sustaining treatments. The situation becomes more pronounced when physicians have little knowledge of what life-sustaining treatments a patient would want or when no one is appointed (or available) to make health care decisions for an incapacitated person.

Uniform Health Care Decisions Act

Maine, Mississippi, New Mexico, and Delaware have adopted versions of a national model statute known as Uniform Health Care Decisions Act (UHCDA). The model represents an attempt by the National Conference of Commissioners on Uniform State Laws to create a comprehensive form that addresses living wills, health care proxies, and surrogate decision-making. It also contemplates decision making by incapacitated persons who do not have a living will or health care proxy, and situations in which incompetent persons do not have a family member to appoint as a surrogate decision maker prior to the onset of incapacity.

The Patient Self-Determination Act

The first significant legislation to address an individual's right to make health care decisions, the federal Patient Self-Determination Act (PSDA) of 1990, was designed to promote the use of advance directives. It mandates that all federally certified health care providers (e.g., hospitals, skilled nursing facilities, home health agencies, and hospice programs) must provide written information to patients about their right under state law to participate in medical decision-making and to formulate advance directives.

This includes (1) providing written information to patients about their rights under state law (whether statutory or recognized by the courts of the state) to make health care decisions, including the right to accept or refuse medical or surgical treatment and the right to formulate, at the individual's option, advance directives; (2) creating written policies and procedures for respecting the implementation of these legal rights, including a clear and precise statement of limitation if the provider cannot implement an advance directive on the basis of conscience; (3) asking each person whether an advance directive has been completed; (4) documenting in each individual's medical record whether an advance directive has been executed; (5) not conditioning the provision of care on the presence or absence of an advance directive; (6) complying with applicable state laws regarding advance directives; (7) educating staff about policy and procedure concerning advance directives; and (8) providing community education about advance directives and documenting efforts regarding same.

LEGAL ISSUES IN CARING FOR COMPETENT OLDER ADULTS

Written Advance Directives

An advance directive is a written instruction, such as a living will or durable power of attorney for health care, recognized under state law (whether statutory or by the courts of the state), relating to the provision of health care when an individual is mentally and/or physically unable to communicate medical preferences or participate in medical decision-making. Many statutes outline the circumstances under which an advance directive is legally valid and communicate witnessing and execution formalities.

A dementia diagnosis does not necessarily mean that the patient is incompetent or unable to initiate a written advance directive. Geriatricians should encourage the older adult to execute advance directives regarding health care and estate planning, especially when the patient is in the early stages of dementia.

How Should a Clinician Determine Patient Capacity to Create an Advance Directive?

Patients must be informed on admission to hospitals and nursing homes of their right to formulate advance directives and are presumed legally competent to establish such directives unless adjudicated incompetent. Joel E. Streim, author of the "Advance Directives" chapter in *Geriatric Secrets,* relates that

> No formal clinical standards exist for determining when a patient's cognitive impairment precludes them from being capable of formulating an advance directive or, conversely, when the situation safely permits a cognitively impaired patient to participate in this process.

> Nevertheless, during discussion regarding the patient's rights and options in formulating advance directives, clinicians

have opportunities to appraise the capacity of patients to:

1. Maintain a stable set of values and goals.
2. Comprehend the relevant information.
3. Reason and deliberate their choices.
4. Appreciate the situation and its possible outcomes.
5. Communicate their choices.

Statutory Forms

Many states have generic statutory living will forms. The forms might assume that all patients would want the administration of food and fluids; define food and fluids as "comfort care;" or focus on other matters such as naming an agent, giving general directions or limiting the liability of those honoring the directive. Some states make use of standardized forms mandatory and discourage writings that are not substantially similar. Generic forms that provide a space for the signature of the attending physician seek to promote physician cooperation in following patient wishes and patient recognition of a physician's conflict with patient desires and concerns.

Limit Health Care Provider Liability

In general, state advance directive statutes, such as those in Alabama, Arizona, California, Delaware, Indiana, Kansas, Minnesota, Montana, New Jersey, Pennsylvania, Tennessee, Utah, and Wyoming, contain specific provisions that exonerate health care providers who honor a directive from all liability or professional discipline so long as actions are undertaken in good faith. While not impossible to imagine a provider's bad faith in refusing to follow an advance directive, there are a few cases highlighting improper motivation. It is fairly easy for the health care institution and/or physician to show the court that advance directive validity, meaning, or even availability was in question at the time of the action at issue. In some situations, state law arguably is unclear, and refusal to remove life-sustaining treatment prior to a court order has been excused on that basis.

The statutes provide a process for creating a directive, but seldom incorporate civil or criminal penalties for failing to enforce or obey a valid, unrevoked directive. A minority of states (e.g., Utah) have penalties for failing to comply with a living will, thus leaving enforcement of an advance directive to the courts.

Litigation in this area is rare but emerging, and may be necessary to enforce a directive; appoint a substitute decision maker if there is no advance directive; halt treatment performed against a patient's wishes; and continue treatment a physician seeks to remove. Causes of action in tort may include battery; failure to obtain informed consent; invasion of privacy (plead in few reported cases); negligence rooted in disagreements regarding treatment provided or the unauthorized administration of treatment, alleged when a physician determines that treatment is futile and seeks to terminate treating the patient, or commenced for a facility's failure to have policies in place regarding end-of-life treatment; negligent infliction of emotional distress asserted by patient or family member where life-sustaining treatment was wrongfully withheld or withdrawn; intentional infliction of emotional distress (also known as the tort of outrage) averred by a third party when treatment performed against a patient' wishes can be deemed outrageous conduct (importantly, courts and jurors are reluctant to find a physician's conduct in administering treatment, even against a patient's wishes, outrageous); wrongful living cause of action claims a diminished quality of life after or while receiving treatment has made life not worth living (again this action is not highly successful because of court reluctance to view the prolonging of life, even against a person's wishes, as a compensable harm); abandonment may be actionable when a physician with a duty to provide treatment unilaterally stops treating the patient without being properly relieved of such duty; and maintaining a cause of action under federal and state law for unwanted medical treatment.

Right Not to Complete Advance Directive

Physicians must respect each person's right not to complete an advance directive. A patient should be informed that he or she will not be abandoned by the physician and/or institution, as well as reassured that he or she will not receive substandard care, if an advance directive is not completed. Note the patient's choice not to formulate an advance directive in the medical record.

Conscience Objections to Advance Directive

The geriatrician is not required to implement an advance directive if, as a matter of conscience, it conflicts with the provider's personal or professional values and state law allows for such conscientious objection. To ensure that patients are given clear warning of any possible conscience-based objections that might be raised by the provider, federal regulations require that a clear and precise statement of limitation be supplied. At a minimum, the statement must (1) clarify any differences between institution-wide conscience objections and those raised by individual physicians, (2) identify the state legal authority permitting such objection, and (3) describe the range of medical conditions or procedures affected by the conscience objection. State laws mandate a good faith effort to transfer the patient to a doctor or facility that will comply with the directive.

Oral Advance Directives

Although a written advance directive is preferable, especially in emergencies, courts view oral advance directives favorably and have enforced or relied on them in adjudicated decisions to forgo life-sustaining treatment. Courts likely will accept oral advance directives if the statements were, among other possibilities, (1) made on serious occasions; (2) solemn pronouncements; (2) routinely repeated; (3) offered by a mature person who understood the underlying issues; (4) consistent with values demonstrated in other aspects of the person's life; (5) spoken shortly before the need for a treatment decision; or (6) specific to the actual condition of the person. Health care providers should document such statements when discussing advance directives or end-of-life treatment preferences.

Living Will-Type Advance Directive

Unfortunately named, a living will-type advance directive, also referred to as an instruction directive, natural death instruction, or advance directive for health care, contains an individual's specific written instructions about wanted, limited, or unwanted life-prolonging health care treatment. Although the language of most living will statutes differ, certain characteristics are true for any living will. First, it applies only when an individual becomes incapacitated. A living will has no legal authority as long as an individual is competent to participate in their health care decision making. Second, statutory language details the varying conditions for withholding or withdrawing life-sustaining treatment. In general, such statutes apply *only* if the patient is declared terminally ill or permanently unconscious and lacks the requisite decisional capacity. Consider, for example, the New Jersey Advance Directive for Health Care Act that permits the withholding or withdrawal of life-sustaining treatment only if the patient is in one of the following defined states: (1) a terminal condition (i.e., a terminal stage of an irreversible fatal illness, disease, or condition); (2) permanent unconsciousness, which includes a persistent vegetative state or an irreversible coma; (3) receiving experimental and futile life-sustaining treatment; or (4) a serious irreversible condition or illness, where it would be inhumane to give treatment contrary to the patient's wishes or where the risk of treatment outweighs the benefit.

A controversial issue that arises with living wills is whether the document can ask for the termination of artificial nutrition and hydration. The American Medical Association and several courts concur that nutrition and hydration are medical treatment and thus fall within the purview of informed consent. Nevertheless, many state statutes do not allow the termination of nutrition and hydration based upon living will language. In the future, expect more legislators, state statutes, and court decisions to recognize that terminating nutrition and hydration is a patient's option.

Health Care Proxy

A health care proxy, also known as a durable power of attorney for health care, is a legally enforceable written document that permits one individual (known as the principal or grantor) to designate *another person* (known as a health care agent, surrogate, health care proxy, or attorney-in-fact) to make health care decisions if he or she loses decision-making capacity. The power delegated may be broad or very specific, as determined by the writing that creates it. For example, an agent may have the right to review medical records; select and discharge health care professionals; make decisions about admission to or discharge from healthcare facilities; grant, refuse, or withdraw consent to the provision of most health care services, treatments, or

procedures (excepting withdrawal of life-support systems or nutrition and hydration); and take any lawful actions necessary to carry out those decisions. As with the living will, health care proxy statutes generally provide immunity to health care providers who act in good faith.

The document becomes effective when the grantor loses competency to make health care decisions. Until that happens, the individual continues to make his or her own health care decisions. To cancel or revoke a durable power of attorney after the grantor is incapacitated, an individual must show the court that the attorney in fact has behaved contrary to an agent's obligation to act solely in the interests of the grantor.

Mental Health Advance Directive

Many older adults suffer from clinical depression, various psychiatric disorders, or Alzheimer's disease. Acting as a very specific advance directive, a mental health advance directive ensures the patient's expression of his or her wishes so that health care professionals can act accordingly. At least 10 states offer mental health advance directives, including Alaska, Hawaii, Idaho, Illinois, Minnesota, North Carolina, Oklahoma, Oregon, Texas, and Utah. These directives also are termed "Ulysses directives," derived from a passage of *The Odyssey.* For example, the Illinois Mental Health Treatment Preference Declaration Act allows any adult of "sound mind" to explicitly declare preferences or instructions regarding mental health treatment. An individual may, for instance, consent to or refuse electroconvulsive therapy or psychotropic medications. The Illinois act permits the designation of an attorney-in-fact who may execute these written preferences or, in the absence of such direction, act in the principal's best interests. The state statutory framework for mental health advance directives may furnish physicians and providers immunity from criminal prosecution, civil liability, and professional disciplinary action as is possible in Alaska, Idaho, Illinois, Hawaii, Minnesota, North Carolina, Oklahoma, Oregon, Texas, and Utah.

Older persons who contemplate mental health advance directives may be subject to fraud and abuse. For instance, a health care provider may seek to condition insurance, treatment, or discharge on the execution of such a declaration. Consequently, at least four states—Idaho, North Carolina, Oregon, and Texas—incorporate provisions into their directives to deter abuse.

Do-Not-Resuscitate Statutes

A few state statutory schemes address "do-not-resuscitate" (DNR) and "do-not-transfer" (DNT) orders. Forty-three states have statutes authorizing some form of nonhospital DNR order, although the District of Columbia and seven states (Delaware, Iowa, Mississippi, Nebraska, North Dakota, Pennsylvania, and Vermont) do not tackle the issue specifically. In some states, such as Alaska, a DNR order issues only if a person is in a certain medical state (e.g., a terminal condition or permanent unconsciousness). Depending on state statute, a DNR order may be used in the acute care and long-term care environments as well as noninstitutional settings (e.g., a person's home) as happens in California, Colorado, Georgia, Montana, New York, Ohio, Oklahoma, South Carolina, Virginia, West Virginia, and Wyoming.

In states with DNR statutes, the approach varies, but usually requires formal execution of a DNR order by the patient's attending physician. While every patient, competent or incompetent, has a right to receive care and comfort, health care professionals are not obligated to provide treatment not medically indicated. Contraindicated treatment may potentially include methods of cardiopulmonary resuscitation (CPR), mouth-to-mouth breathing, bag ball valve, endotracheal intubation, closed-chest cardiac massage, defibrillation, or injection of adrenaline and other stimulants. As with any significant medical decision, an attending physician contemplating a DNR order must determine, in his or her professional judgment, whether resuscitation is medically appropriate and in the patient's best interests. DNR status depends on a patient's medical condition. Hence, the attending physician should periodically reevaluate the continued need for a DNR order as often as clinically necessary. Furthermore, the DNR classification does not apply to therapies (e.g., assisted ventilation) initiated prior to the DNR order.

The decision not to initiate CPR in the event of cardiac or respiratory arrest should be communicated by means of a formal physician's order after discussing the subject with a competent patient who possesses the capacity to consent to the order. The physician should explain the rationale and consequences of the DNR order. Good clinical practice requires that the physician document the substance of this conversation in the patient's medical record.

DNR Orders and Incompetent Patients

Hospitals generally establish DNR protocols and procedures applicable to incompetent patients. In New York, for example, an incompetent person with no health care proxy can have a DNR order under some circumstances. In addition, New York allows appointment of a surrogate to make decisions regarding CPR.

DNR Orders and Emergency Personnel

In most jurisdictions, paramedics and emergency medical personnel have limited authority to refrain from attempting resuscitation. Emergency medical protocols typically mandate resuscitation unless death is unequivocally established. However, if the legal requirements of some state statutes are followed precisely (e.g., Arizona, Arkansas, California, Colorado, Florida, Georgia, Idaho, Illinois, Kentucky, Maryland, Michigan, Montana, New Mexico, New York, Ohio, Pennsylvania, South Carolina, Tennessee, Utah, Virginia, Wisconsin, Washington, West Virginia, and Wyoming), the resulting DNR order permits emergency personnel such as emergency medical services (EMS) workers and hospital emergency room staff to recognize and honor DNR orders.

DNR Orders and Advance Directives

Advance directives may contain instructions concerning authorization of DNR orders. In Arizona and Montana, a patient who strictly complies with statutory provisions can personally direct the withholding of resuscitation by executing a specialized advance directive upon which paramedics can rely. Importantly, the decision belongs to the patient, even though physician confirmation is necessary.

Do-Not-Transfer Orders

A do-not-transfer order prevents transportation (of a nursing home resident, for example) to the hospital for receipt of life-sustaining treatment. New legislation seeks to address this issue in a growing number of states. Advance directives may contain instructions concerning authorization of DNT orders.

LEGAL ISSUES IN CARING FOR INCAPACITATED OLDER ADULTS

If a patient has lost capacity to make health care decisions and has not executed an advance directive or health care proxy, the geriatrician or gerontologist may look to the patient's spouse, family member, or friend to act as surrogate. This should avert the need for court intervention. A surrogate decision maker has to be appointed by the court through a guardianship proceeding if no such options are available.

Guardianship

If there is no advance directive, or the alleged incapacitated person is unable to execute such a document, a guardianship may be required. In such a case, the court is obligated to tailor the guardianship in the least restrictive manner possible and to rule on all health care or placement decisions.

Guardianship is becoming more widespread because individuals age 65 years and older represent the fastest growing segment of the population. This statistic combined with the increased complexity among long-term care choices and the desire by health care providers for legally reliable consent to limit risks of liability contributes to the rising number of guardianship petitions. Guardianship is a legal device by which judgment of a more capable person is substituted by the court for the judgment of an impaired person. It is a matter of state rather than federal law. As a result, variations in guardianship law and its application exist across the United States making knowledge of specific jurisdictional requirements critical. Statutory terminology describing a person's incapacity varies considerably, as do procedures employed and authority granted to a guardian. Two prominent issues in determining a need for guardianship include medical decision making and institutional/residential placement.

The Guardianship Petition

In general, "any person" can file a guardianship petition. However, statutory language also may reference any reputable person, any concerned person, any adult, any interested person, a relative or friend, as well as an interested entity such as a social service agency, hospital, or state agency. The petition is a statement, affirmed under oath, that alleges a need for the appointment of a guardian. It conveys essential information to the court about the matter at issue (e.g., removing a patient from life support or placing the older adult in a nursing home) and identifies the persons involved. State law and local court rules may dictate content, as is the case in California, Nebraska, and New York.

The older adult who is the subject of the guardianship petition is entitled to notice of the guardianship proceeding; time to prepare a legal defense; to participate in the court hearing; to question witnesses, including examiners, who present evidence in favor of guardianship; to present opposing expert opinion, possibly at state expense; and to express a preference about the identity of a guardian and the scope of the guardian's authority. An advisor to the court, called a guardian *ad litem*, may be appointed to investigate circumstances of the petition.

Obtaining Guardianship

To justify creation of a guardianship in the context of medical decision-making, a court must find that the individual alleged to be incapacitated lacks the requisite decisional capacity. The categories of decision-making authority are statutorily defined and may be broad or narrowly detailed.

The expert examination conducted by the court to assess capacity varies from state to state. Statutory requirements may govern who performs the examination and evaluation of the older adult and reports findings to the court. A physician is used in Alabama, Colorado, Connecticut, Georgia, Hawaii, Idaho, Kansas, Maine, Maryland, Michigan, Virginia, Washington, West Virginia, and Wisconsin. Other states select a psychologist to perform this function solely or in tandem with a physician or other statutorily identified professional. A mental health professional works with a physician in Idaho, and may be the single evaluator in Michigan. Arizona teams a registered nurse with a physician and psychologist. Connecticut requires a report from a social worker accompanied by statements from one or more physicians.

Most states minimally require medical and psychological examinations conducted by in-person interviews, resulting in written reports specifying the objective findings and likely implications. The patient's attending physician may be required to submit an affidavit certifying the lack of decisional capacity as a medical mater. The medical report may serve as the foundation of the guardianship petition and as such merits careful scrutiny by the court.

The evidence before the court, then, consists of the allegations featured in the petition, expert reports on the older adult's decision-making capacity and assistance needs, and usually the investigation report prepared by a guardian *ad litem*.

A guardian has a fiduciary duty (i.e., a high degree of responsibility based on trust) to act in the older adult's best interests. Many statutes require specific authority from a court or such important decisions as long-term institutionalization or psychosurgery. Powers not transferred to the guardian by the court can still be exercised by the ward.

Standards for Surrogate Health Care Decisions

There are three primary ethical standards that impact a patient's right to self-determination. The standards by which surrogates make health care decisions on behalf of incapacitated patients include the (1) subjective standard, (2) substitute judgment standard, and (3) best interest standard.

The first is the preferred standard because it relies on a patient's specific intent. The subjective standard compels proof of what the person had actually decided about medical care while competent, rather than what they would do under the circumstance, as in the substituted judgment standard.

The next-favored standard is the substitute judgment standard that directs the surrogate to choose what the surrogate believes the patient would have decided as inferred from direct and indirect evidence (e.g., person's wishes, philosophical views, religious beliefs, or conduct pertaining to medical care) as manifested when the person was competent. Courts articulate assorted factors to consider, such as age; probable treatment side effects; chance or cure, either permanent or temporary; whether the planned treatment is painful; and patient's ability to tolerate the treatment without undue fear or pain.

If the surrogate decision maker has no knowledge of what the patient would want in a given situation, then the surrogate chooses a course of treatment that is in the patient's best interest, based upon what a reasonable person would elect in the same circumstance. Surrogates faced with difficult decisions and unclear parameters on which to base their decisions often appeal for advice from, among other options, health care professionals, attorneys, and ethics committees. The patient's medical condition influences the surrogate's decision. The best interest standard differs, for example, if a person is terminally ill or in a persistent vegetative state.

Family Consent Statutes

A majority of states have family consent laws that designate a legal hierarchy of family members who can make health care decisions for an incompetent patient when the patient has not executed a health care proxy. The practice of seeking family consent for care is one of long-standing in the medical profession, but until recently, such consent had no specific legal significance. Family consent provisions (which may be integrated into health care proxy statutes) designate a hierarchy of family members to make health care decisions if the patient's completed advance directive does not provide instructions. The list of authorized family members varies somewhat from state to state, although typically it includes, in order, the spouse, adult children, siblings, and parents. Some states prefer a legal guardian as the first decision maker; some allow a cohabitant to make decisions if no family member does so. If no one in a higher classification is available or willing to make a decision, the authorization passes to members of the next classification. If there is more than one member of a classification, the members typically must come to a consensus to implement a care decision without seeking a court order.

ADULT PROTECTIVE SERVICES

Each of the 50 states has some form of statutory adult protective services program that is designed to investigate reports of abuse, neglect, or exploitation, and to assist in obtaining protective services for endangered adults. The level of protection and the quality of such programs vary from state to state. Forty-two states require mandatory reporting of suspected or actual abuse. Penalties for violations of the adult protective services schemes vary. Alabama, California, Georgia, Michigan, and Rhode Island, for example, provide for civil fines and/or jail time. Violators in Arkansas, Arizona, New Hampshire, and Texas are guilty of a misdemeanor.

REPORTING ELDER MISTREATMENT

All states have statutory provisions governing voluntary and mandatory reporting of elder mistreatment (i.e., physical, emotional, sexual, and financial abuse) (also see Chap. 125). Mandatory reporting provisions fall into two categories: those requiring universal reporting (i.e., by all citizens) and those requiring reporting by statutorily identified categories of individuals. For example, the universal reporting requirement under Texas law applies "without exception to a person whose professional communications are generally confidential, including an attorney, clergy member, medical practitioner, social worker, and mental health professional." Statutorily identified persons who must report might include physicians, nurses, social workers, clergy, law enforcement officers, nursing home administrators, and mental health professionals. Other types of health care and home-care workers who suspect that an older adult is being mistreated may be required to report this to the appropriate state agency. Attorneys, accountants, trustees, guardians, and conservators also may be statutorily required to report mistreatment.

Special Relationships

Courts recognize an affirmative duty to act where a special relationship exists. Arguably, the relationship between the patient and health care professional gives rise to an affirmative duty to, at a minimum, detect and report mistreatment.

Circumstances that Trigger Reporting

State statutes differ as to what circumstances trigger the duty to report of elder mistreatment. In Hawaii, for instance, health-related professionals including, but not limited to, physicians, physicians in training, psychologists, dentists, nurses, osteopathic physicians and surgeons, optometrists, chiropractors, podiatrists, and pharmacists who "know or have reasons to believe that a dependent adult *has been abused or is threatened with imminent abuse* shall promptly report the matter orally to the department of human services." For comparative purposes, consider Delaware's reporting requirement that any person having reasonable cause to believe that an adult person is in need of adult protective services must report same to the state department of health and social services. The reporting trigger in Missouri involves "reasonable cause to suspect that an eligible adult presents a likelihood of suffering serious physical harm and is in need of protective services." A "substantial cause to believe that an adult is in need of protective services" prompts reporting in the District of Columbia. In Arkansas, the observation by a physician, surgeon, coroner, dentist, osteopath, resident intern, registered nurse, social worker, case manager, mental health professional, law enforcement officer, nursing home employee, firefighter, and emergency medical technician, among other statutorily specified persons, "that an endangered or impaired adult has been *subjected to conditions or circumstances which would reasonably result in abuse,* sexual abuse, neglect, or exploitation" is sufficient basis to require report of the mistreatment. Similarly, Nebraska law requires a report of elder mistreatment when any physician, psychologist, physician assistant, nurse, nursing assistant, other medical, developmental disability, or mental health professional, law enforcement personnel, or caregiver or employee of a caregiver, among other possibilities, "has reasonable cause to believe" or observes that a vulnerable adult has been "subjected to conditions or circumstances which would result in abuse."

Immunity from Civil and/or Criminal Liability

Each state has at least one statute providing immunity from civil and/or criminal immunity that might otherwise be imposed for anyone who, in good faith (as opposed to bad faith or with malicious purpose), reports elder mistreatment. Most statutes also note that the immunity does not apply if the person who makes the report also is the person who committed the mistreatment.

Sanctions for Failing to Report

The sanctions for failing to report elder mistreatment vary depending on the state involved. Persons who are statutorily required to report elder mistreatment and who fail to do so may be found guilty of a misdemeanor and receive a monetary fine, imprisonment, or both. Criminal liability may hinge on a willful or knowing failure to report. A person who must report abuse but does not do so may be personally liable in some states for damages incurred by the victim. In addition, some statutes specify that a mandated reporter who is a licensed professional risks being reported to the appropriate licensing authority for failure to report. Penalties range from loss of the right to practice professionally in that state to criminal prosecution, with a fine or imprisonment if convicted. Notably, some states impose no sanctions for a failure to report.

LIABILITY FOR SUBSTANDARD CARE

Institutional and Professional Liability

Litigating elder injury cases is an evolving area of litigation that combines the subspecialties of elder law, personal injury litigation and medical malpractice litigation. Tort liability exposure is a multibillion dollar per year cost to the nursing home industry. Average claim size tripled from $67,000 in 1990 to $219,000 in 2001. Long-term care facilities incur 11 claims per year for every 100 occupied skilled nursing facility beds. Three of 5 (62 percent) Florida nursing homes were sued in 2001. The Mississippi long-term care industry witnessed a 190 percent increase in lawsuits between 1997 and 2001.

Annual insurance premium levels have increased on average 130 percent between 2000 and 2001, often with reduced coverage. Average long-term care general liability/professional liability cost per annual occupied skilled nursing bed increased at an annual rate of 24 percent from $240 in 1990 to $2,360 per bed in 2001. Forty-seven percent of the total amount of claims costs paid for general liability/professional liability claims in the long-term care industry pays for costs associated with litigation.

Common liability issues that may trigger a lawsuit include malnutrition, dehydration, pressure ulcers, choking, feeding tube management, wandering and elopement, falls and fall-related injuries, physical restraints and bed side rails, chemical restraint, medication errors, and physical/sexual abuse. On average, 60 percent of suits against nursing homes result in damage awards for the plaintiff. Four percent of the awards are greater than $10 million dollars, while 12 percent average $200,000 to $299,000, and 10 percent are in the $100,000 to $149,000 range. One of the most frequently occurring liability situations for nursing homes involves physical/sexual abuse. In fact, plaintiff recovery probability is at 74 percent and settlement ranges between $45,000 and $1,250,000, with a mean of $406,500.

Tort lawsuits usually are financed on a contingency fee basis. That is, the attorney who takes the case receives compensation only if there is a settlement or court award to the plaintiff. Typically, the attorney who files, investigates, and negotiates with the defendant receives one-fourth to one-third of a settlement. If the attorney takes the case to trial, the contingency fee might be up to one-half of the jury award. Such a system sometimes is criticized for bringing to court cases in which a jury is swayed by sympathy rather than a sense of conviction that negligent harm has occurred. On balance, the contingency system allows people who have suffered harm but who cannot afford substantial legal fees to seek compensation in the courts.

The tort, or noncriminal wrong, of negligence is the legal concept that usually serves to define a patient's or client's claim for harm caused by a professional or an institution. To have a claim, an individual must show that the health care provider had a duty arising from a professional relationship. To have a legal claim, the claimant must also show that the professional breached the legal duty. In general, if the professional fails to fulfill a duty to provide care and causes harm, the person harmed may sue seeking monetary compensation.

Common types of harm for which monetary damages are awarded include the cost of otherwise unnecessary health care, including psychological care, before and after the lawsuit, and lost wages during recuperation and as result of any change in occupation due to long-term disability. Noneconomic damages also may be awarded (i.e., a money award that cannot be justified in an accounting sense but is intended to compensate the individual for great personal difficulties). Noneconomic damages include pain and suffering, loss of enjoyment or consortium (i.e., the interaction of a healthy persons with close family members), and sometimes emotional distress. If the professional has engaged in egregious negligence (i.e., often harm that appears to verge on the intentional), some courts will award punitive damages.

Professional harm in rare instances results in criminal charges. Such cases are brought by the state rather than the individual who suffered harm, who as a witness generally receives little or no tangible compensation for participation. Rare criminal cases in geriatrics have included charges against nursing home administrators for allowing life-threatening conditions to exist in their facilities.

Medical Negligence

Every state has enacted a statute setting specific legal standards for the tort of medical negligence. Most such statutes apply to podiatrists, chiropractors, and dentists, as well as to allopathic and osteopathic physicians.

The standard of care required to avoid liability for medical negligence generally is met by providing the generally accepted treatment or response, regardless of any bad outcome resulting from the unique, unforeseeable traits of the patient or the lack of knowledge by the field as a whole. A physician might alternatively provide such care as would be provided by a respectable minority of practitioners or a reasonable and prudent physician under similar circumstances. Usually, differences among the standards are slight, but state case law may favor one standard over another.

Many medical malpractice statutes require plaintiffs to fulfill specific procedural requirements to ensure the validity of a claim, such as pretrial screening by a panel of experts. Most set limits on the time allowed for bringing suit, termed statute of limitations. Finally, a number of state statutes cap the amount of noneconomic damages the individual can receive.

Nursing Home Litigation

A nursing facility is not an insurer that residents will be free from harm. A facility must have and adhere to care and documentation practices that meet regulatory requirements and are of a quality considered acceptable in the industry.

Pressure Ulcers

The risk of litigation for negligent care involving pressure ulcers increased dramatically beginning in the 1990s. A disproportionate number of cases hail from California, Florida, Illinois, and Texas, four of the seven states with the most number of older adults. Interestingly less than 10 percent of all cases reviewed by outside medical experts go to trial. Most claims settle before a case is filed, and many settlements are confidential and unreported. Thus, the total number of cases annually is assumed to be in the thousands.

Not every pressure ulcer that develops results in litigation, and not every pressure ulcer case commands a win for the plaintiff. Common factors that produce decisions favoring the defendant nursing homes include:

- Supporting documentation in the medical record reflects rigorous adherence to the standard of care for pressure ulcers;
- Verifying underlying disease and complications that made bedsore development inevitable;
- Developing and implementing aggressive and comprehensive bedsore prevention and treatment programs;
- Demonstrating preexisting weakness or frailty;
- Alleging contributory negligence (e.g., the resident refuses to comply with a care plan, for example);
- Highlighting contributing medical conditions (e.g., a resident who is unable to lie in a position to alleviate pressure on her skin because emphysema requires that the resident maintain a sitting position); and
- Pressure sore(s) originated in another setting (e.g., hospital or during home care).

Falls and Fall-Related Injuries

Falls and fall-related injuries are a leading cause of lawsuits against nursing homes. Although falls involving older adults in hospitals and nursing homes are common, a fall in and of itself does not indicate that there is a viable claim against the facility. In some cases, a facility's alleged failure to protect a person from falling has been considered ordinary negligence; in other instances health care malpractice. The standard of care used to evaluate a falls case must be based on the regulations and clinical standards of practice in effect at the time of the fall.

Tube Feeding

Lawsuits involving tube feeding allege inadequate staff training and education in, among other areas, tube feeding types and equipment use, feeding techniques, need to complete the tube-feeding treatment record, and failing to assess for potential complications (e.g., aspiration, gastric distension, or diarrhea); failing to identify potential negative outcomes (e.g., self-extubation); failing to provide care and treatment to prevent complications; incorrect tube size;

knotted nasogastric tube; malpositioned tube; and failing to detect and correct tube displacement.

Medication Errors

Some of the most successful litigation against nursing homes concerns medication administration errors. Approximately 95 percent of all nursing home residents receive medication. Over- or underuse of a drug, administration of the wrong medication, failing to monitor the resident for side effects, inappropriate medication prescription, and incorrect prescription dispensing by a pharmacist may result in serious injury or death.

Wandering and Elopement

Many types of problematic behaviors are encountered among the older adult population, including wandering and elopement. Injuries may occur when residents wander around in or wander away from the facility itself. Most of the injuries sustained outside the facility result from exposure to the elements or from being struck by a moving vehicle. In addition, some persons wander away from the facility and are never found.

Physical Restraints

A major legal and clinical issue in acute and long-term care settings is the use of physical restraints. Federal law prohibits using physical restraints for discipline or convenience and when not necessary to treat medical symptoms or to ensure the physical safety of the patient/resident or other patients/residents. Historically, physicians viewed restraints as a "common-sense" intervention to prevent falls and injuries. The legal community possessed similar beliefs and older court opinions favored the facility or physician who applied the "protective" restraint. Today, most clinicians know that no empirical evidence demonstrates the effectiveness of restraint in preventing falls and routinely include restraints in their risk analysis of falls and injuries. The evolving legal standard of care was influenced by passage in 1987 of landmark legislation, the Nursing Home Reform Act, designed to reduce, if not eliminate, physical restraint use. Today, restraint use does not reduce physician or institutional liability particularly in circumstances involving restraint-related positional asphyxiation where a patient is suspended by a restraint from a bed/chair and their ability to inhale is inhibited by gravitational chest compression.

Bed Side Rails

Side rails may be physical restraints when employed to prevent a person from leaving bed when he or she wants to exit the bed environment. The older adult may perceive the side rail as a barrier and fall while attempting to go over, under, around, or through the rail. In addition, the older patient may become entrapped between the mattress and rail, rail and head/footboard, or between split rails, and die. Judgments are being entered against hospitals, nursing homes, and physicians (among other possible named defendants) with increasing frequency for misusing these devices.

Pain Management

Liability for Inadequate Treatment of Pain

A verdict returned in 2001 will forever change the way health care providers view the legal significance of effective pain care. In *Bergman v. Eden Medical Center*, No. H205732 (Cal. Super. Ct. Alameda Cty., jury verdict June 13, 2001), California jurors awarded the surviving children of a lung cancer patient $1.5 million on charges the treating physician committed elder abuse by undertreating his 85-year-old hospital patient's pain.

The *Bergman* decision signals a new type of liability for physicians in an area where they have not been held accountable previously and likely will prompt pain management lawsuits in other states. Physicians will need to be current on pain management issues because the result achieved in the *Bergman* case should empower hospital patients and nursing home residents to insist that physicians treat their pain and other symptoms at the end of life.

Standard of Care Addressing Pain Management

Successful prosecution of a medical malpractice claim usually requires the plaintiff to prove that the care provider deviated from or failed to comply with the customary standard of care. Pain management is becoming an accepted medical practice as evidenced by state pain polices, voluntary accreditation requirements concerning pain management issues, and clinical practice guidelines addressing pain management.

Clinical Practice Guidelines on Pain Management

Although clinical practice guidelines supply an authoritative and settled statement of the standard of care for a specific treatment or illness, they have no force of law and represent suggestions for conduct only. While clinical practice guidelines have been formulated in the area of pain management, they have not yet influenced the custom and practice of physicians to any significant degree. However, some courts may consider such guidelines as "neutral and unbiased" evidence of the appropriate standard of care under the circumstances. In practice, medical expert testimony introduces presumptive evidence of the care standard, establishes its source, and conveys its relevancy. Clinical practice guidelines also are used to impeach an expert's opinion. In 2002, the American Geriatrics Society published *The Management of Persistent Pain in Older Persons*. Good patient care and effective risk management demand geriatricians to become conversant with and make a concerted effort to comply with such guidelines when caring for patients with pain.

CONCLUSION

The high proportion of chronic, debilitating and dementia-related illnesses among older adults requires considerable legal planning. True informed consent among the older population remains an ongoing challenge for the health care community. Although advance directive use is now commonly seen in geriatric practice, the extent of the directive's scope is frequently limited in nature and may not address all issues important to the patient. Patient autonomy and self-determination may be in conflict with physician-ordered treatment, especially when psychoactive medications are involved. The expanding use of tube feedings also has raised many ethical issues, especially when their use is in direct conflict with previously expressed desires of the patient expressed in a "living will" and a family member insists on their utilization. While the designation of health care proxies and guardians is ideal in the care of an incompetent older adult, such individuals are often chosen in times of emergency crisis.

Attention to the legal aspects of geriatric medicine has increased dramatically during the last decade given the avalanche of litigation against long-term care facilities. In nursing home care, many medical conditions, such as depression, dehydration, and urinary incontinence, remain misdiagnosed or untreated and routine onsite medical evaluation of acute medical illness is often not available. This may lead to subsequent litigation if an untoward outcome results. Pain is often undertreated both in the community and long-term care settings and remains an unmet goal of health care practitioners. Liability issues and risk management in caring for older persons require systematic use of state of the science geriatric medicine principles.

REFERENCES

Begley TD, Herina Jeffreys JA: *Representing the Elderly Client.* Panel Publishing, 1999; Suppl. 2001.

Bennett RG: The increasing medical malpractice risk related to pressure ulcers in the United States. *J Am Geriatr Soc* 48:73, 2000.

Braun JA (ed): *Long-Term Care Litigation.* 2001.

Braun JA: Rights of long-term care facility residents, in Braun JA (ed): *Elder Law Portfolio Series.* 2001.

Braun JA: Nursing home litigation, in Margolis HS (ed): *Elder Law Portfolio Series.* 2000.

Braun JA, Capezuti EA: The legal and medical aspects of physical restraints and bed side rails and their relationship to falls and fall-related injuries in nursing homes. *DePaul J Health Care Law* 4:1, 2000.

Braun JA, Capezuti EA: A medico-legal evaluation of dehydration and malnutrition among nursing home residents. *Elder L J* 8:239, 2000.

Braun JA, Capezuti EA, Levine JM: Elder mistreatment: Legal-medico aspects of abuse, neglect and financial exploitation, in Braun JA (ed): *Elder Law Portfolio Series.* 2001.

Capezuti EA, Braun JA: Medico-legal aspects of hospital side rail use. *Ethics Law Aging Rev* 7:25, 2001.

Fleming RB: *Elder Law Answer Book.* 2000; Suppl 2001.

Furrow BR: Pain management and provider liability, no more excuses. *J Law Med, Ethics* 29:28, 2001.

Morgan RC, Sabatino CP: Advance planning and drafting for health care decisions. *Probate Prop* 15:35, 2001.

Rich BA: A prescription for pain: The emerging standard of care for pain management. *William Mitchell L Rev* 26:1, 2000.

Streim JE: Advance directives, in Forciea MA et al. (eds): *Geriatric Secrets* 2nd ed. 2000, p 137.

Weinberg AD: *Risk Management in Long-Term Care: A Quick Reference Guide.* 1998.

Spirituality and the Elderly

CHARLES J. FAHEY

Both professional and popular literature refer to the nexus of spirituality, religion, and health with regularity. Health and sickness, as well as healing, curing, and caring, involve the whole person. How spirituality and religion influence health and longevity is a matter of some dispute, although there is increasing interest in this question. It is clear that spirituality and religion constitute coping mechanisms for some persons and that a person's physical and emotional health (or lack thereof) are elements in one's *spiritual life*. Thus, it is appropriate that the health professional consider a patient's spiritual life in caring for and interacting with the patient.

This discussion of spirituality and the elderly is divided into three sections:

- Description of Spirituality
- The Third Age
- The Spiritual Dimension: Implications for the Health Care Team

DESCRIPTION OF SPIRITUALITY

A Definition

While the word *spirituality* is used widely, it is hardly unambiguous, admitting a variety of definitions and descriptions. "Of breathing or air" is the classical Latin meaning of *spiritualis,* the ancestor of the word *spiritual*. The dictionary defines *spiritual* as "of the spirit or the soul as distinguished from the body or material matters." *Ruach* is the Hebrew word for spirit, and as Oregon State University's Hundere Distinguished Professor of Religion and Culture, Marcus Borg, explains:

> *Ruach* also means wind and breath. The associations of both are suggestive. Both are invisible yet manifestly real. We cannot see the wind, though its presence and effects are felt; it moves without being seen. When it blows, it is all around us. Breath is like wind inside the body. For the ancient Hebrews (as for us), it was associated with life.

Thus *spirituality*, the quality of being spiritual, is nonmaterial and as essential and accessible to us as air, breath, and wind. Spirituality is an understanding that a vital aspect of life itself transcends the material and the visible and that there is much more to life than what we can see, taste, hear, touch, and smell. Knowing that a vital, nonmaterial aspect of life is operative can lead to a sense of meaning, a state of comfort and ease with self and the world, and a perception of homeostasis, especially during times when all is not well with our material selves and/or our material world.

Capacity for Spirituality

Spirituality is based on the capacity of an individual to be conscious and aware, to reflect and remember, to imagine and discern, to react to and make decisions, and to alter both one's interior responses and external behaviors. Spirituality is rooted in one's physiologic systems but transcends them in such a way as to constitute a unique human person. To use a computer analogy, the physiologic systems are the hardware for spirituality.

Spiritual may refer to one's philosophy, that is, a person who is spiritual looks beyond the material world. Spirituality may refer to a systematic approach to using these capacities, as in Christian "Ignatian spirituality," the calling of Muslims to *salat* and *falah* five times a day, and the Eightfold Path of the Buddhists. Spirituality involves a system of beliefs about the self and the world and a consequent pattern of behaviors based on this system.

A person's spirituality may not be apparent but is always there, at least potentially. On the other hand, it may be highly visible and central to one's approach to life. Essentially it involves a sense of the nonmaterial aspect of self *and* of this part of self in relation to all else outside of it.

Spirituality: Natural and Religious

For some, spirituality is based entirely on a relationship with the unseen mystery of the seen and experienced world. This can involve a profound sense of connectedness and oneness with the universe. This connectedness may or may not generate a sense of wholeness and comfort as a person's internal drives, hopes, and instincts become integrated with that which transcends the material and the visible. For the purposes of this chapter, we will call this *natural spirituality* as contrasted with *religious spirituality*. In reality they are closely associated, part of a continuum with the latter building on the former.

Religious spirituality explicitly involves an appreciation of and interaction with a Transcendent Reality many call God, who is perceived as not only *in* all things but also the *creator* of all things. In religious spirituality, all things are seen to be instinctively or consciously directed to God, for example, as expressed in the Alpha and Omega of Christianity, the unity of life central to Hinduism, and the submission to God's will stressed in Islam. Religious spirituality and natural spirituality can give rise to similar emotional responses both positive (peace, tranquility, sense of self-worth, and even ecstasy) and negative (guilt, anger, and depression).

Religious spirituality does not equate with membership in a formal religious organization; conversely, belonging to a religious group does not of necessity mark a person as spiritual. Formal religion involves a series of beliefs, values, practices, and visible structures. A religious person affirms and participates in these. However, this formal membership may entail little reflection or religiously informed spirituality even as some people may have a deep sense of the Transcendent without a formal religious affiliation.

Many people have found their spirituality rooted in religious traditions and even in particular approaches within specific religions, such as the Sufis within Islam, the Hasidim within Judaism, the Mahayana within Buddhism, and the Franciscans within Catholicism. Central elements in religious spirituality include a discernment of "what God wants of me" and a corresponding shaping of one's behavior. Religious spirituality may include certain *mystical* or psychological states, but any of these states should be the result of an intense realization of union with God rather than sought in and of itself.

Religious Spirituality and Healing

The degree to which religious spirituality is healing or curative is a matter of controversy, though the subject of increasing inquiry. Harold G. Koenig, of Duke University's Center for the Study of Religion/Spirituality and Health has written that

> belonging to an emotionally supportive spiritual community gives people a sense of life satisfaction and transcendental purpose. Involved in religion's indirect effect on health are the enriching support of a person's network of concerned friends, the strengthening of marriage and family bonds, and the mitigation of life stress, anxiety, and depression.

The feature article of a recent Infoaging.org Research Spotlight on Spirituality, Religion, and Healthy Aging referred to a study by Dr. William Strawbridge and other researchers appearing in the *American Journal of Public Health* in 1997. In this study, the researchers found that

> People with a strong personal faith who regularly attend religious services generally have lower blood pressure; are less likely to suffer from depression; have a greater sense of

well-being; have stronger immune systems; and live longer— 23% longer. ... (Chippendale, 2001, http://www.infoaging. org/feat9.htm)

That religious spirituality is important to many older persons is validated by experience and at least some recent research. A longitudinal study conducted by researchers Idler, Kasl, and Hays showed that religion is very important for older people. The study found that although attendance at religious services may decline as a person gets close to death, this was because of increasing frailty rather than a diminishment of religious spirituality. Those near death showed either "stability or a small increase in feelings of religiousness and strength/comfort received from religion."

THE THIRD AGE

Biological/Social Construct

To serve the older patient well, the health care professional must understand not only physiology and the impact of various diseases and traumas, but also the patient's life situation. While each person's history and social circumstances are unique, there are cultural and social structures that have an impact not only on individuals but also an entire class. The class in which we have a particular interest is those who we categorize as old. One of the ways to gain insight about the old is to consider them within a biological/social construct of personhood we might describe as separate ages. Each of the ages has the following set of characteristics:

- Physiologic development
- Emotional development
- Intellectual development
- Social roles
- Social status
- Life events
- Moral sphere

For human beings, the norm had been two ages until the latter part of the twentieth century, each with individual and social tasks. The first age spans the initial moment of existence until reproductive capacity was developed, while the second age involves reproduction and contribution to the species. Although there were exceptions, death generally occurred shortly after the reproductive function was completed. Historically the length of life was a function of the needs of the species for continuity. We might characterize these as the First and Second Ages.

The First and Second Ages Today

We can still speak of a First and Second Age in the twenty-first century. The First Age is marked by physiologic, emotional, and intellectual development. The person is viewed as a learner gaining the knowledge and skills to reproduce and make contributions to society. Societies develop structures and rituals, for example, schools, confirmations, and bar mitzvahs to mark passage through this period.

People's status and accompanying sense of self-worth are closely aligned with the way in which they succeed or fail in developmental tasks and roles. Their moral sense is developing as well, though initially with the example and prompting of those persons such as parents and institutions most significant in their lives. During this period, people develop not only a sense of self but also the stirrings of spirituality closely aligned with their newfound sense of identity and relationship to the world around them.

The Second Age begins as individuals move into new relationships, parenting, and work. The Second Age marks the high point of physiologic capacity corresponding to the demands of the new roles as spouses, parents, and workers. Much of emotional life is tied to these roles. Moral life focuses on family, work, and society. Spirituality can evolve but is in competition with the intellectual and emotional demands associated with this period. The Second Age has a number of cultural markers such as graduating from school, marrying, becoming employed, and establishing a home.

The Third Age, A Uniquely Human Experience

Until the latter part of the twentieth century, the normal life course for humans had two ages, although there were always exceptional persons who lived long lives. For most, life had often been short, painful, and uncertain. For all too many, especially in developing countries, those realities continue to prevail.

During the past 50 years, the application of knowledge to the human condition generally, and to public health and medicine specifically, seems to have brought about an aberration in the law of natural selection and the survival of the fittest. In those areas of the world applying the positive fruits of development, premature death has been curtailed and a Third Age has become normal. Pharmacologic agents, prosthetic devices, and changing societal attitudes are enabling even persons having chronic diseases or suffering from various traumas to live longer, less painful, and potentially more productive and satisfying lives.

Challenges of the Third Age

The latter part of the twentieth century experienced the development of a Third Age, an age necessary neither for production nor reproduction. While a triumph for science and often for the individual, the Third Age challenges every individual and social structure: the family, the economy, civic and political life, and, of course, the helping professions.

Society tends to equate older age with retirement, although advocates from the distinguished prizewinner Robert Butler to the editors of *Modern Maturity* emphasize health and "productive aging." While there is a recognition of chronic illnesses and the necessity to manage them better, little attention seems to be given to the latter part of life as a period of gradual but inexorable system decline. This decline is not in itself an illness, but nonetheless is associated with illnesses as well as a concomitant decrease in physiologic capacity and energy. The Third Age is a period marked by sometimes gradual, sometimes precipitous decline in functional capacity. In turn, these decrements and associated frailty interact with the person's psychological and spiritual well being.

There is some evidence that in the latter part of the twentieth century we have also seen some compression of morbidity as well as an extension of life expectancy. In the April 2001 issue of *Aging/Clinical and Experimental Research*, J.A. Brody and M.D. Grant suggest that it is too early to come to a definitive conclusion despite some studies that give a reason to hope that such is the case.

What Do We Know About the Third Age?

The Third Age remains largely a terra incognita. Societies have yet to fully respond to the new reality. Those in the Third Age are part of a new social reality without well-established norms or markers, with the exception of retirement, death of a spouse, dependency (for many), and death (for all). Societal structures that evolved over the centuries in which only two generations were the norm are now challenged by four generations (likely with two in retirement) and continued growth, both in absolute and relative terms, of an older population. The economy, family life, civic life, and public policy, in addition to health care, are faced with the necessity to adapt to a demographic phenomenon that is new. The Third Age has thousands of human faces, ultimately affecting everyone.

Even for those in similar circumstances, there are as many differences as there are similarities. Even in the same culture and society, there are significant individual differences by reason of life experience, social status, personal gifts, and gender. However, there are themes associated with old age that are independent of culture; older persons have had many experiences. Whether they are examined, reflected upon, and made the basis for a better life for themselves or others is another matter. As in the other stages of life, there are positives and negatives. Often individuals are freed from primary family and work responsibilities. On the negative side, people may become frail, poor, dependent, and otherwise marginalized.

By definition the Third Age is a period of the life journey through which all aspire to pass. It is an interval of time, like the other ages, in which there is a progression through various events. It is associated with both personal and social change.

Some persons will have a short Third Age, marked by considerable frailty; others will have a relatively long Third Age of vigor until the moment of death. The normal path is marked by gradual diminishing physiologic capacity, sometimes of psychological and intellectual acuity, and often of social relationships.

For some it is a gifted period filled with possibilities; for others it is a time of new or continued suffering in terms of oppression, illness, poverty, loss, frailty, and loneliness. Paradoxically, from a spiritual perspective, the Third Age is often a graceless period for the former and a time of grace for the latter. An example of grace in oppression, poverty, and loss can be found in Viktor Frankl's very moving book *Man's Search for Meaning*. Dr. Frankl writes about choice of action in the midst of the intense suffering in a Nazi concentration camp, a passage applicable to the accumulation of losses often incurred for the patients in the Third Age:

> We who lived in concentration camps can remember the men who walked through the huts comforting others, giving away their last piece of bread. They may have been few in number, but they offer sufficient proof that everything can be taken from a man but one thing: the last of the human freedoms—to choose one's attitude in any given set of circumstances, to choose one's own way.

In summary, from a societal perspective this is a new phenomenon, just as it is for every person who engages it. It is filled with ambiguity. The Third Age is a time that will certainly test one's spirituality, both natural and religious.

THE SPIRITUAL DIMENSION: IMPLICATIONS FOR HEALTH CARE

Role of Health Care Professionals

Health care professionals play many roles in the lives of persons in the Third Age: contributing to the promotion of health, preventing disease whenever possible, assisting in recovery from disease or trauma, and easing physical and psychological pain, even in situations in which death is approaching. In short, the physician in concert with others is involved in preserving, preventing, restoring, and at all times, caring.

Because diminishing health is so central during a period that can be confusing, frightening, painful, and depressing, all the members of the health care team are key actors in the passage through the Third Age. The complexity of the physical, psychological, economic, social, and spiritual elements of an older person's life requires the skills and commitment of many different professionals: nurses, social workers, physical and occupational therapists, nutritionists, clergy, and pharmacists as well as geriatricians.

As health care professionals consider their interactions with the patient, it is well to recognize that the patient does not exist in a vacuum. Each patient has a unique past with instances of triumph and disappointment, moments of certainty and confusion, and times of generosity and selfishness. The patient's unique journey to the present moment has given him or her a perspective on suffering, loss, mortality, and all the issues of life that are essentially spiritual in nature. This unique journey colors his or her relationships with family, significant others, formal caregivers, and even the health professionals who are so central at this period.

Natural Spirituality

Among common issues faced by all are

- Mortality and morbidity
- Meaning (or perceived lack of meaning) of one's own life
- Unresolved anger and grudges, oftentimes present for many decades of one's life
- Loss of mobility, independence, family, friends
- Unwillingness to forgive or fear of seeking forgiveness
- Guilt
- Sense of disconnectedness
- Dissatisfaction with progressive dependency
- Lack of fulfillment throughout life or at present
- Fear of becoming a burden to others

Religious Spirituality

On the positive side, all those who are part of the healing-curing-caring system strive to help the patient at every stage to have a degree of comfort and ease with self and the world, regardless of the disease of this patient. All must strive to know and understand the patient as a person, including his or her perspective on suffering, loss, and mortality.

Health care professionals are not spiritual directors in the religious sense but should be skilled in understanding the impact for good or ill that the patient's and significant others' spirituality are having on the overall well-being of the patient. Dr. Upinder Singh (personal communication, December 3, 2001), a geriatrician with Loretto in Syracuse, NY, feels that because religious spirituality can help patients cope better with life and lead to more disciplined and healthier lifestyles, this spirituality can play as crucial a role in prevention of health problems as immunization and sanitation. As in instances when a geriatrician and other professional caregivers would call for specialists in a patient's physical or mental care, it is just as appropriate for this geriatrician to seek the assistance of pastoral care personnel.

Spiritually based values are integral to the concept of professionalism. Service to others, the continual acquiring of knowledge and skill, the importance of integrity, and concern for the most vulnerable are the hallmarks of every profession and professional. These values are rooted in a shared perception of the importance and vulnerability of each human being. The sacredness of the helping professions is rooted in the natural spirituality that all share and the religious spirituality that animates many individuals and social interventions. These ideals are the bedrock of the lives of persons such as physicians who daily deal with pain, suffering, and death.

A Concluding Thought

In ancient Israel, the Hebrews had an important tradition to renew the land by letting it lie fallow every 7 years. After seven periods of 7 years, a very long interval of life at that time in history, a Year of Jubilee was to be celebrated. During the Year of Jubilee, in addition to providing for the relationship between the land and the people, the tradition broadened considerably to include relationships among the people themselves. During this year, the Hebrews were to forgive debts, redistribute wealth, and liberate those in servitude.

The Third Age can also be thought of as the time, after a long interval in life, to set relationships aright. Many older people are deeply troubled by ruptured relationships in their lives, especially relationships that were once rich and nurturing. To live into the Third Age gives them an opportunity, perhaps their final opportunity, to forgive and be forgiven. And the *choice* to forgive is always theirs, regardless of whether their forgiveness will be accepted or they will be forgiven in return.

Even when physical curing is not within the range of possibility, the potential for mental and spiritual healing exists for all patients in the Third Age.

REFERENCES

Borg MJ: *The God We Never Knew: Beyond Dogmatic Religion to a More Authentic Contemporary Faith.* San Francisco, Harper, 1997, p 72.

Brody JA, Grant MD: Age-associated diseases and conditions: Implications for decreasing late life morbidity. *Aging Clin Exper Res* 13(2):64, 2001.

Butler RN: *Why Survive? Being Old in America.* New York, Harper and Row, 1975.

Chippendale L: Spirituality, religion and healthy aging. American Federation for Aging Research *Infoaging.org Research Spotlight,* August 25, 2001. Retrieved November 26, 2001, from http://www.infoaging.org/feat9.htm

Cutler DM: Declining disability among the elderly. *Health Affairs* 20(6): 11, 2001.

Frankl V: *Man's Search for Meaning,* 3rd ed. New York: Touchstone, Simon & Schuster, 1984, p 75.

Idler E et al: Patterns of religious practice and belief in the last year of life. *J Gerontol B Psychol Sci Soc Sci* 56B(6):S326, 2001.

Koenig HG et al: *The Healing Power of Faith: How Belief and Prayer Can Help You Triumph Over Disease,* 1st ed. New York, Touchstone, 2001, p 264.

Turner W: *Leviticus Collegeville Bible Commentary on Leviticus 25.* Collegeville, MN, The Liturgical Press, 1985, p 74.

Webster's New World College Dictionary, 4th ed. Foster City, CA, IDG Books Worldwide, 2001, p 1382.

Ethical Issues in Geriatric Medicine: Informed Consent, Surrogate Decision Making, and Advance Care Planning

JASON H.T. KARLAWISH • BRYAN D. JAMES

The competent practice of geriatric medicine relies on mastery of both a body of knowledge about how to diagnose and treat the geriatric syndromes and an ethic to apply this knowledge to the care of patients. In general, the ethics of patient care focus on using the principles of respect for autonomy and beneficence to guide making decisions with patients. Perhaps one of the most important mechanisms to apply these principles is informed consent, that is, the voluntary choice of a competent patient. In these respects, geriatrics is just like fields such as cardiology and endocrinology that have carved out a particular focus of research, education, and practice, and share a common ethic to guide the care of patients.

However, geriatrics differs from other branches of medicine in a number of distinct and ethically substantive ways. Most branches of medicine are largely organized around an organ system, such as the gastrointestinal system, or around a pathology, such as cancer. But geriatrics is organized around a group of persons defined by a label: the elderly. Being elderly does not simply equate to an organ system or pathology. Instead, it describes a stage in a life course whose beginning is indeterminate and constructed out of a matrix of biological, social, political, and cultural conditions. For example, geriatric patients are often defined as persons age 65 years and older. This age cut-off, while precise, is constructed out of the legislation that defines eligibility for state retirement and healthcare benefits.

Of course, all medical practice is in some manner bound to social, political, and cultural conditions. For example, concepts of mental illness are influenced by ideas of sin and morals. Older persons, however, are a group suspended between normal and disease. Geriatricians face the challenge

of negotiating the fungible boarders between illness and normal aging, and between living and dying. This means that mastery of the common ethic of medicine is necessary, but it is not sufficient. This chapter addresses the ethics of medicine focused on the care of elderly persons. The focus is an ethic that addresses the relationship between the patient and physician—informed consent—and particular issues in informed consent that are important for the competent practice of geriatric medicine: advance care planning, quality of life, refusal of treatment, withdrawal and withholding of treatment, and surrogate decision making. We also discuss the conditions that underlie decisions, namely voluntariness and the system of care.

DECIDING WITH PATIENTS

The ethical foundation of making decisions with patients is informed consent, that is, the voluntary choice of a competent patient. Competency is an essential guidance principle to assure that physicians strike a proper balance between protecting patient autonomy and promoting patient welfare. In other words, competency provides a tool to balance the two ethical principles of respect for autonomy and beneficence. A competent patient should be allowed to choose even if the choice is harmful or "goes against medical advice." In contrast, an incompetent patient is not allowed to choose. This denial of choice is not because the physician objects to the patient's choice, but because the patient cannot make a choice. Chapter 10 defines and discusses how to assess competency and decision-making capacity; the point of this section is to address three challenges in the practice of informed consent.

The origins of informed consent are largely surgical cases as follows. A patient suffers harm after an intervention such as lower extremity paralysis after an aortic angiogram. The patient argues that when she agreed to the intervention the physician did not tell her about the chance of hemiplegia and had the physician told her, she would not have agreed to the intervention. From these surgical cases grew an ethical model of informed consent applicable to all of medical practice. The model is that a physician provides the patient facts about the procedure, verifies that the patient has adequate decision-making abilities to use these facts to make a decision, and then practices care based on the patient's choice. This model describes a patient who desires information, control over the decision, and her care guided by her values. Informed consent is seen as a remedy to unilateral physician decisions for patients based on the physician's preferences and values, that is, paternalism.

Informed consent is a vital ethic to guide medical care. In certain kinds of decisions, informed consent facilitates decision making. These decisions include a choice between interventions with very different kinds of risks and benefits (such as surgery versus medical therapy versus watchful waiting for prostate cancer), decisions that are highly personal and value laden (such as advance care planning which is discussed in more detail below), and decisions that are not part of the physician–patient relationship (such as enrollment in research). As useful as informed consent is, there are at least three challenges to its practice.

First, informed consent may not be the ethic that patients want to follow. Specifically, patients describe an asymmetry between their desire for information and their desire to make their medical decisions. In particular, elderly patients often indicate that they want their physician to give them information but they want the physician to make the decision. This asymmetry is often greatest in the case of decisions about the management of serious and life-threatening situations. In these cases, patients will describe decision making built on trust and identification with their physician.

The second challenge to the practice of informed consent is the effective communication of medical information. Much of medical information is probabilistic. This means that the occurrence of an event, such as a fall, is bounded by a chance. Such information can be expressed numerically using figures such as an odds ratio or percentage, or qualitatively using expressions such as "rare" or "likely." Each of these presents challenges to the practice of informed consent. People (both patients and physicians) have difficulty with quantitative expressions. This numerical illiteracy means that people may misunderstand information. Related to this is the ambiguity of qualitative expressions such as "rare." These are subject to widely different meanings: "rare" can mean 1 percent to one person and 0.001 percent to another person. Finally, biases often influence people's decisions. Biases describe implicit cognitive processes that introduce error into a decision.

Related to the challenge of communicating medical information is a third challenge: patients may have impairments in their cognition as a result of geriatric syndromes such as dementia and delirium. These impairments can limit a patient's abilities to understand, appreciate, and reason to the degree that the patient is not competent.

Table 29-1 summarizes these challenges to the practice of informed consent and suggests strategies to address them. A general strategy to guide the practice of informed consent is to reject a "consumer model" of informed consent wherein the patient is the "informed customer" and the physician a kind of "service provider." A more useful strategy is one grounded in the relationship between physician and patient. In this relationship, doctor means "teacher" (from the Latin *doctore*) and consent means "to feel together" (from the Latin *con* plus *sentire*). Together these concepts mean the geriatrician's practice should recognize that patients, like students, have different kinds of learning needs and skills. Some individuals are quick studies who take charge of the task, while others need careful tutoring and even prompting. Some individuals simply cannot be taught or do not want to be taught. In all of these cases, the goal is to create a shared understanding of the relevant facts and the patient's values. These skills are essential for all of medical decision making. The issue is not that some patients are more or less intelligent than others, but that some patients, even very intelligent ones, choose not to control decision making. Below, we discuss additional skills necessary to address the challenges of making decisions with patients including advance care planning; quality of life; refusing, withdrawing, and withholding treatment; and decisions at the end of life.

Advance Care Planning

Elderly patients often have chronic and ultimately fatal illnesses. The care of patients in the severe to terminal stages of these illnesses typically involves decisions that require trade-offs between different kinds of symptoms, or the quality versus the quantity of life. The patients are often unable to make decisions. One strategy to make these difficult decisions is to make them when the patient is competent; that is, advance care planning. The term describes a competent patient and her physician discussing and then documenting the patient's preferences for future medical care. This preserves a patient's self-determination even after she has lost decision-making capacity. The classic mechanism to do this is an advance directive.

An advance directive is a set of instructions indicating a competent person's preferences for future medical care should she become incompetent or unable to communicate. Advance directives typically focus on the conditions of being terminal, comatose, or in a state of irreversible suffering. However, there is no reason why an advance directive cannot address periods of incapacity as a result of other conditions, such as the years spent in the moderate to terminal stages of dementia or a period of delirium that might follow a planned surgery. For example, persons whose religious beliefs proscribe the receipt of blood products can have an advance directive that instructs healthcare providers not to give them a blood transfusion.

There are two types of advance directives: a living will and a durable power of attorney. A living will is a document

development of an acute confusional episode or frank delirium. Adverse changes in cognitive function will often prolong a hospital stay and worsen clinical outcomes. Significant age and disease related reductions in skeletal muscle mass (sarcopenia) decrease the capacity of the older patient to make a functional recovery, possibly resulting in a discharge to a subacute or long-term care facility.

The older patient may be unable to adequately communicate concerns or clinical history to a health care provider. Therefore to ensure the best possible surgical outcome for the older patient it may be necessary to maximize the communication and exchange of data between the surgical team and the medical providers. Clinical programs that have fostered a closer relationship between the surgeon and consulting internist have demonstrated a trend for better surgical outcomes and greater functional recoveries. Several groups within the academic community are promoting comprehensive programs to increase geriatric expertise in the surgical and medical specialties by direct education of the surgical and consulting teams in the principles of geriatric medical care. These efforts are likely to further improve operative outcomes for older patients.

In summary, because normal aging does not account for the bulk of operative risk, the clinician's task is to identify underlying illnesses in older surgical patients and assess their impact on perioperative risk. Teamwork and communication between the disciplines often provides the best possible understanding of the patient's clinical situation, helping to mitigate surgical risk.

SPECIFIC CONSIDERATIONS

Cardiac Complications

Coronary artery disease, the primary cause of death for the elderly person, is highly prevalent in older populations. It is estimated that 25 to 30 percent of all perioperative deaths are attributed to cardiac causes. Because older patients are more likely to have significant CAD, they should be carefully screened for signs and symptoms of occult or overt disease. As previously noted, the age-associated increases in vascular and left ventricular stiffness result in a greater sensitivity to volume shifts. Age-related declines in the electrical conduction system place the elderly patient at a greater a risk for drug-induced bradycardia or high-grade atrioventricular (AV) blocks. A prior myocardial infarction or a low ejection fraction is associated with a greater risk of ventricular tachycardia.

Pulmonary Complications

With advancing age the respiratory system demonstrates several changes in function, which may include a loss of pulmonary elastic recoil, decreased diffusion capacity, and reduced cough and gag reflexes, either as a consequence of neurologic injury or of respiratory muscle weakness. Postoperatively, it is common for older patients to experience atelectasis or frank aspiration. It is estimated that 14 percent of older patients will have a major pulmonary perioperative complication (pneumonia, pulmonary edema, or a pulmonary embolus), particularly after an abdominal or a cardiothoracic procedure. Postoperative pneumonia in older patients is associated with a 15 to 20 percent mortality rate and must be treated with aggressive respiratory therapy and appropriate antibiotics. It is helpful to obtain a detailed pulmonary and occupational exposure history prior to surgery that helps to predict impaired respiratory function. Because neurologic events that may impair airway protection are occasionally subtle, obtaining a history of swallowing difficulties or prior aspiration may prompt an early start to postoperative interventions aimed at reducing aspiration risk.

Renal Complications

Renal function is reduced as a result of glomerular and tubular senescence. The progressive sclerosis of glomeruli occurs with increasing age and is typically hastened by comorbid conditions like HTN, diabetes mellitus (DM), and CAD. In the older patient, the serum creatinine often does not fully reflect the reduction in renal function. The age-associated reduction in skeletal muscle reduces creatinine production, so a reduced creatinine clearance is not always as apparent, even in the setting of diminished filtration. There is greater risk for volume and pH disturbances in the perioperative period because of the impaired renal function.

Functional Capacity

Between the ages of 30 and 80 years, healthy subjects may lose 30 to 40 percent of the muscle mass from the legs and back and 30 percent of the arm musculature. Declines in strength and aerobic capacity parallel the decrease in muscle mass. Decreasing physical activity, common in older adults, and the age-associated loss of muscle mass (sarcopenia) contribute to a decline in exercise capacity. When acute or chronic medical conditions develop in older patients, the loss of muscle mass and functional capacity is often greater and more problematic.

Functional impairment is an index of the severity of many chronic diseases and its severity predicts operative risk. For example, poor performance on a bicycle ergometer is a better predictor than the Goldman criteria of surgical outcomes and postoperative pulmonary complications. The metabolic demand of surgery and the physical immobility associated with recovery may promote further declines in strength and function. It is not atypical to find a previously independent older adult becoming so frail postoperatively that rehabilitative care is needed. Promoting clinical services that increases physical activity and rehabilitation during the surgical recovery process may improve the level of functional independence, shorten recovery times, and prevent readmissions.

Emergency Surgeries

Emergency surgeries are associated with a higher overall death rate in all age groups. This is most apparent in older patients who have the highest rates as a consequence of a greater number of complications. The causes for the increased risk are multifactorial and include the fact that the identical surgical disease in the elderly patient may present later in its course. The diagnosis can be delayed because of an atypical presentation. The elderly patient may be treated later by surgeons wishing to correct the associated comorbidities prior to surgery. In the older patient a delay in a needed nonemergent surgery may have a greater risk if there is a chance that the delay could result in an emergent procedure. Therefore, medical providers should be aware that if the time needed to optimize the patient for surgery is excessive, an anticipated elective procedure could become a higher mortality emergent procedure.

Other Concerns

Neurologic events, such as a stroke, may increase the risk of aspiration by making it difficult to swallow, to move food through the esophagus, and to control respiratory secretions. Advancing age is also associated with a decrease in esophageal peristaltic wave amplitude, reduced tone of the lower esophageal sphincter, a greater incidence of hiatal hernias, delayed gastric emptying, and increased gastroesophageal reflux. All are factors that may increase the perioperative aspiration risk. Age-associated changes in the immune system are subtle, but may contribute to a greater risk for infection from organisms that colonize the pulmonary and urinary tracts. Impaired glucose regulation and risk for stress hyperglycemia is common in this age group, and may increase infection risks. Thus careful monitoring to control blood sugars perioperatively may have important benefits.

Taking the time to discuss the surgery with the older patient and their family promotes a clearer understanding of risk and benefits and will help to reduce the chance of false expectations with surgery. Incorporating the common geriatric care format of patient and family conferences in the surgical environment can be very helpful. In such discussions, it is often apparent that an older patient has a different outlook and acceptance of a specific level of care. Shorter-term goals, such as the quality, not quantity, of life may be most important. Additionally, the tolerance of surgery may be different than that of a younger person. The understanding that a longer time to recover may be necessary is often best communicated in this forum. It is also important to inform the patient and family that an intermediate-care program may be needed, such as a subacute care center, a rehabilitation unit, or the extensive use of home care services.

Period of Risk

Anesthesia is generally considered a safe procedure in elderly patients, with a progressive decline in complication rates observed in recent years. Preoperative risk factors are a better predictor of 7-day mortality than is the duration of anesthesia or the experience of the anesthesiologist. The type of anesthesia (e.g., spinal versus inhalational) fails to predict outcomes once the preoperative risk factors are controlled. The greatest period of risk for complications remains the time after surgery, with half of the events occurring within 3 weeks of surgery.

PREOPERATIVE MANAGEMENT

History and Physical

The accurate assessment of risk is focused on a detailed review of the clinical history and physical examination. It is this comprehensive review that guides the patient along the various algorithms and directs the selection of preoperative testing. Underlying changes in cognitive function are particularly important to the risk assessment of the older patient; these changes may reduce the validity of reported signs and symptoms. A discussion with family members should be sought if clinical data is unclear, cognitive impairments are profound, or the responses are misleading.

The assessment should include a review of physical function, cognitive ability, competency, availability of social support, and symptoms of depression. Cognitive impairment places the patient at an increased risk for perioperative delirium and a longer hospital course. Elderly patients should be screened for impairments using the Mini-Mental State Examination or similar standardized screening instrument. An elderly patient with little family or social support who undergoes surgery is likely to have a protracted recovery period. Therefore, a preoperative evaluation by a social worker with experience in geriatric medicine is helpful in structuring a supportive network of resources that will reduce complications during the recovery process. Subacute nursing care facilities may play a particularly helpful role in advancing the frail older patient through the recovery process and back to independence.

The physical examination can be altered by age and disease. For example, a systolic ejection murmur suggesting aortic stenosis may represent aortic valve sclerosis rather than a hemodynamically significant valvular stenosis. Additionally, markers of severe aortic stenosis, a diminished S2, or a delay in the carotid up-stroke, may be less apparent in older patients. When the exam is uncertain, echocardiography and Doppler studies are warranted to establish an accurate cardiac diagnosis, particularly if the murmur is late peaking or radiating to the carotids.

Medications

The preoperative exam is an ideal time to review medication lists and to determine the overall benefit of these drugs for the patient. Aspirin, clopidogrel, nonsteroidals, and other antiplatelet drugs increase the risk of perioperative bleeding and if not required, should be held for a recommended 7 to 10 days. Drugs with anticholinergic properties, such as diphenhydramine or meclizine, are likely to increase the risk of perioperative delirium and should be held. Chronic benzodiazepine use is common and often under recognized. These drugs should be tapered to reduce the risk of withdrawal symptoms when the patient is made NPO. Holding diuretics for 24 to 48 hours prior to surgery should be considered if they are not needed to treat excessive volume or symptoms of pulmonary congestion in patients with congestive heart failure.

Patients on antiepileptic, cardiovascular, and antihypertensive medications typically should take their medications on the morning of surgery with limited amounts of water. Abrupt discontinuation of beta blockers and clonidine are associated with significant cardiovascular complications. Patients using these medications can be effectively managed with intravenous propranolol, metoprolol, or transcutaneous clonidine patches. Oral hypoglycemics are typically held the night prior to surgery to reduce the risk of perioperative hypoglycemia. Insulin-treated diabetic patients typically receive half of their usual dose of intermediate-acting insulin on the morning of surgery and are typically given appropriate amounts of a 5 percent dextrose solution intravenously. Postoperative glucose above 250 mg/dL are safely managed with subcutaneous insulin or short-acting intravenous infusions of insulin, if hemodynamic instability is present (a cause of variable absorption of subcutaneous insulin). Adrenal suppression resulting from chronic steroid use should be treated with stress doses of a steroid, typically 100 mg of hydrocortisone every 6 hours beginning the night prior to surgery and tapering to the maintenance dose in 3 to 5 days as is permitted by their postoperative course.

Preoperative Assessment for Noncardiac Surgery

As 25 to 30 percent of perioperative deaths are attributed to cardiac causes, much of the risk assessment is focused on predicting these cardiac complications. The poor surgical performance of the older patient reflects the high prevalence of CAD, which is often subtle or even silent until the stress of surgery. The current American College of Cardiology and American Heart Association (ACC/AHA) guidelines are a rapidly applied algorithm that is helpful in assessing risk and directing appropriate preoperative testing and management (Figs. 30-1 through 30-3). An in-depth review of the preoperative assessment prior to noncardiac

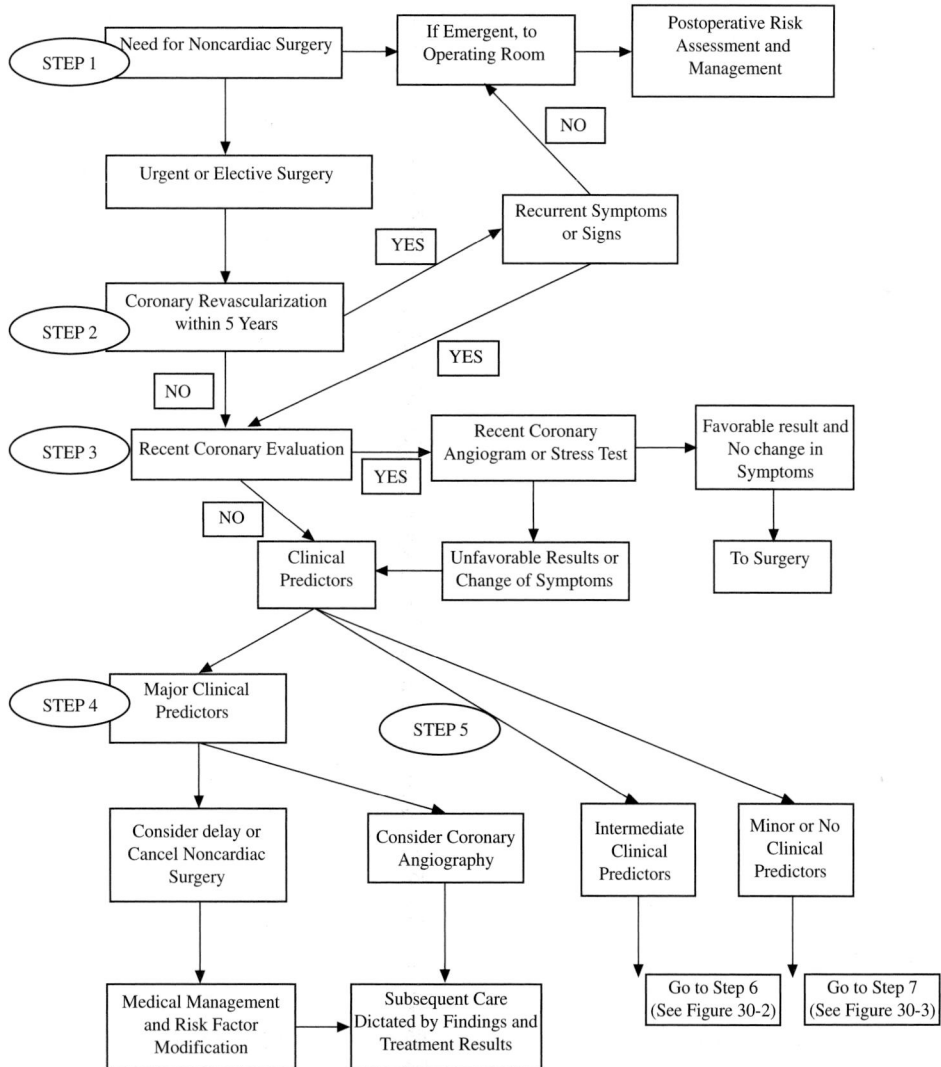

Figure 30-1 Stepwise approach to preoperative cardiac risk assessment. MET, metabolic equivalents of task. †See Table 30-2.

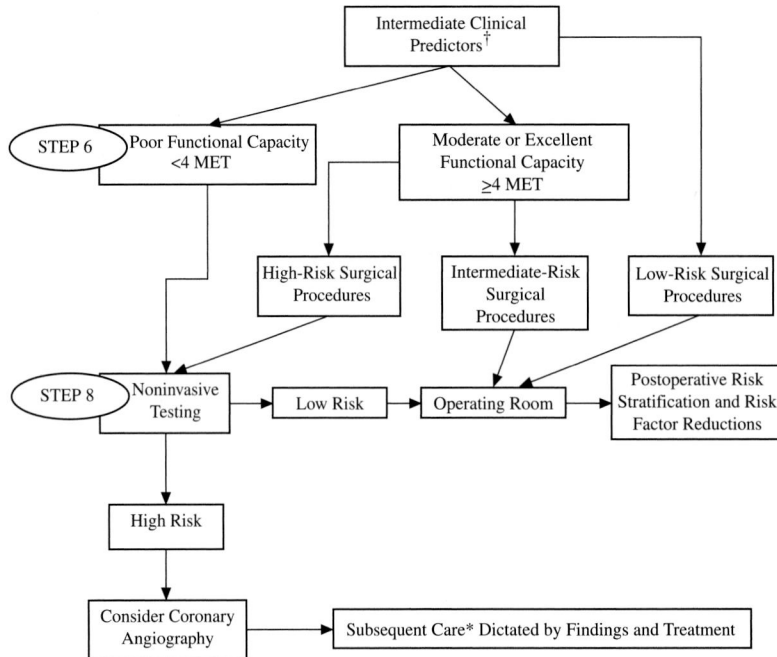

Figure 30-2   MET, metabolic equivalents of task. *Subsequent care may include cancellation or delay of surgery, coronary revascularization followed by noncardiac surgery, or intensified care. †See Table 30-2.

surgery is beyond the scope of this chapter. Nevertheless, the reader should review the published guidelines for a comprehensive understanding of their appropriate use. The aggressiveness of the evaluation is determined by the patient's clinical symptoms. If a surgical emergency exists, appropriate testing and treatment is provided until the time of surgery. On occasion, medical concerns may require the cancellation of surgery.

The initial history, physical examination, and electrocardiogram are helpful in identifying potentially serious cardiac disease such as a prior myocardial infarction, angina, congestive heart failure, conduction abnormalities, or arrhythmias. It is essential to define the severity of the disease, its stability, and any prior treatments before surgery. Clinical factors that are significant tools in assessing risk are functional capacity, age, comorbidities, and the type

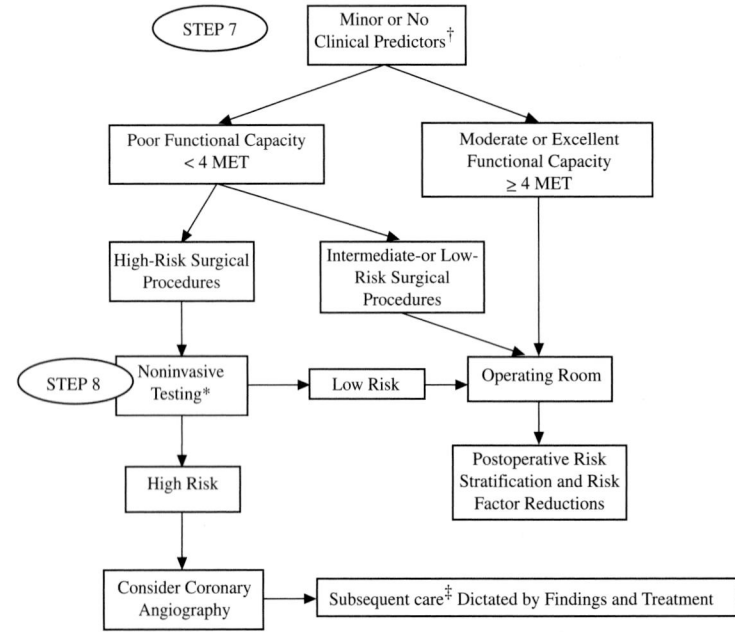

Figure 30-3   Stepwise approach to preoperative cardiac risk assessment. MET, metabolic equivalents of task. *Myocardial perfusion imaging or stress echocardiography. †See Table 30-2. ‡Subsequent care may include cancellation or delay of surgery, coronary revascularization followed by noncardiac surgery, or intensified care.

of surgery. Vascular procedures or prolonged thoracic, abdominal, and head and neck surgeries are considered higher risk.

The benefit of the ACC/AHA guidelines is the stepwise bayesian strategy that uses clinical characteristics to define surgical risk in algorithmic tables (see Figs. 30-1 through 30-3). Eight key questions help to direct the decision process down the flow chart and are briefly reviewed.

- *Step 1. Urgency of surgery:* If a patient has an immediate need for surgery, with a poor likelihood of survival without it, then it is best to provide medical management as needed and permit the surgery without delay (see Fig. 30-1).
- *Step 2. Revascularization:* Has the patient had coronary revascularization in the past 5 years? If yes, have they remained stable or are they currently symptomatic? Further testing is generally not necessary if they have stable symptoms.
- *Step 3. Recent evaluation:* Has there been an evaluation of ischemic symptoms in the past 2 years? If yes, have the symptoms been adequately assessed and the CAD appropriately treated? If it has been appropriately addressed, it is typically not necessary to repeat the workup, unless new symptoms are noted.
- *Step 4. Disease instability:* Does the patient have major clinical predictors (Table 30-2), unstable signs or symptoms that are concerning such as unstable angina, decompensated heart failure, symptomatic arrhythmias, severe valvular heart disease, or a recent myocardial infarction? A yes answer to one of these concerns indicates a significant risk factor that may lead to a delay in surgery until symptoms are addressed and potential interventions are thoroughly considered.
- *Step 5. Intermediate risk:* Does the patient have intermediate clinical predictors of risk (see Table 30-2)?
- *Step 6. Functional capacity:* Patients lacking major risk factors but having intermediate predictors of risk and who have a moderate to excellent functional capacity can routinely undergo an intermediate risk surgery with a small probability of perioperative death or myocardial infarction (see Fig. 30-2). Functional capacity is best assessed in metabolic equivalents of task (MET) and is helpful in predicting risk (Table 30-3). Noninvasive testing is considered for patients with a poor or moderate functional capacity when higher-risk surgery is planned, especially if two or more intermediate predictors are present. Perioperative and long-term cardiac risk is higher in patients unable to meet a 4-MET level of exertion during most daily activities.
- *Step 7. Minor or no clinical predictors:* Noncardiac surgery is generally safe for patients lacking both major and intermediate predictors of risk and who have a moderate or excellent functional capacity (≥4 MET) (see Fig. 30-3). Further testing is considered on an individual basis for patients without clinical markers but with a poor functional capacity who are facing higher risk operations, especially those individuals with several minor clinical predictors who will undergo a vascular surgery. Table 30-4 lists examples of a given surgery's specific risks.

Table 30-2 Clinical Predictors of an Increased Risk for Perioperative Cardiovascular Events

Major clinical predictor of risk (Step 4)
  Unstable coronary signs and symptoms
    Recent myocardial infarction* with ischemic risk by symptoms or testing
    Unstable or severe angina[†] (class III to IV)[‡]
  Decompensated heart failure
  Significant arrhythmias
    High-grade atrioventricular block
    Symptomatic ventricular arrhythmias with underlying heart disease
    Supraventricular arrhythmias with uncontrolled ventricular response
  Severe valvular heart disease

Intermediate predictors of risk (Step 6)
  Mild Angina (class I to II)
  Prior myocardial infarction by history or pathologic Q waves
  Compensated or prior congestive heart failure
  Diabetes mellitus

Minor predictors of risk (Step 7)
  Advanced, age
  LVH, LBBB, ST-T abnormalities on electrocardiogram
  Rhythm other than normal sinus
  Low functional capacity
  History of stroke
  Uncontrolled systemic hypertension

LBBB, left bundle-branch block; LVH, left ventricular hypertrophy

*Recent myocardial infarction is ≥7 days but <30 days.

[†]May include stable angina in those who are very sedentary (e.g., nursing home patients).

[‡]Canadian Cardiovascular Society class.

- *Step 8. Noninvasive testing:* The result of noninvasive testing can be used to determine further preoperative management, which may include further medication or revascularization.

These steps facilitate selecting the appropriate direction on the algorithms. Time should be taken to fully understand how this tool functions. Clinical situations not addressed by these protocols should be reviewed with a consultant cardiologist.

Other Cardiovascular Concerns

Hypertension

Severe HTN should be controlled before surgery as permitted by the clinical circumstances. Continuation of preoperative antihypertensive treatments throughout the perioperative period is critical, particularly if that agent is a beta-blocker or clonidine.

Table 30-3   Estimated Energy Requirements

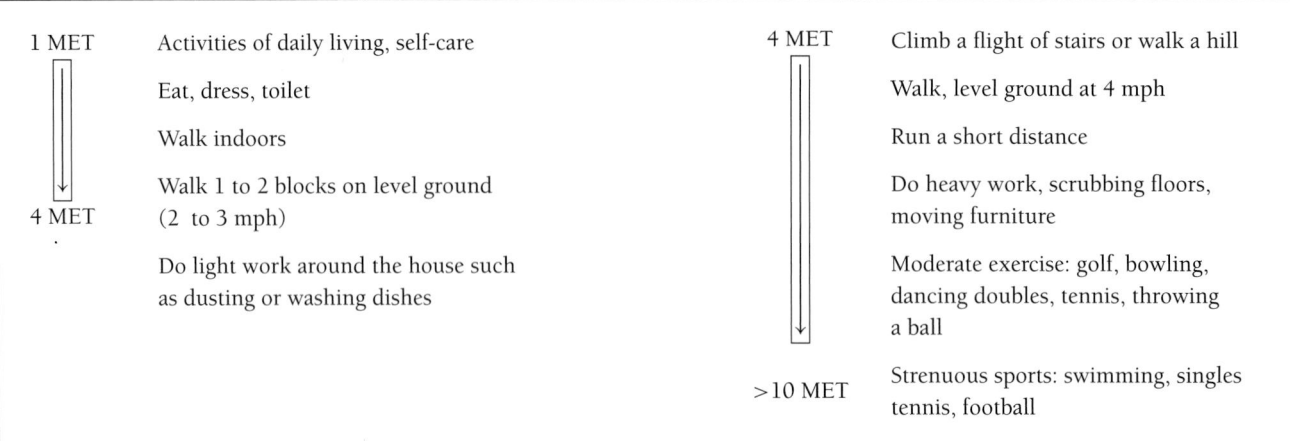

MET, metabolic equivalent of task.

Valvular Disease

Indications for the evaluation and treatment of valvular heart disease are similar to those in the nonoperative setting. Symptomatic mitral or aortic stenosis is associated with significant perioperative risk, severe congestive heart failure, or shock. Patients could be considered for percutaneous valvotomy or valve surgery preoperatively. Symptomatic aortic or mitral regurgitant disease is typically of less risk during surgery when managed with intensive medical therapy and monitoring. The patient with both severe valvular regurgitation and reduced left ventricular function is best managed with the assistance of a consultant cardiologist.

Table 30-4   Cardiac Event* Risk Stratified by Noncardiac Surgeries

High (cardiac risk >5%)
Emergent major operation, especially in the elderly patient
Aortic or major vascular procedure
Peripheral vascular
Prolonged surgeries with large volume shifts and/or blood loss

Intermediate (cardiac risk <5%)
Carotid endarterectomy
Head and Neck
Intraperitoneal and intrathoracic
Orthopedic
Prostate

Low[†] (cardiac risk <1%)
Endoscopic procedures
Superficial procedures
Cataracts
Breast

*Combined incidence of cardiac death and nonfatal myocardial infarction.

[†]Further perioperative cardiac testing is generally required.

Perioperative Beta Blockers

Several reviews recommend the use of beta-blockers perioperatively for all patients at high risk for coronary events who are scheduled for noncardiac surgery, providing contraindications do not exist. When atenolol was given intravenously or orally, beginning 2 days before surgery and continuing for 7 days after, the event-free survival at 6 months was higher in the atenolol group. Ideally, beta-blocker therapy should be initiated several days to weeks prior to surgery. The dose is adjusted to achieve a resting heart rate of no more than 60 beats per minute. The use of shorter-acting agents may be preferable in the elderly patient because it permits greater flexibility in dose titration and allows the opportunity to stop the drug quickly, with less risk of sustained side effects such as symptomatic bradycardias. Beta-blockers should be continued throughout the perioperative period.

Other Preventive Measures

The waiting period before an elective procedure can be used to promote activities that may enhance the recovery from surgery. Patients who receive exercise training twice a week, education, nurse-initiated telephone calls, and an offer to participate in postoperative cardiac rehabilitation have fewer days in the hospital, less time in the intensive care unit, and greater improvements in measures of quality of life. Many surgeons recommend preoperative physical conditioning by encouraging the patient to walk daily for 2 to 3 weeks prior to an elective surgery. This is often coupled with postoperative care plans that encourage early ambulation.

Patients with severe lung disease or who are debilitated should have an introduction to the proper use of incentive spirometry prior to surgery to reduce the risk of pulmonary atelectasis and its associated complications. This is perhaps the most important element in reducing postoperative pulmonary complications, particularly when there is an aggressive education program that encourages the use of these devices in the weeks prior to an elective surgery. Smoking cessation at least 8 weeks prior to surgery may be helpful.

Reactive airway disease should be maximally treated with bronchodilators and possibly steroids prior to surgery.

Intravascular volume status is critical and should be optimized preoperatively. Volume contraction should be avoided because of the older patient's greater dependence on left ventricular preload to maintain cardiac output. Routine hemodynamic monitoring using invasive techniques may prevent a few complications, but its routine use remains highly controversial. The use of an intraoperative pulmonary artery catheter to optimize preload, afterload, and isotropic support is likely of benefit only in selected patients.

Deep venous thrombosis (DVT) is a vexing concern in the postoperative patient. Pulmonary emboli are still thought to be one of the leading causes of in hospital death and may account for one third of the postoperative deaths in the elderly. Procedures commonly performed in the older person, such as hip or knee replacements and urologic or gynecologic procedures, place the older patient at a high risk for this complication. For low-to-moderate–risk procedures, low-dose heparin subcutaneously or external pneumatic compression devices started immediately after surgery is recommended and should be continued until the time of discharge. For higher-risk surgeries low-molecular-weight heparin or warfarin should be considered as a means to prevent postoperative DVT.

Endocarditis remains a risk because of the higher prevalence of valvular disease in older patients. Oral, bowel, urinary tract, biliary, and pulmonary procedures may result in bacteremia and an increased risk for infection if significant valve disease exists. The AHA/ACC recommendations for endocarditis prophylaxis, as well as the preoperative assessment guidelines can be reviewed at the following web sites: www.americanheart.org and www.acc.org.

Do Not Resuscitate Orders

The need for surgery in patients with do not resuscitate (DNR) orders or concerns of medical futility, may be an issue in some elderly patients. Unfortunately, many elderly patients still do not have discussions with their health care providers prior to a hospitalization concerning DNR status, even though this is often mandated. The Patient Self-Determination Act requires that hospitals and other health care facilities inform patients of their right to appoint a proxy or surrogate decision-maker to act on their wishes regarding life-sustaining care should they become incompetent. Focused efforts by nurses, clinicians, and consultants to enhance communication increase the use of advance directives. Debate exists about honoring these orders in the operating suite when patients request a DNR status and still must undergo surgery (e.g., percutaneous feeding tubes). Surgery may hasten a death as the result of an unanticipated complication. Most of the immediate operative causes for a cardiac arrest are more treatable than the causes of an arrest in other clinical settings, such as the nursing home, because they may include correctable conditions such as oversedation, an arrhythmia, hypotension, pulmonary edema, or bleeding. It is a common practice to suspend a DNR order during the procedure and for 24 to 48 hours afterward. If a complication occurs, the patient is treated and the family or those with decision-making responsibilities are consulted. An evaluation of survivability is made and a decision to suspend or continue the interventions is discussed. This process is less clear when there is a concern that the surgical procedure is potentially medically futile (i.e., when a procedure would have only marginal benefit).

Nursing Home Patients

Data that defines surgical outcomes in nursing home patients is sparse. In one review of a nursing care facility, 117 residents required a surgical intervention, totaling 168 procedures. Major abdominal or vascular procedures had a greater rate of death and morbidity by multivariate analysis. Favorable clinical outcomes were less when a diagnosis of CAD, dementia, or an age greater than 70 years was noted preoperatively. The overall survival was poor, indicating that the nursing home population is frail and is often poorly tolerant of surgery. This group of patients should undergo a careful review of the risk-to-benefit ratio prior to a surgical procedure.

POSTOPERATIVE MANAGEMENT

Postoperative management includes the appropriate use of medications for pain, increasing mobilization, proper use of urinary catheters, the treatment and prevention of delirium, and anticoagulation use.

Pain Control

The American Geriatrics Society has published a comprehensive review of pain management in the elderly patient. This report suggests that pain is undertreated in older patients because of the concern of using potent analgesics in older patients and a misconception that pain sensations are diminished in such patients. Postoperative patients should be regularly asked about the severity of their discomfort using analog scales and analgesics should be given according to anticipated needs rather than "as needed." Comments on the management of persistent pain, medication dosing and metabolism, as well as toxicity, are well summarized by the American Geriatrics Society's review of this topic.

Early Mobilization

Prolonged bed rest can adversely affect the elderly patient. Changes notes with prolonged immobility include a decrease in cardiac output and aerobic capacity, baroreceptor desensitization and orthostatic hypotension, skeletal muscle deconditioning, bone loss, hypercalcemia, joint contractures, constipation, incontinence, pressure sores, sensory deprivation, an increased risk for DVT, atelectasis, hypoxemia, and pneumonia. The earliest possible mobilization from bed is vital, helping to reduce the risk for complications. If the recovery process prevents full mobilization, then a physical therapy referral for range or motion exercises and the maintenance of an upright posture (chair) may reduce the frequency and severity of these complications.

Catheters

Postoperative urinary drainage is typically managed by indwelling catheters that predispose to urinary tract infections and the associated complications. Their use should be short, with a goal of the prompt removal by the morning after surgery. If there is a concern for urinary retention or bladder distension, then intermittent catheterization should be considered. The use of urinary catheters beyond 48 hours should be avoided, except when retention is not managed by other means. The use of prophylactic antibiotics for those patients requiring longer-term use of urinary catheters is not recommended.

Postoperative Delirium

Acute confusional states occur in 10 to 15 percent of older patients undergoing general surgery, 30 percent of cardiac surgery patients, and, in one study, up to 50 percent of hip fracture repairs. Making the correct diagnosis of delirium is important. Although the causes are numerous, it is often the result of a postoperative complication that may not be apparent. Delirium is also a marker for worse functional recovery. Older patients with in-hospital delirium are at risk for significant long-term reduction in cognitive function.

Delirium is often subtle and can be easily missed. Clinical factors key to the diagnosis are a rapid onset, a disturbed level of consciousness, decreased attention and environmental awareness, memory deficits, disorientation, perceptual disturbances, and evidence of a condition that contributes to its development. A history of dementia, advanced age, and a prior decline in cognitive function are risk factors for perioperative delirium. As a rule, delirium fluctuates and may not be evident during a single visit. Nursing staff and family members are often the most reliable source for the serial assessments of an at-risk patient.

Delirium often compromises postoperative care. Behaviors can often be controlled with environmental measures, such as a bedside sitter, increased visitations by family, orientation stimuli, minimizing abrupt relocations and permitting patients to return to a more normal day–night cycle. Symptomatic control of agitation to prevent harm is occasionally needed. Unfortunately, no single drug has an accomplished record. High-potency antipsychotics such as Risperidone and Haloperidol may be given slowly and should be cautiously titrated to symptoms. Lower-potency drugs such as chlorpromazine and thioridazine should be avoided because of their anticholinergic and arrhythmogenic effects. If delirium is secondary to alcohol withdrawal, short-acting benzodiazepines are used.

Other Complications

Postoperative surveillance for myocardial ischemia, infarction, arrhythmias, and DVT should ideally lead to a reduction in mortality. Postoperative myocardial ischemia is the strongest predictor of cardiac morbidity. Anginal pain may be masked by narcotics or may be difficult to verbalize during recovery. Currently, no evidence supports the routine use of pulmonary artery catheter monitoring of ventricular performance. Postoperative ST-segment changes are indicative of myocardial ischemia and are an independent predictor of events. They are associated with a worse long-term survival. The optimal surveillance strategy for the diagnosis of postoperative ischemia or infarction has not been defined. In patients without documented CAD, surveillance should be restricted to patients who develop signs or symptoms of cardiovascular dysfunction. In patients with high- or intermediate-risk surgical procedures, an electrocardiogram at baseline, immediately after surgery, and daily for the first 2 days appears to be the most cost-effective strategy. Cardiac troponin measurements should be part of the diagnostic plan for myocardial infarction detection, but additional research is needed to correlate outcomes to the magnitude of an isolated cardiac troponin elevation. As a rule, postoperative myocardial infarctions have a similar pathology to infarction occurring in a nonsurgical patient, the spontaneous thrombosis of the coronary artery. Therefore, when this complication occurs, an aggressive attempt at opening the infarct related artery should be considered in the appropriate postoperative patient.

Postoperative arrhythmias are often caused by correctable noncardiac problems such as infection, hypotension, metabolic abnormalities (hypokalemia, hypomagnesemia), and hypoxia. Ventricular arrhythmias (frequent ventricular ectopic beats or nonsustained ventricular tachycardia) may occur in more than one-third of high-risk patients. Prophylactic use of antiarrhythmics other than beta blockers is currently not justified. Sustained ventricular tachycardia with or without hemodynamic complications requires consultation with a cardiologist. Atrial fibrillation is common; in several surgical trials, 25 percent of the elderly patients developed this rhythm. Age and the type of surgery are strong predictors for the development of atrial fibrillation. The prophylactic use of beta blockers and amiodarone has shown some benefit by reducing the frequency of this rhythm.

Hemoglobin levels often fall after major surgery. Many elderly patients will tolerate hemoglobins below 10 g/dL. Transfusions should be reserved for patients with symptoms and those with levels below 7 g/dL. Controlled trials of oral iron in hip fracture patients demonstrate a lack of benefit and its routine use is not beneficial.

Cognitive declines have been noted following a variety of surgeries. The International Study of Postoperative Cognitive Dysfunction found that 26 percent of patients older than age 60 years who had either intra-abdominal or orthopedic procedures had significant declines in cognitive function 1 week after surgery. Risk factors included older age, greater use of anesthetics and postoperative respiratory and infectious complications. In coronary artery bypass surgery, where the aorta is often cross-clamped and a bypass pump is used, embolization of both gas and particulates occur. Central nervous system ischemic damage is often noted after these procedures. Postoperative infarcts are the likely cause of cognitive declines noted with cardiac surgery. Off-pump coronary artery bypass surgery seems to have a lower rate of short-term declines in cognitive function (21 percent versus 29 percent), but similar declines are noted at 6 months (31 percent versus 38 percent). The risk of further declines in cognitive function should be incorporated into the decision process for patients with underlying dementia who are not undergoing emergent or life-saving surgery. Finally, postoperative critical pathways involving regimens including low-dose opiates, early extubation, and an emphasis on accelerated functional recovery can be safely applied to older patients.

The management of anticoagulants prior to surgery is briefly summarized. For patients on chronic warfarin with an INR goal of 2.0 to 3.0, four scheduled doses should be withheld to allow the INR to normalize to less than 1.5 before surgery. If the INR is typically kept above 3.0, then longer periods without a warfarin dose may be required. The INR should be measured a day before surgery to ensure that it has reached an acceptable range. If the INR is excessive (>1.8), a small dose of vitamin K, 1 mg SQ may be given. When the INR is <2.0 other prophylactic antithrombotic interventions should be considered. Elective surgery is best avoided for a month following a DVT. If this is not possible, then intravenous heparin should be given before and after the procedure while the INR is <2.0. Intravenous heparin should be stopped 6 hours before surgery; restarting it can be considered as soon as 12 hours after surgery, depending on the type of surgery and its result. Patients with a DVT on warfarin for 2 to 3 months need not be on heparin prior to surgery unless there are additional risks. Heparin should be given postoperatively until the INR returns to >2.0. Patients with a DVT on warfarin for more than 3 months may not need preoperative heparin. These patients should receive postoperative prophylaxis with low-molecular-weight heparin until the INR returns to >2.0. These recommendations should be combined with mechanical prophylaxis (gradient compression stockings intermittent pneumatic compression). Elective surgery should be avoided in the first month after an arterial embolism.

SUMMARY

Age alone is not a very good predictor of operative risk and should not be the sole criteria for deciding who should

have surgery. Age is associated with a higher prevalence of chronic diseases, which, in turn, are strong predictors of risk and are determinants of who might benefit from surgery and preoperative testing. The American Heart Association and American College of Cardiology have published revised algorithms that are helpful in preoperative risk assessment. Perioperative care requires a careful medical evaluation and comprehensive postoperative observation that anticipates potential complications.

REFERENCES

AGS Clinical Practice Committee. The use of oral anticoagulation (warfarin) in older people. *J Am Geriatr Soc* 49:224, 2000.

AGS Panel on Persistent Pain in Older Patients: The management of persistent pain in older persons. *J Am Geriatr Soc* 50;S205, 2002.

American Society of Anesthesiologists: Ethical Guidelines for the anesthesia care of patients with do not resuscitate orders or other directives that limit treatment. House of Delegates, American Society of Anesthesiologists, Park Ridge, IL, Oct. 13, 1993.

Auerbach AD, Goldman L: B-Blockers and reduction of cardiac events in noncardiac surgery: Scientific review. *JAMA* 287:1435, 2002.

Auerbach AD, Goldman L: B-Blockers and reduction of cardiac events in noncardiac surgery: Clinical applications. *JAMA* 287:1445, 2000.

Bonow RO et al: ACC/AHA guidelines for the management of patients with valvular heart disease: A report of the American College of Cardiology/American Heart Association task force on practice guidelines (Committee on management of patients with valvular heart disease). *J Am Coll Cardiol* 32:1486, 1998.

Eagle KA et al: ACC/AHA guideline update on perioperative cardiovascular evaluation for non-cardiac surgery—2002. Available at either http://www.acc.org or http://www.americanheart.org.

Fleisher LA, Eagle KA: Lowering cardiac risk in noncardiac surgery. *N Engl J Med* 345:1677, 2001.

Kemper P, Murtaugh CM: Lifetime use of nursing home care. *N Engl J Med* 324:595, 1991.

Solomon DH et al: The new frontier: Increasing geriatrics expertise in surgical and medical specialties. *J Am Geriatr Soc* 48:702, 2000.

Truog RD et al: DNR in the OP: A goal-directed approach. *Anesthesiology* 90(1):289, 1999.

US Census Bureau, Population Projections Branch. Data available at http://www.census.gov/population/www/projections/popproj.html.

Valvona J, Sloan F. Datawatch: Rising rates of surgery among the elderly. *Health Aff* 4:108, 1985.

Zenilman ME. Surgery in the elderly: Cardiac disease as a risk factor and new concepts about prophylaxis. *Advances in Surgery* 34:393, 2000.

Anesthesia for Elderly Patients

G. ALEC ROOKE

Physiologic aging and the comorbid disease so common in older patients make perioperative management more complex. Not only is anesthetic care made more difficult, preoperative preparation and the postoperative care assume greater importance than for young, healthy adults. The best care is provided when anesthesiologists, surgeons, medical specialists, and primary caregivers all contribute to a comprehensive plan for a given patient. It is all too easy for each specialty to view patients from their own perspective and miss the total picture.

MODIFICATION OF ANESTHETIC MANAGEMENT BECAUSE OF AGING

The aging of the organ systems, particularly the heart and lungs, has a significant impact on the response to anesthesia. Equally important are the physiologic changes that affect anesthetic drug action and duration, such as the increase in body fat, decreased glomerular filtration, and reduced hepatic blood flow. Because general anesthesia and regional anesthesia work via different mechanisms, their interaction with physiologic aging will be discussed separately.

General Anesthesia

The distinguishing feature of general anesthesia is that the patient is rendered unconscious, yet much more is involved than just unconsciousness and amnesia. Adjustment of the depth of anesthesia consumes a good deal of the anesthetic manipulations during surgery. How "deep" or "light" the patient is depends heavily on the surgical stimulus. A patient might appear fully anesthetized one moment and then be inadequately anesthetized a moment later if the surgical (painful) stimulus suddenly increases. The effective depth of anesthesia can be monitored through a variety of ways. Certainly patient movement in response to a surgical stimulus suggests an inadequate depth of anesthesia, even though such movement is usually not at a conscious level and is almost never remembered by the patient. If the patient is paralyzed by neuromuscular blocking agents, then movement can no longer be relied upon as a sign of

light anesthesia. Most cases of awareness during anesthesia occur when a light level of anesthesia is used along with muscle relaxation, for example, nitrous oxide plus opioid, but little or no potent gas such as isoflurane. Fortunately, hemodynamic signs of light anesthesia generally appear long before a patient has any chance of "waking up" or of having postoperative recall. A rise in blood pressure and/or heart rate are typically the first signs of light anesthesia and trigger the response of turning up the volatile gas concentration or giving a small bolus of a fast-acting opioid such as fentanyl. A safe strategy is to keep blood pressure at the patient's usual baseline or slightly lower. The risk of awareness/recall is pretty remote under such circumstances. Titration of the depth of anesthesia is typically a matter of balancing the tendency of the surgical stimulus to activate the brain and stimulate the sympathetic nervous system against the anesthetic's ability to depress brain activity and limit the stimulation of the sympathetic nervous system. In fact, the main reason that anesthesia providers desire a stable blood pressure and heart rate is not out of fear of complications such as myocardial infarction or stroke, but merely as a means of titrating the appropriate depth of anesthesia throughout the surgery.

The goal of hemodynamic stability is made much more difficult by the aging process (Table 31-1). General anesthesia lowers the blood pressure in everyone because general anesthesia lowers sympathetic tone, which, in turn, may lower heart rate, decrease systemic vascular resistance and cause peripheral pooling of blood that lowers cardiac preload. There is also some direct depression of the myocardium. These changes produce exaggerated results in elderly patients. First of all, sympathetic nervous system activity increases with age, and the sympathetic nervous system may be more reactive to stimuli than in young people. Chronic hypertension, so common in older patients, further exaggerates the vascular response to changes in sympathetic nervous system activity. The ventricles stiffen with age, as a consequence of changes in connective tissue and, as age stiffens the aorta, in consequence of the ventricular hypertrophy associated with the impedance mismatching between the aorta and the left ventricle in late ejection. Hypertrophy leads to a reduction in the rate of diastolic relaxation that in turn diminishes early diastolic filling. The burden of achieving an adequate ventricular preload now

Table 31-1   Cardiovascular Aging and Anesthetic Implications

Age-Induced Cardiovascular Change	Physiologic Consequence	Anesthetic and Perioperative Implication
Loss of sinoatrial node cells; conduction system fibrosis	1st degree block, occasional sick sinus syndrome	Severe bradycardia when coupled with potent opioids
Stiff arteries	Systolic hypertension	Labile blood pressure
	Impedance mismatching at end-ejection leading to myocardial hypertrophy and impaired diastolic relaxation	Diastolic dysfunction, sensitivity to volume status
Myocardial hypertrophy; connective tissue stiffening	Increased ventricular stiffness	Failure to maintain filling causes an exaggerated decline in cardiac performance; excessive volume more easily increases filling pressures to congestive failure levels
	Ventricular filling dependent on a well maintained atrial pressure	
Decreased β-receptor responsiveness	Limited increases in heart rate and contractility in response to endogenous and exogenous catecholamines	Increased dependency on Frank-Starling mechanism to maintain cardiac performance.
	Impaired baroreflex control of blood pressure	Labile blood pressure
Stiff veins	Decreased buffering of changes in body blood volume impairs ability to maintain constant atrial pressure	Changes in blood volume or body distribution of blood cause exaggerated changes in cardiac filling
		Hypovolemia more easily impairs cardiac performance, whereas hypervolemia more easily leads to symptoms of congestive failure
Increased sympathetic nervous system activity at rest and in response to stimuli	Basal vascular resistance more dependent on basal sympathetic nervous system	Hypotension from anesthetic blunting of sympathetic tone
		Increased blood pressure lability from changes in sympathetic tone in response to the surgical stimulus

shifts to the passive filling produced by the left atrial pressure and the active filling produced by the atrial contraction. Both effects must overcome the increased ventricular stiffness and both effects require a full atrium. Yet atrial blood volume is not so easy to keep constant. The veins stiffen with age, too, and buffer changes in blood volume less effectively, making atrial filling more sensitive to the patient's overall volume status as well as the vagaries of the sympathetic nervous system's control on blood distribution throughout the body. As a consequence, older patients are more prone than young patients to both hypotension and hypertension during surgery.

Management of the inevitable swings in blood pressure can be a challenge. Hypertension is usually managed by increasing the depth of anesthesia with more opioid and/or increasing the anesthetic gas concentration. Unfortunately, the surgical stimulus can increase or decrease faster than the depth of the anesthetic can be manipulated. One approach is to complement the anesthetic with β-blockade to minimize the hemodynamic response to the surgical stimulus. Another approach is to use relatively high doses of opioid and relatively less volatile anesthetic. Opioids produce less intrinsic depression of blood pressure than do volatile anesthetics. If high-dose opioids are used to prevent the hemodynamic response to the surgical stimulus, the primary role of the volatile anesthetic is to produce unconsciousness. This goal requires only approximately half the concentration of gas as would be necessary in the absence of the opioids. Unfortunately, very-high-dose opioids cannot be routinely used because of the need to have the patient breathing spontaneously at the end of the surgery. Yet another approach is to use the maximum amount of opioids compatible with the surgical procedure, and then keep the volatile anesthetic high enough to block the hemodynamic response to the highest level of surgical stimulus. Such a strategy will minimize hypertension, but will also make the patient more prone to hypotension at other, less stimulating, times of the surgery. Sometimes even the minimum level of anesthesia causes an unacceptable depression of blood pressure. In these circumstances, blood pressure needs to be actively supported by the anesthesiologist. Volume administration is often of limited utility in older patients. Volume may restore stroke volume but will not compensate for hypotension caused by severe bradycardia or a low vascular resistance. Bradycardia generally responds to glycopyrrolate, an anticholinergic drug

Table 31-2   Pulmonary Aging and Anesthetic Implications

Aging Induced Pulmonary Change	Physiologic Consequence	Anesthetic and Perioperative Implication
Decrease in bony thorax elasticity	Stiff chest that is hard to move, increasing the work of breathing and making it more difficult to increase minute ventilation Increased residual volume	Increased risk of respiratory failure
Loss of muscle mass	Reduced strength to meet the increased minute ventilation requirements secondary to the metabolic demands after surgery	Increased risk of respiratory failure
Decreased lung parenchymal stiffness	Increased lung compliance Decreased "tethering" of small airways, leading to increased closing volume Impaired ventilation-perfusion matching	Increased risk of atelectasis, hypoxia, and pneumonia
Impaired airway protective reflexes	More frequent aspiration	Increased risk of pneumonia, ARDS
Decreased central nervous system responsiveness	Decreased hypercapnic and hypoxic drives	Increased risk of hypoxia Greater sensitivity to anesthetic agents

that crosses the blood–brain barrier poorly and is presumably less likely to promote postoperative delirium than atropine. Ephedrine stimulates both α- and β-receptors and effectively raises pressure, but tachyphylaxis eventually develops, so it is not used over extended time periods. Phenylephrine, a pure α-agonist, can be conveniently given as either a bolus or a low-dose infusion and effectively maintains blood pressure. On occasion, inotropic infusions (e.g., dopamine) are used, especially if bradycardia doesn't respond to anticholinergics or if there is concern over baseline ventricular function. All pressors have potential adverse effects, of course, but serious problems from their use are infrequent.

Cardiovascular aging makes volume administration more difficult. The stiffness of the venous system exaggerates the response to a given volume excess or deficit. Furthermore, well-anesthetized patients may appear hypovolemic during surgery because of the suppression of sympathetic nervous system activity. Large amounts of crystalloid may achieve what appears to be normovolemia during surgery, but when surgery is over and postoperative pain restores sympathetic activity, that volume may shift back to the central circulation and create a volume overload. One strategy to avoid giving too much fluid is to give minimal maintenance fluid and look for signs of hypovolemia beyond hypotension to dictate volume bolus administration. Useful tools may include a decrease in urine flow, an increase in systolic pressure variation during mechanical ventilation, or a decrease in central venous pressure. Nevertheless, some surgeries, particularly extensive gastrointestinal procedures, may result in severe displacement of fluid to extravascular compartments ("third spacing") of fluid. This phenomenon may extend into the postoperative period as well. Failure to give fluid would result in cardiovascular hypovolemia and impaired cardiac output. In short, volume administration is often unavoidable. The problem comes

when the body recovers from the trauma of surgery and begins to mobilize that "third-space" fluid. The stiffness of the aged venous system, the predisposition toward diastolic dysfunction in older patients, and the diminished capacity of the urinary system to rapidly eliminate the fluid may allow that mobilized fluid to overwhelm the system and produce congestive symptoms even in the presence of normal ventricular function. The key to management is not to point fingers at putative culprits, but to anticipate the event, follow the patient closely, and aggressively diurese the patient at the first sign of fluid overload.

Aging and general anesthesia also have adverse effects on the respiratory system (Table 31-2). Lung closing capacity increases with age because of diminished airway tethering by connective tissue. General anesthesia enhances expiratory muscle tone and diminishes inspiratory muscle tone, thereby decreasing functional residual capacity. Sighs are suppressed. Atelectasis now becomes easier to produce because of the increased closing capacity, decreased functional residual capacity and the loss of sighs. Atelectasis can be easily avoided intraoperatively through the use of large tidal volumes. Mechanical ventilation disturbs the normal pattern of diaphragmatic breathing in the supine patient, disturbing normal ventilation–perfusion matching. Volatile anesthetics reduce the effectiveness of hypoxic pulmonary vasoconstriction. Nevertheless, hypoxia is virtually unheard of in the operating room in the absence of severe pulmonary disease, thanks to the ubiquitous use of pulse oximetry and supplemental oxygen. Both volatile anesthetics and the placement of an endotracheal tube diminish ciliary action of the respiratory tract, an effect that extends into the postoperative period. Opioids diminish the carbon dioxide ventilatory drive. Volatile anesthetics suppress the hypoxic ventilatory drive, even at the low concentrations present postoperatively. Very frail patients are particularly at increased risk for ventilatory failure postoperatively. The increase in body oxygen consumption during recovery from surgery may exceed the ventilatory reserve that is compromised by increased chest wall stiffness and decreased skeletal muscle mass. Finally, silent regurgitation and aspiration are more common in older patients. At-risk patients will be challenged postoperatively by drugs that may further depress the airway protective reflexes and impair gastric emptying. Aspiration is much more likely to occur postoperatively than intraoperatively. It is important to understand, however, that patients who suffer aspiration to a degree that causes clinical signs or symptoms, will present with some evidence of dysfunction (e.g. hypoxia) within a few hours of the aspiration. It is unlikely that a patient will aspirate, function well for many hours, and then develop a clinical problem because of that aspiration.

Intraoperative respiratory management of older patients is basically straightforward. Bronchospasm is probably the most common intraoperative untoward event, and it usually resolves promptly with appropriate treatment. Fortunately, volatile anesthetic gases cause bronchodilation, and it is easy to administer inhaled bronchodilator medications through the endotracheal tube. As implied in the previous paragraph, most pulmonary problems do not become a clinical issue until after surgery. Some degree of hypercarbia is common for at least the immediate postoperative period, especially after considerable opioid administration. This finding usually means nothing more than the presence of good analgesia, so long as supplemental oxygen is administered and the patient can be watched carefully. Supplemental oxygen will likely be necessary for a longer period of time after surgery in older patients, however. Patients with tenuous respiratory function may need ventilatory support until they are past the acute recovery period. Pneumonia remains an important complication and the ability to prevent its development is limited. Deep breathing and vigorous coughing by the patient is thought to help prevent pneumonia, but postoperative pain may impair these maneuvers. Improved pain control may be one mechanism by which epidural analgesia improves perioperative outcome (see "Postoperative Analgesia" later in this chapter). The role of silent aspiration in the development of postoperative pneumonia is unclear and warrants closer examination.

The last major influence of aging on general anesthesia involves administration of intravenous and volatile gas agents. A general rule of thumb is that all drugs will have more dramatic and longer lasting effects in older patients. The mechanisms vary with the drug, but include changes in protein binding, decreases in initial volume of distribution, increases in brain sensitivity (which occurs with volatile anesthetic gases and many drugs), increases in drug volume of distribution, and slowed renal or hepatic metabolism. The therapeutic effect of most intravenous anesthetic agents is not dissipated by metabolism but by redistribution of the drug from the brain to the fat. These drugs are highly lipid soluble and cross membranes rapidly. On initial injection the blood levels are very high compared to what the levels will fall to once the drug has been taken up into fat. The high initial blood levels will promote rapid transfer of the drug into highly perfused organs such as the brain. Even though fat serves as an almost limitless sink for lipid soluble drugs, blood flow to fat is low and transfer of drug into fat takes time. It is that transfer time that largely dictates the duration of the drug's clinical effect. As blood levels decrease, the drug returns to the blood from the vascular organs and is transferred to the fat, thereby eliminating the therapeutic effect. Nevertheless, drug levels in fat are not zero, so neither is the blood level. If large amounts of drug are administered, whether as a large bolus or as multiple small doses, eventually the drug level in fat becomes high enough to sustain a (residual) blood level that produces a therapeutic effect. At this point it will take a long time for the therapeutic effect to wear off, because now the drug must be excreted or metabolized to eliminate the drug from the blood. Metabolism is slow, largely because the drug depot leeches slowly out of the fat.

In the case of most opioids, a certain level of residual analgesia is desirable. Thus a drug such as fentanyl can be given repeatedly to temper the surgical stimulus. So long as too much isn't given, the residual blood levels will provide a head start on the postoperative analgesia without producing the severe respiratory depression that would be present during the redistribution phase of the fentanyl.

From an anesthetic management viewpoint, the pharmacokinetic and pharmacodynamic changes of aging rarely present a major problem. Patient response to drugs is variable at any age, so with the exception of induction, drugs are given in small doses and titrated to effect. The trend in anesthesia practice is to use drugs that are short acting. This goal translates into choosing drugs that have shorter metabolic half-lives, redistribute to yield very low blood levels with minimal residual effects, or both. For example, propofol and thiopental are equally effective induction agents and both are "short acting" because they redistribute rapidly into fat. The residual blood levels of propofol, however, produce less residual sedation than occurs with thiopental, and propofol also has a shorter metabolic half-life. These principles of drug pharmacokinetics apply to patients of all ages, but the ability to use drugs with rapid fat uptake but minimal residual effects are particularly helpful in older patients.

Regional Anesthesia

Included in this category are field blocks ("local anesthesia"), peripheral nerve blocks such as an axillary nerve block, and neuraxial anesthesia (spinal and epidural anesthesia). As a rule, field blocks and nerve blocks have minimal systemic effects unless there is an untoward event during placement, such as intravascular injection of the local anesthetic. Another exception is an interscalene block where the ipsilateral phrenic nerve is invariably blocked, resulting in hemidiaphragmatic paralysis. An ipsilateral Horner syndrome may also be observed in this circumstance. Field and nerve blocks are frequently performed using long-acting drugs such as bupivacaine. This often provides exceptional postoperative analgesia for up to 24 hours. Nerve blocks may be combined with a light general anesthetic, and field blocks are often placed by the surgeon at the operative site prior to or at the conclusion of surgery.

Neuraxial blocks are complete anesthetics in that no other supplement is necessary, although sedation is often provided at the request of the patient. These blocks produce the greatest physiologic effects and will be the focus of this discussion. With spinal anesthesia, the local anesthetic is injected inside the dura and arachnoid, where it quickly diffuses into the spinal nerves. At this location, spinal nerves have minimal connective tissue surrounding them. The local anesthetic effectively blocks all nerve fibers, including motor, touch, and sympathetic nerves. An epidural anesthetic is typically administered through a catheter placed just outside the dura. In the epidural space, spinal nerves are covered with a thick connective tissue sheath. This slows the onset of the anesthetic, and by varying the concentration of the injected local anesthetic, a differential blockade of various nerve types can be achieved. This is important when attempting postoperative analgesia, where partial blockade of pain fibers is desired, but touch and motor nerves are to be spared. Unfortunately, it is not possible to anesthetize pain fibers without also affecting the sympathetic nerves. If used for an anesthetic, a high concentration of the local anesthetic will be used, blocking all nerve types.

The hemodynamic effects of neuraxial anesthesia stem from the blockade of sympathetic nerves. The hemodynamic response depends on many factors, including how many thoracic dermatomes with their sympathetic fibers are affected and how much of a reflex response can be mounted via the vagus and any unblocked sympathetic fibers. In the case of spinal anesthesia, the sympathetic fibers may be at least partially blocked for many dermatomes above the level of blockade as defined by sharp, dull discrimination. It is not uncommon, therefore, to have a near total sympathectomy with spinal anesthesia. The hemodynamic consequences can be dramatic. If one accepts the hypothesis that vascular resistance is increased with age because of increased sympathetic tone, then removal of that tone often results in a large decrease in vascular resistance (Fig. 31-1). Historical data in young adults demonstrate a much smaller decrease in vascular resistance

but a similar decrease in cardiac output. In Fig. 31-1 the sympathectomy also decreased left ventricular filling as blood volume shifted to the legs and mesentery. However, the increase in ejection fraction ameliorated much of the decrease in stroke volume and cardiac output that would have otherwise been expected from the decrease in left ventricular end-diastolic volume.

These results illustrate the potential folly of treating hypotension with volume resuscitation alone. No amount of fluid could ever increase stroke volume enough to restore blood pressure under these circumstances. A better choice may well be a modest infusion of an α-agonist. The goal is not to return blood pressure to its prespinal level, but to increase vascular resistance enough to prevent unacceptably low pressures for that patient.

Choosing Between Regional and General Anesthesia

Many anesthesiologists prefer regional anesthesia over general anesthesia. There is something inherently attractive in providing an anesthetic that just blocks nerves yet avoids direct effects to the brain and other vital organs. Regional anesthesia effectively eliminates the changing surgical stimulus as a mechanism of hemodynamic instability, because the pain pathways are blocked before they can reach the central nervous system and alter autonomic nervous system activity. As noted earlier, however, neuraxial anesthesia alone has profound effects on cardiovascular variables and may require treatment for the induced hypotension.

Whether to perform a regional or a general anesthetic depends on many factors. Obviously the surgery must be compatible with a regional anesthetic technique and the anesthesiologist must be comfortable performing the technique. Occasionally, patient physical limitations, including uncomfortable patient positioning for the surgery, will prevent the use of a regional technique. The presence of coagulopathies or the use of preoperative anticoagulation may preclude the use or regional techniques due to the risk of bleeding and, in the case of spinal or epidural anesthesia, the risk of epidural hematoma (see "Postoperative Analgesia" later in this chapter). The patient must be willing to undergo the regional technique that will invariably involve placing a needle somewhere into the body. Some patients will not accept needles under any circumstance unless they are totally asleep, but for safety reasons most blocks will not be performed under such conditions. Other patients may refuse because of prior bad experiences. On the other hand, many patients welcome the opportunity to avoid a general anesthetic and the attendant postoperative sedation and risk of nausea. All anesthetics should be preceded by a thorough discussion with the patient about anesthetic options, including their benefits, disadvantages, and associated risks. This discussion is best carried out by an anesthesiologist, who is best able to recognize the patient and procedure characteristics that will determine what anesthetic options are appropriate and to explain to the patient the important risks and benefits of each option. As will be discussed in the section on "Perioperative Complications," there is little evidence that regional techniques

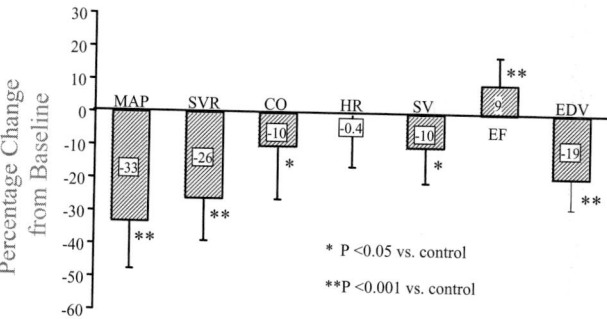

Figure 31-1 The hemodynamic response to high spinal anesthesia is shown in 15 elderly men with cardiac disease. The large decrease in mean arterial blood pressure (MAP) was primarily due to decreases in systemic vascular resistance (SVR) and not decreases in cardiac output (CO). Overall, heart rate (HR) did not change, therefore the decrease in cardiac output was a result of a decrease in stroke volume (SV). The decrease in left ventricular end-diastolic volume (EDV) did not cause a comparable decrease in stroke volume because the ejection fraction (EF) increased. Adapted from Rooke GA et al: Hemodynamic response and change in organ blood volume during spinal anesthesia in elderly men with cardiac disease. *Anesth Analg* 85:99, 1997, with permission.

decrease risk, at least in relatively healthy patients of any age. Thus, the choice of anesthetic technique may be based on patient preference; consequently, it is important to provide patients with comprehensive information and involve them in the decision-making process.

Many patients request sedation during a regional anesthetic, usually because they are not interested in being aware of the activities in the operating room. Almost always this request can be accommodated. Small quantities of midazolam and fentanyl often suffice, but if higher levels of sedation (e.g., sleep) are desired, typically a propofol infusion will be used. Interestingly, older patients commonly fall asleep during spinal anesthesia, even in the absence of any sedative medications. The mechanism behind this phenomenon is unknown, but may involve the loss of sensory input to the brainstem. If sedative and analgesic drugs are used, the risk of airway obstruction increases. The combination of sedation plus spinal anesthesia, for example, produces more postoperative hypoxia than sedation or spinal anesthesia alone. With careful monitoring and skill in airway management, however, the consequences of airway obstruction should be minimal. In unskilled hands, on the other hand, airway obstruction can rapidly lead to hypoxia and patient injury. This risk to the patient forms the basis for the recent Joint Commission on Accreditation of Healthcare Organizations (JCAHO) requirement that trained personnel must be present at procedures performed anywhere in the hospital whenever the patient is likely to be sedated to the point of drowsiness that will require verbal stimuli or more to arouse. The requirements include assigning a person to the sole task of monitoring the patient.

THE ANESTHESIOLOGISTS' PERSPECTIVE ON THE PREOPERATIVE CONSULT

Historically, the apparent purpose of the preoperative consult has been merely to determine whether the risks of surgery outweighed the benefits. Consults dutifully listed the patient's medical problems and severity, then quoted The Goldman Index or Detsky Score as a purported estimate of cardiac risk. To anesthesiologists, this process seemed to be a yes or no proposition, with little effort devoted to what can be done to lower the patient's risk.

Admittedly, a good deal of the problem has been a lack of communication among the involved parties including the internist, the surgeon, the anesthesiologist, and, eventually, the patient. Expectations were rarely made clear and most discussions occurred via chart notes. Fortunately, these attitudes and approaches appear to be changing, and anesthesiologists have become much more involved in the preoperative evaluation and preparation of the patient. Surgeons usually request anesthesia involvement well in advance of surgery because the surgeon doesn't have to second-guess what needs to be done prior to surgery. Internists may also be spared unnecessary and tedious consults. Nevertheless, there will be times when the internist needs to be involved and can have a significant positive impact.

Before a consult can be initiated, someone needs to look at the patient in total. The medical history should be

To: General Medicine Consult Service
From: General Surgery

Mr. DD is a 71 y/o man scheduled for resection of a recurrent dermatofibrosarcoma of the right clavicle. He has diet-controlled adult onset diabetes. He also has a history of a "racing heart" previously evaluated with a Holter 8 months ago revealing brief runs of asymptomatic atrial tachycardia. Today's EKG shows atrial flutter with variable block, and a ventricular rate of approximately 90. Please evaluate his arrhythmia and clear for surgery so anesthesia doesn't cancel him.

To: General Surgery
From: General Medicine Consult Service

The patient reports no new symptoms over the past several months. He describes some shortness of breath on exertion, but denies past or present angina, MI or symptoms of CHF. According to ACC guidelines, he has intermediate clinical predictors (diabetes) and is undergoing a low-risk surgical procedure.
Recommend:
1. Beta-blockade to limit the heart rate response to surgical stress.
2. Proceed with surgery.
3. Subsequent outpatient evaluation/treatment for his atrial fibrillation (Echocardiogram, TSH level, anticoagulation and a trial of cardioversion).
Thank you for this interesting consult.

Figure 31-2 An example of a consult request from a surgical service to a medical service.

summarized and there should be an emphasis on current status. The preoperative management of the medical problems should be determined, such as changes in medication regimen prior to surgery. This process could be performed by the surgeon, the anesthesiologist, or the patient's primary hospital provider. The discipline of the physician principally involved doesn't matter, so long as that individual has a good understanding of the issues that need to be addressed and how they should be handled. Protocols are often very useful when agreed upon ahead of time by the surgeons, anesthesiologists, and internists. The more the preoperative evaluator knows and understands, the less often the need for a consultant. As an anecdotal example, when my institution initiated a preoperative clinic staffed by an internist who also received training from the surgeons and anesthesiologists, the number of consults to cardiology decreased abruptly by more than 75 percent.

Nevertheless, sooner or later greater expertise will be needed, and so a consultation is requested. When made, the request should clearly define the issues that need to be addressed and the expected role of the consultant. The example shown in Fig. 31-2 illustrates a reasonable delineation of the problem to be addressed, even if the motives can be questioned.

In the process of evaluating the patient, there are a number of issues that both the preoperative evaluator and the consultant may want to keep in mind. The most important goal is not risk assessment, but the improvement of the patient's medical status prior to surgery. Occasionally the assessment of risk will determine that the proposed surgery is not warranted, but most of the time risk assessment is necessary to decide how aggressive one should be in preparing the patient for surgery. What should be done for a given medical problem will depend on the severity of disease, the expected stress generated by the surgery, and the potential risks of the proposed intervention. The most developed example of this process is the American College of Cardiology/American Heart Association (ACC/AHA) guidelines for the evaluation of cardiac disease. The guidelines attempt to integrate severity of comorbid disease, exercise tolerance, and surgical severity into a rational plan in order to determine who needs to enter a process that could lead to procedures with a risk greater than what might be associated with the proposed surgery itself. As an aside, it should be pointed out that the ACC/AHA guidelines were developed specifically to limit the number of patients subjected to noninvasive cardiac testing, based on the perception that such tests were being overused. Also, the ACC/AHA guidelines are just that—guidelines. They have never been tested, nor are they meant to supplant clinical judgment. For cardiac problems or any other medical issue, the salient point is that low risk does not equal no risk, and so long as the therapy doesn't involve excessive risk, ways to improve the patient's medical status should be considered.

With most medical problems, clinical judgment is important because few guidelines exist and the impact of optimization of medical conditions on postoperative outcome is usually unknown. Examples include better control of high blood pressure, a steroid taper for a patient with a current exacerbation of reactive airways disease, better control of blood sugar, or considering further therapy for a patient with angina that, although stable, might permit better exercise tolerance if the antianginal medications were adjusted. Clearly the best example of medical optimization leading to improved outcome is the use of β-blockade for patients with known or suspected coronary heart disease. Although these studies documented few adverse effects of that β-blockade even when initiated moments before surgery, an argument can be made to start the therapy well in advance of surgery should that opportunity present itself. If nothing else, it provides more opportunity to find the optimal dose for a given patient.

Disagreements between internists and anesthesiologists on preoperative management occasionally arise when patients present with medical conditions that have not been fully evaluated. The question is usually whether or not planned diagnostic tests can be delayed until after the surgery. The consult shown in Fig. 31-2 provides an example. At first glance, atrial flutter is not a contraindication to surgery, so why should its evaluation delay surgery? The opposing argument states that if tests are to be performed, and if the tests might provide useful information about the patient's medical status or even lead to some intervention that will improve the patient's status, then the patient will be better off having the tests done prior to elective surgery. In the example in Fig. 31-2, an echocardiogram provides useful information, even if it turns out to be normal. Given that it is to be performed at some point, it should be done before surgery, unless surgical urgency dictates otherwise. Furthermore, if the patient is being considered for elective cardioversion, this treatment should be done before surgery. Control of heart rate in the operating room and postoperatively is much easier to achieve in a patient with sinus rhythm.

There are many ways that an internist can provide important patient care in the perioperative period. These aspects of care are especially important in geriatric patients with multiple medical problems. Not infrequently, an older patient may have no identified caregiver in charge of integrating all their problems into one unified care plan. The preoperative and postoperative period offers the opportunity to review the full picture and optimize management. Do they need all those medications? Is the patient experiencing side effects from the drugs or their interactions? Are there medical problems heretofore unrecognized? Examples where geriatricians are generally far more skilled than the average anesthesiologist or surgeon include screening for alcohol or substance abuse, recognizing elder abuse, assessing activities of daily living and instrumental activities of daily living to help determine the level of home care needed after hospital discharge, and diagnosing impaired cognitive skills, including the determination of competency. In short, the preoperative period is an opportunity for the geriatrician to function as a patient advocate as well as improve the medical status of the patient prior to surgery.

The internist should also consider being involved with the postoperative care of the patient. Certainly, there will be aspects of treatment that require consensus between the surgeon and internist, but much of the care of the patient's chronic disease may well be better handled by the internist. Part of the challenge in the perioperative care of the older patient is to find an appropriate way to reward the internist for such involvement in patient care, instead of making the preoperative consult and postoperative care a chore to be disposed of in the most expedient way possible.

What about the truly complex patient? How do you handle the 80-year-old patient with symptomatic aortic stenosis who needs his colon cancer resected? Do you perform aortic valve replacement first and risk a significant GI bleed with anticoagulation during bypass, not to mention delay of the colon resection? Do you go ahead and perform the colon surgery first? If so, how will a safe anesthetic be delivered to the patient? How will postoperative pain and methods to control pain interact with the aortic stenosis? What if the patient was also a Jehovah's Witness and refused blood products? It can be asserted that truly challenging patients cannot have their management determined by one specialist alone. Such situations require the internist, surgeon, and anesthesiologist to make independent assessments of the patient, then get together and discuss options. Once a plan is determined that may include several alternatives, the patient should be consulted and the final plan agreed upon by all parties.

A special comment must be made about the patient with do not resuscitate (DNR) orders or any sort of advanced care directive. Many patients have, in consultation with their primary care physicians, elected to forgo resuscitative measures because of fears that resuscitation will lead to a poor postresuscitation quality of life, or because they feel that resuscitation measures will be futile. These fears are supported by repeated studies that demonstrate that cardiac arrest in the hospital carries a very poor prognosis, because arrests are often not witnessed, and may be a direct consequence of the patient's advanced disease state. In contrast with other in-hospital cardiac arrests, however, most cardiac arrests in the operating room carry a very favorable prognosis, largely because arrests are often a result of reversible causes such as hemorrhage or drug effects. Furthermore, they are witnessed events and resuscitation is instituted in seconds. In the setting of surgery, a patient's DNR order must be reconsidered in light of the different prognostic implications of cardiac arrest during surgery. Regardless of what agreement is reached, DNR orders require review and discussion with the patient. While the anesthesiologist should have such discussions with the patient, input from the patient's primary care physician can be invaluable.

Lastly, there is one important "don't" in the preoperative evaluation, at least from the anesthesiologist's perspective. The geriatrician/internist should not offer advice on anesthetic management. More likely than not, such advice will be wrong. Oftentimes the difficulty stems from the lack of understanding of the surgical procedure and the stress it will likely impose on the patient. This stress can be highly variable because of vagaries associated with the disease, or even the surgeon. Examples of bad advice include suggesting a pulmonary artery catheter be placed for what in reality is a pretty trivial surgery. Sometimes the advice is based on misconception. An example is the "clearing" of a patient for a procedure provided that it is performed with local or regional anesthesia, but not with general anesthesia. As is discussed in the section "Surgical Stress and Anesthetic Technique", there are no good data clearly showing that regional anesthesia is safer. Also, what if the regional anesthetic fails? Does that mean the surgery must be canceled instead of proceeding with a general anesthetic? There are also surgeries where local anesthesia may be feasible, but not preferable, either because of patient characteristics, including apprehension or positioning issues, or because it is difficult to achieve adequate anesthesia with local anesthesia alone. In such circumstances, a general anesthetic may well reduce the total stress to the patient. It is also ill advised to have physicians disagreeing in the medical record. The best strategy is to provide the most complete description possible about the extent of the patient's disease, including information on management that has proven successful. Then let the anesthesiologist integrate that information into the operative plan.

THE CONTRIBUTION OF ANESTHESIA TO PERIOPERATIVE COMPLICATIONS

Anesthetic risk is difficult to quantify, because few people receive an anesthetic in the absence of a procedure. For healthy patients, the risk of death purely because of the anesthetic is estimated to be as low as 1 in 250,000. Such a figure is trivial in comparison to the 1 in 500 risk of death associated with surgery and anesthesia overall. Mortality is dependent on patient age (Fig. 31-3) and is strongly influenced by the type of surgery. Even in patients older than 90 years of age, minor surgeries carry a near zero 30-day mortality, although major abdominal, thoracic, and vascular surgeries can be associated with a 20 to 30 percent mortality. Clearly, comorbid disease, the effects of surgical trauma, and presumably the anesthetic must interact in some way to increase risk, even if the mechanisms underlying adverse events are poorly understood. The popular concept is that age and comorbid disease reduce physiologic reserve and make the body less able to withstand the various stresses associated with surgery such as pain, a hypermetabolic state, and altered neuroendocrine hormones.

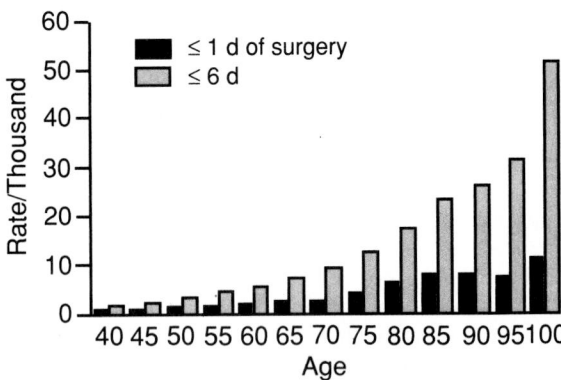

Figure 31-3   Perioperative death rates in the United States (1979–1984 data). More patients die after postoperative day 1 than before postoperative day 2. Modified from Lichtor JL: Sponsored research reveals post-operative mortality stats. *Anesth Patient Safety Found Newsletter* 3(1):9, 1988.

When perioperative complications have been stratified by age and the number of concurrent chronic diseases, the data supports this hypothesis (Fig. 31-4). What is particularly interesting about the data is the apparent interaction between disease and age to increase risk. Although at any age risk is increased by disease, age primarily increases the complication rate in the presence of comorbid disease. In patients with no or at most one chronic disease (Fig. 31-4), increasing age is associated with only a modest increase in risk, whereas patients with two or more chronic diseases demonstrate a dramatic influence of age on complications.

Surgical Stress and Anesthetic Technique

The concept that the "stress" of surgery somehow leads to complications intersects with the long-standing controversy over the safety of regional anesthesia over general anesthesia. Plasma markers of stress, such as cortisol, catecholamines, and cytokines, become elevated during and after surgery with a general anesthetic. Spinal and epidural anesthesia markedly attenuate these changes during surgery, and much of the attenuation will continue after surgery if epidural analgesia is continued postoperatively. The presumption has been that the reduction in stress would translate into a reduction in morbidity and mortality, but it has been surprisingly difficult to prove this hypothesis. Early studies that examined the benefits of postoperative analgesia typically employed an epidural catheter infused with a dilute local anesthetic plus opioid. These studies employed random group assignment but enrolled small numbers of patients (40 to 60 each). Perhaps because a high-risk population was recruited, several of the studies demonstrated lower mortality and morbidity with respect to cardiac and pulmonary complications. Other studies have demonstrated additional benefits of regional anesthesia, including less blood loss during hip replacement surgery, a decreased incidence of deep vein thrombosis and pulmonary emboli, and a reduction in early graft thrombosis in peripheral vascular surgery. Not all studies demonstrate consistent benefits, however.

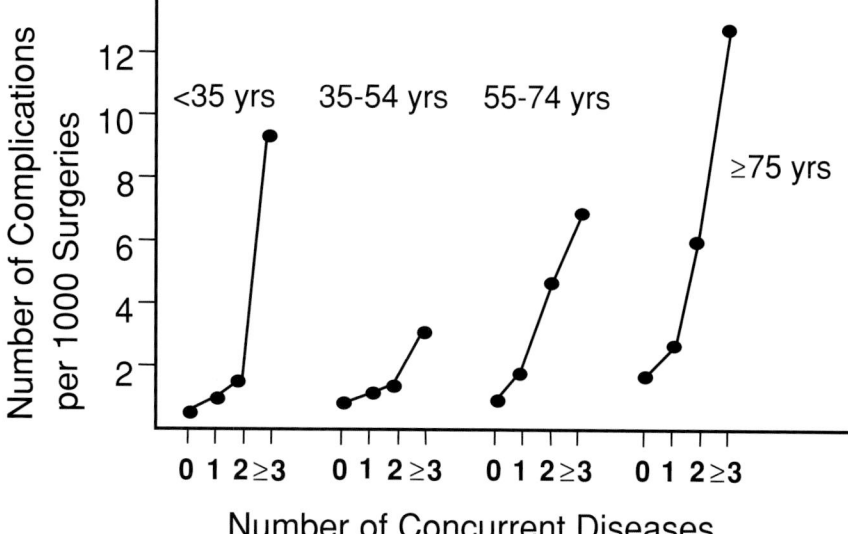

Figure 31-4 The interaction of age and concurrent disease on the incidence of perioperative complications. A retrospective analysis of more than 198,000 surgeries identified 268 major complications. For each age bracket, increasing numbers of concurrent disease was associated with rapidly increasing risk of complications. The effect of age is best assessed by comparing points of equivalent illness. Relative good health (0 to 1 chronic illnesses) demonstrates only a modest increase in complications with increasing age. Poor health (2 or more chronic illnesses) is associated with a much more dramatic increase in complications with age. Adapted from Tiret L et al: Complications associated with anaesthesia—A prospective survey in France. *Can Anesth Soc J* 33:336, 1986, with permission.

To circumvent the problem of small patient enrollment, a meta-analysis was performed on 141 studies that had employed randomized assignment to general anesthesia versus spinal or epidural anesthesia. In approximately half of the studies, the regional anesthetic was accompanied by a general anesthetic. When an epidural catheter was employed (75 percent of the neuraxial blocks), postoperative epidural analgesia was also frequently administered. Thus, group comparison is somewhat muddled. Nevertheless, the results were strongly in favor of the regional technique with deaths from all causes reduced by 30 percent. Decreases in myocardial infarction, pneumonia, and pulmonary embolism (but not stroke) were also demonstrated.

These encouraging results must be tempered by two prospective studies, each involving approximately 1000 patients randomly assigned to general anesthesia alone with parenteral opioids for postoperative analgesia versus a combined general plus epidural anesthesia with postoperative epidural analgesia. In one study the epidural group demonstrated a decreased incidence of respiratory failure. The other study found a lower incidence of adverse events in the epidural group only in the subset of patients undergoing repair of an abdominal aortic aneurysm. Therefore neither study found overwhelming evidence of improved outcome from the addition of epidural anesthesia/analgesia.

It is apparent, then, that current evidence of the benefit of postoperative epidural analgesia is weak, as is the evidence of the superiority of neuraxial anesthesia over general anesthesia as the primary anesthetic technique. Nevertheless, better pain relief is often achieved by regional techniques, and it is still possible that some medical benefits exist. Therefore, these techniques continue to be used, at least in selected circumstances.

Given the difficulty in proving a difference in outcome between regional and general anesthesia, it would be surprising if any study could demonstrate a difference in mortality or major morbidity when comparing, for example, different types of general anesthesia.

Common Perioperative Complications in Older Patients

An exhaustive discussion of complications that may occur in association with anesthesia and surgery is beyond both the scope and goals of this chapter. Nevertheless, it is worth commenting on a few complications.

Cardiac events are the most common form of complications. The risk of myocardial infarction increases with the prevalence of coronary disease in the patient population examined. In a relatively high-risk group, such as patients undergoing peripheral vascular surgery, the incidence of myocardial infarction (MI) is approximately 4 percent and congestive heart failure is approximately 9 percent. Among patients with a prior history of myocardial infarction, a perioperative MI is still associated with approximately 30 percent mortality. The most common time when myocardial infarctions are detected is 2 days after surgery and the same for congestive failure.

Curiously, many physicians, including many anesthesiologists, become greatly concerned when a patient demonstrates even a brief episode of perioperative myocardial ischemia. Patients with coronary disease have ischemic events during ordinary life. Why should perioperative ischemia raise the concern of a myocardial infarction and lead to hospitalization and tests for a myocardial infarction when that same ischemic event outside the hospital would be passed off as the patient's typical angina? It can be argued that isolated, brief (e.g., less than 30 minutes) ischemic events in a patient with known ischemic disease is probably not an indication for major concern. Most ischemic events are not related to intraoperative stress. The humoral stress response is highest during surgery and anesthesia, but the incidence of ischemic events is much lower during anesthesia than pre- or postoperatively. On the other hand, it can be argued that there is a greater likelihood of having an MI in the perioperative period than during ordinary life. The reason for this is not fully understood, but is probably related to the fact that most MIs are thrombotic in origin. Surgery enhances coagulation and impairs fibrinolysis, so it is not too speculative to suggest that patients with coronary disease are at increased risk of forming a clot whenever coagulation is enhanced. It can be argued that perioperative ischemia should be taken seriously primarily when clot could be the likely mechanism. As that determination is not easily made, judgment must be exercised, but it is logical to consider an ischemic event as not clot related if the event is brief and responds as expected to therapy such as hemodynamic control and/or nitroglycerin.

Stroke is a less frequent, but greatly feared, complication of surgery. Perioperative stroke occurs much more frequently than would be expected for the same population in the absence of surgery. The most common cause of stroke in medical patients is ischemic, and there is no indication that it is any different perioperatively. In all likelihood, the same coagulopathic changes that increase the risk of myocardial infarction perioperatively are responsible for the increased risk of stroke. What is not a likely cause of stroke, however, is hypotension. Intraoperative hypotension is certainly not uncommon in older patients, although it rarely is allowed to persist for long periods of time. It is irrational to blame a stroke on a brief period of intraoperative hypotension. First of all, the vast majority of strokes occur after the patient recovers from anesthesia and demonstrates an unchanged neurologic exam. If brief periods of hypotension caused strokes, then extended periods should, too. Yet no study involving deliberate hypotension for control of blood loss has reported an associated stroke. The best such study, involving 235 patients with an average age of 72 years who were randomly assigned to have mean arterial pressure maintained between 45 and 55 mmHg or 55 and 70 mmHg during surgery, demonstrated no strokes. In addition, comprehensive cognitive testing revealed no differences between the two groups in assessments performed before and after surgery. Patients who suffer profound hypotension (with cardiac arrest) may demonstrate global anoxic change, but rarely focal deficits. Lastly, when strokes occur perioperatively, the location of the stroke is no more likely to occur in a border zone perfusion area than anywhere else. Of much greater concern than hypotension as a mechanism for stroke is atrial fibrillation and emboli of cardiac origin, again, perhaps, accentuated by hypercoagulability. The degree to which atrial fibrillation is a risk factor is not well understood, but it raises the issue of how to manage patients who take warfarin chronically for atrial fibrillation or artificial valves. Based on the low risk of stroke in the absence of anticoagulation, it seems statistically safe to stop warfarin 4 days before surgery. A heparin infusion does not need to be used unless the patient has a history of arterial embolus or deep vein thrombosis within the previous 3 months. Warfarin therapy should be reinstituted postoperatively as soon as feasible.

Hepatitis is not a common perioperative complication in older patients. The reason for mentioning hepatitis is to clarify the incidence and mechanism of "halothane hepatitis." Anesthetic-induced hepatitis is an autoimmune-mediated event. A liver metabolite of halothane binds to liver proteins forming a trifluoroacetylated protein. Antibodies then develop to these proteins in susceptible individuals. On reexposure to some volatile agents, the antibodies are activated and cause massive hepatic destruction. Hepatitis induced by halothane has an incidence of 1 in 6000 to 35,000 anesthetics. Halothane is rarely used in adults now. The incidence with other volatile anesthetics, such as isoflurane, is much lower than with halothane, and the phenomenon cannot occur with sevoflurane because it does not yield trifluoroacetylated metabolites. Postoperative jaundice sometimes occurs from activation of already present viruses, but for most cases of elevated liver enzymes, the cause is unknown, and recovery is the rule.

Postoperative delirium is a common complication in older patients, is frequently undiagnosed, and may have a long-term adverse impact on the patient. The incidence may be as high as 60 percent in select surgical populations (e.g., undergoing major orthopedic procedures). As with hospital-acquired delirium in medical ward patients, surgical patients usually develop delirium after a few days of hospitalization. What is different about the two groups is that about one-third to one-half of the cases of delirium in medical patients are present at admission, in comparison to only 7 percent in hip fracture patients. This finding implicates acute illness as a risk factor for delirium. The hip fracture patients presumably were healthy prior to the fracture, and reached the hospital quickly before the delirium could develop. In fact, many mechanisms likely contribute to delirium in both medical and surgical patients, although classification of mechanism appears to be more clearcut in medical patients, and surgical patients are more likely to show recovery by the time of hospital discharge. Certainly some drugs, such as meperidine and anticholinergics, should be avoided, but the risk from opioids is not clear, especially when failure to use such drugs could lead to increased pain and decreased sleep. One might expect general anesthesia to be a major risk factor for delirium, but multiple studies have all failed to demonstrate any differences between general and regional anesthesia, even when tests of cognitive function are included. Perhaps by the time patients become vulnerable, the drugs used during surgery are essentially gone. Besides drugs, sleep disturbance, an unfamiliar environment, sensory loss (lack of glasses, hearing aids), and metabolic disturbance may contribute to delirium. If it is present at any time in the hospitalization, delirium is associated with prolonged hospital stay and a decrease in function (e.g. instrumental activities of daily living) on hospital discharge. The diagnosis and management of postoperative delirium represents a prime example of a problem where the geriatrician can provide much needed assistance.

An even less well understood central nervous system complication of surgery is that of long-term cognitive decline. Until recently, only anecdotal reports appeared in

Table 31-3   Guidelines for Epidural Catheters in Anticoagulated Patients[a]

Medication	Recommendations
Warfarin	Do not place needle or remove catheter if prothrombin levels are therapeutic. Discontinuation of warfarin must be of sufficient duration to restore all prothrombin factors, not just factor VII. If warfarin is initiated prior to needle placement or catheter removal, check the prothrombin time even if only one dose of warfarin has been given.
Intravenous heparin	Do not place needle or remove catheter if partial thromboplastin time is elevated. Heparin therapy should not be initiated until at least one hour after needle placement or catheter removal. Catheter removal should be preceded by heparin discontinuation for 2–4 hours and evaluation of the coagulation status.
Subcutaneous (mini-dose) heparin	Needle placement and catheter removal is not contraindicated, but it may be wise to avoid doing so at the peak heparin effect at around two hours after injection.
Low molecular weight heparin	Needle placement and catheter removal should occur at least two hours before, and at least 10 hours after, once a day LMWH therapy. Twice a day LMWH dictates holding one dose, and waiting 20–24 hours after the last dose.
Non-steroidal anti-inflammatory drugs	No evidence of increased risk.
Combination therapy	Little data, but risk may be increased, especially if low molecular weight heparin is one of the therapies.

[a]For full set of recommendations of the American Society of Regional Anesthesia Consensus Statement, see http://www.asra.com/items_of_interest/consensus_statements

LMWH, low molecular weight heparin.

the literature. In 1998, a prospective study tested surgical patients before and three months after surgery. A matched set of control subjects not having surgery were selected and tested as well. At 3 months 10 percent of the surgical patients had demonstrable cognitive decline, in comparison to only 3 percent of the control subjects. Unpublished follow-up suggests these deficits persist at least 1 year after surgery. It is not known whether postoperative delirium is related to the cognitive decline.

POSTOPERATIVE ANALGESIA

The options for postoperative analgesia have expanded considerably in the past 15 years. Patient-controlled analgesia (PCA) offers the patient the opportunity to obtain pain medication without having to wait for a busy nurse, or endure the cycle of heavy sedation with the initial peak effect, followed by a period of alertness and reasonable analgesia, and ending with increasing pain and anxiety until the next dose comes due. Patient-controlled analgesia allows the patient to finely titrate the analgesia against the opioid side effects, including nausea, sedation, dysphoria, and itching. Peripheral nerve blocks performed with long-acting local anesthetics provide up to 24 hours of postoperative analgesia. Placement prior to surgery provides two additional benefits. First, the ability of the surgical stimulus to produce hemodynamic change is minimized and the decrease in nociceptive input to the central nervous system reduces the amount of general anesthetic that must

be used. Second, blocking the nociceptive barrage to the spinal cord provides preemptive analgesia. Intense spinal cord nociceptive input sensitizes the interneuronal pathways in the spinal cord. The sensitization makes it easier for pain signals, or even nonpainful stimuli, to trigger the ascending pain pathways. By blocking the pain input during their highest period of activity (intraoperatively and for roughly the first day after surgery), pain will be reduced on subsequent days even after the regional block has worn off. Sensitization also occurs at the sensory nerve endings as well. Preemptive analgesia by blocking peripheral sensitization is the purpose of a local anesthetic field block prior to surgery. Nonsteroidal anti-inflammatory medications may produce preemptive analgesia, too. Because of the potential anticoagulant effects of these drugs, however, they are not often given prior to surgery, or even immediately after surgery. In general, adjunct medications, including most nonsteroidal antiinflammatory agents, improve pain relief in the older patients after surgery and often reduce the dependence on opioid therapy.

The most elaborate technique for postoperative analgesia is provided through epidural catheters. Given the time involvement for catheter placement and management and the uncertainty of enhanced outcome, this technique is used selectively. Initially, epidural analgesia was nothing more than boluses of morphine given through a lumbar catheter. Now the typical formula is low concentrations of both a local anesthetic and an opioid that are infused continuously through a catheter placed at the dermatome most central to the incision, be it thoracic or lumbar in location. When the surgery is not appropriate for epidural anesthesia alone, a general anesthetic is also administered and the epidural catheter is used not only for postoperative analgesia, but also intraoperatively to provide preemptive analgesia.

There are significant risks to epidural catheter use. The most likely problem is failed placement. The next most likely problem is inadvertent dural puncture. As epidural catheters are placed with large-bore needles, the risk of a spinal headache is relatively high. Fortunately, the risk of postdural puncture headache decreases with age. If a thoracic catheter is placed, dural puncture could also lead to direct spinal cord trauma. This complication is rare. The most feared complication is the development of an epidural hematoma. The epidural space has many veins that are occasionally punctured. Generally, any bleeding stops spontaneously and quickly, but if it does not, an epidural hematoma may develop that causes cord compression. Permanent paraplegia is likely at that point, as the success of emergency laminectomy is poor once symptoms appear. Retrospective analysis of spinal and epidural anesthetics suggests that the intrinsic risk of paralysis is less than 1:150,000. Patients who have abnormal coagulation, however, are thought to be at greater risk. Most reports of epidural hematoma have been in patients who were anticoagulated when the block was performed or when heparin therapy was instituted less than an hour after the needle placement. The relative risk because of anticoagulation is unknown, as all reports are anecdotal and do not include a denominator. In the case of epidural catheters, epidural hematomas develop almost as often on catheter removal as on insertion, so the catheter removal must be considered an at-risk event as well. There are case series reports on spinal or epidural block performed in anticoagulated patients, but the largest series involved 1000 patients and is too small to be meaningful despite a zero incidence of hematoma. At its peak effect at around 2 hours, even subcutaneous heparin can provide enough anticoagulation to increase risk. Particularly distressing has been the high number of epidural hematomas reported in patients receiving low-molecular-weight heparin. Many of the hematomas developed after catheter removal. In response to these reports of epidural hematoma, it is recommended that any patient with an epidural catheter be given frequent neurologic checks if they receive anticoagulants (warfarin, heparin, low molecular weight heparin). Guidelines for catheter placement and removal have been formulated (Table 31-3).

REFERENCES

ACC/AHA guidelines for perioperative cardiovascular examination for non-cardiac surgery. *Circulation* 93:1278, 1996.

Barash PG et al (eds): *Clinical Anesthesia*, 3rd ed. Philadelphia, Lippincott-Raven, 1997.

Kearon C, Hirsh J: Management of anticoagulation before and after elective surgery. *N Engl J Med* 336:1506, 1997.

Liu S et al: Epidural anesthesia and analgesia—Their role in postoperative outcome. *Anesthesiology* 85:1474, 1995.

Mangano DT et al: Effects of atenolol on mortality and cardiovascular morbidity after noncardiac surgery. *N Engl J Med* 335:1713, 1996.

McLeskey CH (ed): *Geriatric Anesthesiology*. Baltimore, Williams & Wilkins, 1997.

Moller JT et al: Long-term postoperative cognitive dysfunction in the elderly: ISPOCD1 study. *Lancet* 351:857, 1998.

Muravchick S: *Geroanesthesia*. St. Louis, Mosby, 1997.

Park WY et al: Effect of epidural anesthesia and analgesia on perioperative outcome. *Ann Surg* 234:560, 2001.

Recommendations for neuraxial anesthesia and anticoagulation. *Reg Anesth Pain Med* 23(6 Suppl 2), 1998.

Rigg JRA et al: Epidural anaesthesia and analgesia and outcome of major surgery: A randomised trial. *Lancet* 359:1276, 2002.

Rodgers A et al: Reduction of postoperative mortality and morbidity with epidural or spinal anaesthesia: results from overview of randomised trials. *BMJ* 321:1493, 2000.

Rooke GA et al: Hemodynamic response and change in organ blood volume during spinal anesthesia in elderly men with cardiac disease. *Anesth Analg* 85:99, 1997.

Silverstein J (ed): Geriatric Anesthesia. *Anesthesiol Clin North Am* 18, 1, 2000.

Tiret L et al: Complications associated with anaesthesia—A prospective survey in France. *Can Anesth Soc J* 33:336, 1986.

Vandermeulen EP et al: Anticoagulants and spinal–epidural anesthesia. *Anesth Analg* 79:1165, 1994.

Warner MA et al: Surgical procedures among those ≥90 years of age. *Ann Surg* 207:380, 1988.

Williams-Russo P et al: Randomized trial of hypotensive epidural anesthesia in older adults. *Anesthesiology* 91:926, 1999.

Surgery in the Elderly Population

MIKA SINANAN • LILLAN KAO • PHILIP A. VEDOVATTI

Elderly persons represent an increasingly large proportion of the population, and surgery is integral to their care. Increased longevity exposes this population to a greater risk of illness of all kinds, including those best treated surgically. More than one-third of all surgical procedures in the United States are currently performed in patients older than 64 years of age.

Medicare data from the 1990s show that the most common causes of death in the elderly population are heart disease, cancer, and stroke, accounting for 60 percent of all deaths in the older-than-age-65-years group. Based on current trends, it is anticipated that by 2020, 70 percent of all cancer will be diagnosed in patients older than age 65 years, with the highest prevalence in lung, breast, prostate, and colorectal carcinoma. Surgery for curative or palliative treatment of cancer, cardiac valvular procedures, and both cardiac and peripheral revascularization procedures are critical elements in the management of these common disorders. Surgical intervention is the only choice for many acute surgical disorders such as a perforated viscous, acute appendicitis, cholecystitis, visceral bleeding, or obstruction from cancer, all of which affect the elderly. Medicare data also highlight gastroesophageal reflux disease (GERD) and peptic ulcer disease as other potentially surgically treatable disorders in this population. These are common problems in elderly patients, many of whom bring a past medical history of ongoing comorbid factors to the equation. These observations emphasize that despite improvements in medical management, surgery will continue to play an important therapeutic role in this population.

In addition to the specific medical issues that affect the elderly, technological factors have also promoted surgical options for treatment. Technical advances in perioperative care and in the technology of surgery are thought to have improved both the safety and efficacy of surgery in the elderly population, especially among the very old. Broadening the definition of a "surgical" procedure to include percutaneous and transcatheter treatments by interventional radiologists and cardiologists, recent innovation has contributed to the treatment of peripheral vascular disease and myocardial ischemia syndromes with stent–grafts and endovascular techniques. Other aspects of the minimally invasive revolution in surgical treatment include specialized instruments, video cameras, scopes, access ports, and fiberoptic lights sources. Use of these newly developed devices and innovative, minimally invasive techniques in the hollow organs of the urinary tract, joints spaces, and in the chest or abdomen where a real or virtual working space can be created, offers the option for definitive surgical treatment with much less pain and disability, and without the prolonged recovery inherent in more traditional open surgery.

Despite advances in the technology and art of surgery, surgical interventions in the elderly appear to be inherently riskier than in a younger population. Medicare data from 1994 to 1999 show increasing mortality with age following elective major vascular (Fig. 32-1) and cancer procedures (Fig. 32-2). In this study, mitral valvuloplasty and pneumonectomy were associated with 10 and 13 percent mortality, respectively, in patients older than age 65 years, with overall surgical mortality doubling from the 65- to 69-year-old age group to those older than age 80 years. Other studies exploring this issue have shown, however, that when comorbidity factors (which vary with age) are factored into the analysis, age is no longer an independent variable.

For many disorders, both medical and surgical options exist and must be considered for each patient on an individual basis. Careful assessment of comorbid factors, relative potential benefit, patient longevity, and physiologic cost must be made. Comorbid factors that influence the risk of surgical treatment are summarized by the American Society of Anesthesia (ASA) classification and show slow increases in perioperative morbidity for all ASA classes of persons from ages 40 to 70 years, then a rapid rise in morbidity of persons older than age 70 years. For example, the risk of major complications doubles for ASA class 1 and 2 patients between ages 40 and 70 years, reaching 6 percent overall for those age 80 years and higher. For ASA class 4, the corresponding increase in major complications is from 6 to 15 percent between the ages of 40 and 80 years. Efforts to "tune" the medical condition of the patient, controlling comorbidity and ASA risk, contribute to the quality and safety of surgical care in the elderly population.

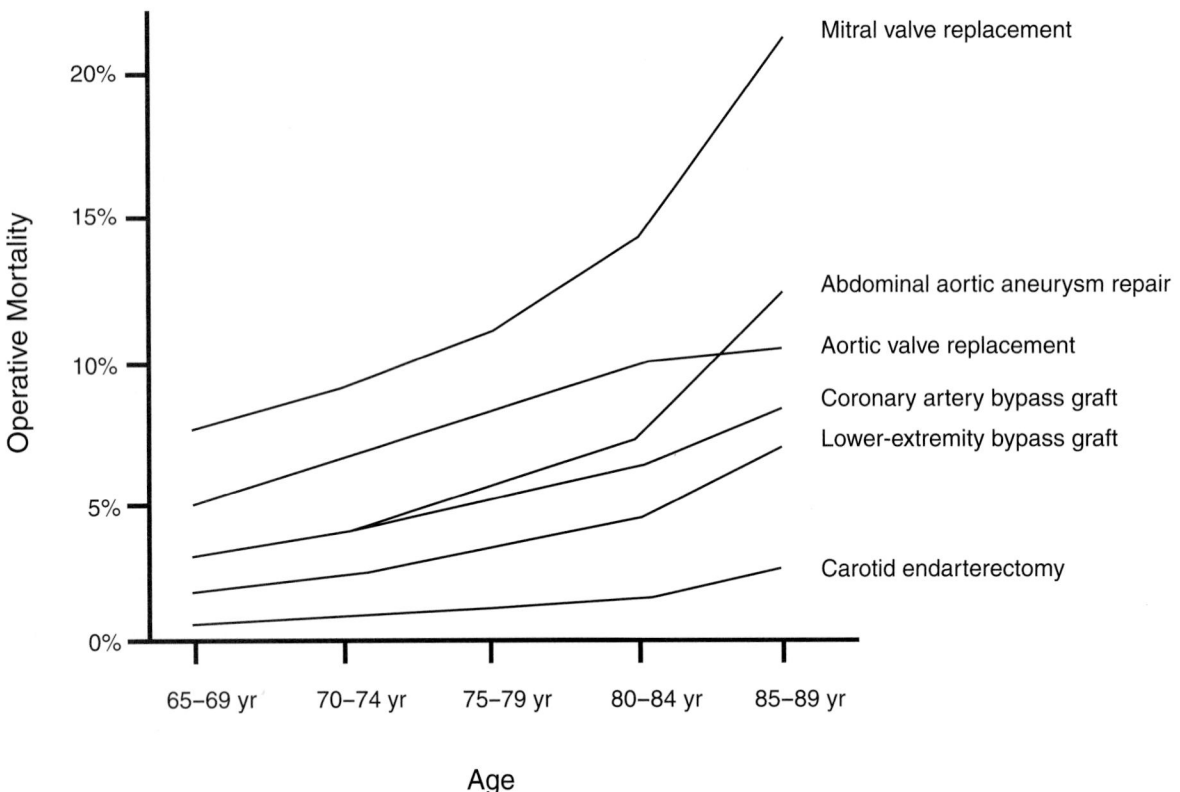

Figure 32-1 Relation between age and operative mortality in major cardiac and peripheral vascular surgical procedures. Data are derived from MEDPARS, the national Medicare claims database for patients older than age 65 years. Note the significant rise in operative mortality for all procedures after age 80 years. Reproduced with permission from Finlayson EV, Birkmeyer JD: Operative mortality with elective surgery in older adults. *Eff Clin Pract* 4:172, 2001.

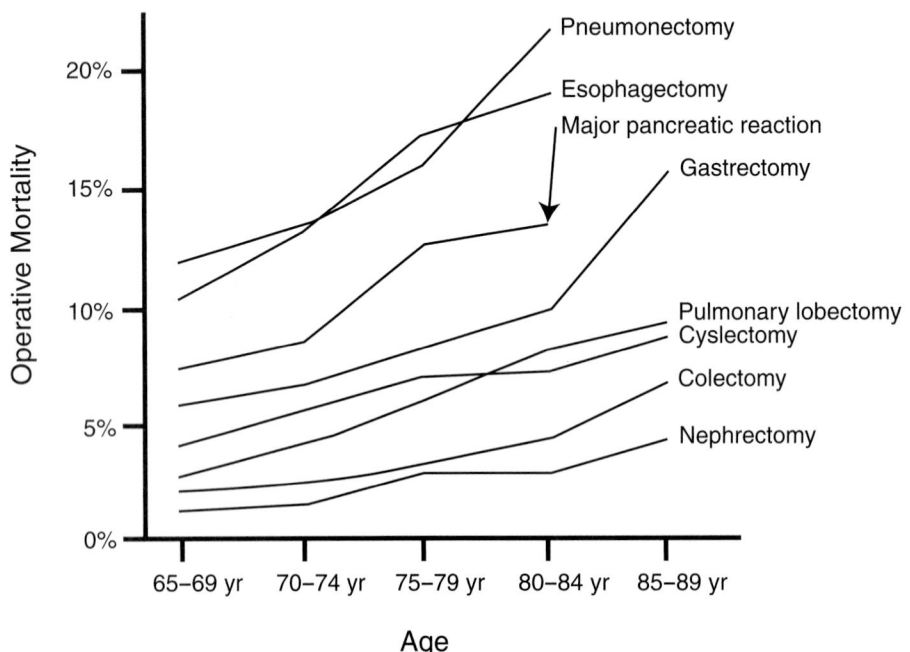

Figure 32-2 Relation between age and operative mortality in major cancer procedures. Data are derived from MEDPARS, the national Medicare claims database for patients older than age 65 years. Note the increase in mortality in all categories at all age ranges. Reproduced with permission from Finlayson EV, Birkmeyer JD: Operative mortality with elective surgery in older adults. *Eff Clin Pract* 4:172, 2001.

PREOPERATIVE PREPARATION

Preparing the elderly patient for surgery requires coordination between several disciplines, particularly if the patient has complex or multiple preexisting medical problems. This preparation involves clinical risk assessment, perioperative interventions to reduce surgical and anesthetic risk, and planning for adverse events that may arise. Clear communication between the medical provider, anesthesiologist and surgeon is critical to ensuring a coordinated plan of care intent on minimizing complications.

Preoperative medical evaluation and care in the geriatric patient is often accomplished by the patient's primary care provider or other medical consultant. While older age alone is not necessarily an indication for preoperative medical consultation, elderly patients with significant medical illness or poor functional capacity should undergo medical evaluation prior to major surgery. Perioperative medical management is discussed in Chap. 30.

Immediate Preoperative Issues: The Day of Surgery

The day of surgery represents one of the many "interface" situations when the principal care of a geriatric patient may overlap or pass from one service to another; it is these instances that highlight the importance of a coordinated transition of care. For example, elderly patients with eyeglasses or hearing aids should be instructed to bring these items with them to the hospital. It can be difficult for patients to participate in their recovery from surgery if communication is hampered by hearing or vision loss. Two key aspects of the immediate perioperative period bear mention, as they are pertinent to not only the internist or geriatrician, but to the anesthesiologist and surgeon as well.

Medications: Take or Skip?

Patients undergoing elective surgery nowadays increasingly present to the hospital on the day of surgery. This trend shifts responsibility of many aspects of immediate preoperative preparation from medical providers to the patient. Because older patients are often taking multiple outpatient medications, they require concise instructions as to which medicines should be taken on the morning of surgery and which should be withheld. In patients with memory impairment or those on complicated regimens, instructions should be written.

In general, essential medications such as antihypertensives, cardiac and antiepileptic medications, and medications which would have an adverse effect by their withdrawal should be taken on the morning of surgery with a small sip of water. Because of the potential for hypotension with administration of anesthetics (and the need for concomitant fluid administration), diuretics are typically held on the day of surgery in the absence of severe heart failure. Inhaled medications, transdermal agents, and the oft-forgotten eye drops may be taken as usual on the day of surgery for most surgical procedures. Patients with significant chronic obstructive pulmonary disease (COPD) may benefit from a bronchodilator given in the preoperative staging area just prior to surgery.

Optimally, patients with diabetes mellitus should be scheduled for surgery early in the day. Oral diabetes agents should be withheld on the morning of surgery. There are various effective regimens for managing diabetes perioperatively, which vary depending on the extent and duration of surgery, the degree of preoperative glucose control, and preexisting insulin requirements. Most regimens for insulin-treated type 2 diabetes patients undergoing major surgery involve taking one-third to one-half of their usual intermediate-acting insulin on the morning of surgery, followed by supplemental short acting insulin intra- and postoperatively as needed. Patients with type 1 diabetes, or with type 2 diabetes with marginal or poor glucose control generally benefit from a continuous insulin and glucose infusion regimen until normal oral intake is established postoperatively. One oral agent for diabetes that requires special mention is metformin. Renal or hepatic insufficiency increases the risk for rare but potentially fatal metabolic acidosis with this agent. It is recommended that metformin be held for 48 hours following major surgical procedures and only be resumed once persistently normal renal function is confirmed.

Pacemakers and Implanted Defibrillators

The incidence of implantable cardiac pacemaker insertion is highest among patients aged 75 years and older, and it is expected that the implantation rate of these devices will continue to rise sharply. Iatrogenic electromagnetic interference during surgery can have serious detrimental effects on implanted cardiac devices, including accidental reprogramming, pulse generator damage, and inducement of ventricular fibrillation. Electrocautery, internal defibrillation, radiation therapy, and lithotripsy procedures have all been associated with pacemaker damage or related complications. Implantable defibrillators additionally carry the risk of unintended discharge during surgery if not deactivated. Implantable defibrillators should therefore be *deactivated* prior to surgery, and reactivated immediately following surgery. External defibrillator pads should be placed on these patients while the device is inactive, and the pads should be placed distant from the implanted generator if possible. For the pacemaker-dependent patient, it is recommended that the pacer be programmed to an asynchronous, nonsensing mode (VOO or DOO) prior to surgery, and reprogrammed to original parameters following the procedure. Electrocautery grounding pads should be placed physically far from the generator, and efforts to prevent current flow across the device should be made. In patients whose pacemakers have not been programmed to VOO or DOO, the surgeon should use relatively short bursts with the electrocautery devices. The pacemaker may misinterpret the electrical energy from the electrocautery devices as cardiac activity, thus suppressing their function. As such, prolonged electrocautery in these circumstances can result in asystole in susceptible individuals. Reprogramming is not usually required for non–pacemaker-dependent patients, although the device should be interrogated following surgery involving exposure to electromagnetic interference.

CARDIOTHORACIC SURGERY

Cardiothoracic surgery comprises procedures on the heart, mediastinum, including great vessels and esophagus, lungs, and chest wall. Coronary vascular disease, degenerative disease of the heart valves and thoracic aorta, as well as cancers of the lung and esophagus, commonly occur in older patients and often require surgical therapy.

Coronary Artery Bypass Grafting

Atherosclerotic coronary vascular disease (ASCVD) is very common in elderly persons, affecting 27 percent of men and 17 percent of women older than age 80 years. The prevalence of ASCVD in the aged population results in an annual incidence of initial coronary events of 2.6 percent in men and 1.2 percent in women older than age 65 years. Medical management, angioplasty with coronary stent placement, and surgical revascularization (coronary artery bypass grafting [CABG]) have emerged as alternatives in the management of ASCVD. In 1995, 573,000 CABG procedures were performed on 363,000 patients, about half the number who underwent percutaneous coronary angioplasty (PTCA). In 1999, 322,000 CABG procedures in the United States were performed in patients age 65 years old and older, comprising more than 50 percent of all bypass procedures done.

Controversy continues regarding use of CABG in the elderly population. Appropriate candidates for CABG according to the American Heart Association include patients with three-coronary-vessel (left anterior descending, circumflex, and right coronary artery) disease especially if associated with left ventricular dysfunction, angina with rest, or minimal exertion despite optimal medical therapy, and those who are not candidates for or who have failed PTCA. Much of the controversy derives from the fact that major, multiinstitutional studies of CABG prior to 1995 supported the efficacy of surgical treatment over medical management but excluded patients older than 65 years of age and included few women. These studies suggested that the survival benefit from CABG peaked 5 years after surgery, as compared to medical therapy and the survival curves from medical and surgical treatment that converged after 10 years.

Factors that may impact on the choice of CABG in elderly patients include the increased operative mortality of CABG in patients older than age 65 years (estimated in 2000 to be three to seven times greater than in patients younger than age 65 years), the three times increased perioperative stroke risk (6.1 percent in patients older than age 70 years versus 1.9 percent in patients younger than age 70 years), the increased number of women in this age group for whom survival may be different, and the limited longevity of older patients for whom 5- and 10-year survival might not apply. In light of these issues, the relative

Table 32-1   Risk Factors Predictive of Perioperative Mortality in Elderly Patients Undergoing CABG

Emergent surgery	Decreased left ventricular function
Obstructive pulmonary disease	Mitral regurgitation
Left main coronary artery stenosis	Previous coronary bypass operation
Age	Renal insufficiency
Cardiogenic shock	

benefit of CABG in elderly patients has been challenged. However, a number of newer studies suggest that cautious use of invasive revascularization procedures may provide benefit with acceptable risk.

The inherent risk of coronary disease in the elderly population has been emphasized by comparison studies of medical, PTCA, and surgical treatment. Table 32-1 lists the risk factors predictive for mortality following coronary bypass surgery. In contrast to younger patients, these preoperative risk factors carry greater significance in the outcomes of elderly patients undergoing CABG. When elderly patients with significant comorbid illness are excluded, however, in-hospital mortality decreases to 4.2 percent. While greater age alone appears to be a significant independent risk factor, procedural mortality rates in elderly patients without comorbid illness are approaching levels seen in younger individuals. Octogenarians undergoing coronary bypass are more likely to have emergent surgery, which is strongly associated with higher perioperative mortality, than their younger counterparts. They are also more likely to be women, to be admitted with acute myocardial infarction (MI), and have cerebrovascular disease or congestive heart failure—all of which have been associated with higher perioperative mortality. Interestingly, the risk factors associated with CABG-related complications are similar to those in younger patients; the greater prevalence of these risk factors in geriatric populations likely contributes to the increase in perioperative CABG mortality.

Despite the increased perioperative risk, CABG in selected patients at all ages results in better long-term survival. One Canadian study showed improved survival, with a relative benefit of CABG to medical therapy reaching 17 percent in the older-than-age-80-years population at 4 years, a finding confirmed by other recent clinical studies. Sustained improvements in quality of life, physical activity, and relief from angina after CABG in the elderly population have been documented and offer perhaps the most compelling argument for considering elective CABG for relief of symptomatic coronary vascular disease.

Elderly patients with emergent symptoms, ventricular failure, or prior CABG are at highest risk for complications. Atrial arrhythmias, respiratory failure, neurologic events, acute renal failure, and perioperative MI are most common and contribute to both prolonged hospitalization and mortality. Technical improvements in recent years may reduce perioperative complications, especially the stroke risk and cognitive impairment. One such approach is off-pump or "beating-heart" bypass, during which the heart is never stopped, retaining physiologic blood flow to the brain and periphery. Revascularization using internal mammary (IMA) grafts was previously less-commonly performed in the elderly population because of concerns of increased morbidity and mortality. Newer studies suggest improved long-term survival in elderly patients receiving unilateral IMA grafts, similar with those in younger groups. Other innovations include the expanding field of minimally invasive coronary surgery, so-called "mid-CAB" procedures done through a small chest incision, or thoracoscopic procedures for vessel harvest and bypass. Innovation in anesthetic management and the use of transesophageal echo imaging for continuous monitoring of cardiac function have also reduced perioperative morbidity. These innovations to reduce the pain and distress from a major chest incision and avoid the physiologic consequences of hypothermic cardiac arrest have already demonstrated improved survival and reduced complications, especially in the elderly population.

Valvular Disease

Cardiac murmurs are present in 40 to 60 percent of the population older than age 65 years, but hemodynamically significant valvular disease is much less common. The largest segment of patients undergoing valve replacement surgery is older than age 65 years, accounting for roughly 56,000 procedures in the United States in 1999. As the population ages, it is expected that older patients will continue to be the dominant recipient of this type of surgery.

As reviewed in Chap. 36, the two most common acquired valvular disorders in the elderly are aortic stenosis (AS) and mitral annular calcification resulting in regurgitation (mitral regurgitation [MR]). Calcific aortic sclerosis as a consequence of aging is present in 29 percent of the elderly population and is the most common cause of AS. Aortic insufficiency is also an indication for valve surgery, but it is much less common in older patients. Degeneration of a congenital bicuspid aortic valve causes aortic stenosis in 70 percent of patients born with that abnormality. Historically, rheumatic valvular disease was the most common cause of MR. At present, myocardial ischemic disease or myxomatous degeneration are the most common causes of chronic MR, affecting 6 percent of patients older than age 60 years. Patients can present with both AS and chronic MR.

Some elderly patients with AS or MR tolerate it poorly. As atrial fibrillation is commonly present, loss of ventricular compliance and the supplementary atrial "kick" accelerates development of symptoms. Myocardial infarction and sudden cardiac death are common, resulting in a 50 percent 1-year survival in elderly patients with significant AS and associated left ventricular dysfunction. Patients with symptomatic AS, and those with MR associated with significant cardiac dilation, are candidates for surgical repair. In any individual patient, comorbid factors, anticipated longevity, response to medical therapy, and performance status must be factored into the decision for surgical therapy. Age is a

Table 32-2 Accepted Indications for Valve Replacement in Aortic Stenosis

Symptomatic severe aortic stenosis

Moderate or severe aortic stenosis at the time of bypass surgery

Asymptomatic aortic stenosis with left ventricular systolic dysfunction

Asymptomatic severe aortic stenosis if:

- Patient desires high level of physical exertion or lives in area remote from medical care
- Elective procedure in patient with severe stenosis due to patient preferences

SOURCE: Adapted from Aikawa K, Otto CM: Timing of surgery in aortic stenosis. *Prog Cardiovasc Dis* 43:477, 2001.

factor only insofar as it is associated with a higher incidence of comorbid factors. A number of retrospective studies suggest that many symptomatic elderly patients with aortic stenosis are not referred for surgery, despite existing evidence that severe symptoms or left ventricular dysfunction are indications, rather than contraindications, to surgical intervention.

Valvular prosthetic replacement may require long-term anticoagulation to avoid embolic complications from the valve, depending on the type of valve used and valve location. Bioprosthetic (tissue) valves that do not need anticoagulation may be a more appropriate alternative for elderly patients because their eventual failure is of less concern in those with a limited life span. Technical factors, patient life expectancy, the risks of anticoagulation, and patient desires should be factored into the final decision regarding type of prosthesis. Accepted indications for valve replacement in aortic stenosis are similar to those in younger populations, and are listed in Table 32-2.

Perioperative mortality from elective aortic valve repair in the elderly population is reported to range from 5 to 20 percent, but in the last 10 years has significantly improved. Mitral valve surgery carries an even higher risk. Mitral regurgitation is more commonly accompanied by aortic disease in the elderly population, which increases operative mortality and reduces functional outcome. Adverse risk factors that increase both perioperative morbidity and morbidity include heart failure, chronic lung or kidney disease, multivalve repair, and associated CABG, although combined procedures are increasingly common. Common surgical complications include bleeding, arrhythmias, cardiac failure, and stroke. However, successful aortic valve replacement for AS is associated with excellent control of symptoms and a 60 to 70 percent 5-year survival, essentially equal to age-matched controls. Long-term survival after mitral valve replacement in the elderly has been poorer, because many patients have concomitant heart failure at diagnosis or undergo combined CABG and mitral valvuloplasty procedures. Innovative minimally invasive approaches to cardiac valvuloplasty have been described and hold promise for improving the perioperative risks currently associated with conventional open heart surgery.

Lung Cancer

Lung cancer is the most common cause of cancer deaths in men, and the second most common cause of cancer deaths in women. More than 60 percent of lung cancers occur in patients older than 60 years of age, usually with a smoking history. Most lung cancers in this group are of squamous origin and stage 3 or higher at presentation, rendering curative treatment impossible.

For those diagnosed with early, stages 1 and 2 lung cancer, treatment is primarily surgical. Until recently, elderly patients, especially those older than age 80 years, had an unacceptably high surgical complication and mortality rate. A series of recent studies have shown acceptable operative mortality of 4 to 5 percent with resection and a perioperative morbidity of 10 to 25 percent, although pneumonectomy (removal of an entire lung) and poor preoperative lung function (forced expiratory volume in one second [FEV_1] and forced vital capacity [FVC] <60 percent of predicted) predispose to higher risk. Limited experience with thoracoscopic lung resection suggests that this technique has benefit in the elderly with an acceptable cure rate while reducing perioperative risk. Unfortunately, long-term survival, even with apparently curative resection, remains poor. Five-year survival in elderly patients undergoing surgical resection is 35 to 50 percent with intervening mortality from cancer recurrence, second primary cancers, other malignancies, and cardiovascular events. Apparently successful treatment of a lung cancer should prompt vigorous and ongoing surveillance for other cancers or cardiovascular risks, especially given the common risk factor of cigarette smoking. It can be anticipated that the declining rates and social acceptability of smoking should eventually reduce the risk of this and other smoking-related diseases.

MINIMALLY INVASIVE SURGERY

In younger patients, laparoscopic surgery is touted as conferring the benefits of a shorter hospital stay, decreased pain, less post-operative ileus, and faster return to work. In elderly patients, these potential benefits must be balanced against the hemodynamic effects of pneumoperitoneum, longer operative times, and a requirement for general anesthesia. While several studies have demonstrated that laparoscopic procedures can be performed safely in elderly patients, a degree of caution should be exercised in patients with underlying cardiac disease or with hemodynamic instability, as in emergent operations.

The physiologic effects of laparoscopy are related to the carbon dioxide insufflation and increased abdominal pressure associated with pneumoperitoneum, as well as to patient positioning. With abdominal insufflation, carbon dioxide is absorbed and converted to carbonic acid in the bloodstream. The patient may become acidotic secondary to the increased carbonic acid and may require hyperventilation in order to compensate. The increased

intraabdominal pressure results in an increased mean arterial pressure, increased systemic vascular resistance, increased pulmonary capillary wedge pressure, and increased inferior vena caval pressure. An increase in heart rate may occur as a result of both the increased partial pressure of carbon dioxide and the decrease in stroke volume as a result of pneumoperitoneum. Cardiac output may thus either be maintained as a result of the increased heart rate or may decrease. Patient positioning, in particular the Trendelenburg position (head down), may increase right heart-filling pressures and thus also affect cardiac output.

As will be described in the following section, laparoscopic operations can be performed safely in elderly patients. However, older patients tend to have more advanced disease at the time of presentation and to have associated comorbidities that may preclude a laparoscopic approach. The benefits of smaller incisions and faster postoperative recovery must be weighed against the patient's ability to tolerate pneumoperitoneum. Invasive monitoring may be appropriate for patients with underlying cardiovascular disease.

GASTROINTESTINAL SURGERY

With an expanding population of elderly patients in the United States, the number of older patients presenting with both benign and malignant abdominal disorders is increasing in frequency. Of those patients presenting to the emergency department with abdominal pain, elderly patients are twice as likely to require urgent surgical intervention and have a ninefold increase in mortality over their younger counterparts. Overall, however, the morbidity and mortality of abdominal operations performed on elderly patients have decreased over the past several decades.

Challenges in determining the etiology of abdominal pain in older patients are a result of several factors. History may be difficult to elicit given either a depressed mental status or declining memory. Physical examination may not be reliable, as elderly patients can present with minimal peritoneal signs. Medications in this population such as nonsteroidal antiinflammatory drugs (NSAIDs) or steroids may further mask potential signs or symptoms. Laboratory evaluation may reveal the lack of a leukocytosis, which does not eliminate the possibility of an acute surgical problem. As abdominal pain in the elderly patient has a wide differential, the diagnostic work-up can be both challenging and time-consuming. Once a diagnosis has been established, careful pre- and perioperative management must ensue as many older patients have multiple comorbidities. Ethical considerations regarding informed consent and quality of life may also need to be taken into account.

The following section discusses various benign and malignant conditions of the gastrointestinal tract that may warrant surgical intervention.

Hepatobiliary and Pancreatic Disorders

Cholelithiasis

Elderly patients have an increased incidence of gallstones, a fact that may be partially attributable to changes in anatomy and function of the biliary tract with age. The common bile duct has been noted to be increased in size in asymptomatic older patients, and may be related to an increased replacement of the myocytes with connective tissue. While there is no net change in gallbladder contractility, older patients have a decreased responsiveness to cholecystokinin but increased circulating levels after meals. There is also an increased lithogenicity of bile with age secondary to increased cholesterol and decreased bile acid synthesis. All of these factors may play a role in the development of biliary tract disease in the elderly population.

In addition, the older population has an increased risk of developing complications from gallstones such as biliary pancreatitis, gangrenous or emphysematous cholecystitis, choledocholithiasis, or gallstone ileus from a cholecystenteric fistula. Nonetheless, as in younger patients, treatment is reserved for those with symptoms. While nonoperative therapies such as ursodeoxycholic acid or extracorporeal shock wave lithotripsy (ESWL) have been investigated, their efficacy is limited and use should be limited to a select subgroup of patients.

The standard treatment for uncomplicated symptomatic cholelithiasis in older patients is laparoscopic cholecystectomy. Multiple studies demonstrate comparable morbidity rates for laparoscopic cholecystectomy in elderly patients, as compared to younger patients. In addition, for uncomplicated gallstones, the conversion rate to an open procedure appears to be similar to that for younger patients. In reasonable candidates, early laparoscopic cholecystectomy should be performed for symptomatic gallstones given the increased morbidity associated with an emergent procedure. However, given the increased incidence of cardiovascular comorbidities in older patients and the hemodynamic effects of pneumoperitoneum, careful preoperative assessment and intraoperative monitoring should be performed.

Choledocholithiasis

When compared to younger cohorts, elderly patients have an increased incidence of choledocholithiasis. While historically the mortality of open surgical intervention in the older patient has been high, percutaneous and endoscopic techniques have improved over the past several years to allow for safe, nonoperative diagnosis and treatment of common bile duct stones. Endoscopic retrograde cholangiopancreatography (ERCP) is the diagnostic modality of choice for detecting common bile duct stones, and endoscopic drainage is safe and effective with a morbidity rate of 3 percent and an efficacy of 96 to 98 percent. In expert hands, ERCP has a complication rate of less than 5 percent, principally pancreatitis, bleeding, and perforation after sphincterotomy. For purely diagnostic evaluations, less invasive imaging modalities such as magnetic resonance cholangiography (MRC) and endoscopic ultrasonography (EUS) are increasingly accurate methods of detecting biliary obstruction caused by choledocholithiasis.

Prior to the advent of advanced endoscopic and radiologic techniques, choledochoduodenostomy was advocated for all elderly patients with common bile duct stones to avoid having to perform operative reexploration of the biliary tract. Currently, endoscopic drainage followed by cholecystectomy is preferred. In one non-randomized study of treatment of acute cholangitis in elderly and younger patients, endoscopic drainage had the least morbidity and mortality, followed by percutaneous drainage. Morbidity and mortality were higher in the older patients in all arms. In elderly patients with endoscopically irretrievable stones, biliary stenting has been reported as a temporizing measure. Endoscopic treatment alone may be sufficient in patients with significant comorbidity or limited longevity.

Acute Cholecystitis

Older patients are more likely than younger patients to present with complicated gallstone disease such as emphysematous or gangrenous cholecystitis. In addition, perforation is more common, possibly as a result of ischemic changes of the gallbladder secondary to atherosclerotic disease.

Elderly patients can present with atypical symptoms for cholecystitis, but usually abdominal pain is present. Fever, nausea, and emesis may also be noted. Cholecystitis in the aged can present as sepsis of unknown origin or mental status changes alone. Therefore, a low threshold of suspicion for cholecystitis must be entertained in patients who present with sepsis without a determined etiology. Leukocytosis and elevated liver function tests may also be present. Ultrasonography is the diagnostic test of choice.

The treatment of choice for acute cholecystitis consists of antibiotic therapy and cholecystectomy. Overall, laparoscopic cholecystectomy can be performed safely in elderly patients. However, studies evaluating laparoscopic cholecystectomy for acute cholecystitis in the aged demonstrate an increased likelihood of conversion to an open procedure secondary to adhesions and inflammation. In addition, length of hospital stay and rate of complications are increased in the elderly population, as a result of both their comorbidities and their complicated presentations.

In patients who are high risk for immediate surgical intervention, either ultrasonography or computerized tomography (CT)-guided percutaneous cholecystostomy is a safe and effective alternative. Placement of a cholecystostomy tube may allow for the resolution of the acute phase of the illness in critically ill patients and can serve as a temporizing measure prior to subsequent elective cholecystectomy. In addition, percutaneous cholecystostomy placement may be definitive treatment in patients with acalculous or even calculous cholecystitis. Further study regarding the necessity of elective cholecystectomy in this situation is needed.

Acute Pancreatitis

Increasing age is a poor prognostic factor for acute pancreatitis. The etiology of pancreatitis in older patients is less likely to be alcohol related as compared to their younger counterparts. Rather, gallstone disease is responsible for 65 to 75 percent of cases of acute pancreatitis in the elderly. Other common causes include drugs, malignancy, ischemia, and ERCP.

Diagnosis is based upon clinical presentation and elevation in amylase and/or lipase. Symptoms are similar to those in younger patients, including epigastric pain radiating to the back, nausea, and vomiting. More severe manifestations of pancreatitis such as shock, acute renal failure, respiratory distress, and hypocalcemia may also develop. Ultrasonographic examination is useful in the diagnosis of gallstones, and CT scanning is indicated for patients with a predicted severe course of pancreatitis, suspected pancreatic necrosis, persistent leukocytosis or fever, or failure to improve clinically.

Treatment of acute pancreatitis in the elderly is supportive, as in younger patients. Bowel rest, intravenous analgesics, and hydration with correction of electrolytes are indicated in mild forms of pancreatitis. For more severe pancreatitis with necrosis, there is increasing evidence for the use of prophylactic antibiotics in decreasing infectious complications and mortality.

Based on four randomized controlled trials, the current recommendation for patients with gallstone pancreatitis and a predicted severe course is ERCP with sphincterotomy. Persistent jaundice and evidence of cholangitis are also indications for early endoscopic intervention. Typically, patients should undergo laparoscopic cholecystectomy at the end of the hospitalization prior to discharge. However, in elderly patients with multiple comorbidities, sphincterotomy alone may be sufficient.

Models for predicting severity of acute pancreatitis include age as a prognostic indicator, such as Ranson's criteria and the acute physiology and chronic health evaluation (APACHE) II scoring system. Despite advancements in critical care and interventional techniques, mortality from severe acute pancreatitis remains high, especially in the older population. Mortality in patients older than age 70 years with necrotizing pancreatitis has been reported as 25 percent, as compared to less than 10 percent in the younger population. In one series of patients older than 80 years of age, all patients with necrotizing pancreatitis died regardless of treatment strategy.

Esophageal Disorders

Gastroesophageal Reflux Disease

GERD is a common disorder among the elderly population. While the symptoms are similar in both younger and older patients, the latter tend to have less-severe complaints. The milder clinical presentation may be the result of multiple factors including decreased pain perception with age and decreased acidity of the refluxed contents caused by gastric mucosal changes. Other physiologic changes related to aging that may predispose to GERD include decreased esophageal peristaltic pressures, increased incidence of hiatal hernias, and a decreased salivary bicarbonate concentration. In addition, while age itself does not contribute to decreasing lower esophageal sphincter pressures, medications associated with comorbid diseases may be contributory.

The clinical presentation of GERD is similar to that in younger patients including symptoms such as retrosternal chest pain, acid regurgitation, dysphagia, or odynophagia (pain with swallowing). In addition, extraesophageal manifestations of GERD are more common such as laryngitis, asthma, pulmonary fibrosis, and aspiration pneumonia. The work-up for GERD is similar to that in younger patients and can include 24-hour pH probe monitoring, esophageal manometry, endoscopy, and barium swallow. One essential difference in older patients is a lower threshold for endoscopy caused by both the milder disease presentation and the increased incidence of complications such as esophagitis or Barrett's esophagus.

As in younger patients, the first line of therapy includes lifestyle modifications. Medical therapy consists of prokinetic agents, H_2 blockers, and proton pump inhibitors. Given the more severe presentation of disease and decreased hepatic and renal clearance in many older patients, a proton pump inhibitor is often the drug of choice. Surgical treatment of GERD is a laparoscopic Nissen fundoplication. This procedure has been demonstrated to be safe and effective in elderly patients with GERD.

Barrett's esophagus, a condition characterized by intestinal metaplasia of the columnar-lined esophagus, increases in incidence in patients older than age 60 years. Because of the increased risk of development of adenocarcinoma, patients with Barrett's esophagus should be enrolled in a strict endoscopic surveillance program.

Paraesophageal Hernia

Paraesophageal hernias, which are characterized by herniation of the stomach into the chest, are increasingly common with advanced age. Depending upon the absence or presence of a sliding hiatal hernia component, they are classified as type II or III hiatal hernias, respectively. Small paraesophageal hernias may be asymptomatic. Larger hernias may present with retrosternal chest pain that mimics cardiac ischemia, heartburn, nausea, vomiting, weight loss, or dysphagia. The conventional wisdom has been that all patients with a paraesophageal hernia should undergo repair in order to avoid major complications, which are reported to occur in up to 45 percent of patients. More recent studies suggest that in the older fragile patient without major symptoms or chronic ulceration and bleeding, some smaller paraesophageal hernias can be followed safely. Giant paraesophageal hernias, virtually unique to the elderly population, are associated with a high risk of gastric strangulation and a 50 percent mortality rate, and should all be electively repaired if possible.

Repair of a paraesophageal hernia can be performed through a thoracotomy, laparotomy, or laparoscopically. The main tenets of paraesophageal repair are reduction of the hernia, repair of the diaphragmatic crural defect, and fixation of the stomach in the abdomen. Use of a concomitant antireflux procedure is controversial, but has been justified to reduce postoperative reflux and to fix the stomach in the abdomen. The reported mortality rate in open and laparoscopic series of elective paraesophageal hernia repairs is 1 to 2 percent. Unfortunately, the morbidity remains high, with a range of 13 to 27 percent in open repairs and 28 percent in laparoscopic repairs. Recurrence because of failure of the crural repair occurs in up to 7 percent of patients, with an even higher risk of gastric wrap herniation, prompting ongoing refinements to the procedure.

Referring physicians may be loath to recommend repair to some elderly patients given their comorbidities. An alternative, less-invasive approach has been reported for patients unable to withstand an open or laparoscopic repair. Reduction of the hernia is performed endoscopically or laparoscopically and fixation of the stomach in the abdomen is performed with a percutaneous endoscopic gastrostomy (PEG) tube. No attempt is made to restore the gastroesophageal junction into the abdomen or to perform an antireflux procedure. This technique aims to prevent problems of incarceration and strangulation.

Esophageal Cancer

Adenocarcinoma of the distal esophagus and gastroesophageal junction is the malignancy with the most rapidly rising incidence in the United States. Many, if not most, of these cancers arise in the setting of chronic GERD and Barrett's esophagus. Surgical resection of the esophagus for cancer or for Barrett's with high-grade dysplasia is the only treatment at present with proven curative potential. In one of the largest evaluations of esophagectomy for cancer in the elderly, Poon et al. found a 14.4 percent mortality in the first 30 days, most a result of complications of surgery. Cardiac and pulmonary complications predominated with an anastomotic leak rate of 3 percent. Median cancer-specific survival was 33 months with 1- and 5-year cancer-specific survival after curative surgery of 81 percent and 36 percent. Palliative resection only yielded a mean of 6.7 months. This series included the classic combined abdominal epigastric and right thoracotomy for complete esophagectomy (Ivor Lewis) and transhiatal esophagectomy using blunt technique. More recently, minimally invasive laparoscopic and thoracoscopic approaches to esophagectomy have been described. Once refined and validated as an effective cancer operation, use of the minimally invasive approach should minimize cardiopulmonary complications and reduce perioperative mortality.

Gastroduodenal Disorders: Peptic Ulcer Disease

Although the incidence of peptic ulcer disease is not increased in the elderly, there is a higher rate of complications such as perforation and hemorrhage. Not surprisingly, elderly patients have a higher morbidity and mortality rate associated with these complications. Multiple factors can contribute to the predisposition of elderly patients to complications from peptic ulcer disease such as a prior history of ulcer disease, the presence of medical comorbidities, an increased use of contributory medications such as NSAIDs and steroids, and a higher incidence of infection with *Helicobacter pylori*. In terms of pathophysiology, there is evidence that elderly persons may have decreased mucosal protection secondary to decreased prostaglandin secretion, as well as impaired repair mechanisms with decreased cellular proliferation.

The clinical presentation of peptic ulcer disease is often atypical in older patients. In fact, the manifestation of a complication of ulcer disease is the initial presentation in as high as 50 percent or more of elderly patients. While nonoperative therapy can be employed initially in many instances, the indications for surgical intervention are perforation, hemorrhage, obstruction, and intractability. In fact, delay in diagnosis and greater than 12 hours between presentation and operative intervention are associated with increased mortality from peptic ulcer disease in the elderly population. In addition, several studies report higher morbidity and mortality with nonoperative treatment, particularly in association with upper gastrointestinal bleeding. Older patients who present with a bleeding peptic ulcer tend to have an increased risk of rebleeding, have more severe bleeding requiring more transfusions, and are more likely to need operative intervention.

The operative strategy depends upon multiple factors including the patient's clinical presentation, hemodynamic status, and medical comorbidities. Operative experience of the surgeon may influence surgical approach as well. More recently, a laparoscopic approach has been described for perforated peptic ulcer disease, as well as for ulcers refractory to medical therapy. There is no clear advantage to laparoscopic treatment of perforated ulcer disease, but further prospective studies are needed.

Mortality from complications of peptic ulcer disease in the elderly ranges from 25 to 50 percent, with a higher mortality associated with perforations. In addition, gastric ulcers are associated with increased mortality, as well as an increased risk of infectious complications and a longer length of stay. A potential malignancy should be considered in patients presenting with non-healing or complicated gastric ulcers.

Small-Bowel Disorders

Small Bowel Obstruction

Small bowel obstruction is the most common surgical disorder of the small intestine in the elderly population. The three main causes of obstruction are abdominal wall hernias, adhesions, and neoplasms. The clinical presentation usually consists of nausea, vomiting, abdominal pain, and distension. The diagnosis can be made based on plain films demonstrating air–fluid levels, distended proximal loops of small bowel, and a paucity of bowel gas distally. Computed tomography has been increasingly used to assist in determining the location, underlying etiology, and severity of a small bowel obstruction. Initial treatment in the absence of peritoneal signs, leukocytosis, or hemodynamic instability is nonoperative with nasogastric decompression, intravenous hydration, and serial observation. Operative intervention is indicated for peritoneal signs or failure to improve with medical therapy.

Gallstone Ileus

Although a rare cause of small-bowel obstruction overall, gallstone ileus has been reported to account for up to

25 percent of small bowel obstructions in patients older than 65 years of age. The pathophysiology is usually caused by gallstone passage through a cholecystoduodenal fistula with subsequent obstruction of the bowel. Although the terminal ileum is the most common location of obstruction, the gallstone can also become impacted in the duodenum, and fistulous disease can develop between the gallbladder and colon as well.

The diagnosis of gallstone ileus can be suggested from findings on plain films by pneumobilia, a right upper quadrant calculus, and a small bowel obstruction. Treatment consists of correction of electrolyte abnormalities, fluid hydration, bowel rest, and operative extraction of the stone. The concomitant treatment of the cholecystoduodenal fistula in a one-stage procedure is controversial. Proponents state that a one-stage procedure is feasible and safe. However, opponents cite a low incidence of recurrence of complications of gallbladder disease and an increased morbidity and mortality associated with a one-stage procedure.

Acute Mesenteric Ischemia

Acute mesenteric ischemia must be considered in the differential diagnosis of elderly patients presenting with acute abdominal pain and potential risk factors such as recent myocardial infarction, cardiac arrhythmias, valvular disorders, congestive heart failure and, hypotension or shock. The patient's medication profile should also be examined for vasoconstricting agents that could potentiate mesenteric ischemia. There are three main mechanisms for acute mesenteric ischemia including superior mesenteric artery (SMA) occlusion with a thrombus or embolus, nonocclusive mesenteric ischemia, or mesenteric venous thrombosis. An SMA embolus accounts for half of the cases of acute mesenteric ischemic followed by nonocclusive ischemia and then venous thrombosis. Given a 70 percent historical mortality rate, early diagnosis is essential but can often be challenging.

Presenting symptoms can include nausea, vomiting, anorexia, pain, distension, diarrhea, or hemoccult-positive stools. The classic presentation is that of pain disproportionate to exam, although in the early stages of ischemia, pain may not be present. Up to 25 percent of patients do not manifest abdominal pain. The presence of peritoneal signs suggests progression to bowel infarction. Laboratory values and radiologic images are often negative early in the disease. Leukocytosis, acidosis, or hyperkalemia may not be present until the late phases of the disease, often beyond the window of opportunity for revascularization. Advanced findings on plain film include "thumbprinting" (mucosal edema), evidence for small bowel obstruction, or perforation. Other diagnostic modalities include computed tomography, duplex ultrasonography, and magnetic resonance angiography. The latter two modalities are not as sensitive in detecting distal emboli or low-flow ischemia.

In patients without peritoneal signs, selective mesenteric angiography is the diagnostic examination of choice in order to confirm the diagnosis and to evaluate the splanchnic vasculature. Thrombolytic drugs and intraarterial vasodilators have been used therapeutically in select patients with emboli distal to the ileocolic artery and with nonocclusive lesions. However, in patients with peritoneal signs or suggestion of infarction, exploratory laparotomy is the treatment of choice. Angiography prior to emergent exploration is controversial. Intraoperative assessment of the intestinal blood flow can be performed using fluorescein dye or Doppler ultrasonography. Embolectomy or thrombectomy is indicated with revascularization as necessary. Necrotic bowel should be resected and second-look laparotomy to evaluate bowel with questionable viability should be planned in 24 hours.

Although mortality still remains high, early diagnosis within the first 12 hours of symptoms increases the likelihood of intestinal viability. In addition, studies demonstrate that an aggressive approach to a diagnostic work-up, including the liberal use of angiography, increases survival to 54 percent. A high clinical suspicion and a low threshold for diagnostic angiography is essential to changing the mortality of this devastating disease.

Colorectal Disorders

Appendicitis

Although acute appendicitis is typically considered to be a disease of the young, a second peak in the incidence of appendicitis occurs in the elderly population. Historically, the morbidity and mortality associated with appendicitis in patients older than 50 years of age are increased, as compared with younger patients, largely because of delays in presentation to a physician, time-consuming diagnostic work-ups, associated comorbidities, and complicated appendicitis at the time of admission. Even with the growing use of CT scans and diagnostic laparoscopy over the past 10 years, the morbidity and mortality of appendicitis in the elderly population has remained largely unchanged.

The clinical symptoms of acute appendicitis in elderly patients are generally similar to that in younger patients. However, fever and leukocytosis are not reliably present in elderly patients, although a left shift has a positive predictive value for appendicitis. In addition, the duration of symptoms prior to presentation tends to be longer. The work-up of abdominal pain in this age group can be time-consuming given a wide differential diagnosis that can include mesenteric ischemia, right- or left-sided diverticulitis, pancreatitis, obstruction, or acute cholecystitis.

Appendicitis in the elderly person is more likely to present at an advanced stage with associated perforation and intraabdominal abscess. The pathophysiology of perforated appendicitis in older patients is postulated to be a result of increased risk of rupture caused by a fibrotic, thinned appendix and decreased vascularity. The alternative explanation is that the increased incidence of advanced appendicitis is secondary to delay in presentation. The current strategy for advanced appendicitis with a nonviable appendiceal base is ileocolectomy with primary anastomosis. The necessity of performing a diverting ileostomy with mucous fistula is rare. Because of the advanced presentation of appendicitis, the length of hospital stay is longer for the elderly population.

The morbidity and mortality for appendectomy in the elderly population is several-fold higher than that for younger patients. In a population-based analysis of patients undergoing appendectomy in Sweden over a period of 10 years, the case fatality rate increased by a factor of three for each decade of age older than 40 to 49 years. The most common causes of mortality are cardiovascular disease and perforated appendicitis.

Clinicians should maintain a low threshold for considering appendicitis in elderly patients with abdominal pain, despite a normal temperature or white blood cell count. Prompt surgical evaluation should be performed whenever appendicitis is clinically suspected. In addition, malignancy should always be ruled out as an underlying factor leading to perforation.

Diverticulitis

Diverticulitis increases in prevalence with increasing age, although 80 to 85 percent of patients are asymptomatic. Complications of diverticular disease requiring surgical intervention in the elderly patient include recurrent episodes of diverticulitis, complicated diverticulitis (abscess, phlegmon, fistula, obstruction), and lower gastrointestinal bleeding.

The clinical presentation of diverticulitis can include left-lower-quadrant pain, a tender mass, fever, leukocytosis, and nausea or vomiting. As with other causes of acute abdominal pain in the elderly patient, however, classic signs may not always be present. CT scanning is the imaging modality of choice and may demonstrate pericolic fat stranding, thickened bowel wall, or abscess. Early CT scanning should be initiated in older patients because the symptoms do not always correlate with the severity of the disease. Barium enemas and endoscopy are generally contraindicated in the acute setting.

Management of diverticulitis depends upon several factors including the severity of the disease, patient comorbidities, ability to tolerate oral intake, and available patient support. In general, elderly patients with diverticulitis should be hospitalized if they have high fevers or leukocytosis, nausea and vomiting, or significant comorbidities, are older than 85 years of age, or have inadequate support systems. Patients with mild diverticulitis can be treated conservatively as an outpatient with oral antibiotics, with the caveat that close follow-up should be available. Patients with complicated diverticulitis should be managed with intravenous antibiotics, bowel rest, percutaneous drainage of abscesses if clinically stable, and surgical intervention as needed. For patients with recurrent episodes of diverticulitis, surgical resection is indicated after the second episode or after the first episode if immunosuppressed.

In emergent settings, sigmoid resection with colostomy is recommended for left-sided diverticulitis. Elderly patients are more likely than younger patients to remain with a permanent colostomy. In nonemergent resections, a preoperative work-up with a barium enema or colonoscopy to rule out the presence of concomitant colonic pathology is necessary. Laparoscopic sigmoid resection in the elderly appears to reduce pain, length of stay, complications, and time to resumption of preoperative activities. In patients with sequelae of diverticulitis such as fistulae or strictures who are poor surgical candidates, attempts at nonoperative management may be preferable. Mortality associated with elective sigmoid resection is less than 4 percent, but increases to 20 to 30 percent in cases of emergent operation.

Ischemic Colitis

Ischemic colitis is the most common vascular disorder affecting the intestines, and while most commonly seen in the elderly population, is not limited to this age group. Risk factors that predispose elderly persons to ischemic colitis include atherosclerosis, shock, congestive heart failure, and aortoiliac surgery. Although all colonic segments can potentially be affected, watershed areas such as the splenic flexure and the junction between the sigmoid colon and rectum are commonly affected. The severity of the illness extends from a transient self-limited episode with or without further sequelae to full-thickness necrosis requiring surgical resection. Not to be confused with acute mesenteric ischemia, colonic ischemia has a good prognosis. Two-thirds of patients do not require surgical intervention, and only 5 percent of patients have a recurrent episode.

The clinical presentation is often that of sudden onset of a cramping abdominal pain without any identifiable precipitating factors. Bright red blood per rectum or bloody diarrhea may occur within 24 hours of the onset of pain. Patients generally do not appear toxic or severely ill as with acute mesenteric ischemia. Diagnosis can be suggested by barium enema or CT and confirmed by colonoscopy with biopsy.

Initial treatment of the patient with suspected ischemic colitis in the absence of peritoneal signs is nonoperative with intravenous antibiotics, bowel rest, hydration, and correction of underlying hemodynamic abnormalities. Failure to improve within 48 hours and the development of peritoneal signs, fever, or leukocytosis suggest transmural infarction with or without perforation and necessitate operative exploration. Most symptoms of ischemic colitis improve within 24 to 48 hours, and radiologic evidence of improvement lags behind clinical improvement by 1 to 2 weeks. A potential complication of ischemic colitis is the development of a stricture that typically manifests 3 to 4 weeks subsequent to the initial episode. Strictures can be treated with endoscopic dilatation or surgical resection.

Large Bowel Obstruction

There are multiple etiologies of large bowel obstruction in the older population, including both malignant and benign causes such as colon carcinoma, diverticular or ischemic stricture, volvulus, and colonic pseudo-obstruction. The treatment of colon cancer is discussed later in this section.

Colonic volvulus in the United States occurs more commonly in males, and predominantly affects elderly patients. The location of the volvulus is most frequently in the sigmoid colon, and then in the cecum, transverse colon, and splenic flexure, in order of descending frequency. Patients with colonic volvulus present with signs and symptoms of large bowel obstruction including abdominal distension, nausea, vomiting, constipation, and abdominal pain.

If bowel necrosis is present, peritoneal signs may also be detected on physical examination. Diagnosis is often suspected on plain abdominal films. Sigmoid volvulus is suggested by an inverted U-shaped gas pattern, and cecal volvulus is typified by the "kidney" or "coffee bean" gas pattern. Barium enema has also been used to confirm the diagnosis of volvulus.

The treatment of sigmoid volvulus is initially colonoscopic decompression with inspection of the bowel for viability. Because the recurrence rate for endoscopic detorsion alone is greater than 40 percent, surgical resection is conventionally recommended in reasonable candidates. Ideally, resection is performed electively at the same hospital admission in order to prevent recurrence. The mortality of resection ranges from 12 to 38 percent when performed emergently for necrosis or perforation. There have been several reports of endoscopic fixation techniques for patients with multiple comorbidities. For example, percutaneous placement of a colostomy tube or T-fasteners has been described. The treatment of cecal volvulus is typically surgical. If there is no evidence of bowel necrosis after detorsion, surgical options include cecostomy tube, cecopexy, and right hemicolectomy.

Acute colonic pseudo-obstruction is a severe form of adynamic ileus characterized by large bowel distension in the absence of mechanical obstruction. Because the mortality rate of an associated perforation of 50 percent, colonoscopic decompression is often recommended. However, the recurrence rate is as high as 40 percent. More recently, neostigmine, an acetylcholinesterase inhibitor, has been used in the treatment of acute colonic pseudo-obstruction with good success. Rarely, if conservative measurements fail, surgical decompression is required, but is associated with increased mortality.

Inflammatory Bowel Disease

Both ulcerative colitis and Crohn's disease are more common in younger patients, but do occur in elderly patients as well. Historically, inflammatory bowel disease has been thought to have a bimodal distribution with a second peak in the elderly population. More recently, however, this second peak has been questioned as inaccurately reflecting patients with underlying ischemic or infectious etiologies rather than inflammatory bowel disease.

New-onset ulcerative colitis occurs in 10 to 20 percent of ulcerative colitis patients older than age 50 years. Some studies suggest that the course of ulcerative colitis in older patients is more aggressive and severe with an increased incidence of life-threatening complications. However, other studies report a more favorable course in the elderly ulcerative colitis patient. The reasons for these discrepancies are unclear.

In general, the signs and symptoms of ulcerative colitis, namely bleeding and diarrhea, are similar across age groups. However, older patients tend to have more left-sided disease and proctitis than do their younger cohorts. The mainstays of medical therapy remain the same across age groups, but particular care must be maintained in the elderly patient in terms of drug interactions and other medical comorbidities. Surgical therapy in younger patients typically consists of total proctocolectomy with ileoanal pouch anastomosis as indicated for refractory disease, dysplasia, or toxic megacolon. Likewise, this procedure can be performed safely with minimal morbidity and mortality in select elderly individuals. Postsurgical fecal incontinence and retrograde ejaculation may be more of a concern in the elderly population.

In the elderly patient, the presenting signs and symptoms of Crohn's disease are similar to those of their younger cohorts. The main age differences cited include increased likelihood of limited colonic involvement, decreased abdominal pain on presentation, and decreased familial association in elderly patients. As with ulcerative colitis, medical therapy is similar to that in younger patients. Surgical intervention is warranted for bowel obstruction, perforation, fistulas, and intractability. Studies demonstrate that laparotomy for Crohn's disease can be performed in the elderly patient with similar anastomotic leak rates and mortality, as compared to those in younger patients. However, there is an increased risk of cardiopulmonary complications.

ABDOMINAL WALL DISORDERS: HERNIAS

Hernias are common in the elderly population as a result of both decreased strength of the abdominal wall musculature and an increased incidence of disorders leading to increased intraabdominal pressure such as benign prostatic hypertrophy. In patients older than 50 years of age, hernias tend to present more commonly as emergent problems such as strangulation or small bowel obstruction. The combination of increased comorbidities and an increased incidence of emergent surgeries leads to higher morbidity and mortality rates in the elderly population.

While physicians may be reluctant to refer elderly patients for elective hernia repair, studies demonstrate that elective hernia repair can be performed safely and effectively in the older population. The anterior tension-free mesh repair is typically the operation of choice. The anesthetic technique used for hernia repair influences outcome. Elderly patients tend to do well without major complications with local anesthesia. General or spinal anesthesia can be associated with major cardiovascular or pulmonary complications. Laparoscopic hernia repair can be performed safely and effectively, but requires general anesthesia and has not been studied extensively in older patients.

Up to 40 percent of hernia repairs in the elderly population are performed for emergent indications. The morbidity and mortality of an emergent repair are greater than 50 percent and 8 to 14 percent, respectively. Surgical outcome is adversely influenced by coexisting cardiopulmonary disorders, ASA classification, and delayed presentation. Morbidity and mortality also increase with the need for concomitant bowel resection and with greater than 48 hours of incarceration. In this population that tends toward delayed presentation and diagnosis, prompt surgical intervention should be performed for incarcerated hernias to minimize complications. In fact, elective surgery should be encouraged in elderly patients with reasonable life expectancy to prevent the need for emergent operation.

VASCULAR SURGERY

Vascular disorders requiring surgical intervention occur primarily in the elderly population. These disorders are a source of substantial disability, degrading the quality of life for many elderly patients. Stiffer vessel walls and reduced inhibition of local platelet aggregation associated with aging, may predispose to atherosclerotic plaque formation, vascular wall degeneration, and symptoms from reduced blood flow, aneurysmal degeneration, or embolic disease. These effects on the vascular integrity manifest as claudication or limb-threatening ischemia in patients with peripheral vascular disease, abdominal aortic and peripheral aneurysms in patients with arterial degeneration, and carotid disease leading to transient or permanent cerebral ischemic events. Amplified by the effects of male gender, cigarette smoking, hyperlipidemia, hypertension, diabetes mellitus, and genetic factors, peripheral vascular occlusive disease is present in 20 to 30 percent of patients older than age 65 years and is severe enough to cause claudication symptoms in many of these patients. Abdominal aortic aneurysm, defined as a dilation of the abdominal aorta to more than 1.5 times normal, is found in 3 to 7 percent of patients older than age 60 years. Between one-third and one-half of these patients will have an associated popliteal aneurysm. Stenosis (>50 percent) of one or both carotid arteries occurs in 5 percent of elderly patients and is highly correlated with the presence of coronary artery disease. Although the incidence of stroke in patients with 50 percent stenosis is only approximately 1 percent per year, one in five of these patients will progress to high-grade (>75 percent) stenosis, with an increasing annual rate of ipsilateral neurologic events that approaches 20 percent when the stenosis is >80 percent.

Peripheral Vascular Disease

Surgical management of peripheral vascular disease in the elderly patient is usually a last resort for uncontrolled symptoms or limb-threatening ischemia. As described in Chap. 39, lifestyle changes, including diet, cessation of smoking, exercise, and medication, are effective at controlling the symptoms of intermittent lower-extremity claudication for most patients. Claudication progresses to limb-threatening ischemia at the rate of 1.4 percent per year. Noninvasive techniques, particularly vascular duplex scanning, now provide a precise map of the vascular anatomy and can be used to follow patients closely. Interventional techniques including angioplasty, stent placement, and atherectomy may offer effective nonsurgical alternatives for limited, largely proximal, large-vessel disease at the level of the iliac and femoral vessels. Only 30 percent of patients will eventually require surgical revascularization of the lower extremity and of this group, 10 percent will progress to requiring an amputation within 5 to 10 years.

In the elderly patient with progressive ischemic symptoms, the outcome of surgical revascularization using native or prosthetic materials to bypass sites of obstruction is variable, depending on the level of the bypass, whether the patient is still smoking, and the nature of vascular runoff beyond the bypass, but not related to age. Such patients must be carefully assessed for perioperative cardiovascular risk to limit immediate surgical mortality. For very proximal lesions treated with aortoiliac or aortofemoral bypass, operative mortality is 2 percent. Graft patency rates greater than 90 percent at 2 years are commonly reported, with persistent symptomatic relief in 77 percent. Surgical treatment for chronic limb-threatening ischemia caused by femoral–popliteal disease is the most common bypass procedure performed. Most vascular surgeons employ saphenous vein in situ or reversed as a conduit and report primary and secondary (with thrombectomy and revision as necessary) patency of 50 to 70 percent and 65 to 80 percent, respectively, at 5 years, with corresponding limb salvage in more than 80 percent of patients. Femoral–distal bypass, again usually employing autogenous tissue, is associated with even poorer patency and limb salvage caused by the nature of the underlying disease. Beyond limb salvage, long-term survival for all patients with peripheral vascular disease is limited by the associated myocardial ischemia risk and resulting mortality in this population.

Abdominal Aortic Aneurysm

The abdominal aorta is the most common site of aneurysmal disease in the elderly; more than 95 percent are infrarenal, extending down to and involving the iliac arteries in 20 percent of patients. Indications for repair of an abdominal aortic aneurysm in an elderly patient include symptoms, rapid expansion defined as an increase in diameter of 0.5 cm/3 months or more, or size greater than 5 cm. Symptoms may develop because of pressure on surrounding structures, rupture, distal embolization, and thrombosis, but only occur in 25 percent of patients. Minor symptoms predict the development of more severe complications, often rupture. Aneurysm less than 5 cm in diameter have an annual incidence of rupture of 4.1 percent, which rises to 6.6 percent in aneurysms between 5 and 5.7 cm. Those larger than 7 cm in diameter have a 19 percent per year incidence of rupture, essentially rupturing in all patients within 5 years. Mortality with elective repair overall is 2 to 7 percent, while the overall mortality after rupture is 75 to 90 percent, with many patients succumbing before any intervention can be made. In patients with a contained, retroperitoneal rupture of an aneurysm who survive until an attempted repair, the reported perioperative mortality ranges from 30 to 70 percent, with hypotension and renal failure, but not age, as independent predictors of mortality. Quality of life and long-term survival in the elderly population who survive repair of an abdominal aortic aneurysm are equal to that of an age-matched population. Development of new, endovascular techniques for the percutaneous repair of an abdominal aortic aneurysm by using stent–grafts holds great promise for reducing the risk and mortality associated with elective abdominal aortic aneurysm repair, a technologic development that may prompt earlier repair of smaller aneurysms to reduce the risk and mortality of a ruptured abdominal aortic aneurysm.

Carotid Disease

Longitudinal studies of patients with asymptomatic carotid disease show that the presence of a carotid bruit is associated with a 0.7 to 1.5 percent annual incidence of stroke, while the combination of a bruit and high-grade stenosis increase the annual stroke rate to 6 percent. Both symptomatic carotid artery disease leading to transient or limited neurological ischemic events and high-grade (70 to 99 percent), asymptomatic carotid stenosis should prompt consideration for treatment because of the high risk of stroke. One in three patients with symptomatic extracranial carotid disease or an asymptomatic carotid bruit has severe, concomitant coronary artery disease that must be factored into their treatment, often prompting a coronary revascularization procedure.

Two of three elderly patients undergoing carotid endarterectomy have symptomatic carotid disease. Endarterectomy is associated with a perioperative stroke in 2 percent of patients, but reduces the actuarial 5-year risk of stroke from native disease progression by 27 to 48 percent, depending on the severity of preoperative carotid stenosis. In patients with severe (>79 percent) stenosis, carotid endarterectomy spares one stroke for every 15 patients undergoing the procedure and although weaker, this relative benefit was also found in patients with moderate stenosis (70 to 79 percent). In asymptomatic patients with lesser degrees of stenosis (<70 percent), carotid endarterectomy did not reduce the risk of stroke. The Leapfrog Initiative has highlighted the importance of adequate surgical volume in complex aortic and carotid artery procedures to achieve best practice and to match the most-favorable published incidence of complications, thereby justifying prophylactic surgical intervention in these fragile patients.

TRANSPLANT SURGERY

In the past, organ transplantation surgery was primarily limited to younger populations. In many cases, advanced age alone was considered a contraindication to organ replacement. Improvements in transplant medicine and surgery have allowed greater numbers of older individuals to become transplant recipients. In addition, as our population ages, growing numbers of people with previously transplanted organs are now surviving longer and into old age.

As a result of limited financial resources and fewer donors than recipients, significant controversy, both medical and ethical, exists regarding selection of elderly patients for organ transplantation. The prevailing opinion, however, is that with careful patient selection, organ transplantation is relatively safe, with outcomes comparable to younger patients. In the case of renal transplantation, an advantage

in survival, cost, and quality of life is seen in the elderly population, as compared with dialysis therapy in patients with end-stage renal disease. Likewise, low-risk elderly patients undergoing liver or heart transplantation have similar short-term graft and patient survival outcomes to those in younger groups.

As patients age, the relative risk of acute organ rejection decreases as a consequence of changes in immunocompetence over time. Conversely, the risk of posttransplant infection rises, as well as intolerance to immunosuppressive medications. Elderly posttransplant patients therefore require closely monitored, individualized immunosuppression therapy, as well as a heightened vigilance for infectious complications. The development of malignancy, as well as infection, in posttransplant elderly patients is a significant cause of mortality.

Partly as a result of donor shortages, eligibility criteria are expanding to include the elderly as organ donors. While this may improve the size of the donor pool, the medical end result of transplanting older donor organs is yet to be determined. As the fields of transplant surgery and geriatric medicine increasingly intermingle, further study into the medical, economic, and ethical consequences of organ transplantation in the elderly will no doubt intensify.

TRAUMA

Although elderly patients comprise a minority of trauma cases, they account for one-third of the health resources used for trauma care. In addition, elderly persons have a longer length of stay and higher mortality rate than younger age groups. With the number of elderly patients expected to double by the year 2030, the potential financial impact of trauma care for this population is staggering. Special considerations must be taken into account in the treatment of the injured elderly patient. From a medical standpoint, associated comorbidities, multiple preinjury medications, and poor physiologic reserve all contribute to an increase in morbidity and mortality. From an ethical standpoint, issues regarding quality of life and withdrawal of care can be of particular importance. Lastly, these patients require special attention in regards to rehabilitation and posthospital care.

The majority of injuries in the elderly population are caused by blunt trauma such as from falls and motor vehicle collisions. Injured elderly patients have a higher risk of dying from a motor vehicle collision than do their younger cohorts. Age, injury severity score (ISS), and male gender are all independent predictors of mortality. Despite the higher rate of mortality in trauma patients older than age 75 years, studies demonstrate a favorable long-term outcome for patients discharged from the hospital, arguing for aggressive treatment of elderly patients.

Resuscitation of the elderly patient begins with rapid evaluation in the emergency department with a low threshold for transfer to the intensive care unit for optimization of hemodynamic status. Because the ability to increase heart rate with stress wanes as a result of aging, elderly patients may appear to have normal hemodynamics initially despite a decreased cardiac output. Survival is linked to the ability to increase cardiac output with resuscitation, and a fixed cardiac output is associated with increased mortality.

The initial work-up of blunt abdominal trauma should be performed rapidly in the emergency room using an accepted diagnostic modality such as diagnostic peritoneal lavage, ultrasonography, or CT. Historically, the management of solid-organ injuries has been operative, but recently, the trend has been toward nonsurgical management in hemodynamically stable patients. The exception, based on several small studies, has in the past been in patients older than 55 years of age. However, more recently, larger retrospective studies suggest that age alone should not be a contraindication to nonoperative management of solid-organ injury, and that older patients can be managed safely nonoperatively.

Blunt chest trauma is associated with increased morbidity and mortality in the elderly. Myocardial infarction can present in a delayed fashion as congestive heart failure upon mobilization of the initial resuscitation fluids. Pulmonary complications such as pulmonary contusion, pneumonia, and adult respiratory distress syndrome (ARDS) are more common in the elderly population, with resultant increases in time on the ventilator, length of stay in the intensive care unit, hospital length of stay, and mortality. Because rib fractures are also associated with an increased morbidity and mortality, aggressive pain management should be undertaken in elderly patients with rib fractures.

Only 5 to 10 percent of elderly trauma patients suffer from penetrating injury. One study compared the outcome after penetrating trauma in patients younger than and older than 65 years of age. Although elderly patients had more associated comorbidities and an increased length of stay, their complication rate was no higher than that of their younger counterparts. Compared to elderly patients recovering from blunt trauma, they were less likely to require continued care after discharge from the hospital.

REFERENCES

Alexander KP et al: Outcomes of cardiac surgery in patients aged 80 years: Results from the National Cardiovascular Network. *J Am Coll Cardiol* 35:731, 2000.

Aune S et al: The influence of age on operative mortality and long-term relative survival following emergency abdominal aortic aneurysm operations. *Eur J Vasc Endovasc Surg* 10:338, 1995.

Bauer JJ et al: Restorative proctocolectomy in patients older than fifty years. *Dis Colon Rectum* 40:562, 1997.

Birkmeyer JD et al: Volume standards for high-risk surgical procedures: Potential benefits of the Leapfrog initiative. *Surgery* 130:415, 2001.

Borzellino G et al: Emergency cholecystostomy and subsequent cholecystectomy for acute gallstone cholecystitis in the elderly. *Br J Surg* 86:1521, 1999.

Bouma BJ et al: To operate or not on elderly patients with aortic stenosis: The decision and its consequences. *Heart* 82:143, 1999.

Boyd WD et al: Off-pump surgery decreases postoperative complications and resource utilization in the elderly. *Ann Thorac Surg* 68:1490, 1999.

Bradley BA et al: Elderly transplant recipients may require less immunosuppression. *Transplant Proc* 33:1115, 2001.

Chaikof EL et al: Endovascular repair of abdominal aortic aneurysms: Risk stratified outcomes. *Ann Surg* 235:833, 2002.

Cina CS et al: Carotid endarterectomy for symptomatic carotid stenosis. *Cochrane Database Syst Rev* CD001081, 2000.

Conti B et al: Major surgery in lung cancer in elderly patients? Risk factors analysis and long-term results. *Minerva Chir* 57:317, 2002.

Fernando HC et al: Thoracoscopic and laparoscopic esophagectomy. *Semin Thorac Cardiovasc Surg* 12:195, 2000.

Finlayson EV, Birkmeyer JD: Operative mortality with elective surgery in older adults. *Eff Clin Pract* 4:172, 2001.

Graham MM et al: Survival after coronary revascularization in the elderly. *Circulation* 105:2378, 2002.

Halpern VJ et al: Factors that affect the survival rate of patients with ruptured abdominal aortic aneurysms. *J Vasc Surg* 26:939, 1997.

Herlitz J et al: Mortality, risk indicators for death, and mode of death in younger and elderly patients during five years after coronary artery bypass graft. *Clin Cardiol* 23:421, 2000.

Jamsen T et al: Results of infrainguinal bypass surgery: An analysis of 263 consecutive operations. *Ann Chir Gynaecol* 90:92, 2001.

Kerdiles Y et al: Results of carotid surgery in elderly patients. *J Cardiovasc Surg (Torino)* 38:327, 1997.

Kulah B et al: Emergency hernia repairs in elderly patients. *Am J Surg* 182:455, 2001.

Pessaux P et al: Laparoscopic cholecystectomy in the elderly: A prospective study. *Surg Endosc* 14:1067, 2000.

Poon RT et al: Esophagectomy for carcinoma of the esophagus in the elderly: Results of current surgical management. *Ann Surg* 227:357, 1998.

Richter JE: Gastroesophageal reflux disease in the older patient: Presentation, treatment, and complications. *Am J Gastroenterol* 95:368, 2000.

Stamou SC et al: Beating heart surgery in octogenarians: Perioperative outcome and comparison with younger age groups. *Ann Thorac Surg* 69:1140, 2000.

Sugiyama M, Atomi Y: Treatment of acute cholangitis due to choledocholithiasis in elderly and younger patients. *Arch Surg* 132:1129, 1997.

Trus TL et al: Laparoscopic antireflux surgery in the elderly. *Am J Gastroenterol* 93:351, 1998.

Uomo G et al: Influence of advanced age and related comorbidity on the course and outcome of acute pancreatitis. *Ital J Gastroenterol Hepatol* 30:616, 1998.

PART III

ORGAN SYSTEMS AND DISEASES

CARDIOLOGY

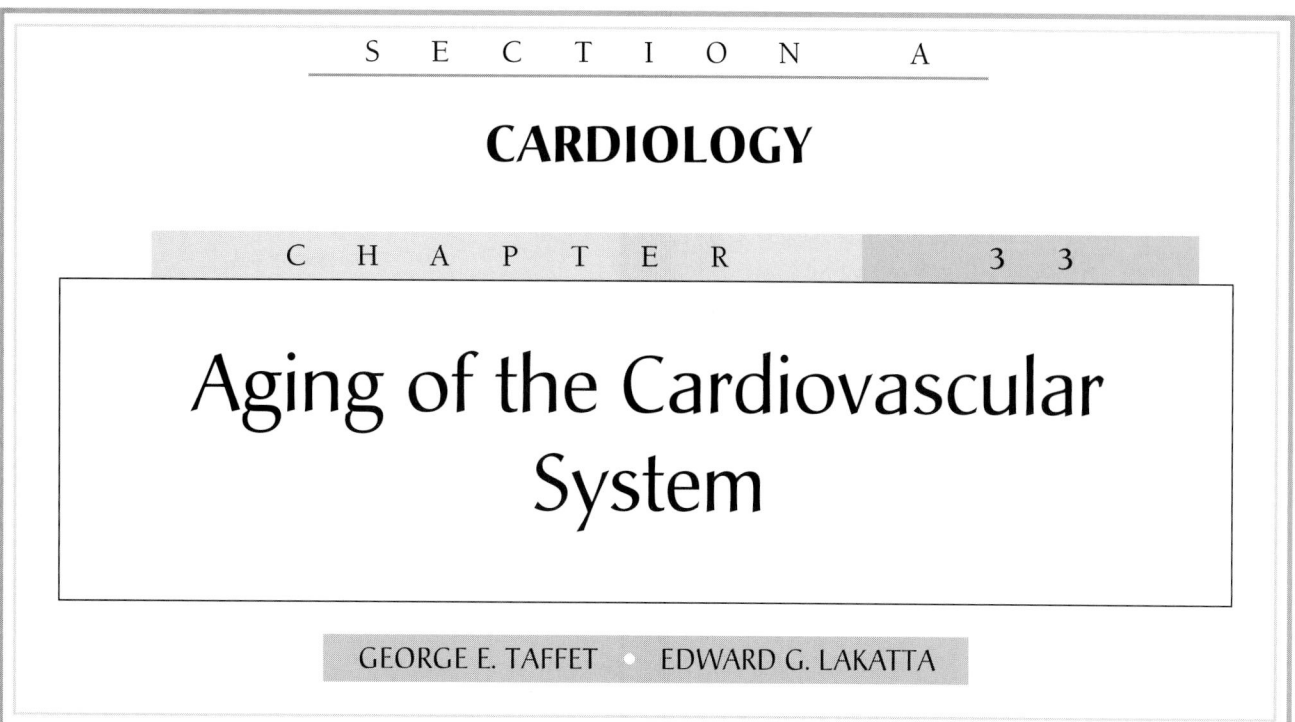

C H A P T E R   3 3

Aging of the Cardiovascular System

GEORGE E. TAFFET   •   EDWARD G. LAKATTA

This chapter focuses on the changes in the cardiovascular system that occur with normal aging and, insofar as possible, excludes those changes caused by disease except as they facilitate the development of disease or alter its presentation. It is tempting, as others have done, to minimize these normal changes for two reasons. First, with normal aging, we experience no dramatic changes in heart rate, left ventricular ejection fraction, or cardiac output at rest. This, as we demonstrate, speaks to the adequacy of the compensatory mechanisms available and employed by the aging heart and vessels to maintain cardiovascular homeostasis rather than to a lack of modification with age. Unfortunately, those compensatory mechanisms, once depleted or invoked, become no longer available to the older person to respond to acute additional stresses as they might be in a younger person, so-called homeostenosis. For this reason, understanding the age-related changes in the cardiovascular system requires examination of both rest and challenged conditions, including, but not limited to, exercise.

The second reason that primary aging effects on the cardiovascular system are often discounted is the high prevalence of atherosclerotic cardiovascular disease and hypertensive cardiovascular disease in Western populations. For example, autopsy data from the 1950s and 1960s showed significant coronary artery stenoses in roughly three-fourths of men older than age 50 years and women older than age 60 years. It remains unclear whether recent trends in diet, smoking, obesity, physical activity, cholesterol and blood pressure management, and the like, have increased or decreased the high prevalence of cardiovascular disease since those studies were performed. What evidence

exists, however, does not suggest a decline in arteriosclerotic disease in the oldest age groups. Furthermore, it is unclear whether the unstable, often troublesome, soft and nonocclusive atherosclerotic plaques now implicated in many myocardial infarctions and strokes were recognized by these early investigators, so their analysis was likely an underestimate. As is discussed below (Aging and Atherosclerosis), although atherosclerosis clearly is a major health problem and its development may be facilitated by age, it does not reflect normal aging. Furthermore, the clinical manifestations of atherosclerosis have substantially higher morbidity and mortality in the elderly population, in large part because of the truly age-related changes rather than modifications in the extent of their disease or the clinical care of its manifestations. Thus, those elderly persons without atherosclerosis or hypertension demonstrate aging in isolation, so-called successful aging. Those with these common diseases, on the other hand, manifest the impact of those conditions superimposed on aging and their clinical consequences in older persons.

Additionally, the clinical manifestations of cardiovascular diseases and altered physiology in the elderly population are tremendously varied, reflecting the variance in efficiency of various organ systems in a given aging individual. This increasing heterogeneity is also apparent within age cohorts. One reason for the increasing heterogeneity is that aging does not occur in a vacuum, and lifestyle choices strongly impact apparent "age" effects. These factors include physical activity, diet, alcohol consumption, smoking, personality characteristics, and the like. The impact of such lifestyle variables on aging processes is gradually

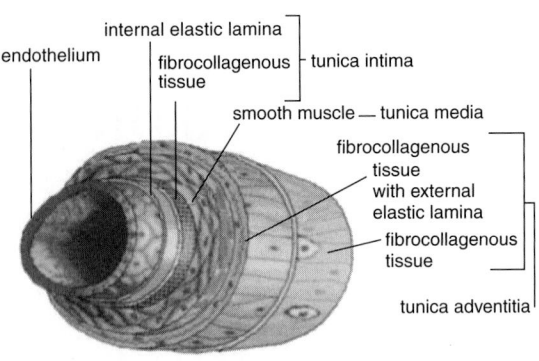

Irregularities in size and shape of
endothelial cells
Fragmentation of elastin in
internal elastic lamina and media
Calcification of media
Increased lumen diameter, vessel
length, wall thickness
Collagen increases, cross-linking,
especially in subendothelium
Subendothelium thickened with
connective tissue and cells
Decreased basal and stimulated
NO production
Increase in systolic and pulse
pressures

Figure 33-1   This figure summarizes the major anatomic and biochemical age-related changes in the elastic arteries and provides an orientation. The IMT (intimal-medial thickness) measures from the lumen to the adventitia.

becoming defined. For example nutritional habits may result in changes in arterial structure and function.

Physical activity is a very important consideration for all studies of aging. The average daily physical activity level declines progressively with age. The magnitude of the physical-conditioning effect on the changes seen with age can be so great that studies that attempt to investigate to what extent aging alters cardiovascular function must control for the physical activity status, or at least consider it in the interpretation of the results. The same confounders present for humans also occur in laboratory animals, in which husbandry practices may limit the opportunity and motivation for exertion. So in many cases it is difficult to segregate the impact of sedentary lifestyle from aging per se.

In earlier editions of this book, the age-associated increase in large artery stiffness was implicated as a primary stimulus for the maladaptive changes in the heart. Therefore, while this hypothesis remains unproven, this exposition starts with changes in the vasculature before examining the cardiac changes.

CHANGES IN VASCULAR STRUCTURE AND FUNCTION WITH AGE

The vascular tree includes multiple components, from the largest of arteries to the capillaries and then back to the large veins. Each of these is altered by age; the changes are not uniform and our knowledge of the changes is quite incomplete. We begin with the large arteries, move progressively through the circulation, and end with the largest of veins. The pulmonary vasculature is discussed last.

Age-Related Structural Changes in Large Arteries

There are a number of anatomic and biochemical changes with aging in the large arteries and their overall impact is the increase in arterial stiffness with age. The changes are summarized in Figure 33-1. These changes are significantly different from those seen in atherosclerosis (Table 33-1). With aging there is gradual elongation and stiffening of the aortic wall, traditionally attributed to fragmentation of

elastin fibers and a relative increase in collagen content. The extent of elastin and collagen modifications with age may be altered by at least one polymorphism in each gene. Both long-lived structural proteins, collagen and elastin, form glucose-mediated cross-links after nonenzymatic glycosylation, which increase their rigidity and strength. While decreasing glucose concentration is extremely effective in decreasing the extent of collagen cross-linking in vitro, the relevance of this maneuver in vivo is uncertain.

In mice, for example, caloric restriction results in lifelong reductions in serum glucose concentrations and reduced collagen-associated fluorescence, a marker of advanced glycosylation end products, but arterial stiffness has not been measured in these animals directly. However, the advanced glycation cross-link end-product–breaking drug, ALT-711, decreases arterial stiffness without changing mean blood pressure in older rats and decreases pulse pressure in aged monkeys. After treatment, cardiac output was increased in the animals perhaps by decreasing arterial stiffness or increasing cardiac distensibility. Importantly, there were also effects on peripheral vascular resistance in

Table 33-1   Summary of Differences Between the Age-Associated Changes in the Elastic Artery Contrasted to Those Associated with Advanced Atherosclerosis

• Atherosclerosis	• Age-associated changes
– Unique to (Western) man	– Occur in many species
– Heterogenous, patchy	– Uniform in large arteries
– Compromises lumen	– Lumen enlarges
– Severity related to turbulence and shear stresses	– Not localized to sites of stress
– Has inflammatory component	– No white cells or others participate
– Cholesterol is cofactor	– Independent of cholesterol

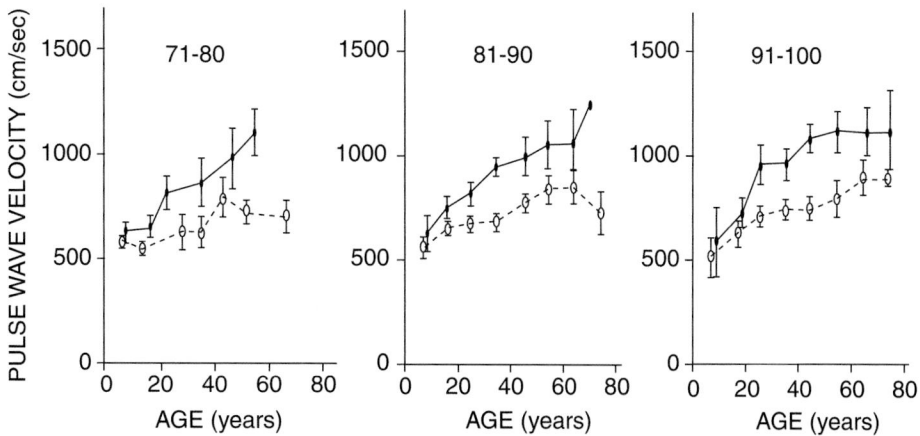

Figure 33-2 Data shows that at all mean blood pressures (71 to 80, 81 to 90, and 91 to 100) there is an increase in pulse wave velocity with age for both urban Chinese people (*filled circles, solid lines*) and for rural, low salt-consuming Chinese people (*open circles, dashed lines*). Reproduced with permission from Avolio AP et al: Effects of aging on changing arterial compliance and left ventricular load in a northern Chinese urban community. *Circulation* 68(1):50, 1983.

animals, implying the effects of ALT-711 were on both the large arteries and resistance vessels.

Similar qualitative effects on large artery stiffness have been seen with ALT-711 in studies of older persons, as reported by Lakatta. No changes were seen in diastolic blood pressure or resting cardiac output but there was a significant decrease in pulse pressure (see below). This agent may thus define a promising way to intervene to decrease age-associated arterial stiffening.

In humans, together with elongation of the aorta with age, the luminal diameter also increases as the tissue expands in all directions. The aortic root diameter increases by 20 percent from age 30 to 70 years, sufficient that nomograms for aortic root diameter should probably be adjusted for age. As the length and luminal diameter of the aorta increase with age, its volume increases substantially. This tends not only to decrease pulse pressure but also to increase the amount of blood whose flow must be accelerated with each systole. Perhaps, as described below, this adaptation may increase cardiac work and act as one stimulus for cardiac hypertrophy with aging. Increasing luminal diameter is an adequate adaptation to keep pulse pressure minimally changed with age up until age 60 years. But beyond this age, the volume adaptation of the aorta appears to be insufficient, and the pressure increase per volume added ($\Delta P/\Delta V$) in the aorta increases rapidly. Therefore the increase in aortic stiffness leads to higher systolic blood pressures and pulse pressures beyond age 60 years, and this may also stimulate cardiac hypertrophy with advancing age. The presence of an increased aortic diameter with unchanged or decreased blood flow velocity leads to decreased shear stress and reduction in its deleterious consequences.

The endothelial cells enlarge and become irregular in size, shape, and contour. Medial hypertrophy, with an increase in both matrix and cellular elements, contributes to increased wall thickness, but whether the medial smooth muscle compartment increases is debatable. The subintima thickens with increases in collagen and smooth muscle cells and subintimal calcification, as reported by Cooper et al. As discussed below, these changes all are integrated to increase the intima medial thickness, a marker of vessel aging

and atherosclerosis. Calcification may markedly increase arterial stiffness. The sum of these changes contributes to an increment in aortic stiffness in the unchallenged state and in humans, the increase in intimal thickness is much greater than the increase in medial thickness, as reported.

Taking the biochemical and morphologic information provided above, it is tempting to directly link the collagen and elastin changes to the increase in arterial stiffness, but evidence may not support this. Avolio et al. found that while arterial stiffness and systolic blood pressure were increased with age in a rural, low salt-consuming, Chinese population, the age-associated increases were even higher in a high salt-consuming, urban, ethnically similar population. At all ages, even at similar blood pressures, the urban persons had stiffer vessels than the rural ones (Fig. 33-2). Two years after a low-salt diet was instituted as an intervention for urban Australians, arterial stiffness decreased significantly, independent of blood pressure. Others report nitroprusside, directly inducing smooth muscle relaxation, acutely decreased aortic stiffness in older people with heart failure with minimal effect on blood pressure. Of the many age changes in the vasculature, one might not expect collagen content or cross-linking, subintimal calcification, medial hypertrophy, elastin fragmentation, and the like to respond to such relatively short-term manipulations. Therefore, it is possible that the increase in arterial stiffening with age is not strictly dependent upon the changes in the long-lived proteins, elastin and collagen. The potential lack of dependence of stiffness in vivo on collagen changes is not totally surprising. In vitro, strain is transferred from elastin to smooth muscle to collagen as the vessel is distended further and further. At normal diameters and pressures scarcely any collagen is engaged; only at high degrees of distension is most of the load placed on the stiff collagen. As distending pressure increases, this results in an inflection point above which stiffness increases dramatically. This point may coincide with the pressure at which the elastic tissue is fully stretched and at which further distention is limited by collagen. It occurs at diastolic pressures that would not be well tolerated in vivo.

The smooth muscle compartment rather than collagen is more likely to impact pulse wave velocity (PWV) at physiologically relevant blood pressures. So the potential role of increased smooth muscle tone in age-related aortic stenosis has been suggested and efforts to address arterial stiffening in aging humans should also consider smooth muscle tone. Normalizing PWV for blood pressure actually increases the correlation between stiffness and age.

The same constellation of large arterial changes that occurs in humans is also observed in the normal mouse, rat, and monkey aorta, which do not develop atherosclerosis. For example, aging increases aortic wall thickness and collagen concentration in mice. Normotensive old mice have been reported to have markedly more smooth muscle in the walls of their aortas than young mice or those treated with enalapril, implying that there is either pressure or hormonal regulation of this process. However, many of the other anatomic changes described above, including the age-related increase in lumen diameter, were unaffected by inhibition of the angiotensin-converting enzymes in these animals. Therefore, significant changes in structural proteins, including cross-links because of nonenzymatic glycation, and smooth muscle that occur with aging in the aorta, once considered inevitable and irreversible, now appear to be potentially modifiable.

The anatomic changes in the vessel wall are assayed by ultrasonic measurement of intimal-medial thickness (IMT) (Fig. 33-3). The increase in IMT with aging in humans is primarily a result of an increase in the intimal thickness caused by increased collagen and matrix proteins, as well as invasion by smooth muscle cells. However, atherosclerotic plaques develop in the intima and media and are frequently also assayed in the IMT measurement. Thus, IMT is further increased in atherosclerotic disease and is decreased by cholesterol-lowering agents such as statins and a colestipol–niacin combination. Surprisingly, however, lifelong exercise may not alter carotid IMT. The increased IMT has been given a dual role as a marker of vascular aging and a sign of atherosclerosis. The association of an IMT greater than 1 mm with atherosclerotic disease likely reflects the compounding of vessel aging and the atheroma itself. These issues and criteria to discriminate aging from disease in the interpretation and utility of IMT assessments need to be developed.

Functional Implications of Age-Related Arterial Stiffening

The load of the heart is attributable to two vascular properties: resistance and impedance. Resistance relates to laminar flow and impedance relates to pulsatile flow. For simplicity, resistance is primarily a function of small vessels especially at the arteriole level where the flow is essentially laminar while impedance is primarily determined by the large, elastic arteries.

Systolic blood pressure, primarily a manifestation of large-artery stiffening, increases steadily with age in most studies of human and animal aging. The noncompliant older aorta is less able to buffer the pulsatile output of the heart. In youth, much of the energy during ejection is stored by the elastic tissue of the aortic wall and then released during diastole. This "windkessel function" is markedly impaired with age. Figure 33-4 shows typical data from the Framingham Heart Study and a number of other studies. The resting systolic blood pressure of healthy 20-year-old men in this population was less than 120 mmHg, and this increased to 140 mmHg by age 70 years. Diastolic pressure also tended to increase from age 20 years to age 60 years, and then plateau or gradually decrease from age 60 years to age 80 years. For women, the age-related increase in

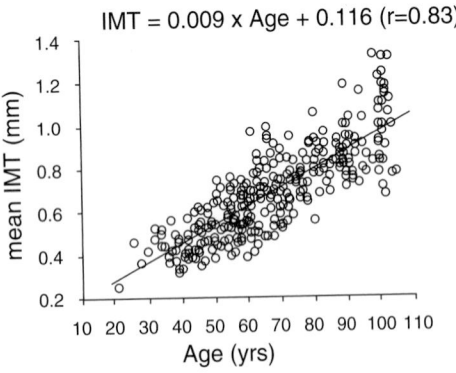

IMT = 0.009 x Age + 0.116 (r=0.83)

Figure 33-3 Data examining carotid intimal-media thickness (IMT) in healthy subjects from Japan. There is clear evidence of increase in IMT with age that extends to the centenerian populations. Reproduced with permission from Homma S et al: Carotid plaque and intima-media thickness assessed by B-mode ultrasonography in subjects ranging from young adults to centenarians. *Stroke* 32:830, 2001.

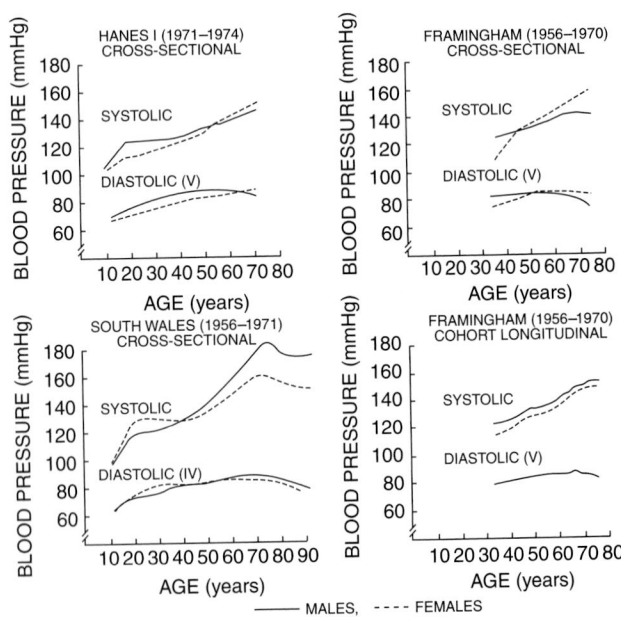

Figure 33-4 Cross-sectional data from Health and Nutrition Examination Survey (HANES) I (*top left*), cross-sectional data from south Wales (*lower left*), and cross-sectional (*top right*) and cohort longitudinal data (*bottom right*) from the Framingham Heart Study document the steady increase in systolic blood pressure with age and the shallow inverted U-shape relationship of diastolic blood pressure and age. In all these cohorts, diastolic pressure decreases subtly beyond age 70 years.

systolic blood pressure was even more dramatic than that seen for men. Within limits, the same pattern of increase in systolic pressure and in diastolic pressure is present in whites, blacks, and Hispanics. Similar trends, albeit at lower absolute values, are seen in the rural Chinese population discussed earlier where sodium intake is consistently low, but in a few rural populations where the average sodium intake is less than 1 g/d there may be no age-related increase in systolic blood pressure.

Consistent with the decreased systemic compliance, the sodium (and intravascular volume) dependence of blood pressure is increased with aging, as evidenced by a reduction of the stroke volume to pulse pressure ratio with age. Pulse pressure (systolic pressure–diastolic pressure) is a manifestation of arterial stiffness (decreased volume compliance). If blood pressure is measured centrally, then the early return of reflected pressure waves also is contributory. As such, pulse pressure is a reasonable marker for large artery stiffness. Pulse pressure is a strong risk factor for many cardiovascular pathologies.

These functional implications of normal aging changes are one reason why isolated systolic hypertension supersedes diastolic hypertension as the dominant type of hypertension present in the elderly population. Furthermore, the inability to tolerate increments in volume may explain why systolic blood pressure increases in healthy older persons with exercise or other maneuvers that increase cardiac output in older persons. There is a gender difference in this response.

In addition to the increase in pulse pressure, there are other, direct means to assess arterial stiffening. PWV is the rate at which pressure waves travel in the wall of the vessel. This is an important measure because it determines the balance between whether returning pressure wave reflections increase impact cardiac work or help perfuse the coronaries. If the pulse wave velocity is low, pressure waves go out to the periphery, are reflected at bifurcations such as the aortic bifurcation into the iliac arteries, and return back to the heart while the aortic valve is closed, augmenting the coronary perfusion pressure. This is beneficial to cardiac efficiency. As the PWV increases, however, the pressure waves return earlier and earlier until they reach the point where they return while the aortic valve is still open, increasing the afterload and perhaps over time stimulating cardiac hypertrophy. This may not be beneficial, in that the loss of the pressure increase during diastole may lead to decreased diastolic coronary blood flow.

The augmentation index is the percentage of increase in the central systolic pressure caused by the pressure reflections. In youth, the augmentation index is less than 5 percent, but in elderly people it can be 20 percent or more. This means that the afterload is increased by this extent in the older person. The augmentation index and pulse wave velocity are highly correlated, but these indices do not reflect the exact same arterial properties.

Elevated PWV is an independent risk factor for stroke and coronary artery disease. Over the next few years, measuring PWV may become routine in the assessment of arterial stiffening as a risk factor for vascular events. While PWV has rapidly become a standard measure of vessel stiffness because of its relative simplicity, the relationship

between PWV and arterial stiffening is not straightforward, and much of the data need to be interpreted with caution. PWV depends both on the mean blood pressure and the stiffness of the vascular wall, in part because of different relative amounts of elastin, smooth muscle, and collagen engaged in each cycle. In fact, PWV increases and decreases though the cardiac cycle as distending pressure varies between systolic and diastolic pressures. PWV increases in the aorta as one gets further from the heart and is greater still in subsequent branches. Muscular artery PWV, that is, brachial or femoral, does not change with age.

In multivariate analysis, age is the strongest correlate of aortic PWV, followed by blood pressure, serum lipids, and gender. In healthy, normal Baltimore Longitudinal Study volunteers, PWV increased threefold from age 20 years to age 80 years, correlating strongly with maximum oxygen consumption. Exercise-trained older men have much-reduced PWV as compared to healthy, age-matched sedentary controls. Highly physical active postmenopausal women also have lower PWV than age-matched controls, but the data are sparse above age 70 years. As reported by Vaitkevicius et al., these data suggest that exercise training or high physical activity of age and aerobic capacity in healthy adults may blunt the age-associated effect on arterial stiffening. Therefore arterial stiffening, at least as measured by PWV, appears to be a modifiable age-related process.

Large-artery compliance, as measured by other techniques, also decreases with age. Using invasive techniques to measure compliance, aortic compliance decreased by 50 percent from age 40 years to age 80 years in the Baltimore studies. Many others have corroborated this finding. In human cadaveric aortas, studied after the smooth muscle component was likely to no longer be functional, retraction was greater for a younger group as compared to an older group.

Large-artery stiffness also increases with age in animals. In animal studies, the same increases in large-artery stiffness as occur in humans are seen. Aged beagles, which develop no clinically significant atherosclerosis, also have reduced systemic arterial compliance. The aorta is also stiffer in old mice. Finally, in vitro studies also confirm the increase in stiffness with age. Isolated rat thoracic aortas from old animals have decreased distensibility. Age-related differences have been shown to be markedly accentuated when the vessels are stretched to lengths above the inflection point where collagen would be engaged.

As noted above, smooth muscle tone may contribute to in situ arterial stiffness. Arterial tone is the net result of factors causing smooth muscle contraction and those stimulating relaxation. Increases in tone may be caused by increases in vasoconstrictors, and/or decreases in relaxing factors, and there is evidence for both in aging. Basal serum levels of catecholamines (epinephrine and norepinephrine) are elevated in the elderly population. Exercise training, which decreases PWV, decreases sympathetic nervous system activity in the elderly population. Additionally, age-related changes in receptor sensitivity or postreceptor efficacy may be important. While α-adrenergic responses (vasoconstrictor) are relatively preserved, β-adrenergic responses (vasodilator) decrease with age in most studies of large artery function (reviewed in Cooper). While much of the data on the molecular changes in receptors are generated in animal studies and await confirmation in humans, messenger ribonucleic acid (mRNA) and protein for α_1-adrenergic receptor may double in the arterial tree of older people, which is consistent with the preserved vasoconstrictor response.

The renin-angiotensin system (RAS) is another regulatory system for vascular smooth muscle tone. The RAS is suppressed and circulating renin and aldosterone levels are decreased at baseline in euvolemic older people. In response to sodium restriction, an impairment in plasma rennin response is also seen in elders. The RAS is also important locally, stimulating local fibrosis. Whether the system is attenuated at the tissue level with age is unclear.

Additionally, and likely of great clinical significance, is the decreased production by vascular endothelium of the potent vasodilator nitric oxide (NO). This decrease is quite dramatic with age in both the unstimulated and stimulated states. Aortic smooth muscle from senescent rats is less responsive to the vasodilator acetylcholine. The decreased relaxation of aortic strips from old rats to atrial natriuretic peptide (also NO dependent) is restored by a cyclic guanosine monophosphate (cGMP) phosphodiesterase inhibitor. Soluble guanylyl cyclase is decreased in aged rat aortas. NO is known to work via a cGMP-dependent pathway. When isolated from the aorta of old rats, the expression of endothelial nitric oxide synthase (eNOS) mRNA in aortic endothelial cells have been reported to be reduced.

The magnitude of the vasodilatation in response to adenosine declines significantly with age, but the sensitivity (concentration needed to produce a 50 percent effect) is preserved. Adenosine appears to use both NO-dependent and NO-independent pathways to produce vessel relaxation. Additionally, no matter what the stimulus, when arterial smooth muscle hyperplasia and hypertrophy occur, arterial wall hyperactivity may result. Perhaps as a net effect of the changes in vasoconstrictor and vasodilator balance, cellular calcium concentrations may also be elevated in the aged smooth muscle consistent with increased tonic contraction of vascular smooth muscle cells. In summary, animal data suggest multiple deficits appear to contribute to tip the balance towards tonic vasoconstriction of the aortic wall smooth muscle.

AGING AND ATHEROSCLEROSIS (SEE ALSO CHAP. 34)

While atherosclerosis is not a normal aging phenomenon and large artery changes caused by atherosclerosis are clearly different from those associated with aging alone (see Table 33-1), there are a number of reasons why atherosclerosis may be so prevalent and aggressive in the susceptible elderly person. NO appears to have an antiatherogenic effect and endothelial NO production is decreased with age. NO also inhibits the proliferation of smooth muscle cells, decreases the influx of lipid into the vessel wall, and may modify platelet–vessel interactions, all key steps in atherogenesis.

In animal studies, smooth muscle cells isolated from old aortas proliferate more rapidly than those from young aortas. Therefore, as reported by Li et al., old vascular smooth muscle cells may be more likely to respond to growth factors, and become a component of the atherosclerotic plaque. This facilitated proliferation is a result of factors intrinsic to the old artery, as exaggerated intimal hyperplasia still occurs when old rat aortas are transplanted into young rats and then injured. There is some evidence that the endothelial cells may have decreased proliferative potential as they approach replicative senescence in old vessels. They are less able to maintain the integrity of the endothelium at sites of turbulence where the turnover of endothelial cells might be expected to be highest. The loss of integrity of the endothelium may allow access by growth factors to the underlying cells, stimulating their replication. Age-related alterations in the matrix including increased expression of adhesion molecules may facilitate the invasion of macrophages into vessel walls. Macrophages are another key constituent of the atherosclerotic plaque. Older rabbits exposed to atherogenic diets have more rapidly progressive atherosclerotic disease than young animals placed on the same diets. However, aging, while clearly facilitating the process, does not absolutely dictate the development of atherosclerotic vascular disease.

Small and Muscular Arteries

While impedance is a large-artery phenomenon, small arteries down to capillaries affect peripheral vascular resistance (PVR) to the greatest degree, primarily impacting diastolic blood pressure. If the impedance changes described above occurred without changes in the smaller vessels, then a decrease diastolic blood pressure would occur, and, indeed, in most human studies, diastolic blood pressure decreases subtly with age beyond age 60 years. Therefore, PVR changes in many, but not all, aging individuals, and decreases in muscle mass and capillary density with age may be key determinants of this change. In general, the increase with age in PVR is more robust in women than in men.

In contrast to the central arteries, the small arteries are less structurally modified by age. In healthy older individuals, the radial artery has both greater wall thickness and luminal diameter, but no age-related differences in distensibility have been observed. The radial artery wall is primarily smooth muscle. A similar lack of significant correlation between age and distensibility has been observed at the femoral artery. The PWV measured in the radial or femoral arteries is not significantly modified by age.

Basal whole-limb blood flow and vascular conductance in the legs decrease progressively with advancing age in healthy men. It is unclear whether or not the reductions are caused by decreases in limb fat-free mass and oxygen consumption. Interestingly, habitual aerobic exercise does not appear to alter either the age-related reductions in basal limb blood flow or vascular conductance. The endothelin responsiveness of femoral arteries is preserved with age, unlike in the aorta. However, like the aorta, the old femoral artery has decreased basal NO release. The mammary artery has increased α_1-adrenergic receptors with age.

Forearm blood flow has been used as an integrated vascular response system. In this model, the results are similar: a lack of NO under basal conditions and in response to stimuli limits the vascular response. Additionally, administration of NO (as nitroprusside) produces prompt vasodilatation in young and old subjects without age differences; hence the assumption that the main lesion is in signal recognition or transduction. Similarly, the ability of old skin to dissipate heat is limited, in part by the inability of cutaneous vessels to maximally dilate in response to parasympathetic and other stimuli.

For the major intracranial arteries there are anatomic age-related changes. These are primarily in relative quantity of connective tissue elements in the intima. The appearance of type 3 pseudoelastic and/or collagen fibers occurs consistently with age and is frequently associated with loss of elasticity of the vessel wall. Therefore, changes seen in large elastic arteries are not uniformly present throughout the more distal components of the arterial system.

Renal artery blood flow declines progressively after age 30 years at rates of up to 10 percent per decade. Intrarenal vessel vasoconstriction and decreases in vasodilatory prostacyclins are implicated. In both monkey and rats, the vasodilation responsiveness of the renal arteries from older animals to atrial natriuretic peptide (ANP), acetylcholine, and isoproterenol is reportedly reduced, but is preserved in response to nitroprusside, nifedipine, and potassium.

Finally, an impairment in new vessel formation in response to ischemia is seen in old animals. This may reflect diminished responsiveness to stimulatory factors like platelet-derived growth factor (PDGF) or vascular endothelial-derived growth factor (VEGF). As reported by Rivard et al., angiographies performed after femoral artery resection show significantly less collateral vessel formation in older animals as compared to young animals. In the older animals, little VEGF was elaborated in response to the ischemia and the level of vascularity increased in response to exogenous VEGF, implicating inadequate signaling rather than an inability to respond.

Capillaries

The number and density of capillaries appears to decrease with age in many organs. While much of the data have been derived from older animals, the capillary-to-fiber ratio is also significantly lower at in vastus lateralis of old healthy men. During aging in mice to 18 months, capillary density in the ears of hairless mice was reduced to approximately 40 percent. In response to exercise training, there are clear increases in capillary density.

In both animals and humans, the process of aging from adult to senescence does not, in itself, cause any significant vessel remodeling, but is associated with a decrease of nutritive perfusion at the capillary level in response to stimuli such as ischemia or heat stress. For example, a 2-minute period of ischemia induced an appropriate hyperemic response during late juvenile and adult life. This response was markedly reduced during senescence.

At the microscopic level there are structural changes in the capillaries. The percentages of capillaries showing basement membrane thickening and deposits of collagen in the basement membrane were determined semiquantitatively in monkeys. Aberrations in the basement membrane are few in young subjects, but increased in frequency during

the aging process in the monkeys. An aging-associated increasing number of capillaries showing depositions of collagen fibrils was seen, rather than local thickenings of the basement membrane. There are indications that new vessel formation occurs at all ages but only at the capillary level. Similar changes in microvascular integrity are observed in humans.

Veins

There is relatively little known about the venous system and age. Beginning in patients at age 60 years old, the common femoral vein shows a significant decline in both diameter and blood velocity at rest. Because older age is associated with both decreased diameter and velocity, the flow is reduced dramatically in the leg. Venous compliance in the calf and capacitance function of the leg vessels are both decreased with age, but there is no age-effect on α-adrenergic receptors. Using lower-body negative pressure (LBNP), venous compliance was found to be reduced by 45 percent in older persons. As reported by Olsen et al., there is a reduction in capacitance response limit reserves available to the older person in response to acute hypovolemic circulatory stress. Consistent with this, aging is associated with a reduction in α_2- and β-adrenoceptor–mediated responses in dorsal hand veins.

PULMONARY VASCULATURE

Relatively little is known about the aging changes in the pulmonary vasculature. Despite the relatively low pressures experienced in the pulmonary circulation, endothelial changes reminiscent of those seen in the systemic vasculature are seen at autopsy in older people . Similarly, intimal thickening is apparent in muscular pulmonary arteries from older individuals.

Reports include mean pulmonary artery pressures increasing up to 60 percent from age 40 years to age 70 years. As reported by Davidson and Fee, the effect of age appears independent of gender, smoking status, or changes in the systemic circulation. Thus, the pulmonary vasculature shares some of the changes of aging with the systemic circulation. However, the data available from the different studies recruited different types of subjects of different ages and gender, limiting their reliability.

In older animals, the regulation of blood flow in the lung is impaired with age. There is a decrease in the β-adrenergic receptor-mediated relaxant responses of ring preparations of pulmonary artery preparations from aged rats. Hypoxic pulmonary vasoconstriction has been reported to be less in aging rats during hypoxic exposures. In contrast, in rat pulmonary arteries studied in vitro, initial rates of NO release, as well as peak NO concentrations, did not change with age between young and old rats.

Ventricular Vascular Coupling in Aging

Arterial stiffening may have significant impact on the heart by increasing cardiac work as described above (Functional Implications of Age-Related Arterial Stiffening). This coupling is much tighter than most recognize—both the left

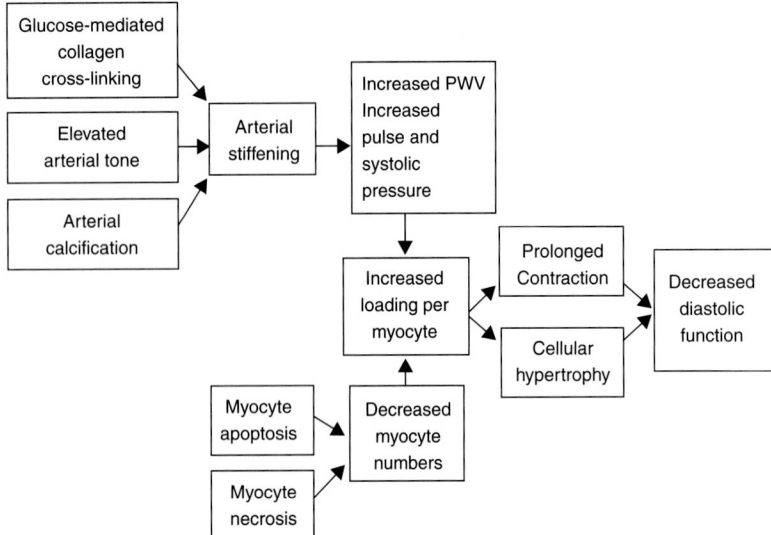

Figure 33-5   Schematic of the pathogenesis of age-related diastolic dysfunction shown with key roles given to age-associated arterial stiffening and myocyte loss.

ventricle and the arterial tree change in concert, both in efforts to optimize function in response to the changes seen in the partner. Consistent with this, acute increases in aortic stiffness increase myocardial O_2 use without changing cardiac output. The increase in afterload produced by the pressure wave reflection and the dilation of the aorta may stimulate cardiomyocyte hypertrophy and thus be one of the major stimuli for the development of left ventricle wall thickening in the aged heart (Fig. 33-5).

THE HEART: ANATOMIC CHANGES IN THE HEART WITH AGE

The old heart shows evidence that it has remodeled and changed in response to either intrinsic or extrinsic signals. The extent of left ventricular hypertrophy is mild when viewed on the level of the whole heart, but this is significant when individual myocytes are studied. This implies that the number of myocytes has decreased and the remaining myocytes have enlarged. Left ventricular myocytes from older subjects have larger volumes as a result of increases in both length and cross-sectional area. In some studies, the extent of the cellular hypertrophy and apoptosis are greater in men than in women. When corrected for body surface area, the thickness of the left ventricular (LV) wall during systole increases up to 50 percent from age 20 years to age 80 years, and a similar hypertrophy is also present in diastole. In certain populations, the prevalence of LV hypertrophy reaches 80 percent in 85-year-olds.

As reviewed by Kitzman and Edwards, at autopsy cardiac mass is more strongly correlated with age in women than in men, even after correcting for body mass. The atria, especially the left atrium, are also enlarged with age during both systole and diastole.

The aged heart becomes more fibrotic. The fibrous tissue forms a patchy network of collagen between cells, not the confluent scar that might be seen after myocardial infarction. Hydroxyproline is increased in both the septum and

the free wall of the left ventricle to approximately similar extents. Collagen subtypes change with age such that subtype I filaments increase in number and thickness in older humans. Calcification of the left heart may be present but is usually limited to the annuli of the valves and the septum. Other changes in the extracellular matrix are also seen in older mouse hearts. In addition to increased collagen content, fibronectin and integrins are increased in the older heart.

The innervation of the heart also decreases significantly. As noted below, decreases in parasympathetic neurons and influence are present, but there may also be a similar decrease in sympathetic neurons especially in the conduction pathways.

As to cardiac valves, with advancing age changes in the valves are noticeable, particularly in the aortic and mitral valves, both of which increase in thickness. Calcification and fibrosis account for this increase, which may subsequently cause enhanced valvular stiffness and also interfere with tight closure. A possible consequence of aortic valve calcification may be aortic stenosis, the most common indication for aortic valve replacement in elderly subjects. However, only in rare instances do the fibrosis and calcification of normal aging lead to functional impairment of the valves. Trivial aortic regurgitation is seen in the majority of those older than age 90 years. One clear factor in this is the dilation of the aortic root discussed above (Age-Related Structural Changes in Large Arteries). Overall, the aortic valve seems to be more greatly affected than the mitral valve with age. This may suggest that the higher pressure in the aorta is responsible for its preferential deterioration. Aging does not seem to lead to significant changes in tricuspid or pulmonic valve function, consistent with the facilitating role of pressure.

In many elderly individuals, cardiac amyloid deposition is found. This is most often limited to the atria. An autopsy study of persons from Japan and Czechoslovakia reported that more than 90 percent of those older than age 80 years had atrial amyloid deposits. Biochemical analysis of these deposits of isolated atrial amyloid disclosed that the major subunit is α-atrial natriuretic peptide, which is synthesized by the atrial muscle cells. Amyloid fibrils in isolated atrial amyloid are seen in the interstitium of the atrial myocardium, in dilated transverse tubules of the cardiomyocytes, and in coated and uncoated secretory vesicles in isolated atrial amyloid. While such isolated atrial amyloid is likely functionally benign, it may be associated with the increased tendency of the elderly population to develop atrial fibrillation. The atrial amyloid, when exposed to the blood in the atrium, may also be thrombogenic, leading to atrial clot formation.

This "normal" amyloid is distinct from senile cardiac amyloid, which is a degradation product of transthyretin, a serum protein that transports thyroid hormone and retinoic acid. Certain polymorphisms of transthyretin are much more amyloidogenic, with deposition in the ventricle and elsewhere. Thus, the ventricular amyloid seen in senile cardiac amyloidosis is not part of normal aging.

In almost all cardiomyocytes there is an accumulation of the brown "age pigment," lipofuscin. Lipofuscin, an end product of lipid metabolism, is thought to have no functional impact on the myocyte.

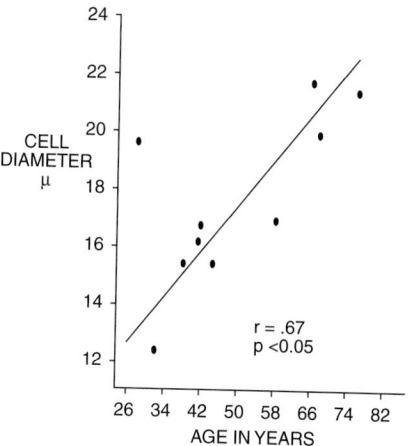

Figure 33-6   Data from ventricular biopsies showing marked age-associated increase in cell diameter. All had normal cardiac history, physical examination, and noninvasive tests of left ventricular function, and underwent ventricular endomyocardial biopsy prior to cancer chemotherapy. Reproduced with permission from Unverferth DV et al: Aging of the human myocardium: A histologic study based upon endomyocardial biopsy. *Gerontology* 32(5):241, 1986.

Myocyte Dropout and Hypertrophy in the Aging Heart

By age 70 years, a healthy man has lost approximately 30 percent of his cardiac myocytes as a result of aging alone. Estimates of this loss are up to 38 million myocytes per year by the left ventricle. This myocyte dropout is independent of any cardiovascular disease. This may occur to a lesser extent in women. Their lesser myocyte loss may help explain why some very old women develop significant concentric hypertrophy that essentially ablates the ventricular cavity. The presence of myocyte dropout has been confirmed in the aging rat and mouse. The magnitude of the dropout in rodents is similar or perhaps even greater than that reported in man, and the rate of myocyte loss increases with increasing age.

There are two mechanisms by which this dropout can occur, apoptosis or necrosis. If the cell is overwhelmingly damaged with depletion of adenosine triphosphate (ATP), then necrosis occurs with its associated inflammatory response. By contrast, if the damage is less drastic but the damage perceived as irreparable, active programmed cell death involving specific cleavage of the deoxyribonucleic acid (DNA) between the nucleosomes and loss of mitochondrial voltage gradient may ensue. Such apoptotic death produces less immune activation. Whether the myocyte dropout seen in both humans and animal models of aging is primarily caused by necrosis or apoptosis is an important question because preventive interventions might differ between the two processes.

In animal studies, using techniques that label single- and double-strand DNA breaks and DNA laddering (which looks at intranucleosomal DNA cleavage, a characteristic of apoptosis), age-associated increases in the number of TUNEL (in situ DNA nick end labeled) cells and amount of "laddered DNA" were observed. This suggests

that apoptosis increases with aging in the rat heart. There were clear increases in both markers with age in the LV free wall. Others have confirmed the increased frequency of TUNEL myocytes in old rat hearts and aged mice, but at a much lower rate. There was no apoptosis of myocytes in the septum or right ventricle in these rodents, implying that changes in cardiac loading may stimulate apoptosis in the heart and allow cross-talk between the two pathogenic arms of Figure 33-5. Thus the potential exists for arterial stiffening to stimulate myocyte dropout by apoptosis.

The loss of functional cells is most impressive in the sinoatrial (SA) node, where 90 percent of functional pacemaker cells may have disappeared by age 75 years. The SA node becomes infiltrated with fat and connective tissue. The extent of these changes is much less prominent in the rest of the conduction system. Perhaps as a result of the loss of pacemaker cells, the intrinsic sinus rate slows with age, as is further discussed below and as reviewed by Bharati and Lev. The escape rate of the heart is also slower in the elderly person.

Because left ventricular mass does not decrease with normal aging (it either increases or remains unchanged) and the expansion of connective tissue is relatively modest, the remaining myocytes must hypertrophy to compensate for the myocyte dropout. Biopsies taken from hearts of people about to receive adriamycin for lung cancer but who were without any evidence of cardiac disease had a strong age-related, nearly 100 percent increase in cardiomyocyte width (Fig. 33-6). Similar age-related increases in cell size are found at autopsy in unselected people, especially men.

In rat hearts, myocytes isolated from 24-month-old animals had a 25 percent increase in length and 100 percent or greater increase in cellular volume, as compared to young animals. In contrast, others have not found myocyte hypertrophy in aged Sprague–Dawley rat hearts. The majority of the evidence supports that in normohypertensive humans and animals, aging results in a heart with smaller numbers of increasingly large myocytes. The hypertrophied myocytes may indeed reach a size where they can hypertrophy no further. Takahashi et al. proposed that the lack of hypertrophic response to aortic banding-induced pressure overload in old rat hearts was because myocytes were already at maximum size. Myocyte width increased 50 percent between 9 months and 18 months of age just by age in this study. There was no further increase in cell size after banding at age 18 months. By comparison there was a 30 percent increase in myocyte width in the young rat in response to the afterload increase. Interestingly, when right ventricular outflow was banded, there was also attenuated hypertrophy in the old rat heart. However, the old heart appears to be able to hypertrophy in response to exercise training, so-called physiologic hypertrophy, where sarcomeres are added in series, not in parallel. Thus the cellular hypertrophy present in the old heart may be similar to that seen in response to hypertension. Furthermore, this cellular hypertrophy can be associated with cardiac dysfunction, "the cardiomyopathy of overload," including the functional changes leading to age-related diastolic dysfunction.

FUNCTIONAL CHANGES IN THE AGING HEART AT REST

There are many functional changes that characterize the aging human heart. However, there are no changes in resting left ventricular ejection fraction, resting heart rate, or cardiac output, as reviewed by Lakatta. Some studies have reported subtle (10 percent) decreases in resting heart rate, which are accompanied by increases in left ventricular end-diastolic volume of similar magnitude. The ability to develop pressure or isometric force is well maintained until very old age, when slow pacing conditions are employed, but maximum rates of pressure development (+dP/dt [upstroke pattern on apex cardiogram]) in vivo in humans or peak rate tension development in isolated papillary muscle from old animals is compromised (Fig. 33-7). There is no decrement in maximum tension generated. As was noted more than 50 years ago, "as the heart grows older, it lifts its load more slowly," but it lifts its load nonetheless. Contraction time is prolonged, but left ventricular ejection fraction does not decline in normal aging. Emax (maximum ventricular elastance) derived from simultaneous invasive pressure volume measurements is decreased in the

old rat, but similar studies still yield conclusive results in healthy older people. If the age-related cardiac adaptations described below are designed to maintain systolic function, then the adaptations are remarkably successful.

In contrast, diastolic function, both its passive and active components, is significantly impaired with age. Early diastolic filling of the left ventricle is diminished, primarily by impaired relaxation. In vivo, early filling of the left ventricle and isovolumic relaxation time (IVRT) are highly dependent on active relaxation, and are both significantly impaired with aging. The impairment seen on Doppler echocardiography of left ventricular filling is almost entirely dependent upon age and not on LV mass, ejection fraction, or filling pressures. The noninvasive measurements are also impacted by other factors, but as reviewed by Lakatta, invasive parameters (tau, time constant of relaxation, and –dP/dt, peak rate of pressure decline) are also slower with age in humans, as well as in animal models.

Isolated muscles are used to remove the confounding effects of loading conditions. Under isometric conditions, papillary muscles from old rats require 50 percent longer to dissipate tension (active relaxation). The impairment in active relaxation is associated with decreased sarcoplasmic reticulum calcium uptake, as reported by Tate et al. In compensation for the decrease in early diastolic filling, the reliance on left atrial systole for filling is increased in old people (Fig. 33-8). In youth, atrial systole contributes only 10 to 20 percent of total left ventricular filling. This contribution increases to 40 percent or more at age 80 years. This may explain why atrial fibrillation, where effective atrial contraction is lost, is poorly tolerated in many elderly persons. Similarly, in young people with increased cardiac demand, such as in response to exercise, atrial systole becomes an increasing contributor as the cardiac output and heart rate increase. This adaptation is less available to the older person.

Because diastolic filling happens at relatively low pressures, the process may be very sensitive to nonuniformity

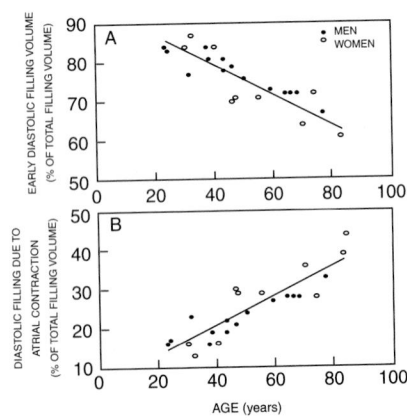

Figure 33-8 Data from using Doppler echocardiography to assess the percentage of left ventricular filling during early diastole (*top panel*) and as a result of atrial systole in late diastole (*bottom panel*). With increasing age, the reliance upon atrial systole for left ventricular filling increases dramatically. Adapted from Swinne CJ et al: Age-associated changes in left ventricular diastolic performance during isometric exercise in normal subjects. *Am J Cardiol* 69(8):823, 1992.

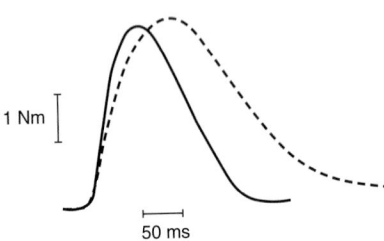

Figure 33-7 Typical isometric contractions of isolated rat papillary muscles from young (*solid line*) and old (*dashed line*) showing maintenance of force generation, but slower development and dissipation of force at low stimulation rates. Reproduced with permission from Lakatta, 1995.

of relaxation of the ventricle. Using regional analysis of time to peak filling rate as a marker of diastolic function, these regional variations are much wider in older, than in younger, people. Furthermore, in the studies of Bonow et al., those subjects with the widest variations had the slowest overall filling rate and the greatest dependency on atrial systole for ventricular filling. Subtle increases in left ventricular end-diastolic pressure may contribute to the age-related increase in circulating brain natriuretic peptide (BNP) levels. Nevertheless, given adequate time, such as under resting conditions, the left ventricular end-diastolic volume (or index) is slightly increased with age. Thus, at rest, the compensations are adequate.

Early diastolic filling (peak E) may be one of the key determinants of the age-related decrease in maximum oxygen consumption, and manipulations that improve early diastolic filling in the short-term improve exercise tolerance, as reported by Vanoevershelde et al. Clearly, age-related diastolic dysfunction is not benign. However, aging, while increasing the likelihood of developing diastolic heart failure, is inadequate to produce diastolic heart failure without other factors, as reviewed by Kitzman.

The data are not as clear for the passive stiffness properties of the aged ventricle, although these studies are limited to aged animals. Early studies with isolated rat papillary muscles showed passive stiffness was not significantly modified by age despite the collagen changes described above. However, passive filling in vivo does not occur with the muscle totally flaccid. There is always some calcium cycling in the myocyte, so actin and myosin are interacting to some extent at all times. Thus the in vivo data obtained with pressure volume loops reveal increased stiffness as volume compliance decreased in the old heart (pressure increase is greater for an increment in volume). Increases in diastolic calcium with age contribute to this increase in active stiffness. This has important implications when cardiac output is increased such as with exercise (see Cardiovascular Performance During Exercise).

PROTEIN AND GENE EXPRESSION CHANGES IN THE AGING HEART

In general, protein and gene expression (and the functional) changes that occur with aging are similar to those that occur in hypertrophy associated with hypertension, but most of the data have been generated from older animals and need to be confirmed in older humans. In contrast, physiologic hypertrophy occurs with endurance exercise training, which results in increased ventricular mass and augmented diastolic function, which is not what is seen with age. Age-related diastolic functional changes are neither inevitable nor immutable. Endurance exercise training prevents or reverses these changes in aged rats. However, this intervention gives no insight into the pathogenesis of age-related diastolic dysfunction in humans, because the data as to whether exercise improves diastolic filling in humans are still equivocal.

Decreased mRNA for the SERCA2a (cardiac sarcoplasmic reticulum [SR] Ca²⁺ATPase) and mitochondrial cytochrome oxidase and increases in mRNA for ANP are seen in the aged rat left ventricle. Decreased SERCA2a

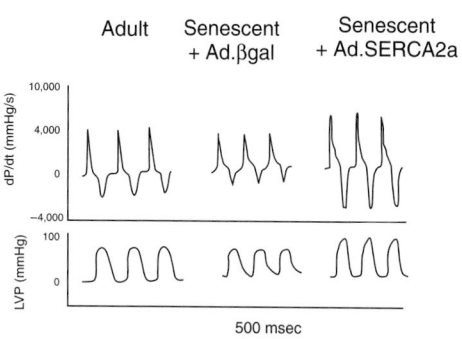

Figure 33-9 Cardiac function in rat hearts showing pressure development (*below*) and its derivative (*above*) for adult (6-month-old) senescent animals given adenovirus with the control protein, β-galactosidase, and senescent animals given a gene to encode the sarcoplasmic reticulum Ca²⁺ATPase (SERCA2a). With this gene therapy, there was marked increase in developed pressure and the rate of pressure development. Importantly there was also more rapid relaxation (improved −dP/dt) after introduction of the SERCA2a gene. Reproduced with permission from Schmidt U et al: Restoration of diastolic function in senescent rat hearts through adenoviral gene transfer of sarcoplasmic reticulum Ca²⁺−ATPase. *Circulation* 101(7):790, 2000.

expression is also seen in pressure-induced hypertrophy and in types of congestive heart failure in rats. Importantly, the SR Ca²⁺ATPase protein, the SERCA2a gene product, is decreased by about 40 percent in the old rat heart, consistent with the decrease in sarcoplasmic reticulum calcium uptake. When a viral vector is used to deliver the SERCA2a gene to the old rat heart, the content of this pump protein is increased and diastolic (and systolic) function improves as well (Fig. 33-9), as reported by Schmidt et al. Similarly, when old animals are exercise trained, the result is increased SR Ca²⁺ATPase, augmented calcium handling, and improved cardiac relaxation. This suggests that the SERCA2a may be the actual cap on age-associated early (or active) diastolic function. Similar decreases in this protein are reported from left atria from older persons, but no data are available yet from ventricles (Fig. 33-10). This also highlights that gene therapies may hold promise for addressing the functional limitations of the aging cardiovascular system independent of disease.

The mRNA for angiotensinogen and angiotensin-converting enzyme are also increased with age, both of which have significant hypertrophic and proapoptotic effects and are characteristic of pressure overload hypertrophy. The mRNAs for both the AT-1 and AT-2 receptors are elevated with age. In contrast, fetal isoforms of troponin I and troponin T, seen in pressure-induced hypertrophy, are not seen in the 24-month-old rat heart. Therefore, on a molecular basis, the hypertrophy associated with aging in the rat heart may be distinct from, although similar to, the pressure hypertrophy seen in response to hypertension.

While for the most part there are great similarities between the rat and the human heart with aging, differences also exist. In rodent models of aging, a gradual change in cardiac myosin isotype occurs such that the fast cardiac α-myosin (V1 myosin heavy chain) predominates in the young ventricle and the slower β-myosin (V3 myosin heavy chain) predominates in the old heart. Analyzing samples

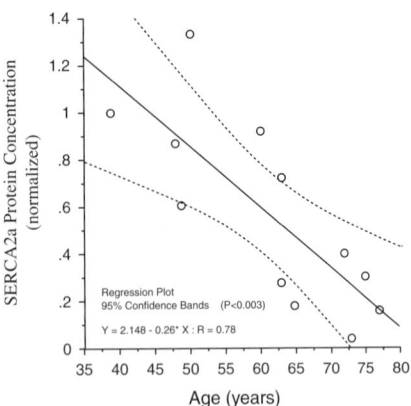

Figure 33-10 Data from left atrial tissue showing a marked decrease in sarcoplasmic reticulum Ca²⁺ATPase (SERCA2a protein) in tissue isolated from older individuals. Reproduced with permission from Cain BS et al: Human SERCA2a levels correlate inversely with age in senescent human myocardium. *J Am Coll Cardiol* 32(2):458, 1998.

from young to middle-aged heart-donor ventricles, there is a strong age-related decrease in mRNA for the cardiac α-myosin. Importantly, the correlation between mRNA and protein is very weak. In humans, even though the vast majority (>95 percent) of the myosin is already slow (V3) shortly after birth, it remains possible that a further increase in the slow myosin isoform with adult aging, could lead to decrements in function such as are observed in heart failure.

Unlike some models of heart failure, there appear to be no extensive subtype changes in the β-adrenergic receptor with age, but like heart failure, there are elevations of ANP in the serum as it is released by the left atrium and the left ventricle. As noted above, ANP is the main component of isolated atrial amyloid, but it also is a molecular marker of myocyte hypertrophy when expressed in the ventricle. Elevations in circulating ANP at rest, or after increases in intravascular volume, are markers of the overall reduced compliance of the aging cardiovascular system and may be used as a predictor of dysfunction, as reported by Davis et al. Furthermore, even in aged groups, those with cardiovascular disease have higher ANP levels than do those in a healthy group of subjects of similar age.

BNP has become an important serum marker for the evaluation and treatment of congestive heart failure. For BNP, age-associated increases are seen, but they also are smaller than those associated with heart failure. It is likely that both subtle increases in left ventricular filling pressures and decreased clearance of the peptide contribute to the observed increases in the elderly person.

Calcium Flux in the Old Myocyte

The protein changes in calcium-handling proteins are a consequence or a cause of modified calcium ion flux in the old myocyte. As a consequence of the decrease in SR Ca²⁺ATPase, the SR may be less able to serve as the predominant source of calcium to activate contraction (Fig. 33-11). The SR Ca²⁺ATPase, regulated by phospholamban, is not obviously modified by age, although its phosphorylation may be decreased as part of the lessened β-adrenergic response described below. In the cardiomyocyte, the amount of calcium entering the cell is generally inadequate to produce contraction; rather the calcium entering triggers the SR to release calcium for contraction. The changes in the old heart include increased calcium flux through the L-type calcium channels on the sarcolemma and decreased calcium release from the SR for each contraction. The flux through sarcolemmal calcium channels is increased primarily because of altered heterogeneity in the opening and closing states of the L-type channel. The net effect is that the inactivation of L-type calcium channel current measured as the ensemble of individual Ca²⁺ channel is slowed. During relaxation in the old myocyte there is a decrease in reuptake by the senescent SR and increased extrusion of the sodium–calcium exchanger relative to the young myocyte, and the relaxation is slower. The sodium–calcium exchanger is increased with age, and elevations in cytoplasmic calcium may increase the flux through this exchanger. Evidence suggests that it can function bidirectionally, not only extruding calcium but also admitting calcium into the cell. As noted above, in old animals, when the content of the SR Ca²⁺ATPase protein is increased back to levels typically seen in young animals with exercise training or gene therapy, the calcium flux is improved and cardiac relaxation is normalized.

In part because of the slower calcium flux, the relative and absolute refractory periods are longer in muscle from old hearts. The shortest interval between contractions in the old heart or old myocyte is up to 40 percent longer than in the young. The average calcium concentration may be higher in the old heart not only because of slower calcium fluxes but also because oscillations in calcium concentration from spontaneous local release by the sarcoplasmic reticulum are reduced. The frequency of this spontaneous release of calcium or calcium waves is significantly increased in myocytes isolated from old rat hearts.

MOLECULAR CORRELATES OF THE POOR TOLERANCE OF STRESS BY THE AGED HEART

Mortality after myocardial infarction is increased dramatically with increasing age, and it is clear that this increase is not a result of larger or more prior infarcts in the older patients. In addition to the limited ability to hypertrophy in the old heart, it is likely that impaired ability to recognize and respond to stress contributes to this elevated mortality.

Under normoxic conditions no age differences are present for contractile function of human atrial tissue. However, hypoxic tissue from old (age 70 to 89 years) and middle-age groups (age 60 to 69 years) studied in vitro showed reduced recovery of developed force as compared with that found in tissue from a younger group. Similar age-associated impairments in recovery after ischemic or hypoxic insult are seen in animal models of aging, differences that are most apparent when the insult is more subtle. Protection from ischemic damage (as well as other types of damage) is afforded, in part, by the heat shock proteins

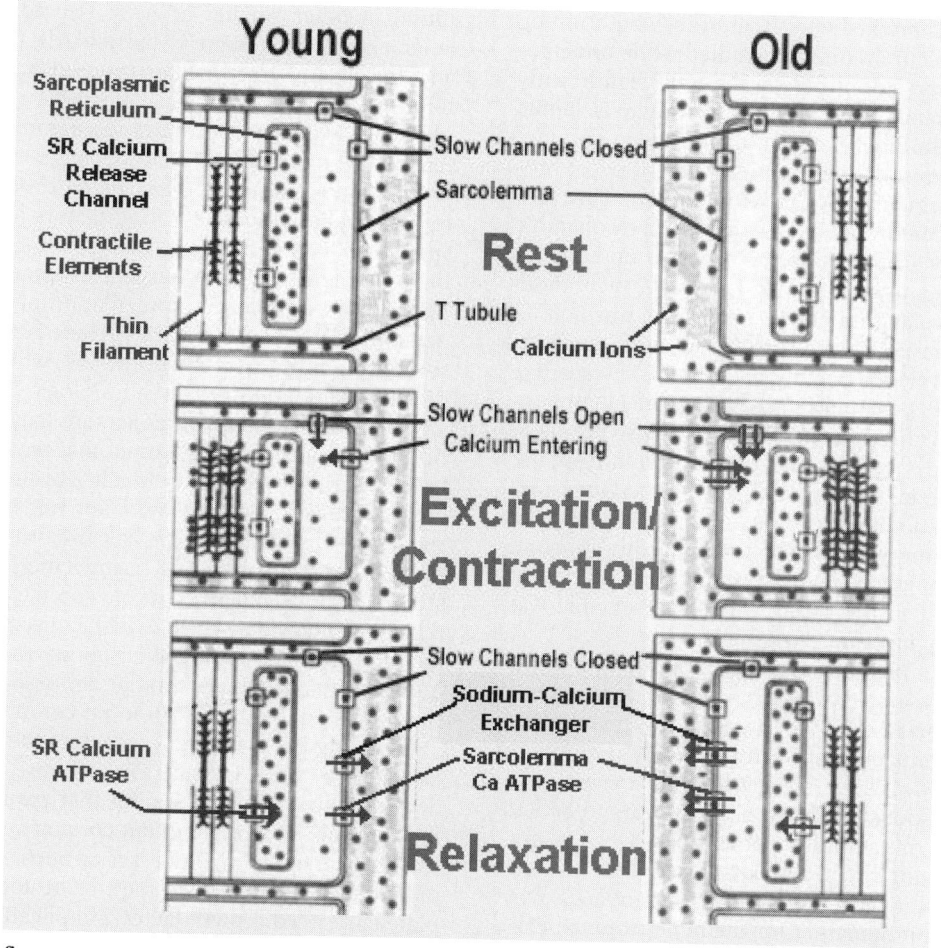

Figure 33-11 This figure summarizes the age-associated changes in myocardial calcium flux. There are small differences at rest as a consequence of spontaneous calcium release from the sarcoplasmic reticulum (SR), such that the resting stores may be decreased with age. With excitation there is increased calcium entry through the slow, L-type calcium channels and relatively less activator calcium released from the SR. For relaxation to occur, calcium must be resequestered away from the contractile elements. The amount of calcium taken up into the old SR by the Ca^{2+}ATPase is less than that of the young heart, and the calcium extruded primarily through the sodium calcium exchanger is increased in the old heart.

(hsps). The content and response of hsp72, one of the most important HSPs in the heart, is decreased in old rat hearts, as compared to young rat hearts. Therefore, the old heart may be less able to recover after ischemic events.

Age-associated differences in gene expression may increase the probability of apoptosis in the old heart after an insult. Because the ratio of Bcl-2 and other antiapoptotic factors to Bax and other proapoptotic factors is a key determinant of the likelihood of undergoing apoptosis, the observation by Liu et al. that expressions of both Bcl-2 and Bax are increased in old hearts, is not in itself enlightening. However, although the Bcl-2 to Bax ratio appeared not to change with age, apoptosis peaked more rapidly after coronary occlusion in the old, suggesting old hearts may be primed towards this mode of cell death. This may be a result of changes in some of the other regulators besides Bcl-2 and Bax. Nitahara et al. have provided evidence that the elevations in intracellular calcium in the aged myocyte might directly trigger DNAase II and induce apoptosis independent of other regulatory systems. In contrast, others report no changes in Bcl-2 or Bax in aged rat hearts. The

insult of ischemia after coronary occlusion may be generalizable, implying that cells in the old heart may be more likely to undergo apoptosis in recognition of damage from any stress.

Oxidative damage is one stimulus for apoptosis. However, there are discrepancies in the extent of protein and lipid damage present in the old heart. While oxygen free radical generation may be higher in mitochondria isolated from old hearts than young ones, some of the protective, antioxidant enzymes are also increased with age. Evidence of lipid peroxidation, protein carbonyl formation, and protein peroxynitration have been noted to be increased in old hearts. Additionally, after an acute bout of exercise where oxygen utilization is clearly increased, the amount of oxidative damage is greater in the old heart than in the young. This is in contrast to the long-term benefits of exercise training discussed below. All these changes, oxidative damage to lipids, and/or proteins may be signals for apoptosis.

Ischemic preconditioning is another stress-protective adaptation. If a heart has a few brief episodes of ischemia as a prelude, then the damage from a subsequent prolonged ischemic episode is markedly less than if the conditioning episodes did not occur. In humans studied while undergoing cardiac catheterization, preconditioning significantly enhanced the tolerance of the heart to subsequent ischemia in adults but not in older patients. Clinically, in younger patients, anginal episodes will provide some level of protection from subsequent myocardial infarction. This protection does not occur in elderly persons with a comparable extent of coronary artery disease, as reported by Longobardi et al. However, as reported by Lee et al., nicorandil, a mitochondrial potassium channel activator, was able to reverse impaired responsiveness in the old heart, suggesting an important role for the mitochondrial ATP-sensitive potassium (K[ATP]) channels in the aging defect.

The loss of ischemic preconditioning that also occurs in old rats parallels decreased hsp72 elaboration in response to heat stress. Exercise training has been reported to restore ischemic preconditioning in old rats. In these studies, and in others in vitro, the age deficit was most readily apparent if the preconditioning stimulus was mild and tended to become equivalent to the young when the ischemia was prolonged or the temperature was higher.

The response to pressure overload is attenuated in the old rat heart. And as noted by Takahashi et al., gene expression of the old heart in response to acute pressure overload is remarkably attenuated, especially the early protooncogenes (c-fos, c-jun), which are markers for the onset of a hypertrophic response. The old heart appears to be less able to respond to this stimulus, perhaps because of its myocytes already having reached maximal size. This may explain why the protooncogene response is attenuated, why the ANP expression (a marker for the hypertrophied cell) is elevated at baseline, and why little additional cellular enlargement was seen in response to pressure overload in these animals.

DNA ALTERATIONS IN MITOCHONDRIA FROM THE OLD HEART

Mitochondrial DNA (mtDNA) deletions and mutations reportedly occur with aging in various tissues. Mitochondria are likely to have oxidative damage and DNA deletions because the repair mechanisms are less-well developed within the organelle than, for example, the nucleus. No age-associated reductions of mtDNA copy number occurred in studies of hearts isolated from old rats as compared to younger ones. Mitochondrial-encoded cytochrome COX subunit I and III transcript levels, and COX enzyme activity also remained unchanged in the aging heart in these studies. Finally, in hearts isolated from old rats, the content of high-energy phosphates (ATP + creatine phosphate) is only modestly changed from the young. Therefore, mitochondrial DNA changes, while intriguing, have not yet been shown to alter the performance of the aged heart or to reflect the adequacy of the energetic adaptation of the aged heart.

CORONARY ARTERIES

In the absence of atherosclerosis, the changes in the coronary arteries that occur with age are reminiscent of those found in other smaller arteries. Degradation of the vascular extracellular matrix, particularly the elastin fibers, and the loss of elastin fiber integrity may lower the arterial wall elasticity, increasing arterial rigidity. Stiffening of collagen fiber network and thickening of arterial walls may also contribute to rigidity. Changes in shape and axial orientation are also seen. Enhanced contractile responses to endothelial vasoconstricting factors and decreased response to NO-dependent vasodilators are seen, which increase the risk of coronary vasospasm in older people. This occurs despite the upregulation of endothelial NOS in the old rat coronary arteries. There is preserved responsiveness to nitrates or nitroprusside, which are direct NO donors and to arginine, the physiologic NOS substrate.

Coronary arteries in older persons have a marked reduction in one specific ion channel that regulates the tension in the arterial smooth muscle cell. This Ca^{2+}-activated $K+$ channel, MaxiK, which plays a key role in regulating arterial tone, was decreased by half in coronaries form older people. The decrease in this channel increases the vasoconstrictor responsiveness of the old coronary artery. Such age-related changes may have drastic consequences in elderly individuals by impairing their ability to adapt to stresses imposed by challenges. Similar age-associated changes in the MaxiK channel are seen in rat coronary arteries.

In young people there is an ability to remodel the coronary artery tree of the heart in response to ischemia, thus developing a collateral supply that partially protects the myocardium from subsequent coronary events. Angiogenesis is decreased in older age groups. However, in the old mouse, angiogenesis may be restored by providing platelet-derived growth factors, implicating an inadequate signal rather than an inability to respond to growth factors. Whether the ability to remodel is one of the reasons that myocardial infarction has a higher mortality in the old is uncertain, however.

THE ELECTROCARDIOGRAM AND ELECTROPHYSIOLOGY

There are no significant differences in resting heart rate with age, but in highly screened older populations sitting heart rate decreases up to 1 beat per minute per decade may be detected. However, the intrinsic heart rate, the rate at which the heart beats when both parasympathetic and sympathetic influences are blocked, decreases significantly with age, as reported by Craft and Schwartz. At rest, the young person has significant parasympathetic tone, slowing down the heart. In contrast, the extent of parasympathetic influence is very small in the old; hence the effects of atropine on heart rate are smaller in the normal older person. This use of a reserve mechanism just to maintain resting heart rate contributes to limiting the increase in heart rate available to respond to challenges.

The other impact of the loss of parasympathetic tone may be decreased heart rate variability in older persons. Monitoring heart rate over hours or days allows analysis of the variability of R-R intervals. In the most robust systems, under multiple influences, the extent of complexity is greatest. As the number of influences decreases or the extent of these influences decreases, the systems become

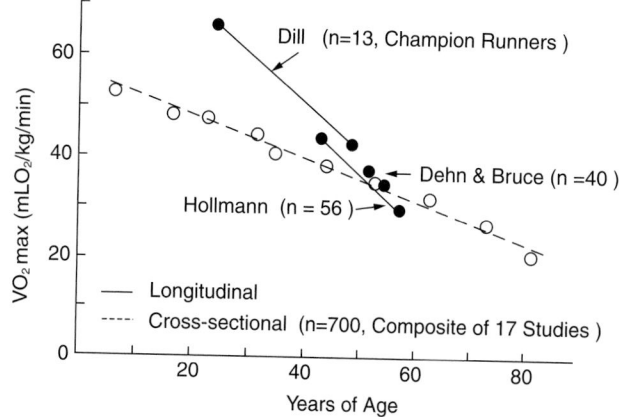

Figure 33-12 A composite of multiple studies that demonstrate the age-associated decrease in VO_2 max (mL O_2/kg/min) in cross-sectional as well as longitudinal studies. The decline was present in all studies, although the steepness of the decline varied with the group studied.

less complex and less robust. This is true of many physiologic systems: they lose complexity with age. For heart rate variability, the decrease in parasympathetic tone is clearly implicated, as the low frequency component decreases with age. The loss of sinus arrhythmia with age is another reflection of this same process. Determining the complexity of systems and the implications of changes with aging as an index of physiologic vitality is still in development but holds the potential to be a very sensitive means of estimating homeostatic reserve.

Also apparent on continuous electrocardiogram (ECG) sampling is that healthy older persons are more constricted in their range of typically attained heart rates. The lowest rate of the day is faster and the highest rate reached is lower than in healthy young persons. Perhaps the age-associated changes in the SA node and conduction pathway contribute to the changes in the resting electrocardiograms of elderly individuals. The duration of the PR interval is increased, the orientation of the electrical axis of the QRS complex is shifted, and the morphology of the atrial and ventricular complexes is also modified. The upper limits of normal for the P-R interval is 220 ms in those older than age 65 years, as compared to 200 ms in the young, and the PR interval increase is a result of prolongation of the atria–His bundle interval, likely in the AV junction. Importantly, second- and third-degree block are not normal aging findings; sinus rhythm is the only normal rhythm in the elderly person. Right bundle-branch block or left anterior fascicular block on the resting ECG may not be normal aging, but these do not have the association with coronary disease in the elderly patient that they have in the young patient. It is not clear whether the QT interval either measured directly or corrected for heart rate (QTc) is prolonged in the normal older heart. This finding has been observed in relatively unscreened populations. Other changes, which may be normal are those involving ventricular repolarization, with a specific flattening of the ST segment and a decreased magnitude of the T wave.

On long-term monitoring, premature atrial contractions are seen in almost all elderly individuals screened to exclude those with common cardiac diseases. Atrial ectopy is correlated with the increase in atrial size described above. Although the incidence of atrial fibrillation increases almost 200-fold from age 30 years to age 80 years, this also is

not a normal finding. The dependence of atrial fibrillation on left atrial size is very strong even in people older than 75 years of age. Ventricular ectopy, usually isolated premature ventricular complexes, are also seen in more than 75 percent of those older than age 75 years without heart disease. However, more complex or frequent ectopy is not likely to be a part of normal aging.

CARDIOVASCULAR PERFORMANCE DURING EXERCISE

A decline in the maximal capacity of the cardiovascular system can be seen with increasing age in healthy physically inactive individuals as well as those who are highly trained. This contributes to the age-related decline in VO_2max (maximum oxygen consumption), although the extent is still unclear and may vary from individual to individual as well as by testing conditions (Fig. 33-12). The factors that have been implicated in the decrease in VO_2max include the decreases in maximal heart rate, maximal stroke volume (and therefore maximum cardiac output), muscle mass, circulating blood volume, and pulmonary function. Maximum cardiac output (the product of heart rate and stroke volume) declines with age. In serial studies of both highly trained individuals and sedentary individuals who start training, there is no modification by training in the age-related decrease in maximum heart rate (Fig. 33-13). Recent studies by Tanaka et al., however, produced slightly less-steep relationships of 0.7 to 0.8 beats per minute lost each year (for example, 208 − 0.7 × age). As shown in the schematic (Fig. 33-14) there are three important factors contributing to the loss in maximum heart rate: (1) the decrease in intrinsic heart rate with age discussed above; (2) vagal tone is less in the resting state and therefore there is little effect on heart rate as the remainder of vagal tone is removed as exercise commences; (3) finally, there is a decrease in chronotropic, inotropic and lusitropic (facilitating relaxation) responses to sympathetic stimulation (and hence a decrease in the bradycardic effect of β-adrenergic antagonist agents, which occurs in humans and rats).

In the rat, during stress, the response of I_{CaL} (the current through the L-type slow calcium channels) to β-adrenergic

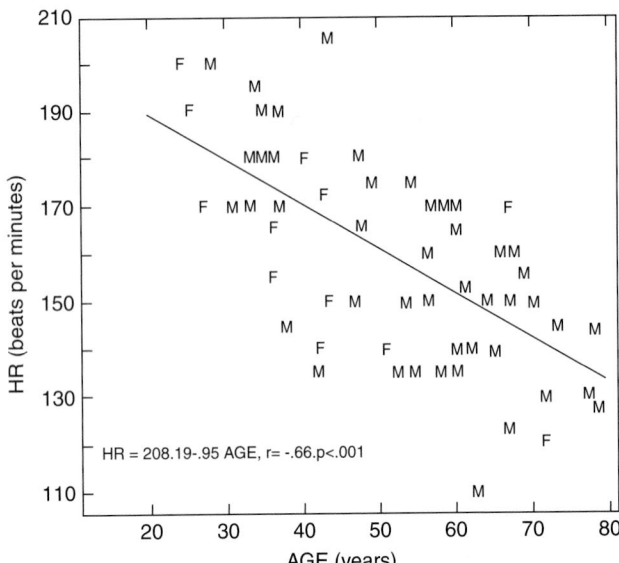

Figure 33-13   These data from the Baltimore Longitudinal Study demonstrate the age-associated decrease in maximum heart rate attained with maximum exercise.

receptor stimulation is markedly reduced, which may be an important cause of the age-related decrease in cardiac reserve function. Of special interest, a similarly age-related decrease in maximum heart rate in response to stress is found in *Drosophila*, underscoring the primary nature of the phenomenon. Overall, the result is a large decrease in maximum heart rate with aging, as a consequence, in part, of using reserve mechanisms to maintain resting heart rate at appropriate levels.

Because older persons cannot increase heart rate to the same extent as in youth, they must depend upon increasing stroke volume to increase cardiac output. As the inotropic responsiveness to sympathetic nervous system stimulation is also decreased with age, the older person may use the Starling relationship to a greater degree than the younger person, increasing filling pressures to increase end-diastolic volume. In contrast, increasing left ventricular filling pressures to increase stroke volume may not occur in healthy young persons (see Fig. 33-14). The timing of the invocation of the Starling mechanism in the elderly has not been uniform across studies, so it may be important to consider gradations of effort rather than just focusing on peak values. Additionally, the young person given β-adrenergic antagonists has a strong resemblance while exercising to the older person studied in the absence of β-adrenergic blockade.

Overall, the cardiac efficiency of the older person is just as great as in the young one; that is, the ratio of cardiac output to work performed is unchanged by age. In the old dog, the relationship between oxygen utilization and

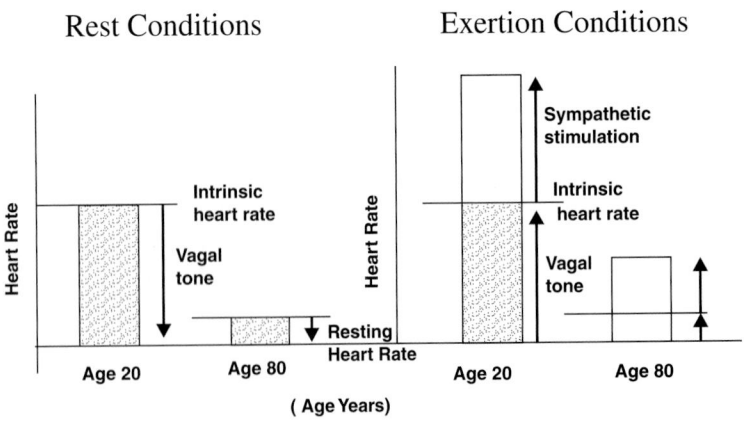

Figure 33-14   This schematic describes the influences that result in the decrease in maximum heart rate with exercise. Under rest condition there is a relatively small age-related decrease in heart rate, but the intrinsic heart rate, that when the sympathetic and parasympathetic influences are blocked, is markedly decreased with age. Thus the vagal tone at rest is much less in the older person. With exertion, first the vagal tone is removed, increasing heart rate, but to a lesser extent in the older person. Then sympathetic stimulation contributes; the chronotropic responsiveness to sympathomimetic agents is also decreased with age. The net result is a lesser maximum heart rate in the older person.

cardiac output is fairly linear and is exactly the same as in the young dog. The young dog, of course, can perform more work and attain a higher peak oxygen utilization and maximum cardiac output. The same is true for persons 20 years of age as compared to those in their sixties.

The mechanisms for the decreased responsiveness of the old heart to sympathetic nervous system stimulation and sympathomimetic drugs remain unclear. Circulating levels of catecholamines are increased in the elderly person under both stimulated and basal conditions, which could induce receptor desensitization. However, evidence of receptor desensitization is lacking. Adenosine is released as an antagonist of the inotropic and chronotropic effects of sympathetic stimulation. Adenosine is released in greater quantities by the old heart than by the young one, and some of the age-associated differences in responsiveness to sympathetic stimulation can be ablated with adenosine antagonists. This is likely to be only one of the important mechanisms contributing to this diminished adrenergic responsiveness.

There is competition between the stimulatory and inhibitory G proteins and some, but not all, reports note an increase with in certain inhibitory G proteins in old rat hearts. There may be decreases in the density of receptors, but no marked changes in the ratio of the β_1 to β_2 receptors have been reported. One early report found altered affinity of the β_1 receptor for agonists but not for antagonists. Post–β-receptor, cyclic adenosine monophosphate (cAMP) is generated by adenyl cyclase. The activity of this enzyme is decreased in the basal state and in response to receptor activation. Muscarinic receptors antagonize the activation of adenyl cyclase, and this antagonist activity may be enhanced with age. The net effects, either increasing cellular cAMP or augmenting calcium signals or target protein phosphorylation, are decreased in the old heart. This area continues to be the focus of significant attention in aging animal models, as increasing sympathetic responsiveness could increase performance in the older individual.

These data do not imply that the old heart is simply generally unresponsive. The inotropic response to dobutamine may be preserved with age, as in hearts isolated from old rats have the same responses to dopamine infusions as those from younger rats. Isolated papillary muscles from old animals have a response to changes in tissue bath calcium identical to that from young animals. Results in humans differ. The sites of the limitation appear to be those of greatest importance in increasing cardiac output in response to exercise. Again, the similarities in response to exercise among the older person, the young person given β-adrenergic antagonists, and the orthotopic heart transplant recipient (where innervation is often not present) are quite remarkable, suggesting a central role of adrenergic responsiveness in the age-related changes observed.

Exercise-induced arrhythmias, including ventricular premature complexes, occur with greater frequency in the elderly population but may have little association with the presence or absence of coronary artery disease or myocardial ischemia. These "benign" exercise-induced arrhythmias are probably limited to unifocal ventricular beats.

RESPONSE TO ORTHOSTATIC STRESS

Clinically significant postural hypotension (orthostatic symptoms or a fall in systolic blood pressure of 20 mmHg or more upon standing) is uncommon in normotensive independent older individuals. In normal healthy individuals, the ability to maintain adequate perfusion of the brain is preserved with aging. However, that ability appears to be in a highly compensated state and therefore more likely be compromised with additional stresses. As noted above, the aging vasculature is less compliant, and increases in blood pressure accompany increases in volume. The same dependence is true for decreases in volume, which translate into decreases in perfusion pressure.

Baroreceptor function is compromised with age. After an acute increase in blood pressure the decrease in heart rate is larger in the young than in the old. Similarly, the increase in heart rate after an acute decrease in pressure is smaller in the old. Baroreceptor modulation of the sympathetic drive to the peripheral circulation is impaired in older persons, primarily in the speed of reflex adjustments to normal and abnormal stimuli. This decreased sensitivity and responsiveness may contribute to the higher frequency of orthostatic blood pressure decreases in the old person.

Techniques that measure the change in carotid artery lumen, instead of the change in blood pressure as the independent variable, show that function of the baroreceptor is unchanged with age. In contrast, studies using phenylephrine to increase pressure and monitor the heart rate response frequently find large age effects. This implies that the stiffer arterial wall stretches less in response to increased pressure, and thus the receptor cells are deformed less in the older person. Importantly, the baroreceptor cells are thought to sense pressure indirectly by sensing changes in cell deformation. Consistent with this concept are many reports of strong correlations between baroreceptor function and large artery stiffness in aging, as noted by Ford. Overall, young people have cardiovagal baroreflex sensitivity (change in R-R interval in milliseconds/change in systolic pressure in mmHg) that is four times greater than in older persons, when given an agent to increase blood pressure and the parasympathetic nervous system slowing the heart is the effector arm. However, correction for the stiffness of the sensing vessels removes any age-related effect in this specific paradigm. This stiffening of the sensing vessels also contributes to the increase in systolic blood pressure with age. Thus, studies that correct for systolic blood pressure may find no "age" effect, perhaps because they have removed it. In applying this correction. And hence if the stimulus sensed by the baroreceptor is decreased because of vessel stiffening, then one would expect all the components of the response to orthostasis to be decreased, which appears to be the case.

Clinically, the more important arm of the response is the reaction to decreases in perfusion pressure to the brain associated with standing up (or experimentally with negative pressure applied to the lower half of the body). Whereas orthostatic hypotension is decidedly uncommon in active, healthy, elderly persons, their venous compliance of the calf and the arm is decreased, the stimulus sensed by their baroreceptors is diminished, and their compensatory response to a change to upright posture is lessened. Specifically, the older person also takes longer to attain his maximum response. However, as the increase in heart rate is less in the older person, the change in stroke volume index is also less than in the young. This is primarily because the older person does not decrease left ventricular diastolic volumes to the extent seen in the young, so the cardiac output is relatively maintained in the healthy older person.

Adding to the complexity of the situation, the baroreflex is not as simple as described above. Changes in the brain, altering central processing, will alter the baroreceptor sensitivity, such as with cerebrovascular accidents or emotional stress.

Finally, the interpretations of these studies are not clearcut, and conflicting data are easily found. What is clear is that the healthy older person, by using compensations and reserves available, is able to tolerate changes in position and volume when at baseline. However, prolonged bed rest, dehydration, cardiovascular drugs, or intercurrent illnesses may easily tax this steady state and produce falls, dizziness, or other symptoms.

EFFECTS OF CHRONIC PHYSICAL TRAINING ON CARDIOVASCULAR AGING

While there are many benefits of regular exercise, expected improvements in cardiac function are an important reason to recommend training to older patients. Sedentary older people who start training experience remarkable increases in VO_2max, the functional equivalent of turning the clock back 20 years. Training does improve (or maintain) stroke volume in people. In studies of initially sedentary old men reported by Levy et al., 6 months of aerobic training improved left ventricular filling. More intense and brief exercise training may also improve ventricular filling and exercise performance.

Nevertheless, maximum cardiac output and VO_2max still decrease with age, even in those who train actively their entire lives. Most specifically, the change in maximum heart rate does not appear to be altered by training. However, as reported by Katzel et al., in athletes who show no changes in the extent of training over the years, the decline in maximal venous oxygen (MVO$_2$) may be minimized, implying that some of the decrease in VO_2max with age in athletes may be a result of subtle decreases in their training regimen or of the important permissive role of the cardiovascular system for exercise.

Exercise training will improve large-artery compliance and the regulation of homeostasis by maintaining the sensitivity of the baroreceptor. Apparently the improvement in baroreceptor function is directly related to the increases in compliance of the carotid and aorta arteries. Specific effects of high physical activity include the preservation of ischemic preconditioning in both humans and animals. Exercise training of even very old animals will decrease collagen content and cross-linking of left ventricular collagen. Therefore, exercise training will improve both the active and passive diastolic function of the older left ventricle.

Exercise training of old rats selectively improved the β-adrenergically mediated facilitation of relaxation, as reported by Taffet et al. There were no training effects on maximum heart rate. β-Adrenergic antagonists will ablate the gains made by training, so it appears that some of the benefits of exercise training are mediated by enhanced responsiveness to the sympathetic nervous system.

EFFECTS OF CALORIC RESTRICTION ON CARDIOVASCULAR AGING

Caloric restriction decreases age-related changes in rodents and likely also in many systems in nonhuman primates. While only a few studies have been completed, caloric restriction appears to improve diastolic filling in old mice, restores the age-related loss of ischemic preconditioning, and decreases the extent of nonenzymatic glycation of aortic proteins and subsequent formation of advanced glycation end products. However, caloric restriction appears to have little effect on age-related changes in peripheral vascular resistance and aortic impedance in rats. Similarly, caloric restriction does not increase systolic function in old mice, nor does it appear to modify the myosin isozyme changes with age in rats. Caloric restriction does attenuate the age-associated increase in plasma ANP. Overall, the effects of caloric restriction on cardiovascular aging are not uniform but warrant further study.

IMPLICATION OF CARDIOVASCULAR AGING CHANGES ON CLINICAL EXAMINATION OF THE ELDERLY PATIENT

On physical exam there are clear implications of these aging changes. When one assesses the carotid pulse in trying to assess the severity of aortic stenosis, this may be misleading in the older person with stiff arteries. The pulse may feel full even with diminished output. The stiff ventricle and increased reliance on atrial systole for filling makes the S4 an almost universal finding on auscultation of older patients in sinus rhythm.

Importantly, interpretation of the pulse rate in an older person needs to take account of the diminished chronotropic responsiveness to stress that accompanies normal aging. A young man who presents with pneumonia and a heart rate of 150 beats per minute is clearly ill. The same relative degree of tachycardia is present in an 85-year-old woman with a heart rate of 96 beats per minute, reflecting a similar extent of activation and presumably equal severity of illness (and an even more ominous prognosis).

Lying, sitting, and standing blood pressure are obtained routinely, but uncertainty exists as to what is acceptable in older persons. A decrease of 20 mmHg upon standing, in the absence of symptoms, may be considered within normal limits; however, this response may fluctuate over time and may become great enough to produce symptoms.

The physical examination is normally performed with the patient at rest. We have attempted to underscore that even significant age-related changes in the cardiovascular system appear to have minimal impact on physiologic parameters in the resting state, and hence are likely to be ignored under exam conditions. This should in no way be construed to suggest that these changes are trivial, but rather that the adaptations to them are adequate to maintain homeostasis at rest. Fortunately, most of life is spent off the table out of the examination room, and this is where the adaptations may be less adequate and age-related changes more apparent.

The reader is strongly urged to pursue the topics introduced in this chapter by exploring the comprehensive reviews by Lakatta and Sollett and by Nichols and O'Rourke.

REFERENCES

Avolio AP et al: Improved arterial distensibility in normotensive subjects on a low salt diet. *Arteriosclerosis* 6:166, 1986.

Bharati S, Lev M: The pathologic changes in the conduction system beyond the age of ninety. *Am Heart J* 124(2):487, 1992.

Bonow RO et al: Effects of aging on asynchronous left ventricular regional function and global ventricular filling in normal human subjects. *J Am Coll Cardiol* 11:50, 1988.

Cooper LT et al: The vasculopathy of aging. *J Gerontol A Biol Sci Med Sci* 49:B191, 1994.

Craft N, Schwartz JB: Effects of age on intrinsic heart rate, heart rate variability, and AV conduction in healthy humans. *Am J Physiol* 268:H1441, 1995.

Davidson WR Jr, Fee EC: Influence of aging on pulmonary hemodynamics in a population free of coronary artery disease. *Am J Cardiol* 65:1454, 1990.

Davis KM et al: Atrial natriuretic peptide levels in the elderly: differentiating normal aging changes from disease. *J Gerontol A Biol Sci Med Sci* 51:M95, 1996.

Ford GA: Ageing and the baroreceptor. *Age Ageing* 28:337, 1999.

Homma S et al: Carotid plaque and intima-media thickness assessed by B-mode ultrasonography in subjects ranging from young adults to centenarians. *Stroke* 32:830, 2001.

Kass DA et al: Improved arterial compliance by a novel advanced glycation end-product cross-link breaker. *Circulation* 104(13):1464, 2001.

Katzel LI et al: A comparison of longitudinal changes in aerobic fitness in older endurance athletes and sedentary men. *J Am Geriatr Soc* 49:1657, 2001.

Kitzman DW: Normal age-related changes in the heart: Relevance to echocardiography in the elderly. *Am J Geriatr Cardiol* 9:311, 2000.

Kitzman DW, Edwards WD: Mini-review: Age-related changes in the anatomy of the normal human heart. *J Gerontol* 45:M33, 1990.

Lakatta EG: Cardiovascular system, in Masoro EJ (ed): *Aging: Handbook of Physiology*. New York, American Physiology Society, 1995, 413.

Lakatta EG, Sollott SJ: Perspectives on mammalian cardiovascular aging: Humans to molecules. *Comp Biochem Physiol A Mol Integr Physiol* 132:699, 2002.

Lee TM et al: Loss of preconditioning by attenuated activation of myocardial ATP-sensitive potassium channels in elderly patients undergoing coronary angioplasty. *Circulation* 105:334, 2002.

Levy WC et al: Endurance exercise training augments diastolic filling at rest and during exercise in healthy young and older men. *Circulation* 88:116, 1993.

Li Z et al: Enhanced proliferation and migration and altered cytoskeletal proteins in early passage smooth muscle cells from young and old rat aortic explants. *Exp Mol Pathol* 64(1):1, 1997.

Liu L et al: Bcl-2 and Bax expression in adult rat hearts after coronary occlusion: Age-associated differences. *Am J Physiol* R315, 1998.

Longobardi G et al: "Warm-up" phenomenon in adult and elderly patients with coronary artery disease: Further evidence of the loss of "ischemic preconditioning" in the aging heart. *J Gerontol A Biol Sci Med Sci* 55:M124, 2000.

Nichols WW, O'Rourke MF: *McDonald's Blood Flow in Arteries*, 4th ed. New York, Oxford University Press, 1998.

Nitahara JA et al: Intracellular calcium, DNAase activity, and myocyte apoptosis in aging Fischer 344 Rats. *J Mol Cell Cardiol* 30:519, 1998.

Olivetti G et al: Cardiomyopathy of the aging human heart, myocyte loss, and reactive cellular hypertrophy. *Circ Res* 68:1560, 1991.

Olsen H et al: Cardiovascular response to acute hypovolemia in relation to age. Implications for orthostasis and hemorrhage. *Am J Physiol Heart Circ Physiol* 278:H222, 2000.

Rivard A et al: Age-dependent impairment of angiogenesis. *Circulation* 99:111, 1999.

Schmidt U et al: Restoration of diastolic function in senescent rat hearts through adenoviral gene transfer of sarcoplasmic reticulum Ca(2+)-ATPase. *Circulation* 101:790, 2000.

Taffet GE et al: Exercise training improves lusitropy by isoproterenol in papillary muscles from aged rats. *Appl Physiol* 81:1488, 1996.

Takahashi T et al: Age-related differences in the expression of proto-oncogene and contractile protein genes in response to pressure overload in the rat myocardium. *J Clin Invest* 99:939, 1992.

Tanaka H et al: Age-predicted maximal heart rate revisited. *J Am Coll Cardiol* 37:153, 2001.

Tate CA et al: Enhanced calcium uptake of cardiac sarcoplasmic reticular in exercise-trained old rats. *Am J Physiol* 258:H431, 1990.

Vaitkevicius PV et al: Effects of age and aerobic capacity on arterial stiffness in healthy adults. *Circulation* 88:1456, 1993.

Vanoeverschelde J-LJ et al: Contribution of left ventricular diastolic function to exercise capacity in normal subjects. *J Appl Physiol* 74:2225, 1993.

Aging and Atherosclerosis

WILLIAM R. HAZZARD • MARY Y. CHANG • ALAN CHAIT

Atherosclerosis is perhaps the quintessential age-related disease process. Its clinical complications in coronary heart disease (CHD), stroke, and peripheral vascular disease underlie the close parallel between advancing age and both all-cause and cardiovascular disease (CVD) mortality in the United States, where CVD (preponderantly atherosclerotic CVD) accounts for nearly half of all American deaths in middle age and beyond.

As a prototypical gerontologic disease process, atherosclerosis challenges the geriatric clinician to recognize the inherent complexity of the atherogenic process. This requires appreciation of the respective and dynamic contributions of the multiple factors that contribute to and modulate this disease: (1) aging at its most basic level, (2) atherosclerotic CVD risk (and protective) factors and their trajectories with age, (3) the role of the passage of time per se and escape from competing causes of morbidity and mortality that permits survival into old age, and (4) the interactions of all these factors, which converge to establish atherosclerotic CVD as a prime concern of geriatric medicine and gerontology.

In Chapter 35 the changes in cardiovascular structure, physiology, and function with aging were segregated insofar as possible from those attributable to atherosclerosis and other age-related CVD by focusing on data derived from aging subjects free of clinical CVD, notably those in the Baltimore Longitudinal Study of Aging (BLSA), and relevant nonhuman models of cardiovascular aging. In contrast, this chapter is centered on atherosclerosis and its relationship to aging across the human life span, a process that culminates in CVD, both clinical and subclinical, in more than three-quarters of Americans older than age 80 and that is virtually universal by the end of life in the "oldest old" (those who survive beyond 85 years).

ATHEROSCLEROSIS AND AGING: INEXTRICABLY INTERTWINED?

Like all classic age-related disease processes, atherosclerosis has a multifactorial etiology. It crosses the clinical horizon to become manifest through its well-known complications at different ages and different stages in the human life cycle according to the rate of its pathogenesis in the individual patient of advancing age. At the one extreme, clearly rooted in major genetic mutations, are the rare instances of atherosclerotic CVD that present in children, for example, in those (one in a million) with homozygous familial hypercholesterolemia (FH). Persons with this mendelian simply inherited disorder lack functional low-density lipoprotein (LDL) receptors, and as a result their LDL cholesterol (LDL-C) levels average at least four times the normal values. Consequently they usually develop coronary and vascular heart disease in the second decade of life through marked acceleration of this time-related (and perforce age-related) process. At the other extreme of the life span is the far more common, indeed normative, scenario in which clinical atherosclerotic CVD presents in old age, either de novo or (with increasing frequency in contemporary American society with advances in the treatment of and survival of CVD clinical events) as recurrent myocardial infarction, stroke, or other extracoronary atherosclerotic CVD. These events often culminate in life-threatening arrhythmias or end-stage ischemic cardiomyopathy and congestive heart failure (subjects of succeeding chapters). In between these extremes are the still numerous cases of atherosclerotic CVD presenting prematurely (i.e., before old age). However, as the age distribution of the US population shifts progressively upward in the twenty-first century and deaths from CVD prior to old age continue to decline (attributable in roughly equal proportions to more effective and widespread adoption of preventive strategies and to more effective treatment of clinical CVD), atherosclerotic CVD will increasingly become a disease of old age: Already 85 percent of persons dying of CHD are age 65 and older, and "geriatric cardiology" has become a mainstream focus in both medical and surgical CVD subspecialties.

THE PATHOGENESIS OF ATHEROSCLEROSIS

The atherogenic process begins with the adherence of circulating monocytes and adhesion molecules expressed on activated endothelial cells at the site of a future arterial lesion (Figure 34-1). Through diapedesis between endothelial cells, these monocytes migrate to the subendothelial space where they are transformed into macrophages. Subsequently they become engorged with lipoprotein cholesteryl

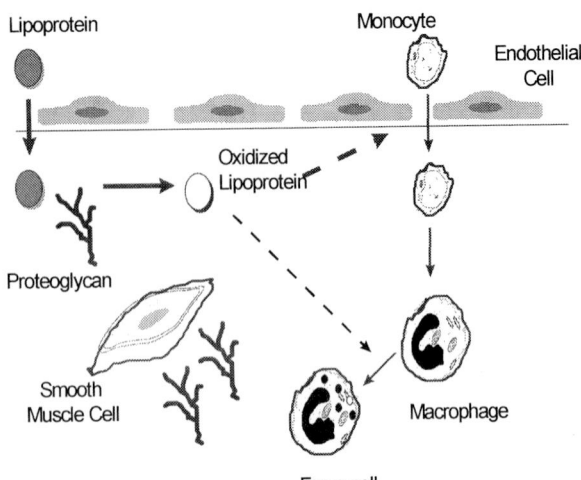

Figure 34-1 Schematic depicting the early events in atherosclerotic lesion development. Transcytosis of low-density lipoprotein (LDL) from the arterial lumen across the endothelial layer of blood vessels leads to binding and retention of LDL by extracellular matrix proteoglycans. This trapped LDL is susceptible to oxidative modification within the subendothelial space, leading to the generation of oxidized LDL. Oxidized LDL can stimulate a variety of atherogenic responses, including the recruitment of blood-derived monocytes into the arterial wall, where they differentiate into macrophages. These macrophages then can actively scavenge oxidized LDL, resulting in the formation of lipid-laden foam cells.

esters via their membrane scavenger receptors, a process not regulated by intracellular cholesterol stores. (This contrasts with the situation in hepatocytes, where such cholesterol accumulation is prevented by the coordinated downregulation of both the LDL receptors and intracellular cholesterol synthesis in response to lipoprotein cholesterol uptake.) This engorgement produces a foamy histologic appearance, giving rise to the apt description "foam cells." As lesions develop, smooth muscle cells may migrate into the subendothelial space, take up cholesterol, and also be transformed into foam cells. Both types of cells respond especially to transcytosed plasma LDLs that bind to the exposed subendothelial matrix and undergo oxidation. This process in turn attracts additional monocytes and smooth muscle cells to the site in a self-perpetuating, self-accelerating cycle of events. As the cholesterol-laden cells accumulate and time passes, the overlying endothelium becomes deformed and discontinuous, serving to further expose the underlying foam cells and extracellular matrix to circulating platelets, which may adhere, aggregate, and also release various factors that contribute to the atherogenic process at the site of the developing lesion.

Mitogenic substances released by platelets (notably platelet-derived growth factor [PDGF]), endothelial cells, and monocytes also stimulate replication of the subjacent smooth muscle cells, adding to the progressive enlargement of the atherosclerotic nidus at the site. The extracellular matrix also becomes progressively expanded at this locus and enriched with lipid-rich material released by dying cells and the continued inspissation of plasma-derived lipoproteins and their oxidation products in situ. Whereas

much of the initial lesion expansion is directed toward the adventitia and is compensated there by arterial wall remodeling to preserve the flow capacity of the overlying vessel, ultimately the lesion may come to encroach on the arterial lumen, limiting blood flow and producing ischemia in downstream tissues.

The process that ultimately results in occlusion of the affected vessel and necrosis of ischemic tissues (Figure 34-2) is far more dynamic, however, than that which was historically described as a slow, inexorable, progressive accumulation of lipids and a reduction in arterial diameter. For the atherosclerotic process also impairs the ability of the arterial wall to respond to stimuli that would normally permit increased blood flow via dilatation, enlargement mediated by endothelium-derived relaxing factors, and changes in autonomic regulation (e.g., during exercise); instead, the atherosclerotic artery may undergo paradoxical vasoconstriction in response to such stimuli and, at least transiently, produce symptoms referable to ischemia.

Moreover, as the lesions mature, their character may change. Early lesions, called fatty streaks, contain only macrophage foam cells and do not cause arterial narrowing. Present as early as in childhood, many of these lesions regress entirely. However, others progress, especially those at sites of arterial bifurcation (notably on low-pressure surfaces of affected arteries). As such lesions progress, a fibrous cap develops, and smooth muscle proliferation may become a prominent feature of the atherogenic process. Advanced lesions are yet more complicated, with a necrotic core of lipids and proteins and calcification at the site produced by a process quite similar to bone ossification. Such calcification, notably at the edges of the fibrous caps, appears to weaken the arterial wall at such sites and predisposes to lesion rupture (see below). Lesions may also vary widely as to degree of cellularity and the relative contributions of macrophages and smooth muscle cells, and the latter may arise from clonal expansion in a neoplastic-like manner.

Rupture of such atherosclerotic plaques (those rich in lipids are especially vulnerable)occurs most frequently at the shoulders of lesions that abut the fibrous caps and at sites of extraordinary shear stress related to the degree of calcification. When this takes place, the circulating blood is exposed to tissue factors from the underlying intima and media, and thrombosis rapidly ensues. Such thrombosis may in turn suddenly occlude the overlying lumen, leading to myocardial infarction, thrombotic stroke, or peripheral artery occlusion. More than 90 percent of myocardial infarcts proceed from such arterial thrombosis at sites of preexisting atherosclerotic lesions; however, as a retrospective review of previous angiograms has disclosed, such sudden occlusions often occur at sites previously manifesting less advanced atherosclerosis (55%–60%) of lumen encroachment, underscoring the role of thrombosis as the final step in the atherosclerotic CVD process. Thrombosis has also been shown to occur at sites of endothelial cell erosion overlying atherosclerotic lesions. However, not all such thromboses are complete or produce tissue necrosis. The thrombosis also triggers fibrinolysis. Thus if the thrombus is only partially occlusive, it may produce unstable angina pectoris and, as the reaction-to-injury reparative

Typical Atherosclerotic Plaque Development
Time and Aging

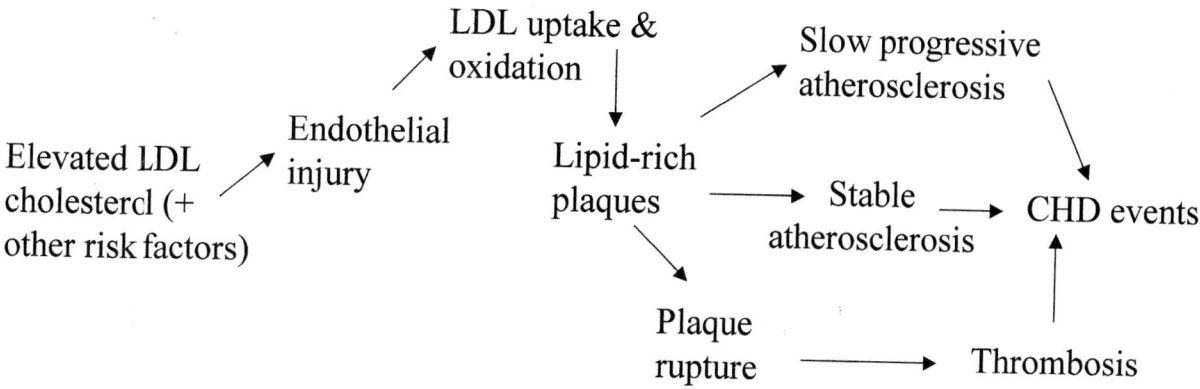

Three types of lesions (plaques):

1. Lesions that gradually progress over time
2. Lesions that remain stable over many years
3. Lesions that rupture and lead to acute coronary events

Figure 34-2   Schematic of the sequential stages in the development of atherosclerotic plaques in aging persons.

process occurs, become incorporated into the lesion as it further progresses. In other instances platelet aggregates may produce only momentary occlusion (and associated chest pain) but rapidly resolve without continuing damage, likewise producing unstable angina. Nevertheless, the net effect of all these interacting processes is generally an increase in the total burden of coronary atherosclerosis with the passage of time (and aging).

PROTEOGLYCANS IN ATHEROGENESIS

The vascular extracellular matrix, which is an intricate meshwork of extracellular macromolecules, is a major site of lipid accumulation in the arterial wall. Although several matrix molecules have been reported to interact with LDLs, proteoglycans are hypothesized to play a key role in the lipoprotein-binding process within atherosclerotic lesions (Figure 34-3). Evidence for this includes the following. (1) Lipoproteins colocalize with proteoglycans in the extracellular matrix; (2) lipoprotein–proteoglycan complexes have been extracted from human and experimental atherosclerotic lesions; (3) LDLs are selectively retained by proteoglycans of altered composition at vascular sites prone to developing atherosclerotic lesions; (4) animals with LDLs defective in the capacity to bind to proteoglycans have demonstrated delayed lesion formation.

Proteoglycans are found intracellularly, on the cell surface, and in the extracellular matrix. In normal arteries, they are present in only minor amounts. However, certain proteoglycans accumulate in atherosclerosis-prone regions and are a major component of atherosclerotic plaques. These structurally diverse, complex macromolecules are composed of a core protein to which one or more glycosaminoglycan chains are covalently attached. The glycosaminoglycan chains are linear polymers of repeating chondroitin sulfate, dermatan sulfate, or heparan sulfate disaccharides, and each contains negatively charged carboxylate and/or sulfate esters. Accordingly, the three major families of proteoglycans are (1) chondroitin sulfate proteoglycans, (2) dermatan sulfate proteoglycans, and (3) heparan sulfate proteoglycans (HSPGs). However, only the first two are present in increased amounts in atherosclerotic tissue (HSPGs are actually decreased in number). Proteoglycans are of particular importance because of their high affinity for LDL, which increases the retention of this lipoprotein in the arterial intima, especially once it is oxidized.

The binding interaction between LDLs and proteoglycans is electrostatic in nature. LDLs are large, spherical particles consisting of a single apolipoprotein B (apo B) molecule embedded in a surface of phospholipid surrounding a core of cholesteryl ester and triglyceride. The numerous positively charged amino groups of apo B can interact

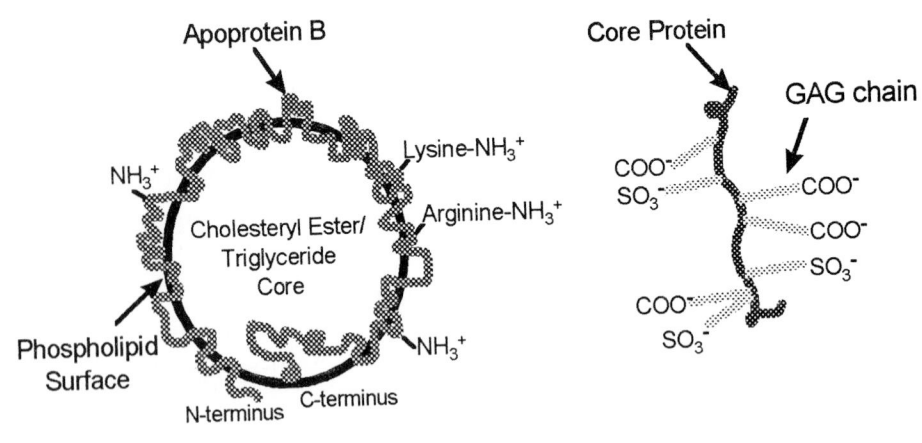

Figure 34-3 Schematic showing the electrostatic nature of the interaction between low-density lipoprotein (LDL) and proteoglycans. Proteoglycans bind LDL via charge-mediated interactions that occur between the positively charged amino groups on the apoprotein B molecule of LDL and the negatively charged sulfate or carboxylate esters on the glycosaminoglycan (GAG) chains of proteoglycans.

with the negatively charged carboxylate and/or sulfate esters of proteoglycans.

OXIDATIVE MODIFICATION OF LIPOPROTEINS

According to the response-to-retention hypothesis, lipoprotein oxidation is an expected consequence of lipoprotein retention and, perforce, increased residence time in the arterial intima. The oxidation of LDLs is a free radical–driven lipid peroxidation chain reaction (Figure 34-4). The process begins when an initiating free radical removes a hydrogen atom from one of the polyunsaturated fatty acids in an LDL lipid. This free radical is generally a reactive oxygen species (e.g., superoxide, hydrogen peroxide, or the hydroxyl radical) potentially generated by a variety of essential metabolic pathways such as electron transport and phagocytosis. The newly generated lipid radical can in turn react with molecular oxygen to generate a lipid peroxyl radical. This radical can then remove a hydrogen atom from another lipid molecule, generating a lipid

Reaction 1: Initiation

$$LH + X^{\cdot} \rightarrow L^{\cdot} + XH$$

Reaction 2: Addition of molecular oxygen

$$L^{\cdot} + O_2 \rightarrow LOO^{\cdot}$$

Reaction 3: Propagation

$$LOO^{\cdot} + LH \rightarrow LOOH + L^{\cdot}$$

Figure 34-4 Schematic of the major events occurring during low-density lipoprotein (LDL) oxidation. LH is any lipid containing a polyunsaturated fatty acid. X®MDSU = X• is any free radical, usually a reactive oxygen species, that can remove a hydrogen atom from LH. L®MDSU = L• is a carbon-centered lipid radical. LOO®MDSU = LOO• is a lipid peroxyl radical. LOOH is a lipid hydroperoxide.

hydroperoxide and a new lipid radical. This chain reaction is self-propagating, and a single initiating event can generate a significant amount of lipid hydroperoxide.

The net amount of lipid hydroperoxide that accumulates depends on the free radical–scavenging capacity of the host's antioxidant defense system, which consists of both enzyme and molecular antioxidants. Enzyme antioxidants, such as catalase, superoxide dismutase, and glutathione peroxidase, act by scavenging specific activated oxygen species. Molecular antioxidants, such as ascorbic acid (vitamin C), α-tocopherol (vitamin E), and β-carotene, act in a more general manner to prevent the propagation of free radicals. HDLs also have a considerable capacity for binding oxidized lipids (representing another antiatherogenic role of HDLs in addition to their contribution to reverse cholesterol transport).

On the basis of a variety of in vitro studies (summarized in Table 34-1), oxidatively modified LDL is believed to be injurious and proatherogenic. In vitro, LDL complexed to proteoglycans is more susceptible to oxidative modification. This oxidized LDL is rapidly internalized by macrophages, which at low levels might enhance the clearance of oxidized lipids and lipoproteins. On the other hand, if this internalization becomes excessive, lipid accumulation and foam cell formation may ensue. Furthermore, oxidized LDL has numerous biological effects in vitro, such as stimulation of monocyte adhesion, chemotaxis, activation and differentiation, and regulation of several growth factor and cytokine genes that may be involved in atherogenesis.

These in vitro studies are supported by evidence that lipoprotein oxidation does occur in vivo and is likely to play an important role in atherogenesis in humans: (1) LDL extracted from atherosclerotic lesions has physical and biological properties similar to those of LDL oxidized in vitro; (2) antibodies generated against oxidized LDL recognize epitopes in atherosclerotic lesions but not in normal arterial tissue; (3) oxidized lipids are found in atherosclerotic tissue; (4) circulating autoantibodies to epitopes of oxidized LDL have been reported; and (5) epidemiologic

Table 34-1   Potential Mechanisms by Which Oxidized LDL may be Atherogenic

Stimulates macrophage foam cell formation

Chemotactic for monocytes

Activates monocytes

Regulates endothelial adhesion molecules

Stimulates smooth muscle cell proliferation

Cytotoxicity

Regulates growth factors and cytokines in vascular cells

Immunogenicity

Alters coagulation pathways by tissue factor and platelet activation

Regulates vascular tone

LDL, low-density lipoprotein.

studies show an inverse relationship between dietary intake of antioxidants or serum levels of antioxidants and the prevalence of CHD.

ATHEROSCLEROSIS IN DISORDERS OF ACCELERATED AGING AND METABOLISM

As a time-related process, atherosclerotic and disease risk increase with age, in part because it generally takes a long time for lesions to develop. The effects of years of exposure to environmental and lifestyle factors (such as a lipid-rich diet and consequently an increased LDL/HDL ratio) and intrinsic aging processes (such as loss of the ability to repair damage from oxidative processes) combine with as yet undiscovered genetic factors to result in the gradual progression of atherosclerotic lesions according to the pathogenetic sequence described above.

As previously noted, genetic metabolic alteration may accelerate atherogenesis and result in premature clinical expression of this time- and age-related process. Alternatively, genetic and metabolic alterations that fundamentally accelerate the aging process per se may produce premature atherosclerosis as part of a progeroid syndrome. Such conditions, for example, Werner's syndrome, provide a caricature of the interaction between aging and atherogenesis that lends insight into the more normal association between the two.

WERNER'S SYNDROME

Werner's syndrome is a very rare autosomal recessive disease of premature aging (progeria) that produces a characteristic "aged phenotype" that begins at a relatively young

age. This phenotype includes the premature onset of several age-related diseases, including diabetes mellitus and atherosclerosis. Prominent atherosclerosis has been observed in most cases, and the majority of deaths, usually by the fourth decade, are attributed directly to CVD. The anatomic findings of extensive atherosclerosis and calcification of the aorta and coronary arteries are similar to those associated with aging (albeit in normal persons of far more advanced age).

Several defects have been described that might account for the accelerated development of atherosclerosis in Werner's syndrome. Among these are hyperlipidemia (with elevated triglyceride levels), hyperinsulinemia, and hypercoagulability (due to increased amounts of tissue plasminogen activator and decreased levels of thrombomodulin). Defects in lipoprotein metabolism by macrophages have also been found. The abnormal accumulation of cholesteryl ester (due to enhanced cellular uptake, lyosomal hydrolysis, and reesterification of free cholesterol) may cause accelerated conversion of macrophages to lipid-laden foam cells in Werner's syndrome.

The gene responsible for Werner's syndrome has been identified, the protein product of which is a helicase. Such enzymes are involved in unwinding DNA, a process required for DNA transcription, repair, replication, and recombination. Mutations in this gene product lead to defects in DNA metabolism or inefficient repair of damaged DNA. It is well known that oxidation causes DNA damage, as well as the lipid and protein damage described above. Thus, the inability of helicase to repair oxidatively damaged DNA might also contribute to the accelerated atherosclerotic development seen in Werner's syndrome.

DIABETES MELLITUS

Diabetes mellitus (see also Chapter 67) is a far more common and more general model of accelerated aging that is also associated with an increased rate of atherogenesis and risk of atherosclerotic CVD. Diabetes and atherosclerosis are strongly linked, particularly in elderly patients. Atherosclerosis associated with aging is more extensive and accelerated in diabetes, and the majority of deaths in patients with type 2 diabetes are attributable to atherosclerosis (and its macrovascular complications). With or without the development of frank type 2 diabetes, impaired glucose tolerance is also a predisposing factor for atherosclerosis, and age is a significant factor in the frequent decline in glucose tolerance seen in older persons. Common features that may be important to the development of accelerated atherosclerosis in type 2 diabetes are dyslipoproteinemia, hypertension, and a hypercoagulable state. The direct toxic effects of glucose may also play a role.

All these factors are commonly linked via decreased sensitivity to insulin and are clinically expressed in the "metabolic syndrome," which is a subject of intense contemporary interest as diabetes increasingly becomes an issue in CVD at all ages but especially in elderly people. This syndrome also includes increased hepatic triglyceride accumulation and obesity, which itself diminishes insulin sensitivity and is accentuated by the increase in adipose tissue that accompanies aging. This syndrome is especially likely to emerge when such acquired adiposity is concentrated centrally in the upper body in the "apple-shaped" or "android" distribution. A more detailed discussion of aging and adiposity is provided in Chapter 91.

DYSLIPOPROTEINEMIA IN DIABETES

The dyslipoproteinemia that occurs in diabetes is characterized by abnormal composition and metabolism of all classes of lipoproteins. It includes hypertriglyceridemia, low levels of HDL-C, and alterations in the composition of all lipoprotein classes that might affect their function. Hypertriglyceridemia is related, at least in part, to the degree of insulin deficiency (lipoprotein lipase is an insulin-dependent enzyme), hence varies with the degree of diabetic control. Diabetic hypertriglyceridemia is also associated with a shift in the size distribution of very low-density lipoprotein (VLDL) particles toward smaller, denser particles, some of which may be atherogenic remnants of the precursor triglyceride-rich lipoproteins. The mechanism by which hypertriglyceridemia increases the risk of atherosclerosis in patients with diabetes is complex, but it might be related to increased cellular cholesterol uptake from these smaller, denser remnant lipoprotein particles. Also, HDL-C levels are inversely related to triglyceride concentrations (in both diabetic and nondiabetic patients), and because triglyceride levels are often increased in diabetic patients, their HDL levels are frequently low, especially those of the more cholesterol-rich, antiatherogenic HDL_2 particles. LDL-C levels are not usually increased in diabetes. However, the composition of the LDL particles is altered, with an increase in small, dense, more atherogenic LDLs (versus larger, buoyant LDLs). The increased cellular uptake and matrix binding or oxidative modification of these particles also might explain the association of small, dense LDLs with increased atherosclerosis in the general population.

Whereas all these alterations in lipoprotein metabolism are most apparent in persons with frank diabetes, they are often present (though to a somewhat lesser degree) in patients with the metabolic syndrome who do not yet manifest hyperglycemia of a magnitude conferring a diagnosis of diabetes.

HYPERTENSION IN DIABETES

Hypertension is a risk factor for the development of atherosclerosis in nondiabetic as well as in diabetic patients and frequently precedes the advent of glucose intolerance in those with insulin resistance and the metabolic syndrome. However, hypertension occurs yet more commonly in subjects with frank type 2 diabetes. Chronically elevated blood pressure may promote atherosclerosis by several mechanisms: (1) altering the permeability of the endothelium of blood vessels, thus facilitating increased lipoprotein transport into the arterial wall; (2) stimulating smooth muscle cell proliferation and synthesis of extracellular matrix molecules, leading to thickening of the arterial wall; and (3) changing vasoreactivity.

HYPERGLYCEMIA IN DIABETES

Mechanisms of atherogenesis related to impaired glucose tolerance and hyperglycemia also include modifications of lipoproteins and other proteins by nonenzymatic glycation and increased oxidation. Evidence for lipoprotein glycation in vivo includes (1) demonstration of a twofold increase in glycated apo B in LDL from subjects with diabetes and (2) the finding that the extent of glycation of LDL is correlated with other indicators of glycemic control such as mean plasma glucose and total plasma protein glycation.

Mechanisms by which glycated LDL might be atherogenic have been explored in vitro. Glycation of LDL reduces its ability to bind to the classic LDL receptor in most cells, leading to a reduced rate of catabolism and hence an increased residence time in plasma and, potentially, increased LDL oxidation. In addition, LDL modified by advanced glycation end product (AGE) is chemotactic for monocytes and is taken up by specific AGE receptors on macrophages, resulting in the stimulation of several cytokines that may promote the atherosclerotic process.

The glycation of other proteins in diabetes might also contribute to atherogenesis via several different mechanisms that impact cellular function. Glycated albumin leads to albuminuria and endothelial cell dysfunction; glycated red blood cell membranes are less deformable; glycated HDL is less able to transport cholesterol out of cells; glycated collagen stimulates platelet aggregation; and glycated fibrin and platelet membranes negatively affect vascular homeostasis.

Oxidative modification of LDL also plays an important role in atherogenesis, as discussed earlier. There are several ways in which LDL oxidation might be accelerated in diabetes: (1) Protein glycation generates reactive oxygen species such as superoxide, which can initiate oxidative processes; (2) glucose can autoxidize, resulting in the generation of reactive oxygen species such as hydrogen peroxide or the highly reactive hydroxyl radical, which can oxidatively modify LDL; and (3) the small, dense LDL particles that are prominent in patients with type 2 diabetes and the metabolic syndrome are more susceptible to oxidative modification than LDL from insulin-sensitive nondiabetic patients.

ATHEROGENESIS AND NORMAL AGING

All the atherogenic processes described above in diabetes occur in nondiabetic patients as well, although they generally proceed at a slower pace. This is seen in the population changes in atherogenic risk factors that begin in childhood and progress with increasing age. They are described in greater detail in chapters that focus on hypertension (Chapter 40), dyslipoproteinemia (Chapter 68), diabetes (Chapter 67), gender differences in longevity

(Chapter 97) and, in the most general sense, preventive gerontology (Chapter 6). Thus even as atherogenesis is an aging- and time-related process, many of the forces that accelerate this process are themselves aging- and time-related. Average blood pressure levels rise progressively beyond adolescence, and the incidence of hypertension accordingly increases with advancing age, especially systolic hypertension, which rises exponentially in old age. Similarly, population mean and especially postglucose challenge blood glucose levels rise progressively with advancing age, and the incidence of glucose intolerance and frank diabetes grows. Lipid levels and distributions change following adolescence, with average LDL-C values rising progressively until about age 50 in men and age 60 in women (the mean LDL-C level in men exceeding that in women until menopause, when a crossover occurs). However, HDL-C levels are lower in males than in females from puberty through old age, both alterations presumably reflecting the effect of physiologic estrogen and androgen secretion on lipoprotein metabolism at different ages.

Apart from alterations attributable to sex hormone changes, these trends with increasing age appear to be mediated importantly by the increase in population mean adipose mass that characterizes aging in Western societies and the associated reduction in insulin sensitivity (though it is important to note that similar changes also occur in other aging species, notably rodents and nonhuman primates with ad libitum feeding patterns). Thus, contemporary worldwide changes in eating behavior and caloric expenditure are likely to accelerate age-related atherogenesis as well as the incidence of age-related risk factors. Ironically, even the current movement toward a reduction in smoking may contribute to these trends as the effect of nicotine in decreasing adiposity becomes less prevalent; however, the net effects of widespread smoking cessation should still be markedly positive in reducing both atherogenesis and oncogenesis.

DETECTION AND DIAGNOSIS OF ATHEROSCLEROSIS IN ELDERLY PATIENTS

Details of the detection and diagnosis of atherosclerosis are well addressed in other chapters in this section and in the contemporary literature on cardiology. Technologic advances made in the past several decades have allowed the detection of atherosclerosis by both invasive and noninvasive methods at ever earlier stages of the disease process in adults of all ages. This trend has been powerfully reinforced by the demonstrated efficacy of both mechanical and pharmacologic (as well as lifestyle) interventions that can treat and even prevent atherosclerosis and its complications. Together with the progressive aging of the population and the predicted increase in its age-associated atherosclerotic burden, these developments ensure that the diagnosis and management of CVD in the elderly population will consume a substantial proportion of health care resources in the coming decades.

The magnitude of this age-associated atherosclerotic burden was demonstrated in the recent (and ongoing)

Cardiovascular Health Study (CHS), a 10+–year, population-based, cross-sectional and longitudinal study of CVD in four American communities involving more than 6000 subjects older than 65 years (65–101 years old, with two-thirds 65–74 years old and 4% older than 85 years). As reported by Psaty et al, this study suggests that in the United States nearly 80 percent of men and two-thirds of women older than 65 years have atherosclerotic CVD either clinically, or subclinically by noninvasive evaluation (electrocardiography, carotid ultrasonography, and echocardiography). Moreover, in this study subclinical CVD was as powerful in predicting future clinical events as clinical disease was (as well as was its absence in predicting the absence of clinical events, i.e., continued freedom from CVD for an average of 5 years of follow-up). The CHS confirmed the value of traditional risk factors (with the exception of LDL-C, which was predictive only at high levels). However, all such risk factors, alone or in combination, were less powerful in predicting future events than the presence, at entry, of clinical or subclinical atherosclerotic CVD.

THE PREVENTION AND TREATMENT OF ATHEROSCLEROSIS IN ELDERLY PATIENTS

The relative contributions of traditional risk factor assessment, application of noninvasive technologies (including carotid ultrasound, echocardiography, electron beam spiral computed tomography [CT] for the detection of coronary calcification, and intravascular ultrasound for the evaluation of coronary anatomy and plaque configuration and composition), and invasive approaches to coronary and extracoronary atherosclerosis detection and management remain controversial in the elderly population . However, regardless of the approach selected, the importance of CVD in aging (of the population and of the individual) will become paramount as the number and average age of elderly individuals increases.

An example is the approach to decision analysis regarding the use of lipid-lowering strategies recommended by the National Cholesterol Education Program Adult Treatment Panel III (NCEP-ATP III) released in 2001. This latest version of the NCEP guidelines recommends employing data from the Framingham Heart Study to formulate individualized lipid-lowering treatment decisions, with lower LDL-C goals (<100 mg/dL) for those whose estimated 10-year risk of CVD events is 20 percent or more (including those with existing clinical coronary or noncoronary CVD and all with diabetes) (Chapter 68). These data from Framingham clearly underscore the dominant role of age (and, less so, gender) in the treatment decision, with aggressive lipid lowering recommended for virtually all men and most women 80 years or older—even as the contribution of LDL-C levels to risk declines to near zero.

The irony and paradox of this circumstance cannot escape the attention of any thoughtful clinician who contemplates preventive CVD intervention in any given elderly patient. While the risk of CVD in the elderly population rises exponentially with age, the risk attributable to

LDL remains stable or declines with age, and yet agents, notably statins, that lower LDL seem efficacious in studies on both primary and secondary CVD prevention that have included subjects older than age 65. The association of statin use with decreased CVD incidence was also reported from the CHS which, as noted above, failed to identify LDL-C as a risk factor except at high levels. This paradox underscores the likelihood, currently under active investigation, that statins may lower risk by a mechanism related only in part to their lipid-lowering actions (perhaps through an anti-inflammatory effect).

This paradox also illustrates the dilemma faced by clinicians who care for elderly patients and their historically wide practice variation in CVD prevention and treatment in these individuals. These issues are addressed in detail elsewhere in this volume in the chapters related to specific domains of CVD and risk factor management. Here we shall summarize the factors that contribute to (and perhaps justify) this inconsistency, all of which underscore the need for well-designed, formal studies involving persons who by virtue of their age and burden of age-associated disease and degree of frailty might be considered "truly geriatric" (generally at least older than 75 years).

1. Few studies to date have been designed explicitly to examine elderly patients in appropriate numbers with a degree of complexity that is truly representative of such a population. Patients with "limited life expectancy" (generally, however, without explicit criteria for such assignment), competing major threats to survival or independence, cognitive dysfunction, or insufficient social support and functional capacity that would hinder full participation and compliance have generally been excluded from clinical trials (explicitly or implicitly). This exclusion has especially been applied to subjects who reside in long-term-care institutions, persons who comprise a substantial proportion of patients cared for by geriatric clinicians who focus their care on older persons.

2. Although many studies reported to date on CVD prevention have included a significant fraction of subjects older than 65 years, these studies have not been explicitly designed or analyzed to examine the efficacy of interventions in subgroups of older patients as classified by, for example, age or functional status. Instead the "elderly" population has generally been considered a single homogeneous group (although advancing age is generally associated with increasing heterogeneity). And when the ages of enrollees have been presented in such studies, participants are generally found to be concentrated at the lower end of the above-65 age spectrum, with few older than 75 years and even fewer older than 80 or 85 years. Thus conclusions (and consequently recommendations) regarding elderly individuals have generally been based on extrapolations from results obtained from studies on persons of middle age and on smaller "young-old" groups of participants.

3. These limitations have led to acknowledgment (in NCEP-ATP III, for example) that the treatment of older patients may require more complex clinical judgment, with due attention to issues of patient social and functional status, comorbidities, competing risks of morbidity and mortality, and risks and costs of drugs and other interventions that make decision making more complex in treating the elderly patient.

Despite these limitations, nihilism regarding CVD prevention in elderly people cannot be justified any more than an unthinkingly aggressive approach can. Indeed, the data acquired to this point regarding prevention, detection, and treatment of atherosclerotic CVD in the truly elderly population are in general most promising, most notably in the treatment of hypertension (e.g., the SHEP study) but more recently in studies on other risk indices as well. This information is detailed in other chapters in this text and has been well summarized in a report on CVD databases on elderly patients by Cheitlin et al. Most studies to date—whether clinical trials, case-control studies, or clinical reports—have generated positive reports regarding the safety and efficacy of treatments in older patients, with no clear upper age limit beyond which net benefit is lost. And lending a sense of urgency to the belief that effective CVD prevention in even the oldest and most frail patients is an issue of high priority are the all too familiar devastating consequences following a stroke or myocardial infarction, which may trigger a tragic, downhill, unstoppable cascade of progressive frailty, dependency, and death.

Thus at least cautious optimism seems justified in approaching atherosclerotic CVD prevention and treatment at all ages and all evolutionary stages, for it seems likely that carefully designed, well-executed studies will yield further advances in prevention and management of CVD in even the oldest segments of the population.

REFERENCES

Berliner JA: The role of oxidized lipoproteins in atherogenesis. *Free Radic Biol Med* 20:707, 1996.

Camejo G: Proteoglycans and lipoproteins in atherosclerosis. *Curr Opin Lipidol* 4:385, 1993.

Chait, A, Bierman EL: Pathogenesis of macrovascular disease in diabetes, in Bussy RK (ed): *Joslin's Diabetes Mellitus*, 13th ed. Malvern, PA, Lea and Febiger, 1993.

Cheitlin MD, Geistenblith G et al: Do existing databases answer clinical questions about geriatric CVD and stroke? *Am J Geriatr Cardiol* 10:207, 2001.

Cheitlin MD, Gerstenblith G et al: Executive summary of the third report of the National Cholesterol Education Program (NCEP) expert panel on detection, evaluation, and treatment of high blood cholesterol in adults (adult treatment panel III). *JAMA* 285;2486, 2001.

Corti MC: Lipoprotein alterations and atherosclerosis in the elderly. *Curr Opin Lipidol* 8:236, 1997.

Gray MD: The Werner syndrome protein is a DNA helicase. *Nat Genet* 17:100, 1997.

Jackson, RL: Glycosaminoglycans: Molecular properties, protein interactions, and role in physiological processes. *Physiol Rev* 71:481, 1991.

Lemaitre, RN, Psaty, BM et al: Therapy with hydroxymethylglutaryl coenzyme A reductase inhibitors (statins) and associated risk on incident cardiovascular events in older adults: Evidence from the Cardiovascular Health Study. *Arch Intern Med* 162:1395, 2002.

Lopes-Virella MF: Modification of lipoproteins in diabetes. *Diabetes Metab Rev* 12:69, 1996.

Munford, RS: Statins and the acute phase response. *N Engl J Med* 2010, 2001.

Psaty BM, Furberg CD et al: Traditional risk factors and subclinical disease measures as predictors of first myocardial infarction in older adults: The Cardiovascular Health Study. *Arch Intern Med* 159:1339, 1999.

Reaven PD: The role of oxidation of LDL in atherogenesis. *Endocrinologist* 5:44, 1995.

Ross R, Fuster V: The pathogenesis of atherosclerosis, in Fuster V et al (eds): *Atherosclerosis and Coronary Artery Disease.* Philadelphia, PA: Lippincott-Raven, 1996.

Vokonas PS: Diabetes mellitus and coronary heart disease in the elderly. *Clin Geriatr Med* 12:69, 1996.

Williams KJ: The response-to-retention hypothesis of early atherogenesis. *Arterioscler Thromb Vasc Biol* 15:551, 1995.

Wolff SP: Protein glycation and oxidative stress in diabetes mellitus and ageing. *Free Radic Biol Med* 10:339, 1991.

Coronary Heart Disease

ERIC PETERSON • DANIEL R. BENSIMHON

Coronary heart disease (CHD) is the leading killer of both men and women in the United States. And with the growth of our elderly population, the prevalence of CHD has now reached epidemic proportions. Improvements in preventing premature coronary disease and treating existing CHD, while certainly welcome, have further fueled the epidemic of CHD in the elderly. So while those aged 65 years or older constitute only 13 percent of the US population, they account for more than 60 percent of all acute myocardial infarctions (MIs) and 85 percent of all MI deaths. Similarly, persons aged 75 years or older make up 6 percent of the population, but account for 34 percent of MIs and 45 percent of all MI deaths.

Given these statistics, it is important for all MD's to understand the major issues relevant to the appropriate diagnosis and treatment of elderly patients with CHD. While many definitions have been used for the term, "elderly," for the purpose of this chapter, we will define "elderly" as those age 75 yrs or older unless otherwise specified. While many of the care strategies for CHD are similar in young and old patients, there are age-related differences that must be appreciated. These include differences in disease presentation, changes in drug pharmacokinetics, more complex disease management due to comorbid illness, and finally, differences in patients' health expectations and preferences for care relative to those in younger patients. As a result, when treating an elderly patient with known or suspected CHD, heavy emphasis must be placed on creating a *patient-centered* plan of care.

EFFECTS OF AGING ON THE CARDIOVASCULAR SYSTEM (SEE ALSO CHAPS. 33 AND 34)

The development of CHD is multifactorial and can be influenced by genetic predisposition and comorbid conditions such as diabetes, as well as by environmental and lifestyle determinants such as diet, smoking, and physical exercise. Not surprisingly, as these factors vary among individuals, one's likelihood for developing CHD also varies. While it is often believed that CHD is inevitable with advancing age, autopsy studies have found that 40 percent of those persons in their nineties will not have occlusive coronary disease. Thus, the *chronologic* age of a patient tends to be a poor surrogate for the *physiologic* age of his or her vascular system.

With this patient-to-patient variability noted, certain cardiovascular changes are seen more commonly with advancing age. Damage to the endothelium accumulates and results in increasing numbers and severity of atherosclerotic plaques (Fig. 35-1). The composition of these lesions also changes with age, with reduction in the soft lipid core, and an increase in calcification and fibrosis. While more advanced calcified plaques are actually less likely to rupture, the sheer increase in lesion numbers leads to an increased overall likelihood for CHD events in the elderly patient.

When a plaque ruptures, platelets and thrombin aggregate at the site, forming a thrombus. If the clot completely occludes the vessel, the patient suffers an acute MI and an injury pattern (e.g., ST elevation) is often seen on the electrocardiogram (ECG). In contrast, patients with plaque rupture can also form a nonocclusive thrombus resulting in subendocardial myocardial ischemia. These patients often have an acceleration of chest pain symptoms (unstable angina) and may have more subtle changes on the ECG (e.g., flipped T waves or ST depression). Longer-term, the ruptured plaque tends to heal but may leave the patient with a flow-limiting stenosis and symptoms of chronic angina. As occlusive disease progresses, coronary flow reserve is lost and an elderly patient becomes at risk for *demand ischemia*, where myocardial damage can occur during periods of high oxygen requirement such as a gastrointestinal (GI) bleed, infection, severe exertion, or major physiologic stressor.

While these cardiac conditions are described as separate diagnoses, they should be appreciated as a continuous spectrum. Thus, CHD is best viewed as a chronic disorder, punctuated by exacerbations (plaque ruptures/demand ischemia) interspersed between longer quiescent periods. It is this uneven nature of the disease that makes it very difficult for clinicians to predict future CHD events.

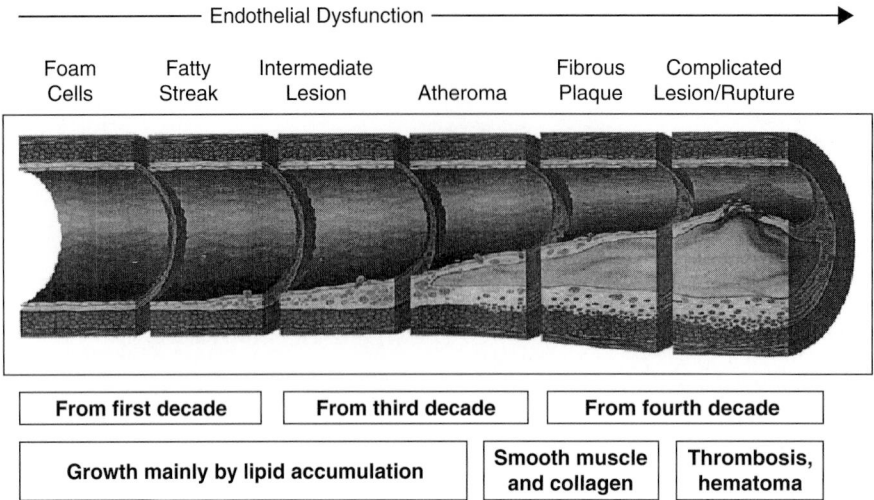

Figure 35-1   Atherosclerosis timeline. Reproduced with permission from Stary et al: *Circulation* 92:1355, 1995.

PREVALENCE

The spectrum of CHD includes asymptomatic (or subclinical) coronary heart disease, chronic stable angina pectoris, unstable angina, and acute MI. In the United States, the prevalence of overt CHD increases in a curvilinear fashion with advancing age in both men and women (Fig. 35-2). Similarly, the annual rate of first heart attack rises with age in all race and gender subgroups. Thus, despite the fact that women typically have a 10-year lag in developing CHD as compared to men, the majority of CHD patients ≥75 years of age or older are women because they typically have a longer life span.

It should also be realized that overt CHD represents just the tip of the coronary disease iceberg and a great number of elderly patients have asymptomatic, subclinical disease. Using a composite measure of MI on ECG or echocardiography and abnormal carotid artery wall thickness or ankle–brachial blood pressure index, researchers for the Cardiovascular Health Study examined the prevalence of both clinical and subclinical cardiovascular disease in a large community-dwelling Medicare population. They found that disease frequency increased from 22 percent in women aged 65 to 70 years to 43 percent in those aged 85 years or older. Similarly, the frequency of subclinical vascular disease in men increased from 33 to 45 percent in these age groups, respectively.

PRESENTATION

The initial manifestation of CHD can change dramatically with age. The elderly are much less likely than younger patients to present with "classic" exertional chest heaviness. Instead, older patients more often complain of a vague feeling of dyspnea, abdominal pain, fatigue, confusion, or malaise that may be misinterpreted as consequences of

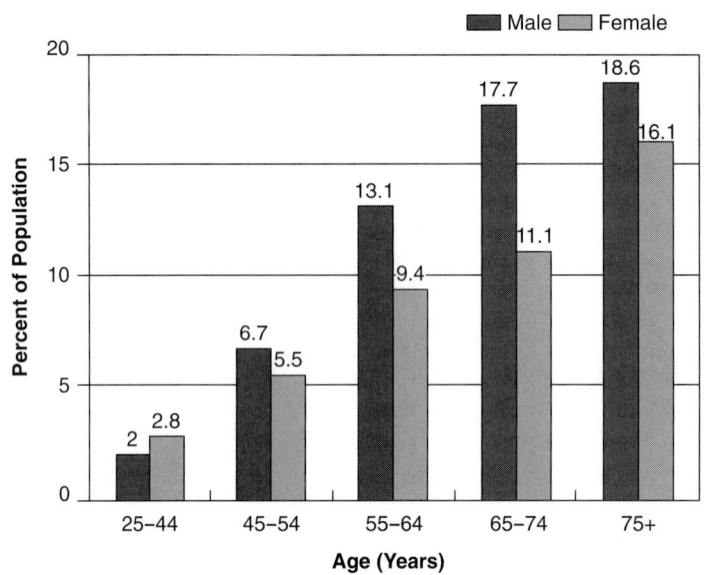

Figure 35-2   Estimated prevalence of coronary heart disease by age and sex in the United States, 1988 to 1994. Reproduced with permission from Vargas et al: *Ann Epidemiol* 7:523, 1997.

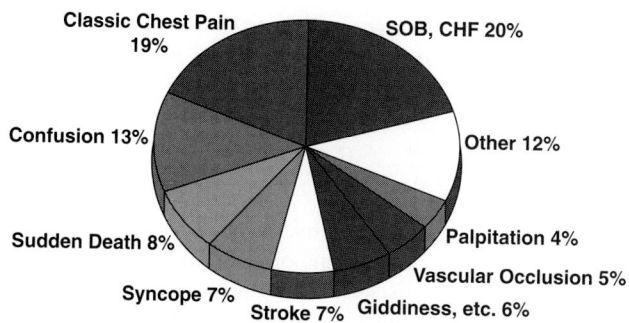

Figure 35-3 Presenting symptoms of acute MI (age >80 years). CHF, congestive heart failure, SOB, shortness of breath. Reproduced with permission from Pathy, *Br Heart J,* 1967.

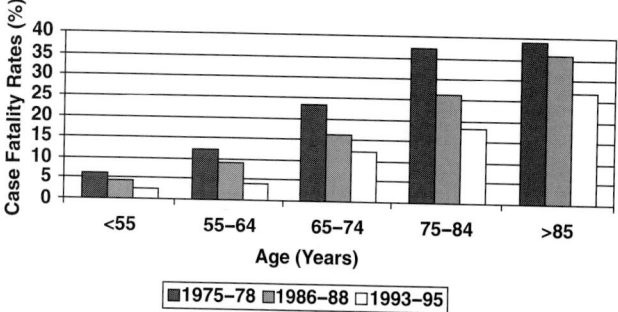

Figure 35-4 Trends in hospital MI mortality by age group.

aging or other comorbid illness (Fig. 35-3). The elderly can also have an impaired ischemia warning system that delays their CHD presentation. In a series of CHD patients undergoing treadmill testing, researchers found that patients aged >70 years took more than twice as long as their younger counterparts to report anginal symptoms after ECG-documented ischemia was noted. Finally, comorbid illnesses such as pulmonary disease, arthritis, or claudication can reduce an elderly patient's functional capacity and mask CHD until a more advanced stage.

Difficulty in recognizing symptoms contributes to later presentation for acute CHD events in the elderly. In fact, studies show that over two-thirds of MI patients >65 years of age fail to reach an emergency room within 6 hours after the onset of their symptoms. Major predictors of a delay in MI presentation include advanced age, female sex, diabetes mellitus, and social isolation. Importantly, delays in MI presentation have strong prognostic implications and are closely associated with poorer outcomes in elderly patients. Thus, clinicians should proactively discuss with their patients that cardiac symptoms can vary widely and they should seek rapid medical attention if potential ischemic symptoms occur.

PROGNOSIS

Multiple studies document that once CHD is manifested, the risk of morbidity and mortality increase steadily with age. In two very large randomized trials of MI patients with ST elevation, age was the single strongest predictor of both short- and long-term mortality, with the risk of death increasing 6 percent with each year of age. In another large registry population, patients aged 65 to 74 years admitted for an MI were four times more likely to die during the hospitalization than those aged 55 or younger (Fig. 35-4). This risk rose to greater than 10 times higher for patients ≥85 years old. Elderly patients are also much more likely to suffer complications from their MI, including heart failure, cardiogenic shock, atrial fibrillation, stroke, acute renal insufficiency, and pneumonia. Finally, patients aged ≥75 years were three times more likely to be discharged to a nursing facility after an acute MI than were those patients aged 65 to 69 years.

The reasons for increasing MI mortality and morbidity as a function of advancing age are multifold. Elderly patients have less cardiac reserve and more comorbid illness (e.g., pulmonary, renal, cognitive impairment), limiting their ability to compensate for cardiac events. Additionally, the elderly MI patients present later, often receives less aggressive medical care, and undergoes fewer potentially life-saving invasive procedures than younger patients.

DIAGNOSTIC EVALUATION

Given its prevalence and often atypical presentation in the elderly, clinicians must harbor a high index of suspicion for CHD in order to make the correct diagnosis. In taking a thorough clinical history, including to history of previous cardiovascular disease, clinicians must pay close attention to assessing a patient's major cardiac risk factors (smoking, hypertension, diabetes mellitus, lipid status), as well as any symptoms suggestive of CHD. Eliciting the temporal course of these symptoms is also important. Patients with new, progressive, or refractory symptoms typically require an expedited—and possibly inpatient—work-up, in contrast to those patients with chronic stable symptoms. Physicians should also assess the impact of symptoms on the patient's functional status and overall quality of life, as these issues may alter preferences for invasive testing and/or need for coronary revascularization.

The physical exam can provide further clues to the presence of CHD. This may include signs of left- or right-sided heart failure (pulmonary edema, displaced point of maximal impulse, an S3 gallop, mitral regurgitation, or peripheral edema) and those of concomitant vascular disease (carotid, abdominal, or femoral bruits, loss of lower extremity hair, or other ischemic dermatologic changes). Once a thorough history and physical are completed, further diagnostic evaluation should be based on the patient's symptoms as outlined below.

Asymptomatic Elderly Patients

For the asymptomatic elderly individual, risk factors (including blood pressure and lipid screening) should be measured as recommended for all aged patients in the Joint National Committee on Detection, Evaluation and Treatment of High Blood Pressure (JNC) VI and National Cholesterol Education Program (NCEP)–Adult Treatment Panel (ATP) III guidelines (see Chaps. 40 and 68). Obtaining a baseline ECG is also reasonable in the initial patient evaluation because of the high prevalence of "silent" MIs in the elderly population. This information should be summarized into a composite risk assessment using one of the multiple standardized indexes such as the Framingham Risk Score (http://www.nhlbi.nih.gov/about/framingham/riskabs.htm).

Patients with low CHD risk (10-year CHD risk <5 percent) can generally be reassured without further testing, with a plan for reevaluation of their risk factors in 5 years. In contrast, high-risk patients (10-year CHD risk >20 percent) should receive aggressive risk factor intervention to the same degree as if they had already experienced an overt CHD event. Intermediate risk patients (10-year CHD risk, 5 to 20 percent) may benefit from further testing to clarify their CHD risk. In these intermediate patients, laboratory studies including homocysteine, lipoprotein (a), and, most recently, C-reactive protein have been proposed as means of identifying those at higher risk and in need for more aggressive risk-factor modification. However the roles of those "newer risk factors" have yet to be clearly elucidated. Beyond the standard history, physical exam, and simple lab tests, further diagnostic testing (ankle–brachial indices, carotid ultrasound, treadmill tests, echocardiography, or electron-beam computed tomography [CT]) in the asymptomatic elderly patient to detect occult or subclinical CHD remains controversial and is not generally recommended.

Chronic Stable Angina in the Elderly Patient

Elderly patients with symptoms suggestive of CHD should undergo a similar assessment of their likelihood for obstructive coronary disease based on algorithms that take into account symptom characteristics, including angina type (nonanginal, atypical, or typical), its course (stable, progressive, unstable), and its duration (Fig. 35-5). This initial assessment of a patient's "pretest probability of disease" should then guide further diagnostic testing. In particular, clinicians need to be cognizant that, according to Bayesian theory, the predictive value of a test is influenced by the disease prevalence in the population tested. For example, clinicians may interpret a negative stress test in a high-risk elderly women (pretest probability of disease 80 percent) as "ruling-out" the presence of CHD, whereas this patient's posttest likelihood remains more than 60 percent (see Table 35-1). For these reasons, elderly patients with high pretest likelihood for coronary disease should be

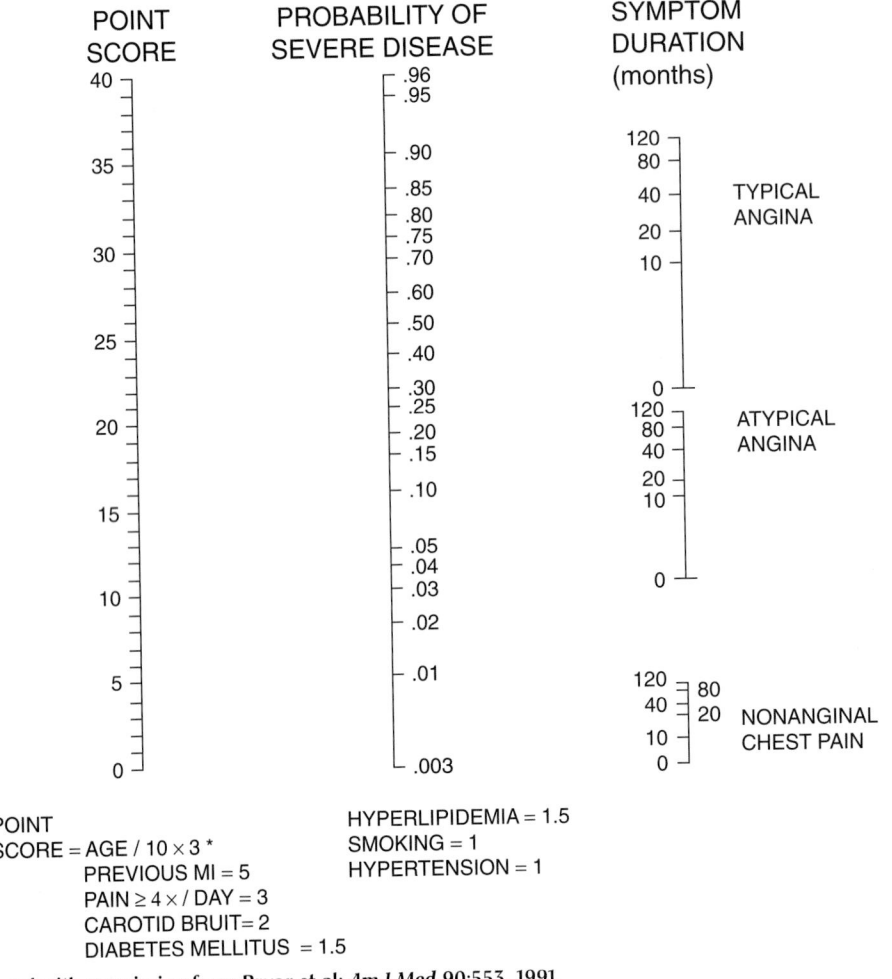

Figure 35-5 Reproduced with permission from Pryor et al: *Am J Med* 90:553, 1991.

Table 35-1 Influence of Age on Predictive Value of Stress Testing (Bayes Theorem)

History	Age (years)	Pretest Likelihood of Significant CAD(%)*	Treadmill Test†	Posttest Likelihood of Significant CAD(%)
Female, typical CP ↑ Lipids	45	30	Positive	56
			Negative	16
	75	80	Positive	92
			Negative	63
Female, atypical CP no RF	45	5	Positive	12
			Negative	3
	75	35	Positive	62
			Negative	18

*Based on the Duke CAD Risk Nomogram (Pryor DB, Ann Intern Med 1993; 118:81–90).

†Sensitivity of treadmill test = 68%, specificity = 77%.

CAD, coronary artery disease; CP, chest pain; RF, risk factors.

considered for direct referral for cardiac catheterization (if revascularization is an appropriate option). At the other extreme, patients with a low pretest probability for CAD <20 percent (i.e., no risk factors, normal ECG, very atypical symptoms), can often be followed clinically and/or be assessed for other etiologies of their symptoms (GI, pulmonary, etc.). Elderly patients with an intermediate pretest probability for CHD (between 20 and 70 percent) are those in whom stress testing tends to have its greatest impact on clinical decision making.

When a stress test is indicated, current guidelines still recommend standard exercise ECG as the test of choice for most patients. These tests provide very important prognostic information (including exercise duration and hemodynamic response), as well as electrocardiographic indications of ischemia (ST depression). Elderly patients, however, frequently experience difficulty with traditional stress-testing protocols because of deconditioning or comorbid illness or disability and may benefit from modified exercise protocols with lower starting levels and slower stage progression. Alternatively, for patients who can't exercise sufficiently, one can use a pharmacologic-based stress test (dobutamine, adenosine, Persantine).

In elderly patients with baseline ECG abnormalities (resting ST depression, left bundle branch block [LBBB], left ventricular hypertrophy [LVH] with strain, or paced rhythms) imaging modalities, such as nuclear perfusion or stress echocardiography, are required. While these modalities significantly add to the cost of the test, they improve the diagnostic accuracy beyond stress ECG alone and provide information as to the location and extent of coronary disease. The published sensitivity and specificity for stress echocardiography and nuclear imaging (80 to 90 percent for each) are nearly identical in most series. Thus, the choice between the two should be based on local availability and expertise.

The use of cardiac catheterization in the elderly patient needs to be based on its potential risk–benefit ratio. While cardiac catheterization has become commonplace and relatively safe in contemporary practice, vascular injury, bleeding, myocardial infarction, stroke, and even mortality can

result, albeit rarely. Advanced age increases these risks slightly; however, the risk to life remains <0.2 percent, and the risk of other serious adverse events is <0.5 percent, even in those aged ≥75 years. Placing a patient even at minimal risk, however, is not worthwhile if the information obtained from a catheterization is unlikely to alter treatment decisions. For example, a cardiac catheterization may have limited impact on the management of an elderly patient who is not a candidate for coronary revascularization, based on medical comorbidity, cognitive decline, or personal preference.

Unstable Angina in the Elderly Patient

Elderly patients who present with ischemic-type symptoms that are rapidly progressive, severe, and refractory, or that occur at rest should be immediately transferred to an emergency care setting for further evaluation. Initial testing for myocardial damage should consist of an ECG and cardiac enzyme or tissue markers. As noted above, however, the ECG in the elderly patient may be difficult to interpret because of baseline abnormalities. As a result of increased sensitivity and specificity, recent care guidelines recommend troponin (I or T) for detection of myocardial damage as compared with creatinine kinase isoforms (CK-MB). However, both CK-MB and troponin assays can be falsely elevated in the elderly patient with renal disease. In such patients, it is often useful to follow serial trends, looking for a typical peak and trough pattern of myocardial injury.

Elderly patients who rule out for MI may need a subsequent evaluation for CHD based on their pretest probability for coronary disease as described previously. Care guidelines recommend that all those diagnosed with an acute MI should have an assessment of both left ventricular function (via echocardiography or other means) and of coronary disease severity. While in the past it had been suggested that "early invasive" (cardiac catheterization) and noninvasive (stress testing) approaches represented equivalent strategies for assessing post-MI patient risk, recent clinical trials

Table 35-2   TACTICS-TIMI 18: Results in Elderly Patients

Age Group (Years)	6-Month Death/MI			
	Number	Relative RR (%)	Absolute RR (Per 1,000 Patients)	NNT to Prevent Event
<55	716	−7	−2	—
55–65	614	18	15	67
65–75	612	27	25	40
>75	278	56	108	9

NNT, number needed to treat; RR, relative risk.

SOURCE: Enhanced benefit of early invasive management of acute coronary syndromes in the elderly: Results from Tactics-Timi 18 arc 104(17); 11–548. Bach RG AHA 2001.

suggest that the early invasive approach might be preferable. Specifically, the Treat Angina with Aggrastat and Determine Cost of Therapy with an Invasive of Conservative Therapy-Thrombolysis in Myocardial Ischemia/Infarction (TACTICS-TIMI) 18 trial, which randomized patients with unstable angina/non-ST elevation MI to one or the other of these strategies, found that those in the early invasive arm (within 48 hours) had nearly 20 percent lower rates of death, nonfatal MI, or rehospitalization at 6 months than did conservatively treated patients. An early invasive strategy was also superior to stress testing in Fast Revascularization during Instability in Coronary Artery Disease (FRISC-II), another randomized trial with similar study design. Importantly, in FRISC-II, 1-year mortality rates were reduced by more than 43 percent in those receiving early invasive therapy. In both trials, the benefits of the early invasive approach were most evident among those at highest risk (e.g., those with positive troponin levels, other high-risk clinical features such as heart failure and ventricular arrhythmias). Preliminary data from the TACTICS trial also demonstrate that the benefits of early intervention were actually accentuated in the elderly relative to younger patients (Table 35-2).

TREATMENT

Because of dramatic advances in medical therapy and percutaneous/surgical revascularization techniques, the death rate from CHD has decreased 24 percent in the last decade alone. In the sections below, a summary of the major age-related issues regarding the safety and efficacy of the available cardiac medications and interventions is provided. However, at the outset it is worth commenting on some general caveats critical to sound decision making in the elderly patient with coronary disease.

Underrepresentation in Clinical Trials

Until very recently, almost all of the national treatment guidelines were based on trials performed predominantly in younger patients, and elderly patients have been routinely and greatly underrepresented. For example, up to 60 percent of cardiovascular (CV) clinical trials performed prior to 1990 explicitly excluded elderly patients. Even among recent studies (i.e., those published since 1995) fewer than 50 percent enrolled a single patient aged 75 years or older.

Altered Pharmacotherapy

Extrapolation of results in younger CHD patients to the elderly patient is potentially fraught with error. A major source of such error can be in the pharmacologic management, since cardiovascular drugs are among the most commonly prescribed in elderly patients. As noted in detail elsewhere (especially in Chap. 19), the elderly can have altered pharmacokinetics (i.e., drug distribution and metabolism [see Chap. 19]). Elderly patients tend to have a smaller volume of distribution and a slower rate of drug clearance than do younger patients. Combined, these factors lead to higher drug concentrations and prolonged half-lives. Dosing for most medications in the elderly patient should, therefore, be initiated at lower doses, dosed less frequently, and be titrated up more slowly than in younger patients.

In addition, pharmacodynamics (i.e., the effect of a drug on a target cell) can be considerably altered with age. For example, increased calcification of the cardiac conduction system can increase an elderly patient's sensitivity to arteriovenous (AV) nodal blocking agents and lead to profound bradycardia. Comorbid illness and frailty can also influence drug selection and safety. For instance, a frail elderly person may have a higher risk of falling, which can markedly increase the likelihood of bleeding complications with anticoagulants. Finally, polypharmacy is often a serious issue in the elderly and can lead to life-threatening drug–drug interactions and poor compliance because of confusion over medications and/or prohibitive costs. It has been estimated that 25 percent of older patients have had at least one adverse drug reaction, and that drug reactions are responsible for 3 to 10 percent of all hospital admissions in the elderly.

Patient Preferences

Beyond physiologic and pharmacologic issues, cardiac treatment plans need to consider the patient's overall heath, as well as his or her health preferences and willingness to accept risk. While some elderly individuals engage in very active, independent lives well into their advanced years, others are frail and suffer from disabling physical and/or mental illnesses. Beyond this variability in health and functional status, there is great diversity in the health values of elderly patients. Some consider illness and disability to be inevitable and have no interest in extensive medical or surgical intervention. In contrast, however, studies directly interviewing elderly patients found a majority view medical care as an important means of maintaining health, and when given a choice, even those in their eighties generally preferred quantity as opposed to quality of life. Thus, it is incumbent on physicians caring for elderly individuals to attempt to directly elicit the elderly patient's treatment goals, while providing the patient with the necessary information regarding potential risks and benefits of each treatment option.

Social/Economic Issues

Finally, in devising a rational treatment plan for the elderly cardiac patient, physicians must consider the patient's social and economic situation. Transportation issues, which are a major limitation for many elderly persons, can disrupt close office follow-up. Many elderly patients live on fixed incomes and may not realize or acknowledge that they cannot afford multiple cardiac medications. The health of an ailing spouse can also substantially impact on an elderly caregiver's personal health and health decisions.

Medical Therapy of CHD in the Elderly Patient

Medical therapy can play a key role in reducing the morbidity and mortality of CHD in all aged patients. In fact, as elderly CHD patients face higher overall risk, the benefits of intervention in absolute terms actually tend to rise with age and the corresponding "number needed to treat" for these therapies falls. The following sections, address the role of specific agents commonly used in CHD management with special emphasis on their safety and efficacy in the elderly patient (Table 35-3).

Aspirin

There is very strong evidence supporting the long-term benefits of aspirin in patients at risk to CHD. In the Physician's Health Study of 44,000 men without known CHD, those randomized to aspirin had a 44 percent lower risk for subsequent MI versus those taking placebo. Observational data from the Nurse's Health Study suggests similar benefits of aspirin for primary CHD prevention in women. These and other studies have led to the recommendation to treat all patients older than age 40 years with one or more CHD risk factors with daily aspirin. Current guidelines recommend a daily dose of 162 mg/d to provide the most benefit while minimizing risk of bleeding. Patients on warfarin should have their aspirin dose reduced to 81 mg/d. Finally, in the small subset of patients who are truly aspirin allergic, a daily dose of 75 mg of clopidogrel can be prescribed as an alternative.

Table 35-3 Strength of Evidence for Commonly Used Pharmacologic Agents for Symptom Control and Reduction of Mortality in Patients with CHD by Age

	Symptom Control	CHD Mortality Benefit by Age		
		<65	65–75	>75
Aspirin	NA	++	++	+
β-Blockers	++	++	++	+
HMG-CoA reductase inhibitors (statins)	NA	++	++	++
ACE inhibitors	NA	++	++	+
Nitrates	++	0	0	0
Calcium channel blockers	++	0/–	0/–	0/–
Angiotensin receptor blockers	NA	0	0	0

– may be harmful
0 no benefit
+ benefit supported by observational data only
++ benefit supported by randomized control data
ACE, angiotensin-converting enzyme;
HMG-CoA, hydroxymethylglutaryl coenzyme A

β-Blockers

Along with aspirin, β-blockers form the cornerstone of therapy for the primary and secondary prevention of CHD in all aged patients. Following JNC VI guidelines, β-blockers should be considered first-line therapy in elderly hypertensive patients without obvious contraindications. For secondary prevention, a meta-analysis of 25 randomized control trials (RCTs) showed a 25 percent reduction from β-blockers in all-cause mortality and reinfarction in patients with prior MI. These long-term benefits are even more remarkable in CHD patients with congestive heart failure and depressed left ventricular function (contrary to the long-standing, previous practice, of avoiding β-blockers in such patients). β-Blockers are also effective antianginal agents, decreasing myocardial oxygen demand and increasing coronary blood flow. Finally, these drugs have potent antiarrhythmic properties and are useful in those with both ventricular and supraventricular arrhythmias.

An adjusted observational analysis recently demonstrated that elderly patients receiving β-blockers following acute MI had a 33 percent reduction in 1-year mortality compared with those not treated. Despite this, many studies demonstrate underuse of β-blockers in CHD patients, particularly in elderly patients. While β-blockers must be initiated with some caution in those with baseline bradycardia, high-degree heart block, or severe reactive airway disease, even these high-risk groups can often tolerate the drug when tested. The selection of a β-blocker in the elderly patient should take into account the drug's route of clearance. Those with impaired creatinine clearance should probably avoid renally cleared β-blockers (e.g., atenolol).

Lipid-Lowering Agents

There are several classes of drugs marketed for lowering serum cholesterol. These include gemfibrozil, niacin, fish oil, and the HMG-CoA (hydroxymethylglutaryl coenzyme A) reductase inhibitors (statins) (see Chap. 68). Of these, statins have the most evidence in support of their efficacy in primary and secondary CHD prevention. Aside from lowering cholesterol levels, the benefit of statins may also come from their antiinflammatory properties. A meta-analysis done with pooled data from five large statin RCTs—two primary prevention and three secondary prevention studies—showed an average 31 percent relative risk reduction in coronary events and 29 percent relative risk reduction in coronary deaths. Unfortunately, of these five trials only one included patients aged ≥ 65 years and none included patients older than 75 years of age. Thus, the question of whether lipid lowering benefited the very elderly remained inconclusive until the recent Heart Protection Study (HPS).

The HPS trial randomized over 20,000 patients aged 40 to 80 years with known CHD or high-risk profiles to 40 mg of simvastatin daily or placebo. After 5 years, patients on simvastatin had a 16 percent relative reduction in cardiovascular deaths and 22 percent relative risk reduction in major cardiovascular events relative to placebo. Most importantly, the benefit of lipid-lowering therapy was independent of age and persisted among those in their middle eighties. Consistent with the results of this recent study, the NCEP guidelines for lipid-lowering therapy do not include age cutoffs or age-specific treatment recommendations. While lipid-lowering drugs are generally safe in elderly patients, routine monitoring of liver function studies are recommended (see also Chap. 34).

Angiotensin-Converting Enzyme Inhibitors

The more angiotensin-converting enzyme (ACE) inhibitors are studied, the greater the number of beneficial uses for these agents are found. ACE inhibitors have strong support as safe and effective treatment of hypertension. They have also been shown to improve survival in post-MI patients with depressed heart function, heart failure, and large anterior MIs. Most recently, the Heart Outcomes Prevention Evaluation (HOPE) Study extended the benefits of ACE inhibitors to nearly all patients with either known CHD or who were at high risk for CHD. In HOPE, CHD patients and other high CHD risk patients (e.g., diabetes plus one or more cardiac risk factor) were randomized to 10 mg of ramipril daily versus placebo. After 5 years, treated patients had a 26 percent lower risk of CHD death than those who were not treated. Rates of MI, congestive heart failure (CHF), stroke, renal dysfunction, and even development of diabetes were lower in the ACE-treated patient group. The treatment effects of ACE inhibition were greater in those patients aged >65 years than in younger

patients. Thus, current guidelines suggest consideration of ACE inhibitors in all CHD patients with depressed ventricular function, diabetes, or hypertension. And many have suggested that these drugs be considered in all patients with known CHD regardless of other risk factors or left ventricular (LV) function. When used in elderly patients, however, one should carefully monitor serum electrolytes and creatinine, as these drugs can cause decreased renal function and hyperkalemia.

Angiotensin Receptor Blockers

Like ACE inhibitors, these relatively new agents exert their effects by blocking the renin-angiotensin-aldosterone cascade. Several RCTs have shown that the angiotensin receptor blockers (ARBs) can slow the progression of nephropathy in patients with diabetes and microalbuminuria in a fashion similar to ACE inhibitors. However, the effect of ARBs on cardiovascular events is much less clear. Two large studies of ARBs in diabetics and hypertensive patients, respectively, found no long-term reduction in MI or CHD events. Thus, when used for primary and secondary prevention of CHD, ARBs should only be considered at this point for those patients who are intolerant of ACE inhibitors (most commonly from troublesome cough). Patients who experience angioedema secondary to ACE inhibitor therapy should not be prescribed ARBs because of the risk of cross-reactivity. As with ACE inhibitors, careful monitoring of serum electrolytes and creatinine is necessary when adding or changing the dose of an ARB in elderly patients.

Nitrates

Nitrates are potent vasodilators and effective antianginal agents. However, these agents do not improve CHD mortality and should not be used routinely in asymptomatic cardiac patients. In those with symptoms, topical and oral agents are equally efficacious, though compliance is typically better with once-a-day agents (patches or long-acting nitrate oral preparations). Many patients with chronic angina also experience improved exercise tolerance by taking one or two sublingual nitrate tablets prior to activity. Caution must be taken when prescribing nitrates to the elderly, as older patients often have orthostatic hypotension that can be exacerbated by nitrate therapy and predispose them to falls. Patients taking sildenafil (Viagra), another potent vasodilator, should not be prescribed nitrates because of the risk of severe hypotension and death with combined therapy.

Calcium Channel Blockers

In general, calcium channel blockers (CCBs) should not be considered first-line therapy for patients with known or suspected CHD, as they have not been shown to reduce cardiovascular mortality and can actually worsen outcomes in patients with LV dysfunction. Nevertheless, when used prudently, they provide an alternative antianginal or rate-controlling agent in those who are intolerant to β-blockers. Short-acting nifedipine should never be used in patients with known or suspected CHD, as it has been clearly associated with an increased mortality in American Cancer Society studies. CCBs should also be used cautiously in elderly patients, because they frequently exacerbate constipation, lower extremity swelling, and orthostatic hypotension.

Hormone Replacement Therapy (See Chaps. 75 and 97 for Further Discussion)

While multiple prior observational studies suggested that hormone replacement therapy (HRT) could decrease risk for CHD events in postmenopausal women, recently completed randomized trials have failed to substantiate this. In the Heart and Estrogen/Progestin Replacment (HERS) trial, a combination of estrogen-progestin had no overall impact on cardiovascular event rates in postmenopausal women with established CHD when compared with placebo (4-year odds ratio [OR] 0.99, 95% confidence interval [CI] 0.80 to 1.22). HRT was actually associated with a 50 percent increased risk for CHD events for the first year of treatment and a 33 percent reduced risk of events after year one. However, longer follow-up of this cohort failed to provide evidence of continuing divergence in outcome between HRT-treated and non–HRT-treated subjects with longer periods of observation. Perhaps most important in this still-evolving area of uncertainty and controversy, the arm of the Women's Health Initiative that compared enrollees with intact uteri taking the estrogen-medroxyprogesterone combination with those taking the placebo failed to demonstrate fewer cardiovascular events or net prevention of various key study end points, leading to premature termination of this component of this massive study (although the estrogen-only arm in women who are status posthysterectomy continues). While further studies are ongoing, current recommendations are that HRT should not be started in postmenopausal women for the purpose of reducing CHD risk.

FIBRINOLYSIS AND PRIMARY ANGIOPLASTY IN ELDERLY PATIENTS

Numerous studies have investigated the role of reperfusion therapy (fibrinolytic therapy or primary angioplasty) in patients presenting with acute ST-segment elevation MIs. A meta-analysis of the major fibrinolytic trials (Fibrinolytic Therapy Trialists' Collaborative) demonstrated a consistent and significant 21 percent relative survival advantage with fibrinolysis versus placebo in all ST elevation MI patients aged <75 years ($n = 6000$) who presented within 12 hours of onset of chest pain. However, in patients aged >75 years the benefit of thrombolysis was significantly reduced, with results showing only a 13 percent relative risk reduction when compared with placebo (29.4 percent versus 26.0 percent, $p = 0.03$).

The possible therapeutic benefits of thrombolysis must be weighed carefully against the risks, especially in the elderly. Data from the Fibrinolytic Therapy Trialists' meta-analysis showed that patients aged >70 years had nearly a threefold higher relative risk of intracranial hemorrhage

after fibrinolysis than those aged <60 years. Bearing this in mind, clinicians should realize that intracranial hemorrhage is a rare event and the absolute risk of this complication after fibrinolysis in those >70 years remains between 0.7 and 2.1 percent in major trials.

In addition, an adjusted observational analysis from two studies using the Cooperative Cardiovascular Project (CCP) database reported that patients >75 years actually had higher 30-day mortality with fibrinolysis than with standard medical therapy. Interestingly, in the one analysis that looked at 1 year outcomes, this early treatment risk in the very elderly reversed itself, and those treated with lysis actually had better survival rates after this interval (OR 0.84, 95% CI 0.79 to 0.89).

Most recently, combination therapy (half-dose fibrinolytic agent with full-dose glycoprotein IIb–IIIa receptor inhibitor treatment) has been proposed as an alternative to fibrinolytics alone as a reperfusion regimen. However, to date, combination therapy is associated with high intracranial hemorrhage rates in elderly patients (i.e., threefold higher risk) relative to full-dose fibrinolytic therapy alone. Thus, at the current time, combination therapy is not favored for treatment of elderly patients.

In contrast with these mixed results for fibrinolysis, reperfusion with acute percutaneous transluminal coronary angioplasty (PTCA) is almost universally associated with improved outcomes in all age groups. For example, a recent randomized study of primary PTCA versus thrombolysis in ST elevation MI patients showed a 40 percent relative risk reduction for death, MI, and stroke in patients treated within 3 hours of presentation with PTCA. Primary PTCA in treatment of MI in the elderly is also supported by a series of observational analyses. In the CCP analysis, acute PTCA was associated with lower 30-day and 1-year mortality when compared to no therapy or thrombolysis among elderly acute MI patients.

The only caveat to the successes of primary PTCA in elderly patients was seen in a trial of very-high-risk MI patients whose course was complicated by hypotension and shock. In this trial, shock patients were randomized to either emergent catheterization and PTCA or to aggressive medical stabilization (with pressor agents and intraaortic balloon pump, if necessary). In the overall trial, those randomized to primary PTCA had significantly higher survival rates; however, this effect was age-dependent, and those >75 years had actually had much higher mortality risk with PTCA.

While not fully resolved, current consensus appears to suggest that primary PTCA is probably the treatment of choice for elderly patients who present within 12 hours with an ST elevation MI at a skilled center that can provide rapid (<90 minute) primary PTCA. This recommendation is clear for those with contraindications to thrombolytic therapy (previous intracerebral insult, recent surgery or major bleeding, or severe hypertension with systolic blood pressure >180). At centers without onsite PTCA, fibrinolytic therapy remains a reasonable alternative for reperfusion, and advanced patient age should not be considered an absolute contraindication. MI patients aged 75 years or older with cardiogenic shock face very high mortality rates (>70 percent) regardless of therapy, and their treatment must be carefully individualized. Finally, as noted above, elderly patients with unstable angina and non-ST elevation MI patients also appear to benefit from a strategy of early catheterization and PTCA if appropriate (Table 35-3).

CORONARY REVASCULARIZATION

A second major challenge in the care of elderly CHD patients is related to who should be considered a candidate for coronary revascularization. In younger patients, randomized clinical trials have simplified this decision-making process by identifying subgroups in which PTCA or coronary artery bypass graft (CABG) surgery improves survival and/or quality of life beyond medical therapy. However, patients older than 75 years were generally not represented in these pivotal trials. Instead, clinicians and patients must rely on a careful comparison between the acute procedural risks and potential long-term benefits.

Procedural mortality rates following revascularization procedures rise dramatically and progressively with advancing age. Figure 35–6 displays the risks for in-hospital mortality following angioplasty and CABG from 123,991 patients in the National Cardiovascular Network Revascularization Database… From these data, it is clear that age-associated risk in procedural mortality is not strictly linear but rises more rapidly beyond the age of 75 years. Additionally, at any age, CABG patients face two- to threefold higher mortality risks than do patients receiving angioplasty. However, technological advances have led to improved procedural success rates and lower risks for both procedures. Thus, despite the fact that procedures were performed on higher-risk patients, the risk of death after CABG in patients aged 65 years or older in the Society for Thoracic Surgery database declined nearly 20 percent between 1990 and 1999 and now rests at just above 4 percent.

Nonfatal procedural complications (stroke, MI, renal failure) also rise in a curvilinear fashion with age and are higher in CABG patients relative to those undergoing angioplasty. Of major importance to many elderly patients are the procedural risks of stroke and loss in mental acuity. CABG patients aged 75 years or older have a reported 3 to 6 percent incidence of permanent overt stroke as compared with a <1 percent incidence for angioplasty. Additionally, by using highly sensitive neurocognitive testing,

Newman and colleagues found that up to 50 percent of patients of all ages undergoing CABG had measurable impairments in neurocognitive function at hospital discharge. Although half of patients with initial impairment recovered by 6 months, cognitive deficits reappeared in many of them during long-term follow-up and portended an impaired functional status. In these analyses, patient age was significantly related to both initial and follow-up cognitive impairment. While increasing age is generally a major risk factor for procedural complications or mortality, it is not the only factor to consider. For example, by using published risk models, one can stratify an octogenarian's likelihood for mortality with CABG from 2 to 3 percent for a "healthy" patient without other comorbidities, to greater than 30 percent for the patient with multiple risk factors such as diabetes or preexisting cerebrovascular disease.

As with reperfusion therapy, the risks of revascularization must be balanced against the potential benefits in terms of prolonged survival, improved functional outcomes, or both. The Alberta Provincial Project for Outcomes Assessment in Coronary Heart Disease (APPROACH) registry examined the care and outcomes of more than 6000 of patients aged 70 to 79 years who underwent cardiac catheterization. Compared with medical therapy, those receiving CABG or PTCA had significantly higher adjusted 4-year survival rates (CABG 87 percent, PTCA 84 percent, medical therapy 79 percent, p < 0.001). These survival benefits of revascularization also held for octogenarians and increased in all aged patients in proportion with the number of diseased vessels and the degree of left ventricular dysfunction. Results from the APPROACH registry have been confirmed in other observational analyses. Together, these studies strongly suggest that elderly patients with multivessel coronary disease have higher survival rates if treated with PTCA or CABG than if they are treated with medical therapy.

Beyond survival, there is also a growing body of literature to support the notion that PTCA and CABG also reduce angina symptoms and improve functional outcomes of elderly patients with CHD. Initially, these results were reported in observational studies that adjusted for treatment-selection issues, as well as other baseline clinical factors. Most recently, similar results have been validated in the Trial of Invasive Versus Medical Therapy in Elderly

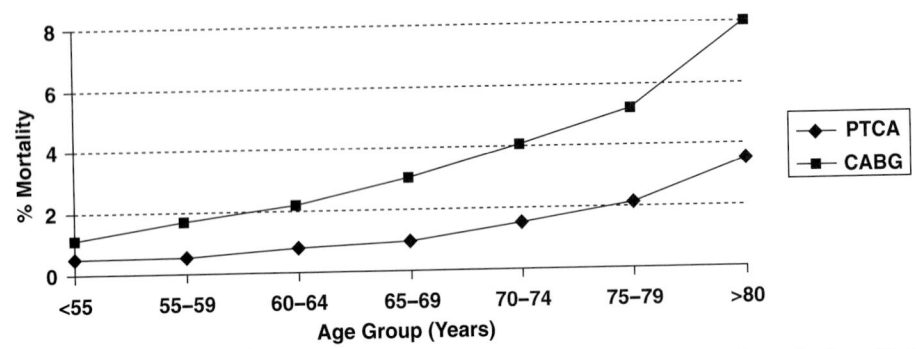

Figure 35-6   In-hospital mortality following coronary artery bypass graft surgery and angioplasty by patient age (National Cardiovascular Network Registry, 1994–1998). Data from Batchelor *J Am Coll Cardiol* 36:723, 2000, and Alexander *J Am Coll Cardiol* 35:731–8, 1999.

Patients with Chronic Symptomatic Coronary-Artery Disease (TIME) trial. The TIME study randomized 305 patients with chronic angina aged 75 years or older to diagnostic catheterization (followed by coronary revascularization as appropriate) or optimized medical therapy with intervention only for those with refractory symptoms. Of those randomized to catheterization and intervention as appropriate, 74 percent underwent CABG or PTCA, while almost 33 percent of the conservative management arm crossed over to revascularization by 6 months. Patients in the early revascularization arm had significantly greater improvement in their symptoms and almost all aspects of functional status and quality of life when compared with medically treated patients. However, clinical end points in the trial were mixed, with a higher 6-month mortality rate but a lower incidence of nonfatal MI in the early invasive arm. While this randomized study was limited in sample size and presented several methodologic challenges, its results do provide further support for the consideration of revascularization in the very elderly patient with CHD. And while we await larger randomized trials, both the American College of Cardiologists (ACC)/American Heart Association (AHA) bypass surgery and percutaneous coronary intervention (PCI) guidelines conclude that age should not be used as the sole criterion to rule out consideration of revascularization.

CARDIAC REHABILITATION

Three large meta-analyses, including more than 50 RCTs, have convincingly shown that cardiac rehabilitation (CR) reduces mortality by 20 to 25 percent in post-MI patients. In addition, patients who participated in CR typically had significant improvements in their anginal symptoms, lipid profiles, functional capacity, and overall quality of life as compared to controls. Recently, a number of observational studies have looked at whether the beneficial effects of CR extend to the elderly CHD patient. These studies have found that elderly patients enrolled in CR generally have marked improvements in functional capacity, quality of life, degree of social isolation, and depression. And given that many elderly patients have a low baseline functional status, CR can often make the difference between a patient maintaining or losing his or her independence.

Despite the overwhelming benefits of cardiac rehabilitation, participation among all groups remains poor, with only about one-quarter of eligible patients enrolling and elderly patients participating at a rate about half that of younger patients. Aside from logistic problems (lacking transportation, having a dependent spouse at home) and increased patient unwillingness to participate, lack of physician referral has been consistently shown to be a major reason why the elderly do not enroll in CR. To minimize the high morbidity associated with CHD in the elderly, all patients with chronic angina, or a recent MI, CABG, or PTCA, should be considered for referral to a comprehensive CR program that includes a monitored exercise, risk-factor modification, disease education and psychosocial counseling.

SUMMARY

Despite remarkable advances in prevention and treatment, CHD remains a major health problem for the elderly in terms of morbidity and mortality. As our population ages, the need for high-quality, well-informed cardiac care for patients aged ≥ 75 years will increase. Fortunately, there has been a groundswell of research interest to explore the safety and efficacy of various prevention and treatment modalities for CHD in the elderly. Preliminary data suggest that many treatment paradigms applied to younger patient groups are appropriate when treating very elderly patients. And in fact, given their greater age-related risks, older patients benefit as much, if not more, from existing therapies than do younger patients. Yet caring for the elderly patient with CHD requires careful individualization of therapy to minimize harm while maximizing benefit.

REFERENCES

Alexander KP et al: Outcomes of cardiac surgery in patients aged >80 years: Results from the National Cardiovascular Network. *J Am Coll Cardiol* 35:731, 2000.

American Heart Association. 2002 Heart and stroke statistical update. Dallas, TX; American Heart Association, 2002. Available at: www.americanheart.org/statistics/medical.html.

Balady GJ et al: Cardiac rehabilitation programs. A statement for healthcare professionals from the American Heart Association. Dallas, TX; American Heart Association, 1994. Available at: www.americanheart.org.

Batchelor WB et al: Contemporary outcome trends in the elderly undergoing percutaneous coronary interventions: Results in 7,472 octogenarians. *J Am Coll Cardiol* 36:723, 2000.

Berger AK et al: Primary coronary angioplasty vs. thrombolysis for the management of acute myocardial infarction in elderly patients. *JAMA* 282:341, 1999.

Braunwald E et al: ACC/AHA guideline update for the management of patients with unstable angina and non-st-segment elevation myocardial infarction: A report of the American College of Cardiology/American Heart Association Task Force on Practice Guidelines (Committee on the Management of Patients With Unstable Angina). Bethesda, MD, 2002. Available at: www.acc.org/clinical/guidelines/unstable/unstable.pdf.

Cheitlin MD et al. Do existing databases answer clinical questions about geriatric cardiovascular disease and stroke? *Am J Geriatr Cardiol* 10:207, 2001.

Eagle KA et al: ACC/AHA guidelines for coronary artery bypass graft surgery: Executive summary and recommendations. A Report of the American College of Cardiology/American Heart Association Task Force on Practice Guidelines (Committee to Revise the 1991 Guidelines for Coronary Artery Bypass Graft Surgery). *Circulation* 100:1464, 1999.

Expert Panel on Detection, Evaluation, and Treatment of High Blood Cholesterol in Adults: Executive summary of the third report of the National Cholesterol Education Program (NCEP) Expert Panel on Detection, Evaluation, and Treatment of High Blood Cholesterol in Adults (Adult Treatment Panel III). *JAMA* 285:2486, 2001.

Gibbons RJ et al. ACC/AHA/ACP-ASIM guidelines for the management of patients with chronic stable angina: Executive summary and recommendations: A report of the ACC/AHA Task Force on Practice Guidelines (Committee on Management of Patients With Chronic Stable Angina). *Circulation* 99:2829, 1999.

Gibbons JG et al: ACC/AHA guidelines for exercise testing: Executive summary: A Report of the ACC/AHA Task Force on Practice Guidelines (Committee on Exercise Testing). *Circulation* 96:345, 1997.

Graham MM et al. Survival after coronary revascularization in the elderly (APPROACH). *Circulation* 105:2378, 2002.

Greenland P et al: Improving coronary heart disease risk assessment in asymptomatic people: Role of traditional risk factors and noninvasive cardiovascular tests. *Circulation* 104:1863, 2001.

Gregoratos G: Clinical manifestations of acute myocardial infarction in older patients. *Am J Geriatr Cardiol* 10:345, 2001.

Krumholz HM et al: National use and effectiveness of β-blockers for the treatment of elderly patients after acute myocardial infarction: Nation Cooperative Cardiovascular Project. *JAMA* 280:623, 1998.

LaRosa JC et al: Effects of statins on risk of coronary disease: A meta-analysis of randomized controlled trials. *JAMA* 282:2340, 1999.

Lee PY et al: Representation of elderly persons and women in published randomized trials of acute coronary syndromes. *JAMA* 286:708, 2001.

Mehta RH et al: Acute myocardial infarction in the elderly: Differences by age. *J Am Coll Cardiol* 38:736, 2001.

Mittelmark MB et al: Prevalence of cardiovascular diseases among older adults: The Cardiovascular Health Study. *Am J Epidemiol* 137:311, 1993.

Pasquali SK et al: Cardiac rehabilitation in the elderly. *Am Heart J* 142:748, 2001.

Pryor DB et al: Value of the history and physical in identifying patients at increased risk for coronary artery disease. *Ann Interb Med* 118:81, 1993.

Ryan TJ et al: 1999 Update: ACC/AHA guidelines for the management of patients with acute myocardial infarction: Executive summary and recommendations: A report of the ACC/AHA Task Force on Practice Guidelines (Committee on Management of Acute Myocardial Infarction). *Circulation* 100:1016, 1999.

Scheifer SE et al: Prevalence, predisposing factors, and prognosis of clinically unrecognized myocardial infarction in the elderly. *J Am Coll Cardiol* 35:119, 2000.

Smith SC et al: ACC/AHA guidelines for percutaneous coronary intervention (revision of the 1993 PTCA guidelines)—Executive summary. A report of the American College of Cardiology/American Heart Association Task Force on Practice Guidelines (Committee to Revise the 1993 Guidelines for Percutaneous Transluminal Coronary Angioplasty). *Circulation* 103:3019, 2001.

The Joint National Committee on Prevention, Detection, Evaluation, and Treatment of High Blood Pressure: The sixth report of the Joint National Committee on Prevention, Detection, Evaluation, and Treatment of High Blood Pressure. *Arch Intern Med* 157:1413, 1997.

The TIME Investigators: Trial of invasive versus medical therapy in elderly patients with chronic symptomatic coronary-artery disease (TIME). *Lancet* 358:951, 2001.

Wei JY: Age and the cardiovascular system. *N Engl J Med* 1735, 1992.

Williams MA et al: Secondary prevention of coronary heart disease in the elderly (with emphasis on patients ≥75 years of age). An American Heart Association scientific statement from the Council on Clinical Cardiology Subcommittee on Exercise, Cardiac Rehabilitation, and Prevention. *Circulation* 105:1735, 2002.

Valvular Heart Disease

JOHN SANTINGA

AORTIC STENOSIS

Aortic stenosis is the most common valvular heart disease in elderly people. The murmur of aortic stenosis is present in more than 50 percent of patients older than the age of 75. Thus, it is important to distinguish patients with significant obstruction from those with a benign lesion. The degenerative changes in the aortic valve may involve fibrosis and thickening of the leaflets, which limits valve opening and produces the systolic murmur. In addition, the aortic side of the valve may develop a mass of calcified fibrotic material often containing lipid, which prevents valve opening and causes obstruction. As the pathology of this valve lesion has many similarities to that of an atherosclerotic plaque, it is not surprising that diabetes and hyperlipidemia are associated with aortic stenosis. In addition, coronary obstructive disease is present in more than 50 percent of patients with aortic stenosis. Decreasing coronary risk factors in the general population could potentially decrease the incidence of this disease in future elderly populations.

Congenital aortic stenosis is a disease of a younger age group. However, a bicuspid aortic valve defect can develop degenerative changes and obstruction later in life. This usually produces symptoms in the 40- to 60-year-old age group, but symptoms may first develop in the elderly age group. Rheumatic heart disease is still present in the elderly population in this country, as well as in patients from other countries where rheumatic fever is more common.

Diagnosis

The medical history is often similar to that of classic aortic stenosis in a younger age group. The symptoms are congestive heart failure, anginal chest pain, and syncope. In elderly people, however, because of decreased physical activity, the symptoms may not appear until the aortic stenosis is far advanced. Fatigue and exertional dyspnea are common early symptoms of aortic stenosis. Syncope, which is often exertional in a younger population, may occur at rest and in settings of vagal stimulation or volume depletion in elderly people. Exertional chest pain may be confused with coronary obstructive disease in this age group. Some patients may present with a low-output state characterized by confusion, weight loss, and debility. This presentation may suggest other chronic diseases such as cancer.

The physical examination is helpful in making this diagnosis. The classic findings of a decreased carotid upstroke, fourth heart sound at the apex, low blood pressure, and systolic ejection murmur at the base are still seen in many elderly patients with this diagnosis. However, some elderly people have associated hypertension, which can lead to a brisk carotid upstroke, S_4, and systolic hypertension, and this may confuse the diagnosis. The systolic murmur is heard in the aortic area and radiates to the carotids. An early-peaking murmur indicates mild obstruction, whereas a late-peaking murmur is associated with major stenosis. Table 36–1 lists the usual physical findings in the three major types of aortic stenosis. Rheumatic aortic stenosis almost always has findings of rheumatic mitral valve disease in addition to the aortic murmurs. In the presence of a low cardiac output, the systolic murmur may be unimpressive. Associated mitral regurgitation also confuses the diagnosis in some patients. The murmur of aortic stenosis in elderly individuals with large chest dimensions may at times be heard only at the apex. The intensity of the aortic stenosis murmur varies more with cycle length than the murmur of mitral insufficiency does.

The electrocardiogram shows left ventricular hypertrophy in two-thirds of patients with symptomatic aortic stenosis. There are ST depressions in the leads with tall R waves such as I, aVL, V_5, and V_6 consistent with concentric left ventricular hypertrophy; left axis deviation and left atrial abnormality are also common findings in aortic stenosis. A left bundle branch block is present in 10 percent of patients with aortic stenosis. The chest radiograph reveals a dilated aortic root (poststenotic dilation) and a boot-shaped heart with left ventricular prominence. Marked cardiomegaly is unusual in patients with aortic stenosis. Aortic valve calcification is difficult to see on a plain chest x-ray film.

Cardiac ultrasound imaging can define the amount of valve calcification and thickening as well as leaflet mobility. The left ventricle can be evaluated for hypertrophy and function. The Doppler velocities across the aortic valve document the amount of obstruction and can also demonstrate the aortic valve area. In addition, the mitral valve can be evaluated for insufficiency, and mitral annular

Table 36-1 Aortic Stenosis

	Rhythm	Heart Sounds	Murmur
Rheumatic	Atrial fibrillation	Normal S_2	Systolic ejection and aortic diastolic murmur
Congenital	Sinus rhythm	Absent S_2, aortic ejection sound	Ejection systolic murmur with diastolic murmur
Calcific	Sinus rhythm	Normal S_2	Ejection murmur

calcification can also be documented. In some patients, a satisfactory surface study cannot be obtained. In these patients, the transesophageal approach gives the necessary information. A peak aortic gradient of greater than 40 mmHg or a mean gradient in excess of 30 mmHg with preserved left ventricular function should raise a concern of significant valve stenosis. An aortic valve area of less than 1.0 cm^2 suggests significant aortic obstruction.

In patients with a decreased left ventricular ejection fraction and low cardiac output, evaluation of the severity of the obstruction may be difficult. The use of a dobutamine echocardiography study may be helpful in this setting. The dobutamine challenge often increases the cardiac output and unmasks severe obstructive aortic disease when the gradients increase and the valve area remains small.

Management

Aortic stenosis is important in three clinical settings. The first is during preoperative assessment for noncardiac surgery. If the diagnostic studies suggest significant obstruction and the proposed surgery will cause cardiac stress, a left-sided catheterization should be considered. If the surgery is urgent, such as following a hip fracture, an aortic balloon valvuloplasty can be performed during the catheterization to improve the operative risk. Calcific aortic stenosis is a progressive disease. Therefore, previous studies on the aortic valve should be made within 1 year to be useful in the preoperative assessment.

The second setting is symptomatic aortic stenosis. Table 36–2 outlines the management of aortic stenosis. Endocarditis is not common in calcific aortic stenosis but is a major risk with the bicuspid valve. Therefore, patients with a harsh ejection murmur (grade III/VI), an ejection sound, or a murmur of aortic insufficiency should receive endocarditis prophylaxis. Diuretics are essential for congestive heart failure, but overdiuresis can drop the left ventricular preload and lead to syncope or to a low-output state. Medications that slow the heart rate, suppress left ventricular function, or cause hypotension should be avoided.

The evaluation of syncope in patients with aortic stenosis should focus on determining the severity of obstruction, volume depletion, vasovagal abnormalities, and,

Table 36-2 Management of Aortic Stenosis

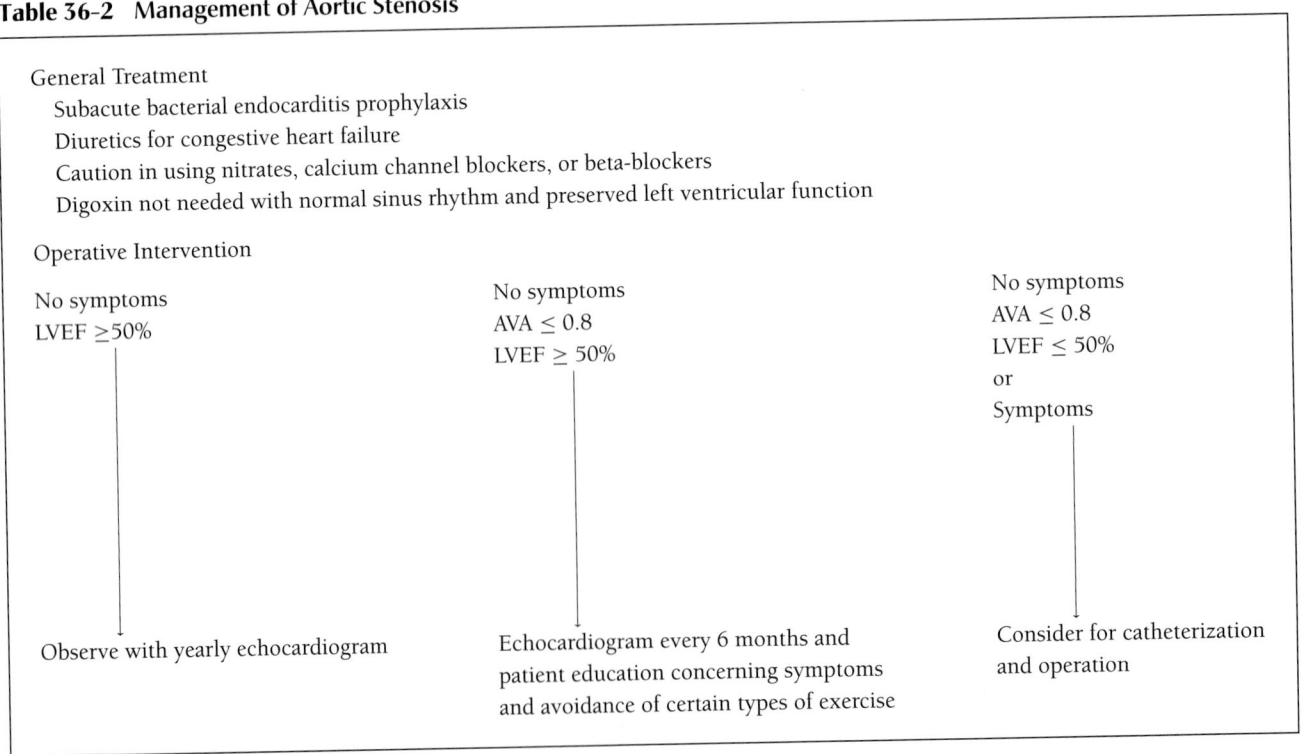

General Treatment
    Subacute bacterial endocarditis prophylaxis
    Diuretics for congestive heart failure
    Caution in using nitrates, calcium channel blockers, or beta-blockers
    Digoxin not needed with normal sinus rhythm and preserved left ventricular function

Operative Intervention

No symptoms LVEF ≥50%	No symptoms AVA ≤ 0.8 LVEF ≥ 50%	No symptoms AVA ≤ 0.8 LVEF ≤ 50% or Symptoms
Observe with yearly echocardiogram	Echocardiogram every 6 months and patient education concerning symptoms and avoidance of certain types of exercise	Consider for catheterization and operation

LVEF, left ventricular ejection fraction; AVA, aortic valve area.

Table 36-3 Factors That Increase Operative Mortality in Surgery for Aortic Stenosis

1. Cardiac factors
    Coronary disease
    Mitral valve disease
    Left ventricular function
    Severe left ventricular hypertrophy

2. Ascending aorta calcification and/or aneurysm

3. Noncardiac factors
    Malnutrition
    Albumin <3.0 gm/dL
    Cholesterol <120 mg/dL
    Creatinine >3.0 mg/dL
    COPD, $FEV_1 \leq 1$ L/min
    Dementia
    Stroke history
    Impaired functional status

FEV_1, Forced expiratory volume in 1 s.

importantly, arrhythmias. Atrial ventricular conduction abnormalities can occur secondarily to aortic root calcification, interrupting the conduction system. In addition, atrial and ventricular arrhythmias are common in severe left ventricular disease. Insertion of a pacemaker or antiventricular arrhythmia treatment may be the correct therapy for certain patients.

Operative intervention is effective in treating symptomatic aortic stenosis. In elderly people, decision making is complex because of age-related issues such as nutrition, dementia, cerebral vascular disease, other comorbidities, and functional ability. The operative mortality often depends more on these noncardiac risk factors than on cardiac disease in this age group. In a review of 46,397 aortic value replacements from the thoracic surgeons' National Cardiac Surgery Database, the operative mortalities for the age groups 65, 70, 75, 80, 85, and 90 or more years were 4.8 percent, 5.2 percent, 7.5 percent, 10 percent, 12.5 percent, and 19 percent, respectively. There has been a decline in operative mortality of 40 percent over the past decade.

Table 36–3 outlines the factors that increase operative mortality. Coronary artery bypass and/or mitral valve surgery double the operative mortality. Ascending aorta calcification increases the chance of intraoperative stroke. The noncardiac factors listed under item 3 in Table 36–3 are very important in estimating operative risk. Common postoperative morbidities include those associated with the use of an intra-aortic balloon assistive device and prolonged intubation, as well as bleeding requiring reoperation and complications such as pneumonia, renal failure, and delirium, well known to the geriatrician. These risks, as well as those of operative mortality, must be discussed with the patient and family.

Valve selection is often an issue. Mechanical valves have good durability but require Coumadin therapy. A tissue valve does not require Coumadin but may malfunction after 10 years. In general, there is an increased use of bileaflet

valves (St. Jude's) in healthy elderly patients. Ball valves are no longer used because of a high stroke risk. Single-disk valves at times offer a hemodynamic advantage, but they require more intensive anticoagulation. A stentless aortic porcine prosthesis has a good orifice area to the exterior size and may be effective in elderly patients with a small outflow tract.

Aortic balloon valvuloplasty initially showed great promise but on follow-up studies has not been shown to change the natural course of the disease. The valve areas after dilation average 0.8 cm^2, which is still in the stenotic range. The procedure has some short-term benefits, mainly in preoperative management for noncardiac surgery.

The third clinical setting is in the treatment of an asymptomatic patient with a murmur of aortic stenosis in whom an echocardiogram study shows a significant gradient. If the ventricular function is normal, these patients should be followed up at regular intervals with a clinical assessment and echocardiography for left ventricular function. If the ejection fraction is below 50 percent, operative intervention is advised. Some elderly patients remain asymptomatic, but the ventricle develops marked hypertrophy with a small chamber size. This may make myocardial protection difficult during noncardiac surgery or other cardiovascular stress situations and thus may be an indication for valve replacement in the absence of symptoms.

In summary, aortic stenosis murmurs are very common in elderly persons. Echocardiographic and Doppler technology have greatly aided in the diagnosis of clinically significant aortic stenosis. Effective treatment is available for most elderly patients with symptomatic aortic stenosis.

AORTIC INSUFFICIENCY

Aortic insufficiency is also common in elderly people. Rheumatic heart disease and syphilis are now rare etiologies for this condition. Patients with Marfan's disease and other hereditary connective tissue diseases are unlikely to survive into the geriatric age group. However, aortic root aneurysm with associated valve insufficiency is not uncommon in elderly individuals. This condition is associated with hypertension and the female gender. Congenital bicuspid aortic valve disease may present with predominantly aortic insufficiency in patients in their late sixties. Patients with rheumatoid spondylitis can present with significant aortic insufficiency.

The pathophysiology of pure aortic insufficiency is volume loading of the left ventricle. The amount of retrograde volume loading is rate-dependent. Some patients have excellent exercise tolerance because the increased heart rate decreases the amount of regurgitation, but at rest with a slow heart rate, the ventricle may be overloaded and symptoms may develop.

Diagnosis

Patients with aortic insufficiency may remain asymptomatic for many years. Symptoms may be absent even though progressive hypertrophy and dilation of the left ventricle are developing. The diagnosis is often made on

Table 36-4   Physical Findings on Examination for Aortic Insufficiency

Accentuated carotid pulsations
Wide pulse pressure
Elevated systolic blood pressure
Diastolic murmur at left sternal border. This may be heard in some patients only at the apex.
When associated with aortic root aneurysm, diastolic murmur may be heard best at the right sternal border.
Loud S_2 with aortic root dilation (tambour sound)
Austin–Flint murmur (soft diastolic murmur at apex) is seldom heard in elderly patients with aortic insufficiency.

physical examination or with cardiac ultrasound. In some patients, the diagnosis may be made with the onset of endocarditis. When symptoms develop, they are usually those of congestive heart failure, but in some patients resting or nocturnal symptoms may be present. Arrhythmias are not common with this lesion. Angina also is rare but may occur at rest in some patients.

A physical examination often discloses an elevated systolic blood pressure, full arterial pulsations, and a diastolic murmur at the left sternal border. The physical findings are outlined in Table 36–4. The murmur of aortic insufficiency may be difficult to hear in elderly patients. A quiet room is essential, and one should use the diaphragm of the stethoscope. The peripheral findings of collapsing arterial pulsations and a low diastolic pressure are not common in aortic insufficiency in elderly individuals. It is rare to hear the low-pitched mitral vibratory diastolic murmur secondary to aortic regurgitation (Flint's murmur) in this age group. It is important to auscultate the right sternal border for the insufficiency murmur because aortic aneurysm is not an uncommon etiology for this lesion, and in this root lesion the murmur may be heard only in this location. In some patients with aortic insufficiency, the murmur can be heard only at the apex in the left lateral position.

Diagnostic studies should include an electrocardiogram, chest radiograph, and echocardiogram. The electrocardiogram may be helpful in predicting the prognosis of patients with aortic insufficiency, as left ventricular hypertrophy, especially with ST depression, predicts symptoms that will occur in the next few years. Voltage criteria for left ventricular hypertrophy are common. ST segment depression is not seen as often as in aortic stenosis. The chest radiograph indicates the degree of left ventricular enlargement. A cardiothoracic ratio in excess of 0.50 also predicts clinical events such as congestive heart failure or angina in the near future. A wide ascending aorta may suggest aortic root dilation, and, rarely, aortic calcification suggests a syphilitic etiology. Long-standing significant aortic insufficiency may lead to massive cardiomegaly clearly seen on the chest radiograph.

An echocardiogram has become an essential part of the evaluation. Aortic root size can be measured, mitral valvular disease is easily evaluated, and, most importantly, the left ventricular size and function can be determined. Mild to moderate aortic valve insufficiency is commonly found by echocardiographic evaluation in elderly people. Usually it is age-related and not clinically important. These patients have normal leaflets on echocardiography and have no murmur on physical examination. Endocarditis prophylaxis is not indicated in this setting.

Management

Endocarditis prevention is important in aortic insufficiency, making the physical examination very important in asymptomatic patients. In those with significant aortic insufficiency and symptoms of congestive heart failure, the usual treatment with digitalis and diuretics is indicated. In addition, an afterload-reducing agent such as nifedipine or an angiotensin-converting enzyme (ACE) inhibitor is advised. There have been reports that these unloading agents can preserve left ventricular function and delay symptoms in asymptomatic patients. Agents such as beta-blockers should be avoided because a slow heart rate increases the backward flow and worsens the congestive failure. If the patient is a surgical candidate, cardiac catheterization to determine the coronary anatomy is indicated prior to surgical intervention. Transesophageal echocardiography is also useful to rule out aortic aneurysm and severe atherosclerotic changes in the aorta that may increase the operative risk.

Patients with major aortic insufficiency may go for many years without symptoms. They may, however, develop dilated cardiomyopathy in the absence of symptoms. This myopathy may not resolve after valve replacement and leads to an increase in postoperative deaths. For this reason, some patients may need aortic valve replacement even without congestive heart failure. Therefore, yearly cardiac ultrasound studies are indicated in asymptomatic patients with significant aortic regurgitation. When the end systolic dimension of the left ventricle exceeds 5 cm and/or the left ventricular ejection fraction falls below 40 percent, aortic valve replacement should be strongly considered. In elderly individuals, the increased operative risk needs to be balanced against the expected benefit. In older high-risk patients, medical management can be very effective in controlling symptoms. Associated aortic root disease such as progressive dilation of the aortic root and/or dimensions in excess of 6 cm or areas of dissection can also be detected with ultrasound studies and may also be indications for surgery in selected patients.

The usual surgical treatment is aortic valve replacement. If the aortic root is large (>6 cm), the surgeon can replace the ascending aorta with a prosthesis and reimplant the coronaries into the graft. Usually, the aortic valve is replaced with a disk or tissue valve. Fortunately, coronary artery disease is less common in these patients than in those with aortic stenosis; so coronary artery bypass is often not needed.

In summary, aortic insufficiency is not rare in the elderly population. It is often associated with degenerative changes in the aortic root. Endocarditis prophylaxis and

Table 36-5   Causes of Mitral Valve Insufficiency in the Elderly

Myxomatous degeneration with valve prolapse and/or chordae rupture
Dilated left ventricle with distortion of the valve support
Papillary muscle fibrosis, often from coronary artery disease
Rheumatic heart disease with dominant insufficiency
Calcified mitral annulus
Rare etiologies including radiation damage, connective tissue disease, and endocarditis.

medical observation are important. In selected cases, effective surgical treatment is available.

MITRAL VALVE INSUFFICIENCY

Mitral valve insufficiency is common in elderly people. It occurs in older patients secondary to left ventricular enlargement, coronary disease with ischemia, infarction of the papillary muscles, or degenerative valvular disease, as summarized in Table 36–5. Some degree of mitral insufficiency on physical examination or cardiac ultrasound is present in the majority of patients older than age 75. A careful evaluation is necessary to separate clinically nonimportant from significant disease.

Diagnosis

With acute valve insufficiency, a patient may present with pulmonary edema. More often, however, the symptoms are fatigue, arrhythmia (atrial fibrillation), and eventually congestive failure. The symptoms may come on slowly, with the patient changing their lifestyle and not realizing their level of disability. Embolism may be the presenting symptom with atrial fibrillation. Endocarditis may also be the first event that calls attention to the valve disease.

A physical examination is helpful in this condition. The rhythm may be irregular if atrial fibrillation is present. The pulse is usually of low amplitude. The cardiac examination reveals a prominent S_2 at the left sternal border. The precordium may be active, with a sharp systolic precordial thrust. This may be caused by right ventricular dilation or from the regurgitant jet expanding the left atrium and pushing the heart forward. The auscultatory findings are listed in Table 36–6. The murmur from rheumatic valve disease is usually pansystolic and often associated with a decreased or absent S_1 and a diastolic murmur. The systolic murmur of nonrheumatic mitral insufficiency may have a late systolic crescendo, which might or might not be associated with a systolic click from mitral valve prolapse.

With anterior leaflet prolapse, the systolic murmur may radiate to the axilla and posterior chest, whereas a

Table 36-6   Auscultatory Findings in Mitral Regurgitation

Severity	S_1	Systolic Murmur	S_3
Mild	Present	Soft (grade I-II)	None
Moderate	Diminished	Loud (grade III)	None
Severe	Absent	Variable	Present

prolapsed posterior valve leaflet often radiates to the left sternal area and upper chest. The common murmur of mitral insufficiency associated with ventricular dilation is soft, is of low frequency, and may vary in intensity through the systolic cycle. This murmur may be confused with an aortic systolic murmur, and often, both murmurs are present in elderly individuals. If there are premature beats, the intensity of the aortic murmur will vary greatly with cycle length, whereas the intensity of the mitral murmur will be better preserved.

Diagnostic studies should include an electrocardiogram, which often shows a left atrial abnormality but less often left ventricular hypertrophy. Atrial fibrillation is common late in the course of this valve defect. A chest radiograph may demonstrate left atrial enlargement in long-standing mitral regurgitation, but with an acute onset of insufficiency, the chest radiograph may still be normal.

An echocardiogram is very helpful in evaluating this valve abnormality. The chamber size of the left ventricle and its function can be determined. The severity of the insufficiency can be evaluated as well as the valve leaflet pathology. If a tricuspid insufficiency jet is present, an estimation of the right ventricular pressure can be obtained.

Management

The question of endocarditis prophylaxis needs to be addressed in patients with mitral valve insufficiency. The evaluation should focus on determining valve pathology versus support abnormalities. Murmurs secondary to ventricular dilation or papillary muscle scarring do not require prophylaxis. Myxomatous mitral valve disease may be present in elderly people and has the usual systolic click with or without a late systolic murmur. If a systolic murmur is present (often late in systole), or the echocardiogram shows significant degenerative valve disease, prophylaxis should be given. A calcified mitral annulus may have associated mitral insufficiency, and endocarditis may develop in this setting. Endocarditis prophylaxis should be provided if significant insufficiency is present, such as a grade III/VI murmur or major mitral regurgitation on echocardiography.

Atrial fibrillation may be present in mitral insufficiency. Embolism is less frequent with major regurgitation, in comparison to atrial fibrillation without valve insufficiency. However, embolism is still two to three times more frequent than in patients with normal sinus rhythm. Therefore, Coumadin therapy is indicated with the international, normalized ratio maintained in the 2 to 3 range. Aspirin should be used if Coumadin is contraindicated. Congestive heart failure therapy might include diuretics, ACE

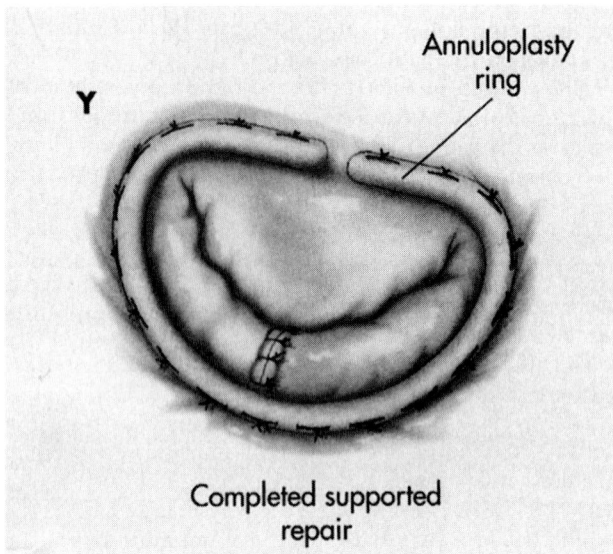

Figure 36-1   Mitral annuloplasty with a supporting ring for repair of mitral insufficiency. From Doty DB: *Cardiac Surgery: Operative Technique.* St. Louis, Mosby–Year Book Inc, 1997, p 259.

antagonists, and digitalis if atrial fibrillation or left ventricular dysfunction is present. Beta-blockade is also useful in preserving left ventricular function. Patients who are asymptomatic but have severe mitral insufficiency should be treated with ACE inhibitors to slow the development of left ventricular myopathy. These patients must be followed with serial cardiac echocardiography studies to monitor left ventricular function.

Surgeons have developed effective operations for this valve lesion. The increasing use of mitral valve repair and an annular support ring has been a major advance. Figure 36–1 shows valve repair with posterior leaflet resection and an annular ring. This procedure can be done with a low operative mortality (1 to 3 percent) even in elderly patients. In addition, this procedure preserves the papillary muscle, which helps maintain left ventricular function. Replacement of the valve with a bioprosthesis or a mechanical valve still remains an option if repair is not possible. However, this procedure has a higher mortality in elderly patients (5 percent to 10 percent) and often leads to a loss of papillary muscle support and left ventricular dilation. Anticoagulation therapy is not needed following mitral valve repair or replacement with a bioprosthesis as long as sinus rhythm is maintained.

The timing of mitral valve repair is an important issue. Symptoms of congestive failure may occur late in the natural history of this valve lesion. Because the left ventricle can unload a portion of its blood volume into the low-pressure left atrium, left ventricular dilation and irreversible myopathy may occur without pulmonary congestion and symptoms. Following repair or replacement of the mitral valve, left ventricular function may deteriorate (with replacement) or remain depressed (with repair), leading to persistent congestive heart failure and a worsening prognosis (Figure 36–2). If an ultrasound study shows an ejection fraction below 55 percent and/or the left ventricular end

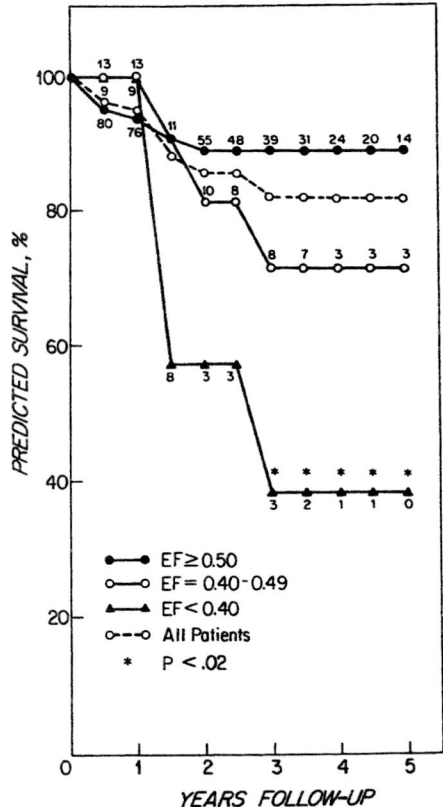

Figure 36-2   The changing frequency of mitral valve repair. From Oury JH et al: Mitral valve reconstruction for mitral regurgitation. *J Cardiac Surg* 1:384, 1986.

systolic measurement is increased to greater than 4.5 cm, surgical repair should be considered. The presence of congestive heart failure is another indication for surgery. When the patient is not a surgical candidate, medical treatment is effective in controlling symptoms. In acute congestive heart failure secondary to chordae tendineae rupture, the symptoms may gradually subside as the left ventricle adjusts to the increased preload. Acute mitral insufficiency secondary to papillary muscle rupture from myocardial infarction should be repaired immediately, if possible. However, the prognosis in elderly patients is grim for this clinical event.

MITRAL STENOSIS

Rheumatic mitral stenosis has been declining in prevalence in the American population. Elderly people, however, remain a population in which this diagnosis may be present. Other etiologies for mitral obstruction in elderly patients are rare. These include congenital stenosis, most often associated with an atrial septal defect, left atrial myxoma, and more commonly, a calcified mitral annulus that causes mitral obstruction. The latter condition is more common in women and in patients with significant renal failure.

Table 36-7 Common Presenting Symptoms in Elderly Patients With Mitral Stenosis

Fatigue

Dyspnea on exertion

Atrial fibrillation

Hemoptysis

Weight loss

Table 36-8 Auscultatory Findings in Mobile and Fibrosed Rheumatic Mitral Valve Disease

	Mobile	Fibrosed
S_1	Loud, snappy	Absent
Opening snap	Present	Absent
Regurgitation murmur	No	Often present
Diastolic murmur	Yes	Yes

Diagnosis

Mitral stenosis may be manifested as acute pulmonary edema, at times associated with significant hemoptysis. This event may be brought on with unusual exertion or with the development of rapid atrial fibrillation. Atrial fibrillation with palpitations is also a common presenting complaint in patients with underlying mitral stenosis. Finally, an embolic event may be the presenting event. Endocarditis is rare in patients with pure mitral stenosis. Common symptoms are listed in Table 36–7. Fatigue is an early and common complaint. It is, however, often better appreciated in retrospect after mitral valve repair. Asthmalike symptoms can often be present years before the diagnosis is made. Underlying lung pathology such as obstructive pulmonary disease or allergic asthma may be made worse by the pulmonary congestion secondary to the obstructive mitral valve disease. Fortunately, the extensive use of cardiac ultrasound has made undiagnosed mitral stenosis uncommon.

A physical examination is helpful in making the diagnosis in mitral stenosis. The pathophysiology and mitral valve anatomy can also be estimated from the examination. The peripheral pulses are often diminished and, if irregular, indicate underlying atrial fibrillation. When the clinician is searching for this condition, the patient should be examined in the left lateral position using the bell or low-frequency setting of the stethoscope. The accentuated first heart sound may often be palpable at the apex. There may be a left sternal thrust from right ventricular dilation. Pulsating neck veins and liver indicate tricuspid insufficiency, which could be secondary to the pulmonary hypertension from the mitral obstruction. There is an accentuated first sound present at the apex and in the absence of atrial fibrillation often associated with a mitral valve opening snap. An increase in the pulmonary closure sound at the upper left sternal border suggest pulmonary hypertension. Rarely, a pulmonary insufficiency diastolic murmur can be heard at the left sternal border; however, this is often is labeled aortic insufficiency, and an echocardiogram may be necessary to make the correct diagnosis.

The anatomy of the mitral valve can be estimated by the auscultatory findings shown in Table 36–8.

An electrocardiogram may have the unusual combination of left atrial enlargement and right ventricular hypertrophy. With right ventricular dilation, there may be Q waves in V_1 through V_3 mimicking a septal infarction.

Atrial fibrillation with coarse fibrillation waves may be present.

A chest radiograph shows right ventricular enlargement and left atrial enlargement. Left atrial enlargement is revealed on the chest radiograph as a double shadow over the right side of the heart, an elevated left main stem bronchus, atrial appendage enlargement, and on the lateral film, a posterior bulge above the left ventricle.

The anatomy of the mitral valve can be estimated by the auscultatory findings shown in Table 36–8 an echocardiogram is essential to understanding the pathophysiology. Table 36–9 lists the information available on an echocardiogram. A transesophageal echocardiogram is very helpful in this setting and can offer clearer echocardiographic windows to help in defining the pathophysiology. Left atrial clots can also be detected with this approach.

Management

Medical treatment includes endocarditis prophylaxis. Coumadin anticoagulation is indicated in the presence of atrial fibrillation, congestive heart failure, or both. The presence of significant mitral stenosis, a left atrial clot, or atrial stroke (slow circulation with coagulopathy) on a transesophageal echocardiogram are also indications for anticoagulation. Heart rate control with digitalis or a beta-blocker is important in the treatment of congestive heart failure. Diuretics are essential in treating heart failure with

Table 36-9 Information from the Echocardiogram in Evaluating Elderly Patients with Mitral Stenosis

Mitral valve thickening and degree of calcification

Severity of stenosis and presence of mitral insufficiency

Chamber size of left atrium, left ventricle, and right ventricle

Ventricular function

Estimate of right ventricular pressure

Presence of other associated valvular disease

Chordal thickening and shortening

mitral stenosis. ACE antagonists are not indicated in this setting.

Determination of the mobility and competency of the valve leaflet is essential in planning valve repair. Balloon valvuloplasty is the procedure of choice for young patients with favorable mitral valve anatomy. Elderly persons, however, often do not have the mobile, noncalcified valves that predict a good outcome with this approach. But because the operative risk is increased in elderly patients, an attempt at valvuloplasty is often indicated. Less than perfect hemodynamic results may still improve the patient's condition enough to avoid surgery. Fortunately, restenosis is not common following balloon valvuloplasty of the mitral valve.

Surgical repair or replacement of the stenotic valve is still successful in the majority of patients. Often, a tissue valve, will be used in this age group. Surgical correction of stenosis from a calcified mitral annulus is very unsatisfactory and should be avoided in this age group.

TRICUSPID INSUFFICIENCY

Tricuspid insufficiency is common in older patients. It is usually secondary to severe left-sided congestive heart failure. Rarely, isolated tricuspid insufficiency is present in primary pulmonary hypertension, atrial septal defect, carcinoid syndrome, and Epstein's anomaly. Treatment should focus on managing the left-sided pathology or correcting the atrial septal defect. Surgical procedures similar to those used in the mitral valve repair are available.

REFERENCES

Astor BC et al: Mortality after aortic valve replacement: Results from a nationally representative database. *Ann Thorac Surg* 70: 1939, 2000.

Bolling SF et al: Mitral valve reconstruction in elderly, ischemic patients. *Chest* 109:35, 1996.

Bonow RO et al: Timing of operation for chronic aortic regurgitation. *Am J Cardiol* 50:325, 1982.

Borer JS et al: Natural history of left ventricular performance at rest and during exercise after aortic valve replacement for aortic regurgitation. *Circulation* 84 (suppl III) III-133, 1991.

Carabello BA: Evaluation and management of patients with aortic stenosis. *Circulation* 105:1746, 2002.

Carbello BA, Crawford FA Jr: Valvular heart disease. *N Engl J Med* 337:32, 1997.

Chizner MA et al: The national history of aortic stenosis in adults. *Am Heart J* 99:419, 1980.

Dajani AS et al: Prevention of bacterial endocarditis: Recommendations by the American Heart Association. *JAMA* 277:1794, 1997.

Enriquez-Sarano M et al: Echocardiographic prediction of survival after surgical correction of organic mitral regurgitation. *Circulation* 90:830, 1994.

Inoue K et al: Clinical application of transvenous mitral commissurotomy by a new balloon catheter. *J Thorac Cardiovasc Surg* 87:394, 1984.

Otto CM et al: Prospective study of asymptomatic valvular aortic stenosis: Clinical, echocardiographic, and exercise predictors of outcome. *Circulation* 95:2262, 1997.

Oury JH et al: Mitral valve reconstruction for mitral regurgitation. *J Cardiac Surg* 1:384, 1986.

Zoghbi WA et al: Accurate noninvasive quantification of stenotic aortic valve area by Doppler echocardiography. *Circulation* 73:452, 1986.

Heart Failure

MICHAEL W. RICH

Heart failure can be defined as an inability of the heart to pump sufficient blood to meet the metabolic needs of the body's tissues or as the ability to do so only at the expense of elevated intracardiac pressures. It is important to recognize that heart failure represents a clinical syndrome rather than a specific diagnosis, and to a large extent it is a geriatric syndrome in much the same way that dementia and incontinence are geriatric syndromes. Indeed, heart failure may be viewed as the quintessential disorder of cardiovascular aging because, as discussed later in this chapter, extensive age-related changes in cardiovascular structure and function, in conjunction with the rising prevalence of cardiovascular diseases with advancing age and the recent decline in premature cardiovascular deaths, all contribute to an exponential rise in the prevalence of heart failure with advancing age. Thus, although the clinical syndrome of heart failure has been recognized by physicians for more than 2000 years, it has only been within the past two decades that it has been identified as a major public health concern, a development which is largely attributable to the aging of the population.

EPIDEMIOLOGY AND ECONOMIC IMPACT

Despite progressive declines in age-adjusted mortality rates from coronary heart disease and hypertensive cardiovascular disease, both the incidence and prevalence of heart failure are increasing, and it is projected that these trends will continue for the next several decades. As shown in Table 37-1, several factors have contributed to the progressive rise in heart failure. Foremost among these is the increasing number of older adults who, by virtue of advanced age and the high prevalence of hypertension, coronary heart disease, and cardiac valvular disorders in older individuals, are predisposed to the development of heart failure. In addition, advances in the prevention and treatment of other acute and chronic cardiac and noncardiac conditions, most notably atherosclerotic heart disease, hypertension, renal failure, cancer, and infectious diseases, have paradoxically contributed to the increasing burden of heart failure. Thus, individuals who 20 years ago might have died in middle age from acute myocardial infarction are now surviving to older age only to develop heart failure

in their later years. Similarly, improved blood pressure control has led to a 60 percent decline in stroke mortality over the last 30 years, yet these same patients remain at risk for the subsequent development of heart failure as a complication of hypertensive left ventricular hypertrophy and age-related diastolic dysfunction.

Heart failure affects approximately 4.9 million Americans, and 550,000 new cases are diagnosed each year. Moreover, both the incidence and prevalence of heart failure are strikingly age dependent (Figs. 37-1 and 37-2). Thus, heart failure is relatively uncommon in individuals under the age of 45, but the prevalence doubles for each decade thereafter and approaches 10 percent in adults older than 80 years of age. Similarly, heart failure mortality rates increase exponentially with advancing age in all major demographic subgroups of the US population (Fig. 37-3).

Heart failure is also a major source of chronic disability and impaired quality of life in older adults, and it is currently the leading indication for hospitalization in individuals older than 65 years of age. In 1999, in the United States, there were 962,000 hospital admissions with a primary diagnosis of heart failure. Of these, 757,000 (78.7 percent) were in patients older than 65 years of age and more than 50 percent occurred in patients 75 years of age or older. The majority of heart-failure patients younger than age 65 are males, but women comprise nearly 60 percent of heart-failure admissions older than age 65, and the proportion of females continues to rise with advancing age. The prevalence of heart failure in older whites and African Americans is similar, but hospital admission rates for heart failure are lower in Hispanics and Asians. Whether this represents a true difference in population prevalence or a cultural difference in the likelihood that affected individuals will seek medical attention is unknown. Heart failure is also a common reason for outpatient physician office visits, with estimates ranging from 3 to 12 million office visits annually for this problem. In this regard, heart failure ranks second only to hypertension among cardiovascular causes for outpatient physician visits.

Because of the high prevalence of heart failure and the resulting need for intensive resource use in both inpatient and outpatient settings, the economic burden of heart failure is staggering. Heart failure is currently the most costly diagnosis-related group (DRG) in the United States, with

Table 37-1   Factors Contributing to the Rising Incidence and Prevalence of Heart Failure

Aging of the population
 Age-related cardiovascular changes
 High prevalence of cardiovascular disease

Improved therapy for coronary heart disease and
hypertension
 Decline in coronary mortality
  Thrombolytic therapy
  Coronary angioplasty and bypass surgery
  Aspirin, β-blockers, converting-enzyme inhibitors
  Hypocholesterolemic agents
  Lifestyle changes (decreased cigarette smoking, diet,
   exercise)
 Decline in stroke mortality
  More widespread use of antihypertensive agents
  Beneficial effects of treating diastolic and isolated
   systolic hypertension
  Anticoagulant therapy for atrial fibrillation
  Hypocholesterolemic agents (statins)

Improved therapy for other disorders
 End-stage renal disease
 Cancer
 Pneumonia, other infections

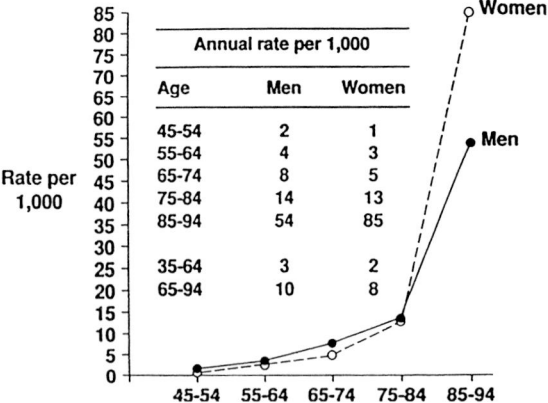

Figure 37-1   Incidence of heart failure by age and sex: 30-year followup from the Framingham Study. Reproduced with permission from Kannel WB, Belanger AJ: Epidemiology of heart failure. *Am Heart J* 121:951, 1991.

estimated total annual expenditures in excess of $20 billion. Indeed, inpatient expenditures for heart failure exceed those for all cancers combined by a factor of 2.4, and for all myocardial infarctions combined by a factor of 1.7.

PATHOPHYSIOLOGY

Heart failure represents the prototypical disorder of cardiovascular aging in that age-related changes in the cardiovascular system in concert with an increasing prevalence of cardiovascular diseases in older age conspire to produce an exponential rise in heart-failure prevalence with advancing age.

Aging is associated with extensive changes in cardiovascular structure and function (see Chap. 33). However, in the absence of coexistent cardiovascular disease, resting cardiac function is well-preserved even at very elderly ages. Thus, the resting left ventricular ejection fraction, an index of left ventricular systolic performance, is unaffected by age in healthy individuals. Similarly, most studies indicate that resting cardiac output is either maintained or declines minimally with normal aging.

From a clinical perspective the changes associated with cardiovascular aging result in an impaired ability of the heart to respond to stress, whether that stress is physiologic (e.g., exercise) or pathologic (e.g., hypertension or myocardial ischemia). Four principal changes in the cardiovascular system contribute directly to the heart's attenuated capacity to augment cardiac output in response to stress. First, aging is associated with reduced responsiveness

to β-adrenergic stimulation. The mechanism underlying this change has not been fully elucidated, but it is not caused by reduced circulating catecholamine levels, decreased β-receptor density on cardiac myocytes, or altered responsiveness to intracellular calcium. In any case, the diminished response to β-adrenergic stimulation limits the heart's capacity to sufficiently increase heart rate and contractility in response to stress, and β_2-mediated peripheral vasodilatation is also compromised.

A second major effect of aging is increased vascular stiffness, primarily caused by increased collagen deposition and cross-linking coupled with degeneration of elastin fibers in the media and adventitia of the large- and medium-sized arteries. Increased vascular stiffness results in increased impedance to left ventricular ejection (i.e., increased afterload), and it also contributes to the increased propensity of older individuals to develop isolated systolic hypertension.

A third major effect of aging is altered left ventricular diastolic filling. Diastole is characterized by four phases: isovolumic relaxation, early rapid filling, passive filling during mid-diastole, and late filling resulting from atrial systole. The first two phases, isovolumic relaxation and early rapid filling, are largely dependent on myocardial relaxation, an active, energy-requiring process, whereas filling during the latter two phases is governed principally by intrinsic myocardial "stiffness," or compliance. Aging is associated with impaired calcium release from the contractile proteins and reuptake by the sarcoplasmic reticulum at the end of systole, leaving the heart in a state of "partial contraction" at the onset of diastole and inhibiting early diastolic relaxation. In addition, increased interstitial connective tissue content and collagen cross-linking reduce ventricular compliance. Compensatory myocyte hypertrophy in response to increased ventricular afterload and myocyte loss caused by apoptosis further compromise left ventricular compliance. Thus, normal aging is associated with important changes that impair both relaxation and compliance, adversely impacting all four phases of diastole and substantially altering the pattern of left ventricular diastolic filling.

Age-related changes in diastolic filling and atrial function can be evaluated noninvasively using Doppler

Age:	50-59	60-69	70-79	80-89
Person-bienniums	20520	19298	8994	2084
Person-bienniums with CHF	166	451	438	190
Percent prevalence	0.8	2.3	4.9	9.1

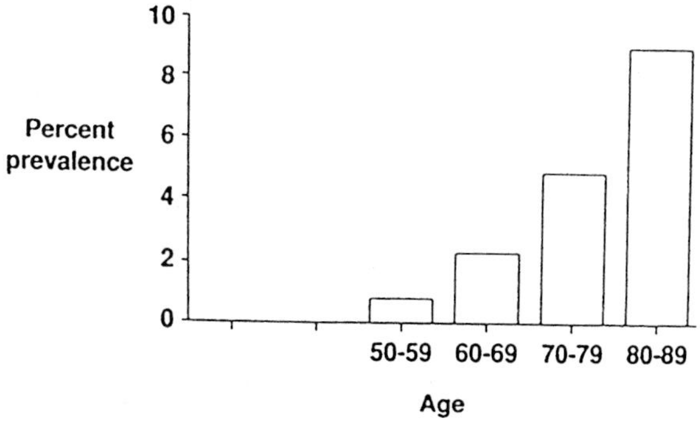

Figure 37-2 Prevalence of heart failure by age: 34-year followup from the Framingham Study. Reproduced with permission from Kannel WB, Belanger AJ: Epidemiology of heart failure. *Am Heart J* 121:951, 1991.

echocardiographic techniques to examine diastolic inflow across the mitral valve (Fig. 37-4). In healthy young persons the transmitral inflow pattern is characterized by a large E-wave with a rapid upstroke representing rapid filling of the ventricle immediately following the opening of the mitral valve and corresponding to active ventricular relaxation (Fig. 37-4A). This is followed by a period in which the rate of filling slows (the downslope of the E-wave), mid-diastolic diastasis, in which left atrial and left ventricular pressures are essentially equal, and a second burst of flow at the end of diastole corresponding to atrial contraction (the A-wave). Importantly, the majority of ventricular filling occurs in the first half of diastole in young individuals, with a relatively small contribution from atrial contraction.

In older persons, alterations in cardiac relaxation and compliance result in characteristic changes in the pattern

of diastolic filling (Fig. 37-4B). Early filling is impaired, and the upstroke of the E wave is delayed. Similarly, the downslope of the E wave is less steep, as it takes a longer time to achieve diastasis. To compensate for increased resistance to ejection, the left atrium enlarges and hypertrophies. This results in a more forceful left atrial contraction and an augmented A wave. As a result of these changes, a greater proportion of filling occurs in the second half of diastole in older individuals, and as much as 30 to 40 percent of left ventricular end diastolic volume may be attributable to atrial contraction. Thus, older individuals become increasingly reliant on the atrial "kick" to maximize left ventricular filling.

A third pattern of diastolic filling, referred to as the restrictive pattern, occurs when the left ventricle's ability to accept blood becomes severely compromised. In this

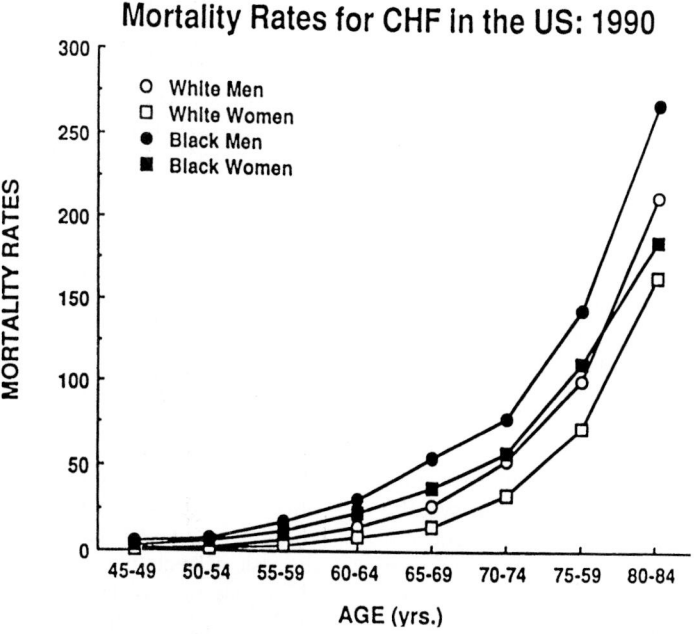

Figure 37-3 Mortality rates for congestive heart failure in the United States by age, sex, and race, 1990. Adapted with permission from Gillum RF: Epidemiology of heart failure in the United States. *Am Heart J* 126:1042, 1993.

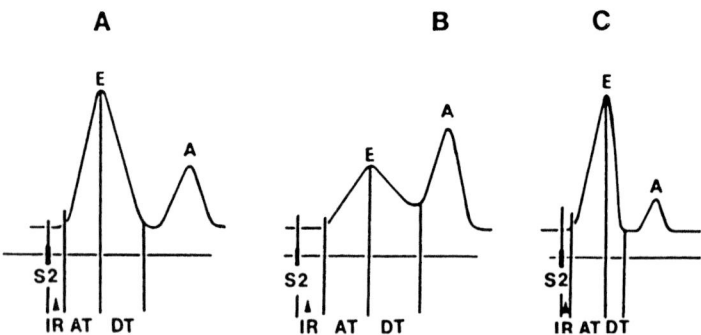

Figure 37-4   Schematic of Doppler echocardiographic mitral valve inflow patterns. See text for details. *A.* Normal pattern. *B.* Impaired filling pattern. *C.* Restrictive pattern. AT, acceleration time; DT, deceleration time; IR, isovolumic relaxation; S2 aortic valve closure. Reproduced with permission from Feigenbaum H: *Echocardiography,* 5th ed. Philadelphia, Lea & Febiger, 1994, p 152.

situation (Fig. 37-4*C*), very little flow occurs after the rapid filling phase in early diastole. This pattern is characterized by a tall, narrow E wave with a rapid downslope as diastasis is achieved early in diastole. Little additional flow occurs during mid-diastole, and the A wave is typically small, with an amplitude that is less than 50 percent of the E wave. A restrictive pattern generally indicates marked elevation of the left ventricular diastolic pressure and it is generally associated with a poor prognosis, particularly in patients with concomitant systolic dysfunction. However, the restrictive pattern usually occurs in patients with advanced cardiac disease, and it rarely results from aging alone.

Age-related changes in diastolic filling have several important clinical implications. First, inability to distend the cardiac myocytes to an optimal fibre length results in a failure of the Frank-Starling mechanism (see Kitzman, 1991), one of the cardinal adaptive responses (along with sympathetic activation) for acutely increasing cardiac output. Second, impaired diastolic filling results in a shift to the left in the normal ventricular pressure-volume relationship; that is, a small increase in diastolic volume is associated with a greater increase in diastolic pressure in older compared to younger individuals. This increase in diastolic pressure is transmitted back to the left atrium, and left atrial myocytes become "stretched." In turn, this increases the likelihood of atrial ectopic beats and atrial arrhythmias, especially atrial fibrillation. This accounts in part for the fact that atrial fibrillation, like heart failure, increases in prevalence with advancing age. In addition, atrial fibrillation itself is a common precipitant of heart failure in older adults for two reasons. First, the absence of a coordinated atrial contraction substantially compromises late diastolic filling due to loss of the atrial "kick." Second, the rapid, irregular ventricular rate associated with acute atrial fibrillation shortens the diastolic filling period, which further attenuates ventricular filling.

A third effect of altered diastolic filling is an increased propensity for older adults to develop diastolic heart failure (i.e., heart failure with normal left ventricular systolic function). As a consequence of the altered left ventricular pressure-volume relation, increases in left ventricular pressure caused by ischemia or uncontrolled hypertension may lead to pulmonary congestion and edema. Moreover, individuals with impaired diastolic function are often "volume sensitive;" that is, small increments in intravascular

volume, as may occur with a dietary salt load or intravenous fluid administration, are poorly accommodated by the noncompliant ventricle. As a result, intraventricular pressure rises abruptly and heart failure ensues. Conversely, intravascular volume contraction, which may arise from poor oral intake or overdiuresis, can cause a marked fall in intraventricular volume, which, in turn, leads to a fall in stroke volume and cardiac output.

The fourth major effect of cardiovascular aging is altered myocardial energy metabolism at the level of the mitochondria. Under resting conditions, older cardiac mitochondria are able to generate sufficient quantities of adenosine triphosphate (ATP) to meet the heart's energy requirements. However, when stress causes an increase in ATP demands, the mitochondria are often unable to respond appropriately. Although the precise mechanism underlying this mitochondrial failure is unclear, the defect adds to the heart's inability to maintain normal metabolic function under stress.

To summarize, four major age-related changes in cardiovascular structure, function, and physiology combine to reduce cardiovascular reserve and to greatly increase the risk of heart failure in older adults. Recalling that cardiac output is determined by four primary factors (heart rate, preload, afterload, and contractile state), and recognizing that each of these factors is adversely affected by one or more of the four major effects of aging on the heart, and also that superimposed upon these changes is the high prevalence of cardiac disease in older adults, it is indeed not surprising that the incidence and prevalence of heart failure rise exponentially with advancing age.

It is also important to note that aging is associated with significant changes in other organ systems that impact directly or indirectly on the development and/or management of heart failure. Aging is accompanied by a decline in glomerular filtration rate that averages 8 cc/min per decade. In addition, the aging kidney is less able to maintain intravascular volume and electrolyte homeostasis. The reduced capacity of the kidneys to respond to intravascular volume overload or dietary sodium excess further increases the risk of heart failure in older individuals. In addition, older patients are less responsive to diuretics and more likely to develop diuretic-induced electrolyte abnormalities than are younger patients, factors that may complicate the management of heart failure in the older age group.

Aging is also associated with numerous changes in respiratory function that serve to diminish respiratory reserve. Some of these effects, such as V/Q (ventilation/perfusion) mismatching and sleep-related breathing disorders, may contribute directly to the development of heart failure by producing hypoxemia or pulmonary hypertension. Other changes reduce the capacity of the lungs to compensate for the failing heart by increasing tidal volume and minute ventilation, thereby contributing to the patient's sensation of dyspnea. In more severe cases of cardiac failure, such as pulmonary edema, acute respiratory failure may ensue, partly as a consequence of the inability of the lungs to maintain oxygenation and effective ventilation.

Age-related changes in nervous system function include an impaired thirst mechanism, which may contribute to dehydration and intravascular volume contraction in patients treated with diuretics, and reduced capacity of the central nervous system's autoregulatory mechanisms to maintain cerebral perfusion in the face of changes in systemic arterial blood pressure. The latter effect may contribute to subtle changes in mental function in older heart-failure patients treated with vasodilators. Aging is also associated with widespread changes in reflex responsiveness. For example, impaired responsiveness of the carotid baroreceptors to acute changes in blood pressure may cause orthostatic hypotension or syncope, and these effects may be further aggravated by many of the drugs used to treat heart failure.

Finally, as is well-recognized, aging is associated with significant changes in the pharmacokinetics and pharmacodynamics of almost all drugs (see Chap. 19). In addition, older patients tend to be at increased risk for both drug–drug and drug–disease interactions because of the high prevalence of comorbid conditions and the use of multiple pharmacologic agents. These factors often lead to alterations in drug efficacy and an increased side effect profile, and these effects must be taken into consideration when designing therapy for older heart-failure patients.

ETIOLOGY AND PRECIPITATING FACTORS

In general, the etiology of heart failure is similar in older and younger patients (Table 37-2), but heart failure in older individuals is more often multifactorial. As in younger patients, hypertension and coronary heart disease are the most common causes of heart failure, accounting for more than 70 percent of cases. Hypertensive hypertrophic cardiomyopathy represents a more severe form of hypertensive heart disease, most commonly seen in older women and often accompanied by calcification of the mitral valve annulus. Such patients often manifest severe diastolic dysfunction and may exhibit dynamic left ventricular outflow tract obstruction indistinguishable from that seen in classical hypertrophic cardiomyopathy.

Valvular heart disease (see Chap. 36) is an increasingly common cause of heart failure in older age. Calcific aortic stenosis is now the most common form of valvular heart disease requiring surgical intervention, and aortic valve replacement is the second most common open heart procedure performed in patients older than 70 years of age

Table 37-2 Common Etiologies of Heart Failure in Older Adults

Coronary artery disease
  Acute myocardial infarction
  Ischemic cardiomyopathy

Hypertensive heart disease
  Hypertensive hypertrophic cardiomyopathy

Valvular heart disease
  Calcific aortic stenosis
  Mitral regurgitation
  Mitral stenosis
  Aortic insufficiency
  Prosthetic valve malfunction

Cardiomyopathy
  Dilated (nonischemic)
    Alcohol
    Anthracyclines
    Idiopathic
  Hypertrophic
  Restrictive (especially amyloid)

Infective endocarditis

Myocarditis

Pericardial disease

High-output failure
  Chronic anemia
  Thiamine deficiency
  Hyperthyroidism
  Arteriovenous shunting

Age-related diastolic dysfunction

(after coronary bypass grafting). Mitral regurgitation in older individuals may be a result of myxomatous degeneration of the mitral valve leaflets and chordae tendineae (mitral valve prolapse), mitral annular calcification, valvular vegetations, ischemic papillary muscle dysfunction, or altered ventricular geometry caused by ischemic or nonischemic dilated cardiomyopathy. Importantly, mitral regurgitation may be acute (e.g., following acute myocardial infarction), subacute (e.g., endocarditis), or chronic (e.g., myxomatous degeneration), and the clinical manifestations may vary widely in each of these settings. In the United States, rheumatic mitral stenosis is a less-common cause of heart failure in older adults, but it is still occasionally seen. Functional mitral stenosis caused by severe mitral valve annulus calcification with encroachment on the mitral valve orifice is an uncommon cause of heart failure, but it is associated with a poor prognosis. Aortic insufficiency may be either acute (e.g., endocarditis or type A aortic dissection) or chronic (e.g., annuloaortic ectasia or syphilitic aortitis), but it is a relatively infrequent cause of heart failure in older adults. Finally, prosthetic valve dysfunction should be considered as a potential cause of heart failure in any patient who has undergone previous valve repair or replacement.

Cardiomyopathies are classified into three categories: dilated, hypertrophic, and restrictive. In older adults, ischemic heart disease with one or more prior myocardial infarctions is the most common cause of dilated cardiomyopathy. Nonischemic dilated cardiomyopathy is less common in older than in younger individuals; when present, it is most often either idiopathic in origin or attributable to chronic ethanol abuse. Less frequently, dilated cardiomyopathy may be caused by anthracycline toxicity or by other causes. Classical hypertrophic cardiomyopathy, once thought to be rare in the geriatric age group, is increasingly recognized in older adults since the advent of echocardiography. Similarly, restrictive cardiomyopathy, most commonly resulting from amyloid deposition (so-called senile cardiac amyloid), is an occasional cause of heart failure. In one autopsy series, cardiac amyloid deposition was thought to be clinically important in approximately 10 percent of individuals 90 years of age or older.

Infective endocarditis is an uncommon but important cause of heart failure in older patients because it is one of the few etiologies for which curative pharmacologic therapy is available. Endocarditis should be strongly suspected in any patient with persistent fever and either a prosthetic heart valve or preexisting valvular lesion. It should also be considered in any patient with fever, recent dental work or other procedure, and a new or worsening heart murmur. It is important to recognize, however, that the clinical manifestations of endocarditis are often protean, and the absence of fever or a heart murmur does not exclude this diagnosis in older individuals.

Myocarditis is a relatively rare cause of heart failure in older adults. It may be infectious (e.g., postviral) or noninfectious (e.g., a result of sarcoid or collagen vascular disease). Pericardial effusions, for which there are numerous etiologies, occasionally present with heart failure symptomatology, including fatigue, exertional dyspnea, and edema. Constrictive pericarditis may be infectious (e.g., tuberculous) or noninfectious (e.g., postradiation), but it is a rare cause of heart failure in older patients.

High-output failure is an uncommon cause of heart failure in older adults, but when present the diagnosis is frequently overlooked. Potential causes of high-output failure include chronic anemia, hyperthyroidism, thiamine deficiency, and arteriovenous shunting (e.g., resulting from a dialysis fistula or arteriovenous malformations).

Finally, in a small percentage of older heart-failure patients, detailed investigation may fail to identify any primary cardiovascular pathology. In cases with normal left ventricular systolic function, heart failure may be attributed to age-related diastolic dysfunction.

Precipitating Factors

In addition to determining the etiology of heart failure, it is important to identify coexisting factors that may have contributed to the acute or subacute exacerbation (Table 37-3). The most common precipitant in patients with preexisting heart failure is noncompliance with medications and/or diet. Indeed, noncompliance may contribute to as

Table 37-3   Common Precipitants of Heart Failure in Older Adults

Myocardial ischemia or infarction

Dietary sodium excess

Excess fluid intake

Medication noncompliance

Iatrogenic volume overload

Arrhythmias
  Atrial fibrillation or flutter
  Ventricular arrhythmias
  Bradyarrhythmias, especially sick sinus syndrome

Associated medical conditions
  Fever
  Infections, especially pneumonia or sepsis
  Hyperthyroidism or hypothyroidism
  Anemia
  Renal insufficiency
  Thiamine deficiency
  Pulmonary embolism
  Hypoxemia from chronic lung disease
  Uncontrolled hypertension

Drugs and medications
  Alcohol
  β-Blockers (including ophthalmologic agents)
  Calcium channel blockers
  Antiarrhythmic agents
  Nonsteroidal antiinflammatory drugs
  Corticosteroids
  Estrogen preparations
  Antihypertensive agents (e.g., clonidine, minoxodil)

many as two-thirds of heart failure exacerbations. In hospitalized patients, iatrogenic volume overload is also an important precipitant of heart failure.

Among cardiac factors, myocardial ischemia or infarction and new-onset atrial fibrillation or flutter are the most common causes of an acute episode of heart failure. Other cardiac causes include ventricular arrhythmias, especially ventricular tachycardia, and bradyarrhythmias, such as marked sinus bradycardia or advanced atrioventricular block. Sick sinus syndrome, which is common in older adults, is a frequent cause of bradyarrhythmias in this population.

As previously discussed, older patients have limited cardiovascular reserve and they are less able to compensate in response to increased demands. As a result, heart failure in older adults is often precipitated by acute or worsening noncardiac conditions. Patients with acute respiratory disorders, such as pneumonia, pulmonary embolism, or an exacerbation of chronic obstructive lung disease, are particularly prone to suffer from deterioration in cardiac function. Other serious infections, such as sepsis or pyelonephritis, may also lead to heart failure exacerbations. In patients with hypertension, inadequate blood pressure control is a common cause of worsening heart failure. Thyroid disease, anemia (e.g., as a result of gastrointestinal bleeding), and declining renal function may also contribute directly or indirectly to the development of heart failure.

Finally, it is important to recognize that numerous drugs and medications may contribute to heart-failure exacerbations. Alcohol is a cardiac depressant and it may also precipitate arrhythmias, especially atrial fibrillation and notably during withdrawal. β-Blockers (including ophthalmologic agents) and calcium antagonists are widely used in older individuals with cardiovascular disease, but both classes of agents are negatively inotropic and may exacerbate heart failure (Hunt et al, 2000). Class Ia (e.g., quinidine, procainamide, disopyramide) and Ic (e.g., flecainide, moricizine, propafenone) antiarrhythmic agents have important myocardial depressant effects that may worsen cardiac function. Nonsteroidal antiinflammatory drugs (NSAIDs), which are widely used by older adults, impair renal sodium and water excretion and may therefore contribute to intravascular volume overload (see Page and Henry). In addition, NSAIDs antagonize the effects of angiotensin-converting enzyme inhibitors, thereby limiting the efficacy of these agents. Corticosteroids and estrogen preparations may cause fluid retention and an increase in total body water. The antihypertensive agent minoxidil also promotes fluid retention, and several other antihypertensive drugs (e.g., clonidine, guanethidine) may have unfavorable hemodynamic effects.

CLINICAL FEATURES

Symptoms

As in younger patients, the most common symptoms of heart failure in older adults are exertional shortness of breath, orthopnea, dependent edema, fatigue, and exercise intolerance. However, there is an increased prevalence of atypical symptomatology in older patients, particularly those older than 80 years of age (Table 37-4). As a result, heart failure in older adults is paradoxically both

Table 37-4   Atypical Manifestations of Heart Failure in Older Persons

Nonspecific systemic complaints
  Malaise
  Lassitude/fatigue/"exhaustion"
  Declining physical activity level

Neurologic symptoms
  Confusion (delirium)
  Irritability
  Sleep disturbances

Gastrointestinal disorders
  Anorexia
  Abdominal discomfort
  Nausea
  Diarrhea

overdiagnosed and underdiagnosed. Thus, shortness of breath and orthopnea in an older individual may be attributed to heart failure when the underlying cause is chronic lung disease, pneumonia, or pulmonary embolism. Similarly, fatigue and reduced exercise tolerance may be a result of anemia, hypothyroidism, depression, poor physical conditioning, or the "frailty syndrome" (see Chap. 116). On the other hand, sedentary individuals and those limited by arthritis or neuromuscular conditions may not report exertional dyspnea or fatigue in the presence of heart failure, and atypical symptoms, such as those listed in Table 37-4, may be the first and only clinical manifestations of heart failure. In such cases, the physician must maintain a high index of suspicion or the diagnosis of heart failure may be readily overlooked.

Signs

As with symptoms, the physical findings in older heart-failure patients may be nonspecific or atypical. The classic signs of heart failure include moist pulmonary rales, an elevated jugular venous pressure, abdominojugular reflux, an S_3 gallop, and pitting edema of the lower extremities. However, pulmonary rales in older individuals may be caused by chronic lung disease, pneumonia, or atelectasis, and peripheral edema may be caused by venous insufficiency, renal disease, or medication (e.g., calcium channel blockers). Conversely, older patients may have an essentially normal physical examination despite markedly reduced cardiac performance. Alternatively, impaired sensorium or Cheyne-Stokes respirations may be the only findings to suggest the presence of heart failure.

Systolic versus Diastolic Heart Failure

The clinical manifestations of systolic and diastolic heart failure are similar, and no single clinical feature can reliably distinguish heart failure patients with intact left ventricular systolic function from those with impaired contractility. Nonetheless, certain features tend to favor one form or the other (Table 37-5). Based on the presence or absence of specific features, the probability of normal or reduced systolic function can be estimated, and there have been several attempts to develop algorithms for distinguishing these two syndromes. Unfortunately, the predictive accuracy of these algorithms has been modest, and additional testing is essential to reliably differentiate systolic from diastolic heart failure.

DIAGNOSTIC EVALUATION

Heart failure may be difficult to diagnose in older patients with multiple comorbid conditions and either vague or nonspecific symptoms and signs. Thus, the first task facing the physician is to establish whether or not heart failure is present. This begins with a careful history and physical examination, giving due consideration to potential alternative etiologies for the patient's findings. As discussed in the previous section, physical signs may be unreliable in older patients. Nonetheless, certain findings, including pulsus

Table 37-5   Clinical Features of Systolic versus Diastolic Heart Failure

	Systolic Dysfunction	Diastolic Dysfunction
Demographics	Age <60 years Male gender	Age >70 years Female gender
Comorbid illnesses	Prior myocardial infarction Alcoholism Valvular insufficiency	Chronic hypertension Renal disease Obesity Aortic stenosis
Presentation	Progressive shortness of breath	Acute pulmonary edema Atrial fibrillation
Physical examination	Normotensive or hypotensive Jugular venous distension Displaced PMI S_3 gallop Pitting edema	Hypertensive Absence of jugular venous distention Sustained PMI S_4 gallop Absence of peripheral edema
Electrocardiogram	Q-waves, prior myocardial infarction	Left ventricular hypertrophy
Chest x-ray	Marked cardiomegaly	Normal or mildly increased heart size

NOTE: PMI, point of maximum impulse.

SOURCE: Adapted from Tresch DD, McGough MF: Heart failure with normal systolic function: A common disorder in older people. *J Am Geriatr Soc,* 43:1035, 1995, and Vasan RS et al: Prevalence, clinical features, and prognosis of diastolic heart failure: An epidemiologic perspective. *J Am Coll Cardiol* 26: 1565, 1995.

alternans, an S_3 gallop, and the presence of jugular venous distension at rest or in response to the abdominojugular reflux maneuver are highly specific signs of heart failure in older patients. In the absence of these findings, the diagnosis often remains in doubt, and additional laboratory studies are required. To establish the presence of heart failure, the chest radiograph remains the single most useful diagnostic tool. In patients with moderate or severe heart failure, the chest film will usually demonstrate typical findings of cardiomegaly, pulmonary vascular engorgement, parenchymal edema, and pleural effusions. However, in patients with mild heart failure or coexisting pulmonary disease, the chest radiograph may be nondiagnostic. In these cases, the diagnosis of heart failure may ultimately rest on clinical grounds. Factors supporting the diagnosis include the presence of significant underlying cardiac disease and a favorable clinical response to diuresis. Conversely, the absence of identifiable cardiac abnormalities and a failure to respond to diuretic therapy should suggest a noncardiac cause for the patient's symptoms. Recently, it was shown that an elevated plasma level of brain natriuretic peptide (BNP) provides high sensitivity and specificity for the diagnosis of heart failure, but the value of this test in older patients requires further investigation (see McDonagh).

Once the presence of heart failure is established, the physician must address two crucial questions, the answers to which will serve as the basis for selecting appropriate therapy:

1. What is the underlying etiology and pathophysiology of heart failure (Table 37-2)?

2. What additional factors, if any, contributed to or precipitated the development of heart failure (Table 37-3)? Often, one or more precipitating factors can be identified, and alleviating these factors may significantly improve symptoms and reduce the likelihood of subsequent heart failure exacerbations.

Additional Studies

In 2001, the American College of Cardiology and American Heart Association Task Force on Practice Guidelines published revised guidelines for the evaluation and management of heart failure (Hunt et al, 2001). Table 37-6 outlines an appropriate initial diagnostic assessment for patients with new-onset heart failure. Class I studies are defined as those which are indicated in most patients, Class II procedures are acceptable in some patients but are of unproven efficacy and may be controversial; Class III studies are not routinely indicated and in some cases may be harmful. Briefly, basic laboratory studies, a thyroid function test, a chest radiograph, an electrocardiogram, and an echocardiogram with Doppler are recommended in all patients. A stress test to evaluate for ischemia is appropriate in patients known or suspected to have significant coronary heart disease if revascularization is a viable therapeutic option. Cardiac catheterization and coronary angiography are appropriate in patients with large areas of ischemia and in those who require surgical correction of a noncoronary cardiac lesion (e.g., aortic stenosis).

The recommendations outlined in Table 37-6 are targeted toward a broad range of adult heart-failure patients,

Table 37-6 Diagnostic Evaluation of Patients with Heart Failure

Class I (indicated in most patients)
  Complete blood count
  Blood chemistries: electrolytes, creatinine, blood urea nitrogen, glucose, magnesium, calcium, liver function tests, albumin
  Thyroid stimulating hormone (TSH)
  Urinalysis
  Chest radiograph and electrocardiogram (ECG)
  Echocardiogram with Doppler
  Stress test in patients with a high probability of coronary heart disease who would be suitable candidates for revascularization
  Cardiac catheterization and coronary angiography in patients with angina or large areas of ischemic or hibernating myocardium; also in patients at risk for coronary heart disease who require surgical correction of another cardiac lesion (e.g., valve surgery)

Class II (acceptable in selected patients; see text)
  Serum iron and ferritin
  Antinuclear antibody and rheumatoid factor
  Assessment for human immunodeficiency virus
  Stress test in all patients with unexplained heart failure who are potential candidates for revascularization (i.e., even if the patient is without angina or there is a low probability of coronary heart disease)
  Coronary angiography in all patients who are potential candidates for revascularization
  Endomyocardial biopsy in patients with suspected myocarditis, anthracycline toxicity, or a systemic illness with possible cardiac involvement (e.g., sarcoid, amyloid, hemochromatosis)

Class III (not routinely indicated, possibly harmful)
  Repeated stress testing or cardiac catheterization in patients without coronary heart disease or objective evidence for ischemia
  Multiple noninvasive studies (e.g., echocardiograms) in the routine followup of patients with stable chronic heart failure
  Routine Holter monitors or signal-averaged electrocardiograms
  Routine cardiac catheterization in patients who are not candidates for revascularization or other cardiac surgery (e.g., valve replacement)
  Endomyocardial biopsy as a routine procedure in chronic heart failure

SOURCE: Adapted from Hunt SA et al. (2001).

and most are applicable in older patients as well. Nonetheless, in older patients it is appropriate to consider the potential risks and benefits of each diagnostic procedure on an individualized basis, taking into account comorbid conditions, the extent of cardiac and noncardiac disability, and the wishes of the patient. For example, in a frail 85-year-old individual with diabetic nephropathy, the risk of precipitating dialysis-dependent end-stage renal disease as a complication of coronary angiography must be carefully weighed against the potential benefits to be derived from a successful revascularization procedure. Similarly, patient autonomy must be respected in all cases, and it is inappropriate to exert pressure on an older patient to undergo a procedure that the patient clearly does not desire. In this regard, it is imperative to discuss the therapeutic implications of specific procedures (especially invasive procedures) with respect to the patient's subsequent care (e.g., need for coronary bypass surgery) prior to performing the diagnostic assessment.

Systolic versus Diastolic Heart Failure

A primary goal of the diagnostic evaluation, apart from determining the etiology of heart failure, is differentiating systolic from diastolic dysfunction, because the management of these two syndromes differs. As noted above, it is difficult to make this distinction on clinical grounds alone, and it is therefore essential to evaluate left ventricular function directly by echocardiography, radionuclide angiography, magnetic resonance imaging, or contrast ventriculography. In general, transthoracic echocardiography is the most useful technique because it is noninvasive, relatively inexpensive, and, in addition to providing information about systolic and diastolic function, it is helpful in evaluating chamber size, wall thickness and motion, valve function, and pericardial disease. Thus, transthoracic echocardiography is appropriate in virtually all patients with newly diagnosed heart failure and in those with an unexplained change in symptom severity. The principal limitation of echocardiography is that the assessment of left ventricular systolic function is only semiquantitative. In addition, adequate visualization of the heart may be unobtainable in a small percentage of patients, although the recent availability of echo-contrast agents has minimized this problem. Alternatively, radionuclide angiography (multigated angiogram [MUGA] scan) can provide an accurate assessment of left ventricular function, as well as information about cavity size and regurgitant valvular lesions. An additional advantage of radionuclide angiography is that it provides an accurate method for quantifying left ventricular ejection fraction. Magnetic resonance imaging provides much the same information as echocardiography and radionuclide angiography, but is less-readily available and more expensive. Finally, for those patients who require cardiac catheterization, contrast left ventriculography is an excellent method for evaluating ventricular function.

Based on the results of echocardiography, radionuclide angiography, magnetic resonance imaging, or contrast ventriculography, heart failure may be classified as being primarily a result of systolic dysfunction, as defined by a left ventricular ejection fraction of less than 40 percent, primarily caused of diastolic dysfunction, as suggested by an ejection fraction of 50 percent or greater, or mixed, as indicated by an ejection fraction of 40 to 49 percent. However, it is important to recognize that systolic and diastolic dysfunction are not mutually exclusive. Indeed, almost all patients with significant systolic dysfunction also have concomitant diastolic dysfunction. Conversely, systolic dysfunction may play a role in the development of heart failure even when the ejection fraction under resting conditions is normal or near-normal. Despite these limitations, the classification of heart failure as systolic or diastolic is useful in guiding therapy.

MANAGEMENT

The primary goals of heart failure therapy are to improve quality of life, reduce the frequency of heart failure exacerbations, and extend survival. Secondary goals include maximizing independence and exercise capacity, enhancing emotional well-being, and reducing resource use and the associated costs of care.

To achieve these goals, optimal therapy in older patients comprises three principal components: correction of the underlying etiology whenever possible (e.g., aortic valve replacement for aortic stenosis or coronary revascularization for severe ischemia), attention to the nonpharmacologic and rehabilitative aspects of treatment, and the judicious use of medications.

As discussed in the section on prognosis, the outlook for patients with established heart failure is poor. Therefore, the importance of effectively treating the primary etiology and all comorbid conditions predisposing to heart failure cannot be overemphasized. Because coronary heart disease and hypertension are the most common causes of heart failure in older adults, primary and secondary prevention of these conditions is critical if heart failure is to be prevented and if the rising prevalence of heart failure is to be forestalled. Indeed, it has now been shown in multiple clinical trials that effective treatment of both systolic and diastolic hypertension can reduce the incidence of heart failure by up to 50 percent (see Moser and Hebert). Similarly, appropriate management of other coronary risk factors, particularly hyperlipidemia and cigarette smoking, will undoubtedly further reduce the burden of heart failure through the primary prevention of coronary heart disease.

Nonpharmacologic Therapy

Despite recent advances in the pharmacotherapy of heart failure, repetitive heart failure exacerbations are common and are more often precipitated by behavioral and social factors than by either new cardiac events (e.g., ischemia or an arrhythmia) or progressive deterioration in ventricular function. In one study, lack of adherence to prescribed medications and/or diet contributed to 64 percent of heart failure exacerbations among urban blacks, while emotional and environmental factors contributed to 26 percent of hospital readmissions. In another study involving 140 patients 70 years of age or older who were hospitalized with heart failure, 47 percent were readmitted at least once during a 90-day follow-up period (see Vinson).

Behavioral and social factors contributing to readmission in this study included medication and dietary noncompliance (15 and 18 percent, respectively), inadequate social support (21 percent), inadequate discharge planning (15 percent), inadequate followup (20 percent), and failure of the patient to seek medical attention promptly when symptoms recurred (20 percent). The findings of these studies suggest that interventions directed at behavioral and social factors could potentially reduce readmissions and improve quality of life in heart failure patients, and this hypothesis has now been validated in several trials.

In the largest study reported to date, Rich et al. (1995) evaluated 282 patients older than 70 years of age (median age 79 years) hospitalized with heart failure. Patients were randomized to receive conventional care either alone or in combination with a nurse-directed multidisciplinary intervention. The intervention consisted of comprehensive patient education using a 15-page teaching guide designed for geriatric patients, individualized dietary consultation, social services evaluation to facilitate discharge planning and to coordinate the transition back to the home environment, a detailed medication analysis designed to simplify and consolidate the medical regimen, and close followup after hospital discharge by the study nurse and home care team. After 90-days of followup, all-cause readmissions were reduced by 44 percent, heart failure readmissions were reduced by 56 percent, non–heart-failure readmissions were reduced by 29 percent, and the number of patients requiring multiple readmissions was reduced by 61 percent among patients receiving the study intervention. Patients in the multidisciplinary care group also exhibited enhanced understanding of their disease, better compliance with both medications and diet, and improved quality of life, as compared to the usual-care group. Overall medical costs were slightly lower in the treatment group during the followup period. Importantly, readmissions for heart failure remained 29 percent lower in the treatment group during the 9-month period following termination of the intervention.

Subsequent studies confirm the validity of the multidisciplinary approach to caring for older heart-failure patients. Table 37-7 lists the components of a comprehensive nonpharmacologic treatment program. As with other aspects of geriatric care, it is important to structure the treatment program to accommodate the needs of each individual patient. Clearly, not every patient will require all of the components listed in Table 37-7. Similarly, the optimal intensity of any given component, for example, patient education or follow-up care, will vary substantially. For these reasons, it is desirable to designate a single individual, such as a nurse case manager, to coordinate all aspects of the patient's care.

Physical Activity and Exercise

Traditionally, patients with heart failure have been advised to restrict physical activity on the grounds that rest is beneficial for the heart and that exercise could potentially worsen cardiac function or precipitate arrhythmias. However, it is now recognized that although some degree of

Table 37-7 Nonpharmacologic Aspects of Heart-Failure Management

Patient education
  Symptoms and signs of heart failure
  Specifics of when to contact nurse or physician about worsening symptoms
  Detailed discussion of all medications
  Emphasize importance of compliance
  Involve family/significant other as much as possible

Dietary consultation
  Individualized and consistent with needs/lifestyle
  Sodium restriction (1.5–2 g/d)
  Weight loss, if appropriate
  Low fat, low cholesterol, if appropriate
  Adequate caloric intake
  Emphasize compliance while allowing flexibility

Medication review
  Eliminate unnecessary medications
  Simplify regimen whenever possible
  Consolidate dosing schedule

Social services
  Assess social support structure
  Evaluate emotional and financial needs
  Intervene proactively when feasible

Daily weight chart
  Specific directions on when to contact nurse or physician for changes in weight

Support stockings to reduce edema

Activity prescription (see text)

Vaccinations
  Annual influenza vaccine
  Pneumococcal vaccine

Intensive follow-up
  Telephone contacts
  Home visits
  Outpatient clinic

Contact information
  Names and phone numbers of nurse and physician
  24-Hour availability

activity restriction may be appropriate, excessive limitation of physical activity may contribute to a progressive decline in functional capacity as a result of cardiovascular and muscular deconditioning. In addition, several small studies have demonstrated that participation in an appropriately structured exercise program may result in significant improvements in functional capacity and quality of life in heart failure patients. As a result, current guidelines for the management of heart failure recommend regular exercise for the majority of heart-failure patients.

The effects of exercise training in patients with heart failure have been reviewed (see McKelvie et al.). McKelvie's report summarized data from 9 trials, ranging in size from 10 to 46 patients. Three of the trials were randomized; the remainder were observational. All but one of the studies excluded patients with preserved left ventricular systolic function, and none of the studies specifically targeted older patients. The average duration of training ranged from 4 weeks to 18 months, and the mode of exercise consisted primarily of walking, jogging, and/or cycling. Exercise capacity improved with training in all but one of the studies, and the magnitude of benefit typically ranged from 10 to 25 percent. These improvements occurred primarily as a result of adaptations in the oxidative capacity of skeletal muscle, and there was no consistent evidence for a beneficial effect on central cardiac hemodynamics. Although the exercise intensity was moderate to heavy in most of these studies, there were no major adverse events attributable to exercise. Nonetheless, many of the participants reported angina or shortness of breath during exercise, and in one study, 41 percent of the patients withdrew from the program.

Since publication of McKelvie's review, several additional studies have shown that low- to moderate-intensity exercise is associated with improved functional capacity and quality of life in heart-failure patients, and in one study mortality and heart-failure admissions were reduced as well (see Belardinelli R et al.). Although none of these studies enrolled elderly subjects, the findings suggest that home-based exercise at low to moderate intensity is safe and feasible, and that it yields important clinical, functional, and quality-of-life benefits. Nonetheless, additional studies are needed to evaluate the safety and efficacy of regular exercise in heart-failure patients older than 75 years of age.

Exercise Prescription

A comprehensive exercise and conditioning program is appropriate for most older heart-failure patients with mild to moderate symptoms and no contraindications to exercise (Table 37-8). Table 37-9 outlines the basic components of such a program. (For more details, see Pollock.) In general, patients should try to exercise every day. A typical session should include some gentle stretching exercises as well as strengthening exercises using elastic bands or light weights and targeting all of the major muscle groups. Suitable forms of aerobic exercise for older patients include walking, stationary cycling, and swimming. The choice of aerobic exercise should be tailored to the patient's wishes and abilities. During the initial phases of an exercise program, the duration and intensity of the aerobic activity should be well within the patient's comfort range. The activity should be enjoyable, not stressful, and after completing the activity the patient should feel "positive" about the experience and not unduly fatigued. For many older heart-failure patients, this may mean starting with as little as 2 to 5 minutes of slow-paced walking. Once the patient feels comfortable exercising, the duration of exercise can be gradually increased over a period of several weeks. Weekly increases of 1 to 2 minutes per session are appropriate for most patients. Once the patient can exercise continuously and

Table 37-8   Contraindications to Exercise in Older Patients

Recent myocardial infarction or unstable angina (within 2 weeks)

Severe, decompensated heart failure (New York Heart Association class IV)

Life-threatening arrhythmias not adequately treated

Severe aortic stenosis or hypertrophic cardiomyopathy

Any acute serious illness (e.g., pneumonia)

Any condition precluding safe participation in an exercise program

comfortably for 20 to 30 minutes, the intensity of exercise may be increased, if desired. For example, if the patient is walking a half-mile in 30 minutes, he or she may gradually reduce the half-mile time to 20 minutes, while maintaining a total exercise duration of 30 minutes.

The two most common techniques for monitoring exercise intensity are the target heart rate method and the patient's subjective assessment of perceived exertion. For patients not taking medications that lower heart rate (e.g., β-blockers), the maximum attainable heart rate in beats per minute (bpm) can be estimated from the formula $220 - \text{age}$. The patient's resting heart rate is then subtracted from this figure to determine the heart rate reserve. A suitable target heart rate for low-intensity exercise can be calculated as the resting heart rate *plus* 30 to 50 percent of the heart rate reserve. For moderate intensity exercise, the target range is the resting heart rate *plus* 50 to 70 percent of the heart rate reserve. For example, an 80-year-old individual has a predicted maximum heart rate of $220 - 80 = 140$ bpm. If the resting heart rate is 80, the heart rate reserve is 60 (i.e., $140 - 80$). For low-intensity exercise, 30 to 50 percent of the heart rate reserve would be 18 to 30 bpm. Adding this to the resting heart rate of 80 would yield a range for the target heart rate of 98 to 110 bpm.

Table 37-9   Exercise Prescription for Older Patients with Heart Failure

Components of conditioning program
　Flexibility exercises
　Strengthening exercises
　Aerobic conditioning

Frequency of exercise: daily, if possible

Duration of exercise: individualized; "start low, go slow"

Intensity of exercise: low to moderate (see text for details)

Rate of progression: gradual over weeks to months

Monitoring: heart rate, perceived exertion (see text)

For many older patients, calculating the target heart rate may be difficult. In addition, it may not be possible to accurately determine heart rate during exercise (unless a heart-rate monitor is used). For these reasons the patient's subjective assessment of perceived exertion is often the most practical method for monitoring exercise intensity. In addition, perceived exertion correlates reasonably well with exercise heart rate. A simple perceived exertion scale comprises five levels: very light, light, moderate, somewhat heavy, and heavy. Older heart-failure patients should begin with very-light exercise, progressing to the light range as tolerated. After several weeks, some patients may wish to increase their perceived exertion level into the moderate range, but more strenuous exercise is not recommended for heart failure patients.

All patients participating in an exercise program should be advised to discontinue exercise if they experience persistent chest discomfort, undue dyspnea or fatigue, dizziness, rapid or irregular heart beats, excessive sweating, or any other symptom suggesting that continuation of exercise may be unsafe. If the above symptoms do not resolve promptly with termination of exercise or if they occur repeatedly, the physician should be notified prior to continuing the exercise program.

Treatment of Systolic Heart Failure

From the therapeutic perspective, heart failure patients with a left ventricular ejection fraction of less than 45 percent may be considered as having predominantly systolic heart failure, while those with an ejection fraction of 45 percent or greater may be considered as having predominantly diastolic heart failure. Although there is considerable overlap between these syndromes, their distinction is helpful in designing therapy.

In general, the treatment of systolic heart failure in older patients does not differ substantially from that in younger patients. Table 37-10 lists currently available therapeutic options for systolic heart failure, and these are discussed in detail below.

Table 37-10   Treatment Options for Systolic Heart Failure

Angiotensin-converting enzyme inhibitors

Angiotensin II receptor blockers

Other vasodilators

β-Adrenergic blocking agents

Diuretics
　Spironolactone

Digoxin

Calcium channel blockers

Antithrombotic agents
　Aspirin
　Warfarin

Angiotensin-Converting Enzyme Inhibitors

Numerous prospective randomized clinical trials using multiple different angiotensin-converting enzyme (ACE) inhibitors in a variety of clinical settings have conclusively demonstrated that these agents significantly reduce mortality and hospitalization rates and improve exercise tolerance and quality of life in patients with impaired left ventricular systolic function, even in the absence of clinical heart failure (see, e.g., SOLVD Investigators, 1991 and 1992). Although none of these studies included patients older than 80 years of age, available evidence indicates that ACE inhibitors are at least as effective in older patients as in younger ones. Based on these findings, ACE inhibitors are now considered first-line therapy for all patients, regardless of age, with left ventricular systolic dysfunction with or without overt heart failure. However, despite these recommendations, ACE inhibitors are substantially underutilized, particularly in older patients.

ACE inhibitors approved for use in the United States for the treatment of heart failure include captopril, enalapril, lisinopril, ramipril, trandolapril, quinapril, and fosinopril. In older patients, therapy should be initiated with a low dose (e.g., captopril 6.25 to 12.5 mg tid-qid or enalapril 2.5 to 5 mg bid), and the dose should be gradually increased as tolerated. In hospitalized patients who are hemodynamically stable, the dose may be increased daily; in outpatients, the dose should be increased weekly or biweekly. Throughout the titration period, blood pressure, renal function, and serum potassium levels should be monitored closely.

For maintenance therapy, ACE inhibitor dosages should be commensurate with those used in the clinical trials. Recommended "target" doses for selected ACE inhibitors are captopril 50 mg tid; enalapril 10 to 20 mg bid; lisinopril 20 to 40 mg daily; ramipril 10 mg daily; trandolapril 4 mg daily; quinapril 40 mg bid; fosinopril 40 mg daily. In patients unable to tolerate full therapeutic doses of ACE inhibitors, lower doses may be used; however, it must be recognized that clinical benefits may be attenuated (see Packer et al., 1999). In addition, although captopril is an excellent agent for use during the titration phase, once the maintenance dose has been reached, it may be desirable to change to a once-daily ACE inhibitor at equivalent dosage for reasons of convenience and compliance.

The most common side effect from ACE inhibitors is a dry, hacking cough, which may be severe enough to require discontinuation of therapy in 5 to 10 percent of patients during long-term use. Less common but more serious side effects include hypotension, a decline in renal function, and hyperkalemia. All of these side effects tend to occur shortly after initiation of therapy and may be aggravated by intravascular volume contraction caused by overdiuresis. As a result, these adverse effects can often be avoided or reversed by reducing the diuretic dosage. Indications for downward-titration or discontinuation of an ACE inhibitor include symptomatic hypotension, persistent increase in serum creatinine of 1 mg/dL or greater, or a rise in the serum potassium level above 5.5 mEq/L. Note that asymptomatic low blood pressure does not mandate dosage reduction.

Although ACE inhibitors are generally well tolerated and can be taken safely in combination with most other medications, it is important to recognize that NSAIDs, which are widely used by older adults (both by prescription and over-the-counter), are potent ACE inhibitor antagonists. In addition, NSAIDs promote sodium and water retention and may adversely affect renal function. Therefore, NSAIDs should be avoided whenever possible in heart-failure patients. The use of aspirin in combination with an ACE inhibitor is controversial, as there is evidence suggesting that aspirin, even at low doses, may attenuate the effects of ACE inhibitors. Although additional study is needed, at the present time it seems prudent to avoid aspirin in patients treated with an ACE inhibitor unless there is a clear indication for its use (e.g., prior coronary bypass surgery, recent myocardial infarction or unstable angina).

Angiotensin II Receptor Blockers

Angiotensin II receptor blockers (ARBs) bind directly to angiotensin II receptors on the cell membrane and provide more complete blockade of the angiotensin system than ACE inhibitors. In addition, unlike ACE inhibitors, ARBs do not inhibit the breakdown of bradykinins, thus eliminating bradykinin-mediated side effects, including cough.

Two recently completed trials evaluated the use of ARBs for the treatment of heart failure, either alone or in combination with an ACE inhibitor. In the second Evaluation of Losartan in the Elderly trial (ELITE-II), losartan 50 mg once daily was compared to captopril 50 mg tid in 3152 patients 60 years of age or older (mean age 71 years) with moderate heart failure and an ejection fraction of 40 percent or less (Pitt et al., 2000). After a mean followup of 18 months, there was no statistically significant difference in mortality between the two treatments, although there were 12 percent more deaths in the losartan group (280 versus 250). As in the smaller ELITE-I trial, losartan was better tolerated than the ACE inhibitor captopril.

In the Valsartan Heart Failure Trial (Val-HEFT), 5010 heart-failure patients with an ejection fraction of less than 40 percent were randomized to valsartan or placebo in addition to standard care, which included an ACE inhibitor in 93 percent of patients and a β-blocker in 35 percent (Cohn et al., 2001). During a 2-year follow-up period, mortality did not differ between patients who were treated with valsartan or with placebo, but there was a significant 24 percent reduction in rehospitalizations for heart failure in the valsartan group, with similar effects in younger and older patients. However, patients receiving both an ACE inhibitor and a β-blocker as background therapy experienced an unexplained increase in mortality when valsartan was added.

Based on available data, ACE inhibitors remain first-line therapy for systolic heart failure, but ARBs are a suitable alternative in patients intolerant to ACE inhibitors because of cough or other side effects. In addition, patients who remain symptomatic despite optimal therapy with ACE inhibitors or other agents may benefit from the addition of an ARB. Ongoing trials scheduled for completion in the next 2 to 3 years should help clarify the role of ARBs in the treatment of heart failure.

Other Vasodilators

In patients who are unable to tolerate an ACE inhibitor or ARB, the combination of hydralazine with oral or topical nitrates provides an acceptable alternative. In the first Veteran's Administration Heart Failure Trial (V-HeFT-I), the hydralazine/nitrate combination was associated with a 36 percent mortality reduction when compared to prazosin and placebo in patients with chronic heart failure and impaired systolic function (Cohn et al., 1986). In a followup study (V-HeFT-II), patients with systolic heart failure were randomized to receive hydralazine/nitrates or enalapril. Although hydralazine/nitrates and enalapril had similar effects on exercise tolerance and quality of life, mortality was lower in the enalapril group (Cohn et al., 1991).

The dose of hydralazine used in the V-HeFT trials was 75 mg qid and nitrates were administered as isosorbide dinitrate 40 mg qid. For older patients, treatment should begin with lower dosages (e.g., hydralazine 12.5 to 25 mg tid-qid; isosorbide dinitrate 10 mg tid-qid), followed by gradual upward titration to achieve the doses used in the V-HeFT trials. The most common side effects associated with hydralazine/nitrates in the V-HeFT studies included headache, dizziness, fatigue, and gastrointestinal disturbances. A small percentage of patients developed arthralgias or other symptoms suggestive of hydralazine-induced lupus.

β-Blockers

Traditionally, β-adrenergic blocking agents have been considered contraindicated in heart-failure patients because of their negative inotropic and chronotropic effects, both of which serve to diminish cardiac output. However, it is now recognized that persistent activation of the sympathetic nervous system is detrimental in heart-failure patients because it exacerbates ischemia, aids in arrhythmogenesis, promotes β-receptor downregulation, and contributes to a progressive decline in ventricular function. These considerations led to the hypothesis that long-term treatment with β-blockers might be beneficial in heart-failure patients, and several large prospective randomized clinical trials have now confirmed that long-term β-blockade improves left ventricular function and reduces both total mortality and sudden cardiac death in a broad range of patients with heart failure and impaired left ventricular systolic function (Packer et al. 1996 and 2001, MERIT-HF 1999, The Cardiac Insufficiency Bisoprolol Study, 1999). Moreover, patients up to age 80 years have been included in these trials, and the absolute benefits of β-blockers have been similar in younger and older patients. As a result, β-blockers are now recommended as standard therapy, along with ACE inhibitors, in almost all patients with symptomatic heart failure in the absence of contraindications.

Carvedilol, metoprolol, and bisoprolol are of proven benefit in the treatment of systolic heart failure, and both carvedilol and metoprolol have been approved for this indication in the United States. Because the initial effect of β-blockade is a reduction in cardiac output, these agents should only be initiated in clinically stable patients receiving appropriate doses of ACE inhibitors, diuretics, and, if indicated, digoxin. Starting dosages are carvedilol 3.125 mg bid, metoprolol 12.5 mg bid (or extended release metoprolol 25 mg once daily), and bisoprolol 1.25 mg once daily. The dose should be gradually increased at approximately 2 week intervals as tolerated to achieve maintenance dosages of carvedilol 25 to 50 mg bid, metoprolol 100 to 200 mg daily, or bisoprolol 10 mg once daily.

Contraindications to the use of β-blockers include severe decompensated heart failure, significant bronchospastic lung disease, marked bradycardia (resting heart rate less than 50 bpm), systolic blood pressure less than 90 to 100 mmHg, advanced heart block (greater than first degree), and known intolerance to β-blockade. In addition, because of the potential for significant adverse effects, it is important to monitor heart rate, blood pressure, clinical symptoms, and the cardiorespiratory examination during initiation and titration of therapy.

Potential side effects of β-blockers during initiation and titration include worsening heart failure, bronchospasm, bradycardia, hypotension, and heart block. Other side effects may include dizziness, syncope, gastrointestinal disturbances, fatigue, low energy level, sleep disturbances, and decreased mood. Patients should be advised that they may experience a modest deterioration in heart failure symptoms during the first few weeks of β-blocker therapy but that in most cases these symptoms resolve and the long-term tolerability of β-blockers is excellent. However, if severe adverse effects occur, dosage reduction or discontinuation of treatment may be necessary.

Diuretics

Diuretics are the most effective agents for relieving pulmonary congestion and edema, and for this reason they remain a key component of heart-failure management. However, neither thiazide nor loop diuretics alter the natural history of heart failure, and their beneficial effects are primarily palliative. In contrast, the aldosterone antagonist spironolactone has recently been shown to reduce mortality in selected patients with advanced heart failure.

In patients with very mild chronic heart failure, a thiazide diuretic (e.g., hydrochlorothiazide 12.5 to 50 mg daily) may be sufficient for relieving congestive symptoms and maintaining fluid homeostasis. However, most patients will require a more potent agent, and the "loop" diuretics, including furosemide, bumetanide, and torsemide, are the drugs most widely used. For optimal effectiveness patients should be instructed to maintain a low sodium diet (1.5 to 2.0 g/d) and to avoid excessive fluid intake. Typical daily doses of "loop" diuretics range from 20 to 160 mg for furosemide, 0.5 to 5 mg for bumetanide, and 5 to 100 mg for torsemide. In patients hospitalized with an acute episode of heart failure, intravenous administration is more effective than the oral route in promoting diuresis, and continuous intravenous infusion is more effective than bolus dosing. In patients who fail to respond adequately to a loop diuretic, the addition of metolazone 2.5 mg to 10 mg daily often leads to a brisk diuresis.

In the Randomized Aldactone Evaluation of Survival (RALES) trial, spironolactone 12.5 to 50 mg once daily reduced mortality by 30 percent and heart failure hospitalizations by 35 percent in patients with New York Heart Association class III or IV heart failure and a left ventricular ejection fraction <35 percent despite therapy with an ACE inhibitor, digoxin, and loop diuretic (Pitt, et al., 1999). Moreover, the beneficial effects of spironolactone were at least as great in older as in younger patients. Based on these findings, low-dose spironolactone is recommended in patients with advanced heart failure symptoms and severe left ventricular systolic dysfunction. Note, however, that spironolactone is contraindicated in patients with significant renal dysfunction (creatinine >2.5 mg/dL) or preexisting hyperkalemia. In addition, older patients may be at increased risk for adverse effects, and renal function as well as serum potassium levels should be monitored closely during initiation and titration of therapy. Furthermore, up to 10 percent of patients receiving long-term treatment with spironolactone may experience painful gynecomastia requiring discontinuation of the drug.

The most common and important side effects of diuretics are electrolyte disturbances, including hypo- and hyperkalemia, hyponatremia, hypomagnesemia, and increased bicarbonate levels indicative of metabolic alkalosis. Because of age-related changes in renal function, as well as a higher prevalence of comorbid illnesses such as diabetes, older patients are at increased risk for serious diuretic-induced electrolyte abnormalities. For this reason, electrolytes should be monitored closely when diuretic therapy is being adjusted. This is particularly true when using metolazone, which can cause life-threatening hyponatremia after relatively short-term use, or spironolactone, which may be associated with a marked rise in the serum potassium level.

Digoxin

Digoxin inhibits the sodium-potassium exchange pump located within the myocyte membrane, producing a rise in intracellular sodium concentration. This facilitates sodium-calcium exchange leading to an increase in intracellular calcium. Calcium binds with troponin C, which initiates the process of contraction by allowing myosin to bind with actin. By increasing calcium availability, digoxin induces a modest increase in the force of myocardial contraction (positive inotropic effect). This effect occurs whether or not heart failure is present, and it does not appear to be affected by advancing age.

In 1997, the Digitalis Investigation Group (DIG) reported the results of a prospective randomized trial involving 6800 patients with heart failure and ejection fractions less than 45 percent. Patients were randomized to receive digoxin or placebo in addition to diuretics and an ACE inhibitor, and the average duration of followup was 37 months (The Digitalis Investigation Group, 1997). Overall mortality did not differ between digoxin and placebo (34.8 percent versus 35.1 percent), but there were 28 percent fewer hospitalizations for heart failure in the digoxin group, and the combined endpoint of death or hospitalization for heart failure was significantly reduced (Fig. 37-5). In addition, the beneficial effects of digoxin were similar in younger and older patients, including

octogenarians (see Rich et al., 2001). These findings confirm that digoxin is beneficial in controlling heart failure symptoms and support the use of digoxin in patients who remain symptomatic despite appropriate dosages of an ACE inhibitor and diuretic. Because digoxin does not prolong life, its value in patients who are well-compensated on standard therapy is less clear.

Side effects from digoxin fall into three major categories: cardiac, neurologic, and gastrointestinal. In the DIG study, side effects that occurred more frequently in patients receiving digoxin included nausea and vomiting, diarrhea, visual disturbances, supraventricular and ventricular arrhythmias, and advanced atrioventricular heart block. Although not reported in the DIG trial, older patients may be at increased risk for digoxin toxicity, especially cardiac toxicity, in part due to a decreased volume of drug distribution as well as reduced glomerular filtration rate.

As a result of age-related changes in renal function and lean body mass, the therapeutic range for digoxin is lower in older adults. Thus, in individuals older than 70 years of age, a serum digoxin concentration of 0.5 to 1.5 ng/mL is appropriate. Higher digoxin levels are not associated with enhanced inotropic effect, but the risk of serious toxicity rises steeply at higher serum levels. Additionally, patients with chronic lung disease, amyloid heart disease, and other conditions may be at increased risk for digoxin toxicity.

In most older patients with relatively normal renal function, a digoxin dose of 0.125 mg daily is usually sufficient to achieve a therapeutic effect. Patients with renal impairment or small body habitus may require an even lower dose. Although routine monitoring of serum digoxin levels is no longer recommended, it is appropriate to maintain a high index of suspicion for digitalis intoxication, and to measure the digoxin level when clinically indicated. Additionally, because diuretic-induced hypokalemia and hypomagnesia potentiate digoxin's cardiotoxic effects, including proarrhythmia, it is important to maintain normal serum concentrations of these electrolytes in all patients receiving digoxin.

Calcium Channel Blockers

First-generation short-acting calcium channel blockers, including nifedipine, diltiazem, and verapamil, are contraindicated in patients with systolic heart failure because each of these agents has been associated with adverse clinical outcomes. In addition, although long-acting formulations of these agents may ultimately prove to be safe and effective, there is currently insufficient information to recommend their use.

The third-generation calcium channel blockers amlodipine and felodipine have each been studied in prospective randomized trials involving heart failure patients with impaired systolic function. Although the initial Prospective Randomized Amlodipine Survival Evaluation (PRAISE) study suggested that amlodipine might be beneficial in patients with nonischemic systolic heart failure (Packer et al., 1996), this was not confirmed in PRAISE-2. Similarly, the V-HeFT-III trial failed to demonstrate a significant benefit in heart failure patients treated with felodipine (Cohn

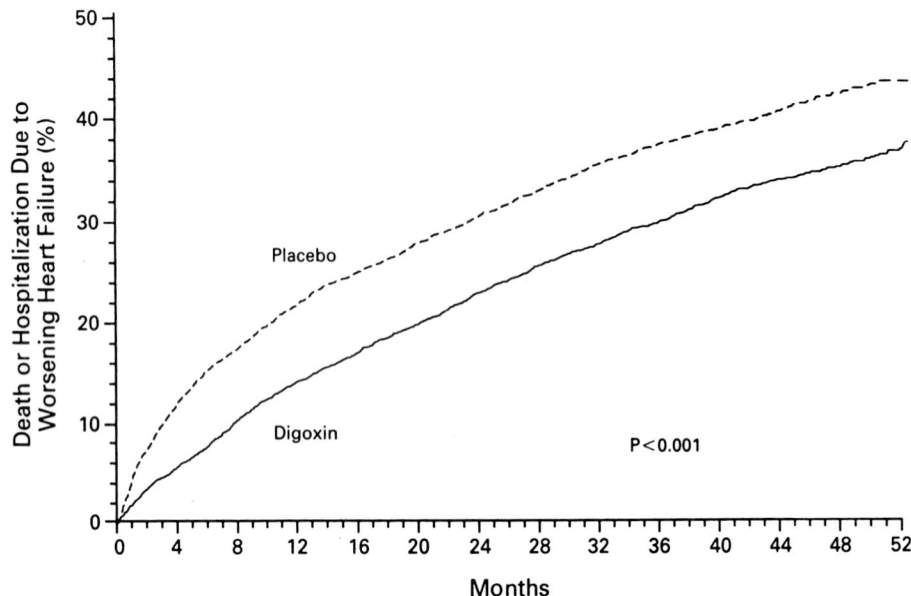

Figure 37-5   Incidence of death or hospitalization as a result of worsening heart failure in patients treated with digoxin versus placebo. The risk for the combined end point was 25 percent lower in the digoxin group. Reproduced with permission from The Digitalis Investigation Group. The effect of digoxin on mortality and morbidity in patients with heart failure. *N Engl J Med* 336:525, 1997.

et al., 1997). In light of these findings, there are no currently approved indications for the use of calcium channel blockers in patients with systolic heart failure, and their use in this condition is not recommended. However, in heart failure patients with active anginal symptoms not controlled with β-blockers and nitrates, the addition of amlodipine or felodipine is reasonable.

Antithrombotic Therapy

Patients with left ventricular systolic dysfunction are at increased risk for thromboembolic events, including stroke. However, in the absence of atrial fibrillation, rheumatic mitral valve disease, or a history of prior embolization, the value of antithrombotic treatment for the prevention of embolic events is unknown. This problem is further complicated by the fact that, as discussed previously, aspirin may attenuate the effects of ACE inhibitors, and warfarin may be associated with a higher risk of bleeding complications in older heart failure patients. Nonetheless, anticoagulation with warfarin to achieve an international normalized ratio (INR) of 2.0 to 3.0 is recommended in high-risk patients without major contraindications. Such patients include those with chronic or intermittent atrial fibrillation or atrial flutter, rheumatic mitral valve disease with left atrial enlargement, prior stroke or unexplained arterial embolus, a mobile left ventricular thrombus (as demonstrated by echocardiography or other imaging modality), or a left atrial appendage thrombus identified by transesophageal echocardiography. Patients with markedly dilated ventricles and severe left ventricular dysfunction (ejection fraction less than 25 percent) may also benefit from warfarin therapy. The ongoing Warfarin Antiplatelet Therapy in Congestive Heart Failure (WATCH) randomized trial is comparing the effects of warfarin, aspirin, and clopidogrel on clinical outcomes in patients with systolic heart failure

and sinus rhythm; the results of this study are anticipated in 2003 or 2004.

Aspirin is justified in patients with known coronary heart disease, particularly those with recent myocardial infarction, unstable angina, coronary angioplasty, or bypass surgery. In addition, aspirin is appropriate in high-risk patients (as listed above) who are not suitable candidates for warfarin. In other situations, routine aspirin use is of unproven benefit, and it should probably be avoided in patients taking an ACE inhibitor.

TREATMENT OF DIASTOLIC HEART FAILURE

Despite the fact that at least 30 to 50 percent of older heart-failure patients have well-preserved left ventricular systolic function, there have been few large-scale clinical trials evaluating specific pharmacologic agents for the treatment of this condition. As a result, therapy for diastolic heart failure remains largely empiric.

Approximately 75 percent of older persons with diastolic heart failure have hypertension, and coronary and valvular heart disease are also highly prevalent in this population. Optimal therapy for diastolic heart failure begins with aggressive treatment of hypertension to target levels, as established by Joint National Committee (JNC) guidelines (The Sixth Report of the Joint National Committee on prevention, detection, evaluation, and treatment of high blood pressure). Myocardial ischemia should be treated with antianginal medications and/or coronary revascularization as indicated. Patients with severe valvular heart disease should be considered for valve repair or replacement, and less severe regurgitant valvular lesions should be treated with unloading agents, such as ACE inhibitors. As with systolic heart failure, nonpharmacologic aspects of therapy should be appropriately addressed.

Diuretics

Diuretics are an essential component of therapy for the relief of pulmonary and systemic venous congestion in patients with diastolic heart failure. However, because patients with diastolic heart failure tend to function on the steep portion of the pressure-volume curve, overly zealous diuresis can precipitate a rapid fall in left ventricular diastolic volume with a resultant decline in stroke volume and cardiac output. This common sequence of events is often manifested by increased fatigue, relative hypotension, and worsening prerenal azotemia. Thus, patients with diastolic heart failure are often "volume sensitive," and diuretics must be prescribed judiciously in order to relieve congestion while avoiding overdiuresis.

β-Blockers

β-blockers have little or no direct effect on diastolic function, but they may improve symptoms in patients with diastolic heart failure by slowing heart rate and lengthening the diastolic filling period. In patients with left ventricular hypertrophy (LVH), long-term β-blockade and effective blood pressure control may aid in the regression of LVH, which, in turn, may be associated with improved diastolic function. Although no large prospective studies have been completed, a small randomized trial involving 158 patients (mean age 81 years) with heart failure, prior myocardial infarction, and an ejection fraction of 40 percent or greater demonstrated that patients treated with propranolol had improved survival when compared to those who did not receive a β-blocker (see Aronow et al.).

The goal of β-blocker therapy in diastolic heart failure is to reduce the resting heart rate to less than 65 beats per minute. With regard to selection of a β-blocker, the β_1-selective agents metoprolol and atenolol may be associated with fewer side effects than some of the nonselective agents (e.g., propranolol, timolol). On the other hand, the mixed α- and β-blockers (e.g., labetalol, carvedilol) may be more effective in controlling blood pressure, although the effect on heart rate may be less pronounced. Regardless of which agent is chosen, the initial dose should be small and titration should be gradual in order to achieve the desired effect on heart rate. In the event that symptoms and exercise tolerance do not improve, alternative therapy should be considered.

Angiotensin-Converting Enzyme Inhibitors

ACE inhibitors may improve symptoms in diastolic heart failure both directly (by improving diastolic function) and indirectly (by promoting regression of left ventricular hypertrophy). The use of ACE inhibitors for the treatment of diastolic heart failure in patients of advanced age is supported by findings from a small, open-label study reported by Aronow et al. in 1993. Compared to controls, patients with an average age of 80 years treated with enalapril for 3 months experienced improvements in exercise capacity and New York Heart Association functional class. In addition, left ventricular mass declined and indices of diastolic function improved in the enalapril group. The ACE

inhibitor perindopril is currently being evaluated for the treatment of diastolic heart failure in a prospective randomized trial. ACE inhibitor dosing and side effects in patients with diastolic heart failure are similar to those for systolic heart failure.

Angiotensin II Receptor Blockers

Angiotensin II receptor blockers may have salutary effects on diastolic function similar to those observed with ACE inhibitors. In a small study, the ARB losartan was associated with improved exercise tolerance and quality of life in older patients with diastolic heart failure. Currently, the ARBs candesartan and irbesartan are being evaluated in clinical trials of diastolic heart failure.

Calcium Channel Blockers

Calcium channel blockers decrease intracellular calcium and may have a modest beneficial effect on diastolic function. Verapamil has been shown to improve symptoms and exercise tolerance in selected patients with hypertrophic cardiomyopathy and normal systolic function. In addition, Setaro et al. studied 20 men, mean age 68 years, with heart failure and an ejection fraction above 45 percent, and found that in comparison with placebo, verapamil at dosages of up to 120 mg tid improved symptoms, exercise capacity, and indices of diastolic function. On the other hand, some patients with diastolic heart failure may experience marked clinical deterioration when treated with verapamil. Moreover, the lack of benefit from calcium channel blockers for the treatment of systolic heart failure tempers enthusiasm for their use in diastolic heart failure. As a result, calcium channel antagonists are not considered first-line agents for the treatment of this condition.

Nitrates

In addition to relieving ischemia, nitrates are effective venodilators and they lower pulmonary capillary wedge pressure. For these reasons, nitrates may serve as a useful adjunct to diuretics in relieving symptoms of pulmonary congestion, particularly orthopnea. However, nitrates have the potential for decreasing venous return to the heart, thereby reducing left ventricular diastolic volume and stroke volume. In addition, tolerance to the hemodynamic effects of nitrates occurs in the majority of patients. As a result, the value of nitrates in the long-term management of diastolic heart failure is uncertain.

Digoxin

Traditionally, digoxin has been considered to be contraindicated in patients with heart failure and normal systolic function. However, digoxin, as well as other inotropic agents, may exert a favorable effect on diastolic function by accelerating calcium reuptake by the sarcoplasmic reticulum at the onset of diastole. Moreover, in the recently completed DIG trial, 988 patients with heart failure and an ejection fraction greater than 45 percent were randomized to digoxin or placebo in an ancillary study. As in the main trial, digoxin had no effect on mortality. However, the combined end point of death or rehospitalization for heart failure was reduced 18 percent in patients receiving digoxin. Although this difference was not statistically significant, it suggests that digoxin may be beneficial in some individuals with heart failure and preserved systolic function. Nonetheless, digoxin is not recommended as routine therapy for diastolic heart failure at the present time.

Thus, optimal therapy for diastolic heart failure is unknown, and the approach to treatment varies widely. The patient's underlying cardiovascular disease should be treated whenever possible, and a diuretic should be administered at low to moderate doses to relieve congestion and edema. In most cases, β-blockers or ACE inhibitors are appropriate first-line agents. If the patient's symptoms improve satisfactorily, the initial therapeutic regimen should be maintained. However, if the patient fails to respond to initial therapy, alternative treatment should be considered. Such therapy might include the use of nitrates, an ARB, a calcium channel blocker, digoxin, or a combination of agents. Again, because none of these agents is of proven efficacy, the clinician should maintain flexibility in designing a regimen which relieves symptoms and improves quality of life while minimizing side effects.

Refractory Heart Failure

Refractory heart failure may be defined as heart failure not amenable to primary corrective measures (e.g., valve replacement or revascularization) and not responsive to aggressive nonpharmacologic and pharmacologic therapy as described above. However, before designating heart failure as refractory, it is important to perform a careful search for potentially treatable causes, to carefully review the patient's medication regimen to ensure that therapy is optimal, and to discuss the patient's diet and medication habits in detail with the patient and family to ensure that an appropriate level of compliance is being maintained. The latter issue is of particular importance, because many cases of refractory heart failure can be traced to nonadherence with dietary restrictions, medications, or both.

In most cases, refractory heart failure simply represents the final common pathway of end-stage heart disease. Under these circumstances, the value of highly aggressive treatment is questionable, and decisions regarding the appropriateness of specific therapeutic interventions must be made on an individualized basis (see also "Ethical Issues and End-of-Life Decisions" later in this chapter).

Table 37-11 lists treatment options for refractory heart failure. In patients with systolic heart failure, intensifying the vasodilator regimen by using high doses of ACE inhibitors (e.g., up to 400 mg/d of captopril or 80 mg/d of enalapril), either alone or in combination with hydralazine/nitrates or an angiotensin II receptor blocker, may result in significant symptomatic improvement. This can often be accomplished in the outpatient setting, but titration must be very gradual with frequent follow-up contacts to avoid adverse events. In patients who fail to respond to these measures, intravenous vasodilator therapy with

Table 37-11   Treatment Options for Refractory Heart Failure

Systolic Heart Failure
Intensive vasodilator therapy
High-dose ACE inhibitors
Combination therapy
ACE inhibitor plus hydralazine/nitrates
ACE inhibitor plus angiotensin II receptor blocker
Intravenous agents (e.g., nitroprusside, nesiritide)
Intensive diuretic therapy
High-dose oral agents, especially in combination
Continuous intravenous infusion
Chronic or intermittent inotropic therapy
Dobutamine
Milrinone
Pacemaker therapy
Dialysis
Short-term or chronic dialysis
Dry ultrafiltration
Investigational agents
Surgical options
Myocardial resection
Cardiomyoplasty
Ventricular assist device
Diastolic Heart Failure
Intensive diuretic therapy (see above)
Empiric trial of inotropic therapy
Dialysis (see above)
AV sequential pacemaker

nitroprusside or nesiritide (recombinant brain natriuretic peptide) may lead to significant clinical and hemodynamic improvements (see Mills et al.).

In patients with persistent pulmonary congestion or peripheral edema, high-dose oral diuretics (e.g., furosemide 200 mg bid or bumetanide 10 mg daily), alone or in combination with metolazone, may be effective. Alternatively, a continuous intravenous infusion of furosemide 5 to 40 mg/h or bumetanide 0.5 to 1 mg/h will often facilitate diuresis (see Howard and Dunn).

The use of intravenous inotropic agents in the management of chronic heart failure is somewhat controversial because these agents have not been shown to improve outcomes and they may increase the risk of life-threatening arrhythmias. Nonetheless, extensive clinical experience indicates that intermittent or continuous outpatient infusions of dobutamine or milrinone may significantly reduce symptoms and improve quality of life in selected patients with refractory heart failure. In most cases, initiation of intravenous inotropic therapy should be conducted in a monitored unit under hemodynamic guidance using a pulmonary artery catheter.

Recently, biventricular or left ventricular pacing was shown to improve symptoms, quality of life, and left ventricular performance in patients with advanced heart failure and left bundle branch block or marked intraventricular conduction delay on the 12-lead electrocardiogram. At present, this procedure should only be performed at specialized centers by experienced electrophysiologists or surgeons.

If the above interventions fail, patients with significant renal dysfunction may benefit from short-term dialysis or dry ultrafiltration to remove excess fluid and stabilize electrolyte homeostasis. If the patient responds to short-term treatment, chronic dialysis may be considered. Finally, in highly selected patients, referral to a tertiary or quaternary facility for investigational medical or surgical treatment may be appropriate.

For patients with refractory heart failure as a result of diastolic dysfunction, therapeutic options are limited (Table 37-11). Intensive diuretic therapy may be attempted, but efficacy is often limited by the development of progressive prerenal azotemia. Similarly, a trial of inotropic therapy or dialysis may be considered, but the clinical response to these interventions is unpredictable. Finally, although preliminary reports have suggested that some patients with diastolic heart failure may benefit from permanent dual-chamber pacing, this procedure remains investigational.

PROGNOSIS

The overall prognosis in patients with established heart failure is poor, and the 5-year survival rate is approximately 50 percent. In elderly patients, the prognosis is even worse, and fewer than 20 percent of heart-failure patients over the age of 80 years survive more than 5 years (Fig. 37-6). In general, the prognosis is worse in men than in women, in patients with systolic rather than diastolic dysfunction, and in patients with an ischemic rather than nonischemic etiology. Patients with more severe symptoms or exercise intolerance, as defined by the New York Heart Association

functional class or as assessed by a 6-minute walk test, also have a less-favorable outlook. Other markers of an adverse prognosis include elevated plasma norepinephrine, atrial natriuretic peptide, brain natriuretic peptide, tumor necrosis factor-α, and endothelin-1 levels; hyponatremia; reduced heart rate variability; and the presence of atrial fibrillation or high-grade ventricular arrhythmias. In patients with chronic heart failure, 40 to 50 percent die from progressive heart failure, 40 percent die from arrhythmias, and 10 to 20 percent die from other causes (e.g., myocardial infarction or noncardiac conditions).

ETHICAL ISSUES AND END-OF-LIFE DECISIONS

As noted above, the prognosis for patients with heart failure is extremely poor, and 5-year survival rates are lower than for most forms of cancer. In addition, once heart failure symptoms have reached an advanced stage (e.g., New York Heart Association class III or IV), quality of life is often severely compromised and therapeutic options are limited. Moreover, even patients with relatively mild or well-compensated heart failure are continually at risk for experiencing sudden cardiac arrest, and if initial resuscitative efforts are successful, questions regarding life support and related issues may arise.

For these reasons, it is incumbent upon the physician to discuss the patient's wishes regarding the intensity of treatment and end-of-life care at a time when the patient is still capable of understanding the issues and making informed choices. In addition, because the patient's views may evolve over the course of illness, these issues should be readdressed at periodic intervals. The development of a "living will" and appointment of durable power-of-attorney should also be encouraged.

A related concern is the extent to which the physician should offer aggressive or investigational therapeutic options that are unlikely to substantially alter the natural history of disease or significantly improve quality of life. This concern applies not only to many of the treatment

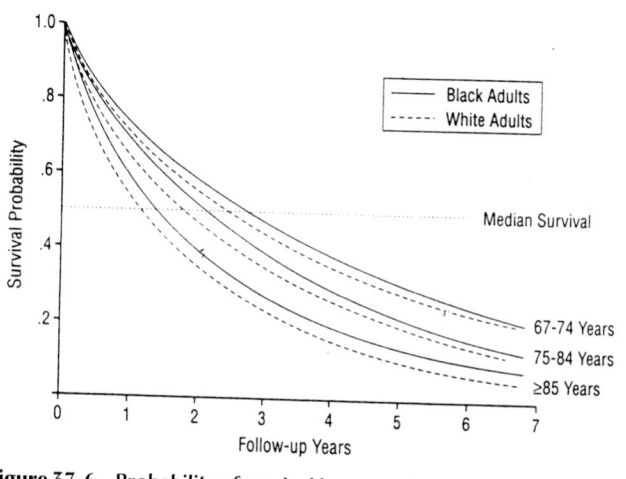

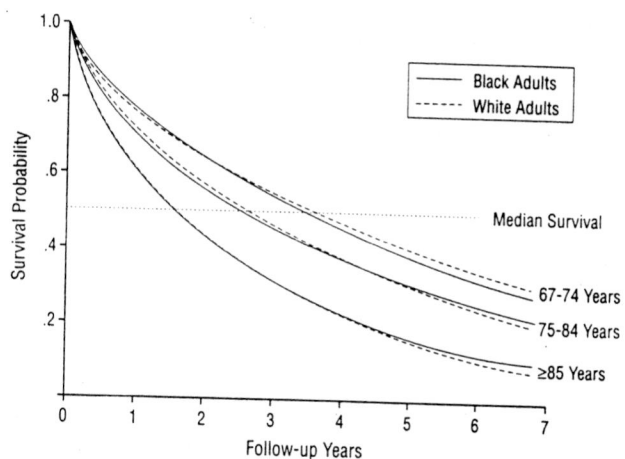

Figure 37-6 Probability of survival by age and race after first hospitalization for heart failure among older men (*left panel*) and women (*right panel*). Reproduced with permission from Croft JB et al: Heart failure survival among older adults in the United States: A poor prognosis for an emerging epidemic in the Medicare population. *Arch Intern Med* 159:505, 1999.

modalities discussed in the refractory heart failure section above, but also to such procedures as endotracheal intubation and intraaortic balloon counterpulsation. In many cases, these interventions not only fail to modify the clinical course, but may actually contribute to the patient's pain and suffering in the terminal stages of disease. Moreover, the suggestion that a given intervention may help stabilize the patient and slow disease progression may create false hopes in the minds of the patient and family, and subsequent failure of the intervention may compound the emotional suffering that both the patient and family are forced to endure. For these reasons, it is essential that the physician realistically appraise the potential benefits and attendant risks, both physical and emotional, prior to offering aggressive therapeutic options which may provide little or no hope of improving the patient's quality of life over a clinically important period of time.

Finally, as the patient approaches the terminal stages of disease, there should be discussions with the patient and family regarding where the patient would like to spend his or her final days. For many patients, the idea of dying at home surrounded by close family is comforting, and this desire should be honored whenever possible. For some patients, a reputable hospice that provides compassionate end-of-life care may be a suitable alternative. For others, the hospital may be the most desirable environment, but an attempt should be made to secure a private room with open visitation hours. The intensive care unit, with its austere, "high-tech" facade, is the least-desirable place to die, and should be avoided whenever possible.

PREVENTION

In view of the exceptionally poor prognosis associated with established heart failure in older adults, it is essential to develop and implement preventive strategies. Appropriate treatment of hypertension has been repeatedly shown to

Table 37-12 Effect of Antihypertensive Therapy on Incident Heart Failure in Older Adults

Trial	Year	Number	Age (Years)	Risk Reduction for Heart Failure (%)
EWPHE	1985	840	>60	22
Coope	1986	884	60–79	32
STOP-HTN	1991	1627	70–84	51
SHEP	1991	4736	≥60	55
STONE	1996	1632	60–79	68
Syst-Eur	1997	4695	≥60	36
Syst-China	2000	2394	≥60	38

EWPHE, European Working Party on Hypertension in the Elderly; SHEP, Systolic Hypertension in the Elderly Program; STONE, Shanghai Trial of Nifedipine in the Elderly; STOP-HTN, Swedish Trial in Old Patients with Hypertension; Syst-China, Systolic Hypertension in China Trial; Syst-Eur, Systolic Hypertension in Europe Trial.

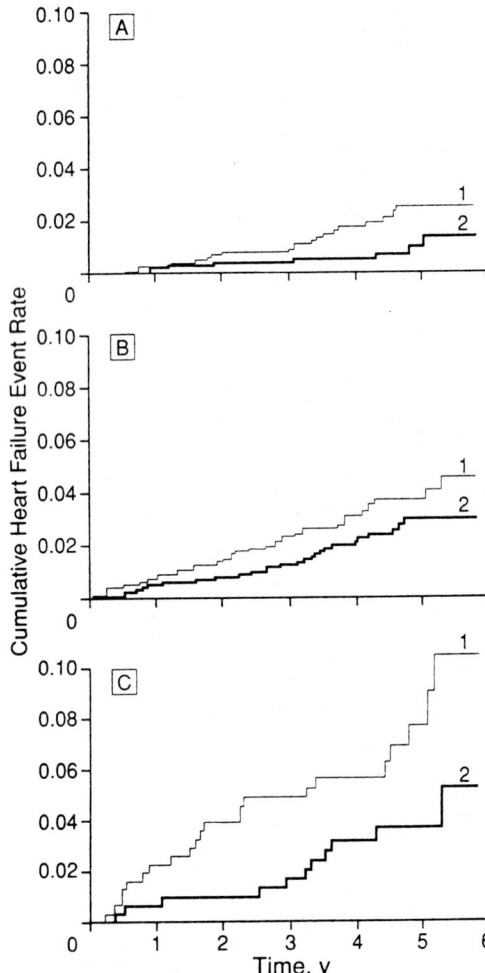

Figure 37-7 Effect of antihypertensive therapy on incident heart failure in patients with isolated systolic hypertension: The Systolic Hypertension in the Elderly Program (SHEP). *Top panel:* age 60 to 69 years; *middle panel:* age 70 to 79 years; *lower panel:* age ≥80 years. Reproduced with permission from Kostis JB et al: Prevention of heart failure by antihypertensive drug treatment in older persons with isolated systolic hypertension. SHEP Cooperative Research Group. *JAMA* 278:212, 1997.

reduce the incidence of heart failure by up to 50 percent (Table 37-12). Moreover, in the Systolic Hypertension in the Elderly Program (SHEP), the greatest benefit was seen in patients older than 80 years of age (Fig. 37-7). Treatment of hyperlipidemia also reduces the incidence of heart failure, most likely through prevention of myocardial infarction and other ischemic events. Likewise, smoking cessation reduces the risk of myocardial infarction and stroke in older adults, and likely has a similar effect on the development of heart failure. Unfortunately, despite abundant evidence that heart failure prevention is feasible through risk factor modification, such strategies are under used, especially in persons older than 80 years of age.

CONCLUSION

Heart failure is an exceedingly common and important clinical problem in older adults, owing in large part to the complex interplay between age-related changes in the cardiovascular system, the high prevalence of cardiovascular and noncardiovascular diseases in the older population, and the widespread use of myriad drugs and other therapies that may adversely affect cardiovascular physiology. As the population of the United States continues to age, heart failure will exact a progressively greater toll on our health care delivery system. In addition, the impact of heart failure on quality of life and independence in the large number of older adults suffering from this disorder is incalculable. Clearly, there is an urgent need to develop more effective strategies for the prevention and treatment of heart failure, with particular emphasis on the geriatric population.

REFERENCES

Aronow WS et al: Effect of enalapril on congestive heart failure treated with diuretics in elderly patients with prior myocardial infarction and normal left ventricular ejection fraction. *Am J Cardiol* 71:602, 1993.

Aronow WS et al: Effect of propranolol versus no propranolol on total mortality plus nonfatal myocardial infarction in older patient with prior myocardial infarction, congetive heart failure, and left ventricular ejection fraction ≥40% treated with diuretics plus angiotensin-converting enzyme inhibitors. *Am J Cardiol* 80:207, 1997.

Belardinelli R et al: Randomized, controlled trial of long-term moderate exercise training in chronic heart failure: Effects on functional capacity, quality of life, and clinical outcome. *Circulation* 99:1173, 1999.

Cohn JN, Tognoni G, for the Valsartan Heart Failure Trial Investigators: A randomized trial of the angiotensin-receptor blocker valsartan in chronic heart failure. *N Engl J Med* 345:1667, 2001.

Cohn JN et al: Effect of the calcium antagonist felodipine as supplementary vasodilator therapy in patients with chronic heart failure treated with enalapril: V-HeFT III. Vasodilator-Heart Failure Trial (V-HeFT) Study Group. *Circulation* 96:856, 1997.

Cohn JN et al: A comparison of enalopril with hydralazine-isosorbide dinitrate in the treatment of chronic congestive heart failure. *N Engl J Med* 325:303, 1991.

Cohn JN et al: Effect of vasodilator therapy on mortality in chronic congestive heart failure. Results of a Vererans Administration Cooperative Study. *N Engl J Med* 314:1547, 1986.

Croft JB et al: Heart failure survival among older adults in the United States: A poor prognosis for an emerging epidemic in the Medicare population. *Arch Intern Med* 159:505, 1999.

Flather MD et al: Long-term ACE-inhibitor therapy in patients with heart failure or left-ventricular dysfunction: A systematic overview of data from individual patients. *Lancet* 355:1575, 2000.

Gottdiener JS et al: Predictors of congestive heart failure in the elderly: The Cardiovascular Health Study. *J Am Coll Cardiol* 35:1628, 2000.

Howard PA, Dunn MI: Aggressive diuresis for severe heart failure in the elderly. *Chest* 119:807, 2001.

Hunt SA et al: ACC/AHA guidelines for the evaluation and management of chronic heart failure in the adult: Executive summary. *J Am Coll Cardiol* 38:2101, 2001. Full text available at: http://www.acc.org/clinical/guidelines/failure/pdfs/hf_fulltext.pdf.

Kannel WB, Belanger AJ: Epidemiology of heart failure. *Am Heart J* 121:951, 1991.

Kitzman DW: Heart failure with normal systolic function. *Clin Geriatr Med* 16:489, 2000.

Kitzman DW et al: Exercise intolerance in patients with heart failure and preserved left ventricular systolic function: Failure of the Frank-Starling mechanism. *J Am Coll Cardiol* 17:1065, 1991.

Maisel A: B-type natriuretic peptide in the diagnosis and management of congestive heart failure. *Cardiol Clin* 19:557, 2001.

McAlister FA et al: A systematic review of randomized trials of disease management programs in heart failure. *Am J Med* 110:378, 2001.

McDonagh TA et al: Biochemical detection of left-ventricular systolic function. *Lancet* 351:9, 1998.

McKelvie RS et al: Effects of exercise training in patients with congestive heart failure: A critical review. *J Am Coll Cardiol* 25:789, 1995.

MERIT-HF Study Group: Effect of metoprolol CR/XL in chronic heart failure: Metoprolol CR/XL Randomised Intervention Trial in Congestive Heart Failure (MERIT-HF). *Lancet* 353:2001, 1999.

Mills RM et al: Sustained hemodynamic effects of an infusion of nesiritide (human b-type natriuretic peptide) in heart failure: A randomized, double-blind, placebo-controlled clinical trial. *J Am Coll Cardiol* 34:155, 1999.

Moser M, Hebert PR: Prevention of disease progression, left ventricular hypertrophy and congestive heart failure in hypertension treatment trials. *J Am Coll Cardiol* 27:1214, 1996.

Packer M et al: Effect of carvedilol on survival in severe chronic heart failure. *N Engl J Med* 344:1651, 2001.

Packer M et al: Comparative effects of low and high doses of the angiotensin-converting enzyme inhibitor, lisinopril, on morbidity and mortality in chronic heart failure. ATLAS Study Group. *Circulation* 100:2312, 1999.

Packer M et al: The effect of carvedilol on morbidity and mortality in patients with chronic heart failure. U.S. Carvedilol Heart Failure Study Group. *N Engl J Med* 334:1349, 1996.

Packer M et al: Effect of amlodipine on morbidity and mortality in severe chronic heart failure. Prospective Randomized Amlodipine Survival Evaluation Study Group. *N Engl J Med* 335:1107, 1996.

Page J, Henry D: Consumption of NSAIDs and the development of congestive heart failure in elderly patients: An underrecognized public health problem. *Arch Intern Med* 160:777, 2000.

Pitt B et al: Effect of losartan compared with captopril on mortality in patients with symptomatic heart failure: Randomised trial—The Losartan Heart Failure Survival Study ELITE II. *Lancet* 355:1582, 2000.

Pitt B et al: The effect of spironolactone on morbidity and mortality in patients with severe heart failure. Randomized Aldactone Evaluation Study Investigators. *N Engl J Med* 341:709, 1999.

Pollock ML: Exercise training and prescription for the elderly. *South Med J* 87:S88, 1994.

Rich MW et al: A multidisciplinary intervention to prevent the readmission of elderly patients with congestive heart failure. *N Engl J Med* 333:1190, 1995.

Rich MW et al: Effect of age on mortality, hospitalizations and response to digoxin in patients with heart failure: The DIG Study. *J Am Coll Cardiol* 38:806, 2001.

Setaro JF et al: Usefulness of verapamil for congestive heart failure associated with abnormal left ventricular diastolic filling and normal left ventricular systolic performance. *Am J Cardiol* 69:1212, 1992.

SOLVD Investigators: Effect of enalapril on mortality and the development of heart failure in asymptomatic patients with reduced left ventricular ejection fraction. *N Engl J Med* 327:685, 1992.

SOLVD Investigators: Effect of enalapril on survival in patient with reduced left ventricular ejection fractions and congestive heart failure. *N Engl J Med* 325:293, 1991.

The Cardiac Insufficiency Bisoprolol Study II (CIBIS-II): A randomized trial. *Lancet* 353:9, 1999.

The Digitalis Investigation Group. The effect of digoxin on mortality and morbidity in patients with heart failure. *N Engl J Med* 336:525, 1997.

The Sixth Report of the Joint National Committee on prevention, detection, evaluation, and treatment of high blood pressure. *Arch Intern Med* 157:2413, 1997.

Vinson JM et al: Early readmission of elderly patients with congestive heart failure. *J Am Geriatr Soc* 38:1290, 1990.

Cardiac Arrhythmias in Elderly People: Advances in Diagnosis and Management

SANJEEV SAKSENA • VIKRAM JALA REDDY

Cardiac arrhythmias are a frequent cardiac disorder in the elderly population, and present in a variety of common clinical syndromes. These range from acute episodes of rhythm disturbances that may manifest as palpitations or worsening of existing cardiac symptomatology, for example, heart failure or angina that can lead to major symptomatic events such as syncope or sudden cardiac death. At the other end of the spectrum are chronic and persistent arrhythmias that can cause intermittent symptoms with minimal disability or prolonged and seriously limiting symptoms.

The entire spectrum of bradycardias and most tachycardias can be seen in the elderly population. Importantly, as distinct from pediatric and younger adult populations, these are generally manifestations of cardiovascular disease or age-related cardiovascular pathology. In addition, systemic disorders may primarily or secondarily impact cardiac rhythms and result in arrhythmias. Thus, while rhythm disturbances in normal hearts can occasionally present for the first time in the elderly person, this is a less-common occurrence than in younger persons.

While genetic disorders resulting in arrhythmias, arrhythmias associated with congenital heart disease, and idiopathic tachycardias have occasionally first become manifest in an elderly patient, this remains an exception. More often, an intercurrent event can trigger an otherwise dormant potential for an arrhythmia. This is often seen in clinical situations such as an induced proarrhythmic event in a patient with preexisting genetic predisposition for the arrhythmia. Thus, common gene sequence variations that increase the risk of life-threatening proarrhythmic drug reactions can be clinically silent before drug exposure. For example, patients with drug-induced long QT syndrome can have sporadic mutations such as a single-nucleotide polymorphism that is commonly seen in approximately 1.6 percent of the general population. In such patients, ion channels are normal at baseline but can be inhibited by drugs that do not affect wild-type channels. Allelic variants

of MiRP1, a subunit of the ion channel that modulates the potassium current IKr, can contribute to drug-induced long QT syndrome.

The commonest rhythm disturbances seen in the elderly population are isolated atrial or ventricular ectopic beats, and the commonest arrhythmia is atrial fibrillation. Other common tachycardias include atrial flutter, ventricular tachycardia, and other supraventricular tachyarrhythmias. Sinus bradycardia and conduction system disease dominates the bradyarrhythmias in this population. Major clinical syndromes leading to the evaluation of the elderly patient for arrhythmias are syncope and near syncope, sudden death, and "unexplained falls or injuries." The diagnosis and evaluation of these conditions are performed using noninvasive and invasive diagnostic techniques, including ambulatory monitoring, evaluation of underlying cardiac disease, and provocative testing for arrhythmias such as electrophysiologic testing. Therapeutic interventions are similar to populations of nonelderly patients and include pharmacologic and nonpharmacologic treatments.

A recent statement from an expert consensus document noted that advanced invasive diagnostic tests and nonpharmacologic therapies have been applied safely in the elderly population, but may be used with less frequency because of comorbidities and inadequate appreciation of the benefits that can be derived in this population.

EPIDEMIOLOGY

Atrial and ventricular ectopy increase with advancing age. The prevalence of isolated atrial ectopic beats on a resting electrocardiogram is seen in more than 5 percent of healthy subjects older than age 60 years and can increase to 10 percent, even in the absence of cardiovascular disease. In the Baltimore Study of Aging, such arrhythmias were seen in 6 percent of subjects on a resting electrocardiogram

(ECG), but in more than 80 percent on 24-hour monitoring. Treadmill exercise can elicit these as well, with 39 percent showing this finding on maximal exercise in one study. In the very elderly population, more than 15 percent may show this at rest and in virtually all individuals on ambulatory electrocardiography. However, these arrhythmias do not appear to have any prognostic significance with respect to cardiovascular risk in these studies.

Short runs of supraventricular tachycardia are most often seen on ambulatory electrocardiography in the elderly population, with nearly 50 percent of men and women older than age 65 years showing these findings, and the prevalence continues to rise through 80 years of age. These are usually brief self-terminating episodes with salvoes ranging from 3 beats to short runs lasting a few seconds. They are often asymptomatic. These rhythms also do not appear to have prognostic significance and rarely require treatment.

Similarly, ventricular arrhythmias show increased prevalence with advancing age in asymptomatic elderly individuals and in hospitalized patients. The prevalence of ventricular premature complexes rises up to 10 percent on a resting ECG by age 80 years, and this is more prevalent if the individual has cardiac disease. In a Finnish study, resting ECGs showed ventricular premature contractions (VPCs) in 5 percent of individuals older than 85 years of age, and this increased to 13 percent if heart disease was present. Ambulatory electrocardiography shows a high prevalence of isolated and complex VPCs, with 4 to 11 percent showing paired beats and 2 to 7 percent manifesting short runs of ventricular tachycardia. In an institutionalized very elderly population, these figures rose to 19 percent and 9 percent, respectively. Exercise testing provokes an increased frequency of these arrhythmias, with 57 percent of the very elderly showing this arrhythmia. However, it remains unclear as to the extent of change that is a result of aging and the contribution that may come from occult cardiac disease. This may account for the varying risk of cardiac death that may be present in association with VPCs in this population. In carefully screened healthy individuals, VPCs may not have prognostic significance, but in other studies where cardiac disease may be present, an increased incidence of sudden death was observed. Aronow et al. reported a doubling of risk in an elderly nursing home population in patients with complex VPCs on ambulatory ECGs. Thus, evaluation of underlying cardiac disease assumes importance when such arrhythmias are detected on routine screening. Further management is dependent on risk stratification of these patients.

Advancing age modifies atrioventricular conduction. The sinus node, atrium, and atrioventricular (AV) conduction system are affected by fatty change and increased fibrosis. Sinus bradycardia and disappearance of sinus arrhythmia are seen, with reduced heart rate variability caused by a reduction in parasympathetic tone. There is also a decreased responsiveness to β-adrenergic stimulation, although heart rates below 40 beats per minute (bpm) are uncommon (4.5 percent in one study), as are sinus pauses longer than 3 seconds (<1 percent). Survival is not usually influenced by these changes in sinus activity, and paced patients experience similar longevity to individuals without these changes. There is a small but significant increase in the PR interval by about 15 to 20 ms with aging. This usually does not produce AV block and has no prognostic significance. The occurrence of first degree AV block increases with age to 0.6 percent in the eighth decade of life. Isolated second-degree AV block type 1 occurs in 6 to 8 percent of octogenarians. A major consideration is whether these are age-related or based in underlying cardiovascular disease. Rarely is treatment required for control of these arrhythmias, because they are generally asymptomatic, or minimally symptomatic and have no prognostic significance in the absence of cardiac disease. More advanced forms of AV block are uncommon in the elderly population and usually occur in conjunction with transient or permanent disturbances of AV conduction. In a community-based population study, third-degree AV block was not observed. However, when present, this is symptomatic as in younger age groups, and requires further evaluation. Finally, a left-axis shift is common with advancing age, with octogenarians developing asymptomatic left anterior hemiblock in increasing numbers. In contrast, bundle-branch block may be a result of cardiac disease, although left bundle-branch block may be observed in 4 percent of healthy octogenarians. In general, this finding should initiate search for underlying cardiac disease.

ATRIAL FIBRILLATION

Atrial fibrillation (AF) is the most common sustained arrhythmia in elderly persons and occurs most often in association with cardiovascular disease. AF is predominantly a disease of elderly persons. In the AF population, 84 percent are older than 65 years of age and 70 percent are between the ages of 65 and 85 years. With advancing age, the prevalence of AF increases from 0.5 percent in individuals 50 to 59 years old to nearly 10 percent of all individuals older than age 80 years. Men develop AF at 1.5 times the incidence in women. Although the age- and disease-adjusted incidence and prevalence of AF are greater in men than in women, because of their greater longevity, approximately one-half of all elderly patients with AF are women.

In the recently completed AFFIRM (Atrial Fibrillation Followup Investigation of Rhythm Management) trial, hypertension was the most common disorder associated with AF. Other risk factors for AF include advancing age and male sex, and diabetes or elevated blood glucose, coronary disease, valve disease, and heart failure. AF can be a manifestation of hyperthyroidism, and apathetic or subclinical hyperthyroidism can be missed in the elderly patient. Alcohol abuse, particularly binge drinking, has long been associated with AF. AF is associated with increased cardiovascular mortality and stroke. Familial AF is undoubtedly rare, but there is provocative evidence that there may be a genetic susceptibility to AF. Echocardiographic predictors for AF include left atrial dilation, impaired left ventricular fractional shortening, and left ventricular hypertrophy. The clinical presentation in the elderly patient can range from no symptoms and detection of AF on routine examination, palpitations, to aggravation of heart failure, stroke, angina, and a low cardiac output state, including syncope or even precipitation of ventricular tachyarrhythmias.

In evaluating AF in the elderly patient, it is necessary to eliminate other disorders as in a younger population; for example, hyperthyroidism, myocardial infarction, or recent cardiac surgery. In addition, the possibility of associated cardiovascular disease should be fully assessed and its management critically examined. Uncontrolled or poorly managed hypertension, cardiac disease, heart failure, or iatrogenic factors, such as electrolyte imbalance, can make rhythm control or rate control difficult in AF. Ischemia may not directly trigger AF, because atrial infarction is often absent in absence of extensive myocardial infarction, but right coronary arterial disease can produce ischemia of the sinus node and right atrium with secondary sinus node dysfunction and AF.

The main goals of AF therapy are to control symptoms, restore sinus rhythm, prevent stroke, and improve heart failure control. Symptoms of AF are mostly caused by rapid ventricular rate, rate irregularity, and lack of ventricular filling as a consequence of the lack of the atrial contribution. These three factors are of varying importance in an individual patient and can influence selection of therapy. For example, in patients with diastolic ventricular dysfunction due to marked left ventricular hypertrophy or hypertrophic cardiomyopathy, cardiac output is highly dependent on atrial filling and contraction. Thus, rhythm control may be preferred to simple rate control in these patients. In contrast, the asymptomatic or minimally symptomatic very elderly patient with AF with marked atrial dilation may respond more favorably to rate control strategies. Treatment strategies for AF are directed either at ventricular rate control or rhythm control to prevent or eliminate AF. In the recently completed AFFIRM study, a large multicenter randomized trial that compared rate control to rhythm control largely by using antiarrhythmic drugs in patients with recent onset atrial fibrillation with background anticoagulation therapy, no difference in mortality or stroke could be demonstrated between these two approaches. Thus, it is reasonable to offer either strategy as a first-line of treatment in new onset AF; however, one or the other approach may be preferred in other AF subpopulations.

In the rate control strategy, AF with a moderate increase in ventricular rate may be handled with outpatient management with beta-blockers or calcium channel antagonist drugs. AF associated with very rapid ventricular rates is best managed with intravenous agents, such as diltiazem, esmolol, verapamil, or amiodarone. Digoxin is widely used but is not especially effective for rate control, particularly during exercise. Recurrent paroxysmal, persistent or permanent AF is often drug-refractory and rate control can be better achieved by radiofrequency ablation of the AV junction with placement of permanent single- or dual-chamber rate-responsive pacemaker. This method offers significant advantages over pharmacologic approaches, including excellent safety, improvement in symptoms and quality of life, superior rate control, and avoidance of adverse drug effects.

The traditional approach to rhythm control starts with antiarrhythmic drug therapy. Safety considerations and tolerance have altered the usage of class 1 drugs. Presently, we prefer to commence therapy with class 3 agents such as sotalol or dofetilide, and we employ amiodarone in the resistant patients or in patients with poor ventricular function and heart failure. Class 1C drugs can be used in patients without significant left ventricular hypertrophy or other structural heart disease, but these agents should be avoided in elderly patients, who frequently have coexisting coronary artery disease. While use of the lowest effective drug dose can improve tolerance, efficacy rates remain modest. At the end of 6 months, 50 percent of patients, on average, can maintain sinus rhythm, and this declines to 30 percent by 1 year for most class 3 and all class 1 agents. Amiodarone may have slightly higher efficacy rates, but its extracardiac side-effect profile leads to serious delayed attrition in efficacy and patient tolerance. Thus, while rhythm control offers hope of avoiding long-term anticoagulation therapy, which is especially desirable in elderly patients, this is often not realized in many of these patients, especially over the long run.

Anticoagulation with warfarin is a mainstay of AF management, but this can be problematic in the very elderly population. Careful attention to the level of anticoagulation is essential to avoid bleeding complications and maintenance of a lower international normalized ratio (INR) level (around 2 rather than 3) may be preferred. Elderly patients with gait disorders, syncope, seizures, or other conditions that could lead to injury must have this therapy and its potential risk/benefit ratio carefully considered prior to implementation. Interaction and potentiation by amiodarone therapy is an important issue and requires drug titration. Cardioversion in the elderly population with AF requires either transesophageal echocardiographic evidence of absence of left atrial thrombus or prethrombotic states, or anticoagulation for 4 weeks prior to conversion. Anticoagulation should be continued for a few weeks after cardioversion because of myocardial stunning and a subsequent predisposition to thrombus development in the atrium.

Nonpharmacologic approaches include the use of device therapy, such as pacemakers or atrial defibrillators, and catheter ablation techniques. The latter are being applied for trigger ablation in the pulmonary veins, or linear compartmentalization of the atrium to reduce available substrate for AF maintenance. Experience with linear atrial ablation in the elderly population is limited, but its safety in the right atrium appears satisfactory. Pulmonary vein ablation is now being attempted in older patients, but this is most often used for lone AF in young patients. Limitations include its technical difficulty, procedural risks, which include left atrial puncture, pulmonary vein stenosis, and other complications, and limited information on long-term efficacy. Atrial pacing, particularly dual-site atrial pacing, has been used in combination with antiarrhythmic drugs in patients with bradycardia and AF or in drug-refractory AF to achieve rhythm control (Fig. 38-1). It is relatively easy to implement, safe, and widely available. In this approach, an additional atrial lead is inserted and placed outside the coronary sinus ostium, permitting simultaneous right and left atrial stimulation to resynchronize the atria and reduce atrial conduction delay. In most elderly patients with AF, bradycardia is common and often observed with drug therapy. Thus, device therapy with multisite atrial pacing is likely to be commonly employed as first-line nonpharmacologic therapy in the elderly patient with AF. In this approach, often referred to as a "hybrid" strategy, serial interventions may be necessary to achieve or maintain rhythm control. However, early experience is very promising, with

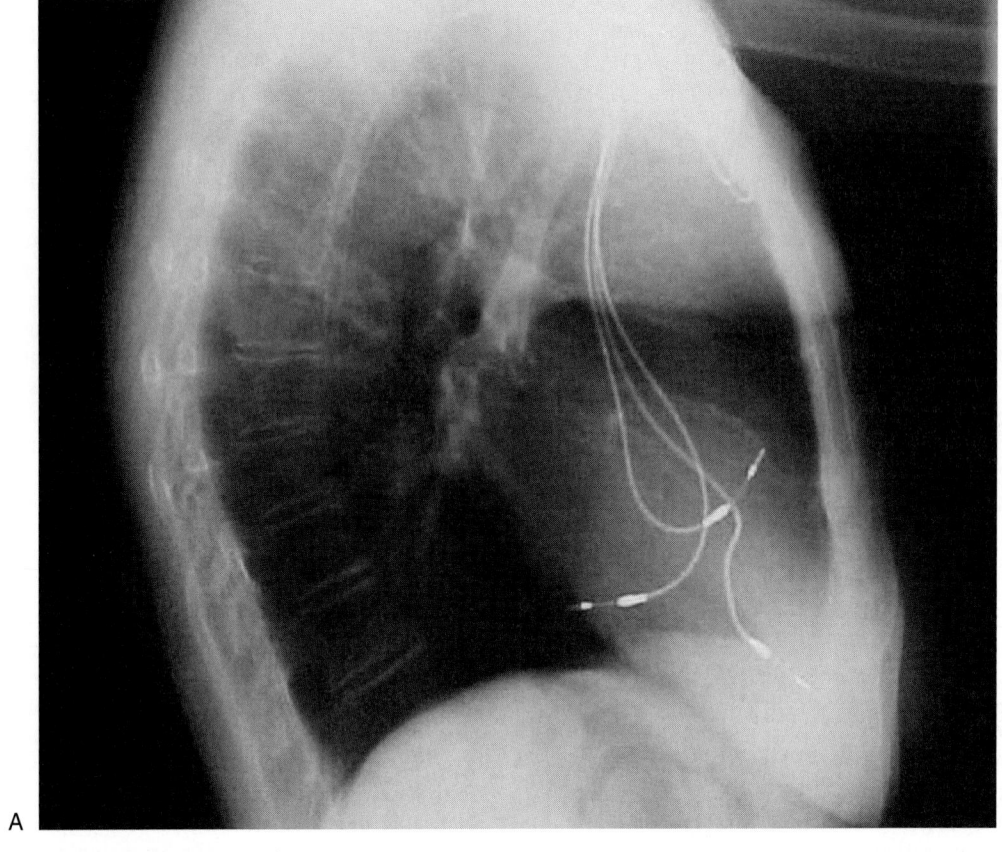

A

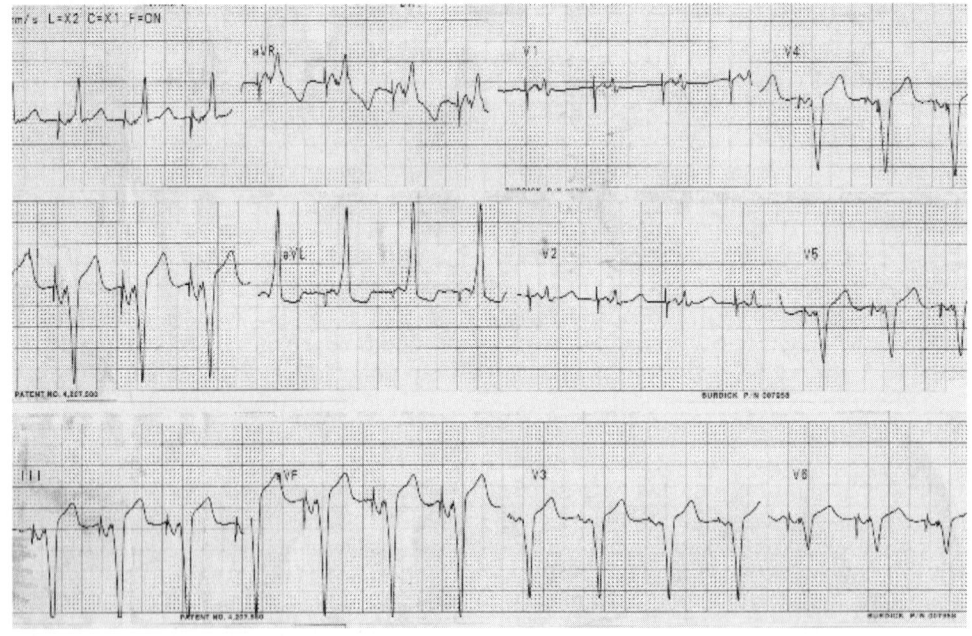

B

Figure 38-1 *(A)* Dual-site right atrial pacing system in an elderly patient with refractory AF. Note the additional lead placed outside the coronary sinus ostium. Reproduced with permission from Saksena et al: *J Am Coll Cardiol* 40:1140, 2002. *(B)* Electrocardiographic pattern of dual-site atrial pacing with inverted or biphasic P waves after the atrial stimulus in the inferior leads. The two atrial locations are simultaneously stimulated using a Y-connector, and right ventricular apical pacing is performed in the conventional manner.

more than 80 percent of these patients achieving long-term rhythm control. In patients without symptomatic or asymptomatic AF recurrences for 1 year, we discontinue antithrombotic treatment. This has been achieved in one-fourth of our population and thromboembolic complications have not increased. This is a major advantage for elderly patients who are at higher risk for complications from warfarin. More advanced pacemaker defibrillators for AF are making their debut and offer patient-activated or automatic atrial defibrillation with backup ventricular defibrillation for patient safety. These devices are ideal for patients with ventricular tachyarrhythmias with AF or persistent AF.

For the resistant and symptomatic AF patient, rate control with catheter ablation of atrioventricular junction with permanent pacemaker insertion can be implemented. This can be an attractive option in patients with comorbidity, avoiding the use of multiple antiarrhythmics with drug-interaction and pharmacokinetic considerations. In patients with AF, this procedure improves quality of life, reduces symptoms, and reduces the left ventricular dysfunction seen with the tachycardia-based cardiomyopathy.

ATRIAL FLUTTER

Atrial flutter is a common arrhythmia in the elderly population. While the true incidence of the arrhythmia is debated, it may coexist in more than 15 percent of patients with atrial fibrillation. The risk of stroke with this arrhythmia was once considered low, but more recent data suggest an intermediate risk as compared to atrial fibrillation. Thus, current guidelines suggest that anticoagulation should be considered in high-risk patients. Its diagnosis, electrophysiologic basis, and management remain similar to those in younger populations. Cavotricuspid isthmus ablation, which has become first-line treatment, is now widely used in elderly patients with common atrial flutter. Ablative therapy should not be unduly withheld from the elderly patient, because the safety of the procedure is now well documented in this population. Atypical flutters are common in the elderly patient and often masquerade as atrial fibrillation. Management options can include antiarrhythmic drugs, antitachycardia devices, or map-guided catheter ablation. Acute termination may be achieved with intravenous ibutilide or procainamide. Rate control is possible to alleviate symptoms using beta-blockers or calcium channel blocker drugs. Antitachycardia devices are likely to become more acceptable in this population, with their increasing versatility and the coexistence of primary or drug-induced bradycardias in this age group. Catheter ablation of atypical flutter is a complex and demanding procedure and is currently not a first line-in management.

PAROXYSMAL SUPRAVENTRICULAR TACHYCARDIA

The spectrum of paroxysmal supraventricular tachycardia (PSVT) includes reentrant tachycardias such as atrioventricular nodal reentrant tachycardia, sinoatrial or intra-atrial reentrant tachycardia, and atrio-ventricular reentrant tachycardia. The emergence or detection of PSVT occurring for the first time in an elderly patient is uncommon (Fig. 38-2). In the example of a patient with "permanent" AF in Figure 38-2, AV nodal tachycardia initiated AF and was successfully ablated. More commonly, these rhythms are unobserved, undocumented, or undiagnosed earlier in life and finally detected in an elderly patient as part of a more comprehensive cardiovascular evaluation. Ectopic atrial

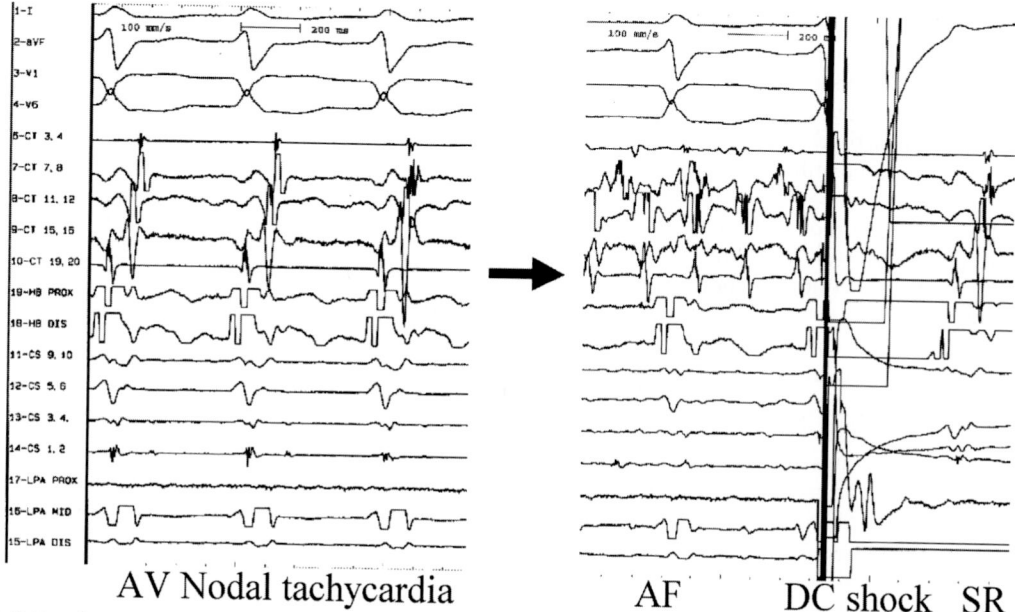

AV Nodal tachycardia   AF   DC shock   SR

Figure 38-2 *Left Panel:* AV nodal reentrant tachycardia detected for the first time after cardioversion of atrial fibrillation in an elderly man with permanent AF. *Right Panel:* AV nodal tachycardia precipitates sustained drug-refractory AF requiring cardioversion in this patient. Abbreviations: CT, crista terminales; CS, coronary sinus; LPA, left pulmonary artery; SR, sinus rhythm; AF, atrial fibrillation.

tachycardia and intra-atrial reentry are often seen with co-existing disease such as chronic lung disease or hypertension in the elderly patient.

The management of these rhythms is similar to that in the younger patient. Management of an acute episode is similar to other patient groups, with intravenous agents such as adenosine, calcium blockers, or beta-blocker therapy. For atrial tachycardias and even other PSVTs, a class 1 drug such as intravenous procainamide may assist in terminating the acute episode. Atrio-ventricular nodal reentry tachycardia (AVNRT) and atrio-ventricular reciprocating tachycardia (AVRT) are best treated with catheter ablation, which is safe and effective, to achieve long-term cure. Efficacy rates exceed 90 percent in skilled hands, and complications now hover around 1 to 2 percent. Serious complications include advanced atrioventricular block and cardiac perforation. The latter is a concern for the elderly patient, in whom the myocardium may be more friable. Nevertheless, no increased risk has been demonstrated in this population.

For the resistant ectopic or intra-atrial reentrant atrial tachycardia, ablation of the atrial focus may be considered. Finally, rate control with catheter ablation of atrioventricular junction with permanent pacemaker insertion can be implemented as a last option. However, atrial tracking with a dual-chamber pacemaker is an important consideration and the device should be programmed to avoid this scenario.

BRADYCARDIAS

Sinus Node Dysfunction

Sinus node dysfunction is the major indication for pacemaker implantation in elderly patient. The spectrum ranges from sinus bradycardia and sinus exit block to frank sinus arrest. Sinus node dysfunction is occasionally asymptomatic but is frequently associated with symptoms (syncope, dizziness, dyspnea) related to inappropriate bradycardia, pauses, and chronotropic incompetence. Furthermore, elderly patients often experience other complications such as atrial tachyarrhythmias, notably AF or atrial flutter with a risk of thromboembolism and precipitating congestive heart failure. Syncope is the main clinical syndrome associated with this bradyarrhythmia, and all degrees of severity can be observed, from minor "gray outs" to syncope with injury. Concomitant conduction system disease is common.

Evaluation of this patient requires assessment of symptoms with arrhythmia correlation. This is often accomplished with ambulatory electrocardiography, event monitors, and stress testing for chronotropic competence. Evaluation for concomitant cardiac or other diseases is necessary, and on occasion, a primary disorder may be uncovered, such as hypothyroidism, or neurologic disorders, such as raised intracranial pressure. Nevertheless, this correlation is often difficult and it is necessary to resort to provocative testing such as electrophysiologic study. Sinus node function tests at electrophysiologic study are highly specific but notoriously insensitive. However, carotid sinus stimulation may elicit pauses and symptoms, and drug testing using atropine alone or with beta-blockers can be

used with greater sensitivity. Finally, neurocardiogenic etiologies for syncope are common in elderly persons and can coexist with sinus node dysfunction or atrioventricular block. Thus, tilt-table testing should be performed in the elderly patient with syncope, even if sinus bradycardia is noted on monitoring. The mainstay of treatment of this disorder is insertion of a permanent pacemaker, which is discussed later in this chapter.

Hypersensitive carotid sinus syndrome is a disease commonly seen in elderly patients. This often occurs with specific activities involving neck motion or stimulation; for example, turning the head, shaving, and tight collars. Cardioinhibitory and/or vasodepressor reflexes result from carotid sinus stimulation and can induce syncope and severe injuries. Carotid sinus stimulation under electrocardiographic monitoring with intravenous access is needed for diagnosis and is one of the most common omissions in the clinical evaluation of the elderly patient with syncope. Symptom relief is usually obtained with permanent pacing. However, approximately 10 percent of implanted patients have recurrent syncope, probably as a consequence of the vasodepressor component of this disease. DDD (dual-mode, dual-pacing, dual-sensing) or DDI pacing with hysteresis and automatic mode conversion is considered the best choice for these patients. New algorithms, such as "rate drop response," which accelerates the heart rate when the device detects a bradycardic episode, are effective in prevention of syncope.

Atrioventricular Block and Conduction System Disease

Atrioventricular block in the elderly patient is secondary to similar pathology, in many respects, as in the younger individual, but the proportion of patients in whom this is related to age-related myocardial pathology (e.g., fibrosis, degeneration, and calcification) is markedly increased. The clinical presentation is similar to that in younger patients, but the elderly patient with paroxysmal AV block may be especially prone to have deceptive symptoms of light-headedness, falls, "gray-out" episodes, or visual blurring that require a high index of suspicion for a transient bradyarrhythmia. Preexisting heart disease worsens the prognosis of the elderly patient with AV block. Advanced ventricular dysfunction and the presence of prior coronary artery disease are also predictors of poorer outcome of permanent pacing for this indication. After acute myocardial infarction in the elderly patient, persistent second- and third-degree AV blocks, especially if symptomatic, are indications for demand pacing.

Bifascicular and trifascicular blocks in the elderly patient are also frequently associated with transient high-degree AV block and sudden cardiac death. Symptomatic patients with these conduction disorders and without other etiologies for symptoms should be considered for permanent pacing. In the asymptomatic individual with bifascicular block, prolongation of H-V interval beyond 80 ms is, in our opinion and in the opinion of other investigators, a marker for potential high-degree AV block. Prophylactic permanent pacing should be implemented in such patients. Other investigators consider prolongation of H-V interval to be a result of underlying heart disease and a marker for increased risk of sudden death.

It is still debated whether dual-chamber pacemaker therapy can improve survival in patients with high-degree AV block and underlying heart disease. The United Kingdom Pacing and Cardiovascular Events Trial (UK-PACE) study addressed this issue and showed no advantage to dual chamber pacing late-(Breaking clinical Trials, American College of Cardiology 2003). In the Canadian Trial of Physiologic Pacing (CTOPP) study, a subgroup of pacemaker-dependent patients demonstrated benefits with respect to mortality and major morbidity, but the remaining patients did not show this finding. Thus, cardiac pacing may offer survival benefit in specific patients and provide alleviation of symptoms in others. Resolution of AV block-related symptoms is observed with demand pacing, but dual-chamber pacing offers advantages of avoiding pacemaker syndrome.

Neurocardiogenic Syncope

Autonomic reflexes primarily mediate this condition, with secondary effects on cardiac rhythm and systemic vascular resistance. This syndrome is common in elderly patients, is aggravated or brought to the clinical horizon by concomitant vasodilator drug therapy or by blood volume contraction by diuretics. Particularly poorly tolerated agents are angiotensin-converting enzyme antagonists, angiotensin receptor-blocking drugs, diuretics, and nitrates. Elimination of these therapies can often ameliorate recalcitrant syncopal events. Head-up tilt-table testing should be performed in the drug-free, hydrated state. The use of a variety of therapeutic approaches is considered in these patients. Most importantly, hydration and improving venous return with support stockings should be considered. Drugs include beta-blockers, anticholinergics, blood volume expanders such as fludrocortisone or erythropoietin, serotonin reuptake inhibitors, theophylline, or α-agonists such as midodrine.

In refractory patients, dual-chamber pacing combined with drug therapy may provide symptomatic improvement. Even if pharmacologic therapy improves symptoms in most patients with vasovagal syncope, some of them still remain severely symptomatic with asystole or severe bradycardias during tilt testing. Initial studies of cardiac pacing in vasovagal syncope show disappointing results even in patients with a mainly bradycardiac mechanism. The hypotensive component of the syncope was incompletely controlled by the pacemaker therapy in these studies, however, and this may explain the recurrence of symptoms. This is in contrast to the efficacy of pacing in carotid sinus syndrome. However, rate drop response algorithms, allowing a faster pacing rate when a vasovagal episode is suspected by the device, give more encouraging results. Benditt et al. observed that 59 percent of patients with vasovagal syncope were recurrence-free with dual-chamber pacing during a mean follow-up of 7 months. In the North American Vasovagal Pacemaker Study, pacing showed definite benefit with early trial termination. In this condition, the challenge is to find the method for appropriate recognition of the onset of the vasovagal episode by the implanted pacemaker device.

Hybrid therapies combining pacemaker and drug therapy will most likely give better results in the future. At our center, studies provide evidence for benefit of dual-chamber pacemaker when combined with drug therapy in patients with drug-refractory neurocardiogenic syncope. We consider device therapy after a minimum of two drug therapies have failed to prevent syncope.

MANAGEMENT OF VENTRICULAR ARRHYTHMIAS

Ventricular Ectopy and Nonsustained Ventricular Tachycardia

Ventricular ectopic beats do not carry any prognostic significance in the absence of cardiovascular disease. While symptomatic palpitations may trouble occasional patients, reassurance is key to management. Symptomatic antiarrhythmic drug therapy is generally inadvisable because of the risk of proarrhythmia and limited benefit. However, in the occasional patient, beta-blocker and calcium blocker therapy may be considered.

More advanced forms of complex ectopy and nonsustained ventricular tachycardia (VT) can prompt efforts at risk stratification. Exclusion of cardiovascular disease and left ventricular dysfunction portend a good prognosis. In the presence of these risk factors noninvasive methods such as ejection-fraction assessment, exercise testing for VT provocation, signal-averaged electrocardiography, and T-wave alternans stress testing can be considered. If a significant risk of sudden death is identified, further invasive electrophysiologic testing is justifiable, particularly in patients with coronary disease and moderate to severe left ventricular dysfunction. In patients with provocable sustained VT, implantable cardioverter-defibrillator (ICD) therapy is recommended, just as in younger populations. In our center's experience, elderly patients derive similar clinical benefit with a shorter time to first ICD therapy (see Fig. 38-5).

Ventricular Tachycardia and Sudden Cardiac Death in Elderly Patients

The presentation of ventricular tachyarrhythmias in general is similar in elderly patients as in younger patients, but hemodynamic tolerance is relatively poorer and syncope may often be associated with sustained ventricular tachycardia in older patients. Recent data from the Antiarrhythmias versus Implantable Defibrillator (AVID) trial indicate that the prognosis of these arrhythmias may approach the severity of malignant ventricular tachyarrhythmias presenting as cardiac arrest. Cardiac arrest in the elderly population remains a major mode of death and a public health problem. It is most often associated with advanced coronary artery disease and heart failure. Evaluation of these arrhythmias or cardiac arrest in the elderly population follows similar guidelines as in other populations. Anatomic definition of the substrate with cardiac catheterization, and electrophysiologic studies to define the arrhythmia or presentation mechanism remain the gold standard of care.

Table 38-1 ACC/AHA 1998–2002 Updated Guidelines for Permanent Pacing in the AV Block

Pacing for Acquired Atrioventricular Block in Adults
Class I

1. Third-degree and advanced second-degree AV block at any anatomic level, associated with any one of the following conditions:

    a. Bradycardia with symptoms (including heart failure) presumed to be due to AV block. (Level of evidence: C)
    b. Arrhythmias and other medical conditions that require drugs that result in symptomatic bradycardia. (Level of evidence: C)
    c. Documented periods of asystole greater than or equal to 3.0 seconds (3) or any escape rate less than 40 beats per minute (bpm) in awake, symptom-free patients. (Levels of evidence: B, C)
    d. After catheter ablation of the AV junction. (Levels of evidence: B, C) There are no trials to assess outcome without pacing, and pacing is virtually always planned in this situation unless the operative procedure is AV junction modification
    e. Postoperative AV block that is not expected to resolve after cardiac surgery. (Level of evidence: C)
    f. Neuromuscular diseases with AV block, such as myotonic muscular dystrophy, Kearns–Sayre syndrome, Erb's dystrophy (limb-girdle), and peroneal muscular atrophy, with or without symptoms, because there may be unpredictable progression of AV conduction disease. (Level of evidence: B)

Class IIa

1. Asymptomatic third-degree AV block at any anatomic site with average awake ventricular rates of 40 bpm or faster, especially if cardiomegaly or left ventricular (LV) dysfunction is present. (Levels of evidence: B, C)
2. Asymptomatic type II second-degree AV block with a narrow QRS, pacing becomes a Class I recommendation. (Level of evidence: B)
3. Asymptomatic type I second-degree AV block at intra- or infra-His levels found at electrophysiologic study performed for other indications. (Level of evidence: B)
4. First- or second-degree AV block with symptoms similar to those of pacemaker syndrome. (Level of evidence: B)

Class IIb

1. Marked first-degree AV block (more than 0.30 seconds) in patients with LV dysfunction and symptoms of congestive heart failure in whom a shorter AV interval results in hemodynamic improvement, presumably by decreasing left atrial filling pressure. (Level of evidence: C)
2. Neuromuscular diseases such as myotonic muscular dystrophy, Kearns–Sayre syndrome, Erb's dystrophy (limb-girdle), and peroneal muscular atrophy with any degree of AV block (including first-degree AV block) with or without symptoms, because there may be unpredictable progression of AV conduction disease. (Level of evidence: B)

Class III

1. Asymptomatic first-degree AV block. (Level of evidence: B)
2. Asymptomatic type I second-degree AV Block at the supra-His (AV node) level or known to be intra- or infra-Hisian. (Levels of evidence: B, C)
3. AV block expected to resolve and/or unlikely to recur (e.g., drug toxicity, Lyme disease, or during hypoxia in sleep apnea syndrome in absence of symptoms). (Level of evidence: B)

Pacing for Chronic Bifascicular and Trifascicular Block
Class I

1. Intermittent third-degree AV block. (Level of evidence: B)
2. Type II second-degree AV block. (Level of evidence: B)
3. Alternating bundle-branch block. (Level of evidence: C)

(*Continued*)

Table 38-1   (*Continued*) ACC/AHA 1998–2002 Updated Guidelines for Permanent Pacing in the AV Block

Class IIa

1. Syncope not demonstrated to be due to AV block when other likely causes have been excluded, specifically ventricular tachycardia (VT). (Level of evidence: B)
2. Incidental finding at electrophysiologic study of markedly prolonged H-V interval (greater than or equal to 100 milliseconds) in asymptomatic patients. (Level of evidence: B)
3. Incidental finding at electrophysiologic study of pacing-induced infra-His block that is not physiologic. (Level of evidence: B)

Class IIb

1. Neuromuscular diseases such as myotonic muscular dystrophy, Kearns–Sayre syndrome, Erb's dystrophy (limb-girdle), and peroneal muscular atrophy with any degree of fascicular block with or without symptoms, because there may be unpredictable progression of AV conduction disease. (Level of evidence: C)

Class III

1. Fascicular block without AV block or symptoms. (Level of evidence: B)
2. Fascicular block with first-degree AV block without symptoms. (Level of evidence: B)

Pacing for Atrioventricular Block Associated with Acute Myocardial Infarction
Class I

1. Persistent second-degree AV block in the His–Purkinje system with bilateral bundle-branch block or third-degree AV block within or below the His–Purkinje system after AMI. (Level of evidence: B)
2. Transient advanced (second- or third-degree) infranodal AV block and associated bundle-branch block. If the site of block is uncertain, an electrophysiologic study may be necessary. (Level of evidence: B)

Class I

1. Persistent second-degree AV block in the His–Purkinje system with bilateral bundle-branch block or third-degree AV block within or below the His–Purkinje system after AMI. (Level of evidence: B)
2. Transient advanced (second- or third-degree) infranodal AV block and associated bundle-branch block. If the site of block is uncertain, an electrophysiologic study may be necessary. (Level of evidence: B)
3. Persistent and symptomatic second- or third-degree AV block. (Level of evidence: C)

Class IIb

1. Persistent second- or third-degree AV block at the AV node level. (Level of evidence: B)

Class III

1. Transient AV block in the absence of intraventricular conduction defects. (Level of evidence: B)
2. Transient AV block in the presence of isolated left anterior fascicular block. (Level of evidence: B)
3. Acquired left anterior fascicular block in the absence of AV block. (Level of evidence: B)
4. Persistent first-degree AV block in the presence of bundle-branch block that is old or age indeterminate. (Level of evidence: B)

AMI, acute myocardial infarction; AV, atrioventricular.

Correction of significant ischemia by using revascularization procedures is an important element of the final therapeutic prescription. This is being increasingly performed using percutaneous coronary interventions in the elderly population. Biventricular pacing can be now applied for treatment of refractory heart failure in specific populations.

Drug therapy of sustained VT or ventricular fibrillation (VF) is currently in disfavor for reasons of limited efficacy and increased proarrhythmic risk in patients with coronary disease or left ventricular dysfunction. Thus, implantation of a cardioverter-defibrillator is the preferred therapy. This is discussed in some detail later. However, in patients with

Table 38-2 ACC/AHA 1998–2002 Updated Guidelines for Permanent Pacing in the Sinus Node Dysfunction

Pacing in Sinus Node Dysfunction

Class I

1. Sinus node dysfunction with documented symptomatic bradycardia, including frequent sinus pauses that produce symptoms. In some patients, bradycardia is iatrogenic and will occur as a consequence of essential long-term drug therapy of a type and dose for which there are no acceptable alternatives. (Level of evidence: C)
2. Symptomatic chronotropic incompetence. (Level of evidence: C)

Class IIa

1. Sinus node dysfunction occurring spontaneously of as a result of necessary drug therapy, with heart rate less than 40 bpm when a clear association between significant symptoms consistent with bradycardia and the actual presence of bradycardia has not been documented. (Level of evidence: C)
2. Syncope of unexplained origin when major abnormalities of sinus node function are discovered or provoked in electrophysiologic studies. (Level of evidence: C)

Class IIb

1. In minimally symptomatic patients, chronic heart rate less than 40 bpm while awake. (Level of evidence: C)

Class III

1. Sinus node dysfunction in asymptomatic patients, including those in whom substantial sinus bradycardia (heart rate less than 40 bpm) is a consequence of long-term drug treatment.
2. Sinus node dysfunction in patients with symptoms suggestive of bradycardia that are clearly documented as not associated with a slow heart rate.
3. Sinus node dysfunction with symptomatic bradycardia due to nonessential drug therapy.

well-preserved left ventricular function (with an ejection fraction of >35 percent), amiodarone may have comparable efficacy. Thus, in an elderly patient with sustained VT or VF who prefers drug therapy or is a poor candidate for ICD insertion, this may be an option. However, the long-term morbidity of amiodarone, particularly its neuromuscular side effects, is an ever-present concern for the elderly patient. Ataxia, loss of balance, difficulty in walking, and falls can accompany this adverse effect.

Antiarrhythmic Device Therapy in the Elderly Patient

Antiarrhythmic device therapy, that is, implantable pacemakers and cardioverter-defibrillators, has provided critical advances in the treatment of cardiac arrhythmias. In specific populations, improvement of patient symptoms, morbidity, and/or mortality has been demonstrated with their application. Decisions to implement device therapy are usually based on the clinical presentation of the patient, the documented arrhythmia, and comorbidities. Indications for these therapies may vary to some extent based on the clinical circumstances of an individual patient.

The paucity of scientific data in this area leads to the obvious question as to whether the elderly patient population can obtain the full advantages of pacemaker and ICD therapies, because advanced age or multiple concomitant illnesses may reduce life expectancy. Physicians, based on subjective evaluations, are often reluctant to initiate ICD

therapy in elderly patients. These issues are discussed in detail below; however, it is to be stressed that age per se is rarely a central issue in the decision as to whether and how to initiate pacemaker therapy. Rather, careful assessment of the patient as to overall condition and degree of frailty or resiliency (including comorbidities) represents the central consideration in this decision.

Indications for Cardiac Pacemaker Therapy

Standard Indications

With increasing age, the probability of developing cardiac conduction disturbances becomes more likely. Abnormalities in the atrial or ventricular substrate resulting from frequent concomitant heart disease in the elderly patient may lead to severe bradyarrhythmias. Even in the absence of heart disease, in many cases idiopathic or isolated conduction system disease may appear in the elderly patient. More than 85 percent of patients receiving pacemaker therapy are older than 64 years old. Prospective and retrospective studies have shown that elderly patients also benefit from the use of sophisticated pacemakers with dual-chamber pacing and rate-response function. These pacemakers improve survival and quality of life as compared with ventricular pacing and non–rate-responsive devices.

Because of the frequent association of sinus node dysfunction with paroxysmal or chronic atrial fibrillation, VVI or VVIR pacing was preferred by many as the primary pacing mode. However, retrospective and prospective studies

Table 38-3   Prevention and Termination of Tachyarrhythmias by Pacing

Class I

1. Symptomatic recurrent supraventricular tachycardia that is reproducibly terminated by pacing after drugs and catheter ablation fail to control the arrhythmia or produce intolerable side effects. (Level of evidence: C)
2. Symptomatic recurrent sustained VT as part of an automatic defibrillator system. (Level of evidence: B)

Class IIa

1. Symptomatic recurrent SVT that is reproducibly terminated by pacing in the unlikely event that catheter ablation and/or drugs fail to control the arrhythmia or produce intolerable side effects. (Level of evidence: C)

Class IIb

1. Recurrent SVT or atrial flutter that is reproducibly terminated by pacing as an alternative to drug therapy or ablation. (Level of evidence: C)

Class III

1. Tachycardias frequently accelerated or converted to fibrillation by pacing.
2. The presence of accessory pathways with the capacity for rapid anterograde conduction whether or not the pathways participate in the mechanism of the tachycardia.

Pacing Recommendations to Prevent Tachycardia
Class I

1. Sustained pause-dependent VT, with or without prolonged QT, in which the efficacy of pacing is thoroughly documented. (Level of evidence: C)

Class IIa

1. High-risk patients with congenital long-QT syndrome. (Level of evidence: C)

Class IIb

1. AV reentrant or AV node reentrant supraventricular tachycardia not responsive to medical or ablative therapy. (Level of evidence: C)
2. Prevention of symptomatic, drug-refractory, recurrent atrial fibrillation in patients with coexisting sinus node dysfunction. (Level of evidence: B)

Class III

1. Frequent of complex ventricular ectopic activity without sustained VT in the absence of the long-QT syndrome.
2. Torsade de pointes VT due to reversible causes.

AV, atrioventricular; SVT, supraventricular tachycardia; VT, ventricular tachycardia.

show the superiority of atrial-based pacing in prevention of AF, but differ with respect to mortality and stroke risk. In the CTOPP study, pacemaker-dependent patients derived mortality benefit with atrial-based pacing, and in the Danish study, AAI pacing benefited all groups of patients with sinus node dysfunction with respect to survival and freedom from chronic AF. Nevertheless, the risk of subsequent AV block, which may be up to 1 to 10 percent during long-term follow-up, limits the AAI approach.

Tables 38-1 to 38-4 list the American College of Cardiology (ACC)/American Heart Association (AHA) practice guidelines published in 1998 and updated in 2002 regarding indications for cardiac pacing. Table 38-1 enumerates indications in atrioventricular block and Table 38-2 in sinus node dysfunction. Class I indications are the conditions for which there is evidence and/or agreement that a given procedure or treatment is beneficial, useful, and effective. Class II indications are conditions for which there is

Table 38-4   Pacing in Hypersensitive Carotid Sinus and Neurocardiogenic Syncope

Recommendations for Permanent Pacing in Hypersensitive Carotid Sinus Syndrome and Neurocardiogenic Syncope
Class I

1. Recurrent syncope caused by carotid sinus stimulation; minimal carotid sinus pressure induces ventricular asystole of more than 3-second duration in the absence of any medication that depresses the sinus node or AV conduction. (Level of evidence: C)

Class IIa

1. Recurrent syncope without clear, provocative events and with a hypersensitive cardioinhibitory response. (Level of evidence: C)
2. Syncope of unexplained origin when major abnormalities of sinus node function or AV conduction are discovered or provoked in electrophysiologic studies. (Level of evidence: C)
3. Significantly symptomatic and recurrent neurocardiogenic syncope associated with bradycardia documented spontaneously or at the time of tilt-table testing. (Level of evidence: B)

Class III

1. A hyperactive cardioinhibitory response to carotid sinus stimulation in the absence of symptoms or in the presence of vague symptoms such as dizziness, lightheadedness, or both. (Level of evidence: C)
3. Recurrent syncope, lightheadedness, or dizziness in the absence of a hyperactive cardioinhibitory response. (Level of evidence: C)
4. Situational vasovagal syncope in which avoidance behavior is effective. (Level of evidence: C)

conflicting evidence and/or a divergence of opinion about the usefulness/efficacy of a procedure or treatment. Class II is divided into two subclasses: Class IIa, for which there is a weight of evidence/opinion in favor of usefulness and efficacy, and Class IIb, for which there is less well-established usefulness and efficacy by evidence and opinion. The conditions for which there is evidence and/or general agreement that a procedure and treatment is not useful and effective and potentially harmful represent Class III. Based on available data, there is no evidence for increased risk of pacemaker implantation in the elderly patient. Tables 38-3 and 38-4 enumerate other less-common indications for cardiac pacing.

Atrioventricular Block   It is now recognized that pacemaker therapy can improve survival, especially in patients with high-degree AV block, with underlying heart disease, and by using dual-chamber pacemakers. While device implantation is faster, easier, and often less expensive with single-chamber ventricular demand pacemakers, VVI pacing as a primary therapy is becoming less and less frequent. AV block-related symptoms resolve with demand pacing in general and DDD pacing in particular. However, the existence of a preexisting heart disease undoubtedly worsens the prognosis of the elderly patient with AV block after pacemaker implantation. Advanced ventricular dysfunction and the presence of prior coronary artery disease are two predictors of poorer outcome for this indication. After acute myocardial infarction in the elderly patient persistent second- and third-degree AV blocks are important indications for demand pacing, especially if associated with symptoms.

Bifascicular and trifascicular blocks are also frequently associated with transient high-degree AV block and sudden death in the elderly patient. Symptomatic patients with such electrocardiographic abnormalities and without other causes explaining the symptoms are candidates for permanent pacing. In the absence of symptoms, prolongation of H-V interval beyond 80 ms is, as stated before, an index of potential high-degree AV block and requires prophylactic permanent pacing.

Sinus Node Dysfunction   Sinus node dysfunction is the most common indication for pacemaker implantation in the elderly patient. Furthermore, patients with this abnormality often experience other complications such as tachyarrhythmias, for example atrial fibrillation. In bradycardia–tachycardia syndrome, VVI or VVIR pacing was once preferred as the primary pacing mode. However, studies show that atrial pacing reduces the incidence of atrial fibrillation. Moreover, new pacemaker technology now allows mode-switching from DDD to VVI or DDI in case of paroxysmal atrial fibrillation episodes, avoiding ventricular tracking by fast atrial rates. We, and others, advocate AAI or AAIR pacing as the best modes in such patients, as these pacing modes provide more physiologic ventricular activation and ease of implantation. Nevertheless, the risk of subsequent AV block should be assessed by testing the Wenckebach rate. In active patients with chronotropic incompetence, rate-responsive pacemakers increase heart rate during physical activity and show clinical benefits.

Supraventricular Tachyarrhythmias   Permanent atrial pacing either in single- or dual-site pacing modes in

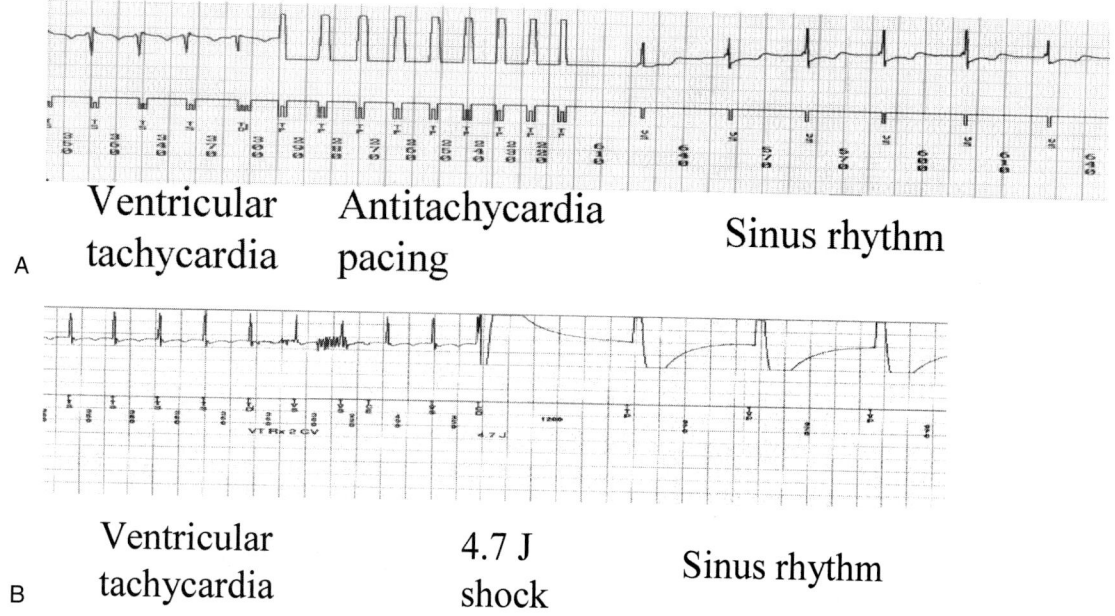

Figure 38-3 *(A)* Termination of sustained VT by implantable cardioverter defibrillator (ICD) by antitachycardia pacing. Reproduced with permission from ACCSAPV. *(B)* Termination of sustained VT by implantable cardioverter defibrillator (ICD) by low-energy cardioversion shock. Reproduced with permission from ACCSAPV.

patients without or with preexisting atrial fibrillation is now recognized to decrease atrial fibrillation recurrences. Single and dual site atrial pacing, included as a standard indication in 1998 ACC/AHA guidelines for prevention of symptomatic AF, have been upgraded to class IIA status. Furthermore, as reported by us and others, atrial multisite pacing can prevent and reduce AF recurrences.

ICD Therapy in the Elderly

ICD therapy has been increasingly used in elderly patients. Most clinical series have included two-thirds of patients older than 65 years of age. Sudden cardiac death caused by ventricular fibrillation or sustained ventricular tachycardia, which are common complications of coronary and other heart diseases in the elderly population. Ventricular tachycardia can be terminated by antitachycardia pacing or low energy shocks (Fig. 38-3). Table 38-5 lists the updated practice guidelines detailing indications for ICD therapy. There is no indication that alludes to special considerations in the elderly patient.

Prior to ICD implantation, the elderly patient should be evaluated for benefits from ICD therapy and surgical risk. Severity of cardiac disease and left ventricular dysfunction are the main parameters influencing life expectancy. ICD implantation risk is increased in patients with high pulmonary capillary wedge pressures and renal failure or azotemia. The benefit of the ICD implant is also potentially impaired in these cases. Biventricular pacing is now available in ICD patients to improve congestive heart failure (CHF) status in patients with left bundle-branch block with or without first-degree atrioventricular block (Fig. 38-4). The benefits and risks of ICD insertion in the elderly patient must be also evaluated in the context of the existence of concomitant disease. ICD insertion is not recommended for patients with life expectancy less than 6 months. Few studies have compared the outcome of ICD insertion in elderly patients with younger patients. Based on available data, prevention of sudden cardiac death by ICD therapy is as effective in the elderly patient as in the younger patient. Panatopoulos et al. reported 100 percent sudden death survival at 4 years in patients older than age 75 years and 97 percent in patients younger than age 75 years. In this particular study, both cardiac and noncardiac mortality were increased in the elderly patients, however, resulting in a lower overall survival in this group. Factors associated with increased mortality were age >75 years, ejection fraction <30 percent, New York Heart Association (NYHA) class III, and appropriate shocks. Tresh et al. compared patient characteristics, surgical complications, and long-term survival rates in elderly and younger patients. Long-term survival curves at 3 years were similar in both groups. We reported the survival and need for device therapy in consecutive patients implanted with transvenous ICD during the period 1989 to 1996 at our center (Fig. 38-5). Remarkably, there was no perioperative mortality with this ICD implant method in the elderly or very elderly patients in our series. The survival from all-cause mortality was 96 percent at 1 year, 87 percent at 3 years, and 73 percent at 5 years (Fig. 38-5A). This was not significantly different among the subgroups categorized by age.

CONCLUSIONS

Specific considerations exist with the management of cardiac arrhythmias in the elderly patient. However, these are related to knowledge of the natural history and

Table 38-5 1998–2002 ACC/AHA Updated Indications for Implantable Cardioverter-Defibrillator Therapy

Class I

1. Cardiac arrest due to ventricular fibrillation (VF) or VT not due to a transient or reversible cause. (Level of evidence: A)
2. Spontaneous sustained VT in association with structural heart disease. (Level of evidence: B)
3. Syncope of undetermined origin with clinically relevant, hemodynamically significant sustained VT or FV induced at electrophysiologic study when drug therapy is ineffective, not tolerated, or not preferred. (Level of evidence: B)
4. Nonsustained VT in patients with coronary disease, prior myocardial infarction (MI), LV dysfunction, and inducible VF or sustained VT at electrophysiologic study that is not suppressible by a class I antiarrhythmic drug. (Level of evidence: A)
5. Spontaneous sustained VT in patients who do not have structural heart disease that is not amenable to other treatments. (Level of evidence: C)

Class IIa

1. Patients with LV ejection fraction of less than or equal to 30% at least 1 month postmyocardial infarction and 3 months postcoronary artery revascularization surgery. (Level of evidence: B)

Class IIb

1. Cardiac arrest presumed to be due to VF when electrophysiologic testing is precluded by other medical conditions. (Level of evidence: C)
2. Severe symptoms (e.g., syncope) attributable to ventricular tachyarrhythmias in patients awaiting cardiac transplantation. (Level of evidence: C)
3. Familial or inherited conditions with a high risk for life-threatening ventricular tachyarrhythmias such as long-QT syndrome or hypertrophic cardiomyopathy. (Level of evidence: B)
4. Nonsustained VT with coronary artery disease, prior MI, LV dysfunction, and inducible sustained VT or VF at electrophysiologic study. (Level of evidence: B)
5. Recurrent syncope of undetermined etiology in the presence of ventricular dysfunction and inducible ventricular arrhythmias at electrophysiologic study when other causes of syncope have been excluded. (Level of evidence: C)
6. Syncope of unexplained sudden cardiac death in association with typical or atypical right bundle-branch block and ST-segment elevations (Brugada's syndrome). (Level of evidence: C)
7. Syncope in patients with advanced structural heart disease in which thorough invasive and noninvasive investigation has failed to define a cause. (Level of evidence: C)

Class III

1. Syncope of undetermined cause in a patient without inducible ventricular tachyarrhythmias and without structural heart disease. (Level of evidence: C)
2. Incessant VT or VF. (Level of evidence: C)
3. VF or VT resulting from arrhythmias amenable to surgical or catheter ablation; for example, atrial arrhythmias associated with the Wolff–Parkinson–White syndrome, right ventricular outflow tract VT, idiopathic left ventricular tachycardia, or fascicular VT. (Level of evidence: C)
4. Ventricular tachyarrhythmias due to a transient or reversible disorder (e.g., AMI, electrolyte imbalance, drugs, or trauma) when correction of the disorder is considered feasible and likely to substantially reduce the risk of recurrent arrhythmia. (Level of evidence: B)
5. Significant psychiatric illnesses that may be aggravated by device implantation or may preclude systematic follow-up. (Level of evidence: C)
6. Terminal illnesses with projected life expectancy less than 6 months. (Level of evidence: C)
7. Patients with coronary artery disease with LV dysfunction and prolonged QRS duration in the absence of spontaneous or inducible sustained or nonsustained VT who are undergoing coronary bypass surgery. (Level of evidence B)
8. NYHA class IV drug-refractory congestive heart failure in patients who are not candidates for cardiac transplantation. (Level of evidence: C)

AMI, acute myocardial infarction; LV, left ventricular; MI, myocardial infarction; NYHA, New York Heart Association; VF, ventricular fibrillation; VT, ventricular tachycardia.

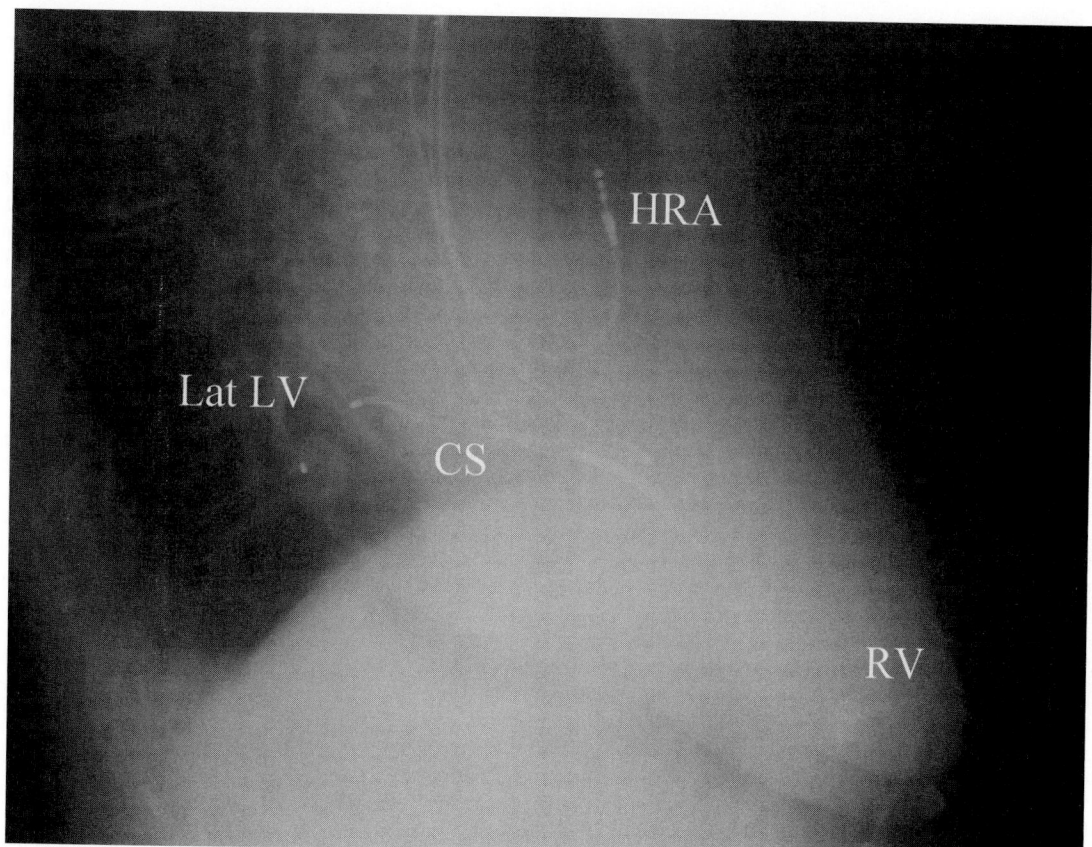

Figure 38-4 Biventricular pacing system in ICD recipient with refractory heart failure, left bundle-branch block, and ventricular tachycardia.

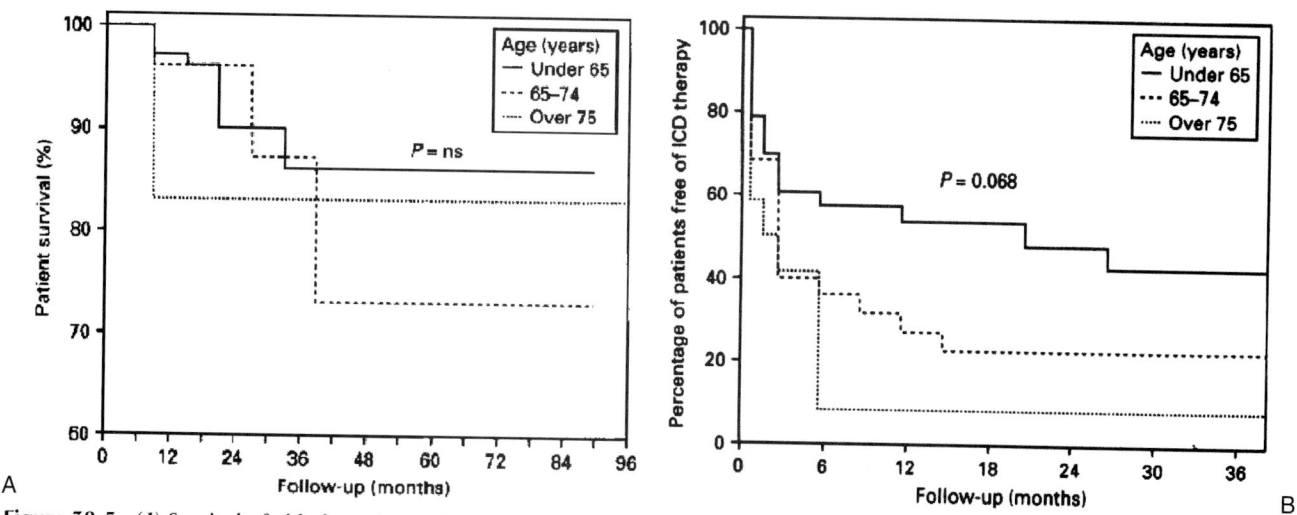

Figure 38-5 (*A*) Survival of elderly patients after ICD insertion compared to other age cohorts. (*B*) Freedom from ICD therapy in elderly patients after ICD insertion compared to younger age cohorts. Reproduced with permission from Circulation online 2003.

presentation of the arrhythmia. Diagnostic evaluations and therapeutic considerations are increasingly similar to those in other adult populations, and interventional electrophysiologic therapies should not be withheld in such patients on the basis of advanced age per se.

REFERENCES

Andersen HR et al: Long-term follow-up of patients from a randomised trial of atrial versus ventricular pacing for sick-sinus syndrome. *Lancet* 305:1210, 1997.

Benditt DG et al: Clinical experience with Thera DR rate-drop response pacing algorithm in carotid sinus syndrome and vasovagal syncope. The International Rate-Drop Investigators Group. *Pacing Clin Electrophysiol* 20:832, 1997.

Bexton RS et al: The rate-drop response in carotid sinus syndrome. *Pacing Clin Electrophysiol* 20:840, 1997.

Brady PA et al: Impact of pacing mode on long-term survival in elderly patients with congestive heart failure. *J Interv Card Electrophysiol* 1:____, 1997.

Cheitlin MD et al: AHA conference proceedings: Do existing databases hold the answers to clinical questions in geriatric cardiovascular disease and stroke? Executive Summary. Database Conference, January 27–30, 2000. Washington, DC, USA. *Circulation* 104(7):E39, 2001.

Coplen SE et al: Efficacy and safety of quinidine therapy for maintenance of sinus rhythm after cardioversion. *Circulation* 82:1106, 1990.

Denes P et al: Sudden death in patients with chronic bifascicular block. *Arch Intern Med* 137:1005, 1977.

Gregoratos G et al: ACC/AHA guidelines for implantation of cardiac pacemakers and antiarrhythmia devices: A report of the American College of Cardiology/American Heart Association Task Force on Practice Guidelines (Committee on Pacemaker Implantation). *J Am Coll Cardiol* 31(5):1175, 1998.

Juul-Moller S et al: Sotalol versus quinidine for the maintenance of sinus rhythm after direct current conversion of atrial fibrillation. *Circulation* 82:1932, 1990.

Kenny RA et al: Carotid sinus syndrome: A modifiable risk factor for non-accidental falls in older adults (SAFE PACE). *J Am Coll Cardiol* 38(5):1491, 2001.

Krol RB et al: New devices and hybrid therapies and new devices for treatment of atrial fibrillation. *J Interv Card Electrophysiol* 4(Suppl 1):163, 2000.

Lamas GA et al: Permanent pacemaker selection and subsequent survival in elderly medicare pacemaker recipients. *Circulation* 91:1063, 1995.

McAnulty JH et al: Natural history of "high risk" bundle-branch block: Final report of a retrospective study. *N Engl J Med* 307:137, 1982.

Moss AJ et al: Improved survival with an implanted defibrillator in patients with coronary artery disease at high risk for ventricular arrhythmia. *N Engl J Med* 335:1933, 1996.

Rosenqvist M et al: Long-term pacing in sinus node disease: Effect of stimulation mode on cardiovascular mortality and morbidity. *Am Heart J* 116:16, 1988.

Saksena S et al: Implantable defibrillator therapy for the elderly. *Am J Geriatr Cardiol* 7:11, 1998.

Saksena S et al: Prevention of recurrent atrial fibrillation with chronic dual-site right atrial pacing. *J Am Coll Cardiol* 28:687, 1996.

Saksena S et al: Improved suppression of recurrent atrial fibrillation with dual-site right atrial pacing and antiarrhythmic drug therapy. *J Am Coll Cardiol* 40(6):1140, 2002.

Scheinman MM et al: Value of the H-Q interval in patients with bundle branch block and the role of prophylactic permanent pacing. *Am J Cardiol* 50:1316, 1982.

Sesti F et al: A common polymorphism associated with antibiotic-induced cardiac arrhythmia. *Proc Natl Acad Sci U S A* 97(19):10613, 2000.

Sgarbossa EB et al: Chronic atrial fibrillation and stroke in paced patients with sick sinus syndrome: Relevance of clinical characteristics and pacing modalities. *Circulation* 88:1045, 1993.

Shen WK et al: Long-term survival after pacemaker implantation for heart block in patients >65 years. *Am J Cardiol* 74:560, 1994.

Stangl K et al: Differences between atrial single chamber pacing and ventricular single chamber pacing with respect to prognosis and antiarrhythmic effect in patients with sick sinus syndrome. *Pacing Clin Electrophysiol* 13;2080, 1990.

Tresh DD et al: Comparison of efficacy of automatic implantable cardioverter defibrillator in patients older and younger than 65 years of age. *Am J Med* 90:717, 1991.

Peripheral Vascular Disease

ANDREW W. GARDNER • JOHN D. SORKIN

DEFINITION

Atherosclerotic cardiovascular disease is the most significant health problem in the United States, as heart and cerebrovascular diseases are leading causes of mortality, and peripheral vascular disease is a leading cause of morbidity in elderly people. Peripheral arterial disease (PAD) is the most typical form of peripheral vascular disease. PAD is characterized by a partial or complete failure of the arterial system to deliver oxygenated blood to peripheral tissue. Atherosclerosis is by far the most common etiology of PAD. However, several other processes can lead to the clinical syndrome (Table 39-1). Although lesions (and symptoms) of PAD can occur in both the upper and lower extremities, they are much more common in the lower extremity, which is the focus of this chapter.

EPIDEMIOLOGY

The ankle–brachial blood pressure index (ABI), defined as the systolic blood pressure measured at the ankle divided by the systolic blood pressure measured in the arm during supine rest, is the most widely used quantitative measure to identify subjects with PAD and to determine PAD severity. The ABI varies widely in the general population and is generally normally distributed with a long tail of low values (Fig. 39-1). The prevalence of PAD is highly dependent on the exact ABI cutpoint used to detect inadequate peripheral circulation. The definition of an abnormal ABI has ranged between <0.80 and <0.97, with a value of ≤0.90 generally considered to be the best reference standard.

The prevalence of PAD is 16 percent in the general population older than 55 years of age when an ABI value of ≤0.90 and symptoms of intermittent claudication and rest pain are used as criteria of PAD. In the Edinburgh Artery Study, approximately 20 percent of the men and women ages 55 to 74 years of age were noted to have an ABI ≤0.90, and thus were diagnosed as having PAD. The prevalence of PAD increases with age, and at all ages is higher in men than in women. At ages 65 to 69 years, the prevalence of PAD in men from the Cardiovascular Health Study was approximately 7 percent, and approximately 5 percent in women. In subjects age 85 years and older, the prevalence was 23 percent in men and 21 percent in women.

PAD and coronary vascular disease (CVD) share risk factors. In addition to age and male sex, risk factors for PAD include smoking, hypercholesterolemia, diabetes, hypertension, hyperhomocystinemia, elevated fibrinogen concentration, having a family history of premature atherosclerosis (suggesting that genetic factors may influence the development of PAD) and being nonwhite. Measures of pulmonary function such as the forced expiratory volume in 1 second (FEV_1) and forced vital capacity (FVC) are related to ABI, reflecting confounding variables caused by smoking. Smoking reduces FEV_1 and FVC, while simultaneously increasing the risk for PAD.

Although PAD can be seen in the absence of clinical CVD, asymptomatic CVD is frequently present in patients with PAD. Every patient presenting with PAD should be considered to have CVD until proven otherwise. Evaluation and treatment for PAD should include evaluation and control of CVD risk factors.

PAD has important implications for function. PAD severity (accessed by ABI) is directly related to 6-minute walk distance, free-living energy expenditure, and steps taken per day. Of particular interest to geriatricians, patients with PAD are more likely to fall than are subjects without PAD.

PAD is not a static disease. Progression from intermittent claudication to rest pain or gangrene can occur in anywhere from 2 to 7 percent of patients per year. Furthermore, PAD is associated with increased risk for mortality, and this risk becomes greater as the severity of PAD increases (Fig. 39-2).

Patients with PAD are at increased risk for coronary heart disease, coronary vascular disease, and all-cause mortality. This risk is independent of traditional risk factors, including age, sex, smoking, systolic blood pressure, plasma lipids, fasting glucose, body mass index, and preexisting clinical cardiovascular disease. Risk for mortality as a consequence of coronary heart disease and cardiovascular disease is three to six times higher in subjects with PAD than in subjects without PAD, even after accounting for traditional risk factors.

Table 39-1   Causes of Peripheral Arterial Disease

Atherosclerosis	Arterial entrapment
Thrombus	Adventitial cyst
Embolism	Fibromuscular dysplasia
Dissection	Trauma
Vasculitis	Vasospasm

PATHOPHYSIOLOGY

The atherosclerotic lesions that lead to PAD tend to form in a few well-defined locations in the vascular tree, and patients often will have lesions in more than one location. Thirty percent of the patients have lesions in the abdominal aorta, 80 to 90 percent have lesions in the femoral and popliteal arteries, and 40 to 50 percent have lesions in the tibial and peroneal arteries. The location of the arterial lesion will determine the clinical presentation. For example, aortoiliac disease (Leriche's syndrome) leads to buttock, hip, and thigh pain along with erectile dysfunction; the more common femoral–popliteal disease leads to symptoms in the calf. The atherosclerotic process is similar to that in other major arteriostenoses and is discussed in Chap. 34.

PRESENTATION

Clinical PAD was recognized as early as 1831, when Jean-Francois Bouley Jeune observed a horse that, when pulling a cabriolet, limped with the hind legs. At autopsy, the horse was noted to have a partially thrombosed aneurysm of the abdominal aorta and occlusion of both femoral arteries.

Two schemes, both based on symptoms and clinical measures, are commonly used to classify the severity of PAD (Tables 39-2 and 39-3). In the early stages of PAD, the

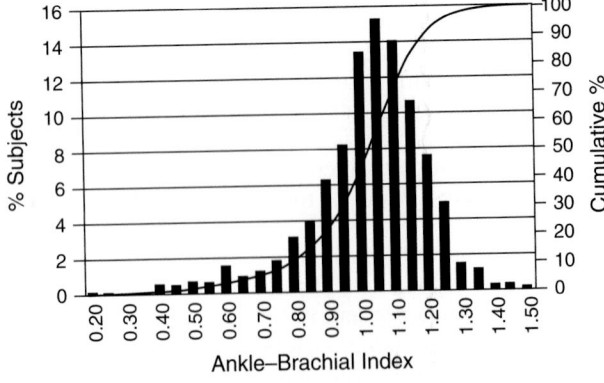

Figure 39-1   Ankle brachial blood pressure index (ABI) in men and women in the Edinburgh Artery Study. The bars and left-hand scale represent the percentage of subjects having a given ABI. The solid line and right-hand scale represent the cumulative percentage of subjects having an ABI at or below the ABIs listed on the abscissa. Adapted from Fowkes FG: Epidemiological research on peripheral vascular disease. *J Clin Epidemiol* 54:863, 2001.

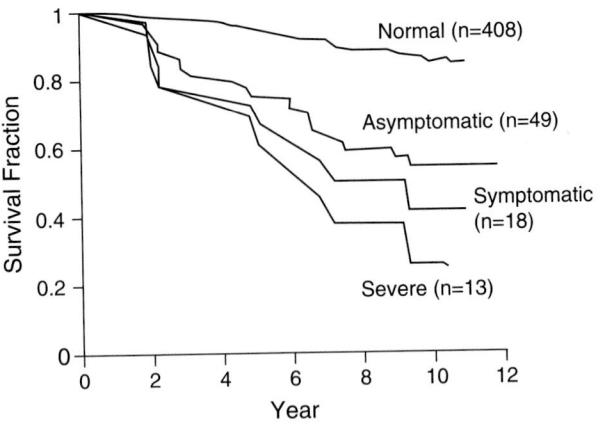

Figure 39-2   Relation of peripheral arterial disease (PAD) severity to mortality in subjects from Rancho Bernardo. Adapted from Criqui MH et al: Mortality over a period of 10 years in patients with peripheral arterial disease. *N Engl J Med* 326:381, 1992.

reduction in blood flow and ABI does not result in any noticeable symptoms (asymptomatic PAD), and is defined as stage I according to the Fontaine classification system and grade I, category 0 according to the Rutherford classification system. As PAD progresses, ischemic pain in the leg musculature occurs when patients walk (intermittent claudication), and is classified as either Fontaine stage II-a or II-b, or Rutherford grade I, category 1, 2, or 3, depending on the walking distance and the change in ABI following walking. In more advanced stages of disease, ABI is reduced to such an extent that pain is experienced even while at rest, classified as either Fontaine stage III or Rutherford grade II, category 4. Further progression of the disease leads to ischemic ulcerations on the lower extremities, gangrene, and tissue loss, classified as either Fontaine stage IV or Rutherford grade II, category 5, or grade III, category 6. Patients in these categories have critical limb-threatening ischemia in which the ischemia endangers part or all of the lower extremity. These patients are candidates for aggressive limb salvage interventions such as percutaneous transluminal angioplasty or bypass surgery.

Table 39-2   Fontaine Classification of Peripheral Arterial Disease

Stage	Symptoms
I.	Asymptomatic
II.	Intermittent claudication
IIa.	Pain-free, claudication walking >200 m
IIb.	Pain-free, claudication walking <200 m
III.	Rest/nocturnal pain
IV.	Necrosis/gangrene

SOURCE: Adapted from Pentecost MJ et al: Guidelines for peripheral percutaneous transluminal angioplasty of the abdominal aorta and lower extremity vessels. *Circulation* 89:511, 1994.

Table 39-3 Rutherford Classification of Peripheral Arterial Disease

Grade	Category	Clinical Description
I	0	Asymptomatic; not hemodynamically correct
	1	Mild claudication
	2	Moderate claudication
	3	Severe claudication
II	4	Ischemic rest pain
	5	Minor tissue loss; nonhealing ulcer, focal gangrene with diffuse pedal ischemia
III	6	Major tissue loss extending above transmetatarsal level; foot no longer salvageable

SOURCE: Adapted from Rutherford RB: Standards for evaluating results of interventional therapy for peripheral vascular disease. *Circulation* 83 (Suppl 2) : 16, 1991.

The presentation of PAD varies widely among patients. PAD can be present without any clinical signs, in which case, diagnosis of PAD can only be made with laboratory tests. With mild disease, the peripheral pulses can be decreased. With more advanced disease there may be an audible bruit or the distal pulses may be absent. The extremity may be pale or cyanotic at rest, upon raising the leg, or with exercise. The skin of the extremity can be cool, smooth and shiny with hair loss, and thickened nails. Dangling the legs following elevating the extremity can lead to delayed return of color to the skin (usual time about 10 seconds), delayed filling of the veins of the feet and ankles (normal about 15 seconds), and the development of a dusky rubor in the legs. Patients with the most severe disease will present with ulcers on their extremity or frank gangrene.

The patient may complain of a sensation of cold or numbness in the foot or toes. Patients with more severe disease will often complain of pain when the extremity is at rest. This pain will often occur at night and will be relieved by dangling the leg over the edge of the bed.

EVALUATION

Pulse Palpation and Rose Questionnaire

A number of noninvasive tests have been used to screen for and to evaluate the extent of a patient's PAD. The most basic clinical test is palpation and auscultation of the peripheral pulses. Little is known about the sensitivity of pulse palpation for the diagnosis of PAD. In situations in which direct examination of subjects is not feasible, such as epidemiologic studies, the Rose Questionnaire is often used to screen subjects for PAD. Rose Questionnaire PAD is defined as leg pain associated with walking that goes away with rest. The sensitivity of the Rose Questionnaire has been reported as being anywhere from 10 to 50 percent.

Noninvasive Vascular Tests

The most common measure to assess the presence and severity of PAD is the ABI. PAD is typically defined by an ABI value ≤ 0.90. The sensitivity of using this cut point of

ABI is >90 percent. Generally, a patient whose ABI is <0.8 will be symptomatic with intermittent claudication during exercise, and a patient whose ABI is <0.30 will generally complain of pain at rest. Very high ABIs, for example, >1.5 are considered invalid because they do not reflect the true ankle blood pressure caused by arteries that have become calcified or noncompressible.

Segmental systolic blood pressure measures in the brachial, upper thigh, lower thigh, and ankle locations have been used to access the extent of PAD. Additional noninvasive tests for PAD include Doppler ultrasonography (i.e., measurement of blood flow velocity), plethysmography (pressure-wave tracing), and measurement of postocclusive reactive hyperemia (PORH). PORH is performed by occluding arterial flow by inflating a blood pressure cuff above systolic pressure at the level of the upper thigh or knee for 3 minutes, followed by measurement of the systolic blood pressure at the ankle or calf blood flow 15 to 30 seconds after releasing the occlusion. When compared to patients without vascular disease, patients with PAD will demonstrate a lower postocclusive ABI and a delayed return to preocclusion pressures. The sensitivity of the postocclusive ABI is >95 percent.

Treadmill Testing

The main effect that PAD has on acute exercise is the development of claudication pain in the leg musculature as a result of insufficient blood flow. As a result, claudication and peripheral hemodynamic measurements obtained from a treadmill test are the primary criteria to assess the effectiveness of an exercise program. The specific claudication variables that are measured to assess the functional severity of PAD include the distances (or times) to onset and to maximal claudication pain. ABI measurements obtained before and after the treadmill test, in addition to claudication measurements, provide a more objective assessment of disease severity.

The primary objective of a treadmill test for patients with PAD is to obtain reliable measures of (1) the rate of claudication pain development, (2) the ABI response to exercise, and (3) the presence of coexisting coronary heart disease. The test should be a progressive test with gradual increments in grade. By having a test with small increases in exercise intensity, claudication distances of patients can be stratified according to disease severity. A highly reliable treadmill tests for patients with PAD uses a constant walking speed of 2 mph and gradual increases in grade of 2 percent every 2 minutes beginning at 0 percent grade. By using this treadmill protocol, typical distances to onset of pain and to maximal pain are approximately 170 meters (3 minutes) and 360 meters (6.5 minutes), respectively. Measurement of the ABI immediately after a treadmill exercise stress test can help diagnose PAD in difficult cases, as well as determine the extent of impairment of the peripheral circulation. Exercise increases systemic blood pressure (i.e., the brachial pressure), while pressure distal to an arterial lesion in the lower extremity falls with exercise as a consequence of dilation of secondary arterioles. As a result, ABI typically drops from a resting value of 0.6 to approximately 0.2 immediately following the treadmill test. The sensitivity of ABI measured after treadmill walking is >95 percent.

Gas-exchange measures during the treadmill test show that PAD patients with intermittent claudication have peak oxygen consumption values in the range of 12 to 15 mL/kg/min, which is approximately 50 percent of age-matched controls. Favorable changes following a program of exercise rehabilitation should include greater walking distances covered before the occurrence of the onset and maximal claudication pain, an increase in peak oxygen consumption, and possibly a blunted drop in ABI and a faster rate of recovery in ABI to the resting baseline value.

Physical Function and Activity

Claudication distance and ABI are the most common measurements obtained in patients with claudication, because previous studies have been done from a vascular surgery perspective. However, a more gerontologic perspective would focus on the improvement in function of PAD, for example, in patients following exercise rehabilitation. Because the typical profile of a PAD patient is that of an elderly person with chronic ambulatory disability, the decline in physical functioning with aging may be accelerated in this population because of the extreme deconditioning brought about from the disease process. Consequently, performance on a 6-minute walk test, as well as measures of gait, walking economy (i.e., efficiency), balance, flexibility, lower extremity strength, and health-related quality of life, may be expected to be worse in PAD patients than in age-matched controls, but should improve after a program of exercise rehabilitation. However, little information is available on these measures in the PAD population.

In addition to laboratory measures of physical function, assessment of the impact that ambulatory and functional limitations have on routine activities performed in the community setting may provide a truer measure of disability. The free-living daily physical activity measured by an accelerometer is one such measure because it quantifies the amount of movement done over an extended period of time. Daily physical activity is approximately 33 percent lower in PAD patients than in non-PAD subjects of similar age, and progressively declines in claudicants with worsening disease severity as measured by ABI. Furthermore, cigarette smoking, which is common in the PAD population, decreases daily physical activity by an additional 30 percent. Thus, PAD patients with intermittent claudication are at the extreme low end of the physical activity spectrum. It is not clear whether the typical improvements in claudication distances following exercise rehabilitation translate into increases in daily physical activity in the community setting. Further research is needed to examine this issue as well as to determine whether functional improvements are related to enhanced quality of life in this elderly, disabled population.

MANAGEMENT

Geriatricians can have their greatest impact on the clinical management of patients who have asymptomatic PAD, intermittent claudication, or residual physical dysfunction following peripheral revascularization caused by the extreme deconditioning process that occurs with critical limb-threatening ischemia. These patients are good candidates for more conservative treatments such as exercise rehabilitation and/or medication therapy. It should be appreciated that if asymptomatic PAD patients can be identified through measurement of ABI, they are ideal candidates for exercise rehabilitation because the atherosclerotic process has not advanced enough to interfere with the ability to exercise.

Effects of Exercise Rehabilitation

In contrast to either drug treatment or surgical procedures, the clinical management of intermittent claudication in patients with PAD can be significantly improved with little cost, morbidity, and mortality through physical conditioning. Significant improvements in claudication pain have occurred following exercise rehabilitation. For example, meta-analysis demonstrated that in 21 exercise rehabilitation studies conducted between 1966 and 1993, the average distance walked on a treadmill to onset of claudication pain increased 179 percent, from a mean of 126 meters to 351 meters following rehabilitation, and the average distance walked to maximal claudication pain increased 122 percent, from 326 meters to 723 meters.

Numerous mechanisms have been proposed to explain the improvement in walking distances to the onset and to maximal claudication pain following exercise rehabilitation. The mechanisms primarily center on hemodynamic and enzymatic adaptations within the exercising musculature of the symptomatic leg(s). These mechanisms include an increase in blood flow to the exercising leg musculature, a more favorable redistribution of blood flow, greater utilization of oxygen because of a higher concentration of oxidative enzymes, improvement in hemorheologic properties of the blood, a decrease in the reliance upon anaerobic metabolism, and an improvement in the efficiency of walking. It is likely that a combination of changes in these factors contribute to the improved walking distances.

Table 39-4 The Effects of Exercise Program Components on Changes in Claudication Pain Distances from 21 Studies

Components of Exercise Programs	Change in the Distance to Onset of Pain (M)	Change in the Distance to Maximal Pain (M)
Exercise duration		
≤30 min/session (n = 8)	143 ± 163*	144 ± 419[†]
>30 min/session (n = 6)	314 ± 172*	653 ± 364[†]
Exercise frequency		
<3 sessions/week (n = 7)	178 ± 130*	249 ± 349*
≥3 sessions/week (n = 11)	271 ± 221*	541 ± 263*
Length of program		
<26 weeks (n = 10)	132 ± 159[†]	275 ± 228[†]
≥26 weeks (n = 11)	346 ± 162[†]	518 ± 409[†]
Claudication pain end point used during training sessions		
Onset of pain (n = 15)	105 ± 91[†]	195 ± 78[†]
Near-maximal pain (n = 6)	350 ± 246[†]	607 ± 427[†]
Mode of exercise		
Walking (n = 6)	294 ± 290*	512 ± 483*
Combination of exercises (n = 15)	152 ± 158*	287 ± 127*
Level of supervision		
Supervised (n = 11)	238 ± 120	449 ± 292
Combination of home and supervised (n = 8)	208 ± 198	339 ± 472

*NOTE: Values for each component are adjusted means ± standard deviations of the change in the distances to onset and to maximal claudication pain after statistically controlling for the other five exercise programs components.
* Significant difference between groups ($P \leq .05$).
[†] $P \leq .01$.
SOURCE: Adapted from Gardner AW and Poehlman ET (1995).

Improvements in psychosocial attitude due to accomplishments that are achieved during exercise rehabilitation may further enhance this effect.

In terms of the peripheral hemodynamic mechanism, calf blood flow under resting and maximal conditions increases on average by approximately 19 percent and ABI increases by approximately 7 percent following exercise rehabilitation. Because the magnitude of change in calf blood flow and ABI does not approach that of the changes in the walking distances to onset (179 percent) and to maximal (122 percent) claudication pain, either a small change in peripheral blood flow yield exponential improvement in claudication pain symptoms, or the other mechanisms mentioned above also contribute to the improved outcome. However, few studies have examined these mechanisms.

Although substantial increases in the average distances to onset and to maximal claudication pain during treadmill walking have been noted following exercise, considerable variability among the studies exists; for example, the increased distance to onset of pain ranges between 73 percent and 746 percent, and the increased distance to maximal pain ranges between 61 percent and 765 percent. Differences in the components of exercise programs (e.g., intensity, duration, and frequency of exercise sessions) may largely account for these widely divergent responses.

To examine the contributions of the components of an exercise rehabilitation program, a meta-analysis was carried out. As displayed in Table 39-4, six components were examined: (1) duration of exercise (minutes per session); (2) frequency of exercise (sessions per week); (3) length of the program (weeks); (4) claudication pain endpoint used in the program (onset versus near maximal pain); (5) mode of exercise (walking versus a combination of exercises); and (6) level of supervision. All of the exercise rehabilitation components had a significant effect on the magnitude of change in the claudication distances except for the level of supervision. For example, programs that exercised patients to near-maximal claudication pain were more effective than programs that exercised patients to only the onset of pain. Additionally, programs consisting of higher exercise duration, higher frequency, greater program length, and walking as the only mode of exercise were more effective than programs consisting of lower exercise duration, lower frequency, shorter program length, and having patients train by a variety of exercise modes. The addition of home exercise to supplement the amount of exercise performed in a supervised setting did not result in additional ambulatory benefit. Of the five components that had an effect on the change in the claudication distances, only three were found to have an independent effect through multivariate analyses. These components were the claudication pain endpoint used in the program, the length of the program, and the mode of exercise. The combination of these components explained nearly 90 percent of the variance in the increase in the walking distances following exercise rehabilitation.

Recommended Exercise Program for Treating Intermittent Claudication

Optimal improvements in claudication symptoms are elicited by having patients walk intermittently beyond the onset of pain for as long as they can safely tolerate, and perform this exercise program for a minimum of 6 months. Although the duration and frequency of the exercise sessions are not independent predictors of the change in claudication pain times, patients should walk for at least 30 minutes per session and for at least three sessions per week, as these amounts were more beneficial than programs using a lower exercise duration and frequency.

A review of only six controlled trials recommends that the optimal exercise program for treating intermittent claudication consists of exercising under supervised conditions for at least 2 months and at high intensity. However, the appropriate exercise intensity to use during training cannot be determined at this time because no study has addressed this issue. There is a common misconception that walking beyond the onset of pain to near maximal pain is an increase in intensity when, in fact, it is merely an increase in duration. The rate of work performed while walking, regardless of the duration, is the important consideration when setting the appropriate exercise intensity. Because heart rate is commonly used as a means to adjust the intensity of exercise, a conservative recommendation for claudicants who are beginning rehabilitation is to walk at an appropriate speed and grade on a treadmill to elicit an intensity of approximately 50 percent of their heart rate reserve, and to gradually increase the intensity to 70 to 80 percent by completion of the program. Table 39-5 summarizes recommendations for an exercise program for patients with PAD.

Pharmacologic Intervention

In addition to exercise rehabilitation, pharmacologic intervention is another medical option to treat intermittent claudication. Pharmacologic therapy for intermittent claudication in the United States is limited to pentoxifylline and cilostazol. Pentoxifylline, which has a hemorheologic effect by improving the flexibility of red blood cell membranes and by reducing platelet aggregation, was first studied in the United States in 1982. It was found to increase the distance to onset of claudication pain by 45 percent and the distance to maximal pain by 32 percent following 24 weeks of treatment. These were significantly greater changes than the 23 percent and 20 percent increases seen with placebo treatment. Although this initial study demonstrated the efficacy of pentoxifylline, its usefulness in treating intermittent claudication has been questioned. Cilostazol is a new medication with more potent vasodilatory and antiplatelet activity than aspirin. Cilostazol was found to

Table 39-5 Recommended Exercise Program for Patients with Peripheral Arterial Disease

Exercise Component	Comment
Frequency	Three exercise sessions per week.
Intensity	Initially, 50% of peak exercise capacity, with gradual progression to 80% by the end of the program.
Duration	Initially, 15 minutes of exercise per session, with gradual progression to 40–50 minutes by the end of the program.
Mode	Weight bearing (e.g., walking, stair climbing). Nonweight-bearing tasks (e.g., bicycling) may be used for warming up and cooling down.
Type of Exercise	Intermittent walking to a claudication pain score of 3 using a 4-point pain scale.
Program Length	Approximately 6 months.

SOURCE: Adapted from Gardner AW: Guidelines for developing an exercise program for elderly patients with peripheral arterial occlusive disease. *Clin Geriatr* 3:41, 1995.

increase the distances to onset and to maximal claudication pain by 40 percent and 42 percent, respectively, which were significantly greater than the 1 percent and –14 percent changes seen with placebo treatment. These studies suggest that pharmacologic intervention may be used to treat intermittent claudication in a large percentage of patients. However, exercise rehabilitation results in greater increases in walking distances in patients who are capable and motivated to walk on a regular basis.

PREVENTION

Risk factors for PAD are typical of those for coronary artery disease, including cigarette smoking, race (nonwhite), diabetes, age, systolic blood pressure, body mass index, high-density lipoprotein cholesterol, total cholesterol, creatinine, and forced vital capacity. Thus, efforts at risk factor reduction make sense in trying to prevent PAD or its progression.

In addition, properties of blood rheology and coagulation also play a role in the development of arterial occlusive disease. Increased blood viscosity and red cell aggregation is associated with an increased risk for PAD. Fibrinogen is an independent risk factor for heart disease and stroke, and disorders of fibrinolysis such as increased plasminogen activator inhibitor are associated with ischemic heart disease. Consequently, fibrinogen and plasminogen activator inhibitor may be independent risk factors for PAD. An emerging body of evidence shows a beneficial effect of exercise training in reducing blood viscosity, red cell aggregation, fibrinogen, and increasing fibrinolytic activity both in healthy subjects and in PAD patients.

Thus, exercise training may improve the more traditionally accepted PAD risk factors (e.g., blood lipids, blood pressure, obesity) as well as measures of blood rheology and coagulation. Finally, because physical activity level is associated with ABI, increasing the activity level may have a preventative role in the development of PAD.

SUMMARY

PAD is a significant health concern in the elderly population, and it will continue to increase in future years. Conservative management of patients with asymptomatic PAD and patients with intermittent claudication is recommended to modify risk factors and improve ambulatory ability, while patients with more severe PAD typically require revascularization of the lower extremities. Exercise rehabilitation is a highly effective, conservative treatment to improve ambulation in patients with intermittent claudication. To date, the primary focus of attention on the benefits of exercise rehabilitation has centered on the increase in walking distances to onset and to maximal claudication pain during a treadmill test. Future research should focus on the improvement in other functional outcomes which may be more representative of everyday activities such as submaximal exercise performance, walking economy, balance, flexibility, and lower extremity strength. Until these measures are obtained, the full benefit of exercise rehabilitation for PAD patients remains undefined.

REFERENCES

Criqui MH et al: Mortality over a period of 10 years in patients with peripheral arterial disease. *N Engl J Med* 326:381, 1992.

Fowkes FG: Epidemiological research on peripheral vascular disease. *J Clin Epidemiol* 54:863, 2001.

Gardner AW et al: Progressive versus single-stage treadmill tests for evaluation of claudication. *Med Sci Sports Exerc* 23:402, 1991.

Gardner AW et al: The effect of cigarette smoking on free-living daily physical activity in older claudication patients. *Angiology* 48:947, 1997.

Gardner AW, Poehlman ET: Exercise rehabilitation programs for the treatment of claudication pain: A meta-analysis. *JAMA* 274:975, 1995.

Gardner AW, Montgomery PS: Impaired balance and higher prevalence of falls in subjects with intermittent claudication. *J Gerontol* 56A:M454, 2001.

Hiatt WR et al: Clinical trials for claudication: Assessment of exercise performance, functional status, and clinical end points. *Circulation* 92:614, 1995.

Hiatt WR et al: Benefit of exercise conditioning for patients with peripheral arterial disease. *Circulation* 81:602, 1990.

Hirsch AT et al: Peripheral arterial disease detection, awareness, and treatment in primary care. *JAMA* 286:1317, 2001.

Kannel WB: The demographics of claudication and the aging of the American population. *Vasc Med* 1:60, 1996.

McDermott MM et al: Asymptomatic peripheral arterial disease is independently associated with impaired lower extremity functioning: The Women's Health and Aging Study. *Circulation* 101:1007, 2000.

McDermott MM et al: Leg symptoms in peripheral arterial disease: Associated clinical characteristics and functional impairment. *JAMA* 286:1599, 2001.

McKenna M et al: The ratio of ankle and arm arterial pressure as an independent predictor of mortality. *Atherosclerosis* 87:119, 1991.

Montgomery PS, Gardner AW: The clinical utility of a 6-minute walk test in peripheral arterial occlusive disease patients. *J Am Geriatr Soc* 46:706, 1998.

Newman AB et al: Ankle-arm index as a marker of atherosclerosis in the cardiovascular health study. *Circulation* 88:837, 1993.

Newman AB: Peripheral arterial disease: Insights from population studies of older adults. *J Am Geriatr Soc* 48:1157, 2000.

Pentecost MJ et al: Guidelines for peripheral percutaneous transluminal angioplasty of the abdominal aorta and lower extremity vessels. *Circulation* 89:511, 1994.

Rutherford RB: Standards for evaluating results of interventional therapy for peripheral vascular disease. *Circulation* 83(2 Suppl):I6, 1991.

Sieminski DJ, Gardner AW: The relationship between daily physical activity and the severity of peripheral arterial occlusive disease. *Vasc Med* 2:286, 1997.

Weitz JI et al: Diagnosis and treatment of chronic arterial insufficiency of the lower extremities: A critical review. *Circulation* 94:3026, 1996.

inhibitors and muscle strength and physical function in older women: An observational study. *Lancet* 359:926, 2002.

Pahor M et al: Health outcomes associated with calcium antagonists compared with other first-line antihypertensive therapies: A meta-analysis of randomised controlled trials. *Lancet* 356:1949, 2000.

Pahor M et al: Therapeutic benefits of ACE inhibitors and other antihypertensive drugs in patients with type 2 diabetes. *Diabetes Care* 23:888, 2000.

Pini R et al: Cardiac and vascular remodeling in older adults with borderline isolated systolic hypertension: The ICARE Dicomano Study. *Hypertension* 38:1372, 2001.

Psaty BM et al: Health outcomes associated with antihypertensive therapies used as first-line agents. A systematic review and meta-analysis. *JAMA* 277:739, 1997.

Randomised trial of a perindopril-based blood-pressure-lowering regimen among 6,105 individuals with previous stroke or transient ischaemic attack. *Lancet* 358:1033, 2001.

Staessen JA et al. for the Systolic Hypertension-Europe (Syst-Eur) Trial Investigators: Morbidity and mortality in the placebo-controlled European Trial on Isolated Systolic Hypertension in the Elderly. *Lancet* 360:757, 1997.

The Systolic Hypertension in the Elderly Program (SHEP) Cooperative Research Group: Prevention of stroke by antihypertensive drug treatment in older persons with isolated systolic hypertension: Final results of SHEP. *JAMA* 265:3255, 1991.

Williamson JD et al: Blood pressure control and incident disability in high-risk older women: Data from the Women's Health and Aging Study. *J Am Geriatr Soc* 49:S137, 2001.

RESPIRATORY SYSTEM

C H A P T E R   4 1

Aging of the Respiratory System

PAUL L. ENRIGHT

This chapter first reviews the changes in lung function with aging that are known to occur in healthy persons (normal, never smokers). Included are the major categories of pulmonary function tests: static lung volumes, maximal expiratory flow, lung mechanics, and gas exchange, plus bronchodilator response and nonspecific airway reactivity. Table 41-1 summarizes these changes. The chapter then adds a discussion of how lung function tests may be used by a clinician to assist in the differential diagnosis of asthma and chronic obstructive pulmonary disease (COPD) in an elderly patient, and to objectively measure the efficacy of asthma and COPD therapy.

STATIC LUNG VOLUMES

Total lung capacity (TLC) is the volume of air within the respiratory system when a subject makes a maximal voluntary inspiratory effort (and the air seen in the lungs on a chest x-ray). It is determined by the balance of forces between the maximally activated inspiratory muscles and the elastic recoil of the lung and chest wall. A nearly constant TLC with aging appears to be the net result of changes in all the factors that determine TLC. In the elderly individual, maximal inspiratory pressure (MIP) decreases with age; however, this measurement is made at residual volume (RV) which increases with age, so respiratory muscles are shorter and less efficient as RV increases.

The static elastic recoil of the lung decreases with aging (just as the skin becomes less elastic), making the lungs easier to expand toward TLC. This reduction of elastic recoil tends to increase TLC; however, the chest wall becomes stiffer with aging, and its inward elastic recoil is increased as the lungs expand, so that a maximal inspiratory effort is not able to achieve a higher lung volume even though

the lungs themselves have become easier to expand. In contrast, the loss of lung elastic recoil caused by smoking-induced emphysema is associated an increase in TLC, and an even larger increase in the residual volume.

Residual volume is the volume of air remaining in the respiratory system when subjects have expired as much air as possible. The RV and RV/TLC ratio increase from middle-age to older age. Because lung elastic recoil

Table 41-1 Effects of Aging on Lung Function

Lower maximal expiratory flows: FEV_1, FEV_1/FVC, FEF 75%
Increased FRC and RV, lower VC, but stable TLC
Lower diffusing capacity (oxygen uptake)
Lower PO_2 and SpO_2 as a consequence of V/Q mismatch (but no change in Pco_2)
Lower respiratory muscle strength and endurance
Stiffer chest wall (less compliant)
Increased lung tissue compliance (loss of lung recoil)
Reduced respiratory drive (for hypoxia, hypercarbia, and resistive loads)
Increased airway reactivity

FEF, forced expiratory flow; FEV_1, forced expiratory volume in one second; FRC, functional residual capacity; FVC, forced vital capacity; Pco_2, partial pressure of carbon dioxide; PO_2, partial pressure of oxygen; RV, residual volume; S_pO_2, arterial oxyhemoglobin saturation; TLC, total lung capacity; VC, vital capacity; V/Q, ventilation/perfusion.

decreases as a consequence of normal aging, the RV increases in healthy elderly persons. Vital capacity (VC) is the difference between the absolute lung volume at TLC and at RV. Because TLC is relatively constant while RV increases with age, the VC decreases with age.

MAXIMAL EXPIRATORY FLOW

Maximal expiratory flow, as seen during spirometry tests, varies as a function of lung volume because higher flows are always possible at a higher lung volume. For forced exhalation beginning from TLC (the usual spirometry maneuver), the initial (peak) flow is determined by the recoil of the lung and chest wall and the degree of effort expended by the patient, as well as by the speed with which the patient's respiratory muscles can generate positive pleural pressure. Once maximal flow is achieved, maximal flow throughout the remainder of the vital capacity is determined by the intrinsic properties of the lung. There are modest decreases of peak expiratory flow (PEF) with age. Larger declines are seen in expiratory flow at lower lung volumes, as shown by the flow volume curve.

SPIROMETRY

Spirometry is the most common test of lung function, and is easily performed by 9 of 10 elderly patients. Modern office spirometers use a flow sensor, connected to a microprocessor that calculates the results (forced expiratory volume in one second [FEV_1] and forced vital capacity [FVC]), and prints the flow–volume curves from the patient's best forced expiratory breathing maneuver. Instrument accuracy and the methods for performing office spirometry are standardized by the American Thoracic Society and the National Lung Health Education Program.

The presence of airways obstruction is determined by a low FEV_1/FVC ratio and visualized on the flow–volume (F-V) curve as concavity toward the volume axis or tail at the end of the maneuver (Fig. 41-1). The descending limb of the F-V curve of healthy young adults is a straight line of about 45 degrees until the end of the maneuver, corresponding to exponential emptying of the lungs. The shape of the F-V curve becomes progressively more curvilinear as a healthy adult becomes older, corresponding to decreases in expiratory flows at low lung volumes. The reduced flow at low lung volumes, even in healthy elderly persons, is a result of a decrease in the mean diameter of small airways. Because the FEV_1 is the average flow during the first second of the maneuver, it includes flows over most of the vital capacity and is also reduced with normal aging.

As in healthy adults older than age 30 years, older adults normally experience a loss in FEV_1 of about one-third liter per decade (Fig. 41-2). The decline in FVC with aging is somewhat less than the decline in FEV1, so that the ratio of FEV1/FVC also declines with age in the elderly population.

Many nonpulmonary factors contribute to the decline in the FEV_1 in elderly persons. All of the factors listed in Table 41-2 are significantly associated with a lower FEV_1. The strongest factors are cigarette smoking; a diagnosis of emphysema, chronic bronchitis, or asthma; and wheezing symptoms—all of which are known to cause airway obstruction (a low FEV_1/FVC ratio). Several of the factors associated with a lower FEV_1 in elderly persons are a result of restriction of lung volumes with a normal FEV_1/FVC ratio; these include obesity, malnutrition, heart disease, and chest wall abnormalities. For a given height, gender, and age, the FVC and FEV_1 of healthy elderly black persons is approximately 12 percent lower than that of healthy elderly white persons, but there is no ethnic difference in the FEV_1/FVC ratio.

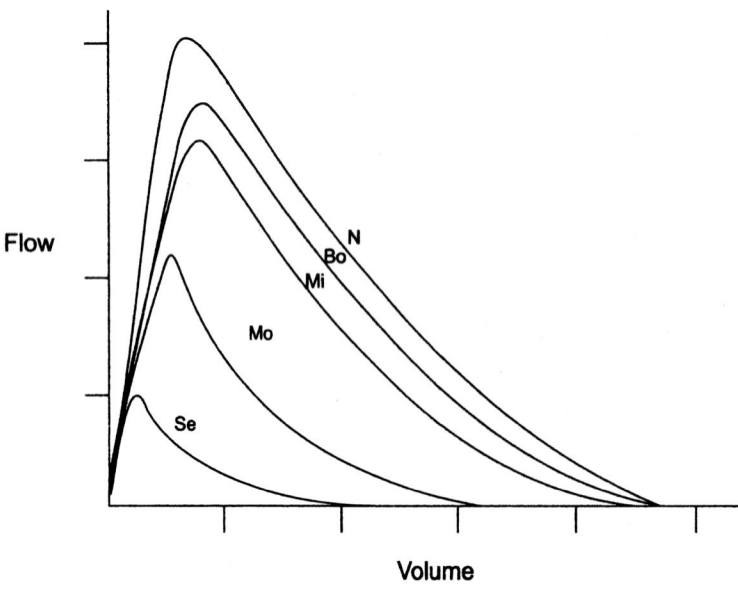

Figure 41-1   Flow-volume curves with increasing degrees of obstruction. Bo, borderline obstruction (85 percent predicted); Mi, mild obstruction (70 percent predicted); Mo, moderate obstruction (60 percent predicted); N, normal (100 percent predicted FEV₁); Se, severe obstruction (35 percent predicted).

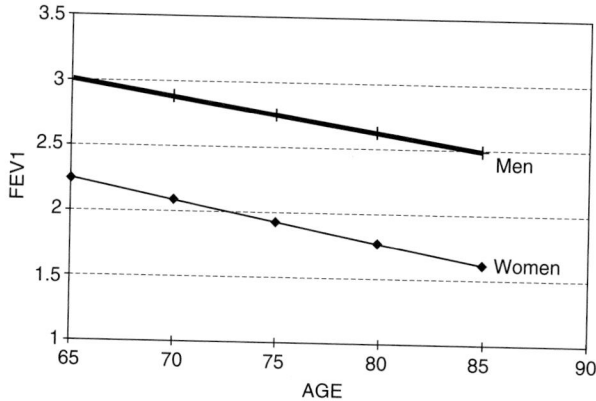

Figure 41-2 The FEV_1 normally declines about 30 mL per year with aging, even in healthy men and women without lung disease.

RESPIRATORY MUSCLE STRENGTH

Another vital component of respiratory function is respiratory muscle strength and endurance. Diaphragm strength is approximately 25 percent lower in healthy elderly persons as compared to young adults. The vital capacity is reduced when the diaphragm is weak, and when the expiratory muscles of the abdominal and thoracic wall cannot empty the lungs below the resting respiratory position. The load on these respiratory muscles increases with aging, because chest wall compliance decreases.

Diaphragm strength may be easily and inexpensively measured in the outpatient office. The patient exhales slowly, then makes a maximal attempt to inhale from a mouthpiece connected to a pressure gauge (-200 cm H_2O range, with a small leak) for 2 seconds. The largest pressure from five such maneuvers (the highest two of which match within 10 percent) is reported as the MIP. Respiratory muscle strength is stronger in men, but declines with aging in both sexes. The mean MIP for healthy 85-year-old men

Table 41-2 Factors Associated with a Lower FEV_1 in Elderly Individuals

Important factors associated with airway obstruction
Cigarette smoking (current, former, and pack-years)
Emphysema or chronic bronchitis
A diagnosis of asthma at any time in the past
Wheezing (during or apart from colds, daytime or nighttime)
A history of workplace exposures to dust, fumes, smoke, or chemicals
Other factors associated with restriction of lung volumes
Dyspnea on exertion
Obesity or malnutrition
Hypertension or hypotension
Major ECG abnormality
Pitting ankle edema
Diabetes, on medication
Prior chest surgery

is approximately 30 percent lower than that for 65-year-old men (65 versus 90 cm H_2O). A lower MIP is associated with many factors, including decreased handgrip strength, a lower FVC, lower body mass index (malnutrition), and current smoking.

ARTERIAL BLOOD GASES

Acid-base balance is tightly controlled, and therefore, normal values for arterial pH and Pa_{CO_2} (partial pressure of carbon dioxide in arterial gas) do not change throughout adult life in healthy persons. However, because of increased nonuniformity of ventilation with aging, mean arterial oxygen tension (PaO_2 [partial pressure arterial oxygen]) declines during middle life even in healthy never-smokers. Mean PaO_2 remains relatively constant at about 80 mmHg from age 65 to 90 years in healthy elderly persons at sea level (Fig. 41-3).

DIFFUSING CAPACITY

A test of the single-breath pulmonary diffusing capacity for carbon monoxide (DLCO) is available at hospital-based pulmonary function laboratories. The 15-minute noninvasive DLCO test is clinically valuable for the differential diagnosis of both airway obstruction and restriction of lung volumes. DLCO is the amount of 3% carbon monoxide that is absorbed into the blood during a 10-second breath-hold.

In smokers with airways obstruction, the DLCO is an excellent index of the degree of anatomic emphysema; a low DLCO correlates highly with a low mean lung tissue density on lung CT scans and the degree of anatomic emphysema. Smokers with airways obstruction but normal DLCO values usually have chronic "obstructive" bronchitis but not emphysema; and nonsmoking patients with asthma and borderline to moderate airways obstruction have normal or high (percent predicted) DLCO values.

In healthy persons, the absolute value of DLCO in adults varies with height, age, gender, and race. Reference values from large population studies are used to obtain percent predicted values for individual patients. DLCO is higher in very obese persons and lower in patients with anemia.

After age 40 years, the DLCO declines with age in healthy individuals, about 5 percent per decade (somewhat more rapidly than does the vital capacity). While men experience a linear decline of approximately 2 DLCO units per decade, women lose only approximately 0.54 DLCO units per decade from age 25 years to 46 years, and subsequently at about the same rate as men as they grow older. This suggests a protective hormonal effect on DLCO decline for women prior to menopause (or a cohort effect).

DIFFERENTIAL DIAGNOSIS OF ASTHMA AND COPD

The differential diagnosis of asthma and COPD in elderly persons is often more difficult than in younger adults because of the higher prevalence of comorbidity. The elderly

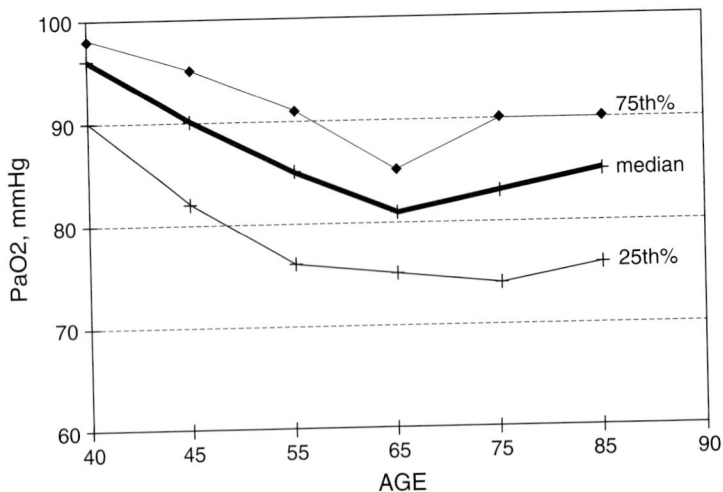

Figure 41-3   Arterial oxygen (PaO$_2$) decreases throughout middle age in healthy persons but stabilizes beyond age 65 years in healthy persons.

are much more likely than middle-aged adults to have COPD and cardiovascular disease, both often a result of cigarette smoking, and both with symptoms which may mimic asthma, increasing the value of objective pulmonary function (PF) tests in the elderly patient.

Because intermittent airway obstruction is the primary physiologic manifestation of asthma, the first (and least expensive) PF test to perform is spirometry, especially if the patient is experiencing symptoms at the time of presentation (Fig. 41-4). If the FEV$_1$/FVC ratio is below the lower limit of the normal range (assuming that appropriate reference equations for elderly patients are used and the quality of the test session was good), the patient has airway obstruction. The degree of severity of the obstruction

is then determined by the percent predicted FEV$_1$. When compared to younger patients with asthma, one will often be surprised by more severe airway obstruction (an FEV$_1$ below 50 percent predicted) in elderly patients with asthma.

If the patient has airways obstruction, repeat spirometry approximately 45 minutes after administration of a combination of albuterol and ipratropium (postbronchodilator [BD] spirometry). A positive (significant) BD response is best defined as an increase of both 200 mL or more and at least a 12 percent improvement in percent predicted FEV$_1$. The mean BD response of groups of elderly patients with asthma is not lower than that of younger adults with asthma.

With good test quality, baseline airway obstruction followed by a BD response helps to confirm asthma in a patient with a history suggesting asthma. However, the lack of a positive BD response is of no help in making the diagnosis (does not rule out asthma), because chronic asthma often leads to airways inflammation that is not acutely reversible. Furthermore, many elderly patients with a history of smoking, current symptoms suggesting asthma, baseline airways obstruction, and a "positive" BD response, still have some "fixed" obstruction (a low FEV$_1$) following aggressive therapy for asthma. Unfortunately, the BD response is frequently not helpful when attempting to separate asthma from COPD, and it is not a good predictor of objective improvement with subsequent chronic bronchodilator or inhaled corticosteroid therapy, nor survival.

Baseline and pre-post–BD spirometry may be normal in patients with a history suggesting asthma. The patient may be asked to return for retesting when symptoms occur; however, methacholine challenge testing can safely be done the next day. This test of bronchial responsiveness has optimal clinical utility when the pretest probability of asthma is intermediate. A high PC-20 (above 16 mg/mL) makes asthma highly unlikely, while a low PC-20 (below 4 mg/mL) in a patient with a history of asthma-like symptoms increases the pretest probability of asthma.

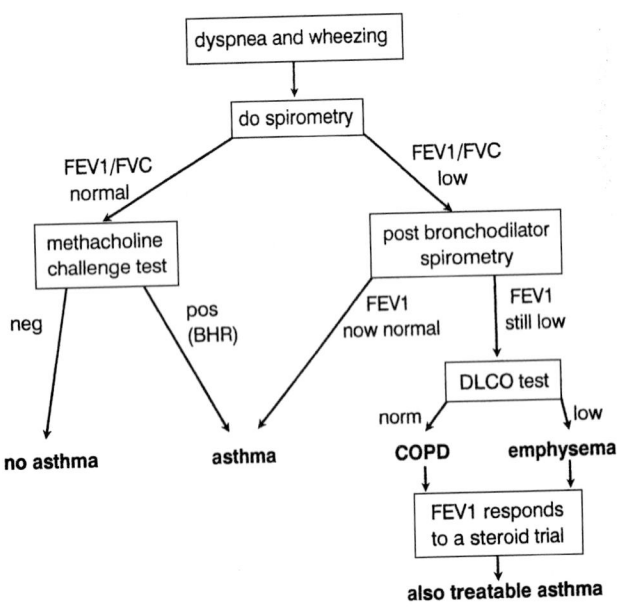

Figure 41-4   The role of PF tests in making a differential diagnosis of asthma versus COPD in a patient with chronic or intermittent dyspnea.

Measurement of the DLCO is quick, safe, and helps to distinguish between emphysema and other causes of chronic airway obstruction: emphysema lowers the DLCO, obstructive chronic bronchitis does not affect the DLCO, and asthma frequently increases the DLCO. A lung CT scan may also differentiate asthma from emphysema in a cigarette smoker. Of course, both diseases may coexist in a smoker.

PF TESTS TO ASSESS RESPONSE TO THERAPY FOR ASTHMA AND COPD

The inhaled corticosteroids used to treat asthma frequently cause thrush, and the long-acting bronchodilator inhalers may cause muscle cramps, tremors, insomnia, and arrhythmias, so these asthma medications should be adjusted upward to maintain asthma control, and then downward a few months later after maximal control is obtained. When oral corticosteroids such as prednisone are necessary to maintain asthma control, serious morbidity frequently occurs because of ocular disease, osteoporosis, and glucose intolerance; therefore, objective measurements of the effectiveness of each newly prescribed asthma medication for each patient is highly desirable.

Two lung function tests are used as asthma therapy outcome measures in the outpatient clinic setting: the pre- or postbronchodilator FEV_1 during a clinic visit, and peak flow measured at home in the early morning. The FEV_1 is more accurate and more sensitive than peak flow for detecting narrow airways, and it is linearly related to the severity of asthma symptoms in groups of elderly patients. Because many elderly patients become tolerant of severe, long-standing airway obstruction and consequently underreport respiratory symptoms, objective measurement of lung function is needed. FEV_1 improvement of more than 20 percent and 200 mL is necessary to be confident that the change was not merely a result of measurement noise. The *postbronchodilator* FEV_1 measures the best lung function that can be achieved on the day of the visit, and therefore, is a more stable measure in asthmatics than comparing visit-to-visit *baseline* FEV_1s.

REFERENCES

American Thoracic Society: Guidelines for methacholine and exercise challenge testing—1999. *Am J Respir Crit Care Med* 161:309, 2000.

Barbee RA, Bloom JW: *Asthma in the Elderly*. New York, Marcel Dekker, 1997.

Camhi SL, Enright PL: How to assess pulmonary function in older adults. *J Respir Dis* 21:395, 2000.

Celli B: The importance of spirometry in COPD and asthma: Effect on approach to management. *Chest* 117:15S, 2000.

Cerveri I et al: Reference values of arterial oxygen tension in the middle-aged and elderly. *Am J Respir Crit Care Med* 152:934, 1995.

Cuttitta G et al: Changes in FVC during methacholine-induced bronchoconstriction in elderly patients with asthma. *Chest* 119:1685, 2001.

Enright PL et al: Reduced vital capacity in elderly persons with hypertension, coronary heart disease, or left ventricular hypertrophy: The Cardiovascular Health Study. *Chest* 107:28, 1995.

Enright PL et al: Correlates of respiratory muscle strength, and maximal respiratory pressure reference values in the elderly. *Am Rev Respir Dis* 149:430, 1994.

Enright PL et al. for the Cardiovascular Health Study Research Group: Under-diagnosis and under-treatment of asthma in the elderly. *Chest* 116:603, 1999.

Ferguson G et al: Office spirometry for lung health assessment in adults. A consensus statement from the National Lung Health Education Program. *Chest* 117:1146, 2000.

Goldstein MD et al: Comparisons of peak diurnal expiratory flow variation, postbronchodilator FEV_1 responses, and methacholine inhalation challenges in the evaluation of suspected asthma. *Chest* 119:1001, 2001.

Hankinson JL et al: Spirometric reference values from a sample of the general US population. *Am J Respir Crit Care Med* 159:179, 1999.

Korenblat PE et al: Effect of age on response to zafirlukast in patients with asthma. *Ann Allergy Asthma Immunol* 84:217, 2000.

Kradjan WA et al: Effect of age on bronchodilator response. *Chest* 101:1545, 1992.

Quadrelli SA, Roncoroni A: Features of asthma in the elderly. *J Asthma* 38:377, 2001.

Sin DD, Tu JV: Underuse of inhaled steroid therapy in elderly patients with asthma. *Chest* 119:720, 2001.

Tolep K, Kelsen SG: Effect of aging on respiratory skeletal muscles. *Clin Chest Med* 3:363, 1993.

Walsh LJ et al: Adverse effects of oral corticosteroids in relation to dose in patients with lung disease. *Thorax* 56:279, 2001.

Chronic Obstructive Pulmonary Disease

SIDNEY S. BRAMAN

In the mid twentieth century, more than 50 percent of adult Americans smoked cigarettes. Following the surgeon general's report on smoking and health in 1964, major public health efforts reduced the rate of adult smokers to 22 percent by the end of the century. Cigarette smoking is the major cause of chronic obstructive pulmonary disease (COPD) in the developed world and, unfortunately, despite causing widespread lung injury, clinical manifestations do not become apparent in the smoker or ex-smoker until many decades have passed. The smoking epidemic of the twentieth century has resulted in a large number of adults with COPD, a largely preventable disease. It has emerged as a major public health problem for the twenty-first century, with more than 16 million Americans currently affected. It has risen to become the fourth leading cause of death in the United States, and globally was responsible for 3 million deaths in the year 2000. It is a disease seen predominantly in the older population in our society (those over 65) and one that causes considerable morbidity in addition to mortality. During the latter part of the twentieth century, smoking increased among American women, which has resulted in a dramatic increase in the prevalence of the disease among older women. The prediction is for a substantial increase in COPD in the twenty-first century with the export of tobacco to developing countries such as India, China, Mexico, Egypt, and South Africa. COPD is projected to rank fifth as a worldwide burden of health within the next 20 years. It has also proven to have tremendous impact as a comorbid condition to many other diseases, often as a silent partner until a serious complication arises. What may begin as a simple elective surgical procedure in an elderly patient may result in a prolonged complicated hospital admission as a consequence of postoperative pneumonia or respiratory failure because of underlying, and often unrecognized, COPD.

The statistics concerning COPD have caused considerable alarm around the world. To address this growing problem, the World Health Organization partnered with the United States National Heart, Lung, and Blood Institute (NHLBI) to form a Global Initiative for Chronic Obstructive Lung Disease (GOLD). In 2001, they offered a global strategy to increase awareness of the disease and offer guidelines for disease prevention and treatment, often referred to as the GOLD Guidelines. These guidelines, as well as those created by several of our national societies, as summarized by McCrory et al., are incorporated into this chapter.

DEFINITION

For many decades COPD has been defined as a disease state characterized by chronic and progressive airflow limitation caused by chronic bronchitis and/or emphysema. Chronic bronchitis is a clinical term referring to the presence of a chronic productive cough for at least three consecutive months in two consecutive years. Other causes of chronic productive cough must be ruled out. Emphysema, on the other hand, has been defined by its pathologic description: an abnormal enlargement of the air spaces distal to the terminal bronchioles accompanied by destruction of their walls and without obvious fibrosis. Contrary to this traditional view, recent data have shown that this destructive process is accompanied by a net increase in the amount of collagen suggesting there is indeed active fibrosis associated with the breakdown of the elastic framework of the lung.

As defined by the GOLD Guidelines, the definition of COPD differs from previous consensus statements. The GOLD Guidelines define COPD as a disease state characterized by airflow obstruction that is not fully reversible and is usually progressive. The disease is caused by an interaction between noxious inhaled agents such as cigarette smoke, industrial and other environmental pollutants, and host factors (genetic, respiratory infections, etc.) that results in chronic inflammation in the walls and lumen of the airways. The pathology of COPD, as well as the symptoms, the pulmonary function abnormalities, and complications all can be explained on the basis of the underlying inflammation.

While the GOLD document does not specifically include chronic bronchitis and emphysema in the definition of COPD, it is clear that they are considered the predominant causes of COPD. In the past, asthma was also included under the umbrella term COPD. As asthma became recognized as an inflammatory disease with a different cellular and inflammatory mediator profile compared to smoking-induced chronic bronchitis and emphysema, it was no longer considered under the term COPD. This has also been justified by two other distinguishing factors of asthma: (1) the airflow obstruction is predominantly reversible and (2) the airways of asthmatics are markedly hyperresponsive to a variety of specific (aeroallergens) and nonspecific (methacholine, histamine, cold air) inhaled substances. While it is still clinically useful to distinguish asthma from COPD (chronic bronchitis and emphysema), it is important to recognize that in many patients these distinctions become blurred.

First, remission rates for adults with asthma are much less than those seen in children, and if remission does occur, the probability of relapse increases with increasing age. Many of such asthmatics, even those who have never smoked, but who are at the age when COPD is most often recognized (older than age 60 years), have evidence of severe poorly reversible airflow obstruction on pulmonary function testing similar to that seen with COPD. This has been caused by a remodeling of the airways with what appears to be permanent changes. This is supported by data from longitudinal studies that have shown that the lung function of many asthmatics declines over a period of years more rapidly than in normals without asthma. It should be noted that many adults with asthma do not show a correlation between their pulmonary function and the duration of their disease. Bronchial hyperresponsiveness—the exaggerated bronchoconstrictive response to nonspecific agonists such as methacholine—is a constant feature in asthmatics that is so important to its pathogenesis it has been incorporated into the definition of asthma.

A second difficulty in distinguishing COPD from asthma relates to the fact that increased responsiveness to constrictors such as methacholine and histamine (but not indirect bronchoconstrictors such as cold air and bradykinin) is seen in the majority of middle-aged smokers with COPD and has even been shown to be a strong predictor of progression of airway obstruction in those who continue to smoke. While it is true that in asthma, bronchial hyperresponsiveness is not related to baseline airway caliber, in COPD, the increased responsiveness to bronchoconstrictors can be explained entirely by the geometric effect of fixed airway narrowing. Clinically, however, this distinction is not useful.

Lastly and perhaps most importantly, many adult patients with asthma are current or former smokers. It is likely that such patients have more than one pathologic process and several pathways of inflammation. These patients are likely to have both COPD and asthma. This has raised a complexity of semantic issues that has not been resolved. One attempt has been to combine two of the major pathologic processes and describe such patients using the term asthmatic bronchitis.

EPIDEMIOLOGY

Over the past decade there has been increasing interest in the pathogenesis and management of COPD as it became recognized that the disease was having a major worldwide impact as summarized by Mannino. It has been calculated that COPD ranks as the twelfth largest disease burden in the world, with projections that it will rank number 5 by the year 2020. In the United States at present, estimates from national interviews taken by the National Center for Health Statistics show that more than 16 million people are afflicted with COPD; approximately 14 million are thought to have chronic bronchitis, while 2 million have emphysema. It is likely that these statistics underestimate the prevalence of COPD by as much as 50 percent, because many patients underreport their symptoms and remain undiagnosed. Results of the National Health and Nutrition Examination Survey (NHANES) III, reported August, 2002, obtained using surveys, physical exams, and pulmonary function testing that generated prevalence estimates based on World Health Organization definitions, show that 23.6 million adults (13.9% of the adult population) have COPD (reported by Mannino et al.). The average number of days of restricted activities reported by patients with COPD is very high, ranking this condition among the highest chronic conditions for this measure of morbidity in the nation. In 1996, COPD was listed as the eighth leading cause of disability-adjusted life-years (DALYs) in men, and the seventh leading cause of DALYs among women. COPD is a leading cause of hospitalizations in the United States. In 1998, nearly 2 percent of all hospitalizations were attributed to COPD and 7 percent had COPD as a contributing cause of hospitalization. More striking are COPD statistics regarding the elderly population. Nearly 20 percent of all hospitalizations in patients older than age 65 years had COPD as a primary or contributing cause.

The magnitude and trend of the mortality rates for COPD have caused considerable concern throughout the world. Over the past few decades the mortality rates associated with other common diseases such as cardiovascular disease and stroke have been declining. However, during the same time period, the mortality rate for COPD was rising at an alarming rate. For example, the US death rate for COPD rose almost 33 percent during the years 1979 to 1991, resulting in COPD becoming the fourth leading cause of death in this country. While the death rate for men with this disease has reached a plateau in recent years, among women it has continued to rise. In 1998, 54,615 men and 51,377 women died from COPD. From 1995 to 1998 the death rate for COPD increased 9 percent for US women.

RISK FACTORS FOR COPD

Table 42-1 lists the major risk factors for the development of COPD. All of these factors have one thing in

Table 42-1 Risk Factors for COPD

Risk	Comment
External factors	
Cigarette smoking	Most important risk factor: 85–90% of cases; 15–20% of 1 pack-per-day smokers and 25% of 2-pack-per-day smokers develop COPD
Pipe and cigars	High risk, but lower than cigarette smokers
Passive smoking	Children of smoking parents have more respiratory symptoms and lower airway function; ? significance for adult COPD
Occupational exposure	Risk in coal miners, gold miners, grain handlers, cement, and cotton workers etc; interacts with smoking
Environmental pollution	Indoor use of biomass fuels for cooking and heating in underdeveloped countries; ? particulate matter from urban pollution
Host factors	
Genetic factor	α_1-Antitrypsin deficiency; >90% caused by homozygous ZZ phenotype
Gender	Males more at risk than females
Socioeconomic	More common with low socioeconomic status
Bronchial hyperresponsiveness	A strong predictor of progressive airway obstruction in smokers
Atopy and asthma	Many adult nonsmoking asthmatics develop fixed airway obstruction; atopy alone not a factor
Childhood illnesses	Low birth weight, respiratory infections, and symptomatic childhood asthma
Dietary influences	Vitamin C and E (tocopherol) deficiencies

common: they are associated with an accelerated decline in FEV_1 (forced expiratory volume in one second) over time. Cigarette smoking leads the list and in most countries is the responsible agent in at least 85 to 90 percent of cases. Because the basic cellular and molecular mechanisms of disease are still poorly understood, the reasons why only certain individuals with a positive exposure history become affected are not known. For example, it is common to see pulmonary function abnormalities reflecting obstruction in the small airways and nonuniform distribution of ventilation in young adults who smoke. These changes are not predictive because only 15 to 20 percent of these heavy smokers will develop an accelerated decline of their FEV_1 over time and clinically evident COPD. The differences in susceptibility to tobacco smoke injury are likely to be related to genetic factors.

Genetic Risk Factors for COPD

α_1-Antitrypsin Deficiency

One genetic abnormality that has been known and well studied is α_1-antitrypsin deficiency. Also called α_1-antiprotease deficiency, this disorder accounts for less than 1 percent of COPD in the United States. α_1-Antitrypsin is a serum protein made in the liver that is capable of inhibiting the activity of specific proteolytic enzymes such as trypsin, chymotrypsin, and neutrophil elastase. If not inactivated by α_1-antitrypsin neutrophil elastase, these enzymes destroy lung connective tissue, particularly elastin, and this leads to the development of emphysema. α_1-Antitrypsin is coded for by a single gene on chromosome 14. The serum protease inhibitor phenotype (Pi type) is determined by the

independent expression of two independent alleles. More than 90 percent of severely deficient patients are homozygous for the Z allele. Such patients are designated Pi ZZ and have a serum α_1-antitrypsin reduced to about 20 percent of the normal level.

Most patients homozygous with the Z allele are of northern European descent. Asian and African Americans are rarely affected. Cigarette smoking is the most important risk factor for the development of COPD in patients with α_1-antitrypsin (AAT) deficiency. Symptoms begin early in adult life (usually by age 40 years) and COPD leads to an early death. On the other hand, Pi ZZ lifetime nonsmokers may develop COPD much later in life. Studies from the Swedish AAT Registry suggest that wheezing symptoms and exposures to gas, fumes, and dust are associated with reduced lung function. Most nonsmokers do not develop any pulmonary symptoms, have a normal life expectancy, and remain undetected unless they are found through family screening. Heterozygotes that are Pi MZ have intermediate levels of α_1-antitrypsin deficiency. Epidemiologic evidence suggests that they are not at increased risk for developing COPD when compared to Pi MM phenotypes. It is generally not important to screen elderly patients for α_1-antitrypsin deficiency, unless a strong family history of COPD points to their diagnosis.

Other Genetic Factors

Studies in relatives of patients with COPD have supported a role for genetic factors in this disease. There are higher rates of airflow obstruction in first-degree relatives of patients with COPD than in control subjects, and a number

Natural History of COPD

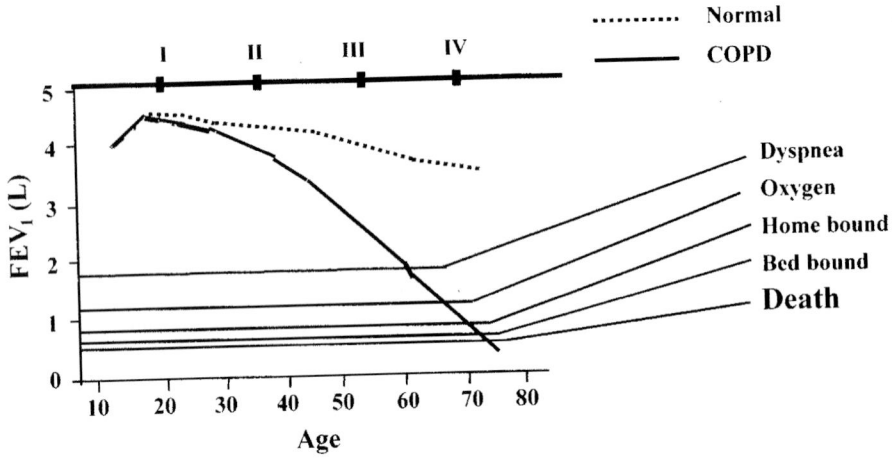

Figure 42-1 The natural history of COPD depicted in four phases (approximation of age group): (1) Age 15–30 years; begins smoking in high school. Inflammatory changes in small airways. No symptoms. Normal pulmonary function tests. (2) Age 30–45 years; chronic productive cough. One or two chest colds each winter. Mild airflow obstruction not clinically detected. (3) Age 45–60 years; dyspnea begins. Airflow obstruction worsens as does quality of life. Frequent exacerbations of bronchitis. (4) Age 60+ years; cor pulmonale develops. Continuous oxygen needed. Homebound, high health care utilization. Adapted from Fletcher C, Peto R: *BMJ* 1:1645, 1977.

of other studies have shown a familial aggregation for chronic bronchitis. It is likely that a number of genetically determined abnormal protective mechanisms against protease, oxidant, and toxic peptide injury are important in the pathogenesis of COPD. For example, polymorphisms of the α_1-antitrypsin gene not associated with deficiency of the protein and polymorphisms in the gene that controls glutathione S-transferases have also been linked to the development of COPD. Glutathione S-transferases are enzymes that play an important role in detoxifying various aromatic hydrocarbons found in tobacco smoke. Genetic polymorphisms of other pro- or antiinflammatory mediators that may alter cellular defenses against cigarette smoke include cytochrome P450, microsomal epoxide hydrolase, and tumor necrosis factor-α. Genotype–environment interactions are also likely to be essential contributors to the development of COPD.

NATURAL HISTORY OF COPD

The natural history of COPD (Fig. 42-1) includes a prolonged preclinical period of approximately 20 to 40 years. During this asymptomatic period there is deterioration of lung function in marked excess of the normal age-related decline. This was first shown in population studies on London working men and reported in the 1970s. It was discovered that the FEV$_1$ declines continuously and smoothly over an individual's life. Nonsmokers without respiratory disease can expect to lose 25 to 30 mL per year of lung function after age 35 years. The rate of decline appears to accelerate slightly with aging, but sudden large irreversible falls are very rare. Although nonsmokers lose FEV$_1$ slowly, they never develop significant airflow obstruction; this is true of most smokers, too. Susceptible smokers, on the

other hand, develop varying degrees of airflow obstruction as they often demonstrate a decline in lung function of 60 mL a year and more. This ultimately causes exertional dyspnea when the FEV$_1$ is between 40 percent and 59 percent of its predicted value and becomes disabling when the FEV$_1$ has declined by approximately 70 percent. Such an inexorable decline may lead to fatality. When the FEV$_1$ falls below 1 L, the 5-year mortality is approximately 50 percent. Smoking cessation in the susceptible smoker will not result in recovery of lost FEV$_1$, but it will slow the rate of decline to normal (Fig. 42-2). Smoking cessation in the patient with early changes of COPD at age 45 years can make the difference between a normal life span and premature death. A prospective multicentered longitudinal study of the effects of smoking cessation in patients identified with mild to moderate airflow obstruction has been conducted in this country and supported by the NHLBI. This Lung Health Study showed that smokers who stopped with the help of an aggressive smoking intervention program significantly reduced the decline in their FEV$_1$ over a 5-year study period when compared to those who continued to smoke. The inhaled bronchodilator ipratropium did not slow the decline of lung function when given over the same time period.

The slowly progressive course of COPD is often interrupted by a sudden change in symptoms and lung function. These acute respiratory illnesses or exacerbations are usually caused by viral or bacterial infections and are heralded by an increase in symptoms. Patients with milder stages of COPD will often develop one to two exacerbations per year; those with more severe disease are likely to have many more. The exacerbations cause a decrease in lung function for up to 90 days and in most are not thought to play a causal role in accelerating the development of chronic airflow obstruction.

Smoking and Lung Function Decline

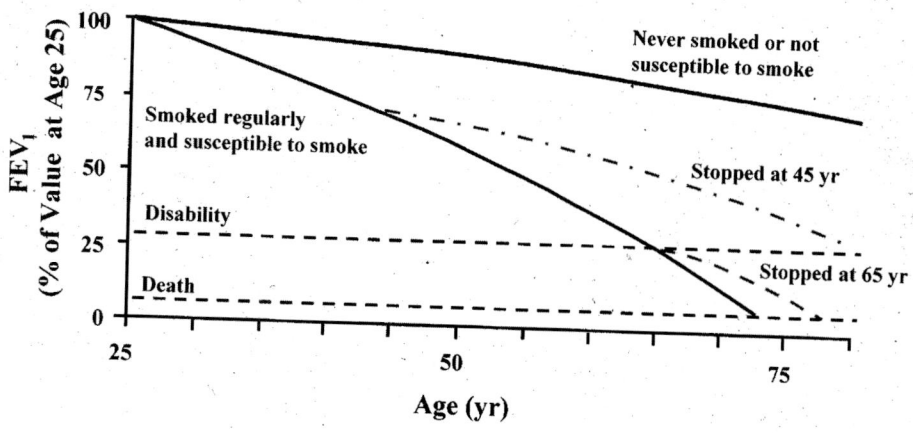

Figure 42-2   Natural history of COPD and effects of smoking cessation. Smoking cessation efforts are helpful at any age, even after age 65 years. Adapted from Fletcher C, Peto R: *BMJ* 1:1645, 1977.

PATHOLOGY AND PATHOPHYSIOLOGY

The pathologic changes in COPD are found in the large and small (less than 2 mm) airways and in the lung parenchyma, a summarized by Saetta et al. (Fig. 42-3). In advanced stages, there are also changes in the pulmonary circulation, heart, and respiratory muscles. Alveolar hypoxia causes medial hypertrophy of vascular smooth muscle with extension of the muscularis layer into distal vessels that do not ordinarily contain smooth muscle. Intimal hyperplasia also occurs in advanced stages. These latter changes are associated with the development of pulmonary hypertension and its consequences, right ventricular hypertrophy and dilatation. Loss of vascular bed also occurs with emphysema in association with the destructive

Mechanisms Underlying Airflow Limitation in COPD

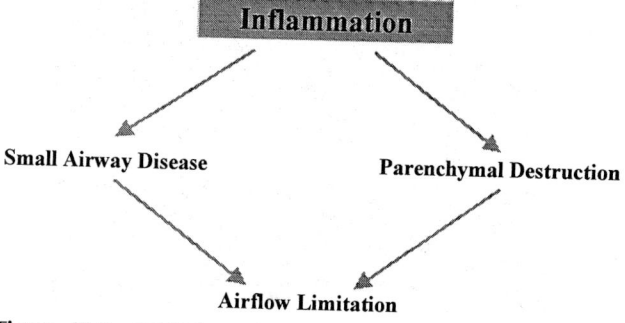

Figure 42-3   COPD is an inflammatory disease causing diffuse changes in small airways of the lung, chronic bronchitis, and diffuse parenchymal destruction (emphysema). Adapted from *Global Strategy for the Diagnosis, Management, and Prevention of Chronic Obstructive Lung Disease*. NHLBI/WHO Workshop Rep, NIH Publication No. 2701, April 2001.

alveolar processes (Fig. 42-4). In some patients with advanced COPD there is atrophy of diaphragmatic muscle.

Changes in the Airways of Smokers

Early structural changes have been described in otherwise healthy smokers even as young as 20 to 30 years old. It is believed that these changes are the precursor to the development of emphysema. The theory supporting this hypotheses has prevailed for more than 40 years. This proteinase–antiproteinase theory proposes that alveolar wall destruction occurs as a result of proteinase activity that digests extracellular matrix. There is considerable experimental animal and human studies to support this concept.

Bronchoalveolar lavage (BAL) studies on smokers have shown an increase in the number of neutrophils and macrophages in the lavage fluid. Macrophages likely play an important role in perpetuating the inflammatory process of COPD and are increased 5- to 10-fold in the BAL when the disease is present. They may release neutrophil chemotactic factors as well as proteolytic enzymes, such as matrix metalloproteinases (MMPs) that damage the epithelial barrier. Neutrophils are also thought to be important in causing the tissue damage of COPD. They release a number of mediators including proteinases such as neutrophil elastase and MMPs, oxidants such as the oxygen free radical H_2O_2, and toxic peptides such as defensins. Proteinases and free radicals can damage the epithelium as well as the basement membrane. The repair process that ensues includes the secretion of antiproteinases, such as secretory leukocyte proteinase inhibitor (SLPI), and tissue inhibitor of metalloproteinases by epithelial cells in order to regulate the proteolytic process. This process may be impaired in patients with COPD. In patients with more advanced airflow obstruction, T lymphocytes and neutrophils are found in the epithelium and T lymphocytes and macrophages are

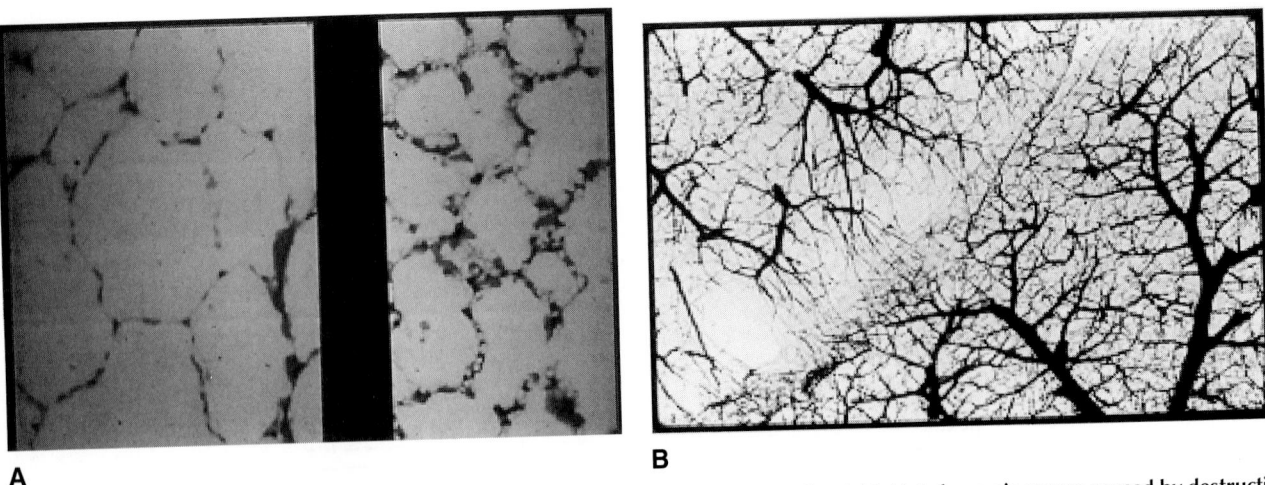

Figure 42-4 (*A*) A comparison of emphysematous lung on the left and normal lung on the right. Note large air spaces caused by destructive changes of intraalveolar septae. (*B*) Notice paucity of vasculature on the left in a patient with COPD when compared to a normal vasculature on the right in the postmortem angiogram.

found in the subepithelium of centriacinar airways where emphysema is most marked. While CD4+ lymphocytes are found in the airways of atopic asthmatics, the T lymphocytes of patients with cigarette-induced COPD are CD8+ cells. These cells are also thought to cause cell damage.

Eosinophilic inflammation of the airways is also a hallmark of asthma and not usually seen in chronic bronchitis, although there is an increase in eosinophilic basic proteins (eosinophil cationic proteins and eosinophil peroxidase) in induced sputum of persons with chronic bronchitis. This may indicate that eosinophils had been present in the sputum, but were destroyed, possibly by neutrophil elastase. The presence of eosinophils in the lung parenchyma and terminal air spaces of surgically resected lungs with emphysema would support this notion. During attacks of acute bronchitis, on the other hand, the number of tissue and sputum eosinophils is markedly increased.

Neutrophils, T lymphocytes, macrophages, and eosinophils are each important contributors to the intense inflammatory response that causes emphysema. Compared with normal lungs, those with severe emphysema contain approximately ten times more of each inflammatory cell. The fact that bronchial biopsies from former smokers show similar inflammatory changes as in the active smoker suggests that the inflammation that causes emphysema may persist in the airway once established. The mechanisms that perpetuate the presence of inflammatory cells long after the stimulus of cigarette smoke has been removed is not known. However, it is known that the peptides released following destruction of alveolar tissue are chemotactic for inflammatory cells and therefore could be responsible for a self-perpetuating process.

A number of extracellular signaling proteins called cytokines are important in the pathogenesis of COPD, as they are thought to mediate the tissue damage and repair induced by cigarette smoking. Increased quantities of certain proinflammatory cytokines, including interleukin (IL)-8, IL-1, IL-6, and tumor necrosis factor (TNF)-α, and the antiinflammatory cytokine IL-10 have been found in

the sputum of smokers and even further increased during an acute exacerbation. Exposure of bronchial epithelial cells to cigarette smoke causes a release of neutrophilic and monocytic chemotactic factors with IL-8 and granulocyte colony-stimulating factor (G-CSF) accounting for increased neutrophilic activity and monocyte chemotactic protein-1 (MCP-1) causing increased monocytic activity. Cytokines may also be involved with tissue remodeling in COPD. Increased expression of transforming growth factor-β (TGF-β) and epidermal growth factor (EGF) may activate fibroblastic proliferation in the airways of patients with COPD.

Other structural changes in the airways of smokers include mucus hyperplasia, bronchiolar edema and smooth muscle hypertrophy, and peribronchiolar fibrosis. These changes result in narrowing of the small airways (less than 2 mm). Recent studies suggest that the inflammatory cellular infiltrate, fibrosis, and muscle in the airway wall show a progressive worsening of pathologic changes when nonsmokers, smokers with mild COPD, and smokers with more severe disease are compared. There is also a progression of the number of airways <400 μm in diameter as the disease worsens. Because the total cross-sectional area of these small airways is so much larger than the cross-sectional area of the central conducting airways (and hence they contribute so little to total airway resistance), dyspnea and changes in the FEV$_1$ are usually absent until the disease is quite advanced. This zone of the lungs is often referred to as the "silent zone," because these pathologic abnormalities usually go undetected by symptom assessment and routine spirometry. As the inflammation and peribronchiolar fibrosis progress, pulmonary functional abnormalities associated with the small airways become evident. In addition to the structural abnormalities seen in the small airways, there is also a loss of alveolar attachments to the airway perimeter. This impairs elastic recoil and favors increased tortuosity and early closure of the small airways during expiration. Several tests, such as frequency dependence of compliance, nitrogen slope of the alveolar plateau, the closing volume, and flow measurements at low lung volume are thought to reflect small airway narrowing. These pathophysiologic abnormalities in airways of 2 mm and less diameter have been referred to as "small-airway disease." Small-airway disease has been described as a distinct clinical entity. It is more important instead to think of the early inflammatory changes in the small airways as the first stage in a protracted process that eventually leads to persistent airflow obstruction and a decrease in the FEV_1.

Pathology of Chronic Bronchitis

The presence of a gel-like mucous in the airways of healthy people is essential for normal mucociliary clearance. This is swallowed and rarely noticed. Smokers with chronic bronchitis produce larger amounts of sputum each day, averaging about 20 to 30 mL per day, and even as high as 100 mL per day. This occurs as a result of an increase in the size and number of the submucosal glands and an increase in the number of goblet cells on the surface epithelium. Mucous gland enlargement and hyperplasia of the goblet cells are, therefore, the hallmark of chronic bronchitis. Goblet cells are normally absent in the small airways, and their presence there (often referred to as mucous metaplasia) is important to the development of COPD. In the larger airways in chronic bronchitis there is a reduction in serous acini of the submucosal glands. This depresses local defenses to bacterial adherence since these glands are known to produce deterrents such as lactoferrin, antiproteases, and lysozyme. Other epithelial alterations seen in chronic bronchitis are a decrease in the number and length of the cilia and squamous metaplasia. The mucociliary abnormalities of chronic bronchitis cause a continuous sheet or blanket of mucous lining the airways instead of discrete deposits of mucous seen on normal airways. Pooling of secretions may also occur. This provides additional cause for bacterial growth, which in turn causes a release of toxins that are further damaging to the cilia and epithelial cells. Bacterial exoproducts are known to stimulate mucous production, slow ciliary beating, impair immune effector cell function, and destroy local immunoglobulins. This cycle is especially apparent in current as opposed to former smokers.

The Pathology of Emphysema

Emphysema is a destructive process that occurs in the gas-exchanging airspaces, the respiratory bronchioles, alveolar ducts, and alveoli. It results in perforations (fenestrae), obliteration of airspace walls, and coalescence of small distinct air spaces into much larger ones. There is permanent enlargement of the gas-exchanging units of the lungs (acini) (see Fig. 42-4A). These pathologic changes cause loss of elastic recoil of the lungs and abnormal gas exchange. Recent studies have shown good correlation between physiologic measurements of lung elastic recoil and diffusing capacity and microscopic measures of airspace wall per unit of alveolar volume and alveolar surface area.

Two morphologic forms of emphysema have been described (Table 42-2). It should be recognized that most

Table 42-2   Pathologic Types of Emphysema

Centriacinar (centrilobular)	Focal destruction of respiratory bronchioles; surrounded by normal lung parenchyma More severe in upper lobes Type most frequently associated with smoking
Panacinar (panlobular)	Uniform destruction of all airspaces beyond the respiratory bronchioles More lower lobe distribution Occurs in smokers earlier in life Associated with α_1-antitrypsin deficiency

smoking-related emphysema has features of both, and the clinical relevance of the difference is limited. Table 42-3 shows the mechanisms by which emphysema and chronic bronchitis cause airflow obstruction.

Pathophysiology

The physiologic hallmark of COPD is the limitation of expiratory flow with relative preservation of inspiratory flow. Reductions in the FEV_1 and FEV_1/FVC (forced vital capacity) percent are characteristic, while the maximal inspiratory flow rate is normal or near normal (Fig. 42-5). The degree of reversibility in COPD is seldom as brisk as it is in asthma. Differences in the degree of reversibility in COPD and asthma may be explained by the fact that in the latter disease, many inflammatory mediators have been implicated, including potent bronchoconstrictors such as histamine, kinins, and prostaglandins. In contrast, there are few bronchoconstrictor mediators released in COPD.

Table 42-3   Mechanisms of Airflow Obstruction in COPD

Emphysema
  Loss of elastic recoil

  1. Less-driving pressure from alveoli to proximal airways
  2. As patency in smaller airways depends on elastic recoil, intraluminal pressure is reduced and airways collapse during forced expiration

Chronic bronchitis
  Airway inflammation and hypersecretion of mucous

  1. Peribronchiolar fibrosis results in narrowing of peripheral airways, loss of alveolar attachments, and loss of elastic recoil
  2. Intraluminal mucous may contribute to airflow obstruction

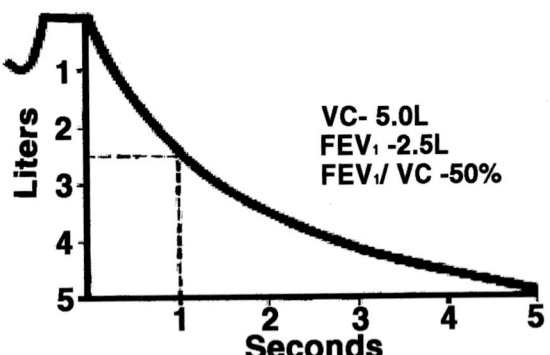

Figure 42-5 A forced vital capacity maneuver is depicted on this spirogram. There is a reduction of the FEV_1 and FEV_1 over FVC expressed as a percent. This is a typical spirogram of moderately advanced COPD.

One important inflammatory mediator found in the sputum of patients with COPD is leukotriene B_4 (LTB_4). It is a potent chemoattractant for neutrophils. The term "partial reversibility" has been used in COPD, although this term has not been adequately defined. Reversibility in COPD patients in response to bronchodilator drugs, can be acute, mainly as a consequence of release of cholinergic tone. It also may occur in response to oral or inhaled corticosteroids, presumably as a result of decreased inflammation. Studies show that the majority of COPD patients will have a small but significant degree of reversibility of airflow obstruction (defined as >12 percent and at least 200 mL improvement in the FEV_1). Some longitudinal studies suggest

that increased reversibility is associated with a higher risk of dying from COPD; however, other studies suggest that the presence of reversibility coupled with close clinical treatment and follow up is associated with better survival rates.

Early in the course of COPD the expiratory flow-volume curve shows a scooped out lower part of the expiratory limb as a result of abnormal flow at low lung volume. In later stages, there is decreased expiratory flow at all lung volumes (Fig. 42-6). Nonuniform ventilation of the lungs is seen even in the earlier stages of COPD and can be demonstrated with the N2 washout test. The multiple inert gas test has been used to quantify the ventilation–perfusion mismatch in the lungs of COPD patients and has also shown these abnormalities in early stages of COPD. The predominant abnormalities detected by this test are low ventilation–perfusion regions. This type of mismatch causes arterial hypoxemia, which progresses as the airflow obstruction deteriorates. There is little right-to-left shunting in COPD. Hypercapnia is also a consequence of severe end-stage COPD. The arterial partial pressure of carbon dioxide (P_{CO2}) usually does not become elevated until the FEV_1 becomes quite reduced, usually below 1 L. Lung and thoracic wall hyperinflation are another consequence of the loss of elastic recoil. This favors expiratory flow. As lung volume increases, elastic recoil pressure also increases and this causes the airways to enlarge. This reduces the airway resistance. The hyperinflation may have a deleterious effect, too. As the chest wall volume expands, the thoracic cage and diaphragm are put at a mechanical disadvantage. This increases the work of breathing and contributes to the sensation of dyspnea.

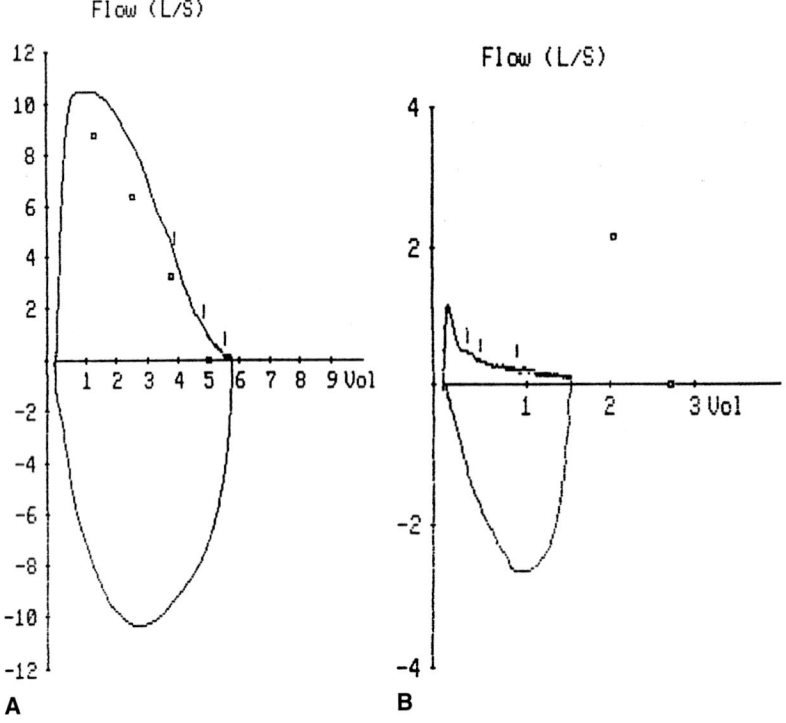

Figure 42-6 Flow volume loop of COPD is compared with a normal patient (*A*). Notice the markedly diminished flow at all lung volumes in the patient with COPD (*B*).

COPD–CLINICAL ASPECTS

Symptoms of COPD

The symptoms that are associated with COPD are usually not present until the patient has been smoking a pack of cigarettes a day for at least 20 years. The patient usually presents in the fifth decade with a chronic cough often worsened after a viral respiratory infection. The second major symptom, dyspnea, usually does not present until the sixth or seventh decade. Over the last two decades, as a result of an intense antismoking campaign, the rate of smoking in the United States has been reduced from approximately one-third of the adult population to its current level of approximately 22 percent. Many susceptible smokers who stopped smoking in midlife delay the onset of COPD symptoms until late in life. It is not unusual to see a patient with COPD present for the first time with symptoms at age 75 years and beyond.

The Physical Exam and Laboratory Tests

The signs of COPD are well known: slow and prolonged expiration, wheezing, chest wall hyperinflation, limited diaphragmatic motion on auscultation, distant breath sounds and heart sounds, and often coarse early inspiratory crackles. The accessory muscles of respiration may be in use and the patient may be using pursed-lip breathing. Signs of cor pulmonale include pedal edema, a tender congested liver, and neck vein distension. The genesis of cor pulmonale in COPD is pulmonary artery vasoconstriction that is caused by alveolar hypoxia. This causes pulmonary hypertension and eventually right heart strain and failure. This sequence usually occurs with severe degrees of arterial hypoxemia and an arterial partial pressure of oxygen (PO_2) below 55 mmHg. Cyanosis may be present, and asterixis, which is associated with severe hypercapnia, may also be evident. The roentgenographic signs of COPD include a low, flat diaphragm, an increased retrosternal airspace, and a teardrop-shaped heart (Fig. 42-7). Pruning of the pulmonary arterial vessels and bullae (Fig. 42-8) are seen in emphysema. The high-resolution computerized tomography (CT) scan has a much better sensitivity and specificity but is not recommended for routine use. It may be helpful when surgery for large bullae is contemplated.

Pulmonary function studies are important for the diagnosis and staging of COPD. Because the best correlate with morbidity and mortality is the FEV_1, proposals for staging have used this test. The American Thoracic Society standards suggest a severity scoring on the basis of the severity of airflow obstruction: stage I is an FEV_1 of 50 percent or greater; stage II is an FEV_1 of 35 to 49 percent predicted; and stage III is an FEV_1 of less than 35 percent predicted. In general, patients with stage I disease have little impairment in their quality of life. Patients with stage II COPD have a significant impairment in the quality of their lives, and this results in a large per capita health care cost. Patients with stage III disease are profoundly impaired, are often hospitalized with severe exacerbations of disease, and, therefore, are high users of health care resources. A new severity scoring system has been introduced by the GOLD guidelines (Table 42-4). It begins staging with an "at-risk" group, stage 0, to emphasize the point that patients with risk factors (cigarette smoking, occupations) who have the symptoms of cough and sputum need to be counseled about COPD even though their screening spirometry is normal. Other stages are modifications of the American Thoracic Society criteria.

COPD MANAGEMENT

Once the diagnosis of COPD is established, pulmonary function testing can be helpful by staging the disease. Pharmacologic intervention is offered according to disease severity and the patient's tolerance for specific drugs. This may be accomplished by improving bronchodilatation, decreasing airway inflammation, and improving mucociliary transport. Because COPD is irreversible in some, and only partially reversible in others, disease management of daily symptoms and other impacts on quality of life are most essential. The patient who still smokes should be encouraged to quit. Preventive therapy with a pneumococcal vaccine and a yearly influenza vaccine is recommended. Vaccination with the flu shot has been shown to result in 52 percent fewer hospitalizations for pneumonia and influenza in patients with COPD. Vaccinated patients also have fewer outpatient visits for respiratory symptoms. The international GOLD Guidelines offer a set of goals that are most useful to follow (Table 42-5).

Smoking Cessation

Cigarette smoking compromises airway function by damaging airway epithelial cells, increasing mucous viscosity and slowing mucociliary clearance. There is a greater bacterial adherence to oropharyngeal epithelial cells in smokers, as compared to nonsmokers. Smokers are prone to attacks of acute bronchitis. As a result, they show increased rates of acute exacerbations, emergency department visits, work absences, and frequency of medication use. They also show greater decline in lung function, worsening of respiratory symptoms, and lower quality-of-life scores than does a comparable group of nonsmoking patients. What is encouraging, and should be mentioned to every elderly smoking patient with COPD, is that smoking cessation can be as effective in stopping the rapid decline in lung function after the age of 65 years as it is in younger smokers (see Fig. 42-2). Unfortunately, the presence of respiratory illness such as COPD in itself does not appear to be a motivator for smoking cessation. However, physician-delivered smoking cessation interventions can significantly increase smoking abstinence rates. An empathetic, nonconfrontational interaction that maximizes patient participation is most effective. The essential elements of a smoking cessation program should include (1) physician intervention (set a quit date) and appropriate follow-up; (2) group smoking cessation programs; and (3) pharmacologic therapy with nicotine replacement, which is needed in highly dependent smokers, as detected by Anthonisen et al. Such smokers can be identified as those who smoke a pack a day or more,

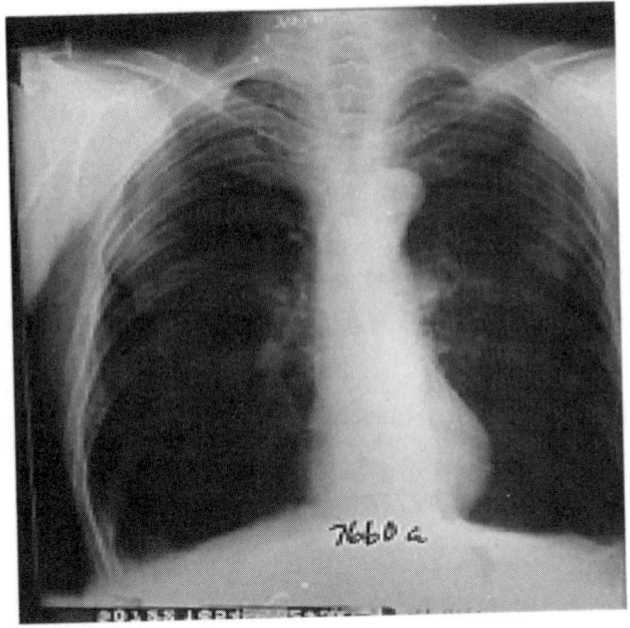

A

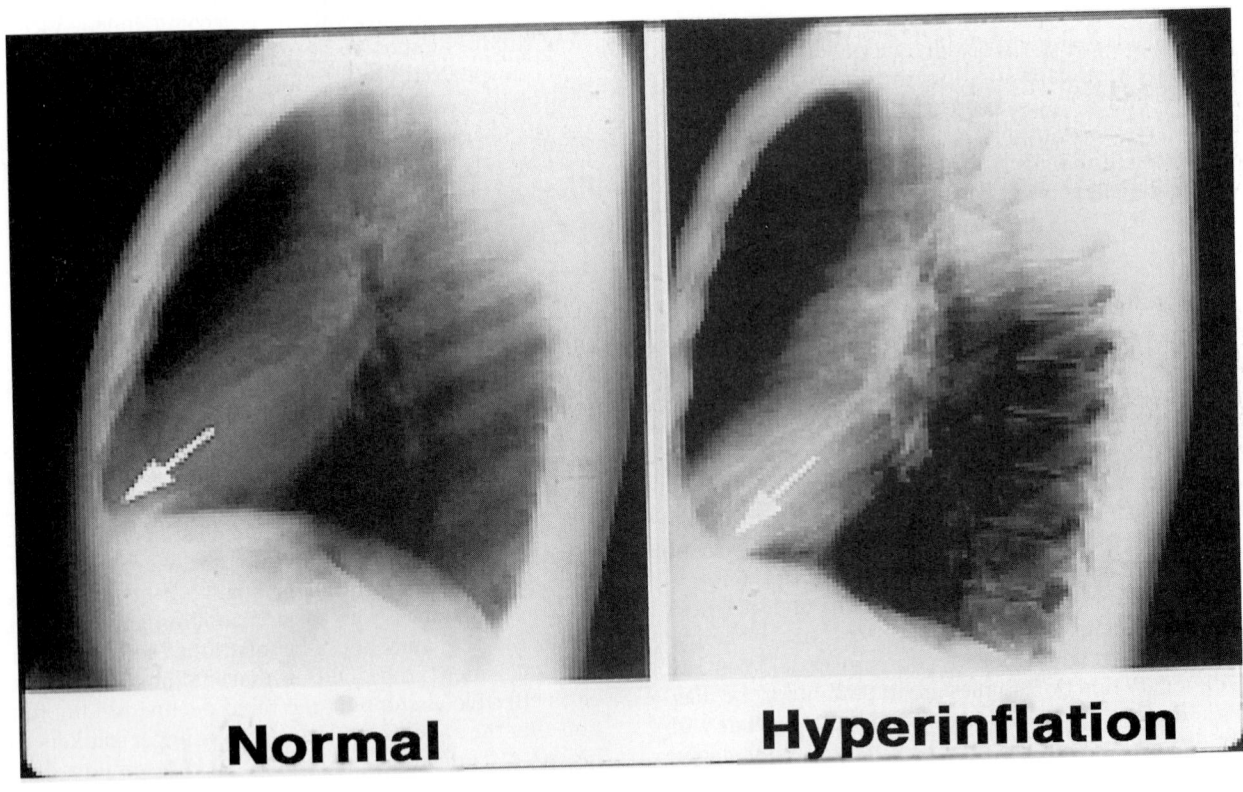

B

Figure 42-7   (*A*) This roentgenogram of a patient with COPD shows a flattened diaphragm and a paucity of lung markings, particularly at the lung bases. Notice the teardrop-shaped heart typical of COPD patients with hyperinflation. Notice the presence of infracardiac air, another abnormal finding. (*B*) On the right is a patient with COPD. The hyperinflation has flattened the diaphragms. This is compared to the normal configuration of the diaphragms at full inspiration on the left.

require their first cigarette within 30 minutes of arising in the morning, and find it difficult refraining from smoking in places where it is forbidden. Therapy with the antidepressant bupropion hydrochloride is also effective, and when used with nicotine replacement can yield quit rates that approach 35 percent. The US Lung Health Study, reported by Anderson et al., showed that despite intensive antismoking efforts, middle-aged smokers with COPD are not likely to quit. Only 22 percent were sustained quitters after a 5-year follow-up. Unfortunately, smoking cessation efforts in the elderly population are frequently even more problematic. Often there have been numerous unsuccessful attempts to

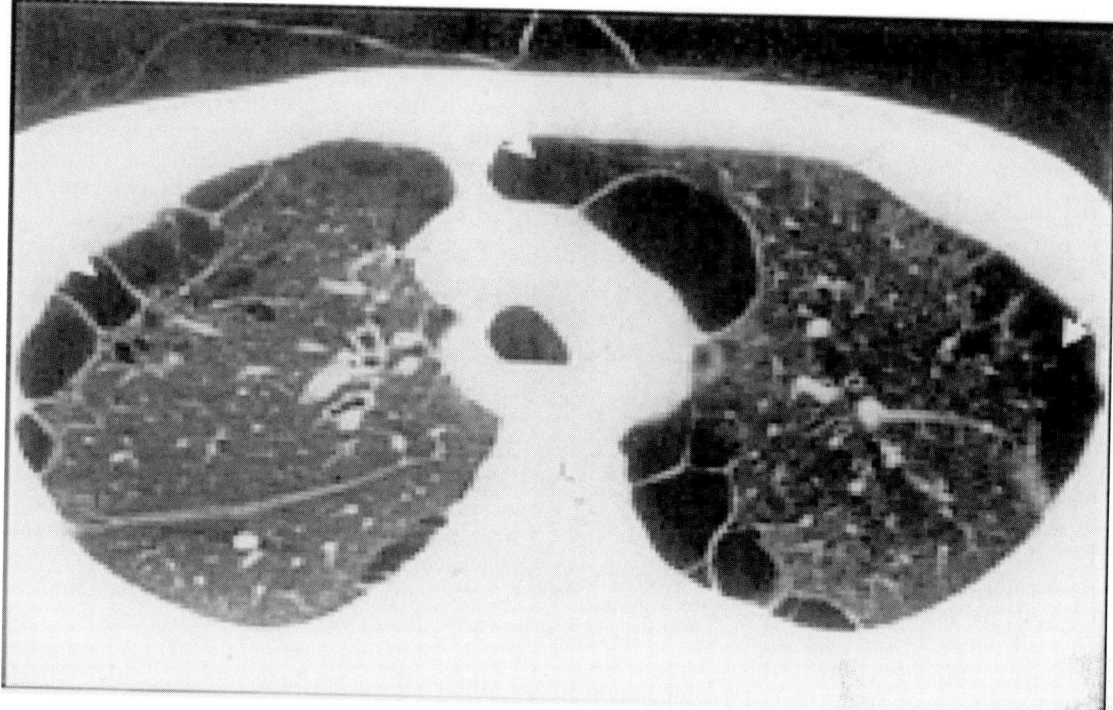

Figure 42-8   A CT scan showing multiple bullas lesions.

quit smoking in the past. This may lead to a defeatist attitude. The elderly patient must be reminded that the average smoker who successfully quits has done so after five to six attempts. The clinician's responsibility is to remember that tobacco addiction is a chronic disease and treatment should be offered at every visit.

Pharmacologic Therapy

Pharmacologic therapy is used to control distressing symptoms, especially poor exercise tolerance, improve overall quality of life, including both physical and emotional distresses, and prevent and control exacerbations of the disease. Unfortunately, no therapy has proven useful in preventing the decline of lung function that occurs as the disease progresses. General pharmacologic therapy is given in a step-like manner in a similar approach as to asthma management. Unlike asthma, where stepdown therapy is often possible, therapies, once initiated, are given for the duration of the illness unless side effects arise. Treatment usually begins with the use of a short-acting β-agonist bronchodilator for instances where sudden shortness of breath occurs. Rapid relief usually occurs within minutes and this can be repeated several times a day. When symptoms become more persistent and begin to interfere with activities of daily living, chronic, longer-acting medications are given.

β-Agonist Therapy

These agents act by relaxing airway smooth muscle by a direct action on the β-adrenergic receptors on the cell surface.

While oral agents are available, their side effect profile makes them less desirable than the inhaled agents. The short-acting β agonists achieve variable degrees of bronchodilatation with a rapid onset of action of a few minutes and a duration of action of 4 to 6 hours. They improve

Table 42-4   GOLD Guidelines: Classification of Severity of COPD

Stage	Characteristics
0: At risk	• Normal spirometry • Chronic symptoms (cough, sputum production)
I: Mild COPD	• FEV_1/FVC <70% • FEV_1 ≥80% predicted • With or without chronic symptoms (cough, sputum production)
II: Moderate COPD	• FEV_1/FVC <70% • 30% ≤FEV_1 <80% predicted (IIA: 50% ≤ FEV_1 <80% predicted; IIB: 30% ≤ FEV_1 <50% predicted) • With or without chronic symptoms (cough, sputum production, dyspnea)
III: Severe COPD	• FEV_1/FVC <70% • FEV_1 <30% predicted or FEV_1 <50% predicted plus respiratory failure or clinical signs of right-heart failure

Table 42-5 GOLD Guidelines: Goals of Effective COPD Management

Prevent Disease Progression

Relieve Symptoms

Improve Exercise Tolerance

Improve Health Status

Prevent and Treat Complications

Prevent and Treat Exacerbations

Reduce Mortality

SOURCE: Global Strategy for the Diagnosis, Management, and Prevention of Chronic Obstructive Lung Disease. NHLBI/WHO Workshop Report, NIH Publication No. 2701. Bethesda, MD, April 2001.

shortness of breath, often help with a distressing cough, and in most patients, improve exercise capacity. Inhaled agents are usually prescribed as a metered dose inhaler (MDI) or with a compressor-driven nebulizer. Despite the minimal systemic absorption seen with these agents, slight tachycardia may be observed. This is presumably a result of vasodilatation, which results from the stimulation of β_2 receptors in vascular smooth muscle. Tremor may also occur and is especially troublesome in the geriatric patient. It is thought to be caused by stimulation of β_2 receptors in skeletal muscle. In general, however, when given three or four times a day, β agonists are safe and effective in all age groups. Higher doses may cause hypokalemia, especially when the patient is taking a diuretic. Cardiac arrhythmias may occur in patients with ischemic heart disease, especially when the coronary disease is unstable. While these agents are not contraindicated in every such patient, careful monitoring is advisable while a thoughtful risk benefit assessment is made.

Long-acting β_2 agonists are helpful for long-term maintenance therapy. Two agents useful in this category are salmeterol and formoterol. Both have a duration of action of 12 hours and therefore improve patient compliance because of twice-a-day dosing. There is also no evidence of tachyphylaxis with these agents. They are capable of improving exercise intolerance, improving quality-of-life measures, and prolonging the time until the next COPD exacerbation. While there is evidence that β receptor function diminishes with age, the short- and long-acting β agonists should be used because of their proven track record.

Anticholinergic Therapy

These agents also act by causing bronchodilatation and are capable of rapidly relieving symptoms. They act by blocking acetylcholine's effect on the M3 receptor. Ipratropium bromide, a commonly used anticholinergic, has a duration of action of 4 to 6 hours and also shows no tachyphylaxis. Its onset of action of 30 minutes is somewhat shorter than those in the β agonist group, and this has made a combination MDI of albuterol, a short-acting β agonist, and the anticholinergic ipratropium bromide very popular.

As these agents are poorly absorbed, the side effects are generally mild. Occasionally, patients complain of a dry mouth or metallic taste. Worsening prostatic symptoms have been reported, but a causal relationship has not been proven with these agents. Mucociliary clearance is not affected, and infection rates are not increased. Rare cases of acute glaucoma have been reported with the use of wet nebulizer solutions caused by direct exposure of the eyes. This can easily be avoided with proper inhalation techniques.

Methylxanthines

Theophylline is the most widely used drug in this class. It is given as a sustained-release preparation and has the advantage of being able to be given once a day. Small improvements in lung function are seen with chronic use and have been associated with improvement in symptoms and exercise capacity in COPD. Its use has diminished over the past decade because of safety concerns, especially in the elderly population. While there is in general a steady decline in drug metabolism from early to late adulthood, theophylline clearance does not appear to be sufficiently altered in the elderly to recommend reducing the dose. The narrow therapeutic range of theophylline, frequency of concomitant illnesses that alter theophylline kinetics, and many drug interactions that affect the clearance of theophylline, make it important to closely monitor the blood theophylline level in older patients. The clinical manifestations of theophylline toxicity have been correlated with blood levels of the drug. With high serum concentrations (>30 μg/mL), life-threatening events may occur. They include seizures and cardiac arrhythmias such as atrial fibrillation, supraventricular tachycardia, ventricular ectopy and ventricular tachycardia. The most common cause for theophylline toxicity is a self-administered increase in medication. There is a stepwise increase in the frequency of life-threatening events caused by theophylline toxicity with advancing age. At comparable theophylline blood levels, patients older than age 75 years have a 16-fold greater risk of life-threatening events or death than do patients younger than age 25 years. The risk of theophylline toxicity can be minimized with careful patient monitoring, including checking blood levels, and patient education. A range of 8 to 15 μg/mL is generally considered therapeutic and gives a margin of error that helps avoid toxicity.

Corticosteroids

Systemic Corticosteroids

The role of systemic steroids in the management of COPD is controversial. In general, they are far less effective in COPD than in asthma, and the side effects are considerable, especially in the elderly population. Complications include cataracts, osteoporosis, secondary infection, diabetes, skin damage, and steroid myopathy, which contributes to respiratory muscle weakness, poor exercise tolerance, and respiratory failure.

In general, long-term treatment with oral corticosteroids is not recommended for COPD unless there is a strong underlying asthmatic component to the disease. Some have advocated giving a short course (2 weeks) of oral corticosteroids to identify which patients will respond to long-term inhaled corticosteroids. There is growing evidence that that such a short-term response is not an effective predictor. Treatment with intravenous or oral corticosteroids is useful for the acute exacerbation of COPD. Treatment of hospitalized patients with high doses has resulted in fewer treatment failures and shorter hospital stays. Two weeks of therapy is a sufficient time; longer courses have resulted in excessive side effects.

Inhaled Corticosteroids

Most studies show minimal effects on lung function. However, there is evidence that these agents may improve exercise capacity and reduce the severity and frequency of COPD exacerbations. Treatment with inhaled corticosteroids therefore has been used for patients with moderate to advanced COPD. As bone mineral loss is a serious problem in this age group, a careful vigilance with bone density studies is warranted.

Inhalation Techniques

The inhaled route of therapy for COPD is preferred over all therapy because it provides quicker action, fewer side effects, and greater bronchodilatation with smaller doses of medication. MDIs are the most commonly used methods for delivery of bronchodilators and corticosteroids. The great majority of the medication delivered by MDIs is deposited in the oropharynx, with only approximately 10 percent of the dose delivered to the lungs. Oropharyngeal deposition causes greater systemic absorption, more local irritation, and for corticosteroids, more likelihood of oropharyngeal candidiasis. The great majority of elderly patients are unable to properly use the MDI, even after proper instruction. Inadequate timing of actuation and inhalation is the most frequent error made. Impaired mental function, weakened or deformed hands, and motor or musculoskeletal diseases are other reasons for inadequate MDI use. There are several solutions to this problem. One may deliver short-acting β agonists, ipratropium, and the inhaled corticosteroid budesonide as aerosolized solutions by pressurized hand-held nebulizers. Alternatively, there is a breath-actuated pressurized MDI that obviates the need to synchronize activation with inhalation. The use of spacer devices fitted to the mouthpiece of the MDI overcome most of the drawbacks of MDI therapy. Spacers decrease oropharyngeal deposition, increase intrapulmonary deposition, improve the pulmonary function of asthmatics that use the conventional MDI inappropriately, and reduce the incidence of oropharyngeal candidiasis. Because drug deposition into the lungs with spacers is greater, the spacers also have the advantage of reducing the number of inhalations of drug needed and, therefore, the cost of drug therapy. Their use in the elderly patient is highly desirable. Lastly, newer dry-powder delivery devices that deliver inhaled corticosteroids and long-acting β agonists provide simple, easy-to-use preparations that do not require coordination or muscle strength.

Mucolytic Agents

These agents have been evaluated as chronic maintenance therapy for COPD and the results are mixed. Some patients with COPD, especially those with viscous sputum, appear to notice improvement. However, overall the benefits are small. Their widespread use is not recommended.

Randomized controlled trials suggest that they are ineffective at shortening the course or improving outcomes of patients with acute exacerbations of COPD.

Oxygen Therapy

Several controlled studies have been done regarding the efficacy of long-term oxygen. These have been summarized by Crockett et al. Long-term oxygen increases the survival time and quality of life of those with advanced COPD and significant arterial hypoxemia. The beneficial effect is related to the duration of oxygen use. For example, patients who receive oxygen for 19 hours or more a day are likely to survive longer than those who use it 12 or 15 hours a day. Patients who use chronic oxygen therapy are likely to have a significant fall in their pulmonary artery pressures and an increase in cardiac output. Table 42-6 provides recommendations for long-term oxygen use in COPD. Long term oxygen therapy does not improve survival in patients with moderate hypoxemia (PaO_2 56 to 65 mmHg) or in patients with nocturnal hypoxemia alone. While oxygen has many beneficial effects in the patient with advanced COPD, the use of uncontrolled oxygen therapy in patients with hypercarbic respiratory failure can be disastrous. A high level of alveolar oxygen can worsen hypercarbia and result in worsening respiratory acidosis and coma. The cautious use of low-flow controlled oxygen and careful blood gas monitoring can often avoid this complication.

Pulmonary Rehabilitation

Pulmonary rehabilitation is a multidisciplinary program for patients with moderate to advanced COPD, especially those who have suffered deconditioning, significant weight loss, depression, and social isolation. These programs attempt to return the patient to the highest functional capacity

Table 42-6 Criteria for Long-Term Oxygen Therapy

- Continuous oxygen therapy $\geq 18/24$ hours:
- PaO_2 ≤ 55 mm Hg
- PaO_2: 56–60 mm Hg
  - Cor pulmonale
  - Pulmonary hypertension
    - Polycythemia (hematocrit >55%)

possible with attention to improving lean body mass, increasing exercise tolerance, and improving dyspnea, because these three factors have each been linked to mortality. The goals of a rehabilitation program are to improve exercise capacity, return the patient to more normal activities of daily living, and improve motivation, psychological well being, and overall quality of life. With the use of lower-extremity exercise training and upper-extremity strength and endurance training, studies prove that pulmonary rehabilitation improves dyspnea and quality-of-life scores and reduces the number of hospitalizations and days spent in the hospital. Some studies also suggest a positive effect on survival.

Weight Loss and Malnutrition

Malnutrition occurs in one-quarter to one-third of patients with moderate to severe COPD and is an independent risk factor for mortality. Both fat mass and fat-free mass are depleted; the latter is caused by depressed protein synthesis. It is believed that weight loss, particularly skeletal muscle mass loss, is associated with a systemic inflammatory response in malnourished patients with COPD, as the proinflammatory cytokines IL-6 and TNF-α are elevated. Recent studies show that leptin, an adipocyte-derived hormone involved in the control of body weight, is decreased in patients with COPD. Serum leptin levels have been correlated with TNF-α levels, thus creating a link between nutritional status and systemic inflammation in COPD. Resting energy expenditure is elevated and contributes to the negative energy balance. Nutritional supplements alone do not reverse the loss; results with anabolic steroids, growth hormone, and the progestational agent megestrol acetate show some effect on appetite and body weight. However, improved exercise tolerance and respiratory muscle function does not always follow, and side effects are often limiting.

Noninvasive Positive Pressure Ventilation

The chronic nocturnal use of noninvasive ventilation for COPD is controversial. There are theoretical advantages. Resting chronically fatigued muscles at night might improve daytime function. COPD patients have a high prevalence of sleep apnea and hypoxemia and hypercarbia at night. They have less rapid eye-movement (REM) sleep and shorter sleep times than do normals. Noninvasive ventilation might be useful for these conditions, too. Trials have revealed conflicting conclusions; patients without CO_2 retention show little gain; patients with severe CO_2 retention, especially those that have severe nocturnal O_2 desaturation, appear to respond more favorably.

Surgery for COPD

Lung volume reduction surgery (LVRS) has emerged as a treatment for far advanced COPD caused by emphysema. It involves resection of functionless areas of emphysematous lung in order to improve lung elastic recoil and lung and chest wall hyperinflation.

Overall mortality with the procedure ranges between 0 and 6 percent within 30 days of surgery and between 0 and 8 percent at 6 months, although in patients with very severe degrees of airflow obstruction and/or hypercarbia the rates are much higher. The range of FEV_1 improvement pre- and postsurgery is approximately 250 to 350 mL and dyspnea scores and distance walked on the 6-minute walk test show improvement. Often patients no longer require oxygen following surgery. It is a modality that is being used in specialized centers.

Resection of large bullae is occasionally necessary. The best results occur when the bullae occupy more than one-third of the hemithorax. Lung transplantation can be life-saving in advanced cases, but is not offered to those of advanced age.

THE ACUTE EXACERBATION OF COPD

Unfortunately, many definitions of the acute exacerbation or "flare" of COPD exist and many authors employ substantially different criteria. The most widely quoted criteria have been referred to as "the Winnipeg criteria," which have also included a staging proposal (Table 42-7). Patients with COPD exacerbation have three changes in their clinical condition: worsening of dyspnea, an increase in sputum volume, and sputum purulence. Patients with type I exacerbations have all of the above symptoms. Patients with type II exacerbations have two of the three symptoms. Type III exacerbations are characterized by at least one of these symptoms and also one of the following clinical criteria: upper respiratory infection in the past 5 days, fever without other apparent cause, increased wheezing, increased cough, and increased respiratory rate or heart rate by 20 percent above baseline. Before the onset of an exacerbation of COPD there is usually a prodromal period of up to 7 days when symptoms of increased dyspnea, cough, sore throat, and the common cold occur. This is not accompanied by a drop in lung function. On the day of the exacerbation, there is a small but significant drop in lung function, including peak flow rates, FEV_1, and FVC. Peak flow rate recovery to baseline values is complete in

Table 42-7   Acute Exacerbation of COPD: The "Winnipeg" Criteria

Severity scale for COPD exacerbation
Three clinical findings:

   (1) worsening dyspnea
   (2) increased sputum volume
   (3) increased viscosity

Type 1 severe exacerbation: all three symptoms
Type 2 moderate exacerbation: two symptoms
Type 3 mild exacerbation: one symptom plus fever/
   upper respiratory symptoms

Causative Agents
in COPD Exacerbations

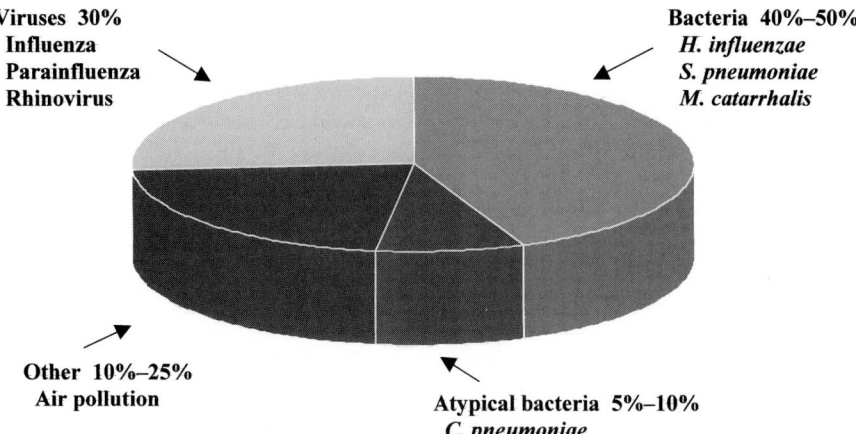

Viruses 30%
Influenza
Parainfluenza
Rhinovirus

Bacteria 40%–50%
H. influenzae
S. pneumoniae
M. catarrhalis

Other 10%–25%
Air pollution

Atypical bacteria 5%–10%
C. pneumoniae

Figure 42-9   The causative agents of COPD include viruses, bacteria, and atypical bacteria such as *Chlamydia pneumoniae*.

75 percent of patients by 1 month. Approximately 7 percent of patients with a COPD exacerbation do not return their peak flow rates to baseline by 3 months. This suggests that following some exacerbations of COPD there is a permanent loss of lung function. If this were to occur repeatedly, it could lead to an accelerated decline in FEV_1 over years.

The most frequent cause of an acute exacerbation of COPD is thought to be respiratory infection (Fig. 42-9). Sputum cultures in patients with mild to moderately severe COPD often show nonpathogenic bacteria (gram-negative and gram-positive bacteria such as *Streptococcus viridans, Neisseria* spp., or *Corynebacterium* spp.). Pathogenic bacteria include *Haemophilus influenzae* (22 percent), *Pseudomonas aeruginosa* (15 percent), *Streptococcus pneumoniae* (10 percent), and *Moraxella catarrhalis* (9 percent). Sputum samples may have limited validity considering the possible contamination from oropharyngeal secretions. Techniques that potentially preclude contamination include transtracheal aspirates, bronchoalveolar lavage, and protected brush sampling during bronchoscopy. Recent studies using these techniques show that patients requiring hospitalization, as compared to those treated as outpatients for an exacerbation of COPD and those outpatients with the most severe degree of airflow obstruction, are more likely to harbor gram-negative enteric organisms. The role of viral infection has been recently revisited using sophisticated methods such as polymerase chain reaction (PCR) viral detection, as well as more standard methods, such as serologic testing and culture. Viruses may be detected in nearly 40 percent of COPD exacerbations using these techniques. These include rhinovirus, respiratory syncytial virus, coronavirus, influenza, and parainfluenza. Evidence for *Mycoplasma* infection has been found in up to one-third of the acute exacerbations of chronic bronchitis in some studies, but in most senses *Mycoplasma* and *Chlamydia pneumoniae* are seen in less than 10 percent of cases. A COPD exacerbation associated with a virus is likely to produce more severe symptoms and the exacerbation is likely to last longer

(13 days). There is also more laboratory evidence of an acute phase response (e.g., elevated levels of IL-6 and fibrinogen) with an associated viral infection. Clearly, environmental factors are also important. Hospital admissions for COPD appear to be high when air pollution levels in the ambient environment are high. Small increases in SO_2 and airborne particles have been shown to cause increases in emergency room visits for COPD during winter and summer seasons by 6 percent and 9 percent, respectively. Whatever the cause of an acute exacerbation of COPD, it is clear that bronchial inflammation is enhanced during this event. Increased levels of myeloperoxidase have been found in the sputum indicating neutrophilic activity, and high levels of IL-8 and LTB_4, well-known neutrophil chemoattractants, are also seen. During recovery, levels of sputum chemoattractants and inflammatory markers rapidly fall.

Diagnostic and Therapeutic Approaches

Often patients present to a local emergency room or hospital with an acute exacerbation of COPD. It is useful to do a chest roentgenogram. The chest roentgenogram may be positive in approximately 15 percent of cases, and in 25 percent of such patients, there is a change of management prompted by the chest roentgenogram result. Spirometry, on the other hand, has not been helpful in decision-making for patients with an acute exacerbation of COPD. There is poor correlation between arterial blood gases and the FEV_1 at the time of presentation. The FEV_1 has not been helpful in predicting need for hospital admission. While severe abnormalities of arterial blood gases and history of prior relapses are helpful, there are no predictive models of adequate sensitivity and specificity to rely on. The best indicators for the need for mechanical ventilation include the blood gas values on admission and the degree of change in pH after initial oxygen therapy. Significant predictors of hospital mortality include older age, lower body mass index, poor functional status prior to admission, lower $PO_2:FIO_2$ (fraction of inspired oxygen) ratio, history of congestive heart failure, low serum albumin, and presence of cor pulmonale.

Most therapeutic interventions for the treatment of the acute exacerbation of COPD have been studied through randomized controlled trials. In general, mucolytic agents are ineffective in shortening the course and improving the outcome of patients. Chest physiotherapy and mechanical percussion of the chest are also ineffective and may be potentially harmful. β_2-Agonists and anticholinergic agents appear to be equivalent in their usefulness and are superior to all parenterally administered bronchodilators including methylxanthines. The addition of a methylxanthine to inhaled bronchodilators has also been carefully examined. There is no solid evidence for lower hospitalization rates or improved outcomes for patients given IV aminophylline in the emergency department. The effect of adding two inhaled bronchodilators has also been carefully studied. There appears to be only marginal improvement with the use of both agents. The side effects of anticholinergic therapy are generally fewer and mild. However, such side effects may be particularly adverse in elderly patients; for example, those with obstructive myopathy. The adverse effects of albuterol in the acute setting include tremors, headache, and palpitations. Changes in heart rate, blood pressure and electrocardiogram tracings are also possible.

The use of systemic steroids for patients with an acute exacerbation of COPD who require hospitalization is helpful. Hospitalization is helpful and a change to oral therapy continues to have a positive effect, but for only two weeks post-hospitalization. The most common adverse effect is hyperglycemia, which may require at least short-term treatment.

Antibiotic therapy has a beneficial effect in patients with an acute exacerbation of COPD, and those with more severe exacerbations (type I, see Table 42-7) are more likely to benefit. The choice of antibiotic is influenced by the age of the patient, the severity of underlying COPD, and the potential for antibiotic resistance, as well as the likelihood that the patient will take the prescribed medication. Patients with severe underlying COPD and an FEV_1 under 35 percent of predicted have a much greater chance of being colonized with gram-negative organisms. Elderly patients, too, need antibiotic coverage for the common pathogenic bacteria, including *Haemophilus influenzae, Streptococcus pneumoniae,* and *Moraxella catarrhalis,* and in such patients, treatment for potential gram-negative organisms should also be strongly considered. There is an increasing prevalence of organisms that produce bacterial enzymes that inactivate traditional β-lactam antibiotics. This has been especially seen with *H. influenzae* and *M. catarrhalis.* Therefore, many of the antibiotics traditionally used for bronchial infections are currently not optimal. It is therefore important to be familiar with local resistance rates of these microorganisms before prescribing. Patient compliance is significantly improved when the antibiotic regimen is give once or twice a day and for shorter courses of time. However, this often means reliance on newer more expensive agents that many elderly on fixed incomes may be unable to afford. The choice of antibiotic coverage should be a decision discussed with the patient to consider all of these important factors.

Noninvasive positive pressure ventilation (NPPV) is beneficial for patients who have a high likelihood of respiratory failure and thus may require invasive mechanical ventilation. The use of NPPV provides a statistically significant difference in the need for intubation, as reported in several clinical trials. Optimal NPPV for the COPD exacerbation requires close patient monitoring, usually in an intensive care setting.

SUMMARY

In the United States, more than 16 million adults have COPD. As the US population ages, the prevalence of this disease will climb even higher. COPD currently accounts for approximately 110,000 deaths per year. There are more than 500,000 hospitalizations in this country for COPD and more than 16 million office visits to physicians. When elderly patients are hospitalized, it is often with an acute exacerbation of COPD. When hypercarbia (>55 mmHg) is present, 11 percent of the patients will die during their hospital stay, and the 60-day, 180-day, 1-year, and 2-year mortality is extremely high (20 percent, 33 percent, 43 percent and 49 percent, respectively). The mean cost of a hospital stay for this condition in the mid 1990s was $7100. Hospitalization costs make up a sizable portion of the more than 30 billion dollars in direct medical costs that the United States spends for the care of COPD. Moreover, after hospital discharge for respiratory failure there is a very high readmission rate. Six months after an admission, almost half the patients are readmitted at least once and some patients are readmitted several times. At 6 months only approximately 25 percent of patients are found to be both alive and well and able to report a good, very good, or excellent quality of life. It is likely that the care of patients around the globe with COPD will consume a growing proportion of

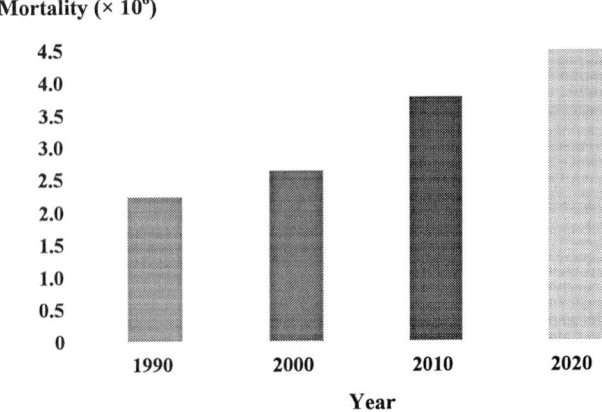

Figure 42-10 Projected global mortality from COPD. Over several decades shown, these statistics were commissioned by the World Health Organization examining the global burden of disease for the twenty-first century. Adapted from Murray CJL, Lopez AW: *Lancet* 349:1498, 1997.

the physician's time for many years to come (Fig. 42-10), at least as long as effects of chronic, heavy cigarette smoking continue to exert their toll on pulmonary physiology and disease.

REFERENCES

ACCP/AACVPR Pulmonary Rehabilitation Guidelines Panel. Pulmonary rehabilitation. *Chest* 112:1363, 1997.

Anderson JE et al: Treating tobacco use and dependence. An evidence-based clinical practice guideline for tobacco cessation. *Chest* 121:932, 2002.

Anthonisen NR et al: Effects of smoking intervention and the use an inhaled anticholinergic bronchodilator on the rate of decline of FEV_1. The lung health study. *JAMA* 272:1497, 1994.

ATS statement: Standards for the diagnosis and care of patients with chronic obstructive pulmonary disease. *Am J Respir Crit Care Med* 152(S):S77, 1995.

Barnes PJ: Medical progress: Chronic obstructive pulmonary disease. *N Engl J Med* 343(4):269, 2000.

Crockett AJ et al: Domiciliary oxygen for chronic obstructive pulmonary diseases. *The Cochrane Library* 2:1, 2001.

Global Strategy for the Diagnosis, Management, and Prevention of Chronic Obstructive Pulmonary Disease. NHLBI/WHO workshop report. *Global Initiative for Chronic Obstructive Lung Disease.* NHLBI Publication No. 2701. 2001.

Kerstjens HAM: Stable chronic obstructive pulmonary disease. *BMJ* 495, 1999.

Mannino DM: Epidemiology, prevalence, morbidity and mortality, and disease heterogeneity. *Chest* 121:121S, 2002.

Mannino DM et al: Chronic obstructive pulmonary disease surveillance—United States, 1971–2000. *MMWR Surveill Summ* 51(SS06);1, 2002.

McCrory DC et al: Management of acute exacerbations of COPD. A summary and appraisal of published evidence. *Chest* 119:1190, 2001.

Saetta M et al: Cellular and structural bases of chronic obstructive pulmonary disease. *Am J Respir Crit Care Med* 163:1304, 2001.

Diffuse Parenchymal Lung Disease in the Elderly Population

VICTOR J. THANNICKAL • GALEN B. TOEWS

The lung brings the ambient air that we breathe into close proximity with the systemic circulation. This allows for its essential function in gas exchange. However, this also exposes the lung to a variety of potentially injurious infectious and noninfectious environmental agents. The normal host response to such insults is to eradicate the etiologic agent and to repair the injury caused either directly by the agent or indirectly by the associated inflammatory process. This complex, but well-orchestrated and tightly regulated host response leads to eventual resolution of injury and restoration of normal lung architecture and function in most cases. However, if the inflammatory and/or repair response is dysregulated, a chronic alveolar/interstitial remodeling process with varying degrees of inflammation and fibrosis ensues. Damage to the pulmonary vascular endothelium via the circulation (e.g., drugs, systemic rheumatic disorders) may produce similar inflammatory/fibrotic reactions in the lung. This results in the restrictive physiology and gas-exchange abnormalities characteristic of the diffuse parenchymal lung diseases (DPLDs). When all potential etiologic agents and associations are considered, the list of DPLDs includes over 150 different clinical entities (Table 43-1). Thus, DPLDs comprise a large and heterogeneous group of diseases that have common features in their clinical, radiographic, and physiologic presentations.

The most prevalent and devastating of all the DPLDs is idiopathic pulmonary fibrosis (IPF), a chronic fibrotic disease of unknown etiology. IPF is primarily a disease of elderly patients. Elderly patients may be particularly susceptible to this disease because of inherent deficiencies in immune function and/or in their inability to mount an appropriate repair response. Alternatively, IPF may present in elderly patients as a result of accumulated insults or because early manifestations of the disease are difficult to recognize. This chapter focuses on emerging new concepts regarding IPF pathogenesis and the challenges facing clinicians taking care of these patients. The chapter also discusses other selected DPLDs that are relatively more common in the geriatric population.

EPIDEMIOLOGY

The prevalence of DPLD is estimated at approximately 20 to 40 per 100,000 general population in the United States. DPLD accounts for 100,000 hospital admissions yearly. The increased use of pneumotoxic drugs to treat malignant and cardiovascular diseases in the elderly population, as well the rising median age of the US population, are likely to contribute to an increased incidence.

IPF was recently reclassified into a group of diseases designated as the idiopathic interstitial pneumonias (IIPs) (see Table 43-1). IIPs are rare in children, but increase with advancing age. IPF, the most common of the IIPs, has a prevalence of 6 to 14.6 per 100,000 persons in different series. In patients older than the age of 75 years, however, the prevalence may exceed 175 per 100,000. The median age of onset of IPF ranges from 50 to 70 years and the diagnosis is almost never made in a patient younger than age 40 years. In contrast, other IIPs such as nonspecific interstitial pneumonia (NSIP) may occur in younger patients.

PATHOGENESIS

Evolving concepts on pathogenesis of the DPLDs suggest different mechanisms and responses of the lung to a variety of insults. This is best illustrated by the wide range of pathologic findings in IIPs. Histopathologically, the IIPs are defined by the pattern and degree of inflammation versus fibrosis, the nature of the underlying inflammatory response (e.g., macrophages versus lymphocytes), and the primary location (alveolar versus interstitial) in which this occurs. Desquamative interstitial pneumonia (DIP) is characterized by intraalveolar macrophage accumulation with little or no fibrosis. NSIP primarily involves interstitial lymphocytic inflammation with moderate fibrosis. Usual interstitial pneumonia (UIP), the histopathologic correlate of IPF, is primarily a fibrotic process involving interstitial and alveolar spaces with minimal inflammation. Thus, the disease "phenotype" represented by the IIPs represents a spectrum

Table 43-1   Classification of Diffuse Parenchymal Lung Disease (DPLD)

Idiopathic interstitial pneumonias
  Idiopathic pulmonary fibrosis (IPF)/usual interstitial
    pneumonia (UIP)
  Nonspecific interstitial pneumonia (NSIP)
  Cryptogenic-organizing pneumonia
    (COP)/bronchiolitis obliterans-organizing
    pneumonia (BOOP)
  Acute interstitial pneumonia (AIP)
  Respiratory bronchiolitis interstitial lung disease
    (RB-ILD)
  Desquamative interstitial pneumonia (DIP)
  Lymphoid interstitial pneumonia (LIP)

Other DPLD (with primary lung involvement)
  Sarcoidosis
  Histiocytosis X
  Lymphangioleiomyomatosis

DPLD associated with systemic rheumatic disease
  Rheumatoid arthritis
  Systemic lupus erythematosis
  Scleroderma
  Polymyositis-dermatomyositis
  Sjögren's syndrome
  Mixed connective-tissue disease
  Ankylosing spondylitis

DPLD associated with drugs or treatments
  Antibiotics
  Antiinflammatory agents
  Cardiovascular drugs
  Antineoplastic drugs
  Illicit drugs
  Dietary supplements
  Oxygen
  Radiation
  Paraquat

**DPLD associated with environmental (occupational)
exposures**
  Organic dusts/hypersensitivity pneumonitis
    (>40 known agents)

  Farmer's lung
  Air conditioner–humidifier lung
  Bird breeder's lung
  Baggasosis
Inorganic dusts
  Silicosis
  Asbestosis
  Coal worker's pneumoconiosis
  Berylliosis
Gases/fumes/vapors
  Oxides of nitrogen
  Sulfur dioxide
  Toluene diisocyanate
  Oxides of metals
  Hydrocarbons
  Thermosetting resins

DPLD associated with "alveolar filling"
  Diffuse alveolar hemorrhage
  Goodpasture's syndrome
  Idiopathic pulmonary hemosiderosis
  Pulmonary alveolar proteinosis
  Chronic eosinophilic pneumonia
  Chronic aspiration syndrome
  Lipoid pneumonia

DPLD associated with pulmonary vasculitis
  Wegener's granulomatosis
  Churg–Strauss syndrome
  Hypersensitivity vasculitis
  Necrotizing sarcoid granulomatosis

Inherited DPLD
  Familial idiopathic pulmonary fibrosis
  Neurofibromatosis
  Tuberous sclerosis
  Gaucher's disease
  Niemann–Pick disease
  Hermansky–Pudlak syndrome

of pathologic lung responses that is likely dependent on several host factors (such as age, genetic susceptibility) and on extrinsic factors (such as cigarette smoking, comorbid conditions) (Fig. 43-1). Alternatively, these same intrinsic and extrinsic factors may influence the progression or lack of progression down "common pathways" leading from injury and inflammation to fibrosis. The validity of this latter conceptual paradigm is difficult to prove without the ability to clearly define the natural history of each of the IIPs. This is further limited by lack of uniform diagnostic criteria, varying clinical presentations, and the reluctance to perform invasive procedures in elderly patients for conditions without proven therapeutic options. The recently

revised classification system for the IIPs (see Table 43-1) may prove helpful in future studies designed to clarify the natural history and interrelationships between the IIPs. The pathogenetic mechanisms that are active *at the time of clinical presentation* are likely to be distinctly different among the IIPs. For purposes of this discussion, we focus on current and evolving concepts of IPF, the most prevalent of the IIPs and the one that carries the worst prognosis.

IPF is localized to the lung parenchyma. Early histopathologic evidence of alveolar epithelial cell injury suggests an inhaled route of entry for the etiologic agent. The temporal and spatial heterogeneity of the fibrotic lesions in UIP suggests that the injury may be recurrent and

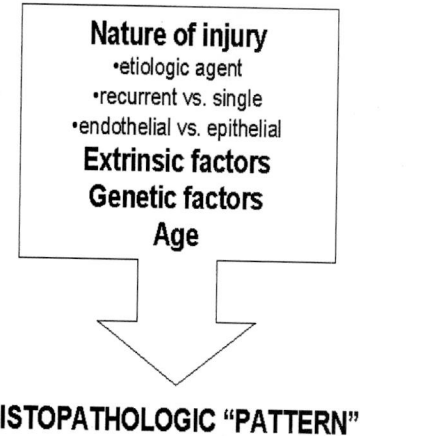

LUNG INJURY

Nature of injury
•etiologic agent
•recurrent vs. single
•endothelial vs. epithelial
Extrinsic factors
Genetic factors
Age

HISTOPATHOLOGIC "PATTERN"

DIP RB-ILD LIP COP NSIP AIP IPF

VARYING DEGREES OF:

Inflammation ◄──────► **Fibrosis**

Figure 43-1 Idiopathic interstitial pneumonias: histopathologic patterns to lung injury. The idiopathic interstitial pneumonias (IIPs) are defined by their histopathologic patterns. IIPs comprise different pathologic responses to lung injury that is likely determined by several factors, including the nature of the injury, extrinsic factors (such as cigarette smoke), genetic susceptibility, and age. These histopathologic patterns represent a spectrum of diseases characterized by varying degrees of inflammation and fibrosis. AIP, acute interstitial pneumonia; COP, cryptogenic-organizing pneumonia; DIP, desquamative interstitial pneumonia; IPF, idiopathic pulmonary fibrosis; LIP, lymphocytic interstitial pneumonia; NSIP, nonspecific interstitial pneumonia; RB-ILD, respiratory bronchiolitis-associated interstitial lung disease.

repetitive, occurring over many years (see Figure 43-1). Although the identity of the putative injurious agent has not been identified, latent viral infections and environmental toxins have been suggested as possibilities.

It is possible that the aging process and the biology of cellular senescence influence tissue remodeling and repair responses. Age-related changes in extracellular matrix composition, expression of cell adhesion molecules, and cellular responses to growth factors have been shown in cells and tissues from various organ systems. Genomic analyses of senescent (aged) fibroblasts demonstrated a pattern of gene expression that mimics inflammatory wound repair and, as such, it has been suggested that senescent cells may contribute to chronic wound pathologies.

Genetic factors are likely to determine the susceptibility to fibrotic sequelae and, perhaps, in the type of pathologic injury and repair that ensues. Complex disorders are influenced by the actions of multiple genes and their interactions with each other and the environment. Familial pulmonary fibrosis appears to be inherited as an autosomal dominant trait with variable penetrance. No systematic assessment has been made of the heritability of IPF in the general population or the risk to relatives of affected individuals. Various forms of fibrotic lung disease have

been associated with gene polymorphisms of interleukin-1–receptor antagonist, tumor necrosis factor-α, and major histocompatability complex loci. Transforming growth factor-β1 gene polymorphisms resulting in increased production of this cytokine are associated with fibrotic lung disease and graft fibrosis after lung transplantation.

Environmental factors modulate the response of the lung to injury. Of these, the most intriguing is the role of cigarette smoke. There is a strong association with cigarette smoking in respiratory bronchiolitis-associated interstitial lung disease (RB-ILD) and DIP; cigarette smoke appears to play an etiologic role in the majority of these cases. Pulmonary histiocytosis X is diagnosed almost exclusively in active smokers. However, there is controversy regarding the role of cigarette smoke in IPF. Previous reports suggested that smoking was an independent risk factor for IPF. However, these studies may have included other types of IIP in addition to IPF/UIP. More recent studies suggest that survival is extended in patients with IPF who are cigarette smokers at the time of initial evaluation when compared with former smokers or never smokers. Interestingly, this "protection" is associated with histopathology that shows less interstitial cellularity and granulation/connective tissue formation but greater alveolar macrophage-predominant inflammation. The effect of cigarette smoke on the progression of IPF may be a result of a factor(s) that negatively regulates fibroblast activation.

A unifying concept predicts that, in susceptible individuals, a fibrotic response to lung injury and repair is dependent on multiple factors that alter homeostasis within the alveolar microenvironment. Animal models of fibrosis suggest the involvement of numerous molecules and regulatory pathways in the inflammation and repair cascade. These alterations include imbalances in profibrotic cytokine production/activation, angiogenesis, eicosanoid synthesis, fibrinolysis, extracellular matrix turnover, and oxidative stress (Fig. 43-2). Such changes in the alveolar microenvironment appears to favor the loss of epithelial cells and accumulation of fibroblasts (and myofibroblasts) within the alveolar and interstitial spaces that leads to an unrelenting, progressive fibrotic process.

DIAGNOSTIC APPROACH

History

The most common presenting symptom is the insidious onset of exertional dyspnea that slowly progresses over many months and, in some cases, years. Initially, dyspnea is mild and the patient often does not seek medical attention. Dyspnea may be attributed to other causes such as being "out-of-shape," normal aging, being overweight, or a viral infection. Patients may initially be misdiagnosed and treated for other ailments (bronchitis, asthma, or heart failure). As the disease progresses, dyspnea occurs at rest. Nonproductive cough and fatigue are also prominent complaints. Cough is a frequent complaint in patients with cryptogenic-organizing pneumonia (COP; also known as bronchiolitis obliterans-organizing pneumonia [BOOP]), eosinophilic pneumonia, RB-ILD and IPF. Pleuritic chest pain may occur

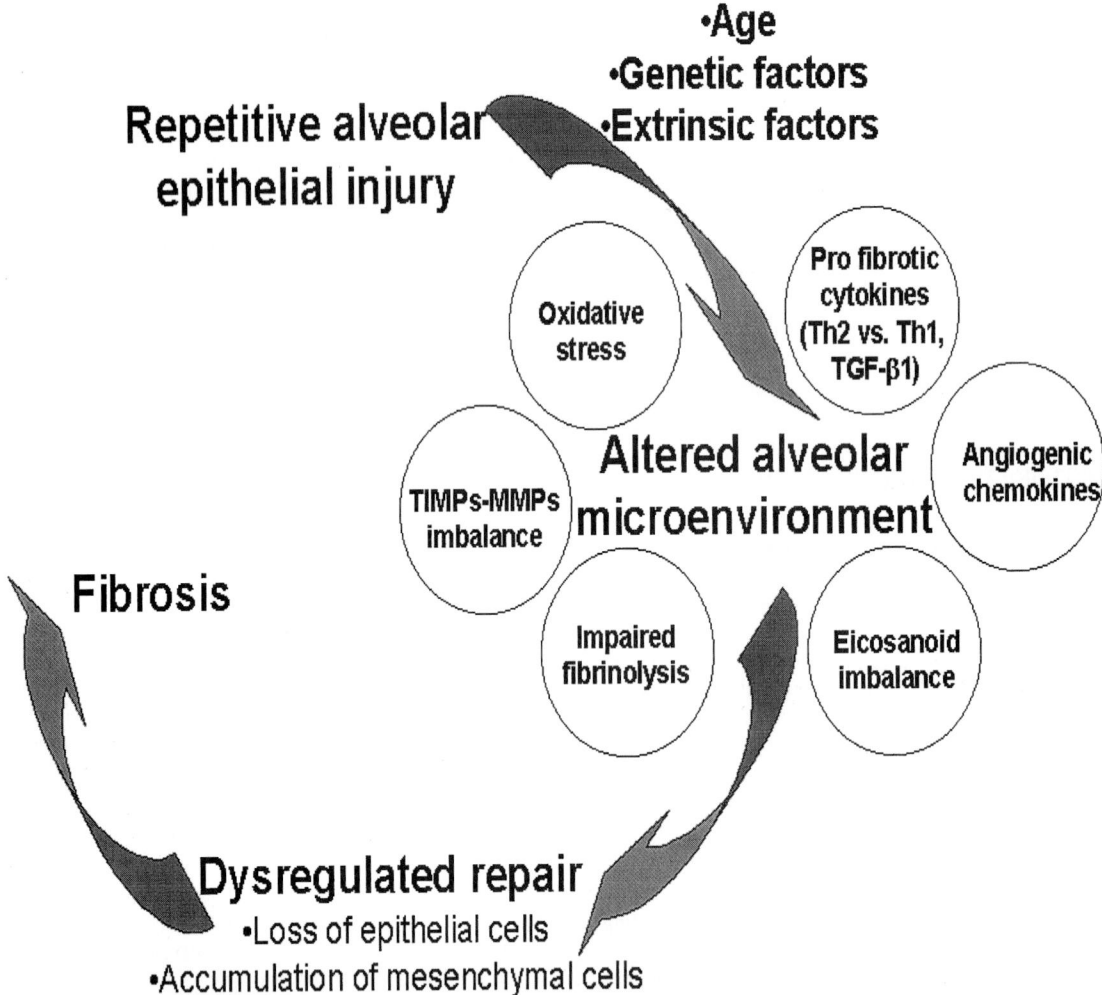

Figure 43-2 Pathogenesis of idiopathic pulmonary fibrosis. Evolving concepts on the pathogenesis of idiopathic pulmonary fibrosis suggest that repetitive alveolar epithelial injury result in aberrant or dysregulated repair responses with ensuing fibrosis. Fibrotic responses are promoted by alterations in the alveolar microenvironment of the lung that includes overproduction/activation of profibrotic cytokines and angiogenic chemokines, imbalances in eicosanoid production, impaired fibrinolytic activity, imbalances in tissue inhibitors of matrix metalloproteinases (TIMPs) production over matrix metalloproteinases (MMPs) and increased oxidative stress. TGF, transforming growth factor; Th, T helper cell.

with DPLDs associated with systemic rheumatic disease and some drug-induced disorders. Pleuritic chest pain and sudden worsening of dyspnea should suggest a spontaneous pneumothorax, a characteristic finding in lymphangioleiomyomatosis, neurofibromatosis, tuberous sclerosis, and pulmonary histiocytosis X. Hemoptysis may be the presenting complaint in patients with diffuse alveolar hemorrhage syndromes or lymphangioleiomyomatosis, but it is infrequent in other DPLDs. Hemoptysis should prompt a search for complications such as malignancy, superimposed infection, or pulmonary embolism.

The history often provides clues to a more specific diagnosis when a DPLD is associated with a systemic rheumatic disorder, an occupational or environmental exposure, or certain drug therapies. Most patients with DPLD associated with rheumatic diseases have an established diagnosis when pulmonary symptoms present or have extrapulmonary manifestations that provide clues to the underlying disorder. A careful history may also reveal

an environmental or occupational exposure. A detailed, lifelong occupational history must be obtained, because DPLDs have long latency periods between exposure and onset of symptoms or radiographic abnormalities. Exposure to agents that cause DPLDs may also occur as a result of hobbies or recreational activities (bird breeder's lung, woodworker's lung, farmer's lung, sauna taker's disease). Accordingly, exposures outside the occupational setting should be explored. An increasing list of both prescribed and over-the-counter medications can cause DPLD. Chemotherapeutic drugs have variable latency periods ranging from a few weeks to many years; therefore, a history of both current and *former* drug therapies must be sought.

Other aspects of the history, although not indicative of a specific etiology, may aid in the diagnostic evaluation. A history of smoking has been strongly linked with histiocytosis X, RB-ILD, and pulmonary hemorrhage associated with Goodpasture's syndrome. In contrast, hypersensitivity pneumonitis and sarcoidosis occur less frequently in active smokers. The role of cigarette smoking in IPF is controversial. It has been reported to be a risk factor for IPF, but recent studies also suggest that IPF patients who are active smokers have a better prognosis. Age and sex are sometimes useful in initial evaluation. IPF is almost exclusively a disease of middle-age and elderly patients. Sarcoidosis, histiocytosis X, lymphangioleiomyomatosis, and the inherited causes of DPLD (see Table 43-1) are generally diagnosed before age 40 years and, thus, are uncommon initial presentations in the geriatric patient. Elderly patients are prone to aspiration; a history of gastroesophageal reflux suggests the possibility of chronic aspiration syndrome. The use of mineral oil nasal drops or petroleum products should raise the possibility of lipoid pneumonia.

Physical Examination

Patients with IPF and other UIP-associated DPLD typically reveal the characteristic bibasilar, crepitant ("Velcro-like") late-inspiratory rales (crackles) on lung auscultation. Wheezing, rhonchi, and coarse rales are occasionally heard. The lung exam can be normal in the early course of the disease. With advanced disease, resting tachycardia and tachypnea may be present. Digital clubbing is relatively common in IPF, but less common in certain other DPLDs such as sarcoidosis. Hypertrophic pulmonary osteoarthropathy is rare. The new appearance of digital clubbing in a patient with known DPLD should prompt a search for complicating lung malignancy. The heart examination may be normal early in the disease. Later, with the onset of pulmonary hypertension and cor pulmonale, an accentuated P2, tricuspid insufficiency, a right ventricular heave, and peripheral edema may be noted. Extrapulmonary findings involving the skin and joints may indicate the presence of a systemic rheumatologic disorder.

Laboratory Tests

Laboratory tests can either confirm or suggest a diagnosis in DPLD, but these studies are seldom diagnostic. Rheumatoid factor and antinuclear antibodies are occasionally present in patients with ILD, but their presence does not necessarily indicate an underlying collagen vascular disorder. Plasma immunoglobulin may be elevated, but this finding is nonspecific. If hypersensitivity pneumonitis is suspected, serum-precipitating antibodies to a limited number of inhaled organic antigens may be measured. Tests for antineutrophil cytoplasmic antibodies (ANCA) should be obtained if Wegener's granulomatosis is suspected. Tests for antibasement membrane antibodies should be obtained when Goodpasture's syndrome is suspected. The electrocardiogram (ECG) is usually normal in DPLD. With progressive loss of alveolar capillary units and cor pulmonale, the ECG may demonstrate a pattern of right atrial and ventricular strain.

Chest Radiography

The chest radiograph is a practical and useful screen for DPLD. The chest radiograph may be normal in up to 10 percent of patients with DPLD detected by high-resolution computed tomography (HRCT). When abnormal, a characteristic radiographic pattern in combination with the appropriate clinical history and physical exam findings may suggest or support a specific diagnosis. In DPLD, the chest radiograph typically reveals bilateral reticular opacities that are predominantly in the periphery and lower lung fields. With more severe disease, cystic dilatation of the distal air spaces ("honeycombing") and traction bronchiectasis with thickened and dilated airways are seen. In other DPLDs, nodular or reticulonodular infiltrates may be more common. Alveolar filling diseases often present with ill-defined alveolar nodules (acinar rosettes) and air bronchograms. A diffuse ground-glass pattern is often seen in diseases characterized by active alveolitis such as DIP, RB-ILD, "cellular" NSIP, and hypersensitivity pneumonitis.

High-Resolution Computed Tomography

HRCT, using thin (1- to 2-mm) sections without the use of contrast, offers many advantages over standard chest radiography in evaluation of DPLD. The improved spatial resolution of HRCT allows characterization of anatomic patterns to the level of the pulmonary lobule. It is useful for the detection of DPLD in cases when the chest radiograph is normal, to quantify the extent and pattern of lung parenchymal involvement and, in a few cases, to make a specific diagnosis with a high degree of certainty. Diseases in which HRCT has been able to detect abnormalities with normal chest radiographs include asbestosis, silicosis, sarcoidosis, and scleroderma. Conversely, the HRCT may be normal in some cases of biopsy-proven DPLD; therefore, HRCT cannot be used to exclude ILD with absolute certainty. In such cases, physiologic data such as gas exchange with exertion may be more sensitive. HRCT is also valuable for following the response to therapy and in identifying a suitable site for transbronchial or open lung biopsy. Recent studies suggest that HRCT data when combined with the clinical information can result in a confident diagnosis of IPF when read by experienced pulmonologists or radiologists; this may obviate the need for a lung biopsy in certain patients.

Pulmonary Function Tests

Physiologic testing can identify the physiologic abnormalities associated with DPLD, determine the severity, and determine the course and response to treatment. The classic physiologic alterations in DPLD include reduced lung volumes (vital capacity, total lung capacity [TLC]), reduced diffusing capacity (DLCO), and a normal or supernormal ratio of forced expiratory volume in 1 second (FEV_1) to forced vital capacity (FVC). Static lung compliance is decreased (decreased lung volume for any given transpulmonary pressure), and maximal transpulmonary pressure is increased (a very high negative pressure must be generated to open fibrotic alveoli). Exceptions to this classic presentation are histiocytosis X, lymphangioleiomyomatosis, neurofibromatosis, sarcoidosis, and tuberous sclerosis, in which airways disease can predominate resulting in an increase in airflow limitation and increased TLC. A mixed restrictive and obstructive pattern is commonly seen in BOOP.

Arterial blood gas analysis typically shows mild hypoxemia. Carbon dioxide retention is rare. Most of the patients with DPLD have marked increases in minute ventilation both at rest and with exercise, resulting in reduced partial pressure of carbon dioxide (Pco_2) and compensated respiratory alkalosis. The increased minute ventilation is accomplished by increases in respiratory rate rather than in tidal volume. Hyperventilation is not a result of abnormalities in acid–base status or to hypoxemia, but rather to an increased stimulation of the respiratory center from neural signals arising from altered mechanoreceptors in the deranged lung parenchyma. Exercise tolerance in DPLD patients is markedly limited. With exercise, arterial partial pressure of oxygen (Po_2) falls and that of carbon dioxide (Pco_2) remains constant. Hypoxemia in patients with DPLD results primarily from abnormal ventilation–perfusion relationships and additionally from diffusion abnormalities with severe disease. The abnormalities in diffusion, which were originally believed to be the result of thickened alveolar walls, are now recognized to be caused by loss of capillary cross-sectional areas and the passage of red blood cells through functioning pulmonary capillaries at a rate that is too rapid to permit full saturation of hemoglobin. Arterial pH is usually normal in DPLD, but can fall with exercise as a result of anaerobic metabolism in oxygen-deprived muscles.

Bronchoscopic Studies

Bronchoscopy should be performed when tissue abnormalities are distributed in the bronchovascular bundle, an alveolar filling disorder is present, or an infectious disease is suspected. The distinctive histologic abnormalities of sarcoidosis, lymphangitic carcinomatosis, and lymphangioleiomyomatosis are usually found in the bronchovascular bundle and transbronchial biopsy may demonstrate their characteristic lesions. Bronchoalveolar lavage (BAL) is diagnostic if an infectious agent or neoplastic cells are noted in the lavage specimen. BAL is also used to analyze the cellular constituents, cellular products, and proteins of the distal air spaces of the lung. A predominance of eosinophils in conjunction with appropriate clinical and radiographic picture can be diagnostic of eosinophilic pneumonia. An asbestos body count of more than 1 per milliliter of BAL fluid documents significant asbestos exposure. In histiocytosis X, ultrastructural studies of BAL mononuclear cells reveal the typical Birbeck granule of the Langerhans cell. Special stains for surfactant may suggest a diagnosis of alveolar proteinosis. However, BAL is usually nonspecific and it is not routinely indicated because of its limited ability to predict the underlying pathology (fibrosis versus inflammation), to stage disease, or to predict response to therapy.

Lung Biopsy

The diagnosis of most DPLDs, and in particular IIPs, depends on histologic studies of lung parenchyma. An open-lung or thoracoscopic biopsy is required to secure a specific diagnosis in the majority of cases when the etiology is unclear. A specific diagnosis can be established in 90 percent of cases by this method. The morality rate for open lung biopsy is less than 1 percent, and the morbidity is less than 3 percent. The benefits of making a definitive diagnosis must be weighed carefully with potential risks, particularly in elderly patients with comorbid conditions. One must also consider the options for meaningful therapy once a diagnosis is made. Currently, for IPF, such options are limited.

THERAPEUTIC APPROACH

The principal aims of therapy are to remove exposure to injurious agents, to suppress any active inflammatory component, and to palliate or treat the complications of these diseases. Avoidance of the etiologic agent, such as drugs and occupational exposures, should lead to resolution or stabilization. A short course of steroid therapy may also be indicated if the patient is symptomatic. In such cases, care must be taken to exclude infectious etiologies before embarking on empiric immunosuppressive therapy. Treatment of DPLDs associated with rheumatologic diseases is directed at suppressing the systemic immune response with prednisone with or without cyclophosphamide (Cytoxan). There are certain other DPLDs such as sarcoidosis and pulmonary vasculitides that are more responsive to such therapies.

The efficacy of antiinflammatory agents in IIPs depends on the specific disease entity. In general, NSIP, COP, RB-ILD, DIP, and LIP are steroid-responsive; whereas, IPF/UIP and acute interstitial pneumonia (AIP) are not. In cases where a lung biopsy cannot be obtained and a process other than IPF is suspected, a trial of antiinflammatory therapy may be initiated. This should be limited to a 3- to 6-month trial of prednisone (or prednisone plus azathioprine) during which time objective improvements in physiologic measures, radiographic findings, and clinical symptoms are assessed. Ten to 30 percent of patients have objective improvement or remain clinically stable with therapy. In general, patients who respond to therapy are younger than 50 years of age; in addition, females respond more frequently than males. In the absence of improvement, therapy with these agents must be discontinued. There appears to be no benefit to more potent antiinflammatory therapy (such as Cytoxan) in steroid unresponsive cases.

Early institution of oxygen therapy for patients with hypoxemia or desaturation (oxygen saturation ≤88 percent) at rest or with exercise is an important aspect of care. Patients who develop pulmonary hypertension and cor pulmonale must be managed supportively with a combination of diuretics, inotropic agents, vasodilator therapy, and anticoagulation. Influenza and pneumococcal vaccines should be administered to these patients.

Lung transplantation may be an option for patients with end-stage DPLD/IIP refractory to medical therapy. Single-lung transplantation is preferred for most patients. Most transplant centers currently do not list patients older than age 65 years. Two-year survival rates range from 60 to 80 percent, with most deaths being a result of infections that complicate immunosuppressive therapy or of chronic allograft rejection.

FUTURE DIRECTIONS

The challenges facing clinicians who care for patients with DPLD, particularly that of the idiopathic variety, include the ability to diagnose patients early in the disease course when the underlying inflammatory processes may be more amenable to therapy and to accurately define the relative degree of inflammation versus fibrosis. In primarily fibrotic processes such as IPF/UIP, antiinflammatory therapies are of limited benefit. A number of "antifibrotic" strategies are now under investigation. Further understanding of the relationships between inflammation and fibrosis and the molecular determinants that result in the varied manifestations of the IIPs may aid in the development of more targeted therapies. Evolving technologies that allow for genotyping and phenotyping of tissue samples may also aid in defining the underlying disease process to allow for more specific therapy and improved prognostication.

REFERENCES

American Thoracic Society. Idiopathic pulmonary fibrosis: Diagnosis and treatment. International consensus statement. American Thoracic Society (ATS), and the European Respiratory Society (ERS). *Am J Respir Crit Care Med* 161:646, 2000.

American Thoracic Society/European Respiratory Society: International multidisciplinary consensus classification of the idiopathic interstitial pneumonias. This joint statement of the American Thoracic Society (ATS), and the European Respiratory Society (ERS) was adopted by the ATS board of directors, June 2001 and by the ERS Executive Committee, June 2001. *Am J Respir Crit Care Med* 165:277, 2002.

Bjoraker JA et al: Prognostic significance of histopathologic subsets in idiopathic pulmonary fibrosis. *Am J Respir Crit Care Med* 157:199, 1998.

Crystal RG et al: Future research directions in idiopathic pulmonary fibrosis: Summary of a National Heart, Lung, and Blood Institute working group. *Am J Respir Crit Care Med* 166:236, 2002.

Flaherty KR et al: Histopathologic variability in usual and nonspecific interstitial pneumonias. *Am J Respir Crit Care Med* 164:1722, 2001.

Gay SE et al: Idiopathic pulmonary fibrosis: Predicting response to therapy and survival. *Am J Respir Crit Care Med* 157:1063, 1998.

Gross TJ, Hunninghake GW: Idiopathic pulmonary fibrosis. *N Engl J Med* 345:517, 2001.

Katzenstein AL, Myers JL: Idiopathic pulmonary fibrosis: Clinical relevance of pathologic classification. *Am J Respir Crit Care Med* 157:1301, 1998.

King TE Jr et al: Idiopathic pulmonary fibrosis: Relationship between histopathologic features and mortality. *Am J Respir Crit Care Med* 164:1025, 2001.

King TE Jr et al: Predicting survival in idiopathic pulmonary fibrosis: Scoring system and survival model. *Am J Respir Crit Care Med* 164:1171, 2001.

Selman M et al: Idiopathic pulmonary fibrosis: Prevailing and evolving hypotheses about its pathogenesis and implications for therapy. *Ann Intern Med* 134:136, 2001.

Toews GB: Interstitial lung disease, in Goldman L, Bennett JC (eds): *Cecil Textbook of Medicine,* 22nd ed. Philadelphia, W.B. Saunders, 2003 (In press).

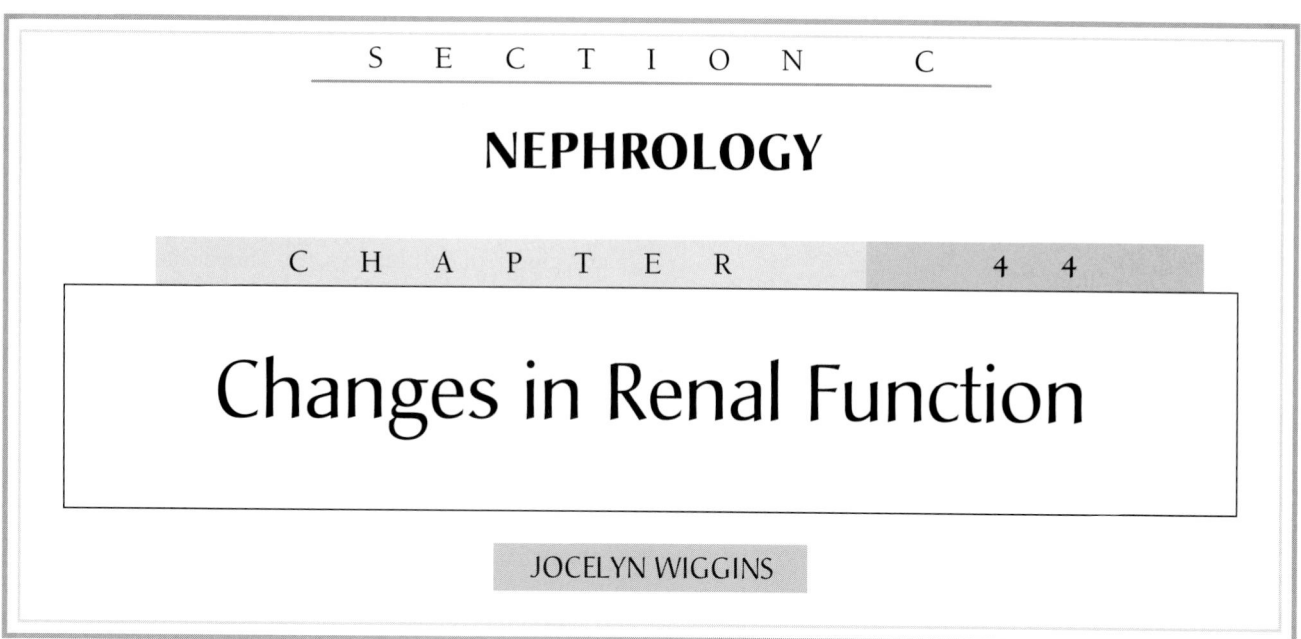

S E C T I O N   C

NEPHROLOGY

C H A P T E R   4 4

Changes in Renal Function

JOCELYN WIGGINS

CLINICAL RELEVANCE

Renal failure is a growing problem in the older population. Data on people reaching end-stage renal disease are collected by the US Renal Data System (USRDS). All dialysis units that receive funding from Medicare are required to file data with the USRDS, so that nationwide data are available on more than 95 percent of people receiving renal replacement therapy. Information published in the 1999 USRDS annual data report shows that approximately 1.3 persons in 1000 older than age 65 years are initiating treatment for end-stage renal disease (ESRD) each year, the highest rate of any age group. The number of older people enrolling for treatment is currently growing at 8 percent per year; this growth rate having peaked in the early 1990s at 17 percent per year. Almost 4 persons in 1000 are currently maintained on renal replacement therapy, with the 75+ years age group growing at 10 percent per year. The peak incidence for ESRD is the 70- to 74-year-old age group, while the peak prevalence falls in the 65- to 69-year-old age group. In contrast, the incidence of ESRD in the 20- to 44-year-old age group has remained flat over the last 10 years, with only 6 percent growth in the 45- to 64-year-old group. Although some of the increase in renal replacement therapy for the older population indicates a greater willingness to offer treatment to older individuals, much of the increase is a result of people surviving to experience the chronic changes that occur with aging. The kidney undergoes significant age-related change. Other common diseases, such as hypertension and diabetes, accelerate these changes.

THE AGING PROCESS

Aging in the kidney is characterized by changes of both structure and function. Many of the aging studies have been performed on laboratory animals, particularly rodents, who demonstrate quite different patterns of aging from humans. For example, kidney weight increases throughout life in rats, while kidney mass and size in humans peaks in the fourth decade and declines thereafter. Care should be taken when reading the literature to keep in mind that changes seen in animal models may not be reflected by parallel changes in humans. Historical data from human postmortems describing changes in the kidney made no effort to exclude patients with renal disease or significant comorbidities. More recently data on aging have been developed from longitudinal studies, such as the Baltimore Longitudinal Aging Study, where the medical histories of volunteers are well documented. There are also data accumulating from the renal transplant population. Older living donors are increasingly being used and are put through a rigorous medical work-up for renal function and comorbid conditions before being accepted as donors. This has allowed acquisition of data on normal aging in the kidney, uncomplicated by the presence of medical comorbidities. Aging in the kidney is generally characterized by spontaneous progressive decline in renal function accompanied by thickening of the basement membrane, mesangial expansion, and focal glomerulosclerosis.

Functional Changes

Changes in renal function with age are well documented, both in human and animal models. Although baseline homeostasis of fluids and electrolytes is maintained with normal aging, there is a progressive decline in renal reserve. This results in a compromise in the kidney's ability to respond to either a salt or water load or deficit. This manifests clinically in patients being vulnerable to superimposed renal complications during acute illnesses. Chronic conditions such as hypertension accelerate this age-related loss of renal reserve and increased vulnerability in these patients should be anticipated. Age-related changes in function will be considered by separate functional domain within the kidney.

Renal Blood Flow

Average renal blood flow decreases about 10 percent per decade, dropping from 600 mL per minute per 1.73 m² to 300 mL per minute per 1.73 m² by the ninth decade. This is accompanied by increasing resistance in both afferent and efferent arterioles. These changes occur independent of cardiac output or reductions in renal mass. This decline in renal blood flow is thought to contribute to the decline in efficiency with which the aging kidney responds to fluid and electrolyte load and loss.

Glomerular Filtration Rate

There is a wide variation in the rate and extent of changes in the kidney within the older population. Approximately 30 percent of the population show no measurable decline in renal function with normal aging. The bulk of the population loses about 10 percent of glomerular filtration rate and 10 percent of renal plasma flow per year after the fourth decade. Between 5 and 10 percent of the population shows accelerated loss, even in the absence of identifiable comorbidities. Because there is also a steady loss of muscle bulk with age, with concomitant reduction in creatinine production, serum creatinine should remain constant. Rises in serum creatinine should therefore be taken seriously and not dismissed as normal aging. As can be seen in Fig. 44.1, serum creatinines at the upper limit of the "normal range" in an older individual represent significant functional decline, and thought should be given to renal dosing of medications. These curves were calculated using the

Cockcroft-Gault equation for a 70-kg man:

$$\text{Creat Cl} = \frac{(140 - \text{age})(\text{wt-kg})}{72 - \text{se creatinine (mg/dl)}}$$

Results for women should be multiplied by 0.85, which shifts the curves downward. In frail older women with very little residual muscle mass, this equation probably overestimates glomerular filtration rates. This steady decline in renal function with age manifests itself clinically as impaired ability to excrete a salt or water load. Extra care should be given when replacing fluids in an older individual to prevent extracellular fluid overload.

Proteinuria

Despite the significant decline in glomerular filtration rate that occurs with aging, proteinuria is not a normal feature of the aging process. Proteinuria is always a pathological finding and requires a full work-up. In contrast, in most rodent models, particularly in the rat, proteinuria is a normal feature of the aging kidney. This difference between humans and rodents should be kept in mind when reading the aging literature.

Tubular Function

Older individuals are well known to be more susceptible to acute renal failure. Much of the information on tubular function comes from animal studies, particularly rat models. Rats spontaneously develop proteinuria with aging, and this protein load is believed to be toxic to the tubule. Because proteinuria is not a feature of normal aging in man, these animal studies may not paint an accurate picture of changes in tubular function in humans. There are also large numbers of studies in experimental animals looking at vasoconstrictive and vasodilatory responses in the older kidney. Impaired response to atrial natriuretic

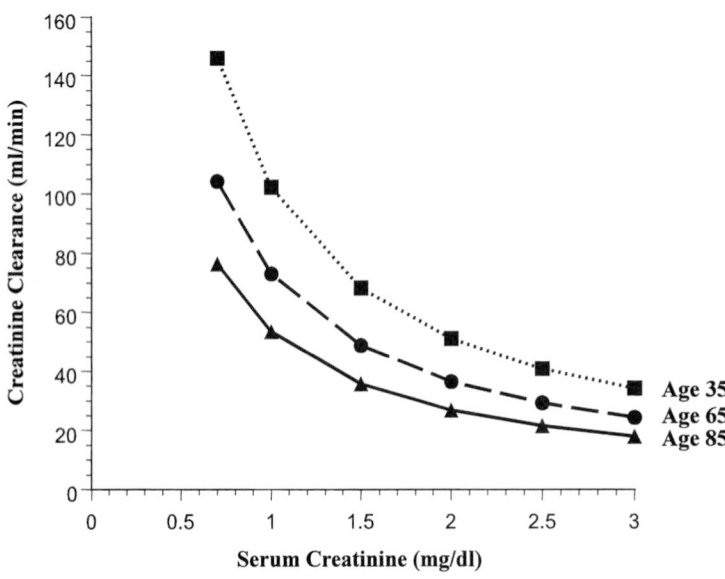

Figure 44-1 Relationship between serum creatinine and calculated creatinine clearance for men aged 35 years, 65 years, and 85 years. Calculations are based on a 70-kg man.

peptide (ANP), acetylcholine, and blunted responses of cyclic adenosine monophosphate to β-adrenergic stimulus have all been implicated. Virtually none of these findings have been confirmed in man. Functional magnetic resonance imaging in older volunteers has demonstrated decreased ability to modulate renal medullary oxygenation. Whether this is a result of fixed vascular changes or changes in renal autocrine systems such as prostaglandins, dopamine, nitric oxide, natruretic peptides, or endothelin is not clear. The result clinically is increased sensitivity to acute ischemic renal failure.

Animal and human studies have shown impaired concentrating ability in the older kidney. Whether this is due to intrinsic defects in the tubular epithelium or impaired response to antidiuretic hormone is not clear. Studies have also demonstrated impaired capacity to acidify urine manifested clinically as reduced excretion of an acid load. Whatever the underlying mechanism, older individuals are less likely to be able to maintain normal homeostasis when challenged. Although there is an age-related decline in tubular functions such as glucose and amino acid transport, these declines closely parallel the decline in glomerular filtration rate and are believed to correlate with the loss of nephrons rather than aging of the tubule. Age-related changes in sodium and potassium homeostasis, acid excretion and water handling are discussed in Chap. 45.

Older individuals are also more sensitive to nephrotoxic injury. Careful thought should be given to the choice and dosing of antibiotics and other nephrotoxic drugs. Increased age is a risk factor for the development of radiocontrast nephropathy. Special care should be exercised before tests requiring radiocontrast are ordered.

Donor Organ Viability

Age also impacts on the viability of kidneys for transplantation. With the steady increase in living related and unrelated donations, more organs have become available for use in the older population. Although nationwide probably less than 5 percent of older individuals reaching end-stage renal disease are being considered for transplantation, many larger transplant programs are routinely offering transplantation to people in their late sixties and early seventies if they are otherwise in good health. Donated organs are commonly coming from a similar aged spouse or family member. Age of the donated organ appears to be an independent risk factor for graft survival. This does not appear to be immune mediated, as older recipients have lower risk of rejection. These organs typically show delayed graft function posttransplant, with chronic allograft nephropathy and result in higher baseline serum creatinines long-term. It has been postulated that this is caused by impaired response to injury in the older kidney, but there is no real scientific evidence to support this at the current time.

Underlying Structural Changes

There is at least 100 years of meticulous research describing the anatomic changes that underlie the functional changes that we see in our patients as they age.

Gross Anatomy

Kidneys grow vigorously from birth through adolescence, reaching their maximum weight and volume during the third decade of life. In humans, although not in most laboratory animals, this weight starts to decline after the fourth decade and continues its decline throughout the remaining life span. Most of the decline in weight and volume appears to happen in the cortex, with relative sparing of the medulla.

The Glomerulus

The young healthy human kidney contains roughly 1 million nephrons. There is no evidence for postnatal nephrogenesis. This underlies the Brenner hypothesis that low-birth-weight babies might have fewer initial nephrons and as a result are more susceptible to renal failure in later life. Although there is some observational data to support this hypothesis, no causal relationship has been proved. There is a steady decline in nephron number with age that starts around the fourth decade, and it this decline that is believed to underlie the decline in glomerular filtration rate discussed above. In studies of kidneys obtained at autopsy from patients with no known history of renal disease, light microscopy showed the development of a focal sclerosing process, accompanied by thickening of the glomerular basement membrane. There was a steady progression with age in the percentage of glomeruli that were scared. By age 50 years, all subjects examined had some evidence of sclerosis, with the percentage of sclerotic glomeruli increasing steadily with age.

Age-related Glomerulosclerosis

Sclerotic glomeruli typically first appear in the fifth decade. This starts as a segmental process with one part of a glomerulus becoming acellular and normal architecture is replaced by extracellular matrix. The glomerular tuft becomes adherent to Bowman's capsule (Fig. 44-2)(Color Plate 1). Gradually an entire glomerulus becomes sclerosed and shrivels down with resultant loss of that nephron and its filtration capacity. It is not known what triggers this pattern of focal sclerosis, which is apparently randomly scattered throughout the cortex. The glomerular tuft increase in size with age. Concomitant with this expansion is an increase in endothelial and mesangial cells, such that the ratio of cell to glomerular area remains constant. Podocytes, the specialized cells that form the filtration barrier in the glomerulus, are postmitotic. They are not able to multiply in response to the increase in tuft volume, and become a progressively smaller percentage of the total cells making up the glomerular tuft. As the filtration area that they have to cover increases, it is believed that they may drop off the basement membrane leaving a denuded area behind. It is this area of bare basement membrane that acts as the trigger for the sclerosing process. Studies of many different experimental models of glomerulosclerosis have concluded that loss of the podocyte and its inability to be replaced is the sentinel event that triggers sclerosis. Studies of the puromycin aminonucleoside model in rats have shown that

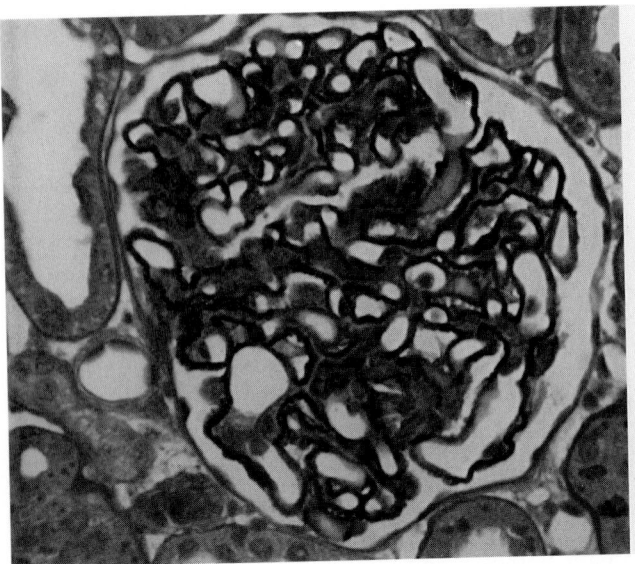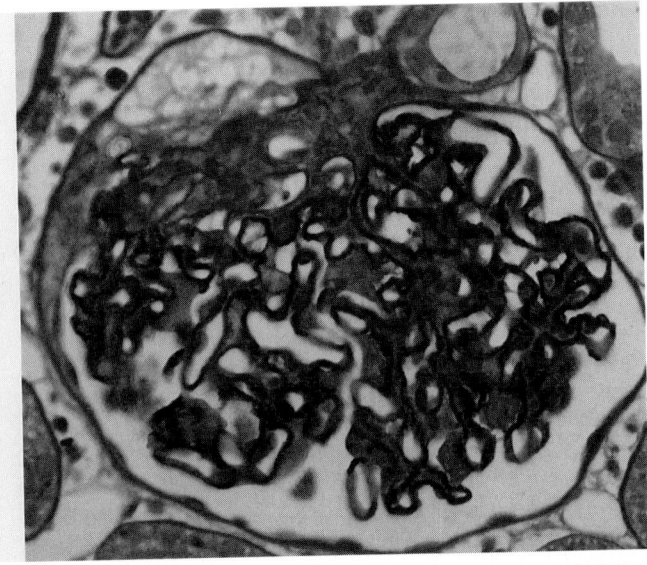

Figure 44-2   Renal glomeruli from a 24-month-old Fischer 344 rat stained with a podocyte marker, GLEPP1, and counterstained with period acid-Schiff. *Left panel:* Normal glomerulus showing normal architecture of the glomerular tuft. *Right panel:* Age-related glomerulosclerosis showing normal cellular architecture replaced by extracellular matrix and adherence to Bowman's capsule.

loss of podocytes precedes the appearance of sclerosis, and podocytes markers can be detected in the urine prior to the development of global sclerosis.

Models of induced glomerular injury, of course, do not exist in man. However, selective loss of podocytes in the kidneys of type I diabetics as diabetic nephropathy progresses has been demonstrated. Podocyte number per glomerulus has been shown to be the best predictor of progression of diabetic nephropathy in Pima Indians with type II diabetes. Extensive studies of the aging process in rat kidneys have noted that a decline in podocyte counts accompanies the appearance of glomerulosclerosis.

Some authors suggest a role for the mesangial cell in initiating the sclerosis process. Certainly with aging, an increase in mesangial matrix and mesangial cell numbers is seen. However, this increase is just as marked in strains of rats that do not develop age-related glomerulosclerosis, as it is in strains that do. Several authors have examined mesangial cell activation in rat models of glomerulosclerosis and found little or none. This suggests that mesangial expansion is a benign manifestation of the aging process rather than a pathologic one.

The Tubule

With the loss of the glomerulus, the tubular section of the nephron usually degenerates and is replaced by connective tissue. Tubular hypertrophy then occurs in the remaining nephrons, principally in the proximal convoluted tubule. This appears to result from both hypertrophy and hyperplasia. With thinning of the cortex there is a decrease in tubule length, and development of diverticula in the distal convoluted tubule. As nephrons are lost, there is generalized tubular interstitial fibrosis. The structure of the distal tubule does not appear to change significantly with age.

The Vasculature

Renal arteries undergo age-related thickening, similar to that seen throughout the circulation. Smaller arteries may become tortuous and show luminal irregularities. When a glomerulus becomes sclerosed, there is frequent formation of an arteriovenous shunt as the afferent and efferent arterioles develop a direct connection, as the glomerular capillary is lost. This shunt is very important in maintaining medullary blood flow. Physiologic studies in both animals and man have documented a decline in renal blood flow and an increase in vascular resistance with age. Studies of renal perfusion in healthy older individuals from a pool of potential kidney donors show steady declines in renal perfusion with age that exceeds the reduction in renal mass, suggesting that declines in blood flow were a significant factor in the changes seen in renal function with age. These changes contribute to the susceptibility of older individuals to acute renal failure, volume overload, and electrolyte abnormalities.

Infarcts may occur in the kidney, just as they do in other tissues of the body. Because one-fifth of the circulating volume passes through the kidney each minute, the kidney is also particularly susceptible to embolization. If other signs of embolization are visible clinically, it is highly probable that the kidney is also undergoing embolization, and embolic disease should certainly be kept in mind in an older individual with widespread vascular disease who demonstrates accelerated loss of renal function.

MECHANISMS UNDERLYING THE DECLINE IN RENAL FUNCTION

There is no clear-cut consensus about what mechanisms underlie the structural and functional changes occurring in the kidney in the older population. It is fairly clear, however, that there are both predisposing genetic and environmental factors that play a role.

Genetic Predisposition

There are as yet no genes known to cause age-related glomerulosclerosis. Accumulating evidence from animals studies, combined with evidence of genetic predisposition in man, has led to a concerted effort to seek genes that may increase susceptibility to renal failure in individuals.

Animal Models

Rats are particularly susceptible to renal failure and much of the work with models of renal disease has been carried out in laboratory rat strains. There are very marked strain differences in susceptibility to age-related glomerulosclerosis. Because these rats are maintained in pathogen-free environments and are fed uniform, scientifically developed diets, this strongly suggests a genetic basis for the development of age-related glomerulosclerosis. The appearance of glomerulosclerosis has been reported as early as 5 months in the Milan normotensive rat, with extensive disease by 10 months of age. This occurs in the total absence of hypertension, and is not ameliorated by administration of angiotensin-converting enzyme (ACE) inhibitors. Wistar rats were used as controls in this study and showed no significant disease during the same time period. In Sprague-Dawley rats, spontaneous age-related glomerulosclerosis first becomes apparent around 9 months of age, and disease becomes widespread by 18 months of age. In Fischer 344 rats, little glomerulosclerosis is seen until almost 2 years of age, with fairly rapid progression thereafter. Other rat strains appear remarkably resistant to renal disease. Brown Norway rats show minimal sclerosis, even at 32 months of age, an advanced age in rat life span.

Human Studies

Clearly these kinds of studies cannot be duplicated in humans. However, there are observational data that would support a similar variation in genetic susceptibility in man. Cross-sectional studies, donor organ data, and longitudinal studies clearly show wide variation in renal function with age. Approximately 5 to 10 percent of the population show accelerated loss of renal function with age, even in the absence of accelerating factors such as hypertension, while 30 percent show no measurable decline. In the presence of predisposing comorbidities, there is also wide variation in the development of renal disease. Some diabetics may never develop nephropathy, while others develop rapidly progressive renal disease early in the course of their diabetes, suggesting an underlying genetic renal susceptibility. Within the African American population, rates of renal disease are much higher than in the white population, independent of the precipitating cause. Within an ethnic group, there are also distinct differences in vulnerability. An African American who develops any predisposing disease, whether it be hypertension, diabetes, or lupus, who has a first-degree relative on renal replacement therapy has a ninefold increased risk of developing renal disease compared to another African American with the same disease burden who has no family history of renal disease. Similarly human immunodeficiency virus (HIV)-associated glomerulosclerosis occurs almost exclusively in the African American population, while HIV-associated mesangial hyperplasia and immune-complex glomerular nephritis occur equally in all ethnic groups. Thus, there is evidence to suggest a genetic predisposition with respect to the development of glomerulosclerosis. Considerable effort and resources are currently being directed towards identifying genes that predisposed to renal disease, so we can expect to have greater understanding of this process soon.

Environmental Predisposing Factors

It has been well known for many years that several diseases predispose to renal failure and will accelerate the progress of age-related glomerulosclerosis. By far, the most frequent of these are hypertension and diabetes, both common disorders in the older population. However, several other mechanisms have been postulated to underlie the aging changes in the kidney.

Diet

One of the most striking aspects of rodent models of age-related nephropathy in the kidney is its complete reversal with calorie restriction. Both the anatomic and functional changes related to aging in the kidney are completely abolished in animals that are fed two-thirds of the calories given to their ad lib fed litter mates. Even though these animals live one-third longer than their ad lib fed littermates, they do not develop age-related glomerulosclerosis. Several explanations have been proffered to account for this observation.

Free Radicals and Lipid Peroxides

One possible explanation for the profound effects of calorie restriction is a reduction in the generation of free radicals and lipid peroxides. There is a wide body of literature discussing the damaging effects of free radicals on cellular systems and the role that this plays in aging. The main consequence of free radical production is lipid peroxidation, which results in damage to cellular proteins, lipids, and nucleic acids. Increased calorie intake is believed to fuel increased free radical production with accelerated aging damage. This hypothesis has generated interest in the role of antioxidants in slowing the aging process. Studies of the effects of supplementing the diets of Sprague-Dawley rats with vitamin E 50 IU/kg, in which investigators were able to measure reductions in markers of oxidative stress and slow the rate of decline in glomerular filtration rate, glomerulosclerosis could not be prevented. Studies in humans with vitamin E have also been disappointing.

Protein Restriction

The benefits of calorie restriction have been attributed to concomitant reductions in dietary protein. There is a large body of older literature on protein restriction in experimental animal models of renal disease. In many of these studies, experimental and control animals were not fed isocaloric diets, and protein restriction also meant calorie restriction. Many of these studies show a slowing in the progression of established renal disease; however, the results were not corrected for total calorie content. Studies of spontaneous age-related glomerulosclerosis in Fischer 344 rats show that protein restriction was much less effective than calorie restriction in preventing age-related declines in renal function. Modest benefits from protein restriction when rats were fed isocaloric diets were demonstrated. Some benefit was also demonstrated when the type of protein in the diet was changed from casein to soy. In contrast, calorie-restricted animals have little or no decline in renal function and no significant glomerulosclerosis, despite significantly increased longevity. Rats that are fed a high protein diet, but restricted to 60 percent calorie intake compared to their ad lib fed littermates, also show dramatic reductions in age-related glomerulosclerosis. Clearly protein restriction does have some benefit in the prevention of age-related nephropathy, but that advantage is small compared to those achieved with caloric restriction. Very few of the studies have looked at changes in sodium, phosphate, and calcium content of the experimental diets. Many of the results of protein restriction can be duplicated by phosphate restriction. The relevance of these studies in humans remains unclear. An observational study, that included individuals up to 80 years of age, compared healthy vegetarians who consume an average of 30 g/d of protein with nonvegetarians who consume an average of 100 g/d. No differences between groups in terms of renal function were shown. There is certainly evidence to support protein restriction in patients with established renal disease to reduce symptoms of uremia, but none to support the role of protein restriction to prevent age-related changes in the human kidney.

Lipids

There is a well-established link between lipids and cardiovascular disease, and restriction of fat intake accompanied by treatment of hyperlipidemia has been shown to be efficacious in preventing or slowing the progress of cardiovascular disease. Certainly, protecting the integrity and function of the vascular supply to the kidney is important to maintaining normal renal function. Evidence for benefits from the manipulation of lipids in renal disease comes mainly from animal models of diabetes. Certainly, animal studies using high-fat diets have shown accelerated progress of renal disease, but in most cases, diets were not corrected for total calorie intake. Lipogenic diets fed to Sprague-Dawley rats resulted in earlier appearance of widespread glomerulosclerosis, compared to standard fed animals. Use of lipid-lowering agents in a variety of animal models of glomerulosclerosis has shown reductions in the incidence of glomerular damage. Clinical studies show that patients with established renal disease, with or without

diabetes, have more rapid deterioration of renal function in the presence of hyperlipidemia. The relevance of lipids to the age-related decline in renal function remains to be established, but it would certainly be reasonable to recommend low-fat diet and lipid management in someone with declining renal function.

Hyperfiltration

The term hyperfiltration is used to describe putative glomerular injury from excessive long-term intraglomerular pressure. Normal age-related loss of glomeruli causes intraglomerular hypertension with hypertrophy of remaining glomeruli. Persistent intraglomerular hypertension causes pressure mediated renal injury. Most of the supporting evidence for this mechanism comes from animal models where one kidney and part of the remaining kidney are removed, leaving a partial kidney remnant. These animals develop a pattern of renal damage in the remnant indistinguishable from age-related glomerulosclerosis, but over an accelerated time course. Clearly, these kinds of studies cannot be duplicated in man. However long-term follow-up over 20 years has not shown accelerated declines in renal function in people who have donated one of their kidneys for transplantation, even though the remaining kidney does undergo hypertrophy.

Nutrition may also play a part in hyperfiltration. After a meal of protein, increases in both renal blood flow and glomerular filtration rate can be demonstrated in animals as well as in man. Excessive intake, particularly of animal proteins, would cause constant hyperperfusion in the kidney, leading to intraglomerular hypertension and accelerated glomerulosclerosis. This would certainly help to explain the benefits so clearly seen with calorie restriction in laboratory animals.

The efficacy of ACE inhibitors in preventing renal hyperperfusion damage early in the course of diabetes and hypertension would also lend support to the hyperfiltration hypothesis. Angiotensin II appears to be important in maintaining glomerular filtration pressure by vasoconstricting the efferent arteriole. ACE inhibition is believed to preserve renal function by blocking the vasoconstriction of the efferent arteriole and reducing intraglomerular pressure. Long-term ACE inhibition dramatically reduces the incidence of age-related glomerulosclerosis in Munich-Wistar rats. However, sufficient doses of ACE inhibitor to significantly lower systolic blood pressure in the treatment group as compared to the control animals was administered in these studies. Whether low doses of ACE inhibitors would help to maintain normal renal function in man, and prevent the appearance of age-related glomerulosclerosis, is a matter for speculation. There is no doubt about their efficacy in preventing progressive decline in renal function when there is underlying disease. It remains to be seen whether they have any role in modifying age-related changes.

CONSEQUENCES OF IMPAIRED RENAL FUNCTION

Patients who show signs of significantly diminished renal function should be managed aggressively, regardless of

Table 44-1 Life Expectancy for Selected Age Groups*

Age	Dialysis	US Population
40–44	6.7–9.2	30.1–40.8
50–54	5.1–6.9	22.5–31.5
60–64	3.7–5.1	16.0–22.8
70–74	2.7–3.5	10.8–15.2
80–84	2.0–2.4	6.9–8.8

*This table compares dialysis patients with general population statistics. Numbers are shown as ranges to accomodate differences by gender and ethnic group.

their age. Individuals who reach dialysis have a mortality rate 4 to 5 times that of age-matched controls (Table 44-1), and are at 10 times the risk of a cardiovascular event. It costs more than $60,000 per annum to maintain someone on dialysis, without including the cost of treatment for any other health problems. Transplantation is also expensive and requires the patient to remain on toxic immunosuppressive regimes for the rest of their life. Patients who show signs of impaired renal function should be managed with the idea of preventing them from reaching end-stage disease. Aggressive measures should be taken to reduce blood pressure with a goal of 125/75 mmHg, if tolerated. A regimen should be used that includes an ACE inhibitor or an angiotensin-receptor blocker. However, it should be kept in mind that neither of these classes of drug will confer significant renal protection in the absence of good blood pressure control. Lipids should also be aggressively managed, as should blood sugar and other potential accelerators of renal decline. Overweight patients should be encouraged to lose weight. Great care should be taken to avoid potential renal toxins, such as aminoglycoside antibiotics, nonsteroidal antiinflammatory drugs, and radiocontrast dyes. Renally excreted medications should be appropriately dosed in amount and frequency. Maintaining residual renal function confers on the patient a greatly superior prognosis when compared to renal replacement therapies. Hopefully, the current emphasis on finding genes that predispose to declines in renal function and the development of age-related glomerulosclerosis will help us to identify those at greatest risk before major losses of function have occurred. As with recent gains in the prevention of cardiovascular disease through control of risk factors, it is anticipated that similar guidelines will be available for the prevention of age-related declines in renal function.

REFERENCES

Abrass CK: The nature of chronic progressive nephropathy in aging rats. *Adv Ren Replace Ther* 7(1):4, 2000.

Clark B: Biology of renal aging in humans. *Adv Ren Replace Ther* 7(1):11, 2000.

Epstein M: Aging and the kidney. *J Am Soc Nephrol* 7:1106, 1996.

Kriz W et al: Progression of glomerular diseases: Is the podocyte the culprit? *Kidney Int* 54:687, 1998.

Lindeman RD et al: Longitudinal studies on the rate of decline in renal function with age. *J Am Geriatr Soc* 33:278, 1985.

Neuringer JR, Brenner BM: Hemodynamic theory of progressive renal disease: A 10-year update in brief review. *Am J Kidney Disease* 22(1):98, 1993.

Striker GE et al: Biology of disease. Pathogenesis of nonimmune glomerulosclerosis: Studies in animals and potential applications to humans. *Lab Invest* 73(5):596, 1995.

United States Renal Data System: *1999 Annual Data Report.* Bethesda, MD, National Institutes of Health, National Institutes of Diabetes and Digestive and Kidney Diseases, April 1999.

Renal Disease

JAMES L. BAILEY • JEFF M. SANDS

The normal aging process induces structural and functional changes in the kidney characterized by progressive development of glomerulosclerosis and interstitial fibrosis. The timing of these changes is highly variable and is not necessarily inevitable, and appears to hinge on associated comorbid factors. Nearly one-third of the elderly population will not demonstrate a decrement in glomerular filtration rate with aging. Nevertheless, the average individual can expect to lose 0.8 mL/min/1.73 m²/year. Because the decline in glomerular filtration rate in individuals with aging is masked by a proportional decline in muscle mass, the serum creatinine generally remains constant. Failure to understand this fact can result in inappropriate dosing of medications with their associated morbidity. It can also result in underrecognition of renal pathology, for even subtle increases in serum creatinine in the elderly can represent a significant loss of renal function. This chapter reviews aspects of renal disease that are prevalent in the geriatric population.

EPIDEMIOLOGY

There has been an increase in the prevalence of renal disease with increasing age as a consequence of improved survival with comorbid conditions that result in renal dysfunction such as congestive heart failure, hypertension, diabetes, and atherosclerotic vascular disease. Currently, more than 20 percent of individuals older than age 65 years who are living in the United States have some degree of renal impairment and 60 percent of the patients with end-stage renal disease (ESRD) who are on chronic dialysis are older than age 65 years. Men and women are affected equally. This is surprising given the higher incidence of renal disease in young men; however, these statistics may reflect the higher survival rate for women in general.

The true incidence of *acute renal failure* in the elderly population is unknown. Multicenter studies from Europe report a threefold increase in the prevalence of acute renal failure in older people. In a recent prospective multicenter European study of acute renal failure involving hospitalized patients, more than 60 percent were older than age 60 years, with about one-third being older than age 70 years. The most frequent causes of acute renal failure were acute tubular necrosis (45 percent), prerenal azotemia (21 percent), acute chronic renal failure (13 percent), and obstructive uropathy (10 percent). Nearly half of the patients who later developed acute renal failure had normal renal function on presentation to the hospital, and the mortality rate was 45 percent. The incidence of prerenal azotemia in the elderly population is probably much higher; data from a series of elderly patients in the United Kingdom and Spain show that of 571 patients with azotemia, approximately 40 percent had evidence of prerenal acute renal failure.

The true incidence of *glomerular disease* cannot be determined in elderly patients because there are no population-based studies. Until recently, glomerulonephritis in geriatric patients received little attention because of fear of an increased risk of morbidity and mortality associated with renal biopsy, and to the more difficult interpretation of histopathologic findings. The increased proportion of elderly people entering renal replacement therapy programs has prompted nephrologists to reconsider the actual prevalence of glomerulonephritis occurring in this population. Referral patterns suggest that proteinuria or renal dysfunction are the most common reasons for renal biopsy. Of these cases, nearly one-third of the renal biopsies performed were for nephrotic syndrome, while another 50 percent were divided fairly equally between evaluation of acute and chronic renal insufficiency. Because of concerns for the safety and efficacy of the biopsy procedure in the past, older studies may not reflect the true incidence of disease. In fact, the Medical Research Council's glomerulonephritis registry in the United Kingdom shows that the percentage of elderly patients in this registry has increased from 6 percent in 1978 to 21 percent in 1990, suggesting that the number of geriatric patients undergoing a renal biopsy for the diagnosis of glomerular disease has also increased. As a result, the incidence of glomerulonephritis in the elderly population may be much higher than previously recognized and is probably higher than in younger groups less than 60 years of age. Idiopathic glomerulonephritis is the most common diagnosis, accounting for 65 to 70 percent of all reported cases. Whatever the histology, a renal biopsy from an elderly individual is more likely to show more than one pathological lesion as well as more evidence of senescence; there is more likely to be more glomerular scarring, interstitial fibrosis,

Table 45-1 Histology of Nephrotic Syndrome in Geriatric Patients

Study No.	Total (n)	NIL (%)	FSGS (%)	Memb (%)	Amyloid (%)	MCGN (%)	Other/Pro (%)	Diabetes (%)	Others (%)
1	63	21	16	33	14	5	5	5	1
2	164	21	3	38	12	5	14	4	3
3	107	2	15	48	10	5	4	5	11
4	317	11	4	37	11	6	13	4	13
5	50	4	4	32	22	4	34	—	—
6	31	6	—	52	—	16	—	—	22
7	35	6	3	43	3	3	23	—	—
8	92	14	0	35	20	11	15	1	2
9	33	27	—	39	9	6	6	—	13
10	87	8	0	34	10	8	15	0	—
11	59	3	6	21	7	4	5	8	5
12	76	25	4	41	13	—	13	—	8
Total	1,114	11.2	7.4	37.7	11.1	6.6	13.3	3.7	9

SOURCE: Adapted from Cameron JS (1996, p 324).

NIL = minimal change; FSGS = focal segmental glomerulosclerosis; memb = membranous; amyloid = amyloidosis; MCGN = membranoproliferative or mesangiocapillary; Other/Pro = other proliferative glomerulonephritis; Diabetes = diabetic nephropathy; Others = non-proliferative glomerulonephritis.

and tubular dropout. Among the glomerulonephritides (Table 45-1), membranous appears to be most common (37.7 percent) while minimal change (11.2 percent), amyloidosis (11.1 percent), focal segmental (7.4 percent), membranoproliferative (mesangiocapillary) (6.6 percent), other proliferative (13.3 percent), and nonproliferative (9.0 percent) account for the bulk of the rest. Because most patients with diabetic nephropathy can be presumptively diagnosed based on certain clinical criteria, its true incidence is underreported. For patients presenting with acute renal failure, crescentic glomerulonephritis (31 percent), acute interstitial nephritis (18.6 percent), acute tubular necrosis with nephrotic syndrome (7.5 percent), atheroemboli (7.1 percent), light-chain cast nephropathy (5.9 percent), and postinfectious (5.5 percent) are the most commonly reported lesions. Longitudinal studies from Italy depict a changing pattern of glomerulonephritis in the elderly population with a much higher incidence of crescentic glomerulonephritis. Elderly patients with chronic renal insufficiency are most likely to have hypertensive nephrosclerosis, focal segmental glomerulosclerosis, interstitial nephritis, or amyloidosis on renal biopsy.

Epidemiologic surveys from England report that the prevalence and incidence of *nephrotic syndrome* in geriatric populations are similar if not higher than those in adult populations of all ages, with about 11 new cases per million people per year. Approximately 18 percent of newly diagnosed adults with nephrotic syndrome are age 60 years or older. The incidence may be higher, but many geriatric patients are not referred for renal biopsy because of age and functional status. This is especially true for patients older than 80 years of age. Geriatric patients with type II diabetes mellitus are also generally underreported in renal biopsy registries because diabetic nephropathy may go unrecognized and because the diagnosis can often be made without the necessity of a renal biopsy. Yet, more than 40 percent of elderly ESRD patients have underlying diabetic nephropathy as the etiology of their ESRD.

The frequency of *renovascular disease* in elderly patients is unknown. It may be an unexpected finding in patients investigated for nonrenal disease, but the prevalence of severe renal artery stenosis increases with age. Autopsy studies show that among those persons older than age 70 years at the time of death, 62 percent had severe renal artery disease. When present, renal artery stenosis was bilateral in 50 percent of cases.

A high incidence of renal artery stenosis among normotensive subjects also has been found in several patient cohort studies undergoing angiography. In one report of patients older than 50 years of age, 69 percent of patients with hypertension and 35 percent without hypertension had identifiable renal artery atherosclerotic disease. A prospective study from Duke University of 1302 patients undergoing elective diagnostic cardiac catheterization showed significant unilateral renal artery stenosis in 11 percent of patients and bilateral stenosis in 4 percent. Multivariate and univariate analyses identified several predictors of increased risk for significant renovascular disease, including older age, multivessel coronary artery disease, and congestive heart failure. Interestingly, a history of hypertension did not predict the presence of renal artery stenosis in this cohort. Other angiographic studies evaluating the prevalence of renal artery stenosis in patients with vascular disease have shown similar findings with a prevalence between 11 and 42 percent. The highest prevalence is found among patients with peripheral vascular and aorto-occlusive disease or aneurysms.

Renovascular disease may also occur in the setting of renal insufficiency. A recent report from Italy of a study that included elderly patients with renal insufficiency of unclear etiology and mild proteinuria (less than 1 g/d) showed a 56 percent prevalence of significant (>70 percent) stenosis at angiography. Other investigators have done angiographic screening of patients older than age 50 years entering renal replacement therapy programs and report finding renal artery stenosis in 11 to 16 percent of these patients.

ACUTE RENAL FAILURE

Definition

Acute renal failure (ARF) is defined as a sudden deterioration in renal function, sufficient to cause retention of nitrogenous waste in the body. The anatomic and physiologic changes occurring in the aging kidney, the presence of comorbid medical conditions, the use of excessive numbers of medications, and the higher prevalence of obstructive uropathy are all contributing factors that can cause ARF in the elderly.

Clinical Presentation

Prerenal azotemia, or functional ARF as a result of extracellular fluid contraction, is the main cause of acute renal failure in the geriatric population (Table 45-2). The reduced renal blood flow and glomerular filtration rate associated with aging leads to a reversible state of acute renal failure in the setting of superimposed volume contraction. Loss of fluids, internal fluid redistribution, decreased cardiac output, and medications are responsible for the majority of cases of prerenal ARF in older individuals. Common medications associated with ARF are nonsteroidal antiinflammatory drugs (NSAIDs), angiotensin-converting enzyme inhibitors (ACEIs) and angiotensin II type 1 receptor antagonist blockers (ARBs). The development of ARF secondary to ACEIs or ARBs in patients with renal artery stenosis is well known. However, recent publications also report cases of ACEIs and ARB-related ARF in patients without renovascular disease. Furthermore, a study from France reported that 67.5 percent of ACEIs-induced cases of ARF in elderly patients occurred in the absence of renal artery stenosis.

NSAID-induced ARF occurs more frequently in the elderly than in the general population, mainly because of the coexistence of conditions associated with decreased effective intravascular volume or true volume depletion. Under these conditions, the kidney is dependent on prostaglandins to maintain renal perfusion. Loss of this important autoregulatory mechanism results in acute renal failure. Advanced age is an independent risk factor for developing ARF in patients taking NSAIDs, presumably because of the normal, aging-related decrease in glomerular filtration rate (GFR).

Parenchymal causes of ARF include acute tubular necrosis (ATN), acute interstitial nephritis, acute glomerulonephritis, and renovascular disease. The most common cause of biopsy-proven intrinsic renal failure in geriatric patients is rapidly progressive glomerulonephritis. Vasculitis and idiopathic crescentic glomerulonephritis make up more than half of these cases.

Acute tubular necrosis results from prolonged renal ischemia or from exposure to nephrotoxins. The causes of ATN are multifactorial, however, the most common cause in elderly patients is volume depletion associated with renal hypoperfusion and ischemia. Complications of major surgery including intraoperative hypotension, postoperative fluid loss, and arrhythmias account for approximately one-third of the cases of ATN in the elderly. Sepsis-induced ATN occurs just as commonly. Nephrotoxic drugs may also cause ATN or acute interstitial nephritis. The former often results from a failure to consider age-related decreases in glomerular filtration rate while the latter is responsible for 10 percent of the cases or ARF. Aminoglycoside nephrotoxicity and radiocontrast-induced ARF are just two examples of drug induced renal failure.

Cholesterol emboli are another important cause of ARF in the geriatric population. Cholesterol crystals can become dislodged from atherosclerotic plaques during intraaortic procedures, or may even arise spontaneously, and cause ARF by obstructing small renal arteries. This entity is important to consider in any patient with ARF following cardiac catheterization or aortic angiography. Rhabdomyolysis, in the settings of acute immobilization, infectious disease, cerebrovascular accidents, crush injury, hyperosmolar conditions, hyponatremia, hypothermia, and falls is being recognized as a prevalent and underdiagnosed cause of ATN in the elderly.

Postrenal or obstructive renal failure is one of the most significant causes of ARF in the elderly and may occur in 5 percent of the cases presenting with ARF. Common causes of obstruction in the geriatric population include: benign prostatic hypertrophy; prostatic carcinoma; retroperitoneal or pelvic neoplasms such as non-Hodgkin's lymphoma, carcinoma of the bladder, cervix, ovaries, or rectum; and neurogenic bladder due to diabetes mellitus. Prompt diagnosis is extremely important because prognosis for recovery of renal function depends on the length of time that the kidney is obstructed. As such, it is considered a true urologic emergency. Therefore, it is imperative to exclude the possibility of obstruction in any elderly patient presenting with ARF, especially in those situations of previous urologic pathology or recent abdominal surgery.

Table 45-2   Acute Renal Failure in the Elderly

Prerenal (acute reversible renal hypoperfusion) ARF
  Hypovolemia
    Fluid loss
      Gastrointestinal
        Diarrhea
        Fistulas
        Vomiting
      Renal
        Diuretic intake
        Salt Wasting
      Redistribution of the extracellular volume
        Shock (septic, cardiogenic), hypoalbuminemia,
          nephrotic syndrome, liver diseases
    Malnutrition
    Hemorrhage
    Inappropriate fluid restriction
    Interference with renal autoregulatory mechanisms
      ACEIs
      Cyclosporine
      NSAIDs
    Cardiac Failure
      Acute
        Acute myocardial infarction
        Arrhythmias
        Cardiac tamponade
        Malignant hypertension
      Chronic: ischemic and hypertensive
        cardiomyopathies
      Valvulopathies

Renal or intrinsic ARF
  Acute glomerulonephritis
    Mesangiocapillary
    Postinfectious
    Rapidly progressive
      Goodpasture's syndrome
      Idiopathic
      SLE
  Vasculitis
    Hypersensitivity angiitis
      Classic
      Hemolytic-uremic syndrome
      Henoch-Schönlein
      Mixed cryoglobulinemia
      Scleroderma
      Serum sickness
      Wegener's granulomatosis
    Polyarteritis nodosa
  Tubulointerstitial nephropathies
    Drugs
      ACEIs
      Allopurinol
      Ampicillin

Analgesics (including NSAIDs)
Cimetidine
Diphenylhydantoin
Methicillin
Thiazides
Infectious: acute pyelonephritis
Infiltrative
  Leukemia
  Lymphoma
  Sarcoidosis
Idiopathic
Intratubular obstruction
  Myeloma proteins
  Myoglobin
  Sulfonamides
  Urates
Hypercalcemia
Hepatorenal syndrome
Vascular obstruction
  Arterial
    Aneurysms
    Atheroembolic disease
  Venous: thrombosis of vena cava
Tubule cell damage
  Nephrotoxin-related
    Antibiotics (aminoglycosides)
    Iodinated contrast media
    IV Immunoglobulin G
    Metals (Hg, Ag, Pt, Bi)
    Organic solvents

Obstructive ARF
  Ureteral and pelvic
    Intrinsic obstruction
      Blood clots
      Fungus balls
      Sloughed papillae
        Diabetics
        Analgesic abusers
      Stones
    Extrinsic obstruction
      Fecal impaction
      Malignancy
      Retroperitoneal fibrosis
  Bladder
    Bladder carcinoma
    Blood clots
    Neuropathic
    Prostatic hypertrophy
    Stones
  Urethra
    Phymosis
    Strictures

ACEI, angiotensin-converting enzyme inhibitor; ARF, acute renal failure; NSAID, nonsteroidal antiinflammatory drugs; SLE, systemic lupus erythematosis.

Source: Modified from Macias-Nunez JF et al. (1996, p. 333).

Diagnosis

A complete history, with special attention to potential nephrotoxic drugs and clinical clues of obstruction, is fundamental in establishing the diagnosis of ARF. Physical findings may be very subtle in the elderly but postural hypotension is usually present in states of true volume depletion. Use of the urinary sodium concentration or the fractional excretion of sodium as markers to differentiate acute prerenal azotemia from established ATN are less reliable in the geriatric population than in the general population. Elderly individuals have a decreased ability to concentrate their urine or respond to sudden changes in sodium and water balance because of aging-related disturbances in the tubular handling of water and/or sodium reabsorption. Thus, geriatric patients with prerenal indices may still have ATN as a result of the physiologic changes associated with aging, and early nephrologic consultation is warranted in any patient with ARF. The most reliable indicator of prerenal azotemia is its reversal following volume repletion, and a judicious volume challenge is indicated if the patient is not volume overloaded.

In the setting of ARF, ultrasonography is the imaging procedure of choice for the diagnosis of obstruction, kidney stones, or renal masses, and for the determination of renal size. Although there are a few case reports of urinary tract obstruction secondary to prior malignancy with minimal or no dilation of the collecting system on ultrasonography, these cases are rare, and duplex Doppler ultrasonography may prove to be a useful diagnostic tool in these instances. Computerized tomography (CT) scans often do not provide any further diagnostic information and should be reserved for those cases where the kidneys are poorly visualized.

Indications for renal biopsy in elderly patients with acute renal failure include the following: (1) prolonged oliguria (3 to 4 weeks); (2) ARF associated with systemic illnesses such as vasculitis; (3) rapidly progressive glomerulonephritis; (4) acute tubulointerstitial nephritis; and (5) anuria in the absence of obstruction. Advanced age alone is not a contraindication for renal biopsy.

Treatment

The management of acute renal failure in the elderly should follow the same principles as in the general population. Maintenance of adequate intravascular volume is paramount in maintaining renal blood flow. Hemodynamic monitoring in critically ill patients is preferable with right-heart catheterization as indicated to measure pulmonary capillary wedge pressure. The routine use of renal dose dopamine for ARF should be discouraged because of the lack of demonstrated efficacy in this setting. Moreover, combinations of α- and β-adrenergic agonists, or colloid and blood transfusions to increase cardiac output to supranormal levels are not helpful in the setting of established acute tubular necrosis. Fenoldopam, a dopamine receptor agonist, is undergoing clinical trials to determine its efficacy as a prophylactic agent for ARF. Medications should

be adjusted for the degree of renal insufficiency and appropriate dietary sodium, potassium and protein restrictions instituted. A Foley catheter should be placed to rule out and treat bladder outlet obstruction. A previously placed Foley catheter should always be replaced, regardless of whether it flushes.

The indication for renal replacement therapy in ARF must be individualized for each patient and depends upon the volume status of the patient and the need for solute clearance. Timely renal consultation early in the course of ARF often obviates the need for dialysis intervention. For those patients with ARF requiring dialysis, the required dialysis dose has not been established and may hinge on volume status and catabolic state. Acute peritoneal dialysis and hemodialysis have been used in elderly patients with ARF with similar results and complications as in younger adult patients. Continuous renal replacement therapy offers the advantages of slow controlled ultrafiltration and represents a potentially promising new technique that needs to be evaluated prospectively in a large multi center trial. Biocompatible membranes are used routinely now because of improved outcomes in patients with ARF.

Nutritional considerations warrant special consideration for any elderly patient with renal disease. There are advantages in early appropriate restriction of sodium, potassium, phosphorus and protein for the elderly patient with acute renal failure. Restricting the dietary protein intake to 0.6 to 0.8 g/kg ideal body weight for those patients not yet on dialysis results in maintenance of nitrogen balance, control of metabolic acidosis, and control of elemental phosphorus normally excreted by the kidney. Potassium and sodium are restricted to 2 g per day based on nutritional requirements. For those patients on dialysis, the dietary protein restriction can be liberalized to 1.0 to 1.2 g/kg ideal body weight for hemodialysis patients and 1.2 to 1.4 g/kg ideal body weight for patients on peritoneal dialysis.

Prognosis

The mortality rate for ARF remains high. For critically ill patients, mortality rates approach 60 percent with sepsis-induced ARF having a worse prognosis than nonseptic ARF. The influence of age on outcome of ARF is debated, however, the elderly patient generally has less renal reserve than a younger individual and is more prone to ARF. As a result, an elderly patient has a moderately worse prognosis than a corresponding younger patient. Nevertheless, age alone should not be used as a discriminating factor in therapeutic decisions concerning ARF.

GLOMERULAR DISEASES

There has been a change in the clinical approach toward patients with acute renal failure or nephrotic syndrome in the geriatric population. Because of the routine use of ultrasonographic guidance for renal biopsies, as well as improvements in the size and accuracy of the biopsy needle, the success rate in obtaining a diagnostic renal biopsy

Table 45-3 Comparison of Mode of Presentation Between Patients Aged Greater than 65 Years and Those Aged 20 to 65 Years at the Time of Biopsy and Reported as Having Idiopathic Glomerulonephritis

| Mode of Presentation | Age | | | |
| | >65 Years | | 20 to 65 Years | |
	(n)	(%)	(n)	(%)
Acute renal failure	37	14	240	11
Asymptomatic urinary abnormality	17	6	841	38
Chronic renal failure	54	20	168	7
Hypertension	4	1	40	2
Nephrotic syndrome	140	52	715	32
Unknown	19	7	226	10
Total number	271	100	2,230	100

SOURCE: Modified from Davison AM and Johnston PA (1993, p 41).

that provides clinically useful information has improved to greater than 90 percent. This is important because ESRD caused by glomerulonephritis currently accounts for approximately 24 percent of patients requiring dialysis in Europe and a higher percentage in the United States. Recent reviews suggest that the clinical features, histopathologic classification, and clinical outcome of glomerulonephritis in elderly patients are comparable to those of younger adults. Based on these observations, a reliable diagnosis and an effective therapeutic plan have to be advocated in elderly patients, similar to the approach taken in younger adult patients.

Clinical Presentation

Elderly patients with biopsy-proven glomerulonephritis usually present with the following major clinical syndromes (Table 45-3): (1) nephrotic syndrome (50 to 60 percent in some series), characterized by heavy proteinuria and a variable tendency toward edema, hypertension, renal failure, and hyperlipidemia; (2) acute glomerulonephritis or acute nephritic syndrome, characterized by the abrupt clinical onset of hematuria, proteinuria, decreased GFR, fluid and salt retention, hypertension, and occasionally, oliguria; (3) rapidly progressive glomerulonephritis, whose clinical pattern includes a more insidious onset, progressive loss of renal function, and, frequently, oliguria; (4) chronic glomerulonephritis, characterized by chronic renal failure accompanied by various degrees of proteinuria, hematuria, and hypertension, and a clinical course that is usually progressive but which may be protracted over several years; and (5) urinary abnormalities with few or no symptoms. Although an asymptomatic urinary abnormality is the single most common clinical presentation in younger patients, it is rarely found in geriatric populations (age ≥60). The reason for this difference may be the aging-related

reduction in renal function, or the lack of routine urine testing in elderly patients even though they are more likely to be seeking advice for medical complaints.

Acute Glomerulonephritis and Rapidly Progressive Glomerulonephritis

These two clinical syndromes often present as acute renal failure in the elderly. The glomerular findings are similar to younger adults presenting with crescentic glomerulonephritis. Indeed, crescentic glomerulonephritis is the most common lesion found on renal biopsy in this group of geriatric patients. With aging, the glomerular basement membrane becomes thickened and the glomerular surface area decreases. As a result, the filtration fraction increases, (glomerular filtration rate/renal plasma flow). These changes tend to render the glomerulus more liable to immune complex mediated damage. In addition, the increased prevalence of autoantibodies and immune-complexes in the elderly increase the risk of immunologically mediated glomerular injury, but these factors may be offset by the reduced renal plasma flow and the aging-associated impairment of cell-mediated immunity. This leads some investigators to believe that there may be other, currently unrecognized factors that increase the risk of developing glomerulonephritis in geriatric patients.

Postinfectious glomerulonephritis is present in approximately 6 to 8 percent of biopsy series of geriatric patients presenting with acute renal failure. The clinical features are similar to those found in younger adults, but the clinical course is associated with a higher incidence of hypertension, azotemia, and end-stage renal disease. Underrecognized is postinfectious glomerulonephritis associated with aortofemoral bypass graft infections, especially those caused by *Salmonella,* which result in increased risk for morbidity and mortality.

Renal biopsies from patients with rapidly progressive glomerulonephritis (RPGN) demonstrate extensive accumulation of cells in Bowman's space (crescents). Although the disorders associated with RPGN can be classified as either primary glomerular disorders or secondary forms associated with infectious processes, multisystem disorders, or drug reactions (Table 45-4), three deserve special attention in the elderly: antineutrophil cytoplasmic antibody (ANCA)-associated renal disease, hepatitis C-associated cryoglobulinemia, and Henoch-Schönlein purpura.

ANCA-associated renal disease presents as a small-vessel vasculitis or as an isolated primary pauci-immune necrotizing and crescentic glomerulonephritis without vasculitis. The clinical manifestations depend on the severity and stage of the underlying renal injury. The light microscopy morphologic findings range from focal sclerosing glomerulonephritis associated with hematuria and/or proteinuria, to more aggressive patterns including necrosis with a few crescents to overt cellular crescentic changes associated with acute nephritis and a rapid loss of renal function. In addition, a few biopsy specimens will depict changes compatible with chronic glomerulonephritis and global glomerular sclerosis associated with slowly progressive nephritis and chronic renal failure.

The most common finding in elderly patients undergoing renal biopsy for the clinical syndrome of RPGN is isolated primary pauci-immune glomerulonephritis. The ANCA is positive in approximately 45 to 55 percent of these cases. Another 20 to 25 percent of patients present with identical histologic findings associated with small vessel vasculitis in an extrarenal location. This group of patients has been classified as microscopic polyangiitis (MPO) according to the Chapel Hill Consensus Conference on the Nomenclature of Systemic Vasculitis. In addition to the renal histologic pattern described above, another 12 to 15 percent of patients present with granulomatous inflammation involving the respiratory tract and will be diagnosed with Wegener's granulomatosis.

The two known staining patterns of ANCA are perinuclear and cytoplasmic. The perinuclear pattern (P-ANCA) is usually associated with specific reactivity against myeloperoxidase and is associated with microscopic polyangiitis in approximately 40 to 55 percent of cases. This pattern is strongly associated with primary pauci-immune crescentic glomerulonephritis in 60 to 70 percent of cases. Finally, approximately 15 to 25 percent of patients with Wegener's granulomatosis present with reactivity to perinuclear ANCA.

The cytoplasmic ANCA (C-ANCA) pattern is associated with reactivity against a serine proteinase (proteinase 3, PR3), and is found in 65 to 75 percent of patients classified as Wegener's granulomatosis, 35 to 45 percent of patients with microscopic polyangiitis, and 30 to 40 percent of patients with primary pauci-immune glomerulonephritis. Ten to 20 percent of patients with one of these three diagnoses are ANCA negative. The treatment of this group of disorders has only been reported in uncontrolled studies.

In addition to testing patients presenting with vasculitis for ANCA, it is important to test for antiglomerular basement membrane (anti-GBM) disease and for systemic lupus erythematosus, because the treatment options for these

Table 45-4 Classification of Rapidly Progressive Glomerulonephritis

Primary diffuse crescentic glomerulonephritis
  Type I: anti-GBM–mediated disease without pulmonary hemorrhage (with anti-GBM)
  Type II: immune complex-associated disease (without anti-GMB or ANCA)*
  Type III: pauci-immune (with ANCA)†
  Type IV: mixed pattern (with anti-GBM and ANCA)
  Type V: pauci-immune (without ANCA or anti-GBM)
Fibrillary and immunotactoid glomerulonephritis
Focal sclerosis (rare)
IgA nephropathy
Mesangiocapillary glomerulonephritis (especially type II)
Membranous glomerulonephritis (with or without anti-GBM)
Superimposed on another primary glomerular disease

Associated with infectious disease
  Hepatitis B and C
  Histoplasmosis
  Infective endocarditis
  Influenza (?)
  Mycoplasma infection
  Poststreptococcal glomerulonephritis
  Visceral abscesses

Associated with multisystem disease
  Carcinoma (lung, bladder, prostate)
  Goodpasture disease (anti-GBM with pulmonary hemorrhage)
  Lymphoma
  Mixed (IgG/IgM) cryoimmunoglobulinemia (hepatitis C)
  Relapsing polychondritis
  Henoch-Schönlein purpura
  Systemic lupus erythematosus
  Systemic polyangiitis
    Churg-Strauss syndrome
    Microscopic polyangiitis (with ANCA)
    Wegener granulomatosis (with ANCA)
    Other variants

Associated with medications
  Allopurinol
  Bucillamine
  D-Penicillamine
  Hydralazine
  Rifampin

*† ANCA, antineutrophil cytoplasmic antibodies; GBM, glomerular basement membrane.
SOURCE: Modified from Glassock RJ (1995, p 682).

two diseases are quite different. Referral to a nephrologist is essential for proper diagnosis and therapy.

Most patients with microscopic polyangiitis or primary necrotizing and crescentic glomerulonephritis achieve remission with therapeutic regimens based on corticosteroids in combination with either intravenous or oral cyclophosphamide. Recent reviews report a long-term remission rate of 60 to 85 percent in patients with these disorders, but relapse occurs in up to 40 percent of patients within 18 months. For those patients with systemic vasculitis such as Wegener's granulomatosis, long-term remission is not possible without the use of cyclophosphamide. The 5-year survival rates cited for patients older than 60 years of age at the time of diagnosis (31 percent) compared with those subjects younger than 60 years of age (83 percent), is partly a result of the reluctance of clinicians to use cyclophosphamide in the elderly patient. Although the toxicity and side effects of steroids and cytotoxic drugs increases with age, these medications should not be necessarily withheld in the elderly patient. Careful examination of the renal biopsy, clinical presentation, and the ANCA reactivity are needed to design an appropriate treatment strategy with the benefits and risks of therapy individualized for each patient. The reader is referred to reference sources listed at the end of this chapter for details about specific therapeutic protocols.

Hepatitis C-associated cryoglobulinemia associated with vasculitis and hepatitis can also present with RPGN. Associated findings include purpuric and necrotizing skin lesions in exposed areas, fever, acroparesthesia, Raynaud's phenomenon, urticaria, neuritis, arthralgia, and hepatosplenomegaly. Some series from Italy report hepatitis C as the second most common cause of secondary glomerulonephritis in the elderly population; amyloidosis is the most common cause. Serum immunoelectrophoresis shows abnormal circulating immunoglobulins that precipitate in the cold with a polyclonal immunoglobulin (Ig) G component and a monoclonal IgM with rheumatoid factor activity (type II cryoglobulinemia). Light microscopic examination of renal biopsies reveal diffuse endocapillary proliferation with a few crescents. Electron microscopic findings of typical intracapillary deposits and subendothelial electron-dense deposits, with a crystalline substructure, confirm the diagnosis.

In the past, immunosuppressive therapy was used for cryoglobulinemia-related vasculitis, but the effect of immunosuppression on chronic hepatitis C infection has not been well defined and could potentially accelerate viral replication. Reduction in the level of cryoglobulins by intensive plasma exchange may be associated with clinical remission, while the administration of interferon-α and ribavirin have the potential to revolutionize therapy for this disease but await future controlled trials.

Henoch-Schönlein purpura presents as a small-vessel vasculitis with IgA-dominant immune deposits, typically involving the skin, gut, and glomeruli, and is frequently associated with arthralgias or arthritis. Potential precipitating conditions in the elderly include alcohol abuse, malignancies, and some medications. This pattern of etiologic agents contrasts with the pattern in younger patients in whom infections are the most common etiologic agent. In general,

Henoch-Schönlein purpura is a benign, self-limited disorder, but the renal dysfunction is significantly worse in geriatric patients than in younger adults. Elderly patients present with a higher prevalence of hypertension, azotemia requiring renal replacement therapy, and histopathologic features of crescentic glomerulonephritis. Improvement in renal function has been noted in some patients after plasma exchange and immunosuppressive therapy, but the small number of cases reported and the lack of a controlled study prevent any firm therapeutic recommendations.

NEPHROTIC SYNDROME

Definition

The nephrotic syndrome consists of urinary protein losses in excess of 3.5 g per 1.73 m^2 body surface area per day in association with hypoalbuminemia, hypercholesterolemia, and peripheral edema. The onset is usually insidious but it can be explosive. As the major clinical manifestation of nephrotic syndrome is generalized edema, many geriatric patients are often misdiagnosed as having congestive heart failure. The etiologies of nephrotic syndrome include the primary glomerular diseases (minimal change disease, focal and segmental glomerulosclerosis, membranous glomerulonephropathy, membranoproliferative glomerulonephropathy), and glomerulonephritis secondary to systemic infiltrative diseases, neoplasms, chronic infectious diseases, atheroembolic disease, or medications.

Clinical Manifestations

The nephrotic syndrome often goes unrecognized in geriatric individuals since it frequently presents in an atypical manner. Because many geriatric patients have poor tissue turgor, edema frequently develops only in dependent portions of the body. Moreover, many geriatric patients with nephrotic syndrome will develop edema at higher plasma albumin concentrations than younger adults, who, in turn, develop edema at higher albumin levels than children. Hypercoagulability is a frequent complication of nephrotic syndrome and is particularly concerning in a geriatric patient who is bedridden. In some series, the proportion of patients who present with a significant complication such as deep venous thrombosis (DVT) or pulmonary embolus (PE) approaches 50 percent. Compared to younger adults, geriatric patients with nephrotic syndrome have a higher incidence of hypertension, hypercholesterolemia, and nonselective proteinuria, a lower value of glomerular filtration rate, and often present with microscopic hematuria. Microscopic hematuria is particularly common in geriatric patients with minimal change disease or hypertensive glomerulosclerosis. Geriatric age individuals with biopsy-proven minimal change disease present with persistent hematuria in 30 percent of cases and with hypertension in 44 percent of cases.

The pathogenesis of coincident nephrotic syndrome and acute renal failure remains obscure. Some investigators suggest that acute renal failure results from an increase in intrarenal pressure and the presence of proteinaceous casts which obstruct tubule lumens. This pathogenetic mechanism suggests that a renal biopsy should be obtained to aid in the management of the nephrotic syndrome in the elderly.

Approximately 5 percent of geriatric patients who present with nephrotic syndrome will have an underlying malignancy or develop one within a year. Of these patients, 33 percent will be diagnosed with membranous glomerulonephritis. In older series, 10 to 33 percent of geriatric individuals with nephrotic syndrome caused by membranous glomerulonephritis were found to have a malignancy, but recent studies suggest that patients with nephrotic syndrome do not have a higher incidence of malignant disease when compared to age-matched individuals without nephrotic syndrome. Currently, most investigators recommend that the only tests that should be performed in all patients presenting with nephrotic syndrome are a chest x-ray, because carcinoma of the lung is the most common malignancy associated with membranous glomerulonephritis, and a stool guaiac, because carcinoma of the colon is the next most common location for an unsuspected malignancy. If no evidence for a malignancy is found on physical examination, chest x-ray, or by occult blood testing, the patient should be carefully followed for the next 15 months for the appearance of a malignancy, and receive routine care thereafter.

The clinical presentation of nephrotic syndrome secondary to another systemic illness does not differ substantially between geriatric and younger adult patients. All patients presenting with nephrotic syndrome should be evaluated for amyloidosis, plasma cell dyscrasias, diabetes mellitus, hepatitis, syphilis, human immunodeficiency virus (HIV), collagen vascular disorders, and cryoglobulins.

Histopathology Findings

The interpretation of the histologic appearance of renal biopsy specimens from geriatric individuals with nephrotic syndrome represents a challenge to the nephropathologist because of the normal aging-related changes that occur in the kidney. Glomerulosclerosis (which can occur in up to 40 percent of remaining glomeruli), vascular changes (especially hypertension-induced changes), and interstitial fibrosis are common findings in normal kidneys from geriatric individuals and must be considered in evaluating renal pathology. However, minimal change disease and membranous glomerulopathy retain their typical histologic appearance and can be diagnosed by an experienced nephropathologist.

Secondary amyloidosis should be distinguished from primary amyloidosis because its prognosis is better and specific therapy aimed at the underlying disease may be available. Special stains including immunofluorescent antibodies against amyloid A protein are useful in diagnosing cases of secondary amyloidosis. Amyloid may be found infiltrating the glomerulus and may also be found infiltrating blood vessels and, occasionally, peritubular spaces. Light-chain glomerulopathy is characterized by the deposition of immunoglobulin light chains in a nodular or diffuse fashion along the basement membranes within the kidney.

Kappa light chains are found more frequently than lambda light chains.

Occasional patients will show histologic findings compatible with nonamyloid fibrillary glomerulopathies. Two categories are recognized on the basis of their ultrastructural appearance: fibrillary glomerulonephritis with extracellular deposits randomly oriented (10 to 30 nm diameter fibrils); and immunotactoid glomerulonephritis characterized by microtubular structures in a parallel array (25 to 45 nm diameter). Because these entities are fairly uncommon, the prognosis and therapeutic interventions remain obscure.

Focal segmental glomerulosclerosis was recently associated with atheroembolic renal disease. The pathologic changes produced by cholesterol atheroemboli show distinctive pathologic findings including glomerular collapse, foot process fusion, podocyte hypertrophy, and frequently, acute tubular injury. Finally, few patients with nephrotic syndrome caused by IgA nephropathy present in the geriatric age group.

Diagnosis

Nephrotic syndrome is often masked by other comorbid conditions in geriatric individuals. The patient evaluation should include microscopic examination of the urine by a nephrologist; serum creatinine; blood urea nitrogen (BUN); albumin; and cholesterol; 24-hour urine collection to quantitatively measure proteinuria and creatinine clearance; serum protein electrophoresis and immunoelectrophoresis; urine protein electrophoresis and immunoelectrophoresis; antinuclear antibody (ANA); antideoxyribonucleic acid (anti-DNA) antibody titer; hepatitis B and C serologies; syphilis serology; complement profile; cryoglobulins; lipoprotein profile; HIV; chest x-ray; and stool guaiac. Renal biopsy is essential for establishing the definitive histopathologic diagnosis.

Treatment and Prognosis

Definitive treatment for the nephrotic syndrome depends upon the histologic type. Regardless of the histology, some generalizations about therapy can be made. Every effort should be made to control the blood pressure. ACEIs and ARBs are rapidly becoming mainstays in treatment because of their efficacy in reducing proteinuria and numerous studies suggesting that they may slow progression of renal disease. If these agents are not tolerated, other agents can be substituted with a goal of maintaining the blood pressure at around 125/75 mmHg. Low-protein diets also have their utility, especially for those patients with heavy proteinuria; and dietary counseling, which is reimbursed by Medicare, can prove to be invaluable. The value of HMG-CoA (hydroxymethylglutaryl coenzyme A) reductase inhibitors remains unproven in patients older than age 75 years, but should be considered for younger patients. Any discussion of therapy should take into consideration the patient's financial status, as some medications may prove to be prohibitively expensive.

The treatment of membranous nephropathy remains controversial because the natural history of the disease includes spontaneous remissions and exacerbations. In general, one-third of patients will be expected to improve; another third will follow an indolent course, while the final third will progress to end-stage renal disease. Risk factors for progression include male sex, poorly controlled hypertension, and heavy proteinuria. Recent reevaluation of data from multiple trials suggest that targeted therapy to those individuals most likely to progress is beneficial. ACEIs and/or ARBs should be considered for control of both hypertension and proteinuria. Likewise, for those individuals likely to progress, a combination of steroids with cytotoxic agents or cyclosporine A should be considered with careful consideration of dose, duration, and other comorbid factors, but treatment with steroids alone is not beneficial. In most instances, it may be more prudent to carefully observe the patient and watch for signs of progression before embarking on a course of steroids and immunosuppressive therapy. Because therapy continues to evolve, nephrology consultation is appropriate.

Geriatric patients with minimal change disease tend to have as favorable a prognosis as younger cohorts and respond equally well to corticosteroid therapy. Moreover, relapses following cessation of prednisone therapy are relatively infrequent. For some individuals, stopping NSAID therapy is the only intervention necessary. Otherwise, patients with minimal change disease should be treated with prednisone for 2 to 4 months before they are diagnosed as corticosteroid-resistant. If a relapse does occur, these patients should be treated in the same way as in younger adults. In steroid-resistant geriatric patients, cyclophosphamide can be used, but the normal age-associated decrease in glomerular filtration rate should be taken into account in determining the appropriate dose. In most instances, a dose of 1 to 2 mg/kg body weight per day that is commonly used in younger patients must be reduced, and the white blood cell count monitored carefully.

The management of amyloidosis remains supportive; there is no specific therapy for primary amyloidosis. For secondary amyloidosis, further amyloid deposition can be prevented if the underlying disease process can be treated. No therapy is available that effects the resolution of amyloid deposits, but treatment that reduces the supply of amyloid fibril precursor proteins can improve survival and preserve renal function. The role of this therapeutic approach, based on cytotoxic agents (e.g., chlorambucil), is difficult to define in geriatric populations since many patients die before any benefit can be seen.

Patients presenting with histologic features of light chain glomerulopathy have a 5-year renal survival of 40 percent. These patients should undergo bone marrow examination to test for the presence of multiple myeloma. Treatment with cytotoxic drugs (melphalan and prednisone) may diminish proteinuria and preserve renal function. However, cytotoxic therapy in the absence of multiple myeloma is controversial. Plasmapheresis, in addition to cytotoxic therapy, should be considered for patients with acute renal failure due to multiple myeloma, but the likelihood of success of this intervention hinges on the blood paraprotein level.

Table 45-5   Categories of Renal Artery Disease

Aneurysms
Arteriovenous malformations
Atherosclerosis
Dissection of the aorta
Embolic disease
Fibrous dysplasia
Kawasaki disease
Neurofibromatosis
Other systemic necrotizing vasculitides
Polyarteritis nodosa
Takayasu arteritis
Thromboangiitis obliterans
Thrombotic diseases
Trauma
Vasculitis involving the renal artery

SOURCE: Modified from Greco BA and Breyer JA (1996, p 3).

RENOVASCULAR DISEASE

Definition

Renovascular disease is an important cause of secondary hypertension and progressive renal insufficiency in the elderly population. The spectrum of diseases that can cause anatomic narrowing of a main renal artery or its branches include many different disease entities (Table 45-5). The two main types of renal arterial lesions are atherosclerosis and fibrous dysplasia, but atherosclerosis accounts for almost 90 percent of cases in the elderly population.

Clinical Features

As mentioned above, the clinical presentation of renal artery stenosis ranges widely from asymptomatic forms to the two well-known clinical syndromes: renovascular hypertension and ischemic nephropathy (Table 45-6). Renovascular hypertension is defined as the secondary elevation of blood pressure produced by any of a variety of conditions that interfere with the kidney's arterial circulation and cause renal hypoperfusion. With the exception of oral contraceptive use and alcohol ingestion, renovascular hypertension is the most common cause of potentially remediable secondary hypertension. Renovascular hypertension has an estimated prevalence of 2 to 3 percent in the general hypertensive population. It is important to differentiate between renal artery stenosis and renovascular hypertension because the diagnosis of the latter requires verification that

Table 45-6 Prevalence of Unsuspected Renal Artery Stenosis (RAS): Angiographic Studies

Study No.	Year	No. of Patients	Indications	% of Patients with >50% RAS
1	1975	190	AAA	22
2	1990	100	PVD	42
3	1992	1302	Cardiac catheterization	11
4	1995	196	Cardiac catheterization	18
5	1994	127	PVD	16
6	1990	395	Aortic/PVD	33–39
7	1990	374	PVD	14
8	1992	450	PVD	23
9	1993	346	AAA/AOD	28
10	1989	118	Cardiac catheterization	23
11	1996	100	PVD	11
12	1990	100	PVD	22

AAA, abdominal aortic aneurysm; AOD, atherosclerotic disease; PVD, peripheral vascular disease; RAS, renal artery stenosis.
SOURCE: Modified from Greco BA and Breyer JA (1996, p 5).

sufficient stenosis (>75 to 80 percent) is present to produce renal tissue ischemia and to initiate the sequence of events leading to hypertension. Clinical clues that might prompt the clinician to diagnose renal artery stenosis in elderly patients are onset of hypertension after the age of 50 years; accelerated or difficult to control hypertension; coexisting diffuse atherosclerotic vascular disease; acute or subacute renal insufficiency after initiation of therapy with ACEIs or ARBs; recurrent pulmonary edema; grades III to IV hypertensive retinopathy; abdominal or flank bruit; hypokalemia in the absence of diuretic use; erythrocytosis; microangiopathic hemolytic anemia; and hyperuricemia. Although renovascular hypertension is thought to occur primarily in white patients, recent cohort studies report a similar prevalence in selected African American and white patients. Whether these racial variations are a result of differences in screening and referral patterns or true differences in the prevalence of renovascular hypertension remains to be determined.

Ischemic nephropathy can be defined as a clinically significant reduction in the glomerular filtration rate resulting from a partial or complete luminal obstruction of the preglomerular renal arteries of any caliber. It occurs in patients with hemodynamically significant stenosis in the renal artery of a solitary kidney or in both renal arteries if two kidneys are present.

Patients with atheromatous renovascular disease may present with different clinical courses. Acute renal failure can be precipitated by treatment of hypertension with ACEIs or ARBs during a period of days to weeks after initiating therapy. This form of acute renal failure may be associated with hypoperfusion of the kidneys caused by inhibition of angiotensin II-dependent autoregulatory pathways in the glomerulus. Nevertheless, many patients with renovascular disease tolerate these agents and are usually not referred for additional noninvasive studies. Thus, the sensitivity of using the response to ACEIs or ARBs as a screening test for the presence of renovascular disease is unknown. Currently available clinical data estimates that 6 to 38 percent of patients with significant renal vascular disease will develop acute renal failure following ACEI or ARB therapy. Other antihypertensive agents have been reported to cause reversible acute renal failure in the setting of ischemic nephropathy. These cases should be distinguished from those hypertensive patients without ischemic nephropathy who develop acute renal failure in the setting of renin dependent decreases in renal perfusion such as intravascular volume depletion or low effective circulating volume states such as congestive heart failure or cirrhosis.

Renovascular disease may also present as progressive azotemia in a patient with suspected or documented renovascular hypertension (Table 45-7) or as recurrent pulmonary edema associated with poorly controlled hypertension and renal insufficiency (23 percent prevalence in some series). Postulated mechanisms include angiotensin II-induced myocardial dysfunction, diastolic dysfunction secondary to left ventricular hypertrophy, and reduced pressure natriuresis in conjunction with subsequent volume expansion. Azotemia in an elderly patient, in the absence of clinical and laboratory signs, that is suggestive of another renal disease, or of unexplained azotemia requiring initiation of renal replacement therapy, should prompt an evaluation for renovascular disease. Because the age of patients with ESRD is increasing, it is possible that a significant proportion of patients on dialysis may suffer from this disease.

Table 45-7   Natural History of Atheromatous Renovascular Disease

Study No.	Year	No. of Patients	Mean Follow-up	Progressive Narrowing of Renal Artery (%)*	Renal Function Deterioration (%)
1	1981	41	36	(?)	37
2	1968	39	27 (?)	36	(?)
3	1984	85	87	44	38
4	1991	48	97	1	(?)
5	1968	30	28	60	19
6	1987	36	48	40	44.4

*On serial angiography.
SOURCE: Modified from Zucchelli P and Zuccala A (1993, p 17).

Atheroembolic renal disease falls into the category of renal insufficiency induced by preglomerular ischemia. This entity has been usually described in patients with clinical evidence of atheromatous occlusive disease following invasive intraaortic diagnostic or therapeutic procedures, although spontaneous embolic episodes have been described. Important clinical clues associated with this disease are the presence of unexplained eosinophilia, purpuric-ischemic skin lesions, and the presence of heavy proteinuria, which can be in the nephrotic range.

Diagnostic Approach

There are three basic steps in making the diagnosis of renovascular hypertension: (1) renal artery stenosis must be demonstrated by angiography; (2) the stenotic lesion must be pathophysiologically significant; and (3) the hypertension is corrected by intervention to relieve the stenosis. In practice, the diagnosis of ischemic nephropathy is almost always made in the context of coexisting hypertension.

In the appropriate clinical setting such as those just described (worsening renal failure, bland urinary sediment, proteinuria <1 g/d, hypertension, and evidence of peripheral vascular disease) the clinician should develop a high index of suspicion for the disease. According to the triage approach proposed by Mann and Pickering, the patient may be classified as having a low (less than 1 percent prevalence), moderate (5 to 15 percent prevalence), or high (>25 percent prevalence) pretesting probability for renovascular disease. Patients classified in the low-risk group should not undergo further work-up. The presence of azotemia in the high-risk group may impair the reliability of the noninvasive tests and may justify performing renal angiography regardless of the results of noninvasive tests. In patients with intermediate probability, noninvasive testing has the most important diagnostic role.

ACEI radionuclide scintirenography is currently the most thoroughly evaluated noninvasive test for the diagnosis of renovascular hypertension. This study should be preceded by measurement of a random morning plasma renin activity (PRA). Evaluation of ACEI renography by using technetium-99m diethylenetriamine pentaacetic acid (^{99m}Tc-DTPA) has shown high sensitivity and specificity (91 to 94 percent) for renovascular hypertension. Currently, renal scintigraphy with Hippuran or Mag3 (renal plasma flow tracers) before and after ACEIs is the functional test of choice to diagnose ischemic nephropathy. Two limitations should be kept in mind: (1) these tests have not been evaluated in patients with azotemia, and (2) while a positive test predicts an improvement in blood pressure, it is not known whether it also predicts an improvement in renal function.

Duplex ultrasound scanning of the renal arteries is a fairly recently described screening tool with promising early results. Duplex ultrasound scanning also allows measurement of kidney size and is not affected by medications or the level of glomerular filtration rate. The reported sensitivity and specificity values are in the low to mid 90 percent range. The main disadvantage of this test is that it is technically demanding and has a steep learning curve for each center that performs this test. Another caveat is that accessory renal arteries are difficult to detect and study.

Another new noninvasive diagnostic modality is magnetic resonance angiography. A recent publication from Italy reports overall accuracy of 97 percent for correct depiction of severe renal artery stenosis when compared head-to-head to conventional angiography (50 percent). Although technical problems such as the detection of significant stenosis in an accessory vessel still need to be overcome, this modality holds promise as a routine screening modality.

The gold standard for diagnosing renal artery stenosis is selective renal angiography. Intraarterial digital subtraction angiography (IA-DSA) or a CO_2 angiogram also provides excellent anatomic detail and requires less contrast than conventional angiography. The technique of intravenous digital subtraction angiography, although less invasive, does not provide comparable resolution to the aforementioned tests because of the high degree of bowel gas and motility artifacts, and usually requires a significantly larger amount of nephrotoxic contrast material.

Table 45-8   Results of Surgical Revascularization for Atherosclerotic Ischemic Nephropathy

Study No.	Year	No. of Patients	No. (%) Improved	No. (%) Stable	No. (%) Deteriorated
1	1992	40	22 (55%)	10 (25%)	8 (20%)
2	1987	91	20 (22%)	48 (53%)	23 (25%)
3	1992	70	34 (49%)	25 (36%)	11 (15%)
4	1992	91	45 (49%)	31 (35%)	15 (16%)
5	1987	161	93 (58%)	50 (31%)	18 (11%)
6	1993	13	9 (69%)	3 (23%)	7 (8%)

SOURCE: Modified from Pohl MA. Ischemic nephropathy. *American Society of Nephrology's Board Review Course Syllabus*, 1996, p 14.

The second step in making the diagnosis of renovascular hypertension is to determine the pathophysiological significance of the lesion. Some of the diagnostic tests already mentioned are also used to assess this issue. Selective renal vein renin measurement is the gold standard for establishing the functional nature of the stenotic lesion and helps predict the blood pressure response to revascularization. In general, a renal vein renin ratio of ≥ 1.5 between the two renal veins is predictive of a beneficial blood pressure response following surgery or angioplasty, but failure to lateralize does not predict a negative response. Overall, the blood pressure response to revascularization cannot be determined with confidence by using renal vein renin measurements. A positive captopril renogram with ^{99m}Tc-DTPA has been reported to accurately predict the blood pressure response to revascularization. The predictive value of all of these tests in terms of the renal function outcome after revascularization is largely unknown and awaits further study.

Treatment

Several studies clearly demonstrate that renovascular disease is a progressive disease. Of patients with the disease, 50 percent can expect their stenosis to worsen, with reported rates varying between 1.5 and 5 percent per year. In general, the rate of progression of renal insufficiency and the likelihood of deterioration of renal function correlates positively with the extent of stenosis at the time of diagnosis. This implies that correction of renal artery stenosis might be worthwhile in preventing renal failure or to improve renal function. This is important because elderly patients with progressive atherosclerotic renal artery obstruction leading to end stage renal disease do not respond well to renal replacement therapy. Of all geriatric patients with ESRD, these patients have the poorest overall survival, with a 27-month median survival rate and only a 12 percent 5-year survival rate.

There is no universally accepted treatment in patients with renovascular disease. Therapy must be individualized and based upon the general status of the patient, the presence of any concomitant disease, and the local surgical or angiographic experience of the center. The role of surgical revascularization in the management of renovascular hypertension was first established by the US Cooperative study 20 years ago. Increasingly good results have been reported (Table 45-8). The combined cured and improved rate is reported approximately 82 percent with a mortality rate of approximately 1 percent when one includes patients of all ages. The results are less favorable in elderly patients with atherosclerotic renal artery stenosis because their prognosis is determined by the extent of atherosclerosis elsewhere and the potential risk of cholesterol embolization during the operation.

Recovery of renal function after surgical revascularization depends upon whether the patient has unilateral or bilateral atherosclerotic renal disease, or a solitary kidney. With regard to unilateral stenosis, revascularization has only a modest beneficial effect on renal function. This occurs mainly because any increase in GFR in the revascularized, poststenotic kidney, is often offset by a decrease in the GFR of the contralateral kidney. Furthermore, when severe azotemia is present in a patient with unilateral stenosis, it is usually a result of severe bilateral nephrosclerosis, that is, bilateral renal parenchymal damage, which will not be improved by revascularization.

In bilateral stenosis, there are two possible clinical presentations. The first is bilateral occlusion of the renal arteries. This situation does not necessarily imply irreversible damage because the viability of the kidneys may be maintained by a collateral blood supply. This is particularly true in patients who have a gradual onset of arterial occlusion. Clinical clues suggesting parenchymal salvageability include the following: angiographic demonstration of retrograde filling of the distal renal arterial system by collateral vessels; renal biopsy showing preserved glomerular architecture; kidney size >9 cm by ultrasound; and function of the involved kidney on renal scintigraphy. Some centers perform kidney biopsies in surgical candidates if their serum creatinine is higher than 4 mg/dL. In patients with serum creatinine less than 3 mg/dL, improved renal function (defined as a reduction in serum creatinine of >20 percent from the baseline value) postrevascularization can be expected in nearly half of patients undergoing this procedure.

The second scenario is bilateral stenosis without total occlusion or stenosis in a solitary kidney. Improvement in

Table 45-9   Ischemic Renal Disease: Outcome of Angioplasty

Study No.	Year	No. of Patients	Angioplasty Outcome			
			No. (%) Improved	No. (%) Stable	No. (%) Worse*	No. (%) Death
1	198	20	7 (35)	10 (50)	3 (15)	0 (0)
2	1983	12	3 (25)	5 (42)	4 (33)	0 (0)
3	1992	17	9 (53)	2 (12)	6 (35)	5 (29)
4	1986	55	26 (47)	19 (35)	10 (18)	NA
5	1993	21	10	38	3	
TOTAL		104	45 (43)	36 (35)	23 (22)	5 (5)

*Includes all deaths; NA, not available

Source: Modified from Pohl MA. Ischemic nephropathy. *American Society of Nephrology's Board Review Course Syllabus*, 1996, p 14.

renal function is frequently seen after reconstructive surgery in 75 to 89 percent of these patients. Unlike cases with total renal occlusion, revascularization to preserve renal function is not worthwhile in patients with severe renal insufficiency (serum creatinine >4 mg/dL) because they usually have advanced underlying renal parenchymal disease (nephrosclerosis and/or atheroembolic disease) which is not improved by revascularization. In older patients, severe atherosclerosis of the abdominal aorta may render an aortorenal bypass technically impossible. In such cases, alternate bypass techniques have been used, such as splenorenal bypass for left-kidney revascularization and hepatorenal bypass for right-kidney revascularization. Considering the significant risks of progressive renal occlusive disease and renal failure that are associated with medical management of this condition in elderly patients, the surgical results showing a favorable influence of revascularization on the natural history of untreated atherosclerotic renal artery disease are of interest and merit further study.

Percutaneous transluminal renal angioplasty (PTRA) has a limited role in elderly patients because of the concomitant presence of aortic atherosclerotic disease making any endovascular procedure hazardous and technically difficult. The currently available data suggest that surgical revascularization has an advantage over PTRA (Table 45-9). Restenosis following dilatation of atheromatous lesions is quite common and a significant number of elderly patients present with osteal lesions which are not amenable to PTRA. The use of endovascular stenting devices is somewhat promising, but its specific role in the prevention of restenosis or maintenance of renal arterial patency awaits further studies and technical developments. One potential advantage of angioplasty over surgery is that it can be undertaken in patients who have prohibitively high surgical risks that are related to systemic atherosclerosis.

TUBULOINTERSTITIAL NEPHRITIS

Tubulointerstitial nephritis involves a heterogeneous group of disorders that primarily affect the renal interstitium and tubules and only secondarily involve the other structures of the kidney. The etiology of these diseases include medications, infectious agents, physical, chemical, immunologic, hereditary, and unknown causes. Elderly patients are predisposed to the development of this entity because of the high prevalence of polypharmacy, comorbid diseases, and impaired immunologic mechanisms to control infections. Interstitial disease in the geriatric patient should be thoroughly investigated. Aging related interstitial changes may precipitate clinical features compatible with tubulointerstitial nephritis but should be considered as a diagnosis of exclusion after other possible underlying conditions are ruled out.

Functional Defects

The pattern of tubular dysfunction will vary depending on the major site of injury. Salt retention, hypertension, edema, and heavy proteinuria are absent in the early phases of the disease. The tubulointerstitial lesions are localized either to the cortex or to the medulla. Cortical lesions can affect either the proximal or distal tubule. Proximal lesions are characterized by Fanconi's syndrome (bicarbonaturia, glucosuria, hyperuricosuria, hyperphosphaturia, and aminoaciduria). Distal lesions are associated with impaired ability to secrete protons (distal tubular acidosis) and potassium, and decreased reabsorption of sodium. Medullary lesions that involve the papilla manifest by sodium wasting and an impaired ability to concentrate the urine maximally.

In addition to abnormalities associated with tubular defects, other clinical features are also suggestive of tubulointerstitial nephritis. Anemia that is out of proportion to azotemia may signify the early failure of erythropoietin synthesis. High levels of parathyroid hormone with mild azotemia may be secondary to reduced tubular generation of the biologically active form of vitamin D, $1,25\text{-}(OH)_2D_3$. Microscopic examination of the urine sediment typically shows leukocytes and white cell casts, but may be surprisingly bland as well. Eosinophiluria, detected by Hansel's stain, may be seen in the setting of drug-induced tubulointerstitial nephritis, especially when it is secondary to β-lactam antibiotics. Despite the number of typical clinical manifestations, early renal consultation should be obtained because the diagnosis of tubulointerstitial disease can only be established by renal biopsy.

Acute Tubulointerstitial Nephritis

Tubulointerstitial nephritis can be divided into acute and chronic forms. Of the etiologies associated with acute tubulointerstitial nephritis, two entities deserve special attention in geriatric populations: acute bacterial pyelonephritis and acute drug-induced hypersensitivity reactions.

Acute Bacterial Pyelonephritis

Infections are a major problem in the elderly population. With advancing age, infections are not only more common, but also more serious. Alterations in host resistance occur with aging, but accompanying chronic diseases are often a relevant, comorbid condition, which increases the incidence and severity of infections. For most, but not all, elderly individuals, the presentation and course of infection involving the urinary tract is no different from that found in younger patients. Bacterial pyelonephritis occurs equally in both sexes and is the most common form of renal disease in the elderly. Prostatic hypertrophy and the decreased antimicrobial properties of prostatic fluid may be the cause of increased incidence in elderly men. In geriatric-aged women, the vaginal pH changes as the epithelium atrophies, resulting in replacement of the usual microbial flora by gram-negative organisms. These changes predispose the patient to infection. Urinary tract infection is strongly correlated with dementia, which may be caused by fecal incontinence and perineal soiling in women, although the reason in men is unknown.

In those patients with an atypical presentation, the disease is a diagnostic challenge. Costovertebral angle tenderness and urinary symptoms may be absent, whereas bacteremia (>50 percent), central nervous system changes, tachypnea, and hypotension are common. There are even case reports of asymptomatic acute pyelonephritis presenting as acute renal failure.

Therapy includes hemodynamic support and eradication of the infection. Uncomplicated pyelonephritis improves within 48 to 72 hours after initiation of adequate antimicrobial agents. Ultrasonographic surveillance is indicated if no improvement is noted in this time frame to exclude obstructive lesions or perinephric abscess.

Drug Hypersensitivity

Drug-induced acute interstitial nephritis has been reported with most medications. The classic description is the one associated with methicillin (and other β-lactam antibiotics). The sulfonamides were the first antibiotics reported to cause acute interstitial nephritis and were followed by the penicillins in the 1950s. Methicillin was implicated in numerous, well-documented, biopsy-proven cases and became the prototype for drug-induced acute interstitial nephritis. Subsequent reports included a vast number of

antibiotics as the cause of this syndrome. Unfortunately, many of the anecdotal reports lack large numbers of cases and do not include biopsy findings, thereby bringing into question the validity of the causal association. A high index of suspicion of acute interstitial nephritis in the clinical setting of acutely deteriorating renal function is the key to diagnosis.

The clinical presentation is characterized by the tetrad of rash, arthralgia, fever, and acute renal failure. The urine sediment shows nonnephrotic range proteinuria, white cell casts, and eosinophiluria in 40 percent of the cases.

The other significant group of drugs causing acute interstitial nephritis in the elderly population are the NSAIDs. All classes of NSAIDs induce this syndrome, with or without minimal change nephropathy. Acute interstitial nephritis has been reported after 2 to 18 months of NSAID therapy and may be sufficiently severe as to require renal replacement therapy. Most cases are reversible after the drug is stopped. Unlike antimicrobial-induced interstitial nephritis, signs of hypersensitivity (fever, rash, eosinophilia, eosinophiluria) are usually absent. Some cases are associated with nephrotic range proteinuria and glomerular lesions similar to minimal change or membranous nephropathy. The most culpable NSAID appears to be fenoprofen, although all NSAIDs induce this pathology.

The best therapeutic option for treating drug-induced acute interstitial nephritis is to identify and withdraw the offending agent, although this may not be obvious in a hospitalized patient on multiple medications. Although there are anecdotal reports of using corticosteroids for treatment, there are no controlled trials showing that their use alters the rate or extent of renal recovery.

Chronic Tubulointerstitial Nephritis

The clinical course of tubulointerstitial disease depends on the primary cause and the magnitude of the renal insult. Sporadic exposure to nephrotoxic materials results in a more indolent clinical course and progressive loss of renal function. Chronic tubulointerstitial nephritis is associated with tubular atrophy and interstitial polymorphonuclear and mononuclear cell infiltrates. The etiologic factors and the pathogenetic mechanisms are essentially the same as in the acute forms of interstitial nephritis. Special considerations in elderly populations are the chronic forms associated with analgesic abuse, neoplasms, and aging-associated interstitial disease.

Analgesic Nephropathy

There are no scientifically acceptable data documenting the safety of NSAIDs on renal structure and function when taken chronically. Epidemiologic data show a ninefold increased relative risk of ESRD in subjects ingesting 5000 or more doses of NSAIDs when compared with age-matched control subjects; however, it has been difficult to demonstrate a cause-and-effect relationship between analgesic use and chronic renal failure or ESRD. In an intriguing study from Sweden, regular use of acetaminophen and aspirin as analgesics was associated with an increased risk of chronic renal failure (CRF). In fact, subjects who chronically took more than 1.4 g of acetaminophen per day had a fivefold increased risk for CRF. The risk was higher in those patients with preexisting CRF. This is particularly germane to the elderly population, which has a high incidence of CRF. Although the incidence of analgesic nephropathy in the ESRD population has declined in those countries where analgesic combinations containing phenacetin were removed from the market, the incidence of this condition appears to be increasing in the elderly population in some countries outside of the United States. The frequency of renal papillary necrosis, the hallmark lesion of analgesic associated nephropathy, as a primary cause or contributing cause of ESRD is unknown because of the infrequent radiographic proof of this diagnosis.

A recent review of the literature that included studies from Europe, Australia, and North America, concluded that the use of NSAIDs in the general population is safe and effective when used in therapeutic dosages for a limited period of time. There are no acceptable epidemiologic or clinical data regarding the risk of NSAIDs for chronic renal failure, renal papillary necrosis, or ESRD. There are also no experimental or clinical data on whether NSAIDs affect the rate of progression of renal disease. Consequently, the National Kidney Foundation recommends the design and implementation of controlled studies on the renal and cardiovascular safety of chronic NSAIDs by themselves, or in the presence of another known cause of renal disease, and the prospective evaluation of combinations of NSAIDs and other analgesics prior to their release onto the market.

Neoplastic Diseases Associated with Interstitial Nephritis

Many neoplastic diseases infiltrate the interstitium of the kidney with variable clinical implications. Leukemias and lymphomas are the most common malignancies associated with direct invasion of the renal parenchyma. Multiple myeloma may affect the kidney by several different mechanisms. One is involvement of the tubulointerstitial structures resulting from the filtration of toxic light chains and the formation of intratubular casts from aggregates of light chains and Tamm-Horsfall mucoprotein. This clinical entity is known as myeloma kidney and may present as an indolent, chronic form of renal failure, or as isolated tubular dysfunction with well-preserved glomerular filtration rate. The clinical manifestations of the tubular involvement include the Fanconi's syndrome, renal tubular acidosis types I or II, and hyperphosphaturia.

The diagnosis of myeloma kidney should be confirmed by kidney biopsy when the clinical picture suggests tubulointerstitial involvement. The presence of tubular involvement has important therapeutic implications. Even though plasmapheresis has been used with rewarding results in the settings of acute myeloma kidney, the role of plasma exchange in chronic tubulointerstitial nephritis secondary to light chain cast nephropathy awaits further investigation and definition. The addition of high intensity chemotherapy has improved survival rates in cases associated with acute renal failure but optimal therapy for chronic tubulointerstitial nephritis is less certain. Prevention is the most effective therapy for myeloma kidney. Institution of effective chemotherapy and prevention of tubular obstruction are fundamental. The role of colchicine to inhibit the intratubular cast formation is still experimental and should be used only in controlled studies.

Aging-Associated Interstitial Disease

Tubulointerstitial nephropathy of the elderly is defined as the decreased renal tubular function associated with aging, including decreased ability to concentrate urine; decreased renin and aldosterone production; and histologic changes, including interstitial fibrosis and mononuclear cell infiltrates. The clinical presentation is essentially identical to any other form of interstitial nephritis. This entity should be considered only as a diagnosis of exclusion.

CHRONIC RENAL FAILURE

The clinical presentation of chronic renal insufficiency as a result of irreversible damage to renal parenchyma in elderly patients includes essentially the same constellation of symptoms and signs as in the general population. Medical management directed to potassium homeostasis, sodium and water balance, acid base status, calcium and phosphate metabolism, anemia, and nutritional support, follow the same guidelines and parameters as described for the general population. The reader is referred to a general nephrology textbook for details.

Renal replacement therapy for geriatric patients has become commonplace within the last decade. United States Renal Data System data analysis from 1999 show that approximately 40 percent of the incident patients receiving a form of renal replacement therapy are older than 65 years of age and 23 percent are older than 75 years of age. Those patients older than 75 years of age constitute the fastest growing segment on dialysis, with their numbers tripling in the last decade. Moreover, it is estimated that 60 percent of all ESRD patients are older than age 65 years. These statistics should not be surprising given the high incidence of hypertension and diabetes mellitus in the elderly, accounting for 40 to 60 percent of the new cases of ESRD. Tubulointerstitial disorders (13.5 percent), obstructive uropathy (11 percent), glomerular disease (10.5 percent), and polycystic kidney disease (2 percent) account for other causes of ESRD.

The selection of the type of renal replacement therapy for a geriatric patient must be individualized and requires a comprehensive evaluation that takes into account the medical and psychosocial problems that affect each individual patient. The fact that life expectancy is limited for the aged population does not justify depriving them of treatment. In fact, in selected populations, octogenarians' 2-year survival rate can exceed 75 percent. Elderly patients with ESRD have multiple therapeutic options available, including center or home hemodialysis, peritoneal dialysis, renal transplantation, and acceptance of death from uremia. Consultation with a nephrologist is essential for counseling the patient on the advantages and disadvantages of the various types of renal replacement therapy; planning for the start of renal replacement therapy, for provision of renal replacement therapy, and for formulating advance directives regarding cessation of renal placement therapy.

HEMODIALYSIS

The primary treatment modality for geriatric patients with ESRD is in-center hemodialysis (78 percent). Despite their complex medical and psychosocial conditions, survival rates and rehabilitation rates are acceptable in elderly dialysis patients. In addition, these patients tend to be more compliant. The risk of death in dialysis patients increases with age and with coexisting diseases. Several studies report that age, diabetes, and cardiovascular disease are associated with a shorter survival. Survival for at least 5 years was 15 percent lower for patients older than 65 years of age at the initiation of hemodialysis than for younger adults in Europe. Early mortality (within the first 90 days after starting hemodialysis) is mainly secondary to comorbid conditions. The principal reported causes of death are acute myocardial infarction, cardiac arrest, sepsis, and malignancies. There are no significant differences in the percentage of deaths as a result of these various causes between geriatric patients and those younger than 65 years of age with the exception of cachexia, which accounts for 10 percent of the deaths in patients younger than age 65 years and increases to 36 percent in geriatric patients. Withdrawal from dialysis has been reported as the leading cause of death in dialysis patients older than 70 years of age. Other important factors associated with the decision to withdraw from dialysis are malnutrition, cancer, and dissatisfaction with the quality of life.

The success rate for vascular access for chronic hemodialysis in the elderly is similar to the rate in younger patients. The US Renal Data System (USRDS) 1997 annual report indicated that the two major types of access for patients older than 65 years of age were arteriovenous fistulas and polytetrafluoroethylene grafts. The elderly experienced more access-related hospital stays than younger patients. Many investigators report a greater number of hospitalization days per year for the elderly hemodialysis patient. This higher morbidity rate in geriatric hemodialysis patients is the result of complications secondary to hypertension, cardiovascular disease, coronary or cardiac insufficiency, or left ventricular hypertrophy. Nevertheless, multiple surveys on geriatric patients with ESRD report a more positive overall satisfaction with life when compared to younger dialysis patients. Other investigators have reported that age has no value as a predictor of quality of life in patients with ESRD.

It is important to note that the quality of hemodialysis has improved markedly during the past decade, due to both new technology and new medications. Thus, historical data on hemodialysis may not be applicable to the way hemodialysis is performed currently in state-of-the-art hemodialysis centers. Technologic improvements include the development of high-flux hemodialysis, improved biocompatible membranes, bicarbonate dialysis, computer-controlled hemodialysis machines, and improved vascular accesses that can produce the high blood flows needed for high-flux hemodialysis. Major medical improvements include the availability of erythropoietin and intravenous iron for treating the anemia of ESRD, and intravenous vitamin D or its analogs for preventing and treating secondary hyperparathyroidism. These advances have resulted in improved hemodialysis with shorter treatment times, less cardiovascular stress during hemodialysis, and an improved quality of life for hemodialysis patients of all ages.

PERITONEAL DIALYSIS

Peritoneal dialysis (PD) has undergone dramatic changes within the last decade with the development and introduction of smaller, portable cycling dialysis machines that introduce and remove dialysis fluid in a timely, programmed manner. This has resulted in alterations in the dialysis prescription such that in most cases, the bulk of the dialysis exchanges can be done mechanically at night, limiting manual exchanges to one a day. The percentage of elderly patients treated with PD varies from country to country; in the United Kingdom 50 percent of elderly ESRD patients are treated with this modality, while in the United States, fewer than 10 percent of the geriatric ESRD patients are on PD.

For the elderly patient, PD has important advantages, including decreased cardiovascular instability and arrhythmias, better maintenance of residual renal function, good control of hypertension, no need for vascular access surgery, efficacy of intraperitoneal insulin therapy (for diabetics), and better clearance of middle molecules. Despite its many advantages, many elderly patients do not choose this mode for psychosocial reasons such as inadequate family support, poor eyesight, and physical and mental impairment. Unlike hemodialysis, peritoneal dialysis must be done daily and does require manual strength to lift 5-kg bags if a cycling dialysis machine is used.

The rate of infectious complications in elderly patients on PD is similar to that of younger patients, but elderly patients tend to have a more protracted course with increased morbidity and longer hospital stays. Unfortunately, the incidence of peritonitis is still unacceptably high and varies from 0.5 to 3 episodes per patient per year. Moreover, more frequent episodes of peritonitis are associated with catheter loss.

As in hemodialysis patients, the incidence of malnutrition is increased in the elderly patient. Causes of malnutrition include comorbid conditions, as well as protein losses of 7 to 15 g/d with the dialysis procedure.

Choice of dialysis modality ultimately hinges on patient preference. Each has its own advantages and disadvantages and optimal rates of survival can be garnered through careful and planned counseling of the pre-ESRD patient.

RENAL TRANSPLANTATION

Despite the high incidence of ESRD in the aged population, the USRDS indicates that fewer than 5 percent of geriatric ESRD patients have a working renal allograft as renal replacement therapy. Previous studies reported a higher mortality rate in older patients receiving a renal transplant. One-year patient and graft survival for patients older than 60 years of age averaged 62 percent and 57 percent, respectively, before the introduction of cyclosporine A. Improved pre- and postoperative management and better immunosuppressive therapy have improved survival to rates equivalent to those obtained in younger transplant populations. The reluctance to transplant elderly ESRD patients is a result of their limited life expectancy. The probability of 10-year patient survival for cadaveric transplant recipients ages 65 to 69 years in the United States is 8 percent, contrasting with 50 to 85 percent 10-year survival rates in patients younger than 44 years of age.

Current data on elderly transplant recipients of cadaveric renal transplant report a 1-year patient survival rate ranging between 80 and 91 percent and 5-year survival exceeding 55 percent. Graft survival has increased to 80 percent at 1 year and 55 to 60 percent at 5 years. Patients dying with functioning renal allografts account for the majority of graft loss in older recipients (50 percent). Review of the USRDS database shows a lower incidence of rejection (accounting for 11 to 28 percent of graft loss at 1 year) when compared with younger renal allograft recipients. This difference may be explained by age-related "tolerance." Living related transplantation offers improved patient and graft survival, and should be investigated in elderly ESRD patients who are suitable candidates for transplantation.

The leading causes of death in elderly transplant recipients are infections and cardiovascular disease. The majority of infections occur in the first 6 months posttransplant and are related to the degree of immunosuppression. Other series report cardiovascular events as the major cause of death in older transplant patients. Underlying cardiovascular disease may be a natural consequence of older age that is exacerbated by transplant-related complications such as posttransplant hypertension and steroid-induced diabetes. Other important causes of death include malignancy (13 to 16 percent) and gastrointestinal hemorrhage (16 percent).

The selection of transplant recipients in the elderly should follow the same clinical practice guidelines dictated for younger patients. In addition, a routine voiding cystourethrogram is recommended for this age group. Careful attention should be given to the effect of transplantation on the quality of life and should ensure that patient's expectations as to benefits of transplantation are realistic.

Attenuated immune responsiveness in elderly transplant patients decreases the likelihood of immunologic rejection, but it is offset by a potentially increased risk of infection. The goal of any immunosuppression protocol in an elderly patient should be to decrease the risk of infection without causing rejection. Acute rejection requires the use of high doses of immunosuppression to prevent graft loss. The optimal immunosuppression regimen, involving cyclosporine A, prednisone, rapamycin, mycophenolate mofetil, tacrolimus, and azathioprine for long-term immunosuppression has not yet been addressed in prospective studies of elderly renal transplant recipients. In addition, new immunosuppressive agents, such as monoclonal antibodies, may confer a greater potential for reducing steroid and other immunosuppressive dosages while retaining excellent graft and patient survival.

REFERENCES

Appel RG et al: Renovascular disease in older patients beginning renal replacement therapy. *Kidney Int* 48:171, 1995.

Becker BN et al: Renal transplantation in the older end stage renal disease patient. *Semin Nephrol* 16:353, 1996.

Cameron JS: Nephrotic syndrome in the elderly. *Semin Nephrol* 16:319, 1996.

Davison AM, Johnston PA: Idiopathic glomerulonephritis in the elderly. *Contrib Nephrol* 105:38, 1993.

Donadio JV Jr: Treatment and clinical outcome of glomerulonephritis in the elderly. *Contrib Nephrol* 105:49, 1993.

DuBose TD et al: Acute renal in the 21st century: Recommendations for management and outcomes assessment. *Am J Kidney Dis* 29:793, 1997.

Fored CM et al: Acetaminophen, aspirin and chronic renal failure. *N Engl J Med* 345:1801, 2001.

Glassock RJ: Syndromes of glomerular diseases, in Massry SG, Glassock RJ (eds): *Textbook of Nephrology*, 3rd ed. Baltimore, Williams and Wilkins, 1995, p. 681.

Grapsa I, Oreopoulos DG: Practical ethical issues of dialysis in the elderly. *Semin Nephrol* 16:339, 1996.

Greco BA, Breyer JA: Natural history of renal artery stenosis. *Semin Nephrol* 16:2, 1996.

Haas M et al: Etiologies and outcome of acute renal insufficiency in older adults: A renal biopsy study of 259 cases. *Am J Kidney Dis* 35:433, 2000.

Jennette JC, Falk RJ: The pathology of vasculitis involving the kidney. *Am J Kidney Dis* 24:130, 1994.

Johnston PA et al: Renal biopsy findings in patients older than 65 years of age presenting with the nephrotic syndrome. A report from the MRC glomerulonephritis registry. *Contrib Nephrol* 105:127, 1993.

Johnson JM II et al: A prospective evaluation of the glomerular filtration rate in older adults with frequent night time urination. *J Urol* 107:146, 2002.

Macias-Nunez JF et al: Acute renal failure in the aged. *Semin Nephrol* 16:330, 1996.

Mandal AK et al: Management of acute renal failure in the elderly. Treatment options. *Drugs Aging* 9:226, 1996.

Moran D et al: Is renal biopsy justified for the diagnosis and management of the nephrotic syndrome in the elderly? *Gerontology* 39:49, 1993.

Novick AZ: Options for therapy of ischemic nephropathy: Role of angioplasty and surgery. *Semin Nephrol* 16:53, 1996.

Pascual J et al: The elderly patient with acute renal failure. *J Am Soc Nephrol* 6:144, 1995.

Ponticelli C et al: Primary nephrotic syndrome in the elderly. *Contrib Nephrol* 105:33, 1993.

Swenson KL et al: Effect of aging on the vasopressin and aquaporin responses to dehydration in Fischer 344/Brown-Norway F1 rats. *Am J Physiol* 273:R35, 1997.

Zent R et al: Idiopathic membranous nephropathy in the elderly: A comparative study. *Am J Kidney Dis* 29:200, 1997.

Zucchelli P, Zuccala A: Ischemic nephropathy in the elderly. *Contrib Nephrol* 105:13, 1993.

End–Stage Renal Disease

RICHARD K. CAPLING   •   WENDY WEINSTOCK BROWN

DEFINITION

End-stage renal disease (ESRD) is a state of irreversible nephron loss. Renal replacement therapy (RRT) becomes necessary when the glomerular filtration rate (GFR) decreases to less than 10 to 20 mL/min. ESRD is associated with the inability to excrete waste products, control serum electrolytes, handle the daily dietary and metabolic acid load, and maintain fluid balance. In addition, there is inadequate production of erythropoietin, deranged calcium and phosphorous metabolism, and difficulties with hypertension.

EPIDEMIOLOGY

Prior to the passage of section 299I of the Social Security Amendments of 1972, which established a near-universal entitlement under Medicare for the treatment of chronic kidney disease by dialysis or transplantation, the therapeutic options for patients with ESRD were limited. There were few dialysis centers and maintenance hemodialysis (HD) was only offered to those individuals who were viewed as "contributing to society," had adequate funds for payment, and had no comorbid conditions. It is not surprising then, that elderly patients were rarely offered dialysis therapy. Since 1972, the criteria for dialysis selection have become more relaxed and older patients are dialyzed and transplanted more frequently. Currently, the average age of patients starting hemodialysis is 61 years old. The greatest increase in incident dialysis rates throughout the 1990s has occurred in the age-65-years-and-older population (Fig. 46-1). This "gerontologizing" of nephrology is occurring despite reports from the 2000 US Census Bureau indicating that the 65-years-of-age-and-older population increased at a slower rate than the overall population for the first time in the history of the census. The most rapid population increase for any age group in the 2000 census report was for the 45- to 54-year-old age group (49 percent), an increase fueled mainly by the "baby boomers". Within the next ten years, as the "baby boomers" enter the 65 years of age and older population, it is likely that the US ESRD population will continue to be dominated by elderly patients.

PRESENTATION

Etiology of ESRD in the Elderly Population

The most common reported causes of ESRD in the elderly population are diabetes and nephrosclerosis that is presumed secondary to hypertension (Table 46-1). This may be misleading because of the reluctance of many nephrologists to biopsy elderly patients even when the usual indications, such as nephrotic range proteinuria or unexplained renal failure, are present. Elderly patients with atypical presentations of ESRD should be evaluated for treatable causes of renal failure just as younger patients.

Comorbidities

Care of the elderly patient with renal dysfunction is particularly challenging for the nephrologist and renal health care team, because of the increased number of comorbid conditions that tend to be present in the elderly patient. In one cohort of adult patients treated with maintenance hemodialysis in the United Kingdom, it was found that 90 percent of patients older than 65 years of age had two or more comorbidities (Table 46-2). Cardiovascular, musculoskeletal, and neurologic problems predominated and adversely affected morbidity, mortality, and quality of life. These findings are in agreement with data from the 2001 United States Renal Data System (USRDS) which show patients 65 to74 years of age have the highest incidence of acute myocardial infarction after the initiation of dialysis (Fig. 46-2). Others have shown a high incidence of gastrointestinal bleeding (22 percent) in patients older than 70 years of age as compared to younger disease-matched controls (7 percent).

Determination of GFR in the Elderly Patient

Serum creatinine is not an accurate reflection of GFR in the elderly. Although there are exceptions, there is, in general, a 10 percent decrease in GFR per decade, after the age of 40 years, without a change in serum creatinine. An 80-year-old with a serum creatinine of 1.0 mg/dL generally has

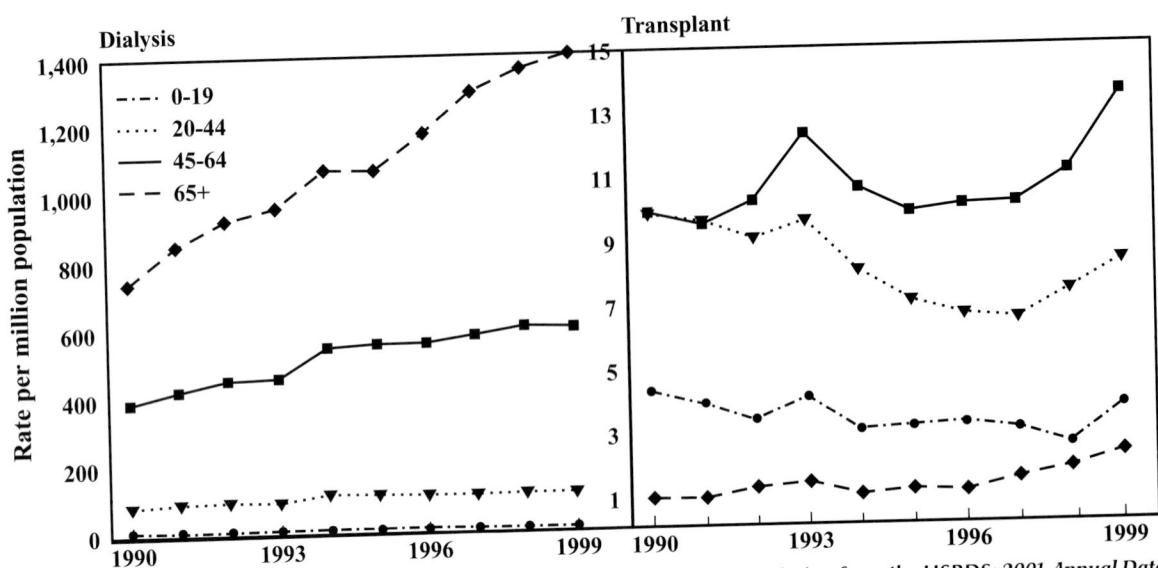

Figure 46-1   Incident rates for 1990 to 1999 by age and first modality. Reprinted with permission from the USRDS: *2001 Annual Data Report: Atlas of End-Stage Renal Disease in the United States.* Bethesda, MD, National Institutes of Health, National Institute of Diabetes and Digestive and Kidney Diseases, 2001, p 562.

a GFR 50 percent of normal. Because GFR is halved every time serum creatinine doubles, the same 80-year-old with a creatinine of 2.0 mg/dL has a profound decrease in renal function, with a GFR approximately 25 percent of normal. It is not unusual for an octogenarian to require renal replacement therapy before their serum creatinine reaches 4.0 mg/dL.

The Cockcroft-Gault formula (Table 46-3), for age-adjusted estimation of creatinine clearance, may be helpful but is only an estimate and not a substitute for careful clinical evaluation. The Cockcroft-Gault formula may underestimate glomerular filtration rate when compared to isotopic measurements in well-nourished patients with stable renal function who were 81 to 96 years of age. One study used iothalamate clearance as the gold standard to compare creatinine clearance, reciprocal creatinine plots, and the Cockcroft-Gault formula in 41 patients 65 to 85 years of age and found poor correlations with all of them. Another equation (Table 46-3), which was derived in the Modification of Diet in Renal Disease study (MDRD), may be better than the Cockcroft-Gault formula for estimation of GFR.

Serious side effects and complications of chronic kidney disease occur at a GFR below 60 mL/min. Patients at

this level of kidney dysfunction should be a referred to a nephrologist for evaluation and co-management. The National Kidney Foundation recently published clinical practice guidelines—the National Kidney Foundation–Kidney Disease Outcomes Quality Initiative (NKF-K/DOQI)—for chronic kidney disease, which includes evaluation, classification, and stratification for purposes of management.

Elderly patients tend to require renal replacement therapy at a higher GFR than disease-matched younger patients (Fig. 46-3). They are particularly susceptible to uremic complications such as protein calorie malnutrition secondary to anorexia and loss of taste, congestive heart failure, and other chronic conditions. They tend to have lower lean body mass, serum creatinine, and blood urea nitrogen (BUN) levels than their younger disease-matched counterparts at initiation of renal replacement therapy (Fig. 46-4).

INDICATIONS FOR INITIATION OF DIALYSIS

The most common symptoms present before initiation of maintenance dialysis in elderly patients tend to be anorexia

Table 46-1   Incident Counts of Reported ESRD Patients, 1996–1999, by Primary Diagnosis and Age

Age (years)	Primary Diagnosis for ESRD (%)					
	DM	HTN	GN	CD	Urologic	Other
65–69	53.1	24.5	6.6	1.7	1.7	12.4
70–79	41.8	34.0	7.2	1.2	2.0	13.8
80+	24.6	47.0	7.4	1.0	2.6	17.4

CD, cystic diseases; DM, diabetes; GN, glomerular nephritis; HTN, hypertension; Other, includes missing data or unknown causes.

SOURCE: Adapted from USRDS (2001).

Table 46-2   Age Related Comorbidity

	% Comorbidity	
Age (years)	35–49	>65
Central nervous system problems	6.4	42.8
Angina/Myocardial infarction	7.5	32.1
Musculoskeletal disorders	6.4	27.4
Gastrointestinal problems	6.4	22.6
Respiratory disease	8.6	19.0
Mental illness	4.3	9.5
Spinal	1.1	8.3

SOURCE: Reprinted with permission from Mallick N and El Marasi A (1999, p 38).

Table 46-3   Estimation of Creatinine Clearance (CrCl)

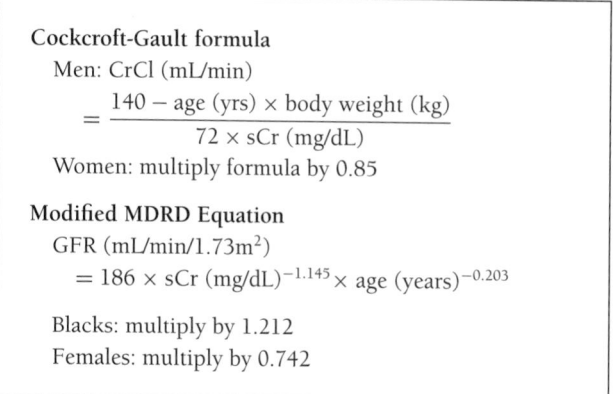

Cockcroft-Gault formula
Men: CrCl (mL/min)
$$= \frac{140 - \text{age (yrs)} \times \text{body weight (kg)}}{72 \times \text{sCr (mg/dL)}}$$
Women: multiply formula by 0.85

Modified MDRD Equation
GFR (mL/min/1.73m^2)
$$= 186 \times \text{sCr (mg/dL)}^{-1.145} \times \text{age (years)}^{-0.203}$$

Blacks: multiply by 1.212
Females: multiply by 0.742

MDRD, Modification of Diet in Renal Disease study; sCr, serum creatinine.

and weight loss, generalized weakness, encephalopathy, and nausea and vomiting. The usual indications for initiation of emergent or acute dialysis therapy in the elderly population vary little from younger patients (Table 46-4). The recognition of uremia in the elderly patient, however, may be more difficult than in the younger patient. Behavioral changes, unexplained dementia, "adult failure to thrive," unexplained worsening of congestive heart failure, or a change in sense of well-being may represent uremia in the geriatric kidney patient. In addition, the decision-making process for initiation of chronic maintenance dialysis in the elderly population is more complex. In addition to the medical indications, it is important to consider the patient's attitude toward life-prolonging measures and the impact of treatment on their quality of life.

Medical Indications for Renal Replacement Therapy

Before 1972, maintenance hemodialysis was usually initiated when the patient developed an acute indication for dialysis. Because of the complications and high mortality associated with urgent dialysis, methodologies have been developed to more accurately predict when renal replacement therapy is necessary. A linear relationship between declines in renal function over time versus the reciprocal of serum creatinine has been demonstrated. Correlation between level of glomerular filtration rate and the development of uremic signs and symptoms is well known. The Center for Medicare and Medicaid Services, CMS, formerly known as the Health Care Financing Administration, bases reimbursement for chronic hemodialysis upon a creatinine clearance below 10 mL/min for nondiabetics and less than 15 mL/min for diabetic patients. Creatinine clearance can

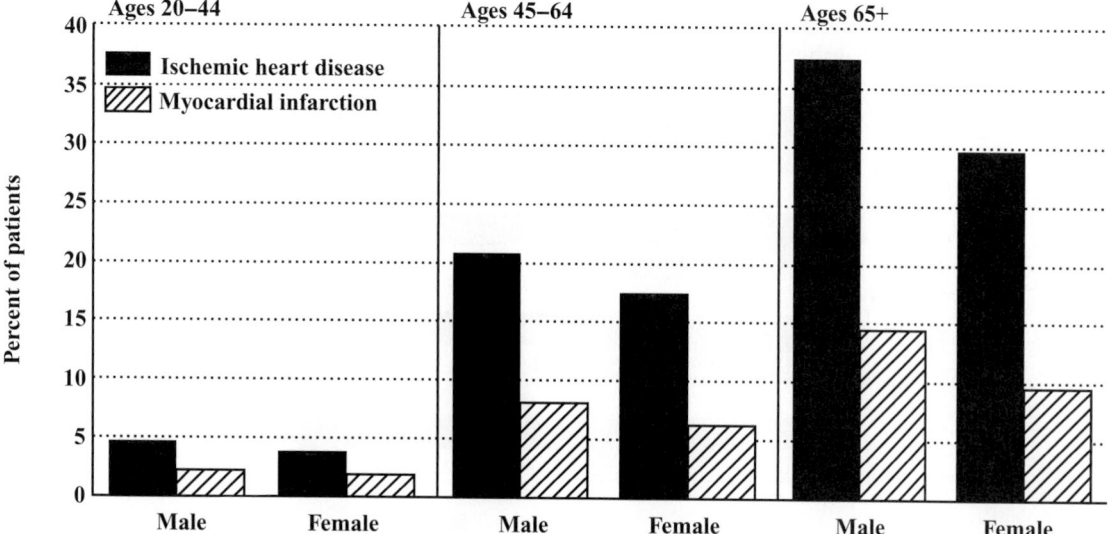

Figure 46-2   History of ischemic heart disease and myocardial infarction at initiation of HD in the year 1999, by gender and age. Reprinted from USRDS: *2001 Annual Data Report: Atlas of End-Stage Renal Disease in the United States.* Bethesda, MD, National Institutes of Health, National Institute of Diabetes and Digestive and Kidney Diseases, 2001, p 562.

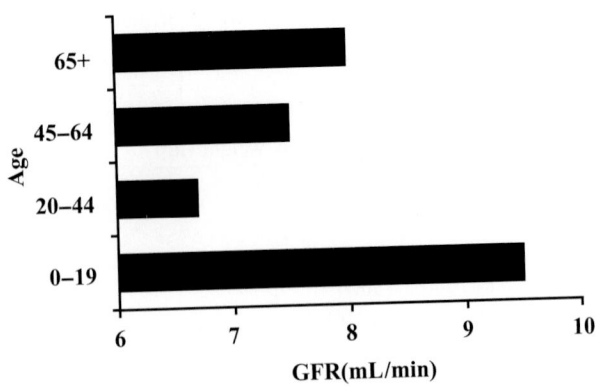

Figure 46-3   Mean glomerular filtration rate (GFR) at initiation of HD by age for incident patients in 1999. Data from USRDS: *2001 Annual Data Report: Atlas of End-Stage Renal Disease in the United States.* Bethesda, MD, National Institutes of Health, National Institute of Diabetes and Digestive and Kidney Diseases, 2001, p 562.

be calculated by using one of the formulas mentioned in Table 46-3 or with a 24-hour urine collection.

Problems arise when patients become symptomatic at a higher glomerular filtration rate. Elderly patients are particularly susceptible to uremic symptoms and may manifest protein calorie malnutrition secondary to anorexia and loss of taste, congestive heart failure, dementia, and other conditions at higher levels of glomerular filtration than younger patients. CMS will reimburse for dialysis if the treating physician can justify early initiation of renal replacement therapy on medical grounds.

Timely initiation of renal replacement therapy not only avoids the need for urgent dialysis, but also is associated with decreased mortality. A strong correlation between "baseline" serum albumin just prior to initiation of dialysis and patient survival has been demonstrated (Fig. 46-5). Although hypoalbuminemia by itself does not necessarily indicate protein-energy malnutrition, it is believed to be a major contributing factor. Analysis of the MDRD study showed that patients tend to adapt to their declining GFR and associated uremic symptoms by reducing their protein intake. Nevertheless, approximately

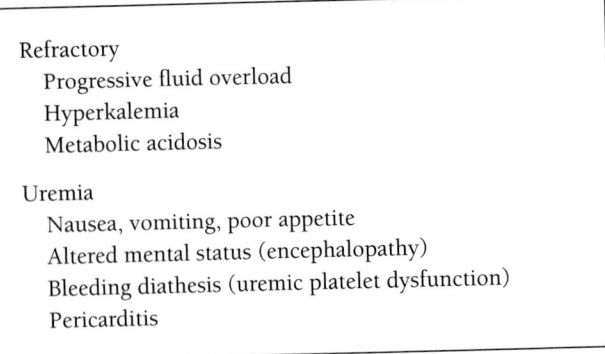

Table 46-4   Indications for Urgent Hemodialysis

Refractory
   Progressive fluid overload
   Hyperkalemia
   Metabolic acidosis
Uremia
   Nausea, vomiting, poor appetite
   Altered mental status (encephalopathy)
   Bleeding diathesis (uremic platelet dysfunction)
   Pericarditis

60 percent of American ESRD patients experience nausea and vomiting at the time dialysis is initiated. NKF-K/DOQI guidelines (Table 46-5) recommend evaluating renal function by monitoring weekly urea clearance (K_rt/V_{urea}). Once the K_rt/V_{urea} falls below 2.0 (equivalent to a creatinine clearance of 9 to14 mL/min/1.73 m^2), there is increased risk for development of uremic anorexia leading to malnutrition, and renal replacement therapy should be initiated.

Medical Contraindications to Renal Replacement Therapy

There are few absolute medical contraindications to renal replacement therapy. Some authors propose that advanced dementia, metastatic cancer, and advanced liver disease are reasons for withholding renal replacement therapy. However, progressive dementia can be confused with uremia-induced delirium in a patient with advanced kidney dysfunction, and a "trial" of dialysis is often justified. It may take as long as 3 to 4 weeks to clear uremic symptoms with dialysis. The patient's family should be aware that if the patient's mental status fails to improve, renal replacement therapy might be inappropriate. Similarly, providing dialysis for a patient with metastatic cancer or end-stage liver disease, may allow the patient to get their affairs in order and spend some quality time with friends and family.

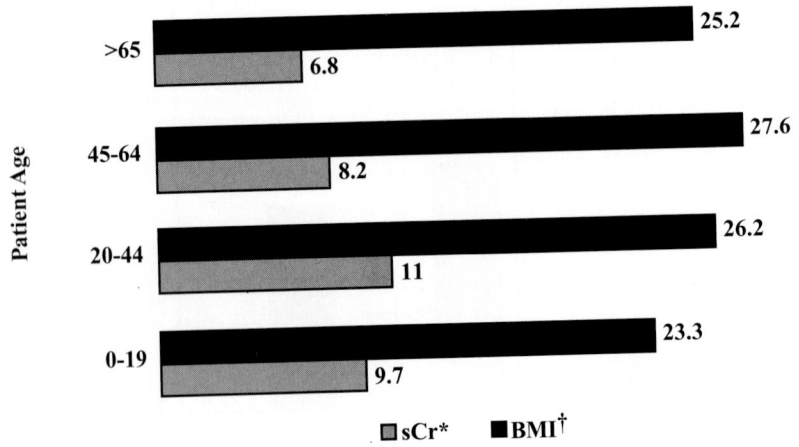

Figure 46-4   Mean body mass index (BMI) and serum creatinine at initiation of dialysis in 1999. *Serum creatinine (mg/dL); †average BMI (weight [kg]/height [m²]). Data taken from the USRDS: *2001 Annual Data Report: Atlas of End-Stage Renal Disease in the United States.* Bethesda, MD, National Institutes of Health, National Institute of Diabetes and Digestive and Kidney Diseases, 2001, p 562.

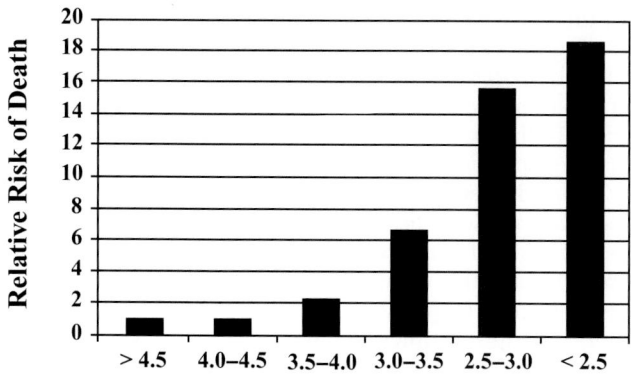

Serum Albumin Concentration (g/dL)

Figure 46-5 Relative risk of death versus serum albumin concentration at initiation of hemodialysis. Values represent risk ratios adjusted for case mix. Adapted from Lowrie EG and Lew NL (1990, p 467).

Time-Limited Trial of Dialysis

When either the patient, family or physician is unsure about the prognosis or the impact that dialysis will have upon the patient's quality of life, it seems reasonable to offer a time-limited trial of dialysis (Table 46-6). If a trial of dialysis is to be conducted, it is important to predetermine a time period (usually 4 to 6 weeks) and to inform all the members of the dialysis team. Such measures will ease withdrawal from dialysis, when appropriate.

Patient Preference

One study in the United Kingdom evaluated elderly patients' attitudes toward dialysis as a life-prolonging measure. Patients who resided in a hospital geriatric ward or a nearby nursing home were provided a short clinical vignette regarding a 75-year-old patient with kidney failure, and asked to give their opinion on choices made by the

Table 46-5 Timely Initiation of Renal Replacement Therapy

RRT should be initiated when
The weekly $K_r t/V_{urea}$ falls below 2.0
Protein-energy malnutrition develops or persists because of decreased nutrient intake without apparent cause for malnutrition

Unless there is
Stable or increased edema-free body weight
Complete absence of clinical signs or symptoms of uremia
Serum albumin within normal range and stable or increasing

SOURCE: Adapted from NKF-K/DOQI Clinical Practice Guideline on Peritoneal Dialysis Adequacy, 1997.

Table 46-6 Indications for Trial of Dialysis in Elderly Patients

- Uremia
- Potentially reversible acute renal failure
- Unexplained dementia
- Unexplained worsening of congestive heart failure
- Personality change
- Irritability/irascibility or newly subdued demeanor
- Adult failure to thrive
- Change in sense of well being

patient about different treatment options. They were then asked what choice they would make if in the same situation. They were also asked what level of symptoms they would tolerate and for their views on cost and treatment allocation. Eighty-four percent of the study patients indicated they would choose dialysis treatment, and 78 percent would agree to be admitted to the hospital, if necessary. Fifty-four percent of the in-patient elderly and 83 percent of the nursing home patients wanted dialysis for ESRD even if physically disabled and living in a nursing home. Seventy-four percent of elderly patients would prefer to have the dialysis performed at home. Only 36 percent of the patients felt that cost was an important factor in determining dialysis allocation for the elderly population. Being independent and free of major symptoms was regarded as important for a good quality of life.

Not all patients have the same attitude toward dialysis and other life-prolonging treatments. It is important to evaluate each patient individually and to ensure that decision-making capacity is not impaired by uremia, acute or chronic pain, treatable depression, or social isolation. Treatment considerations and decisions should involve the patient, their family and/or social support system and the multidisciplinary health care team. The patient, if able, is ultimately the only one who can determine his or her "quality of life" and whether dialysis is beneficial or burdensome. If the patient lacks the decision-making capacity, decisions should involve the patient's health care proxy. It is imperative for the health care team to ensure that the patient and family fully understand the diagnosis, prognosis, and all available treatment options. Options should include a trial of dialysis and all patients should know that they have the right to withdraw from dialysis. If the fully informed patient chooses not to initiate renal replacement therapy, continued supportive management and end-of-life care, such as hospice, should be provided.

Quality of Life

Restoring, maintaining, or improving quality of life is at the heart of all medical interventions. The cardinal tenet in medicine is to do no harm. The degree to which renal replacement therapy affects quality of life is quite variable. A multitude of factors are associated with patients' perceived quality of life. Some of these factors are patient-dependent characteristics (age, race, sex, associated diseases such as

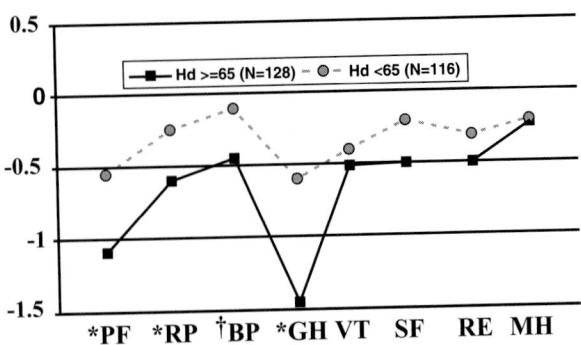

Figure 46-6 Quality of life while on HD, stratified by age, using Short Form-36, standardized mean scores. BP, bodily pain; GH, general health; MH, mental health; PF, physical functioning; RE, emotional; RP, physical; SF, social functioning; VT, vitality. *$P < 0.01$; †$P < 0.05$. Adapted from Rebollo P et al: Is the loss of health-related quality of life during renal replacement therapy lower in elderly patients than in younger patients? *Nephrol Dial Transplant* 16:1678, 2001.

diabetes); others are related to pre-ESRD care (timing of nephrology referral, level of GFR, hematocrit, presence or absence of depression, malnutrition), social factors (income, unemployment, educational level), or type of renal replacement therapy offered (in-center hemodialysis, home hemodialysis, peritoneal dialysis, renal transplantation).

A cross-sectional multicenter study in Spain involving 485 adult hemodialysis and renal transplant patients used the Kidney Disease and Quality of Life Short Form 36 Health Survey (SF-36) to evaluate the effect of ESRD and its treatment on health-related quality of life. In this study, elderly dialysis patients had better physical functioning, lower level of pain, and better general health perception than did subjects of the general population of the same age and gender (Fig. 46-6, Table 46-7). A large Dutch prospective multicenter study (Netherlands Cooperative Study on the Adequacy of Dialysis-2) applied the NKF-K/DOQI guidelines (Table 46.5) for timely initiation of dialysis to 237 new ESRD patients (average age 55 ± 15 years). In this study, 38 percent of patients started dialysis too late, and those patients who started dialysis at the appropriate level of GFR had a better health-related quality

Table 46-7   Quality of Life on Renal Replacement Therapy

	Age <65 Years	Age >65 Years
Hemodialysis patients		
PCS*	39.9 ± 9.65	46.02 ± 8.06
MCS	48.22 ± 12.9	48.49 ± 11
Transplant patients		
PCS*	48.33 ± 8.06	52.55 ± 6.22
MCS	51.37 ± 9.8	54.83 ± 6.33

MCS, mental component summary score; PCS, physical component summary score.

*$P < 0.01$ (student's *t*-test).

SOURCE: Reproduced with permission from Rebollo P et al. (2001, p 1678).

of life when evaluated with the SF-36 at regular intervals during the first 6 months after starting hemodialysis. The "timely starters" had lost their advantage 1 year after starting dialysis, however, and the authors suggested that such early initiation guidelines should not be used. This study did not specifically analyze the potential beneficial effects of timely initiation in the 65 years of age and older population, but a case could be made that for the elderly dialysis population, who have an expected 1.5 to 4.3 years of life remaining after the initiation of dialysis (Table 46-8), an early improvement in quality of life is very meaningful. In addition, the adjusted difference in estimated survival time after 3 years on dialysis treatment was 2.5 months longer (1.1 to 4.0) for the timely starters compared with those with late referral.

MANAGEMENT

Pre-renal Replacement Management

Several studies comparing survival rates for patients treated with various modes of renal replacement therapy (hemodialysis, peritoneal dialysis, or renal transplantation) suggest that the patient's health status prior to initiation of therapy is more important in influencing survival than is the mode of therapy selected. Pre-ESRD care should focus on those issues which improve patient survival and quality of life (timing of nephrology referral, level of GFR, hematocrit, presence or absence of depression, malnutrition).

Early nephrologic referral is important. Late referral patients are more likely to have hypoalbuminemia (56 percent versus 80 percent), hematocrit <28 percent (33 percent versus 55 percent), and predicted GFR <5 mL/min/1.73 m^2 (17 percent versus 40 percent) at the start of dialysis, and are less likely to have a functioning permanent vascular access for their first dialysis treatment (60 percent versus 96 percent).

Alterations in Drug Metabolism in the Elderly Population

Drug disposition in the elderly population is complex and is affected by polypharmacy and concurrent illness and alterations in gastrointestinal absorption, hepatic clearance, protein binding, renal metabolism, and clearance and space of distribution (see Chap. 19). With aging, muscle mass decreases and total body water declines as a percentage of body weight while body fat increases. As a consequence, the space of distribution of water-soluble drugs expands and that of lipid-soluble drugs diminishes, decreasing and prolonging half-lives, respectively. Adverse drug reactions and drug–drug interactions are common. Concurrent illnesses, such as atherosclerosis and heart disease, may be associated with decreased hepatic perfusion metabolism. ESRD patients, of course, have markedly diminished or absent renal metabolism and excretion. It is particularly important to avoid nephrotoxins such as nonsteroidal antiinflammatory agents, and to adjust dosing and frequency of medications for level of GFR.

Table 46-8 Expected Remaining Lifetimes (Years), by Age, Gender, and Race, Period Prevalent Dialysis Patients, 1999

	Dialysis								Transplant							
	White		Black		Native American		Asian		White		Black		Native American		Asian	
Age	M	F	M	F	M	F	M	F	M	F	M	F	M	F	M	F
0–14	17.9	15.9	19.3	16.8	21.6	22.1	29.3	27.0	47.3	46.9	40.6	40.3	50.4	50.8	51.8	54.5
15–19	16.3	14.8	19.0	16.6	18.9	19.1	24.3	23.3	36.3	36.2	33.1	33.0	38.6	39.0	39.5	42.0
20–24	13.6	12.3	16.4	14.3	16.3	16.2	20.8	20.1	32.2	32.3	29.8	29.8	34.4	34.8	35.2	37.6
25–29	11.3	10.2	14.2	12.5	13.8	13.5	17.9	17.5	28.3	28.4	26.5	26.5	30.2	30.6	31.0	33.3
30–34	9.2	8.6	12.1	10.7	11.1	11.4	14.9	14.9	24.3	24.4	23.0	23.2	26.0	26.3	26.7	28.9
35–39	7.9	7.5	10.3	9.4	9.4	9.8	12.6	12.6	20.6	20.9	19.6	19.9	21.9	22.4	22.6	24.6
40–44	6.9	6.6	9.1	8.3	8.1	8.3	10.5	10.9	17.1	17.6	16.4	16.8	18.1	18.5	18.6	20.5
45–49	5.9	5.7	7.7	7.2	6.8	7.2	8.6	9.0	13.9	14.4	13.3	13.7	14.4	14.9	14.9	16.4
50–54	5.0	4.9	6.6	6.2	5.8	6.2	7.1	7.3	10.8	11.3	10.2	10.6	10.8	11.2	11.3	12.5
55–59	4.3	4.3	5.6	5.4	4.9	5.3	5.9	6.1	7.7	8.0	7.4	7.8	7.7	8.1	7.9	8.6
60–64	3.6	3.6	4.6	4.7	4.1	4.6	4.9	5.1	4.3	4.4	4.2	4.3	4.3	4.4	4.3	4.5
65–69	3.1	3.1	3.9	3.9	3.4	3.9	4.1	4.3	—	—	—	—	—	—	—	—
70–74	2.7	2.7	3.3	3.3	2.9	3.4	3.4	3.7	—	—	—	—	—	—	—	—
75–79	2.3	2.3	2.8	2.8	2.4	2.8	2.8	3.0	—	—	—	—	—	—	—	—
80–84	1.9	2.0	2.3	2.3	1.9	2.3	2.3	2.5	—	—	—	—	—	—	—	—
85+	1.6	1.6	1.8	1.9	1.5	1.8	1.8	2.1	—	—	—	—	—	—	—	—

SOURCE: Reprinted from USRDS: *2001 Annual Data Report: Atlas of End-Stage Renal Disease in the United States*. Bethesda, MD, National Institutes of Health, National Institute of Diabetes and Digestive and Kidney Diseases, 2001, p 562.

Choice of Renal Replacement Modality

The most common forms of renal replacement therapy are three times weekly outpatient in-center hemodialysis, chronic ambulatory peritoneal dialysis, chronic cycling peritoneal dialysis, and renal transplantation. A few centers use home hemodialysis, daily or nocturnal hemodialysis, intermittent peritoneal dialysis or hemodialysis, or peritoneal dialysis in a nursing home setting. Patients should be educated regarding the pros and cons of each renal replacement treatment modality and any factors, medical or social, that might impact the appropriateness of their treatment with one form or another. Early discussions allow ample time for the patient to become comfortable with the idea of renal replacement therapy. Most patients who present to the nephrologist emergently are begun on hemodialysis, but it is important discuss other modalities of treatment once the patient is stable.

Hemodialysis

By far, in-center hemodialysis is the predominant form of renal replacement therapy in the United States. Data derived from the USRDS for patients 65 years of age and older show the incident rate of hemodialysis (by first modality) in 1999 was 2336 per 1 million population, representing 50 percent of that population initiating renal replacement therapy. Only 10 percent of patients older than age 65 years were treated with peritoneal dialysis, and 5 percent with renal transplantation.

Many elderly patients tolerate hemodialysis well. In addition, some studies show that older dialysis patients seem to enjoy the scheduled social interaction that in-center dialysis provides them. The two main limiting factors for this treatment modality remain vascular access issues and advanced cardiomyopathies. Vascular access is classified as either temporary or permanent (Table 46-9). Temporary access is usually reserved for acute hemodialysis and is usually via the use of dual-lumen, noncuffed catheters. These catheters are ideal for patients who require renal replacement therapy for fewer than 3 weeks. The femoral vein is the preferred site if dialysis is required for fewer than 72 hours, the patient is supine, and/or there is a coexisting coagulopathy. Otherwise, placement within the internal jugular vein yields fewer infectious complications and allows patient mobility. If temporary access is required for periods longer than 3 weeks, access should be maintained with a cuffed tunneled hemodialysis catheter.

Table 46-9   Vascular Access Options for Hemodialysis

	Location	Disadvantages
Temporary		
Dual-lumen, noncuffed catheter (Quinton®)	IJ > F ≫ SCV	Infection, CVS
Tunneled, cuffed catheter (Permacath®, Vaxcel®, Ash®, Tessio®)	IJ > F ≫ SCV	CVS, clotting, infection
Permanent		
Arterio-venous (AV) fistula	R-C, B-C,	Clotting, infection, CHF
Polytetrafluoroethylene graft (PTFE)	B-C, Fa-Fv, Aa-Av,	Infection, clotting
Tunneled, cuffed catheter (Permacath®, Vaxcel®, Ash®, Tessio®)	IJ > F ≫ SCV	CVS, clotting, infection
Subcutaneous vascular access system (LifeSite®)	IJ > F	CVS, Infection, clotting

NOTE: Av-Aa, axillary artery to axillary vein; B-C, brachial artery to cephalic vein; CVS, central venous stenosis; F, femoral vein; Fa-Fv, femoral artery to femoral vein; IJ, internal jugular vein; R-C, radial artery to cephalic vein; SCV, subclavian vein.

The best permanent dialysis access is a Cimino-Brescia fistula (cephalic vein anastomosed to the radial artery), which has a 75 percent 2-year survival rate. The fistula maturation rate in the elderly patient is slightly better if initial placement occurs at the brachial artery to cephalic vein location . The next preferred type of vascular access is the polytetrafluoroethylene (PTFE) synthetic graft, which has a 2-year complication-free survival rate of 30 percent. Numerous studies have confirmed a decreased incidence of infection, thrombosis and other complications, and increased patency for primary arteriovenous fistulas compared to prosthetic grafts. Access should be placed 6 months or more before the estimated need for dialysis. A primary arteriovenous fistula is the preferred dialysis access whenever surgically possible. If a primary fistula fails to mature, it can be converted to an arteriovenous (AV) graft. Occasionally, permanent access placement is complicated by high-cardiac-output heart failure, limb "steal" syndrome (vascular insufficiency), pseudoaneurysm formation, or venous hypertension.

The least-desirable form of permanent access is use of the cuffed tunneled catheter. This device is designed to provide temporary dialysis access until an AV fistula or graft can be placed. Over time, however, the numbers of suitable veins for adequate maturation of an AV fistula or graft become limited and patients become dependent upon cuffed tunneled catheters as a means of permanent access. Recently, a hemodialysis access device, the LifeSite, was developed. It is a hybrid of the AV graft and the tunneled cuffed catheter. It is a closed system, a button implanted subcutaneously that is accessed via locking needles. It may provide a permanent catheter-based hemodialysis access with infection rates and flow rates similar to an AV graft.

Peritoneal Dialysis

Peritoneal dialysis can be a viable treatment option for the geriatric patient. One study demonstrated that chronic peritoneal dialysis (CPD) is a safe and suitable modality for the treatment of ESRD in the "old old" (>80 years of age) patient. Another study demonstrated that CPD can be performed safely and effectively in the extended care facility (ECF) by ECF staff members with specialized training. The preferred mode of peritoneal dialysis in the ECF setting is continuous cyclic peritoneal dialysis or nocturnal peritoneal dialysis, which requires less nursing time, allows patients to be more fully integrated into social activities, allows interruption-free intensive rehabilitation, and provides better urea clearance (weekly Kt/V). Advantages of peritoneal dialysis include improved blood pressure control, less electrolyte variability, higher hematocrits, less-restrictive diet, and more efficacious large solute removal. Disadvantages may include back pain, peritonitis, hyperglycemia, obesity, hernia formation, inadequate urea clearance (Kt/V) secondary to inadequate peritoneal surface area or membrane transport characteristics, and hypertriglyceridemia.

Renal Transplantation

Transplantation in the elderly patient is no longer out of the question. Many reports over the last decade show renal transplantation to be a safe and efficacious mode of renal replacement therapy inpatients older than 60 years of age. One report reviewed the course of 206 primary renal allograft recipients, aged 60 years or older (mean, 64 years old; range, 60 to 76 years old) and 1640 patients aged 18 to 59 years old to evaluate graft and patient survival in first-time kidney transplant recipients, and to identify pretransplant risk factors that predict clinical outcome. In patients 60 years old or older, graft survival at 1 and 5 years was 86 and 60 percent, respectively, and patient survival at 1 and 5 years was 90 and 68 percent, respectively. Graft and patient survival were decreased when compared to recipients aged 18 to 59 years, but were similar when censored for patient death as a cause of graft loss. A pretransplant history of nonskin malignancy, vascular disease, and a current smoking history were risk factors for decreased graft and patient survival (Table 46-10). In the absence of these risk factors, both graft and patient survival were significantly improved factors and equivalent to that of patients aged 18 to 59 years. The major ethical dilemma facing most transplant centers is rationalizing the allocation of a scarce resource (the cadaver kidney) to a patient population with limited life expectancy.

Table 46-10 Risk Factors for Renal Graft Loss in Patients ≥60 Years of Age

Risk Factor (N = 187)	Risk Ratio	P Value
Pretransplant malignancy	3.9	<0.001
Pretransplant vascular disease	2.1	0.024
Donor age >50 years	2.3	<0.01
Cadaver list <1 year	1.8	0.096
Age 65–70 (vs. 60–64) years	1.7	0.062
Current tobacco use*	8.1	<0.001

*Results for analysis of 155 patients for whom smoking history was available.

SOURCE: Adapted from Doyle et al. (2000).

Management of ESRD on Dialysis

Anemia

The association between hematocrit levels and patient mortality has been evaluated in a retrospective study of a national prevalent Medicare hemodialysis cohort. After adjusting for comorbidity, it was found that patients with hematocrit levels less than 30 percent had a 12 to 33 percent higher risk of all-cause and cause-specific death, when compared to patients with hematocrits in the 30 percent to less than 33 percent range. These data, as well as previous studies, that demonstrated higher hematocrits are associated with improved cognitive function, reduced left ventricular hypertrophy (LVH), increased exercise tolerance, and improved quality of life, support the current NKF-K/DOQI guidelines that recommend a target hematocrit of 33 to 36 percent.

Proper anemia management requires routine analysis and treatment of iron deficiency. Iron levels tend to drop in patients on erythropoietin therapy because of increased iron utilization. All patients, however, should receive routine screening of stool for occult blood and periodic screening colonoscopy. Iron-deficient ESRD patients usually receive intravenous replacement iron at the end of their dialysis treatments, either as dextran, gluconate, or sucrose solution. Because they absorb oral iron poorly, ESRD patients have "functional" iron deficiency when their transferrin falls below 100 ng/mL or their iron saturation is less than 20 percent.

Cardiovascular Disease

Factors that contribute to cardiovascular disease in dialysis patients include older age, diet, male gender, white race, smoking, and underlying conditions such as preexisting nephrotic syndrome or diabetes, hypertension, hyperparathyroidism, hyperlipidemia, anemia, and hypoalbuminemia.

The most common cause of death in dialysis patients is cardiovascular disease. Two-thirds of these cardiac deaths are secondary to left ventricular dysfunction and/or associated arrhythmias, and only one-third are secondary to myocardial infarction. One study of 67 chronic hemodialysis patients older than 65 years of age found that systolic blood pressure, interdialytic weight gain, age, and hematocrit were independent risk factors for increased left ventricular mass index.

Appropriate cardiac evaluation is not different from younger patients or nondialysis patients and includes thallium scans, echocardiography, stress testing, coronary angiogram, percutaneous transluminal coronary angioplasty, or coronary artery bypass surgery, as indicated. It is important to be aware, however, that dialysis patients may be unable to achieve maximal heart rates during exercise stress testing, and that metabolic alterations because of uremia and/or diabetes may affect interpretation of test results.

Calcium, Phosphorous, Hyperparathyroidism, and Bone Disorders

In one study, no difference was found in hyperphosphatemia or severity of renal osteodystrophy in elderly dialysis patients as compared with younger dialysis patients, and no correlation was found between plasma 1,25-dihydroxyvitamin D_3 levels and age in patients with chronic kidney failure. Another study found that elderly female dialysis patients had significantly lower bone mineral content and bone width when compared with younger dialysis patients matched for duration of dialysis. Other studies have noted an increased incidence of pathologic fracture, vascular or metastatic calcification, and bone pain in elderly dialysis patients than in younger patients.

Treatment of renal osteodystrophy and secondary hyperparathyroidism in the geriatric renal patient is similar to the younger patient. Hyperphosphatemia is treated with diet and phosphate binders. Hypocalcemia can be treated with oral calcium, oral or intravenous calcitriol, or higher dialysate calcium. Exercise can be effective in decreasing the effects of reduced physical activity on uremic bone disease and osteoporosis. Estrogen treatment of osteoporosis must be individualized as in the nonrenal patient.

Metabolic Acidosis

The acidosis associated with renal disease is not more severe in the elderly patient despite the decreased ability to handle an acid load seen with normal aging. Because of the adverse metabolic effects of chronic acidosis such as accelerated bone loss and muscle wasting, goals of therapy should be directed at achieving predialysis serum bicarbonate levels of at least 22 mmol/L. If predialysis HCO_3^- levels routinely fall below 22 mmol/L, supplementation can be provided with oral sodium bicarbonate tablets.

Malnutrition

Table 46-11 lists some strategies to enhance good nutrition in elderly dialysis patients. Adequacy of dialysis therapy should be evaluated to avoid the anorexia and nausea associated with underdialysis. Dietary supplements and vitamin and mineral supplements, such as zinc or oral pyridoxine (50 mg/d), might be helpful. It is unclear whether intradialytic parenteral nutrition offers real benefit. There are no controlled studies available, and it is very expensive. Dietary restrictions in the elderly patient should be

Table 46-11 Strategies to Enhance Nutrition in Elderly Dialysis Patients

- Ensure adequacy of dialysis
- Dietary supplements
- Megestrol
- Minimal dietary *restrictions*
- Meals-on-wheels
- Companionship
- Home assistance services
- Metoclopramide
- Adequate dental care
- Treatment of depression
- Treatment of constipation
- Therapeutic nihilism

minimal. Patients with inadequate intake rarely need food restrictions.

Pruritus

Pruritus is more common in the elderly dialysis patient, possibly because of skin changes seen with aging. Treatment consists of keeping the skin moist with baby oil and humectants, oatmeal soap, bathing less frequently and with tepid rather than hot water, and increasing ambient humidity with vaporizers or humidifiers. Antihistamines such as diphenhydramine or hydroxyzine may be used, but may cause sedation or confusion in elderly patients. Increased sun exposure has been recommended.

SPECIAL ISSUES

Survival

ESRD is associated with a decrease in life expectancy for all age groups when compared to age-matched patients. The need for dialysis impacts the risk of death in the patient older than age 75 years to a lesser degree than it impacts patients 45 years of age, with a 3-fold versus 20-fold increased risk as compared to nondialysis patients, respectively.

Multiple studies have identified comorbid conditions or presenting factors associated with poorer outcomes in patients receiving renal replacement therapy. Hypoalbuminemia, mode of renal replacement therapy, low body mass index, and malnutrition have such striking correlation with mortality that they have altered the initiation guidelines for renal replacement therapy. The recent clinical practice guidelines on shared decision making for the appropriate

Table 46-12 Comparative Percent Increase for Death of Eight Factors Studied in Two or More Studies with Multivariate Analysis

Risk Factor	Increased Risk of Death (%)	References	
Age	2–4	Bleyer et al. (1996) Leavey (1998) Lowrie (1995, 1990)	Marcelli (1996) Owen (1998) McClellan (1991)
Race	7–38*	Bleyer et al. (1996) Lowrie (1995, 1990) Owen (1998)	Held (1994) McClellan (1994) McClellan (1991)
Gender	5–73[†]	Leavey (1998) Lowrie (1995, 1990) Marcelli (1996) McClellan (1994)	Held (1994) Owen (1998) McClellan (1991)
Serum albumin	33–81[‡]	Bleyer et al. (1996) Leavey (1998)	Lowrie (1995) Owen (1998)
Cachexia	25–36	Leavey (1998)	Marcelli (1996)
Functional status	52–138 (moderate impairment) 100–216 (severe impairment)	Bleyer et al. (1996) McClellan (1994)	
Diabetes	10–74	Leavey (1998) Marcelli (1996) Owen (1998)	McClellan (1994) Lowrie (1990) McClellan (1991)
Heart disease (CAD/CHF)	11–41	Bleyer et al. (1996) Leavey (1998) Marcelli (1996)	McClellan (1994) Held (1994)

SOURCE: Adapted from Clinical Practice Guideline on Shared Decision-Making in the Appropriate Initiation and Withdrawal from Dialysis. Renal Physicians Association and American Society of Nephrology, Clinical Practice Guideline Number 2, Washington, DC, November 1999.

*Whites vs. Blacks

[†]Men vs. Women

[‡]% increase for every one g/dL decrease in serum albumin

initiation of and withdrawal from dialysis released in 1999 by the Renal Physicians Association and the American Society of Nephrology are an evidence-based review of this topic, and include a comparison table demonstrating the impact of various risk factors. Functional status appears to have the most dramatic impact of all risk factors, with an increase risk of death of 52 to 138 percent for moderate impairment, and 100 to 216 percent for severe impairment (Table 46-12).

Another important factor that influences patient survival while receiving dialysis is the "dose" or "adequacy" of dialysis received. This parameter is most often measured by calculating the urea clearance at a given dialysis session (single-pool Kt/V) on a monthly basis. Factors that influence urea clearance are duration of dialysis treatment, blood flow rate across the dialysis membrane, dialysate flow rate, and the degree of ultrafiltration achieved.

Withdrawal from Dialysis

Stopping dialysis is now one of the most common reasons for death in the US dialysis population, especially for patients 65 years of age or older. Approximately 10 percent of patients are withdrawn or voluntarily withdraw from therapy annually. All dialysis patients should understand that they have the right to stop treatment. As noted previously, however, the health care team should ensure that the patient is not withdrawing because of "burdens" that can be ameliorated. One prospective observational study of 131 adult (average age 70 years) maintenance dialysis patients examined the quality of dying following dialysis termination. Quality of death was evaluated by the use of a quality-of-dying tool that quantified the duration (length of time it took to die), pain and suffering, and psychosocial factors. Death occurred 8.2 ± 0.7 days after the last dialysis treatment. Thirty-eight percent of subjects had a very good death, 47 percent had good deaths, and only 15 percent had bad deaths. However, during the last day of life, 42 percent had some pain (5 percent severe) reiterating the importance end-of-life palliation once the decision to withdraw therapy is made.

Advance Directives

Physicians, patients, and family members often have difficulty with withholding dialysis therapy when a life-threatening complication such as refractory pulmonary edema develops. It is important for advance directives to be discussed with every patient, and it is particularly important for patients with advanced chronic kidney disease. Unfortunately, very few physicians, nurses, or social workers discuss advance directives electively with patients; most discussions occur at the moment of impending death or after deterioration in the patient's health status. It is especially important to discuss advanced directives near the time of diagnosis of chronic kidney disease. Surveys show nephrologists are generally willing to honor advance directives, although one anonymously conducted survey found that 25 percent of nephrologists would have difficulty honoring the directives if they felt it was not in the best interest

of the patient. Patients who decide not to undergo dialysis should have clear documentation in their medical records. It is important for members of the health care team to be informed regarding their wishes. There should be similar documentation of do-not-resuscitate orders, wishes regarding artificial nutrition and other measures, and identification of their health care surrogate.

CONCLUSION

As the ESRD population continues to age, the patient care issues encountered by both the nephrologist and geriatrician will continue to overlap. Unlike the younger ESRD patient, elderly ESRD patients are more physiologically fragile, have an altered ability to maintain homeostasis, and may deteriorate very quickly. It is crucial for both disciplines to be educated about these issues.

REFERENCES

Ahmed S et al: Opinions of elderly people on treatment for end-stage renal disease. *Gerontology* 45(3):156, 1999.

Arora P et al: Prevalence, predictors, and consequences of late nephrology referral at a tertiary care center. *J Am Soc Nephrol* 10(6):1281, 1999.

Bleyer AJ, Tell GS, Evans GW, Ettinger WH, Jr., Burkart JM: Survival of patients undergoing renal replacement therapy in one center with special emphasis on racial differences. *Am J Kidney Dis* 28(1):72–81, 1996.

Brown WW: Hemodialysis in elderly patients. *Int Urol Nephrol* 32(1);127, 2001.

Brown WW: The geriatric dialysis patient, in Henrich WL (ed): *Principles and Practices of Dialysis*, 2nd ed. Baltimore, Williams and Wilkins, 1999, p 460.

Carey HB et al: Continuous peritoneal dialysis and the extended care facility. *Am J Kidney Dis* 37(3):580, 2001.

Chester AC et al: Hemodialysis in the eighth and ninth decades of life. *Arch Intern Med* 139(9):1001, 1979.

Cohen LM et al: Dying well after discontinuing the life-support treatment of dialysis. *Arch Intern Med* 160(16):2513, 2000.

Dimkovic NB et al: Chronic peritoneal dialysis in octogenarians. *Nephrol Dial Transplant* 16(10):2034, 2001.

Doyle SE et al: Predicting clinical outcome in the elderly renal transplant recipient. *Kidney Int* 57(5):2144, 2000.

Galla JH: Clinical practice guideline on shared decision-making in the appropriate initiation of and withdrawal from dialysis. The Renal Physicians Association and the American Society of Nephrology. *J Am Soc Nephrol* 11(7):1340, 2000.

Held PJ, Port FK, Turenne MN, Gaylin DS, Hamburger RJ, Wolfe RA: Continuous ambulatory peritoneal dialysis and hemodialysis: comparison of patient mortality with adjustment for comorbid conditions. *Kidney Int* 45(4):1163–1169, 1994.

Ismail N: Renal replacement therapy in the elderly: An old problem with young solutions. *Nephrol Dial Transplant* 12(5):873, 1997.

Korevaar JC et al: Evaluation of DOQI guidelines: Early start of dialysis treatment is not associated with better health-related quality of life. *Am J Kidney Dis* 39(1):108, 2002.

Leavey SF, Strawderman RL, Jones CA, Port FK, Held PJ: Simple nutritional indicators as independent predictors of mortality in hemodialysis patients . *Am J Kidney Dis* 31(6): 997–1006, 1998.

Lowrie EG, Huang WH, Lew NL: Death risk predictors among peritoneal dialysis and hemodialysis patients: a preliminary comparison. *Am J Kidney Dis* 16(1):220–228, 1995.

Lowrie EG, Lew NL: Death risk in hemodialysis patients: The predictive value of commonly measured variables and an evaluation of death rate differences between facilities. *Am J Kidney Dis* 15(5):458, 1990.

Ma JZ et al: Hematocrit level and associated mortality in hemodialysis patients. *J Am Soc Nephrol* 10(3):610–9, 1999.

Mallick N, El Marasi A: Dialysis in the elderly, to treat or not to treat? *Nephrol Dial Transplant* 14(1):37, 1999.

Marcelli D, Stannard D, Conte F, Helt PJ, Locatelli F, Port FK: ESRD patient mortality with adjustment for comorbid conditions in Lombardy (Italy) versus the United States. *Kidney Int* 50(3): 1013–1018, 1996.

McClellan WM, Anson C, Birkeli K, et al: Functional status and quality of life: Predictors of early mortality among patients entering treatment for end stage renal disease. *J Clin Epidemiol* 44:83–89, 1991.

McClellan W, Soucie JM: Facility mortality rates for new end-stage renal disease patients: implications for quality improvement. *Am J Kidney Dis* 24(2):280–289, 1994.

Mignon F et al: The management of uraemia in the elderly: treatment choices. *Nephrol Dial Transplant* 10(Suppl 6):55, 1995.

National Kidney Foundation: K/DOQI clinical practice guidelines for chronic kidney disease: Evaluation, classification and stratification. *Am J Kidney Dis* 39(Suppl 1):S1, 2002.

Owen WF Jr., Chertow GM, Lazarus JM, Lowrie EG: Dose of hemodialysis and survival: differences by race and sex. *JAMA* 280(20):1764–1768, 1998.

Pastan S, Bailey J: Dialysis therapy. *N Engl J Med* 338(20):1428, 1998.

Rebollo P et al: Is the loss of health-related quality of life during renal replacement therapy lower in elderly patients than in younger patients? *Nephrol Dial Transplant* 16(8):1675, 2001.

Rutecki GW et al: Nephrologists' subjective attitudes towards end-of-life issues and the conduct of terminal care. *Clin Nephrol* 48(3):173, 1997.

USRDS: *2001 Annual Data Report: Atlas of End-Stage Renal Disease in the United States.* Bethesda, MD, National Institutes of Health, National Institute of Diabetes and Digestive and Kidney Diseases, 2001, p 562.

Valderrabaño F et al: Quality of life in end-stage renal disease patients. *Am J Kidney Dis* 38(3):443, 2001.

Zawada ET: Initiation of dialysis, in Daugirdas JT, Blake PG, Ing T, (eds): *Handbook of Dialysis*, 3d ed. New York, Lippincott Williams & Wilkins, 2000, p 3.

Disorders of Fluid Balance

MYRON MILLER

Characteristic of the normal aging process is a decline in physiologic reserve in many body regulatory systems, including those involved in the maintenance of fluid balance. The confluence of normal aging changes, common diseases, and the administration of many classes of drugs can readily lead to clinically evident disturbances of fluid balance, such as water retention or loss and to hyponatremia or hypernatremia with resultant symptomatic consequences. In some individuals, an impaired ability to conserve water may underlie the development of nocturnal urinary frequency as well as urinary incontinence.

The normal regulation of water and electrolyte balance involves the interplay of many homeostatic systems that operate to maintain the composition of fluid and electrolyte compartments within a narrow range. Because of alterations in the normal aging process, these homeostatic systems may be compromised. The key regulatory components of fluid balance include (1) thirst perception, which governs fluid intake, (2) the kidney, which is governed by hemodynamic forces, and (3) hormonal influences of arginine vasopressin (AVP) or antidiuretic hormone (ADH), atrial natriuretic hormone (ANH), and the renin–angiotensin–aldosterone system, which control renal water and electrolyte excretion. Clinicians who are involved in the care of the elderly recognize that disturbances of water and electrolyte balance are common in this age group, especially when older persons are challenged by disease, drugs, or extrinsic factors such as access to fluids or control of diet composition.

EFFECTS OF NORMAL AGING ON FLUID REGULATORY SYSTEMS (TABLE 47-1)

Body Composition

Aging effects on body composition have the potential to contribute to derangements in fluid balance. Normal aging is accompanied by a decrease in lean body mass, an increase in fat, and a decrease in total body water. Thus, total body water declines from the approximate values of 60 percent of body weight in young men and 52 percent in young women to 54 percent and 46 percent, respectively, in individuals

older than age 65 years, primarily through a decrease in the intracellular fluid compartment. The decrease in total body water may place the elderly patient at increased risk for dehydration when challenged by fluid loss or decreased fluid intake and at increased risk for fluid overload and hyponatremia when exposed to excessive oral or parenteral fluid intake.

Thirst and Fluid Intake

The ability to ingest a sufficient volume of fluid to meet body needs requires that thirst perception be present, that a suitable source of fluid be available, and that the individual be physically capable of obtaining and consuming the fluid. Under normal conditions, the requirement for daily fluid intake is approximately 30 mL/kg body weight. This requirement is further increased when there is high environmental temperature, fever, increased gastrointestinal, urinary, or respiratory fluid loss. Older persons may be challenged by increased amounts of fluid by either oral or parenteral routes, especially when they are in institutional acute care or long-term care settings and not in control of their fluid intake. In this circumstance, there is risk of volume overload and hyponatremia.

In healthy individuals, fluid intake is largely controlled by thirst sensation, which is regulated by both extracellular fluid volume and blood tonicity. Blood osmolality is the most important factor in the day to day perception of thirst. Thirst is usually stimulated when plasma osmolality rises to values greater than 292 mOsm/kg. Healthy persons older than age 65 years have shown evidence of an age-associated impairment in thirst perception so that when they were subjected to water deprivation sufficient to raise plasma osmolality to greater than 296 mOsm/kg they exhibited diminished subjective awareness of thirst and consumed significantly less water than young subjects who were similarly water deprived and whose plasma osmolality rose to a lesser level (mean, 290 mOsm/kg). Other studies of elderly patients with cerebrovascular accidents have similarly documented impaired thirst perception in the face of volume depletion and hyperosmolality, both normally being potent stimuli for thirst. Elderly patients with Alzheimer's disease fail to drink adequately when exposed

Table 47-1   Aging Effects on Water and Sodium Regulatory Systems

Body composition
    Decreased total body water
    Decreased intracellular fluid compartment

Fluid intake
    Decreased thirst perception

Renal function
    Decreased kidney mass
    Decline in renal blood flow
    Decline in glomerular filtration rate
    Impaired distal renal tubular diluting capacity
    Impaired renal concentrating capacity
    Impaired sodium conservation
    Impaired renal response to vasopressin

Hormonal systems
    Vasopressin
        Normal or increased basal secretion
        Increased response to osmotic stimulation
        Decreased nocturnal secretion
    Atrial natriuretic hormone
        Increased basal secretion
        Increased response to stimulation
    Decreased plasma renin activity
    Decreased aldosterone production

to water deprivation in spite of the accompanying elevation of blood osmolality to levels above the usual thirst threshold. Further confounding the ability of the elderly person to ingest adequate amounts of fluid is the frequent presence of physical disability (e.g., blindness, arthritis, stroke) and impaired mobility, thus limiting the capacity of the patient to gain access to fluids.

Renal Changes of Normal Aging

Structural and Functional Changes

Normal aging is accompanied by changes in renal anatomy and in renal function. Kidney mass undergoes progressive decline from a normal combined weight of approximately 250 to 280 g in young adults to between 180 and 200 g by age 80 to 90 years, with corresponding decrease in length and volume. Histologically, the number of glomeruli decline by 30 to 40 percent with increasing age and the percent of glomeruli that are hyalinized or sclerotic, increase to 10 to 30 percent. This process accelerates after the age of 40 years, and the residual glomeruli also undergo changes with age. Thus, there is a decrease in effective filtering surface, and an increase in the number of mesangial cells, a decrease in number of epithelial cells, and thickening of the glomerular basement membrane.

As part of the normal aging process, there are changes in the renal vasculature that lead to obliteration of the arteriolar lumen and loss of the glomerular capillary tuft. These changes take place primarily in the cortical glomeruli. In the juxtamedullary area, glomerular sclerosis may lead to anastomosis between afferent and efferent arterioles with direct shunting of blood between these vessels. Blood flow to the medulla, through the arteria rectae, is maintained in old age.

The anatomic changes of the aging kidney are paralleled by alterations in renal function, although a direct relationship between anatomic and functional changes is not firmly established. Renal blood flow declines during the course of normal aging by approximately 10 percent per decade after young adulthood so that by the age of 90 years the renal plasma flow is approximately 300 mL/min—a reduction of 50 percent of the value found at 30 years of age. The decrease in renal perfusion is most extensive in the outer cortex with lesser impairment of inner cortex and minimal effect on the medulla.

Glomerular filtration rate (GFR) remains relatively stable until age 40 years, after which it undergoes decline at an annual rate of approximately 0.8 mL/min/1.73 m². Because there is much individual variability within the elderly population, longitudinal studies show that not all aging persons will undergo a decline in GFR. An estimate of GFR can be made using the Cockcroft-Gault formula for creatinine clearance (for women multiply result by 0.85):

$$\text{creatinine clearance (mL/min)} = \frac{140 - \text{age (years)} \times \text{body weight (kg)}}{72 \times \text{serum creatinine (mg/dL)}}$$

Water Regulatory Capacity

Renal Water Retention   The aging kidney exhibits a modest age-related impairment in the ability to dilute the urine and excrete a water load. The ability to generate free water is dependent on several factors, including adequate delivery of solute to the diluting region (sufficient renal perfusion and GFR), a functional intact distal diluting site (ascending limb of Henle's loop and the distal tubule), and suppression of ADH in order to escape water reabsorption in the collecting duct. The age-related decline in GFR is the most important factor in the aged kidney's diluting capacity. The presence of an age-related diluting defect that is independent of changes in GFR remains controversial.

The diluting capacity of the aging kidney has been evaluated in men by determining the urine osmolality and free water clearance response to acute water loading. In young men (mean age 31 years), minimum urine osmolality was 52 mOsm/kg, whereas in middle-aged men (mean age 60 years) minimum urine osmolality was 74 mOsm/kg, and in the older men (mean age 84 years) it was 92 mOsm/kg. The free water clearance was lowest in the older group. However, when these results were expressed as free water clearance per mL of GFR, the values were not different, suggesting that the defect in diluting capacity was a consequence of an age-related reduction in GFR. In a similar study in which healthy elderly subjects aged 63 to 80 years (mean, 72 years) and healthy young subjects aged 21 to

26 years (mean, 22 years) were administered a water load, the peak free water clearance was 5.7 mL/min in the older group and 8.4 mL/min in the younger group. However, when adjustments were made for changes in creatinine clearance, the difference in these indices was not statistically significant.

Other studies suggest that age-related free water clearance defects persist following correction for a lower GFR. A significantly lower free water clearance/creatinine ratio was found in elderly nursing home residents as compared to healthy younger subjects. The maximal urinary dilution (urinary/plasma osmolality) declined from 0.247 in younger subjects to 0.418 in elderly subjects.

In addition to impaired diluting capacity, the age-related decrease in renal plasma flow and GFR can lead to passive reabsorption of fluid, thereby increasing the risk of water overload and hyponatremia. This effect is clinically evident in elderly patients who have congestive heart failure, extracellular volume depletion, and hypoalbuminemia.

Diuretics, especially thiazides, can decrease renal diluting capacity. In the elderly, this effect becomes especially important when it is superimposed on the already diminished diluting capacity of the aged kidney, thus increasing the risk of developing water intoxication by impairing the ability to excrete excess water promptly.

Renal Water Loss It has been known for many years that there is an age-related change in renal concentrating capacity. In a study of healthy men aged 40 to 101 years who underwent 24 hours of water deprivation, maximum attainable urine specific gravity declined from 1.030 at 40 years to 1.023 at 89 years. Hospitalized men aged 23 to 72 years who underwent 24 hours of dehydration demonstrated a progressive decline in maximum urine osmolality with increasing age. In healthy, active community-dwelling participants in the Baltimore Longitudinal Study of Aging, young subjects responded to 12 hours of water deprivation with a marked decrease in urine flow (1.02 ± 0.10 to 0.49 ± 0.03 mL/min) and a moderate increase in urine osmolality (969 ± 41 to 1109 ± 22 mOsm/kg), whereas elderly subjects were unable to significantly alter urine flow (1.05 ± 0.15 to 1.03 ± 0.13 mL/min) or osmolality (852 ± 64 to 882 ± 49 mOsm/kg). This age-related decline in urine concentrating ability persisted after correction for the age-related decrease in GFR.

The effect of age on renal tubular response to vasopressin has been assessed by measuring the urine-to-plasma insulin concentration ratio in men who ranged in age from 26 to 86 years and who were free of clinically demonstrable cardiovascular and renal disease. The ratio fell from 118 in young men (mean age 35 years) to 77 in the middle-aged group (mean age 55 years) and to 45 in the older men (mean age 73 years). The decreased renal sensitivity to vasopressin with age may be a result of an age-related increase in vasopressin secretion. Animal studies demonstrate that chronic exposure of the kidney to increased vasopressin results in diminished renal responsiveness to the hormone. Thus, an age-related increase in vasopressin secretion may result in downregulation of renal AVP receptors and be the basis for decreased renal concentrating capacity in the elderly.

Sodium Regulatory Capacity

Renal Sodium Retention Several situations may lead to sodium retention and accompanying water overload in the elderly. The previously described age-related decrease in renal blood flow and GFR favors enhanced conservation of sodium. Disease states resulting in secondary hyperaldosteronism, such as congestive heart failure, cirrhosis, or nephrotic syndrome, are common in the elderly. In addition, drugs such as nonsteroidal antiinflammatory agents, which are frequently used in the elderly, may promote sodium retention.

Renal Sodium Loss Elderly individuals are more likely to have exaggerated natriuresis after a water load than are younger subjects. Patients with benign hypertension have an excess of sodium excretion in association with increased age. The aged kidney's response to salt restriction is sluggish so that restriction in sodium intake to 10 mEq/d was followed by a half-time for reduction of urinary sodium excretion of 17.6 hours in young individuals and 30.9 hours in old individuals. These data suggest that the aging kidney is more prone to sodium wasting. Mechanisms underlying this tendency may be multifactorial and are related to the effects of age on ANH, the renin–angiotensin–aldosterone system, and renal tubular function.

Vasopressin System in Normal Aging (Table 47-2)

Neurohypophyseal System

The magnocellular neurons of the hypothalamus where arginine vasopressin is synthesized do not appear to undergo age-related degenerative changes. There is no evidence of the cell destruction, neuronal dropout, or loss of dendritic arborization found in other segments of the aged brain. Moreover, neurosecretory material in supraoptic nuclei (SON) and paraventricular nuclei (PVN) in elderly persons does not appear to differ in amount from that in younger subjects.

Morphologic data provide evidence that these nuclei, in fact, become more active with age. In the human hypothalamic neurohypophyseal system of subjects ranging from 10 to 93 years of age, a gradual increase in the size of the SON and PVN was observed after 60 years of age, suggesting that AVP production increases in senescence. Similar changes have been observed in the nuclear size of AVP neurons. Possibly contributing to the maintenance of normal or increased amounts of AVP in the magnocellular neurons is the observation of a 25 percent reduction in the rate of axonal transport of AVP and its associated neurophysin with advancing age. Thus, it appears that neurosecretory activity of hypothalamic AVP neurons does not decrease but, in fact, remains constant or is elevated with age.

Basal Plasma Vasopressin Levels

There are conflicting data regarding basal concentration of AVP in the blood during normal aging. In young normal

Table 47-2   Aging Effects on the Vasopressin System

Morphology of the neurohypophyseal system
    Normal or increased supraoptic nucleus cell
        number/AVP content
    Normal or increased paraventricular nucleus cell
        number/AVP content
    Decreased suprachiasmatic nucleus cell number/AVP
        content
    Normal extrahypothalamic nuclei cell number/AVP
        content

Hypothalamic vasopressin content
    Normal or increased

Cerebrospinal fluid vasopressin concentration
    Normal

Blood vasopressin concentration
    Normal or increased basal
    Increased after osmotic and pharmacologic stimulation
    Decreased response to volume/pressure stimulation
    Decreased nocturnal secretion

Renal response to vasopressin
    Decreased

Changes are in comparison to values observed in the young.

individuals, there is a diurnal rhythm of vasopressin secretion, with greatest AVP secretion occurring at night. This rhythm appears to be linked to the wake–sleep cycle, rather than to time of day. The sleep-associated peak is absent in the majority of healthy elderly persons. Low AVP levels and the lack of definite diurnal rhythm may, to some extent, explain increased diuresis during the night in some elderly individuals.

Healthy elderly subjects have been found to have basal plasma AVP levels that were significantly lower than in young subjects. In association with the reduced AVP concentration, plasma osmolality was elevated, suggesting that the elderly subjects had a water-losing state similar to partial diabetes insipidus.

Other studies indicate that basal plasma levels of AVP did not differ among young, middle-aged, and elderly healthy individuals who were studied under both supine and ambulatory conditions. Furthermore, there were no differences in plasma osmolality between the groups.

In contrast to the above are reports of elevated basal vasopressin levels in healthy elderly persons as compared with younger individuals. Healthy human subjects aged 20 to 80 years have been observed to exhibit a progressive rise in plasma AVP concentration with age, which become most evident in subjects older than age 60 years. Baseline plasma AVP correlates with serum osmolality in younger adults but not in elderly subjects.

Debate exists regarding a sex-related difference in plasma AVP levels in the elderly population. There are reports of a twofold higher plasma AVP concentration in elderly men as compared to women, while other studies fail to identify a gender effect on basal plasma AVP.

A rise in basal plasma AVP with age cannot be attributed to age-related changes in vasopressin metabolism. No differences were found between young and old subjects in vasopressin half-life, volume of distribution, or clearance. Thus, evidence of increased basal plasma vasopressin most likely reflects age-related changes in central control systems for vasopressin release.

Vasopressin Stimulation

Secretion of AVP normally varies in response to changes in blood tonicity, blood volume, and blood pressure. Hormone release is also affected by other variables such as nausea, pain, emotional stress, a variety of drugs, cigarette smoking, and glucopenia. In recent years, a growing body of information suggests that normal aging affects the way these stimuli act and interact to influence AVP release.

The major physiologic stimulus for vasopressin secretion in humans, plasma osmolality, is regulated by hypothalamic osmoreceptors. Osmoreceptor sensitivity in the elderly population has been assessed by comparing the AVP response to hypertonic saline infusion in healthy elderly persons (age 54 to 92 years) to the response in younger individuals (age 21 to 49 years). Hypertonic saline raised plasma osmolality with a consequent increase in plasma AVP in both groups, but the hormone concentrations in the older subjects were almost double those in the younger subjects. Thus, for any given level of osmotic stimulus, there was a greater release of AVP in the elderly, suggesting that aging resulted in osmoreceptor hypersensitivity.

Use of water deprivation as a stimulus for vasopressin secretion has supported the concept of an age-related enhancement in vasopressin secretion. Water-deprivation for 24 hours in young healthy individuals (age 20 to 31 years) and healthy elderly men (age 67 to 75 years) demonstrated that the older persons responded with higher serum concentrations of AVP than did the younger individuals.

The sensitivity of the hypothalamic-neurohypophyseal axis to volume/pressure stimuli has been studied. In response to acute upright posture after overnight water deprivation, older subjects (age 62 to 80 years) demonstrated the expected changes in pulse and blood pressure but only 8 of 15 older individuals experienced increased plasma vasopressin in contrast to a rise in plasma vasopressin in all young subjects (age 19 to 31 years). This and other studies suggest the presence of an aged-related impairment of volume/pressure-mediated vasopressin release.

The ability of intravenous ethanol infusion to inhibit AVP secretion has been evaluated in young (age 21 to 49 years) and old (age 54 to 92 years) subjects. Younger subjects demonstrated a sustained inhibition of AVP secretion during the infusion of ethanol, whereas there was a paradoxical response in the older group with initial AVP inhibition followed by breakthrough secretion and rebound to twice basal levels. Not only was ethanol less effective in inhibiting AVP release in the elderly, but it eventually lost its suppressive effect entirely as a result of the introduction of a hyperosmotic stimulus resulting from the ethanol-induced constriction in plasma volume.

Metoclopramide can stimulate vasopressin secretion in man through cholinergic mechanisms. Intravenous metoclopramide administration to normal elderly subjects age 65 to 80 years and to normal young subjects age 16 to 35 years produced significantly higher plasma AVP concentrations in the older group with no significant changes in plasma osmolality, blood pressure, or heart rate. Response of AVP to cigarette smoking and insulin-induced hypoglycemia, as well as to metoclopramide, has been evaluated in male subjects aged 22 to 81 years. The AVP response to metoclopramide and to smoking was significantly higher in the older group as compared to two younger groups. In contrast, the AVP response during the insulin hypoglycemia test was identical in pattern and magnitude in all age groups.

The stimulation studies indicate that, in aging, AVP response to osmotic stimuli is increased because of a hyperresponsive osmoreceptor, whereas AVP response to upright posture is reduced because of impaired baroreceptor function. Input from the baroreceptor to the osmoreceptor is usually inhibitory, so that a defect in this reflex arc would result in lesser dampening and consequent heightening of osmotically stimulated ADH release. When coupled with the many alterations in renal function that occur with aging, these changes can increase the risk of elderly persons for hyponatremia by impairing their ability to excrete excess water promptly.

Age-Related Changes in Atrial Natriuretic Hormone Secretion, Regulation, and Action

Atrial natriuretic hormone is synthesized, stored, and released in the atria of the heart. Through its action on the kidney, ANH produces a pronounced natriuresis and diuresis; through its action on blood vessels, it produces vasodilation and decreases blood pressure in both normal and hypertensive individuals. As an important regulator of sodium excretion, ANH may be a significant factor in mediating the altered renal sodium handling of age.

In a comparison of young normal men with elderly male nursing home residents, a fivefold increase in mean basal ANH levels and an exaggerated ANH response to the stimulus of saline infusion has been observed in the elderly group. In response to the stimulus of head-out water immersion, ANH levels in healthy old individuals (age 62 to 73 years), which were twice as high at baseline than in young subjects (age 21 to 28 years), rose to a greater extent than in the young. Healthy male and female subjects age 22 to 64 years have been studied to determine the influence of age on circulating levels of ANH, both under basal conditions and after the physiologic stimulation of ANH release by controlled exercise using a bicycle ergometer to increase heart rate to 80 percent of maximum predicted rate. Subjects older than 50 years of age had higher baseline levels and a greater response to exercise when compared to

subjects younger than age 50 years. Thus, increasing age results in increased ANH basal levels and an increased ANH response to both physiologic and pharmacologic stimuli, perhaps as a consequence of age-related decrease in cardiac muscle compliance.

The renal effects of ANH may be exaggerated in elderly versus young individuals. The natriuretic response to a bolus injection of ANH was higher in older individuals (mean age 52.3 years) as compared with younger subjects (mean age 26 years). No change with age was noted in the blood pressure response to ANH intravenous infusion after correction for higher ANH levels in the elderly.

Atrial natriuretic hormone is known to interact with the renin–angiotensin–aldosterone system. Increases of ANH result in suppression of renal renin secretion, plasma renin activity, plasma angiotensin II, and aldosterone levels, suggesting indirect inhibition of aldosterone secretion by ANH. Minimal increases in ANH within physiologic levels produced by slow-rate ANH infusion can inhibit angiotensin II-induced aldosterone secretion in normal men, suggesting a direct inhibitory effect of ANH on aldosterone release. Thus, ANH may promote renal sodium loss both through inhibition of aldosterone release and through a direct natriuretic action.

ANH may be an important mediator of age-related renal sodium loss. This effect may be the consequence of increased basal ANH levels, increased ANH response to stimuli, increased renal sensitivity to ANH, and ANH-induced suppression of adrenal sodium-retaining hormones.

Renin—Angiotensin—Aldosterone

A substantial body of evidence indicates that the normal aging process affects the renin–angiotensin–aldosterone system. Healthy older individuals (age 62 to 70 years) with normal dietary sodium intake have lower plasma renin activity and aldosterone concentration while in the supine position than do young healthy persons (age 20 to 30 years). Under the stimuli of upright posture and sodium depletion, significant increases in circulating renin and aldosterone occurred in both age groups, but mean values achieved were always significantly lower in the elderly group. The decrease in plasma renin activity in the elderly population is not a result of changes in plasma renin substrate concentration; rather, it is a result of a decrease in active renin concentration, perhaps caused by decreased conversion of inactive to active renin. The decrease in plasma renin activity may also be related to the inhibitory effect of increased amounts of ANH on renin secretion (see above). Decreased aldosterone concentration with age appears to be a direct result of age-related decrease of plasma renin activity and not to aging changes in the adrenal gland because aldosterone and cortisol responses to corticotropin infusion are not altered in the elderly person. It is likely that the age-related decrease in aldosterone concentration is a predisposing factor to renal salt wasting in the elderly person.

Intrinsic renal tubular changes may also play a role in sodium wasting. An impaired capacity to reabsorb sodium

Table 47-3   Clinical Features of Depletional versus Dilutional Hyponatremia

Feature	Depletional	Dilutional

History	Low dietary Na intake
	Na loss
	  Vomiting
	  Diarrhea
	  Nasogastric suction
	
	Use of diuretics
	Diseases
	  Renal
	  Adrenal
		Increased fluid intake (oral, IV)
		Drugs
		Diseases
		  CNS
		  Pulmonary
		  Malignancy

Physical examination	Dry mucous membranes Decreased skin turgor Hypotension, tachycardia, orthostatic changes	Euvolemia or edema Evidence of CNS, pulmonary disease, malignancy
Laboratory evaluation	Increased hematocrit, BUN, creatinine Urinary Na excretion <20 mEq/L	Normal or decreased BUN, creatinine, uric acid, albumin Urinary Na excretion >20 mEq/L

BUN, blood urea nitrogen; CNS, central nervous system.

SOURCE: Reproduced with permission from Miller M: Hyponatremia: age-related risk factors and therapy decisions. *Geriatrics* 53:32, 1998.

has been described along with decreased tubular responsiveness to aldosterone administration. However, a subsequent study failed to find an effect of age on renal tubular sensitivity to aldosterone.

The age-associated decline in the renin–angiotensin–aldosterone system may be linked to alterations in potassium regulation. Hyporeninemic hypoaldosteronism occurs most commonly in elderly persons, especially those with diabetes mellitus. The hyperkalemia characteristic of the disorder responds to treatment with mineralocorticoid and may be the consequence of interaction of chronic renal disease with the hormonal changes of normal aging. The risk of angiotensin-converting enzyme inhibitors in producing hyperkalemia is especially high in elderly persons, and may also be related to the interplay between drug action and physiologic alterations due to aging.

DISORDERS OF FLUID REGULATION

Hyponatremia

Hyponatremia is usually defined as a serum sodium concentration of ≤ 135 mEq/L. It appears when there is an excess of water relative to sodium in the extracellular body fluid compartment and can be the consequence of either a decrease in extracellular sodium content (i.e., sodium depletion) or an increase in extracellular water (i.e., dilutional hyponatremia). In the elderly person, dilutional hyponatremia is the more common mechanism and most frequently is due to the syndrome of inappropriate antidiuretic hormone secretion (SIADH).

Dilutional versus Depletional Hyponatremia

The determination of whether hyponatremia is of dilutional, depletional, or mixed origin can generally be made by history and physical examination and by commonly available laboratory measurements (Table 47-3). The characteristic features of dilutional hyponatremia and SIADH are hyponatremia and serum hypoosmolality with clinical euvolemia and absence of edema, failure of the urine to be appropriately dilute, excretion of sodium in the urine at a concentration of >20 mEq/L and the absence of other hyponatremia-producing disease states such as hypothyroidism, adrenal insufficiency, congestive heart failure, cirrhosis, or renal disease.

Depletional hyponatremia typically results from a prolonged period of inadequate sodium intake and/or from increased gastrointestinal tract or urinary sodium loss. Extracellular fluid volume depletion is often present with physical findings and laboratory values related to hypovolemia.

Epidemiology

Hyponatremia is a common finding in elderly persons. Analysis of plasma sodium values in healthy individuals has shown an age-related decrease of approximately 1 mEq/L per decade from a mean value of 141 ± 4 mEq/L in young subjects. In a population of individuals older than age 65 years who were living at home and who were without acute illness, a 7 percent incidence of serum sodium concentration of 137 mEq/L or less was observed. Similarly, there was an 11 percent incidence of hyponatremia in the population of a geriatric medicine outpatient practice. In

Table 47-4 Risk Factors for Hyponatremia in the Elderly Person

Physiologic changes of normal aging
  Decreased renal sodium-conserving ability
    Altered renal tubular function
    Increased atrial natriuretic hormone secretion
    Decreased renin–angiotensin–aldosterone secretion
  Decreased renal water-excretion ability
    Decreased renal blood flow and glomerular filtration rate
    Decreased distal renal tubular diluting capacity
    Increased renal passive reabsorption of water
    Increased vasopressin secretion

Diseases accompanied by SIADH (See Table 47-5)

Drugs accompanied by sodium loss or SIADH (See Table 47-6)

Increased water intake
  Oral fluids
  Intravenous hypotonic fluids

Decreased sodium intake
  Low-sodium diet
  Tube feeding

Increased sodium loss
  Renal disease
  Gastrointestinal tract
    Vomiting
    Diarrhea
    Gastric suctioning

Idiopathic SIADH of the elderly person
  Age >80 years
  Race other than African American

SIADH, syndrome of inappropriate antidiuretic hormone secretion.

Source: Reproduced with permission from Miller M: Hyponatremia: Age-related risk factors and therapy decisions. *Geriatrics* 53:32, 1998.

hospitalized patients, hyponatremia is even more common. An analysis of 5000 consecutive sets of plasma electrolytes from a hospital population with a mean age of 54 years revealed a mean serum sodium of 134 ± 6 mEq/L, with the values skewed toward the hyponatremic end of the distribution curve. A high prevalence of hyponatremia has been found in patients hospitalized for a variety of acute illnesses, with the risk being greater with increasing age of the patient.

Elderly residents of long-term care institutions appear to be especially prone to hyponatremia. In a study of patients with a mean age of 72 years who resided in a chronic disease hospital, 22.5 percent had repeated serum sodium determinations of less than 135 mEq/L. Of patients admitted to an acute geriatric unit, 11.3 percent were found to have serum sodium concentrations of ≤130 mEq/L. A survey of nursing home residents aged >60 years revealed a prevalence of

18 percent with serum sodium less than 136 mEq/L. When this population was observed on a longitudinal basis over a 12-month period, 53 percent were observed to experience one or more episodes of hyponatremia. Persons with central nervous system (CNS) and spinal cord disease were at highest risk, and water-load testing indicated that most hyponatremic patients had features consistent with SIADH.

Risk Factors (Table 47-4)

Hyponatremia often is a marker for severe underlying disease with poor prognosis and high mortality. A major risk for the development or worsening of hyponatremia is the administration of hypotonic fluid, either as an increase in oral water intake or as intravenous 0.45% saline solution or 5% glucose in water, a finding in 78 percent of nursing home residents with hyponatremia. Low sodium intake coupled with age-associated impaired renal sodium-conserving ability can, over time, lead to sodium depletion with hyponatremia. Many patients whose nutritional support is primarily or entirely provided by tube feeding develop either intermittent or persistent hyponatremia. The underlying cause appears to be sodium depletion because of the low sodium content of most tube-feeding diets. The hyponatremia usually resolves in response to increasing the dietary sodium intake.

Advanced age itself may be a risk factor for hyponatremia. SIADH has been described in elderly individuals, generally older than age 80 years, in whom no identifiable cause for hyponatremia could be found, suggesting that there is an idiopathic form of SIADH that may represent the clinical expression of physiologic changes that take place in the regulation of water balance during aging. Race may play a role because African Americans appear to be at lower risk than whites or Hispanics.

Syndrome of Inappropriate Antidiuretic Hormone Secretion

Diseases Many diseases that are common in the elderly population can cause SIADH (Table 47-5). Almost all central nervous system disorders can lead to dysfunction of the hypothalamic system involved in the normal regulation of AVP secretion with resultant increased secretion of the hormone and consequent risk for water retention and hyponatremia. Such central nervous system disorders include vascular injury (thrombosis, embolism, hemorrhage), trauma with subdural hematoma, vasculitis, tumor, and infection. Malignancies can cause SIADH as a result of autonomous release of AVP from cancer tissue where it is synthesized, stored and discharged in the absence of known stimuli. The malignancy most commonly associated with SIADH in the elderly population is small-cell carcinoma of the lung, in which as many as 68 percent of patients have been found to have evidence of impaired water excretion and elevated blood AVP concentration. Other malignancies include pancreatic carcinoma, thymoma, pharyngeal carcinoma, lymphosarcoma, and Hodgkin's disease. Inflammatory lung diseases can also cause SIADH, perhaps as a result of AVP production by diseased pulmonary tissue, and

Table 47-5   Diseases/Disorders Associated with Hyponatremia in the Elderly Population

Central nervous system disorders
  Vascular diseases (thrombosis, embolism, hemorrhage, vasculitis)
  Trauma (subdural hematoma, intracranial hemorrhage)
  Tumor
  Infectious disease (meningitis, encephalitis, brain abscess)

Malignancy with ectopic AVP production
  Pulmonary (small-cell carcinoma)
  Pancreatic carcinoma
  Pharyngeal carcinoma
  Thymoma
  Lymphosarcoma, reticulum cell sarcoma, Hodgkin's disease

Pulmonary disease
  Pneumonia
  Tuberculosis
  Lung abscess
  Bronchiectasis

Endocrine disease
  Hypothyroidism
  Diabetes mellitus with hyperglycemia
  Adrenal insufficiency

Other
  Acquired immunodeficiency syndrome (AIDS)
  Idiopathic SIADH of the elderly person

SOURCE: Modified with permission from Miller M: Hyponatremia: age-related risk factors and therapy decisions. *Geriatrics* 53:32, 1998.

include such entities as bronchiectasis, pneumonia, lung abscess, and tuberculosis.

Drugs Numerous drugs taken by elderly persons can affect water balance by direct action on the kidney or by altering AVP release from the neurohypophyseal system or its action on the kidney (Table 47-6). In particular, many drugs increase the risk for SIADH.

Hyponatremia with the characteristics of SIADH is recognized as a side effect of several older antipsychotic agents, that is, fluphenazine, thiothixene, and phenothiazine, as well as the tricyclic antidepressants. There is evidence that the selective serotonin reuptake inhibitor (SSRIs) antidepressants can also induce SIADH, with a reported incidence of 3.5 to 6.3 per 1000 people treated per year. Although fluoxetine is the SSRI most commonly reported to produce hyponatremia, other SSRIs, including paroxetine, sertraline, and fluvoxamine, have also been involved. Individuals at highest risk for SSRI-induced hyponatremia are those older than age 65 years in whom the onset of hyponatremia typically occurs within 2 weeks after initiation of drug therapy.

Angiotensin-converting enzyme (ACE) inhibitor use in the elderly population is associated with the development of hyponatremia. In most of the cases, the level of hyponatremia has been clinically significant with serum sodium concentrations as low as 101 mEq/L and with symptoms ranging from confusion to seizures and coma. Although initial reports indicated that the risk was greatest when ACE inhibitors were used in combination with thiazide diuretics, it now appears that the ACE inhibitors alone can precipitate hyponatremia. The hyponatremia appears to be dilutional with features of SIADH and may be mediated by potentiation of plasma renin activity with subsequent increase in brain angiotensin levels, which, in turn, stimulate both release of AVP from the hypothalamus and an increase in thirst. Discontinuing the ACE inhibitor is associated with rapid resolution of the hyponatremia.

Diuretics, both of the loop and thiazide types, can produce hyponatremia. Loop diuretics appear to have a greater natriuretic effect in older persons than in younger persons. Hyponatremia can occur when diuretic-induced sodium and water loss are replaced by hypotonic fluids, resulting in a combined depletional and dilutional hyponatremia. With thiazide diuretics, the induced sodium loss is often accompanied by loss of total body potassium with consequent

Table 47-6   Drug-Induced Changes in Sodium and Water Regulation

Sodium Retention
  Nonsteroidal antiinflamatory agents

Sodium loss
  Thiazide and loop diuretics

Impaired diluting capacity
  Thiazide diuretics

Impaired concentrating capacity
  Lithium
  Demeclocycline
  Potassium-losing diuretics

Syndrome of inappropriate antidiuretic hormone secretion
  Central nervous system agents
    Tricyclic antidepressants
    SSRI antidepressants
    Phenothiazine antipsychotics
    Carbamazepine anticonvulsant
  ACE inhibitors
  Antineoplastic drugs
    Vincristine
    Vinblastine
    Cyclophosphamide
  Chlorpropamide
  Clofibrate
  Narcotics

SOURCE: Reproduced by permission from Miller M: Hyponatremia: age-related risk factors and therapy decisions. *Geriatrics* 53:32, 1998.

Table 47-7 Treatment of Dilutional Hyponatremia

Presentation	Treatment Modality	Potential Adverse Outcomes
Acute	IV 3% saline, 300–500 mL over 4 to 6 hours, followed by 100 mL/h until serum Na reaches ~125 mEq/L at rate of increase of 0.5–1 mEq/L/h (maximum increase 12 mEq/L over 24 hours)	Central pontine myelinolysis, congestive heart failure
	IV furosemide 1 mg/kg body weight	Hypokalemia, hypomagnesemia
Chronic	Correction of underlying cause	
	Fluid restriction to 800–1000 mL per 24 hours	Thirst stimulation, dehydration
	Demeclocycline 600–1200 mg per 24 hours	Photosensitivity, azotemia, nephrotoxicity in patients with hepatic disease or congestive heart failure

SOURCE: Reproduced by permission from Miller M: Hyponatremia: Age-related risk factors and therapy decisions. *Geriatrics* 53:32, 1998.

decrease in intracellular solute content and decreased cell volume. This circumstance can activate hypothalamic pathways leading to increased AVP discharge, water retention and SIADH. This form of thiazide-induced hyponatremia occurs almost entirely in the elderly population and can be reversed by correcting the underlying potassium depletion.

Other drugs associated with development of hyponatremia in the elderly population include the sulfonylurea chlorpropamide, the anticonvulsant carbamazepine, and the antineoplastic agents vincristine, vinblastine, and cyclophosphamide. Analgesics, particularly the narcotics, may be responsible for the occurrence of hyponatremia in the elderly postoperative patient.

Clinical Presentation

The clinical severity of hyponatremia is dependent on both the magnitude of the hyponatremia and the rate at which the serum sodium level has declined. There is often a poor correlation between serum sodium concentration and severity of symptoms. Mild chronic hyponatremia may be asymptomatic. Serum sodium levels <125 mEq/L may be accompanied by lethargy, fatigue, anorexia, nausea, and muscle cramps. With worsening hyponatremia, central nervous system symptoms predominate and range from confusion to coma to seizures. There is substantial risk of death in severely symptomatic patients with serum sodium <110 mEq/L who also have underlying disease with cachexia.

Management (Table 47-7)

Hyponatremia due to sodium depletion is often accompanied by extracellular fluid volume depletion and treatment is directed at correcting the volume deficit with intravenous 0.9% saline. Milder depletional hyponatremia, such as that which occurs in persons whose nutrition is predominantly from enteral feedings, can be corrected by adding saline solution or crushed sodium chloride tablets to the enteral feedings.

The patient with symptomatic dilutional hyponatremia requires prompt intervention and is best managed in an intensive care unit setting. Mildly symptomatic patients with serum sodium >125 mEq/L can be treated with fluid restriction to a level of 800 to 1000 mL/24 h. More severe symptoms should be treated with intravenous 3% saline infusion at a rate sufficient to raise serum sodium by 0.5 to 1 mEq/L/h. The goal is a maximum increase in serum sodium of no more than 12 mEq/L in the first 24 hours, and to a value no higher than 125 mEq/L, in order to avoid central pontine myelinolysis. Occasionally, patients either with fluid overload and pulmonary edema or with symptoms of coma or seizures who have very low serum sodium levels may require initial treatment with intravenous furosemide in a dose 1 mg/kg body weight along with the 3% saline. In this circumstance, attention will need to be given to possible diuretic-induced potassium and magnesium depletion.

Hypernatremia and Dehydration

Hypernatremia, generally defined as a serum sodium of ≥148 mEq/L, most commonly occurs when there is excessive loss of body water relative to loss of sodium in association with inadequate fluid intake. In this circumstance, hypernatremia is accompanied by dehydration. When fluid loss is accompanied by sodium loss, dehydration can occur without associated hypernatremia. In rare circumstances, hypernatremia can be caused by excessive sodium intake without corresponding increased fluid intake and thus be associated with euvolemic or hypervolemic volume status.

Epidemiology

In a study of 15,187 hospitalized patients older than age 60 years, a 1 percent incidence of hypernatremia was reported, with a mean serum sodium concentration of 154 mEq/L. Similarly, a study of elderly residents in a long-term care institution revealed a 1 percent incidence of hypernatremia, which increased to 18 percent over a

Table 47-8 Risk Factors for Hypernatremia in the Elderly Population

Increased water loss
  Renal
    Age-associated impaired concentrating capacity
    Resistance to vasopressin action
      Age-associated
      Acquired (drugs, hypokalemia, hypercalcemia)
    Osmotic diuresis (glycosuria, diuretic-induced natriuresis)
    Renal tubular disease
  Gastrointestinal tract
    Vomiting
    Diarrhea
  Skin (sweating)
  Lung (tachypnea)

Decreased water intake
  Impaired thirst perception
  Impaired cognition (delerium, dementia)
  Impaired access to fluids

12-month observation period. Of 264 nursing home residents in whom acute illness developed requiring hospitalization, 34 percent became markedly hypernatremic with serum sodium concentration greater than 150 mEq/L.

Risk Factors

The renal and hormonal alterations of aging described above are physiologic factors associated with an increased risk for hypernatremia (Table 47-8). Frequent pathologic factors are febrile illness with increased insensible fluid loss, tachypnea with increased water loss from the lungs, diarrhea, and osmotic-induced polyuria from poorly controlled diabetes mellitus or use of loop diuretics. There is a high morbidity and mortality in elderly patients who develop serum sodium concentrations above 148 mEq/L and such elevations of serum sodium are often a consequence of a severe underlying disease process.

Clinical Presentation

The symptoms of moderate hypernatremia may be nonspecific and commonly include weakness and lethargy. More severe hypernatremia, often with serum sodium concentration >152 mEq/L, may be accompanied by obtundation, stupor, coma, and seizures. The clinical signs are those of volume depletion and dehydration with weight loss, decreased skin turgor, dry mucous membranes, tachycardia, and orthostatic hypotension. In addition to the elevated serum sodium, laboratory findings are those of hemoconcentration with increased hematocrit, blood urea nitrogen (BUN), creatinine, and serum osmolality. Urine osmolality may not be greatly increased because of age-related impairment in renal concentrating capacity.

Management

The correction of hypernatremia requires replacement of body water deficits which may be as large as 11 L or 30 percent of total body water. When hypernatremia is due almost entirely from water loss alone, the water deficit can be estimated by means of the following calculation:

$$\text{current total body fluid volume (L)} = \frac{140\,\text{mEq/L} \times \text{basal body weight (kg)} \times 0.45}{\text{current serum Na (mEq/L)}}$$

where 0.45 represents the approximate proportion of body weight that is water. Total body water is subtracted from estimated normal total body water of $0.45 \times$ body weight to give an approximate value for the water deficit.

Modest fluid deficits of 1 to 2 L can be corrected by oral fluid intake. More significant volume deficits require intravenous fluid therapy, preferably starting with 0.9% saline given at a rate sufficient to resolve orthostatic hypotension and tachycardia and to replace approximately 50 percent of the estimated fluid deficit in the first 24 hours and to reduce serum sodium by no more than 2 mEq/L/h. Excessively rapid correction can lead to cerebral edema with consequent brain damage or death. The goal is then to correct remaining volume depletion and hypernatremia over 48 to 72 hours by using 0.45% saline.

Treatment of dehydration without hypernatremia is directed at correction of intravascular volume depletion and involves fluid replacement with intravenous 0.9% saline. Clinical indicators of effectiveness of therapy are correction of orthostatic hypotension and tachycardia and reduction in BUN and serum creatinine concentrations.

Nocturnal Polyuria

In normal young persons, there is a diurnal pattern of vasopressin secretion with highest levels occurring during sleep. This is reflected by a lower rate of urine flow at night than during the daytime so that nighttime urine volume is approximately 25 percent or less of total 24-hour urine volume. In many older persons, there is loss of nocturnal vasopressin secretion and an accompanying reversal of day/night urine production so that nighttime urine flow rate exceeds the daytime flow rate. This alteration in renal function leads to a diabetes insipidus-like nocturnal polyuria. Nocturnal polyuria is considered to be present when any of the following criteria are met: urine production during 8 hours of sleep is ≥33 percent of 24-hour urine production; nighttime urine production rate is ≥0.9 mL/min; 7 P.M. to 7 A.M. urine volume is ≥50 percent of total 24-hour volume (Table 47-9). Nocturnal polyuria is a common finding in community-residing elderly persons with nocturia. The prevalence can be as high as 50 percent in nursing home residents, particularly those with Alzheimer's disease. It is also often seen in patients with central autonomic insufficiency (Shy-Drager syndrome/multiple system atrophy) or spinal cord injury (Table 47-9).

Table 47-9 Nocturnal Polyuria

Definitions
  Urine production during 8 hours of sleep ≥33% of
    24-hour urine production
  Nighttime urine production rate >0.9 mL/min
  7 P.M. to 7 A.M. urine volume ≥50% of total 24-hour
    volume

Causes
  Normal aging
  Multiple system atrophy
  Alzheimer's disease
  Spinal cord injury

Table 47-10 Alzheimer's Disease and Disordered Water Regulation

Alterations in water regulation
  Impaired thirst perception
  Decreased vasopressin secretion
    Basal
    Response to stimulation
    Diurnal pattern

Clinical consequences
  Increased risk of dehydration
  Hypertonicity (increased serum sodium and osmolality)
  Reversal of day/night urine flow rate
  Nocturnal polyuria and incontinence

Both reduced bladder capacity and detrusor instability are commonly present in elderly persons, with prevalence in both men and women increased with increasing age. High nighttime urine production in persons with nocturnal polyuria coupled with these bladder alterations may be a contributing factor to the nocturnal urinary frequency seen so commonly in older persons.

Evaluation

Individuals with nocturia can be evaluated for the presence of nocturnal polyuria by means of a voiding diary in which the time and volume of each void is recorded for a 72-hour period. In addition, urine production during 8 hours of sleep can be measured in a timed urine collection and compared with urine production during the remainder of a 24-hour period. Both approaches allow demonstration of increased nocturnal urine production meeting the above cited criteria.

Management

The vasopressin analog DDAVP (deamino-8-D-arginine vasopressin) may be helpful in treating both nocturnal frequency and nocturnal urinary incontinence. DDAVP can be given either intranasally in a dose of 5 to 20 μg or orally in a dose of 200 to 400 mg taken in the evening. Because DDAVP has a duration of action of 12 to 24 hours, care must be taken to monitor serum sodium to avoid the possible development of dilutional hyponatremia.

Water Balance in Alzheimer's Disease

Persons with Alzheimer's disease are at increased risk for disturbed water regulation (Table 47-10). The secretion of vasopressin may be lower in those with Alzheimer's disease than in comparably aged persons with normal cognitive function and there is absence of the nocturnal rise in hormone secretion. Following dehydration, individuals with Alzheimer's disease show a lesser rise in plasma vasopressin than do age-matched normal subjects. Similarly, pharmacologic stimulation with metoclopramide or physostigmine is accompanied by marked blunting of plasma vasopressin response. These changes contribute to a high prevalence of nocturnal polyuria and nocturia in patients with Alzheimer's disease. In patients with Alzheimer's disease, the cognitive impairment can cause the nighttime polyuria to be clinically expressed as urinary incontinence.

Clinically, patients with Alzheimer's disease are at increased risk for dehydration. Overnight fluid restriction results in greater rise in plasma osmolality, greater water loss, and, in spite of these stimuli for thirst, marked reduction in spontaneous water intake. A direct correlation exists between mini mental status examination score and impairment of water intake.

CONCLUSION

Normal aging is accompanied by many changes in the various regulatory systems involved in the control of sodium and water balance. As a consequence of these alterations, the elderly person has a diminished capacity to withstand the challenges of illness, drugs, and physiologic stresses, and, thus, has an increased risk for the development of clinically significant alterations in sodium and water balance. Awareness of these limitations of homeostasis ability allows the physician to anticipate the impact of illnesses and drugs on volume and electrolyte status of the elderly patient and will lead to a more rational approach to therapeutic intervention and management.

REFERENCES

Anderson RJ et al: Hyponatremia: A prospective analysis of its epidemiology and the pathogenetic role of vasopressin. *Ann Intern Med* 102:164, 1985.

Asplund R, Aberg H: Diurnal variation in the levels of antidiuretic hormone in the elderly. *J Intern Med* 299:131, 1991.

Bauer JH: Age-related changes in the renin-aldosterone system: Physiological effects and clinical implications. *Drugs Ageing* 3:238, 1993.

Espiner EA et al: Natriuretic hormones. *Endocrinol Metab Clinics North Am* 24:481, 1995.

Helderman JH et al: The response of arginine vasopressin to intravenous ethanol and hypertonic saline in man. The impact of aging. *J Gerontol* 33:39, 1978.

Johnson AG et al: Arginine vasopressin and osmolality in the elderly. *J Am Geriatr Soc* 42:399, 1994.

Lindeman RD et al: Longitudinal studies on the rate of decline in renal function with age. *J Am Geriatr Soc* 33:278, 1985.

Miller M: Nocturnal polyuria in older people: Pathophysiology and clinical implications. *J Am Geriatr Soc* 48:1321, 2000.

Miller M: Hormonal aspects of fluid and sodium balance in the elderly. *Endocrinol Metab Clinics North Am* 24:233, 1995.

Miller M et al: Apparent idiopathic hyponatremia in an ambulatory geriatric population. *J Am Geriatr Soc* 44:404, 1996.

Miller M et al: Hyponatremia in a nursing home population. *J Am Geriatr Soc* 43:1410, 1995.

Miller M et al: Physiological changes of aging affecting salt and water balance. *Rev Clin Gerontol* 1:215, 1991.

Ouslander J et al: The dark side of incontinence: Nighttime incontinence in nursing home residents. *J Am Geriatr Soc* 41:371, 1993.

Palevsky PM et al: Hypernatremia in hospitalized patients. *Ann Intern Med* 124:197, 1996.

Phillips PA et al: Reduced thirst after water deprivation in healthy elderly men. *N Engl J Med* 311:753, 1984.

Rowe JW et al: The effect of age on creatinine clearance in man: A cross-sectional and longitudinal study. *J Gerontol* 311:155, 1976.

Snyder NA et al: Hypernatremia in elderly patients. A heterogeneous, morbid, and iatrogenic entity. *Ann Intern Med* 107:309, 1987.

Tsunoda K et al: Effect of age on the renin–angiotensin–aldosterone system in normal subjects: Simultaneous measurement of active and inactive renin, renin substrate, and aldosterone in plasma. *J Clin Endocrinol Metab* 62:384, 1986.

Verbalis JG. Adaptation to acute and chronic hyponatremia: Implications for symptomatology, diagnosis, and therapy. *Semin Nephrol* 18:3, 1998.

Wilkinson TJ et al: Incidence and risk factors for hyponatremia following treatment with fluoxetine or paroxetine in elderly people. *Br J Clin Pharmacol* 47:211, 1999.

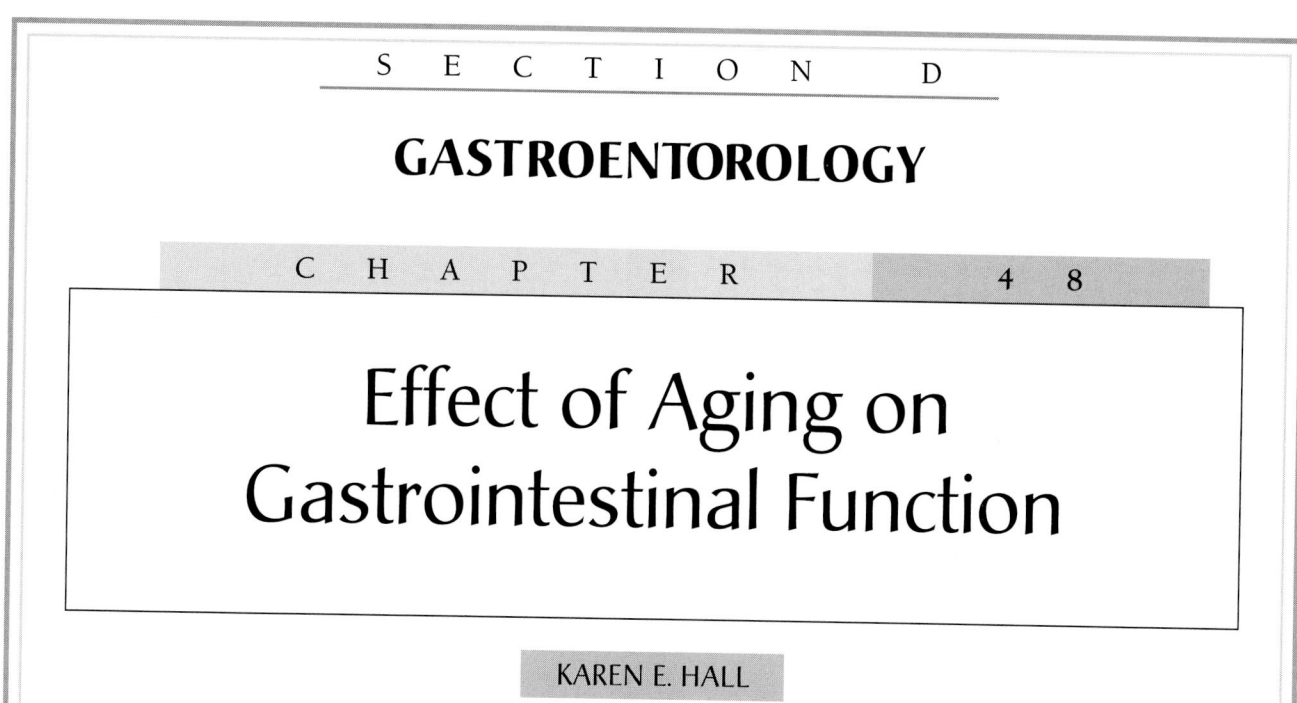

GASTROENTOROLOGY

C H A P T E R 4 8

Effect of Aging on Gastrointestinal Function

KAREN E. HALL

Over the past decade, the view that significant changes in gastrointestinal (GI) function are an expected consequence of normal aging has been revised. It is now apparent that many age-related alterations in gastrointestinal function are associated with intercurrent illnesses, rather than aging per se. The gastrointestinal tract exhibits considerable reserve capacity, and some areas retain normal physiologic function during the aging process (Fig. 48-1). However, certain age-related changes in gastrointestinal function are viewed as dysfunctional by patients and health care providers, a notable example being constipation. There has been a dramatic increase in the amount of clinical data on human aging since the previous edition of this text was published. Such studies have clarified the relative importance of aging versus disease on gastrointestinal function. Animal studies continue to provide important insights into the cellular physiology of aging, despite the issue of species variation. The pathophysiology of neuronal dysfunction in the enteric and central nervous system with aging has been reviewed. A selected subset of recent literature concerning gastrointestinal function in aging is provided in the reference list.

Digestion is complex, and requires integration of neuromuscular motility, luminal secretion, absorption, and assimilation. Thus, age-associated alterations in the luminal gut, exocrine pancreas, liver, and biliary tree have the potential to affect nutrition and maintenance of body systems. In addition to digestion, the gastrointestinal tract has other important functions, such as drug metabolism and immune regulation. There is evidence that substantial variation in gastrointestinal metabolism of drugs occurs in aging. This may have significant implications for drug interactions.

The gastrointestinal tract is an immunologic organ. Lymphocytes residing in the luminal gut produce secretory immunoglobulin A (IgA), an important "frontline" component of the immune system. A substantial population of other immunologically active cells are found in the mucosa and submucosa of the gastrointestinal tract. Age-associated alterations in gastrointestinal immunologic function may contribute to the increased susceptibility observed for infections in the geriatric population.

AGE-ASSOCIATED CHANGES IN OROPHARYNGEAL AND ESOPHAGEAL FUNCTION

As summarized in Chap. 94, the increasing likelihood of dental decay and tooth loss with aging has an obvious effect on the efficiency and completeness of mastication. This contributes to dysphagia, particularly when other mechanisms involved in swallowing are also impaired.

After food is broken up in the mouth by mastication, the act of swallowing moves the food bolus from the oral cavity into the pharynx and esophagus. The oral and pharyngeal stages of swallowing are regulated by cortical input to medullary swallowing centers that innervate skeletal muscle groups in the pharynx (see Chap. 93). The proximal esophagus contains skeletal muscle controlled by nerves from the medullary swallowing centers, whereas the mid- and distal esophagus consists of smooth muscle regulated by intrinsic enteric innervation and extrinsic innervation by the vagus nerve.

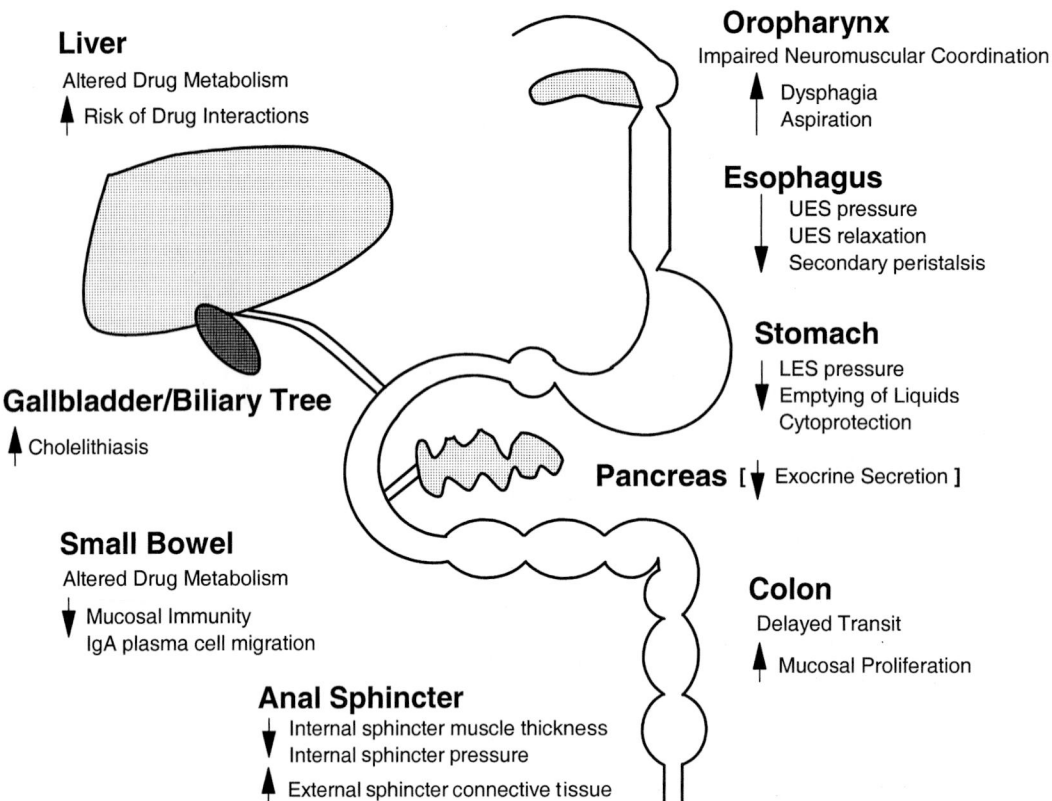

Figure 48-1   Effects of physiologic aging on the gastrointestinal tract. This schematic summarizes significant effects of aging on various divisions of the gastrointestinal tract. *Up arrow,* increased; *down arrow,* decreased; *brackets,* insignificant alteration in function.

Complaints of dysphagia, regurgitation, chest pain, and heartburn are fairly common in patients aged 65 or older, with a prevalence of 35 percent reported in the general population ages 50 to 79 years. As in younger patients, it has been difficult to demonstrate a consistent relationship between symptoms and underlying pathophysiology. There is little data available, particularly in patients older than age 75 years, to indicate whether there is a true difference in the reporting of dysphagia by the geriatric population. Investigation of the symptoms listed above results in demonstrable esophageal abnormalities in only 20 to 30 percent of symptomatic patients. A particular concern in the geriatric population is that symptoms of dysphagia are significantly more likely to have a serious underlying etiology, such as malignancy. Elderly patients also appear to be more susceptible to complications of inadequately treated chronic esophageal disease, such as aspiration, malnutrition, and Barrett's metaplastic disease. Attempts at symptom analysis to identify subgroups at risk for serious underlying disease have met with mixed success. Earlier studies suggested that diminution in esophageal function was a relatively common feature with aging. The term *presbyesophagus* was coined to describe age-related changes in esophageal function, including decreased contractile amplitude, polyphasic waves in the esophageal body, incomplete lower relaxation of the lower esophageal sphincter, and esophageal dilation. The most common alteration in motility observed in older subjects was an increase in rapidity of propagation of the peristaltic wave, together with increased simultaneous contractions. This may be caused by loss of esophageal

inhibitory interneurons, which has been observed in both human and animal models of aging. Despite changes in esophageal motility, most studies of healthy, elderly subjects did not demonstrate any correlation of dysmotility in the body of the esophagus with symptoms. This implies that most symptomatic esophageal motility problems associated with aging are likely related to concurrent medical problems such as diabetes mellitus and neurologic disorders, or the side-effects of medications, rather than aging per se.

A more important factor contributing to the increased prevalence of symptomatic dysphagia in the elderly may be age-associated impairment in transfer of a food bolus from the oral cavity to the pharynx (see Chap. 93). Video fluoroscopy demonstrates abnormal transfer in up to 60 percent of elderly patients without dysphagia. Oropharyngeal swallowing disorders are most commonly observed in patients with cognitive and/or perceptual dysfunction secondary to stroke or dementia, or chronic neurodegenerative diseases that affect the brainstem or motor neurons, such as Parkinson's disease, myasthenia gravis, or amyotrophic lateral sclerosis. Other explanations for the increased prevalence of dysphagia in the elderly population could be anatomic changes in esophageal neuromuscular anatomy or function. Upper esophageal sphincter pressure gradually decreases with age, and is associated with a delay in relaxation after deglutition. It is thought that these changes are related to increased resistance to flow across the upper esophageal sphincter that reflects an age-related loss of muscle compliance. Age-associated changes in the anatomy of the esophageal body appear to be minimal. Thickness of esophageal smooth muscle does not appear to vary significantly between young and aged subjects. The number of myenteric neurons in the esophagus decreases with age; however, the functional significance of this is unclear. Impaired neuromuscular coordination secondary to decreased myenteric innervation might account for some of the observed changes in esophageal function with age.

While the data are conflicting, amplitude of peristaltic contractions appear unaffected by aging. Similarly, the literature contains conflicting reports regarding age-related changes in lower esophageal sphincter (LES) function. Earlier studies reported impaired relaxation or decreased contractions of the LES with aging. However, more recent reports suggest concomitant disease accounts for altered resting pressure of the aged LES.

Symptoms related to gastroesophageal reflux disease (GERD) are a frequent complaint of elderly patients. Risk factors for reflux-induced esophageal damage include decreased esophageal clearance, gastric factors such as decreased emptying or increased gastric pressure, decreased LES pressure, inappropriate LES relaxation, or the presence of a hiatal hernia, and increased gastric acid secretion. A modest increase in the duration and frequency of reflux episodes with age and female sex has been documented in Japanese populations. However, other risks such as increased body weight and hiatal hernia appear to play a more important role. Some studies have demonstrated a significant increase in esophageal acid exposure and longer duration of reflux episodes in the elderly population. This may be caused by decreased occurrence of secondary esophageal peristalsis, an important clearance mechanism for refluxed acid. Other factors, such as gastric emptying and frequency of LES relaxation are relatively unchanged with aging. Concurrent disease and side effects of medications become more important factors in the pathophysiology of GERD in older patients.

AGE-ASSOCIATED CHANGES IN GASTRIC MOTILITY AND LUMINAL FACTORS

Morbidity and mortality associated with peptic ulcer disease is higher in geriatric patients, although the prevalence of ulceration is similar ($\sim$20 percent) as that in younger populations. This increased morbidity does not appear to be caused by excessive secretion of agents that promote mucosal injury, as most healthy older individuals have minimal decreases in acid and pepsin output. A small minority have severe acid hyposecretion (achlorhydria) associated with atrophic gastritis. This may be related to *Helicobacter pylori* colonization, as studies in cohorts of aged Japanese subjects segregated by birth year indicate a decreasing incidence of both *H. pylori* colonization and achlorhydria in individuals born later in the twentieth century, when presumably hygiene and socioeconomic conditions improved. There may be a small reduction in gastric secretion in animal models of aging, such as the Fisher 344 rat. This appears to be a result of decreased antral gastrin release, and is of questionable pathogenesis. Human studies indicate that gastrin

levels tend to rise with age, possibly as a compensatory response to an increased prevalence of gastric autoantibodies and *H. pylori* colonization. The increased prevalence of *H. pylori* carriage in the elderly population does not appear to result in increased rates of duodenal ulceration, but is associated with increased risk of pernicious anemia and gastric lymphoma. Decreased clearance of liquids from the stomach has been documented in older patients, and can be exacerbated by anticholinergic medications. Aging is also associated with decreased perception of gastric distension as measured by subjective fullness during inflation of a gastric barostat balloon. Delayed emptying may prolong the gastric contact time of noxious agents, such as nonsteroidal antiinflammatory drugs (NSAIDs).

It is more likely that the increased susceptibility to gastric mucosal injury from NSAIDs in the elderly population is a result of reduction in gastric mucosal cytoprotective factors. Animal and human studies demonstrate that gastric mucosal prostaglandin content decreases with age, correlating with increasing risk of mucosal injury from acetic acid or aspirin. An alkaline gel layer of gastric bicarbonate provides the first defense against noxious substances such as acid, pepsin, and NSAIDs, and mucous secreted by nonparietal gastric epithelial cells. Human aging is associated with a significant decrease in gastric bicarbonate, sodium ion and nonparietal fluid secretion, and thinning of the mucus gel layer, particularly in *H. pylori*-positive individuals. Similar observations have been reported in rat studies, with decreased gastric luminal pH and bicarbonate output in the stomach, and blunted prostaglandin-mediated increases in gastric acid and bicarbonate secretion. In other animal studies, basal duodenal bicarbonate secretion was unchanged, whereas duodenal bicarbonate response to a fixed load of luminal acid decreased progressively with age.

Gastric mucosal proliferation and regeneration also contributes to gastric mucosal protection. Aging is associated with a decrease in the basal and injury-induced rate of proliferation of stem cells in the neck of gastric glands in rats. Animal studies implicate impaired function of various intestinal growth factors, such as transforming growth factor-alpha (TGF-α) and epithelial growth factor (EGF), although in vitro activation of EGF receptor (EGFR) by membrane-bound TGF-α is actually increased in gastric and colonic mucosa of aged rats.

Mucosal blood flow plays an essential role in maintaining gastric mucosal integrity by supplying oxygen and nutrients, and removing potentially noxious agents. Atherosclerosis of the celiac axis and other major arteries occurs in aging, however, the rich collateral circulation to the stomach and associated organs mitigates the effects of occlusion of a major vessel. In diabetes mellitus, microvascular involvement of vessels within the wall of the gastrointestinal tract does not impair luminal protection. However, in rats, aging is associated with a decrease in basal gastric blood flow associated with impaired healing of acid-induced mucosal lesions. Impaired healing of gastric ulcers has also been associated with underlying impairment in sensory neuron function in several aging models.

Gastric secretion of intrinsic factor is necessary for vitamin B_{12} absorption in the small bowel. Decreased secretion of intrinsic factor in aging is invariably due to atrophic gastritis, not aging per se.

Collectively, these studies indicate that age-related changes in gastric mucosal defense mechanisms, rather than noxious or aggressive luminal factors, may predispose the aged to gastric mucosal injury.

SMALL INTESTINE FUNCTION IN AGING

The small intestine has a large functional reserve capacity, as a result of the substantial mucosal surface area available for secretion and absorption. Impaired absorption of nutrients is not widely observed in the elderly population. Absorption of lactose, mannitol, and lipid in individuals older than 60 years of age revealed no significant impairment in small intestinal mucosal integrity. Animal studies have revealed conflicting results with respect to nutrient uptake as a function of aging. Despite decreased intestinal enzyme production in aged rats, the effect of aging on absorption of many nutrients is minor. However, vitamin D absorption and sensitivity may be significantly impaired with aging. Decreased uptake of folic acid, vitamin B_{12}, calcium, copper, zinc, fatty acids, and cholesterol have also been documented in aged subjects. Absorption of other nutrients, such as vitamin A and glucose, were increased in aged animals. Recommendations by the US Department of Agriculture to increase calcium, B_{12}, and Vitamin D supplementation in persons older than age 70 years reflect this new information.

Intestinal surface area does not appear to change after 6 weeks of age in rats, despite the visual appearance of atrophy noted in the mucosa of the duodenum and jejunum of senescent rats when compared to the same area in young animals. Of interest, no age-associated changes were observed in the ileum, suggesting that region-specific changes in the small bowel may occur in some models of aging. It is unclear whether the specific activity of intestinal disaccharidases and aminopeptidases is affected by aging, as both higher and lower activity has been reported in aged animals, as compared to youthful controls. An enhanced satiating effect of carbohydrates delivered into the small intestine by infusion has been reported in older men. This may reflect alterations in visceral chemosensitivity or hormone responsiveness. Crypt cell proliferation rates in all segments of the small intestine are greater in aged rats compared to their youthful counterparts, probably as a result of increased numbers of crypt cells undergoing cell division. In general, senescence appears to be associated with delayed maturation and expression of brush-border enzymes in small intestinal villus epithelial cells during crypt-to-villus migration. Regional specificity is observed, as epithelial cell maturation and enzyme activity in the ileum does not appear to be significantly affected by aging.

Minor effects of aging on small bowel motility have been described, despite reports that several neuronal subtypes (substance P-, vasoactive intestinal peptide-, somatostatin-, and nitric oxide-containing subtypes) are decreased in aged animals models. The pathophysiology of enteric neuronal loss and efficacy of treatment of aging-associated neuropathy have been reviewed. There appear to be species differences, as studies in cats do not demonstrate significant effects of age on small bowel transit of radiolabeled lipids. In human studies, small bowel transit time measured by breath hydrogen was shorter in elderly males. The latter could be a result of an age-associated decrease in inhibitory nitrinergic myenteric neurons. There was no significant difference between young and elderly women in small bowel transit time. It is of interest that caloric restriction prevents ileal myenteric neuronal loss in Sprague-Dawley rats up to 30 months of age, as caloric restriction delays or prevents neurodegeneration in a variety of aging models.

EFFECT OF AGING ON COLONIC FUNCTION

Aging is associated with a number of diverse effects on the large intestine including alterations in mucosal cell growth, differentiation, metabolism, and immunity. Several disorders are more commonly observed in the elderly population, including colon cancer, diverticulosis, and altered bowel habits. The observation that crypt cell production rate is significantly higher in colonic tissue from aged rats, as compared to youthful animals, may have relevance to these pathologic events. This raises the question of whether normal aging predisposes the colon to malignant transformation. Some studies support the contention that normal aging may increase susceptibility of colonic mucosa to carcinogens. The active metabolite of the colonic carcinogen azoxymethane, methylazoxymethanol, induces a greater stimulation of ornithine decarboxylase activity and tyrosine kinase activity in aged rats compared to their younger counterparts. Similar results have been reported with TGF-α and insulin-like growth factor-1 (IGF-1), both potent mitogens for a variety of tissues in the GI tract, including the colon. In general, aging appears to be associated with increased responsiveness of the colonic mucosa to TGF-α. It is not yet clear whether changes in the expression and/or affinity of TGF-α receptors or altered postreceptor events contribute to this process.

Diverticulosis is an abnormality commonly described in the aging colon, and predisposes to the subsequent development of diverticulitis. Diverticulosis is observed in otherwise healthy individuals, suggesting that some effect of aging on colonic neuromuscular anatomy or function may be responsible. Decreased tensile strength of the muscle wall, and increased intraabdominal pressures required for evacuation have been implicated in the development of diverticula. Human aging is associated with an increase in collagen in the colon wall that is accompanied by a significant decrease in tensile strength, which may predispose to mucosal herniation. Other observations include slow colonic transit and increased frequency of segmenting contractions, resulting in increased water resorption and hard feces. Decreased fiber intake likely also contributes to the production of hard feces and excessive straining, as both animal and human studies indicate that addition of fiber decreases intraluminal pressures in the colon.

Constipation is a common symptom in the elderly population that is often treated with a variety of prescription and over-the-counter medications. Constipation can be variably described as a decrease in the frequency of defecation, or as increasing difficulty with defecation. The latter is usually caused by either stool that is excessively hard or by functional and/or anatomic conditions that prevent normal defecation. Rectal dyssynergy is an example of the latter, and is often a consequence of multiparity and/or difficult deliveries. Medications may contribute to constipation, either as a consequence of anticholinergic properties, or because of neuromuscular injury. Constipation results in increased stool retention times. This may have implications for carcinogenesis, as prolonged retention of ingested carcinogenic compounds, or those formed by metabolism of precursors, may increase the risk of colon cancer.

The regulation of colonic motility is a complex process influenced by the enteric nervous system, neurotransmitter release, and smooth muscle response. While constipation is a common complaint in the elderly population, age-associated alterations in colonic motility have been difficult to demonstrate. Some studies indicate that colonic transient slows with aging, particularly in women. Others found no significant difference in transit times between young and elderly subjects. Altered neuromuscular coordination leading to impaired colonic motility could also be a function of histopathologic alteration of the myenteric plexus. A reduction in the number of neurons in the aged colonic myenteric plexus has been reported, particularly the nitric oxide-containing neurons involved in receptive relaxation. In addition to decreased neuronal numbers, the remaining myenteric neurons may be functionally impaired. Release of the excitatory neurotransmitter acetylcholine was diminished in the colon of aged rats, an effect that appeared to be due to decreased calcium influx. Interestingly, neurotransmitter release from myenteric neurons in the aged colon could be restored to youthful levels by use of calcium ionophores that bypass membrane calcium channels, suggesting that the mechanisms underlying this deficit may be potentially reversible. Impaired calcium signaling may be a fundamental alteration in aging, as it has also been demonstrated in peripheral neurons and muscle.

As chronic laxative use may impair neuromuscular function, inclusion of chronic laxative users in investigations of colonic function in aging should be interpreted cautiously. Chronic use of phenolphthalein results in loss of interneurons that coordinate motility, while other cathartic laxatives, such as senna, may be less injurious.

Epidemiologic studies indicate that fecal incontinence occurs in approximately 10 percent of older patients. This potentially devastating event occurs predominantly in women, particularly those who have a history of complicated peripartum deliveries. There may be a physiologic basis for increased susceptibility to fecal incontinence in women, as several studies suggest that aging is associated with a reduction in anal function. Healthy elderly women demonstrated thinning of the internal anal sphincter, resulting in decreased resting and maximum squeeze pressures in the anal canal. Although thickening of the external sphincter was also observed, this did not correlate with increased ability to maintain continence. In the absence of disease, the effects of aging on male anal sphincter function appear minimal. Other pathologic factors that contribute to fecal incontinence in the elderly person are the presence of neurologic disorders that may predispose to impairment in the recognition of the need to defecate (dementia), or in the ability to coordinate defecation (myasthenia gravis or stroke).

AGE-ASSOCIATED CHANGES IN HEPATIC AND BILIARY FUNCTION

In general, there appear to be no age-specific alterations in conventional liver integrity tests, such as serum concentrations of aminotransferases, hepatic alkaline phosphatase, and bilirubin. However, dynamic assessments of liver function do decrease with aging. In healthy subjects, liver size, blood flow and, perfusion decrease by 30 to 40 percent between the third and tenth decade. Aminopyrine demethylation, galactose elimination, and caffeine clearance decrease in parallel with the reduction in liver volume and blood flow. Studies in isolated perfused livers from young adult and senescent Sprague-Dawley rats indicated age-associated reductions of approximately 50 percent in bile acid-dependent and independent bile flow as well as hepatocellular uptake of taurocholate and rates of bile acid secretion. Tight junction permeability and transcellular transport were decreased modestly in senescent rats. Based on studies of hepatic impairment, including subtotal resection and diseases such as hepatitis or cirrhosis, it is likely that a decrease of greater than 70 percent of the total functional hepatic reserve would be expected to result in clinically relevant impairment of hepatic function in aging. In general, with the exception of some hepatic enzyme systems discussed later in "Aging and Gastrointestinal Drug Metabolism," physiologic aging does not result in this degree of diminution in hepatic function.

However, animal studies suggest that the senescent liver is more susceptible to stress insult than its younger counterparts. The increased susceptibility to stress insult may reflect age-related impairment in liver cell proliferation. Liver injury is associated with a regenerative response characterized by increased hepatocyte mitogen-activated protein (MAP) kinase activity. Animal studies support an age-associated decline in MAP kinase activity and epidermal growth factor-stimulated hepatocytes. Hepatic damage may also be related to accumulation of oxidative metabolites with age, as animal studies indicate that some species have significantly increased hepatic lipid peroxidation by 23 months. It is likely that a number of environmental factors such as diet, alcohol consumption, tobacco use, nutritional status, coexistent diseases, and genetic factors also contribute to increased susceptibility to "stress insult" in the aging liver.

The prevalence of cholelithiasis increases with age. Animal studies indicate that bile appears to be increasingly lithogenic as a function of aging, with precipitation of supersaturated bile and concomitant crystallization of cholesterol or calcium bilirubinate. Much of the available human data has been obtained from subjects younger than age 65 years, therefore it is unclear whether gallbladder function is altered in extreme age. Some studies have demonstrated impaired gallbladder function in older subjects. Fasting and postprandial gallbladder volumes were increased in subjects older than age 35 years, with less-complete emptying following a meal observed in older individuals. A correlation between increased gallbladder volumes in adults in their fifth decade and cholelithiasis has been observed. On the other hand, no difference in fat-induced gallbladder emptying was observed in either male or female subjects older than age 50 years, as compared to younger individuals. As in younger age groups, older females may be more susceptible to impaired gallbladder contractility, with decreased contractile response to acetylcholine in postmenopausal females, as compared to older males. Animal studies in aged guinea pigs suggest that deceased density of receptors for hormones such as cholecystokinin (CCK) and galanin may underlie the decreased gallbladder contractility and increased gallstone formation in this model. Impairment in intracellular calcium mobilization and decreased muscle compliance correlated with decreased CCK responsiveness. The functional significance of these animal studies to humans is unclear, however, as decreased CCK responsiveness in older subjects was apparently compensated by increased CCK release, with no net change in gallbladder kinetics in aging.

AGING AND GASTROINTESTINAL DRUG METABOLISM

An evolving area of interest to clinicians and investigators is the field of age-associated changes in drug metabolism. The cytochrome P450 system plays an essential role in drug metabolism in humans. Recent studies indicate that glucocorticoid-inducible CYP3A, which is expressed in the gastrointestinal tract and liver, is one of the most important isoforms involved in drug metabolism in humans. The CYP3A subfamily appears to be the most abundant form of hepatic cytochrome P450, and has the ability to oxidize a wide variety of clinically and toxicologically important agents. CYP3A plays an important role in the metabolism of xenobiotics. For example, the CYP3A subfamily mediates the hydroxylation of numerous endogenous and exogenous steroids as well as the oxidative activation of certain procarcinogens, including aflatoxins. An important observation regarding CYP3A has been its significant role in the metabolism of numerous therapeutically important drugs including calcium channel antagonists, immunosuppressant agents, cholesterol-lowering agents, benzodiazepines, nonsedating antihistamines, and macrolide antibiotics. The divergent structures of the drugs metabolized by CYP3A indicates the broad substrate specificity of the enzymes. Recent reports of significant morbidity and mortality with the concomitant use of antihistamines, macrolide antibiotics and prokinetic drugs points out the importance of P450 drug metabolism in the elderly. The potential implications to the geriatric population in which a variety of medications are often employed is evident.

The high levels of CYP3A activity present in both the intestinal epithelium and the liver results in significant first-pass metabolism of an orally administered substrate. The presence of CYP3A activity in the intestinal epithelium results in substantial drug metabolism and potentially rapid loss of pharmacologic activity. The extent of elimination by this mechanism depends upon the specific drug and its intrinsic clearance. For example, the relatively low oral

bioavailability of the immunosuppressant cyclosporin does not appear to be related to an absorption problem. Extensive metabolism in the intestinal epithelium results in an extraction ratio (amount of active drug in the circulation) of approximately 60 percent that is followed by hepatic metabolism with an extraction ratio of approximately 30 percent. In other words, CYP3A-mediated metabolism of cyclosporin results in bioavailability of only 18 percent of the ingested dose. CYP3A activity is reduced in aged individuals, reportedly in the range of 25 to 50 percent. Other features of CYP3A expression that are relevant to the clinician include a marked (5- to 20-fold) variability in activity between individuals that is determined by both genetic and nongenetic factors. Superimposed liver cirrhosis may reduce CYP3A activity by 30 to 50 percent. CYP3A activity can be modulated by inducers such as rifamycin and anticonvulsant agents, and by several potent inhibitors such as azole antifungal agents and macrolide antibiotics. Therefore, the potential for drug interactions with these medications and other CYP3A substrates, when given together, is significant. There is considerable effort devoted to developing in vitro and in vivo techniques that will facilitate the identification of potential drug interactions whose clinical significance can be subsequently assessed. For example, CYP3A catalyzes the N-demethylation of erythromycin that led to the development of a noninvasive [^{14}C]erythromycin breath test.

EFFECT OF AGING ON PANCREATIC STRUCTURE AND FUNCTION

The exocrine pancreas possesses adequate reserve to maintain normal digestive capacity during the aging process. Overall, there are not clinically significant decreases in pancreatic exocrine function in elderly humans. Age-related changes in pancreatic anatomy and histology include decreased pancreatic weight after the seventh decade in humans and ductal epithelial hyperplasia, interlobular fibrosis, and acinar cell degranulation. Some studies reported a modest decrease in bicarbonate and enzyme output in response to secretin and cerulein in elderly subjects, as compared to their younger counterparts; however secretin and cerulein (CCK receptor agonist)-mediated stimulation of sphincter of Oddi motor function, pancreatic bicarbonate, enzyme, and volume output were not significantly changed in individuals older than 60 years of age.

Trophic responses of the pancreas to hormonal stimulation have been examined in animal models. In contrast to data obtained from human subjects, these studies suggest that the response of the pancreas to trophic agents is decreased with advanced age in some animal models. Cerulein and secretin administration increased pancreatic weight, protein content, messenger ribonucleic acid (mRNA) expression, enzyme, and polyamine concentrations in young and aged rats, but the magnitude of the responses were significantly greater in young rats, as compared to their aged counterparts.

The pancreas of aged animals demonstrates a diminished capacity to respond to changes in dietary composition. Young rats were able to increase their pancreatic lipase and amylase content in response to a high-fat or high-carbohydrate diet, as compared to their aged counterparts. The pancreas in aged animals may have diminished adaptive capacity under conditions of stimulation with nutrients. This could be important under conditions of refeeding following severe caloric restriction (>50 percent). Studies in rats indicate that aged animals had improved weight gain and increased small intestinal mucosal height with pancreatic extract supplementation, as compared to nonsupplemented age-matched controls. Given the significant reserve capacity of the exocrine pancreas, the clinical significance of these observations to healthy aged individuals is questionable.

AGING AND GASTROINTESTINAL IMMUNITY

The gastrointestinal tract is the largest immunologic system in mammals. Elderly persons are relatively susceptible to infections that enter the body via the gastrointestinal tract. This observation suggests that aging may impair mucosal immunity. Despite its importance as a first-line immune defense, there is limited information concerning the physiology of age-associated mucosal immune function in the gastrointestinal tract.

The gastrointestinal mucosal immune response is a complex process that involves a series of events: (1) Antigen uptake at the mucosal surface by specialized epithelial cells (M cells) overlying Peyer's patches in the small intestine. (2) Presentation of the antigen to specific subpopulations of immunologically competent cells in the Peyer's patches. (3) Differentiation and migration of these cells to the small intestinal lamina propria. (4) Initiation and regulation of local antibody production in the intestinal wall. (5) Mucosal epithelial cell receptor-mediated transport of antibodies to the intestinal lumen. There is a paucity of data concerning the effect of aging on the first two steps, antigen uptake and presentation. No change in the number of Peyer's patches or the yield of lymphocytes per patch was observed in aged rats. However gastrointestinal tract-associated lymphoid tissue (GALT) B- and T-lymphocyte subpopulations are altered with aging. Increased T suppressor/cytotoxic lymphocytes reported in the gut mucosa of aged rats might explain the decrease in lamina propria IgA plasma cells, because of decreased cytokine-mediated differentiation of B-lymphocytes by helper T cells. Animal studies indicate that the third step, differentiation and migration of lymphocytic immunoblasts into the lamina propria is decreased with aging. However, reports on antibody production in the gastrointestinal tract are conflicting. A tissue-specific, age-associated reduction in transport of polymeric IgA across rat hepatocytes has been reported. This may result from decreased synthesis of polymeric immunoglobulin receptor or diminished microtubule-dependent translocation of the receptor-ligand complex.

The increase in incidence and severity of gastrointestinal infectious diseases in the elderly population may represent a relative immunodeficiency state of the gastrointestinal immune system. Other factors that probably contribute to an increased risk of gastrointestinal infection in older patients include improper food storage, decreased taste and smell (problems identifying contaminated food), dementia, reduced gastric acid, and colonic slowing. Diarrhea causes significant morbidity and mortality in older individuals, with 51 percent of deaths caused by diarrhea in the United States occurring in patients older than 75 years. In addition to decreasing exposure to infectious environmental agents, novel interventions aimed at improving gastrointestinal immunity may have a significant impact on morbidity and mortality caused by infectious disease in the elderly population.

SUMMARY

As our understanding of how the aging process affects gastrointestinal function evolves, it is evident that many essential aspects of gastrointestinal function are preserved with aging. A significant amount of gastrointestinal dysfunction in the elderly person can be attributed to the superimposed effects of chronic diseases and environmental/lifestyle exposures (medications, alcohol, tobacco) (Fig. 48-2). A modest decline in function with aging, such as decreased

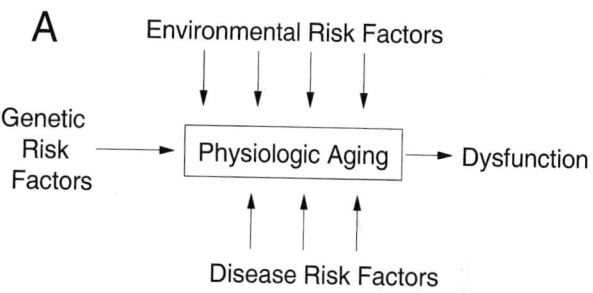

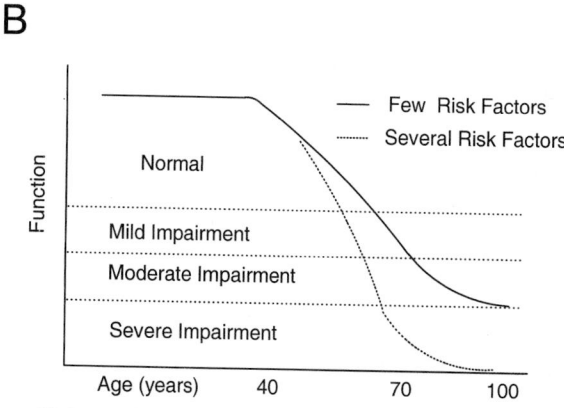

Figure 48-2 *A*. Physiologic aging may be thought of as a baseline state upon which can be superimposed the effects of risk factors such as genetic predisposition, environmental exposure and superimposed disease. The net result is symptomatic dysfunction in senescence that results in impairment. *B*. Physiologic aging of the gastrointestinal tract in individuals with few risk factors (*solid line*) results in minimal alterations in gastrointestinal function in middle age through the sixth decade. Increased risk of gastrointestinal dysfunction may result from a combination of physiologic aging and risk factors such as superimposed disease or environmental stressors (*dotted line*).

gastric mucosal cytoprotection, or decreased esophageal acid clearance, may be significant when superimposed on the side effects of certain medications or concurrent disease. The aging process per se has clinically significant effects on oropharyngeal and upper esophageal motility, colonic function, gastrointestinal immunity and gastrointestinal drug metabolism. Age-related changes in gastrointestinal function will have increasing importance for health care delivery, as the number of elderly individuals increases significantly over the next two to three decades.

ACKNOWLEDGMENTS

I would like to thank Dr. John Wiley for his helpful suggestions, and Marty Ancrum for her expert secretarial assistance. Because of the requirement that citations be limited in number and of recent vintage, many seminal observations have not been specifically referenced. Supported by funding from the Nathan Shock Center and Pepper Centers at the University of Michigan.

REFERENCES

Belai A, Burnstock G: Distribution and colocalization of nitric oxide synthase and calretinin in myenteric neurons of developing, aging and Crohn's disease human small intestine. *Dig Dis Sci* 44:1579, 1999.

Camilleri M et al: Insights into the pathophysiology and mechanisms of constipation, irritable bowel syndrome, and diverticulosis in older people. *J Am Geriatr Soc* 48:1142, 2000.

Cowen T et al: Restricted diet rescues rat enteric motor neurones from age related cell death. *Gut* 47:653, 2000.

El-Salhy M et al: Age-induced changes in the enteric nervous system in the mouse. *Mech Ageing Dev* 107:93, 1999.

Gomes OA et al: A preliminary investigation of the effects of aging on the nerve cell number in the myenteric ganglia of the human colon. *Gerontol* 43:210, 1997.

Hall KE: Neural control of the aging gut: Can an old dog learn new tricks? *Am J Physiol* 283:G827, 2002.

Hall KE et al: Treatment of aged rat sensory neurons in short-term, serum-free culture with nerve growth factor reverses the effect of aging on neurite outgrowth, calcium currents, and neuronal survival. *Brain Res* 888:128, 2001.

Hayashi H et al: Lymphatic lipid transport is not impaired in ageing rat intestine. *Mech Ageing Dev* 113:219, 2000.

Jang I et al: Effects of age and strain on small intestinal and hepatic antioxidant defense enzymes in Wistar and Fisher 344 rats. *Mech Ageing Dev* 122:561, 2001.

Jensen GL et al: Nutrition in the elderly. *Gastroenterol Clin North Am* 30:313, 2001.

Kern MK et al: Comparison of upper esophageal sphincter opening in healthy asymptomatic young and elderly volunteers. *Ann Otol Rhinol Laryngol* 108:982, 1999.

Lee M, Feldman M: The aging stomach: Implications for NSAID gastropathy. *Gut* 41:425, 1997.

Linder JD, Wilcox CM: Acid peptic disease in the elderly. *Gastroenterol Clin North Am* 30:363, 2001.

MacIntosh CG et al: Effect of small intestinal nutrient infusion on appetite, gastrointestinal hormone release, and gastric myoelectrical activity in young and older men. *Am J Gastroenterol* 96:997, 2001.

Majumdar AP et al: Effect of aging on gastrointestinal tract and the pancreas. *Proc Soc Exp Biol Med* 215:134, 1997.

Morihara M et al: Assessment of gastric acidity of Japanese subjects over the last 15 years. *Biol Pharm Bull* 24:313, 2001.

Rayner CK et al: Effects of age on proximal gastric motor and sensory function. *Scand J Gastroenterol* 35:1041, 2000.

Schiller LR: Constipation and fecal incontinence in the elderly. *Gastroenterol Clin North Am* 30:497, 2001.

Schmucker DL et al: Aging impairs intestinal immunity. *Mech Aging Dev* 122:1397, 2001.

Shaker R, Staff D: Esophageal disorders in the elderly. *Gastroenterol Clin North Am* 30:335, 2001.

Xiao ZQ, Majumdar AP: Increased in vitro activation of EGFR by membrane-bound TGF-alpha from gastric and colonic mucosa of aged rats. *Am J Physiol* 281:G111, 2001.

Hepatic, Biliary and Pancreatic Disease

ESTEBAN MEZEY

HEPATIC FUNCTION AND DISEASES

Effect of Age on Liver Function

The liver is the largest and, from a metabolic standpoint, the most complex organ of the body. It has a large functional reserve and there is little evidence of a significant reduction of function with aging. The proportion of liver as 2.5 percent of body weight, constant throughout adult life through middle age, was found to decrease gradually after age 70 years to a mean of 1.6 percent in a group of individuals aged 90 years or older. Liver histology in the aged is more likely to show increases in lipofuscin pigment, giant hepatocytes, large hyperchromatic nuclei, and multiple nucleoli than is found in younger individuals. Ultrastructural changes include a decrease in the number of mitochondria per hepatocyte, but no changes in their integrity, decrease in the endoplasmic reticulum, or increase in the number of lysosomes. Functional studies of the mitochondria in aged rats demonstrate a decrease in membrane potential in association with an increase in mitochondrial size and increase in mitochondrial peroxide generation and a decrease in gluconeogenesis from lactate caused by a decrease in malate export. However, mitochondrial adenosine triphosphate (ATP)/adenosine diphosphate (ADP) remains unchanged. It has been suggested that such changes may be a result of oxidative stress caused by an age-related increase in the generation of oxygen free radicals by mitochondria. No changes in level of serum bilirubin, aminotransferases, and alkaline phosphatase occur with aging in individuals with normal liver histology. Hepatic blood flow decreases because of the decrease in cardiac output that occurs with aging. The most consistent finding in aged individuals is a decrease in the hepatic clearance of drugs, notably those that have a low extraction ratio and whose elimination is dependent on the hepatic activity of drug-metabolizing microsomal enzymes. The hepatic content of cytochrome P450 and the activity of microsomal enzymes are decreased in old as compared to young rats, and these decreases are associated with slower rates of elimination of drugs metabolized by the microsomes. Antipyrine, aminopyrine, chlordiazepoxide, and meperidine are drugs whose hepatic metabolism is decreased in aged individuals. Some of these effects, such as the decrease in antipyrine clearance, appear to be a consequence of an age-dependent effect of smoking, because they are not observed in non-smokers. By contrast, aging has no effect on the rate of clearance of benzodiazepines such as oxazepam and lorazepam, or on morphine, drugs that are primarily metabolized by glucuronidation. Changes in body distribution or protein binding of the drugs that occur during aging also can affect drug clearances. Livers of older donors have lower graft survival in liver transplantation. In one study, graft survival of donor livers age 60 years or older was 52 percent as compared to graft survival of 75 percent with younger donor livers.

Liver Disease

The principal clinical manifestations of liver disease that bring the patient to attention are fatigue, jaundice, and hepatomegaly. Liver disease, however, can also present with nonspecific symptoms of persistent malaise, anorexia, weight loss, and nausea, or may be totally asymptomatic and discovered only during routine examination or by now prevalent multiple automatic laboratory testing of blood samples. In aged patients, there is a relative decrease in the incidence of acute and chronic liver diseases in comparison to increases in the incidence of hepatobiliary tumor and gallstones as a cause of jaundice.

Viral Hepatitis

Viral hepatitis is the most common cause of acute diffuse hepatocellular disease. The four types of viral hepatitis that are well-defined separate entities are designated types A, B, C, and E. Delta hepatitis refers to infection by a defective virus-like particle that is dependent on persistent or concomitant infection with type B virus. Other viruses, such as cytomegalic or Epstein-Barr, only rarely cause clinically

Table 49-1 Comparison of Selected Characteristics of Various Types of Viral Hepatitis

Characteristics	Type A	Type B	Type C	Type E
Hepatitis A antibody	Appearance of or increase in titer	Absent or no change in titer	Absent or no change in titer	Absent or no change in titer
Hepatitis B surface antigen	Absent	Present in early stage of illness	Absent	Absent
Hepatitis C antibody	Absent	Absent	Appears 4–32 weeks (mean of 15 weeks) after onset of hepatitis	Absent
Hepatitis C RNA	Absent	Absent	Present after 10–14 days of onset of hepatitis	Absent
Incubation period	15–50 days	50–160 days	15–160 days	35–40 Days
Route of infection	Oral and parenteral	Usually parenteral, also sexual	Usually Parenteral or sexual	Oral
Age preference	Children	Any age	Any age	15–40 Years
Seasonal incidence	Autumn–winter; epidemic outbreaks	All year	All year	Epidemic outbreaks
Severity	Usually mild	Often severe	Often mild	Mild; severe in pregnancy
Mortality	0.1%	0.1–1.0%	0.1%	0.5% (20% in pregnancy)
Prophylactic value of γ-globulin	Good	Good with hyperimmune hepatitis B globulin	Unclear	Unclear
Hepatitis vaccine	90–100% Efficacy	90% Efficacy	—	—

SOURCE: Mezey E: Diseases of the liver, in Zieve P et al. (eds): *Principles of Ambulatory Medicine.* Baltimore, Williams & Wilkins, 1998.

significant hepatitis. Table 49-1 shows the characteristic features of types A, B, C, and E viral hepatitis. After the age of 60 years there is a lower incidence of hepatitis type A, but an increased incidence of types B and C. This decrease in type A hepatitis is a result of both decreased exposure and increased immunity in older persons. The prevalence of the immunoglobulin (Ig) G class of antibodies to hepatitis A (anti-HA) and of antibodies to hepatitis B surface antigen (anti-HBsAg) increases with age in all populations, reaching a peak in persons age 50 years or older. In white and black populations, the prevalence of antibodies is four times higher in those 50 years of age or older than in those younger than 20 years of age. Chinese Americans have the highest overall prevalences of antibodies to hepatitis A and to hepatitis B surface antigen (76.8 and 74.4 percent, respectively). The increased incidence of types B and C hepatitis in older American populations is principally the consequence of the increased number of blood transfusions received by elderly patients. Many of these blood transfusions were received before screening tests were available to test and exclude donor blood positive for markers of

hepatitis B and C viruses. The present estimated risk of hepatitis infection from transfusion of 1 unit of blood that tests negative for viral hepatitis markers is 1 to 63,000 for hepatitis B and 1 to 100,000 for hepatitis C.

The clinical symptoms of the various types of hepatitis are similar. However, acute viral hepatitis type B is usually more severe, whereas acute viral hepatitis C is usually a mild illness that is very likely to persist and develop into chronic hepatitis. The majority of the cases of hepatitis are endemic; the patients have nonspecific symptoms such as fatigue and nausea, and the disease is often misdiagnosed as a flu-like illness. Initially there is a marked increase in serum aminotransferases. In the anicteric phase the symptoms which usually precede the jaundice are anorexia, fatigue, abdominal discomfort and nausea. In the icteric phase, on physical examination a tender, palpable liver is found in approximately 70 percent of patients. The jaundice usually increases in intensity in the first few days and then begins to decrease, disappearing completely by 2 to 8 weeks after onset. Elderly persons tend to have more severe symptoms, a higher incidence of mental changes, in particular depression, and a more prolonged course of jaundice.

The specific diagnosis of type A hepatitis is made by demonstration of anti-HA antibodies of the IgM class in a titer that rises during the infection and disappears within 3 months after its remission. Type B hepatitis is diagnosed by the detection of hepatitis B surface antigen (HBsAg), which first appears in the blood 1 to 2 weeks before the onset of clinical symptoms and persists for up to 3 months. When HBsAg is no longer detectable, the presence of antibody to hepatitis B core antigen (anti-HBc) is an alternative indicator of infection with hepatitis B virus. Persistence of HBsAg in the serum beyond 3 months after infection suggests that the patient has become a chronic carrier of the hepatitis B virus. The hepatitis Be antigen (HBeAg) appears transiently in the early phase of acute hepatitis B. In chronic carriers of HBsAg, the presence of HBeAg indicates active virus replication and correlates with infectivity. Hepatitis B virus deoxyribonucleic acid (HBV DNA) is also used to detect hepatitis B virus and to obtain information on viral load. Acute delta hepatitis infection is diagnosed by the initial appearance of delta antigen (HDAg), which lasts approximately 10 days, followed by the appearance of delta antibody (anti-HD). Initially, the antibody is of the IgM type, which is followed by the appearance of IgG anti-HD. Acute hepatitis C is diagnosed by the detection of hepatitis C virus ribonucleic acid (HCV RNA), which appears within 10 days of infection and persists during the development of chronic hepatitis. Chronic hepatitis C is diagnosed by detection of HCV RNA or by antibody to hepatitis C (anti-HC) 6 or more months after the onset of the illness. Hepatitis E (HEV) is diagnosed initially by the presence of IgM anti-HEV or, later in the course of the infection, by the appearance of IgG anti-HEV.

Hospitalization may be required in patients older than 70 years of age, because they tend to have a more severe course of illness and because their symptoms may mimic those of biliary obstruction caused by neoplasm or gallstones, which is more common in aged individuals. Acute viral hepatitis usually resolves completely in 1 to 3 months. There is no specific therapy. Bed rest is indicated initially in the symptomatic elderly patient because it often alleviates the symptoms, although there is no evidence that it changes the overall course of the illness. As the patient's symptoms improve, an increase in activity is encouraged as tolerated by the patient. Intake of a normal calorie high protein diet should be encouraged, although it is often difficult for the patient to ingest much food because of nausea and anorexia. However, these symptoms are usually minimal in the morning and hence the patient might be able to eat a large breakfast. In the most extreme cases, intravenous administration of fluids and dextrose, or enteric or intravenous hyperalimentation, may be necessary if the patient has persistent nausea and vomiting. Nausea can be controlled with oral diphenhydramine (Benadryl), 25 mg three times a day, with minimal danger of central nervous system depression. The administration of vitamin K, 15 mg intramuscularly, is indicated if the prothrombin time is prolonged. No sedatives or tranquilizers should be given because they may precipitate hepatic encephalopathy. Corticosteroids are of no value in the treatment of acute

viral hepatitis. Patients can be discharged from the hospital whenever there are indications of clinical improvement and the patient is stable, as long as there is no evidence of encephalopathy, nutrition is adequate, and follow-up is assured. The majority of patients with acute viral hepatitis recover from their illness without any sequelae. Older patients and patients with other medical illnesses, such as diabetes mellitus, are more likely to have a prolonged course and higher mortality. The mortality rate from icteric hepatitis in patients older than age 60 years is 3 to 6 percent, as compared to a mortality of 0.1 to 1.0 percent in younger individuals. The principal cause of death is the development of fulminant hepatitis, which is more common for type B hepatitis. Indications of a poor prognosis are changes in mental status, a nonpalpable liver, which is also small on hepatic scan, or a liver that decreases rapidly in size, and a prothrombin time that is prolonged more than 4 seconds above normal.

Chronic hepatitis develops in approximately 3 to 5 percent of patients with type B hepatitis, and in 60 to 80 percent of patients with parenterally transmitted C hepatitis. It does not occur after type A hepatitis. This complication is to be suspected in patients who continue to have clinical and laboratory evidence of active liver disease after 4 to 6 months following the onset of the acute hepatitis. Elderly patients are more likely to become chronic carriers of HBsAg after acute type B hepatitis than are younger patients. In the population as a whole, approximately 10 percent of patients with type B hepatitis become chronic carriers of HBsAg. By contrast, in one study, 59 percent of patients of mean age 77 years became carriers after an acute outbreak of hepatitis B in a nursing home. The progression of hepatitis C to chronic hepatitis and cirrhosis is more common in patients older than age 50 years than in younger patients. In one study with a mean follow-up of 8 years, 39 percent of patients older than age 50 years developed cirrhosis, as compared with 19 percent of patients younger than age 50 years. Chronic carriers of HBsAg and of hepatitis C RNA have an increased incidence of hepatocellular carcinoma.

Drug-Induced Hepatitis

An increased risk of drug-induced hepatitis occurs in older patients because of their increased intake of medications. Also, increasing age is associated with an increased susceptibility to drug hepatotoxicity. This is best documented by hepatitis caused by isoniazid, which occurs in 0.3 percent of patients between ages 20 and 34 years of age, increasing to 1.2 percent between 35 and 49 years of age, and 2.3 percent at age 50 years or older. Females are more susceptible to drug-induced hepatitis than males. The symptoms, laboratory tests, and findings on liver biopsy of drug-induced hepatitis are indistinguishable from those of viral hepatitis. The hepatitis usually resolves following discontinuation of the drug. However, a mortality rate as high as 12 percent has been reported for severe hepatitis caused by isoniazid. The mortality of fulminant drug-induced hepatitis is increased with age, and most survivors are younger than 40 years of age. Chronic hepatitis can develop if the drug responsible for the hepatitis is continued.

Alcoholic Hepatitis

Alcoholic hepatitis is an uncommon condition in individuals older than age 60 years, probably because of the decrease in alcohol intake that occurs with aging, as well as the early demise of those with severe alcohol abuse. Many of the presenting clinical symptoms of alcoholic hepatitis (such as anorexia, marked fatigue, jaundice, and tender hepatomegaly) are indistinguishable from those of viral hepatitis. However, patients with alcoholic hepatitis are more likely to have fever and leukocytosis. The elevations of the serum aminotransferases are rarely 10 times above normal, and the elevation of the aspartate aminotransferase is characteristically higher than that of the alanine aminotransferase. Liver biopsy differentiates alcoholic hepatitis from drug-induced hepatitis and viral hepatitis and provides an indication of any underlying chronic liver disease. The typical histologic picture of the liver in alcoholic hepatitis reveals hepatocellular necrosis, alcoholic hyaline and an inflammatory reaction that is predominantly polymorphonuclear. The illness of the patient is often more severe than in those with viral hepatitis, and decompensation with hepatic encephalopathy and death may occur. Therapy with corticosteroids may reduce the mortality in selected severely ill patients.

Chronic Hepatitis

Chronic hepatitis refers to chronic inflammation of the liver detected by abnormal liver tests or liver histology that has persisted for longer than 6 months. The principal causes of chronic active hepatitis in the elderly are infection with hepatitis viruses, both types B and C, but not type A, and drugs such as isoniazid, alpha-methyldopa, nitrofurantoin, and sulfonamides. The elderly are at an increased risk of developing chronic hepatitis because they receive more blood transfusions and hence are more exposed to parentally transmitted hepatitis viruses, ingest more drugs, and often have decreased cell-mediated immunity in association with inadequate nutrition or chronic disease. Autoimmune hepatitis is most common in females between the ages 10 and 50 years, but infrequent in the aged. The onset of chronic hepatitis is usually insidious. The patient may be asymptomatic and liver disease may be detected by aminotransferase elevations done on a routine testing or there may be symptoms of malaise, fatigue, anorexia, abdominal discomfort, and jaundice. Physical examination often reveals hepatomegaly and peripheral manifestation of chronic liver disease such as spider angiomata, palmar erythema, and gynecomastia. Elevations of aminotransferases and globulins indicate the activity of the hepatocellular damage, while hyperbilirubinemia, decreases in serum albumin, and prolongation of the prothrombin time reflect loss of hepatocellular function and a poor prognosis. Older male patients are more likely to be positive for HBsAg and to present with an acute onset of illness. The clinical course of patients with chronic active hepatitis is very variable. Patients can be asymptomatic for a long time, have periods of intermittent worsening and remission, or have a progressive course to cirrhosis and death. Lamivudine, a nucleoside analog, in an oral dose of 100 mg/d, results in a decrease in HBV DNA and in normalization of serum aminotransferases in 75 percent of patients. Viral mutants that are resistant to the therapy may appear, which requires that the patient be treated with other newly developed nucleoside analogues. Pegylated interferon alpha2b therapy in combination with oral ribavirin for a period of 6 to 12 months results in a sustained normalization of serum aminotransferases in more than 40 percent of patients with chronic hepatitis C in the population as a whole. The response rates, however, are lower in elderly patients. Corticosteroids are beneficial in patients with autoimmune hepatitis; however, they need to be given with great caution in elderly patients because of the increased incidence and severity of complications such as osteoporosis, glucose intolerance, and cataracts, which occur in older patients.

Cirrhosis

The highest prevalence of cirrhosis is reached between ages 45 and 64 years. The principal causes of cirrhosis in elderly persons are alcoholism and chronic hepatitis C, though some cases are classified as cryptogenic. Nonalcoholic steatohepatitis (NASH) appears to be an important precursor of some cases of cryptogenic cirrhosis. The onset of cirrhosis is usually insidious and associated with nonspecific symptoms such as fatigue, anorexia, weight loss, nausea, and abdominal discomfort. As the disease progresses, signs of hepatocellular failure become prominent. Hepatomegaly and portal hypertension resulting in splenomegaly and venous collateral circulation are common. The most severe complications of cirrhosis are hepatic encephalopathy, ascites, hepatorenal syndrome, bleeding from esophageal and/or gastric varices, and infection. Rapid deterioration of patients with cirrhosis should raise the suspicion of a complicating hepatocellular carcinoma. Infection is a common complication of cirrhosis in the elderly. The principal sites of infection are the urinary tract and ascitic fluid. Analysis and culture of both the urine and the ascitic fluid should be performed routinely in any patient who has worsening clinical symptoms, fever, or recent onset of ascites. The treatment of uncomplicated cirrhosis consists of voluntary restriction of activity if the patient has weakness or fatigue, a diet adequate in protein (a minimum intake of 60 g of protein a day), and abstinence from alcohol. All tranquilizers and sedatives need to be avoided because of the danger of precipitating hepatic encephalopathy. Multivitamins and folic acid, 1 mg/d, may be given if the patient's dietary intake is inadequate or unbalanced. Ascites and edema are treated with sodium restriction (2.0 g of sodium chloride per day) and diuretics. The induced diuresis should be gradual and result in a loss of no more than 5 lb (2.27 kg) of weight per week because of the danger of precipitating electrolyte depletion, hypokalemia, decreased renal function, and hepatic encephalopathy. Diuresis can be initiated with spironolactone, (Aldactone) 100 mg/d, and if necessary, adding furosemide (Lasix) or bumetanide (Bumex) in gradually increasing doses. The dosage of the diuretics should be decreased or the diuretics discontinued altogether if the patient develops hyponatremia or impaired renal function. Patients with ascites unresponsive to sodium

Table 49-2 Treatment of Hepatic Encephalopathy

1. Discontinue and/or avoid all tranquilizers and sedatives.
2. Correct hypokalemia.
3. Search for and manage infection and gastrointestinal bleeding.
4. Restrict or avoid dietary protein depending on the severity of the encephalopathy, but provide protein in the form of oral casein hydrolysates (e.g., Ensure) or by peripheral infusion of amino acids to an optimum of 65 g/d.
5. Continuously give 10% dextrose intravenously in the hospitalized patient with severe encephalopathy to maintain blood glucose.
6. Lactulose enema in patients with severe encephalopathy.
7. Lactulose 30 mL (20 g) every 2–4 hours until diarrhea ensues, then 30 mL po tid to attain two to three soft bowel movements per day.
8. Add neomycin 0.5 g po bid or metronidazole 250 mg qid if response to lactulose is not satisfactory.

restriction and high doses of diuretics may require therapeutic paracentesis, but they should not be subjected to portal systemic shunts because they will almost invariably develop hepatic encephalopathy (see below). Table 49-2 lists the management of hepatic encephalopathy.

Portasystemic shunts for bleeding esophageal varices in patients older than 60 years of age are associated with a very high risk of postoperative encephalopathy and decreased survival. In one study, the incidence of encephalopathy within 6 months following surgery was 63 percent in patients older than age 60 years, as compared to 27 percent in the younger patients. Transjugular intrahepatic portosystemic stent-shunt (TIPS) for esophageal or gastric varices, or for refractory ascites, is also associated with a high incidence of encephalopathy in patients older than 60 years of age. Encephalopathy in the older patient is very hard to reverse, even with optimal medical therapy.

Two other types of cirrhosis that are encountered in elderly persons are primary biliary cirrhosis and hemochromatosis. Primary biliary cirrhosis, which is characterized by progressive intrahepatic cholestasis, is seen most frequently in middle-aged females. Characteristic findings are pruritus, hypercholesterolemia with the formation of xanthoma and xanthelasma, and steatorrhea as a result of decreased delivery of bile acids to the intestine. Antimitochondrial antibodies are found in 95 percent of these patients, and their presence in high titer is virtually diagnostic. Liver biopsy in the early stages reveals injury to the septal and large intralobular bile ducts with surrounding inflammation with plasma cells and lymphocytes and granuloma formation. In the end stages of the disease, cirrhosis develops that is indistinguishable from other causes of non-alcoholic cirrhosis. Treatment consists of the administration of cholestyramine (Questran) for relief of the pruritus, and the administration of fat-soluble vitamins, in particular vitamins A, D, and K, to prevent deficiencies. Osteoporosis, particularly of the vertebra and hip, and leading to bad fractures, is a frequent complication in postmenopausal women with primary biliary cirrhosis. Administration of calcium with vitamin D and estrogen replacement in these women is essential to reduce rates of bone loss. Alendronate sodium (Fosamax), a selective inhibitor of osteoclast-mediated bone resorption, is a new therapy for postmenopausal osteoporosis. Administration of alendronate, 10 mg/d for 3 years, increases bone mass and decreases the incidence of vertebral fractures in postmenopausal women. Treatment with ursodeoxycholic acid reduces bilirubin and aminotransferases, and delays the clinical progression of the disease, although it does not affect the progression of fibrosis.

Hemochromatosis is an inherited disorder of iron metabolism resulting in excess body iron, which is principally characterized by cirrhosis, diabetes mellitus and copperish-grayish pigmentation of the skin. Other symptoms are cardiac failure with arrhythmias, peripheral neuritis, arthritis, and testicular atrophy. Most of the manifestations are caused by iron deposition in the respective organs. Exceptions are the change in the color of the skin, which is caused by increased melanin deposition, and the arthritis, which is caused by calcium pyrophosphate crystal accumulation (pseudogout). The arthritis develops in 25 to 30 percent of patients and initially involves the second and third metacarpophalangeal joints. Thereafter, a progressive polyarthritis involving the wrists, hips, knees, and spine may ensue. The iron overload appears to be caused by an increased absorption of dietary iron, and the mode of inheritance is autosomal recessive. The hemochromatosis (HFE) gene has been identified. The primary mutation in the gene is C282Y (cysteine to tyrosine substitution). Another mutation is H63D (substitution of histidine by aspartate). The homozygous C282Y/C282Y mutation is responsible for 61 to 92 percent of the cases of hemochromatosis. Compound heterozygous C282Y/H63D have a fourfold increased risk of hemochromatosis, as compared with the general population. Homozygous genotype H63D/H63D is not associated with increased iron deposition. The disease usually appears in males older than age 40 years and in females at an older age. The diagnosis is made by demonstration of a high serum iron, a high percent saturation of the iron-binding protein, and increased serum ferritin, often occurring in a patient with a family history of the disease. Finding the genotype C282Y/C282Y confirms the diagnosis. Treatment consists of frequent phlebotomies to decrease iron stores. The principal cause of death is the development of hepatocellular carcinoma, the prevalence of which increases with age. In one study, hepatocellular carcinoma was a finding in more than 60 percent of patients older than age 70 years.

Liver transplantation is only rarely an option in patients with cirrhosis older than 65 years of age, regardless of the etiology of the cirrhosis, because of higher postoperative complications and decreased survival.

Effects of Heart Failure

Heart failure, which is common in the elderly (see Chap. 37), may result in centrolobular hepatic hypoxia and necrosis because of decreased hepatic blood flow, and in hepatic congestion because of decreased venous return to the heart. This combination is often associated with tender hepatomegaly and elevation of serum bilirubin, aminotransferases, and alkaline phosphatase. Marked increases in the serum aminotransferases occur whenever there is severe hypotension and/or hypoxia as a result of cardiac failure or other causes. Characteristically, the abnormal liver tests fall rapidly toward normal following improvement of cardiac failure and correction of hypotension. Cardiac cirrhosis is a very rare consequence of chronic heart failure. It occurs occasionally in patients with rheumatic heart disease and tricuspid insufficiency or in patients with constrictive pericarditis.

Hepatic Tumors

Hepatocellular Carcinoma   The prevalence of hepatocellular carcinoma at autopsy in the United States is 0.27 percent. Much higher prevalences are found in the Bantu tribe in South Africa and among Chinese and Japanese. An underlying cirrhosis is found in approximately 70 percent of cases in the United States, but in only 30 percent of the cases in Taiwan. The most likely types of cirrhosis to be complicated by hepatocellular carcinoma, in decreasing order of frequency, are hemochromatosis, chronic viral hepatitis B and C, and alcoholic cirrhosis. A significant association between hepatocellular carcinoma and the presence of HBsAg in the serum found in various studies suggests that persistent infection with type B hepatitis virus plays a role in the pathogenesis of many cases of hepatocellular carcinoma, particularly in those arising in noncirrhotic livers. By contrast, the increased incidence of hepatocellular carcinoma in patients with hepatitis C occurs principally in association with the development of cirrhosis. The prevalence of hepatocellular carcinoma increases with age and is approximately 10 times more common in males than in females. Usually there is a major tumor with multiple smaller metastases. The tumor spreads via the blood vessels. The major sites of distal metastases, in decreasing order of frequency, are lung, lymph nodes of the porta hepatis, adrenals, bone, spleen, kidney, colon, and pleura. The principal manifestations are weight loss, abdominal pain, and hepatomegaly. The finding of tender hepatic nodules, or a friction rub, or arterial murmur over the liver is highly suggestive of the diagnosis. Leukocytosis and elevation of the serum alkaline phosphatase are found frequently. Erythrocytosis, hypercalcemia, hypoglycemia, or hyperlipidemia is sometimes present. On occasion, these antedate discovery of the tumor. The presence of an elevated serum alpha-fetoprotein in a patient with one or more filling defects in the liver detected by usual scanning techniques is virtually diagnostic. Computerized tomography (CT) scanning with intravenous contrast and magnetic resonance imaging are helpful for differentiating hepatic tumors from cyst, abscess, and regenerating nodules, and for delineating the extent of liver involvement by the tumor. Tissue diagnosis is obtained by directed percutaneous, peritoneoscopic, or open liver biopsy. Surgical resection is the treatment of choice for small, localized hepatocellular carcinomas. Percutaneous ethanol injection or transcatheter arterial chemoembolization (TACE) can cause extensive necrosis of the tumor with a decrease in tumor size, but there is no evidence that it increases survival. However, a decrease in tumor size can make the patient a candidate for liver transplantation.

Metastatic Tumors   The liver is the most frequent organ affected by tumor metastases spread via the blood stream. The patient may present with symptoms caused by the primary tumor or by the liver metastases. The usual symptoms are malaise, anorexia, weight loss, and abdominal discomfort. On examination there is hepatomegaly, often with nodularity. The serum alkaline phosphatase is elevated in approximately 80 percent of advanced cases. Imaging of the liver will show one or more filling defect but will not by itself differentiate metastatic carcinoma from other space occupying lesions such as regenerating hepatic nodules. Directed liver biopsy aided by sonography or CT scanning is used to arrive at a diagnosis.

DISEASES OF THE GALLBLADDER AND BILIARY TREE

Diseases of the gallbladder and biliary tree are more common in old than in young individuals. They are a cause of up to 40 percent of acute abdominal events in patients older than 55 years of age and are the most common indications for abdominal surgery in this age group. The mortality complicating surgical therapy for diseases of the gallbladder and biliary tree is increased in elderly persons. Recent development in laparoscopic cholecystectomy, endoscopic retrograde cholangiopancreatography (ERCP) for removal of gallstones, and decompression of biliary obstruction by stents are particularly applicable to older patients.

Cholelithiasis

The formation of stones in the gallbladder is the cause of almost all diseases of this organ and is a principal cause of obstruction of the common bile duct. Gallstones are a mixture of cholesterol, bilirubin, and calcium. Cholesterol is the principal constituent in most stones, while calcium bilirubinate is the major component of stones in patients with chronic hemolytic anemia or cirrhosis. Cholesterol gallstones form when there is an excess in the proportion of cholesterol relative to the bile acids and phospholipids necessary to keep it in solution in bile. It is estimated that approximately 20 million individuals in the United States have gallstones. The prevalence of gallstones increases gradually with age, and females are twice as likely to have gallstones as males in almost every age group. In the decade of 80 to 89 years of age, the prevalence of gallstones is 22 percent for males and 38 percent for females; this increases to 31 percent in males, but not in females, older than age 90 years. In certain groups of American Indians (e.g., Pimas), gallstones develop at an early age, and the prevalence in women by age 30 years is 70 percent. In these populations, the prevalence is approximately 80 percent for women and 70 percent for men older than 50 years of age. Other factors that are associated with a high prevalence of gallstones are obesity, diabetes, ileal disease or resection, intake of estrogen, intake of a diet enriched in polyunsaturated fatty acids, hyperlipidemia, and clofibrate therapy. In American Indians, the high susceptibility to gallstones results from the high rate of cholesterol output, combined with a diminished bile acid output probably resulting from abnormal feedback regulation of hepatic cholesterol 7-hydroxylase activity, which catalyzes the conversion of cholesterol to bile acids. The mechanism of the increase in gallstone prevalence with aging remains unknown. There is an increased secretion of cholesterol into bile, but no change in bile acid or phospholipid secretion with increasing age in both sexes, resulting in increased cholesterol saturation of bile. The rate of gallbladder emptying after a fat meal is the same in young and old normal subjects. The majority of gallstones remain asymptomatic. A 15-year follow-up of persons with gallstones who had an initial mean age of 54 years revealed the development of biliary colic in 18 percent. Another study demonstrated the development, over a 10- to 20-year follow-up period, of symptoms of indigestion in 27 percent, colic in 19 percent, and mild transient jaundice in 4.5 percent of patients.

Acute Cholecystitis

Acute cholecystitis is usually the result of obstruction of the cystic duct by one or more gallstones. Approximately 5 percent of cases occur in the absence of gallstones. The gallbladder becomes distended, with progressive inflammation of its wall. There is usually a component of bacterial infection as well. The patient presents with severe right upper quadrant pain, vomiting, fever, leukocytosis, and, often, mild hyperbilirubinemia. Although the usual attack may subside within hours, serious complications include perforation with peritonitis, choledocholithiasis, cholangitis, liver abscess, pancreatitis, and fistula from the biliary tree. Symptoms are sometimes associated with passage of a stone into the small intestine, resulting in obstruction (gallstone ileus).

The diagnosis of acute cholecystitis is established by imaging of the liver and biliary tree with[99m] technetium-N-substituted hepatoiminodiacetic acid (HIDA). In acute cholecystitis, this will reveal opacification of the bile ducts but lack of filling of the gallbladder. Ultrasonography demonstrating gallstones further supports the diagnosis.

The initial therapy of acute cholecystitis is discontinuation of oral intake, passage of a nasogastric tube to maintain continuous gastric suction, and correction of dehydration by administration of intravenous fluids and electrolytes. Meperidine (Demerol) is administered for relief of pain.

There is no evidence that the administration of antibiotics in the routine case reduces the incidence of suppurative complications. Cholecystectomy is recommended early in the attack if the patient's clinical status is suitable for general anesthesia. Laparoscopic cholecystectomy has replaced open cholecystectomy as the procedure of choice for the removal of the gallbladder for cholecystitis. Laparoscopic cholecystectomy is performed under general anesthesia. A pneumoperitoneum is established and a laparoscope and three cannulas are inserted through which instruments are placed to remove the gallbladder. Relative contraindications to laparoscopic cholecystectomy include a gangrenous or perforated gallbladder, peritonitis, cholangitis, previous upper abdominal surgery, and morbid obesity. Common duct stones are also a contraindication unless they can be extracted by endoscopic sphincterotomy prior to the cholecystectomy or unless the surgeon is experienced in laparoscopic common duct exploration. Laparoscopic cholecystectomy has the advantage over open cholecystectomy of a short hospital stay of approximately 24 hours with a return to normal activity in 10 to 14 days. In a recent study, laparoscopic cholecystectomy needed to be converted to open cholecystectomy in only 4.7 percent of cases. The common reasons for conversion are severe scarring or acute inflammation that obscures the anatomy, adhesions related to prior surgery, aberrant anatomic features that make dissection difficult, and bile duct or bowel injuries during surgery. Common duct stones encountered during the procedure can sometimes be removed by choledochoscopy, but otherwise these require common duct exploration after conversion to laparotomy. In a reported series, complications occurred in 5.1 percent of cases. The most common complication is wound infection, occurring in 1.1 percent of cases, followed by bile duct injury, occurring in 0.5 percent of cases. Other complications are prolonged ileus, bowel injury, and operative bleeding. Surgical mortality is less than 0.1 percent. However, the mortality of open cholecystectomy for acute cholecystitis increases markedly in elderly patients. In one study, mortality of 9.7 percent was found in patients older than 65 years, as compared to a mortality of 1.6 percent in those younger than 65 years of age. Cardiovascular disease is the principal cause of death in such instances. The morbidity of cholecystectomy is primarily related to superficial wound infections (5 to 7 percent). Wound infection is more common if the operations lasts longer than 2 hours, if the patient is obese or diabetic, and if the patient has acute rather than chronic cholecystitis. Other possible but rare (<1 percent) immediate complications of cholecystectomy are postoperative bleeding, postoperative bile leak, injury to biliary ducts (0.1 percent), and retained common duct stones. A drain may be left in place for 24 to 48 hours after operation. For patients who are very ill and for poor operative risks, the recommended procedure is evacuation of the gallbladder contents by cholecystotomy under local anesthesia followed by continuous drainage. This should be followed at a later time by cholecystectomy whenever possible. In elderly patients who are poor operative risks and who have no evidence of residual stones, the cholecystotomy may be removed. In this case, there is less than a 50 percent recurrence of symptomatic gallstones in 5 years.

Chronic Cholecystitis

In chronic cholecystitis, the wall of the gallbladder is chronically inflamed, stones are almost always present, and the concentrating and emptying functions of the gallbladder are usually lost. Patients may have symptoms of dyspepsia or recurrent attacks of right upper quadrant pain, nausea, and vomiting occurring shortly after meals. Any attack can progress to acute cholecystitis if the cystic duct remains obstructed. The diagnosis is established with 95 percent certainty by demonstration of nonopacification of the gallbladder by oral cholecystography, even after the administration of two doses of iopanoic (Telepaque) dye. Ultrasonography will demonstrate the presence of stones with an accuracy of 90 percent. The therapy of choice for chronic cholecystitis is laparoscopic cholecystectomy as described above. Elective open cholecystectomy has an overall mortality of 0.5 percent in patients younger than 50 years of age, increasing to 1 percent in patients older than 50 years of age. Cholecystectomy may be associated with an increased incidence of development of carcinoma of the colon, particularly of the right colon in females. It is postulated that an increase in secondary bile acids which predominate in the bile after cholecystectomy may have a carcinogenic effect on the colon. Dissolution of gallstones by oral administration of ursodeoxycholic acid is a possible alternative therapy for cholelithiasis and chronic cholecystitis in highly selected elderly patients who prefer not to undergo surgery or who are poor surgical risks. Ursodeoxycholic acid decreases biliary cholesterol excretion by its inhibitory effect on the hepatic enzyme hydroxymethylglutaryl coenzyme A reductase (HMG-CoA reductase), which is rate limiting in the synthesis of cholesterol. The recommended dose of ursodeoxycholic acid for dissolution of gallstones is 8 to 10 mg/kg/d, given in two to three divided doses. Complete stone dissolution can be expected in approximately 33 percent of patients after 2 years of therapy. Mild diarrhea is an occasional side effect. A significant recurrence rate of gallstones is expected after discontinuation of the bile acid therapy.

Choledocholithiasis

Gallstones often enter the common bile duct, and when they block it, gallstones can cause obstructive jaundice, ascending cholangitis, liver abscess, pancreatitis, and, rarely, secondary biliary cirrhosis. Stones are present in the common bile duct in approximately 15 percent of patients who undergo cholecystectomy for chronic cholecystitis with stones. The prevalence of stones in the common bile duct increases with aging and correlates with an increased diameter of the common bile duct that occurs with aging. The symptoms of biliary obstruction include the development of abdominal pain of increasing intensity, nausea, vomiting, and fever, followed by the appearance of dark urine and jaundice. If the obstruction is complete the stools become light in color. Tender hepatomegaly may develop because of the increased pressure in the biliary tree. Ultrasonography is the best initial procedure to determine whether or not the bile ducts are dilated; however, in

biliary obstruction of short duration, the ducts may not yet be dilated. For a more definitive diagnosis, the bile ducts are visualized by either magnetic resonance cholangiopancreatography (MRCP), ERCP, or percutaneous transhepatic cholangiography (PTC). MRCP has the advantage that it is not invasive and is as accurate in the diagnostic aspects as ERCP or PTC, but it lacks the opportunity of therapeutic intervention. Unless the obstruction is relieved spontaneously by passage of the stones to the duodenum, the stones have to be removed either by open cholecystectomy and common duct exploration, or, if possible at the time of ERCP, by endoscopic sphincterotomy. The mortality of this surgery increases with age from 1 percent in patients younger than 50 years of age to 4 percent in those older than 50 years of age. In addition, postsurgical complications consisting of hemorrhage, pancreatitis, cholangitis, and wound infection occur in approximately 30 percent of patients. Removal of stones by endoscopic sphincterotomy is the preferred procedure for elderly patients who are poor surgical risks. This procedure has a low mortality rate and a total complication rate of less than 10 percent, but it has the disadvantage that it leaves behind the diseased gallbladder, which can be a source of subsequent passage of stones. In an 8-year follow-up of patients with endoscopic sphincterotomy, papillary stenosis and/or recurrent bile duct stones occurred in less than 5 percent of cases. On occasion, elderly patients will present with symptoms of lethargy, confusion, and gram negative sepsis resulting from suppurative cholangitis. Both fever and leukocytosis may be absent. The only hope for survival in those patients is emergency surgical relief of the biliary obstruction.

Carcinoma of the Gallbladder

Carcinoma of the gallbladder occurs mainly in elderly individuals. In one study, the average age for the diagnosis of this neoplasm was 73 years. It is four times more common in females than males, and it is found in association with cholelithiasis in 80 percent of cases. The principal clinical manifestations are abdominal pain, jaundice, and weight loss, often in association with upper abdominal mass. The diagnosis is made by laparotomy. Only in situ cancers found incidentally on removal of the gallbladder for chronic cholecystitis are potentially curable. Death occurs within 1 year of the diagnosis in the majority of patients.

Carcinoma of the Extrahepatic Bile Ducts

Primary carcinomas of the bile ducts account for less than 3 percent of all cancer deaths in the United States. They are most common after the age of 60 years, unless associated with inflammatory bowel disease or with sclerosing cholangitis, when they occur at a younger age, and are slightly more common in males than females. They are associated with gallstones in 30 to 50 percent of cases. These carcinomas tend to infiltrate along the wall of the duct and are difficult to distinguish from benign strictures. Patients present with symptoms of jaundice, itching, and weight loss. Abdominal pain is not a prominent feature. The obstruction to the bile duct is demonstrated by either MRCP, PTC, or ERCP. The treatment is surgical. Radical pancreatoduodenectomy (Whipple procedure) performed for tumors of the distal common bile (ampulla of Vater) has the best prognosis; the operation is associated with a mortality of 5 to 10 percent, but results in a cure in 30 percent of cases. Tumors of the more proximal extrahepatic ducts are usually not amenable to removal, and the treatment in this circumstance consists of bypassing the obstruction either by surgical construction of a cholecysto- or choledochointestinal anastomosis or the placement of a stent across the tumor. Biliary decompression by a stent placed by PTC with external or a combination of internal–external drainage for proximal tumors, or by a stent placed by ERCP for distal tumors, is a new approach for relief of biliary obstruction caused by malignancy in high-risk elderly patients. This can be used preoperatively to lower high bilirubin levels (>10 mg/dL), which are associated with a high surgical mortality, or for more permanent palliative relief. The placement of a stent through the obstruction allowing bile to drain into the duodenum, results in prompt decrease or disappearance of pruritus and jaundice. This method or decompression can be maintained for months requiring only replacement of clogged stents.

DISORDERS OF THE PANCREAS

Effects of Age on Exocrine Pancreatic Function

The principal function of the exocrine pancreas is the production and delivery of digestive enzymes to the lumen of the intestine. The functional reserve of the pancreas is great. Significant steatorrhea is only observed after the output of lipase has decreased by 90 percent or more. Pancreatic size remains unchanged with aging. However, the aging pancreas is characterized by a progressive increase in the width of the main pancreatic duct and major branches with the formation of cysts in the interlobular and intralobular ducts. In addition, there is an increased occurrence of protein precipitation and lobular fibrosis. Increased calcification was observed with increasing age in male, but not in female, subjects. Pancreatic secretion after secretin stimulation revealed a decrease in peak volume output in males older than 50 years of age, as compared with younger subjects. A decreased pancreatic reserve with aging is suggested by decreases in the total output of volume, bicarbonate, and amylase after repeated stimulation with pancreozymin and secretin in individuals 61 to 76 years old, as compared with young individuals aged 17 to 33 years. The pancreatic content of pancreatic enzymes such as amylase decreases with age in rats. A decrease in the appearance of chylomicrons in the blood after an oral load of fat was demonstrated in older subjects of a mean age of 82 years, as compared with young subjects of a mean age of 20 years. However, these findings are more likely the result of delayed gastric emptying in the elderly persons rather than because of pancreatic dysfunction or malabsorption, because steatorrhea has not been a finding in the healthy old subjects.

Pancreatic Disease

The principal diseases of the pancreas are pancreatitis and carcinoma. Pancreatitis can be acute or chronic. Acute pancreatitis is characterized by sudden onset of severe episodes of abdominal pain caused by edematous, inflammatory, and sometimes necrotic changes in the pancreas. Chronic pancreatitis is manifested by chronic abdominal pain, mild indigestion, and glucose intolerance caused by narrowing or obstruction of the pancreatic ducts, parenchymal atrophy, and fibrosis. Chronic relapsing pancreatitis is a disorder characteristic of alcoholics in which episodes of acute pancreatitis occur in association with chronic pancreatitis. Pancreatic adenocarcinoma of duct cell origin constitutes more than 90 percent of the neoplasms of the pancreas. Other pancreatic malignancies are acinar and islet cell carcinomas, ampullary carcinomas, cystadenocarcinomas, and other rarer tumors.

Acute Pancreatitis

The most common cause of acute pancreatitis in elderly persons is cholelithiasis. Alcoholism, which is the principal cause of episodes of acute pancreatitis (chronic relapsing pancreatitis) in patients younger than 50 years of age, is a less-frequent cause of acute pancreatitis in older patients. Acute pancreatitis as a result of ischemia, intake of drugs, or following abdominal surgery or obstruction of the pancreatic duct because of carcinoma, are slightly increased in incidence in elderly individuals. The sex ratio in the occurrence of acute pancreatitis changes from a male predominance in the young to a female predominance in older patients. A review of various studies reveals that 59 to 83 percent of cases with pancreatitis occurring in persons age 50 years or older occurs in women. Most likely this is related to the greater prevalence of cholelithiasis in women, as compared to men. The principal symptom of acute pancreatitis is abdominal pain. The pain is usually located to the epigastrium but may progress and involve the entire abdomen and penetrate through to the back. It is almost invariably accompanied by nausea and vomiting. Fever is a finding in approximately 50 percent of patients. The abdomen is tender with guarding, and peristaltic sounds are decreased or absent. Rebound tenderness with absent bowel sounds may require differentiation of acute pancreatitis from intestinal infarction and perforated viscus. Hypotension, which is noted in approximately 44 percent of patients, can lead to complications such as cerebral infarction and renal insufficiency, particularly in elderly persons. Confusion and coma are more common in patients older than age 50 years and are associated with a poor prognosis. An increase in serum amylase is a very sensitive test in detecting acute pancreatitis, but it is also nonspecific because it may also be elevated in patients with acute cholecystitis, intestinal infarction, and other abdominal catastrophes, such as a perforated viscus. In one series, leukocytosis greater than $14,000/mm^3$ was found with pancreatitis in 94 percent of patients older than age 50 years. Transient elevation of the serum bilirubin is frequent, but it rarely exceeds 4 mg/dL. Higher persistent elevations of the serum bilirubin suggest extrahepatic biliary obstruction

Table 49-3 Risk Factory in Acute Pancreatitis Caused by Cholelithiasis

At admission or diagnosis
    Age >70 years
    White cell count >18,000/mm^3
    Blood glucose >220 mg/dL
    Serum lactate dehydrogenase >400 IU/L
    Aspartate aminotransferase >250 IU/L

During initial 48 hours
    Hematocrit fall >10 percentage points
    Blood urea nitrogen rise >2 mg/dL
    Serum calcium <8 mg/dL
    Base deficit >5 mEq/L
    Fluid sequestration >4 L

SOURCE: Ranson JHC: Etiological and prognostic factors in human acute pancreatitis: A review. *Am J Gastroenterol* 77:633, 1982.

as a consequence of a gallstone or neoplasm. Mild hyperglycemia, hyperlipidemia, and hypocalcemia are common. Marked hypocalcemia (serum calcium <7mg/dL) is associated with a poor prognosis. Chest x-ray and plain films of the abdomen often reveal a left pleural effusion and isolated dilated loops of bowel (sentinel loops). Generalized ileus may be present and requires differentiation of pancreatitis from intestinal ischemia or infarction. The presence of trapped gas in the area of the pancreas suggests a pancreatic abscess, while the presence of free gas in the abdomen indicates the presence of a perforated viscus. Table 49-3 lists the factors associated with severity of acute pancreatitis because of cholelithiasis and poor prognosis. Mortality was 1.5 percent with less than three risk factors, and rose to 29 percent when additional factors were present. Medical therapy consists of placing the patient at bed rest, with no oral intake, and the administration of parenteral fluids, electrolytes, and dextrose. In addition, the administration of plasma and whole blood may be required, particularly in elderly patients with hypovolemia. Continuous nasogastric suction is initiated and meperidine (Demerol) is given for relief of pain. Anticholinergic and prophylactic antibiotics are not indicated. Once the abdominal pain subsides and peristaltic sounds return to normal, the nasogastric suction may be discontinued and the patient fed by mouth. Surgical intervention should be contemplated when the diagnosis is in doubt or the case is complicated by abscess or the presence of biliary obstruction because of choledocholithiasis or neoplasm. Surgery for uncomplicated choledocholithiasis or unresolved pseudocysts can be deferred for 4 to 6 weeks after the acute pancreatitis has subsided.

Chronic Pancreatitis

Alcoholism is the principal cause of chronic pancreatitis. There is no good evidence that repeated attacks of acute pancreatitis in association with cholelithiasis results in the development of chronic pancreatitis. In addition, chronic pancreatitis is associated with hyperparathyroidism and occurs in chronically malnourished populations. The principal manifestations of chronic pancreatitis are constant, unremitting abdominal pain, exocrine insufficiency manifested by steatorrhea and weight loss and endocrine insufficiency, manifested by glucose intolerance. Physical examination usually reveals evidence of weight loss and epigastric tenderness. The serum amylase is usually normal unless there is an acute exacerbation of acute pancreatitis. The plain film of the abdomen reveals calcification in the area of the pancreas in about one-third of the patients. The diagnosis can be confirmed by the demonstration of steatorrhea, and an abnormal pancreatic secretion of bicarbonate and digestive enzymes after stimulation of the pancreas with secretin-pancreozymin or a meal. Pancreatic exocrine function can also be assessed by measurement of urinary *p*-aminobenzoic acid after oral administration of the synthetic peptide N-benzoyl L-tyrosyl-*p*-aminobenzoic acid, which is cleaved by chymotrypsin. Patients with chronic pancreatitis demonstrate less than 40 percent recovery of urinary *p*-aminobenzoic acid, as compared to recovery of more than 70 percent in normal subjects. ERCP often reveals intermittent pancreatic duct obstruction characteristic of chronic pancreatitis, and sometimes surgically correctable lesions such as single strictures and cysts. It does not, however, always distinguish strictures caused by chronic pancreatitis from those caused by adenocarcinoma of the pancreas.

The treatment of chronic pancreatitis consists of analgesics for pain; unfortunately, in many cases only narcotics are effective, and narcotic addiction often results. Steatorrhea is reduced by the administration of pancreatic extracts, such as Viokase, 3 to 6 tablets with meals. Administration of cimetidine, 300 mg 30 minutes before each meal, increases the effectiveness of the pancreatic extracts by reducing the gastric acid that inactivates the enzymes in the pancreatic extracts. Insulin may be required for control of diabetes. Resection of 95 percent of the pancreas is effective in controlling pain in 80 percent of the patients, however, this procedure is not recommended for patients older than age 65 years because of the higher surgical morbidity and mortality in elderly patients.

Adenocarcinoma of the Pancreas

Pancreatic cancer has increased in frequency in recent years. The median annual percentage increase in incidence averages approximately 1 percent for both sexes. In the United States, it is now the fourth and fifth most common causes of death from cancer among men and women, respectively. Cancer of the pancreas is about 1.7-fold more common in males than in females, and its incidence increases in both sexes with age. Eighty percent of cases of cancer of the pancreas occur between ages 60 and 80 years. It is uncommon below the age of 45 years, while its occurrence in males older than 75 years is as high as 100 per 100,000, which is 8 to 10 times higher than the occurrence in the general population. Carcinoma of the pancreas is located in the head of the majority of the cases. Ductal cell mucin-producing adenocarcinoma is the most common type of pancreatic cancer. Factors that are definitely associated with a higher prevalence of carcinoma of the pancreas are smoking, chronic pancreatitis, and diabetes mellitus. Other factors that may also be associated with carcinoma of the pancreas are heavy alcohol ingestion, occupational exposure to carcinogens, exposure to radiation, and ingestion of a high-fat diet. However, these associations are far from well established.

The principal symptoms of carcinoma of the pancreas are abdominal pain, weight loss, and jaundice. The pain often radiates from the epigastrium to either upper abdominal quadrant or the back. Weight loss is often marked and associated with anorexia and weakness. Painless jaundice can be a presenting symptom in patients with carcinoma of the pancreas. The jaundice is progressive and frequently associated with dark urine, light colored stools, and pruritus. Mental symptoms of depression and anxiety can be the predominant presenting symptoms, particularly in the elderly. Carcinoma of the pancreas can also manifest by migratory thrombophlebitis or the development of diabetes mellitus in an individual without a genetic predisposition to diabetes.

On physical examination, an enlarged liver and/or gallbladder are found in more than 50 percent of cases. A systolic bruit heard over the abdomen may indicate compression of the splenic vein by tumor of the body or tail of the gland.

Laboratory tests usually show normal serum amylase levels. Elevations of the serum bilirubin and serum alkaline phosphatase, as well as mild elevation of the serum aminotransferases are common; these elevations can be caused by obstruction of the common duct by adenocarcinoma of the head of the pancreas or by liver metastasis. A number of tumor markers have been proposed for the diagnosis of cancer of the pancreas, but none of them are sensitive or specific enough for routine use. Elevated carcinoembryonic antigen (CEA) is found in approximately 62 percent of patients with cancer of the pancreas, but this marker is also detectable in approximately 50 percent of patients with benign disease. Carbohydrate antigen (CA) 19-9 has an 80 percent sensitivity in the detection of pancreatic cancer, but is often normal in early pancreatic cancer and also frequently found in patients with other gastrointestinal cancers or with benign disease. These markers, however, fall after resection of pancreatic cancer, and, hence, can be used for surveillance to monitor for recurrence of the cancer. Genetic markers may prove to be more useful in the detection of pancreatic cancer. K-ras gene mutations were demonstrated in 90 percent of pancreatic adenocarcinoma tissue and found in DNA extracted from duodenal juice collected during secretin stimulation in 9 of 16 (63 percent) patients with pancreatic adenocarcinoma. CT scanning is at present the preferred method for the detection of adenocarcinoma of the pancreas. Ultrasonography is an alternate modality for the examination of the pancreas. The sensitivity and specificity for CT and ultrasonography in the detection of a pancreatic mass or pancreatic carcinoma is approximately 80 percent. ERCP is particularly useful in differentiating pancreatic from ampullary and duodenal carcinomas, which can be visualized as well as biopsied to obtain a definitive diagnosis. The differentiation between pancreatic cancer and chronic pancreatitis by visualization of pancreatic ductal abnormalities is difficult.

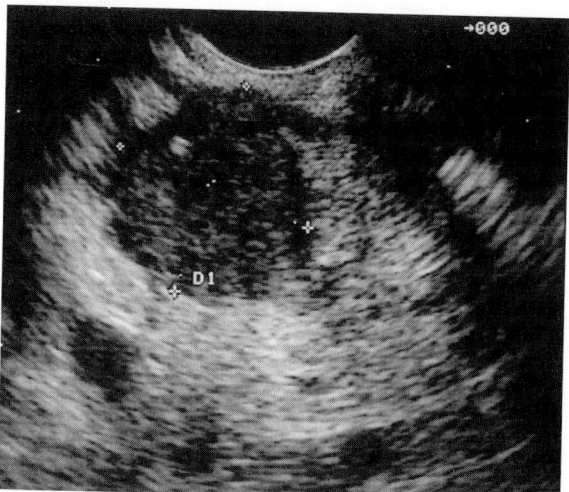

Figure 49-1   Endoscopic ultrasound of a 2-cm pancreatic mass that was not detected by abdominal ultrasonography or by CT scanning. An endoscopic ultrasound-guided fine-needle aspiration of the mass was obtained. The biopsy was positive for adenocarcinoma of the pancreas. Image courtesy of Marcia Canto, MD, of The Johns Hopkins Hospital.

However, cytologic examination of pancreatic secretions obtained during ERCP following secretin stimulation has an 80 percent sensitivity in the diagnosis of pancreatic cancer. Endoscopic ultrasonography is a new technique that is very useful for determining tumor size and extent, lymph node metastases, and involvement of the mesenteric vessels (Fig. 49-1). In addition, selective angiography can be used to localize the tumor, to help differentiate it from other neoplastic lesions, and to determine its potential resectability. Percutaneous guided fine-needle aspiration cytology of the pancreas is a reliable procedure for the diagnosis with positive yields of 80 to 100 percent.

The treatment and prognosis of adenocarcinoma of the pancreas is dismal because by the time the patient presents with symptoms, the tumor is usually widespread and unresectable. Potentially curable tumors are those in the head of the gland that present with obstructive jaundice. In one large study, only 13 percent of 1272 patients with pancreatic adenocarcinoma had lesions amenable to resection with any hope of cure. Radical pancreatoduodenectomy (Whipple procedure) with curative intent in two series was associated with a 16 percent surgical mortality in each, and 5-year survival of 5 and 8 percent. The overall 2-year survival for pancreatic adenocarcinoma in recent years has been approximately 4 percent, and does not vary by race or sex. Palliative relief of biliary obstruction by cholecystojejunostomy performed in unresectable tumors is associated with an operative mortality of 6 percent and a 3-year survival of 2 percent. The preferred method of relief of biliary obstruction in elderly patients is by placement of stents in the biliary tree by PTC or by ERCP, with external or internal drainage. In one study, endoscopic placement of the stent resulted in a greater relief of jaundice, and lower 30-day mortality, as compared to placement of the stent percutaneously, because of the higher complication rate of the latter procedure which sometimes results in bleeding or a bile leak. Control of pain eventually requires the use of opioid analgesics, which often results in marked drowsiness, confusion, nausea, vomiting, and constipation. These side effects of opioid drugs need to be treated with antiemetics and laxatives. Percutaneous coeliac plexus block with alcohol relieves the pain in approximately 80 percent of patients and in some of them this relief lasts until death. However, ethanol injection also has the potential of causing serious side effects such as partial leg paralysis and loss of bladder sphincter control. Radiotherapy combined with chemotherapy (with 5-fluorouracil or, more recently, with gemcitabine) has shown some improvement in survival in unresectable adenocarcinoma.

REFERENCES

Bianchi L et al: *Aging in Liver and Gastrointestinal Tract.* Lancaster, England, MTP Press Limited, 1988.

Collins BH et al: Long-term results of liver transplantation in patients 60 years of age and older. *Transplantation* 70:780, 2000.

Cooperman AM: Pancreatic cancer. *Surg Clin North Am* 81:557, 2001.

Hoofnagle JH, DiBisceglie AM: Drug therapy: The treatment of chronic viral hepatitis. *N Engl J Med* 336:347, 1997.

Kondo Y et al: High carrier rate after hepatitis B virus infection in the elderly. *Hepatology* 18:768, 1993.

Marino IR et al: Effect of donor age and sex on the outcome of liver transplantation. *Hepatology* 22:1754, 1993.

Marcus EL, Tur-Kaspa R: Viral hepatitis in older adults. *J Am Geriatr Soc* 45:755, 1997.

McGinn CJ, Zalupski MM: Combined-modality therapy in pancreatic cancer: Current status and future directions. *Cancer J* 7:338, 2001.

Okuda K: Hepatocellular carcinoma: recent progress. *Hepatology* 15:948, 1992.

Poonawala A et al: Prevalence of obesity and diabetes in patients with cryptogenic cirrhosis: A case-controlled study. *Hepatology* 32:689, 2000.

Purcell RH: Hepatitis viruses: Changing patterns of human disease. *Proc Natl Acad Sci U S A* 91:2401, 1994.

Rosch T et al: Staging of pancreatic and ampullary carcinoma by endoscopic ultrasonography. Comparison with conventional sonography, computer tomography, and angiography. *Gastroenterology* 102:188, 1992.

Rosenthal RA, Andersen DK: Surgery in the elderly: Observations of the pathophysiology and treatment of cholelithiasis. *Exp Gerontol* 28:459, 1993.

The Southern Surgeons Club: A prospective analysis of 1518 laparoscopic cholecystectomies. *N Engl J Med* 324:1073, 1991.

Trevisani F et al: Randomized control trials on chemoembolization for hepatocellular carcinoma: Is there room for new studies? *J Clin Gastroenterol* 32:383, 2001.

Urrutia R, DiMagno EP: Genetic markers: The key to early diagnosis and improved survival in pancreatic cancer? *Gastroenterology* 110:306, 1996.

Warshaw AL, Femandez-Del-Castillo C. Pancreatic carcinoma. *N Engl J Med* 326:455, 1992.

Wynne HA et al: The effect of age upon liver volume and apparent blood flow in health man. *Hepatology* 9:297, 1993.

Upper Gastrointestinal Disorders

AMINE HILA • DONALD O. CASTELL

ESOPHAGEAL DISEASES IN THE ELDERLY

Dysphagia

Symptoms of dysphagia can include difficulty initiating a swallow (oropharyngeal dysphagia) or the sensation of impaired passage of liquid or solid contents from the mouth to the stomach (esophageal dysphagia). Dysphagia is the most common esophageal complaint in the elderly population. Up to 10 percent of people older than age 50 years report troublesome dysphagia, although the majority do not consult a physician for these symptoms. In elderly people, dysphagia is also correlated with important morbidity and even mortality. In one report, 68 percent of 349 residents in a nursing home exhibited signs of dysphagia, and those elderly patients who could eat without help had a significantly lower mortality rate in a 6-month evaluation period than did those patients who required assistance to eat. Increased morbidity and mortality have been found in patients with oropharyngeal dysphagia and associated aspiration.

Dysphagia should be differentiated from odynophagia, defined as painful swallowing, which develops secondary to diseases affecting the esophageal mucosa, particularly inflammatory lesions. Candida, herpes simplex, and cytomegalovirus (CMV) esophagitis, medication-induced esophageal injury, and retropharyngeal abscess are examples of these disorders.

Evaluation of the elderly patient with dysphagia requires a systematic approach, starting with a careful history and physical examination. A thorough history, including medication use and pattern of administration, can lead to an accurate diagnosis in 80 to 85 percent of patients with dysphagia. Figure 50-1 illustrates this diagnostic approach.

Dysphagia in elderly persons may be caused by any of the diseases that can affect the young, as well as by several other diseases unique to elderly persons. It is important to note that eating disorders in elderly persons can result not only from pharyngoesophageal disease, but also from disturbances not associated with the gastrointestinal tract, including cognitive problems, physical disability of the upper limbs, deterioration of the muscles of mastication, dental disease, and osteoporosis affecting the mandible.

As in the young, dysphagia in the elderly person can be divided in two categories: oropharyngeal dysphagia—abnormalities affecting the neuromuscular mechanisms controlling movements of the tongue, pharynx, and upper esophageal sphincter (UES); and esophageal dysphagia—disorders affecting the esophagus itself.

Oropharyngeal Dysphagia

Oropharyngeal dysphagia refers to the inability to initiate the act of swallowing, so that food cannot be transferred from the mouth to the upper esophagus. Patients with oropharyngeal dysphagia generally complain of food sticking in the throat, difficulty initiating a swallow, nasal regurgitation, and coughing or choking during swallowing. Because of associated muscle weakness, they may also have dysarthria or nasal speech. Laryngeal penetration and aspiration may occur in these patients without concurrent choking or coughing. The cough reflex may be diminished from altered sensation related to an underlying neurologic disease or from desensitization from chronic aspiration. Patients with oropharyngeal dysphagia are at much higher risk of developing aspiration pneumonia. In addition, there is a clear relationship between reduced hypopharyngeal sensation and aspiration pneumonia.

Oropharyngeal dysphagia is usually one of several manifestations of a local, neurologic, or muscular disease (Table 50-1).

Causes of Oropharyngeal Dysphagia (Table 50-1)

Central Nervous System Diseases   Normal swallowing is accomplished by a series of neural and muscular events controlled by the brainstem and cranial nerves V, VII, IX, X, and XII. Anything affecting these nerves and associated muscles or the swallowing center in the medulla can cause oropharyngeal dysphagia. Neuromuscular disorders are responsible for approximately 80 percent of cases in elderly patients.

Patients with major strokes often manifest dysphagia as part of their neurologic deficit. Acute cerebral and brainstem vascular events are the neurologic conditions that most commonly produce oropharyngeal dysphagia in

DYSPHAGIA

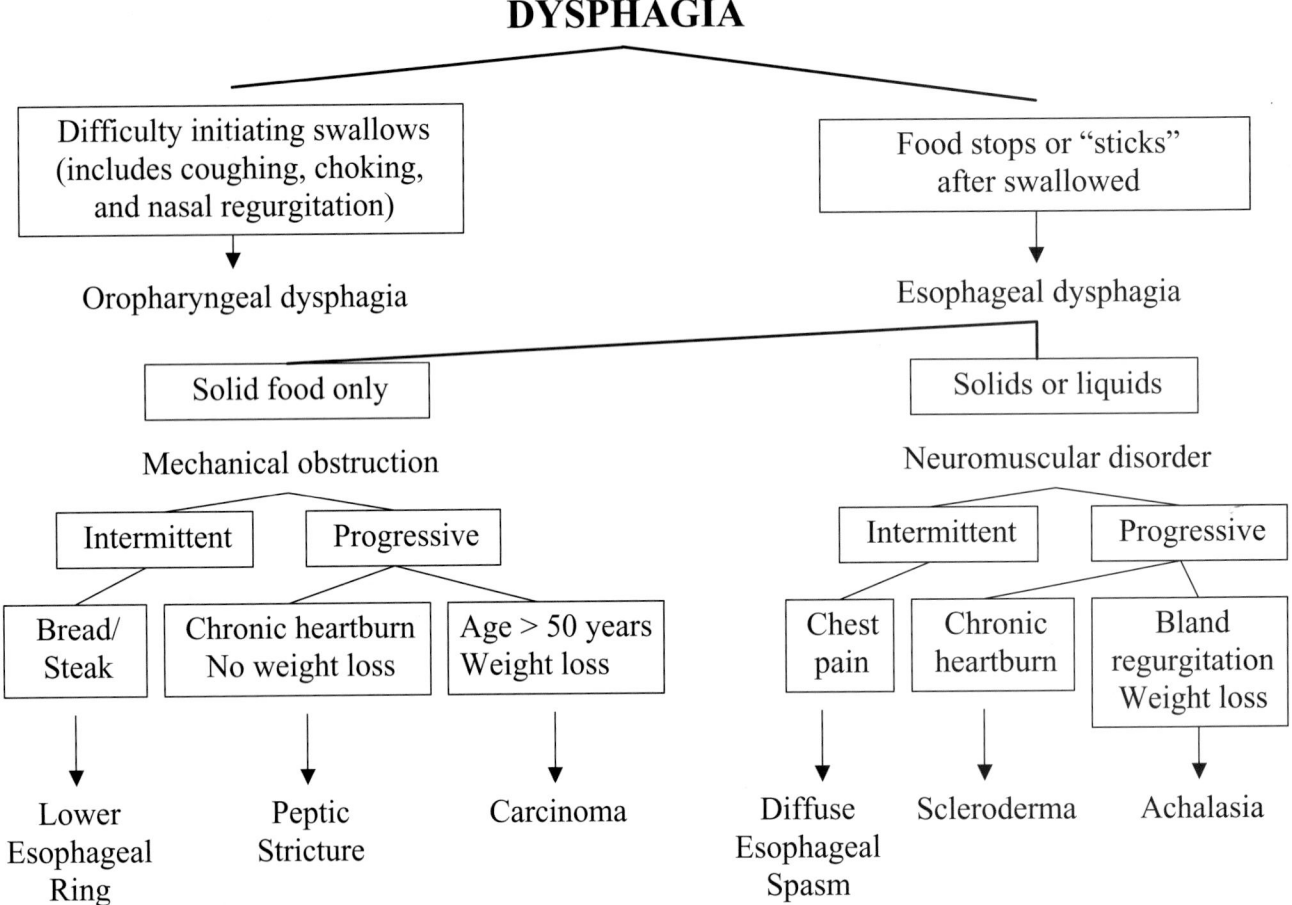

Figure 50-1   Algorithm for evaluating dysphagia in elderly patients.

elderly persons. Symptoms are typically abrupt in onset and are usually associated with other neurologic deficits, particularly of the cranial nerves. The barium swallow may show problems initiating a swallow, generalized motor dyscoordination, reduced pharyngeal peristalsis, and aspiration. Computerized tomography (CT) scan and magnetic resonance imaging (MRI) will often show multiple infarcts of the cerebral hemispheres or brainstem. MRI is more sensitive than CT scan for the evaluation of acute infarcts, small infarcts, and infarcts in the posterior fossa.

The mechanism producing dysphagia with hemispheric strokes is unclear, but brainstem distortion caused by cerebral edema is a likely cause. Reduction of brain edema may lead to resolution of dysphagia within 2 weeks in the majority of affected patients. Aspiration, which may lead to increased morbidity and prolonged hospitalization, is a problem in 20 to 50 percent of patients with strokes, depending on the size and location of the stroke.

In anterior cortical strokes, the motor cortex controlling tongue movement may be affected and thus produce poor oral control of a food bolus. Dysphagia is more likely with larger cortical strokes than with smaller ones. In cortical strokes, lingual and pharyngeal paresis may be unilateral, thus allowing for a compensatory strategy of turning the head to the paretic side so as to exclude the weakened musculature from the path of the food bolus. Dysphagia may

occur in pseudobulbar palsy or in Wallenberg syndrome, a lesion in the distribution of the posterior inferior cerebellar artery.

Brainstem injury caused by vertebrobasilar artery disease secondary to hypertension, or diabetes mellitus often induces dysphagia, usually with obvious cranial nerve involvement. However, small lacunar-type infarcts deep in the brain may produce dysphagia as a sole primary symptom. Brainstem strokes may affect the swallowing center beneath the nucleus of the solitary tract, which coordinates pharyngeal swallowing, or the nucleus ambiguus, which controls the muscles used in swallowing. Bilateral brainstem involvement is more severe and less likely to show recovery than unilateral involvement. Recovery of normal swallowing function is often slower in brainstem strokes as compared to cerebral strokes.

In patients with Parkinson disease, there are no specific motility abnormalities, but dysphagia of some degree is present in as many as 50 percent of these patients, and 95 percent of all Parkinson disease patients have some abnormalities on videofluoroscopy even in the absence of symptoms. In patients with parkinsonism, oropharyngeal dysphagia may result from tremor of the tongue or hesitancy in swallowing. An abnormality of the pharyngeal phase of swallowing is also likely. Although clinically significant dysphagia may appear early in Parkinson disease, it is usually a late complication.

Table 50-1   Common Causes of Oropharyngeal Dysphagia in Elderly Persons

Central nervous system disease
  Stroke
    Anterior cortical
    Wallenberg syndrome
    Pseudobulbar palsy
  Parkinson disease
  Wilson disease
  Multiple sclerosis
  Neoplasms

Other neuromuscular disorders
  Poliomyelitis and postpolio syndrome
  Myasthenia gravis
  Muscular dystrophies
  Polymyositis and dermatomyositis
  Amyotrophic lateral sclerosis
  Hypothyroidism
  Hyperthyroidism
  Hypercalcemia
  Cricopharyngeal dysfunction

Local structural lesions
  Oropharyngeal tumors
  Abscess
  Web
  Thyromegaly
  Cervical osteoarthritis with vertebral osteophytes
  Stricture

Zenker diverticulum

Oropharyngeal dysphagia may also be seen in patients with Wilson disease, multiple sclerosis, amyotrophic lateral sclerosis, and a variety of other congenital and degenerative disorders of the central nervous system. Brainstem neoplasms must also be considered in patients with oropharyngeal dysphagia.

Other Neuromuscular Disorders   Oropharyngeal dysphagia may also result from disorders affecting the peripheral nervous system or muscles involving the tongue, pharynx, or UES. In elderly persons, such disorders include peripheral neuropathy caused by diabetes mellitus, postpolio syndrome, myasthenia gravis, muscular dystrophies, polymyositis, dermatomyositis, hypothyroidism, and hyperthyroidism.

Polymyositis and dermatomyositis are inflammatory myopathies, with 60 to 70 percent of patients having proximal esophageal and UES involvement. They may result in weakness of the muscles controlling pharyngeal function and may lead to nasal regurgitation or aspiration. Radiographic features include poor contraction of the pharyngeal constrictors, pooling and retention of barium in the valleculae, nasal regurgitation, and disordered pharyngeal emptying. These abnormalities may reverse with treatment of

the muscular inflammation. Inflammatory myopathy isolated to the pharynx has also been described.

Two forms of muscular dystrophy involve the striated muscles of the pharyngoesophageal area. Myotonic dystrophy is a rare familial disease characterized by myopathic fasciitis, myotonia, swan neck, muscle wasting, frontal baldness, testicular atrophy, and cataracts. Manometric findings include decreased contraction pressures in the pharynx and upper esophagus and decreased UES resting pressure. Oculopharyngeal dystrophy has similar manometric findings, including abnormal UES relaxation, and frequently presents with dysphagia followed by ptosis.

In amyotrophic lateral sclerosis, oropharyngeal dysphagia is characteristically progressive and severe, resulting in frequent aspiration, which usually signals a preterminal phase of the disease.

Myasthenia gravis is characterized by weakness on repetitive use of certain voluntary muscles, particularly those innervated by motor nuclei of the brainstem. It can occur at any age, with peak incidence for women in the third decade, as compared with the seventh decade for men. Dysphagia occurs in nearly two-thirds of patients and typically presents with dysphagia associated with ptosis or diplopia. In advanced disease, dysphagia may be profound.

In the elderly patient with oropharyngeal dysphagia, it is particularly important to consider a diagnosis of hyperthyroidism, because the clinical presentation may otherwise be occult. Hyperthyroidism exaggerates the normal changes seen with aging by increasing muscle wasting in the elderly. Improvement of dysphagia and UES function have also been observed following treatment of myxedema.

Local Structural Lesions   Anatomic abnormalities causing mechanical obstruction and oropharyngeal dysphagia in the elderly include inflammatory processes, neoplasms, abscess, congenital web, prior surgical resection, thyromegaly, lymphadenopathy, and cervical hypertrophic osteoarthropathy. Although cervical osteoarthritis is frequent in the elderly, oropharyngeal dysphagia as a result of pharyngeal or esophageal compression by hypertrophic spurs of the anterior portion of the cervical vertebrae is unusual. Patients most commonly complain of difficulty when swallowing solids, but on occasion they may also have odynophagia, a foreign-body sensation, cough, hoarseness, and an urge to clear the throat. The diagnosis is made by barium swallow with lateral views with confirmation of delayed transport of tablets or food products by the cervical osteophyte. Endoscopy should be performed to exclude an obstructing neoplasm. Trauma from endotracheal intubation can result in vocal cord weakness, leading to coughing and aspiration during swallowing.

Upper Esophageal Sphincter Dysfunction   The cricopharyngeus and the adjacent hypopharyngeal musculature are responsible for the UES high-pressure zone. Dysfunction of these muscles may produce oropharyngeal dysphagia. Cricopharyngeal dysfunction may result from the inability of the muscles to work in synchrony with other components of the swallowing mechanism or from weakness of the pharyngeal muscles, therefore preventing a bolus from passing the cricopharyngeus muscle. Aging itself is associated with a decrease in UES tone, although age-related decreases in UES tone alone do not appear to result in dysphagia. Primary abnormality of UES relaxation resulting in oropharyngeal dysphagia in elderly persons (i.e., true cricopharyngeal achalasia) is quite unusual.

Zenker Diverticulum   Zenker diverticulum (ZD) is an outpouching in the posterior pharyngeal wall immediately above the UES, between the oblique fibers of the inferior pharyngeal constrictor and transverse fibers of the cricopharyngeal muscle. It is found almost exclusively in people older than age 50 years. The pathogenesis of ZD is thought to relate to decreased compliance of the cricopharyngeus muscle, resulting in decreased ability to relax and increased resistance to the passage of a bolus. The patient may have a history of dysphagia for solids and liquids, cough, fullness and gurgling in the neck, regurgitation of undigested food, recurrent aspiration, bronchitis, halitosis, and recurrent pneumonia. If large enough, a mass in the neck may be seen when eating. This can produce esophageal compression, contributing to and worsening the dysphagia. In some cases, patients learn to perform a variety of maneuvers to empty the diverticulum by applying pressure on the neck and coughing repeatedly. Definitive diagnosis of Zenker diverticulum is usually accomplished by contrast-radiographic examination of the pharynx. Barium swallow with particular attention to the oropharyngeal area is the most helpful procedure, particularly when videoradiography is used. Figure 50-2 illustrates a typical Zenker diverticulum seen on barium swallow. Small diverticula may not a require resection, but if the disease becomes severely debilitating, diverticulectomy with myotomy or endoscopic cricopharyngeal myotomy can be performed.

Evaluation of Oropharyngeal Dysphagia   In evaluating the patient with oropharyngeal dysphagia, a careful history and physical examination may provide clues to the diagnosis. This should focus on a thorough search for evidence of a systemic neurological disorder, including evaluation of the patient's ability to speak and swallow. Gag reflex, the most common test performed, evaluates the afferent activity of the glossopharyngeal nerve, but this is a poor predictor for aspiration. It is important to examine the head and neck carefully, looking for evidence of neoplasm, and possibly by obtaining an ear, nose, and throat (ENT) consultation. A typical history can suggest the diagnosis of ZD. Barium x-ray of the pharynx and UES with videofluoroscopy is the major diagnostic study in the evaluation of oropharyngeal dysphagia. Rapid-sequence pictures must be obtained (i.e., videoradiography) because bolus transfer from the mouth to the upper esophagus requires only approximately 1 second. Use of thick barium and a solid bolus (i.e., a "modified barium swallow") is particularly helpful in assessing the ability of the patient to transfer various foods from the mouth to the esophagus. Transnasal fiberoptic endoscopic examination of swallowing is also used, allowing a direct visualization of the swallow. Manometric studies of the pharynx and UES may also be helpful, particularly in the evaluation of abnormalities of pharyngeal strength and poor UES relaxation or coordination.

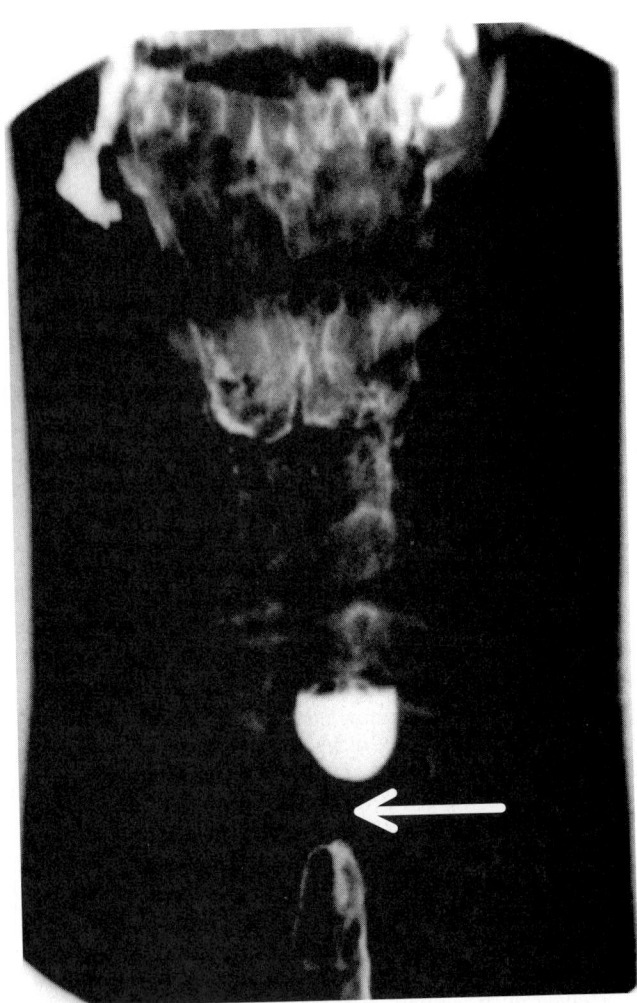

Figure 50-2   Typical Zenker diverticulum as seen on an anteroposterior view during a barium swallow. The *arrow* indicates the location of the cricopharyngeal muscle.

However, because these tests primarily evaluate the motor component of swallowing, the sensory component is not sufficiently evaluated, and if a bilateral sensory deficit is present, it may predispose to aspiration. The fiberoptic endoscopic examination of swallowing (FEES) with sensory testing is a bedside method that combines fiberoptic endoscopic examination of swallowing with a technique that determines laryngopharyngeal sensory discrimination thresholds by endoscopically delivering air-pulse stimuli to the mucosa innervated by the superior laryngeal nerve, which is responsible for laryngeal closure. The application of an air impulse initiates a reflex involving excitation of the superior pharyngeal nerve, which results in provocation of the laryngeal adductor reflex. This new modality of investigation provides adequate measurement of the sensory threshold that is required to maintain a secure airway. This technique is able to detect patients with unrecognized sensory deficit that might present with silent aspiration, and have not been identified by the classical diagnostic modalities.

Treatment of Oropharyngeal Dysphagia   Success in treating oropharyngeal dysphagia is determined by detection of the underlying disorder. The approach should be aimed at identifying and developing safe swallowing techniques, avoiding aspiration, and providing adequate nutritional support. Consultation with a speech pathologist is invaluable at this stage. Oropharyngeal dysphagia associated with systemic diseases, such as Parkinson disease, myasthenia gravis, polymyositis, and thyroid dysfunction, often improves with treatment of the underlying disorder. Oropharyngeal dysphagia associated with amyotrophic lateral sclerosis, multiple sclerosis, myotonic dystrophy, and other neuromuscular diseases is progressive, and little in the way of specific therapy can be offered to these patients. Many patients with oropharyngeal dysphagia from cerebrovascular accidents improve with time. Those with residual defects, as well as the many patients with untreatable neuromuscular diseases, can often be helped by a speech pathologist. The therapist can train patients with impaired tongue function but with an intact swallowing reflex to strengthen their tongue muscles with exercise. They also can optimize head postures to help control the bolus in the oral cavity. Patients with impaired laryngeal closure and aspiration are taught to turn their head to the damaged side, placing tension on the immobile cord and effecting its movement toward the midline. Other strategies include adjustments in food consistency, volume, and delivery rate to maximize the patient's remaining function, strategies based on results of the modified barium swallow. Patients who are alert and motivated are good candidates for therapy.

If aspiration cannot be prevented and nutrition cannot be maintained orally, enteral feeding using either a Dobbhoff, a gastrostomy, or a jejunostomy tube may be necessary on either a temporary or permanent basis.

Neoplasms require resection and, in some cases, chemotherapy or radiotherapy. Unfortunately, treatment itself may also result in dysphagia, because of the removal or loss of function of structures critical to normal swallowing.

Cricopharyngeal myotomy offers relief primarily to patients with ZD or those having disorders resulting in cricopharyngeal dysfunction. In patients with neurologic diseases, including stroke and degenerative conditions, who present with pharyngeal dysphagia, myotomy may be considered, particularly in those in whom manometry has documented incomplete UES relaxation. Limited studies in small groups of patients with oropharyngeal dysphagia reveal good to excellent results with cricopharyngeal myotomy in patients with cerebrovascular accidents, motor neuron disease, head trauma, poliomyelitis, and neoplastic or postsurgical nerve injury. Treatment of ZD usually requires cricopharyngeal myotomy along with pouch resection. The main contraindication to cricopharyngeal myotomy is gastroesophageal reflux disease (GERD), which may increase the risk of aspiration and its consequences.

Injection of botulinum toxin may provide an alternative approach to cricopharyngeal dysfunction, but its exact role in therapy remains to be defined. Passing a large-diameter dilator (18 to 20 mm) may improve dysphagia, particularly in patients in whom manometric studies show high UES pressure or impaired relaxation.

Esophageal Dysphagia

Esophageal dysphagia is the symptom that occurs with a transport problem in which ingested material delivered

Table 50-2 Causes of Esophageal Dysphagia in Elderly Persons

Motility disorders
 Achalasia
 Diffuse esophageal spasm and related disorders
 Scleroderma
 Diabetes mellitus
 Parkinson disease

Mechanical obstruction
 Neoplasms
 Peptic strictures
 Rings and webs
 Vascular lesions (dysphagia aortica)
 Diverticula
 Medication-induced esophageal injury
 Mediastinal adenopathy
 Postsurgical changes

from the hypopharynx is poorly transported down the esophagus into the stomach. A wide variety of mechanically obstructing lesions and neuromuscular (motility) disorders are associated with esophageal dysphagia. A careful history usually allows the physician to place a patient into one of these two main categories. The three most important questions that should be addressed early in the evaluation are (see Fig. 50-1): (1) What kind of food is associated with the symptoms (solids, liquids, or both)? (2) Is the dysphagia intermittent or progressive? (3) Is there associated heartburn? Motility disorders usually produce dysphagia for both solids and liquids, whereas obstructing lesions initially cause dysphagia for solids only. The presence of additional associated symptoms, such as chest pain, and nocturnal symptomatology may also provide helpful clues to the diagnosis. Table 50-2 lists the disorders capable of causing esophageal dysphagia in elderly persons.

Achalasia *Achalasia* means "failure to relax." This is an esophageal motility disorder characterized by a double defect in esophageal function. The lower esophageal sphincter (LES) does not appropriately relax, offering resistance to the flow of liquids and solids into the stomach. In addition, there is loss of peristalsis in the lower two-thirds (smooth muscle portion) of the esophagus. These abnormalities result from a loss of predominantly inhibitory ganglion cells in Auerbach plexuses, causing a functional obstruction at the level of the LES and aperistalsis of the esophageal body.

Achalasia is characterized by slowly progressive dysphagia for solids and liquids and gradual weight loss. The incidence of achalasia is 1 per 100,000 per year in the general population. The onset of symptoms occurs at all ages, including in elderly persons. Achalasia is equally frequent in both sexes. Approximately 15 percent of patients with a new diagnosis of achalasia are older than 60 years of age. Their clinical presentation is similar to that of younger patients, except fewer elderly patients complain of chest pain, and their pain tends to be less severe. For many patients, the symptoms reach a plateau and do not worsen with time;

for others, the symptoms are so severe that weight loss is pronounced. Between 30 and 50 percent of patients have associated retrosternal chest pain, which is precipitated by eating, and between 60 and 90 percent regurgitate undigested food after a meal. Sometimes regurgitation may be induced by the patient to relieve the uncomfortable feeling of chest pain, pressure, or fullness after a meal. Nocturnal coughing is also a frequent symptom. Some patients may initially present with aspiration pneumonia. At the time of diagnosis, symptoms have usually been present for an average of 2 years.

The disease should be suspected after a careful and detailed history. Chest x-rays are normal in early stages of the disease, but in advanced cases a dilated esophagus with an air–fluid level caused by retained food and saliva can be seen. Barium studies typically show a dilated esophagus, with a smooth "bird-beak" narrowing at the gastroesophageal junction (Fig. 50-3). In elderly patients with long-standing achalasia, extreme dilatation and tortuosity of the esophagus may be seen on barium x-ray, the so-called "sigmoid esophagus."

In elderly patients with apparent achalasia, it is important to perform an upper endoscopy (including a retroflexed view of the gastroesophageal junction) with biopsy of any suspicious area, because of the possibility of secondary achalasia caused by a cancer having the clinical, radiologic, and manometric abnormalities associated with idiopathic achalasia. Most commonly, this syndrome is produced by an adenocarcinoma of the gastroesophageal junction. Rarely, pancreatic cancer, lung cancer, breast cancer, mesothelioma, hepatocellular carcinoma, sarcoma, and lymphoma can present in this manner. Other, nonmalignant causes of secondary achalasia, include amyloidosis, sarcoidosis, Chagas disease, pancreatic pseudocyst, and postvagotomy disturbances. Secondary achalasia should be suspected in patients with the clinical triad of age greater than 50 years, dysphagia of less than 1 year's duration, and weight loss of more than 15 lb. However, this triad is not highly specific, because it can also be associated with idiopathic achalasia. Endoscopic ultrasonography may be helpful in detecting small neoplasms at the gastroesophageal junction.

Chagas disease is caused by infection with *Trypanosoma cruzi*, a parasite endemic in South America. Although idiopathic achalasia involves only the esophagus, Chagas disease usually involves the entire gastrointestinal tract and the myocardium. The manometric findings are identical to those occurring in achalasia, including aperistalsis in the distant two-thirds of the esophagus, elevated LES pressure, and incomplete LES relaxation.

Treatment of achalasia is directed to the palliation of symptoms and prevention of complications. It can be either medical or surgical. The choice of the therapeutic modality depends on the preference and expertise of the treating physician, the overall health of the patient, and the patient's preference after being properly apprised of the techniques, risks, and expected outcomes. Pneumatic dilatation, surgical (including laparoscopic) myotomy, and injection of botulinum toxin are the main therapeutic options.

Pneumatic dilatation is a safe procedure in elderly patients, and such patients are less likely to require further

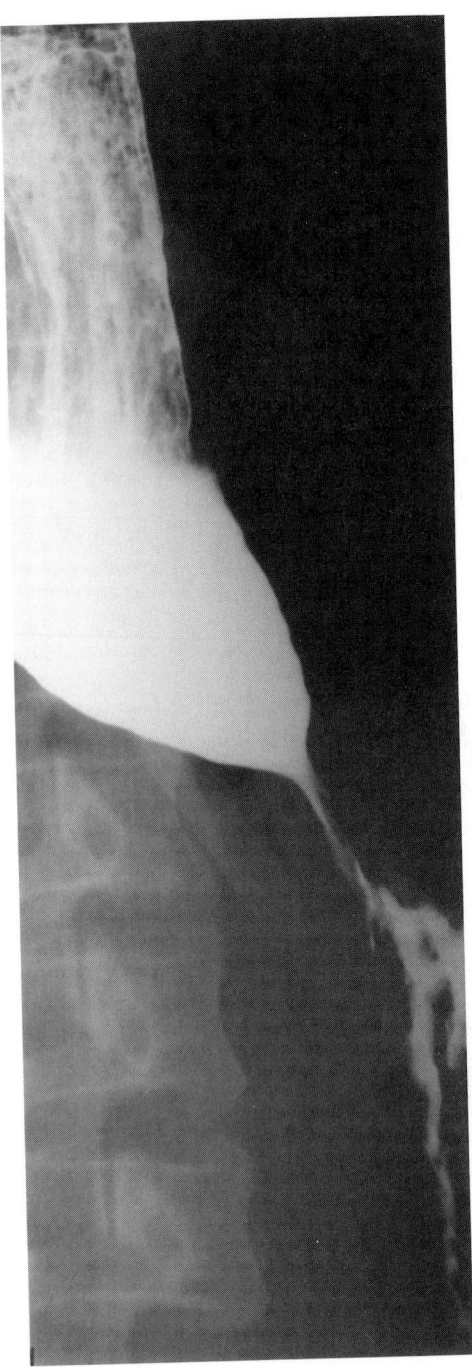

Figure 50-3 Typical achalasia as seen on an anteroposterior view during a barium swallow.

dilatations. Obviously the patient must be a good risk for surgery in the unusual event that a perforation occurs (<5 percent). Even when a perforation does occur, it can usually be managed without surgery. Approximately 85 percent of patients have a good response with pneumatic dilatation, with the highest success rates in the elderly. The modified Heller procedure is successful in approximately 90 percent of patients. However, surgery is generally associated with a higher frequency of side effects, particularly GERD, resulting in the usual practice of adding a partial fundoplication to the area of the myotomy.

In elderly patients with other serious medical problems in whom both pneumatic dilatation and surgery may be associated with a high risk, injection of botulinum toxin in the LES provides effective, albeit temporary, symptomatic relief. Treatment will need to be repeated when symptoms recur (usually in less than 1 year). Medical therapy with smooth muscle relaxing agents, such as isosorbide dinitrate or nifedipine given sublingually before meals, has limited effect in the elderly but occasionally may be helpful. The most recent innovation as an approach to relieve the dysphagia in achalasia patients is sildenafil given orally. This pharmacotherapy relies on availability of local nitric oxide and may have a limited effect due to degeneration of responsible myenteric neurons.

Spastic Esophageal Motor Disorders   Intermittent dysphagia to certain types of foods, particularly hot or cold liquids, and associated chest pain, sometimes resembling angina, suggests a spastic motility disorder of the esophagus. This category includes diffuse esophageal spasm, nutcracker esophagus, and hypertensive LES. Their precise definition requires manometric evaluation, because they have similar clinical presentations. Patients with these disorders also have similar therapeutic options and clinical outcomes. These disorders are of uncertain pathogenesis,

and because their severity rarely progresses, they are less likely to result from a degenerative neural process.

Diffuse esophageal spasm is more common in women and can appear at any age, the average age being approximately 40 years. A barium x-ray may show a highly irregular pattern, which is referred to by a variety of colorful names, including the "corkscrew" esophagus. Esophageal manometry shows normal peristalsis interrupted by simultaneous (nonperistaltic) contractions of prolonged duration (Fig. 50-4). Nutcracker esophagus is characterized by peristaltic contractions of high amplitude (>180 mmHg) with or without increased peristaltic duration, whereas hypertensive LES has an elevated LES pressure (>45 mmHg) with normal relaxation. Both of these have normal esophageal peristalsis.

Treatment is aimed at decreasing esophageal pressure or improving peristalsis to cause symptom reduction, augmented by reassurance that the pain is esophageal and not cardiac in origin. Agents such as nitrates, calcium-channel blockers (specifically nifedipine or diltiazem), anticholinergics, antidepressants, anxiolytics, and even botulinum toxin injection have been helpful in some cases. In cases in which severe dysphagia is the predominant symptom, pneumatic dilatation has been used. In refractory cases with severe dysphagia and weight loss, an extended Heller

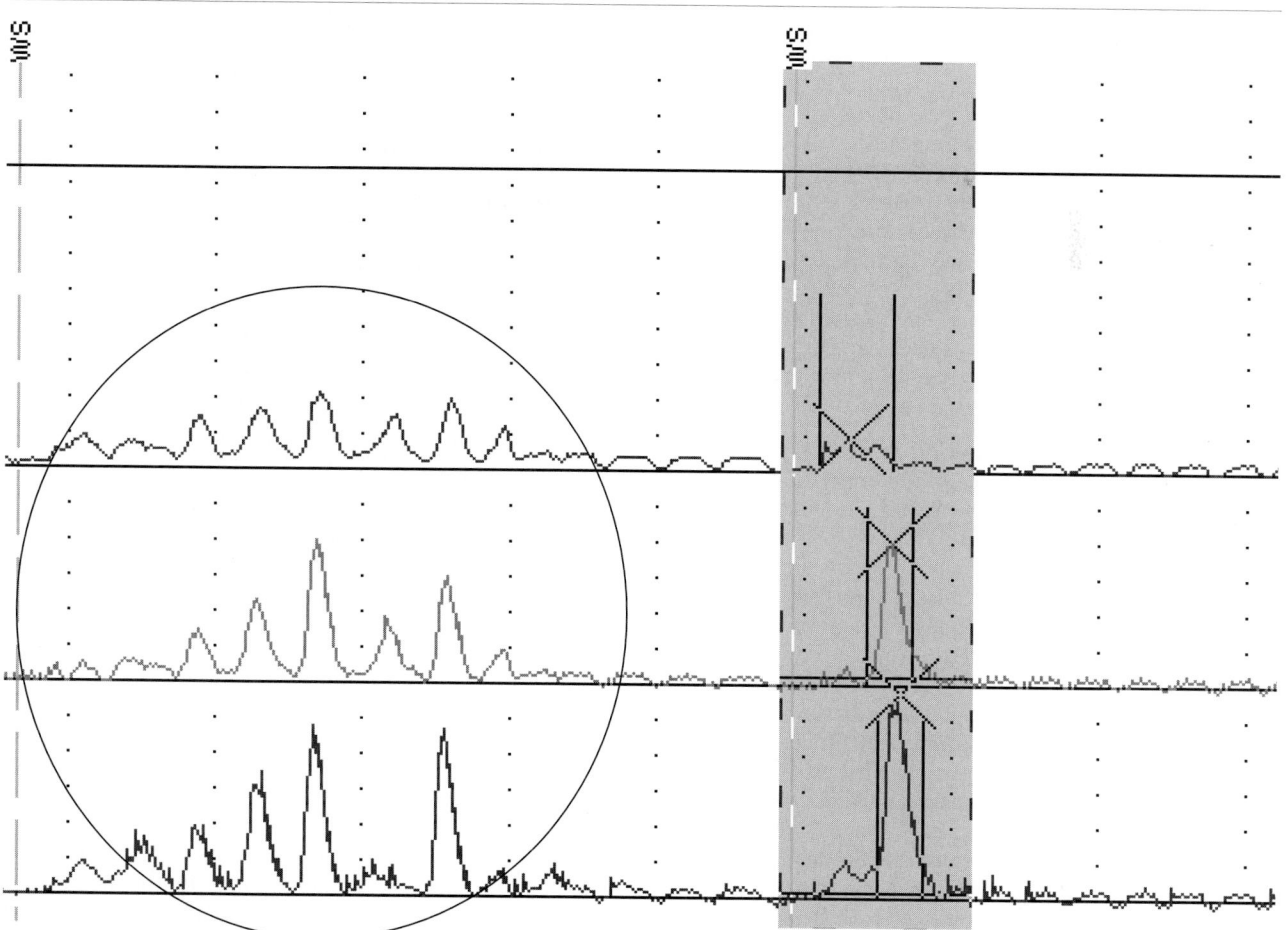

Figure 50-4   Esophageal manometry tracing typical diffuse esophageal spasm. Notice the simultaneous contractions (*circled on the left*), as compared to a normal swallow (*right*).

myotomy may be cautiously considered, ensuring that the circular muscles are cut in the area of the esophageal body shown to be abnormal by manometry. Many patients improve after being reassured that their chest pain is noncardiac in origin.

Scleroderma   The esophagus is involved in more than 80 percent of patients with scleroderma and correlates with the presence of Raynaud phenomenon. The basic process is atrophy of the smooth muscle with fibrosis of the submucosa and muscularis and replacement with collagen, that occurs only in the lower two-thirds of the esophagus. Patients with scleroderma may experience slowly progressive dysphagia for both solids and liquids. Heartburn is a prominent symptom caused by severe gastroesophageal reflux, and up to 40 percent of patients develop either Barrett esophagus or peptic esophageal stricture. Classically, motility studies show low to absent LES pressure, weak to absent distal esophageal peristalsis, but normal upper esophageal and UES function. Dysphagia can arise from the intrinsic motility disorder, but when especially severe, should suggest esophagitis with an associated peptic stricture. The diagnosis is made from the clinical presentation, physical findings compatible with the CREST (calcinosis cutis, Raynaud phenomenon, esophageal motility disorder, sclerodactyly, and telangiectasia) syndrome along with barium radiographs and esophageal manometry. Radiographic studies characteristically show mild esophageal dilatation, aperistalsis of the distal smooth muscle portion, and a patent LES with free reflux.

Unfortunately, there is little available for the treatment of the underlying disease. Gastroesophageal reflux should be identified and aggressively treated, as discussed in "Gastroesophageal Reflux Disease" later in this chapter. Dysphagia without stricture may be reduced by chewing food well, drinking ample fluids, and treating GERD. Stricture formation may require frequent bougienage. In severe cases, antireflux surgery may be necessary, but this should be cautiously undertaken because of the severe motility defect in the esophageal body.

Peptic Stricture   The most common presenting symptom of a peptic stricture is slowly progressive dysphagia for solids in a patient with a long history of heartburn or other symptoms of GERD. Weight loss is seldom noticed with these benign lesions because patients usually have a good appetite. Patients with peptic strictures are usually older than patients with GERD but no stricture, presumably because stricture formation results over a long period of time. Endoscopy always should be performed to rule out malignancy. Barium swallow may suggest the diagnosis (Fig. 50-5). The strictures are typically smooth, tapered, and of varying length. Barrett esophagus may present with a stricture classically higher in the esophagus, representing the proximal extent of the metaplastic tissue.

In most cases, peptic strictures can be managed with intermittent dilatation using standard Maloney or Savary dilators in combination with aggressive long-term antireflux therapy. If the peptic stricture does not respond to conservative therapy, surgical antireflux repair (fundoplication) is indicated.

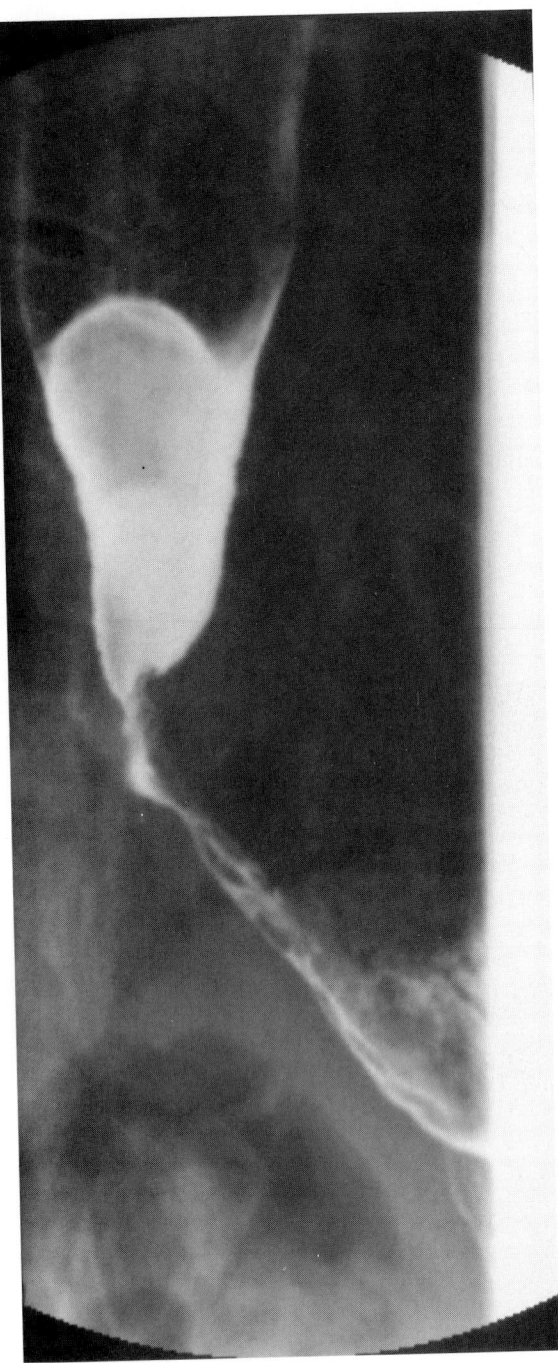

Figure 50-5   Typical esophageal stricture as seen on an anteroposterior view during a barium swallow.

Medication-Induced Esophageal Injury   Elderly patients take more medications than do younger patients, spend more time in a recumbent position, have reduced salivary production in association with poor oral fluid intake, and are more likely to have motility or anatomic disorders of the esophagus. All of these reasons place them at higher risk for medication-induced esophageal injury. As opposed to younger patients in whom antibiotics are the medications most likely associated with esophageal injury, in the elderly patient, potassium chloride, quinidine, nonsteroidal antiinflammatory drugs, and alendronate are the primary culprits. Alendronate, which is currently used to treat osteoporosis especially in elderly women, reportedly causes a severe form of esophagitis. Other medications shown to induce esophageal injury are tetracycline derivatives, emperonium bromide (an anticholinergic agent used to relax the urinary bladder and not available in the United States), and ferrous compounds.

Other factors that predispose to drug-induced esophageal injury include the patient's position at the time the drug is ingested and the volume of fluid ingested with the drug. It has been well established that the likelihood of passage of a pill through the esophagus is reduced when the medication is ingested by a patient in a recumbent position and with less than 15 mL of water. It is thus preferable not to administer drugs at bedtime with small sips of water, even though it is a common practice, especially in the bed-ridden elderly patient. Most patients with medication-induced esophageal lesions have a normal esophagus. The site of injury probably relates to anatomic factors, as injury occurs most frequently in the midesophagus at the level of the aortic arch or distally in the area adjacent to the left atrium or above the LES.

The diagnosis of pill-induced esophageal injury is usually suggested by a history of acute substernal pain, odynophagia, and dysphagia in a patient taking one of the drugs known to cause such injury. Symptoms can present anywhere from hours to weeks after the pill has been taken. A double-contrast barium swallow may identify the lesion and may provide information about possible extrinsic esophageal compression, but the lesions are best seen on endoscopy. These patients have ulcers ranging from pinpoint ulcerations, to circumferential lesions several centimeters long, sometimes with strictures. Lesions in the distal esophagus may be confused with reflux esophagitis, but many times pill-induced lesions spare the squamocolumnar junction. Occasional deaths from hemorrhage and perforation have been reported in patients with potassium chloride-induced esophagitis.

Most medication-induced esophageal lesions heal with discontinuation of the causative agent and short-term therapy with antacids or acid suppression. Occasionally, more aggressive antireflux therapy is required and, in rare instances, resulting strictures must be dilated. Potassium chloride and quinidine preparations are the most likely agents to cause esophageal injury leading to strictures. Older age is a significant risk factor for developing pill-induced strictures.

Esophageal Cancer In any elderly patient with the new onset of dysphagia, cancer should be the initial diagnostic consideration. Squamous cell carcinoma used to be the most common malignancy of the esophagus, particularly in patients with a history of heavy tobacco and/or alcohol use. In the United States, black men have a high risk of developing squamous cell carcinoma of the esophagus, with an incidence four times higher than that of white men. Other potential risk factors include caustic esophageal injury, esophageal webs, squamous cell carcinoma of the nasopharynx, and tylosis (hyperkeratosis of the esophagus, palms, and soles). The principal risk factor for adenocarcinoma of the esophagus is Barrett esophagus as a result of long-standing GERD, and during the past two decades, the incidence of adenocarcinoma of the esophagus has increased faster than that of any other cancer, particularly among white males. It now occurs as frequently as squamous cell carcinoma.

Patients commonly present with dysphagia for solids rapidly progressing to liquids and associated with anorexia and significant weight loss. Pain may be a predominant symptom because of obstruction, infectious esophagitis, or extensive mediastinal metastases. Barium x-ray studies can suggest the diagnosis. Endoscopy with biopsy and cytology is the best method for confirming the diagnosis and is safe and well tolerated in elderly patients. Computed tomography or magnetic resonance imaging of the chest can help to assess the extent of tumor involvement outside of the esophageal lumen. Endoscopic ultrasonography is playing an increasingly prominent role in the staging of esophageal cancer.

The treatment of choice for esophageal cancer is surgical resection, which can usually be performed successfully in selected elderly patients with few or no coexisting medical problems. However, elderly patients are often poor operative risks, and the tumor is often unresectable at the time of diagnosis. Palliation with radiotherapy, chemotherapy, or both may be considered. For relief of dysphagia, bougienage, laser ablation, or endoscopic insertion of an expandable stent are additional options for treating obstructing esophageal lesions. Endoscopic mucosal resection is also proving to be effective in the nonoperative management of focal adenocarcinoma of the esophagus arising in Barrett esophagus. In general, the prognosis of symptomatic esophageal cancer is poor, with a 5-year survival rate of less than 5 percent. Cancer detected during routine endoscopic surveillance of Barrett esophagus has a much better prognosis.

Rings and Webs Esophageal rings and webs are thin, diaphragm-like membranes that interrupt the lumen of the esophagus. They are usually called rings if they are situated at the squamocolumnar junction, and webs if they are located anywhere else along the body of the esophagus. They are often an incidental radiographic or endoscopic finding. Patients with intermittent dysphagia to solids are likely to have a symptomatic ring or web. Unlike dysphagia associated with esophageal cancer, dysphagia caused by rings or webs is typically nonprogressive. The first episode of dysphagia frequently occurs while the patient is eating steak or bread. Often the bolus can be forced down by drinking liquids, but occasionally it must be regurgitated, after which the meal can usually be finished without difficulty. Diagnosis is suggested by compatible history and confirmed by barium studies, with use of a solid test bolus being particularly helpful. Endoscopy is indicated for histologic confirmation.

The two most common types are the cervical esophageal web and Schatzki ring. Webs are thin, transverse membranes of squamous epithelium, composed primarily of mucosa. Their incidence increases with age. A cervical esophageal web is located in the immediate postcricoid area. Women are predominantly affected and may have iron-deficiency anemia, so-called Plummer-Vinson syndrome. The pathogenesis of this entity is unknown. Schatzki ring is composed of invaginated mucosa located at the gastroesophageal mucosal junction. On barium swallow, these rings are seen approximately 3 to 4 cm above the diaphragm. The primary determinant of symptoms is the caliber of the ring. In general, rings with a luminal diameter of less than 13 mm are symptomatic, whereas those larger than 20 mm rarely produce symptoms. Although the association is widely cited, there is only weak evidence that Schatzki ring is related to GERD.

Treatment is usually a one-time esophageal dilatation with a large-caliber bougie. Careful chewing of food may be enough for patients with infrequent symptoms. If patients do not respond to standard bougienage, electrocautery incision of the ring may be offered and is often successful.

Dysphagia Aortica   This disorder is unique to the elderly and presents with dysphagia produced by compression of the esophagus above the gastroesophageal junction, by either a large aneurysm of the thoracic aorta or by a rigid atherosclerotic aorta posteriorly and the heart or esophageal hiatus anteriorly. Occasionally, the esophagus may be compressed by a markedly enlarged left atrium. Rarely, exsanguinating hemorrhage may result from penetration of an esophageal ulcer into an adjacent major blood vessel. Dysphagia aortica is seen predominantly in elderly women because of their predilection to dorsal kyphosis in the postmenopausal years. These patients have solid-food dysphagia, manifested most commonly as substernal fullness and regurgitation. A barium swallow will show impingement of the vascular structure on the esophagus and delayed passage of a solid bolus. Esophageal manometry often shows increased intraluminal pressures with superimposed cardiac pulsations corresponding to the region of aortic impingement.

Infections of the Esophagus   Esophageal infections occur mainly in patients with predisposing diseases, including human immunodeficiency virus (HIV), malignancy (mainly leukemia and lymphoma), and diabetes mellitus, or use of antibiotics, corticosteroids, cytotoxic agents, and immunosuppressive therapy. Otherwise, immunodeficient and malnourished patients are also at higher risk. These infections can occasionally be found in healthy individuals. The two most frequent causative infections are *Candida albicans* (approximately 75 percent of cases) and herpes simplex virus. Odynophagia is the most frequent symptom, but dysphagia can also be present. Definitive diagnosis requires endoscopy with biopsy and cytology. Treatment consists of correcting the underlying predisposing factors and appropriate therapy. Fluconazole is the treatment of choice for candida, with amphotericin B reserved for resistant cases. Herpes simplex infection of the esophagus is less common than candidiasis. Radiographically and endoscopically, herpes is characterized by clean, punched-out ulcerations. Endoscopy, mucosal biopsies with cultures, and brush cytology are often diagnostic. Oral acyclovir is used in mild cases, while intravenous administration is required for severe esophagitis.

Gastroesophageal Reflux Disease

The symptoms of GERD are among the most common complaints attributed to the gastrointestinal tract. It has been estimated that approximately 10 percent of the US population experiences heartburn every day and at least one-third of the population has occasional heartburn. It is also interesting to note that 80 percent of over-the-counter antacids sold in the United States are taken for symptoms of GERD. Several studies show that the prevalence of heartburn, as well as endoscopic esophagitis, increases after age 50 years. GERD may be more difficult to diagnose in the elderly for several reasons, including diminished pain perception (due to visceral autonomic neuropathy), increased gastric pH, and the fact that symptoms are often attributed to known underlying causes such as coronary artery disease.

Changes in Antireflux Mechanism with Age

The LES is the major antireflux barrier. An explanation for the increased incidence of GERD in elderly persons remains unclear, because esophageal function is relatively well preserved with age. In fact, manometric studies of healthy elderly subjects have not shown a consistent decrease in LES pressure with age. However, secondary esophageal peristalsis, an important mechanism to clear refluxed acid, is less consistent in the elderly than in the young. In addition, slight decreases in salivary volume and bicarbonate have been found in healthy elderly subjects and, more importantly, older subjects show a decreased salivary bicarbonate response to esophageal acid infusion.

Although gastric acid secretion does not decrease because of aging per se, gastric acid secretion may decline in the large percentage of elderly persons with long-standing *Helicobacter pylori* infection in whom atrophic gastritis develops. Therefore, refluxed material is often less acidic in elderly patients with *H. pylori* infection when compared to young patients. This may explain in part a lower frequency of heartburn in elderly patients with GERD and the underrecognition of GERD in this population.

The frequency of sliding-type esophageal hiatal hernia increases with age. This condition impairs the diaphragmatic component of the LES and may impede the clearance of refluxed acid from the distal esophagus. Thus, an increased prevalence of hiatal hernia in elderly persons could contribute to an increased prevalence of GERD. On the other hand, the rate of gastric emptying does not appear to change with age.

A possibly important factor in elderly persons is the use of medications known to decrease the LES pressure and thereby increase gastroesophageal reflux. Table 50-3 contains a list of substances suspected to lower LES pressure. Medications listed in that table are more likely to be administered to elderly patients than to young patients, and consequently may contribute to GERD. An increase in body weight (and especially control adiposity) with age may also predispose to GERD.

Presentation of GERD in the Elderly Patient

There is controversy as to whether GERD is more common in elderly persons than in young persons. Many studies show that the prevalence of heartburn but not regurgitation declines with age. Classic symptoms of GERD are heartburn and acid regurgitation. Heartburn is a substernal

Table 50-3 Substances that Reduce Resting LES Pressure

Anticholinergics

Barbiturates

Caffeine

Calcium channel blockers

Chocolate

Coffee

Diazepam

Estrogen

Ethanol

Fat

Meperidine

Nitrates

Progesterone

Somatostatin

Theophilline

burning sensation that typically radiates upward. When the refluxed material reaches the oral cavity, it is called regurgitation. Symptoms of GERD in elderly individuals are often atypical. Dysphagia, chest pain, respiratory symptoms, and vomiting are more common in older patients with GERD than in younger patients. The development of chest pain in an adult patient raises the possibility of ischemic heart disease. However, 10 to 30 percent of patients undergoing coronary angiography will have normal studies. Recent investigations suggest that acid reflux may cause noncardiac chest pain in up to 50 percent of these patients.

In persons older than 80 years, esophagitis may account for a greater percentage of cases of upper gastrointestinal bleeding than in younger persons. Because the severity of symptoms often does not correlate with the degree of esophagitis, diagnostic endoscopy should be considered in all elderly patients with the new onset of symptoms suggestive of GERD. Elderly patients are particularly susceptible to the respiratory complications of GERD. Aspiration of reflux material into the airways may lead to laryngeal and bronchopulmonary manifestations. These include persistent hoarseness, laryngeal granulomas, subglottic stenosis, chronic persistent cough, and recurring aspiration pneumonitis. There is also mounting evidence of an association between reflux disease and obstructive airways disease (asthma), either by microaspiration of acid or via vagally mediated bronchospasm triggered by intraesophageal acid exposure. Elderly patients with GERD have a higher incidence of restrictive pulmonary disease than do similar patients without reflux.

Because GERD is a chronic persistent disorder, it seems likely that the frequency of complications associated with gastroesophageal reflux increases with increasing duration of disease and thus with age. Despite milder heartburn, older patients may be more likely to have severe esophagitis, strictures, and Barrett esophagus. The incidence of Barrett esophagus rises with age. Moreover, elderly patients with Barrett esophagus are less symptomatic than younger patients with Barrett esophagus. Any suspicion of GERD in the elderly patient should be evaluated fully and treated aggressively.

Diagnosis

The diagnostic approach to the patient with possible GERD is multilayered, depending on the presentation. Because the symptoms are believed to be caused by chronic reflux, evaluation should attempt to document this abnormality. In patients presenting with typical symptoms of heartburn and regurgitation, little if any additional information is needed to establish a presumptive diagnosis, and therapy can often be initiated at this point. The patient whose symptoms are less clear or that include atypical manifestations will usually need additional diagnostic testing. The variety of tests and procedures that are available to evaluate the patient with possible GERD can cause diagnostic confusion if not used appropriately. In addition, the ease of administration and the need for technical training, special equipment, expense and discomfort to the patient are important factors in determining the priority with which diagnostic tests are administered.

Although it has limited value, many primary care physicians still use an upper gastrointestinal series to evaluate possible reflux. This test may be helpful, when using air-contrast techniques, to rule out complications of GERD (ulcer, stricture) or other structural abnormalities of the esophagus, stomach, or duodenum. On the other hand, radiographic reflux, the flow of barium from the stomach into the esophagus either spontaneously or induced by various maneuvers, has limited diagnostic value. In recent years, it has become clear that most normal individuals have brief intermittent episodes of reflux (so-called physiologic reflux), particularly on those occasions when the LES will spontaneously relax or open. Hiatal hernias are observed more commonly in reflux patients and may impair both esophageal acid clearance and the antireflux barrier. However, the barium swallow may become the diagnostic test of choice when dysphagia is one of the primary symptoms.

Endoscopy is the diagnostic approach most frequently used to document esophageal injury. Endoscopic findings of erosions, exudate, ulcers, strictures, or Barrett epithelium provide a definitive diagnosis of reflux injury. Unfortunately, these findings may be subtle or absent, even in the presence of specific histologic abnormalities in mucosal biopsy specimens. Only approximately 50 percent of patients with chronic heartburn can be expected to have esophagitis apparent on endoscopy. Mucosal biopsies may improve the diagnostic yield but are unnecessary with clear-cut endoscopic changes of esophagitis. In the absence of macroscopic mucosal changes, endoscopic biopsies may establish the diagnosis of reflux esophagitis if consistent histopathologic changes are present. In addition, when

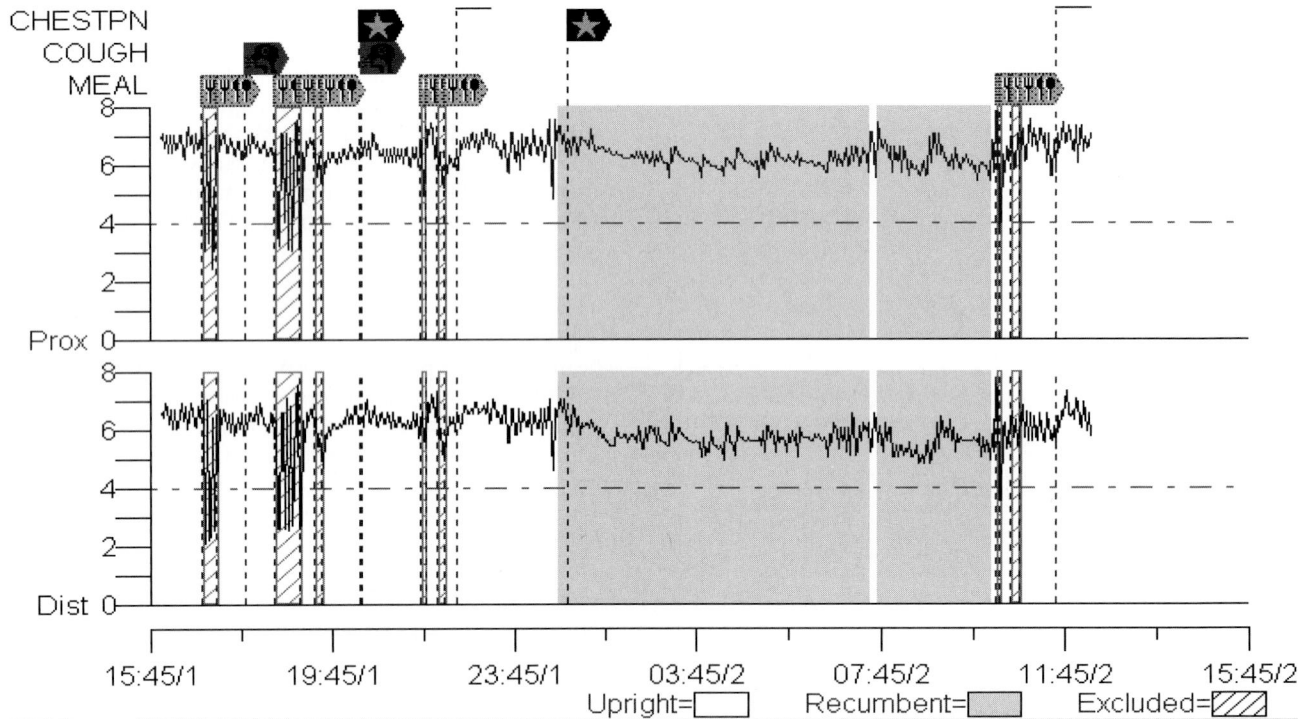

Figure 50-6   Normal 24-hour esophageal pH study.

Barrett esophagus is suspected, mucosal biopsies are necessary to identify the abnormal columnar epithelium in the form of specialized intestinal metaplasia and to evaluate the presence of dysplasia.

The acid perfusion (Bernstein) test, used for many years as a test of acid sensitivity, is rarely performed at present and has been replaced with ambulatory pH monitoring or a trial of acid-suppression therapy. The current gold standard for the diagnosis of GERD is prolonged ambulatory pH monitoring. A pH probe placed 5 cm above the lower esophageal sphincter permits monitoring of esophageal acid exposure time. It provides the most physiologic measurements of acid reflux, incorporating information obtained over an extended time period. Figure 50-6 illustrates a normal 24-hour esophageal pH study, while Fig. 50-7 shows a typical study in a patient with GERD. Ideally, ambulatory pH monitoring is done with the patient in their usual work or home environment. Patients record the time that they experience reflux symptoms during monitoring, thus allowing correlation of intraesophageal pH and subjective symptoms. Clinical indications include patients presenting with difficult diagnostic problems or with atypical reflux symptoms (chest pain, cough, hoarseness), those not readily responding to therapy, or the preoperative and postoperative evaluation of antireflux surgery.

Measurement of LES pressure was previously suggested as a possible means to diagnose reflux disease. The importance of the LES as a major barrier to reflux is well established. An LES pressure of less than 10 mmHg is considered an indication of an incompetent gastroesophageal junction; however, LES pressure variability severely limits the sensitivity and specificity of this measurement as a diagnostic test. Many patients with well-documented esophagitis will have an LES pressure higher than 10 mmHg, and some

asymptomatic subjects with pressures below this value have been studied. Consequently, LES pressure in a given patient is often too imprecise to identify a potential for reflux, even though it is the most measurable part of the antireflux barrier and may distinguish populations of reflux patients from controls. Consequently, manometry should be reserved for patients in whom another diagnosis is suspected (esophageal motility disorder) or prior to antireflux surgery.

Treatment

Therapy of GERD is similar in both the elderly and the young patient. However, care must be taken when prescribing drugs to elderly patients with GERD, because certain medications are more likely to result in adverse effects in elderly patients. In addition, there is a greater frequency of adverse drug interactions in elderly patients, because they are more likely to take a variety of drugs for multiple medical conditions. Patients with symptomatic GERD should be approached from the point of view that this is usually a chronic disorder. An overall medical and surgical approach may be structured by dividing current therapies into three phases.

Lifestyle Modification Therapy   Lifestyle modifications are a frequently underemphasized aspect of medical therapy. They can be effective in controlling episodes of heartburn and dyspepsia in the elderly patient, as well as in the young patient. In fact, emphasis on these approaches may be particularly appropriate in elderly patients, in whom additional drug therapy may be less desirable. The patient should be instructed to eat three meals per day, with the evening meal taken at least 3 hours before bedtime, in order

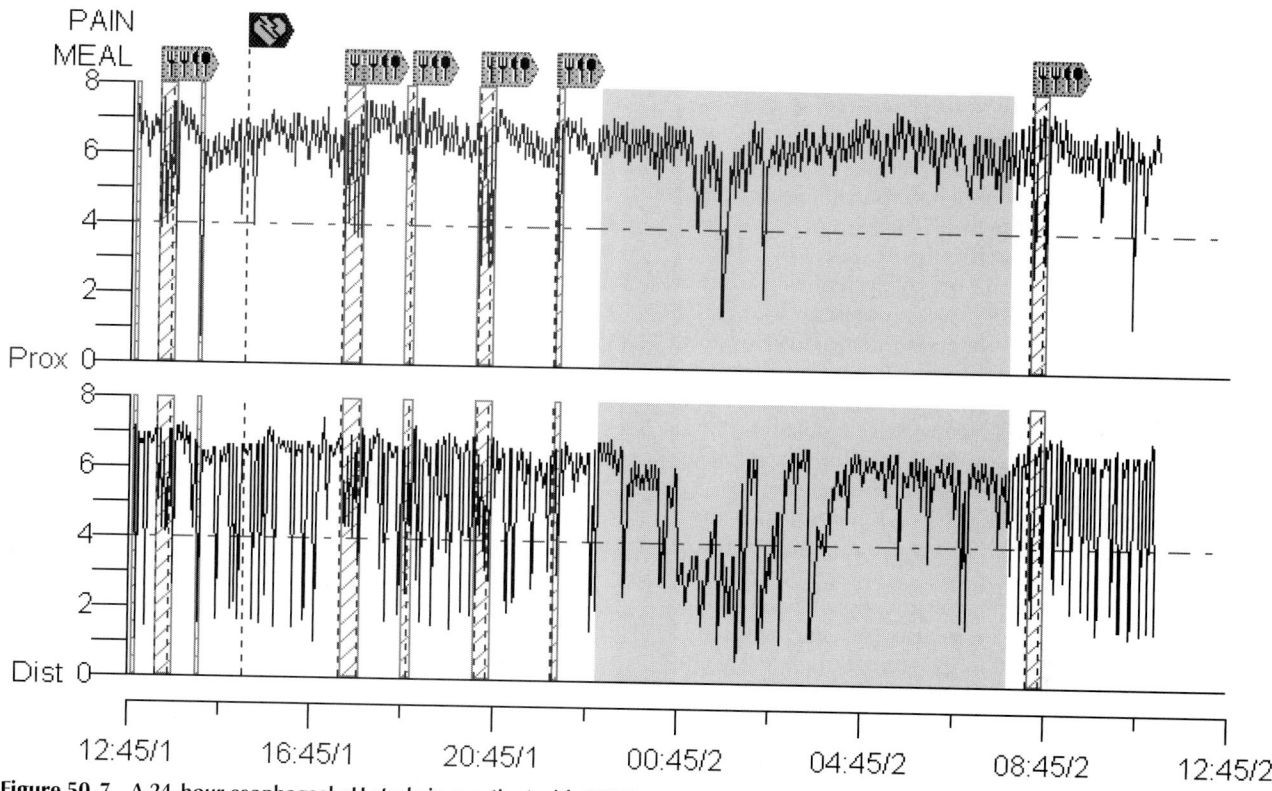

Figure 50-7   A 24-hour esophageal pH study in a patient with GERD.

to avoid recumbency with a full stomach. Patients should be advised to decrease the fat content of their diet. Elevation of the head of the bed on 6-inch blocks significantly decreases nocturnal esophageal acid exposure. Alternatively, placing a foam rubber wedge (10 inches high) on top of the mattress and under the patient's head or preferentially sleeping on the left side may be as effective as elevating the head of the bed and may be more convenient for some elderly patients.

There are at least two potential benefits to diet modification, which are in addition to caloric restriction to reduce being overweight. Certain foods such as fats, chocolates, excessive alcohol, and carminatives decrease LES resting pressure and should be avoided. Agents that may irritate the esophagus such as citrus juices, tomato products, coffee, and probably alcohol should be restricted. Smoking decreases LES pressure and should be discouraged. Drugs that lower LES pressure (Table 50-3), or that interfere with esophageal or gastric emptying, may facilitate reflux. These agents should be avoided in patients with GERD.

The intermittent use of antacids, alginic acid, or over-the-counter H_2-receptor antagonists completes the lifestyle modifications. Antacids are used widely for their acid-neutralizing effect, but they will also increase LES pressure. In clinical practice, antacids appear to be effective in controlling intermittent mild to moderate symptoms of GERD, although they have no role in the treatment of esophagitis. Alginic acid combined with antacids forms a viscous foam that floats on the surface of gastric contents, acting as a mechanical barrier. These preparations may be effective in the relief of reflux symptoms, and some patients prefer them to antacid therapy. Antacids must be used with

caution because of an increased risk of toxicity in the elderly, including salt overload, constipation, diarrhea, hypercalcemia, and interference with the absorption of other drugs.

Pharmacologic Therapy   Most patients with GERD require one or more of the available systemic medications. H_2-receptor antagonists decrease gastric acid production and are the most popular agents available for the treatment of GERD. H_2-receptor antagonists are primarily indicated for mild cases of GERD in combination with lifestyle modifications. Standard doses of H_2-receptor antagonists have no role in severe esophagitis or in patients with Barrett esophagus. In equivalent doses, the H_2-receptor antagonists are equally effective and may be used in patients with symptomatic reflux without mucosal injury. In elderly patients, caution is required in using higher-than-standard doses of H_2-receptor antagonists. Mental status changes have been described in elderly patients, particularly those with renal and liver dysfunction. H_2-receptor antagonists are often the initial agents used in the management of patients with mild to moderate reflux symptoms. Unlike their application in treating ulcer disease, H_2 blockers should be administered in divided doses. Patients with symptoms unresponsive to standard dose H_2 blockers or those with severe esophagitis are preferably treated with proton pump inhibitors.

Prokinetic therapy essentially consists of metoclopramide because cisapride has been restricted. Metoclopramide will increase LES pressure and promote gastric motility, thus decreasing esophageal acid exposure and increasing gastric emptying. Prokinetic drugs are not likely to be effective by themselves if esophagitis is present, and they are usually used in conjunction with a proton pump inhibitor or H_2-receptor antagonist in these patients. Up to 50 percent of patients with uncomplicated GERD may respond to metoclopramide. However, it may cause drowsiness and other neurologic side effects in some patients. It is known to have a potential to cause serious extrapyramidal side effects among elderly patients and therefore should be used with special caution in this age group.

Sucralfate has some appeal for the treatment of GERD in elderly patients because of its lack of systemic absorption and a corresponding lack of systemic toxicity. The major side effect is constipation, which is infrequent. However, sucralfate may also bind to other drugs administered by mouth at the same time and, in the elderly patient, it may be challenging to set up an appropriate schedule for the administration of multiple drugs. Moreover, the efficacy of sucralfate in patients with esophagitis has been disappointing.

Proton pump inhibitors (PPIs) represent the most definitive treatment to achieve near-total control of acid production. Patients usually feel symptomatic improvement shortly after starting these medications. PPIs produce significant increases in the intragastric pH level with rapid healing of esophagitis in 80 to 95 percent of patients. This treatment has to be continued for the long-term. PPIs also positively affect peptic esophageal stricture by decreasing the need for repeated esophageal dilatation. Concern has been expressed that maintenance treatment with PPIs in H. pylori-positive patients with GERD may accelerate progression to atrophic gastritis, a precursor to gastric cancer. However, this is controversial. Although plasma clearance of PPIs decreases with age, no reduction in dose is necessary in elderly patients, even those with impaired renal or hepatic function. It is important to remember to instruct the patients to take PPIs 15 to 30 minutes before meals. Initially, PPIs should be given as a single dose once daily. If this doesn't control symptoms, this can be doubled to twice daily. Because PPIs have gained popularity in recent years and their use has thus markedly increased, a subset of patients has appeared in whom nighttime reflux may continue. Some recent studies suggest that the addition of a dose of H_2-blocker at bedtime will provide better control of gastric acid.

Surgery   The indications for surgical intervention in GERD in the elderly population are similar to those in younger patients, that is, as a reasonable option to medical therapy for long-term care. In the past, failure of medical therapy was the most common reason for antireflux surgery, but with the advent of PPIs this is now less frequent. Surgery can be performed successfully in selected elderly patients who are reasonable operative risks, but should be avoided in patients with concomitant medical problems that make such surgery hazardous. Surgical consideration should also be given for patients with Barrett esophagus and high-grade dysplastic changes, intractable strictures, severe bleeding esophagitis, and severe extraesophageal pulmonary manifestations unresponsive to medical therapy. Laparoscopic Nissen fundoplication is the most commonly performed antireflux surgery. Patients should be carefully investigated with endoscopy, esophageal manometry, and pH monitoring prior to surgery. Surgery initially improves symptoms in more than 90 percent of patients, but the effects of the surgical repair may deteriorate with time.

Barrett Esophagus

Patients with long-standing reflux esophagitis are at increased risk of developing the premalignant condition of Barrett intestinal metaplasia. The initial definition of Barrett esophagus included simply the presence of columnar epithelium above the gastroesophageal junction; however, identification of the risk of adenocarcinoma has clarified that intestinal metaplasia with goblet cells is the "marker" for its malignant potential. The average age of diagnosis ranges between 55 and 65 years. There is a strong male predominance (65 to 80 percent), and the disease is rare in African-Americans. The prevalence of Barrett esophagus in the general population ranges between 0.8 and 3.9 percent; the prevalence is higher in those with symptoms of GERD.

Many patients are entirely asymptomatic, especially those with short segments (<3 cm) of Barrett epithelium. In fact, the metaplastic epithelium is less sensitive to acid exposure than is squamous epithelium. The risk of developing esophageal adenocarcinoma in a patient with Barrett esophagus is 25 times greater than in the general population. The group at highest risk for cancer consists of white men older than age 50 years.

Endoscopic screening for Barrett esophagus should be considered for patients who have chronic symptoms of gastroesophageal reflux disease. Endoscopic examination usually shows salmon-colored mucosa either circumferentially or in tongues or islands extending from the gastroesophageal junction proximally into the esophagus. Histologic examination establishes the diagnosis.

Appropriate treatment for cases with Barrett esophagus is a very controversial issue because there is no evidence that any particular form of antireflux therapy reduces the risk of development of the dysplasia or adenocarcinoma. Some experts recommend acid suppression therapy as needed to maintain symptom relief. This recommendation, however, is confounded by the observations that the metaplastic epithelium is less sensitive to acid exposure and that patients may be asymptomatic despite significant ongoing acid reflux. Other experts recommend aggressive control of esophageal acid exposure, including pH monitoring to document the absence of continuing reflux. This recommendation is based on the accepted belief that Barrett esophagus results from chronic acid reflux over many years. Some surgeons would suggest that all patients with Barrett esophagus should have antireflux surgery as the preferred means to prevent ongoing reflux of acid and other potentially noxious materials such as bile salts and pancreatic enzymes. Finally, questions regarding the appropriate use of endoscopic ablation techniques encompass whether these should be reserved exclusively for high-grade dysplasia or adenocarcinoma or whether these therapies should be extended to low-grade dysplasia or even simply metaplasia.

Reactive hyperplasia secondary to reflux-induced inflammation may interfere with the histologic assessment of dysplasia. Therefore, intensive antireflux therapy for 8 to

12 weeks should be considered prior to endoscopic biopsy to confirm the diagnosis.

The American College of Gastroenterology recommends that endoscopic surveillance be performed every 2 to 3 years in patients without dysplasia, on the basis of an estimated incidence of cancer in patients with Barrett esophagus of 1 to 2 percent per year. Recent studies suggest that the true incidence of cancer is approximately 0.5 percent per year. Therefore, less-frequent surveillance, every 3 to 5 years, may be appropriate in patients without dysplasia. If dysplasia is present, the pathologic slides must be reviewed by an experienced pathologist. For cases with low-grade dysplasia, regular follow-up endoscopy with biopsy is to be done after 6 and 12 months, followed by yearly endoscopy if there is no progression. In case of high-grade dysplasia, it is recommended to perform an esophagectomy in patients healthy enough to withstand this procedure. Intensive endoscopic surveillance may be a valid alternative to immediate esophagectomy for older patients with high-grade dysplasia who can comply with this approach. For patients who are a poor surgical risk or who are unwilling to undergo esophagectomy, endoscopic ablative therapy may be a reasonable alternative. The concept of these modalities is the elimination of the Barrett mucosa by localized superficial destruction of the metaplastic tissue by the application of heat or laser energy, or its removal by endoscopic submucosal resection. This is followed by aggressive acid control to prevent further formation of metaplastic tissue. The concern with such treatment is that it may provide a sanctuary site for the metaplastic tissue to regenerate beneath the healed squamous tissue.

DISORDERS OF THE STOMACH AND DUODENUM IN THE ELDERLY POPULATION

Gastric Function in Old Age

Morbidity and mortality associated with peptic ulcer disease is increased in the elderly population. Although gastric acid and pepsin contribute to mucosal injury, current evidence suggests that aging is not associated with increased secretion of these agents. Gastric acid secretion in humans appears to change little with normal aging, unless there is evidence for coexistent gastric pathology. In fact, recent studies have confirmed that basal acid secretion was not modified in older people, and that, after adjustment for histology, age per se had no independent effect on pentagastrin-stimulated gastric acid secretion. These data were in agreement with histologic studies, which demonstrated that in subjects with normal gastric mucosa, the number of gastric parietal, acid-secreting cells tended to increase with age, while a significant reduction in the acid secreting area of the stomach did occur if an inflammatory or atrophic process was also present. An important pathophysiologic finding in patients with peptic ulcer disease was the absence of a significant change in gastric acid secretion with advancing age. Secretory patterns remained well defined in other gastric ulcer patients, who were generally acid hyposecreters, as well as in duodenal ulcer subjects, who remained hypersecreters. These results correspond with histologic data suggesting that, in comparison with ulcer-free subjects, duodenal ulcer patients had a more developed acid-secreting area in the stomach, even in subjects older than 60 years, while in elderly gastric ulcer patients, the gastric acid-secreting area was reduced, probably as a result of the higher prevalence of intestinal metaplasia and chronic atrophic gastritis.

Recent studies explored the effect of *H. pylori* infection on gastric acid secretion in relation to age. Although the prevalence of *H. pylori* infection is known to increase with the age of subjects studied, gastric acid secretion remained unchanged and was independent of *H. pylori* status, while gastritis with atrophy was the only factor that had an independent negative effect on acid secretion. Conflicting data are present in the literature regarding pepsin secretion in old age. Recent studies seem to indicate that aging is associated with a modest reduction in pepsin output in humans, independent of atrophic gastritis, *H. pylori* infection, or smoking.

Thus, available data do not support the notion that aging per se modifies gastric aggressive factors, such as acid and pepsin secretions. Moreover, pathologic conditions, mainly peptic ulcers or *H. pylori* infection, do not change secretory functions in a different manner in elderly patients than in young patients. Therefore, it is more likely that the increase in susceptibility to gastric mucosal injury observed in the elderly patient, such as that from nonsteroidal anti-inflammatory drug (NSAID) exposure, may result from a reduction in gastric mucosal cytoprotective factors.

Several studies show that gastric mucosal prostaglandin secretion decreases with age. In a study performed in elderly patients with antral erosive gastritis, the gastric mucosal prostaglandin reduction was primarily located in the antrum. Elderly patients with *H. pylori* infection also tended to have higher levels of mucosal prostaglandins than did *H. pylori*-negative subjects. The age associated decrease in prostaglandin secretion correlates with increasing likelihood to develop acetic acid-induced and aspirin-induced gastric mucosal injury.

Gastric bicarbonate and mucus are secreted by nonparietal gastric epithelial cells, providing an alkaline gel layer protective against luminal acid-pepsin and exogenous noxious substances such as NSAIDs. Several studies show that aging is associated with significantly lower gastric bicarbonate secretion. Data on the effect of aging on gastric mucus contents in humans demonstrated no significant differences in acid and neutral glycoprotein concentrations between the healthy young and elderly. A study in healthy subjects demonstrated that the number of gastric mucus cells was reduced in the elderly, with aging having induced a significant increase in the parietal-mucus cell ratio.

Gastric mucosal proliferation and regeneration represents another component of gastric mucosal protection. Animal studies demonstrated that aging was associated with a diminished regenerative capacity of the gastric mucosa secondary to a reduced expression of several growth factors and of enzymes related to growth factor receptors.

An age-related decrease in glutathione content in human gastric mucosa has been reported. Glutathione plays an important role in the cytoprotection of gastric mucosa, particularly in the prevention of acute damage induced by ethanol and drugs. This effect may explain the low gastric mucosal adaptation to NSAIDs in elderly subjects.

Mucosal blood flow plays an essential role in maintaining gastric mucosal integrity and contributes to mucosal repair by supplying oxygen and nutrients and by removing potentially noxious agents. Little data on the effect of aging on gastric blood flow are available in humans. Atherosclerosis of the celiac axis and other major arteries occurs with aging; however, the rich collateral circulation to the stomach appears to protect against occlusion of a major vessel. In diseases noted for microvascular complications, such as diabetes mellitus, microvascular involvement of vessels within the walls of the gastrointestinal tract does not appear to impair luminal protection. Thus available data seem to support the premise that aging is associated with a selective and specific reduction in some gastric mucosal defensive mechanisms.

With aging, there is a physiologic decrease in gastric emptying for liquids, but not for solids. The fact that motility disorders disproportionately affect the elderly is mainly related to the impact of age-associated chronic conditions.

H. pylori Infection in the Elderly Patient

H. pylori is a spiral-shaped, microaerophilic, gram-negative bacterium. The organism's urease, motility, and ability to adhere to gastric epithelium are factors that allow it to survive and proliferate in the stomach. It penetrates the mucous layer and adheres to the gastric epithelial cells and rarely, if ever, invades the cell itself. It secretes a potent urease antigen that ultimately results in increased local ammonia levels. This alkaline milieu protects the organism from gastric acid. The antigen elicits a significant immunoglobulin G and immunoglobulin A response in the host. Those antibodies remain for life in infected patients and for 1 to 2 years after eradication.

H. pylori is the most common chronic bacterial infection in humans. It has been demonstrated worldwide and in individuals of all ages. In fact, every population studied across the world exhibits antibodies against the organism, ranging from 50 to 90 percent in persons older than the age of 60. The prevalence of this infection increases with age worldwide. However, the rates are lower in Western industrialized countries than in developing countries, when infection is acquired at an earlier age. Once acquired, infection persists and may or may not produce gastroduodenal disease. Studies on healthy blood donors in European countries demonstrate that the prevalence of infection is higher in older people, particularly older than 60 years of age. The increased prevalence of infection with age was initially thought to represent a continuing rate of bacterial acquisition throughout one's lifetime. However, epidemiologic evidence now indicates most infections are acquired during childhood even in developed countries. Therefore, the frequency of H. pylori infection for any age group in any locality reflects that particular cohort's rate of bacterial acquisition during childhood years.

The risk of acquiring H. pylori infection is related to socioeconomic status and living conditions early in life. Factors such as density of housing, overcrowding, number of siblings, sharing a bed, and lack of running water have all been linked to a higher acquisition of H. pylori infection. Within a particular country, a decline in prevalence of H. pylori appears to parallel economic improvement. In most industrialized countries, it is projected that a significant decrease in the rate of infection and its associated diseases will occur in the next few decades. In the United States, however, the rate of immigration from both Latin America and Asia may keep the pool of infected persons at its present or slightly increased levels.

The route by which the infection occurs remains unknown. The close correlation among socioeconomic status, overcrowding, and the rate of infection suggests an oral-to-oral or fecal-to-oral mode of transmission. Reinfection with H. pylori following successful bacterial cure is unusual. Recurrence of infection most commonly represents recrudescence of the original bacterial strain.

For many people, advanced age coincides with institutional living and, thus, with an increased risk of infections. In a study, the seroprevalence of H. pylori infection in the asymptomatic elderly persons living in a nursing home for at least 5 years was 86.5 percent. This was not significantly different from the 82 percent serologic prevalence of asymptomatic elderly subjects living at home. No significant correlation was observed between seropositivity and length of stay in the institution, cognitive functions, or self-sufficiency. Moreover, H. pylori infection was not related to modifications of nutritional status or gastric function parameters. Presently, no specific hygienic or behavioral measures are recommended to interfere with H. pylori infection transmission among elderly and professional people in nursing homes.

There are two major categories into which diagnostic tests for H. pylori can be divided: invasive and noninvasive techniques. The techniques may be direct (culture, microscopic demonstration of the organism) or indirect (using urease or an antibody response as a marker of disease). Table 50-4 outlines these different diagnostic methods. The choice of test depends on different factors, but the initial decision depends on the need (or not) for endoscopy. Issues of cost and availability should also be considered. In the elderly population, noninvasive techniques should be used as much as possible to avoid endoscopy if not needed for other indications. Several studies have found that in the elderly population there is a significantly higher prevalence of H. pylori infection as detected by serology when compared to histology. This seems to indicate that a positive antibody titer is not necessarily indicative of the presence of H. pylori in the gastric mucosa. These findings raise the question of validity of the use of serum antibody tests for the detection of H. pylori infection in the elderly patient. Further studies are needed to clarify this issue.

H. pylori infection has become an important subject in the last few years. This is mainly a result of its frequent association with many gastroduodenal pathologies. H. pylori is present in 100 percent of active chronic gastritis, 90 to 95 percent of duodenal ulcers, 60 to 85 percent of gastric

Table 50-4   Diagnostic Tests for *H. pylori* Infection

Test	Sensitivity (%)	Specificity (%)	Cost
Non invasive			
Serum (in office)	88–94	74–88	+
Whole blood (in office)	67–88	75–91	+
ELISA	86–95	78–95	++
Urea breath test	90–100	98–100	+ (14C)
			+++ (13C)
Stool antigen assay	86–94	86–95	++
Invasive			
Urease test	88–95	95–100	++
Histology	95–99	95–99	+++
Culture	80–98	100	+++

ELISA, enzyme-linked immunosorbent assay.

ulcers, and 85 to 95 percent of gastric cancers. The significance of these associations is discussed in more detail later in this chapter.

Over the years, multiple regimens for the eradication of *H. pylori* have evolved. The use of monotherapy or dual regimens is not recommended. The original bismuth triple regimens (bismuth, metronidazole, and either tetracycline or amoxicillin) have eradication rates of 75 to 90 percent. The optimal therapeutic regimen has not yet been defined. Table 50-5 illustrates some of the recommended regimens and their relative effectiveness and cost. The response in a particular patient depends on compliance of the individual, whether the patient is allergic to one or more of the medications, whether antibiotic resistance is present, and whether the cost of therapy is acceptable. Recent combinations have relied on PPIs rather than H_2 blockers for effective eradication of the organism. Their action appears to be related to the maintenance of a neutral pH, enhancing the effectiveness of simultaneous antibiotics as well as

a possible direct bacteriostatic effect on *H. pylori*. At this time, the regimen of choice is triple therapy with a PPI (e.g., lansoprazole 30 mg bid, or rabeprazole 20 mg bid), amoxicillin (1 g bid), and clarithromycin (500 mg bid) for 2 weeks. Metronidazole can be substituted for amoxicillin but only in penicillin-allergic individuals, because metronidazole resistance is common and can reduce the efficacy of treatment. Dual-therapy regimens that use a PPI plus one antibiotic are frequently cited in the literature. However, they cannot be recommended as primary therapy because their eradication rates are significantly lower than the standard regimens. In contrast, there are encouraging data supporting the use of 1-week treatment protocols. If these results are confirmed, recommendations regarding optimal therapy may change. For patients failing one course of *H. pylori* treatment, the choice is either to prescribe an alternate regimen using a different combination of medications, or quadruple therapy consisting of a PPI twice daily and bismuth-based triple therapy for 14 days.

Table 50-5   Examples of Combination Regimens for Eradication of *H. pylori*

Regimen	Eradication Rates (%)	Cost
Triple therapy		
PPI + metronidazole + clarithromycin	80–90	+++
PPI + amoxicillin + clarithromycin	80–90	+++
PPI + metronidazole + amoxicillin	75–90	+++
PPI + bismuth + clarithromycin	85	++
Bismuth + metronidazole + amoxicillin	75–90	+
Bismuth + metronidazole + tetracycline	85–95	+
H_2 blocker + metronidazole + amoxicillin	90	+++
Quadruple therapy		
Bismuth + metronidazole + tetracycline + PPI	94–98	+++
Bismuth + metronidazole + tetracycline + H_2 blocker	84–95	+++

PPI, proton pump inhibitor.

It has been shown that after completion of a dual therapy (amoxicillin plus omeprazole or lansoprazole or ranitidine), patients in whom *H. pylori* was successfully eradicated were significantly older than patients still *H. pylori*-positive, suggesting that the age of patients must be regarded as a major determinant of *H. pylori* therapy eradication rates. Triple-PPI–based therapies are well tolerated. Reports of severe side effects of anti-*H. pylori* therapy in elderly patients related only to the use of tetracycline or to high doses of clarithromycin. Particularly relevant to geriatric medicine is the finding that concomitant diseases and concomitant treatments did not influence the efficacy of anti-*H. pylori* therapy. A 1-year follow-up study performed in elderly patients with peptic ulcer demonstrated that the eradication of *H. pylori* infection significantly improved clinical outcome, reducing ulcer recurrence, symptomatology, and the histologic signs of chronic gastritis activity. The study concluded that the cure of *H. pylori* infection is strongly recommended in elderly subjects with *H. pylori*-associated peptic ulcer disease.

Peptic Ulcer Disease in the Elderly

Peptic ulcer disease (PUD) occurs in approximately 10 percent of US adults. There are an estimated 500,000 new cases and 4 million recurrences each year. This results in about 8 to 10 billion dollars in annual cost. Although the incidence of both gastric and duodenal disease is declining in young and middle-aged patients in developed countries, hospitalization, complications, and mortality related to peptic ulcers have increased significantly in patients older than the age of 65 years. In fact, more than 80 percent of the deaths from PUD in the United States occur in older patients. There has also been a rise in the incidence of PUD in the elderly. This is presumably related to progressive deterioration of protective gastric and duodenal mechanisms, whereas aggressive factors (e.g., NSAIDs, tobacco, alcohol, local ischemia) are taking an increasing toll on the gastric and duodenal mucosa.

Pathophysiology

The pathogenesis of PUD appears to be the result of an imbalance between aggressive and defensive factors. Aggressive factors include acid-induced and pepsin-induced mucosal injury. The two main components of the protective mechanism are the mucous barrier adherent to the gastric epithelium and the integrity of the microvascular supply of the gastric mucosa. Patients with duodenal ulcer disease can have increased or normal gastric acid secretion, decreased duodenal bicarbonate secretion, infection with *H. pylori,* or combinations of the above. The majority of gastric ulcers are associated with NSAIDs or *H. pylori* infection.

Recent studies show that the rates of basal gastric acid secretion, meal-stimulated acid secretion, and gastrin-stimulated acid secretion are unchanged with advancing age. Studies of healthy elderly individuals demonstrate no age-related decrease in acid production, but that reduced acid secretion in the elderly population is a product of their increased incidence of atrophic gastritis. The evidence is also now clear that it is not acid per se that is responsible for the injury, but rather the ability of H^+ ions to penetrate the defense barrier of the gastric and duodenal mucosa and the concomitant activation of pepsin that is ultimately responsible for the digestion of submucosal proteins that results in necrosis and ultimately ulceration.

Endogenous gastroduodenal mucosal prostaglandins are considered to be protective against the development of PUD. Recent studies suggest that prostaglandin levels may decrease with age. There is no effect on gastroduodenal prostaglandins of alcohol, gender, or *H. pylori*. However, cigarette smoking can affect these prostaglandins. Elderly patients who smoke can have up to 70 to 80 percent reduction in prostaglandin production. The integrity of the mucous barrier is dependent on prostaglandins, which enhance the thickness of the layer as well as the secretion of bicarbonate within the layer, raising the pH at the epithelial surface. Furthermore, prostaglandins exert control over the microvascular circulation in the gastric mucosa and submucosa.

H. pylori has been identified as the primary cause of most cases of histologic gastritis and is considered to be an important factor in the development of ulcers. Although almost all patients infected with *H. pylori* develop gastritis, only 15 percent develop PUD. Approximately 9 to 100 percent of patients with duodenal ulcers and 70 to 90 percent of patients with gastric ulcers are infected with *H. pylori*. The lower association with *H. pylori* in the stomach may be related to the degree of gastric atrophy that renders the environment inhospitable for *H. pylori*. Despite the incomplete understanding of the transmission and pathogenesis of *H. pylori* infection, multiple studies demonstrate that eradication of this bacteria is associated with a decrease in ulcer recurrence and may lead to a more rapid and a higher rate of ulcer healing.

Genetic factors may also play a role in ulcer pathogenesis. The concordance for PUD among identical twins is approximately 50 percent. Studies suggest that lifetime probability of developing an ulcer in first-degree relatives of all ulcer patients is approximately threefold greater than that in the general population.

Chronic NSAID use reportedly causes gastroduodenal ulceration. The elderly appear to be at a particular risk for the development of PUD and PUD complications if using NSAIDs. These drugs can produce direct superficial mucosal damage and can reduce mucosal prostaglandin production by inhibiting cyclooxygenase, inhibiting mucosal bicarbonate and mucus secretion, and decreasing mucosal blood flow. It appears that the risk of NSAID complications is greatest during the initial 3 months of therapy. Factors that appear to influence NSAID-induced ulcerations in the elderly include prior history of ulcer disease and medication dose.

Clinical Manifestations

Abdominal pain is the most frequent symptom of PUD, classically a burning sensation localized in the epigastric area occurring 2 to 3 hours after a meal or at night and relieved by food or antacids. This epigastric pain usually recurs episodically for a period of days to weeks. Nocturnal pain may occur in patients with gastric or duodenal ulcers when continuous acid production remains unbuffered through sleeping hours. Although abdominal pain is common, it does not occur in all patients. Nocturnal pain affects only two-thirds of patients with duodenal ulcer and one-third of patients with gastric ulcer. Right posterior subscapular pain suggests penetration of posterior wall duodenal ulcers into the surrounding tissue, mimicking biliary tract or pancreatic pain. Nausea and vomiting suggest pyloric ulcers. Chronic occult blood loss occurs commonly with NSAID-induced ulcers. The resulting iron deficiency anemia may cause symptoms such as fatigue, syncope, shortness of breath, palpitation, or angina pectoris.

PUD presentation in the elderly patient is frequently atypical. Silent ulcerations are common in elderly patients and may present as a catastrophic massive hemorrhage or perforation. It is estimated that pain may not occur in approximately 35 percent of older patients. Approximately half of the patients with PUD who are using NSAIDs do not have ulcer-related discomfort. The lack of pain is attributed to diminished perception as well as the analgesic effect of NSAIDs when taken in therapeutic doses. If pain is present, it can be vague and poorly localized. The presentation of ulcer may be dominated by systemic symptoms related to severe blood loss and anemia in such older patients.

Gastric ulcers in elderly patients are often located more proximally in the stomach as compared to the distribution in younger patients. High gastric ulcers tend to be large and to heal slowly. There is also a higher frequency of complications and death in the patients. Sometimes it is difficult to distinguish between benign and malignant ulcerations. Therefore, gastric ulcers must undergo biopsy to eliminate the possibility of malignancy.

Duodenal ulcers are more common than gastric ulcers in older as well as younger patients. Their presentation in the elderly patient is usually atypical, with a greater incidence of complications. Duodenal ulcers may be large, with ulcers bigger than 2 cm being reported with increased frequency in the elderly. In elderly patients, bleeding from duodenal ulcers is more frequent than in the general population.

Diagnosis

In the elderly patient, dyspeptic symptoms of recent onset should be thoroughly investigated. Empiric use of anti-ulcer medication without diagnostic investigation may be appropriate in young patients with mild or intermittent epigastric symptoms and who are without systemic signs or evidence of complications. However, this approach should not be applied in patients older than 50 years of age, in whom diagnostic studies should be performed. The presence of symptoms suggestive of gastric outlet obstruction or laboratory results consistent with iron-deficiency anemia should result in further work-up in older patients, even if they have an established history of PUD.

Radiologic or endoscopic procedures can diagnose ulcers. The diagnostic procedure chosen is dependent upon the skill and experience of the personnel available. Upper gastrointestinal (GI) barium studies are still commonly ordered. Some findings may have to be further elucidated by endoscopy. Endoscopy as a first study may be preferable when available, because it has a better ability to detect superficial mucosal lesions and allow performance of biopsies and therapeutic interventions if necessary.

Complications

Over the past 20 years, hospitalization for PUD has steadily declined. Nevertheless, the percent of ulcer patients hospitalized who were older than age 65 years has progressively increased, nearing 60 percent of the total. The major complications of PUD are hemorrhage, perforation, penetration, and obstruction. Complications occur in approximately 50 percent of all patients older than 70 years of age. The mortality rate can reach about 30 percent. The high mortality rate may be related to the presence of comorbidity. The increased use of NSAIDs in this population is thought to be responsible for initial presentation with massive hemorrhage or perforation, because 40 to 60 percent are NSAID-induced ulcers.

At present, ulcers refractory to medical therapy are rare, provided dosage and length of therapy are appropriate. A nonhealing gastric ulcer should raise the suspicion of malignancy, even if the original biopsies are benign, because more than 5 percent of gastric ulcers are malignant at the time of presentation. It may be wise to advise surgery for any nonhealing ulcer after 6 weeks of PPI therapy.

Hemorrhage Hemorrhage is the most common complication of PUD. It occurs in approximately 10 to 15 percent of patients. Ulcer hemorrhage is more common in older patients, who have more severe bleeding, require more transfusions, and bleed more often. Ulcers in the elderly are larger and deeper, and bleeding vessels are sclerotic and less likely to form a spontaneous clot.

Ten to 20 percent of patients who bleed from a gastric or duodenal ulcer do not have a previous history of symptoms. Elderly patients who bleed from ulcer disease are more likely to have recurrent bleeding or to need surgery. Elderly patients who bleed are 4 to 10 times more likely to die from such bleeding than are younger patients. The key prognostic indicators in subjects with recurrent bleeding are hypotension and endoscopic stigmata of the recent bleeding; that is, visible vessel or sentinel clot. In the presence of these signs, the risk of rebleeding can increase to approximately 80 percent. Risk factors for death from ulcer bleeding in the elderly include serious comorbidity, the use of NSAIDs, and the need for more than 5 units of blood transfusion. The mortality rate of elderly patients with bleeding ulcers is estimated to be between 30 and 60 percent.

Perforation Perforations are the second most common emergency complication of PUD. They occur in 5 to 10 percent of patients. It is important to know that in the elderly population there can be a delay in seeking medical care because of a lack of symptoms, absence of physical findings, and lack of a history of PUD. Perforation occurs with acute ulcers. Although most elderly patients with perforated ulcers complain of abdominal pain, symptoms are more subdued, and free air under the diaphragm may be absent in 25 percent of cases. If strongly suspected, a CT scan of the abdomen can be helpful.

Perforation occurs approximately five times more frequently in duodenal than in gastric ulcers. Duodenal ulcers tend to perforate anteriorly, whereas gastric ulcers tend to perforate along the anterior wall of the lesser curvature of the stomach. Gastric perforations are more dangerous. In patients older than 75 years, the mortality rate is approximately 50 percent. Delay in early diagnosis is considered to be the major cause of this high mortality. In obtunded patients, the lack of signs of peritonitis may also contribute to delay in diagnosis and surgery. The majority of perforations require prompt surgical intervention, often simple closure. Deeply penetrating ulcers may actually represent contained perforations and should be treated surgically.

Penetration is similar to perforation except that the ulcer crater burrows into an adjacent organ. Duodenal ulcers can penetrate into the pancreas and cause pancreatitis. Gastric ulcers most commonly penetrate into the left lobe of the liver. Gastric ulcers have also been reported to cause colonic penetration, thus creating a gastrocolonic fistula.

Gastric Outlet Obstruction Gastric outlet obstruction has decreased dramatically since the advent and widespread use of H_2 blockers, followed by PPIs, in the past 20 years. This complication occurs in 2 to 5 percent of PUD patients and can be caused by acute inflammation and edema or scarring near the gastroduodenal junction. If the obstruction is a result of inflammation and edema, it usually resolves with medical therapy. If scarring has resulted in outlet obstruction, endoscopic dilatation or surgery may be required. Surgery is usually elective. Thus, it does not carry a higher mortality rate unless the patient is at high surgical risk. Gastric outlet obstruction typically has a lower mortality rate than other ulcer complications. In patients with altered mental status, regurgitation of gastric contents may lead to aspiration.

Treatment

Lifestyle Changes Suggesting lifestyle changes should always be included in the management of PUD. Patients should be advised to stop, or at least to limit, NSAID use, alcohol, caffeine, and tobacco. Alcohol and NSAIDs have the potential to cause direct mucosal damage or worsen existing ulcers. Delay in ulcer healing has been reported with the use of tobacco and caffeine. Certain foods trigger dyspepsia, but there is no evidence that specific foods impair ulcer healing or lead to recurrence of the disease. Bedtime snacks stimulate nocturnal acid secretion. Milk was once a mainstay of therapy for ulcers because of its soothing nature until it was shown to be a strong stimulator of acid secretion, largely because of its calcium and protein content. Milk stimulates more acid secretion than it buffers and is not an effective antacid. However, milk and a bland diet produce subjective benefit in some patients with dyspepsia. Thus, despite a lack of scientific evidence, their use should not be discouraged in patients who find these measures beneficial. However, patients should be cautioned that milk is not specific therapy for their ulcer.

Medical Management Treatment of PUD begins with the eradication of *H. pylori* in infected patients. Antisecretory therapy is the mainstay of therapy in uninfected patients and is appropriate for maintenance therapy in selected cases. Whether NSAIDs should be discontinued or not is discussed in Section V: NSAID. A variety of medications have been proven to be effective in the treatment of gastric and duodenal ulcers. The goals of acute ulcer therapy are to relieve pain, accelerate healing, and prevent complications and recurrences.

Antacids Antacids were the mainstay of ulcer therapy until the development of H_2 blockers. They neutralize gastric acid, resulting in an increase in the gastroduodenal pH. Multiple different formulations exist. Ulcer healing requires frequent dosing, and precautions should be taken in patients who are taking other medications. Potential interference with other drugs can occur through increasing gastric pH, which can alter the drug metabolism by adsorbing or binding drugs, or through increasing urinary pH, affecting the rate of drug elimination. It is particularly important to remember these potential effects in elderly patients, who are often on multiple drug regimens.

It is also important to remember that the sodium content of antacids can be significant. Certain antacids are rich in magnesium, which has a cathartic effect and can cause diarrhea. In addition, magnesium-containing products should be used with caution in known renal dysfunction patients because of the potential hypermagnesemia and its related toxicity. Aluminum-containing antacids can cause constipation and can be associated with osteomalacia, hypophosphatemia, and related toxicity. At the present time, antacids are seldom used as the main therapeutic modality for PUD.

Sucralfate Although it has limited acid-neutralizing capacity, sucralfate helps ulcer healing by forming a protective layer at the ulcer site, developing a barrier to hydrogen ion diffusion, inhibiting the action of pepsin, and adsorbing bile salts. It is minimally absorbed and is excreted primarily in stools. Duodenal and gastric ulcer healing after 4 to 6 weeks of therapy with sucralfate at 1 g qid, is superior to placebo and comparable to cimetidine. Sucralfate can be used for short-term therapy of active ulcers and for maintenance therapy. Sucralfate has minor side effects that rarely necessitate drug discontinuation. Constipation is the most frequent side effect, occurring in approximately 2 percent of patients. In patients with chronic renal failure, this drug should be used with caution because of the potential for aluminum absorption and its associated toxicity. Because of the possibility of its binding to other drugs, sucralfate should be administered at a separate time from other medications, often presenting a practical limitation to its use in elderly patients.

Misoprostol Misoprostol is a synthetic prostaglandin E_1 analog. It has mucosal protective and antisecretory properties. It is used for prevention against NSAID-induced inhibition of prostaglandin synthesis, which can potentially lead to gastric ulcerations. This drug can be prescribed for individuals at high risk of developing NSAID-induced gastric ulcers for the duration of their NSAID therapy. Misoprostol also enhances duodenal ulcer healing at doses of

400 to 800 mg/d. However, it has no advantage over antisecretory agents for ulcer healing and it is not indicated for this purpose. Routine dose adjustments of misoprostol are not recommended for the elderly patient. It is generally well tolerated. Dose-related diarrhea and abdominal pain are the most frequent side effects.

H₂-Receptor Blockers   H₂ blockers are reversible blockers of histamine-induced acid secretion by gastric parietal cells. There are four H₂ blockers available: cimetidine, ranitidine, famotidine, and nizatidine. These drugs are effective inhibitors of gastric acid secretion and are effective in controlling symptoms and preventing complications of PUD. All four H₂ blockers induce healing rates of 70 to 80 percent for duodenal ulcers after 4 weeks of therapy, and 87 to 94 percent after 8 weeks of therapy. They are also effective in gastric ulcer healing. Thus, these agents can be used for short-term treatment and maintenance therapy for duodenal and gastric ulcers.

H₂ blockers have a good tolerance profile and the incidence of side effects is less than 3 percent. Advanced age, hepatic or renal failure, and concomitant diseases increase the risk of developing side effects. All H₂ blockers have similar side effects. However, cimetidine seems to have that highest incidence of antiandrogen and central nervous system (CNS) side effects. Antiandrogen effects are mainly gynecomastia and impotence. CNS effects include confusion, depression, agitation, and anxiety. CNS effects are reversible and typically will occur within 2 to 3 days of starting therapy. They are more frequent in patients who are older than 50 years of age and in patients with renal or hepatic insufficiency. H₂ blockers can affect absorption of drugs that require a gastric acid environment. It is important to remember that cimetidine inhibits the cytochrome P450 oxidase system and thus can impact the metabolism of drugs depending on this system.

Proton Pump Inhibitors   PPIs act by suppressing gastric acid secretion by specific inhibition of the H⁺-K⁺ ATPase (adenosine triphosphatase) enzyme system of the gastric parietal cells (the "proton pump"). Their effect is dose dependent and inhibits both basal and stimulated acid secretion. Elimination rates of omeprazole and lansoprazole are decreased in elderly persons and thus their bioavailability is increased. Nevertheless, dosage changes do not appear to be necessary. Daily doses of omeprazole from 20 to 40 mg induced duodenal ulcer healing in from 63 to 93 percent at 2 weeks and from 82 to 100 percent at 4 weeks. Most studies found that 20 mg daily of omeprazole produced more rapid ulcer healing than did standard doses of H₂ blockers, but this advantage became small after 4 weeks of therapy.

PPIs are generally well tolerated, and ulcer-healing rates and rates of side effects in the elderly are not significantly different than in younger patients. The frequency of side effects with PPIs is similar to that of H₂ blockers. Clinically significant drug interactions with PPIs are theoretically possible but have not been reported. Long-term omeprazole use (>5 years) has been proven to be safe.

Endoscopy and Surgery   In the elderly population, the potential for complications from PUD reinforces consideration of early endoscopy for identification of the disease and possible therapeutic intervention. In patients with bleeding ulcers, endoscopy is useful for identification of endoscopic indicators that help to predict recurrent bleeding and may be a helpful guide for close monitoring and endoscopic intervention.

Effective acid-secretion inhibition with H₂ blockers and PPIs has made surgical intervention for PUD much less frequent. At the present time, surgery is mainly reserved for ulcers refractory to medical management or for PUD complications.

Gastritis and Duodenitis

The words *gastritis* and *duodenitis* are general terms that are used to imply inflammation of the stomach and duodenal mucosa. However, these terms include entities that are quite different from each other pathophysiologically, clinically, and therapeutically. These terms are also often used clinically to describe endoscopic or radiologic characteristics of the gastric or duodenal mucosa, rather than specific histologic findings. In general, the term *gastritis* is used to denote inflammation associated with mucosal injury. However, epithelial cell injury and regeneration are not always accompanied by mucosal inflammation. Epithelial cell damage and regeneration without associated inflammation is referred to as gastropathy. In this section, we discuss some of the most frequent or important types of gastritis and duodenitis.

Acute Erosive Gastritis and Duodenitis

Acute erosive gastritis and duodenitis is an endoscopic diagnosis based on the gross description of intense erythema, submucosal hemorrhage, friability, and multiple erosions of different sizes. The hallmark of this entity is the development of hemorrhagic and erosive lesions shortly after exposure of the gastric mucosa to various injurious substances or a substantial reduction in mucosal blood flow. The lesions can be diffuse or localized to the antrum. These lesions are caused by damage to the surface epithelium, which may be the result of a direct action of injurious agents such as NSAIDs, alcohol use, infection by *H. pylori*, or bile acids. Mucosal hypoxia, such as in trauma, burns (Curling ulcers), prolonged hypotension, or sepsis can also cause acute erosive gastritis and duodenitis. A combination of factors such as with chemotherapy can also cause these lesions.

The approach to treatment and prevention of acute erosive gastritis and duodenitis depends on the cause. The offending agent should be discontinued whenever possible. Antisecretory therapy with H₂ blockers or PPIs is also often used to limit concomitant damage from acid exposure. In case of stress-related erosive gastritis, this can often be controlled with maximal H₂ blockers or PPI therapy. In some cases, endoscopic coagulation of the bleeding erosions or ulcers may be necessary. In high-risk patients, a variety of measures may be effective for prevention, such as antisecretory therapy to prevent stress ulcerations in the intensive care unit.

Chronic Erosive Gastritis

This is an endoscopic entity described in a few patients with dyspeptic symptoms, anorexia, and weight loss. Radiography and endoscopy show enlarged rugae with aphthoid erosions. Biopsy reveals intense infiltration with lymphocytes, suggesting a hypersensitivity reaction to a gastric antigen. It seems possible that *H. pylori* could be the causative antigen in this disease.

Chronic Eosinophilic Erosive Gastritis

Chronic eosinophilic erosive gastritis may be limited to the stomach or as part of multifocal inflammation affecting the small bowel and colon. It is often associated with circulating blood eosinophilia. It has a predilection for the antrum and prepyloric area. Most patients described with this condition have had atopic features, including asthma. Contrast radiology and endoscopic appearances are nonspecific and may include a thickening of antral folds, nodular defects, or frank ulceration. Diagnosis is by endoscopic biopsy, which shows mucosal edema marked by a dense eosinophilic infiltration. With such findings, it is important to exclude intestinal parasitic infection by stool examination for ova and cysts. Corticosteroids appear to be a mainstay of therapy, with good symptomatic response being reported in most, although not all, cases. Elimination diets for potential allergens have also been reported to be successful, as has use of oral sodium cromoglycate.

Chronic Nonerosive Gastritis

Chronic nonerosive gastritis is a histologic diagnosis. There is little correlation between endoscopic findings and the intensity of the inflammatory reaction. A minimum of four biopsies should be obtained to confirm the diagnosis. There is a great deal of controversy about the classification of chronic nonerosive gastritis. The old A and B classification has been replaced by the Sydney system. This system classifies chronic nonerosive gastritis in four major groups:

1. atrophic body gastritis (old type A);
2. antral gastritis (old type B/*H. pylori*);
3. pangastritis (extension of B into A and vice versa); and
4. multifocal atrophic gastritis that begins at the incisura and spreads toward both the cardia and the antrum in a patchy fashion.

Atrophic body gastritis involves the fundus and body of the stomach and can extend into the proximal antrum. The inflammation proceeds from superficial to deep layers. The glands containing parietal and chief cells are originally preserved but eventually destroyed and replaced in patches by pyloric-like mucosa (pyloric metaplasia) or intestine-like mucosa (intestinal metaplasia). Intestinal metaplasia, particularly if the biopsy suggests colonic epithelium, appears to be a precancerous lesion. With progressive atrophy the following changes in gastric function will occur: (1) hypochlorhydria proceeding to complete achlorhydria; (2) a rise in basal serum gastrin; (3) parietal cell antibodies; (4) intrinsic factor antibodies; (5) gradual decrease in blood pepsinogen levels; (6) the development of anemia progressing to the classical syndrome of pernicious anemia; and (7) malignancy of the diffuse type in a small percentage of patients with pernicious anemia (1 to 3 percent). Atrophic body gastritis is thought to be autoimmune in nature because of the multiplicity of antibodies and its association with other autoimmune diseases such as Hashimoto thyroiditis and diabetes mellitus. However, more than 25 percent of patients with this type of gastritis are *H. pylori* positive. Eradication of the bacteria results in definite improvement of the inflammation but no changes in the degree of atrophy, metaplasia, or level of antibodies. Fifty percent of patients with this type of gastritis will develop anemia (mixed B_{12} and iron deficiency) and some will proceed to classical pernicious anemia. Although iron therapy and B_{12} injection alleviate the symptoms of anemia, they have no effect on the gastritis itself and its potential neoplastic transformation.

Antral gastritis is the most common form in the elderly population. It is synonymous with *H. pylori* gastritis and evolves from an intense superficial inflammation to chronic active panmucosal gastritis and eventually to mucosal atrophy with patches of intestinal metaplasia. The inflammation may extend to the body and even fundus but is usually milder in intensity than in atrophic body gastritis. With progressive atrophy, the mucous layer is destroyed and may even completely disappear, resulting in decolonization by *H. pylori*. This may explain the occasional patient with *H. pylori*-negative biopsies and a positive *H. pylori* antibody. Once significant atrophy and intestinal metaplasia are apparent, eradication of the organism does not prevent the neoplastic transformation to adenocarcinoma in some patients.

Multifocal atrophic gastritis is more frequently found in countries with high incidence of gastric carcinoma. The patches of atrophy spread from the incisura both cephalad and distally. Atrophy proceeds to small intestinal and colonic metaplasia and eventually malignancy. It is characterized by hypochlorhydria and a relative hypergastrinemia. No antibodies against parietal cells or intrinsic factor are detected.

Lymphocytic Gastritis

This is a distinctive histologic type of chronic gastritis, characterized by a large number of intraepithelial T lymphocytes. It is seen in 2 to 4 percent of patients with chronic gastritis and affects predominantly the corpus mucosa. Endoscopically, it is often seen as a raised erosive pattern of gastritis. Diagnosis is based on the characteristic histologic appearance. Some patients with this condition are seropositive for *H. pylori*, although organisms are rarely seen on histologic specimens. Lymphocytic gastritis has been treated with steroids and with sodium cromoglycate, although response is variable.

Granulomatous Gastritis

Gastritis characterized by the specific feature of mucosal granulomas is an unusual finding in gastric biopsies. Granulomas are seen in the gastric mucosa in a range of conditions. Most granulomas in the gastric mucosa are a feature of Crohn disease, sarcoidosis, or so-called isolated granulomatous gastritis. There are other rare causes of this type of gastritis, such as those related to the presence of foreign material (e.g., barium, suture material), granulomatous response to adjacent malignancy, or as part of systemic allergic granulomatosis and vasculitis and specific infections such as tuberculosis, syphilis, and histoplasmosis.

Crohn disease involves the stomach usually in combination with disease elsewhere in the gastrointestinal tract. Typically, patients have dyspepsia and symptoms of gastric outlet obstruction. Biopsy shows a patchy active inflammation, with granulomas evident in approximately two-thirds of cases. In most cases, there is concurrent duodenal involvement.

In patients with sarcoidosis, the stomach is usually incidentally involved and does not cause clinical symptoms. The finding of sarcoid-type granulomas in the gastric mucosa should prompt the search for evidence of generalized sarcoidosis.

Ménétrier Disease

This is a rare cause of giant gastric folds that is usually grouped with the gastritides, although there may be little actual mucosal inflammation. Grossly, the rugae are extremely hypertrophied (up to 1 cm) radiologically and endoscopically. This hyperrugosity, described at endoscopy as having the appearance of the cerebral cortex, is confined to the gastric corpus mucosa. Often there is a visible excess of surface mucus. A full-thickness biopsy using a snare is essential to establish the diagnosis. Extreme hyperplasia of the foveolar (mucous gland) layer with concomitant glandular atrophy is the hallmark of this disease. Hypertrophy of the muscularis mucosa and expansion of the submucosa also contributes to the gross rugal thickening. Supervening gastric carcinoma is estimated to occur in approximately 10 percent of cases of Ménétrier disease. Acid secretion is diminished or normal. Gastrin levels are mildly elevated in some cases. Hypoproteinemia is the consequence of the protein-losing gastropathy and the usually slow acid secretion because of reduction in parietal cell mass. The clinical features of Ménétrier disease, when it is symptomatic, usually include epigastric discomfort, hypoproteinemic edema, weight loss, and diarrhea. This disorder usually affects adults, most frequently men in the fifth or sixth decade of life.

Large gastric folds are also common in the Zollinger-Ellison syndrome. This is a hyperplastic gastropathy involving the body and fundus of the stomach. The hyperplastic cell type is the parietal cell, resulting in the hypersecretion of acid in response to the markedly elevated gastrin levels secreted by the pancreatic adenoma. Thus, acid output readily differentiates between these two conditions. Other diseases to consider in the differential diagnosis are lymphoma, malignant carcinoid, sarcoidosis, and lymphocytic and eosinophilic gastritis.

Treatment with antacids, anticholinergics, H_2 blockers, PPIs, and prostaglandins have been generally disappointing. Surgery has been advocated for patients with intractable pain, hypoalbuminemia with edema, hemorrhage, and pyloric obstruction, and for those in whom malignancy cannot be excluded. Surgery can be partial or total gastrectomy. Pain is often relieved and hypoalbuminemia corrected following gastric resection.

Nonsteroidal Antiinflammatory Drugs

More than 30 million people worldwide use NSAIDs daily, and nearly 50 percent of these users are elderly. This increase in NSAID use with age increases the risk of gastrointestinal injuries caused by these drugs, many at the level of the gastroduodenum. These injuries represent various gastroduodenal mucosal lesions, sometimes collectively referred to as NSAID gastropathy. There are two general segments of the geriatric population who use NSAIDs. The first uses aspirin primarily for prophylaxis against cardiovascular or cerebrovascular events and for prevention of colorectal neoplasms. The second uses NSAIDs, generally in higher doses, as therapy for arthritic and other musculoskeletal conditions that disproportionately affect the elderly population. The risk–benefit analysis in the first group is overwhelmingly in favor of the benefits as compared to the risks. In the second, however, the risks are not as acceptable because the benefits can be achieved by other therapeutic regimens without such risks.

Overall, the use of NSAIDs increases the risk of peptic ulcer disease, ulcer complications such as hemorrhage or perforation, and death from ulcer by a factor of between two and four. Although increased NSAID use among the elderly population is an obvious risk factor, epidemiologic data suggest that aging is an independent risk factor for the development of NSAID gastropathy and its complications.

In general, gastric mucosal injury is thought to result when aggressive luminal factors overwhelm local mucosal protective factors. Studies suggest that the production of mucosal lesions by NSAIDs is a result of two independent mechanisms. The first mechanism is a result of topical effects. NSAIDs are all weak organic acids except for nabumetone. As a result, most of the NSAIDs that are not enteric coated are uncharged in the acid milieu of the stomach lumen. They are therefore able to rapidly penetrate the hydrophobic mucous barrier and enter the superficial lining cells. Upon penetrating the epithelial cell, NSAIDs can produce different effects, including changes in the transmembrane permeability, electrical activity, metabolism, and ion transport. These can result in destruction of the epithelial cell within minutes. However, the main action of NSAIDs is systemic, inhibiting cyclooxygenase production and, ultimately, the synthesis of prostaglandin E_2 in the gastric mucosa. Prostaglandin E_2 affects bicarbonate and mucus secretion, proliferation and repair, and microvascular blood flow. Thus, the depletion of gastric mucosal prostaglandins interferes with all elements of the defense barrier, enabling both acid and pepsin to penetrate to the submucosa, which, in conjunction with local vascular ischemia, perpetuate the injury. This cascade of events may culminate in superficial erosions but also can lead to ulcer crater formation.

A variety of symptoms are commonly associated with NSAID-induced gastrointestinal toxicity. Some studies

Table 50-6   Risk Factors for Gastroduodenal Toxicity in NSAID Users

- Increasing age, particularly if older than 60 years
- Past history of peptic ulcer disease
- Past history of gastroduodenal toxicity from NSAIDs
- Higher doses of NSAIDs and their type
- Concurrent use of glucocorticoids, anticoagulants, biphosphonates, or other NSAIDs

show that dyspepsia is the most common problem, affecting up to 50 percent of patients using NSAIDs. Dyspepsia is a frequent reason for discontinuing NSAID therapy. However, in the elderly population complaints of dyspepsia seem to be less frequent, most likely because of altered pain perception, the analgesic effect of NSAIDs, or both. Some patients may also complain of nausea and vomiting, although these symptoms may or may not be directly related to a local mucosal irritation. Esophagitis is a very uncommon problem that can lead to stricture formation. Gastric ulcers are more common than duodenal ulcers, occurring in 10 to 15 percent of NSAID users. Gastric erosions occur in up to 40 percent of NSAID users, with a risk of upper gastrointestinal bleeding. Both gastric and duodenal ulcers are usually asymptomatic, and many do not become clinically significant. The high incidence of gastrointestinal bleeding associated with NSAID-induced lesions is also in part due to their interference with platelet aggregation and, in the case of aspirin, irreversible binding to the platelet. Concomitant warfarin intake increases the gastrointestinal bleeding risk 18-fold. Perforation is the rarest of the NSAID-induced gastrointestinal complications.

A number of factors are associated with increased risk of gastrointestinal toxicity and complications from NSAIDs. Table 50-6 illustrates the most frequent ones. The risk may be additive in patients who have multiple risk factors, who have general debilitation, or who require antacids to control dyspeptic symptoms. The risk of toxicity may not be uniform among the NSAIDs. However, most of the studies that have attempted to stratify individual NSAID risks of gastrointestinal toxicity are difficult to interpret because they compared the effects of different NSAIDs used at varying doses.

The role of *H. pylori* infection in NSAID-induced gastritis or ulcer formation is unsettled. It is not clear that eradication of *H. pylori* in patients with NSAID-induced peptic disease has the same benefit as in patients not taking NSAIDs.

The best prophylaxis against NSAID-induced gastrointestinal complications is their avoidance, particularly in high-risk patients. It is the duty of the physician to weigh the risk versus the benefit of NSAIDs according to the specific needs and health status of the patient. Once the decision is made, the use of concomitant preventive therapy is probably indicated in older patients, as complications may occur within the first week of therapy and at any time in the following months or years.

The risk for NSAIDs induced gastric or duodenal ulcer can be decreased with concomitant use of misoprostol.

Complications of ulcers have also been reduced by this drug. However, the side effects of diarrhea and abdominal pain may limit its acceptance by some patients. Thus, the patient should be instructed not to use concomitant cathartic agents, to stop stool softeners unless absolutely necessary, and then reevaluate the need for these agents after several weeks of therapy. The dose of misoprostol should begin at 100 mg four times daily, then increased as tolerated. Standard doses of H_2 blockers are ineffective for the prevention of NSAID-induced gastric ulcers, although they may be helpful for the long-term prevention of duodenal ulcers. However, high-dose famotidine (40 mg twice daily) may be useful for both types of peptic disease. In fact, at this dose, famotidine has reduced the incidence of both gastric and duodenal ulcers by 50 percent, and it may also decrease the rate of recurrence of NSAID-induced ulcer disease. Proton pump inhibitors may also be useful for the prevention of NSAID-induced duodenal ulcers. Omeprazole 20 mg daily is also reported to be as effective as high-dose famotidine. However, the addition of such prophylaxis to regimens of patients using NSAIDs increases the cost of therapy by an average of 45 to 50 percent.

If a patient develops an ulcer while on an NSAID, this drug should be stopped if possible. Traditional ulcer therapy with H_2 blockers or a PPI should be started. A PPI is preferred in patients with large ulcers. The patient's status regarding infection with *H. pylori* should also be assessed. If positive, appropriate therapy should be instituted to eradicate *H. pylori* infection. There are many patients who must continue NSAID therapy despite the development of ulcers or erosions. These cases require therapy with high doses of H_2 blockers or the use of PPIs. The therapeutic regimens should be instituted for a period of 6 to 8 weeks and have been proven to be effective in 70 to 80 percent of cases. Studies indicate that omeprazole is more effective than misoprostol in these patients. Antisecretory therapy should be continued as a prophylactic measure for as long as NSAIDs are used at the dosage used for ulcer treatment.

Upper Gastrointestinal Bleeding in the Elderly

In the United States, the annual incidence of upper gastrointestinal hemorrhage has been estimated at 50 to 150 per 100,000 population, accounting for more than 300,000 hospitalizations with an overall mortality rate of around 10 percent. The rates of hospital admission for hemorrhage are 4.7 times higher in people older than 65 years of age, and patients with ulcer bleeding who are older than 80 years of age have the highest risk of rebleeding and death. Epidemiologic and clinical studies demonstrate that old age is an independent factor significantly associated with gastrointestinal hemorrhage. Bleeding from the upper gastrointestinal tract is caused by any lesion involving the oropharyngeal cavity, the esophagus, stomach, and duodenum to the level of the ligament of Treitz. Causes of bleeding in the elderly patients with hematemesis or melena are esophagitis (12 to 24 percent), erosive gastritis (21 to 32 percent), PUD (25 to 80 percent), and esophageal or gastric tumors (8 to 8.6 percent). The bleeding can be occult and present as iron-deficiency anemia. The presence of melena implies a blood loss of 300 to 600 mL from the upper gastrointestinal tract. A small amount of emesis of red blood can be associated with a small Mallory-Weiss tear or esophagitis. In the elderly population, hematemesis is the presenting symptom in 80 percent or more of cases with an upper gastrointestinal hemorrhage. In general, patients who hemorrhage from the upper gastrointestinal tract developed systemic manifestations of acute blood loss including diaphoresis, syncope, tachycardia, hypotension, shock, and a drop of the hematocrit within a few hours. The most frequent lesion responsible for this type of hemorrhage is a postbulbar ulcer overlying a large branch of the pancreaticoduodenal artery.

Physical disability and a limitation in activities of daily living are independent predictors of gastrointestinal hemorrhage. As discussed in the previous section, NSAID use is a significant risk factor for peptic ulcer bleeding in subjects older than 60 years of age, as well as the major cause of hospitalization as a consequence of gastric bleeding in patients older than 64 years of age. The risk of gastrointestinal bleeding increases with higher daily doses of NSAIDs. Moreover, in patients older than 64 years of age, upper gastrointestinal bleeding is associated with NSAID use both in patients taking these drugs on a long-term basis and in those who were only recently started on them. Thus, very little therapy may be needed to place the elderly patient at high risk of NSAID-related upper gastrointestinal bleeding. Unexplained iron deficiency anemia with consistently negative fecal occult blood test may be related to remote but significant intake of NSAIDs. The inability of elderly patients to restore their iron stores from food sources alone may account for the persistence of the anemia.

The use of corticosteroids in elderly patients may be associated with severe gastrointestinal hemorrhage, while studies in nonelderly populations report no increase in the risk of bleeding with these drugs. In subjects older than 60 years of age, the use of anticoagulation therapy significantly increases the rate of hemorrhagic complications compared to subjects younger than 60 years of age.

Some lesions causing upper gastrointestinal bleeding are exclusively found in the older patient. Dieulafoy lesion is a dilated aberrant submucosal vessel that erodes the overlying epithelium in the absence of a primary ulcer. It is usually located in the upper stomach in the high lesser curvature near the gastroesophageal junction. This abnormality accounts for less than 1 percent of cases of severe upper gastrointestinal hemorrhage. Bleeding is often self-limited, although it is usually recurrent and can be perfuse. Endoscopy is the diagnostic modality of choice for a Dieulafoy lesion during acute bleeding. In the absence of active bleeding, the aberrant vessel is often not seen. Endoscopic hemostasis is the initial treatment of choice for controlling acute bleeding and preventing rebleeding.

Gastric antral vascular ectasia is a rare cause of upper gastrointestinal bleeding that is often confused with portal hypertensive gastropathy. The diagnosis is based upon the classic endoscopic appearance of "watermelon stomach," derived from the characteristic endoscopic appearance of longitudinal rows of flat, reddish stripes radiating from the pylorus into the antrum that resemble the stripes on a watermelon. Their red stripes represent ectopic mucosal vessels. Histopathologically, watermelon stomach is characterized by vascular ectasia, spindle cell proliferation, and fiber hyalinosis. Endoscopic coagulation obliterates the vascular ectasia and decreases bleeding. Antrectomy prevents recurrent bleeding but is usually reserved for patients who fail endoscopic therapies.

Aortoenteric fistulas are a rare cause of acute upper gastrointestinal bleeding, but they are associated with high mortality if undiagnosed or untreated. The third or forth portion of the duodenum is the most common site for aortoenteric fistulas, followed by the jejunum and ileum. Most patients present with an initial bleed manifested by hematemesis and/or hematochezia. This may be followed by massive bleeding and exsanguination. The most common cause of primary aortoenteric fistulas in the United States is an atherosclerotic aortic aneurysm. The most common cause of secondary aortoenteric fistulas is of prosthetic abdominal aortic vascular graft. Pressure necrosis and graft infection have been implicated in the development of fistulas. Surgical repair of the aortic aneurysm and fistula is the standard treatment regardless of the cause.

Upper gastrointestinal bleeding from portal hypertensive gastropathy occurs equally in younger and older patients.

In the elderly population, it is important to remember that upper gastrointestinal bleeding carries an eventual mortality rate of 25 to 30 percent. Thus, this presentation is to be considered an emergency at the earliest stages of management. Initial placement of a nasogastric tube helps determine the rate and intensity of the bleeding and provides evidence of whether it has stopped spontaneously. Gastric lavage facilitates the suction of small clots. Although nasogastric suction diminishes the likelihood of aspiration of blood and gastric contents, aspiration may occur during the placement of the tube. Also important in the initial phase of therapy is starting resuscitative measures with placement of large-bore venous access and use of plasma expanders. It is particularly important to closely monitor the intravascular fluid status of elderly patients. This may require placement of a Swan-Ganz catheter. The need for transfusions and the number of units required within the first 12 to 24 hours to achieve an acceptable level of hemoglobin, usually >10 g in the elderly patient, is of prognostic significance. Patients requiring 6 units or more will most likely require surgical intervention and incur a high mortality rate. It is important to discontinue the use of NSAIDs or anticoagulants in patients with bleeding. If the prothrombin time is greatly prolonged, the patient should receive injection of vitamin K. As part of the initial phase of therapy, H_2 blockers or PPIs are usually started. However, they appear to be of no value in the final outcome of active hemorrhage, nor do they increase the speed of ulcer healing.

It is incumbent on the treating physician to decide the need for early endoscopy. It is important to consider the status of the patient and the availability of a skilled endoscopist, particularly if the need for endoscopic hemostasis arises. Patients with active bleeding and exhibiting signs of hypovolemia should be considered candidates for early endoscopic intervention. The procedure should not be performed until hypovolemia has been corrected. At the time of endoscopy, the absence of active bleeding or a clean ulcer crater are considered signs of favorable prognosis. There are multiple therapeutic modalities available to the endoscopist, and the choice depends on the type of lesions found and the experience the physician has with each modality. If active bleeding is still present after an endoscopic therapeutic intervention, or if the source of bleeding was not identified, surgical intervention is indicated as soon as possible. Surgery is also indicated in case of rebleeding unless the patient is considered a high surgical risk, in which case another attempt at endoscopic therapy should be considered.

Gastric Emptying Disorders in the Elderly

Pathophysiology

Normal gastrointestinal motor function is controlled by a complex interplay of mechanisms involving an extrinsic nerve supply from the brain and spinal cord, the vagus nerve, the plexus within the wall of the stomach and intestine (the enteric brain), and an even more complex system of hormonal facilitators and inhibitors with feedback loops arising mostly in the duodenum. Abnormalities in any of these factors can lead to delayed gastric emptying.

The primary function of the stomach is to accommodate variable amounts of solids and liquids, to reduce solids to progressively smaller particles by acid and peptic digestion, and to liquefy the meal into a suspension containing solid particles with a diameter of 2 mm or less. These results are achieved by strong antral peristaltic contractions. These contractions continue for 1.5 to 2 hours after the start of a meal, depending on its composition. Several factors can delay gastric emptying, such as a meal with a higher osmolarity, a low pH, or a high caloric content, particularly if it is rich in fat.

During fasting, the stomach participates in the cyclical activity front propagating through the gastrointestinal tract that propel non-digestible solid residue toward the colon. These cyclical motor activities are called migrating motor complexes (MMCs) and are initiated in the stomach. These MMCs are capable of sweeping all intestinal contents through the ileocecal junction in about 60 to 100 minutes. The MMC restarts again at the level of the stomach as long as the stomach is empty.

During a meal, the fundus relaxes during swallowing to start the process of accommodation in which the stomach assumes reservoir functions, facilitating the initial chemical digestion of food before transfer toward the antrum. The antrum produces high amplitude contractions that pulverize solids by physical shearing forces. Solids are reduced in size to particles of 1 to 2 mm; this is called trituration. Once this is achieved, the particles are able to empty through the pylorus. Larger particles are repetitively propelled and retropulsed from the distal stomach by an occluded gastric outlet segment until liquid shearing and chemical digestion achieve trituration. Thus, antral motor function is critical for the grinding, mixing, and emptying of solids from the stomach.

The pylorus is a zone of high resting pressure, 0.6 to 1.6 cm in length, upon which are superimposed phasic contractions at a rate of 3 per minute. These contractions sweep across the antroduodenal junction. The size of the pylorus lumen does not allow the passage of solid particles of more than 2 mm in diameter.

With aging, there is a physiologic decrease in gastric emptying for liquids, but not for solids. The fact that motility disorders disproportionately affect the elderly is mainly related to the impact of age-associated chronic conditions.

Etiology

Delayed gastric emptying can be classified into organic or functional categories. A gastric motility disorder should be considered in patients with underlying diseases with neuromuscular manifestations.

Gastric outlet obstruction as a result of peptic ulcer disease, which is one of the organic causes of gastroparesis, was discussed in an earlier section. In an elderly patient presenting with symptoms of gastroparesis of short duration, it is important to consider the possibility of antral or scirrhous carcinoma.

Gastric emptying delay secondary to functional causes is multifactorial in origin. It is important to first think of medications, especially in elderly patients. Drugs to be considered are particularly those with anticholinergic, dopaminergic, or with opioid analgesic properties such as tricyclic antidepressants, hydrocodone, or β-blockers.

Previous gastric surgery may result in gastric stasis, usually because of intended or accidental injury to the vagus nerve such as with vagotomy, or with Billroth II gastrectomy or fundoplication. Extrinsic vagal denervation or loss of the antrum reduces the capacity of the stomach to empty nondigestible solids during fasting and to triturate and empty digestible food postprandially. Most gastric surgery for peptic ulcer disease was done before introduction of cimetidine in the mid-1970s. Thus, today, postgastrectomy patients are largely concentrated among the elderly. Motility disorders resulting from such surgery are often referred to as "the dumping syndrome," which reflects the effects of rapid gastric emptying and shifts of intraluminal osmolarity and volume status. The Roux stasis syndrome can occur after a Roux-en-Y anastomosis. Stasis results from incoordination of contractions in the efferent Roux limb, which causes stasis either in the gastric remnant or in the Roux limb itself.

Patients with diabetes mellitus may have abnormalities at several levels in the process of gastric emptying. These abnormalities are primarily a result of autonomic dysfunction. However, there may also be a contribution from hyperglycemia itself. Gastroparesis occurs typically in patients who have had diabetes for more than 5 years and who may have concomitant renal, ophthalmologic, or other neurologic involvement.

Diseases affecting primarily the muscle fibers, such as scleroderma, the muscular dystrophies, and other collagen-vascular diseases, are less frequent in the elderly. However, patients with these diseases, especially in their advanced forms, can also present with gastroparesis. Several common neurologic disorders, such as Parkinson disease or multiple sclerosis, can be the cause of gastroparesis. In certain patients, it will not be possible to identify the cause of their disease and it will thus be labeled primary or idiopathic gastroparesis. This is mostly seen in young woman, but a second peak appears in the elderly population.

Diagnosis

Symptoms of delayed gastric emptying are often vague. Patients most commonly present with abnormal pain, nausea, vomiting of undigested material, early or easy satiety, bloating, and weight loss. The character of the abdominal pain is variable. It is most often epigastric and usually described as burning, vague, or crampy. More than half of the patients report exacerbation of their pain after eating.

Abdominal examination may show epigastric distension or tenderness, but no guarding or rigidity. There may be a succussion splash. The physical exam may show findings suggestive of an underlying disorder resulting in gastric stasis.

Routine laboratory testing is not useful for the diagnosis of gastric stasis itself, but it may help to identify associated diseases or to rule out other disorders. A chest x-ray and a plain film of the abdomen are considered part of the initial workup.

All patients require an upper endoscopy or an upper GI barium study to confirm the presence of gastric stasis by the retention of food in the stomach after an overnight fast. These tests also permit the exclusion of mechanical obstruction or mucosal disease as the cause of impaired gastric emptying. In the absence of any lesion, historical evidence of medication intake, diabetes mellitus, or scleroderma is enough to make a presumptive diagnosis.

The diagnosis of gastroparesis is confirmed by a solid-phase gastric-emptying study. Scintigraphic gastric emptying is the most cost-effective, simple, and widely available technique. Documenting the presence and assessing the severity of gastric stasis is best achieved by evaluating the gastric emptying of solids, because liquids often empty from the stomach normally even when solids are abnormally retained. In patients with a known etiologic disorder, such as diabetes mellitus, no further testing is necessary if mechanical obstruction is excluded and scintigraphy confirms gastric stasis.

Gastroduodenal manometry is indicated for patients with evidence of gastric stasis by scintigraphy but who have no known cause for gastroparesis. Manometry is reasonably accurate to differentiate a myopathic from a neuropathic process. In a myopathic process, such as in amyloidosis or scleroderma, manometry typically shows low amplitude contractions. In a neuropathic process, such as diabetes mellitus or idiopathic autonomic neuropathy, manometry typically shows normal amplitude contractions, but the organization of the contractile response is abnormal.

Treatment

Whenever possible, treatment should be directed toward the primary cause. It is important to identify and eliminate possible causative medications. In general, the management of gastroparesis includes supportive measures, optimizing glycemic control in diabetic patients, medications, and, occasionally, surgery.

In patients with gastroparesis, repetitive vomiting and decreased oral intake associated with delayed gastric emptying can lead to various metabolic abnormalities such as hypokalemia, metabolic acidosis, dehydration, or deterioration in the control of diabetes. These patients may also develop essential element, mineral, and vitamin deficiencies. Those who have had previous gastric surgery are particularly at risk for iron and vitamin B_{12} deficiencies, the severity of which is related to the extent of resection. Supplementation of fluids, electrolytes, and nutrients should be achieved by the simplest and least-invasive method possible. If oral supplementation is unsuccessful and gastric stasis is caused by a disorder of gastric motor function, a jejunal feeding tube can be placed. Parenteral nutrition is seldom necessary unless gastroparesis is part of a generalized motility disorder.

In the treatment of delayed gastric emptying, both prokinetic and antiemetic agents may be useful. Intravenous erythromycin, at the dose of 3 mg/kg every 8 hours, is the treatment of choice in patients who cannot take oral medications. Erythromycin induces high-amplitude gastric-propulsive contractions that help to evacuate solid residue from the stomach. It also stimulates fundic contractility. It is important to bear in mind that erythromycin has potential side effects, such as gastrointestinal toxicity, ototoxicity, and pseudomembranous colitis. Because of these potential side effects, the chronic administration of erythromycin is currently restricted to patients who are resistant to other medications.

When it was first introduced, cisapride was considered the drug of choice for patients with gastroparesis who could ingest oral liquids. However, because of its potentially fatal cardiac side effects, its availability is currently severely restricted in the United States.

Bethanecol was the only cholinergic medication available for years. However, because of its limited effect on gastric motility, it should not be considered in gastroparesis. Metoclopramide, a dopamine antagonist, is more effective, acting both centrally and peripherally. Parenteral metoclopramide is an alternative to intravenous erythromycin for patients who cannot take oral medications. This medication can induce diverse side effects such as irritability, anxiety, disorientation, hallucination, galactorrhea, and gynecomastia. It can also cause a Parkinson-like syndrome, especially in an elderly patient. A dystonic reaction caused by metoclopramide is mainly seen in the young.

A variety of antiemetics are used alone or concomitantly with prokinetic agents in patients with gastroparesis. Antihistamines such as diphenhydramine can be used orally or rectally, while phenothiazines, such as prochlorperazine, can be used parenterally or rectally, according to clinical indications.

Surgery is rarely indicated in patients with nonobstructive gastric stasis, except to provide effective decompression or for completion of a subtotal gastrectomy in patients with a previous partial gastrectomy.

REFERENCES

Borum ML: Peptic ulcer disease in the elderly. *Gastroenterology* 15(3):457, 1999.

Fass R et al: Symptom severity and esophageal chemosensitivity to acid in older and young patients with gastroesophageal reflux. *Age Aging* 29:125, 2000.

Friedman LS, Castell DO: Esophageal diseases in the elderly, in Castell DO, Richter JE (eds): *The Esophagus*, 3rd ed. Philadelphia, Lippincott Williams & Wilkins, 1999, p 615.

Fuchs CS, Mayer RJ: Gastric carcinoma. *N Engl J Med* 333(1):32, 1995.

Fulp SR et al: Aging-related alterations in human upper esophageal sphincter function. *Am J Gastroenterol* 85(1):1569, 1990.

Hackelsberger A et al: Role of aging in the expression of *Helicobacter pylori* gastritis in the antrum, corpus, and cardia. *Scand J Gastroenterol* 34:138, 1999.

Lee M, Feldman M: The aging stomach: Implications for NSAID gastropathy. *Gut* 41:425, 1997.

Pilotto A: Aging and the gastrointestinal tract. *Ital J Gastroenterol Hepatol* 31:137, 1999.

Ribeiro AC et al: Esophageal manometry: A comparison of findings in younger and older patients. *Am J Gastroenterol* 93(5):706, 1998.

Sallout H et al: The aging esophagus. *Gastroenterology* 15(3):439, 1999.

Schroeder PL, Richter JE: Swallowing disorders in the elderly. *Semin Gastrointest Dis* 5(4):154, 1994.

Shaker R, Lang IM: Effect of aging on the deglutitive oral, pharyngeal, and esophageal motor function. *Dysphagia* 9:221, 1994.

Staff D, Shaker R: Aging in the gastrointestinal tract. *Dis Mon* 47(3):72, 2001.

Trey G et al: Changes in acid secretion over the years: A 30-year longitudinal study. *J Clin Gastroenterol* 25(3):499, 1997.

Yokoyama M et al: Role of laryngeal movement and effect of aging on swallowing pressure in the pharynx and upper esophageal sphincter. *Laryngoscope* 110:434, 2000.

Common Large Intestinal Disorders

ADIL E. BHARUCHA · MICHAEL CAMILLERI

In the elderly population, lower gastrointestinal (GI) disorders occur commonly, cause significant distress, and account for considerable health care expenditure. This chapter focuses on functional abdominal pain, diverticulosis, ischemic colitis, and lower gastrointestinal bleeding. Constipation and fecal incontinence are discussed in Chaps. 52 and 123. Diagnosis of functional gastrointestinal disorders in elderly patients presents greater challenges than in younger adults, because organic diseases, such as cancer and chronic ischemia, which are more common in the elderly population, may mimic functional disorders; coexisting chronic illness such as Parkinson's disease or chronic renal insufficiency, or the effects of medications may mimic or aggravate functional disorders; and comorbidities affecting mental and functional status and sensory impairment such as poor vision and/or hearing may confuse or disguise the clinical presentation. Understanding the pathophysiology of such disorders facilitates a rational therapeutic approach for their diagnosis and management.

factors; that is, according to the precepts of the biopsychosocial model.

Aging is defined as a series of changes "that occur with time during postmaturational life, that underlie an increasing vulnerability to challenge, thereby decreasing the ability of the organism to survive." At the organ level, aging is associated with metabolic, genetic, neuroendocrine, and immunological changes that may contribute to cell death from apoptosis or phagocytosis. These mechanisms may contribute to neural injury and loss and alterations in smooth muscle function of the large intestine with aging, as summarized in Table 51-1. However, it is unclear whether aging affects the interstitial cells of Cajal, which are the pacemaker cells of the gut. Despite the effects of aging, functional GI symptoms are not inevitable consequences of aging. Perhaps this suggests that the redundancy of neurons (100 million) in the adult mammalian gut provides a functional reserve of surviving neurons, compensating for age-related neuronal loss.

GASTROINTESTINAL AND MOTOR SENSORY FUNCTION

Motility is regulated by coordinated neurohormonal mechanisms that influence smooth muscle contractility. Gut motor activity is primarily controlled by the intrinsic or enteric nervous system. Visceral sensation is conveyed via afferents that travel to the spinal cord and, ultimately, to the cerebral cortex or through the vagus to the brainstem. There is a 10:1 ratio of afferent to efferent fibers in the vagus at the level of the diaphragm. The vagus is primarily concerned with conveying subnoxious messages, while the spinal afferents convey nonnoxious and noxious input. The central nervous system modulates gut motor activity via the extrinsic sympathetic and parasympathetic pathways, while descending pathways in the spinal cord modulate transmission of sensory input from the dorsal horn to supraspinal centers. Functional gastrointestinal disorders result from the combined effect of biological, psychological, and social

Applied Anatomy of Relevance to the Colonic Disorders

Diverticulosis

From the cecum to the rectosigmoid junction, colonic longitudinal muscle is organized in three thick bands, the taeniae, with a thin layer of longitudinal muscle between these bands. At the rectosigmoid junction, the three taeniae broaden to form a uniformly thick layer throughout the rectum. In the anal canal, the longitudinal muscle layer merges with the external anal sphincter while the circular muscle layer extends into the internal anal sphincter. The taenia coli are thought to function as suspension cables upon which the circular muscle arcs are suspended, facilitating efficient contraction of the circular muscle. Diverticula protrude between the taenia coli through weak areas in the bowel wall; these weak areas correspond to points where arteries enter the colon. Regional differences in colonic muscle tone and compliance (discussed below)

Table 51-1   Effects of Aging on Gastrointestinal Neuronal and Smooth-Muscle Structure and Function*

Effect on Gut Neuromuscular Function
Fewer neurons in myenteric plexus–human colon
↓ Amplitude of inhibitory junction potentials; mechanism unclear. Similar concentrations of inhibitory neuropeptides (VIP, PHM, met-Enk), NPY, and somatostatin in colonic smooth-muscle strips from young vs. old persons
↓ Contribution of NO (nitric oxide) to NANC neurotransmission in longitudinal muscle, rat proximal colon
↓ Response to stimuli (acetylcholine, electrical field stimulation)—rat colon
Alterations in L-type calcium currents and calcium-insensitive K^+ current
Increased collagen production → ↑ smooth-muscle thickness. Smaller and more tightly packed fibrils in diverticulosis (human colon)

met-Enk, met^5-enkephalin; No, nitric oxide; NPY, neuropeptide Y; PHM, peptide histidine-methionine; VIP, vasoactive intestinal peptide.
*Specific references for these observations are detailed in Bharucha & Camilleri (references).
SOURCE: Reproduced with permission from Camilleri M et al. (2000).

may determine the predilection for diverticular in specific response of the colon.

Nerve Supply

The colon is innervated by extrinsic and intrinsic nerves. The extrinsic input includes sympathetic and parasympathetic components; the latter are derived from the vagus nerve, which innervates the proximal colon, and sacral (S2-4) segments of the spinal cord that supply the distal colon. After entering the colon, these fibers form the ascending colonic nerves, traveling orad to supply a variable portion of the left colon. The sympathetic fibers originate in the paravertebral "chain" ganglion, segments from the T12 to L4 levels of the spinal cord, and are conveyed to the colon via arterial arcades of the superior and inferior mesenteric vessels. The sympathetic nervous system provides excitatory input to the sphincters and a tonic inhibitory input to nonsphincteric muscle. Norepinephrine is the major neurotransmitter released by sympathetic nerves throughout the small and large intestine. The intrinsic or intramural nerves are organized into myenteric and submucous plexuses and the interstitial cells of Cajal. The myenteric plexus and interstitial cells are primarily responsible for controlling motility; the submucous plexus regulates mucosal absorption. The extrinsic nerves modulate the intrinsic neural activity. For example, the sympathetic nervous system exerts a tonic inhibitory input on colonic motor function, primarily via stimulation of α2-adrenergic receptors, which hyperpolarize cholinergic neurons in the myenteric plexus. Thus, the α2 agonist clonidine decreases colonic tone while the α2 antagonist yohimbine increases colonic tone in humans; clonidine also enhances mucosal absorption of fluid and salt.

Vascular Anatomy

In addition to supplying the small intestine, the superior mesenteric artery also supplies the cecum, ascending and proximal transverse colon via its ileocolic, right, and middle colic branch arteries. Occlusion of the superior mesenteric artery (SMA), which originates at an angle of approximately 30 degrees from the aorta, is frequently catastrophic because there is an inadequate collateral circulation between end branches of this vessel. Because the inferior mesenteric artery (IMA) forms a less-acute angle with the aorta (70 to 90 degrees), IMA embolism is extremely uncommon as compared to SMA embolism. There is an extensive collateral circulation between branches of the superior and inferior mesenteric artery and between the latter and the hypogastric arteries. Colonic ischemia is less common than mesenteric ischemia, with a predilection for affecting the splenic flexure and distal sigmoid colon, watershed areas situated at the junction between two vascular territories. In contrast to ulcerative colitis, ischemic colitis seldom involves the rectum, which is supplied by both portal and systemic circulations. The pericolonic arches formed by these anastomoses supply branches to the colon. Vascular ectasia or angiodysplasia of the colon is attributed to formation of a small arteriovenous communication secondary to an incompetent valvular mechanism between the arterioles and venules.

Applied Physiology of the Colon and Rectum

The human colon serves to absorb water and electrolytes, store intraluminal contents until elimination is socially convenient, and salvage nutrients after bacterial metabolism of carbohydrates that have not been absorbed in the small intestine. These functions are dependent on the colon's ability to control the distal progression of its contents. In healthy adults, colonic transit normally requires several hours to almost 3 days for completion. Although the colon is regarded as a single organ, there are regional differences between the right and left colon, which are indicated in Table 51-2. The clinically important aspects of colonic physiology are described in the following sections.

Fluid and Electrolyte Absorption

The colon absorbs all but 100 mL of fluid and 1 mEq of sodium and chloride from approximately 1500 mL of chyme it receives over 24 hours. Absorptive capacity can

Table 51-2 Comparison of Right and Left Colon

Feature	Right Colon	Left Colon
Embryologic origin	Midgut	Hindgut
Blood supply	Superior mesenteric vessels	Inferior mesenteric vessels
Extrinsic nerve supply		
Parasympathetic	Vagus	Pelvic nerves from sacral S2-4 segments
Sympathetic	Superior mesenteric ganglion	Inferior mesenteric ganglion
Function	Mixing and storage	Conduit

SOURCE: Reproduced with permission from Bharucha AE and Camilleri M (2001).

increase to 5 to 6 L and 800 to 1000 mEq of sodium and chloride daily. In the proximal colon, bacteria ferment organic carbohydrates to short-chain fatty acids (SCFA), predominantly acetate, propionate, and butyrate. There is a low, normal rate of SCFA production from "malabsorbed" carbohydrate (up to 10% of that ingested); diets high in fiber, beans, resistant starches, and complex carbohydrates increase the production of SCFA. SCFA are rapidly absorbed from the colon, augment sodium, chloride, and water absorption, and constitute the preferred metabolic fuel for colonocytes. SCFA may also serve to regulate proliferation, differentiation, gene expression, immune function, and wound healing in the colon. Reduced tonic-sympathetic inhibition impairs net absorption of water and electrolytes and accelerates transit in diabetic neuropathy with diarrhea. Clonidine restores the sympathetic brake, reducing such diarrhea.

Colonic Motility and Transit

In healthy individuals, the average mouth–cecum transit time is approximately 6 hours, and average regional transit times through the right, left, and sigmoid colon are each about 12 hours, yielding an average total colonic transit time of 36 hours. Colonic motor activity is extremely irregular, ranging from quiescence, particularly at night, to isolated contractions, bursts of contractions, or propagated contractions. In contrast to the small intestine, rhythmic migrating motor complexes do not occur in the colon. Contractions are tonic or sustained, lasting several minutes to hours, and shorter, or phasic. Propagated phasic contractions propel colonic contents over longer distances than nonpropagated phasic contractions. High-amplitude propagated contractions (HAPC) are >75 mmHg in pressure occur approximately six times per day, frequently after awakening and after meals, are responsible for mass movement of colonic contents, and frequently precede defecation. Stimulant laxatives such as bisacodyl (Dulcolax), glycerol, and anticholinesterases (e.g., neostigmine) induce HAPCs.

Colonic Tone and Compliance

Tone refers to sustained muscular contractions. In the gastrointestinal tract, tone is a characteristic property of the sphincters, the gastric fundus, and the colon. Colonic tone is relevant to function and augmented after feeding. Colonic tone is reduced by α_2-receptor–mediated sympathetic stimulation and by opiates; excessive colonic relaxation causes colonic dilatation in acute colonic pseudo-obstruction. Colonic compliance (i.e., the "elasticity") of the colon declines with aging, reaching a minimum of 40% of its maximum value by 70 years. Regional differences in colonic compliance may partly explain regional variations in colonic functions; the ascending and transverse colon are more compliant than the descending colon, which, in turn, is more compliant than the sigmoid colon. Under normal circumstances, the highly compliant ascending colon serves as a reservoir, mixing contents, the less-compliant left colon serves primarily as a conduit, while the rectosigmoid colon serves as a conduit and a reservoir before expulsion of stool. The effect of aging on biomechanical properties in vivo requires further study, because diminished rectosigmoid compliance in the elderly person may impair reservoir function, predisposing to frequent evacuation. Moreover, alterations in compliance may also influence visceral sensitivity. A stiff or noncompliant rectum is associated with increased sensitivity to distension in patients with radiation-induced and ulcerative proctitis.

Colonic Response to Feeding

Neurohormonal mechanisms are responsible for increased tonic and phasic colonic motor activity that occur a few minutes after ingestion of a meal of ≥500 Kcal; this response may be sustained for up to 2 hours. The term *gastrocolonic reflex* is a misnomer because this response, induced by gastric distension and chemical stimulation by nutrients, is observed even after a gastrectomy. This response may explain postprandial urgency and abdominal discomfort in patients with irritable bowel syndrome (IBS).

Intestino-Intestinal Reflexes

Peristalsis is a local reflex mediated by intrinsic nerve pathways, characterized by contraction proximal to and relaxation distal to the distended segment. In addition, rectal or colonic distension can inhibit motor activity more proximally in the stomach, small intestine, or colon. These inhibitory reflexes are mediated by extrinsic reflex pathways, which synapse in the prevertebral ganglia independent of the central nervous system. This inhibition may account for delayed left colonic, and/or small intestinal transit in patients with colonic distension, including that associated with obstructive defecation.

FUNCTIONAL ABDOMINAL PAIN

Symptoms consistent with functional gastrointestinal disorders occur commonly in the elderly patient. In a randomly selected sample of elderly residents from Olmsted County, Minnesota, aged 65 to 93 years, the overall age- and sex-adjusted prevalence of frequent abdominal pain (more than six times in the previous year) was 24.3 per 100 persons (95% confidence interval [CI], 19.3 to 29.2). This may be an underestimate of true prevalence because the elderly person may be more reluctant to report pain and the manifestations of functional GI disorders fluctuate over time. Thus, an initial survey of a Danish cohort reported similar figures to the Olmsted County survey, but 50 percent of the Danes did not report IBS symptoms (or functional dyspepsia) when resurveyed 5 years later. Lastly, widespread laxative use in the elderly population confounds interpretation of the unusually high prevalence of diarrhea (14.2 percent) reported in the elderly population on postal questionnaires. Nonetheless, the following overall conclusions can be made:

1. The overall prevalence data are only slightly higher in the elderly population when compared to prevalence rates in younger adults (e.g., diarrhea 17.9 percent, constipation 24.1 percent in Olmsted County) or not different at all (e.g., IBS).
2. Elderly constipated subjects have more symptoms attributable to rectal outlet delay when compared to younger individuals (20.5 percent in elderly versus 11 percent in younger adults). These observations need to be confirmed by physiologic testing because the specificity of straining as a predictor of an evacuation disorder requires further validation.
3. With regard to risk factors, aspirin, other nonsteroidal antiinflammatory drugs , and other constipating medications were associated with a small but statistically significant risk for constipation in the overall group, but not when functional constipation or outlet delay were considered separately. A relationship between physical inactivity and constipation has been reported in homebound subjects, but not in ambulant people in community-based surveys.
4. Functional GI symptoms have a significant impact on quality of life as assessed by a standardized instrument, in the MOS (Medical Outcomes Survey). In particular, patients with IBS and frequent abdominal pain had significantly lower scores on all MOS scales, implying impaired quality of life. When compared to age-matched healthy subjects, patients with frequent abdominal pain had lower scores for physical functioning, mental health, and health perception than for social functioning (e.g., visiting with friends) or role functioning (normal occupation, household duties). Among a normal elderly cohort in Copenhagen, Denmark, functional dyspepsia and IBS reduced functional ability at baseline and 5 years later.
5. In the Olmsted County survey, a majority of elderly subjects did not seek health care for their gastrointestinal symptoms, although frequent abdominal pain (odds ratio [OR] = 2.6; 95% CI, 1.9 to 3.6) or IBS symptoms (OR = 3.1; 95% CI, 2.1 to 4.7) were associated with an increased probability of physician visits.

In contrast to the prevalence data, there is limited information about the incidence of abdominal pain and IBS in the community. The incidence of IBS increased with aging in women, from 0.18 percent in women between 20 and 34 years of age to 0.33 percent in women between 55 and 94 years of age. These data suggest that GI symptoms of recent onset in the elderly patient may be due to a functional gastrointestinal disorder; however, exclusion of organic disease is still essential. In contrast, epidemiologic studies of other chronic painful symptoms reveal that with the exception of joint pains, the overall prevalence of painful conditions, for example, migraine or back pain, peaks between middle-age and 65 years of age, declining thereafter. Indeed the onset of headaches after the age of 55 is strongly suggestive of an organic disorder and calls for careful attention.

Pain in the Elderly Person and Pain Transmission from the Gut

The International Association for the Study of Pain defines pain as "an unpleasant *sensory and emotional experience* associated with actual or potential tissue damage or described in terms of such damage." This definition emphasizes the multidimensional experience of pain. While the actual stimulus may reflect physiologic damage, the pain process is one of sensation and perception of, motivation to avoid, an affective response to that stimulus. Aging influences the sensory, affective and cognitive-evaluative components which contribute to the final pain response.

In humans, research dealing with age differences in pain have focused on pain in the laboratory setting, generally by determining the pain threshold (i.e., the level at which the stimulus is first perceived as painful) to an acute stimulus. Although these studies reveal statistically significant increases in rectal pain threshold, suggesting a reduced pain threshold, they are of questionable relevance to the clinical context. Assessment of pain thresholds involves a well-controlled stimulus with transient emotional reactions and no threat to normal functioning. On the other hand, chronic pain may be associated with a pathologic process, long-term impairment, and profound emotional upheaval. In contrast to the pain threshold, pain tolerance refers to the "lowest stimulation level at which the subject withdraws or asks to have the stimulation stopped." A few studies assessing pain tolerance to somatic stimulation suggest that such tolerance decreases with age, but little is known about visceral pain tolerance and aging. Age-related decline in peripheral nerve functioning of C-fibers, decreases in the amplitude of sensory action potentials, or reduced capacity or speed of central processing of nociceptive stimuli with age do not rationally explain reduced pain tolerance with aging. In the absence of a neurologic explanation for decreased tolerance of pain with aging, we must consider the potential role of psychological factors.

Role of Psychological Factors in Pain in the Elderly Person

A variety of social-psychological processes can affect experience and expression of pain in the elderly person. Factors that may lead to underreporting of pain include a tendency to regard pain as a normal consequence of aging, a manifestation of severe disease, a desire to avoid invasive treatments or dependency, and/or upsetting family members. Conversely, some older people may exaggerate pain to cover functional deficits arising from cognitive or other impairment or to maintain a sick role. The effect of interpersonal relationships on expression of pain is inconsistent; higher rates of pain behavior have been reported either with more supportive or nonsupportive social networks. Lastly, lifelong personality characteristics also influence age-specific interpretations of pain. Chronic pain appears to be more intensive and has more debilitating affective and functional consequences in persons high in neuroticism and hypochondriasis and those low in perceived control. Just as Apley stated "young bellyachers become old bellyachers," it is also true that "old bellyachers become older/elderly bellyachers"!

Pain and Depression—Anxiety in the Elderly Person

A majority of patients with chronic pain have significant depressive symptoms. Conversely, depressed individuals are more likely to report painful symptoms than are nondepressed individuals. However, there are no age differences in the severity or prevalence of depressive symptoms experienced by chronic pain patients (see Chap. 25). These depressive symptoms may not fulfill formal criteria for major depression. The relationship between pain and depression holds true even after adjusting for somatic symptoms (poor sleep, appetite, and activity) that may confound assessments of depression. In clinical practice, the possibility of depression should be considered in patients who have prominent features of depression (early morning awakening, psychomotor agitation or retardation, anorexia, weight loss and pain with a puzzling pattern, onset or distribution), even though these symptoms may be indicative of an organic gastrointestinal illness. Although the effects of anxiety on perception of and tolerance for acute pain has been studied extensively, the role of anxiety in persistent pain syndromes is not well understood.

Pain and Cognitive Impairment

Dementia can impact the sensory, cognitive, and emotional components of the pain experience. The association between dementia and pain is common but hasn't been studied in detail. Assessment of pain in demented people can be difficult. Health care workers tend to underestimate severity of pain. When verbal communication is lost, nonspecific behavioral observations, such as facial expression, are often the only means available to assess severity of pain. Pain must also be considered in the differential diagnosis when patients with dementia seem agitated for unclear reasons. Cognitive impairment limits management to medication or simple physical maneuvers performed by others. Cognitive approaches have no role in patients with more advanced cognitive impairment.

Principles of Management of Abdominal Pain in the Elderly Patient

Patients and physicians are more comfortable when the diagnosis of a functional gastrointestinal disorder is established after excluding organic diseases; this is even more relevant in the elderly population, in whom organic diseases are more prevalent than in young adults. A careful clinical assessment, with consideration of an evacuation disorder, excessive perineal descent, pelvic floor spasm, and painful perianal conditions (e.g., fissure, hemorrhoid) is necessary in patients with constipation. An important caveat is that abnormal findings on investigation such as trivial gastric erosions on endoscopy or diverticulosis on x-ray or endoscopy do not necessarily indicate causality for pain. Uncomplicated diverticulosis and IBS often coexist. To imply that diverticulosis may account for symptoms may negate the impact of conservative therapeutic efforts for IBS and lead to a potentially hazardous decision to resect the colon unless there are complications of diverticulosis.

Having established the diagnosis of functional abdominal pain and reassured patients about the absence of a life-threatening disease, the physician's assessment must include measures of the sensory, cognitive, and affective domains. In some patients a psychologist may be extremely helpful to evaluate these patients thoroughly. The cognitive experience involves measurement of coping strategies, the perceived effectiveness of these strategies, and the perceived ability to control one's pain. The affective consequences are measured in terms of depression and anxiety. It is important to dispel the myth that pain is a normal consequence of aging and therefore not amenable to treatment.

Current management of abdominal pain in the elderly patient is often associated with the need to control other symptoms in the irritable bowel syndrome. Constipation is often relieved by adequate hydration, increased mobility, fiber supplementation (15 to 25 g/d), and an osmotic laxative or stool softener. However, this may sometimes aggravate pain and induce bloating, especially if doses >20 g are used. Diarrhea and urgency can be treated with low doses of peripherally acting opioids, such as loperamide 1 to 2 mg (liquid formula permitting better titration) up to three times per day subject to a maximum of 16 mg/d. Imodium should preferably be taken 30 minutes before eating to reduce the tendency for postprandial symptoms coincident with the gastrocolonic response to eating. A toileting schedule, that is, prompted voiding, may be useful for patients with chronic diarrhea and fecal incontinence.

IBS-related pain may require use of antispasmodics as required for acute episodes or chronic treatment with low-dose antidepressants. The potential benefits of taking antispasmodic medication on a regular schedule include better analgesia, less anxiety, and a lower total analgesic dose. A retrospective chart review of a large (138 patients) series of patients with irritable bowel syndrome treated with tricyclic antidepressants found no significant differences in the clinical response rate between young (35 ± 1 years; mean ± SEM [standard error of mean]) and older patients (61 ± 1 years). In this entire group, patients with predominant pain were more likely to respond to antidepressants, as compared to patients with predominant constipation or diarrhea. Psychological features were not predictive of outcome. However, these medications are to be used judiciously in the elderly population because their anticholinergic side effects may influence cardiac or urinary bladder function or may precipitate glaucoma. Insomnia may be treated by trazodone (Desyrel).

Nonpharmacologic measures may supplement pharmacologic approaches for alleviating abdominal pain, but these measures have not been studied in the elderly population. These nonpharmacologic modalities include exercise, which may raise somatic pain thresholds in younger subjects, and cognitive, cognitive-behavioral, or other approaches (hypnosis, psychotherapy, supportive counseling, stress inoculation techniques, and marital therapy) conducted under the supervision of a psychologist. Behavioral approaches seem particularly worthwhile in elderly patients who already receive many medications and are susceptible to adverse effects of single drugs or polypharmacy. The current trend is to use a cognitive-behavioral approach. Such programs are effective for older people, exploding the commonly held myth that psychological change cannot occur in old age. Multidisciplinary pain management programs should be considered for patients who experience persistent pain and suffering, which are often refractory to standard interventions. In these instances the suffering often assumes a "malignant," all-consuming quality that affects cognition, mood, and behavior. Failure to respond to appropriate therapy may be a result of noncompliance, inadequate dose or duration, or a lack of understanding and/or involvement in the treatment program.

DIVERTICULOSIS

In Western society, acquired diverticulosis affects approximately 5 to 10 percent of the population older than age 45 years and almost 80 percent of those older than age 85 years. Because uninflamed diverticula are asymptomatic, symptoms such as abdominal discomfort and altered bowel habits in patients with diverticulosis should be ascribed to coincident IBS rather than to "painful diverticulosis." Approximately 20 percent of patients with diverticula have an episode of symptomatic diverticulitis. Diverticular hemorrhage is the second commonest cause of colonic bleeding after vascular lesions.

Pathophysiology

Considerations relevant to the pathophysiology of diverticulosis include the orientation of taenia coli, the course taken by perforating arteries supplying the colonic wall, and changes in the biomechanical properties of the colon that accompany diverticulosis (as reviewed by Camilleri et al. [2000]). Colonic diverticula are mucosal pouches that

are pushed out between arcs of circular muscle at weak points; that is, where arteries pierce the muscularis propria in the spaces between the mesenteric taenia and the two antimesenteric taeniae. Thus, diverticula do not occur where the taenia fuse to form a longitudinal muscle layer surrounding the rectum.

A proposed sequence of events, partly evidence-based and partly speculative, leading to diverticulosis is as follows. The colonic circular and longitudinal muscle layers are thickened in diverticulosis. Microscopic observations demonstrate elastin deposition accompanied by shortening of taenia coli. In turn, this causes thickening of the circular muscle layer, which eventually folds upon itself, producing the concertina-like appearance and narrowing of the colonic lumen often observed on barium enema. When the lumen narrows, intraluminal pressures during contractions are higher, predisposing to mucosal outpouching and formation of diverticula, particularly in areas of low colonic compliance, such as the sigmoid colon. It has been speculated that a low-residue diet with diminished fecal bulk predisposes to colonic luminal narrowing and ultimately diverticulosis. However, there is no direct evidence to corroborate a cause and effect relationship between lack of dietary fiber and luminal narrowing or elastin deposition in the taenia coli. Formation of colonic diverticula is attributed to high intraluminal pressures, leading to mucosal protrusion through weak areas in the bowel wall. Epidemiologic studies have demonstrated an association with Western diets high in refined carbohydrates and low in dietary fiber.

Pathology

In the West, diverticulosis predominantly affects the sigmoid colon, but it may also involve the entire colon. Diverticula are formed by mucosal protrusion through weak areas, where the vasa recta penetrate the bowel wall. Consequently, they are arranged in rows, between the mesenteric and lateral taeniae coli. Light microscopy often reveals colonic smooth muscle thickening in diverticulosis. If undigested food blocks the neck of a diverticulum, the latter may distend and perforate; the perforation is generally walled off by the adjacent mesocolon or appendices epiploicae. Colovesical, and less frequently colovaginal and colocutaneous fistulae may occur. In contrast to the situation in colitis, the colonic mucosa is grossly and microscopically normal in acute diverticulitis, despite considerable inflammation of the pericolonic tissue.

Diverticulitis

Classification

Virtually all patients with diverticulitis have a microperforation. Stage I diverticulitis is characterized by small, confined pericolonic abscesses, while stage II disease includes larger, confined pericolonic collections. Stage III refers to patients with generalized suppurative peritonitis ("perforated diverticulitis"); because the diverticular neck is generally obstructive by a fecalith, peritoneal contamination by feces may not occur. In contrast, tearing of an uninflamed diverticulum causes fecal peritonitis or stage IV disease.

Clinical Features

Symptoms of diverticulitis include lower abdominal pain and altered bowel habits, typically diarrhea. While the stool may contain trace blood, profuse lower gastrointestinal bleeding is very uncommon in the setting of acute diverticulitis. Dysuria, urinary frequency, and urgency reflect bladder irritation, while pneumaturia, fecaluria, or recurrent urinary tract infection suggest a colovesical fistula. Physical findings include fever, left-lower-quadrant tenderness, and/or a lower abdominal or rectal mass.

Complications

In elderly patients, initial symptoms and signs may be less pronounced, response to medical therapy is less likely, free perforation is more frequent, and postoperative morbidity and mortality are greater. Rupture of a peridiverticular abscess or uninflamed diverticulum causes peritonitis. Repeated episodes of acute diverticulitis may lead to colonic obstruction. However, small-bowel obstruction occurs more frequently, especially in the presence of a large peridiverticular abscess. Jaundice or hepatic abscesses should raise concern about pylephlebitis. A massively dilated cecum (>10 cm), signs of cecal necrosis on abdominal radiography (i.e., air in the bowel wall), or marked tenderness of the right lower quadrant in the setting of a moderately dilated cecum mandate immediate surgery.

Diagnostic Studies

Contrast x-rays demonstrate diverticula but not diverticular inflammation. Moreover, contrast studies may dislodge an obstructing fecalith, causing a perforation. If the clinical features are highly suggestive of acute diverticulitis, more advanced imaging studies are unnecessary. If the diagnosis cannot be made by clinical features alone, or if an intraabdominal abscess is suspected, computed tomography (CT) is the preferred imaging modality. Moreover, CT-guided percutaneous drainage of an abscess can control systemic sepsis, permitting a single-stage surgical procedure, if necessary, at a later stage. The CT scan is falsely negative in up to 20 percent of cases with acute diverticulitis. While ultrasonography may also reveal diverticular inflammation, it is more operator-dependent than CT. Moreover, abdominal tenderness may preclude application of sufficient external pressure to visualize the intraabdominal contents. A flexible sigmoidoscopy is only necessary to exclude carcinoma or colitis, especially prior to surgery for complicated diverticulosis.

Differential Diagnosis

The clinical distinction between diverticulitis and nonperforating carcinoma is usually obvious, except when diverticulitis is complicated by a stricture or signs of extraluminal compression. Right-sided diverticulitis, which occurs rarely in the West, may mimic acute appendicitis.

Treatment of Acute Diverticulitis

The therapeutic approach is influenced by severity of clinical features, ability to tolerate oral hydration, and prior history of complicated diverticulosis.

Mild First Attack in Patients Who Tolerate Oral Hydration   Outpatient therapy with a liquid diet and a 10-day course of oral broad-spectrum antimicrobial therapy, including coverage against anaerobic microorganisms (i.e., ciprofloxacin and metronidazole). After the acute attack has resolved, a high dietary fiber content and a colonoscopy are advisable to exclude a diagnosis of cancer. Approximately 5 percent of patients will have a second attack within 2 years after medical treatment for the first attack of mild acute diverticulitis; others have noted higher rates of recurrence.

Severe Pain, Inability to Tolerate Oral Hydration, and Persistent Symptoms Despite Adequate Outpatient Therapy   Hospitalization, nothing by mouth, and broad-spectrum intravenous antibiotics. Preferred antibiotics include ampicillin, gentamicin, and metronidazole, or monotherapy with newer broad-spectrum antibiotics such as piperacillin or tazobactam. For pain relief, meperidine is preferred to morphine sulfate, which causes colonic spasm. Imaging studies should be considered if patients do not improve after 2 to 3 days of antibiotic therapy.

Radiologically assisted percutaneous drainage of peridiverticular abscesses more than 5 cm in diameter.

Surgical Intervention   *Emergent* surgery is reserved for generalized peritonitis, uncontrolled sepsis, and visceral perforation. *Urgent* operations are necessary in immunocompromised hosts or when the diagnosis of carcinoma cannot be definitively excluded. Indications for *elective* surgery include fistula formation or recurrent diverticulitis.

If surgical therapy can be deferred until acute inflammation heals, then a single-stage primary resection and reanastomosis procedure, potentially via a laparoscopic approach, can be accomplished with minimal morbidity and less than 1 percent mortality. For emergency indications, the first-stage of a two-stage procedure involves resection of the diseased segment, creation of an end colostomy with oversewing of the distal colonic or rectal stump (Hartmann's procedure). Colonic continuity is reestablished in the second operation; only 30 to 75 percent of the patients who undergo the first-stage resection go on to have colostomy closure.

Diverticular Hemorrhage

Nearly 50 percent of patients who are hospitalized for acute lower gastrointestinal bleeding are bleeding from uninflamed colonic diverticula, generally in the right colon. Diverticular hemorrhage is usually of minor clinical significance, although massive bleeding may occur in 5 percent of patients with diverticulosis. Patients with severe lower gastrointestinal hemorrhage, especially those taking nonsteroidal antiinflammatory medications, should first be examined with emergency upper endoscopy to exclude the possibility of a bleeding duodenal ulcer after fluid resuscitation. Urgent colonoscopy after thorough bowel lavage is indicated to identify stigmata of recent hemorrhage; that is, active bleeding (e.g., arterial spurting), nonbleeding visible vessels appearing as discrete pigmented or nonpigmented protuberances, and focally attached, adherent clots. These stigmata occur in up to 20 percent of patients with acute diverticular hemorrhage, and are associated with a higher risk of recurrent bleeding; endoscopic therapy reduces the risk of recurrent bleeding during the same admission in this group of patients. The risk of recurrent hemorrhage is not known but is estimated to be 20 to 30 percent after one episode, rising to approximately 50 percent after a second diverticular bleed. Emergency angiography and nuclear scanning techniques with ^{99m}Tc sulfur colloid and ^{99m}Tc-tagged red blood cells are alternatives to colonoscopy in patients with brisk (0.5 to 1 mL/min) and low (0.1 mL/min) bleeding rates respectively. Angiography also permits intraarterial infusion of vasopressin or selective embolization; however, the risk of colonic infarction after embolization is as high as 20 percent. Urgent surgery, generally a subtotal colectomy, is indicated for patients with continued severe bleeding and a negative angiogram. Elective colonic resection should be considered after two or more bleeding episodes requiring transfusion, if the source of bleeding has been clearly identified and the operative risk is acceptable. The risk of recurrent bleeding is approximately 20 to 30 percent after the first episode and approximately 50 percent after the second clinically significant episode of bleeding. Colonic resection, generally subtotal colectomy, should be considered after two or more episodes of diverticular bleeding.

COLONIC ISCHEMIA

Colonic ischemia is the most common intestinal vascular disorder in the elderly population; approximately 90 percent of patients are older than age 60 years. The intestines and colon are protected from ischemia by an abundant collateral circulation outside and within the bowel wall. These collateral pathways open in response to arterial hypotension to maintain adequate perfusion. However, prolonged ischemia may induce vasoconstriction, thereby reducing collateral flow. Colonic ischemia encompasses a spectrum of injury that most commonly affect the splenic flexure, descending, and sigmoid colon; systemic low-flow states, local nonocclusive ischemia, and ligation of the inferior mesenteric artery tend to affect the right colon watershed areas, that is, splenic flexure and rectosigmoid, and the sigmoid colon, respectively.

Etiology

Colonic ischemia may occur in association with shock, colon cancer, or after surgical intervention on the aorta or mesenteric vessels. However, in contrast to acute mesenteric ischemia, acute colonic ischemia is often not preceded by hemodynamic instability, and mesenteric angiograms do not disclose vascular occlusion. A recent study by

Koutronbakis et al. found hereditary and acquired thrombotic risk factors in 72 percent of patients with colonic ischemia; mean age was 65 years. These factors include antiphospholipid antibodies, protein C, protein S or antithrombin deficiency, factor V Leiden mutation, prothrombin gene mutations, and methylenetetrahydrofolate reductase C677T. Antiphospholipid antibodies and factor V Leiden mutation were significantly more common in colonic ischemia than in healthy controls and patients with diverticulitis; 25 percent patients had a combination of thrombophilic disorders. Other risk factors, particularly in younger patients, include oral contraceptives, cocaine use, long-distance running, sickle cell disease, and vasculitis. While the proximate cause of acute colonic ischemia is often unclear, the distribution of colonic ischemia, as described above, may provide clues. Nonocclusive injury usually involves longer segments of the colon, while atheromatous emboli, an unusual cause of colonic ischemia, involves shorter segments. Up to 10 percent of patients may have a potentially obstructing benign or malignant colonic stricture which impairs blood flow.

Clinical Features

The typical presenting symptom is acute onset of mild crampy left-lower-quadrant abdominal pain; severe pain may suggest transmural necrosis or small-bowel involvement. Pain is often accompanied or followed by bloody diarrhea or bright-red blood via the rectum. Because blood loss is generally modest, hemodynamically significant bleeding should prompt consideration of another diagnosis such as diverticular bleeding. Physical examination reveals mild to severe abdominal tenderness; persistent peritoneal signs raise the possibility of transmural necrosis or perforation.

Diagnostic Tests

The endoscopic and histopathologic appearances of colonic ischemia, a condition that predominantly affects the mucosa, are generally diagnostic. Endoscopy reveals varying degrees of inflammation, often segmental, within reach of the flexible sigmoidoscope in 50 to 60 percent cases (Fig. 51-1)(Color Plate 3). Overdistension during endoscopy or barium enema must be avoided because intraluminal pressures greater than 30 mmHg can diminish mucosal blood flow, increasing the risk of ischemic damage. Because colon cancer may cause or mimic ischemic colitis, a colonoscopy should be performed at an appropriate time in the course of the illness. Plane abdominal x-rays and barium enemas may reveal thumb printing, reflecting submucosal and mucosal hemorrhage and edema. Stool cultures for *Salmonella, Shigella, Campylobacter,* and *Escherichia coli* O157:H7 should be performed.

Course

In most cases, acute colonic ischemia resolves spontaneously; complete clinical and radiologic healing occurs

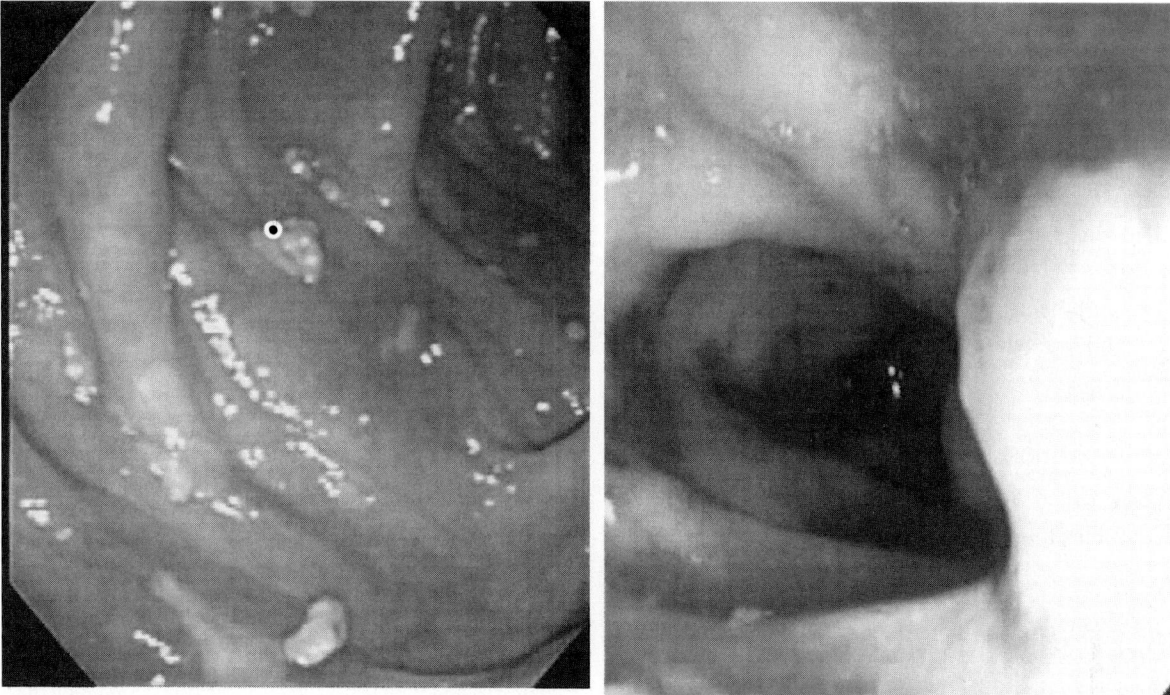

Figure 51-1   Ischemic colitis. Endoscopic appearance is varied, ranging from small ulcers surrounded by an erythematous rim (*left panel*) to a severely ulcerated segmental involvement (*right panel*).

within 1 to 2 weeks, and the condition does not recur. The remaining patients may present with gangrene and perforation, chronic ischemic colitis, or an ischemic colonic stricture.

Management

Management is supportive and includes optimization of cardiac function and bowel rest. Systemic glucocorticoids are of no proven value and may increase the chance of perforation.

Differential Diagnosis

In contrast to ischemic colitis, the rectum is invariably involved in ulcerative colitis. Rectal involvement is obvious at endoscopy. Of the infectious colitides, *E. coli* O157:H7 induces a colitis that mimics or may cause colonic ischemia. Although ischemia may also cause pseudomembranous colitis, *Clostridium difficile* colitis presents with watery, generally nonbloody diarrhea. Infrequently, chronic ischemic colitis may masquerade as a mass and a stricture, which can be distinguished from colon cancer only by an operation.

LOWER GASTROINTESTINAL BLEEDING IN THE ELDERLY PATIENT

By convention, lower gastrointestinal bleeding refers to bleeding distal to the ligament of Treitz. The incidence of lower GI bleeding increases 200-fold from the second to the eighth decade, reflecting the increased prevalence of the commonest causes of nonneoplastic lower GI bleeding; that is, colonic diverticula, angiodysplasia, and ischemic colitis. Lower gastrointestinal bleeding occurs less frequently and generally has a less-severe course than upper gastrointestinal bleeding in the elderly patient. Three questions need to be addressed in the context of lower GI bleeding: Is the bleeding acute or chronic? What is the bleeding location? Does the bleeding warrant urgent or emergency management?

Is the Bleeding Acute or Chronic?

Acute bleeding presenting as melena or hematochezia originates from the lower GI tract in approximately 20% of cases. Chronic bleeding generally manifests as anemia or positive fecal occult blood test results. Even physiologic blood loss from the colon (0.5 ± 0.4 mL/d) may produce a positive fecal occult blood test. However, a blood loss ≥ 10 mL/d is required to generate negative iron balance. Early indices of iron deficiency include absent bone marrow iron stores or a serum ferritin <45 ng/mL. Because ferritin is an acute phase reactant, a threshold of 100 ng/mL should be used in patients with chronic disease. Hypochromic microcytic anemia is a later manifestation of iron deficiency.

What is the Bleeding Location?

Hematochezia indicates bleeding from a colonic source in 90 percent or more of patients. Hematochezia from a more proximal source indicates severe bleeding, which is invariably associated with significant hemodynamic instability. Hematochezia limited to the toilet paper or the stool surface is most suggestive of perianal bleeding. Tenesmus suggests rectal bleeding. When blood is metabolized by bacteria, melena occurs.

Does the Bleeding Warrant Urgent or Emergency Management?

This decision is based on the presence of hemodynamic instability and coexistent morbidity.

Specific Etiologies

Diverticular Bleeding

Diverticular bleeding is covered separately in this chapter.

Angiodysplasia

Angiodysplasia is responsible for 3 to 12 percent of cases of acute lower intestinal bleeding. These lesions occur with equal frequency in men and women older than age 50 years; two-thirds of these lesions are found in patients older than age 70 years. The often-quoted association between bleeding from angiodysplasia and aortic stenosis is unproven. Angiodysplasias are usually multiple lesions, less than 5 mm in diameter, which bleed predominantly from the right colon. Less than 10 percent of patients with angiodysplasia will eventually experience bleeding, presenting either with acute bleeding, or iron-deficiency anemia and occult blood in stool. In more than 90 percent of cases, bleeding stops spontaneously. In an adequately prepared colon, these lesions may be identified during colonoscopy and treated by electrocautery (Fig. 51-2)(Color Plate 2). Angiography may be necessary to identify and treat lesions that are missed at colonoscopy. Other therapeutic options for angiodysplasia include endoscopic ablation of small and large intestinal lesions, and iron repletion and combined estrogen/progesterone therapy, particularly in patients with chronic renal failure.

Neoplasms

Colonic neoplasms may cause acute or occult lower GI bleeding; small-bowel tumors may be an underappreciated cause of frank or occult lower GI bleeding. Other clinical features of small-bowel tumors include weight loss, pain, or obstructive symptoms. Leiomyomas and leiomyosarcomas account for 50 percent of bleeding small intestinal neoplasms. Other small-bowel masses associated with bleeding include malformations such as cavernous hemangiomas or phlebectasias, and tumors such as adenomas or adenocarcinomas, lymphomas, and metastatic disease.

Ischemic Colitis

Ischemic colitis is discussed separately in this chapter.

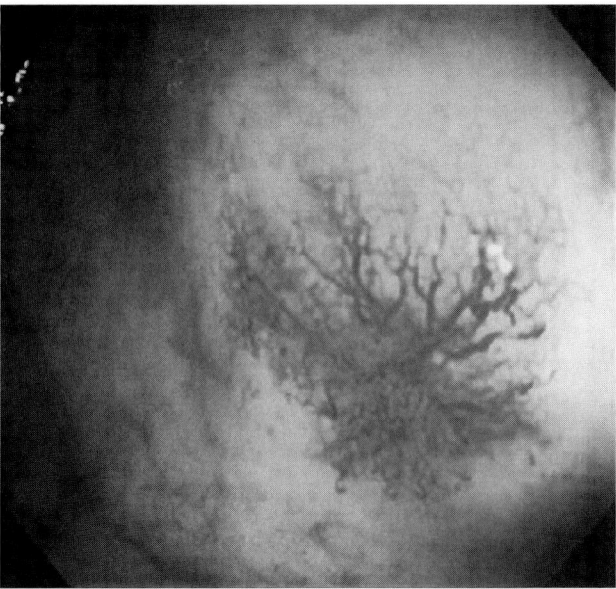

Figure 51-2   Colonic angiodysplasia. Cecal angiodysplasia with the appearance of a spider nevus. The specific nature of a vascular lesion cannot be identified with confidence at endoscopy because several lesions, that is, vascular ectasia, spider angiomas, hereditary hemorrhagic telangiectasia, and angiomas resemble each other.

Other Causes

Patients with infectious colitis, especially *Salmonella* and *E. coli* O157:H7, typically present with crampy abdominal pain and watery diarrhea, followed by bloody diarrhea. Older persons are also more subject to pseudomembranous colitis, in which lower gastrointestinal bleeding is uncommon and generally not severe. *Dieulafoy lesion of the colon* is an unusually large submucosal artery that travels through a tortuous course in the submucosa and erodes through a single 3- to 5-mm defect. The artery appears normal by histology. While *radiation proctitis* generally presents with rectal bleeding 9 to 15 months after radiotherapy, bleeding may be delayed for up to 41 months. Other symptoms of rectal mucosal involvement include transient diarrhea accompanied by tenesmus, mild abdominal cramps, and mucoid or bloody discharge. Sigmoidoscopy reveals characteristic mucosal telangiectases and permits endoscopic treatment of lesions by laser therapy or topical formalin. Patients with chronic proctocolitis may have intermittent bleeding of mild to moderate severity. *Hemorrhoidal* bleeding is generally intermittent and characterized by small amounts of bright-red blood coating the outside of formed stool, in the bowl or on toilet tissue after a bowel movement. Hemorrhoids may occasionally cause severe hemorrhage. *Perianal fissures* most commonly present with blood on the toilet paper or stool surface; they can be distinguished from hemorrhoidal bleeding by symptoms of perianal discomfort and a visible midline mucosal defect or sentinel tag. *Postpolypectomy bleeding* may be either early or delayed (up to 15 days after polypectomy). Early bleeding may occur from a blood vessel in the stalk before adequate hemostasis; delayed bleeding may be attributable to a sloughed off clot. *Stercoral ulcers,* which develop under an adherent mass of hard stool most frequently in the rectosigmoid and sometimes in the transverse colon, may be the source of massive hemorrhage, especially when overlying adherent stool is removed by manual disimpaction. Other causes of lower intestinal bleeding include trauma from an endoscopic procedure or enema catheter, solitary rectal ulcer syndrome, portal colopathy, colonic varices, endometriosis, and bleeding from the appendiceal orifice.

Initial Assessment and Diagnostic Options for Lower GI Hemorrhage in the Elderly Patient

Management includes assessment and intravenous correction of hemodynamic instability, identification of a bleeding source, and cause-tailored therapy. Autonomic dysfunction may exacerbate, while beta-blockers may reduce orthostatic blood pressure and heart rate changes resulting from GI bleeding, respectively. Despite hypovolemia, the hematocrit may be normal initially; serial estimations help guide blood transfusion. Absolute indications for transfusions include continued bleeding despite therapy, shock, low hematocrit (<20 percent or less than 25 percent), or symptoms of poor oxygenation (e.g., angina). Excessive fluid administration may provoke heart failure. A baseline electrocardiogram and chest x-ray are useful for identifying present or future overt or silent myocardial ischemia, congestive heart failure, or pulmonary aspiration. In patients with melena, a rise in blood urea nitrogen is more suggestive of upper GI bleeding; this abnormality, which results from volume depletion and intestinal absorption of protein, is more pronounced in elderly patients.

After colonic lavage, colonoscopy is generally safe and necessary in patients with melena or hematochezia. However, the diagnostic yield and therapeutic utility of colonoscopy is lower as compared to the utility of upper endoscopy in acute upper gastrointestinal bleeding. Not infrequently, colonoscopy reveals altered blood and diverticulosis, sufficing to exclude a colonic tumor and a mucosal process such as ischemic, infectious, or ulcerative colitis in a reasonably prepared colon. In that scenario, the bleeding is likely attributable either to diverticula or a vascular source, typically angiodysplasia, or infrequently, a Dieulafoy lesion. The colonoscopy should be repeated in an adequately prepared colon to identify vascular lesions that may have been missed during the initial examination. Angiography may identify and localize a source, provided bleeding is relatively brisk (>0.5 mL/min); these lesions appear as an ectatic, slowly emptying vein, vascular tuft, or early filling vein. ^{99m}Tc-tagged red blood cell radionuclide scans can detect a bleeding rate as low as 0.1 mL/min. While active bleeding is required for diagnosis, the patient may be scanned repeatedly over 12 to 24 hours to identify intermittent bleeding. The accuracy of bleeding scans is variable, and the false-positive rate for bleeding increases significantly 15 hours after injection. Other options for patients with obscure lower GI bleeding include push enteroscopy with a pediatric colonoscope, permitting examination 40 to 60 cm beyond the ligament of Treitz, specially designed push enteroscopes, which extend the examination for 200 to 250 cm, and Sonde enteroscopy, which is a cumbersome procedure requiring 6 hours or longer to reach the ileum. A recent invention, wireless capsule endoscopy, may be useful for identifying a bleeding source in patients with obscure GI bleeding. Surgical exploration may be necessary for a small group of patients with obscure lower GI bleeding; intraoperative enteroscopy has been reported to identify abnormalities in up to 100 percent of patients. Because melena or hematochezia may be potentially treatable manifestations of an upper gastrointestinal bleeding source, such as a peptic ulcer, an upper gastrointestinal endoscopy should be considered in patients who present with these symptoms.

MEGACOLON

Megacolon means an enlarged colon, which may be acute or chronic. In the *acute* setting, the diagnosis of megacolon is based on a cecal diameter greater than 12 cm. The risk of perforation or ischemia is related to the size and duration of cecal distension. These complications are more likely when the diameter exceeds 12 cm. When the dilatation is persistent or *chronic*, the proposed cutoff is a bowel width above 6.5 cm at the rectosigmoid junction.

Acute Megacolon

Acute megacolon generally occurs in the setting of an intercurrent illness or a surgical operation not necessarily affecting the colon. This syndrome of pseudo-obstruction is named after Ogilvie, who described two patients with constipation, colicky abdominal pain, and dilatation of the right colon. He erroneously attributed colonic dilatation to reduced sympathetic input to the bowel, leaving the parasympathetic action unopposed. Actually, the sympathetic nervous system *inhibits* colonic motility, primarily via α_2-adrenoreceptor–mediated inhibition of acetylcholine release in the myenteric plexus and pelvic parasympathetic plexus. Thus, reflex sympathetic *stimulation* is a potential pathophysiologic mechanism for paralytic ileus and acute colonic pseudo-obstruction.

The precipitating factors for Ogilvie's syndrome, which generally occurs in elderly subjects, include orthopedic surgical procedures or injuries involving the pelvis, hips or knees, pelvic and abdominal surgery, narcotics, obstetric procedures, metabolic imbalance, and neurologic conditions. A high index of suspicion is necessary to make the diagnosis, because patients may not complain of abdominal discomfort and only have modest distension. Flat and upright abdominal radiographs will confirm the diagnosis and disclose whether there is generalized ileus. A Hypaque enema excludes mechanical obstruction and may be therapeutic.

The initial management of hospitalized patients with Ogilvie's syndrome includes treatment of the underlying cause, exclusion of mechanical obstruction, correction of metabolic disturbances, and discontinuation of medications that suppress colonic motility, particularly narcotics and anticholinergic agents. Nasogastric suction, rectal tubes, and frequent changes in the patient's position are often helpful. Until recently, the primary therapeutic

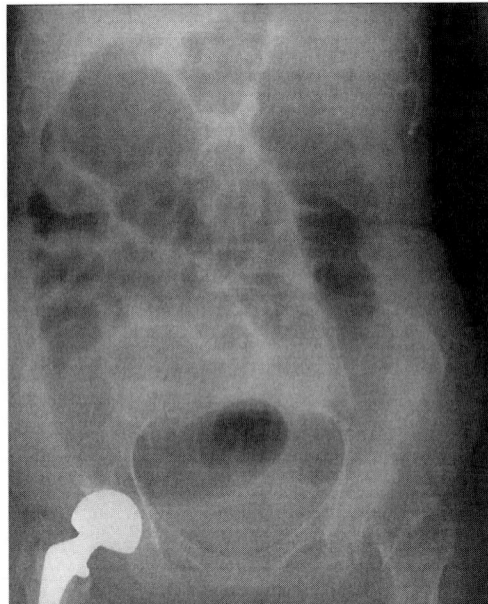 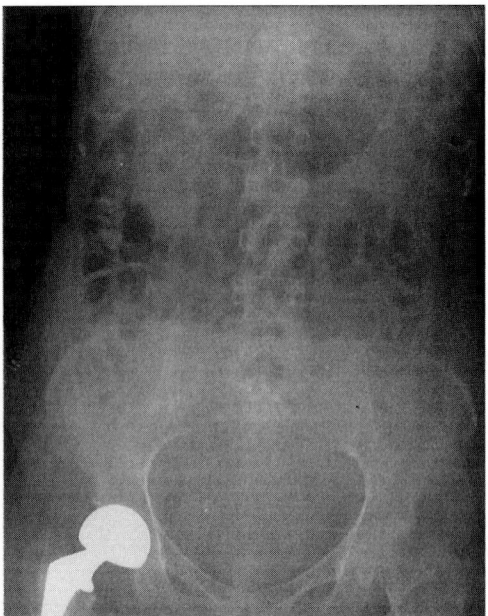

Figure 51-3   Acute colonic pseudo-obstruction. Upright plain x-rays of the abdomen reveal diffuse, but predominantly right colonic distension, with a cecal diameter of 13 cm, that developed after placement of a right hip prosthesis for a fractured femur (*left panel*). Colonic distention resolved shortly after intravenous neostigmine (*right panel*).

option for patients with Ogilvie's syndrome who had not responded to conservative measures was endoscopic decompression of the colon. A placebo-controlled study confirmed the efficacy of the cholinesterase inhibitor neostigmine (1 to 2 mg IV or SQ) in Ogilvie's syndrome (Fig. 51-3). Relative contraindications to neostigmine include a heart rate <50 beats per minute or systolic blood pressure <90 mmHg; sick sinus syndrome or history of second or third degree arteriovenous block without a pacemaker; and active bronchospasm requiring medication. After neostigmine administration, patients should be monitored closely, not necessarily in an ICU setting.

When neostigmine is contraindicated or ineffective, colonoscopic tube decompression enables exclusion of mechanical obstruction and reduces cecal diameter, as measured on plain abdominal radiographs, in 70 percent of patients. The condition will recur in 40 percent of these patients, however, necessitating another colonoscopy. The risk of recurrence may be reduced by placing a drainage tube in the right colon during the initial colonoscopy. Colonoscopy of an unprepared bowel can be technically difficult and complicated by perforation.

The overall prognosis of patients with acute colonic pseudoobstruction is poor, with an in-hospital mortality approaching 30 percent, attributable primarily to the severity of underlying illness. The most dire complication of acute dilatation is colonic perforation, which occurred in 3 percent cases in one retrospective series.

Toxic Megacolon

Toxic megacolon refers to total or segmental nonobstructive colonic dilatation associated with systemic toxicity, generally in patients with idiopathic inflammatory bowel disease or infectious colitis. Less-frequent causes include ischemic colitis, volvulus, diverticulitis, and obstructive colon cancer. Responsible organisms for infectious colitis range from conventional bacterial pathogens, such as shigellosis, to opportunistic pathogens (cytomegalovirus [CMV], protozoa, mycobacteria, fungi) in immunosuppressed patients. CMV colitis may also precipitate toxic megacolon in patients with inflammatory bowel disease. Treatment includes specific medical therapy for the underlying disorder, bowel rest, decompression with nasogastric aspiration, and close monitoring in an intensive care unit by medical and surgical teams. A colectomy is necessary in up to 50 percent of cases; indications for urgent operation include perforation, massive hemorrhage, increasing transfusion requirements, signs of toxicity, and progressive colonic dilatation. Timing an operation for patients with persistent colonic distension who seem to be improving may vary from 48 hours to 7 days.

Chronic Megacolon

Chronic megacolon in the elderly invariably occurs in patients with longstanding constipation of varied etiologies (Table 51-3). Patients with acquired megacolon may also present acutely with sigmoid volvulus. In other forms of chronic megacolon, surgery is occasionally necessary to alleviate refractory constipation or abdominal discomfort unresponsive to conservative measures. Colectomy offers good results with few complications in the treatment of idiopathic megacolon, and an ileorectal anastomosis is the preferred operation.

Table 51-3   Causes of Megacolon

Acute

    Ogilvie's syndrome: secondary to medical or surgical illness

    Toxic megacolon: secondary to inflammatory or infectious colitis

Chronic

    Congenital: Hirschsprung's disease

    Acquired

Idiopathic

    Psychogenic: "institutional colon"

    Neurologic diseases: Parkinson's disease, diabetic and other autonomic neuropathies, multiple sclerosis, intestinal pseudo-obstruction

    Disorders of smooth muscle: scleroderma, amyloidosis, myopathies

    Metabolic: hypothyroidism, hypokalemia, porphyria, pheochromocytoma

    Rectoanal pain: fissures, abscesses

SOURCE: Reproduced with permission from Bharucha AE and Phillips SF (1999).

ACKNOWLEDGMENTS

This study was supported in part by National Institutes of Health grants RO1 DK54681 and K24 DK02638 (Dr. M. Camilleri), and RO1 HD38666 and RO 1 HD-41129 (Dr. A.E. Bharucha).

REFERENCES

Anonymous: American Gastroenterological Association medical position statement: Guidelines on intestinal ischemia [erratum appears in *Gastroenterology* 119:280, 2000]. *Gastroenterology* 118:951, 2000.

Barkin JS, Ross BS: Medical therapy for chronic gastrointestinal bleeding of obscure origin. *Am J Gastroenterol* 93:1250, 1998.

Bharucha AE, Camilleri M: Functional abdominal pain in the elderly, in Friedman LS, Farrell JJ (eds): *Gastroenterology Clinics of North America: Gastrointestinal Diseases in the Elderly.* Philadelphia, WB Saunders, 2001, p 517.

Bharucha AE, Phillips SF: Megacolon: Acute, toxic, and chronic. *Curr Treat Options Gastroenterol* 2:517, 1999.

Camilleri M, Ford M: Review article: Colonic sensorimotor physiology in health, and its alteration in constipation and diarrhoeal disorders. *Aliment Pharmacol Ther* 12:287, 1998.

Camilleri M et al: Insights into the pathophysiology and mechanisms of constipation, irritable bowel syndrome, and diverticulosis in older people. *J Am Geriatr Soc* 48:1142, 2000.

Camilleri M et al: Gastrointestinal sensation: Mechanisms and relation to functional GI disorders, in Camilleri M (ed): *Gastroenterology Clinics of North America, Gastrointestinal Motility in Clinical Practice.* Philadelphia, WB Saunders, 1996, p 247.

Ferzoco LB et al: Acute diverticulitis. *N Engl J Med* 338:1521, 1998.

Gostout CJ: The role of endoscopy in managing acute lower gastrointestinal bleeding. *N Engl J Med* 342:125, 2000.

Jensen DM et al: Urgent colonoscopy for the diagnosis and treatment of severe diverticular hemorrhage. *N Engl J Med* 342:78, 2000.

Koutroubakis IE et al: Role of acquired and hereditary thrombotic risk factors in colon ischemia of ambulatory patients. *Gastroenterology* 121:561, 2001.

Ponec RJ et al: Neostigmine for the treatment of acute colonic pseudo-obstruction. *N Engl J Med* 341:137, 1999.

Rockey DC: Occult gastrointestinal bleeding. *N Engl J Med* 341:38, 1999.

Constipation in Older People

DANIELLE HARARI

Constipation is a frequent health concern for elderly people and their health care providers in outpatient, inpatient, and long-term care settings. The number of physician visits for constipation increases markedly among people older than age 60 years, as does regular use of laxatives. The self-reported symptom of constipation is associated with anxiety, depression, and poor health perception in older people, while clinical constipation in vulnerable individuals may lead to costly complications such as constipation-related hospital admissions, fecal impaction, overflow incontinence, sigmoid volvulus, and urinary retention. This chapter describes the epidemiology, pathogenesis, causes, diagnosis, and treatment of constipation in elderly people. Data sources were a computer-assisted search of the English language literature (1966 to present), systematic review web sites including the Cochrane database, reference lists from recent systematic reviews and book chapters, and expert committee reports and opinion. Strength of recommendations (A to D) are based on recognized evidence levels (Oxford Centre for Evidence Based Medicine) as follows: (A) meta-analysis of randomized controlled trials, or at least one randomized controlled trial; (B) at least one good quality cohort or case-control study; (C) case series (and poor quality cohort or case-control studies); (D) expert committee reports or opinion.

DEFINITION

The applied definitions of constipation in older people in medical and nursing literature are inconsistent. Studies tend to define constipation subjectively by self-report, according to specific bowel-related symptoms, or by daily laxative usage. Few epidemiologic studies of constipation in older people use objective assessment-based definitions. In clinical practice, the feeling of being constipated will often mean different things to different individuals. While the nonspecific and subjective definition of *self-reported constipation* ("Do you suffer from constipation?") provides insight into how individuals perceive their bowel habit, standardized definitions of constipation subtypes based on specific symptoms are more useful for both clinical and research purposes (Rome II criteria, updated 1999) (Table 52-1). These definitions for *functional constipation*

and *rectal outlet delay* are still, however, symptom-based; the definition of *clinical* constipation relies on finding excessive stool retention in the rectum and/or colon by digital rectal examination or plain abdominal radiography.

EPIDEMIOLOGY

Self-Reported Constipation

The generally held belief that constipation is an inevitable consequence of aging stems partly from questionnaire-based studies showing a marked increase of self-reported constipation with age. One community-based study asking the question, "Do you have recurrent constipation?" of persons aged 65 years and older (n = 3166), found a prevalence of 26 percent in women and 16 percent in men; in the 84+ years age group, prevalence was 34 percent and 26 percent, respectively. Age was a strong independent risk factor for self-reported constipation. Other community studies support the relationship of age with self-reported constipation, and show prevalence rates of up to 34 percent of women and 30 percent of men older than age 65 years. The preponderance of women over men reporting constipation tends to attenuate beyond the age of 80 years.

Infrequent Bowel Movements

In contrast, the weekly frequency of bowel movements does not alter with aging alone, with only 1 to 7 percent of both younger and older community-dwelling individuals reporting frequency below the normal range (two or fewer bowel movements a week). This consistent bowel pattern across age groups persists even after statistical adjustment for the greater amount of laxatives used by elderly people. Community-based studies of older people show that among those complaining of constipation, less than 10 percent report two or fewer weekly bowel movements, and more than 50 percent move their bowels daily. Physical frailty in older persons does, however, increase the risk of self-report of infrequent bowel movements: 17 percent of nursing home residents and 14 percent of geriatric day-hospital attendees report two or fewer bowel movements a week. Among

Table 52-1   Definitions of Constipation

Self-Reported Constipation
Patient reports usual bowel habit as being constipated

Functional Constipation
2 or more of the following should be present for at least 12 weeks out of the preceding 12 months: 3 or fewer bowel movements per week Straining at least a quarter of the time Lumpy and/or hard stools at least a quarter of the time Feeling of incomplete evacuation at least a quarter of the time

Rectal Outlet Delay
Feeling of anal blockage at least a quarter of the time *and* Prolonged defecation (>10 minutes to complete bowel movement); *or* Need for self-digitation (pressing in or around the anus to aid evacuation) on any occasion

Clinical Constipation
Large amount of feces in rectum on digital examination *and/or* Excessive fecal retention in the colon on abdominal radiograph

long-term care residents self-reporting constipation, 33 percent have two or fewer bowel movements a week.

Difficult Evacuation

The implication is that bowel-related symptoms other than infrequent bowel movements also drive self-reporting of constipation in elderly persons. These symptoms are primarily straining and passage of hard stools; of older people reporting constipation in a US community study, 65 percent had persistent straining and 39 percent had passage of hard bowel movements. Constipated older people tend to suffer chiefly from difficulties with rectal evacuation, as shown by a prevalence rate of 21 percent for rectal outlet delay among community-dwelling people aged 65 years and older. Thirty percent of nursing home residents report persistent straining.

Constipation Symptoms in the Long-term Care Setting

In a Finnish study, Kinnunen found the prevalence of functional constipation and/or rectal outlet delay to be 57 percent in women and 64 percent in men living in residential homes, and 79 percent and 81 percent respectively in the nursing home setting. The high prevalence of constipation

in the nursing home setting is all the more striking in that 50 to 74 percent of long-term care residents use one or more daily laxative. Advancing age is an independent risk factor for heavy laxative use and symptom-based constipation among elderly nursing home patients. Evidence, mainly from case series, suggests that complications of constipation, such as fecal impaction, overflow, constipation-related hospital admission, sigmoid volvulus, bladder outlet obstruction, and stercoral perforation, are more likely to impact frailer older people.

Table 52-2 provides practice guidance based on evidence from epidemiologic studies of constipation in older people.

PATHOPHYSIOLOGY

Overall, the data suggest that physiologic changes in the lower bowel predisposing toward constipation in older people are not primarily age-related. Extrinsic causes such as reduced mobility, fluid intake, dietary fiber, comorbidities, and medication all impact colonic motility and transit (see below) and influence the pathophysiology of constipation.

Colonic Function

Colonic motility depends on the integrity of the central and autonomic nervous systems, gut wall innervation and receptors, circular smooth muscle, and gastrointestinal hormones. Propagating motor complexes in the colon are stimulated by increased intraluminal pressure generated by bulky fecal content. Studies of total gut transit time (passage of radiopaque markers from mouth to anus, normally 80 percent passed within 5 days), colonic motor activity, and postprandial gastrocolic reflex are no different in healthy elderly people as compared with healthy young people. In contrast, elderly people with symptoms of functional constipation tend to have a prolonged total gut transit time, ranging from 4 to 9 days. Radiologic markers pass especially slowly through the left colon in these individuals, with striking evacuation delay in the rectosigmoid, suggesting that total transit time is prolonged because of segmental dysmotility in the "hindgut." The prolongation in transit time is substantially greater in institutionalized or bedridden patients with constipation as compared with ambulatory elderly patients, with total gut transit time ranging from 6 to more than 14 days. Slow transit results in a cycle of worsening colonic dysfunction by reducing water content of stool (normally 75 percent) and shrinking fecal bulk, which then diminishes the intraluminal pressures, and hence the generation of propagating motor complexes and propulsive activity.

Intrinsic Mechanisms for Colonic Dysfunction in Older People with Constipation

Slower transit in elderly people often results from multiple causes, including chronic illness, immobility, and drugs. However, certain intrinsic mechanisms for altered colonic function in older persons with constipation have been postulated from physiologic studies (Table 52-3). Direct electrophysiologic measurement of colonic motor activity

Table 52-2   Practice Guidance Based on Epidemiological Evidence

Constipation-related symptoms should be routinely enquired about in all patients aged 65 years and over in view of the high prevalence of the condition in this population [B]

Both men and women in their 8th decade and beyond should in particular be regularly screened for constipation symptoms, as the prevalence rate increases with advancing age [B]

A clear understanding of the specific bowel symptoms each older individual has when reporting constipation is important in guiding the health care provider toward appropriate management of this common complaint [B]

Reduced bowel movement frequency is not a sensitive clinical indicator for constipation in older people [B], though it is specific [C]. Difficulty with evacuation and rectal outlet delay should be carefully identified as these are primary symptoms in older individuals [B]

A careful and objective assessment should be undertaken in all frail older individuals self-reporting constipation and/or difficulty with evacuation, as these patients are at increased risk of clinical constipation and associated complications [B]

Periodic objective assessment for constipation in elderly nursing home residents should be incorporated into routine nursing and medical care [B]. Patients unable to report symptoms due to cognitive or communication difficulties should be especially targetted [D]. Such an assessment should occur at a minimum every 3 months (3 monthly incidence rate of new-onset constipation is 7% in nursing home residents), and optimally monthly [C].

All elderly patients being prescribed laxatives on a daily basis should be regularly reviewed for symptoms of constipation and the appropriateness of long-term laxative therapy [C]

The identification of risk factors for constipation in elderly individuals is critical to achieving effective management of the condition [B]

A systematic process for identifying numerous risk factors in vulnerable older people with constipation should be incorporated into good practice guidelines in primary care, acute hospitals and nursing homes [C]

An integrative approach to risk assessment in constipated patients in all healthcare settings involving nursing and medical staff should be established [D]

Patients at increased risk of constipation from recognised causes (see Table 4) should be periodically and objectively assessed for the condition

See text for evidence-based rating scale

in elderly subjects has shown that the sigmoid motor response to intraluminal bisacodyl (a direct stimulant of the myenteric plexus), is diminished in patients who are constipated, implying a deficit in intrinsic innervation. Myenteric plexus dysfunction may partially account for impaired gut motility in elderly persons with constipation, but while neuronal body loss and axonal degeneration have been observed in the colons of younger patients with severe idiopathic constipation, there are no similar histologic studies in elderly patients with functional constipation. Furthermore, the findings from such studies of severely constipated subjects may be confounded by prolonged usage of stimulant laxatives, which in itself may be a possible cause of myenteric plexus degeneration. Another possible intrinsic factor is an age-related deficit in the density of inhibitory nerves, or in the binding sites on smooth muscle for inhibitory gut neuropeptides; in vitro studies of colons across age groups showed an age-related reduction in the amplitude of inhibitory junction potentials, but no decrease in the levels of inhibitory gut neuropeptides. This age-related decline occurs earlier in women as compared with men. Such a decrease in inhibitory nerve input to the circular smooth muscle could result in segmental

motor incoordination, which may lengthen transit time and promote constipation in older persons with other predisposing risk factors. Individuals older than age 60 years have higher plasma concentrations of β-endorphin with increased binding to opiate receptors in the gut wall and myenteric plexus. Higher opiate binding has the effect of relaxing colonic tone, reducing motility, and inhibiting the gastrocolic reflex, and may partly underlie the clinical observation that older people are more susceptible to the constipating effects of exogenous opiates. Parenthetically, recent studies have demonstrated that low-dose naloxone (an intestinal opioid receptor blocker) improves symptoms of constipation and reduces laxative use without reversing analgesia in severely constipated patients receiving opiates for chronic pain.

Anorectal Function

In normal defecation, colonic activity propels stool into the rectal ampulla causing distension and reflexic intrinsically mediated relaxation of the internal anal sphincter followed promptly by reflex contraction of the external anal

Table 52-3 Pathophysiological Mechanisms for Constipation in Older People

Functional Constipation
Intrinsic myenteric plexus dysfunction
Reduced inhibitory nerve input to circular muscle (age-related)
Increased binding of plasma endorphins to gut receptors (age-related)
Prolonged transit due to extrinsic factors (immobility, diet, drugs, comorbidity)

Rectal Outlet Delay
Rectal dyschezia secondary to suppression or disregard of urge to pass stool
Sacral cord dysfunction
Pelvic floor descent
Paradoxical contraction of pelvic floor muscles
Irritable bowel disease
Weak abdominal musculature

sphincter and pelvic floor muscles; these are skeletal muscles innervated by the pudendal nerve. The brain registers a desire to defecate, the external sphincter is voluntarily relaxed, and the rectum is evacuated with assistance from abdominal wall muscle contraction.

Age-Related Changes in Anorectal Function

There is a tendency toward an age-related decline in internal sphincter tone particularly in the eighth decade onward; clinically, this predisposes older individuals to fecal incontinence rather than to constipation. There is a more definite age-related decline (greater in women than men) in external anal sphincter and pelvic muscle strength, which can contribute toward evacuation difficulties. In simulated defecation studies, 37 percent of older subjects without constipation were unable to evacuate a small solid sphere. Consequent prolonged straining may compress the pudendal nerve further exacerbating any preexisting weakness. There appears to be a reduction in rectal motility with normal aging, again in older old age. Rectal sensation does not alter with normal aging.

Anorectal Dysfunction in Older Persons

Older persons with constipation may have one or more of three types of anorectal pathophysiology, all of which may lead to symptoms of chronic straining and rectal outlet delay, and a risk of continuous fecal soiling from chronic rectal impactions.

The most common disorder is "rectal dyschezia" characterized by reduced rectal motility, increased rectal compliance with a variable degree of rectal dilatation, and impaired rectal sensation such that the urge to pass stool is blunted, and an increasing degree of rectal distension is

required to reflexly the defecation mechanism. Such patients tend to have rectal impactions of hard or soft stool on digital examination of which they may be unaware. One postulated primary cause for rectal dyschezia is diminished parasympathetic outflow as a result of impaired sacral cord function, for example, from ischemia or spinal stenosis (Table 52-3). More commonly, the condition may develop secondarily to a persistent disregard or suppression of the urge to pass stool (central neurogenic disinhibition), as occurs in patients with dementia, depression, immobility, or painful anorectal conditions. Some older people will suffer from "pelvic dyssynergia," although this condition is more common in younger women with constipation. There is failure to relax the puborectalis and external anal sphincter muscles during attempted defecation, and manometric studies show paradoxical increases in anal canal pressure on straining. This abnormal expulsion pattern is seen in individuals with symptoms of rectal outlet delay for many years, and in patients with Parkinson's disease. The third type of pathology is "irritable bowel disease" characterized by increased rectal tone and reduced compliance. These patients may complain of difficult passage of small fecal pellets and other symptoms of irritable bowel syndrome, which is often constipation predominant in older people, such as passage of mucus, abdominal distension, and pain.

PREDISPOSING CAUSES OF CONSTIPATION

Thus, the pathophysiologic basis for constipation in older people is not primarily age-related, emphasizing the importance of identifying predisposing causes for the condition in each affected individual. One prospective study examined baseline characteristics predictive of new-onset functional constipation in elderly nursing home patients, using the US Minimum Data Set instrument. Seven percent ($n = 1291$) developed constipation over a 3-month period. Independent predictors were white race, poor consumption of fluids, pneumonia, Parkinson's disease, allergies, decreased bed mobility, arthritis, greater than five medications, dementia, hypothyroidism and hypertension. The authors postulated that allergies, arthritis, and hypertension were associated primarily because of the constipating effect of drugs used to treat these conditions. Other studies have shown that institutionalization itself is an independent risk factor for symptom-based constipation in older people. Table 52-4 summarizes evidence based causes of constipation in the elderly population.

Reduced Mobility

Impaired mobility is a common risk factor for constipation in older people. Greater physical activity is associated with less self-reported and symptom-specific constipation in older people living both at home and in long-term care. Reduced mobility was found to be the strongest independent correlate of heavy laxative use among nursing home residents, following adjustment for age, comorbidity and other relevant clinical factors. Gut transit time in elderly subjects was measured independently as 3 days in the ambulant,

Table 52-4 Causes of Constipation in Older People

Functional Constipation

Medications

Polypharmacy (>= 5 medications)
Anticholinergic drugs (tricyclics, antipsychotics, antihistamines, antiemetics, drugs for detrusor hyperactivity)
Opiates
Iron supplements
Calcium channel antagonists
Calcium supplements
Nonsteroidal anti-inflammatory drugs

Impaired Mobility

Neurological conditions
Parkinson's disease
Diabetes mellitus
Autonomic neuropathy
Stroke
Spinal cord injury or disease

Dehydration

Low dietary fiber
Metabolic disturbances
Hypothyroidism
Hypercalcemia
Hypokalemia

Mechanical Obstruction (e.g. tumor)

Rectal Outlet Delay
Dementia
Depression
Parkinson's disease
Lumbar stenosis
Lack of privacy or comfort
Anorectal disease or prior surgery

Self-Reported Constipation

Misperceptions regarding normal bowel habit
Anxiety/depression

Polypharmacy and Drug Side Effects

Polypharmacy itself increases the risk of constipation in older patients, particularly in nursing homes where each individual takes an average of six prescribed medications per day. Overall, constipation as a drug side effect is likely to be substantially under-reported in the elderly. Certain classes of drugs are particularly implicated in promoting constipation. Drugs with strong anticholinergic properties reduce contractility of the smooth muscle of the gut via an antimuscarinic effect at acetylcholine receptor sites, and in some cases, long-term use may induce chronic colonic dysmotility. In two cross-sectional studies of nursing home residents, anticholinergic antidepressants were independently associated with daily laxative use (following adjustment for age, gender, function, and cognition); anticholinergic neuroleptics and antihistamines were also independently associated in one of the studies. Nonanticholinergic sedatives, however, were not found to be constipating. As described above, older people are highly susceptible to the constipating effects of opiate analgesia. All types of iron supplements (sulphate, fumarate, and gluconate) have the same propensity to cause constipation in adults as the constipating factor is the amount of elemental iron that is absorbed. While slow-release capsules and tablets tend to have a lesser impact on the large bowel, this is because these preparations are likely to carry the iron past the first part of the duodenum into an area of the gut where conditions for elemental iron absorption are poor. Calcium channel antagonists impair lower gut motility, particularly in the rectosigmoid, by inhibition of calcium uptake into smooth muscle cells and alteration of intraluminal electrolyte and water transportation. Severe constipation has been reported in elderly patients taking calcium channel antagonists; nifedipine and verapamil are more potent inhibitors of gut motility than diltiazem and newer agents. Nonsteroidal antiinflammatory drugs (NSAIDs) increase the risk of constipation in older people, most likely through prostaglandin inhibition. In a large case-controlled primary care study, constipation and straining were more common in NSAID users, and constipation was a more common reason for stopping medication than dyspepsia. These studies did not, however, adjust for the possible confounder of arthritis impacting mobility.

Neurologic Conditions

There are a number of neurologic conditions prevalent in older people that are associated with constipation. Parkinson's disease can cause severe constipation symptoms; patients suffer from dual pathologies of primary degeneration of dopaminergic neurons in the myenteric plexus resulting in prolonged transit throughout the colon and rectum, and pelvic dyssynergia resulting in rectal outlet delay and prolonged straining. These symptoms can become prominent even early in the course of the disease, and may significantly impact quality of life.

Diabetes mellitus also causes constipation; a survey of outpatients in a diabetic clinic showed that 60 percent complained of constipation. Patients with autonomic neuropathy are more likely to be affected because of markedly

and 3 weeks in bedridden patients, although comorbid factors are likely to be contributory. A study of healthy young male volunteers, however, showed that after 1 week of bed rest, both transit through the sigmoid colon and stool frequency were reduced. Likewise, it is well-documented that exercise increases colonic propulsive activity ("joggers diarrhea"), especially when measured postprandially.

slowed transit throughout the colon, and impairment of the gastrocolic reflex. Overall gut dysmotility leads to bacterial overgrowth and the clinical presentation of explosive diarrhea; treatment with erythromycin and long-term motility agents such as metoclopramide should be considered in these individuals and in those with autonomic neuropathy due to other causes.

Dementia predisposes individuals to rectal dyschezia, partly through ignoring the urge to defecate. A study in which young men deliberately suppressed defecation resulted in prolonged transit through the rectosigmoid with a marked reduction in frequency of bowel movements. Epidemiologic studies show a significant association between cognitive impairment and nurse-documented constipation in nursing home residents.

Depression, psychological distress, and anxiety are all associated with increased self-reporting of constipation in older persons. In certain cases, the symptom of constipation is a somatic manifestation of psychiatric illness; a careful assessment is required to differentiate subjective complaints from clinical constipation in depressed or anxious patients.

Stroke may cause constipation primarily as a result of secondary effects of impaired mobility and polypharmacy. Weakness of abdominal and pelvic muscles following stroke may also contribute to problems with evacuation. Studies in animals and humans with focal neurologic damage have isolated the defecation and micturition centers to the pons; pontine damage caused by stroke may affect the behavioral response to a full rectum.

Finally, constipation is a significant clinical problem in the majority of people with spinal cord disease or injury. Age and duration of injury interact to promote complications of chronic constipation such as acquired megacolon, which affects over half of patients with spinal cord injury.

Dietary Factors

Numerous dietary factors influence the bowel. Low consumption of wheat bran, fiber, vegetables, fruit, rice, and calories can predispose toward constipation. In a meta-analysis of nonrandomized studies in younger adults with constipation, additional wheat bran was associated with increased stool weight and decreased transit time. Use of fiber in treatment of constipation is summarized under "Nonpharmacologic Treatment" below. Low fluid intake in older adults has been related to symptomatic constipation in epidemiologic surveys, and to slow colonic transit (in an unadjusted analysis). Withholding fluids over a 1-week period in young male volunteers significantly reduced stool output. Elderly people are at greater risk of dehydration because of impaired thirst sensation, less-effective hormonal responses to hypertonicity, limited access with coexisting physical or cognitive impairments, and voluntary fluid restriction in an attempt to control urinary incontinence.

Metabolic Disorders

Metabolic imbalances are remediable causes for often severe constipation. Hypokalemia produces neuronal dysfunction that minimizes acetylcholine stimulation of gut smooth muscle, and so prolongs transit through the gut. Hypercalcemia causes conduction delay within the extrinsic and intrinsic innervation of the gut. Surgical treatment of hyperparathyroidism reverses the neuromuscular bowel dysfunction seen with this condition. Edema of the gut wall with mucopolysaccharide deposition has been documented in myxedema, although whether this contributes to the colonic hypomotility seen in untreated hypothyroidism is uncertain.

Colorectal Cancer

Colorectal cancer is associated with both constipation and use of laxatives, although this risk association is likely to be confounded by the influence of underlying habits. As the prevalence of colorectal cancer increases with age, index of suspicion should be higher in older adults. Abdominal pain, rectal bleeding, recent change in bowel habit, and certainly any systemic features such as weight loss and anemia should prompt further investigations for underlying neoplasm.

PRESENTATION

Table 52-5 lists the important aspects of the bowel history that should be elicited from an elderly person who complains of constipation. It is essential to identify evacuation difficulties where present in order to manage the patient effectively. Patients frequently underestimate the number of bowel movements per week, so it is helpful to have them keep a stool chart for 1 week to document frequency and characteristics of their bowel movements and symptoms associated with evacuation. A recent history of altered bowel habit should prompt an exploration of precipitants (e.g., medications, stroke), and where unexplained, an evaluation for colorectal cancer. Perianal fecal soiling is a common and embarrassing symptom that patients are reluctant to volunteer. In one large nursing home study, 38 percent of elderly individuals who complained of constipation reported fecal soiling of undergarments. Fecal soiling should alert the health care provider to the possibility of stool impaction, or, alternatively, of excessively loose stools caused by inappropriate laxative use, or to other causes of diarrhea. According to the Rome criteria, symptoms relating to irritable bowel syndrome are abdominal distension or pain relieved by defecation, passage of mucus, and feeling of incomplete emptying. While irritable bowel syndrome is often a diagnosis of exclusion in older people, it should be considered particularly in those with a prolonged history of intermittent bowel dysfunction. Rectal pain associated with defecation should alert the physician to rectal ischemia as well as to other more common anorectal conditions. Rectal bleeding should prompt further evaluation for underlying tumor disease, unless examination clearly reveals bright red blood from anal fissure or hemorrhoids.

Importantly, constipation can be underestimated in frail elderly patients. Objective assessment is essential in these individuals (including all nursing home residents), as they may (1) be unable to report bowel-related

Table 52-5   Diagnosis of Constipation in Older People

Bowel History

Number of bowel movements per week
Stool consistency
Straining/symptoms of rectal outlet delay
Duration of constipation
Fecal/urinary incontinence
Irritable bowel syndrome symptoms (abdominal pain,
   bloating, passage of mucus)
Rectal pain or bleeding
Laxative use, prior and current

General History

Mood/cognition
Symptoms of systemic illness (weight loss, anemia)
Relevant comorbidities (e.g. diabetes, neurological
   disease)
Mobility
Diet
Medications

Specific Physical Examination

Digital rectal examination including external and internal
   sphincter tone
Perianal sensation/cutaneous anal reflex
Pelvic floor descent/rectal prolapse
Abdominal palpation, auscultation
Neurological, cognitive and functional examination

Tests

Indications for plain abdominal radiograph

Empty rectum with clinical suspicion of constipation
Evaluation for fecal impaction
Persistent fecal incontinence despite clearing of any rectal
   impaction
Evaluation for abdominal distension or pain (bowel
   dilatation/redundant sigmoid loop/volvulus)

Indications for colonoscopy or barium enema

Systemic illness (weight loss, anemia etc.)
Recent change in bowel habit without obvious risk factors

Indications for anorectal function tests

Severe or persistent symptoms of rectal outlet delay
Persistent fecal incontinence with clinical evidence of anal
   sphincter weakness

symptoms because of communication or cognitive difficulties, (2) have impaired rectal sensation and rectal dyschezia and so be unaware of the presence of a large fecal bolus in the rectum, (3) have daily bowel movements despite having rectal or colonic stool impaction, and (4) have nonspecific symptoms (such as delirium, leucocytosis, anorexia, functional decline) in association with severe fecal impaction.

EVALUATION

Digital rectal examination is recommended in all patients who report constipation; it is useful for revealing rectal impaction (which can be of hard or soft stool) as well as hemorrhoids, anorectal disease, and perianal fecal soiling. Absence of stool on rectal examination does not, however, exclude the diagnosis of constipation. External sphincter tone should be assessed by asking the patient to "squeeze and pull up" around the examining finger. Indicators of reduced internal anal tone are easy insertion of the finger into the anal canal and gaping of the anus on applying gentle traction to the anal margin. The presence of anal sphincter weakness should alert the prescribing physician to avoid causing fecal leakage though excessive laxative-induced softness of stool, and prompt instruction in sphincter strengthening exercises. Absent cutaneous-anal reflex (gentle scratching of the anal margin should normally induce a visible contraction of the anal sphincter) and, in particular, the presence of perianal anesthesia points to significant sacral cord dysfunction with the probability of marked rectal outlet delay. Excessive perineal descent is observed by asking the patient to "bear down" while lying in the lateral position on the examination couch. Rectal prolapse may also be observed with this maneuver, although this condition is best identified by having the patient strain while sitting on a commode. Proctoscopy is simple and quick and useful for diagnosing internal hemorrhoids, and abnormalities of the rectal wall.

In all patients with constipation, a thorough appraisal of predisposing causes should be undertaken by symptom, medication, and dietary history; physical, cognitive, and functional examination; and laboratory measurement of complete blood count, plasma electrolytes, and glucose, and bone, liver, and thyroid profiles.

Clinical diagnosis can often be made on the basis of a thorough history and examination. However, a plain abdominal radiograph is useful in patients without rectal stool in whom colonic fecal impaction is suspected because of a high-risk profile, constipation-related symptoms, or fecal incontinence. It can guide management in those patients who continue to report troublesome constipation-related symptoms despite regular laxative use by showing either absent, or marked stool retention. Marked fecal loading in the descending and sigmoid colon correlates well with prolonged transit time, as does the presence of feces rather than air in the cecum (Fig. 52-1). Dilatation of the colon (>6.5 cm maximum diameter) or rectum (>4 cm) in the absence of acute obstruction points to a neurogenic component to bowel dysfunction, and thus identifies patients at risk of recurrent colonic impactions. Finally, in patients with abdominal distension and/or pain an abdominal

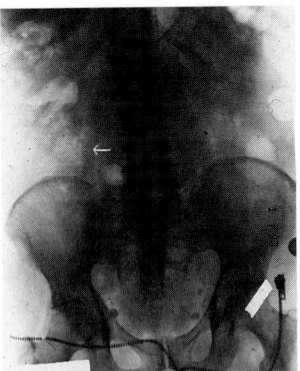

Figure 52-1 Abdominal radiograph of a 73-year-old man with chronic schizophrenia who has taken anticholinergic neuroleptics for many years. This was his third hospital admission for colonic impaction. The arrow points to the cecum, which is full of stool, indicative of slow transit. Fecaliths are visible in the pelvic region.

radiograph may diagnose acute complications of constipation such as sigmoid volvulus and small bowel obstruction secondary to severe impaction.

Further investigation with colonoscopy or barium enemas is warranted if systemic illness or laboratory abnormalities arouse suspicion of colorectal disease. In older patients, colonoscopy is associated with significantly less discomfort than barium enema, as well as being diagnostically more sensitive for conditions such as adenoma, carcinoma, and angiodysplasia. For both procedures, inadequate tests are not uncommon in the elderly because of poor bowel preparation, and this is especially relevant in persons presenting with constipation. Potential nonadherence ("Is the patient able to drink 4 L of GoLYTELY in 24 hours?") should be identified, and unpleasant side effects avoided ("Is the patient's mobility impaired such that the patient will be fecally incontinent prior to reaching the toilet?") during bowel preparation. To improve the tolerability, safety, and efficacy of bowel preparation, the cathartic regimen should be individualized in older constipated individuals according to specific needs (e.g., 1 to 2 L of GoLYTELY daily over 2 to 3 days in those unable to drink 4 L, or use of alternative preparations such as sodium picosulfate). A preprocedure plain abdominal x-ray for evaluation of fecal clearance is also helpful in predicting the adequacy of the test.

Anorectal function tests are mainly useful in patients who report severe and persistent rectal outlet delay, mainly with a view to diagnosing pelvic dyssynergia, as this condition is amenable to treatment by biofeedback, and in individuals in whom fecal incontinence persists despite resolution of coexisting fecal impaction. In the latter group, anorectal function tests can guide management toward conservative treatment (pelvic muscle strengthening exercises and biofeedback therapy), or surgical intervention.

COMPLICATIONS OF CONSTIPATION IN THE ELDERLY (TABLE 52-6)

Constipation is the most important cause of fecal incontinence in older people, as it is treatable, preventable, and frequently overlooked. Few medical symptoms are as

Table 52-6   Complications of Constipation in the Elderly

Fecal straining and incontinence
Fecal impaction
Stercoral perforation
Urinary retention
Sigmoid volvulus
Rectal prolapse
Impaired quality of life

distressing and social isolating for older people as fecal incontinence, a condition that places them at greater risk of morbidity, mortality, dependency, and nursing home placement. All too often, untreated overflow leads to hospitalization of vulnerable older patients. Many older individuals in the community with fecal incontinence will not volunteer the problem to their general practitioner and, regrettably, doctors and nurses do not routinely inquire about the symptom. This "hidden problem" therefore leads to social isolation and a downward spiral of psychological distress, dependency, and poor health. Even when older people are noted by health care professionals to have fecal incontinence, the condition is often poorly assessed and passively managed, especially in the long-term care setting where it is most prevalent. Tobin and Brocklehurst (1986) identified overflow (continuous fecal soiling and fecal impaction on rectal examination) as the underlying problem in 52 percent of frail nursing home residents with long-standing fecal incontinence. A therapeutic intervention consisting of enemas until no further response followed by lactulose achieved complete resolution of incontinence in 94 percent of those in whom full treatment compliance could be obtained. Notably, this study showed that only 4 percent of nursing home residents with long-standing fecal incontinence had been referred to their general practitioner for further assessment of this problem, which may reflect a tendency toward unnecessarily conservative nursing management (e.g., use of pads and pants only).

Fecal impaction is an important cause of comorbidity in older patients, increasing the risk of hospitalization and of potentially fatal complications. Read et al. (1985) reported that fecal impaction was a primary reason for acute hospitalization in 27 percent of geriatric patients admitted consecutively over the course of a year. In frailer patients, the presentation of fecal impaction may be a nonspecific clinical deterioration; more specific symptoms are anorexia, vomiting, and abdominal pain. The findings on physical examination may include fever, delirium, abdominal distension, reduced bowel sounds, arrhythmias, and tachypnea secondary to splinting of the diaphragm. The mechanism for the fever and leucocytosis response is thought to be microscopic stercoral ulcerations of the colon. A plain abdominal radiograph will show colonic or rectal fecal retention associated with lower bowel dilatation (Fig. 52-2). Presence of fluid levels in the large or small bowel suggests advanced obstruction; the closer the fecal impaction is to the ileocecal valve, the greater the number of fluid levels in

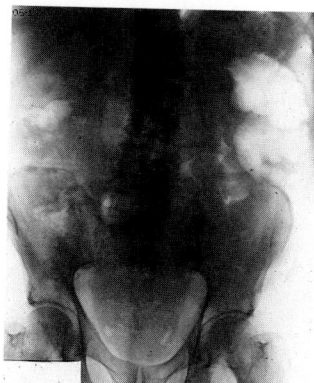

Figure 52-2 Abdominal radiograph of an 83-year-old man with Parkinson's disease and long-standing symptoms of continuous fecal leakage. As his caregiver at home, his wife was changing his clothing up to 6 times a day. The rectosigmoid colon is completely impacted, and the dilated bowel loop implies obstruction. He was briefly hospitalized for disimpaction with enemas and laxatives, resulting in complete resolution of incontinence. He and his wife were educated in regular use of laxatives and suppositories, as well as in lifestyle measures.

the small bowel. Intestinal obstruction increases the risk of stercoral perforation of the wall of the colon secondary to ischemic necrosis, which is associated with a high mortality rate. Stercoral perforation can also occur in chronically constipated persons where pressure from a hard fecaloma produces an ulcer with characteristically necrotic and inflammatory edges; these individuals tend to present with sudden onset of acute abdominal pain. Marked rectosigmoid fecal impaction may impinge on the bladder neck causing some degree of urinary retention; several cases of bilateral hydronephrosis with associated renal failure in older individuals which resolved following disimpaction have been reported in the literature.

Sigmoid volvulus is the third commonest cause of large bowel obstruction in the United States and a complication of slow-transit constipation. Older persons with neurologic conditions such as Parkinson's disease and spinal cord disease, and those on long-term neuroleptics for treatment of psychiatric disease, are at greater risk of volvulus secondary to colonic dysmotility. Subtotal colectomy may be necessary to prevent recurrence of sigmoid volvulus in patients with this clinical profile, who are also more likely to have chronic megacolon or rectum predisposing them to recurrent fecal impaction. Prolonged straining at stool in constipated patients can result in rectal prolapse of varying degrees and may lead to continuous fecal soiling.

Importantly, quality of life and daily living are affected by functional bowel symptoms in older people, even following adjustment for other chronic illnesses.

MANAGEMENT

Pharmacologic Treatment

Laxative and Enema Use and Abuse in Older People

Several researchers have documented an enormous increase in the use of laxatives in older people in the

community with little relation to either frequency of bowel movements or the need to strain. A Food and Drug Administration (FDA) Advisory Panel has registered concern over the widespread overuse of over-the-counter (OTC) laxatives; laxatives are second only to analgesics as the most commonly used OTC medications by the elderly. OTC laxative use is more common in the United States than in other countries, and is encouraged by advertising and popular ignorance of adverse effects. One-fifth to one-third of regular laxative users do not consider themselves to be constipated, and many people take them through a misguided belief in the benefits of regular purgation. One study showed that 78 percent of elderly persons who used laxatives regularly had never gone for more than 3 days without a bowel movement. Habitual rather than surreptitious abuse is more likely to be seen in older individuals; repeated purging empties the colon of stool that would normally descend into and distend the rectal ampulla, thereby removing the urge to defecate, which prompts the patient to take further laxatives.

Although patients in hospitals and nursing homes are at higher risk for clinical constipation, this does not entirely justify the very high levels of cathartic prescribing in these settings. Seventy-six percent of hospitalized elderly and 74 percent of nursing home residents are prescribed at least one type of laxative. Two contributing factors may lead to overprescribing of laxatives to older patients: (1) lack of objective confirmation of the diagnosis by the prescribing physician or nurse, and (2) prescribing patterns of laxatives which are clinically ineffective. For instance, the current pattern of laxative prescribing in older people in US nursing homes shows a predominance of the use of docusate, a fecal softener known to have little or no laxative effect.

Evidence-Based Summary of Laxative, Suppository, and Enema Treatment in Older Persons

Many reported trials of laxative and enema treatment in older people are not of high quality, being limited by unclear definitions for constipation, inconsistent outcome measurement, and underreporting of potential confounding factors during the trial period (e.g., fiber intake). The absence of strong evidence-based guidelines may in part underlie the somewhat empirical way in which laxatives are prescribed to older people. A 1997 systematic review of effective laxative treatment in elderly persons found that the few published randomized controlled trials are potentially flawed due to small numbers and other methodologic concerns. The reviewers nevertheless commented that significant improvements in bowel movement frequency were observed with a stimulant laxative (cascara) and with lactulose, while bulk-laxative psyllium and lactulose were individually reported to improve stool consistency and related symptoms in placebo-controlled trials.

The overall recommendation for use of bowel agents in older people is for an assessment-based stepwise approach, involving the individual in their own treatment where possible, so as to aim for a patient-centered outcome of regular and comfortable defecation. Table 52-7 summarizes the dosage, onset of action, mechanisms of action, potential side effects, and benefits of selected laxatives in current

Table 52-7 Laxative and Enemas Used in Older People With Constipation

Agent and *Type*	Dosage	Onset	Mechanisms of Action, Side-Effects and Benefits
Senna (Sennakot) *Anthroquinone stimulant*	10–30 mg at night	8–12 hrs	Direct stimulation of myenteric plexus, alteration of salt and water transportation, Prostaglandin E-like effect. May cause dose-dependent cramps and diarrhea so titrate dosage. Long-term use associated with melanosis coli, but unlikely to cause 'cathartic colon'. May cause false-positive urine test for urobilinogen Improves propulsive action, softens stool, shortens transit time.
Psyllium (Metamucil) Methyl-Cellulose (Citrucel) Calcium polycarbophil (Fibercon) *Bulk*	1 tblspn/ biscuit qd-tid 2–4 tabs qd	12–72 hrs	Hydrophilic fibers resistant to bacterial degradation, leads to bulkier and softer stool and peristaltic stimulation. May cause transient bloating, flatulence. Good fluid intake needed to avoid colonic fecal retention, avoid use in bedridden or dehydrated patients. Causes more frequent passage of well-formed stools, reduces evacuation discomfort due to hard stools, suitable for long-term use.
Magnesium hydroxide (Milk of magnesia) *Osmotic*	5–30 mls qhs	1/2–3 hr	Stimulates release of cholecystokinin, increases secretion of electrolytes and water into gut lumen. Rapid action may cause watery stool, dehydration, fecal incontinence. Hypermagnesemia in renal insuffiency. Avoid magnesium citrate in elderly, may cause incontinence and colonic pseudo-obstruction Useful in patients with hypotonic colon, not suitable for long-term use.
Lactulose (Chronulac) Sorbitol *Osmolar*	15–30 mls qd-qid	24–48 hrs	Nonabsorbable disaccharides degraded into low molecular weight acids which osmotically draw water into the colon causing reflex gut contractions. May cause abdominal cramps and flatulence, especially if taken with large amount of fruit. Increases transit, softens stool, safe for use in diabetics and patients with renal failure and helpful for long-term use in immobile patients. Sorbitol is cheaper than lactulose and as effective.
Polyethylene glycol (Golytely) *Osmolar*	8–16 oz qd as laxative 0.5–2 L impaction	30–60 mins	Potent hyperosmotic action, shortens transit time. May cause nausea, abdominal cramps, incontinence and loose stool, dose should be titrated against effect. Useful in treatment of fecal impaction (without obstruction), bowel preparation prior to procedures, and long-term use in patients with hypotonic colon.
Colace *Softener*	100 mg bid	24–72 hrs	Stimulates cyclic-AMP increasing fluid secretions, reduces surface tension and promotes penetration of water into stool. Ineffective in treatment of constipation. Risk of fecal soiling in older women. Long-term use alters morphology of gut mucosa.

(Continued)

Table 52-7   Laxative and Enemas Used in Older People With Constipation (*Continued*)

Agent and *Type*	Dosage	Onset	Mechanisms of Action, Side-Effects and Benefits
Enemas Phosphate (Fleets) Soap-sud Mineral oil Tap water	50–500 mls	2–15 mins	Contractile response to gut dilatation, lavage effect. Phosphate: Hyperphosphatemia, tetany, fluid retention, avoid use in renal failure. Soap-suds: Rectal mucosal damage and necrosis, use should be avoided altogether. Mineral oil: useful for acute disimpaction. Tap water: useful for acute disimpaction and impaction prevention in patients with hypotonic rectum and/or colon.
Suppository Bisacodyl (Dulcolax) Glycerine		5–45 mins	Rectal contractile response to increased volume. Daily bisacodyl use may cause rectal burning and cramps. Suppositories helpful for rectal outlet delay, persistent straining, prevention of recurrent rectal impactions.

usage, and the following discussion briefly describes available efficacy and safety data.

Stimulant laxatives   Senna is a cheap and safe agent for use in elderly people with functional constipation. A trial of cascara (a similar plant-derived stimulant laxative) in older hospitalized patients increased bowel movement frequency by an average of 2.6 bowel movements per week as compared to placebo. Administration of 20 mg of senna daily for 6 months to patients older than 80 years of age did not cause any significant losses of intestinal protein or electrolytes, and repeated studies in mice show no evidence of myenteric nerve damage resulting from its use. Senna generally induces evacuation 8 to 12 hours following administration, and should therefore be taken at bedtime. Frail elderly patients may have even slower response times, and may also require several weeks of daily use before achieving regular bowel habit. The dosage of senna should be titrated according to each individual's response. Maintenance therapy with senna is appropriate in patients with recurrent colonic constipation, and it can be used in higher doses for short-term treatment of fecal impaction. In patients with weakened anal sphincters, the moderate stool softening plus laxative effect of senna as a single agent may be sufficient to treat constipation without causing or exacerbating fecal incontinence.

Bisacodyl is more likely to cause side effects as an oral stimulant than is senna (cramping, vomiting, and hypokalemia, especially if taken with antacids). Phenolphthalein and castor oil are not advisable for use in the elderly population because of a high risk of side effects, particularly malabsorption, dehydration, lipoid pneumonia, and, with heavy prolonged use, cathartic colon.

Bulk laxatives   Bulk laxatives are generally underprescribed to older people, despite evidence that they increase bowel movement frequency (by a mean of 1.4 bowel movements per week as compared to placebo), and improve consistency and ease of evacuation. This may partly be because of intolerance in the form of bloating and unpredictable

bowel habit in the first 1 to 3 weeks of taking them, and also of caution on the part of prescribers because of the documented risk of impaction with these agents in frailer patients with poor fluid intake. Bulking agents are, however, useful in older individuals with mild to moderate constipation who are able to tolerate them and who drink sufficient fluids. They have the additional benefit of reducing abdominal pain in patients with irritable bowel syndrome, limiting flare-ups of diverticulitis, and facilitating painful defecation associated with hemorrhoids. Furthermore, psyllium in particular will significantly lower serum cholesterol by binding bile acids in the intestine. Available preparations are natural nonwheat fibers such as psyllium and ispaghula husk, and synthetic compounds such as calcium polycarbophil and methylcellulose. The synthetic compounds tend to be cheaper and are available in more easily administered tablet forms, as compared to reconstituted powder, which can be hard for older patients to swallow. The synthetic bulking agents and the natural fibers are equally effective in increasing stool frequency and volume. It should be noted that bran in tablet form is considerably cheaper than bulk laxatives, but the former may cause even more bloating and unpredictability of bowel habit, and may also, unlike bulking agents, predispose to malabsorption of iron or calcium in elderly people.

Osmotic laxatives   Osmotic laxatives (magnesium salts) are the most commonly prescribed type to elderly in hospital, and magnesium hydroxide comprises 12.5 percent of all over-the-counter laxative sales. There is only one published study evaluating magnesium hydroxide in elderly people, a small trial in nursing home residents, which suggested that this laxative was more effective than a bulking agent in increasing bowel movement frequency and softening stool. Magnesium salts may be favored by physician and patient alike because of their rapid action, but in general, a gradual catharsis is more successful in restoring regular bowel habit in older persons. Their potent catharsis increases the risk of fluid and electrolyte losses, and of causing fecal incontinence in less-mobile people, or in those with weak sphincters. Furthermore, magnesium levels should be monitored in all elderly people who are using magnesium hydroxide on a regular basis, as hypermagnesemia can occur even with normal serum creatinine levels. Long-term use of magnesium hydroxide is contraindicated in renal insufficiency. The more potent salt magnesium citrate carries an even greater risk of side effects, including promoting colonic pseudo-obstruction in frailer patients, and is therefore not recommended for use in the elderly population. Magnesium hydroxide may, however, have a role in treating patients with colonic hypomotility and/or neurologic disease, in whom stimulant agents tend to be less effective, and bulking agents are not indicated as they may cause further stasis.

Hyperosmolar laxatives   Hyperosmolar laxatives are the most rigorously studied laxative type in the current literature in older people. In nursing home residents, lactulose (or the related agent lactitol) versus placebo shortens transit time, increases bowel movement frequency (by an average of 1.9 bowel movements per week), and improves stool consistency. In a comparison study with a bulking/stimulant combination agent, also in nursing home residents, lactulose was a little less effective in influencing bowel pattern and consistency. However, another well-designed trial showed both lactulose and sorbitol to be equally efficacious in treating severe constipation in ambulatory older veterans. The high cost of lactulose makes its use as a long-term laxative less attractive, but sorbitol is a cheaper and equally effective alternative for treatment of functional constipation in older people in all health care settings.

Polyethylene glycol (GoLYTELY), a more potent hyperosmolar laxative, is currently recommended in the United States for bowel preparation prior to colonoscopy and barium enema. There are some recent studies evaluating its use as a treatment for constipation in adults. In a randomized control trial (RCT) of hospitalized patients (mean age 55 years), in comparison to lactulose, polyethylene glycol produced a greater increase in bowel movement frequency and a greater reduction in straining, but at the expense of a higher mean number of liquid stools. Its use in treatment of fecal impaction (in combination with daily enemas) has been evaluated in elderly nursing home residents, showing greater efficacy than lactulose, without the dehydration or hemodynamic-related side-effects. In cases of colonic ± small bowel obstruction secondary to impaction, oral laxatives may worsen abdominal pain and precipitate colonic perforation, so they should not be given until daily application of enemas has relieved the obstruction. The current evidence base suggests that the role of polyethylene glycol in older people is for acute disimpaction (in a hospital or nursing home setting where toilet access is guaranteed), rather than for regular use as a laxative.

Fecal softeners   Docusate sodium has been shown experimentally to have no effect on colonic motility, and little or no laxative action, even at doses of 300 mg/d. In a recent RCT of adults with severe constipation comparing docusate with psyllium, docusate proved significantly

inferior for both softening stools and increasing bowel movement frequency. A recent systematic review of prospective controlled trials evaluating oral docusate in people with chronic illness and constipation showed a small trend toward increased stool frequency, but concluded that there was insufficient evidence to support its use in care of the chronically ill. Nevertheless, docusate is frequently recommended and used in older people as a laxative as well as fecal softener. This is of particular concern in the nursing home and hospital settings, where constipation may as a result be undertreated with an increased risk of fecal impaction. Furthermore, docusate (in combination with the stimulant danthron) increases the risk of fecal incontinence in nursing home residents. Current evidence suggests that docusate is unhelpful in the treatment of functional constipation or chronic evacuation difficulties in frail older people.

Enemas and suppositories   Enemas have a role in both acute disimpaction, and in preventing recurrent impactions in susceptible patients. They induce evacuation as a response to colonic distension, as well as by plain lavage; the commonest reason for a poor result from an enema is inadequate administration. In one study of nursing home residents with overflow incontinence associated with fecal impaction on rectal examination, daily phosphate enemas until no further result was obtained was effective in completely resolving incontinence in 94 percent of patients. Some frail elderly patients with poor mobility, and some individuals with neurogenic bowel dysfunction may present with recurrent stool impactions despite regular laxative and suppository use; these individuals may benefit from weekly enemas as a preventive measure (D). Tap water enemas are the safest type for regular use, although they take more nursing administration time than phosphate enemas, and soapsuds enemas should never be administered to older patients. Arachis oil retention enemas are safe, however, and have practical use in loosening colonic impactions. In patients who have a firm and large rectal impaction, manual evacuation should be performed prior to using enemas or suppositories, using local anesthetic gel if needed to reduce discomfort.

Suppositories are very useful in treatment of rectal outlet delay, or where symptoms of prolonged straining predominate. Regular suppository administration (usually three times a week), is important for effective symptom control in these patients, ideally immediately following breakfast to take advantage of the gastrocolic reflex. A recent study of frail nursing home patients with overflow incontinence found that a regimen of daily lactulose and suppositories plus weekly enemas was only effective in restoring continence when long-lasting and complete rectal emptying was achieved. Consequently, regular use of suppositories is indicated older patients with rectal dyschezia and/or recurrent rectal impactions. With appropriate education, many older people can themselves use suppositories; they are easier to insert and more effective if used blunt end first, and people with impaired dexterity can be helped with suppository inserters designed for spinal cord injured patients. First-line suppository use is with glycerin, a hyperosmolar laxative used solely in suppository form. If ineffective, bisacodyl suppositories (in polyethylene glycol base) should be used, although daily use can sometimes causes symptoms of rectal discomfort or burning. Bisacodyl suppositories have been shown to be effective in treating severe constipation in patients with spinal cord injuries. The onset of action of suppositories varies by individual from 5 to 45 minutes (most likely influenced by the neurogenicity of the rectum), and so patients should be advised to set a quiet time aside for effective evacuation.

Prokinetic agents   Prokinetic drugs are newly developed laxative agents that directly stimulate cellular release of acetyl choline in the myenteric plexus. Cisapride, a drug recently taken off the market because of cardiac side effects, was effective short-term in treating constipation associated with Parkinson's disease, diabetes, and spinal cord injury. Safer alternative drugs within the same class are being developed and may have potential use as adjunctive therapy in constipated older patients with these neurologic conditions.

TREATMENT GUIDANCE

The 1997 systemic review from the United Kingdom concluded that based on the somewhat limited current evidence, older patients should first be prescribed the cheapest laxative, with others given if this treatment fails. Table 52-8 represents a combination of evidence-based and expert opinion in providing treatment guidance, which can be summarized as follows: In ambulant elderly with functional constipation, a daily bulk laxative is appropriate for both rectal outlet delay and slow-transit constipation. If the bulking agent is not tolerated, or proves ineffective, then senna may be substituted (1 to 3 tablets at night) with prn sorbitol (or lactulose) if needed to achieve patient-centered goals of comfortable regular evacuations. In frailer, less-mobile elderly people at higher risk of clinical constipation, a combination of sorbitol and senna should be used with dosage titration. In patients with colonic impaction, oil retention enemas should be administered daily until there are no clinical or radiologic signs of obstruction, and then tap water enemas continued daily until they produce no further result. Where the patient has easy access to a toilet, polyethylene glycol .5 to 2 L daily should then be given with extra fluids for 2 to 3 days, followed by a regular maintenance laxative regimen of senna and lactulose to avoid recurrence of fecal impaction. In cases where toilet access is not so easy (e.g., in a home with stairs), a more gradual clear-out using higher-dose senna and lactulose is appropriate in limiting the risk of incontinence. For rectal outlet delay or a predominant complaint of straining, the first-line approach should be regular use of suppositories, and laxatives should only be given for coexisting symptoms of hard or infrequent bowel movements.

NONPHARMACOLOGIC TREATMENT

More often than not, the consultation between a general practitioner and an older person reporting constipation will result in a laxative being prescribed. Among frailer

Table 52-8   Pharmacological Treatment of Constipation in Older People

Functional Constipation
Bulk laxative 1–3 times daily with fluids in ambulant elderly persons
In individuals with questionable fluid intake or those intolerant of bulk laxatives, give senna 1–3 tablets at bedtime
If symptoms persist, add sorbitol or lactulose 15 mL daily as needed, titrating the dose to achieve regular (>=3 times a week) and comfortable evacuation
In high risk patients (e.g. bedridden individuals, patients with neurological disease, those with history of fecal impaction etc.) give senna 2–3 tablets at bedtime and sorbitol of lactulose 30 mL daily (titrating upwards as needed) long-term

Colonic Fecal Impaction
Daily arachis oil retention enema until clinical or radiological obstruction resolves
Then continue with daily tap water enemas until no further washout result, and give polyethylene glycol $\frac{1}{2}$–2L daily with fluids (for rapid disimpaction e.g. in hospital), or senna 3 tablets at bedtime and sorbitol or lactulose 30 mL twice daily (in patients at risk of anal incontinence due to toilet access difficulties or to weakened anal sphincters)
When impaction resolves, return to maintenence regimen for functional constipation in high-risk patients

Rectal Outlet Delay
Manual disimpaction where necessary, followed by phosphate enema(s) for initial complete clearance of rectal impaction
Glycerine suppository once daily after breakfast for 2 weeks, then use as required to relieve symptoms. For recurrent rectal impaction or overflow FI, use bisacodyl suppositories instead
If stool is hard or infrequent, add daily laxative as for functional constipation

older people, nursing home studies show high rates of self-reported constipation, despite very substantial levels of laxative prescribing. These observations have led to speculation that nonpharmacologic treatments for constipation (e.g., health education and dietary and lifestyle changes) are underused, with laxatives often being a first-line approach in older people. Expert opinion considers that nonpharmacologic measures in older people should be first-line treatment in nonsevere constipation and the mainstay of treatment even when laxatives are deemed necessary. Symptoms of difficult evacuation may be particularly amenable to nonpharmacologic approaches such as stool softening and bulking through increasing fiber and fluid intake, pelvic muscle strengthening exercises, and footstool elevation of the legs during evacuation (see below). There has been little research in this area however; a recent systematic review examining treatment of chronic constipation in older people found no studies evaluating the effect of exercise therapy and only a few nonrandomized trials examining fiber and fluid supplementation. Available data and expert opinion is summarized below.

Education

Education of the elderly person as to what constitutes normal bowel habit, with correction of common misperceptions, should be the initial step in addressing patient complaints of constipation. Patients with no or mild symptoms of constipation should be encouraged to discontinue chronic laxative therapy. Withdrawal may be easier to achieve in the more controlled environment of a nursing home, than in the community where over-the-counter medications are so readily available. Educational interventions promoting lifestyle changes impact older persons' behaviors, particularly in the areas of exercise and diet, with a demonstrable benefit on health outcomes, such as cardiac morbidity and falls. It is helpful to base education interventions for bowel problems on the cognitive Theory of Planned Behavior, which can be summarized as follows: To persuade older people with constipation to change their lifestyle, they need to be convinced that (1) their current behaviors are "bad for their bowels;" (2) bowel-related and general health improvements associated with recommended measures are worth the trouble and expense of changing; (3) it is they who are responsible for what they eat, how much exercise they take, and so on (internal locus of control); and (4) they have the skills and knowledge to modify their own lifestyle to improve their constipation, if they choose to do so (self-efficacy).

It is therefore also important to provide people with clearly written educational materials. For instance, with specific reference to fiber, in a randomized controlled trial, nutrition newsletters sent to older Americans in their homes significantly improved their dietary fiber intake. Another community intervention involved media and social marketing in educational targeting of small retirement communities under the theme "Bread: It's a Great Way to Go," and reported a result of a 49 percent decrease in laxative sales and 58 percent increase in sales of whole meal and whole grain bread.

Diet

The effectiveness of fiber in treatment of constipation in elderly people is equivocal. In one community study, higher fiber intake was associated with lower laxative use among older women, but in another study, higher intake of bran was associated with no reduction in constipation symptoms and greater fecal loading in the colon on abdominal radiography. In older hospitalized patients, daily bran supplementation increased weekly bowel movement frequency and improved overall symptoms as compared with placebo. There have been several small observational nursing home studies reporting that addition of bran fiber to the daily diet increased bowel movement frequency, and reduced laxative intake and the need for nursing intervention in frail older persons, notably without reported side effects. Bias cannot be excluded from these studies, including that of concomitant increased fluid intake contributing significantly to these positive results. Similarly flawed observational studies in institutional settings have also observed beneficial effects on bowel movement frequency, consistency, and laxative costs from the daily introduction of fruit mixtures. Despite these reservations, these observational studies emphasize the potential usefulness of increasing dietary fiber, fluid, and fruit in older people at high risk of constipation. In practical terms, at least 10 g of fiber with additional fluids should be recommended to patients. While coarse bran rather than more refined fiber is more effective in increasing stool fluid weight, it is far less palatable, and is more likely to cause initial symptoms of increased bloating, flatulence, and irregular bowel movements. To promote compliance, fiber should be recommended to older individuals in the form of foods such as whole meal or whole grain bread, fresh fruit, preferably unpeeled, seeded berries, raw or cooked vegetables, beans, and lentils. A minimum of eight large glasses of fluid per day, with increased intake in the summer months, should be recommended to all patients other than those with medical contraindications.

Physical Activity

A program of regular exercise should be encouraged for all ambulatory elderly persons with constipation, within the functional limitations of each individual. A recent review of physical activity interventions in older adults concluded that incorporating exercise naturally into a person's day tends to provide the most effective means for increasing activity levels. Daily exercise in bed and the use of abdominal massage reduce laxative and enema use in chair-fast geriatric long-stay patients, although transit time was unaffected. Positioning immobile elderly patients out of bed and into a chair for up to 60-minute periods with chairlifts at 15-minute intervals, as per Agency for Health Care Policy and Research Guidelines on prevention of pressure ulcers, may have similar beneficial effects.

Toileting Habits

Small nonrandomized studies show that regular toileting habits (scheduled evacuation) restores comfortable

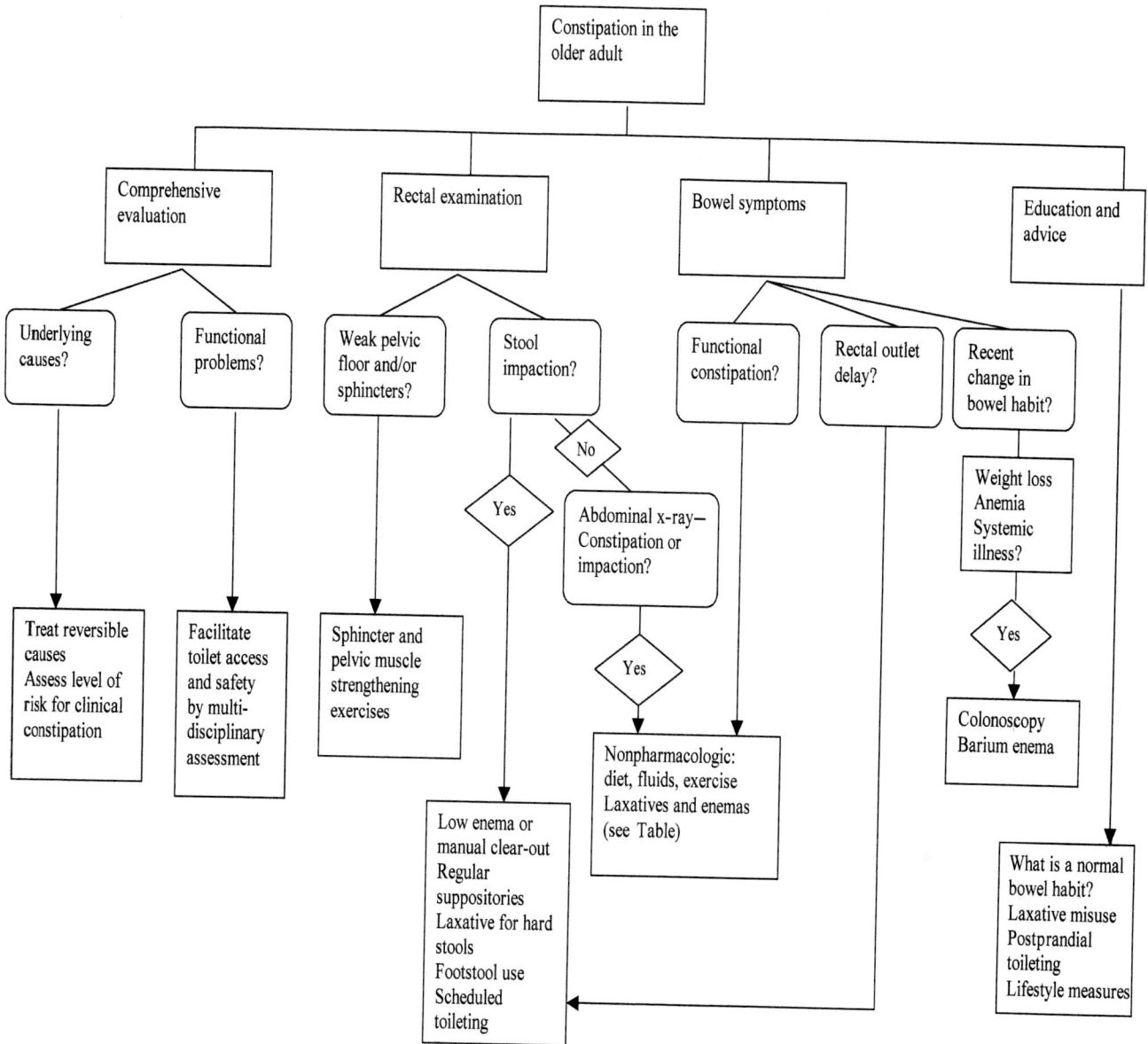

Figure 52-3 A practical approach to assessment and treatment of constipation in older people.

evacuation in stroke survivors (with the assistance of digital stimulation) and in older postoperative inpatients. The preservation of the gastrocolic reflex with aging, supports the rationale for postprandial toilet visits. Where rectal outlet delay and/or persistent straining is associated with excessive pelvic floor descent, pelvic strengthening exercises should be advocated. Care should be given to treating hemorrhoids and any other anorectal condition in these patients. Expert opinion supports the use of footstools during evacuation in individuals with weakened abdominal and pelvic muscles. Facility of toilet access should be assessed particularly in patients with mobility, visual or dexterity impairments, as should bathroom comfort and privacy for individuals in institutional settings.

Medication Review

A careful review of the medication regimen is necessary to eliminate, reduce the dosage, or substitute other medications for those that predispose to constipation. As an example, a selective serotonin reuptake inhibitor may provide an effective therapeutic alternative for elderly patients with depression who exhibit persistent constipation-related symptoms in the setting of tricyclic therapy. Regarding iron supplements, administration of iron sulfate in doses greater than 325 mg/d does not substantially increase iron absorption in elderly persons and may significantly increase gastrointestinal side effects.

PREVENTION

There are only two randomized controlled trials that looked at prevention of constipation in older people; both studies of bran added to the diets of acute hospital inpatients. Neither of these small studies showed a preventive effect; although results from several observational studies of dietary fiber supplementation (done mainly in nursing home residents, discussed earlier) suggest that constipation may be prevented by this intervention. However, these nonrandomized studies are likely to be biased in favor of benefits of treatment.

CONCLUSIONS

Figure 52-3 illustrates a practical algorithmic approach to assessment and treatment of constipation in older people. Health care providers should routinely inquire about constipation symptoms in older people, and be alert to the presence of clinical constipation in individuals unable to communicate. In many older people with constipation symptoms, lifestyle advice (diet, fluids, exercise, toileting habits) will preempt the need for laxative therapy. In higher-risk patients, a stepwise approach to prescribing laxatives, suppositories, or enemas, with the goal of achieving comfortable and regular evacuation. Rectal evacuation difficulties should be specifically addressed. Further research is needed to assess the impact of nonpharmacologic interventions targeting constipation risk factors on bowel and health-related outcomes in older people, to compare the cost-effectiveness of different classes of laxatives in this population, and to explore why the prevalence of constipation in nursing homes is so high despite heavy laxative usage (Is it ineffective laxative prescribing? Is it suboptimal assessment of patients? Is it underuse of nonpharmacologic treatment approaches?). The overall aim in both clinical practice and research should be to develop common evidence-based policies, procedures, guidelines, and targets to promote integrated bowel care for older people within all health care settings.

REFERENCES

Bassotti G et al: Manometric investigation of anorectal function in early and late stage Parkinson's disease. *J Neurol Neurosurg Psychiatriy* 68:768, 2000.

Camilleri M: Gastrointestinal problems in diabetes. *Endocrin Metab Clin North Am* 25:361, 1996.

Chassagne P et al: Does treatment of constipation improve fecal incontinence in institutionalized patients. *Age Ageing* 29:159, 2000.

Donald IP et al: A study of constipation in the elderly living at home. *Gerontology* 31:112, 1985.

Everhart JE et al: A longitudinal survey of self-reported bowel habits in the United States. *Dig Dis Sci* 34(8):1153, 1989.

Harari D et al: How do older persons define constipation? Implications for therapeutic management. *J Gen Intern Med* 12:63, 1997.

Harari D et al: Correlates of regular laxative use in frail elderly persons. *Am J Med* 99(4);513, 1995.

Harari D et al: Constipation: Assessment and management in an institutionalized population. *J Am Geriatr Soc* 42:1, 1994.

Kinnunen O: Study of constipation in a geriatric hospital, day hospital, old people's home and at home. *Aging* 31:161, 1991.

Lederle FA et al: Cost-effective treatment of constipation in the elderly: A randomized double-blind comparison of sorbitol and lactulose. *Am J Med* 89:597, 1990.

Muller-Lissner SA: Effect of wheat bran on the weight of stool and gastrointestinal transit time: A meta analysis. *BMJ* 296:615, 1988.

Passmore AP et al: Chronic constipation in long stay elderly patients: A comparison of lactulose and a senna-fiber combination. *BMJ* 307:769, 1993.

Petticrew M et al: Systematic review of the effectiveness of laxatives in the elderly. *Health Technol Assess* 1(13):i, 1, 1997.

Puxty JA, Fox RA: GoLYTELY: A new approach to fecal impaction in old age. *Age Ageing* 15(3):182, 1986.

Read NW et al: Anorectal function in elderly patients with fecal impaction. *Gastroenterology* 89:959, 1985.

Robson KM et al: Development of constipation in nursing home residents. *Dis Colon Rectum* 43:940, 2000.

Sonnenberg A, Muller AD: Constipation and cathartics as risk factors of colorectal cancer: A meta-analysis. *Pharmacology* 47(Suppl 1):224, 1993.

Szurszewski JH et al: Proceedings of a workshop entitled "neuromuscular function and dysfunction of the gastrointestinal tract in aging." *Dig Dis Sci* 34:1135, 1989.

Talley NJ et al: Constipation in an elderly community: A study of prevalence and potential risk factors. *Am J Gastroenterol* 91:19, 1996.

Tobin GW, Brocklehurst JC: Fecal incontinence in residential homes for the elderly: prevalence, aetiology and management. *Age Ageing* 15:41, 1986.

Varma JS et al: Constipation in the elderly: A physiologic study. *Dis Colon Rectum* 31:111, 1988.

Whitehead WE et al: Constipation in the elderly living at home: Definition, prevalence and relationship to lifestyle and health status. *J Am Geriatr Soc* 37:423, 1989.

ONCOLOGY AND HEMATOLOGY

C H A P T E R 5 3

Oncology and Aging: General Principles of Cancer in the Elderly

HARVEY JAY COHEN

This chapter discusses many of the general relationships of oncology and aging. It focuses on the epidemiologic, basic etiologic, and biologic relationships between the processes of aging and neoplasia, and on the generalizable aspects of management of malignant disease in the elderly patient. This chapter discusses clinical management of individual malignancies only as an example of general principles. The approach to specific malignancies is covered in subsequent chapters related to the appropriate organ system.

It is now well recognized that cancer is a major problem for elderly individuals. It is the second leading cause of death after heart disease in the United States, and 60 percent of all cancers occur in the 12 percent of the population older than age 65 years. What may not be as well appreciated is the magnitude of the problem for the elderly individual as well as for the physicians caring for this population. If one examines incidence and mortality data obtained from the National Cancer Institute's Surveillance, Epidemiology, and End Results (SEER) Program (Fig. 53-1), one sees that the total cancer incidence rises progressively through the middle years and then falls off in the later years. However, the age-specific cancer incidence rises progressively throughout the age range. Thus, while the rate of increase diminishes somewhat in the oldest age groups, and the rate actually falls slightly in the very oldest (perhaps a survivor effect), the overall risk for developing cancer is certainly greatest in the later years. Because the number of people in

this country older than age 65 years is rising rapidly and the oldest of the old, that is, those older than age 85 years, are increasing at the greatest rate, geriatricians, generalists, and internists will be encountering increasing numbers of elderly individuals with cancer in their practices.

Moreover the overall pattern for the incidence of age-specific cancer shows a rise with age, and, overall, 60 percent of cancers occur in those age 65 years or older (Table 53-1), this is not uniform for individual cancers. Moreover, for some malignancies, there is an apparent decrease in incidence in people older than age 80 years. This may be a result of a number of factors, including underreporting or natural selection, which would allow the less-cancer-prone population to survive. However, cohort effects may have the most significant impact. For example, age-specific annual cancer incidence rates from the SEER Program indicate a fall in incidence in the oldest age groups for both prostate and lung cancer. This changes when the data are corrected for certain known risk factors. For prostate cancer when only men are considered in the base population at risk, the incidence continues to rise into the oldest age groups. For lung cancer, an apparent decrease in lung cancer incidence in the older age groups might be explained by a smaller high-risk population because of decreased prevalence of smoking in the older age groups. When data derived from the Lung Cancer Early Detection Project for annual cancer incidence in male

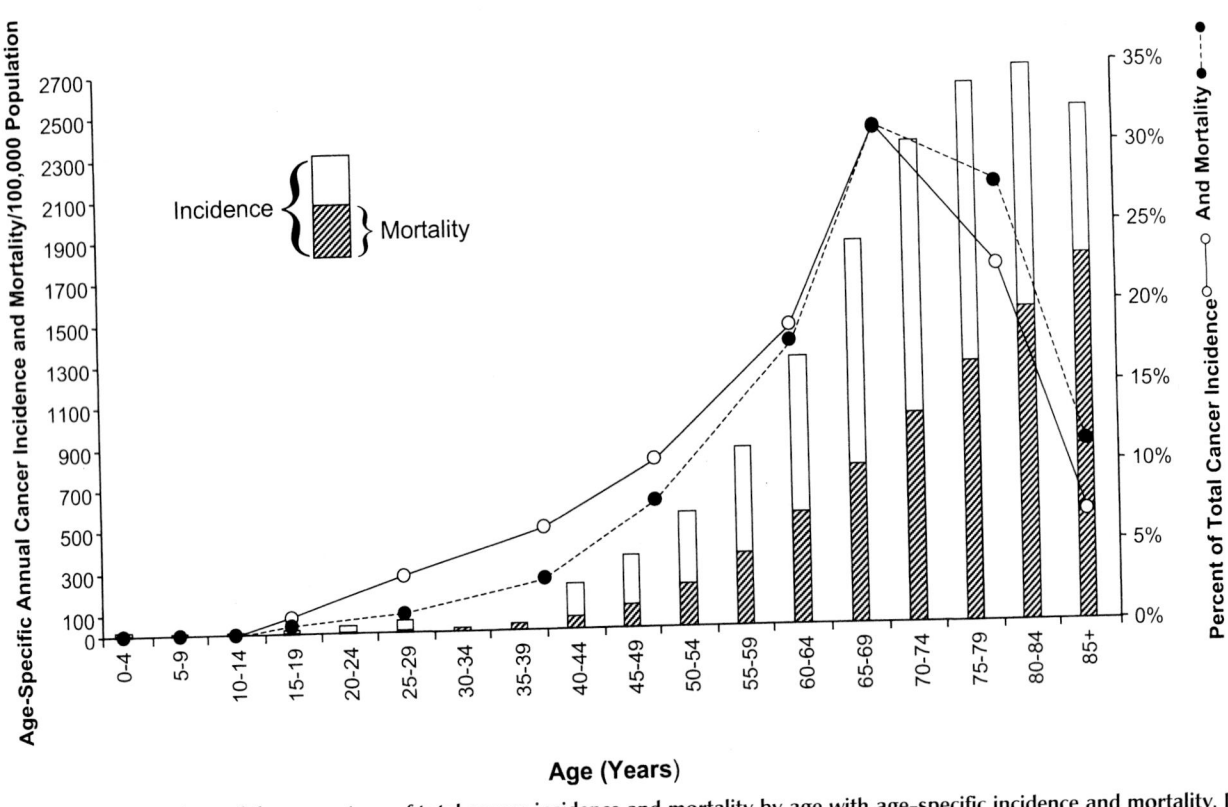

Figure 53-1   Comparison of the percentage of total cancer incidence and mortality by age with age-specific incidence and mortality. Data from *SEER Cancer Statistics Review: 1973–1994*. Bethesda, MD, National Cancer Institute, 1997.

Table 53-1   Percentage of Cancer Patients Age 65+ Years

Cancer	%65+
Prostate	80.9
Colon	73.8
Pancreas	71.8
Urinary bladder	69.9
Stomach	68.5
Rectum	66.0
Lung and bronchus	62.7
Leukemias	56.2
Corpus uteri	55.4
Non-Hodgkin's lymphoma	51.2
Breast	48.2
Ovary	46.2
All Cancers Combined	**59.7**

SOURCE: Data from *SEER Cancer Statistics Review: 1973–1994*. Bethesda, MD, National Cancer Institute, 1997.

smokers older than the age of 45 are used, one notes a continuing increase into advanced age. There is little change in the case of colorectal cancer because the entire population appears to be at risk. For women with breast cancer, data indicate an incidence that continues to rise slowly into advanced age. It has been suggested that data from the most recent survey showing a decrease in breast cancer risk at older ages (>75 years) may be an artifact of recent increases in breast cancer screening in the United States. For other gynecologic malignancies, there does appear to be a decrease, perhaps because of different interactions of hormonal status and neoplasia in hormonally responsive target organs.

Other types of patterns in age-specific incidence may also be seen. For example, Hodgkin's disease has a distinct bimodal distribution in incidence with a peak in the early years and another peak after late middle age. This has led to the suggestion that there actually may be two different diseases involved, one in the young individual and one in the older one, but that they assume similar morphologic features, so with current technologies we are unable to tell them apart. This impression is further substantiated by the markedly different response to treatment in younger and older groups of individuals with this disease. On the other hand, the most common leukemias and lymphomas in elderly patients are those derived from the B-lymphocyte arm of the immune system. These, including chronic lymphocytic leukemia and multiple myeloma, rise dramatically in incidence throughout life, with the real majority of these disorders found in elderly individuals. Whether this dramatic relationship is caused by an enhanced susceptibility of the B lymphocyte to neoplastic transformation in older individuals is a question relevant to the entire issue of the relationship between the aging process and the neoplastic process, a subject that is considered next.

Not only does cancer occur at an increased rate in older individuals, but it makes a significant impact on such people's lives, from the standpoint of both increasing morbidity and mortality. As Fig. 53-1 also demonstrates, the age-specific cancer mortality continues to rise as a function of age, as does incidence. In support of this observation is the report from the SEER Program that 5-year survivals for most types of cancer decrease with advancing age.

RELATIONSHIP OF AGING AND NEOPLASIA

It is difficult to discuss a relationship between two processes—aging (senescence) and neoplastic transformation—both of which are still incompletely understood at this time. To explore the relationship, however, we must first briefly describe the current understanding of the multistep process of carcinogenesis. The first stage of cancer development is known as *initiation.* In this process, chemical or physical carcinogens, or certain viruses, cause a change in the cell that predisposes it to a subsequent malignant transformation. This change appears to be an irreversible lesion in the genomic deoxyribonucleic acid (DNA) of a stem cell; the lesion may remain stable for a long period. It is not clear whether such an initiated cell can be recognized clinically, but certain disorders such as preleukemia, or carcinoma in situ, may be a manifestation of this phenomenon.

The next stage of carcinogenesis is called *promotion* and involves a proliferative phase. *Promoters* are agents that can induce mitogenesis, or cell division, in an initiated cell. This phenomenon includes the activation of a number of growth factors and transcription factors, which promote cell proliferation, and which may arise through the events related to changes in oncogenes or tumor suppressor genes noted later. Whereas it appears that a single initiating event is sufficient to begin the process, promotion appears to be most successful when it is repetitive. This may occur shortly after initiation or after a delay and appears to be dose dependent as well as reversible. For this reason, researchers believe that cessation of cigarette smoking (containing both initiators and promoters) reduces the cancer incidence of former smokers when compared with those who continue to smoke.

The final stage of cancer development in this model is *progression.* This is actually multiphasic itself and involves the transformation of a cell from a premalignant to a malignant state, the potential clonal evolution of a subset of such cells, and the potential development of metastasis. The latter two phenomena are quite important and have led to the concept of tumor cell heterogeneity. Although we believe that tumors arise from a single "clone of cells," tumor cells are genetically more unstable than normal cells, yielding progeny with variable proliferative and metastatic potential. Thus, not all cells within a given tumor are the same. Clinically, this may explain such diversity as variable

chemosensitivity of tumor cells, the selection of resistant cells, the differential behavior of different metastatic lesions compared with the original tumor and with other metastatic lesions, and the sometimes unpredictable behavior of a particular cancer. Other factors relating to the tumor's impact on host tissue may also play an important role at this stage. These include the ability to disrupt stromal elements such as the basement membrane and the ability to promote angiogenesis, which supports further tumor growth.

It is clear that alterations in growth regulatory gene function play a critical role in the development of neoplasia. There are two major classes of such genes—oncogenes and tumor-suppressor genes. *Oncogenes,* or cancer genes, were initially described as viral genes capable of transforming normal cells to malignant ones. It was subsequently found that these viral oncogenes have normal cellular counterparts, that is, a normal cellular gene important to the physiologic regulation of cellular processes. It is now believed that such genes have the potential of causing malignant transformation of a normal cell, if the genetic information is altered or expressed inappropriately, as with the application of mutagenic or carcinogenic stimuli as noted in the previous section.

A large number of oncogenes have been described. They appear to have the potential for growth-enhancing activity at a series of steps along the mitogenic pathway, including activating signal transduction at the cell surface, producing endogenous growth factors at the cytoplasmic level (e.g., *ras*-like), and increasing the sensitivity of the cell to exogenous (or endogenous) growth factors at the nuclear level (e.g., *myc*-like). Another oncogene, *bcl*-2, codes for an inner mitochondrial protein that blocks apoptosis, or programmed cell death. This mechanism may be of particular interest in the context of senescence, as it may operate by increasing cell longevity rather than proliferation. Increased cellular oncogenic expression has been noted in many tumors and can be mimicked experimentally by altering the DNA encoding for the oncogene, usually at or near the promoter. Thus, it is possible that the chromosomal damage noted in neoplasia during the initiation and promotion phases, if it occurred near the region of an oncogene, could result in transformation and clonal evolution of the cancer. The evolutions noted in Burkitt's lymphoma and chronic granulocytic leukemia may be examples of this process. The expression of more than one oncogene is necessary to cause transformation.

A number of *tumor-suppressor genes* have been described, and mutations in such genes as Rb and p53 have been described in many human tumors. The normal function of such genes appears to prevent uncontrolled growth as a result of the action of various growth-promoting factors. It has even been suggested that senescence may act as a form of tumor suppression. In fact, the two tumor-suppressor genes just noted, p53 and Rb, are essential for maintaining the senescent phenotype of cells in culture. Inactivation of either gene extends the replicative life span of such cells and mutations of Rb have been linked to both cancer incidence and longevity in mice. This phenomenon would appear to enhance the likelihood of acquiring further mutations, leading to the ultimate development of

Table 53-2   Theories for Cancer Increase with Age

Longer duration of carcinogenic exposure

Increased susceptibility of cells to carcinogens

Decreased ability to repair DNA

Oncogene activation or amplification

Decrease in tumor suppression gene activity

Telomere shortening and genetic instability

Microenvironment alterations

Decreased immune surveillance

malignancy. Indeed deletions of p53, Rb, or both, are frequently found in common solid tumors, such as lung, breast and colon. Although the inactivation of tumor suppressor genes is important in the development of neoplasia, it is likely that alterations in both oncogenes and tumor-suppressor genes are necessary in many cases to achieve full malignant potential.

How then might the aging process influence the process of neoplastic transformation to result in the markedly increased rates of cancer in older people? General aspects of the aging process were discussed in Chap. 1, and only certain specific aspects relevant to the process under discussion will be reiterated here. Table 53-2 lists the types of theories that appear relevant to an explanation of the striking epidemiologic relationship.

1.   It is possible that aging simply allows the time necessary for the accumulation of cellular events to develop into a clinical neoplasm. There is evidence for age-related accumulation and expression of genetic damage. Somatic mutations are believed to occur at the rate of approximately 1 in 10 cell divisions, with approximately 10 cell divisions occurring in a lifetime of a human being. Certainly, the complex set of events required in the multistep process of carcinogenesis, for example, as described for colon cancer in humans, does occur over time. The passage of time alone, however, is not likely to explain the phenomenon, as the time for a mutated cell to become a malignant cell and then subsequently to become a detectable tumor has been estimated to be approximately 10 to 30 percent of the maximum life span for a given animal species, which may vary from just a few years to more than 100 years.

2.   There may be altered susceptibility of aging cells to a given amount of carcinogenic exposure. Data in this area are somewhat contradictory. In some cases, the incidence of skin tumors in mice produced with benzpyrene has been more related to dose than to age, whereas in other models, accelerated carcinogenesis as a function of age has been demonstrated, as, for example, when dimethyl benzanthracene (DMA) was applied to skin grafts of young and old mice. In addition, an age-related increase in the sensitivity of lymphocytes to cell-cycle arrest and chromosome damage after radiation has been demonstrated. It is also

possible that there are alterations in carcinogen metabolism with age, but the findings from such studies have also been contradictory.

3.   It is possible that damage, once initiated, is more difficult to repair in older cells. A number of studies demonstrate decreased DNA repair as a function of age following damage by carcinogens as well as radiation. Such repair failures may also be reflected in increased karyotype abnormalities in aged normal cells as well as in older patients with neoplastic disease.

4.   Oncogene activation or amplification might be increased in the older host, resulting either in increased action or promotion or in differential clonal evolution. Although evidence is currently limited, there have been observations of increased amplification of proto-oncogenes and their products in aging fibroblasts in vitro as well as evidence for increased c-*myc* transcript levels in the livers of aging mice. Alternatively, such factors as genetic alterations or DNA damage could lead to inactivation of cancer-suppressor genes. Given that age-related mutations frequently appear to result in the loss of function, alterations in tumor-suppressor genes may prove to be an important mechanism.

5.   The function of telomeres and the enzyme telomerase appears to be intimately involved in both the senescence and neoplasia processes. Telomeres, the terminal end of all chromosomes, shorten progressively as cells age. This shortening appears to be causally related to controlled cell proliferation and limitation of population doubling. Because the major function of telomeres is to protect the stability of the more internal coding sequences, the loss of this function may lead to genetic instability, which may promote mutations in oncogenic or tumor-suppressor gene sequences. The function of the enzyme telomerase is to regenerate the telomeres. Generally not expressed in normal cells, telomerase is activated in malignant cells and may play an important role in tumorigenesis. It is possible that p53 or Rb inactivation noted earlier here, or the inactivation of other tumor-suppressor genes, may allow the activation of the telomerase gene and promote cell immortalization and ultimately malignancy.

6.   It has become clear that a number of factors in the tumor microenvironment are critical for the development of the malignant phenotype, especially invasion and metastasis. Thus, senescent cells in the microenvironment may alter the stroma through increased production of enzymes, such as collagenase, to create a more tumorigenic environment. On the other hand, angiogenesis is often retarded in the older host, potentially limiting progression and resulting in greater localization of some tumors in older individuals.

7.   A decrease in immune surveillance, or immunosenescence, could contribute to the increased incidence. This phenomenon is described in detail in Chap. 3. With respect to tumor-related immunity, however, there is a considerable amount of evidence in animal models for a loss of tumor-specific immunity with progressive age. This includes the

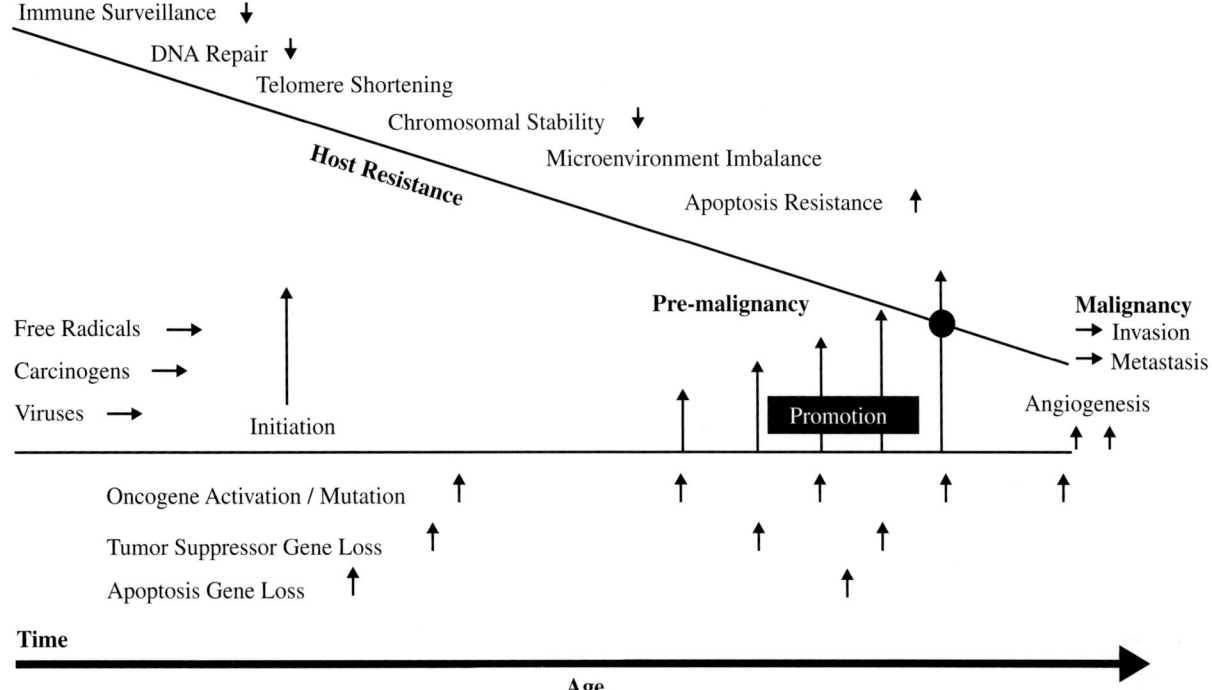

Figure 53-2   Age and cancer susceptibility. This figure presents a model incorporating the various factors that may play a role in the increased incidence of cancer with age.

altered capacity of old mice to reject transplanted tumors, the close relationship between susceptibility to malignant melanomas and the rate of age-related T-cell–dependent immune function decline, and the ability by immunopharmacologic manipulation to increase age-depressed tumoricidal immune function and to decrease the incidence of spontaneous tumors. The evidence linking such data to age-associated immune deficiency and the rise of cancer incidence in humans, however, is mainly circumstantial and not likely to be fully explanatory, as the types of tumors seen in the most striking examples of immune deficiency are very different from those seen in the usual aging human.

Figure 53-2 summarizes in a schematic fashion the potential interaction of these many factors that may be of importance in the increase of cancer with age. It indicates the interface of time and age-related events, such as free radical and other carcinogenic exposure, resulting in initiation, then cumulative promoting events, including mutations and other alterations in critical genes, which alternately exceed a threshold of host resistance factors, which have been progressively reduced during the aging process.

It is possible that the relationship is even more fundamental as suggested by the concept of "negative pleiotropy," which states that functions important for the organism in early life (through the reproductive period) will be selected for, despite the fact that they may be quite injurious in later life. In this case, senescence could be viewed as the price we pay in later life for the rigorous attempt to control proliferation to avoid neoplasia early on. The progressive, and

no doubt multifactorial, loss of the controls with aging ultimately results in an increase in neoplasia in advanced age despite the early control. From the standpoint of natural selection, both of these outcomes would be acceptable, as they tend to occur long after the reproductive life span. It is likely that through research at the basic level concerning the interactions of aging and neoplasia, we will learn a great deal about the fundamental basis of each. It is hoped that such information will enhance our ability to engage in prevention at the primary and secondary levels.

Current information suggests that a large proportion of cancers are potentially preventable. The most obviously available modalities in this regard are avoidance of known and suspected carcinogenic exposures such as tobacco smoke, occupational and environmental chemicals, excessive sunlight, and dietary factors such as excessive fat and smoked, salted, and pickled foods. Although older individuals have potentially acquired a lifetime exposure to such carcinogens, they should still accrue benefits from modifying these behaviors as well as from engaging in positive ones such as the suggested intake of fiber, vitamins, and fresh vegetables. In recent years, there has been increased interest in cancer prevention through chemopreventive intervention approaches. However, results are inconsistent, and some have shown adverse effects. The evidence for tamoxifen as a preventive agent for breast cancer is the strongest but the agent appears to be less effective in elderly women. Currently, there is no compelling evidence for the efficacy of the use of chemopreventive agents among the elderly population, and it still must be considered experimental.

CLINICAL PRESENTATIONS AND DISEASE BEHAVIOR

Screening in Asymptomatic Individuals

The situations in which periodic routine screening are recommended for all individuals regardless of age are relatively few. A number of organizations have made recommendations, and there is some variation among them. It should be recognized that when applied to elderly persons, especially those older than age 75 years, such information is largely empirically derived. These recommendations are directed at mass screening of populations. When applied to individuals within a physician's office or other practice, they serve only as general guidelines for decisions that may be, and often should be, modified by many other factors. Table 53-3 shows the current guidelines of the American Cancer Society relevant to the older adult, those of the US Preventive Health Task Force, a synthesized recommendation by the author, and Medicare reimbursement. Most of these recommendations do not directly address alterations in strategy for people at more advanced ages. Moreover, there is obvious variability in the recommendations. In general, for malignancies for which screening modalities are potentially useful, in the absence of upper age limits, the expectation of 5 to 10 years of life would appear reasonable as a cutpoint. The problem is that assessment of remaining life expectancy for an individual patient may be difficult.

Arriving at a specific recommendation for breast cancer screening in older women has been complicated by several factors. In addition to the lack of specific outcome data for women older than 75 years of age, factors such as increased mammographic detectability of cancers in older women because of the increase in fatty tissue of the breast with age, contrasted with the increased prevalence of comorbid disease, make decision-making difficult. In general, breast cancer screening should be a lifelong activity, although cessation has been suggested if life expectancy is less than 5 years. While there are no specific outcome data to support breast self-examination in older women, if it is practiced, it should be made clear that it is not a substitute for mammography and clinical examination.

In the past, recommendations concerning cervical cancer and the Papanicolaou (Pap) test have been controversial. The effectiveness of this screening modality is widely accepted. Controversy has been centered more around the frequency of testing required and whether testing could be suspended either at a certain age or after a certain number of negative tests. The current American Cancer Society guideline for detection of cervical cancer in asymptomatic women appears to be a consensus position that should adequately address the issue. The guideline states that "all women who are, or who have been, sexually active, or have reached age 18 years, [should] have an annual Pap test and pelvic examination. After a women has three or more consecutive satisfactory normal annual examinations, the Pap test may be performed less frequently at the discretion of her physician."

This recommendation has no specific upper-age limitation, and the discussion of these recommendations contains a reminder that "mature women—those over 65—also require testing." This is considered to be critical if such women have not had a history of regular Papanicolaou testing in their younger years. Thus, we would recommend that for the older patient whose history of previous screening is not clear, Papanicolaou testing be done until the recommendations have been fulfilled.

Recommendations for colon cancer screening center on general agreement over the use of fecal occult blood testing and sigmoidoscopy, with the use of colonoscopy and double-contrast barium enema being more questionable. Prostate cancer screening remains controversial. While some agencies recommend prostrate-specific antigen (PSA) screening, this has been done on the basis only of a demonstration of increased ascertainment. There are yet no data on impact on mortality or even quality of life over long periods. Given the large number of false-positives requiring considerable work-up, and the high incidence of very indolent disease in older men, the US Preventive Services Task Force (USPSTF) decision not to recommend such screening appears reasonable. In any event, if screening is to be considered, a thorough discussion of the risks as well as benefits should first ensue. In such consideration, it would appear that at least a 10-year life expectancy would be required before there is any chance of seeing a positive benefit overall. For ovarian cancer, acceptable screening methods have not been shown to have an impact on tumor-related outcomes. Screening examination for oral and skin cancers is reasonable for high-risk older people as part of an office examination.

For lung cancer, one of the most common malignancies in both genders, specific mass screening is not recommended. This is based on a lack of demonstrated cost–benefit efficacy, even in high-risk smoking groups. However, with the relatively few elderly patients involved in the large screening trials on which these recommendations have been based, and given the very high cancer incidence in the older smoker and evidence (described later in the section on Biologic Behavior of Tumors in the Elderly Host) that this malignancy may present at an earlier stage in older patients, there exists some rationale for the potential usefulness of screening in individual patients in the older age group.

Despite these widely disseminated recommendations, many individuals do not follow them. This appears to relate to both physician- and patient-derived factors. Despite the increased risk of cancer in the older age group, such individuals appear to avail themselves of routine screening even less frequently than their younger counterparts. The physician and other health care professionals should ensure that the older individual is aware of the importance of screening, that the opportunity for such examinations is provided, and that fears and anxieties about these tests are allayed to as great an extent as possible. Screening education materials, made user friendly for the older person, have been developed and should be used.

Initial Presentation

As an extension of the screening concept, the goal for initial cancer detection is to make the diagnosis as early as

Table 53-3 Recommendations for Cancer Screening in Elderly People

Cancer	Test(s)	ACS Guideline	USPSTF Guidelines	Author Guidelines	Medicare Reimbursement
Breast	Mammography (with or without clinical breast examination)	Annually starting at age 40 years for as long as patient is in good health	Annually or biennially between ages 50 and 69 years; consider continuing if patient has reasonable life expectancy	Start biennial screening at age 50 years, continue to offer between 70 and 80 years if life expectancy greater than 5–7 years; explain risks, explore barriers	Yes (1991); annual (2000)
Cervical	Papanicolaou (Pap) test	Annually for 3 years, then less frequently, no upper age limit	Biennially or triennially, may stop at age 65 years if has had regular, normal smears	Biennially or triennially, stop at age 65 years if patient has had regular, normal smears; obtain history of prior Pap smears and risk factors; perform speculum examination before excluding from screening for hysterectomy	Pap and pelvic every 24 months (2001)
Colorectal	FOBT; flexible sigmoidoscopy; colonoscopy; ACBE	At age 50 years, offer: annual FOBT; flexible sigmoidoscopy every 5 years; annual FOBT and flexible sigmoidoscopy every 5 years; colonoscopy every 10 years; or ACBE every 5–10 years	At age 50 years, offer annual FOBT; flexible sigmoidoscopy every 5 years; or annual FOBT and flexible sigmoidoscopy every 5 years	At age 50 years, offer annual FOBT with or without flexible sigmoidoscopy every 5 years; consider 1-time colonoscopy or combined flexible sigmoidoscopy and ACBE	Yes (1997)
Prostate	Digital rectal examination; PSA assay	Both tests annually, starting at age 50 years	Neither test recommended	Neither test recommended except in high-risk patients (e.g., family history of disease, African American)	Yes (2000)
Lung	Chest x-ray; sputum cytology; spiral CT scan; fluorescence bronchoscopy	None of these tests recommended	None of these tests recommended	None of these tests recommended	No
Ovary	Pelvic examination; CA-125 assay; transvaginal ultrasound	None of these tests recommended	None of these tests recommended	None of these tests recommended	No

ACBE, air-contrast barium enema; ACS, American Cancer Society; CT, computed tomography; FOBT, fecal occult blood test; PSA, prostate-specific antigen; USPSTF, United States Preventive Services Task Force.
SOURCE: Modified from Heflin MT and Cohen HJ (2001).

possible, with the hope that treatment at the earliest stages of disease would yield the best survival rates. It is, therefore, of great importance that both patient and physician pay attention to symptoms that may herald the onset of the neoplastic process. Although information on "warning signs of cancer" has been widely disseminated by the American Cancer Society and others, it is often ignored. This is due in part to a lack of knowledge of the implications of such warning signs. Indeed, some have indicated that elderly persons know less about potential cancer symptoms and their significance than do young individuals, which might lead to a delay in presentation. Another factor that might interfere with early diagnosis is what might be called "cancer symptom confusion," that is, a tendency to write off the symptom as simply another change caused by the aging process. Table 53-4 lists examples of such possibilities. Physicians and patients alike may be prone to such assumptions and should be alerted to the fact that a new symptom or a change in symptoms should be appropriately pursued in the elderly individual.

Current evidence suggests that once having noticed a symptom that appears to be related to cancer, older individuals do not delay appreciably in seeking medical help. Thus, in both a study of a Rhode Island population and a population-based study in New Mexico, older individuals were no more likely than younger ones to delay seeking medical attention once the symptom was noted. Physicians, however, may be guilty of delaying further diagnostic pursuits in elderly patients. In one study of factors affecting the delay in the ultimate diagnosis of breast cancer, there was somewhat of a longer delay in diagnosis from the time of presentation for older patients than for younger, but the greatest part of this delay was due to factors for which the physician was responsible, rather than those for which patients were responsible. Part of the problem may lie in a failure to recognize some of the new signs and symptoms in patients with multiple disease processes. It is easy to attribute such symptoms as anorexia, weight loss, or decrease in performance status to social or psychological changes. The increasing prevalence of findings such as anemia in elderly patients may lower the index of suspicion

for attributing the factor to a new specific neoplastic process. The remarkable age-related increase in cancer incidence described earlier in this chapter should be sufficient to promote the maintenance of vigilance in this regard, although it must be balanced by judgment concerning the risk-benefit ratio for diagnostic evaluations in individual patients depending on their other medical status. Thus, the initial discovery of a new symptom in a previously totally well, active 80-year-old may be pursued rather differently than a similar discovery in a severely demented, bed-bound individual with severe congestive heart failure, diabetes, and pulmonary failure.

Biologic Behavior of Tumors in the Elderly Host

The effect of the aging process on the clinical course of cancer, or to put it another way, whether cancer behaves differently in the older individual—is not clear-cut. Although the SEER data noted previously suggested that in many cancers the 5-year survival rate is lower for older people, it is possible that this is related more to comorbid disease and other factors rather than simply to aging per se. On the other hand, there is a widespread belief that cancers may behave more indolently in elderly patients. These are important issues because they may to a considerable degree, affect decisions regarding treatment. Both clinical and experimental evidence support both sides of this issue, and it is likely that there is a spectrum of responses dependent on initial tumor types as well as individual host status. One indicator of the phenomenon is the extent of disease at presentation. For most cancers examined, there has been no consistent difference in the stage of disease or presentation for different age groups. For those that have been determined, the directions are not always the same. For malignant melanoma, older patients have been consistently found to have more advanced-stage local disease with deeper penetrating lesions at presentation. For breast cancer, some studies show a greater proportion of older patients with distant metastatic spread at presentation, whereas for lung cancer the opposite has been found,

Table 53-4 Cancer Symptom Confusion

Symptom or Sign	Possible Malignancy	Aging "Explanation"
Increase in skin pigment	Melanoma, squamous cell	"Age spots"
Rectal bleeding	Colon or rectum	Hemorrhoids
Constipation	Rectal	"Old age"
Dyspnea	Lung	Getting old, out of shape
Decrease in urinary stream	Prostate	"Dribbling"—benign prostatic hypertrophy (BPH)
Breast contour change	Breast	"Normal" atrophy, fibrosis
Fatigue	Metastatic or other	Loss of energy due to "aging"
Bone pain	Metastatic or other	Arthritis: "aches and pains of aging"

and older patients have been noted to present with localized disease in a greater proportion of cases. Uterine and cervical cancers have in some cases been noted to be later in the course of disease at presentation in older individuals. Of course, even these differences might be related to such phenomena as delay in the patient's presenting for diagnosis (which does not appear to be the case), delay in pursuing the diagnosis, intensity of diagnostic endeavors, or a combination of these factors, or, on the other hand, a greater chance for a serendipitous finding because of more frequent visits to physicians.

Another biologic factor that may influence neoplastic behavior in differently aged hosts is the histologic subtype of the tumor. Thus, while thyroid cancer overall appears to behave more aggressively in the older host, it is also true that a larger proportion of thyroid neoplasia in elderly patients is made up by anaplastic carcinoma, which at any age has more aggressive behavior. In addition, however, there may be a poorer overall prognosis for older individuals with thyroid cancer, even independent of histologic type. Similarly, for malignant melanoma, although there is an increased proportion of older people who have melanomas of poor prognostic histologic type and location at presentation, older individuals have a poorer prognosis for survival than do younger ones independent of this phenomenon even for localized disease. Similarly, for lung cancer, the increased proportion of elderly patients with squamous carcinoma of the lung—which is the histologic subset most likely to present as localized disease—partially, but not completely, explains some of the findings just noted. Such biologic differences may be manifested in other ways, as in the case of breast cancer, in which older women have an increased frequency of estrogen-receptor–positive breast cancer, probably related to hormonal influences of the postmenopausal state. An additional factor is the longer tumor doubling time seen in breast cancer cells from older women. Because estrogen-receptor positivity and longer doubling times are associated with better prognosis, with more slow-growing tumors, and with longer disease-free survivals, these phenomena, rather than age per se, might provide the reason why this cancer appears to behave more indolently in an older individual. Despite this, overall cancer related survival is lower in older women, emphasizing the complex interactions of tumor and host that must be considered.

Acute myelogenous leukemia has a much poorer prognosis in older patients, perhaps explained by the higher prevalence of multidrug resistance genes in their cells. Experimental data in animal models likewise show this spectrum in rate of tumor growth and progression as a function of age. In these studies, the ability to contain tumor growth depends on the particular host tumor system used, thus mimicking the clinical situation to some extent. A proposed explanation for the situation in which the older host more effectively controls the rate of tumor is a paradoxical effect of decreasing immune function with age, that is, decreased activity of those cells in the old host's immune system, which, under the stimulation of the neoplastic process, produce tumor-enhancing factors such as angiogenesis factor. When this occurs, tumor growth might

be expected to be diminished. To what extent these various factors play a role in the biologic behavior of neoplasia in the human aging host remains a fascinating puzzle to be unraveled.

MANAGEMENT

This section examines the utility of the major modalities of cancer treatment in the elderly individual. The use of such modalities is heavily conditioned by the initial decision-making process, that is, whether to screen, whether to pursue diagnostic work-ups, whether to treat at all, and how intensively to treat. In such decisions, the physician is often placed in the position of weighing benefits versus risks of diagnostic and therapeutic interventions. This is as it should be, and the physician should take into account the various biologic, psychological, and social factors involved in the patient's well-being. Of great importance in this regard is the patient's own assessment of the value of both quantity and quality of potential survival during and after the treatment for malignancy. In this process, there is a clear need to individualize such decisions, and a decision made for a well elderly patient may be appropriately different than that for a frail elderly patient.

Currently, it would appear that age bias in diagnostic and treatment decisions for older patients with cancer does exist. It has been reported that despite the presentation of older patients with higher proportion of localized lung cancer, such patients more infrequently received potentially curative surgical therapy. Although this study did not address the appropriateness of such decisions, another study of patients with breast cancer did, revealing that older women with breast cancer received appropriate therapy, be it surgical, hormonal, chemotherapy, or another, less frequently than did younger women. Other studies confirm these variations in treatment decisions on the basis of the patient's age. It is not yet clear whether this is based on physician or patient decisions. Differences in decisions may be entirely appropriate in certain situations but must be based on specific individualized patient information not on categorical decisions made on the basis of chronologic age.

We proposed one framework in which the general aspects of such decision making can be considered for the individual patient. This is shown in Fig. 53-3 and is called the Comprehensive Geriatric Model. It graphically presents a number of the concepts critical to the care of the elderly, i.e., that there is a decreased functional reserve and that, as an extension of Engel's Bio-Psycho-Social Model, all of these various aspects of the individual's background must be taken into account when making decisions about the new process, i.e., the cancer. Each of these levels, e.g., biologic or psychological, can create interactions that influence both the cancer and the host, and, likewise, any intervention directed at the cancer may influence both the cancer and each of these levels of the host's function. Conversely, each of these levels of function, when compromised by the aging process or other comorbid diseases, may influence the ability to deliver these various interventions. Thus, in a sense, a conceptual checklist is

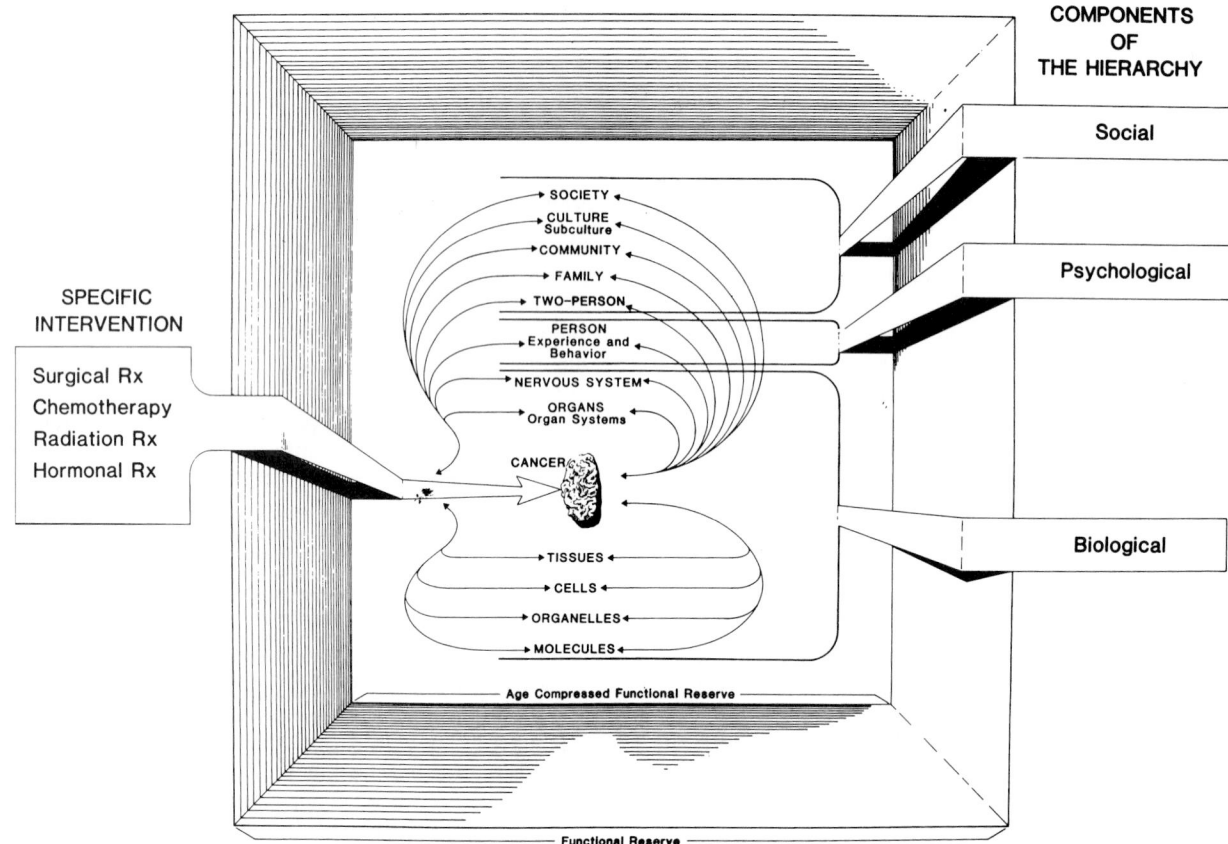

Figure 53-3 The Comprehensive geriatric model. Reproduced with permission from Cohen HJ, DeMaria L: in Lazlo J (ed): *Physician's Guide to Cancer Care Complications.* New York, Dekker, Ch. 10, p. 240, 1986.

presented in which a four-way interaction of various factors can be systematically considered when making decisions. Examples of ways in which physiologic changes occurring with age can impact on cancer treatment are shown in Table 53-5.

The implementation of this concept is through the application of geriatric assessment (as described in detail in Chap. 8) to the elderly cancer patient so that the domains of physiologic status, comorbidity, geriatric syndromes, and functional and cognitive status, can be assessed and define levels of frailty. This information, rather than age per se, should weigh more heavily on subsequent management decisions for use of diagnostic as well as therapeutic technologies for the elderly patient with cancer. The optimal mechanism for practically implementing this approach (e.g., clinic team, inpatient unit, consultation) remains to be determined.

MAJOR THERAPEUTIC MODALITIES

Surgery

Surgery and other invasive procedures are frequently involved in initial diagnostic as well as in therapeutic approaches to the elderly patient with cancer. The general aspects of surgery in the elderly patient are discussed thoroughly in Chap. 32. Suffice it to say here that a number of studies demonstrate that cancer surgery may be

accomplished in elderly patients with mortality and morbidity rates that are often similar to those for younger patients and appear to be conditioned more by the extent of comorbid disease and declines in measurable physiologic functions than by chronologic age. In comparing potential alternative modalities, it is well to remember that the acute and time-limited stress of surgery may be preferable to many older patients than the more chronic or protracted courses of therapy frequently involved in radiation therapy and/or chemotherapy.

Radiation Therapy

Radiation therapy is used in the treatment of malignancies with both curative and palliative intent. In an attempt to cure local or regional disease, given that both radiation therapy and surgery might be considered, one must consider whether the cure rate is equivalent and whether there are differences in morbidity or mortality between the procedures that would favor one over the other. Radiation therapy is generally not contraindicated by associated medical conditions, and it may allow maintenance of function of the organ in which the tumor arises. For example, for an elderly person, radiating laryngeal carcinoma and maintaining speech, rather than requiring the learning of laryngeal speech postoperatively, may be of considerable advantage. On the other hand, radiation treatment frequently involves a protracted course of therapy.

Table 53-5 Aging Physiology and Cancer

Aging Physiology	Cancer Relevance
Cardiopulmonary	
↓ Max CO, VO$_2$ Max	Surgery
↓ Elasticity	C/P toxic drugs
Skin—↓ wound healing	Surgery
CNS—↓ brain weight, cerebral blood flow	Patient interactions CNS toxic drugs
Special senses—↓ taste, smell, salivary flow	Nutrition Radiation therapy
Hematopoiesis—↓ response under stress	Chemotherapy and radiation therapy
Immune system—↓ response	Infection
Body composition—↓ lean, ↑ fat	Drug distribution
Liver—↓ mass and flow	Hepatic drug metabolism
Kidney—↓ GFR	Renal drug excretion

CNS, central nervous system; C/P, cardiopulmonary; GFR, glomerular filtration rate.

Radiation therapy is also used as an effective adjunct to surgery or chemotherapy or both. For those surgical procedures with high operative mortality, using adjunct radiation therapy to reduce the degree of surgery required may be especially attractive to an elderly patient. The results for adjunct radiation therapy and approaches such as quadrantectomy in breast cancer or lymph node excision in head or neck cancer have been demonstrated to be equivalent to more extensive surgical procedures. Radiation is also used in a "neoadjuvant" setting, that is, prior to surgery in an attempt to reduce tumor mass and allow greater operability. Palliatively, radiation therapy can be extremely effective in providing relief from pain from bone metastases, the effects of brain metastases, control of local obstructive symptoms, and spinal cord compromise. Such treatments can frequently be delivered in courses of 1 to 2 weeks' duration rather than the longer courses of therapy that may be more difficult to tolerate. However, short courses of high-dose radiation may be associated with a higher incidence of acute side effects. The results of treatment, as well as the incidence of complications, greatly depend on the technology available and its correct application.

The side effects of therapy may create problems for the older patient. The radiation effect on normal tissue is said to be enhanced approximately 10 to 15 percent in the elderly patient. Logically, those organs with more marked physiologic decline would be at greatest risk. Radiation to the oral pharynx and oral cavity can produce a loss of taste, dryness of mucous membranes, and involution of salivary glands, which when combined with a precarious

nutritional intake in a frail and elderly individual might be lethal, or certainly contribute a considerable amount of morbidity, if not recognized. Moreover, if daily treatment is tolerated poorly owing to nausea or weakness, treatment may be compromised because of the decreased daily doses, the patient's unscheduled absences, or decrease in the total planned dose. Because radiation therapy is frequently used in the treatment of lung cancer, pulmonary complications may be of particular importance. In one study, severe radiation pneumonitis was noted more frequently in elderly individuals than in younger ones, regardless of field size and other therapies. Alterations in schedule can be made and still deliver potentially curative radiation therapy to older individuals. This must be done with care, however; although decreasing the daily fraction has not been shown to be detrimental to local control of neck and head cancer, split-dose schedules are associated with significantly lower control rates for some tumor sites.

Chemotherapy and Hormonal Therapy

A thorough discussion of the principles of pharmacology in elderly persons can be found in Chap. 19. Although still understudied, in recent years there have been more direct studies of the effect of age on the pharmacokinetics of orally or parenterally administered chemotherapeutic agents. In general, absorption of drugs appears to be affected relatively little as a consequence of age but may become more relevant as newer oral agents (e.g., fluorinated pyrimidines) because widely used. Volume of distribution for fat-soluble drugs, such as nitrosoureas, is increased. In people with reduced albumin, volume of distribution for drugs bound to albumin, such as etoposide, is increased and similarly for those with reduced red blood cells, but these changes seem to have little practical impact. Although hepatic metabolism of many drugs is altered with age, this too seems to have relatively little impact. The changes in glomerular function seen with age do have a significant impact on renally excreted drugs and must be carefully considered in dose determinations.

The potential for response and degree of toxicity for various regimens in elderly patients appears to constitute a spectrum depending predominantly on the aggressiveness of the therapeutic regimen. The major limiting factor for most drugs is bone marrow reserve. Decreased reserve capacity has been demonstrated in both experimental animals and humans, but clinical toxicity would depend on the degree to which bone marrow reserve is stressed. Other toxicities, such as the pulmonary toxicity of bleomycin, the cardiotoxicity of doxorubicin, and the peripheral nerve toxicity of vincristine, also appear to be increased somewhat, although, again, depending on the aggressiveness of the regimen. Thus, in one clinical study of treatment for metastatic lung, breast, and colorectal carcinoma, the responses of the elderly patients were equivalent to those of the younger ones with no substantial increase in toxicity. For these relatively unaggressive treatment regimens, excessive toxicity was seen with only two drugs. One was methotrexate. For this drug, however, apparently age-related excesses in toxicity have been shown to be more related to, and reduced by adjustment for, decrements in renal function.

A number of studies of adjuvant chemotherapy indicate similar benefits and toxicities in equivalently selected younger and older patients. When one considers somewhat more aggressive combination chemotherapy, such as for small-cell carcinoma of the lung, equivalent response rates have been obtained for older individuals, but this has come at the cost of increased marrow toxicity. Likewise, multiagent chemotherapy approaches for Hodgkin's disease and for non-Hodgkin's lymphoma are associated with markedly increased toxicity, increased numbers of early deaths, and, therefore, decreased survival for elderly patients. This phenomenon is seen to the maximal extent in elderly patients treated with the most aggressive regimens for acute nonlymphocytic leukemia, wherein excessive early treatment-related deaths severely constrain the use of such approaches. For some of these latter disorders, there may also be intrinsic cellular resistance to therapy in older individuals. For the hormonally responsive cancers, such as prostate cancer and breast cancer, hormonal therapy is purported to be at least as good in elderly patients as it is in younger patients, and it may be actively employed alone or in combination with other modalities for effective palliative treatment.

When approaching decisions about chemotherapy in treating the elderly patient, the clinician should use those modalities that in the prescribed dosages have acceptable responses with acceptable levels of toxicity, whereas in the case of those tumor types that require extremely aggressive therapy, the physician may need to seek modifications and new approaches in order to achieve lower levels of toxicity. Such situations may be amenable to clinical trials, in which elderly subjects are currently under represented, so that the best approaches to therapy can be delineated. We must be wary of the phenomenon of "risk aversion" leading to underdosing, in which, in an attempt to avoid toxicities, we effectively abrogate any chance of a therapeutic response. This occurred in the trials of adjuvant chemotherapy for breast cancer wherein poor results were seen in those elderly women who had lower than the prescribed dosage of adjuvant therapy, presumably in an attempt to avoid toxicities, whereas in those older women who had received doses of therapy equivalent to those of younger women, an equal effect was noted.

Supportive Care

The effects of cancer and its treatment may be devastating to elderly patients and may require substantial supportive care. The goal of such therapy is to maximize the ability of patients to tolerate the treatment as well as the disease. Underlying problems requiring symptomatic relief need to be actively sought by the physician because elderly patients more frequently underreport their symptoms. Many of the specific aspects of supportive care are covered in other chapters and are only mentioned here to stress their importance for the management of the elderly cancer patient. These include the extreme importance of effective pain management (see Chap. 25); maintenance of appropriate

nutritional support (see Chap. 90); the supportive role of nursing (see Chap. 21); the importance of patient, physician, and family discussions concerning decisions regarding terminal care and other issues (see Chaps. 26–29); and the utility of hospice care (see Chap. 26).

One complication frequently seen in treatment of the elderly patient with cancer is nausea and vomiting. These side effects can seriously compromise the ability to deliver effective chemotherapy, and they create a considerable degree of morbidity. It is interesting that elderly patients appear to experience less nausea and vomiting than younger ones. Nevertheless, it is wise to attempt to prevent this occurrence in the first place and to correct it when possible. Patients should be kept well hydrated, and an attempt should be made to eliminate environmental factors, such as food and other odors, that may trigger vomiting. Oral feedings with dry bland foods are generally well tolerated, but high-protein diets are not. Antiemetic drugs may be required for control. For highly emetogenic chemotherapy, such as cisplatin, the serotonin antagonists, such as ondansetron, can be used with great effectiveness and tolerability in elderly patients. Corticosteroids may be a useful adjunct. The substituted benzamides (e.g., metoclopramide), butyrophenones (e.g., haloperidol), and benzodiazepines (e.g., lorazepam) are useful for intermediate emetogenic drugs but have higher toxicity profiles. Phenothiazines are less active and have substantial toxicities. Elderly patients may be particularly predisposed to constipation, especially as a side effect of such drugs as vincristine, and both preventive and treatment approaches to this problem should be borne in mind at all times.

Because of the bone marrow suppressive effects of most cancer chemotherapies, significant cytopenias may result and should be treated with blood products. Because of decreased functional reserve, as well as other comorbid processes, maintenance of an effective and appropriate hemoglobin level should be approached with prophylactic and maintenance transfusion during the period of cytopenia. Hematopoietic growth stimulants such as erythropoietin, granulocyte colony-stimulating factor, and granulocyte-macrophage colony-stimulating factor are receiving increasing attention for the amelioration of such side effects, but their ultimate role in the care of the older cancer patient is yet to be fully established. Erythropoietin effectively maintains higher hemoglobin levels in elderly cancer patients and may help maintain a better quality of life. Although the white cell growth factors have been shown to maintain higher white blood counts and somewhat reduce the incidence of infections during aggressive chemotherapy, they have had little impact on treatment outcomes and on survival. The cost-to-benefit ratios of these therapies must be weighed carefully.

Finally, the all important area of psychological support must be considered. This begins with effective physician-patient communication and acknowledgment of the patient's views and values at every stage of the disease. When appropriate, caregiver involvement can be critical. An assessment of the patient's coping skills and strategies will be very helpful. Acknowledgment and support of those that appear to work best for the patient are important. The patient's spiritual state and use of religious coping strategies are also important to assess and support. It is ironic that despite the increase in physical frailty and other decrements in function with age, older cancer patients appear to cope better with the psychological stress of the illness than do younger patients. This may be a result of the development of effective coping strategies from dealing with many other stressors over the years.

CONCLUSION

Cancer is a disease seen with great frequency in elderly patients. The relationship of cancer to aging poses a challenge to our scientific understanding of these processes as well as to our clinical approach to the elderly patient. Further research is required to resolve the former, but a systematic, logically developed diagnostic and treatment plan can produce effective and gratifying results in the latter.

REFERENCES

Baker SD, Grochow LB: Pharmacology of cancer chemotherapy in the older persons. *Clin Geriatr Med* 13:169, 1997.

Bast RC et al. (eds): *Cancer Medicine,* 5th ed. Hamilton, Ontario, Canada, BC Decker, 2000.

Campisi J: Aging and cancer: the double-edged sword of replicative senescence. *J Am Geriatr Soc* 45:482, 1997.

Fehring RJ et al: Spiritual well-being, religiosity, hope, depression, and other mood states in elderly people coping with cancer. *Oncol Nurs Forum* 24:663, 1997.

Fernandez-Pol JA, Douglas MG: Molecular interactions of cancer and age. Hematol Oncol Clin North Am 14:1:25–44, 2000.

Fox SA, Roetzheim RG, Kington RS: Barriers to cancer prevention in the older person. Clin Geriatr Med 13:79, 1997.

Heflin MT, Cohen HJ: Cancer screening in the elderly. Hospital Practice 36:3:61–69, 2001.

Hershman D, Sundararajan V, Jacobson JS, et al: Outcomes of Tamoxifen chemoprevention for breast cancer in very high-risk women: A cost-effectiveness analysis. J Clin Onc 20:1:9–16, 2002.

Mor V et al: The psychosocial impact of cancer on older vs. younger patients and their families. *Cancer* 74:2118, 1994.

Muss HB, Cohen HJ, Lichtman SM: Clinical research in the older cancer patient, *Hematol Oncol Clin North Am* 14:1:283, 2000.

Naeim A, Reuben D: Geriatric syndromes and assessment in older cancer patients. *Oncology* 15:12:1567, 2001.

Sargent DJ et al: A pooled analysis of adjuvant chemotherapy for resected colon cancer in elderly patients. *N Engl J Med* 345:15:1091, 2001 [see also editorial comment: Older age—not a barrier to cancer treatment. *N Engl J Med* 345:15:1128].

Sporn MB, Lippman SM: Chemoprevention of cancer, in Bast RC et al. (eds.): *Cancer Medicine,* 5th ed. Hamilton, Ontario, Canada, BC Decker, 2000 p 351.

Tyner SD et al: p53 mutant mice that display early ageing-associated phenotypes. *Nature* 415:45, 2002.

Vestal RE: Aging and pharmacology. *Cancer* 80:1302, 1997.

Wright WE, Shay JW: Telomere dynamics in cancer progression and prevention: fundamental differences in human and mouse telomere biology. *Nat Med* 6:8:849, 2000.

Yancik R, Ries LAG: Aging and cancer in America: Demographic and epidemiologic perspectives. *Hematol Oncol Clin North Am* 14:1:17, 2000.

Zachariah B, Balducci L: Radiation therapy of the older patient. *Hematol Oncol Clin North Am* 14:1:131, 2000.

Zagonel V et al: General and supportive care: reducing chemotherapy-associated toxicity in elderly cancer patients. *Cancer Treat Rev* 22:223, 1996.

C H A P T E R 5 4

Breast Disease

GRETCHEN G. KIMMICK ◆ HYMAN B. MUSS

The breast, or mammary gland, is a fibro-fatty organ that produces all the necessary nutrients for a newborn. In women of childbearing age, the breast responds to cyclic hormone production and contains an abundance of epithelial structures and stroma that enable the production of milk. In a postmenopausal woman, declining ovarian function in late menopause leads to regression of these structures. The postmenopausal breast contains a ductal system, but the lobules shrink and collapse, leaving an organ that is composed primarily of fat. Whereas a breast lump in a premenopausal woman is likely to be a benign problem related to cyclic hormonal changes, in a postmenopausal woman, this is not the case. In this age group, the most important breast disease is cancer.

Cancer is the leading cause of death in women ages 55 to 74 years and is second to heart disease in women ages 75 and older. The incidence of cancer increases dramatically with age. In particular, breast cancer, the most common cancer in American women, is a major health concern. According to 2002 American Cancer Society estimates, breast cancer is the most common cancer in women, accounting for 26 percent of all newly diagnosed malignancies (205,600 new cases) and the second leading cause of cancer-related death (40,000 deaths). Moreover, US incidence and mortality data from the 1980s suggest that 12 percent of all women will be diagnosed with breast cancer during their lifetime and that 3.5 percent will die from it.

It has been estimated that almost half the cases of breast cancer occur in women older than age 65 years. In addition, 1984 data from the Surveillance, Epidemiology, and Results (SEER) Program of the National Institutes of Health indicate that the incidence increases dramatically with age (Fig. 54-1) from a rate of 60 per 100,000 in women younger than 65 years to a rate of approximately 320 per 100,000 in women older than 65 years. It is unclear whether increasing age is associated with a worse rate of survival. One major study found that increasing age was associated with higher mortality, but these data were not corrected for the stage of disease at diagnosis. In contrast, SEER data showed similar stage-adjusted 5-year survival for older and younger women. Survival data show that the very young and the very old have the poorest survival rates, but it is unlikely that age alone adversely influences survival.

Breast cancer is a major health concern and will become of even greater importance as the older population grows. Although breast cancer is more common in older women, they are also less likely to be appropriately screened, are more likely to present for care at a more advanced stage and to receive inferior surgical and postoperative management, and are less likely to be entered into clinical trials.

RISK FACTORS AND BIOLOGY

The specific cause of breast cancer is unknown. Many factors associated with increased risk have been identified: increasing age; white race; family history of breast cancer (especially in a first-degree relative); early menarche; late age at birth of first child (older than age 30 years); late menopause; history of benign breast disease (hyperplasia or atypical hyperplasia); heavy radiation exposure; obesity; increasing height; postmenopausal estrogen replacement therapy; and moderate to excessive alcohol use. Most of these factors are associated with relative risks in the range of 1.4 to 2 times the risk in the general female population. There is also geographic variability in breast cancer incidence, with the highest incidence being found in affluent white populations. The reason for these differences is probably related to risk factor distribution as well as

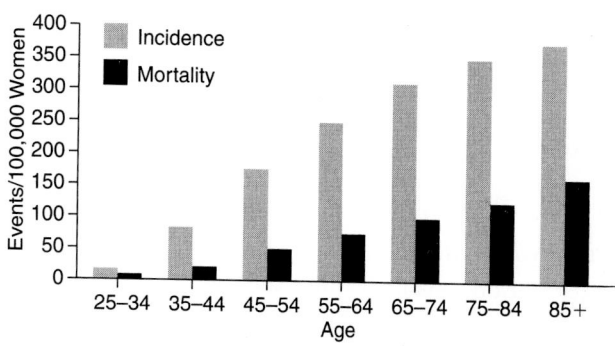

Figure 54-1 Breast cancer incidence and mortality by age. *Modified from Yancik et al: SEER data on 125,000 women from 1973 to 1984.*

genetic and environmental factors. Although breast cancer incidence differs among racial groups, such differences are minimized or lost when racial groups that are at low risk migrate to a high-risk environment.

A family history of breast cancer, implying a genetic defect, may be important in 5 to 20 percent of all cases of breast cancer. Genetic predisposition is particularly important in early onset breast cancer (diagnosed before age 50 years), but is probably not a major factor in the geriatric population. BRCA1 accounts for approximately 2 to 3 percent of breast cancers, but approximately 45 percent of familial breast cancers. Another gene, BRCA2, is responsible for approximately 35 percent of genetic abnormalities in high-risk families. Both BRCA1 and BRCA2 portend increased risks for both breast cancer and ovarian cancer, ranging from 36 to 85 percent for breast cancer and 16 to 60 percent for ovarian cancer. There are probably many modifying factors, including genetic, hormonal, and environmental factors, that determine whether a genetic mutation will lead to cancer.

Most breast cancers originate from ductal epithelium. Comparisons of older and younger patients with breast cancer reveal that infiltrating ductal carcinoma remains the most common histologic type in both groups, accounting for 75 to 80 percent of cases, with lobular carcinoma accounting for approximately 5 to 10 percent. Mucinous carcinoma and papillary carcinoma, histologic types that are associated with a somewhat lower risk of recurrence, are more common in older patients, while inflammatory carcinoma, an aggressive lesion with a poor prognosis, is extremely uncommon in such persons. Older patients are more likely to have well-differentiated and moderately differentiated lesions, positive estrogen and progesterone receptors (60 to 70 percent of patients), lower rates of tumor proliferation (the number of cells synthesizing deoxyribonucleic acid [DNA]), and less frequent expression of the HER-2 oncogene, when compared with younger patients. These data suggest that breast cancer in older patients is biologically less aggressive than it is in younger women. Survival data, however, show that very young and very old (>80 years of age) women have the poorest survival rates. Thus, one might deduce that the lower survival rates in elderly women with breast cancer relate less directly to the biology of their tumors and more to other factors, such as coexisting illness (comorbidity that increases with increasing age).

DIAGNOSIS

Primary Prevention, Screening, and Diagnosis

Primary Prevention

Except for draconian measures such as prophylactic mastectomy (which is not 100 percent effective), there is no known effective means of preventing breast cancer. As the pathogenesis of breast cancer is likely to be related to interactions of estrogens, other hormones, and breast tissue, current research efforts toward prevention focus on the use of antiestrogens. Data from a recent meta-analysis involving 75,000 patients with early stage breast cancer suggest that the use of tamoxifen, an antiestrogen with weak estrogen agonist activities, decreases contralateral breast cancer risk 40 to 50 percent in postmenopausal patients. A national trial (National Surgical Adjuvant Breast Project [NSABP] P1) comparing tamoxifen with placebo as a means of prevention in women at high risk for breast cancer (a risk of 1.66 percent of invasive breast cancer over 5 years) showed that tamoxifen decreased the incidence of invasive breast cancer by 50 percent. Thirty percent of women in this trial were older than age 60 years and 6 percent were older than age 70 years. Tamoxifen, however, was associated with significant increase in the risk of thromboembolism and endometrial cancer. In clinical practice, tamoxifen benefit must be weighed against risk and can be estimated from a model developed from Gail and colleagues. At present the STAR (Study of Tamoxifen Against Raloxifene) trial is comparing raloxifene (which does not increase the risk of endometrial cancer) with tamoxifen in a national trial in postmenopausal women; older patients should be encouraged to participate in this trial.

Screening

Breast cancer screening in a postmenopausal woman includes mammography and a physical examination. After menopause, as estrogen levels diminish, breast glandular tissue and ductal tissue decrease and fat tissue increases. In addition, postmenopausal patients have fewer cysts and fibroadenomas. These biological changes in breast tissue with aging, especially the increased percentage of fat tissue, allow for improved contrast between small foci of malignancy and the surrounding breast tissue, resulting in fewer false-negative mammographic examinations. Several studies show that the routine use of screening mammography in women age 50 through 70 years has improved survival by detecting breast carcinoma at an earlier stage and before metastatic dissemination. Although controversy persists, it is estimated that a 25 to 30 percent reduction in breast cancer mortality could be achieved if all women in this age category received appropriate mammographic screening. Although data are sparse in women older than 70 years of age, a recent overview suggested that mammography is likely to be of major benefit in this group as well. Because the life expectancy of a healthy woman age 75 to 79 years is 10 more years, and for a woman age 85 years it is 7 more years, screening in healthy women appears prudent in women older than age 75 years whose estimated survival exceeds 5 years.

Even with mammography, 10 to 20 percent of all breast cancers are not visualized on a mammogram, and physical examination by health professionals and breast self-examination remain essential and complementary adjuncts to mammographic screening. Several studies show that the most important factor for inducing an older patient to have a screening mammogram is for the physician to personally recommend it to the patient. Medicare law provides for payment for screening mammography on an annual

Table 54-1 Screening Guidelines for Breast Cancer in Women over Age 70

Test	Frequency	Comment
Breast self-examination	Monthly	Value uncertain, but many breast cancers still detected by patient
Physical examination	Yearly	By physician or other health professional; detects 15% of cancers *not* discovered on screening mammograms
Mammography	Every 1–2 years	Value in improving survival in women older than age 75 years unproven, but extrapolation of data from studies in postmenopausal patients suggests benefit

basis. Table 54-1 presents current recommendations for the screening of older women.

Diagnosis

The discovery of a breast mass in a postmenopausal woman requires prompt attention, as the majority of palpable masses in this age group are malignant. Mammography may help define the nature of a mass or find other nonpalpable lesions and is therefore indicated when a breast mass is found, although it is not essential to the diagnosis. All breast masses require biopsy in this patient population.

For lesions that are found on mammography but that are not palpable, biopsy is required, either stereotactic or needle-localization biopsy. Needle-localization biopsy allows for removal of the abnormal lesion for tissue diagnosis. For some patients with mammographic lesions that are likely benign, and after careful discussion, follow-up with physical examination and repeat mammography in several months is appropriate. For most patients, the fear of breast cancer and the possibility that even a low-risk lesion may prove to be malignant provide a compelling motive for lesion biopsy or excision.

For palpable lesions, core-needle biopsy is preferable to fine-needle aspiration (FNA) biopsy because core biopsy can distinguish invasive from in situ lesions in most patients. Although concerns have been expressed that needle biopsy may be associated with tracking of malignant cells and a higher risk of local recurrence, such fears are unfounded. If the core or FNA is negative or inconclusive, unless the mass proves to be a cyst and resolves after aspiration, further biopsy, preferably excision, is necessary. For patients who have a mass that is characteristic of malignancy on physical examination or mammography, initial excision of the lesion or mastectomy, with or without axillary dissection, may be preferable to a two-stage procedure involving a needle, core, or excisional biopsy, followed by definitive surgery. In patients where biopsy is diagnostic of malignancy and in those scheduled for definitive surgery, preoperative evaluation includes a complete history and physical examination, a complete blood count and serum chemistry profile, and a chest x-ray. These studies are generally more helpful in determining the presence of comorbid illness than they are in finding metastases. Bone, computerized tomographic, or magnetic resonance

imaging (MRI) scans should be done to investigate signs or symptoms suggestive of metastases, but are not necessary in asymptomatic patients. Bilateral mammography should be performed on all these patients to evaluate both the ipsilateral breast and the contralateral breast for other nonpalpable lesions.

Again, physicians should be aware that mammography may not image palpable lesions in as many as 20 percent of patients. A palpable lesion in a postmenopausal woman always requires biopsy; mammography is of value mainly for detecting nonpalpable lesions in either the involved or the contralateral breast.

Staging

All patients with breast cancer should have accurate staging as described by American Joint Committee for Cancer (AJCC) guidelines. This system categorizes the extent of malignancy according to the size of the primary lesion (T), the extent of nodal involvement (N), and the occurrence of metastases (M). Table 54-2 presents the AJCC breast cancer staging criteria. Tumor size (the largest diameter of the infiltrating component) and the extent of nodal involvement (the number of axillary nodes removed and the number positive) should be determined from pathologic examination of the specimen and should be included in the pathology report. Less than 5 percent of the time, breast cancer presents as a diffuse infiltrating lesion and cannot be measured accurately. For the extent of nodal involvement to reflect the prognosis accurately, a sample of at least six nodes should be removed. The pathology report should also include histologic type and tumor grade; assessment of vascular or lymphatic invasion, and skin involvement; percentages of ductal carcinoma in situ and invasive carcinoma in the primary lesion; and analysis of estrogen receptors (ERs) and progesterone receptors (PRs) in the primary lesion. Measurement of HER-2 oncogene overexpression (found in about 20 percent of tumors) should also be performed in most patients. Other markers are not of consistent benefit and are not needed on a routine basis. Today, all markers can be accurately assessed on paraffin-embedded tissues. After definitive surgical management, asymptomatic patients who have had an unremarkable preoperative evaluation, including history and physical examination,

Table 54-2   TNM-Pathologic Staging System for Cancer of the Breast: AJCC Criteria-2003

Primary Tumor

TX	Primary tumor cannot be assessed
T0	No evidence of primary tumor
Tis	Carcinoma is situ: ductal carcinoma in situ, lobular carcinoma in situ, or Paget's disease of nipple with no tumor
T1	Tumor ≤2 cm in greatest dimension
T1mic	Microinvasion 0.1 cm or less in greatest dimension
T1a	Tumor more than 0.1 cm but not more than 0.5 cm in greatest dimension
T1b	Tumor more than 0.5 cm but not more than 1 cm in greatest dimension
T1c	Tumor more than 1 cm but not more than 2 cm in greatest dimension
T2	Tumor >2 cm but not >5 cm in greatest dimension
T3	Tumor >5 cm in greatest dimension
T4	Tumor of any size with direct extension to chest wall* or skin (includes inflammatory carcinoma)

Regional Lymph Nodes

NX	Regional lymph nodes cannot be assessed (previously removed or not removed)
N0	No regional lymph node metastases
N1	Metastasis in 1 to 3 axillary lymph nodes, and/or in internal mammary nodes with microscopic disease detected by sentinel lymph node dissection but not clinically apparent [not clinically apparent is defined as not detected by imaging studies, excluding lymphoscintigraphy or by clinical examination].
N1mi	Micrometastasis (greater than 0.2 mm, none greater than 2.0 mm)
N2	Metastasis in 4 to 9 axillary lymph nodes, or in clinically apparent [clinically apparent is defined as detected by imaging studies, excluding lymphoscintigraphy, or by clinical examination] internal mammary lymph nodes in the *absence* of axillary lymph node metastasis
N3	Metastasis in 10 or more axillary lymph nodes, or in infraclavicular lymph nodes, or in clinically apparent [clinically apparent is defined as detected by imaging studies, excluding lymphoscintigraphy, or by clinical examination] ipsilateral internal mammary lymph nodes in the *presence* of 1 or more positive axillary lymph nodes; or in more than 3 axillary lymph nodes with clinically negative microscopic metastasis in internal mammary lymph nodes; or in ipsilateral supraclavicular lymph nodes

Distant Metastases

M0	No distant metastases
M1	Distant metastases

Stage Grouping

Stage 0	Tis	N0	M0				
Stage I (T1 includes T1mic)	T1	N0	M0				
Stage IIA	T0-1,	N1	M0	or	T2,	N0,	M0
Stage IIB	T2	N1	M0	or	T3,	N0,	M0
Stage IIIA	T0-2,	N2	M0	or	T3,	N1-2,	M0
Stage IIIB	T4	N0-2	M0				
Stage IIIC	Any T	N3	M0				
Stage IV	Any T	Any N	M1				

*The chest wall includes the ribs, intercostal muscles, and serratus anterior muscle, but not the pectoral muscle.

Source: American Joint Committee on Cancer: *Manual for Staging of Cancer.* Philadelphia, Lippincott, 1992.

mammography, chest x-ray, complete blood count, and serum chemistries (with liver function tests and calcium), require no further staging procedures. The use of tumor markers such as the carcinoembryonic antigen (CEA) and mucin antigens (CA 27.29 and CA 15.3) in patient management is controversial and is not recommended on a routine basis.

TREATMENT OF BREAST CANCER

Carcinoma in Situ

The more widespread use of screening mammography has led to a major increase in the diagnosis of ductal carcinoma in situ (DCIS). Previously, such lesions were uncommon, usually detected on physical examination, large, and had a cure rate exceeding 95 percent with mastectomy. Currently, most DCIS lesions are nonpalpable and small, and are suggested by microcalcifications found on screening mammography. Mastectomy cures almost all patients, but lesser procedures such as lumpectomy alone or with breast irradiation probably are as effective for patients with lesions less than 2.5 cm.

Axillary dissection finds metastases in less than 1 percent of patients and is generally not recommended. Excision alone, without local radiation therapy, may be appropriate for patients with lesions less than 2.5 cm with generous (>1 cm) margins of normal tissue surrounding the in situ component.

Lobular carcinoma in situ (LCIS) is more common in premenopausal patients, lacks clinical and mammographic signs, is bilateral in 25 to 35 percent of cases, and is usually an incidental finding after breast biopsy. It is not a palpable lesion. Treatment options range from observation to bilateral mastectomy. Of note, 20 to 40 percent of patients with LCIS subsequently develop invasive infiltrating ductal cancer with both the ipsilateral breast and the contralateral breast at similar risk. LCIS serves as a high-risk marker for subsequent invasive cancer, and treatment selection must rest on the desires of the patient. Most experts recommend close follow-up of these patients without aggressive surgery.

Management of Early Localized Lesions (Stages I and II)

Local Management

Breast-conservation procedures result in virtually identical relapse-free and overall survival outcomes compared with more extensive surgical treatment, including simple, modified-radical, and radical mastectomy. Reasonably healthy older women tolerate simple or modified mastectomies as well as younger women do, and should be offered the option of a breast-conserving surgical procedure when clinically appropriate.

Breast Conservation

In general, breast-conservation procedures involve removing the tumor mass with a clear margin of several millimeters of surrounding normal breast tissue (lumpectomy, tylectomy, quadrantectomy, etc.), performing an ipsilateral axillary dissection, and following surgery with local breast irradiation. Concurrent ipsilateral axillary node dissection is recommended by most medical, surgical, and radiation oncologists to provide important prognostic data. Moreover, a carefully done axillary dissection that removes the nodes in the lower two axillary levels reduces the likelihood of axillary recurrence to less than 5 percent. Breast-conserving procedures require close cooperation among the surgeon, pathologist, and radiation oncologist. Although breast irradiation after removal of the tumor mass does not improve survival, it reduces the likelihood of recurrence in the affected breast from 40 percent to less

than 10 percent. Most breast relapses occur in or in close proximity to the previously resected lesion. Other techniques, such as brachytherapy (localized radiation therapy [RT] using implanted radioactive seeds), may prove to be as effective as whole-breast RT and can be completed over a period of several days. Two trials have shown that lumpectomy and tamoxifen confers the same survival benefit as lumpectomy, tamoxifen, and breast RT, but that breast RT is better than tamoxifen in preventing in-breast recurrence. For healthy older patients at higher risk for in-breast recurrence, breast radiation should be strongly considered.

Contraindications to breast-conserving surgery include two or more gross tumors in separate quadrants of the breast, diffuse indeterminate or malignant-appearing microcalcifications, and a history of therapeutic irradiation of the breast region. Relative contraindications include large tumor/breast ratio (mass >5 cm), large breast size, and a history of collagen vascular disease. Connective tissue disease has been reported anecdotally to increase the likelihood of fibrosis associated with radiation. The first three of the relative contraindications are related to the cosmetic result of surgery. It is important, however, not to underestimate the value to a patient of preserving her own breast with sensation intact even if the cosmetic appearance is not perfect. It is now well established that preoperative ("neoadjuvant") chemotherapy for women with large breast cancers can shrink the tumor, allowing breast conservation for many patients.

Breast-conserving procedures may be more costly than mastectomy because of the time, inconvenience, and monetary expense of postoperative RT. Nevertheless, such treatment is preferred by many women irrespective of age. The option of breast-conserving surgery provides motivation for detecting early-stage lesions through screening. In addition, patients who have had breast-conserving procedures have higher self-appraisals of body image and sexuality than do women who have had more extensive surgical intervention.

Mastectomy

For older women who have had a mastectomy, breast reconstruction represents another option for restoring body image. Many physicians, because of personal bias, are unlikely to discuss reconstruction with older patients. This procedure can be done safely in an older patient and should be discussed, with subsequent surgical consultation if desired.

In the past, postmastectomy "adjuvant" irradiation therapy to the chest wall and the contiguous regional lymph nodes (internal mammary, supraclavicular, and upper axilla) was frequently employed. It has been shown that such therapy reduces the likelihood of local recurrence (recurrence in the mastectomy site or contiguous nodal areas) by about 70 percent; recent data also show that overall survival from breast cancer is improved by several percent as well. Because the likelihood of local recurrence is directly proportional to both the size of the primary lesion and the number of axillary nodes involved, postoperative adjuvant irradiation is still frequently recommended for patients with large primary lesions (greater than 5 cm) or four or more positive nodes. Delaying postoperative irradiation for 4 to 6 months to allow the completion of adjuvant chemotherapy is feasible without increasing the risk of subsequent local recurrence.

Axillary Dissections

The role of axillary dissection is being reexamined, and the issue is becoming quite controversial, especially in older women. Tumor size and axillary nodes are the most consistent predictors of the risk of recurrence and therefore are key in making decisions about the risk/benefit ratio of adjuvant treatment. Among women with very small tumors (<1 cm), axillary node involvement has been found in 5 to 37 percent. Physical examination is only of modest benefit in predicting nodal involvement, with false-negative and false-positive rate of 35 percent and 25 percent, respectively. Because arm problems such as swelling (lymphedema), pain, numbness, weakness, and impaired shoulder mobility may all complicate axillary dissection, the argument has been made that its prognostic benefit is not worth the risk of side effects in women with primary tumors less than 1 cm. Moreover, if adjuvant chemotherapy is not a consideration because of physician or patient choice, the risk of axillary dissection may not be worth its prognostic yield regardless of primary tumor size.

To decrease the complication rate of axillary dissection, lymphatic mapping with sentinel node biopsy has become a widely used procedure. This procedure allows identification and sampling of the first node in the lymphatic basin to receive lymphatic flow, that is, presumptive removal of the initial site of metastatic nodal involvement. Although accepted as an appropriate staging procedure by many surgical oncologists, a major clinical trial is in progress comparing sentinel lymph node biopsy and axillary dissection. When the sentinel lymph node(s) is positive, the likelihood of finding further positive nodes after a more complete axillary dissection is approximately 50 percent.

Adjuvant Systemic Therapy

Adjuvant systemic therapy involves preoperative, perioperative, or postoperative administration of endocrine therapy and/or chemotherapy to patients with localized breast cancer to reduce and delay the risk of relapse and improve survival. Such treatment is aimed at eradicating occult, clinically undetectable metastases that may have occurred before diagnosis and treatment of the primary lesion. Figure 54-2 shows 5- and 10-year survival rates for each stage of breast cancer. Adjuvant therapy is chosen on the basis of the risk:benefit ratio. The risk-reduction for metastatic disease is weighed against the risk of toxicity from adjuvant therapy. Estimated improvements in relapse-free and overall survival for adjuvant systemic therapy are provided in the 1998 overview analysis of the Early Breast Cancer Trials Collaborative Group. This landmark analysis calculated 10-year recurrence and mortality data from more than 100,000 women with early-stage breast cancer

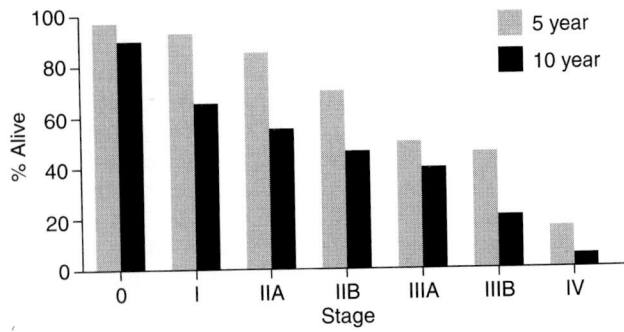

Figure 54-2 Five- and 10-year breast cancer survival by stage. *Modified from Manual for Staging of Cancer, 1992.*

treated with systemic endocrine therapy, chemotherapy, radiation therapy, and/or immunotherapy who were entered in randomized clinical trials. These data clearly confirmed the benefits of adjuvant endocrine therapy and chemotherapy, but not immunotherapy, in significantly reducing the risk of recurrence and death in women with early breast cancer. Table 54-3 summarizes the overview results of adjuvant therapy for postmenopausal patients.

In postmenopausal women, the majority of trials using adjuvant endocrine therapy compared tamoxifen with either no treatment or with chemotherapy. In women older than age 70 years, there was a highly significant decrease in the annual odds of recurrence (54 percent) and death (34 percent) among those treated with tamoxifen. Patients with positive estrogen or progesterone receptors derive greatest benefit from tamoxifen. In addition, tamoxifen significantly decreased the annual odds of developing contralateral breast cancer by approximately 40 percent. Several studies have confirmed that tamoxifen decreases cardiovascular morbidity, lowers cholesterol and low-density lipoprotein levels, and increases or preserves vertebral bone density in postmenopausal women. Currently, 5 years of adjuvant tamoxifen therapy is recommended for most women with estrogen and/or progesterone-receptor node-negative and node-positive early breast cancer.

The overview found a significant decrease in the annual odds of recurrence and death for both node-negative and node-positive women age 50 to 70 years old who where treated with combination chemotherapy (polychemotherapy); unfortunately, not enough data were available to estimate the results of chemotherapy in patients older than age 70 years. Of note, the combination of tamoxifen and chemotherapy was superior to tamoxifen alone in prolonging relapse-free, but not overall, survival. Chemotherapy programs using anthracycline-containing combinations were found to be superior to nonanthracycline regimens in improving both relapse-free and overall survival. Table 54-4 lists commonly used endocrine and cytotoxic agents. Much controversy exists concerning the optimal duration of adjuvant chemotherapy, but short treatment courses of 3 to 6 months appear to be as effective as treatment of longer duration. The dose intensity of chemotherapy (the dose administered during a specific time period) may be a major factor in treatment outcome. Adjuvant chemotherapy regimens that have shown a survival benefit for women age 50 to 70 years also are well tolerated in

Table 54-3 Adjuvant Systemic Therapy in Women Age 50 Years or Older

Comparison	Reduction Annual Odds of[‡]	
	Recurrence %(SD)	Death %(SD)
Tamoxifen for 5 years (ER+)		
Tamoxifen alone versus no adjuvant	46 (4)	22 (5)
Tamoxifen versus same without tamoxifen	50 (4)	28 (5)
Chemotherapy		
Polychemotherapy[†] alone versus nil	22 (4)	12 (4)
Chemotherapy versus no chemotherapy	20 (3)	11 (3)
Tamoxifen plus Chemotherapy		
Tamoxifen plus chemotherapy versus chemotherapy alone	52 (8)	47 (9)
Polychemotherapy plus tamoxifen versus tamoxifen alone	19 (3)	11 (4)

[†]Polychemotherapy given for 2 to 12 months.

[‡]All odds reductions are significant (p <.05).

SOURCE: Modified from *Lancet* 351:1451, 1998; 352:930, 1998:1, 71, 1992.

healthy women older than age 70 years; high-dose regimens with stem cell rescue level have not proven to be superior to current polychemotherapy regimens such as cyclophosphamide, methotrexate, and 5-fluorouracil (CMF), doxorubicin (Adriamycin™) and cyclophosphamide (AC), cyclophosphamide, doxorubicin (Adriamycin™), and 5-fluorouracil (CAF), cyclophosphamide, epirubicin, and 5-fluorouracil (CEF), and AC plus a taxane (paclitaxel and docetaxel). Unlike tamoxifen however, chemotherapy had little effect on the risk of developing contralateral breast cancer in the overview analysis. As a result of the paucity of data, the role of adjuvant chemotherapy in the management of older patients remains unclear. Too few patients have been studied to draw major conclusions; no chemotherapy trial in postmenopausal women has included a large enough cohort of patients older than age 70 years for analysis. Carefully designed trials of chemotherapy for older women are needed and should include drug combinations that provide a dose intensity similar to that of other currently effective therapies. A National Cancer Institute-sponsored trial comparing standard chemotherapy with an oral chemotherapeutic agent (capecitabine) is now in progress and will assess quality of life, comorbidity and toxicity as well as relapse-free and overall survival (Cancer and Leukemia Group B trial 49907; www.calgb.org).

Follow-up for Women with Early Breast Cancer

There is good evidence that close follow-up after diagnosis or adjuvant therapy does not result in improved overall survival, but the detection of early skin or lymph node (soft tissue) recurrence may result in more effective palliation. Mammography is an exception and should be performed yearly to detect new primary lesions. Because a history of breast cancer is a risk factor for another breast cancer, follow-up visits do provide an opportunity for patients to express concerns and for physicians to give them reassurance. Extensive laboratory and radiologic procedures are now available for the detection of metastatic disease, but trials have indicated that a brief, focused history and a limited physical examination (skin, chest, breast, and abdominal examination) detect more than 75 percent of metastases. Because of the growing concern over health care costs, many organizations are formulating guidelines for follow-up. Table 54-5 presents guidelines developed by the American Society of Clinical Oncology. In addition to mammograms and follow-up visits with the oncologist and gynecologist, patients should be educated about the symptoms of breast cancer recurrence so that those symptoms are reported and evaluated promptly.

Treatment of Metastatic Disease

Patients with metastatic breast cancer are currently incurable and have a median survival of approximately 2 years after the discovery of recurrence. Nevertheless, patients may derive major palliative benefit from judiciously chosen therapy. Bone, soft-tissue (skin and lymph nodes), pleural, and pulmonary metastases are the most common sites of breast cancer recurrence. Women with localized symptomatic lesions in brain, skin, lymph nodes, and bone should be considered for palliative radiation therapy, which relieves symptoms in the majority of patients.

Patients with disseminated metastases should be considered for palliative systemic treatment (Table 54-6). Endocrine therapy usually is associated with minimal toxicity, while the toxicity associated with chemotherapy is frequently substantial and in a small percent of patients life-threatening. Provided that metastases are not rapidly progressive or life-threatening, all women with metastases should have a trial of endocrine therapy irrespective of the estrogen and progesterone receptor status of the tumor. Even in receptor-negative patients, endocrine therapy results in complete and partial response (greater than 50 percent shrinkage of the tumor mass) in approximately 10 to 20 percent of those treated. Chemotherapy should

Table 54-4 Endocrine and Cytotoxic Agents Used in the Treatment of Breast Cancer

Class/Agent	Common and Major Toxicities
Endocrine therapy	
Tamoxifen (antiestrogen)	Hot flushes
Megestrol (progestin)	Weight gain
Anastrozole, letrozole, exemestane (selective aromatase inhibitor)	Nausea
Stilbestrol (estrogen)	Nausea and vomiting (N+V), edema, fluid retention
Fluoxymestrone (androgen)	N+V, fluid retention, masculinization
Cytotoxic agents	
Alkylating agents	
Melphalan (L-PAM)	Myelosuppression (M)
Chlorambucil	Myelosuppression
Cyclophosphamide	N, N+V, cystitis
Carboplatin	M, N+V (mild)
Antitumor antibiotics	
Doxorubicin (Adriamycin), Epirubicin	M, N+V, mucositis (MS), alopecia, cardiomyopathy, vesication
Mitoxantrone	M, N+V, mild alopecia, cardiomyopathy
Mitomycin	M, N+V, MS, alopecia, vesication
Antimetabolites	
Methotrexate	M (uncommon), nephrotoxicity, MS
Fluorouracil	M (uncommon), N+V (uncommon), rash (rare)
Capecitabine	Diarrhea, "hand-foot" syndrome
Gemcitabine	M, N+V (mild)
Taxanes	
Paclitaxel	M, hypersensitivity reactions (HR), neuropathy, MS, arthralgia/myalgia, alopecia, MS (rare)
Docetaxel	M, HR (rare), neuropathy, fluid retention, rash, alopecia
Vincas	
Vincristine	Peripheral neuropathy, alopecia, M (rare), vesication
Vinblastine	M, neuropathy (uncommon), vesication
Vinorelbine	M, neuropathy, vesication

be considered when metastases become refractory to endocrine treatment; such a strategy has been shown to be safe and most likely maintains the highest quality of life for the longest time period.

Tamoxifen is the most commonly used endocrine agent for the treatment of metastatic disease with response rates of approximately 30 percent in unselected patients. Recently, aromatase inhibitors, agents that block the synthesis of estrogens in postmenopausal women, have been shown to be as effective as tamoxifen in this setting. Responses to endocrine treatment generally last an average of about 1 year, but in a small percentage of patients they may last many years. Patients with receptor-positive tumors, time intervals greater than 2 years from initial diagnosis to recurrence, soft-tissue or bone metastases, or a prior response to endocrine therapy are the most likely to respond. For patients who have responded to one agent or who have prolonged periods where the tumor does not grow (stable

disease) other agents should be used in succession until it is clear that the metastases are refractory to endocrine therapy. Patients who respond to one endocrine agent are likely to respond to another at the time of progression; the use of successive endocrine agents in patients with minimally symptomatic metastases is an excellent treatment strategy. In addition to tamoxifen and aromatase inhibitors, progestins and estrogens may be effective; moreover, patients who have previously responded or had prolonged stable disease and then had tumor progression may respond to the same agent after being treated with other therapy.

Older patients with metastatic disease, whose general health is otherwise satisfactory, display response and toxicity profiles to chemotherapy similar to those of their younger counterparts. Most cytotoxic drugs are metabolized in the liver with only a select few dependent on renal excretion (methotrexate, carboplatin, and cisplatin); major liver dysfunction probably is required to alter drug

Table 54-5 Follow-up of Early Breast Cancer after Diagnosis and Initial Treatment

	Frequency of Examination		
	0–3 Years	3–5 Years	5+ Years
History and physical examination	Every 3–6 months	Every 6–12 months	Yearly
Breast self-examination	Monthly	Monthly	Monthly
Mammogram*	Yearly	Yearly	Yearly
Gynecologic examination†	Yearly	Yearly	Yearly
Other‡	PRN	PRN	PRN

*In patients treated with lumpectomy and breast irradiation, more frequent mammograms of the radiation-treated breast (every 6 months) may be recommended for the first 3 years.

†Yearly gynecologic exams are recommended; they are required for women on tamoxifen who have an intact uterus.

‡Tumor marker studies, complete blood count, and automated chemistry studies; chest and skeletal x-rays; ultrasound; and radionuclide and computer tomographic scans are not necessary in asymptomatic patients. Appropriate studies should be obtained for patients with signs or symptoms of recurrence.

SOURCE: Adapted from *Recommended Breast Cancer Surveilance Guidelines,* American Society of Clinical Oncology, 1997.

metabolism significantly. Myelosuppression is more common in older patients as a result of diminished bone marrow reserve with aging; nausea and vomiting are seen less frequently than they are in younger patients. Of importance, psychosocial adjustments to chemotherapy appear to be

Table 54-6 Essential Information for the Management of Breast Cancer

Patient characteristics
Significant comorbidities
Complete blood count
Chemistry profile, including liver and renal function
Chest x-ray
Bilateral mammography

Type of initial treatment
Mastectomy or lumpectomy
Radiation therapy—type
Axillary lymph node dissection or sentinel lymph node biopsy

Pathology
Histologic type
Tumor grade
Presence of vascular or lymphatic involvement
Percent of invasive and intraductal cancer
Tumor size (maximum diameter of invasive component)
Number of axillary nodes removed
Number of axillary nodes positive
Estrogen and progesterone receptors

Social environment
Physical and mental function
Access to clinic (transportation)
Family and social support
Financial resources (coinsurance)

better for older than for younger patients. Complete and partial responses to most single chemotherapy agents range from 20 to 30 percent, while responses to combination chemotherapy average 50 to 70 percent. The use of sequential single agents to maximize quality of life yet maintain tumor control is as effective as treatment with several agents in combination and less toxic. Responses generally last an average of 6 to 12 months; response rates to subsequent "salvage" regimens are generally low and last only several months.

Trastuzumab (Herceptin™), a humanized monoclonal antibody targeted against the HER-2 gene product, has been approved by the FDA for use in women with metastatic breast cancer whose tumors over-express the HER-2 gene. It is usually very well tolerated and associated with tumor response rates of about 25 percent. In a pivotal randomized trial, the concomitant use of trastuzumab and chemotherapy was associated with an improvement in response and survival when compared to chemotherapy alone. It is now being tested in the adjuvant setting in women with HER-2 over-expressing tumors.

SPECIAL CONSIDERATIONS

Tamoxifen as Initial Treatment

For many older patients, especially those with advanced but localized lesions (T3 and T4) lesions and those with significant comorbidity or frailty, initial treatment with tamoxifen has been associated with tumor shrinkage in 40 to 70 percent of patients. This treatment is only likely to benefit patients with estrogen or progesterone receptor-positive tumors. Although surgery is more likely to be effective (and potentially curative) in patients with small lesions, several randomized trials comparing surgery with tamoxifen for initial therapy have suggested that long-term survival is not changed by using tamoxifen as the initial treatment and reserving surgical management for patients with tumor progression. Radiation therapy also can be used as "salvage" treatment after tamoxifen failure, but large tumor masses, especially those greater than 3 cm and those with extensive skin involvement, frequently respond only partially. For patients treated with tamoxifen because a comorbidity precludes surgical therapy, radiation therapy should be considered when tumor shrinkage is maximal to try to prolong the duration of local tumor control. In the author's opinion, most older women with localized breast cancer should be offered the same initial treatment options as offered to younger patients; most patients treated initially with tamoxifen fail to achieve complete tumor regression and over time probably will need surgery or other treatments to control the primary lesion. Recently, aromatase inhibitors have been shown to be similar or even more effective than tamoxifen for causing tumor regression in patients with locally advanced estrogen or progesterone receptor-positive breast cancer not amenable to surgery. Unlike tamoxifen, aromatase inhibitors do not increase the risk of endometrial cancer or thromboembolism.

Male Breast Cancer

Male breast cancer is uncommon and accounts for less than 1 percent of all breast cancer incidence. The natural history of male and female breast cancer is similar, but males usually present at a later stage, probably because of a delay in diagnosis. Almost all cases are sporadic except for males with Klinefelter's syndrome (sex chromosomes XXY), in which the prevalence of breast cancer ranges from 3 to 6 percent. Mastectomy with axillary dissection is the standard approach to treatment. Histologically, most lesions are infiltrating ductal carcinomas, and the frequency of estrogen-receptor–positive lesions is 70 to 80 percent. Because of the rarity of male breast cancer, there are few data on the role of adjuvant systemic therapy, and it is unlikely that large randomized trials will be undertaken. Many oncologists use the same guidelines for adjuvant therapy in men that are used in women with a similar stage and receptor status. Uncontrolled trials suggest that such treatment is similar in efficacy to that in women.

Males with metastatic breast cancer are incurable but frequently respond to endocrine therapy, including tamoxifen and orchidectomy; the results with systemic chemotherapy are similar to those in females.

CONCLUSION

Breast cancer is a major gerontologic problem. Both physician education and patient education concerning screening, early diagnosis, and management of breast cancer in this age group are required. The available data indicate that optimal treatment of breast cancer in older women results in outcomes similar to those from treatment of younger

women. Although significant comorbid illness is encountered more frequently in older patients and may complicate breast cancer treatment, most patients can still be managed with judicious "state-of-the-art" therapy. Barriers to the treatment of breast cancer in older women are generic to the treatment of all illnesses in this age group and include access to care, transportation, adequate family and social support, physician bias, and treatment costs. Changes in health care policy, as well as focused research related to cancer in the geriatric population, will be needed to overcome these obstacles.

REFERENCES

Anonymous: Polychemotherapy for early breast cancer: An overview of the randomised trials. Early Breast Cancer Trialists' Collaborative Group. *Lancet* 352(9132):930, 1998.

Anonymous: Tamoxifen for early breast cancer: An overview of the randomised trials. Early Breast Cancer Trialists' Collaborative Group [see comments]. *Lancet* 351(9114):1451, 1998.

Eifel P et al: National Institutes of Health consensus development conference statement: Adjuvant therapy for breast cancer, November 1–3, 2000. *J Natl Cancer Inst* 93(13):979, 2001.

Extermann M et al: What threshold for adjuvant therapy in older breast cancer patients? *J Clin Oncol* 18(8):1709, 2000.

Gail MH et al: Weighing the risks and benefits of tamoxifen treatment for preventing breast cancer [see comments] [published erratum appears in *J Natl Cancer Inst* 2:92(3):275, 2000]. *J Natl Cancer Inst* 91(21):1829, 1999.

Harris JR et al: *Diseases of the Breast,* 2nd ed. Philadelphia, Lippincott Williams and Wilkins, 1999.

Havlik RJ et al: The National Institute on Aging and the National Cancer Institute SEER collaborative study on comorbidity and early diagnosis of cancer in the elderly. *Cancer* 74(7 Suppl):2101, 1994.

Hutchins LF et al: Underrepresentation of patients 65 years of age or older in cancer-treatment trials. *N Engl J Med* 341(27):2061, 1999.

Kimmick GG, Muss HB: Systemic therapy for older women with breast cancer. *Oncology (Huntingt)* 15(3):280, 2001.

Lichtman SM, Skirvin JA: Pharmacology of antineoplastic agents in older cancer patients. *Oncology (Huntingt)* 14(12):1743, 2000.

Mandelblatt JS et al: Breast cancer screening for elderly women with and without comorbid conditions. A decision analysis model. *Ann Intern Med* 116:722, 1992.

Muss HB et al: Clinical research in the older cancer patient. *Hematol Oncol Clin North Am* 14(1):283, 2000.

Olin JJ, Muss HB: New strategies for managing metastatic breast cancer. *Oncology (Huntingt)* 14(5):629, 2000.

Smith TJ et al: American Society of Clinical Oncology 1998 update of recommended breast cancer surveillance guidelines. *J Clin Oncol* 17(3):1080, 1999.

Trimble EL et al: Representation of older patients in cancer treatment trials. *Cancer* 74:2208, 1994.

Welch HG et al: Estimating treatment benefits for the elderly: The effect of competing risks. *Ann Intern Med* 124(6):577, 1996.

Yancik R et al: Effect of age and comorbidity in postmenopausal breast cancer patients aged 55 years and older. *JAMA* 285(7):885, 2001.

Prostate Cancer and the Geriatric Patient

BETH A. HELLERSTEDT • KENNETH J. PIENTA

EPIDEMIOLOGY AND RISK FACTORS

Prostate cancer affects thousands of men annually. In the year 2001, the number of new prostate cancer cases was expected to be 198,100, accounting for 31 percent of new cancer cases in men. According to the Surveillance, Epidemiology, and End Results (SEER) data, the average annual age-adjusted incidence rate of prostate cancer is 61.8/100,000 in the white population and 82.0/100,000 in the African American population; the incidence rates of prostate cancer among African American men are higher than rates for men of *any* other racial or ethnic background. It is more common in the United States and northern European countries, and a relatively rare occurrence in Asia and Africa. It is generally a disease of elderly men, with a median age at presentation of 68 to 70 years. The only undisputed risk factors are older age, African American race, and positive family history.

Although it seems intuitive that testosterone levels may influence the incidence of prostate cancer, no evidence exists to confirm this association. Dihydrotestosterone, the active hormone produced from the conversion of testosterone by the enzyme 5α-reductase, is associated in some studies with increased risk. A prospective, population-based study of 1156 men showed no correlation between 17 different hormones and prostate cancer development, with the possible exception of androstanediol glucuronide. Importantly, no dose–response relationships were seen, suggesting that serum hormone levels may not be useful even in risk stratification.

Dietary fat has been postulated to be a risk factor for prostate cancer. A low-fat diet correlates with a lower incidence of clinically significant disease. This finding is correlated by migration studies: men who change from a low-fat to a high-fat diet also appear to have increased rates of prostate cancer. These studies are complicated by the fact that many of the men migrating from low-fat diet areas also consume green tea and soy. These products contain isoflavones and estrogens, and may act as chemoprotectants against prostate-specific carcinogenesis. A study from Norway with more than 25,000 men did not suggest a correlation between fat intake and prostate cancer, but the cohort was relatively young, and the results relatively immature. A randomized trial evaluating the impact of a low-fat diet in men who have selected watchful waiting in lieu of intervention has been accruing patients since 1997. Currently, 93 men are enrolled, 63 of whom have up to 1 year of follow-up. Although it is still too early to assess the results of the study, there have been no reported adverse events, and adherence to the dietary regimen is reported as $\geq$83 percent.

Agent Orange exposure has also been investigated in a number of studies. Several trials report an association, while others do not. The conclusion of the committee convened by the Secretary of Veterans Affairs, in 1991, categorized prostate cancer as having only limited or suggestive evidence for correlation with exposure.

Smoking is one risk factor that is only loosely associated with risk of developing prostate cancer. Data from the Physician's Health Study and the Australian Anti-Cancer Council suggest no association between current or former tobacco use with the incidence of prostate cancer. Other studies, however, suggest that the combination of smoking and obesity may increase risk. Other factors, including vasectomy, occupational and pesticide exposures, number of sexual contacts, and exposure to sexually transmitted diseases have not been demonstrated to affect the risk of developing prostate cancer.

PREVENTION

Chemoprevention of prostate cancer is an area of ongoing research. In many ways, it is an ideal disease for this approach: relatively slow growing, centered in the elderly population, yet with devastating effects and difficult management after the onset of metastatic disease. Whether the increase in prostate cancer mortality reflects an increase in disease incidence is a matter of intense debate.

When considering the individual patient, whether the rise in mortality represents increasing incidence, earlier detection, or longer life span has no therapeutic significance.

Antiandrogens

Finasteride is a drug that blocks the actions of 5α-reductase, the enzyme that converts testosterone to dihydrotestosterone. The PCPT (Prostate Cancer Prevention Trial) has enrolled 18,000 men since 1993 to study the efficacy of finasteride for decreasing the period prevalence of prostate cancer. It is a randomized, double-blind, placebo-controlled trial. Final results should be available in 2003.

Prostatic intraepithelial neoplasia (PIN) is felt to represent true carcinoma in situ. Autopsy studies confirm that the incidence of PIN increases with age, from 9 percent in the third decade to 20 percent in the fourth decade and 44 percent in the fifth decade. The risk of developing carcinoma after a diagnosis of PIN ranges from 17 to 39 percent. Unfortunately, the development of PIN appears to be a late event in the spectrum of premalignant changes, and preventing the development of invasive cancer may be difficult. The North Central Cancer Treatment Group is currently enrolling patients with PIN on a double-blind, randomized, phase II trial of a low-dose of the antiandrogen flutamide versus placebo. The primary end point of the study is to determine whether flutamide treatment reduces the progression to prostate cancer in men with high-grade PIN.

Vitamin E and Selenium

In recent years, the role of oxidative stress in the development of prostate cancer has been investigated. The damage caused by reactive oxygen species is not limited to deoxyribonucleic acid (DNA); it can encompass lipids and proteins as well. The association of prostate cancer and a high-fat diet may be secondary to the generation of increased fatty acids, which can cause lipid peroxidation.

The two most exciting agents in the area of chemoprevention are selenium and vitamin E. Selenium was initially investigated in the prevention of recurrent basal and squamous cell skin cancers. Although selenium did not show a reduction in the incidence of recurrent skin cancer, an unexpected finding was decrease in the risk of prostate, colorectal, and lung cancer. Remarkably, the incidence of prostate cancer decreased by 65 percent. The antioxidant properties of vitamin E have been studied extensively in a variety of prostate cell lines. Results from human studies are conflicting. In one prospective study, there was no protective association between increased serum levels of vitamin E and the risk of prostate cancer, while other studies have shown a statistically significant positive effect. SELECT (Selenium and Vitamin E Cancer Prevention Trial) is a randomized, prospective, double-blind trial designed to determine whether selenium and vitamin E decrease the risk of prostate cancer in healthy men. It will enroll 32,400 healthy men with a digital rectal examination not concerning for cancer and a prostate-specific antigen (PSA) ≤ 4 ng/mL. The four study arms include: vitamin E + placebo, selenium + placebo, vitamin E + selenium, and placebo + placebo. The primary end point of the trial is the clinical incidence of prostate cancer on a recommended routine clinical diagnostic evaluation. As prostate cancer incidence increases with age, it is important to enroll as many geriatric participants as possible, as the greatest risk reduction may be possible in this group.

PRESENTATION

Most men who present with prostate cancer are asymptomatic. Patients rarely have urinary symptoms, as the majority of cancers arise in the posterior aspect of the prostate. Most men undergo evaluation after routine screening, either elevated serum PSA or abnormal digital rectal exam. Some men are diagnosed at the time of a symptomatic metastasis, usually bony pain.

A difficult task for primary physicians is deciding which patients should undergo screening for prostate cancer. No large, randomized trials show a clear survival advantage from PSA screening. Published guidelines do exist, notably from the NCCN (National Comprehensive Cancer Network). A reasonable approach to screening involves an assessment of the patient's other medical problems and symptoms. Younger men with a family history of prostate cancer and African American men should undergo screening, as the disease prevalence is highest in these groups. If an elderly patient is asymptomatic and has an estimated life expectancy of fewer than 10 years, then screening for prostate cancer is likely unwarranted. Any patient with symptoms that may be referable to prostate cancer (bone pain, hypercalcemia, symptomatic pelvic lymphadenopathy) warrants a PSA evaluation. Clearly, symptomatic patients can enjoy significant improvement with the institution of hormonal therapy. The decision about PSA screening should encompass an active discussion between the physician and patient. An ongoing challenge for the geriatrician is the need to remain current on the development of new treatments. In the future, as more targeted and less toxic therapies are identified, PSA screening may become a routine part of health maintenance for all men.

EVALUATION

The appropriate screening examinations for prostate cancer include a serum PSA and a digital rectal examination. On the basis of an elevated PSA (adjusted appropriately for age; see Table 55-1) or an abnormal digital rectal examination, the patient should be referred for a transrectal ultrasound-guided prostate biopsy. In general, six cores are taken (sextant biopsy) and evaluated; areas that are abnormal on digital rectal examination receive more biopsy attempts. If the biopsy is positive, a Gleason score is assigned. This score is one of the most important determinants of prognosis.

Table 55-1 Age-Adjusted Prostate-Specific Antigen Ranges

Age (Years)	Normal Range (ng/mL)
40–50	0–2.5
51–60	2.5–3.5
61–70	3.5–4.5
71–80	4.5–6.5

To report the Gleason score, the pathologist assigns a numerical value (on a scale of 1 to 5) to the most prevalent and the second most prevalent grades of cancer seen in the specimens. The score is reported on a scale of 2 to 10, with 10 being the most aggressive cancer. The assigned scores should be reported separately, for example, $3 + 4 = 7$, as the primary pathology has prognostic implications.

The staging evaluation for men with known prostate cancer or symptoms that could be attributable to metastatic prostate cancer includes: serum chemistries, PSA, bone scan, and computed tomography (CT) scan of the abdomen and pelvis. These initial tests provide evaluation of the most likely sites of metastatic disease, to avoid inappropriate surgical intervention or radiation therapy. The extent of evaluation for metastatic disease relates to the likelihood of finding disease. A recent prospective survey of 3690 men described the positive yield of a bone scan and CT was <5 percent and 12 percent, respectively, for men with a PSA of 4 to 20 ng/mL. The yield decreased to 2 percent and 9 percent for those who also had a Gleason score of ≤6. Only the combination of a Gleason score of 8 to 10 and PSA >20, or a PSA >50 alone, identified a group of men who had a >10 percent yield on bone scan and a 20 percent yield on CT scan. To stage in an appropriate and cost-effective manner, patients with a low PSAs and low to intermediate Gleason scores do not require evaluation. More risk factors increase the degree of preoperative evaluation. Table 55-2 provides guidelines for preoperative staging. These studies also provide a baseline for follow-up.

Figure 55-1 illustrates a stepwise approach to evaluation, monitoring, and treatment.

MANAGEMENT

Initial

Watchful Waiting

The concept of watchful waiting was first proposed in the 1970s after the results of the Veterans Administration Cooperative Urological Research Group (VACURG) trial suggested that delaying therapy until the onset of symptoms did not increase prostate cancer-specific mortality in patients with locally advanced or metastatic disease. In this study, however, only 41 percent of men died from prostate cancer. As aggressive treatment of other medical conditions has improved life expectancy, it was postulated that this data might no longer be applicable. To evaluate watchful waiting in the modern era, from 1985 until 1993 the Medical Research Council Trial randomized 938 men with locally advanced or asymptomatic metastatic prostate cancer to either immediate or deferred treatment with hormonal therapy. In this study, 67 percent of patients died secondary to prostate cancer, a substantial increase from the findings of the VACURG trial. Overall survival was significantly longer in the patients treated immediately, with the most pronounced difference in men who initially had no evidence of metastatic disease. The rate of complications, such as bone pain, pathological fractures, spinal cord compression, and ureteral obstruction was higher in the deferred group. Additionally, men with metastatic disease at presentation developed an indication for treatment at a median of 9 months of observation, and few remained untreated at the time of death. In these patients, the risks of 9 months of hormonal treatment may be far less than the ravages of unchecked metastatic disease.

Watchful waiting either at the time of initial diagnosis or at the time of progression may still be applicable in a subset of elderly men without metastatic disease. However, if the

Table 55-2 Guidelines for Staging Evaluation

Parameters	Screening	References
PSA <15, Gleason 2–7, clinical stage ≤T2b	No screening	All 237 patients had negative bone scan and all 244 patients had negative CT scans in this category
PSA 15–50, Gleason 2–7, clinical stage ≤T2b	Consider bone scan and perform CT scan of abdomen/pelvis	3 of 308 patients had positive bone scan and 8 of 174 patients had positive CT scan in this category
PSA >50, Gleason 8–10, clinical stage ≥T2c	Perform bone scan and CT scan of abdomen/pelvis	OR for positive CT scan 6.17 for Gleason 8–10 vs 2–6
Symptoms	Appropriate evaluation for symptoms noted	

CT, computed tomography; OR, odds ratio; PSA, prostate-specific antigen.

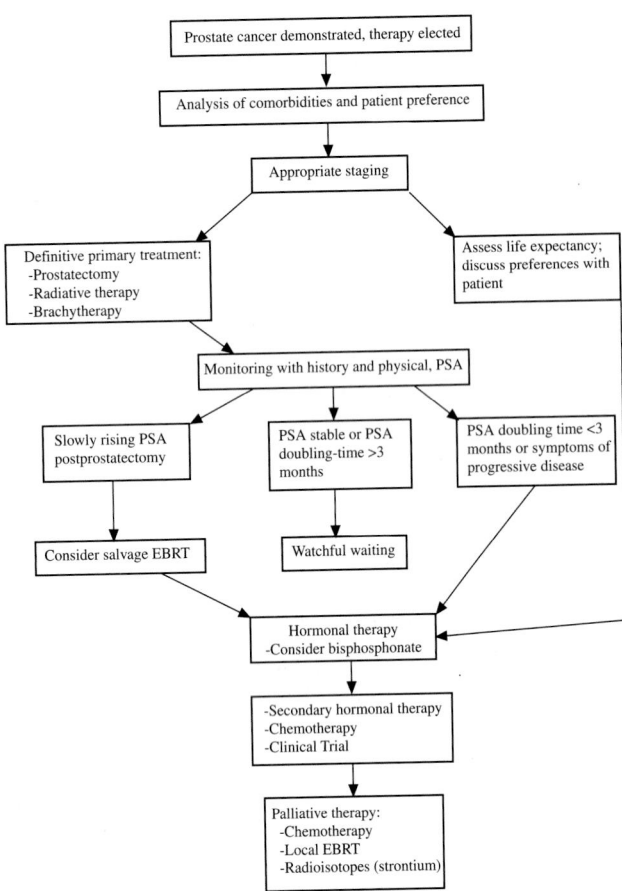

Figure 55-1 Prostate cancer evaluation and management flow-chart. EBRT, external beam radiation therapy; PSA, prostate-specific antigen.

patient is not a candidate for treatment, and has no symptoms attributable to the disease, both the patient and the physician should reflect on why screening was undertaken.

Local Therapy: Surgery, Radiation, or Brachytherapy

Surgery, radiation, or brachytherapy for early stage disease is performed with curative intent. Radical retropubic prostatectomy (RRP), the usual surgical approach, involves removal of the prostate and seminal vesicles, along with pelvic lymph node sampling. External beam radiation therapy (EBRT) usually encompasses 50 cGy to the pelvic bed, with a 20 cGy boost to the prostate. Brachytherapy is performed with radioactive implants, usually radioactive iodine (^{125}I) or palladium (^{103}Pd).

The choice of initial treatment depends upon the input of both the physician and the patient. Several sources have reported outcome comparisons between these modalities. From the data, the choice of treatment depends on the pretreatment assessment of risk for recurrence. A retrospective study of 545 men evaluated biochemical disease-free survival in a group of patients who had undergone prostatectomy, EBRT, or brachytherapy with palladium. For men with low- or intermediate-risk disease (defined as clinical stage T1c, T2a, T2b, PSA ≤20, Gleason score ≤6), there was no difference between modalities in biochemical disease-free survival. Men with high-risk disease (defined

as clinical stage T2c, T3, PSA >20, Gleason score ≥7) treated with prostatectomy had a significant improvement in biochemical disease-free survival. Additionally, men treated with any modality who achieved a PSA nadir of <1 at 1 year had a low likelihood of recurrence. A similar study evaluated 1872 men and found that low-risk patients fared similarly with either modality, while higher-risk patients derived similar outcomes with either prostatectomy or EBRT.

Given similar outcomes between EBRT and prostatectomy, the risk of side effects becomes a deciding factor. Some men may not be candidates for major pelvic surgery, and therefore prostatectomy may not be an option. Quality-of-life studies for postprostatectomy and post-EBRT provide some conflicting results. The Prostate Cancer Outcomes Study evaluated 1291 men 18 months after radical prostatectomy, and found 8.4 percent of patients were incontinent and 59.9 percent of patients were impotent. Older age and non–nerve-sparing procedures were associated with a higher rate of both incontinence and impotence. Two smaller studies reported more incontinence and impotence with prostatectomy, while EBRT was associated with more bowel dysfunction. One study reported lower overall quality-of-life scores for the EBRT group, while the other found no difference in the general health assessments. Primary care providers may want to refer patients to both urology and radiation oncology in order to fully educate patients about their choices. Indeed, a recent study of urologists and radiation oncologists showed that 93 percent of urologists would recommend prostatectomy, while 72 percent of radiation oncologists would offer EBRT to the same patient.

Primary Androgen Deprivation

Patients with unfavorable prognostic factors, or those patients who are not interested in the risk:benefit ratio of local therapy, may choose primary hormonal therapy. Approximately 12.5 percent of the 3486 men in the Prostate Cancer Outcomes Study chose hormonal treatment as initial therapy, considered to be a surprisingly high number. Clearly, there is no chance of cure with this modality, but for some patients the risk of relapse may be too high to pursue aggressive local therapy. There is also scant evidence about the outcomes associated with this approach.

Intermittent Androgen Deprivation

Intermittent androgen blockade has been advocated as a way to decrease side effects from androgen deprivation therapy, and also to, potentially, increase the time to androgen-independence. A recent study of 110 men with clinical stage T1-T3 prostate cancer who refused local therapy were treated with a combination of luteinizing hormone-releasing hormone (LHRH) agonist, antiandrogen, and finasteride. The median duration of induction therapy was 13 months, which was then followed by maintenance with finasteride alone. With a median time of follow-up of 36 months from the start of induction therapy, only 9 patients had a PSA >4 ng/mL. Although most patients had symptoms related to androgen withdrawal,

Lung Cancer

NASIR SHAHAB • MICHAEL C. PERRY

EPIDEMIOLOGY

According to American Cancer Society statistics there will be 169,400 new cases of lung cancer in 2002, accounting for about 13 percent of cancer diagnoses. The incidence rate is declining in men, from a high incidence of 86.5 per 100,000 men in 1984 to 69.8 per 100,000 in 1998, whereas the incidence among women has reached a plateau, with incidence in 1998 at 43.4 per 100,000 men. Among all these cases, 50 percent occur in patients 65 years of age or older. The likelihood of developing lung cancer is 1 in 2500 in men younger than 39 years of age and 1 in 15 in men between the ages of 60 and 79 years.

Although the death rates from lung cancer are falling at a rate of 1.9 percent per year, the vast majority of patients with lung cancer will still die of the disease. It is estimated that 154,900 patients will die of lung cancer in 2002, accounting for 28 percent of all cancer deaths. Among women, the rate of deaths from lung cancer remains high. Since 1987, more women have died from lung cancer than from breast cancer. Despite an enormous effort to find effective therapies for lung cancer, the overall 5-year survival remains only 15 percent. The high mortality rate and low 5-year survival rate are partly the result of an inability to diagnose lung cancer at an early stage, when it is still potentially curable. Only 15 percent of lung cancers are diagnosed at this early stage.

ETIOLOGY

Risk Factors

Tobacco Smoking

Smoking is by far the most common cause of lung cancer. Approximately 85 to 90 percent of lung cancer cases can be attributed directly to tobacco smoking. The risk of lung cancer is directly related to (1) the length of time a person smokes, (2) the number of cigarettes smoked per day, (3) the age at which a person starts smoking, and (4) the amount of tar contained in the cigarettes. The risk of developing lung cancer is 9- to 10-fold higher in an average smoker and up to 25-fold higher for a heavy smoker. However, not all tobacco smokers develop lung cancer. This

may be attributable to differences in an individual's inherited predisposition to cancer development. There is also evidence that nonsmokers exposed to tobacco smoke (passive smokers) have an increased risk of developing lung cancer. It has been estimated that approximately 25 percent of lung cancers in nonsmokers are caused by passive smoking. The risk of lung cancer declines steadily once a person stops smoking, but it can take up to 15 to 20 years for the risk to return to the level of nonsmokers. However, it never reaches this level if they had smoked two packs per day or more.

Other Risk Factors

Other factors reported to cause lung cancer include occupational exposure to arsenic, asbestos, nickel, uranium, chromium, silica, beryllium, and diesel exhaust. Dietary deficiency of vitamins A, C, and E, retinoids, carotenoids, and selenium, and air pollution, lung scars, and oncogenes are all implicated in the causation of lung cancer. Asbestos is the most common occupational cause of lung cancer and increases the risk of lung cancer five fold. Tobacco smoking and asbestos exposure act synergistically, and the risk of lung cancer in smokers who have been exposed to asbestos becomes as high as 80-fold to 90-fold higher than the risk in nonsmokers. Radon, which is produced by the decay of uranium, has a well-established association with lung cancer in underground miners. However, the association between lung cancer and residential exposure to radon is less well established.

SCREENING

Most patients with lung cancer present with advanced-stage disease, when the outcome is dismal. Therefore, there has been an interest in screening high-risk people to detect lung cancers when they are smaller and presumably at earlier and more curable stages. Earlier trials using chest radiography, cytologic examination of the sputum, or both, however, failed to reach the ultimate goal of screening, that is, decreasing disease-specific mortality. These trials have been criticized for their study design, statistical analysis, contamination, and older forms of technology. With

Table 56-1   Lung Cancer Characteristics

	Adenocarcinoma	Large cell	Squamous cell	Small cell
Relative frequency	40%	10%	30%	20%
Growth rate	Variable	Slow	Slow	Rapid
Location	Peripheral	Peripheral	Central	Central
Hormone production	Rare	Rare	Parathyroid hormone	Multiple
Optimal therapy	Surgery	Surgery	Surgery	Chemotherapy/radiotherapy

the development of newer imaging technology, there is a new interest in screening for lung cancer. Two nonrandomized trials from Japan used chest radiography, low-dose computed tomography (CT), and examination of a 3-day pooled sputum sample for screening. The third trial, the Early Lung Cancer Action Project, screened 1000 high-risk smokers over the age of 60 years with chest radiograph and low-dose CT scan. Although these three trials confirmed the superior sensitivity of CT scans over chest radiographs in detecting small lung nodules, the prevalence screening rates for advanced disease on CT scans did not decrease when compared with the earlier dual-screening trials. Therefore, it is assumed that the overall disease-specific mortality would not decrease with the use of low-dose CT. Moreover, the true clinical significance of the small tumors found by screening is unknown. Perhaps these small tumors found by screening are not clinically relevant and if undetected would never have affected the patients. It is also argued that the size of the primary tumor does not correlate with the biologic behavior of the tumor. Therefore, one cannot say that a 5-mm nodule has a better outcome than a 10-mm nodule or even a 30-mm tumor. Tumors may already have demonstrated their potential to remain localized or to metastasize by the time they are visible on CT scan.

Larger trials of screening are currently underway in the United States and Europe, and the final results are pending. The National Cancer Institute (NCI) is sponsoring an American College of Radiology Imaging Network randomized, controlled, multicenter trial that seeks to enroll 7000 high-risk persons. Another future NCI trial to study the effectiveness of CT screening in more than 88,000 participants is planned. Until such trials are completed and their results clearly are in favor of screening, lung cancer will be continue to be diagnosed clinically in the majority of patients.

With better understanding of the molecular pathology of lung cancer, an interesting area of research is to examine the efficacy of molecular and genetic biomarkers in screening high-risk people. Because cancer is a multistep process, identification of these biomarkers in the sputum of high-risk individuals may help to identify the early clonal phase of progression of lung cancer. If this becomes reality, then it may enable detection of cancers earlier than with spiral CT. It could also be complementary to spiral-CT screening.

PATHOLOGY

Based on the light microscopic features, lung cancers are divided into two major groups: small-cell and non–small-cell cancers. The later include squamous cell carcinoma, adenocarcinoma, and large-cell carcinoma (Tables 56-1 and 56-2). Bronchoalveolar carcinoma (BAC) is subclassified under adenocarcinoma. The distinction between small- and non–small-cell histology is important clinically because small-cell histology is more aggressive and, more responsive to chemotherapy and radiation.

In the past, the most common histology was squamous cell carcinoma (SCC) which accounted for 40 percent of lung cancers. However, now only 20 to 25 percent of lung cancers are squamous cell cancers. SCC is the classic lung cancer: central in location, endobronchial in nature, sometimes with central cavitation, and commonly associated with lobar collapse, obstructive pneumonia, or hempotysis, with late development of distant metastases. On the other hand, adenocarcinomas, which in earlier times constituted 20 to 25 percent of all lung cancers, are now the most prevalent histology, accounting for almost 40 percent of all lung cancers. This increase in prevalence has been greater in North America than in Europe, where squamous cell cancer is still the most common type. Changes in smoking

Table 56-2   Histologic Classification of Lung Cancer

Squamous cell (epidermoid) carcinoma
  spindle-cell variant

Adenocarcinoma
  Acinar
  Papillary
  Bronchoalveolar
  Solid tumor with mucin

Large-cell carcinoma
  Giant cell
  Clear cell

Small-cell carcinoma

Adenosquamous carcinoma

Undifferentiated carcinoma

Gastrointestinal Malignancies

SHAHID H. SIAL • SONYA REICHER • VIKTOR E. EYSSELEIN • MARC F. CATALANO

Gastrointestinal malignances are the most common malignancies worldwide. Most gastrointestinal cancers are extremely rare before age of 40 years and have typical onset in the sixth or seventh decade of life. Clinical presentation of gastrointestinal malignancy in elderly patients can be quite subtle. It requires increased awareness of unusual manifestations and familiarity with cancer dynamics on the part of physicians treating the elderly population. Moreover, except for colorectal cancer, widespread screening programs are not efficacious in improving survival. Therefore, to be able to identify high-risk patients, it is the physician's responsibility to obtain extensive knowledge of risk factors and premalignant conditions leading to cancer development.

Over the past decade, our insight into pathogenesis of gastrointestinal cancers has broadened significantly. This new information is complemented by diagnostic and treatment advances that have become available over the past decade. These advances include development of new surgical techniques, new chemotherapeutic regimens, and new palliative approaches such as laser and photodynamic treatments and placement of enteral stents in cases of advanced luminal gastrointestinal malignancies. Other significant advances include development of endoscopic ultrasound as a tool for diagnosis and staging of gastrointestinal malignancies. While accurate gastrointestinal staging is important in any age group, in the elderly population, the significance of accurate diagnosis and staging cannot be overstated. As a result of these advances, modest success has been achieved in the early diagnosis and treatment of gastrointestinal cancer in the elderly patient. Attitudes toward cancer treatment in the elderly population are also changing. There appears to be widespread acceptance of the fact that age itself is not a contraindication to any treatment, including surgical treatment. Treatment decisions should be based on health status and patient's wishes, and the ability to tolerate procedures, not age alone.

ESOPHAGEAL CANCER

Incidence

Esophageal cancer is relatively uncommon in the United States. For year 2000, 12,300 new cases and 12,100 deaths from esophageal cancer were expected. It ranks ninth as a cause of death and sixth as a cause of cancer death worldwide. Most esophageal cancers are squamous cell carcinoma and adenocarcinoma. In the last two decades there has been a significant increase in the incidence of esophageal adenocarcinoma, which now accounts for half of newly diagnosed esophageal cancers and percentagewise is the most rapidly growing cancer in the United States. Men are more affected by esophageal cancer than women. Squamous cell carcinoma is more prevalent in African Americans, and adenocarcinoma is more prevalent in whites. Esophageal cancer accounts for only 5 to 7 percent of all gastrointestinal malignancies. However, its typical onset at the age of 65 to 70 years makes it an important cause of morbidity and mortality among the elderly population.

Risk Factors

Alcohol and tobacco use have long been associated with the development of esophageal squamous cell carcinoma (Table 57-1). The risk rises with the increasing number of cigarettes smoked and is higher among hard liquor than beer or wine drinkers. The rates of esophageal squamous cell carcinoma are higher in the states with higher alcohol intake. In a study of esophageal cancer dynamics among African American men in Washington, DC, alcohol was the main risk factor, accounting for extremely high rates of squamous cell carcinoma in that population. Several other dietary factors have been implicated in the development of

Table 57-1   Risk Factors for Squamous Cell Esophageal Cancer

Dietary factors
Alcohol
Tobacco
Nitrosamines
Betel nut chewing

Esophageal disorders
Achalasia
Chronic strictures (lye, radiation)
Chronic infection (fungal, viral)
Chronic esophagitis

Previous malignancies
History of head and neck cancer
History of gastrectomy
History of radiation therapy

Hereditary disorders
Tylosis
Plummer–Vinson syndrome

squamous cell carcinoma of the esophagus, most notably nitrosamines. Nitrosamines (often found in pickled vegetables) were mutagenic in rats and have been linked to squamous cell carcinoma in endemic areas of China.

A number of esophageal diseases are associated with increased risk for squamous cell carcinoma. These include achalasia and lye-induced strictures. Patients with achalasia have a 16-fold greater risk and develop squamous cell carcinoma a decade earlier than general population. Chronic esophagitis is another condition commonly associated with squamous cell carcinoma. Evidence of chronic esophagitis was found in the majority of squamous cell carcinoma patients in endemic areas.

In contrast to squamous cell carcinoma with its multitude of possible causes, esophageal adenocarcinoma has only one recognizable risk factor—Barrett's metaplasia. Patients with Barrett's esophagus are 30 to 125 times more likely to develop esophageal adenocarcinoma than the general population, with estimated incidence of approximately 0.5 percent per patient, per year.

Clinical Manifestations

Esophageal cancer typically presents quite insidiously. The most common complaint is slowly progressive dysphagia to solids and later to liquids. Patients often recall early symptoms of vague retrosternal discomfort, sensation of friction, burning, slow food passage, or intermittent dysphagia. Weight loss usually accompanies progressive dysphagia. Odynophagia or back pain might be indicative of mediastinal involvement. Persistent cough during swallowing or recurrent aspiration pneumonia are signs of bronchoesophageal fistula; hoarseness is a sign of recurrent laryngeal nerve involvement. Hematemesis can result from

tumor erosions or from aortoesophageal fistula. Malignant ascites, malignant pleural effusions, and hiccups from diaphragmatic irritation are indicative of end-stage disease with distant organ involvement. Squamous cell carcinoma and adenocarcinoma have similar presentations. Extension to diaphragm, liver, and stomach is more frequent in adenocarcinoma, whereas recurrent laryngeal nerve involvement or bronchoesophageal fistula formation are common in squamous cell carcinoma.

Cancer Histology, Dynamics, Prognostic Factors, and Staging

Squamous cell carcinoma usually arises from the middle esophagus. Advanced squamous cell carcinoma is a fungated, ulcerative, polypoid lesion. It typically spreads by direct extension to adjacent organs, as well as hematologically and through lymphatics. Only 8 to 10 percent of squamous cell carcinoma lesions are detected at early stages and up to 30 percent of patients have distant metastasis at the time of diagnosis. Common sites for distant metastasis are liver, lung, and bone. Squamous cell carcinoma arises from the area of dysplasia in esophageal epithelium. Transition to early carcinomatous lesion from severe dysplasia takes 3 to 6 years by some accounts, but once malignant, it progresses to advanced stage in only about a year.

The distal esophagus and gastroesophageal junction is a typical site of esophageal adenocarcinoma. Commonly, adenocarcinoma is a flat or ulcerated lesion, but polypoid or fungating tumors can be found in up to a third of patients. Adenocarcinoma arises from specialized metaplastic columnar epithelium. The time course of low-grade to high-grade dysplasia to invasive carcinoma time is 1.5 to 4 years. On average, adenocarcinoma develops from a high-grade dysplasia lesion in about 14 months.

Several theories have been proposed to account for esophageal cancer progression from dysplastic lesion. It was suggested that cancer arises secondary to acquired genomic instability in Barrett's esophagus, as a result of cell-cycle dysfunction and loss of cell proliferation control. As genetic instability accumulates, abnormal cell clones develop a capacity to invade. In support of this hypothesis, mutations in p53 tumor-suppressor gene have been found in 50 to 85 percent of patients with Barrett's esophagus. Several other factors, such as tumor-associated proteases and protease inhibitors (urokinase-type plasminogen activator, plasminogen activator inhibitors), adhesion molecules (CD44, E-cadherin), and growth factors (epithelial growth factor), are implicated in the development of esophageal cancer, but their roles remain controversial.

The degree of tumor invasion is the most important prognostic factor in esophageal cancer. The TNM (tumor, node, metastases) staging system is widely used to describe tumor burden (Table 57-2). In a T1 lesion, tumor spreads to submucosa; in a T2 lesion, muscularis propria has been invaded; T3 indicates extension to adventitia; and T4 indicates involvement of adjacent organs. N and M stages represent lymph node and distant metastasis, respectively. Distant metastasis and peritoneal carcinomatosis are crucial prognostic indicators. Patients with either finding have

Table 57-2   TNM Staging System for Cancer of the Esophagus

Stage	Description
Primary Tumor (T)	
TX	Primary tumor cannot be assessed
T0	No evidence of primary tumor
Tis	Carcinoma in situ
T1	Tumor invades lamina propria or submucosa
T2	Tumor invades muscularis propria
T3	Tumor invades adventitia
T4	Tumor invades adjacent structures
Lymph Node (N)	
NX	Regional lymph nodes cannot be assessed
N0	No regional lymph node metastasis
N1	Regional lymph node metastasis
Distant Metastasis (M)	
MX	Presence of distant metastasis cannot be assessed
M0	No distant metastasis
M1	Distant metastasis

SOURCE: Modified with permission of the American College of Surgeons from Beahrs O et al: *Manual for Staging of Cancer,* 3rd ed. Philadelphia, JB Lippincott, 1998, p 76.

a median survival of 6 to 12 months irrespective of tumor location or type, with 5-year survival of about 4 percent. In patients without distant disease, the completeness of tumor resection is a major independent determinant of survival. The possibility of complete resection is directly related to cancer stage. In one report, 91 percent of T1 squamous cell carcinoma and 100 percent of T1 adenocarcinoma lesions were successfully resected, in contrast to 19 percent and 54 percent, respectively, of T4 lesions. The number of positive lymph nodes becomes an important prognostic factor in patients who had achieved complete tumor resection. Tumor stage determines the number of lymph node metastases: 20 percent of T2 esophageal cancers have positive lymph nodes, as opposed to 80 to 96 percent of stage T4 tumors. Overall, 5-year survival rate for T1 lesions is 46 percent versus 7 percent for T4 tumors.

Diagnosis

In the last decade, diagnostic modalities for esophageal cancer have been greatly enhanced by the development of endoscopic ultrasonography (EUS). EUS at 7.5 to 12 MHz allows visualization of the esophageal wall as a five-layer structure and at 20 MHz as a seven-layer structure, correlating well with esophageal wall histology. Fiberoptic radial scanning instruments are most widely used. Liner scanning echoendoscopes allow for color Doppler studies and for lymph node biopsies. Nowadays, EUS is used to determine the extent of local tumor invasion and lymph node metastasis. The diagnostic accuracy of EUS is 85 percent with regards to T stage (up to 90 percent for T3 lesions) and 78 percent for regional lymphadenopathy. EUS staging has also been shown to predict survival. Local staging by EUS is commonly combined with computed tomography (CT) for distant metastasis assessment. The accuracy of CT approaches 90 to 100 percent in cases of liver involvement.

Although EUS and CT are critical final steps of esophageal cancer work up, initial evaluation usually involves basic laboratory data and contrast studies. Microcytic anemia (secondary to bleeding), low serum albumin (caused by malnutrition), elevated alkaline phosphatase, total bilirubin, and hypercalcemia (each indicating liver and bone metastases) are all common findings. In contrast radiologic studies, advanced tumors typically present as so-called apple-core lesions because of complete or near complete obstruction. Tumors at earlier stages do not compromise the lumen to the same degree and appear as flat, often ulcerating plaques. Barium swallow is the study of choice if bronchoesophageal fistula is suspected.

Endoscopy with biopsies is the main confirmatory study for the diagnosis of esophageal cancer. It should always be performed, as up to 70 percent of early lesions could be missed on barium swallow. Diagnostic accuracy of endoscopy with multiple biopsies and brush cytology is approaching 100 percent. Up to seven biopsies may be required for diagnosis. Endoscopy is a very safe technique. Contrary to previously held belief, no increase in endoscopic complication rate has been demonstrated among elderly patients. In fact, a recent study of gastrointestinal endoscopy in an extremely elderly patient cohort (median age 87 years) showed no procedure-related mortality or perforations caused by esophagogastroduodenoscopy (EGD), and the rate of cardiopulmonary complications associated with anesthesia was as low as 0.6 percent.

Treatment

Esophageal cancer has long been considered a rapidly terminal illness. In the last decade, significant progress has been made in our understanding of the disease. Morbidity and mortality from esophageal cancer have been decreasing with more therapeutic and palliative options now available. The best example of these changes is in our approach to esophageal adenocarcinoma. Appreciation of adenocarcinoma progression from columnar metaplasia has made prevention possible through endoscopic surveillance for Barrett's esophagus. Patients who undergo routine surveillance have greater survival rates (60 percent versus 20 percent) and their cancer detected at earlier stage with less nodal involvement. All patients with Barrett's esophagus should undergo endoscopic surveillance with the goal of detection of high-grade dysplasia and adenocarcinoma. Previously, patients who were not surgical candidates, such as elderly patients with comorbid conditions, were excluded from surveillance programs. Today, these patients can benefit from photodynamic therapy ablation and should be screened as well. Esophageal adenocarcinoma surveillance is an area of intense debate. There is not yet consensus on what techniques are best to use for endoscopic surveillance biopsies, or what is the appropriate screening interval. Systematic four quadrant biopsies at 2-cm intervals of the involved esophagus are currently recommended. Any irregularities, ulcerations, plaques, nodules, or strictures should be biopsied, since early carcinoma can present without any additional endoscopic abnormalities in Barrett's esophagus. The appropriate screening interval remains unclear. Current guidelines arbitrarily suggest a 2- to 3-year interval for patients without dysplasia, 6-months to 1-year for low-grade dysplasia, and every 3 months until esophagectomy for high-grade dysplasia.

If preoperative staging shows that the esophageal tumor is localized within the esophagus (T1 and T2), without nodal metastases, the patient is regarded as potentially curable. These patients are best treated with esophagectomy en block. The overall 5-year survival rate is 30 percent. In patients who are poor surgical candidates and in patients with early esophageal cancer, endoscopic mucosal resection is an alternative.

Unfortunately, most patients with esophageal cancer present at advanced stages, limiting their chances for complete resection. The use of chemotherapy in such patients could help downstage the primary tumor, decrease distant spread, and thus improve survival. Cisplatin is the most commonly used chemotherapeutic agent and is generally well tolerated. Multidrug regimens (typically, cisplatin in combination with either 5-fluorouracil [5-FU], irinotecan, or paclitaxel) were shown to have response rates superior to single agent regimens. The role of pre- and postoperative chemo-, radiation, or combined therapy has been extensively studied in several randomized controlled studies. Some survival benefit and better local recurrence control was demonstrated for neoadjuvant chemoradiation therapy as compared to surgery alone.

For patients with advanced esophageal cancer, palliation remains the only viable option. Available palliative modalities are directed towards temporary relief of obstruction through laser/electrocoagulation ablation or by placing esophageal stents. Tumor ablation can be achieved with laser or electrocoagulation. The neodymium:yttrium-aluminum-garnet (Nd:YAG) laser has an advantage of protein coagulation and tissue vaporization that allow for hemostasis and relief of obstruction. Short, exophytic, noncircumferential tumors of the middle/distal esophagus are favored for laser treatment. More technically difficult malignant strictures are approached over several sessions and laser treatment can be safely repeated in 48 hours. Procedure-related complication rates are 4 percent, and perforation rates are 2 percent. The specificity of laser therapy can be enhanced with the use of the photosensitizer in photodynamic therapy. A photosensitizer (hematoporphyrin or newer, more specific delta-aminolevulinic acid) accumulates in tumor cells and is activated by laser. This results in release of fluorescence, leading to tumor necrosis. Improved oral intake and life-satisfaction scores, and

longer response to treatment have been shown with photodynamic therapy compared to standard laser. Perforation risk has been less with photodynamic therapy as well, with photosensitivity and sunburn being common complaints. Electrocoagulation applies thermal energy to ablate tumor surface of obstructing lesions. Experience with electrocoagulation is limited; it appears to work best for circumferential, exophytic tumors.

Over the past decade, esophageal stents have been increasingly applied for palliation of malignant dysphagia. They have shown better efficacy in relieving dysphagia compared to chemo- and radiation therapy. Nowadays, the self-expanding metal stent (SEMS) is a preferred esophageal endoprosthesis and provides rapid and lasting relief of dysphagia (Fig. 57-1). Additional applications for SEMS, such as treatment of bronchoesophageal fistulas, benign esophageal strictures, and control of bleeding tamponade, have emerged. Esophageal stent placement includes endoscopic assessment, guide-wire insertion, tumor dilatation, and stent deployment. Esophageal dilatation is usually done prior to stent insertion; exact requirements for dilatation depend on stent type. Currently, prospective randomized controlled studies comparing different stent types are limited. The effectiveness and complication rates appear to be similar among different SEMS, with tumor overgrowth remaining the major obstacle of SEMS use.

Despite significant progress in diagnosis and treatment, esophageal cancer remains a deadly disease with 5-year survival of at best 20 to 30 percent. The future lies in management of this disease, better understanding of the disease process, leading to prevention, and in more accurate diagnostic techniques allowing for patient-tailored and possibly a multimodal approach to esophageal cancer treatment.

GASTRIC CANCER

Incidence

In the United States, almost 22,000 people are affected by gastric cancer yearly; 12,800 died from it in 2001. Worldwide, gastric cancer remains the number two cause of cancer-related death. However, both in the United States and globally, the incidence of gastric cancer has witnessed a dramatic decline. In the last several decades, the United States gastric cancer rates decreased by approximately 30 percent, to 5 to 10 in 100,000 population. Of note, most of this decline is accounted for by a decrease in distal gastric cancer, whereas the incidence of proximal stomach and gastroesophageal junction (GEJ) cancer has been rising sharply. The frequency of gastric cancer varies significantly in different parts of the world: currently, the highest rates are in Japan, the former Soviet Union, and Costa Rica; the lowest, in the United States, India, and southeast Asia.

Gastric cancer is predominantly a disease of the elderly population, as are many other gastrointestinal malignancies. It is rarely found in patients younger than age 40 years, and its incidence is the highest among 70-year-olds. Men are affected twice as commonly as women.

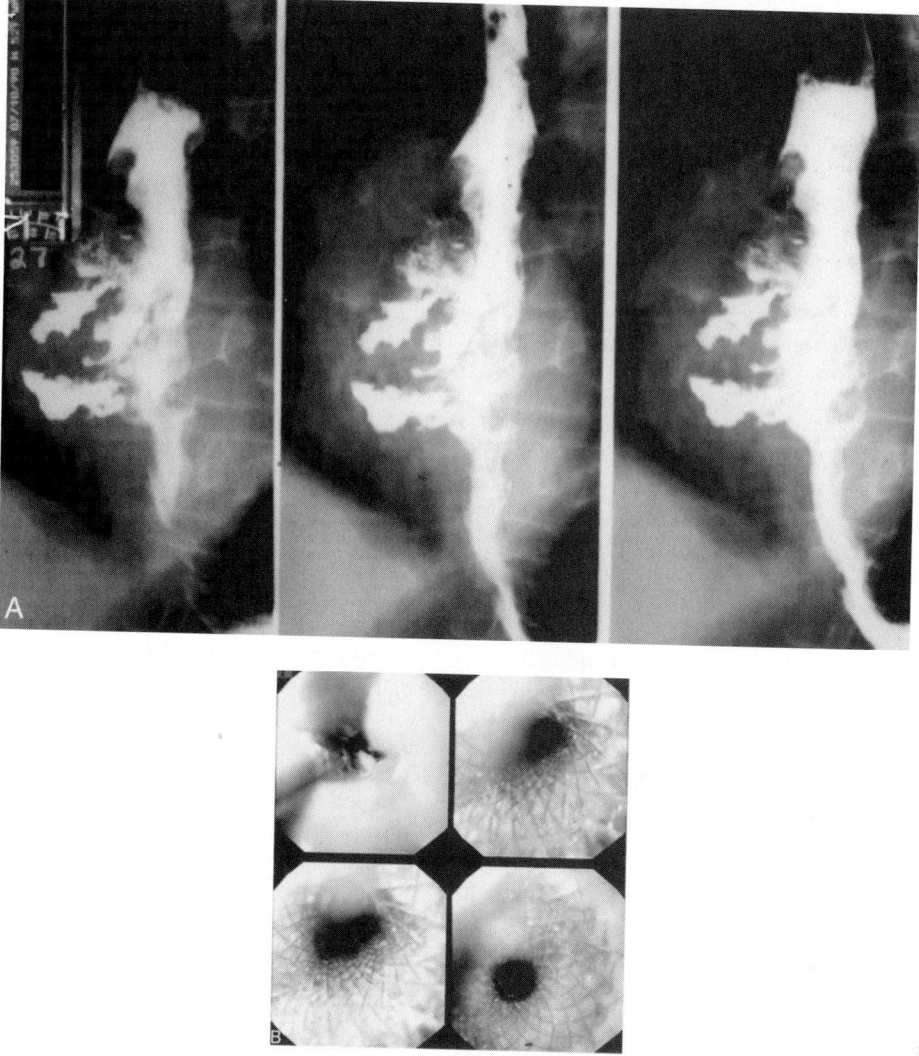

Figure 57-1 *A.* Barium esophagram of an 82-year-old patient presenting with dysphagia to solids and a chronic nonproductive cough and demonstrating a midesophageal irregular esophageal mucosa with two tracheoesophageal fistulas. *B.* Upper endoscopy demonstrates a tracheoesophageal fistula with subsequent deployment of a covered Wallstent. Reproduced with permission from Sial SH, Catalano MF: Gastrointestinal tract cancer in the elderly, in Farrell JJ, Friedman LS (eds): *Gastroenterology Clinics of North America*. Philadelphia, WB Saunders, 2001.

Risk Factors

The pathogenesis of gastric cancer is complex, with both genetic and environmental factors playing a role. The above-stated sharp decline in gastric cancer rates underscores the importance of environmental factors. Some experts explain this dramatic change by variations in environmental exposure over the last several decades. Epidemiologic data demonstrate that this so-called environmental influence has to occur early in life to affect the risk for gastric cancer. In fact, studies on Japanese immigrants to the United States showed that the risk of gastric cancer remained high in the first generation but approached the low US incidence rates by the second or third generation of immigrants. Which environmental factors are important in gastric cancer pathogenesis is difficult to discern from current, largely retrospective studies. It appears that one such factor is diet. A diet rich in fruits and vegetables is associated with lower risk for gastric cancer development, whereas salted, smoked, and poorly preserved foods carry a higher risk. N-nitroso compounds formed from nitrates and nitrites (previously widely used food preservatives) were mutagenic in vitro. Progress in refrigeration and methods of food preservation, as well as increased consumption of fruits and vegetables, is believed to be responsible, at least in part, for the decline in the incidence of gastric cancer. Smoking and alcohol intake are other environmental factors that have been widely studied. The data on the role of smoking and alcohol in gastric cancer development remain, however, largely inconclusive.

In addition to environmental influences, the role of genetic factors in the development of gastric cancer is well documented. A history of gastric cancer in first-degree relatives carries a two- to threefold risk increase. Family clustering of gastric cancer has been described, and the autosomal dominant pattern of inheritance appears to be involved. In several studies, a higher incidence rate of gastric cancer was found in people with blood type A. Some rare hereditary disorders, such as hereditary nonpolyposis colorectal cancer syndrome (Lynch II), are also associated with elevated risk of gastric cancer.

In recent years, a number of conditions have been identified that seem to predispose to gastric cancer; it is unclear what role genetic or environmental factors play in the progression of these predisposing conditions to cancer. In particular, there is mounting evidence connecting *Helicobacter pylori* infection and gastric cancer. *H. pylori* was found to induce gastric adenocarcinoma in animal models. *H. pylori* was isolated from gastric mucosa harboring cancer or precancerous lesions. Large epidemiologic data demonstrate a two- to sixfold gastric cancer increase in populations with high *H. pylori* prevalence. The risk appears to be higher in patients who acquire *H. pylori* infection early in life. By some estimates, *H. pylori* infection is responsible for up to 47 percent of all gastric cancers. Despite significant evidence supporting a causal role of *H. pylori* in gastric cancer pathogenesis, it is unclear whether *H. pylori* eradication reduces the risk of gastric cancer.

The connection between *H. pylori* infection and benign peptic ulcer disease is well documented. However, there are no data conclusively connecting benign peptic ulcer disease and gastric cancer. One recent large study reported a small increase in gastric cancer risk in patients with benign gastric ulcers, the risk being unchanged in patients with prepyloric ulcers and actually decreased in duodenal ulcer patients. On the other hand, partial gastrectomy for benign peptic ulcer disease has definitely been associated with 1.5- to 3-fold elevated risk of gastric cancer.

A number of other predisposing conditions for gastric cancer have been described. Among more common ones is pernicious anemia (a two- to threefold increased risk), which also carries a higher incidence of gastric carcinoid. Adenomatous gastric polyps, particularly those >2 cm in size, have a high malignant potential and are frequently found in pernicious anemia patients. Hypertrophic gastropathy has also been linked to increased gastric cancer risk, although the association is not well defined. Barrett's esophagus is a significant risk factor for gastric cardia cancers, with incidence of malignant transformation of about 2 percent per year.

Clinical Manifestations

The onset of gastric cancer is characteristically slow and insidious. Early mucosal and submucosal lesions are typically asymptomatic. In a recent extensive survey of initial presentations of gastric cancer, weight loss was the most common complaint. Weight loss is usually associated with anorexia, early satiety (secondary to gastric outlet obstruction or gastric stasis) or dysphagia (secondary to gastroesophageal junction obstruction by the tumor). Dysphagia most likely results from tumor infiltration of gastric wall neuronal plexuses. It can be profound, sometimes to the extent of being misdiagnosed as achalasia. In fact, gastric cancer should be always considered as part of a differential for new-onset achalasia, especially, in the elderly patient.

Abdominal pain is almost as frequent a presenting complaint as weight loss. It is typically quite vague early on but increases in severity as the disease progresses. Occult bleeding with or without iron deficiency anemia is another common finding in early gastric cancer. However, melena is only seen in 20 percent of patients and is more frequently associated with leiomyoma or leiomyosarcoma. Palpable abdominal mass is the most common physical exam finding characteristic of more advanced disease.

As gastric cancer evolves, more symptoms and signs of distant spread appear. Textbook findings of lymphatic spread are periumbilical or left supraclavicular lymphadenopathy (Sister Mary Joseph's and Virchow's nodes, respectively). Enlarged ovary (Krukenberg's tumor) or mass in the cul-de-sac area on rectal exam (Blumer's shelf) are indicative of peritoneal involvement. Ascites can be another sign of peritoneal carcinomatosis and liver metastases. Malignant gastrocolic fistula can manifest itself by feculent emesis.

Several systemic paraneoplastic manifestations have been described, although none are specific for gastric cancer. For example, acanthosis nigrans and diffuse seborrheic keratoses are associated with advanced gastric cancer. Microangiopathic hemolytic anemia, membranous nephropathy, and hypercoagulable state (Trousseau's syndrome) have all been noted in connection with gastric cancer.

Cancer Histology, Dynamics, Prognostic Factors, and Staging

More than 90 percent of gastric cancers are adenocarcinomas, followed by non-Hodgkin's lymphomas and leiomyosarcomas.

Grossly, gastric cancer can present in a variety of ways. Signs of early mucosal and submucosal lesions can be quite subtle—protrusions, superficial plaques, mucosal discoloration and ulcerations. Fungating or polypoid tumors are seen at more advanced stages. Superficial infiltrating lesions (linitis plastica) are less frequent.

Histologically, two primary types of gastric adenocarcinoma, described as intestinal and diffuse, have been identified. The major distinction between the two is the ability of malignant cells to form cohesive glandular structures. In the intestinal type, neoplastic cells organize into glands consisting of well-differentiated columnar epithelium with well-developed brush border. In the diffuse type, malignant cells lose their ability to coalesce into glands and therefore do not form a discrete mass. The gross appearance and location of the two types of gastric adenocarcinoma differs as well. The intestinal type lesions tend to ulcerate more often and have a predilection for the distant stomach, whereas diffuse type tumors can occur throughout the stomach but are more frequent in the cardia.

In addition to histologic differences, the two types of gastric adenocarcinoma also have distinct epidemiologic patterns. The intestinal type is more commonly found in the elderly and in endemic areas of gastric cancer. On the other hand, the diffuse type is equally distributed worldwide and predominates among younger patients. The incidence of the intestinal type tumors has been declining, whereas the frequency of the diffuse type has not changed. Of note, intestinal type tumors carry a better prognosis.

In recent years, significant progress has been made in our understanding of genetic alterations leading to gastric cancer. Differences in the molecular mechanisms between the intestinal and diffuse types of gastric adenocarcinoma have also been described. For example, overexpression of epidermal growth factor receptors has been detected in intestinal type tumors but not in the diffuse ones. In contrast, defects in the fibroblast growth factor receptor family are frequently found in the diffuse type lesions. There are reports of decreased production of E-cadherin (a major adhesion molecule responsible for cell–cell contacts) in families with diffuse-type cancer clustering.

Another major difference in the pathogenesis of intestinal and diffuse types of gastric adenocarcinomas is in the occurrence of a precancerous state. The intestinal type is thought to develop over extended periods of time from chronic atrophic gastritis with intestinal metaplasia (precancerous lesion). In contrast, the diffuse type does not appear to arise from such a precancerous state. The current understanding of the stepwise progression of the intestinal type of gastric adenocarcinoma from precancerous lesion can be outlined as follows. *H. pylori* infection, pernicious anemia, or certain diets cause chronic superficial gastritis. With time, atrophic gastritis develops. Loss of parietal cells leads to decreased acid production and increased gastrin levels in an attempt to compensate for achlorhydria. Gastrin is a potent stimulus for gastric cell proliferation. Chronic inflammation is also associated with increased neutrophil infiltration, leading to free radical release and epithelial cell damage. As a result, intestinal metaplasia develops, histologically manifesting itself by the presence of mucin-secreting goblet cells. Clearly, this model is an oversimplification, and other factors must be involved as only 10 percent of patients with intestinal metaplasia ultimately develop cancer.

Although initially the two types of gastric adenocarcinoma behave quite differently, they advance in similar fashion. Cancer progression through the stomach wall is reflected in the TNM staging system. T1 lesion denotes invasion of lamina propria or submucosa, T2 is an extension to muscularis propria, T3 signifies penetration of the serosal layer, and T4 is an invasion of adjacent organs.

The extent of tumor invasion according to the TNM system is the most important prognostic factor. Five-year survival for patients with early stage gastric cancer is approximately 75 percent; it sharply drops to 30 percent with cancer involvement beyond the gastric wall. Lymph node involvement is another prognostic factor. Interestingly, not only the number of affected lymph nodes but also their proximity to the primary lesion has a predictive value. Patients with few positive lymph nodes adjacent to the main tumor have a more favorable prognosis. As mentioned above, tumor location may be one more prognostic factor, with lower survival rates for cardia lesions than for tumors of the distal stomach. On the other hand, histologic grade and tumor gross appearance are poor prognosticators as they depend on tumor stage. Recently, DNA ploidy has been reported as another independent prognostic factor. Aneuploidy was found to be associated with unfavorable

tumor location, aggressive tumor extension, lymph node involvement, and overall less-favorable prognosis.

Diagnosis

Endoscopy with multiple biopsies is the initial step in the diagnosis of gastric cancer (Fig. 57-2). The sensitivity of endoscopy with multiple (up to seven) biopsies for gastric cancer detection approaches 98 percent. It is recommended

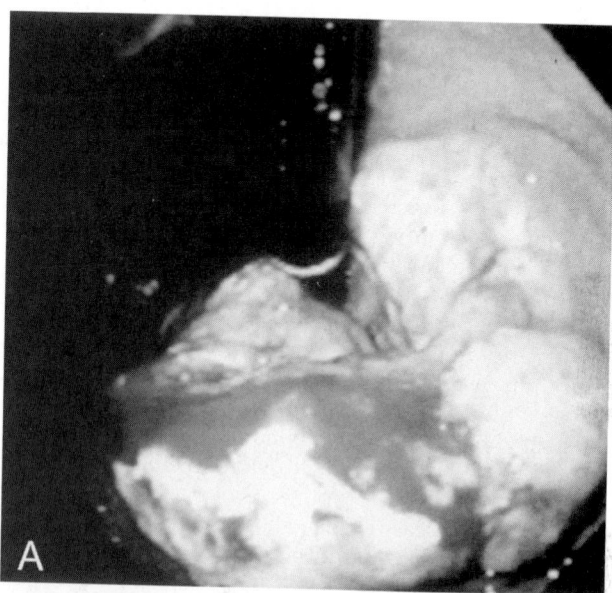

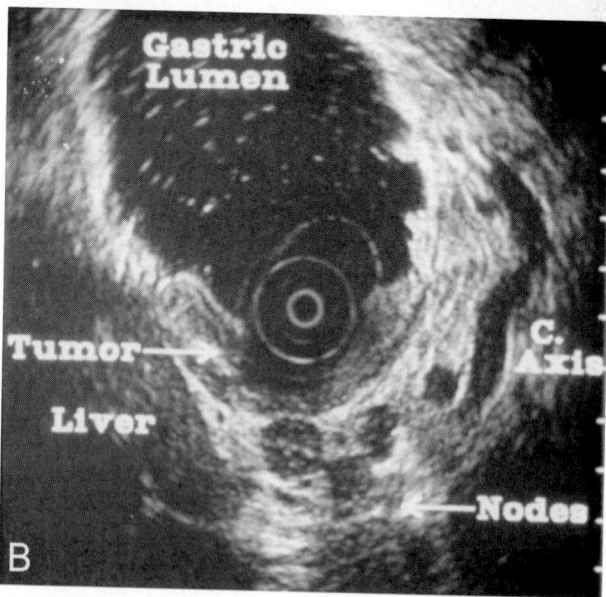

Figure 57-2 *A.* Large ulcerated gastric mass located in the posterior wall of the fundus of the stomach. *B.* Endoscopic ultrasound demonstrates a hypoechoic mass penetrating the serosal layer with adjacent lymphadenopathy (T3N1). Reproduced with permission from Sial SH, Catalano MF: Gastrointestinal tract cancer in the elderly, in Farrell JJ, Friedman LS (eds): *Gastroenterology Clinics of North America.* Philadelphia, WB Saunders, 2001.

that all ulcers, including small and benign in appearance, should be biopsied because 5 percent of malignant lesions can look grossly benign. Biopsy of small ulcers allows diagnosis of gastric cancer at an early stage and therefore improves survival. Endoscopic diagnosis of the diffuse type gastric cancer involving submucosa is quite challenging, as superficial biopsies could be falsely negative. Strip and the bite biopsy technique has been suggested in order to overcome this difficulty if diffuse gastric cancer is suspected. The current standard of treatment advocates routine follow-up endoscopy with biopsies of all unhealed ulcers 8 to 12 weeks after the initial endoscopy. Further studies are needed to confirm the cost-effectiveness of this approach.

Currently available serologic tumor markers have not been particularly useful in diagnosis of gastric cancer because none of them are adequately sensitive and/or specific. Early diagnosis of gastric cancer is crucial because it is the main determinant of survival. The necessity of screening for gastric cancer has been widely debated. In Japan, where gastric cancer incidence is high, an annual screening program with endoscopy and radiography has been established for people older than age 50 years. Early detection is thought to be responsible for declining rates of gastric cancer death in Japan, where 40 to 60 percent of new gastric cancer cases are currently diagnosed at early stages. However, prevalence of gastric cancer in the United States is quite low. Most experts agree that screening in the United States should be done on a case-by-case basis through identification of high-risk individuals. Currently, regular endoscopic screening is recommended for people with a history of gastric adenomas, familial diffuse gastric cancer, and for patients with hereditary nonpolyposis colorectal cancer syndrome (HNPCC) or Barrett's esophagus.

After the diagnosis of gastric cancer is made, further treatment depends solely on tumor stage. In recent years, diagnostic modalities for staging of gastric cancer have expanded significantly. Nowadays, EUS is more commonly used to assess the degree of tumor invasion and lymph node involvement. The accuracy of EUS may be further enhanced through fine-needle aspiration (FNA) of suspicious lymph nodes. In a recent review, EUS correctly identified depth of invasion in 77 percent, and positive lymph nodes in 69 percent of patients. Overstaging is possible secondary to inflammation around the tumor and lymph nodes. EUS evaluation is supplemented by CT to assess the extent of distant spread, in particular, liver metastasis. Laparoscopy can be used to further investigate the presence of distant metastases. It allows direct visualization of liver surface, peritoneum, and local lymph nodes. In one study, laparoscopy led to the detection of peritoneal metastases in 23 percent of patients with CT initially negative for peritoneal spread.

Treatment

Success of complete surgical resection determines to a large degree the long-term survival for gastric cancer patients. In recent years, advances in surgical technique and perioperative care significantly decreased surgery-related morbidity and mortality. Surgical resection serves multiple purposes

in treatment of gastric cancer: it not only provides chance for cure but also allows for effective palliation of nonresectable lesions. Therefore, complete surgical resection should always be attempted unless there is clear evidence of disseminated disease (by noninvasive methods) or the patient is not a surgical candidate because of other comorbidities. The choice of surgical technique is based on tumor location, the extent of tumor invasion, and tumor histology. Gastrectomy is the main surgical approach to gastric cancer lesions. Some early gastric cancers can be removed endoscopically by the technique of endoscopic mucosal resection. The decision on total versus subtotal gastrectomy is mostly made based on tumor location: total gastrectomy is typically done for proximal lesions, whereas subtotal gastrectomy with adjacent lymph node dissection is applied to distal lesions. Several studies demonstrate similar overall survival and perioperative complication rate for subtotal versus total gastrectomy of distal lesions. However, quality of life was significantly better with subtotal than the total gastrectomy of distal lesions. On the other hand, for proximal lesions total gastrectomy is preferred because reflux esophagitis occurs less often and more complete lymph node removal is possible. Usually, linitis plastica and large mid-stomach tumors also require total gastrectomy.

By some estimates, up to 80 percent of patients with gastric cancer face recurrence after complete surgical resection, with 40 percent having local or regional recurrence and up to 60 percent recurring systemically. These grim statistics provide the rationale for adjuvant and neoadjuvant therapy in treatment of gastric cancer, with the aim of decreasing recurrence and prolonging survival. Chemotherapy, radiation, or combined therapy, as well as newer chemoimmunotherapy, have been investigated as potential candidates for adjuvant and neoadjuvant therapy. There are conflicting data on survival benefit of these various modalities. In a recent large trial, only adjuvant chemoradiation therapy with 5-FU and leucovorin was conclusively shown to prolong median survival. A number of chemoimmunotherapy agents have been investigated, including levamisole, bacille Calmette-Guérin (BCG), cimetidine, and protein-bound polysaccharide. However, no conclusions can be drawn from these studies, as the results have not been reproducible across different trials. The data on neoadjuvant therapy in gastric cancer have been even more limited. Preliminary studies, most of which were done outside the United States, show potential survival benefit for neoadjuvant radiation therapy alone or in combination with chemotherapy. Further randomized trials are needed to confirm these preliminary data. New combinations of chemotherapeutic agents for adjuvant and neoadjuvant therapy, such as epirubicin, cisplatin, and 5-FU, or etoposide and doxorubicin, are currently in a number of trials.

Chemotherapy is the standard of care for patients with diffusely disseminated gastric cancer who are not candidates for curable surgical resection with adjuvant therapy. Combination regiments are generally preferred to single-agent treatments. However, although initial response rates are higher with combination regiments, the overall survival is similar. Currently, a combination of epirubicin, cisplatin and infusional 5-FU is most commonly used for advanced

Delayed gastric emptying is a major palliative problem. Up to 60 percent of patients with pancreatic cancer complain of nausea and vomiting related to slowed gastric emptying. The etiology of this phenomenon is unclear, and it is speculated to arise from tumor invasion of neuronal plexuses. Some patients benefit from promotility agents as gastrojejunostomy has not been successful.

Pain has always been a hallmark of advanced pancreatic cancer. Initial pain control is usually accomplished by narcotic analgesics. Recently, EUS-guided celiac plexus block gained popularity because it provides pain control that's superior to the pain control provided by analgesics. Celiac block involves chemical ablation with alcohol of afferents transmitting pain stimuli from abdominal viscera. Treatment of depression (a common complication of advanced pancreatic malignancy) is a crucial part of a comprehensive pain control program. Weight loss and cachexia is another aspect of end-stage pancreatic cancer that is difficult to treat. Several small studies demonstrate moderate improvements in cachexia with pancreatic enzyme supplementation.

HEPATOBILIARY CANCER

Hepatocellular Carcinoma

Incidence

Hepatocellular carcinoma is a source of significant morbidity and mortality worldwide, claiming about 1 million lives yearly. Globally, it ranks as the sixth leading cause of death among men and the eleventh leading cause of death among women. There is a great variability in the frequency of hepatocellular carcinoma throughout the world. In countries with high clustering of hepatocellular carcinoma, such as sub-Saharan Africa and eastern Asia, the incidence approaches 150 per 100,000 population. In contrast, in the United States, hepatocellular carcinoma is quite rare. It accounts for less than 2 percent of all malignancies and occurs at a rate of 1 to 4 per 100,000 population. In the United States, 22,000 people were affected by hepatocellular carcinoma in year 2000. However, despite its low rate, the US incidence of hepatocellular carcinoma has risen dramatically (up to 50 percent by some estimates) over the past decade.

Similar to other gastrointestinal malignancies, the incidence of hepatocellular carcinoma increases with age. Average age of onset is 62 years in the United States. Over the past several years, there has been a shift toward a younger age at initial presentation.

Risk Factors

Liver cirrhosis of any etiology is the major risk factor for hepatocellular carcinoma. Patients with liver cirrhosis have 3 to 5 percent chance per year of developing hepatocellular carcinoma. Reportedly, macronodular cirrhosis compared to micronodular cirrhosis carries a higher risk for hepatocellular carcinoma development. Of note, in more than half of the patients, cirrhosis is first diagnosed at the initial presentation of hepatocellular carcinoma. In the United States, alcohol abuse is the main cause of liver cirrhosis. Several in vitro and epidemiologic studies have linked alcohol to hepatocarcinogenesis but a direct carcinogenic effect of alcohol has not been demonstrated. In addition to alcohol, other causes of liver disease, such as hereditary hemochromatosis and primary biliary cirrhosis, lead to hepatocellular carcinoma solely in the context of liver cirrhosis.

Whereas most cases of hepatocellular carcinoma in the United States can be attributed to alcoholic liver cirrhosis, in countries with high prevalence of hepatocellular carcinoma, chronic hepatitis B infection is the major cause of this disease. A number of large population studies demonstrate dramatically increased risk of hepatocellular carcinoma in hepatitis B surface antigen (HBsAg) carriers (up to 200 times higher than noncarriers). Evidence of previous hepatitis B infection is found in almost 30 percent of hepatocellular carcinoma patients. The risk of hepatocellular carcinoma appears to be even higher if hepatitis B is acquired early in life; for men infected at birth the cumulative lifetime risk is 50 percent.

Chronic hepatitis C infection is another important risk factor for hepatocellular carcinoma development, in particular in areas with a low incidence of hepatitis B carriage. It accounts for 30 to 50 percent of cases of hepatocellular carcinoma in the United States. Hepatitis C virus genotype 1b appears to have an even higher preponderance for hepatocellular carcinoma development and might be an independent risk factor. In contrast to hepatitis B infection, where both carriers and cirrhotic patients are at increased risk, in cases of chronic hepatitis C, hepatocellular carcinoma development is limited to patients with liver cirrhosis. Development of hepatocellular carcinoma is accelerated in patients with combined alcohol abuse and chronic hepatitis C infection or with hepatitis B and C coinfection. The role of hepatitis C in the pathogenesis of hepatocellular carcinoma is not fully understood. Hepatitis C is thought to initiate a cascade of inflammatory response and cellular injury leading to cirrhosis and carcinogenesis.

A number of environmental toxins are associated with hepatocellular carcinoma development. Aflatoxin, a mycotoxin frequently found in corn, soybeans, and peanuts, induces mutations in the p53 gene in in vitro studies. In one report from Taiwan, patients with hepatocellular carcinoma had a higher level of aflatoxin in their diet than matched controls. Betel nut chewing is another dietary factor that appears to be an independent risk factor for hepatocellular carcinoma development according to several case-controlled studies from China.

Clinical Manifestations

As hepatocellular carcinoma typically develops in a setting of chronic liver disease, decompensation of a previously stable liver disease patient should alert one to the possibility of cancer development. New onset of ascites, variceal bleeding, encephalopathy, or jaundice can be subtle indications of tumor progression. Indeed, 15 percent of patients admitted for variceal bleeding and 20 percent of patients admitted with spontaneous bacterial peritonitis are further diagnosed with hepatocellular carcinoma. Hemorrhagic ascites is quite a characteristic finding and is present in 50 percent of patients with hepatocellular carcinoma.

Several symptoms, such as abdominal pain, early satiety, weight loss, jaundice, bone pain, and dyspnea, are typical of fairly advanced disease. For example, persistent right upper quadrant abdominal pain (the most frequent presenting complaint) usually signifies tumor extension to Glisson's capsule. In the case of tumor rupture and bleeding into the peritoneum, abdominal pain can be acute and quite severe, with associated hypotension. Bone pain and dyspnea are related to tumor involvement of the bone and lungs.

A number of paraneoplastic syndromes have been identified in connection with hepatocellular carcinoma. Hypoglycemia is common in end-stage hepatocellular carcinoma, but typically is mild, and most of the patients remain asymptomatic. In rare cases, severe hypoglycemia has been reported secondary to tumor secretion of insulin-like growth factor-II, a potent insulin-like agonist. Some hepatocellular tumors are also thought to produce erythropoietin, and elevated levels of erythropoietin are found in about 20 percent of patients with hepatocellular carcinoma. Watery diarrhea is another common paraneoplastic syndrome and reportedly is a presenting complaint in up to 50 percent of patients 3 months prior to cancer diagnosis. Diarrhea is attributed to a release of vasoactive substances by the tumor, such as gastrin, prostaglandins, and vasoactive intestinal polypeptides. Hypercalcemia is often noted and is most likely a result of parathyroid hormone-related protein production by the tumor.

Cancer Histology, Dynamics, Prognostic Factors, and Staging

Hepatocellular carcinoma represents the majority of primary liver malignancies. Angiosarcoma and hepatoblastoma, other primary liver cancers, are significantly less frequent. Hepatic carcinogenesis is a complex and multistep process, evolving over several years. However, after presenting clinically, hepatocellular carcinoma follows a rapid course, with median survival from the time of diagnosis of 6 to 20 months.

The nodular form is the most frequent type, involving multiple irregular nodules that spread throughout the liver. It usually occurs in the setting of liver cirrhosis. On the other hand, the massive form is typically found in noncirrhotic and in younger patients. Classic presentation of a massive tumor is of a large, well-circumscribed lesion with several smaller satellite nodules. Massive form tumors tend to rupture more often.

In more than half of patients with hepatocellular carcinoma the tumor spreads beyond the liver. Lungs are the most frequent site of distant metastasis (up to 50 percent by some reports), followed by lymph nodes (20 percent). Of note, noncirrhotic patients are more prone to the development of distant metastases than cirrhotic patients. Evidence of portal vein involvement by the tumor is found in 70 percent of cases; spread to hepatic veins and bile ducts is not as common.

In recent years, a number of determinants that can affect hepatocellular carcinoma survival have been identified. It appears that the following factors carry the most prognostic potential: extent of underlying liver disease, size of the tumor, and level of invasion into adjacent organs and distant structures. These prognostic factors are to a varying degree represented in currently available staging systems for hepatocellular carcinoma. The most widely used Okuda system combines tumor size and severity of liver cirrhosis, as judged by the presence of ascites, and albumin and bilirubin levels. However, the Okuda system lacks assessment of vascular and distant tumor involvement. On the other hand, the TNM staging system does take into the account the extent of local as well as distant invasion, but not the severity of underlying liver disease (Table 57-4). The most recently proposed staging system, CLIP (Cancer of the Liver Italian Program) score, considers tumor-based factors and degree of invasion (gross tumor morphology, α-fetoprotein levels, presence of portal vein thrombosis), as well as the extent of associated liver cirrhosis (Table 57-5). Preliminary reports indicate better survival estimates with CLIP score than with Okuda or TNM staging systems.

Several other variables not included into all main staging systems are found to be independent prognosticators. After surgical resection, higher α-fetoprotein levels reportedly carry worse prognosis. This correlation is still present after adjustment for tumor size and histologic grade. Histologic grade appears to be a predictor of survival on its own, with well-differentiated and encapsulated tumors having better prognosis.

Diagnosis

Currently, a widely accepted approach to the diagnosis of hepatocellular carcinoma combines various imaging modalities and serum tumor markers assessment. Ultrasound is usually the first diagnostic tool used, as it is inexpensive and readily available. Classic ultrasonographic appearance of hepatocellular carcinoma is of a lesion with poorly defined margins and mosaic pattern of internal echoes, septum formation and peripheral halo, produced by a fibrotic pseudocapsule. Initially, hepatocellular carcinoma is hypoechoic, but with further growth, the tumor becomes hyperechoic, making it more difficult to distinguish the lesion from underlying liver parenchyma. Ultrasound also allows assessment of hepatic flow and is therefore helpful in determining the extent of vascular invasion by the tumor. The sensitivity of ultrasound for hepatocellular carcinoma detection ranges between 70 and 80 percent, with specificity of 93 percent and positive predictive value of 15 percent.

Because positive predictive value of ultrasound is low, further confirmatory studies are needed to establish the diagnosis. Helical CT is usually the next step in evaluation of a lesion ultrasonographically suspicious for hepatocellular carcinoma. Rapid administration of contrast followed by extremely fast imaging differentiates helical CT technique from the regular CT. Helical CT allows accurate diagnosis of small lesions, in some studies as small as 3 mm. The sensitivity of helical CT has been reported to be 90 percent, compared to the 68 percent sensitivity of regular CT.

Magnetic resonance imaging (MRI) has sensitivity similar to helical CT and is typically used for patients unable to undergo CT because of renal insufficiency or contrast dye

Table 57-4 TNM Staging for Hepatocellular Cancer and Intrahepatic Bile Duct Cancer

Primary Tumor (T)	
T0	No evidence of primary tumor
T1	Solitary tumor 2 cm or less in greatest dimension without vascular invasion
T2	Solitary tumor 2 cm or less in greatest dimension with vascular invasion, or multiple tumors limited to one lobe, none more than 2 cm in greatest dimension without vascular invasion, or a solitary tumor more than 2 cm in greatest dimension without vascular invasion
T3	Solitary tumor more than 2 cm in greatest dimension with vascular invasion, or multiple tumors limited to one lobe, none more than 2 cm in greatest dimension, with vascular invasion, or multiple tumors limited to one lobe, none any more than 2 cm in greatest dimension, with or without vascular invasion
T4	Multiple tumors in more than one lobe, or tumor(s) involve(s) a major branch of the portal or hepatic vein(s), or invasion of adjacent organs other than the gallbladder, or perforation of the visceral peritoneum
Regional Lymph Nodes (N)	
NX	Regional lymph nodes cannot be assessed
N0	No regional lymph node metastasis
N1	Regional lymph node metastasis
Distant Metastasis (M)	
MX	Distant metastasis cannot be assessed
M0	No distant metastasis
M1	Distant metastasis

SOURCE: Modified from *American Joint Committee on Cancer Staging Manual*, 5th ed. Philadelphia, Lippincott-Raven, 1997.

allergy. Another advantage of MRI is its ability to distinguish a hyperplastic nodule from hepatocellular carcinoma in the case of a lesion ambiguous on CT. If no diagnosis can be convincingly made after ultrasound or helical CT studies, CT-guided biopsy may then be attempted. Direct core

Table 57-5 Hepatocellular Carcinoma Clip Scoring System

Variable	Score
Child–Pugh stage	
A	0
B	1
C	2
Tumor morphology	
Uninodular and extension ≤50 percent	0
Multinodular and extension ≤50 percent	1
Massive or extension >50 percent	2
α-Fetoprotein	
<400	0
≥400	1
Portal vein thrombosis	
No	0
Yes	1

SOURCE: Reproduced with permission from Prospective validation of the CLIP score: A new prognostic system for patients with cirrhosis and hepatocellular carcinoma. *Hepatology* 31:840, 2000.

biopsies are preferred to fine-needle aspirates as more tissue can be obtained. The decision about CT-guided biopsy should always be carefully weighed against the potential risks associated with the procedure, particularly the risks of peritoneal cancer seeding, perforation, and bleeding.

α-Fetoprotein is the main serum tumor marker used in hepatocellular carcinoma detection. The generally accepted cutoff value for α-fetoprotein in adults is 20 ng/mL. In addition to hepatocellular carcinoma, α-fetoprotein levels can be also elevated in acute and chronic hepatitis, in certain germ-cell tumors, and in pregnancy. Serum α-fetoprotein levels do not correlate well with size, grade, or stage of the tumor. Up to 40 percent of small hepatocellular tumors have normal α-fetoprotein levels. Nevertheless, α-fetoprotein serum levels higher than 500 ng/mL are very suggestive of hepatocellular carcinoma. Patients with underlying liver disease and persistently elevated α-fetoprotein serum levels should be monitored very closely as they are at increased risk for hepatocellular carcinoma development.

The importance of early diagnosis of hepatocellular carcinoma becomes apparent from the survival statistics. A 3-year survival rate of 83 percent after surgical resection has been reported for the TNM stage I tumors, as compared to a 10 percent survival rate for stage IV (nonmetastatic) lesions. Unfortunately, the experience with screening programs for hepatocellular carcinoma is disappointing. In several large studies of high-risk patients undergoing screening for hepatocellular carcinoma, most tumors were still diagnosed at a late stage, not amenable to surgical resection. Despite the lack of clear evidence supporting screening for hepatocellular carcinoma, most experts recommend regular (every 6 months) assessment of α-fetoprotein serum levels combined with liver ultrasound for patients with established cirrhosis.

Treatment

Treatment for hepatocellular carcinoma is an area of intense research. Multiple treatment modalities, including surgical resection, orthotopic transplantation, locoregional treatments, and systemic chemo- and immunotherapy, are currently being investigated. No one treatment approach is superior and not all treatments are appropriate for every patient. Therefore, careful selection of patients best suited for a particular treatment is crucial. Surgical resectability (similar to other gastrointestinal malignancies) is one of the main determinants of survival. Unfortunately, only 30 percent of patients with hepatocellular carcinoma are considered surgical candidates. To qualify for surgical resection, patients ought to have a solitary tumor less than 5 cm in size, with no evidence of vascular or distant involvement, as well as fairly preserved liver function. Intraoperative ultrasound and laparoscopy are occasionally used prior to surgical resection to enhance staging and assure adequate patient selection. Most of the perioperative morbidity and mortality is related to liver decompensation following the resection. In fact, intraoperative mortality doubles (from 5 percent to 10 percent) in cirrhotic patients with poor liver reserve compared to noncirrhotic patients. Overall, 5-year survival after surgical resection is approximately 30 percent, and the rate of recurrence varies from 40 to 70 percent. However, survival rates can be dramatically increased, in some reports to 50 percent, or even to 90 percent, by careful patient selection.

Orthotopic liver transplantation is another surgical option for treatment of hepatocellular carcinoma. During this procedure, malignant tumor is resected and cirrhotic liver is replaced. Initial results from orthotopic liver transplantation series were quite discouraging, with a high (up to 80 percent) rate of recurrence and a high mortality rate. However, through careful patient selection according to the above-described criteria, promising 4-year survival rates of 70 percent to 90 percent have been achieved. Success of orthotopic liver transplantation requires a short waiting time until the transplant, which is, however, not feasible nowadays, with current waiting times as long as 24 months.

As recurrence rates after surgical resection are quite high, a number of treatment modalities have been proposed as possible adjuvant therapy, with the goal of decreasing recurrence and improving survival. One promising treatment is intraarterial infusion of iodine-labeled lipiodol, a fatty acid ethyl ester derived from poppy-seed oil. In one controlled trial from Hong Kong, patients who received intraarterial radioactive iodine-labeled lipiodol after curative surgical resection had a 50 percent lower recurrence rate and significantly improved disease-free survival. The treatment was well tolerated without any major complications related to angiography.

A number of chemotherapeutic agents have been evaluated for systemic as well as intraarterial adjuvant therapy, however, none increases survival in randomized trials. For patients with small solitary tumors who are not surgical

candidates because of inadequate functional liver reserve, percutaneous ethanol injection (PEI) may be another therapeutic option. This treatment involves percutaneous injection of 95 percent ethanol directly into the tumor, resulting in tumor necrosis. The procedure is relatively well tolerated, with some patients experiencing localized pain as well as generalized peritoneal irritation caused by ethanol leakage. In rare cases, intraperitoneal hemorrhage and hepatorenal failure were reported. Currently, PEI is saved for patients who are unable to undergo surgery because of a lack of liver reserve or because of a surgically inaccessible lesion. PEI may be also an option for patients awaiting orthotopic liver transplantation.

Radiofrequency ablation (RFA) is one more form of locoregional treatment for hepatocellular carcinoma. Thermal energy generated by radiofrequency waves induces tumor necrosis and shrinkage. The advantage of RFA is its ability to treat medium- to large-size tumors. In several prospective trials and series comparing RFA and PEI, the disease-free survival rates were similar between these two modalities, but local recurrence rates were somewhat lower with RFA. Moreover, fewer RFA than PEI sessions were required to achieve similar results. However, RFA was associated with a higher rate of major complications such as hemorrhage, peritoneal cancer seeding, and, ultimately, death.

Treatment options for patients with large unresectable hepatocellular carcinomas are limited to transarterial chemoembolization and systemic chemotherapy. The former involves intraarterial injection of a chemotherapeutic agent with or without lipiodol, followed by hepatic artery occlusion with Gelfoam and plastic particles. Despite the initially reported successes and relatively widespread use, several controlled randomized trials did not find transarterial chemoembolization superior to conservative treatment of patients with advanced hepatocellular carcinoma. Moreover, transarterial chemoembolization was associated with higher rates of major complications, including liver failure and death. Similarly, survival advantage has not been demonstrated with transarterial chemoembolization as neoadjuvant therapy prior to surgical resection or transplantation; mortality rates were higher as well. Currently, recommended use of transarterial chemoembolization is in patients with fairly preserved liver function who are symptomatic with large unresectable tumors and those not amenable to RFA.

Systemic chemotherapy is often the only and the last option for patients who have unresectable hepatocellular carcinoma and are not candidates for locoregional treatments due to large tumor size. Unfortunately, hepatocellular carcinoma is a fairly chemotherapy-resistant malignancy because of high expression of drug resistance genes and a low efficacy and poor tolerance to most of the chemotherapeutic agents in patients with compromised liver function. Some experts recommend cisplatin-based combination regimens with doxorubicin, 5-FU and interferon-α for younger patients with better-preserved liver function, and 5-FU with leucovorin for elderly patients and for patients with more severe underlying liver disease.

Hepatocellular carcinoma is a rapidly progressing disease, with the majority of patients presenting late, at advanced stages not amenable to most of the currently available therapies. Limitations of modern treatment modalities underscore the importance of prevention in management of hepatocellular carcinoma. Vaccination against hepatitis B, and hepatitis C treatment with interferon are two main preventive approaches that can significantly reduce the incidence of hepatocellular carcinoma.

Cholangiocarcinoma

Cholangiocarcinoma, or biliary duct cancer, is a rare and extremely deadly malignancy. Overall 5-year survival is reported to be as low as 5 to 10 percent. Cholangiocarcinoma accounts for less than 3 percent of all gastrointestinal cancers, with 2000 to 3000 cases diagnosed annually in the United States. Incidence of cholangiocarcinoma rises with age, the usual age at presentation being 50 to 70 years. Cholangiocarcinoma is somewhat more prevalent in men than in women. For reasons currently not fully understood, the incidence and mortality from cholangiocarcinoma in the United States has increased over the past two decades.

A number of genetic and environmental conditions and disease states are associated with increased risk for cholangiocarcinoma development. Primary sclerosing cholangitis (PSC) and choledochal cysts are main risk factors in the US population. PSC is an inflammatory disease of biliary ducts, leading to duct fibrosis and stricturing. PSC has well-known strong association with ulcerative colitis, and almost 30 percent of cholangiocarcinomas are diagnosed in patients with both ulcerative colitis and PSC. Patients with PSC have a 10 to 15 percent lifetime risk for cholangiocarcinoma development. The risk is even higher in smokers and alcoholics with PSC. Choledochal cysts also carry increased risk for cholangiocarcinoma development, the degree of which is related to the duration of the disease. Cholelithiasis is another possible risk factor for cholangiocarcinoma, although this association has not yet been firmly established. The incidence of cholangiocarcinoma was found to be much lower in patients with prior cholecystectomy. On the other hand, hepatolithiasis is a well-known risk factor for cholangiocarcinoma development. In patients with hepatolithiasis the incidence of cholangiocarcinoma is 2 to 10 percent, as noted in certain endemic areas of southeast Asia. Liver fluke infection (genera *Clonorchis* and *Opisthorchis*) is associated with chronic inflammation of the bile duct and, therefore, with elevated risk of cholangiocarcinoma development. Certain genetic disorders, particularly primary biliary papillomatosis, carry increased risk for cholangiocarcinoma, as multiple adenomatous polyps found in the biliary duct have high malignant potential. Among environmental factors, the radiologic contrast agent Thorotrast is known to cause cholangiocarcinoma, with malignancy developing as long as 30 years after exposure. Certain occupations, such as in auto, rubber, and wood-finishing industries, are noted to have increased risk for cholangiocarcinoma.

The majority of cholangiocarcinomas are adenocarcinomas, with most tumors located in the upper third of the biliary system, and, commonly, at hepatic duct bifurcation (Klatskin tumors). Most cholangiocarcinomas spread by local invasion; distant metastases are rare. Tumor progression is reflected in the TNM staging system, which is similar to the hepatocellular carcinoma system for intrahepatic lesions but somewhat different in T-stage definition for extrahepatic tumors.

Painless jaundice with weight loss is a textbook presentation of cholangiocarcinoma. Pruritus is another common complaint. Abdominal pain with this tumor is usually localized to the right upper quadrant and is described as dull and constant. Initial laboratory studies typically reveal highly elevated total bilirubin levels (usually, above 10) and increased alkaline phosphatase levels. Liver function is normal at first but can later become compromised with prolonged biliary stasis. Diagnosis of cholangiocarcinoma can be quite difficult, as most currently available modalities lack adequate accuracy. The recommended approach includes initial evaluation with serum tumor markers, such as carcinoembryonic antigen (CEA) and CA19-9, and ultrasonography. Ultrasonographic findings of combined or separate intra- and extrahepatic duct dilation without evidence of cholelithiasis is highly suggestive of cholangiocarcinoma. Suspected lesions are further evaluated by ERCP or percutaneous transhepatic cholangiogram and CT scan. The potential of several newer diagnostic modalities, such as magnetic resonance cholangiopancreatography and endoscopic ultrasonography, has not been fully established. These tests will most likely become useful as noninvasive adjuncts to present techniques in the detection of cholangiocarcinoma.

Surgery is the first line of treatment for patients with potentially resectable tumors. In patients who meet the criteria for resectability (lack of vascular invasion, lymph and distant metastases), the type of surgical procedure mostly depends on tumor location. Distal lesions are typically treated with pancreaticoduodenectomy (Whipple procedure), whereas intrahepatic and perihilar tumors require hepatic resection. Distal tumors have higher resectability rates as compared to proximal lesions, with most perihilar tumors being unresectable. Overall 5-year survival rates after surgical resection range between 8 and 40 percent. Perioperative morbidity is mostly related to the severity of underlying liver disease, with surgical mortality reported at 4 to 8 percent. There are preliminary encouraging reports of improved survival rates with combined regimen of chemo- (5-FU and mitomycin) and radiation therapy after complete surgical resection.

Unfortunately, 50 to 90 percent of patients with cholangiocarcinoma present at advanced stages and are not surgical candidates. Therefore, palliation plays a major role in management of cholangiocarcinoma. End-stage cholangiocarcinoma is associated with debilitating symptoms of biliary obstruction, such as pruritus and pain. Currently available palliative modalities are directed towards relieve of these symptoms. Nowadays, endoscopic placement of expandable metal stents is a preferred approach in palliation of malignant biliary obstruction. Endoscopically placed expandable metal stents have been shown to have better long-term survival and complication rates than bypass surgery or percutaneous stent placement. Photodynamic therapy is another endoscopic technique that recently has been investigated for palliation of malignant biliary obstruction with some promising initial results.

COLORECTAL CANCER

Incidence

In the year 2001, it was predicted that 135,000 new cases of colorectal cancer would be diagnosed and 56,000 patients would die of this disease. Colorectal cancer is the second leading cause of cancer death and the fourth most prevalent cancer in the United States. The average lifetime risk for developing colorectal cancer is approximately 6 percent. Men and women are affected equally. Colorectal cancer is distributed evenly among various racial groups in the United States. However, African Americans and Hispanics have lower survival rates, which can be explained in part by the lack of health care access and a greater percentage of proximal colonic lesions in this population.

Colorectal cancer is a disease of the elderly population. Patients age 50 years and older account for 90 percent of the cases. The onset of colorectal cancer before age 40 years is quite rare, and its incidence progressively increases thereafter to 3.7 per 1000 population per year by the age of 80 years. Furthermore, the prevalence of polyps (two-thirds of which might be precancerous lesions) also increases with age. Polyps are found in 30 percent of patients age 50 years and in 50 percent of patients age 70 years. Although colorectal cancer incidence and mortality has been decreasing slightly in the last several years, it is still a tremendous health care burden, especially among the elderly population.

Risk Factors

Age is the main risk factor for the development of colorectal cancer. As stated above, the age-specific incidence for new cases of colorectal cancer rises sharply from 15 to about 400 per 100,000 population between ages 50 and 80 years.

Colorectal cancer causation is multifactorial, with a number of genetic and environmental factors involved (Table 57-6). Two hereditary disorders with increased tendency for the development of colorectal cancer have been identified. Familial adenomatous polyposis (FAP) and HNPCC were extensively studied in the last decade, and specific gene defects have been determined. Both disorders are inherited in an autosomal dominant fashion. FAP is quite rare and is less than 1 percent of colorectal cancers. On average, patients become symptomatic in their early teens, and 95 percent develop colorectal cancer by age 50 years if colectomy is not performed. Patients with FAP are also at an increased risk for developing upper gastrointestinal tract malignancies. Three variant syndromes of FAP exist. In Gardner's syndrome, adenomas of large and small bowel are associated with desmoid tumors of mesentery and abdominal wall, lipomas, osteomas, and fibromas. In Turcot's syndrome, both colon and brain tumors develop. Cerebellar medulloblastoma is more typical for FAP whereas HNPCC is associated with indolent glioblastoma multiforme. Attenuated adenomatous polyposis coli (AAPC) is another variant of FAP, with fewer adenomas and colon cancer diagnosed at older ages than a typical FAP. The FAP gene defect is a mutation in the adenomatosis

Table 57-6   Risk Factors for Colorectal Cancer

Age >50 years
High-fat, low-fiber diet

Inflammatory bowel disease
    Chronic ulcerative colitis
    Crohn's disease, long-standing

Familial adenomatous polyposis (including Gardner's and Turcot's syndrome)
Hereditary nonpolyposis colorectal cancer
Hamartomatous polyposis syndromes
Peutz–Jeghers syndrome
Juvenile polyposis

Family history
    Colorectal cancer
    Colorectal adenomas

Personal history
    Colorectal adenomas
    Ureterosigmoidostomy
    Breast, ovarian, uterine cancers

SOURCE: Modified with permission from Catalano M, Levin B: Cancer of the colon and rectum. *Clin Geriatr Med* 7:333, 1991.

polyposis coli (APC) gene on chromosome 5. AAPC is also caused by mutations in this gene but at different sites.

HNPCC is a more common disorder than FAP, accounting for 2 to 6 percent of all colorectal cancers. Patients usually present with adenomas in their twenties, and the majority of patients develop colorectal cancer by their fifth decade. HNPCC mostly affects the right colon, with 70 percent of lesions located proximal to the splenic flexure. Patients with HNPCC are at an increased risk for a number of extracolonic tumors, in particular endometrial carcinoma. HNPCC is caused by mutated mismatch repair genes. Genetic mechanisms appear to be also involved in sporadic colorectal cancer development, underscoring the importance of family history. Risk rises with the number of affected first-degree relatives: twofold versus three- to sixfold increase with one versus two first-degree relatives or if one relative is diagnosed before age 50 years. Having two second-degree relatives increases the risk up to twofold. Family history of colonic adenoma seems to have prognostic significance similar to that of colorectal cancer.

Several diseases are associated with increased risk for colon cancer development. Previous history of colorectal cancer and/or of multiple large (>1 cm) adenomatous polyps confers a four- to seven fold increased risk. The relationship between colorectal cancer and inflammatory bowel disease (IBD) is well known. Most of the available data are on chronic ulcerative colitis. The degree of risk depends on the extent and duration of IBD. Frequency of colorectal cancer rises dramatically after 10 years since the initial diagnosis of panniculitis. The incidence of colon cancer is 0.5 percent per year after 10 years of chronic pancolitis and 1 percent per year thereafter. Patients with ulcerative colitis and primary sclerosing cholangitis are at under even greater risk for colorectal cancer. Risk of colorectal cancer is not significantly elevated in patients with proctitis alone. The association between Crohn's disease and colorectal cancer has been less studied, but the risks are assumed to be similar. Some recent evidence suggests that patients with diabetes mellitus have elevated risk for colorectal cancer development. Hyperinsulinemia can explain this association. Insulin and insulin-like growth factors were found to be important stimuli of colonic mucosa proliferation. Acromegaly has also been connected with an increased risk for gastrointestinal malignancies, in particular, proximal colonic adenomas.

A number of epidemiologic studies brought attention to the role of environmental factors in the development of colorectal cancer. For example, the mortality from colorectal cancer differs widely between various countries, with the highest rates in the United States and Canada, and the lowest in Japan. It was suggested that this disparity could be partially accounted for by differences in diet, in particular, the high fat and low fiber intake in the Western world. However, several recent prospective randomized trials did not corroborate this association. Some data from observational studies suggest that folic acid and calcium deficiency might be other risk factors for colorectal cancer. Indeed, folic acid and calcium supplementation appears to somewhat reduce the risk. The benefit from folic acid supplementation becomes apparent after 15 years of use. Sedentary lifestyle is also connected with increased frequency of colorectal cancer.

In recent years, a significant progress has been made in chemoprevention of colorectal cancer. Several drugs have been identified that potentially can reduce the risk for colorectal cancer. In particular, some observational data indicate that hormone replacement therapy reduces the risk of colorectal cancer. One meta-analysis showed a risk reduction of 20 percent, with even greater decrease in current users. HMG-CoA (hydroxymethylglutaryl coenzyme A) reductase inhibitors were also found to have a protective effect. The effects of aspirin and nonsteroidal antiinflammatory drugs (NSAIDs) have been the most studied. NSAIDs decrease the size of adenomatous polyps in patients with FAP. The protective mechanisms of these therapies are not well understood.

Clinical Presentation

Colorectal cancer can be easily called a silent killer, with some reports suggesting that the cancer is present for up to 5 years before becoming symptomatic. To a degree, a patient's presentation depends on tumor location. Because of the wider right colon lumen, proximal lesions grow larger (before announcing themselves) and do not commonly obstruct. Therefore, patients usually present with symptoms mainly caused by anemia, such as fatigue, weight loss, shortness of breath, and lightheadedness. Vague abdominal discomfort is a common complaint indicating further tumor growth. "Mahogany feces" caused by occult bleeding

are occasionally described for right-sided lesions. Obstruction is a common initial presentation for distal lesions. Patients complain of changes in bowel movement pattern (constipation alternating with diarrhea) and postprandial colicky abdominal pain. Hematochezia is common, with blood passed per rectum or coating the stools. Colorectal cancer can lead to obstruction as well, in particular, small bowel obstruction when the ileocecal valve is blocked. Tenesmus is more associated with rectal cancers.

The diagnosis of colorectal cancer is often difficult, especially in the elderly patient. Symptoms are commonly attributed to benign conditions particularly widespread among the elderly population, such as diverticula, hemorrhoids, or constipation. Some of colorectal cancer initial presentations can be quite unusual, further obscuring the diagnosis. In fact, fistulization into adjacent organs such as bladder may be the first sign of colorectal cancer. Bacteremia with *Streptococcus bovis* and *Clostridium septicum* sepsis is indicative of colorectal cancer in 10 to 25 percent of patients. Fever of unknown origin or intraabdominal and retroperitoneal abscess formation is another unusual presentation of colorectal cancer. Up to 6 percent of adenocarcinomas of unknown origin are later found to be colorectal cancer. Considering all of the above, physicians should be particularly attentive to subtle symptomatology in the elderly patient, always keeping in mind the possibility of colorectal cancer.

Cancer Histology, Dynamics, Prognostic Factors and Staging

Adenocarcinomas comprise more than 95 percent of all colorectal tumors, with squamous cell or transitional cell carcinomas limited to the anorectal junction. Histologically, colorectal adenocarcinomas are composed of moderately to well-differentiated glands, which secrete mucin. Gland formation and mucin secretion are less pronounced in poorly differentiated tumors. The gross appearance of colorectal adenocarcinoma depends on tumor location. Proximal lesions are typically large and bulky, often necrotizing. More distal tumors tend to grow circumferentially, producing the classical "napkin ring" constriction. IBD-related colorectal tumors commonly spread intramurally and therefore appear more flat. Precancerous lesions (i.e., adenomatous polyps) also vary in histologic appearance. They are usually divided into tubulous, villous, or tubulovillous, depending on the amount of villous tissue present. Villous adenomatous polyps comprise 5 percent of all adenomas and have the highest malignant potential (15 to 25 percent). Tubular adenomatous polyps are found in 30 percent of older adults but have a low risk for cancer growth (2 to 3 percent). Tubulovillous polyps have variable amounts of villous tissue and therefore carry intermediate risk.

The development of colorectal cancer is a complex process. By some estimates, transformation of normal colonic mucosa into cancer takes 5 to 15 years. It has been proposed that each step in this progression involves specific genetic mutations. In recent years, significant advances have been made in elucidating the molecular mechanisms of colorectal cancer. Somatic mutations in the gene or mutations in

Table 57-7   TNM Staging of Colorectal Cancer

TNM Stage	Primary Tumor*	Lymph Node Metastasis†	Distant Metastasis‡	Dukes Stage
0	Tis	N0	M0	
I	T1	N0	M0	A
	T2	N0	M0	
II	T3	N0	M0	B
	T4	N0	M0	
III				
A	Any T	N1	M0	C
B	Any T	N2, N3	M0	
IV	Any T	Any N	M1	D

*T1 = tumor invades submucosa; T2 = tumor invades muscularis propria; T3 = tumor invades through the muscularis propria into the subserosa or into nonperitoneal pericolic or perirectal tissues; T4 = tumor perforates the visceral peritoneum or directly invades other organs or structures; Tis = carcinoma in situ.

†N0 = no regional lymph node metastasis; N1 = metastases in 1 to 3 pericolic or perirectal lymph nodes; N2 = metastases in ≥4 pericolic or perirectal lymph nodes; N3 = metastases in any lymph node along the course of a named vascular trunk.

‡M0 = no distant metastasis; M1 = distant metastasis.

Source: Modified with permission of the American College of Surgeons from Beahrs O et al: *Manual of Staging of Cancer,* 3rd ed., Philadelphia, 1988, p 75.

DNA repair genes may be early events, leaving the cell susceptible to various environmental mutagens. Subsequently, activation of oncogenes, such as *K-ras,* and deletions in tumor-suppressor genes, such as p 53 or DCC (deleted in colon cancer gene on chromosome 18), leads to further loss of proliferation control and cancerous growth.

Colorectal cancer evolves transmurally, penetrating through the bowel wall into adjacent structures and lymphatics toward distant sites. Liver (via the portal system) is the most common site of distant metastasis. Lungs can also become involved by further spread from the liver. Typically, rectal cancers are more locally invading and spread hematologically to liver, lung, and occasionally to lumbar and thoracic vertebrae. This stepwise invasion of colorectal cancers is reflected in the Dukes staging system. This system underwent a number of modifications and has been widely used in its latest form. Stage A indicates involvement limited to mucosa; B1 lesions penetrate but not through the muscularis propria; B2 tumors invade the bowel wall without lymph node involvement. Category C tumors are characterized by lymph node involvement and are further divided into C1 and C2—with and without bowel wall penetration, respectively. Stage D reflects distant metastasis.

A number of prognostic factors for colorectal cancer development have been identified based on tumor histology, location, clinical presentation, and molecular genetics. The extent of transmural spread and lymph node involvement are the two most critical prognosticators. Five-year survival rates clearly illustrate this relationship, with 98 percent 5-year survival for stage A but only 4 percent for stage D tumors. The degree of bowel wall penetration correlates with the extent of lymph node invasion and with local tumor recurrence after surgical resection. Lymph node involvement is an independent predictor of outcome, with significantly

better prognosis if fewer than four lymph nodes are affected. Distant metastases confer grave prognosis, with the extent of liver involvement being a major determinant of survival in these patients. In contrast with most malignancies, tumor size alone does not correlate well with future survival rates in colorectal cancer. This is in part the reason for a less-common use of the TNM system in staging of colorectal cancer (Table 57-7). Indeed, ulcerating and infiltrating lesions confer a worse prognosis than polypoid, fungated colorectal tumors. There is a correlation between histologic grade and future outcome, with better prognosis for well-differentiated tumors. Lymphocytic infiltration around the tumor appears to pertain some survival benefit, in particular, in HNPCC-related cancers. Location of the tumor is an important predictor, with rectal cancer carrying the worst prognosis at each stage as compared to colon cancer. A number of clinical presentations are associated with decreased survival, in particular, bowel obstruction and perforation. The duration of symptoms per se does not appear to correlate with future outcome.

In recent years, several genetic prognostic markers have been identified. For example, *K-ras*–containing tumors have worse survival and a poorer response to adjuvant chemotherapy. Tumors with p 53 mutations are less responsive to chemo- and radiation therapy. On the other hand, certain mutations in DNA repair genes appear to confer an improved outcome. The exact role of the various molecular factors remains to be elucidated.

Diagnosis

Colorectal cancer is largely a preventable disease. The slow onset of colorectal cancer gives a chance for early detection and treatment of precancerous lesions. Early diagnosis is particularly important in the elderly population because many older patients are not surgical candidates but could be easily treated at the initial disease stages. A number of diagnostic modalities are currently available. However, the exact surveillance strategy remains an area of active debate. Current screening tests most widely used include fecal occult blood testing (FOBT), flexible sigmoidoscopy, barium enema, and colonoscopy.

FOBT is a qualitative color assay with the goal of identifying small amounts of blood in the stools (up to 2 cc of blood is necessary to make the test positive). Sensitivity ranges from 26 to 92 percent, and specificity is 90 to 99 percent. Multiple stool sampling increases sensitivity. Several factors can potentially interfere with FOBT. Benign sources of bleeding (hemorrhoids, rectal fissures) or foods containing nonhuman sources of hemoglobin can lead to false-positive results. Vitamin C and other antioxidants were found to interact with reagents, resulting in a false-negative test. Even a delay in testing can produce a false-negative result. Moreover, adenomatous polyps do not commonly bleed. Two recent randomized controlled trials demonstrated at least a 33 percent reduction in colorectal cancer mortality with annual FOBT. Annual or biennial FOBT was found to decrease the incidence of colorectal cancer after 18 years of follow up.

FOBT is commonly used in conjunction with flexible sigmoidoscopy. A flexible 60-cm sigmoidoscope allows for examination of distal colon up to splenic flexure. Biopsies can be done and small polyps can be removed. Flexible sigmoidoscopy does not require anesthesia and can be done in office setting by a trained primary care physician. Several well-designed case-control studies show a 70 percent decrease in colorectal cancer mortality in the part of the colon examined by flexible sigmoidoscopy. However, a recent study demonstrated that 24 percent of advanced lesions were missed in asymptomatic patients screened with FOBT and flexible sigmoidoscopy.

Double-contrast barium enema is another commonly used surveillance technique. It is relatively safe and the entire colon can be examined. Sensitivity is 80 to 95 percent, with specificity reported around 90 percent. Mucosal irregularities or retained stools can produce false-positive results. Barium enema misses up to 50 percent of polyps larger than 1 cm and approximately 40 percent of all polyps. Data on efficacy of double-contrast barium enema for colorectal cancer prevention is lacking. In theory, combining barium enema and sigmoidoscopy would allow identification of more lesions, but the extent of this additional clinical benefit is unclear.

Colonoscopy is becoming a screening procedure of choice as the incidence of right-sided lesions is increasing and now comprises more than 40 percent of newly diagnosed cases of colorectal cancer (Fig. 57-4). Moreover, the majority of patients with proximal tumors have only benign or no distal lesions, and therefore, no further workup would have been initiated after initial screening with flexible sigmoidoscopy. In several case-control and cohort studies, colonoscopic polypectomy reduced mortality and the incidence of colorectal cancer. Colonoscopy is an extremely safe procedure. In a number of large recent studies, the rate of colonic perforations caused by colonoscopy

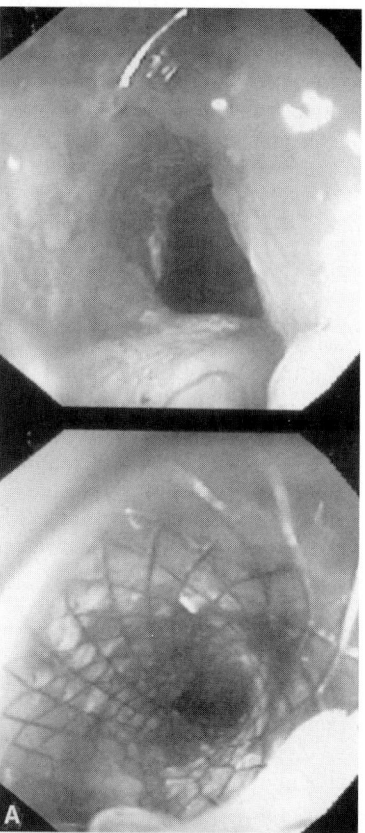

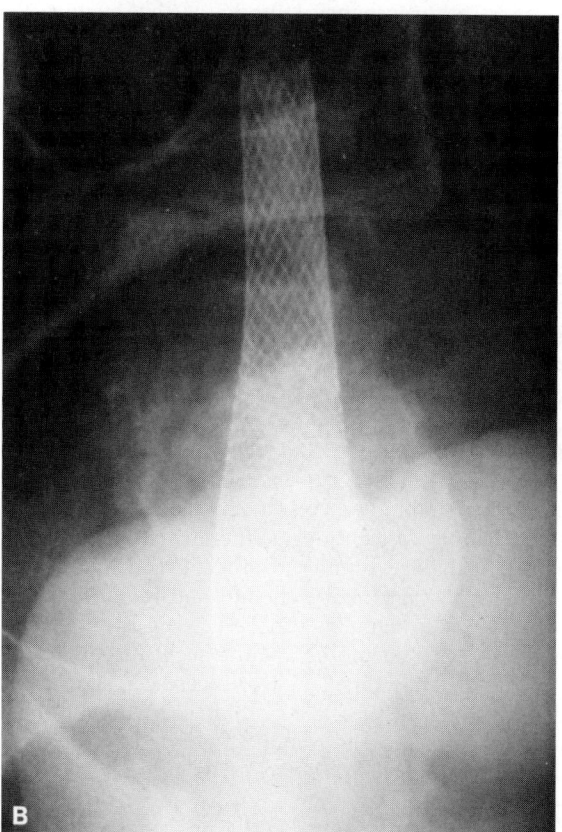

Figure 57-4 *A.* Colonoscopy of a 79-year-old patient with rectal bleeding demonstrating a sigmoid mass and subsequent deployment of a covered Wallstent. *B.* Plain abdominal film demonstrating the position of the Wallstent.

was reported to be less than 0.1 percent. No additional procedure-related complications have been reported in a study on an extremely elderly patient cohort (median age 87 years). Colonoscopy is also a major diagnostic modality, allowing tissue diagnosis in most cases. Double-contrast barium enema is usually done in the 5 to 10 percent of patients for whom colonoscopy is technically not feasible. National guidelines do not provide an upper age limit for colorectal cancer screening for average-risk patients, but some authorities recommend screening limited to persons younger than age 85 years.

Several newer techniques for colorectal cancer diagnosis and screening are currently under development. A more sensitive and specific FOBT designed to detect only lower gastrointestinal bleeds may soon become available. Virtual colonoscopy uses spiral CT to visualize entire colonic mucosa. Certain aspects of this technique remain to be worked out, however, because many patients find it to be even more uncomfortable than the conventional colonoscopy.

Treatment

Treatment of colorectal cancer is usually multimodal. However, surgery remains the mainstay treatment. Surgery is always aimed towards wide resection with 1- to 2-cm negative proximal, distal, and radial margins, and extensive lymphadenectomy including all draining lymph nodes of the excised segment of the bowel. There is no contraindication for en bloc resection even for T4 tumors, as stage by stage, these tumors have equal postsurgical survival and complication rates. The definitive staging is done at the time of surgery as well. There is only a small percentage of liver metastasis that are detected by CT but are missed during surgical exploration. Surgery can also be applied to the treatment of distant metastases. A limited number of liver and lung metastases can be resected with curative intent. Surgery plays an important role in palliative treatment of colorectal cancer. Diverting colostomies or side-to-side anastomosis are typically done to relieve malignant obstruction, and occasionally for bleeding control. Another novel approach is the use of laparoscopy in bowel surgery. Despite its obvious advantages, a number of complications (such as inadvertent bowel injury, resection of wrong bowel segment, and pneumoperitoneum) preclude its wide application.

Colorectal cancer recurrence after potentially curative surgery is thought to be a result of preexisting micrometastases. Postoperative (adjuvant) therapy is directed against this occult disease, aiming to prevent recurrence and increase survival. In theory, chemo- and radiation therapy or combination regimens can be used. 5-FU is the most commonly used chemotherapeutic agent in both cancers. In the last several years, leucovorin has been shown to potentiate the effects of 5-FU. Combined treatment of 5-FU and leucovorin for 6 to 8 months after surgery improves survival in patients with Dukes stage C colon cancer. The use of adjuvant chemotherapy in patients without lymph node involvement (stage B) remains controversial and is not currently considered a standard of care for colon cancer. It is also unclear whether supplementing adjuvant chemotherapy with radiation provides any additional

survival benefit in colon cancer treatment. On the other hand, radiation combined with 5-FU–based regimens reduces mortality in rectal cancer stages B and C. Recently, there have been some promising reports on the use of immunomodulatory therapy in colorectal cancer postoperative treatment. Antibodies to colon carcinoma-associated antigen and autologous tumor cell–BCG vaccine have shown some improvement in survival in the high-recurrence-risk patients.

Diagnosis of advanced colorectal cancer not amenable to surgical resection carries a grave prognosis: such patients have an 8- to 15-month median survival. Systemic chemotherapy is often the only option available to these patients. Average response rates to currently available systemic agents are 20 to 25 percent. Combined regimen of 5-FU, leucovorin, and the new topoisomerase inhibitor irinotecan is currently recommended for metastatic colorectal cancer. Compared to 5-FU/lecovorin alone, the triple regimen has been shown to increase the overall median survival and progression-free survival. Initially, the triple regimen was found to be relatively safe, but a number of later studies demonstrated increased toxicity. The best timing for systemic chemotherapy (early versus late) remains under investigation as well.

In recent years, several new approaches have been developed for local treatment of advanced colorectal cancer (mainly liver metastases). As mentioned above, isolated liver lesions can be resected. Patients who are not surgical candidates can undergo local tumor ablation through cryotherapy, radiofrequency ablation, or microwave coagulation. Finally, if the surgical and ablative approaches fail, local chemotherapy can be attempted. It is usually done via an intraarterial (hepatic artery) catheter with a 5-FU analog. In early studies, initial response rates were better than with systemic therapy but no survival benefit was found.

Colorectal cancer treatment is an area of intense research. New therapies aimed toward specific molecular defects are being developed. With more targeted treatment modalities and a wide, efficient surveillance program, one can hope to see a further decline in colorectal cancer incidence and mortality.

CONCLUSION

Gastrointestinal malignancies encompass a wide variety of diseases, which predominantly strike the elderly population. With continuous aging of population in developed countries, gastrointestinal cancers are expected to occupy an even larger portion of medical care. Over the past decade significant progress has been achieved in the diagnosis and treatment of gastrointestinal malignancies with implementation of new diagnostic techniques, such as endoscopic ultrasound, declines in perioperative mortality after surgical tumor resection, and introduction of new chemotherapeutic agents. Furthermore, the elderly population is not precluded anymore from diagnostic or treatment modalities just based on age. However, prognosis for most of the gastrointestinal cancers remains grim with overall 5-year survival ranging between 20 and 30 percent. Future successes in treatment of gastrointestinal malignancies will come with our deeper understanding of disease progression resulting in the development of novel therapies aimed at molecular targets, improved early detection, and better patient selection criteria for particular therapeutic interventions.

REFERENCES

Aguaya A, Patt YZ: Liver cancer. *Clin Liver Dis* 5:479, 2001.

Ahmad NA et al: Long-term survival after pancreatic resection for pancreatic adenocarcinoma. *Am J Gastroenterol* 96:2609, 2001.

Ahnen DJ: Tissue markers of colon cancer risk. *Gastrointest Endosc* 49:S50, 1999.

Barkin JS, Goldstin JA: Diagnostic approach to pancreatic cancer. *Gastroenterol Clin* 28:709, 1999.

Bond JH: Colorectal cancer update. Prevention, screening, treatment, and surveillance for high-risk groups. *Med Clin North Am* 84:1163, 2000.

Clarke GA et al: The indications, utilization, and safety of gastrointestinal endoscopy in an extremely elderly patient cohort. *Endoscopy* 33:580, 2001.

Cooperman AM: Pancreatic cancer. The bigger picture. *Surg Clin North Am* 81:557, 2001.

De Groen PC et al: Medical progress. Biliary tract cancers. *N Engl J Med* 341:1368, 1999.

Eslick GD et al: Association of *Helicobacter pylori* infection with gastric cancer: A meta-analysis. *Am J Gastroenterol* 94:2373, 1999.

Falk GW: Endoscopic surveillance of Barrett's esophagus: Risk stratification and cancer risk. *Gastrointest Endosc* 49:S29, 1999.

Feldman: *Sleisenger & Fordtran's Gastrointestinal and Liver Disease,* 6th ed. Philadelphia, WB Saunders, 1998.

Fuchs CS, Mayer RJ: Gastric carcinoma. *N Engl J Med* 333:32, 1995.

Giardiello FM et al: American Gastroenterological Association practice guidelines. AGA technical review on hereditary colorectal cancer and genetic testing. *Gastroenterology* 121:198, 2001.

Gold EB, Goldin SB: Epidemiology of and risk factors for pancreatic cancer. *Surg Oncol Clin N Am* 7:67, 1998.

Ince N, Wands J: The increasing incidence of hepatocellular carcinoma. *N Engl J Med* 340:798, 1999.

Lavery IC et al: Treatment of colon and rectal cancer. *Surg Clin North Am* 80:535, 2000.

Lieberman SM et al: Innovative treatments for pancreatic cancer. *Surg Clin North Am* 81:715, 2001.

MacDonald JS et al: Chemoradiotherapy after surgery compared with surgery alone for adenocarcinoma of the stomach or gastroesophageal junction stomach or gastroesophageal junction. *N Engl J Med* 345:725, 2001.

MacDonald JS et al: Postoperative combined radiation and chemotherapy improves disease-free survival and overall survival in resected adenocarcinoma of the stomach and GE junction. Results of intergroup study INT-0116. *Proc Am Soc Clin Oncol* 19:1a, 2000.

Pfau PR et al: EUS predictors of long-term survival in esophageal carcinoma. *Gastrointest Endosc* 53:463, 2001.

Stein HJ et al: Multidisciplinary approach to esophageal and gastric cancer. *Surg Clin North Am* 80:659, 2000.

Wanebo H et al: Cancer of the stomach: Patient care study by the American College of Surgeons. *Ann Surg* 218:583, 1993.

Wiersema MJ et al: Role of EUS in the evaluation of pancreatic adenocarcinoma. *Gastrointest Endosc* 52:578, 2000.

Intracranial Neoplasms in Elderly People

DEBORAH T. BLUMENTHAL • JEROME B. POSNER

Intracranial tumors affect all ages, but malignant gliomas increase with advancing age, and both gliomas and primary central nervous system lymphomas (PCNSLs) are increasing in frequency, especially in the elderly population. In general, the same types of intracranial tumors occur throughout adult life, but those in the elderly population are more likely to be malignant. Elderly persons also differ from their younger counterparts in that some of the classic symptoms and signs of brain tumor (i.e., headache and papilledema) occur less frequently; instead, elderly patients often present with cognitive dysfunction suggesting dementia, or personality changes suggesting depression rather than tumor. Even if a correct diagnosis is made, the treatment may be more complicated in the elderly than in their younger counterparts. Patients may suffer from systemic disease that may make surgery dangerous. In addition, the elderly brain tolerates radiation and chemotherapy less well than does the younger brain. Even if treatment of the tumor is successful, the patient may suffer long-term side effects of the treatment, which may be as disabling as the tumor itself.

This chapter discusses the classification and epidemiology of intracranial tumors, diagnostic considerations, and treatment in the elderly patient. More extensive reviews of the topic can be found elsewhere (see the list of references at the end of the chapter).

CLASSIFICATION AND EPIDEMIOLOGY

Table 58-1 classifies the major intracranial tumors encountered in the elderly population (older than age 65 years) and gives approximate percentages of each. Both primary and metastatic intracranial neoplasms increase in incidence throughout adulthood until approximately age 60 years. An apparent leveling off at age 60 years and a decline in incidence after age 75 years, previously believed to occur, are artifacts of ascertainment. An epidemiologic study from Rochester, Minnesota, demonstrated a decline in incidence of brain tumors in the elderly population, but only

symptomatic intracranial neoplasms were considered. When autopsy data were included, there was an increase in incidence of intracranial tumors throughout the life span. Some of the tumors undiagnosed in the elderly population before death were asymptomatic meningiomas, but others were gliomas in which an incorrect diagnosis of cerebral vascular disease or dementia was made. Such errors are unlikely when magnetic resonance imaging (MRI) scans are performed. "Inapparent" brain tumors are found in approximately 1 percent of elderly patients at autopsy.

A recent report examining brain tumor incidence data from 1983 to 1990 indicates a 5 percent annual rise in the incidence of malignant astrocytomas in those older than age 65 years. The incidence of PCNSL is also increasing independent of age and gender, but PCNSL in the non-acquired immunodeficiency syndrome (AIDS) population is more common in the elderly population. Meningiomas, and probably pituitary adenomas, also increase in incidence with increasing age. With increasing age, low-grade astrocytomas become less common, and more malignant gliomas, particularly glioblastoma multiforme, become more common. Anaplastic astrocytomas comprise 46 percent of malignant gliomas encountered in patients younger than age 40 years, 14 percent in patients ages 40 to 60 years, and only 7 percent of those older than age 60 years. Malignant gliomas have a poorer prognosis in the elderly person than in the young person. The reasons for poorer prognosis may include inherent genetic characteristics, cellular resistance of the tumors associated with increased age, comorbid medical disease, and increased vulnerability to toxic effects of radiation or chemotherapy. Median survivals in the elderly population are shorter even when controlled for the histologic type of glioma. Because patients with malignant glioma die as a result of their tumor, mortality rates correlate with incidence rates for these patients. Riggs suggests that age-specific malignant brain tumor mortality rates are linearly dependent on age group population size. As more older patients live longer, surviving other illnesses that might have caused their death in a less-developed medical setting, more are seen with

Table 58-1　Intracranial Tumors in Elderly People

Primary	39%
Gliomas	49%
Glioblastoma	50%
Other gliomas	50%
Meningioma	34%
Neurinoma	10%
Adenoma	6%
Lymphoma	1–3% (increasing and probably underestimated)
Metastatic	61%
Lung	45%
Breast	15%
Gastrointestinal	13%
Genitourinary	11%
Unspecified and others	16%

Percentages are approximate.

malignant brain tumors, as a consequence of this differential survival phenomenon.

In the elderly population, metastatic brain tumors are more common than primary tumors. Clinical evidence suggests that two thirds to three quarters of metastatic brain tumors are symptomatic during life. Perhaps 10 percent of patients with brain metastases are not known to have cancer and represent a major diagnostic problem.

DIAGNOSIS

Clinical Presentation

Table 58-2 lists some of the symptoms of brain tumors and compares symptomatology in patients older than 60 years of age with those who are younger. The differences in symptomatology between older and younger people probably result from loss of normal brain substance that occurs with aging. This allows tumors to grow larger in the elderly person without raising intracranial pressure. As a result, headache is less common and papilledema is rare. The absence of papilledema probably results not only from lower intracranial pressure but also from fibrosis of the optic nerve sheath with aging, so that intracranial pressure, even when elevated, is less likely to be transmitted to the optic nerve head. Mental changes, including personality change (often mimicking depression), disturbance of memory, and confusion, are more common in the elderly patient than in the young patient. Seizures are less common. Focal findings such as hemiparesis and visual field defects occur with similar frequency in the young and the elderly populations.

Symptoms of brain tumor usually present and progress insidiously. However, in some patients, either an apoplectic onset or paroxysmal symptoms may dominate the clinical picture. As many as 10 percent of patients with malignant glioma may have a sudden or paroxysmal onset of their symptoms. An apoplectic onset may be caused by hemorrhage or vascular obstruction, but in most instances the cause is not known. Paroxysmal symptoms result from seizures originating from irritation of the cerebral cortex surrounding the tumor. Unlike typical epileptic focal or generalized seizures in which positive symptoms (e.g., tonic and clonic movement of extremities) are common, paroxysmal symptoms in patients with brain tumors are often negative (e.g., aphasia, paralysis, episodic confusion) and may have a prolonged postictal phase that lasts hours rather than the usual few minutes.

Thus, the diagnosis of brain tumors in the elderly person may be difficult. When the symptoms begin insidiously as confusion or personality change but without headache or papilledema, the physician may suspect psychiatric disease (e.g., depression) or a degenerative disorder (e.g., Alzheimer's disease). If a careful neurologic examination yields focal motor or sensory changes, one should suspect a brain tumor, but, particularly if the tumor is in the frontal lobe, there may be no such changes. When the symptoms appear abruptly, the physician is more likely to suspect cerebrovascular disease, which is usually sudden in onset and much more common in the elderly population than is brain tumor. Herpes simplex is another diagnosis sometimes made in error. Progression of neurologic symptoms after an apoplectic onset suggests tumor and warrants careful subsequent imaging studies. Paroxysmal neurologic symptoms may mimic transient ischemic attacks that suggest vascular disease. However, paroxysmal symptoms in brain tumors tend to last longer and present with more complex symptomatology (i.e., apraxias and confusion in addition to the usual hemiparesis and aphasia of transient ischemic attacks). Despite these clinical clues, the diagnosis of a brain tumor can often be differentiated from the more common dementing illnesses or vascular

Table 58-2　Some Significant Differences in Symptoms of Intracranial Tumor by Age

	548 Patients Older Than Age 60 Years (%)	2005 Patients Younger Than Age 60 Years (%)
Headaches	48.9	63.1
Disturbances of gait	28.3	21.5
Personality changes	25.2	18.4
Disturbances of memory	19.3	15.1
Confusion	15.5	7.4
Speech disorders	21.0	12.2
Epileptic attacks	17.9	25.0

diseases of the elderly patient only if the physician suspects the presence of a tumor and does appropriate diagnostic tests.

Diagnostic Evaluation

Brain Imaging

The diagnosis of intracranial tumors in all age groups was revolutionized in the 1970s by computed tomography (CT), and more recently by MRI. If the physician suspects an intracranial neoplasm, MRI is the best diagnostic test. Magnetic resonance imaging is more sensitive than CT in detecting parenchymal neoplasms, in examining the posterior fossa and brainstem structures, and particularly in identifying a glioma early in its evolution, when the CT scan is normal. Even small meningiomas that, because of their isodensity with brain, may be difficult to distinguish from normal brain on MRI without contrast become apparent on MRI by intense enhancement after injection of the paramagnetic substance gadolinium. Gadolinium does not cause the allergic reactions that may be seen with iodinated CT contrast, and it does not cause the renal toxicity that contrast dye can. Rarely, when MRI is not available or when the patient is claustrophobic or too restless to tolerate longer scan time, CT performed with and without IV contrast may be preferable.

Although extremely sensitive for detection of brain lesions, neither CT nor MRI specifically proves that an abnormality is a neoplasm, or, if it is a neoplasm, its type. Magnetic resonance spectroscopy (MRS) may help with differentiation of noninvasive tumors versus infectious or demyelinating lesions or even in identifying a tumor by type or grade, although more study needs to be done on this subject before MRS becomes a reliable clinical tool. Positron emission tomography (PET) can be useful in differentiating low-grade from high-grade lesions, as well as active neoplasm from radiation necrosis, by differences in glucose metabolic rates. However, active demyelination or acute radiation necrosis can be misinterpreted for tumor, as all may show increased metabolism. In the appropriate clinical context, lesions identified by CT or MRI that occupy space and are surrounded by edema are likely to be tumors rather than infarcts, abscesses, or inflammatory lesions. Certain other clues help identify the nature of the tumor: multiple lesions within the substance of the brain, particularly if they possess contrast enhancing rings on scan or are each surrounded by extensive edema, suggest metastatic disease. Even single lesions in the cerebellum in the elderly patient suggest metastatic disease because primary tumors of the cerebellum are uncommon in the elderly population. A single lesion with a contrast-enhancing ring of irregular size and shape suggests a malignant glioma. A glioma can also appear as an area of white matter hyperintensity on MRI that does not contrast enhance and is sometimes confused with a cerebral infarct. Such an appearance suggests a low-grade glioma, but high-grade tumors occasionally fail to contrast enhance, and low-grade tumors can contrast enhance. Nonenhancing cerebral masses in older patients are more likely to be anaplastic tumors than low-grade tumors.

A densely and uniformly contrast-enhancing lesion deep in the periventricular white matter suggests primary lymphoma. Primary lymphomas are often multicentric (approximately 30 percent), whereas primary gliomas are usually but not always monocentric (95 percent). Lesions on the surface of the brain (attached to the dura) that uniformly contrast enhance suggest meningioma, although dural-based metastases from carcinomas of the breast, prostate, and other tumors may appear similar.

Metastatic brain tumors are more common than primary brain tumors in the elderly population. Metastasis are multiple in 50 percent of patients, so an elderly patient with more than one brain lesion should be considered to harbor a metastasis until proved otherwise. Metastases from primary systemic tumors above the thorax often metastasize to the supratentorial brain, whereas some primary cancers located below the thorax (such as colonic, prostatic, or gynecologic cancer) more often metastasize to the posterior fossa. However, even an extensive metastatic workup may not identify the primary tumor. If examination of the chest (by CT) or the kidneys (CT or renal sonogram) is negative and if the patient's general physical examination (including rectal examination, stool guaiac, and breast examination) is negative, it is unlikely that a more extensive search will identify a primary lesion. Serum markers such as PSA (prostate-specific antigen), CA125 (ovary), and BRA (breast cancer antigen) sometimes help. If a primary tumor cannot be located, one should consider proceeding to resection or biopsy of the intracranial lesion.

Other diagnostic tests may also yield information of value. Examination of the cerebrospinal fluid may reveal malignant cells, particularly in primary lymphomas of the nervous system or metastatic tumors that have invaded the leptomeninges. Lumbar puncture should not be performed until MRI or CT rules out a large space-occupying lesion that might cause herniation after an inappropriate lumbar puncture.

Arteriography or magnetic resonance arteriography (MRA) can help differentiate vascular disease from tumor. Magnetic resonance arteriography is less invasive, safer, and a more practical modality. If the external carotid artery is injected, the arteriogram (or MRA) will determine whether a tumor is fed by the external carotid circulation, a characteristic feature of meningiomas and dural-based metastases. In both meningiomas and highly malignant gliomas, the vasculature is often abnormal (tumor blush). Vascular embolization can help with the preoperative management of highly vascular tumors, such as some meningiomas.

Biopsy

If CT or MRI reveals a space-occupying lesion suspected of being a tumor, surgical resection or biopsy is the next step. A patient with known cancer and typical metastatic lesion(s) of the brain on scan need not be biopsied, but one should consider that other brain lesions (e.g., glioma, meningioma) can coexist with systemic cancer. Generally speaking, tumors that can be surgically resected, should be; a craniotomy with removal of the tumor both establishes the diagnosis and treats the disease. This approach holds true for most meningiomas, pituitary adenomas, neurinomas, and gliomas. An exception is a malignant lymphoma, which does not benefit by surgical removal. Often, the patient's neurologic symptoms are worsened by attempted removal. It is important to consider the diagnosis of CNS lymphoma preoperatively when the radiographic findings are suggestive, to minimize surgical intervention. In such cases, a frozen preliminary histologic specimen should be examined, before proceeding with a more extensive resection. The same is true of patients with multiple metastatic tumors or surgically inaccessible gliomas. In those instances, because the lesion may not be a tumor and both the treatment of tumor and its prognosis depend on histologic type, an attempt should be made to establish a histologic diagnosis. This can usually be done by stereotactic needle biopsy under CT or MRI guidance. The procedure can be done either under local or general anesthesia, and carries a morbidity of approximately 3 percent. Worsening of neurologic symptoms can result either from hemorrhage into the tumor site or from swelling engendered by the procedure. The morbidity is higher when a malignant tumor is biopsied. A definitive diagnosis can be made in most instances, distinguishing primary from metastatic tumors and both of those from infectious or inflammatory processes that may mimic tumors.

TREATMENT

General Considerations

For the most part, treatment of intracranial tumors is dictated by the tumor type and not the age of the patient. Old age should not prevent surgery. Surgical morbidity and mortality are about the same in the elderly or the young populations. However, at any age, the overall health of the patient is a consideration in determining specific treatment. This is especially true in the elderly population, as coincident coronary artery disease, hypertension, diabetes, chronic obstructive pulmonary disease, venous insufficiency, and other common general medical problems may limit the therapeutic options. With these caveats, the usual brain tumor treatments of adrenal corticosteroids (steroids), surgical extirpation, radiation therapy, chemotherapy, and immunotherapy are available to both young and elderly patients. As a general rule, the physiologic versus chronologic age should be considered. The National Comprehensive Cancer Network senior adult care task force has addressed some of the issues relating to guidelines of cancer care in older patients. The concept of *frailty* in the elderly patient, incorporates not only age, but also criteria of *dependency* for activities of daily living, presence of comorbid conditions, and presence of geriatric syndromes (including dementia, osteoporosis, failure to thrive, and others). The elderly patient meeting such a definition would be a candidate for palliative treatment, rather than more aggressive therapy.

Adrenal Corticosteroids (Steroids)

Steroids have been used in the treatment of brain tumors for more than 30 years. Their beneficial effects result from decreasing the edema that invariably surrounds malignant glial tumors, metastatic brain tumors, and even some meningiomas. The salutary effect on edema appears to be a result of "closing" the blood–brain barrier that has broken down both within and immediately surrounding the tumor. Symptomatic improvement begins in most patients usually within a few hours. The symptoms most likely to respond are those that reflect generalized brain dysfunction (headache, confusion, gait difficulty) caused by cerebral edema, increased intracranial pressure, and brain shifts. Focal signs and symptoms (hemiparesis, aphasia) generally respond less favorably, but are improved in many instances. The most widely used steroid preparation, because of its minimal mineralocorticoid activity, is dexamethasone; it also appears less likely to cause mental changes than are other steroids. The standard starting dose of dexamethasone is 12 to 16 mg/d in divided doses, with increasing doses being used if a patient does not respond to the lower dose. Elderly patients respond to steroids as well as do younger ones. Only 5 percent of elderly patients suffer major side effects, which include psychosis, hyperglycemia, and perforated ulcers. However, long-term use of steroids leads to immunosuppression, osteoporosis, and hypertension, and we have observed severe oral candidiasis and herpes zoster as complications of steroid therapy in the elderly patient. Emotional lability and insomnia are common side effects of steroids. Less common, but potentially disturbing, are side effects of protracted hiccups (which *may* be a dose-responsive effect), or an intense burning dysesthesia in the groin after an intravenous bolus. Steroid myopathy, which selectively effects the type II proximal muscle fibers, can significantly impair functional mobility. Patients who are immune-suppressed from steroids are at heightened risk of infection with *Pneumocystis carinii pneumonia*, a potentially fatal condition. For all these reasons, although steroids are effective in ameliorating the symptoms of brain tumor, they should be used at the lowest possible dose and tapered as soon as definitive therapy permits. Occasionally, patients may experience arthralgias and myalgias from the cessation of steroids, "steroid withdrawal syndrome."

Antiepileptic Drugs

Patients with brain tumors who have seizures should be placed on antiepileptic drugs at therapeutic doses. Carbamazepine, phenytoin, valproate, and lamotrigine are first-line drugs for treatment of partial seizures related to underlying focal lesions. Some newer anticonvulsants may prove effective as adjuncts, including Keppra, Zonegran, Topamax, and Gabitril. Antiepileptic drugs do not decrease the risk of seizure in patients who have not had a previous ictal event. We do not begin antiepileptic drugs in a brain tumor patient who has not had a seizure, other than as a protective measure during the perioperative period. Recurrent seizures, or treatment–refractory seizures, often signal a recurrence or progression of active tumor. Such seizures can be difficult to control, unless tumor growth can be controlled.

Most antiepileptic drugs are primarily metabolized in the hepatic system and can interact with other medications, including anticoagulants, dexamethasone, and chemotherapy agents. These interactions can lead to subtherapeutic treatments or, in some cases, toxicity from increased serum levels caused by slowed metabolism. The medications Keppra and Neurontin are primarily excreted renally and thus not associated with the problems listed above. However, if the elderly patient has renal insufficiency, altered clearance of these antiepileptic drugs may occur. Stevens–Johnson syndrome is a rare but serious and potentially fatal idiosyncratic dermatologic side effect of antiepileptic drugs. Patients with a brain tumor who are beginning radiation therapy and who have started an antiepileptic drug within a month of radiation are at increased risk for Stevens–Johnson syndrome, particularly if steroids are being tapered. Rashes involving the mucosal surfaces, or progressively worsening skin exfoliation are warning signs of Stevens–Johnson syndrome. The likely offending agent, if an antiepileptic drug, should be stopped if Stevens–Johnson syndrome is suspected. If the patient's condition warrants continued antiepileptic drug therapy, phenobarbital, gabapentin, or other benzodiazepines may be used as "bridging" therapy, until the rash has subsided and a substitute antiepileptic can be used, so as to avoid "cross-over sensitivity." A dermatology consultation may be required.

Surgery

Surgical extirpation is the treatment of choice for most intracranial neoplasms. The goal is either to remove the tumor completely, thus obviating recurrence (meningiomas, pituitary adenomas, single metastases), or to remove as much of the lesion as possible (debulk) to allow additional therapy (i.e., radiation and chemotherapy) to be more effective. When a surgical procedure is undertaken, the surgeon should attempt to remove as much of the tumor as is safely possible. Improvements in past decades have enabled greater resections without greater risk to patients. Awake resections with intraoperative monitoring allow mapping of eloquent language and motor areas, to make possible aggressive resections without increasing the risk of functional damage to the patient. Stereotactic computer-guided systems allow for detailed resection planning. Intraoperative MRIs are being used at several centers, and may allow for more complete resections. There is no increase in postoperative morbidity in patients who undergo major resections, as compared with those who undergo lesser resections or biopsies. In fact, the incidence of postoperative herniation is higher in those patients who had minor resections. Survival is substantially better in those patients with malignant gliomas who have little or no residual tumor identifiable on imaging after surgery when compared with those patients in whom substantial residual tumor remains. There is a survival advantage of more than 4 months for patients with glioblastoma who have resection of 98 percent or more of their tumor volume. An MRI within 48 hours of surgery is desirable, to establish a postoperative baseline.

Not all elderly patients in whom a brain tumor is identified require surgery. A small meningioma found either incidentally or after a seizure can be followed up or treated with anticonvulsants. The growth rate may be so slow as not to require surgery before the patient lives out his or her natural life span. Small single metastatic lesions in elderly patients with widespread cancer are probably best treated by focal radiosurgery or standard external-beam radiation therapy because it is often possible to control these tumors beyond the time that the systemic disease incapacitates or leads to the patient's demise.

Radiosurgery

Radiosurgery or gamma knife are noninvasive alternatives to surgical extirpation of a metastatic lesion or circumscribed primary intracranial tumors. For acoustic neuroma, control rates of greater than 89 percent were reported for radiosurgery at University of Pittsburgh, as compared with a less-than-5-percent recurrence rate for gross total surgical resection and a 60 percent recurrence rate for subtotal resection. Neurologic side effects are comparable to those seen with surgery. Radiosurgery may be the treatment of choice for single or two to three brain metastases in a patient who is unwilling or medically unable to undergo surgical resection. Brain metastases from less radiosensitive primary tumors, such as melanoma, renal cell carcinoma, or sarcoma, may be particularly conducive to focal radiosurgical treatment. No randomized prospective trials have evaluated the efficacy of stereotactic radiosurgery over surgical excision for treatment of brain metastases, and retrospective studies differ. Most gliomas are poorly circumscribed and invasive and hence difficult to encompass within a 4-cm treatment circumference. (Treatment to areas larger than 4 cm carries too high a risk of side effects from edema and necrosis.) However, larger areas may be amenable to fractionated radiotherapy treatments. Even if gliomas are of treatable size and dimensions, it is presumed that microscopic malignant cells are present outside of the margins visible on imaging. Treatment-related necrosis and edema that is not responsive to medical treatment with steroids may require surgical decompression for management. Radiosurgery has also been used successfully to treat some meningiomas.

Radiation Therapy

Radiation therapy is a primary treatment for multiple metastatic brain tumors and some pituitary adenomas. Radiation therapy is indicated following surgery in patients with malignant gliomas, meningiomas that cannot be totally resected, and in some cases, after resection of a single intracerebral metastasis. Radiation therapy is not without its complications, and there is some evidence that chronic radiation damage to the nervous system is more severe in the older age group than in patients of a younger age who have received similar radiation therapy. Additionally, older patients with glioblastoma may be less likely to respond to radiation than are younger patients. Small daily doses are safer to the normal brain than are larger doses; however, small doses take more time, and in patients with systemic cancer who have a very limited life span, larger fractions may be more appropriate. Most studies show no difference in response to shorter versus conventional course radiation therapy for poorer performance patients. A Phase II study of 70- to 78-year-old patients with malignant glioma compared short-course (higher fraction per dose) with conventional treatment and showed patients with higher performance status to have a median survival of 10 months, comparable to that with conventional radiation therapy. However, another study showed an advantage to conventional radiation therapy for patients older than age 65 years with higher performance status. Older patients with poor performance may be best treated with an accelerated course. Side effects of radiation therapy are classified as immediate (acute), early delayed, and late delayed. (1) Acute complications include headache, fever, lethargy, and an increase in preexisting neurologic signs; these symptoms respond to steroids. (2) Early delayed complications occur after a delay of weeks with exacerbation of preexisting symptoms and lethargy often responding to steroids or resolving spontaneously. (3) Late side effects appear months to a few years after treatment and are characterized by dementia with or without focal signs; they are usually irreversible, and steroids may provide transient symptomatic improvement or none at all. Isolated reports cite response of radiation-delayed injury (in brain or other tissues) to treatments with anticoagulants, vitamin E, and Trental. The risk of central neurotoxicity is increased by the combination of chemotherapy agents (especially methotrexate) with radiation. Like normal pressure hydrocephalus, which presents with a similar clinical picture, some of these patients may have a transient response to ventriculoperitoneal shunting.

When radiation therapy is prescribed for an elderly patient, the physician and the radiation oncologist should work together to identify the smallest total dose to the smallest brain volume, using conformal techniques, that will control the tumor effectively.

Chemotherapy

Chemotherapy may be an important treatment for patients with primary lymphomas of the brain. Until the mid-1980s, primary radiation was the treatment of choice for PCNSL. However, protocols using combinations of chemotherapy agents and deferring or avoiding radiation show an advantage in increasing long-term survival and in avoiding neurotoxicity that is attributed to radiation therapy, particularly in patients older than age 60 years. Despite improvements for PCNSL survival with chemotherapy regimens, age is a significant negative prognostic factor. Median survival for all patients with PCNSL treated with chemotherapy followed by radiation is 41 months, which compares with median survival of only 29 months for patients older than age 50 years.

There is some evidence that metastatic brain tumors, especially those of chemosensitive primary tumors (small-cell lung carcinoma, breast cancer) may respond to chemotherapy independent of the response to radiation therapy. Chemotherapy added to surgery and radiation therapy appears to prolong the survival of some patients with malignant brain tumors. Elderly patients tend to tolerate chemotherapy somewhat less well than do younger patients, and doses may have to be adjusted to decrease toxicity in the elderly patient.

TREATMENT OF SPECIFIC TUMORS

Malignant Gliomas

The current conventional treatment of malignant gliomas, whether in young or elderly patients, is a maximally feasible resection of the tumor followed by radiation to the tumor site and a 2-cm margin of approximately 60 Gy. Adjuvant chemotherapy with bischloroethyl nitrosourea (BCNU), in a dose of 200 mg/m^2 every 8 weeks, does not appear to significantly increase median survival in elderly patients, but it does increase the long-term survival in 20 to 30 percent of individuals. This small percentage of chemotherapy-sensitive patients may correspond to a subset of patients with malignant brain tumors who have low levels of alkyltransferase. Recent studies of alkyltransferase resistance and correlation of the levels of this enzyme as a possible indicator of sensitivity or resistance to alkylating chemotherapy are now being tested in a Phase III clinical trial using O6-benzylguanine with BCNU.

Multiple other chemotherapy agents have been cited for treatment of primary brain tumors. Most of these are taken from the experience of treatment of systemic malignancies, including alkylating agents such as Matulane (procarbazine) and nitrosoureas, topoisomerase inhibitors such as irinotecan and etoposide, and platinum and tubulin-binding (vincristine) agents.

The most significant recent development in chemotherapy agents used to treat malignant gliomas is the approval of temozolomide. Temodar was approved in 1999 for use in recurrent or PCV (procarbazine, CCNU, vincristine)-refractory anaplastic astrocytoma. It is used widely by neuro-oncologists for front-line treatment of malignant gliomas. This oral chemotherapy is a novel imidazotetrazine with chemical similarities to DTIC (dimethyltriazenoimidazolecarboxamide). It converts spontaneously at normal body pH to an active alkylating agent. It is thought to work by methylation of deoxyribonucleic acid (DNA) which alters the tumor cell's ability to repair mismatched proteins. High levels of O6-alkylguanine alkyltransferase can overcome this effect. Combination with agents that can deactivate the repair mechanism may potentiate the effect of the chemotherapy, and should be studied in future trials.

Oral administration of this drug is an advantage to the older patient, who may have difficulty with intravenous access. Side effects are usually tolerable, and include *noncumulative* myelosuppression, nausea, and fatigue. Most older patients are able to continue with their usual daily routines, affected mostly by mild to moderately increased fatigue. Constipation from serotonin receptor (5-HT specific) antagonist adjuvant antiemetic medications is often significant in the older patient, and should be addressed proactively. Pulmonary fibrosis, a dose-related risk of nitrosoureas, has not been reported with temozolomide, which is an advantage for older patients who may have diminished baseline pulmonary diffusion capacity from cumulative exposures or lung disease unrelated to their brain tumor.

Phase II studies suggest a role for concurrent use of Temodar with radiation therapy, and a large Phase III

European Organization for the Research and Treatment of Cancer (EORTC) trial is underway to evaluate this use.

Irinotecan appears to have a level of activity in malignant gliomas, with some sustained responses. Thalidomide and retinoic acids have been used, and may be more useful as adjunctive agents used in combination with other chemotherapy medications.

Future directions for malignant glioma chemotherapy may focus on "targeted therapy," including increased sensitivity to radiation and chemotherapy for oligodendrogliomas, based on molecular genetics of the tumor; VEGF (vascular endothelial growth factor) expression in malignant gliomas; or antibody-delivered treatments that select the tumor cells and minimize adverse effects upon normal brain cells.

Low-Grade Gliomas

Low-grade gliomas are uncommon in the elderly patient. In patients older than 60 years of age, only 5 percent of gliomas are low grade. When the tumors are symptomatic, conventional treatment involves maximally feasible resection. Radiation therapy, approximately 55 Gy to the tumor, may be helpful, but it is not clear that there is an advantage to radiating early in the course versus deferring treatment until the tumor progresses or becomes malignant. Although the role for radiation in low-grade glioma treatment has not been established, a recent Phase III prospective randomized trial of low- (50.4 Gy) versus high- (64.8 Gy) dose radiation for low-grade adult gliomas found higher toxicity and lower survival for the group treated at the higher dose. Survival was significantly better for patients younger than 40 years of age.

Chemotherapy may be useful for oligodendrogliomas. Chromosomal deletions in loci 1p and 19q associated with many oligodendroglial tumors have been correlated with enhanced chemo- and radiation sensitivity, and better prognosis.

Metastatic Tumors

Single metastasis in patients who are either free of systemic disease as a result of treatment, or whose disease appears to be under control, respond better if the brain tumor is extirpated than if they receive radiation therapy alone. Radiation therapy after the tumor is removed appears to increase the time to recurrence, and thus is probably indicated. For multiple metastatic tumors, radiation therapy is the treatment of choice. If the cancer is widespread, radiation should be delivered in large fractions over a short period (e.g., 3 Gy per 10 days). However, if the patient's systemic disease is under control, and it is likely that the patient will live longer than 6 to 12 months, smaller fractions (e.g., 2 Gy per 20 days) will decrease some of the late-delayed effects of radiation therapy. In rare cases (those with a favorable initial response and delayed recurrence), reirradiation may be helpful, but at high risk of enhanced neurotoxicity. In those patients whose tumors are chemosensitive (for example, carcinoma of the breast, small-cell lung cancer), one

might consider the use of chemotherapy either in addition to or independent of radiation therapy.

Lymphoma

Lymphoma is clearly an immunologically influenced neoplasm. The increased incidence of lymphoma in the elderly population suggests that there may be a not-yet-defined immune deficiency that occurs with aging.

Primary central nervous system lymphoma is sensitive to both radiation and chemotherapy. A significant number of tumors disappear when they are treated with corticosteroids only, often leaving the surgeon nothing to biopsy but giving the oncologist valuable diagnostic information. Most tumors treated with radiation therapy show an initial response, but recur by 14 months and are resistant to further treatment. Most current protocols now call for the use of chemotherapy with high-dose methotrexate, intrathecal methotrexate, and cytosine arabinoside, followed by whole-brain radiation therapy of 45 Gy. Doses >3 g/m^2 penetrate the cerebrospinal fluid (CSF). If these doses are tolerated, some authors would treat without intrathecal drug, particularly if the CSF at initial staging is negative. One of the most controversial questions in the treatment of central nervous system leukemia concerns the role of radiation, specifically for older patients. Because of radiation damage to the brain, particularly in those older than age 60 years, some investigators suggest that radiation be withheld unless chemotherapy fails. Radiation is administered if residual tumor remains after chemotherapy or if the tumor recurs. Retreatment with a methotrexate-based regimen or with other alkylators is also an option. The role of monoclonal antibody treatment for central nervous system leukemia is unclear.

Meningiomas

Surgical resection is the treatment of choice for meningiomas. Radiosurgery may be an option for tumors difficult to access or in a patient who is a high medical risk for surgery. Preoperative embolization can be used in some cases to decrease the vascularity of the tumor and to make surgery easier. When surgical resection is complete, no further therapy is necessary (unless the tumor is found to be atypical or malignant in histology, a rare occurrence). If the surgical resection is incomplete, or if the tumor recurs despite an apparent complete resection, radiation therapy is indicated at the time of recurrence. The radiation should be delivered in doses of about 50 to 60 Gy to a focal port encompassing the tumor. Hydroxyurea is being evaluated as adjuvant chemotherapy for this neoplasm.

Neurinomas

The most common neurinoma in both the young and the elderly patient is the acoustic nerve neurinoma. The treatment is surgical resection or radiosurgery. With modern techniques of surgery and particularly with early detection of acoustic neurinomas, removal may allow preservation of both facial muscle function and hearing. Only large tumors are associated with morbidity involving the central nervous system.

Pituitary Adenomas

Symptomatic adenoma of the pituitary can be treated with a high cure rate and low morbidity by transsphenoidal resection of the tumor. If the tumor cannot be completely resected, or is invasive, postoperative radiation therapy is indicated. Medical therapy with bromocriptine or one of the newer dopamine agents is the treatment of choice in patients with prolactin-secreting tumors. Interference with reproductivity, which can be a complicating factor for the younger patient, is not an issue with the elderly patient. Surgical or radiation therapy may be considered for hormone suppression-refractory adenomas. However, hormonal therapy can cause the tumor to become more fibrotic and more difficult to remove surgically if this becomes necessary at some point. Asymptomatic pituitary tumors can be observed.

CONCLUSION

Elderly patients with brain tumors may present diagnostic and therapeutic challenges to the clinician. Although their prognosis may be worse than that of their younger counterparts, they can still benefit from aggressive treatment and should not be disregarded because of nihilism based on their age alone.

REFERENCES

Abrey LE et al: Long-term survival in primary central nervous system lymphoma. *J Clin Oncol* 16:859, 1998.

Bauman GS et al: A prospective study of short-course radiotherapy in poor prognosis glioblastoma multiforme. *Int J Radiat Oncol Biol Phys* 29:835, 1994.

Amatruda TT et al: Certain endocrine and metabolic facets of the steroids withdrawal syndrome. *J Clin Endocr* 25:1207, 1965.

Barker FG 2nd et al: Age and the risk of anaplasia in magnetic resonance—nonenhancing supratentorial cerebral tumors. *Cancer* 80:936, 1997.

Barker FG 2nd et al: Age and radiation response in glioblastoma multiforme. *Neurosurgery* 49:1288, 2001.

Bernstein M, Parrent AG: Complications of CT-guided stereotactic biopsy of intra-axial brain lesions. *J Neurosurg* 81:165, 1994.

Bindal AK et al: Surgery versus radiosurgery in the treatment of brain metastasis. *J Neurosurg* 84:748, 1996.

Black PM: Hormones, radiosurgery and virtual reality: New aspects of meningioma management. *Can J Neurol Sci* 24:302, 1997.

Black PM, Loeffler JS: *Cancer of the Nervous System.* Cambridge, MA, Blackwell Science, 1997.

Bondy M, Ligon BL: Epidemiology and etiology of intracranial meningiomas: A review. *J Neurooncol* 29:197, 1996.

Braunstein JB, Vick NA: Meningiomas: The decision not to operate. *Neurology* 48:1459, 1997.

Breneman JC et al: Stereotactic radiosurgery for the treatment of brain metastases—results of a single institution series. *Cancer* 79:551, 1997.

Brown PD et al: Stereotactic radiosurgery for patients with "radioresistant" brain metastases. *Neurosurgery* 51:656, 2002.

Conti PS: Introduction to imaging brain tumor metabolism with positron emission tomography (PET). *Cancer Invest* 13:244, 1995.

Deangelis LM: Primary central nervous system lymphomas. *Curr Treat Options Oncol* 2:309, 2001.

Delanian S, Lefaix JL: Complete healing of severe osteoradionecrosis with treatment combining pentoxifylline, tocopherol and clodronate. *Br J Radiol* 75:467, 2002.

Denny BJ et al: NMR and molecular modeling investigation of the mechanism of activation of the antitumor drug temozolomide and its interaction with DNA. *Biochemistry* 33:9045, 1994.

Fleury A et al: Descriptive epidemiology of cerebral gliomas in France. *Cancer* 79:1195, 1997.

Fortin D et al: Oligodendroglioma: An appraisal of recent data pertaining to diagnosis and treatment. *Neurosurgery* 45:1279, 1999.

Freilich RJ et al: Chemotherapy without radiation therapy as initial treatment for primary CNS lymphoma in older patients. *Neurology* 46:435, 1996.

Friedman HS et al: Irinotecan therapy in adults with recurrent or progressive malignant glioma. *J Clin Oncol* 17:1516, 1999.

Furuse K et al: A pilot study of concurrent whole-brain radiotherapy and chemotherapy combined with cisplatin, vindesine and mitomycin in non–small-cell lung cancer with brain metastasis. *Br J Cancer* 75:614, 1997.

Glantz MJ et al: Treatment of radiation-induced nervous system injury with heparin and warfarin. *Neurology* 44:2020, 1994.

Graham K, Caird FI: High-dose steroid therapy of intracranial tumour in the elderly. *Age Ageing* 7:146, 1978.

Halperin EC: Malignant gliomas in older adults with poor prognostic signs. *Oncology* 9:229, 1995.

Hoegler DB, Davey P: A prospective study of short course radiotherapy in elderly patients with malignant glioma. *J Neurooncol* 33:201, 1997.

Kim M, Bernstein M: Current treatment of cerebral metastasis. *Curr Opin Neurol* 9:414, 1996.

Lacroix M, Sawaya R et al: A multivariate analysis of 416 patients with glioblastoma multiforme: prognosis, extent of resection, and survival. *J Neurosurg* 95:190, 2001.

Posner JB: *Neurologic Complications of Cancer.* Philadelphia, F.A. Davis, 1994 p 1.

Prados MD, Russo C: Chemotherapy of brain tumors. *Semin Surg Oncol* 14:88, 1998.

Preul MC et al: Accurate noninvasive diagnosis of human brain tumors by using magnetic resonance spectroscopy. *Nat Med* 2:323, 1996.

Radhakrishnan K et al: The trends in incidence of primary brain tumors in the population of Rochester, Minnesota. *Ann Neurol* 37:67, 1997.

Riggs JE: Rising primary malignant brain tumor mortality in the elderly. A manifestation of differential survival. *Arch Neurol* 52:571, 1995.

Schiff D: Pneumocystis pneumonia in brain tumor patients: Risk factors and clinical features. *J Neurooncol* 27:235, 1996.

Shaw E et al: Prospective randomized trial of low-versus high-dose radiation therapy in adults with supratentorial low-grade glioma: Initial report of a North Central Cancer Treatment Group/Radiation Therapy Oncology Group/Eastern Cooperative Oncology Group study. *J Clin Oncol* 20:2267, 2002.

Stupp R et al: Promising survival for patients with newly diagnosed glioblastoma multiforme treated with concomitant radiation plus temozolomide followed by adjuvant temozolomide. *J Clin Oncol* 20:1375, 2002.

van Roijen L et al: Costs and effects of microsurgery versus radiosurgery in treating acoustic neuroma. *Acta Neurochir (Wien)* 139:942, 1997.

Vecht CJ (ed): *Neuro-Oncology: Part III. Neurological Disorders in Systemic Cancer.* Amsterdam, Elsevier, 1997.

Werner MH et al: The increasing incidence of malignant gliomas and primary central nervous system lymphoma in the elderly. *Cancer* 76:1634, 1995.

Skin Cancer

ARTHUR K. BALIN

More skin cancers occur in the United States than all other cancers combined. Most of these occur in the elderly population. One person dies every hour from malignant melanoma and every 4 hours from nonmelanoma skin cancer in the United States. Accurate data on the number of skin cancers is difficult to obtain because most cancers are treated on an outpatient basis and there is a great variation with latitude so that population studies in a specific geographic area are not applicable to the entire country. It is likely that most of the data on the incidence and prevalence of skin cancer represent an underestimate of the true number. Nevertheless, it is estimated that in 2003 there will be approximately 1.2 million basal cell carcinomas, 400,000 squamous cell carcinomas, 55,000 invasive malignant melanomas, and 40,000 malignant melanomas in situ diagnosed in the United States. There is a worldwide increase in the number of skin cancer cases with the incidence rising by 3 to 20 percent per year.

Several neoplastic conditions that are common in the elderly population are associated with environmental damage to the skin. These conditions include actinic keratoses, Bowen's disease, squamous cell carcinoma, and basal cell carcinoma. The changes that most persons equate with aging of the skin are a result of chronic solar damage. Prolonged exposure to ultraviolet irradiation leads to cutaneous atrophy, alterations in pigmentation, wrinkling, dryness, telangiectasia, and solar elastosis. Ultraviolet B (UVB), at wavelengths between 290 and 310 nm, describes the spectral range that produces sunburn, and it is also thought to be the irradiation mainly responsible for actinic damage to the skin. Some of the strongest evidence that implicates ultraviolet light as being important in the etiology of epidermal tumors comes from epidemiologic data correlating the incidence of tumors with degree of pigmentary protection. The individual principally at risk is light-skinned, easily sunburned, and does not tan. Other strong epidemiologic data correlate an increased incidence of skin tumors with decreasing latitude and increasing sun exposure.

ACTINIC KERATOSES

Actinic keratoses, or solar keratoses, are composed of clones of anaplastic keratinocytes confined to the lower layers of epidermis and occur commonly on sun-damaged skin of elderly individuals. If left untreated, they may progress into squamous cell carcinoma, and atypical cells are then seen histologically at varying levels within the epidermis, termed squamous cell carcinoma in situ. With further progression abnormal cells invade through the basement membrane of the epidermal–dermal junction, thereby becoming invasive squamous cell carcinomas.

Actinic keratoses are extremely common in elderly individuals who have had extensive sun exposure. The National Health and Nutrition Examination Survey investigators found that the prevalence of actinic keratoses in the white population increased with age, irrespective of gender or degree of sun exposure. Male sex and sun exposure, however, predisposed an individual to a larger number of actinic keratoses. This census study found a high prevalence of actinic keratoses in the elderly population of the United States. For example, in the 65 to 74-year-old age group, 55 percent of the males and 37 percent of the females with high sun exposure had actinic keratoses, as compared to 19 percent of the males and 12 percent of the females with low sun exposure. White populations that are subject to greater amounts of sun exposure than the average American population have an even higher prevalence of actinic keratoses. In some Australian cities, up to 80 percent of the elderly women and 95 percent of the elderly men have actinic keratoses. Actinic keratoses usually occur in skin damaged from sun exposure, such as the bald scalp, the face, and the forearms. They are more common in fair-skinned individuals and are almost never seen in African Americans. These observations strongly suggest that chronic exposure to sunlight is an important etiologic factor.

The carcinogenic property of sunlight resides mainly in the UVB range. Experimental evidence indicates that exposure to ultraviolet light causes damage to cellular deoxyribonucleic acid (DNA) by formation of thymidine dimers. If not properly repaired, these dimers may give rise to mutations and transformed cells, which then become cancerous. Skin cancers are particularly common in patients with xeroderma pigmentosum, an inherited condition characterized by defective repair of DNA damage induced by ultraviolet light. Several studies have shown that lymphocytes and skin fibroblasts obtained from people with multiple actinic keratoses have an impaired ability to repair their DNA after an ultraviolet light exposure as compared to those obtained from age-matched controls without actinic keratoses. The etiologic significance of this finding remains uncertain.

Clinical Features of Actinic Keratoses

Actinic keratoses occur as well-demarcated, scaly, rough papules or plaques on sun-exposed skin surfaces. Color varies from tan to red, but sometimes they are the same color as the surrounding skin. As a result, some lesions are more easily palpated than seen (Fig. 59-1)(Color Plate 4).

In some lesions, known as pigmented actinic keratoses, an increased amount of pigmentation renders the lesions a striking brown color. Actinic keratoses are usually small, measuring from a few millimeters to 2 cm in size. Depending on degree of prior sun exposure, a given patient may have one lesion, a few lesions, or hundreds of lesions (Fig. 59-2)(Color Plate 5). There are often other signs of actinic damage in the surrounding skin, including wrinkling, dryness, and yellow discoloration from solar elastosis. Actinic keratoses can occur at the base of cutaneous horns. Solar keratoses have been reported to occur on the conjunctiva (Fig. 59-3)(Color Plate 6).

Spreading pigmented actinic keratosis is an unusual variant of actinic keratosis. Clinically, the lesions in this condition are characterized by large size (greater than

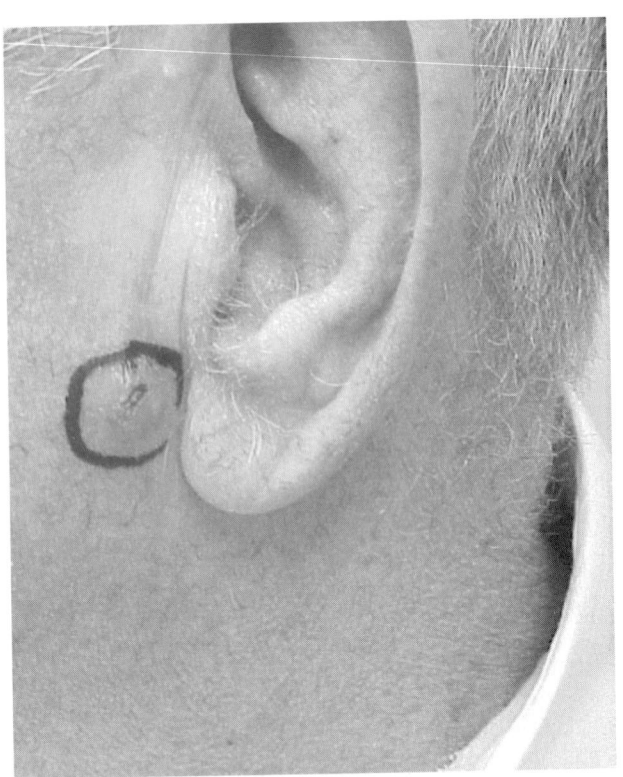

Figure 59-2 Inflamed hypertrophic actinic keratosis. Exuberant hyperkeratosis can result in a palpable lesion. However, induration, erythema, erosion, or increasing size should raise suspicion of the lesion evolving into squamous cell carcinoma.

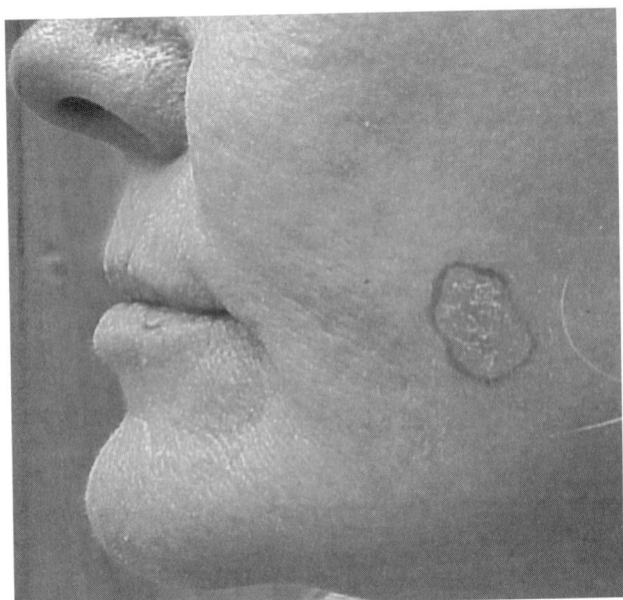

Figure 59-1 Actinic keratosis. An erythematous lesion on the cheek. Early lesions may be perceived by a roughness on palpation before they are clinically evident.

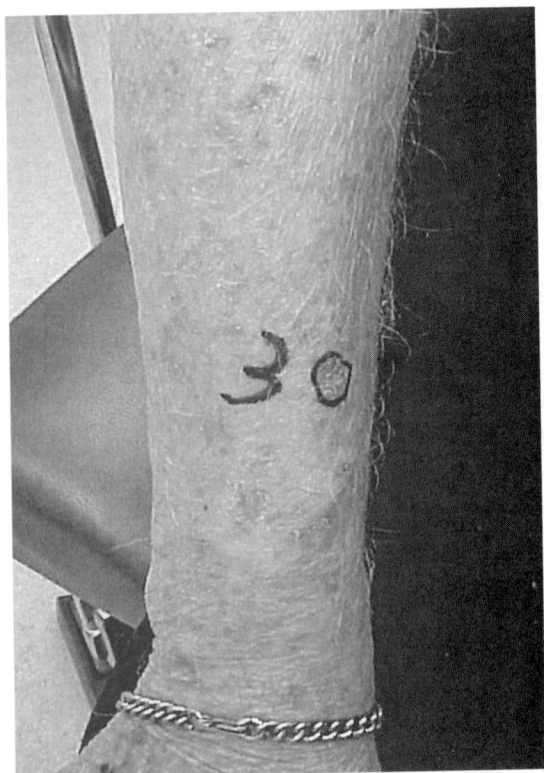

Figure 59-3 Actinic keratosis. The circled erythematous keratotic lesion was an actinic keratosis histologically. There are multiple additional actinic keratoses on this patient's sun damaged arm.

1 cm), brown pigmentation, and a tendency for centrifugal spread. These lesions can mimic lentigo maligna in clinical appearance.

Histologic Features of Actinic Keratosis and Carcinoma in Situ

Histologically, actinic keratoses are well-demarcated islands of abnormal keratinocytes with overlying parakeratosis. Cells of the basal layer and the lower layers of the stratum malpighii show a loss of polarity. The nuclei of the cells are large, irregular, and hyperchromatic, giving rise to a pleomorphic or atypical appearance. These cells produce a nucleated stratum corneum without the formation of a normal intact granular layer. The abnormal cells in the basal layer and in the lower layers of the stratum malpighii have already undergone neoplastic changes and will progress to develop full thickness epidermal atypia and subsequent dermal invasion. By convention, a lesion is referred to as a "premalignant" actinic keratosis when the abnormal cells are confined to the basal layer and the lower layers of the stratum malpighii and as carcinoma in situ when the atypical cells extend through the full thickness of the epidermis. When the neoplastic cells are still in the actinic keratosis stage the epidermal cells of the hair follicles and sweat gland ducts appear normal and keratinize normally. In actinic keratoses and in carcinoma in situ there are changes of solar elastosis present in the underlying dermis.

Progression from Carcinoma in Situ to Invasive Squamous Cell Carcinoma

Progression of actinic keratosis and carcinoma in situ to invasive squamous cell carcinoma occurs when buds of atypical keratinocytes extend deep into the dermis, leading to detached nests of abnormal cells capable of autonomous growth. Clinically, the lesion may become thicker, more indurated, and enlarged. Such signs, however, are not always present and are not substitutes for histologic confirmation of dermal invasion.

Marks et al. (1986) examined 1040 people older than age 40 years and found that 616 (59 percent) had a total of 4746 actinic keratoses. One year later, they reexamined the affected individuals and found that while some of the actinic keratoses had spontaneously resolved clinically, overall there was a 22 percent increase in the total number of actinic keratoses. Most importantly, the study found that the incidence of progression to invasive squamous cell carcinoma was 0.24 percent per actinic keratosis per year. Subsequently, Marks et al. (1988) enlarged upon this study by following 21,905 actinic keratoses for a 1-year period and determining a yearly incidence of progression to invasion of about 0.1 percent per actinic keratosis. Marks et al. found, on average, 7.7 actinic keratoses per person. These figures would indicate that, on average, an individual with actinic keratoses has a likelihood of 1 to 2 percent per year, or 10 to 20 percent in 10 years, of developing an invasive squamous cell carcinoma. This estimate agrees reasonably well with data obtained from a number of pathologic series. Montgomery estimated that in 20 to 25 percent of patients with actinic keratoses, squamous cell carcinoma would develop in one more or the lesions. Graham and Helwig reported results from several series of patients, including 750 patients with actinic keratoses in Philadelphia and more than 5000 patients with actinic keratoses accessioned at the Armed Forces Institute of Pathology. The investigators consistently found that 12 to 13 percent of the patients experience progression of at least one actinic keratosis to invasive squamous cell carcinoma.

In contrast to squamous cell carcinoma arising from burn scars, osteomyelitis sinuses, and chronic wounds, squamous cell carcinomas that originate from actinic keratoses metastasize infrequently. The rate of metastases of squamous cell carcinomas arising in actinic keratoses ranges between 0.5 percent and 6 percent, depending on the series consulted. Moller et al. followed 211 patients with invasive squamous cell carcinoma for 16 to 26 years and found a 3 percent incidence of metastasis in 153 patients with squamous cell carcinoma of the skin; 11 percent of 55 patients with mucous membrane squamous cell carcinoma had metastases. An Australian study that adjusted for life table losses caused by age found that 5.5 percent of patients with cutaneous squamous cell carcinoma develop metastases within 5 years.

Treatment of Actinic Keratosis

A variety of therapeutic methods are available for the patient with actinic keratoses. The optimal choice depends on the number of lesions, the extent of involvement, and the patient's general state of health.

For the patient with a few lesions and little evidence of actinic damage, destructive techniques such as cryotherapy, curettage, electrodesiccation, chemical cauterization with phenol or trichloroacetic acid, or excisional surgery can be successfully employed. A cream or solution of 0.5% (Carac) to 5% 5-fluorouracil (5-FU, Efudex) can be effectively employed topically to treat people with actinic keratoses. This treatment is particularly useful for patients with moderate actinic damage because it can uncover and treat subclinical lesions. Preparations containing 5-FU can be used successfully to treat patients with widespread extensive actinic damage, although adequate treatment is usually a prolonged, uncomfortable, and unsightly endeavor for the patient. In selected patients with extensive involvement and numerous actinic keratoses, dermabrasion may be the treatment of choice. Dermabrasion is extremely effective in eradicating large numbers of actinic keratoses, particularly on the face and scalp. Generally the period of cosmetic incapacitation is longer with 5-FU than with dermabrasion, particularly if the 5-FU is administered with the regional section technique. Additionally, the final cosmetic result with dermabrasion is usually superior to that with 5-FU because dermabrasion destroys the skin uniformly, which then heals uniformly, while 5-FU destroys individual lesions but not surrounding aged skin. A number of experienced dermatologists believe that "5-FU is not as efficacious as dermabrasion in long term prevention of recurrent dyskeratotic and malignant cutaneous disease." UltraPulse CO_2 laser resurfacing is extremely effective in eliminating actinic keratoses, and in recent years has been employed in preference to dermabrasion because it is technically easier to perform and facilitates treatment of periorbital, nasal alae, perioral, and vermillion border areas.

Several additional topical treatments may aid in the therapy of actinic keratoses. Topical tretinoin may be helpful in clearing actinic keratoses and delaying their progression. In particular, it was found to be useful as an adjunct to 5-FU. In order to further define the usefulness of topical tretinoin in treatment of facial actinic keratoses, Balin et al. treated 30 patients with multiple actinic keratoses for 15 months. They found that after 15 months of therapy (consisting of an average of 500 applications of tretinoin, 0.05% or 0.1% as tolerated by the patient), the average number of actinic keratoses decreased to 40 percent of the pretreatment number, and the average lesion size and area decreased to 25 percent of the pretreatment value. They found that improvement was more marked in patients with early actinic keratoses. Advanced lesions responded poorly, and a few progressed to invasive squamous cell carcinoma. Side effects were minor, and the treatment was generally well tolerated. Their data suggest that topical tretinoin may be employed as an adjunctive treatment in the therapy of early actinic keratoses. This treatment seems to delay the progression of actinic keratoses rather than cure the lesions.

A newcomer to the market, topical imiquimod has been reported to facilitate regression of actinic keratosis. Imiquimod is an immunomodulatory agent that generates a host immune response by activating TLR-7, an interleukin (IL)-1–like receptor that upregulates a broad spectrum of type 1 interferons (IFN) and strongly polarizes the immune system in a Th-1 cytokine pattern. Imiquimod also enhances Langerhans cell maturation and migration to the regional lymph nodes, which is required for the development of an immune response. In preliminary studies by Stockfleth et al., with a small number of patients, imiquimod seems to be a promising approach for the treatment of actinic keratoses. In one study, 6 patients were cleared of 1 to 10 actinic keratoses in 8 weeks of treatment, and remained clear for at least 3 months of follow-up.

Diclofenac sodium 3% topical gel (Solaraze) is a cyclooxygenase (COX)-2 inhibitor and has been reported to improve actinic keratosis with 90 days of topical therapy. Thirty percent of patients had clearing of their actinic keratoses, as compared to 10 percent of placebo-treated patients. However, the studies only had 30-day follow-up, so it is not yet clear whether the lesions were cured or simply suppressed. The rationale for this treatment is based on the observations that COX-2 has a tumor promoting function in colorectal carcinogenesis and specific COX-2 inhibitors can reduce the intestinal polyp burden in patients with familial adenomatous polyposis. Additionally, animal studies have shown a chemopreventive effect of selective COX-2 inhibitors in ultraviolet light-induced skin cancer.

Photodynamic therapy is the oxygen-dependent destruction of tissue after photosensitization and subsequent irradiation with visible light. Topical 5-aminolevulinic acid (ALA) selectively induces the production of intracellular porphyrin in epidermal cells, and after irradiation with 635 nm light, leads to singlet oxygen-mediated destruction of tissue. Clinically, the ALA is painted on individual actinic keratoses and 16 hours later the patient is exposed to the light for 20 minutes. Several studies have shown between a 50 to 88 percent response rates. One double-blind study by Ormrod and Jarvis demonstrated that 88 percent of the patients had >75 percent reduction in actinic keratosis at 12 weeks.

BOWEN'S DISEASE

Bowen's disease is another form of squamous cell carcinoma in situ. It may occur anywhere on the skin but is more common on covered surfaces. Three factors are implicated in the etiology of Bowen's disease: exposure to ultraviolet irradiation, arsenic, papovaviruses and oncornaviruses.

Clinically, Bowen's disease appears as a slowly enlarging erythematous patch of scaling skin. It may have a sharp but irregular outline showing little or no infiltration (Fig. 59-4)(Color Plate 7). Within the patch there are areas of crusting. Fifty-five percent of patients have more than one lesion. Lesions of Bowen's disease can occur on the glans penis, the vulva, and the oral mucosa; in these locations, the lesions are called erythroplasia of Queyrat (Fig. 59-5)(Color Plate 8).

Many cases of Bowen's disease develop in persons who ingested inorganic arsenic many years prior to disease presentation. Some persons report that they received Fowler's

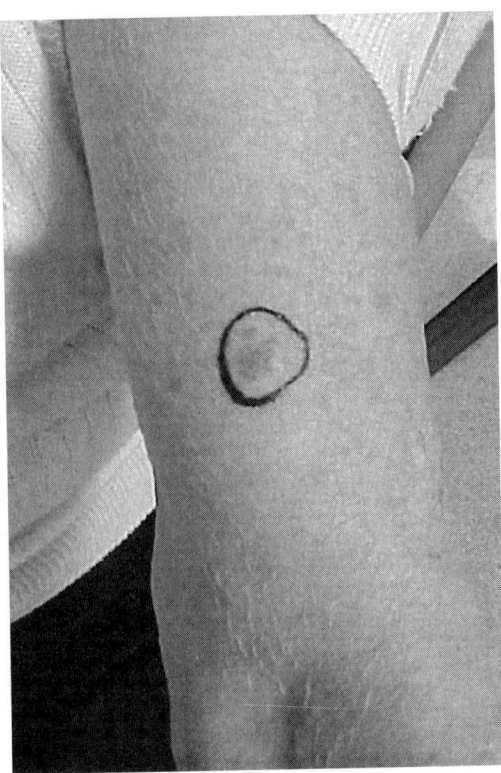

Figure 59-4 Bowen's disease. Sharply demarcated erythematous plaque on arm. Clinical differential diagnosis can include inflammatory (eczema, psoriasis, lichen planus, etc.) and neoplastic processes (amelanotic melanoma, seborrheic keratosis, superficial basal cell carcinoma etc.).

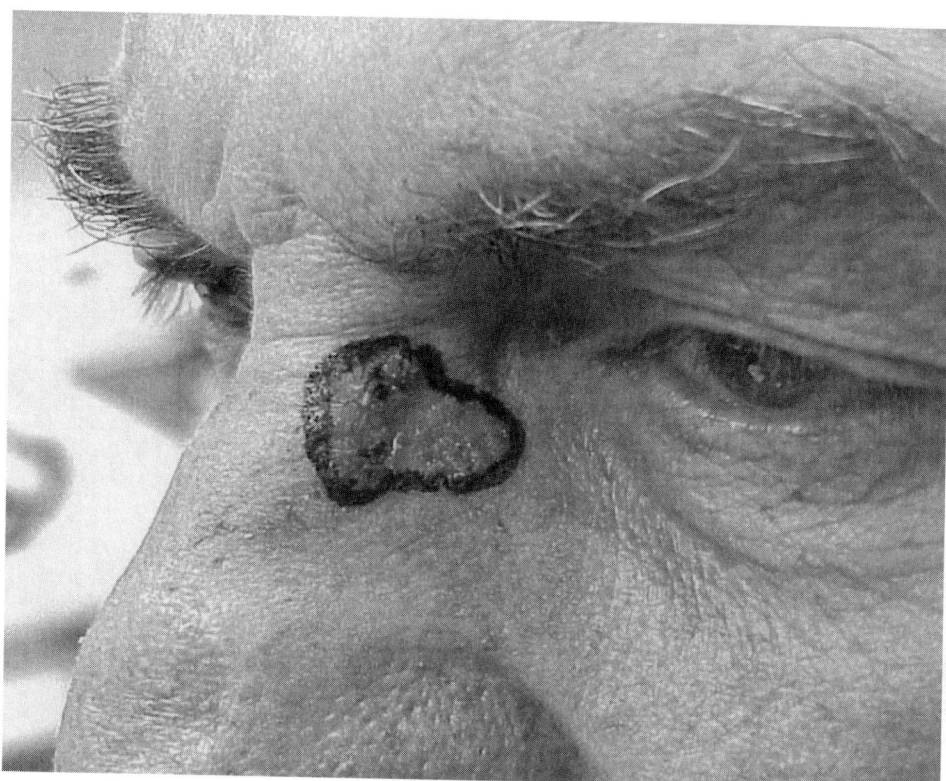

Figure 59-5 Bowen's disease with carcinoma. Scaling hyperkeratotic plaque on the nose. This lesion evolved into invasive squamous cell carcinoma.

solution, which was commonly used to treat asthma and various other medical problems, and which contained 1% potassium arsenite. In other persons, the source of arsenic is thought to have been well water or insecticides. Arsenical keratoses of the palms and soles are verrucous, pale papules without surrounding inflammation. They occur in 40 percent of patients who receive arsenic and histologically are analogous to Bowen's disease. Fifteen to 30 percent of patients with Bowen's disease on a non–sun-exposed site develop internal malignancies; presumably this is caused by exposure to arsenic.

The histologic pattern seen in Bowen's disease is full-thickness epidermal dysplasia. Dysplastic cells often fill the acral portions of the appendages. The dysplastic cells are swollen and clumped and contain markedly atypical mitotic figures. The epidermis shows acanthosis with elongation and thickening of the rete ridges. The thickened horny layer consists largely of parakeratotic cells. Cells throughout the epidermis lie in complete disorder.

SQUAMOUS CELL CARCINOMA

In addition to actinic keratoses and Bowen's disease, conditions predisposing to squamous cell carcinoma include arsenic exposure, radiation exposure, scarring from a previous injury such as a burn or chronic leg ulcer, and exposure to heat. However the majority of cutaneous squamous cell carcinomas arise in actinic keratoses. Squamous cell carcinoma may occur anywhere on the skin or mucous membranes, but it rarely arises from normal-appearing skin.

Ultraviolet light exposure is clearly related to the development of squamous cell carcinoma. The incidence of cutaneous squamous cell carcinoma in white males in New Orleans was 154 per 100,000 in 1980, as compared to 30 per 100,000 in Detroit. The incidence of squamous cell carcinoma (SCC) in Australia is among the highest in the world, and in 1990, there were 250 cases per 100,000. This represents a 51 percent increase in SCC in Australia, when compared to a similar survey 5 years previously. There will be a 2 percent increase in the incidence of squamous cell carcinoma for every 1 percent decrease in atmospheric ozone content. Cutaneous squamous cell carcinoma is approximately twice as common in white men, as compared to white women. This seems to be a result of lifestyle factors such as clothing, leisure activities, lipstick, and hairstyles. The incidence of squamous cell carcinoma increases with age, particularly after the age of 40 years.

A number of other factors also predispose an individual to squamous cell carcinomas. These factors include therapeutic x-ray, viral oncogenesis, immunosuppression, PUVA (psoralen plus ultraviolet A) therapy, arsenic exposure, hydrocarbon exposure, chronic scarring, inflammatory processes, and infrared (heat) radiation.

Ultraviolet-induced mutations of the p53 tumor-suppressor gene interfere with apoptosis of the damaged cells, permitting damaged cells to proliferate. More than 90 percent of squamous cell carcinomas have p53 gene mutations. Nucleotide sequence analysis demonstrates that these mutations are specifically associated with exposure to UVB light.

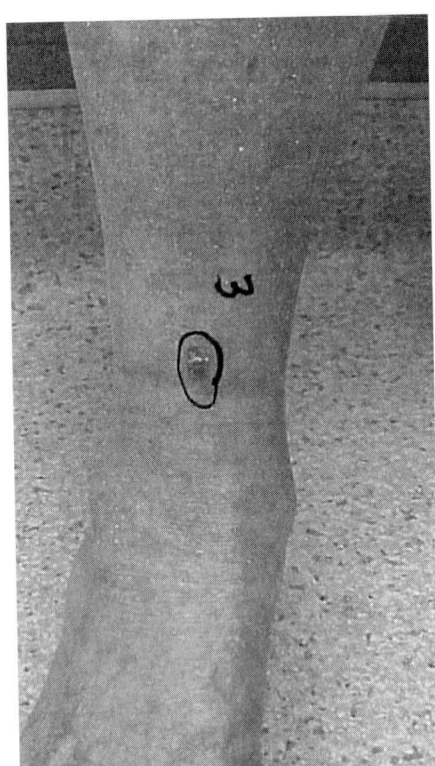

Figure 59-6   Squamous cell carcinoma in situ. Erythematous keratotic lesion on the leg. Clinically often difficult to differentiate from more advanced actinic keratosis. The atypical cells in an actinic keratosis are confined to the lower layers of the epidermis while in a squamous cell carcinoma the atypical cells exist throughout the epidermis.

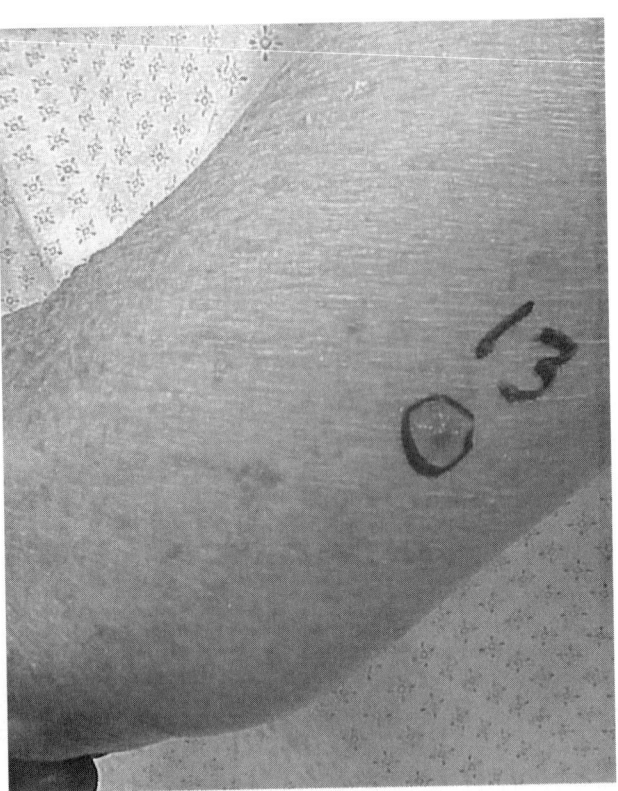

Figure 59-7   Squamous cell carcinoma in situ. Erythematous, keratotic, palpable lesion on arm. Extensive actinic damage and multiple actinic keratoses on arm.

Clinically, squamous cell carcinoma in situ can look similar to actinic keratoses. Often they are thicker than actinic keratoses (Fig. 59-6)(Color Plate 9). They occur as well-demarcated, scaly, rough papules on sun-exposed skin surfaces (Fig. 59-7)(Color Plate 10). Color varies from tan to red, but sometimes they are the same color as the surrounding skin. As a result, some lesions are more easily palpated than seen. Initially, they are usually small, measuring from a few millimeters to 2 cm in size (Fig. 59-8)(Color Plate 11).

Biopsies of the lesions are often required to distinguish squamous cell carcinoma in situ from actinic keratoses. Clinically, as squamous cell carcinoma in situ evolves into invasive squamous cell carcinoma, the lesion becomes more indurated with distinct margins (Fig. 59-9)(Color Plate 12). The growth enlarges and becomes firm with increases in the thickness and the diameter of the lesion. A shallow ulcer may develop surrounded by a wide, elevated, and indurated border. Often the ulcer is covered by a crust that conceals a red, granular base (Fig. 59-10)(Color Plate 13). Continued invasion of subcutaneous tissue forms a nodule that may fix itself to deeper structures. Occasionally raised verrucoid lesions without ulceration occur (Figs. 59-11 and 59-12)(Color Plates 14 and 15).

Squamous cell carcinoma is a malignant, invasive carcinoma. If neglected or improperly treated, tumor cells can invade nerve, muscle, and bone. Histologically, there are irregular masses of epidermal cells proliferating downward and invading the dermis. The invading tumor masses are composed of varying proportions of normal squamous cells

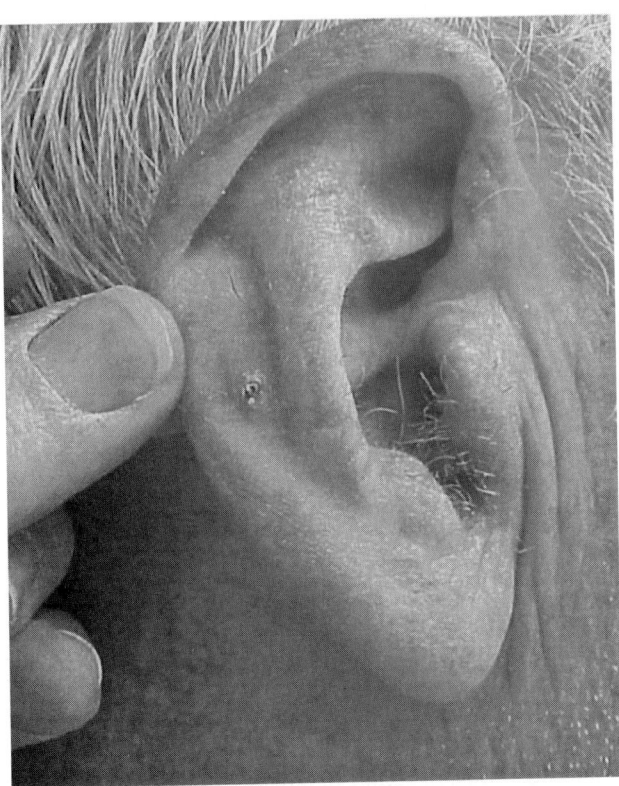

Figure 59-8   Squamous cell carcinoma in situ. Erythematous keratotic lesion on ear. Clinically, this lesion is difficult to differentiate from invasive squamous cell carcinoma.

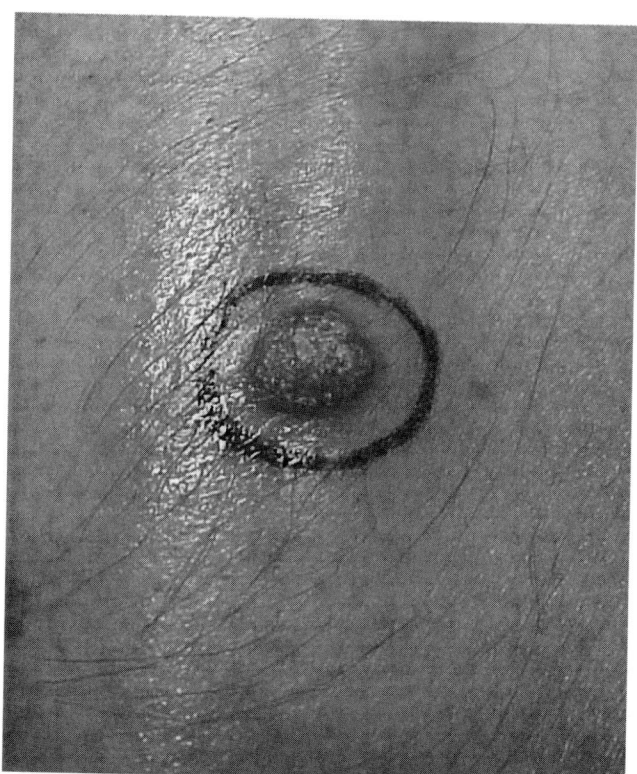

Figure 59-9   Well-differentiated squamous cell carcinoma, superficially invasive. Erythematous keratotic lesion on leg. Continued growth produces increases in the diameter and height of the lesion.

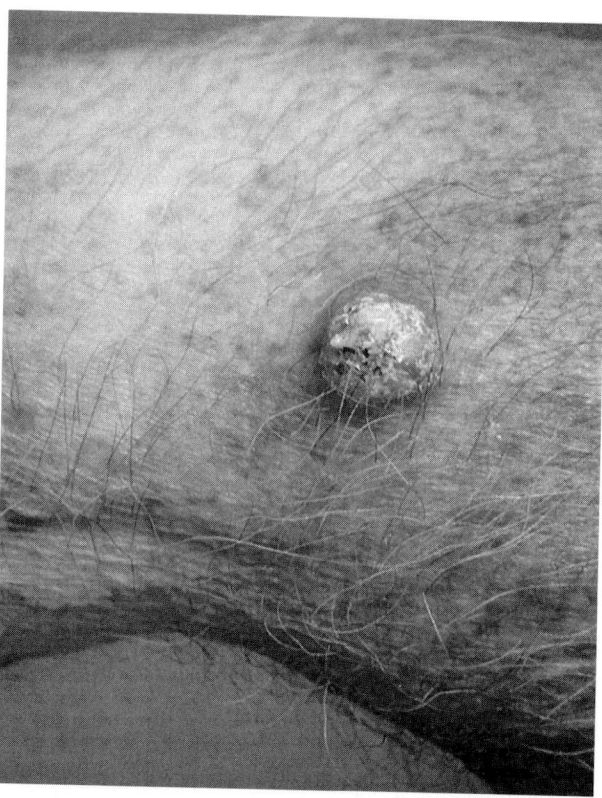

Figure 59-11   Squamous cell carcinoma. Crusted nodular erythematous keratotic squamous cell carcinoma on the wrist. Extensive surrounding actinic damage to skin.

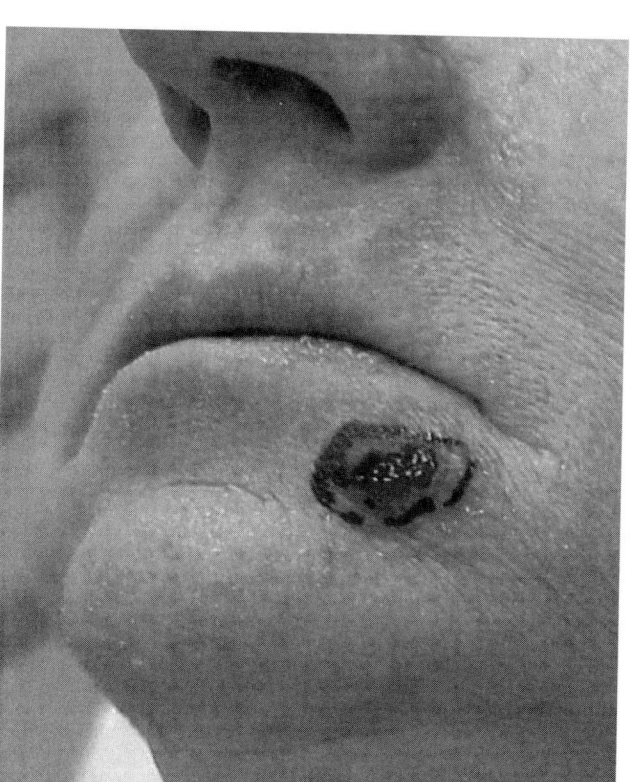

Figure 59-10   Squamous cell carcinoma. Ulceration of the tumor develops sooner in fast-growing lesions. The surface may be granular and bleed easily or may be crusted. The edges are usually elevated and firm.

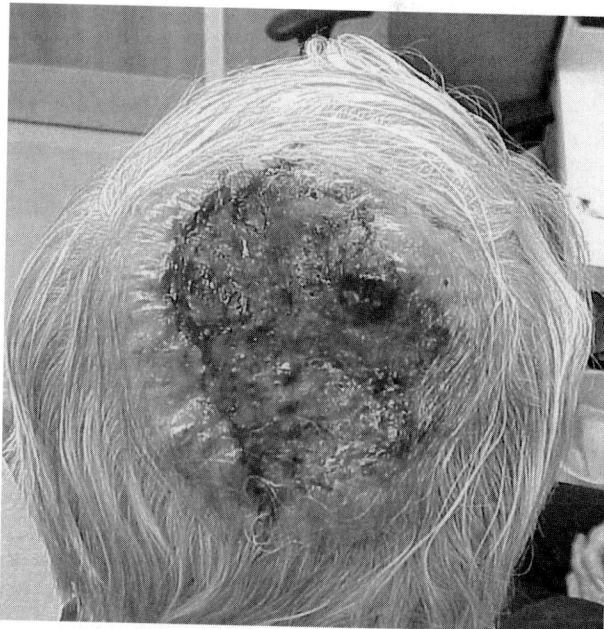

Figure 59-12   Squamous cell carcinoma. This lesion was 2–3 cm in size when it was biopsied 16 months before this photograph was taken. The biopsy revealed invasive squamous cell carcinoma. The patient refused all medical therapy electing instead for herbal treatments. At the time of this photograph the tumor had grown and invaded through the cranium into the brain.

and of atypical cells. These atypical cells demonstrate variations in the size and shape of the cells, hyperchromasia and hyperplasia of the nuclei, absence of intracellular bridges, keratinization of individual cells, and the presence of atypical mitotic figures. In squamous cell carcinoma, differentiation is in the direction of the keratinization. Horn pearls are concentric layers of squamous cells with gradually increasing keratinization toward the center. The dermis often shows a marked inflammatory reaction. Histologic grading of squamous cell carcinoma depends on the percentage of keratinizing cells, percentage of atypical cells, number of mitotic figures, and depth of invasion. The Broders classification system is based on the degree of dedifferentiation of the cells: in grade 1 <25 percent, in grade 2 <50 percent, in grade 3 <75 percent, and in grade 4 >75 percent of the cells are undifferentiated. Tumor grade provides data predicting outcome. The incidence of metastasis varies from 2 to 5 percent in squamous cell carcinomas arising in actinic keratoses to 25 to 30 percent in those arising in a chronic osteomyelitic sinus or in radiodermatitis. Cure rates for squamous cell carcinomas arising from actinic keratosis are high, better than 99 percent when Mohs micrographic surgery is employed to remove the cancer. Treatment failure occurs if the tumor is not completely removed. Five-year survival rates were 50 percent for those cancers associated with chronic radiation and 53 percent for those cancers developing within a scar.

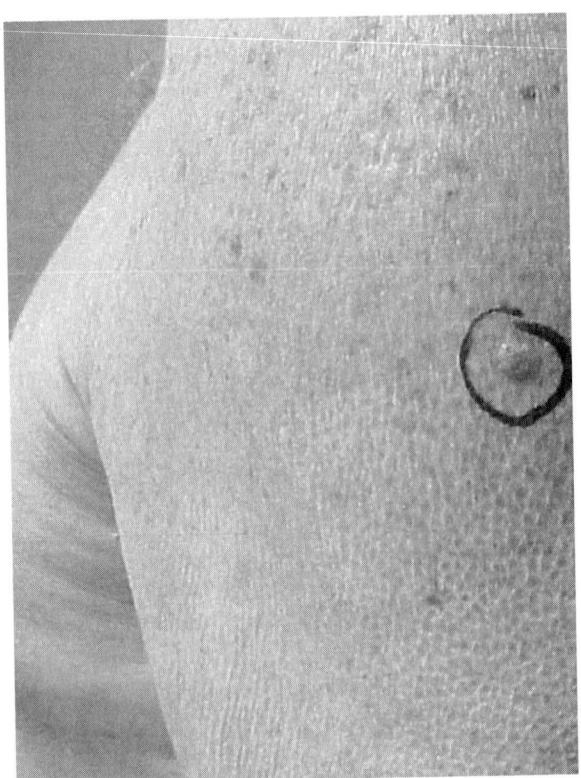

Figure 59-13 Basal cell carcinoma, nodular type. Dome-shaped papule with telangiectatic vessels and a translucent surface on the patient's arm.

BASAL CELL CARCINOMA

The most common skin cancer, and hence the most common cancer in the United States, is the basal cell carcinoma. This type of lesion is found most commonly on the head and neck of men, especially those who sunburn easily and have had chronic sun exposure. These lesions are uncommon in darkly pigmented races. The distribution of lesions on the face, however, does not correlate well with the area of maximal exposure to light. These lesions are common on the eyelids, on the inner canthus of the eye, and behind the ear, and are not so common on the back of the hand or the forearm. Actinic keratoses develop into squamous cell carcinomas but not into basal cell tumors. Basal cell epitheliomas generally occur on hair-bearing skin in adults, usually as single lesions. Predisposing features include chronic sun exposure, exposure to x-irradiation, burn scars, and xeroderma pigmentosum.

Basal cell epitheliomas rarely metastasize but can be quite destructive locally. There are several different clinical types of basal cell epithelioma. Most common is the noduloulcerative basal cell epithelioma, which begins as a small, waxy nodule with small telangiectatic vessels on the surface and a translucent, rolled border (see Fig. 59–12). The nodule increases in size and undergoes central ulceration. The typical lesion consists of a slowly enlarging ulcer surrounded by a pearly, rolled border (Fig. 59-13) (Color Plate 16). This represents the so-called rodent ulcer. Pigmented basal cell carcinomas can contain melanin pigment. The morpheaform, or fibrosing, basal cell epithelioma appears as an indurated, yellowish plaque with an ill-defined border. The overlying skin remains intact for

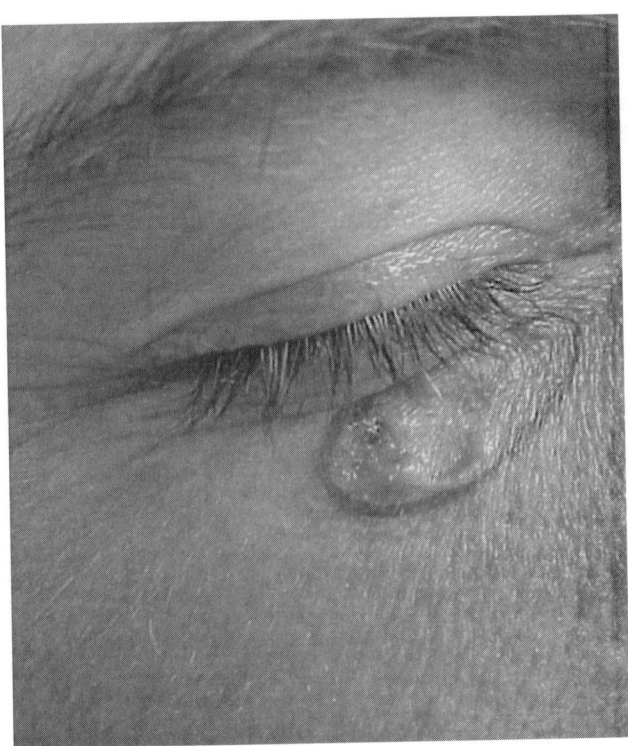

Figure 59-14 Basal cell carcinoma. Rolled, elevated, translucent border in this indurated nodular basal cell carcinoma of the lower eyelid.

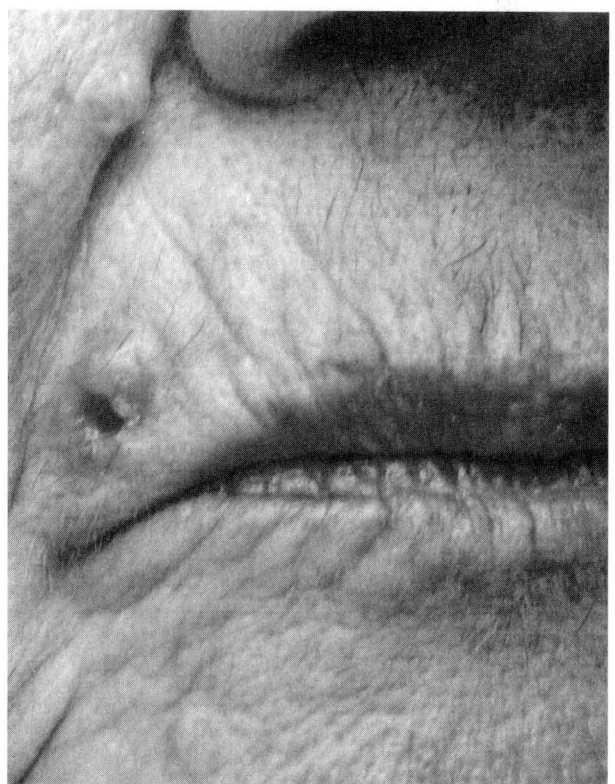

Figure 59-15   Basal cell carcinoma, recurrent. This photograph of a translucent ulcerated nodule on the lip was taken 10 years after a basal cell carcinoma had been treated in this location with electrodessication and curretage. The defect after the cancer was removed by Mohs micrographic surgery measured 3.0 × 2.8 cm and extended to within 1 mm of the inner mucosal surface of the lip.

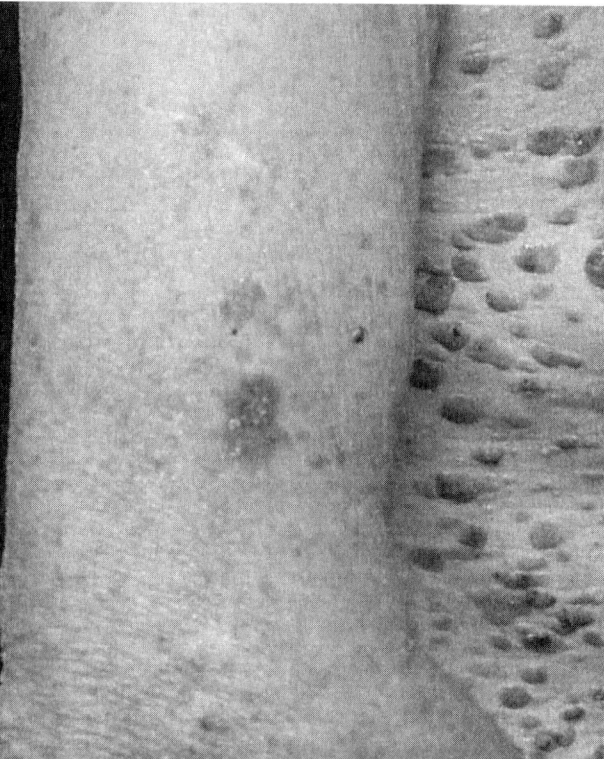

Figure 59-16   Basal cell carcinoma, superficial. This erythematous, scaly plaque on the right arm shows centrifugal growth and may be misdiagnosed as nummular eczema, psoriasis or Bowen's disease. The multiple brownish verrucoid plaques on the chest are seborrheic keratoses.

a long time before ulceration develops (Fig. 59-14)(Color Plate 17).

Superficial, multifocal basal cell epitheliomas consist of one or several erythematous, scaling, slightly infiltrated patches that slowly increase in size by peripheral extension (Fig. 59-15)(Color Plate 18). The patches are surrounded by a fine, thread-like, pearly border and usually show small areas of superficial ulceration and crusting. The center may show smooth, atrophic scarring. Superficial basal cell epitheliomas occur predominantly on the trunk. Morpheaform or sclerosing basal cell carcinomas present as a whitish plaque with poorly defined borders and an indurated consistency. It may seem like a scar and may have wide subclinical extension (Fig. 59-16)(Color Plate 19).

Histologically, the tumor cells have a large oval or elongated nucleus and relatively little cytoplasm. The nuclei are uniform, compact, and dark staining. They do not show variation in size or in staining, nor are there abnormal mitoses. The basal cells at the periphery of the tumor appear to line up, a phenomenon known as peripheral palisading. A connective tissue stroma is always present with the epithelial tumor masses, indicating that a mutual relationship exists between the tumor and its mesodermal stroma. Most basal cell tumors provoke a round cell, lymphohistiocytic inflammatory reaction.

Basal cell tumors are thought to originate from immature pluripotential epidermal cells. The cytokeratin pattern in basal cell carcinoma resembles those found in the outer root sheath of the hair follicle below the isthmus rather than that of the epidermis, supporting a follicular origin for the tumor. These cells can mature and differentiate in a pattern resembling any of the epithelial structures. Their behavior is governed (as that of normal immature cells) by the connective tissue in their proximity. Experimental production of basal cell epitheliomas has been accomplished in rats with chemical carcinogens. Reproduction with exposure to ultraviolet light has not been accomplished.

Each basal cell carcinoma has a unicentric origin. Studies of patients with the basal cell nevus syndrome have identified specific genetic alterations that predispose to the formation of basal cell carcinomas. Inactivation of a tumor-suppressor gene on the long arm of chromosome 9 (9q22) seems to be necessary for the development of basal cell carcinomas. In addition, more than 50 percent of basal cell carcinomas have p53 gene mutations of a type associated with exposure to UVB light.

Several investigators have shown that exposure to ultraviolet light alters the immune system in experimental animals, facilitating the development of fatal skin tumors. This ultraviolet-induced immunologic tolerance of ultraviolet-induced tumors is quite specific, because the animals will continue to reject transplanted tumors caused by oncogenic viruses or chemical carcinogens. It has also been shown that exposure to ultraviolet irradiation causes the development of hapten-specific suppressor T cells. The ultraviolet-induced, abnormal antigen-presenting cell is thought to be an epidermal Langerhans' cell. Alterations in immune function with age and by chronic sun exposure are almost certain to contribute to the development of tumors in exposed skin that are so prevalent in the elderly population.

IMMUNOSUPPRESSION AND SKIN CANCERS

Dermatologists are quite familiar with the large numbers of premalignant tumors (solar keratoses, for example) that can suddenly spring up in an immunosuppressed patient. Moreover, these behave more aggressively and tend to transform into invasive, rapidly growing tumors. Frequent clinical surveillance of the integument is essential in patients who are receiving chemotherapy for cancer or other serious diseases.

It is impossible to exaggerate the contributions of experimental tumor biology to the understanding of human malignancy. Nowhere are these contributions more dramatic than in tumors of the skin. Penn has brought together a vast amount of information relating to the development of skin cancers in immunosuppressed patients. Transplant centers throughout the world are the main source of this important knowledge. Immunosuppressive agents are used to prevent rejection of the homografts. Almost half of the malignancies that arise in patients with impaired immune surveillance occur in the skin. The great majority of these are squamous cell cancers. In Australia, which has the highest incidence of skin cancers, the incidence of these malignancies is increased about 20 times. In New South Wales, a fivefold increase in malignant melanoma has been recorded. The impact of immunosuppression is made clear by the fact that these tumors arise in patients who are much younger than expected for these conditions (approximately a 30-year difference).

The great majority of these iatrogenic tumors occurred in sun-exposed areas, and almost half of the patients had multiple tumors. Some hapless individuals had 30 to 40 carcinomas. Almost 10 percent of skin cancers were associated with internal malignancies.

The tumors are also far more aggressive, tending to metastasize much more rapidly than tumors that arise spontaneously on sun-damaged skin. Thus, a new threat has been added, the high killing capacity of these tumors in immunocompromised subjects. It must be noted, of course, that immunosuppressive agents may be carcinogenic in their own right. Animal studies demonstrate that these drugs greatly potentiate ultraviolet-induced tumors. They can incite new tumors even while curing the original malignancy.

TREATMENT OPTIONS FOR SQUAMOUS CELL CARCINOMA AND BASAL CELL CARCINOMA

There are a number of standard techniques commonly used to eradicate skin cancers: electrodesiccation and curettage (burning), cryosurgery (freezing), radiation therapy (x-ray), surgical excision, and excision by Mohs micrographic surgery. Immunomodulation agents are currently under investigation. Each has advantages and disadvantages.

Burning of the tumor requires electrodesiccation, cautery, or a laser. Burning is quick, and it requires minimal operative skill. The clinician neither has to know how to do incisional surgery nor how to suture wounds.

The major disadvantage of burning the tumor is that one doesn't really know precisely where to burn. One burns the tissue without knowing whether the entire tumor has been destroyed or whether there may be residual tumor cells remaining. Because of that, a certain percentage of these tumors may recur. Five-year recurrence rates after electrodesiccation and curettage of primary basal cell carcinomas were 13.2 percent in a university dermatology clinic and 7.7 percent in a published literature review. A second drawback of burning is that a black scab remains that takes 2 to 3 months to heal. It heals as a depressed and sunken white scar.

A second way to treat a skin cancer is to freeze it with cryosurgery. This technique has the advantage of being quick and easy to perform; often, no injection of anesthesia is required. However, it shares the same disadvantage as burning in that one does not know exactly where to freeze. There is no way to tell if the freezing goes deep or wide enough or if there is residual cancer that has not been destroyed. With cryosurgery, a certain percentage of the tumors will recur. One study reported a 5-year recurrence rate of primary basal cell carcinomas of 9 percent. The freezing procedure leaves a blister that then later forms a scab. It takes 1 to 2 months to heal, and it heals as a flat or depressed white scar.

Freezing involves an extra problem to consider when compared to burning. Freezing a cancer cell does not kill the cell. Viable cells can be preserved for many years by freezing and subsequent storage in liquid nitrogen. However, when the cell thaws, a slow thawing process results in intracellular ice crystals rupturing the cell membrane, causing cell death. Unfortunately, not every cell ruptures as it thaws, only a percentage of them. That is why the freeze–thaw cycle is repeated several times. These spared cells, together with ones that were inadequately treated in the first place, may later produce a recurrence.

X-ray radiation therapy represents a third approach to treating skin cancers. X-rays, of course, kill cancer, but x-rays can also cause cancer to develop. It takes a number of years after exposure to get cancer from x-rays, so x-ray therapy is appropriate for certain patients. A randomized trial of the treatment of primary basal cell carcinomas with radiation therapy revealed a 4-year recurrence rate of 7.5 percent. The recurrence rate for patients followed for 5 years or more is 8.7 percent. One of the more practical problems with x-rays is that patients must receive fractional treatments. The person has to come in for multiple visits to receive a fraction of the dose each time. It is a nuisance to have to return every day for a lesion that otherwise can be taken right off. But for certain selected patients, this is appropriate therapy.

A fourth way to remove skin cancers is standard surgical excision. When a tumor is excised, the surgeon observes the breadth of the lesion then goes a certain distance outside the observed borders, and cuts out the skin. The excised skin is sent to the lab for analysis. A technician cuts a section analogous to slicing a tomato or a loaf of bread and the pathologist checks the vertically cut section for evidence of cancer cells. The trouble is that a 2-cm excision requires four thousand cross-sectional cuts (each slice is 5 microns) to ensure that the entire tumor and any roots are removed. Generally, a lab makes just one slide, or perhaps two to four slides if the piece of skin is large.

Consequently, conventional surgery has two problems. One is that more skin than is necessary is removed. The second is that even if the lab reports that the cancer is entirely removed, one cannot be sure. It all depends on whether or not there happened to be residual cancer at the periphery where the lab cut their section. The cure rates from excisional surgery are similar to or slightly better than electrodesiccation and curettage or cryosurgery, and are approximately 90 percent, depending upon the characteristics of the tumor.

Mohs Micrographic Surgery

Mohs micrographic surgery avoids the problems associated with the aforementioned treatments for skin cancer. Originally developed in the 1930s by Frederick E. Mohs, MD, and later refined from a fixed-tissue to a fresh-tissue technique, the procedure once known as a "chemosurgery" essentially involves excising cancerous tissue serially and examining the undersurface and edges of the section for evidence of remaining cancer. Of all the skin cancer treatments, Mohs surgery offers the highest cure rate (greater that 99 percent), the least likelihood of recurrence, minimal potential for scarring or other disfigurement, and unmatched precision.

Cure rates for removal of basal cell carcinomas with Mohs surgery are reported to be 99 percent for primary lesions and 96 percent for recurrent tumors. This author's personal experience in the removal of more than 11,000 primary and recurrent basal cell and squamous cell skin cancers in the past 12 years has resulted in a cure rate greater than 99.9 percent. Many types of tumors have been excised successfully by using the Mohs technique. Although there is some disagreement among experts about the indications, the procedure is especially appropriate for these cases:

- Large tumors (squamous cell carcinoma >1 cm; basal cell carcinoma >1 cm);
- Tumors with indistinct borders (most tumors have indistinct borders);
- Tumors near vital functional or cosmetic structures; and
- Recurrent tumors for which other treatments have failed.

Mohs Technique

The Mohs surgeon performs a dual role as both surgeon and pathologist. First, the surgeon removes the visible portion of the tumor by excision or curettage. With the scalpel blade held at a 45-degree angle to the skin, the surgeon then excises a layer of tissue from the base of the site. The clinician divides this layer into sections, color codes them with dyes, and makes reference marks on the skin to indicate the source of these sections. This yields a map of the surgical site.

The undersurface and edges of each section are now examined under the microscope for evidence of remaining cancer. If there are cancer cells, the surgeon marks their location on the map and returns to the patient to remove another layer of skin at the corresponding site. This layer is then examined microscopically for additional cancer cells. This process continues layer by layer until there are no detectable cancer cells. This precise technique is well described by Dr. Willis Cottel.

Conventional excision yields specimens that are examined microscopically in broadleaf-type sections, which may not allow accurate examination of the tumor margins. In the Mohs procedure, the orientation and sectioning of the specimens allows examination of the deep and lateral margins of the tumor. This enables detection of subtle microscopic strands of tumor.

The duration of the procedure will vary depending on the size and location of the skin cancer. Another variable is the type of reconstruction needed. Most cases involve one to three surgical stages. The excision itself takes only 10 minutes. The sectioning, marking, and microscopic analysis may take up to 2 hours for each stage.

The size and shape of the final defect will dictate wound treatment. Our approach generally is to suture the wound closed, although some wounds can be allowed to heal by secondary intention. Larger defects may require skin flaps or skin grafts. In cases involving extensive defects, a multidiscipline team approach, working with a reconstructive surgeon may be necessary. Adjunctive radiation therapy may be indicated in cases of deep tumors, extensive perineural spread, and where there is a likelihood of lymphatic spread.

Mohs micrographic surgery is considered the gold standard for removal of cutaneous and mucosal neoplasms. Clinicians can offer patients unmatched long-term cure rates and the best possible cosmetic results. Mohs surgery is superior to all of the other methods of skin cancer removal and patients should be given the option of having their cancer removed by Mohs surgery irrespective of its clinical size or location.

Investigational Therapy

Clinical studies of different therapeutic approaches have been performed with varying degrees of efficacy. Photodynamic therapy has been used for superficial basal cell carcinoma. Immunomodulation with intralesional recombinant interferon-α has been reported to have a maximal cure rate of 80 percent and has not become a standard treatment. Topical imiquimod (discussed above in the section on treatment of actinic keratoses) is under investigation. Treatment of nodular basal cell carcinomas with 5% imiquimod once daily for 6 weeks resulted in a 71 percent cure rate, and for 12 weeks, a 75 percent cure rate. There was an 88 percent cure rate of superficial basal cell carcinomas treated for 6 weeks with 5% imiquimod. These approaches are new and there is no long-term follow-up data on patients treated with this modality. Excising the experimentally treated area and examining the tissue pathologically for evidence of residual cancer established the cure rate data. Thus the patients used in these trials will not be useful to follow for long-term cure data for imiquimod treated cancers. It is worthwhile to remember that some years ago topical 5-fluorouracil was used to treat superficial basal cell carcinoma. Mohs reported a series of basal cell carcinomas treated with topical 5-fluorouracil that lead to disastrous recurrences. In these cases, deep foci of tumor remained and infiltrated widely before clinical recurrence was noted.

DYSPLASTIC NEVI

Atypical nevi or dysplastic nevi are atypical appearing melanocytic nevi. Dysplastic nevi are markers of risk as well as potential precursors of melanoma. Clinically, the lesions vary in color and have irregular, ill-defined borders (Figs. 59-17 to 59-20)(Color Plates 20 thru 23). Histologically the lesions have (1) a proliferation of intraepidermal melanocytes disposed singly and/or in irregular nests in the epidermis in a lentiginous pattern and (2) cellular atypia of the melanocytes. People with dysplastic nevi have a 7- to 70-fold increased risk of developing melanoma and a lifetime melanoma risk of 18 percent. Individuals with dysplastic nevi who have a personal or family history of melanoma have a higher lifetime risk of developing melanoma that approaches 100 percent. One prospective study showed that there was a 57-fold increased risk of developing melanoma in people with dysplastic nevi without a family history of melanoma, and a 400-fold increased risk of developing melanoma if people with dysplastic nevi had a personal or family history of melanoma.

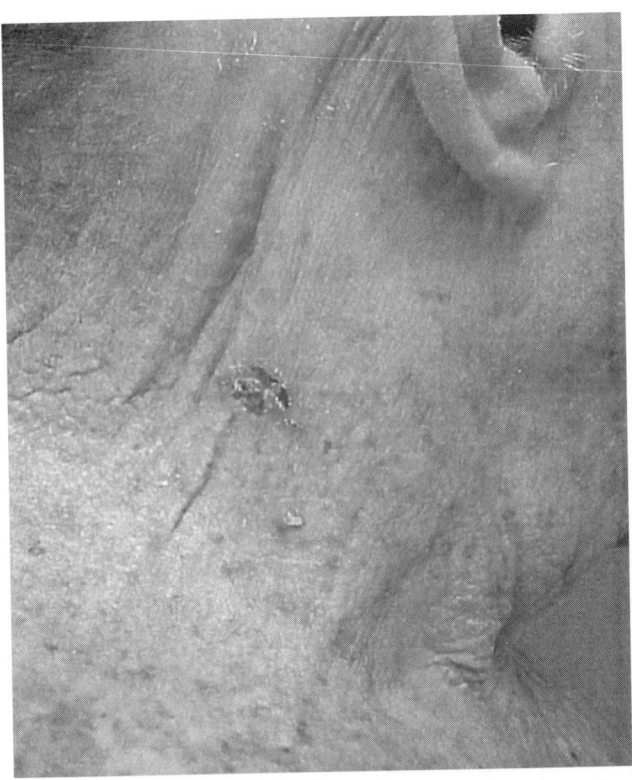

Figure 59-18 Basal cell carcinoma, ulcerated. An ulcerated erythematous indurated basal cell carcinoma on the neck. There is extensive surrounding actinic damage.

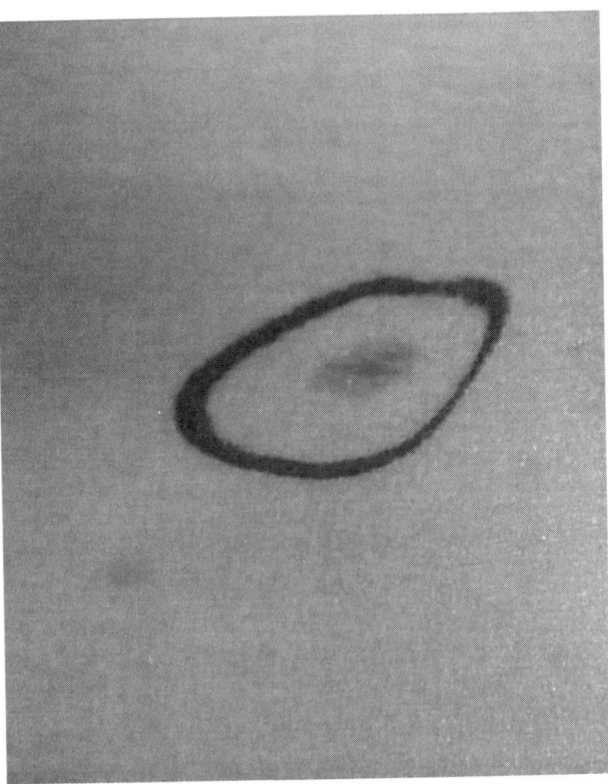

Figure 59-19 Compound melanocytic nevus, atypical. Atypical nevus is the NIH consensus conference's preferred terminology for a dysplastic nevus. Clinically, the lesions have variation in color, and they have irregular ill-defined borders. Histologically, they have architectural disorder and cytologic atypia.

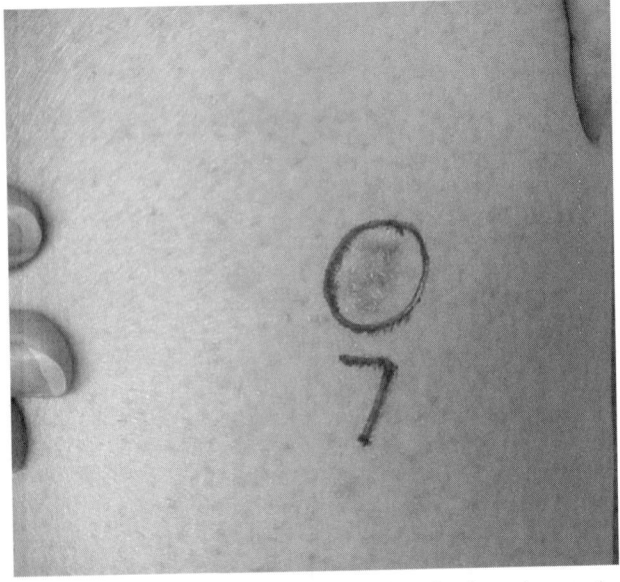

Figure 59-17 A superficial multicentric basal cell carcinoma. An erythematous scaling plaque on the thigh.

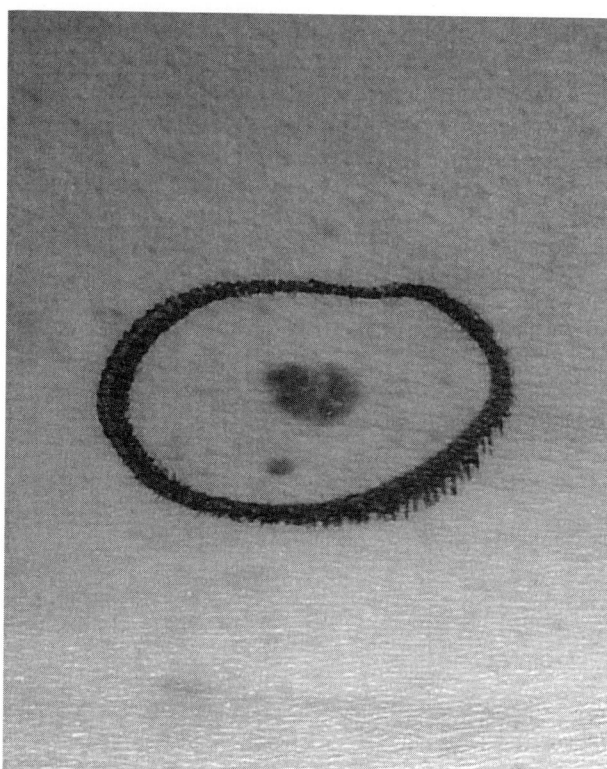

Figure 59-20 Compound melanocytic nevus with architectural disorder and moderate cytologic atypia of melanocytes. Clinically, there is variation in color and irregular ill-defined borders. This lesion requires biopsy to differentiate it from melanoma.

MALIGNANT MELANOMA

Melanoma results from the malignant transformation of melanocytes. Melanoma represents about 3 percent of all cancers by incidence (excluding nonmelanoma skin cancers). It is estimated that there will be 55,000 invasive melanomas and 40,000 melanomas *in situ* diagnosed in 2003 in the United States. The incidence of melanoma is increasing. There is an increasing frequency of newly diagnosed melanoma of approximately 3 to 8 percent per year. The lifetime risk for an individual to develop melanoma has increased in the last century. In 1935, it was 1 in 1500 people; in 1960 it was 1 in 600; in 1980 it was 1 in 150; in 1992 it was 1 in 105; in 1996 it was 1 in 88; and in 2000 it was 1 in 75.

The most frequent sites for melanoma to develop in men are the back, chest, arms, head, and neck. The most frequent sites for melanoma to develop in women are the back, lower legs, arms, head, and neck. Risk factors for the development of melanoma include blue eyes, blond or red hair, and light complexion. A tendency to freckle and sunburn and to tan poorly increases the risk by two to three times. People with dysplastic nevi, changing moles, or congenital nevi have an increased risk of melanoma. People with dysplastic nevi who have a personal or family history of melanoma have a 400-fold increased risk of developing a subsequent melanoma. People who are immunosuppressed have a 10-fold increased risk of melanoma. The main clinical features of melanoma include variation in the color and pigmentation pattern of the lesion and irregularity of the border and presence of notching. Classically an *ABCDE* rule has been established to help diagnose melanomas clinically. *A* stands for asymmetry of the lesion, *B* for irregularity of the borders, *C* for variation in color, *D* for diameter greater than 6 mm, and *E* for elevation of the lesion. However, it must be noted that melanomas are commonly less than 6 mm when diagnosed early, particularly when they develop from dysplastic nevi. Also, melanomas can be completely unpigmented (amelanotic melanoma).

Historically, there are four types of melanoma: lentigo maligna melanoma, superficial spreading melanoma, nodular melanoma, and acral lentiginous melanoma. Although these types of melanomas have been subdivided based on clinical features, it is likely that the biologic behavior of all melanomas can be described by their radial growth phase and vertical growth phase. The radial growth phase is the peripheral spread along the basal layer of the epidermis and upper papillary dermis. The vertical growth phase is the invasion of the papillary and reticular dermis and subcutaneous tissue.

The lentigo maligna melanoma comprises approximately 10 percent of all melanomas and is a pigmented macular lesion with variation in black and brown color. These lesions have irregular outlines and slowly enlarge over many years. They are most common on the sun-exposed areas of the face, arms, or hands. The malignant cells often extend down hair follicles and skin appendages making the lesion difficult to cure by superficial treatments. After many years, a palpable nodule develops that represents entry into the vertical growth phase. Superficial spreading melanoma comprises approximately 70 percent of all melanomas. They are most common on the trunk of males and on the legs of females. They develop as a spreading, pigmented plaque that often has areas of regression (Figs. 59-21 to 59-26)(Color Plates 24 thru 29). This can result in reddish-pink to white area within the black or brown tumor. They

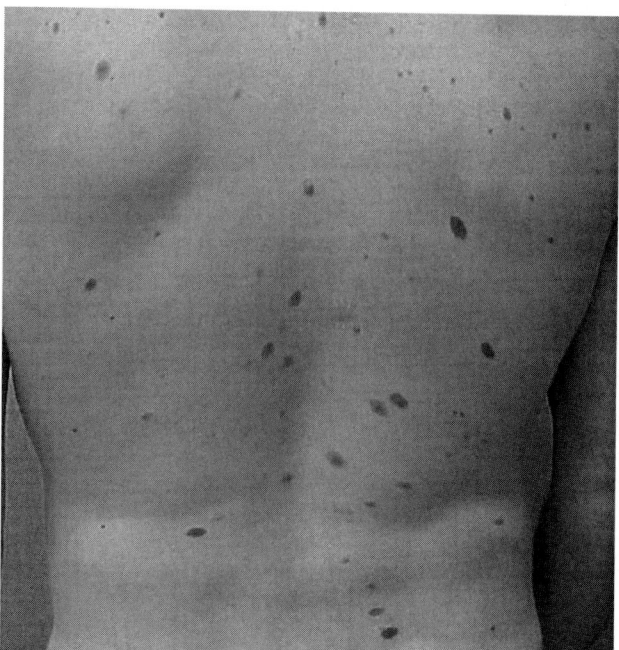

Figure 59-21 Dysplastic nevi, multiple. This patient has multiple two-toned nevi with irregular ill-defined borders.

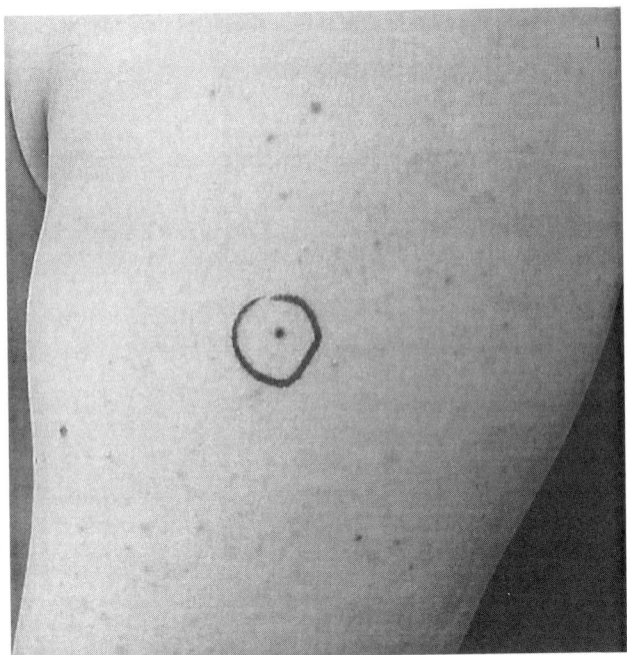

Figure 59-22 Lentiginous junctional melanocytic nevus with architectural disorder and mild cytologic atypia. This atypical nevus on the arm was inflamed. Dysplastic nevi and melanomas can be small (1 to 3 mm).

spread into a vertical growth phase faster than the lentigo maligna.

Nodular melanoma usually arises without evidence of a preexisting lesion. They constitute approximately 20 percent of melanomas and have a minimal radial growth phase. These tumors are more aggressive and often appear as raised or polypoid darkly pigmented lesions, which may become ulcerated. Acral lentiginous melanoma represents approximately 5 percent of melanoma and usually occurs on the hands or feet or beneath the nails. Usually they are flat lesions that show variable pigmentation ranging from dark or brown to light appearance. Melanomas under the nail can show a brown to black discoloration of the nail bed.

Survival prognosis can be estimated by the Clark anatomic level of invasion or the Breslow tumor thickness.

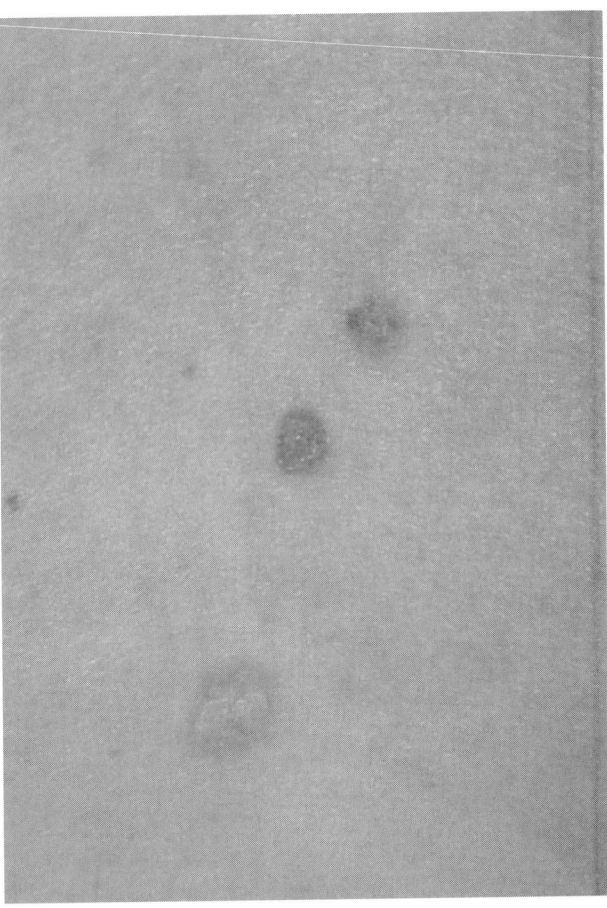

Figure 59-24 Malignant melanoma superficial spreading type (Clarks level III, Breslow 0.73mm) Irregular surface, an irregular border, and variation in color are signs of a superficial spreading melanoma on the back in a man with multiple dysplastic nevi.

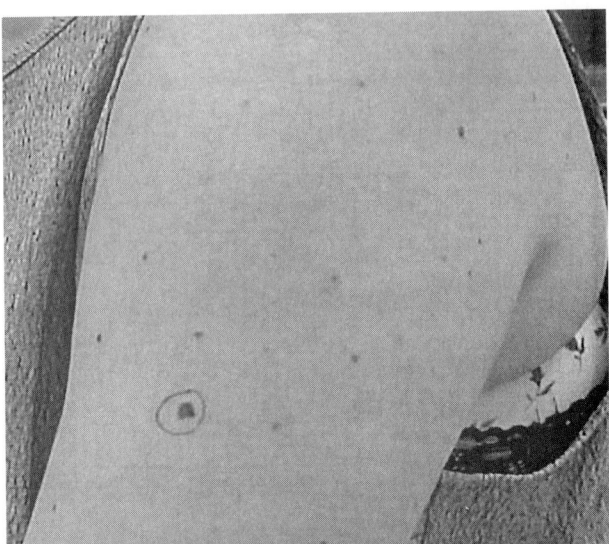

Figure 59-25 Superficial spreading malignant melanoma (Clarks level II, Breslow 0.26 mm). Two-toned lesion with irregular ill-defined borders in a patient with multiple dysplastic nevi and previous melanomas. This lesion did not look as suspicious as som of her other pigmented lesions, which, histologically, were atypical nevi (dysplastic nevi). Excision and histological examination is often required to distinguish dysplastic nevi from melanoma.

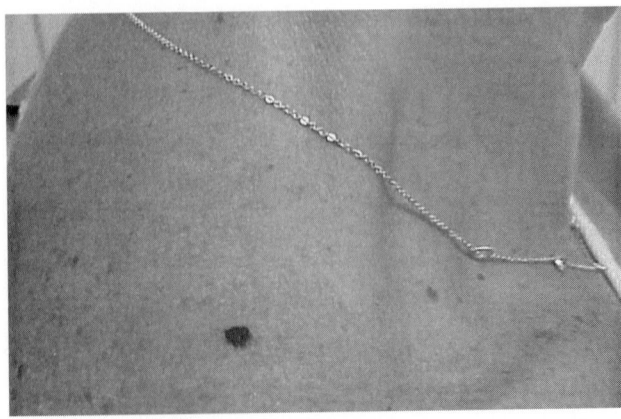

Figure 59-23 Superficial spreading malignant melanoma. (Clarks level III, Breslow 0.62 mm) deeply pigmented lesion with irregular borders on shoulder developing over 6 months.

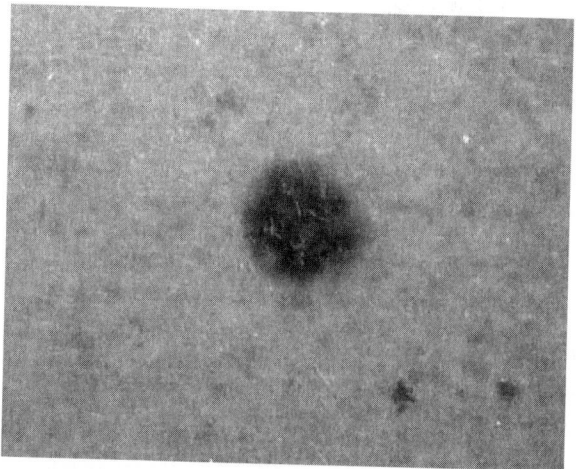

Figure 59-26 Superficial spreading malignant melanoma (Clarks level II, Breslow 0.48 mm). Two-toned lesion with irregular ill-defined border, asymmetry and notching on the back.

In clinical dermatopathologic practice, both measures are usually reported. Clark level I is confined to the epidermis. Clark level II has tumor cells invading into the papillary dermis and has a 99 percent 5-year survival. Clark level III has tumor cells filling the papillary dermis and has a 95 percent 5-year survival. Clark level IV has tumor cells into the reticular dermis and has a 75 percent 5-year survival. Clark level V has tumor cells into the subcutaneous tissue and has a 39 percent 5-year survival.

Five-year survival based on Breslow's tumor thickness measurement is: <0.85-mm thickness, 99 percent survival; 0.85- to 1.69-mm thickness, 95 percent survival; 1.70- to 3.64-mm thickness, 78 percent survival; >3.65-mm thickness, 42 percent survival.

Melanoma in situ may be defined as intraepidermal melanocytic proliferation showing fully evolved cellular atypia that is side-to-side and continuous for a distance of at least two epidermal rete ridges (0.17 mm). Melanoma is feared because of its tendency to metastasize. The risk of metastasis is correlated with the primary tumor thickness: <0.76-mm thickness has a 2 to 3 percent incidence of lymph node metastasis in 3 years; 0.76 to 1.49 mm has a 25 percent incidence of lymph node metastasis in 3 years; 1.5 to 4.0 mm has a 57 percent incidence of lymph node metastasis in 3 years; and >4.0 mm has a 62 percent of lymph node metastasis in 3 years. Melanoma spreads most frequently to the skin, subcutaneous tissue, and lymph nodes. Visceral metastases manifest in the lungs, liver, brain, bone, and intestines.

Treatment of Primary Melanoma

Surgical excision of the primary tumor has been the standard therapy for malignant melanoma. The tumors are usually excised with a 1- to 3-cm margin of normal tissue. In recent years, a number of dermatologic surgeons have employed Mohs micrographic surgery as the treatment of choice for primary melanomas. Examination of the entire periphery of the excised tissue by the Mohs technique permits a narrower 1-cm excision margin in most cases. Approximately 5 percent of primary melanomas and 16 percent of recurrent melanomas will require larger margins as determined by Mohs surgery. Sentinel lymph node mapping to aid in the staging of patients with melanomas greater than 1 mm thick is advocated by some clinicians. In one study, the 5-year disease-free survival rate in patients with a negative sentinel node biopsy was 91 percent, in contrast to 49 percent for patients with a positive biopsy. It is not proven whether sentinel lymph node biopsy has any effect on survival and it adds significantly to the cost of managing a primary melanoma.

UNUSUAL TUMORS

There are a number of less-common cutaneous tumors that are beyond the scope of this chapter. The reader is referred to a standard dermatology text for discussion of

Merkel cell carcinoma
Cutaneous T-cell lymphoma and mycosis fungoides
Cutaneous B-cell lymphoma
Histiocytic tumors
Mast cell tumors
Malignant adnexal tumors

  hair follicle origin: malignant proliferating tricholemmal tumor, tricholemmoma carcinoma, malignant pilomatrixoma
  eccrine gland origin: malignant eccrine poroma, hidradenocarcinoma, malignant chondroid syringoma, malignant spiradenoma, malignant cylindroma, eccrine ductal carcinoma, mucoepidermoid carcinoma, microcystic adnexal carcinoma, eccrine epithelioma, adenoid cystic carcinoma, mucinous carcinoma, aggressive digital papillary adenocarcinoma
  Apocrine gland origin: extramammary Paget's disease, apocrine adenocarcinoma
  Sebaceous gland origin: sebaceous epithelioma, sebaceous carcinoma

Cutaneous sarcoma: fibrosarcoma, malignant fibrous histiocytoma, dermatofibrosarcoma protuberans, liposarcoma, synovial sarcoma, leiomyosarcoma, rhabdomyosarcoma, malignant nerve sheath tumor, angiosarcoma, lymphangiosarcoma, malignant hemangiopericytoma, Kaposi's sarcoma, alveolar soft part sarcoma, epithelioid sarcoma of Enzinger, clear cell sarcoma of tendons and aponeuroses, extraskeletal osteosarcoma, extraskeletal chondrosarcoma
Metastatic cancer to the skin

REFERENCES

Anderson S et al: Relationship between Bowen's disease and internal malignant tumors. *Arch Dermatol* 108:367, 1973.

Baker SR, Swanson N: Complete microscopic controlled surgery for head and neck cancer. *Head Neck Surg* 6:914, 1984.

Balin AK et al: Actinic keratosis. *J Cutan Aging Cosmet Dermatol* 1:77, 1988.

Batra RS, Kelley LC: Predictors of extensive subclinical spread in non-melanoma skin cancer treated with Mohs micrographic surgery. *Arch Dermatol* 138:1043, 2002.

Bernardeau K et al: Cryosurgery of basal cell carcinoma: A study of 358 patients. *Ann Dermatol Venereol* 127:175, 2000.

Cottel W: Mohs surgery, fresh-tissue technique. *J Dermatol Surg Oncol* 8;576, 1982.

Czarnecki D et al: The majority of cutaneous squamous cell carcinomas arise in actinic keratoses. *J Cutan Med Surg* 6;207, 2002.

Engel A et al: Health effects of sunlight exposure in the United States. Results from the first National Health and Nutritional Examination Survey, 1971–1974. *Arch Dermatol* 124:72, 1988.

Freedberg I et al. (eds): *Dermatology in General Medicine,* 5th ed. New York, McGraw-Hill, 1999 p 1.

Field LM: On the value of dermabrasion in the management of actinic keratoses, in Epstein E (ed): *Controversies in Dermatology.* Philadelphia, W B Saunders, 1984 p 96.

Gloster HM, Brodland DG: The epidemiology of skin cancer. *Dermatol Surg* 22:217, 1996.

Graham JH, Helwig EB: Cutaneous premalignant lesions, in Montagna W, Dobson RF (eds): *Advances in Biology of the Skin: Carcinogenesis.* Oxford, Pergamon, 1966 p 277.

Gray DT et al: Trends in the population-based incidence of squamous cell carcinoma of the skin first diagnosed between 1984 and 1992. *Arch Dermatol* 133:735, 1997.

Henriksen T et al: Ultraviolet-radiation and skin cancer. Effect of an ozone layer depletion. *Photochem Photobiol* 51:579, 1990.

Lang PG: Current concepts in the management of patients with melanoma. *Am J Clin Dermatol* 3:401, 2002.

Langley R et al: Neoplasms: Cutaneous melanoma, in Freedberg I et al. (eds): *Dermatology in General Medicine,* 5th ed. New York, McGraw-Hill, 1999 p 1080.

Marks R et al: Malignant transformation of solar keratoses to squamous cell carcinoma. *Lancet* 1:795, 1988.

Marks R et al: Spontaneous remission of solar keratosis: The case of conservative management. *Br J Dermatol* 115:649, 1986.

Mohs FE: Carcinoma of the skin: A summary of therapeutic results, in *Chemosurgery–Microscopically Controlled Surgery for Skin Cancer.* Springfield, IL, Charles C. Thomas Publishers, 1978 p 153.

Moller R et al: Metastases in dermatological patients with squamous cell carcinoma. *Arch Dermatol* 115:703, 1979.

Montgomery H: Keratosis senilis, in Ormsby OS, Montgomery H (eds): *Diseases of the Skin,* 8th ed. Philadelphia, Lea and Febiger, 1955, p 846.

Orengo IF et al: Celecoxib, a cyclooxygenase 2 inhibitor as a potential chemopreventive to UV-induced skin cancer. A study in the hairless mouse model. *Arch Dermatol* 138:751, 2002.

Ormrod D, Jarvis B: Topical aminolevulinic acid HCl photodynamic therapy. *Am J Clin Dermatol* 1:133, 2000.

Penn I: Immunosuppression and skin cancer. *Clin Plast Surg* 7:361, 1980.

Rowe DE et al: Long-term recurrence rates in previously untreated (primary) basal cell carcinoma: Implications for patient follow-up. *J Dermatol Surg Oncol* 15:315, 1989.

Silverman MK et al: Recurrence rates of treated basal cell carcinoma, part 3: Surgical excision. *J Dermatol Surg Oncol* 18:471, 1992.

Stockfleth E et al: Successful treatment of actinic keratosis with imiquimod cream 5%: A report of six cases. *Br J Dermatol* 144:1050, 2001.

Tiersten AD et al: Prospective follow-up for malignant melanoma in patients with atypical-mole (dysplastic nevus) syndrome. *J Dermatol Surg Oncol* 17:44, 1991.

Ziegler A et al: Sunburn and p53 in the onset of skin cancer. *Nature* 372:773, 1994.

Aging of the Hematopoietic System

GURKAMAL S. CHATTA • DAVID A. LIPSCHITZ

NORMAL BONE MARROW FUNCTION

Hematopoiesis is regulated by a complex series of interactions between hematopoietic cells, their stromal microenvironment, and diffusible regulatory molecules that affect cellular proliferation. The orderly development of the hematopoietic system in vivo and the maintenance of homeostasis require that a strict balance be maintained between self-renewal, differentiation, maturation, and cell loss. Within the hematopoietic system, populations of terminally differentiated cells are continually entering the peripheral blood, to be replaced by cells from a transit or amplification compartment. Our understanding of human hematopoiesis has increased exponentially over the last decade. However most of the initial breakthroughs in the biology of hematopoiesis occurred in murine models.

MURINE HEMATOPOIESIS

The earliest morphologically recognizable cells of the myeloid and erythroid series are the myeloblasts and proerythroblasts (Fig. 60-1). These cells are derived from the morphologically unrecognizable progenitors that can only be identified by appropriate in vitro culture techniques. There are two forms of erythroid progenitors: a more primitive precursor, which forms large colonies in cultures containing high concentrations of erythropoietin, and is referred to as a burst-forming unit–erythroid (BFU-E), and a more mature progenitor referred to as the colony-forming unit–erythroid (CFU-E). A committed myeloid progenitor, also known as colony-forming unit–granulocyte/macrophage (CFU-GM), is the immediate precursor of the myeloblast. The committed progenitor cell compartments are supplied, in turn, by a common pluripotent stem cell, which is derived from totipotential stem cells that have the capacity to differentiate into either hematopoietic or lymphoid cells. Figure 60-1 shows the hierarchy of cellular proliferation and differentiation in this pathway. The pluripotent hematopoietic stem cell is also called a colony-forming unit–spleen (CFU-S) by virtue

of its ability to produce colonies in spleens of lethally irradiated mice. The CFU-S is also capable of repopulating the marrow of irradiated recipients and preventing marrow failure. A unique feature of the CFU-S compartment is its ability to both renew and to differentiate. The CFU-S is the earliest hematopoietic cell that can be satisfactorily assayed and constitutes a powerful research tool for studying differentiation and growth control. There is evidence that the number of CFU-S in cell cycle is minimal, but that cycling can be greatly increased if demands for regeneration are increased. Most evidence suggests that regulation of proliferative control is local and is presumably mediated by the environmental milieu.

Effect of Age on CFU-S

A major question with regard to the aging hematopoietic system is whether or not the pluripotent hematopoietic stem cell has a finite replicative capacity. There is evidence that the CFU-S has a heterogeneous self-renewal capacity and an age structure in which a young CFU-S with high self-renewal capacity produces older CFU-S with decreasing self-renewal capacity and increasing differentiation potential. This hypothesis has been strengthened by studies of long-term bone marrow culture, which show that maintenance of hematopoiesis in long-term bone marrow cultures varies inversely with the age of the donor from which the culture was initiated. Additional evidence for a finite replicative capacity for stem cells has been obtained in a series of elegant studies in which stem cell kinetics and myeloid cell production was examined in long-term bone marrow cultures subjected to varying doses of irradiation.

Studies using serial transplantation to assess finite replicative capacity have yielded conflicting results. When cells are subjected to in vivo serial transfer by repeated injection into lethally irradiated recipients, they gradually lose their ability to self-replicate. There is evidence that CFU-S from young donors are better able to repopulate the marrow of irradiated mice than stem cells obtained from old donors. The growth capacity of old stem cells remains

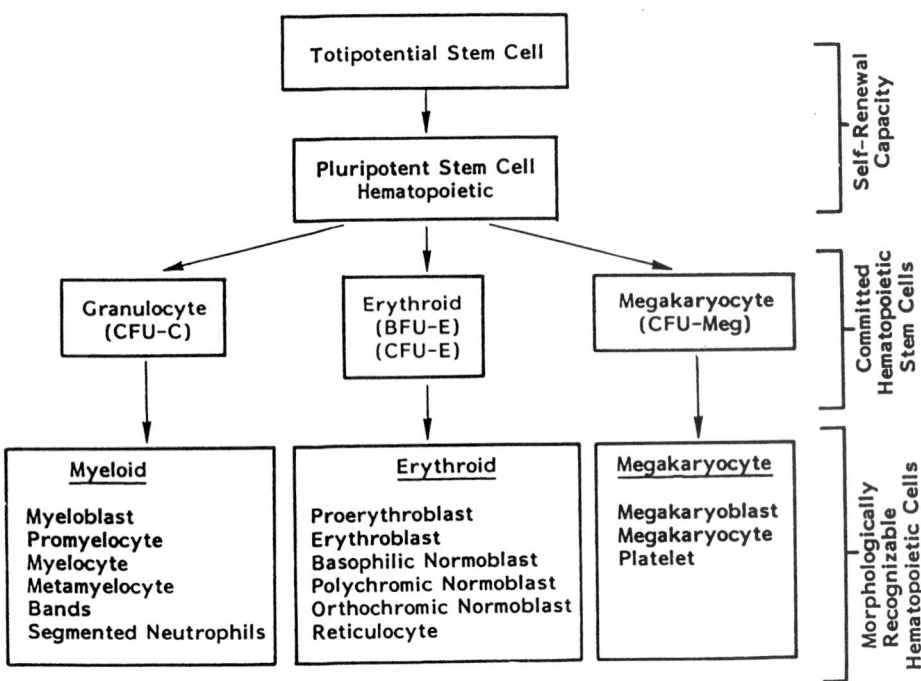

Figure 60-1 The hierarchy and production of hematopoietic precursors from primitive pluripotent stem cells.

characteristically old, even after prolonged self-replication in the bone marrow of young recipients. This fact suggests an intrinsic characteristic of the CFU-S that cannot readily be altered. However, the spleen colony growth capacity of young stem cells can be reduced by allowing them to self-replicate in old recipients. Thus, the rate at which young cells age can be accelerated by allowing them to replicate in old recipients. There are also data that CFU-S decline minimally, or not at all, with age. Recent evidence suggests that results of earlier serial transplant studies were related to methodologic artifact. Given the availability of stage-specific membrane markers, it is now possible to distinguish between long-term (LTR) and short-term (STR) repopulating cells, and thus more accurately dissect the changes in the sub-types of CFU-S with age. Studies on isolated bone marrow cells bearing the phenotype of LTR stem cells, Thy-1^{lo} Sca-1^{hi} Lin^{neg}, from young and old mice revealed that there was a fivefold increase in the frequency of cells with the stem cell phenotype, from older mice. However, their functional capacity was only a quarter of that seen with these cells from younger mice. Even if its life span is finite, it is clear that the CFU-S has a reserve capacity to produce adequate numbers of hematopoietic cells for periods that far exceed the maximum life expectancy of the animal.

Effect of Normal Aging on Bone Marrow Function

The effect of age on committed hematopoietic stem cell number and on the number of differentiated hematopoietic bone marrow cells has also been examined. In mice no age-related reduction in the number of erythroid (BFU-E, CFU-E) or myeloid/macrophage (CFU-GM) progenitor

cells occurs. In addition, the number of differentiated erythroid and myeloid precursors in the bone marrow is unaffected by age in normal animals. Erythrokinetic studies show that red blood cell survival is unchanged with aging, the plasma iron turnover and erythron iron turnover are unchanged, and the red blood cell mass is normal. The apparent anemia frequently observed in aged mice appears to be caused by an expansion of plasma volume. These findings and those of others indicate that no change in basal hematopoiesis occurs with aging. However, the ability of the aged hematopoietic system to respond to increased demands appears to be compromised. For example, older mice recover their hemoglobin values more slowly after phlebotomy than do young mice. Furthermore, when aged animals are placed in a high-altitude chamber, the expected increase in hemoglobin level is more variable and tends to be lower in older, as compared with younger, animals. Interpretation of data with phlebotomy or exposure to high altitude is difficult because many other physiologic variables determine the measured hematopoietic response.

One approach that allows the study of hematopoiesis while minimizing other variables is to induce polycythemia in mice by injecting homologous red cells. This results in a predictable switching off of erythropoiesis that is characterized by marked decreases in the number bone marrow BFU-E and CFU-E. When erythropoietin is injected into these animals, a measurable wave of erythropoiesis occurs. Twenty-four hours after injection, bone marrow CFU-E and proerythroblasts are significantly increased. After 48 hours, polychromic and orthochromic normoblasts are elevated. Between 48 and 72 hours, these cells leave the bone marrow and appear in the blood as reticulocytes. Studies using this model demonstrate that older polycythemic mice develop a smaller wave of erythropoiesis after erythropoietin injection than do younger animals. The decrease in response does not, however, universally affect all erythroid precursors. Thus, the increase in proerythroblasts and normoblasts (differentiated cell) after the injection of erythropoietin is significantly less in old, as compared with young, animals. In contrast, the increase in the committed erythroid progenitor cell number (CFU-E) after erythropoietin injection was identical in both young and old animals, suggesting that a uniform defect in the proliferative response of all cells does not occur with aging.

The fragility of the aged hematopoietic system is further highlighted by studies on mice approaching their maximal life expectancy. The median life span of C57BL/6 mice is 24 months, and the maximum reported life expectancy is 48 months. If 48-month-old mice are housed in individual cages (one animal per cage), no change in hematopoiesis is seen. If, however, they are housed in groups of five animals per cage, a significant alteration in bone marrow function occurs. The animals become more anemic and the number of stem cells in their bone marrow decreases. This observation indicates that a minor stress, which does not affect hematopoiesis in young animals, causes significant abnormalities in aged animals.

THE EFFECT OF AGE ON HEMATOPOIESIS IN HUMANS

Normal Hematopoiesis

The human hematopoietic system derives from a small pool of stem cells that can either self-renew or differentiate along one of several lineages to form mature leukocytes, erythrocytes, or platelets. Marrow progenitors can be enriched on the basis of surface markers expressed at sequential stages of maturation. With respect to the myeloid lineage, the relevant surface markers are CD33 and CD34. CD33 is found on most cells of the myeloid lineage in the marrow, and CD34 is expressed only by more primitive progenitors (1 to 4 percent of the marrow cells). Because CD34+ marrow cells can engraft and reconstitute hematopoiesis in lethally irradiated baboons and humans, surface expression of CD34 on marrow and circulating cells, serves as a surrogate for stem cell function.

Proliferation and differentiation of progenitor cells to become mature blood cells requires intimate contact between stem cells, stromal cells and the extracellular matrix, and is thought to be mediated by the hematopoietic growth factors (HGFs). The HGFs are produced by multiple cell types and, on the basis of their actions, are characterized either as multilineage hematopoietins, for example, stem cell factor (SCF), or mast cell growth factor (MGF), interleukin-3 (IL-3), and granulocyte-macrophage colony-stimulating factor (GM-CSF); or as lineage restricted hematopoietins, for example, granulocyte colony-stimulating factor (G-CSF), macrophage colony-stimulating factor (M-CSF), erythropoietin (EPO), thrombopoietin (TPO), and T cell growth factor (IL-2). In addition to the above growth factors, lymphohematopoiesis is also modulated by an ever-expanding list of other cytokines (Table 60-1). These are produced by diverse cell types, have

Table 60-1   Cytokines Modulating Hematopoiesis

Lymphokine	Major Biological Properties
IL-1	Activates resting T cells; induces fever; activates endothelial cells and macrophages
IL-2	Growth factor for activated T-cells; synthesis of other lymphokines
IL-3	Supports growth of multilineage bone marrow stem cells
IL-6	B-cell growth factor
IL-7	B-cell and T-cell growth factor
IL-12	Differentiation of naive CD4 T cells to the Th1 subset
Stem cell factor (SCF)	Promotes proliferation of primitive progenitors
Granulocyte-macrophage colony-stimulating factor (GM-CSF)	Promotes growth of neutrophilic, eosinophilic and macrophage cell lineages
Granulocyte CSF (G-CSF)	Promotes growth of neutrophilic cells
Macrophage CSF (M-CSF)	Promotes growth of monocytes and macrophage
Erythropoietin (EPO)	Promotes growth of erythroid cells
Thrombopoietin (TPO)	Stimulates megakaryocyte and platelet production

CSF, colony-stimulating factor; IL, interleukin.

wide-ranging biological effects, and participate in a variety of cellular responses. Currently, G-CSF, GM-CSF, EPO, and IL-2 are in common clinical use.

G-CSF is a 24-kilodalton (kDa) glycoprotein that promotes the growth and maturation of myeloid cells and in particular, the proliferation and differentiation of neutrophil progenitors both in vitro and in vivo. There are two recombinant forms of G-CSF currently in use. Filgrastim (produced in *Escherichia coli*) is nonglycosylated, is smaller (19 kDa) in size than the native molecule, but has the same biological activity. Lenograstim is recombinant glycosylated human G-CSF, and at least in vitro, is reportedly more potent than the nonglycosylated form. Phase III studies established the safety and efficacy of recombinant human (rh) G-CSF in ameliorating chemotherapy-related neutropenia in cancer patients and for the treatment of severe chronic neutropenia. G-CSF is also being increasingly used for the purposes of mobilizing peripheral blood stem cells (PBSCs). It is usually administered subcutaneously, is well tolerated, and other than medullary bone pain and a skin rash at the site of injection, no significant side effects have been reported.

GM-CSF is a glycosylated 22-kDa peptide that has a broader range of cellular targets than G-CSF. The two forms of recombinant human GM-CSF currently in use are sargramostim (glycosylated or yeast-derived) and molgramostim (nonglycosylated or *E. coli*-derived). The yeast-derived form is reported to have a lower incidence of causing skin rashes. In clinical trials, the effects of rhGM-CSF both on abrogating neutropenia and in mobilizing PBSCs are very similar to those of G-CSF. However, because of its wider spectrum of biologic effects, GM-CSF has more systemic toxicity and at high dosage levels, the capillary leak syndrome is a particular concern. EPO is a 34- to 39-kDa glycoprotein that selectively acts on the erythroid lineage. The recombinant product (epoetin alfa) has a molecular weight of 30 kDa and has been in clinical use since 1985, particularly in patients with end-stage renal disease (ESRD) on dialysis. It is well tolerated and most of its side effects, that is, thromboembolic phenomena, have been described in the setting of dialysis.

Age-Related Changes in Lymphohematopoiesis

The evaluation of hematopoiesis in older humans is made exceedingly difficult by the complex interaction of environmental variables with the host over extended periods of time. Figure 60-2 illustrates the large number of factors that may modulate erythropoietic function in elderly subjects.

An extensive study performed on a group of carefully selected, hematologically normal (Table 60-2) healthy young and elderly subjects, revealed no significant differences in peripheral blood or ferrokinetic data. Furthermore, quantitation of marrow progenitors and differentiated precursors demonstrated no significant differences between the young and the elderly group. A series of longitudinal studies of hematologic parameters on a group of affluent subjects in New Mexico also demonstrated no obvious hematologic problem, and no abnormalities developed during a 3-year follow-up. Based upon these observations and the animal studies described above, the aging process is thought to primarily affect stimulus-driven hematopoiesis, with little or no impact on the basal state. The blunted hematopoietic response to stress has been ascribed to age-related deficits in marrow progenitor cell numbers, changes in the marrow microenvironment, decreased production of regulatory growth factors, or a combination of these mechanisms. However, in a number of areas the data are conflicting. This is partly a result of the tremendous heterogeneity of the aging process and partly a result of the difficulty in separating the effects of age per se from the effects of occult diseases. The effects of age on lymphohematopoiesis are summarized in the following sections.

Myeloid Lineage
Hematopoietic Progenitors

Studies on marrow hematopoietic progenitors in the gerontologic literature report increased, decreased and no change in colony numbers in aging humans. When isolated

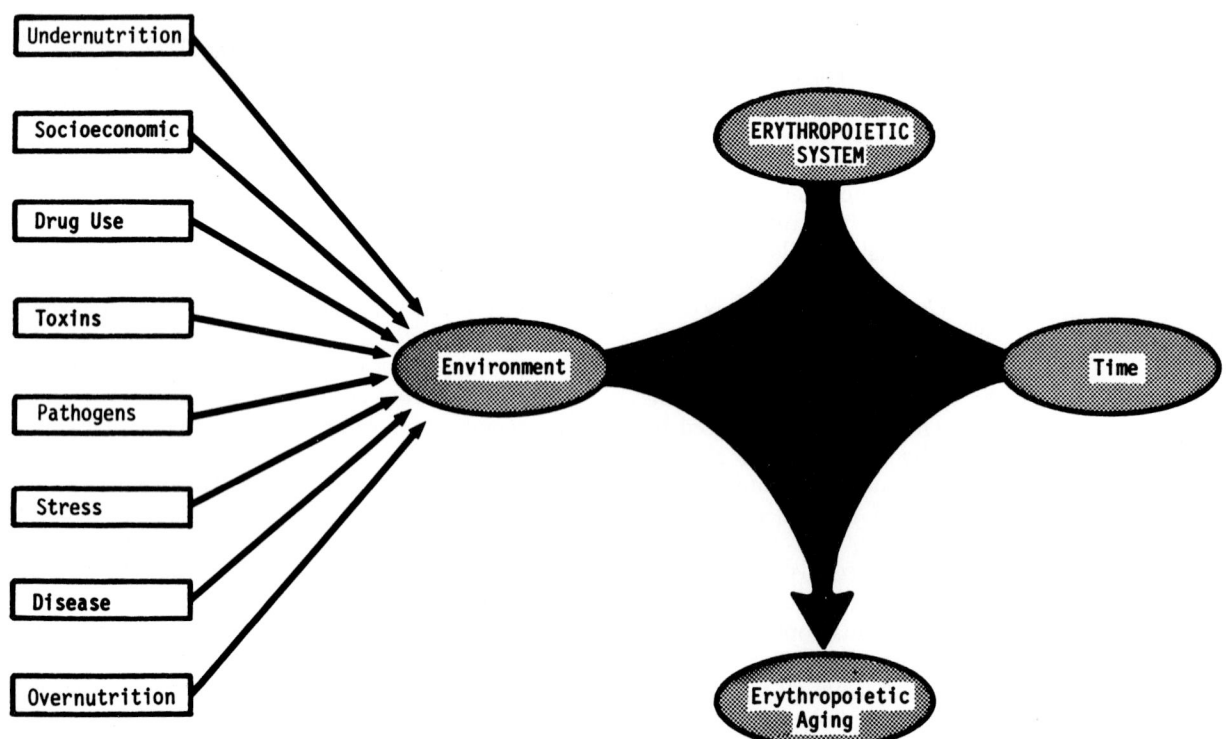

Figure 60-2   External variables likely to modify age-related decrements in erythropoiesis.

Table 60-2   Hematologic Profile in Young and Elderly Hematologically Normal Subjects

	Young	Elderly
Age (years)	34.0 ± 2.0*	78.0 ± 2.0
Hemoglobin (g/dL)	15.4 ± 0.3	15.0 ± 0.2
Mean corpuscular volume (fl)	89.0 ± 0.9	90.7 ± 1.8
Serum iron (μg/dL)	107.0 ± 8.1	93.0 ± 5.0
TIBC (μg/dL)	297.0 ± 10.0	307.0 ± 13.0
Saturation (%)	36.0 ± 3.0	30.1 ± 2.2
Serum ferritin (ng/mL)	126.0 ± 17.0	219.0 ± 26.0
Proto:heme (μmol/mol)	24.4 ± 1.4	22.0 ± 1.8
Vitamin B12 (μg/mL)	476.0 ± 34.0	451.0 ± 34.0
Serum folate (ng/mL)	5.6 ± 0.8	4.8 ± 0.5
Retic index	1.1 ± 0.3	1.0 ± 0.2
Leukocyte (×10³/μL	8.8 ± 0.4	7.6 ± 0.5
Neutrophils (×10³/μL)	5.9 ± 0.3	4.5 ± 0.6
Lymphocyte (×10³/μL)	1.9 ± 0.8	1.9 ± 0.3
Platelet (×10³/μL)	361.0 ± 38.0	277.0 ± 2.1
EIT[†]	0.5 ± 0.1	0.5 ± 0.1
Total myeloid precursors (× 10⁹ cells/kg)	38.0 ± 16.0	40.0 ± 15.0
CFU-C (−10⁶/kg)	0.9 ± 0.3	0.7 ± 0.2

*Mean ± SE.

[†] Erythron iron turnover (mg/dL whole blood per day).

marrow CD34+ cells from the young and elderly persons were assayed in culture, similar proportions of committed marrow progenitors, that is, CD34+ marrow cells, were found in the two groups. However "in vitro" colony formation by marrow CD34+ cells from elderly individuals required a twofold higher concentration of G-CSF to induce equivalent levels of colony formation as the young. In contrast to the reduced sensitivity of the marrow CD34+ cells to G-CSF of elderly persons, there was no age-related difference in progenitor responsiveness to GM-CSF and IL-3. The number of subjects evaluated in all these studies was relatively small, and at present, in humans there are no reports on the effects of age on the very primitive marrow progenitors, that is, CD34+Lin− cells. Compared to marrow progenitors, there is little information on circulating progenitors. However, it has been reported that at least in response to G-CSF, the ability of elderly persons to mobilize peripheral blood colony-forming cells is reduced. This is of potential clinical significance, given the increasing use of cytokine-mobilized PBSC as a part of high-dose chemotherapy protocols.

Telomere length, which is known to correlate with the replication history of somatic cells, has also been investigated in hematopoietic cells: adult CD34+ CD38lo stem cells have shorter telomeres than their counterparts from fetal liver and umbilical cord blood; blood cell telomeres of marrow transplant recipients were 0.4 kilobase (kb) (95% confidence interval [CI] 0.2 to 0.6) shorter than those of their respective donors. This suggests that stem cells in humans probably have a finite replicative capacity, which is further attenuated in the presence of replicative stress: the telomere loss in the marrow recipients in the above study being the equivalent of 15 years of aging.

Differentiated Cells

Polymorphonuclear neutrophils   Polymorphonuclear neutrophils (PMNs) phagocytose and kill bacteria by the generation of a series of toxic radicals and microbicidal halogens and by the release of a series of enzymes located in neutrophil granules. The process of bacterial killing is associated with a 100-fold increase in neutrophil metabolism and oxygen uptake and the reaction is referred to as the respiratory burst. Thus PMN function can be assessed by exposing PMNs to a series of chemotactic peptides or other reagents, which stimulate the respiratory burst and evaluating oxygen metabolism in the cells. Alternatively, the end products of the respiratory burst, that is, the generation of superoxide, can be measured.

Using these approaches, a series of studies revealed that the respiratory burst activity of neutrophils from elderly individuals was decreased and the level of various neutrophil enzymes secreted during degranulation was reduced. PMNs from elderly volunteers had impaired release of the second messengers, inositol triphosphate and diacylglycerol, and as a consequence reduced mobilization of calcium to the cytosol. Further studies demonstrated the prime defect with age to be a decline in the concentration of the metabolically active phosphoinositide precursors of inositol triphosphate and diacylglycerol. This defect in PMN function is not large enough to interfere with the ability of neutrophils from the elderly person to phagocytose or to kill bacteria. However, this diminution in PMN reserve capacity does have relevance. When old mice are made protein-deficient, PMN function decreases to a level where the ability of the PMNs to phagocytose and kill bacteria is severely compromised. This observation maybe a partial explanation for the high prevalence of serious bacterial infections in hospitalized older individuals who are also frequently malnourished.

Other studies evaluating different aspects of PMN function in aging, that is, adherence, chemotaxis, phagocytosis, microbicidal capability, and response to cytokines, report that neither PMN counts nor PMN function at the level of the individual cell are significantly altered with aging. Neutrophil production has been found to be reduced in healthy elderly individuals, as reflected by endotoxin measurements of the bone marrow neutrophil reserves, and others have demonstrated reduced mobilization of marrow neutrophils in the elderly person in response to a steroid challenge. Although the basis of this suboptimal PMN response to endotoxin and steroids is unclear, at least in the healthy elderly person, both neutrophil production and function can be upregulated to levels comparable to young adults with the exogenous administration of G-CSF.

Monocytes and macrophages   Circulating monocytes are transformed into tissue macrophages and are the principle cells for processing antigens. Their number and function are not effected significantly by the aging process. There is little information on age-related changes (if any) in the ability of dendritic cells to process and present antigens.

Red cells   Although unexplained anemia is often seen in healthy elderly people, it is unclear whether baseline counts are affected with aging. However, the erythroid response to hematopoietic stress is known to be blunted in aged animals and thought to be suboptimal in elderly persons.

Hematopoietic Growth Factors

The blunted hematopoietic response to stress has been attributed to age-related decrements in growth factor secretion, particularly by marrow stromal cells. However in humans, available data indicates that at least with severe infections, G-CSF levels can rise to a comparable degree in young and elderly patients. Erythropoietin levels in the anemic elderly patient are also not significantly different from young controls, but altered responsiveness of erythroid precursors has been invoked as a possible cause for the unexplained anemia in the healthy elderly people. Animal data is more compelling for age-associated defects in stimulus-driven hematopoiesis: bacterially challenged, aged mice had blunted myelopoiesis when compared to younger animals challenged in a similar fashion.

The production of certain growth factors, that is, IL-6 has also been reported to go up with the aging process. Hence, according to one view, aging is associated with inappropriate underproduction and overproduction of different cytokines leading to a dysregulated hematopoietic state.

Lymphoid Lineage

Most components of the immune system undergo age-related restructuring, leading to both enhanced as well as reduced function in different components. The effect of aging on cell-mediated and humoral immunity is reviewed in detail in Chap. 3. A brief summary is provided here.

T cells, which are effectors of cell-mediated immunity, are bone-marrow derived and undergo maturation in the thymus. Baseline counts are unaltered with aging, and there is a slight increase in the levels of CD4+ cells in the periphery. A hallmark of T-cell aging is the gradual shift from naïve CD45RA+ cells toward an increase in the CD45RO+ activated or memory cells. There is also a decrease in CD62(L-selectin)+ cells, and an increase in CD44^{hi} cells. Additionally, there is an expansion of the natural killer (NK) subset, and an increase in the repertoire of T cells that coexpress NK-cell markers. Thus, with aging, (1) there is an increase in the number of memory cells that proliferate suboptimally, and (2) the presence of a constricted T-cell repertoire for responding to new antigenic challenges.

B cells are bone marrow derived and mediate humoral immunity. B cell responses to a large measure are regulated by T cell subsets. Derangements in B-cell mediated immunity with aging include (1) reduced antibody responses to T-cell–dependent and T-cell–independent antigens; (2) decrease in isoagglutinins; and (3) a rising incidence of autoantibodies and monoclonal gammopathies (10 percent in individuals older than age 80 years). There is an increase in bone marrow B-cell precursors, and there also tends to be a CD5+ B-cell clonal expansion with aging. There is little or no age-related change in the levels of serum immunoglobulins and the suboptimal antibody response to vaccines is thought to reflect a T-cell, rather than a B-cell effect of the aging process.

Thymic involution was formerly thought to be complete by age 50 years. However, there is recent evidence that even centenarians continue to generate thymic T cells. Using an assay based on the presence of excision circles created during T-cell receptor (TCR) rearrangements, thymic output has been reevaluated. T-cell receptor rearrangements are present exclusively in naïve cells, and their level is diluted with progressive cell replications. High levels of T-cell receptor rearrangements can be detected in elderly people consistent with residual lymphoid mass. However, the output of both naïve T cells and double-positive T cells (CD4+, CD8+) declines with age. There is a concomitant increase in thymic B and T cell precursors. In part, these changes are thought to result from decreased production of IL-7 by the thymic stroma.

Reduced T-cell function occurs secondarily to (1) decreased synthesis of IL-2 receptors, (2) decreased binding of ligand to the CD3/T cell receptor complex on the surface of T cells, (3) decreased IL-2 production, (4) defects in the activation of the protein kinase C dependent transcription factors, and (5) a shift in cytokine profiles of T cells from IL-2 to IL-4 and IFN-γ.

Thus, age-related defects in lymphohematopoiesis are subtle and of the same order of magnitude as other cellular defects known to occur with aging. The concern about hematopoietic exhaustion with aging remains unanswered. But from available data in animals, the proliferative capacity of hematopoietic stem cells, though finite, is thought to be well in excess of the life span of a species.

Hematopoietic Growth Factors in Elderly Persons

There is emerging consensus that aging per se has no appreciable effect on steady state hematopoiesis. Age-related deficits tend to be subtle and are of clinical import either when present cumulatively or under conditions of hematopoietic stress. Relatively few studies have specifically addressed the use of growth factors in the elderly population. The effects of administration of growth factors in the context of cancer chemotherapy, aplastic anemia, myelodysplasia, chronic neutropenia, and anemia, and involving the use of either recombinant GM-CSF, G-CSF, IL-3, or erythropoietin have been studied. When the hemoglobin level and the total neutrophil count were the end points, there was no age-related difference either in the mean time

Table 60-3   Growth Factors in the Elderly

Growth Factor	Molecular Weight	Indications
Granulocyte colony-stimulating factor	24 kD	Chemotherapy-related neutropenia
		Chronic and drug-induced neutropenia
		Peripheral blood stem cell transplantation
		?Myelodysplasia
Erythropoietin	34–39 kD	Renal disease with anemia
		Anemia in cancer patients
		?Myelodysplasia
Granulocyte-macrophage colony-stimulating factor	22 kD	As for G-CSF

to response or in the level of absolute hematopoietic response at different doses of the growth factors.

Recently, in a prospective randomized study, the effects of rhG-CSF on the blood and marrow in 19 young and 19 healthy elderly volunteers were also evaluated. When rhG-CSF was administered subcutaneously to young and healthy elderly volunteers over a 2-week period, rhG-CSF was well tolerated in both age groups, with an equivalent increase in PMN response in both groups. The increase in PMNs in blood was dose dependent, being 5-fold at 30 μg and 15-fold at 300 μg. No age-related compromise, either in the magnitude or in the timing of the PMN response to rhG-CSF, was found. In the marrow, rhG-CSF caused expansion of the mitotic pool primarily at the promyelocyte and myelocyte stage, with no significant change in marrow myeloblasts. This would suggest that G-CSF expands the marrow myeloid pool at or distal to the colony-forming unit granulocyte-macrophage (CFU-GM) stage and that this portion of the myeloid pathway is well preserved in healthy elderly people. The only age-related change observed was the reduced ability of elderly people to mobilize peripheral blood CFU-GM in response to rhG-CSF. The doses of G-CSF used in this study were relatively modest (5 μg/kg). Hence it is unclear whether routinely used mobilization dosages of G-CSF, that is, 10 to 30 μg/kg/d would further accentuate or blunt differences between young and the elderly people.

Thus, on the basis of the available data, the indications for the use of hematopoietic growth factors in the elderly population are no different from the general population. Table 60-3 summarizes the growth factors that have special relevance for use in elderly people. Given the increased susceptibility of the elderly cancer patient to treatment related morbidity and mortality, there may be even more compelling reason for the use of growth factors to obviate complications like bleeding and infections.

SUMMARY

Evaluation of the effect of age on hematopoiesis at the organ or cellular level demonstrates evidence of a diminished reserve capacity. Abnormalities in function, not evidenced in the basal state, become apparent in the stimulus-driven state. In addition to being lower, the aged response tends to be more variable. Given a comparable stress, hematologic abnormalities are likely to occur earlier and to be of greater severity in elderly people as compared to the young. Age-related changes in the early stages of hematopoiesis remain to be elucidated. The impact on hematopoiesis of declining growth hormone and insulin-like growth factor-1 levels with aging is being investigated. The question of hematopoietic exhaustion, particularly under prolonged growth factor stimulation is also pertinent and still unanswered.

REFERENCES

Allen PM et al: In vivo effects of recombinant human granulocyte colony-stimulating factor on neutrophil oxidative functions in normal human volunteers. *J Infect Dis* 175(5):1184, 1997.

Balducci L et al: Hematopoietic growth factors in the older cancer patient. *Curr Opin Hematol* 8(3):170, 2001.

Bronchud MH: Recombinant human granulocyte colony-stimulating factor in the management of cancer patients: Five years on. *Oncology* 51:189, 1994.

Buchanan JP et al: Impaired expression of hematopoietic growth factors: a candidate mechanism for the hematopoietic defect of aging. *Exp Gerontol* 31:135, 1996.

Chatta GS et al. Hematopoietic progenitors and aging: Alterations in responsiveness to recombinant human G-CSF, GM-CSF, and IL-3. *J Gerontol* 48:M207, 1993.

Chatta GS et al. The effects of in vivo rhG-CSF on the neutrophil response in healthy young and elderly volunteers. *Blood* 84:2923, 1994.

Chatta GS et al: Aging and marrow neutrophil reserves. *J Am Geriat Soc* 42:77, 1994.

Chatta GS, Dale DC: Aging and haemopoiesis: Implications for treatment with haemopoietic growth factors. *Drugs Aging* 9(1):37, 1996.

Effros RB: Ageing and the immune system. *Novartis Found Symp* 235:130, 2001.

Globerson A: Hematopoietic stem cells and aging. *Exp Gerontol* 34:137, 1999.

Grant S, Heel R: Recombinant granulocyte-macrophage colony-stimulating factor (rGM-CSF). A review of its pharmacological properties and prospective role in the management of myelosuppression. *Drugs* 43:516, 1992.

Lieschke GJ, Burgess AW: Granulocyte colony stimulating factor and granulocyte-macrophage colony stimulating factor, parts I and II. *N Engl J Med* 327:28, 1992, 327:99, 1992.

Miller RA: The aging immune system: Primer and prospectus. *Science* 273:70, 1996.

Morrison SJ et al: The aging of hematopoietic stem cells. *Nat Med* 2:1011, 1996.

Ozer H: American Society of Clinical Oncology recommendations for the use of hematopoietic colony-stimulating factors: Evidence-based clinical practice guidelines. *J Clin Oncol* 12:2471, 1994.

Rothstein G: Hematopoiesis in the aged: A model of hematopoietic dysregulation? *Blood* 82:2601, 1993.

Rowe JM et al: A randomized Phase III study of granulocyte-macrophage colony-stimulating factor in adult patients (>55 to 70 years of age) with AML: A study of the Eastern Cooperative Oncology Group. *Blood* 86(2):457, 1995.

Spangrude GJ: Biological and clinical aspects of hematopoietic stem cells. *Annu Rev Med* 45:93, 1994.

Stone RM et al: Granulocyte-macrophage colony-stimulating factor after initial chemotherapy for elderly patients with primary acute myelogenous leukemia. Cancer and Leukemia Group B. *N Engl J Med* 332:1671, 1995.

Anemia

GURKAMAL S. CHATTA • DAVID A. LIPSCHITZ

It is generally recognized that anemia is a common clinical problem in elderly people. Studies have shown a high prevalence of anemia in hospitalized older subjects, in patients attending geriatric clinics, and in institutionalized older individuals. However, if stringent criteria are employed for the selection of apparently normal subjects, elderly people should have minimal, if any, decline in hemoglobin values. This chapter reviews the etiology of anemia and presents evidence that declines in hemoglobin levels with advancing age are not necessarily a consequence of the normal aging process. A rational approach to the clinical evaluation of subjects with anemia will be presented.

PREVALENCE OF ANEMIA

Many studies demonstrate a high prevalence of anemia in elderly people. In women older than age 59 years, anemia occurs as frequently as in women of childbearing age. In both men and women, the prevalence of anemia increases significantly with each successive decade. Based upon a lower normal limit of 14 g/dL for hemoglobin concentration, a very large percentage of elderly males would be found to be anemic. This study proposed that the reduction in hemoglobin in males was a consequence of aging, and most likely secondary to a decline in the serum testosterone. Hence, age-specific reference standards for hemoglobin concentration should be adopted and used for diagnosing anemia in elderly people.

There are few reports on the incidence of new cases of anemia in the elderly population. In the general population, the annual incidence of anemia is estimated to be 1 to 2 percent. Compared to this, the incidence of anemia in a well-defined population of elderly (older than 65 years of age) whites attending the Mayo Clinic was reported to be four- to sixfold higher, the incidence of anemia being 13 percent per year in the "oldest-old" (older than 85 years of age). Anemia was diagnosed in accordance with World Health Organization (WHO) criteria, if the hemoglobin concentration was <13 g/dL in men and <12 g/dL in women. In this study, in every age group over 65 years, the incidence of anemia in men was higher than that in women. At the time of diagnosis, <50 percent of the men had a hemoglobin concentration lower than 12 g/dL. Significantly, despite an exhaustive work-up, in 16 percent of elderly individuals, the etiology of the anemia was uncertain.

The above data are consistent with an evaluation of apparently healthy elderly subjects with mild anemia, which also failed to uncover an obvious cause of the anemia. A careful assessment of hematopoiesis in these individuals revealed mild marrow failure, as evidenced by reductions in bone marrow progenitor cell number and modest decreases in peripheral leukocyte counts. A major unanswered question is whether this decline in hemoglobin with advancing age is a consequence of the normal aging process or reflects some yet-to-be-defined abnormality. Of particular importance in this regard is the finding that anemia is extremely rare in an affluent, healthy, elderly population examined in New Mexico. None of the elderly males and females in this group were anemic. Furthermore, longitudinal monitoring of these subjects over a 5-year period failed to demonstrate an increased prevalence of anemia. Based upon this observation and the animal studies of hematopoiesis (see Chap. 60), it seems highly likely that the decrease in hemoglobin seen commonly with advancing age is not a consequence of the normal aging process and is related to some extrinsic variable that remains to be determined.

Inflammation or chronic disease is one likely etiology of apparent age-related anemia (see below for a discussion of this type of anemia). A second possibility is that the anemia has a nutritional basis. This is suggested by a closer examination of data obtained in epidemiologic surveys in which anemia has been shown to be most prevalent in populations that are at a low socioeconomic level, where the prevalence of nutritional deficiencies is high. Further evidence suggesting that a nutritional factor may contribute to the anemia comes from the observation that there is a marked similarity between the alterations in immunologic and hematopoietic function that occur with aging and those that occur with protein deprivation (Table 61-1). This raises the possibility that protein deprivation in some form may contribute to the hematopoietic changes normally ascribed to aging.

There is evidence that correction of protein–energy malnutrition in hospitalized elderly patients can markedly improve hematopoietic function. In these subjects, interpretation of improvements in hematologic status is extremely difficult. Any hospitalized elderly individual has coexisting

Table 61-1   Similarities Between Changes in Immune and Hematopoietic Function Caused by Aging or Protein–Energy Malnutrition

	Aging	Protein-Energy Malnutrition
Cell-mediated immunity		
Delayed cutaneous hypersensitivity	Decreased	Decreased
T-cell number	Decreased	Decreased
Percentage of T-suppressor cells	Decreased	Increased
Blastogenic response to mitogen	Decreased	Decreased
Humoral immunity		
B-cell number	Unchanged	Unchanged
Antibody production	Moderately Decreased	Moderately Decreased
Erythropoiesis		
Hemoglobin	Decreased	Decreased
Marrow erythroid cells	Decreased	Decreased
CFU-E number	Decreased	Decreased
BFU-E number	Normal	Normal
Myelopoiesis		
Granulocyte number	Reduced	Reduced
Granulocytosis after endotoxin administration	Decreased	Decreased
CFU-C number	Decreased	Decreased

BFU-E, burst-forming unit–erythroid; CFU-C, colony-forming unit–culture; CFU-E, colony-forming unit–erythroid.

diseases that can affect hematopoietic function. Thus the overall improvement seen with nutritional rehabilitation may reflect an overall improvement of the patient's medical status. The effect of increased feeding on hematopoietic status has been examined in relatively healthy elderly individuals who lived at home, who were ambulatory but were underweight and had marginal evidence of protein-energy deprivation. By providing polymeric dietary supplements to these subjects between meals, it was possible to correct nutritional deficiencies and obtain weight gain. Despite a positive impact on nutritional status, however, the anemia, invariably present in this population, did not improve.

Some conclusions can be drawn from these observations. It is clear that significant nutritional deficiencies reversibly aggravate the hematologic abnormalities in elderly people. Even in apparently healthy older individuals, it is possible that nutritional factors contribute to hematopoietic changes, but alternative mechanisms other than simple nutritional deficiency must be considered. Marginal reductions of one or more nutrients acting alone or in combination over a prolonged period of time may modulate hematopoietic change usually ascribed to aging. Alternatively, nutrient delivery to the target organ may be altered with aging or changes in nutrient target interaction may occur. These possibilities could account for the higher prevalence of anemia reported in epidemiologic studies. They remain no more than potential hypotheses that require further research.

In contrast to healthy older persons, in whom the prevalence of anemia is relatively low, the disorder is extremely common in hospitalized patients in both acute and chronic care settings. In a survey of hospitalized patients in a Veterans Affairs hospital, 56 percent of patients older than age 75 years had a significant anemia.

EVALUATION OF ANEMIA IN AN ELDERLY PATIENT

For practical purposes, we recommend 12 g/dL as a lower limit of normal for hemoglobin for both elderly men and elderly women. Attempting to define the cause of anemia when the hemoglobin concentration is between 12 and 14 g/dL in elderly men only rarely yields an etiology. Even at a level of 12 g/dL, a decision as to how aggressively to evaluate a patient with borderline low hematocrit must rest on clinical judgment. The complex nature of the problems that present in older individuals, together with the high risk of multiple pathologies occurring simultaneously, makes this decision much more critical. On the other hand, once a decision has been made to investigate a low hemoglobin in an older person, the principles involved in assessment and evaluation are very similar to those that would be used in subjects of any age group. Table 61-2 summarizes the etiologies of the various anemias seen in the elderly population.

Table 61-2   Physiologic Classification of Anemia

Hypoproliferative	Ineffective	Hemolytic
1. Iron-deficient erythropoiesis	1. Megaloblastic	1. Immunologic
a. Iron deficiency	a. Vitamin B_{12}	a. Idiopathic
b. Chronic disease	b. Folate	b. Secondary
c. Inflammation	c. MDS (RA)	
2. Erythropoietin lack	2. Microcytic	2. Intrinsic
a. Renal	a. Thalassemia	a. Metabolic
b. Nutritional	b. Sideroblastic	b. Abnormal Hgb
c. Endocrine	c. MDS (RARS)	
3. Stem cell dysfunction	3. Normocytic	3. Extrinsic
a. Aplastic anemia	a. Stromal disease	a. Mechanical
b. Red blood cell aplasia	b. Dimorphic	b. Lytic substance
	c. MDS	

Hgb, hemoglobin; MDS, myelodysplastic syndromes; RA, refractory anemia; RARS, refractory anemia with rigid sideroblasts.

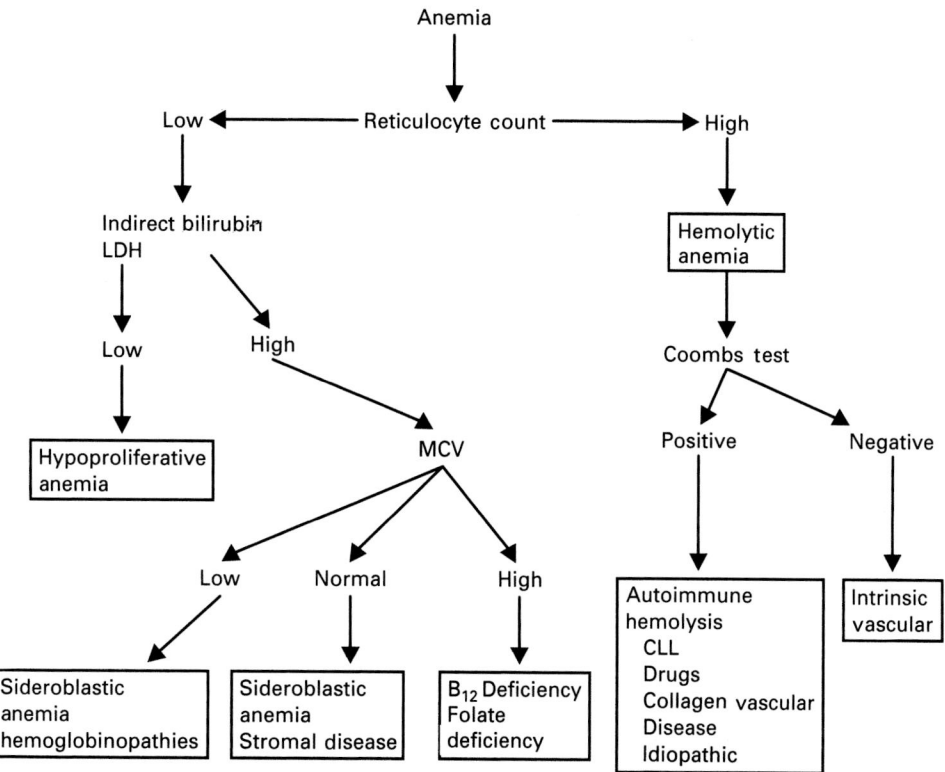

Figure 61-1   A rational strategy for the workup of anemia in the elderly person. The initial approach is to exclude hemolysis and ineffective erythropoiesis. CLL, chronic lymphocytic leukemia.

The initial approach to the patient with anemia must include a complete history and physical examination, as well as a complete blood count (CBC), in order to evaluate the production rate of red blood cells. Microcytosis, defined as a mean corpuscular volume (MCV) of less than 84 (Coulter counter), indicates an impairment of hemoglobin synthesis. Macrocytosis, defined as an MCV of greater than 100, may be caused by reticulocytosis or, more frequently, by an abnormality in nuclear maturation. Red cell production is estimated from the reticulocyte production index. Hemolytic anemia usually has a reticulocyte index greater than 3, whereas a failure of production is indicated by a reticulocyte index of less than 2. Decreased production is caused by the hypoproliferative anemias or by ineffective erythropoiesis. The latter disorder is characterized by marrow erythroid hyperplasia. However, owing to abnormalities in maturation, these erythroid cells are unable to exit the bone marrow and are destroyed by marrow reticuloendothelial cells in a process referred to as intramedullary hemolysis. The disorder may be associated with either macrocytosis or microcytosis. An elevated lactate acid dehydrogenase (LDH) level and indirect hyperbilirubinemia result from the increased destruction of red cell precursors in the marrow and may be used to distinguish ineffective erythropoiesis from hypoproliferative anemia.

Observation may be reasonable for those older individuals who have a mild decrease in hemoglobin (10.5 to 12 g/dL), a normal reticulocyte index, normochromic normocytic indices, no leukocyte or platelet abnormalities, and no occult blood in the stool. Further investigation is indicated if the anemia worsens, or if a change in the peripheral blood pattern occurs. For individuals with mild anemia and hypochromic microcytic indices or more severe anemia with normochromic normocytic indices, a more extensive workup is required. Similarly the presence of macrocytosis warrants additional investigation. Figures 61-1 and 61-2 illustrate a rational approach to the laboratory workup of anemia. A significantly elevated reticulocyte count, indirect hyperbilirubinemia, and elevated LDH are diagnostic of hemolytic anemia. A low reticulocyte count, elevated indirect bilirubin, and elevated LDH suggest ineffective erythropoiesis. In older persons with ineffective erythropoiesis, macrocytosis strongly suggests vitamin B_{12} or folate deficiency, and microcytosis should suggest sideroblastic anemia (Fig. 61-1).

THE HYPOPROLIFERATIVE ANEMIAS

Figure 61-2 illustrates an approach to the workup of hypoproliferative anemia, which accounts for the majority of anemias in elderly people. Iron is the only nutrient that limits the rate of erythropoiesis. Thus inadequate iron supply for erythropoiesis, the commonest cause of anemia in older persons, results in a hypoproliferative anemia. This is diagnosed by the presence of a decreased serum iron and a reduced transferrin saturation (serum iron divided by the total iron-binding capacity [TIBC] expressed as a percent). Absolute iron deficiency (blood loss) is the commonest cause of iron-deficient erythropoiesis in younger subjects. In elderly people, the etiology is more likely to be the "anemia of chronic disease," or anemia associated

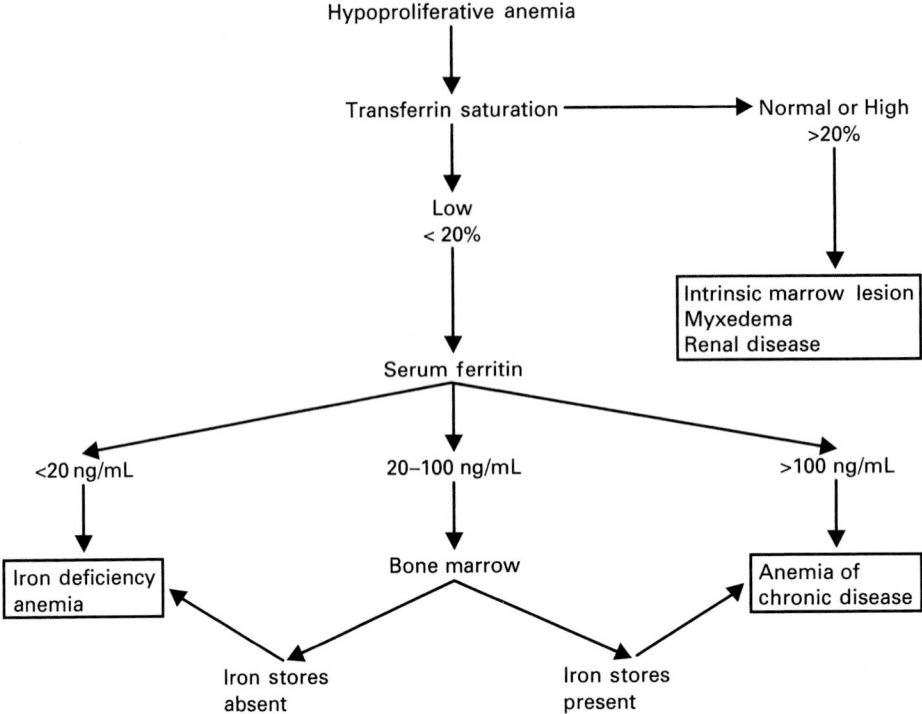

Figure 61-2 The workup of hypoproliferative anemia in the elderly population.

with inflammation. Iron-deficient erythropoiesis in these disorders results from a defective ability of the reticuloendothelial system to reuse iron derived from senescent red cells. Thus, tissue iron stores are normal or increased, resulting in a serum ferritin concentration above 50 ng/mL and reduction in the TIBC. This contrasts with a low serum ferritin and high TIBC, which reflect absent iron stores in blood-loss anemia.

Blood loss, the anemia of inflammation and chronic disease, and that associated with protein-energy malnutrition are the most prevalent anemias in elderly populations. In younger individuals, iron-deficiency anemia is usually caused by either blood loss or nutritional iron deficiency. In both men and women, a progressive increase in iron stores occurs with advancing age. In older men, tissue iron stores average 1200 mg; in women, iron stores increase from a mean of 300 mg to approximately 800 mg over the decade following menopause. Thus nutritional iron deficiency is very rare in the elderly despite the prominence of other nutritional problems. When unexplained iron deficiency does occur, it is almost exclusively caused by blood loss from the intestinal tract, even if bleeding is not detected by repeated stool guaiac determinations. Other routes of bleeding may occur but are easily recognizable (epistaxis, abnormal bleeding from the uterus, hematuria). The causes of blood loss in elderly people include drugs (aspirin) and bleeding as a consequence of a neoplasm. Angiodysplasia of the large bowel and diverticular disease are frequent causes but should only be considered once a neoplasm has been excluded. Rarely, iron deficiency can result from malabsorption or urinary losses of iron which occur in the face of intravascular hemolysis.

Inflammation is another important cause of anemia in elderly people and is perhaps the more frequent. Inflammation may be the result of infection, an immune response, or a neoplastic process. Usually the decrease in hematocrit is moderate. Hematologic findings differ from iron deficiency in that the iron block is less severe and microcytosis is usually minimal. In some instances, these hematologic findings may be present with little or no evidence of inflammation. Inadequate food intake and increased tissue breakdown may also contribute to the severity of the anemia. Treatment is that of the underlying disease. Only rarely is anemia severe enough to require transfusion. Iron therapy is usually ineffective owing to the limited absorption of iron in the presence of inflammation and the trapping of parenteral iron in the macrophage.

The term anemia of chronic disease is often used to explain an anemia associated with some other major disease process. Examples include renal dysfunction, cancer, collagen vascular disorders, rheumatoid arthritis, and inflammatory bowel disease. Occasionally, the anemia may be the initial manifestation of an occult disease. It is critical for the clinician to be aware of this possibility and to assure an appropriate workup. Management of the anemia associated with inflammation or chronic disease consists of ensuring adequate nutrition and treating the underlying disease process.

Decreased EPO production accounts for the anemia of end-stage renal disease. EPO has been in clinical use since 1985 for patients with ESRD. In the elderly patient, the usual dose of EPO is 75 to 100 U/kg administered IV, three times per week, during the last 5 minutes of dialysis. On this dose, 95 percent of patients reach the target hematocrit (>35 percent) in 10 to 12 weeks, have marked reduction in transfusion dependency, and have beneficial cardiac, neurovascular, immunologic, and psychosocial effects. For a normal response to EPO, the patient must have adequate iron stores and red cell folate. Although EPO is well tolerated, dialysis patients on EPO have a higher risk of hypertension, seizures, cerebrovascular disease, and thromboembolic episodes. Because elderly people are more prone to all these diseases, older patients on EPO need to be monitored closely. The indications for EPO treatment in ESRD prior to dialysis are essentially the same. The recommended dose of EPO is 50 to 75 U/kg/wk subcutaneously. The dose can be increased by 1000 U/wk, every 3 to 4 weeks, to a maximum of 40,000 U/wk. At the higher dose, one must exclude hemolysis, blood loss, and iron and folate deficiency. The target hematocrit is approximately 35 percent.

In some instances, the anemia of cancer and chronic diseases is associated with inappropriately low EPO levels. Many cancer patients have anemia independent of any myelosuppressive therapy. The anemia is characterized by an inability to use iron stores, and an inadequate EPO response. In addition, a component of the erythroid suppression is mediated by cytokines like interleukin-1, tumor necrosis factor (TNF)-α, and transforming growth factor (TGF)-β. The precise incidence of cancer-related anemia is not known and even less is known about the frequency of blood transfusions in these patients. However, a number of studies have documented a decrease in transfusion frequency following treatment with EPO. Depending on symptoms, erythroid support is recommended for hemoglobin levels below 11 g/dL. EPO treatment should be instituted after excluding hemolysis and iron deficiency. Typically, the starting dose of EPO ranges between 20,000 and 40,000 units subcutaneously every week. If required, the dose can be escalated to 60,000 U/wk. Conversely, some patients require treatment only every 2 to 3 weeks. Hemoglobin levels should be monitored weekly, to avoid the vascular sequelae of an iatrogenic polycythemia. A target hemoglobin of 12 to 13 g/dL is usually safe. Most patients respond within 4 to 6 weeks. Iron should be added to the regimen if ferritin levels fall below 50 ng/mL. If there is no reticulocyte response after 4 to 6 weeks of EPO treatment, therapy should be discontinued. Although it is difficult to prospectively identify responders, it has been reported that patients with endogenous erythropoietin levels of <200 mU/mL are most likely to respond to treatment with EPO. More recently, EPO was investigated in the setting of cancer-related fatigue (see Cancer, Anemia, and Fatigue below). The level of hemoglobin at which EPO treatment mitigates fatigue, remains the subject of intense investigation.

Nutritional deprivation in elderly people generally results in a normocytic normochromic anemia with an essentially normal peripheral smear. In the hospitalized patient, evidence of iron-deficient erythropoiesis (low transferrin saturation) is common and the serum ferritin is elevated. There is usually a history of weight loss, and laboratory studies indicate a reduced serum albumin and a decreased TIBC (<240 g/dL). This disorder is particularly important, as there is evidence that correction of the nutritional deficiency and its underlying cause can result in significant improvement in the hemoglobin level and other hematopoietic parameters.

Marrow failure because of interference with the proliferation of hematopoietic cells occurs in the elderly population. The disorder is generally associated with suppression of all marrow elements and is suggested by the presence of peripheral pancytopenia. Common causes include drugs, immune damage to the stem cell population, intrinsic marrow lesions, and marrow replacement by malignant cells or fibrous tissue. The latter is usually associated with a myelophthisic blood picture (nucleated red cells, giant platelets, and metamyelocytes on smear) as a reflection of the disruption of marrow stromal architecture. The presence of pancytopenia and the absence of iron-deficient erythropoiesis is an indication for bone marrow aspiration and biopsy. Occasionally, isolated suppression of erythropoiesis occurs, which is referred to as pure red cell aplasia. This disorder may be drug-related or may be caused by benign or malignant abnormalities of lymphocytes, including thymoma. These subjects present with isolated anemia, an elevated serum iron, and absent erythroid precursors on bone marrow examination.

INEFFECTIVE ERYTHROPOIESIS

Macrocytic anemias in elderly people result from vitamin B_{12} and folate deficiency. The prevalence of pernicious anemia increases significantly with advancing age. The disorder results from malabsorption of vitamin B_{12} as a consequence of antibodies against gastric parietal cells and intrinsic factor. Atrophic gastritis and decreased secretion of intrinsic factor occur, resulting in failure of vitamin B_{12} absorption. Pernicious anemia occurs most frequently in subjects older than age 60 years and is more common in women. The anemia may be very severe, presenting with weakness and a lemon-yellow discoloration, although occasionally anemia is absent. Neurologic abnormalities—including peripheral neuropathy, ataxia, loss of position sense, and upper motor neuron signs—are frequent. Behavioral abnormalities and dementia are well described and may occur in the absence of anemia or macrocytosis. Occasionally, there is evidence of a more generalized autoimmune process, manifesting with myxedema, hypoadrenalism, and vitiligo.

The presence of pancytopenia, macrocytosis, hypersegmented neutrophils in the peripheral smear, a decreased reticulocyte index, an increased LDH, and indirect hypobilirubinemia suggests a diagnosis of megaloblastic anemia. The bone marrow classically shows giant metamyelocytes, hypersegmented neutrophils, and enlarged erythroid precursors with more hemoglobin than would be expected from the immaturity of their nuclei (nuclear cytoplasmic dissociation). The diagnosis is made by demonstrating serum vitamin B_{12} concentration of less than 100 pg/mL. However, one study reported that one-third of patients with pernicious anemia had a value >100 pg/mL. Chronic pancreatitis and diseases of the distal ileum (blind loop syndrome) may also cause vitamin B_{12} deficiency. The Schilling test is able to distinguish a deficiency of intrinsic factor (malabsorption corrected by ingested vitamin B_{12} and intrinsic factor) from an abnormality in the ability of the ileum to absorb the vitamin B_{12}–inrinsic factor complex (absorption still impaired with intrinsic factor plus vitamin B_{12}). Treatment consists of weekly or biweekly injection of 1000 μg of vitamin B_{12} until stores are replenished. A maintenance dose at monthly intervals is then adequate.

Epidemiologic studies generally show adequate folate intake in elderly people. Folate deficiency of sufficient severity to cause anemia in the elderly person is most frequently found in association with protein–energy malnutrition and excessive alcohol consumption. Alcohol and various other drugs are also known to interfere with folate absorption and metabolism. Vulnerability to deficiency is significantly greater when folate requirements are increased as a result of inflammation, neoplastic disease, or hemolytic anemia. The hematologic profile is identical to that described for vitamin B_{12} deficiency. The diagnosis is made by the demonstration of significant reductions in the serum (<2 ng/mL) or red cell (<100 ng/mL) folate concentration. Prior to commencement of therapy with folate, it is important to exclude vitamin B_{12} deficiency, as treatment with folate can aggravate the neurologic abnormalities in the latter disorder.

The major causes of ineffective erythropoiesis and microcytosis are thalassemia and the sideroblastic anemias. Although thalassemia is generally diagnosed at an earlier age, there are reports of its initial detection in older people. Mild anemia, a disproportionately low MCV, and the absence of iron deficiency, usually points to a diagnosis of thalassemia trait. This condition is common in African Americans, and is of little or no clinical consequence. Iron supplements have no role in the treatment of thalassemia trait and on the contrary can be detrimental due to potential iron overload.

Acquired sideroblastic anemia is primarily a disease of elderly persons. It is a heterogenous group of disorders characterized by the presence of iron deposits in the mitochondria of normoblasts. The disorder is a consequence of impaired heme synthesis. It usually reflects an intrinsic marrow lesion (idiopathic) but may be secondary to inflammation, neoplasia, or drug ingestion. The common finding is the presence of a dimorphic red cell population, in part markedly hypochromic and in part well filled with hemoglobin. The diagnosis is made by the demonstration of ringed sideroblasts in the bone marrow as well as the presence of maturation abnormalities of myeloid and erythroid precursors. A fraction of elderly patients with sideroblastic anemia show some response to pharmacologic doses of pyridoxine (200 mg three times daily). This dose should be given to all patients until it becomes apparent that a rise in hemoglobin concentration will not occur. For patients who are unresponsive to pyridoxine, the anemia must be treated symptomatically.

The myelodysplastic syndromes (MDS) are a group of stem cell disorders characterized by disordered hematopoiesis, that occur primarily in elderly people. Refractory anemia (RA) and refractory anemia with ringed sideroblasts (RARS), account for 25 to 30 percent of the MDS syndromes. RA commonly presents as a macrocytic anemia with marrow erythroid hyperplasia, and relatively normal myeloid and megakaryocytic lineages. Cytogenetic abnormalities are relatively common in MDS, and one of particular interest in elderly people is 5q– deletion. The median age at presentation is 66 years, and the 5q– syndrome is characterized by (1) macrocytic anemia, (2) modest leukopenia, (3) normal or increased platelet counts, (4) marrow erythroid hypoplasia or hyperplasia, and (5) female preponderance. Treatment of MDS in elderly people tends to be supportive. The 5q– syndrome has a relatively good prognosis with a low propensity for transformation to an acute leukemia.

Di Guglielmo's syndrome is another stem cell disorder that is more common in older people. It presents with anemia, and is characterized by megaloblastic erythroid precursors, dysplastic myeloid cells, and hyperplasia in the marrow. The disease usually evolves into an M6 acute myelogenous leukemia (AML), with an associated pancytopenia and the presence of nucleated red cells, and immature myeloid and megakaryocytic precursors in the circulation. Treatment is usually supportive.

HEMOLYTIC ANEMIAS

The causes of hemolytic anemia in elderly people are somewhat different than those found in younger subjects. Although most patients with congenital disorders will previously have been identified, an occasional patient with congenital hemolytic anemia may present for the first time with symptoms related to cholelithiasis. Autoimmune hemolytic anemia is the commonest cause in the elderly patient; the diagnosis is made by the presence of a positive Coombs' test. In younger subjects, an etiology of the autoimmune hemolysis is only rarely identified. In the elderly person, however, the anemia is more likely to be associated with a lymphoproliferative disorder (non-Hodgkin's lymphoma or chronic lymphocytic leukemia), collagen vascular disease, or drug ingestion. Steroids and splenectomy are usually effective in patients with red cell antibodies of the immunoglobulin (Ig) G type. Patients with red cell antibodies of the IgM variety are more likely to be refractory to such treatment.

A disorder of some importance in elderly people is microangiopathic hemolytic anemia. This is usually associated with severe infections or disseminated neoplasm and presents not only with hemolysis but also a consumptive coagulopathy. The presence of red cell fragmentation, thrombocytopenia, a prolonged partial thromboplastin time, and hemosiderinuria should suggest this diagnosis.

CANCER, ANEMIA, AND FATIGUE

Cancer is primarily a disease of elderly people, with approximately 50 percent of the cancer burden being in individuals older than age 65 years. Depending on the specific cancer, the incidence of anemia in the older cancer patient can be as high as 70 percent while on chemotherapy. Several large studies show that fatigue, depression, and impaired cognitive function are the primary symptoms that account for a diminished quality of life as a result of anemia.

Table 61-3 Diagnosis of Anemia in Patients Older than Age 75 years in an Acute Care Veterans' Hospital

Diagnosis	Percentage
Multiple diagnoses	53
No diagnosis	17
Single diagnosis	30
Anemia of chronic disease	10
Malnutrition	9
Infection	4
Postoperative bleeding	3
Alcohol	1
Iron deficiency	1

Of these, fatigue can be significantly ameliorated by treatment of the anemia, with an improvement in the quality of life. Although an area of intense debate, it is generally believed that a hemoglobin level of ≥ 12 g/dL appears to be optimal for obtaining the best improvements in quality of life.

COMPLEX PRESENTATION OF ANEMIA IN THE ELDERLY POPULATION

The presence of multiple pathologies frequently makes the evaluation of anemia difficult in older persons. As illustrated in Table 61-3, an investigation of hospitalized patients indicated that multiple diagnoses contributed to the anemia in 53 percent. A classic example is a patient with active rheumatoid disease who has lost blood from aspirin ingestion. Similarly protein–energy malnutrition or blood loss will markedly aggravate the anemia associated with neoplasia. Iron deficiency and vitamin B_{12} deficiency may coexist, presenting confusing red blood cell indices. The possibility of a multifactorial etiology—including blood loss, malnutrition, folate deficiency, and hemolytic disease—should always be considered when the anemia of chronic disease or inflammation is associated with a hemoglobin below 10 g/dL. In this circumstance, laboratory investigations frequently give equivocal results; hence a bone marrow examination may be required. Clinical judgment is critically important in deciding how aggressive the workup for anemia ought to be.

REFERENCES

Aapro M et al: Age, anemia, and fatigue. *Semin Oncol* 29 (Suppl 8):55, 2002.

Ania BJ et al: Incidence of anemia in older people: An epidemiologic study in a well-defined population. *J Am Geriatr Soc* 45(7):825, 1997.

Boultwood J et al: The 5q– syndrome. *Blood* 84:3253, 1994.

Carmel R: Pernicious anemia. The expected findings of very low serum cobalamin levels, anemia, and macrocytosis are often lacking. *Arch Intern Med* 148:1712, 1988.

Dicato M et al: The optimal hemoglobin level in the cancer patient. *Semin Oncol* 29 (Suppl 8):88, 2002.

Lindenbaum J et al: Neuropsychiatric disorders caused by cobalamin deficiency in the absence of anemia or macrocytosis. *N Engl J Med* 318:1720, 1988.

Lipschitz DA, Mitchell CO: The correctability of the nutritional, immune, and hematopoietic manifestations of protein calorie malnutrition in the elderly. *J Am Coll Nutr* 1:17, 1982.

Paganini EP et al: Erythropoietin therapy in renal failure. *Adv Intern Med* 38:223, 1993.

Spivak JL: Recombinant human erythropoietin and the anemia of cancer. *Blood* 84:997, 1994.

CHAPTER 62

White Cell Disorders

BAYARD L. POWELL

White blood cells (WBC) provide major host defense mechanisms against invading pathogens through phagocytosis and the immune response. In addition, lymphocytes provide immune surveillance against the development of cancer and are important mediators of disorders of the immune system. White cell disorders are usually the result of overproduction or underproduction of one or more of the WBC series, which include the granulocytes—neutrophils, basophils, and eosinophils—and/or the lymphocytes and monocytes; less frequently, WBC disorders result from WBC dysfunction despite normal numbers of cells. The acuteness and severity of the disorder is related to the number of white cells, the subset(s) of WBC involved, their degree of maturity, and their functional capacity. Initial clinical manifestations of diseases of WBC include signs and symptoms of infectious (e.g., neutrophils; Table 62-1) and neoplastic diseases.

Disorders of WBC, benign or malignant, frequently also involve abnormalities of the red blood cells and platelets. In these situations, the signs and symptoms of disease at presentation may include those related to anemia (i.e., weakness and easy fatigability) and/or thrombocytopenia (i.e., easy bruisability, mucosal or gastrointestinal bleeding, and hematuria). A careful history and physical examination with evaluation of the peripheral blood, and bone marrow when needed, will establish a diagnosis in many cases.

Aging is not associated with significant changes in the peripheral white blood cell count or WBC differential (Table 62-2). Therefore, abnormalities in white cell numbers should be evaluated as a probable sign of an active disease process. Most white cell disorders (Table 62-3) are more common with increased age; apart from neuroplastic causes of leukocytosis (which are usually acute and unsubstantiated), the most common WBC disorders in the elderly are neoplastic diseases. Table 62-3 lists the spectrum of white cell disorders encountered in clinical practice. Full descriptions of these processes are available in textbooks of hematology and oncology. This chapter focuses on these disorders as related to geriatric medicine.

The most common assessment of white cells is quantitative evaluation of their numbers and the distribution of the different types of white cells (WBC differential). Equally important is the microscopic examination of the peripheral blood smear (and bone marrow when needed)

for morphologic changes in the WBC as well as the red cells and platelets. Specific quantitation of WBC subsets by immunophenotyping techniques is important in evaluating many disorders in white cells. Qualitative or functional defects are more difficult to establish with laboratory techniques and are usually strongly suggested by the medical history.

DECREASED WBC

Leukopenia, most frequently neutropenia (Table 62-1), may occur with a broad array of medical problems. Most intrinsic (hereditary/familial) disorders and syndromes are detected during infancy or childhood. Leukopenia in older adults is generally the result of acquired or secondary disorders, either reactive (drugs, nutritional, infections, immune) or malignant.

Drug/Toxin Effects

Elderly patients commonly take a number of prescribed and over-the-counter medications, many of which may have a greater or lesser propensity for isolated neutropenia or pancytopenia. The bone marrow is one of the more rapidly proliferating organs of the body; therefore, it is not surprising that exposure to noxious agents may temporarily or permanently inhibit production of one or more elements of the blood. The list of possible offenders is extensive. Table 62-4 lists some of the more common offenders. In a situation of neutropenia, leukopenia, or pancytopenia, the physician should thoroughly review the patient's medications and the duration of the medications. Short duration does not remove the possibility of a drug-induced cytopenia; it could be an idiosyncratic reaction.

Drug effects on the bone marrow range from mild neutropenias (more common) to agranulocytosis; lymphocytopenia occurs less frequently. The red blood cells (RBC) and platelets may or may not be affected. Drug-induced reduction of the granulocytic series may be a direct toxic effect, as with many cancer chemotherapeutic drugs or may be the result of an immunologic phenomenon wherein a drug–antibody complex reacts with mature neutrophils

Table 62-1   Neutropenia

Absolute Neutrophil Count (ANC) = WBC × %(seg + bands)	
ANC	Infection Risk
≥1000	Essentially normal
500–1000	Slight ↑ risk
<500	"Significant" risk
<100	Severe risk

Table 62-2   Normal WBC Counts for Adults

Test	Range (× $10^3/\mu L$)
WBC	4.5–11.0
Segmental neutrophils	1.6–7.3
Band neutrophils	0.0–0.2
Lymphocytes	1.0–5.1
Monocytes	0.1–0.9
Eosinophils	0.0–0.5
Basophils	0.0–0.5

and their precursors in the bone marrow. Upon withdrawal of the offending agent, there may be a relatively brisk marrow recovery within 14 to 21 days. A bone marrow examination during this recovery period may reveal an increased number of immature elements, which can be confused with a malignant process such as an acute leukemia or myelodysplasia. If this is a possibility, close followup for an additional 2 to 3 weeks will usually provide the answer. The recovering marrow will go on to differentiate, but the malignant marrow will either stay the same or will worsen. Other marrow toxins include a variety of household and industrial chemicals, especially organic

Table 62-3   Disorders of White Blood Cells

I. Lack of production
    A. Drug or toxin suppression, which may be temporary or permanent
    B. Ineffective myelopoiesis secondary to B_{12} or folate deficiency
    C. Bone marrow failure (aplastic anemia)

II. Increased destruction
    Immune neutropenia secondary to rheumatologic disorders, Felty's syndrome, and lymphoproliferative malignancies

III. Increased splenic sequestration
    Congestive splenomegaly with cirrhosis, Gaucher's disease, etc.

IV. Nonneoplastic increases in WBC
    A. Response to stress (e.g., infection)
    B. Response to drug (e.g., corticosteroids, granulocyte colony-stimulating factor)
    C. Other reactive increases (e.g., inflammation, stress)

V. Neoplastic diseases
    A. Primary hematologic
        1. Myelodysplastic syndromes (MDS)
        2. Acute leukemias
            a. Acute myelogenous leukemia (AML)
            b. Acute lymphocytic leukemia (ALL)
        3. Chronic leukemias
            a. Chronic lymphocytic leukemia (CLL)
            b. Chronic myelogenous leukemia (CML)
            c. Hairy-cell leukemia
        4. Other myeloproliferative diseases
        5. Non-Hodgkin's lymphoma (with circulating lymphoma cells)
    B. Cancers metastatic to bone marrow
        Most commonly breast, lung, prostate, and lymphomas

VI. Normal count with impaired function
    A. Diabetes mellitus: impaired polymorphonuclear neutrophil function
    B. Chronic renal failure: Impaired polymorphonuclear neutrophil and lymphocyte function
    C. Drugs (e.g., corticosteroids)

Table 62-4   Agranulocytosis/Neutopenia Caused by Drugs

1. Cancer chemotherapeutic agents

2. Drugs for ulcer disease: H_2 blockers

3. Thiazide diuretics

4. Oral hypoglycemic drugs

5. Anti-inflammatory/antiarthritic drugs:
   Nonsteroidal anti-inflammatory agents
   Penicillamine
   Gold salts
   Colchicine
   Immunosuppressive agents

6. Cardiovascular drugs:
   Procainamide
   Hydralazine
   Quinidine
   Captopril
   Methyldopa

7. Antibiotics:
   Semisynthetic penicillins
   Cephalosporins
   Sulfa drugs
   Vancomycin

8. Phenothiazines

9. Thyroid suppressants

10. Antiepileptic drugs:
    Phenytoin and derivatives
    Carbamazepine

solvents, naphthalenes, insecticides, and herbicides. Inquiries about chemical exposure from hobbies or occupations must therefore be part of history taking. While the hematologic effects of drug and chemical exposure are frequently reversible, some may result in myelodysplastic syndromes or aplastic anemia which, in turn, may evolve into acute myelogenous leukemia.

Nutritional Deficiency

Mild neutropenia may be associated with nutritional anemias secondary to folate or B_{12} deficiency. Older individuals, especially those living alone, may not be attentive to their diet for various socioeconomic, psychological, or medical reasons. The main sources of folates are fresh green vegetables, many fruits, and beans. Cooking and canning destroys folates. The body's folate stores can be depleted after 4 to 5 months of poor dietary intake. Thus, a dietary history may provide an important clue to the diagnosis of the hematologic problem. Dietary folate deficiency may be aggravated by alcoholism and chronic hemolysis. Potential folate deficiency is best evaluated by measuring RBC folate.

In contrast, body stores of vitamin B_{12} are not readily depleted by poor dietary habits alone. It takes 3 to 5 years to deplete the body stores of vitamin B_{12}. However, gastric atrophy is more common with increasing age, and this may lead to failure of gastric secretion of intrinsic factor, which binds to dietary cobalamin—a necessary step in the absorption of vitamin B_{12} in the ileum. Other conditions that cause a B_{12} deficiency include gastrectomy or subtotal small-bowel (ileal) resection. It should be noted that neurologic signs and symptoms of B_{12} deficiency may be confused with other neurologic problems in the elderly patient. These include peripheral paresthesias (peripheral neuritis), loss of balance (posterior column damage), spasticity (lateral column damage), and impaired cognitive function. Any of these neurologic signs and symptoms may be mistakenly attributed to "old age," but if caused by B_{12} deficiency may be corrected with vitamin B_{12} replacement therapy.

Infections

A number of infections can be associated with neutropenia and/or leukopenia in older adults. These infections include viral (e.g., influenza, varicella, hepatitis A, B, or C, cytomegalovirus, human immunodeficiency virus, parvovirus B19), bacterial (e.g., *Staphylococcus aureus*, brucellosis, tularemia), rickettsia, and tuberculosis. The mechanism of leukopenia is usually bone marrow suppression, but in the case of overwhelming bacterial sepsis, can result from exhaustion of bone marrow reserves.

Bone Marrow Failure

Severe and prolonged bone marrow failure may occur in association with drugs, toxins, or infections, but is frequently idiopathic. Aplastic anemia is characterized by severe pancytopenia and bone marrow hypoplasia. Clinical signs and symptoms reflect these cytopenias: infection, bleeding, and/or the signs/symptoms of anemia. Pure white cell aplasia occurs rarely. Treatments for this life-threatening disease include supportive care (transfusion, antibiotics), immunosuppression (antithymocyte globulin, cyclosporine, steroids), and stem cell transplant (limited application in the elderly population).

Increased Destruction

Immune neutropenia may be associated with various rheumatologic conditions such as systemic lupus erythematosus, rheumatoid arthritis, polyserositis, and lymphoproliferative malignancies. In these situations, the neutropenia is caused by the elimination of immunoglobulin-coated granulocytes by the reticuloendothelial system. The neutropenia of Felty's syndrome (rheumatoid arthritis, splenomegaly, and neutropenia) has a complex etiology that includes immune destruction and suppression as well as splenic sequestration. These neotropenias frequently respond to granulocyte colony-stimulating factors (G-CSF) or granulocyte-macrophage colony-stimulating factors (GM-CSF).

Splenic Sequestration

Any condition causing splenomegaly (e.g., hepatic cirrhosis) may lead to sequestration of sufficient neutrophils to cause mild to moderate neutropenia as a component of the pancytopenia of hypersplenism. The mild to moderate neutropenia usually does not predispose to increased infections and often occurs in association with anemia and/or thrombocytopenia.

INCREASED WBC

Benign Causes of Leukocytosis

The most common causes of sustained increases in WBC are neoplastic diseases. However, there are a number of nonneoplastic etiologies for increases in one or more white cell forms. The most common among these is a leukocytosis, specifically neutrophilia, in response to infection. This is associated with a "left shift" in the differential, with increases in bands and other less-mature granulocytes, including metamyelocytes and myelocytes. Such a normal granulocytosis can also be seen in response to an exogenous steroids. Increases in specific subsets of white cells (e.g., eosinophils or basophils) can occur in response to a number of exposures or illnesses. Hereditary and familial (e.g., Down's syndrome) causes of leukocytosis are rare and usually detected early in life.

Infection

Infection stimulates the acute release of neutrophils from the marginated storage pools of the bone marrow. An increase in band neutrophils and metamyelocytes (± myelocytes) occurs, and toxic granules in those cells are frequently present on review of the peripheral blood smear. A dramatic "leukemoid reaction," characterized by a WBC >50,000/μl, a marked left shift with increased immature granulocytes including myelocytes, promyelocytes, and even blasts, may be confused with malignant disorders, especially chronic myelogenous leukemia (CML). Leukemoid reactions are characterized by a high leukocyte alkaline phosphatase (LAP [low in CML]) and absence of the Philadelphia chromosome.

Drug-Induced Leukocytosis

Corticosteroids are the most common medications associated with increases in WBC, primarily neutrophilia. The hematopoietic colony stimulating factors (e.g., G-CSF, GM-CSF) are designed to stimulate neutrophilia, and lithium can induce neutrophilia through similar CSF pathways. Beta-Adrenergic agonists also frequently stimulate acute release of neutrophils from marginated pools.

Other Reactive Leukocytosis

Chronic inflammation may stimulate a modest increase in bone marrow production and release of neutrophils; stress neutrophilia, a mild neutrophilia (WBC 12,000 to 20,000/μl) resulting from release of neutrophils from marginated pools into the bloodstream, may occur after stress, including normal exercise and illnesses (e.g., seizures, heatstroke). Asplenia can also be associated with moderate leukocytosis. Mild to moderate leukocytosis (WBC <30,000/μl) may occur in association with a variety of malignancies without bone marrow involvement.

Isolated increases in WBC subsets occur with or without increase in total WBC. Monocytosis may be associated with inflammatory diseases, specifically infections, autoimmune and granulomatous diseases, and numerous malignancies. Eosinophilia (>600/μl) usually represents a reaction to drugs, infection (e.g., fungi, parasites), allergic disorders, vasculitis, or malignancies. Lymphocytosis, though frequently representing malignancy, may occur in response to infection.

MALIGNANT DISEASE OF THE HEMATOPOIETIC SYSTEM

Hematologic malignancies, although most frequently characterized by elevated WBC, can be associated with low, normal, or high WBC. The WBC differential, as well as the red cell and platelet counts, are usually abnormal.

Malignant diseases of the white blood cells include the four major subtypes of leukemia—acute myelogenous leukemia (AML), acute lymphocytic leukemia (ALL), chronic myelogenous leukemia (CML), and chronic lymphocytic leukemia (CLL); as well as the myelodysplastic syndromes (MDS; preleukemias); the myeloproliferative disorders other than CML; hairy cell leukemia; metastatic cancers to the bone marrow; and circulating non-Hodgkin's lymphoma cells. While the incidence rates of most of the hematologic malignancies have remained relatively stable, the effectiveness of treatments has improved substantially over recent decades for most hematologic malignancies. Unfortunately, the response rates and cure rates in elderly patients have lagged far behind for a number of reasons, including the more common occurrence of chronic leukemias, MDS, and myeloproliferative disease in the elderly person, limited ability of the elderly person to tolerate the more aggressive curative approaches for acute leukemia, and the more common occurrence of multiple poor prognostic factors in elderly patients. The age-specific incidence rates of all leukemias other than ALL increase in the elderly population.

Myelodysplastic (Preleukemia) Syndromes

The myelodysplastic syndromes, frequently referred to as preleukemia, encompass a group of hematopoietic disorders characterized by ineffective hematopoiesis, with peripheral blood cytopenias and hypercellularity of the bone marrow. All the myelodysplastic syndromes are associated with some degree of predisposition to develop AML; however, diseases such as chronic myelogenous leukemia, the other myeloproliferative disorders, and Fanconi's anemia

Table 62-5 Characteristics and Prognosis of Myelodysplastic Syndromes

Subgroup	Peripheral Blood Blasts(%)	Bone Marrow Blasts(%)	Progression to AML(%)	Median Survival (Months)
Refractory anemia	<1	<5	10	70
Refractory anemia with ring sideroblasts	<1	<5	15	65
Chronic myelomonocytic leukemia	<5	≤20	30	10
Refractory anemia with excess blasts	<5	5–20	40	10
Refractory anemia with excess blasts in transformation	≥5	21–30	60	5

that are also associated with an increased risk of AML are not classified as MDS.

The true incidence of myelodysplastic syndromes is not known. About two-thirds of patients with MDS are elderly males. MDS are clearly diseases of aging patients, with a median age at diagnosis of 65 to 70 years. The nomenclature associated with myelodysplastic syndromes is confusing. Terms found in the literature include odoleukemia (threshold of leukemia), subacute myeloid leukemia, smoldering leukemia, dysmyelopoietic syndrome, and preleukemia.

In 1982, the French-American-British (FAB) Cooperative Group established a classification system with five diagnostic categories based on peripheral blood and bone marrow characteristics. These include refractory anemia (RA), RA with ring sideroblasts (RARS), RA with excess blasts (RAEB), RAEB in transformation (RAEBT), and chronic myelomonocytic leukemia (CMML) (Table 62-5). Patients with RA or RARS have <1 percent of such blasts in the peripheral blood and <5 percent of blasts in the bone marrow; reticulocytopenia and dyserythropoiesis are the predominant features for these disorders. RARS is distinguished from RA by the presence of ringed sideroblasts in the bone marrow. The granulocytic and megakaryocytic series are usually relatively normal. Patients with RAEB and RAEBT are distinguished by the percentage of blasts in the peripheral blood and bone marrow. These patients usually have hypercellular marrows with prominent dysgranulopoiesis in addition to abnormalities in the erythrocytic and megakaryocytic series. Patients with RAEB have <5 percent blasts in the peripheral blood, and their bone marrow has 5 to 20 percent blasts. Patients with RAEBT have (1) ≥5 percent blasts in the peripheral blood, or (2) 21 to 30 percent blasts in the bone marrow, or (3) presence of Auer bodies (rods) in granulocyte precursors. Patients with CMML have an absolute monocytosis (≥1000/μl) with <5 percent blasts in the peripheral blood; the bone marrow has ≤20 percent blasts, often with an increased number of monocytic precursors. A common additional finding in patients with MDS is the presence of one or more cytogenetic abnormalities, most frequently involving chromosomes 5, 7, 8, or 20.

The proposed World Health Organization (WHO) classification of MDS (Table 62-6) defines ≥20 percent blasts (RAEBT) as AML; defines CMML as a myelodysplastic/myeloproliferative disease; and adds new categories of MDS. While correlation of clinical course with this new classification system is not yet defined, the WHO classification system incorporates current knowledge about these heterogenous disorders.

The natural history of patients with MDS syndromes is quite variable. Estimates of risk of progression to acute leukemia and median survival for the subgroups are outlined in Table 62-5. Prognostic factors, in addition to FAB subgroup, include the presence of cytogenetic abnormalities or secondary or mutagen-induced MDS, which are associated with a poor prognosis.

The clinical course of patients with RAEB, RAEBT, and CMML is frequently complicated by serious, and sometimes fatal, infection and hemorrhage related to pancytopenia. Patients who develop AML after MDS have a lower frequency and duration of response to standard therapy than patients with de novo AML.

There are few effective therapies for MDS. Therapeutic trials with corticosteroids, androgens, possible cytodifferentiating agents (low-dose cytosine arabinoside, 13-*cis*-retinoic acid, vitamin D analogs), cytotoxic chemotherapy, recombinant hematopoietic growth factors, and stem cell transplantation have produced disappointing results. Supportive care with red cell and platelet transfusions, and antibiotics for infection have long been considered standard therapy for most patients with MDS. Recent publications by Silverman and Kornblith described improvements in survival and quality of life in patients with MDS who received 5-azacytidine (versus observation) in a randomized trial of the national cooperative group Cancer and Leukemia Group B (CALGB). The strongly positive results of this large randomized study support 5-azacytidine as the new standard of care, although this drug is not yet commercially available.

Acute Myelogenous Leukemia

The average annual age-adjusted incidence of acute myelogenous leukemia in the United States is 2.8 per 100,000 population (about 9,500 cases per year) with a mortality rate of 2.3 per 100,000 population. The incidence increases with age in adults older than age 35 years to rates of 6.9 per 100,000 population in persons ages 60 to 64 years; 8.2 per 100,000 population in ages 56 to 69 years; 12.6 per 100,000

Table 62-6   Peripheral Blood and Bone Marrow Findings in Myelodysplastic Syndromes

Disease	Blood Findings	Bone Marrow Findings
Refractory anemia	Anemia No or rare blasts	Erythoroid dysplasia only <5% blasts <15% ringed sideroblasts
Refractory anemia with ringed sideroblasts	Anemia No blasts	≥15% ringed sideroblasts Erythroid dysplasia only <5% blasts
Refractory cytopenia with multilineage dysplasia (RCMD)	Cytopenias (bicytopenia or pancytopenia) No or rare blasts No Auer rods $<1 \times 10^9$/L monocytes	Dysplasia in ≥10% of the cells of two or more myeloid cell lines <5% blasts in marrow No Auer rods <15% ringed sideroblasts
Refractory cytopenia with multilineage dysplasia and ringed sideroblasts (RCMD-RS)	Cytopenias (bicytopenia or pancytopenia) No or rare blasts No Auer rods $<1 \times 10^9$/L monocytes	Dysplasia in ≥10% of the cells in two or more myeloid cell lines ≥15% ringed sideroblasts <5% blasts No Auer rods
Refractory anaemia with excess blasts-1 (RAEB-1)	Cytopenias <5% blasts No Auer rods $<1 \times 10^9$/L monocytes	Unilineage or multilineage dysplasia 5–9% blasts No Auer rods
Refractory anaemia with excess blasts-2 (RAEB-2)	Cytopenias 5–19% blasts Auer rods ± $<1 \times 10^9$/L monocytes	Unilineage or multilineage dysplasia 10–19% blasts Auer rods ±
Myelodysplastic syndrome-unclassified (MDS-U)	Cytopenias No or rare blasts No Auer rods	Unilineage dysplasia: one myeloid cell line <5% blasts No Auer rods
MDS associated with isolated del (5q)	Anaemia Usually normal or increased platelet count <5% blasts	Normal to increased megakaryocytes with hypolobated nuclei <5% blasts Isolated del(5q) cytogenetic abnormality No Auer rods

SOURCE: Reproduced with permission from Brunning et al. (2001).

population in ages 70 to 74 years; and >20 per 100,000 persons ≥ age 75 years. The incidence of AML is higher in white males living in industrialized areas in developed countries, suggesting environmental exposure as a possible cause, but the etiology of most cases of AML remains unknown.

Patients with AML usually present with evidence of bone marrow failure: anemia, bleeding caused by thrombocytopenia, or infection secondary to granulocytopenia. An international classification system (FAB) details subtypes of AML (M1 through M7) based on morphology, histochemical characteristics, and immunophenotyping. The purposed WHO classification of AML (Table 62-7) incorporates morphologic, immunophenotypic, genetic, and clinical features. There are four major categories, each with two or more subtypes described by Brunning et al.

If untreated or unresponsive to chemotherapy, AML may be rapidly fatal (median survival <2 months). The major causes of death are overwhelming infection and hemorrhage related to the disease-associated cytopenias.

Standard induction therapy for AML is combination chemotherapy that includes cytosine arabinoside (ara-C) and an anthracycline such as daunorubicin. These drugs yield complete remissions in 50 to 80 percent of patients, depending upon various prognostic factors. Increased age is an important negative prognostic factor. The poorer prognosis associated with increased age is related to both a higher frequency of fatal infections and hemorrhage during the period of disease and treatment-related marrow hypoplasia (induction deaths), and to chemotherapy failure (residual or resistant leukemia). While complete remission (CR) rates have usually been 60 to 80 percent in

Table 62-7 Classification of Acute Myeloid Leukemia

Acute myeloid leukemia with recurrent genetic abnormalities

Acute myeloid leukemia with t(8;21)(q22;q22); (AML1/ETO)

Acute myeloid leukemia with abnormal bone marrow eospinophils inv(16)(p13q22) or t(16;16)(p13;q22); (CBFβ/MYH11)

Acute promyelocytic leukemia (AML with t[15;17][q22;q12] [PML/RARα] and variants)

Acute myeloid leukemia with 11q23 (MLL) abnormalities

Acute myeloid leukemia with multilineage dysplasia

Following a myelodysplastic syndrome or myelodysplastic syndrome/myeloproliferative disorder

Without antecedent myelodysplastic syndrome

Acute myeloid leukemia and myelodysplastic syndromes, therapy-related

Alkylating agent-related

Topoisomerase type II inhibitor-related (some may be lymphoid)

Other types

Acute myeloid leukemia not otherwise categorized

Acute myeloid leukemia minimally differentiated

Acute myeloid leukemia without maturation

Acute myeloid leukemia with maturation

Acute myelomonocytic leukemia

Acute monoblastic and monocytic leukemia

Acute erythroid leukemia

Acute megakaryoblastic leukemia

Acute basophilic leukemia

Acute panmyelosis with myelofibrosis

Myeloid sarcoma

SOURCE: Reproduced with permission from Brunning et al. (2001).

younger patients with AML, the CR rate in patients ≥age 60 years and older has generally been ≤50 percent (with induction death rates of 20 to 40 percent).

Attempts to improve response rates in older patients with AML have included attenuated doses of standard therapy; these treatments have resulted in decreased induction death rates but without improved CR rates. The role of gemtuzumab ozogamicin (Mylotarg), a monoclonal antibody directed at CD33 has demonstrated substantial activity alone or in combination with ara-C; optimal use of this and other directed therapies are yet to be determined. Patients in the subgroup with acute promyelocyte leukemia (APL; AML-M3) are now treated very effectively with oral all-trans-retinoic acid (ATRA) plus chemotherapy; AML-M3, however, occurs uncommonly in older patients. The role of more aggressive therapies, including stem cell transplantation (high-dose therapy with stem cell rescue), has been limited in elderly patients by the high rates of complications and prohibitive toxicity. However,

improvements in supportive care have allowed for increased investigation of dose intensive therapies in older patients.

The median duration of complete remission is approximately 1 year, and a small percentage (≤15 percent) of older (≥60 years of age) patients will be cured of their leukemia. Patients who achieve complete remissions should be considered for therapy after remission in an attempt to prevent or delay relapse. However, the exact role and optimal type of such postremission therapy in older patients remain poorly defined.

The impact of other prognostic factors (other than age) within the elderly population are not well defined, but poorer functional performance status and the presence of a preceding myelodysplastic syndrome are generally considered indicators of a poor outcome.

Acute Lymphoblastic Leukemia

ALL is primarily a disease of children, but in adults age adjusted incidence increases in the elderly. There are approximately 3200 new cases of adult ALL in the United States annually, with a slight male predominance (1.2:1). With available therapy today, childhood ALL is curable in the majority of patients. ALL in adults is not the same as the childhood disease. First, the frequency of complete response is lower—70 to 75 percent in adults as opposed to more than 90 percent in children. Second, the remission duration and curability using the same therapy is considerably less. Important prognostic features for outcome in the treatment of ALL include age, cytogenetics, and immunophenotype. Poor prognosis is especially associated with the presence of chromosomal translocations such as Philadelphia (Ph) chromosome t(9;22), t(4,11), t(8;14), t(2;8), or t(8;22), and with a phenotype indicating mixed lymphoid-myeloid leukemia (also called biphenotypic leukemia).

The initial goal of therapy for adult ALL is to correct problems secondary to bone marrow failure; that is, to treat anemia with blood transfusions, treat documented or suspected infection, and control bleeding. Specific antileukemia treatment is then directed toward the achievement of a complete remission. Induction chemotherapy therapy for ALL, very different from that for AML, usually includes the use of prednisone, vincristine, daunorubicin, and asparaginase. While these drugs are well tolerated in children, increasing age is associated with poorer drug tolerance. Mortality, usually from infection and/or bleeding during the induction process, may occur in 10 to 20 percent of elderly patients.

In contrast to the treatment of AML, it is widely accepted that patients with ALL require therapy after complete remission. These phases of treatment once the patient is in complete remission have been referred to as intensification therapy and maintenance therapy. The optimal therapy after remission and the duration of such therapy in older patients are not clearly defined. Most programs use multiple drugs administered in a cyclic fashion over a 2-year period; the more intensive therapy is given over about 6 months after CR is achieved (intensification or consolidation), followed by a less-intensive outpatient maintenance regimen for approximately 18 months.

Table 62-8 Immunophenotype of B-cell Neoplasm

Diagnosis	SIg*	CD5	CD10	CD23	CD43	CD103
B-CLL	+	+	−	+	+	−
Splenic marginal zone lymphoma	+	−	−	−	−	−
Hairy-Cell leukemia	+	−	−	−	−	++

*Surface immunoglobulin.

Directed treatment to the craniospinal axis (central nervous system [CNS] prophylaxis) is standard practice in the treatment of childhood ALL. While the incidence of CNS leukemia is lower in adults than in children, treatment to the CNS is also part of ALL therapy in adults. This usually consists of intrathecal methotrexate in conjunction with cranial radiation or high dose systemic therapy such as high-dose methotrexate and ara-C.

With the above intensive treatment plan, the median duration of remission is approximately 2 years, with 35 to 45 percent of adult patients disease-free at 5 years; however, prognosis is poorer for older adults. One contributing feature to this poorer response duration in adults as opposed to children is the inability to deliver optimal chemotherapy at maximal doses due to comorbid diseases.

Chronic Lymphocytic Leukemia

CLL is a disorder of clonal proliferation of mature lymphoid cells in the peripheral blood, bone marrow, and lymphoid organs. CLL occurs predominantly in older adults, with median age at diagnosis of 60 to 65 years. The reported incidence of 3 per 100,000 population in Western countries (about 10,000 new cases per year in the United States) may be an underestimate because many patients are asymptomatic for years; incidence in persons older than age 60 years is about 20 per 100,000 population. There is no racial difference in the United States between blacks and whites, but there are very few cases in the Far East and among persons of Oriental descent; the male:female

ratio is approximately 2:1. Current diagnostic studies, especially immunophenotyping, allow for differentiation of the chronic lymphoid malignancies: B-cell CLL, T-cell CLL, prolymphocytic, circulating non-Hodgkin's lymphomas, and hairy-cell leukemia (Table 62-8).

B-cell CLL

B-cell CLL accounts for over 95 percent of all CLL. Twenty percent of such patients are identified with asymptomatic lymphocytosis during evaluation for other medical problems. In most patients, the disease has a gradual progression spanning several years, and the extent of the lymphoid burden at diagnosis correlates well with length of preexisting disease. In some patients, the disease has a more aggressive course and progression to advanced clinical stages may occur within a few months of diagnosis.

The diagnosis of CLL is based on peripheral blood lymphocytosis >10,000 lymphocytes/μl and a specific immunophenotyping pattern (coexpression of CD5 and CD20/23 with weak expression of surface immunoglobulin) showing a clonal proliferation of lymphocytes. Diagnosis and staging of CLL can usually be established by history, physical exam, CBC with review of the blood smear, and immunophenotyping of the peripheral blood; bone marrow studies are usually not needed. The original Rai classification (Table 62-9) implied an orderly progression from lymphocytosis alone to the successive development of adenopathy, organomegaly, and, eventually, anemia and thrombocytopenia. The prognostic importance of these variables has been confirmed. Pattern of bone marrow

Table 62-9 CLL Rai Clinical Classification

Stage	Risk*	Clinical Findings	Survival (Years)
0	Low	Lymphocytosis only	≥12
1	Intermediate	↑ Lymphs plus ↑ nodes	7–10
2	Intermediate	↑ Lymphs plus ↑ spleen and/or liver ± ↑ Nodes	4–9
3	High	↑ Lymphs plus ↓ Hgb (<11 g/dl) ± ↑ Nodes, ↑ liver, ↑ spleen	1.5–2
4	High	↑ Lymphs plus ↓ platelets (<100, 000/ul) ± ↑ Nodes, ↑ liver, ↑ spleen, ↓ Hgb	1.5–2

*Modified Rai classification.

infiltration and sex have also been identified as prognostic factors.

Therapy for B-cell CLL has been considered palliative and therefore has been reserved for patients who are symptomatic or who have signs of progressive disease by clinical or laboratory criteria. The mainstay of therapy has been oral alkylating agents (chlorambucil or cyclophosphamide) for control of lymphoid proliferation and steroids for autoimmune complications. Leukocytosis alone (stage 0) does not require therapy, because the prognosis of these patients is excellent in the absence of the other poor prognostic factors. The rate of increase of leukocytosis is a better indicator of disease activity than the absolute count. Leukostasis associated with high circulating blast counts in acute leukemias does not generally occur in this condition because most of the lymphocytes are mature, small cells.

Treatment with chemotherapy or local radiation can be used to control symptoms in patients with stage I or II disease; however, symptomatic improvement does not appear to prolong survival. In contrast, when treated with combination chemotherapy, patients with stage III or IV CLL have an improved median survival, which ranges from 1.5 years to more than 4 years. The development of more effective initial therapies for CLL such as nucleoside analogs (e.g., fludarabine) have resulted in an increased number of patients achieving complete remission. It is not yet clear that these remissions result in prolonged survival, although data from recent clinical trials are encouraging. These promising results have encouraged many hematologists and oncologists to institute therapy at an earlier stage. The best way to integrate newer agents such as fludarabine and monoclonal antibodies (e.g., rituximab and alemtuzumab) with each other and/or with more traditional therapies (alkylators and steroids) are not yet well-defined. There are multiple clinical trials currently evaluating different combinations of these medications (concurrent or sequential).

Autoimmune manifestations of CLL are common and include development of antibodies to platelets and red cells (IgG and C3 on direct antiglobulin test) and to erythroid precursors, resulting in red cell aplasia. All these complications are indications for therapy with steroids or intravenous gamma globulin for refractory cases of red cell aplasia.

Recurrent infections are the most common complications leading to death in CLL. Patients with stage 0 CLL have minimal increased risk of infection. In anticipation of gradual deterioration in immune response, however, pneumococcal vaccine and boosters should be administered while the potential for response is still intact. All other patients have higher risks for infection. As the disease advances clinically, immune function becomes progressively compromised, with increased susceptibility to viral, bacterial, and fungal infection. Patients should avoid direct contact with the body fluids of children who have received live-virus vaccines (oral polio, measles-mumps-rubella) for the duration of viral shedding.

B-Cell Prolymphocytic Leukemia

This rare subtype of lymphoid leukemia is characterized by marked lymphocytosis (often >100,000 lymphocytes/μl), extensive bone marrow infiltration, massive splenomegaly, and minimal to absent adenopathy. Prolymphocytes comprise the majority of circulating WBC (>55%; often >90%). The prolymphocyte is about twice the size of a normal lymphocyte, with a characteristic dense border outlining a prominent nucleolus. B-cell prolymphocytic leukemia (B-PLL) cells usually express CD19, CD20, CD22, CD79a, FMC7, and strong surface IgM; CD23 is usually negative.

Most patients with B-PLL have advanced clinical disease at presentation, with a prognosis similar to that of patients with stage III and IV B-cell CLL. Therapy for these patients has included multiagent chemotherapy to control the splenomegaly and leukocytosis, and radiation therapy to palliate splenic engorgement. Patients become increasingly refractory to therapy, with an expected survival of 1.5 years and death caused by uncontrolled disease. Recent data suggest that more aggressive newer agents such as alemtuzumab (CAMPATH-1H) are more effective than previous therapies for PLL, with improved response rates and survival.

T-cell PLL/CLL

T-cell PLL/CLL is a rare subtype that accounts for 2 to 3 percent of all small lymphocytic leukemia ("CLL") cases. Clinical manifestations include lymphocytosis, hepatosplenomegaly, generalized lymphadenopathy, skin infiltration (20 percent), and bone marrow involvement. Immunophenotyping in the peripheral blood shows a clonal proliferation of the malignant T cells—CD2, CD3, CD7 positive with weak CD3; in approximately 60 percent of patients, the cells are CD4+/CD8–, 25 percent are CD4+/CD8+, and 15 percent are CD4–/CD8+. Prognosis is generally poor, with limited responsiveness to therapy though newer agents (e.g. alemtuzumab) appear to be active.

Hairy-Cell Leukemia

Hairy-cell leukemia is rare and almost exclusively seen in men older than age 60 years. The clinical features include massive splenomegaly, absence of adenopathy, and peripheral pancytopenia. The diagnosis is made by the morphologic characteristics of the circulating lymphocytes, which are small and have cytoplasmic projections ("hairs"). Diagnosis, previously made histochemically with the TRAP (tartrate-resistant acid phosphatase) stain, is now made with immunophenotyping that shows positive sIgM, CD19, CD20, CD22, CD79a, CD11c, CD25 and CD103; negative CD5, CD10 and CD23. Bone marrow aspiration usually yields little material (dry tap), and bone marrow biopsy shows increased cellularity with diffuse infiltration by the hairy cells. The spleen is infiltrated with the same clone of cells. Infections with gram-negative and staphylococcal species are the predominant complication.

Splenectomy was the treatment of choice in the past with improvement of neutropenia in about 50 percent of patients for 8 to 10 years. Interferon (IFN)-α produced partial and complete remissions in more than 50 percent of patients, sparing many patients a surgical procedure and the effects of the splenectomy on the immune system. Interferon has now been replaced by the nucleoside analogs, especially cladribine (2-CdA), which is very well tolerated. This yields high remission rates, frequently after only one course of therapy.

Chronic Myelogenous Leukemia

Chronic myelogenous leukemia is a disorder of excess production of mature granulocytes that eventually progresses to a clinical picture similar to acute leukemia with an overgrowth of immature cells (blast crisis). It accounts for 15 percent of all leukemias, with an age-adjusted incidence rate of 1 per 100,000 population without geographic, sex, or racial differences.

Diagnosis is made by the demonstration of granulocytosis in the peripheral blood with a predominance of segmented neutrophils and myelocytes, increased basophils and eosinophils, increased bone marrow cellularity, a low leukocyte alkaline phosphatase (LAP) score, and the presence of the Philadelphia chromosome t(9;22). In the past, the disease was divided into Ph+ and Ph−; it is now felt, however, that the diagnosis of CML should be reserved for those with the Ph chromosome, with the Ph− disorder classified among other myeloproliferative diseases.

The disease characteristically proceeds through three phases; chronic, accelerated, and terminal (blastic) phase. The length of the chronic phase is highly variable, from 1.5 years to 14 years (median duration of 3 years). In the chronic phase, the disease is easily controlled without aggressive therapy. The accelerated phase begins with gradual increases in white cells, platelets, and spleen size. Initially good maturation persists, but eventually more blasts are seen in the peripheral blood, and higher doses of medication are required to maintain control. This phase generally lasts a few months but may extend over 1 year. The terminal phase of the disease is indistinguishable from acute leukemia. The blasts have myeloid surface markers in 85 percent of the patients and lymphoid markers in the remaining 15 percent.

Effective agents for CML in the chronic phase include hydroxyurea, busulfan, and IFN-α; IFN-α was the first drug to change the natural history of CML, decreasing the percentage of cells exhibiting the Ph chromosome and prolonging the chronic phase by 1 to 2 years. Allogeneic stem cell transplantation in the chronic phase, a promising intervention in younger patients, has limited benefit in the elderly patient because of the morbidity and mortality of this treatment. Imatinib mesylate (Gleevec; STI-571) a targeted tyrosine kinase inhibitor designed specifically for the treatment of CML (in oral formulation), has dramatic activity in the blast phase and accelerated phase of CML. In a recently completed trial in chronic phase CML, imatinib mesylate yielded marked improvements in clinical and cytogenetic responses, rates of disease progression, and treatment related toxicity compared to IFN-α plus low-dose ara-C. Based on these results, imatinib mesylate has replaced interferon regimens as the standard of care for patients with chronic phase CML. It is too early to determine the duration of remissions for elderly patients treated with the medication.

Imatinib mesylate should be the initial treatment for both the accelerated and blastic phases of CML if not already used during the chronic phase of disease. Treatment of the blastic transformation (after Gleevec) depends on the cell origin of the blasts. Myeloid blastic states respond poorly to standard AML therapies, and no standard therapy is available. Lymphoid blastic states can be controlled for 6 to 12 months, with standard combination regimens as used for de novo ALL.

Myeloproliferative Diseases

Myeloproliferative diseases include CML (described above), polycythemia vera, myelofibrosis, and essential thrombocytosis. Both polycythemia vera and myelofibrosis can be associated with increased WBC. Polycythemia vera is usually associated with mild increases in white count with a relatively normal differential, while myelofibrosis is frequently associated with immature white blood cells in addition to nucleated RBC's. The leukocytosis associated with polycythemia vera is usually of little consequence and treatment is directed towards the control of the increased red cells. Myelofibrosis can be associated with variable abnormalities in WBC numbers, either increased WBC with circulating immature precursors or decreased WBC's, especially in the present of massive splenomegaly.

Cancers Metastatic to Bone Marrow

Many of the common malignancies have a propensity for metastasis to the bone and bone marrow. These include carcinomas of the breast, lung, prostate, and the lymphomas. Space-occupying lesions in the bone marrow, which crowd out normal hematopoietic elements, are termed myelophthisis. Manifestations of myelophthisis in the peripheral blood include pancytopenia and leukoerythroblastosis. Pancytopenias may be aggravated by nutritional deficiencies, especially folate deficiency.

QUALITATIVE WHITE BLOOD CELL DEFECTS

Congenital disorders of WBC function are usually detected during childhood, though some such as myeloperoxidase deficiency and IgA deficiency may remain clinically silent and be first detected in adulthood.

Patients with severe diabetes mellitus and chronic renal failure may develop impaired polymorphonuclear neutrophil and lymphocyte function. Consequently, they are prone to serious infections. Many medications, especially steroids and other immunosuppressive agents, frequently produce qualitative WBC dysfunction.

REFERENCES

Beutler E et al (eds): *Williams Hematology*, 6th ed. New York, McGraw-Hill, 2001.

Brunning R et al: *Tumors of Hematopoietic and Lymphoid Tissues*. Geneva, World Health Organization, 2001.

DeVita VT et al: *Cancer: Principles and Practice of Oncology*. Philadelphia, Lippincott Williams and Wilkins, 2001.

Hoffman R et al (eds): *Hematology: Basic Principles and Practice,* 3rd ed. New York, Churchill Livingston, 2000.

Jaffe ES et al (eds): *World Health Organization Classification of Tumours. Pathology and Genetics of Tumours of Haematopoietic and Lymphoid Tissues*. Lyon, IARC Press, 2001.

Kornblith AB et al: Impact of azacytidine on the quality of life of patients with myelodysplastic syndrome treated in a randomized phase III trial: A Cancer and Leukemia Group B study. *J Clin Oncol* 20:2441, 2002.

Lenhard RE et al (eds): *The American Cancer Society's Clinical Oncology*. Atlanta, GA, American Cancer Society, 2001.

Silverman LR et al: Randomized controlled trial of azacitidine in patients with the myelodysplastic syndrome: A study of the Cancer and Leukemia Group B. *J Clin Oncol* 20:2429, 2002.

Non–Hodgkin's Lymphoma, Hodgkin's Disease, and Multiple Myeloma

WILLIAM B. ERSHLER

NON-HODGKIN'S LYMPHOMAS

Non-Hodgkin's lymphomas (NHLs) are a varied group of proliferative disorders that have in common the clonal expansion of cells of lymphoid origin. There is a wide clinical spectrum of NHLs, and the appropriate therapy for elderly patients remains controversial. Recent research advances have provided important leads to a better understanding of the mechanisms of molecular pathogenesis and to the development of curative treatment strategies.

Epidemiology

The American Cancer Society estimated that 35,600 new patients with NHL were detected in 1990 and that 18,200 deaths were attributed to this disease. This amounts to an almost 25 percent increase since 1950, which reflects at least two phenomena. First, NHL is one of a few malignancies associated with acquired immunodeficiency syndrome (AIDS), and accordingly, there has been a rise in the incidence of this disease, especially in young and middle-aged males. Second, the median age for NHL is older than 60 years, and more than two-thirds of patients with NHL are older than age 65 (one-third are older than age 70). With the dramatic increase in the number of older people, it is not surprising that NHL is being observed with increasing frequency.

Classification

Since the first description early in the nineteenth century of the conditions now known as Hodgkin's disease (HD) and NHL, several distinct classification systems have been developed. The number of systems has resulted in difficulty in comparing clinical features and assessing treatment outcomes. To remedy this problem, a National

Cancer Institute panel of experts representing all the modern classification schemes proposed a working formulation (Table 63-1) that divides NHL into four basic groups (low grade, intermediate grade, high grade, and miscellaneous). This classification highlights an intriguing paradox observed in lymphoma at all ages but which is nowhere more clearly evidence that in the elderly population. With technical advances in recent years that allow more precise cytogenetic and molecular identification of genetic lesions, important clues regarding the pathogenesis of NHL have been uncovered. Several distinct entities have emerged with common clinical (including prognostic) and pathologic features. However, some of these entities defy classification in the above-mentioned schemes. They include enteropathy-associated T-cell lymphomas, monocytoid B-cell lymphomas, CD30+ anaplastic large-cell lymphoma, mediastinal B large-cell lymphoma, and angiocentric immunoblastic lymphoma. Accordingly, an additional complex classification system, the Revised European-American Lymphoma (REAL) system has been introduced, but it remains to be seen whether it will offer practical advantages over the previously described systems. The development of microarray technology and evidence that the correlation of various patterns of gene expression with different clinical outcomes is comparable to that found with existing histologic classification systems. This suggests that these techniques will, before long, be incorporated into newer iterations of the existing systems (Rosenwald).

Working Group Classification

In general, low-grade lymphomas frequently present with few symptoms but with widespread disease and generally are not curable with the currently available modalities. Intermediate- and high-grade lymphomas present with more constitutional symptoms and at earlier stages and are

Table 63-1　Classification of Non-Hodgkin's Lymphoma

Grade	Working Formulation	Rappaport Classification
Low grade (favorable)	Small lymphocytic Follicular, predominantly small cleaved cell (FSC) Follicular, mixed small cleaved, large cell (FM)	Diffuse, lymphocytic, well differentiated Nodular, lymphocytic, poorly differentiated Nodular, mixed, lymphocytic, and histiocytic
Intermediate grade	Follicular, predominantly large cell Diffuse, small cleaved cell (DSC) Diffuse, small and large cell (DM) Diffuse, large cell (DL): cleaved or noncleaved cell	Nodular histiocytic Diffuse, lymphocytic Diffuse, mixed, lymphocytic, and histiocytic Diffuse histiocytic
High grade (unfavorable)	Immunoblastic (IBL) Lymphoblastic (LL) convoluted or nonconvoluted cell Small, noncleaved cell (SNC): Burkitt's or non-Burkitt's	Diffuse histiocytic Diffuse, lymphoblastic Diffuse, undifferentiated
Miscellaneous	Mycosis fungoides Extramedullary plasmacytoma Composite Unclassifiable	

in some cases curable even at an advanced stage. It is a challenge for those treating lymphomas in elderly patients to assess the likelihood of a meaningful treatment response in view of the enhanced rate and severity of treatment toxicity in the setting of an individualized assessment of a patient's functional status and projected longevity.

Evaluation and Staging

Precise pathologic staging (Table 63-2) of NHLs is not as critical in developing a treatment strategy as it is in HD because experience has indicated that the clinical stage (based on anatomic distribution) does not correlate as well with survival as it does in HD. For example, in low-grade lymphomas, the disease may be stage IV without much of a change in prognosis compared with earlier stages, and in higher-grade lymphomas, systemic treatment is necessary even for disease confined to one anatomic region. Staging laparotomies are rarely indicated for NHL. Systemic symptoms do not have the same dire prognostic significance that they have in HD but still indicate a poorer prognosis. Serum markers such as lactate dehydrogenase (LDH) and interleukin-6 (IL-6) have been shown to correlate with tumor burden, constitutional symptoms, and survival. High-grade lymphomas may require evaluation of the central nervous system (CNS), especially in patients with diffuse histologic findings and bulky abdominal lymphadenopathy. Furthermore, there is a much greater likelihood that NHLs will arise in extranodal tissue such as the stomach, intestine, lung, and brain. Alternative staging systems that use the largest tumor mass and LDH levels higher than 500 IU/L as indicators of tumor bulk may turn out to be more accurate indicators of prognosis. Older patients are more likely to present with more advanced disease, but this may reflect a delay in diagnosis, as has been demonstrated for solid tumors.

In light of the evolution and utilization of different classification schemes and because older patients were for several years excluded from clinical trials and often were not referred to cancer centers, it is difficult to state with confidence whether there are clinical or pathologic features of

Table 63-2　Staging for Hodgkin's and Non-Hodgkin's Lymphoma—Ann Arbor Classification

Stage	Description
I	Single node region
IE*	Single extralymphatic site
II	Two or more node regions on the same side of the diaphragm
IIE	Single node region plus localized single extralymphatic site
III	Node regions on both sides of the diaphragm
IIIE	Plus localized single extralymphatic site
IIIS†	Plus spleen involvement
IISE	Plus localized single extralymphatic site and spleen involvement
IV	Diffuse involvement, extralymphatic organs and/or site node regions
All A stages	Without weight loss, fever, sweats
Stage B	With weight loss, fever, sweats

*E, extranodal.
†spleen involved.

NHL that are unique to older patients. However, in certain series it appears that older patients constitute one-third to one-half of all NHL cases and that they are more likely to have diffuse histologic findings and present with extranodal disease involving gastric or bone marrow sites.

Clinical Features and Therapy

Low-Grade Lymphomas

Low-grade lymphomas (well-differentiated lymphocytic lymphoma and nodular poorly differentiated lymphocytic lymphoma, according to the Rappaport classification) are the most common lymphomas in older persons. These lymphomas are usually of B-cell origin. The median age of patients with these tumors is more than 55 years, and both types of low-grade lymphomas are uncommon before age 40. Most frequently, older patients present with advanced disease with multiple lymph nodes in the neck, axillary, inguinal, mediastinal, and para-aortic areas. Often splenomegaly is also present. A bone marrow biopsy reveals the presence of lymphoma in the majority of cases.

Diffuse well-differentiated lymphocytic lymphoma occurs in patients who are well into their eighties, whereas nodular, poorly differentiated lymphocytic lymphoma occurs rarely after age 70. Initially, there are few symptoms of small-cell lymphomas. Fevers, sweats, and weight loss (typical B-cell symptoms) are uncommon and should prompt a physician to evaluate other potential causes such as infections, histologic conversions, and second malignancies.

NHLs with favorable histologic features are not curable with current therapies, except in the very select case in which a stage I tumor can be cured by radiation therapy. Many investigators consider even these tumors incurable. However, disease progression (or recurrence) is often slow even in older, frail patients, and the median survival with advanced disease is 5 to 8 years. Occasionally these tumors convert to more aggressive large-cell lymphomas (in 1%–10% of cases), often after 5 to 8 years of fairly indolent disease (Richter's conversion). These converted tumors are more resistant to treatment, and the prognosis is adversely affected (median survival is less than 6 months). Commonly, one finds a single node or group of nodes growing out of proportion to other nodes, and a biopsy reveals large-cell lymphoma, with small-cell lymphoma still present in other nodes or in the bone marrow.

Clinically quantifiable immunologic abnormalities are found in most histologic types of low-grade lymphomas except well-differentiated lymphocytic lymphoma, which is similar to chronic lymphocytic leukemia (CLL). In this disorder, hypogammaglobulinemia is common and is associated with a propensity to infection, primarily with encapsulated bacterial organisms but also with common viruses. Monoclonal gammopathies are sometimes seen, and if examined by very sensitive techniques, are common. Circulating tumor cells can be detected by immunoglobulin gene rearrangement studies even when the peripheral lymphocyte counts are not elevated. Hemolytic anemias, especially cold-agglutinin disease (1.7%) and immune thrombocytopenia (0.4%) are uncommon but well-known complications of lymphomas.

Staging of low-grade lymphomas is generally important, but precise staging is much less useful than in HD because curative radiotherapy is not an option. Therefore, staging by physical examination, routine laboratory tests (a complete blood count, and a chemistry panel), a chest radiograph, a computed tomography (CT) scan of the abdomen, and a bone marrow biopsy is generally sufficient to plan treatment and offer prognostic information. Only in rare circumstances are tests such as a liver biopsy, lymphangiography, gallium-67 scanning, positron emission tomography (PET), or a staging laparotomy indicated. Because the stage of the disease is most often III or IV (Table 63-2) and because curative therapy is not an option, further investigations should be based only on localizing symptoms or concern about local complications. Because CNS invasion by low-grade lymphomas is rare, routine evaluation of the CNS (by CT imaging or spinal fluid analysis) is not warranted. However, Richter's conversion lymphomas do invade the CNS, and an evaluation should be done as described below for high-grade lymphomas.

The treatment of indolent lymphomas, although safe and effective, remains controversial. The major continuing questions are whether initial therapy prolongs survival and whether waiting until organ dysfunction or symptoms mandate treatment is sufficient. If the initial treatment is beneficial, it is also not known whether aggressive treatment (regimens used for high-grade lymphomas), less aggressive multiagent chemotherapy such as CVP (cytoxan, vincritistine, and prednisone) or single-agent therapy is the treatment of choice. A published report from Stanford University by Portlock et al comparing chlorambucil with CVP showed a higher complete response rate with CVP, but by 4 years the disease status and survival were equivalent. Other studies have confirmed these findings.

Patients who had no symptoms and slowly enlarging nodes over a period of months were selected for initial observation only in another Stanford study by Rosenberg. Therapy was initiated if symptoms developed, low blood counts resulted from marrow involvement, or the function of a vital organ was threatened. Often therapy was initiated only after a prolonged period, although many patients required therapy within 1 to 2 months of the initial evaluation. It appeared that long-term control and survival were unaffected by this approach.

In young, otherwise healthy patients, investigations into very aggressive treatment have been disappointing because permanent remissions do not seem to occur. Therefore, it appears that such treatment is inappropriate for a patient without significant symptoms or rapidly progressive disease. However, for those who have more virulent tumors, more intensive therapy appears to be beneficial. The COPP regimen (cytoxan, Oncovin, procarbazine, and prednisone) was shown in an Eastern Cooperative Oncology Group (ECOG) study to achieve a 56 percent remission rate, and 57 percent of the patients survived more than 5 years. Whether this regimen improves survival is difficult to evaluate because of the already lengthening median survival for patients with indolent lymphomas. Experience with this regimen shows that it is relatively well tolerated by older patients, in contrast to anthracycline (e.g., Adriamycin) containing regimens, although bowel toxicity caused by vincristine remains a problem. Alternative chemotherapy regimens have been utilized successfully in elderly patients, and when analyzed in the context of patient age, remission rates and survival are comparable.

Recently, there has been a resurgence of interest in biological therapies for lymphoma. Monoclonal antibodies, most notably rituximab (Rituxan), have shown great promise as single agents or in combination with chemotherapy for low-grade NHLs, particularly those with overexpression of the target antigen, CD20. A number of other therapeutic antibodies are under development and may offer an effective treatment strategy with limited toxicity for elderly lymphoma patients.

Intermediate-Grade Lymphomas

Intermediate-grade lymphomas (diffuse mixed lymphoma, diffuse histiocytic lymphoma, and immunoblastic lymphoma) often present with diffuse adenopathy without marrow or other organ parenchymal involvement. Patients with marrow, CNS, liver, or pulmonary involvement along with adenopathy have a poorer prognosis. Also common are lymphomas primary to extranodal sites, such as Waldeyer's tonsillar ring and the stomach, liver, spleen, and CNS. These diseases must be considered separately from primary nodal disease.

Diffuse large-cell (histiocytic) lymphoma, which originally was thought to be a tumor of histiocytes, is now known to be of either B- or T-cell origin. In fact, some of these tumors are true histiocytic lymphomas, but they are quite rare (approximately 1%). The prognosis seems to be independent of the cell of origin. The median age of patients is the late fifties, but there is a wide age distribution, this disease appears to occur more commonly in older individuals. The other intermediate-grade lymphomas are all of B-cell origin. Immunoblastic lymphomas occur in an age distribution similar to that of diffuse large-cell lymphoma, whereas diffuse mixed-cell lymphoma is rare after age 80.

Intermediate-grade lymphomas are now generally considered curable by modern chemotherapy. There remains controversy about whether tumors with diffuse mixed-cell histologic findings are curable, but long-term remissions are achieved in about 30 percent of patients. In contrast to indolent lymphomas, these tumors often present with a rapid increase in nodal masses accompanied by systemic constitutional symptoms such as fever and weight loss, and if untreated, they are often rapidly fatal. For example, patients with untreated diffuse large-cell lymphoma have a median survival of 2 to 3 months. With treatment, median survival is in the range of 3 to 5 years, with some subgroups having better than 50 percent cure rates.

Several studies show that advanced age is a negative prognostic factor in large-cell lymphomas. For example, in a French study involving 73 patients by Solal-Celigny et al, 39 younger than age 60 and 34 older than age 60, the only negative prognostic feature was age. The older patients had a median survival of 18 months, whereas median survival was 48 months for the younger patients. The difference did not appear to be related to the intensity of treatment or its tolerance. The Nebraska Lymphoma Study Group, as reported by Vose et al, used the CAP/BOP regimen (cytoxan, Adriamycin, procarbazine, bleomycin, Oncovin, and prednisone) to treat all patients with diffuse mixed-cell

or large-cell lymphoma. They found a similar overall complete remission (CR) rate of 65 percent in patients older and younger than 60 years; however, patients younger than 60 years had a 62 percent 5-year survival, whereas those older than 60 years had a 35 percent 5-year survival. They found that treatment toxicity was similar and that deaths from apparently unrelated causes accounted for most of the survival difference. CR durability was similar in older and younger groups, as opposed to the results from the French study, in which CR durability was poor in the older populations.

The Southwest Oncology Group (SWOG) studied CHOP (cytoxan, doxorubicin hydrochloride [Adriamycin], vincristine sulfate [Oncovin], and prednisone) chemotherapy with or without bleomycin or immunotherapy in patients of all ages, with an initial dose reduction required for patients older than age 65, as reported by Dixon et al. They found that CR rates declined with age, from 65 percent for those under age 40 to 37 percent for those older than age 65. Survival also declined from 101+ months in patients younger than age 40 to 16 months in those older than age 65. However, when full-dose initial chemotherapy was given to the older patients in violation of the protocol, the differences in the CR and death rates declined in the different age groups, showing that the initial "required" dose reduction might have accounted for part of the survival difference. Toxicity was similar in all age groups. The addition of bleomycin had an adverse effect in older patients. Several recent studies on other intensive chemotherapy regimens have shown poorer survival and increased toxicity in older age groups.

Rituximab, as mentioned above, has also been shown to be of benefit in the treatment of diffuse NHL. For example, Coiffer and colleagues reported that the addition of rituximab to standard CHOP chemotherapy significantly reduced the risk of treatment failure and death (risk ratios 0.58 [95% confidence interval (CI) 0.44 to 0.77] and 0.64 [95% CI 0.45 to 0.89], respectively). Importantly, clinically relevant toxicity was not significantly greater with CHOP plus rituximab.

Aggressive Lymphomas

Burkitt's lymphoma (and the similar undifferentiated non-Burkitt's lymphoma) and lymphoblastic lymphoma are considered aggressive lymphomas. Because lymphoblastic lymphoma is almost completely a disease of adolescence and young adulthood, it is not considered here. In the United States, Burkitt-like lymphomas usually present with rapidly expanding abdominal masses, high LDH and uric acid levels, and systemic symptoms. Without treatment, the median survival is 1 to 2 months, and treatment is often an emergency. Although Epstein–Barr virus is associated with the endemic (African) form, its role in the pathogenesis of Burkitt's lymphoma in the United States is unclear. These tumors arise from relatively mature B cells, as evidenced by the expression of surface immunoglobulin (SIg), B4 (CD19), B1 (CD20), and B3 (CD22). Immunophenotypic differences between the two clinical subtypes of Burkitt's lymphoma (endemic and sporadic) have been reported. The tumor can be identified karyotypically by one of three characteristic chromosomal translocations [t(8:14), t(8:22), and t(2:8)], all of which result in juxtaposition of the c-*myc* proto-oncogene (chromosome 8) to one of the three immunoglobulin heavy-chain genes.

The prognosis is poor in older patients because of the need for extremely aggressive treatment. Often the bone marrow is involved, which makes the disease essentially incurable in an elderly patient. Treatment requires prophylaxis against tumor lysis syndrome (intravenous fluids, alkalinization of the urine, and allopurinol), intensive doses of chemotherapy for several months, and CNS prophylaxis with intrathecal chemotherapy and whole-brain irradiation.

HODGKIN'S DISEASE

Hodgkin's disease has a bimodal age-specific incidence in the United States. The early peak occurs between the ages of 20 and 30, and the later peak between ages 70 and 80, with the incidence starting to increase at about age 50. Men far outnumber women in the later peak. It has been thought that two different etiologic processes may explain the bimodal distribution. MacMahon proposed an infectious etiology for HD in the younger population (ages 15 to 23). The epidemiologic finding of an increased risk in higher socioeconomic classes (similar to that for paralytic polio myelitis) suggests that HD in this age group is the rare result of a common (probably viral) infection that occurs later in life than is usual in lower socioeconomic classes. This effect of socioeconomic class persisted in persons aged 40 to 54 at the time of diagnosis but was absent in those older than age 54. Although an etiologic factor has not been found for either younger or older presentations of HD, these data, as well as the shift in pathologic subtypes outlined below, suggest the possibility of different etiologic mechanisms for younger and older persons who develop HD.

There has been a curious association between Epstein–Barr virus and HD. There is an increased risk for HD in patients with a history of infectious mononucleosis, and Epstein–Barr virus has been demonstrated directly in some cases. However, this association is not found in HD developing in older patients. The contribution of age-associated immune dysregulation to the pathogenesis in late-life HD has theoretical appeal, but no supporting data have been reported to date.

Presentation

Adenopathy is the most common presenting sign of HD in all age groups. Lokich et al found that adenopathy was a more common presentation in younger patients (80%) than in patients older than age 60 (50%), whereas 25 percent of older patients had systemic symptoms, in contrast to only 2 percent of younger patients. Abdominal disease was more prevalent in older patients. A study from the Finsen Institute in Copenhagen by Specht and Nissen found that older patients were more likely to have bulk abdominal disease, whereas younger patients were more likely to have thoracic and nodal disease, independent of histologic findings. In a study from Stanford University by Peterson

et al, unexplained adenopathy was the most common presentation (65%) in patients older than 60 years, and B-cell symptoms were the presenting complaint in 29 percent. Forty-two percent of these patients had significant intercurrent disease, including coronary artery disease or peripheral vascular disease, chronic obstructive pulmonary disease, diabetes mellitus, and hypertension. A staging laparotomy was performed in 48 percent of the patients, including 45 percent of those with intercurrent disease. In the Stanford study, in 75 percent of patients older than 60 years HD was considered to be adequately staged, and 64 percent of patients were considered to be adequately treated by the standards of the time (1982). The experience from this study and others indicates that elderly patients who present with localized HD should undergo a full staging evaluation, including a staging laparotomy.

These studies show that the presentation of HD in older patients is different from that in younger patients. Although some of this difference is accounted for by differences in histologic findings (nodular sclerosis [NS] is more likely in the thorax, and mixed cellularity in the abdomen), other differences are not related to histology and may involve an altered etiology or host response.

Histology

The diagnostic cell for HD is the Reed–Sternberg (RS) cell, a large, binucleated cell with prominent nucleoli. Strict criteria require the presence of an RS cell for a diagnosis of HD; however, on occasion it can be diagnosed if the mononuclear form—the "Hodgkin's cell"—is prominent. Although the RS cell occasionally can be found in other disorders, it is considered to be the malignant cell in HD, and the diagnosis of this condition depends on its histologic demonstration.

The origin of the RS cell remains controversial. It is almost always aneuploid, containing four to eight times the normal cellular content of DNA, and cytogenetic alterations (both random and nonrandom) are common. A number of T-cell surface markers (including CD1, CD2, CD, and CD4) and monocyte markers (including CD15) have been detected on HD cells. However, specific monoclonal immunoglobulin gene J-chain rearrangements also have been observed in some cases (particularly with lymphocyte-predominant histologic findings), suggesting a B-cell origin in these cases.

The Leu-1 antibody recognizes the CD15 molecule, which is generally present on RS cells. However, this molecule also has been detected on the surface of cells in some T-cell NHLs. Similarly, the Ki-1 antibody, which was induced by using RS cells as antigen, has been shown to detect CD30. It was hoped that it would be specific for RS cells, but it is now clear that it is present on the cells of an NHL subtype as well.

Hodgkin's disease has four histologic types: lymphocyte-predominant, NS, mixed cellularity, and lymphocyte-depleted. Of these types, lymphocyte-predominant and NS are generally considered to indicate a better prognosis; however, this advantage largely disappears when the pathologic stage is considered. The malignant cell in HD is thought to be the RS cell, whereas infiltrating

Table 63-3   Influence of Age on Histologic Patterns of Hodgkin's Disease

Histologic Pattern	Specht and Nissen		Peterson et al		Wedelin et al	
	Age <40 (%)	Age >60 (%)	Age <40 (%)	Age >60 (%)	Age <50 (%)	Age >50 (%)
Lymphocyte-predominant	12	12	7	11	12	17
Nodular sclerosing	61	44	30	7	49	21
Mixed cellularity	25	37	42	52	29	46
Lymphocyte-depleted	<1	2	14	20	7	13
Unclassified	2	4	7	11	4	4

lymphocytes, eosinophils, and neutrophils are thought to be reactive phenomena. Histologic findings for aggressive HD show abundant RS cells, whereas those for indolent forms have few.

It is generally thought that subtypes of HD based on histologic patterns occur with different frequencies in older compared with younger patients. The NS histology is found most frequently in adolescents and young adults and is unusual in patients older than 50 years. Several studies comparing histologic patterns in older and younger patients are somewhat contradictory but support a decline in the incidence of NS histology compared with mixed cellularity histology (Table 63-3).

The Finsen Institute study by Specht and Nissen involved 506 unselected patients who were studied for the age distribution of histologic. In the younger groups, NS was the most common; however, in those older than age 60, NS, although less prevalent than in younger patients, was still the most common subtype; it was found in 44 percent of patients, whereas mixed cellularity was found in 37 percent. Lymphocyte-depleted histologic patterns were notably uncommon in this study.

Investigations at Stanford University by Austin-Seymour et al found that 65 percent of older patients had NS histologic findings. However, only 52 of 1169 patients in the study were older than age 60, suggesting a possible referral bias. A report from Cancer and Acute Leukemia Group B (CALGB) published by Newell et al stated that 73 of 385 patients who were older than age 60 were treated for advanced HD. Only 7 percent demonstrated NS histologic patterns, compared with 30 percent of patients younger than age 40. The low percentage is explained by the small likelihood that this histologic pattern occurs in advanced disease. Wedelin et al found that 49 percent of patients younger than age 50 showed NS and 29 percent mixed cellularity, whereas in patients older than age 50, 21 percent showed NS and 45 percent mixed cellularity.

These studies suggest that a shift toward mixed cellularity and away from NS histologic patterns occurs with advancing age. They also reveal that NS histology is not uncommon in older persons and that mixed cellularity is not uncommon in younger populations. Whether these moderate shifts in histologic subtypes with age are indicative of a differing etiology (as mentioned above), the biology of the malignancy, or a differing host response to the malignancy, remains unclear.

Staging

Precise anatomic recognition of all the involved sites is critical in HD management because the best chance for a cure is with the initial treatment, which is predicated on the stage. A suggested plan for staging is found in Table 63-4. A careful medical history and a thorough physical examination are essential. Evaluation of the chest typically involves a chest radiograph and frequently computed tomography (CT) imaging. If the chest radiograph is normal, including the mediastinum, CT scanning may not be necessary. However, the upper abdominal regions are best evaluated by CT imaging, and this can be accomplished at the same time as the chest CT scan with a few additional cuts below the diaphragm. Lower abdominal nodes are still best evaluated by lymphangiography, and bilateral bone marrow biopsies can indicate the presence of marrow involvement in a subset of patients (perhaps 10%) for whom staging

Table 63-4   Staging Recommendations for Hodgkin's Disease

History, with special attention to B-cell symptoms, including fevers, night sweats, and >10% loss in body weight

Physical examination with special attention to node-bearing areas, liver, and spleen

Initial blood work to include a complete blood count with white cell differential and platelet count, serum chemistries including liver function tests, creatinine, albumin, total protein, and erythrocyte sedimentation rate

Radiologic studies to include chest radiography and chest computed tomography (CT) imaging if chest radiograph is abnormal, abdominal and pelvic CT, and bipedal lymphangiogram

Bilateral iliac crest bone marrow biopsies

In selected cases, laparotomy with exploration of lymph node–bearing areas, liver biopsies, and splenectomy; if laparotomy is not to be performed, percutaneous or laparoscopy-guided liver biopsies should be considered to this point did not indicate any suspicion of extranodal disease. In older individuals, the marrow cellularity and evidence for adequate hematopoiesis are of additional value in planning therapy.

For patients with stage IIIA disease or better after the completion of these studies, a staging laparotomy should be considered. This procedure involves careful abdominal exploration with routine biopsies of para-aortic, celiac, splenic hilar, mesenteric, portal, and iliac nodes; wedge and core biopsies of the liver; and splenectomy. A staging laparotomy demonstrates more advanced disease (upstaging) about 35 percent of the time, but in some cases (10–15%) radiographically suspicious lesions are shown to be not HD and downstaging is the result. A staging laparotomy is considered major surgery and may not be well tolerated in elderly patients. The benefits of a more accurate assessment and more precise therapy have to be weighed against the operative risks. Alternative staging approaches, including new visualizing techniques, are being explored. However, for patients in whom radiation therapy is being used with curative intent, a staging laparotomy remains the standard evaluative approach.

Therapy

The therapy for HD has become better defined as a result of clinical trials (Table 63-5). For younger patients, there remain few areas of substantial controversy. Patients with stage IA or IB disease and patients with stage IIA with supradiaphragmatic disease can be cured with involved-field irradiation. Patients with stage IIA nonbulky disease have good relapse-free survival rates with total nodal irradiation, and many who relapse can ultimately be cured with chemotherapy. The treatment of patients with stage IIB HD is an area of controversy, as the relapse rate with radiation is higher than that with chemotherapy, and it is unclear if

Table 63-5   Recommended Therapy for Hodgkin's Disease

Stage	Therapy
I, II (A or B, negative laparotomy results)	Subtotal lymphoid irradiation
I, II (A or B with mediastinal mass >1/3 diameter of chest wall)	Combination chemotherapy followed by irradiation to involved field
IIA$_1$ (minimal abdominal disease)	Total lymphoid irradiation
IIIA$_2$ (extensive abdominal disease)	Combination chemotherapy with irradiation to involved sites
IIIB	Combination chemotherapy
IV (A or B)	Combination chemotherapy

salvage rates with chemotherapy make this approach as beneficial as up-front chemotherapy. Patients with stage IIIA bulky disease and those with stage IIIB, IVA, or IVB disease require chemotherapy. Individuals with early-stage disease with large mediastinal masses (occupying more than 50 percent of the pleural cavity diameter by chest radiograph) have a high relapse rate with radiation therapy alone, and combined-modality therapy is recommended.

Many regimens have been used to treat advanced HD, including MOPP (methotrexate, Oncovin, procarbazine hydrochloride, and prednisone), ABVD (Adriamycin, bleomycin, vinblastine sulfate, and dacarbazine), BCVPP (carmustine [BCNU], cyclophosphamide, vinblastine sulfate, procarbazine, and prednisone), and the alternating regimens MOPP/ABVD and MOPP/ABV. The best regimens have not yet been determined. However, alternating MOPP and ABVD for 8 to 12 cycles (at least 4 cycles beyond documented CR) is an aggressive, reasonable approach. Although BCVPP is better tolerated than MOPP, there are concerns that BCNU is more leukemogenic, and therefore it is now less commonly used.

Toxicity from both radiotherapy and chemotherapy increases with age. The typical side effects of radiation therapy for HD include acute and transient anorexia with occasional nausea, vomiting, diarrhea, transient and occasionally permanent drying of salivary secretions, transient pharyngitis and esophagitis, fatigue, and cytopenias. The long-term side effects include hypothyroidism (common), pneumonitis, constrictive pericarditis, rare endocardial or myocardial fibrosis, skin pigmentation and breakdown, and leukemias. The long-term follow-up of patients who have received radiation therapy to upper mantle areas should include periodic thyroid evaluations.

The side effects of chemotherapy are also enhanced in older patients. However, many of these patients tolerate intensive chemotherapy well. Certain drugs were found by the ECOG to cause more severe toxicity in older patients as reported by Berg et al. Those used commonly in the treatment of HD and NHLs include vinblastine sulfate, methotrexate (possibly because of decreased renal function in older patients, the sole mode of clearance of this drug), VP-16, and doxorubicin (Adriamycin). The liver metabolism of other drugs is probably slowed in older persons. Given the possibility of enhanced toxicity, an older patient with HD can still be treated safely with curative intent. Even those for whom curative treatment is not indicated, significant palliation and prolongation of life can be achieved with localized radiation and single-agent or multiagent chemotherapy.

Response to Treatment and Survival

Many published series have demonstrated poorer survival in older patients with HD, but these series have been difficult to interpret because modern staging and treatment were not applied consistently, and it is now understood that age bias may influence cancer therapy outcomes.

The Stanford study by Peterson et al described earlier reported decreasing freedom from relapse with increasing age in patients treated from 1968 to 1981. The 5-year freedom-from-relapse rate was 81 percent for those younger than age 17; for those aged 17 to 49 it was 70 percent, for those aged 50 to 59 it was 63 percent, and for those aged 60 and older it was 38 percent. Multivariate analysis revealed that age was the most important factor in determining freedom from relapse.

MULTIPLE MYELOMA AND OTHER PLASMA CELL DYSCRASIAS

The autonomous proliferation of plasma cells, unlike that of most other immune cells, is associated with the elaboration of a monoclonal protein—either an intact immunoglobulin or a fragment thereof (usually the light-chain component). The unusual clinical features of plasma cell malignancies in general and multiple myeloma in particular can be explained by:

- The pathophysiologic effects of the abnormal protein
- The production of an osteoclast-activating factor by plasma cells, resulting in bone resorption
- The "crowding out" of normal marrow, with resulting cytopenias.

Epidemiology

Although multiple myeloma is still a rare disease, the incidence is gradually increasing for reasons that are unclear. In the United States there are two or three new cases per 100,000 population per year, which is similar to the incidence of HD and CLL. Myeloma accounts for 1 percent of all malignancies. Although the age range is wide, it is considered a disease of older adults. Cases are rare before age 30, and the peak incidence occurs in the seventh decade. Males are affected slightly more frequently than females, and it is more common in African Americans than in members of other races.

Etiology

Radiation or other carcinogen exposure and antigenic stimulation are involved in causing this disease. Japanese atomic bomb survivors have had a fivefold increase in risk.

In mice, the spontaneous development of plasma cell tumors is less common in animals maintained in a germ-free environment. Additionally, intraperitoneal deposition of mineral oil produces a granulomatous inflammatory response that frequently is followed by activation or over-expression of certain oncogenes (most notably c-*myc* and H-*ras*) and ultimately intra-abdominal plasma cell tumors that produce monoclonal immunoglobulin. Chronic antigenic stimulation therefore is considered a probable etiologic feature in the mouse, but the association in humans is less apparent. Cytokine (particularly IL-6) dysregulation is also an important feature of multiple myeloma. Serum levels of IL-6 are very high and correlate with tumor mass, the extent of bone destruction, and survival. Furthermore, in the murine model mentioned above, plasma cell tumors did not develop in mice genetically engineered to be IL-6-deficient (IL-6 knockouts).

Because of the low fraction of cells in DNA synthesis, few mitoses are usually available to define karyotypic abnormalities, and therefore disease-specific anomalies have not been identified as they have for leukemia and lymphoma. Analysis of the nuclear DNA content by flow cytometry (which does not depend on mitoses) has demonstrated aneuploidy in 80 percent of patients. Chromosomal translocations were found in 10 percent of cases, and interestingly, t(8:14) abnormalities were associated with an immunoglobulin A (IgA)-type myeloma.

Pathogenesis

Hyperviscosity and Other Defects Resulting From High Levels of Circulating Protein

Many of the features of myeloma are due to the high concentration of serum protein. Hyperglobulinemia produces similar effects whether it is polyclonal or monoclonal. Plasma becomes viscous when the IgM level exceeds 2 g/dL (as in Waldenström's macroglobulinemia) and also in IgA myeloma if IgA polymerization occurs and occasionally with high levels of IgG. Hyperviscosity decreases cerebral blood flow, producing headache, nausea, visual impairment, and mental clouding. Decreased renal blood flow may contribute to the renal failure so common in multiple myeloma (Tables 63-6 and 63-7). The blood volume expands, and congestive heart failure may develop. The high concentrations of serum protein interact with

Table 63-6 Plasma Cell Disorders

Disease	Immunoglobulin	Frequency (%)	Prognosis (Months)
Multiple myeloma	IgG	52	29–35
	IgA	21	19–22
	IgD	2	9
	IgE	<0.01	—
	Light chains only	11	10–28
Waldenström's macroglobulinemia	IgM	12	50

Table 63-7   Causes of Renal Failure in Myeloma

Light-chain deposition in tubules ("myeloma kidney")

Hyperviscosity

Hypercalcemia

Hyperuricemia

Infection

Dehydration (especially after an intravenous pyelogram)

Associated amyloidosis

erythrocyte membranes and cause a coinlike stacking of red cells known as rouleaux formation. The coating of platelets results in diminished aggregation and purpura. The high protein level may also interfere with coagulation factors by inhibiting fibrin polymerization, and bleeding may result.

In the absence of glomerular kidney disease, the intact immunoglobulin molecule is too large to be filtered and is therefore not found in the urine. However, immunoglobulin light chains are filtered and then to a variable extent reabsorbed by the proximal tubule and secreted by the distal tubule. Crystals of light-chain protein have been demonstrated in tubular cells, and protein casts often are seen in tubular lumens. These findings are associated with renal tubular dysfunction and overt renal failure in many patients. Monoclonal lambda light chains are more likely to produce tubular injury than are kappa chains. Renal injury may explain the poorer prognosis associated with lambda light chains (median survival, 11 months) versus kappa light chains (median survival, 28–30 months) in patients with light-chain disease.

Bone Erosion Resulting from Osteoclast-Activating Factors (Interleukin-1α and Interleukin-6) and Plasma Cell Tumors

Approximately 70 percent of patients with myeloma intially complain of bone pain. Radiographs reveal either localized punched-out lytic lesions or diffuse osteoporosis, usually in bones with active hematopoietic tissue. In fact, patients with myeloma who do not have radiographic evidence of bone disease are uncommon.

The discrete lytic lesions are characterized by large, numerous osteoclasts on the bone-reabsorbing surface. Myeloma cells grown in culture secrete IL-1α and IL-6, and both these molecules are potent stimulators of osteoclast activity. Thus, bone destruction in myeloma appears to be an exaggeration of the normal bone-remodeling process mediated by these cytokines.

With bone demineralization caused by osteoclast activation and with decreased activity because of pain, hypercalcemia can be expected. The symptoms of hypercalcemia (drowsiness, confusion, nausea, and thirst) are nonspecific, but their occurrence should alert the physician to investigate this possibility. Cardiac arrhythmias, renal insufficiency, and profound CNS depression can develop as hypercalcemia progresses.

Tumor Expansion

In the early stages of multiple myeloma, as many as 10^{11} malignant plasma cells may occur in clusters in the marrow. A single bone marrow sample may not reveal the abnormal cells despite positive results from serum or urine tests. As the disease evolves, however, a random marrow aspirate characteristically reveals large numbers of abnormal-appearing plasma cells (as the total approaches 10^{12}). The normal hematopoietic tissue disappears, and in most cases a normochromic, normocytic anemia develops with moderate neutropenia and thrombocytopenia. Plasma cells also may form a tumor mass that erodes and destroys vertebrae, causing collapse. Extrusion of the mass into the epidural space can lead to spinal cord compression. Infiltration into the liver, spleen, lung, and other vital organs can occur but usually does not compromise their function. Occasionally plasma cells are found in the peripheral blood. IgE myeloma presents a distinct clinical entity—plasma cell leukemia—which, in contrast to multiple myeloma, is characterized by greater tissue and organ involvement, less bone destruction, and a more fulminant course. It resembles acute leukemia more than it does myeloma.

Clinical Features

Multiple myeloma occurs primarily in older patients. In a large series, only 2 percent of the patients were younger than 40 years old, and the greatest incidence occurred in the seventh decade. Bone pain is the most common symptom, as is reported by 70 percent of patients at presentation. However, fatigue, weakness, and recurrent infections also may cause a patient to seek medical attention. Occasionally, a patient is found to have an incidental myeloma when examined for other medical problems. These patients generally develop overt myeloma, although this presymptomatic period may last a decade or longer (and should not to be confused with benign monoclonal gammopathy, as described below). Death from infection, renal failure, or hypercalcemia occurs when the tumor burden reaches approximately 3×10^{12} cells. A bone marrow aspirate or biopsy characteristically reveals more than 20 percent plasma cells, many of which are large, immature, and multinucleated.

Therapy

Effective treatment for patients with myeloma includes chemotherapy, radiotherapy, and the aggressive use of supportive measures. The current standard chemotherapy consists of intermittent oral melphalan (phenylalanine mustard) and prednisone. Cyclophosphamide, nitrosoureas (BCNU), doxorubicin, vincristine, and various forms of interferon all have been used either alone or in combination with variable success. In selected cases, autologous or allogeneic bone marrow transplantation has shown to be beneficial. However, typically, more than a 90 percent reduction in myeloma cells is unusual, and cures do not occur. Focal radiotherapy is used for pain relief and to decrease the risk of fractures.

Originally developed several decades ago as a sedative, thalidomide has been reintroduced into clinical medicine because of its antiangiogenesis and cytokine-inhibiting effects. The impressive activity of this agent, either alone or with dexamethasone, has been demonstrated in patients with myeloma, and the combination is currently under investigation as first-line therapy, particularly for elderly patients.

Measures designed to maintain activity and hydration are also important. Analgesics, orthopedic surgery, and supports facilitate mobilization. With adequate mobilization and fluid intake, the symptom complex of hypercalcemia, dehydration, and renal failure can often be avoided. Objective responses to chemotherapy currently approach 70 percent, and the median survival for new patients is approximately 36 months, which is a marked improvement compared with the survival of myeloma patients before the use of chemotherapy and aggressive medical treatment (less than 12 months).

Other Plasma Cell Dyscrasias Seen in Geriatric Populations

Waldenström's Macroglobulinemia

Waldenström's macroglobulinemia is due to the proliferation of a neoplastic clone of IgM-producing cells called lymphocytoid plasma cells. Bone destruction is not a feature. In many respects, macroglobulinemia resembles a well-differentiated lymphocytic lymphoma (low grade) with infiltration of the marrow by lymphocytes or lymphocytoid plasma cells, lymphadenopathy, and splenomegaly.

The circulating monoclonal IgM (macroglobulin) appears to explain much of the pathophysiology. The macroglobulin coats platelets and interferes with clotting. Oncotic expansion of the plasma volume leads to spurious anemia and may result in congestive heart failure. The hyperviscosity syndrome is common.

Therapy is directed at both the proliferating malignant clone of cells and the abnormal circulating protein. Agents such as chlorambucil have proved effective in prolonging survival. If hyperviscosity causes symptoms, plasmapheresis can produce dramatic, albeit temporary, relief.

Heavy-Chain Disease

Heavy-chain diseases are rare malignancies characterized by the proliferation of plasma cells that produce an abnormal monoclonal heavy chain without associated light-chain synthesis. Like macroglobulinemia, these disorders resemble lymphoma more than they do myeloma. Bone disease does not occur, but lymphadenopathy and hepatosplenomegaly are common. Gamma, alpha, and mu heavy-chain diseases have been described. Alpha-chain disease is usually associated with lymphomas involving the gastrointestinal tract and with malabsorption, whereas mu heavy-chain disease is associated with long-standing CLL. Gamma heavy-chain disease can present as a lymphoma that histologically resembles HD.

Amyloidosis

Amyloidosis is a heterogeneous group of disorders characterized by the deposition of insoluble protein in tissues that eventual compromises the function of the involved organs. Several different proteins have been identified in deposits, but two are common. In type I amyloidosis, the principal protein is on immunoglobulin light chain, whereas in type II amyloidosis a nonimmunoglobulin protein (protein A) is found. In both types the proteins form noncovalent polymers in a fibrillar pattern that can be recognized

Table 63-8 Early Myeloma Versus Benign Monoclonal Gammopathy

	Early Myeloma	Benign Monoclonal Gammopathy
Pathogenesis	Neoplastic plasma cell disorder (malignant)	Disordered immunoregulation (most common) or benign B-cell neoplasm (less common)
Bone marrow	Frequently >10% plasma cells with many bizarre, multinucleated forms	Usually <10% plasma cells, and these appear normal
Bone	Majority have bone erosions or diffuse osteoporosis (even early)	Usually no bone disease
Symptoms	Bone pain, fatigue, weight loss, or those associated with kidney failure	Usually no symptoms
Serum pike	Progressively rising	Stable level IgG <3.5 g/dl, IgA <2.0 g/dl, BJ <1.0 g/24 h (urine)

Table 63-9 Summary Points for the Practicing Geriatrician

General

Older patients present with more advanced disease.

Published cooperative trials on which standard therapy is based include disproportionately few elderly patients.

Older patients are not *a priori* more resistant to chemotherapy. However, end-organ toxicity, especially for heart, lung, and bone marrow, may be greater.

Non-Hodgkin's lymphoma

Increases in frequency with advancing age, especially low-grade lymphomas.

High-grade lymphomas must be treated aggressively or survival will be short.

Hodgkin's disease

Older patients have relatively more unfavorable histologic findings (i.e., mixed cellularity or lymphocyte-depleted).

Chemotherapy has been less successful in achieving cures in older patients, perhaps because of comorbidity.

Multiple myeloma

It is important to differentiate early myeloma from benign monoclonal gammopathy (Table 63-8).

Myeloma should be a consideration for all older patients with persistent bone (especially low back) pain. The average delay in diagnosis from first seeking medical attention is 6 months or more.

on electron microscopy. Different patterns of tissue distribution are associated with the different types of protein deposited.

When amyloidosis is associated with plasma cell dyscrasia (type I), amyloid deposits are found primarily in the muscles (including the heart and tongue), gastrointestinal tract, and skin. In conditions associated with protein A deposition (such as chronic infections and familial Mediterranean fever), amyloid deposition occurs in the kidney, spleen, liver, and adrenals. Mixed patterns, however, are common, and the presenting site of involvement is not sufficient to classify the type of amyloid involved.

Benign Monoclonal Gammopathy

Immunoregulatory functions are affected by the aging process and paraproteinemia, and autoantibodies are observed with increasing frequency with each advancing decade. In general, paraproteinemia (often termed monoclonal gammopathy of uncertain significance) is an indicator of dysregulated B-cell clonal expansion, but it is not considered an antecedent of multiple myeloma. Although it is not thought to be a malignant process itself, patients with monoclonal gammopathy of undetermined significance have their life expectancy shortened by 2 years compared with age-matched, unaffected controls. Furthermore, there is a subset of individuals within the group thought to have benign monoclonal gammopathy (perhaps 15%) who progress to overt myeloma after a prodrome of up to 30 years. Also, because myeloma with a more typical presentation increases in incidence with advancing age, it must be distinguished from the monoclonal gammopathy of undetermined significance. Typically, this is accomplished through examination of the bone marrow, skeletal radiographs, renal function, and serum α-2 microglobulin levels (Table 63-8). Indeed, some cases are early myeloma, whereas others reflect a completely different pathogenesis and do not result in clinically important disease. Early myeloma shows signs of disease progression over the first year or two, whereas benign gammopathy has stable protein readings, no bone disease, and a marrow that may or may not show mild to moderate plasmacytosis but instead shows normal-appearing plasma cell morphology. It is important to make this distinction because benign gamopathy is common and does not require therapy.

REFERENCES

Austin-Seymour M et al: Hodgkin's disease in patients over 60 years old. *Ann Int Med* 100:13, 1984.

Bataille R, Harousseau JL: Age dependence on the early-phase pharmacokinetics of doxorubicin. *Cancer Res* 43:4467, 1983.

Begg CB et al: *A Study of Excess Hematologic Toxicity in Elderly Patients Treated on Cancer Chemotherapy Protocols.* New York: Springer, 1989.

Coiffier B, Lepage E et al: CHOP chemotherapy plus rituximab compared with CHOP alone in elderly patients with diffuse large-B-cell lymphoma. *N Engl J Med* 24;346:235, 2002.

Dixon DO et al: Effect of age on therapeutic outcome in advanced diffuse histiocytic lymphoma: The Southwest Oncology Group experience. *J Clin Oncol* 4:295, 1986.

Ezdinli EA et al: Moderate versus aggressive chemotherapy of nodular lymphocytic poorly differentiated lymphoma. *J Clin Oncol* 3:769, 1985.

Gould J et al: Plasma cell karyotype in multiple myeloma. *Blood* 71:453, 1988.

Gutensohn N: Social class and age at diagnosis of Hodgkin's disease: New epidemiologic evidence of the "two-disease hypothesis." *Cancer Treat Rep* 66:689, 1982.

Harris NL et al: A revised European-American classification of lymphoid neoplasms: A proposal from the International Lymphoma Study Group. *Blood* 84:1361, 1994.

Hellman S et al (eds): *Hodgkin's Disease.* Philadelphia: JB Lippincott, 1989.

Hilbert DM et al: Interleukin-6 is essential for in vivo development of B lineage neoplasmas. *J Exp Med* 182(1):243, 1985.

Kurzrock R et al: Serum interleukin 6 levels are elevated in lymphoma patients and correlate with survival in advanced Hodgkin's disease and with B symptoms. *Cancer Res* 53:2118, 1993.

Kyle RA: Monoclonal gammopathy of undetermined significance and solitary plasmacytoma: Implications for progression to overt myeloma. *Hematol Oncol Clin North Am* 11:71, 1997.

Kyle RA, Rajkumar SV: Therapeutic application of thalidomide in multiple myeloma. *Semin Oncol* 28:583, 2001.

Lokich JJ et al: Hodgkin's disease in the elderly. *Oncology* 29:484, 1974.

MacMahon B: Epidemiology of Hodgkin's disease. *Cancer Res* 26:1189, 1966.

Monfardini S, Carbone A: Non-Hodgkin's lymphomas, in Balducci L et al (eds): *Comprehensive Geriatric Oncology.* Harwood Academic Publishers, Singapore, 1997, pp. 577–594.

Newell GR et al: Age differences in the histology of Hodgkin's disease. *J Natl Cancer Inst* 45:311, 1970.

Peterson B et al: Effect of age on therapeutic response and survival in advanced Hodgkin's disease. *Cancer Treat Rep* 66:889, 1982.

Portlock C et al: Treatment of advanced non-Hodgkin's lymphomas with favorable histologies: Preliminary results of a prospective trial. *Blood* 47:747, 1976.

Radl J: Age-related monoclonal gammopathies: Clinical lessons from the aging C57BL/6 mouse. *Immunol Today* 11:234, 1990.

Robb-Smith, AH. US National Cancer Institute working formulation of non-Hodgkin's lymphomas for clinical use. *Lancet* 2:432–4, 1982.

Robert J, Hoerni B: Age dependence on the early-phase pharmacokinetics of doxorubicin. *Cancer Res* 43:4467, 1983.

Rosenwald A et al: The use of molecular profiling to predict survival after chemotherapy for diffuse large B cell lymphoma. *N Engl J Med* 346:1937, 2002.

Rosenberg SA: The low-grade non-Hodgkin's lymphomas: Challenges and opportunities. *J Clin Oncol* 3:299, 1985.

Silverberg E et al: Cancer statistics. *CA Cancer J Clin* 40:7, 1990.

Solal-Celigny P et al: Age as the main prognostic factor in adult aggressive non-Hodgkin's lymphoma. *Am J Med* 83:1075, 1987.

Specht L, Nissen HI: Hodgkin's disease and age. *Eur J Haematol* 43:127, 1989.

Vose JM et al: The importance of age in survival of patients treated with chemotherapy for aggressive non-Hodgkin's lymphoma. *J Clin Oncol* 6:1838, 1988.

Wedelin C et al: Prognostic factors in Hodgkin's disease with special reference to age. *Cancer* 53:1202, 1984.

Young J et al: *Surveillance, Epidemiology, and End Result: Incidence and Mortality.* Bethesda, MD, National Cancer Institute, 1981.

Thrombotic and Hemorrhagic Disorders

MELISSA MATULIS • MARY ANN KNOVICH • JOHN OWEN

THE HEMOSTATIC SYSTEM

The influence of age on disorders of hemostasis is poorly understood. Certainly age is an important variable in assigning probabilities to specific diagnoses, and age also enters into the equation for determining the appropriate therapy. In addition, age is an independent risk factor for thrombotic, and possibly for hemorrhagic, disease. In the context of diagnosis, age may be a surrogate for other factors, such as an increased risk of malignancy and an increased extent of atherosclerosis. By contrast, congenital severe bleeding disorders are unlikely to manifest initially in the elderly patient. On the other hand, congenital disorders, which predispose to thrombosis, are somewhat different. In these disorders the first thrombotic episode can occur in an older patient. The pathophysiology of bleeding and that of thrombosis usually are viewed in disparate terms; the underlying biochemistry is, however, the same. It is the same hemostatic system that is implicated in venous thrombosis, arterial embolism, and spontaneous hemorrhage. It is thus not surprising that coexisting bleeding and thrombosis can and do occur, nor should it be surprising that "correction" of a bleeding diathesis can predispose a patient to thrombosis. All physicians are aware that the treatment of thrombosis with anticoagulants predisposes to bleeding. This chapter addresses thrombotic and hemorrhagic disorders by means of an appeal to common mechanisms. As far as possible, clinical observations and basic science are reconciled. A limited number of references are included, which can serve as starting points for a more extensive search of the primary literature. For most purposes, a specialized text in hematology will supply adequate further details, but for the more arcane issues, reference to specialized texts in thrombosis and hemostasis may be necessary.

Procoagulant Functions

These are the reactions that lead directly to the formation of a hemostatic plug or a thrombus. Note that these systems are dominated by positive feedback and would be expected to proceed to completion if unopposed.

The Coagulation Cascade

This biochemical construct has served physicians well as a model of the reactions involved in hemostasis. Superficially, the cascade has changed little over the past 20 years. In fact, a great many changes have occurred, and perhaps of equal importance, many details have withstood the test of time. The basic cascade is shown in Fig. 64-1. Note that factor VIIa is shown activating factor IX to IXa, not factor X to Xa. This change reconciles the biochemical pathway with the clinical observation of the severity of the hemophilias (factor VIII or factor IX deficiency). The backbone of this system is composed of the serine proteases, which are converted from inactive zymogens to active enzymes, as signified by the addition of the suffix "a." Factors V and VIII act differently; these are cofactors that serve to accelerate the proteolytic activity of factors Xa and IXa, respectively. The cofactor activity of factors V and VIII is increased markedly by limited proteolysis by thrombin or factor Xa. More extensive proteolysis by either enzyme leads to a progressive loss of cofactor function, but it is the action of activated protein C (aPC) which is the major control agent for the accelerations (Fig. 64-2). Proteolytic cleavage of either factor V or factor VIII by aPC results in complete loss of procoagulant function. Factor VIIa is inactivated by the tissue factor pathway inhibitor in a complex reaction that requires the formation of a complex between factor VIIa, factor Xa, tissue factor, and the inhibitor. The inactivation of the central axis serine proteases is accomplished by complex formation with antithrombin III (AT3). These complexes show no procoagulant activity. The mode of inactivation of factor XIIIa is uncertain.

Platelets

Platelets are important in both hemostasis and thrombosis. The ability of platelets to adhere and their ability to

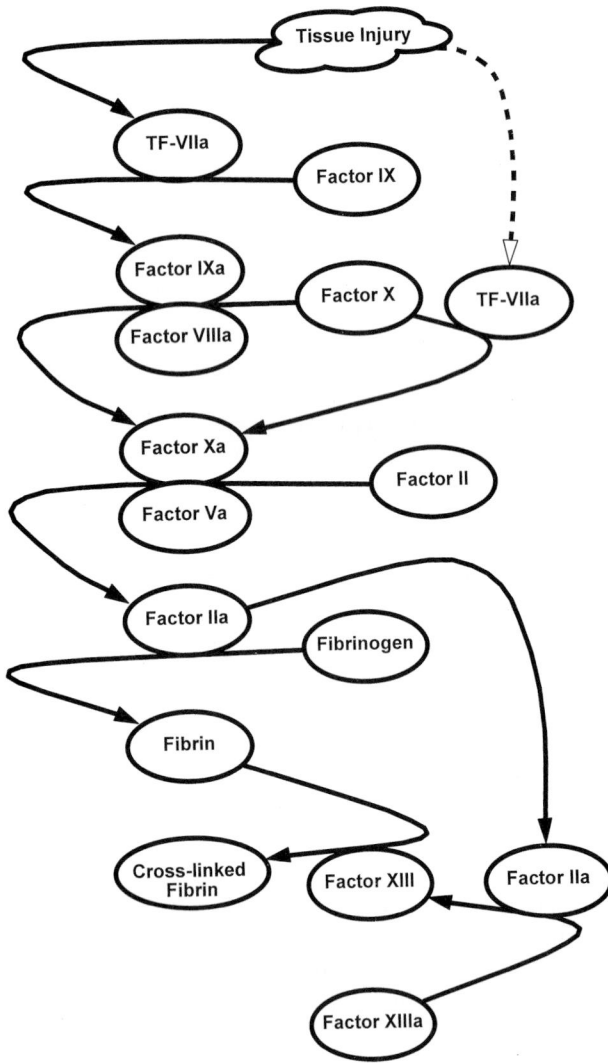

Figure 64-1 The key procoagulant reactions of the coagulation cascade are shown beginning with tissue factor exposure to circulating active factor VII. This produces the tissue factor-VIIa complex, which activates both factor IX and factor X. Factor II is prothrombin and factor IIa is thrombin.

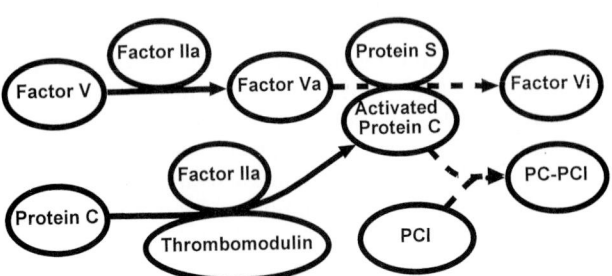

Figure 64-2 The principal reactions of the natural anticoagulant systems. Factor V and factor VIII undergo essentially identical reactions. For simplicity only factor V is shown. Activation is shown with solid lines, and inhibition with dotted lines. Factor Vi = inactivated factor V; PC-PCI, inactivated protein C; PCI, activated protein C inhibitor.

promote coagulation are particularly important. The view of platelets as providing bulk, like stones in concrete, is probably overly simplistic. Activated platelets bind to fibrin and form a focus of coagulant activity. More fibrin is laid down over the platelet, and another activated platelet is attracted to adhere. The platelet-fibrin mass grows, resisting the effects of blood flow. Hemostasis is secured or a thrombus is formed; only the location differs. White clots and red clots have achieved some level of individual recognition. The distinction has much in common with the perennial discussion of brown eggs versus white eggs; it is a superficial distinction. Thrombi formed in flowing blood, particularly in regions of high shear, contain many platelets and few red cells. The platelets adhere to the growing platelet-fibrin mass, and the red cells are swept away. In nonflowing blood, there is no opportunity for nonadherent cells to be swept away, and red cells outnumber platelets 20 to 1. It is not surprising that venous thrombi are mostly red. The critical biochemistry, however, remains the same: Fibrin formation is the central event in hemostasis and thrombogenesis in both the arterial and the venous circulations.

Anticoagulant Functions

The anticoagulant functions are essential in that they provide the only means of limiting the activity of the procoagulant functions. This function is carried out by the serpin AT3 and by the natural anticoagulant system.

Antithrombin III

A major problem with the cascade is that there is no obvious way to turn off the system. It has been suggested that with the first significant trauma to the vasculature, one should convert all blood to clot. This dilemma has been resolved by the integration of the inhibitors and negative regulators of the cascade into the system. The principal inhibitor is antithrombin III. This serine protease inhibitor, which is a member of the serpin family, acts to irreversibly inhibit the activated forms of coagulation factors II, IX, and X. This is achieved by covalent binding to the active center of the serine protease, creating an inactive protease–inhibitor complex. Heparin, which has no intrinsic anticoagulant activity, functions to accelerate the inhibitory action of AT3 against factor IIa (thrombin) and factor Xa. Thus, while in the coagulation lexicon antithrombin III is also known as heparin cofactor, mechanistically it is probably more correct to consider heparin the antithrombin III cofactor.

Natural Anticoagulant System

The second major regulatory system involves protein C and has been referred to as the natural anticoagulant system (Fig. 64-2). Protein C is a serine protease with marked homology to the procoagulant serine proteases. Like factors II, VII, IX, and X, it undergoes vitamin K–dependent posttranslational modification of specific glutamic acid residues. Protein C is activated by a compound enzyme composed of a bimolecular complex of thrombin with thrombomodulin. Thrombomodulin is an integral membrane protein that is found on all endothelial cells. When thrombin is bound to thrombomodulin, it loses the ability to convert fibrinogen to fibrin and acquires the capacity to activate protein C (PC). The resulting aPC converts factors V and VIII to inactive forms. The activated forms of factors V and VIII are preferred substrates for aPC, but preactivation of factors V and VIII is not required for action by aPC. Following the common theme, aPC activity is dependent on the presence of a cofactor. Protein S (PS) is that cofactor and is also a member of the vitamin K–dependent protein family. Protein S shows marked sequence homology with the vitamin K–dependent serine proteases, but PS shows no enzymatic activity. An important part of this system is the means of inactivation. Thrombin (IIa) is inactivated by complexing with antithrombin III, aPC, by forming a complex with the aPC inhibitor.

Resolution

While plasmin is usually thought of as the central effector in this phase of hemostasis, it must be remembered that other systems also are activated. The inflammatory response is one of those systems, and the neutral proteases released from granulocytes are potent fibrinolytic agents. Local infection sometimes is seen as the cause of bleeding from the dissolution of hemostatic plugs. These proteases do not show the same degree of substrate specificity that plasmin shows. The result in some patients with venous thrombosis is destruction of valves in addition to resolution of the thrombotic obstruction. The resulting valvular insufficiency is the dominant long-term consequence of venous thrombosis in such cases.

Fibrinolysis

If PC, PS, and AT3 are thought of as checks in the coagulation cascade, then the fibrinolytic system (Fig. 64-3) should be thought of as its balance. The interplay between coagulation and fibrinolysis is central to hemostatis and thrombogenesis. Plasmin is to fibrinolysis what thrombin is to coagulation. Plasmin is formed from plasminogen through the action of a plasminogen activator. Most commonly this is the tissue type plasminogen activator (t-PA), but urokinase also plays both a physiologic and pharmacologic role. t-PA is released from endothelial cells along with its principal inhibitor, type 1 plasminogen activator inhibitor (PAI-1). In this setting, it is the balance of activator and inhibitor that determines the net activity of the fibrinolytic system. Supranormal activation of the fibrinolytic system follows the activation of coagulation; the balance is maintained with fibrinolysis responding. Hemostatic balance is thus driven by the relative activity of the two systems, but complications occur when the difference in activity of the two systems exceeds some threshold value. Excess thrombin activity predisposes to thrombosis; excess plasmin activity leads to a bleeding diathesis.

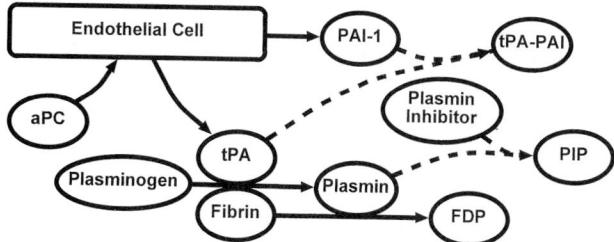

Figure 64-3 Principal reactions of the fibrinolytic system in which fibrin is converted to soluble fibrin degradation products (FDP). Activation steps are shown with solid lines and inhibition is shown with dotted lines. aPC, activated protein C; PAI-1, plasminogen activator inhibitor-1; PIP, plasmin inhibitor–plasmin inactive complex; tPA, tissue plasminogen activator; tPA-PAI, inactive plasminogen activator–inhibitor complex.

BLEEDING DISORDERS

Assessment of a bleeding diathesis demands the integration of laboratory investigation and traditional history and physical examination. A complete history and a physical examination are essential and form the basis for the selection of appropriate laboratory studies. Certain features in the history and physical examination are of particular importance and should be addressed explicitly, in a focused fashion if necessary. Any history of bleeding beyond that expected must be considered significant. Examples include any transfusion given after a simple procedure such as a tonsillectomy. Judgment is required, however. Many elderly patients today may have undergone such procedures in circumstances and in an era that precluded transfusion. Thus, the absence of transfusion does not imply the absence of a bleeding diathesis. In the elderly patient, it is often more useful to inquire about bleeding after a tooth extraction. In general, there is little significance to the reported rate of blood loss. The critical features are the time from onset to cessation of bleeding, whether some form of intervention was required to stop the bleeding, and whether bleeding recurred after completely stopping. There is some diagnostic value to knowing the site(s) of bleeding. Recurrent bleeding at a single site usually is a result of an anatomic defect. Spontaneous bleeding into joints and muscles is always significant. Gum bleeding is often insignificant unless it is profound and of recent onset. Epistaxis, gum bleeding, bruising, and petechiae usually are associated with thrombocytopenia or dysfunctional platelets. Deep muscle hemorrhage and intraarticular bleeding are more commonly seen in disorders of the coagulation system. Neither constellation is sufficiently reliable to use as the sole means of making a diagnosis of the cause of hemorrhage but can be useful in directing the course of the initial laboratory investigation.

Presurgical Assessment of Bleeding Risk

One often is presented with the need to certify a patient's fitness to withstand surgery. Without doubt, the medical history is the most useful and reliable index of bleeding risk. The elderly patient is more likely to need surgery, but fortunately is also more likely to have undergone a surgical procedure in the past. While prior experience does not forecast the future perfectly, history does tend to repeat itself, at least in hemostatic terms. A patient who had major hemostatic problems in two previous operations is likely to have problems again. One who has undergone multiple procedures without a problem probably will have little trouble in the future. These generalizations hold if no major change occurs in the patient's overall condition. When there is no prior exposure, risk is much more difficult to assess. The standard laboratory tests offer more comfort than assurance. The bleeding time is probably the most widely used screening test, but even this has proved unreliable in predicting clinically significant surgical bleeding. How much faith can be placed in the activated partial thromboplastin time (aPTT), a test performed on cell free plasma using reagents made from a chloroform extract of brain and incorporating ground glass as an accelerator? The distance from in vivo hemostasis to these artificial systems is such that it is not difficult to see why they perform poorly as global tests of the efficacy of the hemostatic system.

It is now generally accepted, though less widely practiced, that patients without a history of abnormal bleeding are at low risk of significant bleeding at surgery, provided that the individual has been placed at risk in the past. An individual who has had no prior surgery, no prior tooth extractions, no significant trauma, and has not delivered a child must be considered an unknown entity. Such people are the most likely to benefit from screening tests of hemostatic function, but it is in this very situation that the standard tests are the least informative. It has become the norm in many centers to do a battery of tests as a preoperative screen for occult bleeding disorders. The combination of prothrombin time and partial thromboplastin time, with or without a bleeding time, is particularly popular. We remain skeptical that this approach efficiently or effectively identifies individuals at risk. Individuals with a clear history of abnormal bleeding should be investigated as thoroughly as possible. The greatest risk in this setting is to ascribe the bleeding to the first abnormality uncovered, failing to uncover the presence of a second, more significant abnormality. Once the abnormality is known, risk assessment and appropriate management can be based on a broad body of experience, taking into account the details of the proposed surgical procedure. This approach does not guarantee the outcome for any single patient, but overall it maximizes the benefit obtained from screening and prophylaxis. In general, the approach of using screening tests of coagulation and hemostasis is not a substitute for a history and reasoned judgment.

Approach to a Bleeding Patient

There are a number of critical questions to answer at the outset: How did the bleeding start? When did it start? Has the bleeding ceased at any time, only to restart? What maneuvers have been tried to stem the bleeding, and with what success? Has this ever happened before? Is the patient known to have a hemostatic defect, and what is the defect? This is only a partial list of the significant variables,

and it is immediately obvious that they can be combined in too many ways to treat each combination as a distinct entity. Some simplification is essential, and the mode of presentation forms a useful starting point. In most circumstances all these questions will be addressed in the initial evaluation, as will an assessment of the urgency of the situation. A lifelong problem or a clear, positive family history suggests an inherited disorder; a recent onset suggests an acquired disorder. It is not uncommon, though, for a mild congenital deficiency of factor VIII or factor IX to become evident in later life, a possibility that is easily overlooked when the aPTT is only slightly abnormal. Such individuals nonetheless can experience profound hemorrhage in response to surgical assault. As automation enters the coagulation laboratory, screening tests are becoming more sophisticated and, most importantly, more available. Some form of mixing study which tests the ability of added normal plasma to correct an abnormal prothrombin time (PT) or aPTT is widely available. This test is very useful in distinguishing coagulation factor deficiency from inhibitor. The test, however, may not detect the presence of a mild clinically significant deficiency of either factor VIII or factor IX. Nor will a simple mixing study distinguish a lupus inhibitor with an attendant risk of thrombosis from anti–factor VIII producing acquired hemophilia. An appreciation of the limitations of these tests is crucial in making appropriate decisions regarding diagnosis and intervention.

Petechiae or Minor Bruising

In general, this presentation is associated with defects in the platelet–vessel wall interaction. Thus, thrombocytopenia must be ruled out before one embarks on a costly effort to determine the functional capacity of platelets. Older individuals develop friable skin and have increased capillary fragility. This often manifests as ecchymoses and purpura on the forearms, but the problem may not be confined to this area. The recent onset of thrombocytopenia can be caused by an autoimmune problem but also can be the first sign of a myelodysplastic syndrome or acute leukemia. The template bleeding time is useful in this setting. A normal result provides strong evidence that platelet function is intact, provided that the patient does not have a myelodysplastic syndrome. The bleeding time in patients with a myelodysplastic syndrome is an unreliable and potentially misleading guide to in vivo platelet function. Mild von Willebrand's disease is the most common diagnosis in this group, but the diagnosis is far from simple. The plasma level of von Willebrand factor behaves like an acute phase reactant, leading to considerable variability in test results.

Major Bruising

This presentation is seen most often in patients with deficiencies of one or more coagulation factors. An acquired inhibitor of factor VIII, a vitamin K deficiency, a warfarin overdose, liver disease, and disseminated intravascular coagulation are all possible. The distinction between them requires the use of the laboratory, but the clinical setting can give some clues to the most likely diagnosis. The PT and aPTT are the most useful tests in this setting, though some type of mixing study coupled with specific factor assays may be necessary to make a precise diagnosis.

Epistaxis or Gum Bleeding

Platelet disorders predominate here, though other possibilities must be kept in mind. In addition to primary disorders of the oro- or nasopharynx, primary hematologic malignancy must be considered.

Hemorrhage

It is critically important to distinguish generalized from localized breakdown of the hemostatic system. Localized bleeding almost always is the result of an anatomic defect. Peptic ulcer, tumor, laceration, surgery, and trauma are common. Defects in the hemostatic system, which under normal circumstances are clinically silent, can become major factors. Often, however, correction of the mild hemostatic defect is not practicable and correction of the anatomic defect is required. Thrombocytopenia or platelet dysfunction also can contribute to hemostatic system abnormalities. In general, multiple abnormalities are the rule rather than the exception. Bleeding from multiple sites almost always signifies a profound disturbance of the hemostatic system. Rebleeding at old puncture sites suggests excess fibrinolytic system activity, a common scenario in patients with fulminant disseminated coagulation. Coagulation factor deficiencies more typically are manifest in failure of primary hemostasis or in rebleeding shortly after bleeding appears to be controlled. As with patients who present with major bruising, the PT and the aPTT are the most important tests, but in this case the level of fibrinogen and fibrin(ogen) degradation products becomes important. Thrombocytopenia is seen frequently in this setting, and so a platelet count is essential.

Diagnosis and Treatment of Specific Disorders of Hemostasis

Von Willebrand's Disease

The majority of patients with von Willebrand's disease have the mild variety hemostasis. This mild disorder sometimes is referred to as heterozygous, but the precise genetics of this condition are uncertain at best. The bleeding time is usually prolonged, factor VIIIc is approximately 50 percent of normal, ristocetin-induced platelet agglutination is decreased, ristocetin cofactor level is approximately 50 percent of normal, and immunologic measurement shows the von Willebrand protein to be approximately 50 percent of the normal level. The bleeding diathesis is usually mild and characteristically variable. This diagnosis is often difficult to make with assurance and not infrequently is made in error. It is not a diagnosis of exclusion. Only very rarely is some form of prophylaxis required for these patients on a day-to-day basis. If surgery is needed, the aim is to raise the von Willebrand protein level to normal before the operation. The mainstay of treatment has been the infusion of cryoprecipitate, which remains a viable option.

The best choice today is to administer the vasopressin analog desmopressin (DDAVP), which stimulates the release of von Willebrand factor from endothelial cells, achieving much the same results as does infusing cryoprecipitate. There is clear evidence that DDAVP administration will shorten the bleeding time and adequate evidence that it improves hemostasis. The usual dose is 0.4 μg/kg immediately before surgery. The same dose can be repeated every 12 hours until the patient is safely beyond the risk of bleeding. A larger dose of DDAVP does not produce a higher level of von Willebrand factor, and more frequent administration leads to tachyphylaxis. Occasional patients have one of the variant forms of von Willebrand's disease, including a severe disorder that appears to be much like hemophilia. The diagnosis and treatment of these patients are beyond the scope of this text, and such patients should be referred to a coagulation specialist.

Vitamin K Deficiency

The dietary requirement for vitamin K is about 100 μg per day, and frank deficiency of vitamin K resulting solely from an inadequate diet is extremely rare. A borderline intake of vitamin K can easily be unmasked by any intercurrent illness. Most commonly, the problem manifests in an acute care setting when appetite is diminished or feeding is withheld and antibiotics are being administered. A presumptive diagnosis often can be based on the clinical situation, and confirmation can be obtained by the response to vitamin K administration. Oral administration is almost always adequate, even in the face of all but the most profound fat malabsorption. More commonly, in the acute setting, vitamin K is administered subcutaneously. Intravenous administration is also feasible: not more than 10 mg infused over at least 30 minutes in at least 100 mL of saline. Significant shortening of the PT and aPTT usually is evident within 12 hours, and virtually complete normalization occurs in 24 to 36 hours. The laboratory can be most helpful in confirming the diagnosis by comparing the plasma concentrations of the vitamin K-dependent factors II, VII, IX, and X. The different levels of the factors allow a re-creation of the time frame of development of the deficiency. Comparison with the level of factor V controls for the possibility that the patient suffers from liver dysfunction leading to decreased protein synthesis.

Warfarin Overdose

Again the setting suggests the diagnosis, and the same maneuvers can be tried that were outlined above for vitamin K deficiency. In the elderly population, it is not uncommon to find patients who appear to be exquisitely sensitive to warfarin. It has been suggested that this is a feature of aging, but the "hypersensitivity" disappears when the dietary intake is supplemented with 80 to 150 μg of vitamin K daily. With this steady supplementation, dietary intake of vitamin K becomes a minor component of the equation, and sensitivity to warfarin returns to normal. A patient with a warfarin overdose who is thought to need continuous anticoagulation presents a special problem. The usual pharmacologic dose of vitamin K (10 mg subcutaneously) often

Table 64-1   Idealized Classification of the Stages of Disseminated Intravascular Coagulation

Stage	PT	aPTT	Fibrinogen	D-dimer	Platelet Count
I	Normal	Short	Normal	Slightly increased	Decreased
II	Prolonged	Prolonged	Low	Elevated	Low
III	Prolonged	Prolonged	Low	Marked elevation	Low

makes it difficult to reestablish controlled therapeutic anticoagulation. Consideration must be given to instituting another form of prophylaxis as an interim measure, and subcutaneous heparin is a reasonable choice. When administered by the subcutaneous route, heparin takes many hours to reach its full effect, approximating the time taken for vitamin K to reverse the effect of warfarin. Alternatively, infusion of plasma at a dose of 10 mL/kg body weight will rapidly bring the prothrombin time down to the usual therapeutic range, avoiding the overcorrection effect. As was noted above, borderline vitamin K depletion leads to warfarin hypersensitivity. Some patients, particularly among the elderly population, develop a marked prolongation of the prothrombin time because of the development of vitamin K deficiency and not as a result of a warfarin overdose. These individuals can easily be controlled by the daily oral administration of 80 to 150 μg of vitamin K, as formulated in an ADEK or Geritol Complete multivitamin. A special case is worthy of note. The rat poison warfarin has been reformulated to contain a different coumarin. When it is ingested by humans, the anticoagulant effect lasts for weeks. Accidental poisonings have been reported, and prolonged administration of pharmacologic doses of vitamin K is necessary before the effect disappears.

Disseminated Intravascular Coagulation

No single test can be used to make a diagnosis of disseminated intravascular coagulation (DIC); rather, the diagnosis is based on a constellation of clinical and laboratory findings. At the pathophysiologic center is thrombin activity in the fluid phase of blood. The complications and clinical manifestations can be grouped, giving three rather different syndromes (Tables 64-1 and 64-2). Without being quantitative, one should consider the consequences of

generating different amounts of thrombin in the circulation. At the lowest pathologic rate of generation of thrombin, the principal biochemical effect is to activate components of the coagulation cascade. Factor VIII in particular, but also factor V, becomes activated and behaves as though the plasma concentration had been markedly increased. This increased coagulant potential is promoted by platelets, which also become activated by thrombin. This constellation is prothrombotic and sometimes is referred to as a hypercoagulable state. Such patients benefit from the administration of heparin in low doses, approximately 500 U/h intravenously. While this condition is generally prothrombotic, thrombocytopenia is a common finding. Occasional patients are seen in whom the thrombocytopenia is the dominant feature, and such patients are often refractory to platelet transfusion. Responsiveness to platelet transfusion can be restored in some patients by the administration of low-dose heparin, even though the patient's own platelets may take days to weeks to return to normal numbers.

If the amount of thrombin in the circulation is somewhat higher, the situation changes to one in which there is defective primary hemostasis. Protein C activation occurs; in turn, factors V and VIII undergo proteolytic degradation. The resulting low levels of factors V and VIII are characteristic of "classical" DIC. The PT and aPTT are prolonged, thrombocytopenia is almost always present, and the fibrinogen level is low. Plasma levels of degradation products of fibrin(ogen) are significantly increased, whether measured as crude nonclottable material or as neoantigenic monomeric fibrin. More commonly today some form of D-dimer measurement is the test offered. While there is considerable controversy regarding the nature and mechanism of the generation of the moiety being measured, the tests have proved useful in the clinical arena. Treatment of this variant of DIC centers on replacement of the depleted

Table 64-2   Other Features of Disseminated Intravascular Coagulation

Stage	Dominant Pathophysiology	Typical Clinical Manifestation	Principal Treatment Modality
I	Thrombin activation of factors V and VIII and of platelets	Increased risk of thrombosis	Low-dose heparin
II	Activated protein C-mediated consumption of factors V and VIII	Bleeding from new wounds	Coagulation factor and platelet replacement; consider low-dose heparin after factor replacement
III	Activation of the fibrinolytic system	Spontaneous rebleeding from old wounds	Platelet and coagulation factor replacement; consider giving a fibrinolytic inhibitor, but only after giving heparin

clotting factors. Fresh-frozen plasma has been the mainstay of treatment and remains popular. Platelet transfusions are indicated, especially if the patient is bleeding. Replacement of AT3 may be beneficial in a few subgroups of nonheparinized severely septic patients. Once clotting factors have been replaced, consideration should be given to administering low-dose heparin. Data are unclear in this area, though there seems to be sufficient experience to contraindicate full anticoagulation. Well-reasoned attempts to use full anticoagulation have produced more than an occasional catastrophe.

Even higher levels of thrombin and/or more time leads to a state in which there is activation of the fibrinolytic system and plasminemia. This plasmin serves to digest the fibrin hemostatic plugs in old wounds. The clinical picture is that of spontaneous bleeding from wounds in which hemostasis had initially been secured. This occurs in addition to failure of primary hemostasis. The PT and aPTT are prolonged, fibrinogen levels are frequently below 50 mg/dL and profound thrombocytopenia is almost invariant. Adequate therapy must be able to contain the fibrinolytic response, and it is both rational and appropriate to use an inhibitor of plasmin. Before the introduction of a plasmin inhibitor, it is essential that the excess thrombin activity be controlled by the administration of heparin. Again, only a low dose of heparin is required, but in this setting even a low dose may contribute significantly to the bleeding diathesis. It is therefore essential that missing coagulation factors be replaced first, then low-dose heparin, and finally a plasmin inhibitor. Around the world there are a number of plasmin inhibitors in use or under development; in the United States only ε-aminocaproic (EACA, Amicar) and aprotinin (Trasylol) are available for intravenous use. The usual dose of EACA is 1 g/h by constant intravenous infusion. Some practitioners have given a loading dose of some 4 to 6 g before beginning the constant infusion. There are no data showing the need for a loading dose, but it makes good theoretical sense and certainly produces a therapeutic level much more quickly. Note that hypersensitivity reactions do occur with Trasylol.

Liver Dysfunction

The major problem here stems from failure of the liver to synthesize the components of the hemostatic system. This failure extends far beyond the coagulation factors to include the inhibitors and regulators of the hemostatic system. In general, the parallel reduction in the levels of all components allows a patient with only marginal liver function to suffer only minimal hemorrhagic complications. However, there is little room to maneuver, and minor stress can lead to major consequences. Once it was thought that the majority of patients with severe liver disease had ongoing activation of the coagulation system; the strongest evidence for this was the frequent finding of fibrin(ogen) degradation products in the plasma of such patients. It is now clear that most of these patients have dysfibrinogenemia, and it is this nonclottable molecule that was mistaken for a degradation product. A small number of patients with liver disease do have an ongoing DIC-like syndrome, but they are the exception and not the rule. A common problem is the need to correct the abnormal PT and aPTT before an

invasive procedure in a patient with liver disease. The usual procedure is to transfuse 2 units of fresh-frozen plasma; this rote formula is convenient but not optimal. Patients with only slightly abnormal tests usually are treated this way, although whether the plasma actually reduces the risk of bleeding is not clear. The amount of clotting factor in 2 units of fresh-frozen plasma would at best raise the circulating levels by about 15 percent. Therefore the success of this regimen may be a result of the careful selection of patients who undergo invasive procedures rather than to the prophylactic effect of 2 units of fresh-frozen plasma. At the other extreme is a patient with severe liver disease and markedly low levels of all the coagulation factors produced in the liver. In the acute setting, if the abnormality must be corrected, infusion of coagulation factor concentrates is needed. Prothrombin complex concentrate contains all the vitamin K-dependent factors; cryoprecipitate is a good source of fibrinogen, and platelets provide factor V. Each of these has to be used to give full replacement doses of each factor, with an added benefit being the transfusion of the regulators PC and PS: for the average patient, 3000 units of prothrombin complex, 10 units (bags) of cryoprecipitate, and 8 units of platelets. Now that prothrombin complex concentrates are heat-treated, there is only a small risk of transmitting hepatitis B, hepatitis C, and human immunodeficiency virus. A significant risk is induction of thrombosis, which must be balanced against the need to normalize the levels of the coagulation factors.

THROMBOTIC DISORDERS

Thrombogenesis remains something of a mystery, principally because it is so difficult to observe the initial event. The seminal observation, which was made by Virchow, was that venous thrombogenesis requires that a change in the vessel, a change in the blood, and stasis occur at the same time. The change in the vessel was originally described as inflammatory. It now is believed that some change occurs in the endothelial cells lining the vessel. This change alters the nature of the endothelial cell from antithrombotic to prothrombotic. Indeed, under some conditions the endothelial cell appears to behave much as the platelet does. Prostacyclin, a potent platelet inhibitor, is produced by the endothelial cell. von Willebrand factor is synthesized and secreted. Plasminogen activator and the inhibitor of plasminogen activator are produced and secreted. There are binding sites for coagulation factors, and the surface promotes coagulation; the whole of the pathway from factor XIa action on factor IX to fibrin formation is supported on the surface of the endothelial cell. Thrombomodulin, the cofactor which alters the specificity of thrombin to be become the protein C activator, is an integral membrane protein of the endothelial cell. Knowledge regarding the variety and complexity of endothelial cell function increases daily. It is clear that the endothelial cell can no longer be considered passive in coagulation.

The change in the blood is best seen as a shift in the balance of coagulation and fibrinolysis. This concept was first put forward by Astrup in the 1940s. He suggested that in normal individuals there is constant and ongoing activity of both systems. In recent years, this has become generally accepted, although it has not become dogma. This paradigm of balanced thrombin and plasmin activity predicts that either increased thrombin action or decreased plasmin action will predispose to thrombosis. Both situations are well recognized in clinical practice. Increased thrombin action occurs when there is exposure of the blood to tissue factor or elaboration of tissue factor activity on circulating monocytes. Certain malignant tissues have been shown to produce a procoagulant, and severely hypoxic endothelial cells produce an activator of factor X. Increased thrombin activity also occurs when there is a deficiency of any of the natural anticoagulants, protein C, protein S, or antithrombin III. Decreased plasmin activity occurs when there is decreased activity of plasminogen activator or increased activity of plasminogen activator inhibitor. Similarly, deficiencies of activatable plasminogen predispose to thrombosis, as do antibody inhibitors of the fibrinolytic system. It is worth noting that in patients who develop thrombosis after surgery, changes are evident in the blood as much as 3 days before the thrombus becomes evident on fibrinogen scanning. This opens a window of opportunity both for the detection of the impending thrombus and for intervention to prevent the actual formation of a thrombus.

The role of venous stasis in the genesis of thrombosis is far from clear. Recently it was shown that hypoxic endothelial cells produce an activator of factor X. For some time it has been recognized that intermittent pneumatic compression of the legs reduces the risk of thrombosis. A simple explanation of preventing stasis is called into question by the data of Knight and Dawson , who demonstrated that compressing one leg has a protective effect on the contralateral side. In similar fashion, intermittent pneumatic compression has been shown to alter the balance of thrombin and plasmin activity, particularly in the 2 days after surgery.

Venous Thromboembolic Disorders

Risk Factors for the Development of Venous Thrombosis

In assessing risk factors for venous thrombosis, it is useful to consider three time frames: immediate, short-term, and long-term. The immediate category includes trauma, surgery, and temporary immobility. The short-term category includes the factors listed under immediate risk factors and is extended to include malignancy, pregnancy, and severe illness. Factors predicting long-term risk include an empiric group based on multiple prior episodes of thrombosis and a better-understood group made up of acquired and congenital thrombophilic disorders. The congenital disorders include deficiency of protein C, protein S, antithrombin III, plasminogen, plasminogen activator, some dysfibrinogenemias, the factor V Leiden mutation, the prothrombin promoter mutation, and hyperhomocystinemia. The acquired disorders in this group include autoantibodies that inhibit a step in the fibrinolytic cascade. The lupus anticoagulant, an antibody directed against phospholipid, lies between empiric and understood. There are many

proposed mechanisms for the prothrombotic effect; one of them may well prove to be correct. At this time it is not known which of the many competing explanations will survive. Investigation of an individual with a history of recurrent thrombosis and a clear family history of thrombosis once yielded a clear diagnosis in only 10 to 15 percent of cases, but that number has increased dramatically with the discovery of the factor V Leiden mutation. The factor V Leiden mutation is currently the most common of these disorders and in whites, is responsible for 45 percent of congenital thrombophilias. This disorder involves a mutation in the factor V gene that renders the factor V coagulant protein resistant to inactivation by activated protein C, thus leading to a prothrombotic condition. Heterozygotes with this mutation have a lifetime risk of thrombosis that is close to 10-fold greater than normal. In the homozygous state, the patient has a greater than 90 percent lifetime risk of thrombosis. The age-related risk of thrombosis is still being defined for the thrombophilias. While age is now seen as an independent risk factor for thrombosis, the additional risk factors conferred by hyperhomocystinemia and the prothrombin promotor mutation are not yet known. An approximate rule for heterozygotes for proteins C and S and antithrombin III, as well as for the homozygous factor V Leiden mutation, is that there is a low risk of thrombosis until age 15 to 20, after which about half of these persons will develop thrombosis by age 50 years and about three-quarters will develop it by age 80 years. One-quarter of heterozygotes for factor V Leiden will develop thrombosis by age 50 years, and another 15 percent by age 80 years. Inverting these numbers, one can see that some 15 to 25 percent of these patients will present with the first episode of thrombosis between the ages of 50 and 80 years. Thus, even in the geriatric population, these congenital disorders must be considered. Approximately 10 percent of patients who present with idiopathic deep venous thrombosis (DVT) and nearly 20 percent of patients with recurrent idiopathic DVT eventually develop clinically overt cancer. More than half those patients are older than 60 years of age. Most of these cancers are adenocarcinomas and become evident within the first year after presentation with a DVT.

Presurgical Assessment of Thromboembolic Risk

This question can be better answered than the question of the risk of bleeding. A number of studies have identified significant risk factors for the development of postoperative venous thrombosis. These risk factors have been elaborated into scoring schemes, which allow an assessment of the probable risk of thrombosis. The major impetus for such schemes is the notion that prophylaxis is indicated in those at highest risk but is unnecessary or even contraindicated in those at the lowest risk. The major risk factor is the procedure itself. Some operations carry a low risk of thrombosis, and others a very high risk. Second, the condition of the patient exerts a powerful effect; the adage that sick patients do poorly applies in this setting. The presence of intercurrent illness is significant, particularly a malignancy, and any laboratory evidence of activation of the coagulation system is associated with increased risk. The independent influence of age on the risk of thrombosis is clear. Older hospitalized patients are more likely to have venous thrombosis than are young hospitalized patients, but the frequency of other risk factors is much higher in older patients—heart failure, malignancy, and immobility in particular. Furthermore, older patients in general have a lower tolerance for pulmonary embolism. Finally, the diagnosis of pulmonary embolism may be missed if one ascribes increasing shortness of breath to worsening heart failure. A high level of suspicion is warranted at all times, particularly in the geriatric population.

Diagnosis of Venous Thrombosis and Pulmonary Embolism

It is clearly impractical to screen all patients all the time, and it is equally clear that one needs to identify patients with venous thromboembolism in order to institute therapy. The appropriate diagnostic test depends on the situation, particularly the mode of presentation and any intercurrent conditions. The intercurrent conditions can be reduced to one issue: the strength of the contraindication to using heparin anticoagulation. A patient with a high probability of venous thromboembolism in whom the use of heparin is strongly contraindicated must have the diagnosis of thrombosis established beyond a reasonable doubt before beginning anticoagulation. One must recognize that in general, a contraindication does not mean interdiction and that the presence of thrombosis does not mandate full anticoagulation. Judgment is essential, and there is no formula for balancing the competing risks.

The gold standard for establishing the presence of venous thrombosis remains contrast venography, but sonography is now a realistic alternative. Color Doppler sonography can demonstrate the presence of thrombus with high precision and sensitivity, but only in accessible veins. The abdomen and pelvis remain difficult to probe with noninvasive tools. A patient with a low probability of thrombosis should be approached with noninvasive testing. The use of serial impedance plethysmography has been well established. This approach is possible because a negative study is a reliable way to rule out the presence of significant proximal venous thrombosis in the lower limb. A negative study does not rule out the subsequent development of significant thrombosis, however, so to be confident of the outcome, serial studies are needed. This approach avoids invasive tests but does so at the cost of the inconvenience of repeated testing and significant expense. Efforts have been made to develop blood tests for the diagnosis of venous thrombosis. Most of the proposed tests have been impractical for routine clinical use, but some have shown promise in that negative tests reliably predict those without thrombosis.

Recently, the application of monoclonal antibody technology has enabled the development of assays that are facile and fast. These new tests for specific degradation products of fibrinogen show promise as clinical tools in the diagnosis of patients with thrombosis. Quantitative assays of D-dimers have a good negative predictive value when less than 500 ng/mL. The principal problem with making the diagnosis of pulmonary embolism (PE) is one of clinical impression. A young patient "looks too young to have a PE,"

while an older patient does not "look like the typical case of PE." In this case, too young means that the patient should be older and atypical means that the patient does not fit the classic description of a young person with PE. The second problem to be overcome is the use of the arterial pO_2 as a screening test. It is true that most patients with massive pulmonary embolism have low arterial pO_2, but these are not the difficult diagnostic dilemmas. It is the atypical patient one seeks to identify. The choice of test and the need to pursue further testing if preliminary tests are negative depend on one's degree of suspicion, or pretest probability. Once clinical suspicion has been raised, it is appropriate, when possible, to proceed to radionuclide ventilation and perfusion lung scan. A negative result essentially rules out pulmonary embolism, and for most purposes a scan interpreted as indicating a high probability of pulmonary embolus usually can be taken as an adequate reason to begin therapy. In some studies, high-resolution spiral computed tomography (CT) has been quite specific for PE. Pulmonary emboli occurring in the main, lobar, or segmental vessels can be identified with a high degree of sensitivity. More studies to know whether spiral CT technology can replace ventilation/perfusion lung scans are needed. In cases where stronger evidence, positive or negative, is needed, arteriography is the next step. This procedure should be reserved for the few patients in whom the answer is of paramount importance, but in that small group, it should be pursued aggressively. In the elderly patient, the dye load is often a matter of concern. The load can be lessened by using the radionuclide lung scan to select the most appropriate areas of the lung for selective visualization. The selection depends on the question of ruling in or ruling out thromboembolism.

Treatment of Venous Thromboembolism

In selecting a course of therapy, it is important to keep in mind the objective of treatment. In general terms, these objectives can be considered in three time frames. The first is to gain immediate control of the thrombotic process and overcome the hemodynamic consequences of an embolus. The second is to minimize the short-term risk of new pulmonary embolism. The third is to minimize the long-term risk of further thromboembolism and to reduce the likelihood of the development of the postphlebitic syndrome.

Immediate Therapy For the majority of patients, immediate therapy of DVT or PE will consist of the administration of intravenous unfractionated heparin or subcutaneous low-molecular-weight heparin (LMWH). There are both theoretical and practical arguments that favor the rapid establishment of an effective level of anticoagulation. At the theoretical level, it is recognized that the coagulation system operates under positive feedback. Thus, it is critically important to interrupt this process with an adequate dose of heparin before real control can be established. This phenomenon is in large part responsible for the apparent heparin resistance that is seen at the time of initiating treatment. At the practical level there is evidence that patients who achieve a therapeutic level of anticoagulation within the first 24 hours have a better outcome.

It is not clear, however, whether this is a consequence of more aggressive anticoagulation or a reflection of the underlying disorder. This issue cannot be resolved without a randomized trial, but the implication is that one should try to achieve therapeutic levels of heparin as quickly as is practicable without placing the patient at major risk of hemorrhage from a heparin overdose. Several studies suggest that compared with unfractionated heparin, LMWH may be associated with decreased mortality, fewer major hemorrhages, and less thrombus extension. Thus, LMWH is first-line therapy for DVT. Plasminogen activators for thrombolytic therapy also have been used for DVT and catheter-related thrombosis. In DVT, this therapy results in better clearance of thrombus than does heparin anticoagulation alone, and may decrease the postphlebitic syndrome; however, the risk of hemorrhage may be increased, and therefore treatment must be determined on a case-by-case basis. Thrombolytic therapy for catheter-related thrombosis can result in clearance of thrombus in 95 percent of patients and salvage of the catheter in 85 percent.

Reducing the Risk of New Pulmonary Embolism   For a short time after heparin treatment is started, new embolization is common, but there is only a small risk of further significant pulmonary embolism. In general no other treatment is required. Exceptionally, the consequence of further embolism becomes significant. The presence of severe hemodynamic compromise is perhaps most common, and is particularly seen in older patients. Prevention of embolization by mechanical means then assumes greater importance, particularly the placement of filters in the vena cava. Transvenous placement of filters has brought this tool to the forefront, and the ease of placement has certainly had a major impact on the frequency with which this option is exercised. Caval filters are associated with surprisingly few side effects, and this, coupled with the ease of insertion, has led to the irrational notion that a caval filter is a substitute for anticoagulation. Hemodynamic status determines the consequences of embolization; control of coagulation determines the probability of embolization. Taken together, they define the risk of pulmonary embolism. The determinants of the development of the postphlebitic syndrome are unclear, but the extent of thrombosis is a significant factor. Anticoagulation effectively limits the further growth of thrombus and is the single most effective means of preventing this devastating complication of thrombosis. The substitution of a caval filter for anticoagulation, while effective in the short-term, is likely to predispose the patient to long-term complications. In patients with thrombophilia, a foreign body in the vasculature may act as a focus for further thrombus formation, mandating rather than obviating the need for anticoagulant therapy.

Long-term Prophylaxis   Some period of anticoagulation with warfarin is usually appropriate. Initial studies suggested some 3 months after an acute thrombosis as the high-risk period. These data form the basis for the typical recommendation of 3 to 6 months of anticoagulation after an acute thrombosis. This period frequently is doubled after a second episode and may be extended indefinitely after a third episode. These figures are somewhat arbitrary,

but nonetheless, are useful guidelines for the duration of warfarin therapy. In general, the goal international normalized ratio (INR) in deep venous thrombosis, PE, and atrial fibrillation is 2.0 to 3.0. Anticoagulation issues in patients with cardiac valve replacement are more complex, and specific recommendations are beyond the scope of this chapter. Recommendations are based on risk factors, type of valve, and location of prosthetic valve, and are published by the American College of Chest Physicians. In general, the goal INR for tissue valves is 2.0 to 3.0; for mechanical valves, a higher value of 2.5 to 3.5 is favored.

Note that the recommended intensities are given as INRs. The INR was introduced because different preparations of the reagent used to perform the PT measurement give different degrees of prolongation at the same intensity of warfarin therapy. The international standardization index (ISI) was devised to categorize the reagents in common use and is required to make calculations of INR values. The INR adjusts for the differences in the reagents and allows direct comparison of data obtained from different laboratories and different countries.

This comparability has little impact on the week-to-week management of the anticoagulation dose. Instead, it allows a degree of confidence in the choice of target values. It also should be remembered that these recommendations are not a substitute for judgment but are meant to provide a starting point for an otherwise undifferentiated patient. A patient who has developed thrombosis with an INR of 2.0 may be best served by an increased anticoagulant dose to achieve an INR of 3.0. A patient with a history of bleeding may be better served with a lower INR. In all cases it is important to recognize that it is the balance of risks which is being manipulated; greater protection from thrombosis can be bought at the expense of an increased risk of bleeding.

Specific Disorders

Renal Vein Thrombosis   This usually is seen in patients with protein-losing nephropathy, and the role of urinary loss of antithrombin III has been suggested to be central. While there is no doubting the attractiveness of this notion, there is no compelling reason to assume causation. Deficiency of plasma albumin is just as good as AT3 as a marker of the risk of thrombosis in patients with the nephrotic syndrome.

Hepatic Vein Thrombosis   This is a devastating condition that carries a generally miserable prognosis. The principal risk factors appear to be hematologic, in particular myeloproliferative and myelodysplastic disorders. Intrahepatic microvascular thrombosis (venoocclusive disease) is a well-recognized complication of bone marrow transplantation. Anticoagulation is appropriate in most patients, but all too often the process cannot be reversed and surgical intervention is required. Shunt procedures to reduce portal pressure are appropriate when there is adequate residual liver function. In cases where there is inadequate residual function, liver transplantation offers the only hope.

Superior Vena Cava Syndrome   External compression, often by mediastinal malignant tissue, and the presence of an indwelling central catheter are potent inducers of this syndrome. Because the clinical syndrome is produced by the obstruction to blood flow, appropriate therapy requires an adequate diagnosis. Patients with thrombotic occlusion of the superior vena cava have a significant incidence of pulmonary thromboembolism, and for this reason, anticoagulation is indicated. Catheter-directed thrombolytics are used routinely to treat thrombotic occlusion of the superior vena cava. Success rates as high as 70 percent can be achieved if thrombolytic therapy is begun within 2 days of the onset of symptoms. There is insufficient information at this time to recommend one particular course of action, but anticoagulation is usually valid and thrombolytics should at least be considered, especially in patients with catheter-related superior vena cava syndrome.

Arterial Thromboembolic Disorders

Risk Factors for the Development of Arterial Thrombosis

Many but not all risk factors for venous thrombosis are also risk factors for arterial thrombosis. AT3 deficiency and protein C deficiency have most commonly been associated with venous thrombosis. To some extent this is biased by early studies of these deficiencies, which examined stored plasma samples from patients with venous thrombosis. It is now clear that arterial thrombosis is also a problem in these disorders. Defects in the fibrinolytic system seem to predispose to arterial thrombosis more than to venous thrombosis. Atherosclerosis is a particularly potent risk factor, so much so that many researchers would consider that a causal relationship has been established.

Specific Arterial Thrombotic Disorders

Acute arterial occlusion generally produces immediate and often devastating downstream effects. The slow development of occlusion usually is accompanied by the development of a collateral circulation that minimizes the immediate problems but may still leave significant dysfunction. This is best appreciated by contrasting acute myocardial infarction with chronic stable angina. In general it is necessary to consider the problems of arterial thrombosis and embolism in separate time frames and with due regard for the site of the actual or impending occlusion. In contrast to thrombosis in the venous system, lysis of the offending thrombus is a major goal of therapy in patients with an acute arterial occlusion. Restoration of blood flow is seen as an important and urgent factor in the viability of the organ or limb at risk.

Acute Myocardial Infarction This disorder has been the subject of a great deal of research, both formal and informal. It is now accepted that arteriosclerosis sets the stage and that thrombosis changes stable coronary artery disease into acute myocardial infarction. Further support for this construct is provided by the spectacular success of thrombolytic therapy in reversing the changes of acute myocardial infarction.

Risk Factors Risk factors are well known for the development of coronary artery disease. Dyslipoproteinemia, hypertension, hyperhomocystinemia, obesity, smoking, and lack of exercise are only a sampling of the more than 200 identified risk factors. Less clear are risk factors that relate to the development of thrombotic occlusion in an atherosclerotic vessel. It is tempting to place plasma fibrinogen and factor VII in this category but, to invoke an old saw, correlation doth not causation make. Attempts to demonstrate increased baseline activity of the coagulation system in patients at high risk have been largely unsuccessful. However, coagulation clearly is central to thrombogenesis. These observations are best reconciled by the postulate that thrombosis is a result of episodic activation of the coagulation cascade. Such a construct is strengthened by data obtained in patients with unstable angina. This condition appears to be a drawn-out version of the transition state. The coagulation system is active, and thrombus is continuously being laid down and removed from the coronary arteries.

Treatment of Acute Myocardial Infarction Thrombolytic agents have assumed a central role in the treatment of patients with acute myocardial infarction. The fear of inducing an intracranial bleed has been placed in perspective, and the initial wild enthusiasm for tissue plasminogen activator has been significantly tempered. The GISSI study has forever changed the way such patients are approached. This study clearly demonstrated the benefit of early thrombolytic therapy in the treatment of a patient with acute myocardial infarction. It is, however, the observation that concurrent aspirin administration adds benefit that will make the greatest long-term contribution. This finding constitutes the best evidence to date that platelets are actively involved in thrombogenesis and that control of procoagulant forces is essential for full thrombolytic efficacy.

A full discussion of the relative merits of the three best known thrombolytic agents is beyond the scope of this chapter. There are pros and cons to each. Streptokinase is relatively inexpensive, but there is concern about the development of antistreptokinase antibodies. Tissue plasminogen activator offers some degree of thrombus selectivity and preservation of fibrinogen, but it is expensive and must be given by continuous infusion over a number of hours. Urokinase is a direct activator of plasminogen, but it is also somewhat expensive and offers little or no thrombus selectivity. Single-chain plasminogen activator does offer some selectivity and may act synergistically with tissue plasminogen activator, but the combination is expensive and has not been shown to offer a clinical advantage. The goal now is to develop adjunct therapies to achieve results even better than those obtained with streptokinase plus aspirin. The concern, of course is that greater efficacy will be gained only at the expense of an increased risk of hemorrhage.

Platelet glycoprotein IIb/IIIa inhibitors reduce cardiac complications in patients undergoing cardiac intervention. A recent meta-analysis found that these agents reduce the risk of death or myocardial infarction in patients with acute coronary syndromes not routinely scheduled for revascularization. This reduction is greatest in those patients at highest risk for thrombotic complications.

Prevention of Arterial Thrombosis   It is sometimes thought that the biochemistry of arterial thrombosis is profoundly different from that of venous thrombosis. Specific thrombin inhibitors are potent agents in preventing arterial thrombosis, and patients with deficiencies of AT3 are at increased risk for arterial thrombosis. These observations suggest that while the underlying biochemistry is the same, it is the situation that is different. Platelets appear to be more important in arterial thrombogenesis than in venous thrombogenesis. This probably relates to the ability of the platelet to adhere and focus the activity of the coagulation system. This view is supported by experience with monoclonal antibodies, which block the adherence function and are effective in blocking arterial thrombogenesis. It is not yet clear which approaches will prove the most effective against the thrombotic component of acute myocardial infarction.

The vitamin folic acid is known to decrease plasma concentration of homocysteine, thereby decreasing cardiovascular risk. Homocysteine metabolism also depends on vitamin B_{12} levels, particularly when folic acid is supplemented.

Stroke and Transient Ischemic Attacks   Patients with stroke can be divided into three roughly equal groups according to etiology. One group has intracranial hemorrhage, a diagnosis that is now readily made with the CT scan. A second group has clear evidence of embolism with a plausible source such as a carotid artery or intracardiac lesion most commonly in a patient with atrial fibrillation. The third group has no evidence of intracranial bleeding, and clinically the presentation is that of an embolic event. The interest in this group lies in the absence of an identifiable lesion that could be the source of the embolus.

Risk Factors   The majority of cerebrovascular accidents occur in the context of abnormal vasculature. Aneurysms and arteriovenous malformations predispose to hemorrhage, while arteriosclerosis predisposes to vascular occlusion. Identifiable risk factors for thrombus development have been difficult to ascertain. Deficiency of the natural anticoagulant proteins, particularly PS, has been noted in patients who present with nonhemorrhagic stroke, and individuals who are congenitally deficient in these factors are at increased risk of stroke. However, there are no adequate data that address the question of the predictive value of routine measurements of such factors in the general population.

Treatment   It is important to search for and correct hemostatic abnormalities in patients with hemorrhagic stroke. In the elderly population, there is an increased frequency of vitamin K deficiency, a condition that is easily treated once it is recognized. As was mentioned earlier, the appropriate intervention depends of the urgency with which correction is desired. Parenteral vitamin K is appropriate, but if even faster correction is needed, the infusion of a commercial prothrombin complex concentrate should be considered. Such concentrates contain all the vitamin K-dependent factors and can be used to obtain virtually instant complete correction of the defect induced either by deficiency of vitamin K or by warfarin ingestion.

There is considerable support for the use of anticoagulation in treating thrombotic stroke in evolution. Recently there has been renewed interest in the use of thrombolytic agents to effect removal of the offending thrombotic occlusion. Thrombolytic therapy decreases the number of disabled patients, but an increased risk of intracranial hemorrhage has also been demonstrated.

Prevention   In this setting the best preventive measures are those directed toward reducing the risk of atherosclerosis. Prevention of hemorrhagic stroke in individuals with no known defect in hemostasis is beyond current knowledge. Prevention of thrombotic stroke by interfering with the hemostatic system has been attempted but has had only limited success. Given the central role of platelets in arterial thrombosis, these cells form a logical target for therapy. Aspirin, ticlopidine, and possibly clopidogrel, appear to confer some protection but are ineffective in a significant number of patients. This has led to a reconsideration of anticoagulation with warfarin, a drug that can be used with greater assurance now that intracranial bleeding can be ruled out with confidence by CT. There is definite evidence that warfarin is beneficial in decreasing the risk of stroke in patients with atrial fibrillation and artificial heart valves. It has been shown to be ineffective in preventing ischemic strokes. The use of HMG-CoA (hydroxymethylglutaryl coenzyme A) reductase inhibitors ("statins") in ischemic stroke prevention is encouraging, presumably attributable to low-density lipoprotein (LDL)-cholesterol lowering and stabilization of carotid and intracranial arteriosclerosis.

Peripheral Artery Embolism and Thrombosis   There is little challenge in making the diagnosis of acute peripheral artery obstruction. Chronic obstruction is somewhat more insidious in onset, but even in this setting the diagnosis is usually evident. Therapeutic options are limited to the use of heparin to minimize thrombus extension and thrombolytic agents to restore patency.

Surgical removal of the thrombus is usually the first approach to a patient with acute peripheral artery obstruction. Not infrequently the distal vessel is found to be occluded by a thrombus which cannot be removed effectively by the use of a Fogarty catheter. If the procedure has succeeded in restoring some blood flow, the natural fibrinolytic system may be adequate to remove the remaining thrombus. This may require the use of heparin anticoagulation to prevent further thrombus generation. Some patients will require pharmacologic intervention to resolve the residual thrombus adequately. Such patients respond well to protracted intraarterial infusion of a thrombolytic agent. A small-bore catheter is placed so that the tip is just proximal to the residual thrombus, and a constant infusion of a thrombolytic agent, usually urokinase, is begun. The rate of infusion is typically 50,000 to 100,000 U/h, at which rate there is only minimal systemic activation of the fibrinolytic system. The infusion is continued for as long as 48 hours. Progress can be monitored by radiography with contrast medium injected through the catheter. This approach is highly successful in some patients, but has been singularly unsuccessful in others. At this time there is no good way to select appropriate candidates for the procedure. In general terms, fresh thrombus is more amenable to lysis than is old thrombus, but this has not proved to be as strong a factor as it is for coronary artery thrombosis.

Purple Toe Syndrome   This term has been used for two apparently different conditions, both associated with warfarin therapy. A few patients taking warfarin develop a dusky discoloration of the toes that is not accompanied by any pain, tenderness, or sensory changes and appears to be benign. An entirely different condition involves the onset, usually sudden, of profound discoloration resembling gangrene. The distinction from gangrene is usually straightforward in that sensation is well preserved. Where there is differential involvement of the toes, there may be sparing of the great and fifth toes. This syndrome appears to be due to cholesterol embolization, presumably from an atherosclerotic lesion in a proximal vessel. The emboli induce both spastic and thrombotic changes in the blood vessels. Anticoagulation is useful in minimizing the thrombotic complications while the vasospastic response resolves. There is limited experience with the use of thrombolytic agents delivered via catheter to the affected limb; however, in some patients there has been dramatic resolution of the occlusion with restoration of nearly normal blood flow.

Microvascular Thrombosis

General Considerations

This is a heterogeneous group of disorders in which organ failure is the predominant feature. Histologically and pathophysiologically these disorders are characterized by microvascular occlusion. Not infrequently, there are multiple organs involved, though some conditions have characteristic patterns of involvement.

Specific Conditions

Disseminated Intravascular Coagulation   In this disorder, the occlusions are platelet-fibrin thrombi. The typical picture of purpura fulminans is striking and often is followed by or even accompanied by a breakdown in hemostasis. This two-faced and protean picture can confound the treatment, and the conflicting issues are difficult to resolve. In the absence of life-threatening hemorrhage, treatment of thrombosis takes precedence over treatment of bleeding. Heparin administration is at the heart of such treatment, and suitable attention must be paid to restoring hemostatic function. Fortunately, the thrombotic tendency usually is controlled by the administration of only a small amount of heparin. Unfortunately, however, even this small amount may induce a significant breakdown in hemostasis in a compromised patient. The use of heparin in this setting is extremely valuable but should not be undertaken without a clear understanding of the potential complications.

Thrombotic Thrombocytopenic Purpura   Thrombotic thrombocytopenic purpura (TTP) is a mysterious disease. The widespread organ dysfunction is clearly a result of microvascular occlusion by platelet-fibrin thrombi, but there is no evidence of generalized activation of the coagulation system. Recent evidence supports the presence of an acquired inhibitor to von Willebrand factor-cleaving enzyme in patients with acquired TTP and an absence of this protease in cases of familial TTP as the pathogenic mechanisms. The protease normally functions to cleave high molecular weight multimers of von Willebrand factor, and accumulation of these high-molecular-weight multimers could lead to platelet clumping and fibrin deposition in small vessels. Without treatment, the mortality rate is in excess of 90 percent; with the best available treatment, it is less than 20 percent. This marked difference underscores the importance of making the diagnosis and instituting the appropriate therapy. The paradigm for this disease is a patient with the pentad of thrombocytopenia, microangiopathic hemolytic anemia, renal dysfunction, fever, and fluctuating neurologic dysfunction. In daily practice the paradigm needs to be replaced by a set of minimum criteria. Thrombocytopenia and microangiopathic hemolysis with normal coagulation studies are reasonable minimum criteria. Elevation in the plasma level of lactate dehydrogenase (LDH) is universal in this disease, although typically not to the degree that can be seen in megaloblastic states. Once the diagnosis is made, treatment should begin as soon as possible. Patients with TTP can suffer cardiac arrest without warning, and such patients are extremely difficult, if not impossible, to resuscitate. By contrast, the neurologic dysfunction of TTP is essentially completely reversible. This dissociation of clinical condition from prognosis is nowhere more extreme than in TTP and is the most cogent argument for seeking expert assistance with such patients.

The most important treatment modality is the infusion of plasma. Most centers now use plasmapheresis rather than simple infusion, and this choice is supported by the results of a randomized clinical trial. A great deal of therapy has not been formally tested, and the agents in use include aspirin, dipyridamole, prednisone, and vincristine. Splenectomy was once the principal mode of treatment, but it has been eclipsed by plasmapheresis in recent years. It is not clear whether splenectomy is appropriate for patients who fail to respond to plasma infusion. Presence of an antibody to the cleaving protease in cases of acquired TTP constitutes a rationale for the use of immunosuppressive agents to treat refractory disease.

Hemolytic Uremic Syndrome   Hemolytic uremic syndrome (HUS) bears some similarities to TTP, and some researchers contend that both diseases are part of the same spectrum. Recent evidence showing normal von Willebrand factor-cleaving enzyme levels in HUS patients suggests that the two are different entities with overlapping clinical features. It is clear that the presentation of HUS is usually different from that of TTP. In HUS, there is always marked renal dysfunction, coagulation abnormalities are common, neurologic defects tend to be global rather than focal, and fever is less common. The optimum treatment has not been defined for HUS, but the combination of plasma infusion and antiplatelet agent seems to produce good results in the majority of patients. In a few patients, the coagulation abnormalities overshadow the thrombocytopenia and microangiopathy, and treatment for DIC has to be instituted.

Warfarin-induced Skin Necrosis   This condition is recognized by the sudden onset of patchy skin necrosis, usually at the time of starting warfarin anticoagulation. The pathophysiology is thought to be related to the short half-life of PC in the circulation. The level of this anticoagulant falls rapidly after warfarin is begun, rendering the individual temporarily in prothrombotic imbalance. If there is concomitant activation of the coagulation system, the risk of thrombosis is significant. There is no satisfactory explanation for the predilection for microvascular thrombosis. This pathophysiology predicts that individuals congenitally deficient in protein C would be at particular risk, a prediction borne out in practice. Protein S deficiency also appears to increase the risk of this disorder, presumably through its role as cofactor to activated PC. Patients with a known deficiency of PC and previous skin necrosis have been reanticoagulated successfully with warfarin by a gradual increase in dose or by the use of heparin anticoagulation until the full warfarin effect has developed.

Multiple Organ System Failure and the Sepsis Syndrome
These conditions are the scourge of intensive care, being responsible for the majority of late deaths in a wide variety of primary disorders. The organ dysfunction appears to be due to microvascular occlusion, in most cases by platelet-fibrin thrombi. The morbidity and mortality associated with these conditions are high, and thus far treatment has been largely ineffective. It is fatuous to note that prevention is the best remedy, because these syndromes occur in the face of the best that medical science has to offer. Recent studies demonstrate benefit in the administration of activated protein C in certain patient populations with severe sepsis.

Essential Thrombocytosis   Primary thrombocythemia is a relatively uncommon disorder that predisposes to both bleeding and thrombosis. Typically platelet counts are higher than 1×10^{12}/L, but some patients are symptomatic with platelet counts of only 600×10^{9}/L . Elderly persons are at particular risk of complications because of the common coexistence of vascular diseases. Treatment options include platelet pheresis (in life-threatening situations), low-dose aspirin, hydroxyurea, interferon-α, and anagrelide.

Cryoproteinemia and Cold Agglutinin Disease   These are included here for completeness. In most cases, the vascular occlusion involves the extremities, is transient, is induced by cold exposure, and is resolved by warming. Occasionally, a thrombotic component supervenes and the occlusion does not reverse with warming. These patients may benefit from heparin infusion to limit the progression

of the thrombosis, but loss of tissue often occurs in this setting. The use of thrombolytic agents is attractive but has not been proven in clinical studies.

Heparin-induced Thrombocytopenia/Thrombosis   Heparin-associated thrombocytopenia is a common benign process that is seen in patients on heparin therapy. The mechanism is unclear, but thrombocytopenia is mild and no action in needed. Heparin withdrawal is not required. In contrast, heparin-induced thrombocytopenia/thrombosis is an uncommon disastrous clinical syndrome in which there is an immune-mediated fall in platelet counts in patients treated with heparin. Ten to 25 percent of patients with thrombocytopenia will develop venous or arterial thrombosis and many of these will require amputation as a result. Heparin-induced thrombocytopenia is secondary to immunoglobin (Ig) G antibodies that are formed to platelet factor 4–heparin complexes. Binding of the Fc receptor on the platelet leads to activation of the platelet and clearing by the spleen, accounting for the thrombocytopenia. It is unclear why some patients subsequently develop thrombosis; however, thrombin formation on the platelet surface, microthrombi formed by platelet aggregates, and vascular injury are thought to contribute. Thrombocytopenia is generally seen within 10 to 14 days after the initiation of heparin or within 2 to 3 days in patients with prior heparin exposure. The degree of thrombocytopenia is variable. The current definition suggests that a 50 percent decline in total platelet count or a platelet count of less than 100,000/μL is needed for the diagnosis. We suggest that any platelet count that is half of what is expected should also trigger suspicion of heparin-induced thrombocytopenia/thrombosis. Rarely does the platelet count fall below 20,000/μL. The diagnosis is made by the use of enzyme-linked immunoassay (ELISA), platelet aggregation studies, serotonin release, or flow cytometry. None of these assays is foolproof, and clinical correlation is advised.

Treatment consists of immediate discontinuation of heparin, and initiation of an alternative anticoagulant other than low-molecular-weight heparin or warfarin. There are several alternatives available currently. Cross-reactivity between antiheparin antibodies occurs rarely. Lepirudin (Refludan) is a direct thrombin inhibitor that is FDA approved for the treatment of heparin-induced thrombocytopenia/thrombosis. This agent is also renally cleared. Dosing is weight-based, and activity is measured by the PTT, with a goal of 1.5 to 2.5 times the normal PTT. Antilepirudin antibodies have been described. Argatroban is another antithrombin agent that is hepatically cleared. The dose is based on weight, and adjusted to maintain the PTT 1.5 to 3 times baseline.

Coumadin as a sole anticoagulant is not recommended after discontinuation of heparin because of the rapid decline in levels of protein C and the increased risk of thrombosis. It is important to continue some form of anticoagulation for at least 7 days after discontinuation of the heparin (during the time of platelet activation) to prevent thrombosis. This is true even in those patients receiving heparin for DVT prophylaxis only, who would not require long-term anticoagulation. At this point, after clearing of activated platelets, it is reasonable to continue or resume coumadin if long term anticoagulation is required. The antibody is usually cleared within 100 days after discontinuation of heparin, and absence can be confirmed by one of the above assays. Rechallenge with heparin at a later date is not universally recommended, but extenuating circumstances should be considered on an individual basis. For instance, if a patient with an acute myocardial infarction develops heparin-induced thrombocytopenia/thrombosis and later requires surgery for bypass grafting, short-term heparin use in the absence of a demonstrable antibody may be warranted.

REFERENCES

Barnett HJ et al: Drugs and surgery in the prevention of ischemic stroke. *N Engl J Med* 332(4):238, 1995.

Bernard GR et al: Efficacy and safety of recombinant human activated protein C for severe sepsis. *N Engl J Med* 344(10):699, 2001.

Bertina RM et al: Resistance to activated protein C and factor V Leiden as risk factors for venous thrombosis. *Thromb Haemost* 74(1):449, 1995.

Boersma E et al: Platelet glycoprotein IIb/IIIa inhibitors in acute coronary syndromes: A meta-analysis of all major randomized clinical trials. *Lancet* 359:189, 2002.

Coller BS: Antiplatelet agents in the prevention and therapy of thrombosis. *Annu Rev Med* 43:171, 1992.

Coller BS et al: Deficiency of plasma protein S, protein C, or antithrombin III and arterial thrombosis. *Arteriosclerosis* 7(5):456, 1987.

Furie B, Furie BC: The molecular basis of blood coagulation. *Cell* 53(4):505, 1988.

Hartzler GO et al: Percutaneous transluminal coronary angioplasty with and without thrombolytic therapy for treatment of acute myocardial infarction. *Am Heart J* 106(5 Pt 1):965, 1983.

Hirsh J: Optimal intensity and monitoring warfarin. *Am J Cardiol* 75(6):39B, 1995.

Knight MT, Dawson R: L Effect of intermittent compression of the arms on deep venous thrombosis in the legs. *Lancet* 2 (7998), 1976.

Lind SE: The bleeding time does not predict surgical bleeding. *Blood* 77(12):2547, 1991.

Mohr JP et al: A comparison of warfarin and aspirin for the prevention of recurrent ischemic stroke. *N Engl J Med* 345(20):1444, 2001.

Mughal TI: Primary thrombocythemia: A current perspective. *Stem Cells* 13(4):355, 1995.

Prandoni P et al: Deep-vein thrombosis and the incidence of subsequent symptomatic cancer. *N Engl J Med* 327(16):1128, 1992.

Rasi V, Lintula R: Platelet function in the myelodysplastic syndromes. *Scand J Haematol Suppl* 45:71, 1986.

Rosenberg RD et al: Protease inhibitors of human plasma: Antithrombin-III: "The heparin-antithrombin system." *J Med* 16(1–3):351, 1985.

ENDICRONOLOGY AND METABOLISM

C H A P T E R   6   5

Aging of the Endocrine System and Selected Endocrine Disorders

DAVID A. GRUENEWALD • ALVIN M. MATSUMOTO

PRINCIPLES OF GERIATRIC ENDOCRINOLOGY.

Impaired Homeostatic Regulation

As in other organ systems, the normal aging of the endocrine system is characterized by a progressive loss of reserve capacity, resulting in a decreased ability to adapt to changing environmental demands. This loss of homeostatic regulation reflects important alterations in hormonal synthesis, metabolism and action, but these changes may not be clinically apparent under baseline conditions. In fact, basal plasma concentrations of many hormones and metabolic fuels are essentially unchanged with normal aging. This is illustrated by fasting plasma glucose levels that exhibit little change with normal aging, but after a glucose challenge, glucose levels increase much more in healthy elderly persons as compared to young adults. In some instances, the function of aging endocrine systems is maintained by compensatory changes in secretion of one hormone to offset the loss of function of another hormone in a feedback system, or to compensate for alterations in metabolic clearance. For example, in many elderly men with testosterone levels in the normal range, pituitary luteinizing hormone (LH) secretion and serum LH levels are increased (although levels usually remain within the normal range), partially offsetting a reduction in testicular testosterone secretion. However, in other cases these compensatory mechanisms are inadequate to maintain normal function with aging even under basal conditions. For example, unlike cortisol, adrenal production of aldosterone and dehydroepiandrosterone (DHEA) declines disproportionately to clearance rates with aging, leading to age-related decreases in plasma levels of these hormones even under baseline conditions.

Altered Presentation of Endocrine Diseases

The presenting manifestations of endocrine disorders in elderly patients are often nonspecific, muted, or atypical. For example, hypothyroidism and hyperthyroidism may present similarly with nonspecific symptoms in elderly people, such as weight loss, fatigue, weakness, constipation and depression. Endocrine diseases may also present with signs and symptoms that are classic for older patients yet atypical compared to those commonly observed in younger patients. As illustrations, thyrotoxic elderly patients may exhibit apathy and depression with psychomotor retardation ("apathetic hyperthyroidism"), and diabetes mellitus may present with hyperosmolar nonketotic state, a classic presentation rarely seen in individuals younger than age 50 years (see Chaps. 66 and 67). In addition, with aging, it is increasingly common for illnesses to present without any symptoms, such as hypothyroidism or hypercalcemia secondary to hyperparathyroidism. Finally, the manifestations of endocrine disease may be altered or masked by coexisting illnesses and medications used to treat comorbidities that commonly occur in elderly people. For example, exacerbations of congestive heart failure or angina may be precipitated by hyperthyroidism in older patients with preexisting cardiac disease, but practitioners may mistakenly attribute the symptoms to worsening primary cardiac disease rather than to thyrotoxicosis in such patients.

Changes in Diagnostic and Therapeutic Approach

Based on the above discussion, it is clear that a high index of suspicion for endocrine (and other) diseases is required in older patients with nonspecific signs and symptoms or functional decline. Indeed, the presence of these diseases may be appreciated only upon routine laboratory screening. However, there is no firm consensus on appropriate screening practices for endocrine disorders in asymptomatic elderly adults. Furthermore, even with normal aging, alterations in endocrine system function may have an important impact on the diagnostic evaluation of the older patient. For example, several factors contribute to an age-related decrease in intestinal calcium absorption, including decreased renal production of 1,25-dihydroxyvitamin D (1,25(OH)2D) and reduced intestinal responsiveness to 1,25(OH)2D. In turn, these alterations in vitamin D metabolism and action cause an increase in parathyroid hormone (PTH) levels to maintain calcium homeostasis, and ultimately a reduction in bone mass. As a result of these changes, together with the effects of sex hormone deficiency (a common problem in both elderly women and men), many asymptomatic elderly people require evaluation for osteoporosis. In addition, the presence of concomitant medical problems, medications, and changes in nutritional status and body composition may lead to a mistaken impression of endocrine disease in elderly as well as in younger patients. For example, decreased serum triiodothyronine and thyroxine levels may occur in patients who are systemically ill but euthyroid ("euthyroid sick" syndromes), or thyroxine levels may be increased in others receiving certain medications such as estrogen supplements, falsely giving the impression of an endocrine abnormality (see Chap. 66).

Another factor complicating the evaluation of the older patient is the lack of age-adjusted normal ranges for most endocrine laboratory tests. Normal values for these tests are usually determined in healthy young subjects, or young to middle-aged blood donors, which may or may not reflect normal values in healthy elderly people. Furthermore, most studies of aging and endocrine function are cross-sectional rather than longitudinal. Because interindividual variability and heterogeneity are important concomitants of aging, the usefulness of cross-sectional studies in predicting age-related changes within an individual is limited. Finally, normative studies in older populations are often confounded by the inclusion of subjects with age-associated diseases.

Alterations in the therapeutic approach for geriatric patients with endocrine disease are similar to those required in elderly patients with illnesses involving other body systems. First, treatment plans must take into account coexisting medical illnesses, medications, alterations in clearance rate of hormones and medications, and changes in target organ sensitivity and effects. Second, to minimize the risk of drug toxicity and polypharmacy, dosage levels for hormone replacement and medications must be adjusted for changes in clearance rate with aging, and patients should receive the lowest dose of medication needed to achieve the therapeutic effect. Third, new medications should be initiated at low doses and increased very gradually if needed. Fourth, the medication regimen should be reviewed periodically, and medications should be discontinued if no longer needed. Finally, approaches that improve physical or cognitive function are of paramount importance for elderly people.

NEUROENDOCRINE REGULATION

Neurotransmitters and Neuropeptides

Studies directly assessing parameters of hypothalamic neuroendocrine function have not been performed in vivo in humans. However, age-related effects on hypothalamic function may be studied indirectly by examining alterations in pulsatile secretion of pituitary hormones, which reflect changes in pulsatile secretion of hypothalamic releasing and/or inhibiting hormones. Other indices of the effects of aging on hypothalamic function in humans include pituitary hormonal responses to administration of (1) hypothalamic releasing hormones, (2) agents that block end-organ feedback (e.g., clomiphene and metyrapone), and (3) agents that stimulate hypothalamic/pituitary hormonal secretion (e.g., the use of hypertonic saline to stimulate antidiuretic hormone [ADH] secretion, or arginine to stimulate growth hormone [GH] secretion).

A number of neurotransmitters and neuropeptides within the central nervous system have been found to affect the secretion of hypothalamic and pituitary hormones. Changes in activity of these neurotransmitters and neuropeptides are responsible for many age-related alterations in endocrine system function.

Dopamine

Dopamine released by hypothalamic neurons inhibits pituitary prolactin secretion. In turn, prolactin stimulates hypothalamic dopaminergic neurons, forming a short feedback loop. In humans, to a greater extent than some of the other hypothalamic neurotransmitters, changes in dopamine secretion are indirectly observable with commonly available methods. This is because dopamine is the major regulator of prolactin secretion, and changes in hypothalamic dopamine activity can be inferred through observation of changes in pulsatile prolactin secretion. The frequency of pulsatile prolactin secretion is unchanged with aging, suggesting an intact pulse generator. However, humans become relatively hypoprolactinemic with normal aging. Furthermore, the circadian rhythm of prolactin secretion is altered in elderly men, with a blunted or absent nocturnal rise in prolactin and reduced amplitude of prolactin pulses, as compared to young controls. Metoclopramide, a dopamine antagonist, increases nocturnal prolactin secretion to a greater degree in elderly people than in young subjects, suggesting that this blunted nocturnal elevation in prolactin in older men may be caused by an increase in dopaminergic tone with aging. In turn, these age-related alterations in dopaminergic activity may contribute to alterations in secretion of other anterior pituitary hormones. For example, after administration of the dopamine precursor L-dopa, plasma gonadotropins increase and thyroid-stimulating hormone (TSH) levels decrease in old but not in young male subjects, implying altered dopaminergic regulation of these hormones with aging.

Norepinephrine

Studies of postmortem brain tissue in normal elderly persons demonstrate a modest decrease in the number of noradrenergic neurons in the locus coeruleus, the primary source of noradrenergic innervation within the central nervous system. However, levels of norepinephrine in the cerebrospinal fluid (CSF) of normal older subjects are increased as compared to young adults, both in the basal state and in response to yohimbine, a stimulator of central noradrenergic activity. CSF norepinephrine is thought to be produced by noradrenergic neurons within the central nervous system rather than the peripheral sympathetic nervous system. Taken together with the observation that norepinephrine clearance from the central nervous system is unchanged in older adults, these findings suggest that central noradrenergic neuronal activity is increased with aging.

The noradrenergic neuronal system is thought to exert an important influence on pituitary secretion of a number of hormones, including growth hormone, TSH and LH; therefore, the age-associated increase in central noradrenergic tone may be an important factor underlying age-related changes in the secretion of these hormones.

Opioid Peptides

Endogenous opioid peptides are believed to be important regulators of neuroendocrine systems. The products of proopiomelanocortin metabolism are the most extensively studied of these peptides, including adrenocorticotropic hormone (ACTH), β-endorphin, β-lipotropin, and α-melanocyte–stimulating hormone. β-Endorphin, for example, is thought to exert a tonic inhibitory influence on gonadotropin-releasing hormone (GnRH) secretion, and to be an important regulator of reproductive function. In older men, administration of the opioid receptor antagonist naltrexone causes a smaller increase in LH levels than it causes in young men, and unlike in young men, there is no increase in LH pulse frequency. Taken together, these observations suggest a decrease in opioid tone with aging. However, basal plasma levels of ACTH and β-endorphin are unaffected by normal aging. Furthermore, plasma ACTH, cortisol and β-endorphin responses to physostigmine, a drug that increases central nervous system cholinergic activity, and ACTH and cortisol responses to administration of corticotropin-releasing hormone, are increased in elderly compared to younger adults. Increased responsiveness of β-endorphin and the hypothalamic–pituitary–adrenal axis with aging may cause significant alterations in the function of endocrine systems.

Melatonin

Melatonin is a hormone produced in the pineal gland that is involved in the organization of circadian and seasonal biorhythms. Its synthesis and release are stimulated by darkness and inhibited by light. Therefore, the diurnal rhythm of melatonin secretion mirrors the day–night cycle. This circadian rhythm of melatonin production is controlled by a "pacemaker" in the suprachiasmatic nucleus of the brain, but changes in environmental lighting can alter the timing of this rhythm. For example, light exposure inhibits melatonin release in a dose-dependent fashion, and it is possible to reverse the diurnal melatonin rhythm within a few days by reversing the diurnal pattern of light exposure. Melatonin affects reproductive function in a variety of species, with antigonadotropic effects that are more pronounced in species with marked seasonal variation in reproductive function and breeding patterns. However, even in humans dwelling in the Arctic, conception rates and pituitary–gonadal function are reduced during the winter as compared to the summer. Melatonin levels are increased in women with hypothalamic amenorrhea, and there has been some interest in very-high-dose melatonin (75 to 300 mg) as a potential contraceptive agent, used in combination with a progestin.

During development and aging, melatonin production is negligible in young infants, but rises markedly between 3 months and 1 to 3 years of age, when nighttime levels are at their highest. Most studies have reported that after early childhood, melatonin secretion gradually decreases, with a progressive decline continuing into old age. However, reanalysis of data from earlier studies revealed that most of the age-related decline in melatonin secretion occurred by the age of 30 years. Furthermore, nocturnal and 24-hour melatonin secretion appear to be similar in healthy older men and women free of confounding conditions and medications, as compared to healthy young men.

Melatonin has long been known to have sedative effects, suggesting a role in sleep production. In young adult subjects, melatonin doses of 0.1 to 1 mg decreased the time to sleep onset, and higher doses of 5 mg increased the duration of rapid eye- movement (REM) sleep. In elderly people with insomnia, serum melatonin levels were lower than in age-matched controls without insomnia, suggesting that insomnia in older adults is caused, at least in part, by melatonin deficiency. Elderly people are often exposed to significantly less environmental light than younger adults, a factor that is associated with diminished nocturnal melatonin secretion. Supplementary exposure to bright light during midday increased melatonin secretion in older adults, and tended to improve sleep disturbances in elderly insomniacs. In older insomniacs, administration of melatonin in doses of 0.1 to 6 mg per day for up to 3 weeks improved some measures of sleep quality. However, melatonin had little effect on sleep quality in elderly people without sleep complaints.

Melatonin is a potent free radical scavenger, and it has been proposed that if the age-related decline in melatonin were prevented, then potentially the degenerative changes of aging could also be delayed. However, others have noted that the reported antioxidant effects of melatonin probably occur only at pharmacologic concentrations. In humans, high-affinity melatonin receptors are present on CD4 T lymphocytes, but little additional information is available on the effects of melatonin on the human immune system.

Based in part on the assumption that a decline in endogenous hormone levels constitutes a deficiency needing replacement, there has been considerable enthusiasm in the lay community for supplementation of certain hormones, including melatonin. Melatonin is readily available without a prescription, and many older people are already taking melatonin without physician consultation. It is noteworthy that melatonin dosages of 1 to 5 mg contained in preparations commonly available over the counter in the United States boost nighttime levels 10 to 100 times higher than the usual maximum within an hour after administration, and only very low doses (0.1 to 0.3 mg) achieve peak serum levels within the normal nighttime range. Thus far, no serious side effects have been reported in humans after melatonin ingestion (aside from sleepiness after the dose), even with pharmacologic melatonin doses. However, large, long-term studies of melatonin use are still lacking, and the long-term risks and benefits of melatonin supplementation remain to be determined. Until this information is available, it is premature to advocate its use.

Hormonal Changes in Alzheimer's Disease

Alzheimer's disease is characterized by a profound impairment of cholinergic neuronal function within the central nervous system, but changes in the function of many other neurotransmitter and neuropeptide systems have been described. In turn, these central nervous system alterations are associated with changes in pituitary and peripheral hormone levels. Perhaps the most important endocrine system abnormality observed in patients with Alzheimer's disease is an increase in hypothalamic-pituitary-adrenal axis activity. This is manifested in elevated plasma ACTH and cortisol levels, and in a lack of suppression of cortisol levels by dexamethasone, suggesting decreased glucocorticoid feedback inhibition. In addition, ACTH responses to exogenous administration of corticotropin-releasing hormone (CRH) are blunted, which may be a result of downregulation of pituitary responsiveness to CRH secondary to chronically increased hypothalamic CRH stimulation. Finally, cortisol and ACTH responsiveness to physostigmine, which increases central cholinergic activity, is markedly increased in patients with Alzheimer's disease and normal elderly persons, as compared to young subjects.

This elevated glucocorticoid milieu may play a role in the pathogenesis of Alzheimer's disease. It has been hypothesized that chronically increased glucocorticoid stimulation damages the hippocampal neurons that mediate glucocorticoid feedback inhibition of the hypothalamic–pituitary–adrenal axis, leading, in turn, to a "glucocorticoid cascade" of neurodegeneration in Alzheimer's disease (and to a lesser extent in the aging brain). While controversial, this hypothesis remains under active study to determine whether glucocorticoid levels are a potentially modifiable risk factor for Alzheimer's disease.

Many other alterations in hormone, hormone receptor, neuropeptide and neurotransmitter levels have been reported in plasma, cerebrospinal fluid, and postmortem brain tissue specimens. However, it should be noted that in many instances, studies of hormonal changes in Alzheimer's disease were not well-controlled for the effects of nutritional status, medications, or coexisting medical illnesses and depression. Therefore, it is unclear in these studies whether the reported changes are primarily caused by Alzheimer's disease or by the presence of confounding variables. Well-controlled studies have found that norepinephrine (NE) levels in cerebrospinal fluid are increased in individuals with Alzheimer's disease as they are in normal elderly people. This increase in central nervous system noradrenergic activity is apparently caused by an increase in NE biosynthesis without a change in NE clearance. Because there is a marked loss of noradrenergic neurons in the locus coeruleus of the brain in patients with Alzheimer's disease, these findings suggest a strong compensatory activation of the remaining noradrenergic neurons in these patients.

Anterior Pituitary

Prolactin

Healthy aging is associated with a decrease in prolactin secretion in both men and postmenopausal women, reflecting a decrease in both basal prolactin secretion and the amplitude of pulsatile prolactin release. Mild hyperprolactinemia in older adults may result from any of several underlying causes (Table 65-1), including hypothalamic diseases that interfere with the production of dopamine (prolactin-inhibitory factor). A number of medications commonly used by older adults inhibit dopaminergic activity and increase prolactin levels, and hypothyroidism increases thyrotropin-releasing hormone which stimulates prolactin secretion.

The clinical manifestations of hyperprolactinemia are typically subtle and often unrecognized. Hyperprolactinemia causes secondary hypogonadism and may exacerbate sexual dysfunction. Less commonly, galactorrhea and gynecomastia may occur. In addition, hyperprolactinemia can accelerate age-related bone loss primarily because of the antigonadotropic effects of prolactin and resulting hypogonadism. Thus, measurement of prolactin is important in the evaluation of secondary causes of osteoporosis, especially when hypogonadism is present, and patients with hyperprolactinemia should be questioned regarding other osteoporosis risk factors such as family history of hip fractures, excessive alcohol intake, or thyrotoxicosis. If drugs and hypothyroidism have been ruled out as causes of hyperprolactinemia, it is appropriate to obtain either a computed tomography (CT) scan or magnetic resonance imaging (MRI) to rule out the presence of a pituitary tumor or hypothalamic lesion. Dynamic pituitary testing, for example, thyrotropin-releasing hormone (TRH) testing, is of no value in the diagnosis of this disorder.

If the hyperprolactinemia is secondary to another disorder such as hypothyroidism or a medication, the underlying cause should be corrected if possible, which often results in

Table 65-1   Causes of Hyperprolactinemia in Older Adults

Hypothalamic diseases
   Tumors
      Metastatic disease
      Meningioma
      Glioma
   Granulomatous diseases
      Sarcoidosis
      Tuberculosis
   Irradiation

Hypothyroidism

Pituitary stalk section
   Suprasellar extension of pituitary adenoma
   Trauma

Pituitary prolactinoma

Chronic renal failure

Chronic liver disease

Chest wall lesions
   Herpes zoster
   Surgery

Drugs
   Phenothiazines
   Cimetidine
   Opiates
   Metoclopramide
   Estrogens

normalization of prolactin levels. However, if the etiology is a microadenoma (defined as a pituitary tumor <10 mm in size) or idiopathic hyperprolactinemia, options include watchful waiting or dopamine agonist medications. The natural history of microadenomas is incompletely understood, especially in older adults, but most prolactin-producing microadenomas are stable or involute with time. Accordingly, observation is the most appropriate strategy in many patients, although treatment may be indicated if sexual dysfunction or additional risk factors for osteoporosis are present. Dopamine agonists such as bromocriptine, pergolide, or cabergoline are effective in reducing prolactin levels and normalizing reproductive axis function in most patients, but gastrointestinal, behavioral and other side effects such as hallucinations are common in older patients. These side effects can be minimized by following a "start low, go slow" approach when beginning these medications. Surgery is rarely indicated, but may be necessary in those with macroadenomas (>10 mm) and persistent visual field defects or inability to tolerate dopamine agonists. Alternatively, radiation therapy may be an option for patients with large tumors who are unable to tolerate medical therapy and are not surgical candidates. However, the clinical response to radiation is often delayed for months to years, and anterior pituitary insufficiency eventually occurs in many of these patients.

Age-associated alterations in secretion of other anterior pituitary hormones are discussed below, under the individual hormonal systems.

Pituitary Adenomas

Although the incidence of pituitary tumors increases with aging, symptomatic pituitary tumors are uncommon even in people of advanced age. However, the prevalence of pituitary tumors at autopsy ranges from 8.5 to 27 percent, indicating that the vast majority of these tumors are clinically "silent." In case series of pituitary tumors in older adults, the majority of lesions are apparently nonfunctioning adenomas, whereas 13 to 14 percent are growth hormone-secreting tumors and 5 to 8 percent are prolactinomas. However, many, if not most, apparently nonfunctioning adenomas actually produce quantities of gonadotropins or the α subunit of these glycoprotein hormones.

Nonsecreting tumors and tumors that secrete LH, follicle-stimulating hormone (FSH), or α subunit are usually large at the time of diagnosis, because there are few or no symptoms of hormone overproduction. Gonadotropin hypersecretion from such tumors usually does not result in excessive gonadal hormone secretion, although LH hypersecretion occasionally results in elevated testosterone levels. Clinical manifestations of these tumors are usually a result of a mass effect, including visual field abnormalities, headaches, and panhypopituitarism. Gonadotropin-secreting pituitary tumors are particularly difficult to diagnose in postmenopausal women in whom gonadotropin levels are elevated due to ovarian failure. For these women, exaggerated α, LH-β, and FSH-β subunit responses, and/or intact gonadotropin responses to TRH are useful in diagnosing these tumors. Management of large pituitary tumors usually involves transsphenoidal decompression and debulking, along with assessment of anterior pituitary hormone function and replacement of hormone deficiencies.

Hypopituitarism and the Empty Sella Syndrome

As a pituitary macroadenoma grows, destruction of normal surrounding pituitary tissue occurs, leading ultimately to a predictable loss of gonadotropins and growth hormone followed by TSH and, eventually, ACTH secretion. The resulting panhypopituitarism may present clinically as a constellation of symptoms including postural hypotension, fatigue, weight loss, hypogonadism, and hypoglycemia, but because some of these symptoms are relatively common in elderly patients without panhypopituitarism, a high index of suspicion is required to make the diagnosis.

As brain imaging techniques such as CT and MRI have come into widespread use, it is increasingly common to discover incidentally the presence of both pituitary masses and empty sella syndrome. In a CT study of the pituitary in subjects older than age 75 years, 65 percent were found to have a partially or completely empty sella, and only 24 percent had a completely normal scan. A more recent MRI study of healthy young and elderly subjects confirmed previous studies showing that pituitary height and volume tend to decrease with aging, but empty sella was observed in only 19 percent of subjects, and there was no relationship between pituitary volume and anterior pituitary hormone levels. Most cases of primary empty sella syndrome (i.e., not associated with prior pituitary surgery or irradiation) occur in obese, hypertensive middle-aged women. Clinically apparent pituitary dysfunction is uncommon, although up to 15 percent of subjects may manifest endocrine dysfunction including hyperprolactinemia, hypogonadism or panhypopituitarism. However, the functional significance of an empty sella as an incidental finding on imaging studies in apparently healthy elderly patients is unclear. In such patients, conservative management is appropriate, including visual field testing and serum hormone testing to rule out subclinical pituitary dysfunction and suprasellar involvement.

Posterior Pituitary

Elderly people are at higher risk than young adults for the development of both volume depletion and excess free water states. This is a result of age-related changes occurring in the systems that maintain volume status and osmolality, including ADH secretion, osmoreceptor and baroreceptor systems, renal concentration of urine and hormone responsiveness, and thirst mechanisms. There is evidence for a state of relative ADH excess with aging, with normal to increased basal ADH levels, increased ADH release after an osmotic stimulus such as hypertonic saline infusion, and impaired ethanol inhibition of ADH secretion in elderly persons, as compared with young adult subjects. Furthermore, renal free water clearance decreases with aging in proportion to declining glomerular filtration rate. This age-related reduction in free water clearance, together with relative ADH excess and the increased prevalence of conditions such as congestive heart failure, hypothyroidism, and the use of sulfonylurea and diuretic medication all contribute to the common occurrence of free water excess and hyponatremia in elderly people. When present, hyponatremia in frail older adults is usually mild and asymptomatic, but these individuals may develop more marked symptomatic hyponatremia in the setting of acute illness.

In contrast to the increased osmoreceptor sensitivity to ADH, baroreceptor responsiveness to ADH is decreased with aging, resulting in decreased ADH release in response to hypotension or hypovolemia and increased risk of volume depletion. Furthermore, renal responsiveness to ADH is diminished with aging, possibly because of chronic exposure to elevated ADH levels, leading to a decrease in maximal urine concentrating ability. Decreased aldosterone and increased atrial natriuretic hormone activity with aging contribute to the potential for volume depletion by decreasing the capacity of the kidneys to conserve sodium under conditions of fluid deprivation (see "Renin–Angiotensin–Aldosterone System" later in this chapter). Finally, healthy older adults exhibit decreased thirst and reduced fluid intake in response to fluid deprivation, hyperosmotic stimuli, and hypovolemia, further contributing to the risk of dehydration with aging. Elderly patients with immobility or dementia, such as nursing home residents, are at particularly high risk for severe dehydration.

A number of factors predispose older people to nocturnal polyuria. These include age-related blunting of the circadian rhythm of circulating ADH, with loss of the nocturnal increase in ADH levels, and an increase in nighttime plasma atrial natriuretic hormone levels. Patients with Alzheimer's disease have lower circulating ADH levels than cognitively intact people of the same age, and appear to be particularly prone to nocturnal polyuria. Superimposed on age-related changes in bladder function and mobility, altered ADH regulation can contribute to urinary incontinence. Older patients with nocturnal polyuria may benefit from administration of the ADH analog desmopressin (DDAVP), in addition to other interventions such as detrusor relaxants and behavioral interventions.

THE HYPOTHALAMIC–PITUITARY– ADRENAL AXIS

Physiology

Compared to the other hypothalamic–pituitary–end-organ axis, hypothalamic–pituitary–glucocorticoid function is relatively intact with aging in humans (Table 65-2). The cortisol secretion rate is decreased with aging, but this is matched by a decrease in the cortisol metabolic clearance rate. As a result, basal plasma concentrations of cortisol are unchanged with aging, even in very old subjects. Consistent with intact cortisol secretion, basal ACTH levels are also unaffected by aging. Furthermore, glucocorticoid responsiveness of the hypothalamic–pituitary–adrenal (HPA) axis to stimulation is well-maintained in older adults, with intact cortisol responses to exogenous ACTH stimulation (except at very-low doses of ACTH [0.06 μg]) and normal or slightly prolonged cortisol and ACTH responses to metyrapone, ovine corticotropin-releasing hormone (CRH) and insulin-induced hypoglycemia. ACTH pulse frequency has been reported to be unchanged in healthy young compared to elderly men, suggesting intact hypothalamic regulation of glucocorticoid function.

Table 65-2   Alterations in Hypothalamic–Pituitary–Glucocorticoid Axis Function with Aging

ACTH levels	↔
ACTH response to CRH stimulation	↔
Cortisol production	↓
Cortisol clearance from plasma	↓
Plasma cortisol levels	↔
Cortisol response to stimulation	
ACTH	↔
Metyrapone, hypoglycemia	↔/↑
Surgical stress	↑
HPA axis sensitivity to glucocorticoid feedback	↓

↓, decreased; ↔, unchanged; ↑, increased.

ACTH, adrenocorticotropic hormone; CRH, corticotropin-releasing hormone; HPA, hypothalamic–pituitary–adrenal.

Moreover, the circadian rhythm of ACTH and cortisol secretion is intact in healthy older subjects, although the amplitude of the cortisol rhythm is reduced compared to young adults. In addition, a phase advance of the cortisol rhythm occurs in elderly people, with earlier nadir and peak secretion, as compared to young adults. This phase advance has been attributed to behavioral changes, possibly reflecting an earlier bedtime in older adults.

The most consistently demonstrated age-related abnormality in HPA axis function is the cortisol response to stress. After a stressful stimulus such as surgery, peak cortisol levels are higher and remain elevated longer in older compared to young adult subjects. Furthermore, dexamethasone is less effective in suppressing cortisol levels in older subjects, and in studies using metyrapone to remove endogenous cortisol feedback inhibition, the decline in ACTH levels after exogenous cortisol infusion was blunted and delayed in older compared to young adult subjects. Taken together, these studies indicate that the sensitivity of the HPA axis to glucocorticoid negative feedback is decreased with aging. The clinical implications of this decreased responsiveness to glucocorticoid feedback inhibition are unclear. However, it has been proposed that the resulting increase in glucocorticoid exposure may damage hippocampal neurons regulating glucocorticoid secretion and important to cognitive function, leading to a vicious cycle of further glucocorticoid hypersecretion and damage to mechanisms regulating HPA feedback inhibition.

Laboratory Testing of HPA Axis Function

Although glucocorticoid function is well-preserved with aging, certain factors may interfere with testing of HPA axis function in older patients. For example, excretion of steroids commonly measured in urine is decreased with renal impairment, and measurements are unreliable in patients with a creatinine clearance of less than 50 mL/min. In patients with severe malnutrition, cortisol clearance may be decreased, leading to falsely elevated cortisol levels. Moreover, because the acute cortisol stress response may be higher and prolonged in older patients, testing for Cushing's syndrome should be delayed for at least 48 hours after major stresses such as high fever, trauma or surgery. Finally, medications such as phenytoin and phenobarbital that induce liver metabolism of cortisol and other corticosteroids may result in artificially low measurements of urinary 17-hydroxycorticosteroids, which are sometimes used as indices of cortisol secretion. In addition, these medications may increase dexamethasone metabolism, resulting in failure of normal cortisol suppression by dexamethasone (i.e., a false-positive result on dexamethasone suppression testing; see "Hyperadrenocorticism" later in this chapter).

The ACTH stimulation test is used to screen for both primary and chronic secondary (central) adrenal insufficiency. Expected cortisol responses to the standard dose of 250 μg of ACTH (absolute cortisol level of >20 μg/dL 30–60 minutes after IV bolus) do not change with aging. The rationale for its use in assessing pituitary function is that in patients with chronic pituitary disease, the absence of sufficient stimulation of the adrenal glands by endogenous

ACTH leads to adrenal atrophy and hyporesponsiveness to exogenous ACTH. However, the standard ACTH stimulation test lacks sensitivity for mild secondary adrenal insufficiency. The low-dose ACTH stimulation test, performed with 1 μg of ACTH and measurement of cortisol 30 minutes after injection, has been proposed as a more sensitive test. Although very reliable in detecting mild primary adrenal insufficiency, some experts believe it is less sensitive for mild secondary adrenal insufficiency than traditional "gold standard" provocative tests such as insulin-induced hypoglycemia. In studies of older adults, the low-dose ACTH test accurately evaluated adrenal function in patients following uncomplicated abdominal surgery. However, the test was difficult to interpret in seriously ill postoperative patients with clinical features such as unexplained hypotension suggesting relative adrenal insufficiency. Furthermore, optimization of test sensitivity (to minimize the occurrence of false negative results) requires establishment of the criteria for an abnormal test in each laboratory.

Based on the foregoing, the low-dose ACTH test may offer greater sensitivity and diagnostic accuracy than the standard ACTH test for chronic secondary adrenal insufficiency. However, additional dynamic testing of adrenal axis function may be indicated for borderline abnormal test results. Furthermore, the ACTH stimulation test should never be used in cases of acute or recent onset of hypopituitarism, because the adrenal glands may still be able to respond normally to any ACTH challenge.

The cortisol response to insulin-induced hypoglycemia is a reliable test for primary or secondary adrenal insufficiency, but may be inappropriate in frail older patients because of the potential risks associated with severe hypoglycemia. In patients with a normal response to ACTH stimulation, the metyrapone test can be used to confirm suspected secondary adrenal insufficiency. Metyrapone inhibits 11β-hydroxylase, the final step in cortisol synthesis, and in normal individuals, ACTH secretion increases, stimulating adrenal secretion of 1L-deoxycortisol. However, oral metyrapone may cause dizziness, nausea, and vomiting in some older patients, and it has been suggested that intravenous metyrapone infusion is safer and better tolerated in elderly people.

Hyperadrenocorticism

Cushing's syndrome is an eponym for the constellation of signs and symptoms of chronic corticosteroid excess, including central obesity; catabolic effects on muscle, skin, and bone; glucose intolerance; and hypertension. The most common cause of Cushing's syndrome in older adults, as in other age groups, is the administration of glucocorticoids. The undesirable effects of glucocorticoid treatment are similar in older and younger patients, but in elderly people glucocorticoids may cause major adverse effects upon function (Table 65-3). When it is necessary to use pharmacologic doses of glucocorticoids, older patients should receive the minimum necessary dosage, and the dosage requirement should be reviewed at frequent intervals. Bone densitometry measurements using dual-energy x-ray absorptiometry (DXA) should be performed prior to initiating

Table 65-3   Adverse Effects of Glucocorticoids in Elderly Patients

Central nervous system
  Impaired cognition
  Emotional lability
  Depression
  Psychosis

Bone
  Osteoporosis
  Fractures

Muscle
  Proximal muscle wasting
  Weakness

Fluid and electrolytes
  Sodium retention
  Hypokalemia

Metabolic
  Obesity
  Hyperglycemia
  Hypertriglyceridemia

Cardiac
  Congestive heart failure
  Hypertension

Gastrointestinal
  Peptic ulcer disease

Skin
  Fragility
  Impaired wound healing

Vision
  Cataracts
  Glaucoma

Immune system
  Decreased cell-mediated immunity
  Increased risk of infections

Functional
  Impaired ambulation and transfers
  Falls
  Loss of independence

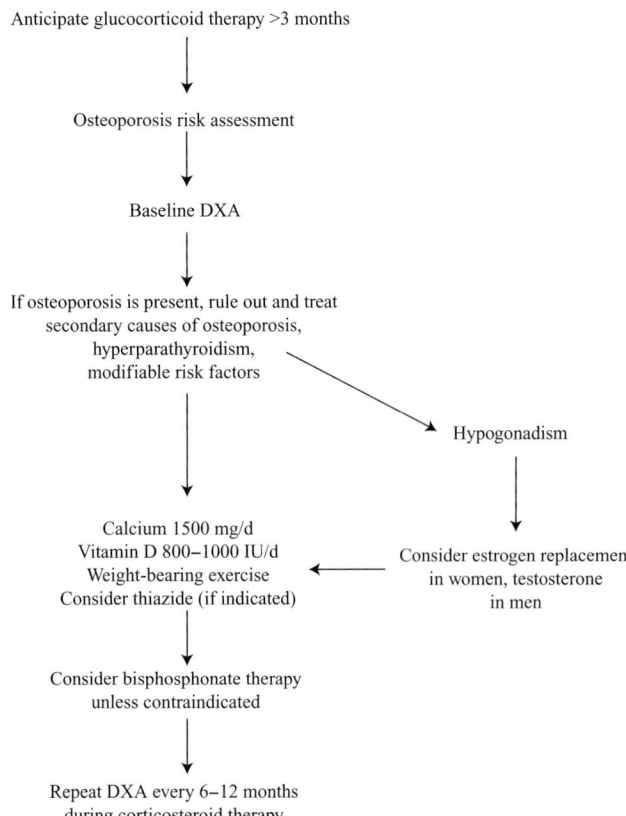

Figure 65-1   Management of glucocorticoid-induced osteoporosis. DXA, dual-energy x-ray absorptiometry.

long-term corticosteroid therapy and after 6 to 12 months of therapy (Fig. 65-1). As for the evaluation of osteoporosis not associated with corticosteroid use, all patients should be assessed for modifiable osteoporosis risk factors, secondary causes of osteoporosis, hyperparathyroidism, and vitamin D deficiency.

Some of the adverse effects of corticosteroid use in older people can be minimized with other interventions (Fig. 65-1). For example, because corticosteroids decrease intestinal calcium absorption and increase urinary calcium losses, ensuring an intake of at least 1500 mg elemental calcium per day together with 800 to 1000 IU/d of vitamin D helps to minimize bone loss. Alternatively, high-dose vitamin D (ergocalciferol 50,000 IU once or twice weekly) or calcitriol (0.5 μg/d) may be used, but follow-up of both serum and urine calcium levels is required. Furthermore, dietary sodium restriction (2 to 3 g/d) and thiazide diuretics (e.g., hydrochlorothiazide, 25 mg/d) are useful to reduce the hypercalciuria associated with corticosteroid use, although their effects on bone density have not been adequately determined in patients receiving corticosteroids.

Hormone replacement therapy can be considered to counteract corticosteroid-induced suppression of sex hormones. Estrogen supplementation (e.g., conjugated estrogens 0.625 mg/d with medroxyprogesterone acetate 2.5 to 5.0 mg daily for women with an intact uterus) may help postmenopausal women taking corticosteroids, but its use is controversial. Men with hypogonadism should receive androgen-replacement therapy (e.g., testosterone enanthate or cypionate, 100 to 200 mg IM every 2 weeks, or daily transdermal application of a testosterone patch or gel). Bisphosphonates should be considered as first-line therapy for patients who will be taking the equivalent of prednisone 7.5 mg per day or more for at least 3 months, because clinically significant bone loss may occur with this dose and duration of therapy. Meta-analyses of bisphosphonates for prevention and treatment of corticosteroid-induced osteoporosis have reported increased bone mineral density at the lumbar spine and hip, and a reduction in the risk of fractures of the vertebral spine. Appropriate bisphosphonate choices include cyclical etidronate 400 mg daily for 2 weeks repeated at 3-month intervals, alendronate 10 mg daily or 70 mg weekly, and risedronate 5 mg daily. Calcitonin (e.g., 200 IU intranasally per day) preserves bone mass at the lumbar spine but not at the femoral neck in patients taking glucocorticoids. However, its efficacy in fracture prevention in these patients has not been established.

Corticosteroid-induced myopathy is characterized by weakness and atrophy of the muscles of the hip, thigh, and proximal upper extremities, which may result in an increased risk of falls in older people with age-related loss of muscle mass. The best approach for this difficult problem is to minimize the dose of corticosteroid or to eliminate it altogether if possible. For those who require ongoing corticosteroid therapy and cannot be tapered off these drugs, resistance and endurance exercise, and androgen-replacement therapy in men, may help to prevent glucocorticoid-induced muscle atrophy. However, the effectiveness of these approaches in preventing functional decline in older patients has not been determined.

Cushing's disease, or hypercortisolism caused by excessive pituitary ACTH secretion, is most common in persons between 20 and 40 years of age. Accounting for approximately two-thirds of cases of endogenous hypercortisolism in younger adults, Cushing's disease is a much-less-common cause of cortisol excess in elderly people, although its exact prevalence in older adults is unclear. In contrast, the ectopic ACTH syndrome is more common in older people, most of whom have obvious neoplasms such as small cell lung cancer, although other tumors may be clinically undetectable as in the case of some bronchial carcinoid tumors. Patients with the ectopic ACTH syndrome caused by small-cell lung cancer or other rapidly growing tumors typically present with cachexia rather than central obesity, hypertension, and metabolic disturbances including hypokalemia, metabolic alkalosis, and hyperglycemia. Cortisol-producing adrenal carcinomas are more common in older people than in young adults, with a bimodal peak incidence in children and in people older than age 60 years. These tumors may produce severe Cushing's syndrome with virilization in women and mineralocorticoid excess, although many of these tumors are nonfunctioning and do not cause symptoms of Cushing's syndrome. Adrenocortical carcinomas are typically large (>100 g) and palpable, unlike benign adrenal adenomas which are usually 10 to 20 g (size 1 to 6 cm) at presentation.

If there is a clinical suspicion of Cushing's syndrome, a 24-hour urinary free cortisol or a low dose dexamethasone suppression test (DST) is performed to confirm the diagnosis (Fig. 65-2). False-positive results are common with the low-dose DST in elderly people, even in apparently normal individuals, therefore urinary free cortisol measurements are usually preferred to differentiate normal older individuals from those with Cushing's syndrome. However, the urinary free cortisol test may be confounded by inadequate urine collections or the presence of renal insufficiency. If the low-dose DST is used, after oral ingestion of 1 mg of dexamethasone at 11 P.M. for the overnight test, or 0.5 mg every 6 hours for 48 hours, measurement of serum cortisol normally shows suppression to less than 5 μg/dL, whereas

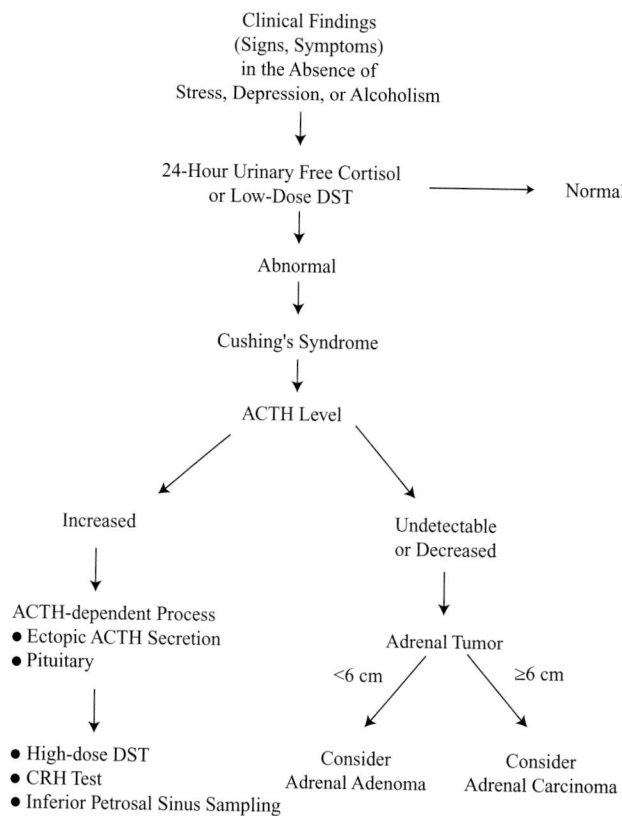

Figure 65-2 Diagnostic approach to evaluate possible Cushing's syndrome. ACTH, adrenocorticotropic hormone; CRH, corticotropin-releasing hormone; DST, dexamethasone suppression test.

those with Cushing's syndrome fail to suppress. In addition, several conditions commonly encountered in older adults may present diagnostic problems. Obesity, medications such as phenytoin, depression, active alcoholism, or other coexisting stressful illnesses may be associated with dexamethasone nonsuppression and elevated urinary cortisol levels. In these instances of "pseudo-Cushing's syndrome," other approaches are necessary to clarify the diagnosis. Obese patients may exhibit increased 24-hour urinary free cortisol levels, but these elevations are generally modest compared to patients with Cushing's syndrome. Patients receiving medications such as phenytoin that increase dexamethasone clearance may require concomitant plasma dexamethasone and cortisol measurements to ensure that an adequate dexamethasone level is achieved. Finally, patients with pseudo-Cushing's syndrome as a consequence of a variety of disorders, including active alcoholism, depression, obesity, and poorly controlled diabetes mellitus, may exhibit elevated urinary free cortisol levels, but retain normal circadian variation in serum cortisol levels despite increased cortisol secretion. A single midnight serum cortisol level >7.5 μg/dL was reported to distinguish patients with Cushing's syndrome from those with pseudo-Cushing's syndrome with 100 percent specificity and 96 percent sensitivity, and is probably the test of choice in this situation. In any event, abnormalities in cortisol secretion in patients with pseudo-Cushing's syndrome usually normalize with remission of the underlying condition.

After the diagnosis of Cushing's syndrome is established, simultaneous plasma ACTH and cortisol levels are obtained to determine whether the cortisol excess is ACTH-dependent or ACTH-independent. If ACTH and cortisol levels are increased, the hypercortisolism is ACTH-dependent, usually reflecting a pituitary adenoma (Cushing's disease) or, less commonly, ectopic ACTH secretion. Most patients with ectopic ACTH syndrome have extremely high ACTH levels that do not suppress with high-dose dexamethasone, but 10 to 20 percent of these patients show significant suppression that may be misleading. Infusion of CRH is useful to distinguish ectopic ACTH secretion from Cushing's disease; most patients with a pituitary tumor will show an increase in cortisol and ACTH levels after CRH, whereas patients with ectopic ACTH-secreting tumors will not. Stringent criteria have been proposed for interpretation of the high-dose dexamethasone suppression and CRH stimulation tests to maximize their specificity for Cushing's disease (greater than 90% suppression and greater than 50% rise in cortisol, respectively). However, this increase in test specificity sacrifices test sensitivity, and many patients with Cushing's disease do not meet the stringent response criteria for one or both tests. Accordingly, further testing such as venous sampling from the inferior petrosal or cavernous sinus is still required in these cases, and referral to an endocrinologist is usually indicated. If ACTH levels are undetectable or low and cortisol levels are high, then an ACTH-independent process is present, suggesting an adrenal tumor. In this case, CT scanning of the adrenals is indicated to confirm the diagnosis.

In patients with Cushing's disease, transsphenoidal surgery is the treatment of choice, although radiotherapy and the steroidogenesis inhibitor ketoconazole are alternatives in those who are unable to undergo surgery. When possible, surgical tumor removal is also indicated for most patients with functional adrenal adenomas or the ectopic ACTH syndrome, although for those who are not surgical candidates, aminoglutethimide, mitotane, or metyrapone and spironolactone may be useful in reducing the symptoms of glucocorticoid and mineralocorticoid excess, respectively.

Adrenal Insufficiency

Primary adrenal insufficiency is less common in elderly persons than in young adults; less than 10 percent of patients with adrenocortical failure are older than age 60 years at initial presentation. As in younger patients, most cases of adrenal insufficiency in elderly people are a result of acute stress or rapid withdrawal of glucocorticoids in patients with suppressed adrenal function caused by chronic glucocorticoid administration. Autoimmune adrenocortical insufficiency is rare in older patients, but other causes of adrenal insufficiency, including tuberculosis, adrenal hemorrhage, and metastatic disease, are much more common in elderly persons than in young adults. Tuberculous involvement of the adrenals is nearly always associated with evidence of past or current tuberculosis infection elsewhere in the body, and may manifest with large calcified adrenal glands on plain x-rays or CT scans. Adrenal

hemorrhage typically presents acutely in anticoagulated patients with symptoms such as nausea, vomiting, hypotension, and tachycardia, and is likely to be the cause if bilateral adrenal enlargement is demonstrated on CT scan. Metastatic disease involving the adrenals occurs most commonly with lymphomas and carcinomas of the lung, colon, and prostate, although even when metastases are present, it is unusual for cortisol secretion to be impaired.

The presentation of chronic adrenal insufficiency is usually vague and nonspecific in older patients, often with symptoms of "failure to thrive" including weight loss, anorexia, confusion, weakness, and decreased functional status. Examination findings may include orthostatic hypotension, supine hypotension, cachexia, and hyperpigmentation, and laboratory testing may reveal hyponatremia, hyperkalemia, azotemia and hypoglycemia. However, one third of older patients with primary adrenal insufficiency are not hyperkalemic at initial presentation, and hyperpigmentation, hyperkalemia and orthostatic hypotension are not present in patients with secondary adrenal insufficiency. These signs and symptoms are common in elderly people and are easily attributable to another condition. Consequently, it is important to suspect this diagnosis in older patients with worsening functional status and vague symptoms. Unfortunately, adrenal insufficiency has historically been more commonly fatal in older people and more likely to be diagnosed only at autopsy, as compared to younger patients.

Once the diagnosis is suspected, the evaluation is the same as for younger patients; the ACTH stimulation test establishes the diagnosis. However, it is important to rule out common nonautoimmune causes of adrenal insufficiency, especially tuberculosis. Treatment is also the same as in young adults. In patients with primary adrenal insufficiency and less-severe mineralocorticoid deficiency, replacement doses of hydrocortisone may provide sufficient mineralocorticoid activity. However, those with absent mineralocorticoid function (manifested by orthostatic hypotension and electrolyte abnormalities such as hyperkalemia and hyponatremia) also require fludrocortisone, titrated to normalize electrolyte abnormalities. These patients should be monitored closely to avoid volume overload and hypertension. During minor illnesses or other stresses, maintenance glucocorticoid doses should be doubled for 2 to 3 days, whereas for major surgery or trauma, much higher doses of hydrocortisone (e.g., 100 mg intravenously every 8 hours) are usually administered initially.

Patients with adrenal insufficiency may benefit from replacement of the adrenal androgen DHEA, with improvement in mood, fatigability, sexuality, and sense of well-being. However, it is unclear whether DHEA also has important effects on physiologic parameters such as body composition, glucose and lipid metabolism, or functional capacity (see Chap. 103 for detailed discussion of DHEA and androgen-replacement therapy).

Chronic glucocorticoid therapy suppresses HPA axis function and results in adrenal atrophy because of the loss of ACTH stimulation. As a result, cessation of corticosteroids may be associated with a prolonged period of decreased pituitary ACTH secretion and adrenal responsiveness to ACTH. However, recovery of HPA axis responsiveness is variable and may not occur for months in some individuals. Elderly people may be particularly at risk to develop adrenal insufficiency as a consequence of withdrawal of steroid therapy for several reasons. For example, older adults may forget medicines or become confused about their medicines because of a complicated regimen or associated cognitive impairment. Other patients may discontinue medicines abruptly without consulting their physician because of expense or unacceptable side effects. The clinical features of adrenocortical insufficiency secondary to withdrawal of glucocorticoids (or hypopituitarism) are nonspecific and similar to those of primary adrenal sufficiency, although findings suggesting mineralocorticoid insufficiency (orthostatic hypotension, hyperkalemia, hyperpigmentation) are usually absent. Based on the foregoing, a high index of suspicion is necessary to detect adrenocortical insufficiency in elderly people caused by cessation of chronic glucocorticoid therapy. It is appropriate to perform the ACTH stimulation test in such patients, and those with persistent adrenocortical insufficiency should receive glucocorticoid coverage for major surgery or other stresses as described above until HPA axis function has returned.

Adrenal Androgens and Aging

In contrast to cortisol, levels of the adrenal androgens DHEA and its sulfate decline progressively and markedly with aging. These steroids circulate in high concentrations in young adults, and it has been hypothesized that this decrease in adrenal androgens such as DHEA may contribute to the deterioration of a variety of physiologic functions with aging.

In women, androgens such as androstenedione and testosterone are secreted by both the adrenal glands and the ovaries, whereas DHEA is produced almost exclusively by the adrenal glands. Total circulating androgens decline with aging as a result of both ovarian failure and a decrease in adrenal production of androgens and androgen precursors. However, in contrast to estrogen deficiency, the decline in androgens is more gradual, typically beginning in the decade before menopause. This relative androgen deficiency is associated with a decline in sexual functioning, loss of energy, depression, and loss of bone mass, suggesting that age-related androgen deficiency may contribute to these problems in women.

Androgens are thought to be important in maintaining libido in older women. Estrogen replacement in surgically menopausal middle-aged women with loss of libido improves vasomotor symptoms, vaginal dryness and general well-being but does not restore libido, whereas addition of androgens to the regimen has been demonstrated to improve some aspects of sexuality including sexual drive, arousal, and satisfaction. Furthermore, androgens may play an important role in maintaining bone mineral density in older women. Indeed, in one study bone mineral density was positively correlated with percent free testosterone in postmenopausal women, whereas no relationship between bone mineral density and free estradiol was found. Finally, androgen deficiency may be important in the pathogenesis of vulvar lichen sclerosis, a pruritic dystrophic skin condition of the vulva usually affecting postmenopausal women.

Adrenal androgen-replacement therapy is discussed in Chap. 103.

Adrenal Neoplasms

Benign adrenal neoplasms are common, with autopsy studies identifying these masses in approximately 6 percent of cases. Adrenocortical nodularity increases with aging, and the probability of identifying an adrenal "incidentaloma" on computerized tomography of the abdomen increases from 0.2 percent in people between 20 and 29 years of age to 6.9 percent in people older than 70 years of age. Most of these are adrenocortical adenomas, but adrenal carcinomas and pheochromocytomas also occur. The goals of assessment are to determine whether the incidentaloma is functional (hormone-secreting), and to characterize it as benign or malignant.

Appropriate screening tests to determine whether the tumor is functional include a 24-hour urine collection for metanephrines and catecholamines or vanillylmandelic acid (VMA) to rule out pheochromocytoma, and in hypertensive patients, a morning plasma aldosterone concentration to plasma renin activity ratio. Androgen-secreting tumors are rare, and endocrine screening for androgen overproduction is not indicated in the absence of clinical signs and symptoms of hormone excess. Screening for corticosteroid hyperfunction is controversial. Increasing evidence indicates that many adrenal cortical adenomas have a degree of functional autonomy. In 57 patients (mean age 59 years) with adrenal incidentalomas screened with a 2-day low-dose DST, 12 percent had serum cortisol levels of 5 to 7.8 μg/dL, 67 percent had values of 1 to 5 μg/dL, and cortisol was undetectable in only 21 percent, whereas all control subjects suppressed cortisol to undetectable levels. Furthermore, higher cortisol levels after the DST were associated with larger adrenal incidentaloma size, higher midnight cortisol levels, and lower basal ACTH levels. Moreover, hypertension and obesity are significantly more prevalent in people with adrenal incidentalomas than in the general population. Indeed, some middle-aged patients with incidentalomas and cortisol nonsuppression after low-dose DST experienced improvement in hypertension, obesity, and diabetes control after adrenalectomy.

These data suggest that subtle autonomous glucocorticoid secretion is common in adrenal cortical adenomas, and that this secretory activity may be clinically significant. However, tests of glucocorticoid function, such as the low-dose DST, have a high sensitivity but a relatively low specificity, therefore screening all elderly people with adrenal incidentalomas for subclinical Cushing's syndrome would result in a large proportion of false-positive results. Furthermore, the long-term outcomes of adrenalectomy versus medical management of hypertension, diabetes, and obesity in older patients with adrenal cortical adenomas are unknown. Therefore, it may be prudent to restrict screening for corticosteroid hyperfunction to younger patients and those with a symptom complex including weight gain, muscle weakness, osteoporosis, hypertension, diabetes mellitus and skin atrophy suggesting Cushing's syndrome. However, screening is indicated in patients with adrenal incidentalomas who are scheduled for major surgery, because postoperative adrenal crisis may occur in patients with unrecognized subclinical Cushing's syndrome.

The other major issue in the evaluation of adrenal incidentalomas is assessment of malignancy risk. The size of the mass is a useful indicator of risk, with benign adenomas usually ranging in size from 1 to 6 cm, and adrenal carcinomas usually greater than 6 cm in diameter. In one large survey of 1004 patients with adrenal incidentalomas, a size cut-off of 4 cm yielded optimal sensitivity but low specificity for malignant adrenal lesions. However, patients with carcinoma were significantly younger than were patients with adenoma. Imaging characteristics other than size may also be helpful in assessing malignant potential, including image attenuation on noncontrast CT, enhancement with contrast media, and magnetic resonance signal intensity on T2-weighted images. Although an increase in mass size has been considered suggestive of malignancy, excision of enlarging masses has generally identified benign underlying pathology. Indeed, studies of the natural history of adrenal incidentalomas indicate that with long-term follow-up, most of these lesions remain clinically insignificant and hormonally and morphologically unchanged. Furthermore, aggressive evaluation and management of adrenal incidentalomas in all older adults would be cost-prohibitive.

Based on the foregoing, a conservative approach is warranted in the management of most elderly people with apparently nonfunctioning adrenal incidentalomas. In surgical candidates, functioning tumors and lesions larger than 6 cm should generally be removed. Masses less than 3 cm in size probably do not need further evaluation or follow-up. Lesions between 3 and 6 cm without other imaging characteristics suggesting malignancy may be followed with serial imaging studies, although the benefits of serial imaging have been questioned.

THE SYMPATHOADRENAL SYSTEM

Physiology

Norepinephrine is the primary neurotransmitter released by sympathetic postganglionic neurons. After release, most of the NE is taken up again into the presynaptic and postsynaptic axon terminals, whereas only a small fraction diffuses into the circulation. The adrenal medulla contains specialized postganglionic sympathetic neurons that enzymatically convert NE into epinephrine, the major secretory product of these cells.

There is a general consensus that sympathetic nervous system (SNS) activity is increased with aging in humans. Basal plasma NE levels are increased in elderly people, because of an increase in NE secretion and, to a lesser extent, because of a decrease in clearance. Furthermore, plasma NE responses to various stimuli such as upright posture, cold pressor tests, exercise, and hand grip are also increased with aging. By comparison, adrenal medullary function is relatively unchanged until 75 to 80 years of age. Clearance of epinephrine is increased with aging. However, in subjects younger than age 75 years, increased clearance appears to be balanced by a proportionate increase in epinephrine

secretion, with no change in circulating epinephrine levels. However, in people older than age 80 years, levels of epinephrine were increased both at baseline and after cold-pressor testing, suggesting important effects of advanced age on both the sympathoneural and the sympathoadrenomedullary components of the SNS.

Although SNS tone is increased with aging, physiologic responses to adrenergic receptor-mediated stimulation generally decrease with aging. For example, the increased NE levels in older subjects do not increase basal heart rate, and stimulation of β-receptors by isoproterenol produces less of an increase in heart rate and contractility in aging, as compared to young individuals. Furthermore, aging subjects exhibit decreased α-receptor–mediated chronotropic responses to stimuli such as hypoxia, and decreased arterial vasoconstrictor responses to α-adrenergic stimulation. This decreased responsiveness to catecholamines appears to be a result of changes at both the receptor and the postreceptor level, including reduction in receptor number, decreased receptor affinity, and receptor-effector uncoupling.

Clinical

Hypertension

Clinical consequences of this age-related hyperadrenergic state may include the development of hypertension. Several studies report unchanged α-mediated arterial vasoconstriction with normal aging. Based on these studies, together with observations that β-adrenergic–mediated vascular smooth muscle relaxation is decreased with aging, it has been hypothesized that older people are predisposed to develop hypertension as a result of relatively unopposed α-adrenergic tone. However, this hypothesis was cast into doubt by other studies in vivo that found a decrease in arterial α-adrenergic responsiveness to NE in normal elderly people, implying an appropriate compensatory response to elevated SNS tone with aging. More recent studies show that when compared with older normotensive people, elderly hypertensive subjects exhibit an increase in vascular α-adrenergic receptor responsiveness despite equal or greater SNS activity. Therefore, a combination of an increase in systemic SNS tone and enhanced α-adrenergic receptor responsiveness may contribute to essential hypertension in older adults.

Autonomic Insufficiency

Other SNS abnormalities associated with aging are the product of disease states rather than normal aging. Autonomic insufficiency may result from primary peripheral nervous system failure, coexisting diseases such as diabetes mellitus or Parkinson's disease, or drugs that interfere with SNS function. The most common clinical manifestation of these conditions is orthostatic hypotension, defined as a decrease in systolic blood pressure of at least 20 mmHg, or a fall in diastolic blood pressure of at least 10 mmHg after several minutes of upright posture. In addition, the pulse rate may fail to increase despite a significant fall in blood pressure in more advanced cases. Aside from these clinical observations, and the identification of underlying disorders such as diabetes mellitus, routine laboratory testing of SNS function is not indicated. Management options include elimination or reduction of medications associated with postural hypotension or effects on SNS function if possible, dangling the legs for several minutes prior to arising from bed, avoiding dehydration, increasing venous return with elastic support stockings, expanding plasma volume with dietary sodium or fludrocortisone, and initiating a trial of midodrine, an α_1-adrenergic receptor agonist with few cardiac or central nervous system side effects.

Pheochromocytoma

Pheochromocytoma is a rare tumor, with an incidence of less than 1 percent in patients with hypertension. Most cases in some series have been reported in young and middle-aged adults, but epidemiologic and autopsy data indicate a progressive increase in the age-specific incidence rate. It is unclear whether some pheochromocytomas diagnosed at autopsy are nonfunctioning and of no clinical significance, or whether the disease is underdiagnosed in elderly patients. However, based on the foregoing discussion, the age-related decrease in responsiveness to catecholamines may result in a muting or an absence of symptoms of excessive adrenergic stimulation such as diaphoresis and palpitations. Therefore, a high index of suspicion is necessary to make this diagnosis in patients with refractory or severe hypertension or a paradoxical response to antihypertensive medications.

The diagnosis depends on the documentation of elevated 24-hour urinary free catecholamines, metanephrines or VMA, plasma metanephrines or plasma catecholamines in a patient who is hypertensive or symptomatic at the time of specimen collection. There is debate regarding the relative merits of the various tests, but the diagnostic yield may be improved by using a combination of tests such as urinary catecholamines and metanephrines. Preoperative localization of tumor should be undertaken using abdominal CT or MRI scanning, with localization of extra-adrenal foci using iodine-131–labeled metaiodobenzylguanidine (MIBG) scintigraphy. An additional benefit of MIBG scintigraphy is that the compound is taken up by adrenergic cells, confirming that the mass is adrenergic in cases where biochemical studies are indeterminate. 6-[18F]fluorodopamine positron emission tomography scanning may be valuable in cases where conventional imaging modalities fail to locate the tumor despite compelling biochemical and clinical evidence of pheochromocytoma.

Preoperative management typically includes blood pressure control with combined α- and β-receptor blockade. However, β-receptor–blocking agents should not be given until after α blockade is achieved, to avoid an increase in blood pressure induced by unopposed α activity. In addition, patients with pheochromocytoma have a contracted plasma volume, and liberal salt intake is indicated for moderate volume expansion. Surgical intervention is indicated in elderly patients with resectable pheochromocytomas, in view of the potential for surgical cure and the poor prognosis with medical management. Occasionally, a pheochromocytoma will present as an adrenal incidentaloma with normal urinary metanephrines and VMA and negative MIBG scintigraphy, but during surgery its intraoperative behavior and subsequent histologic findings

Table 65-4   Effects of Aging in Hormonal Regulation of Fluid and Sodium Balance

Antidiuretic hormone (ADH)	
Basal ADH levels	↑
ADH release after osmoreceptor stimulation	↑
ADH release after baroreceptor stimulation	↓
Renal responsiveness to ADH	↓
Aldosterone	
Basal aldosterone levels	↓
Aldosterone release after sodium depletion	↓
Aldosterone release after postural challenge	↓
Aldosterone release after ACTH stimulation	↔
Atrial Natriuretic Hormone (ANH)	
Basal ANH levels	↑
ANH responses to stimuli	↑

↓, decreased; ↔, unchanged; ↑, increased.

indicate pheochromocytoma. It is important to take prophylactic measures during surgery for this possibility, including placement of an arterial line and arrangement for immediate access to intravenous nitroprusside.

THE RENIN–ANGIOTENSIN–ALDOSTERONE SYSTEM

Although aldosterone secretion and clearance rates are both decreased with aging, basal plasma aldosterone levels are not maintained at normal levels in persons of advanced age, declining by 30 percent in healthy octogenarians compared to younger adults (Table 65-4). Aldosterone secretion is also reduced after stimuli such as sodium depletion or upright posture. However, these changes do not appear to be secondary to adrenal dysfunction, because aldosterone responsiveness to ACTH is intact with aging. The primary defect responsible for these changes in aldosterone secretion is thought to be a reduction in plasma renin activity, which is decreased by 50 percent in elderly persons, as compared to younger adults. This decline in active renin concentration is thought to be a result of diminished conversion of inactive to active renin. In addition, age-related increases in atrial natriuretic hormone secretion contribute to the suppression of aldosterone secretion with aging, both directly and by inhibiting renal renin secretion, plasma renin activity, and angiotensin II levels.

The clinical consequences of decreasing aldosterone levels with aging include a predisposition to renal sodium wasting, which, in combination with reduced thirst and decreased renal ADH responsiveness, further increases the potential for volume depletion and dehydration in geriatric patients. Furthermore, this state of relative hyporeninemic hypoaldosteronism places older adults at increased risk of hyperkalemia, especially patients with diabetes mellitus and renal insufficiency (Table 65-5). The addition of aldosterone antagonists, β-blocking agents, nonsteroidal antiinflammatory drugs, or heparin may lead to potentially lethal hyperkalemia in such patients.

Table 65-5   Risk Factors for Hyperkalemia in Older People

Diabetes mellitus*
Renal insufficiency or failure

Intravascular volume depletion

Adrenocortical insufficiency

Acidosis

Medications
  Aldosterone antagonists ("potassium-sparing" diuretics)
  Angiotensin-converting enzyme inhibitors
  Angiotensin antagonists
  β-Adrenergic blocking agents
  Nonsteroidal antiinflammatory agents

Potassium-containing salt substitutes

Tissue injury with rapid release of potassium from cells
  Crush injury
  Tumor lysis syndrome
  Hemolysis

*Multiple contributors, including insulin deficiency, renal insufficiency, hyporeninemic hypoaldosteronism, type IV renal tubular acidosis, and use of angiotensin-converting enzyme inhibitors.

THE GROWTH HORMONE AXIS

Physiology

Secretion of growth hormone (GH) from the pituitary is regulated by the hypothalamic peptides growth hormone-releasing hormone (GHRH) and somatostatin. These two peptides exert an opposing effect on GH secretion, with GHRH stimulating and somatostatin inhibiting GH secretion by the pituitary somatotropes. Experimental evidence suggests that GH secretion is primarily controlled by a tonic inhibitory effect of somatostatin, and that pulsatile GH secretion occurs in response to GHRH when somatostatin tone is decreased. In turn, insulin-like growth factor-1 (IGF-1 or somatomedin C), which is secreted by the liver and other peripheral tissues in response to GH, mediates most of the actions of GH. Furthermore, IGF-1 exerts a negative feedback effect on GH secretion through a direct effect at the pituitary level and indirectly by increasing somatostatin production. Secretion of GH is pulsatile, generally with very-low circulating levels except for several pulses occurring during the first few hours of sleep, after meals or exercise, or without apparent cause. In young adult men, most of the GH is secreted within the first 4 hours after sleep onset, with large amplitude pulses occurring during slow-wave sleep, whereas in contrast, IGF-1 levels remain fairly constant over a 24-hour period.

GH release is affected by numerous other factors, including other neurotransmitters and neuropeptides, medications, hormonal influences, blood glucose levels, degree of obesity, and physiologic states such as sleep and exercise.

For example, the neurotransmitter dopamine and central nervous system (CNS)-active dopaminergic agonists such as bromocriptine exert a stimulatory effect on GH release by promoting hypothalamic GHRH release. Norepinephrine and α-adrenergic agonists also increase GHRH and GH release, whereas β-adrenergic agonists and dopamine- or α-receptor–blocking agents inhibit GH secretion. Furthermore, the GH-releasing effects of other stimuli such as exercise, stress, hypoglycemia, and arginine are thought to be mediated via α-adrenergic stimulation. Estrogens stimulate GH release, and premenopausal women have higher peak GH levels with exercise, arginine, and insulin-induced hypoglycemia than age-matched men. In contrast, GH secretion is inhibited in those treated chronically with glucocorticoids. Hyperglycemia is associated with decreased GH levels and GH responses to GHRH. Similarly, obese subjects exhibit decreased spontaneous GH secretion and reduced GH responsiveness to pharmacologic stimulation compared to nonobese subjects, although IGF-1 levels are typically within normal limits. GH levels are acutely elevated during exercise, and there is indirect evidence that regular exercise may enhance GH secretion over the long-term.

GH secretion reaches maximum levels at puberty, followed by a gradual but progressive decline with age. In adult men, GH secretion declines by approximately 14 percent per decade, such that by age 70 to 80 years, about half of all individuals have no significant GH secretion during a 24-hour period. Plasma IGF-1 levels exhibit a corresponding decline of 7 to 13 percent per decade, and by age 70 to 80 years, approximately 40 percent have plasma IGF-1 levels in the range found in GH-deficient children. In addition, serum levels of IGF-binding protein-3 (IGFBP-3) decline with aging in healthy adults, but it is unclear whether this affects the metabolic activity of IGF-1 with aging. Collectively, these decreases in pituitary secretion of GH and circulating IGF-1 levels are known as the somatopause. The age-related decrease in GH production appears to be primarily caused by a decrease in hypothalamic GHRH secretion and an increase in hypothalamic somatostatin release, rather than an attenuation in pituitary responsiveness to GHRH. Accordingly, GH secretion and IGF-1 levels can be normalized with exogenous GHRH administration.

Growth Hormone Deficiency in Adults with Hypothalamic–Pituitary Disease

GH deficiency in adults with established hypothalamic–pituitary disease is associated with reduced lean body mass, muscle strength and exercise capacity; decreased psychological well-being; increased total body adiposity; higher waist-to-hip ratio of fat distribution; reduced bone density; adverse effects on lipid metabolism; and increased risk of death from cardiovascular disease, despite adequate replacement of other hormones including thyroxine, cortisol, and sex steroids. Many of these effects can be improved or corrected with GH administration, and the use of GH has been approved in the United States for this indication in adults with hypopituitarism and GH deficiency. Improvements in cardiac function, muscle strength, body composition, bone mass, and metabolic indices have been sustained in trials lasting up to 5 years, and treatment has generally been well tolerated. The most commonly reported adverse effects of GH treatment in adults with hypopituitarism are fluid retention, arthralgias, and myalgias. These symptoms are most likely to occur in people who are elderly or obese, and are more common in those with the greatest increase in IGF-1 levels during treatment. However, these symptoms often resolve spontaneously during treatment, and disappear with treatment cessation. Concerns have been raised regarding a worsening of glucose tolerance over 30 months of treatment, that potentially could precipitate diabetes in some susceptible patients. However, others have reported improvements in glycosylated hemoglobin and triglyceride levels that were observed only after several years of treatment.

The diagnosis of GH deficiency in adults is suggested clinically by the presence of multiple pituitary hormone deficiencies. However, laboratory criteria for distinguishing older adults with organic GH deficiency from those with normal age-related reductions in GH secretion have not yet been clearly defined. Furthermore, assessment of GH function is complicated by the need for GH stimulation tests, the lack of adequate normative data for many laboratories, assay variability, and the unavailability of appropriate age-adjusted normal values for diagnostic tests. Static GH levels are unsuitable for diagnosis, because GH is secreted episodically. IGF-1 levels decline during normal aging and are not a reliable indicator of GH deficiency secondary to pituitary disease in people over 40 years of age, although normal IGF-1 levels are helpful to exclude GH deficiency. The insulin tolerance test is considered the most definitive test for GH deficiency in adults, but this test may be dangerous in older patients with ischemic heart disease. Arginine-induced GH secretion remains intact with normal aging, and the arginine stimulation test has been proposed as a safer yet reliable alternative to distinguish GH deficiency secondary to hypopituitarism from normal age-related reductions in GH secretion.

Compared to younger adults, elderly people with GH deficiency related to hypopituitarism also appear to benefit from GH replacement. GH-deficient adults older than age 65 years receiving GH replacement therapy for at least 6 months experienced significant improvements in total and low-density lipoprotein cholesterol levels, diastolic blood pressure (males only), and quality-of-life scores. However, the GH replacement dose in older GH-deficient adults is lower than that required by younger adults. In one study, a dose of 0.5 mg of GH per day resulted in elevated serum IGF-1 levels in half of older subjects, and 25 percent developed side effects on this dose. Most elderly subjects maintained IGF-1 levels within the normal range on 0.17 to 0.33 mg per day. By contrast, younger adults commonly require doses up to 1 mg per day. Treatment should begin at a low dose (e.g., 0.15 mg per day) with titration at no more than monthly intervals based on clinical and biochemical responses. Serum IGF-1 levels should be maintained within the normal adult range, to optimize the beneficial effects of GH replacement while minimizing the potential for side effects such as carpal tunnel syndrome, arthralgias, fluid retention, and gynecomastia.

Reduced Growth Hormone Secretion in Elderly People Without Hypothalamic–Pituitary Disease

Normal aging is associated with alterations in body composition similar to those in GH-deficient younger patients, including decreased muscle mass and strength, reduced bone mass, and increased adiposity. In turn, declining strength and bone mass are associated with increasing risk for falls and fractures in elderly people. These observations suggest that the reduction in GH secretion associated with aging (the somatopause) may contribute to alterations in body composition and increased frailty in older adults, and that GH supplementation, GHRH, or GH secretagogue treatment might be clinically useful in preventing or reversing these age-related changes. GH supplementation for the somatopause is discussed in Chap. 103.

THE HYPOTHALAMIC–PITUITARY– TESTICULAR AXIS

Physiology

Significant age-related changes occur in male reproductive function with aging, including a decrease in sexual activity, libido, and fertility rates. However, in contrast to the relatively rapid and complete loss of gonadal function in women at the time of menopause, these changes in aging men occur gradually, vary considerably between individuals, and often do not result in severe hypogonadism. Many healthy older men exhibit a degree of primary testicular failure, with decreases in total and free or bioavailable testosterone levels, testosterone responses to exogenous gonadotropin administration, and daily sperm production, together with increased serum gonadotropin levels. Occasionally, community-dwelling elderly men present with overt testicular failure with total testosterone levels well below normal and symptoms of androgen deprivation including hot flashes, decreased libido and gynecomastia. However, it is more common to see older patients with mildly decreased testosterone levels and relatively nonspecific symptoms such as impotence, loss of libido, osteopenia and muscle weakness. In contrast, more marked testosterone deficiency is common in frail elderly men. For example, in male nursing home residents, it has been reported that 45 percent exhibit testosterone levels within the hypogonadal range.

Several factors contribute to this decrease in testosterone levels with aging. First, testicular testosterone production is markedly reduced with aging, which is reflected in the decreased number and volume of Leydig cells in the aging testis. This reduction in testosterone production capacity may manifest as a more severe and prolonged depression of testosterone levels during intercurrent illness or other stresses in older men. Second, both production rates and metabolic clearance of testosterone are reduced in aging men, but in contrast to adrenal cortisol secretion and metabolism, the decrease in testosterone production is not completely offset by a decrease in clearance. Third, the normal circadian variation in testosterone levels observed in young men, with highest levels in the morning, is lost with aging, resulting in reduced serum testosterone concentrations. Fourth, the concentration of the major testosterone binding protein, sex hormone-binding globulin (SHBG), increases with aging, therefore, serum free or non-SHBG–bound (bioavailable) testosterone concentrations decline to a greater extent than total testosterone with aging. Finally, impairment of testicular function is associated with medical illnesses, medications and alcohol which are commonly present in aging men. However, hypogonadism does not occur in all aging men; many healthy men older than age 80 years maintain serum testosterone levels within the normal young adult range.

In addition to these deficits in testicular function, hypothalamic/pituitary control of testicular function is also impaired with aging. Although gonadotropin levels increase with aging, they usually remain within normal limits, and the hormonal profile of a low testosterone and normal gonadotropin levels is consistent with aging-related secondary hypogonadism. Even in men with elevated levels of LH and FSH, the increases in gonadotropins are sometimes inappropriately low in comparison to younger men with similar reductions in testosterone levels. Furthermore, the ratio of bioactive to immunoreactive LH and FSH is decreased in elderly men, indicating that gonadotropin levels measured by radioimmunoassay may underestimate the extent of gonadotropin deficiency. Finally, healthy older men exhibit intact LH and FSH responsiveness to prolonged exogenous pulsatile GnRH administration but an inappropriately normal or decreased LH pulse frequency (an indicator of hypothalamic GnRH pulse-generator activity), as compared to young men. Based on the above evidence, it appears that age-related hypogonadism is a consequence of both testicular and hypothalamic dysfunction.

The physiologic significance of the decrease in testicular androgen production associated with aging (the "andropause") is uncertain. However, as testosterone levels decline with aging, various functional changes occur in androgen-dependent body tissues. In the testes, there are significant age-related decreases in the number of Sertoli cells, volume of seminiferous tubules, daily sperm production, and to some extent testicular volume. In studies controlled for the increased length of time between ejaculations in older men, sperm concentrations were unchanged with age, but older men exhibited lower ejaculated volume, decreased sperm motility, and a higher percentage of abnormal spermatozoa. However, these parameters remained within normal limits in most of the older subjects. Sperm fertilizing capacity by in vitro testing remains intact in healthy older men. Male fertility is thought to decrease with aging, mostly as a result of reduced sexual activity and sexual dysfunction. The causes of declining libido and sexual activity with aging are multifactorial, including the presence of chronic illnesses such as diabetes mellitus, vascular or neuropathic disease of the penis, medications, and depression (see Chap. 102).

As with estrogens, androgens are thought to affect cognitive function. For example, several studies have demonstrated differences between men and women on tasks involving spatial cognition. Reports of the relationship between testosterone levels and spatial cognition have been inconsistent, but testosterone supplementation in older men improved some aspects of spatial cognition and verbal memory. In women, some evidence suggests that postmenopausal estrogen deficiency may play a role in the development of Alzheimer's disease, but it is unknown whether the more gradual development of a milder sex hormone deficiency plays an analogous role in aging men.

Androgens are also important in the maintenance of bone mass, muscle mass, and strength in men. Bone mass declines progressively with age in men, and hypogonadism in men is associated with premature osteoporosis and an increased risk of fractures. Moreover, androgen receptors are present in osteoblasts, and androgens affect a number of osteoblast functions, suggesting that bone is an androgen-dependent tissue. Similarly, hypogonadal men exhibit excessive adiposity and reduced lean body mass that are reversible with testosterone replacement, and supraphysiologic doses of testosterone increase muscle strength and lean body mass in healthy young men.

The role of testosterone in the development of coronary artery disease in men is controversial. Males have an increased incidence of coronary artery disease compared to females of similar age, suggesting that androgens may predispose men to the development of coronary heart disease. However, most epidemiologic studies have found either a neutral or favorable effect of testosterone and other androgens on coronary heart disease in men.

Laboratory Diagnosis of Hypogonadism

The best approach to the laboratory diagnosis of age-related testosterone deficiency is controversial. Total testosterone measurements do not fully reflect age-related reductions in biologically active testosterone. Therefore, elderly men with symptoms or signs consistent with androgen deficiency should be evaluated with a free or bioavailable (non-SHBG–bound) testosterone level, either measured directly or calculated from measurements of total testosterone and SHBG. However, the convenient and widely used "analog" free testosterone assays are affected by alterations in SHBG levels. These assays may underestimate androgen deficiency in elderly men and overestimate androgen deficiency in men with low SHBG (e.g., moderately obese men), and are not recommended. Additionally, the laboratory evaluation of men with suspected hypogonadism should include serum LH and FSH levels, as well as a prolactin level if gonadotropins are inappropriately low-normal or low in the presence of reduced testosterone levels. Hyperprolactinemia inhibits hypothalamic GnRH secretion, resulting in a decrease in LH and FSH secretion, and could indicate the presence of a pituitary adenoma or a hypothalamic disorder. In patients with secondary hypogonadism suspected on the basis of low or inappropriately normal gonadotropins, additional studies may be warranted, including magnetic resonance imaging of the pituitary fossa, measurements of other pituitary hormones such as growth hormone and thyroid hormone levels, and an ACTH stimulation test. Furthermore, bone densitometry measurement is indicated in hypogonadal men to evaluate for asymptomatic osteoporosis.

Androgen-Replacement Therapy

Androgen deficiency is only one of several factors to be considered in the evaluation of age-related sexual dysfunction. The role of androgens in the evaluation and management of erectile dysfunction in older men is considered in more detail in Chap. 102. Androgen replacement therapy is discussed in Chap. 103.

OTHER ENDOCRINE DISORDERS

Menopause and the clinical manifestations of estrogen deficiency and estrogen replacement therapy are discussed in Chap. 99. Androgen-replacement therapy for women is discussed in Chap. 103. Age-related alterations in the hypothalamic–pituitary–thyroid axis (Chap. 66), parathyroid and calcium metabolism (Chaps. 69 and 75), obesity and lipid metabolism (Chaps. 68 and 91), and carbohydrate metabolism and diabetes mellitus (Chap. 67) are discussed in subsequent chapters in this section or in the following sections.

REFERENCES

Gotherstrom G et al: A prospective study of 5 years of GH replacement therapy in GH-deficient adults: Sustained effects on body composition, bone mass, and metabolic indices. *J Clin Endocrinol Metab* 86:4657, 2001.

Hernandez FC et al: A five-year report on experience in the detection of pheochromocytoma. *Clin Biochem* 33:649, 2000.

Homik JE et al: A meta-analysis on the use of bisphosphonates in corticosteroid induced osteoporosis. *J Rheumatol* 26:1148, 1999.

Hunt PJ et al: Improvement in mood and fatigue after dehydroepiandrosterone replacement in Addison's disease in a randomized, double-blind trial. *J Clin Endocrinol Metab* 85:4650, 2000.

Klee GG, Heser DW: Techniques to measure testosterone in the elderly. *Mayo Clin Proc* 75:S19, 2000.

Miller M: Nocturnal polyuria in older people: Pathophysiology and clinical implications. *J Am Geriatr Soc* 48:1321, 2000.

Mishima K et al: Diminished melatonin secretion in the elderly caused by insufficient environmental illumination. *J Clin Endocrinol Metab* 86:129, 2001.

Monson JP et al: Growth hormone deficiency and replacement in elderly hypopituitary adults. KIMS Study Group and the KIMS International Board. Pharmacia and Upjohn International Metabolic Database [see comments]. *Clin Endocrinol (Oxf)* 53:281, 2000.

Matsumoto AM: Andropause: Clinical implications of the decline in serum testosterone levels with aging in men. *J Gerontol A Biol Sci Med Sci* 57:M76, 2002.

Papanicolaou DA et al: A single midnight serum cortisol measurement distinguishes Cushing's syndrome from pseudo-Cushing states. *J Clin Endocrinol Metab* 83:1163, 1998.

Raskind MA et al: Patterns of cerebrospinal fluid catechols support increased central noradrenergic responsiveness in aging and Alzheimer's disease. *Biol Psychiatry* 46:756, 1999.

Reincke M: Subclinical Cushing's syndrome. *Endocrinol Metab Clin North Am* 29:43, 2000.

Richards ML et al: The rapid low-dose (1 μg) cosyntropin test in the immediate postoperative period: Results in elderly subjects after major abdominal surgery. *Surgery* 125:431, 1999.

Supiano MA et al: Sympathetic nervous system activity and alpha-adrenergic responsiveness in older hypertensive humans. *Am J Physiol* 276:E519, 1999.

Toogood AA et al: The diagnosis of severe growth hormone deficiency in elderly patients with hypothalamic–pituitary disease. *Clin Endocrinol (Oxf)* 48:569, 1998.

Tsagarakis S et al: The low-dose dexamethasone suppression test in patients with adrenal incidentalomas: Comparisons with clinically euadrenal subjects and patients with Cushing's syndrome. *Clin Endocrinol (Oxf)* 48:627, 1998.

Turner HE et al: Pituitary tumours in the elderly: A 20-year experience. *Eur J Endocrinol* 140:383, 1999.

Wilkinson CW et al: Human glucocorticoid feedback inhibition is reduced in older individuals: Evening study. *J Clin Endocrinol Metab* 86:545, 2001.

Young WFJ: Management approaches to adrenal incidentalomas. *Endocrinol Metab Clin North Am* 29:159, 2000.

Thyroid Diseases

SIMA HASSANI • JEROME M. HERSHMAN

Thyroid disorders in the elderly population are common, often challenging diagnostically, and frequently overlooked. The clinical presentations of thyroid diseases may be subtle, with nonspecific signs and symptoms that are attributed to other illnesses or to a normal aging process. Thyroid function tests can be misleading in the presence of concurrent acute or chronic diseases and may be affected by some medications. This chapter describes the most common thyroid disorders encountered in the elderly population.

THE AGING HUMAN THYROID

Anatomy

The thyroid gland is the largest endocrine organ in the human body, and weighs approximately 12 to 20 g in adults. The structural and functional changes of the thyroid gland that occur with aging are controversial. Some investigators report that there were no size or weight changes, others found increases to twice normal size after age 70 years, whereas other reports indicated that the thyroid gland undergoes atrophy, fibrosis, and decrease in weight. The thyroid gland is also more nodular with advancing age, and there is an increase in fibrosis and lymphocytic infiltration. Despite these changes, normal thyroid function is maintained by the vast majority of the elderly population. Estimation of the thyroid size and its palpation may be difficult in elderly patients because of cervical kyphosis, obesity, or chronic pulmonary disease.

Physiology

Iodine, an essential substrate for synthesis of thyroid hormone, is absorbed from the diet and enters the circulation as inorganic iodide that is distributed in extracellular fluids as well as in salivary, breast, and gastric secretions. The average daily iodine intake is about 250 μg/d in the United States. A 24-hour urinary iodine measurement is an index of dietary iodine intake.

Iodide is actively concentrated by the thyroid gland or cleared from the plasma by the kidney. The thyroid gland, compared with the kidneys, is the active participant in the competition for plasma iodide and adjusts the rate of entry of iodide into the thyroid tissue based on the changes in thyroid hormone synthesis rather than renal avidity for iodide ion. The active transport of iodide from plasma to follicular cell is carried out by the sodium-iodide symporter, a transport protein on the follicular cell plasma membrane. The extracellular fluid iodide concentration is usually very low because of the rapid clearance of iodide from extracellular fluid by the thyroidal uptake and renal clearance.

Table 66-1 summarizes the aging effects on thyroid function. The renal and thyroidal iodide clearance rate diminishes with advancing age. Thyroid iodide clearance, estimated by a 24-hour radioactive iodine uptake by the thyroid gland, decreases in euthyroid subjects after age 60 years. Urinary iodine excretion also was found to be significantly reduced in subjects older than 80 years of age.

In the thyroid cell, the iodide is oxidized by the peroxidase enzyme and incorporated into tyrosine to form the thyroid hormone precursors monoiodotyrosine (MIT) and diiodotyrosine (DIT). The iodinated tyrosine is incorporated into a large protein, thyroglobulin, that serves as a substrate for coupling of monoiodotyrosine and diiodotyrosine to produce thyroxine (T_4) and triiodothyronine (T_3). In the plasma, the main binding protein is thyroid-binding globulin (TBG), which binds about 70 percent of serum T_4 and T_3. The other binding proteins are transthyretin and albumin. Only 0.02 percent of T_4 and 0.3 percent of T_3 are free and metabolically active because only the free hormone is rapidly transported into cells. Total serum T_4 and T_3 are readily measured. Free T_4 (FT_4) and free T_3 (FT_3) concentrations also can be measured to evaluate thyroid function.

The daily production rate of T_4 is about 85 μg/d and that of T_3 is about 30 μg/d in normal adults. About 80 percent of T_3 production is derived from T_4-to-T_3 conversion by 5′-deiodinase, a selenoprotein (Fig. 66-1), in extrathyroidal tissues such as the liver, muscles, and kidneys. The other 20 percent of T_3 production is that secreted directly by the thyroid gland. Selenium deficiency results in reduced 5′-deiodinase activity and serum T_3 concentration. Reverse T_3 (rT_3), inactive biologically, differs from T_3 because it is missing an iodine from the inner or tyrosyl ring of T_4 rather than from the outer ring or phenolic ring. T_4 is converted

Table 66-1   Age-Related Changes in Thyroid Physiology

Renal iodide clearance ↓
Thyroid iodide clearance ↓
Total T_4 production ↓
T_4 degradation ↓
Serum T_4 concentration ↔
Serum TBG concentration ↔
T_3 concentration ↓
Reverse T_3 concentration ↔
TSH response to TRH ↑ ↔↓
Diurnal variation of TSH ↓ ↓

↓, Decreased; ↑, Increased; ↔, unchanged.
T_3, triiodothyronine; T_4, thyroxine; TBG, thyroid-binding globulin; TRH, thyrotropin-releasing hormone; TSH, thyroid-stimulating hormone.

to rT_3 by 5′-deiodinase in peripheral tissue. Total T_4 production and degradation decline with aging, but T_4 concentration and TBG concentration remain unchanged in healthy individuals throughout adult life. In contrast, the concentration of T_3 was reported to decrease by 10 to 20 percent with advancing age. This finding suggests that 5′-deiodinase activity decreases with increasing age. There is no change in rT_3 concentration with aging.

Thyroid hormone regulation is through a negative feedback loop involving the hypothalamus, the anterior pituitary, and the thyroid gland (Fig. 66-2). Thyrotropin-releasing hormone (TRH), synthesized and stored within the hypothalamus, stimulates the release of thyroid-stimulating hormone (TSH) from the anterior pituitary gland. TSH binds to the TSH receptor located on the outer side of the thyroid cell plasma membrane and increases thyroid hormone synthesis and secretion. In turn, T_4 and T_3 from the serum feed back on the pituitary and the hypothalamus to inhibit TSH and TRH production and secretion.

The secretory response of TSH to TRH stimulation in aging men has been reported to be decreased to 38 percent of the values in young men. This may be an adaptive mechanism to the reduced need for thyroid hormone in old age. However, other reports of TRH-stimulated TSH secretion with aging have shown an unchanged or even increased response.

The serum TSH concentration has been either unchanged, lowered, or increased with aging in various reports. The heterogeneity of the populations studied may explain some of these discrepancies. Studies employing sensitive TSH assays have raised the question of whether the abnormal TSH reflects the prevalence of thyroid disorders or physiologic changes related to aging. In a random selection of the community-based population followed in the Framingham Heart Study, euthyroid older persons were found to have the same level of TSH as younger persons, although older euthyroid women had a slightly lower serum TSH level than middle-aged women. In another study of healthy centenarians (age range, 100 to 110 years), the median serum TSH level was lower than that of older

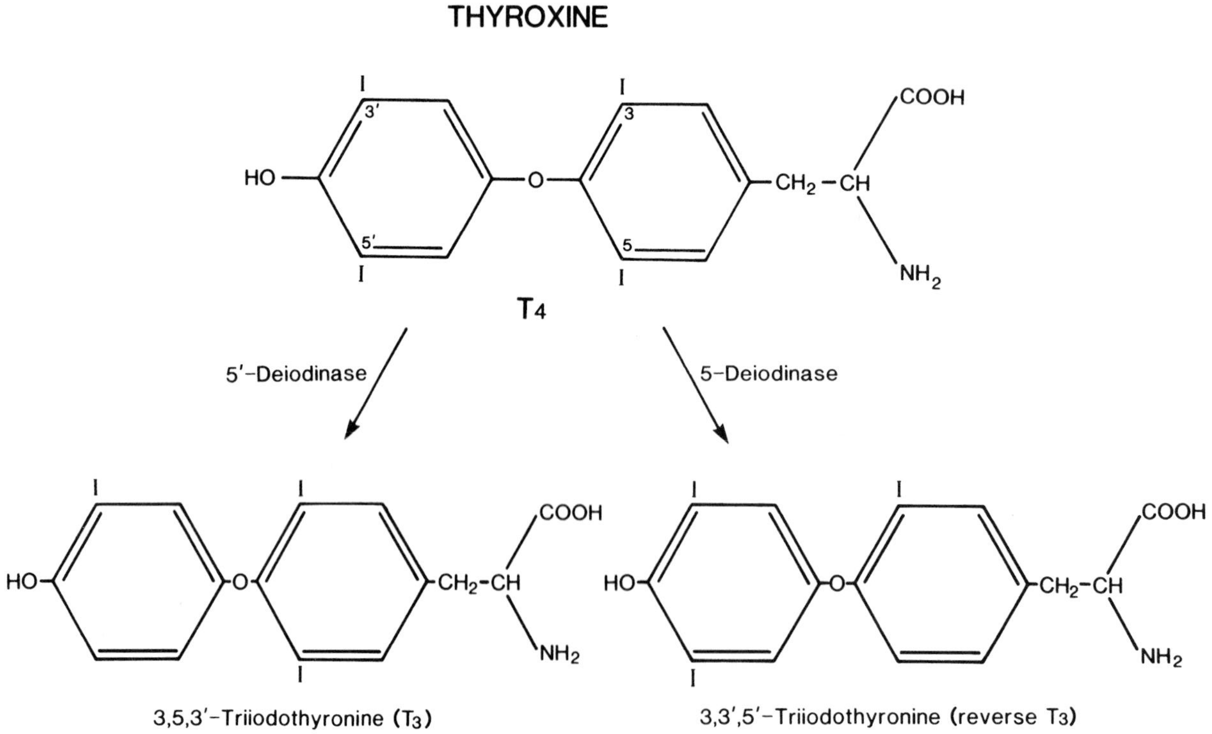

Figure 66-1   Structures of T_4 and the enzymatic pathways for deiodination of T_4 to its major active metabolite, T_3, and to reverse T_3 in peripheral tissues.

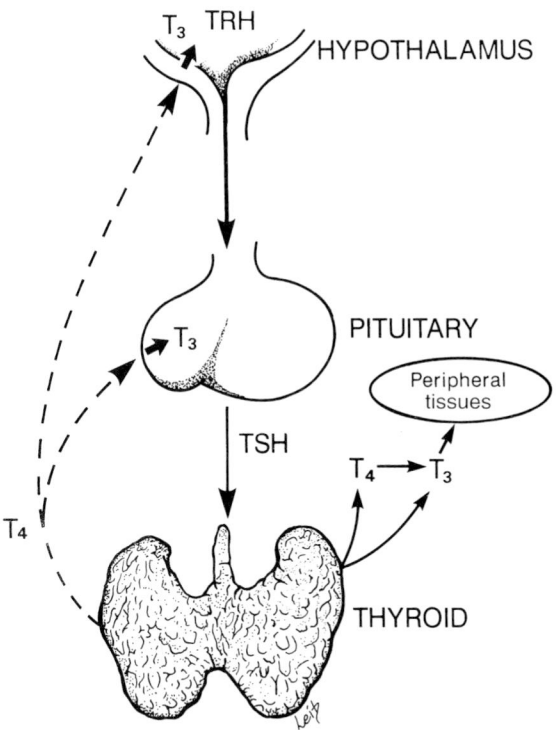

Figure 66-2 Feedback regulation for control of thyroid function that involves the hypothalamus–pituitary–thyroid axis. Arrows represent positive feedback; dashed lines denote the inhibitory feedback of T_4 and T_3 on pituitary thyroid-stimulating hormone (TSH) and hypothalamic thyrotropin-releasing hormone (TRH) secretion.

individuals (age range, 65 to 80 years). The data of this study were consistent with TSH being well preserved until the eighth decade of life in healthy elderly subjects, whereas a decline in TSH occurs in extreme senescence over 100 years of age. TSH levels rise about 50 percent in the late evening before the onset of sleep. Sleep attenuates this nocturnal peak of TSH secretion, and sleep deprivation exaggerates nocturnal TSH secretion. The diurnal variation of TSH levels has been reported to be absent in the elderly. The data from the healthy centenarians and individual older than age 65 years also showed an age-related blunting of the nocturnal TSH peak.

An increased prevalence of thyroid autoantibodies is associated with human aging. The thyroid autoimmune phenomenon is not a consequence of the aging process but rather an expression of age-associated disease.

SCREENING FOR THYROID DISEASE

The practice of preventive medicine in the community for patients older than 65 years of age involves using laboratory tests for screening and diagnosis of various diseases including thyroid disorders. To be cost-effective in early diagnosis of thyroid disease, the clinician must consider the clinical condition of the patient. Screening thyroid function tests are not indicated for patients with acute medical or psychiatric illnesses admitted to the acute care medical ward or intensive care unit. However, the elderly patients admitted

to specialized geriatric units for failure to thrive, depression, and/or chronic disability may benefit from screening for thyroid dysfunction. Epidemiologic surveys suggest that therapy of asymptomatic elderly patients with thyroid disease improves well-being, function, and some objective parameters. The potential benefits of treating mild thyroid failure include prevention of progression to overt hypothyroidism, reduction of elevated serum cholesterol level induced by subclinical hypothyroidism, and improvement in the quality of life in these patients. The American Thyroid Association recommends screening all adults older than age 35 years for thyroid dysfunction and every 5 years thereafter by measurement of TSH. Screening serum TSH should be carried out in patients with a prior history of thyroid disease, autoimmune disease, unexplained depression, cognitive dysfunction, or hypercholesterolemia. However, the American College of Physicians does not recommend routine screening of asymptomatic patients because of presumed lack of demonstrated efficacy or proven benefit in treatment of subclinical thyroid disease. An epidemiologic study indicated that every-5-year screening of women older than 35 years of age for mild thyroid failure was cost-effective. In our opinion, the high prevalence of hypothyroidism in patients older than 65 years of age justifies periodic screening for hypothyroidism in both women and men.

NONTHYROIDAL ILLNESS

The terms *sick euthyroid syndrome* or *nonthyroidal illness* (NTI) refer to altered serum thyroid hormone concentrations secondary to the physiologic stress of severe illness. By definition, patients with NTI have no apparent intrinsic thyroid disease. The types of illnesses responsible for thyroid function abnormalities include sepsis, surgery, trauma, burns, infections, malignancy, and chronic metabolic diseases such as malnutrition, starvation, and poorly controlled diabetes mellitus. An understanding of the effect of nonthyroidal illness on thyroid function tests is important, especially in the elderly patient who has multiple other underlying medical problems.

The effects of NTI on thyroid function have been described as the low T_3 and low T_4 states. The low T_3 state is associated with a decrease in extrathyroidal T_3 production resulting in a low serum total T_3 level and usually low free T_3 level with a normal serum TSH concentration. With more severe illness, the serum T_4 level decreases. In severe NTI, the decreases in T_4 and T_3 may be an adaptation to spare the patient from the catabolic effect of thyroid hormone during the periods of extreme stress. A reduction in serum T_3 concentration is the most common change of thyroid function tests in NTI with a frequency of 25 to 50 percent. The severity of the underlying illness correlates with the degree of the fall in serum T_3 concentration. The mechanisms responsible for low T_3 concentration are (1) a decrease in the peripheral conversion of T_4 to T_3 either because of inhibition of the 5′-deiodinase that is responsible for this conversion or because of a deficiency of a cofactor, such as glutathione, that is necessary for the activity of 5′-deiodinase; (2) a decrease in T_3 secretion from the thyroid gland; and (3) a decrease in tissue uptake of T_4 that limits the conversion of T_4 to T_3 in the extrathyroidal tissues. The serum rT_3 is increased in NTI because of the impaired rT_3 clearance as a consequence of the decreased activity of 5'-deiodinase with illness. The central question is how does the body maintain a euthyroid state when serum T_3 is reduced? The basis for an apparent euthyroid status in NTI is still unclear. There are several possible explanations: (1) T_3 concentrations may remain normal in the intracellular compartment even though serum T_3 level is decreased; (2) T_3 may be converted to triiodothyroacetic acid (Triac), which is metabolically active; and (3) studies of patients with various acute illnesses showed an increase in T_3-receptor messenger ribonucleic acids (mRNAs) and T_3-receptor protein that results in an increase in production of proteins that express the action of thyroid hormone, hence maintaining a euthyroid state in NTI.

The patients with the low T_4 state, also known as a low T_3/T_4 state, exhibit a low serum thyroxine level as well as low T_3 with a normal serum TSH concentration. Low serum total T_4 correlates with a poor prognosis. The mortality of critically ill patients with NTI is inversely related to serum T_4 concentration and has been reported to be as high as 84 percent in patients with serum T_4 concentration less than 3.0 μg/dL. There is no clear mechanism to fully explain the low T_4 state; however, possibilities include (1) reduced TBG concentration as a consequence of reduced hepatic protein synthesis; (2) inhibition of serum T_4 binding to TBG, probably by a substance released by injured tissue, or an acquired structural alteration of TBG that reduces its affinity for T_4; (3) alterations in hepatic uptake and metabolism of T_4; and (4) reduced secretion of

T_4 caused by alteration in the structure of TSH resulting in decreased biologic activity. Proinflammatory cytokines produced by the mononuclear cells (macrophages, lymphocytes, and monocytes) of the immune system in patients with NTI are probably responsible for the changes in thyroid function tests. Administration of proinflammatory cytokines such as tumor necrosis factor (TNF)-α and interleukin (IL)-1 to experimental animals made the animals sick and reduced serum T_4, T_3, and TSH concentrations. These cytokines inhibit thyroid iodide uptake by reducing the activity and transcription of the sodium-iodide symporter, and they inhibit T_3 production by reducing the activity and transcription of 5'-deiodinase.

Recovery from the underlying illness results in improvement of the low T_3 and T_4 states. Serum T_4 level returns to normal faster than serum T_3 level. Serum TSH concentration usually remains normal except in those patients receiving pharmacologic doses of dopamine or glucocorticoids, which reduce serum TSH levels. During the recovery stage, serum TSH usually remains in the normal range, but it may transiently increase above the normal range. Figure 66-3 diagrams the changes in thyroid hormone and serum TSH levels in NTI.

The effects of thyroid hormone replacement in NTI have been studied. Treatment of the low T_3 state with replacement doses of T_3 was found to be detrimental in a fasting model of NTI, resulting in an increase in protein catabolism and possibly muscle breakdown. T_3 given intravenously to cardiac patients undergoing open-heart surgery improved cardiac performance, but this was not confirmed in randomized trials. T_4 therapy in severe NTI had no beneficial effects and did not improve survival.

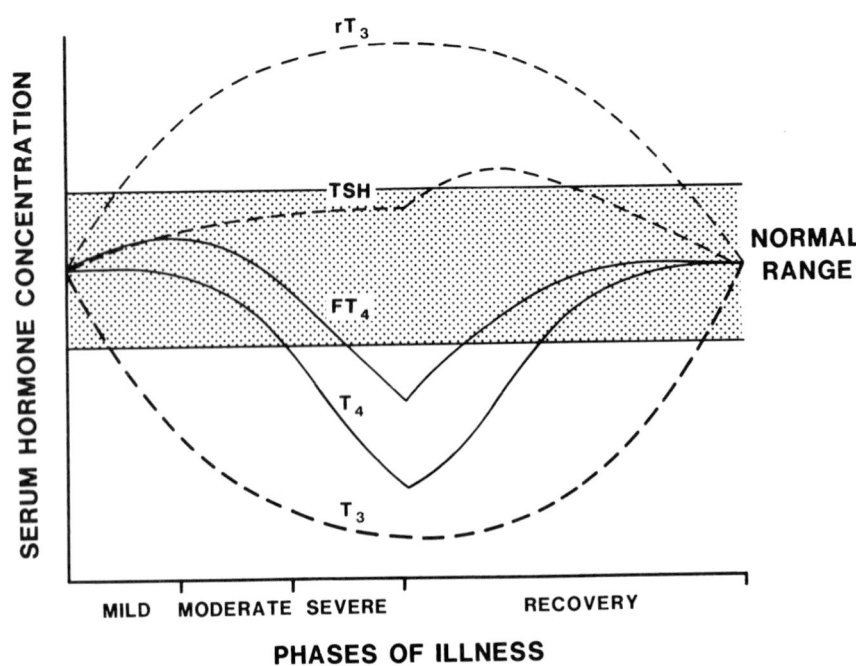

CONTINUUM OF THYROID HORMONE AND THYROTROPIN PROFILES IN NONTHYROIDAL ILLNESS AND RECOVERY

Figure 66-3 The relative changes in serum thyrotropin and thyroid hormone concentrations with increasing severity of nonthyroidal illness and with recovery. Serum T_4 and free T_4 falls with more severe illness, whereas serum T_3 is subnormal in mild illness. The recovery is generally a reverse of the illness pattern with a slight elevation of serum TSH in many instances.

DRUGS AND THYROID FUNCTION

Many elderly patients are on multiple medications, which may affect thyroid hormone secretion rate, thyroid function tests, and levothyroxine therapy (Table 66-2). Knowledge of drug effects on thyroid economy and the site of the drug interaction enable the clinician to anticipate changes or abnormalities of the thyroid function tests in evaluation of patients with thyroid dysfunction. Altered sensitivity to drugs is particularly relevant in elderly patients with thyroid diseases. The metabolism and secretion of many drugs are attenuated in hypothyroidism and accelerated in thyrotoxicosis. Hypothyroidism results in increases in the plasma half-life of digoxin, insulin, glucocorticoids and morphine; consequently, sensitivity to the toxic effects of these drugs increases and the maintenance doses need to be decreased.

Table 66-2 Drugs that Affect Thyroid Function

Decrease TSH secretion
Dopamine
Glucocorticoids
Octreotide
Bexarotene
Increase thyroid hormone secretion
Iodine
Amiodarone
Interferon alpha
Decrease thyroid hormone secretion
Lithium
Iodine
Amiodarone
Aminoglutethimide
Decrease T$_4$ absorption
Calcium
Cholestyramine, Colestipol
Aluminum hydroxide
Ferrous Sulfate
Sucralfate
Increase serum TBG
Estrogen
Tamoxifen
Fluorouracil
Heroin
Methadone
Decrease serum TBG
Androgen
Anabolic steroids (danazol)
Glucocorticoid
Increase hepatic T$_4$ and T$_3$ metabolism
Phenobarbital
Rifampin
Phenytoin
Carbamazepine
Sertraline

Opposite metabolic changes in hyperthyroidism result in increased maintenance doses of these drugs. Resistance to the anticoagulant effect of warfarin in hypothyroidism is a result of slower-than-normal clearance of vitamin K-dependent coagulation factors; an augmented response is seen in hyperthyroidism.

The most common cause of an increase in serum TBG and T$_4$ concentration in postmenopausal women is estrogen-replacement therapy. The serum TBG concentration is increased by 30 to 50 percent in women receiving 0.625 mg of conjugated estrogen daily for 4 to 8 weeks. Serum total T$_4$ and T$_3$ are increased, but free T$_4$, free T$_3$, and TSH remain normal. In contrast, patients taking androgen, anabolic steroid or glucocorticoid have a lower serum TBG concentration and slightly decreased serum T$_4$ level.

The activity of the hepatic microsomal enzymes that metabolize T$_4$ and T$_3$ is affected by phenobarbital, rifampin, phenytoin, and carbamazepine. Hypothyroid patients treated with levothyroxine may become hypothyroid again when rifampin or phenobarbital is administered. In patients without thyroid disease, serum total and free T$_4$ and T$_3$ concentrations are decreased by 20 to 40 percent while on phenytoin or carbamazepine.

Therapy with interferon-α is associated with the development of antimicrosomal antibodies in 20 percent of patients and may precipitate hypothyroidism, thyrotoxicosis, or the biphasic pattern of hyperthyroidism followed by hypothyroidism seen in silent thyroiditis. Patients with antithyroid antibodies are at higher risk of developing thyroid dysfunction during treatment with interferon-α.

HYPOTHYROIDISM

Definition

Hypothyroidism results from an insidious process of thyroid failure and a state of decreased thyroid hormone availability to peripheral tissues. Mild thyroid failure with an elevated serum TSH level and normal FT$_4$ concentration is referred to as *subclinical (biochemical) hypothyroidism*. A serum TSH level that is greater than 50 percent above the normal range is sufficiently abnormal to define subclinical hypothyroidism. The combination of a low serum FT$_4$ level and elevated serum TSH level together with clinical findings of hypothyroidism is defined as *overt hypothyroidism*.

Prevalence

The prevalence of hypothyroidism varies based on the population under study (i.e., geriatric inpatient versus primary care setting), ethnicity, and iodine content of the diet. Among the patients admitted to a geriatric unit, the prevalence of hypothyroidism has been reported as 2 to 7.4 percent. In patients older than 60 years of age in the general population, the incidence of overt hypothyroidism is 2.3 to 10.3 percent. High TSH values were more common in women (11.6 percent) than in men (2.9 percent), and antithyroid antibodies were found in 60 percent of patients with high TSH levels older than 60 years of age in the United Kingdom. The most recent National Health and

Nutrition Examination Survey in the United States found that 12 to 14 percent of the population older than age 70 years had high serum TSH, as compared with approximately 2 percent of the population younger than age 40 years. The prevalence of autoimmune thyroid disease is low in regions with low dietary iodine. In a comparative study of healthy elderly female patients, the prevalence of hypothyroidism in Regio Emilia, Italy, where there is low dietary iodine intake, was 0.9 percent, whereas a prevalence of 14 percent was found in Worcester, Massachusetts, where the dietary iodine is much higher.

Etiology and Pathogenesis

Table 66-3 lists the causes of hypothyroidism. Primary hypothyroidism accounts for the vast majority of cases of thyroid failure, and less than 1 percent of cases are caused by secondary hypothyroidism.

In the areas of adequate iodine intake, chronic autoimmune (Hashimoto's) thyroiditis is the most common cause of primary hypothyroidism in the elderly population and is more common in women. Chronic autoimmune thyroiditis is characterized by a focal or diffuse lymphocytic infiltration of thyroid parenchyma, damaged or atrophic follicles, and the presence of autoantibodies in the serum. The thyroid may be enlarged or atrophic. Thyroid atrophy has been attributed to blocking antibodies that bind to the TSH receptor and inhibit the action of TSH.

Autopsy reports from the United Kingdom and the United States reveal the presence of focal thyroiditis in 40 to 50 percent of women and in 20 percent of men with no prior history of thyroid diseases. The incidence of chronic autoimmune thyroiditis was significantly higher in white than in black Americans in the same study. The prevalence of more severe thyroiditis was 5 to 15 percent in women and 1 to 5 percent in men. Antithyroid peroxidase

Table 66-3   Causes of Hypothyroidism in the Elderly Population

Primary hypothyroidism
  Chronic autoimmune thyroiditis
  Radiation
    [131]I therapy for hyperthyroidism
    Radiation therapy for head and neck cancer
  Surgical thyroidectomy
  Drugs
    Iodine-containing drugs: amiodarone, iodinated glycerol (Organidin)
    Antithyroid drugs (propythiouracil, methimazole)
    Lithium

Secondary hypothyroidism
  Hypothalamic tumors or granuloma
  Pituitary tumors
  Pituitary surgery
  Radiation

(antimicrosomal) or antithyroglobulin antibodies are present in greater than 90 percent of patients with chronic autoimmune thyroiditis. The prevalence of positive thyroid antibodies increases with age, with frequencies as high as 33 percent in women older than 70 years of age. Positive antithyroid antibodies do not always correlate with development of overt hypothyroidism; however, they may be used as a risk factor for its development or as a predictor of progression of the disease.

The second most common cause of hypothyroidism is treatment with radioiodine or thyroid surgery. Radiation-induced hypothyroidism is caused by either radioactive iodine treatment of hyperthyroidism or by external radiation therapy of head and neck cancer. Hypothyroidism has been reported in 76 percent of hyperthyroid patients treated with radioiodine and 20 to 47 percent of patients receiving radiotherapy for treatment of various malignancies of the head and neck region. This may take many years to develop, so patients having received radiation treatment at a young or middle age may develop overt hypothyroidism in old age.

Hypothyroidism in the elderly person may be precipitated by certain drugs listed in Table 66-3. Patients with underlying autoimmune thyroid disease are more susceptible to develop iodine-induced hypothyroidism. This effect is a result of iodine-induced inhibition of thyroid hormone synthesis. Amiodarone, an iodine-containing drug, is commonly used for treatment of arrhythmias in the elderly population. It inhibits conversion of T_4 to T_3 peripherally and slows the metabolism of thyroxine. The incidence of amiodarone-induced hypothyroidism varies with the environmental iodine intake, with frequency of 10 to 20 percent in the United States. Lithium carbonate, a drug used to treat manic-depressive states, inhibits thyroid hormone release and synthesis. Hypothyroidism develops in approximately 15 percent of patients taking lithium chronically and is more frequent in those with positive antithyroid antibodies.

Central hypothyroidism, resulting from an anatomic or functional disorder of the pituitary gland or the hypothalamus or both, is relatively rare. Thyroid hormone secretion is reduced secondary to deficient stimulation of the normal thyroid gland by thyrotropin. The impairment of TSH secretion is caused by either primary or metastatic pituitary tumors, external radiotherapy, infection, or surgery.

Clinical Manifestations

Many of the signs and symptoms of hypothyroidism in older persons tend to be nonspecific because of the insidious onset of the disease and its slow progression over months to years. In one report, a definite diagnosis of hypothyroidism was established by clinical examination in only 10 percent of patients with laboratory evidence of the disease. In another study of patients with hypothyroidism, the diagnosis was not suspected by the examining physicians even though some of the signs and symptoms were present at the time of examination. Table 66-4 lists the common clinical features of symptomatic hypothyroidism. Table 66-5 compares signs and symptoms of overt hypothyroidism between elderly and younger patients. The mean serum TSH and FT_4 levels and duration of evolution

Table 66–4 Clinical Features of Hypothyroidism in Elderly Patients

Cutaneous
  Dry skin
  Hair loss
  Edema of face and eyelids
  Cold intolerance

Neurologic
  Paresthesia (carpal tunnel syndrome)
  Ataxia
  Dementia

Psychiatric and behavioral
  Depression
  Apathy or withdrawal
  Psychosis
  Cognitive dysfunction

Metabolism
  Weight gain
  Hypercholesterolemia
  Hypertriglyceridemia
  Peripheral edema

Musculoskeletal
  Myopathy
  Arthritis/arthralgia

Cardiovascular
  Bradycardia
  Pericardial effusion
  Congestive heart failure

Table 66–5 Comparison of Clinical Features of Overt Hypothyroidism in Elderly versus Young Patients

Symptoms and Signs	Elderly, ≥70 Years (%)	Young, ≤55 Years (%)
Bradycardia	12	19
Fatigue	68	83
Weight gain	24	59
Cold intolerance	35	65
Depression	28	52
Disorientation	9	0
Hypoactive reflexes	24	31
Weakness	53	67
Paresthesia	18	61
Dry skin	35	45
Hair loss	12	28
Reduced hearing	32	25
Muscle cramps	20	55
Snoring	18	22
Constipation	33	41

at the time of diagnosis were similar between two groups of patients. This study showed that the classic signs of overt hypothyroidism such as cold intolerance, paresthesia, weight gain, and muscle cramps were less frequent in older patients. In many cases, hypothyroid patients present to other specialists for specific complaints: to neurologists for paresthesia and symptoms of carpal tunnel syndrome; to dermatologists for dry skin or hair loss; and to psychiatrists for depression, dementia, or mental confusion. Weight loss with a decreased appetite was reported in 13 percent of elderly patients with hypothyroidism.

Carpal tunnel syndrome is the most frequent type of peripheral neuropathy in patients with hypothyroidism. Nerve entrapment in carpal tunnel syndrome presents as nocturnal paresthesia and pain in a median nerve distribution. Cerebellar ataxia or unsteady gait, another neurologic manifestation of hypothyroidism in the elderly population, causes difficulty in locomotion so that patients may require assistance to stand or walk. Cerebellar motor function is restored to normal with T_4 treatment.

The dermatologic manifestations of hypothyroidism involve not only the epidermis and the dermis layer of the skin but also the sweat glands and the hair follicles. Thyroid hormone deficiency results in decreased cell division and protein synthesis at the epidermal layer and decreased

sweat eccrine gland secretion resulting in rough, scaly, and dry skin. Myxedema, the nonpitting edema of the extremities, and puffiness of the face, especially around the eyes, are related to deposition of mucopolysaccharides and hyaluronic acid in the dermal layer of the skin. In severe hypothyroidism, myxedema affects the subcutaneous tissue, the tongue, and the laryngeal and pharyngeal mucous membranes, resulting in thick, slurred speech and hoarseness. Alopecia in hypothyroid patients is secondary to inhibition of the growth cycle of the hair follicle.

The neuropsychiatric features of hypothyroidism in the elderly population are initially nonspecific. Patients may report slowing of thought processes. As the patient becomes less motivated and responsive to others, disoriented, and less interested in usual activities, the diagnosis may be confused with that of depressive mood disorder. Older people who present with a deterioration in personality, retardation of thought or action, apathy, and global loss of intellectual function should be evaluated for hypothyroidism. As hypothyroidism becomes more severe, paranoia, delusions, hallucinations, and psychosis may develop.

In a population of patients with dementia, the incidence of hypothyroidism was the same as in the general population. In a study of demented patients, 2.3 percent were found to have hypothyroidism, of whom only 25 percent improved with treatment.

Abnormalities in plasma lipids are among the most important metabolic changes that occur in hypothyroidism. In the majority of overt hypothyroid patients, hypercholesterolemia (plasma cholesterol level >250 mg/dL) is present. A reduction in cholesterol uptake because of reduced number of low-density lipoprotein (LDL) receptors results in an increase in low-density cholesterol-carrying apolipoprotein concentration. The synthesis rate of free fatty acids and triglycerides is normal in hypothyroidism; the hypertriglyceridemia is caused by a decreased fractional removal rate of triglycerides.

Thyroid hormone deficiency causes several cardiac abnormalities. Cardiomegaly is secondary to hypothyroid-induced pericardial effusion, bradycardia, diastolic hypertension, and atherosclerosis. Pericardial effusion is found in approximately 30 to 50 percent of patients with overt hypothyroidism. The volume of the effusion correlates with the severity of the disease. The electrocardiogram may show ST and T wave changes, QT prolongation, and more often low-amplitude QRS complexes or a low voltage that is a result of pericardial effusion rather than a myocardial conduction defect. Cardiac tamponade and hemodynamic compromise are very rare. Bradycardia results from the effects of thyroid hormone deficiency on the cardiac conducting system. The slowing of the heart rate is moderate, and its role in the development of fatigue in hypothyroid patients is unclear. Hypothyroidism may mask typical symptoms of coronary artery disease by causing depressed myocardial contractility and bradycardia, resulting in reduced myocardial oxygen consumption.

Exertional dyspnea and reduced exercise tolerance are present in 50 percent of elderly patients with overt hypothyroidism and may be related to skeletal muscle dysfunction rather than impaired cardiac function. Anginal chest pain was reported in 25 percent of patients with overt hypothyroidism, suggesting an increased prevalence of coronary heart disease in these patients. Patients with a long-standing history of hypothyroidism are especially at risk of developing atherosclerotic vascular disease that may have been induced by diastolic hypertension and hypercholesterolemia. Hypothyroidism predisposes to diastolic hypertension by impairment of the diastolic relaxation phase. Approximately 1 percent of patients with diastolic hypertension may have hypothyroidism as the cause. Blood pressure normalizes with thyroid hormone replacement therapy in such patients.

Patients with hypothyroidism may present with joint pain and stiffness. The articular pain may involve the large and small joints of the extremities. Joint effusions are often present, and the synovial fluid aspirate is viscous due to increased hyaluronic acid.

The myopathy of hypothyroidism causes proximal muscle pain and stiffness. The muscular symptoms result from increased muscle volume and slowness of contraction, which makes movements mildly painful. There is an associated muscular weakness. In a study of 20 patients with primary hypothyroidism, 40 percent were found to have scapular and pelvic muscle weakness without atrophy or hypertrophy. The electromyographic alterations were improved in 1 to 8 weeks after treatment of hypothyroidism. The arthralgia and myopathy of hypothyroidism are similar in presentation to those with polymyalgia rheumatica or polymyositis. The musculoskeletal manifestations of hypothyroidism are reversible with thyroxine therapy, which highlights the significance of including hypothyroidism in the differential diagnosis of myopathy.

Hypothyroidism is a well-known cause of sleep apnea. The proposed mechanism is upper airway obstruction resulting from myopathy of the pharyngeal skeletal muscles and the respiratory muscles. Studies show a significant improvement in sleep apnea after thyroxine therapy.

Anemia, either microcytic, normocytic, or macrocytic, is a well-characterized hematologic feature of hypothyroidism. Mild anemia may be present in 30 to 40 percent of patients with overt hypothyroidism caused by reduction in erythropoiesis. Macrocytosis may be associated with vitamin B_{12} deficiency or folic acid deficiency. Patients with hypothyroidism induced by an autoimmune process have an increased incidence of pernicious anemia and parietal cell intrinsic factor antibodies.

Central hypothyroidism is most often a part of hypopituitarism that affects the secretion of other anterior pituitary hormones such as luteinizing hormone, follicle-stimulating hormone, adrenocorticotropin, and growth hormone. The clinical features vary in severity. The skin is cool and pale, rather than coarse and dry as in primary hypothyroidism. Other features of hypopituitarism may be present. Hypogonadism results in diminished axillary, pubic, and facial hair in addition to impotence and testicular atrophy in men and atrophy of the breasts in women. Adrenocorticotropic hormone (ACTH) deficiency usually presents later in the course of the hypopituitarism and can result in weakness, hypotension, and depigmentation of the areola and other normally pigmented areas of the skin.

Diagnosis

An elevated TSH level suggests thyroid failure, and the FT_4 level determines the degree of failure. Any degree of primary thyroid gland failure, either subclinical or overt hypothyroidism, can be identified with sensitive assays of serum TSH. Serum T_3 concentration is normal in about one-third of overtly hypothyroid patients and is therefore an insensitive test for assessment of primary hypothyroidism. An elevated serum TSH level also may be seen during the recovery period from nonthyroidal illness. Therefore, the serum TSH measurement must be interpreted in the context of the clinical situation. Central hypothyroidism results in low serum T_4 and T_3 levels with a low or normal serum TSH concentration. The paradoxically normal serum TSH is attributed to secretion of TSH with reduced biologic activity.

Treatment

The purpose of treatment of hypothyroidism, regardless of its cause, is to achieve a euthyroid state that is indicated by normal thyroid function tests. Synthetic levothyroxine is the preferred preparation for treatment of hypothyroidism because of its long half-life (approximately 7 days), reliable absorption, and relatively constant serum T_4 concentration after single daily doses. The replacement therapy dose of levothyroxine depends on the weight and age of the patient. The thyroxine requirements are decreased in the elderly person because of a decline in the metabolism of thyroid hormone. The average requirement of T_4 in elderly patients is 25 percent less than in young adults. This decrease results from the age-related decrease in fractional thyroxine degradation rate.

In elderly patients with coexisting cardiovascular disease, starting treatment with full replacement doses can result in exacerbation of angina and worsening of the underlying heart disease. Therefore, it is crucial that the starting dose of thyroxine should be small, such as 12.5 to 25 μg/d. The replacement dose titration needs to be done cautiously with close monitoring of the patient's symptoms and thyroid function tests. The dose should be adjusted at 6-week intervals by an increment of 12.5 to 25 μg until the patient is euthyroid and the serum TSH is in the mid-normal range. Once the serum TSH level is within the normal range, its measurement may be done every 6 to 12 months to monitor the dose and compliance. Patients with central hypothyroidism should be monitored by free T_4 measurement and not serum TSH.

Angioplasty or coronary bypass graft can be safely performed before starting thyroxine administration in patients with coronary artery disease. Calcium channel blockers are more suitable than beta blockers for controlling angina in hypothyroid patients receiving thyroxine.

There are a number of drugs that may interfere with levothyroxine absorption or clearance (see Table 66-2). Drugs that block its absorption are calcium carbonate, ferrous sulphate cholestyramine, colestipol, sucralfate, and aluminum hydroxide. This malabsorption of thyroxine can be avoided to a large extent by instructing the patient to allow a time interval of at least 4 hours between the ingestion of the two drugs. Rifampin, carbamazepine, phenytoin, and sertraline (Zoloft) accelerate serum T_4 clearance and increase the serum TSH level in patients on previously ideal replacement doses. Therefore, a higher levothyroxine replacement dose is required. Estrogen therapy may also cause an increased thyroxine replacement dose.

Subclinical Hypothyroidism

Subclinical hypothyroidism is the term applied to the state in which serum TSH concentration is raised while free T_4 and T_3 concentrations are normal in a patient with no clinical features of hypothyroidism. Serum TSH concentration bears a logarithmic relation to free T_4 level; small decrements in free T_4 concentration result in large increases in serum TSH concentration. The prevalence of TSH elevation is both age and sex dependent. Multiple studies show that older women are at greatest risk for hypothyroidism. In England, in the Whickham survey, the prevalence of subclinical hypothyroidism was 17.4 percent in women older than age 75 years. In a survey in the United States, the prevalence of serum TSH elevation was 8.5 percent in women and 4.4 percent in men older than age 55 years.

The common causes of subclinical hypothyroidism are the same as the causes of overt hypothyroidism (see Table 66-3). The majority of patients have chronic autoimmune thyroiditis with positive antithyroid peroxidase antibodies. Those patients with high titers of antithyroid antibodies and more than twice the upper limit of serum TSH are most likely to develop overt hypothyroidism, defined as a low serum free T_4 level. In the 20-year follow-up study of patients with subclinical hypothyroidism in the Whickham Survey, the annual rate of thyroid failure was 4.3% in those with positive thyroid antibodies, as compared to 0.3% in thyroid-antibody-negative patients. The common reversible causes are drug therapy with lithium carbonate or amiodarone.

A survey of elderly women in Rotterdam showed that subclinical hypothyroidism increased the risk for myocardial infarction two- to threefold. Cardiovascular abnormalities associated with mild thyroid failure include left ventricular diastolic and endothelial dysfunction. The cardiac structure and function remain normal at rest, but ventricular function, cardiovascular and respiratory adaptation is impaired during exercise. Left ventricular ejection fraction is similar to the euthyroid state at rest, but reduced with exercise. These changes are reversible when the euthyroid state is established.

To evaluate the efficacy of thyroid hormone therapy in the treatment of subclinical hypothyroidism, serum lipid concentrations, cognitive function, and psychiatric status should be assessed. Subclinical hypothyroidism can contribute to increased low-density lipoprotein-cholesterol (LDL-C) and decreased high-density lipoprotein-cholesterol (HDL-C). Levothyroxine therapy in such patients results in decreased LDL-C and apolipoprotein B level and a decrease in the ratio of the cholesterol to HDL-C, which may reduce the risk for the development of coronary artery disease.

Replacement therapy is recommended for all patients with serum TSH concentrations of greater than 8 to 10 mU/L (more than twice the upper limit of normal). It is also recommended if there are any clinical features of depression, fatigue, hyperlipidemia, or goiter. The goal of therapy is to normalize the serum TSH concentration. In older people, 12.5 to 25 μg levothyroxine is recommended as the initial dose. With minimal TSH elevation and absence of clinical features, patients should be followed at intervals of 6 months.

The central nervous system appears to be affected by hypothyroidism at an early stage. However, only 25 percent of the patients with subclinical hypothyroidism scored better in psychometric and neurophysiologic testing during hormonal therapy.

Myxedema Coma

Myxedema coma is a rare syndrome that represents the result of severe untreated hypothyroidism. Most patients are older than 60 years of age. It is characterized by lethargy, progressive weakness, stupor, hypothermia, hyponatremia, cardiovascular shock, and coma. The mortality rate is very high in older patients, approximately 80 percent in untreated cases. Myxedema coma may be precipitated by exposure to cold weather; drugs such as narcotics, sedatives, analgesics, anesthetics or tranquilizers; pulmonary or urinary tract infections; and other coexisting medical conditions such as cerebrovascular accidents and congestive heart failure.

The patient may have a history of a previous thyroid disease, radioiodine therapy, or thyroidectomy. The medical history is of gradual onset of progressive weakness and impaired cognitive function, depression, and stupor. Physical findings include marked hypothermia, bradycardia, hoarseness, delayed reflexes, dry skin, and periorbital edema. Laboratory evaluation may indicate hyponatremia, elevated creatine phosphokinase level, neutropenia with a left shift, elevated serum cholesterol level, increased cerebrospinal fluid protein, carbon dioxide retention, and hypoxia. Serum tests will reveal a low FT_4 level and a markedly elevated TSH concentration, except in central hypothyroidism, in which case an increased serum TSH would not be found.

Treatment of myxedema coma is an acute medical emergency; 500 μg levothyroxine should be given by intravenous bolus because such patients absorb drugs poorly through the gastrointestinal tract. This is followed by daily administration of 50 μg thyroxine intravenously. Because the possibility of concomitant adrenal insufficiency (because of autoimmune adrenal or pituitary insufficiency) may exist, hydrocortisone hemisuccinate 100 mg intravenously should be administered followed by 50 mg every 6 hours. A serum cortisol level should be obtained prior to hydrocortisone infusion. If the serum cortisol level is greater than 20 μg/dL, then the corticosteroid can be discontinued. The patient's renal function, fluid status, and cardiopulmonary status must be monitored closely.

HYPERTHYROIDISM

Prevalence

There is a considerable variation reported in the prevalence of hyperthyroidism. Based on different ethnic and geographic regions and the criteria used for diagnosis, the prevalence varies from 0.5 to 2.3 percent in the elderly population. Approximately 10 to 17 percent of all hyperthyroid patients are older than age 60 years. Using sensitive TSH assays, patients with subnormal serum TSH levels had a 12 percent predictive value for eventually developing hyperthyroidism.

Etiology and Pathogenesis

The most common cause of hyperthyroidism in the elderly population is Graves' disease, or diffuse toxic goiter. The reported frequency of Graves' disease as the cause of hyperthyroidism in patients older than age 75 years has been 84 percent. Graves' disease, an autoimmune disorder, results from the action of a thyroid-stimulating antibody on TSH receptors. Antibodies that bind to the TSH receptor may be either TSH-stimulating or TSH-blocking. TSH receptor antibodies are detectable in the serum of approximately 80 to 100 percent of untreated patients with Graves' disease.

The cause of the extrathyroidal manifestations of Graves' disease, such as ophthalmopathy and dermopathy, is unknown. The proposed mechanism for the ophthalmopathy is the development of retrobulbar autoimmune inflammation caused by the release of cytokines, thickening of extraocular muscles, and swelling of orbital contents.

Toxic multinodular goiter is more common in the elderly population and has been reported in about one-half of older patients with hyperthyroidism, especially in regions of relative iodine deficiency. It occurs more prevalently in patients with a long-standing history of multinodular goiter. The etiologic factor causing the transition from nontoxic to toxic multinodular goiter is unclear. However, there is generation of new follicles within the gland with functional autonomy independent from TSH stimulation. Autonomously functioning thyroid nodules synthesize and secrete thyroid hormones despite suppression of TSH secretion. In one study, 55 percent of hyperthyroid patients older than 60 years of age were found to have autonomous functioning thyroid nodules. Thyrotoxicosis can be precipitated in patients with nontoxic multinodular goiter by administration of a large iodine load such as radiocontrast agent. Some autonomously functioning thyroid adenomas have a mutation in the TSH receptor that results in chronic activation of the follicular cell.

Thyroiditis, either acute or subacute, occurs with less frequency in the aged as compared with younger patients with hyperthyroidism. Thyrotoxicosis results from extensive destruction of follicular cells by either an inflammatory or infectious process and release of T_4 and T_3 into the circulation. Amiodarone may cause destructive thyroiditis and thyrotoxicosis. Hyperthyroidism resulting from a TSH-secreting pituitary adenoma or pituitary resistance to thyroid hormone is very rare.

Clinical Manifestations

Absence of the typical manifestations of hyperthyroidism in the elderly patient was first described in 1931 by Lahey as "apathetic hyperthyroidism," in which there was only slight evidence of hypermetabolism. The diagnosis of hyperthyroidism may be overlooked because of apathy, or the dominant clinical findings may be weight loss or cardiac or gastrointestinal manifestations. Table 66-6 lists the signs and symptoms of hyperthyroidism in the elderly patient. Recognition of these important clues will facilitate detection of the disease at an earlier stage.

Table 66-7 compares clinical findings of hyperthyroidism in elderly and young patients independent of etiology. The thyroid hormone levels were similar in both groups, and there was no correlation between serum TSH and FT_4 levels and the prevalence of signs and symptoms of hyperthyroidism. The results of this study confirm that the presentation of hyperthyroidism in older patients is associated with fewer classic signs or symptoms and increased frequency of anorexia, atrial fibrillation, and a lack of goiter. Interestingly, palpable goiter is absent in approximately 50 percent of the older patients with hyperthyroidism, whereas 80 percent of the younger patients have thyroid enlargement on physical examination.

Table 66-6   Clinical Features of Hyperthyroidism in Elderly Patients

Cardiovascular
    Palpitations
    Chronic or intermittent atrial fibrillation
    Congestive heart failure

Psychiatric and behavioral
    Depression
    Apathy
    Lethargy
    Irritability

Gastrointestinal
    Decreased appetite
    Weight loss
    Nausea
    Constipation

Musculoskeletal
    Proximal muscle weakness
    Muscle atrophy

Table 66-7   Comparison of Clinical Features of Hyperthyroidism in Elderly versus Young Patients

Symptoms and Signs	Elderly, >70 Years (%)	Young, <50 Years (%)
Tachycardia	71	96
Fatigue	56	84
Weight loss	50	51
Tremor	44	84
Dyspnea	41	56
Apathy	41	25
Anorexia	32	4
Nervousness	31	84
Hyperactive reflexes	28	96
Weakness	27	61
Depression	24	22
Increased sweating	24	95
Diarrhea	18	43
Muscular atrophy	16	10
Confusion	16	0
Heat intolerance	15	92
Constipation	15	0

The cardiovascular manifestations of thyrotoxicosis may predominate. Palpitation and tachycardia are experienced by a majority of thyrotoxic patients. However, in the elderly population, the initial cardiac manifestation can be atrial fibrillation or supraventricular tachycardia. Occult hyperthyroidism should be ruled out in any elderly patient with a new onset of tachyarrhythmias. Patients with atrial fibrillation are at risk for systemic embolization and stroke. Older patients with concurrent heart disease have a higher prevalence of embolism.

The excessive amounts of thyroid hormones increase myocardial oxygen demand and may unmask coronary artery disease or exacerbate underlying cardiac conditions such as angina pectoris or congestive heart failure. Elderly patients with thyrotoxicosis and evidence of cardiac contractile dysfunction caused by hypertension, coronary artery disease, valvular heart disease, or atrial fibrillation are at higher risk of developing congestive heart failure.

Dyspnea on exertion and exercise intolerance are also common complaints of thyrotoxic patients. These symptoms can be caused by weakness of the skeletal and respiratory muscles rather than compromised cardiac function. Marked weakness and atrophy of muscles may have an insidious onset and slow progression in some elderly patients with thyrotoxicosis that has been long-standing as a result of delayed diagnosis because of its atypical presentation. Weakness involves mostly the proximal muscles, especially those of the shoulder girdle and the pelvis.

The classic gastrointestinal signs and symptoms are increased appetite, rapid intestinal transit resulting in more frequent defecation, and weight loss. However, some elderly patients with apathetic hyperthyroidism present with weight loss, anorexia, nausea, vomiting, and constipation. In a group of 880 patients with Graves' disease, weight loss became a major diagnostic finding in 80 percent of patients older than age 70 years. This weight loss is secondary to increased metabolic demands and reduced appetite.

The neurobehavioral and psychiatric changes associated with hyperthyroidism in young adults include anxiety, emotional lability, insomnia, lack of concentration, restlessness, and tremulousness. In contrast to these features, apathy, lethargy, pseudodementia, and depressed mood frequently are present in older people with hyperthyroidism. Patients with an atypical depression (an increased prevalence of somatic complaints, anxiety, and fewer complaints of sadness or guilt) later in life should be evaluated for hyperthyroidism.

Diagnosis

The serum T_4 level is elevated in 86 percent of elderly hyperthyroid patients, so this test is reasonably sensitive for screening for hyperthyroidism. However, there are hyperthyroxinemic patients without hyperthyroidism, indicating low specificity of the serum total T_4 assay. The preferred approach to diagnosis of hyperthyroidism is the combination of free thyroxine or free thyroxine index level and a sensitive TSH assay. Serum TSH level is suppressed in hyperthyroidism, but a suppressed TSH alone in a geriatric patient is not generally indicative of hyperthyroidism. Most elderly subjects with suppressed serum TSH levels are not hyperthyroid (see "Subclinical Hyperthyroidism" later in this chapter). Medications such as dopamine or glucocorticoids and conditions such as hypothalamic or pituitary disorders may cause suppression of the serum TSH level.

An elevation of serum T_3 level in addition to an elevated serum T_4 level is a strong confirmation of hyperthyroidism. The serum T_3 level is not increased in every elderly patient with hyperthyroidism and was found to be elevated in only 50 percent of such patients between 75 and 95 years of age. The relative absence of T_3 elevation may be a reflection of less conversion of T_4 to T_3 peripherally in the aged population.

Hyperthyroid patients with a low serum TSH and normal FT_4 levels should have the T_3 level measured to identify T_3 thyrotoxicosis, a condition seen in 1 or 2 percent of hyperthyroid patients in the United States. T_3 thyrotoxicosis is more common in elderly patients with a solitary adenoma or with early toxic multinodular goiter.

Once hyperthyroidism is detected, a 24-hour radioactive iodine uptake should be done to exclude the conditions causing thyrotoxicosis with low thyroid uptake: thyroiditis, exogenous intake of thyroid hormone, or iodine-containing drugs.

Treatment

The preferred mode of therapy in the elderly is radioactive iodine-131. To avoid postradiation release of preformed thyroid hormone from glandular stores and subsequent thyroid storm, severely affected patients should be treated with antithyroid drugs for at least 3 months to achieve a near-normal serum T_4 level or a euthyroid state prior to use of ^{131}I. The usual doses are 5 to 15 mCi of radioactive ^{131}I for Graves' disease and 15 to 50 mCi for large multinodular glands. The antithyroid drugs should be discontinued 7 days before administration of the radioiodine dose and restarted 7 days after ^{131}I treatment. Beta blockers are often used as an adjuvant, especially in cases of symptomatic tachycardia, and should be continued until the patient is euthyroid. The incidence of hypothyroidism in the first year after radioiodine treatment varies from 10 to 30 percent, and hypothyroidism continues to develop in subsequent years. Therefore, the patient should be monitored regularly for the development of hypothyroidism, and thyroxine therapy should be started promptly after the diagnosis of hypothyroidism is established.

Definitive therapy with thionamide antithyroid drugs is appropriate for otherwise healthy elderly patients. Propylthiouracil and methimazole are the antithyroid drugs in the United States. Retrospective analysis of the therapeutic response to antithyroid drugs in patients with hyperthyroid Graves' disease has shown that euthyroidism was achieved in 2 to 3 months in patients older than age 60 years after treatment with methimazole. In a 4-year follow-up after methimazole was discontinued, the recurrence rates were found to be the highest (27 percent) in patients younger than age 30 years and were significantly less with advanced age. In patients 51 to 60 years old, the recurrence rate was 5.6 percent, whereas no recurrence took place in patients older than 61 years of age.

Patients should be warned about the side effects of antithyroid drugs, especially agranulocytosis, which occurs in 1 in 250 Japanese patients, but only in 1 in 3000 English patients. If the patient develops sore throat, chills, or fever, the antithyroid drug should be stopped until the patient is assessed clinically and the white blood cell count is found to be normal. Fortunately, the agranulocytosis is reversible.

Surgery is only advised if there are obstructive symptoms from a large goiter or the presence of a nodule that is suspicious for malignancy. Preparation for thyroidectomy includes using a beta-adrenergic antagonist drug for several weeks before surgery in doses sufficient to lower the resting pulse rate to less than 90 beats per minute. If surgery must be done urgently, then sodium iopanoate has been reported to be safe and effective when given for 5 days together with a β-adrenergic antagonist. Although the mortality from subtotal thyroidectomy is very low, the complications of recurrent laryngeal nerve damage and hypoparathyroidism can result in lifelong disability. Because of the complications, surgery is rarely advisable in the elderly patient.

Atrial fibrillation in the context of hyperthyroidism may resolve once euthyroidism is achieved. Approximately 8 percent of the hyperthyroid patients with atrial fibrillation may develop embolic stroke; therefore, such patients should be given anticoagulation unless there is a contraindication.

Subclinical Hyperthyroidism

Subclinical hyperthyroidism is defined as a state of suppression of serum TSH with normal free thyroxine (FT_4) and triiodothyronine (T_3) levels in a patient who lacks clinical features of thyrotoxicosis. Table 66-8 lists the causes of subclinical thyrotoxicosis.

The prevalence of suppressed TSH, using a sensitive TSH assay, has been reported to range from 1 to 14 percent based on the patient population. The prevalence of subclinical hyperthyroidism was found to be less than 1 percent when those on exogenous thyroid hormone were excluded from the study and a third-generation TSH assay was used. In a study of patients older than 55 years of age, 0.7 percent had

Table 66-8   Common Causes of Subclinical Hyperthyroidism

Thyroid hormone suppressive therapy for thyroid malignancy or thyroid nodules
Excess thyroid hormone replacement
Graves' disease

Autonomously functioning thyroid
    Multinodular goiter
    Hyperfunctioning adenoma (hot nodule)

endogenous subclinical hyperthyroidism. The progression of subclinical hyperthyroidism to overt thyrotoxicosis is independent of thyroid antibody status and does not increase with advancing age. In patients with multinodular goiter, the rate of progression to overt hyperthyroidism is 5 percent each year, and much higher with increased dietary iodine in areas of endemic goiter.

Most of the available data on pathophysiologic effects of TSH suppression have been derived from patients with either thyroid carcinoma or nontoxic nodular goiter on levothyroxine suppressive therapy. Mild thyroid hormone excess in this situation is associated with increased bone turnover rate; the bone resorption rate exceeds the formation rate, and bone loss results. Multiple studies in postmenopausal women with suppressed TSH have shown an accelerated bone loss in the hip, lumbar spine, and distal radius, whereas other studies have failed to demonstrate this. Two meta-analysis studies found a significant 10 percent loss of bone density in postmenopausal women with suppressed serum TSH. Subclinical hyperthyroidism caused by multinodular goiter in postmenopausal women results in 2 percent bone loss each year. This is reversible by treatment and restoration of the thyrotropin level to the normal range. There is inconclusive evidence that exogenous subclinical hyperthyroidism is a risk factor for osteoporosis except in post-menopausal women. Estrogen and calcium replacement therapy attenuates bone loss in this group of patients.

Atrial fibrillation may be a consequence of subclinical hyperthyroidism. In the Framingham Heart Study of patients older than 60 years of age with subclinical hyperthyroidism, 28 percent of patients developed atrial fibrillation in a 10-year follow-up, as compared to 11 percent of the elderly population with normal TSH levels. Even with adjustments for other known risk factors, this study shows that a low serum TSH concentration is associated with a threefold higher risk of development of atrial fibrillation in the subsequent decade. In one Italian study, long-term thyroxine suppression therapy increased left ventricular mass index and caused diastolic dysfunction and reduced ventricular compliance, but a similar study in the United States did not find cardiac dysfunction. A subsequent study by the Italian group showed that administration of a cardioselective beta blocker induced significant regression of cardiac hypertrophy and improved diastolic dysfunction. The effects of subclinical hyperthyroidism on lipid levels include a reduction of LDL cholesterol by 6.4 percent and triglycerides by 4.1 percent.

Subclinical hyperthyroidism is associated with an increased frequency of nervous symptoms. An increased risk of dementia and Alzheimer's disease was reported among patients who were 55 years of age or older with antithyroid antibodies and endogenous subclinical hyperthyroidism.

Therapy should be considered in any patient with subclinical hyperthyroidism who has mental symptoms, osteoporosis, atrial fibrillation or cardiac disease. A trial of antithyroid drugs to normalize the serum TSH level is warranted. In patients with more severe features, such as atrial fibrillation, ablation of the hyperfunctioning thyroid with radioactive ^{131}I must be considered.

THYROID NODULES

Prevalence

Thyroid nodules, either solitary or multiple, increase in frequency with advancing age. It has been estimated that 90 percent of women older than age 60 years and 60 percent of men older than age 80 years have a nodular thyroid gland. The lifetime risk of developing a palpable thyroid nodule is estimated to be 5 to 10 percent in the United States based on a prospective follow-up of more than 5000 patients in the Framingham, Massachusetts, population study. The prevalence of thyroid nodules was found to be higher in women than in men, approximately 5:1, in the same study. Thyroid nodules in asymptomatic individuals ("incidentalomas") are identified more frequently by ultrasonography as compared with palpatory examination of the gland. The prevalence of incidentalomas was 67 percent by high-resolution ultrasonography, and only 21 percent by neck palpation in North American subjects. The lateral location of some nodules and deep lesions with overlying normal tissue contributed to the lower frequency of identification of nodules by palpation. Autopsy examination commonly has revealed thyroid nodules. A large autopsy series indicated that 50 percent of the population with no known history of thyroid disease had discrete nodules, 35 percent of whom had nodules greater than 2 cm in diameter.

Clinical Evaluation

In formulating an effective management of a patient with a thyroid nodule, a careful history and physical examination should be done to assess the risk of malignancy. The patient's age and gender are important risk factors for malignancy. Although thyroid nodules are found more frequently in women, the likelihood of a thyroid nodule being malignant is higher in men than in women. The proportion of malignant nodules was sixfold higher in male patients older than age 70 years according to a 10-year follow-up study of more than 5000 patients with a diagnosis of cold thyroid nodule.

The history of radiation exposure during childhood is important because thyroid nodule or thyroid carcinoma can develop years later. Most patients received radiation therapy for treatment of benign conditions such as tonsillitis, acne, tinea capitis, impetigo, sinusitis, or an enlarged thymus. The earlier the age of exposure, the higher was the likelihood of cancer development. However, the latency period probably does not exceed 50 years, so the chance of radiation induction from childhood exposure is very low in the elderly person.

A family history of thyroid cancer suggests familial medullary thyroid cancer as a component of multiple endocrine neoplasia (MEN) type 2. However, patients with MEN usually present in childhood or early adulthood, rather than in the geriatric age group. A history of goiter in the family may be reassuring of a benign disorder.

Most thyroid nodules do not cause symptoms. Many are found incidentally during a procedure such as carotid

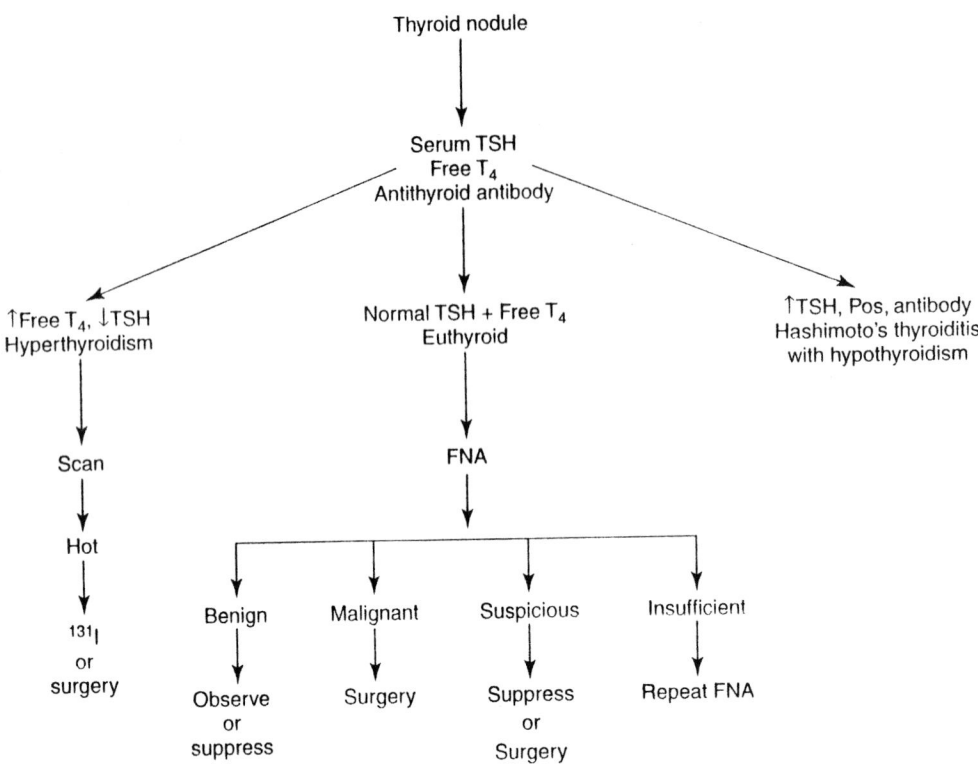

Figure 66-4 Algorithm for evaluation and management of patients presenting with nodular thyroid disease.

ultrasonography or computed tomography (CT) scan or magnetic resonance imaging (MRI) of the neck in the elderly person, giving rise to the term *incidentaloma*. Pain may occur with a hemorrhage into a preexisting colloid nodule or a benign adenoma. Symptoms of rapid nodular growth over a period of weeks or months are suspicious of malignancy. Other symptoms that suggest malignancy are persistent hoarseness or change in voice consistent with recurrent laryngeal nerve dysfunction.

The physical examination of the patient with a thyroid nodule should include careful palpation of the neck with attention to the size and consistency of the nodule and the presence of adenopathy. The location of the nodule within the thyroid gland and the anatomy of the patient's neck may be the limiting factors in palpatory examination of neck. In general, most nodules larger than 2 cm in diameter are easily recognized on palpation. A hard and fixed nodule is more likely to be malignant, but many papillary carcinomas or follicular tumors are soft or cystic. Lymphadenopathy is strongly suggestive of malignancy; therefore, after finding a thyroid nodule, the neck should be examined carefully for the central and deep cervical lymph nodes.

A distinction between solitary and multinodular gland by neck examination may be limited. In approximately 50 percent of patients with a clinically solitary nodule on palpation, the lesion subsequently was found to be a dominant nodule in a multinodular goiter on histologic examination. The relative risk of cancer in solitary versus multinodular thyroid glands has been controversial. Many studies have reported lower rates of thyroid carcinoma in palpable multinodular glands (5 to 13 percent) as compared with solitary nodules (9 to 25 percent), but other studies have found similar incidences of cancer in palpable multinodular and single nodule glands.

Diagnostic Tests

Laboratory and radiographic evaluation of thyroid function is useful to assist in determining whether a nodule is benign or malignant. Figure 66-4 illustrates a recommended approach to diagnostic evaluation. Nearly all patients with either thyroid carcinoma or a benign nodule are euthyroid. An abnormal thyroid function test in a patient with a thyroid nodule does not rule out thyroid cancer but may make thyroid carcinoma a less likely possibility. Low serum TSH concentration in the setting of a nodular goiter suggests the presence of either an autonomously functioning adenoma or a toxic multinodular goiter. Elevated antiperoxidase and antithyroglobulin antibody titers indicate lymphocytic thyroiditis, which may present as a nodule. The serum thyroglobulin level is not a useful test to distinguish benign from malignant nodules because it is increased with any goitrous process.

By thyroid scans with radioiodine, nodules are classified into hyperfunctional or "hot" nodules, nonfunctional or "cold" nodules, or normal functioning or "warm" nodules. This classification is based on the extent of radioiodine incorporation into a nodule compared with the rest of the gland. In a study of more than 5000 patients with thyroid nodules undergoing preoperative scanning, approximately 85 percent of the nodules were cold, 10 percent were normal, and 5 percent were hot. These patients underwent thyroidectomy regardless of the scan result. Thyroid cancer was found in 16 percent of patients with cold nodules, in 9 percent with warm nodules, and in 4 percent with hot nodules. The last figure is higher than expected because most other studies show that a hot nodule is rarely malignant. The finding of a cold nodule has relatively low specificity because the majority of both benign and malignant solitary thyroid nodules appear hypofunctional relative to adjacent normal thyroid tissue. The malignant potential in cold nodules is related to age, sex, and iodine intake. The frequency of cancer with cold nodules is greatest after age 60 years; the incidence of cancer in women was 4.2 percent, and 8.2 percent in men. Because the thyroid scan generally is not useful for diagnosis of malignancy, it is not recommended in the initial evaluation of a thyroid nodule.

Thyroid ultrasound is a noninvasive test that discriminates cystic from solid lesions. It is useful for differentiating thyroid from nonthyroid neck masses and for localizing nodules deep within the gland. In such cases, it can be used to guide fine-needle aspiration biopsy. Thyroid ultrsonography is capable of identifying impalpable solid nodules as small as 0.3 mm in diameter and cystic nodules of 0.2 mm. The clinical significance of small nodules detected by ultrasonography remains uncertain. Ultrasonography does not help in the overall diagnosis of malignancy. Cystic nodules constitute 15 to 25 percent of all thyroid nodules with a malignancy rate of 17 percent.

Positron emission tomography (PET) was used recently to differentiate benign from malignant solitary tumors in patients with thyroid nodular disease. More studies are needed to confirm an increased uptake of the glucose analog [18F]2-deoxy-2-fluoro-d-glucose in the malignant thyroid nodules.

Fine-needle aspiration (FNA) biopsy is the most important diagnostic technique. It reliably identifies thyroid nodule cytology and is the most effective method to diagnose malignancy. In experienced hands, it is safe, with accuracy, sensitivity, and specificity of 98 to 99 percent. Use of FNA has been reported to result in reduction in thyroid nodule management costs by 25 percent, and the number of patients requiring surgery declined by more than 40 percent. Results of FNA biopsies are divided into four basic categories: (1) benign, (2) suspicious (includes aspirates with some features of thyroid carcinoma but not conclusive), (3) malignant, and (4) insufficient. In a large series of patients with FNA biopsy of the thyroid, benign cytology was found in 69 percent (mainly colloid goiter), malignant cytology in 3.5 percent, and suspicious cytology in 10 percent. The suspicious category consists of variants of follicular neoplasm, but follicular adenomas are about tenfold more common than follicular carcinomas. The insufficient or nondiagnostic cytology was reported as an average of 17 percent in the same report and has been attributed to lack of operator experience, nodular vascularity, or a small or posteriorly located nodule. Those patients with a nondiagnostic or "insufficient" cytologic diagnosis should have a repeat biopsy. An adequate specimen is obtained in 30 to 50 percent of repeat aspiration of nodules. Ultrasonography-guided FNA is used for sampling of a small nodule and the solid component of cystic nodules.

In patients with nodules that are follicular lesions, radioiodine scan should be performed. Hot or functional nodules are rarely malignant. The presence of nuclear atypia in a follicular lesion gives a 44 percent prevalence of malignancy, and absence of nuclear atypia denotes a benign lesion. Positive immunostaining for galectin-3 correlates with malignancy; it is likely that immunostaining for galectin-3 and other proteins will improve the differential diagnosis of suspicious lesions.

Solitary incidentalomas larger than 1.5 cm should probably be biopsied under ultrasonographic guidance. Those with a diagnosis of cancer should be removed, but it is not practical or cost-effective to biopsy or surgically excise all nonpalpable nodules. In patients with incidentalomas smaller than 1 cm, the risk of thyroid cancer is very low.

Management

Treatment of the thyroid nodule depends on the functional state of the nodule and cytologic diagnosis with FNA biopsy (see Fig. 66-4). The hyperfunctioning "hot" nodule is treated with radioiodine ablation or surgery. Patients treated with ^{131}I ablation become euthyroid in a few months, and hypothyroidism develops in only a small proportion of such patients.

The vast majority of thyroid nodules are benign and should be managed medically. Medical management with thyroid hormone suppressive therapy is based on the assumption that growth of the nodule depends on TSH. Spontaneous regression of thyroid nodules may occur. L-Thyroxine suppressive therapy is useful for nodules that do not decrease in size over several months of initial observation. Suppressive therapy in the treatment of benign thyroid nodules has been challenged in the past few years by failure of some studies to show a significant decrease in nodule size and concern about reducing mineral bone density. However, several recent studies showed greater than 50 percent reduction in nodular size in 40 percent of patients with a single nodule. Generally, patients are followed by palpation at intervals of 3 months. Ultrasonographic examination can be performed to assess growth or shrinkage of a nodule if more objective documentation is required.

If the cytologic diagnosis indicates malignancy or is strongly suspicious for malignancy, the nodule should be removed surgically. In the 10 percent of "suspicious" cytologic findings for malignancy by FNA, approximately one-fourth of patients who go to surgery are found to have a malignant lesion. Altogether, only approximately 5 percent of thyroid nodules are malignant.

THYROID CANCER

Thyroid cancer accounts for 1.6 percent of all cancers in the United States. Mortality from thyroid cancer is 0.4 percent of all cancer deaths. Epidemiologic studies during the last two decades report an increased incidence of thyroid carcinoma in the United States because of improved diagnosis; however, the mortality has decreased because of earlier detection and improved treatment, in addition to a decline in incidence of anaplastic thyroid carcinoma.

Thyroid carcinoma is classified into five major types: papillary, follicular, medullary, and anaplastic and thyroid lymphoma. Most thyroid cancers are indolent and grow slowly over years, whereas a few grow aggressively and cause death in a year. Thyroid carcinomas tend to be more aggressive clinically and poorly differentiated in elderly patients compared with younger individuals.

Papillary Thyroid Carcinoma

Papillary carcinoma, the most common type of thyroid cancer, accounts for 80 percent of all thyroid tumors. In autopsy studies, the prevalence of occult papillary carcinoma (<1 cm) was found to be 7 percent in patients older than 80 years of age. Papillary carcinoma arises from follicular thyroid cells and is often indolent and slow growing. The tumor tends to invade lymphatics and metastasize to the regional lymph nodes and the lungs. Hematogenous spread also can occur to the bone and the central nervous system. The disease is more aggressive in the older patients.

The prognosis of papillary thyroid carcinoma depends on the age of the patient at the time of initial diagnosis, the size of the primary lesion, local invasion, and the degree of metastases. Death rates are greater in adults older than 45 years of age. In a 12-year follow-up of patients older than 47 years of age with papillary thyroid carcinoma, the death rate was 70 percent in patients with distant metastases, versus 0.8 percent in patients with intrathyroidal disease. Thyroid tumors smaller than 1.5 cm in diameter rarely metastasize to distant sites, whereas larger tumors are associated with higher mortality rates. Extension of the tumor through the thyroid capsule and into the surrounding structures is associated with poorer prognosis. Cervical lymph node metastases occur in about 50 percent of patients diagnosed with papillary carcinoma and carry only a slightly higher rate of recurrence and mortality.

Surgery, either near-total or total thyroidectomy, is the initial treatment of choice for patients with papillary carcinoma. Near-total thyroidectomy is performed for extensive unilateral tumors with local metastases. Total thyroidectomy is performed for patients with extensive multifocal disease with metastases to the cervical lymph nodes, contiguous neck structures, or distant sites. The main disadvantage of total thyroidectomy is the higher incidence of hypoparathyroidism.

Radioiodine therapy is used as an adjunct to surgery to treat patients with residual or recurrent papillary cancer in the neck. The prophylactic use of radioactive iodine after surgery reduces the mortality rate and increases survival in such patients.

In order to scan and treat patients with ^{131}I, thyroxine therapy must be withheld for 4 to 6 weeks to allow serum TSH levels to rise. Alternatively, patients can be placed on 25 μg triiodothyronine (liothyronine) twice daily for 1 month instead of thyroxine; then the triiodothyronine is stopped for 2 weeks before administration of ^{131}I. This alternative procedure shortens the period of symptomatic hypothyroidism. Thyroid hormone in a suppressive dose is given after thyroidectomy to reduce thyroid cancer recurrence rates. TSH stimulates thyroid tumors, which contain TSH receptors. The dose of thyroxine should be adjusted to keep the TSH suppressed without causing clinical thyrotoxicosis. The degree of suppression should be based on the staging of the patient. In patients with a good prognosis, TSH should be suppressed to the slightly subnormal range. In patients with worse prognosis, which includes many of the elderly, TSH should be suppressed to less than 0.05 mU/L without causing clinical thyrotoxicosis.

Recombinant human TSH (rhTSH) may be used to stimulate radioiodide uptake in scanning patients with well-differentiated thyroid cancer while they continue to take levothyroxine. This avoids the symptoms of hypothyroidism that occur after withdrawal of levothyroxine. rhTSH stimulates radioiodine uptake and thyroglobulin secretion in normal and abnormal thyroid tissue. A clinical trial comparing 48-hour ^{131}I whole-body scan results showed 89 percent concordance in patients receiving rhTSH, as compared to the withdrawal of levothyroxine therapy. Of the discordant results, 8 percent of scans were superior after levothyroxine withdrawal, while 3 percent were superior after stimulation with rhTSH (no significant difference).

Follicular Thyroid Carcinoma

Follicular thyroid carcinoma accounts for about 5 to 10 percent of all thyroid cancers in the United States. It occurs more frequently in elderly people. Approximately 80 percent of follicular cell neoplasms are benign. Larger follicular cell neoplasms are more likely to be malignant, especially in men and patients older than age 50 years. Follicular thyroid carcinoma is slightly more aggressive than papillary carcinoma. With minimally invasive follicular carcinoma, there is usually invasion of small vessels, whereas with maximally invasive tumors there is vascular and capsular invasion and penetration into the surrounding tissue, causing a poorer prognosis. Hürthle cell carcinoma is considered a variant of follicular thyroid carcinoma and carries an even worse prognosis.

Follicular carcinoma also metastasizes to the lung, bone, central nervous system, and other soft tissues with higher frequency than papillary carcinoma. Tumor recurrence in distant sites is seen more frequently with follicular than with papillary carcinoma and occurs with higher prevalence in highly invasive tumors.

Treatment includes total thyroidectomy and ^{131}I therapy to ablate residual tumor. Radioiodine is the principal treatment of metastatic tumors. If the tumor does not concentrate the isotope, external radiation may be effective. As with papillary carcinoma, thyroxine therapy should be given to suppress serum TSH levels to the subnormal range.

Medullary Thyroid Carcinoma

Medullary carcinoma accounts for 2 to 4 percent of thyroid cancers and is derived from the calcitonin-secreting cells or parafollicular cells. Elevated serum calcitonin levels establish the diagnosis and correlate with tumor mass. Approximately 20 percent are familial tumors and are associated with other endocrine neoplasias (MEN type 2A or 2B). The recognition of point mutations in the *ret* protooncogene on chromosome 10 has enhanced the ability to detect these neoplasms at an early and potentially curable stage in suspected family members. Approximately 80 percent of medullary carcinoma is sporadic and diagnosed later in life, mostly after age 50 years.

Immunohistochemical studies demonstrate the presence of calcitonin in the tumor that is also able to synthesize calcitonin gene-related peptide, ACTH, serotonin, prostaglandin, histamine, and carcinoembryonic antigen. Diarrhea occurs in 30 percent of patients with advanced disease and correlates directly with the tumor mass. Recurrence rate increases in frequency with age. About two-thirds of patients older than age 70 years have persistent disease or a higher recurrence rate after surgery.

Anaplastic Thyroid Carcinoma

Anaplastic carcinoma of the thyroid, the most aggressive and lethal neoplasm, accounts for 2 percent of all thyroid carcinomas. It may be derived from a well-differentiated thyroid carcinoma. The peak occurrence of this tumor is in the seventh decade of life; three-quarters of patients are 60 years of age or older. Treatment includes surgery, followed by external radiation and chemotherapy, which may result in disease-free intervals of 1 to 5 years.

Thyroid Lymphoma

Thyroid lymphoma accounts for about 1 percent of thyroid malignancies. It is always accompanied by chronic lymphocytic thyroiditis. At the time of presentation with lymphoma, the patient is usually older than 60 years of age. There is a female preponderance. This tumor always arises from B-cell lymphocytes. It usually invades the walls of blood vessels and extends outside the thyroid gland. The usual clinical presentation is a rapidly enlarging thyroid mass in a patient with long history of a goiter or diagnosis of Hashimoto's thyroiditis that was treated with thyroid hormone. The patient may complain of neck pressure, local swelling of the thyroid gland, hoarseness, and dysphagia. Fine-needle aspiration may suggest the diagnosis, but

definitive diagnosis usually requires an open biopsy. Surgical removal of the lymphoma by total thyroidectomy is unwise. Treatment with external radiation and four to six courses of chemotherapy nearly always produces a permanent remission.

REFERENCES

AACE/AAES medical/surgical guidelines for clinical practice: Management of thyroid carcinoma. *Endocr Pract* 7:203, 2001.

Bagchi N et al: Thyroid dysfunction in adults over age 55 years. *Arch Intern Med* 150:785, 1990.

Belfiore A et al: Cancer risk in patients with cold thyroid nodules: Relevance of iodine intake, sex, age, and multinodularity. *Am J Med* 363:363, 1992.

Bemben DA et al: Thyroid disease in the elderly: I. Prevalence of undiagnosed hypothyroidism. *J Fam Pract* 38:577, 1994.

Biondi B et al: Cardiac effects of long term thyrotropin-suppressive therapy with levothyroxine. *J Clin Endocrinol Metab* 77:334, 1993.

Cooper DS: Subclinical hypothyroidism. *N Engl J Med* 345:260, 2001.

Hershman JM et al: Serum thyrotropin and thyroid hormone levels in elderly and middle-aged euthyroid persons. *J Am Geriatr Soc* 41:823, 1993.

Kahaly GJ: Cardiovascular and atherogenic aspects of subclinical hypothyroidism. *Thyroid* 10:665, 2000.

Ladenson PW et al: American thyroid association guidelines for detection of thyroid dysfunction. *Arch Intern Med* 160:1573, 2000.

Langton JE, Brent GA: Non-thyroidal illness syndrome: Evaluation of thyroid function in sick patients. *Endocrinol Metab Clin North Am* 31:159, 2002.

Lin JD et al: Characteristics of thyroid carcinomas in aging patients. *Eur J Clin Invest* 30:147, 2000.

Mariotti S et al: Complex alteration of thyroid function in healthy centenarians. *J Clin Endocrinol Metab* 77:1130, 1993.

Mazzaferri EL: Management of a solitary thyroid nodule. *N Engl J Med* 328:553, 1993.

Mazzaferri EL: Using recombinant human TSH in the management of well-differentiated thyroid cancer: Current strategies and future directions. *Thyroid* 10:767, 2000.

Shapiro LE et al: Minimal cardiac effects in asymptomatic athyreotic patients chronically treated with thyrotropin-suppressive doses of L-thyroxine. *J Clin Endocrinol Metab* 82:2592, 1997.

Toft AD: Subclinical hyperthyroidism. *N Engl J Med* 345:512, 2001.

Trivalle C et al: Differences in the signs and symptoms of hyperthyroidism in older and younger patients. *J Am Geriatr Soc* 44:50, 1996.

Wong TK, Hershman JM: Changes in thyroid function in nonthyroid illness. *Trends Endocrinol Metab* 3:8, 1992.

Yamada T et al: Age-related therapeutic response to antithyroid drugs in patients with hyperthyroid Graves' disease. *J Am Geriatr Soc* 42:513, 1994.

Diabetes Mellitus

JEFFREY B. HALTER

Diabetes mellitus is a common metabolic disorder affecting elderly people. Although it is recognized by its effects on carbohydrate metabolism to cause hyperglycemia, diabetes mellitus usually also affects lipid and protein metabolism. With time, effects of diabetes on the cardiovascular system, the kidneys, the retina, and the peripheral nervous system, often referred to as long-term complications of diabetes, substantially increase mortality and morbidity in older adults. In general, diabetes mellitus in older adults is underdiagnosed and undertreated. A growing body of evidence assessing outcomes of interventions and an increasing number of therapeutic options for diabetes management have increased the importance of making a diagnosis and offering appropriate intervention strategies to elderly patients who have this potentially devastating disorder.

DEFINITION AND CLASSIFICATION

Diabetes mellitus is a heterogeneous set of disorders affecting multiple body systems; however, diagnostic criteria are based on documentation of elevated circulating blood glucose levels. Because glucose levels vary during the course of the day, and even in the fasting state form a continuous variable in populations, the definition of a single cut-point that separates normal from abnormal is somewhat arbitrary. The challenge of establishing appropriate diagnostic criteria for elderly subjects is made more difficult by well-described effects of aging on glucose metabolism (summarized later in this chapter in the section on Effects of Aging). Similar to criteria for hypercholesterolemia and hypertension, the diagnostic criteria for diabetes mellitus are based on values that predict poor outcomes in population studies.

Table 67-1 summarizes the currently accepted diagnostic criteria, which were established by an expert panel convened by the American Diabetes Association (ADA) and published in 1997.

Type 1 Diabetes

Type 1 diabetes is a condition characterized by destruction of the insulin-producing beta cells of the endocrine pancreas, resulting in absolute deficiency of insulin.

While evidence of cell-mediated autoimmunity is a hallmark of type 1 diabetes, some patients develop a type 1 diabetes phenotype with evidence of severe insulin deficiency and episodes of diabetic ketoacidosis (DKA) with no detectable autoimmunity. Such individuals have idiopathic type 1 diabetes. Although the incidence of new-onset type 1 diabetes in older adults is very low, effective treatment of type 1 diabetes may prevent or delay the development of long-term complications and increased mortality. Thus, people who develop type 1 diabetes earlier in life may live to old age and therefore become a part of the spectrum of diabetes mellitus in an older adult population.

Type 2 Diabetes

Approximately 90 percent of older adults with diabetes have type 2 diabetes mellitus. Hyperglycemia, often asymptomatic, is the hallmark and DKA is not part of the clinical syndrome. Obesity is often present, and resistance to insulin's metabolic effects is a characteristic feature. Impaired insulin secretion is also part of the picture, but severe absolute insulin deficiency is not. While there is a strong genetic predisposition to development of type 2 diabetes, its etiology is currently unknown and is likely to be highly heterogeneous. The interaction between genetics, lifestyle factors, and aging in the development of type 2 diabetes is discussed later in this chapter in the section on Pathophysiology of Diabetes.

Other Specific Types of Diabetes

The 1997 ADA classification for diabetes mellitus identifies a number of specific conditions that lead to development of diabetes mellitus, each of which is relatively uncommon. One group of disorders includes genetic defects of the pancreatic beta cell. The clinical phenotype for these genetic disorders is maturity-onset diabetes of youth (MODY). These genetic disorders have autosomal dominant inheritance with first presentation of asymptomatic hyperglycemia early in life. Patients with MODY can live to old age, however, and therefore can be a part of the spectrum of diabetes in an elderly population. The metabolic disorder in some affected individuals may be mild, whereas

Table 67-1   1997 American Diabetes Association Diagnostic Criteria for Diabetes Mellitus and Impaired Glucose Tolerance

Diabetes mellitus
  Classic diabetes symptoms plus a random glucose level ≥200 mg/dL (11.1 mmol/L)
  Fasting* glucose level ≥126 mg/dL (7.0 mmol/L)†
  Glucose level ≥200 mg/dL (11.1 mmol/L) at 2 hours during a standard OGTT†

Impaired glucose tolerance (IGT)
  Glucose level ≥140 mg/dL (7.8 mmol/L) and <200 mg/dL (11.1 mmol/L) at 2 hours during a standard OGTT

Impaired fasting glucose (IFG)
  Fasting glucose level ≥110 mg/dL (6.1 mmol/L) and <126 mg/dL (7.0 mmol/L)

OGTT, oral glucose tolerance test.
*No caloric intake for at least 8 hours.
†Either of these criteria should be confirmed on a separate day to establish a diagnosis of diabetes mellitus.

others may develop symptomatic hyperglycemia and long-term complications of diabetes mellitus similar to patients with typical type 2 diabetes. Another type of genetic defect has been identified in a few families in which insulin processing prior to secretion is impaired, which can predispose to development of hyperglycemia.

Other families have genetic defects affecting insulin action. Severe insulin resistance results, and when it is not adequately compensated for by increased insulin secretion, hyperglycemia occurs. Diseases of the exocrine pancreas can lead to damage to pancreatic beta cells, diminished insulin secretion, and hyperglycemia. Hyperglycemia also can occur in patients with excessive secretion of hormones that adversely affect carbohydrate metabolism, such as in acromegaly, Cushing's syndrome, glucagonoma, and pheochromocytoma. Similarly, tumors making aldosterone can cause hyperglycemia as a result of hypokalemia-induced inhibition of insulin secretion. A number of drugs or toxins can impair insulin secretion or insulin action and lead to the development of hyperglycemia. Table 67-2 lists such drugs. Several genetic neuromuscular disorders are associated with diabetes mellitus, but they are rare in the older adult population.

Gestational Diabetes Mellitus

Gestational diabetes mellitus (GDM) is a separate category in the 1997 ADA classification and refers to the first identification of an alteration in glucose metabolism during pregnancy. While GDM per se is not part of the spectrum of diabetes in older adults, a history of GDM may be part of the background of an older woman presenting with type 2 diabetes mellitus. As GDM has been aggressively sought for and treated, increasing numbers of women reaching the geriatric age group will have this history, as GDM complicates approximately 4 percent of all pregnancies in the United States. The hyperglycemia in these individuals generally goes away postpartum, but there is a substantial rate of subsequent development of overt diabetes.

Diagnostic Criteria

The rationale for the circulating glucose level criteria shown in Table 67-1 is based on prediction of risk for diabetes-related complications. Thus, a 2-hour value during the oral glucose tolerance test (OGTT) greater or equal to 200 mg/dL is a strong predictor of diabetes complications, even when the fasting glucose level is less than 126 mg/dL. Individuals who meet the 2-hour OGTT criterion for diabetes but who do not meet the fasting glucose criterion are described as having isolated postchallenge hyperglycemia (IPH).

There is no age adjustment in the recommended criteria for the diagnosis of diabetes mellitus because the same glucose level cut points that predict complications appear to apply regardless of age. There is no current criterion for diagnosis of diabetes mellitus based on measurement of glycosylated hemoglobin, as no level of glycosylated hemoglobin accurately identifies people who meet glucose level diagnostic criteria.

The 1997 ADA criteria shown in Table 67-1 also identifies an intermediate category of altered glucose metabolism

Table 67-2   Drugs That May Increase Glucose Levels

Diuretics

α-Adrenergic agonists

β-Adrenergic blockers

Alcohol

Ca^{2+} channel blockers

Caffeine

Glucocorticoids

Growth hormone

Nicotine

Nicotinic acid

Nonsteroidal antiinflammatory drugs

Oral contraceptives (estrogen/progesterone)

Pentamidine

Phenytoin

to the manifestation and severity of diabetes related complications. Diabetic patients who also have hypertension are at greater risk for renal disease and for macrovascular disease than diabetic patients without hypertension. Similarly, neuropathy is more likely in a diabetic patient who is exposed to a neurotoxic agent.

Presentation

The classical clinical hallmarks of diabetes are symptoms associated with marked hyperglycemia, including polydipsia, polyuria, polyphagia, and weight loss. Patients with type 2 diabetes may present with such symptoms, although it is relatively uncommon for them to do so. With the profound insulin deficiency of type 1 diabetes, mobilization of fatty acids occurs leading to accelerated production of ketoacids, potentially resulting in life-threatening DKA. Although type 1 diabetes usually occurs in early life, it can occur at any age, including first presentation in an elderly patient.

Development of DKA is the classic form of presentation for a patient with type 1 diabetes, but it is now recognized that people with type 1 diabetes may have long periods of abnormal circulating glucose levels before the development of DKA. Furthermore, with early detection of such hyperglycemia and appropriate diabetes management, an episode of DKA might never occur. Older people in particular may be more likely to present with an indolent course of type 1 diabetes.

The most common presentation for type 2 diabetes is from detection of an elevated glucose level on routine laboratory testing of an asymptomatic person. Some of these patients may have sufficient hyperglycemia to cause mild symptoms, while others may have had gradual unexplained weight loss. Because type 2 diabetes may go undetected for years, some older adults first present with symptoms or findings related to diabetes complications, such as visual loss with classic retinopathy on exam, proteinuria, or symptomatic peripheral neuropathy.

EVALUATION

Diabetes mellitus is a complex disorder that can have effects on many body systems, and its treatment may require a complex program including medication plus lifestyle changes. The choice of intervention strategies and the patient's capability to adhere to a diabetes treatment program may be limited by the presence of other health problems, as well as by the patient's living situation, economic status, availability of caregiver support, and the like. A comprehensive geriatric assessment (Chap. 8) is highly appropriate to provide the basis for developing a treatment plan for an older person with diabetes mellitus.

Medical Evaluation

Once a diagnosis of diabetes is established, a thorough medical evaluation is needed. Because the risk for developing diabetes complications is related to the duration of hyperglycemia, effort should be made to pinpoint the time of onset. Unless patients at risk have been followed up carefully with yearly measurement of a fasting glucose level, as currently recommended by the ADA, it may be difficult to establish a time of onset for type 2 diabetes mellitus in a given patient. Because of the usual uncertainty about time of onset, a careful search for existing diabetes complications is warranted even when a new diagnosis is made in an older adult. Such an evaluation is even more justified in a patient with a multiyear history of diabetes mellitus who is establishing a new relationship with a health care system or primary care provider. The evaluation for eye complications of diabetes should be carried out by an ophthalmologist with a detailed retinal examination, as early signs of diabetic retinopathy can easily be missed.

Evaluation of diabetic nephropathy should include a screening serum creatinine level. An elevated serum creatinine is a poor prognostic sign, suggesting that substantial kidney damage has already occurred and that an irreversible course of progressive renal insufficiency has already started. Depending on the patient's overall situation, referral to a nephrologist may be warranted to assess other potential causes of renal insufficiency. Urine screening for proteinuria should be carried out to detect earlier stages of diabetic nephropathy that are amenable to intervention. A positive qualitative urine for protein (dipstick method) indicates gross proteinuria. If confirmed on repeat testing, this finding in itself is an indication for treatment intervention. However, a negative qualitative urine protein test does not rule out early diabetic nephropathy. If the qualitative dipstick test is negative, a spot urine sample should be sent for quantitative measurement of urine protein and creatinine. A value greater than 30 mg/g, often referred to as microalbuminuria, suggests early diabetic nephropathy. Such a test should be repeated twice in subsequent months for confirmation. If two of three tests are positive, intervention is warranted.

A careful neurologic examination should be carried out for signs of diabetic neuropathy. This examination should include monofilament testing. This is a qualitative test with a 10-g nylon monofilament carried out at different points along the foot with simple yes or no responses by the patient about feeling the pressure of the monofilament. Vibration sense should also be tested with a tuning fork. This neuropathy evaluation should be carried out in conjunction with a careful foot examination to identify possible structural abnormalities that might contribute to risk for skin breakdown and damage.

The medical evaluation of an older patient with diabetes should also include information about other coexisting risk factors including hypertension, hyperlipidemia, and use of cigarettes. These conditions interact with diabetes to increase risk of adverse cardiovascular events and therefore need to be addressed in an overall patient management program. Blood pressure should be assessed both in the supine position and with upright posture, as an orthostatic drop in blood pressure may be another marker of diabetic neuropathy and is often associated with supine hypertension. The genitourinary system should also be assessed, as patients with diabetes may be prone to bladder dysfunction associated with autonomic neuropathy, thereby increasing risk for urinary tract infection and kidney damage. Sexual dysfunction has been reported in a high percentage of older men with diabetes, suggesting an interaction between aging, neuropathy, and vascular disease in this population.

A thorough evaluation of the cardiovascular system also should be carried out, given the high rate of vascular disease in older people with diabetes mellitus. The history and physical examination should carefully assess evidence for cerebrovascular disease, coronary heart disease, and peripheral vascular disease. Suggestive history or physical findings should be documented with more in-depth testing including Doppler evaluation for carotid artery stenosis or extremity blood flow, or cardiovascular stress testing if there is any suggestion of coronary artery disease. Silent ischemia and myocardial infarction appear to be more common in people with diabetes mellitus. Thus, the threshold for stress testing should be rather low.

The drug history of an older patient with diabetes is important both to identify drug therapy that may be contributing to the patient's hyperglycemia (see Table 67-2), as well as to identify potential drug interactions that may affect diabetes management. The initial assessment should also include a diet history, a review of potential nutritional problems, and an oral health assessment, as dietary intervention is a key component of a treatment program for virtually all patients with diabetes. The assistance of a nutritionist who has a particular interest in diabetes is often very helpful for this part of the evaluation. Particular attention should be paid to dietary habits, ethnic food preferences, and meal patterns.

Other Evaluation Components

Diabetes Knowledge

Because of the complexity of diabetes management, usually requiring both lifestyle and medication interventions, the patient or caregivers must be actively involved in their own care and take responsibility for its many aspects. It is particularly important to review the patient's knowledge base regarding diabetes and its complications. Standardized diabetes knowledge tests are available, or an interview with a diabetes educator or suitably trained nurse can establish the status of the patient's knowledge base. The diabetes education program that becomes part of the treatment plan can then provide this base for new patients or fill in needed gaps for existing patients.

Functional Status

A review of activities of daily living and instrumental activities of daily living should also be a part of comprehensive assessment of an elderly patient with diabetes mellitus. Diabetes puts the patient at increased risk for functional deficits. Such functional limitations must also be considered in developing a diabetes treatment program. In addition to general assessment of functional status, the ability of the patient and caregiver to carry out diabetes-specific functional tasks needs to be evaluated. For example, the ability

to carry out home glucose monitoring or self-injection of insulin requires certain functional abilities.

Cognitive and Psychosocial Status

Given the complexity of diabetes management programs, an assessment of a patient's cognitive status is essential to developing an appropriate treatment plan. A screening cognitive test should be carried out, with more detailed testing as indicated by the screening test or a history of cognitive decline. Cognitive function may be affected directly by diabetes as a result of cerebrovascular disease, postulated direct effects of hyperglycemia to cause subtle impairments of cognition, as well as by diabetes treatment, which can result in hypoglycemia. Complex cognitive skills are required for a number of aspects of diabetes treatment. Similarly, the presence of other psychiatric disorders such as depression or bipolar disorder could have a major impact on the decision about diabetes treatment interventions.

The patient's socioeconomic and living situation can also have an important impact on the diabetes treatment plan. The availability of caregivers in the home or nearby can compensate for some limitations in the patient's self-care abilities and influence lifestyle factors that can affect diabetes management. Economic issues may affect the patient's ability to adhere to a costly medical regimen, and cultural influences may need to be considered as a treatment plan is developed. The availability of a social worker or suitably trained nurse to assist in this aspect of the patient evaluation can be extremely helpful.

Overall Health Status

The presence of other medical problems needs to be documented, as decisions about the extent of intervention for diabetes need to be put in the context of the patient's overall health situation, disease burden, and prognosis in terms of functional status and estimated longevity. The presence of a coexisting illness such as congestive heart failure or uncontrolled cancer, which would substantially limit a patient's future life expectancy, will influence the decision about intensity of diabetes management.

DIABETES MANAGEMENT

General Approach

The first key step in developing a diabetes management program for an elderly patient is to establish the treatment goals. The overall treatment goal of a basic diabetes care plan is to prevent metabolic decompensation and to control other risk factors that may contribute to long-term complications in any patient with diabetes. Control of hyperglycemia as a means to reduce what some have termed glucose toxicity as a contributing factor to long-term diabetes complications is one part of an overall strategy of risk reduction. Such a strategy must also include intensive effort at identifying and controlling hypertension, lipid disorders, and cigarette smoking (also see Chap. 6). Thus,

Table 67-4   Factors to Consider in Setting a Diabetes Treatment Goal for Elderly Patients

Patient's estimated remaining life expectancy

Patient's preference and commitment

Beliefs of the primary care provider (e.g., whether glycemic control can prevent complications)

Availability of social support and services

Economic issues

Coexisting health problems

Major psychiatric disorder
Major cognitive disorder
Diabetes complications
Major limitation of diabetes functional status

Complexity of medical regimen

a complex, multifaceted treatment program is important for many older patients with diabetes.

It may be neither feasible nor appropriate to attempt to achieve such a complex diabetes management program for some patients. Table 67-4 lists some of the factors to consider when deciding whether to strive for a treatment goal designed to minimize risk for diabetes complications. It is true that a limited remaining life expectancy shortens the time for long-term complications to develop and progress. Given the increasing life expectancy of older adults, only the very oldest segment of the population or those with coexisting illness that markedly shortens remaining life expectancy should be excluded from consideration for an aggressive treatment program. For example, it would be hard to justify abandoning risk reduction goals in an otherwise healthy 75-year-old woman with a recent diagnosis of diabetes mellitus, as such a person's remaining life expectancy may be 15 years or more. Given the complexity of treatment programs designed to minimize diabetes risks, the commitment on the part of an adequately informed patient is clearly critical. Availability of a supportive environment including a strong diabetes treatment team and adequate economic support for an intensive treatment program are also important. Such a treatment goal is also difficult to achieve without commitment of the health care team, which must believe that achievement of the treatment goal will really make a difference in the patient's long-term health.

Any decision about an intensive treatment program must take into account coexisting conditions and the overall complexity of the patient's medical regimen. For example, the existence of advanced diabetes complications in an elderly patient may provide a rationale for less strict control of hyperglycemia. A significant psychiatric or cognitive disorder may also preclude an intensive management program. On the other hand, some older adults are able to devote a substantial amount of time to their own health care and are able to manage complex multidrug interventions

for multiple health problems. Based on the initial comprehensive patient assessment as described here, many older adults with diabetes may fit in a category for which an intensive treatment goal is appropriate.

Management of Cardiovascular Risk Factors

Management of hypertension and abnormal lipid metabolism is discussed in Chaps. 40 and 68, respectively. Because of the high risk status of patients with diabetes, a target goal of 130/85 for blood pressure control is advocated in the *Sixth Report of the Joint National Committee on Detection, Evaluation and Treatment of High Blood Pressure* and a goal of 130/80 is recommended by the ADA. As described in Chap. 68, many diabetic patients have a dyslipidemia, requiring that attention be paid to triglycerides as well as cholesterol levels. Diabetes is considered a cardiac disease equivalent. Thus, an aggressive target for intervention (low-density lipoprotein [LDL] cholesterol <100 mg/dL) is recommended by the ADA and the National Cholesterol Education Program (NCEP), even in the absence of a known cardiac history.

Use of aspirin reduces cardiovascular risk in patients with diabetes. Thus, older patients with diabetes should be treated with one aspirin per day unless there is a contraindication. Alternative approaches may be developed to reduction of systemic glucose toxicity other than simply lowering circulating glucose levels. There have been efforts to develop drugs that inhibit formation of advanced glycosylation end products, although none are yet available clinically. In addition, aldose reductase inhibitors have been tested and continue to be under investigation.

Prevention of Microvascular Complications

Angiotensin-converting enzyme (ACE) inhibitors and angiotensin receptor blockers reduce the rate of progression from microalbuminuria to overt proteinuria and diabetic nephropathy. An ACE inhibitor or angiotensin receptor blocker should be added to a treatment program for any patient who has evidence of nephropathy. Also, rigorous blood pressure control is particularly important for such individuals.

Laser therapy reduces the rate of visual loss in patients with diabetic retinopathy. Thus, early detection is critical. Despite clear evidence of efficacy of retinopathy screening by ophthalmologic examination and appropriate intervention, only 50 percent or fewer of diabetes patients receive recommended annual screening for retinopathy.

Other Diabetes Complications

Prevention of amputation in older people with diabetes requires careful attention to peripheral vascular disease, neuropathy, and foot care. While microvascular disease and peripheral neuropathy may contribute to skin damage and impaired healing, it is clear that patients with diabetes can benefit from treatment of large vessel disease, which is the

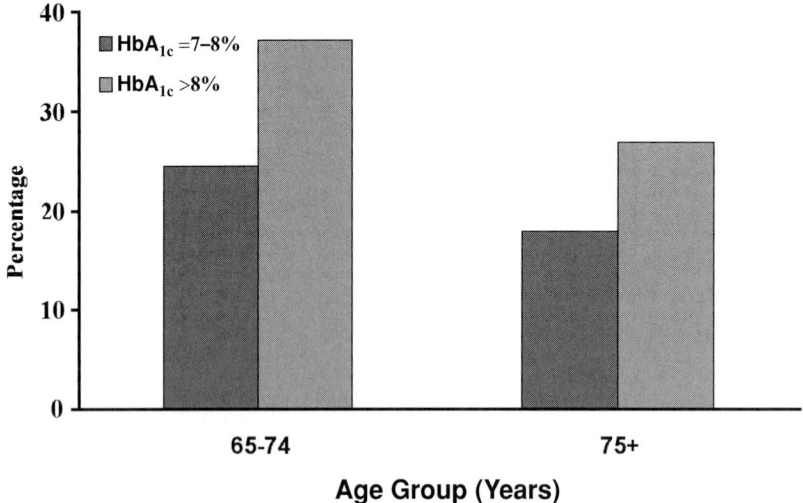

Figure 67-5 Percentage of elderly diabetes patients in NHANES III who did not achieve the level of hemoglobin A_{1c}(HbA$_{1c}$) recommended by the American Diabetes Association (HbA$_{1c}$>7 percent). Patients were analyzed by age group and according to whether their HbA$_{1c}$ was in the range at which the ADA recommends therapeutic action (>8 percent) or not (7 to 8 percent). Adapted from Shorr RI et al: Glycemic control of older adults with type 2 diabetes: Findings from the Third National Health and Nutrition Examination Survey, 1988–1994. *J Am Geriatr Soc* 48:264, 2000.

primary factor responsible for lower-extremity ischemia in people with diabetes mellitus. As the development of neuropathy is insidious, patients should be instructed to examine their feet carefully on a daily basis, and a foot examination should be a routine part of a diabetes clinic visit. Although there is no current therapeutic approach to reduce the rate of development of neuropathy other than reducing glucose levels toward normal, a number of drugs are under development that target neuropathy.

Painful neuropathy is a common complication of diabetes and may be very difficult to manage. A range of therapeutic options are available, none of which are particularly satisfactory. Pain management should start with acetaminophen, as it is least likely to cause harmful side effects. Opioid analgesics may be necessary at times. Nonsteroidal antiinflammatory drugs may also be helpful, but these should be avoided in patients with diabetic nephropathy who are being treated with an ACE inhibitor. Other drugs that have been used include tricyclic antidepressants, Dilantin, and locally administered capsaicin cream.

Management of Hyperglycemia

A major challenge in diabetes management is to set a treatment goal for hyperglycemia. One target that has been set by the ADA is a fasting glucose less than 120 mg/dL and a hemoglobin $A_{1C} \leq 7\%$. Such a treatment goal of near normoglycemia is based on the concept that its achievement will markedly reduce, if not eliminate, the risk for diabetes complications. The ADA's recommendation is broad and not limited to a specific type of diabetes or to any age group. Because of the difficulty in measuring the rates of these complications and the long time it takes for them to develop, a detailed picture of the relationship between

the degree of hyperglycemia and rate of development of complication has not been completed. A growing body of evidence from studies such as the National Institutes of Health's Diabetes Control and Complications Trial in people with type 1 diabetes and the United Kingdom Prospective Diabetes Study in people with type 2 diabetes has established that intensive diabetes management designed to achieve near normal glucose levels can reduce the rate of development of the microvascular complications of diabetes. At this point there is also no evidence that the fundamental mechanisms contributing to diabetes complications differ between type 1 and type 2 diabetes. Until further information becomes available, the recommendations of the ADA seem reasonable for many elderly patients. Unfortunately, as in other patient groups, only a minority of older people with diabetes achieve these goals for hyperglycemia treatment, as illustrated in Figure 67-5.

Regardless of whether a decision is made to try to prevent diabetes complications with intensive hyperglycemia management, a basic set of objectives should be part of the treatment plan for virtually all patients with diabetes. Metabolic decompensation with weight loss, muscle wasting, and a catabolic state is unlikely to occur if the average circulating glucose level is in the range of 200 mg/dL. This seems like a reasonable target goal for basic diabetes care. Such a goal translates to a fasting glucose level in the range of 160 mg/dL and a hemoglobin A_{1c} value of 8–9 percent.

Basic Care

All patients with diabetes should receive a basic diabetes education about what diabetes is; what the long-term complications are and the importance of periodic evaluation for them; as well as basic lifestyle modifications that can improve risk and assist with diabetes management, including basic principles of diet and exercise. Basic diabetes care should include yearly follow-up and reevaluation for the development of diabetes complications, and intervention for those complications as appropriate. Recognition and treatment of hypoglycemia should also be part of the basic diabetes education program for any patient treated with insulin or a sulfonylurea drug.

Aggressive Care

Individuals who are selected for an aggressive treatment program should also receive all aspects of basic diabetes care. While the ADA recommended treatment goal of achieving a hemoglobin A_{1c} of 7 percent may require considerable effort and attention, it is important not to forget about aggressive detection and treatment of hypertension, dyslipidemia, and cigarette smoking. Regular monitoring for diabetes complications and institution of complication-specific interventions should also be carried out. In addition to basic diabetes education, the patient participating in an aggressive treatment program should be trained to carry out home blood glucose monitoring on a regular basis and should become familiar with various treatment approaches for hyperglycemia including diet, exercise, and medications. Such patients should participate in a formal diabetes education program to cover this material thoroughly. Access to a multidisciplinary diabetes care team should be part of an aggressive treatment program.

Specific Interventions for Hyperglycemia

A decision about setting a goal for either basic diabetes care or an aggressive treatment program should be made for each older person with diabetes. Once this decision has been made, a growing range of therapeutic options enables the diabetes treatment program to be individualized according to the specific situation of the individual patient, as determined in part by the initial comprehensive assessment carried out.

Diet

Dietary intervention has long been a cornerstone of diabetes management. Fundamental to any dietary recommendation is ensuring that essential dietary needs are met with adequate provision of vitamins and minerals. Over the years, dietary supplements have been proposed to assist in diabetes treatment such as vitamins C, E, or B complex, or minerals such as zinc or chromium to replace possible diabetes-related losses, thereby improving the metabolic state and possibly reducing the rate of various complications. There is, however, no convincing evidence that any of these dietary supplements improves diabetes control or influences diabetes complications. Two aspects of diet need to be addressed in any dietary program: the total caloric intake, which is a key to maintenance of body weight or weight reduction; and dietary composition, or the distribution of fat, carbohydrate, and protein calories.

Caloric Intake   Caloric restriction is usually part of the initial approach to management of overweight patients with diabetes mellitus. Because it is generally desirable to maintain muscle and bone mass, the target of caloric restriction is reduction in adiposity, particularly the central adiposity that seems to be critical in mediating obesity-related insulin resistance. One criterion for obesity is a BMI of 30 kg/m². A serious effort at weight reduction should be considered for any patient with a BMI in excess of 30. A BMI greater than 25 is used as a marker of overweight and may also be an indication for caloric restriction. As reviewed in Chap. 91, because of an age-related decline in lean body mass, older individuals may have increased adiposity and central adiposity without being overweight by usual BMI criteria. Documentation of central adiposity by waist measurement or computed tomography may suggest a role for caloric restriction in such individuals. Relatively normal-weight people with central adiposity likely already have diminished lean body mass, which will be further threatened by caloric restriction. For individuals who are not overweight and who do not have central adiposity, there is no role for caloric restriction as part of the diabetes treatment program.

Although many types of diets are successful in the short-term in achieving weight reduction, long-term maintenance of weight reduction continues to be a major challenge. Some individuals are able to lose a significant amount of weight and maintain it. Therefore patients should be offered assistance with caloric restriction and supported for a weight loss program. In general, behavioral modification to change dietary habits is the most successful approach long-term. Relatively modest weight reduction can have a significant impact on the degree of insulin resistance and on control of glucose levels. Part of the approach should be to set a realistic goal of no more than 5 to 10 percent reduction of body weight, even if that will not achieve a normal BMI of less than 25 kg/m². The role for medications to assist weight loss in an older person with diabetes mellitus is uncertain. With the current explosion of knowledge about regulation of food intake in relation to obesity, it is likely that new medications will appear on the market to assist in weight reduction. These should be integrated into diet treatment if justified by results of clear studies of efficacy and risks in an older adult population, evidence lacking to date for any pharmacological weight loss agent.

Diet Composition   The average American diet includes approximately 45 percent of calories as carbohydrate, 40 percent as fat, and 15 percent as protein. Current recommendations by the ADA are consistent with those of the American Heart Association and other groups, all of which recommend a diet relatively low in fat (approximately 25 to 30 percent of calories from fat). This recommendation for patients with diabetes especially makes sense given the very high rate of atherosclerosis-related complications in this patient population. Given the limited ability to increase protein content in the diet, a reduction in fat intake means an increase in carbohydrate intake to 60 to 65 percent of total calories. It could be argued that increasing carbohydrate intake may adversely affect diabetes control by increasing circulating glucose levels postprandially. While this could happen in theory, it appears as though such a change in carbohydrate intake generally has little affect on overall glucose control, particularly in patients who are receiving hypoglycemic drug treatment as well. A diet relatively low in cholesterol and saturated fat should also be considered, consistent with a heart healthy type of diet. There should not be any conflict in diet prescription if there is coexisting dyslipidemia that needs management as well. The recommendation for dietary composition for patients with diabetes is not designed to improve control of hyperglycemia, but is more oriented toward prevention of cardiovascular complications.

Consistency of dietary intake in terms of meal composition and timing is particularly an issue in patients treated with insulin. The ADA's diet exchange program is one means of providing guidance to such patients to maintain consistency of dietary intake. Nutritional counseling can be particularly helpful in assisting patients to adhere to a dietary program.

Dietary Issues in Older People   As summarized in Table 67-5, there are a number of special issues to consider in dietary management of older adults with diabetes. Older adults with a significant mobility limitation may be relatively inactive and have low caloric utilization. Thus, caloric intake may need to be limited to rather low levels to achieve significant weight reduction. The potential benefit of caloric restriction and weight reduction under such circumstances needs to be balanced against the potential risk for complications related to undernutrition. Such patients also may have difficulty with access to food both in terms of food preparation and shopping to bring food in. Furthermore, dietary habits established for a lifetime and often with a cultural background may be particularly difficult to modify. Older persons, especially men living alone, may have limited food preparation skills. The presence of impaired cognitive function may make following a dietary prescription particularly difficult. Any of these issues can be modified if there is sufficient caregiver support and/or social services that can assist with providing meals in the home setting.

Problems with taste and oral health, which are common in older people, may further limit adaptation to a prescribed diet. Oral health problems can be exacerbated by diabetes, which may increase the rate of periodontal disease. This may be a growing issue as more older adults are keeping their teeth for longer periods. Xerostomia is also more common in older people owing to decreased salivary gland flow, sometimes exacerbated by coexisting medication use.

Exercise

An exercise program may be an important adjunct to diabetes management. By increasing caloric expenditure, an exercise program can facilitate the effectiveness of a weight reduction program for overweight people with diabetes mellitus. It may also help prevent reaccumulation of weight following caloric-restriction facilitated weight loss. Simple increases of physical activity, such as with stretching exercises or walking, while potentially useful to improve overall functional capability, will have only a very modest effect

Table 67-5   Dietary Therapy: Special Considerations for Older Adults with Diabetes Mellitus

Access to food
Functional disability
Poor meal preparation skills
Lack of formal or informal support to obtain food
Limited financial resources
Food intake
Decline in taste and smell appreciation
Poor dentition and/or xerostomia
Ingrained dietary habits
Past experience and ethnic food preference
Impaired cognitive function

on total caloric expenditure. There is, however, a growing body of evidence that exercise training can also enhance sensitivity to insulin by improving insulin-mediated glucose uptake. Thus, exercise training may have a beneficial affect beyond simply enhancing the effectiveness of a weight reduction program. Furthermore, patients with diabetes may benefit from the effects of exercise training to enhance cardiovascular function, lower blood pressure, and improve the lipid profile. A more detailed discussion of the effects of exercise training in older individuals is provided in Chap. 72.

Exercise training alone has not had consistent effects to improve circulating glucose levels in patients with diabetes mellitus. For all the reasons just indicated, exercise may be a useful adjunct to drug therapy and may well contribute to enhanced effectiveness of glucose-lowering agents. Given the high prevalence of coronary artery disease in older patients with diabetes mellitus, which may be asymptomatic or atypical in symptoms, it is important for such patients to have medically supervised stress testing before entering any challenging exercise training program. An additional issue to consider in an older person is the potential for foot and joint injury with upright exercise such as jogging. Particular attention should be given to the foot examination in an older person prior to and during the course of exercise training. Finally, because of its effects to enhance glucose uptake by muscle, exercise training may contribute to risk for hypoglycemia in patients treated with hypoglycemic agents. Issues related to hypoglycemia in older patients with diabetes are discussed in more detail later in the section on Hypoglycemia in this chapter.

Oral Agents

A growing number of oral medications are available for management of older adults with diabetes mellitus. Table 67-6 lists the available drugs and summarizes some of the dosage and mechanism of action information. As the different classes of drugs have different mechanisms of action, there is increasing opportunity to individualize therapy as

Table 67-6 Oral Agents for the Management of Diabetes Mellitus

Generic Name	Brand Name	Usual Daily Dose	Mechanism of Action
Sulfonylureas (Second Generation)			Enhance insulin secretion
Glimepiride	Amaryl	1–8 mg once	
Glipizide	Glucotrol	10–20 mg once or divided	
Glipizide, sustained release	Glucotrol XL	5–20 mg once or divided	
Glyburide	Diabeta, Micronase	2.5–20 mg once or divided	
Glyburide, micronized	Glynase	1.5–12 mg once or divided	
α-Glucosidase inhibitors			Decrease glucose absorption
Acarbose	Precose	25–100 mg tid	
Miglitol	Glyset	25–100 mg tid	
Biguanide			Decrease hepatic glucose production
Metformin	Glucophage	1500–2550 mg divided	
Thiazolidinediones			Enhance insulin sensitivity
Pioglitazone	Actose	15–45 mg once	
Rosiglitazone	Avandia	2–8 mg once or divided	
Meglitinide			Enhance insulin secretion
Repaglinide	Prandin	0.5–2 mg tid (before meals)	
D-Phenylalanine Derivative			Enhance insulin secretion
Nateglinide	Starlix	60–120 mg tid (before meals)	

more is learned about the heterogeneity of type 2 diabetes. All of these oral agents are effective in lowering glucose levels in clinical trials of patients with type 2 diabetes mellitus. Some of them may also assist in lowering glucose levels as an adjunct to insulin therapy in patients with type 1 diabetes. The effectiveness of these agents must be considered in relation to the treatment goal set for the patient. For example, these agents are frequently successful in achieving the basic goal of hyperglycemia management; that is, to achieve an average glucose level in the range of 200 mg/dL and avoid the catabolic effects associated with very poor diabetes control. These drugs have been much less successful in achieving the goals of aggressive hyperglycemia therapy, that is, a Hgb A_{1c} ≤7% and a fasting glucose level close to the normal range. In fact, even in carefully conducted clinical trials of relatively short duration, only a minority of patients with type 2 diabetes are able to achieve such rigorous goals for hyperglycemia management with one of these agents alone or even in combination. Thus, a therapeutic trial of one or more of these agents for older patients who have not achieved their goal for hyperglycemia management with lifestyle modifications in diet and exercise is warranted. Such therapeutic trials should be instituted over a limited time frame without losing sight of the overall therapeutic goal. For the substantial number of patients for whom such a trial does not successfully achieve the treatment goal, both the patient and health provider team should be prepared to move forward to a more aggressive regimen including treatment with insulin.

Sulfonylurea Drugs Sulfonylurea drugs have been on the market for many years and have been historically the predominant oral agents used in the elderly diabetes population. As first-generation sulfonylureas are now rarely used (and chlorpropamide is relatively contraindicated in older people), Table 67-6 only includes second-generation agents. Because of their long history, there is a substantial body of knowledge about the mechanism of action and side-effect profile of sulfonylureas. Their primary mechanism of action is to enhance insulin secretion by the beta cells of the endocrine pancreas. Indeed, there is a sulfonylurea receptor on pancreatic beta cells that is closely linked to the signaling mechanism for glucose-induced insulin secretion. There is also some evidence that sulfonylurea drug treatment can enhance sensitivity to insulin in peripheral tissues. While enhancement of insulin action may be a direct effect of sulfonylureas on peripheral tissues, it is more likely that improved sensitivity to insulin is secondary to lowering of glucose levels, as hyperglycemia per se appears to contribute to insulin resistance in patients with diabetes mellitus.

Sulfonylurea drugs have established a long record of safety, with hypoglycemia being the main side effect about which to be concerned. Glyburide has been associated with hypoglycemia in older people; however, it is also the sulfonylurea most frequently prescribed and is somewhat more potent than the other agents. These drugs should not be used in patients with renal insufficiency or with significant liver disease, as they depend on the liver for metabolism and the kidney for excretion. Hyponatremia has also been observed as a complication in some patients. Because of similar risk with use of thiazide diuretics, the combination of thiazide and sulfonylurea drugs should be avoided if hyponatremia is a concern.

α-**Glucosidase Inhibitors**   These agents work by inhibiting the key gastrointestinal (GI) enzyme responsible for breakdown of carbohydrates prior to absorption. They are particularly helpful to reduce postprandial increases of glucose levels and may be a useful adjunct to therapy with other agents. The major side effect is local to the GI tract because these drugs are not absorbed to any significant degree; however, 20 to 30 percent of patients may develop diarrhea. To some degree, this may be a welcome side effect in some elderly people with chronic constipation, and other patients may tolerate it without much discomfort.

Biguanide   Metformin appears to work primarily by suppressing hepatic glucose production. Increased hepatic glucose production is an important contributing factor to fasting hyperglycemia in patients with diabetes mellitus. The precise mechanism by which metformin affects the liver is unknown, and there is some evidence for a small effect of metformin to enhance peripheral sensitivity to insulin as well. Metformin has a different mode of action that complements the other classes of drugs available. The most common side effect of metformin is some GI discomfort, which in some patients can be associated with decreased appetite and modest weight loss. While some have viewed this as a potential benefit for a patient on a weight-reduction program, this effect needs to be balanced against the degree of symptoms and the appropriateness of decreased caloric intake and weight loss in a given individual. The biguanide class of drugs is also known to be associated with development of life-threatening lactic acidosis under some circumstances. Although this complication appears to be rare in patients using metformin, this drug should be avoided in situations that may put people at risk for development of lactic acidosis. The drug should not be used in patients with chronic congestive heart failure, and it should be withheld during acute hospitalization for any major illness that could result in decreased tissue perfusion as a precipitating factor for lactic acidosis. Metformin also should be avoided in patients with significant liver disease or renal insufficiency (a creatinine level >1.5 mg/dL).

Thiazolidinediones   This class of drugs appears to work primarily by enhancing peripheral tissue sensitivity to insulin, although the specific molecular mechanism is not known. This mechanism of action complements that of the other drug classes available. As peripheral resistance to insulin is a key part of the metabolic syndrome that predisposes to development of diabetes, use of a drug that targets this abnormality is attractive. These drugs have been well tolerated in initial clinical trials that have included older adults. One disadvantage is economic, as this is the most expensive class of drugs available and widely used for treatment of diabetes mellitus. As one thiazolidinedione, troglitazone, was withdrawn from the market because of rare cases of severe hepatic toxicity, these drugs should not be used in patients with preexisting liver disease, and any patient treated with one of these drugs should have periodic monitoring of liver enzymes. These drugs may cause fluid retention and so should not be used in patients with heart failure.

Meglitinides   Repaglinide enhances insulin secretion, but by a mechanism that differs from the sulfonylureas. Repaglinide acts rapidly to enhance insulin secretion, and is designed to be used immediately before meals. It is of moderate potency and is currently expensive. No specific information is yet available regarding its use in older patients. If used as additive therapy with sulfonylureas, repaglinide could presumably increase the risk of hypoglycemia. The role of repaglinide in older diabetes patients awaits further clinical use and testing.

D-**Phenylalanine Derivative**   Nateglinide acts directly on pancreatic beta cells to rapidly stimulate insulin secretion. Because of the rapid onset and short duration of action, it was developed to address mealtime needs for insulin secretion. It is to be taken shortly before a meal at a standard dose of 120 mg, although a 60 mg dose is also available. Because of the glucose level dependency of its effect on insulin secretion and its short duration of action, its use has been associated with a low rate of hypoglycemia when used alone or in combination with other agents such as metformin. There are currently no known drug interactions and nateglinide can be used in patients with renal insufficiency.

Combination Therapy   Combinations of these oral agents or a combination of one of these agents with insulin are theoretically attractive because of the different modes of action of the various classes of drugs. Thus combination therapy addresses various aspects of the pathophysiology of hyperglycemia in diabetes, offering the possibility of synergism in therapeutic efficacy without synergism in toxicity. Overall, the effects of such combinations are additive.

For elderly patients, the logic of combination therapy must be balanced against incremental costs and incremental risks of side effects with each additional drug. Furthermore, the potential for polypharmacy for multiple coexisting conditions such as hypertension, hyperlipidemia, osteoarthritis, and coronary artery disease needs to be considered. The overall treatment goal for the patient must also be kept in mind. Adding a second or even third oral agent without achieving the target goal of near normoglycemia must still be considered a failure of oral agent therapy and an indication to proceed to use of insulin.

Insulin

Use of insulin is required in patients with type 1 diabetes mellitus. Insulin is also often used in patients with type 2 diabetes either as a primary hypoglycemic agent or to maintain reasonable glucose control in the hospital setting during acute stressful illness or in the perioperative period when oral agents may be less acceptable or useful.

Advantages of Insulin   There are now more than 75 years of clinical experience with use of insulin since its discovery in 1922 and the dramatic demonstration of its effectiveness to save lives of patients with type 1 diabetes in DKA. Many formulations of insulin with varying duration of action allow individualization of treatment plans. Insulin is the natural hormone that is deficient in relative or absolute terms in diabetes, so its use fits with the overall concept of hormone replacement for endocrine deficiency syndromes. Virtually all forms of insulin currently in use are identical to human insulin or with only slight molecular modifications, so the incidence of allergic reactions is very small. There are virtually no known drug interactions, at least from a pharmacokinetic point of view, and virtually no absolute contraindications to insulin use.

With appropriate dosage modification and monitoring of glucose levels, insulin can be used safely for patients with renal or hepatic insufficiency, patients unable to eat, and during major illness. Insulin itself is relatively inexpensive, although the overall program of insulin treatment, including frequent glucose monitoring, may become expensive. While appropriate insulin use can be a complex challenge, it encourages active self-care by the patient and/or caregivers. Finally, and perhaps most important from the point of view of achieving treatment objectives, insulin can effectively lower glucose levels in virtually any patient and in sufficient dosage has at least the potential to normalize circulating glucose levels if the regimen intensity is sufficient.

Disadvantages of Insulin   One major disadvantage of insulin is that it requires injection to be effective. While an intensive effort has been devoted to development of inhaled or orally available forms, these are not yet approved for use. Injection may represent an insurmountable psychological barrier for a small number of patients. For others, insulin injections may not be feasible owing to functional limitations or insufficient caregiver support. Many older adults can, however, be trained to use insulin appropriately. Insulin is a potent agent, and the dose must be carefully measured to minimize risk of hypoglycemia. Accidental overdosage is a risk. The most common issue to address with insulin management is risk for hypoglycemia, which is discussed in more detail later in the chapter in the section on Hypoglycemia.

A range of therapeutic options is available for insulin, which can make a treatment program complex. If, however, a basic hyperglycemia treatment program is the goal for the patient, this can often be achieved with a single injection a day or two injections of intermediate-acting insulin in a patient with type 2 diabetes. Patients with type 1 diabetes may need three or four injections a day with mixtures of intermediate-acting and short-acting insulins to achieve even a basic treatment goal. Some patients with type 2 diabetes can also achieve an aggressive management goal with one or two injections of intermediate-acting insulin per day as long as a sufficient overall dose is provided. Mixtures of short- and intermediate-acting insulin, as well as increased frequency of insulin dosing, may be needed to meet an aggressive treatment goal in some patients with type 2 diabetes.

Newer, modified insulin preparations may help to target therapy. Insulin glargine (Lantus) is modified to slow degradation. It has a stable time course of action over 24 hours, so can be given once daily for basal insulin replacement. Insulin aspart (NovoLog) or insulin lispro (Humalog) were developed as agents with a very rapid onset of action and short duration. These insulins are used

for injection prior to meals and are less likely to result in postmeal hypoglycemia than is longer-acting regular insulin. Thus a combination of once-daily insulin glargine plus premeal injections of short-acting insulin may be used for intensive hyperglycemia management, with potentially similar results as with use of a subcutaneous insulin pump system delivering a continuous insulin infusion plus bolus injections prior to meals.

Initiation of Insulin Therapy   In developing an insulin treatment regimen for an older adult, it is useful to keep in mind a target total dose range per 24 hours, even though the initial starting dose may be substantially lower. An estimate of 0.5 to 1.0 units per kilogram for a thin patient with type 1 diabetes and 1.0 to 2.0 units per kilogram for a typical type 2 diabetes patient with insulin resistance represent reasonable targets. Of course, there will be substantial variation among individuals in total dose needed, depending on the target treatment goal, patient adherence to lifestyle modification recommendations, degree of insulin resistance, and individual variation of insulin dose pharmacokinetic patterns. Thus, a low starting dose of a single injection of intermediate-acting insulin 10 to 20 units per day before breakfast, depending on the degree of obesity, is reasonable. Initiation of insulin treatment is usually done as an outpatient and in conjunction with a diabetes education program for the patient and family members.

Frequent follow-up should be provided initially to ensure that the treatment program is progressing smoothly and that hypoglycemia does not occur early on. Given the metabolic stability of most older patients with type 2 diabetes, there is no need to escalate the insulin dose rapidly. Doses can be adjusted in 3- to 5-unit increments every 3 to 5 days while glucose levels are being monitored. Patients should be prepared from the outset to progress to at least two injections per day, although some patients may achieve the treatment goal with a single dose. Once the single morning dose reaches approximately 40 units per day, it is wise to add a second dose administered before the evening meal.

As insulin doses continue to be gradually adjusted upward, an obese patient with type 2 diabetes may need a total well in excess of 100 units per day to achieve an aggressive treatment goal. Also, as doses are increased, it makes sense to include a combination of short-acting insulin with intermediate-acting insulin to help cover meal-related increases of glucose levels. It is also wise to set a target of approximately 6 months to achieve an aggressive treatment goal so that there are opportunities to check the glycosylated hemoglobin at 3-month intervals and make appropriate adjustments. This time frame also can help to limit frustration by the patient who may be hoping to see rapid normalization of blood glucose levels.

As glucose levels are reduced, insulin sensitivity will likely improve owing to amelioration of the direct effects of hyperglycemia. Thus, an overweight older patient who appears relatively unresponsive to a moderate dose of insulin initially may begin to respond dramatically to modest further increases of insulin dose. In fact the patient may progress to having episodes of hypoglycemia even with reduction to a total insulin dose that previously was not very effective. It is apparent that close follow-up with the diabetes care team, careful attention to glucose monitoring, and coaching about symptoms of hypoglycemia are all critical to a successful treatment program. A suitably trained diabetes nurse can play a particularly critical role during this phase of treatment.

Combination of Insulin and an Oral Agent   Combination therapy of insulin with one or more oral agents has also been considered, although there are little data available in older adults. One regimen is use of an evening injection of an intermediate-acting insulin such as NPH (neutral protamine Hagedorn) to target control of the fasting glucose level plus oral agents for daytime use. There are theoretical advantages to combining insulin with an agent that enhances insulin sensitivity in a patient with insulin resistance or with an agent that reduces meal-related glucose excursions. However, the combination of insulin and a thiazolidinedione should generally be avoided because of potential additive effects on fluid retention. Furthermore, insulin dose adjustments can achieve remarkably similar control of hyperglycemia as combinations of lower doses of insulin with an oral agent. Given the minimal incremental cost of additional insulin to a patient already on insulin and the potential for adverse drug reaction with any addition of a therapeutic agent, the practical gain of such combination therapy remains unclear.

There is also a theoretical argument that high doses of insulin may have adverse cardiovascular effects. Such concerns are based in part on epidemiologic studies demonstrating that (in people without diabetes) higher circulating insulin levels are associated with coronary artery disease. There is also some evidence for direct effects of insulin on the cardiovascular system, some of which might be detrimental. There are, however, no convincing data linking dose of insulin in patients with diabetes to adverse cardiovascular effects.

Another concern about using a high dose of insulin is the potential for weight gain with an intensive insulin treatment program. For patients for whom the indication for insulin is a period of substantial weight loss due to decompensated diabetes, insulin therapy should be expected to cause weight gain back toward baseline with accompanying restoration of lean body mass. For other patients, it may be necessary to balance the potential risk of weight gain versus the benefit of substantial lowering of circulating glucose levels. In general, weight gain with insulin therapy is modest (in the range of a few kilograms) except for those individuals who have lost substantial weight prior to insulin therapy. By emphasizing and reinforcing lifestyle modifications as insulin therapy is instituted, substantial weight gain can generally be avoided.

Follow-up Care

Diabetes mellitus is a chronic disease that requires long-term follow-up. Frequency and intensity of follow-up depend on the treatment goal for the patient and the type of treatment program that the patient is on. At a minimum, a patient should annually have a dilated retinal examination by an ophthalmologist, screening for early nephropathy, a foot examination and testing for neuropathy, measurement of circulating lipids, reassessment of blood pressure and smoking status, and review of key aspects of diabetes self-management and education. Measurement of glycosylated hemoglobin is a very useful way of assessing overall diabetes control and should be performed every 3 to 6 months for most patients. At regular follow-up visits, which can vary from monthly to every 3 months depending on the patient's situation, body weight and blood pressure should be assessed, a review of lifestyle components of the treatment program should be carried out, home glucose monitoring data should be evaluated, interim health problems and psychosocial problems should be reviewed, and appropriate adjustments in the overall treatment plan should be made. For patients with type 1 diabetes, or type 2 diabetes with an aggressive treatment goal or with multiple diabetes complications, participation by a specialized diabetes care team in the overall management program should be carefully considered.

Prevention

Type 2 diabetes is a gradually progressive disorder of carbohydrate metabolism that develops over a long period of time. It has been estimated that abnormalities of glucose regulation can be detected 8 to 10 years before the clinical diagnosis of type 2 diabetes is made. The importance of lifestyle factors in the pathophysiology of type 2 diabetes and the epidemiological associations of healthy lifestyles with reduced risk for diabetes suggest that lifestyle interventions might prevent the development of diabetes. Given the progressive nature of impairments of glucose regulation, there is great interest in trying to identify people early in this course who are at high risk and therefore candidates for intervention to prevent progression. There are now a number of studies that demonstrate that high risk individuals can be identified and that progression to type 2 diabetes can be delayed. Populations which appear to benefit from such interventions include people with IGT and obesity, and individuals from high-risk ethnic groups or who have a history of GDM.

In the largest of these studies, the multicenter Diabetes Prevention Program (DPP) in the United States, an effort was made to recruit older adults with IGT. A lifestyle intervention program including both caloric restriction and exercise was shown to be remarkably effective in reducing the rate of progression to type 2 diabetes, even though only 5 to 7 percent weight reduction was achieved. In the DPP, the lifestyle intervention program was even more effective in people older than age 60 years than in younger people at risk, reducing progression to diabetes by more than 70 percent as compared to a control group. Drug interventions have also been tested. Metformin was used in the DPP and was effective in slowing progression in younger adults, but had surprisingly little effect in people older than age 60 years. A thiazolidinedione successfully slowed progression in people with previous GDM, but has not been tested yet in older adults.

As more is learned about the genetics of type 2 diabetes, it may be possible to identify high-risk individuals early in life based on genotype and to effectively target interventions. The success of the initial intervention trials to prevent progression has raised the question, not yet resolved, about whether and how screening should be carried out to identify high risk individuals for more widespread clinical interventions.

SPECIAL ISSUES

Hypoglycemia

Hypoglycemia is the primary short-term risk of a hyperglycemia treatment program, particularly one that is targeted at achieving near-normal control of glucose levels. Multiple mechanisms exist to maintain adequate circulating glucose levels because glucose is a fuel particularly targeted to meet the needs of the brain and other tissues that are not dependent on insulin for glucose uptake. The major peripheral tissues, muscle and fat, have a glucose transport system that primarily depends on insulin for activation. Brain cells, however, have a different type of glucose transporter molecule that is continually expressed on the cell surface and does not depend on insulin for activation. Thus, when insulin levels are low, as after an overnight fast, the brain does not have to compete with other major tissues for access to glucose. This is in contrast to fat-related fuel such as free fatty acids and ketones, which have ready access to muscle and fat tissue and therefore are less available to the brain. Because of the brain's dependency on glucose as a fuel, it is particularly vulnerable to injury from hypoglycemia, a fact that must be carefully considered as the overall benefits and risk of a diabetes treatment program are reviewed.

Hypoglycemia Counterregulation

Table 67-7 lists factors that are important in recovery from hypoglycemia. The major source of endogenous glucose is the liver. The liver contributes to recovery from hypoglycemia by increasing glucose production under the influence of counterregulatory hormones. As the insulin effect fades during insulin-induced hypoglycemia, there is a decline in peripheral glucose uptake, preserving more circulating glucose for recovery. The degree of fall of glucose levels determines the magnitude of counterregulatory

Table 67-7   Factors Affecting Recovery from Hypoglycemia

Hepatic glucose production
Glucose uptake by tissues
Degree of hypoglycemia
Wearing off of drug effect
Counterregulatory hormone responses
Behavioral responses

responses and the speed with which normal glucose levels can be restored. Normally, there is a hierarchy of responses to hypoglycemia with release of counterregulatory hormones such as epinephrine and glucagon occurring before a patient becomes symptomatic and aware of hypoglycemia. The initial symptoms are caused by autonomic nervous system activation with tachycardia, nervousness, and a sweating response, all of which can alert the patient to the need to seek exogenous sources of glucose to facilitate recovery. Hunger is often a part of this behavioral response. However, as glucose levels fall lower and brain cell function becomes compromised, confusion, lethargy, and progression to coma can occur. Fortunately, the response to glucose administration is quick, and dramatic recovery normally occurs.

It is now recognized that the history of the glucose level that the brain is exposed to influences the counterregulatory response mechanisms, perhaps by affecting the brain glucose transport system. For example, there appears to be adaptation to chronic hyperglycemia in patients with diabetes, with resulting elevation of the glucose level at which counterregulatory responses begin to occur. Thus, a patient with diabetes may begin to develop symptoms of hypoglycemia at a glucose level in the range of 80 to 100 mg/dL, well above the symptomatic threshold in nondiabetic individuals of 50 to 60 mg/dL. Conversely, the brain appears to adapt to low glucose levels as well, with a shift downward of the glucose threshold for activation of counterregulatory responses. Prior exposure to hypoglycemia leads to diminished counterregulatory hormone responses. This can set up a vicious cycle by which patients are less able to counterregulate hypoglycemia and have more recurrent episodes. A key issue seems to be that as the glucose threshold for counterregulation drops, it becomes perilously close to glucose levels that can adversely affect brain function. Thus a patient may have a very narrow margin for error, proceeding from relatively normal function without symptoms to profound hypoglycemia and loss of consciousness. This so-called hypoglycemia unawareness syndrome is in part iatrogenic in origin and generally responds to strict avoidance of hypoglycemia.

Hypoglycemia in Elderly Patients

Table 67-8 summarizes a number of risk factors for hypoglycemia in an older patient with diabetes. As counterregulatory hormone responses are important for both symptom recognition and hypoglycemia counterregulation, impairment of autonomic nervous system reflexes can contribute to risk for hypoglycemia. In addition to risk of the hypoglycemia unawareness syndrome, some older patients may have autonomic neuropathy because of longstanding diabetes or other causes, and many older patients are treated with antiadrenergic agents for cardiovascular diseases. For example, β-adrenergic blocking drugs can potentially interfere with counterregulation of hypoglycemia. Given the substantial benefit of β-adrenergic blockade to patients with cardiovascular disease, a combination with hypoglycemic drug therapy should not be viewed as an absolute contraindication, but only as a concern to keep in mind and share with the patient.

Table 67-8   Risk Factors for Hypoglycemia in Older Diabetic Patients

Impaired autonomic nervous system function
Diminished glucagon secretion
Poor or irregular nutrition
Cognitive disorder
Use of alcohol or other sedating agent
Polypharmacy
Kidney or liver failure

Fortunately, the counterregulatory system is redundant. Glucose counterregulation can be maintained quite well as long as there is an adequate glucagon response even when the adrenergic nervous system is blocked. However, some patients may have impaired glucagon secretion as well, particularly patients with longstanding type 1 diabetes or those with diabetes caused by inflammatory disease of the exocrine pancreas. Patients who have relatively poor nutrition and an irregular meal pattern are at increased risk of hypoglycemia, in part because of inadequate maintenance of muscle and liver glycogen stores. Use of alcohol or a sedating agent should be avoided in patients receiving hypoglycemic agents, particularly if an aggressive treatment program is being pursued. Clearly, a cognitive disorder will interfere with recognition of hypoglycemia and possibly affect decisions about responding to hypoglycemia. Patients with underlying renal or hepatic insufficiency may have problems eliminating hypoglycemic agents, particularly an issue for sulfonylurea drugs. Insulin is partly cleared by the kidney, and the insulin dose must often be reduced substantially in patients with renal insufficiency. A patient with severe hepatic insufficiency may have difficulty mobilizing a counterregulatory increase of glucose production. Finally, any complex drug regimen may include agents that influence the pharmacokinetics of hypoglycemic agents, or counterregulatory or behavioral responses to hypoglycemia, and therefore should be an issue when considering risk for hypoglycemia.

Despite all of these issues and concerns, many older patients with diabetes can be treated aggressively with low risk for hypoglycemia. By providing a strong educational program focused on hypoglycemia recognition and treatment and considering the risk factors outlined in Table 67-8, severe hypoglycemia can generally be avoided. Only subtle alterations of hypoglycemia counterregulatory mechanisms have been identified in healthy older adults, and patients who are hyperglycemic actually have elevated thresholds for counterregulation. Patients with type 2 diabetes are at less risk for severe hypoglycemia than are intensively treated patients with type 1 diabetes.

Hyperosmolar Coma and Diabetic Ketoacidosis

Diabetic ketoacidosis and hyperosmolar coma are the extreme examples of impaired metabolism in patients with diabetes mellitus. DKA is relatively uncommon in older people, but it can occur in an older patient with type 1 diabetes mellitus. As in younger people, the hallmarks of DKA are substantial hyperglycemia, hyperosmolarity, and volume depletion, and the presence of systemic acidosis due to marked elevation of ketoacids. Ketoacids result from metabolism of elevated free fatty acids released by lipolysis as a result of severe insulin deficiency. Diabetic ketoacidosis can occur in a patient with type 1 diabetes when insulin is inappropriately discontinued, but in an older adult, this may be a result of a major underlying illness that interferes with the patient's self-care capability. In the setting of severe coexisting major illness in an older individual and decreased tissue perfusion, lactic acidosis may occur in the setting of hyperglycemia. It is important to document the presence of significant ketonemia to ensure that DKA is contributing to the systemic acidosis observed. Treatment of DKA should focus on immediate insulin replacement to inhibit lipolysis and reverse the ketoacidosis, vigorous replacement of fluids and salt to replace losses, and a thorough evaluation to identify underlying illness. Careful monitoring is required to ensure response and particularly to monitor the cardiovascular system for signs of failure.

Hyperosmolar coma, which occurs primarily in older people, is characterized by marked hyperglycemia, hyperosmolality, severe volume depletion, and associated renal insufficiency. The mortality rate is high because there is often a severe underlying illness such as pneumonia or a cardiovascular accident. Metabolic acidosis is notably absent, or, if present, it is caused by lactic acid rather than ketoacids. The reason for failure to mobilize fatty acids despite severe insulin deficiency in these patients is unclear. While insulin should be provided as part of the initial therapy, the focus should be on volume and sodium replacement and on identification and intervention for major underlying illness. In fact, as volume status is corrected, in the presence of recovering renal function, glucose levels can fall precipitously. Therefore attention must be paid to avoidance of hypoglycemia.

Diabetes in Long-Term Care

Diabetes mellitus is very common among nursing home residents. Because of the overall disease burden, degree of disability, and limited life expectancy of these patients, basic diabetes care should usually be the goal. As undernutrition may be a much more important health problem than obesity in this situation, diet therapy should focus on matching caloric intake to meet nutritional needs rather than restriction of calories. Furthermore, for a nursing home patient with limited remaining life expectancy, the priority should be to stimulate the patient's appetite and take advantage of opportunities for the patient to enjoy this aspect of life, rather than introduction of unnecessary dietary restrictions. Consistency of caloric intake is important for a patient treated with insulin and may be a particular challenge in a disabled nursing home resident.

Careful attention to skin and foot care are clearly important to avoid problems with healing and infection. Similarly, intensive exercise may not be appropriate for a nursing home resident. Efforts should focus on constructive leisure time activity. Given the staff support available, reliable insulin treatment should be available for a nursing home patient, and nursing home staff can also carry out glucose monitoring as needed. Staff needs to be trained to recognize symptoms of hypoglycemia, carry out testing as appropriate, and provide rapid intervention when hypoglycemia is present. In nursing home patients already at high risk for developing urinary tract infection, diabetes may increase this risk because of bladder dysfunction secondary to autonomic neuropathy. Particular attention should be paid to keeping the bladder free of infection and carrying out intermittent catheterization as needed.

REFERENCES

American Diabetes Association. Standards of medical care for patients with diabetes mellitus. *Diabetes Care* 25:S33, 2002.

Blaum CS et al: Characteristics related to poor glycemic control in NIDDM patients in community practice. *Diabetes Care* 20:7, 1997.

Caruso LB et al: What can we do to improve physical function in older persons with type 2 diabetes? *J Gerontol A Biol Sci Med Sci* 55A:M372, 2000.

Clark CM, Lee DA: Prevention and treatment of the complications of diabetes mellitus. *N Engl J Med* 332:1210, 1995.

Funnell MM, Herman WH: Diabetes care policies and practices in Michigan nursing homes, 1991. *Diabetes Care* 18:862, 1995.

Halter JB: Carbohydrate metabolism, in Masoro EJ (ed): *Handbook of Physiology, Volume on Aging.* New York, Oxford University Press, 1995 p 119.

Harris MI et al: Prevalence of diabetes, impaired fasting glucose and impaired glucose tolerance in US adults. *Diabetes Care* 21:518, 1998.

Hays LM, Clark DO: Correlates of physical activity in a sample of older adults with type 2 diabetes. *Diabetes Care* 22:706, 1999.

Lewis EJ et al: The effect of angiotensin-converting-enzyme inhibition on diabetic nephropathy. *N Engl J Med* 329:1456, 1993.

National Diabetes Data Group (eds): *Diabetes in America.* 2nd ed. Bethesda, MD, National Institutes of Health, National Institute of Diabetes and Digestive and Kidney Diseases, 1995.

Resnick HE et al: American Diabetes Association diabetes diagnostic criteria, advancing age, and cardiovascular disease risk profiles: Results from the Third National Health and Nutrition Examination Survey. *Diabetes Care* 23:176, 2000.

Shorr RI et al: Glycemic control of older adults with type 2 diabetes: Findings from the Third National Health and Nutrition Examination Survey, 1988–1994. *J Am Geriatr Soc* 48:264, 2000.

Shorr RI et al: Incidence and risk factors for serious hypoglycemia in older persons using insulin or sulfonylureas. *Arch Intern Med* 157(15):1681, 1997.

Sinclair AJ et al: Mortality in older people with diabetes mellitus. *Diabet Med* 14:639, 1997.

The Diabetes Control and Complications Trial (DCCT) Research Group: Effect of intensive diabetes management on macrovascular events and risk factors in the diabetes control and complications trial. *Am J Cardiol* 75:894, 1995.

The Diabetes Control and Complications Trial Research Group: The effect of intensive treatment of diabetes on the development and progression of long-term complications in insulin-dependent diabetes mellitus. *N Engl J Med* 329:977, 1993.

The Diabetes Prevention Program Research Group: Reduction in the incidence of type 2 diabetes with lifestyle intervention or metformin. *N Engl J Med* 346:393, 2002.

Tuomilehto J et al: Effects of calcium-channel blockade in older patients with diabetes and systemic hypertension. *N Engl J Med* 340:677, 1999.

Tuomilehto J et al: Prevention of type 2 diabetes mellitus by changes in lifestyle among subjects with impaired glucose tolerance. *N Engl J Med* 344:1343, 2001.

UK Prospective Diabetes Study Group. Intensive blood-glucose control with sulphonylureas or insulin compared with conventional treatment and risk of complications in patients with type 2 diabetes (UKPDS 33). *Lancet* 352:837, 1998.

Vijan S et al: Screening, prevention, counseling and treatment for the complications of type 2 diabetes mellitus. *J Gen Intern Med* 12:567, 1997.

Dyslipoproteinemia

LESLIE I. KATZEL • ANDREW P. GOLDBERG

Coronary heart disease (CHD) is the leading cause of death in older men and women. Despite secular declines in mortality rates from CHD because of the aging of the population since 1950, the number of CHD deaths in the United States has actually increased in people 65 to 74 years of age, and has more than doubled in those older than age 75 years. As a consequence of the age-associated increase in CHD incidence and prevalence, in contrast to the portrayal of middle-aged men as the prototypical CHD patient, 80 percent of the deaths from CHD occur in people older than age 65 years. Based on demographic projections, particularly the rapid growth of the population older than age 85 years by 2030, there will be a huge increase in the burden of CHD.

Dyslipidemia is clearly a risk factor for CHD in the "young" old (<75 years), but there is less certainty about this relationship for the "old" elderly (>75 years). Many older individuals have metabolic abnormalities that promote atherosclerosis, but are not detected by routine lipid panels or blood chemistries. These include the apolipoprotein (apo) E4 genotype, elevated levels of lipoprotein (Lp) (a), increased levels of apoB, the atherogenic low-density lipoprotein (LDL) pattern B phenotype, insulin resistance, elevated levels of C-reactive protein (CRP) and other inflammatory markers, and elevated levels of homocysteine. These disorders are more common in both the general population and older CHD patients than familial heterozygous hypercholesterolemia, familial hypertriglyceridemia, and familial multiple lipoprotein (combined) hyperlipidemia. Given the high prevalence of dyslipidemia, obesity, physical inactivity, hypertension and type 2 diabetes in the elderly population, the geriatrician must understand the pathogenesis and treatment of disorders of lipoprotein metabolism in the geriatric population. This chapter reviews the epidemiology and mechanisms underlying age-associated changes in lipoprotein lipid concentrations, evidence that hyperlipidemia is a risk factor for CHD in the elderly population, and controversies regarding the screening and treatment of hyperlipidemia in the elderly population.

OVERVIEW OF LIPOPROTEIN SUBCLASSES AND METABOLISM

Triglycerides (TG) and cholesterol of exogenous (dietary) and endogenous origin are transported in the blood stream as part of lipoprotein particles. These lipoprotein particles contain TG, cholesterol, cholesterol esters, phospholipids, and apolipoproteins. Historically, the lipoprotein particles in the plasma are classified on the basis of their density or by their electrophoretic mobility. By using ultracentrifugation, five major classes of lipoproteins are separated in plasma on the basis of their density. These five classes, in ascending order of density, include chylomicrons, very-low-density lipoproteins (VLDLs), intermediate-density lipoproteins (IDLs), low-density lipoproteins (LDLs), and high-density lipoproteins (HDLs). Lp(a), composed of particles of LDL complexed to glycoprotein apo A, is also present in variable amounts in the plasma. The major classes of lipoproteins are in turn comprised of subpopulations of lipoproteins that differ in composition, metabolic function, and atherogenic potential based on their lipid and apolipoprotein composition (Table 68-1).

Lipoprotein metabolism involves the processing of exogenous dietary fat in the GI tract, and the endogenous synthesis and secretion of TG-rich lipoproteins by the liver. The physiologic regulation of this process provides an understanding of the pathogenesis of atherosclerosis and the metabolic mechanisms by which therapies can target key regulatory sites to reduce CHD risk. In summarizing this process, we highlight 10 key regulatory sites of normal and abnormal metabolic regulation (Fig. 68-1). Strategies for drug and dietary treatments for hyperlipidemia should be directed at these key regulatory sites of lipoprotein metabolism. A more detailed review can be found in Scriver.

During the past several decades, increased knowledge of the metabolic regulation of the lipoprotein subclasses by enzymes, cofactors, and transfer proteins, and various receptors has provided a framework for understanding the pathogenesis of disorders of lipoprotein metabolism. These disorders arise either from accelerated synthesis,

Table 68-1   Characteristics of the Major Classes of Lipoproteins in Plasma

Lipoprotein Class	Density (g/mL)	Diameter (mm)	Electrophoretic Mobility	Major Lipids	Major Apolipoprotein
Chylomicrons	~0.93	75–1200	Remains at origin	Dietary TG	AI, AII, AIV, B48, CI
VLDL	0.93–1.006	30–80	Prebeta	Endogenous TG	B48, CI, CII, CIII, E
IDL	1.006–1.019	25–35	Slow prebeta	Cholesteryl esters, TG	B100, CIII, E
LDL	1.019–1.063	18–25	Beta	Cholesteryl esters	B100, CII, E
HDL	1.063–1.210	5–12	Alpha	Cholesteryl esters	AI, AII, CI, II, III, D; E
Lp(a)	1.040–1.131	25–30	Slow prebeta	Cholesteryl esters, free cholesterol, TG, phospholipids	Apo(a)

Source: Adapted from Havel RJ and Kane JP (2001).

decreased degradation of the lipoproteins, or both. The dyslipoproteinemias can be either primary, or secondary to other systemic disorders such as diabetes, renal disease, and hypothyroidism (Table 68-2). Some of the primary dyslipoproteinemias are the result of biochemical defects that can result from single-gene mutations, whereas other disorders are polygenetic, or multifactorial.

Age, environmental factors, diet, and other lifestyle factors affect the phenotypic expression of both the single-gene and polygenetic disorders. The prevailing dogma is that dyslipidemias that arise from single-gene mutations have both an earlier age of onset and clinical manifestations of atherosclerosis at a younger age than the polygenetic disorders. For example, individuals with familial hypercholesterolemia, both the homozygous and heterozygote genotypes, can be identified in childhood. Familial multiple lipoprotein hyperlipidemia might not be phenotypically manifest until after puberty, but is usually clinically and biochemically diagnosed by the fourth or fifth decade. Familial hypertriglyceridemia and other disorders associated with increased TG production and decreased clearance may not become clinically apparent until middle-age when age-associated increases in adiposity, physical inactivity and the development of insulin resistance enhance the expression of the metabolic defects. It is important to note that most older individuals presenting to the geriatrician with hypercholesterolemia have polygenetic disorders in whom the development of hyperlipidemia is multifactorial. In these individuals, age-associated increases in adiposity, decreased fitness, decreased number/and or function of the LDL receptor, and hormonal changes associated with menopause act in concert with polygenetic factors to raise LDL-C concentrations in middle age or old age. Similarly, the interaction of genetic, lifestyle, and environmental factors increases the age-associated prevalence of the atherogenic LDL pattern B phenotype. Early detection and treatment of hyperlipidemia is critical for primary and secondary prevention of CHD in these individuals.

EPIDEMIOLOGY OF AGE-ASSOCIATED CHANGES IN LIPIDS

A recurring theme in the examination of the aging process is the attempt to distinguish changes caused by biological aging (primary aging) from those caused by lifestyle (secondary aging) and those caused by disease (tertiary aging). To address this question, many cross-sectional studies have examined age-associated changes in lipoprotein concentrations in both men and women. The knowledge of longitudinal changes in lipoproteins is less comprehensive primarily because of the inherent difficulties in following cohorts of individuals over extended periods of time, and methodologies that limited widespread measurement of HDL-C and apolipoproteins prior to the mid 1970s. In general, the cross-sectional studies demonstrate that total cholesterol, LDL-C, and TG concentrations increase in both men and women from the third to seventh or eighth decades of life, with a more pronounced increase in LDL-C levels in women (Fig. 68-2). Typically, there is a decline in LDL-C and total cholesterol levels in oldest age. In National Health and Nutrition Examination Survey (NHANES) III, the mean total cholesterol levels was 205 mg/dL for men older than age 75 years. In the Honolulu Heart Study, total cholesterol levels were 8 percent lower in men older than age 85 years, as compared to men aged 71 to 74 years. This decline in cholesterol levels in the population older than age 75 years could reflect selective mortality, or be caused by changes in body composition, coexistent comorbid diseases, and poor nutrition. Indeed, longitudinal change in body weight over an 8-year period of time was an independent predictor of changes in total cholesterol, LDL-C, and HDL-C in older men and women in Rancho Bernardo, California.

There also may be age-related changes in the LDL subclass population distribution that affects the atherogenicity and susceptibility of LDL to oxidation for uptake into the arterial wall by macrophages. The prevalence of individuals with a predominance of small, dense apoB-enriched LDL

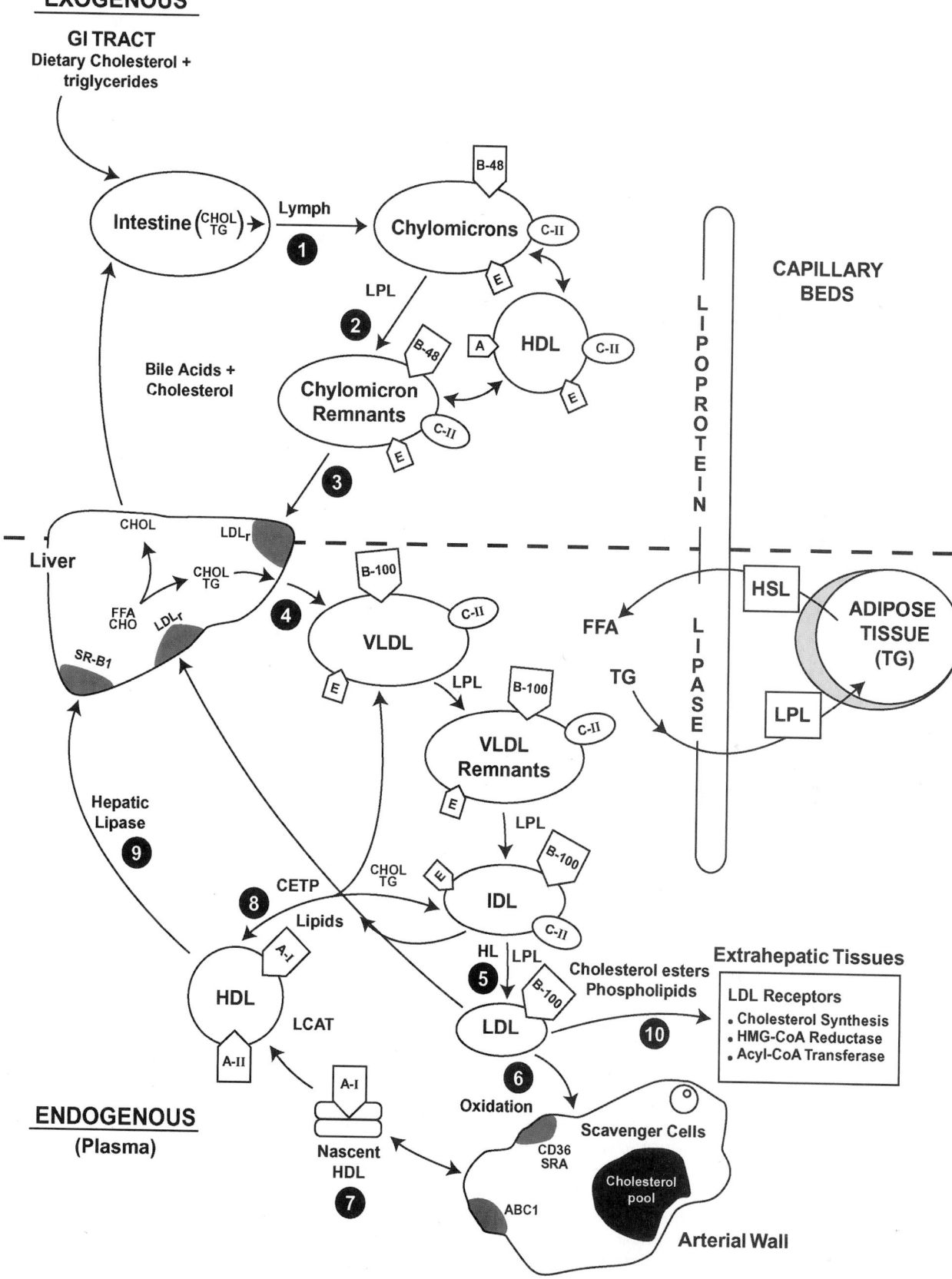

Figure 68-1   Schematic overview of exogenous and endogenous lipoprotein metabolism. Adapted from Havel RJ, Kane JP: Introduction: Structure and metabolism of plasma lipoproteins, in Scriver CR et al. (eds): *The Metabolic and Molecular Bases of Inherited Disease,* 8th ed. Vol. II. New York, McGraw-Hill, 2001 p 2705 and Santamarina-Fojo S et al: Lecithin-cholesterol acyltransferase: Role in lipoprotein metabolism reverse cholesterol transport and atherosclerosis. *Curr Opin Lipidol* 11:267, 2000.

particles (atherogenic LDL pattern B phenotype) increases with aging. In women, there may be marked changes in lipoprotein concentrations and composition associated with menopause. In the Framingham Offspring Study, postmenopausal women had 16 percent higher values of total cholesterol, 62 percent higher TG, 23 percent higher LDL-C, and smaller LDL particles than premenopausal women. These changes in LDL composition adversely impact CAD risk, and are not detected by routine methods for measurement of lipoproteins.

Aging is also associated with increases in plasma TG levels, and there is a change in HDL-C levels across the age span in both men and women. In men, at puberty, there is a drop in HDL concentrations. The HDL-C level then remains fairly constant until the sixth or seventh decade of life, at which time there may be an increase in the HDL-C concentration. This increase in HDL-C concentrations at older age noted in cross-sectional studies also may be a result of selective morbidity and mortality, as opposed to true age-associated changes in HDL metabolism. In the Lipid Research Clinics study, HDL-C levels tended to increase across the age span in women. However, a number of other studies, including the Framingham Offspring Study, report 8 percent lower HDL-C levels in postmenopausal women. Analogous to LDL, there are also compositional changes in the HDL subfractions associated with menopause that result in smaller HDL particles that also may increase CHD risk.

Interpretation of the longitudinal and cross-sectional studies of age-related changes in lipoprotein concentrations is confounded by secular and cohort effects. For example, a comparison of normative data from the National Health Examination Survey of 1960 to 1962, and from the NHANES III of 1988 to 1991 demonstrated that secular changes in diet and other factors resulted in lower total cholesterol levels across the age span. This fall in cholesterol levels could have a significant impact on CHD morbidity and mortality. Conversely, secular changes resulting in an increased prevalence of obesity may raise TG levels, and lower HDL concentrations in the elderly population.

As a result of the age-associated changes in cholesterol metabolism, the prevalence of hypercholesterolemia increases markedly, particularly in older women. Using the diagnostic criteria of a total cholesterol level above 240 mg/dL for hypercholesterolemia, in NHANES III, 39 percent of women age 65 to 74 years had hypercholesterolemia, as compared to 8 percent of women age 20 to 34 years. In men, the corresponding percentages are 22 percent for men age 65 to 74, as compared to 9 percent for men age 20 to 34 years. It is noteworthy that the prevalence of hypercholesterolemia in the elderly population varies considerably in different populations. For example, in the Framingham Offspring study, 21 percent of individuals age 60 to 69 years had hypercholesterolemia, whereas in the Bronx study, 55 percent of women age 75 to 85 years had hypercholesterolemia.

As a result of the marked age-associated increase in the prevalence of hypercholesterolemia, in conjunction with the high prevalence of CHD, and other CHD risk factors in the elderly population, based on the prior National Cholesterol Education Program Adult Treatment Panel (NCEP ATP II) guidelines, approximately 2 million adults older than age 65 years with established CHD, and 3.1 million older than age 65 years without overt CHD might be candidates for cholesterol-lowering drugs. An even larger number of individuals older than age 65 years with LDL-C >130 mg/dL and coexistent CHD risk factors, or known

---

Figure 68-1 (*Continued*) Lipids in the diet are hydrolyzed in the small intestine, and the fatty acids and monoglycerides repackaged with apoB-48 into TG-enriched chylomicron particles and secreted by capillary endothelial cells into the lymphatics (*site 1*). Dietary chylomicrons bypass the liver to enter the plasma via the thoracic duct. They acquire apoE and C-II from HDL and are hydrolyzed by lipoprotein lipase (LPL) to smaller TG-depleted, cholesterol-rich chylomicron remnants (*site 2*). These remnants are taken up by the liver primarily by the LDL receptor-related protein receptor (LDL-R), degraded and their products affect endogenous TG synthesis and secretion (*site 3*). Endogenous TG is synthesized in the liver from carbohydrate and free fatty acid (FFA) derived from adipocyte hydrolysis by hormone-sensitive lipase (HSL) precursors, assembled in the Golgi with apoB-100, E, C-II, and C-III, and secreted as TG-rich very-low-density lipoproteins (VLDL-TG) (*site 4*). VLDL-TG are hydrolyzed by LPL to VLDL remnants and intermediate-density lipoproteins (IDL), which are taken up by scavenger cells or apoE-specific hepatic receptors and degraded in the liver. VLDL remnants are removed irreversibly or hydrolyzed further by LPL and hepatic lipase to cholesterol-rich LDL particles (*site 5*). LDL then has its cholesterol removed from plasma by the LDL receptor, or is oxidized and taken up by class A or CD36 scavenger receptors on macrophages to generate an intracellular cholesterol pool (*site 6*). The hydrolysis of TG from VLDL-TG by LPL also generates free cholesterol, phospholipids (PL), substrates for lecithin cholesterol acyltransferase (LCAT).

Nascent HDL interacts with the ATP-binding cassette transporter-1 (ABC1) to remove excess cholesterol from cells and then binds with apoAI, the principal activator of LCAT, to esterify cholesterol forming large, spherical cholesterol ester-rich HDL2 particles (*site7*). Cholesterol is transported back to the liver directly by HDL or via transfer to the apoB- containing VLDL or IDL by the cholesterol ester transfer protein (CETP) (*site 8*). Hepatic lipase (HL) stimulates HDL cholesterol ester uptake by the hepatic scavenger class B type 1 receptor (SR-B1). However, if there is excess VLDL-TG production or dietary fat intake, CETP exchanges cholesterol from HDL with TG from VLDL, raising the TG and lowering the cholesterol composition of HDL (*site 9*). Hepatic lipase hydrolyzes HDL-TG and phospholipid, converting HDL2 to smaller HDL3 particles, reducing the efficient clearance of cholesterol from cells. Cholesterol is also synthesized endogenously from acetate precursors, regulated by the enzyme HMG-CoA (hydroxymethylglutaryl coenzyme A) reductase. Excessive accumulation of intracellular free cholesterol suppresses intracellularly cholesterol synthesis by inhibiting HMG-CoA reductase, the rate-limiting enzyme in cholesterol synthesis, stimulates cholesterol reesterification by acyl-CoA (acylcoenzyme A):cholesterol transferase, and downregulates LDL receptor synthesis (*site 10*). Excess cholesterol might then be resecreted into the circulation from the liver on VLDL via increased endogenous VLDL synthesis, excreted directly into the bile, or converted to bile acids for reabsorption (enterohepatic circulation) or excretion in stool and bile. Genetic abnormalities at each of these sites may lead to inherited forms of dyslipoproteinemia.

Table 68-2 Classification of the Hyperlipoproteinemias

A. Primary Dyslipoproteinemia Plasma Lipoprotein Pattern	Synonym	Primary Biochemical Defect	Relative Frequency	Atherogenicity
Exogenous hyperlipdemia (↑ chylomicrons)	Type I	Deficiency of lipoprotein lipase	Rare AR (1 in 5,00O)	None
		Deficiency of apoCII		None
Hypercholesterolemia (↑ LDL)	Type IIa	Deficiency of LDL receptor	1 in 500 (AD)	+++
Combined hyperlipidemia (↑ LDL + VLDL)	Type IIb	Familial multiple lipoprotein hyperlipidemia	1 in 100 (AD)	+++
Remnant hyperlipidemia (↑ chylomicron remnants IDL)	Type III	Abnormal apoE VLDL metabolism associated with apoE2/2 genotype	Rare (AR, AD)	+++
Endogenous hyperlipidemia (↑ VLDL)	Type IV	Unknown, some may have familial hypertriglyceridemia (mild form)	1 in 200 (AD)	+
Mixed hyperlipidemia (↑ chylomicrons + VLDL)	Type V	Unknown, some may have deficiency of lipoprotein lipase or deficiency of apoCII	Rare	+

B. Secondary Dyslipoproteinemia Pathophysiology	Relation to Aging	Clinical Findings	Therapy
↓ Chylomicron removal (exogenous hyperlipidemia)	↑ Obesity diabetes	Eruptive xanthomas, pancreatitis	low fat diet, fibrates
Defective LDL clearance (hypercholesterolemia)	↑ Liver and renal disease, hypothyroid, menopause	Tendon xanthomas	HMG-CoA reductase inhibitor, bile-acid resin, niacin
↑ ApoB VLDL and LDL production (combined hyperlipidemia)	↑ Obesity, steroids, type 2 diabetes, uremia nephritic syndrome	Tendon xanthomas	HMG-CoA reductase inhibitor, bile-acid, resin, niacin
↑ VLDL production ↓ IDL (remnant clearance) (remnant hyperlipidemia)	↑ Obesity, hypothyroid, uremia, estrogen status, nephritic syndrome	Palmar and tuberous xanthomas	Fibrates
↑ VLDL production (endogenous hyperlipidemia)	↑ Obesity (central), diabetes, alcohol, steroids	Eruptive xanthomas	Fibrates, niacin
↓ Chylomicron clearance, ↑ VLDL production (mixed hyperlipidemia)	↑ Obesity, diabetes, uremia, steroids, alcohol	Eruptive xanthomas	Fibrates, niacin

AD, autosomal dominant; AR, autosomal recessive; HMG-CoA, hydroxymethylglutaryl coenzyme A.

CHD would be candidates for pharmacologic therapy under the more recent NCEP ATP III guidelines. Judicious application of the NCEP guidelines by the medical community, and continued effort by older individuals to reduce their dietary intake of saturated fat and cholesterol and body weight to recommended levels, and increase physical activity should reduce plasma cholesterol and TG levels and raise HDL-C. The important question is whether such changes will lower CHD morbidity and mortality in patients older than 65 years of age.

MECHANISMS UNDERLYING THE AGE-ASSOCIATED CHANGES IN LIPIDS

A number of mechanisms have been proposed to account for the age-associated changes in lipoprotein concentrations, particularly for changes in LDL-C levels. These mechanisms include age-associated increases in dietary fat content and adiposity, declines in physical activity and physical fitness, and decreases in the number and or function of the hepatic LDL receptor. The evidence

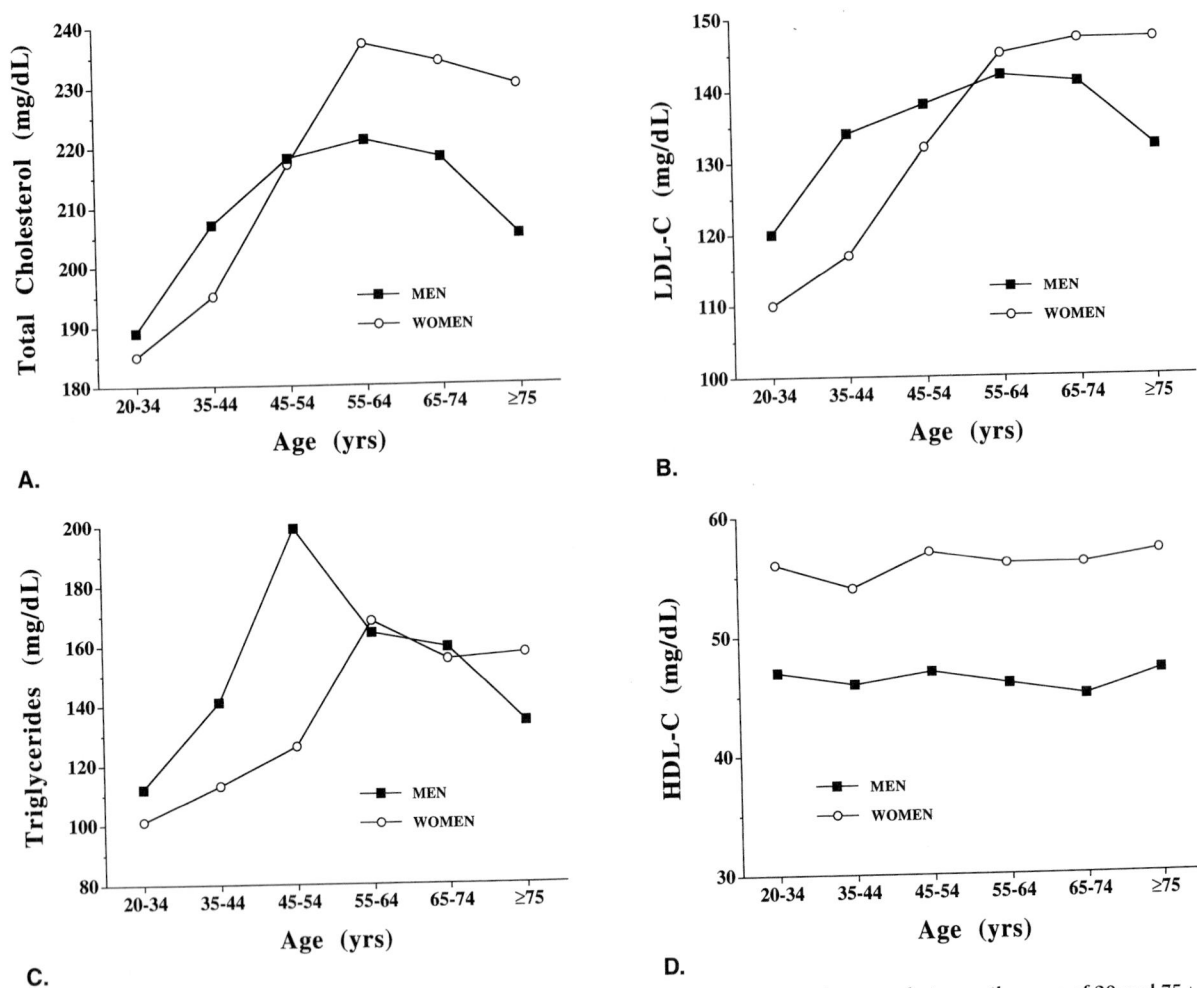

Figure 68-2   Mean American population total cholesterol, TG, LDL-C and HDL-C in men and women between the ages of 20 and 75+ years. Data from National Health and Nutrition Examination Survey (NHANES) III. (Johnson CL, et al: Declining serum total cholesterol levels among US adults. The National Health and Nutrition Examination Surveys. *JAMA* 269:3002, 1993.)

supporting some of these mechanisms is reviewed in this section.

Age-Associated Changes in Diet

Age-associated changes in dietary content are reviewed in Chap. 90. In men in the Baltimore Longitudinal Study of Aging (BLSA) total caloric intake, cholesterol intake, the percent of calories obtained from fat, and the percent of calories obtained from saturated fat declined with age. Such age-associated changes in dietary content would be expected to result in lower levels of total and LDL-C, a result that is opposite to the commonly observed age-associated increase in these parameters.

Age-Associated Increases in Total and Central (Truncal) Adiposity

The prevalence of obesity increases with aging, with a preferential accumulation of fat in central (truncal) sites (see Chap. 91 for details). This is associated with hyperinsulinemia and the development of a syndrome of metabolic risk

factors for CHD. Recent data from the Italian Longitudinal Study on Aging showed that higher insulin levels in a cohort of 5632 people aged 65 to 84 years were associated with low HDL-C and apoAI levels, higher TG and glucose, hypertension and higher body mass index, but not high total or LDL-C. Among the diabetic subjects, TG levels were higher but HDL-C levels did not differ across insulin quartiles; however, total and LDL-C levels were lower and white blood cells higher in diabetic women with high insulin. Longitudinal follow-up and the assessment of mortality will determine the relationship of hyperinsulinemia and the metabolic syndrome to CHD risk in this cohort.

Age-Associated Declines in Physical Fitness

Physical activity has a significant effect on plasma lipoprotein concentrations. Older athletes have higher HDL-C and lower TG and LDL-C levels than their age-matched sedentary counterparts, lipoprotein profiles that are often more similar to their younger counterparts. The interpretation of these cross-sectional comparisons is confounded by differences in body composition that exist between the sedentary and trained populations, as the trained subjects are significantly leaner than the untrained population. The differences in obesity contributed the most to the difference in TG and HDL-C concentrations between older athletes and their sedentary counterparts, but the differences in maximal aerobic capacity (VO_2max) did account for a small, but statistically significant percentage of the variance in these lipoproteins. These studies suggest exercise training, by reducing body fatness and raising VO_2max can prevent the age-associated increase in TG and LDL-C, and reduction in HDL-C. (See chap. 72 for details)

Age-Associated Changes in Lipoprotein Metabolism

In pooled data examining the relationship between the fractional catabolic rate of LDL and age in both healthy men and women, and in individuals with heterozygous familial hypercholesterolemia, the fractional catabolic rate of LDL decreased with aging, in both normal individuals, and in individuals with hypercholesterolemia, whereas the LDL production rate did not change with aging. The age-related rise in LDL-C has been attributed to an acquired defect in LDL receptor function or in hepatic LDL receptor expression. Kinetic studies employing stable isotopes suggest that the age-associated increase in VLDL apoB-100 is a result of an increased rate of production, whereas the age-associated increase in LDL apoB-100 is a result of increased residency time. These studies did not control for differences in body weight and physical activity among the age groups. Obesity and physical deconditioning may elevate free fatty acid concentrations, glucose and insulin levels in the older subjects, thereby raising the hepatic production of VLDL-apoB. Many of the purported age-related changes in lipoprotein levels may reflect interactions between primary age-related changes in LDL metabolism and the effects of secondary aging on TG and HDL-C caused by obesity, physical inactivity, diet, and other lifestyle habits.

HYPOCHOLESTEROLEMIA IN THE ELDERLY

Older individuals with hypocholesterolemia, typically defined as total cholesterol levels <160 mg/dL (6th percentile Multiple Risk Factor Intervention Trial [MRFIT]) are at increased risk for adverse events. Hypocholesterolemia is associated with increased death from intracranial hemorrhage, lymphatic and hematopoietic cancers, chronic obstructive pulmonary disease, particularly in smokers, and cirrhosis. In free-living populations, chronic liver disease, chronic obstructive pulmonary disease, pneumonia, and other chronic conditions, including failure to thrive, are associated with low cholesterol levels. Biologically plausible mechanisms of low total cholesterol as a cause of death include alterations in cell membrane structure and function, abnormalities in steroid hormone metabolism, and fat and vitamin deficiency.

The examination of the reasons for the association between low cholesterol and subsequent morbidity and mortality are confounded by the presence of active or occult disease in the study population. To minimize this bias, longitudinal analyses can be performed after excluding individuals with early deaths who may have had undiagnosed active disease. In data pooled from 19 cohort studies, men and women with cholesterol levels <160 mg/dL were at a 40 to 50 percent higher risk for noncardiovascular deaths that occurred more than 5 years after baseline measurement than were individuals with cholesterol levels of 200 to 239 mg/dL. In men, the pooled data demonstrated a U-shaped relationship between total cholesterol levels and mortality as a consequence of a positive relationship of cholesterol with CHD death, and an inverse relationship with deaths caused by some cancers, respiratory disease, digestive diseases, and residual death. In women, there was a relatively flat relationship between total cholesterol levels and CHD death.

Low-normal cholesterol levels, and declining cholesterol levels may be markers for increased morbidity and mortality, even in apparently healthy community-dwelling older people. In the Honolulu Heart Study, persistence of low cholesterol levels over a 20-year period of time was associated with increased risk of death. In that study, the earlier in life that the patients start to have low cholesterol levels, the greater the risk of death. Based on their findings, the authors questioned whether it was advisable to lower cholesterol levels below 4.65 mmol/L (180 mg/dL) in elderly people.

When evaluating an older patient with hypocholesterolemia, the geriatrician must consider the time course of the relationship between cholesterol levels and the change in cholesterol levels with the development of disease. There are important questions concerning the natural history of patients with hypocholesterolemia: (1) Is cholesterol low in those individuals who will develop disease (causality)? (2) Is low cholesterol a marker for those with cancer or other diseases, clinically inapparent or overt? (3) Do cholesterol levels drop gradually throughout stages of a developing disease, or drop precipitously at a given stage?

Because hypocholesterolemia may be a marker for occult malignancy and other diseases that result in increased morbidity and mortality, the questions arises as to the appropriate diagnostic evaluation and therapeutic intervention. Unfortunately, there are no firm guidelines for the recommended evaluation of patients with hypocholesterolemia. Some investigators advocate the performance of routine cancer evaluations, colonoscopy, pelvic examination, and the like, in otherwise healthy community-dwelling individuals with hypocholesterolemia. Randomized clinical trials are needed to determine the efficacy of aggressive nutritional intervention in older patients with hypocholesterolemia.

LIPOPROTEIN RISK FACTORS FOR CHD IN ELDERLY PERSONS

Many case-control and prospective studies examining lipoprotein risk factors for atherosclerosis have focused on the impact of the traditional lipoprotein risk factors, that is, total cholesterol, LDL-C, and HDL-C. There is also substantial evidence that many older individuals have abnormalities in lipoprotein metabolism that are not detected by routine lipid profiles. These dyslipidemic syndromes include the apoE4 genotype, elevated levels of Lp(a), and the atherogenic LDL pattern B phenotype. These disorders of lipoprotein metabolism are more common than familial heterozygous hypercholesterolemia and familial multiple lipoprotein hyperlipidemia in both the general population and CHD patients, and may play major roles in the pathogenesis of CHD in older individuals. In this section, the evidence that dyslipidemia is a risk factor for CHD in the elderly population is reviewed.

Elevated Total and LDL-C Concentrations

There is convincing evidence that elevated levels of total cholesterol and of LDL-C increase the risk for CHD in middle-aged men. The evidence supporting elevated levels of LDL-C as a risk factor for CHD in the elderly population, particularly elderly women, is mixed. In pooled data presented at a National Heart, Lung, and Blood Institute (NHLBI) conference, in 21 of 24 studies of men age 65 years and older, the relative risk was >1.00 for total cholesterol concentrations >240 mg/dL, as compared to cholesterol levels <200 mg/dL. The pooled relative risk was 1.32. By comparison, for women age 65 years and older, in 10 of 16 studies, the relative risk was >1.00 for cholesterol >240 mg/dL, as compared to cholesterol levels <200 mg/dL. The pooled relative risk was 1.12. Although statistically significant, the relative risk for CHD in older individuals with hypercholesterolemia is lower than the relative risk than that observed in studies of men younger than 65 years of age.

There are many factors that may account for the disparities between the studies that have examined the relationship between cholesterol levels and CHD in the elderly. One explanation may be a nonlinear relationship between cholesterol levels, CHD events, and total mortality, that is, a J- or U-shaped curve. In this situation, individuals with the highest or lowest cholesterol levels are at increased risk for CHD, as compared to those with intermediate levels. Another confounder in the association between cholesterol levels and CHD outcomes in the elderly person is that cholesterol levels measured at a given time may not accurately reflect the lifelong average exposure to plasma cholesterol, leading to spurious conclusions. For example, at age 70 years, the measured total cholesterol level may be 220 mg/dL, whereas the average cholesterol level over the adult life span could have been 180 or 250 mg/dL. As a result, longitudinal studies that examine both the baseline cholesterol level, and its change over time are needed to provide insight into the predictive values of cholesterol levels for subsequent CHD and all cause mortality in the elderly population. For example, in a Finnish 30-year longitudinal study, there was a U-shaped relationship between the change in cholesterol level and coronary and all-cause mortality.

The majority of studies report data on the relative risk of hypercholesterolemia for CHD morbidity and mortality. However, some investigators suggest that the attributable risk is a more useful parameter for making clinical decisions concerning treatment of hypercholesterolemia in the elderly patient. In this context, the attributable risk is the

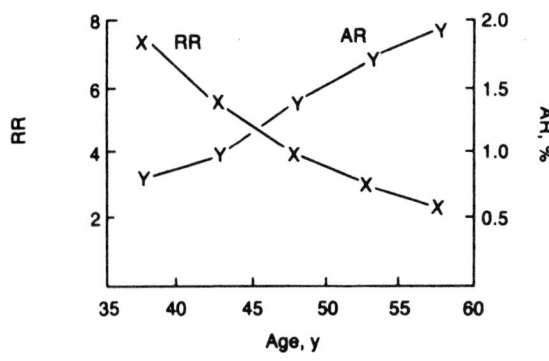

Figure 68-3   The effect of age on the relative and attributable risk of hypercholesterolemia for CHD death in patients of the Multiple Risk Factor Intervention Trial (MRFIT). Although the relative risk (RR) for CHD death for individuals with hypercholesterolemia declines with aging, as a consequence of age-associated increases in the absolute death rate from CHD, the attributable risk (AR) for CHD in the upper versus lowest quintile increased progressively with age. Reproduced with permission from Malenka DJ, Baron JA: Cholesterol and coronary heart disease: The importance of patient-specific attributable risk. *Arch Intern Med* 148:2247, 1988.

difference in the absolute risk of death or morbidity from CHD between individuals with high levels versus those with low levels. Thus, the attributable risk provides an estimate of the absolute probability that risk of CHD would be lower if the putative risk factor were maximally lowered or eliminated. Unlike the relative risk, the attributable risk estimates are strongly determined by the absolute rates of death from CHD in the population. For example, in MRFIT, the relative risk for CHD death for a man in the upper quintile of the population declined from greater than 7 in men age 35 to 39 years to 2 for men age 55 to 59 years (Fig. 68-3). However, because of age-associated increases in the absolute death rate from CHD, the attributable risk for CHD in the upper versus lowest quintile increased progressively with age; 0.7 percent for men age 35 to 39 years, as compared to 1.9 percent for men age 55 to 59 years. Given the high prevalence of CHD events in elderly patients, the attributable risk for increased total or LDL-C may be even higher than observed in MRFIT. Because of the age-related increase in the population-attributable risk for hypercholesterolemia, there may be a substantial public health benefit by treating hypercholesterolemia in the elderly population. Furthermore, the number of subjects needed to treat with pharmacologic therapy to prevent cardiovascular end points is substantially lower in older populations than in younger populations. Thus, pharmacologic interventions to decrease morbidity and mortality from CHD may be more cost-effective in older people, as compared to younger people.

Reduced Concentrations of HDL-C

Because the relative risk for CHD with elevated total cholesterol levels declines with aging, the question arises as to whether the HDL-C concentration provides additional information on CHD and stroke risk in the elderly patient. A number of studies suggest that HDL-C concentrations, and the ratio of total cholesterol to HDL-C are useful in predicting CHD risk in the elderly population. In the Framingham Study, 4-year and 12-year follow-up data demonstrated inverse relationships between HDL-C levels and incident CHD in subjects age 50 to 79 years. For men, the relative risk of death for those with HDL-C <35 mg/dL was 1.9, as compared to those men with HDL-C >54 mg/dL, and risk of CHD death was 4.1. In women, the relative risk for death was 1.5 for women with HDL-C <45 mg/dL, compared to those women with HDL-C >69 mg/dL, and the risk of CHD death was 3.1. In data pooled from the three Established Population for the Epidemiologic Study of the Elderly (EPESE) sites, low HDL-C was a risk factor for CHD in persons older than age 70 years. In addition, the pooled data demonstrated that high total cholesterol was associated with CHD death in women, but not in men. Low HDL-C levels are also a risk factor for ischemic stroke in the elderly population. Therapy aimed at raising HDL-C levels by using gemfibrozil reduced the risk of stroke in older men with prevalent CHD. These studies support the use of measurement of HDL-C along with total cholesterol to predict CHD and stroke risk in older individuals.

Atherogenic LDL Pattern B Phenotype

The atherogenic LDL pattern B phenotype, is a metabolic syndrome characterized by a predominance of small, dense, enriched apoB-containing LDL particles, mildly elevated TG, and reduced HDL concentrations, as well as hypertension and other manifestations of the insulin-resistance syndrome. Some consider the LDL B phenotype to be a biochemical marker for the insulin resistance syndrome. Most, but not all, studies demonstrate an association between LDL pattern B and increased risk for CHD. In the Physicians' Health Survey, LDL pattern B was prospectively associated with a threefold increased risk of CHD, independent of total cholesterol, HDL and body mass index. The prevalence of the atherogenic LDL pattern B phenotype increases markedly with aging; in one study, the prevalence increased from 10 to 15 percent in young men to 30 to 35 percent in middle-aged men, and from 5 to 10 percent in young women to 15 to 25 percent in postmenopausal women. Thus, this syndrome is very prevalent in older populations. Several investigators propose that the atherogenic LDL pattern B phenotype may be the most common abnormality in lipoprotein metabolism that predisposes to CHD.

The etiology of LDL pattern B is multifactorial. Family studies suggest that LDL pattern B may be inherited as a mendelian dominant or polygenetic trait interacting with other genes to increase apolipoprotein B production. The phenotypic expression of the pattern is affected by age, visceral obesity, diet, sedentary lifestyle, and the presence of type 2 diabetes. There appears to be a linkage of LDL pattern B to a number of genetic loci, but there is no consensus as to which of these, if any, is responsible for the syndrome.

Individuals with the LDL pattern B have a different metabolic response to drug and dietary interventions than those individuals with the "normal" LDL pattern A phenotype. Differential lipoprotein lipid response between subjects with LDL patterns B and A have been reported for dietary interventions, weight loss, and drug therapy with a variety of different agents including statins, niacin, bile acid-binding resins, gemfibrozil and clofibrate. Certain classes of drugs are more effective than other drugs at lowering the levels of the small, dense LDL particles, and in several angiographic trials, reduction in the concentration of these particles was associated with decreased coronary artery disease (CAD) progression or regression. For example, in the St. Thomas' Atherosclerosis Regression Study (STARS), small, dense LDL was significantly reduced in the groups showing regression, and dense LDL concentration was the best predictor of arteriographic outcome. Similarly, in the Helsinki Trial, the subset of subjects characterized by elevated TG levels and low HDL-C, that is, patients who presumably were LDL pattern B, received substantial clinical benefit from gemfibrozil. Consequently, the clinician must realize that lipid-lowering drugs can have significantly different effects on the lipoprotein subclasses that are not detected by routine measurements of TG, LDL-C, and HDL-C. This differential response, in turn, could affect the decision of which drug therapy should be implemented for the prevention or regression of atherosclerosis in given patient. Advancements in technology may make measurement of the lipoprotein subfractions and apolipoproteins part of the routine lipoprotein profile. This would permit more targeted and specific therapy to address the underlying metabolic abnormalities.

Apolipoprotein E4 Allele

Apolipoprotein E is a constituent of chylomicrons, VLDL, and HDL, and modulates the metabolism of the apoB-containing lipoproteins. The gene that codes for apoE is polymorphic with single amino acid substitutions that result in three common alleles designated E2, E3, and E4. These alleles determine the six common apoE genotypes: E2/2, 2/3, 2/4, 3/3, 4/3, and 4/4. The relative frequencies of the E2, E3, and E4 alleles in adult populations are approximately 8 percent, 78 percent, and 14 percent, respectively. LDL-C cholesterol levels are in part determined by the apoE gene locus. Individuals with the apoE2/3 genotype on average have LDL-C levels 20 percent lower than the common apoE3/3 genotype, whereas subjects with apoE4/3 have LDL-C levels 10 percent higher than apoE3/3. In addition, some individuals with apoE2/2 genotype have defective clearance of lipid remnants (remnant hyperlipidemia, type III hyperlipidemia).

The apoE4 allele is a risk factor for CHD. In the Framingham Offspring Study, the apoE4 was a determinant of CHD risk, independent of age, gender, hypertension, cigarette use, obesity, diabetes, or the concentrations of LDL-C and HDL-C. The odds ratio for men was 1.53; for women, it was 1.99. Given its prevalence, apoE4 allele may be the most common genetic lipid abnormality associated with CHD. The mechanism underlying the increased CHD for individuals with apoE4 allele is not known with certainty, but is partly a result of changes in LDL metabolism. Patients with the apoE4 allele also tend to have lower

HDL-C levels and higher TG levels than do individuals with the common apoE3/3 genotype.

The apoE4 allele also is associated with increased mortality, and decreased survival into older age. This may be partly a result of an association between the apoE4 allele and Alzheimer's disease (refer to Alzheimer's disease in Chap. 107). The frequency of the E4 allele seems to be lower in older populations than in younger populations. In one cross-sectional study, the apoE4 frequency declined progressively across the age span; 0.198 in young adults to 0.116 in nonagenarians. Similarly, in another study, the frequency of the E4 allele was lower in older women (0.098) than in younger women (0.122), whereas the allele frequency of apoE2 was higher and associated with lower total and LDL-C levels in the older cohort.

These cross-sectional studies are supported by results of longitudinal studies. In older Finnish men (mean age at entry 72 years), the death rate from CHD over 5 years of follow-up of men with the apoE4 allele was double that of men with the other apoE genotypes. In the Baltimore Longitudinal Study of Aging, in multivariate analyses, apoE4 was an independent predictor of coronary events (relative risk of 2.9) in middle-aged and older men over 20 years of longitudinal follow-up. These studies strongly suggest that the E4 allele is associated with increased all-cause mortality and death from CHD, while the E2 allele is advantageous for longevity. Hence, selective mortality probably accounts for some of the decline in the prevalence of the E4 allele with aging. It is not known whether lifestyle or pharmacologic interventions specifically targeted for older individuals with the E4 allele would reduce morbidity and mortality from CHD, and all-cause mortality. Ethical issues related to genetic screening, employment, and health insurance will need to be addressed prior to widespread measurement and treatment based on the apoE genotype in clinical practice.

Elevated Lp(a)

Lipoprotein(a) is a cholesterol-rich lipoprotein particle similar to LDL. Structurally, Lp(a) is assembled from apolipoprotein(a) that is covalently linked to apolipoprotein B. The genetic locus for apolipoprotein (a) is polymorphic and there is a large number of genetically determined isoforms of Lp(a). Genetic studies indicate that Lp(a) levels are highly heritable. One study estimated that 98 percent of the variance in Lp(a) levels could be explained by the apolipoprotein (a) locus. As a result, Lp(a) levels are essentially constant across the life span.

The pathogenicity of Lp(a) is attributed in part to the strong homology of apolipoprotein (a) to plasminogen, thereby providing a link between atherosclerosis and thrombosis. The Atherosclerosis Risk in Communities (ARIC) study showed that over a 10-year period, Lp(a) along with LDL-C, HDL-C, HDL3-C, and TG levels were independent predictors of CHD events in middle-aged subjects, whereas apoB, apoAI, and HDL2-C were not. Lp(a) levels were higher in subjects who developed CHD, but added only a small predictive value above that provided by LDL, HDL, and TG, and was not a predictor in black men. Lp(a) levels are refractory to most lipid-lowering pharmacologic agents including resins, fibrates, and HMG-CoA (hydroxymethylglutaryl coenzyme A) reductase inhibitors. However, niacin appears to lower Lp(a) levels. There are contradictory reports of the effects of estrogen replacement therapy on Lp(a) concentrations.

Knowledge of a patient's Lp(a) level might provide the clinician with additional insight into the patient's risk for CHD, complementing the information provided by the standard lipoprotein profile. Unfortunately, there is no universally accepted standardization program, thus limiting its utility due to the lack of reproducibility and reliability of measurement.

Elevated Homocysteine Levels

Elevated levels of plasma homocysteine are associated with increased risk for CHD, stroke, and vascular disease. Increasing age, male gender, elevated serum creatine levels, and reduced concentrations of blood folate and serum B_{12} are independently associated with elevated plasma homocysteine levels in older subjects. Treatment with folate lowers plasma homocysteine levels. Intervention data indicates that folate supplementation reduces the rate of restenosis after coronary angioplasty. Ongoing clinical trials are examining the effect of vitamin supplementation on the primary and secondary prevention of CHD and stroke.

Summary

Despite impressive advances in our understanding of the pathogenesis of atherosclerosis, there are several ongoing questions to be resolved concerning the lipoprotein risk factors for CHD in the elderly population: (1) Do lipoprotein subfractions (Lp(a), LDL, HDL) predict CHD morbidity and mortality, as well as total mortality in the elderly? (2) What impact does the age of lipoprotein measurement have on disease prediction? (3) How do longitudinal changes in lipoprotein lipid concentrations impact on the prediction of CHD? (4) Would genetic screening for high CHD risk-associated polymorphisms identify individuals for whom early therapy might reduce CHD risk and prolong survival?

INTERVENTION TRIALS

Over the past 25 years more than 50 clinical trials employing a number of pharmacologic therapies demonstrate that lowering LDL-C concentrations decreases rates of CHD events in individuals younger than age 65 years. In general each 10 percent reduction in total cholesterol reduces the incidence of CHD by approximately 22 percent after 2 to 5 years of therapy, and a 10 percent reduction in all-cause mortality for each 10 percent reduction in cholesterol. In general, however, individuals older than age 65 years, particularly older women, were often excluded from these trials. Therefore, the value of cholesterol-lowering interventions, particularly in the primary prevention of CHD in the elderly population, has been questioned. This section

Table 68-3 Effect of Lifestyle and Pharmacologic Interventions on Lipoprotein Profiles

Intervention	Anticipated Effect*	Comment
Lifestyle		
AHA Step I diet	5–10% decline in TCHOL, LDL-C, and HDL-C; TG effect variable	Greatest absolute improvement in hyperlipidemia. Universality of AHA Step I diet questioned in primary prevention of CHD in individuals >75 years, and in some individuals with type 2 diabetes.
Weight loss (WL)	10–15% decline in TCHOL, LDL-C; 10–15% increase in HDL-C	Ideal body weight guidelines remain controversial. Beneficial effect of WL on other risk factors. WL enhances the effect of AHA diet and AEX on CHD risk factors.
Aerobic exercise (AEX)	5–10% decline in TCHOL, LDL-C; 0–15% increase in HDL-C	Much of the effect of AEX on lipids is a result of concomitant WL. AEX has beneficial effects on other CHD risk factors and quality of life.
Drugs		
Fibrates	35% reduction in TG; 10% reduction in LDL-C; 10% increase in HDL-C	For hypertriglyceridemic patients. May need to add resin for multiple lipoprotein hyperlipidemia. Often have coexistant insulin-resistance syndrome.
Statins	20–40% reduction in TCHOL, LDL-C; 5–15% reduction in TG;5–10% increase in HDL	For hypercholesterolemic patients. Well tolerated. More potent than resins in lowering LDL. Growing body of evidence for use of statins for both primary and prevention of ↓ CHD in 60- to 75-year old individuals. Monitor for liver toxicity, myopathy.
Resins	15% reduction in TCHOL, LDL-C; increases TG, HDL-C	For hypercholesterolemic patients. Often used as a second-line drug or in combination with statins and fibrates. Causes bloating, constipation, ↑ TG.
Niacin	20% reduction in TCHOL, LDL-C; >20% increase in HDL-C	Effective for multiple lipoprotein hyperlipidemia, ↑ TG, low HDL-C, liver toxicity with sustained-release formulation, contraindicated in liver disease, diabetes, peptic ulcer, gout.

*Consensus of literature assuming weight loss results in a 10% reduction in weight, exercise a 10% improvement in maximal aerobic capacity, and mid range dosage of medications.

AEX, aerobic exercise; AHA, American Heart Association; HDL-C, high-density lipoprotein cholesterol; LDL-C, low-density lipoptotein cholesterol; TCHOL, total cholesterol; TG, triglyceride; WL, weight loss.

reviews the effects of lifestyle and pharmacologic interventions on cholesterol profiles and on the primary and secondary prevention of CHD in the elderly person.

Lifestyle

Diets reduced in saturated fat and cholesterol (American Heart Association Step I diet), weight loss, and aerobic exercise training are widely advocated for the initial treatment of hyperlipidemia. In obese individuals, moderate weight loss alone, or in combination with aerobic exercise, can decrease total cholesterol and LDL-C concentrations by 10 to 15 percent, increase HDL-C by 15 percent, improve glucose tolerance, and lower blood pressure (Table 68-3). Moreover, the lipid-lowering response to lifestyle interventions is related to the initial lipoprotein profiles. Individuals with the highest baseline cholesterol concentrations show the greatest improvements with weight loss and AHA Step I diet interventions. However, it should be recognized that the beneficial effects of low fat diets on reductions in total and LDL-C concentrations are tempered by the reductions in HDL-C which are often of the same magnitude as the reduction in LDL-C. Without concomitant weight loss, the ratio of LDL-C to HDL-C may actually increase, not decrease when individuals are placed on diets low in saturated fat and cholesterol. This suggests that the AHA Step I diet might not be optimal for older women in whom HDL-C concentrations are a major determinant of CHD risk, but the beneficial effects of reduced atherogenic LDL-C concentrations may outweigh any putative harmful effects of reductions in HDL-C.

The 2000 American Heart Association Dietary Guidelines advocate a balanced diet consisting of: >5 servings per day of fruits and vegetables, >6 servings per day of whole grains, >2 servings of fish per week, lean meats, poultry, legumes, soluble fiber and non- or low-fat dairy products; caloric intake to maintain a healthy weight; <30 percent daily calories from fat by limiting saturated fat to <10 percent total calories and cholesterol <300 mg/d to keep LDL-C <100 mg/dL; <6 g salt per day; and <1 alcoholic drink per day. These recommended changes in dietary content should result in lower levels of total and LDL-C and greater protection from CHD.

We advocate lifestyle interventions consisting of the AHA Step I diet, moderate weight loss, and low-intensity exercise in older individuals with overt manifestations of atherosclerosis, or in higher risk asymptomatic individuals with multiple CHD risk factors. Clinical trials with long-term follow-up can determine whether these lifestyle interventions will decrease CHD and overall morbidity and mortality.

Pharmacologic Trials

A key issue is whether lowering of LDL-C levels results in improved outcome. Although definitive evidence is lacking in men and women older than age 75 years, there is now data supporting beneficial effects of cholesterol lowering in the men and women age 65 to 75 years. As noted previously, the majority of the outcome data comes from secondary prevention trials.

In the Scandinavian Simvastatin Survival Study (4S), men older than age 65 years randomized to the simvastatin arm had significant reductions in death (relative risk, 0.65) and major coronary events (relative risk, 0.69), as compared to the placebo group. For women older than age 65 years randomized to the simvastatin arm, the relative risk for major coronary events (0.66) was similar to that observed in men. However, there were too few deaths to assess the effects of simvastatin on mortality in women. It is relevant that cholesterol lowering with simvastatin produced similar relative reductions in CHD events in men and women older than age 65 years as in those younger than age 65 years.

A number of clinical trials have employed pravastatin as the therapeutic intervention. In a subgroup analysis of pooled data from the Pravastatin Limitation of Atherosclerosis in the Coronary Arteries (PLAC I) and the Pravastatin, Lipids, and Atherosclerosis in the Carotid Arteries (PLAC II) trials, among patients older than age 65 years, over 3 years of follow-up, pravastatin therapy was associated with a 79 percent reduction in coronary event incidence (2 of 63 versus 11 of 75), and an 86 percent reduction in nonfatal myocardial infarction (1 of 63 versus 8 of 75). By comparison, in patients younger than age 65 years, the coronary event incidence and nonfatal myocardial infarctions were reduced by 53 percent and 42 percent, respectively. Subgroup analysis of the Long-Term Intervention with Pravastatin in Ischemic Disease (LIPID) study data demonstrated a 15 percent reduction in death in coronary patients aged 70 to 75 years, whereas there was a 28 percent reduction in patients aged 65 to 79 years.

The Cholesterol and Recurrent Events (CARE) trial examined the effects of pravastatin on recurrent cardiovascular events in patients age 21 to 75 years with prior myocardial infarction and baseline cholesterol values below 240 mg/dL. Subset analyses were performed that examined the response in patients aged 65 to 75 years, as compared to the younger subjects. Overall, there was a 32 percent reduction in major coronary events (coronary death, nonfatal myocardial infarction, angioplasty, or bypass surgery) and stroke in the older treated patients, as compared to controls. The number of older patients needed to treat for 5 years to prevent a major coronary event and to prevent a coronary death were 11 and 22, respectively. Considering all cardiovascular events, 225 events would be prevented for every 1000 older patients treated for 5 years as compared to 121 in younger patients.

The West of Scotland Coronary Prevention Study (WOSCOPS) was a primary prevention trial that examined the effectiveness of 40 mg of pravastatin in reducing morbidity and mortality from CHD in men age 45 to 64 years who never had a myocardial infarction. Overall, there was a 31 percent reduction in cardiac end points in the pravastatin group. This trial therefore complements the results of the secondary prevention trials.

Each of these trials included relatively modest numbers of older individuals. The Prospective Pravastatin Pooling Project combined outcome data from the WOSCOPS, CARE, and LIPID trials. In this analysis, individuals in all three age groups examined, younger than age 55 years, age 55 to 64 years, and age 65 to 75 years, demonstrated substantial benefit from treatment. Furthermore, there was no evidence for an age effect on the reduction in events. Collectively, these intervention studies support the use of cholesterol-lowering drugs in older individuals younger than age 75 years, particularly in those with prevalent CHD. The NCEP ATP III recommends that using prudent clinical judgment, older people are candidates for cholesterol-lowering drugs for primary prevention.

Hormone Replacement Therapy

Given the accelerated incidence of CHD in postmenopausal women, it is highly relevant whether estrogen replacement therapy can reduce CHD morbidity and mortality in postmenopausal women. There are more than 40 observational epidemiologic studies that demonstrate that postmenopausal women who use estrogen are at a lower risk for CHD than are women who do not. Indeed, this is biologically plausible as small intervention trials demonstrate that estrogen therapy decreases LDL-C, raises HDL-C, and reduces Lp(a). Estrogen therapy also has adverse effects of CHD risk factors, including raising triglyceride levels, and has prothrombotic effects.

Unfortunately, the observational data is not supported by clinical trials, which indicate that hormone-replacement therapy does not decrease the risk for future cardiac events in women with established CHD. For example, in the Heart and Estrogen/Progestin Replacement Study (HERS) conducted in women with established CHD, there was no difference in coronary death or nonfatal myocardial infarction in treatment versus placebo groups. There was actually a 50 percent increase in CHD events during the first year of treatment in the estrogen group that was offset by a subsequent decrease in risk. A similar pattern of increased short term risk for CHD after initiation of hormone replacement therapy use followed by a decreased rate of CHD events with long-term use was also noted in postmenopausal women with previous myocardial infarction or documented atherosclerosis participating in the observational Nurse's Health Study. Combined hormone-replacement therapy with estrogen plus progesterone also failed to lower the risk of CHD events in postmenopausal women without prevalent CHD in the Women's Health Initiative (WHI). This component of the WHI was stopped

Table 68-4 Considerations of Factors for and Against Treatment of Hyperlipidemia in the Elderly Patient

Factors favoring treatment of hyperlipidemia

CHD is the most common cause of death in old age.

Attributable risk increases with age.

Atherosclerosis is pathologically indistinguishable in elderly and middle-aged persons.

Hypolipidemic drugs appear to be as efficacious in elderly persons as in middle-aged persons.

Numerous clinical trials of lipid-lowering therapy found substantial reductions in cardiac morbidity and mortality in the "young" old (age 65–75years).

Factors against treatment of hyperlipidemia

Lack of evidence that primary or secondary prevention decreases CHD morbidity and mortality in individuals older than age 75 years.

Drug side effects may be greater.

There may be a lag time (2 years) between the initiation of therapy and the reduction of morbidity and mortality from CHD.

Cost for elderly persons on fixed incomes with limited insurance.

The presence of other multiple comorbid diseases might limit life span or the quality of life.

Polypharmacy and risk of drug side effects.

prematurely because putative cardiovascular benefits did not outweigh risks of adverse outcomes.

SCREENING AND TREATMENT CONTROVERSIES AND RECOMMENDATIONS

The screening of older individuals, particularly those without overt CHD for hyperlipidemia, and the treatment of hyperlipidemia in older individuals remain controversial. It is evident that the older the individual, the less supporting data is available. Therefore, in patients who are in their mid-seventies and older, extrapolation from data obtained in younger individuals becomes an issue. Table 68-4 summarizes Some of the arguments for and against the treatment of hyperlipidemia in the elderly patient. These arguments, both for and against screening and treatment of hyperlipidemia in the elderly patient fail, however, to take into consideration several secular changes that affect the approach to the older patient.

1. First and foremost, all the published guidelines assume that the clinician is faced with the de novo decision of whether an elderly patient should be screened for hyperlipidemia without taking into consideration prior evaluations that these individuals may have had when younger. Indeed, given that cholesterol profiles are routinely obtained as part of the automated battery of laboratory tests in patients admitted to the hospital, and that over the past 20 years there has been widespread cholesterol screening, many older individuals, particularly the "young" old, and those with CAD, have already had measurements of their cholesterol profiles.

2. Given secular increases in the use of hypolipidemic drugs for both the primary and secondary prevention of CHD in middle-aged and older individuals, an increasing number of older patients presenting to the geriatrician will already be on lipid-lowering medications. The geriatrician will have to decide on the appropriateness of continuing therapy. It will be difficult to discontinue medications in patients with overt CHD, and in those with multiple risk factors for CHD, unless there are compelling reasons.

3. There is growing emphasis on maintaining or increasing functional independence and quality of life for the elderly person. The avoidance of coronary or vascular events that contribute to disability in the elderly population must be factored into any decision on the screening and treatment of hypercholesterolemia.

4. Given the large number of clinical trials in progress, it is likely that there will be a growing body of evidence that will support the use of pharmacologic interventions for primary and secondary prevention of CHD in older individuals. Delaying therapy while awaiting definitive evidence in support of therapy may be untenable.

The approach to the management of hyperlipidemia in older persons (men age ≥ 65 years; women age ≥ 75 years) was extensively modified in the most recent National Cholesterol Education Program Adult Treatment Panel III report. This report recommends the calculation of the Framingham risk score as the primary means of identifying older persons at increased risk for coronary events (Table 68-5). Based on the overall Framingham risk score, older people are stratified into four main risk categories (Table 68-6) with different recommendations for cholesterol management: (1) older people with prevalent CHD or CHD risk equivalents (diabetes, stroke, peripheral vascular disease, etc.) with a 10-year risk >20 percent; (2) older people with multiple (2+) risk factors with a 10-year risk of 10 to 20 percent; (3) older people with multiple (2+) risk factors and a 10-year risk <10 percent; and (4) older people who have no risk factors other than their age with an absolute 10-year risk <10 percent.

There are different treatment recommendations and therapeutic goals for the different risk categories with the most aggressive therapy directed at patients with the highest risk. For individuals with CHD or CHD risk equivalents, the treatment goal for LDL-C is <100 mg/dL. NCEP ATP III recommends therapeutic lifestyle changes for LDL-C ≥ 100 mg/dL, and consideration of drug therapy for those

Table 68-5 Framingham Risk Score

Estimate of 10-Year Risk for Men	Estimate of 10-Year Risk for Women

(Framingham Point Scores)

Men

Age	Points
20–34	9
35–39	4
40–44	0
45–49	3
50–54	6
55–59	8
60–64	10
65–69	11
70–74	12
75–79	13

Total Cholesterol	Age 20–39	Age 40–49	Age 50–59	Age 60–69	Age 70–79
<160	0	0	0	0	0
160–199	4	3	2	1	0
200–239	7	5	3	1	0
240–279	9	6	4	2	1
<280	11	8	5	3	1

	Age 20–39	Age 40–49	Age 50–59	Age 60–69	Age 70–79
Nonsmoker	0	0	0	0	0
Smoker	8	5	3	3	1

HDL(mg/dL)	Points
>60	−1
50–59	0
40–49	1
<40	2

Systolic BP (mmHg)	If Untreated	If Treated
<120	0	0
120–129	0	1
130–139	1	2
140–159	1	2
≥160	2	3

Point Total	10-Year Risk %
<0	<1
0	1
1	1
2	1
3	1
4	1
5	2
6	2
7	3
8	4
9	5
10	6
11	8
12	10
13	12
14	16
15	20
16	25
≥17	≥30

10-Year risk _____%

Women

(Framingham Point Scores)

Age	Points
20–34	−7
35–39	−3
40–44	0
45–49	3
50–54	6
55–59	8
60–64	10
65–69	12
70–74	14
75–79	16

Total Cholesterol	Age 20–39	Age 40–49	Age 50–59	Age 60–69	Age 70–79
<160	0	0	0	0	0
160–199	4	3	2	1	1
200–239	8	6	4	2	1
240–279	11	8	5	3	2
≥280	13	10	7	4	2

	Age 20–39	Age 40–49	Age 50–59	Age 60–69	Age 70–79
Nonsmoker	0	0	0	0	0
Smoker	9	7	4	2	1

HDL(mg/dL)	Points
>60	−1
50–59	0
40–49	1
<40	2

Systolic BP (mmHg)	If Untreated	If Treated
<120	0	0
120–129	1	3
130–139	2	4
140–159	3	5
≥160	4	6

Point Total	10-Year Risk %
<9	<1
9	1
10	1
11	1
12	1
13	2
14	2
15	3
16	4
17	5
18	6
19	8
20	11
21	14
22	17
23	22
24	22
≥25	≥30

10-Year risk _____%

U.S. Department of Health and Human Services; Public Health Service; National Institute of Health; National Heart, Lung and Blood Institute; NIIT Publication No. 01-3305 May 2001. (Wilson PW et al: Prediction of coronary heart disease using risk factor categories. *Circulation* 97:1837, 1998.)

Table 68-6 Special Considerations for Cholesterol Management in Older Persons (Men ≥65 Years of Age; Women ≥75 Years of Age)

Risk Level	Special Considerations*
CHD and CHD risk equivalents 10-year risk >20% LDL goal <100 mg/dL	Sizable number of older persons were included in secondary prevention statin trials. Older persons respond similarly in risk reduction as do middle-aged persons. Guidelines for use of LDL-lowering drugs thus are similar in older and middle-aged persons for secondary prevention. Prevalence of diabetes, a CHD risk equivalent rises markedly in the older population.
Multiple (2+) risk factors 10-year risk 10–20% LDL goal <130 mg/dL	Risk assessment by standard risk factors probably less reliable in older persons; emerging risk factors (e.g., noninvasive assessment of subclinical atherosclerosis) may assist in risk estimation. LDL-lowering drugs can be consider in older persons when multiple risk factors are present and when LDL-C is ≥130 mg/dL after therapeutic lifestyle changes. Management of other risk factors (e.g., smoking, hypertension, diabetes) has priority in older persons.
Multiple (2+) risk factors 10-year risk <10% LDL goal <130 mg/dL	LDL-C can be a target of drug therapy when LDL-C ≥160 mg/dL to reduce short-term risk. However, risk assessment by standard risk factors is probably less reliable in older persons; emerging risk factors (e.g., noninvasive assessment of subclinical atherosclerosis) may assist in risk estimation. Emphasis should be given to dietary changes that promote overall good health.
0–1 risk factors 10-year risk <10% LDL goal <160 mg/dL	Persons in this category have no risk factors other than age. Absolute short-term risk is relatively low. Very high LDL-C, 190 mg/dL after therapeutic lifestyle changes, justifies consideration of drug therapy. High LDL-C (160–189 mg/dL) makes drug therapy optional.

*Clinical judgment assumes increases importance in choice of LDL-lowering therapies in older persons; see number needed to treat for benefit in older persons (Table 68-7).
Source: Adapted from NCEP ATP III, section VIII-6 (2001).

with LDL-C ≥130 mg/dL, with drug therapy optional for LDL-C levels of 100 to 129 mg/dL. For individuals with multiple risk factors without prevalent CHD or CHD risk equivalents, the goal for LDL-C is <130 mg/dL. Note that the 10-year risk estimate affects the approach to the treatment of individuals with multiple risk factors (risk categories 2 and 3), but not the treatment goal. Therapeutic lifestyle changes are recommended for individuals with two or more risk factors for LDL-C ≥130 mg/dL. For individuals with a 10-year risk of 10 to 20 percent, NCEP ATP III recommends initiation of pharmacologic therapy at LDL ≥130 mg/dL, whereas for individuals with a 10-year risk <10 percent, the LDL-C level to consider drug therapy is ≥160 mg/dL.

There is considerable controversy concerning the management of hyperlipidemia in older individuals who have no risk factors other than their age. For individuals in the fourth risk category, the LDL goal is <160 mg/dL. NCEP ATP III recommends the initiation of lifestyle changes for LDL-C >160 mg/dL, and pharmacologic therapy for LDL-C ≥190 mg/dL with drug therapy optional for LDL-C levels of 160 to 189 mg/dL. The NCEP ATP III acknowledges that clinical judgment plays a crucial role in determining the appropriate management of hyperlipidemia in the elderly patient.

In general, for patients without CHD or CHD equivalents, patients are initially started on diet and activity modification to lower LDL-C, and if LDL-C goals are not reached in 3 months, then LDL-lowering drugs are started. We begin with low to moderate doses of HMG-CoA reductase inhibitors (statins) or fibrates, which are better tolerated than bile acid sequestrants or niacin. Although statins are well-tolerated, patients must be monitored for liver toxicity and myopathy. After 6 weeks of therapy, the lipoprotein lipid levels are remeasured. If the LDL-C goal is not met, we increase the dose, or consider combined therapies of statins with niacin or bile sequestrants, not fibrates. Liver, renal, and muscle toxicity should be checked monthly for 3 months, then every 6 months on statin therapy, but quarterly when drug combinations are prescribed. When prescribing lipid-lowering medications, the geriatrician also needs to carefully assess potential interactions with other prescribed medications, over-the-counter medications and vitamins with the hypolipidemic medications. Supplemental antioxidant vitamin therapy may interfere with the potential benefits of lipid-lowering therapy of statins and niacin.

The approach to the management of hypertriglyceridemia was extensively modified in NCEP ATP III. The goals is for TG levels to be <150mg/dL. Borderline-high

Table 68-7 Number Needed to Treat with Statin Therapy for 15 Years to Prevent CHD Events by Age 80 Years Starting at Age 65 Years

10-Year Risk for Hard CHD	Number Need to Treat to Prevent CHD Events (15 Years of Drug Therapy)		
	CHD Death	Hard CHD	Total CHD
10%	42	21	10
20%	20	10	5
30%	13	13	3
40%	10	10	1–2

*The results in this table assume that statin therapy reduces relative risk for all CHD events by one-third.

Hard CHD includes myocardial infarction + CHD death; Total CHD includes myocardial infarction, CHD death, unstable angina, and coronary procedures (angioplasty and coronary bypass surgery).

SOURCE: Adapted from NCEP ATP III, section II-49 (2001).

TG is defined as 150 to 199 mg/dL, high TG is 200 to 400 mg/dL and very-high TG is >500 mg/dL. Although it is still controversial whether elevated TG levels are independently associated with increased risk for CHD, caused by the increased prevalence of obesity and CHD risk associated with the metabolic syndrome of visceral obesity, hyperinsulinemia, type 2 diabetes, low HDL-C, hypertension, and prothrombic state in older individuals with elevated TG levels, most would advocate therapeutic interventions for elevated TG levels. Treatment is weight loss and exercise in the borderline-to-high category, but when levels are higher and associated with the metabolic syndrome, we add fibrates or niacin along with treatments for medical conditions associated with insulin resistance. Adherence to lifestyle therapy may reduce TG and the need for medication. If LDL-C levels and TG are both high, atorvastatin is the preferred drug, but fibrates or niacin are often effective. Secondary causes for hyperlipidemia, especially diabetes, thyroid, and renal disease should be considered when multiple lipoprotein classes are abnormal in the elderly patient.

Low HDL-C is redefined in NCEP ATP III as <40 mg/dL for both men and women. After maximizing dietary and activity lifestyle changes, and drug therapy to lower LDL-C and TG levels, niacin may be added to raise HDL-C levels. However, drug interactions with statins and fibrates increase risk for liver, renal, and muscle toxicity, especially in the elderly population. The potential for side effects related to drugs is especially high in the elderly population, who, in general, are more susceptible to toxicity because of reduced clearance and polypharmacy.

Despite evidence that lipid-lowering therapy can reduce CHD risk and progression in older patients, risk for toxicity is higher and compliance may be poor. Careful monitoring for liver, renal, muscle, and hematologic side effects is paramount, and adherence can be improved by (1) simplifying drug regimens to once per day dosage, combination pills, and timing to early morning or bedtime; (2) recommending prompts and family assistance; (3) providing clear instructions; and (4) reinforcing good behaviors of lifestyle change and drug compliance.

As noted earlier, the relative risk of hyperlipidemia for CHD is lower in the elderly population than in younger people because of competing causes of mortality and cumulative effects of comorbid diseases. However, as a consequence of both the high absolute risk in the elderly population, and the high attributable risk for CHD events, a given therapeutic treatment such as statin therapy will prevent a greater number of events in older people than in younger people. NCEP ATP III estimates that the number needed to treat with statin therapy for 15 years to prevent CHD events by age 80 years, starting at age 65 years, is only 10 for a 65-year-old with a 10-year risk for hard CHD of 10 percent (Table 68-7). The number needed to treat for a 65-year-old with a 20 percent 10-year risk for hard CHD is 5. Thus, because of their high absolute and attributable risk, elderly patients with CHD and those with multiple risk factors would be expected to particularly benefit from pharmacologic therapy.

In summary, there is substantial evidence to support the use of lifestyle and pharmacologic interventions to treat hyperlipidemia in the "young" elderly. Based on the available evidence, we believe that in the elderly older than age 75 years, in general, pharmacologic treatment should be reserved for individuals with overt CHD or atherosclerotic vascular disease, or those with multiple CHD risk factors in whom the potential risks and costs must be balanced against the potential benefit. Finally, primary prevention may be philosophically tenable in the vigorous "older" elderly person.

REFERENCES

Burke GL et al: Factors associated with healthy aging: the cardiovascular health study. *J Am Geriatr Soc* 49:254, 2001.

Grundy SM et al: Cholesterol lowering in the elderly population. *Arch Intern Med* 159:1670, 1999.

Havel RJ, Kane JP: Introduction: Structure and metabolism of plasma lipoproteins, in Scriver CR et al. (eds): *The Metabolic and Molecular Bases of Inherited Disease*, 8th ed. Vol. II. New York, McGraw-Hill, 2001 p 2705.

Jacobs D et al: Report of the conference on low blood cholesterol: Mortality associations. *Circulation* 86:1046, 1992.

Johnson CL et al: Declining serum total cholesterol levels among US adults. The National Health and Nutrition Examination Surveys. *JAMA* 269:3002, 1993.

Kelly DT: Our future society. A global challenge. Paul Dudley White international lecture. *Circulation* 95:2459, 1997.

Kervinen K et al: Apolipoprotein E and B polymorphisms—Longevity factors assessed in nonagenarians. *Atherosclerosis* 105:89, 1994.

Lewis SJ et al: Effect of pravastatin on cardiovascular events in older patients with myocardial infarction and cholesterol levels in the average range. Results of the Cholesterol and Recurrent Events (CARE) Trial. *Ann Intern Med* 129:681, 1998.

Manson JE, Martin KA: Postmenopausal hormone-replacement therapy. *N Engl J Med* 345:34, 2001.

Millar JS et al: Impact of age on the metabolism of VLDL, IDL and LDL apolipoprotein B-100 in men. *J Lipid Res* 36:1155, 1995.

National Cholesterol Education Program Expert Panel on Detection, Evaluation, and Treatment of High Blood Cholesterol in Adults

(Adult Treatment Panel III): National Cholesterol Education Program Adult Treatment Panel III Report. 2001. (http://www.Nhlbi.Nih.gov/guidelines/cholesterol/atp3full.pdf)

O'Leary DH et al: Carotid artery—Intima and medial thickness as a risk factor for myocardial infarction and stroke in older adults. *N Engl J Med* 340:14, 1999.

Proceedings of the National Heart, Lung, and Blood Institute of the National Institutes of Health: Cholesterol and heart disease in older people and in women. *Ann Epidemiol* 2:1–176, 1992.

Sacks FM et al: Effect of pravastatin on coronary disease events in subgroups defined by coronary risk factors. *Circulation* 102:1893, 2000.

Santamarina-Fojo S et al: Lecithin-cholesterol acyltransferase: Role in lipoprotein metabolism reverse cholesterol transport and atherosclerosis. *Curr Opin Lipidol* 11:267, 2000.

Scandinavian Simvastatin Survival Study Group: Randomized trial of cholesterol lowering in 4444 patients with coronary heart disease: The Scandinavian simvastatin Survival Study (4S). *Lancet* 344:1383, 1994.

Scriver CR et al (eds): *The Metabolic and Molecular Bases of Inherited Disease,* 8th ed. Vol. II. New York, McGraw-Hill, 2001.

Stampfer MJ et al: A prospective study of triglyceride levels, low-density lipoprotein particle diameter and risk of myocardial infarction. *JAMA* 276:882, 1996.

Wilson PW et al: Prediction of coronary heart disease using risk factor categories. *Circulation* 97:1837, 1998.

Hyperparathyroidism and Paget's Disease of Bone

KENNETH W. LYLES

HYPERPARATHYROIDISM

Background and Epidemiology

Hyperparathyroidism is a common disorder of calcium, phosphorus, and bone metabolism caused by increased circulating levels of parathyroid hormone (PTH). This disease is important to geriatricians because it occurs with increasing frequency in older patients. Widespread use of multiphasic biochemical screening tests led to an increase in the incidence of cases of primary hyperparathyroidism. In the population in Olmstead County, Minnesota, which is served by the Mayo Clinic, the annual incidence rose from 16 per 100,000 people before 1978 to a peak of 112 per 100,000 people 7 years later, then the rate declined. Now such screening tests are used less frequently and the incidence has fallen to 4 per 100,000 people. It is not clear why the incidence of hyperparathyroidism is decreasing, but it is postulated that there is decreased exposure to ionizing radiation, or better supplementation with vitamin D.

Primary hyperparathyroidism may occur at any age but is found most commonly between the ages of 40 and 65 years. The incidence is approximately 1 per 1000. The disease affects women more than men by almost 2:1, and in women, this usually occurs in the first decade after menopause. In the United States, approximately 80 percent of patients with primary hyperparathyroidism have no signs or symptoms that are referable to their disease. With the development of sophisticated and specific technologies during the past 15 years, it has become feasible to evaluate patients with asymptomatic primary hyperparathyroidism in ways that have helped to establish prudent guidelines for surgical or medical management.

In hyperparathyroidism, PTH is inappropriately secreted by single or multiple glands in the presence of increased serum calcium levels. The disease is considered primary when autonomous hypersecretion of PTH is caused by a single adenoma, diffuse hyperplasia, multiple adenomas, or, rarely, a parathyroid carcinoma. Secondary hyperparathyroidism occurs when there is a prolonged hypocalcemic stimulus, as in cases of vitamin D deficiency or chronic renal failure. Tertiary hyperparathyroidism occurs in patients with chronic secondary hyperparathyroidism who develop autonomous hypersecretion of PTH and hypercalcemia, e.g., patients who undergo successful kidney transplants. This chapter focuses on primary hyperparathyroidism only.

Etiology and Pathology

The etiology of primary hyperparathyroidism is unknown. When calcium is infused into hypercalcemic hyperparathyroid patients, there is a failure to suppress the PTH levels. Furthermore, when cells from hyperparathyroid glands are incubated in vitro, higher levels of ionized calcium in the medium are required to suppress PTH release than are required to suppress PTH release from cells from normal glands. These data suggest that, in part, the abnormality occurring in the parathyroid gland is an elevation of the set point at which ionized calcium levels suppress PTH release. The receptor that is responsible for calcium-sensing in parathyroid glands has been cloned; it is a guanosine triphosphate (GTP) binding protein that has a seven-amino-acid transmembrane domain. Mutations in this receptor are rare in primary hyperparathyroidism.

In most cases of hyperparathyroidism, no etiologic agent can be identified; these represent sporadic cases. Previous neck exposure to ionizing radiation is associated with an increased incidence of hyperparathyroidism. Lithium, when used for therapy of bipolar disorders, is associated with hypercalcemia and increased PTH levels in up to 10 percent of patients. Thiazide diuretics can cause hypercalcemia, but the persistence of hypercalcemia 6 weeks after stopping a thiazide usually means the agent has unmasked primary hyperparathyroidism. A few causes of hyperparathyroidism, usually parathyroid hyperplasia, are familial disorders that have an autosomal dominant mode of transmission, such as (1) familial hyperparathyroidism, (2) multiple endocrine neoplasia type I (Werner's syndrome: hyperparathyroidism, islet cell tumors, and pituitary tumors), and (3) multiple endocrine neoplasia type II (Sipple's syndrome: medullary carcinoma of the thyroid, pheochromocytoma, and hyperparathyroidism). Only rarely does hyperparathyroidism occur in multiple endocrine neoplasia type IIB or III (medullary carcinoma of the thyroid, pheochromocytoma, mucosal neuromas, and marfanoid body habitus).

The pathologic abnormality in the parathyroid gland(s) may be an adenoma, four-gland hyperplasia, multiple adenomas, or carcinoma. Single adenomas cause 80 percent of cases of hyperparathyroidism. Hyperplasia of all four glands is found in 15 percent of cases; parathyroid carcinomas and multiple adenomas comprise the remainder. Determining whether a single gland is an adenoma or chief cell hyperplasia is often difficult to do by histologic features alone, so the gross pathology seen at operation is necessary to classify the disease. An adenoma is diagnosed when only one abnormal gland is found (all other glands are normal). Chief cell hyperplasia is diagnosed when more than one abnormal gland is found. Controversy currently exists regarding whether it is possible to have multiple adenomas. In several studies, enlargement of only two glands was documented, with the remaining two being normal. A rarer form of parathyroid hyperplasia is called "water-clear cell" hyperplasia, in which large, membrane-lined vesicles fill the cytoplasm. Finally, parathyroid carcinoma is diagnosed by finding mitotic figures in the gland or finding capsular or vascular invasion in pathological specimens obtained during surgery.

Signs and Symptoms

Patients with primary hyperparathyroidism can present with a varying spectrum of signs and symptoms ranging from a total lack of symptoms to acute hypercalcemic crisis. The diagnosis is most frequently made by routine calcium measurements with multichannel screening chemistries in a patient with either no symptoms or only weakness or easy fatigability. Acute hypercalcemic crisis is now a rare form of presentation.

Osteitis fibrosa cystica, with radiographic features of osteopenia, subperiosteal bone resorption, brown tumors, bone cysts, and "salt and pepper" skull, is rare. Patients with hyperparathyroidism show evidence of increased bone remodeling on bone biopsy, with increased amounts of osteoid surface and eroded surface when compared to normal subjects. However, dynamic parameters of bone remodeling show that the mineral apposition rate is unchanged. Although radiographic evidence of hyperparathyroid bone disease in hand films—with subperiosteal resorption and loss of the distal tuft of the phalanges—is rare in cases of primary hyperparathyroidism now, it is found in patients with secondary hyperparathyroidism from chronic renal failure.

Because osteoporosis is such a major health problem in older patients, attention has been directed at determining PTH's effect upon bone mass. With improved techniques to measure bone mass, it is possible to assess changes in both trabecular and cortical bone envelopes. Several early cross-sectional studies suggested that hyperparathyroid subjects have decreased amounts of trabecular bone in the vertebrae. More recent work shows that cortical bone as measured in the forearm or femur is reduced in affected patients. Thus, elevated levels of PTH seem to have different effects upon cortical bone. Four studies suggest that patients with hyperparathyroidism have an increase in vertebral compression fractures, but one study found no evidence of an increased incidence of vertebral fractures. A study in Sweden of more than 1800 patients reported no increase in hip fractures in women with hyperparathyroidism, but there was an increase in hip fractures in men.

Nephrolithiasis occurs in 20 percent of hyperparathyroid patients. Of patients with kidney stones, approximately 5 percent have hyperparathyroidism. PTH causes a proximal renal tubular acidosis, increasing bicarbonate loss and decreasing hydrogen ion excretion, as well as lowering the phosphate reabsorption threshold. These changes cause a hyperchloremic metabolic acidosis, and 30 percent of patients will be hypophosphatemic. Hyperparathyroidism can cause nephrocalcinosis and a subsequent decline in the glomerular filtration rate. Hypercalcemia can lead to nephrogenic diabetes insipidus because the renal tubule becomes unresponsive to the action of antidiuretic hormone. Asymptomatic patients with primary hyperparathyroidism have defects in their ability to concentrate urine.

Most other signs and symptoms of hyperparathyroidism can be attributed to the resultant hypercalcemia or, more specifically, the elevated ionized calcium level. *Gastrointestinal* disorders include anorexia, nausea, vomiting, and constipation. Peptic ulcer disease occurs with increased frequency, and, rarely, it may be the first clue to a multiple endocrine neoplasia type I syndrome (hyperparathyroidism, islet cell tumors, especially gastrinoma, and, finally, pituitary tumors). Pancreatitis can also occur or be exacerbated by the hypercalcemia. *Central nervous system* disorders include impaired cognition, recent memory loss, anosmia, depression, lethargy, and coma. Thus, hypercalcemia and hyperparathyroidism are rare but important considerations in the differential diagnosis of depression and dementia in the elderly. *Neuromuscular* disturbances include a proximal weakness, more prominent in lower than in upper extremities. Many patients complain of malaise and fatigue. Rarely, pruritus can be caused by metastatic calcification in the skin. *Articular* disturbances include pseudogout from calcium pyrophosphate crystal deposition in articular cartilage, calcific tendinitis, and chondrocalcinosis. The main *cardiovascular* disturbance is an increased frequency of hypertension. Stefenelli et al. report that patients with surgically confirmed primary hyperparathyroidism showed a high incidence of left ventricular hypertrophy (82 percent) and aortic and/or mitral valve calcifications (46 percent and 39 percent, respectively). At 41 months after successful parathyroidectomy, there was regression of the left ventricular hypertrophy. Further studies are needed to confirm and expand upon these observations.

Physical signs are unusual in hyperparathyroidism. Soft-tissue calcification can cause pseudogout or cutaneous calcification. When present in the eye, deposits of calcium phosphate crystals can cause conjunctivitis. In the cornea, band keratopathy (a vertical line of calcium phosphate deposition parallel to and within the ocular limbus) is best appreciated with a slit lamp examination. Enlarged parathyroid glands are difficult to palpate in the neck; generally, when a nodule is found in the neck of a suspected hyperparathyroid patient, it represents thyroid rather than parathyroid tissue.

Diagnosis

Primary hyperparathyroidism is diagnosed by elevated serum calcium levels and, frequently, associated hypophosphatemia, without any other apparent disease or drug causing the abnormalities. The serum calcium should be measured fasting on several occasions with minimal or no venous stasis. Techniques for measuring PTH have improved significantly, making it possible to diagnose hyperparathyroidism directly, rather than by exclusion as had been done previously. Thus, to prove hyperparathyroidism, serum PTH levels should be measured directly. Early assays measured the carboxy terminal portion of PTH. Because this fragment is cleared by the kidney, the diagnosis of hypercalcemia in patients with renal insufficiency was confounded. With improvement in assay techniques for the intact PTH molecule, using immunoradiometric (IRMA) and immunochemiluminescent (ICMA) assays, it is possible to show PTH elevations in 90 percent of patients.

Most clinical PTH assays have been validated so that the laboratory provides a range reflecting previous experience with the assay and showing where the patient's PTH and serum calcium levels fall in relation to the laboratory's other cases of hyperparathyroidism. In most nonparathyroid causes of hypercalcemia, PTH levels are suppressed, except in the unusual case of a malignant neoplasm that produces PTH. As is discussed in the section on Differential Diagnosis, malignancy-associated hypercalcemia is always a concern in the differential diagnosis of hypercalcemia, but neoplasms that are actually proved to produce active PTH are unusual, most such cases being renal, pancreatic, ovarian, or hepatic carcinomas. In such instances, the PTH-related peptide secreted by the tumor does not usually cross-react with PTH of parathyroid origin in the immunoassays employed in most laboratories.

Serum phosphate levels may be low in hyperparathyroidism, but they can be normal, especially if there is renal impairment. Although PTH does cause phosphaturia, other factors such as dietary intake and time of day may affect renal phosphate handling. Furthermore, patients with malignancy-associated hypercalcemia can have a decrease in the renal phosphate reabsorption threshold from hypercalcemia per se or from the tumor-derived peptides which produce the hypercalcemia. Other serum electrolyte abnormalities, such as elevated chloride, low bicarbonate, and low magnesium levels, are not specific enough to be of diagnostic value. Both an elevated serum alkaline phosphatase level and increased urinary hydroxyproline level suggest significant skeletal involvement from hyperparathyroidism.

Patients who are being evaluated for hyperparathyroidism should have a 24-hour urine calcium and creatinine excretion measured. Patients with a calcium:creatinine ratio of 0.1 may have familial hypercalcemic hypocalciuria, a disorder with normal PTH levels that does not require surgery.

Routine use of preoperative localization of abnormal parathyroid tissue in hyperparathyroidism should not be part of the diagnostic evaluation because noninvasive imaging techniques require further development before being valid for such application. Some centers are evaluating the use of technetium-99m sestamibi scans or ultrasonography, but they should not be used routinely in evaluating patients for parathyroidectomy. Arteriography and selective venous catheterization looking for "stepped-up" levels is a technically difficult procedure and should be performed by experienced hands only when hyperparathyroidism persists after a failed neck exploration.

Differential Diagnosis

The differential diagnosis of hyperparathyroidism is that of hypercalcemia, which can be caused by a diverse group of diseases and drugs (Table 69-1). A major concern when hypercalcemia is encountered is whether it is due to a neoplasm. The clinical setting must be considered. Most patients with malignancy-associated hypercalcemia have obvious neoplastic disease on thorough examination and routine diagnostic workup. Thus, a chest x-ray a mammogram, and a serum and urine protein electrophoresis should be ordered when evaluating hypercalcemia. Since primary hyperparathyroidism is a common disease in older women, an elderly female with hypercalcemia without obvious evidence of malignant disease will be more likely to have primary hyperparathyroidism than occult malignancy.

Familial hypocalciuria hypercalcemia (FHH) should be considered in an evaluation of hypercalcemia. Although uncommon, FHH can present with hypercalcemia, but there is usually a family history reflecting an autosomal dominant mode of inheritance, and 24-hour urinary calcium:creatinine excretion ratio of 0.1 is highly suggestive. At present, no adverse effects of the hypercalcemia have been reported from affected kindreds under supervision, and parathyroidectomy does not alter the hypercalcemia.

Drugs that cause hypercalcemia, such as thiazide diuretics and calcium supplements, can be excluded by withdrawing them for 4 weeks and making sure that serum calcium levels return to normal. Hypercalcemia caused by vitamin D intoxication can be diagnosed by measuring 25-hydroxyvitamin D levels and finding a level above 120 ng/mL. Hypercalcemia can be found in sarcoidosis, tuberculosis, and chronic fungal infections. The mechanism in all these diseases is believed to be increased production of 1,25-dihydroxyvitamin D by the granulomatous tissue, which causes increased calcium absorption from the gastrointestinal tract. Other diseases causing hypercalcemia, such as hyperthyroidism, adrenal insufficiency, and vitamin D intoxication, should be diagnosed by their historical or clinical features.

Therapy

Treatment of hyperparathyroidism depends upon the way in which the patient presents to the physician. Because most cases are asymptomatic at presentation, no immediate therapy is usually necessary, and a thorough diagnostic evaluation can be undertaken. When the patient presents with a hypercalcemic crisis (e.g., obtunded with serum

Table 69-1   Differential Diagnosis of Hypercalcemia

A. Primary hyperparathyroidism

  1. Solitary adenoma
  2. Hyperplasia
  3. Multiple endocrine neoplasia

B. Malignancy-associated hypercalcemia

  1. Local osteolytic hypercalcemia
  2. Humoral hypercalcemia of malignancy
  3. $1,25(OH)_2D$–mediated hypercalcemia

C. Granulomatous disorders

  1. Sarcoidosis
  2. Berylliosis
  3. Tuberculosis
  4. Histoplasmosis
  5. Coccidiomycosis
  6. Candidiasis
  7. Eosinophilic granuloma
  8. Silicone implants

D. Medications

  1. Vitamin D and A intoxication
  2. Lithium
  3. Thiazide diuretics
  4. Estrogens/antiestrogens
  5. Theophylline

E. Immobilization plus

  1. Juvenile skeleton
  2. Malignancy
  3. Paget's disease of bone
  4. Primary hyperparathyroidism
  5. Renal failure

F. Milk alkali syndrome
G. Parenteral nutrition
H. Familial hypocalciuric hypercalcemia
I. Hypophosphatemia
J. Renal failure
K. Idiopathic hypercalcemia of infancy
L. Hyperthyroidism
M. Addison's disease
N. Hyperproteinemia

with potassium phosphate (Neutra-Phos-K), etidronate disodium (Didronel), or oral cellulose phosphate with dietary calcium restriction may lower serum calcium levels, while other aspects of the disease may progress. The second-generation bisphosphonates, alendronate, and risedronate can lower serum calcium levels, but long-term studies are needed to document their benefits. Therefore, long-term management of hyperparathyroidism must involve a decision about whether to intervene surgically or to follow the patient until there is an indication for surgery.

Because many cases of hyperparathyroidism are asymptomatic and without any potential complications of the disease at diagnosis, immediate surgery is not necessary, and some patients may never need an operation. A National Institutes of Health (NIH) consensus conference points out that because surgery is the only effective therapy for this disorder, the patient and the physician must realize that meticulous, long-term follow-up is necessary. Understanding of long-term complications is incomplete, and no study has randomized asymptomatic patients to surgery or medical follow-up.

There are indications for surgery in asymptomatic patients with primary hyperparathyroidism: (1) markedly elevated serum calcium (above 12.0 mg/dL); (2) history of life-threatening hypercalcemia; (3) reduced creatinine clearance (below 30 percent for age-matched normals); (4) nephrolithiasis; (5) markedly elevated 24-hour urinary calcium excretion (above 400 mg); and (6) reduced bone mass as measured by direct measurement (more than 2 standard deviations below age-matched normals). Surgery should be considered strongly in the following circumstances: (1) the patient desires surgery; (2) meticulous, long-term follow-ups are unlikely; (3) coexistent illness complicates management; and (4) the patient is young (younger than age 50 years). After successful surgery, recovery is rapid. Serum calcium levels normalize within hours to several days. There is a 90 percent reduction in recurrent renal stones in patients with nephrolithiasis. Bone mass also improves after surgery; patient can gain 12 to 20 percent of their femoral or lumbar density respectively in 4 years.

Patients with serum calcium levels below 11.0 mg/dL and no other evidence of disease may be safely followed. There is agreement that malaise and fatigue are associated with hyperparathyroidism, but no prospective studies are available to show that these complaints improve with surgery. This is also true for neuropsychiatric disturbances in patients with serum calcium levels below 11.0 mg/dL. At present, no markers are available in lieu of direct measurements to suggest who will lose bone, develop nephrolithiasis, or have a decline in glomerular filtration rate. Therefore, patients with asymptomatic hyperparathyroidism require close follow-up; in addition, they should be educated about the signs and symptoms of hypercalcemia. These patients should have yearly serum measurements of calcium and creatinine, determination of creatinine clearance, and yearly kidney–ureter–bladder radiography searching for nephrolithiasis. Most experts believe that bone mass measurements (spine, hip, and possibly radius) should be followed annually for 2 to 3 years until stable. Thus, if physician and patient decide not to operate for hyperparathyroidism, education and long-term follow-up are necessary.

calcium levels of greater than 12 mg/dL), management of the hypercalcemia must take precedence over diagnostic studies. Most hypercalcemic patients are dehydrated and may require several liters of parenteral fluids to lower the serum calcium into the 11.0 mg/dL range. Once hydration has been reestablished and the patient is stable, further decisions about therapy can be made.

At this time, there is no effective medical therapy for primary hyperparathyroidism. Beta blockers, estrogen therapy in postmenopausal women, phosphate supplementation

For patients who require surgery, the most important aspect is referral to a surgeon who is experienced in neck dissections and identification of parathyroid glands. With an experienced surgeon, parathyroidectomy is usually not a major procedure unless the sternum must be split to find a substernal gland. All four glands should be identified and biopsied for histologic confirmation. Because 80 percent of the cases of hyperparathyroidism are caused by a single adenoma, removal of the offending gland is curative. When hyperplasia is identified, most surgeons remove 3.5 glands, marking the remaining portion of gland so it can be identified if necessary in the future. Transplantation of parathyroid tissue into the forearm after removal of all of the glands from the neck is used by some surgeons, especially when they anticipate removing more tissue should hyperplasia become a problem at a later time (e.g., with chronic renal failure).

Postoperatively, patients should be watched closely for 72 hours for signs of hypocalcemia. Nervousness, tingling, and a positive Chvostek or Trousseau sign may indicate hypocalcemia, which should be confirmed by total or ionized serum calcium levels. Many patients have transient hypocalcemia, and additional calcium should be given only if the level is below 8.0 mg/dL. Intravenous calcium as the chloride or gluconate salt may be given for several days, but persistent hypocalcemia requires oral calcium in a dose of 1000 to 1200 mg daily. If hypocalcemia is severe, 1, 25-dihydroxyvitamin D (calcitriol) can be added at 0.5 to 1.0 μg/d in doses divided every 12 hours. Because calcitriol can cause hypercalcemia and hypercalciuria, serum and urine levels must be monitored. Patients who have developed hypocalcemia from skeletal uptake of calcium and phosphorus with healing of osteitis fibrosa cystica ("hungry bones") have normal or low serum phosphorus levels. This complication is currently rare because of early detection of the disease; treatment with calcium supplements and calcitriol can be necessary for up to 3 months. Permanent hypoparathyroidism is a rare complication of parathyroidectomy (when performed by experienced surgeons), but it can occur. Hypocalcemia with persistent hyperphosphatemia postoperatively suggests hypoparathyroidism. This can occur transiently from bruising of the glands as they are identified and biopsied at surgery, so follow-up is required to determine whether parathyroid function returns over time. Finally, hyperparathyroid patients can have low serum magnesium levels, another cause of hypocalcemia. Thus, the serum magnesium level should be checked if hypocalcemia develops postoperatively. Because serum magnesium levels may not reflect tissue stores, patients should receive parenteral magnesium if a low normal level is found.

PAGET'S DISEASE OF BONE

Epidemiology

Paget's disease of bone is a focal disorder of accelerated skeletal remodeling, first described by Sir James Paget in 1877. In his original description, Paget described six patients with enlarged skulls, hearing loss, bowed extremities, and kyphotic spines. He called the disease osteitis deformans and proposed an inflammatory basis to the lesion, which he said led to the progressive deformity of the affected bones over the lifetime of an individual.

Paget's disease is a disease of older people. In the United States and England, the disease reportedly occurs in 1.5 to 4.0 percent of people older than 50 years of age. Its prevalence increases to 10 to 15 percent by the ninth decade of life. Paget's disease affects men and women equally. The disorder is rarely recognized before age 40 years. The incidence and severity of Paget's disease of bone appears to be declining in New Zealand and Great Britain. Further studies are needed to confirm these observations in other parts of the world where the disease is common.

There are clear geographic distributions of Paget's disease. The disorder is most prevalent in England, Western Europe, the United States, Australia, and New Zealand, but is uncommon in Scandinavia, China, Japan, and India.

Etiology

Although the etiology of Paget's disease of bone is unknown, there are two hypotheses currently promulgated that are not mutually exclusive: one, a viral etiology, and the other, a genetic susceptibility. Since the early 1970s, studies have suggested that paramyxoviruses may have a role in this disorder. Studies also document familial clusters of Paget's disease, suggesting a genetic component to this disorder.

Several paramyxoviruses (measles virus, respiratory syncytial virus, and canine distemper virus) are postulated to play a role in the etiology of Paget's disease. This hypothesis was based on finding nucleocapsid-like structures and antigens in osteoclast nuclei and cytoplasm. In addition, measles virus messenger ribonucleic acid (RNA) was found in osteoclasts and mononuclear cell progenitors. However, no virus has been cultured from pagetic cells, and despite use of sensitive techniques no direct evidence of any type of paramyxovirus RNA or of virus infection has been found. In three other skeletal disorders—osteopetrosis, pyknodysostosis, and osteoclastoma—nuclear inclusions bodies have been identified. Until the nature of nuclear inclusions is definitely determined, the role of paramyxoviruses in Paget's disease will remain controversial.

Increased interleukin-6 (IL-6) levels have been reported in bone marrow plasma and the peripheral blood of pagetic patients, and IL-6 increases osteoclast formation when added to normal marrow cells. Cytokines in the marrow microenvironment are postulated to influence the development of osteoclast precursors and thus limit the lesions to local sites once the initial lesion occurs. What is still unknown is how the initial lesion begins.

The hypothesis that Paget's disease has a genetic etiology is supported by work showing that 15 to 30 percent of patients have a positive family history of the disorder. In one study from Spain, 40 percent of pagetic patients had an affected first-degree relative. An autosomal dominant mode of transmission of the disease has been described. Subjects with a positive family history have an earlier onset of the disease and a greater prevalence of bone deformity than those subjects with a negative family history. Several groups have reported the association of Paget's disease with various histocompatibility locus antigen (HLA) groups, but no consistent pattern has been confirmed with repeated studies. Finally, possible candidate susceptibility loci for Paget's disease have been reported for five different regions on chromosomes 2, 5, 6, 10, and 11. Such data suggest that a number of chromosomal sites will be found for Paget's disease(s).

Pathophysiology

Because Paget's disease of bone is a localized disorder of accelerated bone remodeling, it is useful to briefly review the normal remodeling process (see Chap. 75). All areas of the skeleton must be remodeled throughout life to repair acquired microfractures and to strengthen parts of the skeleton placed under new or increased mechanical loads. The process begins when osteoclasts from bone marrow colony-forming units of the macrophage lineage come to a surface that needs remodeling. They excavate a cavity 50 μm in depth over a 2- to 4-week period and then undergo apoptosis. A new series of cells, osteoblasts, derived from bone marrow colony-forming units of fibroblast lineage, appear in the resorption cavity and fill it with layers of osteoid tissue known as *lamellae*. The cavity is filled with osteoid tissue and the osteoblast also form hydroxyapatite crystals on the collage, which provides strength to the matrix. The process of bone remodeling is tightly coupled so that increases or decreases in rates of bone resorption are followed an increase or decrease in bone formation. Through this coupling process, it is possible for most people to maintain their skeleton as a serviceable, lightweight frame throughout life. We now know that the coupling process is mediated by cytokines and growth factors released by osteoblasts and osteoclasts which serve to control the remodeling process. Factors such as interleukin-6 and transforming growth factor-β play a role in modulating bone turnover.

In pagetic lesions, the primary abnormality is in the osteoclast. A major histologic feature is the increased number and size of the osteoclasts and their nuclei. Normal osteoclasts have 10 nuclei while osteoclasts from areas of the skeleton with Paget's disease have up to 100 nuclei. There is a compensatory increase in the number and size of the osteoblasts in the areas of increased remodeling activity, which leads to large amounts of new bone formation. The increased rate of bone turnover disrupts the normal lamellar pattern of the osteoid tissue and results in immature woven or mosaic bone. This bone has increased amounts of fibrosis and vascularity as well as enlarged haversian canals. Thus, although the bone appears denser radiographically, it is more subject to fracture, can bow with weight bearing, and, especially in the skull, can enlarge as long as the remodeling activity is increased.

Clinical Manifestations

Patients with Paget's disease of bone present with a wide array of symptoms. Many patients have the diagnosis made incidentally when an elevated serum alkaline phosphatase level is found on a multiphasic chemistry screening panel

or radiography is performed that shows an asymptomatic bone lesion. The disease may affect any bone and can be monostotic or polyostotic. Symptoms depend on the bone(s) and the part of the bone involved as well as the activity of the bone remodeling. Many patients with radiographic evidence of Paget's disease have no symptoms.

In patients with symptomatic Paget's disease, bone pain can be mild to severe. The pain is usually not related to physical activity. The pain can be variously described as dull aching, burning, or boring in nature. Acute pain may develop as a consequence of a pathologic fracture in an affected bone. Bone pain may also arise from increased vascularity or from stretching of the periosteum due to the increased amount of new bone from the disorganized bone remodeling. Periarticular pain may be the presenting symptom in 50 percent of cases and is an important diagnostic problem because Paget's disease commonly affects bone around major joints such as the hip and knee, as well as those of the spine, with narrowing of the joint spaces and formation of osteophytes.

Bowing of weight-bearing bone is another common feature, occurring most commonly in the femur, tibia, humerus, and ulna (Fig. 69-1). The bowing seen in the

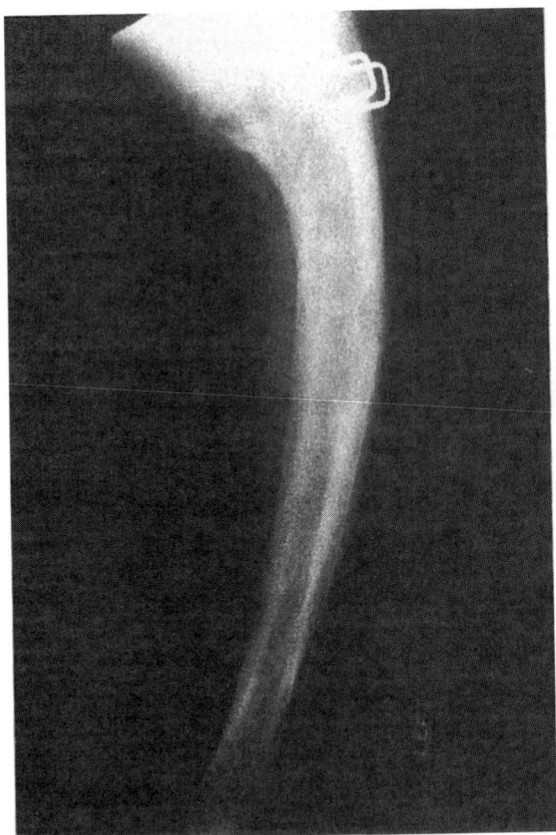

Figure 69-1 Left anteroposterior tibia and fibula radiograph from a 78-year-old woman with Paget's disease of bone involving the tibia. At the proximal portion of the tibia are staples from a failed osteotomy 25 years before. Note the lateral bowing of the tibia. There is the characteristic increase in cortical bone size from the abnormal remodeling process. In the distal portion of the tibia is seen the advancing lytic disease front, sometimes called a blade-of-grass lesion.

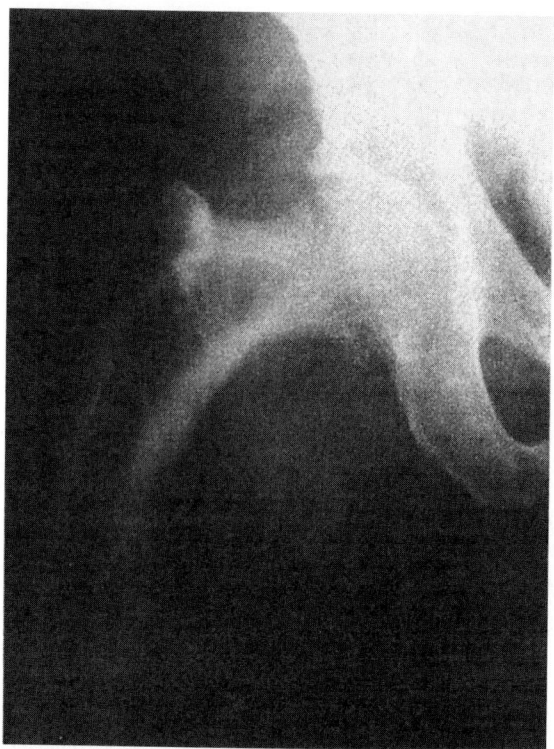

Figure 69-2 Right proximal femur and pelvis radiograph of a 68-year-old man with Paget's disease of bone involving both the femur and ilium. The angle of the femoral neck and femur are decreased as the bone is less strong, a coxae vera deformity. Also note the lateral bowing of the femur with the stress fractures on the convex side of the femur.

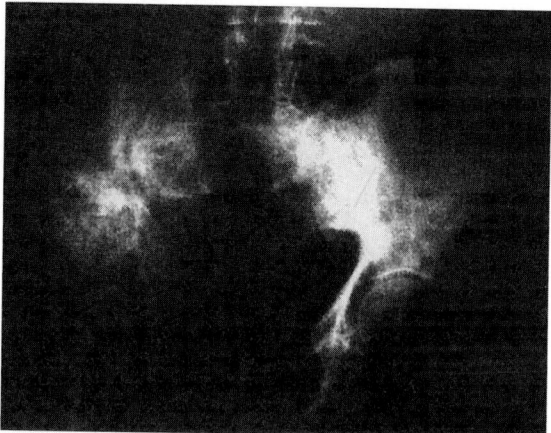

Figure 69-3 Anteroposterior pelvis radiograph from a 72-year-old man with Paget's disease of bone involving the entire pelvis. Femurs are not involved with Paget's disease, but the right side of the pelvis has marked protrusio acetabuli.

femur and tibia is often associated with stress fractures on the convex surface of the bowed bone (Fig. 69-2). Bone deformity alters force transmission through the adjacent joint causing premature loss of articular cartilage and secondary osteoarthritis especially in the hip and knee. In addition to deformities, the affected bone can enlarge. Degenerative arthritis in joints contiguous to pagetic lesions causes juxta-articular enlargement and altered subchondral bone support. Patients also develop osteoarthritis in unaffected knees as a result of favoring the non-pagetic knee. Protrusio acetabuli occurs in some patients with disease involving the ilium (Fig. 69-3).

Neurologic complications reflect the predilection of the disease to affect the axial skeleton. Disease in the skull can cause nonspecific headaches, possibly from increased blood flow. Patients with skull involvement can develop deafness. Pagetic involvement of the temporal bone can cause conductive hearing loss. Involvement of the cochlea results in mixed sensory and conductive deafness. Occasionally, the optic or trigeminal nerves may be involved, resulting in visual loss or tic douloureux. Skull deformity may result in enlargement of the vault, with a characteristic appearance particularly of the forehead (frontal bossing) or of the maxilla (leontiasis osseum). Basilar invagination of the skull can cause symptoms from internal hydrocephalus or long tract signs from brainstem compression. Bone enlargement of vertebrae can cause spinal stenosis, resulting in spinal radiculopathy or cauda equina syndrome.

Increased blood flow to the highly vascular pagetic bone has been postulated to provoke a "steal syndrome." In this situation, blood is shunted away from the neural elements, exacerbating the neurologic symptoms and signs accompanying the stenosis.

Pagetic bone fractures more easily because it is formed more rapidly than normal bone. In addition to incomplete fissure fractures on convex surfaces of bowed long bones, complete transverse fracture can occur with minimal trauma (Fig. 69-4). These fractures are called chalk stick fractures because the bone breaks evenly as a piece of chalk would, rather than with jagged fragments as normal bone does. Such fractures also have a higher rate of non-union, between 10 and 40 percent, occurring most commonly in the femur.

A serious but rare complication of Paget's disease (less than 0.1 percent of affected patients) is the development of malignant neoplasms. Osteosarcomas, chondrosarcomas, fibrosarcomas, and tumors of mixed histologic characteristics may develop, almost always in a preexisting pagetic lesion. Primary giant cell tumors and secondary spread of other cancers to existing pagetic lesions also occurs. When malignant neoplasms occur, they are very aggressive and unless the neoplasm can be removed totally (usually limb amputation), the disease is rapidly fatal. At present, there is no data showing that treatment of Paget's disease of bone reduces the occurrence of malignant neoplasms.

With high rates of bone remodeling, some patients with Paget's disease can develop nephrolithiasis. Occasionally, when patients with active polyostotic disease must be put in bed, for example, after a fracture, they can develop hypercalcemia and hypercalciuria. When this occurs, antiresorptive agents must be initiated on an emergent basis to reduce calcium release from bone resorption. Hyperuricemia and gout are reported to occur in patients with Paget's disease of bone. It is unclear whether abnormal purine metabolism is caused by the elevated bone remodeling or whether gout and Paget's disease are just two common diseases occurring in the same patient.

High-output cardial failure has been reported to occur in patients with Paget's disease. Generally, patients have

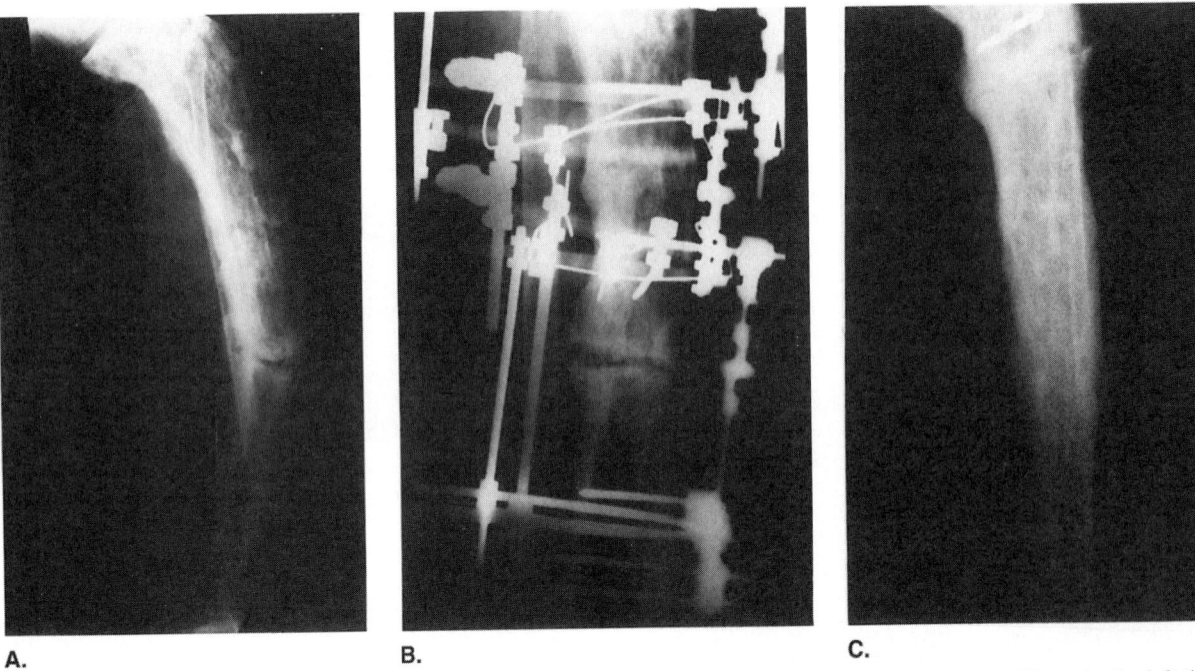

A.   **B.**   **C.**

Figure 69-4   A series of left anteroposterior tibial radiographs from a 74-year-old man with Paget's disease of bone in the left tibia. *A,* The patient's tenth fracture; note chalk stick nature. The fracture did not heal with casting over 6 months. *B,* The patient underwent tibial straightening with two osteotomies. He also wore an Ilizarov external fixation device for 1 year and received 6 months of alendronate 40 mg daily. *C,* The left tibia is much straighter. The patient now walks with a clamshell leg brace.

more than one-third of their skeleton involved with bone turnover lesions; however, documented occurrences are rare.

A series of fibrosing or inflammatory disorders are reported to occur with Paget's disease: Dupuytren's contractures, Peyronie's disease, and Hashimoto's thyroiditis. Whether these inflammatory/fibrotic disorders are only associated with Paget's disease or in some fashion caused by the release of cytokines from the areas of increased turnover awaits further study. Angioid streaks and peripapillary chorioretinal atrophy are associated with Paget's disease of bone but are more frequently with pseudoxanthoma elasticum, another connective tissue disease.

Diagnosis

All patients with Paget's disease of bone should receive a thorough history and physical examination. Because 30 to 50 percent of patients have the diagnosis made serendipitously, it may be necessary to reevaluate the patient, seeking symptoms and signs of the disease. All patients with Paget's disease should have a total-body bone scan using a technetium-labeled bisphosphonate. Areas of rapidly remodeling bone will appear as hot spots and this technique is the most sensitive method for localizing pagetic areas. Areas that are hot on bone scan should then have radiographs to confirm the presence of abnormal remodeling. Radiographs of painful or deformed bones are usually diagnostic, showing the characteristic mixed appearance of areas of lysis from increased osteoclastic resorption with sclerotic areas from excessive osteoblastic bone formation as well as cortical thickening. In the early stages of the disease, the changes may be predominantly lytic with flame-shaped resorption fronts in long bones or osteoporosis circumscripta in the skull. A characteristic appearance that distinguishes Paget's disease from other conditions radiographically is the increased size and diameter of affected bones, particularly those of the spine or shafts of long bones. If spinal stenosis, hydrocephalus, or brainstem compression from basilar skull invagination is suspected, computed tomography (CT) or magnetic resonance imaging (MRI) scans may be necessary to confirm these diagnoses.

Measurement of a serum alkaline phosphatase level is the most useful biochemical test for Paget's disease. This enzyme is located in the plasma membrane of osteoblasts, and levels are elevated above the normal range in 90 percent of affected patients. Alkaline phosphatase activity reflects the number and functional state of osteoblasts in patients with the disease. The serum level of alkaline phosphatase correlates roughly with the extent of skeletal involvement as established by radionucleotide bone scans. Serial determinations of alkaline phosphatase provide useful, simple, and inexpensive biochemical indices of skeletal activity. Serum alkaline phosphatase levels do vary from day to day, so that for a change in levels to represent a change in disease activity or a response to therapy, the level should increase or decrease by 25 percent to be clinically significant. Because 10 percent of patients with Paget's disease have normal serum alkaline phosphatase levels, it can be helpful to measure bone specific alkaline phosphatase. This isoenzyme of alkaline phosphatase can be elevated when total alkaline phosphatase levels are normal and can also be useful in patients with coexisting liver disease. Measurement of serum osteocalcin level, a vitamin K-dependent protein made by osteoblasts, has not been useful in diagnosing or following patients with Paget's disease.

Increased bone resorption is the initial abnormality in Paget's disease. Bone resorptive activity can be assessed by measuring urinary excretion of pyridinoline cross-links or n-telopeptide levels. The samples can be collected for 2 or 24 hours, and a urine creatinine level should always be measured to assess adequacy of the collection and allow for normalization for glomerular filtration rates. These measurements reflect the breakdown rate of bone collagen. Markers of bone resorption change within a day to a week after the initiation of therapy for Paget's disease while it may take 1 to 2 months before serum alkaline phosphatase levels show a response to therapy. Once a diagnosis of Paget's disease has been made and the extent of the bone involvement quantitated, only serum alkaline phosphatase levels need to be followed. In some patients, bone pain can reoccur after successful suppression or disease activity with therapy. When this occurs, and serum alkaline phosphatase levels are normal, measurement of urinary levels of pyridinoline cross-links or n-telopeptide levels can show an increase in bone resorption activity.

Table 69-2 lists the diseases that should enter into the differential diagnosis of Paget's disease. These diseases can be categorized as either causing an elevated serum alkaline phosphatase level or causing a radiographic lesion similar to Paget's disease.

In most cases, the diagnosis of Paget's disease is not difficult. An asymptomatic or symptomatic bone lesion with an elevated serum alkaline phosphatase level can be easily resolved with the clinician and a radiologist. Occasionally, the author has seen an isolated skeletal lesion in the ilium or in a vertebral body that may not have the classical

Table 69-2 Differential Diagnosis of Paget's Disease of Bone

Causes of elevated serum bone alkaline phosphatase level
Metastatic neoplasm to the skeleton
Osteomalacia
Hyperparathyroidism with osteitis fibrosa cystica
Idiopathic hyperphosphatasia
Causes of skeletal lesions with similar radiographic appearance
Metastatic neoplasm to the skeleton
Vertebral hemangioma
Fibrous dysplasia
Chronic osteomyelitis
Metaphyseal dysplasia (Engelmann's disease)
Familial expansile osteolysis
Sternocostal clavicular hyperostosis

SOURCE: Modified from Crisp AJ (1993).

radiographic appearance of Paget's disease and the markers of bone turnover; serum alkaline phosphatase, urinary pyridinoline crosslinks, or n-telopeptide levels are all normal. In these cases, a closed or open bone biopsy is necessary to rule out a neoplasm. Rarely, a patient with Paget's disease of bone may develop a metastasis from another cancer that is in a preexisting pagetic lesion. The author saw a man whose first recurrence of an adenocarcinoma from his lung primary appeared 2 years after resection of the primary lesion as a bone metastasis to an area of Paget's disease in his ilium. Finally, fibrous dysplasia can cause diagnostic confusion with Paget's disease because the lesion appears hot on bone scan. An experienced skeletal radiologist or a bone biopsy may be required to clarify this diagnosis.

Therapy

As with any chronic disease, patient education about Paget's disease is the first and most important aspect of disease management is education of the patient about their illness. The Paget Foundation for Paget's Disease of Bone and Related Disorders, 120 Wall Street, New York, NY 10007, is helpful in providing information to patients and health care professionals, the web site is http://www.paget.org/.

With current knowledge, not all patients with Paget's disease require treatment. In some cases, the symptoms that cause the patient to seek medical care are caused by an associated disorder. Thus, careful consideration of the symptoms and the physical and radiographic findings are necessary to determine whether treatment of the Paget's disease is indicated.

Patients with bone pain from associated osteoarthritis should be treated with aspirin, acetaminophen, or nonsteroid antiinflammatory agents (NSAIDs). Because many patients are elderly, care should be taken to avoid renal and gastrointestinal toxicity from NSAIDs. Some patients with severe joint destruction from Paget's disease who are not candidates for joint replacement may require narcotics to control their pain.

Patients who develop deformities or gait disturbances from their Paget's disease should be evaluated to correct or improve these impairments. A cane can be a very important therapeutic device for patients with disease in the pelvis or lower extremities. If the patient has a leg-length deformity, our group tries to correct the deformity with a shoe lift to 50 percent of the leg length discrepancy over 3 to 4 months. When this has been accomplished, the patients find they ambulate better. Patients with hearing impairments should be referred to an audiologist. When patients have maxillary or mandibular disease, they should be evaluated by a dentist.

Patients should be followed, once they are stable, semiannually or annually. An alkaline phosphatase should be checked annually, and radiographs performed when symptoms indicate a change in the disease.

The ultimate goal of therapy for Paget's disease is to restore bone remodeling to normal levels so that all new bone formed is normal. At present, all available therapies

Table 69-3　Recommendations for Antiresorptive Therapy in Patients with Paget's Disease

1. Treatment is recommended for symptoms caused by metabolically active Paget's disease: bone pain referable to a pagetic site or fatigue fracture, headache in an involved skull, back pain from involved pagetic vertebrae, pain from pagetic radicudopathy or arthropathy, or other neurologic syndromes associated with pagetic skeletal changes.
2. In patients who will undergo elective surgery on a pagetic site (e.g., elective total hip replacement), treatment is indicated to attempt to minimize the increased blood flow in metabolically active pagetic bone (those patients with an elevated alkaline phosphatase level) and reduce perioperative blood loss by decreasing hypervascularity.
3. Treatment is recommended for the management hypercalcemia that can occasionally occur with immobilization of a patient with polycystic disease and an elevated serum alkaline phosphatase level.
4. Treatment is recommended to attempt to decrease local disease progression and to reduce the risk of future complications in asymptomatic patients whose sites of disease and degree of elevated bone remodeling place them at risk of progression and further complications.

Source: Modified from Lyles KW et al. (2001).

only control the abnormal remodeling rates and do not cure the disease.

Two classes of drugs—bisphosphonates and calcitonins—are available to treat Paget's disease. Although both of these types of drugs control the increased bone remodeling by inhibiting bone resorption, bisphosphonates are more effective in controlling the increased remodeling rates. Now, calcitonin therapy is used when patients are allergic to bisphosphonates. Any patient who has pain or other symptoms or an asymptomatic patient with a pagetic lesion that give a risk of complications should receive antiresorptive therapy. Table 69-3 lists recommendations for the types of patients who should receive therapy. No controlled clinical trials have been performed to support these guidelines and such trials may never be performed. The recommendations are generally accepted by experts who treat large numbers of patients.

The development of potent "second-generation" bisphosphonates has made these agents the drugs of choice for the treatment of Paget's disease. Bisphosphonates are analogs of inorganic pyrophosphate. Pyrophosphate binds avidly to the surface of the calcium phosphate mineral phase of bone and modulates the rate and extent of mineralization. Bisphosphonates have a carbon atom substituted for the oxygen atom in pyrophosphate. Bisphosphonates bind to bone mineral but are resistant to hydrolysis. Different side chains on the central carbon atom confer different activities to bisphosphonates. Bisphosphonates bind to bone mineral and are potent inhibitors of osteoclasts. The earliest bisphosphonate etidronate inhibited osteoclast activity, but it also impaired bone mineralization. Prolonged use of etidronate was associated with the development of osteomalacia.

There are now five bisphosphonates approved for the treatment of Paget's disease in the United States: alendronate, risedronate, tiludronate, pamidronate, and etidronate. Alendronate is given in doses of 40 mg daily for 6 months. More than 60 percent of patients who receive this drug normalize their serum alkaline phosphatase levels. Orally administered alendronate cause gastrointestinal (GI) disturbances in 17 percent of patients; in some,

esophagitis can be severe enough to cause discontinuation of the drug. Risedronate is given at a dose of 30 mg orally for 60 days. At this dose, 70% of patients experience normalization of their alkaline phosphatase levels. Although esophagitis can occur with risedronate, it is believed to occur less frequently than with alendronate.

Tiludronate is more potent than etidronate, but less potent than alendronate or pamidronate. It is given 400 mg orally for 3 months. This regimen is well tolerated and will normalize alkaline phosphatase levels in 40 percent of patients. Pamidronate is another second-generation bisphosphonate that has been used in Europe for 15 years, but is approved in the United States only as an intravenous preparation. The approved regimen is 30 mg intravenously over 4 hours on three consecutive days. A second course of pamidronate may be administered as needed. The advantage of pamidronate is that it can be given intravenously and thus GI toxicity is avoided. Approximately 20 to 30 percent of patients who receive this drug have an acute phase response 24 to 72 hours after receiving the medication. This reaction can be controlled with aspirin or acetaminophen and is self-limited.

Etidronate was the first bisphosphonate to be used for therapy and is given for 6 months at a dose of 5 mg/kg. It is not as potent an inhibitor of osteoclastic bone resorption as the other bisphosphonates and is now used less frequently. It does inhibit resorption, but it impairs bone formation with equal potency. Thus, it is only given for 6 months at a time.

All patients treated with bisphosphonates should receive oral calcium supplements of 1200 to 1500 mg daily as well as 800 IU of vitamin D. Also, 20 percent of patients treated with bisphosphonates may have a transient exacerbation of pain in their pagetic lesions with initiation of therapy. Usually, aspirin or acetaminophen will control this pain, but short-term narcotics may be needed to control this pain which does resolve.

Calcitonin is a safe and effective treatment for Paget's disease. Salmon calcitonin must be administered subcutaneously, usually daily at first, and after 1 to 2 months, it is given three times a week. Calcitonin can normalize bone turnover indices in mild cases of Paget's disease, but it is clearly not as potent an antiresorptive agent as the bisphosphonates are. Usually, the biochemical response is partial, with about a two-thirds reduction in serum alkaline phosphatase levels. In approximately 20 percent of patients, resistance to chronic salmon calcitonin develops after a successful initial treatment period. Neutralizing antibodies develop to calcitonin, but it is not clear whether these antibodies are responsible for the resistance. Side effects occur in approximately 20 percent of patients treated with either salmon or human calcitonin. These include nausea, facial flushing, and polyuria. Recently, nasal salmon calcitonin was approved by the FDA for treatment of postmenopausal osteoporosis. It is not recommended for use in Paget's disease because only 40 percent of the drug is absorbed from the nasal mucosa, and, thus, does not provide a high enough dose of medication. If calcitonin is discontinued, exacerbation of biochemical abnormalities and symptoms usually occurs in 1 year.

Plicamycin and gallium nitrate are two other drugs that have been used to treat Paget's disease. Both are approved for use in treatment of hypercalcemia of malignancy and are effective antiresorptive agents. They are not approved by the FDA for use in Paget's disease and have been supplanted by the more effective second-generation bisphosphonates.

Patients with Paget's disease may need emergency or elective orthopedic surgical procedures because of complications of their Paget's disease. Fractures may require open reduction and internal fixation. Before any operative orthopedic procedure, it is desirable to reduce the remodeling activity to reduce excessive blood loss. Such a reduction in remodeling activity can be obtained with intravenous pamidronate or calcitonin if the surgery is emergent. Oral bisphosphonates may be used if the procedure is elective. A goal of this form of therapy is to reduce alkaline phosphatase levels to normal. Surgery for spinal stenosis can be effective in relieving symptoms, but most experts suggest a course of bisphosphonates or calcitonin to try to improve symptoms before undertaking a decompression procedure. Total joint replacement especially for the hip is a highly effective way to control pain and improve mobility in patients with advanced Paget's disease and degenerative arthritis of the femur or ilium. Tibial osteotomy is effective in relieving knee pain in patients who have severe tibial bowing if the associated osteoarthritis is not too severe. Recently, an external fixation device (Ilizarov) has been used in patients with tibial Paget's disease, which allows an osteotomy to be performed and then gradual changes in external pressure to be used to straighten the bowed tibia or to allow a non-union fracture to heal (see Fig. 69-4). When any orthopedic procedure is performed, it is important to maintain the patient on antiresorptive medication after surgery so that prostheses will not loosen with accelerated remodeling or straightened limbs will not rebow.

ACKNOWLEDGMENTS

The author appreciates the help of Sandra D. Giles in preparation of this chapter. Support for this work came from the VA Medical Research Service, AG11268 from NIA, and RR-30 from the Division of Research Resources, General Clinical Research Centers Program, NIH.

REFERENCES

Consensus Development Panel: Diagnosis and management of asymptomatic primary hyperparathyroidism: Consensus Development Conference statement. *Ann Intern Med* 114:593, 1991.

Cooper C et al: The epidemiology of Paget's in Britain: Is the prevalence decreasing? *J Bone Miner Res* 14:192, 1999.

Crisp AJ: Paget's disease of bone, in Maddison PJ et al. (eds): *Oxford Textbook of Rheumatology*. Oxford, Oxford University Press, 1993 p 1025.

Delmas BD, Meunier PJ: The management of Paget's disease of bone. *N Engl J Med* 336:558, 1997.

Good D et al: Familial Paget's disease of bone: Nonlinkage to the PDB1 and PDB2 loci on chromosomes 6p and 18q in a large pedigree. *J Bone Miner Res* 13:33, 2001.

Helfrich MH et al: A negative search for a paramyxoviral etiology of Paget's disease: Molecular immunological and ultrastructural studies in UK patients. *J Bone Miner Res* 15:2315, 2000.

Hocking L et al: Familial Paget's disease of bone: Patterns of inheritance and frequency of linkage to chromosome 18q. *Bone* 26:577, 2000.

Kenny AM et al: Fracture incidence in postmenopausal women with hyperparathyroidism. *Surgery* 118:109, 1995.

Khosla S et al: Primary hyperparathyroidism and the risk of fracture: A population-based study. *J Bone Miner Res* 14:1200, 1999.

Larsson K et al: The risk of hip fractures in patients with primary hyperparathyroidism: A population-based cohort. *J Intern Med* 234:585, 1993.

Lyles KW et al: Peyronie's disease is associated with Paget's disease of bone. *J Bone Miner Res* 12:929, 1997.

Lyles KW et al: A clinical approach to the diagnosis and management of bone. *J Bone Miner Res* 16:1379, 2001.

Miller PD et al: A randomized, double-blind comparison of risedronate and etidronate in the treatment of Paget's disease of bone. *Am J Med* 106:513, 1999.

Mirra JM et al: Paget's disease of bone review with emphasis on radiologic features. Part I and Part II. *Skeletal Radiol* 24:163 and 173, 1995.

Rao DS et al: Effect of vitamin D nutrition on parathyroid adenoma weight: Pathogenic and clinical implications. *J Clin Endocrinol Metab* 85:1054, 2000.

Reddy SV et al: Bone marrow mononuclear cells from patients with Paget's disease contain measles virus nucleocapsid messenger ribonucleic acid that has mutations in a specific region of the sequence. *J Clin Endocrinol Metab* 80:2108, 1995.

Silverberg S, Bilezikian JP: Primary hyperparathyroidism: still evolving? *J Bone Miner Res* 12:856, 1997.

Stefenelli T et al: Cardiac abnormalities in patients with primary hyperparathyroidism: Implications for follow-up. *J Clin Endocrinol Metab* 82:106, 1997.

van Staa TP et al: Incidence and natural history of Paget's disease of bone. *J Bone Miner Res* 17:465, 2002.

MOBILITY AND MUSCULOSKELETAL SYSTEM

C H A P T E R   7 0

Aging of the Muscles and Joints

RICHARD F. LOESER • OSVALDO DELBONO

Aging-related changes present in the tissues which make up the musculoskeletal system contribute to a number of common chronic conditions seen in older adults. In fact, musculoskeletal disease is the most common cause of chronic disability in people older than age 65 years. This is attributable both to the prevalence of diseases affecting the musculoskeletal system and the central role of the musculoskeletal system in physical function. Despite the prevalence of musculoskeletal disease, however, there is still much to learn about the pathogenesis of these diseases, including the role of aging in their development.

A number of diverse tissues, including muscle, tendon, ligament, cartilage, and bone comprise the musculoskeletal system. Aging-related changes, as well as changes secondary to disuse, have been noted to occur in all of these. As in other systems, it is often difficult to separate aging from disuse from disease. Because the musculoskeletal tissues must function in concert for normal joint motion and thereby appropriate movement to occur, it is easy to see why physical function so commonly declines with age. However, it is also clear that regular submaximal stress to the musculoskeletal system through exercise can prevent or slow the age-related decline in physical function as well as improve function of diseased tissues.

There are a number of age-related changes common to tissues of the musculoskeletal system which have also been noted in other tissues within the body (Table 70-1). Because of the relatively slow turnover rate of cells and matrix components in musculoskeletal tissues, aging-related changes such as the accumulation of advanced glycation end-products and oxidative damage to cells and matrix components can have particularly profound affects on the

aging musculoskeletal system. This chapter reviews aging in each of the major components of the musculoskeletal system including cartilage, muscle, ligaments and tendons, and intervertebral disks. Although bone is a key player in the musculoskeletal system, aging changes in this tissue are discussed in more detail elsewhere in this book in the section entitled "Bone and Mineral Metabolism."

ARTICULAR CARTILAGE

Normal Structure and Function

Articular cartilage is the tissue present on the ends of bones that comprise diarthrodial joints (Fig. 70-1). This cartilage serves to provide a smooth surface with a very low coefficient of friction necessary for rapid, painless, and smooth joint motion. During joint motion, the opposing cartilage surfaces, separated by a thin layer of viscous and slippery synovial fluid, easily glide over each other. In addition to providing a form of lubrication for the joint surface, the synovial fluid also provides a large portion of the nutrition for the articular cartilage, which is an avascular and aneural tissue.

When a load is placed across the joint surface, such as occurs in the knee joint during ambulation, the thin gel-like cartilage is compressed. Compression of the cartilage helps to distribute the load evenly to the underlying bone, where force can be absorbed. Cartilage is too thin to absorb any substantial amount of force itself. Rather, the force of joint loading is absorbed by the muscle and bone associated with the loaded joint. This concept is relevant to

Table 70-1   General Mechanisms of Musculoskeletal Tissue Aging

Accumulation of modified and degraded extracellular matrix components

Increased collagen cross-linking by advanced glycation endproducts

Decreased numbers of mesenchymal stem cells to replace lost cells

Decreased mitogenic response to injury

Decreased synthetic capacity in response to growth factor stimulation

the pathogenesis of diseases occurring in weight-bearing joints. If changes occur in muscle or bone that limit their ability to absorb mechanical loads, then the articular cartilage may experience abnormal stresses, which could adversely affect the tissue.

Complete compression of cartilage during joint motion is resisted by forces within the tissue generated primarily by the highly negatively charged proteoglycans. Proteoglycans are composed of a core protein to which are attached chains of glycosaminoglycans containing negatively charged sulfate groups. In articular cartilage a large proteoglycan called aggrecan is present. Aggrecan is bound at its aminoterminus to a long strand of hyaluronic acid (Fig. 70-2). Many aggrecan molecules are bound to a single strand of hyaluronic acid to form a large complex that is quite hydrophilic. Cartilage is approximately 70 to 75 percent water, and much of this water is bound to the negatively charged groups on proteoglycans, forming a gel-like substance. Water is partially extruded from the cartilage matrix during compression, resulting in exposure of negative charges that, as they are brought closer together, resist further compression. As the force is released, the proteoglycans reexpand and water is drawn back, bringing with it nutrients from the synovial fluid. The role of joint motion in providing cartilage nutrition may be very relevant to changes occurring in cartilage with disuse.

In addition to proteoglycans, a number of other matrix proteins are responsible for the physical properties of cartilage, including several types of collagen (predominantly types II, VI, IX, and XI) and glycoproteins (including fibronectin and cartilage oligomeric protein). Collagen is quite abundant in cartilage, comprising about half of the dry weight of the tissue. The majority of the collagen in cartilage is type II collagen. Type II collagen forms long fibrils that provide the tensile strength of the tissue, while the proteoglycans provide the resiliency. The collagen fibers appear to hold aggrecan complexes in place and prevent the proteoglycan gel from complete expansion, which results in the generation of swelling or osmotic pressure within the tissue. Thus, in normal cartilage the osmotic pressure generated by proteoglycans is balanced by the tensile force provided by the collagen fibrils. The exact function of the other collagen types and other matrix proteins in cartilage is not

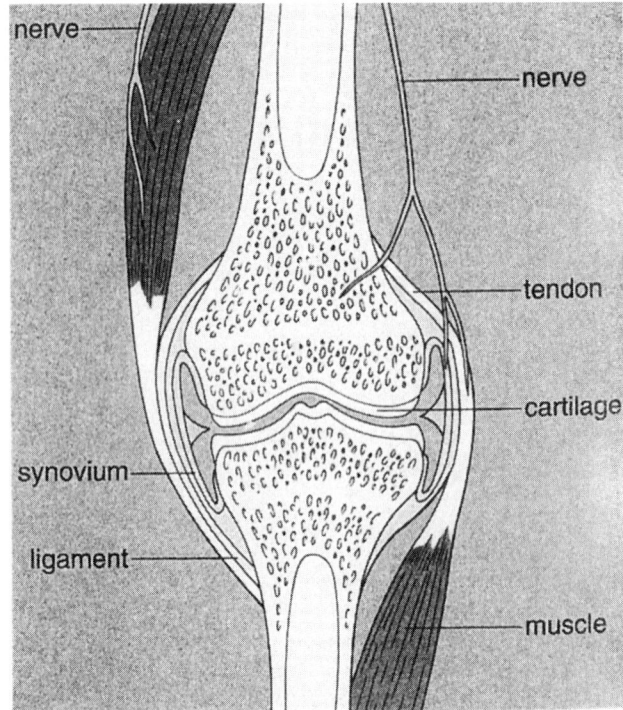

Figure 70-1   Components of the musculoskeletal system that comprise the joint include bone, cartilage, muscle, tendon, ligament, synovium, and meniscus (not shown). Note that the nerve supply to the joint does not include cartilage, and, therefore, age- or disease-related changes in cartilage are not directly responsible for joint pain. Reproduced with permission from Bullough PG: *Atlas of Orthopedic Pathology*, 2nd ed. New York, Gower Medical Publishing, 1992, p 9.4.

clear, but they are thought to be involved in the organization and maintenance of the collagen fibrillar network, in structural interactions between collagen and proteoglycans, and in mediating interactions between the chondrocytes and the extracellular matrix.

Chondrocytes, the only cells present in cartilage, control the composition and organization of the cartilaginous matrix through the synthesis and degradation of selected extracellular matrix (ECM) components. Together, the processes of synthesis and degradation result in ECM repair and remodeling. From studies performed in a number of tissues, including cartilage, it is becoming clear that ECM proteins can bind to cell surface receptors such as the integrin family of receptors (Fig. 70-2), which, along with growth factors and cytokines, send signals to the cell to regulate matrix synthesis and degradation.

Several different types of enzymes capable of degrading cartilage ECM proteins are produced by chondrocytes, including the metalloproteinases, serine proteases such as elastase, and the cathepsins. The matrix metalloproteinases (MMPs) are prominent players in mediating cartilage catabolism. These include collagenases (MMP-1, MMP-8, and MMP-13), which cleave fibrillar collagens, the gelatinases (MMP-2 and MMP-9), which degrade denatured collagen, and stromelysin (MMP-3), which degrades proteoglycans. Other important MMPs in cartilage are the membrane-type (MT-MMPs), the ADAMs (a disintegrin

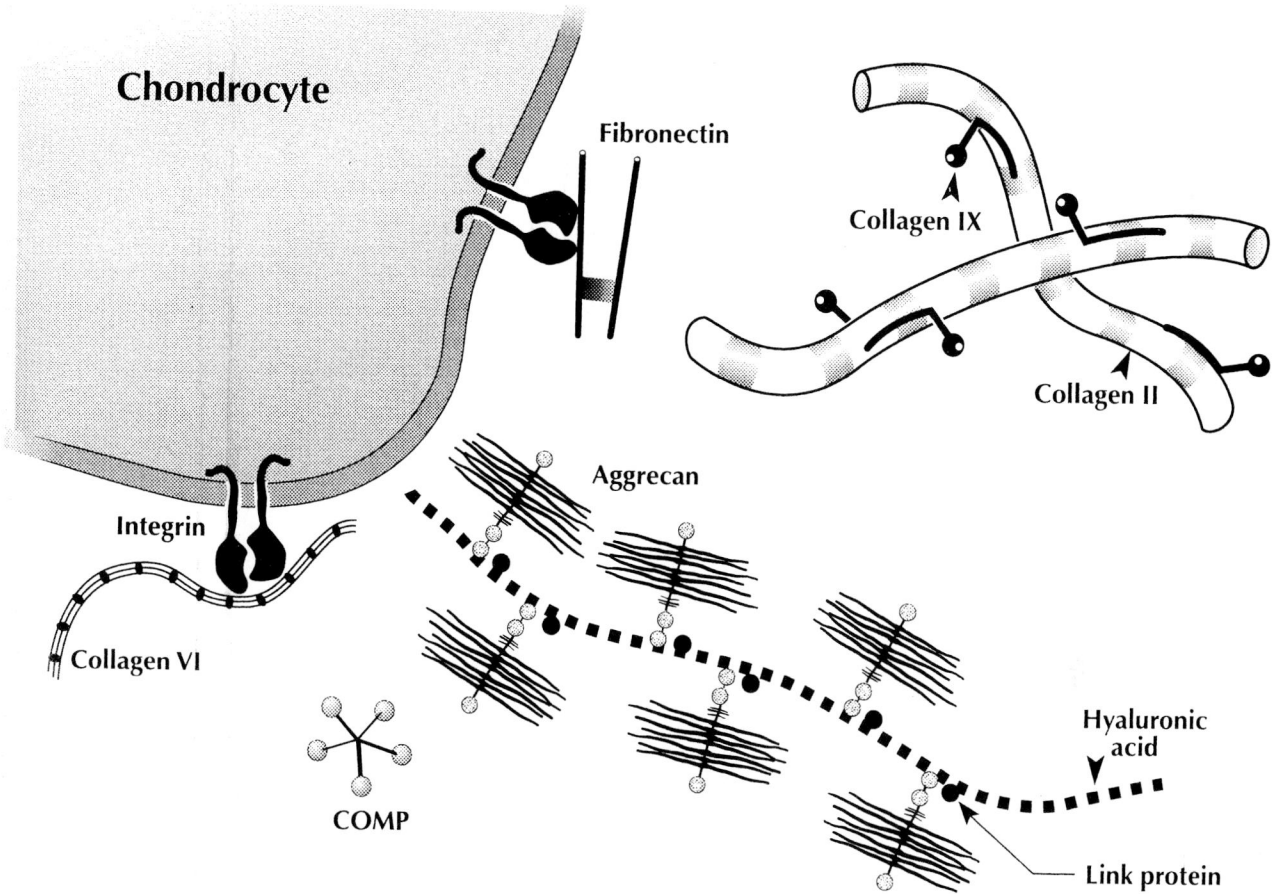

Figure 70-2   Articular cartilage consists of chondrocytes that are surrounded by an abundant extracellular matrix composed of a network of collagen, proteoglycans (aggrecan), and other glycoproteins, including fibronectin and cartilage oligomeric protein (COMP). The binding of aggrecan to long strands of hyaluronic acid is stabilized by link protein. These large complexes function in providing resiliency, and the collagen fibers provide the tensile strength of the tissue. Several of the matrix proteins can directly interact with the chondrocyte via cell surface receptors. Shown is the binding of fibronectin and type VI collagen to integrin receptors.

and a metalloproteinase) and the ADAMTSs (a disintegrin and a metalloproteinase with a thrombospondin motif). The MT-MMPs are bound to the chondrocyte surface through transmembrane domains and can serve to activate other MMPs at the cell surface. An ADAM found in cartilage is ADAM-17, also known as TACE (tumor necrosis factor-α–converting enzyme), which functions to cleave tumor necrosis factor (TNF)-α to an active form. The ADAMTSs use the thrombospondin motif to interact with proteoglycans that can serve as substrates for these enzymes. ADAMTS-4 and ADAMTS-5 are aggrecanases that cleave the large proteoglycan aggrecan. The activity of the MMPs in cartilage is controlled in part by proteins called tissue inhibitors of metalloproteinase (TIMP). There is evidence for a reduction in the levels of TIMPs relative to the increased levels of MMPs in osteoarthritic (OA) cartilage.

A number of growth factors and cytokines are present in cartilage. These serve to regulate anabolic and catabolic processes involved in repair and remodeling (Table 70-2). In general, growth factors stimulate matrix synthesis, whereas the inflammatory cytokines inhibit synthesis and stimulate degradation. Insulin-like growth factor-1 (IGF-1) and osteogenic protein-1 (OP-1) appear to play

a prominent role in regulating adult articular cartilage metabolism. They are expressed in cartilage and act in a paracrine and autocrine fashion to stimulate cartilage matrix synthesis as well as inhibit cytokine-stimulated matrix degradation. IGF-1 also appears to promote chondrocyte survival in conjunction with signals from the matrix. As discussed later in this chapter, there is growing evidence that chondrocytes from older individuals are less responsive to growth factor stimulation than those from younger persons. This could contribute to aging-related changes in the tissue, as well as to disease progression with age.

The mitogenic properties of growth factors noted in cell culture studies may not be relevant to normal adult cartilage homeostasis in vivo. In the normal tissue, adult articular chondrocytes do not appear to proliferate or do so at such low rates that proliferating cells are not detected. Chondrocytes, however, are not postmitotic cells. When removed from cartilage by enzymatic digestion of the tissue and placed in cell culture, human chondrocytes will proliferate. Proliferation of chondrocytes in situ occurs during the development of OA, when the presence of clusters or "clones" of chondrocytes is a common pathologic finding. These clusters of cells are thought to represent an attempt at repair of damaged and lost tissue (Fig. 70-3).

Table 70-2 Major Growth Factors and Cytokines Active in Cartilage

Growth Factor/Cytokine	Activity
IGF-I	Promotes cell survival, stimulates matrix synthesis
OP-1 (BMP-7)	Stimulates matrix synthesis, inhibits some catabolic pathways
TGF-β	Mitogenic, stimulates matrix synthesis, stimulates chondro-osteophyte production
bFGF	Mitogenic, stimulates matrix synthesis, potentiates IL-1 induced protease release, may be more important in fetal and growth plate cartilage than adult
IL-1β	Inhibits matrix synthesis and stimulates matrix degradation
TNF-α	Similar to IL-1β
LIF	Stimulates matrix degradation
IL-6	Inhibits proteoglycan synthesis
IL-8	Neutrophil chemoattractant
MCP-1	Monocyte chemoattractant; stimulates MMP production

bFGF, basic fibroblast growth factor; BMP-7, bone morphogenic protein-7; IGF-1, insulin-link growth factor-1; IL-1β, interleukin-1β; IL-6, interleukin-6; IL-8, interleukin-8; LIF, leukemia inhibitory factor; MCP-1, monocyte chemotactic protein-1; MMP, matrix metalloproteinase; OP-1, osteogenic protein-1; TNF-α, tumor necrosis factor-α; TGF-β, transforming growth factor β.

Normal articular cartilage in the adult contains fully differentiated cells and does not contain its own source of undifferentiated mesenchymal cells available to repair or replace damaged or lost tissue. However, mesenchymal stem cells capable of differentiating into chondrocytes are present in the bone marrow, synovium, and periosteum. Current research is trying to use these cells for repair of cartilaginous lesions because endogenous repair responses in cartilage are inadequate to replace significant amounts of lost matrix, particularly after damage to the collagen network has occurred. The potential role of aging in the failed repair response in cartilage is discussed in the following sections.

Age-related Changes in Cartilage

A number of studies have examined age-related changes in articular cartilage by using tissue collected from various animal species or human tissues obtained either at autopsy or from surgical specimens. When surgical specimens are studied, they usually are obtained from subjects undergoing hip or knee replacement surgery for arthritis, in which case the tissue is taken from grossly normal appearing areas but may not be truly normal. Tissues have also been obtained during hip replacement surgery after femoral neck fracture, which is usually associated with osteoporosis. In these cases, the cartilage is felt more likely to be normal because osteoporosis and OA tend to occur in different patient populations, although this is not always true.

Problems in interpreting the results of cartilage aging studies include translating the biology from lower species of animals to humans and separating disease effects from aging effects. In addition, a number of changes have been reported to occur in cartilage when comparing immature versus middle-aged animals. These changes are probably best considered to be developmentally related rather than

aging related. With the above caveats in mind, there do appear to be a number of changes occurring in cartilage that can be related to aging and, importantly, many of the aging-related changes can be contrasted to changes seen in disease (Table 70-3).

Structurally, fibrillation of the articular cartilage surface becomes more prevalent with age. This change could represent the presence of early OA, although other pathologic changes of OA are not always present. An extensive pathologic study, reported in 1942 by Bennett et al., was performed on cadaver and amputated knees from 63 individuals ages 1 month to 90 years who did not have a history of joint symptoms. This study revealed some degree of cartilage "degeneration" in every subject older than age 15 years. The earliest changes were roughening of the cartilage surface in areas of the joint that receive the greatest stress, such as regions of the tibial condyles not covered by the menisci and the lateral facet and vertical ridge of the patella. The morphologic changes became more common and more extensive with advancing age of the subjects. Although all knee joints of subjects in the sixth decade of life demonstrated some gross or microscopic change, the variation in the degree of changes was great, suggesting that factors other than age were responsible for the progression of pathologic changes.

In this same study, changes in the menisci were also seen with age, beginning with slight fraying in the second decade. This appeared to advance more slowly than the changes in articular cartilage, with meniscal fibrillation appearing around the sixth decade, particularly in the medial meniscus. Meniscal deterioration was more severe in the seventh decade, and by the eighth decade, menisci were thin and frayed and often calcified as well.

This study also found that morphologic changes in the synovial membrane did not appear until the eighth decade of life, when villous hypertrophy and condensation of

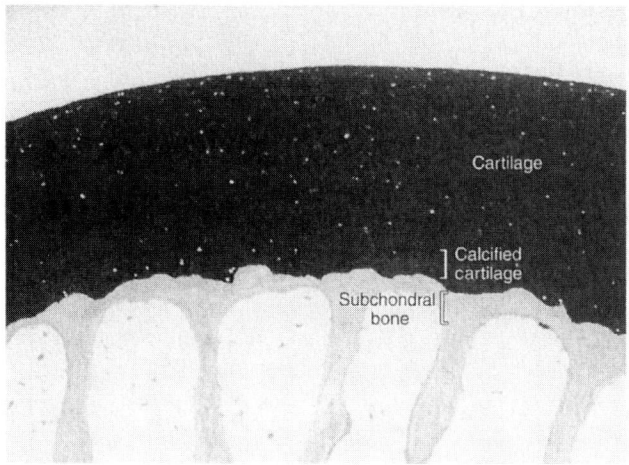

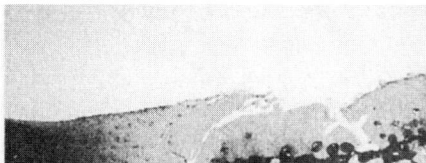

A.

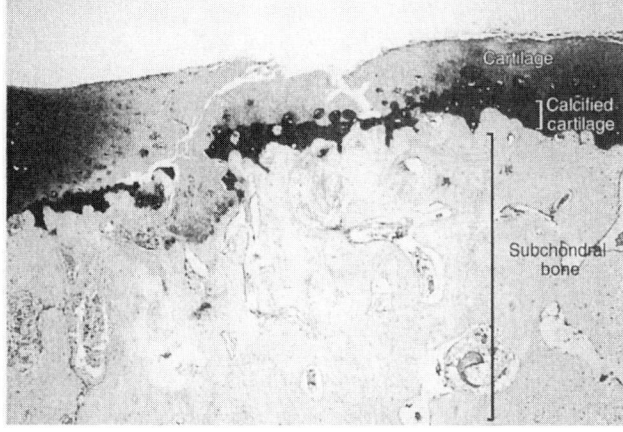

B.

Figure 70-3 Normal (*A*) and osteoarthritic (*B*) cartilage. These sections from monkey knee joints are stained with toluidine blue, which binds to the negatively charged proteoglycans that are abundant in cartilage. In the osteoarthritic tissue, there is a loss of cartilage matrix staining resulting from loss of proteoglycans. Other changes include fibrillation and cleft formation, presence of chondrocyte clusters, and a marked thickening of the subchondral bone. Photographs are courtesy of Dr. Cathy S. Carlson.

fibrous tissue in the subintimal layers were noted. It appeared that the gradient of change in both the synovium and menisci was greater than the changes in articular cartilage by the ninth and tenth decades. No histologic evidence of synovial inflammation was detected. This could be one reason why the subjects did not have known symptoms of joint disease despite the histologic changes in their cartilage. Because cartilage is aneural, joint pain requires pathology at other joint structures that contain nerve endings such as the synovium, joint capsule, or neighboring bone (see Fig. 70-1).

Unlike the knee, the ankle joint is rarely affected by OA. Studies of ankle cartilage from tissue donors have revealed a much lower prevalence of age-related fibrillation and ulcer formation. This could be related to differences in mechanical stresses between the two joints, although cellular and biochemical differences appear to exist as well. Further comparisons of cartilage from the knee and ankle

Table 70-3 Contrasting Differences Between Aging and Osteoarthritis

Aging	Osteoarthritis
Decreased cartilage hydration	Increased cartilage hydration
Proteoglycans	Proteoglycans
Normal quantity	Decreased quantity
Smaller size	Smaller size
Ratio of CS 4/6* decreased	Ratio of CS 4/6* increased
Collagen	Collagen
Normal quantity	Decreased quantity
Increased stiffness	Decreased stiffness
Increased cross-linking	Cross-links lost during degradation
Chondrocytes	Chondrocytes
No or reduced proliferation	Increased proliferation
Reduced metabolic activity	Increased metabolic activity
No change in subchondral bone	Increased subchondral bone thickness

*Ratio of CS 4/6 is the ratio of chondroitin sulfate containing sulfate groups on either the fourth or sixth carbon.

SOURCE: Adapted and modified from Hamerman D: The biology of osteoarthritis. *N Engl J Med* 320:1322, 1989.

may provide important information needed to understand why knee OA is so prevalent in the aging population.

There appears to be a slight decline in the number of chondrocytes present in cartilage with age. Early studies of cartilage from the femoral head noted a 30 percent fall in cell density between the ages of 30 and 100 years. But more recent studies of knee joints have noted much lower cell loss, with normal aging in the range of 1 to 2 percent. Cartilage from older individuals has also been noted to have microcracks in the calcified layer. The significance of these cracks is not clear, but if they extend to the underlying subchondral bone, they could provide a mechanism for the exchange of cytokines and growth factors between the two tissues; and if vascular invasion occurs, they could mediate remodeling of subchondral bone, which is a characteristic feature of OA.

A consistent biochemical finding in cartilage is an age-related decrease in hydration. A decrease in hydration could explain recent evidence from magnetic resonance imaging that some thinning of knee cartilage occurs with age, particularly at the femoral surface. The decrease in cartilage hydration is likely related to changes with age in the proteoglycans that bind the majority of the water in cartilage. The total proteoglycan content does not appear to change significantly, instead, changes in proteoglycan structure have been reported that could affect its biophysical properties. Aggrecan molecules become smaller with age and are structurally altered as the result of proteolytic modification in the core protein as well as changes in the length and abundance of the attached glycosaminoglycan chains. Hyaluronic acid, to which the aggrecan molecules bind to form large aggregates, is also decreased in size with age. In addition, proteolysis of the aggrecan core protein between the G1 and G2 domains results in increased levels of molecules bound to hyaluronic acid that contain only the G1 region and therefore lack the remainder of the aggrecan molecule necessary for normal function. The half-life for the free binding region is calculated to be as long as 25 years, consistent with its accumulation in cartilage with aging. By occupying and competing for space on the hyaluronic acid strands, the bound G1 domains may reduce the number of newly synthesized aggrecan molecules bound to hyaluronic acid.

As with the proteoglycans there does not appear to be a significant reduction in the total amount of collagen present in cartilage with age. However, important changes in collagen structure and function have been noted. The collagen network appears to become stiffer with age. The increased collagen stiffness is thought to be a result of increased collagen cross-linking. There is evidence for nonenzymatic glycosylation in cartilage from older adults that results in the formation of pentosidine residues that can cross-link collagen molecules. An age-related accumulation of advanced glycation end-products (AGEs) has been noted in cartilage (Fig. 70-4). Pentosidine and other AGEs have been found in collagen, as well as in aggrecan. The accumulation of pentosidine is reported to be greater in collagen than aggrecan because of the exceptionally long half-life of collagen in cartilage, which is calculated to be approximately 117 years.

In addition to increased cross-linking from the accumulation of advanced glycation end products, collagen fibril diameter tends to increase with age, and this may also contribute to changes in collagen stiffness. Increased collagen network stiffness could contribute to the decrease in hydration, as stiffer collagen would tend to cause greater proteoglycan compression and thereby push out more water from the matrix. Biomechanical studies suggest that the stiffer network is more prone to fatigue failure. With age there is a decrease in the tensile strength of cartilage as well as a decrease in overall tensile stiffness. Therefore, age-related changes in the overall composition of the cartilage matrix result in a tissue that is less capable of handling mechanical stress.

In addition to changes in type II collagen and aggrecan, age-related changes in several of the other less-abundant cartilage matrix proteins have been reported. These include a decrease in type IX collagen, a protein that may be important in holding together adjacent collagen fibers and an increase in link protein, the protein that helps bind aggrecan molecules to hyaluronic acid. While link protein is increased with age, it also appears to undergo proteolytic modification with age that could affect its function.

Changes in the proliferative and synthetic capacity of chondrocytes with age have been noted. There is evidence for an age-related decreased mitogenic response to serum and growth factor stimulation. In addition, a reduction in proteoglycan and protein synthesis in response to growth factor stimulation has been in seen in cartilage from older animals, including non-human primates.

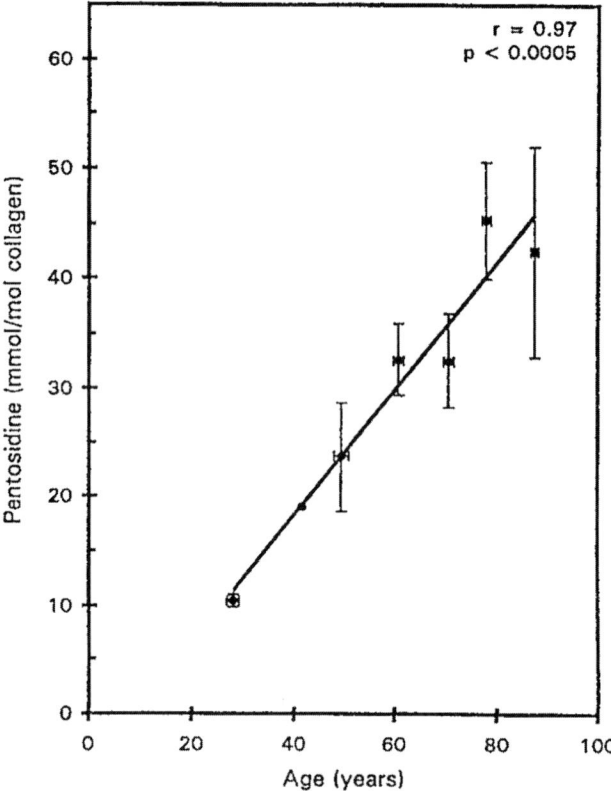

Figure 70-4   Age-related accumulation of advanced glycation end-products in cartilage. Pentosidine levels were measured in cartilage samples from 36 donors clustered into 10-year age intervals. Results shown are mean ± SEM (standard error of mean). Reproduced with permission from DeGroot et al: Age-related decrease in proteoglycan synthesis of human articular chondrocytes: The role of nonenzymatic glycation. *Arthritis Rheum* 42:1003, 1999.

Likewise, decreased proteoglycan synthesis in response to serum stimulation has been noted in human cartilage from older adults. In the human samples the decreased serum response correlated with the presence of advanced glycation end-products. Other studies also suggest that a decline in cell signaling in response to growth factors is responsible for the decreased mitogenic and synthetic responses.

A reduction in response to growth factor stimulation with age, disease, or both, could be significant in the development of OA, where catabolic processes are greater than anabolic. Senescent dermal fibroblasts have been shown to have increased expression of collagenase and stromelysin accompanied by a fall in TIMP expression, but studies have not determined whether this change occurs in chondrocytes as well. In addition, studies are needed to determine whether replicative senescence occurs in cartilage in vivo.

An age-related finding in cartilage, one which is also observed in many other soft tissues, is an increased prevalence of crystals and calcification. It is difficult to determine the relative effects of age and disease on cartilage calcification. Calcification or crystal formation within cartilage is a common feature of OA, particularly in advanced disease and, like OA, age is the strongest risk factor for the development of crystal-associated arthritis. Cartilage from older individuals often contains crystals composed of calcium pyrophosphate dihydrate or hydroxyapatite. Studies with animal tissues show that the increase in the formation of calcium pyrophosphate crystals may be caused by an age-related increase in the activity of transglutaminase, an enzyme that is involved in the biomineralization process. Also chondrocytes from older individuals produce more inorganic pyrophosphate in response to transforming growth factor-β stimulation, despite a decreased proliferative response to this and other growth factors.

Currently, there are insufficient data concerning the effect of age on the biomechanical properties of cartilage, which makes it difficult to come to any definite conclusions about the effect of the age-related biochemical changes on cartilage function. Overall, it appears that the changes that occur in cartilage with age alone are minor as compared with the changes that occur with disease, such as OA. The link between the observed aging changes and the development of OA has not yet been established. The available information would suggest that factors other than age are important in the initiation of this disease, but that aging changes may contribute to OA progression. This hypothesis would be consistent with the findings of early "OA-like" changes in autopsy studies of young adult humans and animals.

Aging and the Development of Osteoarthritis

Although aging and OA are not one and the same, the changes noted in cartilage with age almost certainly must contribute to the incidence and prevalence of OA, which increase directly with age (Fig. 70-5). OA is a condition that is not seen clinically in children or adolescents and is rare in young adults, but becomes increasingly common in those older than age 55 years. In the Framingham cohort of subjects, radiographic knee OA was present in 27 percent of those ages 63 to 70 years and in 44 percent of those ages 80 years or older. Radiographic hand OA is even more common and can be seen in upwards of 80 percent of people in the oldest age groups. Even so, not everyone develops OA with age; all joints are not equally affected by OA; and, perhaps most importantly, not every joint or every individual with radiographic or even pathologic evidence of the disease is symptomatic. Clearly there are factors, in addition to age, that contribute to the development of the disease and to the expression of symptoms and disability.

As is the case with all diseases that are common in old age, osteoarthritis is really a group of diseases of various etiologies resulting in common pathologic changes within diarthrodial joints. Pathologically, OA is characterized by changes in both cartilage and bone (see Fig. 70-3). Fibrillation and loss of articular cartilage by degradation are accompanied by hypertrophic changes in the subchondral bone, resulting in subchondral thickening and in osteophyte formation at joint margins. There is also evidence for some degree of synovial inflammation in most patients with symptomatic OA, although the amount of synovial inflammation is much less than that found in more inflammatory forms of arthritis such as rheumatoid arthritis. Other pathologic changes include thickening of the joint capsule and, in advanced OA, degeneration of the menisci.

OA is often described as a "wear and tear" degenerative disease because the cartilage changes are most severe in the areas that receive the greatest mechanical stress. But the pathobiology of OA is much more complicated than either simple joint aging or wear and tear from repetitive use. Unlike an automobile part that can simply wear out with time, the tissues that comprise the joint contain living and metabolically active cells. The cells themselves are responsible for the destruction of the cartilage, likely under the influence of biomechanical forces, as well as for dynamic processes involved in continual regeneration, repair, and remodeling.

The cartilage changes found in OA appear to be caused by an imbalance between anabolic and catabolic activity. In OA, the chondrocytes are synthetically active producing increased amounts of a number of matrix proteins most likely as an attempt at repairing the damaged matrix. However, OA chondrocytes also produce increased amounts of degradative enzymes that overwhelm the repair response. Increased levels of several of the MMPs, including MMP-1, 2, 3, 9, and 13, as well as the aggrecanases (ADAMTS-4 and -5), have been noted in OA cartilage and appear to play a key role in matrix degradation. Cytokines, including interleukin-1 (IL-1), tumor necrosis factor-α, and others, are also increased in OA cartilage and may be responsible for the increased production of MMPs. Other factors associated with inflammation such as prostaglandins and nitric oxide are also increased in OA cartilage. The increased local production of cytokines and inflammatory mediators in OA cartilage indicates that OA is really a process that involves cartilage inflammation.

Another characteristic of OA cartilage is the appearance of clusters of chondrocytes resulting from cell proliferation, thought to be part of the attempt at matrix repair. But

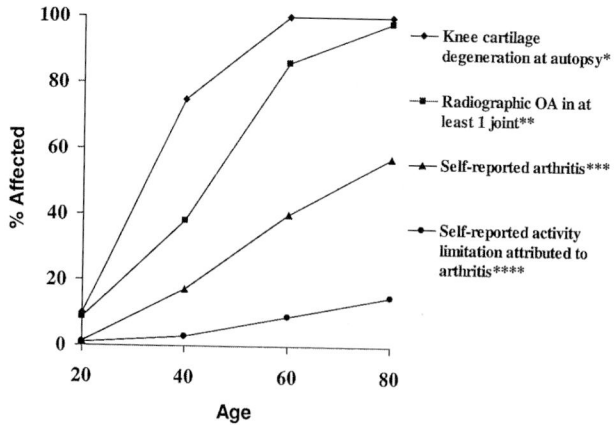

Figure 70-5   Effect of age on the prevalence of arthritis. *Knee cartilage degeneration at autopsy is the prevalence of significant histological changes of degeneration. **Radiographic evidence of OA (Kellgren and Lawrence Grade 2 or greater) present in at least one joint site (hands, feet, spine, knees, and hips) in a population survey in northern England. ***Self-reported arthritis and ****activity limitation attributable to arthritis derived from the National Health Interview Survey--US, 1989–1991. Reproduced with permission from Loeser RF: Aging and the etiopathogenesis and treatment of osteoarthritis. *Rheum Dis Clin North Am* 26:547, 2000.

areas practically devoid of cells can be seen adjacent to areas containing cell clusters. The overall number of cells in OA cartilage appears to decline, especially in the advanced stages of the disease. This decline is associated with the appearance of apoptotic chondrocytes, indicating that cell death is occurring, although significant cell death has not been confirmed at earlier stages of the disease. Therefore, it is not clear whether an imbalance between cell proliferation and death plays an important role in the development of OA. If it does, then aging changes that reduce the proliferative capacity of the cells and changes which make the cells more susceptible to dying would contribute to the development of OA in older adults.

Similar to findings suggestive of a reduced response to growth factor stimulation with age in normal cartilage, recent studies indicate that chondrocytes from OA cartilage are also less responsive to growth factor stimulation. A lack of an anabolic response to IGF-I has been noted in several studies of OA chondrocytes. The decrease in response to IGF-I in OA may be related to increased levels of IGF-binding proteins, also noted in OA cartilage, which could decrease the amount of free IGF-1 available to bind to cell receptors. Although serum levels of IGF-1 decrease with age, there is no evidence that local levels in cartilage decrease. In fact, in OA cartilage levels of IGF-1 appear to be increased. If the cells maintain responsiveness to cytokines such as IL-1 while losing responsiveness to growth factors such as IGF-1, this could sway the balance of cartilage synthesis and degradation toward the catabolic side.

Like many of the changes seen in cartilage, the changes in bone appear to be in opposite directions when comparing aging and OA (see Table 70-3). Thickening of the subchondral bone is a consistent finding in OA, whereas decreasing bone mass is commonly seen with age, at least in cortical and particularly in trabecular bone. However, studies of aging in bone have not specifically assessed the region of the subchondral bone. The subchondral bone can remodel in response to mechanical loading, and this bony remodeling may play an important role in the OA disease process. It has been hypothesized that thicker and stiffer subchondral bone would place additional stress on the overlying cartilage during joint loading, resulting in mechanical failure of the cartilage. There is much debate about whether OA actually starts with changes in the subchondral bone rather than in cartilage. The answer as to which comes first may depend on the circumstances by which OA has developed. The importance of the subchondral bone to the OA disease process has been emphasized by a recent study that shows that activity in this region, detected by technetium bone scans, can predict disease progression in OA.

Given the discrepancy between aging and OA changes found in cartilage as well as in bone, it is apparent that although OA is clearly an age-related disease, it is not due to simple aging of the joint. Instead, OA is a disease process that usually develops slowly over a long period and becomes manifest in the later years of life. Most likely the process leading to OA is initiated earlier in life under the influence of factor(s) specific to each individual, such as obesity, joint injury, and genetically abnormal cartilage matrix proteins. These factors act by either directly altering the structure or metabolism of cartilage or bone or indirectly

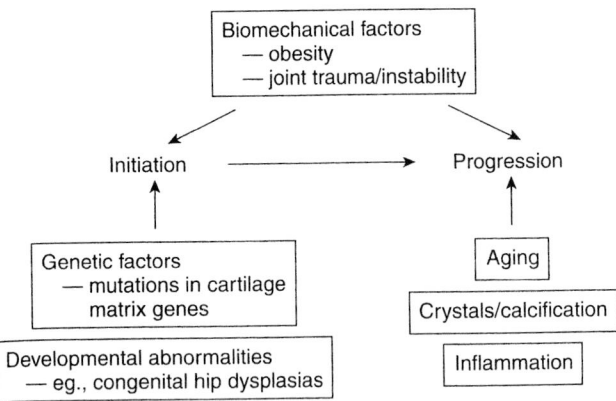

Factors contributing to the initiation and progression of osteoarthritis.

Figure 70-6   Factors contributing to the initiation and progression of osteoarthritis.

affecting the tissues by altering joint biomechanics (Fig. 70-6). Additional factors, including aging-related changes in the tissues, affect the rate of progression of the disease. The disease remains asymptomatic until sufficient damage occurs to structures capable of producing pain or results in changes in joint function. An additional level of complexity is added by the physical, psychological, and sociological factors that contribute to the development of symptoms such as pain. The end result is a multifactorial, heterogeneous group of diseases in which symptoms do not always correlate with pathologic changes as visualized using methods such as plain radiographs.

SKELETAL MUSCLE

Skeletal Muscle Structure and Function

The entire skeletal muscle is enclosed by a sheath of connective tissue called epimysium. Bundles of muscle fibers and individual contracting units of muscle fibers are surrounded by partitions of the connective tissue constituting the perimysium and the endomysium, respectively. Blood vessels, lymphatics, and nerves reach all the muscle compartments by way of these fibrous partitions. The connective tissue merges into stronger structures such as tendons, aponeuroses, raphes, the reticular layer of dermis, or the periosteum that provide support for muscle insertion and contraction.

Matured single muscle fibers are long multinucleated and cylindric units separated from other cells and surrounded by a membrane, the sarcolemma. Muscle fibers contain myofibrils made up of the contractile proteins myosin, actin, tropomyosin and troponin and the structural supportive proteins actinin and titin. The particular spatial arrangement of the thick and thin contractile proteins is responsible for the characteristic cross-striations in skeletal muscle. Differences in the refractive index of the muscle fiber determine the alternation of light I band and dark A band (Fig. 70-7). Z lines in the middle of the I bands are the limits of a sarcomere. The thick filaments are made up of myosin, whereas the thin filaments are made up of actin, tropomyosin and troponin.

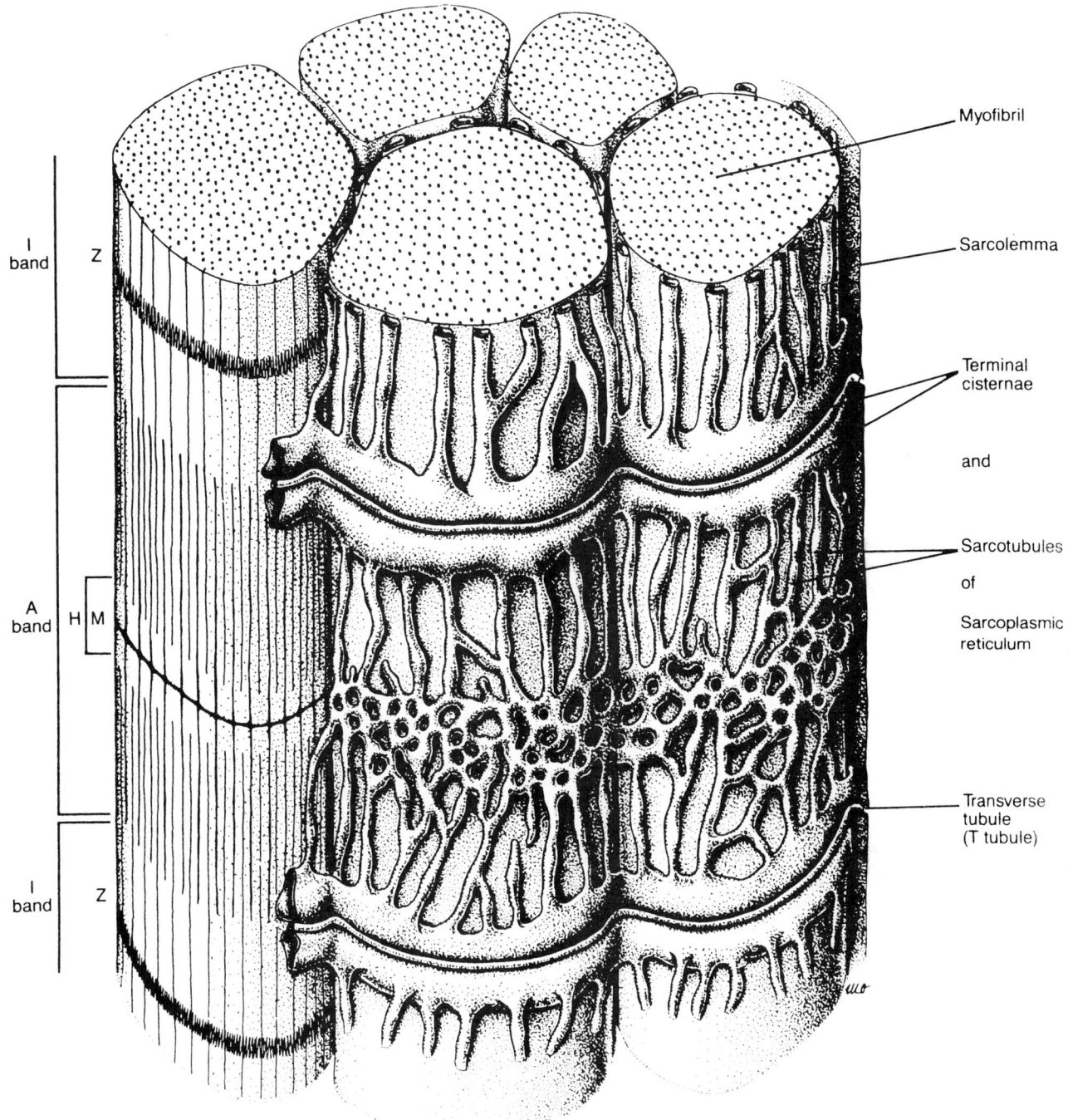

Figure 70-7   Diagram of a skeletal muscle fiber illustrating the spatial arrangement of contractile proteins and surrounding membrane system. Reproduced with permission from Cormack DH: *Ham's Histology*, 9th ed. Philadelphia, Lippincott, 1987, p 402.

Myosin is an actin-binding protein provided with a catalytic site that hydrolyzes adenosine triphosphate (ATP), the source of energy for muscle contraction. Actin molecules polymerize in long, thin double-helix filaments, forming a groove where tropomyosin molecules are located. Troponin molecules are located at regular intervals along the tropomyosin molecules. Troponin has three components: troponin T binds the other components to tropomyosin, troponin I inhibits the interaction of myosin with actin, and troponin C contains the binding sites for calcium that initiate muscle contraction.

The Motor Unit

Lower spinal cord motor neurons provide a common pathway for transmitting neural impulses from upper motor levels of the central nervous system to the skeletal muscle. This information is directed to skeletal muscles via the ventral roots, peripheral nerves and cranial nerves. Each motor neuron innervates muscle fibers within a single muscle and the motor neurons innervating a single muscle are grouped in the spinal cord, forming the motor neuron pool for that muscle. During development, polyinnervated muscles become innervated by a single motor neuron. Axonal branches establish synapsis with multiple muscle fibers of a single muscle. The activation of a motor neuron brings all the muscle fibers with which it establishes synapsis to the mechanical threshold; therefore, a single motor neuron and its associated muscle fibers constitute the motor unit that is the smallest that can be activated to induce movement. On the basis of the speed of contraction, three types of motor units can be distinguished: fast-fatigable motor units, fatigue-resistant motor units, and slow-motor units that are in between the first two subtypes in terms of time for fatigue initiation. These differences in motor unit performance are based on physiologic and biochemical characteristics of their constituent muscle fibers.

Events in Muscle Contraction and Relaxation: Skeletal Muscle Excitation–Contraction Coupling

Skeletal muscle contraction is initiated by generation and conduction of action potentials by the motor neuron, release of acetylcholine at the motor end-plate, and binding to nicotinic acetylcholine receptors, and an increase in sodium and potassium conductance in the end-plate membrane. End-plate potentials at the muscle membrane lead to generation of action potentials and their conduction to the sarcolemmal infoldings (T-tubules).

The transduction of changes in sarcolemmal potential into elevations in intracellular calcium concentration is a key event that precedes muscle contraction. The muscle electromechanical transduction requires the participation

of a protein located at the sarcolemmal T tubule, the dihydropyridine receptor (DHPR), in the early steps of this signal-transduction mechanism. The DHPR is a voltage-gated L-type Ca^{2+} channel (dihydropyridine-sensitive), and its activation evokes Ca^{2+} release from an intracellular store, the sarcoplasmic reticulum (SR) through ryanodine-sensitive calcium channels (RyR1) into the myoplasm. Figure 70-8 illustrates the typical arrangement of DHPR and RyR at the skeletal muscle triadic junction. The functional consequence of alterations in the number, function, or interaction of these receptors is a reduction in the amount of intracellular calcium mobilization and in the development of force. Calcium is bound to troponin C, leading to formation of cross-linkages between actin and myosin and sliding of thin on thick filaments, which produces shortening. Muscle relaxes as a result of calcium pumping back to the sarcoplasmic reticulum, release of calcium from troponin, and cessation of interaction between actin and myosin filaments.

Muscle Fiber Subtypes and Types of Contraction

Muscle fiber types can be determined using immunostaining or the ATPase (adenosine triphosphatase) stain based on the pH dependence of myosin ATPase activity, which relates closely to antigenic differences in myosin between fast- and slow-twitch muscles. Specific monoclonal antibodies for types I, IIA, and IIB fibers are commercially available. An antibody against IIX fibers was recently reported. According to the histochemical classification, muscle fibers are divided into type I and type II (A, B, and C) (Table 70-4). Human muscles fibers are classified into fast- and slow-twitch based on their contractile properties in response to brief stimulation (action potential). Fast-twitch fibers (type II, glycolytic, white) contract for less than 10 ms and are primarily concerned with fine, precise, and rapid movements. Slow-twitch fibers (type I, oxidative, red) exhibit twitch durations up to 100 ms and are involved in strong, gross, and sustained movements. Muscle fibers are integrated into motor units and are classified into fast-fatigable, fast-fatigue-resistant, and slow motor units

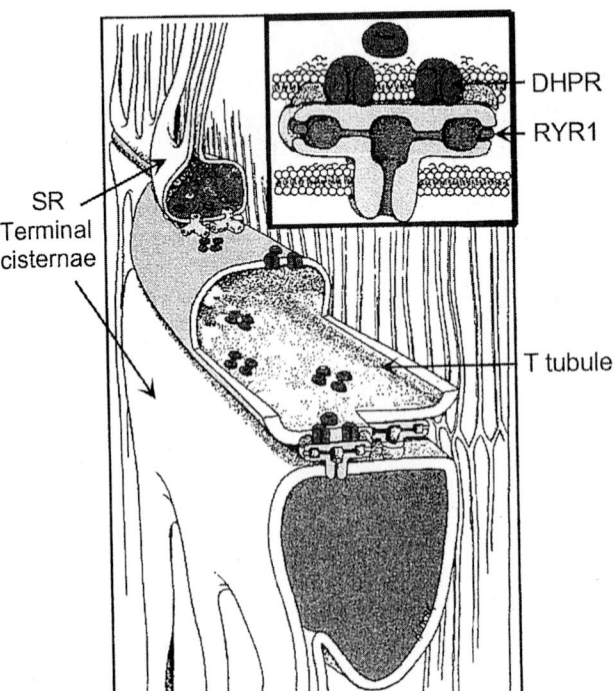

Figure 70–8 Schematic of the interaction between the dihydropyridine receptor (DHPR) and ryanodine receptor (RyR1) and their location at the sarcolemmal tubular system and sarcoplasmic reticulum terminal cisternae, respectively. Redrawn from Rios E, Pizarro G: Voltage sensor of excitation-contraction coupling in skeletal muscle. *Physiol Rev* 71(3):890, 1991.

Table 70–4   Histochemical Classification of Muscle Fibers

Muscle fiber subtypes	Functional and histochemical characteristics	ATPase stain		
		PH 9.4	pH 4.6	pH 4.3
Type I	Slow twitch, oxidative	Light	Dark	Dark
Type IIA	Fast twitch, oxidative-glycolytic	Dark	Light	Light
Type IIB	Fast twitch, glycolytic	Dark	Dark	Dark
Type IIC	Fetal	Dark	Dark	Dark

according to their speed of contraction, maximum tension generated, and degree of fatigue.

Mechanisms Underlying Skeletal Muscle Weakness in Old Age

Age-related decreases in skeletal muscle mass and quality contribute to physical disability and loss of independence in the elderly population. In addition to decreased muscle mass, aging muscle is characterized by decreases in contractile force or weakness that have been reported to occur with age in several mammalian species including humans. Age-related weakness may be associated with fatigue, weakness discerned as an absolute decrease in muscle force, and fatigue as a progressive decline in force with prolonged physical activity. Muscle weakness is associated with limitations in activities of daily living, such as climbing stairs or rising from a chair, that lead to loss of independence. Muscle weakness is a risk factor for falling and also increases the risk for fractures resulting from a fall. Reduced heat and cold tolerance, impaired glucose homeostasis, and obesity have been also related to aging skeletal muscle. Decline in muscle performance with aging has been quantified in untrained and highly trained individuals. These studies showed that although the individuals with higher levels of physical activity were stronger, the rate of decrease in the level of muscle performance in both groups was similar. These results suggest that age-related deficits largely inevitable and in addition to those secondary to decreases in physical activity.

Despite the importance of muscle strength in preventing disability, the biological mechanisms responsible for these phenomena are poorly understood. Cellular and molecular aspects have been explored both in human and more extensively, in animal models of aging. The conclusions included in this section arise from investigations in human and nonhuman aging skeletal muscle. Factors that determine skeletal muscle impairment with aging can be divided into four groups: (1) neurogenic, (2) myogenic, (3) a combination of neural and muscular alterations, and (4) general mechanisms that involve skeletal muscle (Table 70-5).

Neurogenic Mechanisms of Skeletal Muscle Impairment with Aging

The neurogenic mechanisms include reduction in the number and/or size of spinal cord motor neurons and alterations in axonal flow and the neuromuscular junction. Each of these factors, individually or in combination, leads to chronic muscle denervation and motor unit remodeling. Some older persons present electromyographic evidence of muscle denervation suggestive of motor neuron alterations. These patients never develop classical amyotrophic diseases (e.g., amyotrophic lateral sclerosis). Muscle denervation is associated with reinnervation, as demonstrated by the presence of muscle fiber grouping in histologic sections. Cycles of muscle denervation associated with reinnervation lead to motor unit remodeling.

The functional significance of motor unit remodeling still needs to be determined. The relative histologic

Table 70-5   Suggested Pathogenesis of Skeletal Muscle Impairment with Aging

I. Neuronal alterations

   A. Spinal cord motor neurons

      1. Reduction in number
      2. Reduction in size

   B. Alterations in axonal flow
   C. Neuromuscular transmission alterations

      1. Decrease in nerve terminal numbers
      2. Reduced neurotransmitter release
      3. Decrease in acetylcholine receptor numbers

II. Primary muscle alterations

   A. Contraction-induced injury
   B. Alterations in muscle signal transduction (trophic factor/hormone resistance)

III. Combined neurogenic-muscular mechanism

   A. Muscle unloading
   B. Excitation—contraction uncoupling

IV. General mechanisms that involve skeletal muscle

   A. Oxidative stress
   B. Mitochondrial deoxyribonucleic acid mutations
   C. Age-related vasculopathy

areas corresponding to fast- and slow-twitch muscle fibers change with aging, becoming predominantly slow muscle fibers. Age-related remodeling of motor units appears to involve denervation of fast muscle fibers with reinnervation by axonal sprouting from slow fibers. Therefore, motor unit remodeling leads to changes in fiber-type distribution in mixed fiber-type muscles.

Reinnervation of muscle fibers tends to compensate for denervation; however, a net loss of fibers across age has been detected. This obviously occurs when the rate of muscle fiber denervation surpasses the rate of axonal sprouting and reinnervation. Indirect studies show a decrease in the total number of fast-motor units and enlargement of the remaining motor units with age. Direct neuronal counting shows a reduction in the number and/or size of ventral spinal motor neurons at the cervical or lumbar regions with aging. Whether alterations in motor neuron, nerve terminal, or axonal transport account for muscle denervation is not clear.

Studies on conduction velocity in peripheral nerves do not show significant changes with aging. This would suggest that alterations in myelin or severe reductions in nerve axonal composition do not occur with age. Although denervation has been suggested as a contributing factor to aging skeletal muscle, the extension of denervation in individual muscles and its effect on human muscles remain to be determined. In addition, it is becoming apparent that denervation does not explain a significant deficit in specific maximum isometric tetanic force (muscle force normalized to cross-sectional area) recorded in aged skeletal muscles. Also, decreases in the number of spinal cord motor neurons occur after the eighth decade, when the loss in muscle mass and strength is already well established.

Myogenic Mechanisms of Skeletal Muscle Impairment with Aging

Primary muscular or myogenic factors refer to a group of alterations including contraction-induced injury and alterations in muscle signal transduction (trophic factor/hormone resistance). The phenomenon of contraction-induced injury is related to increased mechanical frailty and decline in muscle restorative capacity with age. Muscles from older individuals or animals become injured when undergoing lengthening contractions. Also, older muscles recover more slowly and do not exhibit complete recovery when compared with those in younger controls. Eccentric contraction injury has also been demonstrated in older individuals. Insulin and IGF-1 resistance in aging skeletal muscle have been reported. The influence of weight and physical activity on trophic factor/hormone resistance, are currently under investigation.

Combined Neurogenic–Muscular Mechanism

Combined mechanisms include muscle unloading and excitation–contraction uncoupling. Muscle unloading associated with sedentary lifestyle is a major determinant of muscle atrophy in the elderly population. The decrease in physical activity is a combined process in which the lower the nerve activation, the lower the muscle contraction. This process leads subsequently to muscle atrophy. However, not all the motor units within a muscle seem to be affected to the same extent. Predominant atrophy of type II fibers has been reported in aging muscles from rodents; however, the clinical significance of this finding is uncertain because there are very few type IIB fibers in human muscles.

Alterations with age in muscle fiber signal transduction such as sarcolemmal excitation–sarcoplasmic reticulum calcium release uncoupling and impaired IGF-1–dependent modulation of muscle calcium channels have been demonstrated. Studies in muscle fibers deprived of sarcolemma (skinned muscle fibers) demonstrated that the force generated per unit cross-sectional area does not differ in adult and old mice during isometric contractions. These results suggest that muscle atrophy does not explain entirely the age-related decline in muscle strength. A deficit in specific contractile force (force normalized to muscle cross-sectional area) in aging skeletal muscle has been described in the literature. However, the significance of this finding in terms of the etiology and therapeutics of the age-related decline in muscle force has not been sufficiently investigated.

The deficit in specific force is a widespread phenomenon involving fast- and slow-twitch fibers in different muscles. Several mechanisms have been postulated to explain the skeletal muscle weakness associated with aging. However, whether the loss of specific and absolute force share common mechanisms is not known at the present time. It appears that the age-related impairment in muscle force is only partially explained by the loss in muscle mass.

Therefore, both the loss in specific and absolute forces contributes to the muscle weakness measured in the elderly and in animal models of aging.

Successful interventions aimed at counteracting age-associated functional deficits will require better insight into the mechanisms underlying the decline in muscle-specific force. Alterations in several mechanisms of signal transduction operate in aging skeletal muscles. Two of them these mechanisms in particular are directly involved in development of muscle force. These are excitation-induced elevations in intracellular calcium and the mechanism of energy conversion from ATP into a mechanical response. It seems that changes in phosphorus metabolites involved in energy transduction (phosphocreatine, adenosine diphosphate [ADP], and ATP) and myosin isoforms do not change with aging. However, alterations in excitation–contraction coupling have been demonstrated in human quadriceps.

Physiologic activation of the muscle membrane elicits elevations in intracellular Ca^{2+} that, in turn, induce muscle contraction by interaction with contractile proteins. Impairments in the mechanism of transduction of muscle activation into intracellular Ca^{2+} mobilization lead to decreases in muscle tension, clinically manifested as muscle weakness. The basic mechanism underlying excitation–contraction uncoupling with aging is a molecular unlinkage between the two calcium channels, one that functions at the external membrane (sarcolemma) as a voltage-sensor the other that mediates calcium release from intracellular stores (sarcoplasmic reticulum). Alterations in excitation–contraction coupling result from significant changes in either or both the number and regulation of these molecules.

General Mechanisms that Involve Skeletal Muscle

General mechanisms that may adversely affect skeletal muscle directly or indirectly are oxidative deoxyribonucleic acid (DNA) damage, mitochondrial DNA (mtDNA) mutations, and age-related vasculopathy. Superoxide radical and hydrogen peroxide that are continuously produced in aerobic cells undergo metal ion-catalyzed conversion into hydroxyl radicals. These hydroxyl radicals can cause oxidative damage, which, in turn, may be related to the development of mutations in mtDNA. Mitochondrial DNA mutations are associated with ischemic heart disease, late-onset diabetes, Parkinson's disease, Alzheimer's disease, and aging. The accumulation of damage to mtDNA by oxidation may be the basis for defects in oxidative phosphorylation capacity with age. A decline in oxidative phosphorylation capacity would become symptomatic when tissue energetics fall below the threshold of an organ.

A group of factors that deserve attention are subclinical inflammation, vascular pathology and muscle perfusion. Subclinical inflammation has been suggested as a mechanism for loss in muscle mass and weakness in the elderly, often called sarcopenia. Such inflammation-related loss may be mediated by tissue increases in tumor necrosis factor-α, interleukin-6, interleukin-1α, and/or interleukin-1β. Some evidence suggests that subclinical inflammation may contribute to the debilitating muscle atrophy associated with congestive heart failure, renal failure, or rheumatoid arthritis. In the extreme, this may lead to cachexia, generalized loss of muscle as well as fat mass, aggravated by the anorexia associated with starvation, acquired immunodeficiency syndrome, or advanced cancer. Thus, the involuntary decline in muscle mass characteristic of old age may represent a continuation in degree and rate of development with inflammation, subclinical or clinical, as an important mediating mechanism. The existence of an altered capillary bed in aging skeletal muscle is controversial at the present time. Reduced or increased numbers of capillaries have been reported in the literature. Less is known about muscle perfusion in physiologic conditions.

Clinical and Experimental Interventions Aimed at Delaying or Preventing Age-Associated Changes in Skeletal Muscle Composition and Function

We are just beginning to identify the specific changes in muscle with age. Withdrawal of anabolic stimuli to skeletal muscle, including decline in estrogen/androgen, growth hormone, insulin, or IGF-1 may lead to both loss in muscle mass and impairment in the intrinsic capacity of the muscle fiber to generate force. A key question to be addressed at this time in studies of both muscle and cartilage is: Does a cell-signaling impairment with aging result from tissue resistance to trophic factors? Increasing evidence supports this concept. However, understanding this process requires further insight into a more general phenomenon, the role of trophic factors in mature tissue maintenance and restoration.

In healthy individuals, deficiency with aging in spontaneous and stimulated growth hormone secretion, as well as circulating IGF-1 and IGF-binding protein-3 levels, is associated with decreased lean body mass, decreased protein synthesis, and increased percent body fat. Administration of recombinant human growth hormone or growth hormone secretagogues improves nitrogen balance, increases lean body mass, and decreases body fat in older people with low IGF-1 levels. However, the effects on muscle strength do not seem to be proportional to the improvement in muscle mass with such replacements.

IGF-1 is a peptide structurally related to proinsulin which has a primary role in promoting skeletal muscle differentiation and growth. In skeletal muscle, IGF-1 potentiates calcium current through L-type calcium channels in adult fibers but not in muscles from aging mammals, probably because of IGF-1 resistance. Using a transgenic mouse model overexpressing IGF-1 in skeletal muscle, increases in the number of DHPR have been reported. IGF-1 also has an effect on muscle mass, inducing hypertrophy in transgenic models or preventing atrophy in aging rodents. Virally mediated overexpression of IGF-1 in muscle prevents the age-related loss in type IIB fibers and contractile force in rodents. In summary, IGF-1 prevents excitation–contraction uncoupling, changes in fiber type composition, and loss in absolute and specific force. One of the main stumbling blocks for IGF-1 application to human therapeutics is the need to design a strategy for safe delivery of IGF-1 in a sustained fashion.

Exercise is clearly one of the most effective interventions in reducing muscle impairment in the elderly. Exercise interventions such as resistance training are being used in an attempt to restore muscle force in the elderly. Strength training in sedentary young and sedentary older individuals improves muscle force, improves metabolic capacities, increases glycogen storage, and enhances oxidative enzyme activity. Aerobic training involving high-repetition, low-intensity muscle contractions leads to minimal strength gain when compared to the low-repetition, high-intensity stimulus of resistance training in which both strengthening as well as endurance activities are included. Further studies on the use of trophic factors and on the use of specific exercise interventions are needed to determine the best means of preventing or reversing the decline in muscle function with age.

TENDONS AND LIGAMENTS

Tendons and ligaments are composed of dense connective tissue that has a high content of fibrillar collagen to provide tensile strength. Tendons attach muscle to bone, while ligaments attach bone to bone. The integrity of these attachments is important for normal joint function. Ligaments serve to stabilize the joints, and tendons transmit the forces of muscle contraction to bone. There appears to be a general decline in joint range of motion with age that may be related, at least in part, to changes in tendons and ligaments.

The percent reduction in range of motion varies with the joint studied and is greatly influenced by both disuse and disease. In general, declines in the range of 20 to 25 percent have been reported. In addition to effects on joint motion, aging-related changes in tendons and ligaments may contribute to the development of injuries to these structures, resulting in conditions ranging from tendonitis to tendon and ligament tears or rupture. Although these injuries certainly occur in younger individuals, the amount of trauma required to produce them is reduced with age. In addition, ligamentous ruptures from injuries in younger individuals can predispose the affected joint to the development of OA later in life as a result from joint instability altering joint biomechanics.

Biomechanical studies reveal that the strength of tendons and ligaments and their insertions to bone are reduced with age. In one study, it took approximately one-third less loading to cause failure of the anterior cruciate ligament attachment in cadaver knees from individuals ages 60 to 97 years, as compared with a younger group individuals ages 22 to 35 years. A twofold decrease in the strength of the anterior longitudinal ligament of the spine has also been noted in subjects between the ages of 21 and 79 years in cadaver studies.

Shoulder problems are quite common in older adults and may be related to aging changes in the rotator cuff tendons. Changes with age including calcification, microtears, and fibrovascular proliferation have been reported in the region where the tendons attach to bone. These changes would result in a weakening in the attachment, predisposing the tissue to injury after minor trauma.

Biochemical studies of aging in tendons and ligaments have been limited but have shown changes with age, some of which are similar to changes noted in cartilage. Like cartilage, the tensile strength of these tissues depends on the collagen fibers, although the primary fibrillar collagen is type I rather than the type II found in cartilage. There is no clear evidence that collagen content in ligaments or tendons changes with age, but changes in cross-linking have been reported with the appearance of nonreducible cross-links with age, including cross-links formed by nonenzymatic glycation. Increased cross-linking may cause increased stiffness of the collagen and make it more prone to fatigue failure. Like cartilage, there appears to be a decrease in the water content of tendons and ligaments with age, but there is little information on changes in proteoglycans that, if altered, could explain the reduced water content as discussed earlier with respect to cartilage proteoglycans.

INTERVERTEBRAL DISCS

Imaging studies of normal subjects without recent back pain, as well as morphologic studies of autopsy material, show that disc degeneration increases directly with age, with at least some degree of degeneration universally present by the sixth decade of life. Because the presence of disc degeneration does not correlate well with symptoms of pain, it is often difficult to determine the clinical significance of these findings. Magnetic resonance imaging evidence of disc bulging and herniation increases with age but is often asymptomatic. On the other hand, disc herniation associated with extrusion of disc material is more likely to be associated with symptoms, particularly if the disc material extends beyond the posterior longitudinal ligament. It is also generally agreed that degenerative changes in the intervertebral discs likely contribute to a variety of conditions seen in older adults, including osteoarthritis, spondylosis and spinal stenosis.

The intervertebral discs consist of an outer fibrous ring of dense connective tissue referred to as the annulus fibrosus and an inner gel-like material called the nucleus pulposus. The annulus fibrosus is composed of approximately 70 percent collagen by dry weight, whereas the nucleus pulposus is approximately 20 percent collagen and 50 percent proteoglycan. The superior and inferior boundaries of the discs are formed by end-plates consisting of a thin layer of cortical bone covered by hyaline cartilage that directly connects with the vertebral bodies. Aging changes occur within all these regions but are probably most pronounced in the nucleus pulposus.

The most common age-related change in the disc is dehydration. There is a marked decrease in water content, particularly in the nucleus pulposus, which becomes fibrotic, and, starting in young adults, contains fissures and cracks. Tears also become common in the outer annulus in young adults. These can lead to disc herniation, which has a peak incidence at about age 40 to 50 years. With advancing age the nucleus pulposus becomes more dehydrated and less likely to herniate. The decrease in water content is likely related to a decrease in proteoglycans in the nucleus pulposus as well as an increase in collagen cross-linking which, by making the collagen network stiffer, allows for less expansion of the proteoglycans. Similar to articular cartilage, there is evidence that increased collagen cross-linking with age is due to the accumulation of advanced glycation end-products.

Many of the age-related changes noted in intervertebral discs are thought to be attributable to a decline in the diffusion of nutrients to the disc cells. Cells in the nucleus pulposus derive their nutrition by diffusion from vessels in the outside layers of the annulus and from the vertebral end plates. There appears to be a decline in the number of vessels in these regions with age, a disease which can be made worse by conditions including atherosclerotic vascular diseases and diabetes. There is a dramatic decline in the number of viable cells in the nucleus pulposus with age. This is associated with evidence of apoptotic cell death, likely because of the lack of nutrients.

Apoptotic cell death has also been noted in the endplates. These structures become increasingly calcified with age. This contributes to the development of sclerosis. Because the facet joints of the spine are intimately linked with the end-plates and the discs, the age-related changes in these structures contribute significantly to the development of osteoarthritic changes in the spine. Degenerative disc disease accompanied by vertebral osteophytosis results in spondylosis, which, when severe, can cause spinal stenosis.

There is still much that is not known about aging in the intervertebral discs as well as in cartilage, muscle, ligaments, and tendons. It is necessary to continue to try to separate normal aging from changes in these tissues that lead to disease so that appropriate interventions can be designed to prevent and treat musculoskeletal disease in older adults.

REFERENCES

Bennett GA et al: *Changes in the Knee Joint at Various Ages.* New York, The Commonwealth Fund, 1942.

Buckwalter JA et al: Soft-tissue aging and musculoskeletal function. *J Bone Joint Surg* 75A:1533, 1993.

DeGroot J et al: Age-related decrease in proteoglycan synthesis of human articular chondrocytes: The role of nonenzymatic glycation. *Arthritis Rheum* 42:1003, 1999.

Jarvik JG, Deyo RA: Imaging of lumbar intervertebral disk degeneration and aging, excluding disk herniations. *Radiol Clin North Am* 38:1255, 2000.

Loeser RF: Aging and the etiopathogenesis and treatment of osteoarthritis. *Rheum Dis Clin North Am* 26:547, 2000.

Pelletier J-P et al: Osteoarthritis, an inflammatory disease: Potential implication for the selection of new therapeutic targets. *Arthritis Rheum* 44:1237, 2001.

Renganathan M et al: Overexpression of IGF-1 exclusively in skeletal muscle prevents age-related decline in the number of dihydropyridine receptors. *J Biol Chem* 273:28845, 1998.

Roubenoff R, Hughes VA: Sarcopenia: Current concepts. *J Gerontol* 55A:M716, 2000.

Verzijl N et al: Effect of collagen turnover on the accumulation of advanced glycation end products. *J Biol Chem* 275:39027, 2000.

Wang Z-M et al: Sustained overexpression of IGF-1 prevents age-dependent decrease in charge movement and intracellular calcium in mouse skeletal muscle. *Biophys J* (In press).

Weindruch R: Interventions based on the possibility that oxidative stress contributes to sarcopenia. *J Gerontol A Biol Sci Med Sci* 50:157, 1995.

Zheng Z et al: Charge movement and transcription regulation of L-type calcium channel alpha-1S in skeletal muscle cells. *J Physiol (Lond)* (In press).

Biomechanics of Mobility in Older Adults

JAMES A. ASHTON-MILLER • NEIL B. ALEXANDER

PREVALENCE OF MOBILITY PROBLEMS AMONG OLDER ADULTS

Problems with mobility in older adults are common. In the United States, among noninstitutionalized persons age 65 years and older, approximately 13 percent have difficulty in performing activities of daily living. Approximately 9 percent have difficulty with bathing; 8 percent have difficulty with walking; and 6 percent have difficulty with bed or chair transfers. The rate at which these problems occur increases progressively after age 65 years and climbs sharply after age 80 years, so that, for example, more than 34 percent of noninstitutionalized persons who are age 85 years or older have mobility problems.

AGE AND GENDER DIFFERENCES IN FALLS AND FALL-RELATED INJURY RATES

Perhaps the most serious problem of mobility impairment is the tendency of older adults to fall and to be injured by falls. Death rates from falls per 100,000 persons in 1999 were 9.1 for those between 65 and 74 years of age, 31.7 for those between 75 and 84 years of age, and 109.7 for those age 85 or more years old. For comparison, in those aged 75 years and older, the death rate from falls (67.9 per 100,000) is more than double that from motor vehicle accidents (29.8 per 100,000). Falls and fall injuries are of substantial concern because of their frequency and because of their physical, psychological, and social consequences. Even when a fall does not result in injury or death, it can have a substantially adverse effect on an older person's self-confidence, mobility, and independence. Fear of falling, which can accompany decreased mobility, can lead to avoidance of social activities because of the possibility of embarrassment as well as injury in connection with a fall.

Older females are substantially more prone to fall and to be injured in a fall than are older males. Three studies of rates of falls, involving more than 4500 adults age 65 years or older, found those rates to range from 137 to 690 falls per 1000 persons per year, with older females falling from 1.3 to 2.2 times more often than older males. Three studies of rates of fall injuries requiring medical attention, involving more than 38,000 adults, found that fall injuries leading to hospital admission or death occurred in males and females at rates per 1000 persons per year of 1.88 and 0.83, respectively, for those ages 20 to 29 years and increased steadily with age to 6.97 and 15.58, respectively, for those ages 70 to 79 years. Correspondingly, female-to-male ratios of these serious fall injury rates increased with age from 0.44 to 2.24.

In 1996, there were 340,000 hip fractures requiring hospital admission. The direct medical and other costs for the injury have been estimated as being at least $16,300 in the first year following the injury. With current trends, approximately 500,000 hip fractures are expected to occur in the year 2040 with an associated total annual cost of $240 billion. Most hip fractures occur in older adults, and more than 95 percent of those hip fractures result from a fall; the remainder fracture spontaneously during a physically stressful activity or prior to the fall.

Hip fractures can be devastating, particularly in older women. In 1998, there were 863 hip fractures per 100,000 adults older than age 65 years (1056 and 593 per 100,000 in women and men, respectively), with the highest rate in white women age 85 years and older (2690 hip fractures per 100,000). Approximately 20 percent of women who fracture their hip do not survive the first year after fracture, and another 20 percent do not regain the ability to walk unassisted. The incidence of hip fractures rises much faster with age than that of falls. This increase in hip fractures with age is not fully accounted for by increases in the number of falls or decreases in bone mass of the hip with age. Therefore, other factors must increase susceptibility to hip fractures. The biomechanics of the fall arrest responses are likely to be among these factors. More than 85 percent of wrist fractures involve falls. The incidence of wrist fractures rises from age 50 to 65 years and then reaches a plateau after age 65 years, but why this occurs is not yet known.

Most falls (78.3 percent) in those age 65 years and older occur in or within the immediate vicinity of the home. Much is known about the epidemiology of falls, but little is known about the mechanisms responsible for the remarkable increase with aging in falls and fall-related injury rates. Diagnosis of specific diseases does not discriminate elderly fallers from elderly nonfallers. Individual risk factors for falls may be grouped into intrinsic factors and extrinsic factors. Intrinsic factors include decreased level of physical activity, cognitive impairment, depression, visual deficits, sensory and strength deficits in the lower limbs, previous stroke, dizziness, medications, abnormal balance and gait, use of assistive devices, and age older than 80 years. Extrinsic factors include environmental factors including stairs and obstacles in the gait path that can cause trips or slips. The presence of multiple risk factors substantially increases the risk of a fall. Little is known about the changes with age in impending fall response biomechanics that must in part be responsible for the rate changes. For example, tripping is commonly self-reported by older persons as a cause of falls: in a 1-year study of 1042 persons older than 65 years of age, tripping was reported to be the cause of the fall in 53 percent of the 356 falls that were documented. Whatever the underlying neurologic and physiologic mechanisms, responses to trips are ultimately expressed in terms of biomechanical factors.

FALL-RELATED-INJURY BIOMECHANICS

There probably are a number of factors that determine whether a fall will result in an injury: the initial conditions under which the fall begins, the biomechanics of the response during the fall, the passive and active mechanisms for dissipating energy upon impact with the ground or other surfaces, and the proneness to injury of the hard and soft tissues that are impacted. However, the biomechanics of fall arrests and of fall-related injuries have received little attention. Clear need exists to examine them, in order to improve assessments of risk and programs for both intervention and prevention.

THE BIOMECHANICS OF HIP FRACTURES

The risk of bony fracture has been defined by Hayes and colleagues as the ratio of the magnitude of the force applied to the bone divided by the force necessary to cause fracture. A fall from standing height directly onto the greater trochanter carries a 21-fold higher risk for hip fracture than landing on another body part. This is because the loss in potential energy associated with such a fall is an order of magnitude greater than the average energy required to fracture the proximal femur in elderly cadaver specimens. Hence, falls in a lateral direction, which carry a higher risk for landing on the hip than other directions, must be avoided if possible. This is particularly true in an individual with reduced bone mineral density and reduced body mass index. Reductions in the latter are associated with less soft tissue over the hip to dissipate the impact energy. Hip pad protectors are effective in reducing the risk of hip fracture

in frail ambulatory elderly persons. By diverting the impact energy to adjacent tissues, the impact force on the hip may be more than halved. However, patient compliance is problematic because the pads are uncomfortable to sleep with and the garment in which they are located can impede dressing and undressing.

THE BIOMECHANICS OF WRIST FRACTURE

Once a fall is initiated, fall arrests have two post-initiation phases: a preimpact phase and an impact phase. In a fall from standing height the preimpact phase lasts approximately 0.7 seconds as the body falls to the ground. The impact phase lasts only tens of milliseconds for structures near the impact site (Fig. 71-1) to a few tenths of a second at more proximal body sites further from impact. Thus, for structures near the impact site, like the hands and elbows in a forward fall, short and long-loop neuromuscular reflexes are simply too long to be able to alter the fall arrest strategy during the impact phase.

The hands and arms are commonly used to protect the head and torso during a fall. The primary factors that determine the risk of Colles fracture, the most common upper extremity fall-related injury, are the height of the fall and the compliance of the surface. However at impact the relative velocity of the hand as it strikes the surface, the elbow flexion angle, and the angle of the lower arm with respect to the ground, and forearm bone mineral density status also play a role. There is almost always time for older women or men to deploy their upper extremities in the event of a fall. But

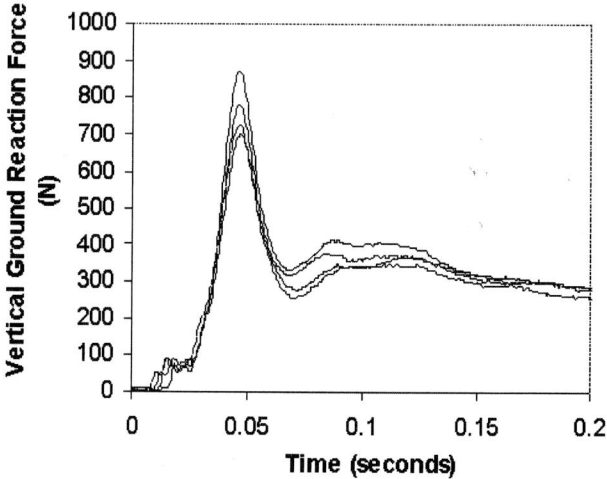

Figure 71-1 Example of the measured wrist impact force (in N) plotted versus time for one hand in four consecutive forward falls onto both arms for a young subject weighing 620 N. The subject fell onto a lightly padded surface from a shoulder height of 1 m. Note that (1) the time-to-peak-force is less than any upper extremity neuromuscular reflex, rendering reflexes unable to protect the wrist, and (2) the magnitude of the peak impact force on one hand exceeds as much as one body weight (620 N) for a brief time, mainly as a result of the ground arresting the downward momentum of the upper extremity over a relatively short distance. Data from De-Goede KM, Ashton-Miller JA: Fall arrest strategy affects peak hand impact force in a forward fall. *J Biomech* 35:843, 2002.

a fall by an older woman from 25 cm or more onto a stiff surface, landing with a straight arm, will almost certainly break the wrist. However, falling onto a slightly flexed arm will reduce this risk, although triceps and shoulder muscle strength is required to prevent the elbow from buckling. This is one important justification to encourage maintenance of upper extremity muscle strength in older adults.

AGE CHANGES IN COMPONENTS OF BIOMECHANICAL CAPABILITY

The biomechanical factors that underlie mobility impairments among older adults in general, and falling and fall injuries in particular, are not well understood. To come to that understanding, examination of the changes in biomechanical capabilities that occur with natural aging and with disease is merited. This section discusses the changes that occur in myoelectric latencies, reaction times, proprioception, joint ranges of motion (ROM), and muscular strengths and the rapid development of those strengths.

Myoelectric Latencies

The myoelectric latency or premotor time is the delay from a test stimulus cue to the onset of the first measurable change in myoelectric activity in a muscle. Myoelectric activity refers to the electrical signals sent through the nerves to initiate or modify the muscle contraction process. At the latency time, the muscle will not have yet developed any significant contractile force or, if already contracted, changed that force.

Myoelectric latencies typically range from 30 to 50 ms for myotatic reflexes involving the muscle spindles; 50 to 80 ms when cerebellar or cortex neural pathways are involved; 80 to 120 ms when afferent receptors and higher motor centers are involved; and 120 to 180 ms for volitional actions.

Reaction Times

Reaction time refers to the delay from a stimulus signaling a needed reaction to making a movement or developing a force. Reaction time is longer than myoelectric latency because it includes both the myoelectric latency and the finite time required for a muscle to develop or change its force magnitude after myoelectric activity begins. This additional time interval is called the *motor time*.

Reaction time is defined in different ways. For example, in studies of postural control, reaction time is often defined as the delay between stimulus onset and the first measurable change in the forces exerted by the feet on the floor support. This reaction force is usually measured with an instrumented force plate. This force development reaction time incorporates the myoelectric latency and the motor time required for the muscles to contract in order to alter the body configuration enough to change the support force. This happens with little discernible foot movement or limb segment acceleration. Reaction time has also been defined to be the delay from stimulus onset until the first

detectable acceleration of a body segment. This might be termed *segment acceleration reaction time*. Reaction time has also been defined as the delay from stimulus onset until a limb has been moved to a target. This movement-to-target reaction time incorporates myoelectric latencies, body segment acceleration reaction times, and body segment movement times.

Movement reaction times depend on how far body segments have to be moved. Reaction times also depend on how many choices a subject has in responding to a cue. Simple reaction times are those exhibited when no choices are given the subject. Choice reaction times are those exhibited when the subject must decide between two or more courses of action, depending on which of two or more cues is presented. Choice reaction time increases in proportion to the logarithm of the number of choices to be made. Choice reaction times are typically considerably longer than simple reaction times. Speed–accuracy tradeoff is also found in reaction time measurements. As the accuracy requirement of the task is increased, reaction time increases.

These differing definitions of reaction time and differing circumstances in which it is measured make it difficult to compare results from different studies of reaction times. Meaningful data on group differences in reaction times seem best obtained by comparing those times among different groups performing the same task, with the reaction time measure defined in the same way among the different groups.

Age and Gender Group Differences in Latencies and Reaction Times

Myoelectric latencies are typically 10 to 20 ms longer in healthy old adults than in young adults, but no gender differences, have been observed.

Age systematically increases force development reaction times. Older, as compared with younger, adults require perhaps 10 to 30 ms longer to volitionally develop modest levels of ankle torque from rest or to begin to take a step upon loss of balance. Systematic age differences in movement-to-target reaction times are often found. They increase on the order of 2 ms per age decade between the second and tenth decades. Age differences increase when subjects are not warned several seconds in advance of the cue that it is imminent. Much larger increases with age occur in choice reaction times than in simple reaction times. For example, in 10-choice button pushing tasks, where choices were identified by letter or color or both, choice reaction times increased 27 percent to 86 percent more in subjects ages 65 to 72 years, as compared with those ages 18 to 33 years. No notable gender differences in reaction times have been reported.

Biomechanical Effects of Age Differences in Latencies and Reaction Times are Minor

Despite these statistically significant age differences of 10 to 20 ms in latencies and of 15 to 30 ms in some reaction times, they seldom seem critical to mobility function. Even rapid responses in time-critical situations take place over perhaps 200 to 500 ms, so these latency and reaction time differences, when compared with the task execution times, are not large. For example, among healthy older adults, the time required to fully contract a muscle is on the order of 400 ms. The time to lift a foot in order to take a quick step is on the order of 200 to 400 ms. Adults need warning times on the order of 400 to 500 ms to be able to stop before reaching or to turn away from obstacles that come suddenly to attention.

Reaction times, which include muscle latencies, are task and strategy dependent. They are modifiable by central command. Reaction times of older adults are not always slower than those of young. Moreover, reaction times do not necessarily predict performance on complex mobility tasks. For example, one of our studies found that simple reaction times in lifting a foot immediately upon a visual cue did not predict how well the same young or older subjects could avoid stepping on a suddenly appearing obstacle during level gait. In fact, age-group differences in simple reaction times were substantially larger than age-group differences in the response times needed to avoid the obstacles successfully.

Proprioception

Proprioception describes awareness of body segment positions and orientations. Relatively few studies have examined changes with aging in proprioception. One study found joint position sense in the knee to deteriorate with age. Joint angles could be reproduced to within 2 degrees by 20-year-olds, but only to within 6 degrees by 80-year-olds. Twenty-year-olds could detect passive joint motions of 4 degrees, but 80-year-olds could detect only motions larger than 7 degrees. Other studies have found no major decline with age in motion perception in finger and toe joints but have found declines with aging in sensing vibration. Proprioceptive acuity at a joint is significantly better when muscles at the joint are active than when they are passive. Proprioceptive thresholds during weight bearing are at least an order of magnitude lower than those typically reported during non–weight-bearing tests.

Studies exploring the effect of age on thresholds for sensing ankle rotations show that healthy adults can sense quite small rotations in the sagittal and frontal planes under the weight-bearing conditions of upright stance. The probability of successful detection of rotation increases with increasing magnitude and speed of imposed foot rotation. A 10-fold reduction in the angular threshold was observed on increasing the speed of rotation from 0.1 to 2.5 degrees per second, but thresholds did not further reduce at higher speeds. In healthy adults between the third and eighth decades, age, rotation angle, and rotation speed also significantly affected the threshold for sensing the direction of foot rotation. Threshold angles were three to four times larger in older females than in younger females.

Individuals with central or peripheral proprioceptive impairments can exhibit articular pathology. Examples include Charcot changes occurring in the upper or lower extremities because of central nervous system damage caused by syringomyelia over several levels of the spinal cord, and changes in the foot or ankle because of lower extremity peripheral neuropathy often associated with diabetes. Peripheral neuropathy increases the proprioceptive threshold at the ankle nearly fivefold as compared with age-matched healthy controls. This increased threshold adversely affects postural stability and raises the risk of obstacle contact during gait, suggesting one mechanism that might underlie the 20-fold increase in fall risk and the 6-fold increase in fall-induced fractures that these patients have.

Joint Ranges of Motion

Body joint ROM have generally been found to diminish with age, but not all findings are consistent. For example, studies report approximately a 20 percent decline between ages 45 and 70 years in hip rotation and 10 percent declines in wrist and shoulder ROM. Comparisons of the ROM of lower-extremity joints for young and middle-age adults with those for older adults showed declines ranging from negligible to 57 percent. At age 79 years, one-fifth of a large group of subjects had restricted knee joint motion and two-thirds had restricted hip joint motion. Among more than 3000 blue-collar workers with ages ranging from 20 to 60 years of age, a 25 percent decline with age was found in ability to bend to the side, and a 45 percent decline in shoulder motion. Declines of 25 to 50 percent have been found in various ROM of the lumbar spine between ages of 20 and 80 years. However, a comparison between two groups with mean ages of approximately 65 and 80 years found no significant differences in 28 different joint ROM. At least one study suggests that passive or active stretching exercises can increase hip extension ROM in young adults by 8 to 17 degrees, and another study suggested that exercises with a focus on stretching improve spine flexibility in older adults.

The effects of decreased ROM on abilities to perform activities of daily living are not well understood in young or old adults. One study of adults with arthritis found that the ability to move around in one's environment correlated well with ROM in knee flexion, the ability to bend down correlated with hip flexion ROM, and the abilities in activities requiring use of hands and arms correlated well with ROM of the upper extremities. Another study found that restricted knee motion in 79-year-olds correlated with disability in entering public transport vehicles but that ROM impairment did not generally associate with commitment to institutional care. A third study found the majority of a group of 134 people age 79 years to have enough spinal mobility to perform common activities of daily living.

Muscle Strength and Power

The loss of strength with age, even in healthy and physically active older adults (Table 71-1), has long been recognized. Isometric strengths peak at about age 25 years and then decline. The loss is approximately one-third by age 65 years. Isometric strength is more reliably measured, and considerably greater values are recorded, when the patient exerts force on a fixed force transducer, rather than one held by

Table 71-1   Literature Values for Joint Torque Strengths (Nm)

Data Source	Young Adults*		Older Adults†	
	Females	Males	Females	Males
Ankle dorsiflexors				
Oberg et al.	49			
Sepic et al.	44	78	46	74
Thelen et al.	28	43	22	37
Ankle plantarflexors				
Oberg et al.	188			
Gerdle and Fugl-Meyer			78	139
Falkel	58	87		
Sepic et al.	100	129	82	131
Thelen et al.	130	181	88	137
Knee flexors				
Knapic et al.	87	195		
Borges	100	155	65	109
Murray et al.	78		50	
Knee extensors				
Knapic et al.	160	250		
Dannenskiold et al.			75	120
Aniansson et al.			108	191
Borges	183	289	128	188
Murray et al.	176		110	
Hip flexors				
Markhede and Grimby		120		
Cahalan et al.	66	108	51	89
Hip extensors				
Markhede and Grimby		248		
Cahalan et al.	126	204	110	203
Shoulder flexors				
Murray et al.	50	104	38	84
Shoulder extensors				
Murray et al.	53	80	35	74

*Mean ages approximately 25 to 30 years.

†Mean ages approximately 60 to 80 years.

SOURCE: Modified from Schultz AB: Mobility impairment in the elderly: Challenges for biomechanics research. *J Biomech* 25:519, 1992. Data sources are cited in that paper. Most values quoted are for isometric strengths, but a few are for low-rate isokinetic strengths.

an examiner. To express the strength developed about the joint in units of torque, the force (in Newtons) developed by the limb segment against a force-measuring transducer is multiplied by its lever arm (in meters) about the joint being tested. It has long been recognized that mean strengths of female adults of any age are on the order of one-third lower than those of male adults (Table 71-1). However, when those strengths are normalized by body size (for example, by dividing by body weight times body height), then that difference is reduced to 20 percent for the hip and knee muscles. At more distal joints there is often no longer a significant gender difference in normalized strengths.

Reports of strength values vary widely because they depend on many factors such as on which subjects are measured (substantially), at which joint angles, whether under isometric or constant velocity conditions, and, at constant velocity, whether muscle shortening or lengthening is occurring. Thus, for the hip flexor muscles, which are needed to recover balance after tripping by swinging a leg forward rapidly, maximum hip flexor torque decreases linearly with increasing hip flexion angle, and, additionally, with increasing hip flexion speed. The capacity to move a limb segment or limb rapidly can best be measured by the maximum power developed about the relevant joint. Because power is defined as the product of torque times angular velocity, high hip flexion power values would be attained by being able to develop a large torque about the joint at a high rotational velocity. Maximum power usually occurs in a shortening muscle at about one-third of the maximum movement velocity. Older adults are particularly prone to loss of torque at high velocities because of the irreversible loss of the largest (and fastest) motor units with age. The current methods for measuring maximum power developed at speeds over 250 degrees per second, however, leave much to be desired because of substantial measurement artifacts. Age differences in strength have been reported to be smaller when muscles lengthen than when they shorten.

A prevalent casual belief is that many of the mobility impairments that arise in the elderly population are a result of declines in muscular strength. This belief warrants careful consideration. Studies described subsequently suggest that the joint torques needed to maintain postural balance and even to rise from a chair are often well below the joint torque strengths that healthy older adults have available.

The decline with aging in the ability of muscles to produce power is perhaps well illustrated by records of elite athletic performances. In short-distance races, male elite runners older than age 70 years run approximately one-third slower than do elite young adult male athletes. In long-distance races, male elite runners older than age 70 years old run approximately half as fast as elite young adult male athletes. In rodent muscle, power outputs decline with aging approximately 30 percent in absolute terms and 20 percent on a per-unit-muscle-mass basis. Age-related changes in muscle morphology and physiology are widely reported. The maximum speed of unloaded shortening and contraction times for specific fiber types do not seem to change significantly with aging, but fast/slow fiber innervation ratios do seem to do so. Muscle power reduction with aging may also be caused by systemic factors, such as declines in cardiopulmonary function. It is thus likely that to maintain muscle function in older adults, the focus should be on the assessment and training of power, rather than isometric joint torques.

Rapid Development of Joint Torque Strengths

Upon a substantial perturbation of standing balance, as already noted, fewer than 500 ms are often available for the critical initial phase of balance restoration, yet 300 to 400 ms can be required to develop maximum joint torques. Even older adults who are healthy and physically active have diminished abilities to develop large joint torques rapidly, compared with young adults. Moreover, older females have lower torque development rates than do older males. For example, in one study, the mean total time required to develop 60 Nm of ankle plantarflexion torque, when subjects were asked to develop maximum torque as fast as possible, was 311 ms in young adult females and 472 ms, or 161 ms (52 percent) longer, in older females. Corresponding times for males were 270 and 313 ms (16 percent longer), respectively (Fig. 71-2). Maximum rate of torque development tends to correlate highly with maximum voluntary torque strength, with correlation

coefficients on the order of 0.8. Owing to slowing in peak rate of joint torque development abilities, capacities of even healthy old adults to recover balance or to carry out other time-critical actions that require moderate-to-substantial strengths, such as those required to avoid obstacles that come suddenly to attention, may be considerably reduced.

Source of Age Differences in Rapid Strength Development

Measurements of myoelectric signals in ankle dorsiflexor and plantarflexor muscles during rapid isometric and isokinetic exertions have been used to explore the extent to which this age-related slowing in rapid torque development might be attributed to neural factors; that is, those processes that precede the initiation of muscle contraction. In one study, latency times, muscle activation rates, and myoelectric activity levels of agonistic and antagonistic muscles were quantified. There were few marked age differences in the latencies or in the onset rates or magnitudes of agonistic or antagonistic muscles activities during maximum isometric and during isokinetic exertions. Myoelectric latency times were statistically associated with age, but in the mean, they were only approximately 10 to 25 ms longer in the elderly. Given the outcomes of this study, the differences observed in rapid torque development abilities in healthy elderly adults, as compared with healthy young adults, seem largely a result of differences in muscle contraction mechanisms once contraction is initiated, rather than to differences in the speeds of stimulus sensing or central processing of motor commands or to differences in the muscle recruitment decisions that precede contraction initiation.

AGE DIFFERENCES IN PERFORMANCE OF SIMPLE MOBILITY TASKS

To reach a better understanding of the biomechanical mechanisms that underlie mobility impairments in general, and falling and fall injuries in particular, attention is merited on how the changes in biomechanical capabilities that occur with natural aging and with disease affect the performance of individual mobility tasks. This section discusses age differences in performance of common mobility tasks, such as walking, rising from chairs, beds, and floors, and regaining standing balance when it is disturbed. Age-related declines in mobility task performances are seen in tasks that are physically and/or cognitively very challenging long before any declines are seen in tasks easily performed. Physical and cognitive capacities can decrease substantially without leading to any impairment if task performance demands are modest because they do not tax the functional reserve. Once capacity falls to the point at which task demand begins to equal capacity, performance ability begins to decline substantially. In healthy adults the consequences of a decrement in capacity are unlikely to be seen in performances of easy tasks but are likely to be seen in performances of demanding tasks, accompanied perhaps by compensatory changes in performance strategies.

Plantarflexion

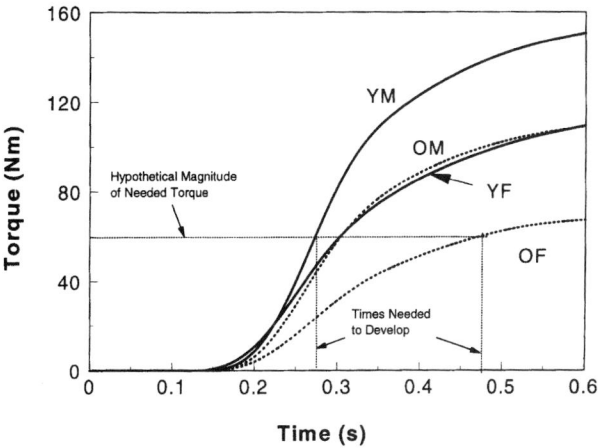

Figure 71-2 Age and gender differences in rapid development of ankle plantarflexor torque. The subjects tested were healthy younger and older (Y, O) females and males (F, M). Time is measured from a light flash cue signaling the subjects to push against a pedal as hard and as fast as possible. The four subject groups exhibited nearly the same mean reaction times, approximately 160 ms. However, the mean time needed to develop a given magnitude of torque varied substantially among the four age/gender groups. For example, were a plantarflexion torque of 60 Nm required to regain balance upon the initiation of a fall, YM would need approximately 275 ms to develop that torque, and OF would need approximately 475 ms. Data from Thelen DG et al: Effects of age on rapid ankle torque development. *J Gerontol Med Sci* 51A:M226, 1996.

Assessment of Mobility Function

Mobility does associate with decrements in biomechanical variables. For example, in community-dwelling older adults, self-reported difficulty with chair rise, ascending and descending stairs, and fast walking was associated with a reduction of isometric knee extensor strength capacity below 3 Nm/kg body weight. A number of performance-based test batteries have been developed to globally assess a patient's mobility function, including that in changing positions, controlling upright posture, and walking. These batteries are designed to detect clinically significant changes that might, for example, place an individual at risk for falls or for developing mobility disability. Not all of these batteries are sensitive to the subtle age-related changes in performance found among healthy adults. Some do not include tasks that are sufficiently demanding. Others use rating systems that are not quantitative enough. Such batteries serve well for assessing more impaired older adults, but healthy older adults can often perform without difficulty all of the tasks the batteries include.

Batteies are available that can elicit subtle age-related effects because they rate performance sensitively enough and include tasks with sufficient demand. For example, in one test patients are asked if health problems or physical impairments have resulted in adaptation in the way daily tasks are performed; are tested for the ability to balance on one leg for 10 seconds; and are measured for average gait speed relative to a 0.5 m/s standard. For example, if a patient has altered the way he or she performs daily tasks, cannot balance for 10 seconds on one foot, and walks at less than 0.5 m/s, then their risk of developing mobility disability in the next 18 months is greater than 55%. A recent review of fall risk assessment measures showed that certain measures showed good sensitivity and specificity in acute care settings (e.g., STRATIFY, Fall Risk Assessment Tool), others performed well in extended care settings (e.g., Morse Fall Scale, Timed Up and Go Test), while yet others performed best in outpatient settings (e.g., Elderly Fall Screening Test, Timed Up and Go Test).

Ascribing Functional Decline Fully to Insufficient Motivation, Activity, or Training is Questionable

Performance records of elite older athletes suggest that physical inactivity, lack of motivation, and lack of training cannot fully explain functional decline in healthy older adults. Declines with age in physical performance abilities can be seen among even highly trained and highly motivated athletes. As already noted, top running speeds of short- and long-distance older elite runners are notably lower than those of younger adult elite runners.

Gait

In older adults free of overt neurologic, musculoskeletal, cardiorespiratory, or cognitive problems, comfortable gait speed declines minimally until approximately age 60 years and then declines by 1 to 2 percent per year through age 80 years; however, there is substantial variability among studies of age changes in comfortable gait speed (Fig. 71-3).

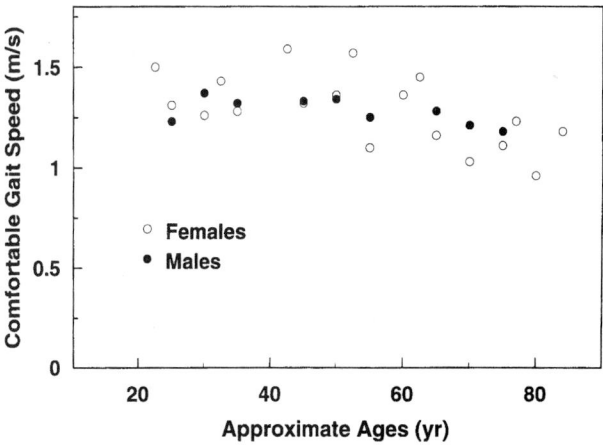

Figure 71-3 Age and gender differences in self-selected comfortable gait speeds. These data are graphed using those abstracted by Bohannon et al. from seven earlier literature reports. The mean speeds reported vary substantially. Nonetheless, the general trend is for comfortable gait speed to decline minimally until approximately age 60 years and then to decline by 1 to 2 percent per year through age 80 years.

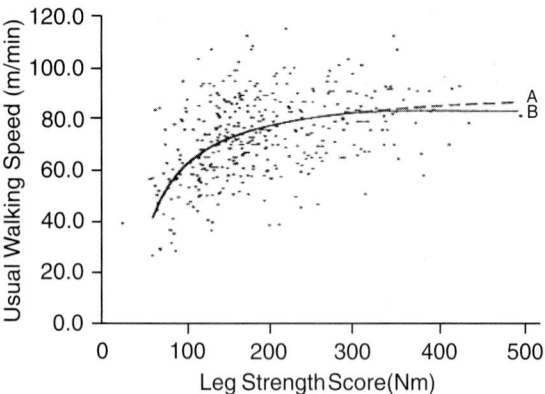

Figure 71-4 Comfortable gait speed is nonlinearly related to leg muscle strength score in a population-based sample of more than 400 adults between the ages of 60 and 96 years. The strength score was formed from the summed isokinetic right knee and ankle flexor and extensor muscle strengths. The regression curve 'A' represents the fit for an average age of 76 years and average weight of 71 kg. ('B' represents an alternative regression model.) Data from Buchner DM et al: Evidence for a non-linear relationship between leg strength and gait speed. *Age Ageing* 25:390, 1996.

The causes of gait slowing with age are a subject of controversy. They may be multifactorial, including subtle age-related changes in joint stiffness, leg strength, and energy conservation strategies. Independently of age, comfortable walking speed associates nonlinearly with muscle strength (Fig. 71-4) and maximum aerobic power. Much of the decline in speed is attributed to reductions in step length. The earliest studies of gait in older adults found that men in their sixties demonstrated significantly shorter step and stride lengths and decreased ankle extension and pelvic rotation when compared with younger males.

Other studies confirm those findings, but not without exception. One study found no significant age group differences in step and stride lengths, velocity, or movements of the ankles, pelvis, and total-body-mass center. Another concluded that increased variability in gait should not be regarded as a normal concomitant of old age. Still another found that among older adults, more than 40 percent of the variance in normal walking speed can be accounted for by differences in height, calf muscle strength, and the presence of health problems such as leg pain. A prospective study in older women showed that those with the poorest knee strength and balance scores were five times more likely to develop severe walking disability than those with normal function.

There is little evidence of an association between age-related reductions in stride length and gait speed and a tendency to fall. On the other hand, increased stride time variability is associated with a fivefold increase in the risk of falling.

Rising from Chairs, Beds, and Floors

The mechanical demands of rising from a regular chair impose the largest strength demands on the knee and hip extensor muscles: a healthy older individual is required to develop approximately 30 percent and 25 percent of his or her maximum knee and hip extensor strengths, respectively. It is instructive to think about how disease or impairments that affect muscle strength can affect the ability to rise from a chair. With bilateral symmetry in function and their young adult body weight, knee strength would have to be reduced by 70 percent before becoming inadequate. Thus, healthy elderly persons have considerable functional reserve. However, if their body weight has doubled from their young adult weight, the older individual's knee strength would only have to fall 35 percent below age norms before knee extensor strength is inadequate to rise from a chair without arms. Likewise, a complete unilateral loss in knee extensor strength would mean that a healthy older individual could only tolerate a 35 percent loss in remaining knee strength before it becomes inadequate. In general, healthy older adults do rise more slowly than young adults, but the time differences for bed and chair rises are 2 seconds or less. When rising from the floor, age differences are larger, with older adults tending to take twice as long as young. Characteristic age-related changes in trunk, arm, and leg motions used to rise may account for these differences.

When rising from a chair, particularly without the use of hands for assistance, healthy old persons flex their necks, trunks, and legs and extend their thighs more than young persons, resulting in a more anterior placement of their floor reaction force than young adults demonstrate. In one study of graded difficulty chair rising tasks, healthy younger and older adults did not differ in the leg joint torques that they used to perform the series of tasks. Both younger and older adults had enough strength to perform even the most challenging task. However, old persons generally used a greater percentage of their available knee strength to rise from a chair, using near-maximum levels in challenging situations. Some of the older adults failed to rise when their postural control was challenged by a lowered seat and by a narrow foot support base. So, there are situations in which older adults have adequate strength to rise from a chair but are limited by other factors, such as difficulty with postural control.

While rising from a bed, older adults, as compared with younger adults, tend to lengthen the time of contact of their arm with the bed surface. They are more likely to rotate and laterally flex their trunks, bear weight on their hip/gluteal area, and use their elbow to help pivot while rising. Declining trunk strength may account for some of these findings.

Many healthy older adults are unable to sit up in bed without the use of their hands. When rising from the floor, older adults tend to use key intermediate positions, such as getting to an all-fours positions, in order to reduce the strength requirements and to enhance postural stability. In general, intermediate postures that reduce physical demands (for example, knee extensor strength required) can be used as part of task-specific exercises to improve the ability to rise from the floor. Improvements as a result of these interventions, quantifiable biomechanically (such as increased momentum during the rise) and clinically (such as in time), are modest.

Restoration of Standing Posture Upon its Modest Disturbance

There is evidence of deterioration in many of the sensori-motor systems underlying postural control, even in elderly populations without obvious signs of disease. However, aging alone does not account for the heterogeneity of postural control problems in the elderly population. Moreover, responses to postural perturbations are task and perturbation specific, so that a single assessment technique may not serve as a true indicator of the overall integrity of the balance control system.

Sway while standing generally increases with age during adulthood. Age-related changes in postural control in healthy adults are minimal through age 70 years under situations of low task demand. Examples of low-demand tasks are standing on two feet with eyes open, or maintaining stance when it is perturbed by modest movements of the support surface or by gentle backward pushes. When task demand increases, age-group differences in postural control abilities become more apparent. For example, when a sway response no longer suffices to recover balance in the face of a perturbation, young adults tend to resort to a single step, whereas older adults tend to employ multiple steps in order to recover their balance. Task demand can be increased by decreasing visual input or by making the support surface more compliant.

The most striking age-related differences often occur when several different demands are increased simultaneously. For example, when both the support surface and the visual surround were rotated in phase with body sway, 50 percent of older adults lost their balance on their first attempt to maintain stance, as compared with 9 percent of younger controls. There is evidence that the age-group differences may increase after age 70 years. The mean time for standing on one leg with eyes open before losing balance for 20- to 29-year-olds was at least twice as long as that for 70- to 79-year-olds and nearly seven times longer with eyes closed. In contrast, mean stance time for 60- to 69-year-olds, as compared with 20- to 29-year-olds, was only 20 percent less with eyes open and only three times less with eyes closed (Fig. 71-5).

It is not known why these changes in postural control abilities occur with age. One-leg stance time differences might result from reduced ankle joint lateral muscle strength or endurance, increased muscle latency times, decreased cutaneous or joint proprioception, or decreased willingness to allow the center of the floor reaction to deviate from the center of the foot support area. The few studies to date that have analyzed whole-body response biomechanics, or even the body-segment motions that are used or the joint torques developed in response to postural disturbances, report that the required motions and torques are generally modest compared with the literature-reported capacities of healthy old adults.

Cognitive and Other Psychological Factors

Cognitive demand relative to cognitive capacity substantially influences physical task performance. As mobility

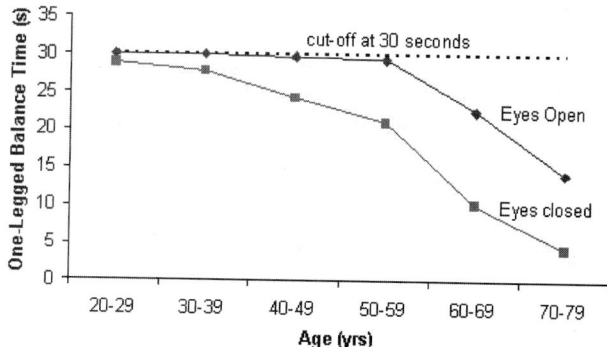

Figure 71-5   Age differences in ability to stand on one leg. Healthy adults were asked to balance on one leg for up to 30 seconds, with eyes open and then with eyes closed. The *y* axis shows the time until balance was lost. Difficulty in performing the eyes open task did not arise until after age 50 years, but when the eyes were closed, even the younger subjects had some difficulty. The older subjects had substantial difficulty with both tasks. Data from Bohannon RW et al: Decrease in timed balance scores with aging. *Phys Ther* 64:1067, 1984.

task complexity increases, so do the cognitive demands placed on the individual. The need to perform two tasks simultaneously or to divide attention degrades performances of healthy elderly persons more than for healthy young persons. For example, in a study of abilities to step over suddenly appearing obstacles while walking, the attention of groups of healthy younger and older adults was divided by having them simultaneously respond in two reaction time tasks. Both young and old adults had a significantly increased risk of obstacle contact while negotiating obstacles when their attention was divided, but attention division diminished obstacle avoidance abilities of the old more than it did in the young. These results suggest that diminished abilities to respond to physical hazards present in the environment when attention is directed elsewhere may partially account for high rates of falls among the elderly population.

In our studies of relationships between neuropsychological status and physical performance, relatively minimal associations have been found in performance of simple tasks, such as in assessments of proprioception, joint ROM, and strengths. With tasks of increasing complexity, such as in chair rising, ambulation, and postural maintenance, visual attention abilities and psychomotor speed were found to be good predictors of performance. In performance of mobility tasks of substantial complexity, such as avoiding obstacles when attention is divided or stepping accurately under adverse conditions, measures of problem-solving ability and mental flexibility, along with psychomotor speed and attention, become performance predictors.

Difficulties in walking seem to relate to cognitive impairment. Demented older adults have shorter step lengths, lower frequencies of stepping, more step-to-step variability, and lower gait speed. A geriatric rehabilitation program led to greater gains in walking speed in subjects with normal cognition than it did in those with impaired cognition. Moreover, walking speed appeared to be closely related to ability to rise from a chair and to be a powerful predictor of patient placement upon discharge from the rehabilitation

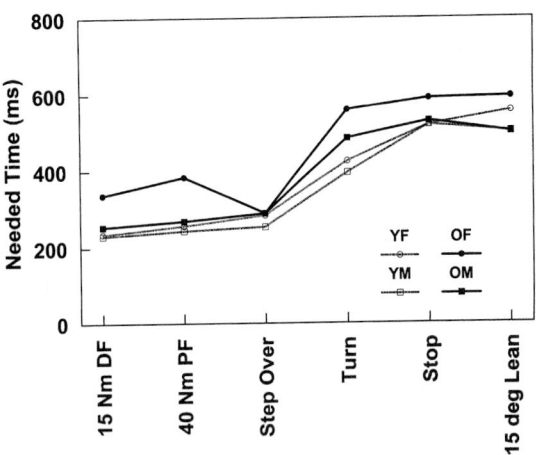

Figure 71-6 Summary of age and gender differences in times needed for various quick responses. Mean values across groups of healthy older females (OF), older males (OM), young females (YF), young males (YM) of the times required for six different responses are shown. The responses are indicated by the horizontal axis labels. Each of the situations being responded to is further described in the text of this chapter. From left to right, the responses are the development of, respectively, (1) 15 Nm of ankle dorsiflexor flexor torque, or (2) 40 Nm of ankle plantarflexor torque, as fast as possible; the achievement of a 50% rate of success in avoiding suddenly-appearing obstacles by, respectively, (3) stepping over the obstacle, (4) turning away before reaching the obstacle, or (5) stopping before reaching the obstacle; and (6) the replacement of the stepped foot on the ground when recovering balance by taking a single step up on sudden release from a 15 deg whole-body forward lean. The data points are connected by lines only to help distinguish the four subject groups. Data are replotted from the authors' own studies.

program. Of 116 older adults studied, none were able to live alone or even in a rest home if they were discharged with a walking speed of less than 0.15 m/s. Many frail elderly persons are aware of the difficulty of dividing one's attention while walking, as demonstrated by the ability of the simple but effective Stops Walking When Talking Test to predict impending falls in these patients.

AGE DIFFERENCES IN PERFORMANCE OF TIME-CRITICAL MOBILITY TASKS

Times Needed for Quick Responses to Maintain or Recover Balance

As already noted, the time available in which to recover from a substantial disturbance of upright balance or to safely arrest a fall is often less than 1 second. For example, when walking forward at 1.3 m/s, the comfortable walking speed typically self-selected by healthy young and old adults, only 200 to 300 ms may be available in which to make initial responses appropriate for balance recovery when tripping over an obstacle. If a large obstacle in the gait path, such as a moving vehicle, suddenly comes to attention 1 m ahead while walking at this speed, then a turn

away from the obstacle or a stop before reaching it would have to be accomplished within approximately 750 ms. The term "time-critical" is used here to refer to such situations. Differences in abilities to respond appropriately in at least some time-critical situations (Fig. 71-6) may help explain age and gender differences in rates of falls and fall-related injuries.

Studies of Time-Critical Obstacle Avoidance Tasks

Avoiding Obstacles by Stepping Over Them

The abilities of healthy and physically active young and older adults, who were walking forward at approximately 1.3 m/s, to step over an obstacle that suddenly appeared at seemingly random times and locations in front of them have been examined. The appearance of this obstacle was arranged to give the subjects available response times that varied from 200 to 450 ms before they would have stepped on it. This task is a time-critical one, but because avoidance requires relatively minor changes in stepping pattern and relatively minor redistributions among segments of kinetic energies and forward momenta, the strength requirements of the task likely are modest. Few young or old persons could avoid obstacles if only 200 ms were available. Most young and old persons reliably avoided obstacles that appeared so as to give 450 ms warning time. Over all available response times used, old persons had lower avoidance success rates than did young persons, but in biomechanical terms, it was estimated that they would have needed only 30 ms more warning time to have the same success rates as young persons. No significant gender differences in avoidance abilities were found.

Avoiding Obstacles by Turning Away Before Reaching Them

In a study of abilities to make sudden turns to avoid previously unseen obstacles, healthy elderly adults were substantially less successful than young adults when available response times were short. For example, for an available response time of 450 ms, mean success rates in completing the turn without colliding with the obstacle were 68 percent in young adults, and 27 percent in older adults. Moreover, males had substantially better success rates for given available response times than did females in corresponding age groups. This task is a time-critical one. Avoidance requires complete arrest of forward momenta and quick development of lateral momentum, but relatively minor redistributions among segments of kinetic energies. Therefore, the strength requirements of the task likely are moderate.

Avoiding Obstacles by Stopping Before Reaching Them

In a similar study of abilities to make sudden stops to avoid previously unseen obstacles, healthy old adults again were substantially less successful than young adults when available response times were short. For example, for an available response time of 525 ms, mean success rates in stopping before passing forward of the obstacle were 58 percent for young female and male adults and 51 percent for older males, but only 23 percent for older females. This task is also a time-critical one. Avoidance requires complete arrest of forward momenta and total dissipation of body kinetic energy. Thus, the strength requirements of the task likely are substantial.

Studies of Time-Critical Balance Recovery Tasks

Once a fall begins, quick recovery of balance may be needed to avoid injury. In one set of studies by Grabiner and coworkers, forward falls were induced in healthy older adults by an unexpected trip or backward movement of the support surface. Factors associated with a failure to recover balance were one or more of the following: too short a recovery step, slower response time, greater trunk flexion angle at toe-off, greater trunk flexion velocity at recovery foot contact with the ground, and buckling of the recovery limb.

We have studied the ability to recover from a forward fall by rapid step-taking. Subjects were released from a forward-leaning position and instructed to regain standing balance by taking a single step forward. Lean angle was successively increased until a subject failed to regain balance as instructed. This task is a time-critical one, likely requiring the use of maximum strengths. It was found that the mean maximum lean angle from which older males could recover balance as instructed, 23.9 degrees, was significantly smaller than that for the young males, 32.5 degrees. Corresponding angles for the females were 16.2 degrees and 30.7 degrees, but those numbers do not include 5 of the 10 older females who could not recover balance from even the smallest lean angle at which they were tested, approximately 13 degrees. Maximum lean angles were well correlated with the average forward step velocity and inversely correlated with the time required to unload the stepping foot, but were unrelated to myoelectric response latencies of ~70 msec in both young and elderly persons.

A gender difference has been found in torques used for recovery of balance. None of the males needed to use their maximum ankle, knee, or hip torque capacities; but the young females used maximal hip flexion torques, and the older females used maximum plantarflexor, knee flexion, hip flexion, and extension torques. The results suggest that reduced abilities of healthy older adults to recover from a forward fall result from an inability to move body segments fast enough, rather than from delayed initiation of response.

Mechanisms Underlying Age and Gender Differences in Performance of Time-Critical Tasks with High Strength Demands

Some of the studies discussed in the section on Age Differences in Performance of Time-Critical Mobility Tasks suggest that the source of both age and gender differences in performance of tasks that are both time critical and have high strength requirements lies primarily in strengths and speeds of muscle contraction, rather than in sensory processing or motor planning abilities. As pointed out earlier in this chapter, studies of myoelectric latencies for rapid ankle torque development have found no significant gender group differences. They have found statistically significant age group differences, but the differences in the mean latencies were only approximately 10 to 20 ms, whereas the total times needed to develop near-maximum torques were on the order of 400 to 600 ms. They showed that age group differences in the use of co-contraction were not responsible for the age group differences in torque development rates. Studies of mean reaction times have also found statistically significant age group differences in those times. However, those differences were only approximately 10 to 20 ms, whereas the total response times ranged approximately from 400 to 800 ms. No substantial gender differences were found in those reaction times. This suggests that among healthy older compared with young adults and among females compared with males, differences in rapid torque development abilities, noted earlier in this chapter (see Rapid Development of Joint Torque Strengths), and differences in performance of tasks that are both time critical and have high strength requirements, seem largely a result of differences in strengths and speeds of muscle contraction once contraction is initiated, rather than to delays in initiating contraction.

The outcomes of these and other studies suggest that healthy older adults, when compared with young adults, and healthy older females, when compared with older males, are more at risk for injury in tasks that are both time critical and have high strength requirements. Time-critical obstacle avoidance tasks involve rapid visual processing, rapid triggering of preplanned strategies, and rapid execution of movements, during which whole-body balance must be maintained. Among healthy adults, the times needed for the visual processing and response triggering phases are a few hundredths of a second longer for old than for young. In contrast, the times needed for movement execution are a few tenths of a second longer for old than for young persons. Almost exclusively because of these longer movement execution times, the warning times that older adults, as compared with younger adults, need to perform successfully time-critical tasks with high strength requirements are a few tenths of a second longer. Although differences of a few tenths of a second in abilities to respond are not usually important, circumstances leading to needs for time-critical, high-strength responses probably combine at random. Sometimes the consequence of needing a few tenths of a second longer to execute avoidance or recovery maneuvers may not be small, and that need, when circumstances combine unfavorably, may substantially lower the probability of regaining balance or avoiding a fall-related injury. The ability to perform these avoidance and recovery maneuvers usually involves stepping, but well-established clinical tests of these time-critical stepping responses do not yet exist. Tests of voluntary maximal distance and high-speed stepping are being evaluated.

CONCLUSIONS

Studies of the biomechanics of mobility among healthy older adults suggest the following:

1.   In activities such as ambulation, chair and bed rise, and postural responses to small perturbations, performances of healthy older adults are often remarkably similar to those of young adults. Age group differences among healthy adults that seem biomechanically significant have been found in only certain kinds of tasks.

2.   Age differences in performances of many tasks apparently seldom arise from limitations in joint ROM. Only a few physical tasks present substantial joint ROM requirements.

3.   Similarly, those differences apparently arise only in some circumstances from limitations in joint torque strengths. The strength requirements of many daily tasks, excluding time-critical tasks requiring high strengths and certain kinds of transferring tasks, are modest compared with the available strengths of healthy old adults.

4.   There are substantial age and gender differences in abilities to develop joint torques rapidly, but these differences generally seem to be of importance chiefly in performing time-critical tasks requiring high strengths.

5.   When significant age differences in responses have been found, those differences appeared seldom to depend in major ways on age differences in latencies or reaction times. Under many circumstances, the age differences that do exist in sensing and neural processing times are small compared with total response times.

6.   In performing time-critical tasks requiring high strengths, for which major age differences arise, they presumably arise because of age differences in the muscle contraction physiology underlying the biomechanical response execution.

7.   Cognitive and other psychological factors, such as risk-taking preferences, have a substantial role in mobility task performance.

8.   Age-related declines in mobility function appear during performances of tasks that are physically and/or cognitively very challenging at much younger ages than they appear in tasks that are easily performed.

REFERENCES

Alexander NB et al: Muscle strength and rising from a chair in older adults. *Muscle Nerve Suppl* 5:S56, 1997.

Alexander NB et al: Task-specific resistance training to improve the ability of ADL-impaired older adults to rise from a bed and from a chair. *J Am Geriatr Soc* 49:1418, 2001.

Bohannon RW et al: Walking speed: Reference values and correlates for older adults. *J Orthop Sports Phys Ther* 24:86, 1996.

Chen HC et al: Stepping over obstacles: Dividing attention impairs performance of old more than young adults. *J Gerontol Med Sci* 51A:M116, 1996.

DeGoede KM, Ashton-Miller JA: Fall arrest strategy affects peak hand impact force in a forward fall. *J Biomech* 35:843, 2002.

Faulkner J et al: Skeletal muscle weakness in old age: Underlying mechanisms. *Ann Rev Gerontol Geriatr* 10:147, 1990.

Fitzpatrick R, McCloskey DI: Proprioceptive, visual and vestibular thresholds for the perception of sway during standing in humans. *J Physiol* 478:173, 1994.

Greenspan SL et al: Fall direction, bone mineral density, and function: Risk factors for hip fracture in frail nursing home elderly. *Am J Med* 104:539, 1998.

Leon J, Lair T: Functional status of the noninstitutionalized elderly: Estimates of ADL and IADL difficulties. National Medical Expenditure Survey Research Findings 4. Rockville, MD: Agency for Health Care Policy and Research, DHHS Publication No. PHS 90-3462, 1990.

Luukinen H et al: Incidence rate of falls in an aged population in northern Finland. *J Clin Epidemiol* 47:843,1994.

Malmivaara A et al: Risk factors for injurious falls leading to hospitalization or death in a cohort of 19,500 adults. *Am J Epidemiol* 138:384, 1993.

Medell JL, Alexander NB: A clinical measure of maximal and rapid stepping in older women. *J Gerontol* 55A:M429, 2000.

Pavol MJ et al: Influence of lower extremity strength of healthy older adults on the outcome of an induced trip. *JAGS* 50:256, 2002.

Richardson JK, Ashton-Miller JA: Peripheral nerve dysfunction and falls in the elderly. *Postgrad Med* 99:161, 1996.

Schultz AB et al: What leads to age and gender differences in balance maintenance and recovery? *Muscle Nerve Suppl* 5:S60, 1997.

The American Geriatrics Society Panel of Falls in Older Persons: Guideline for prevention of falls in older persons. *J Am Geriatr Soc* 49:664, 2001.

Thelen DG et al: Effects of age on rapid ankle torque development. *J Gerontol Med Sci* 51A:M226, 1996.

Tideiksaar R: *Falling in Old Age: Prevention and Management,* 2nd ed. New York, Springer, 1997.

Exercise in Elderly People: Physiologic and Functional Effects

ROBERT S. SCHWARTZ • WENDY M. KOHRT

AGING, DISUSE, AND DISEASE

A common belief among the lay public, as well as among many health care professionals, is that much of the disease and loss of function that commonly accompanies aging is inevitable and a result of the "aging process" itself. However, it has become clear that at least some of the physical decline and reduced physiologic reserve previously blamed on aging is in fact caused by the complex interactions of true genetically determined aging, disease (often subtle or subclinical), and disuse.

The myriad of possible interrelationships among true aging changes, disease, and disuse make it difficult to ascribe specific causality for the loss of physical vigor or function in many cases. Thus, for example, preconceived societal notions about aging may predispose to greatly reduced expectations with regard to physical as well as mental performance. Such preconceptions may promote inactivity and disuse in women at an even earlier age than in men. With years of ensuing inactivity, disuse not only exaggerates and enhances the true age-related loss of endurance, strength, and flexibility, leading to further inactivity and disuse, but may also exacerbate previously subtle or subclinical diseases such as intraabdominal obesity, glucose intolerance, osteopenia, hypertension, dyslipemia, and coronary artery disease. These physiologic disorders, the drugs used in their treatments, and the associated functional impairments can, in turn, further limit activity and continue the vicious downhill spiral. Although not conclusive, evidence that activity level is inversely related to the risk for mortality and is associated with a greater average life span (about 2 years in human studies) supports this concept.

This chapter reviews the physiologic effects of aging and exercise training on the most common measures of physical fitness: (1) endurance, or maximum aerobic exercise capacity; (2) skeletal muscle strength and power; and (3) body composition. Next, it investigates the theoretical relationship between fitness and functional status, reviewing the available, albeit somewhat limited, data on the effect of increased activity on functional performance. The chapter then reviews the effects of aging and activity on several disorders commonly observed in geriatric patients. Last, the risks associated with exercising are discussed and some suggestions are made with respect to prescribing an exercise program for older individuals.

While we and others commonly discuss health benefits of "exercise training," it is now abundantly clear that many benefits can be accrued by merely leading a more active lifestyle, without the need for formal "training." This concept may be especially helpful in trying to encourage older individuals who may feel unable or unwilling to engage in exercise training but can and will increase their physical activity.

AGING AND EXERCISE

Endurance (Aerobic) Exercise Capacity

Aging-Associated Changes in Endurance Exercise Capacity

The best physiologic measure of an individual's endurance work capacity is the amount of oxygen consumed at maximal exercise (maximal aerobic power or $\dot{V}O_2max$). Cross-sectional studies have repeatedly demonstrated a significant age-related decrement in $\dot{V}O_2max$ in both men and women. Together, these cross-sectional data suggest that exercise capacity declines by approximately 1 percent per year when $\dot{V}O_2max$ is expressed as milliliters of oxygen consumed per minute and corrected for kilograms of body weight (e.g., $mL/min^{-1}/kg^{-1}$). Longitudinal data in this area are somewhat more confusing, probably owing to (1) variation in the initial level of fitness of the

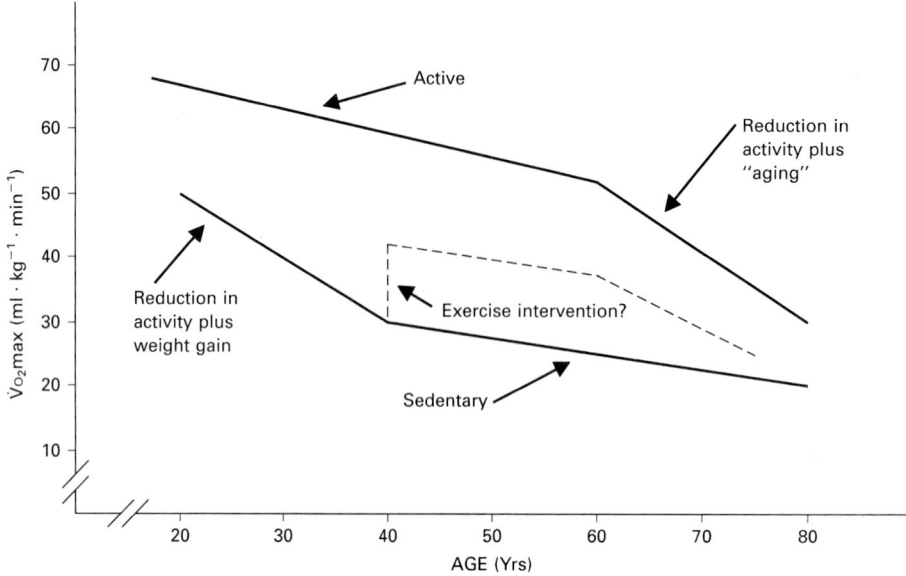

Figure 72-1 Possible interindividual differences in the age-related decline in $\dot{V}O_2$max. The possible effects of regular physical activity (or lack thereof) and the inevitable decline at advanced age are depicted. Reproduced with permission from Buskirk.

subject populations, (2) spontaneous modifications in activity level between test periods, (3) alterations in body weight and composition, and (4) intervening illness. It is possible that the data are further influenced by a nonlinear decline over time (Fig. 72–1), with a more rapid decline in $\dot{V}O_2$max in early adulthood in sedentary individuals followed by a less-steep decline later in life. Recent longitudinal studies in both men and women demonstrate approximately a 0.5 mL/min^{-1}/kg^{-1} decline per year after a 4-year follow-up period. Almost half of this decrement could be accounted for by independent changes in adiposity and self-reported physical activity.

Both cross-sectional and longitudinal approaches have been used to determine whether habitual endurance training slows the age-related decline in $\dot{V}O_2$max. Cross-sectional comparisons of younger and older endurance athletes and normally active controls indicate that the slope of the regression line for age-related decline in $\dot{V}O_2$max is not as steep in athletes as in their more sedentary counterparts. In fact, these comparisons suggest that habitual exercise may reduce the rate of decline in $\dot{V}O_2$max with aging by up to 50 percent (0.5 versus 1.0 percent per year). Three longitudinal studies of older endurance-trained men, followed over 10 to 22 years, all indicate that the slower decline in $\dot{V}O_2$max occurs only in men who continue to train vigorously for competition. Only one study followed both sedentary and trained men, and the average rate of decline in $\dot{V}O_2$max was higher in the athletes than in the nonathletes (–2.9% versus –1.5% per year). When athletes were characterized by the level of exercise training they maintained, the rate of decline was –0.3% per year in those who trained vigorously, –2.6% per year in those who trained moderately, and –4.6% per year in the low-training group. However, even in the low-training group, $\dot{V}O_2$max remained higher at follow-up (33.8 mL/min/kg; age 74 years) than in the sedentary controls (25.8 mL/min/kg; age 70 years). Thus, the higher fitness levels of active individuals may afford them protection later in life by allowing them to remain above the threshold of exercise capacity necessary to remain functionally active.

The Peripheral Components of Endurance Exercise Capacity

$\dot{V}O_2$max is equal to the product of maximal cardiac output (Qmax) and the maximal ability of muscle to extract oxygen from the blood (a-VO$_2$ difference), and thus is determined by both central (cardiovascular) and peripheral (primarily muscle) components. Studies have almost uniformly detected significant changes in body composition associated with aging (see the following section on body composition), including increases in fat mass, and decreases in fat-free mass (FFM) or lean body mass (LBM). Furthermore, with aging, muscle mass comprises a lesser percentage of what is usually measured as FFM. Several studies of carefully screened older subjects confirm that differences in FFM can explain some of the age-related differences in $\dot{V}O_2$max. In one cross-sectional study of very healthy men and women between 22 and 87 years of age, muscle mass, as reflected by 24-hour creatinine excretion, was found to decline 23 percent between ages 30 and 70 years. When normalized for this decrease in muscle mass, the slope of the decline in $\dot{V}O_2$max with age flattened significantly, and thus, the predicted decline in $\dot{V}O_2$max between the ages of 30 and 70 years was lessened in both men (39 percent versus 18 percent) and women (30 percent versus 14 percent). In this study, approximately half of the original age-related decline in $\dot{V}O_2$max was explained by the age-associated loss of muscle mass. It must be stressed, however, that muscle mass and $\dot{V}O_2$max are not independent and that individuals who are more active are likely to develop and/or maintain a larger muscle mass. Additional peripheral mechanisms might also account for some of the age-related decrement in $\dot{V}O_2$max by attenuating the a-VO$_2$ difference, including a reduced ability to direct blood flow

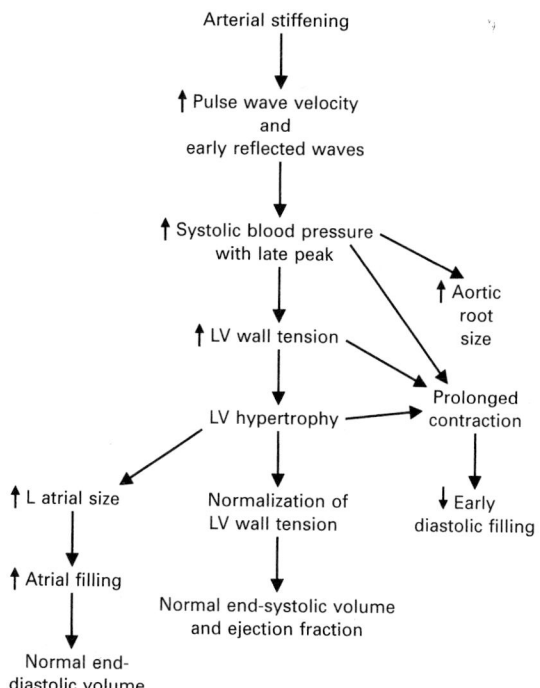

Figure 72-2 The interplay of vascular changes and adaptive cardiac changes that occur to varying degrees with aging in otherwise healthy individuals. Reproduced with permission from Lakatta.

to the working muscles or a diminished ability of muscle cells in older (inactive) individuals to use oxygen.

The Central (Cardiovascular) Component of Endurance Capacity (See Chap. 33)

Deficits in the central (cardiovascular) component contribute substantially to the age-related reduction in $\dot{V}O_2$max. In the absence of hypertension or coronary artery disease (clinical or asymptomatic), studies consistently find that resting cardiac output, heart rate, and heart size are normal in older individuals. However, as illustrated in Figure 72-2, a number of age-related changes in resting cardiac function have been defined. These cardiovascular changes detected at rest in the elderly person are quite similar to those observed with hypertension. Indeed, it has been hypothesized that mild vascular stiffness and ensuing subclinical hypertension may initiate this group of compensatory responses noted at rest.

As with most age-related abnormalities, alterations in cardiovascular physiology are most apparent and most clinically relevant during stress, such as physical exercise. In the setting of maximal exercise, and a three- to four-fold increase in cardiac output, striking differences between young and older individuals become apparent. By far the most salient and consistent Lakatta EG, Eur Heart J 11 (suppl C): 22, 1990 is a marked decline in maximal heart rate with age. Beyond this one finding, however, there is little agreement. While some studies suggest that most of the age-related decrement in $\dot{V}O_2$max is explained by a decline in cardiac output, others detect decrease in maximal cardiac output with age.

Studies that find no significant decline in maximal cardiac output support a compensatory increase in stroke volume mediated by the Frank–Starling mechanism and an increase in left ventricular end-diastolic volume, a physiologic profile similar to that observed with β-adrenergic blockade. This explanation is appealing, given the plethora of data demonstrating reduced cardiovascular responses to β-adrenergic-agonist stimulation in elderly people. These findings suggest that most of the decline in $\dot{V}O_2$max in elderly people is related to peripheral mechanisms. These findings may differ from other studies that detect a diminished cardiac output with age, because subjects with occult heart disease were meticulously excluded. However, data from our laboratory, using similar stringent screening criteria, found a substantial difference in peak cardiac index between healthy young and older men despite no significant differences at baseline. In fact, the majority of studies now support the concept that diminished central responses to maximal exercise substantially contribute to the reduced $\dot{V}O_2$max with aging. The degree to which this defect can be explained by a lower maximal heart rate or a reduced stroke volume response to exercise remains unclear, as does the role of diminished β-adrenergic sensitivity.

The Physiologic Effects of Endurance Exercise Training

Effect on $\dot{V}O_2$max

Certain individuals (e.g., master athletes) can maintain a reasonably high endurance exercise capacity into old age. However, the results of initial endurance training studies in previously sedentary older individuals had been quite variable. This was understandable in light of the numerous factors that can affect the response to a training program, including (1) the intensity and duration of the program, (2) the baseline health of the subjects, (3) the testing methods used, and (4) subjects' baseline level of fitness. It is now clear that the fitness response to an endurance training program in previously sedentary, healthy older individuals is comparable to that in younger subjects. Depending on the type and duration of exercise employed, the improvement in $\dot{V}O_2$max varies between 10 and 30 percent, with similar responses in both men and women. Furthermore, when young and older subjects are trained in the same program at the same relative intensity, the increments in $\dot{V}O_2$max are similar.

Healthy older individuals can tolerate supervised endurance training at relatively intense levels (e.g., 85 percent of heart rate reserve; HHR = 0.85 [(HR max − HR rest) + HR rest) with acceptable attrition rates and few if any significant injuries. Indeed, it appears that speed is a more important determinant of injury than the actual intensity of the exercise. However, few choose to maintain this rigorous training intensity on their own and a clinically more salient question is whether qualitatively similar adaptive responses can occur with lower-intensity training. Although not all studies agree, it appears that cardiovascular improvement can be obtained with low- to moderate-intensity programs, where subjects train at about 50 percent of HRR. In addition, metabolic improvements can occur with low- to moderate-intensity exercise that is maintained over a sufficient period of time (see below).

Effect on Body Composition

As noted above, with aging there is a significant loss of FFM or LBM, mostly caused by a reduction in skeletal muscle mass. This decline has been estimated to be approximately 6 percent per decade between ages 30 and 80 years. Despite the loss of LBM, body weight may be sustained or increase as a result of the accumulation of adipose tissue. More importantly, with age, fat is preferentially accumulated in a central distribution. This centralization of body fat seems to occur continuously with age in adult men, but in most women, a significant increase in central adiposity first occurs following menopause. This central distribution of adipose tissue mass is a major risk factor for many obesity- and age-related metabolic abnormalities, and in many studies is independent of relative weight or other measures of obesity.

In cross-sectional studies comparing highly physically active older individuals with more sedentary controls, body adiposity in the active group is consistently lower and, in fact, similar to active younger individuals. This is true for both men and women, with the physically active groups having approximately 10 percent less body fat than sedentary controls. Furthermore, there is an inverse correlation between $\dot{V}O_2max$ and central adiposity, as defined by waist:hip ratio, within a population of healthy older men. However, relatively little difference in FFM or LBM has been observed in active, as compared to sedentary, healthy elderly persons. Therefore, even highly endurance-trained older individuals have significantly less LBM than do younger individuals.

Longitudinal endurance training studies in previously sedentary individuals support these cross-sectional findings. Endurance training has consistently produced small but significant decrements in percent body fat and overall fat mass in older men and women. In two studies a loss of 2.5 percent body fat and 1.5 to 3 kg of fat mass followed a 6- to 12-month intensive endurance-training program in older subjects. Associated with this modest decrement in overall adiposity was a preferential decrease in the central distribution of fat. In fact, following endurance training in older men, we demonstrated not only a small fall in waist:hip ratio, but also a 20 percent decline in intraabdominal fat as measured by computed tomography. In contrast to the modest but consistent decrement in adiposity, little or no change in overall FFM has been detected following even intensive endurance training in the elderly population. The lack of improvement in overall FFM may be countered by significant changes in specific muscle groups. Thus, in our study, cross-sectional mid-thigh muscle mass, measured by computed tomography, increased 10 percent in older men, despite no change in overall FFM. This finding suggests a redistribution of FFM with intensive endurance training in older men. The lack of accretion of FFM with endurance exercise in older individuals may reflect a reduced anabolic hormonal milieu, with lower levels of sex steroids, growth hormone, and insulin-like growth factor I.

Although highly trained athletes are leaner than less-active controls, the loss of weight or fat with endurance training is small when compared to dieting with caloric restriction. As noted above, however, the effect of exercise may be magnified by the preferential loss of central and specifically intraabdominal fat with endurance training. Endurance training can increase the usually low resting metabolic rate in the elderly person by approximately 10 percent, even when corrected for any observed change in FFM. It should be noted that vigorous exercise in older subjects might be associated with a compensatory decrement in activity during nonexercising periods and, thus, no increment in overall energy expenditure. Concomitant exercise training is associated with a lower rate of long-term recidivism in subjects participating in a dietary weight reduction program. Exercise may mitigate the drop in resting metabolic rate, lipolysis and fat oxidation that usually accompany dietary restriction and which would lead to rapid regain of lost weight. While there are fewer data available, it appears that strength training has many of the same effects of endurance training on adiposity.

Effect on Cardiac Function

While cross-sectional studies suggest a significant age-related decline in cardiac output (see previous discussion), training status appears to positively affect this end point, with a greater maximal cardiac output found in well-trained older men and women when compared to matched sedentary controls. In fact, most of the higher $\dot{V}O_2max$ in trained older individuals can be explained by their higher maximal cardiac output. In turn, a larger stroke volume explains the higher cardiac output, whereas no difference in maximal heart rate is detected between trained and untrained individuals. The relation between $\dot{V}O_2max$ and left ventricular performance seems to be linear over a wide range of fitness levels, suggesting that similar improvements could be expected with training no matter what the initial fitness level.

Longitudinal studies of endurance training in previously sedentary older subjects have provided conflicting results. Initially some found no improvement in estimated cardiac output following either low- or high-intensity endurance training. However, studies using more sensitive methods and more vigorous exercise training interventions provide evidence of enhanced left ventricular systolic and diastolic function. There is some evidence for a sex- and age-specific difference in the left ventricular response to endurance training, with an improvement in diastolic function demonstrated in young and older men and possibly only in young women. Others have been unable to show significant differences in left ventricular diastolic filling dynamics between older trained and sedentary men, with both being reduced compared to young controls.

The finding in some studies that older women do not increase maximal cardiac output in response to endurance exercise training, but that older men and young women and men do, raises the question of whether estrogens are involved in this adaptation. When older women, either on or not on hormone replacement therapy (HRT), underwent a 20-week endurance-exercise program of stationary cycling, both groups of women had similar increases in estimated cardiac output at peak exercise in response to training. This contradicts previous findings, but it should be noted that the methodology used to evaluate cardiac function was not as sophisticated in this study as in the others that found that maximal cardiac output did not increase in older women not on HRT. The role that estrogens play in the cardiovascular adaptations to exercise therefore remains uncertain.

SKELETAL MUSCLE STRENGTH AND POWER

Strength can be defined as the maximum force exerted by a muscle, and power is the rate of force development. Strength and power are not determined by muscle mass alone but also by intact neurological function. Consequently, as discussed in more detail below, strength and power can be increased by improving muscular function (e.g., muscle cell hypertrophy) or by improving neurologic function (e.g., learning).

Strength assessment depends upon the conditions of measurement, specifically the speed of muscular contraction, whether the muscle is shortening (concentric) or lengthening (eccentric) during the contraction, and the conditions of mechanical leverage. Muscle strength can be measured during isometric, isotonic, or isokinetic contractile activity. Isometric strength is the force generated against a fixed object and isotonic strength is the force generated against a moving object (i.e., free weights, most resistance-exercise machines). Isokinetic strength also involves the generating force against a moving object, but in this case, the speed of movement is controlled and constant. Muscle power can be determined simultaneously with the assessment of either isotonic or isokinetic strength by measuring the speed of movement.

Aging-Associated Changes in Muscle Strength and Power

For more than 100 years, cross-sectional studies have demonstrated that strength declines with age. After peak strength is reached sometime around age 40 years, cross-sectional studies show approximately a 30 to 40 percent reduction in strength by age 80 years. Longitudinal studies suggest that the true rate of decline is underestimated by the cross-sectional data. For example, a longitudinal study estimated a 60 percent loss of handgrip strength between ages 30 and 80, while a cross-sectional analysis of the same data estimated loss at only 40 percent. Strength loss appears even more rapid at greater ages. Longitudinal studies have found approximately a 10 to 25 percent loss in quadriceps strength within only 5 to 7 years in 70-year-old adults. In the majority of these studies, muscle power was not measured. However, there is growing evidence that the rate of decline in muscle power is even greater than the decline in strength. Measurements of muscle strength and power over 10 years in the Baltimore Longitudinal Study on Aging indicated that the decline in muscle power was approximately 10 percent greater than the decline in strength.

Evidence is accumulating that the decline in muscle power is a stronger determinant than muscle strength of physical functional status in old age. This is not surprising

if the decline in power is, indeed, more pronounced than the decline in strength. Leg muscle power was reduced in older women prone to falling, as compared with nonfallers, and was a stronger predictor than strength of self-reported functional status in elderly women. These findings suggest that intervention strategies should be aimed not only at preserving muscle mass and strength with aging, but also muscle power.

Muscle Mass

A close relationship exists between the size of a muscle, measured as cross-sectional area, and its ability to generate force. One would predict, then, that a 40 percent decline in muscle strength should be accompanied by a decline in muscle mass of a roughly equal amount—approximately 30 to 40 percent. This is the case, and just as strength loss is more rapid at greater ages, loss of muscle mass is also reported as becoming more rapid with age. In laboratory animals, there is also an age-related decrease in muscle-specific force, which is the peak force per cross-sectional area. Single muscle fiber characteristics of tissue obtained from younger and older men and older women also indicate that the reduction in the capacity to generate force with aging is not solely a result of the reduction in fiber size or muscle mass and raise questions about how muscle fiber function and composition change with aging.

Muscle Fibers

Skeletal muscle is comprised of bunches of individual muscle fibers. These contain myofibrils, which are, in turn, composed of a number of myofilaments. The myofilaments contain the proteins actin and myosin and are arranged to form sarcomeres—the contractile units of muscle.

There are two major types of muscle fibers: slow-twitch and fast-twitch. Furthermore, there are at least three subtypes of fast-twitch fibers: a, b, and c. The fast-twitch fibers are variously referred to either as FTa, FTb, and FTc or as type 2a, type 2b, and type 2c. The slow-twitch fibers are referred to as ST or type 1 fibers. Type 1 fibers can sustain tension for long periods, are slow to fatigue, and have high oxidative (aerobic) capacity. Type 2 fibers can rapidly develop high tension, but only for short periods of time, and have high glycolytic (anaerobic) capacity. Type 2a, type 2b, and type 2c fibers all differ in their relative oxidative capacity.

The evidence that muscle mass decreases with aging is unequivocal. There is less certainty regarding the extent to which this is caused by a loss of muscle fibers versus a decrease in fiber size. There is a loss in the number of muscle fibers with age, but whether some fiber types are lost more rapidly with age is controversial. Some evidence suggests that type 2 fibers are lost more rapidly than type 1 fibers. Opposing evidence suggests a more rapid reduction in type 2 fiber size with age but not a more rapid reduction in the total number of type 2 fibers. One factor that may contribute to the variation in these findings is the tremendous plasticity of skeletal muscle. Fiber cross-sectional area, and even the relative proportion of fiber types, may reflect the response to existing or recent physical activity patterns. That is, type 2 fiber loss and/or atrophy could be caused by an age-related change in activity patterns. As older adults perform fewer activities requiring rapid development of muscular force, they may have selective reduction in the type 2 fibers that are required for such activities.

Motor Units

Muscle function depends on the coordinated activity of groups of muscle fibers and the motor neuron that innervates them, i.e., the motor unit. The motor neuron appears to control the size, contraction time, resistance to fatigue, and enzyme activity of the muscle fibers it innervates. Hence, neuronal mechanisms could account for many age-related changes in muscle fibers. There is growing evidence that the number of motor units decreases with age. This conclusion is supported by electromyographic studies that suggest a loss of functional motor neurons with age. Indeed, the loss of motor units may even exceed the loss of neurons.

Muscle Quality

The concept that the quality as well as the quantity of muscle declines with aging has emerged in recent years, although there is no consensus regarding the factors that determine muscle quality or how it should be measured. It has been suggested that muscle quality encompasses many factors (e.g., structural composition, innervation, contractility, capillary density, fatigability, intramuscular fat content, protein metabolism, mitochondrial function, oxidative damage, and glucose metabolism). In general, there is an age-related deterioration in most factors that are thought to influence muscle quality. However, whether these are inevitable consequences of aging seems unlikely, as almost all respond favorably to increased physical activity.

Disuse versus Aging

There is some epidemiologic evidence that regular physical activity may prevent some of the age-related loss in strength. However, when activities are classified as to their expected effects on muscle strength, epidemiologic studies have probably focused on a relatively narrow range of activity near the middle of the continuum. At one end of the continuum is bed rest. Bed rest is associated with a dramatic loss of strength—estimated as high as 1 to 5 percent per day. At the other end of the continuum is vigorous strengthening exercise (discussed below), which produces substantial gains in strength in older adults.

It is this perspective, integrating findings from studies of bed rest, epidemiology, and experimental interventions, that most clearly suggests that age-related losses in strength are mainly a result of age-related changes in physical activity. As a corollary, epidemiologic studies of adults with similar activity at all ages should show little or no loss in strength. Indeed, a cross-sectional study of workers at a machine shop showed no decline in grip strength between the ages of 20 and 60 years. But aging per se appears to

have some role in loss of strength, as, at some point during life, strength will begin to decline despite continued activity patterns.

The Physiologic Effects of Strength Training

Strength training (resistance exercise) can be done in several ways. Unfortunately, at present there is no standard and little agreement on a preferred method. In general, resistance exercise regimens typically involve either a high number of repetitions at a moderate level of resistance or a few repetitions at a high level of intensity. The former is aimed more at improving muscle endurance while the latter is aimed more at increasing muscle strength. Analogous to the way in which strength can be measured, strength training can involve isometric, isotonic, or isokinetic exercises. The majority of equipment used for resistance training (i.e., free weights and machines) involve isotonic contractions. The relative level of intensity is usually based on the maximal weight that the subject can lift only one time (called the one-repetition maximum or 1RM).

A standard resistance-training program therefore involves performing a prescribed number of sets (usually 1 to 3) of each exercise, with a prescribed number of repetitions in each set, at a prescribed percentage of the 1RM. The number of repetitions that can be performed depends on the relative intensity. For example, at an intensity of 70 percent of the 1RM, people can typically perform 10 to 12 repetitions of an exercise, but at 80 percent of the 1RM usually only 6 to 8 repetitions can be completed. When multiple sets of each exercise are performed, the relative intensity may be fixed for each set (e.g., 80 percent), increase with each set (70 percent, 80 percent, 90 percent), or decrease with each set (90 percent, 80 percent, 70 percent); whether one method is more effective is equivocal. With progressive resistance-exercise training, once a subject can do a full set at 85 to 90 percent of the 1RM, the resistance is increased by determining a new (higher) 1RM, and the number of repetitions and percent of 1RM are gradually increased.

Effect on Muscular Strength and Power

Historically, the majority of exercise intervention studies in older adults involved endurance exercise. More recently, there has been a dramatic increase in the number of resistance training studies. These have been primarily isotonic, fixed-resistance exercise programs lasting 2 to 6 months. Although almost all studies report that resistance training increases the strength of older adults, there is tremendous variability in the magnitude of the reported strength gains (from a few percent to almost 200 percent). A number of factors likely contribute to the variability, including the method of measuring strength, the duration of training, the exercise intensity, and baseline characteristics of the study sample. Not surprisingly, the largest relative improvements in strength have been reported in frail elderly people in whom a small absolute increase in strength represents a large relative improvement because of their low initial strength levels.

A meta-analysis suggests that intensity of training is the most important factor affecting study results. Some studies used low- and moderate-intensity resistance training and reported only modest increases (10 to 25 percent) in strength. Other studies of healthy adults, physically unfit adults, and even frail adults have used more vigorous strength training, where resistance is typically set at 80 percent of the 1RM. These studies report substantially larger strength gains (50 to 200 percent). Expressed in terms of the cross-sectional distribution of strength in the study samples, subjects improve from 1.0 to 3.5 standard deviations in strength over just a few months with these vigorous training protocols.

Duration of training also affects strength gain. Studies report weekly measurements of 1RMs, and strength continues to increase throughout the training interval, at least up to 6 months. Most studies of strengthening exercise fail to comment on the fact that their results show substantial variability in how older adults respond to strength training. The observed variability occurs despite the use of standard training protocols administered in supervised research settings. The causes of this observed variability remain to be explained.

Few studies have measured the extent to which older individuals can increase muscle power with resistance-exercise training. One study reported that the relative increase in power was not as great as the increase in strength. Another study found that the relative increase in muscle power with resistance training was similar in younger and older individuals, but higher in men than in women. Because power is a velocity-dependent measurement, it is likely that the effectiveness of resistance exercise training to increase muscle power depends on the rate at which lifting activity is performed. It will be important to determine whether the rate of lifting is a determinant of improvement in muscle power, and also whether increases in power translate into improved functional performance. In one recent study, the gain in physical function following strength training was closely correlated to improvement in anaerobic power. The potential for injury may also be increased with faster rates of lifting.

Physiologic Mechanisms Explaining Gains in Strength with Exercise

Resistance exercise causes muscular hypertrophy in older adults, and muscle biopsies show hypertrophy of both type 1 and type 2 fibers. However, moderate (10 to 20 percent) increases in fiber size or whole-muscle cross-sectional area have been reported to be accompanied by much larger (50 to 200 percent) increases in strength. This situation apparently violates the "rule" that muscle cross-sectional area is highly correlated with muscle strength. Actually, it is true in both older and younger adults that, after short-term strength training, there is a discrepancy between the increases in strength and muscle cross-sectional area. Some attribute the increase in strength that cannot be accounted for by hypertrophy as being caused by increased neural discharge. In younger adults, the discrepancy appears to be transient, as highly trained individuals show the predicted ratio of strength to cross-sectional area. In older adults, it is unclear how the ratio of strength to cross-sectional area

changes over the course of prolonged strength training. However, even very old individuals maintain the capability of increasing the synthesis rate of muscle contractile proteins in response to resistance exercise, suggesting that strength gains in elderly people are mediated both by neural mechanisms and by muscle hypertrophy.

Exercise, Physical Activity, and Functional Limitations

The question "Can regular physical activity prevent and/or reverse functional limitations and disability in older adults?" is of great public health importance. In discussing this question, we adopt the terminology and framework of the Nagi model of disablement (from the book *Disability in America*). In the model, etiologic factors (risk factors) include genetic, behavioral, and environmental factors. The effects of these factors on the disabling process can be measured at four distinct levels:

1. Measurements of disease or pathology are made at the cell and tissue level.
2. Measurements of physiologic impairment (e.g., muscle strength, $\dot{V}O_2$max) are made at the organ and organ system level.
3. Measurements of functional limitations are made at the behavioral, whole-organism level. Measures of functional limitations range from assessing simple movements (e.g., pushing with the foot), to more complicated movements (e.g., ability to walk as measured by gait speed), and to sequences of movement (e.g., ability to stand, walk, turn, and sit down).
4. Measurements of disability are made at the level of the interaction of the whole-organism with the physical and social environment. For example, a person using a wheelchair is disabled if stairs are the only means of getting inside, and not disabled if there is a ramp.

In this framework, risk factors cause disease, which causes physiologic impairment, which causes functional limitations, which causes disability. (The model also includes the possibility of feedback loops and more complicated causal pathways.)

The discussion also makes a distinction between physical activity and exercise. Physical activity can be defined as any movement of the body produced by skeletal muscles that causes energy expenditure. Exercise is a subset of physical activity, and can be defined as planned, structured, and repetitive body movement done specifically to improve fitness.

Evidence that Exercise Improves Functional Limitations

It is intuitive that adults who remain physically active are less likely to experience problems in performing activities of daily life, such as climbing stairs, walking, gardening, and housework. In the framework of the Nagi model, physical inactivity (risk factor) causes muscle weakness and low

$\dot{V}O_2$ max and other physiologic impairments, which then cause functional limitations.

This intuition regarding the importance of physical activity in helping to maintain activities of daily life is supported by a growing number of epidemiological studies. For example, in the Established Populations for Epidemiologic Studies of the Elderly (EPESE), older adults who were physically active at the baseline examination were significantly less likely to experience mobility impairments during several years of follow-up. But the crucial issue is whether increasing physical activity levels in normally inactive older adults achieves the same health benefits found in naturally active older adults. A growing number of randomized trials address this issue.

The emerging consensus is that exercise improves functional limitations in older adults. However, not all well-designed randomized trials show a beneficial effect of exercise. To illustrate how results vary among studies, consider the following randomized trials. A study of adults age 75+ years, which compared resistance training and balance training, found that balance training, but not strength training, improved functional balance tasks. A study that compared strength training, aerobic training, and combined training found no effects of exercise on functional limitations. In a study of adults age 68 to 85 years, walking exercise improved gait speed and SF-36 (Kidney Disease and Quality of Life Short Form 36 Health Survey) role–physical scores, while aerobic movement and cycling exercises did not. In a study of older adults with knee osteoarthritis, aerobic exercise and strengthening exercise caused similar, modest improvements in functional limitations over 18 months. Also, few studies have assessed whether regular physical activity (as opposed to exercise) affects functional limitations. This is important, as most adults who are sufficiently active according to public health guidelines do not also participate in regular, structured exercise programs.

The situation may be explained by the plausible argument that the effects of exercise on functional limitations should differ according to (1) type, frequency, duration, and intensity of exercise, (2) the functional limitations of interest, (3) the method of measuring limitations, and (4) the target population. In particular, the effects of exercise on functional limitations should differ by target population because of a complicated, nonlinear relationship between physiologic impairment and functional limitation.

Nonlinear Relationship Between Physiologic Impairment and Functional Limitation

Note that nonlinear relationships and thresholds are implicit in the Nagi model. Healthy humans have excess physiologic capacity not tapped during most daily activities, so humans can lose a fair amount of physiologic reserve before functional limitations occur. Recent epidemiologic studies confirm a nonlinear relationship, for example, between leg strength and walking speed. This nonlinear relationship is actually intuitive. After all, if strength were linearly related to walking speed, highly trained weight lifters would walk ridiculously fast (16 to 30 km/h) because they are several times as strong as normal adults, who walk at around 5 to 8 km/h. That is, above a certain threshold level of adequate physiologic reserve, function is normal; below the threshold, function is impaired (Fig. 72–3). The exact shape of the curve depends upon the task and the physiologic capacity of interest. The figure may oversimplify the situation, because most tasks have multiple physiologic determinants that may interact to affect behavioral ability.

To illustrate the concepts of thresholds, consider that in steady-state measures of oxygen consumption, walking

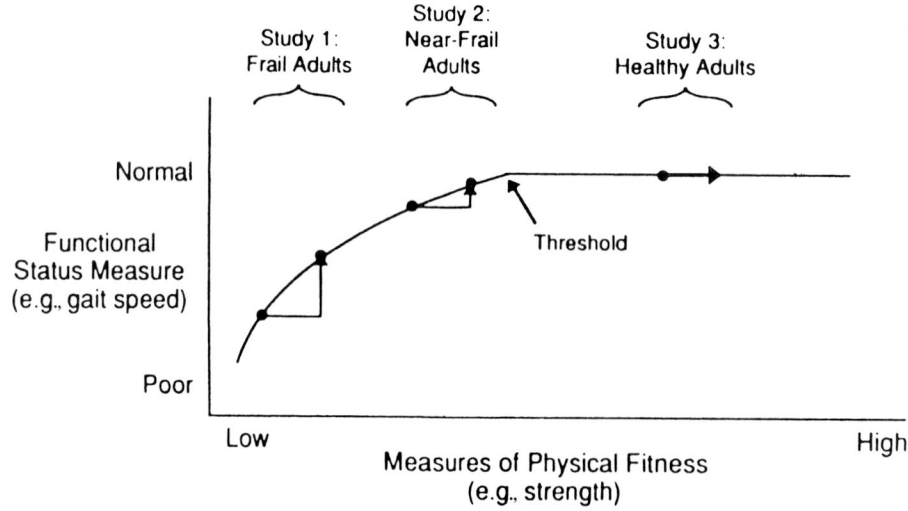

Figure 72-3 Theoretical relationship between physical fitness and functional status. The curvilinear relationship shows a threshold effect: above the threshold level of fitness, functional status is normal; below it, function is impaired. A curvilinear relationship implies that the benefit from exercise depends upon the target group. Three hypothetical exercise studies are shown. Each study produces the same absolute improvement in fitness. In the frail adults of study 1, exercise produces a large improvement in functional status. In the healthy adults of study 3, no benefit is seen. Study 2 shows intermediate benefits. Reproduced with permission from Buchner DM et al: Evidence for a non-linear relationship between leg strength and gait speed. *Age Ageing* 25:386, 1996.

on a level grade at 5 km/h requires 3.2 METS (1 MET = 3.5 mL $O_2/kg^{-1}/min^{-1}$). With illness or inactivity, aerobic capacity falls below the level required for daily tasks. Because exercise can increase aerobic capacity, it should improve functional status when aerobic capacity is below the threshold needed for normal daily function. However, aerobic exercise would not affect ability to walk at 5 km/h in adults whose aerobic capacity already greatly exceeded 3.2 METS.

The implication of this model is that the effect of exercise on functional limitations depends upon the target group. In frail adults with little or no physiologic reserve, exercise theoretically produces a large improvement in function. In general, well-designed studies of exercise in frail adults report improvements in functional limitations with exercise. A randomized trial of 3 months of weight lifting in frail, very old nursing home residents found improvements in gait velocity and stair climbing. Even a 3-month supervised low-intensity exercise program produced a small improvement in physical performance in a group of frail older adults when compared to home-based flexibility training. Similarly, a 3-month task-specific resistance training program improved both the ability and speed of bed and chair rises in a group of older patients living in a congregate care setting. In contrast, in healthy older adults, exercise would be expected to have much smaller effects on functional limitations, at least in basic activities of daily life. In general, the well-designed studies that do not report an effect of exercise training on functional limitations have enrolled relatively healthy older adults.

It follows that, if exercise has effects on functional limitations in healthy adults, effects will mainly occur with more difficult tasks, and a sensitive measurement tool may be required to ascertain the effects. One randomized trial of general exercise in healthy older adults suggests this conclusion is true. The trial used , the Continuous-Scale Physical Functional Performance, which is sensitive to changes in functional limitations in the range of difficult tasks. In this study, there was a significant improvement in function noted in generally healthy older individuals following mixed endurance and strength exercise training.

EXERCISE AND COMMON GERIATRIC DISORDERS

Insulin Resistance and Glucose Intolerance

Aging is frequently associated with inactivity, increased adiposity, and a central distribution of fat. Because each of these potentially interrelated parameters can be associated with insulin resistance and glucose intolerance, the importance of aging alone has been unclear (see Chap. 67). Indeed, when secondary factors such as relative weight (e.g., body mass index), central adiposity, and hypertension were statistically accounted for, age itself was not a significant independent determinant of the insulin resistance and/or glucose intolerance associated with "aging."

Immobilization or inactivity is known to be associated with a decline in insulin sensitivity and glucose tolerance.

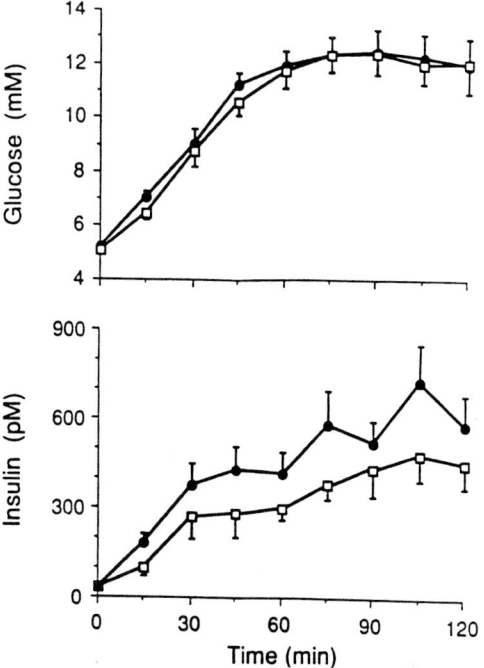

Figure 72-4 Glucose and insulin responses after a 100-g oral glucose load in 13 older subjects before and after 6-month exercise training. Data points, means ± standard errror. Reproduced with permission from Kahn.

An important effect of physical activity on glucose and insulin metabolism with age is supported by cross-sectional studies finding normal or near-normal insulin sensitivity and glucose tolerance in physically well-trained older individuals. Prospective studies have investigated the effects of endurance exercise training on glucose and insulin metabolism in older individuals. For example, following a 6-month intensive endurance training program, no change in fasting glucose or the oral glucose response curve was observed (Fig. 72–4). However, both fasting insulin and the insulin response to the oral glucose challenge declined, suggesting improved insulin sensitivity. Although quantitative measurement demonstrated a 36 percent improvement in insulin sensitivity, the sensitivity of the older men remained 30 to 60 percent lower than that of normal young controls. Because the improvement in insulin sensitivity was balanced by a reciprocal change in insulin secretion, overall glucose tolerance was unchanged. While both endurance exercise and weight loss may reduce insulin resistance in nondiabetic obese men, only weight loss appears to improve oral glucose tolerance. Strength training in older subjects may similarly enhance insulin action.

There are few studies that have evaluated the effect of endurance exercise training in older patients with type 2 diabetes mellitus. In one study of patients ages 55 to 75 years old, no improvement in either glycosylated hemoglobin or insulin sensitivity was found after 26 weeks of endurance training. It should be noted, however, that no significant training effect was detected in the exercise group at the end of the study (following a 14-week unsupervised training period), and even short periods of detraining may significantly reduce the metabolic effects of exercise. It is now generally agreed that most of the metabolic effects of exercise training are transitory and that most of the observed changes are related more to the effects of repeated acute bouts of exercise rather than a more sustained training effect. Studies in middle-aged patients suggest modest improvements in glucose tolerance associated with increased insulin sensitivity. A modest (7 percent) but significant decline in glycosylated hemoglobin was also detected in patients with type 2 diabetes following a 3-month strength-training intervention.

One potentially important role for exercise is in the prevention of type 2 diabetes mellitus in at-risk subjects, such as those with a strong family history of type 2 diabetes, personal history of gestational diabetes, central obesity, impaired glucose tolerance, hyperinsulinemia, hypertension, or a sedentary lifestyle. Large, long-term prospective studies have detected significant reductions in the transition to type 2 diabetes in subjects with impaired glucose treated with a lifestyle intervention (diet and exercise). The Diabetes Prevention Program followed more than 3000 nondiabetic individuals with impaired glucose tolerance randomized to placebo, metformin, or lifestyle treatment for an average of approximately 3 years. The incidence of developing type 2 diabetes was 11.0, 7.8, and 4.8 cases per 100 person-years in the placebo, metformin, and lifestyle groups, respectively. While both the metformin and lifestyle groups reduced the incidence of type 2 diabetes as compared to placebo, the incidence rate with lifestyle intervention was 39% lower than with the metformin intervention group. These impressive reductions in the incidence in type 2 diabetes with the lifestyle intervention occurred with an average of only 6 kg of weight loss and an increase in leisure-time activity of only 6 MET-hr/wk^{-1}. While this study was not specific to older individuals, approximately 16 percent of the subjects were greater than 60 years old. It should be noted that the lifestyle intervention was even more effective in the older subjects.

Thus, it appears that endurance training in older individuals produces a response similar to that noted in younger subjects. Insulin sensitivity is improved, as reflected by a decline in plasma insulin levels. Glucose tolerance improves modestly in type 2 diabetic patients but little or not at all in older subjects with normal or impaired glucose tolerance. Although there are fewer data for strength training, the qualitative and quantitative responses appear to be similar. It is as yet unclear whether these changes are related indirectly to alterations in body fat, fat distribution, and/or FFM, or whether they are directly related to the training itself through changes in muscle capillary density or blood flow, fiber type, enzymes, or glucose transporters. Despite relatively unimpressive effects of exercise on overall adiposity or glucose tolerance, exercise-induced changes could be important in the long-term, given the accumulating data linking insulin resistance and hyperinsulinemia to diabetes mellitus, hypertension, dyslipemia, and atherosclerosis. Exercise may play a major role in the prevention or delay in the onset of type 2 diabetes in subjects who are at high risk for its development. The topic of the role of exercise in the treatment and prevention of type 2 diabetes was recently reviewed in a position paper by the American College of Sports Medicine.

Dyslipidemia

Dyslipidemia is common in the elderly population (see Chap. 68). However, it is not known to what degree this may be related to inactivity; secondary factors such as abnormal body composition; pathologic processes such as diabetes mellitus, thyroid, renal, or liver disease; or drugs such as thiazide diuretics, β-adrenergic blockers, or glucocorticoids. Furthermore, the relationship between measured plasma lipid abnormalities and mortality may be more complicated with age.

Higher levels of physical activity are associated with less atherogenic lipoprotein profiles in cross-sectional studies in young and middle-aged individuals. Reduced plasma triglyceride (TG), very-low-density lipoprotein (VLDL) TG concentrations, and higher high-density lipoprotein (HDL)-C, HDL2-C, and apolipoprotein A-I levels are consistently observed in trained subjects, when compared to sedentary controls. Of interest is the apparent lack of effect of activity on total and low-density lipoprotein (LDL) cholesterol levels in many studies. These cross-sectional findings are supported by studies of enforced inactivity as well as prospective endurance training studies in young and middle-aged subjects. Large cross-sectional studies in young and middle-aged individuals support a dose–response relationship between HDL-C and exercise for subjects running more than 10 miles/wk but no effect for lower mileage. However, the duration and frequency of the training regimen may affect the relationship between exercise intensity and HDL-C. One study found no increase in HDL-C in older men and women who exercised vigorously or moderately for 1 year. After 2 years of participation, small but significant increments in HDL-C were noted at both exercise intensities. In fact, the increases were somewhat greater in the group that exercised more frequently (5 versus 3 times per week) at a lower intensity. While not all studies agree, many suggest that weight loss (or fat loss) is necessary to attain an increase in HDL-C with exercise training. The discrepancies between studies in this regard may be explained by the particular importance that intraabdominal fat may play in the increase in HDL-C with exercise. This small but metabolically important fat depot may be preferentially affected by exercise with little or no measurable loss of overall weight or adiposity.

It is noteworthy that there appears to be a difference in the effect of training on plasma lipoproteins between men and women, with women often demonstrating little or no improvement, especially with regards to HDL levels. The reason for this gender-related difference in response is not entirely clear but may relate to more favorable baseline lipoprotein concentrations in premenopausal women, or to differences in training effects on body composition or intraabdominal fat depots between men and women.

The effect of vigorous exercise with and without HRT has been examined in postmenopausal women. While endurance exercise was associated with a 9 percent drop in LDL-C but no change in HDL-C, HRT produced a 17 percent decline in LDL-C, a 21 percent increase in HDL-C, and a 42 percent increment in TG. The combined (exercise and HRT) group had a 20 percent fall in LDL-C and a 17 percent increase in HDL-C, but no increment in TG. The observed changes were not related to changes in weight adiposity or waist circumference. Thus, there were independent effects of exercise and HRT, and exercise mitigated the elevation in TG associated with HRT alone.

There are at present no published studies on the effects of strength or resistance training on lipoprotein profiles in elderly individuals. In general, strength-training studies in young and middle-aged individuals show little if any lipoprotein response.

Hypertension

Drug treatment of hypertension in the elderly population produces long-term benefits, with reductions in stroke, atherosclerotic cardiovascular disease, or both (see Chap. 40). Despite the known benefits of antihypertensive therapy, the side-effect profile of many drug therapies, especially in elderly people, has led to a resurgence of interest in nonpharmacologic treatments (e.g., weight loss, low-sodium diet, and endurance exercise), especially in patients with mild to moderate hypertension. The effect of exercise on blood pressure has been the subject of many individual studies as well as several good reviews. The majority of cross-sectional and cohort studies find modestly lower systolic and diastolic blood pressures (about 5 to 10 mmHg) in active subjects, but the magnitude of the difference is dependent on the type and intensity of exercise, as well as the position in which the blood pressure was measured (with greater differences when the subject is supine). As a whole, studies also suggest a greater exercise effect in older subjects and those with mild to moderate hypertension.

Two large prospective cohort studies demonstrated that both leisure-time activity and increased fitness, measured by $\dot{V}O_2$max testing, were protective against the development of hypertension, with the effect being independent of age, obesity, and family history. In these studies there tends to be a dose–response effect with the lowest risk of developing hypertension in the most active groups. In a cohort study of nearly 3000 middle-aged men and women, the relative risk of developing hypertension over the 10-year follow-up period was 1.7 in the least, as compared to the most, active group of men. A quantitatively similar but non-significant trend was noted for women. A 25-year follow-up of a prospective cohort study of men born in Malmo, Sweden, in 1914, found that hypertensive men who regularly exercised vigorously had an adjusted relative risk of 0.43 for total mortality and 0.33 for cardiovascular mortality.

Exercise intervention studies have frequently demonstrated small decrements in blood pressure after chronic endurance training. However, some of these had no true control group and are difficult to interpret given the well-known blood-pressure-lowering effect of participating in a study in control groups. A meta-analysis of 54 randomized controlled studies found a 3 to 4 mmHg decline in both systolic and diastolic blood pressure with standard endurance training programs. While the number of studies comparing different intensities of exercise is small, it appears that the blood pressure lowering response to low- to moderate-intensity exercise is at least as good, if not superior, to

that of more vigorous exercise. Indeed, even light T'ai Chi exercise can reduce blood pressure in sedentary older hypertensive patients. While older subjects with orthostatic hypotension must be careful of the hypotensive effect of an acute bout of strenuous exercise, chronic endurance exercise training may be useful in the treatment of patients predisposed to orthostatic dizziness and presyncope.

The blood-pressure-lowering effects of exercise are also found when ambulatory blood pressure monitoring is measured in older hypertensive patients, although it appears that most of the effect occurs during the daytime hours. Using ambulatory blood pressure monitoring, it appears that there is a positive relationship between blood pressure lowering (amount and duration) and the intensity of an acute bout of exercise.

There is at present no agreement on the possible etiology of any of the exercise-related effects on blood pressure in older individuals, although changes in body composition, fat distribution, sympathetic nervous system activity, and insulinemia have all been postulated. Newer work has demonstrated effects of both salt restriction and exercise on arterial stiffness measures, with a threefold greater effect from salt restriction as compared to exercise. Similarly, most studies have found that weight loss alone or combined with exercise provide greater blood pressure lowering than exercise alone. Exercise also appears to restore the age-associated decline in cardiovagal baroreflex sensitivity in sedentary older subjects.

The available data on the effect of strength training on blood pressure is more limited and at present there is no consensus. A meta-analysis of randomized controlled trials of progressive-resistance-training effects on blood pressure revealed a 3 mmHg drop in both systolic and diastolic blood pressure, but one study failed to show an effect of resistive training on ambulatory blood pressure in young subjects. Because of the relatively small number of studies and lack of consistent findings, this form of exercise cannot be recommended for treatment of hypertension at present.

Atherosclerotic Cardiovascular Disease and Overall Mortality

An important effect of increased activity in reducing the risk of atherosclerotic cardiovascular disease is supported by (1) population studies demonstrating a low prevalence of ischemic heart disease in extremely active societies; (2) retrospective studies comparing rates of heart disease in workers with active versus sedentary jobs; and (3) studies where activity mitigated the deleterious effects of a diet high in saturated fat and cholesterol in monkeys. Several large prospective cohort studies in humans also support this hypothesis. Paffenberger's classic study of Harvard alumni found a greater than 50 percent reduction in the risk for heart attack in subjects expending more than 2000 kcal per week in leisure-time physical activity. Furthermore, it was present, not college, activity level that was inversely related to risk. Published multiyear follow-up studies of men who were middle-aged at baseline confirm the importance of activity in protecting against cardiovascular disease

(CVD) and reducing all-cause mortality. The 16-year follow-up of the Multiple Risk Factor Intervention (MRFIT) Study found excess CVD and all-cause mortality (29 percent and 22 percent, respectively) when comparing the least active (5 minutes of leisure time physical activity per day) with to those with light to moderate activity levels (23 minutes per day) and found no additional protection from more vigorous activity schedules. This study strongly supports the excess risks inherent with a sedentary lifestyle and suggests that even low to moderate activity can ameliorate much of this risk. The 20-year follow-up of the Goteborg Primary Prevention Study evaluated both leisure and workplace-related activity in men ages 47 to 55 years at baseline. They detected higher all-cause mortality in men with the greatest work-related activity that was accounted for by smoking, alcohol and occupational hazards. Leisure-time activity was associated with a relative risk of approximately 0.7 for both CVD and overall mortality when comparing the most- and the least-active groups. This protective effect of leisure-time activity was independent of other major risk factors. A 12-year follow-up of the Honolulu Heart Study in 707 nonsmoking Japanese men living in Hawaii (ages 45 to 68 years at baseline) also noted a 50 percent increase in overall mortality in subjects who walked <1 mile/d, as compared to those who walked >1 mile/d. The cumulative all-cause mortality at 12 years in the group walking >2 miles/d (approximately 20 percent) was reached by the most sedentary group by 7 years of follow-up. At 12 years the cumulative mortality in the sedentary group was twice that in the most active group (43/100 versus 21/100).

Most of the older studies assessing the protection of activity against CVD and overall mortality were completed in male populations. Similar data have now been published in a 7-year follow-up of more than 40,000 postmenopausal women (ages 55 to 69 years at baseline). Those reporting regular physical activity had a relative risk of death of 0.77, as compared to those who reported none. While a dose–response effect was noted for increasing frequency of moderate activity, moderate activity as seldom as once a week was protective.

A study of nearly 16,000 healthy Finnish twins (ages 25 to 64 years at baseline), evaluated the effect of physical activity on mortality while controlling for possible hereditary influences. When subjects were classified as "conditioning" (6 bouts of leisure-time exercise per month equivalent to 30 minutes of brisk walking), "sedentary" (no reported leisure-time activity) or "occasional exercisers" (the rest), there was a significant trend for a reduced mortality risk with more vigorous exercise. In addition, when the total volume of exercise was estimated, there was also a trend toward a protective effect of increasing volumes of exercise. A 5 percent reduction in the hazard ratio was found for each quintile of increasing exercise volume. In twin pairs who were discordant for death during the follow-up period, the odds ratio for dying was .44 in the conditioning group and .66 in the occasional exercising group, when compared to the sedentary controls. When adjusted for smoking, occupation, and alcohol, these odds ratios did not quite reach significance, but the trend between the three activity categories remained significant.

While there is little argument about the positive effects of exercise on CVD and all-cause mortality, there remains some discrepancy about whether or not there is a threshold below which little protective effect is noted. It appears that the continuous inverse relationship between activity level and mortality is more easily detected when fitness level ($\dot{V}O_2max$) is used, rather that just a physical activity questionnaire. While activity questionnaires are clearly important in large population-based studies, they are more valid for either high-intensity activity or sedentary lifestyle, and are less reliable for low or moderate levels of activity. In addition, it is possible that older studies that have used leisure-time physical activity questionnaires have consistently underestimated low to moderate levels of activity in women by failing to ascertain the activity involved in housework.

When fitness is used, not only is a continuous gradient of effect noted on mortality but the relative risk for mortality in the least-fit group (1.5 for men and 2.1 for women) is quite similar to the effect of smoking. Furthermore, when fitness level was measured at a mean interval of 5 years, an improvement in fitness (in a previously sedentary group) was associated with reduced mortality. For every minute increment in maximal treadmill time, there was an 8 percent decline in mortality risk. It should be noted that all of the above studies involved endurance exercise, and we are aware of no published studies assessing the relationship between CVD or all-cause mortality and strength training. The relationship between low cardiorespiratory fitness and CVD death was confirmed in an 11-year prospective follow up of a cohort of nearly 1300 middle-aged Finnish men. Men in the low-fitness group ($\dot{V}O_2max$ <27.6 mL/kg or <8 METs) were threefold more likely to have a CVD-related death than the high-fitness group ($\dot{V}O_2max$ >37.1 mL/kg or >10.5 METs) when adjusted for age, smoking, and alcohol. This excess CVD death in the low-fitness group remained significant even when adjusted for lipids, diabetes, blood pressure, fasting insulin, and plasma fibrinogen. While there appeared to be a continuous effect of fitness on overall mortality, the major benefit seemed to occur for fitness levels above 9 METs. Low fitness was also found to be an important risk factor for non-CVD death, with a relative risk of 2.6, as compared to the high-fitness group. In this study, fitness was at least as good a predictor of both overall and CVD-related death as blood pressure, obesity, smoking, or diabetes. In a study of fitness, obesity, and mortality, existing baseline CVD was the greatest predictor of overall mortality in the entire population, but low fitness conferred similar risk in the obese men.

Arthritis

Arthritis is an important cause of functional impairment in older adults. A description of age-related changes in joint function and the impact of arthritis on function in older adults is given in Chap. 78. Despite concerns that exercise could be harmful to arthritis patients, several randomized controlled trials have demonstrated that exercise, even vigorous exercise, is beneficial in arthritis. These studies have enrolled both young and older adults and have included functional status outcomes. Exercise has included endurance training, such as riding a stationary bicycle, and strength training by using weights.

The exercise trials in arthritis patients report a 10 to 25 percent improvement in functional status outcomes. Improvements include faster gait, improve physical function performance, lower depression scores, less subjective pain, and less-frequent use of pain medications. Improvements have persisted as long as 9 months after discharge from supervised exercise classes. As a group, these studies provide strong evidence of a beneficial effect of exercise on functional status in patients with mild to moderate arthritis (both rheumatoid and osteoarthritis). In one study, endurance and strength training were directly compared, and similar positive effects were found. In a recent study using this same population, both resistance (RR = 0.6) and endurance (RR = 0.53) exercise reduced the loss of activities of daily living.

Osteoporosis

The decline in bone mineral density with age is well recognized (see Chap. 75). A fracture threshold is hypothesized, and many older adults are below this theoretical threshold. The result is an epidemic of osteoporotic fractures that affects women more than men and that primarily involves vertebral, wrist, and hip fractures. The extent to which the decline in bone mineral density with aging is a result of reduced physical activity is unknown.

The concept that mechanical loads are important to the integrity of the skeleton is more than 100 years old. Animal studies confirm the importance of mechanical strain to bone modeling and remodeling, and have also identified the characteristics of loading forces that produce the greatest increase in bone mass. These studies demonstrated that (1) the osteogenic response to mechanical loading is optimized with relatively few repetitions of high magnitude forces; (2) the application of force must be in a dynamic, rather than static, fashion; and (3) fast strain rates are more osteogenic than slow strain rates. Furthermore, the osteogenic response to mechanical loading is mediated locally in skeletal regions subjected to the strain, rather than systemically, highlighting the need for exercises to specifically target regions of the skeleton at risk for fracture. Studies of laboratory animals suggest that bone cells become progressively less responsive to mechanical loading with repetitive loading cycles. For example, 4 sets of 90 load applications per day was more osteogenic than 1 set of 360 loading cycles, and interposing an 8-hour recovery period between loading sessions resulted in a greater osteogenic response than when the recovery period was 0.5 hour. These concepts remain to be evaluated in humans.

There are numerous cross-sectional studies of the effects of exercise on bone mass, comparing athletes who participate in different sports or physically active versus sedentary people. Interpretation of many of these studies is limited, because the area of bone density measurement frequently did not correspond to the bones that would be expected to receive the bulk of the mechanical stress from the given exercise. Because there is no known systemic

effect of mechanical stress, measurement of radial bone mass in runners versus nonrunners is unlikely to be informative. However, one well-conceived study found that the humerus in the dominant arm of tennis players had approximately 30 percent greater cortical bone thickness when compared to the nondominant arm. Studies using more sensitive and reproducible methodologies, capable of assessing weight-bearing bone (hip and spine), have found roughly 5 to 10 percent higher trabecular bone density in eumenorrheic runners when compared with eumenorrheic control women. Athletes who participate in muscle-building activities (e.g., weight lifting, body building) and in activities that involve jumping or vaulting (e.g., volleyball, gymnastics) also tend to have elevated bone mineral density. These data suggest that exercise in younger individuals may increase peak bone mass—an important negative risk factor for osteopenia in older women.

Several prospective studies of the effects of exercise on bone mass in postmenopausal women have been difficult to interpret because of the small numbers of subjects, short duration of the intervention, or, as noted above, a mismatch between the area of measurement and the bone that is loaded by the intervention. However, studies of postmenopausal women, using better designs and measurement techniques, have detected exercise-related increases in bone mineral density of up to 5 percent, as compared to noexercise controls, with average increases generally only 1 to 3 percent. The majority of the prospective studies have used a weight-bearing, endurance exercise intervention. Although there are theoretical reasons why strength training may be a preferable intervention to increase bone mass, the few published studies to date suggest that the magnitude of increase in bone mineral density in response to either resistance exercise or weight-bearing endurance exercise is similar.

Cancer

Studies describing higher rates of cancer deaths in sedentary workers dates back at least to the early 1960s, but these findings may have been skewed by greater alcohol and tobacco use in the higher-paid office workers. Subsequent studies investigated possible links between activity and risk for several different kinds of cancers, including breast, colon, rectum, endometrium, ovary, prostate, testis, and lung. Indeed, one recent study demonstrated a dose–response relationship between fitness level and overall cancer death. At present, the most compelling data involve the relationship between activity and breast or colon cancer.

Studies of the association between inactivity and colon cancer have included both cohort as well as case-control studies. These have been carried out in both men and women in a number of different ethnic populations. Most but not all studies have found a reduced relative risk of colon cancer when comparing the most to the least active groups (range of relative risk, 0.4 to 0.9) although this finding was not uniformly statistically significant. In general, controlling for other cancer risks including tobacco, alcohol, age, obesity, and diet does not diminish the relationships. Evidence for a relationship between activity and rectal cancer appears to be substantially weaker. A negative result was reported from the Physicians Health Study, where no level of reported physical activity was associated with a protection form colon cancer.

The risk for breast cancer has been linked to inactivity in 17 of 22 studies with relative risks ranging from 0.20 to 0.89 when comparing the most active to the least-active groups. These associations remain even after adjusting for potential confounding factors such as age, body mass index (BMI), reproductive history, tobacco, and diet. The association holds for both pre- and postmenopausal women, although the risk factors for breast cancer in these two populations are felt to be different.

In the 12-year follow-up of the Honolulu Heart Study, nearly one-third of the 208 deaths were from cancer. There was an inverse relationship between the distance walked and the risk of death from any cancer. The relative risk of cancer death was 2.4-fold greater in the sedentary group (<1 mile walked per day) when compared to the group walking >2 miles per day.

The possible explanation for the link between cancer and inactivity remains obscure. It is well known that the immune system declines with aging (see Chap. 3). Moderate physical exercise can have a significant immune-modulating effect with enhancement of programmed cell death. Some of the changes that have been describe include greater proliferative responses to antigenic stimulation, higher production rates of interleukin 2 and 4, and elevation in macrophage and natural killer cell concentrations. Exercise may reduce intestinal transit time by prostaglandin mediated effects and thus confer some protection to the colon from contact with potential carcinogens. Another possible biological explanation may be through the link between obesity, with excess peripheral conversion of estrogenic steroids, and cancer risk. Because adjusting for obesity does not eliminate the association of cancer with inactivity in most studies, it is possible that excess central or intraabdominal fat depots might confer risk through their relationship to insulin resistance, and subsequent changes in sex hormone binding proteins and free sex hormone levels.

Other Chronic Medical Disorders

While exercise rehabilitation has long been used in the treatment of patients with coronary artery disease, more recently, trials have begun to assess the effectiveness of exercise rehabilitation for the treatment of other common cardiovascular disorders. Exercise has also been found to provide improved functional outcomes in patients with peripheral arterial disease and claudication. In a randomized control trial, 6 months of endurance exercise improved distance walked until the onset of claudication (134 percent), distance to maximal claudication (77 percent), and walking economy (12 percent). Even more importantly, the daily physical activity in the trained group increased by almost 40 percent. While the most effective training appears to be walking, strength training may also provide some benefits.

Similarly, exercise rehabilitation has been shown effective in the treatment of some patients with congestive heart failure (CHF). Not only have increments in exercise duration and peak $\dot{V}O_2max$ been found in these patients, but there may also be some improvement in the skeletal muscle myopathy that has been described in CHF patients. Patients with chronic obstructive lung disease have been shown to benefit from exercise training with the ability to do more absolute work, and also to sustain a constant submaximal workload for a longer duration and with a lower minute ventilation.

Subjects who exercise regularly frequently report an improved sense of well-being and reduced tension and anxiety. Indeed, similar responses occur acutely and persist for several hours after a single bout of exercise. There is also considerable evidence that exercise can ameliorate some of the symptoms of depression and anxiety. Cohort studies have found a dose–response relationship between exercise at baseline and the development of depression at a later time. While almost all of these studies involve endurance exercise, a randomized controlled trial found that resistance training was also of benefit in a group of older depressed patients. In this study, the intensity of training was independently related to the decline in the Beck depression score.

RISKS ASSOCIATED WITH EXERCISE

Despite the recognition of exercise as a major public health concern and objective for our entire population, there has been little systematic assessment of the health risks of exercise. This lack of information may be a result of the complex interplay of factors that may or may not predispose to injury: (1) host factors such as age, sex, fitness level, gait, balance, health status, and body weight; (2) exercise factors such as frequency, intensity, speed, duration, competition, and proper use of warm-up/cool-down periods; and (3) environmental factors such as surface, location, temperature, weather conditions, and use of proper supportive and protective equipment.

By far, the majority of injuries are caused by "overuse" and involve soft tissues. Approximately 10 percent of individuals (ages 16 to 65 years) participating in active sports or recreation reported having an injury within the last 4 weeks, with half of the incidents causing limitations in activity and 15 percent causing a hospital visit. Although the number of injuries might be expected to be reduced with less-intensive and noncompetitive activity, it is also likely to be greater with increasing age. As noted previously, the speed of an activity may be a greater risk for injury than the intensity of the activity. Thus fewer injuries would be expected from walking uphill as compared to jogging on a flat surface. Evidence also suggests that eccentric exercise (e.g., lowering a weight that has been lifted) may predispose to excess muscle injury. Patients with osteoporosis are at increased risk for fracture if they fall while exercising.

A rigorous review of the potential exercise risks in an older population is outside the scope of this chapter, but two specific areas require comment. The risk of an untoward cardiovascular event has been carefully addressed in studies which found a significant transient increase in the risk of sudden death occurring during a bout of vigorous exercise, especially in previously sedentary individuals. However, the reduction in risk during the nonexercising period of the day more than makes up for the transient increase during exercise, producing an overall risk of sudden death in active men that is 30 percent of that in sedentary men. These data are supported by studies describing lower cardiovascular-related and overall mortality in active individuals. It should be emphasized that the relationship between the type, intensity, and duration of exercise and the reduction in cardiac risk remains unclear.

Exercise in older patients with diabetes mellitus also deserves additional comments. Careful attention to the possibility of both immediate and delayed episodes of exercise-induced hypoglycemia are critical, because of the sustained improvement in insulin sensitivity (24 to 48 hours) associated with vigorous exercise. Transient worsening of orthostatic hypotension can also occur following vigorous exercise, especially in hot weather. Meticulous foot care and supportive, well-fitted shoes are particularly critical for the exercising diabetic patient. Patients with proliferative retinopathy should avoid anaerobic (specifically isometric) exercise, such as power lifting, because of the increased ocular and systemic pressure occurring with the Valsalva maneuver. Diabetes is an important risk factor for ischemic heart disease, and its presence also puts the diabetic patient in a higher risk category with respect to exercise-associated cardiovascular events.

RECOMMENDATIONS

There is now ample evidence strongly supporting the beneficial effects of exercise in older individuals on several important health-related end points. It is also clear, however, that we do not yet know enough about different types of exercise regimens to accurately prescribe a specific program which can be aimed at a specific disorder. Several large prospective cohort studies as well as smaller clinical trials have demonstrated a dose response relationship between the intensity of exercise and the improvement in most outcome measures (blood pressure being one possible exception). This gradient of effect seems even clearer when fitness is substituted for physical activity. However, it has also been shown that significant cardiovascular and metabolic improvements can be obtained when less-intense exercise is maintained over sufficiently long periods of time and that less-intense exercise regimens are generally more acceptable (especially to older individuals) and appear to make long-term compliance more likely. Low-intensity programs may be necessary in frail populations, such as those with strokes, congestive heart disease, and chronic lung disease, in which more-intensive exercise is not tolerated. While there is some data to suggest that multiple short bouts of exercise (5 to 10 minutes each) may be effective in improving certain outcome measures, the data remain scanty and thus longer sessions remain preferable if tolerated. Another potential disadvantage of vigorous exercise in older individuals is that it has been shown to have little effect on total daily energy expenditure and may reduce overall activity during nonexercising periods.

After a thorough review of the types and amounts of exercise required for promotion of health and prevention of disease, a distinguished panel, representing the Centers for Disease Control and Prevention and the American College of Sports Medicine, published a consensus recommendation. This states that every adult should accumulate 30 minutes or more of moderate-intensity physical activity on most, if not all, days of the week. This public health message emphasizes the need for individual modifications in any given exercise programs and attempts to foster a change that can be sustainable within the individual's lifestyle. In addition, it clearly emphasized the terrible medical toll of being totally sedentary in our society.

For reasons of safety, most experts strongly recommend a preexercise assessment, including a complete history and physical examination, as well as an exercise stress test for men older than age 40 years and women older than age 50 years. However, the substantial cost of such an evaluation would affect the practicality of using exercise as a public health measure and could limit the participation of many older individuals in an exercise program. Furthermore, many older individuals have safely participated in community-based exercise programs for years with no such prior evaluation. The American College of Sports Medicine suggests that for those without symptoms of coronary disease, a formal medical examination and exercise testing may not be necessary if moderate noncompetitive exercise is performed in a supervised setting. The geriatric medicine axiom of "start low and go slow" should always be applied to beginning an exercise program. It is certainly appropriate for patients to notify their physicians of their intent to begin an exercise program, because adjustments in medications or dosages may be necessary.

An appropriate structured exercise program for an elderly population might start with heart rate monitoring at a target heart rate starting at 50 percent of maximum and increasing gradually, as tolerated, every 2 to 4 weeks, up to 70 to 80 percent of maximum heart rate. The maximum heart rate can be most accurately obtained during a maximal exercise test, but it can also be estimated from the formula "220 minus age." Endurance exercise should involve large muscle groups in large arcs and can potentially be complemented by low-resistance, high-repetition strength training. Appropriate warm-up and cool-down periods, as well as emphasis on stretching and flexibility, are likely to be especially important in reducing soft-tissue injury in an older population.

As discussed earlier, there are compelling reasons why an activity plan for older adults should also include activities which maintain and/or increase muscle strength. The Surgeon General's report on physical activity affirmed the accumulating evidence of the health benefits of strength-developing exercises.

Changes in lifestyle are difficult to maintain at any age and recidivism rates for exercise programs are high. This problem may be reduced by (1) careful attention to warm-up periods and slow progression in an effort to reduce early injuries; (2) enthusiastic leadership; (3) regular assessment of improvement with personalized feedback and praise; (4) spousal and family support for participation; (5) flexible goals (time rather than distance) set by the participant; and (6) use of distraction techniques such as music. Because it is inevitable that a participant will at some time have a setback, it is important to provide strategies for coping with this stress at the beginning of any exercise program.

REFERENCES

Albright A et al: Exercise and type 2 diabetes. *Med Sci Sports Exer* 32:1345, 2000.

Blair SN et al: Influences of cardiorespiratory fitness and other precursors on cardiovascular disease and all-cause mortality in men and women. *JAMA* 276:205, 1996.

Buchner DM et al: Evidence for a non-linear relationship between leg strength and gait speed. *Age Ageing* 25:386, 1996.

Cress ME et al: Exercise effects on physical functional performance in independent older adults. *J Gerontol* 54A:M242, 1999.

Diabetes Prevention Program Group: Reduction in the incidence of type 2 diabetes with lifestyle intervention or metformin. *N Engl J Med* 346:393, 2002.

Ettinger WH et al: A randomized trial comparing aerobic exercise and resistance exercise with a health education program in older adults with knee osteoarthritis. The fitness arthritis and seniors trial (FAST). *JAMA* 277:64, 1997.

Gill T et al: Role of exercise testing and safety monitoring for older persons starting an exercise program. *JAMA* 284:342, 2000.

Haapanen N et al: Association of leisure time physical activity with the risk of coronary heart disease, hypertension, and diabetes in middle-aged men and women. *Int J Epidemiol* 26:739, 1997.

Hurley BF, Roth SM: Strength training in the elderly: Effects on risk factors for age-related diseases. *Sports Med* 30(4):249, 2000.

Kujala UM et al: Relationship of leisure-time physical activity and mortality. *JAMA* 279:440, 1998.

Kushi LH et al: Physical activity and mortality in postmenopausal women. *JAMA* 277:1287, 1997.

Laukkanen JA et al: Cardiovascular fitness as a predictor or mortality in men. *Arch Intern Med* 161:825, 2001.

Lexell J, Dutta C (eds): Sarcopenia and physical performance in old age: National Institute on Aging Workshop. *Muscle Nerve Suppl* 5, 1997.

Marcus R: Role of exercise in preventing and treating osteoporosis. *Rheum Dis North Am* 27:131, 2001.

Mazzeo RS, Tanaka H: Exercise prescription for the elderly: Current recommendations. *Sports Med* 31:809, 2001.

Mazzeo RS et al: ACSM position stand: Exercise and physical activity for older adults. *Med Sci Sports Exerc* 30:992, 1998.

Schwartz RS et al: The effect of intensive endurance training on body fat distribution in young and older subjects. *Metabolism* 40:545, 1991.

Spirduso WW, Cronin DL: Exercise dose-response effects on quality of life and independent living in older adults. *Med Sci Sports Exerc* 33(6 Suppl):S598, 2001.

US Department of Health and Human Services. Physical activity and health: A report of the surgeon general. Atlanta, GA: US Department of Health and Human Services. Center for Disease Control and Prevention, National Center for Chronic Disease Prevention and Health Promotion, 1996.

Mobility

STEPHANIE STUDENSKI

Mobility problems are pervasive in older adults. Mobility limitations have a direct and immediate effect on personal independence, need for human help, and quality of life. Like other geriatric syndromes, mobility disorders are caused by diseases and impairments across many organ systems. Multiple perspectives and disciplines can be useful for evaluation and management. Mobility status is a potent predictor of future health, function, and survival. Providers of health care for older adults should be able to assess mobility status and know the natural history of mobility limitations. They should be familiar with the physiologic and biomechanical mechanisms underlying normal and abnormal mobility, the differential diagnosis of the causes of mobility disorders and approaches to management of mobility problems.

DEFINITIONS AND METHODS OF CLASSIFICATION

Defining Mobility

Mobility is the ability to move one's own body through space. At a biomechanical level, mobility requires force production and feedback control systems to navigate the mass of the body through a three-dimensional environment. In the framework of disablement processes (see Chap. 24), mobility problems are *functional limitations* caused by impairments in organ systems that are themselves a result of disease, disuse, and aging. In the disablement process, mobility limitations result in disabilities in activities of daily living and handicaps in social roles. Disablement can be modified by psychological, social, and environmental factors; in addition, disablement has bidirectional effects. For example, reduced mobility can worsen impairments such as strength or endurance. Walking is the fundamental mobility task for human life. Mobility also includes a wide range of other important activities that require moving one's body, from turning over in bed to climbing stairs. Mobility tasks have an inherent hierarchical order based on the biomechanical and physiological demands made on

the body. This orderedness is apparent in the developmental tasks of infancy and childhood, when mobility independence is first achieved. The simplest and first mobility task is turning over in bed, followed by sitting upright, transfers from lying to sitting and sitting to standing, locomotion with an increased base of support (like crawling or using a walker), to independent two-legged walking, and then more challenging tasks like ascending and descending stairs, running, climbing ladders, and sports.

Classification of Mobility

Mobility classification is often driven by a tacit assumption of orderedness. It is not realistic for any single instrument to assess the full range of mobility from the lowest levels of rolling over to the highest levels of endurance and coordination required for athletics or dance. Mobility assessment for older adults can generally be assigned to one or more of three levels; nonambulatory, ambulatory, and vigorous, corresponding broadly to Tinetti's levels of frail, transitional, and vigorous. While mobility abilities can fluctuate over hours to weeks, people generally tend to remain in one level unless a major event has occurred. For the nonambulatory, bed mobility, self-transfer skills, and wheelchair mobility affect independence in personal care activities, and thus have strong implications for care needs and demand for human help. Very limited mobility or immobility also directly affects health by contributing to problems such as pressure ulcers. Mobility assessment at the advanced level may be important for distinguishing "usual" from "successful" aging. It may also help estimate "physiologic reserve" as a marker of ability to tolerate physiologic stressors such as acute illness, surgery or periods of reduced activity.

Similar to other functional tasks, mobility can be classified along dimensions of amount of difficulty with task performance (e.g., none, some, much, unable), need for help (e.g., independent through completely dependent or unable), or means of performance (e.g., walk with/without assistive device, use wheelchair). These varying dimensions are reflected in the following sections.

EPIDEMIOLOGY

Prevalence

The epidemiology of mobility can be considered from the perspective of basic or higher level mobility. Examples of basic mobility problems include getting around inside the home and transfers from bed or chair. Examples of higher-level mobility problems include getting around outside the home, ability to walk one-quarter or one-half mile, and ability to climb stairs. Basic mobility problems are uncommon among the entire population of community-dwelling older persons, but are very frequent in institutionalized older people. Among community-dwelling persons age 65 years and older, 4.7 percent are dependent in getting in and out of a chair or bed, and 7.5 percent are dependent in getting around inside. Among institutionalized persons older than age 65 years, 78 percent are dependent in getting in and out of a chair or bed, and 82 percent are dependent in getting around inside. In the community, mobility disability increases dramatically with age; dependence in getting around inside increases from 5 percent of persons ages 65 to 74 years to 30.3 percent of persons ages 85+ years. Women tend to have higher rates of mobility disability than do men, and nonwhites have higher rates than whites. In institutionalized older persons, mobility disability does still tend to increase with age and, to a more modest degree, occur in women more than in men, while the effect of race disappears.

Higher-level mobility includes components such as the ability to go outside the home without help, ability to walk distances such as one-quarter to one-half mile and ability to climb stairs. United States census data on the community-dwelling population estimates that 13 percent of Americans older than age 60 years have difficulty going outside the home alone, including those with and without self-care limits. There is a marked decrease in outside the home mobility with age. There is also geographic variation; the highest proportions of older Americans reporting mobility limits live in the Southern United States. Higher-level mobility disability, defined as difficulty walking a quarter mile or climbing stairs, is more common in women than men and appears to be decreasing over recent decades (Table 73-1).

The prevalence and incidence of higher-level mobility disability was assessed in a recent population-based study of community-dwelling older Americans. Higher-level mobility disability at baseline increased at age 70 years from 22 percent in women and 15 percent in men, to 65 percent in women and 43 percent in men at age 85 years. The annual incidence of new higher disability increased with age and remained higher in women than in men (11 percent for women age 70 years, 7 percent for men age 70 years, 33 percent for women age 85 years, 25 percent for men age 85 years). Prevalence of disability is influenced by incidence, mortality, and recovery. The higher prevalence in women was most affected by incident mobility disability until approximately age 90 years when mobility recovery, which was higher in men, had a greater effect. Mortality differences between men and women had only a modest impact on the gender effect.

Table 73-1 Percentage of Noninstitutionalized Americans Age 70 Years or Older with Higher-Level Mobility Limitations

	1984	1995
Men		
Walk one-quarter mile	12.9%	12.3%
Climb 10 steps without resting	9.3%	8.2%
Women		
Walk one-quarter mile	20.9%	17.8%
Climb 10 steps without resting	16.0%	12.3%

SOURCE: Second supplement on aging in older Americans 2000: Key indicators of well being. Federal interagency forum on aging-related statistics: disability. Available at: http://www.agingstats.gov/chartbook2000/default.htm.

Consequences

Mobility problems have serious consequences. Mobility status can predict mortality risk. Older people with difficulty walking 2 kilometers (1.2 miles) or climbing one flight of stairs are twice as likely to die over the next 8 years as compared to those with no difficulty, after controlling for age, chronic conditions, smoking, marital status, and education. Mortality risk is even higher among those who have both mobility difficulty and are physically inactive. Poor mobility performance is an independent predictor of death and nursing home placement. In a population based study of community dwelling older adults, baseline physical performance score was associated with a twofold increase of death and nursing home placement after adjusting for age, disability in basic activities of daily living, and higher-level mobility disability.

Poor mobility performance is an independent predictor of new basic and mobility disability, even in persons with no self-reported disability at baseline. Among community-dwelling persons older than age 70 years with no baseline disability in activities of daily living and no higher-level mobility disability as measured by ability to walk one-half mile and climb stairs, baseline physical performance score was a powerful predictor of incident disability in both activities of daily living and in higher-level mobility disability. Mobility self-report and performance do predict mortality and disability in many populations including Mexican Americans, Japanese, Chinese, and Swedes.

Poor mobility performance is an independent predictor of hospitalization. In a population-based study of older adults who reported no disability, poor baseline physical performance score was associated with a twofold increased risk of hospitalization and more days in the hospital over 4 years. The increased hospitalization risk was independent of baseline health status. The increased risk was mostly associated with hospitalization for geriatric conditions, such as dementia, pressure ulcer, hip fractures, other fracture, pneumonia, and dehydration.

Mobility may be part of an underlying constellation of core areas that link multiple outcomes associated with aging. Poor mobility as measured by timed chair stands is

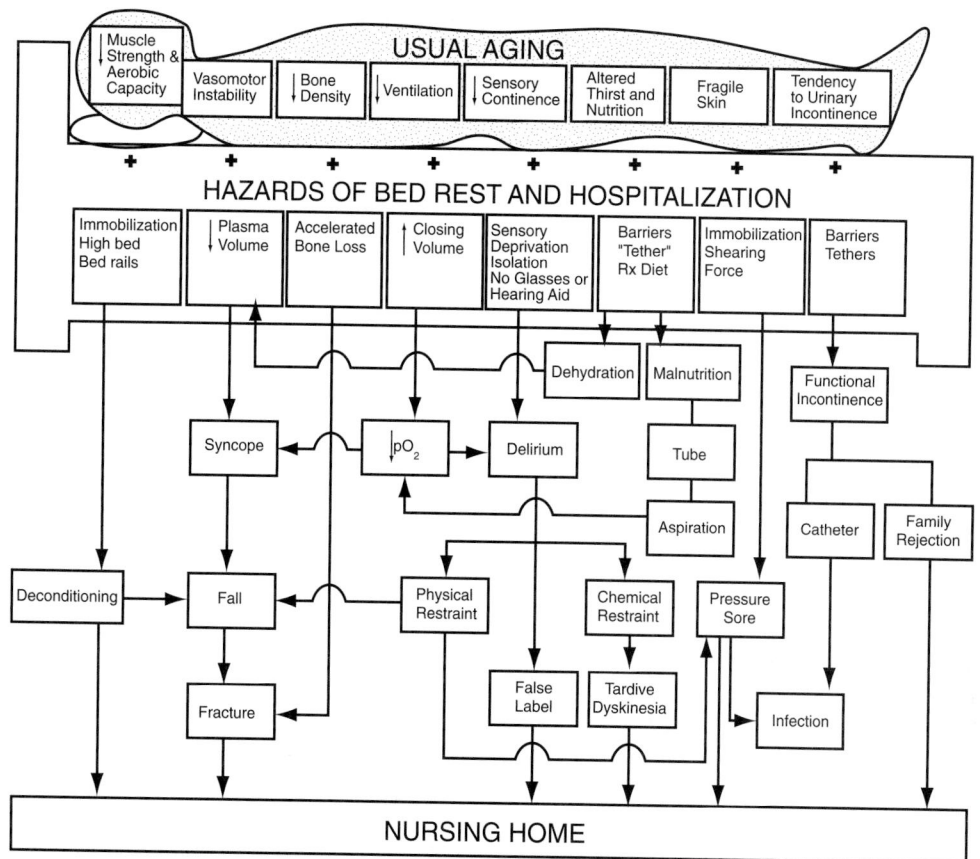

Figure 73-1   Bed rest, in combination with physiological changes of aging and acute illness, affects numerous organ systems and increases the risk of poor outcomes. Reproduced with permission from Creditor MC: Hazards of hospitalization of the elderly. *Ann Intern Med* 118:219, 1993.

one of four factors proposed to be common risk factors for geriatric syndromes including incontinence, falls and functional decline. Conversely, good mobility, along with good cognition and nutritional status is an independent predictor of recovery of independence after a period of disability.

Severe mobility disability, or immobility has widespread and devastating consequences (Fig. 73-1). It accelerates impairments in multiple organ systems, including bone, muscle, heart, circulation, lung, skin, blood, bowel, kidney, nutrition, and metabolism. Loss of organ system function can be rapid and severe; muscle strength can decline by 1 to 5 percent per day of enforced bed rest. Skin breakdown and pressure ulcer start to occur after only hours of persistent and unrelieved pressure. Major consequences of clinical significance include decreased plasma volume, orthostatic hypotension, accelerated loss of bone density, weakness, decreased pulmonary ventilation, and constipation leading to fecal impaction. When even temporary bed rest is combined with the increased vulnerability of aging and acute illness, there is a marked increased risk of death, disability, and institutionalization.

PATHOPHYSIOLOGY

The causes of mobility problems are complex. Unique and complementary etiologic perspectives contribute to a

better understanding of mobility. Three perspectives are presented here: epidemiologic, biomechanical, and biomedical. Each has advantages and disadvantages for the clinician and researcher.

Epidemiologic Perspective: Risk Factors

Epidemiologic risk factors for the onset of higher level mobility disability include demographics, health behaviors, and diseases. In a population-based cohort study of community-dwelling older adults, the cumulative incidence of higher-level mobility disability was 36 percent. Demographic factors associated with increased risk were advancing age, lower income, and lower educational level. Behavior-related risk factors included current smoking, alcohol abstention, low physical activity, and high body mass index. Psychological factors that influence mobility included ageist expectations, fear of falling, and emotional vitality. Physical activity, a health behavior that is key to mobility, is, in turn, influenced by multiple psychological, social, and environmental factors. Common reasons given by older adults for limiting or avoiding physical activity include lack of an exercise companion, lack of interest, fatigue, fear of falling, weather, and safety. Self-reported conditions associated with increased risk of higher level mobility disability include baseline and incident heart

Human Walking

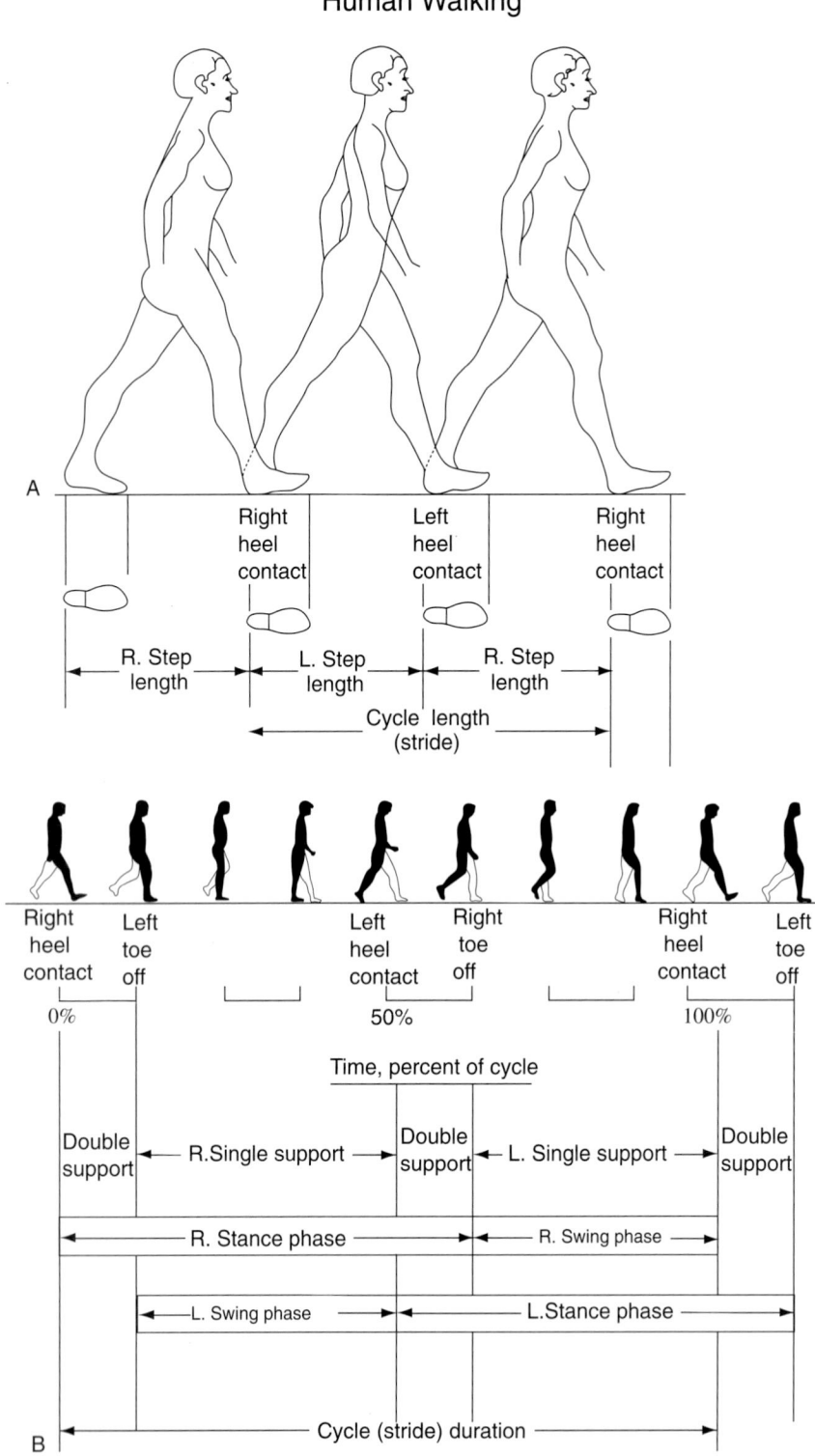

Figure 73-2 Basic elements of the walking cycle. Reproduced with permission from Inman VT et al: *Human Walking*. Baltimore, MD, Williams and Wilkins, 1981 p 26.

attack and stroke, baseline hypertension, diabetes, angina, dyspnea, and exertional leg pain, and incident cancer and hip fracture. Self-reported conditions identified as major barriers to activity by older adults include arthritis and past injury. Walking speed, one legged balance, self-report of modification of mobility tasks, and stair-climbing speed, were each associated independently with new mobility disability, after controlling for age, chronic diseases, depression, and knee strength, in the Women's Health and Aging Study.

Biomechanical Perspective: Direct Assessment of the Body in Motion (see also Chapter 71)

Age affects the biomechanics of walking. Normal gait can be defined in terms of the gait cycle with two main phases; stance and swing. (Fig. 73-2). A normal cycle begins with a push off from the forefoot, then a swing through and heel strike, timed tightly to be followed by the push off of the other leg. There are well-defined normal patterns of foot, ankle, knee, hip, pelvis, trunk, and arm motions. With age, gait speed slows, step length decreases, and the proportion of the gait cycle when both feet are in contact with the ground increases. These changes are attributable to alterations in muscle power, motor control, and flexibility. During gait, older people, as compared to young adults, tend to have more thoracic kyphosis, more anterior pelvic tilt, increased hip flexion, and greater external rotation of the foot. Older people tend to generate less power about the ankle and use hip flexion to compensate more than young adults. When older people walk, they must choose a strategy that best combines energy efficiency, stability, and safety, given their physiologic and psychological resources. Sometimes, a choice that maximizes stability or velocity can compromise gait efficiency. A biomechanical perspective can be applied more broadly to problems of mobility and balance based on an ordered increasing biomechanical demand placed on the body in motion. Typically, tasks are considered more challenging as the base of support narrows and transfers of mass over the base become more demanding. A biomechanical approach to postural alterations and body segment movement abnormalities can be useful for identifying causes of, and solutions to, mobility problems. Specific abnormalities can be addressed by targeting rehabilitative programs, the type of assistive devices or the design of environmental adaptations.

Physiologic Perspective: Using Organ System Impairment to Link Function and Disease

The causes of mobility limitation can be assessed from a physiologic perspective. There are two main physiologic components of mobility; balance control and force production. In walking, balance includes the ability to remain upright and the ability to generate a stepping pattern. Balance control and force production are like the steering and engine of a car. The physiologic elements of mobility can be assigned to three main components, namely sensory inputs, central processing and effector factors. Force production factors, such as endurance, pain, and flexibility, have less often been integrated into ideas about balance, but they are important for mobility. The physiologic components of mobility can be defined at the impairment or organ-system level, which can then be linked to distinct diseases, conditions, and pathologic processes. The cooccurrence of more than one impairment can increase the risk of mobility problems. Interventions can be built around controlling or treating the underlying conditions that are causing the impairment, directly treating the impairments, or creating compensations and adaptations. Ferrucci created a

framework that identifies six main physiologic subsystems of the ability to walk: central nervous system, perceptual system and peripheral nervous system, muscles, bones, joints, and energy production (Table 73-2). A physiologic approach offers a constructive way to connect mobility assessment to a biomedical model of diagnosis and treatment.

EVALUATION AND MANAGEMENT

Strategy for the Clinical Encounter

There are no established standards for the overall evaluation and treatment of mobility problems in older adults. At this point in time, the best strategy is to build on approaches that have been used for other geriatric syndromes. These approaches are based on a biopsychosocial model that incorporates biomedical, rehabilitative and psychosocial elements and a multidisciplinary team. Geriatric syndromes can be caused by a single major deficit that is often clinically obvious, a dominant deficit with several coimpairments, or by a series of modest impairments that accumulate to cause functional limitations and disability. The initial goal of assessment is to classify the mobility problem into one of three large groups; nonambulatory, ambulatory, or vigorous (Fig. 73-3). For the person who presents in a wheelchair or bed, one can screen for ability to stand or walk with assistance. For ambulatory individuals, a quick sorting strategy is to observe gait. Because most gait parameters are highly interrelated, abnormal gait can be grossly distinguished from normal by a few simple characteristics such as use of an assistive device, gait speed less than 1 meter per second (or step length less than twice foot length), or step asymmetry. Persons with normal gait can be assessed for higher level fitness by use of one or more screening tests for higher level abilities such as single-foot stand for 30 seconds, ability to tandem walk, or ability to walk more than 450 to 500 meters in 6 minutes. Persons with normal walking but inability to perform higher level tasks might be good candidates for exercise programs for well elders or for further evaluation if the mobility change is recent or causing problems. Further assessment of nonambulatory patients or for those with abnormal gait depends in part on the treatment goals. The team can select a basic strategy: either to try to improve mobility or to compensate for irreversible mobility loss (Fig. 73-3). This decision is based on the time course of the mobility loss, the potential to reverse impairments, the ability of the patient to participate in treatment, and the preferences of the patient. For example, a person with severe cognitive deficits or severe long-standing motor paralysis might be considered more appropriate for compensation than for interventions to improve mobility. Planning for compensation might target mobility care needs and resources.

For the person considered to have potential for improving mobility, the major decisions are the timing and value of interventions directly on mobility (usually through exercise and rehabilitation) and on underlying impairments (usually through medical team care). In some cases, it is clear that a person requires medical intervention first. For

Table 73-2 Subsystems of the Ability to Walk

Tests used in In-CHIANTI to evaluate the degree of impairment in each of the six subsystems that influence walking performance.

Bone

- Trabecular and cortical bone density estimated from pQTC images obtained from right lower leg
- Biomarkers of bone metabolism included circulating levels of calcium, bone-specific alkaline phosphatase, vitamin D, parathyroid hormone, and 24-hour urinary excretion of calcium and c-telopeptide of type I collagen
- Participants who reported foot pain while standing or walking were evaluated by an expert podiatrist who performed an objective and instrumental examination to establish the causes of such pain and estimate the chances of effective treatment
- Spinal mobility evaluated as absolute change in the distance between the spinous processes of the C7 and S1 vertebrae when moving from upright position to maximal trunk flexion, and the distance between C7 and the wall while the person was standing straight with the back touching the wall

Joints

- Goniometric measures of the passive range of motion of the hip (abduction, adduction, flexion, extension, and external rotation), knee (flexion and extension), ankle (flexion and extension), and shoulder (abduction and elevation)
- Clinical joint examination
- Pain in the lower back, hips, and knees and its severity evaluated using standard instruments

Muscle

- Lower leg muscle mass, intramuscular fat, and subcutaneous fat estimated from pQTC images
- Isometric muscle strength using a hand held dynamometer (Nicholas Manual Muscle Tester, Model #BK-5474, Fred Sammons, Inc., Burr Ridge, IL) on eight muscle groups of the lower extremity (abduction, adduction, flexion, and extension of hip; flexion and extension of knee and ankle) and two of the upper extremity (abduction and elevation of the shoulder)
- Lower extremity explosive muscle power (physical work delivered to the external environment in a unit of time) evaluated using the device proposed by Bassey
- Biomarkers of muscle metabolism including circulating levels of myoglobin and creatinine and 24-hour urinary excretion of creatinine and 3-methylhystidine, and the characterization of polymorphisms for myostatin

Peripheral nervous system and perceptual system

- Nerve conduction velocity evaluated in the right peroneal nerve by standard surface electroneurography
- Proprioceptive and vibration sensitivity assessed in the lower extremity by standard methods
- Tactile sensitivity assessed using von Frey's monofilaments of predefined rigidity
- Symptoms attributable to peripheral neuropathy and vestibular dysfunction investigated using specific questionnaires
- Near (30 cm) and far (3 m) visual acuity, contrast sensitivity, and three-dimensional perception investigated by standard methods

Central nervous system

- Screening of cognitive impairment performed by the Mini-Mental State Examination. Participants who screened positive underwent a comprehensive clinical and neuropsychological assessment to establish the diagnosis of dementia based on the DSM-IIIR criteria
- The psychological component of mobility was assessed in terms of depressive symptoms and personal mastery by, respectively, the Center for Epidemiologic Studies Depression Scale (CES-D) and selected questions from the Hopkins Symptoms Checklist
- Ability to maintain balance for 10 seconds in progressively more challenging positions (free position, feet under the anterior iliac spines, feet side by side, semitandem, tandem, one leg)
- Detailed neurologic examination specifically designed to detect even minor signs of neurologic impairment such as tremor, pathologic reflexes, subcortical reflexes, delay in movement initiation, manual dexterity, coordination, ability to perform rhythmic repetitive movements.

Energy production and delivery

- Daily intake of various macro- and micronutrients assessed by the EPIC questionnaire
- Circulatory and respiratory function evaluated by standard medical examination
- Venous insufficiency and thrombosis evaluated using color-Doppler scan
- Arterial circulation assessed by measuring ankle–brachial index

DSM-IIIR, *Diagnostic and Statistical Manual of Mental Disorders,* 3rd ed. revised; EPIC, European Prospective Investigation into Cancer and Nutrition.
SOURCE: Reproduced with permission from Ferrucci et al. (2000).

A clinical strategy for the assessment and management of mobility limitations

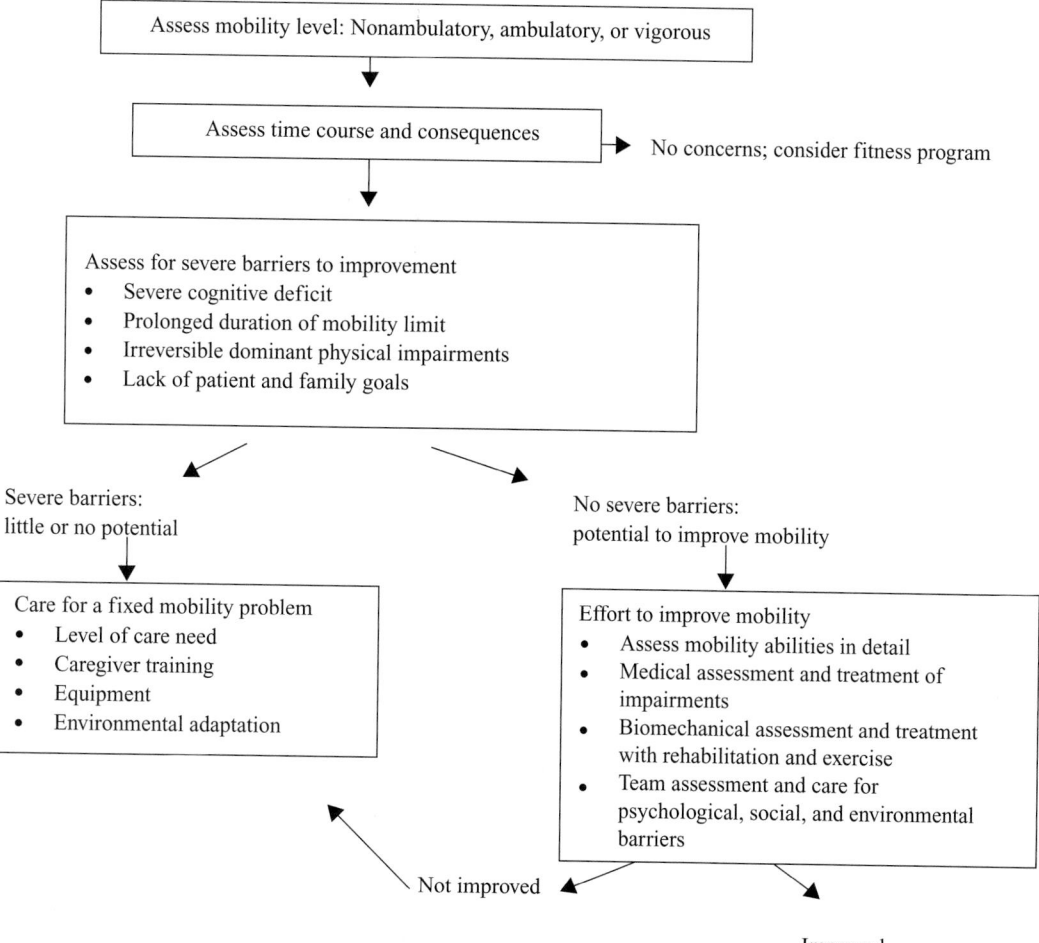

Figure 73-3   Screening, triage and many interventions are feasible in primary care. Comprehensive mobility assessment requires a multidisciplinary team.

example, in a person with poorly controlled congestive heart failure, medical treatment for symptom control probably needs to occur prior to rehabilitation. In other cases, it can be difficult to predict whether intervention on multiple impairments should occur before or during rehabilitation efforts. For example, in a person with depression, low vision, and peripheral neuropathy, one could intervene with rehabilitation and exercise simultaneously with vision correction and antidepressants or one could try to correct the impairments first. This decision is based in part on whether the impairments are felt to create significant barriers to the success of rehabilitation. One could argue that in the absence of obvious barriers, a "trial" of rehabilitation should be started. Treatment can be initiated for impairments that cause barriers along the way. Alternatively, one could argue that it is more efficient to eliminate barriers prior to starting therapy. Because the time and effort of comprehensive mobility assessment and rehabilitation are both substantial, it is a challenge to determine where to apply efficiencies. Older adults with mobility problems often have numerous impairments identified as part of comprehensive assessment, some of which may be barriers and some may not. The process is likely to be inefficient, and like comprehensive geriatric assessment, hard to use in routine clinical practice. To the extent that there are "high payoff" areas based on prevalence or responsiveness to intervention, it may be possible to prioritize and streamline the process. The most common abnormalities found in people with gait disorders in several case series were musculoskeletal and neurologic in origin. In primary care, the provider can offer a screening and triage function by recognizing mobility disorders and assessing potential for intervention. The primary provider can also identify and treat overt clinical impairments that can be detected quickly in the clinic, like weight-bearing pain caused by osteoarthritis or dyspnea caused by congestive heart failure. When the cause of the mobility problem is less obvious, a referral to multidisciplinary team for comprehensive mobility assessment can be considered. Because the potential causes range across many organ systems, this strategy might be more efficient than referral to several organ system based specialists. Because research into mobility problems is an active and high-priority area in aging, in the future, efficient clinical practice and referral may be better informed by evidence. (See Chap. 24, for further discussion.)

Table 73-3   Instruments Used to Screen and Assess Mobility

Instrument Type	Instrument name, References	Items	Range	Comments
Self-report	Rosow–Breslau	Walk $1/2$ or $1/4$ mile, climb stairs	Ambulatory to vigorous	Used as single items
	SF-36 physical function	10 items, many directly related to mobility, from walking 1 mile to walking across a room	Ambulatory to vigorous	Score 0–100 US adult, mean 84.2; older adult, mean 52.0; insensitive at lower levels of mobility
	Long-term care survey	Walking inside and bed/chair transfers	Nonambulatory to ambulatory	Used as single items
	Mobility modifications	Self-report of changing the way one walks, one-half mile of climbing stairs	Ambulatory	Used as single items
	Avlund mobility	Fatigue and need for help in six mobility activities, from transfer to stairs and walking outside	Nonambulatory, ambulatory, and vigorous	Scores 0–6
Professional assessment	Barthel mobility items	Walking (or wheeling), transfers, stairs	Nonambulatory, ambulatory, and vigorous	Mobility items integrated into total score
	Functional Independence measure (FIM)	Transfers and locomotion (walk, wheelchair, stairs)	Nonambulatory, ambulatory, and vigorous	Seven-level scoring of need for assistance with items. Mobility items are integrated into total score
	MDS	Bed mobility, transfers, locomotion (includes wheelchair mobility) walking	Nonambulatory to ambulatory	Used as single items
Performance	EPESE battery	Timed walk, chair rises, tandem stands	Ambulatory	Score 0–12 Scores of 10–12, 7–9, and 4–6 associated with increasing risk of poor outcomes
	Gait speed	Timed walk, varying distances, instructions, procedures	Ambulatory	Healthy older adult >1.0 m/s Slow <0.6 m/s Very slow <0.4 m/s
	Timed up and go	Time to rise from chair, walk 10 feet, turn, walk back and sit down	Ambulatory	<10 seconds - normal; <20 seconds - able to move in community; >30 seconds—needs assistance for mobility
	Six-minute walk	Distance covered in 6 minutes	Ambulatory to vigorous	Healthy older adult mean >500 meters older adults in assisted living <300 meters

(Continued)

Table 73-3 (*Continued*) **Instruments Used to Screen and Assess Mobility**

Instrument Type	Instrument name, References	Items	Range	Comments
	Health ABC	Walking endurance: 400-meter walk time, distance in 2 minutes	Ambulatory to vigorous	Supplements EPESE battery by expanding differentiation among healthy older adults.
		Expanded EPESE battery: longer tandem stands, one-foot stand, narrow walk time		Useful for persons with scores of 10–12 on EPESE battery; score range 0–4

EPESE, Established Populations for the Epidemiologic Study of the Elderly; MDS, Minimum Data Set.

The comprehensive approach to the clinical assessment of treatable causes of mobility is currently a specialized referral function that is resource intensive (see Chap. 8). Evaluation starts with the clinical assessment of the severity, course and consequences of mobility limitation and the determination of potential to improve mobility. Mobility performance is assessed in more detail, including biomechanical aspects of functional limitations during movement. Potential contributing factors are identified based on physiological impairments, and evidence is sought for psychosocial and environmental influences.

Evaluation

Methods of Mobility Assessment

Mobility can be assessed by self-report, professional observation or direct measurement. Instruments to assess mobility using all three methods have been developed (Table 73-3). Each has advantages and disadvantages. These tests have been used to estimate the incidence and prevalence of mobility disorders, as well as for screening and classification of care needs. More detailed instruments have been developed specifically for sorting out causes and mechanisms. Measures have varying strengths and limitations based on characteristics such as reliability and validity, respondent burden, feasibility and convenience of use, and assessor skill required. Self-report measures can be easier to obtain from large populations, represent the opinion of the person most affected and can integrate fluctuating ability over time. Self-report measures may be limited by problems with reliability, accuracy, and nonresponse. As self-report measures are usually ordinal scales, they lack ability to discriminate small but important differences. Professional report measures can provide the opinion of an experienced assessor, can integrate over time and may be more feasible when the person cannot respond accurately or cooperate with formal performance testing. Professional report measures may be limited by problems with reliability and the need for assessor experience and training. Because they are usually ordinal scales, they have somewhat limited ability to discriminate small but important differences. Performance testing can be somewhat more independent of opinion, and can produce quantitative results that show

small but important or subclinical differences. Performance measures require direct observation, examinee cooperation and standardization of instruction and procedures. For example, there are no current standards for the technique to determine gait speed. Walk distances can range from 8 feet to 50 feet, instructions from usual to maximum speed and timing can begin with gait initiation or when a constant velocity is achieved. This lack of standardization is reflected in the wide range of gait speeds reported for normal older adults. The need for examinee cooperation can lead to problems with non-response. Performance measures do not account well for short-term fluctuations over hours to weeks. Furthermore, performance testing assesses mobility under standardized conditions that may or may not correlate with mobility during usual daily activities. Despite these limitations, performance testing may have direct applications in clinical settings because it can provide useful information and is brief and quantitative.

Clinical Assessment of Mobility Performance

Gait, balance and a range of mobility tasks can be assessed clinically from a biomechanical perspective (Table 73-4). Gait can be examined for general characteristics such as path deviations or a widened base of support and for altered motion of the component parts: trunk, hip, knee, ankle, and foot. Mobility tasks can be examined for performance difficulty or altered movement patterns as task demands increase. Sometimes, the finding of an abnormal body segment movement or gait characteristic suggests a specific impairment or disease. More often, the abnormality is nonspecific, but is amenable to direct intervention in rehabilitation.

Clinical gait assessment tools that include many of these biomechanical elements include the Performance-Oriented Mobility Assessment (POMA) and the gait-abnormality rating scale (GARS). A tool for analyzing the elements of bed mobility from the perspective of body segments has been proposed. Mobility and balance assessments can be based on a hierarchy of task difficulty. The Berg balance scale assesses 14 tasks of progressive difficulty from sitting balance to one-leg standing, and rising onto a step. Some scales are designed to discriminate mobility capacity among the nonambulatory. The Hierarchical

Table 73-4   A Biomechanical Assessment of Common Gait Abnormalities

Gait Component	Gait Abnormality	Possible Causes
Lower extremity segments		
Ankle and foot	Forefoot strikes floor simultaneously with initial heel contact (foot slap)	Weak ankle dorsiflexors
	Initial contact is by forefoot	Leg-length discrepancy, plantar flexion contracture, painful heel
	Heel and toe leave floor together during push off	Fixed ankle, weak plantar flexors, painful forefoot
	Forefoot drags during swing (foot drop)	Weak ankle dorsiflexors
Knee	Knee flexed at initial contact	Painful knee, weak knee extensors, leg-length discrepancy
	Decreased knee extension during swing	Knee pain or decreased range
Hip	Decreased hip flexion at initial contact	Weak hip flexors, decreased range
	Increased hip flexion during swing (steppage gait)	Compensation for foot drop
	Decreased hip extension during late stance	Hip flexion contracture
	Hip circumduction with lateral movement of entire limb	Weak hip flexors, inability to flex leg
Gait pattern		
Gait initiation	Hesitation	Parkinson's disease, frontal lobe disorders, normal pressure hydrocephalus
Stance width	Increased	Cerebellar disorders, peripheral neuropathy
Path	Weaving	Vestibular disorders

SOURCE: Adapted from Rothstein JM et al: *The Rehabilitation Specialists Handbook.* Philadelphia, FA Davis, 1991 p 699; Alexander NB: Gait disorders in older adults. *J Am Geriatr Soc* 44:434, 1996; and Nutt JG et al: Human walking and higher level gait disorders, particularly in the elderly. *Neurology* 43:268, 1993.

Assessment of Balance and Mobility assesses mobility, transfers, and balance, and detects multiple levels within the bed and chair fast. The Physical Disability Index has eight mobility tasks, including six items for nonambulatory persons. Mobility task scales usually have a functional rather than a biomedical perspective and are not designed to detect specific impairments. These scales can be used to identify areas for task practice or adaptation in rehabilitation and to assess the effects of treatment.

Differential Diagnosis Based on a Physiologic Perspective

A clinical schema derived from Ferrucci, Tinetti, and the author's own work is proposed in Table 73-5. Many impairments are detectable through the usual geriatric clinical history and physical examination. Some sensory systems are amenable to clinical evaluation. Vision can be assessed for acuity by Snellen chart and fields by confrontation, dark adaption by history, and depth perception with a low-cost portable device resembling a shoe box with two pointers attached to cords. Peripheral sensation can be assessed by proprioception, vibratory threshold, and filaments. Some central systems can be assessed clinically. Perfusion can be assessed by history of orthostatic symptoms or presyncope and by direct assessment of orthostatic blood pressure change. Reaction time can be assessed by timed finger and foot tapping, or grossly by observation of rapid alternating movements. Frontal lobe function can be assessed using the Trail Making B test or by a dual task such as walking and carrying a glass of water. Postural responses can be assessed by a test of the righting reflex. This test can be performed as a sternal nudge or rapid pull on the pelvic rim, with the goal to displace the center of mass sufficiently to require a displacement of the base of support, which generates a need to take a step. A normal response is a single brisk step backward. A grossly abnormal response is the "timber reaction" in which no lower extremity movement occurs. An equivocal response is several small steps. Because older adults can unexpectedly lack righting reflexes, it is essential to be positioned to catch the individual during this test. Absent righting reflexes are found in Parkinson's disease, in association with cogwheel rigidity. Absent or decreased righting reflexes can also be found in other poorly defined central nervous system conditions. Poor trunk control, dysmetria, and a wide base of support in standing are seen in cerebellar disorders. Musculoskeletal and neurologic effector factors that can be assessed in the clinic include simple assessments of strength by manual muscle testing and by maneuvers that require the individual to move his own body mass, like chair rise, standing on the toes (with hands on exam table for stability) and squatting. Focal or asymmetric weakness is pathologic may be caused by central, spinal cord, or peripheral nerve disorders. Flexibility can be assessed by

Table 73-5   Assessment and Treatment of Physical Impairments that Cause Mobility Problems

Area	Organ System	Impairment	Assessment	Related Causes	Treatment
Sensory	Eye	Acuity	Near and far by Snellen chart	Presbyopia, cataracts	Lenses, surgery
	Eye	Peripheral vision	Confrontation	Glaucoma, stroke	Prisms
	Eye	Depth	Depth testing	Monocular	Lighting, contrast, avoid multifocals when walking
	Eye	Dark adaption	Self-report	Miotic agents for glaucoma	Change medications, lighting
	Vestibular	Otoliths	Ability to perceive vertical	Benign positional vertigo	Vestibular rehabilitation
	Vestibular	Semicircular canals	Ability to perceive rotation and acceleration	Ménière's disease	Medications, vestibular rehabilitation
	Peripheral nerve	Neuropathy	Filaments, vibratory sense	Diabetes, peripheral vascular disease	Haptic enhancement, footwear
Central	Circulation	Decreased brain perfusion	Hypotension, orthostasis	Medications, arrythmias Postprandial hypotension dehydration	Change medications, antiarrhythmics or pacemaker; alter intake fluid
	Brain	Motor processing	Level of consciousness, timed tapping, trail B, timed up-and-go with hand-carrying task	Medications	Change medications
	Brain	Postural reflexes	Righting reflexes	Parkinson's disease; other central nervous system diseases	Parkinson medications
Effector	Muscle	Strength	Manual muscle tests, strength based motions (chair rise, squat)	Multiple neurologic conditions, inactivity	Exercise
	Musculoskeletal	Flexibility	Contractures, ROM	Injury, arthritis, inactivity	Active and passive ROM, orthotics
	Heart endurance	Cardiomyopathy	Dyspnea at rest or on exertion, fluid retention, echocardiogram	Systolic or diastolic dysfunction	Standard care for systolic and diastolic dysfunction
	Lung endurance	Hypoxia or air flow	Dyspnea rest or on exertion, hypoxia, decreased peak flow	COPD, asthma, other lung	Standard pulmonary care, oxygen
	Circulation endurance	Peripheral vasculature	Leg pain on exertion, decreased pulses, bruits	Arteriosclerosis, venous insufficiency	Medical and surgical, exercise
	Muscle endurance	Sarcopenia	Leg fatigue on exertion	Inactivity	Exercise

(Continued)

Table 73-5   (*Continued*) Assessment and Treatment of Physical Impairments that Cause Mobility Problems

Area	Organ System	Impairment	Assessment	Related Causes	Treatment
	Musculoskeletal pain	Bone and joint deficits	Weight-bearing pain	Osteoarthritis, osteoporotic fractures Periarticular conditions, Foot problems	Pain medications, injections, assistive devices, orthoses, exercise
	Neurologic pain	Spinal cord, roots, nerves,	Leg and back pain with activity	Spinal stenosis, radiculopathies, peripheral neuropathies	Injections, surgery, medications

COPD, chronic obstructive pulmonary disease; ROM, range of motion.

range of motion. Flexibility in the neck and spine, as well as in the lower extremities affect mobility. Weight-bearing pain and pain in the chest, back, or legs during motion or exertion can be assessed by history and maneuvers that reproduce the symptoms. Endurance can be assessed in part by history and examination of the heart, peripheral circulation and lungs. A 6-minute walk test in the clinic might be feasible during comprehensive assessment.

Some impairments are hard to detect in the clinic and require further testing. Vestibular testing may be helpful when there is unsteadiness that is not well explained by other impairments or when specific vestibular symptoms are present. Electrodiagnostic testing of nerve conduction velocity or abnormal muscle activity may be indicated when neurologic findings are suspicious. Exertional chest pain or dyspnea requires appropriate cardiac and pulmonary testing. Leg pain on exertion suggests testing for peripheral vascular disease or lumbar stenosis (see Chap. 79).

Psychosocial and Environmental Assessment

Mobility limitations are influenced by psychological, social, and environmental factors (Table 73-6). Depression, self-confidence (efficacy), and fear of falling can have powerful effects on the desire to be mobile. Screens for these conditions should be part of a comprehensive mobility assessment. Apathy and lack of motivation are a common concern in geriatric rehabilitation. Formal and informal social support resources can be critical for the person with mobility limitations. Cultural and financial factors can influence attitudes toward disability and resources for addressing the problem. The safety and accessibility of the living environment can be a barrier or facilitator for persons with mobility problems. A home visit for assessment can offer many opportunities for creative problem solving.

Management

Intervening Directly on Mobility

Interventions directed at functional limitations are often rehabilitative in nature and involve exercise, adaptive equipment and environmental modifications. Mobility limitations can be addressed through mobility task practice, and exercise to improve strength, balance, endurance, and flexibility. Because deconditioning is almost always present as a direct consequence of reduced mobility and inactivity, and deconditioning has been found to be treatable in many older adults who are sick or frail, general conditioning programs of exercise are frequently indicated. Assistive and orthotic devices can improve stability and reduce weight-bearing pain. The evidence for the effectiveness of rehabilitation and exercise interventions is growing and has been examined in older adults with varying levels of mobility limitations. Chapters 24 and 72 present these interventions in more detail.

Treating Impairments

Some impairments can be linked to diseases and pathological processes that are amenable to treatment and some impairments can be improved directly regardless of pathologic cause (see Table 73-5). Visual function for mobility can be modified by prisms, lenses that expand the visual field, and lighting. Some vestibular disorders are amenable to rehabilitation. Peripheral sensory disorders are often not correctable but compensation can be achieved through the use of lighting to improve visual information, appropriate footwear (thin soles and high box) to maximize proprioceptive input, and use of a cane to enhance haptic perception. Haptic perception is demonstrated by the remarkable decrease in sway with eyes closed seen in persons with peripheral sensory or vestibular disorders when they are allowed even minimal, nonsupporting contact with a stable surface such as a table or wall. It appears that another sensory input source can be used by the brain to provide information about body position when information from the feet is lost. In this case, the cane is providing information to the hand about body position and is not used as weight-bearing device. Interventions for orthostatic hypotension include medication adjustment, compression stockings, increased fluid intake, and, in some cases, salt loading or medication such as fludrocortisone or milrinone. Delayed movement speed can be reduced if medications that exacerbate the problem are removed. The slowed gait of Parkinson's disease can be responsive to medication, although the

Table 73-6 Psychosocial and Environmental Assessment and Management of Mobility

Domain	Type	Assessment	Management
Psychological	Depression	Standard screen	Antidepressants, counseling
	Self-efficacy	Interview	Counseling
	Apathy	Interview, observation	Stimulants, social therapies
Social	Emotional and instrumental supports	Interview	Community programs, family engagement
	Culture	Interview	Cultural consultation
	Finances	Interview	Community resources
Environmental	Physical barriers	Home visit	Environmental adaptations
	Access	Interview and home visit	Community programs

balance disorder is not. Parkinson patients may move faster and thus increase their risk of fall injury when medications are initiated. Cardiac and pulmonary symptoms that limit endurance may be managed medically. Strength and endurance are amenable to exercise training. Pain may be managed using medications, injections, orthotics, exercise, and sometime surgery.

Attention to Factors that Modify Behavior and Environment

The modifiable psychosocial factors that influence physical activity may offer opportunities to intervene (see Table 73-6). Depression can be managed medically. In postacute care settings, methylphenidate has been used short-term to treat apathy. Social support and encouragement can be promoted through group activities. Physical environmental adaptations in the home include ramps and railings, bathroom modifications, and strategic placement of stable furniture items. Further modifications are often indicated in institutional settings.

Care for the Immobile Person

Interventions to reduce the consequences of immobility include determining the level of care need and living setting, training others to properly position and move the patient, implementing a mobilization plan, use of pressure-reducing devices to prevent pressure ulcers, and sometimes using equipment to aid in transfers. Persons who are responsible for carrying out transfers of immobile patients, including health aides and family caregivers, need training in proper techniques that reduce injury to the patient and the assistant. Absolute bed rest is almost never indicated and should be discouraged in all settings. An exception for humanitarian reasons to routine mobilization is under active discussion in geriatrics. When an individual is actively dying, routine mobilization might cause suffering without associated benefit. In this case, discontinuing it might be justifiable. Mobilization rather than bed rest during hospitalization for acute illness has been one of the most consistent interventions in acute care of the elderly units.

SUMMARY

Mobility disorders are widespread in older adults. Mobility limitations constrain many functions required for independent living and are powerful indicators of future problems. Mobility can be classified using simple screens. Evaluation starts with a triage function. Screening, referral, and management of many common impairments that contribute to mobility loss can be managed in primary care settings. A comprehensive mobility evaluation is resource intensive and requires a multidisciplinary team. Evaluation and management include a biomechanical approach to function, a biomedical approach to the physiologic components of mobility, and a psychosocial and environmental approach to modifying factors.

REFERENCES

Alexander NB et al: Bed mobility task performance in older adults. *J Rehabil Res Dev* 37:633, 2000.

Allen C et al: Bed rest: A potentially harmful treatment needing more careful evaluation. *Lancet* 354:1229, 1999.

Avlund K et al: Tiredness in daily activities at age 70 as a predictor of mortality during the next 10 years. *J Clin Epidemiol* 51:323, 1998.

Black FO et al: Outcome analysis of individualized vestibular rehabilitation. *Am J Otol* 21:543, 2000.

Connell BR: Role of the environment in falls prevention. *Clin Geriatr Med* 12:859, 1996.

Ferrucci L et al: Subsystems contributing to the decline in ability to walk: Bridging the gap between epidemiology and geriatric practice in the In CHIANTI study. *J Am Geriatr Soc* 48:1618, 2000.

Fried LP et al: Preclinical mobility disability predicts incident mobility disability in older women. *J Gerontol Med Sci* 55A:M43, 2000.

Gerety M et al: Development and validation of a physical performance instrument for the functionally impaired elderly: The physical disability index (PDI). *J Gerontol Med Sci* 48:M33, 1993.

Gill TM et al: Assessing risk for the onset of functional dependence among older adults: The role of physical performance. *J Am Geriatr Soc* 43:603, 1995.

Guralnik JM et al: Lower-extremity function in persons over the age of 70 years as a predictor of subsequent disability. *N Engl J Med* 332:556, 1995.

Harper CM, Lyles YM: Physiology and complications of bed rest. *J Am Geriatr Soc* 36:1047, 1988.

Jeka JJ: Light touch contact as a balance aid. *Phys Ther* 77:476, 1997.

Lundin-Olsson L et al: Attention, frailty, and falls: The effect of a manual task on basic mobility. *J Am Geriatr Soc* 46:758, 1998.

Maino JH: Visual deficits and mobility. *Clin Geriatr Med* 12:803, 1996.

Peeters P, Mets T: The 6-minute walk as an appropriate exercise test in elderly patients with chronic heart failure. *J Gerontol Med Sci* 51A:M147, 1996.

Penninx BWJH et al: The protective effect of emotional vitality on adverse health outcomes in disabled older women. *J Am Geriatr Soc* 48:1359, 2000.

Penninx BWJH et al: Lower extremity performance in nondisabled older persons as a predictor of subsequent hospitalization. *J Gerontol Med Sci* 55:M691, 2000.

Podsiadlo D, Richardson S: The timed "up and go": A test of basic functional mobility for frail older persons. *J Am Geriatr Soc* 39:142, 1991.

Rantanen T et al: Co impairments as predictors of severe walking disability in older women. *J Am Geriatr Soc* 49:21, 2001.

Satariano WA et al: Reasons given by older people for limitations or avoidance of leisure time physical activity. *J Am Geriatr Soc* 48:503, 2000.

Simonsick EM et al: Measuring higher level physical function in well-functioning older adults: Expanding familiar approaches in the health ABC study. *J Gerontol Med Sci* 56A:M644, 2001.

Tinetti ME et al: Shared risk factors for falls, incontinence and functional dependence. *JAMA* 273:1348, 1995.

Tinetti ME: Performance-oriented assessment of mobility problems in elderly patients. *J Am Geriatr Soc* 34:119, 1986.

Wolfson L et al: Gait assessment in the elderly: A gait abnormality rating scale and its relation to falls. *J Gerontol Med Sci* 45:M12, 1990.

Osteoarthritis

LIANA FRAENKEL • DAVID FELSON

DEFINITION AND CLASSIFICATION OF OSTEOARTHRITIS

Osteoarthritis (OA), also commonly called degenerative arthritis, refers to a group of overlapping diseases that share clinical and pathologic features. These features include joint pain after joint use and failure of many structures within the joint including, but not limited to, wearing away of hyaline articular cartilage. OA is most commonly classified as primary (idiopathic) or secondary, the latter referring to syndromes associated with an identifiable cause (Table 74-1). This disorder can also be classified by anatomic location, either by the site of primary involvement or by the number of joints affected (localized versus generalized). The joints frequently involved in primary OA are depicted in Figure 74-1. In secondary OA, joint involvement depends on the underlying disease or the site of injury. Routine clinical, laboratory, and radiographic criteria permit accurate classification of the most commonly involved joints, namely, the knees, hips, and hands (Table 74-2).

EPIDEMIOLOGY OF OSTEOARTHRITIS

Overview

Osteoarthritis is the most common form of arthritis and a leading cause of disability in older persons. More than 80 percent of individuals older than 55 years have radiographic evidence of OA, and up to 20 percent of affected individuals are significantly disabled. In fact, knee and hip OA limit mobility more than any other chronic disease. The quality of life of elderly patients with OA, as assessed by the SF-36® (a well-validated health-related quality of life survey), is significantly poorer than that of healthy controls, especially in domains associated with physical function. Musculoskeletal disorders, of which OA is the most common, result in significant economic costs, accounting for 1 percent to 2.5 percent of the gross national product in the United States. In older adults, most of these costs are associated with hospitalization for total joint replacement. In middle-aged patients, indirect costs due to premature retirement may be substantial.

Incidence

A large-scale study from a Massachusetts health maintenance organization found that the incidence of symptomatic knee OA (new occurrences of disease) was 240 per 100,000 person-years; hip OA, 88 per 100,000 person-years; and hand OA, 100 per 100,000 person-years (Figure 74-2). As can be seen in Figure 74-2, the incidence of OA increases with age and is more common in older women than in older men. Given the projected increase in the segment of the population older than 65 years, by 2020 the estimated number of persons with arthritis is expected to increase by 57 percent, and the disability associated with this condition by more than 65 percent.

Risk Factors for Osteoarthritis

Nonmodifiable Risk Factors

Age, gender, and race Age is one of the strongest risk factors for OA in both men and women (Figure 74-2). The prevalence of symptomatic knee OA, defined as almost daily pain and characteristic findings on radiographs, is 6 percent in adults 30 years and older and rises to 11 percent in adults 65 years and older. After age 50 years, women are more commonly affected by OA than men at every site except for the hip.

Studies examining ethnic differences in rates of OA suggest that although the prevalence in African Americans may be comparable to that in whites, African Americans are more likely to have severe, disabling disease. Elderly people in China have higher rates of knee OA but lower rates of hand and hip OA than white Americans. In Chinese Americans, hip OA is rare. These ethnic differences in disease prevalence and severity may be due to genetic factors or, in some cases, to a higher likelihood of joint overuse and injury.

Genetics Twin and family studies have estimated the heritable component of OA to be between 50 percent and 65 percent, with larger genetic influences for hand and hip OA than for knee OA. Potential genetic abnormalities that could increase susceptibility to OA include abnormalities in bone or cartilage metabolism and/or structural defects

Table 74-1   Classification of Osteoarthritis

I.   Primary (idiopathic) osteoarthritis

II. Secondary osteoarthritis
     Developmental
          Congenital dysplasias
          Congenital dislocation of the hip
          Leg length inequality
     Traumatic, for example,
          Major joint trauma (e.g., fracture)
          Joint surgery (e.g., meniscectomy)
          Chronic injury (e.g., occupational overuse)
     Metabolic
          Hemochromatosis
          Acromegaly
          Ochronosis
     Inflammatory
          Any inflammatory arthritis, including
               crystal-induced, rheumatoid, and septic arthritis
     Other
          Paget's disease
          Avascular necrosis
          Slipped capital femoral epiphysis

involving molecules in cartilage such as collagen. Specific candidates currently being explored include genes encoding minor forms of collagen, genes encoding enzymes required for cartilage synthesis and/or breakdown, and genes that regulate the transcription of these and other factors. It is likely that more than one OA susceptibility gene will be found.

Modifiable Risk Factors

Weight   Overweight individuals are at high risk for developing knee OA. Compared to men, the relationship between obesity and knee OA is stronger in women, in whom body weight is linearly related to knee OA risk. Furthermore, among those who already have knee OA, obesity is a risk factor for disease progression. The relationship between obesity and hip OA is not as strong, nor as consistent, as that demonstrated for knee OA.

Increased knee loading is probably the main mechanism by which obesity causes knee OA. During walking, each pound of excess weight exerts the equivalent of 3 to 6 extra pounds of knee loading. Interestingly, there is evidence that weight may be a risk factor for hand OA, suggesting that the increased risk for OA due to obesity is partially mediated by metabolic factors.

Injury   Major trauma and repetitive activities that stress the joints can increase the risk for subsequent OA. In a large population-based study, men with a history of a major knee injury had a 3.5-fold increased risk, and women a 2.2-fold increased risk, for developing subsequent knee OA. In joints that are rarely affected by OA, such as the

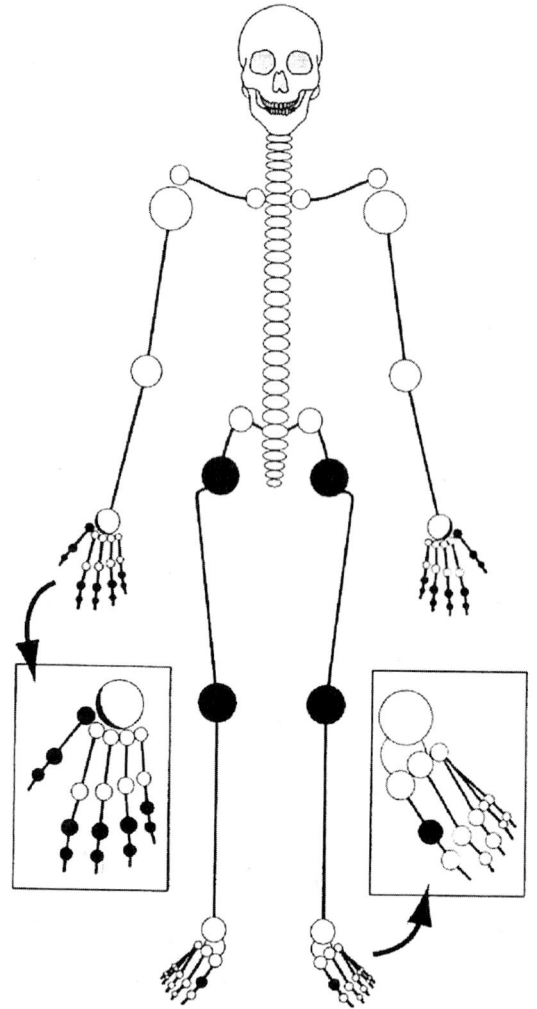

Figure 74-1   Joints affected by primary osteoarthritis. Reprinted with permission from Brandt KD: *Diagnosis and Nonsurgical Management of Osteoarthritis.* Caddo, OK, Professional Communications, p. 72, 2000.

ankles and elbows, major injuries account for a large proportion of disease.

Certain occupational groups are at high risk for OA in overused joints. For example, farmers have a high prevalence of hip OA, jackhammer operators a high prevalence of disease involving upper extremity joints, and miners a high prevalence of OA in both knees and spine. The increased risk for OA conferred by occupational overuse appears to be related to repeated excessive mechanical joint stress. For example, workers whose jobs require repeated knee bending have a higher incidence of knee OA.

Studies examining the relationship between sports activities and subsequent OA have produced conflicting results, in large part because of inadequate adjustments for major injury. Sports activities associated with a high incidence of injury and those involving repetitive torsional loading (activities that involve loading and concurrent twisting) may increase the risk for subsequent knee OA. In the absence of an acute injury, recreational (moderate) long-distance running and jogging do not appear to increase the risk for subsequent OA. However, elite

Table 74-2 Classification Criteria for Osteoarthritis of the Hips, Knees, and Hands

Hand Osteoarthritis	Knee Osteoarthritis	Hip Osteoarthritis

Hand pain, aching, or stiffness plus at least three of the following criteria:
  Hard tissue enlargement of two or more of 10 specified joints*
 	
  Hard tissue enlargement of two or more distal interphalangeal joints
  Fewer than three swollen metacarpophalangeal joints
  Deformity of one or more of 10 specified joints*
	Knee pain plus at least one of the following criteria:
	  Age greater than 50 y
	  Stiffness less than 30 min
	
	  Crepitus plus osteophytes on radiograph
		Hip pain plus at least two of the following criteria:
		  ESR <20 mm/h
		  Radiographic femoral or acetabular osteophytes
		  Radiographic joint-space narrowing

Sensitivity 84%	Sensitivity 91%	Sensitivity 89%
Specificity 87%	Specificity 86%	Specificity 91%

*Ten specified joints: second distal interphalangeal joints, third distal interphalangeal joints, second proximal interphalangeal joints, third proximal interphalangeal joints, first carpometacarpal joints.

Source: Reprinted with permission from Altman R, Asch E et al: Development of criteria for the classification and reporting of osteoarthritis: Classification of osteoarthritis of the knee. *Arthritis Rheum* 29:1039, 1986. Altman RD: Classification of disease: Osteoarthritis. *Semin Arthritis Rheum* 20 (suppl 2):40, 1991.

long-distance runners, such as nationally competitive athletes, may be at high risk for the development of subsequent knee and hip OA.

Mechanical factors Varus and valgus deformities of the knee joint are commonly seen in patients with knee OA

(Figure 74-3). In a varus deformity, increased forces are transmitted across the medial compartment of the tibiofemoral joint, whereas in a valgus deformity, increased forces are transmitted across the lateral compartment. In patients with OA, those with varus deformities are at a high risk of developing structural progression in

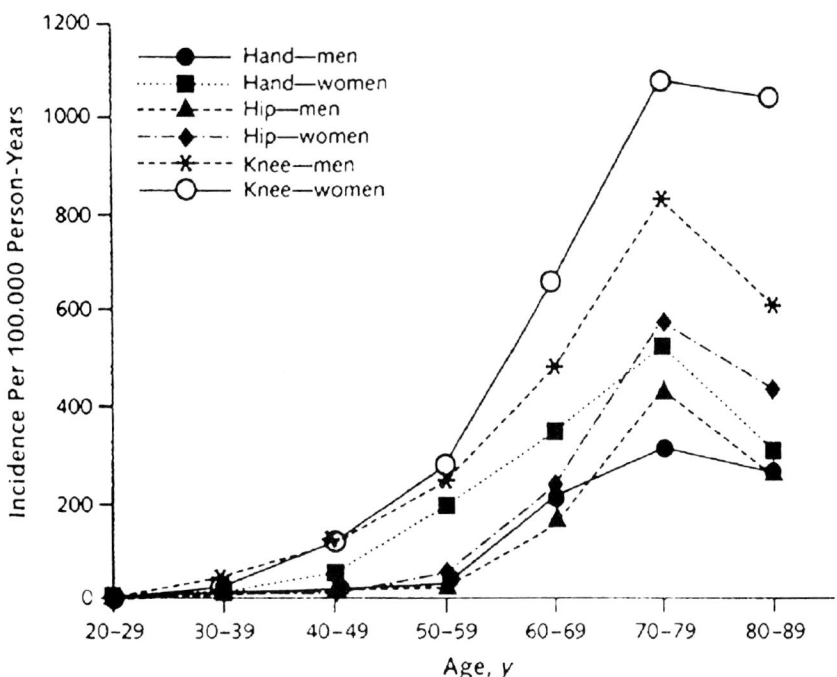

Figure 74-2 Age- and gender-specific incidence rates of osteoarthritis. Solid circles: hand, men; solid squares: hand, women; solid triangles: hip, men; solid diamonds: hip, women; asterisks: knee, men; open circles: knee, women. Reprinted with permission from Oliveria SA et al: Incidence of symptomatic hand, hip, and knee osteoarthritis among patients in a health maintenance organization. *Arthritis Rheum* 38:1134, 1995.

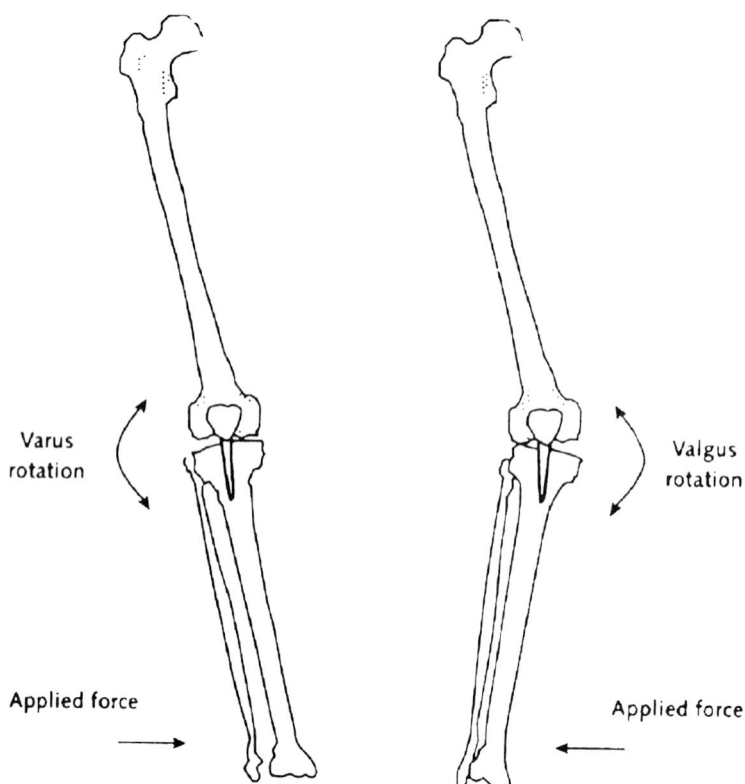

Figure 74-3   Varus and valgus deformities of the knee. Reprinted with permission from Sharma L et al: Does laxity alter the relationship between strength and physical function in knee osteoarthritis? *Arthritis Rheum* 42:25, 1999.

the medial compartment, whereas lateral compartment progression is likely in those with a valgus deformity. In addition, persons with varus and valgus malalignment are at higher risk of subsequent disability than those with a more neutral alignment. Mild acetabular dysplasia increases the incidence of hip OA in elderly women, suggesting that subclinical deformities may also increase the risk for OA, perhaps by distorting the forces normally transmitted across the involved joint.

Intact proprioception (position sense) is required to maintain joint stability. Proprioceptive acuity decreases with age, especially in elderly persons with limited mobility. In a cross-sectional study, proprioceptive accuracy was worse in both arthritic and nonarthritic knees of patients with OA compared to the knees of age-matched controls, suggesting that decreased proprioception increases the risk for disease.

Muscle weakness   Quadriceps muscle weakness is very common in patients with arthritis. This is particularly true in older persons, as aging is associated with a generalized decrease in muscle strength. Furthermore, joint swelling inhibits the contraction of muscles that bridge involved joints, and inactivity due to pain leads to disuse atrophy.

Although muscle weakness has generally been thought to be a consequence of knee OA, in a recent study involving women without evidence of radiographic OA at baseline, those with weaker quadriceps were more likely to develop radiographic OA after 30 months than their counterparts. This finding suggests that, in women, quadriceps weakness increases the risk for developing new OA.

Bone mass   In cross-sectional studies, women with higher bone mass were much more likely to have knee and hip OA compared to women with lower bone mass. Two longitudinal studies found that higher bone mass was associated with an increased risk for new-onset knee OA but, ironically, a decreased risk for radiographic progression in those with established disease.

Estrogen   The high incidence of OA occurring in women just after menopause (Figure 74-2) suggests that a deficiency in estrogen may have a role in the pathogenesis of this disease. This hypothesis is supported by observational studies demonstrating a protective effect of estrogen replacement therapy on radiographic OA. In the Heart Estrogen/Progestin Replacement Study, however, 4 years of combined hormonal replacement therapy had no significant effect on knee pain and disability.

Nutritional deficiencies   Nutritional factors have been examined as potential OA risk factors because of either their antioxidant properties or their role in maintaining normal bone metabolism. Observational studies suggest that patients with knee OA with low levels of plasma 25-hydroxyvitamin D are at high risk for knee and hip OA progression. One study has suggested that patients with low intakes of vitamin C are at higher risk for radiographic progression of their disease compared to those with higher intakes. Vitamin C is an antioxidant and might protect cartilage against reactive oxygen species–mediated damage. The association with vitamin D and OA progression may reflect the importance of this vitamin in maintaining normal bone metabolism.

Table 74-3 Magnetic Resonance Image Findings in Patients With Knee Osteoarthritis With and Without Pain

Magnetic Resonance Finding	Knee OA Subjects With Pain	Knee OA Subjects Without Pain	p Value
Any bone marrow lesion (%)	77.5	30.0	<.001
Large bone marrow lesion (%)	35.9	2.0	<.001
Moderate or large effusion (%)	54.6	15.6	<.001
Synovial thickening (%)	73.6	21.4	<.001

OA, osteoarthritis.

SOURCE: Reprinted with permission from Felson DT et al: The association of bone marrow lesions with pain in knee osteoarthritis. *Ann Intern Med* 134:541, 2001. Hill CL, et al: Knee effusions, popliteal cysts, and synovial thickening: Association with knee pain in osteoarthritis. *J Rheumatol* 28:1330, 2001.

Risk factors for disability in patients with osteoarthritis
Not all patients with radiographic evidence of OA have pain or functional limitations. The best-established predictor of disability in patients with OA, especially knee OA, is muscle weakness. In fact, quadriceps weakness has been shown to be a stronger predictor of lower limb disability than knee pain. The risk for disability is higher in women with OA than in men with OA. Other factors that increase the likelihood of disability in OA include decreased proprioception, malalignment, limited range of motion, aerobic deconditioning, and comorbidity. Many of these conditions are modifiable and may therefore present an opportunity to decrease the impact of OA.

PATHOGENESIS

Osteoarthritis results from dynamic processes involving all components of the joint (synovium, cartilage, and adjacent bone) in response to mechanical and/or inflammatory insults. OA may develop in a setting of excessive forces acting on a normal joint or normal forces acting on abnormal cartilage and surrounding tissues.

Hyaline articular cartilage loss is characteristic of OA and results from an imbalance of catabolic (lysosomal proteases, neutral metalloproteinases, and collagenases) and anabolic factors. In early disease, chondrocytes are hyperactive, producing excess amounts of cartilage matrix molecules and synthesizing higher quantities of metalloproteinases, which break down matrix. In advanced disease, chondrocytes produce less matrix.

Despite the increased activity of chondrocytes in early OA, the products produced (collagen, proteoglycan, and hyaluronan) do not function normally, and the resulting cartilage has inadequate biomechanical properties to deal with normal loading. As the disease progresses, catabolic proteins driven by interleukin-1 and other cytokines, coupled with repeated excess joint stress from maldistributed loading, overwhelm the attempts of chondrocytes to make repairs, resulting in fibrillation and erosion of cartilage and eventual exposure of underlying bone.

Calcium-containing crystals, including calcium pyrophosphate dihydrate and basic calcium phosphate, may play a role in the pathogenesis of OA. These crystals are commonly found in the synovial fluid of patients with OA, and patients with OA who have evidence of calcium deposition in their joints have more severe disease than patients without it. The synovial fluid of patients with OA and crystals demonstrates greater chondrolytic activity compared to that of patients with OA and without crystals, suggesting that crystals might accelerate cartilage breakdown, which is reflected clinically by more rapidly progressive and severe OA.

Although OA is commonly thought of as a degenerative, noninflammatory disease, mild synovial inflammation occurs in many patients with OA. The etiology of this synovitis is unknown, but it is present in animal models of OA caused by joint injury, suggesting that the release of factors from injured cartilage stimulates the inflammation of cells lining the joint.

In contrast to a normal joint, which is typified by smooth articular surfaces and surrounding bone, an OA joint is characterized by loss of cartilage and bony overgrowth, which are seen as joint-space narrowing and osteophytes on plain radiographs. At the individual patient level, however, the correlation between radiographic changes and symptoms is poor.

Pain in patients with OA may be due to synovitis, to abnormal forces on innervated soft tissue structures including the ligaments and joint capsule, to increased intraosseous pressure in adjacent subchondral bone, and/or to injury of adjacent muscles, tendons, and bursae attributable to abnormal biomechanics of the involved joints. A magnetic resonance imaging study found that bone marrow lesions, synovial thickening, and effusions were significantly more common in patients with knee OA with pain than in those without pain, suggesting that these pathologic features may be an important source of pain in OA (Table 74-3).

Once OA begins to develop in a joint, many factors potentiate the progression of disease. The wearing away of cartilage increases joint laxity, and joint swelling inhibits muscle contraction, creating weakness. Altered anatomy secondary to the focal loss of cartilage increases loading stresses on isolated joint areas, leading to further damage. Synovitis produces cytokines that prevent cartilage repair. Many of these vulnerabilities—weakness, laxity, decreased proprioception—occur naturally as part of aging and may explain why elderly people are at especially high risk for OA. In addition, evidence indicates that normal cartilage in elderly people responds poorly to anabolic stimuli, suggesting an intrinsic vulnerability with aging.

CLINICAL PRESENTATION

Symptoms

The onset of OA is almost always insidious, with patients reporting a gradual onset of symptoms over weeks to months (Table 74-4). The most common symptom associated with OA is pain, especially during or just after activity. For knee and hip OA, the activities that most often cause pain are getting up out of a chair, going up and down stairs, and walking. Patients with hip OA may have trouble putting their shoes and socks on and getting out of a car. Advanced disease is characterized by rest pain and eventually nocturnal pain.

A sensation of stiffness associated with inactivity, often referred to as "gelling," is also a common complaint of patients with OA. Gelling refers to difficulty in initiating movement of an involved joint after a period of rest and usually lasts for only a few minutes. Patients may also describe having early morning stiffness that, in contrast to stiffness in patients with rheumatoid arthritis, usually lasts less than 30 minutes. A reduced range of movement, due to either pain or mechanical factors (e.g., bony overgrowth and capsular tightening), is common in OA and may result in substantial disability. Many patients with knee OA experience knee instability and may report that their knees have given way or buckled. Unlike the situation in younger patients with ligament injuries, the feeling of instability is probably related to muscle weakness and not to actual ligament damage.

Signs

An OA joint is characterized by bony swelling, tenderness of the joint margins and surrounding periarticular soft tissues, crepitus, and deformity (Table 74-4). Enlargement of the involved joint is usually due to bony overgrowth and not synovitis. Synovial effusions do occur in some pa-

Table 74-4   Symptoms and Signs of Osteoarthritis

Symptoms
   Pain with or after activity localized to the affected
      joint(s)
   Less than 30 min morning stiffness
   Gelling
   Instability and buckling (most commonly with knee
      osteoarthritis)
   Functional limitations
Signs
   Bony enlargement
   Soft tissue swelling
   Joint tenderness
   Periarticular tenderness
   Decreased range of movement
   Crepitus
   Deformity
   Effusions (most commonly with knee osteoarthritis)

tients, particularly those with knee OA. In patients with moderate to large knee effusions, an accumulation of synovial fluid may protrude posteriorly, causing the development of a popliteal or Baker's cyst. Ruptured popliteal cysts dissect into the soft tissues of the calf, causing pain and swelling, and may be confused with deep venous thrombosis. Heberden's and Bouchard's nodes are characteristic localized swellings occurring over the distal and proximal interphalangeal joints, respectively. They begin as painful cystic structures that over time become firm and less tender. Palpable coarse crepitus is a characteristic finding in OA. In patients with more severe disease, crepitus may be audible.

Joint deformities characterize advanced disease. For example, in OA of the thumb base, there is squaring of the radial wrist due to bony enlargement of the carpometacarpal joint; in distal interphalangeal and proximal interphalangeal joint OA, there is lateral subluxation of the bone distal to the affected joints; in hip OA, joint narrowing creates a leg length discrepancy; and a varus deformity of the knee develops as a consequence of medial joint involvement. A valgus deformity associated with OA of the lateral tibiofemoral joint may also occur, but it is less common, at least in the United States.

Diagnosis and Differential Diagnosis in Osteoarthritis

The diagnosis of OA is based on clinical and radiographic features. Characteristic radiographic changes in established disease include cysts and sclerosis in the bone deep to the articular cartilage, osteophytes, and asymmetric joint-space narrowing. However, radiographs may be normal in patients with early disease.

Laboratory parameters are most useful in ruling out comorbid conditions that may affect the safety of OA treatments, such as renal or hepatic disease. When effusions are present, joint aspiration is helpful to rule out coexisting inflammatory disease such as crystal-induced arthritis. Effusions consistent with OA are noninflammatory; that is, they appear clear and have less than 2000 white blood cells/mm^3, of which fewer than 50 percent are polymorphonuclear leukocytes.

Complications in the clinical assessment of patients with OA most commonly occur when new or worsening joint symptoms are mistakenly attributed to OA. For example, middle-aged women with established knee OA presenting with worsening knee pain might have superimposed crystal-induced arthritis, anserine bursitis, spontaneous osteonecrosis of the knee, or worsening OA. Similarly, a patient with known OA of the carpometacarpal joint might have worsening thumb pain because of de Quervain's tenosynovitis. Consideration of a broad differential diagnosis is important in patients with established OA to ensure an accurate diagnosis and appropriate therapy.

MANAGEMENT OF OSTEOARTHRITIS

The management of OA is aimed at decreasing symptoms and improving or maintaining function. Nonpharmacologic, pharmacologic, and surgical interventions are

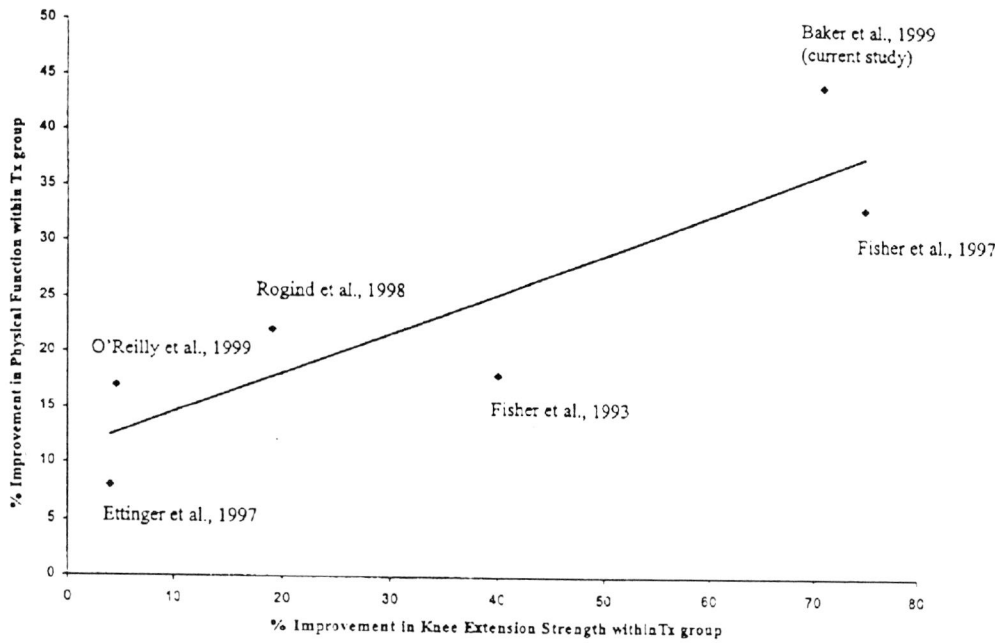

Figure 74-4   Effect of quadriceps-strengthening exercises on physical function in knee osteoarthritis trials. Physical function is self-reported; *r* = .877, *p* = .02. Reprinted with permission from Baker KR et al: The efficacy of home-based, progressive strength training in older adults with knee osteoarthritis: A randomized controlled trial. *J Rheumatol* 28:1655, 2001.

available as possible therapies for patients with symptomatic OA. Except for total joint replacement, each modality is only modestly effective. Treatment plans, therefore, generally combine both nonpharmacologic and pharmacologic measures.

Nonpharmacologic Therapies

Weight Loss

Evidence shows that combined programs of weight loss and exercise lead to improvement in pain and self-reported measures of physical function in older obese adults with knee OA. Furthermore, the combination of weight loss and exercise is more efficacious than either alone.

Exercise

Controlled trials have demonstrated that, compared to educational interventions, aerobic exercise is an effective means of maintaining function and decreasing pain in patients with knee OA. In a large trial, patients randomized to aerobic exercise (3 months of group-supervised exercise followed by 15 months of home-based exercise with limited supervision) had improvement in function compared to those in a control group whose function progressively declined. Isometric quadriceps strengthening exercises followed by progressive resistance training also decreases pain and improves function in patients with knee OA (Figure 74-4).

It is not clear which type of exercise is better. Exercise interventions that combine multiple modalities may improve symptoms more than unimodal interventions. Maintaining adherence to exercise is challenging, especially for patients who have no history of regular physical activity. Guidelines and videos demonstrating appropriate range-of-motion and flexibility exercises, muscle strengthening, and aerobic exercises for older adults with arthritis are readily available (Chapter 72).

Joint Protection Techniques

Joint protection techniques decrease the loading forces transmitted across painful joints. Examples of these techniques include the use of proper shoes with well-cushioned soles, the use of assistive devices such as canes (which can decrease forces transmitted across contralateral joints by 50%), and the avoidance of positions or activities associated with excessive mechanical stress such as sitting on low chairs, kneeling, and squatting. Joint protection techniques may be very helpful for older adults with all types of chronic arthritis.

Braces and Orthotics

Supportive devices that immobilize or limit motion in the joint may be of use in the treatment of patients with knee OA. A randomized controlled trial involving 170 patients found that the use of an elastic knee brace was more effective in decreasing pain than standard care. A second trial found that patients with medial knee OA—randomized to either a rigid brace (that pushed the knee into a more valgus alignment) or a neoprene sleeve—had less pain on a 6-minute walking test compared to patients receiving standard medical care (Figure 74-5).

Other potentially useful techniques include medial taping of the patella for patients with patellofemoral OA and splinting of the carpometacarpal joint for patients with

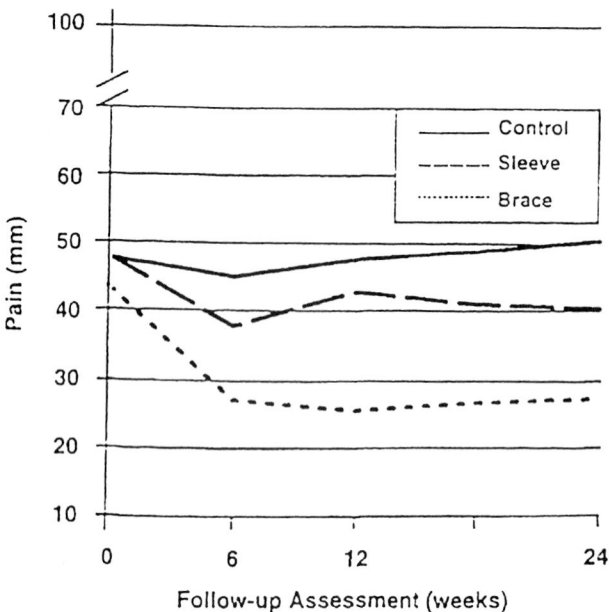

Figure 74-5   Effect of bracing on knee osteoarthritis pain and function. Graph showing the mean absolute scores for pain on a 6-minute walking test. (The worst possible score is 100 mm.) Solid line, control; dashed line, sleeve; dotted line, brace. Reprinted with permission from Kirkley A et al: The effect of bracing on varus gonarthrosis. *J Bone Joint Surg Am* 81A:539, 1999.

painful OA of the thumb base. Uncontrolled trials suggest that wedged insoles designed to correct varus knee stress decrease pain and improve function in knee OA. A recent controlled trial, however, showed that these insoles had no effect.

Ambulatory and Adaptive Aids

Ambulatory aids can act to both increase stability and decrease loading forces across painful joints. A cane, when used correctly, can increase a patient's sense of security and decrease pain. Crutches or walkers should be used for patients requiring further support.

Adaptive aids can also minimize the disability associated with OA. For example, a reaching aid might allow someone with hip OA to put on his or her socks. High stools or chairs facilitate tasks that require prolonged standing, and raised toilet seats and shower benches might allow patients to remain independent in performing basic functions. These interventions, although not aimed at alleviating symptoms, may significantly improve function and quality of life.

Acupuncture

The results of studies examining the effectiveness of acupuncture in decreasing pain due to OA are conflicting, in part, because of small sample sizes and poor study design. A trial using sham acupuncture as a placebo found that patients with OA randomized to the acupuncture arm had significantly greater pain relief compared to those in the control group. A large multicenter National Institutes of Health (NIH)-sponsored trial is currently underway

to examine the efficacy, safety, and cost-effectiveness of acupuncture for patients with OA.

Behavioral Interventions

Behavioral interventions are an effective means of improving health care and outcomes for patients with OA. For example, telephone-based counseling programs improve functional status and decrease the need for future health care services. Group education programs, such as the Arthritis Self-Management Plan, improve health status and moderately reduce pain. Cognitive-behavioral therapy and didactic education programs also improve pain and function. Studies suggest that a common theme underlying effective behavioral interventions is an improvement in self-efficacy, a sense by patients that they have control over the symptoms and impact of their disease.

Pharmacologic Therapies

The only current indication for drug therapy in patients with OA is pain. There are no disease-modifying drugs currently approved to prevent the structural progression of OA, as there are for rheumatoid arthritis. Pharmacologic therapy should always be added to nonpharmacologic measures. This is especially true given the modest efficacy associated with available drugs and the increased risk of drug toxicity in older adults.

Nonopioid Analgesics

Acetaminophen is the nonopioid analgesic most commonly used in treating older adults with OA. Although it is generally well tolerated, chronic use of acetaminophen has been associated with an increased risk of renal insufficiency. In addition, acetaminophen must be used cautiously in patients with known liver disease and avoided by patients who consume excessive amounts of alcohol because of the increased risk of hepatotoxicity associated with these conditions.

Opioid Analgesics

Opioid analgesics are an alternative when inadequate pain control is achieved with acetaminophen. Tramadol is a synthetic opioid agonist that inhibits the reuptake of norepinephrine and serotonin. Common adverse effects include nausea, constipation, and drowsiness. Seizures are a rare side effect and have been reported in patients taking doses above the recommend range, in patients with known seizure disorders, and in patients taking concomitant medications that lower the seizure threshold.

Other opioid analgesics may also be effective in patients with OA. In a randomized trial, controlled-release oxycodone was superior to a placebo in reducing pain and improving enjoyment of life, mood, and sleep in patients with moderate to severe OA but caused frequent side effects, which often led to drug discontinuation. Therefore, although moderately effective, adverse effects commonly limit the use of opioid preparations in older patients.

Table 74-5 Risk Factors for Peptic Ulcer Disease Induced by Nonsteroidal Antiinflammatory Drug Use

Age

Previous history of peptic ulcer disease

Dose and duration of NSAID use

Concomitant use of more than one NSAID

Use of corticosteroids

Use of anticoagulants

Alcohol use

Poor health status

NSAID, nonsteroidal antiinflammatory drug.
*Including low-dose (81 mg/d) or enteric-coated aspirin.

Nonsteroidal Antiinflammatory Drugs

Nonsteroidal antiinflammatory drugs (NSAIDs) are among the drugs most commonly prescribed for OA. Multiple randomized controlled trials have demonstrated that NSAIDs are superior to a placebo in decreasing pain and stiffness related to OA. A well-designed, large, controlled trial found that NSAIDs were also more efficacious than acetaminophen in patients with knee OA. The major concern related to the use of NSAIDs is the risk of toxicity. Chronic NSAID use causes 16,500 deaths annually in patients with arthritis in the United States. Each year, up to 2 percent of older adults using NSAIDs on a chronic basis present to hospitals with a serious upper gastrointestinal tract complication such as bleeding or perforation. Between 20 percent and 30 percent of all peptic ulcer–related hospitalizations and deaths are attributable to NSAIDs in patients older than 65 years. In fact, age is one of the strongest risk factors for the development of clinically significant NSAID-induced ulcer disease. Other risk factors are listed in Table 74-5.

For patients obtaining clinical benefit from NSAIDs, there are several strategies available to practitioners to decrease the risk of gastrointestinal toxicity. Misoprostol at doses of 200 μg three to four times a day decreases the risk of both gastric and duodenal ulcers, as well as serious ulcer complications. Adverse effects related to misoprostol, including abdominal discomfort and diarrhea, are common. Proton pump inhibitors are as effective or more effective than misoprostol in preventing endoscopic ulcers. Histamine-2 receptor antagonists are efficacious in decreasing duodenal ulcers but not the more common NSAID-induced gastric ulcers.

Currently two classes of antiinflammatory agents are available for patients with OA. Both inhibit cyclooxygenase (COX), the enzyme responsible for converting arachidonic acid to prostaglandins and thromboxanes. COX exists in two isoforms: COX-1 and COX-2. Nonselective NSAIDs inhibit both isoforms, whereas the newer agents (COX-2 inhibitors) selectively inhibit COX-2.

Cyclooxygenase-1 is constitutively expressed in almost all tissues, most notably the gastrointestinal tract, kidneys, endothelial cells, and platelets. The COX-2 isoform is constitutively expressed in the brain, kidney, and female reproductive tract and is upregulated at sites of inflammation. COX-2 synthesis is stimulated by interleukin-1, tumor necrosis factor α, lipopolysaccharide, and growth factors.

Cyclooxygenase-1 is required to maintain the normal gastrointestinal mucosa. Inhibition of this isoenzyme explains the increased risk for peptic ulcer disease caused by nonselective NSAIDs. In contrast, COX-2 inhibitors do not inhibit COX-1 at therapeutic doses and therefore do not interfere with maintenance of the normal gastrointestinal mucosa.

There is no evidence suggesting that COX-2 inhibitors have superior therapeutic efficacy compared to nonselective NSAIDs. However, compared to NSAIDs, COX-2 inhibitors are associated with a significantly lower risk of endoscopic ulcers as well as serious ulcer complications. In a combined analysis of eight trials evaluating the efficacy of rofecoxib (a COX-2 inhibitor) in patients with OA, the relative risk (95 percent confidence interval) of serious gastrointestinal adverse effects was 0.51 (0.26 to 1.00) for rofecoxib versus NSAIDs.

It is not known whether the combination of NSAIDs and proton pump inhibitors is as safe as COX-2 inhibitors, but one study found similar rates of recurrent gastrointestinal complications in high-risk patients randomized to either celecoxib (5.2 percent) or the combination of lansoprazole and naproxen (3.5 percent). The risk of renal toxicity associated with COX-2 inhibitors is comparable to that expected with nonselective NSAIDs.

Cyclooxygenase-2 inhibitors, unlike NSAIDs, inhibit prostacyclin without a commensurate blocking of platelet thromboxane, leading to concerns that they might increase the risk for vascular thrombosis. Evidence supporting this possibility, however, is conflicting. Ibuprofen, when administered before low-dose aspirin, reduces aspirin's antithrombotic effect by competing for the binding site for aspirin on platelets. Other NSAIDs and COX-2 inhibitors do not have similar effects on aspirin platelet effects. Thus, for a patient taking low-dose aspirin, ibuprofen should either be avoided or be administered after aspirin tablets are ingested. It should be noted, however, that low-dose aspirin is associated with an approximately twofold increased risk for peptic ulcer disease and that this risk is further increased with the addition of a NSAID.

Glucosamine and Chondroitin Sulfate

Glucosamine and chondroitin are both compounds that occur naturally in joint cartilage. Numerous, mostly industry-sponsored, randomized controlled trials have demonstrated that these agents decrease pain in patients with OA. A meta-analysis has suggested that the quality of most of these trials was poor and that there are small null trials for which the results have not been published. Nonetheless, the preponderance of evidence available suggests that both agents are moderately effective in decreasing pain in patients with OA (Figure 74-6). Preliminary evidence suggests that glucosamine might also delay the progression of

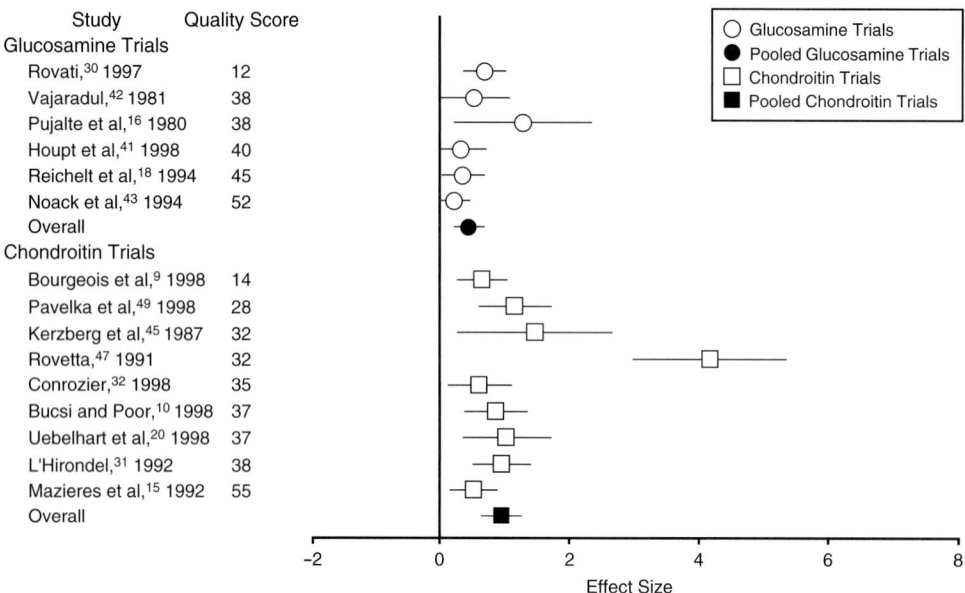

Figure 74-6   Forest plot of effect sizes for trials and pooled effects. Open circles, glucosamine trials; solid circles, pooled glucosamine trials; open squares, chondroitin trials; solid squares, pooled chondroitin trials. The 95 percent confidence intervals are shown using lines extending from the symbols. Effect size: 0.8 = large effect, 0.5 = moderate effect, 0.2 = small effect. Reprinted with permission from McAlindon TE et al: Glucosamine and chondroitin for treatment of osteoarthritis: A systematic quality assessment and meta-analysis. *JAMA* 283:1469, 2000.

radiographic OA. Patients typically experience few if any adverse effects related to either glucosamine or chondroitin sulfate use. Stomach upset has been reported but at rates comparable to those found in patients taking a placebo. A multicenter randomized NIH-sponsored controlled trial is currently being conducted to determine the efficacy of glucosamine and chondroitin sulfate, either alone or in combination, in patients with knee OA.

Topical Agents

The use of topical analgesics may also benefit patients with OA. Based on trial evidence, applying capsaicin cream four times daily significantly improves pain in hands and knees compared to a placebo. Adverse effects are restricted to localized burning, which decreases or disappears with subsequent applications.

Intraarticular Drugs

Intraarticular corticosteroids   Intraarticular corticosteroids are widely used in patients with OA, most commonly in those who have recurrent effusions. Controlled trials have found that this treatment modality may be effective in providing short-term pain relief (up to 4 weeks). In clinical practice, however, some patients have a sustained response to intraarticular steroids. There are no clinical, radiographic, or laboratory markers that accurately predict which patients are most likely to respond to intraarticular corticosteroid injections.

Hyaluronic acid   Hyaluronic acid is a linear polysaccharide found in normal synovial fluid. Three preparations of hyaluronic acids, which differ primarily in molecular weight, have been approved for use in knee OA. The

procedure is generally safe, but up to 20 percent of patients experience a transient joint flare after the injection. The mechanism of action may be improved joint viscosity through the stimulation of endogenous synthesis of hyaluronate (because the treatment remains in the joint only briefly), inhibition of synovial prostaglandins or other anti-inflammatory effects, and/or preventing the degradation of cartilage proteoglycans.

Randomized controlled trials examining the efficacy of hyaluronic acid have yielded conflicting results, in part because of poor study design, unblinded assessment of outcomes, significant dropout rates, and large, sustained placebo responses. Intent-to-treat analyses of the largest trials have shown the compound to have no effect when compared to a placebo. Based on the weak efficacy data available, some experts recommend that this modality be reserved for patients who have not responded to conventional therapy. Further research is required to better clarify whether, and under what circumstances, hyaluronate injections are efficacious in decreasing the symptoms associated with OA.

Surgical Interventions

Several surgical options are available for patients who have an inadequate response to medical therapy.

Arthroscopy

Arthroscopic surgery has long been used as a therapeutic modality for patients with knee OA, but clinical trials have demonstrated that arthroscopic knee lavage is not more efficacious than sham arthroscopy, at least after 24 months. Although arthroscopy may be indicated for patients with acute tears or ligamentous injuries in the knee, arthroscopy should probably no longer be offered as a therapeutic option for unselected patients with knee OA.

Cartilage Transplantation

Cartilage transplantation is increasingly being performed in clinical practice. Although the results are encouraging, especially when growth factors are used to encourage cell growth of chondrocytes, the procedure is currently reserved for patients with localized cartilage defects and is therefore not appropriate for patients with OA who have much more extensive cartilage, subchondral bone, and surrounding soft tissue involvement.

Total Joint Replacement

Total joint replacement is the most effective intervention available for patients with OA in the knee or hip. This procedure significantly improves function and in many cases eliminates pain. According to a meta-analysis, almost 90 percent of patients have a favorable outcome after total knee replacement. Joint replacement surgery also improves the quality of life for patients with OA and has been shown to be highly cost-effective.

Postarthroplasty physical function is dependent on the level of disability prior to surgery, and patients with severe disability at the time of joint replacement do not respond as well as those with milder levels of functional limitation. Age does not appear to adversely affect outcomes following total joint replacement, with patients older than 80 years recovering just as well as those between the ages of 55 and 79 years. However, patients aged 70 years and older with severe OA disability may be much less likely to be offered the operation than younger patients. Total joint arthroplasty procedures for joints other than the knee and hip are still under development, and outcomes related to these interventions have not been as favorable.

Others Therapies

Many other therapies have been reported to be useful in OA, some of which have been shown to be effective in at least one randomized controlled trial (Table 74-6). Further studies regarding the possible mechanisms of action, safety, and effectiveness of these interventions will be required before specific recommendations regarding their use in older patients can be made.

Future Treatments

Current areas under investigation include the development of disease-modifying drugs whose objective is to decrease the rate of progression of structural damage in OA. A 3-year placebo controlled trial found that 51 percent of patients with hip OA taking diacerein, a derivative of rhubarb, had less cartilage loss (as indicated by a diminution in progressive joint-space loss) than patients taking a placebo. Twenty-five percent of patients randomized to diacerein

Table 74-6 Osteoarthritis Treatments With One or More Placebo-Controlled Trial Demonstrating Efficacy

Avocado/soybean extract

Vitamin E

Niacinamide

Dextrose intraarticular injections (10%)

Oral enzymes

S-Adenosylmethionine

Acupuncture

Spa therapy

Energy
  Narrow band light
  Low-level laser
  Pulsed magnetic fields
  Pulsed electrical stimulation

withdrew because of adverse effects, the most common being diarrhea, urine discoloration, and a rash. Diacerein may slow OA progression by inhibiting interleukin-1, a central degradative cytokine in cartilage. This compound has also been shown to decrease pain and disability in patients with both hip and knee OA in short-term trials.

Therapies to limit cartilage loss are under widespread development. Most, including novel compounds and older drugs such as tetracyclines, focus on preventing metalloproteinase-mediated cartilage degradation.

Therapies that replace or repair cartilage and underlying bone, menisci, and/or ligaments are under development and may result in arthroscopic OA treatments that address localized pathology. These procedures are most likely to be effective in relatively young individuals with early disease.

PREVENTION

Osteoarthritis is a major cause of disability in older adults. As the population ages, this disease will have an even greater impact on society. The modification of risk factors could decrease the incidence of and disability associated with OA. There are three levels of prevention: primary, preventing incident or new-onset disease; secondary, preventing progression in people with early disease; and tertiary, preventing disability in patients with established disease.

Obesity is the strongest known modifiable risk factor for knee OA. Eliminating obesity could decrease the incidence of knee OA by up to 50 percent in women, in whom the relationship is strongest. From the individual patient's perspective, an overweight woman of average height (body mass index greater than 25) can decrease her risk of developing subsequent symptomatic knee OA by 50 percent if she loses 5 kg. Weight loss can also significantly decrease pain and improve function in patients with established disease.

Table 74–7   Strategies to Prevent the Onset, Progression, and Disability Associated With Osteoarthritis

Primary Prevention	Secondary Prevention	Tertiary Prevention
Weight loss	Weight loss	Exercise
Prevent injury	Muscle-strengthening exercises	Analgesic medications (topical, oral, intraarticular)
Modify job environment	Improve alignment	Total joint replacement
Muscle-strengthening exercises	Vitamin D	Behavioral strategies
Improve joint stability		

Although difficult in practice, eliminating major joint injuries and overuse activities that injure the joint more insidiously might be extremely important in preventing OA. In a study involving older male workers, occupational knee bending accounted for more subsequent knee OA than obesity. Epidemiologic data predict that preventing knee injuries could decrease the incidence of knee OA by up to 25 percent and that eliminating repeated knee bending and carrying of excessive loads could decrease the incidence of knee OA by up to 30 percent.

Longitudinal data suggest that muscle strengthening might decrease the risk of incident knee OA in women. Table 74-7 summarizes the prevention strategies available for OA patients.

REFERENCES

American College of Rheumatology Subcommittee on Osteoarthritis Guidelines: Recommendations for the medical management of osteoarthritis of the hip and knee. *Arthritis Rheum* 43:1905, 2000.

Dougados M et al: Evaluation of the structure-modifying effects of diacerein in hip osteoarthritis. *Arthritis Rheum* 44:2539, 2001.

Ettinger WH et al: A randomized trial comparing aerobic exercise and resistance exercise with a health education program in older adults with knee osteoarthritis. *JAMA* 277:25, 1997.

Felson DT et al: Osteoarthritis, new insights, Part 1: The disease and its risk factors. *Ann Intern Med* 133:635, 2000.

Felson DT et al: Osteoarthritis, new insights, Part 2: Treatment approaches. *Ann Intern Med* 133:726, 2000.

Felson DT et al: Weight loss reduces the risk of symptomatic knee osteoarthritis in women: The Framingham Study. *Ann Intern Med* 116:535, 1992.

Guccione AA et al: Specific diseases and their effects on functional limitations in elders in the Framingham Study. *Am J Public Health* 84:351, 1994.

Hawker G et al: Health-related quality of life after knee replacement. *J Bone Joint Surg Am* 80:163, 1998.

Hawker GA et al: Differences between men and women in the rate of use of hip and knee arthroplasty. *N Engl J Med* 342:1016, 2000.

Kirkley A et al: The effect of bracing on varus gonarthrosis. *J Bone Joint Surg Am* 81-A:539, 1999.

McAlindon TE et al: Relation of dietary intake and serum levels of vitamin D to progression of osteoarthritis of the knee among participants in the Framingham Study. *Ann Intern Med* 125:353, 1996.

McAlindon TE et al: Glucosamine and chondroitin for treatment of osteoarthritis: A systematic quality assessment and meta-analysis. *JAMA* 283:1469, 2000.

Oliveria S et al: The incidence of symptomatic hand, hip, and knee osteoarthritis in a health maintenance organization. *Arthritis Rheum* 38:1134, 1995.

Pelletier JP et al: Osteoarthritis, an inflammatory disease: Potential implication for the selection of new therapeutic targets. *Arthritis Rheum* 44:1237, 2001.

Poole AR et al: Changes in cartilage metabolism in arthritis are reflected by altered serum and synovial fluid levels of the cartilage proteoglycan aggrecana: Implications for pathogenesis. *J Clin Invest* 94:25, 1994.

Sharma L, Felson DT: Studying how osteoarthritis causes disability: Nothing is simple. *J Rheumatol* 25:1, 1998.

Sharma L et al: The role of knee alignment in disease progression and functional decline in knee osteoarthritis. *JAMA* 286:188, 2001.

Simon LS: Viscosupplementation therapy with intraarticular hyaluronic acid: Fact or fantasy? *Rheum Dis Clin North Am* 25:345, 1999.

Slemenda C et al: Quadriceps weakness and osteoarthritis of the knee. *Ann Intern Med* 127:97, 1997.

Spector TD et al: Genetic influences on osteoarthritis in women: A twin study. *BMJ* 312:940, 1996.

the hip, anteroposterior spine, lateral spine, calcaneus, and wrist can be measured using this technology. Quantitative computerized tomography (QCT) is also used to measure BMD of the spine. Specific software can adapt CT scanners for BMD measurement. The advantages of DXA over QCT include lower cost, lower radiation exposure, and better reproducibility over time. The cost of DXA is approximately $200, and Medicare will cover approximately $125 of these costs. Newer techniques, such as peripheral DXA (measures wrist BMD) or ultrasonography of the calcaneus, may be useful for general osteoporosis screening, and they have the advantage of reduced cost and portability. In a recent study, peripheral bone densitometry (performed at the heel, finger or forearm) was highly predictive of hip, spine, wrist, rib and forearm fractures over the subsequent 12 months. Current recommendations for measurement of BMD are (1) all postmenopausal women under age 65 years with one or more additional risk factors (other than menopause); (2) all women over 65 years, regardless of additional risk factors; (3) all postmenopausal women who present with fracture (to confirm diagnosis and determine severity); (4) women considering therapy for osteoporosis, if BMD testing would facilitate the decision; and (5) women who have been on hormone replacement therapy (HRT) for prolonged periods of time (even with long-term HRT, women may have low BMD). A recent study of more than 200,000 postmenopausal women from more than 4000 primary care practices in 34 states reported that approximately 50 percent of this population had low BMD that was previously undetected, including 7 percent of women with osteoporosis. This study suggests that efforts should be made to increase BMD measurements in postmenopausal women; however, further study is required to determine the usefulness of various clinical decision rules in medical practice.

BMD may also be used to establish the diagnosis and severity of osteoporosis in men, and should be considered in men with low-trauma fracture, radiographic changes consistent with low bone mass, or diseases known to place an individual at risk for osteoporosis. Data relating bone mineral density to fracture risk were originally derived from studies completed in women, but recent data suggest that similar associations may be valid in men as well.

Biochemical Markers of Bone Turnover

Serum and urine biochemical markers of bone turnover have been used successfully to assess rapid turnover states such as Paget's disease and primary hyperparathyroidism. Bone turnover changes in osteoporosis are generally smaller and require more sensitive methods. Markers are available that reflect collagen breakdown (or bone resorption) and bone formation. Increased levels of markers have been associated with increased hip fracture risk, decreased bone density, and increased bone loss in older adults. In addition, markers of bone resorption and formation decrease in response to antiresorptive treatment and increase in response to PTH, a treatment with anabolic properties. The use of markers in clinical practice, however, is controversial because of the substantial overlap of marker values in women with high and low bone density

or rate of bone loss. Furthermore, few studies have compared the response of a particular marker (or combination of markers) and bone density to therapy in order to determine the magnitude of decrease of a biochemical marker necessary to prevent bone loss or, more importantly, fracture. Be that as it may, markers are most useful in assessing the response of an individual patient to treatment. Urinary deoxypyridinoline cross-links, N- and C-telopeptides of type I collagen, and serum N-telopeptides of type I collagen are commercially available markers of bone resorption that may be useful in monitoring response to treatment in older women. The advantage of the serum versus urinary markers is that the intrapatient variability tends to be lower with serum markers, thus reducing error.

MANAGEMENT

Osteoporosis develops in older adults when the normal processes of bone formation and resorption become uncoupled or unbalanced, resulting in bone loss. Osteoporosis prevention and treatment programs, then, should focus on strategies that minimize bone resorption and maximize bone formation as well as strategies that reduce falls. A number of nonpharmacologic and pharmacologic options are available to health care providers. Modification of risk factors (see Table 75-4) is an important first step in preventing osteoporotic fractures in older adults.

Nonpharmacologic:

Exercise

Exercise is an important component of osteoporosis treatment and prevention programs. Data in older men and women suggest a positive association between current exercise and hip BMD. Among regular exercisers, those who reported strenuous or moderate exercise had higher BMD at the hip than did those who reported mild or less-than-mild exercise. Similar associations were seen for lifelong regular exercisers and hip BMD. In a randomized study of women at least 10 years past menopause, the group receiving calcium supplementation plus exercise had less bone loss at the hip than did those assigned to calcium alone. Furthermore, high-intensity strength training effectively maintains femoral neck BMD as well as improves muscle mass, strength and balance in postmenopausal women compared to nonexercising controls, suggesting that resistance training would be useful to help maintain BMD and to reduce the risk of falls in older adults.

Marked decrease in physical activity or immobilization results in a decline in bone mass; accordingly, it is important to encourage older adults to be as active as possible. Weight-bearing exercise, such as walking, can be recommended for older adults who should be encouraged to start slowly and gradually increase both the number of days, as well as the time, walked each day. Physical therapy is an important part of osteoporosis treatment programs, especially after acute vertebral compression fracture. The physical therapist can provide postural exercises, alternative modalities for pain reduction, and can suggest changes in body mechanics that may help prevent future fracture.

Nutrition

Calcium and vitamin D are required for bone health at all ages. A consensus conference recommended 1200 mg per day of elemental calcium for postmenopausal women and men older than age 65 years in order to maintain a positive calcium balance. The amount of vitamin D required is between 400 and 800 IU per day. Calcium plus vitamin D at different doses increases or maintains bone density in pre- and postmenopausal women and prevents hip and other nonvertebral fractures in older adults. Furthermore, women with acute hip fracture have lower 25(OH) vitamin D levels and higher PTH levels than do women admitted for elective hip replacement with or without osteoporosis by BMD, supporting a role for vitamin D deficiency and secondary hyperparathyroidism in hip fracture. In a recent study, the beneficial effect of calcium supplementation on BMD and femoral medullary expansion in older men and women was demonstrated; vitamin D alone was more effective in men and women with lower vitamin D levels. Thus, adequate calcium and vitamin D should be recommended to all older adults, regardless of BMD, in order to maximize bone health.

Additional nutritional aspects may also play a role in bone loss and fracture in older adults. Two recent prospective studies examined the effect of various nutritional factors on bone loss and fracture risk in older adults. From the Framingham Osteoporosis Study, higher baseline magnesium, potassium, and fruit and vegetable intakes were associated with higher baseline BMD; none of these parameters were associated with bone loss in women. In men, increased potassium and magnesium intake were associated with lower bone loss at the femoral neck. Baseline BMD values were not associated with protein intake. Lower baseline protein intake or percent of total energy from animal protein, however, was associated with greater bone loss at the femoral neck and lumbar spine. In another prospective cohort study, the Study of Osteoporotic Fractures, BMD was not associated with the ratio of animal to vegetable protein intake, but a higher ratio of animal/vegetable protein intake was associated with greater femoral neck bone loss and increased risk of hip fracture. These studies suggest that nutritional factors other than calcium and vitamin D are important for bone health in older adults. Prospective randomized studies are indicated to further elucidate the role of nutrition in prevention and treatment of osteoporosis in older adults.

Pharmacologic

Estrogen Replacement Therapy (see Chap. 97)

Estrogen replacement therapy (ERT) is an important choice for prevention of osteoporosis. In case control and cohort studies, estrogen replacement therapy is associated with 30 to 70 percent reduction in hip fracture incidence. Multiple studies demonstrate that postmenopausal estrogen use will prevent bone loss at the hip and spine when initiated within 10 years of menopause and other studies suggest that older women with low initial bone mass gain more bone than younger women. However, there have been few prospective studies of ERT and fracture prevention. One was a small study that demonstrated a reduction in vertebral fractures in postmenopausal women with transdermal estradiol, compared to placebo. The Women's Health Initiative is an ongoing randomized, placebo-controlled study of the effect of ERT (conjugated equine estrogen 0.625 mg/d) on hip fracture in postmenopausal women.

Few studies have evaluated the use of estrogen in women in older than age 70 years. Observational data, however, from the Study of Osteoporotic Fractures support a protective effect of current estrogen use against hip fracture, even in the oldest women. Furthermore, small short-term studies suggest that older women are responsive to estrogen treatment and a recent study demonstrated that ERT increased BMD of the spine and hip in frail, older women with just 9 months of treatment. Other studies suggest that low-dose estrogen in combination with calcium and vitamin D have an additive effect on bone turnover in women older than 70 years of age. Recent data suggest that lower doses of estrogen are effective in reducing bone resorption and bone loss in older women; the lower doses also result in fewer side effects than the usual replacement doses typically used by clinicians. In a randomized placebo, controlled study, 0.25 mg/d was as effective as 0.5 mg/d and 1.0 mg/d of 17β-estradiol in reducing biochemical markers of bone turnover in 75-year-old women, compared to placebo. In this study, the side-effect profile of 0.25 mg/d was similar to placebo and significantly different from the two higher doses. In a longer-term study, 0.3 mg/d conjugated equine estrogen (CEE) plus 2.5-mg/d medroxyprogesterone acetate (MPA) increased bone density of the hip and spine in older women who were vitamin D replete. Table 75-6 lists the various preparations of estrogen are listed, along with dosing regimens. Estrogen may be given in either continuous or cyclical fashion, depending on the preference of each woman.

Bisphosphonates

Alendronate   Alendronate sodium, a bisphosphonate, is an FDA-approved treatment for osteoporosis treatment and prevention. Alendronate increases bone density of the spine and hip, as well as decreases vertebral fracture rate in women with osteoporosis, compared to placebo. In women with decreased bone mass at the hip and prevalent vertebral fractures, a decrease in both vertebral and hip fracture was seen with alendronate, compared to placebo. Women with two or more vertebral fractures at baseline had the best response to alendronate therapy, suggesting that alendronate is effective in preventing fractures in women at highest risk for fracture. In women with low hip bone mass without previous vertebral fracture, bone density of the spine and hip also increased, and asymptomatic vertebral fracture rate decreased by 51 percent with alendronate, as compared to placebo. However, clinical fractures, the primary outcome in this study, did not decrease in the group overall, but only in those women with t-scores <−2.5. Another study in women 60 to 85 years of age indicated that an even lower dose of alendronate might be effective

Table 75-6 Approved Medications Used for the Prevention and Treatment of Osteoporosis

Medication	Dose	Special Considerations
Estrogen Replacement Therapy		In older women, continuous administration is usually preferred; lower doses effective in older (>70 years) women
(1) Conjugated equine estrogen (Premarin)	0.3–0.625 mg/d*	
(2) 17β-estradiol (Estrace)	0.5–1.0 mg/d	For prevention only
(3) Transdermal estrogen (Estraderm)	0.05–0.1 mg biweekly	
Alendronate (Fosamax)	10 mg/d for treatment 70 mg/wk for treatment 5 mg/d for prevention	Strict adherence to dosing instructions required
Risedronate (Actonel)	5 mg/d for treatment and prevention	Strict adherence to dosing instructions required
Raloxifene (Evista)	60 mg/d for treatment and prevention	Deep venous thrombosis is main serious adverse effect; breast cancer incidence reduced
Parathyroid hormone (Forteo)	20 μg/d by injection	Second-line agent for severe osteoporosis; in rats treatment associated with osteosarcoma
Calcitonin, nasal spray (Miacalcin)	200 IU/d	1 spray gives daily dose; alternate nostrils each day; injectable useful in some patients
Calcitonin, injection (SQ or IM) (Miacalcin, Calcimar)	50–100 IU 3–5 times per week	

*For cyclical therapy, estrogen is given days 1 to 25 and then stopped. In women with a uterus, progesterone must be given with the estrogen to prevent endometrial hyperplasia. Medroxyprogesterone (Provera) is given 2.5 to 5.0 mg/d continuously, or 5 or 10 mg/d days 16 to 25 for cyclical treatment. Micronized progesterone is also available (200 mg/d days 16 to 25; continuous dose probably lower but no studies).

in older women. Alendronate may also be given weekly; 70 mg/wk increases bone density of the spine and hip as effectively as the daily dose (10 mg) and is more convenient for most patients and probably has fewer side effects. Alendronate has also been approved for prevention of osteoporosis in early postmenopausal women. The dose for prevention is a lower dose than that given for the treatment of osteoporosis (see Table 75-6). Combination therapy with alendronate plus estrogen replacement therapy appears to have a slight additive effect on bone mass, as compared to either alone. There are no published data addressing fracture outcomes for combination therapy. Alendronate is also an approved treatment for men with osteoporosis. In a 2-year randomized, placebo-controlled study, alendronate (10 mg) increased lumbar spine and hip bone density, as compared to placebo, and reduced vertebral fracture incidence in men with osteoporosis. Approximately one-third of men had low serum-free testosterone levels at baseline; these men also benefited from alendronate therapy. Finally, alendronate prevented bone loss, reduced biochemical markers of bone turnover, and vertebral fractures in men and women on at least 7.5 mg/d of prednisone.

The major side effects of alendronate are gastrointestinal, including abdominal pain, dyspepsia, esophagitis, nausea, vomiting, diarrhea; musculoskeletal pain may also

occur. Esophagitis, particularly erosive esophagitis, may be seen most frequently in patients who do not take the medication properly. For this reason, it is extremely important to provide specific and detailed instructions for patients receiving alendronate therapy.

Risedronate Another bisphosphonate, risedronate, is approved for prevention and treatment of osteoporosis. Risedronate is a pyridinyl bisphosphonate that effectively treats Paget's disease and multiple myeloma. Risedronate (5 mg/d) prevented lumbar spine bone loss, compared to placebo, in early postmenopausal women; similar but smaller effects were seen at the hip. In a larger study, risedronate (5 mg/d) effectively reduced cumulative incidence of vertebral fractures by 41 percent and nonvertebral fractures by 30 percent, compared to placebo, in postmenopausal women younger than 85 years of age (mean, 69 years) with at least 1 vertebral fracture at baseline. Bone mineral density of the lumbar spine, hip, and wrist also increased in women receiving risedronate, as compared to placebo. In this study, all women received 1000 mg/d of calcium and women with low 25(OH) vitamin D levels at baseline also received cholecalciferol supplementation. The effect of risedronate on hip fractures in

70- to 79-year-old women with osteoporosis (t-score <−4 or t-score <−3 + nonskeletal risk factor for fracture) and women at least 80 years old with at least one nonskeletal risk factor for fracture or low bone density (t-score < −4 or <−3+ hip axis length >11.2 cm) was investigated. These women were randomly assigned to treatment with placebo, 2.5 mg/d or 5 mg/d for 3 years. All women received 1000 mg/d calcium supplementation and women with 25(OH)D levels <16 ng/mL at baseline also received 500 IU vitamin D supplementation. In women 70 to 79 years of age with osteoporosis, risedronate decreased the risk of hip fracture by 40 percent, as compared to calcium and vitamin D alone; the effect was seen in women with prevalent vertebral fracture at baseline (60 percent decreased risk for hip fracture) but not in women without baseline vertebral fractures. In women at least 80 years of age, risedronate did not significantly reduce hip fracture incidence. These women were selected primarily on the basis of clinical risk factors rather than BMD criteria. This study demonstrates that even in older women, BMD measurement and assessment of previous vertebral fractures are needed to identify those women for whom the treatment will be the most effective. In the two large studies on risedronate previously mentioned, the drug was well tolerated, with all adverse events being similar in the treated and placebo groups. Two uncontrolled studies demonstrated that weekly risedronate (30 mg) increased lumbar spine and hip BMD by 4 percent and 2 percent, respectively, over 1 year; these increases are similar to that seen with daily risedronate. Data from a 1-year randomized, placebo-controlled study suggested that the combination of risedronate and estrogen replacement therapy had a greater additive effect on appendicular bone density sites than on axial sites. Risedronate also prevented bone loss and vertebral fractures in men and women on glucocorticoid therapy. Like alendronate and other bisphosphonates, risedronate must be taken on an empty stomach with plain water and patients must wait at least 30 minutes before ingesting food or other beverages. Preliminary data suggest that risedronate has fewer gastrointestinal side effects than alendronate; however, these findings need to borne out in further studies.

Zoledronic acid, a new, intravenous bisphosphonate, is currently being tested in trials in the United States and other countries. A recent study demonstrated that zoledronic acid, given at various doses and intervals, decreased bone turnover, as estimated by biochemical markers, and increased bone mineral density of the hip and spine, as compared to placebo. The three groups received 0.25, 0.5, and 1 mg every 3 months for 1 year; another group received 2 mg every 6 months and another 4 mg given once. All women in this study were postmenopausal with spine BMD t-score <−2 at baseline. The change in bone turnover parameters and bone density were similar in magnitude to oral bisphosphonates that have already been approved for prevention and treatment of osteoporosis.

Calcitonin

Calcitonin is a peptide hormone that is used to treat osteoporosis. It is available as a subcutaneous injection and as a nasal spray. The advantages of a nasal spray over injectable calcitonin are fewer reported side effects and greater patient acceptance. Calcitonin has been shown to increase bone density in the spine and to reduce vertebral fractures. In epidemiologic studies, calcitonin reduces hip fractures, although in clinical trials hip bone density does not increase. A recent 5-year study demonstrated a decrease in vertebral fracture in women on nasal spray calcitonin (200 IU/d), as compared to those women on placebo; in this study, 400 IU and 100 IU did not have any significant effect on vertebral fracture rate. Bone density at any site and markers of bone turnover did not change, compared to placebo, in this study. Nasal spray calcitonin does not appear to be as effective in preventing fractures as other approved agents; therefore its use should be limited to those women who are unable to tolerate other treatments. In some studies calcitonin therapy has also been associated with an analgesic effect in acute compression fractures, in Paget's disease of bone and in bone pain due to metastatic disease.

Selective Estrogen Receptor Agonists

The selective estrogen receptor modulators (SERM) are agents that act as estrogen agonists in bone and heart, but act as estrogen antagonists in breast and uterine tissue. These medications have the potential to prevent osteoporosis or heart disease without the increased risk of breast or uterine cancer. Tamoxifen, an agent used in breast cancer treatment, has been shown to have beneficial effects on bone in several studies, but has stimulatory effects on the uterus; it is not approved for treatment or prevention of osteoporosis. Raloxifene, a nonsteroidal benzothiophene, is a newer SERM that has been approved for prevention and treatment of osteoporosis in postmenopausal women. In one study of postmenopausal osteoporotic women, raloxifene resulted in decreased bone turnover and increased BMD of the hip, spine and total body bone density, as compared to placebo. Furthermore, raloxifene did not increase endometrial thickness over 2 years and had positive effects on the lipid profile. A later study examined the effect of 60 mg/d or 120 mg/d raloxifene on fractures. Raloxifene decreased the risk of new vertebral fractures (relative risk [RR] 0.5 [0.4 to 0.8] to 0.7 [0.6 to 0.9]). There was no difference in nonvertebral fracture incidence in the raloxifene treated groups, as compared to placebo. Bone mineral density of the lumbar spine and femoral neck increased in both raloxifene treated groups compared to placebo. Interestingly, the BMD increases with raloxifene were modest in this study yet the reduction in vertebral fracture risk was clinically significant suggesting that antiresorptive agents have effects on bone that are not reflected in BMD measurement. The major serious adverse effect of raloxifene was an increase in venous thromboembolic events, including deep vein thrombophlebitis and pulmonary embolism events (RR 3.1 [1.5 to 6.2]). However, raloxifene-treated women in this study had a reduced risk of breast cancer incidence (RR 0.3 [0.2 to 0.6]). In a 6-month study, raloxifene had effects on bone histomorphometry and bone turnover that were similar in direction to CEE, but were lower in magnitude.

Parathyroid Hormone

Parathyroid hormone, while leading to increased bone resorption when chronically elevated, increases bone mass, trabecular connectivity, and mechanical strength in rodents when administered intermittently, and, in uncontrolled studies, increases spinal BMD in osteoporotic men and women. In a 3-year randomized study of postmenopausal women with osteoporosis, the group receiving estrogen plus intermittent PTH had continuous increase in spinal bone mass over the study period, as well as decreased rate of vertebral fracture. Bone mass of the hip and total body also increased significantly in the estrogen + PTH group, compared to estrogen alone. In another randomized control trial, women randomly assigned to daily injections of 20 or 40 μg PTH experienced reduced new vertebral fractures and nonvertebral fractures, as compared to placebo. There was also a dose-dependent increase in BMD at the hip, spine, and total body, as compared to placebo. The side effects that occurred more frequently in the PTH-treated groups were headache, nausea, dizziness, and hypercalcemia. Permanent withdrawal of the study drug because of hypercalcemia was required in one woman on placebo, one in the 20-μg group, and 9 in the 40-μg group. In a small controlled study, daily subcutaneous injection of PTH (400 IU, roughly equivalent to 40 μg/d), compared to placebo, increased BMD of the spine and hip and increased bone turnover in men with idiopathic osteoporosis over 18 months, suggesting that PTH may also be beneficial in men. PTH may also be beneficial to postmenopausal women on chronic corticosteroids. PTH increased osteocalcin, a marker of bone formation, more rapidly than deoxypyridinoline crosslinks, a marker of bone resorption, suggesting early uncoupling of the bone remodeling cycle and providing a potential mechanism for an anabolic effect of PTH on bone. Further study is needed before the clinical role for PTH is determined.

Other Agents

Fluoride Use of fluoride to treat osteoporosis is appealing, because fluoride results in a large increase in spine bone density; however, the increase in BMD is not associated with a decrease in vertebral fractures. In fact, the group receiving fluoride had a higher rate of appendicular fractures. Although slow-release intermittent fluoride is associated with an increase in spine BMD, as well as with decreased incidence of vertebral fractures, further studies are required before slow-release fluoride can be recommended for treatment of osteoporosis.

Statins Statins are used in the management of hypercholesterolemia and inhibit the enzyme (3-hydroxy-3-methylglutaryl coenzyme A reductase) of the first step of the mevalonate pathway, which is involved in cholesterol synthesis. Amino bisphosphonates inhibit bone resorption by acting in the same pathway but on a different enzyme (farnesyl diphosphate synthase). Thus, it was suggested that statins might also inhibit osteoclast action. Subcutaneous administration and oral dosing of statins increased bone density in mice. The effect of statins on fracture occurrence has been inconsistent in observational studies. Present data do not support the use of statins for management of osteoporosis, although prospective studies in adults at high risk for osteoporotic fractures are needed.

Tibolone Tibolone is a synthetic compound with tissue-specific effects on bone, breast, endometrium, and the cardiovascular system. The tissue-specific effects are thought to occur through enzymatic conversion of steroids within various tissues to more or less bioactive forms. Several studies demonstrated that tibolone (2.5 mg/d) maintained BMD in postmenopausal women. Endometrial hyperplasia, endometrial cancer, and vaginal bleeding all occurred more frequently in the tibolone treated groups in year 1, as compared to placebo. Further study of this medication is required before its use can be recommend in prevention and treatment of osteoporosis.

Isoflavones Phytoestrogens, a group of nonsteroidal compounds found in plants, bind to estrogen receptors in animals and humans. There are several classes of phytoestrogens; the classes associated with health benefits are lignans and isoflavones; isoflavones include genistein, daidzein, glycitein, biochanin A, and formononetin. Soybeans are the richest source of isoflavones and epidemiologic studies report decreased hip fracture incidence as well as lower rates of breast and prostate cancer in Asian countries where the daily isoflavone intake ranges from 20 to 80 mg/d. In contrast, the average US intake of isoflavones is 1 to 3 mg/d. A recent consensus panel of the North American Menopause Society suggested that establishing the safety and efficacy of isoflavones at different stages of life and determining whether health benefits are attributed to isoflavones or the other components of soy foods are important areas of future research. Few human studies have examined the effect of soy protein with and without isoflavones on bone. In one study, after 6 months of treatment, the women receiving soy protein with 90 mg/d isoflavones had an increase in spine, but not hip, BMD. BMD did not change in the group receiving soy protein containing 56 mg/d of isoflavones. In another recent study women who received isoflavone rich soy protein ($N = 24$) did not lose spine BMD while those on whey ($N = 24$) did lose spine BMD. The group that received isoflavone-deficient protein ($N = 21$) demonstrated a trend toward bone loss ($p = 0.97$). A more recent short-term study in pre- and early postmenopausal women did not demonstrate any effect of isoflavones on markers of bone turnover. Prospective studies are underway to determine the effect of isoflavones on bone in older women.

REFERENCES

Amin S et al: Association of hypogonadism and estradiol levels with bone mineral density in elderly men from the Framingham Study. *Ann Intern Med* 133:951, 2001.

Black DM et al: Randomised trial of effect of alendronate on risk of fracture in women with existing vertebral fractures. Fracture Intervention Trial Research Group. *Lancet* 348(9041):1535, 1996.

Chen CL et al: Hormone replacement therapy in relation to breast cancer. *JAMA* 287:734, 2002.

Chesnut CH 3rd, Silverman S, Andriano K, et al: A randomized trial of nasal spray salmon calcitonin in postmenopausal women with established osteoporosis: the prevent recurrence of osteoporotic fractures study. PROOF Study Group. *Am J Med* 109(4):267, 2000.

Cummings SR, Black DM, Thompson D, et al: Effect of alendronate on risk of fracture in women with low bone density but without vertebral fractures. *JAMA* 280:2077, 1998.

Ducy P: Cbfa 1: A molecular switch in osteoblast biology. *Dev Dyn* 219:461, 2000.

Ettinger B et al: Reduction of vertebral fracture in postmenopausal women with osteoporosis treated with raloxifene: Results for a 3-year clinical trial. *JAMA* 282:637, 1999.

Gallagher JC et al: Prevention of bone loss with tibolone in postmenopausal women: Results of two randomized, double-blind, placebo-controlled, dose-finding studies. *J Clin Endocrinol Metab* 86:4717, 2001.

Gold DT: The nonskeletal consequences of osteoporotic fractures. *Rheum Dis Clin North Am* 27:255, 2001.

Harris ST et al: Effects of risedronate on vertebral and nonvertebral fractures in women with postmenopausal osteoporosis. *JAMA* 282:1344, 1999.

Kholsa S: Minireview: The OPG/RANKL/RANK system. *Endocrinology* 142:5050, 2001.

Lane NE: An update on glucocorticoid-induced osteoporosis. *Rheum Clin North Am* 27:235, 2001.

Lindsay R et al: Risk of new vertebral fractures in the year following fracture. *JAMA* 285:320, 2001.

Little RD et al: A mutation in the LDL receptor-related protein 5 gene results in the autosomal dominant high bone mass trait. *Am J Hum Genet* 70:11, 2002.

Manolagas SC: Birth and death of bone cells: Basic regulatory mechanisms and implications for the pathogenesis and treatment of osteoporosis. *Endocr Rev* 21:115, 2000.

McClung MR et al: Effect of risedronate on the risk of hip fracture in elderly women. *N Engl J Med* 344:333, 2001.

Mosca L et al: Hormone replacement therapy and cardiovascular disease: A statement for healthcare professionals from the American Heart Association. *Circulation* 104:499, 2001.

Neer RM et al: Effect of PTH on fractures and bone mineral density in postmenopausal women with osteoporosis. *N Engl J Med* 344:1434, 2001.

NIH Consensus Development Panel on Osteoporosis Prevention, Diagnosis, and Therapy: Osteoporosis prevention, diagnosis, and therapy. *JAMA* 285(6):785, 2001.

Nuttall ME, Gimble JM: Is there a therapeutic opportunity to either prevent or treat osteopenic disorders by inhibiting bone marrow adipogenesis? *Bone* 27:177, 2000.

Orwoll E et al: Alendronate for the treatment of osteoporosis in men. *N Engl J Med* 343(9):604, 2000.

Peacock M et al: Effect of calcium or 25OH vitamin D_3 dietary supplementation on bone loss at the hip in men and women over the age of 60. *J Clin Endocrinol Metab* 85:3011, 2000.

Prestwood KM et al: The effect of low dose micronized 17β-estradiol on bone turnover, sex hormone levels and side effects in older women: A randomized, double-blind placebo-controlled study. *J Clin Endocrinol Metab* 85:4462, 2000.

Reid IR et al: Intravenous zoledronic acid in postmenopausal women with low bone mineral density. *N Engl J Med* 346:653, 2002.

Reid IR et al: Effect of pravastatin on frequency of fracture in the LIPID study: Secondary analysis of a randomized controlled trial. *Lancet* 357(9255):509, 2001.

Schnitzer T et al: Therapeutic equivalence of alendronate 70 mg once-weekly and alendronate 10 mg daily in the treatment of osteoporosis. *Aging (Milano)* 12:1, 2000.

Siris ES et al: Identification and fracture outcomes of undiagnosed low bone mineral density in postmenopausal women. *JAMA* 286:2815, 2001.

Teitelbaum SL: Bone resorption by osteoclasts. *Science* 289:1504, 2000.

Togerson DJ, Bell-Syer SEM: Hormone replacement therapy and prevention of non-vertebral fractures. *JAMA* 285:2891, 2001.

Villareal DT et al: Bone mineral density response to estrogen replacement therapy in frail elderly women: A randomized controlled trial. *JAMA* 286:815, 2001.

Hip Fractures

LINDA A. RUSSELL

DEFINITION

An insufficiency fracture is a fracture sustained after a fall from a standing position. This excludes high-impact fractures, such as those obtained in a pedestrian–motor vehicle accident. Insufficiency fractures of the hip remain the most devastating fractures, both to the individual who sustains the fracture and to society at large.

Overall, patients who sustain a hip fracture have a 20 percent chance of mortality within 1 year after the fracture. For elderly patients with a hip fracture, the risk of mortality is greater. In addition, many patients lose their independence. Some become household ambulators, when they had previously been community ambulators. Others are forced to reside in assisted-living arrangements, when they had previously lived alone. The psychological impact is often great. Patients often become depressed as they begin to feel "old" and helpless. Isolation because of the physical inability to get to prior social events, as well as fear of walking outside, all contribute to the frequent decline after a hip fracture.

Society suffers a huge economic burden as a result of hip fractures. One recent prospective study demonstrated that the costs of treating a hip fracture are about three times greater than the costs of caring for a patient without a fracture. Patients may lose their ability to work. Other family members may lose time at work while caring for an ill family member. Patients may require costly long-term care in addition to the exorbitant acute costs associated with the repair of a hip fracture.

EPIDEMIOLOGY

There are approximately 30 million falls per year in the United States. One percent of all falls results in hip fractures, accounting for approximately 300,000 hip fractures per year in the United States. More than 90 percent of hip fractures are the result of falls. Others are the result of even less trauma, that is, twisting injuries. The risk of hip fracture is greater in women than in men primarily because of lower bone mineral density in women and associated decreased bone strength. Men do have an increased risk of fracture with aging, but the risk begins at slightly older ages than for women (5 to 10 years later.) In Australia and Northern Europe, the female-to-male age-adjusted hip fracture incidence ratio is approximately 2. There are a greater number of elderly women, as compared to men, and this contributes to the larger number of hip fractures occurring in women. It is estimated that approximately 30 percent of all hip fractures occur in men. As men often suffer from hip fractures at an older age, these patients have more overall morbidity and often do not fair as well as their female counterparts. A recent study noted that low bone mineral density at the hip in men was a strong independent predictor of all-cause and cardiovascular mortality in men.

Many studies have examined the risk factors for hip fractures. A recent case-control study examining 174 women who fell and had a resultant hip fracture identified several risk factors, including lower-limb dysfunction, various neurologic conditions, barbiturate use, and visual disturbance. A retrospective study performed in Oslo, Norway, examining 1316 fractures noted no seasonal variation in fracture rate. Seventy-eight percent of all hip fractures occurred in women. Older age was an independent risk factor. The incidence had not changed significantly over the past decade and was among the highest in the world. The age-adjusted fracture rates per 10,000 for those older than 50 years of age were 118.0 and 44.0 in 1996–1997, in women and men, respectively.

Long-term intake of diet high in retinol (vitamin A) may promote the development of osteoporotic hip fractures in women. Fluoride treatment for osteoporosis increases the risk of microfractures and stress fractures. One study that examined the level of fluoride in a public water supply found a small but significant increase in the rate of hip fracture in both men and women who were exposed to artificial fluoridation at 1 part per million.

A study designed to specifically examine the risk of hip fracture among black women noted that low weight, use of aids in walking, and alcohol consumption are associated with increased risk of hip fracture. One study that examined marital status and socioeconomic status demonstrated that women who were gainfully employed and married had a lower rate of hip fracture as compared to their unemployed, single counterparts. Studies examining risk of hip fracture and prior lactation have not demonstrated a substantial risk of hip fracture in women with a history of breast-feeding. One study has examined the rate of

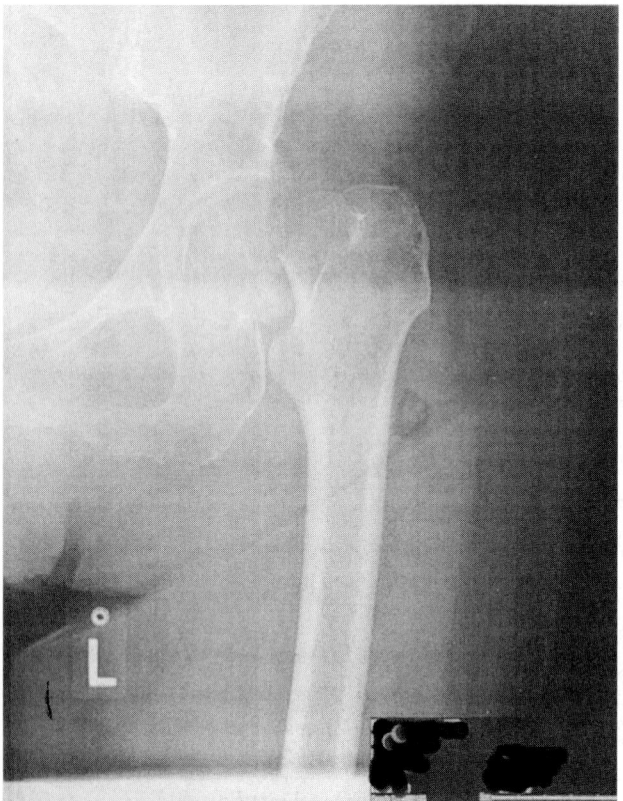

Figure 76-1   Radiograph depicting a displaced, intracapsular fracture of the left hip.

childhood growth and risk of hip fracture. A reduced growth rate in childhood does seem to correlate with risk of fracture later in life. This may be the result of many factors including childhood lifestyle, genetic background, or intrauterine exposures.

Thiazide diuretics decrease the urinary excretion of calcium. Clinically, the use of thiazide diuretics may occasionally be associated with mild hypercalcemia. Studies examining the risk of fracture in patients maintained on a thiazide diuretic have revealed mixed results with some suggesting a decrease in risk of hip fractures and others demonstrating no effect on the risk of hip fracture. Loop-diuretics such as furosemide promote hypercalcuria and have been associated with an increased risk of hip fracture. A recent study noted that low bone mineral density at the hip in men was a strong independent predictor of all-cause and cardiovascular mortality in men.

PATHOPHYSIOLOGY

There are many classification schemes for hip fractures. In patients with osteoporosis, fractures are often classified as either intracapsular or intertrochanteric. This is illustrated in Figs. 76-1 and 76-2. In intracapsular fractures, the fracture is within the hip capsule. These fractures are problematic because the fracture often puts the blood supply at risk. The Garden classification grades the hip fracture in a 4-stage system (Table 76-1). Stage I fractures are not displaced and the capsule is intact; the fracture is incomplete. Stage II fractures are complete, nondisplaced, but

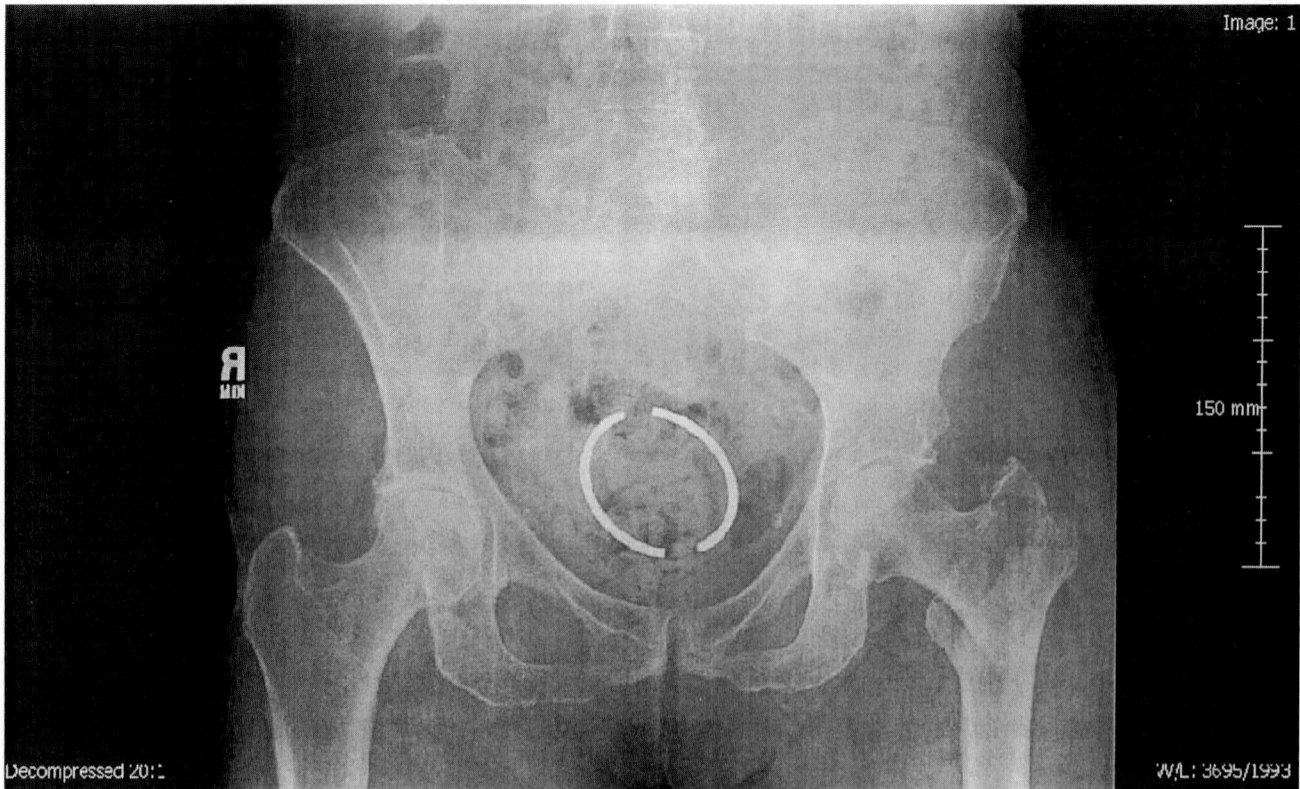

Figure 76-2   Radiograph depicting an intertrochanteric fracture of the left hip. A pessary is evident.

of perioperative antibiotics is even more critical when hardware is being placed, as infections involving the hardware are very difficult to treat without removal of the pin or prosthesis. For orthopedic procedures, cefazolin 1g IV is given. Vancomycin 1g IV can be substituted in patients allergic to cefazolin.

In many elderly patients who sustain hip fractures, malnutrition is present. This may have contributed to the patient's overall fragility and been a significant factor contributing to the fall that resulted in the fracture. This was recently demonstrated in the National Health and Nutrition Examination Survey (NHANES) I epidemiologic follow-up study data. Weight loss from a maximum reported body weight in women ages 50 to 64 years and 65 to 74 years increased their risk of hip fracture, especially among those who were relatively thin. The relative risks were 2.54 and 2.04, respectively. A poor nutritional status hinders wound healing and contributes to postoperative complications. Aggressive postoperative protein supplementation in patients hospitalized for a hip fracture has been associated with weight gain, shorter hospitalizations, and fewer postoperative complications. Thus, hospitalization for hip fracture is an important time to address causes of malnutrition and intervene so to improve the acute need and to hopefully contribute to falls prevention in general. High-calorie liquid protein supplementation is often ideal in the postoperative setting.

Postoperative delirium is a common problem in the elderly patient with hip fracture. If this occurs, the patient should be evaluated for treatable causes, including hypoxia, infection, metabolic disturbances, neurologic events, and medication reactions. Often the cause is multifactorial and related to the patient's preoperative functional status. In orthopedic procedures, postoperative delirium may be related to fat emboli. During the fracture or during orthopedic repair, fat enters the vasculature. If a right-to-left shunt exists, fat may enter the intracranial vasculature causing sedation and confusion. Fat may also enter the pulmonary vasculature causing hypoxia. Care is supportive and usually symptoms resolve over 3 to 7 days.

After the patient is stable and the fracture repaired, attention must focus on the treatment of the underlying bone deficiency. Causes of osteomalacia should be considered. Vitamin D deficiency is increasingly being recognized in the elderly population. The level can be checked and appropriate replacement prescribed. Osteomalacia can be considered in patients with abnormalities in serum calcium, phosphorus, or alkaline phosphatase. Alkaline phosphatase will be elevated immediately after a fracture. Parathyroid hormone can be checked in appropriate patients. All patients should be instructed to consume 1500 mg of calcium per day (divided tid) and 400 to 800 IU vitamin D. For patients older than age 70 years, 600 IU of vitamin D per day is recommended.

If the patient has not had a bone density measurement, or if it was done more than 1 to 2 years prior, it is recommended that the patient have a dual-energy x-ray absorptiometry (DXA) bone scan. This will help establish the diagnosis and offer a baseline study, so that response to therapy can be monitored. A few practitioners have argued that in the elderly patient, the diagnosis of osteoporosis is

made based on the occurrence of an insufficiency fracture. Having a hip fracture therefore establishes the diagnosis of osteoporosis. No testing is needed; the patients should simply be started on therapy. This may have merit in the frail institutionalized elderly patient, but in general, it is helpful to use the bone density to follow a response to therapy.

There are several FDA-approved therapies for the treatment of osteoporosis (see Chap. 75). Of the therapies FDA-approved for osteoporosis, not all reduce the incidence of hip fractures. Those that do include the oral bisphosphonates alendronate and risedronate. Although the studies involving alendronate and risedronate were not exactly comparable, most feel that the effect on hip fracture reduction is fairly comparable between these two agents. Specifically, risedronate decreases the rate of hip fractures in elderly women with confirmed osteoporosis. Alendronate increases hip bone mineral density (BMD) and reduces the rate of new hip fractures by close to 50 percent. Parathyroid hormone is FDA-approved for the treatment of osteoporosis. This may prove to be the most potent agent in terms of increasing BMD and reducing the risk of hip fracture. In a recent study involving 1637 women with prior vertebral fractures, receiving 20 or 40 μg of subcutaneous parathyroid hormone daily was associated with an increase in BMD of 3 and 6 percent, respectively, over a median duration of 21 months. There was a statistically significant decrease in vertebral and nonvertebral fractures as compared to placebo.

Large prospective studies evaluating the effects of hormone replacement therapy (HRT) on the incidence of hip fractures are not available. Analysis of available data does suggest that the use of HRT helps prevent hip fracture. The benefit of the oral bisphosphonates and parathyroid hormone are felt to be greater. The use of HRT is increasingly being scrutinized because of potential risks, and at this time the use of HRT should not be considered first-line therapy for the prevention of a hip fracture.

Some agents are FDA-approved for use in osteoporosis but do not reduce the risk of hip fracture. These agents include raloxifene and calcitonin. Raloxifene increases hip BMD, but does not reduce the risk of hip fracture. The use of these agents should be individualized to the patient at risk for fracture based on their BMD, risk factors for fracture, and comorbidities.

In postmenopausal women, the use of appropriate supplementation with calcium and vitamin D does not reduce the risk of hip fracture in those women with low bone mass. Conversely, elderly patients in institutional settings have had decreased hip fracture rates when supplemented with calcium and vitamin D in this patient population. This is felt to relate to elderly patients having a lower baseline level of calcium and vitamin D. Many studies document the prevalence of vitamin D deficiency and associated secondary hyperparathyroidism in the elderly.

The effects of the bisphosphonates on fracture healing have increasingly been studied. Initially, there was a concern that the use of bisphosphonates may slow fracture healing because of the effect on bone resorption. Early studies suggest that this is not so; in fact, the fracture callus may be larger in those on bisphosphonate therapy. Further study is needed in this area.

Stress fractures must be evaluated by an orthopedist. Depending on the patient's age, bone quality, and location of the fracture, a determination for the need for surgery is made.

Unfortunately, osteoporotic bone may not heal quickly or with sufficient structural integrity and surgery is often needed even for stress fractures. Nondisplaced pelvic fractures are often managed conservatively. Patients are instructed to weight bear as tolerated. Analgesia is provided as needed. Pain often resolves in 6 to 8 weeks.

PREVENTION

Despite the increasing awareness of osteoporosis, many studies demonstrate that practitioners are not diagnosing and treating those with osteoporosis appropriately. In a study involving bone density analysis in postmenopausal ambulatory care patients, almost half of these patients had previously undetected low bone density. Most distressing is the fact that even if a patient presents with an insufficiency fracture, few are being evaluated and begun on appropriate therapy. An audit of patients attending a tertiary teaching hospital with an incident fracture revealed that only 32 percent subsequently had a bone mineral test and only 39 percent were offered treatment. The risk of another insufficiency fracture after one insufficiency fracture is quite high.

In addition to medication therapy, many nonpharmacologic interventions can be made to reduce the risk of hip fractures. Falls prevention should be a focus of the health care team. An evaluation of the home environment can be done with special attention to lighting, rugs, and objects that might be tripped over. Patients should be encouraged to ask for help when needed. This is most critical at night. If patients awake to use the bathroom, they should be encouraged to turn on lights and to wear appropriate footwear. Care should be taken to avoid medications that might alter the sensorium promoting lightheadedness, dizziness, or confusion. All of these considerations are even more important if the patient at risk is in a new environment, such as a hospital or a relative's home.

Many studies demonstrate the benefit of exercise in falls prevention. Exercise that promotes improved balance, agility, and improved muscle strength is critical in reducing falls. There have been several studies demonstrating the benefit of Tai Chi. Exercise programs also improve confidence, which has a marked impact on quality of life. Exercise programs should be generalizable, safe, easily adaptable, simple to implement, and not cost prohibitive. Physical therapists can be guided to instruct patients in weight-bearing exercise programs that patients can then do on their own. Many patients who have been inactive feel that they do not know what exercises to do and are hesitant to begin a program on their own. The benefit of exercise is primarily in falls prevention and not in improvement in bone density. It is possible to improve bone density with an intense high-impact exercise regime; this has been demonstrated best in professional athletes. For most older people, the amount of impact activity needed to increase bone density is prohibitive. In addition, for those with

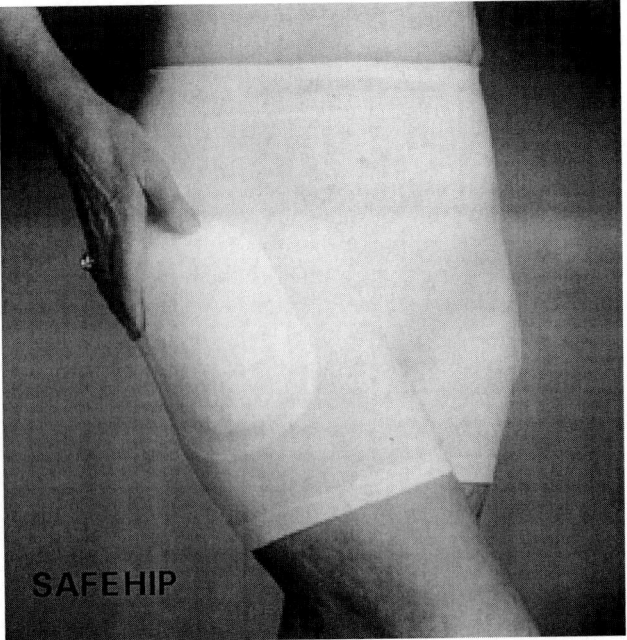

Figure 76-8   Picture of a hip protector (SAFEHIP). Reprinted with permission.

osteoporosis, high-impact activities are relatively contraindicated for fear of causing a fracture. It is also recognized that bed rest is associated with rapid bone loss; patients who become immobile should be targeted for prevention strategies to help reduce bone loss, muscle mass, and strength. One study examined the level of activity in older people living in an institutional-like setting; the level of activity was minimal. Those with increased hours of physical activity per week had fewer hip fractures. Emphasis should be placed on exercise in older individuals living in institutional-like settings.

Hip protectors reduce the risk of hip fractures, if worn properly (Fig. 76-8). In more than 90 percent of cases, hip fracture is the result of impact on the greater trochanter, often with a force or 3400 N. Rigid hip protectors disperse the force from the trochanter to the hip protector and surrounding tissues. Several studies demonstrate a 50 percent reduction in hip fractures when hip protectors are worn. In most of the studies, the rate of protection would have been greater had the participants wore the device more regularly. The device consists of a short pant containing two rigid, snug-fitting inserts. The device may be washed and comes in different sizes. Patients often find the devices expensive (approximately $90 each) and cumbersome, although others appear to become easily accustomed to them. A recent study evaluated acceptance of hip protectors by recipients in 20 nursing homes in Switzerland. One hundred and sixty-four patients were randomly selected into the control group and 384 into the intervention group. Of the patients in the intervention group 138 (35.9 percent) wore the hip protector for the whole 10 months duration, 124 (32.3 percent) quit after the initial wearing period, and 122 (31.8 percent) refused to wear them at all.

In summary, the best strategies for preventing hip fractures include the prevention of osteoporosis; this must focus on men and women of all ages, including children, adolescents, and adults. Exercise and fitness must be emphasized throughout the lifetime, without ignoring the elderly person. Falls prevention must be emphasized. Hip pads should be considered in all patients with osteoporosis felt to be at risk for hip fracture. Newer hip pads are under development with the hope of being better tolerated and less expensive.

SPECIAL ISSUES

Patient Preference

Many elderly patients are reluctant to use assistive devices for ambulation because they feel there are certain stigmata associated with using a cane or walker. Patients with poor gait patterns should be encouraged to use assistive devices. A physician, nurse, or physical therapist can teach the proper use of an assistive device. The size must be correct and physical therapists are often best suited to this task. When used properly, an assistive device can improve balance, confidence and reduce falls.

Comorbidity

Underlying psychiatric illness does increase the risk of mortality after hip fracture. One study examining 731 participants with hip fracture found that dementia, delirium, and depression all increased the risk of mortality. A meta-analysis examining 19 studies confirmed this finding. The studies also suggest that people with underlying psychiatric illness have an increased incidence of hip fracture. It has been proposed that screening for underlying psychiatric illness be done in those admitted with hip fracture. Once recognized, a plan should be developed that coincides with rehabilitation. This will hopefully improve both the patient's recovery and quality of life.

Care Settings

Functional ability to ambulate and to perform necessary activities of daily living often decreases after a hip fracture. After discharge from the hospital, patients can be transferred to one of numerous settings including home, a subacute rehabilitation facility, an acute care rehabilitation facility, a nursing home, or an assisted-living environment. Transition from one level of care to another can be both physically and mentally taxing. Emphasis should be placed on providing patients with speedy transition to a level of care that will be tolerated by the patient and provide the best chance for a complete recovery. The safety of the patient must always be considered. The appropriate level of rehabilitation must take mental status into account and the ability to participate in a rehabilitation program. Controlling pain after hip fracture may improve chances of functional recovery. As our population ages, more emphasis will need to be placed on care in the home in order to prevent hip fractures and to allow patients to return home after injury, as most patients would eventually prefer to live independently.

REFERENCES

Chapuy MC et al: Vitamin D₃ and calcium to prevent hip fracture in elderly women. *N Engl J Med* 327(23):1637, 1992.

Haentjens P et al: The economic cost of hip fractures among elderly women. *J Bone Jt Surg* 83A(4):493, 2001.

Hubacher M, Wettstein A: Acceptance of hip protectors for hip fracture prevention in nursing homes. *Osteoporos Int* 12:794, 2001.

Kiel DP et al: Hip Fracture and the Use of Estrogens in Postmenopausal Women. *N Engl J Med* 317(19):1169, 1987.

Langlois JA et al: Weight loss from maximum body weight among middle-aged and older white women and the risk of hip fracture: The NHANES I epidemiologic follow-up study. *Osteoporos Int* 12:763, 2001.

McClung MR et al: Effect of risedronate on the risk of hip fracture in elderly women. *N Engl J Med* 344(5):333, 2001.

Neer RM et al: Effect of parathyroid hormone (1–34) on fractures and bone mineral density in postmenopausal women with osteoporosis. *N Engl J Med* 344(19):1434, 2001.

Pols HAP et al: Multinational, placebo-controlled, randomized trial of the effects of alendronate on bone density and fracture risk in postmenopausal women with low bone mass: Results of the FOSIT study. *Osteoporos Int* 9:461, 1999.

Shah MR et al: Outcome after hip fracture in individuals ninety years of age and older. *J Orthop Trauma* 15(1):34, 2001.

Smith M, Ross W, Ahern MJ: Missing a therapeutic window of opportunity: An audit of patients attending a tertiary teaching hospital with potentially osteoporotic hip and wrist fractures. *J Rheum* 28:2504, 2001.

Myopathies, Polymyalgia Rheumatica, and Giant Cell Arteritis

KENNETH S. O'ROURKE

The contributions made by healthy muscle to maintaining basic metabolic and functional activities cannot be underestimated. Muscle disease symptoms and myopathies are not uncommon in the elderly population, and when present, they are superimposed upon the natural age-related decline in muscle function. The combination of inherent muscular compromise over time with the acquired burden of disease-related muscular pain, stiffness, and or weakness can lead to profound disability in an elderly individual. This chapter surveys the more common myopathies seen in the elderly population, highlighting the differences in presentation and or therapy between elderly and younger adults, and reviews the closely related diseases of polymyalgia rheumatica and giant cell arteritis. The discussion of these inflammatory and noninflammatory conditions is based upon a review of the changes that occur in muscle with aging, and how these changes can affect the results of the standard assessments of muscle disease symptoms in the elderly person.

CLINICAL EVALUATION OF MUSCLE DISEASE SYMPTOMS IN THE ELDERLY PATIENT

The age-unrestricted differential diagnosis of conditions that can cause muscle disease symptoms is extensive (Table 77-1). Although not all of these disorders present in elderly patients, a comprehensive history (including a thorough review of systems) and physical examination is necessary to narrow the list of possible etiologies and to exclude causes of generalized weakness and/or fatigue (e.g., heart failure, systemic infection, malignancy). A focused evaluation of myopathic symptoms is further developed, supplemented by laboratory tests, electromyography (EMG), and muscle biopsy. This approach is not age-specific, but the results must be interpreted in light of age-related variation that can be seen in each component of the process.

History

As most extremity muscle bulk is proximal, symptoms of myopathic weakness tend to be associated with shoulder and hip girdle motions, such as reaching above the head, hair brushing, or stair climbing. Patients may report either the inability to perform a specific task because of weakness, or poor stamina in performing tasks once readily accomplished. Independence with activities of daily living (ADLs), maintenance of balance and gait, and freedom from falling should be addressed as all are sustained in part by maintenance of muscle strength. Muscle pain is an uncommon symptom of a primary myopathy, and in the elderly patient, should suggest polymyalgia rheumatica, or a regional or generalized musculoskeletal disorder (see Chap. 81).

Examination

Documenting the severity of initial and serial assessments of muscle strength should be accomplished by using the Medical Research Council (MRC) grading scale of 0 to 5, where 0 represents no muscle contraction, 1 represents trace muscle contraction without movement of the part, 2 represents active movement with gravity eliminated, 3 represents active movement against gravity, and 5 represents normal power. A score of 4, representing movement against some resistance, is often subdivided to indicate movement against slight (4−), moderate (4), or strong (4+) resistance. The healthy elderly person should be able to sustain muscle contraction against full resistance for the 2 to 4 seconds normally allotted to test individual muscles. More physiologically complex yet standard functional assessments, such as arising from a chair without the use of the arms, measuring the time necessary to perform this maneuver 5 to 10 times, or squatting from

Table 77-1   Differential Diagnosis of Myopathies—An Abbreviated List

Collagen Vascular
    Idiopathic inflammatory myopathies
    Polymyalgia rheumatica—giant cell arteritis
    Rheumatoid arthritis
    Systemic lupus erythematosus
    Scleroderma
    Vasculitis
 	
Neurologic
    Amyotrophic lateral sclerosis
    Myasthenia gravis
    Eaton–Lambert syndrome
    Guillain–Barré syndrome
    Muscular dystrophies
 	
Pharmacologic
    Alcohol
    Cocaine
    Colchicine
    Cyclosporine
    Glucocorticosteroids
    Lipid-lowering agents
    Others
 	
Endocrine
    Hyperthyroidism
    Hypothyroidism
    Hyperparathyroidism
    Cushing's syndrome
    Addison's disease
    Aldosteronism
    Amyloidosis
    Osteomalacia
	Metabolic
	    Uremia
	    Hepatic failure
	
	Malabsorption
	    Hypoxic states
	
	Electrolyte imbalance
	    Hypo- or hypernatremia
	    Hypo- or hyperkalemia
	    Hypo- or hypercalcemia
	    Hypomagnesemia
	
	Infectious
	    Viruses (influenza, coxsackie)
	    Toxoplasmosis
	    Trichinella
	    Bacterial toxins (staphylococcal, streptococcal, clostridial)
	
	Chronic infections (tuberculosis, endocarditis, osteomyelitis)
	
	Cancer-related
	    Disseminated carcinomatosis
	    Paraneoplastic syndromes (Eaton-Lambert, neuromyopathy)
	    Myositis
	
	Inherited errors of metabolism
	
	Glycogen storage diseases
	    Lipid storage diseases
	    Myoadenylate deaminase deficiency
	
	Other conditions
	    Sarcoidosis
	    Fibromyalgia
	    Chronic fatigue syndrome
	    Hysteria

SOURCE: Adapted from *Bull Rheum Dis* 43(6) 1994. Used by permission of the Arthritis Foundation. For more information, please call the Arthritis Foundation information line 1-800-283-7800 or log on to www.arthritis.org. Wortmann RL: Muscle disease symptoms: Evaluation and significance.

the standing position and then arising without assistance, should be accomplished without difficulty by normal younger adults but may be difficult even for the healthy elderly person. The distribution of weakness may provide clues as to broad categorical etiologies: symmetric proximal extremity weakness with a normal neurologic exam suggests a myopathy, whereas distal weakness, distal and proximal weakness, or asymmetric weakness, particularly with abnormal neurologic findings, suggests an underlying neuropathic problem. Compared with objective muscle weakness, muscle tenderness is a less-common finding in most primary myopathies. Muscle tenderness in the elderly person, without demonstrated significant weakness, is seen with polymyalgia rheumatica (symmetric proximal extremities), fibromyalgia (diffuse muscle tender points), or regional musculoskeletal disorders (focal findings) (see Chap. 81).

Laboratory Markers

Routine laboratory measurements of electrolytes and muscle enzymes are an essential component of muscle disease evaluation. Muscle contraction is dependent on the homeostasis of sodium, potassium, calcium, magnesium, and phosphorous, abnormalities in any of which can lead to muscle weakness. An elevated serum level of creatine kinase (CK) is the most sensitive indicator of muscle cell injury, but aldolase, aspartate aminotransferase (AST), lactate dehydrogenase (LDH), and, rarely, alanine aminotransferase (ALT) may also be increased. In the elderly population, there is an age-related decrease in CK and aldolase specific activity per unit deoxyribonucleic acid (DNA) in muscle, and up to a 20 percent decline in the mean value of CK as compared to a young population. Despite this fall in mean CK levels with age, the diagnostic accuracy of an elevated CK level in the elderly patient with histologically proven myopathy is equal to that of younger adults. The ability of CK to be detected in standard assays is a function of extracellular glutathione in vivo: glutathione prevents excessive oxidation of CK, preserving it for its average lifetime in the circulation (22 hours). During states of extracellular glutathione depletion (multiorgan failure or critical illness), serum CK levels can drop to levels below the lower limit of normal, despite ongoing muscle wasting. CK levels must be interpreted with caution in patients with myopathic illness under these circumstances. Autoantibody testing is not a component of the usual assessment of myopathic symptoms but may be helpful to categorize subsets of patients with proven inflammatory myopathies (see below).

Electromyography

Neurophysiologic testing by EMG through needle electrode assessment of voluntary motor unit action potentials (MUAPs) and spontaneous muscle electrical activity can categorize muscle symptoms as arising primarily from either muscle or nerve. EMG provides information on the distribution, severity, and if done serially, the progression of myopathic changes. MUAP duration best distinguishes between a myopathy and neuropathy: total duration increases in neuropathies but decreases in myopathies. Other myopathic findings include MUAPs of small amplitude, and polyphasic composition. Increased needle insertional activity (increased in damaged muscles, decreased in muscles replaced by fat or scarring), and spontaneous activity (fibrillation potentials [a degenerating muscle fiber with an unstable membrane fires spontaneously at a regular rate] and positive sharp waves [needle-touching damaged, degenerating fibers]) are features of an inflammatory myopathy. In the elderly population, there is a slight tendency toward prolonged MUAP duration above the age of 55 years, and a small increase in the proportion of polyphasic potentials. These changes are a result of the process of denervation followed by intramuscular axonal spouting from neighboring axons and reinnervation described above. This process occurs slowly, and thus the typical features of active degeneration—fibrillations and positive sharp waves—are not seen with aging alone. EMG assessment of a cool limb will also produce a higher percentage of increased duration, polyphasic potentials, as well as reduced spontaneous activity. This must be taken into account during EMG testing in the elderly, who are at increased risk for cool limbs from circulatory insufficiency and reduced insulation (subcutaneous fat).

Muscle Biopsy

History, exam, laboratory assessments, and EMG infrequently provide a diagnosis of a specific muscular disorder. Muscle biopsy is then necessary to make or confirm a diagnosis and to provide a basis for therapy. In most clinical circumstances, satisfactory muscle samples for evaluation can be provided by either open or percutaneous techniques. A combination of complementary tissue stains is chosen to evaluate general muscle morphology and fiber typing and distribution, and screening tests are chosen for evaluating enzyme deficiencies and storage diseases. Further enzymatic studies and/or electron microscopy are performed based on these initial results and clinical data. Based on autopsy and muscle biopsy studies, muscle biopsy specimens from the elderly population show an increased frequency of type II muscle fiber atrophy, neurogenic changes (including fiber type grouping, angular atrophic fibers, target or "targetoid" fibers), ragged red fibers (the hallmark of mitochondrial dysfunction), and fibers staining negative for cytochrome *c* oxidase. Findings of necrosis, cytoplasmic bodies, ring-fibers, and fibers with increased central nuclei have been noted in muscle specimens from those older than age 70 years. Clinically, the diagnostic accuracy of muscle biopsy findings for inflammatory myopathy in patients aged 65 years and older approximates that of younger adults.

MYOPATHIES IN THE ELDERLY PATIENT

Table 77-2 provides a more specific list of conditions that should be considered in the elderly patient suspected of

Table 77-2 Myopathies More Specific for the Elderly Patient

Primary muscle diseases
    Idiopathic inflammatory myopathies
        Sporadic inclusion body myositis
        Polymyositis
        Dermatomyositis
    Late onset muscular dystrophies
        Facioscapularhumeral dystrophy
        Oculopharyngeal dystrophy
        Late onset limb girdle dystrophy
    Late onset mitochondrial myopathy
    Axial myopathies
        Thoracolumbar kyphosis (bent spine syndrome; camptocormia; cormoptosis)
        Dropped head syndrome

Diseases or conditions of extramuscular origin with proximal muscle weakness
    Endocrine/Metabolic diseases
        Thyroid disease
        Osteomalacia
    Amyloid myopathy
    Drug-induced myopathies
        Corticosteroids
        Alcohol
        Colchicine
        Lipid-lowering agents

having a myopathy. These diseases, both primary muscular diseases and diseases or drug-related syndromes with symptomatology in the muscular system, represent a more focused list of inflammatory and noninflammatory conditions and assumes a comprehensive evaluation has excluded electrolyte disturbances and organ failure syndromes as causes of weakness. These disorders can also be separated into those causing primarily proximal muscle weakness or spinal weakness. The following discussion surveys these diseases, highlighting clinical findings of presentation or therapy that are more distinctive in older patients.

Idiopathic Inflammatory Myopathies

As a group the idiopathic inflammatory myopathies (IIM) are the most common cause of primary myopathy in the elderly patient. These diseases—polymyositis (PM), dermatomyositis (DM), and sporadic inclusion body myositis—share findings of slowly progressive muscle weakness, which is usually symmetric and involves primarily proximal muscles in a limb, elevated serum levels of muscle enzymes, characteristic changes of an inflammatory myopathy on EMG, and abnormal muscle pathology, with degenerating and regenerating myocytes, and inflammatory cells in and around muscle cells and sometimes around vessels. Extramuscular manifestations in common include constitutional symptoms and dysphagia; polyarthralgias/polyarthritis and cardiopulmonary involvement are more likely to occur in PM and DM. Other unique features that serve to define the clinical subsets of IIM include certain demographic characteristics, skin manifestations, myositis-specific antibodies, and pathologic criteria. In up to 20 percent of cases of IIM, a second connective disease is present in an individual patient. Systemic lupus erythematosus, rheumatoid arthritis, Sjögren's syndrome, scleroderma, and mixed connective-tissue disease are the most commonly diagnosed associated diseases.

Sporadic Inclusion Body Myositis and the Hereditary Inclusion Body Myopathies

The term *inclusion body myositis* (IBM) was first used in 1971 to describe patients with IIM whose muscle biopsies displayed degenerating muscle fibers with rimmed vacuoles and unique, tubulofilamentous nuclear and cytoplasmic inclusions. The inclusions have been further characterized by electron microscopy as 15- to 18-nm diameter paired helical filaments. Patients with IBM are now separated into two distinct sets based on patterns of inheritance, clinical findings, muscle biopsy changes at the light- and electron-microscopic levels, and immunoreactivities demonstrated in the filaments: sporadic inclusion body myositis (s-IBM) and the hereditary inclusion body myopathies (h-IBM).

Patients with h-IBM present in their twenties and thirties with slowly progressive weakness, which, in some, may include early involvement of distal limb muscles. This heterogeneous group of patients, clustered by certain religious backgrounds and countries of origin, are further classified according to pattern of inheritance (autosomal recessive or dominant) and whether or not the quadriceps muscle is involved (in the autosomal recessive group). A specific gene for all patient subsets has not been identified, but some are linked to a locus on chromosome 9p1-q1. Patients share similar features on muscle biopsy, but unlike in s-IBM, there is an absence of inflammatory changes in muscle biopsy specimens, hence the term inclusion body "myopathies" and not "myositis"

s-IBM is the most common inflammatory myopathy in patients older than age 50 years. As contrasted against PM and DM, s-IBM affects males two to three times as frequently as females, and is more common in whites than in other races. The course of painless, proximal muscle weakness develops insidiously, commonly over years, but distal limb muscle involvement is seen in 50 percent, occurs early, and may predominate in up to a third of patients. Muscle weakness is more commonly asymmetric than in PM or DM. A characteristic pattern of finger and wrist flexor, knee extensor, and ankle dorsiflexor weakness has been described and may be specific enough to make the diagnosis even when rimmed vacuoles and other characteristic histologic muscle biopsy findings are absent. Impaired distal limb strength may lead to difficulty with fine motor movements and suggest a neuropathy. The prominent involvement of the hip flexors and quadriceps muscles may be severe enough in some patients that patellar reflexes are diminished, simulating an underlying neuropathy. Quadriceps weakness and knee giving-way may lead to an increased frequency of falling. Muscle enzymes are normal in approximately 20 percent of patients and elevated no more than 12 times normal in most patients. EMG findings are atypical in 30 percent of patients, including the absence of inflammatory changes or the presence of a prominent neuropathic component. Up to 16 percent of patients may have an associated autoimmune disease. Table 77-3 lists proposed diagnostic criteria for IBM (s-IBM) incorporating pathologic and clinical findings.

A physical therapy program of strength training should be prescribed for all patients with s-IBM. Reported clinical outcome in patients with s-IBM using standard medical therapy for IIM, corticosteroids with or without immunosuppressive agents, is generally disappointing. The lack of improvement with therapy has been described as a clinical hallmark of the disease. More recent reports describe a small subgroup of patients with s-IBM who have mild to modest improvement or stabilization of findings with standard therapy, either in CK levels and degree of muscle fiber inflammatory changes histologically, or in strength. Common findings noted in many of these responding patients include coexistence of an associated autoimmune disease (e.g., systemic lupus erythematosus), higher CK levels or degree of inflammation noted histologically at baseline, and the absence of significant replacement of muscle by fat and fibrosis. The limited number of clinically improved patients in these studies, and the variable durations of patient improvement and documented follow-up, does not allow for subgroup analysis sufficient to recommend that a therapeutic trial is warranted for any specific combination of clinical and laboratory findings. However, because of the possibility of improvement, and if the risks in an individual patient

Table 77-3   Proposed Diagnostic Criteria for Inclusion Body Myositis by J. Mendell and Colleagues

I. Inclusion criteria
   A. Clinical features
      1. Duration >6 months
      2. Age of onset >30 years
      3. Muscle weakness: affecting proximal and distal muscle of arms and legs, and
         a. Finger flexor weakness
         b. Wrist flexor > wrist extensor weakness
         c. Quadriceps weakness ≤ grade 4 (MRC scale)
   B. Laboratory features
      1. Serum CK <12 times normal
      2. Muscle biopsy
         a. Mononuclear cell invasion of nonnecrotic muscle fibers
         b. Vacuolated muscle fibers
         c. Either
            (i) Intracellular amyloid deposits, or
            (ii) 15–18-nm tubulofilaments by electron microscopy
      3. EMG changes of an inflammatory myopathy
   C. Family history: rarely sporadic inclusion body myositis is observed in families

II. Associated disorder: presence of an associated disorder does not exclude inclusion body myositis if criteria below are fulfilled

III. Diagnostic criteria for inclusion body myositis
   A. Definite: all muscle biopsy features exhibited
   B. Possible: muscle inflammation without other biopsy features, and criteria A1, A2, A3, B1, and B3

SOURCE: Reprinted with permission from Griggs RC et al: Inclusion body myositis and myopathies. *Ann Neurol* 38:705, 1995.

with s-IBM are acceptable, a medication trial with corticosteroids with or without immunosuppressives is probably indicated (see "Polymyositis and Dermatomyositis" later in this chapter). Failure to respond after 3 months of corticosteroids (at up to 1 mg/kg/d), followed by a 3-month trial of an additional agent such as methotrexate in patients with marked chemical or biopsy features of inflammation at onset, should lead to discontinuation of immunosuppressive therapy. A growing number of case reports and small uncontrolled series of patients, as well as small and short-term controlled trials of intravenous immunoglobulin (IVIg) therapy for s-IBM demonstrate mild but inconsistent benefit, and suggest the need for larger, longer controlled trials before this form of therapy can be universally recommended.

It has been noted that steroid and immunosuppressive therapy can improve serum and pathologic markers of muscle inflammation in s-IBM, but not retard the progression of clinical weakness, and muscle fiber vacuolization and amyloid deposition. This finding suggests that s-IBM is a primary degenerative disorder of muscle with secondary inflammation. Inflammation as a secondary finding can also be seen in certain muscular dystrophies, and in the brain of patients with Alzheimer's disease, which, shares certain ultrastructural similarities to muscle tissue in patients with s-IBM (Table 77-4). It has been postulated that muscle fiber abnormalities in IBM are either a direct cause of, or associated with, oxidative stress in muscle, derived from the overexpression of amyloid precursor protein within the

cyto-milieu of aging muscle. The trigger for these events remains unknown, but may include products of mutated genes (in the case of h-IBM) or some other agent, perhaps a virus (in s-IBM).

As patients with IBM have generally less visceral involvement, they have a better survival rate (>90 percent) than the estimated 80 percent rate 5 years postdiagnosis seen in patients with PM and DM. However, presumably because of the progressive nature of muscle degeneration, patients with IBM have a poorer functional outcome than do those with PM or DM.

Polymyositis and Dermatomyositis

Clinical Subsets   The clinical and laboratory findings that lead to a diagnosis of either PM or DM are not age specific and are based on criteria initially set forth by Bohan and Peter in 1975: symmetric limb-girdle and anterior neck flexor muscle weakness, skin rash (in patients with DM), elevation of skeletal muscle enzymes, EMG evidence of an inflammatory myopathy, and muscle biopsy evidence of an inflammatory infiltrate, cellular necrosis, and regeneration. These criteria describe a heterogeneous group of disorders that lead to chronic muscle inflammation. Recent advances in autoantibody detection have identified clinical subgroups of patients with either PM, DM, or myositis associated with malignancy or connective tissue disease with antibodies directed at aminoacyl–transfer ribonucleic acid (tRNA) synthetases, nonsynthetase cytoplasmic antigens,

Table 77-4   Comparison of Selected Pathologic Changes Between Muscle in IBM and Brain in Alzheimer's Disease (AD)

Cellular Phenotype	IBM in Muscle	AD in Brain
Congophilia, associated with amyloid-β	Small intracellular "plaquettes"	Large extracellular plaques
Amyloid-β in filaments, diameter	6–10 nm	6–8 nm
Other amyloid-β precursor epitopes accumulated	Yes	Yes
Presenilin 1 accumulated	Yes	Yes
Paired helical filaments	Yes, in bundles	Yes, in neurofibrillary tangles
Paired helical filaments contain:		
Phosphorylated τ	Yes	Yes
Ubiquitin	Yes	Yes
Apolipoprotein E (Apo E)	Yes	Yes
Presenilin 1	Yes	Yes
Heme-oxygenase-1 (HO-1)	Yes	Yes
Nitrotyrosine	Yes	Yes
Malondialdehyde	Yes	Yes
Apo E mRNA increased	No	Yes, in astrocytes
Superoxide dismutase-1 accumulated	Yes	Yes
HO-1 accumulated	Yes	Yes
Nitrotyrosine accumulated	Yes	Yes
Non-Alzheimer accumulations		
Prion (normal cellular type?)	Yes	No
Prion mRNA (normal cellular type)	Yes	No

mRNA, messenger ribonucleic acid.

SOURCE: Reprinted with permission from Askanas V and Engel WK (1998).

or nuclear antigens. These myositis-specific autoantibodies define more homogeneous populations within the spectrum of the IIM, each with distinct clinical findings, prognosis, and immunogenetic associations (Table 77-5), and have been included in newer proposed criteria for the diagnosis of an IIM (Table 77-6). The syndromes marked by these autoantibodies are more commonly seen in younger adults, with mean age at diagnosis between 36 and 46 years, but there is insufficient published data to state that they cannot be seen in the elderly population.

Epidemiology   Incidence rates of PM-DM are bimodal, peaking in childhood, and again in adults of mean age of 45 to 64 years. The mean age is higher (60 years) for those with malignancy-associated myositis, and conversely, the elderly population with PM-DM have a higher incidence of malignancy. Three retrospective studies of patients identified clinically with either PM or DM, two by hospital records and one study of both outpatients and inpatients, specifically addressed the frequency of age >65 years at diagnosis. Of the 380 patients represented in these reports, 76 (20 percent) were 65 years or older (range, 6.5 percent to 29 percent). The gender distribution in these 76 patients was 47 females and 29 males, for a ratio of 1.6:1, slightly less than the range of 2 to 2.5:1 in younger adults with PM-DM.

Clinical Findings   Symmetric, proximal-limb muscle weakness that evolves over weeks to months is the most common presentation. The myositis is usually painless. Neck flexor muscles can be involved, but more cephalad muscular involvement in the face or ocular muscles is very rare. Involvement of striated muscles in the pharynx and upper esophagus can cause cervical dysphagia symptoms, aspiration, nasal regurgitation, and voice alterations.

Skin manifestations are mandatory for a diagnosis of DM. Most commonly seen cutaneous findings include the pathognomonic Gottron's sign (a macular erythematosus rash occurring over the knuckles and other extensor surfaces such as the knees and elbows) and Gottron's papules (which show additional scale and plaque changes, in a similar distribution; Fig. 77-1) in 60 to 80 percent, and a heliotrope periorbital rash (erythematosus or violaceous eyelid color change usually with lid edema) in up to 50 percent. Less-common skin changes include macular erythema over the anterior chest (V-neck sign) or shoulders and upper back (shawl sign; Fig. 77-2), nail fold capillary changes similar to those that may occur in patients with scleroderma (cuticle dystrophy with periungual capillary tortuosity, dilation, or infarct; Fig. 77-3), and "mechanics hands" (fissuring and cracking over the lateral aspects of the fingers and finger pads). Subcutaneous calcinosis

Table 77-5 Associations of the Myositis-Specific Autoantibodies.

Myositis-Specific Autoantibody (Frequency in Myositis)	Clinical Manifestations	Onset of Myositis			Response to Therapy	Five-year Survival Rate	HLA
		Rate	Severity	Season			
Antisynthetase[†] (20–25%)	Arthritis, interstitial lung disease, fever, mechanic's hands, Raynaud's phenomenon	Acute	Severe	Spring	Moderate flares with Rx taper	70%	DR3 DRw52 DQAI*-0501
Antisignal recognition particle (anti-SRP) (<5%)	Cardiac involvement with palpitations, myalgias; mostly African American women	Very acute	Very severe	Fall	Poor; some improve with aggressive chemo-therapy	25%	DR5 DRW52 DQA1*-0301
Anti–Mi-2[‡] (5–10%)	Classic dermatomyositis with V sign, shawl sign, and cuticular overgrowth	Acute	Mild	Unknown	Good; rash may persist and require additional Rx	Approx-imately 100%	DR7 DRw53 DQA1*-0201

[†]Antibody directed at the enzyme (synthetase) that binds an amino acid with its specific tRNA. Examples include anti–Jo-1 (histidyl tRNA synthetase), anti–PL-7 (threonyl tRNA synthetase), anti–PL-12 (alanyl tRNA syntheatse), anti–EJ (glycyl tRNA synthetase), anti–OJ (isoleucyl tRNA synthetase), and anti-KS (asparaginyl tRNA synthetase).
[‡]Anti–Mi-2 autoantibodies immunoprecipitate a nuclear complex composed of five proteins.
HLA, human leukocyte antigen.
SOURCE: Data adapted from Miller FW: Myositis-specific autoantibodies. Touchstones for understanding the inflammatory myopathies. *JAMA* 270:1846, 1993. Reprinted with permission.

occurs less frequently in adults with DM than in children. Typical skin findings may occur in the absence of clinically detectable muscle involvement. When this combination of findings is present for 2 years, patients are said to have *dermatomyositis sine myositis* or *amyopathic dermatomyositis*. Although their long-term prognosis is good, early reports noted an association of malignancy with this subset of patients.

Major extramuscular sites of inflammation in patients with PM or DM include joints, lungs, and the heart. Joint pain or a mild, small joint, symmetric polyarthritis similar in distribution to rheumatoid arthritis, is seen in 25 to 50 percent of patients, but is more destructive and is more common (90 percent) in patients with the antisynthetase syndrome (see Table 77-5). Pulmonary involvement includes abnormal pulmonary function tests in up to 50 percent of patients, respiratory muscle weakness, aspiration pneumonia from pharyngeal muscle dysfunction, diffuse acute alveolitis, or interstitial lung disease (ILD) in 5 to 10 percent of patients. ILD is present in up to 80 percent of those patients with an antisynthetase syndrome. The most common cardiac manifestations are conduction defects and dysrhythmias, with abnormal electrocardiograms seen in up to 40 percent of patients. Diastolic dysfunction, and rarely pericarditis, and myocarditis with secondary heart failure are seen in patients with advanced disease.

Laboratory and Biopsy Findings CK levels are typically elevated with active disease, to as high as 50-fold, and may precede symptoms of weakness by 4 to 5 weeks. CK levels

were falsely low or normal in the setting of active disease in up to 30 percent of patients in one series. Reasons for falsely normal CK levels include the presence of other severe illness causing depletion of glutathione as noted above, marked muscular atrophy, or the current use of corticosteroids or immunosuppressive agents. Elevated CK levels may respond slower to therapy than clinical improvement in strength, and thus should not be used as the sole indicator when deciding on therapy. CK-MB (myocardial muscle creatine kinase isoenzyme) bands may be transiently elevated during active myositis and unrelated to cardiac involvement, as regenerating skeletal muscle produces all three isoforms of CK. Biochemical evidence of rhabdomyolysis is usually lacking, given the typical slow progressive nature of the muscle degeneration. A positive antinuclear antibody is found in 40 to 80 percent of patients, but the presence of a myositis-specific antibody is highly specific for an inflammatory myopathy, and serves to delineate subgroups with common clinical features and prognoses (see Table 77-5). EMG findings of an inflammatory myopathy are seen in affected muscles, but a falsely normal test is seen in up to 10 percent of patients. EMG testing of paraspinal muscles may pick up abnormalities indicative of an inflammatory myopathy before such changes are seen in limb muscles. Testing should be done on one side of the body to preserve the untested limb muscles for possible muscle biopsy. Typical muscle biopsy findings include combinations of muscle fiber degeneration, regeneration, necrosis, phagocytosis, and interstitial infiltrate of lymphocytes. In PM (and s-IBM) the lymphocytes are predominately CD8+

Table 77-6   Proposed Classification Schemes for Polymyositis and Dermatomyositis

	Proposed Criteria (Lead Authors and Year of Publication)		
	Bohan and Peter (1975)	Tanimoto (1995)	Targoff (1997)
Clinical Criteria			
1. Symmetric proximal muscle weakness	+	+	+(or abnormal MR scan of muscle)
2. Muscle pain on grasping or spontaneous pain		+	
3. Nondestructive arthritis or arthralgias		+	
4. Rashes of dermatomyositis	+	+	+
5. Elevated serum muscle enzymes	+	+	+(or abnormal MR scan of muscle)
6. Myositis-specific antibody		+(anti–Jo-1)	+(any)
7. Systemic inflammatory signs (fever, elevated acute phase reactants)		+	
8. EMG findings of an inflammatory myopathy	+	+	+
9. Inflammation on muscle biopsy	+	+	+
Diagnostic subsets			
Polymyositis			
Definite	Criteria 1, 5, 8, 9	Four of criteria 1–3, 5–9	Four of criteria 1, 5, 6, 8, 9
Probable	Three of criteria 1, 5, 8, 9		Three of criteria 1, 5, 6, 8, 9
Possible	Two of criteria 1, 5, 8, 9		Two of criteria 1, 5, 6, 8, 9
Dermatomyositis			
Definite	Criteria 4 and three of criteria 1, 5, 8, 9	Criteria 4 and four of criteria 1–3 and 5–9	Criteria 4 and three of criteria 1, 5, 6, 8, 9
Probable	Criteria 4 and two of criteria 1, 5, 8, 9		Criteria 4 and two of criteria 1, 5, 6, 8, 9
Possible	Criteria 4 and one of criteria 1, 5, 8, 9		Criteria 4 and one of criteria 1, 5, 6, 8, 9

T cells that participate in direct cytotoxic attack on muscle cells throughout the fascicle. In DM, the filtrates are composed predominately of B cells and CD4+ T cells that preferentially target blood vessels at the periphery of a fascicle, causing perifascicular atrophy secondary to local ischemia.

Few studies address the differences in clinical manifestations, response to therapy, and prognosis between the elderly and younger adults with PM-DM. In the most comprehensive review of an elderly cohort to date, Marie and colleagues retrospectively analyzed 79 consecutive patients with PM-DM presenting to a university's clinic or hospital over a 14-year period. Twenty-three (29 percent) of the patients were 65 years of age or older (9 men and 14 women; median age 69 years), 11 who had dermatomyositis, and 12 with polymyositis. Comparing the elderly patients to the younger patients, there were no differences in the duration of symptoms prior to diagnosis, and the frequencies of distribution of PM to DM diagnoses, Raynaud's phenomenon, dysphonia, cardiac impairment, interstitial lung disease,

nor peripheral neuropathy. There was a statistically higher frequency (p <0.05) in the elderly patients of esophageal dysfunction (35 percent versus 16 percent) and bacterial pneumonia (21 percent versus 5 percent), as well as a trend ($p = 0.12$) toward ventilatory insufficiency. Aspiration from esophageal dysfunction combined with ventilatory insufficiency were postulated to lead to the higher frequency of pneumonia. The diagnostic accuracy of an elevated CK or aldolase, myopathic EMG findings, and characteristic inflammatory changes on muscle biopsy was similar to that in younger patients, but older patients had a statistically higher frequency of acute phase reactants and lower levels of hemoglobin, total protein, and albumin. These latter findings may be owing to concurrent malignancy.

Relationship to Malignancy   The frequency of malignancy in patients with PM-DM increases with age and is supported by the study of Marie: 11 of the 23 elderly

Table 77-8 Published Diagnostic Criteria for Polymyalgia Rheumatica.

Clinical Criteria	Bird (1979)	Jones (1981)	Hunder (1982)	Healey (1984)
Age, in years	>65	NM	≥50	>50
Duration of symptoms	2 weeks	≥2 months	1 month	1 month
Distribution of pain	Shoulder	Shoulder and pelvic girdle	2 of 3: neck or torso, hip or proximal thigh, shoulder or proximal arm	2 of 3: neck, shoulders, pelvic girdle
Morning stiffness (in hours)	>1	Present	NM	>1
Lab findings (ESR in mm/h)	ESR >40	ESR >30 or CRP >6 mg/dL	ESR >40	ESR elevated
Response to steroids	NM	Prompt and dramatic	NM	Rapid (dose ≤20 mg/d prednisone)
Other requirements	Depression ± weight loss; proximal arm tenderness	No RA or inflammatory arthritis; no muscle disease; no cancer	Exclude other disease, but GCA allowed	Negative RF and ANA
Required for diagnosis	3 of the above	All of above	All of above	All of above

Column spanning header: Proposed Criteria (Lead Authors and Year of Publication)

ANA, antinuclear antibody; NM, not mentioned; RF, rheumatoid factor.
Bird HA et al: An evaluation of criteria for polymyalgia rheumatica. *Ann Rheum Dis* 38:434,1979.
Jones JG Hazleman BL: Prognosis and management of polymyalgia rheumatica. *Ann Rheum Dis* 40:1, 1981.
Hunder reference (Hunder is the 2nd author): Chuang T-Y, Hunder GG et al: Polymyalgia rheumatica: A 10-year epidemiologic and clinical study. *Ann Intern Med* 97:672, 1982.
Healy LA: Long-term follow-up of polymyalgia rheumatica: Evidence for synovitis. *Semin Arthritis Rheum* 13:322, 1984.

is pathognomonic for the disease. A number of diagnostic criteria have been proposed (Table 77-8).

Treatment

The mainstay therapy for PMR is systemic corticosteroids. An initial dose of 10 to 15 mg of prednisone per day usually leads to prompt improvement, if not complete remission, of subjective symptoms within hours to days. Despite rapid clinical improvement, further tapering of the dose is done slowly in order to prevent relapse. Once the ESR normalizes and symptoms resolve, but usually after 4 to 8 weeks, the dose is reduced in small decrements: by 2.5 mg every 2 to 4 weeks until 10 mg every day is reached, then by 1 mg every 4 weeks. The lowest dose that controls symptoms should always be used. If exacerbations occur during taper, the dose can be increased (although not necessarily to the starting level), and the tapering then recommenced once the symptoms have come under control. Patient symptoms rather than the ESR level alone are the main parameter to follow. Alternate-day dosing of steroids is less effective than a daily schedule. A course of steroids under these guidelines may take a minimum of 12 to 18 months to complete. By 2 years, 75 percent of patients are off steroid therapy

altogether. Persistent elevation of the ESR, rise of the ESR after initial fall and symptom improvement during therapy, or failure to improve with low-dose corticosteroids, may indicate the presence of GCA and consideration for temporal artery biopsy or an alternate diagnosis. Patients should be evaluated for signs and symptoms of GCA at every visit, and if present, referred for temporal artery biopsy even while on corticosteroid therapy. All patients receiving corticosteroids should be started on measures to prevent osteoporosis and be closely monitored for other metabolic side affects.

A percentage of patients, ranging from 10 to 30 percent, depending on the reported series, may require longer courses of corticosteroids or chronic daily doses (e.g., prednisone at 5 mg or less per day) to maintain symptom control. The benefits of such prolonged therapy should be weighed against the serious risk of steroid-induced side effects in the elderly patient. Alternative therapies are not well supported by conclusive clinical trials. Nevertheless, hydroxychloroquine, methotrexate, azathioprine, and other cytotoxics have been used as steroid-sparing agents in PMR, albeit with only limited success. Analgesics may be added to improve pain symptoms. A nonsteroidal anti-inflammatory drug (NSAID) or cyclooxegenase-2 inhibitor may be used as initial therapy in very mildly affected patients but should be changed to corticosteroids if marked improvement is not seen in 2 to 4 weeks. NSAIDs do not alter ESR levels nor suppress subclinical GCA if present. More frequently, these agents are used as a means of providing adjunctive antiinflammatory therapy to ongoing steroid therapy. Their use must be balanced against the risk of eliciting renal, cardiovascular, gastrointestinal, and hematologic side effects in an elderly patient.

Giant Cell Arteritis

GCA is a systemic, granulomatous vasculitis usually focused along the internal elastic lamina of medium- and large-sized extracranial arteries. The aorta and branch vessels from the aortic arch are most frequently involved. Disease manifestations are generally the result of tissue–organ ischemia or necrosis downstream from the site of vascular occlusion. This disease is steroid-responsive but requires higher doses at the initiation of therapy, as contrasted with the treatment for PMR.

Epidemiology and Pathogenesis

As in PMR, GCA is seen in patients older than age 50 years, most commonly in whites, women, and in those of Scandinavian ancestry. The disease is rare in African Americans and those of Hispanic descent. The incidence rate for GCA is two to three times less than PMR, approximately 17 to 27 cases per 100,000 persons older than age 50 years. The associated prevalence rate for GCA is about 200 per 100,000 persons older than age 50 years.

The cause of GCA is unknown, but histologic and biochemical evaluations of affected arteries suggest that it is an antigen-driven disease with a cell-mediated immune response. Association with a HLA-DRB1 gene polymorphism parallels that seen in the immunogenetics of patients with PMR, and the cellular infiltrate throughout the vessel wall mirrors that seen in the synovium of patients with active PMR. Activated CD4+ T cells and macrophages comprise the predominant cell types, and B cells are absent. Destruction of the arterial wall is centered on the elastic fibers of the internal elastic lamina. The cytokine milieu, supported by locally elevated concentrations of interferon–γ and IL-2, promotes the further development of a granulomatous reaction in the vessel. Multinucleated giant cells are found in 50 percent of specimens. Secondary smooth muscle and matrix proliferation contributes to vascular occlusion.

Clinical Features and Diagnostic Criteria

Most patients have clinical findings attributable to involved arteries at some time during the illness. The most prevalent symptoms include headache (65 percent) in the distribution of either the temporal or occipital arteries, visual disturbance (30 percent), permanent visual loss (15 percent), jaw claudication symptoms (45 percent), dysphagia or swallowing claudication (8 percent), tongue claudication (6 percent), limb (usually arm) claudication (4 percent), and persistent cough or sore throat (4 percent).

Headaches may be severe, acute, and associated with scalp sensitivity in temporal and or occipital artery distributions. Typical PMR is seen in 40 to 60 percent and may be the presenting finding in 25 percent. Constitutional symptoms are common and may exist as the sole manifestation of disease. These include weight loss or anorexia (50 percent), fever (which may be prolonged and meet the criteria for fever of unknown etiology; 45 percent), fatigue (40 percent), and depression. Overall, the nonspecific nature of many of the aforementioned symptoms contributes to the delay before diagnosis is made—which could take weeks.

Examination reveals signs related to affected arteries in up to two-thirds of patients. Scalp artery tenderness (27 percent) was a less-frequent finding than a decreased temporal pulse (46 percent) in one study. A swollen, nodular or erythematous scalp artery is detected with equal frequency as a large artery bruit (20 percent). Involvement of the thoracic or abdominal aorta may lead to aneurysmal dilation and possibly rupture, usually occurring years after the onset of disease during a time when most patients are not otherwise thought to have active disease. Hypertension from renovascular involvement is rare. Involvement of the ophthalmic, central retinal, and posterior ciliary arteries to the eye can cause optic nerve ischemic lesions (either anterior or posterior ischemic optic neuropathy, the former the commonest lesion and associated with partial or complete visual loss) or retinal ischemic lesions (either central retinal or cilioretinal artery occlusions, which may also lead to severe visual loss). Visual loss may be sudden, without warning, and risk for permanent loss is increased in patients with prior transient loss. Less-common findings in patients with GCA include peripheral neuropathy, scalp necrosis, cerebral infarction and lesions that may mimic central nervous system vasculitis, tinnitus and deafness.

The ESR is usually markedly elevated, not uncommonly to 80 to 100 mm/h or higher. A normo-to-hypochromic anemia may be seen and can be accompanied by reactive thrombocytosis. Other acute phase reactants such as C-reactive protein, haptoglobin, and α_2-macroglobulin can be elevated. A mild hepatic transaminase or elevation and an increased alkaline phosphatase can occur. The presence of anticardiolipin antibodies at presentation may be an ominous prognostic marker for the subsequent development of vascular complications.

Radiographic investigations can help define the extent of disease, but alone they are rarely sufficient to make the diagnosis of GCA. Angiography of the aorta and its proximal major branches can demonstrate the vascular occlusions responsible for limb claudication, and computed tomography of the chest and abdomen is useful to evaluate for clinically suspected aortic involvement. Doppler ultrasonography of the temporal arteries may show edema of the vessel wall and decreased blood flow and velocity as noninvasive diagnostic signs of active inflammation, but this is not currently recommended as an alternative to diagnostic arterial biopsy.

As clinical features are not specific, temporal artery biopsy remains the gold standard diagnostic test. The yield is increased when the artery to be biopsied is palpably or visibly abnormal. As the pathologic changes in an involved artery tend to occur as skip lesions along its length, a biopsy specimen of at least 4 cm is preferred. The artery should be sectioned at 3- to 5-mm intervals prior to microscopic examination. The need for biopsy should not delay steroid therapy, but biopsy should be performed within the first few days of steroid use. Prior or ongoing therapy with steroids (e.g., in a patient with PMR) should not prevent a decision to confirm the diagnosis by biopsy if the patient has active signs and symptoms of GCA. The temporal artery is the preferred site for biopsy, although a diagnosis can be confirmed by biopsy from a symptomatic occipital artery. An initial negative biopsy may be present in up to a third of patients and should first lead to careful reevaluation of the specimen. Biopsy of the contralateral artery only infrequently provides pathologic confirmation when the initial biopsy is negative, but that should be pursued in a patient for whom the diagnosis remains in doubt, especially if systemic symptoms predominate. A negative biopsy does not preclude a diagnosis of GCA if sufficient other clinical findings are present.

The 1990 American College of Rheumatology classification criteria for GCA have become de facto diagnostic criteria in clinical practice (Table 77-9). These criteria provide a structured approach to making the diagnosis if artery biopsy is either not available or a temporal artery abnormality is not present. In the original derivation, the criteria had a sensitivity of 94 percent and a specificity of 91 percent.

Treatment

The risk of acute visual loss mandates that corticosteroid therapy should be initiated in anyone suspected of having GCA. Initial doses of 40 to 60 mg of prednisone per day in a single morning dose, higher than starting doses for PMR, are standard. Even higher doses, 2 to 3 mg/kg/d, through intravenous administration of methylprednisolone if necessary, are suggested for patients with visual symptoms, whereas in those at high risk for steroid side effects and no visual symptoms, or with mainly constitutional symptoms, a dose of 20 to 40 mg may be initiated. The starting dose is maintained for 4 to 8 weeks to suppress clinical symptoms and to normalize the ESR, and then is slowly tapered over months. Most patients require an average of 2 years of therapy to control symptoms. One suggested schedule for tapering is to reduce the initial dose by 10 mg every 2 to 4 weeks until 40 mg daily is reached, then by 5 mg every 2 to 4 weeks until 20 mg daily is reached, followed by a reduction of 2.5 mg every 2 to 4 weeks until 10 mg per day is reached. Thereafter, the dose is tapered following the pattern for patients with PMR, by 1 mg every 2 to 4 weeks. Disease exacerbations during tapering of steroids or after completion of therapy occur in up to two-thirds of patients and require a transient increase or resumption in dose followed by further attempts at weaning. The are no clinical predictors for those at risk for relapse. The ESR is an imperfect indicator of disease activity and must be used in combination with clinical symptoms for assessment of disease and adjustment of therapy. Persistent elevation of ESR despite absence of clinical disease activity may indicate silent large-vessel disease (e.g., aortitis) or be associated with another condition such as an unrecognized infection masked by steroid use. The utility of methotrexate as a steroid-sparing agent is under debate. Initial reports of a steroid-sparing effect from limited studies contrast with results from a recent multicenter, randomized placebo-controlled trial showing no additional benefit from the addition of moderate dose methotrexate to prednisone in terms of control of disease activity, and the ability to reduce cumulative dose and toxicity of corticosteroids in patients with GCA.

Although the life expectancy of patients with GCA is similar to that of the age-matched general population,

Table 77-9 Criteria for the Classification of GCA.

For purposes of classification, a patient shall be said to have GCA if at least 3 of the 5 criteria are present:

Criterion	Definition
1. Age at onset ≥50 years	Development of symptoms or findings beginning at age 50 years or older
2. New headache	New onset of or new type of localized pain in the head
3. Temporal artery abnormality	Temporal artery tenderness to palpation or decreased pulsation, unrelated to arteriosclerosis of cervical arteries
4. Elevated ESR	Erythrocyte sedimentation rate (ESR) ≥50 mm/h by the Westergren method
5. Abnormal artery biopsy	Biopsy specimen with artery showing vasculitis characterized by a predominance of mononuclear cell infiltration or granulomatous inflammation, usually with multinucleated giant cells.

SOURCE: Adapted from Hunder GG et al: The American College of Rheumatology 1990 criteria for the classification of giant cell arteritis. *Arthritis Rheum* 33:1122, 1990. Reprinted with permission.

morbidity from the disease itself and its therapy may be substantial. Twenty to 50 percent of patients develop toxicities from corticosteroids. The impact from disease manifestations and the side effects of therapy impact should not be underestimated in the elderly population.

REFERENCES

Askanas V, Engel WK: Sporadic inclusion-body myositis and its similarities to Alzheimer disease brain. Recent approaches to diagnosis and pathogenesis, and relation to aging. *Scand J Rheumatol* 27:389, 1998.

Bohan A, Peter JB: Polymyositis and dermatomyositis (parts 1 and 2). *N Engl J Med* 292:344, 403, 1975.

Cantini F et al: Inflamed shoulder structures in polymyalgia rheumatica with normal erythrocyte sedimentation rate. *Arthritis Rheum* 44:1155, 2001.

Cherin P: Treatment of inclusion body myositis. *Curr Opin Rheum* 11:456, 1999.

Evans JM, Hunder GG: Polymyalgia rheumatica and giant cell arteritis. *Rheum Dis Clin North Am* 26:493, 2000.

Gaist D et al: Lipid-lowering drugs and risk of myopathy: A population-based follow-up study. *Epidemiology* 12:565, 2001.

Hoffman GS et al: A multicenter, randomized, double-blind, placebo-controlled trial of adjuvant methotrexate treatment for giant cell arteritis. *Arthritis Rheum* 46:1309, 2002.

Janssen I et al: Low relative skeletal muscle mass (sarcopenia) in older persons is associated with functional impairment and physical disability. *J Am Geriatr Soc* 50:889, 2002.

Marie I et al: Influence of age on characteristics of polymyositis and dermatomyositis in adults. *Medicine* 78:139, 1999.

Mazzeo RS et al: ACSM position stand on exercise and physical activity for older adults. *Med Sci Sports Exerc* 30:992, 1998.

McGonagle D et al: Comparison of extracapsular changes by magnetic resonance imaging in patients with rheumatoid arthritis and polymyalgia rheumatica. *J Rheumatol* 28:1837, 2001.

Mitch WE, Goldberg AL: Mechanisms of muscle wasting. The role of the ubiquitin-protease pathway. *N Engl J Med* 335:1897, 1996.

Morley JE et al: Sarcopenia. *J Lab Clin Med* 137:231, 2001.

Oerlemans WGH, de Visser M: Dropped head syndrome and bent spine syndrome: Two separate clinical entities or different manifestations of axial myopathy. *J Neurol Neurosurg Psychiatry* 65:258, 1998.

O'Rourke KS: Myopathies in the elderly. *Rheum Dis Clin North Am* 26:647, 2000.

Pascuzzi RM: Drugs and toxins associated with myopathies. *Curr Opin Rheum* 10:511, 1998.

Reginato AJ et al: Musculoskeletal manifestations of osteomalacia: Report of 26 cases and literature review. *Semin Arthritis Rheum* 28:287, 1999.

Salvaranic et al: Polymyalgia rheumatica and giant-cell arteritis. *N Engl J Med* 347:261, 2002.

Sivakumar K, Dalakas MC: Inclusion body myositis and myopathies. *Curr Opin Neurol* 10:413, 1997.

Tanimoto K et al: Classification criteria for polymyositis and dermatomyositis. *J Rheumatol* 22:668, 1995.

Targoff IN et al: Classification criteria for the idiopathic inflammatory myopathies. *Curr Opin Rheumatol* 9:527, 1997.

Weyand CM et al: Corticosteroid requirements in polymyalgia rheumatica. *Arch Intern Med* 159:577, 1999.

Zachwieja JJ, Yarasheski KE: Does growth hormone therapy in conjunction with resistance exercise increase muscle force production and muscle mass in men and women aged 60 years or older? *Phys Ther* 79:76, 1999.

Zantos D et al: The overall and temporal association of cancer with polymyositis and dermatomyositis. *J Rheumatol* 21:1855, 1994.

Rheumatoid Arthritis and Other Autoimmune Diseases

RAYMOND YUNG

Rheumatoid arthritis and other autoimmune diseases are prevalent in the elderly population. The past decade has seen exciting new developments in our understanding of the pathogenesis and treatment of these diseases. This chapter summarizes these new advances, with specific references to the geriatric population.

RHEUMATOID ARTHRITIS

Definition

Rheumatoid arthritis (RA) is a chronic systemic inflammatory disease that preferentially affects diarthrodial joints. The current classification criteria for rheumatoid arthritis was developed in 1987, based on the study of predominantly middle-aged patients attending hospital outpatient clinics (Table 78-1). While the criteria set is useful for diagnosing established and active disease in younger patients, its usefulness in detecting early disease and elderly onset (>60 years old) rheumatoid arthritis (EORA) has not been established. This is important because the disease presentation in EORA is often different from that of young-onset RA (YORA).

Epidemiology

Unlike other common arthritides which may have existed in this country for thousands of years, there is evidence that RA may be a relatively new disease in America, brought on after the crossing of the Atlantic Ocean around the fifteenth century. Although the overall incidence and severity of RA may be declining in recent years, it is still the most prevalent autoimmune disease, afflicting 0.5 to 2 percent of the Western adult population. Gender and age are important factors in RA. Overall, two to three times more women are affected by the disease than men. However, this gender parity disappears in old age. The prevalence of rheumatoid arthritis increases with age and is commonest in the most elderly group studied (often 65 years and older or 70 years and older). The incidence of rheumatoid arthritis also increases with age with the peak incidence occurring in the sixth to eighth decades (Fig. 78-1). The reason for the age-associated increase in disease susceptibility is currently unknown. With the "graying" of America, RA is of considerable importance because of the rising number of new cases in the elderly population and because more people with RA are surviving into old age.

Pathophysiology

Although the inciting agent for RA remains elusive, investigations in recent years have yielded important insights into the pathogenesis of this disease. This has led to some of the most important advances in RA therapy.

The concordance rate for monozygotic twins is between 12 percent and 15 percent, approximately three times that of dizygotic pairs and much higher than that of the background prevalence rate of the general population. The fact that most monozygotic twins are discordant for RA illustrates the importance of environmental factors. The association between RA and human leukocyte antigen (HLA) has been refined to alleles coding for a "shared" epitope (the sequences QRRAA or QKRAA) on the HLA-DRB1 genes. The presence of the DRB1*04 (DR4) allele (especially if both alleles are present) is a marker for increased susceptibility and severe disease. Population differences in the prevalence of the "shared epitope" may help to explain in part the geographic variation in the prevalence of RA.

An infectious etiology for RA has been postulated for more than half a century. (1) The onset of RA can be heralded by polyarthralgias, fever, and malaise that are indistinguishable from an acute infection. (2) The joints are known targets for diverse microorganisms from gonococci to *Borrelia burgdorferi* and *Mycobacterium tuberculosis*. (3) Acute and chronic "reactive" arthritis can follow specific gastrointestinal or genital urinary infection. (4) A

Table 78-1 Classification Criteria for Rheumatoid Arthritis* (R₃A₄)

Rheumatoid factor	Using a method with positive results in <5% of normal controls.
Rheumatoid nodules	Subcutaneous nodules over bony prominences, extensor surfaces, or in juxtaarticular regions.
Radiographic changes	Typical changes of RA on hand and wrist radiographs, including erosions or unequivocal bony decalcification localized in or adjacent to the involved joints.
Arthritis of the hand joints	Swelling of wrist, metacarpal phalangeal (MCP), or proximal phalangeal (PIP) joints for at least 6 weeks.
Arthritis in 3 or more joints	Soft-tissue swelling or fluid present simultaneously for at least 6 weeks. Possible areas include PIP, MCP, wrist, elbow, knee, ankle, metatarsal phalangeal joints.
Arthritis that is symmetrical	Simultaneous involvement of the same joint areas on both sides of the body for at least 6 weeks.
AM (morning) stiffness	Morning stiffness in and around the joints, lasting at least 1 hour before maximal improvement at anytime in the disease course.

*Requires at least four criteria for the classification of rheumatoid arthritis.

SOURCE: Modified from Arnett FC et al: The American Rheumatism Association 1987 revised criteria for the classification of rheumatoid arthritis. *Arthritis Rheum* 31:315, 1987.

transient RA-like illness can be seen in viral infections including parvovirus B19, Epstein–Barr virus (EBV) and human T-lymphotropic virus type 1 (HTLV-1).

Tantalizing evidence of a potential pathogenic role for microorganisms in RA includes: (1) retroviral-like particles have been observed in RA synovial fluid. (2) Viral or bacterial superantigen can reawaken a latent or subclinical disease in animal models of inflammatory arthritis. (3) Heat shock proteins (viral and cellular) can act as autoantigens. Interestingly, both the dnaJ class of bacterial heat shock

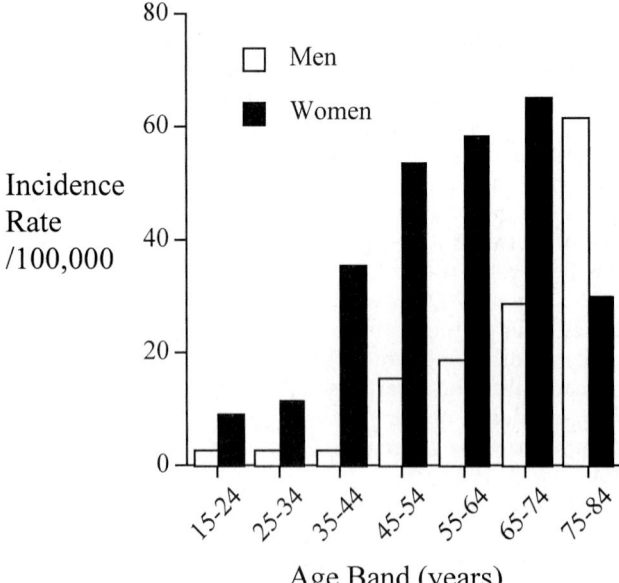

Figure 78-1 Age-related incidence of rheumatoid arthritis. Adapted from Symmons DPM et al: The incidence of rheumatoid arthritis in the United Kingdom: Results from the Norfolk Arthritis register. *Br J Rheumatol* 33:735, 1994.

protein and the gp110 capsid protein of EBV have the QKRAA "shared epitope" amino acid sequence.

Despite these observations, a direct role for infection in the pathogenesis in RA has not been proven. It is possible that transient exposure of the joints to microorganism protein with homology to normal antigen could attract lymphocytes to the synovium. This, in turn, may set up an autoimmune response through a molecular mimicry mechanism without requiring the presence of the inciting organism (the "hit and run" theory). Recent studies suggest that RA synovial cells may have defective apoptosis and a transformed phenotype. This opens up the possibility that environmental agents, including viruses, may transform synovial or lymphoid cells to cause inflammation and tissue destruction without requiring the presence of the inciting agent.

The higher female incidence in RA is likely a result of gender-related differences in reproductive hormones. The risk of developing new-onset RA during pregnancy is lower than that expected in age-matched controls. In addition, patients with existing RA often have a milder disease course during their pregnancy. Interestingly, the first year after delivery is associated with an increased risk for a flare-up, as well as the development of new RA. Nulliparity and breastfeeding have been suggested as additional risk factors. However, supporting data for these assertions are less convincing.

The linkage of RA to specific major histocompatibility complex (MHC) alleles, the abundance of specific T-cell subsets in synovial tissue and fluid, and other evidence from animal models of inflammatory arthritis all point to a central role of T lymphocytes in the immunopathogenesis of this disease. RA is considered to be a Th (T helper) 1-mediated disease based on the cytokine and more recently the chemokine receptor profile of T cells in synovial joints. Although it is tempting to postulate that

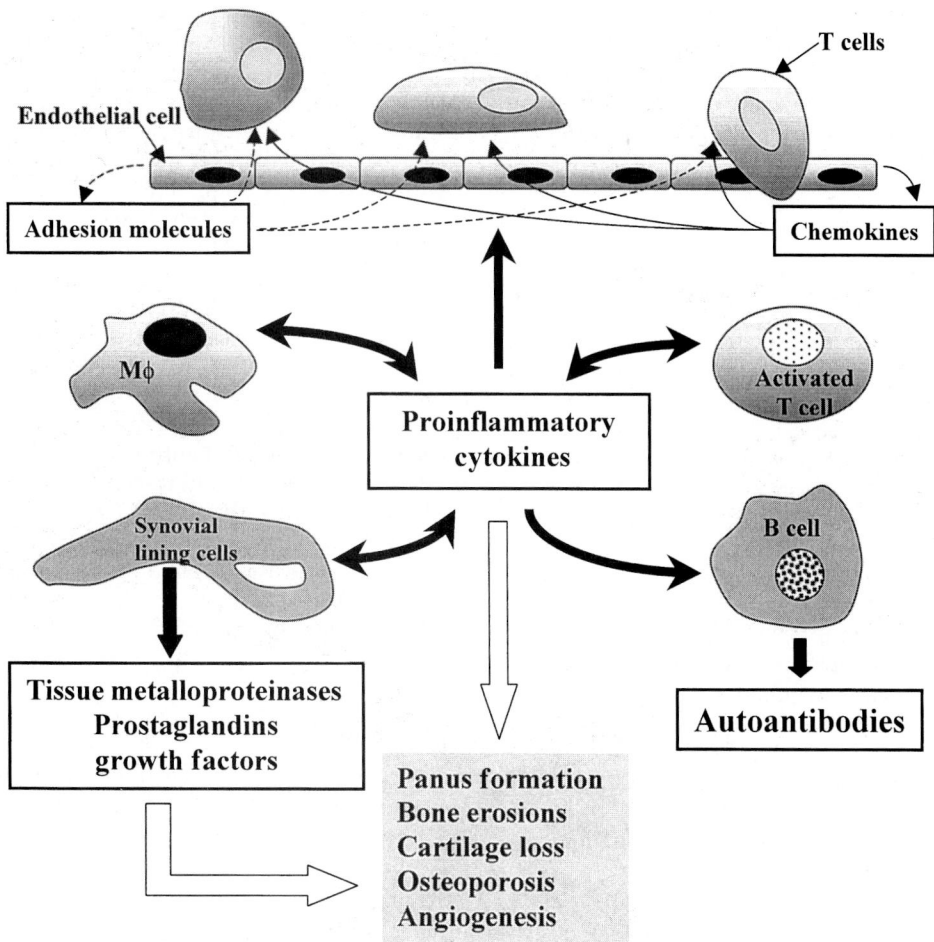

Figure 78-2   The inflammatory cascade in rheumatoid arthritis.

RA-associated DRB1 epitope triggers disease by presenting an arthrogenic peptide to T cells, extensive search of unique peptides that are displayed selectively by RA-associated HLA molecules has so far been unsuccessful. Costimulatory molecules, including CD28 and CD60, may play a role in activating T cells in RA joints. However, their precise role in human disease is unclear. Signal transduction through the T-cell receptor (TCR) is defective in RA, suggesting that non–TCR-activating pathways may be important in T-cell activation in this disease.

Activation and recruitment of T cells into the RA joint set into motion a complex cascade of inflammatory responses (Fig. 78-2). This, in turn, leads to synovial proliferation, pannus formation, localized osteoporosis, bone erosions, and destruction of periarticular structures that are characteristic of this disease. Interaction between T cells, macrophages, synovial cells, and vascular endothelial cells leads to the production of proinflammatory mediators that act in an autocrine and paracrine fashion. These include cytokines (interleukin [IL]-1, -6, -13, -15, tumor necrosis factor [TNF]), metalloproteinases (stromelysin, collagenases, gelatinases), transforming growth factor-β (TGF-β), granulocyte colony-stimulating factor, and activated complement components.

The reason for the age-associated increase in RA susceptibility is unclear. The traditional view that aging is associated with a "decline" in immune response does not explain the high incidence and severe onset of this autoimmune disease that is commonly seen in older adults. Decline in sex hormone production in postmenopausal years also cannot account for the high incidence of RA in elderly females. Unlike their younger counterparts, EORA occurs with equal frequency in males and females. However, the rising incidence of RA in postmenopausal women suggests that while reproductive hormones may influence the disease manifestation, they are unlikely to play a major pathogenic role in the elderly population.

Animal studies suggest that aging is accompanied by a shift from a Th1 to a predominantly Th2 cytokine profile. However, such changes cannot explain the high incidence of RA, a predominantly Th1-mediated disease, in the elderly population either. Studies on the effect of age on the adenovirus vectors (AV) model of inflammatory arthritis have yielded conflicting results, with some strains showing more chronic and destructive arthritis in older female animals. The enhanced production of proinflammatory cytokines, including TNF-α and IL-1, in aging, may contribute to the clinical features of EORA. The recruitment and retention of T cells in the RA synovial joint are complex processes determined by the interaction of leukocyte adhesion molecules and chemokine receptors interacting with their respective ligands expressed by synovial and vascular endothelial cells. T cells from aged animals may express high levels of selective chemokine receptors that are important in the recruitment of T cells to RA joints. These lines of research may eventually provide the explanation for the increased susceptibility and severity of RA in the elderly.

Presentation

Whether EORA is a different disease from YORA is controversial. The clinical studies that address the issue were mostly descriptive or cross-sectional studies done in the 1950s and 1960s that have significant methodologic problems. The older definition of RA used in these studies also allowed terms, such as "classical," "definite," and "probable" RA, that are no longer used today. As mentioned before, the most widely accepted classification of RA currently in use has not been validated in the elderly population.

Table 78-2 summarizes the features of EORA. In general, patients with EORA have a more equal gender distribution. The large joints, including the shoulder joint, are more often involved at presentation in EORA. Whether this is a result of concomitant rotator cuff disease that is prevalent in this age group is unclear. Symptoms in the proximal girdles have led to the belief that EORA may present with a polymyalgia rheumatica-like illness. Erythrocyte sedimentation rate (ESR) normally increases with age especially in females. Elevated ESR is also more common in EORA. The prevalence of rheumatoid factor (RF) similarly increases after the age of 60 years, reaching 30 percent by age 90 years. Earlier reports suggest a lower frequency of RF in EORA than YORA. However, this has not been confirmed in more recent studies. As in younger patients, EORA patients who are seropositive for RF have more severe clinical disease, more bony erosions on x-ray, worse functional outcome, and increased mortality. Whether seropositive EORA patients have worse prognosis than do their younger counterparts is unclear. It is possible that the poor prognosis of EORA reported in some studies reflects the greater number of comorbid conditions that are present in older patients.

Table 78-2   Clinical Features of Elderly Onset Rheumatoid Arthritis

Age of onset >60 years
Male: female ~1:1
Acute presentation
Oligoarticular (2–6 joints) disease
Involvement of large and proximal joints
Systemic complaints, e.g., weight loss
Absence of rheumatoid nodules
Sicca symptoms common
Laboratory: high erythrocyte sedimentation rate; often negative rheumatoid factor

"Benign polyarthritis of the elderly" person occurs in up to a third of EORA patients. They have a more explosive disease onset associated with systemic features such as fever and night sweats. The clinical features have led some to describe the disease as "infectious-like." The disease is called benign because its general prognosis is good, with most people going into remission within 1 year with or without treatment. Within this group can be included a peculiar syndrome unique to the elderly population called the RS$_3$PE (remitting, seronegative, symmetric synovitis with pitting edema) syndrome. This typically affects elderly men (2 to 3:1, male:female ratio) and is characterized by acute onset of symmetric polyarthritis/tenosynovitis with pitting edema involving both upper and lower extremities. As the name implies, these patients generally have negative rheumatoid factor and antinuclear antibody (ANA). They often have high ESR and respond to low-dose prednisone. The association with HLA-B7 has been reported inconsistently. RS$_3$PE may occasionally be associated with other rheumatic diseases, including polymyalgia rheumatica, spondyloarthropathies, psoriatic arthritis, rheumatoid arthritis, and sarcoid, and, rarely, malignancies.

Evaluation

The assessment of RA in older adults is different from that of the younger age group. The nonspecific symptoms and signs of RA are prevalent in the geriatric population. Rheumatic diseases that can mimic EORA, such as polymyalgia rheumatica, osteoarthritis, and crystal-induced arthritis, are prevalent in the elderly population. Arthritis associated with malignancy can be misdiagnosed as RA before the correct diagnosis is made months or years later. Other differential diagnoses of RA in the elderly population include inflammatory (erosive) osteoarthritis, late-onset spondyloarthropathy, endocrinopathy (e.g., hypothyroidism, hyperparathyroidism, diabetic cheiroarthropathy), amyloidosis, and the edematous phase of scleroderma. Conditions such as sarcoidosis, adult Still's disease, hemochromatosis, and glycogen storage diseases can mimic RA, but are unlikely to present for the first time so late in life.

In addition to the above considerations, the initial evaluation of an elderly patient with RA should include a careful assessment of the patient's living condition, social support, and cognitive and functional status. Many elderly patients have the misconception that there is no effective treatment for arthritis and they should accept their physical suffering as part of normal aging. Older adults are often embarrassed about their arthritis pain. They may minimize their symptoms by using terms such as "aching" and "stiff" instead of pain. Unfortunately, many clinicians also do not take their symptoms seriously, resulting in the patients frequently feeling that their care resembles "a lick and a promise." Because pain is by far the commonest presenting symptom of RA, pain assessment should be an integral part of the patient's evaluation at presentation and in subsequent office visits. This can be difficult in the elderly patient who has significant cognitive or verbal impairment. Information from caregivers, nonverbal pain behavior, physical evidence of active joint inflammation, and decline in functions

Table 78-3 American College of Rheumatology 1991 Revised Criteria for the Classification of Global Functional Status in Rheumatoid Arthritis

Class I	Completely able to perform usual activities of daily living (self-care, vocational, and avocational)
Class II	Able to perform usual self-care and vocational activities, but limited in avocational activities
Class III	Able to perform usual self-care activities, but limited in vocational and avocational activities
Class IV	Limited in ability to perform usual self-care, vocational, and avocational activities

SOURCE: Adapted from Hochberg MC et al. (1992).

are important clues that more aggressive therapy may be necessary.

American College of Rheumatology published a useful classification system for assessing the functional status of RA patients in 1991 (Table 78-3). This is a quick assessment tool that is useful for describing the global functional status and allows patients to be grouped for studies. RA patients with the worst (class IV) functional status were reported to have extremely poor prognosis, with survival similar to patients with multiple vessel coronary artery disease and stage IV Hodgkin's lymphoma. Many clinicians now feel that the prognosis for RA has improved with the advent of better therapeutic regimens for RA in the past two decades. Whether this translates into prolonged survival remains to be determined. Concomitant medical conditions affecting the patient's hearing, eyesight,

continence, and balance need to be addressed to optimize functional ability and to prevent falls. Current and past medical histories are important elements of the initial evaluation. This information is important in determining the selection of specific treatment (see Management). In contrast, family history is not as helpful in assessing elderly patients with RA.

In addition to excluding diseases mentioned above, a new patient suspected of having RA should be tested for the presence of anemia, cytopenia, liver or renal dysfunction, rheumatoid factor, and elevated ESR. The presence of extremely high rheumatoid factor should prompt the clinician to consider the possible diagnosis of cryoglobulinemia. Some patients have negative rheumatoid factor but positive ANA. These patients tend to have more severe disease, similar to the rheumatoid factor positive patients. A work-up for secondary Sjögren's syndrome should be done in patients with concurrent sicca symptoms (dry eye, dry mouth). In general, ESR is a better indicator of disease activity than changes in the titer of rheumatoid factor. For some patients C-reactive protein level may more closely parallel their clinical course than ESR.

Radiographic joint examination is an integral part of the evaluation of RA patients. Elderly patients with RA for more than 10 years are at particular risk for cervical spine disease and atlantoaxial joint instability. This is an important consideration before a patient is submitted to a surgical procedure as overextension of the cervical spine during intubation may compromise the brainstem or spinal cord. Early x-ray changes include soft-tissue swelling and regional osteoporosis around the joint. Typical erosions in hands and feet involve the juxta-articular "bare areas" of bone not covered with cartilage (Fig. 78-3). Isolated erosions in the first and second metacarpophalangeal (MCP) joints may prompt the clinician to search for occult calcium pyrophosphate depositive disease (CPPD) disease, hyperparathyroidism, or hemochromatosis. Erosions are

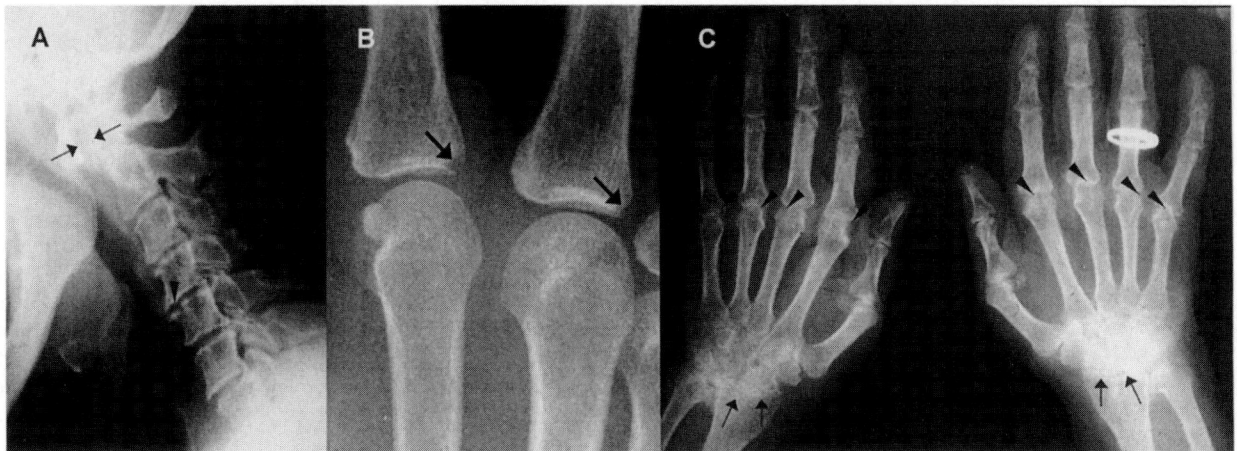

Figure 78-3 Radiographic changes of rheumatoid arthritis. (*A*) X-ray of the cervical spine in the flexed position showing severe atlantoaxial joint subluxation in a patient with chronic rheumatoid arthritis, with *arrows* highlighting the abnormal distance between the posterior surface of the anterior arch of the atlas and the anterior surface of the odontoid process. *Arrowhead* points to the erosion on the surface of C5. (*B*) Early erosive changes in the metacarpal phalangeal joints affecting the "bare area" of the bone not protected by cartilage. (*C*) Bilateral hand x-ray with advanced rheumatoid arthritis. Some of the features include juxtaarticular osteoporosis, collapse of the carpal bones, radial deviation of the radiocarpal joint of the wrist (*arrows*), and erosion and destruction of metacarpal phalangeal joints (*arrowheads*). Note also the symmetric nature of the disease. Courtesy of Curtis Hayes, MD, University of Michigan.

less common in the knee and hip joints. At these sites, RA typically causes cartilage loss and joint-space narrowing. Joint-space narrowing occurring predominantly in the lateral compartment of the knee and diffusely in the hip without bony proliferation are helpful features for distinguishing RA from osteoarthritis. To assess for joint-space narrowing of the knees, clinicians should request semiflexed weight-bearing films.

There is no evidence that EORA patients are more likely to develop extraarticular disease, as compared to those with YORA. However, the elderly population may be disproportionately affected because extraarticular manifestations are more common in chronic RA. High titer of rheumatoid factor is a risk factor for extraarticular RA, especially in male patients. Rheumatoid nodules are the most characteristic extraarticular manifestation of RA and are present in up to 40 percent of seropositive white patients. They are most commonly found in areas of pressure such as the elbows, heels, and sacrum. Their presence does not correlate with disease activity, and may increase in number during methotrexate therapy when synovitis is improving. Rheumatoid vasculitis affects vessels of all sizes. This complication may present as cutaneous vasculitis, mononeuritis multiplex, nail fold infarcts, or deep "punched-out" ulcers at atypical sites that fail to respond to conventional therapy. Pleuritis and pericarditis are found in 20 to 30 percent of RA patients and do not usually cause any symptom. Other respiratory complications of RA include pulmonary granuloma (often in the upper lobes), Caplan's syndrome, fibrosing alveolitis, and bronchiolitis obliterans. Felty's syndrome (RA with splenomegaly and neutropenia) typically occurs in white patients with long-standing, chronic erosive RA. These patients are at increased risk of developing lymphoproliferative malignancies. Thrombocytopenia may occur, in part, because of splenic sequestration. Mild to moderate normochromic, normocytic anemia is extremely common in patients with chronic RA. Iatrogenic causes (e.g., nonsteroidal antiinflammatory drugs [NSAIDs], methotrexate) of anemia need to be excluded in all RA patients with anemia.

Management

Nonpharmacologic Therapies

Successful management of RA involves patient participation in his/her care. In addition, family, social, and psychological support are critical in maintaining the patient's independence. Establishing a good rapport, gaining the trust of the patient and the family, providing information about the nature of the disease, and setting realistic goals are all important elements of the initial management of RA. Many patients and their relatives also find it helpful to seek out support groups in their local area. Increasingly, elderly patients and their families are turning to the internet, health magazines, and other nontraditional sources for information about treatments options including over-the-counter complementary therapies. It is important that health care professionals be aware of the pros and cons of these options. In this regard, resources such as *The Arthritis Foundation's Guide to Alternative Therapies*

can be helpful. Unfortunately, the unexpected side effects of over-the-counter medications are increasingly being recognized. The latest information is often not available in traditional textbooks. Directing the patients to reputable web sites such as that offered by the National Institute on Aging can be useful for more up-to-date information.

Nonpharmacologic therapies are crucial components of the total care of the RA patient that should be emphasized throughout the treatment course. In addition to their inherent usefulness, participation in these treatment modalities often provides the patients and their families with a sense of control over their chronic illness. The team approach that typifies geriatric medicine is eminently suitable for treating elderly patients with chronic arthritis. Physical and occupational therapy should be offered to every RA patient including those with mild and early disease. Education about rest/activity, use of cold/heat, massage, adaptive devices (to improve function and to prevent/correct joint deformity) are important. Performing exercises to strengthen muscles and ligaments for joint protection, gait training and fall prevention can make a big difference in the life of RA patients. Community-based exercise programs such as PACE (Patients with Arthritis Can Exercise, the Arthritis Foundation) are a good resource for those who are able to participate. Psychological counseling and support groups are often helpful, especially to those who are socially isolated because of their arthritis. Depression is increasingly recognized as a common problem in the elderly and in those with chronic illness. Adequate treatment will help break the vicious cycle of pain, depression, and disability. Although nonpharmacologic therapies have not been shown to affect the course of RA, they can improve the patient's quality of life and help to reduce the requirement for pain medications that have significant potential for side effects in this vulnerable population.

Pharmacologic Therapies

Recent years have seen an exciting explosion of new drugs available for the treatment of RA. Pharmaceutical companies have increasingly included the geriatric population in pre- and postmarketing clinical trials. Although this provides some reassurance to clinicians, knowing that these agents may be efficacious in the elderly population, it is important to remember that subjects participating in these studies rarely mirror the patients geriatricians see in their clinic who have multiple comorbidities and who already suffer from polypharmacy. The costs of these new agents may be out of reach for patients who do not have prescription coverage. Because of the complexity of modern treatment regimens, coupled with the need to monitor many potentially serious side effects, drug therapy for RA should ideally be instituted in consultation with a rheumatologist. Involvement of physicians experienced in the use of immunosuppressive therapies (e.g., hematologists and oncologists, or a gastroenterologist in the case of infliximab) will be helpful in patients living in isolated communities where there may not be a local rheumatologist.

The gradualism of the "pyramid approach" to RA treatment in the 1980s has been replaced with the widespread belief that rheumatoid inflammation should be suppressed as completely and as soon as possible once the diagnosis is confirmed. This change in philosophy is, in part, a result of the recognition that joint damage occurs much sooner than was previously believed. Results of well-designed clinical trials in the past decade have persuaded many that this new standard is attainable with more aggressive drug regimens. In the American College of Rheumatology updated *2002 Guidelines for the Management of Rheumatoid Arthritis*, it is suggested that the majority of patients with newly diagnosed RA should be started on disease-modifying antirheumatic drug (DMARD) therapy within 3 months of diagnosis.

Although NSAIDs are useful adjunct therapies for RA, many geriatricians are reluctant to prescribe this class of medication because of concern that elderly persons are vulnerable to the potential serious toxicity that can occur in almost every major organ system in the body. Meta-analysis of epidemiologic studies published in the 1990s found that NSAID use is associated with a 5- and 3.5-fold increased risk of serious upper gastrointestinal (GI) tract disease in women and men, respectively. Age alone is a risk factor for upper GI bleeding (relative risk of 4.5 in age 70 to 80 years group, and 9.2 in those older than age 80 years). Because of the high background rate of upper GI events in the elderly population, the relative risk for GI bleeding only increases modestly in elderly patients on NSAID. Not surprisingly, elderly patients with history of GI bleeding are at the greatest risk for serious GI complications when they are placed on a NSAID. The concurrent use of glucocorticoids further increases the risk of GI bleeding.

The introduction of selective cyclooxygenase-2 (COX-2) inhibitors represents an important advance in NSAID therapy because of their low incidence of GI events and because they do not significantly affect platelet function. However, COX-2 inhibitors still have significant renal toxicity, including hypertension, peripheral edema, and rising serum creatinine. NSAID-induced renal complications are more likely to occur in patients who are on concurrent diuretics or angiotensin-converting enzyme (ACE) inhibitors. There is also the unresolved concern that their use may be associated with an increased risk of cardiovascular events. This may be caused by the unopposed thromboxane pathway when the COX-2 pathway is inhibited. The use of a COX-2 inhibitor is not a substitute for aspirin cardioprotection. A recent study showed that prolonged dosing of ibuprofen blocked the platelet inhibition effects of aspirin. Although other NSAIDs tested so far do not appear to have the same problem, this raises the concern that the aspirin/ibuprofen combination may not be ideal for RA patients with cardiovascular risk factors. Concurrent use of low-dose (≤325 mg/d) aspirin increases the already high risk for GI events in elderly patients taking traditional NSAIDs and may negate most of the GI-sparing effect of COX-2 inhibitors. At present, it appears that most at-risk elderly RA patients requiring a traditional NSAID or a COX-2 selective agent plus aspirin should receive GI cytoprotection.

Low-dose glucocorticoid is effective for short-term symptom control in patients with active RA. There is also intriguing data showing that prednisone in early disease may be "disease modifying." Unfortunately, elderly patients commonly develop significant side effects, but become functionally dependent on the drug. The lowest dose, and if possible, alternate-day dosing should be prescribed. Assessment, prophylaxis, and treatment of osteoporosis, cardiovascular risk factors, diabetes, and GI complications are important. Judicious use of intraarticular steroid injections may provide local (and systemic) symptom relief, and may be safer than oral glucocorticoids in elderly patients with poorly controlled diabetes, severe osteoporosis, and congestive heart failure.

Antimalarials including hydroxychloroquine and chloroquine are useful in mild cases of RA and are most often prescribed as part of a combination regimen. Hydroxychloroquine is often preferred over chloroquine because it has a lower incidence of ocular complications. Approximately 50 percent of hydroxychloroquine is protein-bound in the plasma, a property that is important in elderly patients with low serum albumen and who are taking other highly protein-bound drugs. The mechanism of drug action is uncertain, but is postulated to include changes in intracellular pH that in turn affect antigen presentation by immune cells. An added benefit in RA patients who are at increased risk for coronary heart disease is the drug's favorable effect on serum cholesterol level. The major side effect of hydroxychloroquine and chloroquine is retinal (macular) toxicity with the classical "bull's-eye" lesion. The patients most susceptible to this complication are those older than age 70 years who are on >6.5 mg/kg daily dose or who have a cumulative dose of >800 g of the drug.

Sulfasalazine is only occasionally used as monotherapy in the United States, although there is data showing that the drug may slow the progression of radiographic damage in RA. Its mechanism of immunosuppression is unclear but may include reducing immunoglobulin levels, suppressed T and B cell proliferative response, and cytokine inhibition. Cytopenias (particularly leukopenia), GI symptoms (nausea and vomiting, dyspepsia), and skin rashes are the commonest side effects. In addition to monitoring for hematologic toxicity, some experts recommend that liver enzyme levels should be tested regularly as well.

Methotrexate, an analog of folic acid, is the most commonly prescribed DMARD for RA in the United States. More than 50 percent of patients on methotrexate continue the drug beyond 3 years, longer than any other DMARD. The drug and its metabolites are potent inhibitors of dihydrofolic acid reductase (DHFR) and other distal enzymes in the folic acid metabolic pathway. The immunosuppressive effects may be partly a result of folate-dependent inhibition of lymphocyte proliferation. Methotrexate has also been reported to reduce the production of leukotriene B_4 and to directly alter phospholipase A_2 activity. Common side effects include cytopenias (particularly anemia), liver toxicity (fibrosis and cirrhosis), hypersensitivity pneumonitis, infections, mucosal ulceration, and alopecia. The elderly population is particularly susceptible to these side effects because methotrexate is excreted primarily by the kidneys and renal impairment is common in this group. Great caution and dose adjustment are therefore needed when using the drug to treat elderly RA patients and those with a history of hepatitis. In addition, folic acid (1 to 3 mg/d) or folinic acid (leucovorin, 2.5 to 5 mg given 24 hours after the methotrexate) supplementation reduces the incidence of many of methotrexate side effects and should be used routinely.

Leflunomide is an inhibitor of pyrimidine synthesis and has been available for the treatment of RA in the United States since 1998. The oral medication is rapidly metabolized to an active metabolite that is partially excreted in the bile and reabsorbed by the enterohepatic circulation. The plasma half-life of leflunomide is approximately 14 days. However, the excretion can be accelerated by oral cholestyramine. In clinical studies, leflunomide has been shown to be equal to methotrexate in efficacy. It is also the first drug to receive an FDA-approved label indication to retard structural damage in RA as evidenced by x-ray erosions and joint-space narrowing. The commonest side effects include diarrhea (20 percent), reversible alopecia (10 percent), and elevated liver function enzymes. The long-term infection risk with the drug is not known.

Treatment of RA has entered into the new era of biologic response modifiers. At the time of this writing three anti-TNF and one anti–IL-1 drugs have been approved for RA in the United States, with a number of other similar agents in various stages of drug development. Etanercept is a recombinant soluble p75 TNF receptor fused to the Fc portion of human immunoglobulin (Ig) G_1. The drug is usually given by subcutaneous injection twice a week, with or without concomitant methotrexate. Infliximab is a chimeric (mouse–human) anti-TNF monoclonal antibody that is given to patients intravenously every 4 to 8 weeks, usually in combination with methotrexate. Adalimumab, a fully human anti-TNF antibody, is usually given subcutaneously every two weeks, usually with methotrexate. Anakinra is a recombinant human form of IL-1 receptor antagonist (IL-1ra) that blocks the binding of IL-1α and β to the IL-1 receptor. The drug is administered daily by subcutaneous injection with or without methotrexate. The advantages of these agents include rapid onset of action, with many patients experiencing improvement within a few weeks of treatment. To date, there is no head-to-head study comparing the long-term safety and efficacy of the different biologic agents.

While there is little doubt about the potential efficacy of the biologics in RA, there remains significant concern about their side effects especially in vulnerable populations such as elderly RA patients with multiple comorbidities. In addition, the significant cost associated with these drugs is prohibitive to elderly patients without prescription coverage. TNF is involved in host defense against foreign pathogens and in tumor surveillance. Anticytokine therapy is associated with increased risk of developing common and opportunistic infections including fungal, tuberculosis, and atypical mycobacterial infections. Most cases of tuberculosis appear to be reactivation of latent infection. There have been reports of sepsis and death in patients receiving these drugs. Rare cases of demyelinating disorders, aplastic anemia, lupus-like illnesses and depression have also been associated with anti-TNF therapies. Finally, the long-term consequence of anticytokine suppression is unknown. Whether these agents affect cancer development can only be answered by a large epidemiologic study.

A number of other DMARDs are occasionally used as monotherapy for RA. Clinicians are often reluctant to use them because of their limited efficacy, high dropout rate, and potential serious side effects, especially in the elderly. These include cyclosporin, azathioprine, gold, and penicillamine. Staphylococcal protein A immunoabsorption column may be useful in a small subset of RA patients with refractory disease. However, difficulty in administering treatment and high cost have prevented the treatment from being used widely.

Most combination therapies involve adding one or more DMARD to methotrexate. The triple therapy of methotrexate, hydroxychloroquine, and sulfasalazine is more efficacious than methotrexate alone. Similarly, patients treated with methotrexate and leflunomide experienced better outcomes than methotrexate alone. Interestingly, although methotrexate plus hydroxychloroquine is the commonest combination used in this country, its efficacy, as compared to methotrexate, has not been examined systematically. The main advantage of using combination therapy over the anti-cytokine treatments is cost. The argument that biologics may be cost-effective because they reduce work disability may not apply to elderly, retired patients. However, whether the elderly tolerate combination therapies as well as monotherapy is uncertain. As many as 60 percent of patients receiving both methotrexate and leflunomide develop elevated liver enzyme levels. Combining methotrexate with a nephrotoxic drug such as cyclosporin has been used successfully in the treatment of RA but is potentially hazardous in the elderly patient who may already have underlying renal insufficiency and hypertension.

Surgical Interventions

Surgeries can be useful to restore function and in many cases reduce pain in end-stage RA joints. These procedures include small-joint arthroplasty, joint fusion, and resection of metatarsal heads. Improvements in surgical techniques, prosthetic materials, perioperative care, and rehabilitation in the past two decades have resulted in much better outcomes in patients undergoing surgical treatments. In addition, synovectomy and tendon repairs are important to prevent and to treat tendon rupture that can have disastrous functional consequences in RA patients. Careful planning and timing of various joint procedures in RA patients are important. For example, it may be wise to first correct upper-extremity deformities before lower-extremity surgery is performed to allow the use of the upper extremities to assist in transfer, rising from a chair, and stair climbing during rehabilitation.

Prevention

A major problem in attempting to prevent the disease is identifying those who are at risk for developing the disease in the first place. Although genetic studies provide some clues as to which segment of the population may be at risk, the available information is not precise enough to be of practical use. There is some evidence that oral contraceptive pill and hormone replacement therapy may reduce the risk of developing RA. Conversely, epidemiologic data suggest that smoking is associated with a slightly increased risk for the disease. Over the past decade there has been considerable interest in developing T-cell receptor peptide vaccines for RA. This approach has shown some promising results in an animal model of chronic inflammatory arthritis. Whether this will eventually lead to useful human vaccine is unclear.

Special Issues

Patient Preference and Comorbidity

The choice of therapy should be made in conjunction with the patient and the caregivers. Unfortunately, some elderly patients are reluctant or unable to perform regular exercises, especially if they have lived an inactive lifestyle for many years. In these situations, emphasizing the positive aspects of exercise (physical, psychological, and social), setting realistic goals, and recommending exercise programs specially tailored for the elderly population are helpful.

The importance of assessing a patient's risk of developing GI, renal, cardiac complication, and osteoporosis prior to starting NSAIDs and corticosteroids has already been emphasized. Patient preference is important when deciding on a specific DMARD. Elderly patients with poor eyesight are often reluctant to begin antimalarials out of fear of potential ocular complications, however small the risk may be. These drugs are contraindicated in elderly patients who cannot be monitored for retinal toxicity, including individuals with macular degeneration or untreated cataract. Older adults who do not want to give up drinking alcohol may choose not to take methotrexate. Some older women have refused to take methotrexate because the drug was part of their breast cancer chemotherapy in the distant past. Intramuscular methotrexate can be used in elderly patients who experience dyspepsia or who have difficulty swallowing. Methotrexate and biologic response modifiers must be used with extreme caution or not at all in patients with chronic or active infection. Elderly RA patients should have received all the appropriate immunizations prior to receiving DMARDs. Whether elderly patients with chronic lung disease taking DMARDs should receive *Pneumocystis carinii* prophylaxis is unclear. Assessment of the patient's tuberculosis status should be done prior to beginning anticytokine therapy.

Care Settings

The physician's choice of therapy has to take into account the patient's overall state of health and mobility, and the care setting. In most cases, home laboratory monitoring for DMARD toxicity can be arranged for patients with significant mobility problems. Instead of DMARDs, the use of corticosteroids (oral, intraarticular, or parenteral; low- or high-dose "pulse" treatment) may be a good option in RA patients with active disease in the end stages of their lives.

SYSTEMIC LUPUS ERYTHEMATOSUS

Systemic lupus erythematosus (SLE) is a prototypic autoimmune disease that predominantly affects the female population. The incidence of lupus has been increasing in the past few decades with a quarter of a million patients now with the disease in this country. Late-onset lupus (LOL), defined as symptoms beginning after the age of 55 years, accounts for up to 10 percent of all cases of lupus. In addition, improved therapies have resulted in more lupus patients surviving into old age.

Diagnosis

The diagnosis of SLE is based on the presence of signs, symptoms, and laboratory features of autoimmunity. The 1982 American College of Rheumatology Classification Criteria for SLE was recently revised to include the presence of antiphospholipid antibodies (Table 78-4). It is important to recognize that these criteria were designed for research purposes and have not been validated in LOL. Low-titer ANA may be present in up to one-third of the elderly. Positive ANAs (titer $\geq$1:160) have high sensitivity but poor specificity for SLE when measured by indirect immunofluorescence using the standard Hep-2 substrate.

Table 78-4   Revised Classification Criteria for SLE

Serositis	Pleuritis, pericarditis, or peritonitis
Oral or nasal ulceration	Oral ulcers are often painless and occur in unusual parts of the oral cavity
Arthritis	Nonerosive polyarthritis involving the small joints
Photosensitivity	Skin rash when exposed to sunlight
Blood dyscrasia	Hemolytic anemia, leukopenia/lymphopenia, or thrombocytopenia
Renal disease	Proteinuria ($>$0.5 g/d), cellular casts, unexplained hematuria
ANA	$\geq$1:160 titer in the absence of lupus-inducing drug
Immunologic abnormalities	Anti-dsDNA, anti-Sm, or antiphospholipid antibody
Neuropsychiatric illness	Seizures or psychosis
Malar rash	Tends to spare the nasolabial folds
Discoid rash	Often scarring

ANA, antinuclear antibody; dsDNA, double-stranded deoxyribonucleic acid; Sm, Smith (antigen).
Source: Adapted from Berney SM (1998).

In contrast, the presence of anti-dsDNA (double-stranded deoxyribonucleic acid) or anti-Sm (Smith) antibodies is highly specific for SLE. However, these antibodies are only detected in 31 to 86 percent and 0 to 24 percent of LOL patients, respectively.

Pathogenesis

The cause of SLE is unknown. The concordance rate of SLE in monozygotic twins is between 25 percent and 50 percent, suggesting that genetic and environmental factors are both important. Human SLE is a polygenic disease. Genetic studies have identified multiple susceptibility loci in human and murine lupus (e.g., *sle*1, 2, 3). A defect or deficiency in gene product(s) regulating immune complex clearance, such as in some cases of inherited complement (C1, C4, C2) deficiencies, is associated with a high likelihood of the development of SLE. Variability in the Fcγ receptor alleles is believed to play a role in determining the susceptibility to SLE in some racial and ethnic populations. Defective apoptosis as a consequence of mutations of the Fas or Fas-ligand gene is the central mechanism responsible for the lupus-like disease seen in the MRL/*lpr* and MRL/*gld* mice. However, such defects are exceedingly rare in humans, and when present, they cause a much more limited autoimmune disease (the Canale–Smith syndrome).

Hormonal factors are important in the pathogenesis of SLE. The disease principally affects females of childbearing age. The decline in female sex hormones in postmenopausal years is believed to be an important reason for the low incidence of SLE in this age group. Conversely, there is data showing that exogenous estrogens (hormone replacement therapy and oral contraceptive pill) may impose a (small) risk for developing lupus. Similar to other autoimmune diseases, an inciting role for microbial organisms has been postulated but not proven.

Presentation

Because of the lack of awareness of this disease in older people, the average time it takes from the onset of symptoms to the diagnosis of LOL is long, averaging between 2 and 3 years. The female:male ratio of LOL is approximately 4:1, much lower than the 9:1 ratio seen in the younger age group. It has been reported that the high prevalence of SLE in African Americans is not so apparent in LOL. However, whether this merely reflects the demographics of the study locations is unclear.

The clinical features of LOL patients are quite different from those who develop their lupus at a younger age (Table 78-5). The LOL patients tend to have a milder disease and are less likely to develop alopecia, malar rash, photosensitivity, oral/nasal ulceration, glomerulonephritis and lymphadenopathy. LOL patients may be more prone to develop cytopenias, serositis, and interstitial pneumonitis. Interestingly, the incidence of cancer, with the exception of non-Hodgkin's lymphoma, may be lower in LOL than in younger lupus patients. The cause of death in LOL patients

Table 78-5   The Frequency of Symptoms and Signs of SLE in the Older Adults

Symptoms/Signs	Frequency (%)
Arthritis/arthralgia	60
Rash	47
Cytopenias	45
Interstitial pneumonitis	41
Serositis	32
Raynaud's phenomenon	28
Neuropsychiatric	25
Peripheral neuropathy	25
Glomerulonephritis	24

SOURCE: Adapted from Kammer GM, Mishra N (2000).

is usually related to complications of treatment such as infections, cardiovascular disease, and stroke.

Management

The choice of therapy is largely dictated by the specific disease manifestations. Antimalarials are useful for many lupus symptoms including arthritis, serositis, mucositis, and skin disease. Available evidence strongly supports the long-term use of antimalarials in lupus patients. Quinacrine, available from many compounding pharmacists, does not cause retinal damage and may be used in elderly patients who cannot take potentially retinotoxic drugs. NSAIDs are used by the majority of lupus patients for symptomatic relief of arthralgias, myalgias, serositis, fever, and headaches. Their use in elderly patients must be weighed against their potential side effects. This class of drugs is best avoided in lupus patients with renal involvement.

Local corticosteroid treatments such as (short-term) topical or intradermal injections can be helpful in cutaneous lupus. Systemic steroids are often reserved for more severe disease such as lupus pneumonitis, carditis, hemolytic anemia, or new onset renal disease. Intravenous "pulse" methylprednisolone in doses of 1 g/d for up to 3 consecutive days can be lifesaving in rapidly progressive or fulminant disease.

The use of cytotoxic drugs such as cyclophosphamide has significantly reduced the morbidity and mortality associated with lupus nephritis. Monthly intravenous pulse cyclophosphamide is generally well tolerated and has fewer side effects than does daily oral administration of the drug. Azathioprine, chlorambucil, or nitrogen mustard may be used in lupus patients with renal disease who are unable to tolerate high-dose corticosteroids or cyclophosphamide. Cytotoxics should not be withheld from elderly lupus patients with major organ involvement. The use of alkylating agents is associated with an increased risk of future cancer development. However, this may be a more important consideration in younger patients with a longer life expectancy.

SJÖGREN'S SYNDROME

Definition

Sjögren's syndrome is a chronic inflammatory autoimmune disease characterized by progressive lymphocytic and plasma cell infiltration of the exocrine glands, leading to dry mouth (xerostomia) and dry eye (keratoconjunctivitis sicca). The syndrome can occur in isolation (primary) or in association with other autoimmune diseases (secondary) such as rheumatoid arthritis, systemic lupus erythematosus, or polymyositis. In addition to the sicca symptoms (dry eyes and mouth) serologic evidence of autoimmunity and objective assessment of oral and ocular involvement need to be documented before the diagnosis of Sjögren's syndrome is made. The Schirmer test, in which a strip of Whatman No. 41 filter paper is placed in the lower conjunctival sac, is considered positive if less than 5 mm of the paper is wet after 5 minutes. Ocular involvement can also be documented by staining the conjunctiva with 1% Rose Bengal stain and slit lamp eye examination. Minor salivary gland biopsy is the most commonly performed test used in diagnosing salivary gland involvement in Sjögren's syndrome. The test is considered positive when there is more than one focus (aggregate of ≥ 50 lymphocytes) per 4 mm^2 of biopsy specimen. Biopsy of the parotid, rather than of a minor salivary gland, should be done in patients complaining of parotid gland swelling. Saliva production is measured after overnight fasting without oral stimulation (brushing of teeth, smoking, etc.). A normal person should produce at least 1.5 mL of saliva in 15 minutes. Parotid sialography and salivary gland scintigraphy are alternate procedures for documenting salivary gland involvement.

Epidemiology

Depending on the definition and the age of the population studied, the prevalence of Sjögren's syndrome has been estimated to be between 0.04 percent and 4.8 percent, making it the second commonest autoimmune disease after RA. The disease is likely underdiagnosed as patients often fail to discuss their symptoms with their physicians, or believe that the symptoms are part of the inevitable consequence of aging. One study on a geriatric population suggests that subclinical disease may occur in up to 3 percent of the nursing home population. Although the prevalence of sicca symptoms increases with age, the peak incidence of primary Sjögren's syndrome occurs in the fourth and fifth decades of life, with a 9:1 female:male ratio.

Pathogenesis

Most cases of Sjögren's syndrome occur sporadically, although that are also examples of familial aggregation. An

association with HLA antigens has been reported including HLA-DR3, HLA-DR2, HLA-DRw52 in white populations. In addition, HLA-DR3 and HLA-DQw2.1 are linked to the development of anti-Ro antibodies. Like most other autoimmune diseases, an environmental or viral trigger has been proposed for Sjögren's syndrome. One theory suggests that autoimmune lymphocytes are "homed" to salivary and lacrimal glands. This is followed by clonal expansion of the autoreactive cells in the glands, upregulation of major histocompatibility complex (MHC) and adhesion molecules by epithelial cells and secretion of proinflammatory cytokines by lymphocytes and epithelial cells. Defective apoptosis causing the failure to delete autoreactive cells has been proposed as a central mechanism explaining the lymphoid aggregates seen in the exocrine glands. α-Fodrin, a cytoskeletal protein, was recently identified as a candidate autoantigen in Sjögren's syndrome. Interestingly, neonatal immunization with this antigen can prevent the development of the disease in an animal model of Sjögren's syndrome.

Presentation and Clinical Features

Most patients with Sjögren's syndrome have a slowly progressive and benign course. The onset of the disease is insidious and it may take up to 10 years for the full blown disease to develop. Older patients with Sjögren's syndrome usually present with sicca symptoms. They may complain of difficulty chewing and swallowing dry foods, the frequent need to drink liquid especially at night, difficulty wearing dentures, abnormal taste, sore/burning sensation in the mouth, and intolerance to spicy foods. Xerostomia also predisposes these patients to dental decay and the development of oral candidiasis. Instead of the classical white candida plaque, Sjögren's syndrome patients may have erythematous oral candidiasis. In addition to the feeling of dryness in the eyes, patients with ocular involvement may complain of an itching or burning sensation, the feeling that there is a foreign body in the eye, and photosensitivity. Unilateral or bilateral parotid gland swelling occurs in one-third of all primary Sjögren's syndrome patients, and is more commonly seen in the younger age group. The differential diagnosis of unilateral or bilateral parotid gland swelling includes viral (including HIV-1) and bacterial infections, sarcoidosis, salivary gland ductal obstruction, and neoplasm.

Approximately 60 percent of Sjögren's syndrome patients develop extraglandular disease (Table 78-6). Nonerosive arthritis/arthralgia is the commonest extraglandular manifestation, and may precede sicca symptoms. Any part of the pulmonary tree from the trachea to the pleural lining may be involved causing cough, hoarseness, and shortness of breath. Pseudolymphoma and lymphoma should be suspected when an unexplained pulmonary nodule or lymphadenopathy is seen on chest radiograph. Patients with Sjögren's syndrome may experience dysphagia because of dryness of the oral pharynx or abnormal esophageal motility. Chronic atrophic gastritis, gastric lymphoma, vitamin B$_{12}$ deficiency, and antibodies to parietal cells have all been described in this disease. Autoimmune

Table 78-6 Extraglandular Manifestations of Sjögren's Syndrome

Cutaneous	Xerosis (including dryness of nasal passage, skin, and vagina); Raynaud's phenomenon; cutaneous vasculitis
Pulmonary	Dessication of the tracheobronchial tree; lymphocytic infiltration (alveolitis, interstitial pneumonitis, pseudolymphoma, lymphoma); pleuritis/pleural effusion; vasculitis; pulmonary hypertension
Gastrointestinal	Dysphagia; atrophic gastritis; malabsorption; pancreatic dysfunction and pancreatitis; hepatomegaly and hepatitis; primary biliary cirrhosis
Renal	Interstitial nephritis; glomerulonephritis; distal renal tubular acidosis; kidney stones
Hematologic	Anemia; cryoglobulinemia
Neruromuscular	Sensory and trigeminal neuralgia; vasculitis; mononeuritis multiplex; neuropsychiatric disorders; seizures; encephalopathy; myelitis; aseptic meningitis; dementia; myopathy and myositis
Endocrine	Autoimmune thyroid disease

thyroid disease is present in 13 to 45 percent of patients with Sjögren's syndrome. Sjögren's syndrome patients often have elevated liver enzyme profile, especially if antimitochondrial antibodies are present. Interestingly, sicca symptoms are present in 50 percent of patients with primary biliary cirrhosis. Renal disease occurs in approximately 10 percent of patients with Sjögren's syndrome. Lymphocytic infiltration and immune complex deposition, proximal tubular acidosis with Fanconi syndrome, renal stones, electrolyte imbalance, and cryoglobulinemia have all been reported.

The association of RA and Sjögren's syndrome was first described by Henrik Sjögren in 1933. Although it is believed that RA is the commonest cause of secondary Sjögren's syndrome, its true prevalence in RA is unknown. Patients with secondary Sjögren's syndrome have milder disease with primarily sicca symptoms (dry eyes and dry mouth). Systemic complications such as salivary gland swelling, central nervous system disease, renal disease (interstitial nephritis or glomerulonephritis), and lymphoproliferative disease are uncommon.

Patients with Sjögren's syndrome often have polyclonal hypergammaglobulinemia, as well as selective increased production of specific autoantibodies. ANA and rheumatoid factors are present in more than 75 percent and 66 percent of Sjögren's syndrome patients, respectively. Anti-Ro and anti-La antibodies are detected in 70 percent and 40 percent of the affected patients. Interestingly, anti-La antibodies are less common in the secondary form of the disease.

Management

Simple lifestyle changes such as air humidification and avoidance of cigarette smoke are helpful. Nasal dryness can be treated with saline drops or gel. Vaginal dryness can be reduced using water-soluble lubricants and estrogen cream. Dry skin can be improved by using moisturizers and bath oil. Lipstick and lip balm can be used to reduce lip dryness. Meticulous oral hygiene and frequent dental visits are important to prevent complications such as dental decay and oral candidiasis. Frequent fluid replacement, topical fluoride treatment, the use of non–alcohol-based mouthwash, and sugarfree chewing gum can all be helpful. Unfortunately, artificial saliva substitutes that are currently available are not very helpful. Oral candidiasis can be treated with a prolonged course (1 to 4 months) of a noncariogenic antifungal drug (e.g., nystatin vaginal tablets 100,000 units two to three times a day), with separate treatment of dentures.

The mainstay of treatment for dry eye remains artificial tears. Newer preparations now available can penetrate better into the epithelial cell layer and last longer. However, they may occasionally cause blurring and leave residue on eye lashes. Because Sjögren's syndrome patients generally require long-term tear replenishment, preservative-free artificial tears should be used. Tear drainage can also be reduced by the placement of occlusive elements (e.g., silicon implants) in the puncta or permanently by laser or thermal cautery. Soft contact lenses may be used to protect the cornea especially in the presence of keratitis filamentosa. Because the contact lenses require wetting, the patient needs to be careful not to introduce infection to the eyes. Plastic wrap or swimming goggles can be used at night to reduce tear evaporation.

Whenever possible, drugs with significant cholinergic side effects should be discontinued. Muscarinic agonists (pilocarpine, cevimeline) may be helpful in alleviating dry mouth symptoms in Sjögren's syndrome patients. Topical cyclosporine may be helpful to treat severe ocular inflammation. Systemic corticosteroid and immunosuppressive drugs (e.g., cyclophosphamide) are sometimes used for severe extraglandular diseases such as interstitial pneumonitis, interstitial nephritis, and vasculitis. Musculoskeletal symptoms are often alleviated by the judicious use of NSAIDs, hydroxychloroquine, or sulfasalazine. Interferon-α may improve salivary flow in a subset of Sjögren's syndrome patients.

DRUG-INDUCED RHEUMATIC SYNDROMES

Polypharmacy and iatrogenic diseases are important geriatric issues. Medications are also increasingly recognized as common causes of rheumatic syndromes. These can be broadly categorized into drug-induced lupus (DIL), drug-induced myopathy/myositis (DIM), and drug-induced vasculitis (DIV).

Drug-Induced Lupus

More than 100 drugs have now been implicated in DIL (Table 78-7). Compared to the idiopathic disease, patients with "classical" DIL have a milder illness and a more restricted autoantibody profile. The incidence of DIL has been estimated to be approximately 15,000 to 20,000 per year with between 30,000 and 50,000 patients currently affected in the United States.

Procainamide (procainamide-induced lupus, PIL) and hydralazine (hydralazine-induced lupus, HIL) are the drugs most frequently associated with DIL. DIL patients are usually older and more likely to be men, reflecting the age and sex of the population receiving these drugs. One-third of patients receiving procainamide for more than a year will develop symptoms, and almost all will become ANA-positive after 2 years. In contrast, fewer than 20 percent of hydralazine-treated patients will develop DIL. The

Table 78-7 Drugs Implicated in Drug-Induced Lupus

Acebutolol	Interferon (α, γ)	Phenylethyacetylurea
Aminoglutethimide	Interleukin-2	*Phenytoin*
Amiodarone	*Isoniazid*	Practolol
Amoproxan		Prazosin
Anthiomaline	Labetalol	Primidone
Atenolol	Lamotrigine	Prinolol
	Leuprolide acetate	*Procainamide*
Benoxaprofen	Levodopa	Promethazine
	Levomeprazone	Prophythiouracil
Canavanine (L-)	Lithium carbonate	Psoralen
Captopril	Lovastatin	Pyrathiazine
Carbamazepine		Pyrithoxine
Chlorpromazine	Mephenytoin	
Chlorprothixene	Mesalazine	*Quinidine*
Cimetidine	Methimazole	Quinine
Cinnarazine	*Methyldopa*	
Clonidine	Methylsergide	Rifamycin
Clozapine	Methylthiouracil	
COL-3	Metrizamide	*Sulfasalazine*
	Minocycline	(5-amino) salicylic acid
Danazol	Minoxidil	Simvastatin
Diclofenac		Spironolactone
1,2-Dimethyl-3-hydroxypyride-4-1 (Ll)	Nalidixic acid	Streptomycin
Disopyramide	Nitrofurantoin	Sulindac
	Nomifensine	Sulfadimethoxine
Estrogens		Sulfamethoxypyridazine
Etanercept	Oral contraceptives	
Ethosuximide	Olsalazine	Terbinafine
	Oxyphenisatin	Tetracycline
Flutamide		Tetrazine
Fluvastatin	Para-aminosalicyclic acid	Thionamide
	Penicillamine	Thioridazide
Gold salts	Penicillin	Timolol eye drops
Griseofulvin	Perazine	Tolazamide
Guanoxan	Perphenazine	Tolmetin
	Phenelzine	Trimethadione
Hydralazine	Phenopyrazone	
Hydrazine	Phenylbutazone	Zafirlukast
Ibuprofen		
Infliximab		

Drugs with the strongest associations are in italic.
SOURCE: Adapted from Yung RL, Richardson BC (2002)

risk for developing HIL is dose dependent and is highest in patients taking more than 200 mg/d, and in those who have taken more than 100 g cumulative dose. Compared to idiopathic lupus patients, PIL and HIL patients have fewer renal, neuropsychiatric, and skin manifestations. Pleuropulmonary complaints are particularly common in PIL, while immune cytopenias are uncommon in DIL in general. By definition all patients with DIL are ANA-positive (mostly homogenous pattern). More than 90 percent of PIL and HIL patients have antihistone antibodies, and 20 to 40 percent are rheumatoid factor-positive.

Up to 19 percent of interferon-α (IFN-α)-treated patients develop some form of autoimmunity. Approximately 12 percent of patients receiving this drug develop positive ANA, and between 0.15 percent and 0.7 percent will develop a lupus-like illness. Anti-dsDNA antibodies occur in 8 percent, and almost all the patients with IFN-α–induced lupus have elevated anti-dsDNA antibodies. The development of autoimmunity appears to be dependent on the dose and duration of treatment. Other rheumatic syndromes associated with IFN-α include rheumatoid arthritis, polymyositis, psoriatic arthritis, Reiter's syndrome, and sarcoidosis. Autoimmune thyroid diseases are common following IFN-α treatment. It is important to differentiate this from idiopathic hypothyroidism that is prevalent in the elderly population.

Patients receiving TNF antagonists often develop serologic evidence of autoimmunity. In one study, new ANA and anti-dsDNA antibodies were found in 33 percent and 9 percent of infliximab recipients, respectively. However, there is clear discordance between the development of autoantibodies and clinical autoimmunity with only a handful of symptomatic patients reported. Approximately 13 percent of patients exposed to infliximab develop infliximab-specific antibodies. Patients receiving concurrent immunosuppressants such as methotrexate or azathioprine are less likely to develop these antibodies. The presence of antibodies to infliximab increases the likelihood of an infusion reaction but does not predict the development of autoantibodies or DIL.

Drug-Induced Myopathy/Myositis

Drug-induced muscle diseases include myopathy/myositis and rhabdomyolysis. In addition, drugs that impair consciousness (e.g., sedatives and hypnotics) and those that cause seizures (e.g., theophylline), hyperthermia (e.g., halothane, cocaine), malignant neuroleptic syndrome (e.g., haloperidol, phenothiazines), and dystonia (e.g., butyrophenones) can also result in muscle necrosis and elevated creatine phosphokinase (CPK).

Hydroxymethylglutaryl coenzyme A (HMG-CoA) reductase inhibitors (the "statins") are well known to cause myalgias and occasionally myopathy and rhabdomyolysis. The incidence of statin-induced myopathy (defined as a greater than 10-fold increased in CPK and muscle pain or weakness) is approximately 1 in 1000 patients taking the drug. The risk is greater when these drugs are used in conjunction with gemfibrozil, cyclosporin, niacin, erythromycin, itraconazole, and diltiazem. Other risk factors include renal insufficiency, hypothyroidism, advanced age, and serious infection. The mechanism of statin-induced myopathy is unclear. These agents may interfere with mitochondrial metabolic pathways. Myopathy associated with one statin does not predict the development of a similar problem with a different statin. However, there are rare reports of statin-induced rhabdomyolysis in patients with a previous history of statin-induced myopathy.

A number of drugs rheumatologists prescribe can cause significant muscle disease. Neuromyopathy occasionally develops in patients receiving colchicine. Older patients and those with renal impairment may develop this complication even if they are taking conventional doses of the drug. Patients receiving either chloroquine or hydroxychloroquine are at risk for developing a proximal myopathy and rarely cardiomyopathy. Steroid myopathy usually occurs when greater than 20 mg of prednisone is prescribed. The onset can be acute or insidious involving the proximal muscle groups (especially the thighs and hip girdle). Serum creatinine kinase level is usually normal but urine creatine may be elevated. Biopsy of the affected muscle classically shows type 2b fiber atrophy. Corticosteroid use is also associated with rhabdomyolysis when it is administered in the intensive care unit, often in the setting of concurrent paralytics or sedatives ("critical care myopathy"). Penicillamine used in the treatment of rheumatoid arthritis and Wilson's disease may cause polymyositis, myasthenia gravis, and other autoimmune disorders, including lupus, pemphigus, and Sjögren's syndrome.

Interest in over-the-counter "complementary" medicine has exploded in recent years. Several of these oral supplements have now been linked to the development of musculoskeletal syndromes. The best example is the eosinophilia-myalgia syndrome, believed to be caused by one or more contaminant(s) (the identity of which is still unclear) introduced during the manufacturing process of L-tryptophan by a single manufacturer from Japan. Patients who consumed the product developed peripheral eosinophilia, incapacitating myalgias and tight skin and/or fasciitis. DL-Carnitine is sold in health food stores and is being promoted as a supplement to increase muscle strength. Although L-carnitine may improve fatigue and muscle strength in some individuals, the DL-carnitine preparation may rarely cause muscle weakness and a myasthenia-like syndrome.

Drug-Induced Vasculitis

Ingestion of a number of drugs is associated with the development of antineutrophil cytoplasmic antibody (ANCA)-positive vasculitis, including hydralazine, propylthiouracil, methimazole, penicillamine, and minocycline. Renal involvement is surprisingly common. The ANCAs often lack specificity and may have activity against myeloperoxidase (MPO), elastase, or anti-proteinase 3 (PR-3). Discontinuation of the offending drug results in resolution of the clinical disease and a fall in the ANCA titer. DIV should be differentiated from drug-induced ANCA production, which is much more common.

Administration of hematopoietic growth factors including granulocyte colony-stimulating factor (G-CSF) and granulocyte-macrophage colony-stimulating factor (GM-CSF) has been associated with the development of cutaneous and rarely systemic vasculitis. Interestingly, there is a particularly high prevalence of vasculitis among patients with chronic benign neutropenia receiving these growth factors. The risk of vasculitis increases when the absolute neutrophil count (ANC) rises above 800/mm^3, and the problem almost always subsides with decreasing ANC. A number of vasculitis mimics may also develop in association with hematopoietic growth factors, including Sweet's syndrome and pyoderma gangrenosum. Finally, the use of colony-stimulating factors in the settings of Felty's syndrome and malignancies is associated with a flare of preexisting rheumatoid arthritis.

There are numerous reports of postvaccination vasculitic syndromes (Table 78-8). Symptom onset usually occurs within days or weeks. Most cases resolve spontaneously or with steroid therapy. Some of these cases may be related to an infectious agent or coincidental primary/idiopathic disease. It is also possible that vaccination may trigger the onset of an underlying autoimmune process. The overall incidence of vaccination-induced vasculitis appears to be low. Clinicians should not withhold the appropriate vaccination from patients with preexisting autoimmune diseases or vasculitis based on these reports.

There are a number of reports linking the development of Churg–Strauss syndrome with the use of leukotriene inhibitors (particularly Zafirlukast) in asthma patients. Onset of Churg–Strauss syndrome is often associated with exposure to the offending drug during a steroid taper. It is therefore possible that these cases represent unmasking of undiagnosed Churg–Strauss syndrome with tapering of the steroids, rather than a drug-induced disease. Nevertheless, in the absence of further information, it remains possible that some cases of Churg–Strauss syndrome represent

Table 78-8 Vaccines Associated with Vasculitis

Hepatitis B	Takayasu's, PAN, cutaneous, Churg–Strauss, cryoglobulinemia, GCA
Influenza	PMR, GCA, HSP, cryoglobulinemia, microscopic polyangiitis, cutaneous
Pneumococcus	Cutaneous
Varicella	Hypersensitivity vasculitis
Measles	HSP
BCG	PMR, GCA, urticarial vasculitis, Kawasaki's disease
Tetanus	GCA
Menningococcal C	HSP

GCA, giant cell arteritis; HSP, Henoch-Schoenlein purpura; cutaneous, cutaneous leukocytoclastic vasculitis; PAN, polyarteritis nodosa; PMR, polymyalgia rheumatica.

an idiosyncratic eosinophil-based response to leukotriene inhibitors.

RHEUMATIC SYNDROMES AND CANCER

Clinicians are often concerned that a patient's rheumatic complaints may represent the early systemic presentation of an occult tumor. Patients with autoimmune diseases are also at higher risk for developing cancers. Finally, immunosuppressive therapies used for treating autoimmune diseases may predispose the patients to malignancies as well.

Musculoskeletal Symptoms Associated with Cancer

An extensive search for an occult malignancy is not recommended in patients with most rheumatic syndromes unless there are specific findings suggesting the possible presence of a tumor. Nevertheless, the possibility of metastatic disease should be considered in an elderly patient presenting with severe pain in or around a joint. Metastatic joint disease caused by lung or breast cancer is usually monoarticular or oligoarticular (two to five joints). Pain and synovitis are caused by synovial inflammation in response to tumor cells in and around the joint. Large joints (e.g., knee, hip) are most commonly affected. However, asymmetric polyarthritis can occur at the late stages of cancer. The vertebral column is a common place for metastatic disease. A malignancy work-up should be done if an elderly patient presents with intractable or nocturnal back pain that is increasing in severity, and if the patient has constitutional symptoms such as fever or weight loss. Multiple myeloma frequently causes lytic lesions and pathologic fractures. Light-chain amyloidosis occurs in 15 percent of these patients and is associated with a symmetric small-joint arthropathy. In addition, amyloid infiltration in the shoulder joint produces the classical "shoulder pad sign." Hyperuricemia and gout may develop in patients with large tumor bulk, especially during chemotherapy.

Hypertrophic osteoarthropathy is the most common rheumatic syndrome associated with malignancy and is almost always caused by metastatic lung cancer in the Western world. Ankles, wrists, knees, and fingers are the sites most frequently affected. The cause is unknown but a neurally mediated mechanism is suggested by improvement with vagotomy and atropine. Carcinomatous polyarthritis can precede or follow the diagnosis of the underlying cancer, most commonly breast in women and lung in men. The classical description is an acute onset asymmetric seronegative polyarthritis in an elderly patient that resembles elderly onset rheumatoid arthritis. The arthritis often improves with cancer therapy and may relapse with tumor recurrence. A polymyalgia rheumatica-like disease has been linked to metastatic cancer. This is suggested by a younger age of onset, prominent constitutional symptoms, asymmetric involvement of proximal muscle groups, a relatively low sedimentation rate, and an incomplete response to prednisone. The Lambert-Eaton syndrome is characterized by an antibody-mediated defect in acetylcholine release at the neuromuscular junction. It is most commonly associated with small cell carcinoma of the lung. Ptosis, distal muscle involvement, and characteristic electromyogram findings distinguish the disease from common inflammatory myopathies. The combination of palmar fasciitis and polyarthritis is associated with gynecologic tumors, in particular, ovarian carcinoma. This is usually associated with late metastatic disease and carries a poor prognosis. Panniculitis with synovitis and serositis is a well-known accompaniment of pancreatic cancer. Finally, there are sporadic reports of steroid-resistant eosinophilic fasciitis associated with hematologic malignancies.

Rheumatic Diseases and Cancer

Patients with autoimmune diseases are at an increased risk for the development of a variety of malignancies. This tendency may be exacerbated by the use of specific immunosuppressive drugs. Patients with RA have a two- to fivefold increased risk of developing hematologic malignancies including Hodgkin's and non-Hodgkin's lymphomas. The risk is even higher if secondary Sjögren's syndrome or a serum paraprotein is present. An increased risk for oral–pharyngeal cancers has been described in geographic locations where these tumors are prevalent. Interestingly, there are epidemiologic data showing that RA patients may be at a lower risk for developing colorectal cancer. Whether this is related to the regular use of NSAIDs in this population is unknown. Sjögren's syndrome patients are 44 times more likely to develop lymphoma than are age-, sex-, and race-matched normal subjects. The risk may be higher if the patient is anti-Ro or anti-La positive. In some of these patients, there appears to be a progression from benign exocrinopathy to pseudolymphoma to lymphoma. These tumors are almost exclusively B-cell lymphomas with a high frequency of a t(14;18) chromosomal translocation. The malignant transformation is likely the result of chronic B-cell stimulation. The presence of a monoclonal IgM spike on serum protein electrophoresis may herald the transformation to malignant lymphoma. Hypogammaglobulinemia and loss of autoantibodies may eventually occur when the lymphoma cells replace the normal antibody-producing plasma cells.

Patients with polymyositis have a twofold increased risk of developing cancer, particularly in the 1 to 5 years following the diagnosis of the muscle disease. The risk of cancer in dermatomyositis patients is much higher (four to five times) and the cancer may be discovered years before or after the muscle disease is diagnosed. Older age, the presence of digital vasculitis, and normal serum creatinine kinase level have been cited as possible risk factors for cancer development in patients with inflammatory myositis. Patients with overlap syndromes and those with myositis-specific antibodies do not appear to have a higher incidence of cancer than other patients with polymyositis or dermatomyositis. The cancers associated with inflammatory myositis are those that are commonly seen including breast, lung, gynecologic, and gastrointestinal malignancies. Interestingly, nasopharyngeal carcinomas are the dominant cancers

associated with myositis in countries that have a high prevalence of these malignancies.

It is controversial whether patients with other autoimmune diseases are more likely to develop cancer. Some reports have described an increased risk of lymphoma (particularly non-Hodgkin's lymphoma) and possibly lung, breast, and cervical cancers in patients with systemic lupus erythematosus. Scleroderma patients may be predisposed to skin cancer, and systemic sclerosis patients with pulmonary fibrosis are at risk for developing lung cancer.

Risk of Cancer with Immunosuppression

Epidemiologic studies have reported that rheumatoid arthritis patients treated with methotrexate may be at increased risk for developing cancer and lymphoma. This is unclear, however, because most studies only examined the relative risk compared to that of the general population. Nevertheless, there are a large number of case reports or case series linking the occurrence of lymphoma (mostly diffuse, large-cell non-Hodgkin's lymphomas) in RA patients receiving low-dose weekly methotrexate. In most cases, cessation of therapy is associated with complete regression of the lymphoid cancer, suggesting a causative relationship. DNA analysis shows that approximately 50 percent of these lymphomas harbored the Epstein–Barr virus genome. It is therefore possible that the drug regimen may promote the malignant transformation of normal lymphoid tissue by the oncogenic virus. RA patients on azathioprine and cyclosporin A have a twofold increased risk of lymphoma relative to control RA patients. A real association between the use of immunosuppressive therapy and the development of lymphoproliferative disorders is also supported by studies of patients with organ transplantation. The incidence of non-Hodgkin's lymphoma is 50-fold greater in renal transplant patients, especially if they receive cyclosporin A as part of their immunosuppressive regimen.

Cyclophosphamide is commonly used to treat severe lupus manifestations, including nephritis and cerebritis. Lupus patients on cyclophosphamide are more likely to develop bladder cancer, lymphoma (primarily non-Hodgkin's lymphoma), and possibly skin cancer. A small increased cancer risk has also been reported in RA patients treated with the drug.

REFERENCES

American College of Rheumatology Subcommittee on Rheumatoid Arthritis Guidelines: Guidelines for the management of rheumatoid arthritis: 2002 update. *Arthritis Rheum* 46:328, 2002.

Berney SM: Systemic lupus erythematosus. *Hosp Physician* 1(3):2, 1998.

Catella-Lawson F et al: Cyclooxygenase inhibitors and the antiplatelet effects of aspirin. *N Engl J Med* 345:1809, 2001.

Drosos AA et al: Prevalence of primary Sjögren's syndrome in an elderly population. *Br J Rheumatol* 27(2):123, 1988.

Haneji N et al: Identification of α-fodrin as a candidate autoantigen in primary Sjögren's syndrome. *Science* 26:604, 1997.

Hernandez-Diaz S, Rodriquez LAG: Association between nonsteroidal antiinflammatory drugs and upper gastrointestinal tract bleeding/perforation. *Arch Intern Med* 160:2093, 2000.

Hochberg MC et al: The American College of Rheumatology 1991 revised criteria for the classification of global functional status in rheumatoid arthritis. *Arthritis Rheum* 25:498, 1992.

Kammer GM, Mishra N: Systemic lupus erythematosus in the elderly. *Rheum Dis Clin North Am* 266:475, 2000.

Kremer LM: Rational use of new and existing disease-modifying agents in rheumatoid arthritis. *Ann Intern Med* 134:695, 2001.

Leandro MJ, Isenberg DA: Rheumatic diseases and malignancy—Is there an association? *Scand J Rheumatol* 30:185, 2001.

MacGregor AJ: Classification criteria for rheumatoid arthritis. *Bailliere Clin Rheumatol* 9:287, 1995.

Moreland LW et al: Treatment of rheumatoid arthritis with a recombinant human tumor necrosis factor receptor (p75)-Fc fusion protein. *N Engl J Med* 337(3):141, 1997.

Naschitz JE et al: Rheumatic syndromes: Clues to occult neoplasia. *Semin Arthritis Rheum* 29:43, 1999.

O'Dell JR et al: Treatment of rheumatoid arthritis with methotrexate alone, sulfasalazine and hydroxychloroquine, or a combination of all three medications. *N Engl J Med* 334(20):1287, 1996.

Perez-EB et al: Autoimmune thyroid disease in primary Sjögren's syndrome. *Am J Med* 99(5):480, 1995.

Savage P, Waxman J: Post-transplantation lymphoproliferative disease. *QJM* 90:497, 1997.

Symmons DPM et al: The incidence of rheumatoid arthritis in the United Kingdom: Results from the Norfolk Arthritis register. *Br J Rheumatol* 33:735, 1994.

Yung RL: Changes in immune function with age. *Rheum Dis Clin North Am* 26(3):455, 2000.

Yung RL, Richardson BC: Drug-induced rheumatic syndromes. *Bull Rheum Dis* 51(4):1, 2002.

Back Pain and Spinal Stenosis

LEO M. COONEY, Jr.

EPIDEMIOLOGY

Low back pain, often considered a problem of middle-aged individuals, remains a common, and often disabling, condition in the older person. It is the third most frequent cause for physicians' visits for those over 65 years. A recent survey indicated that 23 percent of women and 18 percent of men 65 years and older experienced low back pain during any given year; prevalence rates declined with increasing age. The prevalence of back pain was assessed among surviving members, aged 68 to 100 years, of the Framingham Heart Study. Respondents were asked if they had pain, aching, or stiffness in their back on most days. A total of 22.3 percent of respondents, including 25.6 percent of females and 16.5 percent of males, gave a positive response to this question. The prevalence did not change with advancing age among this cohort.

Back pain is thus a common problem for older individuals, for which they frequently seek the help of a physician. The Iowa 65+ Rural Health Survey reported that low back pain caused limitation of walking, sitting, bending over, and performing household tasks in 15 to 40 percent of individuals with this pain, and difficulty with sleep in 21 percent. In a study of disabled women aged 65 years and older, back pain was the major cause of disability in 16 percent. Women with severe back pain were three to four times more likely than women without back pain to have difficulty with light household tasks or shopping. Back pain also was associated with reporting an increased likelihood of difficulty with mobility tasks and basic activities of daily living (ADLs). No association was found, however, between back pain and the inability to perform these tasks.

PATHOPHYSIOLOGY

A single, discrete etiology of back pain can be determined in only a small percentage of older persons. To date, there are no studies that describe the etiology, natural history, and response to interventions of back pain in older persons. The physician must thus deduce the most likely cause(s) of pain, recognizing changes in the anatomy of the lumbar spine that occur with aging (Table 79–1).

The lumbar spine, and supporting structures, change with age. The water and proteoglycan content of the center of the intervertebral disc, the nucleus pulposus, decreases with age. By age 50 years, 97 percent of persons have degenerative changes in their vertebral discs at autopsy. As these discs deteriorate, the vertebrae move closer together, the articular cartilage of the apophyseal joints degenerate, and osteophytes form (Table 79–1). In addition to changes in the support structure, osteoporosis of the vertebral bodies increases with age. Anatomic abnormalities alone, however, may have a limited role in determining the specific cause of an older person's back pain.

While a specific etiology often cannot be determined in older patients, there are signs, symptoms, and imaging findings suggestive of specific categories of back pain. Recognition of the usual history, physical examination, and laboratory and diagnostic imaging presentation of mechanical back pain, for example, can alert the clinician to tumors and infections, which deviate from these patterns.

CLASSIFICATION AND PRESENTATION

Back pain in older individuals can be classified into mechanical, osteoporotic, and systemic causes. The common mechanical problems that produce back pain in older patients are degenerative disc disease with intervertebral instability, lumbar spinal stenosis, and disc displacement causing sciatica. Osteoporosis causes osteoporotic vertebral compression fractures and osteoporotic sacral fractures. Systemic conditions which can cause back pain in older individuals are primary and metastatic tumors and infections of the vertebral body and disc space (Table 79–2).

Mechanical Causes of Back Pain

Unstable Lumbar Spine

A frequent cause of back pain in younger individuals is displacement of the outer annulus fibrosis or inner nucleus pulposus of the intervertebral disc. The disc does not contain pain fibers. The perivertebral structures with the most sensitive pain fibers are the posterior longitudinal ligament

Table 79-1   Changes in Lumbar Spine with Aging

Water and proteoglycan content of nucleus pulposus decreases

Intervertebral disc degenerates

Vertebrae move closer together

Loss of articular cartilage of apophyseal joint

Apophyseal osteophytes encroach on lumbar spine canal

Table 79-3   Characteristics of an Unstable Lumbar Spine

Intermittent sharp back pain

Pain comes on and subsides rapidly

Pain ongoing from lying to sitting and with bending.

Asymmetric loss of motion of lumbar spine

Weakness of L4,L5, and L5,S1 innervated muscles

and the dura mater, which lie posterior to the vertebrae and discs. The sinuvertebral nerve innervates these structures. Irritation of this nerve causes reflex spasms of the paravertebral muscles of the lumbar spine. It is thus logical to assume that soft tissue displacement in this area will cause pain and limitation of some, but not all, of the planes of movement of the lumbar spine, spasm of the paravertebral muscles, and subtle weakness of the muscles innervated by the corresponding nerves roots (L4, L5, and S1 in most cases).

In a young lumbar spine, the central nucleus pulposus often herniates outside the annulus fibrosis, indents the pain sensitive posterior longitudinal ligament and dura mater, producing pain which often lasts for several weeks, and occasionally causing sciatica because of nerve root irritation. Because of decreased water content, however, the nucleus pulposus becomes less gel-like as one ages, and rarely herniates after the age of 55 years.

Older patients often have a syndrome of sharp pain in the lumbar area, worsened with bending movements, which comes on and subsides rapidly, but recurs frequently. On physical examination, these patients often have asymmetric loss of range of motion in the lumbar spine, paravertebral muscle spasm, weakness of the L4, L5, and S1 innervated muscles, and pain going from the flexed to the erect position. Clinicians often use the term "unstable lumbar spine" to describe this syndrome, although the evidence for specific mechanical instability is lacking (Table 79-3). Patients with this condition often have one intervertebral disc space which is narrowed and sclerotic out of proportion to other disc spaces, and anterior displacement of one vertebra on

Table 79-2   Classification of Back Pain in Older Persons

Mechanical
   Unstable lumbar spine
   Lumbar spinal stenosis
   Sciatica

Osteoporosis
   Vertebral compression fracture
   Osteoporotic sacral fracture

Systemic
   Tumor
   Infection

the other, an entity known as spondylolisthesis. Maneuvers such as going from lying to sitting and bending forward often produce pain. Before considering major interventions, it is important to distinguish this condition, in which pain results from movement of the lumbar spine such as lying to sitting, from lumbar spinal stenosis, in which pain results from prolonged extension of the spine during standing and/or walking.

Lumbar Spinal Stenosis

Osteoarthritis, a condition of loss of articular cartilage with accompanying osteophytes at the margin of the cartilage, affects central as well as peripheral joints (see also Chap. 74). These osteophytes, when present in the facet or apophyseal joints of the lumbar spine, encroach on the lumbar spinal canal in which the roots of the cauda equina travel. Anatomic changes in the canal are quite common. These abnormalities have clinical significance only if the typical history of lumbar spinal stenosis is present (Table 79-4).

Changes in spinal dynamics with movement explain some of the clinical features of lumbar spinal stenosis. Flexion of the lumbar spine decreases the intraspinal protrusion of the disc, decreases the bulge of the yellow ligaments within the canal, and stretches and decreases the cross sectional area of nerve roots, resulting in an increase in spinal canal volume in relation to nerve root bulk. Extension of the lumbar spine causes bulging of the disc into the canal, enfolding and protrusion of the yellow ligaments into the spinal canal, and a relaxation and increase of cross-sectional diameter of nerve roots. Extension of the spine thus produces a decreased volume of the spinal canal in relation to nerve root bulk.

These changes in dynamics fit the clinical picture of lumbar spinal stenosis. Positions that extend the spine such as standing, walking, walking downhill, prone lying, and extending the back, worsen symptoms. Positions that flex the spine, on the other hand, including sitting, bending forward, or lying in a flexed position relieve the symptoms.

Patients with lumbar spinal stenosis present with pain, either in the lower back or legs, which comes on with prolonged standing and walking, and is relieved with sitting. Individuals with this condition will often bend their spine more as they walk ("Simian stance"), and find that they can walk further in a grocery store, supported by a cart. The leg pain can present with a classic picture of sciatica, pain radiating from the posterior aspect of the buttock down to the foot, or with isolated pain in the calf after walking.

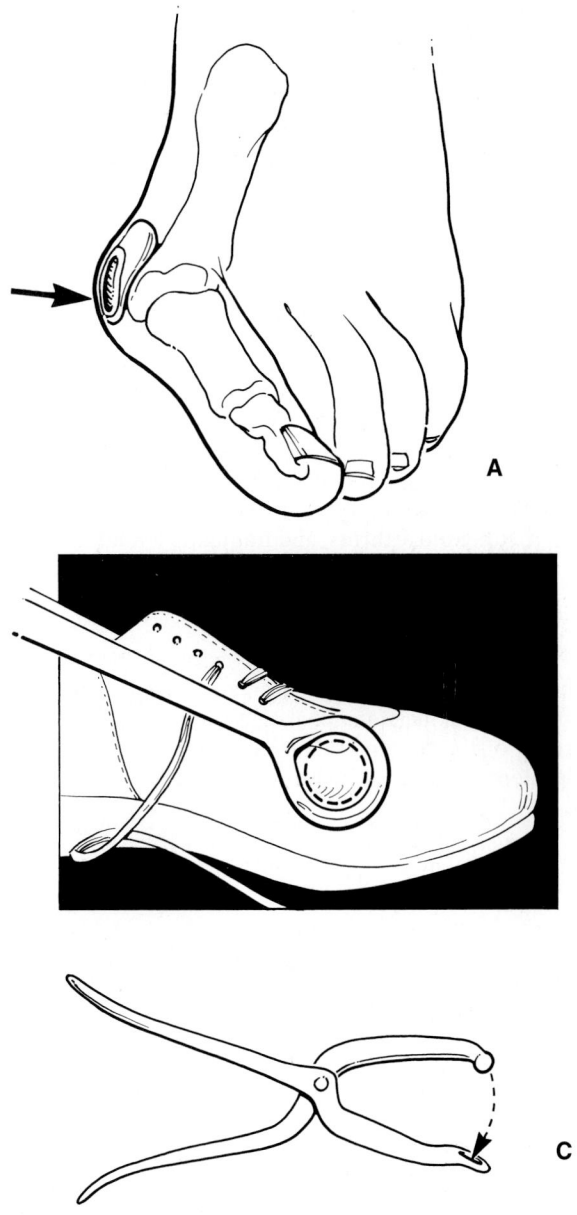

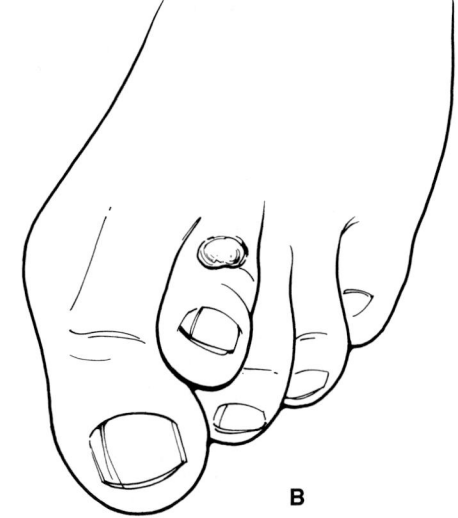

Figure 80-2   *A.* Bunion with painful callosity and bursitis. *B.* An overlapping second toe from crowding in a patient with bunion deformity of the great toe. *C.* Ball-and-ring stretcher used to accommodate the prominent first metatarsal head in a patient with a bunion.

callosity and underlying bursitis (Fig. 80-2*A*). Metatarsus primus varus (medial deviation of the first metatarsal) is often an associated condition, and in some cases, the head of the metatarsal is rounded or its base inclined. This deformity occurs most often in the pronated foot. There is a familial tendency toward the development of this condition, but no true genetic link exists. Shoe wear has been shown to contribute to its development, with pointed, narrow-toeboxed, high-heeled shoes being the primary culprit.

Signs and Symptoms

Patients will complain of pain over the medial eminence of the metatarsal head and also of inability to fit into their shoes. The deformity is obvious on physical examination, but the treating physician also must examine the foot for transfer metatarsalgia, the degree of first metatarsopha-

langeal motion, and the presence of a second-toe hammer deformity (overlapping second toe). The secondary hammertoe may present with a painful dorsal corn (see Fig. 80-2*B*).

Treatment

No surgical treatment is necessary if the bunion deformity is asymptomatic and the patient accepts required footwear modifications. Initial management steps include conservative measures of patient education and acceptance, shoe modification, and occasionally bunion pads. The shoe should have a wide, high toe box to accommodate the deformity. A ball-and-ring stretcher (see Fig. 80-2*C*) may mold the leather over the prominence to provide even further space. The shoe occasionally may need to be cut out to accept the deformity.

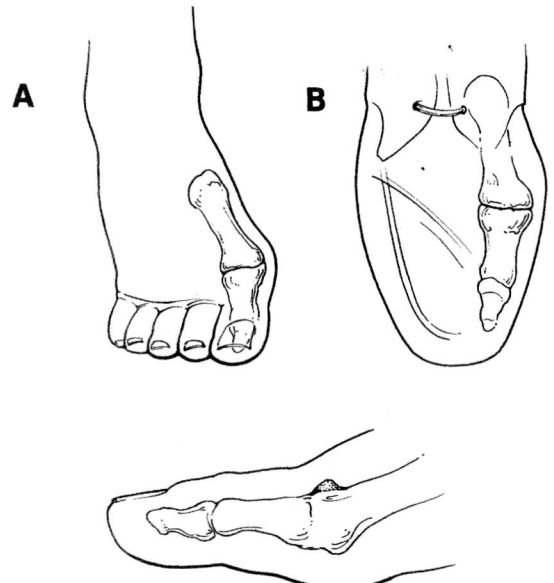

Figure 80-3   *A.* Hallux rigidus with dorsal osteophyte formation on the first metatarsal head. *B.* Oblique shoe crease from transfer of weight to the lateral side of the foot.

One must be willing to address the problems often associated with a bunion. The second-toe hammer deformity can be addressed with daily filing of the dorsal proximal interphalangeal joint corn and soft pads. Transfer metatarsalgia is often responsive to a metatarsal pad. Surgical treatment is reserved for those patients who are unresponsive to conservative measures and in those feet with significant deformity and adequate blood supply.

Hallux Rigidus (or Limitus)

Etiology

This disorder is characterized by painful and limited range of motion of the first metatarsophalangeal joint, predominantly in dorsiflexion. Repetitive microtrauma leads to a degenerative process that manifests with a proliferation of dorsal bone, limiting toe dorsiflexion (Fig. 80-3A).

Signs and Symptoms

Patients will complain of pain in the first metatarsophalangeal joint with walking and an inability to wear heels. They may note an oblique shoe crease that is secondary to decreased first metatarsophalangeal joint motion (see Fig. 80-3B). A palpable dorsal osteophyte is often present, and the patient will have pain with forced plantar flexion of the great toe. Secondary lateral ankle pain from a shifting of weight away from the great toe and toward the lesser digits during toe-off may develop.

Treatment

The initial aims of treatment should include conversion to a rocker-bottom-sole shoe to allow easier transition from stance into toe-off. A steel shank in the sole of the shoe also may dissipate the need for the great toe to achieve plantar flexion forcibly in walking. An enlarged toe box may limit excessive pressure on the dorsal bone.

Surgical intervention should be entertained if other measures fail. Cheilectomy (removal of the bump), fusion, and arthroplasty (resection versus silastic implant) are all options.

Hammer Toe/Claw Toe/Mallet Toe

Etiology

Lesser toe deformities (Fig. 80-4) are often the result of crowding inside the shoe. There are, however, many other etiologies for the development of these conditions. Muscle imbalance following a neurologic event (e.g., cerebrovascular accident, head injury), peripheral nerve damage, diabetes, rheumatoid arthritis, and traumatic tendon disruption can all lead to the development of the these conditions.

Signs and Symptoms

The hammertoe (Fig. 80-5A) is primarily a hyperextension deformity at the metatarsophalangeal joint plus a flexion deformity of the proximal interphalangeal joint. Early in the development of these deformities, patients may have a

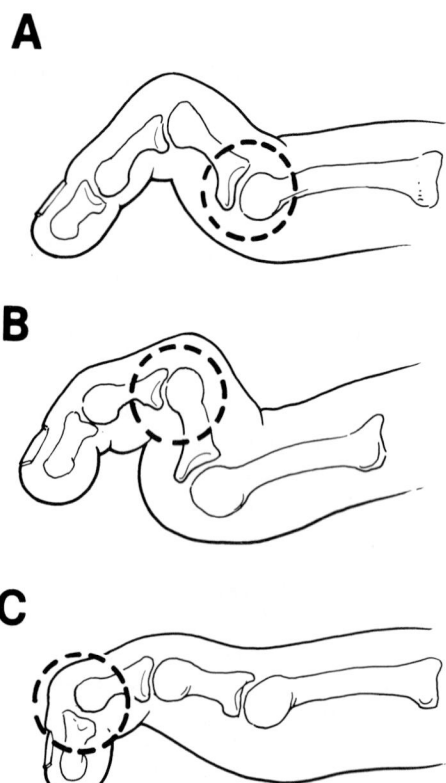

Figure 80-4   *A.* Hammertoe with primary hyperextension deformity of the metatarsophalangeal joint. *B.* Claw toe with primary hyperflexion deformity of the distal interphalangeal joint. *C.* Mallet toe with primary hyperflexion deformity of the distal interphalangeal joint.

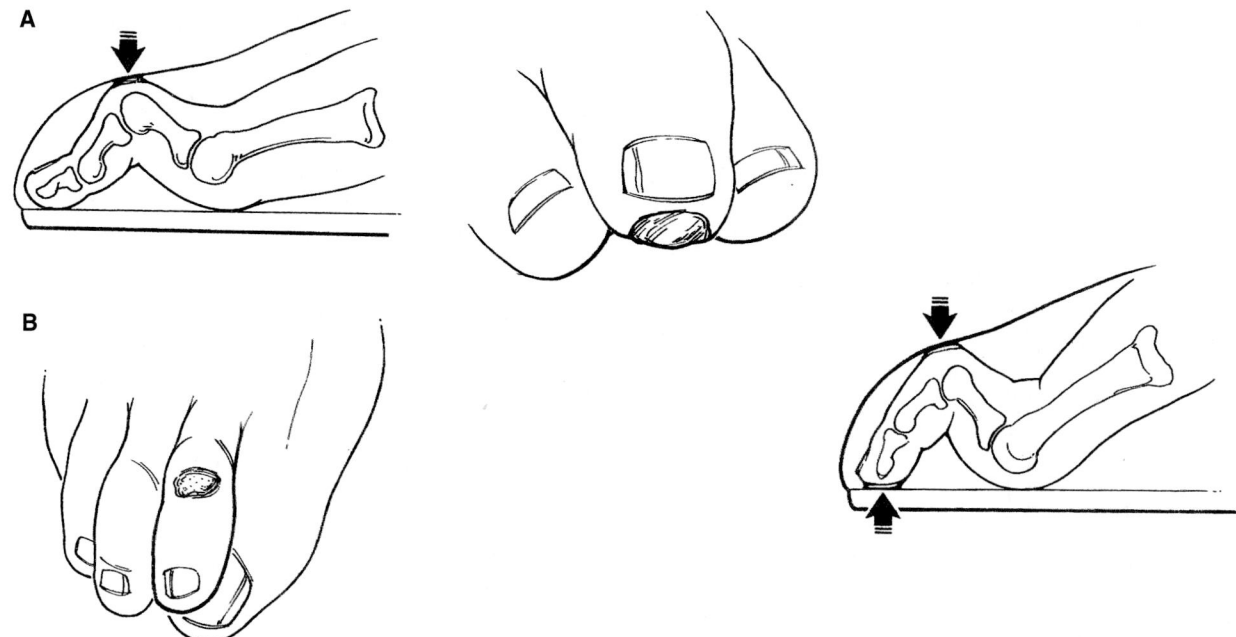

Figure 80-5 *A.* Hammering of the second toe with dorsal proximal interphalangeal callosity secondary to bunion deformity. *Arrow* illustrates callosity formation. *B.* Clawing of the toe with painful distal phalangeal corn. *Arrow* illustrates callosity formation.

mildly painful metatarsophalangeal synovitis. As the disease progresses, painful corns above the proximal interphalangeal joint develop as a result of continuous rubbing against the overlying shoe. Development of intractable plantar keratosis is often not far behind.

The claw toe (see Fig. 80-5*B*) is primarily a hyperextension deformity at the metatarsophalangeal joint, with flexion of both the distal interphalangeal and proximal interphalangeal joints. Corns form both over the dorsal proximal interphalangeal and at the tip of the distal phalanx.

The mallet toe is primarily a flexion contracture of the distal interphalangeal joint. This deformity results in weight being borne by the tip of the toe and may result in an exquisitely tender end-bearing callus.

Treatment

When the lesser toe deformity is flexible, conservative measures may suffice. Shoe modification with inlay orthotics, callus soaking and filing, metatarsal pads for associated intractable plantar keratoses, comma crest pads for distal calluses, and passive stretching with taping are all modes of attack in treatment. Surgical intervention of these lesser-toe deformities is reserved for patients with intractable flexible toe deformities or symptomatic rigid lesser toe pathology.

Bunionette

Etiology

The flat splayfoot with associated bunion deformity of the great toe may predispose to the development of the tailor's bunion or bunionette of the fifth metatarsal. The prominent fifth metatarsal head prompts irritation from the overlying shoe, and a secondary callus and bursa develop (Fig. 80-6).

As in the more common great-toe bunion deformity, the overgrown, inflamed tissue can be either bony or soft in origin.

Signs and Symptoms

Patients will have pain over the firth metatarsal head with a prominent callus over the lateral aspect of the toe. Occasionally, the metatarsal head will be plantar-flexed, and

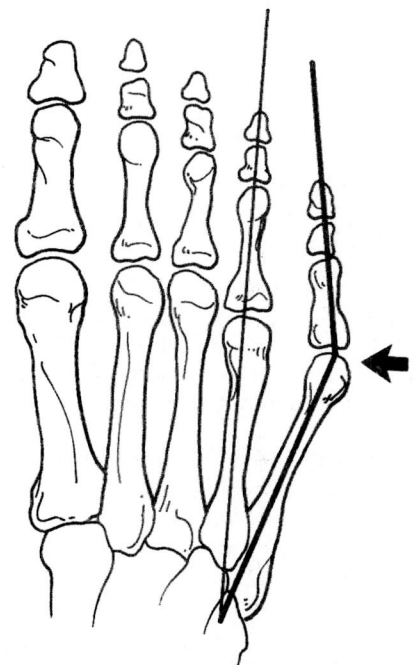

Figure 80-6 Bunionette deformity with deviated fifth metatarsal in a splay foot. *Arrow* illustrates callosity formation.

an area of intractable plantar keratosis may present on the sole of the foot.

Treatment

Conservative measures are aimed at accommodating the deformity. A ball-and-hook stretcher can soften leather shoes over the prominence. Simple shoe modifications to include a wide toe box is often all that is necessary. Many surgeries—ranging from simple bone and soft-tissue removal to metatarsal shaft osteotomy—have been advocated in unresponsive patients. By way of an oblique osteotomy, the metatarsal head may be shifted both medially and dorsally to relieve associated intractable plantar keratosis.

METATARSALGIA

There is a constellation of foot problems that presents to the physician with metatarsalgia (pain under the forefoot). The following is a discussion of the more common causes of metatarsalgia in elderly patients. Not included in this section are discussions of systemic inflammatory processes and the cavus or high-arched foot, which also can contribute to or cause metatarsalgia.

Morton's Neuroma

Etiology

Repetitive microtrauma of the common digital nerves leads to a cycle of inflammation, accumulation of perineural fibrosis, and enlargement of the neurolemma. This is not a true neuroma but an irritation and scarring of tissue surrounding the nerve. The microtrauma is thought to originate from traction of the interdigital nerve as it passes around the intermetatarsal ligament. Compression from adjacent metatarsal heads also may initiate the pathologic process, and often the swelling is located adjacent to the metatarsal heads as the nerve bifurcates (Fig. 80-7).

Signs and Symptoms

Women are affected four times more often than men because they more often wear tight, confining shoes (pumps). The neuromas are unilateral in 85 percent of patients, are most frequent in the third web space (>85 percent), but occasionally are found in the second web space (<15 percent). This problem rarely, if ever, occurs in the first and fourth web spaces.

Patients complain of a burning type of pain at the third and second web spaces, with radiation into the tips of the involved toes. Weight bearing exacerbates the symptoms, whereas shoe removal and massage often relieves the pain. Physical examination reveals tenderness to palpation at the involved web space and symptoms with compression of the involved metatarsals. The neuroma may be palpable and often may be "pushed" back and forth between the involved toes, causing a clicking sensation. Diminished interdigital toe sensation may be demonstrated by light touch testing.

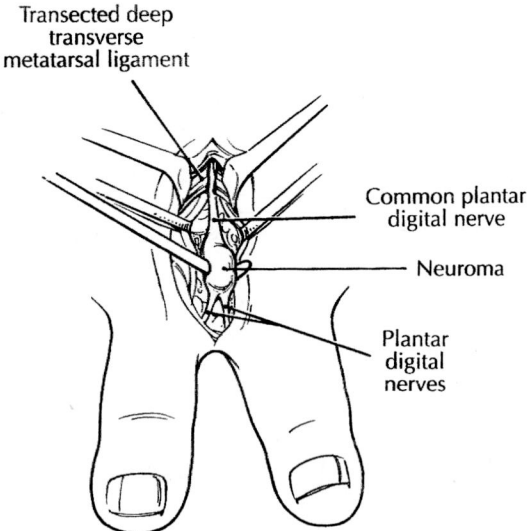

Figure 80-7   Intraoperative diagram of a Morton's neuroma between two adjacent metatarsal heads. The neuroma is adjacent to the nerve bifurcation.

Symptomatic relief can result from common digital nerve block with local anesthetic. This also serves as an excellent diagnostic test.

Treatment

Metatarsal pads are the first line of defense. By acting to spread the metatarsal heads and decompress the nerve, they may bring relief. Steroid injection and antiinflammatory medications may interrupt the cycle of chronic inflammation/fibrosis. Neuroma resection is advised in recalcitrant cases that meet diagnostic criteria. The procedure does cause some loss of sensation, and it is important that patients be aware of this preoperatively.

Metatarsophalangeal Joint Instability (Dislocated Toe)

Etiology

Instability of the metatarsophalangeal joint can involve the second and occasionally the third toes, causing forefoot pain. Women are most often affected. Use of high-heeled shoes with pressure put on the prominent second metatarsophalangeal joint causes instability and inflammation. Continued dynamic pressure against the lengthened plantar plate may allow the toe to dislocate at the metatarsophalangeal joint (Fig. 80-8A).

Signs and Symptoms

The patient will complain of pain in the forefoot region, but it is mostly at the metatarsophalangeal joint of the second toe. The subluxation test (see Fig. 80-8B) of the joint is helpful in reproducing the pain and making the diagnosis. Holding the foot firmly with one hand and then clasping the dorsal and plantar aspects of the proximal phalanx

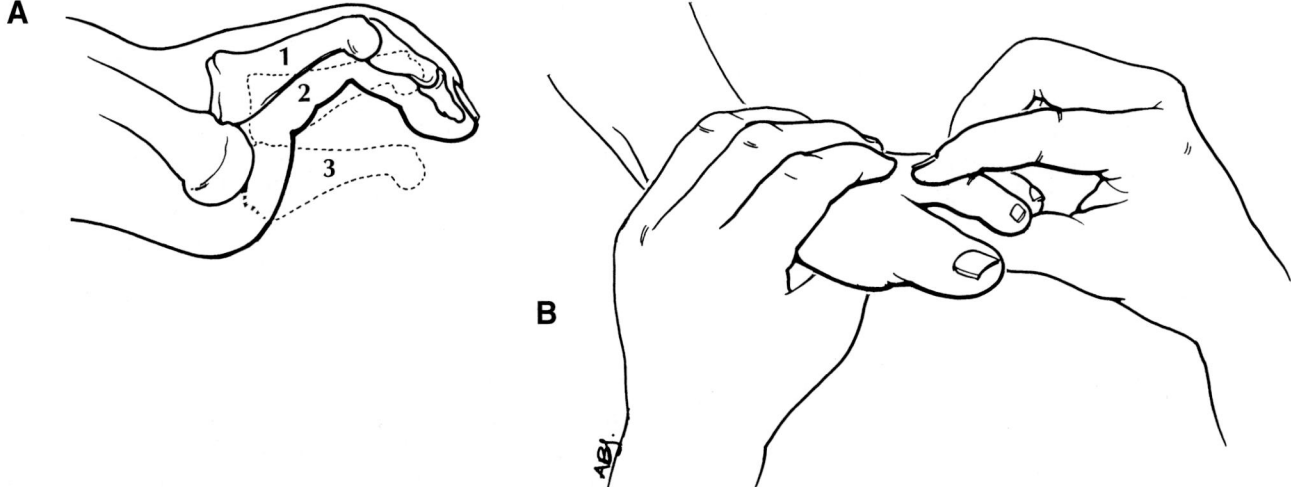

Figure 80-8   *A.* Continued dynamic pressure against the lengthened plantar plate may allow the toe to dislocate at the metatarsophalangeal joint. *B.* The subluxation test of the joint is helpful in reproducing the pain and making the diagnosis.

with the other, the metatarsal is stabilized and the proximal phalanx is subluxed dorsally and relocated plantarward with repetitive motion. The patient usually states that this reproduces the pain being experienced.

Treatment

Restriction of activities, orthotics, a stiff-soled shoe, and antiinflammatory medications are used initially to treat metatarsophalangeal joint instability. An injection of steroid into the joint also can alleviate the pain. Various surgical options have been entertained for this common condition when the toe has become dislocated. Resection of the base of the proximal phalanx of the second toe (painful toe) alleviates the pain.

Second-Toe Metatarsalgia

Etiology

The foot with a relatively long second metatarsal is predisposed to excessive plantar forces with ambulation. The disorder is often associated with a great-toe bunion and the classic "transfer metatarsalgia" (Fig. 80-9*A*).

Signs and Symptoms

There is a large, diffuse plantar centered over the second metatarsal head. The first metatarsal cuneiform joint is often hypermobile, and occasionally there is an associated bunion. Radiographs may show an elongated second metatarsal.

Treatment

The first-line of treatment is a metatarsal pad or custom inlays (see Fig. 80-9*B*) with a medial forefoot post. In addition, treatment should include attention to the great-toe bunion deformity. Surgical osteotomy of the second metatarsal is the preferred treatment when pads fail. This

can be combined with a corrective bunion procedure when indicated.

Intractable Plantar Keratosis

Etiology

Often a pressure point on the plantar surface leads to a callosity on the sole of the foot. When this hypertrophied

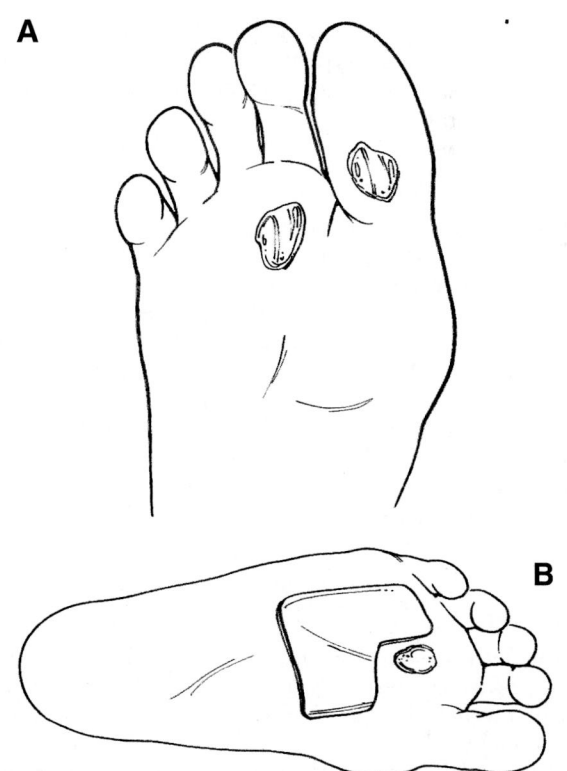

Figure 80-9   *A.* Transfer metatarsalgia (second-toe metatarsalgia) in a patient with bunion deformity. *B.* Padding to alleviate point pressure on the prominent second metatarsal head.

skin becomes trapped, a discrete seed callus develops. The condition is associated with prominent fibular condyles of the lesser metatarsal heads, prominent tibial sesamoid under the first ray, tailor's bunion, hammertoe, or a prominent whole metatarsal head adjacent to a previously osteotomized metatarsal.

Signs and Symptoms

The sole of the foot will have a discrete, isolated callus. There is associated pain, which can be exquisite. Paring of these lesions seldom causes bleeding. Radiographs may demonstrate a bony prominence as the source of the point pressure.

Treatment

Callus shaving sometimes will reveal a keratin pearl. Metatarsal pads, custom inlays, and felt relief pads may be satisfactory treatment. When this fails, operative correction of the primary process (i.e., bony abnormality) is the goal of interventional treatment.

Stress Fractures

Etiology

Stress fractures of the metatarsal shaft occur in the elderly population. The second metatarsal is involved most frequently, followed closely by the third metatarsal. The etiology is felt to be recurrent microfractures of the bone produced by chronic repetitive stressful activity.

Signs and Symptoms

The most common complaint is pain. There is usually a direct relationship to activity. Relief of pain occurs when the foot is elevated and protected from activity. Physical examination includes tenderness, swelling, and ecchymosis over the shaft of the involved metatarsal. Point tenderness over the location on the metatarsal shaft where the fracture has occurred is diagnostic. The patient often will have a limp. Radiographs of the foot may be normal initially. About 2 to 3 weeks following the development of pain, callus at the fracture site may be noted. A bone scan may be helpful in the initial diagnosis.

Treatment

The majority of stress fractures can be treated with a combination of decreased activity, limited weight bearing, and the use of a well-molded arch support with or without taping (strapping).

The use of a short-leg walking cast for 4 to 6 weeks, followed by a well-molded arch support, should be reserved for patients with severe pain and an inability to ambulate.

Sesamoiditis

Etiology

The sesamoid bones are contained in the two tendons of the short great-toe flexor muscle (flexor hallucis brevis). They articulate with the underface of the great toe metatarsal head. Symptoms involving the great toe sesamoids may originate from osteochondritis, microfracture, or avascular necrosis. Inflammation and irritation in this weight-bearing area that is a source of toe-off power can result in a constellation of symptoms.

Signs and Symptoms

Patients often will have vague complaints of pain over the involved sesamoid that is worsened with activity. The pain may be quite severe and radiate into the great toe. Tenderness can be elicited with direct palpation, and pain can occur with forced dorsiflexion of the great toe. The examination will demonstrate point tenderness under the involved sesamoid, with occasional associated metatarsophalangeal joint swelling. Radiographic evidence of fragmentation or collapse of the sesamoid often can be demonstrated on special views. The bone scan is frequently positive and can be used to pinpoint areas of inflammation with pinhole columnation.

Treatment

Nonoperative treatment may take 2 years to improve the condition and should be pursued as a first-line of therapy. Metatarsal pads or cutout inlays can relieve pressure under the sesamoid.

Operative removal of the involved sesamoid is associated with a significant complication rate and should be considered a last resort. Medial sesamoid removal may lead to hallux valgus deformity, lateral removal to hallux varus, and removal of a "cock-up" deformity.

Plantar Warts (Verrucae)

Etiology

The papovaviruses are etiologic in the formation of plantar warts. Subacute viral infection leads to scarring and papule formation with heaping of the skin.

Signs and Symptoms

These well-circumscribed, hyperkeratotic papules may be exquisitely tender. The pain is associated with weight bearing. The lesions may be isolated or in clusters. They bleed freely with attempts at paring (unlike intractable plantar keratoses).

Treatment

Many plantar warts will resolve with time (50 percent at 1 year, 75 percent at 2 years) and no treatment. Preparations containing salicylic acid may alleviate symptoms, and local lidocaine injection also may be of benefit. Surgical removal of plantar warts is contraindicated in most cases, since this process can replace the painful wart with a painful scar. Cryotherapy and CO_2 laser are ways of removing the warts with minimal scarring.

SOFT PARTS

Clavus (Soft Corn)

Etiology

A clavus forms in response to the abutment of one toe against a prominent bony condyle of the opposing toe. A hyperkeratotic lesion forms on the inner surface (web space) between the toes (Fig. 80-10A). The skin often will macerate and cause problems with local infection and tenderness. The underlying digital nerve may become compressed by the same process. Tight shoes have been implicated in the etiology of this process.

The two most common locations for clavuses to occur are (1) deep in the fourth web space, where a prominent

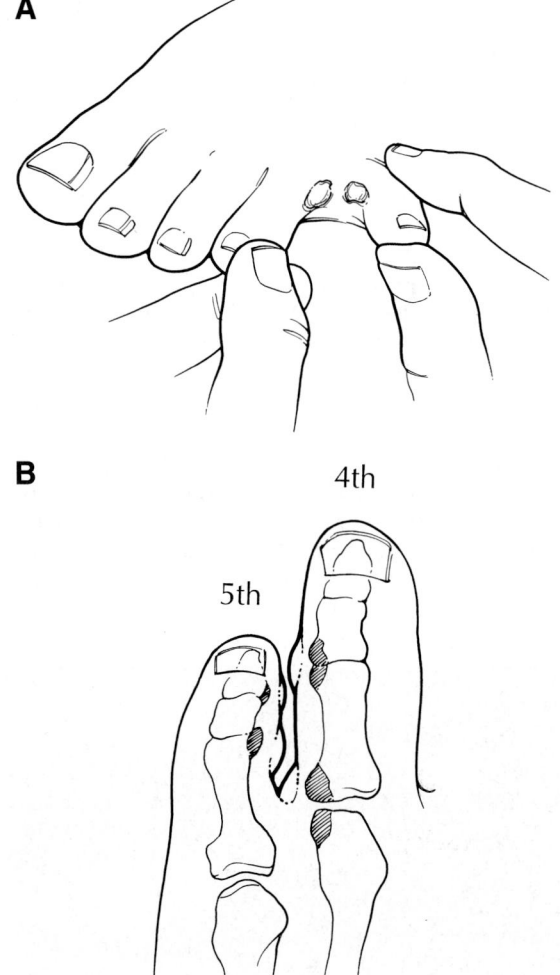

Figure 80-10 A. Soft corns in the fourth web space. B. Areas of bony abutment between the fourth and fifth toes predisposing to formation of soft corns.

lateral base of the fourth proximal phalanx abuts with a prominent fifth proximal interphalangeal joint (see Fig. 80-10B), and (2) on the medial side of the second proximal interphalangeal joint as it rubs against the great toe interphalangeal joint.

Signs and Symptoms

An area of raised skin in the web space is apparent on clinical examination. The overlying skin may be macerated, and signs of local infection are not uncommon. Patients will have extremely painful soft corns when the underlying digital nerve becomes involved.

Treatment

Primary treatment is directed at reducing pressure on the overlying skin by padding with lamb's wool. Shoes with a wide toe box relieve lateral compression. Trimming of the corn also may be of benefit. If conservative therapy fails, surgical intervention through decompression of bony prominences by condylectomy is often indicated. This is a modest but very successful procedure.

Heloma Duram (Hard Corn)

Etiology

Hypertrophic skin changes generally are associated with pressure in a specific location. Often exostoses are found lying deep to the cutaneous lesion and are easily palpated.

Signs and Symptoms

Hard corns are present most commonly on the dorsolateral aspect of the fifth toe. These are thickened, hyperkeratotic areas that are extremely painful, especially when accompanied by a small bursa that often forms as a result of the lesion.

Treatment

Padding of the affected toe relieves pressure, redness, and pain. Surgical excision of an underlying exostosis will lead to a more permanent correction of the problem.

Posterior Tibial Tendinitis/Tendon Rupture

Etiology

Chronic and recurrent tenosynovitis of the posterior tibial tendon leads to its attenuation and degeneration with age. Attritional rupture of the tendon is not uncommon. The attenuation or rupture is commonly located at the level of the medial malleolus, where its blood supply is limited and the tendon tunnel is narrowest.

Signs and Symptoms

Patients complain of pain and swelling over the medial aspect of the ankle. They also may complain of a change in the shape of the foot or instability with ambulation.

When the tendon is significantly attenuated or ruptured, the patient will demonstrate a significant valgus deflection of the heel, loss in height of the medial longitudinal arch, and abduction of the forefoot, with a positive "too-many-toes sign" (appearance of more toes lateral to the ankle when comparing the feet from behind). Radiographs can demonstrate a flat foot with talonavicular sag and valgus deflection of the os calcis. Magnetic resonance imaging is most helpful in diagnosing rupture or degeneration of the posterior tibial tendon.

Treatment

Conservative treatment includes shoe modification with a quarter-inch medial heel wedge and a medial arch support. Antiinflammatory medication and patient education on limiting activity are also helpful. Surgical reconstruction of the posterior tibial tendon in the elderly patient is rarely indicated. In selected long-standing cases, limited fusions including tarsonavicular and triple arthrodesis may be warranted.

TOENAILS

Ingrown Toenail

Etiology

Extrinsic pressure on the toe can trap the sharp corner of an improperly cut nail into the medial or lateral soft tissues. Continuous irritation of the soft parts by the nail leads to inflammation, infection, and hypertrophic granulation tissue. Factors predisposing to the development of ingrown toenails include improper trimming, heredity, improper shoe fit, and obesity. The nail of the great toe is most commonly involved (Fig. 80-11A).

Signs and Symptoms

Patients will complain of pain of the involved toe while walking or wearing tight shoes. They occasionally may have drainage associated with local bacterial infection.

Treatment

Early, local cases may respond to warm soaks, antibiotics, and elevation of the nail corner with wisps of cotton placed beneath the spicule of the nail. Most cases, however, require that the offending nail be removed. This can be combined with matrixectomy (see Fig. 80-11B).

Onychomycosis

Etiology

Fungal or dermatophyte infections of the toenail begin with an area of localized discoloration beneath the nail that begins at the tip, moves proximally, and ultimately enters through the nail plate itself. The etiologic agents

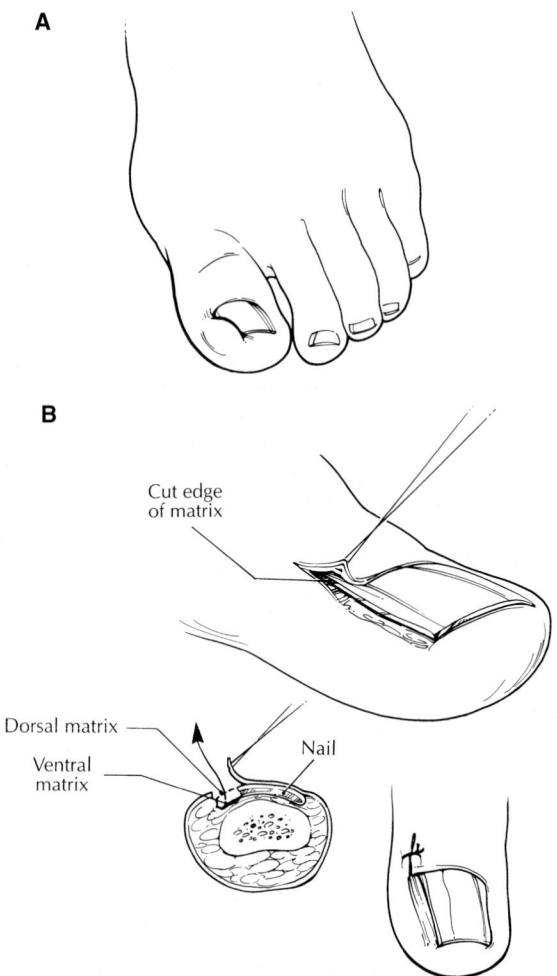

Figure 80-11 *A.* Ingrown toenail with hypertrophic granulation tissue. *B.* Removal of involved nail plate and underlying matrix in patient with ingrown toenail.

are *Trichophyton mentagrophytes*, *Candida albicans*, and *Trichophyton rubrum*. As the nail bed becomes chronically irritated from persistent local inflammation, an accumulation of hyperkeratotic debris leads to thickening, cracking, and brownish-yellow discoloration.

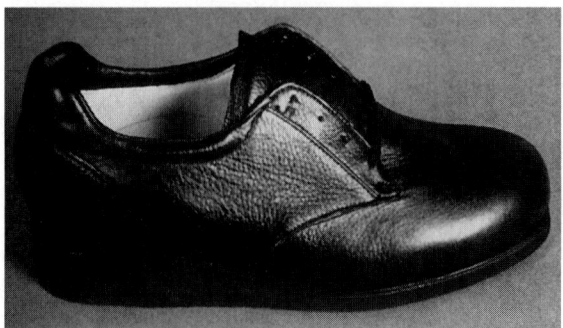

Figure 80-12 Proper shoe wear with ample toe box, soft rocker-bottom sole, padded shoe tongue, leather construction, light weight, and a well-molded Achilles pad.

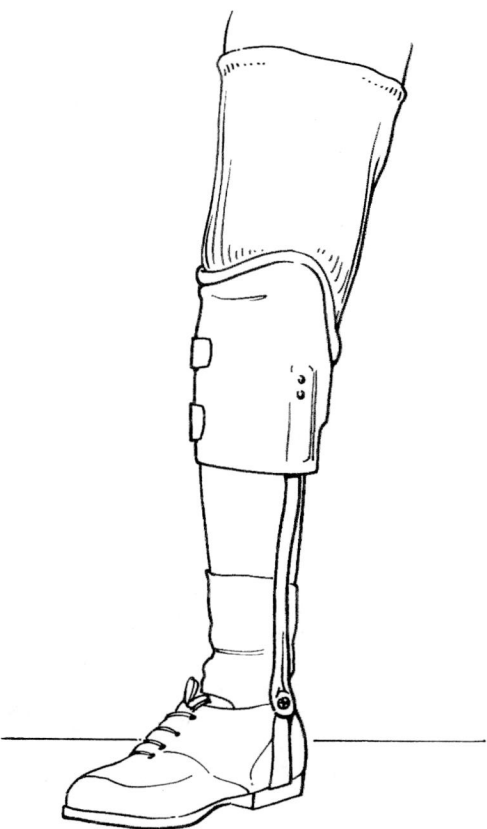

Figure 80-13   Double upright patellar-tendon–bearing in patient with chronic malperforans ulcerations.

Signs and Symptoms

The enlarged nail may make it difficult for patients to find comfortable shoes. Patients also may express concern about local spread to other toenails as well as cosmetic appearance of the foot. The infection itself is asymptomatic.

Treatment

Nail trimming is the mainstay of treatment for the enlarged, thickened nail. Medical management, including oral griseofulvin for 12 months coupled with a local antifungal agent (e.g., clotrimazole) applied beneath the nail plate, may eliminate the infection. Resistant cases should be managed with nail removal and nail matrix destruction.

SPECIAL CONSIDERATIONS

Care of the Diabetic Foot

The prevention and early detection of foot problems in the diabetic patient population are critical. The number of elderly diabetic patients continues to increase. Secondary manifestations of the diabetic disease process are also becoming more prevalent. It is the responsibility of the treating physician to emphasize the importance of daily foot care in this patient population. Periodic examination by the physician and daily examination by the patient must be encouraged. Selection of proper shoe wear, including ample toe box, soft rocker-bottom sole, padded shoe tongue, leather construction, light weight, and a well-molded Achilles pad, should be recommended (Fig. 80-12).

Peripheral diabetic neuropathy predisposes the foot to clawing of the toes and loss of sensation. This contributes to the development of malperforans ulceration adjacent to the prominent metatarsal heads. These ulcers are painless, rimmed by callus, and less necrotic than vascular ulcerations.

The diabetic patient is also vulnerable to infection. Altered chemotaxis and other factors predispose the diabetic patient to bacterial processes. The location of malperforans ulceration predisposes the metatarsal heads to the development of osteomyelitis. Broad-spectrum antibiotics with aggressive incision and débridement, including amputation in advanced cases, are the recommended treatment of such patients.

Fragile defense mechanisms, coupled with the potential for disastrous foot problems in the diabetic population, mandate the need for early detection and active participation of the foot care team. When inspection discovers early malperforans ulceration, wound care, orthotics, total contact casting, patellar-tendon–bearing bracing (Fig. 80-13), and ultimately, surgery may be required. Infected ulcers need even more aggressive treatment. Most important in this population is taking the time to educate the patient in daily foot care and prevention.

REFERENCES

Baxter DE et al: Chronic heel pain. *Orthop Clin North Am* 20:563, 1989.

Bordelon RL: Orthotics, shoes and braces. *Clin Orthop* 20:751, 1989.

Cimino WR: Tarsal tunnel syndrome: Review of the literature. *Foot Ankle* 11:47, 1990.

Glover MG: Plantar warts. *Foot Ankle* 11:172, 1990.

Gould JS: Metatarsalgia. *Orthop Clin North Am* 20:553, 1989.

Harrelson JM: Management of the diabetic foot. *Orthop Clin North Am* 20:605, 1989.

Hawkins BJ, Haddad RJ: Hallux rigidus. *Clin Sports Med* 7:37, 1988.

Jahss MH: *Disorders of the Foot and Ankle: Medical and Surgical Management.* Philadelphia, Saunders, 1991.

Johnson KA: *Surgery of the Foot and Ankle.* New York, Raven Press, 1989.

Johnson KA, Strom DE: Tibialis posterior tendon dysfunction. *Clin Orthop* 239:196, 1989.

Kwong PK et al: Plantar fasciitis: Mechanics and pathomechanics of treatment. *Clin Sports Med* 7:119, 1988.

A major goal of examination is to differentiate rotator cuff tendinitis from glenohumeral arthritis. Examination with tendinitis reveals tenderness over the cuff: laterally, either at its insertion at the greater tuberosity of the humerus or in the subacromial space, or just inferior to the lateral part of the clavicle as the cuff is rotated anteriorly with passive arm extension. Pain is noted on active more than passive abduction between 60 and 110 degrees, and increased with resistance to active abduction. Resisted internal rotation generally leads to more pain than resisted external rotation. Impingement signs—forced passive movements that evoke pain as the cuff is impinged under the roof of the subacromial space—may be seen: pain at any time during forward arm flexion from 0 to 180 degrees, or pain during internal rotation with the arm forward flexed and abducted 90 degrees. Pain from glenohumeral arthritis occurs with smaller arcs (30 to 45 degrees) of passive arm motion, and may be elicited over the joint line anteriorly, located 1 cm inferior and lateral to the coracoid process. Loss of motion and pain with minimal movement may be seen with severe rotator cuff tendinitis and lead to confusion with signs from a potential intraarticular problem. The injection of 5 mL of 1% lidocaine into the subacromial space should lead to marked improvement within minutes of painless passive arm motion, and assist in confirming tendinitis as the source of a patient's symptoms.

Radiographs of the shoulder are not necessary in all patients, as most therapy should begin following a diagnosis based on a thorough history and physical examination. Radiologic studies to evaluate shoulder pain should be limited to patients who have sustained trauma; those in whom arthritis or bony lesions are suspected; to plan for surgical therapy; or to evaluate for unsuspected lesions in patients responding poorly to initial medical management. Shoulder radiographs are usually normal in the acute stages of rotator cuff tendinitis. Chronic tendinitis leads to irregularity and sclerosis of the greater tuberosity and the formation of a degenerative sulcus between the tuberosity and the articular surface. Calcification may be seen in the subacromial space at the insertion or along the length of the supraspinatus tendon or within the space occupied by the subacromial bursa. The presence of calcifications correlates poorly with symptoms. Radiographs may also detect osteophytes off the inferior surface of the acromioclavicular joint, which may serve as the source of impingement as they project into the subacromial space.

Therapy begins with patient education. Identification and modification of those activities that either precipitate or aggravate pain is important in preventing recurring symptoms. This may include restructuring living quarters to include lowering shelves or placing heavier objects on lower shelf levels to reduce repetitive overhead arm motions. Strenuous activities may also need to be modified or restricted.

In the acute stages, rotator cuff tendinitis is treated with relative rest from function (but not from submaximal movement) and avoidance of overhead arm motion. Limited courses of antiinflammatory therapy with NSAIDs are appropriate for mild symptoms. For moderate to severe pain, mild pain that is chronic, or pain with functional limitation, the subacromial injection of a corticosteroid–anesthetic mixture may be added.

A home exercise program should begin once pain is controlled. Patients should be instructed first on range-of-motion and stretching exercises. These exercises include gentle full abduction in the scapular plane (70 degrees from the forward plane) holding for 30 seconds times 5 repetitions; stretching by placing the abducted arm against a wall and gently leaning the body into the wall for 30 seconds times 5 repetitions; wall push ups; and rotation both internally and externally with the elbow flexed 90 degrees and held against the side for 25 repetitions while holding 1 to 2 pound weights. Pendulum (Codman's) exercises further assist in shoulder mobilization: patients rotate the dependent arm in 12-inch-diameter circles while leaning to the side and holding 1 to 5 pound weights. A formal program of physical therapy should be prescribed for those affected patients with persistent loss of motion or strength, repeated episodes of rotator cuff tendinitis, or lack of compliance with a home exercise program.

The course of rotator cuff tendinitis is variable. Younger patients and those with acute symptoms have a more favorable prognosis, with a good outcome from treatment in nearly all by 6 weeks. Older patients have a higher prevalence of persistent problems despite therapy, because of the usual underlying factors responsible for the generation of symptoms (chronic overuse/repetitive impingement and inherent tendon degeneration as discussed above). Up to one-third of patients will have impairment of personal care or pain on movement 3 years following an initial course of treatment. Consequently, close follow-up reevaluations are essential to measure progress and to adjust therapeutic plans as necessary. Patients who do not respond to intensive medical therapy, including up to three corticosteroid injections in a year, should be referred to an orthopedist for consideration of arthroscopic decompressive surgery with acromioplasty.

Rotator Cuff Tear

Normal tendons do not rupture. Partial or complete tears of the rotator cuff tendon occur primarily as a consequence of the same factors that predispose to rotator cuff tendinitis; less than half of patients can recall a specific traumatic episode, and in those that do, the trauma serves to extend a previously undiagnosed small or incomplete tear. In asymptomatic adults the prevalence of partial- or full-thickness tears of the rotator cuff, as detected by ultrasound, increases markedly after the age of 50 years: changes are present in the dominant shoulders of as many as 50 percent of those older than age 70 years, and in 80 percent of those older than age 80 years.

Tears of the rotator cuff may be classified as acute or chronic, and complete (full-thickness vertically oriented rent of variable size, but not necessarily complete front-to-back rupture, leading to communication between the glenohumeral joint and subacromial bursa) or partial (at least one layer of tissue separates the joint and bursa). In acute complete tears, patients may feel a snap, followed by severe pain. A coexistent fracture or dislocation may be present. Patients may be unable to raise the arm or sustain abduction when the arm is passively elevated. In chronic complete tears, symptoms are more variable: patients may experience severe pain with little weakness or no pain and marked weakness. The duration of symptoms may be difficult to describe. Partial tears of the rotator cuff are more difficult to diagnose, but these should be suspected in patients with night pain, recurrent rotator cuff tendinitis, or poor response to subacromial corticosteroid injection.

Physical examination may reveal signs of rotator cuff tendinitis and impingement. Weakness is present on active abduction or external rotation, and chronic tears may lead to loss of active motion and muscle atrophy. The drop arm test assesses the integrity of the tendon: a positive test occurs when the patient is unable to maintain the arm in 90 degrees of passive abduction after support is withdrawn. A large tear is likely if the test remains positive after the subacromial injection of a short-acting anesthetic. Large tears are associated with superior migration of the humeral head, giving the shoulder a "squared-off" appearance.

The radiographic correlate of a squared shoulder is a reduction in the acromiohumeral distance to less than 6 mm on an anterior shoulder film. Small or partial tears may not produce changes on plain radiographs. Ultrasonography for diagnosing tears of the rotator cuff is a more sensitive examination but is operator dependent. Prior to widespread use of magnetic resonance imaging (MRI), the gold standard radiologic evaluation was the arthrogram: in the presence of a complete tear, dye will enter the subacromial space from the glenohumeral joint. However, MRI of the shoulder has replaced the arthrogram in many centers, as it is noninvasive and renders images of the rotator cuff, joint capsule, and other soft-tissue structures with high sensitivity and specificity.

Therapy for rotator cuff tears varies according to the extent of the lesion, the degree of disability, and the patient's premorbid activity level. Initial therapy includes NSAIDs, analgesics, and thermal modalities, followed by shoulder range of motion and then strengthening exercises. Subacromial corticosteroid–anesthetic injection may provide adjunctive relief of pain and inflammation but there should be limited numbers of such injections because they may cause further tendon degeneration. Surgical intervention, by either arthroscopic or open technique, encompassing débridement of the cuff and subacromial space and possible cuff repair, should be restricted to patients unresponsive to 6 months of conservative therapy or who have acute, complete tears associated with marked disability.

Bicipital Tendinitis

The diagnosis of bicipital tendinitis implies involvement of the long head tendon of the biceps muscle, which originates from the superior bony lip of the glenohumeral joint on the scapula and superior portion of the joint capsule, passes under the supraspinatus tendon and then anteriorly down the humerus in the bicipital groove to join with the short head from the coracoid process. There is a small hypovascular area in the tendon, similar to that of the supraspinatus tendon, near the head of the humerus. The long head

tendon is covered by tenosynovium and may join with the anterior edge of the subacromial bursa. Symptoms from bicipital tendinitis may thus overlap with those of rotator cuff tendinitis or subacromial bursitis, and physical findings of each may coexist.

Bicipital tendinitis may be acute or chronic. A history of repetitive motion involving forearm supination (e.g., tightening jar lids or using a screwdriver), elbow flexion, or overhead activity may be elicited. Anterior shoulder pain is the main symptom. Examination reveals tenderness over the long head tendon in the bicipital groove. Tenderness can also be elicited with passive arm extension, resistance to active forearm supination with elbow flexion and forearm pronation (Yergason's sign), or resistance to forearm supination and elevation of the humerus to 60 degrees with the elbow extended (Speed's test). Fibrotic or nodular thickening of the tendon may be palpable in patients with chronic symptoms. Palpable discontinuity of the tendon and distal muscle with elbow flexion denotes tendon rupture, which usually occurs in the hypovascular zone as an uncommon consequence of chronic tendinitis and degeneration.

Therapy of mild bicipital tendinitis includes relative rest, application of thermal modalities, and the use of NSAIDs, followed by passive stretching of the tendon to regain motion by placing the arm in gradually increasing arcs of extension. The adjunctive use of peritendinous corticosteroid injection is useful in more symptomatic patients. Care must be taken to avoid intratendinous injection and its long-term sequelae of secondary tendon rupture. As the tendon is held in the bicipital groove by a connective tissue retinaculum, the peritendinous sheath in the proximal humerus can be bathed with a corticosteroid–anesthetic mixture by directing the tip of a 25-gauge needle to the bony floor of this tunnel, parallel with the tendon, then withdrawing the needle 1 to 2 mm before injecting. Inability to push the syringe plunger indicates an intratendon position.

ADHESIVE CAPSULITIS

Also termed frozen shoulder, shoulder periarthritis or periscapulitis, adhesive capsulitis is a poorly understood syndrome of capsular fibrosis and generalized shoulder pain with progressive restriction of active and passive motion in all planes. The condition is self-limiting but runs a prolonged course. Affecting females slightly more than males and occurring most frequently between the ages of 40 and 70 years, adhesive capsulitis is bilateral in up to one-third of patients, although up to 7 years may pass before the contralateral shoulder is affected. Fibrosis is thought secondary to an inflammatory reaction in the synovium and or capsule, yet there is considerable variation in the reported degree of synovitis and presence of capsular adhesions as seen during shoulder arthroscopy and in the intensity of inflammation in histologic specimens. Adhesive capsulitis may be primary (idiopathic) or secondary to a number of diverse conditions including other regional shoulder disorders (trauma, chronic impingement); bony lesions (avascular necrosis of the humeral head, fracture); glenohumeral joint involvement of inflammatory arthritides;

disorders associated with shoulder pain or prolonged immobilization or arm dependency (cerebrovascular accidents, myocardial infarction, cervical spine disease with radiculopathy, intrathoracic conditions including tumors, postmastectomy with axillary lymph node dissection); and other fibrosing disorders and medical conditions (scleroderma, diabetes mellitus, thyroid disease).

Shoulder pain develops insidiously over weeks to months, and patients often cannot remember an inciting event. Pain develops over the anterolateral shoulder and upper arm, but may also be felt laterally and posteriorly. Rest and night pain are common, and the pain is exacerbated with any shoulder motion. Progressive shoulder stiffness, voluntary guarding, and disuse lead to a marked reduction in all movement; during this process, pain may subside and be limited to the end range of motion. Examination elicits pain in all motions, especially external rotation (as contrasted against rotator cuff tendinitis, which is more painful with resisted internal rotation). Both active and passive motion in all directions is reduced, again most notably in external rotation; a careful exam will note that passive movements are limited by mechanical restriction more so than pain. Tenderness may be elicited with palpation over the rotator cuff as well as other periarticular structures and over the glenohumeral joint capsule. Findings may suggest impingement, although the diagnostic subacromial injection of anesthetic does not improve motion.

Radiographs of the shoulder are usually negative but are useful to exclude findings of potential etiologic conditions arising from the glenohumeral joint or bony structures. Arthrography is painful and should be limited to patients in whom clinical findings are equivocal or there exists the possibility of a rotator cuff tear. Reduced capsular volume with obliteration of axillary and subscapular recesses with normal tendon structures confirms the diagnosis of adhesive capsulitis.

The goal of treatment for adhesive capsulitis is to restore glenohumeral motion, which is best accomplished through a comprehensive program of pain control and extensive (and often prolonged) rehabilitation. Measures to reduce pain and facilitate physical therapy include the use of analgesics and NSAIDs, thermal modalities including ultrasound, intraarticular and periarticular corticosteroid injections (more effective earlier in the course of the syndrome), stellate ganglion or suprascapular nerve block, and in some patients, transcutaneous electrical nerve stimulation. Therapy begins with painless gentle pendulum motions and passive stretching exercises of the capsule by using the contralateral arm to bring the affected arm across the chest to the point of a pulling sensation but not pain. Hand wall-walking, arm rotation, and abduction and overhead stretching exercises are added as motion improves, but vigorous or forceful exercises are avoided as pain may be exacerbated by tearing of capsular adhesions. As contrasted to exercise regimens for other regional shoulder disorders, the course of therapy for adhesive capsulitis may last many months, and supervised physical therapy is more often required in order to prescribe the appropriate intensity, frequency, and duration of the therapy, and to insure compliance with the rehabilitation program. Only rarely do patients require referral for more invasive procedures such as saline joint distension, shoulder manipulation under anesthesia, or open capsulotomy. Most patients regain functional motion. The mean recovery time may be as long as 2 years. However, elderly patients have a higher incidence of residual motion loss.

TRIGGER FINGER

The lifetime prevalence of trigger finger in nondiabetic adults older than age 30 years is estimated at 2 percent. Although most commonly seen in patients in their fifties and sixties, the condition is frequently reported in patients in their seventies and eighties. Women are more frequently affected than men. The thumb is most commonly involved, followed by the middle and ring fingers. Most patients are symptomatic with single rather than multiple affected digits. Patients present with the gradual onset of finger stiffness, clicking, snapping and/or locking as they try to extend a flexed finger. The ability to flex the finger is usually not impaired owing to the relative greater strength of finger flexors over extensors. The condition may be intermittent, and pain, when present, does not radiate. Rupture of the flexor tendon in this condition is not reported. When untreated, the condition is generally chronic and progressive, but spontaneous recovery may occur in as many as 25 percent of patients.

Triggering occurs when the digital flexor tendon is entrapped by a thickened, fibrous, retinacular ligament called a pulley. The flexor tendon is normally covered along its course in the palm and finger by a series of intermittent ligaments running transverse (annular or A pulleys) or at an angular crossing (cruciate or C pulleys) over the tendon. These structures allow the tendon to flex the finger at the metacarpophalangeal (MCP), proximal interphalangeal (PIP), and distal interphalangeal (DIP) joints without bowstringing. The annular pulleys occur at the palmar plates of these joints, and are subjected to the greatest tendon forces. The most common site of tendon entrapment is at the volar aspect of the MCP head where the flexor tendon canal is compromised by an abnormal thickened A1 pulley, although tendon gliding may be compromised anywhere along its course from the carpal tunnel to the more distal digital compartments. Histologically, the pulley (and occasionally the contiguous flexor tendon) undergoes degenerative changes with an increase in fibrous tissue as well as fibrocartilaginous metaplasia, with minimal, if any, inflammatory changes. Secondary tendon changes may include focal swelling and granulation tissue formation. Nodular tendon swelling may occur as a secondary finding, or a primary factor in triggering when occurring in the setting of systemic disease such as rheumatoid arthritis.

Examination may elicit the clicking, snapping or triggering with either passive or voluntary finger flexion and extension. The presence of palpable swelling or tenderness along the tendon or at the A1 pulley site is variable. Pain can at times be further elicited with resisted finger flexion, or passive stretch of the tendon through finger extension. Further examination of the hand should look for evidence of associated diseases such as rheumatoid arthritis, large osteophytes of osteoarthritis, Dupuytren's disease (contraction of the palmar fascia, with or without nodular swelling, characteristically along the fourth and fifth finger rays), and carpal tunnel syndrome. Laboratory tests, when ordered, are done to evaluate for possible secondary causes such as diabetes mellitus, rheumatoid arthritis, amyloidosis, and hypothyroidism.

Conservative treatment involves prolonged splinting of the affected digit. Thermal modalities, as well as either phonophoresis or iontophoresis, may be considered as an adjunct, and in some patients, a nonsteroidal antiinflammatory agent may be useful. Local corticosteroid injection by a skilled operator into the flexor tendon sheath and/or into the stenosed fibroosseous canal at the A1 pulley may hasten improvement, and is indicated in patients unimproved by more conservative care or with severe symptoms at onset. Resistant cases require surgical release of the A1 pulley. As long as the palmar aponeurosis and A2 pulley (just distal to the A1 pulley) are intact, the loss of the A1 pulley does not lead to functional compromise of finger flexion.

ENTHESITIS AND SPONDYLOARTHROPATHIES

Enthesitis

The enthesis is the area of insertion of tendon, ligament, joint capsule, or fascia into bone. Although this region can be involved in tendinitis syndromes, typically associated with chronic repetitive overuse, acute tendon overload, or direct tendon injury (see Fig. 81-2) as noted above, spontaneous inflammation can occur and is termed enthesitis. These insertional sites can be dispersed over a wide area of bone, may be intraarticular, may be situated deep to connective tissues or be closely related to other structures such as bursae, and thus be difficult to detect clinically when inflamed. Enthesitis is a cardinal feature of the spondyloarthropathies.

Anatomically, entheses are of two types: fibrous, and fibrocartilage. The fibrous entheses are located at the metaphyses and diaphyses of long bones where dense fibrous connective tissue bundles of tendon attach to bone. Fibrocartilage entheses are located at sites of joint movement and have an additional layer of fibrocartilage between connective tissue and bone. The function of the fibrocartilage is thought to assist in dissipating mechanical stress. Entheseal regions are well innervated, and are perfused by periosteal, bone marrow, and tendon sources of vasculature. They are capable of a high rate of tissue turnover in response to continual mechanical stimulation.

The etiology of spontaneous enthesitis is not understood. Pathologic studies demonstrate the presence of inflammatory cell infiltrates and pannus formation, soft-tissue inflammation, and bony destruction at entheseal insertions. Secondary new bone formation is an important feature of this process and leads to reduced mobility, such as can be seen with the ankylosis of a finger joint in a patient with psoriasis or the spine in a patient with ankylosing spondylitis. Entheses are numerous near to, or within, the synovial joints commonly involved in the

spondyloarthropathies, and thus can explain many, if not all, of the clinical findings. Through the use of highly sensitive imaging procedures (e.g., fat-suppressed MRI), even early, large-joint synovitis (knee) in patients with spondyloarthropathy has been shown to be associated with entheseal abnormalities not seen in patients with active rheumatoid arthritis. This suggests that enthesitis may be the source for not only periarticular inflammatory changes, but also the synovitis (as a secondary feature) typically seen in the extremity joints of patients with spondyloarthropathies. It is postulated that the local production of cytokines and growth factors from sites of enthesitis initiate such synovitis in neighboring joints.

Clinical sites of pain from enthesitis include the nuchal crests at the base of the skull; the manubriosternal joint; the costochondral joints; the greater tuberosity and the epicondyles of the humerus; along the iliac crests and the anterior–superior and posterior–superior iliac spines of the pelvis; the ischial tuberosities; the greater trochanteric prominence and condyles of the femur; the tibial tuberosities; the fibular head; the insertions of the Achilles tendon and the plantar fascia into the calcaneus; and the spinous processes along the entirety of the spine.

Spondyloarthropathies

The spondyloarthropathies are a heterogenous group of inflammatory disorders characterized by inflammatory back pain, peripheral inflammatory arthritis (often asymmetric and oligoarticular), enthesitis, variable involvement of other organ tissues, and a tendency toward familial aggregation (through human leukocyte antigen [HLA]-B27 and likely other contributing genetic markers). Table 81-4 summarizes the clinical findings of ankylosing spondylitis, reactive arthritis, psoriatic arthritis, and enteropathic arthritis.

These "classical" spondyloarthropathies only rarely present for the first time in the elderly person. More commonly, the clinician is responsible for assessing and directing management of elderly patients with the sequelae of long-standing disease, including inflammatory arthritis, and extraarticular manifestations such as inflammatory ocular disease, or cardiopulmonary involvement such as aortic insufficiency and fibrocavitary lung abnormalities that can occur after long-standing ankylosing spondylitis. The principles of therapy are similar to those for the treatment of patients with rheumatoid arthritis (see Chap. 78), and rely on a close working relationship between clinician and therapists skilled in the physical, occupational, and rehabilitative care of patients with arthritis. Therapy to promote the maintenance of posture, as well as back strengthening and flexibility is a critical adjunctive measure to pharmaceutical therapy. Drug therapy includes analgesics and nonsteroidal antiinflammatory agents for mild joint disease, corticosteroids for more aggressive arthritic symptoms (in a pattern of therapy as per the treatment of rheumatoid arthritis) and uveitis, and disease-modifying antirheumatic drugs (DMARDs) for persistent arthritis. Methotrexate and sulfasalazine are the most commonly used DMARDs. Tumor necrosis factor-α blockers have been used with success

Table 81-4   Clinical Findings of the Common Spondyloarthropathies

Characteristic	Ankylosing Spondylitis	Reactive Arthritis (Reiter's Syndrome)	Psoriatic Arthritis*	Enteropathic Arthritis[†]
Usual onset age	Adult <40	Young–middle-aged adult	Young–middle-aged adult	Young–middle-aged adult
Sex ratio	Males 3:1	Predominately males	F = M	F = M
Usual onset type	Gradual	Acute, 1–4 weeks after gastrointestinal or genitourinary infection	Variable	Gradual
Sacroiliitis or spondylitis	Virtually 100%	<50%	20%	<20%
Symmetry of sacroiliitis	Symmetric	Asymmetric	Asymmetric	Symmetric
Peripheral joint involvement	25%	90%	95%	15–20%
HLA-B27–positive (in whites)	90%	75%	<50%[‡]	<50%[‡]
Eye involvement[§]	25–30%	50%	20%	≤15%
Cardiac involvement	1–4%	5–10%	Rare	Rare
Skin or nail involvement	None	<40%	Virtually 100%	Uncommon
Role of infectious agents as triggers	Unknown	Yes[¶]	Unknown	Unknown

*Approximately 5-7% of patients with psoriasis develop extremity arthritis, and psoriatic spondylitis accounts for approximately 10% of all patients with psoriatic arthritis. Other nonspondylitic forms are oligoarticular asymmetric; DIP joint disease (frequently associated nail disease); polyarthritis (joint distribution like rheumatoid arthritis); and arthritis mutilans (gross destruction of bones as well as joints).

[†]Associated with chronic inflammatory bowel disease (ulcerative colitis and regional enteritis or Crohn's disease).

[‡]B27 prevalence is higher in those with spondylitis or sacroiliitis.

[§]Mainly conjunctivitis in reactive and psoriatic arthritis, and acute anterior uveitis in ankylosing spondylitis and enteropathic arthritis.

[¶]Includes reports of *Campylobactr jejuni, Chlamydia trachomatis, Neisseria gonorrhoeae,* Salmonella species, *Shigella flexneri, Yersinia enterocolitica* and *Yersinia pseudotuberculosis.*

for psoriatic arthritis, and in limited patients with ankylosing spondylitis and enteropathic arthritis.

Despite the categorization of spondyloarthropathy patients into the above specific diagnostic entities, it is increasingly recognized that many patients have either atypical or incomplete forms of disease. In order to recognize that patients with spondyloarthropathies encompass a population with a wide spectrum of findings, a newer classification system has been proposed (Table 81-5). This system encompasses patients with what is now termed an undifferentiated spondyloarthropathy, and is meant to represent patients with an early phase of a more definitive spondyloarthropathy, arrested forms of a spondyloarthropathy not progressing to the established disease, syndromes of overlapping features of more than one spondyloarthropathy, and heretofore undescribed spondyloarthropathies awaiting future delineation. In contrast to the very uncommon occurrence of "classical" spondyloarthropathies in older adults and elderly persons, late-onset undifferentiated spondyloarthropathy occurs more frequently. Patients with late-onset undifferentiated spondyloarthropathy usually have combinations of two or more findings from those listed in Table 81-5, although some present with only one abnormality that may persist for many years before the addition of an additional clinical variable. The presence of distal upper extremity joint synovitis with pitting, dorsal hand edema, similar to that which may occur in patients with polymyalgia rheumatica, is more frequent in patients with late-onset than early adult or childhood undifferentiated spondyloarthropathy.

ENTRAPMENT NEUROPATHIES

Nerve entrapment syndromes are the result of focal injury to a peripheral nerve and are more common in the upper extremities (Fig. 81-4). Damage is produced by mechanical forces (internal or external [traumatic] compression,

Table 81-5 European Spondyloarthropathy Study Group (ESSG) Criteria for the Classification of Spondyloarthropathy*

Variable	Definition
1. Inflammatory spinal pain	Past or present back, dorsal, or cervical pain, with at least 4 of the following: onset before age 45 years, insidious onset, improved by exercise, associated with morning stiffness, at least 3 months duration
2. Synovitis	Past or present asymmetric arthritis or arthritis in the lower limbs
3. a. Positive family history	First-degree or second-degree relative with ankylosing spondylitis, psoriasis, acute uveitis, reactive arthritis, or inflammatory bowel disease
b. Psoriasis	Past or present, diagnosed by a physician
c. Inflammatory bowel disease	Past or present Crohn's disease or ulcerative colitis diagnosed by a physician and confirmed by radiologic examination or endoscopy
d. Urethritis, cervicitis, or acute diarrhea within 1 month before arthritis	Nongonococcal urethritis or cervicitis
e. Alternating buttock pain	Past or present alternating between right and left gluteal regions
f. Enthesopathy	Past or present spontaneous pain or tenderness at examination of the site of the insertion of the Achilles tendon or plantar fascia
g. Sacroiliitis	Bilateral radiographic grade 2–4 or unilateral grade 3–4 (0 = normal; 1 = possible; 2 = minimal; 3 = moderate; 4 = ankylosis)

*For classification purposes, patients must have either 1 or 2, and one or more of the findings in 3.

SOURCE: Adapted from Dougados M et al: The ESSG preliminary criteria for the classification of spondyloarthropathy. *Arthritis Rheum* 34:1218, 1991.

stretch, friction, or angulation), and leads to variable symptoms of pain, tingling, numbness, and/or weakness in the distribution of the affected nerve. A careful history and exam is usually sufficient to make a presumptive diagnosis. Electrophysiologic testing (e.g., nerve-conduction velocity testing), the gold standard for diagnosis, is not necessary in the initial evaluation of all patients, but is useful to confirm an uncertain diagnosis, to exclude other superimposed neuropathies, to document the severity of nerve damage, and to follow the course of therapy. Conservative therapy may include splinting or cushioning vulnerable anatomic sites to reduce mechanical irritation, and oral or injectable antiinflammatory medications. Surgical release of nerve compression is considered for those patients failing conservative therapy, with acute severe symptoms, or with significant sensory or motor function loss.

Carpal Tunnel Syndrome

Compression of the median nerve at the wrist is the most common entrapment neuropathy, and results in the carpal tunnel syndrome (CTS). The carpal tunnel or canal is a relatively inelastic closed compartment formed by the dorsolateral bony carpal arch and the palmar transverse carpal ligament. The median nerve runs just underneath the ligament, on the radial side of the palmaris longus tendon (when present), accompanied in the canal by the long flexor tendons to the fingers. The median nerve supplies sensation to the palmar aspect of the first through third fingers and the radial half of the fourth finger, and innervates most of the muscles of the thenar eminence and intrinsic lumbrical

muscles of the index and middle fingers. Compression of the median nerve occurs when the carpal tunnel is narrowed or its contents increase in size. Aging is associated with narrowing of the canal, as well as an increased prevalence of slowed median nerve sensory conduction velocity as measured electrodiagnostically.

CTS is more common in women than men, and more than three-fourths of all cases occur in individuals older than age 40 years. Up to half of those affected have bilateral symptoms, and one-third of patients with unilateral symptoms have electrodiagnostic abnormalities on the asymptomatic contralateral side. An associated condition can be identified in fewer than half of patients, and includes median nerve compression from localized processes at the wrist (e.g., fracture, osteophytes, ganglions, lipoma) and systemic conditions (e.g., inflammatory arthritides such as rheumatoid arthritis, diabetes mellitus, myeloma, thyroid disease, amyloidosis). Although CTS secondary to cumulative trauma from repetitive motion (particularly flexion and forceful grasping) is generally an occupational disorder, symptoms may be provoked by avocational pursuits or during activities of daily living such as driving, knitting, or writing.

Symptoms at presentation are more prominent in the dominant hand, and include rest or use-related tingling, numbness, and pain of the palmar aspect of the radial three and a half fingers. Nocturnal pain relieved by shaking the hand is a classic symptom; pain may also be present in the wrist, and, less commonly, radiate proximally to as high as the shoulder, or involve the entire hand. Patients may complain of hand stiffness or clumsiness with pinch or fine motor activities, and that they drop objects. Hand sensory

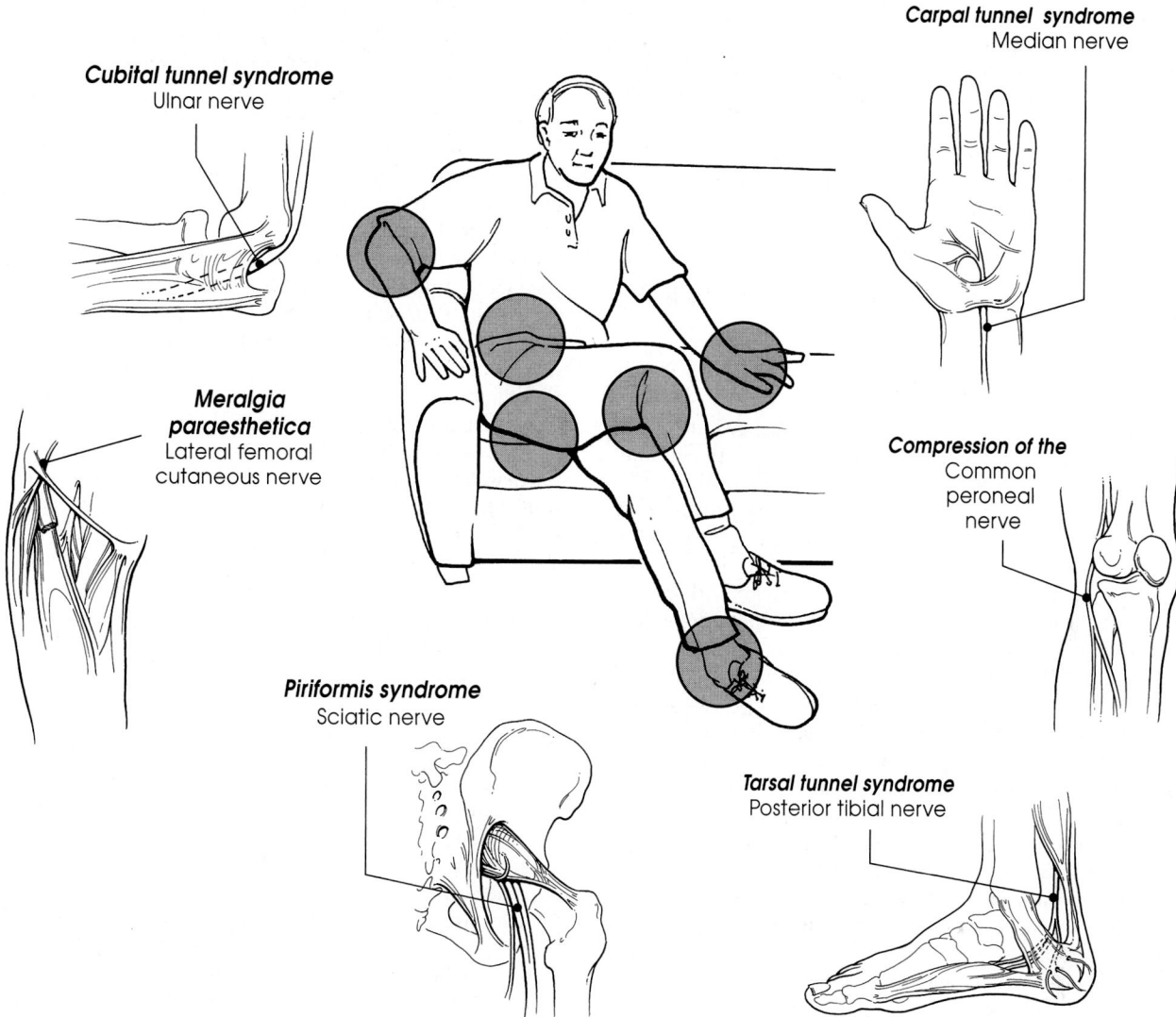

Figure 81-4   The major entrapment neuropathies.

and motor examination in patients with early symptoms may be normal; the earliest sensory loss seems to occur at the volar tip of the third finger. Atrophy and weakness of the muscles of the thenar eminence (opponens muscle measured by resisting opposition of the thumb against the fifth finger tip, and abductor pollicis muscle measured by resisting motion of the thumb away from the palm) are late signs. Provocative tests for median nerve compression include maneuvers that produce paraesthesias in the distribution of the median nerve: Tinel's sign by gentle percussion over the median nerve at the wrist creases and has a sensitivity and specificity of 60 percent, and Phalen's sign is produced by a 60-second sustained wrist flexion, and has a sensitivity of 75 percent and specificity of 47 percent. Electrodiagnostic testing is not necessary in all cases, but is useful to exclude other causes of hand and arm pain such as peripheral neuropathies, cervical radiculopathies (most often C6) or median nerve compression proximal to the wrist, or in making the diagnosis of CTS when history and exam findings are equivocal. The most sensitive electrodiagnostic sign is an increased distal sensory latency,

which is the amount of time required for a sensory impulse to cross the wrist from the fingers.

Initial conservative therapy is indicated for all patients without motor weakness, muscle atrophy, or acute CTS from trauma. Treatment of mild or intermittent symptoms and acute flares begins with wrist rest to include avoidance of precipitating activities and the use of splints that place the wrist in 0 to 15 degrees of dorsiflexion to maximize the diameter of the carpal canal. Splints may be worn at night and as needed during the day. Persistent symptoms may be treated by the addition of a NSAID or a short course of oral steroids; a limited trial of diuretics can be considered if fluid retention is a major contributing pathogenic factor. Injecting the carpal tunnel with corticosteroids is a useful adjunctive therapy for patients who do not respond to rest and oral medication. This subligamentous injection is easily performed with a short 25-gauge needle at the proximal wrist crease, placed lateral to the palmaris longus and at a 30-degree angle to the skin. Care should be taken to avoid injection into the median nerve, tendons, or vessels. Conservative therapy controls symptoms in up to two-thirds of patients. Factors that correlate with a higher rate of failure of conservative medical management include older than age 50 years, symptoms for longer than 10 months, constant paraesthesias, thenar atrophy, and a positive Phalen's test within 30 seconds.

Surgical therapy to decompress the carpal tunnel by release of the transverse carpal ligament is indicated for patients with acute CTS and those who fail medical therapy or have persistent sensory loss. Outcome is best for patients with primarily sensory loss and pain, whereas those with thenar atrophy and motor function loss uncommonly regain function.

Cubital Tunnel Syndrome

Ulnar nerve compression at the elbow is the second most common entrapment neuropathy and results in the cubital tunnel syndrome. The ulnar nerve passes relatively unprotected into the cubital tunnel along the groove formed by the medial humeral epicondyle and olecranon; the floor of the tunnel is the ulnar collateral ligament and the roof the aponeurosis of the flexor carpi ulnaris muscle. With elbow flexion the floor of the tunnel bulges into the groove and the aponeurosis becomes taught, narrowing the tunnel and compressing the ulnar nerve. The ulnar nerve may also be damaged because of trauma acutely or from prolonged direct pressure from resting the elbow on a flat surface, as can occur with arm immobilization (e.g., from neurologic disorders or restraints) or chronic placement of the elbow on tables or wheelchair armrests.

Cubital tunnel syndrome produces tingling and numbness on the ulnar side of the hand, including the fifth finger, extending no more than a few centimeters proximal to the wrist crease. Sensory symptoms may mimic those from a cervical radiculopathy or ulnar nerve lesions proximal or distal to the elbow; sensory symptoms that increase with elbow flexion implicate nerve entrapment at the elbow. Medial elbow pain radiating to the hand may be present. Motor loss is a late finding and can lead to weakness of finger and thumb abduction, pinch, and loss of control over fine finger motion.

Conservative therapy for cubital tunnel syndrome consists of avoidance of direct elbow pressure and repetitive elbow flexion. Foam elbow pads and splinting the elbow in extension are useful in selected patients. Short courses of a NSAID or corticosteroid injection into the cubital tunnel may be tried but are less successful as contrasted to their use for carpal tunnel syndrome. Similar to the situation with the carpal tunnel, syndrome surgical release of the cubital tunnel is most effective in patients who have failed conservative management but do not have significant motor dysfunction or muscle atrophy.

Meralgia Paraesthetica

Entrapment of the purely sensory lateral femoral cutaneous nerve produces a syndrome of anterolateral thigh symptoms termed meralgia paraesthetica. The nerve may be compressed as it passes under or through the inguinal ligament at its attachment to the anterior superior iliac spine or just distally as it passes through the aponeurosis of the sartorius muscle and then the fascia lata. This syndrome is more common in men than women, and in obese individuals.

Symptoms of anterolateral thigh tingling or numbness are commonly exacerbated by coughing, prolonged standing and walking, all of which cause a downward pull of the inguinal ligament in relation to the nerve. Examination may reveal sensory loss on the anterolateral thigh, but the lack of muscle weakness and knee reflex abnormalities differentiate the syndrome from lesions of the lumbar nerve roots. Symptomatic relief from the local injection of anesthetic medial to the anterior superior iliac spine confirms the diagnosis.

Meralgia paraesthetica is usually self-limiting. Patients should be advised to restrain from aggravating activities, participate in exercises to strengthen the abdominal wall muscles, and to lose weight and restrain from wearing tight-fitting garments if indicated. Local injection of a corticosteroid–anesthetic mixture deep and medial to the anterior superior iliac spine may be a useful measure for short-term relief. Only rarely will patients require decompressive surgery for persistent pain.

Piriformis Syndrome

Piriformis syndrome is an entrapment neuropathy of the sciatic nerve as its two major branches pass, either together or divided, around or through the piriformis muscle at the sciatic notch. Irritation of the sciatic nerve from piriformis muscle contraction or compression can lead to a syndrome that mimics sciatica, and this accounts for approximately 5 percent of such presentations. Patients describe variable degrees of buttock, paralumbar, and leg pain. Men may also complain of scrotal pain or numbness, and women of pelvic pain or dyspareunia. Symptoms can be aggravated by direct compression from prolonged sitting on a hard surface, and excessive leg activities requiring rotation of the hip.

Piriformis muscle tenderness may be elicited with palpation just lateral to the sciatic notch and during rectal and pelvic examination. The straight-leg-raising test may be positive, and pain is exacerbated during passive internal or resisted external rotation of the hip. Electrodiagnostic testing and imaging studies such as computed tomography and MRI are useful to exclude other causes of sciatica when history and exam findings are not diagnostic.

Most patients respond to conservative therapy. Physical therapy includes correction of posture and gait abnormalities, ultrasound-mediated thermal application, piriformis stretching, and then hip abductor straightening. NSAIDs and analgesics are useful to treat pain. More resistant symptoms can be treated with a local injection of a corticosteroid–anesthetic mixture into the piriformis muscle, piercing the skin at a point midway between the posterior superior iliac spine and the greater trochanter of the hip. Once a primary from of therapy, surgical release of the piriformis muscle is now limited to patients who fail conservative therapy.

Common Peroneal Neuropathy

Injury to the common peroneal nerve at the neck of the fibula is the most common lower extremity compression neuropathy. The nerve at this site rests fixed on the bony fibula and other than for skin and subcutaneous tissue is completely unprotected from direct pressure. Compression most commonly occurs from chronic leg crossing as the nerve is pressed on the contralateral patella but may also be caused by tight stockings or bandages, during prolonged leg immobilization, or from excessive nerve stretch from prolonged squatting.

Patients complain of tingling and numbness over the dorsum of the foot and inability to raise the foot. A dimple in the skin may be present if compression is chronic, and a Tinel's sign can be elicited at the fibular neck over the nerve. Motor weakness is limited to ankle dorsiflexion and eversion; the patient may have a muscle atrophy in the anterolateral leg and a slapping gait. The presence of impaired ankle inversion excludes common peroneal nerve compression, and suggests an L5 radiculopathy as the source of foot drop.

Most patients recover with conservative therapy to include avoiding aggravating behaviors, ankle range of motion exercises, and splinting to maintain mobility and provide foot protection. Surgical release is indicated only for persistent or progressive motor weakness.

Tarsal Tunnel Syndrome

The tarsal tunnel syndrome is an entrapment neuropathy of the posterior tibial nerve behind the medial malleolus of the ankle. The tunnel is formed by the groove between the malleolus and calcaneus, is covered by a fibrous flexor retinaculum, and also contains the posterior tibial, flexor digitorum longus, and flexor hallucis tendons. Within the tunnel, the nerve divides into medial and lateral plantar nerves to the sole of the foot; the third division to the calcaneus usually does not cross the tunnel. Tarsal tunnel syndrome produces pain and sensory dysfunction in the plantar aspect of the foot and toes. Nocturnal pain is common, and relief is attempted by shaking or dangling the foot. Foot weakness is generally not reported. Women are more commonly affected than men, and patients with a pronated forefoot with either valgus or varus heel, or flexor tenosynovitis, such as from trauma or rheumatoid arthritis, are at increased risk.

Examination may reveal sensory loss on the sole of the foot. Motor loss may be demonstrated more by loss of muscle bulk over the medial arch and dorsolateral aspects of the foot rather than weakness. A Tinel's sign and tenderness over the nerve at the tarsal tunnel can be elicited. Electrodiagnostic testing revealing motor and sensory abnormalities in the distribution of the plantar nerve branches can confirm the diagnosis.

Therapy begins with a trial of ankle splinting and as needed shoe modifications to correct foot deformities. NSAIDs may be tried as well as corticosteroid injection into the tarsal tunnel. Failure to improve after 2 months or worsening interval symptoms are indications for surgical referral.

NOCTURNAL LEG CRAMPS

Nocturnal leg cramps are a common complaint among elderly persons, occurring in as many as 70 percent at some time. The cramps are random, sudden, involuntary painful contractions of the calf and occasionally foot muscles, lasting seconds to minutes, rarely hours, that occur with recumbency and often awaken the person from sleep. The cramp leads to visible and palpable muscle contractions that patients massage and attempt to stretch for relief. The etiology of nocturnal leg cramps is unclear, but affected individuals have a higher prevalence of peripheral vascular disease or peripheral neurologic deficit. Lack of lower extremity, particularly knee bending, activity, leading to muscle and tendon shortening, may contribute to nocturnal leg cramping. There is no relation of nocturnal leg cramps to abnormalities of sleep.

Initial history and examination should be directed to exclude other causes for leg cramping or calf pain, including claudication from peripheral vascular disease, neurogenic claudication from spinal stenosis, lower motor neuron disease, peripheral neuropathy, restless leg syndrome (subcutaneous crawling sensations in the legs relieved by leg movement), certain systemic conditions (thyroid disease, diabetes mellitus, fluid and electrolyte alterations), and alcohol and other drugs (diuretics and calcium channel blockers). In the absence of an observed cramp, the exam is usually unremarkable.

Treatment of acute leg cramps involves muscle massage and stretching. Calf muscles can be stretched by manually forcing the foot into dorsiflexion, or by pressing the heel onto the floor with the knee extended while leaning onto a wall from a distance of 2 to 3 feet. Prophylaxis against recurrent attacks should begin with calf stretching exercises performed three times daily. A footboard may also be used to promote this stretching and to keep the ankle from passive plantar flexion during sleep. Patients failing exercise therapy can be considered for a trial of pharmacologic management. A number of drugs have been reported to improve symptoms, most in uncontrolled short-term trials, including quinine sulfate, calcium channel blockers, vitamin E, carbamazepine, orphenadrine, and diphenhydramine. Meta analysis has shown that the short-term (2 to 4 week) use of quinine can reduce the frequency but not severity or duration of nocturnal leg cramps. Care must be taken in the prescription of quinine for elderly patients, who are at increased risk of toxicity because of the prolonged half-life of the drug. A 1-week trial at 200 mg at bedtime is usually sufficient to assess efficacy. Toxicities include thrombocytopenia, hypoglycemia, and the development of cinchonism. The earliest signs of cinchonism, tinnitus and decreased hearing, may be masked in the elderly patient because of presbycusis. Later signs include nausea, vomiting, and disturbed vision, followed by abdominal pain, blindness, delirium, and cardiac dysrhythmias.

Table 81-6   The American College of Rheumatology 1990 Criteria for the Classification of Fibromyalgia

For classification purposes, criteria 1 and 2 must be satisfied

1. History of widespread pain for at least 3 months:

    *   Left and right side of body
    *   Above and below waist
    *   Axial pain must be present (cervical spine or anterior chest or thoracic spine or low back)

2. Pain on 11 of 18 tender points on digital palpation (4 kg of force). Patient must state that the palpation was painful. "Tender" is not to be considered "painful":

    *   Occiput: bilateral, at suboccipital muscle insertions
    *   Low cervical: anterior aspects of the intertransverse spaces, C5–C7
    *   Trapezius: bilateral, midpoint upper border
    *   Supraspinatus: bilateral, at origins above scapular spine near the medial border
    *   Second rib: bilateral, upper surfaces, just lateral to costochondral junctions
    *   Lateral epicondyle: bilateral, 2 cm distal to the epicondyles
    *   Gluteal: bilateral, in the upper outer quadrants of buttocks in anterior fold of muscle
    *   Knee: bilateral, medial fat pad proximal to joint line

SOURCE: Adapted from Wolfe F et al: The American College of Rheumatology 1990 criteria for the classification of fibromyalgia: Report of the Multicenter Criteria Committee. *Arthritis Rheum* 33:160, 1990.

FIBROMYALGIA

Although not a regional musculoskeletal disorder, the prevalence of fibromyalgia in the community in general, and in the elderly population in particular, mandates inclusion in a review of musculoskeletal disorders. Fibromyalgia is a syndrome of widespread pain, decreased pain threshold, and diffuse tenderness. Despite clinical reports in the early 1900s of patients with compatible symptomatology, the criteria for the modern construct of the syndrome were not described until 1975. In 1990, the American College of Rheumatology described classification criteria for fibromyalgia (see Table 81-6), listing 18 specific common muscular tender points, which have become the de facto diagnostic criteria. It should be noted however that patients with fibromyalgia are tender all over, not just in these described tender point regions. The tender points merely represent areas where the majority of patients have relatively low pain threshold. Patients may be diagnosed with fibromyalgia with fewer than the minimum 11 tender points provided they have chronic widespread

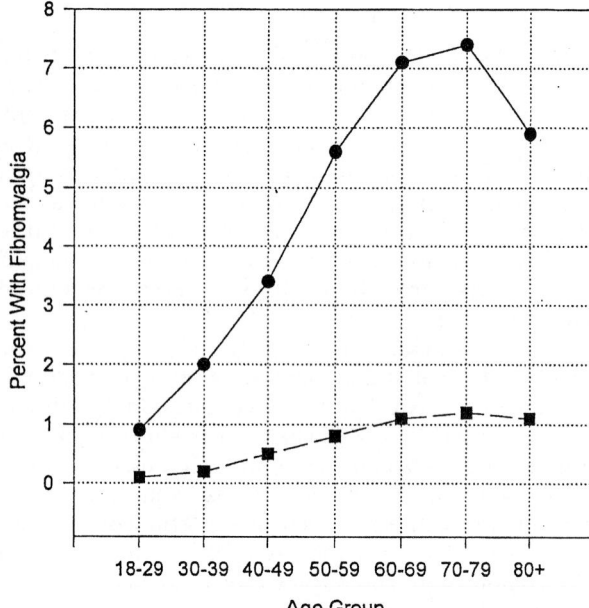

Figure 81-5   Prevalence of fibromyalgia, by age and sex (*circles* = women, *squares* = men) for the Wichita, KS, population ages 18 and older. Reprinted with permission from Wolfe M et al: The prevalence and characteristics of fibromyalgia in the general population. *Arthritis Rheum* 38:19, 1995.

pain and many of the characteristic symptoms of the syndrome.

Fibromyalgia is more common in women than in men at all age groups, including in the elderly population. The ratio of women to men is reported to be as high as 10:1. The true prevalence of fibromyalgia in the community is unknown, but is estimated to be 2 percent. The prevalence increases with age, more for women than men, with prevalence estimates for women older than age 60 years as high as 8 to 9 percent (Fig. 81-5). There are insufficient data for the elderly population to judge the impact of other chronic medical illnesses on the prevalence and severity of fibromyalgia, although one small study has shown an increased odds ratio of having coronary artery disease as compared to elderly patients without fibromyalgia.

Fibromyalgia is a clinical diagnosis based on the presence of chronic widespread pain of at least 3 months duration and the presence of tender points. In the elderly population, the syndrome is underrecognized, underdiagnosed, and a frequent cause of inappropriate corticosteroid therapy. The diagnosis is best made in the context of longitudinal observation. Other commonly associated features include fatigue (80 percent), paraesthesias (up to 60 percent), chronic headaches, Raynaud's syndrome (15 percent), and sleep and mood disturbances. Polyarthralgias (up to 40 percent) and subjective stiffness greater than 15 minutes (75 percent) are in some patients severe enough to simulate symptoms of an inflammatory arthritis. Patients may also exhibit symptoms of irritable bowel syndrome (30 to 80 percent), "irritable bladder" syndrome, and restless leg syndrome and leg cramps (20 to 30 percent). As compared to younger adults, limited studies demonstrate elderly

bacteremias, often with more resistant organisms (e.g., *Enterobacter* spp.), can also result in PVE.

Endocarditis is difficult to diagnose in the elderly patient. Fever and leukocytosis are less common (55 percent and 25 percent, respectively, for elderly patients versus 80 percent and 60 percent, respectively, for younger patients). The prominence of degenerative, calcific valvular lesions and prosthetic valves lowers the sensitivity of transthoracic echocardiography (TTE) to 45 percent in the elderly compared with 75 percent for younger patients. Transesophageal echocardiography (TEE) may be more sensitive, and in at least one study, TEE improved the diagnostic yield by 45 percent over that of TTE. Age alone is not a major risk for mortality, with a 2-year survival of 75 percent for IE in all age groups unless major comorbidities exist.

Antibiotic treatment of IE is directed at identified pathogens or the most likely causes if blood cultures are negative (Table 82-2). Therapy is administered intravenously for 2 to 6 weeks. Combination regimens with aminoglycosides are particularly problematic in the elderly patient because of toxicity (both renal and ototoxicity), but is occasionally unavoidable in certain circumstances (e.g., enterococcal IE). Surgical therapy is required only when specific criteria are met, primarily recurrent embolic events or worsening heart failure.

Antibiotic prophylaxis is available for bacterial endocarditis for all "at-risk" patients and should be provided for dental, upper respiratory tract, GI, or GU procedures. Although the evidence supporting this practice is relatively weak, it has become the standard of care. Current recommendations for IE prophylaxis are available in sources listed in the references.

Bacteremia and Sepsis

Bacteremia rates are much higher in elderly patients than in younger patients, comprising up to 14 percent of all admissions in some geriatric units. Older patients with bacteremia are less likely than younger patients to have systemic signs such as fever, chills, or diaphoresis. Bacteremia in the elderly patient is more likely to arise from a gastrointestinal or genitourinary source than in young adults. Thus, the causative agent is more likely to be a gram-negative rod.

Despite a similar initial cytokine response to that of young adults with sepsis, the prognosis of sepsis in the elderly is worse. The 28-day mortality for sepsis in young adults is 26 to 33 percent versus 35 to 42 percent in adults older than age 65 years. Nosocomial gram-negative bacteremia carries a mortality rate of 5 to 35 percent in young adults, but 37 to 50 percent in older adults. A major contributing factor is reduced physiologic reserve because of age and comorbidities that reduce the ability of older adults to recover from a septic episode.

Management of bacteremia and sepsis in the elderly patient is similar to that of younger adults. The first immunomodulatory/adjunctive therapy for sepsis, activated protein C, was recently approved for use by the Food and Drug Administration (FDA) after many prior failed trials with nonsteroidal antiinflammatory agents, corticosteroids, antiendotoxin antibodies, IL-1 receptor antagonist, and anti-TNF antibodies. In a subset analysis of the trial that led to FDA approval for activated protein C, elderly persons appeared to benefit as much as young persons.

Prosthetic Device Infections

As the prevalence of the US population older than age 65 years has increased, permanent implantable prosthetic devices have become common. Prosthetic joints, cardiac pacemakers, artificial heart valves, intraocular lens implants, vascular grafts, penile prostheses, and a variety of other devices are primarily placed in the elderly. Foreign bodies interact with bacterial and host immune factors, often leading to infection. While it is impossible to review all prosthetic device infections in this chapter, several general concepts are presented. Prosthetic device infections are usually categorized by causative agents that typically present early (<60 days from implantation) or late (>60 days). Early infections are primarily caused by contamination at the time of surgery or events associated with the implantation hospitalization (e.g., bacteremia caused by IV or urinary catheters). Thus, the causative organisms for early prosthetic device infections are primarily skin and nosocomial flora. Coagulase-negative staphylococci predominate; *S. aureus* and diphtheroids are common as well. Gram-negative bacilli, fungi, or polymicrobial infection rarely cause early infection except when the material itself or associated products such as dressing material are contaminated. Late infections tend to be caused by the same organisms that cause community-acquired bacteremia in the elderly population. Staphylococci, including coagulase-negative staphylococci, are the exception to this rule, playing a major role in prosthetic device infections in both the early and late periods. Thus, empiric antistaphylococcal therapy is imperative in either early or late prosthetic device infection.

It is difficult to cure prosthetic device infections (i.e., eradicate the organism) with the device in place. However, in some instances, early antibiotic intervention combined with aggressive surgical débridement may result in cure without removing the device. Because prosthetic device infections often include biofilms and occur in the setting of other factors that limit antibiotic efficacy (e.g., poor circulation), it is preferable to use bactericidal antibiotics, and combinations with a second agent that penetrate these areas well (e.g., rifampin) may be most effective. If early, aggressive therapy is ineffective in controlling the infection, it is imperative that the device be removed. Two-stage procedures, where the device is removed and antibiotics given for an extended period (usually 6 weeks for bone involvement) with delayed reimplantation, have the highest success rate. However, for lifesaving devices, such as mechanical valves or implantable defibrillators, this is not an option.

A recent analysis of surgical débridement and long-term suppressive antibiotics versus two-stage removal/reimplantation for prosthetic hip infection used functional assessment, not just cure rate, as an important indicator

Table 82-2   Suggested Empiric Antimicrobial Therapy for Common Infections in Older Adults

Infection	Therapy	Comments
Community Acquired		
Outpatient Therapy		
Acute sinusitis	Amoxicillin	Amox/clav or new macrolide if refractory
Chronic bronchitis	Amoxicillin	Infectious exacerbations only
Pneumonia	[Azithromycin or Clarithromycin + 2nd gen Ceph or Amox/clav] or Resp-FQ	Smoker/COPD most common
Cellulitis	Amox/clav or Dicloxacillin or Cephalexin	
Infected neuropathic ulcer	Amox/clav	Initial outpatient treatment of diabetic foot infection
Symptomatic UTI	FQ, TMP-SMX	Uncomplicated cystitis or pyelonephritis
Infectious diarrhea	FQ	Oral rehydration is key
C. difficile diarrhea	Metronidazole	Elevated white blood cell count common
Inpatient Therapy		
Pneumonia	[Ceftriaxone + Azithromycin or Clarithromycin] or Resp-FQ alone	Seriously ill (intensive care unit) combination therapy may be best; can't exclude Legionella, consider Pseudomonas if severe COPD or structural lung disease
Pyelonephritis (no catheter)	3rd gen Cephalosporin or FQ	
Urosepsis (with catheter)	3rd gen Cephalosporin + ampicillin or vancomycin	Catheter-related urosepsis often polymicrobic; have to consider enterococcal species, in addition to gram-negative bacilli
Acute meningitis	Ceftriaxone + Vancomycin	Vancomycin needed because of small percent of ceftriaxone-resistant S. pneumoniae
Intra-abdominal infection	[Ampicillin/sulbactam + Gentamicin] or Ampicillin + Gentamicin + Metronidazole] or Pip/tazo or carbepenem	Surgery often indicated for appendicitis, cholecystitis, ischemic colitis, abscess drainage; rarely required for diverticulitis
Native valve endocarditis	Penicillin + Nafcillin	Vancomycin for penicillin-allergic patient
Infected diabetic foot ulcer	Ticar/clav or Pip/tazo	3rd gen Ceph and clinda for penicillin allergy
Cellulitis	Ampicillin/sulbactam	Add clinda if high suspicion for GAS; vancomycin + FQ for β-lactam allergy
Septic shock syndrome; with no obvious focus	Carbepenem; add clindamycin if GAS suspected	Aggressive supportive care; ? activated protein C
Nursing Home Acquired		
Infected pressure ulcer	FQ + clindamycin (po); ticar/clav or Pip/tazo (IV)	Pressure-relieving devices, nutrition, débridement essential; culture/x-ray to identify osteomyelitis or MRSA
Pneumonia	Resp-FQ or Ceftriaxone + Azithromycin or Clarithromycin	Consider tuberculosis
Urosepsis	Ciprofloxcin (po) Ceftriaxone (IM/IV)	Add enterococcal coverage if catheter
C. difficile colitis	Metronidazole	Close attention to infection control as nosocomial spread documented
Nosocomial/Hospital		
Pneumonia	Cefepime or carbepenem or pip/tazo	Decision influenced by numerous factors: underlying medical conditions, mental status, respiratory support, prior antibiotic exposure, aspiration, risk of MRSA (add vancomycin)

(continued)

Table 82-2 Suggested Empiric Antimicrobial Therapy for Common Infections in Older Adults (continued)

Infection	Therapy	Comments
Catheter-associated urosepsis	Ampicillin plus 3rd gen ceph or FQ	Culture to guide subsequent therapy
Intravenous catheter-associated infection (cellulitis, phlebitis, abscess, bacteremia)	Vancomycin	If immunocompromised, add cefepime or ceftazidime; surgery required for septic thrombophlebitis
C. difficile-related diarrhea	Metronidazole	Discontinue the implicated antimicrobials if possible; attention to infection control
Postoperative wound infection; incision/deep with cellulitis, abscess, or bacteremia	Cefazolin (mild infection) Vancomycin + 3rd gen ceph (severe infection)	Reopen and explore wound; definitive therapy guided by smears/cultures

2nd gen, second generation; 3rd gen, third generation; Amox/clav, Amoxicillin-clavulanate; Carbepenem, imipenem-cilastatin or meropenem; ceph, cephalosporin; clinda, clindamycin; COPD, chronic obstructive pulmonary disease; FQ, Fluoroquinolone; GAS, group A streptococci (*S. pyogenes*); MRSA, methicillin-resistant *S. aureus*; Pip/tazo, Piperacillin-tazobactam; Resp-FQ, respiratory fluoroquinolone (gatifloxacin, levofloxacin, moxifloxacin); Ticar/clav, ticarcillin-clauvulanate; TMP-SMX, trimethoprim-sulfamethoxazole; vanco, vancomycin.

outcome. Using Markov modeling, the two-stage procedure was preferred if the relapse rate in the débridement strategy was assumed to be >60 percent or the age of the patient with the infected arthroplasty was <79 years (Fig. 82-2). However, débridement and suppressive antibiotics strategy were favored when these conditions were not met. Relapse rates of the débridement/retention with long-term antibiotic strategy are approximately 30 percent overall, but depend on the organism, duration of symptoms, which joint is infected, the susceptibility of the organism, and many other factors known and unknown. This model gives some guidance, but allows clinicians freedom to adjust 12, 53]. All costs were converted to 1999 dollars by means of

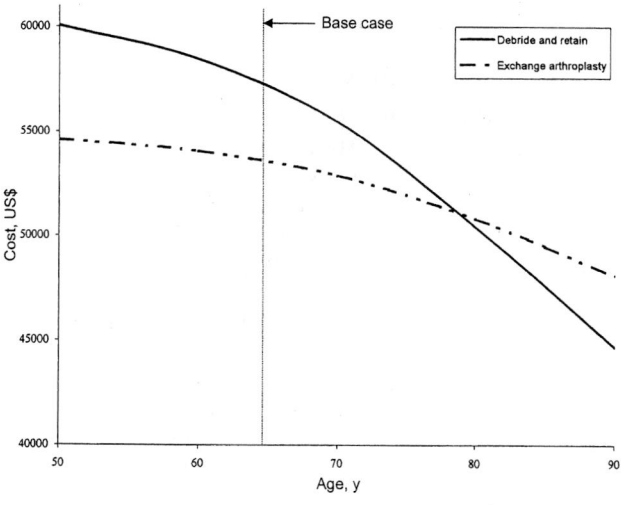

Figure 82-2 Markov model for cost-effectiveness of joint replacement therapy versus a débridement/retention strategy in older adults with an infected hip prosthesis. QALY, quality-adjusted life year. After age 79 years, débridement/retention is cost saving. Reprinted with permission from Fisman, et al.

strategy based on baseline functional status and infecting agent.

Prevention of prosthetic device infection is facilitated by the use of clean air systems and/or personal isolator systems in the operating room. Although there are limited data for efficacy, typical antimicrobial prophylaxis for clean surgery seems appropriate; prophylaxis other than at the time of surgery remain contentious. Perioperative antimicrobial prophylaxis for dental, GI, and GU procedures is clearly indicated for prosthetic valves and is frequently employed for vascular grafts, particularly within the first few months after placement. There is no evidence to demonstrate benefit for prophylaxis in patients with prosthetic joints, intraocular lens implants, intracoronary artery stents, cerebrospinal fluid shunts, breast implants, or other less-commonly used prostheses. The American Dental Association (ADA) recommends "considering" antibiotic prophylaxis for patients with prosthetic joint at "high risk," which the ADA define as joints within 2 years of placement, immunosuppressed patients (including immune compromise as a result of diabetes mellitus, rheumatoid arthritis, and malnourishment), or those with a previous joint infection.

Fever of Unknown Origin

Fever of unknown origin (FUO), classically defined as temperature >101°F °(38.3°C) for at least 3 weeks and undiagnosed after 1 week of medical evaluation, has different causes in elderly adults and in young adults (Table 82-3) that should influence the diagnostic work-up (Fig. 82-3). The cause of FUO can be determined in virtually all cases and approximately one-third of cases will have treatable infections (e.g., intraabdominal abscess, bacterial endocarditis, tuberculosis, or occult osteomyelitis). In contrast to young adults, connective-tissue disease (CTD) is a more frequent cause of FUO in adults older than age 65 years. A compilation of several recently published series suggests that 25 percent of all FUOs in the elderly patient are caused by CTDs. However, whereas the CTD most likely to cause FUO in young adults is systemic lupus

Table 82-3 Fever of Unknown Origin (FUO) in the Elderly Patient

Major Causes	% of Cases*
Infections	35
Intraabdominal abscess	12
Tuberculosis	6
Infective endocarditis	10
Other	7
Collagen vascular disorders	28
Temporal arteritis/polymyalgia rheumatica	19
Polyarteritis nodosa	6
Other	3
Malignancy	19
Lymphoma/other hematologic	10
Solid tumors	9
Other (pulmonary emboli, drug fever)	10
No diagnosis	8

*Percentages represent pooled data from three studies of FUO in the elderly patient.

erythematosus (SLE), SLE was absent in series of elderly patients and replaced by temporal arteritis (TA) and polyarteritis nodosa (PAN). Neoplastic disease accounts for another 20 percent, most often a result of hematopoietic malignancies (e.g., lymphoma and leukemia). Drug fever is a common cause of FUO in the elderly, and Wegener's granulomatosis, deep venous thrombosis with or without recurrent pulmonary emboli, and hyperthyroidism occasionally cause FUO in older adults.

A reasonable approach to FUO in the elderly can be inferred from the most likely causative entities (Fig. 82-3). A thorough history and physical examination; basic laboratory evaluations of complete blood counts and differential, serum chemistries and hepatic enzymes, thyroid function studies, erythrocyte sedimentation rate (ESR), placement of a purified protein derivative, a chest x-ray, and initial blood and urine cultures should begin the search. If the diagnosis continues to be elusive and the ESR is elevated, temporal artery biopsy even in the absence of objective physical findings should be strongly considered. If the source remains obscure, or if there is a low suspicion for temporal arteritis, abdominal imaging with computed tomography (CT) or magnetic resonance imaging (MRI) should be performed. Further invasive diagnostic procedures, such as bone marrow and liver biopsy, or laparoscopy, should be considered in specific cases, but are low yield unless there are significant clues for involvement (e.g., cytopenias or hepatomegaly).

IMMUNIZATION OF THE ELDERLY

Immunization recommendations for older adults are constantly being updated. The latest consensus recommendations can be found on-line at the Centers for Disease Control (CDC) web site at: www.cdc.gov/nip/publications/ACIP-list.htm.

Pneumococcal Vaccine

Many reviews and meta-analyses have been performed to help assess the benefit of pneumococcal immunization in older adults. Although many have failed to reach statistical significance indicating benefit, the confidence intervals of negative studies have not ruled out benefit, particularly when only invasive disease end points (i.e., bacteremia and meningitis) were the outcomes selected. Some of the lack of clear benefit may be a result of waning of efficacy at the extremes of old age (>85 years), unrecognized immune compromise in many older adults, and the fact that the pneumococcal vaccine is really 23 different vaccines (i.e., 23 serotypes) and failure of any one serotype is considered a failure of the vaccine. Despite these ongoing scientific discourses, pneumococcal immunization for persons age 65 years and older has become standard practice, as well as for many patients under age 65 years with comorbid conditions. If >5 years has elapsed since the first dose and the patient was vaccinated prior to the age of 65 years, repeat vaccination is recommended and safe (Fig. 82-4). The 23-valent polysaccharide vaccine, when given to adults older than age 65 years, is similar in cost-effectiveness to many procedures commonly employed in older adults (e.g., multiple screening procedures, angioplasty and coronary artery bypass grafting), even when one limits consideration of efficacy to only invasive disease (i.e., blood-borne infection), making no assumption for any benefit with regard to pneumonia. Pneumococcal vaccine can be given concurrently with other vaccines at a different anatomic site.

Implementing current pneumococcal vaccine recommendations remains the greatest obstacle to prevention of fatal *S. pneumoniae* disease in the elderly. According to CDC estimates, approximately 30 percent of eligible elderly persons receive pneumococcal vaccine. Many unvaccinated elderly patients diagnosed with invasive pneumococcal disease saw a medical practitioner within the prior 6 to 12 months. The CDC and its Advisory Committee on Immunization Practices (ACIP) have outlined several strategies for improving vaccine administration including (1) age-based: review immunizations in all persons at age 50 years, vaccinating those with qualifying comorbid conditions; (2) organizational (e.g., standing orders): routine administration in elderly and at-risk patients in office, nursing home, and hospital settings by a blanket order for all patients (this is the single most-effective strategy); (3) community-based: public health promotions focusing on underserved, often inner-city populations and community outreach programs (senior centers, civic organizations, etc.); and (4) provider-based: physician-reminder systems (chart checklists, computer "flags," prehospital discharge, etc.).

Protein-polysaccharide conjugate pneumococcal vaccines may be more effective and are approved for use in children. Conjugate vaccines reduce nasopharyngeal carriage of pneumococcus, thus reducing the incidence of both mucosal (i.e., otitis media) and invasive disease in

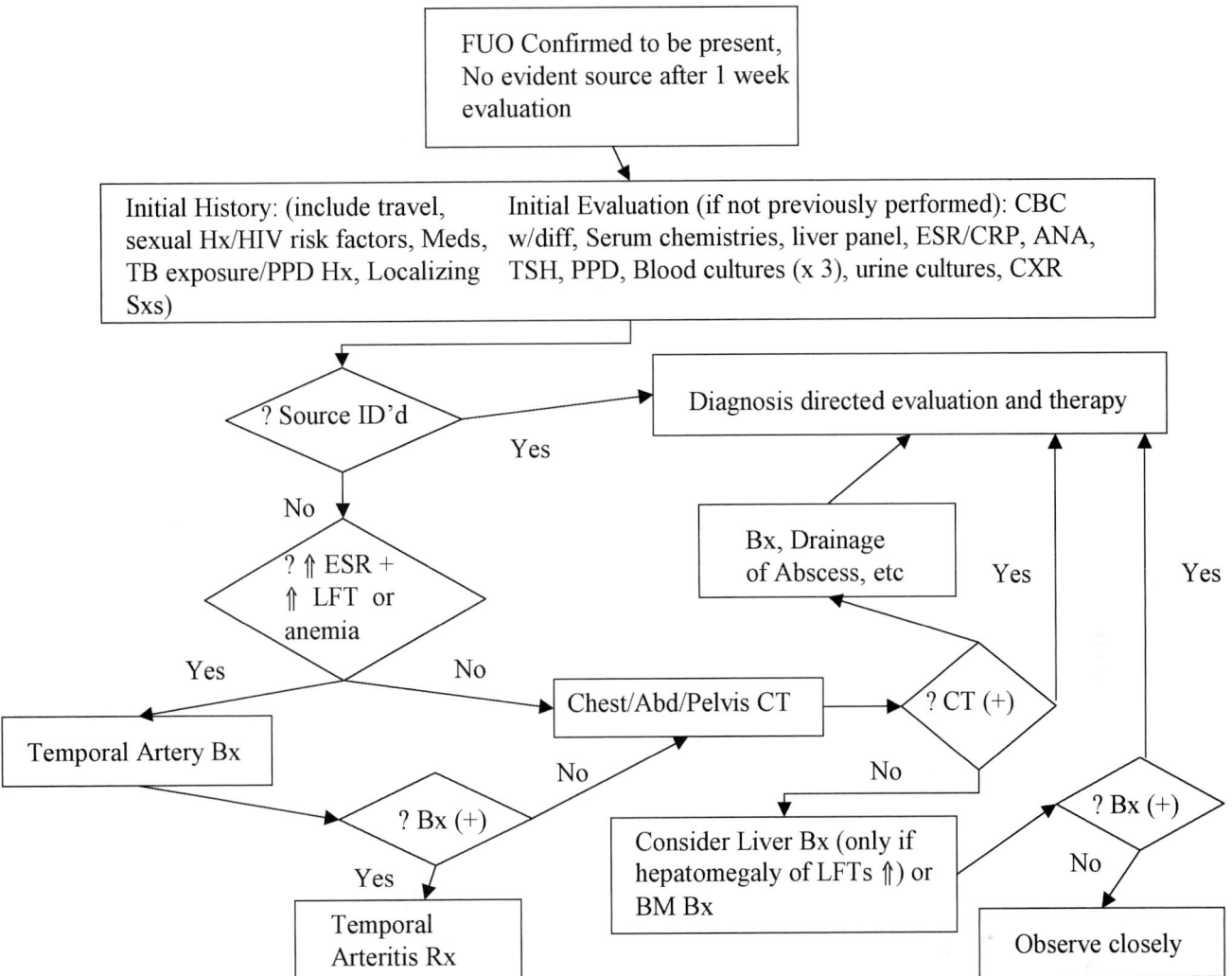

Figure 82-3 Recommended algorithm for evaluation of fever of unknown origin in older adults. ANA, antinuclear antibody; BM, bone marrow; Bx, biopsy; CBC, complete blood count; CRP, C-reactive protein; CT, computed tomography; CXR, chest x-ray; ESR, erythrocyte sedimentation rate; FUO, fever of unknown origin; HA, headache; HIV, human immunodeficiency virus; ID, identify; LFTs, liver function tests; PPD, purified protein derivative; Rx, therapy; TB, tuberculosis; TSH, thyroid stimulating hormone.

children, and potentially could have benefit by reducing both invasive and noninvasive illnesses (sinusitis, bronchitis) in adults. However, these conjugate vaccines have not yet been adequately tested in older adults to determine whether there is greater benefit with these vaccines than with the current polysaccharide vaccine, particularly because only 7 serotypes are represented in the conjugate vaccine and the cost is much higher.

Influenza (For Detailed Information, See Chap. 89)

The current influenza vaccine is a killed virus that is modestly immunogenic with estimated efficacy rates of 60 percent for illness and 50 to 60 percent for mortality. Annual influenza immunization reduces rates of respiratory illness, hospitalization, and mortality in the elderly population, and current ACIP recommendations are for all patients over the age of 50 years or with underlying medical

illnesses to be immunized just prior to influenza season each year. Medical personnel and caregivers for high-risk patients should also be immunized to reduce transmission to those at increased risk for complications. A live, attenuated influenza vaccine has been under development for years and appears to be more effective, but has not yet been approved for widespread use.

Other Vaccines

The elderly population is the group most at risk for tetanus in the United States, with older women being particularly susceptible because of a lower likelihood of receiving boosters associated with minor/moderate trauma. Subprotective levels of tetanus antibody (<0.01 U/mL) have been found in 43 to 61 percent of men and in 48 to 71 percent of women older than age 50 years. A complete vaccine series is indicated for persons with an uncertain history of tetanus immunization and for those who have received

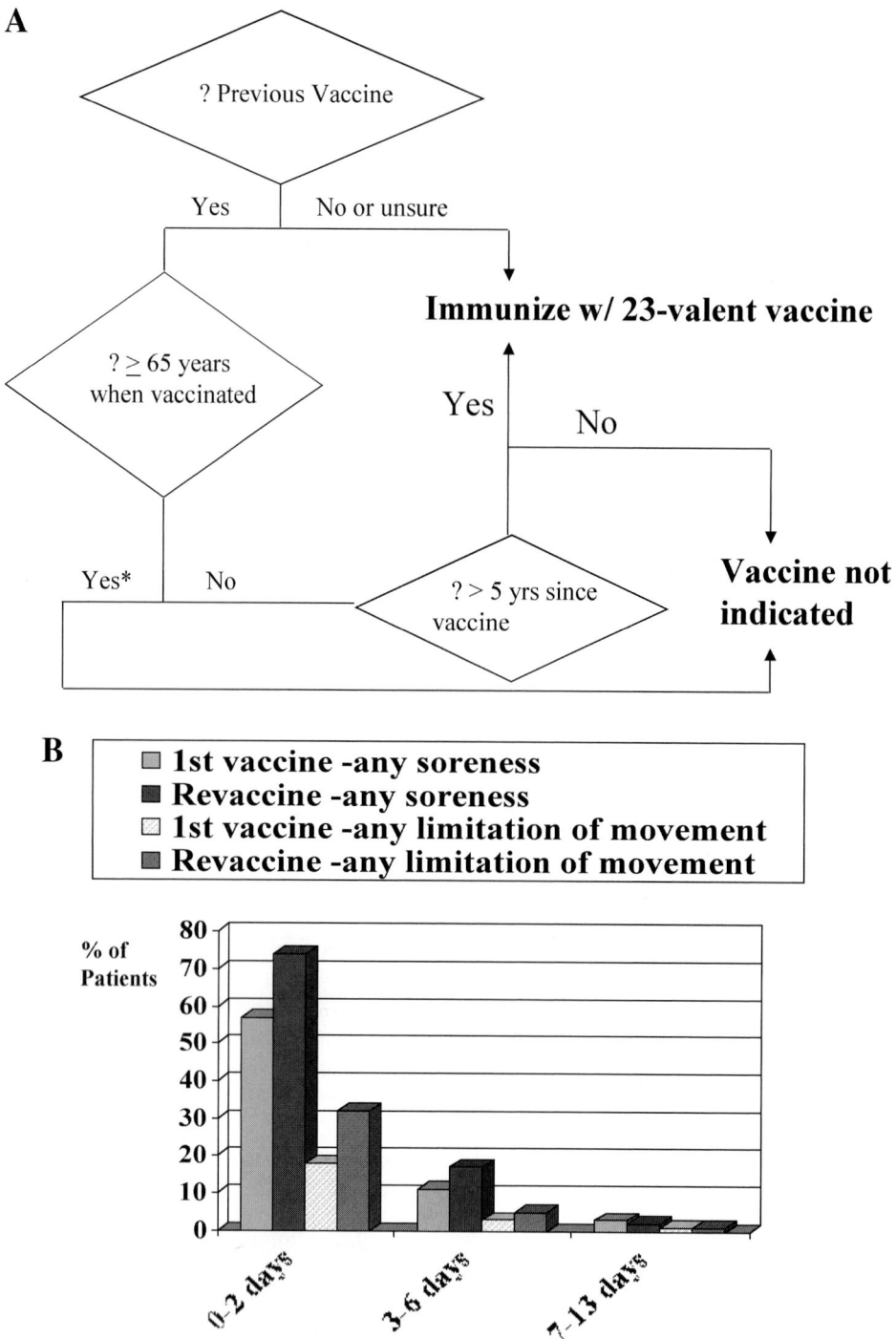

Figure 82-4 **A.** Decision analysis for pneumococcal vaccine per current Advisory Committee on Immunization Practices recommendations. **B.** Adverse events associated with primary or reimmunization with pneumococcal vaccine. Data from Jackson et al: Safety of revaccination with pneumococcal polysaccharide vaccine. *JAMA* 281:243, 1999. *re-vaccination not indicated for persons vaccinated at age ≥65 yrs.

fewer than three doses. Boosters should be given at 10-year intervals, or more frequently with high-risk injuries such as burns, puncture wounds, or extensive soft-tissue injury.

Hepatitis vaccines may also be considered for the elderly patient under certain circumstances. Hepatitis B vaccine is indicated for all persons at risk for percutaneous or mucosal

exposure to infected blood or body secretions. Older adults may have comorbidities (e.g., renal failure) that place them at risk, but they also commonly volunteer at healthcare facilities and should be considered at risk if they engage in any patient contact. Hepatitis A vaccine is indicated in more limited circumstances such as chronic hepatitis C, travel, and for men who have sex with men.

Finally, varicella vaccine may become important in the elderly person. A large, multicenter study of the live-attenuated vaccine of varicella-zoster virus (VZV) is underway to determine its efficacy for preventing zoster. The results of this trial should become available within the next 3 to 5 years.

TRAVEL RECOMMENDATIONS FOR THE ELDERLY PERSON

Elderly persons are among the most widely traveled members of our society. Many countries require cholera and yellow fever vaccines prior to entry, but a specific note of caution must be sounded for elderly adults. The yellow fever vaccine is a live-virus vaccine and recent data suggest that older adults are six times more likely than young adults to experience a serious adverse event. Furthermore, although still quite rare, reactions requiring hospitalization or resulting in death are 3.5- and 9-fold higher in adults age 65 to 74 and older than 75 years, respectively, when compared to young adults. Because the incidence of yellow fever in travelers is very low, particularly when travel is limited to urban centers, a compelling case to administer the vaccine should be elicited prior to administering yellow fever vaccine in older adults. Often the most compelling reason is that countries may deny access to those who cannot prove recent immunization, but a physician's letter of exemption is often acceptable.

Other recommended immunizations include hepatitis A vaccine which has replaced intramuscular immunoglobulin as the preferred method of prevention for hepatitis A. Hepatitis A immunization is strongly encouraged for individuals anticipating prolonged travel (usually longer than 3 weeks) in areas where water and sanitary conditions are uncertain. Similarly, typhoid vaccine may be indicated for travel for extended periods of time to rural areas with poor sanitation. Other considerations include rabies, hepatitis B, Japanese encephalitis, and meningococcal vaccines.

Malaria chemoprophylaxis can be difficult in the elderly. Side effects are more common for many agents (e.g., mefloquine may produce dizziness, change in mental status, and bradycardia or prolonged QT intervals), and coadministration may be difficult in those taking cardiac medications or with significant heart disease. There are multiple alternative regimens for malaria prophylaxis but recognition of current resistance patterns is critical. Clinicians are directed to the CDC web site (www.cdc.gov/travel) for the most up-to-date information.

Diarrhea occurs in 25 to 50 percent of travelers to developing countries. Primary treatment consists of fluid and electrolyte replacement, but antimicrobial therapy with a quinolone is indicated when diarrhea is accompanied by fever, bloody stools, or is prolonged. Antimotility agents are safe when coadministered with antibiotics.

REFERENCES

Advisory Committee on Immunization Practices: Prevention of pneumococcal disease. *MMWR Morb Mortal Wkly Rep* 46(RR-8 Supple):1, 1997.

American Dental Association Report: Antibiotic prophylaxis for dental patients with total joint replacements. *J Am Dent Assoc* 128:1004, 1997.

Bentley DW et al: Practice guideline for evaluation of fever and infection in long-term care facilities. *Clin Infect Dis* 31:640, 2000.

Berk S, Myers JW: Prosthetic device infections, in Yoshikawa TT, Norman DC (eds): *Infectious Disease in the Aging: A Clinical Handbook.* Totowa, NJ, Humana Press, 2001 p 197.

Bradley S: Issues in the management of resistant bacteria in long-term care facilities. *Infect Control Hosp Epidemiol* 20:362, 1999.

Castle SC: Clinical relevance of age-related immune dysfunction. *Clin Infect Dis* 31:578, 2000.

Castle SC et al: The SENIEUR Protocol after 16 years: A need for a paradigm shift? *Mech Ageing Dev* 122:127, 2001.

Castle SC et al: Lowering the fever criteria improves detection of infections in nursing home residents. *Aging Immunol Infect Dis* 4:67, 1993.

Chintanadilok J, Bender BS: Sepsis, in Yoshikawa TT, Norman DC (eds): *Infectious Disease in the Aging: A Clinical Handbook.* Totowa, NJ, Humana Press, 2001 p 33.

Conte HA et al: A prognostic rule for elderly patients admitted with community-acquired pneumonia. *Am J Med* 106:20, 1999.

Dajani AS et al: Prevention of bacterial endocarditis: Recommendations by the American Heart Association. *JAMA* 277:1794, 1997.

Evans R, Stoddart G: Producing health, consuming health care. *Soc Sci Med* 31:1347, 1990.

Fisman DN et al: Clinical effectiveness and cost-effectiveness of 2 management strategies for infected total hip arthroplasty in the elderly. *Clin Infect Dis* 32:419, 2001.

Graat JM et al: Effect of daily Vitamin E and multivitamin-mineral supplementation on acute respiratory tract infections in elderly persons, a randomized controlled trial. *JAMA* 288:715–721, 2002.

High KP: Nutritional strategies to boost immunity and prevent infection in elderly individuals. *Clin Infect Dis* 33:1892, 2001.

Jackson LA et al: Safety of revaccination with pneumococcal polysaccharide vaccine. *JAMA* 281:243, 1999.

Leder K et al: Travel vaccines and elderly persons: Review of vaccines available in the United States. *Clin Infect Dis* 33:1553, 2001.

Lim W-S, Macfarlane JT: Defining prognostic factors in the elderly with community acquired pneumonia: A case-controlled study of patients aged >75 yrs. *Eur Respir J* 17:200, 2001.

Marcus EL et al: Ethical issues relating to the use of antimicrobial therapy in older adults. *Clin Infect Dis* 33:1697, 2001.

Marik PD, Zaloga GP: The effect of aging on circulating levels of proinflammatory cytokines during septic shock. Norasept II Study Investigators. *J Am Geriatr Soc* 49:5, 2001.

Norman DC, Yoshikawa TT: Fever in the elderly. *Infect Dis Clin North Am* 10(1):93, 1996.

Werner GS et al: Infective endocarditis in the elderly in the era of transesophageal echocardiography: Clinical features and prognosis compared with younger patients. *Am J Med* 100:90, 1996.

Wilson WR et al: Antibiotic treatment of adults with infective endocarditis due to streptococci, enterococci, staphylococci, and HACEK microorganisms. *JAMA* 274:1706, 1995.

Yoshikawa TT: Aging and infectious diseases. Past, present and future. *J Infect Dis* 176:1053–1057, 1997.

Pneumonia

THOMAS J. MARRIE

DEFINITIONS

From the viewpoint of the pathologist, pneumonia is an inflammatory response in the lung caused by an infectious agent that involves the alveoli and terminal bronchioles. It is manifested by increased weight of the lungs, replacement of the normal lung sponginess by consolidation and alveoli filled with white blood cells, red blood cells, and fibrin (Figs. 83-1 and 83-2).

The clinician defines pneumonia as a combination of symptoms (fever, chills, cough, pleuritic chest pain, sputum), signs (hyper- or hypothermia, increased respiratory rate, dullness to percussion, bronchial breathing, egophony, crackles, wheezes, pleural friction rub), and an opacity (opacities) on a chest radiograph (Fig. 83-3). In addition, laboratory findings, such as increased white blood cell count and decreased level of oxygen saturation, may also be part of the definition.

The epidemiologist or clinical trialist defines pneumonia as two or more of the symptoms listed above, one or more of the physical findings listed above, and a new opacity on chest radiograph that is not caused by a condition other than pneumonia (such as congestive heart failure, vasculitis, pulmonary infarction, atelectasis, or drug reaction).

Pneumonia may also be categorized according to the site of acquisition: community, hospital (nosocomial), or nursing home. Some authorities categorize nursing home-acquired pneumonia as community-acquired, while others insist it more closely resembles nosocomial pneumonia and should be labeled institutionally acquired. However, nursing homes or long-term care facilities have residents who range from fully functional to those who are bedridden. I prefer to consider nursing home/long-term care facility acquired pneumonia as a separate category.

It is useful for the practicing clinician to remember definitions for the certainty with which an agent can be implicated as the cause of the pneumonia. An agent is said to be the definite cause of pneumonia if it is isolated from blood (although some blood isolates, such as coagulase-negative staphylococci, are usually contaminants and not pulmonary pathogens), pleural fluid, or pulmonary tissue; if it isolated from sputum and is a pathogen that does not colonize the upper airway (such as *Mycobacterium*

tuberculosis, Legionella species, Nocardia species); or if antigen is detected in urine (*Streptococcus pneumoniae, Legionella pneumophila*). An agent is the presumptive cause of pneumonia if it is isolated from a sputum sample that has >25 polymorphonuclear leucocytes per low-power field and <10 squamous epithelial cells, or if there is a fourfold or greater rise in antibody titer between acute and convalescent serum samples.

EPIDEMIOLOGY

Pneumonia is a common and often a serious illness. It is the sixth leading cause of death in the United States. About 600,000 persons are hospitalized with pneumonia each year and there are 64 million days of restricted activity because of this illness. The overall mortality rate for patients with community-acquired pneumonia (CAP) who require admission to hospital ranges from 6 to 15 percent. For those who require admission to an intensive care unit for treatment of pneumonia, the mortality rate ranges from 45 to 57 percent. The annual per capital cost of pneumonia from an employer perspective is five times higher than the costs for typical beneficiaries. For elderly patients, there is a burden of care for family.

Approximately 80 percent of adults with CAP are treated on an ambulatory basis. The mortality rate for those who are ≥65 years of age treated on an ambulatory basis is approximately 4 percent. The 20 percent of patients with CAP who require admission to hospital account for more than 80 percent of the total costs of treating pneumonia. The mean age of patients with CAP requiring admission to hospital was 55 years in 1955; by year 2001, it was 71 years. The admission rate for pneumonia is subject to considerable variation from region to region within a province or state, and even from hospital to hospital within a single city. This variation cannot be explained on the basis of severity of illness and likely reflects variation in physician practice. However, admission rates for pneumonia consistently increase with increasing age. In Alberta, 1.33/1000 adults in the 18- to 44-year-old age group are admitted to hospital for treatment of CAP each year. The rates for the 45 to 64, 65 to 74, 75 to 84, and the 85 and older age groups are 3.12, 10.84, 26.03, and 51.59 per 1000 adults, respectively.

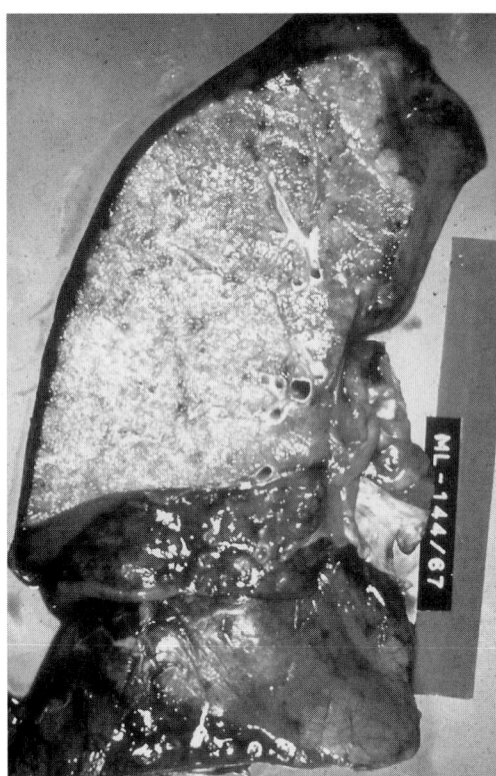

Figure 83-1   Photograph of a lung with pneumonia (white area) involving the entire upper lobe.

In a population-based study in a Finnish town, 14/1000 persons per year who were >60 years of age developed pneumonia. Seventy-five percent of these cases were community-acquired. In this study, independent risk factors for community-acquired pneumonia were alcoholism, relative risk (RR) 9; asthma, RR 4.2; immunosuppression, RR 1.9; age >70 versus age 60 to 69 years, RR 1.5. In another approach to determining the risk factors for pneumonia, investigators studied 101 patients aged ≥65 years who were admitted with CAP. Each patient with pneumonia was and age and sex matched with a control subject who arrived at emergency within ±2 days of the case and was subsequently admitted. By multivariate analysis the following were identified as risk factors for pneumonia: suspected aspiration, low serum albumin, swallowing disorder, and poor quality of life. Significant predictors of a fatal outcome were bedridden state prior to onset of pneumonia; temperature ≤98.6°F (37°C); presence of a swallowing disorder; respiratory rate ≥30 breaths per minute; shock; creatinine greater than 1.4 mg/dL; and ≥three or more lobes involved on chest radiograph.

The attack rate for pneumonia in adults is highest among those in nursing homes with rates of 1.2 episodes of pneumonia per 1000 resident days. Pneumonia is the leading cause for transfer of nursing home patients to hospital. In many areas, nursing home/long-term care facility acquired pneumonia accounts for 10 to 18 percent of all pneumonia admissions. Lower respiratory tract infections are the fourth most common infection among residents of long-term care facilities, affecting 2.1 percent of the residents. In a nursing home population, old age (odds ratio [OR] 1.7), male sex (OR 1.9), swallowing difficulty (OR 2), and inability to take oral medication were significant risk factors for pneumonia. In another study, profound disability (Karnofsky score of <10), bedfast state, urinary incontinence, presence of a feeding tube, or deteriorating health status were risk factors for pneumonia in this setting.

In one study, the average length of stay (LOS) for patients hospitalized with pneumonia was 3.5 days for those <15 years old and 6.9 days for those >65 years of age. In the six hospitals in Edmonton, Alberta, Canada, the mean LOS for adult patients with CAP ranged from 6.2 to 9.9 days. Six percent of the patients stayed 22 days or more, accounting for 31 percent of all inpatient days for patients

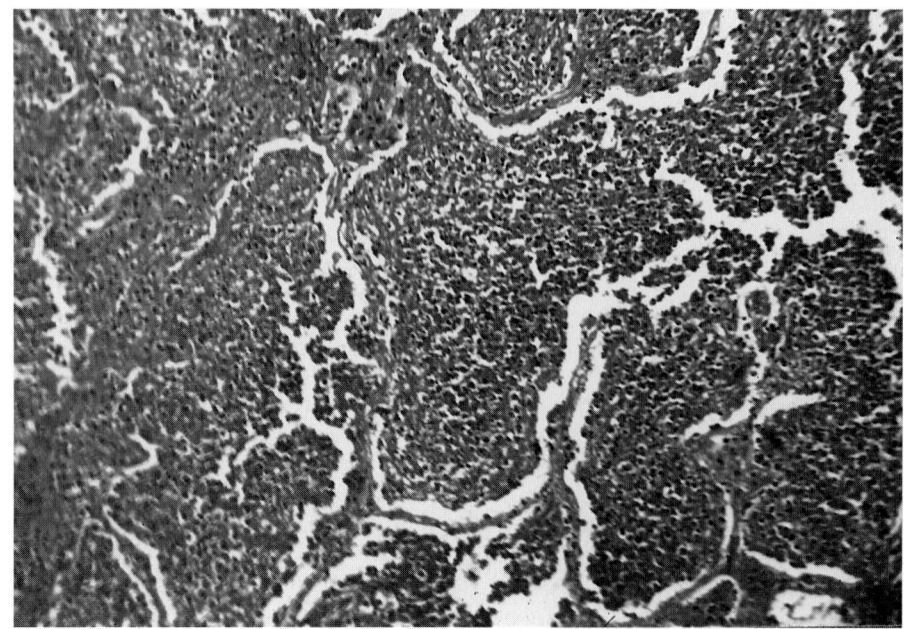

Figure 83-2   Photomicrograph of lung showing alveoli filled with inflammatory exudate. Magnification × 445.

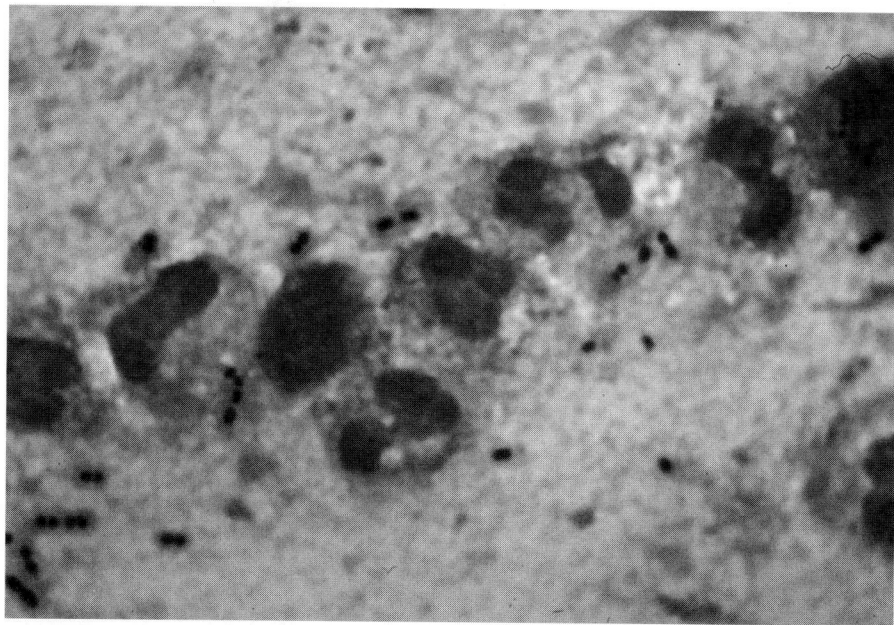

Figure 83-3 Gram stain sputum showing many polymorphonuclear leucocytes and gram-positive diplococci (*Streptococcus pneumoniae* was recovered on culture of this specimen). Magnification × 1000.

with pneumonia. Most of these patients were elderly and had multiple comorbid illnesses.

For specific etiologies of pneumonia, risk factors may differ from those for pneumonia as a whole. Thus dementia, seizures, congestive heart failure, cerebrovascular disease, tobacco smoking, and chronic obstructive lung disease are risk factors for pneumococcal pneumonia. Fifty percent of patients with bacteremic pneumococcal pneumonia were homozygous for $Fc\gamma$RIIa-R31, which binds weakly to immunoglobulin (Ig) G_2, as compared with 29 percent of uninfected controls, suggesting that genetic factors may also be important risk factors for pneumococcal pneumonia.

Among human immunodeficiency virus (HIV)-infected patients the rate of pneumococcal pneumonia is up to 41.8 times higher than age-matched patients who are not HIV-infected. Risk factors for Legionnaires' disease include male gender, tobacco smoking, diabetes, hematologic malignancy, cancer, end-stage renal disease, and HIV infection.

There is a seasonal variation in the rate of pneumonia. Both attack rates and mortality rates are highest in the winter months.

ETIOLOGY

There are more than 100 microbial (bacteria, viruses, fungi, protozoa, and other parasites) causes of community-acquired pneumonia. *Streptococcus pneumoniae* is the most common cause of CAP, accounting for about 50 percent of all cases. Table 83-1 gives the most common causes of CAP. Table 83-2 identifies clues that might be obtained from the history to suggest a particular organism(s) as the cause of the pneumonia. It is important to remember that the relative frequency of each pathogen may vary geographically and seasonally. Many elderly persons travel for pleasure, placing them at risk for a variety of pathogens (Table 83-2). Vacations in the sun to Arizona or parts of California can

result in acquisition of the fungus *Coccidioides immitis* by inhalation. In most instances, the infection is asymptomatic. However, atypical pneumonia, hilar adenopathy, or lung nodules may result. The latter are often misdiagnosed as carcinoma and the nodules excised. Elderly women who are receiving hormone replacement therapy may be at greater risk for the pulmonary nodule presentation of coccidioidomycosis.

Table 83-1 Most Common Causes of Community-Acquired Pneumonia in the Elderly Population

Streptococcus pneumoniae
Chlamydia pneumoniae
Enterobacteriaceae
Legionella pneumophila
Haemophilus influenzae
Moraxella catarrhalis
Staphylococcus aureus
Influenza A virus
Influenza B virus
Respiratory syncytial virus
Legionella species
Mycobacterium tuberculosis
Pneumocystis carinii
Nontuberculous mycobacteria
Mycoplasma pneumoniae

Table 83-2   Clues to the Etiology of Pneumonia

Factor	Possible Agent(s)
Travel	
Southeast Asia	*Burkholderia pseudomallei (melioidosis); Mycobacterium tuberculosis*
Many countries	*M. tuberculosis*
Arizona, parts of California	*Coccidioides immitis*
Occupational history	
Health care workers	*M. tuberculosis*, acute HIV seroconversion with pneumonia (if recent needlestick injury from an HIV-Positive patient)
Veterinarian, farmer, abattoir worker	*Coxiella burnetii*
Host factor	
Diabetic ketoacidosis	*Streptococcus pneumoniae, Staphylococcus aureus*
Alcoholism	*S. pneumoniae, Kelbsiella pneumoniae, S. aureus*, oral anaerobes; *Acinetobacter spp.*
Chronic obstructive lung disease	*S. pneumoniae, Haemophilus influenzae, Moraxella catarrhalis*
Solid organ transplant recipient (pneumonia occuring >3 months after transplant)	*S. pneumoniae, H.influenzae, Legionella* species, *Pneumocystis carinii, cytomegalovirus, Strongyloides stercoralis*
Sickle cell disease	*S. pneumoniae*
HIV infection and CD4 cell count of <200/μL	*S. pneumoniae, P. carinii, H. influenzae, Crytococcus neoformans, M. tuberculosis, Rhodococcus equi*
Dementia, stroke, altered level of consciousness	Aspiration pneumonitis
Structural lung disease (bronchiectasis)	*Pseudomonas aeruginosa*
Environmental factors	
Exposure to contaminated air-conditioning cooling towers, hot tub, recent travel stay in a hotel, exposure to grocery store mist machine, or visit to, or recent stay in a hospital with contaminated (by *Legionellaceae*) drinking water	*Legionella pneumophila* or other Legionellaceae
Exposure to mouse droppings in an endemic area	Hantavirus
Pneumonia after windstorm in an area of endemicity	*C. immitis, C. burnetii*
Outbreak of pneumonia in shelter for homeless men or jail	*S. pneumoniae, M. tuberculosis*
Outbreak of pneumonia occurs in military training camp	*S. pneumoniae, Chlamydia pneumoniae*, adenovirus
Outbreak of pneumonia in a nursing home	*C. pneumoniae, S. pneumoniae*, respiratory syncytial virus, influenza A virus; *M. tuberculosis*
Pneumonia associated with mowing a lawn in an endemic area	*Francisella tularensis*
Exposure to bats, excavation or residence in an endemic area (Ohio and Mississippi River valleys)	*Histoplasma capsulatum*
Exposure to parturient cats in an endemic area	*C. burnetti*
Sleeping in a rose garden	*Sporothrix schenckii*
Camping, cutting down trees in an endemic area	*Blastomyces dermatitidis*

Streptococcus Pneumoniae

Worldwide *S. pneumoniae* continues to be the most common cause of CAP. It accounts for approximately 50 percent of all cases of pneumonia requiring admission to hospital for treatment and for 60 percent of all cases of bacteremic pneumonia. Although there are 90 capsular polysaccharide types of *S. pneumoniae*, 80 percent of the strains that cause invasive disease are present in the 23-valent-pneumococcal vaccine.

One problem facing clinicians treating patients with CAP is drug-resistant *S. pneumoniae*. If an isolate is resistant to penicillin, it is likely also that it is resistant to three or more drug classes (multidrug resistant). Currently, 12 to 25 percent of *S. pneumoniae* isolates in North America are resistant to penicillin—about half demonstrate low-level resistance (minimal inhibitory concentration [MIC] 0.1 to 1.0 mg/L) and half have high-level resistance (MIC ≥ 2 mg/L). In many communities, the levels of penicillin resistance are much higher than this. In the United States and Canada, approximately 20 percent of isolates of *S. pneumoniae* are resistant to erythromycin and the other macrolides. This resistance may be caused by an efflux pump mechanism or to alteration of the target site of erythromycin action through a mutation in the *erm* gene. Approximately 70 percent of pneumococcal erythromycin resistance in North America is a result of an efflux pump mechanism and these isolates may respond to treatment with a macrolide. Isolates that are resistant because of target site modification will not respond to treatment with a macrolide. Risk factors for penicillin-resistant *S. pneumoniae* include β-lactam antibiotic use within the previous 6 months; residence in a nursing home; residence in a day care center or being a parent of a resident in a day care center; and immunocompromised state. Age ≤ 5 years and nosocomial acquisition of the infection were independent predictions of macrolide resistance. Resistance among isolates of *S. pneumoniae* is also beginning to appear to fluoroquinolones, although at present it is uncommon with a 1 to 2 percent level of resistance. Risk factors for fluoroquinolone-resistant *S. pneumoniae* are presence of chronic obstructive pulmonary disease, nursing home residence, fluoroquinolone use within the last 12 months, and nosocomial acquisition of the infection. More than 30 percent of *S. pneumoniae* isolates are resistant to trimethoprim-sulfamethoxazole, and approximately 15 percent are resistant to tetracycline. In general, third-generation cephalosporins can be used to treat patients with drug-resistant *S. pneumoniae*. If central nervous system infection complicates the pneumonia, vancomycin should be added. Cefixime, ceftibuten, cefaclor, and loracarbef have poor activity against *S. pneumoniae* and should not be used to treat pneumonia caused by this microorganism.

Early mortality (within the first 3 or 4 days) in patients with bacteremic pneumococcal pneumonia may not be influenced by antibiotic therapy. An APACHE II (the acute physiology and chronic health evaluation scoring system) score of ≥ 28 is associated with a mortality rate of 80 percent in patients with bacteremic pneumococcal pneumonia.

Chlamydia Pneumoniae

C. pneumoniae is commonly implicated serologically as a cause of CAP. It is more frequent in those with chronic obstructive pulmonary disease. In the elderly population, it usually manifests as reactivation of previous infection, while in younger adults it can be a primary infection. It is not necessary to include diagnostic studies for *C. pneumoniae* in working up a patient with CAP because in more than 50 percent of cases it is a copathogen and patients recover without specific treatment directed at *C. pneumoniae*.

Mycoplasma Pneumoniae

This microorganism is usually a cause of pneumonia in young adults; however, it can also cause pneumonia in older adults. It has rarely been responsible for outbreaks of pneumonia in nursing homes. *M. pneumoniae* has a number of extrapulmonary manifestations, including cold agglutinin-induced hemolytic anemia, leukoerythrophagocytosis, encephalitis, cerebellar ataxia, stroke-like syndromes, arthritis, erythema multiforme, and a maculopapular rash.

Legionnaires' Disease

The most common cause of Legionnaires' disease is *Legionella pneumophila* serogroup 1, although just under half of the over 40 recognized species in the Legionellaceae family can cause Legionnaires' disease. *Legionella* spp. often cause a severe pneumonia with a high mortality rate. Epidemiologically, there is frequently a history of exposure to a contaminated water source. Outbreaks of pneumonia caused by *Legionella* spp. appear to be uncommon in nursing homes and are more likely to occur in a community or hospital setting. Severe headache combined with hyponatremia are features that should raise a clinical suspicion of Legionnaires' disease although the clinical features are usually not distinctive.

Enterobacteriaceae

Enterobacteriaceae are commonly isolated from the sputum of elderly patients with CAP. The problem is distinguishing colonization from infection because these microorganisms commonly colonize the upper airway of elderly persons. Elderly patients who are bacteremic (usually secondary to pyelonephritis), with *Escherichia coli* in particular, may have secondary seeding of the lungs.

Mycobacterium Tuberculosis

Nursing home residents account for 20 percent of cases of tuberculosis in older people. In the 1980s, approximately 12 percent of persons entering a nursing home were tuberculin positive, and active tuberculosis developed in

1 percent of isoniazid (INH) treated tuberculin-positive patients compared with 2.4 percent of those who did not receive INH. The incidence of active tuberculosis among nursing home patients is 10 to 30 times greater than among community-dwelling elderly adults.

Aspiration Pneumonia

Aspiration pneumonia denotes two distinct clinical entities: (1) aspiration pneumonitis, which is aspiration of gastric contents (usually sterile as long as there is gastric acid present) into the lungs with a resultant inflammatory response, and (2) pneumonia, which is aspiration of oropharyngeal flora into the lung with resultant bacterial infection.

In studies of Medicare patients, it was noted that the diagnosis of aspiration pneumonia increased 93.5 percent between 1991 and 1998. The mortality rate for patients with aspiration pneumonia was 23.1 percent as compared with 7.6 percent for pneumococcal pneumonia. In elderly patients with CAP, there is a high incidence of silent aspiration. In one study, 71 percent of elderly patients aspirated during sleep, as compared with 10 percent of control subjects. In another study, just over 28 percent of patients with Alzheimer's disease and 51 percent of those with a stroke aspirated when swallowing was tested using videofluoroscopy. Furthermore, feeding tube placement in patients shown to aspirate on videofluoroscopy was associated with increased rates of pneumonia and death over those who aspirated but did not receive such a tube. The manifestations of aspiration pneumonia vary according to the volume and the nature of the material aspirated. Gastric acid results in a chemical pneumonitis that can be very severe requiring assisted ventilation. There is an acute onset of dyspnea, tachypnea, bronchospasm, and cyanosis. The chest radiograph often shows diffuse opacities. Many elderly patients are achlorhydric, so this presentation may not occur in the elderly. Indeed, clinically, aspiration pneumonitis is often indistinguishable from pneumonia in this population. A history or a witnessed account of an aspiration event (one or more events of vomiting, coughing while eating, displacement of a feeding tube, vomitus, or tube feeding on bed clothes or on the patient within 24 hours of the diagnosis of pneumonia) is present in only 40 percent of definite aspiration events among residents of a long-term care facility.

In the setting of aspiration of oropharyngeal contents, if there is poor dental hygiene, anaerobic bacteria may also be present and lung abscess is not uncommon. Particulate matter may be aspirated resulting in mechanical obstruction of the airway.

Outbreaks

Outbreaks of pneumonia caused by influenza A or B viruses, respiratory syncytial virus, *Streptococcus pneumoniae, Legionella* species, *M. tuberculosis,* and *Chlamydia pneumoniae* have occurred in nursing homes and in the community.

PATHOPHYSIOLOGY

There are three routes whereby pathogens gain access to the pulmonary parenchyma: hematogenous, airborne, and microaspiration. The latter is most common. Hematogenous spread may occur in the elderly patient bacteremic from a urinary tract source with secondary seeding of the lung. Most viruses and *Coxiella burnetii* cause infection via the airborne route. *Legionella* species may gain access to the lower respiratory tract via the airborne route or aspiration.

Once a pathogen is in an alveolus an inflammatory response is triggered. The pathogen serves as a chemoattractant for polymorphonuclear leucocytes. Proinflammatory mediators (tumor necrosis factor-alpha interleukins 1 and 6) are liberated from the leucocytes amplifying the inflammatory response. Red blood cells, fibrin and leucocytes fill the alveoli resulting in consolidation of the lung (Fig. 83-1 and 83-2). This inflammatory response results in fever, cough, purulent sputum, myalgia, and arthralgia, and if blood levels of the proinflammatory cytokines are high enough, septic shock ensues. In due course, antiinflammatory mediators, especially interleukin (IL)-10, are released leading to resolution of the inflammatory response.

Consolidation of the lung leads to dyspnea (caused by decreased compliance) and hypoxemia. Hypoxemia is caused by ventilation–perfusion mismatch (consolidated lung is perfused but not ventilated).

PRESENTATION

Pneumonia may present with a sudden or insidious onset of symptoms. Table 83-3 gives the frequency of each symptom or sign of pneumonia at the time of presentation. Extrapulmonary symptoms, such as nausea, vomiting, diarrhea, myalgia, and arthralgia, are common. Older patients with pneumonia complained of fewer symptoms than did younger patients: patients aged 45 to 64, 65 to 74, and ≥75 years old had 1.4, 2.9, and 3.3 fewer symptoms, respectively, than did patients aged 18 to 44 years.

Pneumonia can be one of the causes of insidious or nonspecific deterioration in general health and/or activities, for example, confusion or falls in the elderly; infection, including pneumonia, should also be considered as a cause of sudden deterioration of, or a slow recovery from, an existing primary disease in this group of patients. While these latter presentations are emphasized in teaching the care of the elderly, there are no data to indicate what percentage of elderly patients with pneumonia present in this fashion. A diagnosis of pneumonia based on physical examination has a sensitivity of 47 to 69 percent and a specificity of 58 to 75 percent; thus, a clinical diagnosis of pneumonia should be confirmed with a chest radiograph. Crackles, wheezes, and the signs of consolidation (dullness to percussion, bronchial breathing and egophony) may be found. The most sensitive sign of pneumonia in an elderly adult is an increased respiratory rate (provided it is counted for 1 minute), with a respiratory rate of >28 breaths per minute indicating severe pneumonia.

Canadian Infectious Diseases Society and the Canadian Thoracic Society. *Clin Infect Dis* 31:383, 2000.

Medina-Walpole IS, Katz PR: Nursing home-acquired pneumonia. *J Am Geriatric Soc* 47:1005, 1999.

Meehan TP et al: Quality of care, process, and outcomes in elderly patients with pneumonia. *JAMA* 278:2080, 1997.

Metlay JP et al: Influence of age on symptoms at presentation on patients with community-acquired pneumonia. *Arch Intern Med* 157:453, 1997.

Naughton BJ et al: Outcome of nursing home-acquired pneumonia: Derivation and application of a practical model to predict 30-day mortality. *J Am Geriatr Soc* 48:1292, 2000.

Nichol KL et al: The efficacy and cost effectiveness of vaccination against influenza among elderly persons living in the community. *N Engl J Med* 31:778, 1994.

Riquelme R et al: Community-acquired pneumonia in the elderly. A multivariate analysis of risk and prognostic factors. *Am J Respir Crit Care Med* 154:1450, 1996.

Tuberculosis

SHOBITA RAJAGOPALAN • THOMAS T. YOSHIKAWA

At the turn of the twenty-first century, tuberculosis (TB) remains the leading infectious cause of mortality worldwide. In 1997, 3.81 million TB cases were reported to the World Health Organization (WHO) with an estimated current case-detection rate of 39 percent, suggesting that approximately 10 million new cases occur each year. Estimates of mortality from TB vary widely, but reliable sources report an approximate 2 to 3 million deaths per year. Projections based on skin-test surveys suggest that up to a third of the world's population, that is, 2 billion people, are currently infected with quiescent but viable tubercle bacilli. The causative agent is *Mycobacterium tuberculosis*, a formidable perpetrator that has been well described to escape immune surveillance at the earliest stages of immune compromise. As a result, TB has become an important infectious complication of immune deficiency diseases, for example, human immunodeficiency virus (HIV) infection. Other contributing factors to the persistence of TB include complex social structure, rising homeless population, international migration, and the immense challenge encountered by the public health infrastructure to ensure identification, treatment, cure, and prevention of TB. The emergence of multiple-drug–resistant (MDR) *M. tuberculosis* strains, which may result in disease refractory to all of the available antituberculous agents, has posed an additional therapeutic dilemma. Overall, older adults across all racial and ethnic groups and both genders are at particular risk for *M. tuberculosis* infection, perhaps because of both biological (compromised nutrition and immune status, underlying disease, medications, and possible racial susceptibility to *M. tuberculosis*) and socioeconomic factors (poverty, living conditions, and access to health care). Especially vulnerable are the elderly residents of nursing homes and other long-term care facilities, and persons who are at risk for reactivation of latent TB and are susceptible to new TB infection. Because of the communicable potential of *M. tuberculosis*, it is not surprising that endemic transmission between residents and from resident to staff has been documented in such facilities.

In 1989, the original *Strategic Plan for the Elimination of TB in the United States* (subsequently updated in 1999) was published and included the necessary actions to meet the Centers for Disease Control and Prevention's (CDC) goal of elimination of TB by the year 2010, defined as a case rate of less than 1 per 1 million population per year. However, this goal suffered a setback, because of an increase in TB cases associated with the HIV and acquired immunodeficiency syndrome (AIDS) epidemic. The Institute of Medicine report, *Ending Neglect: The Elimination of TB in the US*, undertaken through sponsorship from the CDC, reviews the lessons learned from the neglect of TB between the late 1960s and the early 1990s, and reaffirms commitment to a more realistic goal of elimination of TB in the United States.

This chapter reviews the epidemiology, pathogenesis, and immunologic aspects, unique clinical characteristics, diagnosis, treatment, and prevention of *M. tuberculosis* infection in community-dwelling and institutionalized aging adults, and highlights the recently published guidelines for targeted tuberculin skin testing and treatment of latent TB infection.

EPIDEMIOLOGY

Population-based surveys of both TB infection and TB disease reveal that the overwhelming burden of disease and the highest annual risk for infection are borne by those living in developing countries. (TB infection refers to contained and asymptomatic primary infection with a positive tuberculin skin test reaction; TB disease indicates overt clinical manifestations of TB). More than 95 percent of all incident cases and more than 98.6 percent of all TB deaths occur in countries where TB is endemic. The increasing proportion of all cases of TB reported in low-prevalence regions in Europe and North America are diagnosed among patients born in high prevalence countries. In the United States, for example, almost 40 percent of all culture-positive TB cases are diagnosed in foreign-born persons. Consequently, and as expected, in regions characterized by high rates of immigration, a disproportionately high number of TB cases are diagnosed among foreign-born individuals. The WHO estimates that 19 to 43 percent of the world's population is infected with *M. tuberculosis* and that more than 8 million new cases, and 2 million deaths occur from TB each year. Ninety-five percent of TB cases occur in developing countries, resulting from limited available resources that ensure adequate treatment and where HIV infection may be common. Developed nations, including the United States, report an estimated 380 million persons infected with *M. tuberculosis;* approximately 80 percent of infected persons in Europe are 50 years of age or older. Similar increases in the incidence of TB with advancing age have been demonstrated in other regions of the world, such as Southeast Asia. Although a significant percentage (80 to 90 percent) of TB in the elderly occurs in community dwellers, there is a two to three times comparatively higher incidence of active TB in nursing home residents. The enhanced efficiency of TB transmissibility within congregate settings such as prisons, nursing facilities, chronic disease facilities, and homeless shelters has raised concerns about TB infection and disease in the institutionalized elderly. Positive tuberculin reactivity associated with prolonged stay among residents of long-term care facilities for the elderly has been demonstrated, implying an increasing risk of TB infection.

PATHOGENESIS AND IMMUNOLOGIC ASPECTS

TB is an airborne communicable disease spread primarily via tiny airborne particles (droplet nuclei) expelled by an actively infected individual. Droplet nuclei containing a relatively low inoculum of one to three viable tubercle bacilli are able to reach the alveolar spaces by inhalation. The number of bacilli necessary to initiate infection is unknown, but certainly both the virulence of the inhaled organism and the microbicidal activity of the host's neutrophils and alveolar macrophages, the first line of alveolar defense, are important factors. Nevertheless, it is estimated that human infection requires 5 to 200 inhaled bacilli.

Four stages of TB infection have been described. In the first stage, scavenging (nonspecifically activated) macrophages ingest the tubercle bacilli and transport them to the regional lymph nodes (most often hilar and mediastinal). The bacilli then multiply or are inhibited or destroyed, depending on the organisms' virulence and the macrophages' innate microbicidal ability. Infected macrophages release chemotactic factors such as complement component C5a, which attract additional macrophages and circulating monocytes to the infected area; monocytes transform into macrophages at the tissue level. Macrophages containing multiplying bacilli may die, releasing more bacilli and cellular debris that also attract monocytes. The second stage, or "the symbiotic stage" or "the stage of logarithmic growth," occurs from day 7 to day 21. The balance between microbial virulence and host defense results in macrophages, still not specifically activated, that harbor multiplying organisms. As a result, the number of organisms increases logarithmically. Monocytes continue to migrate to the site of infection during this stage. The third stage, which occurs after 3 weeks, is characterized by the onset of cell-mediated immunity (CMI) and delayed-type hypersensitivity (DTH) responses, the latter associated with a positive dermal reactivity to standard-dose tuberculin. Alveolar macrophages, which are now lymphokine activated by T lymphocytes (the T helper I subset), demonstrate an increased ability to destroy intracellular tubercle

bacilli. The result is formation of the characteristic tubercle granuloma or the Ghon complex, which consists of organized collections of epithelioid cells, lymphocytes, and capillaries; caseous necrosis may occur with ultimate healing. The fourth stage represents the reactivation (secondary or post primary) stage of TB. In this final stage, hydrolytic enzymes liquefy the caseum, and bacilli multiply in great numbers in the extracellular environment, with ultimate cavity formation caused by continued delayed-type hypersensitivity responses. Tubercle bacilli seed the bloodstream with hematogenous dissemination to distant sites. The tubercle bacilli often remain at a steady state of dormancy indefinitely, as long as the host immune integrity remains intact. About 10 percent of infected persons may develop TB disease at some time in their lives, but the risk is considerably higher in persons who are immunosuppressed, especially those with HIV infection, who use illicit drugs, or who are aging. Other factors such as poor nutrition, homelessness, imprisonment, or alcoholism also increase the susceptibility to TB disease.

Although it is likely that the increased frequency of TB in the elderly could partly be caused by cell-mediated immunity that is impaired by senescence (shown in murine models), other concomitant age-related diseases (diabetes mellitus, malignancy), chronic renal failure, and renal insufficiency, poor nutrition, and immunosuppressive drugs may also contribute to this increase. Approximately 90 percent of TB disease cases are caused by reactivation of primary infection in the elderly population. Persistent infection without disease may occur in 30 to 50 percent of individuals. Some elderly persons previously infected with *M. tuberculosis* may eventually eliminate the viable tubercle bacilli and revert to a negative tuberculin reactor state. These individuals are thus at risk for new infection (reinfection) with *M. tuberculosis.* Consequently, there are three subgroups of older persons potentially at risk for TB: one subgroup never exposed to TB that may develop primary TB disease, a second subgroup with persistent and latent primary infection that may reactivate, and a third subgroup that is no longer infected and consequently at risk for reinfection.

UNIQUE CLINICAL CHARACTERISTICS

The elderly population accounts for the largest reservoir of *M. tuberculosis* infection. The majority of these infected older persons are asymptomatic, although they harbor potentially viable *M. tuberculosis* organisms. They acquired their infection at a young age during the early 1900s. An estimated 80 percent of the US population was infected with *M. tuberculosis* by the age of 30 years during that time period. Although only 15 to 30 percent of the survivors of this cohort currently remain infected with the organism, they account for the majority of cases of TB disease in the elderly population. TB chemoprophylaxis is often withheld even when indicated because of concern about adverse drug reactions in the elderly patient; however, successful treatment could be accomplished by careful monitoring of these patients for adverse drug effects. Clinicians should take an especially aggressive approach to the diagnosis, treatment, and prevention of TB in older patients in keeping with the national objective of elimination of this potentially curable disease.

A major concern with TB disease in the elderly is the failure to recognize or diagnose the disease. TB disease in the elderly may not exhibit the classic features of TB, that is, cough, hemoptysis, fever, night sweats, and weight loss. Clinical presentations in this population may include anorexia, chronic fatigue, cognitive impairment, unexplained prolonged low-grade fever, or changes in functional capacity (e.g., activities of daily living).

Pulmonary Tuberculosis

Most older patients (75 percent) with *M. tuberculosis* infection manifest active disease in their lungs. Because a significant number of these patients may exhibit minimal pulmonary symptoms, a high index of suspicion for TB disease in the presence of unexplained constitutional symptoms, as mentioned in the previous paragraph, should be exercised. The chest radiographic characteristics of pulmonary TB in the elderly are discussed in a separate section of this chapter.

Miliary Tuberculosis

As seen with other forms of disseminated TB, miliary TB in older patients is relatively common and, unfortunately, frequently diagnosed only at autopsy. A hematogenous form of miliary TB seen in geriatric patients consists of repeated episodes of low-grade *M. tuberculosis* bacillemia and a slowly progressive protracted illness, associated with fever without localizing symptoms or signs, and radiographic evidence of miliary mottling. A nonreactive form of miliary TB has also been described in older and immunosuppressed patients; this is an overwhelming tuberculous infection consisting of numerous small caseous lesions with large numbers of replicating bacilli, minimal neutrophilic infiltrate, and little or no granulomatous reaction. Clinical presentation includes fever, weight loss, and hepatosplenomegaly; elderly patients may occasionally present as a "fever of unknown origin."

Tuberculous Meningitis

Older adults may develop tuberculous meningitis as a consequence of reactivation of a latent primary focus or from miliary seeding of the meninges in primary, disseminated TB. This form of TB in general is associated with high mortality and severe neurologic sequelae in survivors. Elderly persons may present with unexplained obtundation and dementia, or, similar to younger individuals with this form of TB, with fever, headache, confusion, and weakness.

Bone and Joint Tuberculosis

Skeletal TB most commonly involves the thoracic and lumbar spines; cervical involvement rarely occurs. Paravertebral (cold) abscesses may be associated with spinal infection. Tuberculosis of the spine is a common extrapulmonary form of this disease in the elderly, particularly in the United States and Europe. Presenting manifestations consist of pain over the involved spine, fever, weight loss, and constitutional symptoms, and, in advanced cases, neurologic deficits or sinus tract formation. Involvement of larger weight-bearing joints such as the hips may occur with TB infection. Older persons can sometimes present with *M. tuberculosis* involvement of other peripheral joints such as the knees, ankles, wrists, and metatarsophalangeal joints. Tuberculosis infection of these smaller joints may be overlooked as a consequence of preexisting and concomitant degenerative joint disease in these patients.

Genitourinary Tuberculosis

This relatively common form of TB in older adults may involve any part of the genitourinary tract. The kidney is one of the major sites of involvement in genitourinary TB. Although localizing symptoms such as flank pain, dysuria, or hematuria may occur, approximately 20 to 33 percent of patients are asymptomatic. Sterile pyuria is a frequent finding. Genital structures may be involved with scrotal or pelvic masses or draining sinuses and, occasionally, the absence of symptoms.

Tuberculosis at Other Sites

Regardless of age, extrapulmonary TB, can involve virtually any organ in the body. Infection of lymph nodes, pleura, pericardium, peritoneum, gall bladder, small and large bowel, the middle ear, and carpal tunnel have been described in the literature.

DIAGNOSIS

TB disease is a frequently overlooked diagnosis in older patients. A high index of suspicion for this fully treatable infectious disease is crucial for the identification of and treatment of these infected individuals.

Tuberculin Skin Testing

The Mantoux method of tuberculin skin testing using the Tween-stabilized purified protein derivative (PPD) antigen remains the diagnostic modality of choice for TB infection, despite its potential for false-negative results. In the elderly patient, because of the increase in anergy to cutaneous antigens, the two-step tuberculin test is suggested as part of the initial geriatric assessment in order to avoid overlooking potentially false-negative reactions. The American Geriatrics Society recommends routine two-step tuberculin testing as part of the baseline information for all institutionalized elderly. The two-step tuberculin skin test involves initial intradermal placement of 5 tuberculin units of PPD, and the results are read at 48 to 72 hours. Patients are retested within 2 weeks after a negative response (induration of less than 10 mm). A positive "booster effect," and therefore a positive tuberculin skin test reaction, is a skin test of 10 mm or more and an increase of 6 mm or more over the first skin test reaction. It is important to distinguish the booster phenomenon from a true tuberculin conversion. The booster effect occurs in a person previously infected with *M. tuberculosis* but who has a false-negative skin test; repeat skin test elicits a truly positive test. Conversion (not to be confused with the booster phenomenon) occurs in persons previously uninfected with *M. tuberculosis* and who had a true negative tuberculin skin test but who become infected within 2 years as demonstrated by a repeat skin test induration that is positive 10 mm or more during this period. Several factors influence the results and interpretation of the PPD skin test. Decreased skin test reactivity is associated with waning delayed-type hypersensitivity with time, disseminated TB, corticosteroids and other drugs, and other diseases, as well as the elimination of TB infection. False-positive PPD results occur with cross-reactions with nontuberculous mycobacteria and in persons receiving the bacillus Calmette-Guérin (BCG) vaccine, the latter having been administered to some foreign-born elderly persons, which has an unpredictable effect on the PPD skin test reactivity and is presumed to wane after 10 years.

Chest Radiography

Chest radiography is indicated in all individuals with suspected TB infection, regardless of the primary site of infection. In the elderly population, 75 percent of all TB disease occurs in the respiratory tract and largely represents reactivation disease; 10 to 20 percent of cases may be as a result of primary infection. Although reactivation TB disease characteristically involves the apical and posterior segments of the upper lobes of the lungs, several studies show that many elderly patients manifest their pulmonary infection in either the middle or lower lobes or the pleura, as well as present with interstitial, patchy, or cavitary infiltrates that may be bilateral. Primary TB can involve any lung segment, but more often tends to involve the middle or lower lobes, as well as mediastinal or hilar lymph nodes. Thus, caution must be exercised in dismissing the radiographic diagnosis of pulmonary TB in the elderly because of the atypical location of the infection in the lung fields.

Laboratory Diagnosis

Sputum samples must be collected from all patients, regardless of age, with pulmonary symptoms or chest radiographic changes compatible with TB disease and who have not been previously treated with antituberculous agents. In elderly patients unable to expectorate sputum, other diagnostic techniques such as sputum induction or bronchoscopy should be considered. Flexible bronchoscopy to obtain bronchial washings and to perform bronchial biopsies has diagnostic value for TB disease in the elderly; however, in the frail and very old patient, the risk of such a procedure must be carefully balanced against the benefits of potentially making a definite diagnosis of TB. In the case of pulmonary and genitourinary TB, three consecutive early morning sputum or urine specimens, respectively, are recommended for routine mycobacteriologic studies. Sputum samples are examined initially by smear before and after concentration and then cultured for *M. tuberculosis*. Smear tests for *M. tuberculosis* are designed to detect acid-fast bacilli (AFB) and require a minimum of 10^{4-5} AFB per milliliter to be seen by light microscopy. Because routine mycobacterial culture methods may require up to 6 weeks for growth of *M. tuberculosis,* many laboratories now use radiometric procedures for the isolation and susceptibility testing of this organism. Radiometric systems using ^{14}C-labeled liquid substrate medium may identify the organisms as early as after 8 days. Sterile body fluids and tissues can be inoculated into liquid media such as oleic acid–albumin broth of Dubos and Middlebrook, which also allow the growth and detection of *M. tuberculosis* 7 to 10 days earlier than the solid-media techniques. Histologic examination of tissue from various sites, such as the liver, lymph nodes, bone marrow, pleura, or synovium, may show the characteristic tissue reaction (caseous necrosis with granuloma formation) with or without AFB, which would also strongly support the diagnosis of TB disease. Other diagnostic methods for TB that have been clinically evaluated include serology (e.g., enzyme-linked immunosorbent assay [ELISA], radioimmunoassay, latex particle agglutination assay) and gas chromatography assay for tuberculostearic acid. When applied to serum samples alone, however, these tests have not been considered sensitive and specific enough to be used as the sole diagnostic procedure for TB. Nucleic acid amplification may facilitate rapid detection of *M. tuberculosis* from respiratory specimens. The CDC recently updated the interpretation and use of these tests. Similar techniques that use deoxyribonucleic acid (DNA) probes can be used to track the spread of the organism in epidemiologic studies, and may be used to predict drug resistance prior to the availability of standard results. The rapid diagnosis of TB is especially important in elderly patients, as well as HIV-infected persons, and patients with MDR-TB.

TREATMENT

Despite much concern over the emergence of MDR isolates of *M. tuberculosis* and the complex issue of TB in HIV-infected persons, it is fortunate that the vast majority of cases of TB in the elderly population is caused by drug-sensitive strains of *M. tuberculosis*. Past evidence suggests that most cases of active TB in the elderly result from reactivation of a latent infection. These individuals presumably acquired the infecting organism during the time prior to the availability of effective antituberculous chemotherapy. Hence, unless the older patient is from a country or region with a high prevalence of drug-resistant *M. tuberculosis*, had previously been inadequately treated with *M. tuberculosis* chemotherapy, or had acquired the infection from a known MDR-TB contact, most TB cases in the elderly population will be highly susceptible to isoniazid and rifampin. Because of the rise of MDR-TB cases, the TB treatment recommendations have been modified (Table 84-1). In areas where isoniazid resistance is 4 percent or less, or if the population in question has a low risk for drug resistance such as most older persons, the empiric four-drug regimen

Table 84-1 Treatment Regimens of Tuberculosis

Option 1	Isoniazid, rifampin, pyrazinamide and ethambutol or streptomycin for 8 weeks followed by isoniazid and rifampin for 16 weeks daily or 2–3 times/week (DOT)[1]
Option 2	Isoniazid, rifampin, pyrazinamide and ethambutol or streptomycin for 2 weeks followed by 2 times/week administration of the same drugs for 6 weeks (DOT), then 2 times/week administration of isoniazid and rifampin (DOT)
Option 3	Isoniazid, rifampin, pyrazinamide and ethambutol or streptomycin 3 times a week (DOT) for 6 months. Consult a TB medical expert if patient is still symptomatic, or smear or culture positive after 3 months

Reference: American Thoracic Society. *Am J Resp Crit Care Med* 1994; 149: 1359–74. In areas where primary isoniazid resistance is less than 4%, omit fourth drug; streptomycin is not recommended for the elderly.

[1]Directly observed therapy

is not necessary. In such cases, if active TB is suspected and appropriate diagnostic tests are performed, antituberculous therapy with standard doses of isoniazid (300 mg/d) and rifampin (600 mg/d) for 9 months is an appropriate option for the elderly. A regimen initiated by an intensive phase with isoniazid (300 mg/d), rifampin (600 mg/d), and pyrazinamide (30 mg/kg/d up to 2 g) for 2 months, followed by a continuation phase with 4 months of isoniazid and rifampin only, is also an effective option for older patients. The latter regimen potentially has greater drug toxicity and adds another drug in a patient population already burdened with polypharmacy. Conversely, shorter course, more-intensive regimens, particularly when administered by directly observed therapy, are increasingly preferred, to avoid the emergence of drug resistance resulting from poor compliance with antituberculous drug regimens.

Treatment of MDR-TB is complex and often needs to be individualized, requiring the addition of a minimum of two additional antituberculous agents to which the organism is presumably susceptible, preferably in consultation with a TB expert who is familiar with *M. tuberculosis* drug resistance. Alternate drugs such as capreomycin, kanamycin, amikacin, ethionamide, and cycloserine, as well as the newer quinolones, may have to be used for treatment in such cases.

Monitoring of Response to Drug Therapy

Patients with active pulmonary TB should be monitored on a monthly basis with sputum examination until conversion to negative by culture is achieved; this usually occurs within 3 months in 90 percent of cases. Continued positive sputum cultures for *M. tuberculosis* beyond 3 months of initiation of therapy should raise the suspicion for drug resistance or noncompliance; such patients should have sputum culture and susceptibility repeated and started on directly observed therapy pending results of these data. Follow-up chest radiography is indicated 2 to 3 months after initiation of drug therapy. Older patients are at greater risk for hepatic toxicity from isoniazid. Although isoniazid therapy poses a small but significant risk for hepatitis, the hepatitis is relatively low in frequency and mild in severity. It would appear, therefore, that with careful monitoring of the older patient, antituberculous chemotherapy is a relatively safe intervention in this population. Clinical

assessments as well as baseline liver function tests are recommended before the administration of isoniazid and rifampin (and pyrazinamide) in older patients.

Monthly clinical evaluations and periodic measurements of the serum glutamic-oxaloacetic transaminase (SGOT) level should be performed in the elderly. If the SGOT rises to five times normal or if the patient exhibits symptoms or signs of hepatitis, isoniazid (as well other hepatotoxic drugs) should be discontinued. After clinical symptoms improve, or the SGOT level normalizes, or both, isoniazid may be resumed at a lower dose (e.g., 50 mg/kg/d) and gradually increased to a full dose if symptoms and the SGOT level remain stable. In case of relapse of the hepatitis with the isoniazid challenge, the drug should be replaced with an alternative regimen. There is some disagreement among clinicians regarding the monitoring of liver function tests in older patients on isoniazid. Because frail, elderly patients may often be asymptomatic in the presence of worsening hepatitis and may not be able to communicate symptoms, laboratory monitoring seems prudent. The frequency of such monitoring (e.g., monthly or every 2 to 3 months) remains less clear. Rifampin, in addition to hepatitis, is also associated with orange discoloration of body fluids. Ethambutol may cause loss of color discrimination, diminished visual acuity, and central scotomata; consequently, older patients receiving this drug should have frequent evaluation of visual acuity and color discrimination. Streptomycin is associated with irreversible auditory and vestibular damage and generally should not be prescribed in the elderly. Adverse effects of pyrazinamide include hyperuricemia, hepatitis, and flushing. Dose adjustment of antituberculous drugs is necessary with streptomycin, when used in the presence of renal impairment; however, no adjustment is needed for isoniazid, rifampin, or pyrazinamide in most elderly patients.

Treatment of Latent TB Infection

Table 84-2 outlines the revised criteria for positive tuberculin skin test reactivity by size of induration necessitating drug treatment. Drug therapy for latent TB (based on tuberculin skin test reactivity) substantially reduces the risk of progression of TB infection to TB disease. Certain conditions heighten the risk of developing TB disease in the setting of prior latent TB infection. These include known or

Table 84–2   Skin Test Criteria For Positive Tuberculin Reaction (MM Induration)*

≥5 mm
1. HIV-positive persons
2. Recent contacts of person(s) with infectious tuberculosis
3. Persons with chest radiographs consistent with tuberculosis (e.g., fibrotic changes)
4. Patients with organ transplants and other immunosuppressed hosts receiving the equivalent of >15 mg/d prednisone for >1 month

≥10 mm
1. Recent arrivals (<5 yr) from high-prevalence countries
2. Injection drug users
3. Residents and employees of high-risk congregate settings: prisons, jails, nursing homes, other health care facilities, residential facilities for AIDS patients, and homeless shelters
4. Mycobacteriology laboratory personnel
5. High-risk clinical conditions: silicosis; gastrectomy; jejunoileal bypass; ≥10% below ideal body weight; chronic renal failure; diabetes mellitus; hematological malignancies (e.g., lymphomas, leukemias); other specific malignancies (carcinoma of the head or neck, and lung)(alcoholics are also considered high risk)

≥15 mm
1. Persons with no risk factors for TB

Chemoprophylaxis recommended for all high-risk persons regardless of age Persons otherwise low-risk tested at entry into employment, ≥15 mm induration is positive.
Reference: American Thoracic Society. Am J Resp Crit Care Med 2000; 161:1376–95.
HIV: Human Immunodeficiency Virus
AIDS: Acquired Immunodeficiency Syndrome

suspected HIV infection, intravenous drug use with negative HIV serology, close contact with a known case of active TB, chest radiographic evidence for previous TB without adequate treatment, recent tuberculin conversion, and certain medical diseases or disorders (silicosis; diabetes mellitus; lymphoreticular and other hematologic malignancies; head and neck malignancies; prolonged corticosteroid therapy or other immunosuppressive therapy; end-stage renal disease; intestinal bypass or gastrectomy; chronic malabsorption syndromes; and less than 90 percent ideal body weight). The recent therapy guidelines for latent TB infection in adults including the elderly, is shown in Table 84-3. The isoniazid daily regimen for 9 months recently replaced the previously recommended 6-month schedule for treatment of latent infection. Randomized, prospective trials in HIV-negative persons indicate that a 12-month regimen is more effective than 6 months of treatment. Subgroup analyses of several trials indicate that the maximal beneficial effect of isoniazid is likely to be achieved in 9 months, with minimal additional benefit gained by extending therapy to 12 months. Although the 9-month regimen of isoniazid is preferred for the treatment of latent infection, the 6-month course also provides substantial protection and is superior to placebo in both HIV-positive and -negative persons. Hence, clinical judgment must be exercised based on local conditions, health departments or providers' experience, cost, and compliance issues. In a community-based study conducted in Bethel, Alaska, persons who took <25 percent of the prescribed annual dose had a threefold higher risk for TB than did those who took more than 50 percent of the annual dose. However, a more recent analysis of the study data indicated that the efficacy decreased significantly if less than 9 months of isoniazid was taken. In instances of known exposure to drug-resistant organisms, alternative

preventive therapy regimens may be recommended. Despite the fact that these new recommendations do not specifically address aging adults, one has to extrapolate the concept of targeted skin testing and latent infection treatment of high-risk populations to include the elderly. Elderly persons receiving isoniazid should continue to be monitored for hepatitis and peripheral neuropathy induced by the drug.

PREVENTION

Prevention of transmission of TB in any health care environment is of utmost importance for both patients and health care workers. The primary goal of an infection-control program is to detect TB disease early and to isolate and promptly treat persons with infectious TB. Enhanced awareness of drug-resistant TB has prompted public health agencies to institute strict TB identification, isolation, treatment, and prevention guidelines. The TB infection control program in most acute care, as well as long-term care facilities should consist of three types of control measures: administrative actions (i.e., prompt detection of suspected cases, isolation of infectious patients, and rapid institution of appropriate treatment), engineering control (negative-pressure ventilation rooms, high efficiency particulate air filtration, and ultraviolet germicidal irradiation), and personal respiratory protection requirements (masks). The Advisory Committee for the Elimination of Tuberculosis of the CDC has established recommendations for surveillance, containment, assessment, and reporting of TB infection and disease in long-term care facilities. Health care professionals, administrators, and staff of such extended care programs should be alerted to these recommendations.

Table 84-3   Recommended Drug Regimens For Treatment Of Latent TB Infection in Adults

Drug	Interval and duration	Comments	Rating* HIV−	Rating* HIV+
Isoniazid (INH)	Daily for 9 months	In HIV+ persons, INH can be given with nucleoside reverse transcriptase inhibitors (NRTI's), protease inhibitors (PI's), or non-nucleoside reverse transcriptase inhibitors (NNRTI's)	A(II)	A(II)
	Twice weekly for 9 months	Directly observed therapy (DOT) must be used with twice weekly dosing	B(II)	B(II)
Isoniazid	Daily for 2 months	Not indicated for HIV+, fibrotic lesions on chest X-ray, or for children DOT with twice wkly dosing	B(I)	C(I)
	Twice weekly for 6 months		B(II)	C(I)
Rifampin+Pyrazinamide (PZA)	Daily for 2 months	May also be offered to persons with INH resistant, rifampin susceptible TB	B(II)	A(I)
	Twice weekly for 2–3 months	In HIV+ persons, PI's or NNRTI's should generally not be administered with rifampin; rifabutin can be used with indinavir, nelfinavir, amprenavir, ritonavir, efavirenz, nevaripine or soft gel saquinavir DOT with twice wkly dosing	C(II)	C(I)
Rifampin	Daily for 4 months	Intolerance of PZA INH-resistant, rifampin–susceptible TB with intolerance of PZA	B(II)	B(III)

*Rating: A = Preferred; B = Acceptable alternative; C = Offer when A and B cannot be given.
Reference: American Thoracic Society. *Am J Resp Crit Care Med* 2000; 161:S221–47

Recent proceedings from the International Symposium on TB Vaccine Development and Evaluation suggest that, although the development of novel vaccines for TB prevention is currently an area of renewed interest to scientists, pharmaceutical companies, and public health agencies, to date there has been minimal success in developing a vaccine more effective than BCG.

REFERENCES

Adler JJ, Rose DM: Transmission and pathogenesis of tuberculosis, in Rom WN, Garay SM (eds): *Tuberculosis*, 1st ed. New York, Little, Brown and Company, 1996.

American Thoracic Society: Diagnostic standards and classification of tuberculosis in adults and children. *Am J Resp Crit Care Med* 161:1376, 2000.

American Thoracic Society: Targeted skin testing and treatment of latent tuberculosis infection. *Am J Resp Crit Care Med* 161:S221, 2000.

Centers for Disease Control and Prevention: Nucleic acid amplification tests for tuberculosis. *MMWR Morb Mortal Wkly Rep* 49:593, 2000.

Centers for Disease Control and Prevention: Tuberculosis elimination revisited: Obstacles, opportunities, and renewed commitment. Advisory Council for the Elimination of Tuberculosis. *MMWR Morb Mortal Wkly Rep* 48(RR-9):1, 1999.

Centers for Disease Control and Prevention: Prevention and control of tuberculosis in facilities providing long-term care to the elderly: Recommendations of the Advisory Committee for the Elimination of Tuberculosis. *MMWR Morb Mortal Wkly Rep* 39;(RR-10):7, 1990.

Comstock GW: How much isoniazid is needed for prevention of tuberculosis among immunocompetent adults? *Int J Tuberc Lung Dis* 3:847, 1999.

Dannenberg AM: Pathogenesis of tuberculosis: Native and acquired resistance in animals and humans, in Leive L, Schlessinger D (eds): *Microbiology*. Washington, DC, American Society for Microbiology, 1984, p 344.

Geiter L (ed): *Ending Neglect: The Elimination of Tuberculosis in the United States*. Washington, DC, National Academy Press, 2000, p 1.

Perez-Guzman C et al: Does aging modify pulmonary tuberculosis? A meta analytical review. *Chest* 116:961, 1999.

Rajagopalan S: Tuberculosis and aging: A global health problem. *Clin Infect Dis* 33:1034, 2001.

Rajagopalan S, Yoshikawa TT: Tuberculosis in long-term care facilities. *Infect Control Hosp Epidemiol* 21:611, 2000.

Stead WW et al: Tuberculosis as an endemic and nosocomial infection among the elderly in nursing homes. *N Engl J Med* 312;1483, 1985.

Tort J et al: Booster effect in elderly patients living in geriatric institutions. *Med Clin (Barc)* 105:41, 1995.

World Health Organization: *The world health report. Making a difference.* World Health Organ Tech Rep Ser 3:310, 1999.

Yoshikawa TT: Tuberculosis in aging adults. *J Am Geriatr Soc* 40:178, 1992.

Zuber PLF et al: Long-term risk of tuberculosis among foreign-born persons in the United States. *JAMA* 278:304, 1997.

URINARY TRACT INFECTIONS IN THE ELDERLY

LINDSAY E. NICOLLE

Urinary infection is the most frequent bacterial infection in elderly populations. Urinary infection in the elderly person is usually asymptomatic. However, symptomatic infection occurs frequently, with associated morbidity including hospitalization and, rarely, mortality. Optimal management of urinary infection in the elderly patient remains a challenge in the face of current concerns of excess antimicrobial use and increasing antimicrobial resistance in both the community and nursing home. Current limitations in knowledge and management approaches for this problem must be appreciated. In addition, the heterogeneity of elderly populations means approaches may be different for different groups. The impact and management of urinary infection differs for women and men, and differs for the institutionalized and noninstitutionalized elderly person. There are also unique considerations for the subgroup of institutionalized elderly persons with chronic indwelling catheters. The discussion in this chapter is relevant to individuals without long-term indwelling catheters, unless stated otherwise.

The bladder is normally sterile. While bacteriuria is always abnormal, it is not necessarily detrimental. "Bacteriuria" is used interchangeably with "asymptomatic urinary tract infection" in this chapter. The majority of elderly individuals with asymptomatic urinary infection, or bacteriuria, have evidence for a local host response. Some authors use the term "bladder colonization" in discussing asymptomatic bacteriuria. This term does not have clinical or biologic relevance in elderly populations, and is not used in this discussion.

Recurrent urinary infection, which may be either reinfection or relapse, is frequent. Reinfection is recurrent urinary infection with an organism isolated following antimicrobial therapy which differs from the pretherapy isolate. Relapse is recurrent urinary infection with the organism isolated posttherapy similar to that which was present prior to therapy. When relapse occurs, the organism usually remains sequestered within the urinary tract, and is not eradicated with antimicrobial therapy. Superinfection is a new urinary infection (i.e., a reinfection) that occurs in the presence of existing bacteriuria, without an intervening episode free of bacteriuria.

EPIDEMIOLOGY

Asymptomatic Infection

There is a marked increase in the prevalence of asymptomatic bacteriuria with increasing age in women. The prevalence of bacteriuria is 2 to 3 percent in young women, and increases to more than 10 percent for women older than age 65 years (Table 85-1). Bacteriuria is uncommon in younger men. With aging, particularly coincident with the development of prostatic hypertrophy, the prevalence of bacteriuria increases substantially, and approximately 5 percent of men older than age 70 years living in the community have bacteriuria. There are few studies of the incidence of asymptomatic urinary infection in elderly ambulatory populations. In one study of 209 initially nonbacteriuric elderly ambulatory male outpatients of a veterans hospital, 10 percent had at least one episode of bacteriuria during a mean of 2.8 years followup. Three-quarters of these episodes resolved spontaneously.

The prevalence of asymptomatic bacteriuria in institutionalized elderly populations is remarkably high (Table 85-1). Women have a somewhat higher frequency than men, with 25 to 50 percent of women being bacteriuric, as compared to 15 to 40 percent of men. The variation in reported prevalence is primarily determined by characteristics of the institutionalized population. Within institutionalized populations, there may be an increased prevalence with increasing age, although this is not consistent among studies. In fact, bacteriuria in the very elderly, those older than age 90 years, may be somewhat lower. The incidence of asymptomatic infection amongst institutionalized populations is also high. In a group of previously bacteriuric women, new infections occurred at a rate of 87 infections per 100 patient years. In men resident in a veterans

Table 85-1   Prevalence of Asymptomatic Bacteriuria in Elderly Populations

Population	Positive Urine Culture (%)	
	Women	Men
Community >70 years of age	10–18%	4–7%
Long-term care	25–55%	15–37%

hospital with urine cultures obtained every 2 weeks, an incidence of infection of 45 infections per 100 patient years was observed, with 10 percent of previously nonbacteriuric residents becoming bacteriuric in every 3-month period.

The high frequency of asymptomatic bacteriuria in elderly institutionalized populations has also been described by repeated prevalence surveys, with observations reported as both acquisition and loss of bacteriuria between surveys. Acquisition of bacteriuria in 1 month was 11 percent and 12 percent for nonbacteriuric men and women, respectively, in one study, and 8 percent of women acquired bacteriuria by 6 months and 23 percent by 1 year in another study. Reversion to negative urine cultures was observed in 22 percent of bacteriuric men at 1 year, and for women, 12 percent at 1 month, 31 percent at 6 months, and 27 percent at 1 year. Resolution of bacteriuria is often coincident with antimicrobial therapy. While the overall prevalence of asymptomatic bacteriuria may remain stable in a given institutionalized population, bacteriuria is dynamic, with continuous acquisition of bacteriuria by nonbacteriuric subjects, and resolution of bacteriuria in previously bacteriuric subjects.

Symptomatic Urinary Infection

Clinically diagnosed urinary infection in a community-living American population older than 65 years of age was reported to be 13 per 100 person-years, 10.9 per 100 years in men and 14 per 100 years in women. The rate was 15 per 100 years in those aged 65 to 74 years, but 12 per 100 years in those older than age 75 years. The frequency of symptomatic infection was 0.17 per 1000 days in a cohort of 29 ambulatory elderly male veterans with bacteriuria. In women with asymptomatic bacteriuria, resident in a geriatric apartment, the incidence of urinary symptoms was 0.9 per 1000 days during 6 months follow-up. For more severe presentations of urinary infection, hospitalization for acute pyelonephritis in subjects older than age 70 years was 10 to 15 per 10,000 population in one Canadian province, with hospitalization for women 1.3 times more frequent than men.

The incidence of symptomatic urinary infection in long-term care facilities varies from 1.0 to 2.4 per 1000 resident days. Definitions to identify symptomatic urinary infection are, however, often imprecise, and variable among studies. The reported incidence of symptomatic infection is only 0.1 to 0.15 per bacteriuric year for men or women when restrictive clinical definitions, which require localizing genitourinary symptoms, are used. The incidence of fever caused by urinary infection in noncatheterized subjects in nursing homes is reported to be 0.5 to 1 per 1000 resident days, using restrictive clinical or serologic criteria for identification of invasive urinary infection. Urinary tract infection is also the most frequent reason for prescribing antimicrobial therapy in long term care facilities. A substantial proportion of antimicrobial courses are, however, given for asymptomatic infection.

Morbidity and Mortality

For symptomatic infection, morbidity may be measured along a continuum of limited discomfort with voiding to disruption in daily activities or to hospitalization. For the institutionalized population, deterioration in functional status may also be a measure of morbidity, but has not been rigorously evaluated. From 8 to 30 percent of transfers to an acute care facility from long-term care are necessitated by acute urinary infection. No long-term adverse outcomes have been attributed to asymptomatic bacteriuria in the absence of symptomatic infection. Persistent asymptomatic urinary infection is not associated with an increased risk of development of renal failure or hypertension. In addition, despite a high prevalence of infection with urease-producing organisms such as *Proteus mirabilis*, complications from renal stone disease are not a common problem in institutionalized populations.

Studies from Greece and Finland in the 1970s reported an association between asymptomatic bacteriuria and decreased survival for both elderly men and women. Subsequent studies in both community and institutionalized elderly populations in Finland, the United States, and Canada have not confirmed this observation. Thus, current evidence does not support an association between asymptomatic bacteriuria and decreased survival for elderly populations. In addition, symptomatic urinary infection is rarely identified as a direct cause of mortality in the institutionalized population.

PATHOGENESIS

Route and Site of Infection

Urinary infection occurs by the ascending route. Organisms that colonize the periurethral area ascend the urethra into the bladder. Infecting organisms may subsequently reach the kidney, with renal infection determined by virulence characteristics of the infecting organism, or the presence of genitourinary abnormalities such as obstruction or reflux in the host. For men, ascending infection may also lead to prostatic infection. Thus, urinary infection may be localized to the bladder, may involve the kidneys as well as the bladder, and, for men, may also be localized in the prostate. Infection of the upper tract (kidney) is present in 50 percent of elderly women with asymptomatic infection. Renal localization is more frequent with increasing age, and in residents of nursing homes. The proportion of men with a prostatic site of infection is unknown, but is

Table 85-2   Distribution of Infecting Bacteria Isolated from Elderly Populations with Asymptomatic Urinary Infection

Organism	Population (% of isolates)			
	Community		Institutionalized	
	Women	Men	Women	Men
E. coli	68	19	47	11
P. mirabilis	0.8	4.7	27	30
Klebsiella pneumoniae	10	4.7	6.8	5.9
Citrobacter spp	—	—	2.6	2.5
Enterobacter spp	—	1.7	0.9	1.7
Providencia spp	—	—	6.8	16
Morganella morganii	—	—	1.7	2.5
Pseudomonas aeruginosa	—	4.7	5.1	19
Group B streptococci	10	—	—	1.7
Enterococcus spp	4.8	25	6.0	5
Coagulase-negative staphylococci	5.6	39	0.9	1.7
Staphylococcus aureus	—	—	—	2.5

likely substantial. Men with prostatic infection may present with recurrent episodes of symptomatic or asymptomatic urinary infection due to recurrent relapse in the urinary tract from a prostate source.

The reservoir for infecting organisms is usually the gastrointestinal flora. In the institutionalized population, transfer of organisms which colonize the perineum between patients may occur, especially with the use of indwelling or external catheters. Rarely, infection may be hematogenous rather than ascending, with urinary infection secondary to bacteremia from a nonurinary source.

Microbiology

The most frequent infecting organism isolated from urinary infection in ambulatory elderly women is *Escherichia coli* (Table 85-2). In men, gram-negative organisms other than *E. coli* and gram-positive organisms are isolated more frequently. For the institutionalized population, *E. coli* remains the most frequent infecting organism in women, although less frequently isolated than in noninstitutionalized women, and *P. mirabilis* is most frequent in men. *E. coli* may be more common in bacteremic infection than other gram-negative uropathogens. *E. coli* is also more likely to persist in women with asymptomatic bacteriuria than are other organisms. Many other gram-negative organisms are frequently isolated in the institutionalized population, including Enterobacteriaceae such as *Klebsiella pneumoniae*, *Serratia* spp., *Citrobacter* spp., *Enterobacter* spp., and *Morganella morganii*, as well as *Pseudomonas aeruginosa*.

Providencia stuartii is an organism isolated virtually only from institutionalized subjects. When this organism is isolated from residents with urinary infection in an institution, it will frequently be the predominant organism in the ward or facility. Thus, it has a unique propensity for spread within the institutional setting. Gram-positive organisms include group B streptococci, especially in diabetic subjects, and *Enterococcus* spp. Coagulase-negative staphylococci are frequently isolated in men, but are seldom associated with symptomatic infection.

Bacteria isolated from urinary infection in institutionalized populations are characterized by a higher frequency of antimicrobial resistance than are organisms isolated from urinary infection in the community population. This is a consequence of intense exposure to antimicrobials resulting in colonization with more resistant organisms, together with facilitation of transmission of organisms amongst patients in the institutional setting. Polymicrobial bacteriuria is also frequent in both male and female residents in institutions, occurring in 10 to 25 percent of bacteriuric subjects.

Host Factors

Several host factors contribute to the high frequency of urinary infection in elderly populations (Table 85-3). In the well elderly population in the community, some changes of normal aging contribute. Loss of the estrogen effect on the genitourinary mucosa in postmenopausal women results in increased colonization of the vagina with potential uropathogens, and may contribute to the high prevalence

Table 85-3   Factors Contributing to the High Prevalence of Bacteriuria in Elderly Populations

Women	Loss of estrogen effect on genitourinary mucosa
	Changes in colonizing flora
	Cystoceles
	Increased residual volume
Men	Prostatic hypertrophy
	Bacterial prostatitis
	Prostatic calculi
	Urethral strictures
	External urine collecting devices
Both	Genitourinary abnormalities
	Bladder diverticulae
	Urinary catheters (intermittent, indwelling)
	Associated illnesses
	Neurologic disease with neurogenic bladder dysfunction
	Diabetes

of urinary infection. Prostatic hypertrophy is the most important factor in elderly men. Prostatic hypertrophy causes obstruction and turbulent flow within the urethra which facilitates ascension of organisms into the bladder or prostate. Once bacteria are established in the prostate they are difficult to eradicate because of poor diffusion of antimicrobials into the prostate and the increasing likelihood of prostate stones with age. These stones provide a nidus from which it may be impossible to eradicate bacteria. Frequent relapse of urinary infection from a prostatic source is common, although months or even years may intervene between episodes. Current evidence does not support a role for immunologic changes of aging being important contributors to the high frequency of urinary infection.

In the normal genitourinary tract, intermittent, complete voiding is the preeminent host defense against urinary infection. Any structural or functional abnormality which impairs voiding will increase the likelihood of urinary infection. Structural genitourinary abnormalities such as urethral or ureteric strictures, bladder diverticulae, and cystoceles occur with increased frequency in older populations, and contribute to bacteriuria. Whether an increased residual urine volume is an expected concomitant symptom of normal aging is currently unknown.

The prevalence of asymptomatic bacteriuria in the institutionalized elderly population increases with the extent of functional impairment. The bacteriuric institutionalized elderly population are characterized by incontinence of bladder and bowel, immobility, and dementia. Impaired bladder emptying and ureteric reflux frequently accompany neurologic diseases, which also precipitate institutional care, such as Alzheimer's disease, Parkinson's disease, and cerebrovascular disease. These voiding abnormalities promote the occurrence and persistence of urinary infection. An association of bacteriuria with other chronic diseases, such as diabetes, or with specific medication use, has

not been documented, but further evaluation of these and other potential contributing factors is necessary.

The use of external condom collecting devices for management of incontinence in men also promotes bacteriuria. Men who have incontinence managed with the use of these devices have a twofold increased prevalence of bacteriuria when compared to men with incontinence in whom external catheters are not used. The initiation of condom catheter drainage is also frequently temporally associated with onset of bacteriuria in a previously nonbacteriuric resident. In men with external catheters, bacteria colonize the periurethral area in high concentrations and may ascend into the bladder, particularly if there is kinking or obstruction of the drainage tube.

Thus, the high prevalence and incidence of urinary infection in elderly populations is multifactorial. The relative importance of potential contributing factors differs for men and women, and is dependent on associated comorbidity. Host factors that predict symptomatic rather than asymptomatic infection have not been defined. Trauma to the genitourinary mucosa or obstruction of the genitourinary tract in the presence of asymptomatic urinary infection may certainly lead to fever or bacteremia from a urinary source. Beyond this, host determinants of symptomatic infection require further study.

Immune and Inflammatory Response

There is an immune and inflammatory host response for most bacteriuric elderly subjects. More than 90 percent of institutionalized men or women with asymptomatic bacteriuria have pyuria. Approximately 30 percent of institutionalized subjects without bacteriuria, however, also have pyuria, which is assumed to be caused by other inflammatory processes of the genitourinary tract. Urinary antibody to the infecting organism is elevated compared to nonbacteriuric controls in most bacteriuric subjects, and markedly elevated in more than one-third of subjects. Cytokines, such as interleukin (IL)-1α, IL-6, or IL-8, are measurable in the urine in a significantly higher proportion of bacteriuric than nonbacteriuric subjects. Finally, at least one-third of subjects with asymptomatic bacteriuria have markedly elevated serum antibody levels to their infecting uropathogens, and these elevated levels persist while bacteriuria persists. Thus, most individuals with asymptomatic bacteriuria have evidence for a local host response, and a substantial proportion have evidence of a systemic response. The clinical significance of the presence or degree of this response in asymptomatic subjects is currently unknown.

The response to symptomatic urinary infection in the elderly population is, generally, similar to that described for younger populations. There is evidence of local inflammation within the genitourinary tract as evidenced by pyuria and elevated urinary cytokine levels and urine antibody. For febrile urinary infection, including pyelonephritis, there is a systemic antibody response to the infecting organism, and elevation of serum IL-6 and C-reactive protein levels. All these variables decline with treatment of the infection and resolution of systemic symptoms.

Table 85-4 Clinical Presentations of Symptomatic Urinary Tract Infection in Elderly Populations

Probable urinary infection:
  Acute lower tract irritative symptoms (frequency, dysuria, urgency, increased incontinence)
  Acute pyelonephritis (fever, flank pain, and tenderness)
  Fever with urinary retention or obstruction of the urinary tract
  Fever with chronic indwelling urethral catheter

Unlikely caused by urinary infection
  Fever without localizing genitourinary signs or symptoms
  Gross hematuria
  Nonspecific symptoms of clinical deterioration

Not caused by urinary infection
  Chronic incontinence
  Other chronic genitourinary symptoms

CLINICAL PRESENTATION

Symptomatic Urinary Infection

Asymptomatic bacteriuria is the most frequent presentation of urinary infection in the elderly. Clinical presentations of symptomatic infection may be similar to those in younger populations (Table 85-4). Acute lower tract infection (cystitis) presents with frequency, urgency, suprapubic discomfort, and dysuria. New or increased incontinence may also be a common presenting symptom in the elderly. Acute pyelonephritis presents with the classic triad of fever and costovertebral angle pain and tenderness, with or without associated lower urinary tract symptoms.

The clinical diagnosis of symptomatic urinary infection in the highly functionally impaired institutionalized elderly population is frequently problematic. Difficulties in communication because of mental impairment or hearing loss, and the presence of chronic symptoms associated with comorbid illnesses, complicate the assessment of changes in clinical status. Chronic genitourinary symptoms are common. With the expected high prevalence of bacteriuria amongst the institutionalized population, many subjects with chronic genitourinary symptoms have a positive urine culture. These chronic genitourinary symptoms are not associated with bacteriuria, and are not improved by antimicrobial therapy. Thus, chronic genitourinary symptoms should not be attributed to urinary infection, even if the urine culture is positive.

Clinical Deterioration without Localizing Symptoms

Fever without localizing signs or symptoms presents a diagnostic dilemma. As the usual prevalence of positive urine cultures in the institutionalized population is as high as 50 percent, attributing fever to urinary infection because of an associated positive urine culture will usually be an incorrect diagnosis. Only approximately 10 to 15 percent of episodes of fever without localizing genitourinary symptoms in bacteriuric institutionalized subjects are from a urinary source. The positive predictive value of a positive urine culture for a urinary source of fever in the absence of associated genitourinary symptoms is only 12 percent. Currently, however, clinical features that discriminate between a urinary and nonurinary origin have not been identified.

Several other clinical presentations are sometimes attributed to urinary infection in the elderly population. It has been suggested that urinary infection should be a consideration in any elderly resident with "nonspecific" decline in clinical status, even without fever. Again, with a high prevalence of positive urine cultures the norm in the institutionalized population, a positive urine culture is not sufficient for a diagnosis of symptomatic urinary infection. In the absence of localizing genitourinary symptoms, a diagnosis of urinary infection to explain general decline should be entertained with skepticism. Further study defining clinical presentations of urinary infection in the functionally impaired elderly person are needed.

Finally, an unpleasant urinary odor caused by polyamine production in the urine by infecting organisms is frequently a concomitant of urinary infection. However, not all malodorous urine is bacterial infection, and infected urine is not universally malodorous. The appropriate approach to managing malodorous urine is through incontinence management rather than infection management.

Hematuria

Gross hematuria in institutionalized subjects occurs more frequently in men than in women. The majority of subjects with hematuria are bacteriuric, approximately 75 percent in one study. However, urinary infection is seldom the direct cause of hematuria. The most frequent causes are bladder stones, tumors, or trauma associated with an indwelling catheter. Bacterial hemorrhagic cystitis is uncommon, with a reported incidence of only 6.3 per 100,000 resident days. Hematuria in the presence of an infected urinary tract may, however, lead to secondary systemic urinary infection. As many as 30 percent of institutionalized subjects presenting with gross hematuria will subsequently become febrile, presumably from the urinary source.

LABORATORY EVALUATION

Microbiologic Diagnosis

A definitive diagnosis of urinary infection requires isolation of appropriate quantitative counts of uropathogens from an optimally collected urine specimen (Table 85-5). While a positive urine culture cannot differentiate symptomatic from asymptomatic infection, a negative urine culture obtained prior to initiating antimicrobial therapy effectively

Table 85-5 Quantitative Urinary Microbiology for Diagnosis of Urinary Tract Infection

Clinical Presentation*	Quantitative Microbiology
Asymptomatic urinary infection	Same organism(s) $\geq 10^5$ CFU/mL on two consecutive cultures
Pyelonephritis or fever with localizing genitourinary symptoms	$\geq 10^4$ CFU/mL
Acute lower tract symptoms	$\geq 10^3$ CFU/mL of uropathogen
Specimen collected from:	
External collecting device (men only)	$\geq 10^5$ CFU/mL
Aspirated indwelling catheter	$\geq 10^3$ CFU/mL

*For both women and men unless otherwise stated.

CFU, colony-forming units.

excludes a diagnosis of urinary tract infection. When symptomatic urinary infection is a diagnostic consideration, a urine specimen for culture is essential to confirm the diagnosis as well as to ascertain the antimicrobial susceptibilities of the infecting organism.

For asymptomatic urinary infection, two consecutive specimens with the same organism(s) isolated at $\geq 10^5$ colony-forming units (CFU)/mL are necessary. For symptomatic infection, a single specimen with $\geq 10^5$ CFU/mL is consistent with infection. In men with symptomatic infection, and for men or women with the clinical presentation of acute pyelonephritis, lower quantitative counts of $\geq 10^4$ CFU/mL of a single organism are generally considered sufficient for a microbiologic diagnosis of urinary infection. In the presence of renal failure, diuretic therapy, or with certain uncommon infecting organisms (e.g., *Candida albicans*) even lower quantitative counts may also be consistent with infection. Rarely, with unusual pathogens (e.g., *Haemophilus influenzae* or *Ureaplasma urealyticum*), or with infection proximal to a complete obstruction, the urine culture may be negative. The urine culture, of course, may also be negative if the specimen for culture is obtained after antimicrobial therapy has been initiated.

Functionally impaired elderly subjects may not be able to cooperate for optimal collection of a voided urine specimen. In this situation, urine specimens may be contaminated with colonizing genital organisms, which will interfere with interpretation of the culture result. Contamination with periurethral flora is less frequent in men than in women, and a clean-catch urine specimen can usually be obtained from men with voiding. Urine specimens may be collected from external urine collecting devices in men who cannot cooperate for specimen collection. A standard approach of cleaning of the glans, and using a clean, freshly applied condom and collecting bag should be used

for specimen collection when using this approach. When urine specimens are collected through external devices, a quantitative count of $\geq 10^5$ CFU/mL is necessary for diagnosis. Lower quantitative counts should be interpreted as contamination with colonizing periurethral organisms.

Women may be unable or unwilling to cooperate in the collection of voided urine specimens. The use of "pedi bags" or bedpans has been proposed, but such collection methods are subject to bacterial contamination, and require further validation before they can be accepted as methods of specimen collection. In-and-out catheterization should be used for urine specimen collection where a specimen is required and a woman cannot provide a voided specimen. A bacterial quantitative count of $\geq 10^3$ CFU/mL is diagnostic for such a catheterized specimen. Catheterization should only be used where urine specimen collection is essential for clinical management as this procedure, itself, will precipitate bacteriuria in up to 5 percent of episodes.

Other Diagnostic Tests

Several urine-screening tests have been proposed and evaluated in elderly populations as surrogate markers for identification of bacteriuria. The most widely used is the leukocyte esterase test, a marker for pyuria rather than bacteriuria. Other screening tests include nitrate- and antigen-detection tests. These tests generally have low sensitivity for bacteriuria and, if positive, cannot differentiate symptomatic from asymptomatic infection. A negative leukocyte esterase screen test, however, has high specificity and may be useful in excluding urinary infection. None of these surrogate tests for bacteriuria have been demonstrated to have clinical utility in elderly populations, and they cannot currently be recommended for use in the management of urinary infection.

MANAGEMENT

Asymptomatic Infection

Antimicrobial treatment of asymptomatic bacteriuria in the institutionalized elderly is not beneficial. Therapy for asymptomatic urinary infection does not decrease episodes of symptomatic urinary infection or improve survival. Chronic incontinence in bacteriuric subjects is not improved with antimicrobial therapy, and the prevalence of bacteriuria in a long-term care population is not decreased by efforts to eradicate bacteriuria in asymptomatic residents. Antimicrobial therapy for asymptomatic bacteriuria is, however, associated with an increased occurrence of adverse drug effects, increased emergence of resistant organisms, and increased cost. Thus, for the institutionalized population, asymptomatic bacteriuria should not be treated with antimicrobial therapy. The only exception would be the circumstance where an invasive genitourinary procedure is planned, and prophylactic antimicrobial therapy is indicated to prevent postprocedure bacteremia and sepsis. Similarly, the presence of pyuria in the absence of symptoms is not an indication for therapy.

Table 85-6   Oral Antimicrobial Regimens for Treatment of Acute Urinary Tract Infection

Agent	Dose*
First line	
Nitrofurantoin	50–100 mg qid
Trimethoprim/sulfamethoxazole	160/800 mg bid
Trimethoprim	100 mg bid
Amoxicillin†	500 mg tid
Other	
Amoxicillin/clavulanic acid	500 mg tid
Norfloxacin	400 mg bid
Ciprofloxacin	250–500 mg bid
Ofloxacin	200–400 mg bid
Lomefloxacin	400 mg od
Gatifloxacin	400 mg od
Cephalexin	500 mg qid
Cefaclor	500 mg qid
Cefadroxil	1 g od or bid
Cefixime	400 mg od
Cefuroxime axetil	250 mg bid
Cefpodoxime proxetil	100–400 mg bid

*Assumes normal renal function.

†For susceptible gram-positive organisms.

Few studies have evaluated antimicrobial therapy for asymptomatic urinary infection in the elderly living in the community, and further studies are needed in this population. Until evidence to support improved outcomes with treatment of asymptomatic infection is available, treatment is not warranted. It follows that screening for bacteriuria in asymptomatic elderly populations is also not indicated.

Symptomatic Urinary Infection

Treatment of symptomatic urinary infection requires optimal use of urine culture for diagnosis, appropriate antimicrobial selection, and an appropriate duration of therapy. A urine specimen for culture should be obtained prior to antimicrobial therapy for all institutionalized residents, for all men, and for women with a clinical presentation consistent with pyelonephritis. Pretherapy urine culture may not be uniformly needed for ambulant women presenting with lower tract symptoms consistent with cystitis who have not recently been treated with antimicrobial therapy. Pretherapy culture should be obtained from all women, however, in whom the diagnosis is uncertain, or with early symptomatic recurrence following therapy. The results of the urine culture are necessary to confirm the diagnosis and to assist in appropriate antimicrobial selection based on susceptibilities of the organisms isolated.

Antimicrobial selection for treatment of urinary infection is similar for elderly and younger populations. Consistent alterations in antimicrobial pharmacokinetics are observed in the elderly, including increased volume of

distribution and decreased renal clearance. These changes are not, however, of sufficient consistency or magnitude that differences in selection or dosing of antimicrobials is recommended routinely on the basis of age alone. Therapy may be given either orally (Table 85-6) or, when oral administration cannot be tolerated or absorption is uncertain, by parenteral therapy (Table 85-7). The specific antimicrobial selected is determined by appropriateness of the agent in treatment of urinary infection, known or presumed susceptibilities of the infecting organism, whether oral or parenteral therapy is indicated, tolerance of the patient, and renal and hepatic function. Antimicrobial cost will also usually be a factor, especially for institutionalized populations.

The preferred oral therapy of urinary tract infection for susceptible gram-negative organisms would usually be nitrofurantoin or trimethoprim-sulfamethoxazole, as these are relatively inexpensive agents with which there is extensive clinical experience. Concerns about sulfa allergy have led some countries, including Sweden and Great Britain, to restrict the use of trimethoprim-sulfamethoxazole. However, there is long experience with this antimicrobial and it seems premature to remove such a useful agent from our armamentarium. Where sulfa allergy precludes use of the combination, trimethoprim alone may be used. There is,

Table 85-7   Parenteral Antimicrobial Regimens for the Treatment of Urinary Tract Infection

Agent	Dose*
Preferred	
Gentamicin	1–1.5 mg/kg q8h or 4–5 mg/kg q24h
Tobramycin	1–1.5 mg/kg q8h or 4–9 mg/kg q24h
Ampicillin†	1 g q4–6h
Cefazolin	1–2 g q8h
Other	
Trimethoprim-sulfamethoxazole	160/800 mg q12h
Amikacin	5 mg/kg q8h or 15 mg/kg q24h
Piperacillin	3 g q4h
Piperacillin/tazobactam	4 g/500 mg q8h
Cefotaxime	1–2 g q8h
Ceftriaxone	1–2 g q24h
Cefepime	2 g q12h
Ceftazidime	0.5–2 g q8h
Aztreonam	1–2 g q6h
Imipenem/cilastatin	500 mg q6h
Vancomycin†	500 mg q6h or 1 g q12h
Ciprofloxacin	200–400 mg q12h
Ofloxacin	400 mg q12h
Lomefloxacin	400 mg qd

*Assumes normal renal function.

†For gram-positive organisms.

however, an increasing occurrence of trimethoprim resistance in some populations, and knowledge of local susceptibilities of organisms is necessary in selecting optimal empiric therapy. Nitrofurantoin should not be used for renal infection, *P. mirabilis* infection, or in patients with renal failure. Effective, but more costly agents, often with a wider bacterial spectrum, include amoxicillin/clavulanic acid and quinolone antimicrobials. These are most appropriately reserved for treatment of infections with organisms resistant to first-line agents, or in individuals who cannot tolerate alternate antimicrobials. Amoxicillin is indicated for the treatment of infections with susceptible gram-positive organisms, such as group B streptococci or enterococci. It is not first-line therapy for gram-negative organisms because of a high frequency of antimicrobial resistance and, for kidney infection, it is less effective than antimicrobials with a mechanism of action other than cell wall inhibition. Many cephalosporins are also effective in the treatment of urinary infection, but are not recommended as first-line agents because of their broad spectrum activity and cost.

When initial treatment with parenteral therapy is indicated, aminoglycosides such as gentamicin or tobramycin remain the antibiotics of choice. Ampicillin or vancomycin may be added if enterococcal infection is a concern. Ototoxicity and nephrotoxicity with aminoglycoside therapy are unlikely when therapy is limited to 48 to 72 hours duration. After assessment of the initial response to therapy, and when the pretherapy urine culture and susceptibility results are known, a decision may be made whether it is appropriate to continue aminoglycoside therapy, change to alternate parenteral therapy, or complete the therapeutic course with oral therapy. Many other parenteral antimicrobials are also effective, but these are more costly and, again, there are concerns with promoting antimicrobial resistance.

Duration of Therapy (Table 85–8)

The optimal duration of therapy for lower tract infection in elderly women is not determined. Treatment of symptomatic lower urinary infection in elderly women is less effective than for younger women. This is consistent for all durations of therapy, but shorter courses of therapy, such as

Table 85-8   Recommended Duration of Antimicrobial Therapy for Treatment of Symptomatic Urinary Tract Infection

Clinical Presentation	Duration
Women	
Acute cystitis	3–7 days
Acute pyelonephritis	10–14 days
Men	
Acute cystitis	14 days
Acute pyelonephritis	14 days
Relapsing infection (likely prostatitis)	6–12 weeks

single dose or 3 days, are likely proportionately less effective than 7-day courses in older women. Despite this, the majority (>50 percent) of postmenopausal women with acute cystitis will be cured by 3 days therapy. For treatment of acute cystitis in postmenopausal women, a 7-day course of therapy may be preferred. Further comparative studies, specifically of 3- and 7-day courses of therapy, are necessary to define the optimal duration in this population.

Women with renal infection and men with acute urinary infection should receive 10 to 14 days of therapy. If early recurrent infection from a prostatic source occurs in men, retreatment with prolonged therapy of 6 or 12 weeks will achieve higher cure rates, and is indicated.

More prolonged antimicrobial therapy is appropriate in selected, uncommon, clinical situations. Ongoing suppressive antimicrobial therapy may be considered where persistent or recurrent morbidity is occurring and bacteria cannot be eradicated from the urinary tract. Such circumstances include recurrent invasive infection in the presence of an underlying genitourinary abnormality that cannot be corrected, persistent infected stones where suppressive therapy may prevent further stone enlargement, or frequent symptomatic recurrences from a prostatic source. The antimicrobial selection should be based upon susceptibilities of the infecting organism, and may need to be continued indefinitely. Suppressive therapy is seldom indicated. When this therapeutic approach is used, the therapy should be reevaluated regularly to ensure it remains appropriate and the antimicrobial chosen is effective.

Outcome Following Therapy

Bacterial cure rates of 70 to 80 percent at 4 to 6 weeks posttherapy are anticipated for ambulatory elderly women treated for symptomatic infection. Recurrence may be symptomatic or asymptomatic. For ambulatory men with prostatic infections, cure rates are only 40 to 50 percent at 4 to 6 weeks, even with more prolonged therapy. Prostatic infection may also be associated with very late relapses, occurring up to a year or more after therapy.

The expected outcomes of treatment of urinary infection for both men and women in the institutionalized population are similar to those for populations with complicated urinary infection. Recurrent infection, either relapse or reinfection, occurs by 4 to 6 weeks following at least 50 percent of therapeutic courses. Thus, high microbiologic failure rates are the norm in treatment of urinary infection in the institutionalized elderly. The goal of treatment is to ameliorate symptoms, not to sterilize the urine. Posttherapy urine cultures should be obtained only if symptoms persist or recur.

PREVENTION

Asymptomatic Infection

The extraordinary frequency of urinary infection in elderly populations is primarily attributable to aging changes and associated comorbidities in the elderly. Prevention of urinary infection on a population basis would require modification of these contributing factors. Certainly, optimizing management of comorbid illnesses is desirable, but the potential impact on bacteriuria is unknown. It seems unlikely, at present, that there are opportunities for intervention which would substantially decrease the prevalence of bacteriuria.

Some interventions to prevent urinary infection have been evaluated in selected elderly populations. Ingesting large quantities of "natural" urinary antiseptics, particularly cranberry juice, has been a popular approach. The urinary antiseptic properties of cranberry juice may be mediated through interference with bacterial adherence, or through the high concentration of hippuric acid. In one study, female residents of a long-term care facility who drank large quantities of cranberry juice had a decreased prevalence of bacteriuria with pyuria, but not bacteriuria, nor symptomatic episodes. Thus, the clinical significance of this intervention is not clear. While there is no reason to discourage drinking cranberry juice, it is premature to endorse this as a means of preventing urinary infection or its complications.

As previously noted, devices used for management of incontinence contribute to acquisition of bacteriuria. These include external urine collecting devices, intermittent catheterization and, of course, indwelling urethral catheters. Avoidance or limitation of use of these devices will be effective in decreasing the frequency of bacteriuria. This may not, however, be an achievable goal in the individual elderly subject. In subjects in whom intermittent catheterization is used for bladder emptying, the frequency of bacteriuria and antimicrobial treatment for urinary infection are similar in subjects whether sterile or clean technique is used for catheterization. Thus, in the long-term care setting a clean technique is appropriate, and less costly.

Symptomatic Infection

The determinants of symptomatic urinary infection in elderly populations are not well studied. Because elderly subjects with an increased prevalence of asymptomatic infection also have an increased occurrence of symptomatic infection, strategies to prevent or decrease asymptomatic infection will likely also be effective in decreasing symptomatic infection. In addition, there is an increased risk for invasive urinary infection in the presence of obstruction within the genitourinary tract, such as the elderly man with prostatic obstruction. Where obstruction is possible, evaluation and early intervention to provide adequate urine drainage should be effective in decreasing systemic infection.

Some elderly women will experience frequent recurrent episodes of acute cystitis, similar to younger women. Where such episodes are of sufficient frequency to be distressing to the patient or to interfere with daily routine, symptomatic episodes may be prevented through the use of long-term low-dose prophylactic antimicrobial therapy (Table 85-9). Prophylactic therapy is usually taken at bedtime, and initially continued for 6 months or 1 year. This approach is indicated for otherwise well women in the

Table 85-9   Antimicrobial Regimens for Prophylaxis of Acute, Recurrent, Symptomatic Lower Tract Infection in Ambulatory Women

Antimicrobial	Regimen*
Preferred	
Nitrofurantoin	50–100 mg daily
Trimethoprim-sulfamethoxazole	80/400 mg daily or three times weekly
Trimethoprim	100 mg daily
Second line	
Cephalexin	125 mg daily
Norfloxacin	200 mg daily or three times weekly
Ciprofloxacin	125 mg daily

*Medication taken at bedtime.

Topical estrogen use may prevent recurrent symptomatic infections in postmenopausal women.

Patients with recurrent infections should be evaluated for a structural lesion (see text).

community, but would seldom be appropriate in women resident in long-term care facilities with neurologic impairment of bladder emptying. Topical vaginal estrogen therapy may also decrease the frequency of acute symptomatic infection in selected women. The relative effectiveness and tolerance of this therapeutic intervention as compared to antimicrobial therapy has not been studied.

Prophylactic antimicrobial therapy is also indicated where bacteriuria is present and an invasive genitourinary procedure likely to be associated with mucosal trauma is performed. Examples include cystoscopy in men and transurethral resection of the prostate, but not uncomplicated replacement of a long-term indwelling urethral catheter. Antimicrobial therapy must be initiated prior to the invasive procedure, preferably within 1 hour, and usually does not need to be continued beyond the duration of the procedure. Several studies suggest a single dose of antimicrobial selected on the basis of the infecting bacteria and susceptibilities is adequate.

LONG-TERM INDWELLING CATHETERS

Between 5 and 10 percent of elderly residents of institutions have urinary voiding managed with long-term indwelling catheters. The major indications for catheterization are retention and continence control. A higher proportion of women have chronic indwelling catheters. Subjects with long-term indwelling catheters are always bacteriuric, usually with two to five organisms at any time. Morbidity from urinary infection is increased in the presence of a long-term indwelling catheter. Symptomatic presentations include febrile urinary infection and complications such as stone formation and urethral abscesses. There is a greater frequency of renal inflammation consistent with acute pyelonephritis at autopsy compared to elderly individuals with bacteriuria without an indwelling catheter. Catheter obstruction occurs frequently in some patients. Obstruction is usually secondary to struvite formation by urease producing organisms such as *P. mirabilis* or *P. stuartii*. Mucosal trauma may occur with catheter change, and in the presence of infected urine may lead to fever. However, this occurs in less than 10 percent of episodes of catheter change. Residents with an indwelling urinary catheter also have an increased mortality compared to noncatheterized residents, but this is likely attributable to underlying population differences rather than catheterization. In view of the increased morbidity, chronic indwelling catheters should only be used when indications are compelling, and the need for continued use should be repeatedly reassessed.

Currently, there are no specific interventions identified to decrease the frequency of bacteriuria or complications of urinary infection in elderly subjects with chronic long-term indwelling catheters. Maintenance of a closed drainage system for the catheter and tubing delays prevents onset of bacteriuria in subjects with short-term indwelling catheters, but whether this benefits the universally infected patient with a long-term indwelling catheter has not been studied. Routine catheter change, periurethral catheter care, or catheter irrigation do not decrease the frequency of urinary infection and are not recommended.

Antimicrobial therapy given to subjects with a chronic indwelling urethral catheter will encourage emergence of resistance in infecting urinary organisms. The catheter is a foreign body within the urethra which becomes coated with a bacterial biofilm within which organisms exist in an environment where they are relatively protected from both antimicrobials and the host immune response. Urine specimens obtained for culture through the catheter reflect the bacteriology of the catheter biofilm, rather than bladder urine. The biofilm provides a persistent source of organisms that may cause relapsing infection after antimicrobial therapy. For these reasons, it is recommended that the indwelling catheter be changed prior to initiating antimicrobial treatment. Catheter replacement prior to antimicrobial therapy also leads to a more prompt resolution of fever and to less frequent symptomatic relapse.

Symptomatic urinary infection in subjects with an indwelling urethral catheter is most frequently manifested by fever. There may be associated local findings such as obstruction or leaking of the catheter, or evidence of trauma to the mucosa, such as hematuria. In the absence of such localizing findings, the diagnosis of urinary infection is problematic. Fever without localizing signs or symptoms is more likely from a urinary source in a patient with a long-term indwelling catheter than in a bacteriuric resident without an indwelling catheter. However, the urinary tract is the source of fever in only approximately 20 to 30 percent of such episodes.

When symptomatic urinary infection is diagnosed in a subject with a chronic indwelling catheter, antimicrobial therapy should be selected on the basis of the known or presumed infecting organisms, and patient tolerance. The antimicrobial agent selected for therapy is similar to those indicated in subjects without indwelling catheters. The duration of antibiotic therapy should be for as short a period as possible, so as to limit the emergence of resistant organisms. Generally, only 5 to 7 days therapy is recommended. There are no clinical studies, however, that define the optimal length of therapy, and clinical judgment is necessary.

REFERENCES

Abrutyn E et al: Does asymptomatic bacteriuria predict mortality and does antimicrobial treatment reduce mortality in elderly ambulatory women. *Ann Intern Med* 120:827, 1994.

Boscia JA et al: Therapy vs no therapy for bacteriuria in elderly ambulatory non-hospitalized women. *JAMA* 257:1067, 1987.

Mims AD et al: Clinically inapparent asymptomatic bacteriuria in ambulatory elderly men: Epidemiological, clinical, and microbiological findings. *J Am Geriatr Soc* 38:1209, 1990.

Nicolle LE et al: Infections and antibiotic resistance in nursing homes. *Clin Microbiol Rev* 9:1, 1996.

Nicolle LE: The chronic indwelling catheter and urinary infection in long-term care facility residents. *Infect Control Hosp Epidemiol* 22:316, 2001.

Nicolle LE: Urinary tract infection in long term care facility residents. *Clin Infect Dis* 31:757, 2000.

Nicolle LE: Asymptomatic bacteriuria in the elderly. *Infect Dis Clin North Am* 11:647, 1997.

Nicolle LE et al: Bacteriuria in elderly institutionalized men. *N Engl J Med* 309:1420, 1983.

Nicolle LE et al: Hospitalization for acute pyelonephritis in Manitoba, Canada, during the period from 1989 to 1992. Impact of diabetes, pregnancy, and aboriginal origin. *Clin Infect Dis* 22:1051, 1996.

Nicolle LE et al: Gross hematuria in residents of long-term care facilities. *Am J Med* 94:611, 1993.

Nicolle LE et al: The association of bacteriuria with resident characteristics and survival in elderly institutionalized males. *Ann Intern Med* 106:682, 1987.

Nicolle LE et al: Prospective randomized comparison of therapy and no therapy for asymptomatic bacteriuria in institutionalized elderly women. *Am J Med* 83:27, 1987.

Nicolle LE, SHEA Long Term Care Committee: Urinary tract infections in long-term care facilities. *Infect Control Hosp Epidemiol* 22:167, 2001.

Nordenstam G et al: Bacteriuria in representative population samples of persons aged 72–79 years. *Am J Epidemiol* 130:1176, 1989.

Orr P et al: Febrile urinary infection in the institutionalized elderly. *Am J Med* 100:71, 1996.

Ouslander JG et al: Does eradicating bacteriuria affect the severity of chronic urinary incontinence in nursing home residents? *Ann Intern Med* 12:749, 1995.

Ouslander JG et al: External catheter use and urinary tract infections among incontinent male nursing home patients. *J Am Geriatr Soc* 35:1063, 1987.

Raz R et al: Recurrent urinary tract infection in post-menopausal women. *Clin Infect Dis* 30:152, 2000.

Raz R et al: Chronic indwelling catheter replacement prior to antimicrobial therapy for symptomatic urinary infection. *J Urol* 164:1254, 2000.

Raz R, Stamm W: A controlled trial of intravaginal estriol in post-menopausal women with recurrent urinary tract infections. *N Engl J Med* 329:753, 1993.

Infections of the Nervous System

CHERYL A. JAY

Infections of the nervous system are important diagnostic considerations for many neurologic syndromes. Fever, craniospinal pain, and focal or diffuse dysfunction of the nervous system are typical clinical features, but these may also indicate systemic infection in a patient with baseline neurologic impairment. Moreover, fever may be less prominent or absent in older individuals. Hence diagnosis of these disorders in the elderly can be particularly challenging, requiring a high index of suspicion and skillful use of serologic, microbiologic, and neurodiagnostic testing. Antibiotics and adjunctive medical management, sometimes supplemented by surgical intervention, and always combined with meticulous supportive care and expectant management of common complications, constitute the mainstays of therapy. Coordinated efforts across numerous specialties may be required. This chapter reviews the clinical approach to the patient with suspected infection of the nervous system, then surveys the clinical features, diagnosis, treatment, and prognosis of disorders particularly relevant to elderly patients.

PATHOGENESIS AND CLINICAL APPROACH

The diverse clinical manifestations of infectious diseases depend on a relatively simple pathogenetic scheme. An individual encounters a microorganism that manages to evade host defenses, multiply, and cause disease locally or by dissemination. Host defenses include the immune system and anatomic barriers. The latter are quite formidable for the central nervous system (CNS), and include the skin, skull, spine, and meninges, as well as the blood–brain barrier, which is formed by capillary tight junctions unique to the CNS. Viruses, typical and atypical bacteria, fungi, and parasites, in turn, employ diverse strategies to elude host defenses. The host–pathogen relationship thus plays a central role in the development of infections, and is dynamic. For example, *Staphylococcus aureus* rarely causes meningitis, unless trauma or neurosurgery has disrupted the substantial anatomic barriers protecting the brain and spinal cord. Patients with defective cell-mediated immunity from human immunodeficiency virus (HIV) infection or cytotoxic agents become vulnerable to serious infection

with unusual pathogens such as cytomegalovirus (CMV), which rarely causes invasive disease in normal hosts.

Once established, infectious agents injure the nervous system by forming mass lesions, directly infecting neurons or glia, causing inflammation with secondary vasculopathy or neuronal damage, or, rarely, elaborating neurotoxins. Cerebral infections may be complicated by hydrocephalus, edema, and seizures, which may cause further neural injury. Finally, complications of sepsis, such as hypotension, multiple organ failure, and coagulopathy, can lead to additional neurologic dysfunction.

Diagnostic evaluation seeks to assess the host-pathogen interaction and define the neurologic infectious syndrome (Table 86–1). Relevant host factors, such as travel history, recent antibiotic use, immune status, and craniofacial surgery or trauma, should be systematically assessed. Examination establishes the baseline against which treatment response is measured. Computed tomography (CT) and magnetic resonance imaging (MRI) have revolutionized diagnosis of focal cerebral infections such as brain abscess and encephalitis, as well as spinal epidural abscess. Pre- and postcontrast images should be obtained when these diagnoses are suspected. Noncontrast CT or MRI can detect hydrocephalus and stroke, which can complicate cerebral infections. Microbiologic and serologic studies of blood and cerebrospinal fluid (CSF) help identify specific pathogens. Blood tests include cultures, acute and convalescent antibody determinations, antigen titers, and toxin assays. CSF protein, glucose, and cell count confirm the diagnosis of meningitis and narrow the list of likely causes. Additional studies, such as direct examination, culture, serologic testing, and polymerase chain reaction (PCR) can establish the diagnosis of specific infections. Skin testing may indicate exposure to mycobacteria or certain fungi, or reveal cutaneous anergy. Biopsy of extraneural tissues such as lymph nodes or bone marrow may document disseminated infection with an organism also responsible for the neurologic syndrome. Surgical intervention may be necessary, either for treatment, as in the case of brain abscess, or for diagnostic purposes, as sometimes becomes necessary in chronic meningitis. Specimens must be handled properly in order to maximize the yield of microbiologic and neuropathologic evaluation.

Table 86-1   Diagnosing Neurologic Infections

Assess host–pathogen interaction: host defenses and likely pathogens
  History: Travel, medications (antibiotics, antipyretics, immunosuppressants), associated medical conditions (diabetes, alcoholism), HIV risks, head trauma or neurosurgery, chronic care resident or recent hospitalization
  Examination: General appearance; craniofacial infection, trauma, or surgery; evidence of systemic infection; rash; stigmata of chronic medical illness
  Studies: Peripheral white count, HIV serology, skin testing

Define clinical syndrome: neurologic involvement and specific organism
  History: Tempo of illness, focal cerebral dysfunction, photophobia, and other symptoms of meningeal irritation
  Examination: Meningismus, spine tenderness, level of consciousness, focal cerebral (visual field deficit, aphasia, neglect, hemiparesis, reflex asymmetry, hemisensory deficit), spinal cord (paraparesis or quadriparesis, sphincter dysfunction), or peripheral nerve abnormalities
  Studies: Cranial CT or MRI (pre- and postcontrast if focal cerebral dysfunction suggests encephalitis or abscess), spine MRI or CT-myelography, CSF examination (protein, glucose, cell count, smears and culture, antigen or antibody titers, PCR for selected pathogens), blood tests (culture, acute and convalescent serologies, toxin assays), surgical specimens (abscess material, neural or extraneural biopsy)

Identify early complications: medical and neurologic
  History: Seizures, bowel or bladder dysfunction
  Examination: Blood pressure, pulse, papilledema
  Studies: Electrolytes, platelet count, coagulation, CSF pressure

CSF, cerebrospinal fluid; CT, computed tomography; HIV, human immunodeficiency virus; MRI, magnetic resonance imaging; PCR, polymerase chain reaction.

Treatment (Table 86–2) often begins before the diagnosis is established unequivocally. Empiric antibiotic therapy depends on likely pathogens in a given clinical setting, local resistance patterns, and allergies. For CNS infections, it is important that selected agents cross the blood–brain barrier and kill pathogens, rather than simply inhibit their growth. Hyperimmunoglobulin or antitoxins are administered in some circumstances. Most cerebral and spinal abscesses require neurosurgical intervention. Other indications for neurosurgical consultation include hydrocephalus or the need for intracranial pressure (ICP) monitoring. Associated craniofacial infection often requires concurrent eye, head and neck, or dental procedures to eradicate a primary infectious focus. Prophylaxis against complications of immobility such as decubiti, venous thromboembolism, and contractures, and attention to nutritional, fluid, and electrolyte status are also important. Because initial therapy is often empiric, close neurologic monitoring is essential. Deterioration may suggest inadequate antimicrobial coverage or systemic or secondary neurologic complications. Finally, management often extends beyond the patient. Many of these disorders require notifying public health authorities. In some instances, close contacts, including health care providers, as well as family and friends, may require prophylaxis.

INFECTIOUS NEUROLOGIC SYNDROMES

Meningitis

Bacterial meningitis (Table 86–3) occurs most commonly at the extremes of life. US surveillance data document increasing incidence among individuals age 65 years and older.

Case series in the elderly population indicate that signs and symptoms can be much more subtle than the classic acute febrile illness with prominent headache, neck stiffness, and altered mentation. In particular, the absence of one of these features cannot be used in geriatric patients to exclude bacterial meningitis on clinical grounds. Focal cerebral findings are noted in more than 25 percent of patients. Neurosurgery, alcoholism, malignancy, steroid therapy, sinusitis, and diabetes predispose to bacterial meningitis, which is frequently accompanied or complicated by pneumonia in elderly patients.

Diagnosis depends on CSF examination, which typically reveals elevated pressure and protein, hypoglycorrhachia, and polymorphonuclear pleocytosis. In most cases, CSF obtained prior to antibiotic therapy yields positive Gram's stain, culture, or both in most case. Blood cultures identify a causative organism in about half of cases. Antigen-detection techniques such as latex agglutination can quickly identify common meningeal pathogens, but are too insensitive to exclude bacterial meningitis if negative. The differential diagnosis includes the many causes of chronic meningitis (discussed later in this section), viral encephalitis, and parenchymal or extra-axial cerebral abscess (also discussed later in this chapter in the section on Focal Intracranial Bacterial Infections).

Therapy consists of prompt administration of intravenous antibiotics. When focal cerebral findings or papilledema warrants head CT prior to CSF examination in a patient with suspected bacterial meningitis, empiric antibiotic therapy should be started after blood cultures are obtained, and prior to lumbar puncture. The procedure should be performed as soon as possible after CT, because CSF profile confirms the diagnosis and cultures remain positive for several hours after antibiotics are begun.

Table 86-2 Managing Neurologic Infections

Primary infection
Medical
   Antimicrobials:
     Consider ability to reach infected site at adequate concentration.
     Choose cidal over static agent.
     Select empiric therapy to cover likely pathogens given clinical setting, refining therapy when culture and sensitivity data
      available.
   Adjunctive therapy: hyperimmunoglobulin, antitoxins
Surgical
   Neurosurgery: cerebral and spinal abscesses
   Eye, head, and neck, dental surgery: contiguous craniofacial infection
   General: soft-tissue débridement (tetanus)

Secondary complications
Neurologic
   Seizures: antiepileptic drugs
   Hydrocephalus: ventricular drainage
   Increased ICP: head elevation, osmotic agents, steroids
   Stroke: ? steroids in selected situations (tuberculous meningitis)
Medical
   Acute severe infection: sepsis, DIC, stress ulcer, malnutrition
   Cerebral dysfunction: aspiration pneumonia, diabetes insipidus, syndrome of inappropriate antidiuretic hormone secretion
   Immobilization: pressure sores, venous thromboembolism

Public health issues
   Notify authorities of reportable infections.
   Ensure appropriate assessment and prophylaxis for contacts.

DIC, disseminated intravascular coagulation; ICP, intracranial pressure.

Common pathogens among elderly patients with community-acquired bacterial meningitis include *Streptococcus pneumoniae, Neisseria meningitidis, Listeria monocytogenes,* and gram-negative bacilli. Empiric initial therapy has changed with the emergence of penicillin-resistant pneumococcus. Ampicillin covers *Listeria,* and third-generation cephalosporins such as ceftriaxone and cefotaxime cover most gram-negative rods. However, while both β-lactam antibiotics typically cover meningococcus, neither may be adequate for some resistant strains of pneumococcus, and thus many authorities recommend adding vancomycin or rifampin until culture and sensitivity results are known. Steroids, administered just before antibiotics, improve outcome in infants and children with bacterial meningitis. The data are less clear for adults. When meningococcus meningitis is suspected, prophylaxis should be considered for close contacts.

Parenteral antibiotics are typically given for 14 days, although longer courses are customary for gram-negative bacilli or *Listeria.* Repeat lumbar puncture does not need to be performed routinely, but should be considered if blood and CSF cultures are negative or if the patient does not appear to be improving clinically. The clinical features of bacterial and chronic meningitis sometimes overlap, and empiric therapy for *Mycobacterium tuberculosis* (TB), fungi, or both, may be appropriate for patients who fail to improve after several days of antibacterial treatment.

With antibiotics, more than 70 percent of patients survive bacterial meningitis, as compared with fewer than 10 percent in the preantibiotic era. In most studies, depressed level of consciousness at presentation and advanced age emerge as poor prognostic signs. Case fatality rates are higher in elderly patients. Neurologic sequelae are common in survivors, and range from deafness, mild cognitive impairments, and epilepsy to hemiparesis or the persistent vegetative state.

The aseptic meningitis syndrome is less common among the elderly than bacterial meningitis, and is defined as an acute illness with symptoms, signs, and CSF profile suggesting meningeal inflammation, but without evidence of typical bacterial pathogens. Notably absent is evidence of parenchymal dysfunction such as altered mentation, seizures or focal cerebral dysfunction. CSF reveals normal to slightly elevated pressure, elevated protein, normal glucose, and lymphocytic pleocytosis. The course is benign and self-limited. Most cases are viral, although atypical bacteria (syphilis and other spirochetes, *Rickettsia, Legionella*), partially treated bacterial meningitis, parainfectious causes (endocarditis, parameningeal infection), drugs (nonsteroidal anti-inflammatory drugs, sulfa, gamma globulin), neoplasms, collagen vascular disorders and sarcoidosis also can cause the syndrome. Many of these can be excluded by history and examination, supplemented by routine blood tests, chest radiography, and serum and CSF syphilis serologies. Freezing serum collected during acute

Table 86-3 Bacterial Meningitis

Key clinical features: Classic acute febrile illness with headache, stiff neck, and altered mental status may not be fully expressed in elderly patients.

Diagnosis:
  CSF
    Classic profile: elevated pressure (>200 mm H₂0) and protein (>50 mg/dL), low glucose (<40 mg/dL or CSF/serum <0.31), polymorphonuclear pleocytosis (10–10,000/mm³)
    Gram's stain; antigen detection tests helpful if positive
    Culture positive in most cases, without prior antibiotic therapy
  Blood cultures positive in about half of cases

Important pathogens: Pneumococcus, meningococcus, gram-negative bacilli, *Listeria* in community-acquired cases; *Staphylococcus aureus* in head trauma or neurosurgical patients

Therapy: High-dose intravenous antibiotics emergently to cover likely pathogens, or based on Gram's stain or antigen-detection testing results.

Consults to consider:
  Infectious disease for most cases
  Otolaryngology, oral surgery, or ophthalmology if relevant adjacent head and neck, dental, or eye infection
  Neurosurgery if prior surgery or head trauma
  Neurology for seizures, stroke, or increased ICP

Practical points:
  If CSF examination delayed by need to obtain CT first, draw blood cultures, begin antibiotics, and perform LP as soon as possible after CT.
  Consider penicillin-resistant pneumococcus in selecting antibiotic therapy.
  Assess need for prophylaxis of close patient contacts in meningococcal meningitis.
  Reassess for causes of chronic meningitis (see Table 86-4) if no improvement after several days of treatment.

CSF, cerebrospinal fluid; CT, computed tomography; ICP, intracranial pressure; LP, lumbar puncture.

illness for subsequent determination may be helpful. The major clinical challenge is distinguishing aseptic meningitis, with its good prognosis, from the early stages of chronic meningitis, with its more ominous causes, which include TB, fungal infection, and malignancy.

Occasionally, CSF in early viral meningitis demonstrates polymorphonuclear pleocytosis. Empiric antibiotic therapy may be started until blood and CSF cultures are negative. Alternatively, patients may be closely monitored without antibiotics, with repeat CSF examination in 6 to 12 hours to confirm the expected shift to CSF lymphocytosis. Recurrent episodes of aseptic meningitis may indicate a treatable etiology and should be evaluated fully, usually with guidance from infectious disease and neurology consultants.

Chronic meningitis (Table 86–4) has been defined as a syndrome in which symptoms and signs of meningeal inflammation and cerebral dysfunction, accompanied by abnormal CSF, persist for more than 4 weeks. Patients typically come to medical attention well before this, but the definition highlights the distinction between chronic meningitis and the aseptic meningitis syndrome. The differential diagnosis of both disorders overlaps, with two major distinctions. First, except for HIV, viruses rarely cause chronic meningitis. Second, TB, fungi, and neoplasm are more prominent diagnostic considerations for chronic

meningitis than aseptic meningitis. In older patients, carcinomatous meningitis may be a particularly important consideration. Patients with chronic meningitis frequently require extensive diagnostic evaluation, and may require empiric therapeutic trials with antituberculous or antifungal agents or steroids. Prognosis varies with the underlying cause.

Focal Intracranial Bacterial Infections

Although peak incidence of brain abscess is in the second and third decades, older patients are also vulnerable. Progressive headache and focal cerebral deficit or altered mentation suggest an expanding mass lesion, the most typical presenting syndrome. Fever, nausea, or vomiting is noted in only half of patients. Brain abscess develops most commonly by spread from an infected contiguous site, such as sinuses, ear, orbit, teeth, or skull base; related predisposing conditions include head trauma or neurosurgery. Multiple abscesses without these risk factors may suggest hematogenous spread of infection, with endocarditis or chronic dental or pulmonary infection being potential primary sources. Most brain abscesses are mixed infections, consisting of *Streptococcus* spp., *S. aureus*, anaerobes, and gram-negative bacilli. Except for pneumococcus, abscess and meningitis

Table 86-4   Chronic Meningitis

Key clinical features: Persistent or progressive headache, fever, and meningismus

Diagnosis:

　CSF shows normal or elevated pressure, elevated protein, normal or low glucose, lymphocytic pleocytosis. Obtain syphilis serology, cryptococcal antigen, TB and fungal smears and culture, cytology

　Cranial CT or MRI (pre- and postcontrast)

　Other tests: CBC, ESR, chemistry profile, collagen vascular screen, chest film, skin testing for TB and fungi

Important pathogens: Mycobacterium tuberculosis, spirochetes (syphilis, Lyme), other bacteria (anaerobes, *Actinomyces,* among others), fungi (*Cryptococcus, Histoplasma, Cocciodiodes,* among others); parainfectious and noninfectious causes

Therapy: Depends on specific cause

Consults to consider: Infectious disease, neurology

Practical points:

　Consider parainfectious causes: endocarditis, parameningeal focus (chronic craniospinal infection), partially treated bacterial meningitis

　Consider noninfectious causes: medications (NSAIDs, sulfa, azathioprine, gamma globulin, among others), carcinomatous meningitis, collagen vascular disorders, sarcoidosis, unrecognized subarachnoid hemorrhage

CBC, complete blood count; CSF, cerebrospinal fluid; CT, computed tomography; ESR, erythrocyte sedimentation rate; NSAIDs, nonsteroidal antiinflammatory drugs.

share few pathogens. Differential diagnosis includes primary brain tumors or cerebral metastases, as well as other cerebral infections such as meningitis or encephalitis. In immunosuppressed patients (discussed later in this chapter in the section on HIV and Acquired Immunodeficiency Syndrome), atypical pathogens, such as fungi and parasites, and primary or metastatic lymphoma are additional diagnostic considerations. Cranial CT or MRI, with and without contrast, is the test of choice, and demonstrates ring-enhancing lesions with surrounding edema. Lumbar puncture is usually contraindicated because of the risk of herniation. Moreover, CSF profile is nonspecific and cultures are rarely positive, unless the abscess has ruptured into the subarachnoid space or ventricles.

Typical antibiotic regimens include metronidazole, for its excellent penetration across the blood–brain barrier and anaerobic coverage, and third-generation cephalosporins, with additional coverage for *S. aureus* in head trauma or neurosurgical patients. Many patients require surgical drainage, either stereotactically or by open craniotomy, hence neurosurgical, as well as infectious disease, consultation should be obtained in all patients with suspected brain abscess. Coexisting craniofacial infection requires subspecialty consultation, as orbital, dental, or head and neck surgery may be required to eradicate a primary site. Operative specimens should be sent for smears and cultures for aerobes and anaerobes, as well as for mycobacteria and fungi in most cases. Increased ICP and seizures should be anticipated and managed aggressively. Improved neuroimaging and neurosurgical techniques over the past two decades have significantly decreased mortality from brain abscess.

Although far less common, subdural empyema and cranial epidural abscess share many aspects of pathogenesis, clinical presentation, diagnosis, and management. These extra-axial bacterial infections develop most typically as unusual complications of craniofacial infection, trauma, or neurosurgery. CT or MRI assists in the diagnosis. With antibiotics and aggressive neurosurgical intervention, more than half of patients survive these otherwise relentlessly fatal infections.

Viral Encephalitis

Classically, viral encephalitis (Table 86–5) presents as an acute febrile illness with altered mental status, headache, and focal cerebral deficits, seizures, or other evidence of parenchymal brain involvement. The differential diagnosis includes brain abscess, bacterial meningitis, and postinfectious encephalomyelitis. Viral encephalitis may occur sporadically or in epidemics. Important pathogens include arboviruses, herpesviruses, enteroviruses, and paramyxoviruses. Arboviruses, arthropod-borne pathogens, may cause summer outbreaks. The recent spread of West Nile encephalitis to North America illustrates how modern travel can lead to outbreaks far from usual areas of distribution. As with many forms of viral encephalitis, cerebral involvement is an infrequent complication of otherwise minor systemic infection. For West Nile, the elderly population appears to be at particular risk for developing encephalitis.

In the United States, herpes simplex virus (HSV) type I causes 10 percent of viral encephalitis, about half of which occur after age 50 years. Personality changes may precede the acute febrile illness by up to a week. Temporal or orbitofrontal lesions, sometimes enhancing, hemorrhagic or both, are often seen on cranial CT or MRI. Electroencephalogram (EEG) may reveal periodic lateralized epileptiform discharges which, while not specific for HSV

Table 86-5   Viral Encephalitis

Key clinical features: Acute febrile illness with early evidence of parenchymal cerebral involvement (lateralizing signs, seizures)

Diagnosis:
   Cranial CT or MRI: focal hemorrhagic necrosis or enhancement
   CSF: normal or elevated pressure, normal or low glucose, lymphocytic pleocytosis, PCR for HSV-I
   EEG helpful in HSV encephalitis
   Acute and convalescent serum viral titers do not provide diagnostic information quickly enough to influence therapy of individual
      patients, but may be important for public health surveillance

Important pathogens: Herpesviruses, arboviruses, paramyxoviruses, enteroviruses

Therapy: High-dose IV acyclovir *for all patients with suspected viral encephalitis*

Consults to consider: Infectious disease, neurology

Practical points:
   HSV encephalitis may be preceded by personality changes for up to a week before the acute illness
   Notify public health authorities, and consider storing acute phase serum
   Monitor renal function in patients on IV acyclovir

CSF, cerebrospinal fluid; CT, computed tomography; EEG, electroencephalogram; HSV, herpes simplex virus; IV, intravenous; MRI, magnetic resonance imaging; PCR, polymerase chain reaction

encephalitis, suggest the diagnosis in the appropriate clinical setting. CSF shows increased pressure and protein, normal to borderline glucose, mononuclear pleocytosis, and sometimes red blood cells or xanthochromia. Each of these tests may be minimally abnormal in very early HSV encephalitis and may need to be repeated in the first week of the illness. It is important to consider the diagnosis, as high-dose intravenous acyclovir significantly decreases morbidity and mortality. Acute and convalescent titers do not yield results rapidly enough to affect therapy, but can be important for surveillance purposes. Because early therapy is important, acyclovir should be given empirically to all patients with suspected viral encephalitis. PCR for HSV nucleic acids from CSF has largely replaced brain biopsy for establishing the diagnosis. Age greater than 30 years and depressed level of consciousness at presentation portend a poor outcome. Relapse occurs in 5 to 10 percent of patients.

Spinal Infections

Spinal epidural abscess (Table 86–6) is a neurosurgical emergency that presents as fever and back pain with local spine tenderness, variably accompanied by symptoms and signs of root or cord compression. Infection develops by direct extension of vertebral osteomyelitis or paraspinous soft tissue infection or by hematogenous spread. A history of skin infection can be obtained in approximately half of patients, and diabetes appears to be a risk factor. Local spine tenderness is an important diagnostic clue. The major pathogen is *S. aureus,* with streptococci or gram-negative bacilli in some cases. Peripheral white count and sedimentation rate are typically elevated, and blood cultures usually correlate well with abscess cultures. Emergent MRI or CT-myelography establishes the diagnosis. Lumbar puncture

should be avoided because of the risk of spinal herniation and spreading infection to the subarachnoid space. Emergent neurosurgical consultation is mandatory, as surgical intervention is often indicated to decompress the spinal cord, obtain cultures, or both. Prognosis for neurologic recovery depends on the duration and severity of cord dysfunction. Recovery is unlikely if motor involvement is severe or present for longer than 24 hours prior to surgery.

Table 86-6   Spinal Epidural Abscess

Key clinical features: Fever, back pain with spine tenderness, and radiculopathy or myelopathy

Diagnosis: Emergent spine MRI or CT-myelography (LP almost always contraindicated), blood cultures, smears, and cultures of abscess material

Important pathogens: Staphylococcus aureus, streptococci, gram-negative bacilli

Therapy: Surgical decompression in many cases, parenteral antibiotics

Consults to consider:
   Emergent neurosurgical consultation in all cases
   Infectious disease

Practical points:
   Most case series note high frequency of delayed diagnosis.
   Optimal neurologic outcome depends on early intervention.

CT, computed tomography; LP, lumbar puncture; MRI, magnetic resonance imaging

SELECTED PATHOGENS

Neurosyphilis

Neurologic disease may develop throughout the entire course of syphilis. The various neurosyphilis syndromes figure in the differential diagnosis of lymphocytic meningitis, stroke, dementia, psychiatric syndromes, myelopathy, neuropathic leg pain, and cerebral mass lesions. In 1992, 3 percent of primary and secondary syphilis cases in the United States were diagnosed in individuals older than age 55 years. The late parenchymal forms of neurosyphilis, general paresis and tabes dorsalis, develop 10 to 20 years after primary infection. General paresis presents as chronic, progressive cognitive decline that may be accompanied by psychotic features. Tabes dorsalis manifests as lancinating leg pains with progressive proprioceptive loss, leading to the wide-based, slapping gait of sensory ataxia. For both disorders, the Argyll-Robertson pupil, which reacts poorly to light, but well to accommodation, may provide a useful diagnostic clue.

With public health interventions and broader use of antibiotics, these classic neurologic forms of tertiary syphilis are now uncommon. In a recent practice guideline on evaluation of dementia, the American Academy of Neurology did not recommend routine serologic screening for syphilis in the absence of clinical suspicion for neurosyphilis. The Centers for Disease Control (CDC) recommends CSF examination for patients with ocular or tertiary syphilis or who fail treatment, as well as for patients with positive serum serologies and neurologic disease. In HIV-infected patients, the CDC also recommends lumbar puncture for late latent syphilis or syphilis of unknown duration.

The limitations of serum and CSF screening and treponeme-specific serologies complicate clinical decision making. In nonbloody CSF, the Venereal Disease Research Laboratory (VDRL) test is quite specific for neurosyphilis, but may not be highly sensitive, and pleocytosis may be the only CSF abnormality. Hence in both symptomatic and asymptomatic neurosyphilis, positive serum serologies and CSF pleocytosis may indicate the need for parenteral penicillin, even if CSF VDRL is negative. The CDC recommends that treated patients be followed with serial clinical evaluations, serum serology and CSF examinations, to ensure efficacy of therapy.

Herpes Zoster and Postherpetic Neuralgia

The incidence of herpes zoster (shingles) (Table 86–7) increases with age, particularly after age 50 years. Varicella-zoster virus (VZV) remains latent in sensory ganglia after primary infection (chicken pox). VZV may reactivate in response to waning cell-mediated immunity related to immune senescence or immunocompromise caused by HIV infection, cancer, or cytotoxic drugs. Shingles typically begins with painful paresthesias in one or two adjacent cranial or spinal dermatomes, sometimes associated with flu-like symptoms. Any region may be affected, although thoracic dermatomes and the ophthalmic division of the trigeminal nerve are most commonly involved. In most cases, a

Table 86-7 Herpes Zoster

Key clinical features: Pain, paresthesias, and vesicular eruption in 1–2 adjacent cranial or spinal dermatomes. Postherpetic neuralgia may follow, and is particularly common and severe in elderly patients

Diagnosis: Based on clinical features

Pathogen: Varicella-zoster virus

Therapy:
  Acute zoster: Acyclovir, famcyclovir, or valacyclovir within 72 hours of rash onset shortens course. Steroids may be beneficial if not otherwise contraindicated.
  Provide adequate pain relief through acute illness
  Postherpetic neuralgia: Tricyclic antidepressants, carbamazepine, gabapentin, topical lidocaine or capsaicin, opiates, TENS (transcutaneous electrical nerve stimulator) unit, biofeedback

Consults to consider:
  Ophthalmologic consultation for trigeminal (ophthalmic division) zoster
  Pain management specialist for postherpetic neuralgia

vesicular eruption develops within days to weeks in the affected area, which may be left with scarring and persistent sensory abnormalities.

Postherpetic neuralgia (PHN), defined as pain persisting more than 6 weeks after onset of rash, develops with increasing frequency with advancing age. Oral acyclovir, famciclovir, or valacyclovir decreases acute zoster pain if begun within 72 hours of onset of rash; 7- to 10-day courses are typically prescribed. Whether these agents significantly decrease the incidence, duration, or severity of PHN is less certain. In patients without contraindications, many clinicians would also prescribe a short course of corticosteroids, although data on their efficacy are conflicting. Providing for adequate pain relief is a frequently neglected aspect of acute zoster care; opioids may be necessary, with appropriate dietary and medical intervention to prevent constipation.

PHN poses considerable therapeutic challenges, particularly given the increased risk of medication side effects in the elderly population. Systemic agents include tricyclic antidepressants, the anticonvulsants carbamazepine and gabapentin, and opiates. Topical agents include the lidocaine patch and capsaicin ointment. Transcutaneous electrical nerve stimulation units and biofeedback may be useful adjuncts. A recent study demonstrated benefit of intrathecal methylprednisolone for established PHN. The high prevalence of acute zoster among the elderly population and the significant disability associated with PHN have generated interest in effective preventive strategies. The varicella vaccine boosts VZV immune responses in adults, and trials are in progress to determine whether it is effective in preventing acute zoster and, thus, PHN.

Tetanus

Waning immunity among the elderly population also contributes to tetanus being largely a geriatric disease in the United States. With routine immunization of infants combined with missed booster injections among adults, more than half of American tetanus cases occur after age 60 years. Deep, necrotic wounds, such as decubitus ulcers and chronic skin or dental infections, favor the growth of *Clostridium tetani,* a strictly anaerobic, spore-forming gram-positive bacillus. *C. tetani* produces the neurotoxin tetanospasmin, which causes the motor, reflex, and autonomic hyperactivity seen in tetanus. Trismus is a common early manifestation, followed by generalized muscle rigidity, reflex spasms, and autonomic instability. Differential diagnosis includes hypocalcemia, dystonic reaction, seizure, strychnine poisoning, and meningoencephalitis. Tetanus immunoglobulin, wound débridement, and metronidazole neutralize circulating toxin and eliminate its source. Maintaining a quiet environment, early tracheostomy, sedation with parenteral benzodiazepines or barbiturates, and neuromuscular blockade help decrease spasms and maintain ventilation. Dysautonomia may require pulmonary artery catheter placement and therapy with beta-blockers, pressors, or both. Complications include hemodynamic collapse, infection, venous thromboembolism, stress ulcer, ileus, urinary retention, decubiti, contractures, fractures, and joint dislocation. Mortality exceeds 50 percent after age 80 years. Tetanospasmin causes clinical illness at extremely low serum concentrations, and clinical tetanus does not ensure immunity. Consequently patients should receive a primary immunization series or booster as appropriate. Better attention to tetanus immunization status in emergency departments, primary care settings, and chronic care facilities could significantly decrease the incidence of this devastating illness.

Postpolio Syndrome

International vaccination programs have nearly eliminated paralytic poliomyelitis, an acute febrile illness of infants and children. However, survivors of the polio epidemics of the 1940s and 1950s may come to medical attention for postpolio syndrome, a somewhat controversial disorder. After decades of neurologic stability, patients may develop late functional impairment, including fatigue, muscle and joint pain, cramps, atrophy, and increased weakness. Patients should be evaluated for other conditions that can cause similar symptoms, including cervical or lumbar spondylosis, entrapment neuropathies, depression, sleep disorders, and thyroid disease. Electromyography may show acute and chronic denervation, perhaps caused by premature motor neuron loss or normal aging superimposed on a motor neuron pool already depleted by acute polio. Subtle abnormalities in muscle histology and CSF have been interpreted as supporting an infectious or immunologic etiology for postpolio syndrome. Neurologic consultation can supplement general medical evaluation to exclude treatable conditions that can cause late functional deterioration in polio survivors. While occasional postpolio syndrome patients develop progressive impairment, most do not, and most patients respond well to rehabilitation programs. Occasionally, patients may benefit from orthopedic intervention to correct spine or joint deformities.

Creutzfeldt–Jakob Disease

Atypical infectious agents called prions cause Creutzfeldt–Jakob disease (CJD), a human transmissible neurodegenerative disorder, as well as similar disorders in animals, such as bovine spongiform encephalopathy. Classically, CJD manifests in the sixth or seventh decade of life as rapidly progressive dementia with myoclonus. Neuroimaging and CSF examination typically reveal nonspecific findings, although CSF 14-3-3 protein may be a helpful diagnostic test. EEG shows background slowing, with characteristic periodic complexes in many patients, particularly in the middle stages of the disease. Neurologic consultation can help confirm the characteristic clinical syndrome. There is no effective treatment, and CJD progresses inexorably over months to death, usually from intercurrent infection. Brain biopsy remains the gold standard for premortem diagnosis. However, prions resist routine disinfection methods, and special precautions are necessary in processing pathologic specimens and surgical instruments from proven or suspected CJD cases. For routine patient care, universal precautions are recommended. CJD has been transmitted by dural grafts, corneal transplant, cadaveric growth hormone, and contaminated neurosurgical instruments. In England, bovine spongiform encephalopathy has crossed the species barrier to humans. Compared to CJD, patients with so-called new variant CJD are younger, and experience a more protracted course, often heralded by behavioral symptoms resembling psychiatric illness.

THE IMMUNOCOMPROMISED PATIENT

Infections of the nervous system occur frequently in immunocompromised patients. The same immune deficiency that predisposes to these life-threatening disorders also results in atypical clinical presentations, which may be particularly difficult to detect among the complex medical problems that often attend immunocompromised states. Early diagnosis thus depends on a high index of suspicion and familiarity with the clinical syndromes seen with specific immune deficiency disorders.

HIV and Acquired Immunodeficiency Syndrome

HIV infection is increasing among the elderly, with persons age 50 years or older accounting for approximately 10 percent of US acquired immunodeficiency syndrome (AIDS) patients. Clinically apparent neurologic disease develops in about half of HIV-infected patients (Table 86–8). Opportunistic infections and malignancies, HIV effects,

Table 86-8 Overview of HIV-Related Neurologic Disorders

Focal cerebral disorders
  Key clinical features: Lateralizing symptoms and signs
  Common causes: Toxoplasmosis, primary CNS lymphoma, progressive multifocal leukoencephalopathy
  Important studies: Pre- and postcontrast CT or MRI, serum toxoplasma IgG titer, CSF PCR for EBV and JC virus; brain biopsy
    in selected cases

Diffuse cerebral disorders
  Key clinical features: Globally impaired cognition or alertness, without lateralizing symptoms or signs
  Consider: Medications, metabolic derangements (electrolyte disturbances; respiratory, renal or hepatic failure)
  Common causes: HIV-associated dementia (alertness normal), cryptococcal meningitis
  Important studies: Pre- and postcontrast CT or MRI, CSF examination including cryptococcal antigen

Neuromuscular disorders
  Peripheral neuropathy
    Pain prominent: HIV neuropathy, nucleoside (ddI, ddC, d4T) neuropathy, herpes zoster
    Weakness prominent: CMV polyradiculitis, demyelinating neuropathies, mononeuritis multiplex
  Myopathy
    Key clinical features: Myalgia, proximal weakness, elevated creatine kinase
    Causes: HIV-associated polymyositis, zidovudine mitochondrial myotoxicity

*Consider neurologic consultation for HIV-infected patients with suspected neuropathy and motor involvement.
CMV, cytomegalovirus; CSF, cerebrospinal fluid; CT, computed tomography; EBV, Epstein-Barr virus; HIV, human immunodeficiency virus; IgG, immunoglobulin G; MRI, magnetic resonance imaging; PCR, polymerase chain reaction.

medications, and complications of serious systemic illness may all cause neurologic dysfunction. These disorders may involve any level of the neuroaxis and become more prevalent as HIV infection advances. Characterizing the neurologic syndrome—diffuse or focal cerebral dysfunction or neuromuscular disease—in the context of the stage of HIV infection, as defined by CD4 count, underlies evaluation of HIV-infected patients with nervous system dysfunction.

Focal cerebral disorders present with lateralizing symptoms and signs, warranting expeditious evaluation with pre- and postcontrast CT or MRI. In advanced HIV infection, when CD4 count falls below 200/mm^3, the most common causes are toxoplasmosis, primary CNS lymphoma (PCNSL), and progressive multifocal leukoencephalopathy (PML). Toxoplasmosis, a reactivated infection by the parasite *Toxoplasma gondii,* typically presents with headache, fever, and focal cerebral dysfunction developing over days to weeks. Neuroimaging reveals one or more ring-enhancing lesions with surrounding edema. These improve, along with neurologic symptoms and signs, after 10 to 14 days of pyrimethamine, sulfadiazine, and folinic acid. Chronic suppressive therapy with lower doses of these agents was necessary before highly active antiretroviral therapy (HAART); whether this is still so in the era of HAART remains uncertain. Most patients with toxoplasmosis have positive serum toxoplasma immunoglobulin (Ig) G titers. The patient with enhancing brain lesions and negative titers or who does not improve with empiric antitoxoplasma therapy may have PCNSL. In HIV-infected patients, Epstein–Barr virus (EBV) genome can be found in all of these high-grade B-cell tumors, and EBV PCR from CSF may be a less-invasive diagnostic alternative to brain biopsy. Radiotherapy and steroids extend mean survival from several weeks to several months. When focal cerebral

dysfunction is not accompanied by headache and fever, and MRI shows white matter lesions without enhancement or mass effect, PML, a reactivated infection of oligodendroglial cells by the papovavirus JC, is likely. JC virus PCR in CSF may further support the diagnosis. There is no specific therapy, although many HIV clinicians attempt aggressive HAART in an effort to slow or arrest the disease.

Diffuse cerebral dysfunction manifests as global impairment of alertness or cognitive function without lateralizing signs such as aphasia or hemiparesis. Medication effects, electrolyte disturbances, or organ failure may cause such symptoms but are easily ruled out by history and routine blood tests. Neuroimaging excludes unusual presentations of the focal brain disorders just discussed. Particularly in patients with CD4 counts less than 200/mm^3, CSF should be examined to exclude cryptococcal meningitis. Meningeal symptoms and signs are often minimal in AIDS patients with this opportunistic fungal infection. CSF protein, glucose, and cell counts may be only minimally abnormal. Interpretation of CSF profile is complicated further by the high frequency of asymptomatic protein elevation and lymphocytic pleocytosis in HIV-infected patients. Fortunately, CSF cryptococcal antigen testing is highly sensitive when compared to the gold standard of fungal culture. Initial therapy consists of amphotericin B. Acute mortality approaches 25 percent, with symptomatic increased intracranial pressure being an ominous clinical feature at presentation. As for toxoplasmosis, the necessity for chronic suppressive therapy in the HAART era remains uncertain. Relapse was the rule prior to HAART, with fluconazole typically used as secondary prophylaxis.

HIV-associated dementia is another important cause of cognitive impairment with preserved alertness, in later HIV infection. Advanced age increases the risk for this primary

HIV effect on brain. Early symptoms include apathy and social withdrawal, resembling depression. Memory impairment, gait disorder, motor slowing, and hyperreflexia follow. Dementia often coexists with myelopathy and neuropathy, the other neurologic syndromes due primarily to HIV. MRI is superior to CT in revealing symmetric, ill-defined, anterior predominant white-matter lesions that support, but do not establish, the diagnosis. Many clinicians favor aggressive combination antiretroviral therapy that includes zidovudine, which crosses the blood–brain barrier, and has been showed to ameliorate dementia, although at doses two to three times higher than those currently used. Other antiretrovirals that cross the blood–brain barrier include stavudine, abacavir, nevirapine, and indinavir. Dementia progressing over months rather than years is atypical for Alzheimer's disease and should prompt inquiry into HIV risks and consideration of HIV testing.

Neuromuscular disorders commonly complicate HIV infection, and can significantly impair quality of life. Polyneuropathy affects at least a third of HIV-infected patients and result either from advanced HIV infection or the "d-drug" nucleoside antiretrovirals didanosine (ddI), zalcitabine (ddC), stavudine (d4T). Minimizing these and other neurotoxic exposures such as ethanol, isoniazid, pyridoxine, dapsone, metronidazole, hydroxyurea, and vincristine should be attempted. Weakness is minimal, but pain can be severe. Tricyclic antidepressants must be used cautiously, because cognitively impaired patients can be particularly vulnerable to their anticholinergic side effects. Although an off-label use, the newer anticonvulsant gabapentin offers effective pain relief without untoward drug interactions, and is usually well-tolerated.

A rare, but distinct syndrome of very advanced AIDS (CD4 $<50/\text{mm}^3$) is CMV polyradiculitis, which presents with paresthesias and weakness in the legs, accompanied by sphincter dysfunction. The CSF profile is distinctive, and resembles bacterial meningitis, with elevated protein, low glucose, and polymorphonuclear pleocytosis. Ganciclovir, foscarnet, or both, can be lifesaving, and PCR for CMV in CSF confirms the diagnosis. Shingles is common in midstage and advanced HIV disease and may require chronic suppressive therapy with acyclovir. Myopathy also complicates HIV infection, although mild proximal weakness can be difficult to recognize as primary muscle disease in the context of a debilitating illness. An inflammatory myopathy, resembling polymyositis, can develop throughout the course of HIV infection and may require steroid therapy if functionally limiting. Zidovudine treatment for more than 6 months can cause a toxic mitochondrial myopathy that gradually improves with stopping the drug.

Other Immunocompromised States

Patients receiving chronic steroid therapy, with lymphoma, or who have undergone organ transplantation have impaired cell-mediated immunity. The spectrum of opportunistic pathogens resembles, but is not identical to, those seen in HIV infection. As is the case in AIDS patients, symptoms and signs may be subtle, and a low threshold for evaluating headache, minor cognitive changes, or focal cerebral disturbance is prudent. *Aspergillus, Nocardia, Toxoplasma gondii,* or PCNSL cause cerebral mass lesions, which should be biopsied in lieu of the empiric antitoxoplasma therapy often attempted in HIV-infected patients. Common causes of meningitis or meningoencephalitis include *Listeria, Cryptococcus,* TB, CMV, and VZV. Impaired humoral immunity renders patients with myeloma or chronic lymphocytic leukemia vulnerable to infection with encapsulated organisms such as pneumococcus, *Haemophilus influenzae,* and meningococcus. Defective granulocyte function, as occurs during cancer chemotherapy, is associated with meningitis caused by *Pseudomonas* or *Enterobacter,* and fungal abscesses from *Candida, Aspergillus,* or *Mucorales.*

REFERENCES

Anderson M: Management of cerebral infection. *J Neurol Neurosurg Psychiatr* 56:1243, 1993.

Brock DG, Bleck TP: Extra-axial suppurations of the central nervous system. *Semin Neurol* 12:263, 1992.

Centers for Disease Control for Prevention: 1998 Guidelines for treatment of sexually transmitted diseases. *MMWR Morb Mortal Weekly Rep* 47(No. RR-1):28, 1998.

Chiao EY et al: AIDS and the elderly. *Clin Infect Dis* 28:740, 1999.

Choi C: Bacterial meningitis. *Geriatr Clin* 8:889, 1992.

Clifford DB: Human immunodeficiency virus-associated dementia. *Arch Neurol* 57:321, 2000.

Durand ML et al: Acute bacterial meningitis in adults: A review of 493 episodes. *N Engl J Med* 328:21, 1993.

Ernst ME et al: Tetanus: pathophysiology and management. *Ann Pharmacother* 31:1507, 1997.

Gilden DH et al: Neurologic complications of the reactivation of varicella-zoster virus. *N Engl J Med* 342:635, 1998.

Hook EW, Marra CM: Acquired syphilis in adults. *N Engl J Med* 326:1060, 1992.

Kidd D et al: Poliomyelitis. *Postgrad Med J* 72:641, 1996.

Knopman DS et al: Practice parameter: Diagnosis of dementia (an evidence-based review). *Neurology* 56:1143, 2001.

Kotani N et al: Intrathecal methylprednisolone for intractable postherpetic neuralgia. *N Engl J Med* 343:1514, 2000.

Mackenzie AR et al: Spinal epidural abscess: the importance of early diagnosis and treatment. *J Neurol Neurosurg Psychiatry* 65:209, 1998.

Marra CM: Encephalitis in the 21st century. *Semin Neurol* 20:323, 2000.

Mastrianni JA, Roos RP: The prion diseases. *Semin Neurol* 20:337, 2000.

Mathisen GE, Johnson JP: Brain abscess. *Clin Infect Dis* 25:763, 1997.

Quagliarello VJ, Scheld WM: Treatment of bacterial meningitis. *N Engl J Med* 336:708, 1997.

Roos KL: Encephalitis. *Neurol Clin* 17:813, 1999.

Rotbart HA: Viral meningitis. *Semin Neurol* 20:277, 2000.

Rubin RH, Hooper DC: Central nervous system infection in the compromised host. *Med Clin North Am* 69:281, 1985.

Schmader K: Herpes zoster in the elderly: issues related to geriatrics. *Clin Infect Dis* 28:736, 1999.

Simpson DM, Tagliati M: Neurologic manifestations of HIV infection. *Ann Intern Med* 121:769, 1994.

Wilhelm CS, Marra CM: Chronic meningitis. *Semin Neurol* 12:234, 1992.

Human Immunodeficiency Virus/Acquired Immunodeficiency Syndrome

AMY C. JUSTICE

Aging and human immunodeficiency virus (HIV) infection were once consider mutually exclusive conditions. Older people did not "get AIDS" (acquired immunodeficiency syndrome) and the younger people who did never had a chance to grow old. Now, thanks to the substantial success of multiclass combination antiretroviral therapy, many people are living with HIV infection into their fifth, sixth, seventh, and even eighth decades of life. As the prevalence of HIV infection grows in older population groups, the risk of new HIV infections is also likely to increase in this age group.

Several factors may place older people at higher risk of HIV transmission given exposure. First, age-associated erectile changes make condom use difficult. Second, postmenopausal women may consider condoms unnecessary as there is no risk of pregnancy. Third, postmenopausal vaginal changes may put older women at higher risk. Finally, age-associated decline in immunity may also place older individuals at higher risk.

Research in age, aging, and HIV has focused on comparing outcomes among persons age 50 years and older to their younger counterparts. This particular cut point is supported in HIV for both sociologic and medical reasons: people age 50 years and older with HIV state they feel marginalized because of age and this group experiences a shortened survival and greater burden of comorbid disease. People older than 50 years of age are contracting HIV infection through homosexual and heterosexual contact and intravenous drug use, and account for 10 percent of newly diagnosed AIDS cases each year.

Few geriatricians are likely to choose to manage antiretroviral agents in their older patients with HIV infection, but geriatricians need to be aware of the possibility of HIV infection. Furthermore, geriatricians will be increasingly needed to comanage the effects of aging and the many comorbid medical and psychiatric conditions and drug toxicities common in older people with HIV infection.

Finally, the study of HIV infection among aging individuals may help improve our understanding of the multifaceted problems of aging racial and sexual minority groups among whom HIV infection is more common. These groups are often ignored or understudied when more common conditions of aging are addressed. There is growing evidence to suggest that older members of these minority groups practice sexual, alcohol, and drug use behaviors that place them at substantial risk of HIV infection and other complications. At the same time, physician's knowledge of these behaviors is poor.

CLINICAL PRESENTATION

Little is known about the presentation of acute HIV infection in older patients. In younger patients, acute infection may be completely asymptomatic or present as a flu-like syndrome. Like older HIV-negative individuals, older people with HIV infection underreport symptoms as compared to younger individuals, and this underreporting may be especially pronounced in older African Americans. In addition, the symptoms associated with HIV infection are common among older patients without HIV infection.

Among those persons 50 years of age and older who are chronically infected with HIV and in care, the most common self-reported symptoms are fatigue, peripheral neuropathy (pain in hands or feet), problems sleeping, myalgias or arthralgias (muscle or joint pain), and problems with having sex. Thus, unless the clinician has a high index of suspicion in the older patient, it may be difficult to identify mildly or moderately symptomatic HIV-positive individuals.

Like the symptoms just discussed, most of the medical diagnoses seen in older people with HIV are not unique to HIV infection. The most common AIDS-related conditions among veterans age 50 years and older are peripheral

Table 87-1   AIDS-Related and Comorbid Diagnoses Among Older People with HIV Infection

Diagnosis	HIV or General Medical	Percent with Condition (n = 802)		P Value
		Age <50 years	Age ≥50 years	
Chemical hepatitis	General medical	54	51	0.36
Hypertension	General medical	18	33	<0.001
Hyperlipidemia	General medical	14	22	0.001
Peripheral neuropathy	HIV	16	17	0.59
Oral candidiasis	HIV	25	16	0.001
Herpes zoster	HIV	16	15	0.74
Diabetes	General medical	8	15	0.001
Bacterial pneumonia	HIV	14	13	0.78
Pulmonary disease	General medical	10	12	0.35
Pneumocystis pneumonia	HIV	13	10	0.16
HIV wasting	HIV	9	8	0.57
Renal insufficiency/failure	General medical	5	8	0.14
Tuberculosis	HIV	4	7	0.12
Non-HIV cancer	General medical	2	6	0.006
HIV dementia	HIV	4	5	0.91
Pancreatitis	General medical	3	5	0.16
Myocardial infarction/CAD	General medical	2	5	0.05
Stroke/TIA	General medical	1	5	<0.001
Kaposi's sarcoma	HIV	2	4	0.13
Bacterial sepsis	HIV	2	4	0.19
Congestive heart failure	General medical	1	4	0.006
Enteric parasites	HIV	2	3	0.4
Peripheral vascular disease	General medical	1	3	0.02
Mycobacterium	HIV	3	2	0.93
Cryptococcus	HIV	3	2	0.5
CMV retinitis	HIV	2	2	0.85
Liver failure/cirrhosis	General medical	2	2	0.92
Toxoplasmosis	HIV	1	1	0.35
Histoplasmosis	HIV	1	1	0.96
Lymphoma	HIV	1	1	0.83
Coccidiomycosis	HIV	<1	0	0.4

CAD, coronary artery disease; CMV, cytomegalovirus; TIA, transient ischemic attack.

Table 87-2   Short Sex and Drug History to Use with Older Adults

I now need to ask you some questions about some possible activities that may put you at risk for infectious diseases. Do you mind if we discuss your sexual health and other possible risks?

- Do you have sexual or intimate contact with another man or woman? If yes, with men, women, or both?
- Do you take disease precautions? If yes, explain your precautions? If no, why not?
- Do you take any recreational drugs that involve the use of needles? If yes, do you share needles? If yes, how do you clean them?
- Have you ever had a sexually transmitted disease? If yes, how was it treated?
- Do you drink alcohol before sex? Do you use any illicit drugs or other substances before sex?

Do you have any questions that you would like to ask me about your sexual health and practices? Specifically, do you have any questions about AIDS or sexually transmitted diseases?

SOURCE: Adapted from Linsk NL (2000).

neuropathy, oral candidiasis, shingles, bacterial pneumonia, and *Pneumocystis carinii* pneumonia (Table 87-1). Of these, only *Pneumocystis* is uncommon among older individuals without HIV infection.

DIAGNOSIS

Both physicians and their older patients are likely to underestimate the older patient's risk of HIV infection. The patient may be misinformed or in denial. The physician may mistakenly believe that the patient is not sexually active or using illicit drugs. Any patient, regardless of age, who reports multiple sexual partners and unprotected sex, who has had a prior diagnosis of gonorrhea, syphilis, chlamydia, or trichomonas, or who reports illicit drug use should be tested for HIV infection. Intravenous drug use is a risk factor by itself; illicit drug use, IV or otherwise, is commonly associated with risky sexual behavior. Alcohol abuse is also an important risk factor for unprotected sex. Because older patients may be less forthcoming with reports of these behaviors and conditions, physicians should routinely ask (Table 87-2).

Similarly, any patient with unexplained peripheral neuropathy, oral candidiasis, widespread herpes zoster, recurrent bacterial pneumonia, or any of the more traditional AIDS-associated conditions (*Pneumocystis carinii* pneumonia, Kaposi's sarcoma, atypical mycobacterium, or tuberculosis) should be tested for HIV. One should also consider testing patients with lymphoma or significant unexplained anemia. Furthermore, any patient for whom more common causes of debilitating fatigue or weight loss have been eliminated should be tested for HIV. The blood test is simple, accurate (sensitivity and specificity >99.9 percent), and widely available. The first test is a screening enzyme immunoabsorbent assay for HIV antibody. If this test is positive, a Western blot is used to confirm the diagnosis. Even in low-risk populations such as blood donors, the false-positive rate of these combined tests is low (<0.001 percent).

PROGNOSIS

Survival without treatment from the time of first AIDS-associated diagnosis is on the order of 1 to 2 years (median).

Survival with current multiclass, combination antiretroviral treatment has not been fully characterized, but estimates suggest that current treatments confer a minimum of 4 to 6 additional years of survival, perhaps more.

Throughout the epidemic, age at seroconversion has been strongly associated with survival. Even though all individuals with AIDS are living longer than in the past, the age-associated difference in survival rates has grown (the hazard ratio for death among those 50 years of age and older as compared to their younger counterparts grew from 1.3 in 1982 to 1.75 in 1994). This is, in part, explained by delays in treatment. A much larger proportion of AIDS diagnoses are made within 90 days of death among those 50 years of age and over than among younger patients with AIDS (during the period 1993 to 1994, 27 percent of those younger than 50 years of age in the United States and 41 percent of those age 50 years and older were diagnosed within 90 days of death; $p < 0.001$). However, when treated, older people appear to respond as well as younger individuals and adhere to multiclass, combination antiretroviral treatment better than their younger counterparts. It is not yet known whether older individuals are more susceptible to short- or long-term adverse drug effects from antiretroviral therapy.

OVERLAPPING COMPLICATIONS AND COMORBIDITIES

The majority of patients with HIV infection have complicating conditions and comorbidities (Fig. 87–1). These include HIV and related conditions; aging and associated medical and psychiatric conditions; and effects of substance use and abuse; and beneficial and harmful effects of HIV treatment. Each of these is discussed below. The total burden of disease experienced by the patient is the sum of effects from all these conditions and not from HIV infection alone. In fact, non-HIV conditions explain as much of the variance in quality of life, survival, and health care use as do HIV-associated conditions and older people with HIV infection are much more likely to have comorbid conditions. We are now challenged to develop diagnostic strategies and team-management techniques to convert what was once a rapidly fatal disease to a well-tolerated (and well-managed) complex chronic disease.

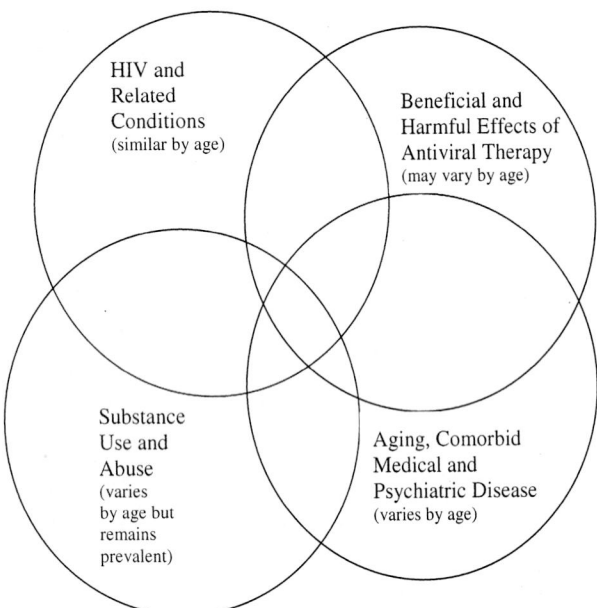

Figure 87-1   Outcomes among people aging with HIV infection.

HIV and Related Conditions

Most HIV-associated comorbid conditions do not vary significantly in prevalence when older patients are compared with their younger counterparts. It is, however, important to note that the prevalence of these conditions has dropped significantly in the era of multiclass combination antiretroviral treatment. Furthermore, the conditions that are most prevalent are no longer *Pneumocystis carnii* pneumonia, Kaposi's sarcoma, or atypical mycobacterium infection. They are instead conditions that commonly occur in people without HIV infection such as peripheral neuropathy, herpes zoster, and bacterial pneumonia. This change makes the clinical recognition of HIV in the older patient even more challenging.

Substance Use and Abuse

As a group, patients infected with HIV who are older than age 50 years are also more likely than the average 50-year-old to have consumed hazardous amounts of alcohol, used illicit drugs, and smoked cigarettes. As a result of these behaviors, these patients are also more likely than the general aging population to be coinfected with hepatitis C or B and to have liver, lung, and heart disease. Among patients who continue to drink hazardously and or to use illicit drugs, ongoing organ injury and adherence to antiretroviral therapy are likely to be important issues. Patients should be asked directly about alcohol, cigarette, and illicit drug use, and encouraged to stop or curtail ongoing use. Any patient reporting current drug or alcohol use should be questioned closely regarding treatment adherence. Current research is attempting to determine whether even moderate levels of alcohol consumption may be hazardous in this group.

Aging and Comorbid Medical and Psychiatric Disease

No one is immune from HIV infection. Nevertheless, HIV infection occurs more commonly among the homeless, members of inner-city minority or sexual minority populations, or those suffering from psychiatric illness as compared to the general population of people older than age 50 years. General medical comorbidities such as hypertension, diabetes, and chronic obstructive pulmonary disease are common in these populations. Depression and severe mental illnesses such as psychosis and post-traumatic stress disorder are also more common among older people with HIV infection than among the general population of people older than age 50 years. Their risk for many forms of cancer may be elevated as well. Finally, older people with HIV infection may have multiple reasons to have cognitive dysfunction, whether it be from cognitive diseases of aging (multi-infarct dementia or Alzheimer's disease) or from HIV (minor cognitive motor disorder or HIV-associated dementia).

Thus, even before contracting HIV infection and receiving antiretroviral therapy, older people with HIV infection may be at greater risk of comorbid medical and psychiatric disease. Clearly, the prevalence of general medical comorbid conditions is high among HIV positive patients receiving antiretroviral treatment (see Table 87–1). The most common general medical conditions include hepatitis (51 percent), hypertension (33 percent), hyperlipidemia (22 percent), diabetes (15 percent), and pulmonary disease (12 percent).

Benefits and Harms of Antiretroviral Treatment

It is not easy to determine the degree to which the current burden of comorbid medical disease experienced by people with HIV infection is a result of concurrent, preexisting, or cumulative disease or to what extent it is caused by treatment toxicity. Geriatricians are familiar with the concept that those who have prior organ injury are the most susceptible to adverse drug effects. This rule may be especially true in HIV treatment. Early reports from Phase I and II trials of antiretroviral therapies substantially underestimated the rates of toxicity probably because of the exclusion of individuals with prior organ injury from the trials. Longer term, postmarketing surveillance studies of populations receiving these drugs are beginning to describe the degree to which the earlier studies underestimated these effects.

Common adverse antiretroviral drug effects include gastrointestinal intolerance (gas, bloating, nausea, and vomiting), diarrhea, chemical hepatitis, hyperlipidemia, hyperglycemia, peripheral neuropathy, bone marrow suppression (anemia, thrombocytopenia, neutropenia), fat redistribution, nephrolithiasis, lactic acidosis, and bleeding diathesis. There is growing evidence that these are substantially more common among individuals with prior injury from comorbid conditions. Thus, aging individuals who are more likely to have renal insufficiency, prior hepatic injury, and preexisting hyperlipidemia or glucose intolerance may be at especially high risk for adverse effects of antiretroviral therapy. Longer-term observation is required to determine whether HIV treatment also incurs increased risk for subsequent cancers.

MANAGEMENT

Generalist, emergency room physicians, and geriatricians must begin to screen for sexual and drug use behavior in their older patients and to include HIV infection in their differential diagnosis of unexplained conditions.

Because of the overlapping complications and comorbid medical and psychiatric disease experienced by most patients with HIV infection, comprehensive care requires a team approach. No one specialist or generalist can hope to stay on top of optimal care in all these domains. HIV specialists need to turn to generalists and geriatricians when determining the best way to manage overlapping comorbid medical disease and to psychologists, psychiatrists and social workers when managing psychiatric diseases. The management of alcohol and drug abuse also requires the insights of generalists familiar with the medical complications of these behaviors and of psychiatrics, psychologists, and social workers familiar with methods of managing these behaviors. Generalists and geriatricians will need careful guidance from HIV specialists in determining when to start antiretroviral treatment, choosing optimal drug combinations and in determining when to stop or change therapy. For those who must manage patients far from specialty services, frequent telephone conferencing with specialists in HIV and with those experienced in the management of comorbid conditions recommended.

REFERENCES

Babiker AG et al: Age as a determinant of survival in HIV infection. *J Clin Epidemiol* 54:S16, 2001.

Dunbar-Jacob J, Mortimer-Stephens MK: Treatment adherence in chronic disease. 54:S57, 2001.

Engels EA. Human immunodeficiency virus infection, aging, and cancer. *J Clin Epidemiol* 54:S29, 2001.

Goodkin K et al: Aging and neuro-AIDS conditions and the changing spectrum of HIV-1–associated morbidity and mortality. *J Clin Epidemiol* 54:S35, 2001.

Hinkin CH et al: Neuropsychiatric aspects of HIV infection among older adults. *J Clin Epidemiol* 54:S44, 2001.

Justice AC, Weissman S: The survival experience of older and younger adults with AIDS: is there a growing gap? *Res Aging* 20:665, 1998.

Justice AC et al: Justification for a new cohort study of people aging with and without HIV infection. *J Clin Epidemiol* 54:S3, 2001.

Justice AC, Whalen C: AIDS and aging: Aging in AIDS [editorial]. *J Gen Intern Med* 11:645, 1996.

Kahana E, Kahana B: Successful aging among people with HIV/AIDS. *J Clin Epidemiol* 54:S53, 2001.

Kilbourne AM et al: General medical and psychiatric comorbidity among HIV-infected veterans in the post-HAART era. *J Clin Epidemiol* 54:S22, 2001.

Linsk NL: HIV among older adults: Age-specific issues in prevention and treatment. *AIDS Reader* 10(7):430, 2000.

Zingmond DS et al: Differences in symptom expression in older HIV-positive patients: The VACS and HCSUS experience. J Acquir Immune Defic Syndr (*in press*).

Zoster

JACK I. TWERSKY • KENNETH SCHMADER

DEFINITION

Herpes zoster is a neurocutaneous disease that is caused by the reactivation of varicella-zoster virus (VZV) from a latent infection of dorsal sensory or cranial nerve ganglia. VZV is a double-stranded deoxyribonucleic acid (DNA) herpes virus. Genes are divided into early and late based upon when they are activated in the life cycle of the VZV. Early genes encode proteins that are important in viral replication, such as virus-specific DNA polymerase and viral thymidine kinase. These are the genes that are the target of current anti-VZV therapy. Late genes encode structural nucleocapsid proteins and membrane glycoproteins. These gene products serve as targets for the immune system.

VZV spreads from person to person when a virus-naïve individual is exposed to the vesicular rash of varicella or herpes zoster. The virus establishes a latent infection within sensory nerve cells for the lifetime of the host and maintains the ability to reemerge as herpes zoster. During reactivation, VZV overwhelms cellular immune control and spreads in the affected sensory nerves to the skin. VZV reactivation is most likely to occur in the elderly population, partly because of age-related decline in specific cell-mediated immune responses to VZV, and in individuals with cellular immune deficiency. VZV reactivation and subsequent herpes zoster puts elderly patients at risk for chronic pain, or postherpetic neuralgia (PHN), which has been defined as pain after 1 month or 3 months after rash onset.

EPIDEMIOLOGY

Age is a very important risk factor for VZV and PHN. Figure 88-1 illustrates this correlation. The lifetime incidence of herpes zoster is estimated to be 10 to 20 percent in the general population, and may be as high as 50 percent among those surviving to age 85 years or older. Patients who are immune compromised are at increased risk for developing herpes zoster. This includes patients with human immunodeficiency virus (HIV) infection, Hodgkin's disease, non-Hodgkin's lymphomas, leukemia, bone marrow and other organ transplants, systemic lupus erythematosus, and those taking immunosuppressive medications. Other risk factors include white race, psychological stress, and physical trauma. Exposure to VZV has not been shown to precipitate new attacks of herpes zoster and second episodes of herpes zoster have about the same chance as if there were no first attack. Risk factors for PHN, besides being elderly, include the presence of prodromal pain, severe pain during the acute phase of herpes zoster, greater rash severity, more extensive sensory abnormalities in the affected dermatome, and, possibly, ophthalmic nerve involvement. Patients with herpes zoster are contagious during the vesicular phase of the rash, but they do not transmit VZV when the rash is crusted over.

PATHOPHYSIOLOGY

During primary infection, VZV passes from skin and mucosal lesions into the associated sensory nerves. The virus then proceeds dromically through the sensory fiber to the sensory ganglia where it establishes a latent infection. Herpes zoster distribution is related to the original infection, that is, it occurs most often in dermatomes in which the original virus achieved the highest density and was most clinically apparent. Common sites for herpes zoster include the first (ophthalmic) division of the trigeminal nerve and spinal sensory ganglia from T1 to L2. Herpes zoster can also reemerge at the site of a prior varicella vaccination. The mechanism that operates to reactivate the virus is unknown At some point when the host is vulnerable, the virus multiplies and spreads within the ganglia resulting in neuronal necrosis and an inflammatory reaction which can manifest as neuralgia. VZV spreads antidromically and is released around the sensory nerve ending in the skin and mucosa where it presents as vesicles. Limited hematogenous spread produces a few scattered vesicles at a distant site from the dermatome infected by the virus. This often occurs near the affected dermatome. The virus can also spread proximally along the posterior nerve root to the meninges resulting in leptomeningitis and segmental myelitis. Extension of the infection can result in meningoencephalitis and transverse myelitis. Infections of motor neurons in the anterior horn and the motor neuron cause local palsies. The infection stimulates an anamnestic immune response that limits spread and kills the reactivated

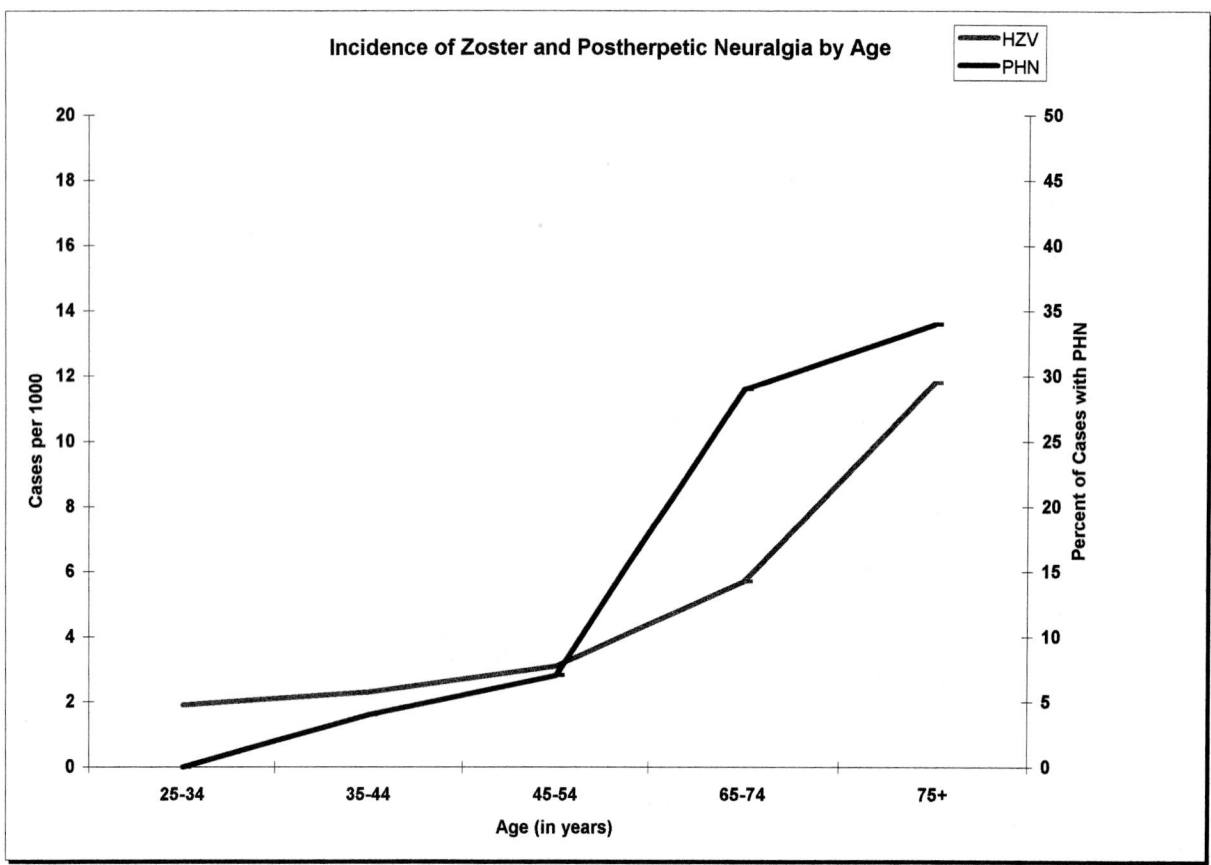

Figure 88-1   The increases in the incidence of herpes zoster (HZV) per 1000 persons and the percentage of those patients with post-herpetic neuralgia (PHN) by age.

virus. VZV may spread down sensory nerves and cause dermatomal pain without a rash, a phenomenon known as zoster sine herpete. This is thought to be the result of neutralization of the virus before it is able to reach the skin or other mucosal surfaces. Zoster sine herpete is demonstrated by a rise in the titer of antibody to VZV.

The pathogenesis of PHN involves viral, inflammatory, and pain-related excitotoxic damage to the peripheral nerve and neurons in the spinal cord and ganglion early in the course of herpes zoster. First, affected primary afferent nerves may become spontaneously active and hypersensitive to peripheral stimuli and also to sympathetic stimulation. Second, excessive afferent nerve activity may sensitize central nervous system neurons, producing prolonged and augmented central responses to innocuous as well as noxious stimuli. Finally, the loss of afferent input to second-order dorsal horn neurons may cause deafferentation pain, in which input from normally non–pain-transmitting neurons becomes painful. Clinically, these mechanisms may result in constant aching or burning pain, intermittent shock-like pain and/or in allodynia (pain elicited by stimuli that are normally not painful, e.g., light touch).

PRESENTATION

The first symptoms of herpes zoster frequently precede the vesicles by several days. The symptoms in the involved dermatome range from a superficial itching, tingling, or burning to severe, deep, boring, or lancinating pain, paresthesia, and hyperesthesia. The pain can be constant or intermittent. Zoster sine herpete is characterized by the painful symptoms without ever having vesicles. The symptoms are a result of the neuronal inflammation, hemorrhage, and destruction. The symptoms without signs are often perplexing to the patients and physicians. It may be mistaken for many other conditions particularly in the patients with cognitive impairment. These conditions include pleurisy, myocardial infarction, cholecystitis, appendicitis, renal colic, collapsed intervertebral disk, glaucoma, trigeminal neuralgia, or unappreciated trauma. One clue to the presence of zoster-induced pain is sensitive skin in the affected dermatome. The prodromal symptoms usually last a few days, although it has been reported to last weeks and even months.

The initial cutaneous presentation of herpes zoster is a unilateral red, maculopapular eruption, usually with vesicles, and most commonly involves the T1 to L2 or V1 dermatomes. Adjacent dermatomes frequently have a few vesicles. Because the vesicles contain VZV, people that have not been exposed can become infected. However individuals who have been exposed to VZV are not at risk for reacquiring disease nor are they at risk for activating latent virus. Typically, the vesicles crust over in 7 to 10 days and at that point the patient is no longer contagious. Most patients also experience pain in a dermatomal pattern caused by acute neuritis. This neuritis may be described as a burning, deep aching, tingling, itching, or stabbing that ranges from mild to severe in intensity. The vesicles may develop superinfections complicated by scaring and even septicemia. These disseminated complications are more frequent among immunocompromised hosts.

Between 10 and 15 percent of cases involve the ophthalmic division of the trigeminal nerve. This may present with impaired vision as a result of local inflammation and even cerebral vascular accident caused by granulomatous arteritis of the internal carotid artery. In 30 to 40 percent of cases of ophthalmic zoster there is involvement of the nasociliary branch, which also innervates the side and tip of the nose so symptoms on the nose should immediately lead to a thorough search for involvement of the eye. Complications of ophthalmic zoster include neurotrophic keratitis and chronic ulcerations. Secondary bacterial infections can cause panophthalmitis and enucleation. The stroke symptoms present as contralateral hemiplegia weeks to months after the episode of ophthalmic zoster. Arteriograms show segmental narrowing of cerebral arteries ipsilateral to the ophthalmic zoster. The mortality rate is reported to be 15 percent for the granulomatous arteritis.

Herpes zoster can affect the second and third division of cranial nerves and other cranial nerves. Lesions can involve the mouth, pharynx, and larynx. Seventh and eighth cranial nerve involvement or Ramsey Hunt syndrome, is characterized by facial palsy in combination with herpes zoster of the external ear or tympanic membrane. Symptoms include tinnitus, vertigo, deafness, problems with balance, and facial paresis. Motor paralysis may be seen in 1 to 5 percent of herpes zoster cases. It is a manifestation of destruction of motor neurons in the anterior horn or a motor radiculitis. The paralysis is seen within 2 weeks of the onset of herpes zoster and involves the muscle groups that are associated with the corresponding dermatome. Herpes zoster myelitis and meningoencephalitis are rare events. Although they usually follow the cutaneous presentation by 7 to 10 days, they may precede the rash by as much as 2 months. Most patients fully recover, but many have PHN and motor palsies.

PHN may occur in as many as 70 percent of patients older than age 80 years. The more severe the presentation of the herpes zoster, the more likely the development of PHN. Pain is described as constant burning, aching or throbbing, intermittent lancinating, and allodynic. Allodynia is particularly problematic. A cold wind, clothes, or bed sheets may cause debilitating pain. PHN is associated with depression, fatigue, sleep problems, and social isolation. Instrumental and basic activities of daily living may all be compromised by PHN. Although most people eventually have relief of pain, many are refractory to all treatments and some may get worse over time.

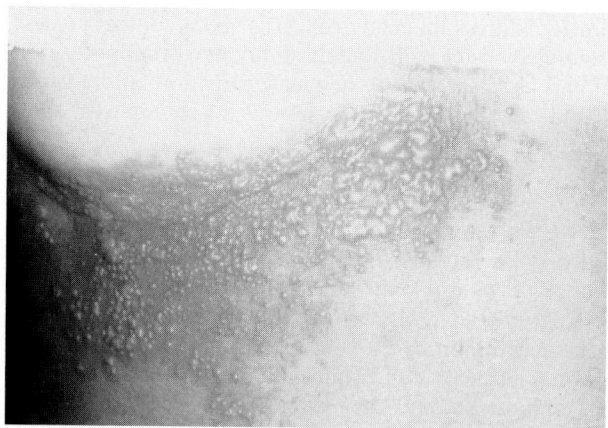

Figure 88-2   A patient with herpes zoster illustrates a range of lesions (e.g., large pustules, erythematous papules, and crusting).

noted above. Localized cutaneous sensory hyperesthesias or dysesthesias and lymphadenopathy are suggestive of a herpes zoster presentation. The absence of vesicle eruption is not reliable because patients may present with zoster sine herpete. During the rash phase, herpes simplex has the most similar presentation to herpes zoster. Evidence supporting herpes simplex includes a higher likelihood of presenting in a younger population, the multiple recurrences of lesions, and the absence of chronic pain. The lesions themselves are more difficult to distinguish, particularly when herpes simplex occurs in areas affected by herpes zoster.

Diagnostic testing is most helpful for differentiating herpes zoster from herpes simplex, for determining suspect organ involvement (particularly central nervous system), and for atypical presentations. The diagnostic tests include viral culture, immunofluorescent antigen (IFA) detection, polymerase chain reaction (PCR), and serology. VZV isolation in culture of vesicular fluid is the "gold standard," but it is slower than other tests and not very sensitive as only 30 to 60 percent of vesicle culture specimens are positive. VZV is almost never isolated from crusts in viral culture. VZV antigen detection by IFA tests of vesicle scrapings or tissue biopsies takes hours to get results and is both specific and sensitive. For these reasons, it is the most useful test when specimens are available. PCR is highly sensitive and specific and may be used to test crust or other unusual samples. Acute and convalescent VZV immunoglobulin (Ig) M and IgG levels may be useful in making a retrospective diagnosis when there are no peripheral lesions or specimens are inadequate. Tzanck smears suggest herpes zoster when multinucleated giant cells and intranuclear inclusions are seen on slides but this does not differentiate herpes zoster from herpes simplex.

EVALUATION

Herpes zoster is easily diagnosed when an elderly patient presents with the typical dermatomal vesicular rash and pain (Fig. 88-2). However, zoster's pain presentation before vesicle eruption may be mistaken for other causes as

MANAGEMENT

Herpes Zoster

The principle goal of the treatment of herpes zoster in the elderly is to decrease the length of the acute attack and to reduce or eliminate pain. Reassurance and education directly address the many concerns about contagiousness, prolonged zoster pain, and disability. Social support, mental and physical activity, adequate nutrition, and a caring attitude are important interventions for coping with a herpes zoster attack.

Antiviral Agents

The first-line of drug therapy is aimed at VZV. The guanosine analogs, acyclovir, famciclovir, and valaciclovir, are phosphorylated by viral thymidine kinase to a triphosphate form that inhibits VZV DNA polymerase and VZV replication. Valaciclovir and famciclovir are prodrugs and have greater bioavailability than acyclovir. The advantage for the prodrugs are the higher blood levels previously achieved by intravenous acyclovir and less frequent dosing schedule. Randomized controlled trials indicate that oral acyclovir (800 mg five times a day for 7 days), famciclovir (500 mg every 8 hours for 7 days), and valacyclovir (1 g three times a day for 7 days) reduce acute pain and the duration of chronic pain in elderly herpes zoster patients who are treated within 72 hours of rash onset. Fifteen to 30 percent of patients may have pain for more than 6 months, even if the receive timely antiviral treatment. Topical antiviral therapy is not an effective treatment. Ophthalmic zoster requires ophthalmologic consultation and oral antiviral therapy. The kidneys excrete these medications and the dose should be adjusted for renal insufficiency. They are safe and well tolerated among the elderly. The most common adverse effects are nausea, vomiting, diarrhea, and headache. The data from current clinical trials indicate that all three drugs are acceptable agents with factors other than efficacy determining the choice, such as cost and dosing schedule. The effectiveness of antiviral agents is doubtful if more than 72 hours have elapsed since the onset of rash, except perhaps for patients who have ophthalmic zoster or continue to have new vesicle formation.

Anti-inflammatory Drugs

There is some controversy over the use of corticosteroids. Randomized, controlled clinical trials demonstrate that corticosteroids do not prevent PHN when compared to placebo or acyclovir. However, one trial showed benefits in improvement in time to uninterrupted sleep, return to routine activities, and cessation of analgesic medications in patients with an average age of 60 years and no relative contraindications to corticosteroids. In the trial, prednisone was administered orally at 60 mg/d for days 1 to 7, 30 mg/d for days 8 to 14, and 15 mg/d for days 15 to 21. Corticosteroids are used to treat VZV-induced facial paralysis and cranial polyneuritis. Topical steroids are used to treat keratitis and uveitis, but there are no randomized studies that demonstrate their effectiveness. The most common adverse effects of corticosteroids are dyspepsia, nausea, vomiting, edema, and granulocytosis.

Topical Treatments

Cool compresses, calamine lotion, cornstarch, or baking soda may help to reduce local symptoms and speed the drying of the vesicles. When the vesicles have crusted over, a bland ointment or olive oil may help separate the adherent crusts. Occlusive ointments and topical steroids should be avoided.

Analgesics and Pain Management

Opioid and nonopioid analgesia are a standard of care for the acute pain syndrome. There is a tendency among many clinicians to undertreat the pain and to use opioid analgesia sparingly. The choice of medication depends upon the severity of pain and the response to the medication. There are good data to justify the use of opiates such as oxycodone to provide adequate pain relief. Assessment of appropriate analgesia should include the ability to sleep and manage routine activities, as well as to provide sufficient relief. Regional and local anesthesia blocks may be used if pain is poorly controlled with opioid analgesia. Uncontrolled severe acute pain is a risk factor for PHN. The effectiveness of well-managed opiates, gabapentin, and tricyclic antidepressants during the acute phase of herpes zoster in preventing or reducing PHN is not known.

Postherpetic Neuralgia

The treatment for PHN is more vexing because the pain may last from months to a year or more and be associated with a prolonged decline in activities and quality of life. Based on evidence of effectiveness from clinical trials, the current front-line treatments for PHN include topical lidocaine, tricyclic antidepressants, gabapentin, and opiates. Topical treatments include the lidocaine patch and EMLA (eutectic mixture of local anesthetics) cream. One or more patches may be applied over the affected area for 12 hours a day. EMLA is applied under an occlusive dressing. It may take up to 2 weeks for these treatments to reach full effectiveness. Systemic lidocaine toxicity has not been reported from these topical products. Capsaicin, trans-8-methyl-N-vanillyl-6-nonenamide, is an extract of hot chili peppers. It is known to deplete substance P, an endogenous neuropeptide that is involved in the transmission of nociceptive impulses from the sensory nerve endings to the central nervous system. Although this treatment can be effective, it takes days to deplete substance P, and many patients are unable to tolerate the burning it causes.

Tricyclic antidepressants modulate nerve transmission. They provide moderate to good pain relief in more than 50 percent of elderly patients with PHN. The preferred agents are nortriptyline and desipramine. Amitriptyline should be avoided because of its more prominent anticholinergic effects. Nortriptyline and desipramine medicines have fewer anticholinergic effects, resulting in less sedation, constipation, and risk for cognitive impairment and orthostatic hypotension. A dosing regimen of nortriptyline for PHN begins with 10 mg at night and increases the dose every 4 to 7 days by the same amount until reduction in pain or intolerable side effects. At least 4 weeks of therapy is required.

Gabapentin is a very popular treatment partly because a randomized study showed that 43 percent of patients had moderate or greater improvement in their pain as compared to 12 percent of placebo recipients. The dosing schedule in the trial was an initial dose of 300 mg and then titration over a 4-week period to 300 mg tid, 600 mg tid, 900 mg tid, and 1200 mg tid, or until intolerable adverse effects. Frail elderly patients often need small doses because of problems with tolerating higher doses. Doses should be adjusted for creatinine clearance. Adverse effects include somnolence, dizziness, and ataxia. Cognitive impairment is also seen in elderly patients.

There is a growing literature and clinical experience that indicates that PHN pain is opiate responsive in a subset of patients, which supports the use of opiate analgesia for PHN. For example, in a randomized, crossover trial showing significant pain relief with oxycodone, 67 percent of patients expressed masked preference for oxycodone, as compared to 11 percent of placebo recipients. Although oxycodone is an effective treatment, equianalgesic doses of other opiates are likely to be as effective. The most frequently reported adverse effects were constipation, nausea, and sedation.

PREVENTION

The live, attenuated varicella vaccine is safe and effective in preventing varicella and is currently licensed for use in the United States. The Centers for Disease Control reported that varicella incidence declined by approximately 80 percent when compared to prevaccination incidence rates in varicella surveillance areas in the year 2000, with the greatest decline among children 1 to 4 years of age. Vaccine uptake among children aged 19 to 35 months in the United States was 67 percent in 2000, and many states now mandate the vaccine for school entry. These remarkable results indicate that the varicella vaccine is having a dramatic impact on the epidemiology of varicella in the United States. The effect of widespread use of the varicella vaccine and primary prevention of varicella on the incidence and natural history of herpes zoster will not be known for years. However, millions of latently infected older adults are at risk for herpes zoster for the foreseeable future. A more potent formulation of the varicella-zoster vaccine than the currently licensed vaccine does boost cellular immunity to VZV in the elderly person and is well tolerated. A randomized, double-blind, placebo-controlled Veterans Affairs Cooperative Studies Program trial is in progress in the United States to evaluate the effects of the stronger formulation of the vaccine on herpes zoster and PHN in the elderly population.

REFERENCES

Dworkin RH, Portenoy RK. Pain and its persistence in herpes zoster. *Pain* 67:241, 1996.

Dworkin RH, Schmader KE: The epidemiology and natural history of herpes zoster and postherpetic neuralgia, in Watson CPN, Gershon AA (eds): *Herpes Zoster and Postherpetic Neuralgia,* 2nd ed. Amsterdam, Elsevier, 2001, p 51.

Esmann V et al: Prednisolone does not prevent postherpetic neuralgia. *Lancet* 2:126, 1987.

Galer BS et al: Topical lidocaine patch relieves postherpetic neuralgia more effectively than a vehicle topical patch: Results of an enriched enrollment study. *Pain* 80:533, 1999.

Gilden DH et al: Varicella-zoster virus reactivation without rash. *J Infect Dis* 166(Suppl 1):S30, 1992.

Hardy IB et al: The incidence of zoster after immunization with live attenuated varicella vaccine: A study in children with leukemia. *N Engl J Med* 325:1545, 1991.

Hope-Simpson RE: Postherpetic neuralgia. *J Royal Coll Gen Pract* 25:571, 1975.

Hope-Simpson RE: The nature of herpes zoster: A long-term study and new hypothesis. *Proc Royal Soc Med (London)* 58:9, 1965.

Kanazi GE et al: Treatment of postherpetic neuralgia. An update. *Drugs* 59:1113, 2000.

Oxman MN: Immunization to reduce the frequency and severity of herpes zoster and its complications. *Neurology* 45:S41, 1995.

Rowbotham M et al: Gabapentin for the treatment of postherpetic neuralgia: A randomized controlled trial. *JAMA* 280:1837, 1998.

Schmader KE: Herpes zoster in older adults. *Clin Infect Dis* 32(10):1481, 2001.

Straus S et al: Varicella and herpes zoster, in Freedberg IM et al. (eds): *Fitzpatrick's Dermatology in General Medicine,* 6th ed. New York, McGraw-Hill, 2003, in press.

Watson CPN, Babul N: Efficacy of oxycodone in neuropathic pain: A randomized trial in postherpetic neuralgia. *Neurology* 50:1837, 1998.

Whitley RJ et al: Acyclovir with and without prednisone for the treatment of herpes zoster: A randomized, placebo-controlled trial. *Ann Intern Med* 125:376, 1996.

Wood MJ et al: Oral acyclovir therapy accelerates pain resolution in patients with herpes zoster: A meta-analysis of placebo-controlled trials. *Clin Infect Dis* 22:341, 1996.

Wood MJ et al: A randomized trial of acyclovir for 7 days or 21 days with and without prednisolone for treatment of acute herpes zoster. *N Engl J Med* 330:896, 1994.

PART IV

CROSS CUTTING DOMAINS

S E C T I O N   A

NUTRITION

C H A P T E R   9 0

NUTRITION AND AGING

DENNIS H. SULLIVAN • LARRY E. JOHNSON

Throughout life, nutrition is an important determinant of health, physical and cognitive function, vitality, overall quality of life, and longevity. The quantity and variety of available foods, as well as the meaningfulness of the social interactions provided by meals, are important to psychological well-being. The composition of the diet and the amount of food consumed are strongly linked to physiologic function. When a well-balanced diet is not maintained, malnutrition may develop, with consequent detrimental effects on health and well-being.

Malnutrition can have many manifestations. As outlined in Chapter 92, a diet that is deficient in one or more of the required nutrients (e.g., calories, protein, minerals, fiber, or vitamins) can lead to a state of nutritional deficiency. The greater the magnitude and duration of nutritional deprivation and the more fragile the individual, the more likely the occurrence of noticeable body compositional changes, functional impairments, or overt disease caused by nutritional deficits. Even borderline dietary deficiencies can have important health consequences, such as producing subtle organ system impairments, causing diminished vitality, or increasing an individual's susceptibility to disease. Protein and protein-energy undernutrition are two of the most common, frequently unrecognized, and potentially serious forms of nutritional deficiency. The prevalence of these conditions is particularly high in chronically ill older individuals and in those in hospitals, nursing homes, and other institutional settings. Although there is a complex interrelationship among nutrition, disease, and clinical outcome, protein and protein-energy undernutrition appears to be a significant contributor to disease-related morbidity and mortality in these populations. At the other end of the spectrum, the persistent consumption of excess quantities of one or more nutrients can have similar untoward consequences. Forms of malnutrition that result from excess consumption include hypervitaminosis and obesity. Studies indicate that obesity is the most common nutritional disorder of advanced age in western societies, with a high prevalence among noninstitutionalized free-living elderly people. Many obese older individuals have other nutritional disorders as well. In chronically ill or functionally debilitated obese older people, protein undernutrition is a common, serious, and frequently unrecognized problem that can develop for many reasons including an imbalanced diet, disease, and inactivity.

Recognizing and maintaining an optimally balanced diet is an important challenge, particularly as people age. The challenge is particularly great for older people who already are malnourished, especially if they have a nutritional disorder that developed earlier in life such as obesity, osteoporosis, or protein undernutrition. Even healthy individuals often fail to maintain an optimal diet because of a lack of knowledge, resources, or will power. The process of aging can introduce other factors, including acute and chronic disease, physical disabilities, social isolation, the use of multiple medications, depression, impaired cognitive ability, and dysregulation of appetite control, that can contribute further to poor eating habits and to the development or exacerbation of nutritional disorders. In turn, inappropriate dietary intake and poor nutritional status can impact the progression of many acute and chronic diseases such as coronary heart disease, cancer, stroke, diabetes, and osteoporosis, which are among the 10 leading causes of death in the United States. The 1988 Surgeon General's Report on Nutrition and Health noted that two-thirds of all deaths in the United States are due to diseases associated with poor diets and dietary habits.

Assessing the quality of the diet of elderly persons is critical to addressing issues relevant to their health and nutritional status. Such an assessment must be based on knowledge of what constitutes a balanced diet for a given individual. The goal of this chapter is to identify an approach to nutrition evaluation and management that takes into account the unique needs, limitations, and desires of each elderly individual. The chapter starts out by examining the interrelationship among nutrition, activity, disease burden, and health outcomes and then focuses on age-related changes in body composition, lifestyle, and appetite regulation that affect nutritional status and nutrient requirements. Also included is a discussion of specific dietary considerations related to optimal health requirements.

THE INTERRELATIONSHIP AMONG NUTRITION, ACTIVITY, AND DISEASE

Although nutrition is a vital component of good health, it cannot be evaluated in isolation. The relationship between nutrient intake and health is influenced by other factors, most notably activity level, disease burden, and advancing age. A basic understanding of these interrelationships is essential in order to assess the potential benefits and limitations of nutritional interventions.

Nutrition—Activity Interrelationship

Nutrition and physical activity are closely linked, each having vitally important interacting effects on body composition, functional ability, and well-being. The balance between nutrient intake and physical activity is particularly important in determining muscle mass and strength, body fat content and distribution, and bone density and resilience. To preserve existing muscle mass and strength, it is necessary to maintain both an adequate level of physical activity and a balanced diet that includes sufficient protein, energy, vitamins, and minerals to meet metabolic demands and prevent a negative nitrogen balance (as discussed in detail below). It is not known precisely what level of physical activity is needed to prevent the loss of existing muscle mass and strength in older adults. However, studies indicate that even a few weeks of bed rest or a similar degree of activity restriction can result in a noticeable loss of muscle mass, strength, and function even when the diet is adequate and the individual is otherwise healthy. Whereas the combination of inadequate diet and inactivity can result in an accelerated loss of muscle, overfeeding does not prevent muscle atrophy associated with inactivity and may exacerbate the functional consequences because the excess nutrients are converted to fat.

To increase muscle strength, size, or endurance, the average daily level of exertion has to increase significantly. Aerobic exercises are most effective in improving the oxidative capacity of muscles and are the mainstay of endurance training. High-intensity progressive resistance training, such as weight lifting, is needed to build strength and mass. Nutrition alone is not an effective method of restoring muscle mass or improving strength or endurance in frail older individuals who have experienced a recent loss of weight. Efforts at repletion should focus on increasing both nutrient intake and exercise. Studies on healthy elderly men suggest that the combination of progressive resistance muscle strength training and a high-protein diet (containing up to 1.6 g of protein per kilogram of body weight per day [g/kg/d]) may be the most effective method of improving muscle mass.

Exercise can have an important effect on body fat content and distribution. In obese older individuals, it can play a synergistic role with caloric restriction in promoting weight loss and preventing further weight gain. With weight loss, visceral fat is mobilized at a rate two to five times that for other fat stores. Even when total body weight does not change, exercise can induce a significant decrease in intra-abdominal fat in both obese and nonobese individuals. The preferential mobilization of fat stores has important metabolic implications for the prevention and treatment of the insulin resistance syndrome because it is predominantly excess visceral fat that is associated with the derangements of dyslipidemia, elevated fibrinogen, hyperinsulinemia, and hypertension.

Exercise and nutrition also play a critical role in the maintenance of optimal bone density and strength. As discussed in Chapter 75, the nutrient needs of bone include the correct balance of protein and energy and an adequate intake of vitamins and minerals, especially vitamin D and calcium. The amount of exercise needed for optimal bone health has not been defined. However, it is known that people who exercise regularly have higher bone density than more sedentary age-, race-, and gender-matched controls. Randomized controlled trials involving postmenopausal women demonstrated that those assigned to progressive resistance muscle strength training or weight-loading aerobic exercise programs attained a 1 percent to 1.6 percent greater bone mineral density in both the lumbar spine and femoral neck regions per year compared to the controls. It is also known that bed rest and weightlessness are associated with a rapid decline in bone mineral density. Consequently, osteopenia can develop despite an optimal diet if exercise or other weight-bearing activities are not adequate. Because of its apparent beneficial effects on bone mineral density, exercise should be combined with an appropriate diet for both the prevention and treatment of osteoporosis and fracture-related disabilities.

Having both direct and indirect effects on numerous metabolic processes within muscle, bone, and adipose tissues, exercise has a major impact on how nutrients are utilized by the body during health and illness. By inducing an increase in the mass and metabolic capacity of muscle, exercise affects energy expenditure, glucose metabolism, and the size of protein reserves in a manner that counteracts some of the effects of aging and thus has important nutritional implications for individuals as they grow older. Total energy expenditure (TEE) is the sum of basal energy expenditure, postprandial thermogenesis, and energy expenditure of activity (EEA). Muscle not only represents the primary source of energy expenditure during physical activity but is also the primary contributor to basal energy expenditure, which may be 50 percent to 80 percent of TEE. With advancing age, there is a parallel decline in muscle mass and in both basal and daily TEE that may be partially or fully accounted for by the fact that people tend to become more sedentary as they grow older. A study involving master athletes demonstrated that men who maintained a vigorous weekly routine of weight training throughout their lives had muscle mass and energy capacity comparable to that of healthy 30-year-old males. Older men who do not exercise have significantly less muscle mass than their younger counterparts.

Exercise-induced increases in muscle size or protein content result in greater body protein reserves, which can be critical to survival during the episodes of nutritional deprivation that usually accompany profound physiologic stress such as that caused by trauma, sepsis, or other acute disease. Such acute physiologic insults trigger an acute inflammatory response that causes ketogenesis to be suppressed, leaving glucose as the primary energy source available to the body. The problem is invariably compounded by the reduced nutrient intake resulting from anorexia and gastrointestinal tract dysfunction induced by the inflammatory response. With the nutrient intake suppressed, gluconeogenesis becomes the predominant source of glucose. Because the primary substrate for gluconeogenesis is provided by the catabolism of skeletal muscle, lean body mass becomes an important determinant of survival. Once the lean body mass falls below a critical level, the chance of surviving a serious acute illness diminishes dramatically. Studies conducted in the Warsaw Ghetto, hospital intensive care units, and other settings suggest that a loss of more than 40 percent of baseline lean mass is incompatible with life. Other studies indicate that very few healthy people have a lean body mass less than 70 percent of the mean value for adults aged 20 to 30 years.

In addition to inducing muscle hypertrophy, exercise also affects insulin sensitivity, glucose disposal, and high-density lipoprotein (HDL) levels directly, and plays a synergistic role with diet in maintaining a healthy weight and a sense of well-being. These effects of exercise can be important adjuncts to good nutrition in the prevention and treatment of hypertension, diabetes, dyslipidemia, and osteoporosis.

Nutrition–Disease Interrelationship

There is a complex interrelationship among nutrition, health status, and clinical outcomes. Although a full discussion of this topic is beyond the scope of this chapter, it is important to emphasize several key points. Nutrient requirements and the ability to metabolize select nutrients are influenced by many disease states. In addition, many diseases compromise the ability of older individuals to consume adequate amounts of all nutrients. This can be caused by a number of mechanisms including disease-induced suppression of appetite, alteration of the normal swallowing mechanism, maldigestion or malabsorption, and a loss of self-feeding ability. Because these potentially deleterious effects of disease can be difficult to predict, older individuals with one or more acute or chronic health problems should have frequent reassessments of their nutritional status and their nutritional care plan revised as necessary.

AGE-RELATED CHANGES THAT AFFECT NUTRITION

Changes in Body Composition

With advancing age, there are significant changes in body composition that affect the nutritional needs of an individual. According to data obtained primarily from cross-sectional studies, weight increases steadily in most people from age 30 to 60 years. An increase in total body fat accounts for a majority of this weight gain. After age 60, weight usually stabilizes and then begins to decline. The improved survival of nonobese individuals during middle age and cohort effects may account for some of the decline in weight with age reported in cross-sectional studies. However, weight maintenance becomes increasingly difficult in the advanced years of life. The incidence as well as the potential causes of weight loss increase with age, particularly beyond age 75.

Regardless of whether or not weight changes, advancing age is characterized by a progressive loss of lean body mass, a relative increase in fat mass, and a redistribution of fat from peripheral to central locations within the body. Data from cross-sectional studies indicate that all these changes begin in the third decade and increase at an accelerated rate after age 65. This late accelerated phase may be a threshold effect brought about by the loss of lean body mass and the increased prevalence of chronic disease in old age. The loss of lean body mass consists predominantly of skeletal muscle, particularly type II or fast-twitch fibers. Central lean body mass, such as the liver and other splanchnic organs, is relatively preserved. Some studies indicate that muscle mass may decline by up to 45 percent between the third and eighth decades of life (Figures 90-1 and 90-2). The few longitudinal studies that have been reported indicate that the loss of muscle mass with age may be greater in men than in women; however, this remains controversial.

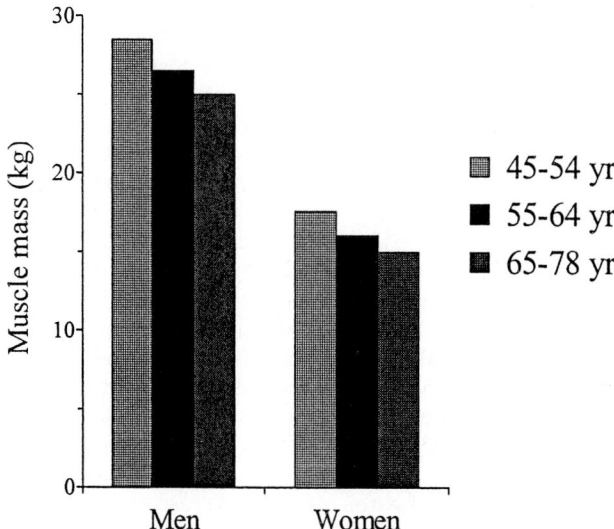

Figure 90-1 Declining muscle mass with increasing age. Reproduced by with permission from Frontera WR, Hughes VA et al: A cross-sectional study of muscle strength and mass in 45- to 78-yr-old men and women. *J Appl Physiol* 71:644, 1991.

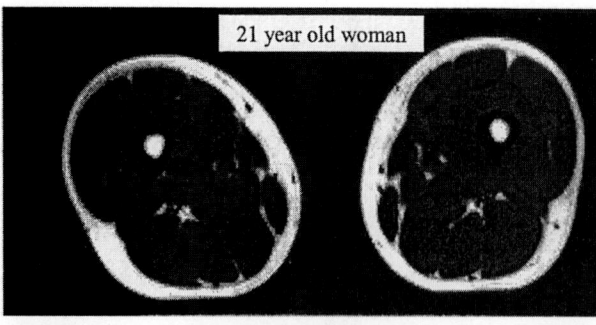

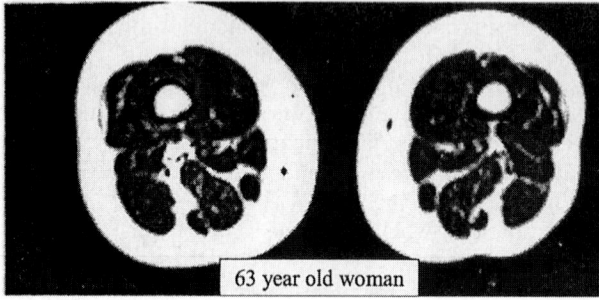

Figure 90-2 Cross-sectional computed tomography images of the midthighs of a younger and an older woman demonstrating the decline in muscle mass and relative increase in fat mass with age.

The loss of muscle mass with age appears to be the result of multiple interrelated factors including age-related changes in metabolism, function, or structure of organ tissues; disease; and the behavior and lifestyle choices of the individual. Notable age-related changes that appear to contribute to a loss of muscle include a progressive loss of alpha motor units in the spinal column, a diminution in the intrinsic muscle protein synthetic capacity, and a decline in the production of multiple hormones including testosterone, estrogen, and insulin-like growth factors. Other age-related changes detrimental to muscle include the increased production and delayed inactivation of catabolic mediators and a change in liver protein metabolism that may decrease the availability of amino acids to axial muscles. The decrease in nutrient consumption and the decline in activity level that often accompany advanced age are possibly modifiable contributors to the loss of muscle mass. Many diseases accelerate the age-related decline, particularly degenerative diseases of the central nervous system and those affecting any part of the motor pathway. An accelerated loss of muscle mass can occur when a serious illness is accompanied by low nutrient intake and the need for prolonged bed rest. In all individuals, the loss of muscle mass with age is closely linked with a reduction in muscle strength and exercise capacity, a decline in one causing further loss of the other. When exercise capacity falls below that required to comfortably perform the basic activities of daily living, physical activity often becomes very limited, causing a rapid acceleration of the downward spiral. The loss of muscle mass and exercise capacity is also linked to the development of coronary artery disease, diabetes, and other diseases that contribute further to the decline.

Parallel with the loss of lean body mass, there is an increase in the relative amount and distribution of body fat with advancing age. Between the second and ninth decades of life, the percentage of body weight that is fat increases by 35 percent to 50 percent in females and to an even greater extent in males. In one cross-sectional study of 500 healthy individuals between the ages of 18 and 85 years, fat mass as a percentage of body weight increased across the age range of the sample from 33 percent to 44 percent in females and from 18 percent to 36 percent in males. Whether or not the total body weight changes, intra-abdominal (visceral) fat increases quantitatively and proportionally more than peripheral fat mass. In females, the accumulation of intra-abdominal fat accelerates at menopause and represents primarily a shift from peripheral sites. In males, the increase in intra-abdominal fat with age represents primarily an increase in total body fat mass.

Numerous factors have been cited as potential contributors to the changes in adipose tissues with advancing age. Some studies suggest that much of this change can be accounted for by the reduction in both the quantity and oxidative capacity of skeletal muscle that also occurs at the same time. With advancing age, fat oxidation is reduced at rest, following a meal, and during exercise. This reduced rate of fat metabolism with age promotes the accumulation of fat at both peripheral and central locations. The decline in total skeletal muscle mass that occurs with age correlates with, and may be responsible for, the decreased rate of metabolism of fat at rest. Likewise, the decline in the maximal oxidative capacity of muscle may cause the reduction in fat metabolism with exercise. The decline in physical activity resulting from the loss of muscle with age contributes to the increase in intra-abdominal fat. Other factors that may also contribute to the increase in intra-abdominal fat with age include declining testosterone levels in men, estrogen withdrawal or increased testosterone levels in females, the decline in growth hormone levels, increased resistance to leptin, and the increased secretion of cortisol in both genders. Studies indicate that subjects with abdominal obesity tend to secrete greater quantities of cortisol in response to small psychosocial stressors than do controls. This exaggerated stress response appears to contribute to the development of central obesity through the actions of cortisol.

Changes in Appetite and Energy Intake Regulation

Maintenance of a stable weight requires a steady balance between nutrient intake and energy expenditure. With advancing age, the metabolic, neural, and humoral pathways that normally maintain this delicate balance by regulating appetite and hunger begin to lose their compensatory responsiveness to changes in energy demands. Psychological, socioeconomic, and cultural influences and numerous disease processes further contribute to the dysregulation. From the third to seventh decade of life, these factors integrate to create an imbalance usually favoring a tendency toward weight gain and increased fat deposition, at least in societies where food is plentiful and the physical demands of life are light. However, after age 70, the risk of losing weight increases steadily with each year of survival. This observation correlates with findings from numerous studies indicating that low dietary energy intake is common in both healthy and frail elderly people.

factors that influence their serum concentration. More details regarding the interpretation of laboratory tests in nutritional assessment are provided in Chapter 92.

Assessment of Nutrient Intake

Although frequently difficult to obtain, a detailed nutrient intake assessment is often the most critically needed part of a nutritional assessment. In the outpatient setting, where both over- and undernutrition may be a concern, a 24-hour recall or a 3-day food intake diary can be an effective tool for estimating nutrient intake and identifying where dietary modifications are needed, especially if a dietitian or a comparably skilled health care provider gives the patient and the family adequate instructions on how to collect the needed data. The employment of more accurate methods of measuring nutrient intake is often necessary within hospitals and nursing homes. Several recent studies demonstrate that many older patients are maintained throughout their hospitalization on nutrient intakes that are far less than their estimated maintenance energy requirements. Contributing to the problem, the attending health care team often overestimates how much food an older patient is consuming. In one study, more than 20 percent of nonterminally ill older hospitalized patients had an average daily nutrient intake that was less than 50 percent of their maintenance energy requirements. This lack of adequate nutrient intake was associated with a significant deterioration in their protein-energy nutritional status by discharge and a sevenfold increased risk for mortality. Low nutrient intake may be an even more widespread problem within nursing homes. Only by carefully monitoring each older individual's nutrient intake during their institutional stay can this problem be avoided.

REFERENCES

1. Campbell WW, Crim MC et al: Increased protein requirements in elderly people: New data and retrospective reassessments. *Am J Clin Nutr* 60:501, 1994.
2. Ewing JA: Detecting alcoholism: The CAGE questionnaire. *JAMA* 252:1905, 1984.
3. Frontera WR, Hughes VA et al: A cross-sectional study of muscle strength and mass in 45- to 78-yr-old men and women. *J Appl Physiol* 71:644, 1991.
4. Jula A, Marniemi J et al: Effects of diet and simvastatin on serum lipids, insulin, and antioxidants in hypercholesterolemic men: A randomized controlled trial. *JAMA* 287:598, 2002.
5. McGee M, Jensen GL: Nutrition in the elderly. *J Clin Gastroenterol* 30:372, 2000.
6. National Research Council. *Recommended Dietary Allowances*, 10th ed. Washington, DC, National Academy Press, 1989.
7. Roberts SB, Fuss P et al: Control of food intake in older men. *JAMA* 272:1601, 1994.
8. Roubenoff R. Sarcopenia and its implications for the elderly. *Eur J Clin Nutr* 54(suppl 3):S40, 2000.
9. Schatzkin A, Lanza E et al: Lack of effect of a low-fat, high-fiber diet on the recurrance of colorectal adenomas. Polyp Prevention Trial Study Group. *N Engl J Med* 342:1149, 2000.
10. Schiffman SS, Graham BG. Taste and smell perception affect appetite and immunity in the elderly. *Eur J Clin Nutr* 54(suppl 3):S54, 2000.
11. Starling RD, Poehlman ET. Assessment of energy requirements in elderly populations. *Eur J Clin Nutr* 54(suppl 3):S104, 2000.
12. Sullivan DH: What do the serum proteins tell us about our elderly patients? *J Gerontal Med Sci* 56A(2):M71, 2001.
13. World Health Organization/Food and Agriculture Organization/ Energy and protein requirements. *WHO Tech Rep Ser* 724:1, 1985.
14. Willett WC, Stampfer MJ: Clinical pratice. What vitamins should I be taking, doctor? *N Engl J Med* 345:1819, 2001.

Weight and Age: Paradoxes and Conundrums

TAMARA B. HARRIS

The evaluation of weight in an older person is representative of the challenges of geriatric medicine, requiring integration of information on normative biologic change with age and past individual health behaviors to assess future risk. Although weight is one of the easiest clinical measures to obtain, interpretation of weight in the geriatric patient and assessment of the need for intervention on weight is far more difficult. This chapter provides a rationale and recommendations for an approach to weight in older patients.

SHOULD THE HEALTH PRACTITIONER BE CONCERNED ABOUT WEIGHT IN AN OLDER PATIENT?

From both a practical and theoretical viewpoint, body weight is an important contributor to health in old age. However, health practitioners are often skeptical about evaluating weight in older patients because it seems unlikely this evaluation will change clinical treatment, except in the event of clear-cut weight loss. In fact, the health practitioner caring for older patients is already concerned with issues related to weight. Clinically, weight stability is used as a sign of general health status. Many of the health conditions requiring chronic care are weight-related, even in the frail elderly person. Weight is a contributor to the most problematic areas in geriatric medicine, particularly comorbidity contributing to hospitalization and physical and cognitive decline, and resulting health care costs. With development of new drugs for symptomatic relief of weight-related conditions such as osteoarthritis and with extension to older persons of established preventive treatments for hypertension and hyperlipidemia, polypharmacy is increasingly a weight-related health issue as well. Caring for older patients involves dealing with weight-related issues on a daily basis, even if not explicitly recognized as such.

Apart from weight-related diseases, change in body composition with age, particularly the loss of muscle and bone and the increase in fat, may independently contribute to decline in functional status and loss of independence.

Osteoporosis is an important risk factor for fracture. The loss of muscle with age, termed sarcopenia, is hypothesized to contribute to disability. The increase in fat mass with age may contribute as well. Adipose tissue is now known to produce multiple endocrine factors, including proinflammatory cytokines such as interleukin-6 (IL-6). IL-6 has been shown to be associated with body fat, independent of weight-associated health conditions, and is also an independent risk factor for physical disability and death. Thus even accounting for body weight, change in body composition with age may independently contribute to risk.

Lastly, research in the biology of aging has shown caloric restriction to be the only intervention that consistently promotes longevity in laboratory animals, even when restriction is instituted in adult life. Restricted animals are thinner and weigh less, reflecting their lower calorie intake, but lower weight alone does not explain the protection from disease and the survival advantage. Caloric restriction studies of nonhuman primates suggest regulation of insulin and energy metabolism may be critical, but the underlying mechanism is unknown. Nonetheless, these studies suggest lower body weight mediates fundamental physiologic change associated with health and longevity.

LIFETIME WEIGHT HISTORY: CURRENT WEIGHT AND RECENT WEIGHT CHANGE AREN'T ENOUGH

Only a small proportion of people, probably less than 10 percent of the population, remain approximately at the same weight over their lifetime. As a result, the clinician cannot assume the current weight is representative of a life-long pattern. Although weight tends to fluctuate very little day-to-day, longitudinal studies show that for most people, weight increases gradually with age, peaking in the seventh decade, and then declines. However, there is a great deal of variation in the timing of the peak weight and the decline. Risk of disease, disability and mortality in old age has been associated with change in weight from early adult

Lifetime Weight Patterns Based on Percentile Distributions in 3,611 Japanese-American Men

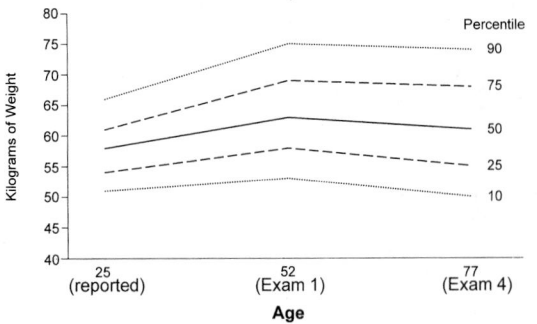

Figure 91-1 Lifetime weight patterns based on percentile distributions in 3611 Japanese American men from the Honolulu Heart Study cohort. Weight was measured at examination 1 (1965–1968) and at examination 4 (1992–1994); weight at age 25 years was reported at examination 1.

weight (age 25 years) or from midlife, and with the difference between maximum and minimum weight. In addition to current weight and recent weight change over the prior 6 months, these four weights constitute a reasonable weight history.

Data from Japanese American men participating in the Honolulu Heart Program, a lean and long-lived cohort, indicate the average pattern of weight change with age to be a steady increase from young adulthood to a plateau in late middle age with a decline in old age (Fig. 91-1). However, the average disguises the heterogeneity in this

Lifetime Weight Patterns Based on 5% Weight Change in 3,611 Japanese-American Men
(Means within groups)

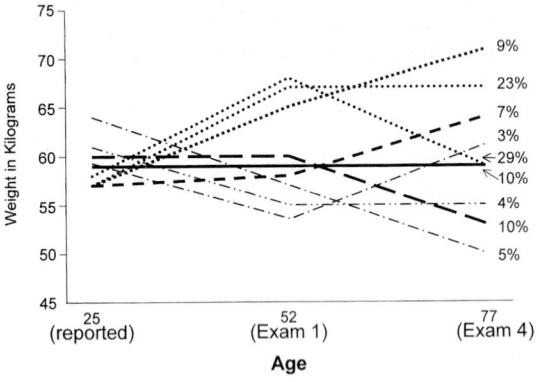

Figure 91-2 Weight patterns across the lifetime from age 25 years to old age based on 3611 Japanese American men in the Honolulu Heart Study cohort. Each *line* represents one of nine weight patterns over the lifetime, with the percentages on the *right side* of the figure indicating the frequency of each pattern. These patterns were determined by using weight at examination 1 as the base; the position of the line for age 25 years and examination 4 was based on whether weight at that time was less than, greater than, or within 5 percent of weight at examination 1. Ten percent of the men (*solid line*) were within 5 percent of their mean weight at examination 1 on reported weight at age 25 years and at examination 4. Twenty-nine percent had gained 5 percent or more from age 25 years and then lost at least that much, whereas 23 percent had gained 5 percent or more from age 25 years and maintained that weight.

pattern as subgroups continue to gain and lose weight over the entire lifetime (Fig. 91-2). Longitudinal studies of weight from middle age to old age show that thinner older people were often heavier earlier in life. Conversely, among heavier older people, many have gained weight since middle age (Fig. 91-3).

The most important determinants of change in weight over the lifetime are likely to be behavioral, particularly related to physical activity and caloric intake. Only a small proportion of the US population engages in regular exercise. This lack of exercise, coupled with a small average increase in caloric intake, leads to the deposition of extra body weight over time (as little as a 1% excess caloric intake over expenditure daily for a year would result in an increase of approximately 2.5 pounds in that year). Weight gain with age may be linked to changes in lifestyle, such as becoming less physically active or quitting smoking. Controlled feeding studies in older and younger men suggest that appetite in the old may be relatively insensitive to imbalance between calories and energy output.

Weight loss is associated with a diverse set of factors including depression, cancer, pulmonary disease, and inflammatory arthritides. Weight loss may also be associated with diseases thought of as associated with overweight, including diabetes, coronary heart disease, and stroke, all of which may have a wasting phase. Stressful life events, such as care giving or deaths of significant others, may also play a role in either weight gain or loss. Periods of weight loss are important also as accelerators of loss in lean mass. The issue of weight loss in older people is reviewed in greater depth in Chap. 90 and in Chap. 92

FAT AS A FACTOR IN THE AGED BODY

Even if weight is maintained constant over life, the body becomes relatively fatter with age, with increases in total fat and losses in lean mass and bone. Fat redistributes centrally with growth of the visceral fat compartment reflected as an increase in waist circumference. In many tissues, including in muscle and bone marrow, there is a gradual replacement of tissue by fat. At any weight then, older people will have relatively more fat, less muscle, and less bone than will younger people.

Gain in weight and increases in body fat are associated with metabolic and physiologic alterations that affect health and level of physical function. Cardiovascular risk factors of blood pressure, lipids, and glucose reflect increased weight and fat. Higher levels of intraabdominal fat are associated with insulin resistance, which may cause metabolic abnormalities even in the absence of overt overweight. Intramuscular fat may also contribute to these metabolic abnormalities.

Fat may also play an important role in promotion of inflammation and health-related effects. Until recently, fat was regarded primarily as an energy storage tissue primarily active in production of sex-steroids and glucocorticoid metabolism. It is now known that adipocytes actively produce and secrete a number of hormones and proteins, termed *adipokines*, which may have both local and systemic effects. These factors include leptin, angiotensin, resistin, adiponectin, plasminogen-activator inhibitor 1, and the

Weight Pattern Groups within Tertiles of BMI at Exam 4
(Japanese-American Men)

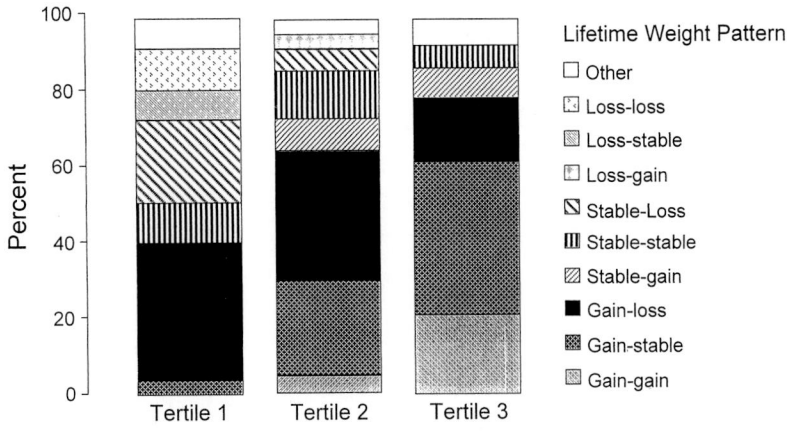

Figure 91-3 The weight patterns across the lifetime from Figure 91-2 are shown within each tertile of the population based on increasing body mass index as measured in old age at examination 4. The legend refers to the type of change between reported weight at age 25 years and measured weight at examination 1 and change between measured weight at examinations 1 and 4. Men in the lowest third of body mass index in old age had lost weight (the most common patterns are gain-loss and stable-loss), whereas men in the highest third of body mass index had generally gained weight over time (the most common patterns are gain-gain and gain-stable).

cytokines IL-6 and tumor necrosis factor-α. Many of these substances have been associated with cardiovascular morbidity, disability or risk of mortality. As the importance of these and other newly identified molecular metabolic regulators is identified for obesity, we may come to understand more about physiologic function in old age. For instance, leptin is highly correlated with body fat even in old age, and was thought to primarily regulate fat mass. Leptin may also play a role in the regulation of bone metabolism and in the vascular system.

An imbalance between calories and activity is not the complete explanation for body composition changes with age. Even master athletes who maintain a high level of physical activity tend to lose muscle mass with age, albeit at a slower pace than inactive people. On the other hand, resistance training can increase strength and muscle mass even in very old age, suggesting that the loss of muscle mass may be partially reversible and mediated to some extent by biomechanical or neurohumoral factors. Hormone changes with age affecting estrogen, testosterone, and growth

NHANES III – Race-adjusted BMI Categories for Males

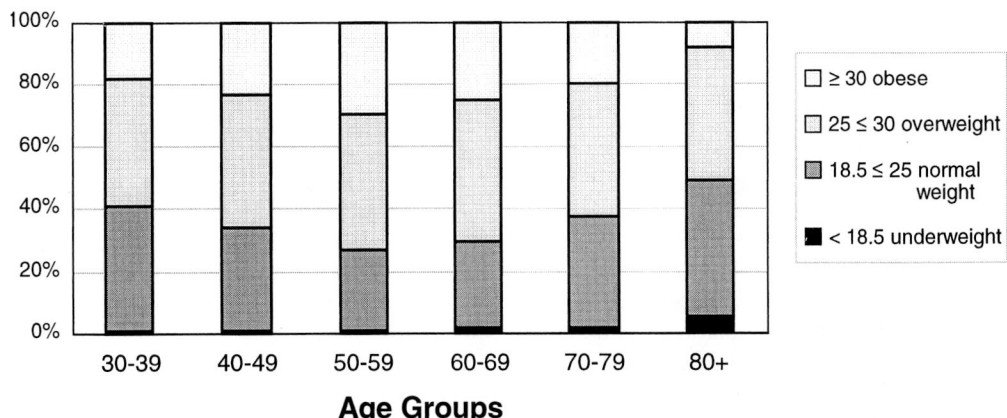

Figure 91-4 Data for body mass index (BMI) categories for noninstitutionalized US males aged 30 years and older from the National Health and Nutrition Examination Survey (NHANES) III. With age, the proportion obese (BMI greater or equal to 30) increases and then decreases in old age, while the proportion in the normal weight category follows an opposite pattern, decreasing to middle age and then increasing with age. Of those aged 80 years or older, 5% are underweight and 8% are obese.

NHANES III – Race-adjusted BMI Categories for Females

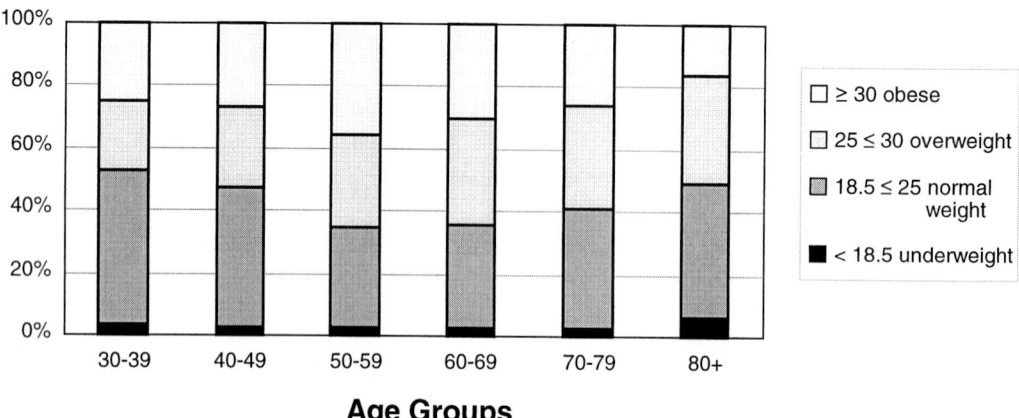

Figure 91-5 Data for body mass index (BMI) categories for noninstitutionalized US females aged 30 years and older from the National Health and Nutrition Examination Survey (NHANES) III. With age, the proportion obese (BMI greater or equal to 30) increases into middle age. The proportion in the normal weight category decreases into middle age and then increases again in old age. Of those aged 80 years or older, 6% are underweight and 16% are obese.

hormone are often cited as principal contributors to change in body composition. Genetic factors likely contribute to body composition and change with age, interacting with behavioral factors even late in life. For instance, although sarcopenia is common in old age, both men and women with preserved muscle mass and little infiltrating fat can be identified, representing a spectrum of genetic predisposition to muscle loss with age. Cigarette smoking also affects weight and body composition. Smokers are generally thinner, as smoking is associated with increased metabolic rate coupled with decreased appetite; smokers tend to gain weight when they stop smoking. Paradoxically, current smokers have relatively higher waist

circumferences, which indicates preferential deposition of intraabdominal fat.

STANDARDS FOR OVERWEIGHT AND OBESITY: RIGHT FOR OLDER PATIENTS?

Current guidelines define overweight as a body mass index (weight in kilograms divided by height in meters squared) of 25 kg/m² or more and obesity as a body mass index of 30 kg/m² or more. Normal weight extends to a body mass index of 20 kg/m².

Overweight by these standards is common in both men and women, even in older people (Figs. 91-4 and 91-5). Earlier data, using a slightly different cutpoint, show that the prevalence of obesity in old age is increasing over time, especially in men (Figs. 91-6, 91-7), reflecting changes in the US population.

There is controversy whether the same guidelines for weight should apply across all age groups or whether there should be age-specific guidelines liberalized for older people. While data on morbidity related to weight show consistently that overweight increases risk in old age, the data on mortality are less consistent, suggesting there may be a trade-off in risks. The data are discussed below; in terms of recommendations, the appropriateness of the guidelines for geriatric patients is likely health status specific. In healthier individuals these guidelines are appropriate and good clinical practice. In more frail older persons, different considerations are relevant.

Trends in the Prevalence of Overweight in Men
1960-1991

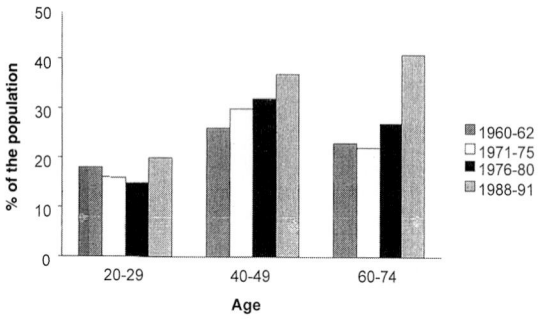

Figure 91-6 These are data from the National Health and Nutrition Examination Surveys, which show the proportion of men with body mass index (weight in kilograms/height in meters squared) of 27.8 kg/m² in the US population over time. For men, the proportion overweight is increasing over time. Reprinted with permission from Kuczmarski RJ et al: Increasing prevalence of overweight among US adults. The National Health and Nutrition Examination Surveys, 1960 to 1991. *JAMA* 272:205, 1994.

RISKS ASSOCIATED WITH UNDERWEIGHT

In the frail elderly, undernutrition is more likely an issue than overnutrition. Undernutrition is associated with poor

Trends in the Prevalence of Overweight in Women
1960-1991

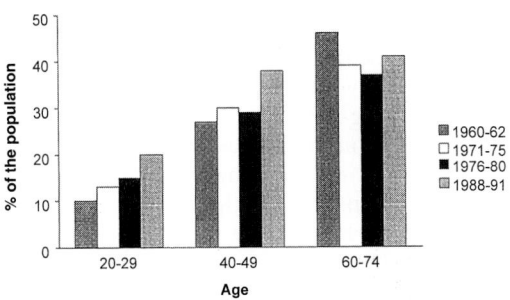

Figure 91-7 These are data from the National Health and Nutrition Examination Surveys , which show the proportion of women with body mass index (weight in kilograms/height in meters squared) of 27.3 kg.m² in the US population over time. The proportion overweight is high but stable over time. Reprinted with permission from Kuczmarski RJ et al: Increasing prevalence of overweight among US adults. The National Health and Nutrition Examination Surveys, 1960 to 1991. *JAMA* 272:205, 1994.

health and weight loss. Older people who are underweight are often found in situations of dependency at home, in hospitals, or in long-term care facilities. Risks associated with undernutrition are generally related to depletion of protein stores and are exacerbated by episodes of illness. These issues are reviewed in greater depth in Chaps. 90 and 92.

RISKS ASSOCIATED WITH OVERWEIGHT

Morbidity and Disability

Overweight in old age is associated with the same risk factors and diseases as in younger populations. Overweight is a major contributor to osteoarthritis of knees and hips. In postmenopausal women, overweight and weight gain are associated with risk of breast cancer, and with poorer outcomes for the cancer; overweight increases the risk of colon cancer. Studies of coronary heart disease risk in older men and women show an increased risk in heavier older persons, particularly when weight change in earlier life is accounted for, and overweight is associated with incidence of diabetes. There is some evidence that waist circumference, independent of level of weight, also contributes to risk of diabetes and coronary heart disease. The diseases of overweight are exacerbated by weight gain. Thus, available evidence suggests that overweight remains an important risk factor for increased morbidity in old age. Given the association of overweight with these diseases, it is not surprising that disability risk is also associated with overweight, particularly in women.

In terms of body composition, evidence supports both fat and lean mass influencing function. The New Mexico Aging Study showed lower lean mass is associated with disability, while other studies suggest that only higher fat mass is associated with disability. These are surprising results given that clinical trials show improved functional outcomes associated with increased strength and muscle

mass. It is possible that heavier weight and greater body fat may contribute to disability risk over a wide range of body weight, but that muscle mass is associated with a threshold of risk such that only those individuals below that threshold will be affected. Heavier individuals may also have relatively less muscle mass than expected on the basis of size, termed sarcopenic obesity, but risk would likely be attributed to body fat rather than muscle.

Mortality Risks

In younger populations, overweight is associated with risk of death. Some studies of older people are consistent with this result, particularly those studies in which midlife weight is used to estimate risk of death in old age, or where those with significant weight loss are excluded. However, most studies of weight and mortality in old age show a U-shaped association with increased risk associated with both lower and heavier weight. Other studies, particularly of people older than age 75 years, report either an increase in deaths, primarily in underweight individuals, or no relationship at all between weight and mortality. What might explain these results and should these studies affect the approach to the geriatric patient?

Several explanations contribute to these differing results among studies and between older and younger populations. For thinner individuals, a number of factors have been suggested. Cigarette smokers are both thin and at high risk of death secondary to smoking. Those who are ill and losing weight are overrepresented among the thinner populations and at increased risk of death. The critical factor contributing to risk of death may be low protein reserves. The loss of lean mass with age would exacerbate the risk in thinner people and the risk associated with thinness would increase with age, which is what is observed.

Among the heavier older people, there are at least theoretical protective benefits in terms of mortality risk. Heavier weight is associated with higher bone mineral density and with lower fracture risk. Heavier weight is associated with greater lean mass, and under catabolic stress, heavier weight may supply a functional nutritional reserve. Heavier weight is often associated with never having smoked which may be an advantage in terms of pulmonary function; in addition, these individuals were often with substantially thinner midlife weight. When risk of death in old age is estimated on the basis of weight in middle age, risk of death is consistently increased in the group whose middle age weight was heavier.

The mortality risk in old age may relate to fat distribution rather than body fatness per se. Several studies have shown increased risks of disease and mortality with larger waist circumference, even when there was no increased risk observed with weight alone. Future studies using body composition should yield even better estimates.

However, without strong evidence supporting any of these hypotheses, there is no a priori reason to assume that the relationship between heavier weight and poor health outcomes is different in old age. The most important issue is to judge the weight of older persons in the context of their weight trajectory and their current health status.

INTERVENTIONS AND RECOMMENDATIONS

Body Composition

Regardless of level of weight, interventions to change body composition hold promise, although it is unclear at present which method will prove most effective. Ideally, these interventions would increase lean mass and decrease body fat, particularly visceral fat. Interventions attempted have included increased physical activity, which tends to decrease body fat with concomitant improvement in metabolic parameters associated with overweight, but has little effect on lean mass. Clinical trials for older patients with strength training have demonstrated increases in muscle mass, increased strength, and improvement in level of physical function. Whether these gains can be sustained over time and translated into programs applicable to larger, less-selected populations of older people is being tested. These studies have encouraged many older people to become involved in regular exercise and strength training. These interventions are reviewed in Chap. 72. Interventions to alter body composition by using various trophic factors and pharmacologic agents show promise but are also problematic. This topic is reviewed in Chap. 103. Trials of these agents, either alone or in combination with exercise or strength interventions, are likely to inform the next generation of efforts to control body fat and increase muscle mass and strength in old age.

Overweight and Weight Reduction

What should we counsel older patients about weight reduction? A history and physical examination related to weight should include a survey of weight-related health conditions, particularly those that are treatable with weight reduction, including hypertension, hyperlipidemia, type 2 diabetes, arthritis of the knees and hip, and peripheral vascular disease. A detailed weight history should be part of the initial evaluation of all geriatric patients and should include early adult weight, midlife weight, maximum and minimum weight, and recent weight change. In the absence of major cognitive impairment, reported weight history is reasonably accurate. Even in an overweight patient, recent unexplained weight loss should raise the need for a careful evaluation for contributory medical, psychological, or functional factors. Prevention of weight gain may be another consideration, particularly for older smokers who decide to quit or those who become disabled with diminished mobility. All older persons should be encouraged to participate in regular physical activity, including some resistance training and stretching. This can be tailored to the level of initial fitness and function, and can be adapted over time to reflect gains in capacity.

Overweight, accompanied by metabolic abnormalities or difficult-to-control symptomatic disease or polypharmacy, suggests the need for a weight-loss program. Will weight reduction benefit the older person? Short-term clinical trials of weight loss in older people show that weight loss can be achieved and results in improvements in hypertension, diabetes, and symptomatic relief of osteoarthritis of the knee. Most of the studies in which weight loss is associated with poor health outcomes are observational studies in which the weight loss was likely to be involuntary. In one of the few studies in which voluntary and involuntary weight loss could be differentiated, there was no increase in adverse outcomes with voluntary weight loss. In the absence of relevant long-term clinical trial data on outcomes with weight reduction, advice on weight loss should be guided by symptoms related to the overweight, anticipated short-term health benefits, and the general level of health status of the patient. In a patient on multiple medications for weight-related health conditions, weight reduction may be an important adjunct in weaning the patient off of the medications.

The goal of a weight reduction program should be to achieve a modest weight loss resulting in improvement in the target weight-related health condition. Little is known about how to best achieve and maintain weight loss successfully in older adults. Efforts to increase physical activity and to decrease caloric intake are preferable to drug therapy for obesity and overweight. Drugs should be considered when it proves impossible to control the metabolic consequences of obesity (e.g., sustained hypertension or prolonged inadequate diabetic control) or under circumstances in which the obesity would constitute a major deterrent to approaching other health problems, for example, knee-replacement surgery. The current set of drugs for weight reduction is limited, but active drug development is under way.

If a weight reduction program is undertaken, whether by caloric restriction or by drug intervention, it is important to recognize that bone and muscle will be lost during the weight-loss period. Older persons lose weight in similar proportions of fat and muscle as in younger people; however, because they start with less lean mass as a result of age-related changes in muscle and bone, continued losses may result in falling below thresholds of risk for fracture and loss of strength. Efforts should be made to preserve bone and muscle in the face of weight loss, including aerobic and resistance exercise components, or other short-term antiosteoporotic therapy. In addition, caloric restriction needs to be supplemented to insure adequate intake of nutrients and vitamins during a period of dieting.

The physician caring for older people also needs to identify particular times when older people are likely to be at high risk for loss of body weight, especially lean mass. These include major episodes of illness, whether inpatient or outpatient, that result in a significant period of bed rest or recuperation; changes in patterns of daily activities, such as retirement, caring for a sick spouse or friend, or minor injuries such as strains or sprains, that limit usual activity; or new medications that may prevent full activity secondary to sensory or cognitive effects including mild sedation or increased instability in balance. Encouragement of specific activities to return to the former baseline is desirable. These may include nutritional intervention, short-term physical therapy, change in medication, and an exercise prescription. It is likely far easier to intervene when the patient appears relatively healthy and can assist in a program to regain and stabilize body weight and mass than when the patient has become frail and in clear need of rehabilitation.

CONCLUSIONS

Weight concerns remain important in old age but become increasingly complex. There is no simple set of tables that give appropriate ideal weight for older people, especially considering that what may be ideal as a predictor of one outcome (e.g., mortality) may be quite different from what may be ideal for another outcome (functional ability). Further developments in the field will incorporate measurements of body composition and fat distribution as well as information about neuromodulation of weight to assist clinicians in rational management of this complicated problem. For the present time, most important is recognition and control of symptomatic weight-related health conditions and attention to precipitants of involuntary gains or losses in weight.

REFERENCES

Ahima RS, Flier JS: Adipose tissue as an endocrine organ. *Trends Endocrinol Metab* 11:327, 2000.

Allison DB et al: Hypothesis concerning the U-shaped relation between body mass index and mortality. *Am J Epidemiol* 146:339, 1997.

Andres R et al: Impact of age on weight goals. *Ann Intern Med* 103:1030, 1985.

Baumgartner RN et al: Epidemiology of sarcopenia among the elderly in New Mexico. *Am J Epidemiol* 47:755, 1998.

Ensrud KE et al: Weight change and fractures in older women. Study of Osteoporotic Fractures Research Group. *Arch Intern Med* 157:857, 1997.

Felson DT et al: Weight loss reduces the risk of symptomatic knee osteoarthritis in women. The Framingham Study. *Ann Intern Med* 116:535, 1992.

Folsom AR et al: Body fat distribution and 5-year risk of death in older women. *JAMA* 269:483, 1993.

Gallagher D et al: How useful is body mass index for comparison of body fatness across age, sex, and ethnic group? *Am J Epidemiol* 143:228, 1996.

Goodpaster BH et al: Attenuation of skeletal muscle and strength in the elderly: The Health ABC Study. *J Appl Physiol* 90:2157, 2001.

Harris TB et al: Associations of elevated interleukin-6 and C-reactive protein levels with mortality in the elderly. *Am J Med* 106:506, 1999.

Kuczmarski MF et al: Descriptive anthropometric reference data for older Americans. *J Am Diet Assoc* 100:59, 2000.

Kuczmarski RJ et al: Increasing prevalence of overweight among US adults. The National Health and Nutrition Examination Surveys, 1960 to 1991. *JAMA* 272:205, 1994.

Lean MEJ et al: Impairment of health and quality of life in people with large waist circumference. *Lancet* 351:853, 1998.

Losonczy KG et al: Does weight loss from middle age to old age explain the inverse weight mortality relation in old age? *Am J Epidemiol* 141:312, 1995.

Morley JE et al: Sarcopenia. *J Lab Clin Med* 137:231, 2001.

Roberts SB et al: Control of food intake in older men. *JAMA* 272:1601, 1994.

Seeman TE et al: Predicting changes in physical performance in a high-functioning elderly cohort: MacArthur Studies of Successful Aging. *J Gerontol* 49:M97, 1994.

Stevens J et al: The effect of age on the association between body-mass index and mortality. *N Engl J Med* 338:1, 1998.

Visser M et al: Reexamining the sarcopenia hypothesis. Muscle mass versus muscle strength. Health, Aging, and Body Composition Study Research Group. *Ann N Y Acad Sci* 904:456, 2000.

Wallace JI et al: Involuntary weight loss in older outpatient: Incidence and clinical significance. *J Am Geriatr Soc* 43:329, 1995.

Whelton PK et al: Sodium reduction and weight loss in the treatment of hypertension in older persons: A randomized controlled trial of nonpharmacologic interventions in the elderly (TONE). *JAMA* 279:839, 1998.

Williamson DF et al: Prospective study of intentional weight loss and mortality in never-smoking overweight US white women aged 40–64 years. *Am J Epidemiol* 141:1128, 1995.

Malnutrition and Enteral/Parenteral Alimentation

JEFFREY I. WALLACE

MALNUTRITION

Definition

Protein-energy malnutrition, the primary focus of this chapter, is present when insufficient energy and/or protein is available to meet metabolic demands. Protein-energy malnutrition (PEM) may develop because of poor dietary protein or calorie intake, increased metabolic demands as a result of illness or trauma, or increased nutrient losses.

Epidemiology

Maintenance of nutrition is an essential component of comprehensive geriatric care, particularly in the acute care setting where the presence of malnutrition is clearly associated with increased complications and other adverse health outcomes. Prevalence data, relying on a variety of measures of nutritional adequacy, suggest that deficiencies in macronutrients (protein-energy intake) and micronutrients (vitamins and minerals) are very common among older adults. National survey data indicate that 40 to 50 percent of noninstitutionalized older adults are at moderate to high risk for nutritional problems, and that up to 40 percent have diets deficient in three or more nutrients. Prevalence estimates in selected populations over sixty-five years old indicate that 9 to 15 percent of older persons seen in outpatient clinics, 12 to 50 percent of hospitalized elderly persons, and 25 to 60 percent of older persons residing in institutional settings have one or more nutritional inadequacies—with protein-energy malnutrition being the most common. Physical and psychosocial factors that may lead to inadequate nutrition are listed in Table 92-1.

Energy intake does decline significantly with aging, attributable to the decrements in lean body mass and physical activity that often accompany aging. A still greater reduction in caloric intake well below the Recommended Dietary Allowance (RDA) has been a consistent finding of nutritional surveys conducted among community-dwelling elderly. In the National Health and Nutrition Examination Surveys (NHANES I and II) the mean daily energy intake was approximately 1600 kcal for men (70 percent of the RDA) and 1200 kcal for women (63 percent of the RDA), and more than 15 percent of the elderly consumed less than 1000 kcal/d. Even if this limited energy intake met the caloric needs of less-active older adults, it is unlikely that all noncaloric nutrient needs (vitamins and minerals) would be met unless the diet was extremely diverse and rich in nutrients. Although micronutrient deficiencies are common when PEM is moderate to severe, it is the PEM that tends to have the greater clinical impact. Accordingly, this section focuses primarily on PEM, with particular attention to prevention and management of PEM in the acute care setting.

Poor nutritional status and PEM are associated with altered immunity, impaired wound healing, reduced functional status, increased health care use, and increased mortality. Despite the confounding effect of coexisting nonnutritional factors, many studies indicate that poor nutrition remains an independent source of increased morbidity and mortality after adjustment for nonnutritional factors. Similarly, the efficacy of nutritional support to improve outcomes in many circumstances is unproved, but data is accumulating suggesting that there are measurable benefits from interventions to correct or prevent nutritional deficits.

Pathophysiology

Protein-energy malnutrition may occur as a consequence of inadequate intake alone (i.e., starvation) or in association with disease-activated physiologic mechanisms that affect body metabolism, composition, and appetite (i.e., cachexia). In the former (primary caloric deficiency state) the body adapts by using fat stores while conserving protein and muscle, and the resulting physiologic changes are often reversible with resumption of usual intake and activity. Cachexia is marked by an acute phase response that is associated with elevated inflammatory mediators (e.g., tumor necrosis factor-α and interleukin-1) and increased

Table 92-1 Factors Contributing to Inadequate Nutrition in Older Adults

Socioeconomic	Physiologic
Fixed income	Impaired strength/aerobic capacity
Reduced access to food	Impaired mobility/dexterity (arthritis, stroke)
Social isolation	Impaired sensory input (smell, taste, sight)
Inadequate storage facilities	Poor dentition
Inadequate cooking facilities	Malabsorption
Poor knowledge of nutrition	Chronic illness (via anorexia, altered metabolism)
Dependence on others	Alcohol
Caretakers Institutions	Drugs (e.g., serotonin reuptake inhibitors, digoxin, narcotics, xanthines, antibiotics, NSAIDs, others)
Psychological	**Acute Illness/Hospitalization**
Depression	Failure to monitor dietary intake and record weights
Bereavement	Failure to consider increased metabolic requirements
Anxiety, fear, paranoia	Iatrogenic starvation (e.g., npo for diagnostic tests)
Dementia	Delay in instituting nutritional support

NPO, nothing by month; NSAIDs, nonsteroidal antiinflammatory drugs.

protein and muscle degradation that may not be readily reversed by refeeding. Although cachexia is usually associated with specific chronic disease conditions (e.g., cancer, infection, inflammatory arthritis) this state may develop in older persons without obvious disease. However, to some extent these physiologic changes are adaptive and caution is necessary when devising strategies to interrupt the cycle of lean body mass loss and functional decline that often accompanies cachexia.

Presentation and Evaluation

Despite its apparent clinical importance, physician recognition of malnutrition is often lacking, and a number of studies suggest that even when recognized, appropriate steps to attempt to correct malnutrition are often not taken.

Effective management of frail or ill older adults mandates an evaluation of nutritional status to better allow for early recognition of PEM and consideration of appropriate nutritional interventions. Assessment of nutritional status by standard anthropometric, biochemical, and immunologic measures can be complex, as both nutrient intake and nonnutrition-related factors can affect these parameters. The use of such measurements (e.g., body-mass index, skinfold thickness, muscle circumferences, serum concentrations of proteins, lymphocyte counts, and presence of anergy) to detect the presence of poor nutrition is often advocated, but may not result in earlier or more effective intervention than can be achieved by a careful history and physical examination. The close monitoring of body weight, a readily obtainable measure that reflects imbalance between caloric intake and energy requirements, may be the simplest and most reliable way to screen for malnutrition, particularly in the outpatient setting. Body weight should be recorded at all patient visits. Weight change should be expressed as a percentage of change from past to current weight, because proportional weight change helps account for variability in baseline weight and appears to be the most clinically relevant measure. Although weight gain caused by excessive energy intake is a common form of malnutrition, only undernutrition and weight loss caused by deficits in energy balance are considered here. Weight loss of 5 percent or more of usual body weight, a degree that has been associated with increased morbidity and mortality in the outpatient setting, should prompt investigation. Illness-related weight loss exceeding 10 percent of preillness weight is associated with functional decline and poor clinical outcomes. Weight loss of 15 to 20 percent or more of usual body weight implies severe malnutrition.

In the hospital setting, where acute illness or injury often coexists with inadequate intake, alterations in nutritional parameters associated with PEM may develop rapidly. Elevated levels of inflammatory mediators appear to be responsible for the greater losses in lean body mass and the rapid declines in albumin that often accompany PEM in physiologically stressed patients relative to PEM which is primarily a result of inadequate caloric intake in the absence of acute illness. While serial weight measures remain clinically relevant, early detection and correction of PEM in acutely ill hospitalized patients is enhanced by determination of dietary intake relative to metabolic requirements. Although registered dietitians often provide this information, physicians should routinely monitor dietary intake and can readily estimate caloric and protein requirements using formulas presented in Table 92-2. Biochemical and immunologic measures (i.e., albumin, prealbumin, transferrin, lymphocyte counts) are useful adjuncts in the assessment of nutritional status and can provide prognostic information, but their lack of specificity limits their utility as markers of PEM. Anthropometric measures of fat stores (skinfolds) and muscle mass (midarm muscle area) may help in the assessment of PEM, but clinicians are generally not well versed in obtaining these measures and interrater variability can be high. Although less sensitive, clinical evaluation for loss of skin turgor and the presence of atrophy in hand interosseous or head temporalis muscles can help assess for losses in subcutaneous fat and muscle

Table 92-2 Estimation of Daily Energy and Protein Needs

I. Daily energy requirements (kcal/d)

    A. Quick estimate: maintenance 25–30 kcal/kg; stress 30–40 kcal/kg; sepsis 40–50 kcal/kg (tends to overestimate requirements for the elderly and obese)

    B. Estimates based on resting metabolic rate (RMR, kcal/d):

        1. First estimate RMR (using either equation below)

            a. Harris–Benedict: $RMR_{women} = 655 + [9.5 \times wt(kg)] + [1.8 \times ht(cm)] - (4.7 \times age)$
                                        $RMR_{men} = 66 + [13.7 \times wt(kg)] + [5 \times ht(cm)] - (6.8 \times age)$

            b. Schofield: $RMR_{women} = [Wt (kg) \times 9.1] + 659$
        (age >60 years) $RMR_{men} = [Wt (kg) \times 11.7] + 588$

        2. Then multiply RMR by adjustment factor to estimate total energy requirement:

        Total daily energy requirement = RMR × 1.3 for mild illness/injury
                                      = RMR × 1.5 moderate illness/injury
                                      = RMR × 1.7–1.8 severe illness/injury

II. Daily protein requirements (g/d) (may overestimate if patient obese)

RDA healthy adult age 51 + years	0.8 g/kg
Minimally stressed patients	1.0 g/kg
Injury/illness	1.2–1.4 g/kg
Severe stress/sepsis	1.4–1.8 g/kg

mass. Because all of these parameters may be affected by nonnutrition-related factors, an effective assessment of nutritional status requires synthesis of information provided from the dietary history, physical exam, and biochemical data. Although there are no definitive criteria for classifying degrees of PEM, when weight loss exceeds 20 percent of premorbid weight, serum albumin is less than 21 g/L, transferrin is less than 1 g/L, and total lymphocyte count is less than 800/μL, PEM is generally considered to be severe.

Assessment for Remediable Causes of Weight Loss

Initial management of patients with PEM and/or weight loss should include a thorough evaluation to identify underlying causes, and if found, to aggressively attempt to correct potentially remediable disorders. In the acute care setting the cause(s) of malnutrition are often readily evident, although depression may be a contributing factor that is frequently overlooked. In contrast, reasons for poor nutrition and weight loss among community-dwelling elderly persons may be multiple and not as readily discernible. Data available from studies on the causes of involuntary weight loss suggests that depression, gastrointestinal maladies (most often peptic ulcer or motility disorders), and cancer are the three most common causes of weight loss in older adults (Table 92-3). In these studies, when cancer was the cause of weight loss, the diagnosis was rarely obscure. Most diagnoses were made readily after standard evaluations which included a careful history and physical examination and basic screening lab tests (urinalysis, complete blood count, electrolyte, renal, liver and thyroid

function tests, stool hemoccults, and a chest radiograph), with additional tests only as directed by signs and symptoms. If this initial basic evaluation is unrevealing, it is best to enter a period of "watchful waiting" rather than pursue more extensive undirected testing. A diagnostic algorithm (Fig. 92-1) focusing first on verifying actual weight loss (patients may inaccurately report a history of weight loss) and then on whether caloric intake is adequate can help guide an appropriate workup.

Management

General Considerations

Older persons who are not meeting their protein and caloric requirements through oral intake should be considered for nutritional support. Table 92-4 outlines approaches to nutritional support and factors to consider in deciding whether to pursue specific interventions. The urgency for nutritional interventions relates to the degree of protein-calorie depletion at the time of diagnosis coupled with the expected magnitude and duration of inadequate nutrition. In the hospital setting, clinicians must consider that patients may have been suffering from PEM for some time prior to admission. Therefore avoidance of delays in instituting appropriate nutritional support while waiting for improved intake is desirable. One approach is to intervene after a period of 5 to 7 days of severely limited intake, or for weight loss more than 10 percent of preillness weight in hospitalized patients. However, attempts should be made to prevent PEM rather than wait for this degree of PEM to develop because weight loss and undernutrition are associated with worse clinical outcomes and recovery of lost lean

Table 92-3 Diagnostic Spectrum of Involuntary Weight Loss

	Study (Study Size)					
	Marton et al (N = 91)	Rabinovitz et al (N = 154)	Huerta et al (N = 50)	Lankisch et al (N = 158)	Levine (N = 107)	Thompson et al (N = 45)
Study population	70% Inpatient	Inpatient	Inpatient	Inpatient	Outpatient	Outpatient
Weight loss definition*	≥5%/6mos.	≥5%/not stated	≥10%/6mos.	≥5%/6mos.	≥5%/6mos.	≥7.5% /6mos.
Mean age (range)	59 ± 17†	64 (27–88)	59 (18–83)	68 (27–92)	62 (17–91)	72 (63–83)
Gender (% male)	100%	45%	64%	44%	53%	33%
Diagnosis (n[%])						
Neoplasm	18(19%)	56(36%)	5(10%)	38(24%)	6(6%)	7(16%)
Gastrointestinal	13(14%)	26(17%)	9(18%)	30(19%)	6(6%)	5(11%)
Psychiatric	8(9%)	16(10%)	21(42%)	17(11%)	24(22%)	8(18%)
Endocrine	4(4%)	6(4%)	5(10%)	18(11%)	5(5%)	4(9%)
Cardiopulmonary	13(14%)	–	1(2%)	16(10%)	9(9%)	–
Other medical dignoses	16(18%)	14(9%)	4(8%)	13(8%)	17(16%)	10(22%)
Unknown	24(26%)	36(23%)	5(10%)	26(16%)	38(36%)	11(24%)

*Weight loss study definition: percent body weight lost per time interval in months.
†Mean age in years ± SD (age range not reported).
‡Neurologic, infectious, alcohol, medication, renal, inflammatory disease, multifactorial.

body mass is often difficult. This is particularly important in severe stress states (e.g., sepsis, major injury) where protein catabolism can lead to losses of lean body mass that approach 0.6 kg/d. In support of early intervention when the development of PEM is likely, a trial of enteral nutrition among patients with major injury found that early (within 24 hours) enteral feeding had clinical benefits over tube feeding started later in the course of hospitalization.

Specific indications for providing nutrients by enteral (gastrointestinal) or parenteral (intravenous) routes are not yet defined.

Patient Preference

The effect of the planned intervention on the patient's quality and/or quantity of life should be addressed before

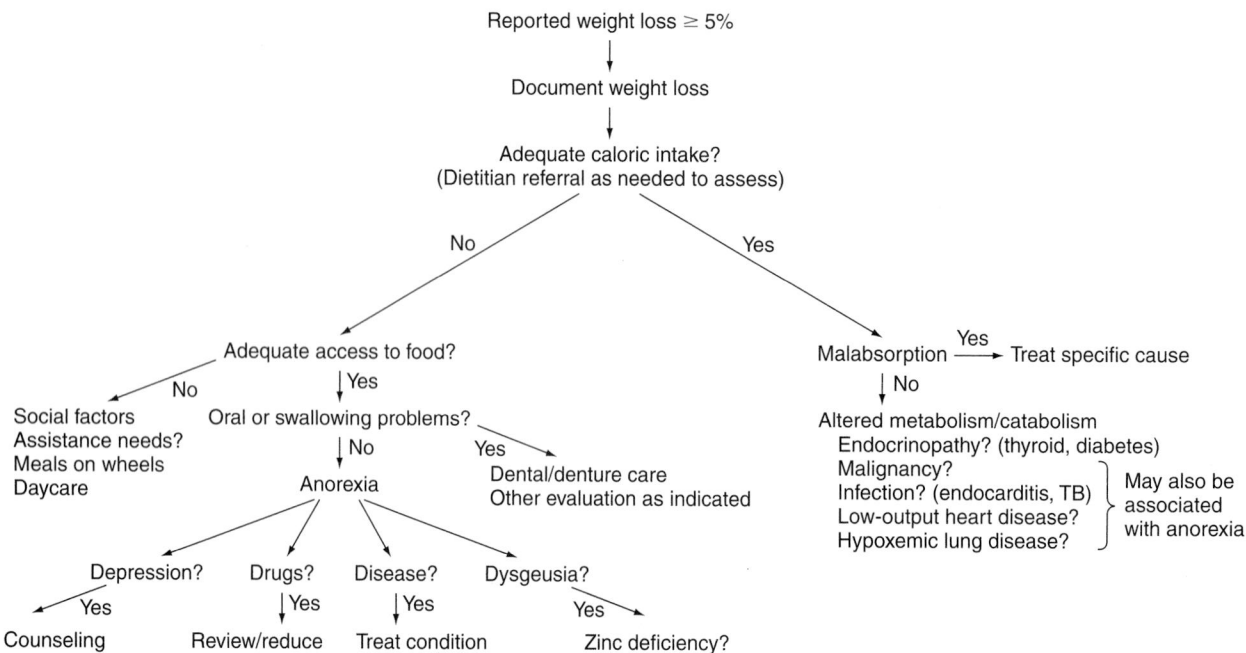

Figure 92-1 Weight-loss evaluation algorithm.

Table 92-4 Approaches to Implementing Nutritional Support

Available Interventions	Factors to Consider
Enhance oral intake	Degree of baseline protein-calorie depletion
Frequent meals, snacks	Current intake relative to requirements
Enhance food flavor	Expected duration of
Provide favorite foods	inadequate nutrition
Protein-calorie supplements	Effect of intervention on clinical outcomes
Multivitamins	Potential benefits
Appetite stimulants	Potential adverse effects
Anabolic agents	Potential for reversibility
Enteral nutrition	Quality of life
Parenteral nutrition	Patient/family care preferences

proceeding with nutritional support. Although nutritional support interventions may improve weight and other nutritional parameters, evidence demonstrating their ability to improve clinical outcomes is still limited, particularly when PEM is associated with serious (e.g., critically ill intensive care unit patients) or irreversible underlying disease (e.g., cancer). While most agree that efforts to improve nutrition, even in patients with serious underlying disease, are warranted, late in the course of disease appropriate palliative care may include, if not mandate, discontinuing such efforts. Determination of the care preferences of the patient and family is a critical component of the decision-making process. Patient and family counseling prior to implementing nutritional support should include a review of the interventions being considered and their potential for adverse, as well as beneficial, effects. Figure 92-2 shows an algorithm to help guide nutritional support decisions.

Enhancing Oral Intake

Nonpharmacologic Although it is uncommon for elderly persons with PEM to be able to increase their food consumption sufficiently to correct their nutritional deficits, short trials of strategies to improve voluntary intake are reasonable for stable patients with mild PEM (no definitive criteria exist, but parameters consistent with mild-moderate PEM include weight 85 to 90 percent of premorbid weight, albumin 25 to 30 g/L, transferrin 1.5 to 2.0 g/L, total lymphocyte count 800 to 1200/μL). As previously outlined, underlying causative or contributing condition(s) to PEM should be considered and addressed. Strategies to overcome anorexia and improve oral intake include assessing and meeting food preferences as best as possible and providing frequent small meals and snacks (dietitians may aid greatly in these efforts).

The use of favorite high-calorie foods (i.e., sweets) may help overcome anorexia and reverse PEM in some hospitalized patients. High-calorie snacks and oral nutritionally complete supplements are generally recommended. Randomized trials provide some evidence that oral nutritional supplements can improve dietary intake, prevent or lessen weight loss, improve immunocompetence, and improve functional status of older adults with, or at risk for, malnutrition. Higher-calorie "plus" variety nutritional supplements (1.5 to 2.0 kcal/mL) are preferred over standard (1 kcal/mL) formulas. Costs are only slightly higher and because they deliver higher calorie content per milliliter ingested, patients need not drink as much volume to improve caloric intake. Supplements should be provided between, rather than with, meals as this appears to result in less compensatory decreases in food intake at mealtime, thereby more effectively increasing total daily caloric intake. However, even if total caloric intake is only marginally improved, the provision of energy from nutritionally dense supplement sources may be beneficial due to improved micronutrient intake.

A standard multivitamin supplement should also be considered for all older adults with poor intake. Evidence suggests that improving micronutrition with multivitamins can improve clinical outcomes (particularly infection). Increased physical activity is an important adjunct that can increase lean body mass, increase metabolism, improved appetite and sense of well-being, thereby leading to improved caloric intake and micronutrient status.

Drugs Pharmacologic approaches to stimulate appetite and promote weight gain may be considered on an individual basis with the knowledge that the few agents

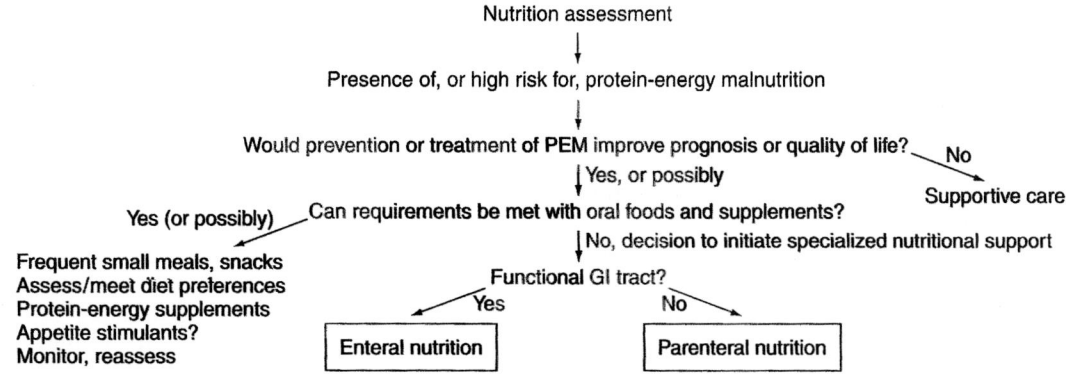

Figure 92-2 An algorithmic approach to nutritional support.

(megestrol acetate, dronabinol, cyproheptadine) that have been shown to improve intake in some patient populations (e.g., cancer, human immunodeficiency virus) have not been well studied in older adults and have the potential to cause important side effects. Megestrol acetate and dronabinol show some promise in relatively small studies conducted in nursing home patients, and a recent head-to-head comparison trial in cancer patients found megestrol acetate to be more effective than dronabinol in improving appetite and promoting weight gain. Megestrol acetate's mechanism of action may involve suppression of inflammatory cytokines (interleukin-6 and tumor necrosis factor-α) and catabolic enzymes, consistent with the observation that this agent appears most effective in subjects with elevated cytokine levels. If initiated, megestrol acetate may not have a demonstrable effect on appetite for several weeks, but if no effect is seen by 8 weeks, megestrol acetate should probably be discontinued. If positive effects are demonstrated without significant side effects, megestrol acetate should be continued for at least 12 weeks. Potential megestrol acetate side effects include fluid retention, nausea, glucose intolerance, and venous thrombosis. Treatment for more than 12 weeks can suppress the adrenal–pituitary axis, resulting in adrenal insufficiency if acutely withdrawn. Only very preliminary data exists for dronabinol use in older adults, and although potential benefits of this agent include positive effects on pain, mood, and nausea, as well as appetite, further study is needed to clarify its efficacy and safety in this population. Delirium is the major side effect of concern from dronabinol.

If depression is felt to be a likely, or possible, contributing factor to poor intake, a trial of therapy is probably warranted. Although selective serotonin reuptake inhibitors (SSRIs) are often chosen as first-line antidepressant agents, and can improve appetite by improving depression, mirtazapine and tricyclic antidepressants (e.g., nortriptyline) may increase appetite independent of their effects on mood and might be considered earlier when anorexia/weight loss is a prominent presenting symptom.

Anabolic hormones (e.g., growth hormone, testosterone, oxandrolone, nandrolone) have received considerable attention in the search to find strategies to help preserve or increase lean body mass in patients with malnutrition and weight loss. Although adequate nutrition is essential for patients with weight loss, a physiologically stressed catabolic patient may lose significant lean body mass despite aggressive nutritional support (and the weight gain that does occur with nutritional support and appetite stimulants may be primarily fat and water). Studies of growth hormone in intensive care and congestive heart failure patients have yielded disappointing results (with cost, need for injection, and potential side effects further limiting clinical use of this agent). Testosterone increases muscle protein synthesis mass and strength, and improvements in functional outcomes have been observed in small controlled trials in selected male populations (e.g., older men after knee replacement surgery, deconditioned older men on a Geriatric Evaluation and Management unit). Although testosterone might be considered in men with documented hypogonadism, its role in the setting of malnutrition and/or cachexia remains to be clarified. Oxandrolone, a synthetic anabolic agent with an increased anabolic to androgenic effect ratio, shows some utility for patients with weight loss in association with acquired immunodeficiency syndrome (AIDS)/human immunodeficiency virus (HIV) or burns, and preliminary data also suggests benefit in patients with chronic obstructive pulmonary disease (COPD). This agent can cause hepatitis, hirsutism, and fluid retention, and is contraindicated in patients with breast or prostate cancer. Further research is needed to define the clinical role of oxandrolone as a pharmacologic intervention to be used in combination with nutrition therapy in older adults.

NUTRITIONAL SUPPORT

Enteral Nutrition

Enteral nutrition, defined here as the nonvolitional delivery of nutrients by tube into the gastrointestinal tract, is the preferred method of nutritional support for patients with, or at high risk for PEM who cannot meet their requirements through oral intake. Enteral nutrition requires a functional gastrointestinal (GI) tract and is contraindicated in patients with inadequate bowel surface area, intestinal obstruction, paralytic ileus, or severe pancreatitis. Although purported benefits of enteral tube feedings relative to parenteral nutrition include the maintenance of gastrointestinal structure and function, more physiologic delivery and use of nutrients, ease and safety of administration, and lower costs, recent reviews suggest such advantages are more theoretical than actual. Increased risk of sepsis associated with parenteral nutrition may have been caused by overfeeding and hyperglycemia, while problems with enteral nutrition, including frequent delivery complications and inadequate nutritional intake, may have been underestimated. Although enteral nutrition is recommended when gastrointestinal function is felt to be adequate, enteral nutrition and parenteral nutrition should not be considered mutually exclusive. For patients who are unable to fully meet their nutritional requirements with enteral feedings, a mixture of parenteral nutrition and enteral nutrition is preferable to moving to parenteral nutrition alone.

Efficacy

Enteral nutrition can improve prognostically important intermediate nutritional parameters and may improve clinical outcomes. One study comparing young and old severely undernourished patients, found that nocturnal tube feedings were well-tolerated and improved nutritional parameters in both age groups. Several prospective studies, including a randomized, controlled trial among older patients with hip fracture, have provided evidence that enteral nutrition can improve both nutritional parameters and clinical outcomes such as length of stay, infectious complications, and mortality. However, further study is needed to determine which elderly hospitalized patients might benefit most from aggressive nutritional support. In the interim, sufficient rationale exists to use enteral nutrition for patients who cannot meet their nutritional needs with oral intake and are deemed appropriate candidates for nutritional support as outlined above.

Tube Placement

The route selected for tube feeding depends on the anticipated duration of feeding, the potential for aspiration, and the condition of the gastrointestinal tract (e.g., esophageal obstruction). Nasogastric or nasointestinal tubes provide the simplest approach for patients requiring relatively short-term enteral nutrition (weeks). Patient comfort and tolerance is best when a small-diameter, soft feeding tube is used rather than a standard large-bore nasogastric tube. The use of longer specialized feeding tubes also allows the tube to reach beyond the pylorus into the small intestine, which is the preferred site of placement to decrease the risk of aspiration. Methods to promote passage of the tube past the pylorus and into the duodenum or jejunum include ensuring adequate tube length, having the patient lie on their right side, and prescribing metoclopramide. If these methods fail and the risk of aspiration is felt to be high, tube placement into the duodenum or jejunum can be performed under fluoroscopic guidance. After placement, the desired tube position should be verified radiologically before starting feedings. Tubes should also be marked at their exit point to help identify if movement has occurred, and tube position may need to occasionally be reconfirmed (by x-ray, pH testing) if proper placement is in doubt.

Percutaneous tube placement (gastrostomy, gastrojejunostomy, jejunostomy) is indicated when long-term tube feeding is anticipated (months). However, they may also be appropriately considered earlier, especially when enteral nutrition is likely to exceed 2 weeks, because they are usually better tolerated than nasointestinal tubes. Percutaneous placement of gastrostomy tubes (G-tubes) can be performed either endoscopically or under radiographic guidance. The risks of major complications with either procedure are generally low, but infection, hemorrhage, and peritonitis have each been reported at rates of 1 to 3 percent in some series. Insufficient data are available to clearly favor one method over the other in terms of safety and efficacy, but one meta-analysis suggested that radiologic placement had slightly higher success rates and slightly lower complication rates. Radiologic placement does offer advantages in terms of ability to navigate tubes into the jejunum or past near-total proximal obstructions (e.g., head and neck or esophageal cancers that endoscopes cannot get past), whereas endoscopic placement offers added diagnostic capabilities and possibly lower overall costs. Radiologically placed gastric tubes advanced into the jejunum appear to have a lower risk for displacement back into the stomach than endoscopically placed gastrostomy-jejunostomy (G-J) tubes.

Tube feeding may be associated with risk for aspiration pneumonia. However, most aspiration pneumonias are the result of difficulty handling endogenous (oral or gastric) secretions rather than aspiration of material introduced through tube feeding. Distal feeding tube placement does not appear to lower the risk of aspiration pneumonia, as two trials found no differences in aspiration pneumonia rates in patients with gastrostomy versus jejunostomy tubes. Placement of feeding tubes directly into the jejunum may be required for patients with abnormal or inaccessible stomachs (e.g., gastrectomy, duodenal obstruction) or when aspiration is a major problem despite the preceding approaches.

Although direct jejunostomy tube (J-tube) placement can be accomplished at some institutions using percutaneous radiologic methods, J-tubes traditionally require an open surgical procedure and are often placed at the time of laparotomy when the need for prolonged nutritional support is anticipated. Endoscopically placed G-J tubes and direct J-tubes tend to have smaller diameters and are more prone to clogging.

Formula Selection

Adult enteral formulas fall into one of the following categories: general use, high nitrogen, high nitrogen and high calorie, fiber enriched, disease specific, and elemental (Table 92-5). All consist of varying mixtures of protein (often casein), carbohydrate (often cornstarch), and fat (usually vegetable oils), and most do not contain lactose. Formula variability includes digestibility, availability of nutrients, nutritional adequacy, viscosity, osmolality, and cost. Costs tend to be 2- to 3-fold higher for disease-specific specialty formulas, and up to 10-fold higher for critical care and elemental specialty formulas. Isotonic general-use formulas with caloric densities of 1 to 1.2 kcal/mL and ratios of nonprotein calories to nitrogen around 130:1 are usually the initial products of choice (with or without added fiber). The importance of the ratio of nonprotein calories to nitrogen intake relates to the maintenance of positive nitrogen balance. For ingested amino acids to avoid catabolism and be available for protein synthesis, higher ratios (approaching 150:1) are necessary. However, for highly stressed patients (e.g., critically ill, burns, healing wounds, trauma), increasing protein intake can enhance nitrogen balance as long as energy intake is adequate. Higher caloric density formulas (1.5 to 2.0 kcal/mL) may be useful when volume restriction is paramount, but their higher viscosity increases the risk of tube clogging and their higher osmolalities increase the likelihood of diarrhea. Formulas with higher fiber content can be useful for preventing or decreasing tube-feed–related diarrhea.

Disease-specific/specialty formulas are available for patients with renal failure, liver failure, diabetes mellitus, pulmonary disease, gastrointestinal dysfunction, and critical illness. Renal disease formulas are low in protein, low in electrolytes, and dense in calories to assist in fluid restriction. These formulas may be useful before dialysis but are not necessary for most patients once on dialysis. Some formulas have been developed for diabetic patients, but use of cheaper standard formulas with adjustments in glucose control regimens as necessary is adequate for most diabetic patients. Formulas for pulmonary patients have higher fat content, because energy utilization from fat results in less carbon dioxide production relative to the metabolism of carbohydrate energy sources. Although possibly useful for patients being weaned from ventilators, these formulas are of questionable clinical importance for most patients with chronic lung disease. Hepatic formulas have specific amino acid mixtures (high in branched-chain, low in aromatic amino acids) that clinical trials have shown to be less likely to cause or exacerbate hepatic encephalopathy. They are indicated when, in spite of appropriate medical therapy, hepatic encephalopathy limits the delivery of adequate protein to a patient with liver disease.

Table 92-5   Approximate Composition of Standard and Disease Specific Enteral Nutrition Products

Product Type (Brand Examples)	Caloric Density (kcal/mL)	Protein (g/L)	NonPro Kcal:N*	Percent energy from CHO†	Fat	Protein
General use formula (Osmolite, Ensure, Jevity)	1.0	35–45	≥125:1	55%	30%	15%
High nitrogen (Promote, Replete, Sustacal)	1.0	62	75:1	50%	25%	25%
High nitrogen, high calorie (Nutren 1.5, "Plus" products‡)	1.5	60	≥130:1	50%	35%	15%
Very-high nitrogen, very-high cal (Magnacal, Nutren 2.0)	2.0	70–80	≥130:1	45%	40%	15%
Renal disease						
Predialysis (Suplena, AminAid)	2.0	20–30	≥350:1	50–75%	20–45%	5%
Dialysis (Nepro)	2.0	70	150:1	43%	43%	14%
Diabetes (Glucerna)	1.0	70	125:1	33%	50%	17%
Pulmonary disease (Pulmocare, Nutrivent)	1.5	60–70	≥125:1	27%	55%	18%
Critical care (AlitraQ, Impact)	1.0	50–70	variable	55–65%	15–25%	20%
Gastrointestinal dysfunction/elemental (Vivonex, Vital HN)	1.0	40	≥125:1	75%	5%	20%

*Ratio nonprotein calories to nitrogen.
†Carbohydrate.
‡For example, Ensure Plus, Resource Plus, Sustacal Plus.

A number of specialty formulations have been designed for critically ill patients and patients with decreased digestive and absorptive capacity. Some of these products are enriched with glutamine, an amino acid associated with improvements in nitrogen balance, gut barrier function, decreased infections, and decreased length of hospital stay when delivered parenterally in clinical trials. In elemental formulas, carbohydrates are supplied primarily as oligosaccharides and proteins have been partially or fully hydrolyzed to free amino acids. Although they are promoted for patients with diminished ability to digest nutrients, it is uncommon for patients to be incapable of digesting and absorbing standard formulas unless they have significantly impaired gastrointestinal function (assuming appropriate adjustments are made in rates of feedings, osmolality, and fiber content). Elemental diets can also cause, rather than reduce, diarrhea because of their high osmolality.

Administration Guidelines

After desired tube placement is confirmed, tube feeds can be started at a rate of 25 to 50 cc/h. Isotonic formulas can be started at full strength, whereas elemental/hyperosmolar formulas are usually diluted to half strength to improve initial tolerance. Gastric residuals should be monitored every 2 to 4 hours until the desired rate, which should be based on estimates of the patient's total protein and energy needs (see Table 92-2), is established. Feeding rates can be advanced 25 cc every 8 to 12 hours based on individual tolerance. Feedings should be held if residuals are more

than 1.5 times the hourly rate. Once daily requirements are reached, further adjustments to deliver nutrients primarily at night may be desirable to allow more freedom of movement during the day (nocturnal feeds probably offer little benefit in terms of decreased satiety and improved intake during the day relative to continuous feeds). Larger-bore nasogastric and gastrostomy tubes allow for intermittent feedings without requirement of a pump. Although this offers convenience advantages, intermittent bolus feedings generally should be avoided because they increase the risk of diarrhea, vomiting, and aspiration pneumonia. Attention must also be paid to patients' water and electrolyte requirements. Basal free water requirements for hospitalized patients are 30 to 35 mL/kg per day, or about 1 cc/kcal delivered. Free water will need to be increased if excess fluid loss is occurring as a consequence of diarrhea or urinary or increased insensible losses. For patients with fever, an additional 300 to 400 cc of water may be needed for each degree centigrade of temperature elevation. Monitoring of weight and electrolytes can help clarify any needed adjustments, with additional free water given in divided boluses three or four times a day.

Risks and Complications

Proper consideration of whether to proceed with enteral nutrition entails an understanding of common adverse effects (Table 92-6). Nasogastric (NG) tubes are often not well tolerated, with patient agitation and self-extubation being particularly common among patients with cognitive

Table 92-6   Adverse Effects of Enteral Nutrition and Management Approaches

Adverse Effects	Management
Poor tolerance	Consider
Frequent self-extubation	Parenteral nutrition
Agitation	Percutaneous gastrostomy tubes
Pulmonary	Elevate head of bed ≥30°
Aspiration	Monitor gastric residuals, ↓ rate as needed
	Nasointestinal, G-J, J-tubes
Gastrointestinal	
Gastric retention	Low-fat formula, metaclopramide
Nausea/vomiting	Nasointestinal, G-J, J-tubes
Diarrhea	↓ Delivery rate, ↑ fiber, antidiarrheals
Metabolic complications	
Hyperglycemia	Routine monitoring glucose, electrolytes
Fluid and electrolytes	Monitor weight, volume status, free water
Refeeding syndrome*	Monitor phosphate, magnesium, potassium
Mechanical Problems	
Insertion site irritation/infection	Local skin care
Tube plugging	Regular flushing, cola/cranberry flushes
G-tube, J-tube extubation	See text
Nasopharyngitis, sinusitis, local pain, epistaxis	Use small-bore flexible tube and avoid prolonged nasal intubation (<4–6 weeks)
Drug interaction considerations	
Tube feeds ↓ bioavailability (e.g., ciprofloxacin, azithromycin)	Hold feedings 15 minutes before and after medications
Frequent medications interrupt nutrition	Alternate medication routes (IV, IM, rectally, transdermal)

*Abrupt, often large drops in serum potassium, phosphorous, magnesium, which may accompany initiation of nutritional support in malnourished patients.

impairment or delirium. The subsequent need for physical or chemical restraints can increase complications and appropriately dampen enthusiasm for NG tube feedings. Also, enteral nutrition in actual practice often involves delayed and inadequate nutritional support because of frequent problems with tubes (e.g., self-extubation, plugging) or GI intolerance (e.g., high residuals, bloating, diarrhea). These factors may explain why attempts to provide elderly persons with enteral nutrition are often abandoned after only a short course of therapy. Some have advocated an early switch to, or starting with, parenteral nutrition, particularly if patients are confused or delirious and the expected duration of therapy is short (1 to 2 weeks). If longer-term support is likely, early use of percutaneous gastrostomy tubes, which tend to be better tolerated by uncooperative or confused patients, may be considered (along with a reevaluation of overall patient care preferences and goals before proceeding with this more invasive approach).

Pulmonary aspiration is a relatively common and serious complication of enteral nutrition. Patients with gastric retention, decreased gag reflex, and altered levels of consciousness are at increased risk for aspiration, and mechanically ventilated patients should not be considered protected by the presence of an endotracheal cuff. The risk of aspiration can be reduced as outlined in Table 92-6. Gastric retention problems may respond to a change to a low-fat formula or to pharmacologic intervention with metoclopramide. Diarrhea is another gastrointestinal problem that frequently complicates enteral nutrition. When significant diarrhea occurs, infectious causes (particularly *Clostridium difficile*) must first be excluded. The possibility of intolerance to formulas with high fat content also should be considered. Interventions to reduce diarrhea include slowing the rate of infusions, diluting hypertonic formulas, increasing formula fiber content, and the use of antidiarrheal agents. In addition to the electrolyte abnormalities that can occur due to diarrhea, hyperglycemia and other metabolic abnormalities may develop related to tube feedings. Potassium and phosphorous requirements can be very high in the first few days after nutritional support is started because of extracellular to intracellular shifts that accompany nutrient utilization, particularly among cachectic patients ("refeeding syndrome"). Fluid-retention problems are also not uncommon in older adults with impaired renal or cardiac function. To minimize these problems, monitoring protocols should include frequent evaluations of gastrointestinal tolerance, daily weights, and daily monitoring of glucose and electrolytes (including phosphorus, calcium, and magnesium) until stable.

Increased problems with tube clogging often occur when more viscous higher-calorie formulas and medications (especially fiber and calcium supplements) are passed via small-bore (smaller than no. 10 French) catheters. Tube maintenance with regular flushing every 4 to 8 hours for patients on continuous feeds, and before and after the delivery of intermittent tube feeds or medications (with 30 cc warm water) can reduce clogging problems. When possible, give medications by mouth rather than by feeding tube. Use of cola, cranberry juice, or meat tenderizer in solution may help open clogged catheters. Another common mechanical problem is the replacement of gastrostomy or jejunostomy tubes that have fallen out. Feeding tube fistula tracts are generally not well established for at least 1 to 2 weeks after placement (and often longer given malnutrition's effect on wound healing). Tubes that come out early (in the first 2 to 3 weeks after placement) require replacement by the original specialist. If the fistula tract is well established, patients or care providers should be able to gently replace tubes that have fallen out, and delay in doing so for more than 6 to 12 hours risks spontaneous closure of the tract. However, feeding should not be resumed until proper tube placement is confirmed.

Parenteral Nutrition

Total parenteral nutrition (TPN), the delivery of all required nutrients by vein, is essential for survival in patients who cannot eat for extended periods of time and who are not candidates for enteral support. To preserve nutritional status and prevent starvation-induced complications, TPN should be considered for even well-nourished, minimally stressed patients who are anticipated to be unable to eat for more than 10 to 14 days. TPN should also be considered to prevent starvation-induced complications in critically ill or severely stressed patients in whom enteral intake is precluded for 5 to 7 or more days. TPN indications established in clinical trials include patients with major trauma, bone marrow transplant recipients, and perioperatively for major surgical procedures for severely malnourished patients (defined in the reference study by a low nutritional risk index score, which generally was reached if weight loss exceeded 10 to 15 percent and albumin was <33 g/L, or, in the absence of weight loss, if serum albumin was <28 g/L). To be effective, preoperative TPN needs to be given for at least 7 to 14 days.

Efficacy

Evidence that TPN can improve clinical outcomes comes primarily from studies demonstrating that TPN reduces complications in severely malnourished (defined in the paragraph above) patients undergoing major elective surgery and improves outcomes in selected patient populations (e.g., organ transplant recipients, malnourished critically ill patients, and patients with major trauma). There is a paucity of studies and many unanswered questions about the efficacy and safety of TPN in elderly individuals. Data such as a pooled analysis indicating that routine TPN for cancer chemotherapy patients is associated with detrimental clinical outcomes, along with the cost and level of invasiveness of TPN, suggest that risks and benefits must be reviewed carefully for each patient. That TPN may be of some benefit when used in cancer patients who are severely malnourished affirms the importance of patient selection and the identification of clear goals of therapy before instituting TPN.

Administration Guidelines

Intravenous access TPN requires the use of hypertonic solutions that can only be tolerated when delivered into large venous vessels, preferably into the superior vena cava.

Because peripheral veins are limited to solutions containing lower concentrations of amino acids and dextrose (<10% dextrose), peripheral parenteral nutrition (PPN) usually cannot deliver nutrients in sufficient quantity to meet all requirements. The infusion of lipids can improve energy delivery and vessel tolerance to PPN, making PPN occasionally useful for short-term support or as adjunctive therapy for patients with limited tolerance of enteral nutrition support. Central catheter placement has traditionally been accomplished via subclavian or internal jugular veins with associated operator-dependent risks of insertion complications that include pneumothorax, inadvertent arterial puncture, and hemorrhage. Central venous access for long-term use (weeks to months) can also be obtained via catheters advanced through peripheral vessels (usually median cubital, basilic, or cephalic veins). Peripherally inserted central lines (PICCs) offer reduced risks of the aforementioned central placement complications and may have a reduced risk of infectious complications. Complications that may be increased with PICCs include early mechanical phlebitis, catheter occlusions, and catheter tears, although the latter two problems can be minimized with proper line maintenance. One nonrandomized study of TPN delivered through PICCs versus through subclavian vein-inserted central catheters found no difference in complication rates and concluded that PICC lines can be used safely and effectively for TPN. Regardless of the placement method used, proper line position needs to be confirmed by x-ray before initiating TPN.

TPN composition Standard TPN solutions contain carbohydrate (dextrose) and protein (amino acid) concentrates, fat emulsions (soybean or safflower oil with egg phospholipids), micronutrients, and electrolytes. Knowledge of usual TPN formula composition can help provide a working framework (Table 92-7) but macronutrient and electrolyte content in particular must be individualized. Energy and protein content should be based on estimates of patient requirements (see Table 92-2). Electrolyte requirements are highly variable and often require adjustments as they are influenced by the patient's underlying disease (e.g., heart failure, renal dysfunction) and factors such as renal or gastrointestinal fluid losses. Standard packages of vitamins and trace elements are added to TPN solutions daily to prevent the development of micronutrient deficiencies. Because patients on warfarin should not receive vitamin K, it is not included in standard vitamin packages and must be given separately in doses of 5 to 10 mg/wk. Patients with large gastrointestinal fluid losses may require additional zinc, whereas patients with severe renal dysfunction may need their supplements reduced.

The optimal proportions of fat and carbohydrate to meet energy needs are controversial. All standard formulas contain hypertonic glucose (10% to 70% dextrose before mixing), but because glucose tolerance declines with age, slow upward titration in delivery rates are necessary in older adults. Glucose infusion rates should not exceed 5 mg/kg/min (about 500 g/d for a 70-kg person on continuous TPN) because the rate at which stressed patients can metabolize glucose as energy is limited. Overfeeding with glucose results in increased risks of hyperglycemia,

Table 92-7 "Average" TPN Formula Composition and Parameters for Daily Vitamin, Mineral, and Electrolyte Requirements

Macronutrients*	Protein 15%	Carbohydrate 55–60%	Fat 25–30%
Vitamins			
Vitamin A	3300 IU	Pantothenic acid (B$_5$)	15 mg
Vitamin D	200 IU	Pyridoxine (B$_6$)	4 mg
Vitamin E	10 IU	Biotin (B$_7$)	60 μg
Thiamine (B$_1$)	3 mg	Folic acid (B$_9$)	400 μg
Riboflavin (B$_2$)	3.6 mg	Cobalamin (B$_{12}$)	5 μg
Niacin (B$_3$)	40 mg	Vitamin C	100 mg
Trace Elements			
Zinc	5 mg	Manganese	0.5 μg
Copper	1 mg	Selenium	60 μg
Chromium	10 μg		
Electrolytes			
Sodium	60–150 mEq	Magnesium	16 mEq
Potassium	70–150 mEq	Acetate	20–40 mEq
Chloride	Equal to sodium	Calcium	10 mEq
Phosphorus	10 mmol/1000 kcal		

*Percent of total calories

increased carbon dioxide production, and the conversion of excess glucose calories into fat (which requires energy and contributes to fatty liver changes).

Lipids in the form of 10 to 20 percent fat emulsions are added to TPN as a source of concentrated energy and to supply essential fatty acids. A minimum of 2 to 4 percent of total calories as linoleic acid is required to prevent essential fatty acid deficiency. This usually can be accomplished with the delivery of fat emulsions two to three times a week. Fat emulsions are isotonic and are generally well tolerated, but patients occasionally have difficulty with hyperlipidemia and, less frequently, with allergic reactions (usually to the egg phospholipid component). Increasing the proportion of energy supplied by fat can reduce hyperglycemia and carbon dioxide production, but fat delivery should not exceed 2.5 g/kg/d (or 50 to 60 percent of nonprotein calories) to avoid possible adverse consequences associated with fat overload. The fat overload syndrome is characterized by hyperlipidemia with diffuse fat deposition that can cause organ and reticuloendothelial system dysfunction, impaired immune function, and increased risk of sepsis. Lipid formulations enriched with medium-chain triglycerides may have less potential for these side effects and improve nitrogen balance relative to long-chain triglycerides, but studies have not demonstrated consistent benefits and their proper role in nutritional support remains unclear.

TPN formulas with special amino acid compositions are available for patients with severe renal or hepatic disease. The renal formulas consist primarily of essential amino acids to allow delivery of necessary proteins while minimizing nitrogen loads. Their use should be restricted to predialysis renal failure patients. The hepatic failure formulas have increased ratios of branched-chain amino acids to aromatic amino acids. They can reduce problems with hepatic encephalopathy, but because of their expense,

they should be reserved for patients who develop hepatic encephalopathy with standard TPN formulas.

Formula delivery Initial infusion rates should be at a rate of 25 to 50 cc/h and increased every 8 to 12 hours as metabolic status allows until fluid and nutrition goals are met. At some institutions carbohydrate, fat, and protein TPN components are mixed together into a single bag (total nutrient admixture or three-in-one formula). Although this simplifies administration the admixed product is less stable, and concerns have been raised that the haziness imparted to the admixture by the lipids makes it difficult to detect problems that can occur with calcium and phosphorous precipitation. Such precipitation, which can have dire clinical consequences, is relatively easy to detect with the traditional delivery system that infuses the lipid emulsion separately from the bag containing all the other TPN components. In most circumstances, daily TPN volumes are infused continuously over the full 24 hours. This allows slower delivery of carbohydrate (which can help reduce hyperglycemia), and the continuous flow may decrease the risk of catheter occlusion while avoiding interruptions that might lead to hypoglycemia. Shorter infusion schedules with brief periods off TPN (cyclic TPN) are occasionally desirable, but this is more of an issue for long-term TPN in the home care setting. Because TPN formulas (especially the lipid component) can suppress appetite, it may be desirable to reduce or hold lipid emulsions for a few days to help improve intake prior to planned discontinuation of TPN.

Patient monitoring and complications Elderly persons receiving TPN should be monitored closely (Table 92-8). Table 92-9 details common complications and their prevention and/or treatment. Correction of dehydration and volum depletion can most readily be accomplished with standard intravenous fluids, which can be infused

Table 92-8   Guidelines for Monitoring Patients on TPN

Clinical Data	Laboratory Data
Vital signs three times per day until stable	Glucose chemsticks qid until stable
Daily weights	Daily: Electrolytes, glucose, creatinine, blood urea nitrogen, calcium, phosphorus, magnesium until stable, then twice weekly
Daily fluid input and output	
Daily line and skin inspection	
Efficacy of nutritional support	Weekly: LFTs, albumin, CBC, PT, triglyceride

CBC, complete blood count; LFTs, liver function tests (alanine and aspartate aminotransferase, alkaline phosphatase, bilirubin) PT, prothrombin time.

Table 92-9   TPN Complications and Potential Corrective Measures

Condition	Prevention/Management
Metabolic	
Fluid overload	Restrict fluid by ↑ macronutrient concentrations
Hyperglycemia	↓ Carbohydrate delivery (rate, concentration), insulin IV; consider ↑ proportion energy from fat
Hypoglycemia	Avoid sudden cessation/interruption of TPN
Refeeding syndrome	Start/titrate TPN slowly, avoid overfeeding
Hypertriglyceridemia	↓ Fat infusion rates and/or frequency of lipids
Hyperchloremic metabolic acidosis	↑ Acetate/↓ chloride; consider renal/gastrointestinal causes
Metabolic alkalosis	Consider renal/gastrointestinal causes; replete K+;↓ acetate
Respiratory (hypercarbia)	↓ Total calories, ↑ proportion energy from fat
Nonmetabolic	
Line infection	Single-lumen catheter; dedicated TPN; line; aseptic line care; rule out other fever sources
Hepatic	
Steatosis/↑ LFTs	Avoid carbohydrate overfeeding; rule out other causes
Biliary (cholestasis)	Enteral feed if possible; rule out other causes
Catheter occlusion	Regular flushes; no line blood draws; urokinase

LFTs, liver function tests

separately or added to TPN bags for convenience. Fluid overload can be managed by using higher concentrations of macronutrients to limit total volumes infused, with diuretics added as needed. Although insulin may be added directly to TPN solutions as needed to control hyperglycemia, it is best to give intravenous insulin separately until caloric delivery and glucose control are stabilized. Intravenous insulin is preferred over subcutaneous insulin owing to the latter's potential for erratic absorption in malnourished patients. Infection and volume depletion need to be considered if hyperglycemia is a persistent problem. As with enteral nutrition, potassium and phosphate must be monitored closely because they may drop precipitously after initiating TPN in malnourished patients. In most cases, electrolyte requirements stabilize within 1 week. The relative amounts of chloride (which can lead to metabolic acidosis) and acetate (which can be metabolized to bicarbonate and lead to metabolic alkalosis) can be adjusted as needed depending on the patient's acid–base balance. Patient monitoring should also include clinical (e.g., weight, functional status) and laboratory (e.g., albumin, prealbumin) assessment of the efficacy of nutritional support. Because lean body mass gains rarely are greater than 1 kg/wk, weight gain in excess of this indicates a positive fluid balance rather than the accrual of lean body mass.

Infection of the access line is uncommon in the first 72 hours, so early fevers are usually a result of other causes. The risk of infection can be reduced with proper aseptic line care, and the line site should be monitored daily for erythema, tenderness, or discharge. Positive line cultures in the absence of other sources are usually an indication for line removal. The increased rates of sepsis that have been observed in some trials of TPN can be ascribed to overfeeding (often causing hyperglycemia). It appears that this risk of TPN has been exaggerated.

Another concern regarding TPN that may have been previously overstated is its potential adverse effect on the gastrointestinal tract that includes decreased brush border hydrolase and microvillus height and increased mucosal permeability. In humans, TPN does not cause gastrointestinal mucosal atrophy or increased bacterial translocation. Liver abnormalities that can occur with TPN include fatty liver with elevated liver function tests (often occurs early, may be related to carbohydrate overfeeding, generally benign/reversible) and cholestasis (tends to occur later, after 3+ weeks). Enteral nutrition, even in small amounts, may reduce problems with cholestasis.

Special Issues
Comorbidity

Responses to nutritional support efforts may vary substantially owing to heterogeneity in underlying disease states associated with PEM (particularly the presence and severity of inflammatory/catabolic states). Limited data on the interaction between nutritional support and specific comorbid conditions and care settings include the following.

Hip fracture As many as half of all older patients who present with hip fractures are malnourished. Undernutrition may directly contribute to hip fracture events via increased presence of osteoporosis, increased risk of falls as a consequence of reduced lean body mass and strength, and reduced fat to "cushion" a fall. Seven randomized trials of postoperative nutritional treatments (oral supplements or enteral nutrition) have been conducted in hip fracture patients and a recent analysis performed by the Cochrane Library concluded that there is evidence of benefits ranging from decreased complications to reduced length of hospital stay to faster rehabilitation. Although limited, available data is consistent in suggesting the utility of such nutritional support for hip fracture patients.

Chronic obstructive pulmonary disease Prevalence estimates of malnutrition in patients with COPD range from 20 to 70 percent. Increased inflammatory activity probably contributes to catabolic processes that combine with undernutrition to cause weight loss and loss of lean body mass. Although a recent meta-analysis concluded that energy supplementation does not have significant effects in patients with *stable* COPD, another review indicated that 10 of 12 randomized-controlled trials have noted positive effects of nutritional support (mostly oral supplements providing 400 to 1000 kcal/d) on anthropometric, immune, muscular strength and respiratory function outcome measures. Given the relative low cost and potential for benefit, nutritional support might be considered for patients with COPD and evidence of PEM.

Nursing home care setting Very high prevalence rates of PEM and weight loss (up to 50%) have been documented in nursing home settings. Because conditions associated with reduced intake are common in nursing home residents (e.g., dental, chewing, swallowing problems, depression, cognitive impairment and dependence on others for feeding) it is likely that the proportion of patients with PEM caused by reduced intake (without inflammatory/cachexia states) is higher than in hospitalized patients. Studies demonstrate that simple interventions, such as high-calorie snacks and nutritional supplements, can improve nutritional parameters and help to stabilize weight in the nursing home setting. Although it is not clear that improvements in these intermediate measures translate to improved clinical outcomes, such interventions are likely reasonable and appropriate for most nursing home residents.

Dementia A number of recent reviews have addressed the difficult subject of tube feeds in patients with advanced dementia. Evidence from observational studies suggests that tube feeds in such patients do not appear to have utility for improving nutritional status, decreasing pressure sores or infections, reducing aspiration problems, or improving functional status or survival. Potential adverse effects of tube feeds in these patients include increased risk of aspiration, discomfort and complications from tube placement, potential for increased pressure ulcers from increased urine and fecal output (and possibly increased use of restraints), and diminished quality of life from decreased interaction at mealtime and loss of gustatory pleasure from food intake. Although controversial, some suggest that the lack of proven benefits combined with considerable potential for harm, argues against the use of feeding tubes in patients with severe dementia who can no longer meet their nutritional requirements through oral intake.

Future Directions

Despite aggressive nutritional support it is often difficult to attenuate the catabolic response to illness or injury. Also, anthropometric measures indicate that when body weight does increase with nutritional support, gains are mostly in the form of fat and water, whereas greater increases in lean body mass might lead to better functional and overall clinical outcomes. In addition to previously mentioned anabolic agents, other strategies under investigation to better prevent protein catabolism and/or promote anabolism include enriched delivery of certain macronutrients (e.g., glutamine, arginine, and omega-3 fatty acids) that may have positive immunomodulating action independent of their role as nutritional substrates. Glutamine and arginine are conditionally essential amino acids that have been studied primarily as additives to parenteral nutrition and have been added to some critical care enteral products. Glutamine, an important intermediate for many metabolic pathways and the primary fuel source for enterocytes and other rapidly dividing cells, is probably the best studied. In some clinical trials, patients whose TPN solutions were supplemented with glutamine had improved nitrogen retention, decreased infections, and decreased hospital days. One review suggested that immunonutrition in critically ill patients may reduce infectious complication rates but does not appear to impact overall mortality. This review concluded that physiologic inconsistencies and concerns regarding study methodologies leave the role of glutamine and arginine in nutritional support unclear. Other agents with anticatabolic/anticytokine activity that have the potential to be useful for patients with acute stress response reactions include pentoxifylline, thalidomide, and melatonin. However, to date no convincing data exists for the utility of these drugs in patients with cachexia. Although promising, strategies to increase anabolism and/or decrease catabolism require further study to better define their efficacy and safety in various disease states before considering widespread use.

REFERENCES

Akner G, Cederholm T: Treatment of protein-energy malnutrition in chronic nonmalignant disorders. *Am J Clin Nutr* 74:6, 2001.

Finucane T et al: Tube feeding in patients with advanced dementia. *JAMA* 282:1365, 1999.

Hebuterne X et al: Acute renutrition by cyclic enteral nutrition in elderly and younger patients. *JAMA* 273:638, 1995.

Heyland D et al: Should immunonutrition become routine in critically ill patients? *JAMA* 286:944, 2001.

Huerta G, Viniegra L: Involuntary weight loss as a clinical problem. *Rev Invest Clin (Spanish)* 41(1):5, 1989.

Jeejeebhoy K: Total parenteral nutrition: Potion or poison? *Am J Clin Nutr* 74:160, 2001.

Klein S et al: Nutrition support in clinical practice: Review of published data and recommendations for future research directions. *Am J Clin Nutr* 66:683, 1997.

Kotler D. Cachexia. *Ann Intern Med* 133:622, 2000.

Lankisch PG et al: Unintentional weight loss: Diagnosis and prognosis. *J Intern Med* 249:41, 2001.

Levine MA. Unintentional weight loss in the ambulatory setting: Etiologies and outcomes. (Personal communication and abstract) *Clin Res* 39(2):580A, 1991.

Marton KI et al: Involuntary weight loss: Diagnostic and prognostic significance. *Ann Intern Med* 95:568, 1981.

Ng P et al: Peripherally inserted central catheters in general medicine. *Mayo Clin Proc* 72(3):225, 1997.

Potter J et al: Routine protein energy supplementation in adults: Systematic review. *BMJ* 317:495, 1998.

Rabinovitz M et al: Unintentional weight loss. *Arch Int Med* 146:186, 1986.

Souba W: Nutritional Support. *N Engl J Med* 336:41, 1997.

Sullivan D: The role of nutrition in increased morbidity and mortality. *Clin Geriatr Med* 11(4):661, 1995.

Thompson MP, Morris LK: Unexplained weight loss in the ambulatory elderly. *J Am Geriatr Soc* 39:497, 1991.

Woodcock N et al: Enteral versus parenteral nutrition: A pragmatic study. *Nutrition* 17:1, 2001.

Yeh S et al: Improvement in quality of life measures and stimulation of weight gain after treatment with megestrol acetate oral suspension in geriatric cachexia. *J Am Geriatr Soc* 48:485, 2000.

Disorders of Swallowing

JOANNE ROBBINS • STEVEN BARCZI

Demographic changes related to aging necessitate that clinicians have the resources to address eating and swallowing difficulties present in older adults. The capacity to effectively and safely eat or swallow is one of the most basic human needs and see other satisfying social activities. Therefore the loss of this capacity can have far-reaching implications. Many would argue that swallowing is one of the cardinal behaviors needed to sustain life. The process of swallowing requires orchestration of a complex series of psychological, sensory, and motor behaviors that are both voluntary and involuntary. Dysphagia refers to difficulty in swallowing that may include oropharyngeal or esophageal problems. More specifically there may be difficulty in oral preparation for swallowing and/or moving material from the mouth to the esophagus and from the esophagus to the stomach. Although age-related changes place older adults at risk for dysphagia, an older adult's swallow is not inherently impaired. Presbyphagia refers to characteristic changes in the mechanism of swallowing of otherwise healthy older adults. Clinicians need to be able to distinguish among dysphagia, presbyphagia, and other related diagnoses such as globus hystericus to avoid overdiagnosis and overtreatment of dysphagia. Older adults appear to be more vulnerable, and with additional stressors such as acute illness and certain medications, they can cross over from having a healthy older swallow to being dysphagic. This chapter reviews dysphagia outcomes, normal and altered swallowing with aging, multidisciplinary approaches to diagnosing and managing dysphagia, and newly recognized rehabilitation strategies for dysphagia care.

THE IMPACT OF DYSPHAGIA

Estimates indicate that 15 percent to 40 percent of individuals older than 60 years have dysphagia. The prevalence depends on the specific population sampled, with community-dwelling and more independent individuals having rates near 15 percent. This figure is in agreement with the prevalence rates for several other "geriatric syndromes." Upward of 40 percent of people living in institutional settings such as assisted-living and nursing homes are dysphagic. Based on the 15 percent prevalence rate and 1998 US census data, it is estimated that 6 million adults

have dysphagia. With the projected growth in the number of individuals living in nursing homes, there is a stated need to address dysphagia not only in ambulatory and acute care settings but also in long-term-care settings.

The consequences of dysphagia vary from social isolation because of the embarrassment associated with choking or coughing at mealtime to physical discomfort (e.g., food sticking in the chest) to potentially life-threatening conditions. The more ominous sequelae include dehydration, malnutrition, and both overt and silent aspiration. For the purposes of this chapter, aspiration is defined as the entry of material into the airway *below* the level of the true vocal folds. Silent aspiration refers to the circumstance in which a bolus comprising saliva, food, liquid, or in fact any foreign material enters the airway below the vocal folds *without* triggering overt symptoms such as coughing or throat clearing. Both overt and silent aspiration may lead to pneumonitis, pneumonia, exacerbation of chronic lung disease, or even asphyxiation and death. To gain a better understanding of the effect these consequences have on older adults and the impact of dysphagia interventions, research in this area has aimed to develop more meaningful outcome measures. Assessments focused on pathophysiology, function, and health services are now being conducted to create more evidence-based practices in dysphagia care.

Insofar as dysphagia is a biomechanical disorder of bolus flow, signs of flow abnormality, using videofluoroscopy, have been well detailed. These include (1) the duration, direction, and completeness of bolus flow; (2) the duration and extent (range) of anatomic structural movements; and (3) the relationship between bolus flow and structural movements. Other clinical outcomes of dysphagia have become important endpoints in assessing interventions that aim to make it possible for patients to eat and drink adequately and safely. These include measures of hydration, nutrition, and aspiration episodes. Additionally, pneumonitis, overt aspiration pneumonia, and additional forms of evidence of pulmonary damage are monitored. Nonetheless, it has been difficult to attribute mortality directly to dysphagia because it is often a secondary rather than a primary diagnosis.

Other measures have been developed that target what and how dysphagic adults eat and drink. Most of these

Table 93-1   Summary Descriptions of Selected Tools for Assessing Eating and Drinking Function *Semin Sp Path*

Tool	Components
American Speech Language Hearing Association Scale (1996)	1. Oral versus nonoral 2. Need for supervision 3. Need for special techniques 4. Need for extra time
Rehabilitation Institute of Chicago Clinical Evaluation of Dysphagia (Cherney et al, 1986)	1. Oral versus nonoral 2. Need for and type of supervision 3. Need for special techniques 4. Type of diet 5. Episodes of choking
Amyotrophic Lateral Sclerosis Severity Scale (Hillel et al, 1989)	1. Oral versus nonoral 2. Type of diet 3. Time to eat 4. Patient symptoms 5. Choking
Dysphagia Disability Index (Silbergleit et al, in progress)	1. Emotional reactions 2. Time to eat 3. Need for compensations 4. Need for special food and liquid 5. Coughing 6. Choking 7. Other influences on behavior
Dysphagia Severity Rating Scale (Waxman et al, 1990)	1. Findings from videofluoroscopy 2. Oral versus nonoral 3. Time to eat 4. Consistency of food and liquid 5. Need for cueing and compensation
Functional Outcome Swallowing Scale (Salassa, 1997)	1. Findings from videofluoroscopy 2. Variety of medical consequences 3. Oral versus nonoral 4. Coughing, choking, and other symptoms
Functional Outcome Assessment of Swallowing (Wisconsin Speech and Hearing Association, 1996)	1. Percent oral and nonoral 2. Food/liquid consistency 3. Need for cueing 4. Need for strategies 5. Time to eat

SOURCE: Adapted from McHorney CA, Rosenbeck JC: Functional outcome assessment of adults with oropharyngeal dysphagia. *Semin Speech Lang* 19 (3):235, 1998.

scales are directly applicable to older adults. More than seven recognized scales exist, and Table 93-1 summarizes some of their features, components, and endpoints. Among the common components of all these tools are the distinction between oral and nonoral eaters, the time to eat, the need for special techniques or compensations, and the presence of coughing and choking during eating.

Dysphagia is felt to profoundly influence quality of life (QOL). Patients with swallowing difficulties, especially those who relinquish oral eating, manifest significant changes in psychosocial status, functional status, and emotional well-being. Eating and drinking are social events that relate to friendship, acceptance, entertainment, and communication. As such, major adjustments in the process of feeding and eating can lead to distressing responses such as shame, anxiety, depression, and isolation. Only recently have dysphagia-specific, comprehensive, QOL measures been developed. SWAL-QOL is a 44-item tool that assesses 10 dysphagia-specific QOL concepts, and SWAL-CARE is a 15-item tool that assesses quality of care and patient satisfaction. By monitoring functional outcomes with tools like SWAL-QOL in clinical practice, physicians and other health care providers may be able to better assess and adjust their treatment of dysphagia.

THE SWALLOWING PROCESS

Although most people never think about swallowing until a bit of food or a pill is caught in the throat, or until a sip of liquid is aspirated, swallowing is a highly complex "balancing act." Approximately 30 oral and pharyngeal muscles and multiple nerves must perform precisely on cue so that the upper aerodigestive tract is reconfigured from a mechanism that channels air for breathing and speaking (Figure 93-1) to a food-propelling mechanism that accomplishes ingestion (Figure 93-2). The four morphologic regions serving these purposes are the oral cavity, pharynx, larynx, and esophagus. Of these, the first three collectively are termed the upper aerodigestive tract because they also serve the airway-dependent functions of respiration and speech production. In humans, with our upright posture, it is the adjacent position of the anatomy for breathing to the anatomy for food passage that facilitates gravitational influences on food to flow into an unprotected airway. Such anatomy and physiology require precision and a delicate balance between swallowing physiology and breathing—each a life-sustaining function that must

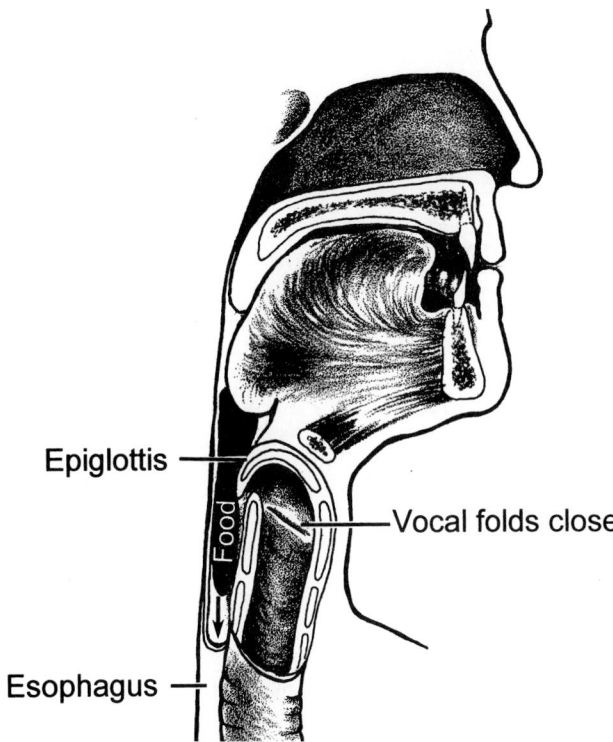

Figure 93-2 Aerodigestive tract reconfigured from an air channel to a food-propelling mechanism. The tongue propels food into the throat; the epiglottis covers the larynx, which is the airway entrance; and the vocal folds close to protect the trachea and lungs from foreign material. Adapted with permission from Weihofen D et al: *The Easy to Swallow, Easy to Chew Cookbook.* New York, John Wiley and Sons, 2002.

occur during cessation of its counterpart. Thus, a basic understanding of the relationship between the anatomic components and the functional interaction of this mechanism is essential to an understanding of normal swallowing and the effects of age and age-related diseases on it.

Normal Swallowing

Swallowing is an integrated neuromuscular process consisting of a combination of volitional and relatively automatic movements. Although normal swallowing is usually conceptualized as a continuous sequence of events, the process of deglutition has been conveniently described as occurring in two, three, or four phases or stages. Moreover, the system engaged in swallowing can be divided into two basic structural subsystems, horizontal and vertical (Figure 93-3), that mirror the direction of bolus flow and the potential for gravitational influence on it.

Horizontal Subsystem

The oral cavity components comprise the horizontal subsystem. As such, this subsystem is involved in the initial, largely volitional, processing and transport phases of swallowing—the swallow preparatory phase and the oral

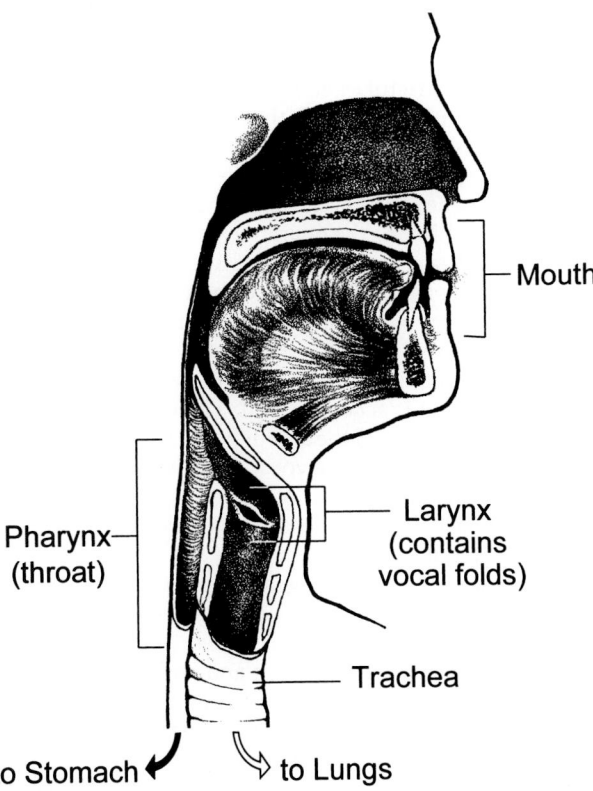

Figure 93-1 Aerodigestive tract channeling air for breathing from the nose and mouth through the open larynx into the lungs and back up and out. For speaking, air is channeled similarly, but the vocal folds vibrate to produce voice. Adapted with permission from Weihofen D et al: *The Easy to Swallow, Easy to Chew Cookbook.* New York, John Wiley and Sons, 2002.

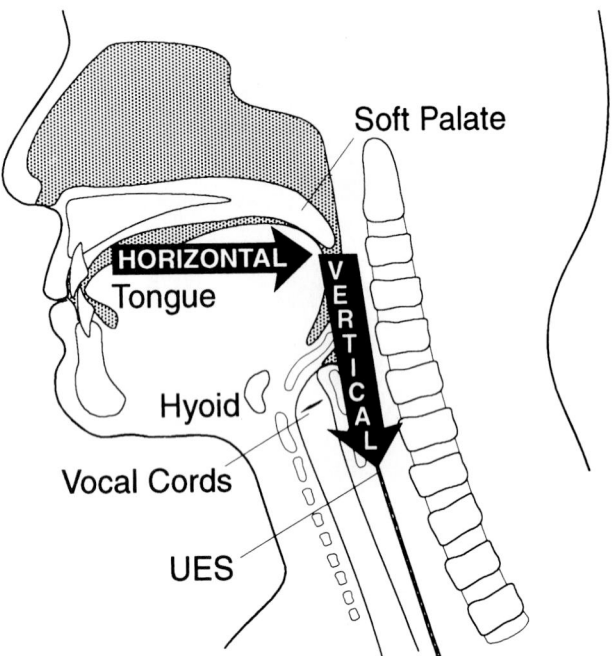

Figure 93-3 The oropharyngeal swallowing mechanism can be divided into two basic structural subsystems, horizontal and vertical, that mirror the direction of bolus flow. UES, upper esophageal sphincter. Adapted with permission from Robbins JA: Normal swallowing and aging. *Semin Neurol* 16(4):309, 1996.

transport phase. The swallow preparatory phase is characterized by food acceptance, containment, and manipulation. The lips and the buccal musculature act in complex patterns, varying the size and shape of the oral opening to allow acceptance and/or containment of food within the oral cavity. The process of chemically changing the material requires that numerous labial and lingual glands secrete into the oral cavity an enzyme-rich fluid that maintains and lubricates the mucosa and is directly incorporated into the food. This textural manipulation of food and the mechanical formation of a bolus are accomplished largely by the tongue. The tongue positions the bolus between the teeth and moves in a complex three-dimensional chewing pattern if the bolus requires mastication. The moistening of the food in the oral cavity is essential for normal bolus transit and/or flow and clearance, particularly because gravity provides no assistance until the vertical phases of swallowing.

The oral transport phase comprises movement of the cohesive bolus (masticated if necessary) posteriorly (and horizontally when the subject is in a normal upright seated posture) to the inlet of the superior aspect of the vertical subsystem, the pharynx (Figure 93-4). The intrinsic tongue muscles change the shape of the tongue, forming grooves along its body and anterior and lateral seals to facilitate containment. This occurs along with lowering and raising of the tip of the tongue, thereby beginning constriction of the passage anteriorly to the bolus while opening the passage posteriorly to provide direction for the bolus. The extrinsic tongue muscles also change the position of the tongue within the oral cavity and assist in changing its shape. This includes confining the bolus to the anterior portion of the oral cavity by elevating the dorsum in a

ramplike posture, which is referred to as loading the bolus (Figure 93-4A), and then progressively arching the tongue posteriorly to transport the bolus to the vertical subsystem (Figures 93-4B and C).

Vertical Subsystem

The pharyngeal and laryngeal components, in conjunction with the tongue dorsum, comprise the superior aspect of the vertical subsystem, where gravity begins to assist in the transport of the bolus. The anatomic juxtaposition of the entrance to the airway (laryngeal vestibule) and the pharyngeal aspect of the upper digestive tract demand biomechanical precision to ensure simultaneous airway protection and bolus transfer or propulsion through the pharynx. To this end, the pharyngeal transport phase is characterized by a sequence of rapid, highly coordinated neuromuscular events that cause pressure changes critical to bolus transport or transit in a safe, timely, efficient manner.

Linguapalatal contact sequentially moves the bolus against the posterior pharyngeal wall, contributing to the positive pressures imparted to the bolus and propelling it downward. Simultaneously, the pharyngeal constrictors begin to contract in a descending sequence, first elevating and widening the entire pharynx to engulf the bolus (Figure 93-4D and E). A descending peristaltic wave then cleanses the pharynx of residue. Although the tongue is the primary propulsive mechanism responsible for plunging the bolus into the vertical subsystem by virtue of its contact with the pharyngeal constrictor or constrictors, several other events occur just milliseconds apart that also contribute to pressure gradients facilitating the bolus transfer.

Velar movements may occur earlier during the volitional swallow sequence, however, tight closure of the velopharynx is achieved during the pharyngeal transport phase. Closure provides a seal at the superior aspect of the vertical system, preventing nasal leakage of the bolus and contributing to the generation of high positive pressures which are applied to the bolus.

Several mechanisms ensure the redundancy by which airway protection is accomplished. Three levels of sphincteric closure include (1) the aryepiglottic folds, (2) the false vocal folds, and (3) the true vocal folds, with closure of the true vocal folds (the lowest of the three sphincters) providing "the last line of defense" to prevent aspiration of invasive material.

Additionally the hyolaryngeal complex is lifted upward and forward by the combined contraction of the suprahyoid muscles, thyrohyoid muscles, and pharyngeal elevators. This hyolaryngeal elevation and anterior movement, coupled with retraction of the tongue base, covers the laryngeal vestibule and diverts the bolus laterally around the airway. Timely relaxation and opening of the upper esophageal sphincter (UES) permits continuous vertical passage of the bolus into the esophagus, and the pharyngeal transport stage terminates when the UES returns to its hypertonic, closed resting state. The UES functions as a mechanical valve. For it to open normally, four criteria must be met: (1) relaxation of muscle tone, (2) compliant tissue, (3) traction force provided by sufficient hyolaryngeal excursion, and (4) pulsion force imparted by the bolus.

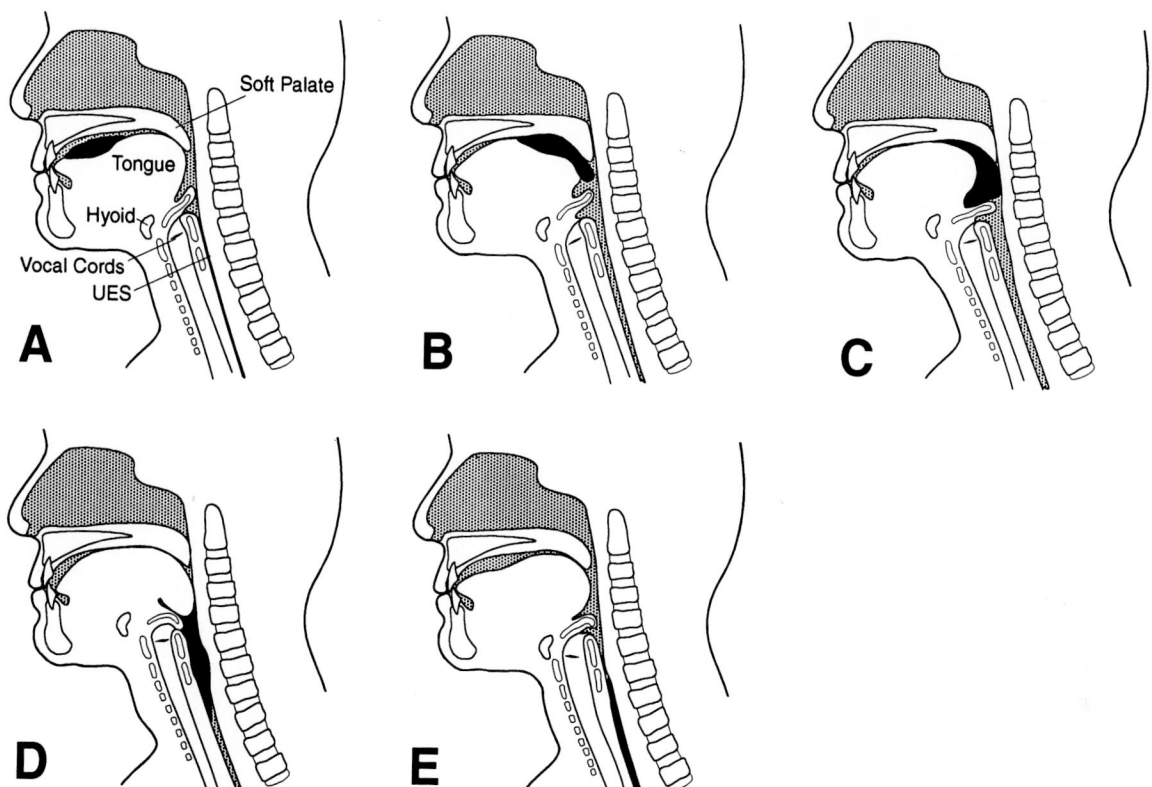

Figure 93-4   Lateral view of the propulsion of a bolus (black mass) during swallowing. UES, upper esophageal sphincter. (A) Voluntary initiation of the swallow by tongue "loading." (B) Bolus propulsion by the tongue dorsum and UES opening in anticipation of bolus arrival. (C) Bolus entry into the pharynx associated with downward tilting of the epiglottis, hyolaryngeal excursion, and UES opening. (D) Linguapharyngeal contact facilitating bolus passage through the pharynx. (E) The UES and the completion of oropharyngeal swallowing when the entire bolus is in the esophagus. Adapted with permission from Robbins JA: Normal swallowing and aging. *Semin Neurol* 16(4):309, 1996.

In normal swallowing UES relaxation and opening occur *prior to* bolus arrival at the hypopharynx. In fact, anticipatory opening of the UES produces subatmospheric pressure at the bottom of the pharynx, providing a suction force from below to in effect "pull" the bolus into the esophagus as it is being plunged from above.

As the bolus volume increases, so do the magnitude and duration of the anterior and superior hyolaryngeal excursion and the related UES opening and relaxation. Bolus consistency also affects the temporal organization of the ensuing swallow. The importance of bolus characteristics indicates that swallowing events during the oral phase influence pharyngeal events downstream and suggest the presence of feed*back* and feed *forward* mechanisms in the swallowing neural circuitry that have important clinical implications.

Neurophysiology of Oropharyngeal Swallowing

Historically, swallowing was largely viewed as a sequence of pharyngeal and esophageal events and was defined as reflexive. The findings from quantitative temporospatial studies on normal swallowing conducted in the last two decades, and current knowledge of the underlying neural substrates, have provided new insights into oropharyngeal

swallowing showing that it is a patterned response rather than a traditional reflex.

Sensorimotor control of swallowing requires the coordinated activity to be distributed across both the cranial and spinal nerve systems, including the peripheral nerves, their central nuclei, and their neural centers. More specifically, the neural control of swallowing involves five major components: (1) afferent sensory fibers contained in cranial nerves, (2) cerebral and midbrain fibers that synapse with the brainstem swallowing centers, (3) paired swallowing centers in the brainstem, (4) efferent motor fibers contained in cranial nerves and the ansa cervicalis, and (5) muscle and end organs. Indeed, this neural network spans all levels of the neuraxis from the cerebrum superiorly to the brainstem and spinal nerves inferiorly and muscles and end organs at the periphery. This relatively diffuse network is designed to integrate and sequence both the volitional and automatic actions of swallowing.

Healthy persons depend on a highly automated neuromuscular sensorimotor process that intricately coordinates the activities of chewing, swallowing, and airway protection. To accomplish a normal swallow in 2 seconds or less, the muscles of chewing interact with 26 pairs of striated pharyngeal and laryngeal muscles. The muscles involved in chewing include the masseters, temporalis, and pterygoids (innervated by cranial nerve V); the lip and buccal musculature, the orbicularis oris, and the buccinator (innervated

A

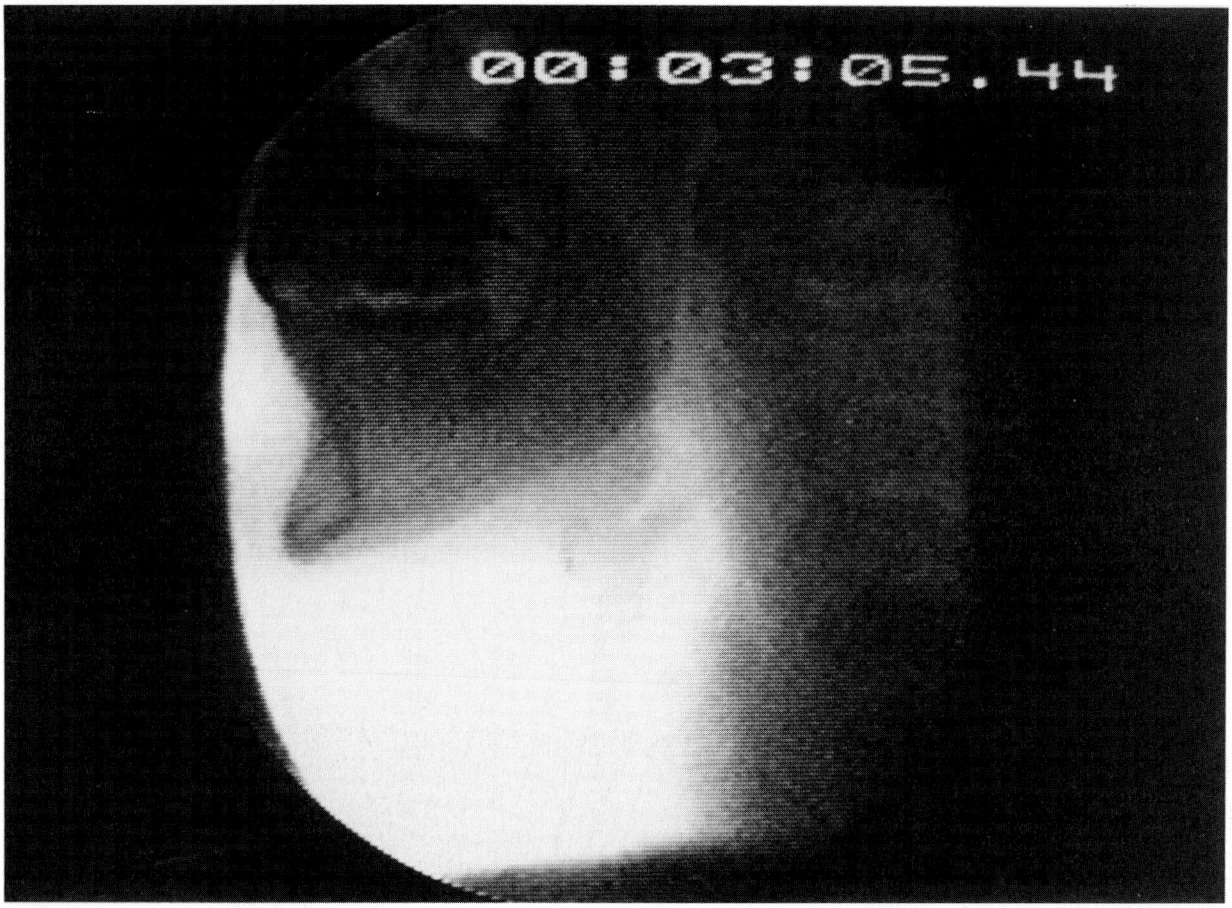

00:03:05.44

B

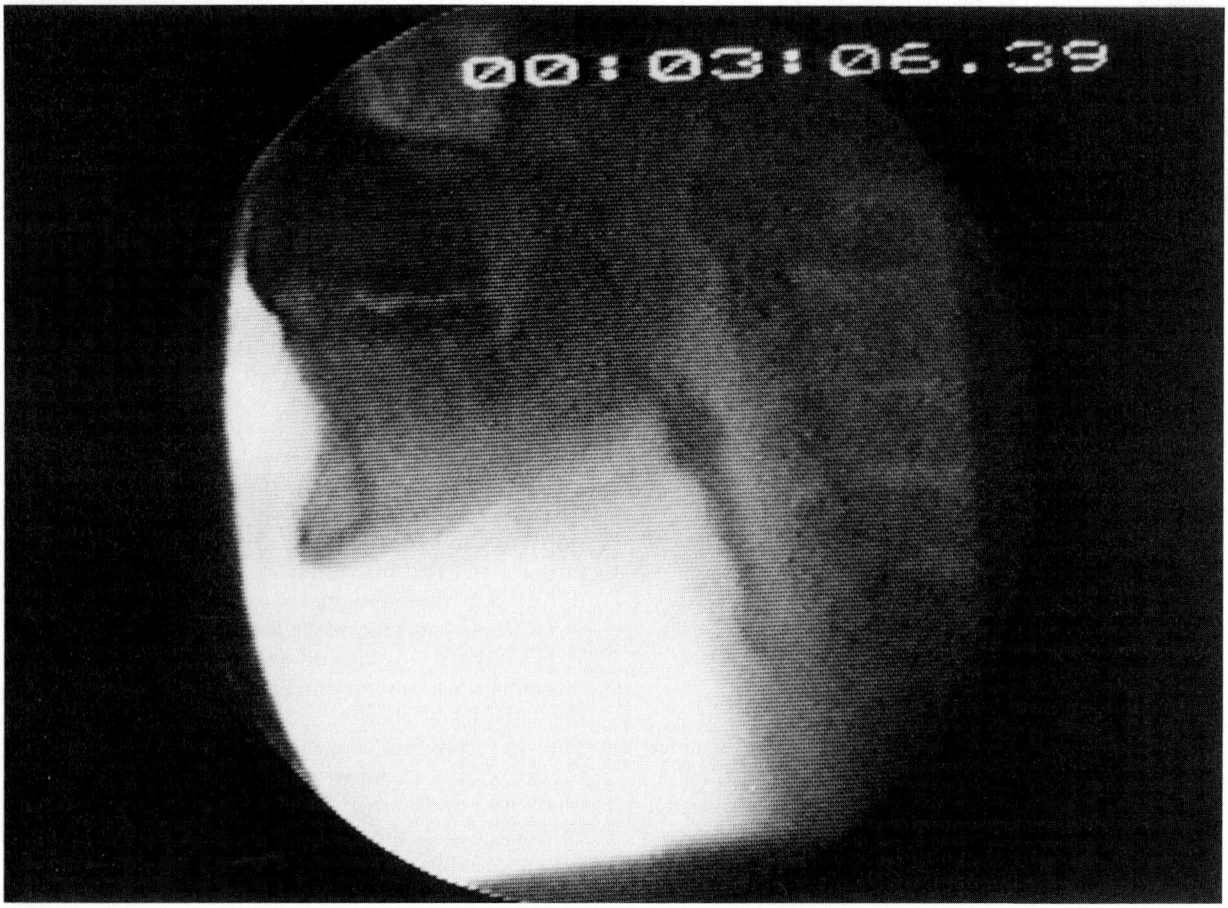

00:03:06.39

C

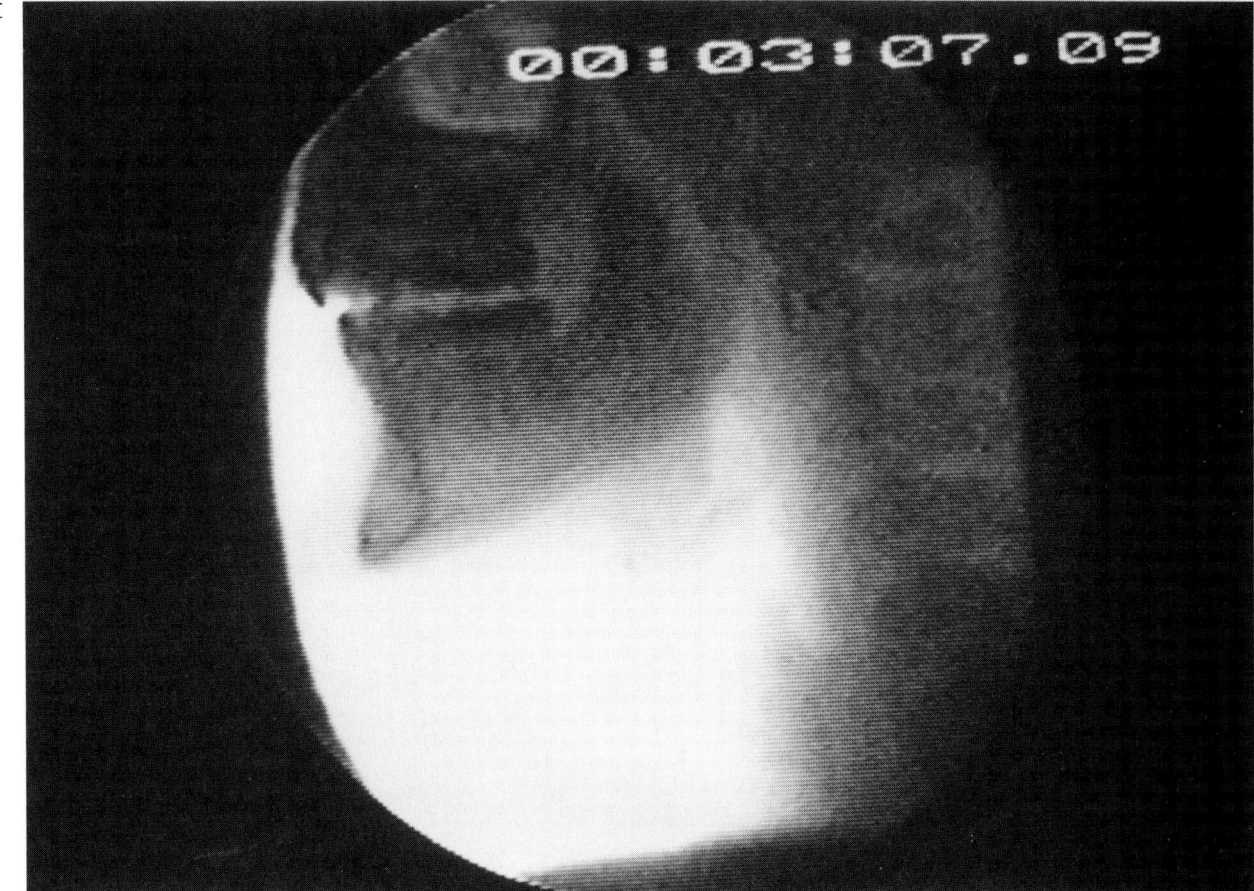

Figure 93-5 Healthy young swallowing documented with videofluoroscopy. (A) Bolus in oral cavity, ready to be swallowed. (B) Bolus appears as a "column" of material swiftly moving through the pharynx. (C) Oropharynx cleared of material when the swallow is completed. Adapted with permission from Robbins JA: Normal swallowing and aging. *Semin Neurol* 16(4):309, 1996.

by cranial nerve VII); and the intrinsic and extrinsic lingual muscles (innervated by cranial nerve XII). Optimal structural integrity and precise neural mediation result in continuous, rapid bolus flow from the mouth to the esophagus (Figure 93-5) that accommodates variations in bolus size, texture, and temperature and the individual's intent to swallow, chew, or just hold the bolus in the mouth.

Research on swallowing neurophysiology over the past decade has begun to reveal complex underlying neural substrates that may provide an understanding of how willful control during the early stage of swallowing allows access to the patterned response. Behavioral and sensory interventions attempting to modify a response certainly have more treatment potential than if they are aimed at a reflex.

SENESCENT SWALLOWING

Traditional thinking suggests that the causes of dysphagia are always disease-related, with direct or indirect damage to effector end-organ systems of swallowing. More recently, research has indicated that swallowing changes occur even with healthy aging. This work, focused primarily on the anatomy and physiology of the oropharyngeal swallowing mechanism, describes a progression of change that may

put the older population at increased risk for dysphagia. This research is particularly relevant when an older healthy adult, whose functional reserve is naturally diminished, is faced with increased stressors such as central nervous system (CNS)-altering medications, mechanical perturbations (e.g., a nasogastric [NG] tube or a tracheostomy), or chronic medical conditions (e.g., frailty) that might not elicit dysphagia in a less vulnerable individual. Translation of this work into clinical practice will provide safeguards against the overdiagnosis and overtreatment of dysphagia in the elderly population.

Age-associated Changes in Swallowing

A major characteristic of older healthy swallowing is that it occurs more slowly. More time is required for initiation of the more automatic pharyngeal phase of the swallow. In people older than 65 years, the initiation of laryngeal and pharyngeal events, including laryngeal vestibule closure, maximal hyolaryngeal excursion, and upper UES opening, takes significantly longer than in adults younger than 45 years. Although the specific neural underpinning has not been confirmed, oral events may become uncoupled from the pharyngeal response. Thus, in older healthy adults the bolus may remain adjacent to an open airway by pooling or

A

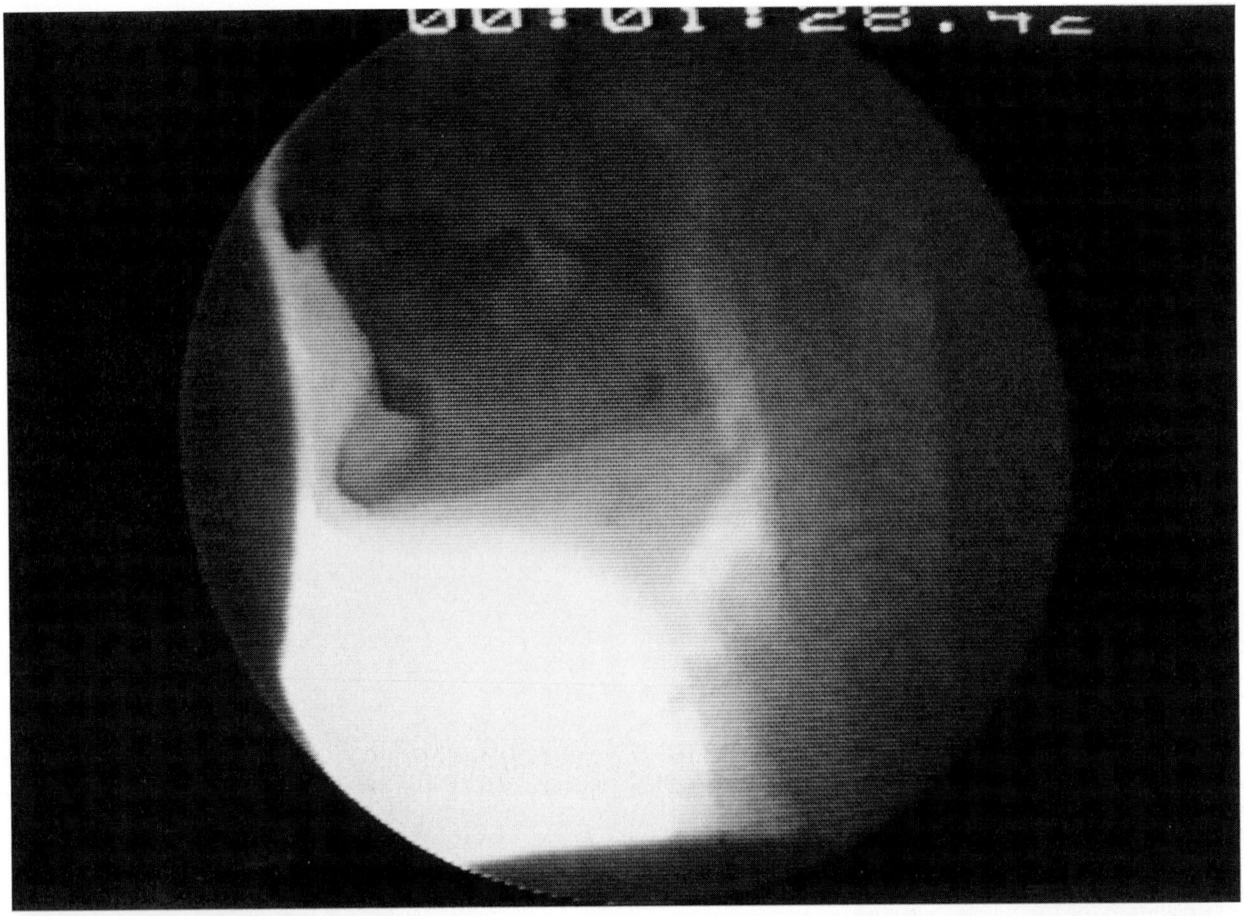

B

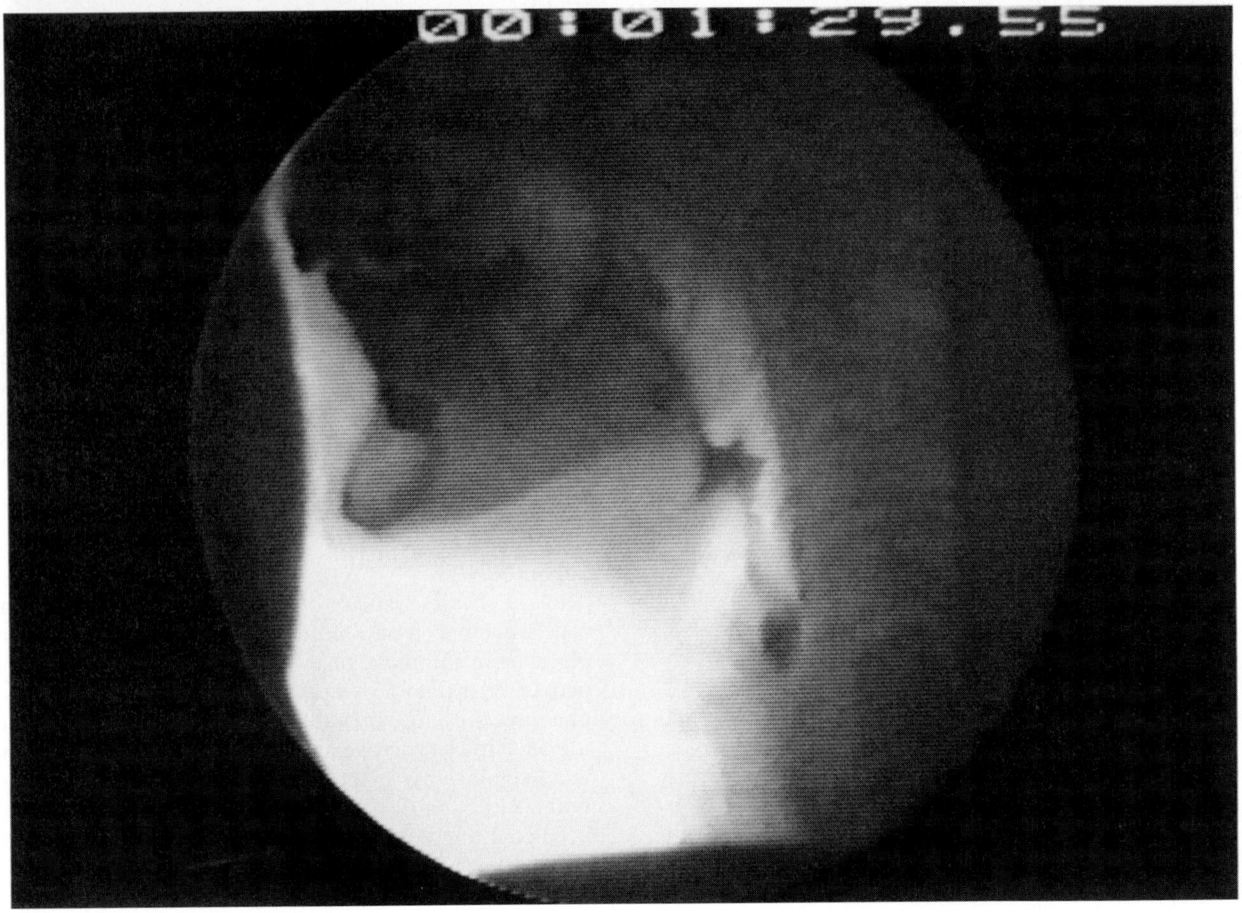

C

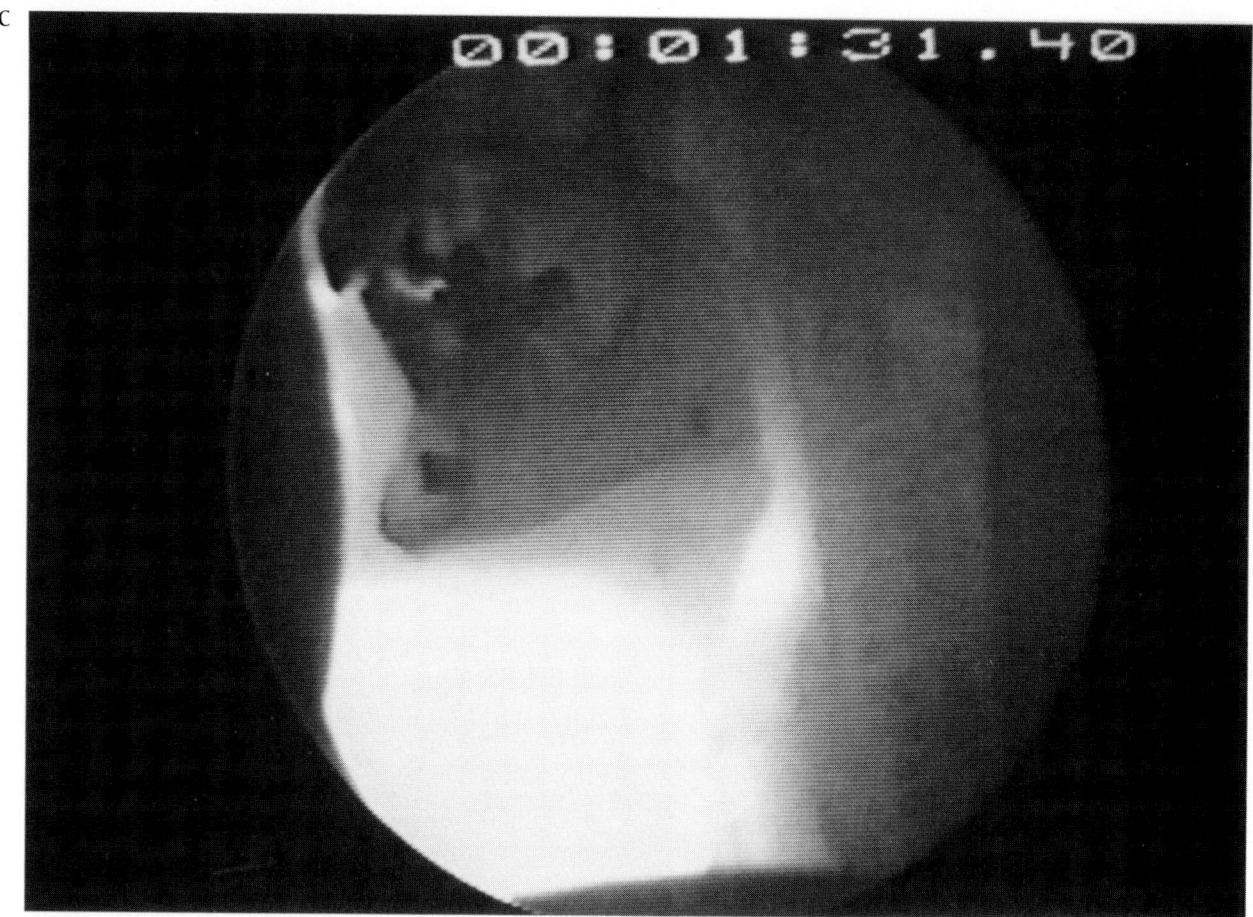

Figure 93-6   Healthy old swallowing documented with videofluoroscopy. (A) Bolus in mouth ready for swallowing. (B) Bolus pooled in vallecula and pyriform sinus during delayed onset of pharyngeal response. (C) Bolus cleared of material when the swallow is completed. Adapted with permission from Robbins JA: Normal swallowing and aging. *Semin Neurol* 16(4):309, 1996.

pocketing in the pharyngeal recesses longer than in younger adults (Figure 93-6).

Whereas older adults tested during swallowing demonstrate that pharyngeal events, including opening of the UES, are delayed from initiation of the swallow, an equally critical finding may be that the *range* of the UES opening is diminished. Scintigraphic studies have shown increased pharyngeal residue with age, possibly related to the limited UES opening, which indicates that the glottis is exposed to the swallowed bolus longer in older individuals.

Aspiration and airway penetration are believed to be the most significant adverse clinical outcomes of misdirected bolus flow, as reflected in the high rates of pneumonia with increasing age and disease. However, airway invasion in healthy adults is largely absent. The use of an eight-point scale (Table 93-2) that discretely quantifies the occurrence, the depth, and the person's reaction to airway penetration or aspiration found no significant difference between young (21- to 32-year-old) and old (63- to 84-year-old) age groups in scale scores.

Using simultaneous videofluoroscopy and manometry (manofluoroscopy) and a tube through the nasopharynx similar in size to a "garden variety" NG tube, a significant interaction was found for tube by age. That is, liquid penetrated the airway significantly more frequently when

the tube was in place only in the *oldest* group of men and women (older than 70 years). Thus, it appears that under stressful conditions (e.g., the perturbation caused by a tube through the nasopharynx), older individuals are less able to compensate and are more at risk for aspiration. Findings such as these characterize presbyphagia or "old swallowing" which is *not* abnormal swallowing in the elderly population.

Age-related changes in the generation of lingual pressure also define presbyphagia. Healthy older individuals have reduced isometric tongue pressures compared with younger individuals. In contrast, the generation of maximal lingual pressure during swallowing (which requires submaximal pressures) remains "young" in magnitude. Because the peak lingual pressures used in swallowing are lower than those generated isometrically, healthy older individuals manage to achieve the pressures necessary to effect a successful swallow. The relationship between maximum isometric pressure and peak swallowing pressures can be considered an indication of the functional reserve available for swallowing. As people get older, slower swallowing may allow time to recruit the necessary number of motor units required for pressures critical for adequate bolus propulsion through the oropharynx. Thus, therapeutically speeding up an older swallow may result in less than sufficient

Table 93-2 Multidimensional Depth of Airway Invasion and Residue, Single-digit Scoring System for the Penetration-Aspiration Scale

Category	Score	Description
No penetration or aspiration	1	Contrast does not enter the airway
P E N E T R A T I O N	2	Contrast enters the airway, remains above vocal folds, no residue
	3	Contrast remains above vocal folds, visible residue remains
	4	Contrast contacts vocal folds, no residue
	5	Contrast contacts vocal folds, visible residue remains
A S P I R A T I O N	6	Contrast passes glottis, no subglottic residue visible
	7	Contrast passes glottis, visible subglottic residue despite patient's response
	8	Contrast passes glottis, visible subglottic residue, absent patient response

Rosenbek JC, Robbins JA, Roecker EB, Coyle JC, Woody GL: A penetration aspiration scale. *Dysphagia*, 11: 93–98, 1996.
Robbins JA, Coyle JC, Roecker EB, Rosenbek JC, Woody Differentiation of normal and abnormal airway protection during swallowing using the penetration aspiration scale. *Dysphagia*, 14(4):228–232, 1999.

swallow pressures and therefore may be contraindicated as a therapy technique.

Neurophysiologic Correlates of Senescent Swallowing

A slowing of performance in fine and gross motor tasks is well documented in elderly persons. The reaction time to sensory stimuli declines with increasing age. Magnetic resonance imaging (MRI) is highly sensitive in detecting periventricular white-matter hyperintensities (PVHs) in cerebral white-matter tracts. Neuroimaging studies using cranial MRI in normal adults show a relationship between slower swallowing and an increase in the number and severity of PVHs in the brain, supporting the concept that voluntary control of swallowing is mediated by corticobulbar pathways traveling within the periventricular white matter. The occurrence and degree of PVHs increase with age and may explain, at least in part, the relatively asymptomatic decline in oropharyngeal motor performance observed in older people.

Changes in the periphery also occur with age and may be a function of changes in various sensory mechanisms or caused by muscle atrophy. Similar to the age-related loss of limb skeletal muscle, are the changes with age in fiber density, muscle tension, muscle strength, and muscle contraction in facial, masticatory, and lingual musculature.

Thus, the differences in the swallowing function between elderly and young individuals appear to be dependent on age-associated changes in both central and peripheral mechanisms. Rather than reflecting CNS deterioration, slowed swallowing that remains coordinated and effective, as found in most healthy old people, may represent a compensatory strategy for achieving pressure-generation values that may be critical to successful bolus propulsion. Progress in elucidating the biological basis of presbyphagia may have far-reaching significance for approaches to intervention in and prevention of age-related dysphagia. For example, lingual exercise protocols may reduce the probability that environmental demands will exceed the remaining functional capacity in older swallowers.

DIFFERENTIAL CONSIDERATIONS FOR DYSPHAGIA AND ASPIRATION

Etiologies

Older adults are at increased risk for developing dysphagia because of a number of age-associated phenomena. Several factors contribute to and several comorbid processes also increase the chances that older adults will suffer the adverse consequences of dysphagia—dehydration, malnutrition, and aspiration pneumonia. By targeting high-risk groups and intervening with acceptable compensatory and rehabilitative approaches, it is hoped that the ultimate burden of dysphagia on the geriatric population will decline.

A decreased physiologic reserve can combine with a number of age-related, disease-related, or iatrogenic changes to transform an at-risk individual into an older adult with dysphagia. The concept of homeostenosis, or decreased physiologic reserve, is being recognized as a crucial covariable with dysphagia. Frailty or sarcopenia may be outward manifestations of this poor reserve. Several anatomic or pathologic perturbations occurring throughout the orobuccal cavity, the laryngopharyngeal region, and the esophagus must also be acknowledged as important cofactors in the onset of dysphagia.

Age-related Conditions

Age-related changes throughout the upper aerodigestive tract can influence swallowing integrity. Oral risks are also discussed in Chapter 94. During the oral phase, the food bolus may be inadequately prepared because of poor or absent dentition, periodontal disease, ill-fitting dentures, or inappropriate salivation caused by xerostomia. Musculoskeletal factors such as weakness of the muscles of mastication, arthritis of the temporomandibular joint or larynx, osteoporosis of the jaw, or changes in tongue strength and coordination of the oropharyngeal events can deter efficient swallowing. Sensory input for taste, temperature, and tactile sensation changes in many older adults. This disruption of sensory-cortical-motor feedback loops may interfere with proper bolus formation and timely response of the swallowing motoric sequence and detract from the pleasure of eating. Sensory discrimination thresholds in the oral cavity and laryngopharynx increase with age, interfering with initiation of the natural swallowing reaction when pharyngeal pooling of liquid or saliva occurs. Controversy exists regarding the predictive value of an absent gag reflex for aspiration, but many clinicians still use this criterion to screen for altered pharyngeal sensation.

Material can penetrate into the upper airway in normal individuals if the bolus is not properly prepared, if the timing of the swallow is delayed, or if the intake is too rapid. Important risk factors for aspiration include altered level of attention during feeding (e.g., delirium), altered sensory discrimination in the oropharynx, feeding problems, mechanical ventilation, and feeding tube placement. In the latter circumstance, the rate of tube feeding, the position of the patient, altered intestinal transit times, and the ability of the patient to protect their airway all influence the occurrence of reflux and aspiration and are discussed in detail in Chapter 92. Gastroesophageal reflux due to lower esophageal sphincter (LES) incompetence also predisposes individuals to micro- or macroaspiration.

Age-related Disease

Neurologic and neuromuscular disorders are one of the principal risks for dysphagia (Table 93-3). Neurologic diseases rise in prevalence in older cohorts of the population. Stroke, head injury, Alzheimer's disease and other dementia syndromes, and parkinsonism all place older adults at increased risk for dysphagia with its incipient consequences.

Because cognitive function and/or communication may be impaired, it is important for the practitioner to note the warning signs associated with dysphagia and a risk of aspiration (Table 93-4). Between 50 percent and 75 percent of patients who have had a recent acute stroke develop eating and swallowing problems, with ensuing complications of aspiration developing in 50 percent, malnutrition in 45 percent, and pneumonia in 35 percent. Other adverse consequences have also been reported, with up to 15 percent of patients who have suffered a cerebrovascular accident (CVA) developing pneumonia within 1 year of the acute insult. Brainstem or bilateral hemispheric strokes produce dysphagia, but unilateral lesions can contribute to dysphagia. Daniels and colleagues identified six clinical features associated with an increased risk for aspiration poststroke. These included (1) an abnormal volitional cough, (2) an abnormal gag reflex, (3) dysarthria, (4) dysphonia, (5) a cough following a trial swallow, and (6) a voice change following a trial swallow. The presence of any two of these findings had a sensitivity of 92 percent and a specificity of 67 percent in predicting that there would be penetration and aspiration of material as evidenced with videofluoroscopy.

A host of common problems involving the head and neck can directly damage the effector muscles of swallowing and increase the risk for dysphagia. Head and neck injury, carcinoma, complex infections and thyroid

Table 93-3   Neurologic Disorders Causing Dysphagia

Stroke

Head trauma

Parkinsonism and other movement and neurodegenerative disorders

Progressive supranuclear palsy
   Olivopontocerebellar atrophy
   Huntington's disease
   Wilson's disease

Torticollis
   Tardive dyskinesia

Alzheimer's disease and other dementias

Motor neuron disease (amyotrophic lateral sclerosis)

Guillain-Barré syndrome and other polyneuropathies

Neoplasms and other structural disorders
   Primary brain tumors
   Intrinsic and extrinsic brainstem tumors
   Base of skull tumors
   Syringobulbia
   Arnold–Chiari malformation
   Neoplastic meningitis

Multiple sclerosis

Postpolio myelitis syndrome

Infectious disorders
   Chronic infectious meningitis
   Syphilis and Lyme disease
   Diphtheria
   Botulism
   Viral encephalitis, including rabies

Myasthenia gravis

Myopathy
   Polymyositis, dermatomyositis, inclusion body
     myositis, and sarcoidosis
   Myotonic and oculopharyngeal muscular dystrophy
   Hyper- and hypothyroidism
   Cushing's syndrome

Iatrogenic conditions
   Medication side effects
   Postsurgical neurogenic dysphagia
     Neck surgery
     Posterior fossa surgery
     Irradiation of the head and neck

conditions, and diabetes are associated with age-related dysphagia. Although vertebral osteophytes are common, these bony growths alone rarely cause dysphagia. Dysphagia more commonly results from the presence of osteophytes in conjunction with neuromuscular weakness or

Table 93-4 Warning Signs Associated With Dysphagia and Aspiration Risk

Decreased alertness or cognitive dysfunction
 Stupor, coma, heavy sedation, delirium, "sundowning," dementia, agitation
 Playing with food, inappropriate size of bites, talking or emotional lability during attempts to swallow

Changes in approach to food
 Avoidance of eating in company
 Increase in amount of food remaining on plate
 Special physical preparation of food or avoidance of foods of specific consistency
 Prolonged mealtime, intermittent cessation of intake, frequent "wash downs"
 Compensatory measures (head and neck movements)
 Laborious chewing, repetitive swallowing
 Coughing and choking on swallowing, increased need to clear throat

Manifestations of impaired oropharyngeal functions
 Dysarthria
 Wet, hoarse voice and other voice changes
 Dysfunction of focal musculature (facial asymmetries, abnormal reflexes or dystonia, dyskinesias or fasciculations)
 Drooling or oral spillage, pooling and pocketing of food
 Frequent throat clearing

Patient complaints or observations of
 Difficulty initiating a swallow
 Sensation of obstruction of bolus in the throat or chest
 Regurgitation of food or acid
 Inability to handle secretions
 Unexplained weight loss
 Impaired breathing during meals or immediately after eating
 Pain on swallowing
 Leakage of food or saliva from a tracheostomy site

Table 93-5 Mechanisms by Which Common Medications Contribute to Dysphagia

Xerostomia
Anticholinergic effects
 Tricyclic antidepressants
 Antipsychotic agents
 Antihistamine drugs
 Antispasmodic drugs
 Antiparkinsonism drugs
 Antimetic drugs
Other mechanisms
 Antihypertensives (e.g., diuretics, calcium channel blockers)

Reduction in esophageal and/or laryngeal peristalsis
Antihypertensive drugs (e.g., dihydropyridine calcium channel blockers)
Antianginal drugs (e.g., nitrates)

Delayed neuromuscular responses
Drugs that promote delirium (e.g., anticholinergic agents, opiates, benzodiazepines)
Drugs that have extrapyramidal side effects (e.g., antipsychotic drugs)

Esophageal injury and/or inflammation
Drugs that relax the lower esophageal sphincter (e.g., calcium channel blockers, nitrates)
Large pills that have incomplete esophageal transit

---

discoordination, probably caused by combinations of several underlying conditions such as diabetes, chronic obstructive pulmonary disease, congestive heart failure, renal failure, an immunocompromised status, and/or cachexia.

Sometimes dysphagia can be a direct consequence of a treatment provided for another disease process. Health care interventions can result in drug-induced delirium, protracted hospital stays, and ultimately malnutrition. Indwelling NG tubes, airway intubation, and medication effects may all predispose a frail older adult with borderline airway protection to develop frank aspiration. Understanding the iatrogenic causes of dysphagia can alter medical practice and may reduce its incidence and complications.

Older adults are much more likely to be taking medications for multiple medical conditions. Many of these agents can influence salivary flow, intestinal peristalsis,

cognition, or psychomotor status, thereby interfering with normal oropharyngoesophageal function or altering airway protection. More than 2000 drugs can cause xerostomia or reduced salivary flow via anticholinergic mechanisms. The list is extensive and can include common antidepressants, antihistamines, antipsychotics, and antihypertensive agents. Likewise, a number of delirium-promoting therapies exist and similarly produce adverse consequences through either anticholinergic or other central mind-altering effects. Certain agents can directly relax the LES and increase acid reflux and esophageal problems. Finally several psychotropic drugs can produce delayed neuromuscular responses or extrapyramidal effects, thereby influencing the tongue and bulbar musculature. Table 93-5 provides a partial list of these agents and how they can contribute to dysphagia.

An altered level of attention and cognition may also produce special concerns with regard to safe eating and swallowing. As described elsewhere in this book, delirium is frequently underrecognized and undertreated in both hospital and institutional settings. In general, testing an inattentive adult for dysphagia results in the poorest evaluation. If swallowing is assessed during one of these episodes, aspiration is likely to occur. If a staff member at a hospital or nursing home feeds a patient during one of these intervals, the outcome may be disastrous.

Several different treatments can either directly or indirectly damage swallowing effector organs as described previously. Head and neck cancer surgeries, some spinal cord surgeries, thyroid surgeries, and any intervention that can jeopardize the recurrent laryngeal nerve may result in dysphagia. A number of chemotherapy and radiotherapy regimes can cause oropharyngeal injury. The prospective outcome of dysphagia should be incorporated into the risk–benefit discussions of these procedures.

Symptoms

Medical history plays a critical role in establishing a diagnosis of dysphagia (Table 93-6). A detailed history can elucidate the proper diagnosis in some dysphagic adults and is an important first step in the evaluation process. Recognizing the classic complaints associated with dysphagia and differentiating them from symptoms of common age-related diseases can be challenging. Nevertheless, a careful history may avert increased testing and potential iatrogenic complications in frail older patients. Dysphagia may also present in a more subtle fashion, without symptoms, but with recurring exacerbations of an underlying disease such as chronic obstructive pulmonary disease.

In an institutional setting the medical history can be obtained from the patient, a caregiver, or even a nurse's aide. Patients may initially complain of difficulty in swallowing liquids, solid food, or pills. Caregivers or nursing personnel may note "pocketing" of pills within the oral cavity. The patient or the patient's family members may complain of the increased time needed to complete a meal. The patient or the practitioner may identify weight loss without any other localizing explanation. However, clinicians must distinguish these dysphagia or aspiration symptoms from a myriad of other common health problems that may mimic dysphagia in older adults. For example, in frail individuals depression or early parkinsonism may be manifested solely by weight loss and slowed eating. Without a complete history, these patients may be sent for a dysphagia work-up before an attempt is made to manage their "root problem."

Certain symptoms may help identify difficulties in specific phases of the swallowing sequence. Symptoms of oral preparatory or oropharyngeal dysphagia can include food spillage and excessive drooling. Difficulty in initiating the swallow, nasal regurgitation, or residual food in the oral cavity following the swallow can signify oral transit problems. Other commonly described symptoms indicating changes in the oropharyngeal swallow include immediate choking, coughing, and alteration of voice quality during or after meals. Important, albeit more subtle, associated symptoms suggesting oropharyngeal dysphagia include a nasal voice or new snoring. Both these findings correlate with weakness of the palatal muscles and perhaps tongue musculature as well. In individuals with cognitive impairment or dementia, the only sign of dysphagia may be refusing food or retaining food in the mouth after extended chewing. In advanced dementia, patients may even appear to forget how to eat or swallow without significant cueing. Whether the motor pattern for swallowing has been forgotten or whether the problem is more of the nature of swallowing apraxia secondary to dementia is yet to be determined.

Table 93-6   Historical Data Used for Clinical Diagnosis of Dysphagia

Site or timing of impairment
  Oral (problems with chewing, bolus gathering, initiation of swallow)
  Pharyngeal (problem immediately on swallowing, choking after a long delay, suggestive of passage of residue from the pharynx into the larynx)
  Esophageal (seconds after swallow, behind chest bone)

Onset, frequency, and progression
  Duration, sudden onset related to a specific event (stroke, pill impaction, etc.), or gradual
  Frequency (constant, intermittent)
  Progression and severity (including more and more foods and impairing nutrition and hydration?)

Aggravating factors and compensatory mechanisms
  Food consistency (solids and/or liquids)
  Temperature
  Usefulness of sucking, turning, and tilting of head, and so on
  Intermittent, constant, or fatiguing symptoms

Associated symptoms
  Change in speech or voice
  Weakness; lack of control of musculature, particularly of the head and neck
  Choking or coughing
  Repetitive swallows or increased need to clear the throat
  Regurgitation (pharyngeal and nasal, or esophageal and gastric; immediately on swallow, or long delay, undigested food, putrefied or secretions?)
  Fullness/tightness in the throat (globus sensation)
  Pain, localized or radiating
  Odynophagia (pain on passage of bolus)

Ancillary symptoms and evidence of complications
  Loss of weight or loss of energy (including from dehydration)
  Change in appetite; attitude toward food, toward eating in company; preparation of foods
  Respiratory problems (cough, increased sputum production, shortness of breath, pneumonias and other respiratory infections)
  Sleep disturbances (secondary to secretion management or regurgitation)
  Changes in salivation (water brash or dry mouth)

Symptoms of esophageal dysphagia include food "hanging up" behind the sternum, neck pain, chest pain, and heartburn. This issue is also addressed in Chapter 50, which includes a discussion of esophageal disorders. A specific problem with solid food dysphagia suggests a mechanical obstruction. If the symptoms are intermittent, a lower esophageal ring may be present. If the symptoms are progressive, a peptic stricture or carcinoma is more likely. If there are difficulties in ingesting solids and liquids, a neuromuscular or dysmotility etiology must be considered.

SCREENING ACROSS A CONTINUUM OF CARE SETTINGS

Dysphagia evaluation varies depending on the clinical setting. The comprehensive diagnostic approaches available for hospitalized older patients with dysphagia are often not logistically feasible for bed-bound nursing home residents. Likewise, interdisciplinary dysphagia teams are frequently available only in an academic setting or in larger hospital systems. When such a team is not available, the responsibility for screening for swallowing problems falls on the primary provider or the hospital staff. Speech language pathologists, who are usually the swallowing therapists, are well trained to conduct bedside (also referred to as noninstrumental) examinations that include history taking, oral motor assessment, voice evaluation, and assessment of trial swallows. Prior to this referral, though, clinicians can provide a focused secondary screening during their encounter with the patient. A number of attempts have been made to identify a simple screening tool for use in ambulatory clinics or at the patient' s bedside. None of these maneuvers has proven altogether effective, but certain approaches warrant mention.

A 3-oz water swallow test can be performed at the bedside. The clinician auscultates over the patient's trachea before and after the water is swallowed. Overt coughing, choking, or a change in the character of breath sounds suggests aspiration. While this test identified 80 percent of poststroke patients in a rehabilitation unit who aspirated during a subsequent videofluoroscopic swallow study, it provides no information for identifying the underlying pathophysiology of the swallow or for selecting specific interventions.

Because swallowing difficulties are very common in geriatric patients, some mechanism of primary screening should also take place within a primary care clinic setting. An example of a dysphagia screening form is provided in Table 93-7. Because swallowing is not something a patient usually mentions, it may be necessary to ask related questions until a particular word or phrase triggers an association with the patient's experience (e.g., swallowing, chewing, moving food to the throat, coughing, choking).

Many forms of comprehensive geriatric assessment now include nutritional screening, which can be used as a surrogate screening for dysphagia. Some geriatric clinics now incorporate questions about difficulties with eating or swallowing that are included in periodic screening exercises. The simple question, Do you have difficulty swallowing food? was reported to have 100 percent sensitivity and 75 percent specificity in detecting swallowing difficulties in patients with parkinsonism. Alternatively, a practitioner's recognition of the relationship among symptoms of weight loss, cough or respiratory decompensation, and dysphagia may serve as a start in addressing this common problem. Nonetheless, once dysphagia is suspected, a more complete assessment is necessary not only to validate its presence but also to define and construct a treatment plan that modifies the underlying sensorimotor pathophysiology.

THE TEAM APPROACH TO DYSPHAGIA

Interdisciplinary health care teams play an important role in the care of complex older adults with dysphagia. This cross-disciplinary focus helps to address not only the medical but also the functional and psychosocial consequences of this problem. The team approach offers the stated advantage of a more efficient comprehensive assessment with shared responsibility for interventions and often makes timely consultation possible. Although team care has been demonstrated to control treatment costs of at-risk older adults in managed organizations, similar studies relating to dysphagia care have not, to date, been conducted. Dysphagia teams aim to restore or maximize functional swallowing and nutritional intake. The responsibilities of team members are often divided among disciplines and can include reviewing health issues, obtaining pertinent swallowing history and an examination (which may include instrumental studies), providing education and counseling to the patient and to the family or the care provider, conducting psychosocial screening, and reviewing advance directives. Teams can be either formal or informal in composition. Formal teams exist across a spectrum of settings including dysphagia clinics, inpatient nutrition services, head and neck cancer programs, stroke programs, and nursing homes. Core teams frequently include a speech language pathologist, a dietitian, and either a physician or a nurse practitioner.

Focused Assessment of Swallowing

A major function of the swallowing team is to perform a thorough assessment of the swallowing mechanism and its function. Most commonly, the speech language pathologist plays a major role, performing a two-part examination consisting first of a clinical (bedside) noninstrumental evaluation often followed by an instrumental assessment of swallowing. A brief description of both methods follows.

Noninstrumental Swallowing Assessment

The clinical evaluation is noninstrumental and although often referred to as a "bedside" procedure can be performed in a variety of environmental settings including an outpatient office. It usually involves four types of assessment: (1) history taking; (2) voice assessment; (3) oral motor assessment; and (4) performance on trial swallows. The specific methods and measures preferred and most frequently used by clinicians when working with dysphagia of neurogenic origin, which is frequently the case in older patients, are shown in Table 93-8.

Although a noninstrumental assessment provides a breadth of information, it can only increase the suspicion of aspiration through findings such as increased secretions

Table 93-7 Dysphagia Screening Form University of Wisconsin and Madison GRECC

Patient Name: _____

Medical record # _____ or Social security # _____

Primary Diagnosis: _____

1. Do you have difficulty swallowing? Yes No Chewing? Yes No
2. Do you have difficulty moving food/liquid out of your mouth into your throat to swallow? Yes No
3. Does food/liquid remain in your mouth after you finish swallowing? Yes No
4. Do you cough or choke when drinking or eating? Yes No
   If so, how often does this occur: Infrequently
                                            Once a day
                                            1 or more times per meal
5. Does food/liquid feel like it remains in your throat after you finish swallowing? Yes No
6. Does food/liquid feel like it stays in your chest (esophagus) after you finish swallowing or eating a meal? Yes No
7. Do you bring back up food or liquid after you've swallowed it? Yes No
   If so, how many minutes or hours after swallowing does it come back up?
8. Do you have any pain when swallowing? Yes No If so, where?
9. Is your mouth dry? Yes No
10. Any difficulty swallowing your saliva? Yes No
11. Have you noticed any drooling? Yes No Wet pillow in the morning? Yes No
12. Is it taking longer to eat a meal? Yes No
13. Do you eat everything you want to eat? Yes No
14. What have you stopped eating because of difficulty?
15. What type of foods are easiest for you to swallow:

    A. All kinds of foods
    B. Soft solids (e.g., pasta, soft vegetables)
    C. Pureed
    D. Liquids

16. Are you hungry? Yes No
17. Current weight: _____
    Occurrence of weight loss over past 3 months: Yes No
    If so, please specify amount: _____
18. Are you congested in your chest, throat, nose? Yes No
    How often do you have a head cold or chest cold?

or a wet and/or gurgly voice quality. Given the possibility of silent aspiration due to decreased cognition or diminished sensation in older people, coughing and throat clearing, which are the characteristic signs of aspiration, may be absent. To rule out aspiration with an acceptable level of confidence, an instrumental assessment is often necessary. Moreover, effective dysphagia intervention relies on an accurate diagnosis of the specific pathophysiology. That is, the underlying movement disorder that results in disordered bolus flow in terms of direction, duration, and clearance, must be defined and remediated in order to eliminate or minimize the dysphagia. Most frequently, instrumental methods are necessary to clarify the aspects of the swallowing sequence that must be modified to effect safe and efficient bolus flow. Although clinicians must pursue a complete oropharyngeal and esophageal assessment of many dysphagic patients, this section focuses on oropharyngeal dysphagia and the reader is referred to Chapter 50 for a discussion of the esophagus.

Instrumental Examination

If a patient's complaints and/or symptoms involve the oral and/or pharyngeal aspects of swallowing, useful information can be obtained from an examination of the structure and function of the upper aerodigestive tract. Often the cause of dysphagia is obvious from the medical history, in which case the examination is used not to establish a medical diagnosis but to document and confirm the diagnosis as well as to describe the pathophysiology of the swallowing function. The examination sets the stage for treatment recommendations and follow-up planning. Treatment plans are often formulated after consultation with a variety of clinicians. Good documentation of the physical examination, sensorimotor findings, and the results of initial therapeutic interventions are helpful in the conference setting. Videotape recordings of the examination and still photographs may be available with most methods and are exceptionally helpful.

Table 93-8 Clinical and Bedside Swallowing Methods and Measures

History	Oral motor
Patient report of problem	Tongue strength/range of motion
Family report of problem	Lip seal/pucker
History of pneumonia	Jaw strength/lateralization
Type of neurologic insult	Soft palate movement/symmetry
Nutritional status	Dysarthria
Gastrointestinal anomaly	Speech intelligibility
Structural abnormality	Oral apraxia
Previous surgery	Volitional cough
Other disease	Ability to follow directions
Medications	Management of secretions
Voice	**Trial swallows**
Breathiness	Thin liquid
Harshness	Thick liquid
Wet/gurgly	Puree
Strained/strangled	Solid
Overall dysphonia/aphonia	Oral transit estimate
Resonance	Estimate swallow duration
	Laryngeal elevation
	Voice quality after swallow
	Ability to feed self
	Swallows per bolus
	Spontaneous cough
	Estimate of penetration/aspiration
	Estimate of oral stasis
	Observation of meal

SOURCE: Adapted from McCullough GH et al: Clinicians' preferences and practices in conducting clinical/bedside and videofluoroscopic swallowing examination in an adult/neurogenic population. *Am J Speech Lang Pathol* 8(2):149, 1999.

To obtain the most useful and valid representation of swallowing, a diagnostic test should

1. Depict soft tissues, air, fluid-filled cavities, and surrounding bone
2. Produce clear images of functional changes in multiple planes and real time
3. Allow viewing of the entire swallow
4. Be noninvasive and risk-free
5. Detect and quantify aspiration
6. Allow objective and repeatable measurements
7. Estimate prognosis and treatment potential.

A variety of imaging methods are available for studying the swallow, including ultrasound, MRI, computed tomography scanning, and scintigraphy. The two most commonly used techniques are described in the following sections.

Oropharyngeal Videofluoroscopic Swallowing Evaluation

An oropharyngeal videofluoroscopic swallowing evaluation is most commonly used to assess the integrity of the oropharyngeal anatomy, swallowing physiology, and bolus flow. Structural abnormalities and mucosal lesions are identified by the barium that is swallowed and used to outline the soft tissue structures it passes. In this manner, webs, pharyngeal diverticula, masses, and other soft tissue anomalies are revealed. Of course, structural anomalies such as postsurgically modified anatomy, scar tissue, and osteophytes can be elucidated by radiographic means. Perhaps, the two greatest strengths of the videofluoroscopic swallow evaluation are that the swallow is recorded *in motion* and preserved on a videotape for replay.

This method permits viewing of the dynamic swallow. That is, all oropharyngeal structures can be examined with regard to their contribution to the coordinated (or uncoordinated) swallow in terms of timing and range of motion. Their impact on bolus flow is made apparent. Therefore, the specific pathophysiology and its impact on bolus flow is clarified and can be targeted for treatment.

An oropharyngeal videofluoroscopic swallow study is not designed simply to determine if a patient is aspirating or even why a patient is aspirating or retaining residue. It is designed also to assist a clinician in determining if a patient can safely receive oral nourishment and tests proposed interventions to maximize their efficacy and safety. In fact, during the study the clinician often varies bolus characteristics sufficiently to be able to offer a diet recommendation (such as thickened liquid or semisolid). Additional recommendations may be simple postural adjustments, such as tucking the chin, that are shown under fluoroscopy to improve direction or efficiency of bolus flow.

Although videofluoroscopy is the instrumental method most commonly used to assess swallowing, it is limited in the following ways.

1. The amount of information obtained is restricted to a few minutes in an effort to limit radiation exposure.
2. The environment can be distracting for patients with cognitive deficits.
3. The material ingested is barium, not food, and may not simulate the swallow evoked when real food is used as a stimulus (taste, smell).

Despite these limitations, videofluoroscopy is preferred for the breadth of information it provides with regard to anatomy, physiology, bolus flow, and assessment of trial intervention.

In addition, a fluoroscopic examination can easily be extended to the esophagus when indicated. A number of patients with oropharyngeal symptoms (such as "food sticks in my throat") may demonstrate no difficulty during an oropharyngeal swallow study. These and an entire subgroup of patients with dysphagia who have no or minimal dysphagia findings in an oropharyngeal videofluoroscopic swallow study likely have an esophageal swallowing disorder often in addition to oropharyngeal dysphagia. In fact, there is a clinical phenomenon known as "referred sensation" that patients experience. Patients may sense swallowing symptomology in the throat or sternal area when in fact an extensive instrumental assessment extending to the LES reveals an explanation more distally in the esophagus. Merging of the videofluoroscopic swallow study directly into esophagraphy, which results in a distinct third test referred to as an oropharyngeal esophagram, may reveal anatomic or physiologic findings for the referred sensation. Findings may include a Schatzki's ring, an esophagus-narrowing web or stricture, a delay in LES opening or esophageal stasis, or other esophageal etiologies for the dysphagia. Thus, an oropharyngeal esophagram permits a more organized, efficient, cost-effective process for professional personnel and for the patient. Most importantly it optimizes the potential for comprehensive findings and facilitates immediate intervention.

Fiberoptic Endoscopic Evaluation of Swallowing

Fiberoptic endoscopic evaluation of swallowing (FEES) is second to videofluoroscopy in frequency of use with elderly patients. It combines the traditional endoscopic examination, in which the flexible scope allows direct visualization of the nasal cavity, the entire nasopharynx, the oropharynx, the larynx, and the hypopharynx, with dynamic recording of swallowing. Although FEES permits only limited observation of the pharyngeal swallow with details of the phases of the swallow, it provides a valuable alternative to a noninstrumental clinical assessment. It is being used with increased frequency in long-term care facilities where videofluoroscopy is unavailable. Other advantages are its repeatability, the use of real food and fluid during the assessment, and its potential as a biofeedback tool.

The limitations of FEES involve risks related to endoscopy, which include nosebleed, mucosal injury, gagging, allergic reaction to the topical anesthesia, laryngospasm, and vasovagal response. Laryngospasm is reported most often as patients are being extubated or by a sudden flow of refluxed gastric contents. Aspiration of food or liquid also might trigger laryngospasm. Patients with a history of significant aspiration, patients who require supplemental oxygen, and patients with acute mental status depression may be at increased risk if they are functioning on the edge of adequate respiratory status and cannot tolerate the minor laryngopulmonary trauma caused by the endoscope. Finally, a vasovagal response, commonly manifested as fainting, is a fairly uncommon event but can be dangerous. The unlikely possibility of encountering an adverse reaction during a flexible endoscope examination must be balanced against the daily risks faced by patients with dysphagia.

Summary of Swallowing-Focused Assessment

From a swallowing-focused assessment performed by a speech language pathologist, the following information should be made available.

1. Whether and how patients can continue to eat orally
2. An estimate of the risk for prandial aspiration or obstruction

3. Recommendations for food textures and fluid viscosities
4. Compensatory strategies such as postural adjustments and the need for adaptive feeding equipment
5. Whether assistance is required for eating
6. Rehabilitative strategies such as exercise
7. When reassessment and monitoring are recommended.

DYSPHAGIA INTERVENTION

Dysphagia clinicians and researchers have historically felt most comfortable with physiologic outcomes (movement parameters such as range of motion) and the effect on bolus flow direction, duration, and clearance as indicators of the success of an intervention. Attitudes are changing as reflected by increased concern about Quality of Life (QOL) and the development of SWAL-QOL, a dysphagia-specific patient-centered QOL instrument. Through focus group methodology, SWAL-QOL was designed to represent the patient's perspective in measuring QOL attributable to dysphagia. The questionnaire, comprising 10 domains, is completed by patients in 10 minutes on average.

The intent is for advances in QOL measurement such as SWAL-QOL to fill a void in dysphagia care, including understanding how variations in treatment affect the human experience of living with a swallowing difficulty and documenting the effectiveness of any given treatment in terms of both physiologic function and QOL. Once data are obtained clarifying how QOL varies with treatment, the dysphagia-specific tool can be used to facilitate decision making by patients and clinicians and to monitor the longitudinal course of individual patient treatment outcomes.

Treatment for dysphagia is usually either rehabilitative or compensatory in nature. Rehabilitative interventions have the capacity to directly improve dysphagia at the biological level. That is, aspects of anatomic structures (e.g., muscle) or neural circuitry are the targets of therapy that may have a direct influence on physiology, biomechanics, and bolus flow. On the other hand, compensatory interventions avoid or reduce the effects of impaired structures or neuropathology and resultant disordered physiology and biomechanics on bolus flow. Examples are presented in the following section.

Compensatory Dysphagia Interventions

Traditionally, interventions for dysphagia in elderly patients are most often compensatory in nature and are directed at modifying bolus flow by targeting neuromuscularly induced pathobiomechanics or by adapting the environment. Compensatory strategies are believed by clinicians to be less demanding on the patient in terms of effort, and many of these strategies can be imposed on a relatively passive patient. A nonexclusive sampling of compensatory strategies includes postural adjustment, slowing the rate of eating, limiting bolus size, adaptive equipment, and the most commonly used environment adaptation, diet modification.

Postural Adjustments

Postural adjustments are relatively simple to teach to a patient, require little effort to employ, and can eliminate misdirection of bolus flow through biomechanical adjustment. A general postural rule for facilitating safe swallowing is to eat in an upright posture so that the vertical phase of the oropharyngeal swallow capitalizes on gravitational forces at work when the patient is sitting with the torso, and neck at a 90° angle to the horizon and the head in line with the horizon. This posture also can assist in precluding early spillage of food or liquid from the horizontal oral phase into the pharynx and a potentially open airway as well as diminishing the probability of nasal regurgitation. A less obvious postural adjustment is useful for patients with disease-specific hemiparesis resulting from a unilateral stroke. For this group of patients, a common strategy is a head turn toward the hemiparetic side, effectively closing off that side to bolus entry and facilitating bolus transit through the nonparetic pharyngeal channel. On the other hand, if the pathophysiologic condition is the uncoupling of the oral from the pharyngeal phase of the swallow, a simple chin tuck (45°) reduces the speed of bolus passage, thereby giving the neural system the time it needs to initiate the pharyngeal and airway protection events prior to bolus entry. Other postural adjustments facilitate safe swallowing and are designed to specifically compensate for pathophysiologic conditions analyzed and treated by a swallowing clinician on referral for a swallowing assessment and treatment.

Food and Liquid Rate and Amounts

Although we live in a "fast food" society, older individuals and especially those with dysphagia take longer to eat. Eating an adequate amount of food becomes a challenge not only because of the increased time required to do so but also because fatigue frequently becomes an issue. Typically, smaller amounts per swallow are less likely to enter or block the airway, but in individuals who experience a sensory loss in the mouth or throat, larger amounts of food or liquid may be necessary to trigger a swallow. To promote a safe, efficient swallow in most individuals with swallowing and chewing difficulties, the following recommendations are useful.

- Eat slowly and allow enough time for a meal.
- Do not eat or drink when rushed or tired.
- Take small amounts of food or liquid into the mouth—use a teaspoon rather than a tablespoon.
- Concentrate on swallowing—eliminate distractions like television.
- Avoid mixing food and liquid in the same mouthful.
- Place the food on the stronger side of the mouth if there is unilateral weakness.

Adaptive Equipment

Eating and drinking aids can assist in placing, directing, and controlling the bolus of food or liquid and in maintaining proper head posture while eating. For example, modified cups with cutout rims (placed over the bridge of the nose) or straws prevent a backward head tilt when drinking to the bottom of a cup. A backward head tilt, which results in neck extension, should be avoided in most cases because when the head is tilted back, food and liquid are more likely to be misdirected into the airway. Spoons with narrow, shallow bowls or glossectomy feeding spoons (spoons developed for moving food to the back of the tongue) are useful to individuals who require assistance in placing food in certain locations in the mouth. More importantly, these utensils and devices promote independence in eating and drinking. A speech pathologist or swallowing clinician can make suggestions regarding appropriate aids for optimizing swallowing safety and satisfaction. Occupational therapists are experts in the area of adaptive equipment and can be helpful in obtaining products that are often available only commercially.

Diet Modification

The most common compensatory intervention is diet modification, a totally passive environmental adaptation. Withholding thin liquids such as water, tea, or coffee, which are most easily aspirated by older adults, and restricting liquid intake to thickened liquids is almost routine in nursing homes in an attempt to minimize or eliminate thin-liquid aspiration, presumably the long-term related outcome of which is pneumonia. Despite the huge impact these seemingly unappealing practices may have on patient QOL, they are commonly implemented in the absence of efficacy data. In keeping with the current call for evidence-based practice in health care, a National Institutes of Health (NIH)-funded clinical trial is underway to determine the efficacy of the latter practice for patients with dementia with or without Parkinson's disease. With the recent appearance of SWAL-QOL on the clinical scene, some of these ongoing practices can be evaluated from the patient's perspective as well as by the clinicians who recommend them with good intent. Additional diet modifications include a soft food diet in which the bolus maintains itself in a cohesive mass during transit. The use of sauces and gravies to minimize the formation of dry particles that may easily be misdirected into the airway is a common practice. Other strategies within this category as interventions are available, and the dietitian should work closely with the team to ensure that the safest diet is provided and that it is effective in maintaining adequate nutrition and hydration for patients.

Knowing the Heimlich Maneuver

Educating care providers and family members about the signs of choking and the standard first-aid technique for clearing the airway, namely, the Heimlich maneuver, is essential. While in fact the Heimlich maneuver can be self-administered, it is recommended that individuals with dysphagia eat in the company of someone who knows this first-aid technique. Family members should be trained in emergency techniques for clearing the airway.

Rehabilitative Dysphagia Interventions

Rehabilitative exercises are, by nature, more active and rigorous. Often a rehabilitative approach to dysphagia intervention is withheld from elderly patients because such a demanding activity is assumed to deplete any limited remaining swallowing reserve, thus potentially exacerbating dysphagia symptoms. Sufficient treatment efficacy data are unavailable, and so assumption-based patterns of practice prevail.

Although progressive resistance training appears to be safe and effective for limb musculature in older adults, such training has only begun to be systematically applied to the muscles of swallowing. A description of two different exercise regimens that are supported with efficacy data for improving swallowing-related function in the elderly follow.

One is a simple isotonic/isometric neck exercise performed over a 6-week period in which the patient simply lies flat on his back and lifts his head (keeping shoulders flat) for a specified number of repetitions. The improved physiologic outcome of UES opening that affects swallowing is speculated to result from strengthening the mylohyoid/geniohyoid muscle groups and possibly the anterior segment of the digastric muscle.

Lingual resistance exercise has been used to strengthen the tongue, which as mentioned earlier is a key to successful oropharyngeal swallowing. Elderly patients have demonstrated increased lingual strength, improved timing of the swallowing components, and broadened their dietary intake seemingly as a function of this exercise.

Such findings suggest that older individuals are able to benefit from rehabilitative exercises focused on bulbar-innervated head and neck musculature. The methods hold promise for not only influencing safe, efficient bolus flow with significant functional gains but also may restore health and improve QOL as well.

OPTIMIZING SWALLOWING AND RELATED HEALTH THROUGH PREVENTION

The prevention of dysphagia and its sequelae, such as pneumonia, can be pursued actively in several ways. As described above, preventative exercises for retaining maximum functional reserve appear promising.

Medications

Minimizing medications that may, most often in combination, put a patient at risk for dysphagia is an important goal. Furthermore, pills are often described by patients as being difficult to swallow. Patients should be informed about medications that can be crushed, can be mixed with foods, or are available in liquid form. Pill-induced damage to the esophagus can occur if pills are taken when lying down or with inadequate amounts of liquid.

On the other hand, some medicines can enhance the swallow. For example, in parkinsonism, the timing of medication can be adjusted to allow it to achieve the greatest effect in improving swallowing coordination at mealtimes.

Oral Hygiene

Poor oral hygiene is a risk factor for pneumonia, and aspiration of saliva, whether or not it is combined with food

or fluid, can increase the likelihood of infection. Therefore, patients should be encouraged to perform oral hygiene several times a day and undergo periodic dental examinations. Furthermore, products to relieve oral dryness, as well as alcohol-free mouth care products, can be recommended.

Mealtime Atmosphere

Optimizing the mealtime atmosphere is critical to successful swallowing for many older adults. Individuals with swallowing problems may have to utilize a series of strategies or compensations in order to swallow more easily. For instance, a chin tuck while taking smaller sips of fluid is a common, useful combination. In order to ensure that a sequence of strategies is implemented, or merely to permit the additional concentration that a reduced reserve capacity demands for optimal performance, a quiet, distraction-free atmosphere while eating is important to promote safe swallowing and enhance intake. Reducing noise and eliminating distractions such as television, radio, and telephone calls is helpful. Limiting conversation during the meal is also important. Any techniques for maximizing the powers of concentration and minimizing distraction during mealtime are encouraged.

TuBe or Not TuBe —Oral Versus Nonoral Intake

Oropharyngeal dysphagia is potentially life-threatening. In the older population, critical decisions often must be made that impact on the patient's safety, health, and QOL. Among these perplexing issues is the question of continuing oral intake or providing nonoral enteral or parenteral nutrition. This dilemma is also reviewed in Chapter 92.

Enteral nutrition, the delivery of nutritive products to the digestive system through nonoral means, is often selected for the temporary prevention of aspiration in acutely ill patients. It also is chosen for longer-term nutritive supplementation or permanent replacement in patients whose disease process results in confirmed or suspected swallowing-related aspiration or malnutrition and dehydration. In the case of the latter, older patients whose chronic disease processes are overlaid on a system with a reduced functional reserve for safe, sufficient swallowing, the clinician's impressions often direct decisions relating to tube feeding for weeks, months, or even years. Rabenek et al wrote: "No explicit guidelines for percutaneous endoscopic gastrostomy (PEG) tube placement are available to guide clinical decision-making. In the absence of such guidelines, the decision to place a PEG tube focuses mainly on the patient's ability to take food by mouth." However, it would clearly be narrow and short-sighted to make decisions with such an impact solely on the basis of empirical swallowing abilities or even instrumental physiologic and bolus flow test results. For an issue that may be a critical source of a patient's sense of autonomy, self-respect, dignity, and QOL, swallowing ability is merely one factor in a decision-making formula that is yet to be determined. Unfortunately the current situation remains as stated by Logemann: "An important decision is whether the patient should continue to be fed orally, or be placed on a nasogastric tube or given some type of gastrostomy or jejunostomy. At this time, there are no absolute guidelines the clinician can use to make the decision."

Therefore, both published evidence and the practitioner's own clinical experience must contribute to such decision making. One study involving an elderly population followed for 11 months documented the incidence of complications of tube feeding. At 2 weeks postintubation, 43 percent of patients fed by NG tube and 56 percent of those fed by gastric (G) tube had been diagnosed with aspiration pneumonia. Sixty-seven percent of patients fed by NG tube and 44 percent of those fed by G tube had become agitated and/or self-extubated, requiring restraints or sedative medications to maintain the integrity of enteral nutrition. Late complications in patients in the NG tube group included a 44 percent incidence of aspiration pneumonia and a 39 percent incidence of self-extubation, whereas a 56 percent incidence of aspiration occurred in the gastrostomy group.

These data and others have led to comparisons between the outcomes of parenteral (intravenous) and enteral modes of feeding. Findings suggest advantages in safety and somewhat equivocal physiologic and clinical outcomes, whereas costs may be less for the latter mode.

In summary, while oropharyngeal dysphagia may be life-threatening, so are the alternatives, particularly for frail elderly patients. Therefore, contributions by all team members are valuable in this challenging decision-making process, with the patient's family or care provider's point of view perhaps being the most critical. The state of the evidence calls for more research, including randomized clinical trials in this area. Until (and perhaps after) these data are in and have been analyzed, the many behavioral, dietary, and environmental modifications described in this chapter and being further refined are compassionate and, in many cases, preferred alternatives to the always present option of tube feeding.

REFERENCES

Barczi SR et al: How should dysphagia care of older adults differ? Establishing optimal practice patterns. *Semin Speech Lang* 21(4):347, 2000.

ECRI: *Diagnosis and Treatment of Swallowing Disorders (Dysphagia) in Acute-Care Stroke Patients*. Evidence Report/Technology Assessment 8. Prepared by the ECRI Evidence-Based Practice Center under contract 290-97-0020, AHCPR Publication 99-E024. Rockville, MD, Agency for Health Care Policy and Research, 1999.

Gunter-Hunt G et al: Team evaluation of older patients with dysphagia. *Fed Pract* 30–37, October, 1997.

Howard L, Malone M: Clinical outcome of geriatric patients in the United States receiving home parental and enteral nutrition. *Am J Clin Nutr* 66:1364, 1997.

Hudson HM et al: The interdependency of protein-energy malnutrition, aging and dysphagia. *Dysphagia* 15:31, 2000.

Langmore SE: Risk factors for aspiration pneumonia. *Nutr Clin Pract* 14:S41, 1999.

Logemann J. *Evaluation and Treatment of Swallowing Disorders*. Austin, TX, Pro-Ed, 1998.

McHorney CA, Rosenbek JC: Functional outcome assessment of adults with oropharyngeal dysphagia. *Semin Speech Lang* 19(3):235, 1998.

Mitchell SL: The risk factors and impact on survival of feeding tube placement in nursing home residents with severe cognitive impairment. *Arch Intern Med* 157:327, 1997.

Nicosia MA et al: Age effects on temporal evolution of isometric and swallowing pressure. *J Gerontol Med Sci* 55A:M634, 2000.

Rabenek L et al: Ethically justified, clinically comprehensive guidelines for percutaneous endoscopic gastronomy tube placement. *Lancet* 349:396, 1997.

Robbins JA: Old swallowing and dysphagia: Thoughts on intervention and prevention. *Nutr Clin Pract* 14:S21, 1999.

Robbins JA et al: Lingual isometric and swallowing strength in the elderly: Is intervention warranted? *Gerontology* 38:6, 1998.

Robbins JA et al: Differentiation of normal and abnormal airway protection during swallowing using a penetration-aspiration scale. *Dysphagia* 14:228, 1999.

Robbins JA et al: Oropharyngeal swallowing in normal adults of different ages. *Gastroenterology* 103:823, 1992.

Shaker R et al: Augmentation of deglutitive upper esophageal sphincter opening in the elderly by exercise. *Am J Physiol* 272(6 pt 1); G1518, 1997.

Ship JA et al: Geriatric oral health and its impact on eating. *J Am Geriatr Soc* 44:456, 1996.

The Oral Cavity

JONATHAN A. SHIP

The oral cavity serves three essential functions in human physiology: (1) the production of speech, (2) the initiation of alimentation, and (3) protection of the host. A discussion of the status of the oral cavity during the aging process must consider the impact of any disturbance of these functions on an older person's life.

In order to speak, process food, and protect the host from pathogens and trauma, many specialized tissues have evolved in the oral-facial region (Table 94-1). The teeth, the periodontium, and the muscles of mastication exist to prepare food for deglutition. The tongue occupies a central role in communication, and is also a key participant in food bolus preparation and translocation. Salivary glands provide a secretion with multiple functions. Saliva, in addition to lubricating all oral mucosal tissues to keep them intact and pliable, moistens the developing food bolus, permitting it to be fashioned into a swallow-acceptable form. All these tissue activities are finely coordinated, and a disturbance in any one tissue function can significantly compromise speech and/or alimentation and diminish the quality of a patient's life (Table 94-2).

The oral cavity is exposed to the external world and is potentially vulnerable to a limitless number of environmental insults. Extensive mechanisms have evolved to protect the mouth and permit normal oral function. The oral cavity is richly endowed with sensory systems that contribute to the enjoyment of food and alert an individual to potential problems. These systems include mechanisms for taste (and its inextricable relationship with smell); thermal, textural, and tactile sensation; and pain discrimination. Also, saliva plays an important protective role and contains a broad spectrum of antimicrobial proteins that modulate oral microbial colonization. Other proteins maintain the functional integrity of the teeth by keeping saliva supersaturated with calcium and phosphate salts and in effect repairing incipient caries (tooth decay) by a remineralization process.

The use of dental services among older cohorts has improved over the past 40 years in the United States. However, findings from several national surveys indicate that a significant proportion of the elderly population does not see a dental professional on a regular basis and may thus be at risk for developing severe oral medical problems. For example, patients of all ages report more physician visits per year than dental visits, and this difference increases with greater age. More than 25 percent of the US population aged 65+ years has not seen a dental professional in the past 5 years. In addition, elderly persons who wear complete dentures are four times less likely to visit a dentist than are those with remaining teeth. However, because of improved oral health earlier in life, future cohorts of older persons are more likely to seek dental care than in the past. Nearly one-third of the elderly population are edentulous, but the prevalence of edentulousness has been decreasing steadily for the past four decades. This has resulted in an increased retention of the natural dentition, and therefore dental caries and periodontal diseases will remain substantial oral health concerns for older individuals in the future.

Persons with oral prostheses often experience multiple problems related to those appliances, including the development of oral fungal infections, yet are less likely to see dentists than are dentate older adults. Oral and pharyngeal cancers develop in both dentate and edentate older adults, especially individuals with long-term alcohol and tobacco use, and regular cancer screening examinations are essential to diagnose and treat these tumors at early stages. Therefore, adequate oral health care for the elderly should include preventive dental treatment and increased availability and use of dental health services. Most oral diseases are preventable and treatable at every age.

Accordingly, physicians, nurses, and aides who care for older patients need either to recruit dental expertise routinely as part of the overall assessment or to familiarize themselves with the appearance of oral health and disease states. Patient well-being is optimized when nondentists detect oral disease and recommend preventive and interventive services. Similarly, dentists should refer patients to physicians for previously undiscovered or inadequately controlled medical problems (e.g., diabetes, hypertension, cardiovascular disease). Communication is critical between dental and medical practitioners regarding medically compromised patients who may need individualized health care planning to maintain oral health at minimal risk.

This chapter focuses on specific oral tissues and their functions. It summarizes "normal" oral physiologic status in older adults and explains how common systemic disease and its treatment may affect the oral tissues

Table 94-1 Oral Tissues and Their Functions

Oral Tissue	Function
Teeth	Mastication, bone regeneration
Periodontium	Mastication, bone regeneration, host defense
Salivary glands	Lubrication, buffering acids, antimicrobial activity, mechanical cleansing, mediation of taste, remineralization of teeth, oral mucosal repair
Taste buds	Taste, host defense
Oral mucosa	Host defense, mastication, swallowing, speech
Muscles of mastication and facial expression	Mastication, swallowing, speech, posture

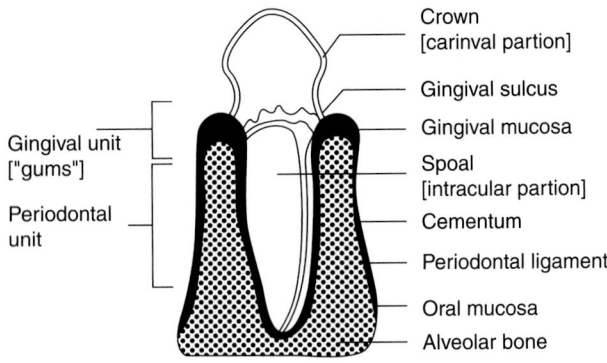

Dental and periodontal anatomy

Figure 94-1 Dental and periodontal anatomy.

during aging (Table 94-3). It also briefly reviews the evaluation and management of oral disorders frequently encountered in the elderly population. Additional information on the diagnosis and treatment of these disorders is available in several comprehensive reviews cited in the reference section.

THE DENTITION

The loss of teeth has long been associated with aging. National health surveys demonstrate that approximately one-third of Americans older than age 65 years are edentulous. Although the prevalence of edentulous adults has decreased dramatically since the first National Health Survey in 1957–1958, the population older than age 65 years still has an average of 11 missing teeth. Advances in dental treatment, disease prevention, increased availability of dental care, and improved awareness of dental needs have resulted in significant gains in dental health.

Tooth loss is attributed to two major etiologic processes: dental caries and periodontal diseases (see below). Caries affects the exposed dental surfaces, and periodontal diseases are confined to the supporting bony and ligamentous dental structures. With the current trends toward increasing tooth retention in aging populations, there is a correspondingly greater risk for the development of both of these disease entities.

A tooth consists of several mineralized and nonmineralized components supported by the periodontal ligament and the alveolar bone (Fig. 94-1). The outer dental structure is enamel and is the hardest, most mineralized component, consisting of ~90 percent hydroxyapatite. Enamel covers the coronal aspect of the tooth and is the first hard tissue exposed to caries-causing bacteria. Dentin constitutes the main portion of the tooth structure, extending almost the entire length of a tooth. It is covered by enamel

on the crown and by cementum on the root. Cementum is the least mineralized of the three components (50 percent) and is the component most susceptible to caries-causing bacteria. The central, nonmineralized portion is the dental pulp, which houses the vascular, lymphatic, and neuronal supply to the tooth.

Tooth loss in children and young adults is caused predominantly by dental caries, whereas in middle-aged and older adults, periodontal diseases play a greater role in the loss of teeth. Longitudinal studies of generally healthy adult males have found that the principal cause of tooth extraction is dental caries. Furthermore, caries activity continues throughout life and is not a phenomenon confined to any single period.

There are two classifications of dental caries, depending on the dental surface affected. Coronal caries, which is characteristic of caries in young adults and children, occurs when the enamel and dentin of the coronal portion of the tooth are affected. In older adults, if gingival recession or periodontal disease causes the root surfaces of the tooth to become exposed to the oral environment, root surface or cervical caries may occur.

The primary caries-causing microorganism is *Streptococcus mutans;* oral *Streptococcus, Actinomyces,* and *Lactobacillus* organisms are also associated with coronal and cervical lesions. These bacteria reside on the tooth surface in dental plaque, a soft, firmly adherent mass that contains bacteria, food debris, desquamated cells, and bacterial products. Acid production by plaque bacteria dissolves the mineral content of the enamel, dentin, or cementum. The exposed protein constituents are destroyed by hydrolytic enzymes, and caries results. Dental plaque is considered a primary etiologic factor in dental caries, as well as a principal source of pathogenic organisms in periodontal diseases.

As a dentate individual ages, there is susceptibility to coronal caries as a result of recurrent decay around existing restored surfaces, and the prevalence of root surfaces caries increases. For example, there is an 18-fold increase in the average number of tooth surfaces with root caries between persons age 20 years and those age 64 years (thus, root caries often begins well before old age). There are many risk indicators for cervical caries: increased age, decreased exposure to fluoride, coronal caries, periodontal attachment loss, and several medical, behavioral, and social factors.

Table 94–2   Clinical Manifestations of Oral Infections

Disease	Oral Manifestations
Dental and periodontal infections	
Dental caries	Soft to hard discolored defect on tooth surface
Gingivitis and periodontitis	Erythematous, edematous, and hemorrhagic gingiva, which may be accompanied by gingival recession and tooth mobility
Viral infections	
Primary herpes simplex infection	Clear to yellow vesicles that rupture and form shallow, painful ulcers on all mucosal surfaces; gingival tissues inflamed, edematous, and painful
Recurrent herpes simplex infection	Burning or tingling prodrome in lesion sites (lip, hard palate, attached gingiva); whitish-gray vesicles rupture to form painful ulcers, which then develop a crust
Herpes zoster	Unilateral vesicular eruptions in areas following the distribution of ophthalmic, maxillary, or mandibular divisions of trigeminal sensory nerves
Cytomegalovirus	Mononucleosis-like symptoms, petechial hemorrhages, enlarged salivary glands, pharyngotonsillitis
Fungal infections	
Pseudomembranous candidiasis	Soft, white or yellow plaques that can be wiped off to expose an underlying erythematous mucosa
Erythemic or atrophic candidiasis	Painful erythematous oral mucosal lesions; tongue appears "bald"; diffuse inflammation of denture-bearing areas
Hyperplastic candidiasis	Leukoplakic or keratotic lesions that cannot be removed by scraping
Angular cheilitis	Erythematous cracked or fissured lesions at the lip commissures
Salivary gland infections	
Acute sialoadenitis	Tender salivary gland swelling with purulent discharge on palpation of the gland duct
Chronic sialoadenitis	Recurrent, tender swellings of salivary gland progressing to a firm and atrophic gland

Studies in the United States reveal an increase in the mean number of decayed and restored teeth among dentate adults in the older age cohorts over the last 40 years. These trends probably reflect the increased retention of the natural dentition and a greater use of dental services by older adults; it is unlikely that they represent a true increase in dental caries activity. However, epidemiologic projections suggest that significant increases in the prevalence of root surface caries will occur in aging populations in the future.

For an older person with teeth, caries is a significant concern and may be a source of pain, infection, and dysfunction. Dental caries will appear as darkish lesions that frequently are associated with dental plaque. Long-standing caries ultimately results in the destruction of the tooth with the possibility of a disseminated infection. Once teeth have been destroyed (from dental caries or periodontal disease), mastication, phonation, and deglutition may be perturbed. Also, social contact and nutritional status may be affected in a substantially edentulous aging individual.

The prevention of dental caries in an older adult is no different from that in a younger individual—fluoride is the primary agent. Adult tooth surfaces can become resistant to decalcification and decay through repeated exposure to fluoride in water supplies, toothpaste, rinses, and gels. However, even resistant tooth surfaces can become carious when oral hygiene is inadequate and there are dietary sources of fermentable carbohydrate. When detected early, caries can be débrided from a tooth, and the missing tooth structure can be restored with a wear-resistant, insoluble dental material (e.g., amalgam or composite resin). Untreated dental caries, however, in most circumstances progresses to severe or even total loss of tooth

Table 94–3   Oral–Pharyngeal Processes in Older People

Process	Healthy Older People	Medically Compromised Older People
Taste	Unaffected	Diminished
Smell	Diminished	Diminished
Food enjoyment	Unaffected	Diminished
Salivary output	Unaffected	Diminished
Chewing efficiency	Slightly diminished	Diminished
Swallowing	Slightly diminished	Diminished

structure and possibly pain, abscess formation, cellulitis, and bacteremia.

THE PERIODONTIUM

The periodontium consists of the tissues that invest and support the tooth. It is divided into the gingival unit (gums) and the attachment apparatus (cementum, periodontal ligament, and alveolar bony process) (see Fig. 94-1). Gingivitis occurs when the gingival unit is inflamed. Periodontitis (or periodontal disease) exists when there is inflammation and an appreciable loss of the attachment apparatus as a result of the presence of pathogenic microorganisms. Microbial species (e.g., *Bacteroides, Fusobacterium, Prevotella, Actinobacillus, Capnocytophaga, Streptococcus*) cross the gingival epithelium and enter subepithelial tissues, where they activate specific host defense mechanisms. Eventually this causes tissue destruction, including bone loss and tooth morbidity.

Certain periodontal changes occur in aging individuals. For example, cross-sectional studies demonstrate that older adults show an increase in dental plaque, calculus (calcified dental plaque), and the frequency of bleeding gingival tissues. Older persons also experience greater gingival recession and loss of periodontal attachment. Longitudinal studies report that periodontitis is more prevalent and usually more extensive among black people, subjects with less education, those who have not seen a dentist recently, and those with gingivitis and certain pathogenic organisms. Currently, it is believed that periodontal disease proceeds through a series of episodic attacks rather than occurring as a slowly progressing continuous process. It is not known whether older age cohorts are more susceptible to periodontal destruction than are younger populations. Recent longitudinal studies demonstrate that among healthy adults, periodontal attachment loss occurs at small increments in all age cohorts and does not occur in greater amounts in older healthy adults. However, many systemic diseases and therapeutic regimens commonly found in older individuals may affect adversely periodontal health. Therefore, an older medically compromised adult is especially susceptible to developing periodontal diseases and is at risk for associated dental-alveolar infections, pain, and tooth loss.

Several classes of medications commonly prescribed for older people are associated with gingival enlargement and hyperplasia, a condition that if left untreated predisposes to both caries and destructive periodontitis. The family of calcium channel blockers can cause this unwanted drug side effect, which may require periodontal surgery for definitive treatment. The antiseizure medication phenytoin and the immunosuppressant cyclosporine also have also been associated with gingival enlargement.

Periodontal diseases have oral and systemic effects on health. They are directly associated with halitosis, gingival bleeding, tooth mobility, and tooth loss. Untreated periodontitis has been reported to interfere with blood glucose control in diabetic patients, and recent investigations suggest associations between cardiovascular disease and periodontitis after controlling for traditional risk factors such as weight, gender, tobacco use, age, and blood lipid levels. Gram-negative bacteria are implicated in the pathogenesis of periodontal disease, and colonization of the oropharynx with gram-negative bacilli predisposes a patient to pneumonia. Aspiration pneumonia can occur when oropharyngeal secretions are aspirated into the lungs, causing infection. Periodontal bacteria from the gingival sulcus in dentate individuals have been isolated from patients with pneumonia. Risk factors for aspiration pneumonia include older age, immunocompromised state, mechanical ventilation, feeding problems and/or feeding tubes, and deteriorating health status. Importantly, many debilitated older patients have received inadequate oral hygiene and are therefore highly susceptible to aspiration pneumonia.

For an older person with teeth, periodontal diseases can cause pain, difficulty with mastication, and infection. Gingivitis may be detected by the presence of erythematous and/or edematous gingival tissues with occasional hemorrhage. Gingival recession produces exposed dental root surfaces, a sign of periodontitis. This ultimately causes tooth mobility, a condition that necessitates definitive treatment. The systemic health of an already compromised individual may be further threatened by bleeding and suppurating gingiva, dental alveolar infections, and the potential transmission of oral bacteria via bacteremias and/or oral–pharyngeal secretions.

Treatment of gingivitis and periodontitis starts with regular oral hygiene in the form of toothbrushing and flossing after each meal. Electric toothbrushes and mechanical irrigation systems can assist older patients who have motor and/or cognitive disorders. Periodontal therapy ranges from conservative (e.g., dental prophylaxis) to surgical techniques (e.g., débridement, excision of hyperplastic tissue), depending on the extent of periodontal infection and bony destruction. Numerous antimicrobial and anticollagenase pharmaceuticals have been approved for treatment as well: oral rinses (e.g., chlorhexidine 0.12%), subgingival irrigants (e.g., doxycycline extended-release liquid 50 mg/500 mg blended formulation), short-term antimicrobials (e.g., clindamycin 300 mg qid or metronidazole 400 mg tid for 7 to 10 days), or long-term anticollagenases (e.g., doxycycline 20 mg). While periodontal healing after surgery tends to be slower even in healthy older persons, the long-term results of periodontal therapy are indistinguishable from those in younger adults. The decision either to save the dentition and restore periodontal health or to extract teeth with moderate periodontal disease should be determined after all oral and systemic factors have been evaluated. Therefore, the health of a person, rather than age per se, should determine the extent of periodontal treatment.

SALIVARY GLANDS

There are three major pairs of salivary glands (parotid, submandibular, and sublingual) and numerous groups of minor glands (e.g., labial, palatal, and buccal), all of whose principal function is the exocrine production of saliva. Each gland type makes a unique secretion derived from either mucous or serous cell types, forming the fluid in the mouth termed *whole saliva*. Saliva includes many constituents that are critical to the maintenance of oral health. Its most important functions are lubrication of the oral mucosa, promotion of the remineralization of teeth, and protection against microbial infections. Although the role of saliva in digestion is limited, saliva helps prepare the food bolus for deglutition and is responsible for dissolving tastants and delivering them to taste buds.

It was previously thought that salivary output diminishes with increasing age. This was based on the clinical observation that older individuals frequently have a dry mouth and complain of xerostomia. However, investigations reveal that, in general, there is no substantial diminution in salivary production across the human life span in healthy adults. Thus, in the absence of complicating factors (e.g., certain systemic diseases, medications), there is no generalized age-related perturbation in the production of salivary fluid. In addition, there appear to be no significant alterations in the composition of saliva in older, healthy persons.

These physiologic findings contrast with the morphologic changes seen in aging salivary glands. Major salivary glands lose ~30 percent of their parenchymal tissue over the adult life span. The loss primarily involves acinar components, while proportional increases are seen in ductal cells and in fat, vascular, and connective tissues. Because acinar components are primarily responsible for the secretion of saliva, it is not known why, in the presence of a significant reduction in the gland acinar volume, total fluid production does not diminish with increasing age. It has thus been deduced that salivary glands possess a functional reserve capacity that enables them to maintain fluid output throughout the human adult life span. Furthermore, it is hypothesized that older adults are more vulnerable to salivary gland insults (e.g., anticholinergic medications) compared to younger adults. Therefore, salivary hypofunction and complaints of a dry mouth (xerostomia) should not be considered to be normal sequelae of aging but instead are indicative of oral and systemic diseases and/or their treatment (Table 94-4). The most common etiology of salivary gland dysfunction is iatrogenic. Many medications taken by older persons reduce or alter salivary gland performance. In addition, radiation for head and neck neoplasms and cytotoxic chemotherapy can have direct and dramatic deleterious effects on salivary glands.

The single most-common disease affecting salivary glands is Sjögren's syndrome, an autoimmune exocrinopathy that occurs predominantly in postmenopausal women. Alzheimer's disease, diabetes, dehydration, rheumatoid arthritis, and cerebrovascular accidents may also affect salivary output. Furthermore, several oral inflammatory and obstructive salivary gland disorders (e.g., bacterial infections, sialoliths, trauma, neoplasms) result in salivary dysfunction.

A clinician is likely to encounter many older patients with oral complaints related to salivary gland dysfunction. A brief clinical examination should include palpation of all major glands and inspection of the duct orifices to ensure patent glands, and the application of a mild solution of citric acid or lemon juice to the tongue can help determine whether a patient's salivary glands will respond

Table 94-4   Conditions Associated with Salivary Dysfunction in Older People

Category	Examples
Medications	Anticholinergics
	Antidepressants
	Antihistaminics
	Antihypertensives
	Anti-Parkinson
	Anxiolytics
	Diuretics
Oncological therapy	Cytotoxic chemotherapy
	Head and neck radiotherapy
Oral diseases	Bacterial and viral infections
	Salivary gland obstructions
	Traumatic lesions
	Neoplasms
Systemic diseases	Alzheimer's disease
	Cerebrovascular accidents
	Diabetes mellitus
	Dehydration
	Parkinson's disease
	Sjögren's syndrome
	Systemic lupus erythematosus

to a gustatory stimulus. Regardless of etiology, any of the major oral physiologic roles influenced by saliva (see Table 94-1) may be affected adversely. With gland dysfunction, increased dental caries will ensue rapidly, increasing the possibility of tooth loss. The oral mucosa can become desiccated and cracked, leaving the host more susceptible to microbial infection. Furthermore, salivary dysfunction can lead to difficulty in swallowing or speaking at length, pain (which may arise from either the teeth or the oral soft tissues), impaired denture use, altered taste, and diminished food enjoyment.

Treatment of salivary dysfunction starts with identification of the etiology. Medication-induced salivary problems can be eliminated by stopping unneeded drugs, modifying drug use and dose, or substituting one drug with another drug that has fewer anticholinergic side effects. Even when no reduction in the daily dose is recommended, the splitting of a dose into several smaller and more frequently taken doses may alleviate or diminish the sensation of oral dryness. To enhance salivary production, gustatory (sugarless mints, candies), masticatory (sugarless gums), and pharmacologic (pilocarpine 5 mg tid and qhs, cevimeline 30 mg tid) stimulants can be useful in a patient who has remaining salivary function. Salivary substitutes, rinses, and moisturizing gels can assist a patient who has little or no remaining salivary function. Prevention of dry-mouth problems is essential and can be achieved with the frequent use of sugarless beverages, topical fluoride, and regular oral hygiene after meals. Removable prostheses must be kept clean and out of the mouth during sleeping hours.

Frequent lubrication of the lips helps prevent lip cracking and infections.

SENSORY FUNCTION

Many reports suggest that food enjoyment, recognition, and sensory function decline as a function of age and that this can produce significant nutritional deficits. It has been suggested that there is a true anorexia (loss of appetite) associated with aging, although this is confounded by the many comorbidities that cause anorexia, and which are so common in the elderly population, as well as other social and psychological factors that may reduce oral food and fluid intake. Perturbations in taste, smell, and other oral sensory modalities can occur with age and reduce the rewards of eating, thus contributing to a diminished interest in food among many elderly persons.

The taste receptors of the human gustatory system are distributed throughout the oropharynx and are innervated by three cranial nerves: VII, IX, and X. It appears that the number of lingual taste buds does not diminish with age. The registration of a taste phenomenon is complex, because multiple factors are involved: gustation, olfaction, and central nervous system function. The ability to taste is often evaluated at two levels: (1) *threshold,* the most common measure, a "molecular-level" event, which reflects the lowest concentrations of a tastant that an individual can recognize as being different from water, and (2) *suprathreshold,* a measure that is reflective of the ability to taste the intensity of substances at functional concentrations encountered in daily life. In addition to detection, recognition, and intensity, the normal sensation of taste involves a hedonic component: the degree of pleasantness.

Many earlier studies citing a higher frequency of taste complaints among older persons examined institutionalized individuals rather than the healthy elderly. It now appears that subjective reports of taste function among generally healthy, community-dwelling persons demonstrate that only modest changes occur with increased age, in comparison to studies revealing a threefold increase in the frequency of subjective complaints among older persons who take prescription medications. Objective threshold and suprathreshold evaluations of gustatory function in healthy older adults have been reported for all four taste qualities (sweet, sour, salty, and bitter), and in general the decremental changes detected with increased age have been modest and taste-quality-specific. For example, the ability of older persons to detect salt decreased slightly with age, while no change in the detection threshold for sucrose (sweet) was noted. The importance of medication usage and place of residence in the evaluation of taste dysfunction has been confirmed in clinical studies in which institutionalized persons and those using more prescription medications had significantly elevated taste thresholds.

Older individuals perform less well in the more complicated problems of flavor perception, food recognition, and food preference. This is probably a result of diminished olfactory performance rather than the modest changes that accompany taste function with aging. The available data on olfactory performance clearly indicates declines in thresholds, suprathreshold intensity judgments, and odor recognition in both men and women with increasing age. Among older adults, average thresholds are higher, the ability to perceive suprathreshold intensities is blunted, odor recognition is impaired, and the judgment of pleasantness is reduced compared with younger subjects. Moreover, longitudinal studies demonstrate that as people get older, recognition decrements become even more severe.

However, in the real world, people do not typically taste a single tastant in aqueous form and foods that contain solely olfactory cues are not consumed. Foods are chemosensory mixtures, and the most relevant but most difficult to obtain measures of gustatory and olfactory function involve the use of complex food analogs. In one study, younger subjects were significantly better than were elders at recognizing stimuli in blended food. However, when younger persons repeated the test with their nasal airways occluded, their performance dropped to the level of elderly individuals. One conclusion from this finding is that the daily life chemosensory functions of older individuals are handicapped by diminished olfactory performance. Moreover, it has been suggested that for many persons the "anorexia of aging" can be reduced or reversed by adding flavor enhancers to foods.

Many other sensory cues (temperature, texture, pressure) participate in the experience of food enjoyment. Little research attention has been dedicated to these phenomena. One study demonstrated no age-related changes in the ability of subjects to distinguish fluids of varying temperatures and viscosities; however, a specific decline was observed in the perception of localized lingual pressure.

Normal chemosensory function cannot operate independently of good oral health. Numerous oral conditions can directly or indirectly affect smell and taste by altering the underlying biology of the taste or smell system or by introducing exogenous stimuli into the mouth or nose. Many oral conditions, including infections, lesions, salivary gland hypofunction, poorly fitting prostheses, and oral manifestations of systemic diseases, can cause chemosensory dysfunction. For example, inadequate removal of food particles can allow their breakdown or metabolic conversion by oral microorganisms to noxious, unpleasant substances. Periodontal diseases can result in accumulations of putrefied acidic materials that may leak into the oral cavity and alter taste sensation. Similarly, periapical dental infections with subsequent fistula formation may contribute continuously low levels of purulent matter in the mouth.

The complaint of a smell or taste problem may be indicative of a chemosensory disorder or could be the manifestation of an oral and/or systemic medical problem. For example, the sudden loss of either smell or taste may be a sign of a brain tumor. Alternatively, gradual diminishment in food enjoyment may be related to multiple sources (e.g., a poorly fitting removable prosthesis, an oral fungal infection, decreased smell identification, a drug). Older subjects are more likely to have chemosensory complaints, but unfortunately those complaints are very poor predictors of olfactory dysfunction. A patient should be asked if he or she can specifically identify the four basic tastants and distinguish between different odorants; such patients can be given the University of Pennsylvania Smell Identification Test. A thorough multidisciplinary approach is required for a patient presenting with chemosensory complaints because of the wide range of potential oral, systemic, physiologic, cognitive, and pathologic factors that are involved in oral sensory functioning.

ORAL MUCOSA

The soft-tissue lining of the mouth may be characterized by three general types: (1) well-keratinized tissue with a dense layer of connective tissue and firmly attached to underlying bone (e.g., marginal gingiva, palatal mucosa), (2) slightly keratinized and freely movable tissue (e.g., labial and buccal mucosa, floor of the mouth), and (3) specialized mucosa (e.g., dorsum of the tongue). The primary function of the oral mucosa is to act as a barrier to protect the underlying structures from desiccation, noxious chemicals, trauma, thermal stress, and infection. The oral mucosa plays a key role in the defense of the oral cavity.

Aging frequently is associated with changes in the oral mucosa similar to those in the skin, with the epithelium becoming thinner, less hydrated, and thus supposedly more susceptible to injury. The reasons for these changes (if they are normally a sequela of aging) could be complex and may include alterations in protein synthesis and responsiveness to growth factors and other regulatory mediators. Cell renewal (i.e., mitotic rates) and the synthesis of proteins associated with oral mucosal keratinization occur at a slower rate in aging individuals, but the normal tissue architecture and patterns of histodifferentiation, which probably are dependent on complex interactions with the underlying connective tissue, do not display any changes with age. Overall, changes in the vascularity of oral mucosa probably contribute to an alteration in mucosal integrity because of reductions in cellular access to nutrients and oxygenation. Mucosal, alveolar, and gingival arteries demonstrate the effects of arteriosclerosis. Varicosities on the floor of the mouth and the lateral and ventral surfaces of the tongue (comparable to varicosities on the lower extremities) are also observable in geriatric patients.

The maintenance of mucosal integrity depends on the ability of the oral epithelium to respond to an insult. Insults can be due to physical factors, exposure to chemical or microbiological toxins, and oral and/or systemic conditions. Many studies have documented that the immune system undergoes a decline with age (Chap. 3) and it is likely that this decline extends to mucosal immunity. Therefore, the oral mucosa may be more susceptible to transmission of infectious diseases as well as delayed wound healing. Similar findings have been reported for healing gingival tissues.

Cross-sectional studies have demonstrated that age *per se* has no effect on the clinical appearance of the oral mucosa. However, considerable evidence suggests that the use of removable prostheses has a potentially adverse effect on the health of the oral mucosa. The denture-bearing mucosa of aged maxillary and mandibular ridges shows significant morphologic changes. Ill-fitting dentures can produce mechanical trauma to the oral tissues as well as cause mucosal hyperplasia. Oral candidiasis frequently is found on denture-bearing areas in an edentulous individual, often occurring with angular cheilitis (deep fissuring and ulceration of the epithelium at the commissures of the mouth). Therefore, the clinician should ask the patient to remove all removable prostheses before conducting an adequate oral examination.

Oral mucosal alterations in an older person are often a result of multiple oral and systemic factors (Table 94-5). Numerous medications have been associated with oral

Table 94-5 Conditions Associated with Oral Mucosal Changes

Classification	Disease/Disorder	Examples
Oral conditions	Infections	Candidiasis, herpes simplex, herpes zoster
	Ulcerative conditions	Recurrent aphthous stomatitis
	Periodontal diseases	Gingivitis, periodontitis
	Prosthodontic problems	Poorly fitting dentures
	Salivary gland dysfunction	Dessicated oral tissues
	Food allergies	Cinammon allergy
	Social habits	Tobacco and alcohol consumption
	Trauma	Traumatic fibroma, mucocele
Systemic diseases	Dermatological disorders	Systemic lupus erythematosus, lichen planus, pemphigus vulgaris, cicatricial pemphigoid, erythema multiforme
	Endocrine disorders	Diabetes mellitus
	Cancer	Oral and pharyngeal cancers
	Neurologic disorders	Alzheimer's, Parkinson's, CVA
	Immunocompromising disorders	HIV, AIDS, rheumatoid arthritis
Medical therapies	Medications	Diuretics, calcium channel blockers, antibiotics, antiseizures, immunomodulating drugs
	Head and neck radiotherapy	Head and neck radiotherapy
	Cytotoxic chemotherapy	Methotrexate, 5-FU, cyclosporin

AIDS, acquired immunodeficiency syndrome; CVA, cerebrovascular accident; 5-FU, 5-fluorouracil; HIV, human immunodeficiency virus.

mucosal changes. For example, long-term use of antibiotics frequently results in oral candidal infections, while drugs with xerostomic side effects (see above) increase the potential for mucosal injury. Drugs commonly used in older patients for arthritic conditions, hypertension, cardiac arrhythmias, seizures, and dementia are associated with lichenoid reactions. The withdrawal of a causative drug usually results in complete resolution of the lesion within 2 to 3 weeks, but if there is no clinical improvement, a definitive diagnosis should be obtained with a biopsy specimen.

Numerous oral mucosal disorders affect the elderly population, ranging from benign (e.g., recurrent aphthous ulcers and traumatic lesions) to malignant (e.g., squamous cell carcinomas). The diagnosis of mucosal diseases requires a detailed history and a thorough head and neck and oral examination, including all mucosal tissues. For vesiculobullous and erosive diseases, a simple three-item classification is helpful: (1) acute multiple lesions (e.g., erythema multiforme, herpes simplex, herpes zoster, allergic reaction), (2) recurring oral ulcers (e.g., recurrent aphthous stomatitis, traumatic ulcer), and (3) chronic multiple lesions (e.g., pemphigus vulgaris, cicatricial pemphigoid, lupus erythematosus, lichen planus, dysplasia, squamous cell carcinoma). If a lesion does not resolve after 2 to 3 weeks, a tissue biopsy is required. For lesions that are suspected to be oral manifestations of autoimmune connective tissue disorders (e.g., pemphigus, pemphigoid, lichen planus), biopsies should also include specimens for direct immunofluorescence. If trauma from an injury or an ill-fitting denture is suspected, removal of the etiology should allow the lesion to heal. Many of these conditions have an immunological etiology, and therefore management strategies involve topical and/or systemic immunomodulating agents (Table 94-6).

The oral mucosal disease with the greatest potential morbidity and mortality is cancer. According to the National Cancer Institute's Surveillance, Epidemiology and End Results Program (SEER), 2.2 percent (more than 30,000 cases) of all cancers in 2000 were in the oral cavity and pharyngeal region, resulting in nearly 8000 deaths per year. The three greatest risk factors for developing oral cancer are age, alcohol, and tobacco use; nearly half of all oral cancers occur in persons older than 65 years of age. The average age at the time of diagnosis is approximately 60 years, and males are more than twice as likely to develop oral cancer than are females. While attempts to diagnose and treat oral cancer have improved in the last 30 years, 5-year survival rates have not improved dramatically, and the average 5-year survival rate is only ~50 percent.

Neoplasms may arise in all oral soft and hard tissues and in the oropharyngeal and salivary gland regions. The clinical appearance of an oral carcinoma is quite diverse (ulcerative, erythematous, leukoplakic, papillary) and may be innocuous as well as asymptomatic. If a patient presents with an unusual and suspicious lesion with no readily apparent etiology (such as a denture sore), the patient should be referred to a specialist more familiar with the appearance of the oral mucosa. Carcinoma should be considered part of the differential diagnosis of any oral lesion.

Table 94-6 Treatment of Common Vesiculobullous and Erosive Diseases in Older People

Medication	Regimen
Topical treatments[a–d]	
Fluocinonide gel 0.05%	Apply to affected regions
Triamcinolone acetonide in gel base 0.1%	tid and qhs
Clobetasol propionate gel 0.05%	
Oral rinses[b,c,e]	
Dexamethasone elixir 0.5 mg/5 mL	Rinse and spit 10 mL qid for 5 min
Diphenhydramine elixir 12.5 mg/5 mL	
Dyclonine HCL 1%	
Systemic medications[b,f]	
Prednisone 5 mg	12 tabs qod × 2 days, decreasing by 2 tabs every other day
Azathioprine 50 mg	1 tab bid

[a] If extensive gingival lesions are present, use with a custom-fabricated tray.

[b] Oral candidiasis may result and concomitant antifungal therapy may be necessary.

[c] Taper as indicated by clinical response.

[d] Can be combined in a 1:1 mixture with orabase.

[e] Can be combined in a 1:1 mixture with sucralfate, kaopectate, or maalox.

[f] Dose and duration depend on severity of disease and concomitant systemic diseases. Azathioprine in combination with prednisone permits use of lower doses of prednisone.

The treatment of oral cancers involves oral, head, and neck surgery; radiotherapy; chemotherapy; or a combination of any of these three modalities, depending on the tumor's histopathology and stage. Before receiving definitive therapy, the patient should have a comprehensive oral examination so that focal areas of infection or potential infection (dental caries, periodontal disease, dental-alveolar infections, soft and hard tissues lesions) can be treated before surgery, radiotherapy, or chemotherapy. The patient must be educated about many potential risks: surgery-related sensory, aesthetic, and functional problems; radiotherapy-induced mucositis, salivary gland dysfunction, and osteoradionecrosis; and chemotherapy-induced mucositis and immunosuppression.

MOTOR FUNCTION

The oral motor apparatus is involved in several routine yet intricate functions (speech, posture, mastication, and swallowing). Regulation of these activities may occur at three levels: the local neuromuscular unit, central neuronal pathways, and systemic influences. In general, aging is associated with changes in neuromuscular systems. Animal studies strongly suggest that age-associated deficiencies in motor function are not related to the composition and contractile function of skeletal muscles. Instead, these changes probably are related to other factors, such as neuromuscular transmission and propagation of nerve impulses.

Studies of oral motor function have shown that some alterations in performance (mastication, swallowing, oral muscular posture, and tone) can be expected with increased age. These changes appear to be more common among predominantly edentulous persons than among those with a natural dentition. The most frequently reported oral motor disturbance in the elderly population is related to altered mastication, and even fully dentate older persons are less able to prepare food adequately for swallowing than are younger individuals. Older persons are more likely to be partially or completely edentulous than are persons in other age groups, and therefore the geriatric population is susceptible to altered chewing. It also has been reported that older persons tend to swallow larger-sized food particles than do younger adults. This suggests that there is a diminution in masticatory efficiency that can be further exacerbated among individuals with a compromised dentition. It also suggests that older individuals may be more susceptible to aspiration pneumonia resulting from chewing problems in addition to periodontal pathogens. In summary, the majority of research findings suggest that dentition, not age *per se*, has a direct influence on mastication.

After mastication, a food bolus is ready for swallowing. A thorough review of swallowing and swallowing problems in older people is provided in Chap. 93. Normal aging has minor adverse effects on swallowing, although in a healthy older person, advanced age *per se* does not appear to cause any clinical dysfunction. However, patients with neuropathies may have oral swallow times four- to sixfold longer than those in healthy controls, and these persons may not even be able to produce the recognizable characteristics of an oral swallow. Furthermore, neurovascular conditions (e.g., cerebrovascular accidents, dementia, motor neuron disease) are likely to cause dysphagia and predispose a person to the danger of aspiration. Therefore, swallowing changes in older persons are usually caused by sensory, muscular, and neurologic deterioration.

The temporomandibular joint (TMJ) is located between the glenoid fossa and the condylar process of the mandible, and exhibits a functionally unique gliding and hinge-like movement. It is of particular interest to clinicians, for it is the focus of several craniofacial pain disorders. Using radiographic and postmortem evaluations, several studies have reported that various components of this joint undergo degenerative alterations with increasing age. However, data does not confirm TMJ functional impairment as a "normal" age-associated event. Conversely, many oral and systemic conditions commonly seen in the elderly population are linked with temporomandibular disorders (TMD). Orofacial pain in the elderly patient may be due to a variety of chronic systemic diseases, as well as to problems of the oral–facial complex, making diagnosis and treatment challenging and frequently requiring a multidisciplinary approach.

In general, two types of pathology are associated with the TMJ: *articular*, related to the joint itself, and *nonarticular*, pathology occurring in structures unrelated to the joint but causing similar or referred symptomatology. Several articular abnormalities common to all joints also affect the TMJ, including trauma, ankylosis, dislocation, and arthritis. Nonarticular disorders may result from a variety of clinical entities, including trigeminal neuralgia, dental pulpitis, otitis, and masticatory myalgia. Orofacial habits (e.g., jaw clenching and tooth grinding) and poor head and neck posture can produce muscle fatigue and subsequent spasm. Moreover, psychological conditions (stress and depression) can exacerbate underlying articular and nonarticular disorders. Clinically, the patient will present with pain in the TMJ; the temporal, cervical, or neck region; the masticatory muscles; and the oral cavity. Limited jaw opening (less than 40 mm from the maxillary central incisor to the mandibular central incisor) and pain on mastication or during jaw movements may be indicative of TMD. Treatment, as with other arthritic or muscular disorders, requires the elucidation of an appropriate diagnosis and ranges from conservative and reversible regimens (antiinflammatories, analgesics, muscle relaxants, physical therapy, oral bite splints) to more invasive procedures for unresolved painful conditions (e.g., TMJ surgery).

Results from the 1989 National Health Interview Survey indicate that older adults report considerable amounts of orofacial and TMJ pain. The estimated prevalence rates among adults 75 years and older were 1.2 percent for burning mouth pain, 1.6 percent for face pain, 3.4 percent for toothache, 3.9 percent for jaw joint pain, and 6.2 percent for oral sores. While toothaches, oral sores, and jaw joint pain decreased with age, face pain was age-independent, and burning mouth pain increased with age. Results from the same survey indicate that similarly aged adults are approximately five times more likely to visit a physician than a dentist in a year. This finding suggests that people may be more likely to visit a physician even for orofacial problems and/or that a considerable number of older adults may not seek stomatological treatment from dentists for their pain.

Speech production is another function subserved by the oral structures, and it undergoes some changes with increasing age, including statistically significant alterations in activities such as tongue shape and function during specific phoneme production and frequency variability. However, among healthy older persons these changes do not compromise or alter speech in any perceptible way. Tongue strength undergoes decreases with age, even among healthy adults, yet tongue endurance is similar between younger and older persons. There are also age-associated alterations in intraoral and maxillofacial posture. Drooping of the lower face and lips in the elderly person results not only from the loss of supporting hard tissues, but also from a diminished tone of the circumoral muscles. The latter changes may elicit esthetic concerns and can lead to embarrassment from drooling or food spills caused by the inability of an older individual to close the lips competently while eating or speaking. Often, drooling caused by reduced circumoral muscle tone can result in complaints of excess salivation.

Significant oral motor disorders also may result from a number of therapeutic drug regimens, such as the frequent association of tardive dyskinesia with phenothiazine therapy. These dyskinesias may include diminished performance and speech pathoses as well as alteration in movement (chorea, athetosis).

SUMMARY

The health of the oral cavity and its ability to fulfill its function of communication, nutritional intake, and host protection can be impaired in older adults. Age alone does not appear to play a strong role in the impairments. Instead, oral and systemic diseases and the treatment of medical problems compromise oral health and function. This will predispose an older person to develop oral microbial infections, pain, altered chemosensation, dysphagia, difficulty chewing and speaking, greater risk for disseminated systemic infections, and, importantly, a diminished quality of life. All health care providers should attempt to identify older persons at risk for developing oral diseases, be able to recognize existing oral diseases, and either treat or refer patients who have stomatologic disorders.

REFERENCES

Chavez EM, Ship JA: Sensory and motor deficits in the elderly: Impact on oral health. *J Pub Health Dent* 60(4):297, 2000.

Ettinger RL: The unique oral health needs of an aging population. *Dent Clin North Am* 41(4):633, 1997.

Ghezzi EM, Ship JA: Systemic diseases and their treatments in the elderly: Impact on oral health. *J Pub Health Dent* 60(4):289, 2000.

Robbins J: Normal swallowing and aging. *Semin Neurol* 16(4):309, 1996.

Shay K, Ship JA: The importance of oral health in the older patient. *J Am Geriatr Soc* 43(12):1414, 1995.

Ship JA et al: Xerostomia and the geriatric patient. *J Am Geriatr Soc* 50(3):535, 2002.

Ship JA: The influence of aging on oral health and consequences for taste and smell. *Physiol Behav* 66(2):209, 1999.

Ship JA et al: Oral facial pain in the elderly, in Lomranz J, Mostofsky DI (eds): *Handbook of Pain and Aging*, 1st ed. New York, Plenum, 1997 p 321.

Ship JA et al: Geriatric oral health and its impact on eating. *J Am Geriatr Soc* 44(4):456, 1996.

Silverman SJ: *Oral Cancer*, 4th ed. Hamilton, ON, Canada, The American Cancer Society, 1998.

Squier CA, Hill MW (eds). *The Effect of Aging in Oral Mucosa and Skin*, 1st ed. Boca Raton, FL, CRC Press, 1994.

SENSORY FUNCTION

C H A P T E R   9 5

Assessment and Rehabilitation of Older Adults with Low Vision

GALE R. WATSON

DEMOGRAPHICS

Estimates of the number of people with visual impairments per 1000 persons demonstrate the dramatic increase in visual impairments with age. An estimated 6.07 per 1000 persons ages 0 to 54 years, but 104.1 in 1000 persons ages 55 to 84 years, and 216 in 1000 persons ages 85 years and older were visually impaired in 1990. An estimated 364,000 (26 percent) of the 1.4 million nursing home residents in the United States older than age 65 years have visual impairments. Another 9 percent had unknown visual status, because it could not be estimated. Much of this visual impairment is undiagnosed and not well managed in these settings, adding to other functional disabilities.

Age-related visual impairment is not only challenging to the person who develops it, but also affects society as a whole. The Alliance for Eye and Vision Research estimated that 22 billion dollars is the annual price of visual impairment in older persons in the United States. The National Advisory Eye Council addressed age-related vision loss in its Five-Year Plan, stating:

> Effective treatment of even 25 percent of all cases can lead to significant savings to society and a decrease in the number of Social Security and other disability payments, with savings far outweighing the costs of clinical management and treatment.

The most prevalent age-related causes of visual impairment in the United States are macular degeneration, diabetic retinopathy, glaucoma, and cataract. In addition, visual impairment is commonly related to other health impairments.

Approximately 60 percent of persons with visual impairments who are not institutionalized have one or more additional impairments, including the loss of hearing, impaired mobility, decreased energy and stamina from respiratory and heart disease, cognitive changes resulting from stroke or dementia, and chronic illness, such as failure of the endocrine system. Vision loss has been ranked third, behind arthritis and heart disease, among the most common chronic conditions that require persons who are older to have assistance with activities of daily living. Because the majority of people with visual impairments have useful vision, rehabilitation services and vision enhancing techniques and devices offer opportunities to increase their visual and general functional capacity.

AGING AND LOSS OF VISION

Normal Age-Related Changes in Vision

Every older person experiences age-related changes in vision. Table 95-1 summarizes the age-related changes that cause functional declines for older persons. Decreased transmission of the ocular media, increased scatter in the cornea, lens, vitreous body and retina as well as decreased pupil size are related to anatomic changes in the aging eye. The age-related changes discussed here are those that have the greatest impact on function in daily life. These common changes in vision function must be taken in account when considering the daily living, quality of life, and the design of facilities for all older persons.

Table 95-1 Normal Age-Related Changes in Vision

Changes	Reason	Implications for Daily Life
Loss of accommodation	• Crystalline lenses lose flexibility • Ciliary muscles lose tone	Increasing inability to focus on close targets beginning around age 45 years. Plus lenses prescribed in a bifocal, reading glasses, or contact lenses; required to compensate for loss of accommodative ability.
Loss of low-contrast acuity	• Decreased transmission of ocular media • Decreased pupil size	Functional loss of acuity under glare or low lighting may cause small targets to be missed, bumping or tripping into low-lying objects.
Increased sensitivity to glare	• Increased light scatter in cornea, lenses, vitreous body, and retina	Discomfort even in low glare conditions such as cloudy days. High glare causes decreased acuity and difficulty in seeing targets in the environment. Sunlenses, hats, visors, and umbrellas provide more comfort outdoors; tinted lenses may be prescribed for indoors.
Increased difficulty with dark adaptation	• Losses in ocular transmittance and papillary miosis	Difficulty moving from bright to dim environments. Risk for stumbling or falling is greater under these circumstances. Fear of balance problems or falling may cause compensatory behaviors such as shuffling, reaching for hand-holds, etc. Change environmental lighting to avoid light/dim areas.
Loss of color discrimination	• Smaller pupil diameter, reduced light transmission through the lens, changes in photoreceptors and neural pathways	Difficulty detecting differences in dark colors and pastels; adding lamps or identifying matching colors near a sunny window helps.
Loss of attentional visual field	• Decline of higher order visual processes such as selective and divided attention and rapid processing speed	Risk factor for balance and mobility problems and vehicle crashes in driving. Training improves performance.
Increased difficulty with visual reading ability	• Related to attentional visual field and low contrast acuity and slower saccadic performance in eye movements.	Reading speed of older readers reduced by one-third that of younger readers; text navigation skills decline with age. Training improves performance.

The ability to accommodate for focus on visual targets from distance to near, which is dependent on a flexible crystalline lens and the ciliary muscle, is altered with age, beginning around age 45 years. During this change, an increasing amount of plus in a concave lens (usually prescribed in bifocal lenses or reading glasses) is required to boost the focusing power of the eye to compensate for the loss in refracting ability of the lens.

The visual acuity of normally sighted older persons show only a modest decrease under high-contrast conditions, but reducing the illumination of an acuity chart, reducing the contrast of the acuity chart, and/or adding surrounding glare, produce drastic age-related acuity losses, as compared to young observers. For example, in a sample of 900 older observers, for those at age 82 years the median high-contrast visual acuity was 20/30, low-contrast high-luminance acuity was 20/55; low-contrast, low-luminance acuity was 20/120; and low-contrast acuity in glare conditions was 20/160. A young observer loses only about one line of acuity under similar conditions.

Because of anatomic changes in the eye and media, older persons are more sensitive to glare in the environment, more likely to experience disabling glare, and have reduced glare recovery time. This may have the most impact on activities such as walking outdoors or driving, but may also affect indoor activities as well, if very bright and dim environments are adjacent, such as restaurants, movie theaters, and atriums. Visual discomfort may arise because of glare, and disabling glare may hide important targets that must be viewed for safety's sake.

Attentional visual field, the visual field area over which one can use rapidly presented visual information, declines with age. Unlike conventional measures of visual field that assess visual sensory sensitivity (such as static flashing lights), attentional visual field relies on higher-order processing skills such as selective and divided attention and rapid processing speed. Decreased attentional visual field has been correlated to a greater incidence of driving accidents and is related to a greater risk for balance and mobility problems for normally sighted older persons. Attentional visual field can be improved with training, but such training is not widely available.

Visual reading ability decreases with age as well. The reading rate of older persons who are normally sighted and have good high-contrast visual acuity decreases by as much as a third of that of young readers. Accuracy of reading, however, can remain comparable to that of younger readers. Reading performance among older persons with good acuity (20/30) is highly correlated with attentional visual field; those with good reading performance into very old age also retain good attentional fields as well. Low-contrast visual acuity is also correlated with reading performance for this population; older persons with poor low-contrast acuity tend to read more slowly. Even when high-contrast acuity is good, older persons, especially the oldest old, are at risk for reading difficulties that may arise from a combination of reduced attentional visual field, slower saccadic performance in eye movements, and poor low-contrast visual acuity. Reading rate for normally sighted older adults with good high-contrast acuity and good comprehension skills can be improved with training. Training in reading efficiency that emphasizes improvements in eye movements for reading similar to those exercises used to improve reading for school children has given good results for this population. Such training, however, is not widely available.

Color discrimination is another aspect of vision that declines with advancing age. Persons who are older have greater difficulty detecting differences between dark colors such as brown, black, or navy, and also have difficulty with pastels. Loss of color vision in old age is related to smaller pupil diameter, reduced light transmission through the lens, and changes in photoreceptors and neural pathways.

Finally, dark adaptation declines due to losses in ocular transmittance and pupillary miosis resulting from the aging process. Difficulty with dark adaptation can be limiting to older adults moving from light to dim environments and vice versa. The risk for stumbling or falling may be greater under these circumstances.

PREVALENT AGE-RELATED CAUSES OF VISUAL IMPAIRMENT

Age-Related Macular Degeneration

Functional vision loss because of age-related macular degeneration may include metamorphopsia (visual images appear distorted and wavy), relative scotomas, and, finally, result in dense central scotomas for those whose pathology progresses to visual impairment. Individuals with central scotoma usually develop a strongly preferred retinal locus (PRL) that performs as the primary fixation reference, although the patient may not always be aware that there is a scotoma present. The loss of central visual field results in loss of visual acuity and contrast sensitivity. The ability to use the PRL that develops for fixation may be difficult for many persons. The effects of macular degeneration on daily life include difficulty with reading print, inability to recognize faces (that can lead to reluctance to participate in social activities), difficulty with distance and depth cues (that adversely affect safe mobility) and loss of color and contrast sensitivity (that interfere with a variety of household and work/leisure tasks) (Table 95-2).

Diabetic Retinopathy

The progression of diabetic retinopathy includes macular edema that may cause blurred vision if the fovea is involved, retinal hemorrhages (and/or laser treatments), which may result in scattered central, peripheral or midperipheral scotomas, and retinal detachment, which can cause larger areas of field loss if not reattached. Diabetic retinopathy can progress to total blindness. Loss of function can include decreased visual acuity, scattered field loss over the retina, metamorphopsia across the retina, increased sensitivity to glare, loss of color and contrast sensitivity. If the fovea is lost to scotoma, then a preferred retinal locus will develop. Vision fluctuations can be manifested over time as macular swelling increases or subsides, and can also be related to hemorrhage. Sudden vision loss is common following hemorrhage, with the patient describing episodes of smoky vision, a dropped veil over the eye(s), or seeing black or red strings across the field of view. Treatment and absorption of blood can improve acuity, though not usually to normal levels. The effects on daily life include difficulty reading print materials, difficulty recognizing faces, increased sensitivity to glare and light/dark adaptation, difficulty with distance and depth cues, loss of color and contrast sensitivity, and fluctuating vision.

Cataract

Age-related cataract is manifested by gradual opacity of the lens which interferes with the passage of light, causing reduced visual acuity, light scatter, sensitivity to glare, altered color perception and image distortion (straight lines appear wavy). Persons with cataracts may experience trouble with glare and loss of contrast, may have decreased acuity, and report areas of metamorphopsia or small scotomas in the visual field. When the cataract has begun to interfere with lifestyle, surgery may be performed to remove either the entire lens, or the posterior portion. Correction for the removal of the lens is provided through intraocular lens implants, eyeglasses, or contact lens. Cataract surgery is the most common major surgical procedure done for persons older than age 65 years who are receiving Medicare. Cataract surgery with lens implantation is associated with improved objective and subjective measures of function in

Table 95-2   Age-Related Causes of Visual Impairment

Condition	Common Clinical Presentation	Implications for Rehabilitation
Macular degeneration	• Reduced visual acuity • Loss of central visual field and contrast sensitivity	Difficulty with tasks requiring fine detail vision such as reading, inability to recognize faces, distortion or disappearance of the visual field straight ahead, loss of color and contrast perception, mobility difficulties related to loss of depth and contrast cues.
Diabetic retinopathy	• Reduced visual acuity • Scattered central scotomas • Peripheral and midpheripheral scotomas • Macular edema	Difficulty with tasks requiring fine detail vision such as reading, distorted central vision, fluctuating vision, loss of color perception, mobility problems because of loss of depth and contrast cues.
Cataract	• Reduced visual acuity • Light scatter • Sensitivity to glare • Altered color perception • Loss of contrast sensitivity • Image distortion • Possible myopia	Usually remedied by lens extraction and implant, except in extreme cases. If not managed by implant, difficulty with detail vision, difficulty with bright and changing light, color perception, decreased contrast perception, some mobility problems due to loss of perception of depth and distance, sensitivity to glare and loss of contrast.
Glaucoma	• Degeneration of optic disc • Loss of peripheral visual fields	Mobility and reading problems because of restricted visual fields, people suddenly appearing in the visual field seen as "jack in the box."

activities of daily living, as well as improved levels of vision to normal acuity in most cases.

Glaucoma

Glaucoma is an increase in intraocular pressure caused by an abnormality in flow of aqueous fluid from the anterior chamber. It can cause a degeneration of the optic disc, loss of visual fields, and severe visual impairment. When left untreated, or if treatment is not successful, glaucoma results in a loss of peripheral fields, and can lead to blindness. The effect of peripheral field loss on daily life is most problematic in safe ambulation. Because of field restrictions the patient may not see objects in the path and may bump into objects that fall outside the field of view in any direction (street signs, tree branches, etc.). In addition, a person outside the patient's field of view may suddenly be seen as a "jack-in-the-box" and create a startle effect. Peripheral field loss may also create problems in reading and writing as only a small portion of the page can be see at once.

THE ROLE OF THE GERIATRICIAN IN VISION REHABILITATION

After diagnosis and medical management of the patient's vision loss by an ophthalmologist, the geriatrician can play an important role in assuring that visually impaired persons receive rehabilitation services that are of high quality, are

sought in a timely manner, and provide all the benefit that the patient might be able to derive from them.

A geriatrician can provide the following services for their patients related to vision rehabilitation:

1. A visual acuity evaluation. Current best practice includes the use of a logarithmic visual acuity chart.
2. A contrast sensitivity function evaluation. The Pelli–Robson chart is recommended for its ease of use and reliability.
3. A referral to a low vision eye care specialist (ophthalmologist or optometrist) for the appropriate prescription of magnification devices for tasks the older person can no longer perform such as reading, writing, watching television, and recognizing street signs.
4. A referral to vision rehabilitation professionals for assessment and instruction of vision and magnification devices for literacy, activities of daily living, and safe travel. These therapists can also provide environmental analyses and teach the use of environmental cues.
5. Assistance to patients in preparing for rehabilitation by providing information and encouraging them to consider the goals they would like to achieve. The National Eye Institute: Visual Functioning Questionnaire–14 is a modified 14-item questionnaire that is effective in assessing the impact of vision loss on quality of life, and is helpful in assisting patients in setting goals for rehabilitation.
6. Counseling or referral for coping with psychosocial issues related to visual impairment. Patients may not

be forthcoming about these issues, so the doctor must ask. Adjustment disorder and depression are associated with visual impairment for older persons. When patients are dealing with loss of independence and control, poor self-esteem, and strained social relations, counseling and/or psychotherapy may be recommended for both patients and family members.

7. Reinforcement of simple strategies, such as the use of saturated colors and contrast in the home environment, and the use of simple devices, such as sun lenses outdoors and bright indoor environments.

8. Information to the patient and family about the variable nature of low vision, its effect on daily life tasks, and the variable nature of visual abilities according to fluctuations of light and contrast.

9. Sponsorship of, or referral to, support groups where older persons with vision loss and their families can discuss problems, coping, and rehabilitation strategies they have learned with other patients.

10. Assistance in community awareness efforts about the prevalence, treatment, and rehabilitation of visual impairment among older persons.

Patients likely to benefit from vision rehabilitation include those with reduced acuity of less than 20/50, central or peripheral field loss with intact acuity, reduced contrast sensitivity, glare sensitivity, and/or light/dark adaptation difficulties. Candidates for cataract surgery with macular disease might also benefit from preoperative low-vision assessment and coincident rehabilitation training that enhances postoperative visual performance and satisfaction with a cataract procedure.

ADAPTATIONS OF CLINICAL AND FUNCTIONAL EVALUATIONS FOR OLDER ADULTS

The clinical and functional low-vision examinations for older persons should distinguish aging from treatable disease processes; focus holistically; be multidisciplinary and incorporate family and caregiver support; and identify and set realistic goals to improve functional status and quality of life.

In health care service delivery to older adults with low vision, certain aspects of the examination sequence will need to be adapted to accommodate these principles.

Case History Interview

Because most age-related visual impairments result in a central scotoma, most patient complaints will be related to the loss of acuity, the loss of central visual field, and resultant decrease in contrast sensitivity and color sensitivity. Patient goals for rehabilitation will usually include reading, writing, activities of daily living such as meal preparation, management of glare and other illumination concerns, and safe independent travel.

This information may be taken by a preexamination telephone interview to lessen the amount of time a first visit

might require. Because low vision rehabilitation requires a great deal of energy and motivation from the patient, it will be guided by his or her personal goals for rehabilitation, those tasks that are difficult or impossible to perform because of low vision. In this regard, the intake interviewer may find that some education is necessary in order to set reasonable goals for low-vision treatment. Because most low-vision interventions are "task specific," it is important to state treatment goals as specifically as possible.

Because of the nature of the older person's vision loss, professionals should become familiar with some of the courtesies and accessibility issues that assist in providing quality health care. Unless there is a problem with the person's hearing, always speak directly to the older adult with visual impairment. Allow the older adult to take your arm when moving from place to place in the environment, and use appropriate sighted guide techniques. Say your name when first coming into the room, and tell the older adult when you are leaving the room. Do not leave the older adult with low vision standing alone in a hallway or room without a wall or furniture near to touch for orientation and balance. Avoid using directional cues that are visual in nature such as pointing or giving directional references that are unclear to those with low vision. For example, instead of saying, "take that chair over there," say, "take the red chair against the white wall to your immediate right."

The Clinical Low-Vision Evaluation

The low-vision eye-care specialist (who may be an ophthalmologist or an optometrist) will find that in order to provide the best low-vision service to older adults, flexibility and the ability to adapt to a variety of different environments, schedules, and communication styles may be necessary. The conventional pattern of the low-vision examination will be followed including distance and near acuities; internal and external ocular health examination; retinoscopy; tonometry and slit-lamp biomicroscopy; ophthalmoscopy; ophthalmometry; determination of central and peripheral fields; color vision and contrast-sensitivity testing; glare testing; and near and distance testing of vision-enhancing devices, including optical, electronic, and nonoptical devices. For many older adults, especially those in long-term care facilities, a careful refraction and updating conventional spectacles may provide significant improvement in vision. Table 95-3 summarizes the aspects of the clinical low-vision examination.

Because of the nature of medical and long-term care service delivery to older adults it is often necessary to take the low-vision examination and therapeutic intervention out of the office or clinical setting. There is a growing trend of providing low-vision services as a part of outpatient hospital care, comprehensive outpatient rehabilitation facilities, and long-term care facilities, such as nursing homes, and the private homes of older adults.

Nursing Homes

Despite the fact that an estimated 26 percent of persons in nursing homes have visual impairment, few nursing home

Table 95-3   Clinical Low Vision Examination

Alternative settings	• Long-term care facilities • Individual's home • Community service agency • Rehabilitation center
Aspects of the examination	• Distance/near acuities • Internal/external health exam • Retinoscopy • Tonometry • Slit-lamp biomicroscopy • Ophthalmoscopy • Ophthalmometry • Central/peripheral fields • Color vision testing • Contrast-sensitivity testing • Evaluation of low vision • Devices (optical, nonoptical, and electronic)

residents receive low-vision care. For example, one study found only approximately 25 percent of visually impaired patients at a long-term care facility who were in need of vision rehabilitation were referred by their attending ophthalmologists. Another study found there was no difference in the referral rate for vision services for nursing home residents between those who complained about their vision and those who did not. Another study found that only 11 percent of all residents in 19 nursing homes had received eye examinations in the last 2 years. Providing information about vision and vision impairment to the nursing home staff is important for assisting residents in using their remaining vision effectively. Because stroke is another common medical condition requiring rehabilitation for older adults, it is important that the low-vision team work closely with those professionals who diagnose, treat, and rehabilitate older adults with cerebrovascular accident. A curriculum in low vision for in-service training for long-term care staff has been developed and is effective in increasing staff knowledge and positive outcomes for patients.

Hospital Settings

Low-vision care is routinely provided to older veterans in the hospital system of the Department of Veterans Affairs. In the Blind Rehabilitation Centers, the veteran who is legally blind is seen for up to 16 weeks of rehabilitation, including low vision rehabilitation. Preliminary results from a national outcomes study indicate positive outcomes and veteran satisfaction from these programs. The Visual Impairment Centers to Optimize Remaining Sight provide low-vision services to veterans who have low vision but who are not legally blind. In addition, low vision is routinely provided at outpatient eye clinics in VA medical centers. Outcome studies of all VA vision rehabilitation services indicate that veterans who are provided low

vision services regain their ability to perform instrumental activities of daily living independently and become active community participants. Hospitals in the private sector are increasing services to older persons as a part of outpatient services, and low-vision rehabilitation is often provided.

Community Service Agency Settings

The Older Americans Act mandates the provision of supportive community resources for older adults. State Units on Aging and Area Agencies on Aging were created under the auspices of the Administration on Aging, a branch of the Department of Health and Human Services. Some examples of community agency settings include senior centers, nutrition centers, senior clubs, adult daycare centers, and senior rehabilitation centers. These services may be contacted through the local telephone book yellow pages. For example, in Atlanta, the services are clustered in the Bell-South Yellow Pages under the heading, "Senior Services." The explanation of the local county services contracts is provided, and a contact number for each county is listed. Low-vision services might be provided onsite at these community service settings because of the prevalence of visual impairment among older adults.

Private Home Settings

Almost 71 percent of the older population requiring long-term care reside in the community. Senior residential retirement centers have increased in number. Most frail older persons requiring care are living at home with family members, and not in long-term care facilities. Interactions with family members and caregivers become very important in these situations. It is crucial that family members and caregivers understand the sometimes contradictory nature of visual impairment; for example, visual performance varies widely under different levels of illumination, and can decline if the older person is fatigued. This understanding will help the family in supporting the older adult achieve his or her goals for vision rehabilitation.

Functional Visual Assessment

Whenever possible the functional assessment should take place in the older adult's daily environment. Specific goals stated by the older adult will guide the functional assessment to discover what visual target size, target distance, and visual skills are required to achieve that goal. For example, if the patient's goal is to read the newspaper again, the target size requires approximately 20/40 or better vision with magnification, the target distance will be determined by the magnification device, and the visual skills required are precise fixation and saccades while maintaining the focal distance of the magnification device. The functional assessment can also uncover the need to address other goals, the need for environmental assessment and modification, and provide ongoing opportunities to educate the older adult and his or her significant others about vision and

Table 95-4   Key Aspects of the Functional Visual Assessment

Functional visual acuities	Distance and lighting required for discriminating detail of objects in the environment
Functional visual fields	Ability to perceive objects in the environment in central and peripheral quadrants of the visual field at near and distance
Color/contrast discrimination	Ability to detect objects, their color, and contrast with the background at varying distances
Ocular motor skills	Ability to maintain fixation and move the eyes/head/body to scan, track, and localize targets in the environment
Lighting	Analysis of the usefulness of environmental lighting; need for illumination and control
Use of visual and nonvisual cues	Availability and use of visual and nonvisual cues in the environment for task performance
Performance of activities of daily living and instrumental activities of daily living that are affected by vision	Observe for ability to perform, ease and speed of performance, comfort and stress level, safety

rehabilitation. Table 95-4 presents the key aspects of the functional vision assessment.

The functional low-vision assessment may be completed by a wide variety of rehabilitation professionals. Traditionally, the functional low-vision assessment of older persons has been provided by a low-vision therapist, a rehabilitation teacher for the visually impaired, an orientation and mobility specialist, or some other professional from the field of visual impairment. Now, as low vision is increasingly a part of hospital services and comprehensive outpatient rehabilitation facilities, the functional assessment may be provided by a rehabilitation nurse, an occupational therapist, or some other rehabilitation professional who has received specialized training in low vision.

Regardless of the background of the rehabilitation professional, he or she should be well versed and experienced in basic optics of the eye; lenses and low-vision devices; methods of observation and evaluation of visual skills for all activities of daily living; the causes and functional implications of visual impairments; basic techniques of sighted guide and orientation and mobility; assessment of reading; assessment of the environment; and basic techniques of assessing and using technology such as low-vision devices (e.g., magnifiers, spectacles, monoculars) and electronic devices (e.g., Braille writer, Kurzweil reader, closed-circuit television system). The rehabilitation professional providing the evaluation may also be the rehabilitation therapist, in which case he or she must be familiar with techniques of teaching visual-motor skills for all activities of daily living (ADLs) and instrumental activities of daily living (IADL) with and without low-vision and electronic devices, task analysis, teaching basic orientation and mobility, and teaching basic techniques of reading with low-vision devices. The professional must also be familiar with tools and techniques that do not require the use of vision, in order to assist the older person with low vision in developing other

mechanisms for performance when using vision is not the safest or most efficient mechanism (e.g., slate and stylus that are used for writing Braille). This rehabilitation professional will work closely with the eye-care specialist providing the clinical low-vision examination, and the low-vision team may also include a counseling professional, and any other professionals who are providing care associated with the use of vision. Because many older persons are at risk for multiple impairments, this team may also include other doctors, such as a geriatrician or physiatrist, orthopedist, speech, physical, respiratory, and recreational therapists, other nurses, and technicians.

MANAGEMENT OF LOW VISION

Developing a Vision Rehabilitation Plan

The clinical low-vision examination and functional visual assessment culminates in a vision *rehabilitation plan* that summarizes the information obtained in the evaluations into clearly stated goals and objectives. In some cases, family members also may be involved. The implementation of the vision rehabilitation plan should emphasize a process using the principles of andragogy, or adult learning, that incorporates the older person's values, beliefs, attitudes, and life experiences.

Following the clinical examination and functional assessment, the low-vision team will recommend low-vision devices (including optical, electronic, nonoptical, and environmental modifications) that will be evaluated to assess their usefulness to the older adult. There should be additional focus on the rehabilitation program and its adaptation for older individuals. Successful use of low-vision devices is related to the intensity of the instructional program. Research shows that specialized therapy in the use of visual skills and low-vision devices improves the abilities of low-vision individuals who are older to a greater extent than do the services provided by eye-care specialists alone.

Instruction and Guided Practice Using Remaining Vision and Low-Vision Devices

Working with a low-vision therapist will provide an opportunity for the older adult to develop the appropriate visual skills, as well as learn the benefits, limitations, and uses of low-vision devices, and apply principles of color, illumination, and contrast that make the environment as conducive as possible to the use of remaining vision. It is important to assist caregivers in understanding how remaining vision and low-vision devices aid the older adult in accomplishing visual tasks. Family members and caregivers can provide important social support in this regard, but must understand the process in order to be most helpful. In a study of visually impaired older veterans, a supportive caregiver was the most strongly correlated variable to continued use of low-vision devices 2 years after they were prescribed. If at all possible, pertinent low-vision devices should be loaned for use in the daily environment, to assure that they are useful to older adults, before they are prescribed.

Some aspects of instructing the use of vision and devices are particularly important when working with older persons with low vision. Because of the potentially devastating consequences of falling, the low-vision therapist must be certain to address safety issues related to using low-vision devices that will prevent falls. Nausea, dizziness, and other aspects of motion sickness are common side effects of using magnification, and reducing these effects is an important aspect of instruction. Monoculars and binoculars should be used as spotting devices only, and older adults must never attempt to walk while viewing through them.

Another factor to be explored in the use of low-vision devices for older adults is hand tremor. Hand tremor may be severe enough that hand-held magnifiers or telescopes are not useful. The low-vision team may want to explore spectacle-mounted devices to avoid the difficulty of maintaining focus if hand tremor is problematic.

Postural support and ergonomic considerations are an important aspect to using devices for persons who are older. Because of the prevalence of back and neck pain, as well as limited stamina, it is important that the therapist be able to keep the learner as comfortable as possible. The low-vision therapist will evaluate and teach the use of appropriate ergonomic devices such as the appropriate chair and table, lumbar and cervical support, footstool, lamps and reading stands.

Finally, illumination is an important aspect of the instruction. Most older persons need more light, but some may be extremely sensitive to light. An evaluation of a variety of lamps and overhead lighting situations is necessary, with the use of illuminations controls that are individually recommended such as filters, absorptive lenses, hats with brims, pinhole glasses, and side shields.

Low-Vision Devices

Low-vision devices are optical devices, electronic devices, or other tools that enhance the use of vision. Some devices, such as those optical devices that incorporate refractive correction, require special prescription. Others are more simple and straightforward in their assessment and recommendation, such as lamps, reading stands, or large-print books. During the clinical evaluation and functional assessment, the low-vision team will discover whether magnification, minification, or other nonoptical devices will be useful for enhancing the vision. Table 95-5 summarizes the types of devices available and their uses.

Devices are prescribed based on the goals of the older person, and most persons require instruction and practice in their use.

Magnification devices may be categorized as four types: relative distance, relative size, angular, and electronic. Relative distance magnification is provided by bringing the device to be viewed closer to the eyes. Often older adults who want to recognize someone will move more closely to the face they want to see, exhibiting this type of magnification. Spectacle-mounted magnifiers focus the target image, such as print for reading, at ranges closer than the older eye can accommodate, and allow very close distances to be maintained. These lenses must be prescribed by an eye-care specialist experienced in low vision in order to incorporate the refractive correction of the older person. Typically, these devices require a close focal distance and a short depth of focus. Depending on the power and focal distance, they can be used for near tasks such as reading, writing, and viewing photographs.

Magnification may also be provided by stand or hand-held magnifiers, which are often more familiar to older adults who may have used them previously for maps or coins. These devices do not require a close eye-to-lens distance, but the closer to the eye the lens is held, the wider the field of view. Some are available with built-in illumination, which overcomes the problem of illuminating the target the older adult is viewing. Hand-held magnifiers require a steady hand to maintain focus and may be fatiguing to use for long periods. Older adults who use stand magnifiers must wear their bifocal correction for visual accommodation, as the lens is set slightly inside the true focal distance of the lens in order to provide a better optical image at the periphery of the lens.

Relative size magnification is used whenever a target to be viewed is made physically larger. Examples of this are phone dials with enlarged numbers or large print in magazines and newspapers. Environments such as older adult high-rise apartments or condominiums and planned communities may also used enlarged signage, another example of relative-size magnification.

Telescopic devices provide angular magnification by the use of a positive and negative lens in housing (galilean) or by the use of two positive lenses with an erecting prism (keplerian). Older adults may have used monoculars or binoculars in the past for sporting or other events, and may have developed basic skills in their use. Older adults use telescopic devices for identifying targets that are further away, such as street signs or television. The telescope

Table 95-5 Low-Vision Devices

Type of Device	Typical Use
Stand or hand-held magnifiers	Short-term reading or writing tasks such as checking a price tag or recipe, signing a check
Spectacle-mounted magnifiers	Long-term reading such as newspaper; used for writing in low powers
Hand-held monoculars or binoculars	Traffic or street signs, spectator events
Spectacle-mounted monocular or binocular telescope	Television viewing, spectator events, possible driving Short-focus telescope can be used for cards, reading music, games, woodworking, etc.
Closed-circuit television system	Reading, writing, independent activities of daily living With distance camera, can be used like a telescope
Field-expansion devices: • Reverse telescope • Field-expansion prisms • Hemianopic mirrors	Field expansion for ambulating or obstacle detection, identification, and/or avoidance Best with normal or near-normal acuity
Nonoptical devices: • Lamps • Illumination control devices • Handwriting implements • Posture and focal distance support • Large print • Color/contrast aids	 Provide brighter illumination, primarily used as task lighting Control glare: sunlenses, hats, visors, colored filters Felt-tip pens, bold-line paper, check- and letter-writing stencils, allow user to stay on line and write legibly Upright reading stand, footstool, chair with arms and high back Cervical and lumbar support: provide comfort and allow user to read or write for a longer period Large-print books and news, large phone dials, etc., to enhance visibility Brightly colored tape/paint for marking dials, edge of steps, etc., to enhance visibility and safety

may be hand-held, or may be mounted into spectacles for hands-free viewing. Mounted short-focus telescopes may be used for tasks that are closer, such as reading music from a stand or identifying cards on a table. Some older adults who meet visual and driving requirements may use mounted telescopes for driving.

The closed-circuit television system (CCTV) is an example of electronic magnification. The CCTV provides a camera to focus on the visual task and the older adult sees the image projected onto a monitor. The visual task may be reading and writing from a desktop, or the camera may be positioned for visual tasks at a greater distance such as seeing the minister and choir at church. The advantages of the CCTV include more magnification than any other device, a wider field of view, and contrast enhancement via reversed polarity. CCTV offers a mechanism for the development of new technologies such as miniaturization, head-worn devices, contrast enhancement, and image remapping.

A variety of software and hardware packages have been developed that produce enlarged print on the computer screen. Computer use in conjunction with CCTV can use multiple cameras to provide split-screen images for designing a workstation that simultaneously accesses computer, print viewing, word processing, and distance viewing.

Expanded field devices are helpful to older adults who maintain normal or near-normal acuity while experiencing decreased field of view, such as that caused by glaucoma or hemianopsias. Expanded field devices provide the ability to find targets by increasing the perceived view of a scene. For example, an older adult with restricted fields wishes to find the arriving and departing flight monitors in an airport. By using a field-expansion device, these monitors can be more easily located, and then an older adult moves closer to them in order to read the information without the device. A reverse telescope functions similar to a peephole in a door, but with better optics. Another type of field-expanding device minifies in the horizontal meridian only. The visual field may also be expanded by the use of base-out prisms incorporated into spectacles. The base-out prism shifts the image in, allowing a small eye movement to see the expanded field. Small mirrors attached to spectacles may also be used for field expansion.

Nonoptical devices that enhance the use of vision may also enhance the use of optical and electronic devices. Illumination controls in the form of lamps, filters, absorptive sun lenses, and environmental lighting are of vital importance to visual functioning for older adults. Setting up kitchen and living room "workstations" for visual activities that include ergonomic considerations enhances the use of vision and all devices. Simple devices that use large features, large print, and judicious use of bold color and contrast can enhance the vision and independence of older adults.

Instruction in the Use of Low-Vision Devices

A sequence of instructional procedures covers several areas:

- Use of visual skills without low-vision devices
- Use of visual skills with low-vision devices
- Use of vision and low-vision devices for individualized functional tasks that lead to the accomplishment of defined goals.

Instruction in the use of visual skills without devices covers fixation, spotting, localization, scanning, tracing, and tracking. Individuals with maculopathy (such as age-related macular degeneration or diabetic retinopathy) may require additional instruction in the development and maintenance of visual skills using the preferred retinal locus.

Instruction in the use of visual skills with low-vision devices includes integrating unaided visual abilities with the unique demands of a low-vision device such as maintaining the focal distance or focusing the device, and adjusting eye and head movements to compensate for a restricted field of view through the lens. If the individual is using eccentric viewing (the use of a preferred retinal locus other than the fovea), the instructor assures that the device selected allows the opportunity to maximize field and acuity in the eccentric position.

Reading with Low-Vision Devices

Reading is a task that is so fundamental to our society and so disrupted by age-related visual impairment that it is the primary goal for vision rehabilitation among older adults. Readers with low vision can develop visual skills that are well-adapted to reading if they receive appropriate intervention. Most readers develop a strongly preferred retinal locus following the onset of central scotoma. The PRL is an area that will take over the function of fixation in an eccentric, nondamaged area of the retina. The reader may require instruction and practice in using the PRL for reading, especially because of the demands of using magnification to compensate for acuity loss. A Swedish study found that 71 percent of older adults with low vision could read the newspaper following rehabilitation, although at a 3-year follow-up that number had dropped to 48 percent. However, the number of fluent readers (70 words per minute or better) had increased from 41 percent to 48 percent over the 3-year period. These results indicate that those older adults with vision loss who persevere with rehabilitation strategies are able to continue improving their skills over time. In another study, persons with macular loss who had a PRL below the scotoma exhibited faster reading rates, and the size of the atrophic area in the macula was the predominant limiting factor in reading; the larger the atrophy, the lower the reading rate. Reading rate is also related to window size (number of characters available in the field of view) and the reserves of acuity and contrast sensitivity provided by the visual system and low vision device. Accuracy of word identification and comprehension of reading, however, can remain near normal for readers with macular loss, despite their slow rates. Readers with low vision often supplement visual reading with speech output devices such as spoken computer programs and books on audiotape. They may also have normally sighted readers who assist in handling bills, mail, or other reading requirements.

ENVIRONMENTS FOR OLDER PERSONS

The onset of visual impairment for older adults can make even the most familiar environment seem strange and hazardous. It is important that older adults be oriented to familiar and unfamiliar environments, and that the environment be as "user-friendly" as possible to increase independence and safety. There are a variety of rehabilitation techniques that assist in accomplishing this. Table 95-6 presents the basic strategies.

Improving the Lighting

Most older persons require two to three times more light than do younger persons for the same tasks, but those with cloudy media (cataract, keratoconus, vitreous floaters, etc.) are more sensitive to glare. The challenge is to get enough light without creating glare, which can be disabling. For example, the glare from a sunny window onto a waxed floor, tabletops, and picture glass could cause objects in the dining room of a senior community to be obscured. An older person with low vision might function as if blind in that environment and be unable to find a chair, recognize his friends, serve his plate, or even see the food in a buffet line.

In an environment that is conducive for the function of older persons, it is important to manage not only light, but also shadow, which can be conducive to function, for example, a triangular shadow at the end of a step indicates the height and depth of the step as well as how many steps there are. But shadow can also be hazardous, such as the shadow of a garden wall that obscures a sidewalk curb, causing a person to trip or fall.

Lighting is best if controllable, no matter what type it is. Most older persons with low vision will require task lighting that can be positioned closer to reading material or craft activity. Because the intensity of light is inversely related to the squared distance from its source, adding light at ceiling height will not provide adequate task illumination for older viewers. Task lights must be used that can be positioned closely, and therefore flex-armed lamps are best in this regard.

There are a variety of different types of bulbs that are useful and recommended for older viewers with low vision.

Table 95-6   Ways to Make an Environment More Visually Accessible

Change the real or perceived size of objects to be viewed	For loss of detailed vision: • Increase size (large print) • Move closer (move chair closer to the television) • Use magnification For loss of peripheral fields with normal acuity: • Minify image (reverse telescope) • Move further away • Use field-enhancement devices such as mirrors
Improve lighting	Use appropriate environmental lighting to decrease glare and increase overall light level; use illumination controls such as sunlenses, hats with brims, visors, colored filters; use task lighting such as flex-arm lamps
Increase contrast between objects and background	Eliminate busy background patterns, mark down steps with contrasting color on risers; increase contrast between furniture, china, and background
Use bright, clear colors	Mark light switches, dials, etc. with colored tape; use large areas of bright color for discrimination of objects
Organize the environment for ease and safety	Doors completely open or closed, chairs under table when not in use, furniture against the wall, organize clothing for color and function, etc.
Consider alternative strategies that do not use vision	Use of other senses for task performance, such as audiotaped reading materials, use of long cane for safe travel, olfactory cues for doneness of food, etc.

• Fluorescent lighting spreads evenly, is inexpensive and energy efficient, but provides less contrast because of that evenness, and produces less shadow. It is a harsh light and flickers, and may be bothersome to some viewers, causing headache and eye strain. Covering or shading fluorescent bulbs or bouncing the light from the ceiling to the eye may be helpful.

• Incandescent light is easily directed and provides more contrast and shadow. But the light can pool, if provided by one bulb suspended from the ceiling, causing pinpoint glare or pools of light within relative darkness. Using multiple incandescent fixtures can eliminate this problem. Incandescent lamps are good for task lighting such as reading, sewing, or hobbies.

• Halogen light uses the glow of halogen gas, as well as the incandescent filament to create a brighter light. The light is more blue, and therefore may require filtering. Ultraviolet or blue light may generate superoxide and hydroxide free radicals that may be related to damage in the eye. Although controlled clinical studies have not been done, blue light has been suggested as increasing risk of cataract and macular degeneration. Subsequent studies have not shown a correlation to visible light exposure and risk, but many rehabilitation services are cautious about "blue light hazard." An Australian study suggests that persons with less melanin (i.e., light-colored iris, fair skin) are at more risk from light.

• Neodymium oxide and incandescent bulbs are currently touted as "full-spectrum lighting." These bulbs emit fewer ultraviolet and infrared rays and provide a sharp drop in the emission of yellow light. The effect is a more vivid "true" color, similar to sunlight, so contrast is increased.

These types of lighting can be mixed to achieve effects that are most pleasing and comfortable for older viewers with low vision. A recent study exploring these types of lighting in reading lamps found strong preferences among older readers with low vision, but no differences in reading performance based upon the type of light. Thus, informed reader choice should guide the selection of the type of light for older readers.

Light/dark adaptation is another aspect of environmental lighting that must be considered. Most older persons have difficulty traveling from bright areas to dim ones because their dark adaptation is not as efficient as in young adults. Persons with severely restricted field loss (e.g., advanced glaucoma) become functionally blind in dim lighting. Avoiding light/dark areas in the environment such as a bright dining room and dim hallway is helpful. When these areas are unavoidable, the older person could use illumination controls such as sunglasses or brimmed hats to assist with light/dark adaptation.

Increasing Contrast

Light/dark contrast is produced by the amount of light that is reflected from different surfaces (a light object is brighter than a dark one). A greater contrast between objects and their backgrounds make them easier to see. Therefore, providing an area of dark background and an area of light background in the bathroom, kitchen, and bedroom can help a person more easily identify possessions. For example, if a comb and brush are a light color, they may be kept on a dark tray. Most TV remotes are black, so they should be placed on a very light background. Similarly, marking the edge of stairs with contrasting colored tape makes each step more visible.

Using Color

The ability to identify colors, especially darks and pastels diminishes with age. Certain visual impairments, especially those that affect the cones, such as macular degeneration, also reduce color vision. However, bright, clear colors can be seen by most older persons with low vision. For example, yellow against navy blue is very visible, because it combines both color and contrast cues.

Use Organizational Strategies

Organization can be extremely helpful for the person with low vision. For example, always making sure that doors are never left partially open and placing chairs under the table when not used increases the safety of the environment. Organizing and labeling clothing by color and function in closets and drawers and organizing the kitchen can assist an older person in continuing to live independently. Learning new ways of performing daily tasks can make the loss of vision less of a problem in independent living. For example, retrieving a pair of spectacles that have fallen onto a light carpet might be difficult for some older adults. Learning a visual scanning pattern that begins at the site where the spectacles seem to have fallen and then continues in a circular pattern outward until they are found will assist in retrieving them.

Using color coding can be helpful as well. For example, chicken soup cans could be marked with wide yellow rubber bands, and tomato soup cans could be marked with wide red rubber bands. These markers could be quickly identified, avoiding the necessity for identifying the soup with a magnifier each time a can is retrieved from the cabinet.

Alternative Strategies

Even when an older adult with low vision retains useful vision for a wide variety of tasks, it is sometimes helpful to use alternative techniques that do not require the use of vision because vision may not be the most efficient way of accomplishing some tasks. For example, even though an older adult may have useful vision for traveling, he may find it best to use a long cane in order to detect drop-offs, so that vision can be used to seek landmarks for orientation. An older adult with low vision may use speech output (a program that speaks symbols or words) for most computer word processing, so that limited stamina for reading and writing may be used for reading mail, which must be done visually. Knowledge of a wide variety of rehabilitation strategies and tools will assist older adults with low vision in developing a repertoire of techniques and devices that allows them to complete tasks efficiently and effectively.

Orientation to a new setting requires some basic alternative techniques that can be used anywhere. Some older adults may be able to use all of the techniques, some may only need one or two. It is important to remember not to rush the older adult in orientation, whether it's a long-term care facility or doctor's office. These exercises may be repeated as often as necessary. Teaching family members these techniques may be helpful when new environments come up in the future. Table 95-7 presents an overview of these techniques.

PSYCHOSOCIAL CONSIDERATIONS

Adaptation to Vision Loss

Anxiety and depression are common reactions to loss, and age-related visual impairment is complicated by the other losses associated with aging. There are two schools

Table 95-7 Orientation to a New Setting

Using a starting/ending point	Begin at one starting/ending place in the room, such as the door. Have the older adult reach out and feel both sides of the doorway, then describe the contents of the room, while leading him around the room via sighted guide and trailing and allowing him to feel features. Give simple names to the walls using some feature of the wall (example, the wall to the right is the bed wall, the wall opposite is the window wall).
Using compass directions or clock face	Some older adults will be more familiar with compass directions. Using the same starting points as previously explained, use north wall, south wall, east wall, and west wall to name the four sides of the room. Proceed using compass directions as the way of finding and naming locations in the room. Use clock face numbers in a similar manner for those who can more easily understand them.
Using landmarks and cues	Use familiar landmarks for orientation to a new environment, for example, the smell of food is a landmark for the dining room. The audible hum and red glow of a soft-drink machine may be another landmark.

of thought on the timing of rehabilitation related to adaptation. Some rehabilitation professionals subscribe to a "loss theory" of psychological adjustment. This theory proposes that the person must "die" as a sighted person, and be "reborn" as a visually impaired person, incorporating the visual impairment into the sense of self. According to this theory, attempting rehabilitation would be fruitless until the process is complete. Others subscribe to the theory that anxiety and depression are related to a person's negative stereotypes about visual impairment and a lack of confidence and motivation to attempt rehabilitation, but that if rehabilitation is successful, depression and anxiety should be reduced.

Older adults may hold many negative stereotypes associated with visual impairment: increased helplessness, inhabiting a world of darkness, increased vulnerability to crime, the perception that use of devices mark them as different or to be pitied. Older adults with low vision may attempt to pass as fully sighted in order to avoid having others project these negative stereotypes onto them. But attempting to pass as fully sighted may cause other difficulties. For example, older adults with low vision do not recognize faces well, and the lack of a friendly hello when passing acquaintances may be interpreted as unfriendliness. Failure to use alternative techniques for identifying targets and moving in the environment may lead to falls, burns, or other safety hazards.

Support groups and peer counseling for older adults with low vision can be extremely helpful in coping with vision loss. Support groups may be found through local multiservice agencies for persons who are visually impaired, or may be started by senior citizen's centers or other groups. Short-term professional counseling in conjunction with rehabilitation may be very helpful.

Family and Social Support

In a recent study of low-vision device use among veterans, most of whom were older males with macular degeneration, family support was the most powerful predictor of continued use of devices up to 2 years following their prescription. Providing information and support to family members who are experiencing the impact of the elder's vision loss can be powerful. Visual impairment is experienced by the entire family or caregiving system, not just by the older person, and both social and psychological concerns must be addressed. The loss of vision by one family member can disrupt roles in the family, create economic demands, and add stress when tasks previously performed by the older adult must be performed by someone else.

For family members who understand the functional implications of visual impairment, understanding the behavior of their older adult with low vision is easier. For example, understanding the effect of changing lighting conditions, the effects of glare, the adaptation times when traveling from dim light to bright and vice versa, can help explain behaviors like shielding the eyes, shuffling the feet, hesitation, and fear of falling. The fact that an older adult with restricted visual fields may pick up a dime from the floor, then bump into a partially open door seems contradictory, but is perfectly explained by the functioning field of view.

Assisting older adults with low vision in continuing social activities, such as hobbies, crafts, games, and traveling can aid them in maintaining important contacts with family and peers. Social support and contact is associated with less depression in older adults with low vision. Support groups can assist older adults with low vision in completing and using their rehabilitation, as well as facilitating adaptation to vision loss. Peer support, or mutual aid groups who meet regularly to share their mutual concerns may be especially beneficial for older adults who may be overprotected, abused, or treated paternalistically by those who do not understand visual impairment or aging. Facilitating assertiveness for older adults with low vision is recommended because it is linked to less depression and more social support. Social skill training in assertiveness for older adults with low vision has been shown effective in decreasing depression, and deriving greater satisfaction in life.

FUNDING FOR LOW-VISION REHABILITATION

Traditionally, vision rehabilitation services have been funded through private pay, or through vocational rehabilitation services for individuals who were preparing for the work force. Funding for services to older adults with vision impairment has been a critical health care issue in the United States. Public funding for the Independent Living Services for Older Individuals Who are Blind program under the Rehabilitation Act is minimal, approximately $20 million nationally in fiscal year 2000. These funds provide services in the traditional "blindness" system, state or private agencies for the visually impaired that are serving persons of all ages who have visual impairments. Prior to 2002, only older veterans with low vision who served in the US military and whose disability is service-connected have full access to comprehensive blindness and low-vision services through the Department of Veterans Affairs Medical Centers. However, most visually impaired veterans have age-related vision loss, and their income is such that a copay is required from them or from their private insurance carrier.

Vision-rehabilitation services were developed initially to meet the needs of blinded veterans returning from World War II. Young war-blinded men had few other medical problems, so efforts to rehabilitate them for the work force spawned the professions of orientation and mobility instructors, rehabilitation teachers for the blind, and low vision therapists in order to meet their unique needs. This specialized "blindness and low-vision" rehabilitation was not considered part of the broader medical rehabilitation. Credentialing of vision-rehabilitation professionals developed separately from occupational or physical therapists, and their practice was autonomous, requiring neither medical referral nor supervision. As a result, many medical professionals are unaware of their services, and do not understand the "blindness" rehabilitation system in which their practice began. The Department of Veterans Affairs model of service delivery in vision rehabilitation continues today in the same vein. Services are provided nationally by teams of professionals. Ophthalmologists or optometrists provide the medical services, and the rehabilitation professionals are orientation and mobility specialists, rehabilitation teachers, and low-vision therapists. This model is also implemented in most state agencies for the visually impaired.

The dramatic increase in the numbers of older adults with vision impairment has forced professionals to seek more traditional sources of medical funding to cover the increasing costs of vision rehabilitation services for the rising numbers of older persons. The US health care system has provided rehabilitation to restore functional independence following the onset of other disabling conditions such as stroke or hip replacement. Medicare sets patterns that other insurers follow, so low-vision practitioners have petitioned for funding for vision rehabilitation services, including clinical low-vision evaluations, instruction in the use of vision and adaptive equipment, provision of adaptive devices, mobility training for safe travel, and training in adaptive techniques for communication, home, and personal management.

Practitioners have been reimbursed most successfully if they have been recognized by the traditional medical rehabilitation health care field, that is, MDs (ophthalmologists or physiatrists), optometrists and occupational therapists (OTs). OTs as low-vision providers have been criticized as being unable to provide adequate services because their education and training do not address in-depth the particular needs of people who have visual impairments, especially the needs of those who are functionally blind. OTs have countered, however, that their training as generalists in rehabilitation provides them with basic abilities, and their training in providing rehabilitation for other disabilities related to aging, as well as their pervasive numbers, especially in rural areas, make them likely candidates as low-vision rehabilitation service providers. In managed care health care plans, however, these arguments are likely moot, as the use of paraprofessionals and physician assistants to primary care physicians are most likely to provide services, and vision-related services are rarely covered. Physical therapists have not entered a national dialog, and have not, so far, been key providers in vision rehabilitation.

On May 29, 2002, the Centers for Medicare & Medicaid Services (CMS) released a national program memorandum (Change request 2083, Pub. 60AB, Transmittal AB-02-078) to alert the provider community that Medicare beneficiaries who are blind or visually impaired are eligible for physician-prescribed rehabilitation services from approved health care professionals on the same basis as beneficiaries with other medical conditions that result in reduced physical functioning. The end date for this program memorandum is May 31, 2003. This memorandum was issued in response to the committee report accompanying the FY 2002 Labor/Health and Human Services/Education appropriations bill. The memorandum stated that an evaluation of the patient's level of functioning and implementation of a therapeutic plan should be implemented by an occupational therapist or physical therapist.

The memorandum further directed that the patient receiving services must have a potential for restoration or improvement of lost functions, and must be expected to improve significantly within a reasonable and generally predictable amount of time. The rehabilitation that is covered was short-term and intense; maintenance therapy was not covered. Applicable Health Care Common Procedural Coding System therapeutic procedures are outlined in the memorandum, as are applicable International Classification of Diseases (ICD)-9 codes that support medical necessity. Only services are covered; adaptive equipment, such as low-vision devices, is not.

The effect of the program memorandum has been to increase the visibility of Medicare provisions for vision rehabilitation, but it is not a national coverage decision. Medicare carriers are not compelled by the memorandum to develop a Local Medical Review Policy as a result, and are still able to deny all claims that the local carrier does not deem medically reasonable or necessary.

Soon to be introduced in the 108th Congress, the *Medicare Vision Rehabilitation Services Act* will provide Medicare Part B access for vision rehabilitation services for older adults who are blind or partially sighted that are not dependent on Center for Medicare/Medicaid Service policy or Medicare carrier discretion. Legislation was introduced in the 107th Congress (Representative Capuano, D-MA: HB2484, and Senator Kerry, D-MA: S1967) and was cosponsored by 136 Representatives and 14 Senators representing bi-partisan support. The Act has been endorsed by more than 70 national organizations representing medicine, aging, health care, organizations for consumers who are blind and visually impaired, and vision rehabilitation professionals. Sponsoring organizations include the American Academy of Ophthalmology, the National Alliance on the Aging, and the American Optometric Association. The Congressional Budget Office has not yet scored the legislation, but an independent assessment by the Lewin Group, Inc. has found that the estimate of five-year gross costs to Medicare from additional Medicare beneficiaries receiving vision rehabilitation services due to the proposed benefit standardization is $10.8 million. The Lewin Group, Inc. Report estimates from data in the Framingham Eye Study that hip fractures are experienced by approximately 18 percent of persons with impaired sight. Each fracture costs approximately $35,000 in medical expenses resulting in annual costs of more than $2.2 billion. If only one in five of these fractures could be prevented each year by providing vision rehabilitation services, the annual cost savings to Medicare would be more than $440 million.

REFERENCES

Brabyn JA et al: The Smith–Kettlewell Institute longitudinal study of vision function and its impact among the elderly: An overview. *Optom Vis Sci* 78:264, 2001.

De l'Aune WR et al: Outcome assessment of the rehabilitation of the visually impaired. *J Rehabil Res Dev* 36:273, 1999.

Elner SG: Gradual painless visual loss: Retinal causes. *Clin Geriatr Med* 15:25, 1999.

Hersen M et al: Assertiveness, depression, and social support in older visually impaired adults. *J Vis Imp Blind* 89:524, 1995.

Kendrick R: Gradual painless visual loss: Glaucoma. *Clin Geriatr Med* 15:95, 1999.

Magione CM et al: Development of the "activities of daily vision scale," a measure of visual functional status. *Med Care* 30:1111, 1992.

Nelson KA, Dimitrova E: Statistical brief #36: Severe visual impairment in the United States and in each state, 1990. *J Vis Imp Blind* 87:80, 1993.

Owsley C et al: Visual processing impairment and risk of motor vehicle crash among older adults. *JAMA* 279:1083, 1998.

Schuchard RA, Fletcher DC: Preferred retinal locus: A review with applications in low-vision rehabilitation. *Ophthalmol Clin North Am* 7:243, 1994.

Silverstone B et al (eds): *The Lighthouse Handbook on Vision Impairment and Vision Rehabilitation.* New York, Oxford University Press, 2000.

Valluri S: Gradual painless vision loss: Anterior segment causes. *Clin Geriatr Med* 15:87, 1999.

Watson GR et al: A national survey of veterans' use of low-vision devices. *Optom Vis Sci* 74:249, 1997.

Age-Related Changes in the Auditory System

JOHN H. MILLS

TERMINOLOGY

Age-related hearing loss, or the hearing loss associated with increased chronologic age, is also called *presbyacusis* or *presbycusis*. Sometimes these terms are used loosely to describe a seemingly endless list of genetic, environmental, and disease states that can cause or be associated with a hearing loss in an older person. Other times, the term *presbycusis* is used to refer to a hearing loss caused purely by the natural process of aging. More often, hearing loss is considered to be presbycusis if the person is beyond the fifth decade, without consideration of disease, genetic, or other factors.

More precision and less uncertainty can be achieved by use of the terms *presbycusis, socioacusis,* and *nosoacusis*. Socioacusis is defined as the hearing loss produced primarily by exposure to nonoccupational noise in combination with lifestyle factors such as diet, exercise, smoking, use of vitamins and antioxidants, and alcohol consumption. Nosoacusis is the hearing loss attributable to diseases with otologic consequences. Presbycusis has a generic definition: age-related hearing loss or age-related threshold shift that is the effect of increased chronological age combined with socioacusis and nosoacusis. A more precise and restrictive definition of presbyacusis is the hearing loss associated with increased chronologic age and is attributable to "aging" per se. This "purely aging" hearing loss probably has a largely genetic basis and may very well be highly correlated with age-related deterioration or declines in other senses, especially smell, taste, touch, and vision. Thus, the hearing loss assessed in a person into the fourth or fifth decade and beyond may be the combined result of aging, socioacusis, nosoacusis, and, possibly, for many persons, exposure to occupational noise as well. For medical and legal reasons it may be important to differentiate presbycusis from socioacusis, nosoacusis, and occupational hearing loss.

EPIDEMIOLOGIC AND DEMOGRAPHIC FACTORS

Currently, of the 28 million hearing-impaired individuals in the United States, approximately 75 percent are older than age 55 years. Moreover, the population of persons older than age 55 years is increasing much more rapidly than is the younger population. The three most prevalent handicapping conditions associated with aging are arthritis, hypertension, and hearing loss. Indeed, age-related hearing loss is the most prevalent of chronically handicapping conditions among males age 65 years and older, and ranks third behind arthritis and hypertension (National Center for Health Statistics) when data for males and females are combined. This combination of facts suggests that the demands placed upon hearing health care professionals in the coming years will be substantially increased.

Age-related hearing loss in the United States has been well characterized by surveys such as the Framingham Heart Study, Baltimore Longitudinal Study of Aging, and Epidemiology of Hearing Loss Study of the adult residents of Beaver Dam, Wisconsin. Data from many parts of the world have been collated to form an international standard (see International Organization for Standards). Figure 96-1 combines data from the Framingham Study (ages 60 years and older) in the United States with data (ages 30 to 60 years) of an international standard (International Organization for Standards). Figure 96-1 shows a systematic increase in hearing levels (threshold shifts) with increases in chronologic age. Small changes in hearing thresholds are measured in both males and females even at age 30 years. At high frequencies, thresholds are higher (poorer) for males than for females. The prevalence of hearing loss ranges from about 42 to 47 percent, depending upon the study with hearing loss defined as average thresholds exceeding 25 dB in the poorer ear; however, prevalence varies greatly with age and gender, ranging from 10 percent

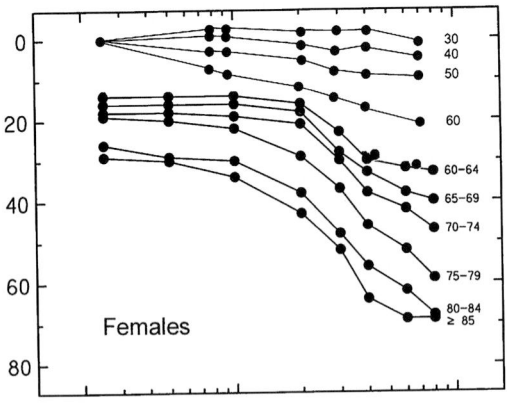

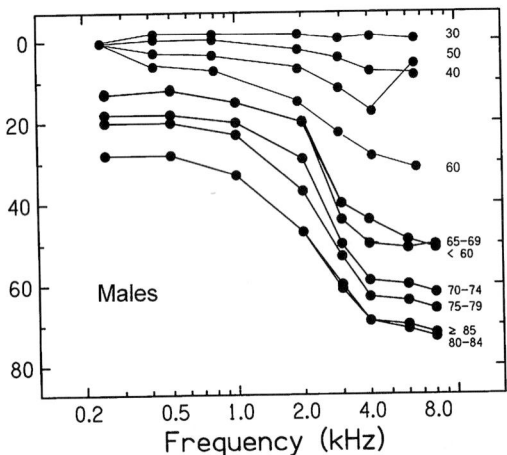

Figure 96-1 Mean pure-tone thresholds (hearing levels in dB) for the better ear of males (*lower panel*) and females (*upper panel*) in the Framingham Heart Study (age groupings 60 to 64 years and older) and from Data Base A of International Organization for Standards 1990 (age groupings 30, 40, 50, and 60 years). Upper panel modified from Moscicki EK et al: Hearing loss in the elderly: An epidemiologic study of the Framingham Heart Study Cohort. *Ear Hear* 6:184, 1985.

for females 48 to 52 years of age to 97 percent for males older than 80 years of age. Variance between studies with respect to prevalence is oftentimes attributable to sampling, especially the elimination of subjects who have a history of significant noise exposure or otological disease. A second factor is the operational definition of hearing loss. For example, the American Medical Association/American Academy of Otolaryngology–Head and Neck Surgery includes only the test frequencies from 0.5 to 3 kHz in the definition of hearing handicap, and the average hearing level at 0.5, 1, 2, and 3 kHz must exceed 25 dB for the hearing loss to be considered a handicap. Others include audiometric results at test frequencies of 4 kHz, and sometimes higher, in their assessments of the prevalence of hearing handicap or impairment.

A noteworthy and remarkably consistent age-related hearing loss occurs at frequencies of 8 kHz and higher, and begins well before the age of 30 years. Figure 96-2 shows hearing levels in the conventional (0.25 to 8 kHz) and extended high frequencies (greater than 8 kHz) for younger and older adults, grouped according to average thresholds from 1 to 4 kHz (Matthews et al.). Thresholds

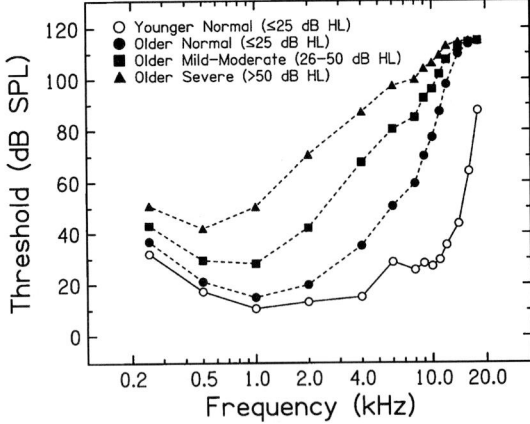

Figure 96-2 Mean pure-tone thresholds at frequencies from 0.25 to 18 kHz for three groups of subjects 60 to 79 years of age, grouped by pure-tone average at 1, 2, and 4 kHz (normal, mild-moderate, and severe), and one group of younger subjects with normal hearing. Adapted from Matthews LJ et al: Extended high-frequency thresholds in older adults. *J Speech Lang Hear Res* 40:208, 1997.

are elevated substantially at 8 kHz and higher, even for individuals with essentially normal hearing below 4 kHz. Clearly, there is a dramatic age-related decline in hearing levels at very high frequencies. Several sets of data suggest that this high-frequency loss begins in the 16 to 20 kHz region in the second decade of life and spreads slowly but systematically throughout life to lower frequencies.

Interpretation of the data in Figures 96-1 and 96-2 is not straightforward. One point of view is that these age-related changes in hearing thresholds are genetically determined, age-dependent events. That is, these age-related events are totally endogenous in origin. They are independent of exogenous events such as diet, exposure to environmental noise (socioacusis), and disease (nosoacusis). As part of the Framingham Heart Study, Gates and colleagues estimated the role of genetics in age-related hearing loss. Their heritability estimates suggest as much as 55 percent of the variance associated with age-related hearing loss is attributable to the effect of genes. These heritability estimates of age-related hearing loss are similar in magnitude to those reported for hypertension and hyperlipidemia, are much stronger in women than in men, and can be used to support the point of view that age-related changes in the ear and hearing reflect the combined effect of genetics, socioacusis, and nosoacusis. In some views of presbycusis, socioacusis is given a major role, almost surely because of the famous Mabaan study.

A hearing survey of Mabaans, a tribe located in a remote and undeveloped part of Africa, showed exceptionally good auditory sensitivity for males and females in their sixth to ninth decades. In addition to the lack of exposure to occupational noise, no exposure to firearms, and exposure only to very low levels of environmental noise, the Mabaans were reported to lead a low-stress lifestyle, have a low fat diet, and a very low prevalence of cardiovascular disease. This study was quoted widely in lay and professional publications, and became the scientific basis for the thesis that persons in Western industrialized societies were at risk of hearing losses because of socioacusis. Later analysis of the Mabaan data indicated very few differences between hearing levels of Mabaans and hearing levels of well-screened individuals from industrialized societies. One possible exception was that the hearing levels of Mabaan males older than age 60 years were slightly better in the high frequencies than their Western male counterparts. Additional criticism of the original Mabaan data involved the accuracy of the age of the Mabaan subjects. Apparently, the exact ages of the Mabaan subjects could not be confirmed. Lastly, important epidemiologic details of the Mabaan sample could not be determined, thus the validity of the sampling was questionable, that is, a highly biased sample. It is possible, for example, that only the healthiest subjects were available and that these subjects also had the best hearing. Thus, the Mabaan data are equivocal in their support of the thesis of profound effects of socioacusis and nosoacusis on age-related hearing levels.

Experiments with aging laboratory animals strongly support the idea of an age-related hearing loss that is independent of socioacusis, nosoacusis, and exposure to occupational noise. Variance in epidemiologic data in Figures 96-1 and 96-2 is substantial and is usually attributed to sampling error and the inclusion or exclusion of persons with a significant history of noise exposure or otologic disease. An alternative indicator of variance in age-related hearing loss comes from experiments with laboratory animals. Figure 96-3 shows age-related threshold shifts in gerbils who were born and reared in an environment that was under control of the experimenter. That is, the vivarium was acoustically controlled so that sound levels did not exceed 40 dB. Diet, room temperature, humidity, and other environmental variables were identical for each animal. In other words, the hearing losses shown on Figure 96-3 can be attributed to the aging processes rather than to the aging processes interacting with a number of known and unknown exogenous factors. The variability shown on Figure 96-3 is dramatic. Hearing losses range from 5 dB to greater than 60 dB in a group of animals in which all known major variables were under experimenter control. Such variability suggests that there is a strong genetic component to age-related hearing loss in quiet-reared gerbils, and that age-related hearing loss can occur and be

of a substantial magnitude independently of socioacusis, nosoacusis, or exposure to occupational noise.

In light of the complexities of age-related hearing loss, there are several ongoing efforts to develop valid animal models. An appropriate animal model may allow the identification and control of many pertinent variables as well as systematic studies of the biology of age-related hearing loss. It is also important to examine and conduct laboratory studies with humans and to make comparisons with laboratory animal data when possible.

BIOLOGICAL BASES OF AGE-RELATED HEARING LOSS

Basics of the Anatomy and Physiology of Hearing

Although the entire auditory system, from the external ear to the auditory cortex, undergoes age-related changes, the most significant changes occur within the inner ear or cochlea. Before detailing the most significant age-related effects, it may be worthwhile to very briefly discuss the basics of the anatomy and physiology of the ear.

The external ear consists of the pinna and external auditory canal. The canal acts as a resonator and alters sound transmission. The acoustic properties of the head and the external ear are important, particularly by providing cues for localizing sources of sound. In regard to aging, the external ear may present with cerumen impaction. Also, because of age-related cartilaginous changes the external auditory canal may collapse with the placement of earphones for audiologic testing. This problem is solved with the use of insert earphones. Although not involved in auditory function or age-related hearing loss, the pinna is a common site for both squamous and basal cell carcinomas. Indeed, nearly 90 percent of squamous cell carcinomas occur on the face or ears of older adults.

The middle ear acts as a transformer between air and the fluid-filled inner ear (cochlea) and provides a pressure gain of 25 to 30 dB. The combined effect of the acoustic properties of the head, external ear, and middle ear, as well as the input impedance of the cochlea, determines the frequency range of human hearing, 20 Hz to 20 kHz. Although the structures of the middle ear undergo age-related changes, there appears to be very little effect, if any, on the physiology of the middle ear or on audiometric tests. Data suggest strongly that the acoustic properties of the middle ear are largely unaffected by the aging process.

Whereas the middle ear is a passive device with a linear response for signals up to 130 dB sound pressure level (SPL) and is essentially unaffected by the aging process, the cochlea (inner ear) is an active device with nonlinear characteristics and is dramatically affected by the aging process. Accordingly, the cochlea is discussed in some detail.

The cochlea is a coiled bony tube approximately 35 mm in length that is divided into three compartments: scala tympani, scala vestibuli, and scala media (see Fig. 96-4). Scalae tympani and vestibuli contain perilymph, which have a high sodium concentration and are connected through the helicotrema at the apex of the cochlea. Scala

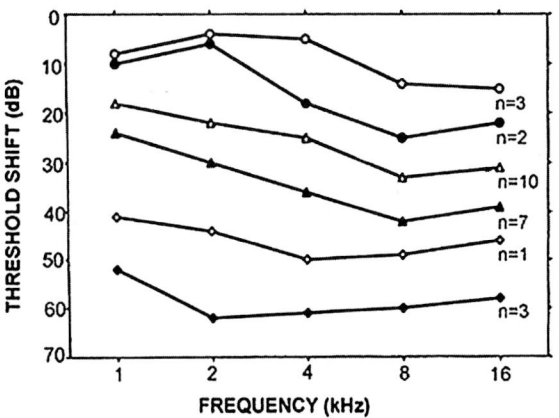

Figure 96-3 Variability of age-related hearing loss in old animals (Mongolian gerbil) who were born and reared in a "quiet" facility. Diet, room temperature, and humidity were controlled. Adapted from Mills JH et al: Age-related changes in auditory potentials of Mongolian gerbil. *Hear Res* 46:301, 1990.

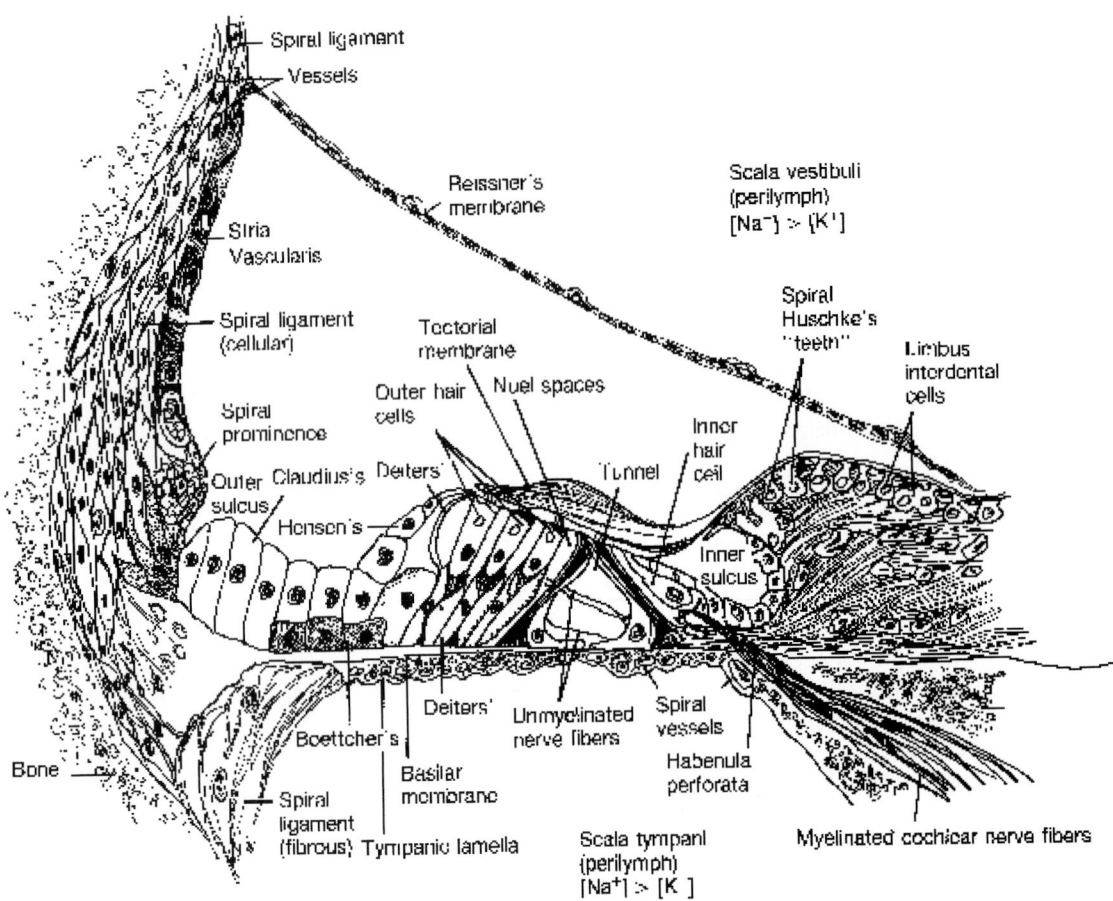

Figure 96–4 Midmodiolar sections of the cochlea.

media contains endolymph with a high concentration of potassium. A direct current (DC) resting potential of 80–90 mV is measurable in scala media.

This large DC resting potential arises from Na,/K-ATPase pumps in the stria vascularis located on the lateral wall of the cochlea. This region of the cochlea (including the blood supply) and the DC resting potential are seriously affected by the aging process and are discussed in more detail later.

The auditory transducer is the organ of Corti, which contains sensory cells (three rows of outer hair cells and one row of inner hair cells). Deflection of stereocilia (hairs) of the sensory cells by a mechanical traveling wave initiates the transduction process. A traveling wave along the basilar membrane, moving from the base toward the apex of the cochlea, arises in response to the piston-like movements of the stapes in the middle ear. The traveling wave has a sharply tuned peak that is located basally for high-frequency sounds and progresses apically as the frequency is decreased. Deflection of stereocilia by the traveling wave opens and closes ion channels, resulting in a current flow (K+) into the sensory cell. The potassium flux arises from the +80- to +90-mV endocochlear potential of scala media added to the negative intracellular potential of outer and inner hair cells. The resulting depolarization causes an enzyme cascade, releasing chemical transmitters and subsequently activating afferent nerve fibers. Although the notion of the cochlea and the organ of Corti as an active

rather than passive organ is no longer debated, specific details of the "cochlear amplifier" and the biological basis of its operation are under active investigation.

One approach attributes the cochlear amplifier to the ability of hair cells to contract and lengthen in response to electrical signals, a property called *somatic motility*. A protein named prestin has been identified in outer hair cells and is considered to be the motor protein of outer hair cells and the driving force of electromotility of hair cells. A second approach focuses on rapidly acting potassium and calcium ion channels, which are presumed to be the basis of the cochlear amplifier and its regulation. A third approach suggests a collection of motor proteins within a hair cell can generate oscillations that depend upon the elastic properties of the cell. All of the above approaches are nonlinear models involving rapidly acting calcium channels. The specification of the biological basis of the cochlear amplifier is important inasmuch as many forms of hearing loss involve the loss or malfunction of the cochlear amplifier, and it is this amplifier with its nonlinear properties that allow the inner ear to respond to a wide range of intensities with excellent frequency specificity.

The auditory nerve contains approximately 30,000 neurons connecting the sensory cells to the auditory brainstem (cochlear nucleus). Dendrites connected to sensory cells, spiral ganglion cells or cell bodies of the auditory nerve are located in the modiolus or central core of the cochlea, and the axons course centrally to the brainstem. The auditory

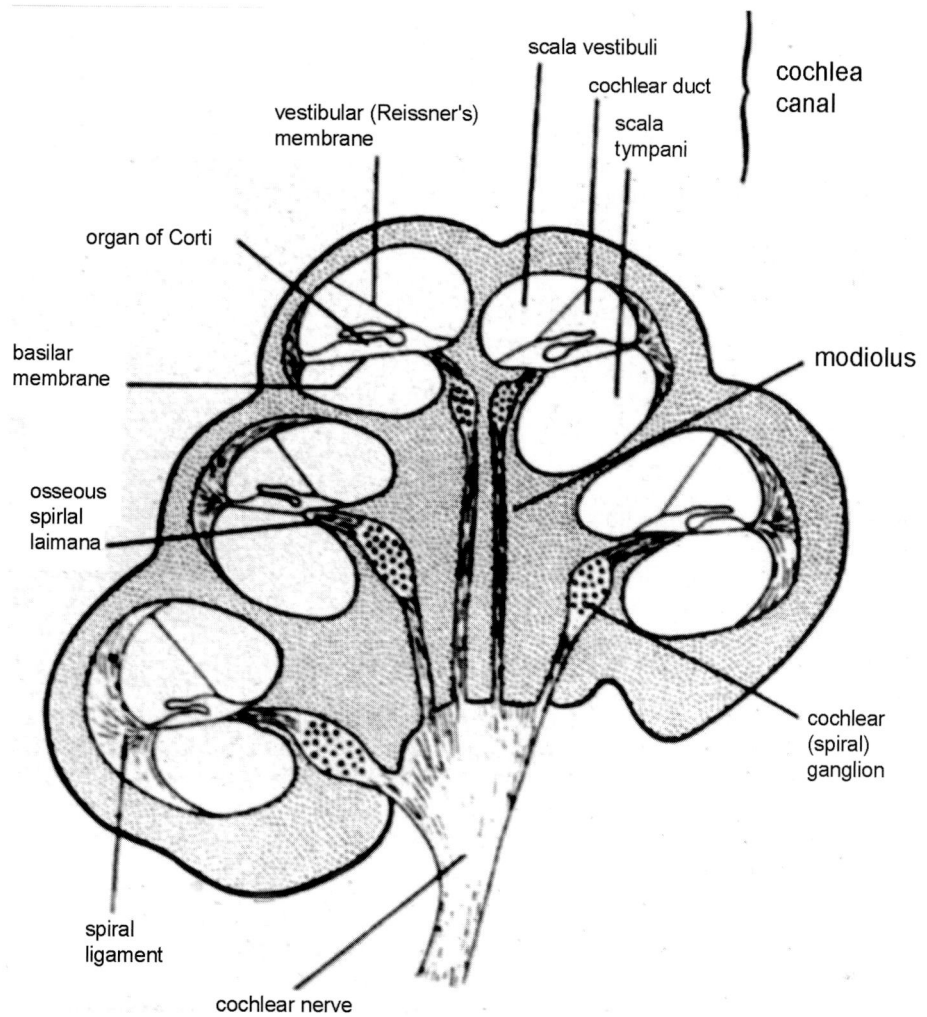

Figure 96-4 (*Continued.*)

nerve is characterized by two types of fibers. Type I are large, myelinated bipolar neurons that synapse with inner hair cells. Ninety to 95 percent of type I fibers (radial nerve fibers) innervate inner hair cells. The remaining 5 to 10 percent are type II fibers (outer spiral fibers), which are small, unmyelinated neurons that synapse with outer hair cells.

Pathologic Anatomy and Physiology of Age-Related Hearing Loss

Perhaps the most quoted and most extensive data on age-related hearing loss comes from the histopathologic studies of human temporal bones reported by the late Harold F. Schuknecht and his colleagues at the Harvard Medical School. From a large number of studies starting in 1953, Schuknecht and colleagues identified four major types or categories of presbycusis: sensory presbycusis; neural presbycusis; strial/metabolic presbycusis; and mechanical or cochlear conductive presbycusis.

Sensory presbycusis is characterized by atrophy and degeneration of the organ of Corti, that is, outer and inner hair cells and supporting cells. Degeneration and cell loss begins at the base of the cochlea, proceeds apically, and is most pronounced for outer hair cells; *neural presbycusis* is typified by a significant loss of neurons with or without an accompanying loss of sensory cells; *strial/metabolic presbycusis* is characterized by degeneration of the lateral wall of the cochlea, especially the stria vascularis; in *mechanical or cochlear conductive presbycusis,* the physical properties of the inner ear change, particularly the mechanical properties of the basilar membrane, and thereby produce an inner ear conductive loss. Each of these categories was considered to have a particular audiometric configuration (i.e., sloping audiogram, flat audiogram) and, therefore, to be of diagnostic significance. In subsequent studies over the years, considerable difficulty was encountered in correlating the audiometric configuration with histopathologic observations and in differentiating one type of presbycusis from another on the basis of the audiometric configuration. The problem is that the audiometric configurations of older persons do not form clearly defined categories, and histopathologic changes at the level of light and electron microscopy are almost always observed at multiple sites in a specific aging ear.

In 1993, Schuknecht and Gacek revised the traditional categories of presbycusis described above. The revision is based upon hundreds of observations of human temporal bones and is summarized by the quote "(1) sensory cell losses are the least-important type of loss; (2) neuronal losses are constant and predictable expression of aging; (3) atrophy of the stria vascularis is the predominant lesion of the aging ear; (4) no anatomical correlate for a gradual descending hearing loss . . . reflects a cochlear conductive loss; (5) 25 percent cannot be classified using light microscopy." This conclusion by Schuknecht and Gacek is important for at least two reasons: first, the significance of sensory cell losses is deemphasized in presbyacusis; second, the dominance of strial degeneration is emphasized. These two points bring a consensus to human temporal bone results and those obtained from experiments with animals.

Neural Presbycusis

Most laboratory studies with animals and clinical histopathologic studies with humans show age-related declines of spiral ganglion cells that may occur independently of any loss of inner or outer hair cells. In humans, degeneration of the auditory nerve apparently begins at a young age (younger than age 20 years) and continues throughout the lifetime of the individual. Loss and shrinkage of spiral ganglion cells is diffuse, involving all regions of the cochlea. The impact of primary degeneration of the auditory nerve on the audiogram and on tests of word recognition is highly variable, ranging from no measurable effects to significant hearing loss and poor word recognition scores. In general, spiral ganglion cell loss/shrinkage must exceed at least 20 to 30 percent (or possibly more) to have audiometrically measurable effects.

In experimental animals (gerbils) raised in a quiet environment (as described for Fig. 96-3) there is a 15 to 30 percent loss/shrinkage of spiral ganglion cells, which is distributed throughout the cochlea. The distribution of the loss of spiral ganglion cells is unrelated to the small loss of outer hair cells observed in the apex of aging animals. There is no loss of inner hair cells. Inasmuch as 95 percent of the afferent nerve fibers synapse with inner hair cells, age-related degeneration of spiral ganglion cells, in both animals and humans, reflects primary degeneration of the auditory nerve.

For animals as for humans, the relation or correlation between degeneration of the auditory nerve and audiometric effects is not straightforward. It is clear, however, that more than 50 percent loss/shrinkage of the spiral ganglion cells is required before there are measurable audiometric effects.

Strial/Metabolic Presbycusis

Degeneration of the stria vascularis is probably the most prominent/dominant form of age-related hearing loss. Laboratory studies with animals and histopathologic studies of human temporal bones, largely by Schuknecht and colleagues, are consistent in showing age-related degeneration of the stria vascularis. The degeneration usually originates in both the base and apex of the cochlea, extending to midcochlear regions as age increases. In some cases, the degeneration is patchy. In addition to age-related, systematic

degeneration of marginal and intermediate cells of the stria vascularis, there is a loss of Na,K–adenosine triphosphatase (ATPase). Sometimes the loss of this important enzyme, which is detectable using immunohistochemical techniques, occurs when the stria vascularis appears normal under light microscopic examination. Thus, a normal appearing stria vascularis in an older ear is no assurance that the stria vascularis is normal. Accordingly, the prevalence of "metabolic presbyacusis" may prove to be substantially higher in humans when the appropriate immunohistochemical techniques are applied to the study of temporal bones of older humans.

Age-related degeneration of the stria vascularis has a profound influence on the basic physiology of the cochlea, especially on the endocochlear potential (EP). As mentioned earlier, the EP is an 80- to 90-mV DC resting potential measured in scala media. Its generation and maintenance depend upon a healthy stria vascularis. Figure 96-5 shows age-related reductions in EP at different regions in the cochlea (apex, low-frequency sounds to basal, high-frequency).

The parameter is an estimate of functioning stria remaining as indicated by a loss of immunostaining for the enzyme Na,K–ATPase and from measurements of strial area and strial capillary area. Figure 96-5 shows a reduction in EP throughout the cochlea and that the reduction is related to the magnitude of strial degeneration. As much as 20 to 30 percent of the stria may degenerate with only a 20-mV reduction in the EP. As strial degeneration exceeds 50 percent, EP values drop substantially.

The stria vascularis and underlying spiral ligament have a prominent role in generating electrochemical gradients and regulating fluid and ion homeostasis in the cochlea. As mentioned above, these tissues undergo age-related changes in a number of species including humans. In accordance with its name, the stria is heavily vascularized and has an extremely high metabolic rate. Conceivably, alterations in strial microvasculature could compromise cochlear blood flow and lead ultimately to strial degeneration. Physiologic changes in cochlear blood flow in aging ears are inconsistent. Histopathologic studies on aging gerbils, on the other hand, have provided strong evidence for vascular involvement in age-related hearing loss. Morphometric analyses of lateral wall preparations stained to contrast blood vessels (Fig. 96-6) have revealed losses of strial capillary area in aged animals. The vascular pathology first presented as small focal lesions mainly in the apical and lower basal turns and progressed with age to encompass large regions at both ends of the cochlea. Remaining strial areas were highly correlated with normal microvasculature and with the endocochlear potential. Not surprisingly, areas of complete capillary loss invariably correlated with regions of strial atrophy. Subsequent ultrastructural analysis has revealed a significant thickening of the basement membrane which is accompanied by an increase in the deposition of laminin and an abnormal accumulation of immunoglobulin as shown histochemically. Thus, considerable support exists for the major involvement of strial microvasculature in age-related degeneration of stria vascularis; however, the question of what constitutes the initial injury remains unanswered. Although it is tempting to speculate that atrophy of the stria vascularis occurs

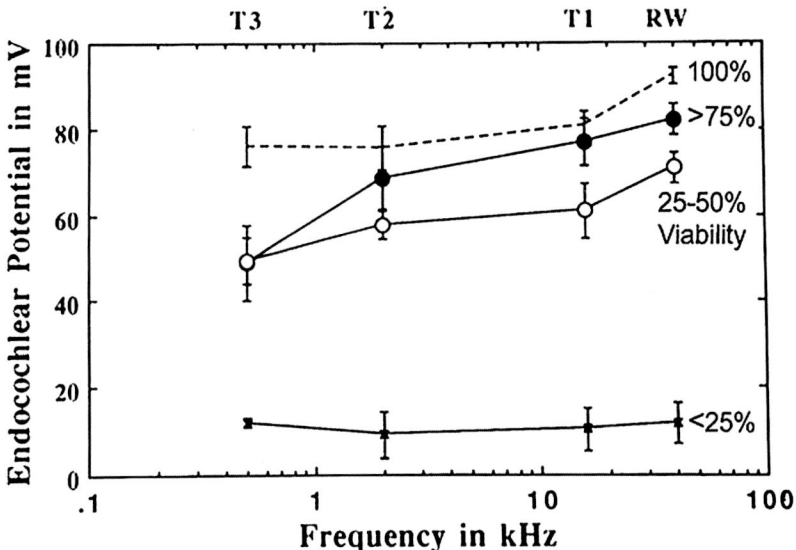

Figure 96-5   Mean values of endocochlear potentials recorded near the round window and at three locations in the cochlea from young control animals and from three groups of old gerbils. The parameter is the percentage of remaining stria vascularis immunostained for Na, K–ATPase. Note that the endocochlear potential does not decrease to less than 20 mV until less than 25 percent of the stria vascularis remains. Adapted from Schulte BA, Schmiedt RA: Lateral wall Na, K–ATPase and endocochlear potential decline with age in quiet-reared gerbils. *Hear Res* 61:35, 1992.

secondarily to vascular insufficiency resulting from capillary necrosis, the reverse could very well be true.

In addition to the age-related decrease in the EP of scala media, there are other changes in the physiologic properties of the aging cochlea and auditory nerve. One is losses of auditory nerve function as indicated by increased thresholds of the compound action potential (CAP) of the auditory nerve. Slopes of input–output functions of the CAP in aging animals are decreased, even when the loss of auditory thresholds is only 5 to 10 dB. In other words, as the signal intensity is increased the amplitude of the CAP increases by a fraction of that observed in young animals with normal hearing or young animals with noise-induced or drug-induced hearing losses. These shallow input–output functions of the CAP are also reflected in shallow input–output functions of physiologic potentials arising from the auditory brainstem. Thus, what appears to be abnormal function of the auditory brainstem in older animals, reflects

only the abnormal output of the auditory nerve. The reduced amplitudes of action potentials observed in aging ears are probably reflective of asynchronous or poorly synchronized neural activity in the auditory nerve. The pathologic basis of asynchronized activity in the auditory nerve is unknown, but probably involves the nature of the synapse between individual auditory nerve fibers and the attachment to the inner hair cell, primary degeneration of spiral ganglion cells, and reductions in the endolymphatic potential. It remains difficult to separate malfunctions of the auditory nerve caused by a reduced EP from malfunctions caused by degeneration of spiral ganglion cells.

There is a perhaps unique feature of the aging cochlea with its characteristic strial degeneration; that is, in an aging animal with a 40- to 50-dB hearing loss and an EP of 20 mV rather than 90 mV, hearing thresholds can be improved 20 to 25 dB by introducing a DC voltage into scala media and raising the low endolymphatic potential (20 mV) to a value approaching 60 to 70 mV. This experimenter-introduced DC voltage into scala media not only returns the EP to nearly normal values, it reduces the magnitude of the hearing loss as indicated by the threshold of the CAP and significantly increases the amplitude of the CAP produced by moderate- and high-level signals. Degeneration of the stria vascularis, the "battery" of the cochlea, with the resultant decline in the endocochlear potential has given rise to the "dead battery theory of presbyacusis."

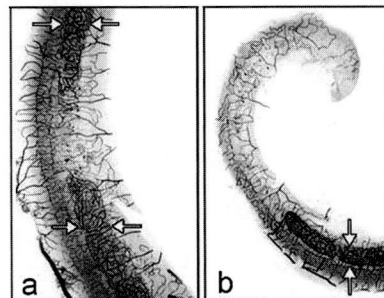

Figure 96-6   Surface preparation of lateral wall dissections from an old gerbil stained to contrast blood vessels. *(A)* The strial capillary bed (between the *arrows*) overlies vessels of the spiral ligament. The cochlea in *(A)* shows a focal area of strial capillary atrophy whereas *(B)* shows a complete loss of strial capillaries throughout the apical turn. *(A)*   40×; *(B)*   20×. Photo courtesy of Michael Ann Gratton and Bradley A. Schulte.

Sensory Presbycusis

This category is controversial. Some studies with animals and with humans, particularly Schuknecht and colleagues, suggest that sensory cell loss is not a significant factor in age-related hearing loss. Other data suggest otherwise. It is my belief that significant age-related loss of sensory cells in some animals, especially C57 mice and other highly inbred strains, is not relevant to age-related hearing loss in many other mammals, including humans. In many of the human studies showing age-related histopathologic effects on sensory cells, it is my belief that much of the observed pathology reflects exposure to noise and other ototoxic agents rather than aging per se.

The issue of sensory cell loss in age-related hearing loss has implications for auditory physiology, especially the presence of nonlinear phenomena such as two-tone rate suppression and otoacoustic emissions. The nonlinear phenomenon of two-tone rate suppression, that is, activity of the auditory nerve elicited by one tone is suppressed or eliminated by the addition of a second tone of different frequency, is characteristic of a perfectly intact organ of Corti, including outer and inner hair cells. In ears of quiet-reared aging animals, the mechanism of two-tone rate suppression appears to remain intact. In contrast, in noise-induced or drug-induced injury of the cochlea, a reduction or complete loss of two-tone rate suppression may be the first indicator of injury of the cochlea, usually outer hair cells. These data are an excellent indicator that the pathologic basis of age-related hearing loss is fundamentally different from the pathologic basis of most forms of noise-induced or drug-induced hearing loss.

Otoacoustic emissions, both transient-evoked and distortion-product, are nonlinear phenomenon which are assumed to reflect the integrity of sensory cells, especially outer hair cells. Given this assumption, one would expect to find very high correlations between loss of outer hair cells and changes in otoacoustic emissions; however, inconsistent relations among distortion products, threshold measures, and sensory cell pathology have been reported from widely different types of experiments. Indeed, there are reports of normal emissions in the presence of missing outer hair cells as well as reduced emissions in the presence of a complete complement of outer hair cells. In the aging ear of experimental animals with a minimal, if any, loss of outer hair cells, distortion product emissions are reduced somewhat in amplitude, but are clearly present and robust. In aging human ears, transient otoacoustic emissions are present in approximately 80 percent of persons with a pure-tone average hearing level better than 10 dB; present in about 50 percent with pure-tone average of 11 to 26 dB, and absent in approximately 80 percent with a pure-tone average greater than 26 dB. Thus, the presence of a transient otoacoustic emission suggests excellent hearing levels for most persons whereas the absence of transient acoustic emissions is difficult to interpret. It may suggest an age-related loss of sensory cells or a history of noise exposure with a loss of sensory cells.

A recent development is the association of mitochondrial deoxyribonucleic acid (mtDNA) deletions with sensorineural hearing loss and age-related hearing loss. DNA specimens extracted from peripheral blood leukocytes showed a higher rate of mtDNA deletions in patients with sensorineural hearing loss than in controls. In a study using aging rats, mtDNA deletions were related to hearing loss, and mtDNA was related to reactive oxygen metabolites (ROM). That is, ROM are highly toxic molecules that can damage mitochondrial DNA resulting in the production of specific mtDNA deletions. Thus, compounds that block or scavenge ROM should attenuate age-related hearing loss. Rats were assigned to treatment groups including controls, caloric restriction, and treatment with several antioxidants including vitamins E and C, and allowed to age in a controlled environment. The caloric-restricted groups maintained the best hearing, the lowest quantity of mtDNA deletions in brain and ear tissues, and the least amount of outer hair cell loss. The antioxidant-treated subjects had better hearing than the controls and a slight trend for fewer mtDNA deletions. The controls had the poorest hearing, the most mtDNA deletions, and the most outer hair cell loss. These data suggest that nutritional and pharmacologic strategies may prove to be an effective treatment that would limit age-related increases in ROM production and reduce mtDNA deletions, thus reducing age-related hearing loss. ROM (or ROS, reactive oxygen species) and oxidative stress are also implicated in noise-induced hearing loss and ototoxic hearing loss, and to cumulative injury that presents as age-related hearing loss. It is speculated that there is a genetic impairment of antioxidant protections which leads to the production of both age-related and noise-induced hearing loss by placing the cochlea into a state of vulnerability. An age-related hearing loss gene has been identified in C57 mouse, the murine Ahl mutation, and mapped to the proximal end of chromosome 10. The discovery of the molecular/genetic basis of presbyacusis, noise-induced hearing loss, and sensory neural hearing loss in general is currently undergoing a monumental effort.

Age-Related Changes in the Auditory Central Nervous System

There is a large literature detailing age-related changes in the auditory central nervous system (CNS). In general, at all levels of the CNS—from the cochlear nucleus to the auditory cortex—histopathologic studies show age-related neuronal degeneration characterized by loss of neurons, shrinkage of cell bodies, and loss of dendrites. Age-related alterations of the CNS may be most prominent in the auditory cortex, particularly in the superior temporal gyrus. In general, histopathologic changes of the aging CNS are subject to wide variations across individuals and across different levels of the CNS. The functional significance of age-related pathology of the auditory CNS is not well established and is discussed further in relation to auditory evoked responses.

Auditory-evoked potentials are a series of positive and negative voltages (waveforms) that can be recorded from the scalp of awake humans in response to a series of auditory signals including clicks, tones, and speech. The potentials reflect the function of neural generators at several sites within the CNS. With the development and refinement of straightforward, noninvasive techniques to measure evoked potentials arising from the auditory nerve, brainstem, and auditory cortex, there has been significant progress in evaluating the aging auditory nervous system of human subjects.

The auditory brainstem response (ABR) is composed of approximately seven "wavelets" occurring in the first

10 msec after the onset of a short, auditory signal. Wave V is most easily recorded and has the most clinical utility. It arises near the level of the lateral lemniscus/inferior colliculus. In regard to the ABR, most studies show large, age-related declines in the amplitude of wave V. These age-related declines in ABR amplitude, however, are also present in the amplitude of potentials arising from the auditory nerve. Thus, age-related declines in the ABR have been interpreted to reflect peripheral (cochlear) hearing loss rather than age-related changes in the brainstem near the inferior colliculus. Even in older persons with excellent hearing levels, ABR waveforms are of "poor quality" and reduced amplitude probably reflecting pathology of the cochlea and auditory nerve as well as a reduction in synchronized neural activity. For young subjects with normal and abnormal hearing, auditory thresholds measured behaviorally are approximately 10 dB better than auditory thresholds estimated from the ABR. For aging subjects, this behavioral/ABR disparity is 20 dB, reflecting the poor quality/low amplitude of the ABR.

Most other evoked potentials are generated in or near the auditory cortex. Middle-latency response (MLR) is a series of wavelets that occurs approximately 15 to 50 msec after the onset of a short, auditory signal. The MLR is probably generated at multiple sites including the auditory cortex (posterior temporal lobes) and thalamocortical pathways. Whereas the ABR and CAP are reduced dramatically in older persons, the amplitude of the MLR is increased. This result has been confirmed in several studies. Increased amplitudes of evoked potentials have also been observed in the N100-P200 potential, which is generated in the primary auditory cortex 90 to 250 msec after the auditory signal. As with the MLR, the amplitude of the N100-P200 appears to be larger in older subjects than in younger subjects. The P300 potential, a long-latency potential arising from the auditory cortex that is elicited by "surprising" or novel auditory stimuli, shows age-related declines that are small but suggestive of reduced selective attention.

Two other potentials, the amplitude-modulated following response (AMFR) and the frequency-modulated following response (FMFR), are both generated in the auditory cortex in response to long duration AM or FM signals. They are considered to be correlated with the auditory behavioral capabilities of amplitude and frequency discrimination. The AMFR from older subjects has clearly normal amplitudes, thus suggesting that the AMFR may remain unaffected by aging. In contrast, the FMFR is larger in older subjects than in younger subjects. Although much of this research is in progress, it appears that evoked potentials produced by short-duration signals (onset responses such as ABR and CAP) are dramatically decreased in amplitude in older subjects with and without threshold changes, whereas those evoked potentials (except P300) produced at higher levels in the CNS by long-duration signals are increased in amplitude or have normal amplitude, as in the case of the AMFR. Behavioral correlates of increased amplitudes of cortical evoked potentials have not been reported.

Age-related increases in the amplitude of cortical evoked potentials could reflect several factors including efforts by the CNS to compensate for age-related changes in the auditory periphery, or age-related changes in the excitatory/ inhibitory balance of the auditory CNS. An outstanding candidate to affect excitatory/inhibitory balance in the aging CNS is the neural inhibitory transmitter γ-aminobutyric acid (GABA), which is found throughout the CNS and declines with age. Age-related changes in other inhibitory neurotransmitters such as glycine also may be affecting the physiology of the CNS.

In summary, animal experiments conducted under strict conditions show age-related declines in auditory function that indicate a "pure aging" hearing loss. Most of the pathologic anatomy associated with this "pure aging" hearing loss is in the cochlea, where the dominant pathology is degeneration of the stria vascularis, and primary degeneration of the auditory nerve. In experimental animals, most of the hearing loss can be accounted for by anatomic, physiologic, and biochemical changes in the auditory periphery. Indeed, there is no need to include the auditory CNS in an explanation of age-related hearing loss, even when the criterion measure of age-related hearing loss is derived from potentials arising from the auditory brainstem. Nearly all changes observed in auditory brainstem potentials can be explained by alterations in the auditory periphery.

Explanations of age-related changes in auditory brainstem potentials in terms of alterations in the auditory periphery run counter to the current dogma that there is a significant, perhaps dominant, component of presbyacusis that involves degeneration of the auditory CNS. Indeed, there are significant, age-related changes in the auditory CNS involving subtle to gross changes in anatomy and neurochemistry; however, the behavioral correlates of age-related changes in the auditory CNS remain elusive, poorly documented, controversial, or speculative.

PERCEPTION OF AUDITORY SIGNALS AND SPEECH

In addition to age-related declines in auditory sensitivity as shown in Figures 96-1 and 96-2, there are age-related declines in differential sensitivity for intensity, frequency, and time (_i, _f, and _t, respectively) as well as many other psychoacoustic phenomenon. Until recently, these age-related declines in the basic properties of the ear and hearing were almost always measured in older persons with significant hearing losses. Thus, it was nearly impossible to separate the effects of a hearing loss from the effects of aging. Recently, however, both _i and _f, as well as many other auditory phenomenon usually involving temporal discriminations (temporal order, duration discrimination, gap duration discrimination) have been shown to decline with age and to do so independently of any hearing loss. These results are important because they show age-related declines in auditory behavior measured in the presence of normal auditory thresholds, and may very well represent age-related declines in information processing capability. It remains unclear whether these age-related declines represent age-related effects attributable to the auditory periphery, to the auditory CNS, or to both.

The term phonemic regression was coined to describe a disproportionate difficulty in speech perception relative to

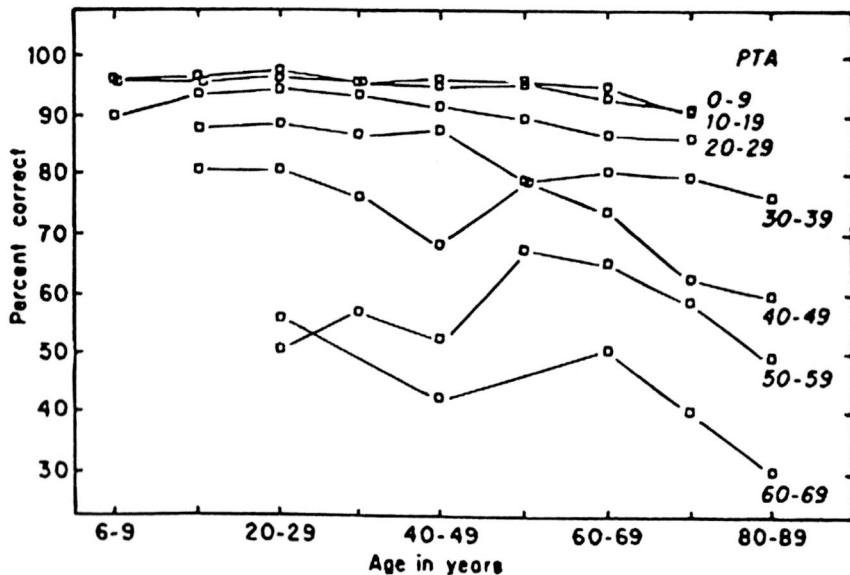

Figure 96-7 Speech discrimination as a function of age with average hearing loss at 0.5, 1, and 2 kHz (pure-tone average) as the parameter. (Adapted from Jerger J: Audiological findings in aging. *Adv Otorhinolaryngol* 20:115, 1973.

the magnitude of hearing loss of older persons. Indeed, in almost all discussions of age-related hearing loss, one reads that older persons have difficulty understanding speech in noisy situations. Later, many studies of speech discrimination and other complex listening tasks showed results with older subjects that were difficult to explain solely on the basis of the audiogram alone. With the ready availability of many published papers showing degenerative changes in the auditory brainstem and cortex of older persons, there evolved a viewpoint that a significant component of age-related hearing loss is attributable to the decline of the auditory CNS. Almost everyone would agree that the auditory CNS is involved in age-related hearing loss; however, the extent of the involvement of the CNS in presbyacusis is currently receiving much debate. Here, we should like to examine the CNS issue and the dogma that old people have difficulty in understanding speech in noisy situations.

Perhaps the largest qualitative/quantitative description of speech discrimination as a function of age and hearing loss is provided by Jerger from the clinical records of 2162 patients. Figure 96-7 shows percent correct on phonetically balanced words as a function of chronologic age. The parameter on the figure is the puretone average of 0.5, 1, and 2 kHz. Figure 96-7 shows that speech discrimination declines systematically as a function of chronologic age; however, the decline with age is dramatically dependent upon hearing loss. That is, for subjects with very little hearing loss (less than 30 dB) the decline with age is measurable but small through age 70 years. On the other hand, for subjects with moderate to severe hearing losses, the decline with age is noteworthy, particularly for persons between the ages of 45 and 85 years with hearing losses of 40 to 49 dB, 50 to 59 dB, and 60 to 69 dB. In different words, when hearing loss as indicated by the puretone average is held constant, speech discrimination scores decreased between the ages of 40 and 80 years for moderate (greater than 40 dB) to severe (60 dB) hearing losses. In contrast, age had very little effect as long as the pure-tone average

is less than about 30 to 39 dB. A remarkable, and perhaps the most noteworthy, feature of Figure 96-7 is that persons older than the age range of 50 to 80 years perform as well as 25-year-olds as long as their average hearing loss at 0.5, 1, and 2 kHz is less than 35 dB or so. This fact runs counter to the stereotype of 70- to 80-year-old persons.

Performance on several tests of speech discrimination by older persons is shown (Fig. 96-8) for phonetically balanced words, three measures taken from the Speech Perception in Noise (SPIN) test, and synthetic sentence identification (SSI). Subjects were placed into three age groups

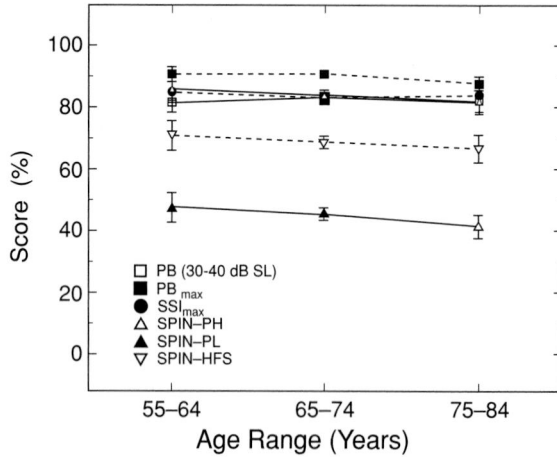

Figure 96-8 Speech discrimination scores on six tests for subjects over the age range of 55 to 84 years, where hearing thresholds are equal for subjects of different age groups. The six measures are word recognition for NU-6 monosyllabic words (PB); maximum word recognition (PBmax); maximum synthetic sentence identification (SSI max); keyword recognition for high-context (SPIN-PH) and low-context (SPIN-PL) sentences of the Speech Perception in Noise (SPIN) test; and "percent hearing for speech" (SPIN-HFS). Adapted from Dubno JR et al: Age-related and gender-related changes in monaural speech recognition. *J Speech Lang Hear Res* 40:444, 1997.

over the range from 55 to 84 years where hearing levels were nearly identical (± 3 dB); however, statistical analysis of the speech discrimination data showed that performance on all tests was not affected by age. That is, when hearing levels were equated, there were no age-related declines in performance on tests of speech discrimination in persons over the age range of 55 to 84 years. In an additional analysis using partial correlations, significant gender effects were observed, that is, significant declines with age for males in word recognition, SSI, and SPIN in high-context sentences. Age-related declines were not observed for females.

There are many additional studies of speech discrimination using background noises, degraded speech signals, reverberation, and other variations, which resulted in a more difficult listening task than the usual speech discrimination test that is done in quiet listening conditions. Many of these studies show age-related effects; however, the interpretation of many of these data showing age-related declines in auditory behavior are not straightforward because the subjects usually have significant hearing loss as indicated by the audiogram. Accordingly, some persons believe there is a large CNS component to presbyacusis, whereas others believe and have shown that speech discrimination by older persons is predictable given the audiometric hearing loss, and the audibility of the speech material. Indeed, as much as 95 percent of the variance in speech discrimination results can be accounted for on the basis of the audiogram. In other cases where predictions of performance by older persons under noisy listening conditions are in error by 20 to 25 percent, it is still not necessary to invoke the involvement of the CNS, although this is usually the interpretation.

Although there are large individual differences in auditory behavior among individuals that are predictable by individual differences in auditory thresholds, there are many age-related declines in auditory behavior that are not strongly associated with auditory thresholds. This is most evident with monaural listening tasks involving temporal properties of the acoustic signals and in binaural listening tasks conducted under acoustically stressful conditions. In many binaural experiments using older subjects, age-related declines are observed that appear to be independent of peripheral hearing loss; however, it is oftentimes difficult to separate truly central processing disorders from disorders initiated by a pathologic input from the aging cochlea.

In a series of studies on age-related hearing loss Jerger and associates have statistically identified factors which explain individual differences in age-related hearing loss. Hearing loss (threshold shifts) including magnitude and audiometric configuration were significant; however, the remaining factors were unrelated to the audiogram with two factors related to speech understanding and the last to perceived auditory handicap.

The assessment of perceived hearing handicap is important and provides a supplement to pure tone thresholds and other audiologic measurements. The Hearing Handicap for the Elderly (HHIE), a self-report questionnaire, has been used to compare older individuals' assessment of their auditory communication abilities and objective measures of hearing and to threshold based estimates of hearing handicap such as that recommended by the American Academy of Otolaryngology–Head and Neck Surgery. Discrepancies between HHIE and objective (audiologic) measures can be substantial, and variance in pure-tone thresholds within hearing handicap categories (none, mild to moderate, severe) is large. Thus, whereas hearing loss is among the most prevalent chronic conditions of aging, the impact of hearing loss on auditory communication skills and daily activities varies greatly among older individuals and is not accurately predicted by the audiogram. Clearly, even though most of the variance in monaural tests of speech discrimination can be accounted for by the audiogram, the story of age-related hearing loss is just not that simple.

ALLEVIATION/TREATMENT

Assuming a complete and competent otologic/audiologic work-up, assuming any problems with the external and middle ear are diagnosed and treated, assuming other medical issues are under control, and assuming a diagnosis of presbyacusis in the general sense, the best treatment currently available is a hearing aid supplemented with aural rehabilitation. There is no known medical or surgical treatment for age-related hearing loss.

The successful use of hearing aids by older persons and hearing impaired individuals in general is mixed. There is a literature of substantial magnitude that reports on the successful or unsuccessful use of hearing aids by the elderly population. Many older persons who would clearly benefit from an aid do not use one. The major reasons for not using an aid or being a dissatisfied user include cost, stigma of a hearing handicap and of being old, difficulty in manipulating controls, and too little benefit, particularly in the presence of background noise.

In a large group of older persons ($N = 516$) who are participants in our longitudinal study of age-related hearing loss, 53 percent ($n = 272$) are candidates for a hearing aid. Candidacy by very conservative audiologic criteria is an speech threshold greater than 30 dB in the better ear, or hearing level greater than 40 dB at 3 and 4 kHz in the better ear. Using these criteria, 48 percent ($n = 131$ of 272) of those who are considered to be excellent candidates have never tried a hearing aid, and only 38 percent ($n = 104$ of 272) of candidates were successful hearing aid users. For one or several reasons, 37 persons were dissatisfied hearing aid users. Of those who did not meet the conservative criteria for a hearing aid ($n = 244$), our clinical judgment suggested that at least 40 to 50 percent of these persons would benefit from an aid. The numbers from our participants, while dismally low, are substantially higher than those reported for participants in the Framingham and Beaver Dam studies wherein fewer than 20 percent were hearing aid users. In some European countries, the number of hearing aid wearers may be less than 10 percent. Clearly, older persons are uninformed about hearing aids, poorly served, or underserved. Hearing loss is a primary determinant of functional health status and psychosocial well being and has an impact similar to that of other chronic conditions. Thus, untreated hearing loss can have a negative effect on the quality of life well beyond that due to poorer auditory communication skills. Indeed, it is our opinion that as a result of excellent advances in hearing aid technology in combination with improved fitting techniques, nearly every older hearing impaired person should be considered a potential candidate for a hearing aid.

MEDICAL–LEGAL ASPECTS

An ongoing medicolegal issue is the assessment of hearing loss in older (and younger) persons and determining the amount of hearing loss that is a result of occupational noise. This undertaking is oftentimes associated with a claim for worker's compensation or with litigation involving product liability. In different words, what are the rules for combining hearing loss caused by exposure to noise (occupational or nonoccupational) from the hearing loss associated with aging or with disease (viral infections, ototoxic drug usage, etc.)? Is it possible to separate the effects of presbycusis from socioacusis, from nosoacusis, and from exposure to occupational noise?

Some laboratory (animal) studies and field studies suggest that hearing losses caused by exposure to noise are additive (in decibels) with the hearing loss associated with aging. For example, a small hearing loss of 25 dB at age 25 years seemingly has little social or medical significance; however, by age 70 years, a hearing loss of 25 dB, presumably caused totally by the aging process (no noise exposure or nosoacusis between age 25 and 70 is assumed), is added to the existing sensorineural hearing loss. The result is a loss of 50 dB, 25 dB caused by aging and 25 dB caused by occupational noise exposure that ended 45 years earlier. Thus, a seemingly minor hearing loss at age 25 years has the potential to become a severe loss when the effects of presbycusis become operative. Although this additivity rule is used in recently developed international and United States noise standards, there are both laboratory and field data that support a different approach that significantly reduces the combined effect of hearing loss caused by noise and hearing loss associated with aging. In this case, a noise-induced hearing loss of 25 dB and an age-related hearing loss of 25 dB combine to form a hearing loss of 28 dB, not 50 dB as in the additivity rule.

For medical–legal reasons or for diagnostic–rehabilitative reasons, the precise quantitative separation of presbycusis from socioacusis, nosoacusis, and exposure to occupational noise requires precise acoustical and medical information, as well as serial audiometry. Oftentimes, this information is not available. In its absence, qualitative judgments can be made and less-than-precise estimates can be formulated. Statistical procedures for deriving quantifiable estimates of hearing loss caused by occupational noise rather than by presbycusis and other factors are given by Dobie (1993) for use in litigation involving hearing loss and workers' compensation cases. The application of these procedures in both legal and other applications remains controversial.

SUMMARY

Age-related hearing loss is the most prevalent of the chronic conditions of aging among males 65 years and older, and

the third most prevalent when male and female data are combined. To varying degrees, age-related hearing loss is the combined effect of aging, exposure to environmental noise (socioacusis), otologic, and other diseases (nosoacusis), and possibly occupational exposure to noise as well. Epidemiologic studies show the prevalence of hearing loss (average pure-tone thresholds greater than 25 dB from 0.5 to 4 kHz) to vary greatly with gender and age, ranging from 10 percent for females ages 48 to 52 years of age to 97 percent for males 80 to 92 years of age. There is a significant genetic component to age-related hearing loss with heritability coefficients indicating that as much as 55 percent of the variance of hearing thresholds in older persons is genetically determined. Heritability coefficients are higher for women than for men, and are comparable to those reported for hypertension and hyperlipidemia.

Although the pathologic anatomy associated with age-related hearing loss occurs from the external ear with collapsing ear canals to the auditory cortex, cochlear degeneration is overwhelmingly dominant and not amenable to medical or surgical treatment. The primary pathology of the aging ear is degeneration of marginal and intermediate cells of the stria vascularis/lateral wall of the cochlea with significant involvement of the strial microvasculature. It is likely that degeneration of the stria occurs secondarily to vascular insufficiency resulting from capillary necrosis. Accompanying stria degeneration is a reduction in the DC endolymphatic potential of scala media from 80 to 90 mV to voltages as low as 10 to 20 mV. In addition to strial degeneration, there is significant loss/shrinkage of spiral ganglion cells which are the cell bodies of the auditory nerve. Loss/shrinkage of the cell bodies of the auditory nerve represents primary degeneration of the auditory nerve inasmuch as such cell loss/shrinkage occurs throughout the cochlea in the absence of any observable pathology of inner hair cells. The role of sensory cell loss in age-related hearing loss is not clear. Some human and animal data suggest that loss of outer and inner hair cells is more likely to reflect exposure to noise or ototoxic agents than age-related hearing loss. Thus, age-related hearing loss can be viewed as a metabolic/vascular neural hearing loss rather than the traditional sensorineural hearing loss. Although most age-related changes in hearing can be accounted for by changes in the cochlea and auditory nerve, there are many age-related changes in the neuroanatomy, neurophysiology, and neurochemistry of the CNS. The effects of these changes on auditory behavior are largely unknown.

In addition to the pure-tone audiogram, perhaps the most important measures of age-related hearing loss are speech discrimination in quiet and in noisy backgrounds, supplemented by a subjective measure of hearing, the HHIE. This questionnaire provides subjective information that is not predicted accurately from audiologic measures. Although current dogma is that older persons have great difficulty understanding speech in noisy environments, some data show otherwise. Indeed, 75 to 90 percent of the variance in monaural speech discrimination may be accounted for by variance in the audibility of speech. In other words, when hearing levels of older subjects are equated with hearing levels of younger subjects, speech discrimination scores are equal for the two groups. For listening situations that are more complex than monaural in a noisy background, age-related differences in speech discrimination may become more apparent.

Older persons with hearing loss can obtain dramatic improvements in their auditory communication skills and in their emotional well-being by the use of a hearing aid; however, more than 70 to 80 percent of older individuals who are highly likely to benefit from a hearing aid do not use one. The potential benefit to listening skills and quality of life, coupled with new hearing aid fitting options and improved technology, strongly suggests that older adults should be encouraged to try a hearing aid.

ACKNOWLEDGMENTS

Preparation of this chapter was supported by NIH (P01 DC00422). Nancy Smythe assisted in preparation of the figures and final document.

REFERENCES

American Academy of Otolaryngology: Guide for the evaluation of hearing handicap. *Otolaryngol Head Neck Surg* 87:539, 1979.

Caspary DM et al: Central auditory aging: GABA changes in the inferior colliculus. *Exp Gerontol* 30:349, 1995.

Committee on Hearing, Bioacoustics, and Biomechanics (CHABA): Speech understanding and aging. *J Acoust Soc Am* 83:859, 1988.

Cruickshanks KJ et al: Prevalence of hearing loss in older adults in Beaver Dam, Wisconsin. The Epidemiology of Hearing Loss Study. *Am J Epidemiol* 148:879, 1998.

Dobie RA: *Medical-Legal Evaluation of Hearing Loss*. New York, Van Nostrand Reinhold, 1993.

Dubno JR et al: Age-related and gender-related changes in monaural speech recognition. *J Speech Lang Hear Res* 40:444, 1997.

Fitzgibbons PJ, Gordon-Salant S: Age effects on duration discrimination with simple and complex stimuli. *J Acoust Soc Am* 98:3140, 1995.

Frisina RD: Anatomical and neurochemical bases of presbycusis, in Hoff PR, Mobbs CV (eds): *Functional Neurobiology of Aging*. San Diego: Academic Press, 2001 p 531.

Gates GA et al: Genetic associations in age-related hearing thresholds. *Arch Otolaryngol Head Neck Surg* 125:654, 1999.

Gordon-Salant S, Fitzgibbons PJ: Temporal factors and speech recognition performance in young and elderly listeners. *J Speech Hear Res* 36:1276, 1993.

Gratton MA, Schulte BA: Alterations in microvasculature are associated with atrophy of the stria vascularis in quiet-aged gerbils. *Hear Res* 82:44, 1995.

He NJ et al: Frequency and intensity discrimination measured in a maximum-likelihood procedure from young and aged normal-hearing subjects. *J Acoust Soc Am* 103:553, 1998.

Humes LE, Christopherson LA: Speech identification difficulties of hearing-impaired elderly persons: The contributions of auditory processing deficits. *J Speech Hear Res* 34:686, 1991.

Humes LE et al: Factors associated with individual differences in clinical measures of speech recognition among the elderly. *J Speech Hear Res* 37:465, 1994.

International Organization for Standards: *Acoustics, 1990: Determination of Occupational Noise Exposure and Estimation of Noise-Induced Hearing Impairment*. Geneva, International Organization for Standards, 1999.

Jerger J: Audiological findings in aging. *Adv Otorhinolaryngol* 20:115, 1973.

Jerger J, Chmiel R: Factor analytic structure of auditory impairment in elderly persons. *J Am Acad Audiol* 8:269, 1997.

Matthews LJ et al: Extended high-frequency thresholds in older adults. *J Speech Lang Hear Res* 40:208, 1997.

Mills JH et al: Age-related changes in auditory potentials of Mongolian gerbil. *Hear Res* 46:301, 1990.

Moscicki EK et al: Hearing loss in the elderly: An epidemiologic study of the Framingham Heart Study Cohort. *Ear Hear* 6:184, 1985.

National Center for Health Statistics: *Prevalence of Selected Chronic Conditions, United States 1979–1981*. Vital and Health Statistics Series 10, No.155. OHHS Pub. No. (PHS) 86-1583. Public Health Service. Washington, DC, US Government Printing Office, 1986.

Rosen S et al: Presbyacusis study of a relatively noise-free population in the Sudan. *Ann Otol Rhinol Laryngol* 71:727, 1962.

Schuknecht HF: *Pathology of the Ear*. Cambridge, Harvard University Press, 1974.

Schuknecht HF, Gacek MR: Cochlear pathology in presbycusis. *Ann Otol Rhinol Laryngol* 102:1, 1993.

Schulte BA, Schmiedt RA: Lateral wall Na,K–ATPase and endocochlear potential decline with age in quiet-reared gerbils. *Hear Res* 61:35, 1992.

Weinstein BE: *Geriatric Audiology*. New York, Thieme Press, 2000.

Willott JF: *Aging and the Auditory System: Anatomy, Physiology, and Psychophysics*. San Diego, Singular Publishing, 1991.

SECTION C

GENDER AND SEXUALITY

CHAPTER 97

Sex and Gender Across the Human Life Span: Implications of the Sex Differentials in Longevity and Health for the Care and Welfare of the Elderly

WILLIAM R. HAZZARD

John Anderson, My Jo*

John Anderson, my jo, John,

When we were first aquent:

Your locks were like the raven,

Your bonie brow was brent.

But now your brow is beld, John,

Your locks are like the snaw;

But blessings on your frosty pow,

John Anderson, my jo.

John Anderson, my jo,

We clamb the hill thegither;

And mony a cantie day, John,

We've had wi' ane anither;

Now we maun totter down, John,

And hand in hand we'll go,

And sleep thegither at the foot,

John Anderson, my jo.

Robert Burns, 1789

A visit to almost any long-term care facility will prompt an obvious question from even the most casual observer:

*joy

1253

"Where are the men?" This chapter attempts to answer this intriguing question on the basis of both practical and theoretical considerations and extrapolate its conclusions and speculations to considerations of the health and social care of the elderly in this century of an unprecedented "age wave" in America and the world at large.

The principal issues addressed in this chapter include:

- What is the magnitude of the sex differential in longevity in the United States?
- How universal is this differential among different populations–ethnic groups in the United States? Among different nations, especially by degree of socioeconomic development?
- Has this differential always existed? If not, when did it emerge? And why?
- Are there genetic determinants of this differential? Are these mediated by sex hormones? How do these change across the life cycle?
- What are the extragenital consequences of the sex differential in sex hormone physiology at various stages in the life cycle? What are these consequences, notably in the:
  - Nervous system?
  - Endocrine/metabolic system?
  - Immune system?
  - Cardiovascular system?
- What are the social, psychological, and behavioral implications of these differentials at various stages in the life cycle?
- What are the age-specific mortality rates of men and women (and commonly expressed as the ratio between the two)—both all-cause and cause-specific?
- What are the age-specific morbidity rates in men and women—both all-cause (especially as expressed in functional status) and cause-specific?
- How do these differentials affect the lives of older persons, with specific implications for the duration and quality of life for elderly men and women? For the prevalence and duration of widowhood? For the health—physical, psychological, social, functional, and financial—social care, and living circumstances of elderly widows and widowers?

- Are these trends changing? If so, how and why? And if so, what are the implications of those changes for the lives of elderly Americans in the twenty-first century?
- And, on a more macro level, what are the planning and policy implications of those changes (with special reference to health care and long term care)?

DEFINITIONS

Throughout this chapter the following definitions are used, conforming to the recommendations of the Committee on Understanding the Biology of Sex and Gender Differences formed by the Board on Health Sciences Policy of the Institute of Medicine of the National Academy of Sciences as put forth in their landmark 2001 report, *Exploring the Biological Contributions to Human Health: Does Sex Matter?*:

- Sex: The classification of living things, generally as male or female according to their reproductive organs and functions assigned by chromosomal complement.
- Gender: A person's self-representation as male or female, or how that person is responded to by social institutions based on the individual's gender presentation. Gender is rooted in biology and shaped by environment and experience.

It is noteworthy that to clarify use of the terms *sex* and *gender* was one of the principal recommendations of this report. As will become evident, this distinction is important in consideration of the central issues in this chapter, for both contribute significantly to the longevity, function, and quality of life of elderly Americans and must be considered in responsible planning efforts for their health and social care in the twenty-first century.

DIMENSIONS OF THE SEX DIFFERENTIAL IN LONGEVITY

The sex differential in longevity from birth in contemporary American society is currently nearly 6 years (Table 97-1). However, this has not always been so. At the beginning of the twentieth century, when the United States was still a developing nation, this differential was just 2 years, and the overall age-adjusted male:female mortality ratio was

Table 97-1 Life Expectancy at Birth, Age 65, and Age 75 Years, United States, All Races, 1998

Age	Life Expectancy (Years)		Difference (Female minus Male)	Percent Difference*
	Males	Females		
At birth	73.8	79.5	5.7	7
At age 65	16.0	19.2	3.2	17
At age 75	10.0	12.2	2.2	18

*Percent difference equals (life expectancy for females minus life expectancy for males) divided by life expectancy for females.

SOURCE: Adapted from National Center for Health Statistics (2000a). Reprinted with permission from Institute of Medicine, *Exploring the Biological Contributions to Human Health: Does Sex Matter?* Washington DC, National Academy Press, 2001.

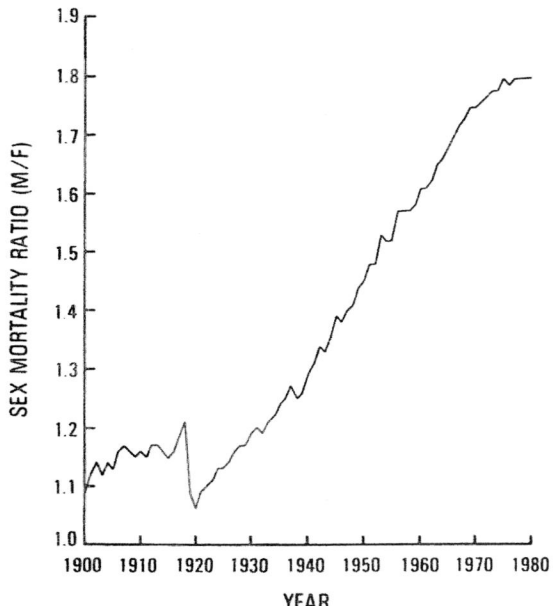

Figure 97-1 Gender mortality ratio (M/F), United States 1900–1980. Based on mortality rates age-adjusted to the 1940 total U.S. population. From Wingard DL: The gender differential in morbidity, mortality, and lifestyle. *Ann Rev Public Health* 5:433, 1984.

Table 97-2 Average Life Expectancy at Given Ages for Adult Whites, United States, 1980, Presented by Gender

	Life Expectancy, (Years)		Male/Female Ratio, %
	Male	Female	
At birth	70.7	78.1	90.5
At 60 years	17.5	22.4	78.1
At 65 years	14.2	18.5	76.8
At 70 years	11.3	14.8	76.4
At 75 years	8.8	11.5	76.5
At 80 years	6.7	8.6	77.0
At 85 years	5.0	6.3	79.4

SOURCE: Adapted from Wylie CM: Contrasts in the healths of elderly men and women: An analysis of recent data for articles in the United States. *J am Geriatr Soc* 32:670, 1984.

only 1.1 (Fig. 97-1). Throughout the first 70 years of the century that ratio climbed steadily (except for a brief decline to near unity during the period 1918 to 1919, which was attributable to the greater female mortality during the influenza pandemic of that era). This increase translated into a sex differential in expected longevity at birth that reached its maximum at 7.5 years during the period 1969 to 1971. During those seven decades the country experienced progressive and dramatic socioeconomic development, a series of cataclysmic wars, and major changes in the roles of men and women in society. The social progress of women in the post-World War II and Viet Nam war era and the rise of the feminist movement led some cynics (mostly men) to predict that women would begin to suffer the health and mortality consequences of the lifestyles and social roles historically considered as "masculine." In this author's experience, all persons, both lay and professional, have strong opinions as to why women outlive men. These opinions, however, are more often rooted in their personal biases and perspectives than in any objective scientific consideration. Illustrative of this point, a 1996 survey of more than 500 college-aged students confirmed a distinct sex difference in attribution of the sex differential in longevity: young males ascribed the difference to the traditionally greater physical labor of men and the less stressful life of women, while the females attributed it to better self-care and attention to health by women.

While there is very little evidence to support this predicted deterioration in health or longevity of women in the present climate of changing lifestyles and occupational status (women in the workforce generally experience considerably fewer health problems and seek medical attention substantially less often than women who are not employed), there can no longer be any doubt that the sex differential in longevity in America has begun to narrow

and, in retrospect, has been doing so progressively over the past 30 years. Harbingers of this trend were apparent in mortality data from the late 1960s, when a plateau in the previous progressive rise in the sex differential in age-specific death rates emerged (see Fig. 97-1), and the absolute difference between the sexes in expected longevity subsequently began to decline. However, this reflected a greater gain among males than females (compare Table 97-2 with Table 97-1), even as both sexes have experienced continuing increases to unprecedented average longevity. If this pattern continues, it will introduce an important change in demography of the aging population, with significant implications for strategies on both individual and societal levels to enhance longevity in both sexes. If successful, these strategies should in turn reduce the burden of widowhood on survivors and hence the vulnerability of those survivors, especially widows, to loss of independence and consequent institutionalization (discussed further below).

Nevertheless, a certain minimum sex differential in longevity appears to be a fundamental and perhaps immutable principle of human gerontology. In America, this appears to hold true across ethnic groups with a broad range of average longevities. Nor is this phenomenon confined to the United States: the gap that developed in the United States in the twentieth century simultaneously emerged in all nations that underwent similar socioeconomic development, with accompanying increases in average longevity of both sexes. These increases are attributed principally to improvements in nutrition, education, housing, transportation, sanitation, public health, and health care, all leading to reductions in the diseases and conditions that predispose to the vastly premature deaths of infants and children. Those developments also reduced the deaths of women of reproductive age associated with child-bearing (including reduced numbers of pregnancies and deliveries). Those same societies also generally experienced simultaneous advances in the status of women in general, a trend that appears to parallel reductions in premature mortality of women wherever it occurs. Thus, in the early twenty-first century, America and other developed nations may be entering the hypothesized fourth and final stage in the evolution of the sex differential in longevity presented by Lopez in the volume edited by Ory and Warner.

WHEN DOES THE SEX DIFFERENTIAL IN MORTALITY BEGIN?

The sex differential in mortality (Fig. 97-2) appears to begin at conception, when the ratio of male to female zygotes may be as high as 170 to 100 (for reasons that remain unclear, Y-bearing sperm are more likely to fertilize an egg than are sperm with the X-chromosome). Because of greater in utero male fetal death, however, by 10 to 12 weeks of gestation (as determined in abortuses), the gender ratio has declined to approximately 130:100. This decline in male survival continues throughout fetal life such that by birth this ratio has decreased yet further to 106:100 (see chapter by Neel in the volume edited by Ory and Warner).

This trend continues throughout the remainder of the human life span, albeit less dramatically with advancing age. And because the sex ratio of the population at every age is the product of the cumulative survival of the sexes from each preceding birth cohort, the sex differential among survivors progressively favors females over males with every passing year of life. After the initial 6 percent excess of males over females at birth, the continued surplus of male deaths produces parity in numbers between

the sexes during adolescence. However, at every age beyond that era women outnumber men with an ever-growing sex disparity. This leads to a progressive rise in the ratio of women to men with advancing age, a pattern that appears to grow almost exponentially in old age, to a female:male ratio of approximately 3:2 among community-dwelling elderly persons older than age 85 years.

Somewhat paradoxically, this sex differential in the population grows with age in spite of a progressive narrowing in the gap in expected remaining longevity between the sexes, especially beyond middle age. This dwindles to little more than 2 years at age 75 years (see Table 97-1) and 1 year at age 85 years. Of practical utility to clinicians (in counseling aging couples), the ratio of remaining expected longevity between men and women remains relatively constant beyond middle age, stabilizing at approximately 80 percent (men compared with women) even as the absolute difference narrows with each passing year of survival. Thus to minimize the duration of widowhood, men must survive youth and middle age, the phases of life in which their greater vulnerability to premature death contributes most to the protracted widowhood of their spouses.

By contrast with the situation among community-dwelling older persons, however, the sex ratio among residents of long-term care facilities (except those in the Veterans Affairs system) is far higher than 3:2. Ratios of 6:1 or 7:1 are not unusual in community nursing homes. This reflects in part the more vulnerable functional status of elderly women, as compared with men of similar age (and even in nursing homes measures of the performance of activities of daily living display lower average scores in female than male residents—one of many paradoxes raised in the sex/gender/longevity domain—in spite of the greater risk of death in the men in such facilities). Thus older women demonstrate greater musculoskeletal weakness and disability than do men of comparable age. Women older than age 85 years also have a greater prevalence of dementia, a pervasive disorder among the elderly that greatly increases their risk of institutionalization and often has devastating consequences to function and quality of life in the nursing home environment.

However, just as important, the social circumstances of elderly women, who often live alone, also contribute to their preponderance in long-term care institutions. This reflects their more frequent single marital status: while approximately 80 percent of American men older than age 65 years are married, only 40 percent of women older than age 65 years are married, and the widow to widower ratio is 4:1, all figures that grow by the year with advancing age. Thus, given that for both sexes the person most likely to provide close and continuing support for a vulnerable older individual is the spouse, the elderly man who requires social and health care support to remain in the community is much more likely to have the help and companionship of his wife (who is also usually younger and more vigorous). However, the elderly woman who requires such support is much less likely to have an able spouse in attendance, often having outlived her husband, and she is a candidate for long-term institutional care unless alternative sources of social and health care support can be identified. Widowhood is the normative last phase of life for women: it

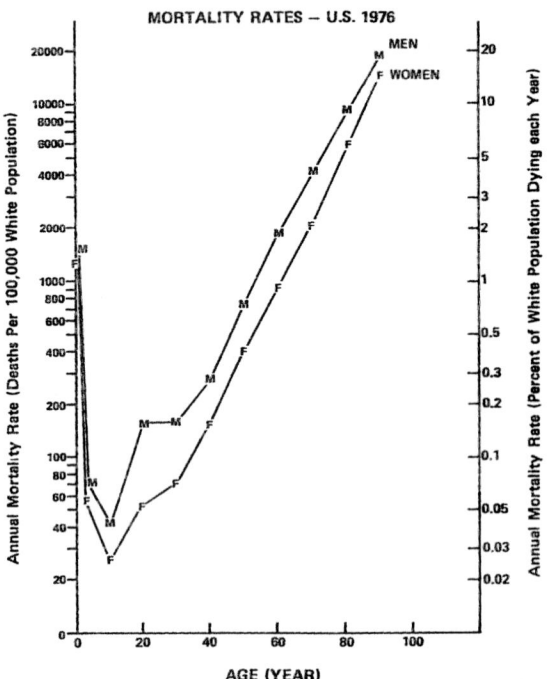

Figure 97-2 Mortality rates by gender, United States, 1976. Compiled from data presented in Gee EM, Veevers JE: Accelerating sex differential in mortality: An analysis of contributing factors. *Soc Biol* 30:75, 1984.

often lasts more than a decade and is a reality that deserves serious consideration in responsible planning for the care and welfare of older persons.

This differential in care-giving needs and provision of care to elderly men and women is an example of how the terms *sex* and *gender,* as defined earlier, differ in a meaningful way: care-giving is culturally (as well as, arguably, genetically and hormonally) determined; the care provided by wives to their husbands represents an extension of their traditional and normative female nurturing role, a role that carries major implications for the care and welfare of aging persons both male and female.

THE BIOLOGICAL BASIS OF THE SEX DIFFERENTIAL IN LONGEVITY

The universal nature of the sex differential in mortality across ethnic and geographic lines suggests that this phenomenon may be rooted in the biology as well as the sociology of the human species. This hypothesis is reinforced by the observation that the greater longevity of the female versus the male appears to be virtually universal in zoology. An important and instructive caveat prevails here, however: to observe this phenomenon, the environment must mitigate the harsher consequences of "survival of the fittest" according to strict darwinian principles (that arguably prevail in the earlier evolutionary stages in sex differential in mortality); this, in turn, will permit survival of both sexes to an age approaching the maximum lifetime potential of the species. This is notably the case in zoos, in which aged animals are protected from inimical forces such as predation and malnutrition, and where females tend to outlive males.

BASIC MOLECULAR GENETICS OF SEX DIFFERENCES (SEE TABLE 97-3)

The sex chromosomes constitute but approximately 5 percent of the human genome (Fig. 97-3). The Y chromosome is much smaller than the X and codes for only about two dozen different genes. Of those, the SRY gene determines development of the male gonadal phenotype, while spermatogenesis is related to a small number of other genes, mutation or deletion of which has been associated with certain cases of male infertility. Another class of Y chromosomal genes code for ribosomal proteins in Y-bearing cells (RPS4Y in Fig. 97-3) , while homologous genes on the X-chromosome code for those proteins in XX cells; thus certain ribosomal proteins throughout the organism differ between male and female cells. However, the functional consequences of these differences remain to be determined.

Male and female genomes differ in another important respect: females have twice the dose of X-chromosomal genes. The X chromosome has approximately 160,000 deoxyribonucleic acid (DNA) base pairs encoding an estimated 1000 to 2000 genes (see Fig. 97-3), only a few of which, the "pseudoautosomal," have homologues on the

Table 97-3 Genetic Factors that May Differentially Affect the Basic Biochemistry of Male and Female Cells

Female specific:

- Expression of some genes from both X chromosomes
- Defect in initiation or maintenance of X chromosome inactivation
- Changes in estrogen-responsive genes (e.g., the HER2 gene in breast cancer) in germ line or somatic cells

Male specific:

- X-chromosome-linked recessive mutations
- Expression of Y-chromosome-specific genes
- Changes in androgen-responsive genes in germ line or somatic cells

SOURCE: Reprinted with permission from Institute of Medicine, *Exploring the Biological Contributions to Human Health: Does Sex Matter?* Washington DC, National Academy Press, 2001.

Y chromosome. Products of these genes, like those on the autosomes, play a role in virtually every aspect of cellular function, metabolism, development, and control of growth and turnover. Especially germane to this discussion are those that play specific roles in particular tissues at particular points in development, several of which have been demonstrated to play critical roles in gonadal differentiation.

The twofold increase in X-chromosomal genes in females is in general nullified by X-chromosomal inactivation, a complex, carefully regulated process unique to female cells marked in each by one of the two X-chromosomes becoming heterochromatic (identifiable on microscopy as the Barr chromatin body in the nucleus of female cells). This process renders genes on the inactivated X-chromosome functionally silent. It occurs in every somatic cell of XX females but not in XY males. Thus, not only must XX cells maintain the state of cell-specific X-inactivation throughout life but also, because the same X-chromosome is not inactivated in every cell, XX females are "epigenetic mosaics." Not surprisingly, the process of X-inactivation is itself controlled by multiple factors, including genes. However, this may vary widely; in some families sisters may show nearly identical patterns of X-inactivation, whereas in other studies of female identical twins, such patterns differ widely within twin pairs.

Germane to the focus of this discussion, female mosaicism underlies the dramatic sex difference in the severity and risk of death from diseases that are transmitted in a sex-linked recessive mode. For whereas a mutation in a gene on the X-chromosome will be expressed in every cell of an affected male, only half of the cells of the female will experience the consequences of that mutation, and her heterozygous state may carry no functional significance. However, given the rarity of X-linked recessive diseases with major physiologic consequences (e.g., classical hemophilia), the aggregate contribution of all the premature deaths of males from such sex-linked autosomal recessive diseases to the sex differential in longevity is miniscule.

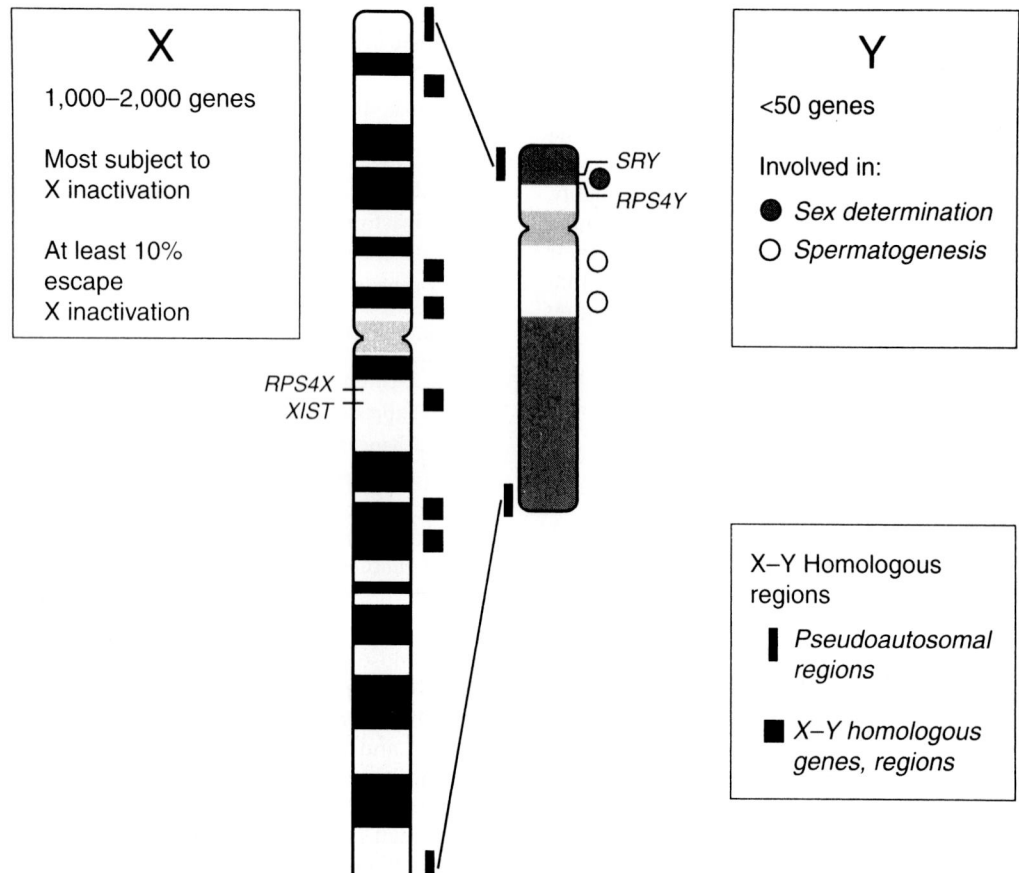

Figure 97-3 The human sex chromosomes. Reprinted with permission from Institute of Medicine, *Exploring the Biological Contributions to Human Health: Does Sex Matter?* Washington DC, National Academy Press, 2001.

Perhaps more germane, however (at least theoretically), it appears in cells grown in culture that at least 10 to 15 percent of X-linked genes appear to be expressed from the inactive chromosome and hence have "escaped" X-inactivation, contributing to a net increase in activated X-chromosomal gene products in females. This differential X-inactivation may have implications for vulnerabilities to certain diseases in affected individuals; for example, the suspected relationship between gastrin-releasing peptide receptor and smoking-related lung cancer, which is released by both active and inactive X chromosomes, with elevated levels hypothesized to lead to increased risk of lung cancer in women smokers. And, at the purely theoretical level, is X-inactivation maintained constantly throughout life? Could reactivation of the silenced X provide "back-up" genetic resiliency for women in later life?

SEX DIFFERENTIALS DURING FETAL, CHILDHOOD, AND ADOLESCENT DEVELOPMENT

All humans—XX, XY, or with an atypical sex chromosome configuration—begin development from a common starting point in utero, with similar, phenotypically female genitalia until 6 to 7 weeks of gestational age. After that

point expression of the SRY gene on the Y chromosome in males induces development of the testes. At about 9 weeks this results in the secretion of testosterone. This, in turn, as modulated by multiple genes (at least 70 on sex chromosomes and autosomes), results in the development of the reproductive tract and masculinization of the male fetus as expressed most notably in the genitalia and the brain. Absent testosterone, the female phenotype is expressed; ovarian hormones are not required for this development. Moreover, animal studies and research on human dizygotic twins have suggested that testosterone secreted by a male fetus can exert a masculinizing influence on adjacent female fetuses, with anatomic, physiologic, and behavioral consequences. Thus events during intrauterine life, especially the secretion of testosterone by the fetal testis, exert powerful and enduring effects on postnatal life.

During late fetal life and infancy the hypothalamic–pituitary–gonadal axis is largely suppressed, giving rise to relative hormonal stability throughout childhood (the "juvenile pause"). Adolescence, the gradual coming of age that transpires during most of the second decade of life, is the next phase of development during which the sex and gender differentials in growth and behavior are dramatic. Within that life phase puberty constitutes the transitional period between the juvenile state and adulthood during which the adolescent growth spurt occurs, secondary sexual traits appear (which produce the dramatic sexual dimorphism between adult men and women), fertility is initiated, and profound psychological changes also occur. This tends to be conceptualized as a series of changes arising from reactivation of the hypothalamic–pituitary–gonadal axis.

However, despite the relative hormonal quiescence during the juvenile phase, small pulsatile patterns of follicle-stimulating hormone (FSH) and leuteinizing hormone (LH) can be detected as harbingers of coming adolescence in prepubertal children, and a striking eightfold difference in estradiol levels is demonstrable in girls. This is associated with a 20 percent advancement in bone age in girls versus boys and may be related to their earlier onset of puberty. The development of breasts, which begins in white girls at an average age of 10.6 years, is under the control of estrogen, whereas growth in axillary and pubic hair is influenced by androgens secreted by the adrenals and ovaries. The age at which the benchmarks of pubertal development appear is also influenced by ethnicity (breast development begins about a year earlier on average in African American girls than in white girls). Whether or not there has been an earlier age of breast development in recent decades remains a subject of controversy, while, contrary to much popular opinion, the average age of menarche appears not to have changed in at least four decades. In boys, the beginning of puberty is marked by an increase in testicular size, which begins at a mean age of approximately 11 years (in both white and African American boys).

One of the most striking sex differentials associated with puberty is the earlier onset of the growth spurt in girls (Fig. 97-4), in whom it may actually begin prior to breast development or growth of axillary or pubic hair. In boys, peak height velocity is reached approximately 2 years later than in girls, although boys are taller than girls at the onset of the spurt and finish, albeit later, with a mean height that is 12.5 cm greater. This differential reflects the greater prepubertal growth of boys, their taller status when their pubertal growth spurt takes off, and their greater growth during that pubertal phase. The principal hormonal determinants of the growth spurt are growth hormone, insulin-like growth factor-1(IGF-1), and triiodothyronine in the prepubertal phase (accounting for 50 percent of the height increase during the subsequent pubertal phase), while estradiol is the main sex hormone involved in the pubertal phase in boys as well as in girls (the estrogen in boys arising principally by extragonadal conversion from testosterone).

Another hormonal feature of puberty is the phenomenon of adrenarche, which begins before age 8 years and is marked by progressive increases in adrenal androgen secretion and plasma dehydroepiandrosterone (DHEA) and DHEA-sulfate. Adrenarche is independent of the mechanisms that regulate the secretion of sex steroids from the gonads (gonadarche). Clinically adrenarche is signaled by the appearance of axillary and pubic hair and is considered premature when it occurs in white girls before age 7 years and in African Americans before age 5 years. In contrast to the circumstance in boys, in whom premature adrenarche is a benign variant of normal puberty, in girls it is associated with a 10-fold increased risk of the polycystic ovary syndrome (PCOS) and its associated (and pathophysiologically important) features of insulin resistance and ovarian hyperandrogenism. These lead to an

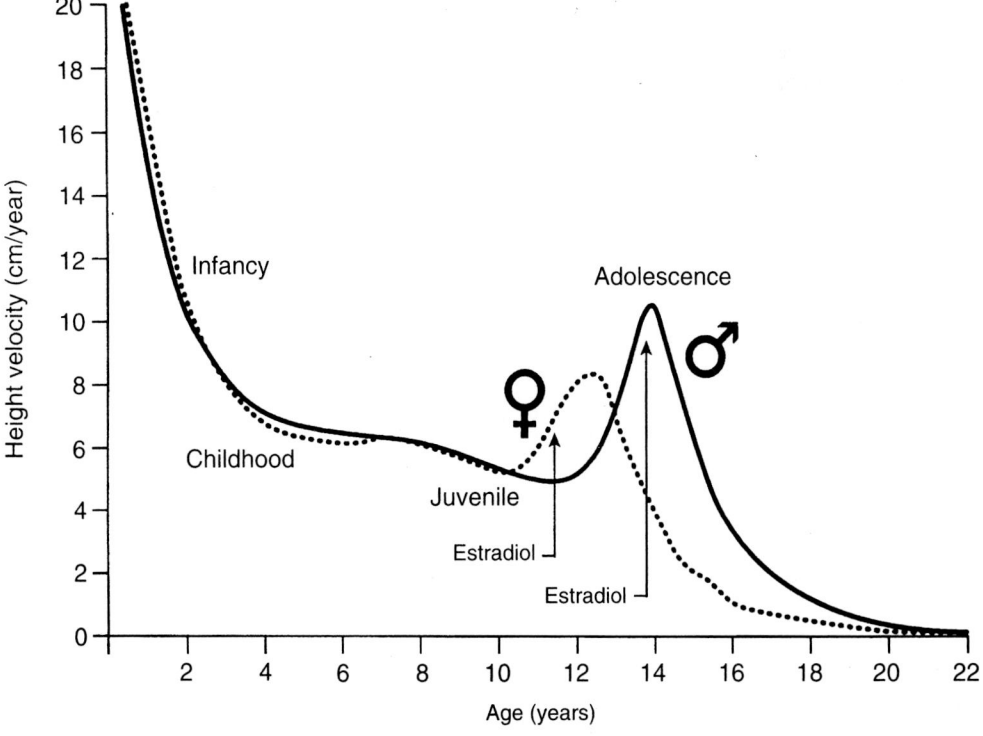

Figure 97-4   The relationship between age and height velocity through adolescence in human females and males. Reprinted with permission from Institute of Medicine, *Exploring the Biological Contributions to Human Health: Does Sex Matter?* Washington DC, National Academy Press, 2001.

increased incidence of central obesity, type 2 diabetes, hypertension, and dyslipidemia (with the pattern of higher low-density lipoprotein [LDL] and lower high-density lipoprotein [HDL] cholesterol levels typical in men prior to the era of the menopause), all cardinal features of the "metabolic syndrome." PCOS, which has been estimated to occur in as many as 10 percent of women, appears to attenuate the sex-specific relative immunity to cardiovascular disease (CVD) otherwise enjoyed by women. As such, its understanding may provide special insights into the mechanism whereby men are at increased CVD risk, as compared with women, and the role of hormones, including sex hormones, in mediating that sex differential. Such insight may also provide opportunities to intervene with both behavioral and pharmacologic strategies to prevent premature CVD in men (and potentially in women as well, especially those with PCOS).

Of special relevance to the premise of this chapter that the sex differential in longevity originates in events in the life cycle long before old age, an increasing body of evidence suggests that there is an association in girls between retarded in utero growth, the risk of premature adrenarche, and their subsequent development of PCOS; recent studies suggest that girls with antenatal growth retardation and low birth weights have fewer primordial ovarian follicles and a smaller uterus and ovaries at puberty and subsequent hyporesponsiveness to FSH, which may mediate (or at least be a marker for) the pathophysiology of PCOS. Thus, PCOS may be a classic example of a disorder of adolescence and adulthood that is programmed during fetal life, but which holds important implications for health and longevity in middle and late life—as well as providing major insight into the general mechanism whereby nonandrogenized women enjoy longer (and more CVD-free) lives than their male counterparts.

These hormonal and physical changes at puberty also hold important implications for the sex differences in behavior during adolescence that are the subject of such intense contemporary public interest and concern. Some of these differences appear to proceed from the direct effects of gonadal hormones on the brains of adolescent boys and girls. For example, in studies of early adolescents, increasing levels of testosterone were associated with increasing aggression and social dominance in boys, while changes in estrogen levels correlated with changes in behavior patterns in girls during the pubertal transition. In various studies, certain behaviors appear to relate to absolute levels of sex hormones, others to the ratio of testosterone to estrogen, and still others to fluctuations in hormone levels. Still other studies reported changes in sex hormones in response to behaviors, such as increases in testosterone following athletic successes.

Such changes may have important, even life-altering, effects on the adolescents who experience them. Earlier maturation by girls, for instance, has been associated with social adjustment problems during puberty, earlier initiation of sexual activity and pregnancy, and later problems with eating disorders, depression, and substance abuse.

Boys may not have the same extent of social and behavioral problems, partly because of the recognition they receive from precocious physical strength and athleticism.

However, there can be little doubt but that the risk-taking behavior of adolescent and young adult males contributes importantly to the stark contrast in mortality rates between young men and women (see below), and it seems logical to attribute such behaviors to hormonally mediated sex differentials across the adolescent transition. These become manifest not only in differentials mediated by sex in the sense of the definition urged by the Institute of Medicine report, but, importantly, also in how adolescents present themselves to the world and how its social institutions respond to them; that is, their gender manifestations. Again the physical, psychological, behavioral, and social sex and gender differentials that present such stark contrasts during adolescence are rooted in the antecedent genetic, hormonal, and environmental lives of those boys and girls and also continue to modulate individual and group sex and gender differentials in health and longevity throughout adolescence and the remainder of the life span.

A practical consideration regarding the earlier maturation of girls than boys is also germane to the central theme of this chapter: that the duration of widowhood is an important determinant of the long-term care needs of elderly persons, especially women who have outlived their husbands. Because there is a normative sex differential in the age at marriage of bride and bridegroom (generally about 2 years, likely reflecting the earlier maturation of females), this adds a commensurate period to the duration of widowhood, which may average nearly a decade (2 to 3 years difference in age at marriage plus approximately 6 to 7 years in the sex differential in longevity).

SEX AFFECTS NEURAL ANATOMY AND FUNCTION

A fundamental strategy of gerontologic investigation looks to biological integrating systems for insights into the aging process. This strategy examines how changes with aging in those systems render the organism progressively vulnerable to insults from the environment in a stochastic cascade that limits survival of the individual and determines average and maximum longevity of a given species. Hence, consideration of the determinants of the sex differential in longevity (as well as of the causes of morbidity at various stages of the life cycle) have focused upon modulation of the neuroendocrine and immune systems by sex hormones across the lifespan and how these might explain that differential.

As introduced in the immediately preceding sections and well-summarized in the recent Institute of Medicine report, fundamental differences in genetics and physiology between males and females result in important differences in neural anatomy and circuitry, as well as in cognition and behavior at all points across the life span. While these begin during fetal life, they are amplified and modulated continuously at each age and stage in a fashion that interacts dynamically with the environment, including the different "male" and "female" cultures in which boys/men and girls/women develop and live.

These sex and gender differences can increasingly be demonstrated in the central nervous system and brain as investigative techniques in neuroanatomy, physiology, and imaging become more sophisticated. The brain is increasingly appreciated as an endocrine organ, too, with behavioral and anatomical consequences of exposure to hormones, including sex steroids, especially testosterone (e.g., greater aggression in male than in female mice). Such exposures are also being examined in relation to the gender identity of children. For example, case studies report that certain children with an XY-karyotype raised as girls because of mutilated or ambiguous genitalia may develop a male gender identity, presumably because of their intrauterine testosterone exposure. This challenges the belief that individuals are born with the potential to develop either male or female gender identity as determined by the sex of rearing.

Other sex differences in human behavior are also becoming increasingly documented in studies of males and females at various stages across the human life span. Many have focused on childhood play behavior and related activities and interests, personality (such as aggression and interest in babies), nonverbal communication, and cognitive abilities. These differences carry over into adult life. Here there are well-documented sex differences in frequency of visits to health professionals, use of complementary medicine, both higher in women than men, and incidence and course of certain mental disorders, notably depression, also substantially more frequent in women, and substance abuse, notably of tobacco and alcohol, which is far more common in men.

These sex differences also apply to cognition, differences that are more marked at the extremes of the distribution of any given ability. In general, women more often demonstrate greater abilities in the verbal domain: verbal fluency, speech production, the ability to decode a language, spelling, and perceptual speed and accuracy. Women also generally excel in fine motor skills. Men, on the other hand, more frequently demonstrate better performance on tests of spatial and quantitative abilities, as well as gross motor strength. These sex differences may be reflected in the performance of certain tasks highly relevant to certain conditions common in old age (e.g., dementia), because women typically perform better than men in tests of working memory of both verbal and nonverbal information. Mathematical abilities of males are greatest at the highest levels of performance (e.g., boys outperform girls on the mathematics SATs by 2:1 at a score of 500 and above, 5:1 at 600 and above, and 17:1 at 700 and above). However, such differentials are confounded by the important contribution of experience to performance on such tests, and because boys are enrolled in advanced mathematics courses far more often than girls, their superior performance, especially at the highest levels, may reflect that exposure more than their sex, gender, or sex hormone physiology (a general caveat for interpreting all such studies).

Demonstrating the continuing importance of sex hormone exposures on cognition and behavior in adult life, variations in performance, especially verbal skills, have been observed in women across the menstrual cycle; for example, during the preovulatory phase, when estrogen levels are high, women have demonstrated deterioration in spatial abilities, while manual coordination and skills in articulation improved.

Recent technologic imaging advances are translating these descriptive studies into visual images of differential performance in cognitive tasks between men and women. For example, functional magnetic resonance imaging (fMRI) studies of cerebral blood flow during performance of certain activities differ between the sexes: men rely upon the left inferior frontal gyrus (Broca's area) to carry out phonologic processing, while women employ both left and right frontal gyri (extrapolated perhaps to why women may experience less loss of speech function than men after a stroke involving the left frontal gyrus).

Another area of differential neural function with major implications for health and function of women versus men across the life span that was a focus of the Institute of Medicine report is the reported increased perception of pain by women (Table 97-4). This bears much further investigation but clearly impacts morbidity in old age and the care of the elderly. Not only are older persons preponderantly women but women also have a greater prevalence of many of the disorders listed in Table 97-4, the management of which falls into the domain of the geriatric clinician.

SEX AFFECTS IMMUNE FUNCTION

Just as there is a general "domino hypothesis" of aging and longevity regarding general physiological regulation across the lifespan, there is an analogous hypothesis regarding the immune system and aging: involution of the thymus, which begins at puberty, is associated with a reduced thymic cellular output that leads to fewer naïve T cells contributing to the peripheral T-cell pool. In the steady state, the number of T cells within that pool is held constant within narrow limits by homeostatic mechanisms. These induce the proliferation and extend the survival of resident T cells to fill niches left by declines in naïve T cells. According to this hypothesis, however, with the passage of time (and aging), as T-cell population is maintained constant through proliferation, an increasing fraction of T cells reach their replicative limit. This, in turn, renders the organism vulnerable to infections and certain cancers as the immune response to those challenges progressively fails. Relevant to the theme of this chapter, comparison of sex differences in life span and death rates at each age from infectious and parasitic diseases suggests that the immune system works more efficiently and is effective longer in females than males (implying in turn that thymic involution occurs at a more rapid rate in males).

This sex differential applies more to the adaptive than the innate immune system (granulocytes and their products). The adaptive system includes activation and suppression of T and B lymphocytes, macrophages, and dendritic cells; secretion of their cytokine products; production of immunoglobulin antibodies; and activation of the complement and coagulation systems. As a rule, estrogens upregulate and androgens downregulate these systems, although the sex differential in these functions is relatively narrow. Accordingly, modest variation in these functions can be seen at various phases of the menstrual cycle. In general these differences have been sufficiently

Table 97-4 Sex Prevalences of Some Common Painful Syndromes and Potential Contributing Causes

Female Prevalence	Male Prevalence
Head and neck	
Migraine headache with aura	Migraine without aura
Chronic tension headache	Cluster headache
Postdural puncture headache	Posttraumatic headache
Cervicogenic headache	Paratrigeminal syndrome*
Tic douloureux	
Temporomandibular disorder	
Occipital neuralgia	
Atypical odontalgia	
Burning tongue	
Carotodynia	
Temporal arteritis	
Chronic paroxysmal hemicrania	
Limbs	
Carpal tunnel syndrome	Thromboanglistis obliterans†
Raynaud's disease	Hemophilic arthropathy‡
Chilblains	Brachial plexus neuropathy
Reflex sympathetic dystrophy	
Chronic venous insufficiency	
Piriformis syndrome	
Peroneal muscular atrophy‡,¶	
Internal organs	
Esophagitis	Pancoast tumor§,**
Gallbladder disease**	Pancreatic disease
Irritable bowel syndrome	Duodenal ulcer
Interstitial cystitis	
Proctalgia fugax	
Chronic constipation	
General	
Fibromyalgia syndrome	Postherpetic neural
Multiple sclerosis, T††	
Rheumatoid arthritis, T	
Acute intermittent porphyria‡	
Lupus erythematosus, T	

*Raeder's syndrome.

†Buerger's disease.

‡Sex-linked inheritance is a potential contributory cause.

¶Charcot–Marie–Tooth disease.

§Bronchogenic carcinoma.

**Lifestyle is a potential contributory cause.

††T, autoimmune.

SOURCE: Berkley and Holdcroft (1999). Sex prevalence information is mainly from Merskey and Bogduk (1994) and was cross-checked by using MedLine and other search sources. Reprinted with permission from Institute of Medicine, *Exploring the Biological Contributions to Human Health: Does Sex Matter?* Washington DC, National Academy Press, 2001.

subtle as to present a challenge to provide mechanistic insights through research. And whereas studies of animals in controlled circumstances have demonstrated that males are more susceptible to infections with parasites, bacteria, fungi, and viruses than females, this has not been clearly demonstrable in humans, in whom the sex differentials in such infections have generally been attributed to sex differentials in exposures rather than in the individual's response to those exposures.

In contrast to the relatively subtle hypothesized greater vulnerability of males to infections, the far higher risk of females to diseases of autoimmune origin stands out as a

Table 97-5 Female/Male Ratios Associated with Common Autoimmune Diseases

Disease	Female:Male Ratio
Hashimoto thyroiditis	10
Primary biliary cirrhosis	9
Chronic active hepatitis	8
Graves' hyperthyroidism	7
Systemic lupus erythematosus*	6
Scleroderma	3
Rheumatoid arthritis	2.5
Idiopathic thrombocytopenic purpura*	2
Multiple sclerosis	2
Autoimmune hemolytic anemia	2
Pemphigus	1
Type I diabetes*	1
Pernicious anemia	1
Ankylosing spondylitis	0.3
Goodpasture nephritis/pneumonitis	0.2

NOTE: Not all diseases are predominant in females.

*Age specific.

SOURCE: Reprinted with permission from Institute of Medicine, *Exploring the Biological Contributions to Human Health: Does Sex Matter?* Washington DC, National Academy Press, 2001.

major cause of the greater morbidity of women than of men from these afflictions (summarized in Table 97-5). Indeed, as well-summarized and referenced in the recent Institute of Medicine report, autoimmune diseases may well constitute the prototypical domain of greatest contrast between the sexes and provide unique insights into mechanisms of the sex differential in many other diseases as well as in overall morbidity and longevity. However, research to date demonstrates great complexity of the determinants of the sex differential in this domain as well, with sex differentials in exposure at different stages of the life cycle and hormonal modulation (including that related to pregnancy in females) playing important roles. Especially germane to the sex differential in health and function across the life span, because those autoimmune diseases with greatest female preponderance arise in young adulthood and generally carry over throughout the remainder of life (e.g., rheumatoid arthritis), the contribution of those disorders to the greater lifelong morbidity of women and their greater burden of chronic illness in old age is substantial. However, as is proving to be the case in most diseases that differ by sex, the role of sex hormones in their pathophysiology and management is not clear; for example, many of the autoimmune diseases appear to be ameliorated during pregnancy and not aggravated by female hormone replacement

therapy. Thus a simple, cohesive theory to explain the sex disparity is lacking, and caution is urged in attributing the difference to either physiologic or pharmacologic effects of the sex hormones.

SEX AFFECTS SEX HORMONE PHYSIOLOGY ACROSS THE ADULT LIFE SPAN

Review of the changes in sex hormone physiology across the adult life span is distributed among several other chapters in this textbook, notably, regarding the aging of the endocrine system (Chap. 65), menopause (Chap. 99), male hormone replacement therapy (Chap. 103), and female HRT for osteoporosis prevention and treatment (Chap. 75). These chapters focus on aspects with implications for the aging process and approaches to hormone replacement therapy (HRT) as part of a strategy to mitigate some of the associated declines in physical and functional status.

Female HRT is also addressed in this chapter in the section devoted to that subject as related to thromboembolism and cardiovascular disease, cancer, and gall bladder disease. For details of other aspects of sex hormone physiology such as reproductive function the reader is referred to standard textbooks of endocrinology (e.g., *Williams Textbook of Endocrinology,* 9th ed.) Suffice it to summarize here that such changes are likely to influence the physiology and pathophysiology of human aging across the entire adult life span. Such differentials in sex hormone physiology are also likely to underlie much of the sex differential in longevity, as well as the health status of elderly adults in cumulative, complex patterns in multiple organ systems and diseases of those organs. However, it must be stressed that sex differences in the physiology of sex hormone regulation and the attributed effects of those differences on the function, health , and longevity of men and women cannot be not legitimately extrapolated to HRT (for either women or men), which differs from physiologic hormone regulation both quantitatively and qualitatively. Attempts to obviate the changes in sex hormone physiology with aging through HRT remains a controversial approach, an "antiaging" strategy that lacks consistent validation through rigorous research and evidence-based practice. Indeed, a lesson of history learned over again in the recent early termination of the Women's Health Initiative is that HRT—as with all such hopeful gerontologic interventions—must be formally tested in randomized clinical trials before any such treatment can be recommended for widespread clinical use, and HRT is currently quite definitely not recommended for this purpose.

THE SEX DIFFERENTIAL IN LONGEVITY

An empirical approach to the sex differential in human longevity begins with inspection of the all-cause sex ratio in longevity across the life span in the United States. This displays a bimodal pattern, with a peak of approximately 3:1 at age 20 years and a plateau of approximately 2:1 in late middle age (and a decline toward unity in old age). A similar

Table 97-6 Gender-Specific Mortality Rates and Gender Differentials for the 12 Leading Causes of Death, United States, 1980*†

Cause	Age-Adjusted Mortality Rate		Gender Ratio (M:F)	Absolute Gender Difference (M:F)	% of Difference
	Males	Females			
Diseases of the heart	280.4	140.3	1.99	140.1	40.7
Malignant neoplasms	165.5	109.2	1.51	56.3	16.3
Respiratory system	59.7	18.3	3.43	41.4	12.0
Cerebrovascular diseases	44.9	37.6	1.19	7.3	2.1
Accidents	64.0	21.8	2.93	42.2	12.2
Motor vehicle	34.3	11.8	2.90	22.5	6.5
Other	29.6	10.0	2.96	19.6	5.7
Chronic obstructive pulmonary disease	26.1	8.9	2.93	17.2	5.0
Pneumonia and influenza	17.4	9.8	1.77	7.6	2.2
Diabetes mellitus	10.2	10.0	1.02	0.2	0.1
Cirrhosis of the liver	17.1	7.9	2.16	9.2	2.7
Atherosclerosis	6.6	5.0	1.32	1.6	0.5
Suicide	18.0	5.4	3.33	12.6	3.7
Homicide	17.4	4.5	3.86	12.9	3.7
Certain causes in infancy	11.1	8.7	1.27	2.4	0.7
All other causes	98.5	63.5	1.55	35.0	10.1
All causes	777.2	432.6	1.79	344.6	—

*Rank based on number of deaths.

†Per 100,000, direct standardization to the 1940 total US population.

SOURCE: Calculated from data from the National Center for Health Statistics, 1983.

pattern is seen in nearly all developed nations (although the ratios under the peak and plateau vary by country), with the late sex mortality ratio being notably higher (and more in a dome-like configuration) in the nations of Eastern Europe and the former Soviet Union, where male mortality rates are increasing at an alarming rate. Perhaps providing insight to the genesis of this "spike and dome" configuration, it seems likely germane to note that this pattern emerged in the United States and these other nations in the twentieth century in parallel with their socioeconomic development as well as their involvement in major international military conflicts.

To pursue the possible mechanisms of the evolution of the sex longevity disparity at the next level of inquiry, the sex ratio for the top 12 causes of death in 1980 (Table 97-6 and Fig. 97-5) can be reviewed. This exercise reveals that men have a higher age-adjusted death rate than do women for nearly all causes. Diabetes is the one clear exception to this rule; men and women are at virtually identical age-adjusted mortality risk. However, such inspection also readily allows grouping of those causes of death into those that are frequent in adolescence and young adulthood—notably, those related to violence and the risks of a youthful lifestyle—and those that are prevalent in middle and

old age, the chronic and progressive "degenerative" diseases of complex etiology. In the first group, neurobehavioral gender differentials appear clearly causative—"macho" behavior involving considerable risk constituting the most obvious factor increasing male vulnerability. There is increasing acknowledgment that such behavior is determined at least in part by hormonal factors, although modulation—exaggeration or dampening—by sociocultural forces is clearly also important (i.e., sex plus gender issues). This risk-taking behavior also extends to sex differentials in drug abuse and sexual practices, with consequences that could have a dramatic impact on the sex differential in longevity if the human immunodeficiency virus (HIV) epidemic continues to affect more men than women (see Chap. 87). However, narrowing in the sex differential in HIV-related deaths recently became apparent as the viral infection spreads to women by heterosexual contact and intravenous drug abuse. Indeed, HIV disease is now the fastest-growing cause of death in young American women.

The causality of the diseases clustered under the plateau of greater male mortality in late life, which in the aggregate account for approximately 90 percent of the sex differential in longevity, is more complex and certain to prove

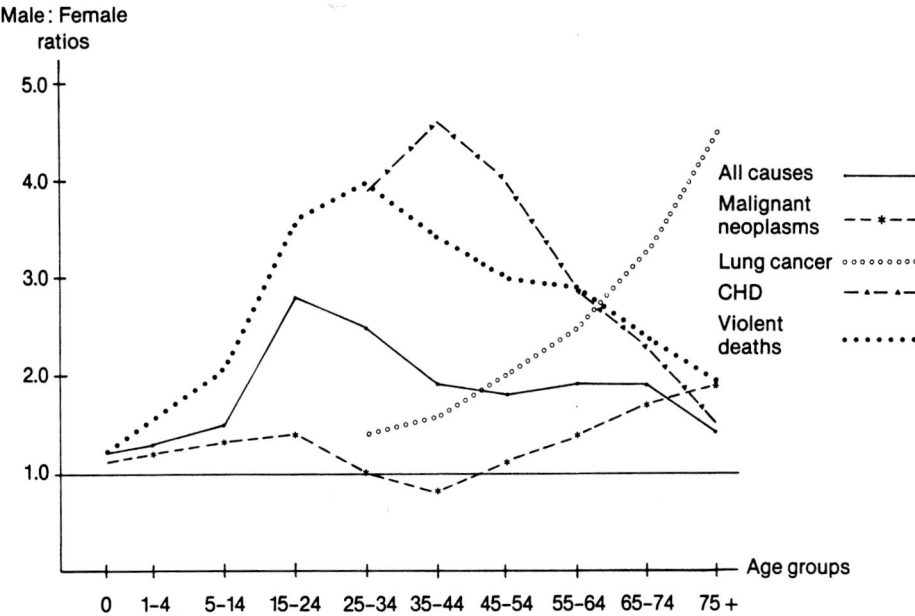

Figure 97-5 Sex mortality ratios for specific causes of death by age in the United States according to World Health Organization (WHO) statistics. *World Health Statistics Annual: Vital Statistics and Causes of Death.* World Health Organization, Geneva 1986. CHD, coronary heart disease. Reprinted with permission from Johnasson S: Longevity in women, in Douglas P (ed): *Heart Disease in Women.* Philadelphia, Davis, 1989, p 8.

multifactorial. An attractive hypothesis advanced principally by social scientists, has, as with the spike in youth, focused on behavioral–cultural factors. Men in western societies traditionally adopted lifestyles with greater risk to their health: more miles driven, more cigarettes smoked, less focus on health promotion, disease prevention, and early detection. Men also traditionally made fewer visits to physicians and take fewer prescription drugs. Indeed, as reported by Courtenay, these differences in attitudes and health behaviors that undermine men's health often serve as signifiers of masculinity and instruments that men use in the negotiation of social power and status. Put another way, denial of their vulnerability to disease and death is part of the masculine tradition and gender identity, an attribute that presents a cultural and behavioral barrier to strategies of "preventive gerontology" for men (see Chap. 6).

These phenomena have tended to confound the issue of sex/gender and health, introducing another paradox: women experience greater morbidity (often reported in terms of numbers of encounters with the health care system), but men have higher mortality rates. The bases for these sex and gender differentials in health behavior have been widely investigated (although with relatively little correlation with quantitative biomarkers of disease risk or measurements of sex hormone physiology or effects). These have been reviewed elsewhere (see especially chapters by Wingard and by Nathanson in the volume edited by Ory and Warner and the recent Institute of Medicine report edited by Wizemann and Pardue).

The behavior with the greatest potential impact on the sex differential in longevity—and that behavior currently in greatest flux—is cigarette smoking. To illustrate this point, it was reported by Waldron in the Ory and Warner volume that mortality in middle-aged nonsmoking men exceeds that in nonsmoking women by only

30 percent, as compared with a male excess of greater than 120 percent for the total population studied (put another way, nonsmoking men and smoking women have more equal age-adjusted mortality rates). Cigarette smoking became fashionable in the United States in the twentieth century, and until recently, was predominantly a masculine habit—men started earlier in life and smoked more heavily than women. This behavioral sex differential was reinforced by the encouragement of cigarette smoking by servicemen during the world wars. The clear parallel between increases in male cigarette smoking and the rising sex ratio in mortality in the twentieth century would seem causally related. Review of the sex ratios in mortality from the leading causes of death in America (see Table 97-6) strongly suggests that the historical sex differential in cigarette smoking constitutes a major factor in the majority of such causes, notably vascular disease, both coronary heart disease (CHD) and stroke, cancer, especially lung cancer, and nonmalignant lung disease. Indeed, it was estimated by consensus at the conference that produced the volume by Ory and Warner that the historical sex differential in cigarette smoking behavior might account for as much as 4 years of the 7-year sex differential in longevity at birth that reached its peak in 1970.

In this context, it is relevant to examine recent trends in cigarette smoking in both sexes and parallel trends in mortality rates from diseases related to smoking. Cigarette smoking reached its peak prevalence in the United States shortly after World War II, when nearly half of the adult population were smokers. At that time not only did more men than women smoke, but also heavy cigarette use was far more prevalent in men. From that time until the present, cigarette smoking has declined progressively in the United States (although recent reports disclose that this trend is slowing, especially in younger persons and notably in younger women). The beginning of this decline closely paralleled the release of the first Surgeon General's Report on Smoking and Health in 1963, the first clear public statement linking cigarette smoking with lung cancer and other feared diseases. Initially, the decline in smoking appeared to be greater in men than women, but by the late 1960s women were also giving up smoking at a comparable rate. The decline has been most notable among those older than age 35 years in both sexes. When the decrease in CHD mortality first received public attention in the early 1970s (the "epidemic" having reached its peak at the time of the Surgeon General's report), a significant proportion of that reduction was attributed to the decline in cigarette smoking. This decline, which has continued to the present, has generally been equivalent, as expressed in relative (percentage) terms in both genders. However, because the previous absolute levels of CHD mortality were far greater in men, their absolute decrease in CHD deaths has been greater. In parallel fashion, because the level of cigarette smoking in men was far higher, their absolute reduction in cigarette consumption has been greater (see especially the chapter by Nathanson in the volume edited by Ory and Warner). Hence, recent trends show a decrease in the difference in the number of CHD deaths in men versus women, in parallel with the decrease in the number of cigarettes smoked by men as compared with women. That women are as vulnerable as men to the untoward effects of cigarette smoking—given the lag between exposure to tobacco carcinogens and the onset of lung cancer—is evident in the narrowing of the historical sex differential in lung cancer, which surpassed breast cancer as the most common cause of cancer-related death in women in the 1980s (see Fig. 97-5), as well as in other smoking-related diseases, such as chronic obstructive lung disease and peptic ulcer disease. However, these trends appear likely to stabilize as cigarette smoking rates become equivalent in both sexes, and both men and women, especially those of higher income and educational levels, adopt healthier lifestyles in response to the widespread public health educational campaigns against cigarette smoking.

THE SEX DIFFERENTIAL IN ATHEROSCLEROSIS

Review of the sex differential in the leading causes of death (see Table 97-6) clearly places atherosclerosis and its clinical consequences—CHD, cerebrovascular disease, and peripheral arterial disease—at the center of any consideration of the sex/gender gap in longevity: in the aggregate, these diseases account for more than 40 percent of the total. Moreover, it has been estimated that elimination of all atherosclerotic disease could add up to 10 years to average longevity beyond age 65 years in the United States, raising the mean age at death to nearly 85 years (a popular estimate of the maximum possible average human longevity according to the essays by Fries and by Olshansky et al.). Furthermore, by deferring death among men to beyond middle age, when the sex ratio is highest, a reduction in ages at death between marriage partners would be important by-products.

SEX DIFFERENTIAL IN CVD RISK FACTORS

Although sex differentials may exist in the most basic aspects of atherogenesis (e.g., arterial intimal integrity, vasomotor response, lipoprotein uptake, or other aspects of arterial wall biology—see Chap. 34), evidence for all such possibilities must at present be considered preliminary, albeit intriguing. A more practical approach is to review the sex differentials in the traditional atherosclerosis risk factors across the life span during stages as defined in general and convenient terms by the author: childhood and adolescence (infancy to age 25 years); middle age (ages 25 to 75 years, conveniently bisected at age 50 years into first and second halves [approximately the age of menopause for women]); and old age (older than age 75 years).

Here population studies suggest at least subtle differences at each stage that provide the pathophysiologic basis for earlier expression of cardiovascular disease in men. These studies demonstrate that the sex differentials begin in childhood and adolescence, as well documented in the Bogalusa community studies led by Berenson (which also demonstrated early atherosclerosis in the arteries of adolescents from this community killed in vehicular accidents). In middle age, blood pressure, both median systolic and diastolic, are lower in women than men during the first half, beyond which a crossover occurs such that hypertension (especially isolated systolic hypertension) is more common in older women than men. Regarding control of blood glucose levels, glucose tolerance tests applied to population samples (e.g., in Tecumseh) demonstrate a pattern of change in efficiency of glucose disposal with age also favoring women until midlife, with convergence between the sexes beyond middle age. This carries over into an overall age-adjusted excess male prevalence of diabetes of greater than 10 percent, a disparity still evident in old age. Regarding median levels of blood lipids (cholesterol and triglyceride), these change with age in a biphasic pattern, increasing in both sexes (albeit at a lower rate in women) until the midpoint of middle age, when a plateau is reached, and declining thereafter (Fig. 97-6). Except for the abrupt increase in cholesterol levels in women older than age 50 years (the "postmenopausal overshoot"), these changes in lipids, blood pressure, and glycemic control in the first half of middle age may be mediated by gains in relative body weight, which normatively continue until the middle of middle age, when a plateau is reached (although adiposity may continue to accrue, it is offset by decreases in lean body mass). A decline in median relative body weight during old age ultimately follows, perhaps signaling the onset of frailty and terminal decline (the continued increases in blood pressure and blood glucose beyond middle age require a different explanation).

Close inspection of such curves reveals patterns that are subtly different between men and women, the middle-aged weight plateau being achieved approximately a decade later in women than in men (during their sixties rather than their fifties). Thus, a slower accretion of weight and a later achievement of peak weight in women than men may partly explain the more favorable CVD risk profile of women prior to age 50 years and the infrequency of clinical CVD prior to that age, a benefit that may carry over into

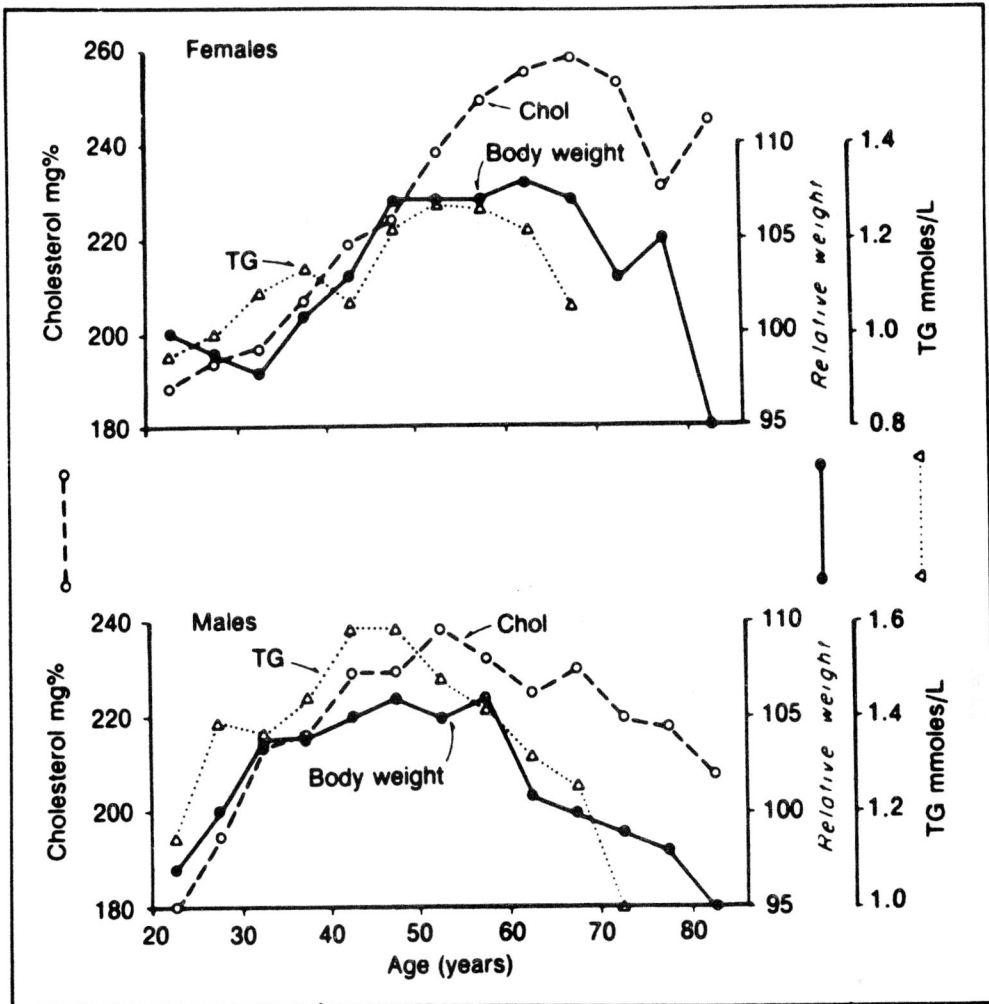

Figure 97-6 Median plasma cholesterol (Chol), triglyceride (TG), and relative body weight values as a function of age in Tecumseh (cholesterol and relative weights) and Stockholm (TG) community studies. Reprinted with permission from Williams RDH (ed): *Textbook of Endocrinology,* 5th ed. Philadelphia, Saunders, 1974.

the succeeding postmenopausal era by virtue of the slower rate of atherogenesis to that point.

A sex differential in regional patterns of midlife weight gain is another possible explanation of the lower CVD risk in women (see also Chap. 92). Beyond adolescence women prototypically gain more adipose mass about the hips and buttocks (producing "lower body," "pear-shaped," or "gynoid" obesity), whereas adult men add fat about the waist (leading to "upper body," "apple-shaped," or "android" obesity). The latter confers extra CVD risk, exaggerating the known interaction between relative body weight and the traditional risk factors in population studies such as in Framingham. Moreover, those atypical women who develop upper-body obesity—especially those with hyperandrogenism and the polycystic ovary syndrome—have CVD risk profiles resembling those of men, and they are at substantially increased risk of type 2 diabetes (presumably because of increased insulin resistance and compensatory hyperinsulinism) and its attendant increased risk of atherosclerosis and its complications.

Additional insight into the role of sex hormones in mediating the sex differential in atherosclerosis differential

may be afforded by inspection of the sex ratio in cardiovascular mortality across the adult life span (see Fig. 97-5). After the peak in this ratio is reached in the premenopausal era, there occurs a major, progressive decline with advancing age, from nearly 5:1 at age 35 years to but 1.2:1 at age 85 years (it never drops below unity). Viewed from another perspective, women enjoy an approximately 10-year relative immunity to CVD, as compared with men (the rate in women ages 55 to 65 years, for instance, is equivalent to that in men ages 45 to 54 years).

Consideration of this delay in women reaching equivalent CVD mortality risk as men is important in resolving an apparent paradox in popular media presentations on population aging and especially the wave of post-World War II female baby boomers currently passing through the menopause and contemplating hormone replacement therapy (see discussion on hormone replacement therapy below). Whereas at any given age women are at lower risk to CVD mortality than are men, CHD remains the leading cause of death in women beyond reproductive age. However, because of their greater longevity, the percentage of women dying of CHD ultimately equals that of men (nearly

50 percent in both sexes). Moreover, because with advancing age the population becomes progressively skewed toward surviving women, the annual numbers of women who succumb to CHD death may actually come to exceed those in men. As death rates from CHD progressively decline, those deaths will occur in older and older persons (already the majority of CHD events occur in Medicare recipients, older than the age of 65 years), and cardiology will focus on progressively older patients and especially older women.

THE ROLE OF SEX HORMONES IN MEDIATING THE SEX DIFFERENTIAL IN CHD RISK

Population studies such as from Framingham, which have reported a higher prevalence of CHD in pre- versus postmenopausal women of comparable age, suggested a physiologic role for sex hormones (specifically estrogen and progesterone) in mediating the sex differential in CHD between women and men. Other population studies, such as those of the early 1970s of the Lipid Research Clinics, carefully examined average cholesterol levels (total, LDL, and HDL) in males and females who were not taking hormone replacement therapy between childhood and old age (Fig. 97-7). Lipid levels are equivalent between the sexes until puberty. At that point (and in parallel with the Tanner stage of pubertal development) HDL concentrations begin to decline in boys, and average levels of HDL remain relatively stable at lower concentrations in men than women (by approximately 10 mg/dL) from the twenties through the seventies. This suggests that this gap is principally attributable to an HDL-lowering effect of testosterone in men. This hypothesis is supported by studies of the effect of testosterone replacement in hypogonadal men, which suppressed HDL levels. This hypothesis has also received direct experimental support in studies of normal men rendered hypogonadal with a gonadotropin-releasing hormone (GnRH) agonist, in whom HDL levels rose (a rise that could be prevented with simultaneous testosterone administration). However, this consequence of testosterone therapy is not a pure androgenic effect, because a substantial fraction of testosterone is converted to estrogen by aromatase in various tissues. Treatment with testosterone with coadministration of aromatase inhibitors results in a greater decrease in HDL levels. Moreover, androgenic anabolic steroids, which are incapable of conversion to estrogen, produce a profound suppression of HDL levels: experimental studies of women given such agents for osteoporosis or endometriosis have demonstrated a 50 percent reduction in total HDL levels, especially marked (85 percent) in the more antiatherogenic HDL2 subfraction.

On the other side of the coin, prospective studies of HDL levels in women followed across the menopause (Chap. 99) have also disclosed a slight average decline (especially in HDL2) coincident with ovarian failure. This suggests at least a mild effect of endogenous estrogen in raising HDL and specifically HDL2.

With regard to LDL, whereas mean levels rise in both sexes between puberty and the menopause (perhaps attributable to increasing adiposity), they remain substantially lower in women than men until the menopausal

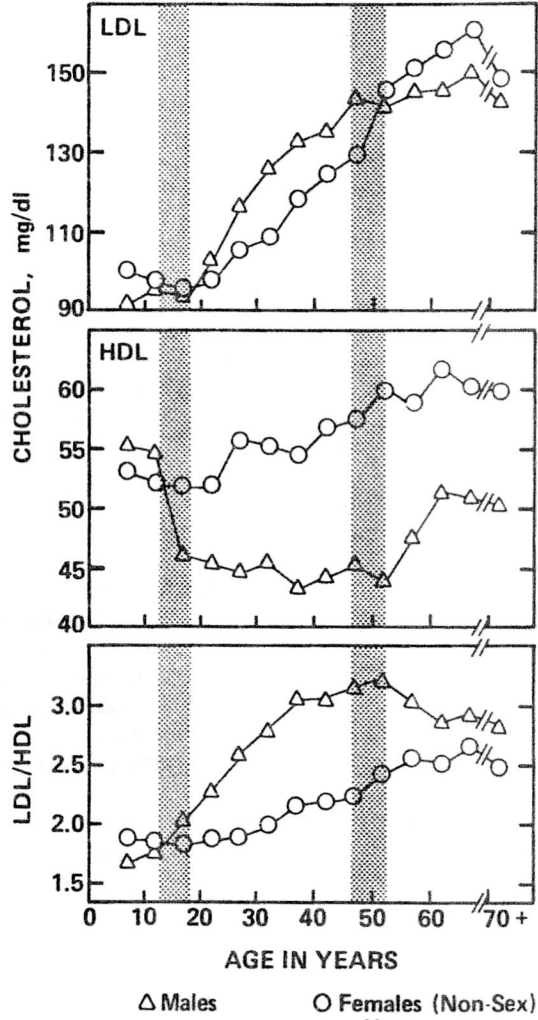

Figure 97-7 Median North American population high-density lipoprotein (HDL) cholesterol, low-density lipoprotein (LDL) cholesterol, and the ratio between the two versus age in white subjects. Data from The Lipid Research Clinics: *Population Studies Data Book*, vol. 1: *The Prevalence Study*. DHHS (NIH) 80:1527, 1980.

era, when they rise significantly, average levels in postmenopausal women actually coming to exceed those in men of comparable age. These trends in women seem most likely to be attributable to the physiological effects of estrogen in premenopausal women and the lack of estrogen beyond the menopause.

The net effect of these changes in lipid levels across the adult lifespan produces a more favorable pattern in women than men at all stages, with the lower HDL levels in men overriding the higher LDL levels in postmenopausal women as to associated CHD risk. However, the sex differential in the LDL:HDL ratio (a convenient single index of lipid-associated risk) is greater in the premenopausal era, when the sex differential in CHD is also the greatest, declining following menopause in parallel with the declining magnitude of that differential.

However, the mechanism of these putative effects of endogenous, physiologic sex hormones on plasma lipids remains largely conjectural, since there is a nostable lack of association between plasma levels of those hormones and plasma lipoprotein concentrations in either population-based or carefully controlled metabolic investigations. Further investigations may reveal correlations with mechanistic implications for atherogenesis beyond lipoprotein metabolism, as suggested in analyses of the American Atherosclerosis Risk in Community (ARIC) cohort study by Golden et al. However, these may prove counterintuitive. In the ARIC study of carotid atherosclerosis, for example, intimal–medial thickening was inversely related to testosterone levels in postmenopausal women.

Thus mechanistic conclusions to date are largely extrapolated from results of pharmacologic interventions, which at best produce but a caricature of the effects of endogenous sex hormones and their physiologic regulation. Perhaps the most insightful of these on a population basis were the same Lipid Research Clinic Prevalence studies (Fig. 97-8). Compared to women not taking hormone supplements, in premenopausal women taking oral contraceptives, average LDL levels were higher, while HDL concentrations were equivalent. However, closer examination of the data revealed that women consuming contraceptives with more powerful androgenic progestational components had lower HDL than those taking contraceptives containing less androgenic progestins. In the postmenopausal women taking HRT (in that era, almost all ingesting unopposed conjugated equine estrogens in a dose of 1.25 mg/d) average LDL levels were lower and HDL levels clearly higher than in women not taking estrogens.

These population studies have been widely confirmed in the intervening decades. Furthermore, careful metabolic studies of post-menopausal women such as those reported by Applebaum-Bowden et al. have quantitatively documented the powerful effects of exogenous estrogens in both lowering LDL levels and raising HDL (and selectively HDL2) levels.

Other studies have identified multiple additional mechanisms by which exogenous HRT in postmenopausal women might sustain their relative immunity to CHD. Indeed, for several decades population studies suggested that the changes in lipid levels seen with HRT were insufficient to account for the degree of protection enjoyed by women. Such studies reported beneficial effects of estrogens in decreasing arterial wall LDL uptake, perhaps retarding LDL oxidation and hence atherogenic potential, and protecting against the paradoxical vasoconstrictive effects of such agents as acetylcholine in the presence of atherosclerosis (likely mediated by enhanced NO synthesis by arterial endothelial intimal cells).

SEX DIFFERENTIAL IN ATHEROSCLEROTIC CARDIOVASCULAR DISEASE

Thus a biological rationale for a slower rate of atherogenesis in women as compared to men would seem to emerge from their more favorable CVD risk profile, especially in the premenopausal era, and the demonstrated effects of sex hormones in mediating the lipoprotein dimension of that differential—albeit clearly demonstrable only with exogenous sex steroid administration.

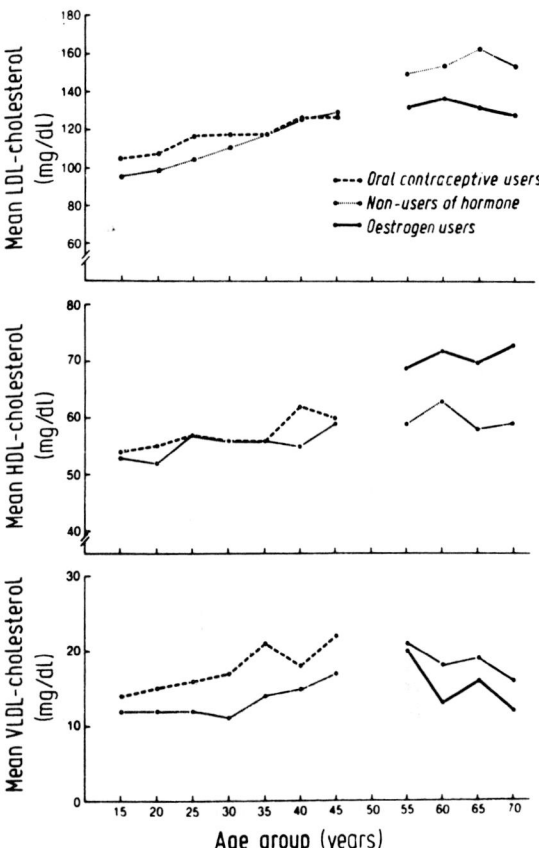

Figure 97-8 Plasma lipoprotein cholesterol levels in users and nonusers of oral contraceptives and estrogens. Reprinted with permission from Wallace RB et al: Altered plasma lipid and lipoprotein levels associated with oral contraceptives and oestrogen use. *Lancet* 2:11, 1979.

Other studies of subclinical atherosclerosis, such as the 15-year prospective population study of the middle-aged men and women of Tromso, Norway, as reported by Stensland-Bugge et al., have confirmed a sex differential in progression of atherosclerosis as reflected in ultrasound measurements of carotid artery intimal–medial thickness. Here age, blood pressure, total and HDL cholesterol, and body mass index were independent long-term predictors of intimal–medial thickness in both sexes, while triglycerides were predictive in women only and physical activity and smoking predictive in men only (though the trend was also apparent in women with heavy smoking exposures). Moreover, as in many other studies of CVD risk factors, CVD risk was associated with the number of such factors in a stepwise fashion. Of note with regard to the central message of this chapter, in this study the mean intimal–medial thickness was less in women than men at all cholesterol levels. Thus women may be relatively spared by factors in addition to their more favorable lipid profiles.

Similar trends were apparent in the ARIC studies reported by Chambless et al. Conducted in four populations of middle-aged subjects (45 to 64 years of age) over an 11-year period, these studies demonstrated that carotid intimal–medial thickness changes were associated with baseline diabetes, HDL-cholesterol, pulse pressure, white

Table 97-7 Prevalence of Cardiovascular Disease in the Cardiovascular Health Study

Prevalence (%)	Men		Women	
	Blacks	Whites	Blacks	Whites
Any clinical CVD	37.2	37.2	36.4	28.2
Subclinical CVD	43.7	41.9	39.7	41.3
Neither	19.1	20.9	24.9	32.5

CVD, cardiovascular disease.

blood cell count, and fibrinogen levels, as well as with changes in LDL-cholesterol (most dramatic in women passing through menopause), triglycerides, and new-onset diabetes and hypertension.

Most germane to geriatric medicine, these trends seem to carry over into old age.

This was demonstrated in the Cardiovascular Health Study (CHS), a longitudinal, population-based study of men and women older than age 65 years from four communities (Table 97-7). This epidemiologic research disclosed detectable, significant CVD in up to 80 percent of the men, but in only 67 percent of the women, by using a combination of clinical disease and indices of subclinical atherosclerosis (including carotid ultrasound and ankle–brachial blood pressure index). Of special note, in this study subclinical disease carried a prognostic significance equal to that of clinical disease in predicting incident CVD events in the 5-year follow-up (while conversely, the absence of atherosclerosis predicted a continued low risk of such events, even in the oldest segments of the cohort). Thus, even as atherosclerosis comes to affect the great majority of American elderly persons, women continue to enjoy a relative, albeit modest, protection compared with their male counterparts of comparable age.

HORMONE REPLACEMENT THERAPY

Despite the biological plausibility of an important role for sex steroids in mediating the relative immunity of women to CVD and the clear effect of exogenous HRT in sustaining and even magnifying the putative role of endogenous estrogen in conferring more favorable lipid profiles, this does not translate into HRT being recommended for postmenopausal women for either primary or secondary prevention of CVD. As with all studies based upon epidemiologic associations, these must be confirmed in formal clinical trials before such recommendations can be justified. The recent dramatic change in the trend toward widespread postmenopausal HRT is a case in point, as well-summarized in the reviews by Manson and Martin and the landmark report from the Women's Health Initiative Writing Group.

At the time these reports were released, it was estimated that approximately 38 percent of US postmenopausal women were using HRT. This was not only for relief of menopausal symptoms, where the benefit remains clear,

but also in the belief that such therapy would reduce the burden of several chronic diseases in the remaining one-third of their lives spent in the postmenopausal state. Such putative benefits included reductions not only in CVD, but also all cancer, osteoporosis (see Chap. 75)—where the benefit also remains clear—and even cognitive impairment (although associated increased risks of breast cancer, thromboembolism, and gall bladder disease gave pause to many women contemplating HRT). This hopeful, pleiotropic preventive strategy was increasingly embraced by the "age wave" cohort of midlife baby boomers, notably the more highly educated and health-conscious women from higher socioeconomic strata who were more likely to receive such supplements. Their enthusiasm for HRT was buttressed by numerous (more than 40) clinical and observational epidemiologic studies that reported substantially less CVD in women taking HRT. As reviewed earlier, such benefit from HRT is biologically plausible, estrogen exerting effects at multiple levels from the genome to whole populations that, on balance, might support their widespread use in postmenopausal estrogen replacement (as reviewed by Mendelsohn and Karas). Randomized clinical trials (RCTs) confirmed that estrogen reduces LDL cholesterol by 10 to 14 percent and increases HDL cholesterol by 7 to 8 percent. Estrogen was also shown to favorably affect other indices of CVD risk: lipoprotein(a) levels are reduced, LDL oxidation is inhibited, and plasminogen-activator inhibitor-1 (PAI-1) levels are reduced. However, other indices appear to be adversely affected: triglyceride levels rise; coagulation is promoted through increases in factor VII, prothrombin fragments 1 and 2, and fibrinopeptide; and—perhaps most germane to CVD in old age—C-reactive protein (CRP), a marker of immune system activation, is increased (by oral HRT). Thus at the level of basic biology, a mixed scorecard in support of HRT for CVD prevention was being assembled even as more and more post-menopausal women elected to take such agents (Table 97-8).

The wisdom of this trend began to engender skepticism among professionals and the lay public alike when the results of the Heart and Estrogen/Progestin Replacement Study (HERS) were reported in 1998 by Hulley et al. HERS was an approximately 4-year RCT of HRT, comparing continuous daily conjugated equine estrogen (Premarin) combined with medroxyprogesterone acetate (Provera) versus placebo in 2673 women with established CHD. This study demonstrated no overall effect of the HRT on coronary death rate and nonfatal myocardial infarction. In the first year of the trial, however, there was a 50 percent greater incidence of coronary events in the women taking HRT. Nevertheless, by the termination of the study this had abated, and even a trend toward a later benefit of HRT appeared to emerge in years 3 through 5, suggesting a biphasic pattern of response to the hormones. During subsequent unblinded follow-up, however, this potential later benefit did not prove sustained. Thus after 6.8 years neither net benefit nor increased risk of HRT for secondary prevention of CHD was apparent. This disappointing outcome was subsequently echoed in the Estrogen Replacement and Atherosclerosis (ERA) secondary prevention trial of estrogen alone or in combination with progestin on angiographically

Table 97-8 Benefits and Risks of Postmenopausal Hormone-Replacement Therapy (HRT)

| Variable | Effect | Benefit or Risk | | Source of Data |
		Relative	Absolute	
Definite Benefits				
Symptoms of menopause (vasomotor, genitourinary)	Definite improvement	>70–80% decrease		Observations studies and randomized trials
Osteoporosis	Definite increase in bone mineral density; probable decrease in risk of fractures	2–5% increase in bone density; 25–50% decrease in risk of fractures	172 fewer hop fractures (402 vs. 574) per 100,0000 woman-years	Observation studies and limited data from randomized trials
Definite Risks				
Endometrial cancer	Definite increase in risk with use of unopposed estrogen; no increase with use of estrogen plus progestin	Increase in risk by a factor of 8 to 10 with use of unopposed estrogen* for >10 years; no excess risk with combined estrogen-progestin	Excess of 46 cases (52 vs. 6) per 100,0000 woman-years of unopposed estrogen use (>10 years of use); no excess with use of combined therapy	Observational studies and randomized trials
Venous thromboembolism	Definite Increase in risk	Increase in risk by a factor of 2.7	Secondary prevention: excess of 390 cases per 100,000 woman-years; primary prevention: excess of 20 cases per 100,000 woman-years	Heart and Estrogen/Progestin Replacement Study Observational studies
Probable Increase in Risk				
Breast cancer	Probable increase in risk with long-term use (>5 years)	Overall increase in risk by a factor of 1.35 with HRT use of >5 years	Excess of 20 cases per 10,000 women using HRT for 5 years; 60 excess cases after 10 years of use; 120 excess cases after 15 years of use	Meta-analysis of 51 observational studies
Gallbladder disease	Probable increase in risk	Increase in risk by a factor of 1.4	Excess of 360 cases per 100,000 woman-years	Heart and Estrogen/Progestin Replacement Study
Uncertain Benefits and Risks				
Cardiovascular Disease				
Primary prevention	Could range from net benefit to net harm	Uncertain	Uncertain	Observational studies and randomized trials[†]
Secondary prevention	Probable early increase in risk	Uncertain	Uncertain	Observational studies and randomized trials
Colorectal cancer	Possible but unproven decrease in risk	20% decrease	24 fewer cases (96 vs. 120) per 100,000 woman-years	Observational studies
Cognitive dysfunction	Unproven decrease in risk (inconsistent results)	Uncertain	Uncertain	Observational studies and randomized trials

*The term "unopposed estrogen" refers to the use of estrogen without medroxyprogesterone acetate.

[†]Observational data suggest a decrease in risk of 35 to 50 percent, whereas randomized trial data show no effect or a possible harmful effect during the first 1 or 2 years of use. Most studies have assessed conjugated equine estrogen alone or in combination with medroxyprogesterone acetate.

SOURCE: (Reproduced with permission from Manson JE, Martin KA: Postmenopausal hormone replacement therapy. N Engl J Med 345:34, 2001).

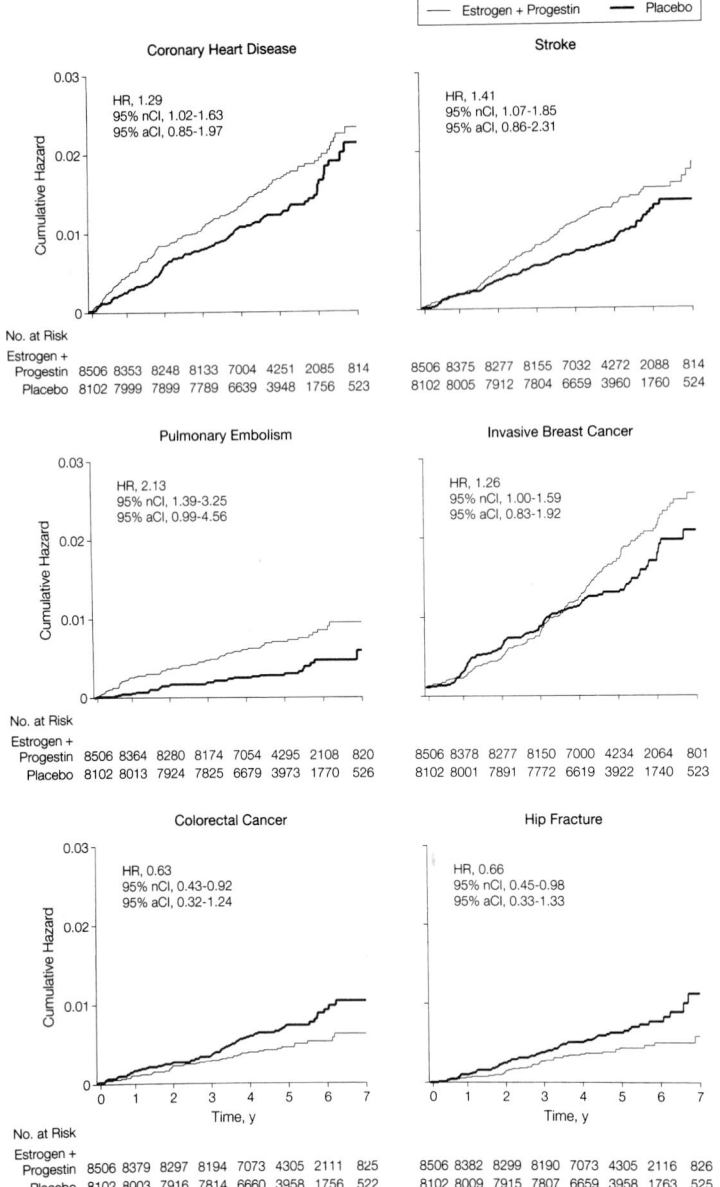

Figure 97-9 Kaplan–Meier estimates of cumulative hazards for selected clinical outcomes of the Women's Health Initiative randomized controlled trial. Writing Group for the Women's Health Initiative: Risks and benefits of estrogen plus progestin in healthy postmenopausal women. Principal results from the Women's Health Initiative randomized controlled trial. *JAMA* 288:321, 2002. (Reproduced with permission).

quantified coronary atherosclerosis: no net effect was seen. Moreover, a review of 22 primary prevention trials of HRT, albeit mostly small and of short duration, also failed to disclose net benefit.

However, the impact of these limited trials, especially as related to the potential for primary CHD prevention, was overwhelmed in 2002 when the first principal results of the Women's Health Initiative (WHI) of the effect of HRT on all-cause and cause-specific morbidity and mortality were released. This arm of the WHI was a large, community-based, placebo-controlled, randomized clinical trial of continuous conjugated equine estrogens (0.625 mg/d) plus medroxyprogesterone acetate (2.5 mg/d). Involving 16,608 postmenopausal women ages 50 to 79 years (average age 63 years, including 21 percent older than age 70 years)

recruited to 40 clinical centers in 1993 to 1998, the study had a planned duration of 8.5 years. The primary favorable targeted outcome was CHD (nonfatal myocardial infarction and CHD deaths), with invasive breast cancer as the primary adverse predicted outcome. A global index was also developed reflecting these two primary outcomes plus stroke, pulmonary embolism, endometrial cancer, colon cancer, hip fracture, and death from other causes.

However, after just 5.2 years of average follow-up, the study was terminated prematurely because the test statistic for invasive breast cancer exceeded the stopping boundary and the global index statistic indicated that the risks exceeded the benefits of the HRT (Figs. 97-9 and 97-10). The estimated hazard ratios (HRs) and nominal 95% confidence

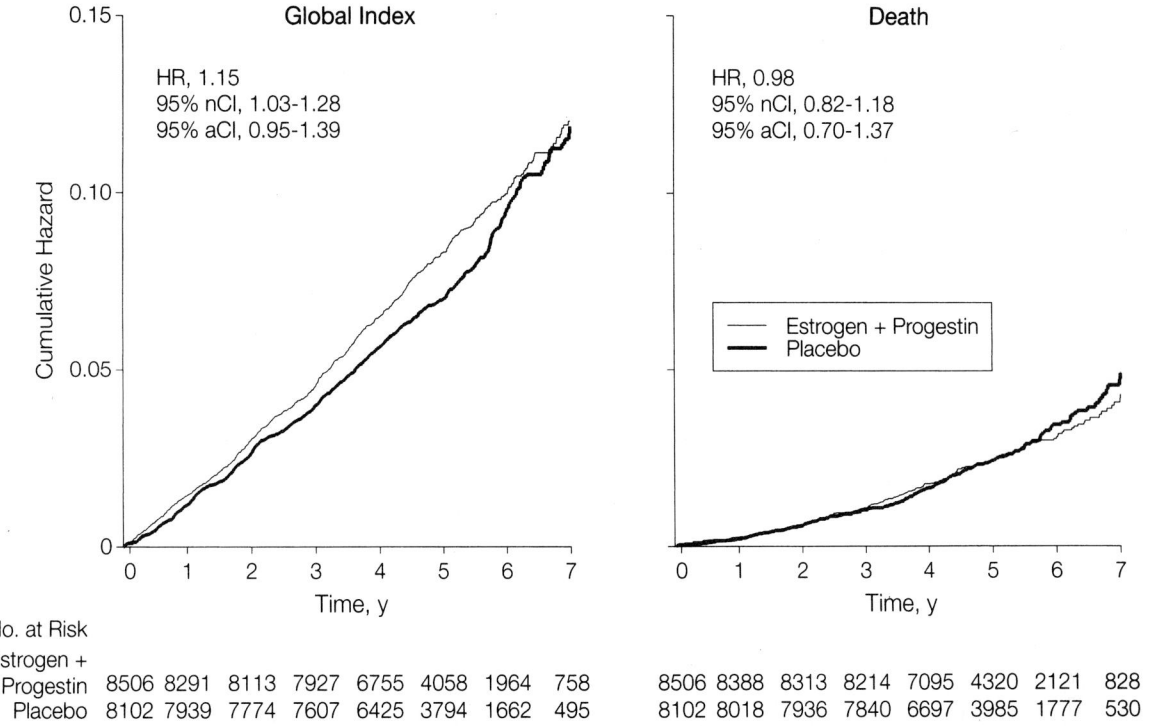

Figure 97-10   Kaplan-Meier estimates of cumulative hazards for global index and death, Women's Health Initiative randomized controlled trial. Writing Group for the Women's Health Initiative: Risks and benefits of estrogen plus progestin in healthy postmenopausal women. Principal results from the Women's Health Initiative randomized controlled trial. *JAMA* 288:321, 2002.

intervals (CIs) (in parentheses) included CHD 1.29 (1.02 to 1.63); breast cancer 1.26 (1.00 to 1.59); stroke 1.41 (1.07 to 1.85); pulmonary embolism 2.13 (1.39 to 3.25); colorectal cancer 0.63 (0.43 to 0.92); endometrial cancer 0.83 (0.47 to 1.47); hip fracture 0.66 (0.45 to 0.98); and death due to other causes 0.92 (0.74 to 1.14). The corresponding HRs and CIs for composite outcomes were total CVD (arterial and venous) 1.22 (1.09 to 1.36); total cancer 1.03 (0.90 to 1.17); combined fractures 0.76 (0.69 to 0.85); total mortality 1.02 (0.82 to 1.18); and global index 1.15 (1.03 to 1.28). Absolute excess risks per 10,000 person-years attributable to the combination HRT were 7 more CHD events, 8 more strokes, 8 more cases of pulmonary embolism, and 8 more invasive breast cancers; while absolute risk reductions per 10,000 person-years were 6 fewer colorectal cancers and 5 fewer hip fractures. The absolute excess risk of events in the global index was 19 per 10,000 person-years. The WHI writing group concluded that "this regimen should not be initiated or continued for primary prevention of CHD."

Thus for both primary and secondary prevention of CHD, combination HRT cannot presently be recommended, especially in the form of continuous treatment with conjugated equine estrogens and medroxyprogesterone acetate in a woman with an intact uterus. However, individualized regimens for women at increased risk for, for example, colon cancer or osteoporosis, may be prescribed. And doubtless many women will elect at least short-term HRT for control of menopausal symptoms; some may even choose long-term treatment because of strongly-held beliefs as to the long-term benefits of HRT (and perhaps

especially estrogen alone in the posthysterectomy state, the study of which continues as another arm of the WHI).

Moreover, the relative immunity to CHD enjoyed by women, especially premenopausally, continues to suggest that a regimen of postmenopausal HRT more accurately reflecting premenopausal female hormone physiology might provide enduring benefits to women over their remaining life span. Indeed, the discrepancies between endogenous physiology and exogenous HRT suggest that important mechanistic insights might be provided by careful examination of the differences. For example, current research in atherosclerotic CVD is focusing on the role of inflammation in the pathogenesis of this disease, with special emphasis on the CRP and other proinflammatory markers as possible mediators. Here research suggesting opposite effects of oral and transcutaneous or vaginal estrogens are especially intriguing, as reported by Modena et al. Oral estrogens, subject to magnification of their effect on hepatic metabolism by their "first pass" exposure, induce increases in CRP, while transdermal estrogens, which enter the systemic circulation directly, actually suppress CRP levels in healthy postmenopausal women.

All in all, however, for at least the present, long-term, combination estrogen-progestin HRT cannot be generally recommended for prevention of postmenopausal CVD, although this is certain to continue to be an area of controversy and active investigation. Specifically in the realm of geriatric medicine—for example, in women older than age 75 years—the paucity of current or contemplated future research regarding HRT for CHD prevention seems certain to remain an area of uncertainty for the indefinite future.

THE SEX DIFFERENTIAL IN LONGEVITY IS DECLINING

By the end of the 1960s, the progressive rise in the sex differential in average American longevity that marked the first seven decades of the twentieth century had begun to abate (see Fig. 97-2). Subsequently, this trend converted to a clear and progressive decline in the differential (see Table 97-1), even as the expected longevity of both sexes continues to rise (albeit at a slower rate in women than in men). Thus by the advent of the twenty-first century, the United States (and other developed countries) were entering the "posttransitional" stage of convergence in longevity by sex hypothesized in the chapter by Nathanson in the Ory and Warner volume.

The reasons for this convergence remain uncertain and controversial. As suggested earlier in this chapter, these are perhaps most focused in the narrowing sex ratio in cigarette smoking exposure in the past four decades, and hence in the various disease risks attributable to that exposure. Of those CVD contributes the greatest proportion of that decrease: the decline in CHD in the United States in both sexes during that interval has been continuous and cumulatively profound. In the ARIC surveillance study of more than 360,000 men and women ages 35 to 74 years in the four communities as reported by Rosamund et al, for example, the reduction in CHD applied both to hospital admissions and deaths caused by CHD both in and out of the hospital. Between 1987 and 1996 the age-adjusted CHD mortality rate fell 3.2 percent in men (CI 2.0 to 4.3) and 3.8 percent in women (CI 1.9 to 5.6). However, this produced a somewhat greater reduction in the absolute number of such deaths in men than women (adjusted for age) because of the greater risk in men at the beginning of the study. The reductions in both hospitalizations and in-hospital mortality were consistent with earlier studies of national data that attributed declines in CHD mortality equivalently to improved population preventive strategies and risk factor profiles as well as more effective treatment of CHD once clinically manifest. It should also be noted, however, that these reductions were more evident in the earlier years of the ARIC study, 1987 to 1991, than subsequently. This raises the question as to whether the decline in CHD will continue indefinitely or whether and when a floor effect will be observed, below which further decreases may not be possible, especially perhaps in an aging population.

This question also applies to the more general issue as to whether the greater advances in longevity among men than women in the past three decades reflect greater relative improvements in health behaviors and medical interventions in men over that time span or the reality that women are approaching the upper limit of the average potential longevity of the human species, the "barrier to immortality" described by Fries as 85 ± 5 years (recently modified in a personal communication at 85 ± 7 years, with a preterminal phase of "compressed morbidity" of 2 to 3 years).

However, that the sex differential in longevity in the United States is declining is no longer a subject of debate. Perhaps the most encouraging aspect of this closure in the sex/gender longevity gap are its implications for institutional long-term care services in the upcoming decades.

As men live longer, couples can expect to live together independently longer, the duration of widowhood will decline, and the need for long-term care services will decline. There is already mounting evidence that this hopeful sequence of events has begun. Even as the number of persons most likely to require such services continues to increase (notably those older than age 85 years), the nursing home bed capacity has reached a plateau in America. Nor is this trend confined to the United States. Other nations at comparable levels of socioeconomic development (e.g., Sweden and Australia) are experiencing a similar relative decline in long-term institutional care. Careful deconvolution of the curves of decline has fractionated these trends into multiple components, including those that reflect improved health and reduced age-adjusted disability of the population as well as the development of noninstitutional alternatives to nursing home care. Clearly these changes are occurring, especially in the United States, where serial studies of aging populations have disclosed progressive decrements in disability among the elderly, especially those older than age 80 years, as well as declining mortality rates for both sexes in this age group. However, such studies have identified that the greater longevity gains in men than women in recent decades may well be the predominant factor contributing to the decline in nursing home utilization, particularly in the 1990s.

This optimistic trajectory is also likely to continue well into the twenty-first century in developed nations. This prediction is reinforced by the association between enhanced longevity of both sexes and increased educational level, because the cohort of elderly citizens with low levels of educational attainment born in the first half of the twentieth century will be succeeded by later cohorts with higher average educational levels. This might also disproportionately favor men, given the relationship between attained educational level and the adoption of more healthy lifestyles and the probability that men of higher educational level (and often higher socioeconomic status) seem more likely to embrace health attitudes and behaviors (such as decreased cigarette smoking) consistent with the practice of effective "preventive gerontology" (see Chap. 6).

Thus the poetic dream of Robert Burns in the preamble to this chapter may yet become reality in a future wherein average longevity of both sexes might approach the maximum lifetime potential of our species.

Nevertheless, given the evidence and theoretical projections gathered to date, as a gerontologist, geriatrician, and endocrinologist, I would predict that because of fundamental and immutable biological differences between the sexes, women will always outlive men. However, in the steady state, the gap will be substantially narrower than at present—perhaps 2 to 3 years (the estimate of Kranczer for the year 2025).

REFERENCES

Applebaum-Bowden D et al: Lipoprotein, apolipoprotein, and lipolytic enzyme changes following estrogen administration in postmenopausal women. *J Lipid Res* 30:1895, 1989.

Berenson GS et al: Association between multiple cardiovascular risk factors and atherosclerosis in children and young adults. *N Engl J Med* 338:1650, 1998.

Chambless LE et al: Risk factors for progression of common carotid atherosclerosis: The Atherosclerosis Risk in Communities Study. *Am J Epidemiol* 155:38, 2002.

Cheitlin MD et al: Do existing databases answer clinical questions about geriatric cardiovascular disease and stroke? *Am J Geriatr Cardiol* 10:207, 2001.

Couternay WH: Constructions of masculinity and their influence on men's well-being a theory of gender and health. *Soc Sci Med* 50:1385, 2000.

Fries JF: Aging, natural death and the compression of morbidity. *N Engl J Med* 303:130, 1980.

Golden SH et al: Endogenous postmenopausal hormones and carotid atherosclerosis: A case control study of the atherosclerosis risk in communities cohort. *Am J Epidemiol* 155:437, 2002.

Grady D et al: Cardiovascular disease outcomes during 6.8 years of hormone therapy: Heart and Estrogen/Progestin Replacement Study follow-up (HERS II). *JAMA* 288:49, 2002.

Hodis HN et al: Estrogen in the prevention of atherosclerosis. *Ann Intern Med* 135:939, 2001.

Hulley S et al: Randomized trial of estrogen plus progestin for secondary prevention of coronary heart disease in postmenopausal women: Heart and Estrogen/Progestin Replacement Study research group. *JAMA* 280:605, 1998.

Humphrey LL et al: Postmenopausal hormone replacement therapy and the primary prevention of cardiovascular disease. *Ann Intern Med* 137:273, 2002.

Kranczer S: Continued United States longevity continues. Metropolitan Insurance Companies. *Stat Bull* 80:20, 1999.

Manson JE, Martin KA: Postmenopausal hormone replacement therapy. *N Engl J Med* 345:34, 2001.

Mendelsohn MM, Karas RH: The protective effects of estrogen on the cardiovascular system. *N Engl J Med* 340:1801, 1999.

Modena MG et al: Effects of hormone replacement therapy on C-reactive levels in healthy postmenopausal women: Comparison between oral and transdermal administration of estrogen. *Am J Med* 113:331, 2002.

Olshansky SJ et al: In search of Methuselah: Estimating the upper limits to human longevity. *Science* 250:634, 1990.

Ory MG, Warner HR (eds): *Gender, Health, and Longevity*. New York, Springer, 1990.

Rosamund WD et al: Coronary heart disease trends in four United States communities. The Atherosclerosis Risk in Communities (ARIC) study 1987–1996. *Int J Epidemiol* 30(Suppl 1):S17, 2001.

Stensland-Bugge E et al: Sex differences in the relationship of risk factors to subclinical carotid atherosclerosis measured 15 years later: The Tromso study. *Stroke* 31:574, 2000.

Wallace JE: Gender differences in beliefs of why women live longer than men. *Psychol Rep* 79:587, 1996.

Wingard DL: The sex differential in morbidity, mortality, and lifestyle. *Ann Rev Public Health* 5:433, 1984.

Wizemann T, Pardue ML (eds): *Exploring the Biological Contributions to Human Health: Does Sex Matter?*, National Academy Press, Washington, DC 2001 .

Writing Group for the Women's Health Initiative: Risks and benefits of estrogen plus progestin in healthy postmenopausal women. Principal results from the Women's Health Initiative randomized controlled trial. *JAMA* 288:321, 2002.

Sexuality and Aging

ROBERT N. BUTLER   •   MYRNA I. LEWIS

Many people worry about what happens to the body sexually as it ages. It is reassuring to know that aging itself does not lead to sexual problems.

Indeed, if one is reasonably healthy and has a healthy and interested partner, one's sex life can remain active and satisfying. When problems do occur, the principal culprits are medical, and to a lesser extent, psychological problems, as well as the absence of a partner as a result of loss of a spouse or companion.

The United States lacks population-based studies of sexuality and aging. The Kinsey studies (now outdated), the physiologic investigations of Masters and Johnson (involving very few older persons), and the findings of the Duke Longitudinal Studies and the Baltimore Longitudinal Study on Aging constitute the limited information currently available. Most other research beyond these classic data tends to be conducted on convenience samples recruited through organizations or clinic populations, limiting their value. For example, clinic populations may overrepresent medical conditions that cause erectile dysfunction. Information obtained through phone or mail surveys may overrepresent less inhibited or more sexually assertive individuals. All in all, much remains to be learned about the precise nature and frequency of sexual activity among older people.

The major physiologic change that occurs in human sexuality in the course of normal aging relates to a gradual slowing of physical response time (affecting erections in men and vaginal lubrication in women). It takes more time to achieve sexual arousal, to complete the sexual act and to become rearoused for further sexual activity. This contrasts with sexual activity among the young, typified by intense excitement and rapid arousal, discharge, and recovery. The slower tempo characteristic of the later years can be emotionally frightening if it is misunderstood as a sign of sexual decline rather than normal aging changes that can be compensated for. This is particularly true for men. But the slower pace also has attractions, especially perhaps for heterosexual women, who may be pleased that their partners requires more time during sexual activity.

OLDER WOMEN

Older women are more subject to anxiety about changes in physical appearance with aging, in contrast to older men, who focus more on sexual performance. Because of their greater longevity (currently more than 5 years longer) as compared to men, women are also more frequently left without a partner or with one who has become infirm. Nonetheless, in the absence of ill health, many older women's sexual capacity continues throughout life. Although sexual activity tends to mirror individual patterns established earlier, some women actually become more sexually active after menopause, as concerns about pregnancy disappear.

Nonetheless, the loss of estrogen during menopause can present major physical and, at times, related psychological impacts for a proportion of women. (For a full discussion of menopause, see Chap. 99.) It has been estimated that approximately 25 percent of all women have menopause-related symptoms that lead them to seek medical care. These usually involve hot flashes (with accompanying sleep deprivation that is a frequent cause of irritability and depression) and other acute symptoms. Later, more chronic problems can occur that also affect sexual functioning. Estrogen loss reduces the usual acidity of vaginal secretions, increasing the likelihood of infection as well as causing burning, itching, and discharge. This has been called estrogen-deficient, atrophic, or "senile" vaginitis and is treatable. Allergies, trichomoniasis, and yeast and fungus infections, especially in diabetic women, are other causes of itching and discomfort.

A thinning of the vaginal walls may be problematic, resulting in both the bladder and the urethra becoming less protected and more likely to be irritated during intercourse. Physicians must be aware that pain during sexual intercourse may be a result of other factors as well, such as a fixed or retroverted uterus, a prolapsed ovary, or water in the fallopian tubes (hydrosalpinx). The evaluation of symptoms should also include a Papanicolaou test to rule out the possibility of a tumor.

The clitoris may gradually become slightly reduced in size, and the labia less firm. The covering of the clitoris and the pad in the pubic area lose some fatty tissue, especially in late life, leaving the clitoris less protected and more easily irritated. The shape and size of the vagina may change, especially in the absence of regular sexual intercourse (typically seen during widowhood or other loss of partners). Masturbation, if personally acceptable, may help to protect sexual functioning when a partner is not available.

Hormone replacement therapy counteracts many of the sexual effects of estrogen loss during and after menopause. Its risks and benefits are covered elsewhere in this volume (see Chap. 75). For our purposes, It is often quickly effective against hot flashes, as well as ameliorating and even preventing the longer term consequences of menopause. Oral administration of estrogen is the most common approach but other strategies may also be useful. Vaginal estrogen cream applied directly into the vagina aids in counteracting vaginal dryness and atrophy, but is rapidly absorbed and so acts somewhat systemically as well as locally.

Perhaps the most frequent complaint of women is a lessening of vaginal lubrication. This lubrication, produced by congestion of the blood vessels in the vaginal walls during sexual activity, is the physiologic equivalent of erection in men. Lubrication begins to take longer as women grow older and may disappear altogether, particularly in the early stages of sexual arousal. As mentioned, estrogen replacement therapy is particularly effective in relieving symptoms. But in addition to or in place of estrogen, individuals experiencing discomfort may be advised to use simple, over-the-counter, water-based lubricants (Lubrin, K-Y jelly, HR Lubricating Jelly, Gyne-Moistrin, and others), as well as moisturizing gels such as Replens. Oil-based lubricants, including petroleum jelly and mineral oil, should not be used, because they do not dissolve in water and can be a vehicle for vaginal infections.

OLDER MEN

Older men frequently worry about erectile dysfunction or impotence, the temporary or permanent incapacity to have an erection that allows a man to carry out sexual intercourse. As described earlier, it is most important to reassure men that aging itself does not produce impotence. Relatively healthy men do not lose the capacity for erections and ejaculations as they age. When problems occur, a medical examination should be sought in order to identify precipitating physical, and less frequently, psychological conditions. Treatment and reversal of sexual difficulties is often possible. Because occasional erectile problems are so common and often self-correcting, the diagnosis of erectile dysfunction should not be made unless it occurs in at least 25 percent of sexual encounters with the same partner. (See Chap. 102 for further discussion of erectile dysfunction.)

The gradual slowing of physical reaction time described earlier constitutes the most common physical change with aging. Men may begin to notice this already in their forties, although for many it is not apparent until later in midlife. Reassurance that this is normal and predictable is critical for both men and their partners in order to avoid the fear and anxiety that may ensue in the face of lack of such information. A simple solution is available. Most men respond well to increased manual (or other) stimulation of the penis and genital area, either by their partners or themselves, and are thus able to achieve a firm erection. A lengthening of the period of foreplay is also recommended. Some also find visual stimulation useful in the arousal phase, including sexually explicit films and videos.

Aside from a slowing speed of reaction time, there are other changes that older men should be aware of, again with the reassurance that these changes do not imply impending erectile dysfunction. Erections may become somewhat less firm than in younger years, but still maintain the capacity for satisfactory intercourse. The lubrication from the Cowper's gland that appears before ejaculation decreases or disappears completely; however, this has little effect on sexual performance. The volume of seminal fluid decreases. Men younger than age 50 years produce 3 to 5 mL of semen every 24 hours on average, while men older than age 50 years produce 2 to 3 mL. Ejaculation may be less forceful, and the semen is propelled a shorter distance. While the contraction is less powerful, an older man can still experience satisfying orgasmic pleasure.

Male fertility, the capacity to father children, may diminish, usually in the middle seventies, although there are instances where it continues into the nineties. Therefore birth control is important if the partner is a younger woman and pregnancy is not desired.

Despite media pronouncements, there is no "male menopause." It has not been easy to define a male climacteric, sometimes called andropause or viropause, because unlike female menopause, it is not distinct and predictable. Administration of testosterone should be undertaken only after careful testing to determine an actual deficiency. This is particularly important because of testosterone's possible interaction with incipient prostate cancer.

It is possible that sexual functioning for older people may improve in the future as health care professionals learn to differentiate the diseases and psychological impairments of late life from aging processes per se and become better able to prevent and treat them. For example, much that is attributed to aging today may be a result of physical changes such as atherosclerosis, which limits blood flow to the pelvic area but may ultimately be preventable and treatable.

COMMON MEDICAL PROBLEMS

Health conditions, both acute and chronic, may impact on sexuality. The most obvious example is heart disease. A myocardial infarction (MI) may lead couples to give up sexuality altogether because of fears of another MI or even a cardiac death. Yet such occurrences are extremely rare. A study by James E. Muller of Harvard Medical School found that for those who had already had an MI, the chance of a second MI during sexual activity is only 2 in 1 million. The general medical consensus is that most individuals who have had an MI can safely resume sexual activity after a waiting period of 8 to 14 weeks, depending on general fitness and conditioning.

In average sexual activity, the heart rate ranges from 90 to 160 beats per minute, about equal to the rate resulting from light to moderate physical activity. The systolic blood pressure may double from 129 to 240, and the respiratory rate rises from 16 or 18 to about 69 breaths per minute. These signs increase slightly more in men than in women, perhaps in part because of the customary sexual position of the man on top. Thus the increase in vital signs can be moderated by a side-to-side position or a bottom position for the person with the heart condition. For most couples, the oxygen usage during the sex act is about equal to climbing one or two flights of stairs or walking rapidly at a rate of 2 to 2.5 miles per hour; therefore the ability to walk briskly for three blocks without chest distress, pain, palpitations, or shortness of breath is a rough indicator of readiness to resume sexuality. A program of physical conditioning (such as brisk walking and/or swimming) under a doctor's guidance as well as a fitness trainer is useful, in part because such conditioning can lower the pulse-rate rise during sex. If chest discomfort occurs, the use of coronary dilators such as nitroglycerine and a pattern of sexual activity after a period of rest are desirable. (Remember that sildenafil citrate/Viagra should never be used with nitrates.)

Episodes of congestive heart failure may require a period of 2 to 3 weeks of treatment and stabilization before sexual activity is resumed. With coronary bypass surgery, the sternum usually takes about three months to heal adequately enough for sexual intercourse to comfortably and safely continue. Medications such as beta-blockers may cause a decrease in sexual desire and erectile functioning. Switching to other medications with fewer sexual side effects, such as calcium channel blockers, may be possible and should be discussed with patients.

For cardiac patients, short-term treatment for anxiety and depression with appropriate medication may be helpful, but these medications, too, can interfere with sexual functioning. In the long run, reassurance and information from physicians and other health care providers about their cardiac condition, as well as sexual counseling, and individual, couples, or group psychotherapy are usually more effective treatment directions.

Patients with mild to moderate hypertension need not restrict themselves sexually. However, hypertension should be well-controlled by diet, exercise, weight control, and appropriate medication as indicated. With severe, uncontrolled hypertension medical management is a priority and sexual activity should be postponed until the blood pressure is improved. It is important to note that up to one-third of men with untreated hypertension report erectile dysfunction. Females have been less-well studied.

Unless a cerebrovascular accident causes severe trauma to the brain, sexual desire after this event often continues, although physical performance may be affected. Men tend to have erectile and ejaculatory difficulties, whereas women may experience problems with vaginal lubrication. Readjustments in one's expectations and experience are likely to be important and sexual couples counseling can be most helpful. Even if paralysis has occurred, appropriate sexual positions and bed boards can often be used to compensate for physical limitations. Above all, couples should be assured that sexual activity has *not* been found to be a factor in bringing on a stroke or causing more damage to those who have already had a stroke.

It is common for diabetic men and women to experience sexual dysfunction, and this may even be the first symptom of the disease. Diabetic men are three times more likely to experience erectile dysfunction than is the general population, and this is likely to affect patients an average of 10 to 15 years earlier than occurs in the general population.

Indicators for erectile problems in diabetic men older than age 60 years include prior alcohol intake and the degree to which the diabetes was initially controlled.

Diminished sexual desire in men may be associated with chronic prostatitis. There may be pain in the perineal region and at the end of the penis upon urination and ejaculation. Treatment includes antibiotics and warm sitz baths. Alcohol should be avoided.

Arthritis, a very common condition in older people, strikes women twice as frequently as it strikes men. Rheumatoid arthritis commonly begins between ages 25 and 50, and osteoarthritis in the later years. Hip discomfort is the arthritic problem that affects sexual activity most frequently. Patients should be encouraged to experiment with new sexual positions that do not aggravate pain in sensitive joints. A program of exercise, rest, and warm baths reduces arthritic discomfort. Exercise, including a full range of motion for stretching the joints and strengthening the muscles, can ease the discomfort. The use of heat both before undertaking an exercise program and before sex relaxes muscle spasms. Timing is important, since pain and stiffness may diminish at certain times of the day. For example, those with osteoarthritis usually find the morning most desirable and least uncomfortable, whereas those with rheumatoid arthritis experience greater pain and stiffness in the morning. It is reassuring to know that most drugs used to treat arthritis, with the exception of corticosteroids (which may produce at least temporary erectile difficulties), do not interfere with sexual desire or performance. There is also some evidence that regular sexual activity may provide a measure of relief for a period of time from the pain of rheumatoid arthritis.

Women who experience recurrent cystitis and urethritis after intercourse can take comfort in the fact that even long-standing conditions can often be evaluated and cured. Medication, surgical correction, education concerning sexual techniques and positions, and pain management can all help.

Stress or urge incontinence is a common factor for many women (approximately 20 percent of women older than age 40 years), especially those who have borne children, and can interfere with sexual function. Control and even total elimination of these problems are often possible. Mild conditions can often be resolved through the use of Kegel exercises. See Chap. 123 for a full discussion of the diagnosis and treatment of urinary incontinence.

Parkinson's disease commonly causes depression and may include problems of sexual dysfunction, including the loss of sexual desire. It has been found, however, that L-dopa improves sexual performance, largely because of an increased sense of well-being and greater mobility.

Peyronie's disease, which is found in men, produces an upward bowing of the penis with the shaft angled to the right or left. There is a fibrous thickening of the walls of the blood vessels or corpora cavernosa of the penis. Its causes are unknown, and it can make intercourse painful for approximately 50 percent of men who have it. Therapies include *p*-aminobenzoate, surgical removal of plaque formation, and cortisone injections. The application of ultrasound to the fibrous area of the penis can be helpful for men who have not had the disease for a long period.

Although no therapy has been universally successful, sexual activity usually can continue.

The pelvic steal syndrome is an example of erectile dysfunction resulting from circulatory changes. A man with this syndrome loses his erection as soon as he enters his partner and begins pelvic thrusting, redirecting the blood supply from the penis to the muscles in the buttocks which have been activated by the thrusting. If men lie on their back, they can alleviate this syndrome. A side position also may work.

Shortness of breath caused by chronic emphysema and bronchitis can hinder physical activity, including sex. Resting at intervals or the use of bronchodilators before sexual activity may help.

For persons with hernias, straining of any kind during sexual intercourse may increase hernia symptoms; although it is rare, this can lead to strangulation, resulting in a true emergency. Many surgeons recommend corrective hernia surgery early on rather than waiting for such an emergency to occur.

SURGERIES

Surgery that involves the sex organs frequently produces apprehension and worries about sexual consequences. Hysterectomy and mastectomy may have the psychological effects of causing a woman to feel that she is "less of a woman." Even a partial mastectomy can have understandable psychological implications. Men, on the other hand, tend to believe that prostate surgery means the end of their sex lives altogether. Patients should be reassured their fears are unlikely to be realized as long as their surgeons are skilled, knowledgeable about possible problems, and sensitive to their patients' interest in preserving sexual functioning. Both patients and their partners should be part of medical and psychological counseling by physicians and others before and after surgery.

Hysterectomy seldom causes sexual problems per se. Clitoral and vaginal sensations are not affected as long as wound repair from the hysterectomy is done carefully. However, some women do notice a change in the feeling of orgasm, because the uterus and cervix are no longer present and their rhythmic contractions are therefore absent. Overall, women are generally advised to wait 6 to 8 weeks after surgery before resuming sexual activity.

There is no known physiologic change in sexuality with mastectomy. However breast loss can have profound psychological implications for women and their partners. There is now a vast pool of knowledge on how to support women through their adjustment to breast loss, ranging from individual and couples counseling to group support through organizations such as Reach to Recovery and other programs designed specifically for this purpose.

Men who have a noncancerous prostatectomy find that potency is rarely affected, and, in fact, may improve with the alleviation of prostate symptoms. Transurethral prostatectomy, the least traumatic and safest surgical procedure, seldom affects potency. However, older men may also face the possibility of more extensive prostate surgery for cancer. Such surgery results in some degree of erectile dysfunction for approximately 60 percent or more of patients. Nerve-sparing surgery offers a much greater chance of preserving sexual potency. Oral sildenafil (Viagra) may be helpful for postprostate surgery sexual dysfunction. However, testosterone treatment must be avoided in patients with prostate cancer. Treatment of metastatic cancer of the prostate that involves orchiectomy, either medical or surgical, secondarily will cause impotence in most cases. Emotional preparation before and counseling after surgery are imperative.

EFFECTS OF ALCOHOL AND DRUGS

Drugs, including alcohol, can cause serious sexual problems for both men and women. Alcohol is an exceptionally common culprit that adversely affects sexual capability. Because of its nicotine content, tobacco is also a drug which may cause sexual difficulties through vasoconstriction. Regular use of opiates such as morphine and heroin is often sexually impairing, and those who are addicted usually develop chronic problems. Medications that counteract insomnia must be included here, because the majority of people older than age 50 years have some form of sleep disturbance. Although sleep deprivation itself can induce problems, the use of medication in treatment must be weighed against its untoward sexual effects. Nonmedical remedies should be tried first, such as relaxation exercises, meditation, warm baths, and the like.

Tranquilizers, antidepressants, anticholinergic, and certain antihypertensives have all been implicated in leading to sexual problems in men. The effects in women are less-well understood, largely because measures of female sexual response have been less-well developed.

Antihypertensive medications are the most common cause of impaired erection. Methyldopa (Aldomet) reduces the flow of blood into the pelvic area and inhibits erection. Guanethidine (Ismelin) may inhibit ejaculation. Angiotensin-converting enzyme (ACE) inhibitors, calcium channel blockers, and peripheral vasodilators appear to have few or no adverse effects on sexuality. Tranquilizers such as Mellaril (thioridazine) and other phenothiazines may cause failure to obtain an erection or ejaculate. Xanax and Valium, both minor tranquilizers, can have adverse effects on sexual capacity.

Depression is a common cause of sexual dysfunction. Not only are depressed individuals less likely to be sexually active, but many antidepressants (including the selective serotonin reuptake inhibitors [SSRIs]) that are frequently prescribed to alleviate depressive symptoms, have the side effect of inhibiting sexual arousal and orgasmic capacity. Depression also can be a result of inability to engage in satisfying sexual activity. Changes in medication may be possible. Drugs such as Remeron, Serzone, Wellbutrin, and possibly Celexa reportedly have fewer negative sexual side effects. In addition, reductions in antidepressant dosages, taking "drug holidays" (only possible with some medications and for some patients), and using another medication as an antidote may be options (for example, using Wellbutrin in addition to a person's regular antidepressant). Viagra is showing promise in several small studies. Surprisingly, even caffeine may be helpful.

SEXUALLY TRANSMITTED DISEASES

Among all persons with acquired immune deficiency syndrome (AIDS), 10 percent are older than 50 years of age and 4 percent are older than age 70 years. While most have received the human immunodeficiency virus (HIV) through blood transfusion, there are instances of older persons acquiring AIDS through intravenous drug use and through sexual intercourse. In addition, older men and women, especially those without partners, may seek paid sex, which can expose them to AIDS and other conditions. Therefore, safe sex, including latex condom use, should be de rigueur for older as well as younger people who are in nonmonogamous relationships. Older women are more vulnerable than older men because of vaginal thinness and the possibility of skin tearing. With the advent of protease inhibitors that extend the life expectancy of AIDS patients, there probably will be more older persons with AIDS. All other sexually transmitted diseases—genital herpes, gonorrhea, chlamydia, syphilis, and hepatitis B—can also occur in older persons. Early detection and treatment are essential. Hepatitis B is the only sexually transmitted virus that is preventable by vaccine.

PHYSICAL FITNESS

The maintenance and promotion of health—especially exercise, a moderate diet, adequate rest, and control of stress—also help to maintain sexual activity and contributes to continued attraction between partners. Specific exercise regimens may be indicated as well. For example, many women develop weakened pelvic muscles that can cause continence problems as well as lessen the capacity for a gripping response during sexual intercourse. Kegel exercises (described in Chap. 102) performed several times per day in a sitting or standing position can help greatly to improve this situation. These exercises may also help men treat or prevent prostatitis.

COMMON EMOTIONAL PROBLEMS

Up to now most attention has been directed toward the physical basis of sexuality. Most physical problems are associated with emotional reactions, and it is appropriate to assist patients with a psychological as well as a physical approach.

Sexual guilt and shame may still be operative in older persons, who may shy away from sexual activity such as masturbation or, if widowed, may find it difficult to date. There may also be problems between partners such as boredom, anger, grief, and the like. Individual psychotherapy or couple or group therapy can help. At times sexual therapists are necessary, following the contributions of William Masters and Virginia Johnson, who initiated a three-stage method of "sensate focus." This method is now used in many forms of sex therapy to teach people to relax and slowly move each other into a state of sexual arousal that eventually results in sexual pleasure and release.

Performance anxiety is common in older men and is often a result of the equation of masculinity with speedy and explosive sexual prowess. A man may become so preoccupied by his performance that his confidence and capacity are undermined and result in erectile dysfunction. Physical appearance changes with age are analogous concern, especially for women. Both of these situations can be alleviated through a variety of forms of information, support, and counseling.

WIDOWED AND SINGLE OLDER PERSONS

Women live on average 5.4 years longer than men and most women eventually become widowed. There are approximately 150 women for every 100 men older than age 65 years and 250 women for every 100 men older than age 85 years. This is a great disadvantage for women who are interested in relationships in their later years. Ultimately, medical science and public health programs are aiming at equalizing the life expectancies of men and women. In the meantime, older women themselves are adapting in a number of ways; by challenging negative social stereotypes; by learning to take the initiative in building friendships and a social life; and by redefining their own sexuality to include a wider range of options for satisfying intimacy and sexual release, including relationships with younger men.

The 5 percent of persons older than age 65 years, again mostly women, who live in homes for the aging, chronic disease hospitals, and other long-term care institutions are often denied the opportunity for a private, social, or sexual life. In fact, although federal regulations issued in 1978 provide some right to privacy, it is limited to married couples and to nursing homes and homes for the aging that participate in federal Medicare or Medicaid programs. These regulations are not uniformly enforced, but failure to observe them constitutes grounds for legal action.

LESBIAN, GAY, BISEXUAL, AND TRANSGENDER RELATIONSHIPS

It has been commonly held that life becomes increasingly bleak and lonely as a lesbian, gay, bisexual, or transgender (LGBT) person grows older. In reality this is an inaccurate assumption. An estimated 5 percent or more of all Americans characterize themselves as LGBT (a relatively new term designed to capture the full range of experience) and, like the heterosexual population, many are in long-term relationships that are emotionally stable and successful through the later years.

LGBT couples, of course, may face the same interpersonal problems that confront heterosexual couples. In addition, they many find themselves isolated and without support in the larger society. Often hospitals and other institutions do not recognize such relationship in terms of visitation rights and consultations with medical personnel. Legal rights are still often unclear and unprotected. For example, relatives of the deceased can and do contest wills that leave property to the unmarried partner of the deceased. There is now a growing sense of community and advocacy among the upcoming generations of LGBT persons. Specific organizations that address issues of LGBT aging have been formed around the country. An example is SAGE (Senior Action in the Gay Environment), which offers a variety of social services to older members in the New York metropolitan area. In San Francisco, New Leaf Outreach to Elders has a program of services for elders.

ADULT CHILDREN

At times, the adult children of older persons become vehemently opposed to a widowed parent's resumption of a sexually active life. They may be especially resistant to thoughts of a parent living with a new partner or remarrying. There are multiple reasons for these responses, including loyalty to a deceased parent, a negative relationship with the remaining parent, a willful personality, or a concern about inheritance. Prenuptial legal planning can help offset the latter concern. Family councils and heart-to-heart talks can often resolve other issues. Professional counseling may be necessary. The bottom line is that older persons have an inherent right to live their own lives and their children must eventually be led to accept this fact.

WHERE TO GO FOR HELP

Historically, it has not been easy to find physicians and other health providers who are knowledgeable about sexuality in general and sexuality among the aging in particular. Few medical and other professional schools teach the subject matter; therefore, most practitioners must learn on their own. In terms of specific health conditions, however, such as sex after an MI or surgery or the impact of medications, many physicians are becoming more aware of sexual implications and more skilled in helping to avoid or treat problems. Of course, some specialties such as urology have developed a good deal of expertise in dealing with problems like erectile dysfunction. Older people may need to be coached as to pertinent questions to ask health professionals. If satisfactory help is not forthcoming or knowledge is lacking, it will be necessary to search further for help.

For psychological or sexual counseling, most current information is now available quickly and in an up-to-date manner on the Internet. The American Association of Sex Educators, Counselors, and Therapists certifies sex counselors/therapists and has a national roster of providers. The Sex Information and Education Council of the United States (SIECUS) is an additional source of information and referral. The American Association for Marriage and Family Therapy, the National Institute of Mental Health's Public Information Office, the American Psychological Associations Aging Section and the National Association of Social Workers Aging Section are other referral resources, among others.

Organizations that offer support to individuals coping with a specific ongoing conditions include the Crohn's and Colitis Foundation, the United Ostomy Association, Reach to Recovery, and the like. Nearly every medical and psychological condition has a support group offering information, counseling and referral. The Internet also serves as an efficient way to locate resources.

CONCLUSION

Human intimacy is life-affirming and valid across the entire life span, with youth a time for exciting exploration and self-discovery, middle age a time for gaining skill and confidence, and old age a time for bringing the experience of a lifetime and the unique perspective of the final years of life to the art of loving another person. Indeed, younger persons have much to learn from those who have over the years personally mastered this complex and wonderful art.

REFERENCES

Butler RN, Lewis MI: *The New Love and Sex after Sixty: A Guide for Men and Women in Their Later Years,* 4th ed. New York, Ballantine, 2002.

Carson D et al: *Textbook of Erectile Dysfunction.* Oxford, Isis Medical Media, 1999.

Consumer Reports: *When Sex and Drugs Don't Mix.* Consumers Union of the United States, Yonkers, NY, December 1998 p. 9.

Derogatic LR Conklin-Powers B: Psychological assessment measures of female sexual functioning in clinical trials. *Int J Impot Res* 10:S1111, 1998.

Goldstein I et al: Oral sildenafil in the treatment of erectile dysfunction. *N Engl J Med* 338:1397, 1998.

Gwenwald M: The SAGE model of serving older lesbians and gay men, *Journal of Homosexuality* 20(3/4):53–61, 1991.

Laumann EO et al: Sexual dysfunction in the United States: Prevalence and predictors. *JAMA* 281:537, 1999.

McCullough AR: Management of erectile dysfunction following radical prostatectomy. *Sex Dysfunct Med* 2(1):2, 2001.

Muller JE et al: Triggering myocardial infarction by sexual activity. Low absolute risk and prevention by regular physical exercise. *JAMA* 245(18):1405, 1996.

Richardson JP, Lazur D: Sexuality and the nursing home patient. *Am Fam Physician* 51:121, 1995.

Rosen R: Effects of SSRIs on sexual function: A critical review. *J Clin Psychopharmacol* 19:65, 1999.

Schover L: *Sexuality and Cancer: For the Woman Who Has Cancer and Her Partner.* Atlanta, GA, American Cancer Society, 2001.

Schover L: *Cancer: For the Man Who Has Cancer and His Partner.* Atlanta, GA, American Cancer Society, 2001.

Siipski ML, Alexander CJ (eds): *Sexual Function in People with Disability and Chronic Illness: A Health Professional's Guide.* Gaithersburg, MD, Aspen Publishers, 1997.

Wolfe D: *Men Like Us: The GMHC Complete Guide to Gay Men's Sexual, Physical, and Emotional Well-Being.* New York, Ballantine Books, 2000.

Menopause and Midlife Health Changes

KAREN A. MATTHEWS • JANE A. CAULEY

The menopause is the permanent cessation of menses as a consequence of ovarian aging. Menopause is clinically diagnosed after 12 months of amenorrhea. Why is there a chapter on menopause and midlife health changes in this volume on geriatrics? First, because menopause is a clear milestone in a woman's life, indicating exposure to declining levels of ovarian hormones. Second, because midlife is a time of substantial risk factor changes in women, which provide the basis of the development of later debilitating diseases. Third, because midlife and the perimenopausal transition are optimal times for clinical intervention as most midlife women are not disabled, are open to information about preventive care and risk factor screening, and often seek care for menopausal symptoms.

This chapter begins by discussing some of the methodologic issues that have to be considered in understanding the effects of menopause in the context of midlife aging. It then reviews the demography of aging women and its relation to the menopausal transition; the endocrine basis of the menopause and associated symptoms; and the effects of the menopause and midlife aging on women's health defined broadly. The benefits and risks associated with hormone replacement therapy are reviewed elsewhere (see Chap. 97).

METHODOLOGIC ISSUES IN THE STUDY OF MENOPAUSE

Untangling the effects of menopause from aging of other systems has been difficult. Some studies have approached the study of menopause and midlife by using chronologic age as a proxy for menopause. However, the variation in age at menopause is substantial, and this approach is not sufficiently precise. A second, more precise approach is to use the date of the last menstrual period, but it is subject to memory distortions if information on bleeding patterns is not collected prospectively. A third approach uses prospective assignment of bleeding patterns and then compares the rate of change in women who change from pre- to postmenopause with age-adjusted changes in women who remain premenopausal. While this approach has been useful, the data it yields must also be interpreted with care because age at the menopause is associated with important sociocultural characteristics and health behaviors that challenge the interpretation of any data. Furthermore, these designs compare changes in women who have an early menopause with those who have a late menopause. Finally, changes in bleeding patterns are an approximate marker of ovarian aging, but are the best available at present for use in large-scale studies.

Several other challenges are noteworthy. Most of the large-scale epidemiologic studies recruited women who have been at least in their mid-forties. Consequently, a substantial number of younger women who had already ceased bleeding by their mid-forties were not included. Perhaps more importantly, because rates of hysterectomy peak in the early forties, many women who have had a surgical menopause prior to their mid-forties would not be eligible to be in the study. If women who are ineligible for the study because of surgical menopause are sicker or have a more adverse set of psychological symptoms or risk factors, the remaining women who experience a natural menopause may have little adverse response because they are healthier. In addition, there are marked ethnic differences in the rate of hysterectomy, which may result in selective exclusion of one group from these studies. An increasing number of women are electing to use hormone replacement therapy during the late perimenopausal and early postmenopausal periods, which may mask some of the effects of ovarian aging. Ovarian aging does not cease with the last menses.

Because of the above issues, some investigations have used hormone replacement therapy trials to make inferences about the effects of endogenous estrogens on diverse systems. While these investigations are useful in understanding the effects of replacement therapy on women's health, they do not allow strong inferences about the effects of ovarian aging. This is because types of estrogen and androgens administered, dosages, routes of administration, and the like, have substantial effects and hormone replacement therapy is not necessarily designed to mimic the menstrual cycle. Furthermore, studies of short-term use may yield different results than studies of long-term use. Finally, selection factors for hormone use are well established. Women who chose to go on hormones are, for example, thinner, more educated, less likely to smoke, and healthier, all of which could influence the results of these studies.

In our review below, we emphasize those studies that used the best available methodology, that is, prospective, longitudinal studies based on reasonable sample sizes and prospective measures of menstrual patterns. When such studies are not available, we note the methodologic constraints for interpreting the data. Finally, most of the data on the menopause has come from studies of white women, predominantly European and North American. It has been shown in several instances that the physiologic changes that accompany menopause differ in African American women and white women. Explanations for these discrepancies are currently unknown. Now, we turn to a description of the cohort of women approaching the menopausal transition.

DEMOGRAPHY OF AGING WOMEN AND AGE AT MENOPAUSE

The life expectancy of women born in 2000 in the United States is approximately 80 years, with life expectancy estimated to increase 4.3 years by the year 2050. A very large cohort of women born after World War II is in or approaching midlife (Fig. 99-1) and will result in an increasing number of women seeking treatment for symptoms associated with the menopause and for chronic conditions common in midlife.

The current cohort of US women entering midlife is unique. Around the turn of the century, approximately 20 percent of women were working outside the home. These women were usually single or widowed—very few were in career paths. By the year 2001, 76 percent of women ages 25 to 54 years were in the labor force. Women have fewer children at home than in previous generations. The number of live births per 1000 women aged 15 to 44 years has declined from the mid-1950s, when it was 120 to the approximate rate of 68 in 2000. Finally, women have more education than ever before. At the turn of the century, very few women had even a high school education, whereas now, among persons 25 to 29 years of age, 30 percent of women have received a 4-year undergraduate degree, as compared to 28 percent of men.

In contrast to substantial differences in labor force participation rates, family size, and education experienced by the current cohort of women approaching midlife relative to earlier cohorts, the current cohort may not experience a different median age at menopause. A natural menopause is estimated to occur at a median age of 51 years, with historical records dating back thousands of years suggesting 50 years as an approximate age of the menopause. However, most of the data are based on self-reported age of menopause from cross-sectional surveys, with less-than-optimal accuracy; sometimes it is not clear whether the definition is age at last menses or age at last menses plus 1 year, or if women who had a surgical menopause are included in the estimates. Finally, this cohort has also had relatively unique exposures. For example, it is likely to represent the first cohort to have potentially been exposed to oral contraceptives during the premenopausal period. It

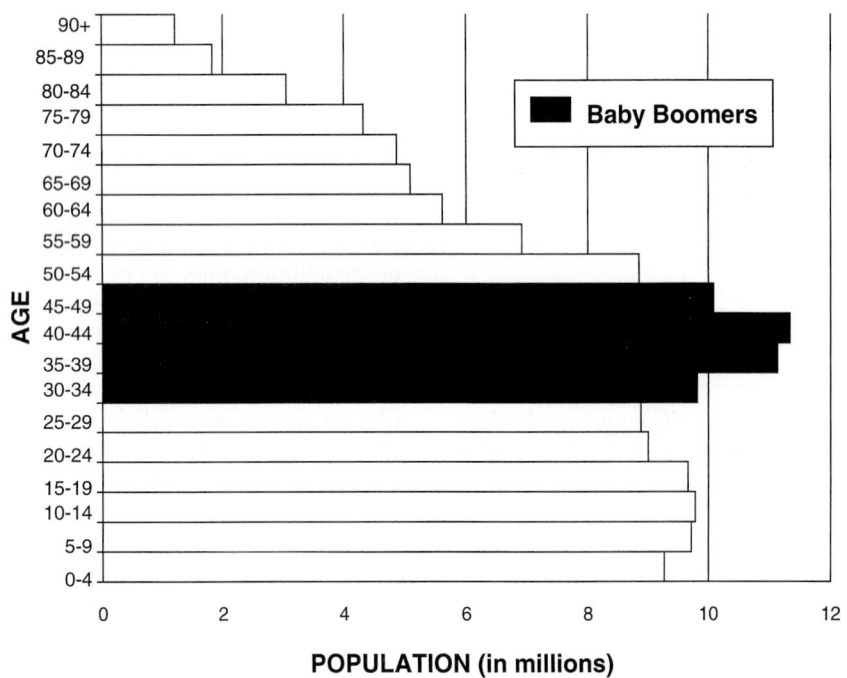

Figure 99-1   Age distribution of women in the United States in 2000. Source: US Census of Bureau, 1992.

Table 99-1 Percent Probability of Menopause According to Duration of First Amenorrhea and Age

Length of First Amenorrheal Interval in Days	Age Group		
	45–49 Years	50–52 Years	≥53 Years
60–89	6.0	21.6	35.2
90–119	12.8	30.4	47.4
120–149	25.1	42.4	56.2
150–179	39.5	56.4	65.6
180–209	45.5	65.2	71.9
210–239	55.3	73.1	78.4
240–269	63.5	81.5	85.3
270–299	74.1	86.3	88.6
300–329	83.0	90.3	89.5
330–359	88.2	92.5	92.9
360+	89.5	93.6	95.5

Source: Wallace et al. (1979).

is unknown if prior exposure to oral contraceptives will influence the menopausal experience. In one study, an increase in breast cancer among long-term postmenopausal hormone users was only observed among women who had used oral contraceptives for 10 or more years.

Menopausal status can only be determined accurately after retrospective review of the patterns and absence of menses collected prospectively. Not surprisingly, the probability of menopause increases with increasing duration of amenorrhea. After 6 months of amenorrhea, the probability that a woman is menopausal ranges from 46 percent to 72 percent, depending on her age. More than 90 percent of women are menopausal after 12 months of amenorrhea. Table 99-1 shows the association between length of amenorrhea and likelihood of being menopausal according to age groups 45 to 49, 50 to 52, and 53 years and older.

The perimenopausal transition is defined as the period of time prior to permanent cessation of menses that is characterized by menstrual cycle irregularity. The transition is highly variable in length, ranging from 2 to 8 years. Early perimenopause is thought to occur when the neurohormonal systems that govern ovulation dysregulate without evidence of overt changes in menstrual cycle patterns. Middle to late perimenopause is characterized by more overt changes in menstrual cycles including irregularity and cycle length. In the Massachusetts Women's Health Study of women ages 45 to 55 years, a median of 3.8 years elapsed between the first time a woman reported changes in menstrual regularity and menopause, defined as 12 months of amenorrhea. Ten percent of the women ceased cycling immediately after the first change in menstrual regularity. Figure 99-2 shows the percentages of women who were peri- and postmenopausal at 45 to 55 years of age in this study.

There is a wide variation in age at natural menopause, with ages 40 to 55 years considered to be typical. Factors that are related to early age at a natural menopause include smoking, lean body weight, low social class, nulliparity or having few children, short cycle length, and African American ethnicity. Smoking, the most established risk factor for an early menopause, may cause an earlier onset because smoking may affect the rate of the metabolism of estrogen and accelerate follicle aging and estrogen-receptor binding.

Environmental factors, however, explain only a modest portion of the variance around the age at menopause. Heritability estimates for age at natural menopause in a population-based sample of sisters range from 0.71 to 0.87, indicating a major genetic role in determining age at menopause. Although the exact genes that contribute to age at menopause are unknown, it is likely that multiple genes contribute, each with small to modest effects.

OVARIAN AGING AND ASSOCIATED SYMPTOMS

The number of follicles remaining in the ovary is a major determinant of the timing of both the perimenopause and menopause. There is a 10-fold difference in the number of ovarian follicles between regularly menstruating women and perimenopausal women. The factors that precipitate the decline in follicles is unknown. However, it has been hypothesized that elevations in follicle-stimulating hormone (FSH) in the decade preceding menopause may contribute to the acceleration in the loss of ovarian follicles.

The menopausal transition is accompanied by marked endocrine changes both in the period leading to complete cessation of menses and the period following cessation of menstruation. There have been relatively few longitudinal studies of the hormonal changes across menopause. The available studies are limited to white women.

Dramatic endocrine changes in a large number of hormones occur during the peri- and postmenopausal periods, but the magnitude, pattern, and timing of these changes are uncertain. This uncertainty reflects the difficulty in carrying out longitudinal studies of women undergoing a natural menopause. Methodologic issues include the difficulty in standardizing the blood draw for specific menstrual days, especially as a woman's cycle becomes more irregular.

In a 6-year longitudinal study of 150 women who experienced a natural menopause, FSH levels started to increase approximately 2 years before the last menstrual period, increased most rapidly within 10 months before the last menstrual period, and had plateaued by 2 years. In a similar fashion, estradiol levels began to decrease about 2 years prior to the final menstrual period, to decline most rapidly around the time of menopause, and to plateau also by 2 years after the last menstrual period. This stabilization in estradiol was also observed by Longcope et al. (Table 99-2), although data from Sweden suggested that the decline in serum estrogen might continue for up to 8 years after cessation of menses. Furthermore, several studies indicate that the estradiol level may be fairly stable in the early

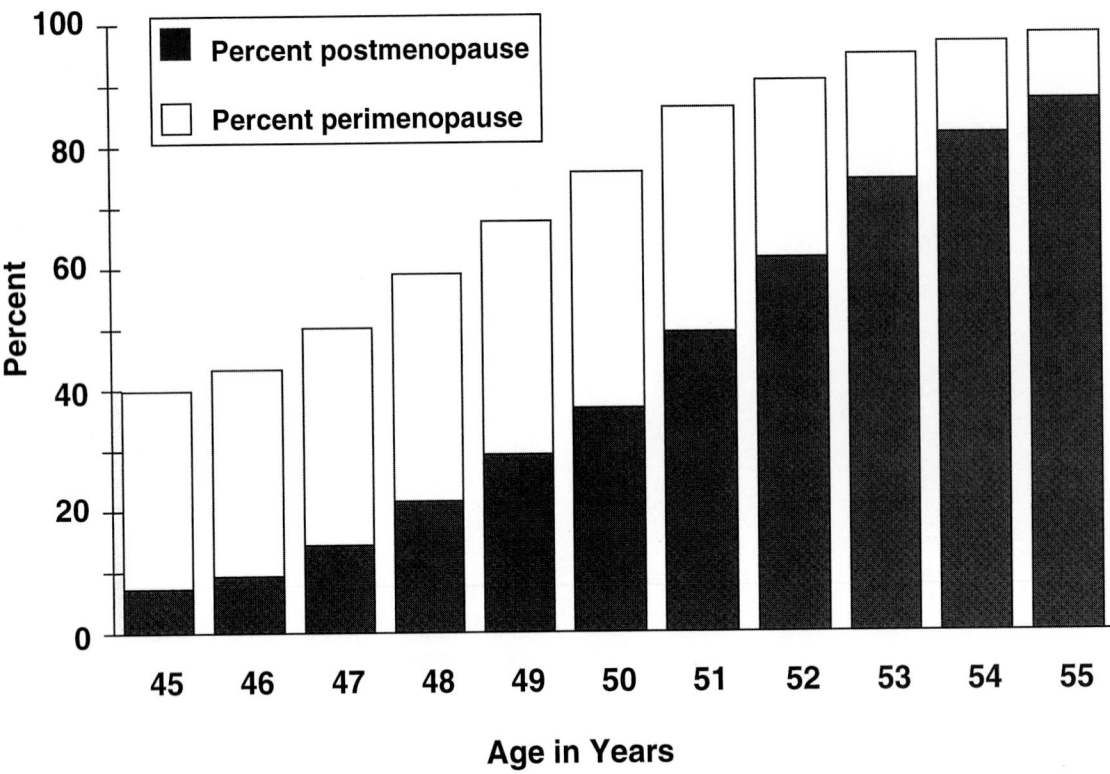

Figure 99-2 Massachusetts Women's Health Study (MWHS) proportion of women who are peri- and postmenopausal at ages 45 to 55 years. (Percentage distributions, by age, at T_0 for two menopausal transitions, excluding surgical menopause: MWHS 1981–82 (n = 5547). Median age at inception of perimenopause = 47.5 years; median age at menopause (last menstrual period) = 51.3 years.) Adapted from McKinlay et al. The normal menopause transition. *Maturitas* 14:103, 1992.

perimenopause at a time when anovulatory cycles are common, leading to a hyperestrogenic state. It has been speculated that an unopposed estrogenic state may lead to excessive bleeding in the perimenopause.

Progesterone levels declined with cessation of menses and leveled off in the Longcope study (Table 99-2). There was little change in serum testosterone and androstenedione levels around the menopausal transition in this

study. It has been postulated that the decline in androgens may precede the decline in the estrogens, and hence could not be characterized. It is possible, however, that the postmenopausal ovary continues to secrete testosterone, thereby maintaining its concentration.

Premenopausally, the major source of estrogen is ovarian secretion and the predominant estrogen is estradiol. Postmenopausally, the major source of estrogen is the

Table 99-2   Mean Concentrations of Serum Hormones and Gonadotrophins According to Months From Last Menses

Months From Last Menses	Estrone (pg/mL)	Estradiol (pg/mL)	Progesterone (ng/mL)	Testosterone (pg/mL)	Androstenedione (ng/mL)	Luteinizing hormone (mIU/mL)	Follicular stimulating hormone (mIU/mL)
0–0.9	78 ± 55	92 ± 83	1.61 ± 3.65	0.19 ± 0.10	0.59 ± 0.36	13 ± 13	17 ± 17
1–1.9	69 ± 50	88 ± 89	0.56 ± 0.62	0.18 ± 0.09	0.44 ± 0.26	32 ± 20	38 ± 29
2–5.9	64 ± 64	79 ± 108	0.36 ± 0.39	0.22 ± 0.12	0.45 ± 0.28	38 ± 20	49 ± 23
6–11.9	50 ± 42	45 ± 57	0.23 ± 0.14	0.17 ± 0.08	0.49 ± 0.32	36 ± 19	56 ± 25
12–17.9	34 ± 12	28 ± 16	0.21 ± 0.17	0.18 ± 0.10	0.45 ± 0.29	42 ± 16	75 ± 24
18–23.9	45 ± 24	35 ± 30	0.34 ± 0.39	0.20 ± 0.11	0.50 ± 0.26	38 ± 12	65 ± 24
24–35.9	34 ± 14	24 ± 11	0.29 ± 0.26	0.21 ± 0.12	0.52 ± 0.34	40 ± 17	78 ± 29
36–80	34 ± 14	21 ± 10	0.26 ± 0.21	0.17 ± 0.08	0.53 ± 0.46	34 ± 12	64 ± 20

SOURCE: Longcope et al. (1986).

Table 99-3 Percentage of Women Reporting Symptoms in Previous 2 Weeks at Baseline and Peri- or Postmenopausal Examination

	Examination		
	Baseline	Perimenopausal	Postmenopausal
Forgetful	41	53*	45
Headache	56	47	48
Constipation	18	25*	26
Heart pounding	14	25*	19
Trouble sleeping	24	33	38
Aches in neck/skull	29	38*	26
Joint pain	27	43*	39*
Crying spells	23	21	16
Depressed	42	35	35
Hot flashes	19	59*	64*
Cold sweats	4	16*	13

*$p < .05$ compared to Baseline percentage.

SOURCE: Adapted with permission from Matthews et al. (1990 and 1994).

aromatization of androstenedione to estrone, which primarily occurs in fat tissue. Estrone, although a biologically weaker estrogen, is the predominant estrogen. Postmenopausally the estrone to estradiol ratio is about 2:1. The peripheral aromatization of androstenedione to estrone is twofold higher and the aromatization of testosterone to estradiol is threefold higher among postmenopausal women older than age 60 years as compared with regularly menstruating women younger than age 40 years. The interconversions of androstenedione to testosterone and estrone to estradiol do not appear to vary in pre- and postmenopausal women.

The perimenopausal transition is associated with hot flashes (or flushes), sweats, and perhaps insomnia. It appears that a long transition, that is, a long interval between the inception of the perimenopause and the cessation of menses, is associated with a greater risk of vasomotor symptoms. Approximately 10 to 20 percent of regularly menstruating midlife women report hot flashes in the last 2 weeks of the menstrual cycle, peaking at 50 to 60 percent of perimenopausal women reporting hot flashes. Reporting of hot flashes is associated with low levels of serum estradiol and estrone. More generally, it appears that the early perimenopause is associated with a greater number and diversity of symptoms than is the early postmenopausal period. Table 99-3 shows the percentages of women in the Pittsburgh Healthy Women Study reporting symptoms when still menstruating, when perimenopausal was defined as no menses for 3 to 5 months, and when postmenopausal was defined as no menses for at least 12 months. Comparisons of the percentages of women reporting symptoms at the perimenopause or postmenopause, compared to the premenopause, showed more types of symptoms associated with the perimenopause than with the postmenopause.

A recent cross-sectional survey of ethnically diverse women of varying health status has also confirmed that being perimenopausal is associated with elevated risk of experiencing hot flashes and night sweats in the previous 2 weeks as well as urine leakage, vaginal dryness, stiffness, forgetfulness, and difficulty sleeping. Being African American, obese, a smoker, having low educational attainment, or physical inactivity was associated with elevated rates of vasomotor symptoms.

The above conclusions regarding menopause-induced symptoms are based on studies of women who have a natural menopause. Hysterectomy is second only to cesarean section as the most frequently performed major operation in the United States. By age 60 years, more than one-third of US women have undergone hysterectomy, with the rates of hysterectomy peaking between ages 40 and 44 years. Ninety percent of hysterectomies are elective, with 30 percent for uterine leiomyomas, 20 percent for dysfunctional uterine bleeding, 20 percent for endometriosis, and 15 percent for genital prolapse. Excessive bleeding is the symptom shared by the first three conditions. Excessive bleeding may be exacerbated by the menopausal transition. In addition, high rates of hysterectomy during the period of rapid ovarian aging may be related to issues of quality of life after the usual childbearing years.

Hysterectomy resulted in marked improvements in a range of symptoms, including pelvic pain, urinary symptoms, fatigue, psychological symptoms, and sexual dysfunction after 1 year in the prospective Maine Women's Health Study of hysterectomy. Most frequent new problems among hysterectomized women in this study were hot flashes and weight gain, reported by 12 percent and 13 percent, respectively. Women who had a bilateral salpingo oophorectomy reported most of the hot flashes. Vasomotor symptoms among hysterectomized women are correlated with other symptom complaints. Hormone replacement therapy can reduce vasomotor symptoms among women who have had oophorectomy and should be considered, even among overweight women.

MIDLIFE AGING AND CHRONIC CONDITIONS

Quality of Life and Mental Health

Health-related quality of life refers to freedom from emotional and physical disorders that allow women to carry out important life tasks of work, family, and relationships. An important clinical issue is the extent to which menopausal symptoms lower overall quality of life. Women who report severe vasomotor symptoms also report many other symptoms not thought to be related to the natural menopause, but it is not clear if the vasomotor symptoms interfere with quality of life or if the associations reflect a more general style of symptom reporting. Decline in exposure to estrogen is thought to affect sexuality in midlife. Estrogens stimulate the synthesis, maturation, and turnover in collagen, leading to dermal atrophy. Collagen loses its flexibility as fibrillar cross-links develop. Attenuation of sexual activity may result in part because of the atrophic endothelial changes in the vagina. Atrophic changes in the vagina include a decrease in lubrication accompanying sexual arousal, thinning of the endothelium, and loss of rogation, which are associated with dyspareunia. Libido and sexual activity, however, have not been studied in longitudinal studies of the menopause, so the extent of estrogen-dependent alterations in sexual interest and behavior is unknown. Small clinical studies suggest that estrogen administration alleviates symptoms associated with atrophic changes in the vagina and dyspareunia, but testosterone, not estrogen, may be related to sexual interest. A sexually interested partner and the quality of the women's relationship with her partner are of obvious importance.

Sleep problems are twice as common among women than among men. The number of women reporting sleep disturbances increases in their forties and plateaus by the end of the fifth decade. In the Pittsburgh Healthy Women Study, 42 percent reported some type of sleep disturbance and trouble sleeping was correlated with higher levels of anxiety, depressive symptoms, and stress. Several small clinical studies have shown that estrogen replacement therapy can reduce sleeping difficulties in patients experiencing substantial sleep disturbance due to severe vasomotor symptoms.

Historically, menopause was thought to cause poor mental health, especially depression and anxiety. At one time, involutional melancholia or menopausal depression was a distinct clinical depressive entity and a definition for it was included in the second edition of the *Diagnostic and Statistical Manual* (the classification and definition of psychiatric disorders). In the late 1970s, Weissman demonstrated that there was no empirical evidence of a unique menopausal

depressive disorder and the classification was omitted from subsequent editions of the manual.

Recent epidemiologic investigations of prevalence rates of psychiatric disorders do not show that women in midlife have elevated rates of depression. Only one prospective study has included psychiatrist-diagnosed "mental disability" and showed no increased risk among menopausal women. Other longitudinal studies of increases in depressive symptoms also show no direct effect of menopausal status. Rather, it appears that chronic stress and life events common in midlife, for example, illness and death of parents, and a history of previous depression are the most important determinants of increases in depression. There is no evidence that the "empty nest syndrome" leads to depression. In a cross-sectional analysis of depressive symptoms in the Pittsburgh Healthy Women Study participants, those whose children had moved out of the home in the previous 6 months had lower rates of symptoms than those who remained at home.

Cognitive Function

The influence of aging on cognitive function has been the subject of extensive investigation (see Chap. 105). However, only a few longitudinal studies of normal aging provide the basis for strong conclusions. In general, these studies show that different types of cognitive ability appear to decline at different ages. The cognitive ability that is most likely to change in midlife is the ability to retain a large amount of new information, or secondary memory function. Other abilities appear to be altered later in the life course.

The influence of ovarian aging specifically on cognitive function has rarely been studied. Women during the perimenopause and early postmenopause do report being forgetful, but it is not clear whether this is an effect of ovarian aging. Studies of the effects of hormone replacement therapy provide indirect clues as to the effects of declining ovarian hormones on cognitive function. Although not entirely consistent, available longitudinal data from large-scale studies suggest that hormone replacement therapy does not prevent age-related deficits in cognitive function. A number of early observational studies and a few small clinical trials indicate that women who use estrogen replacement therapy are less likely to be diagnosed with Alzheimer's disease than are nonusers. More recent studies fail to support this hypothesis, including a randomized clinical trial of 120 women with mild to moderate Alzheimer's disease. It has been suggested that estrogen may delay the initiation of neurodegeneration, as opposed to the progression of Alzheimer's' disease. Several ongoing large clinical trials, including the Women's Health Initiative–Memory Study, will provide more definitive data in the future. At present, there is not sufficient scientific evidence to recommend hormone replacement therapy on a routine basis to prevent or delay Alzheimer's disease.

Body Composition

Obesity is a major public health problem in midlife. National surveys have documented a dramatic increase in the proportion of overweight (defined as body mass index [BMI] of ≥ 25 kg/m^2) and obese (defined as BMI of ≥ 30 kg/m^2) individuals in the United States over the past two decades. Based on National Health and Nutrition Examination Survey (NHANES) III data, nearly 38 percent of women ages 40 to 49 years and 42 percent of women ages 50 to 59 years are overweight. The age-adjusted prevalence of overweight is even more striking among African American and Mexican American women with approximately half being classified as overweight. Several studies suggest that midlife, particularly menopause, is associated with significant weight gain in women. However, weight gain during the perimenopausal transition appears to be attributable more to chronologic aging, as opposed to ovarian aging. Among women enrolled in the Pittsburgh Healthy Women Study, the average weight gain during the initial 3 years of the study was about 2 kg. Of importance, there was no difference in the amount of weight gained between women who remained premenopausal and those who transitioned during the 3-year period. Although the number of African Americans in this study was relatively small, the data suggested that the weight gain was greater among this ethnic group. Women who experienced the greatest weight gain also reported the greatest decline in physical activity.

Body weight consists of several compartments, including fat mass, fat-free mass, skeletal mass, and a fluid compartment. Examination of weight change through the menopause could mask important changes within each compartment. Changes in body composition could impact on a woman's risk of a number of chronic health conditions as well as contribute to the onset of functional disability, independent of her total body weight. Resting metabolic rate represents the largest portion of the daily energy expenditure, accounting for approximately 60 to 75 percent. It has been reported that resting metabolic rate declines during menopause, likely due to the concomitant decrease in metabolically active lean (skeletal) mass that occurs. Energy expenditure from physical activity may also decrease during the menopause. Thus, small changes in daily energy expenditure from physical activity and resting metabolic rate without a proportionate decrease in energy intake could adversely influence changes in body composition.

Changes in body composition with aging have been fairly well characterized by using a variety of assessment and imaging techniques. In general, cross-sectional and longitudinal studies in women show an increase in total body fat with age. Accumulation of adipose tissue in the trunk and in the intraabdominal area occurs. Fat-free mass or lean mass declines. Extracellular fluid increases with age as the proportion of the total body fluid. Bone mass also declines.

Few studies have examined changes in body composition longitudinally through the menopausal transition. However, it appears that age-related changes begin around the median time of menopause in women. Both cross-sectional and longitudinal studies have documented a loss of lean mass and accumulation of central body adiposity with menopause. A well-controlled longitudinal study demonstrated that over 6 years of follow-up, women who experienced menopause lost more fat-free mass than

age-matched women who remained premenopausal (mean = -3.0 ± 1.1 kg and -0.05 ± 0.5, respectively). Women who became menopausal also experienced greater declines in their resting metabolic rate and greater increases in fat mass, particularly in the abdominal region. Of interest, leisure time physical activity declined in the menopausal group. A 4.5-year follow-up study observed increases in fat mass (including waist-to-hip ratio) along with decreases in lean mass among middle-aged women approaching menopause. Physical activity in these women was associated with preservation of lean mass. Both studies only recruited white women. The results of these studies, if confirmed in larger samples of ethnically diverse women, suggest that the hormonal changes associated with the menopause may precipitate adverse changes in body composition as part of a complex metabolic process that occurs during this transitional period.

Differences in fat mass are smaller between endurance trained older and younger athletes compared to older and younger sedentary individuals. Similar patterns have not been consistently observed for fat-free mass. Studies show that women who gain weight or experience a gain in fat mass and a loss in lean mass in midlife report decreases in leisure time physical activity. Although many reasons besides optimization of body composition provide encouragement for women to maintain their physical activity as they age, these studies suggest that increases in physical activity could partially offset the potentially detrimental changes in body composition that accompany menopause.

Bone Mineral Density

Albright et al. first described a link between the decline in estrogens at menopause and bone loss in 1940. However, the rate, duration and quantity of loss, and the timing of onset have not been definitively established, especially across several skeletal sites and particularly those that are most prone to fracture. Some, but not all studies have suggested that bone loss may begin prior to the menopause, perhaps as early as the third decade. However, cross-sectional and longitudinal studies have reported mixed results.

The work of Ahlborg et al. confirms the acceleration of bone loss during the first 5 years of menopause. In a sample of white women followed prospectively for 16 years, the rate of radial bone loss 1 year premenopause to 5 years postmenopause approximated 2.4 to 2.6 percent per year compared to 0.4 to 1.9 percent per year 5 to 11 years postmenopause. In contrast to other studies, age at menopause did not seem to significantly influence bone mineral density at age 64 years (Fig. 99-3).

Several reports have summed the total amount of postmenopausal bone loss. For the hip, the average bone loss after the first 5 years at menopause was 9 to 13 percent; after 20 years, 17 to 30 percent. For the radius, the average bone loss 8 years after menopause was 16 percent. Patterns of loss may differ for axial and appendicular sites. These values are averages, but the rate of bone loss varies markedly within individuals ranging from a 50 percent loss to a gain of 5 percent (Fig. 99-4). The individual variability

Spine BMD Relative to Baseline

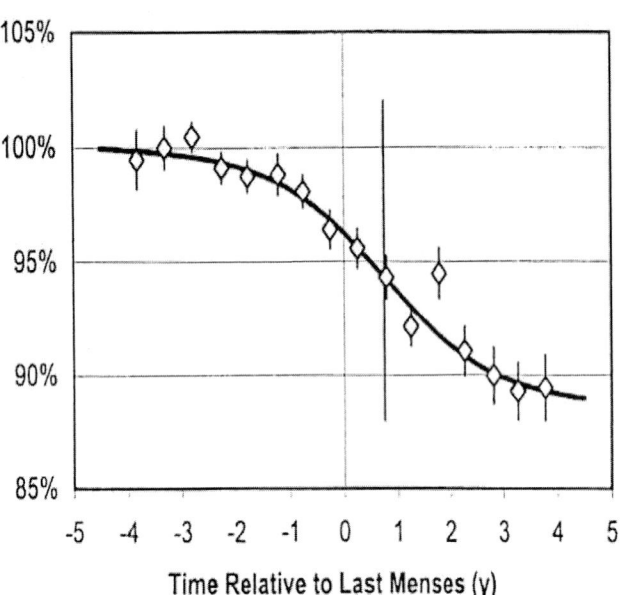

Spine BMD Relative to Baseline

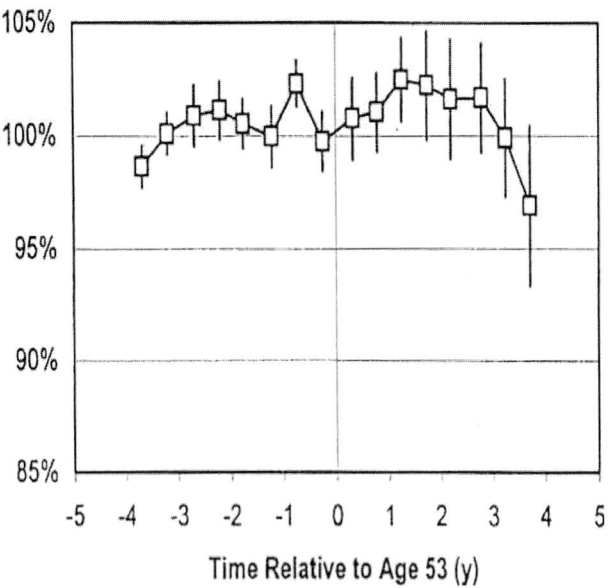

Figure 99-3 Time course of spine bone mineral density (BMD) relative to baseline. Bone loss is expressed as a percentage of the baseline value, defined at the age of last menses for postmenopausal women, and for estrogen replete women, corresponding to the average age of last menses for the postmenopausal women. Postmenopausal women experienced an estrogen-dependent loss of spine (10.5 percent) BMD that began 2 years prior to the last menses and continued for 3 to 4 years after the last menses Adapted from Recker et al: Characterization of perimenopausal bone loss: A prospective study *J Bone Miner Res* 15(10):1970, 2000. Used with permission of author.

in bone loss is present even among women 10 years after menopause, ranging from a loss of 22 percent to a gain of 6 percent.

Osteoporosis is characterized not only by loss of bone mass, but also by microarchitectural deterioration of bone tissue. Provocative data from Japan using peripheral quantitative computed tomography (QCT) measures of the distal radius demonstrated a significant increase in the number of trabecular perforations among women within the first 5 years after the menopause. The lack of difference in bone mineral density between premenopausal and early postmenopausal women in this sample may suggest that the trabecular bone disconnectivity may precede significant bone loss. Quantitative ultrasound measures of bone are believed to reflect not only the density of the bone but also the quality of the bone and are lower among postmenopausal Japanese women. Assessment of bone microarchitecture may be more sensitive to early menopausal changes in bone than traditional bone mineral density measures.

Hip fractures are the most serious consequence of osteoporosis. The average age at hip fracture in women is 80 years; thus, there is an average of 30 years between when a woman goes through menopause and when she is likely to fracture her hip. Bone mineral density predicts hip fracture over the short-term in postmenopausal women, but it is unknown if bone mineral density measurements at the menopause or rates of bone loss at menopause predict subsequent risk of hip fracture. Black and colleagues developed a model that estimates a woman's risk of fracture from a measurement of radial bone mass at age 50 years. A 50-year-old white woman has a 19 percent lifetime risk of hip fracture if her radial bone mass is in the 10th percentile for her age and an 11 percent lifetime risk if her bone mineral density is in the 90th percentile. In a 15-year study, a high rate of bone loss during the early postmenopausal period, along with low bone mineral density at menopause, predicted subsequent risk of wrist and spine fracture. Thus, measures of bone mineral density at menopause and information about the rate of bone loss in the first 2 years after menopause may identify high-risk women and could assist clinicians and patients in the decision to begin various therapies to prevent osteoporotic fractures.

In summary, there is growing evidence primarily from longitudinal studies that bone loss at several key skeletal sites begins early and accelerates in the late perimenopausal period and continues into the early postmenopausal period. The rate of loss tends to decelerate 10 years after menopause. The total amount of bone loss is estimated at 16 to 20 percent. Of importance, there are marked individual differences in the rate of bone loss. It is unknown which factors contribute to this wide individual variability. Preliminary models developed using appendicular bone mineral density suggest that bone mineral density measured at menopause may identify women at higher risk of hip fracture. Because hipbone mineral density predicts hip fracture better than radial bone mineral density, future models based on hipbone mineral density are needed. More research is also needed to evaluate the predictive value of measures of bone microarchitecture and rates of bone loss in determining future risk of fracture.

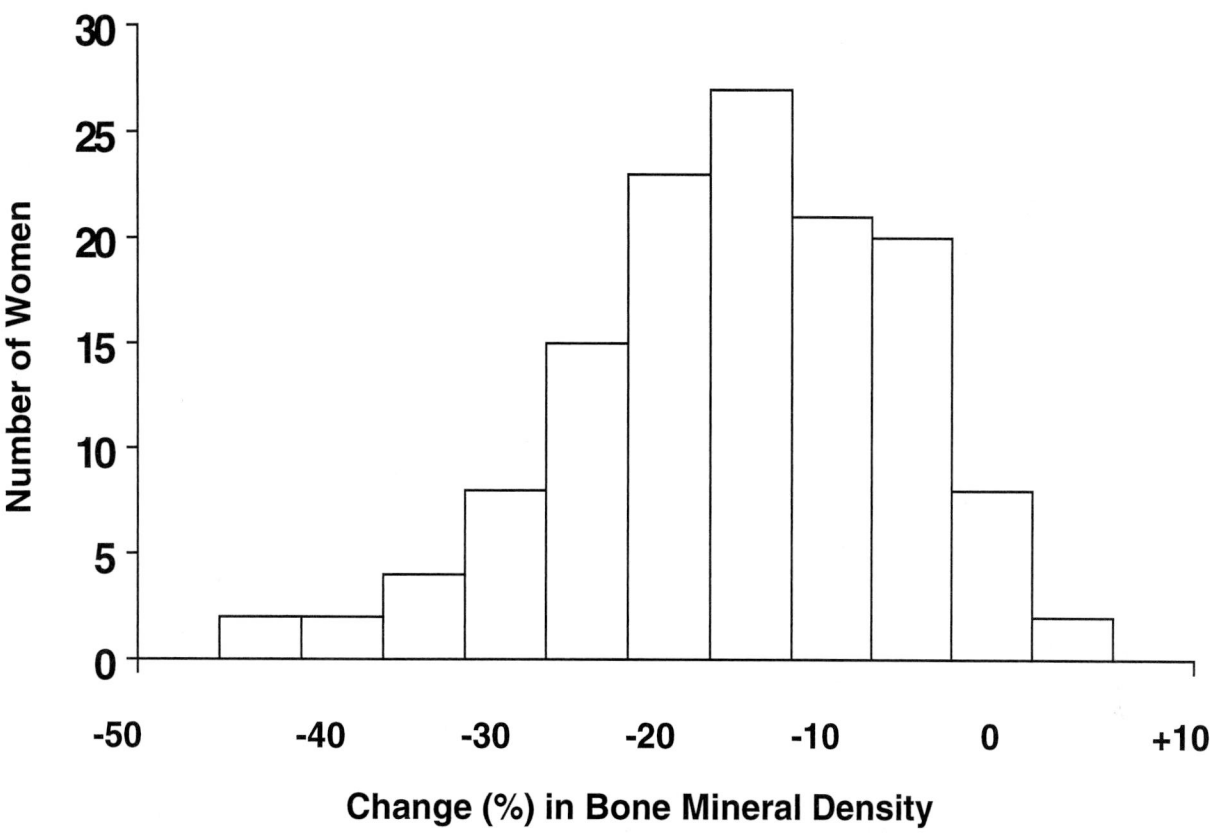

Figure 99-4 Number of women with a change in midshaft radius bone density from 13 to 24 months premenopausal to 73 to 96 months postmenopause. Adapted from Rannevik et al: A longitudinal study of the perimenopausal transition: Altered profiles of steroid and pituitary hormones, SHBG, and bone mineral density. *Maturitas* 21:103, 1995.

Osteoarthritis

Osteoarthritis is the most common rheumatic disease and a major cause of pain, physical disability and loss of independence in older adults. The evidence that sex steroid hormones may play a role in the etiology of osteoarthritis comes from several observations. Osteoarthritis is more common in women than men, a gender difference that begins around the time of menopause. After the age of 50 years, women appear to be affected more often than men, with greater severity and more joints involved. A specific type of "menopausal arthritis" has been described consisting of rapidly progressing hand osteoarthritis. As noted in Table 99-3, joint pain is commonly reported by women as they transition.

Hormone replacement therapy is associated with a lower risk of hip and knee osteoarthritis in some studies, but not in all studies. There have been few randomized trials. As part of the Heart Estrogen/Progestin Replacement Study, 4 years of hormone replacement therapy had no effect on knee pain or related disability. This study did not, however, include direct measures of radiographic changes. Hormone users may have a lower risk of hip or knee osteoarthritis, but this lower risk may reflect a lower risk profile, for example, less obesity among estrogen users.

There are few studies of endogenous hormones and osteoarthritis, and their results are conflicting. For example, no association was obtained between endogenous estrogen concentrations and prevalent hand osteoarthritis among older women. However, only total estradiol was measured. Observations of an association between sex hormone-binding globulin and osteoarthritis suggest a need to measure the biologically active form of estradiol. The observations of an increase in cytokine activity at menopause and the ability of estrogen to reverse or oppose this increase suggest a complex interaction between inflammatory actions and endogenous hormone concentrations. Changes in body composition across menopause, in particular, a possible loss of lower extremity lean mass, may also contribute to the increase in osteoarthritis around menopause. Finally, estrogen receptors have been identified in articular cartilage and several polymorphisms in both estrogen receptors may contribute to the development of osteoarthritis. Other cytokine and growth factor genes may also play a role in osteoarthritis and could influence the expression of osteoarthritis at menopause.

In summary, the degree to which menopause and, by inference, sex hormones contribute to either the development or progression of osteoarthritis has not been established. Longitudinal studies of changes in cartilage with age and across the menopause using more sensitive techniques such as high-resolution magnetic resonance imaging could identify earliest measurable changes in cartilage and subchondral bone and identify the risk factors both hormonal and nonhormonal that contribute to these changes.

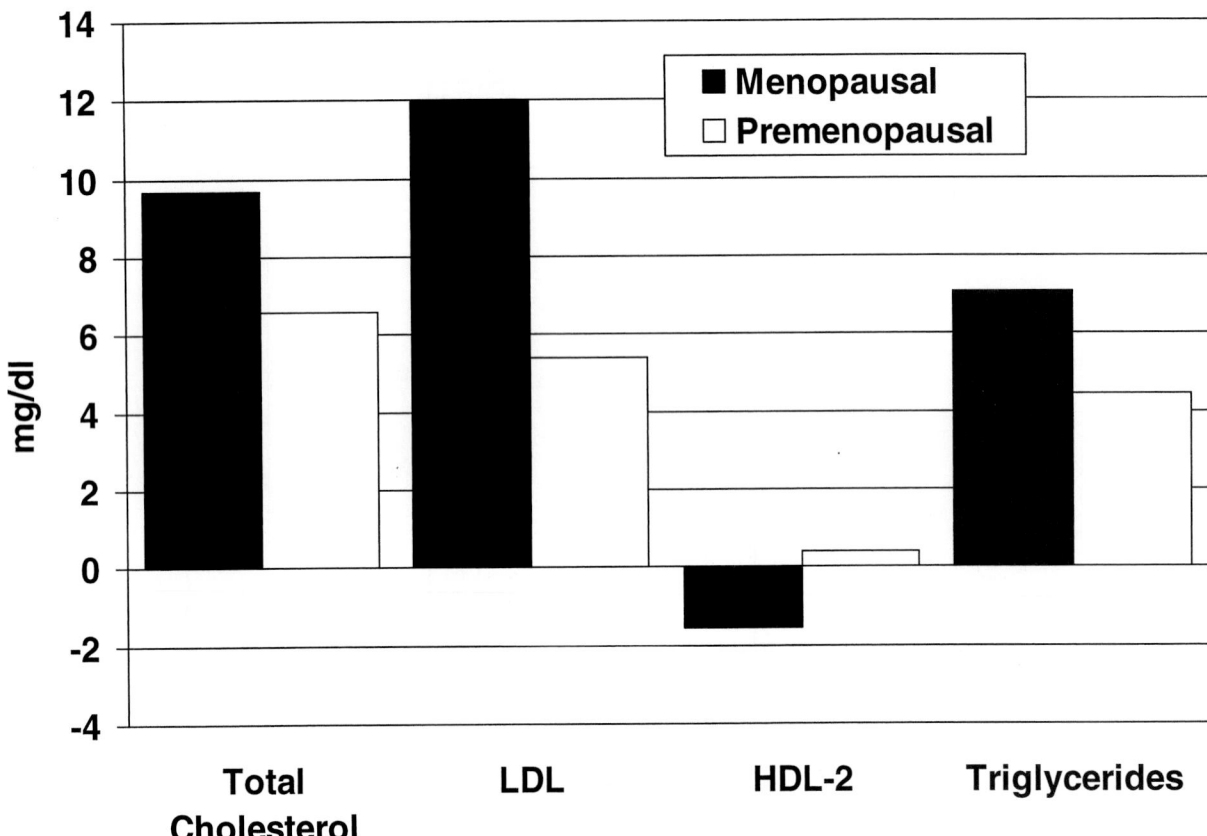

Figure 99-5   Changes in cholesterol and lipid levels for premenopausal and menopausal women in Healthy Women Study. Adapted from Matthews et al. Menopause and coronary heart disease risk factors. *N Engl J Med* 321:641, 1989. Used with permission of author.

Cardiovascular Function and Risk Factors

Bilateral salpingo oophorectomy is associated with heightened risk for cardiovascular disease, especially when it occurs relatively early and without hormone replacement therapy as treatment. An early natural menopause is also associated with heightened risk for cardiovascular disease, although statistical adjustments for other cardiovascular risk such as age and smoking can eliminate the association of age at natural menopause and cardiovascular disease. Atherosclerosis in the abdominal aorta is more likely among women who have a bilateral oophorectomy or early natural menopause than among premenopausal women.

Prospective studies of the natural history of cardiovascular risk factors have attempted to disentangle the effects of ovarian aging versus aging in other systems. With the exception of a study of Japanese women, participants in the available studies were European whites. It is well known that cardiovascular risk factors differ by ethnic groups. Thus, the influence of ovarian aging on risk factors in whites should not be generalized to other ethnic groups. Nonetheless, it appears that ovarian aging is associated with alterations in lipids and lipoproteins, but not blood pressure or weight gain (see Fig. 99-5) above alterations expected based on chronological aging. For example, in the Pittsburgh Healthy Women Study, women who

changed from pre- to postmenopausal status during the first 2.5 years of the study experienced a twofold increase in low-density lipoprotein (LDL)-cholesterol and a small decline in high-density lipoprotein (HDL) cholesterol, as compared to women remaining premenopausal during the same period of time (Fig. 99-5). The lipid changes were most apparent in women who declined the most in estradiol levels, and were smaller among women using hormone replacement therapy.

A longer follow-up of participants in the Pittsburgh Healthy Women Study compared the magnitude of change in risk factors from premenopause to 5 years postmenopause and correlated those changes with carotid disease measured 5 to 8 years after the menopause. Increases in LDL cholesterol and triglycerides and declines in HDL cholesterol were substantially greater during the perimenopause, that is, between the premenopausal and first year postmenopausal evaluations, than during the early postmenopause, that is, between the first and fifth years postmenopausal evaluations. Increases in blood pressure and fasting glucose levels were greater during the postmenopause than the perimenopause. Premenopausal levels of systolic and pulse pressure, LDL and HDL cholesterol, triglycerides, and body mass index strongly predicted carotid disease approximately 9 years later, suggesting that women in midlife, well before the menopause-induced changes in risk factors occur, can be targeted for early prevention of cardiovascular disease. The importance of early prevention is heightened by results from recent primary and secondary prevention trials showing no benefit of estrogen therapy for women with coronary disease.

Blood pressure rises in midlife are correlated highly with weight gain. Population data show a gradual increase in systolic blood pressure and a constant or gradual decline in diastolic blood pressure in midlife and beyond. The development of isolated systolic hypertension should be monitored beginning in midlife.

Clotting and lytic factors are increasingly recognized for their importance as risk factors in atherosclerotic cardiovascular disease. Factor VII coagulation activity, factor VII antigen, plasminogen activator inhibitor (PAI)-1 levels, C-reactive protein, and fibrinogen levels have all been associated with cardiovascular disease risk and are higher in postmenopausal women than in premenopausal women in cross-sectional studies. There are no direct data on ovarian aging and clotting and lytic factors, although studies of the effects of estrogen replacement therapy suggest both beneficial and detrimental effects.

Lipoprotein(a) (Lp[a])is thought to have both atherogenic and thrombotic properties. Postmenopausal women have higher levels than premenopausal women and Lp(a) concentrations increase after bilateral oophorectomy, whereas they do not change after hysterectomy alone.

Cardiovascular function may also change during the menopause. Indicators of myocardial contractility, blood flow in the internal carotid artery and in the aorta, are associated with time since menopause. Among hypertensives, change from pre- to postmenopausal status is associated with a decrease in compliance or an increase in stiffening of the aortic root. Nonhuman primate studies show that ovariectomy leads to altered vasomotion in the coronary arteries and that poor ovarian function is associated with coronary atherosclerosis. Taken together, these findings suggest that the perimenopausal period may be a time of accelerated change in hemodynamic function.

CONCLUSIONS

What can be concluded about aging in midlife generally and ovarian aging specifically? The endocrine changes that accompany menopause occur over a long period of time, the length of which is highly variable within individuals. The menopausal period is characterized by unpredictability with respect to both menstrual patterns and hormones between individuals as well as within an individual. Vasomotor symptoms are a hallmark of the perimenopausal transition, but not all women experience them. To the extent women experience adverse symptoms during the menopause, they will occur early in the transition and women will likely seek treatment for symptom relief at that time. Clinical studies show that short-term use of hormone replacement therapy will relieve severe vasomotor symptoms but not eliminate them.

Midlife is a time of small, but significant changes in a number of systems, including blood pressure, glucose, insulin, lipids, heart function, symptoms, sleep patterns, bone, joints, and verbal memory. Weight gain in midlife is

small on an annual basis, but over midlife can be quite substantial and has important effects on other systems. Maintenance and increasing physical activity may prevent some of these effects. Ovarian aging specifically appears to be associated with alterations in lipids, bone, and body composition.

These conclusions are based on studies composed largely of white women. It is likely that other ethnic and racial groups will show some different effects of ovarian aging, given that they differ from whites in weight, preventive practices such as use of hormone replacement therapy and physical activity, cultural factors affecting symptom reporting, and use of the health care system. It is also likely that Baby Boomers have higher expectations about quality of life than earlier generations, and will actively seek information and treatment for early signs of the menopausal transition, given that they are better educated, more often in the labor force, and have smaller families, relative to previous generations. Midlife is an optimal time to introduce women to a life-long orientation to prevention of disease and promotion of health during the postmenopausal years.

REFERENCES

Ahlborg HG et al: Bone loss in relation to menopause: A prospective study during 16 years. *Bone* 28:327, 2001.

Albright TF et al: Postmenopausal osteoporosis. *Trans Assoc Am Physicians* 55:298, 1940.

Avis NE, Crawford SL: Menopause and weight. *Menopause* 8:23, 2000.

Baumgartner RN: Body composition in healthy aging. *Ann N Y Acad Sci* 904:437, 2000.

Black DM et al: Appendicular bone mineral and a woman's lifetime risk of hip fracture. *J Bone Miner Res* 7:639, 1992.

Burger HG et al: Prospectively measured levels of serum follicle-stimulating hormone, estradiol, and the dimeric inhibins during the menopausal transition in a population-based cohort of women. *J Clin Endocrinol Metab* 84:4025, 1999.

Carlson KJ et al: The Maine Women's Healthy Study: I. Outcomes of hysterectomy. *Obstet Gynecol* 83:556, 1994.

de Bruin JP et al: The role of genetic factors in age at natural menopause. *Hum Reprod* 16:2014, 2001.

Gold EB et al: Relation of demographic and lifestyle factors to symptoms in a multi-racial/ethnic population of women 40–55 years of age. *Am J Epidemiol* 152:463, 2000.

Longcope C et al: Steroid and gonadotropin levels in women during the peri-menopausal years. *Maturitas* 8:189, 1986.

Manson JE, Martin KA: Postmenopausal hormone-replacement therapy. *N Engl J Med* 345:34, 2001.

Matthews KA et al: Influence of the perimenopause on cardiovascular risk factors and symptoms of middle-aged healthy women. *Arch Intern Med.* 154:2349, 1994.

Matthews KA et al: Influences of natural menopause on psychological characteristics and symptoms of middle-aged healthy women. *J Consult Clin Psychol* 58:345, 1990.

McKinlay SM et al: The normal menopause transition. *Maturitas* 14:103, 1992.

Nevitt MC et al: The effect of estrogen plus progestin on knee symptoms and related disability in postmenopausal women: The Heart and Estrogen/Progestin Replacement Study, a randomized, double-blind, placebo-controlled trial. *Arthritis Rheum* 44:811, 2001.

Poehlman ET et al: Changes in energy balance and body composition at menopause: A controlled longitudinal study. *Ann Intern Med* 123:673, 1995.

Rannevik G et al: A longitudinal study of the perimenopausal transition: Altered profiles of steroid and pituitary hormones, SHBG, and bone mineral density. *Maturitas* 21:103, 1995.

Recker R et al: Characterization of perimenopausal bone loss: A prospective study. *J Bone Miner Res* 15:1965, 2000.

Sowers MF et al: Longitudinal changes in body composition in women approaching the midlife. *Ann Hum Biol* 23:253, 1996.

US Bureau of the Census: *Current Population Reports, P251092. Population Projections of the United States by Age, Sex, Race, and Hispanic Origin: 1992 to 2050.* Washington, DC, US Government Printing Office, 1992, p 48.

Wallace RB et al: Probability of menopause with increasing duration of amenorrhea in middle-aged women. *Am J Obstet Gynecol* 135:1021, 1979.

Wing RR et al: Weight gain at the time of menopause.*Arch Intern Med* 151:97, 1991.

Gynecologic Disorders

TOMAS L. GRIEBLING

Demographic data clearly show that a dramatic population shift with an increase in the number of older adults is occurring in the United States. It is estimated that by the year 2030, at least 20 percent of the total population will be older than 65 years of age. Because women have a longer life expectancy than men, they constitute a disproportionately larger segment of the population of older adults. Gynecologic disorders represent a substantial and important part of geriatric health care for older women. A wide range of both benign and malignant problems can occur. Sensitive clinical evaluation and routine preventive management may help to alleviate many of these problems and prevent additional morbidity and mortality.

GYNECOLOGIC HISTORY AND PHYSICAL EXAMINATION

Gynecologic symptoms such as pain, bleeding, itching, and masses are common in older women. However, elderly women may be reluctant to discuss these issues with their health care providers because of embarrassment or fear. It is important that providers specifically ask about symptoms related to gynecologic and urologic conditions, including sexual health, as part of routine clinical care. Serious health problems may develop if conditions remain untreated for an extended period of time.

The history should include questions about voiding symptoms because many older women who experience urinary incontinence do not seek medical attention for the problem. Problems with defecation should also be assessed, including fecal urgency or incontinence. The past history should include a discussion of any prior pelvic surgery or radiation therapy. Review of the patient's obstetric history is important to identify any prior birth trauma or other risk factors that could predispose to a decrease in pelvic floor support. The use of exogenous hormone replacement therapy should be identified. The patient should also be questioned about her breast health and any changes or problems she has recently experienced. A breast examination should be performed as part of the routine physical exam.

The general consensus is that pelvic examination should be performed at baseline evaluation and then every 1 to 2 years, or if the patient develops new gynecologic symptoms such as postmenopausal vaginal bleeding, pain, or a significant change in voiding habits. The pelvic examination may be difficult for some older women because of physical limitations such as stenosis of the vaginal introitus or limitations of hip flexion. Patients with osteoarthritis or osteoporosis may be unable to comfortably assume the traditional dorsal lithotomy position. In these cases, the left lateral decubitus position may be used. This generally provides adequate exposure to the genitals and perineum. Both a speculum exam and a bimanual exam can be performed in this position. In long-term care or hospital settings, the examination may need to be performed with the patient in bed.

Visual inspection of the external genitalia may reveal a number of changes that are considered a normal part of the aging process. Pubic hair may be gray or diminished, and there may be a decrease in fat content of the mons pubis and labia majora. The clitoris may be prominent in some hypoestrogenic women because of a relative predominance of circulating androgens. Any suspicious vulvar lesions, including ulcerations or pigmented lesions, should be noted. Biopsies are generally indicated to rule out evidence of malignant disease. Palpation of the inguinal region should be performed to evaluate for lymphadenopathy or hernia. A neurologic examination should be performed to assess light touch sensation in the labia majora and perianal region. These areas correspond to the lower lumbar (L4–L5) and sacral (S2–S4) dermatomes. Alterations in sensation, including asymmetry, may be associated with voiding, defecation, or sexual dysfunction.

A speculum examination should be performed and if needed, a Papanicolaou (Pap) smear obtained. Narrowing of the vaginal introitus may necessitate the use of a smaller speculum. Lubrication may be helpful to improve comfort and ease of examination. However, artificial lubrication should be avoided if a Pap smear is to be obtained because the lubricant can alter cytologic morphology. The vaginal epithelium and cervix should be examined for any masses or lesions. Atrophic vaginitis is common in older women and appears as a pale discoloration or thinning of the vaginal epithelium with loss of rugations. Inflammation of the vaginal mucosa may also be present.

Bimanual examination is used to evaluate for adnexal tenderness or mass, and the position and mobility of the cervix and uterus. Pelvic floor support is assessed to identify any evidence of prolapse. Use of a single-blade speculum helps facilitate visualization. In patients who have undergone hysterectomy, the support of the apical vaginal cuff should be assessed. The perineum should be examined for masses or tenderness. A rectovaginal exam should also be performed to identify any rectal masses or lesions in the rectovaginal septum. Sphincter tone is assessed and a bulbocavernosus reflex may be checked as part of the neurologic examination. A stool guaiac test may also be obtained at this time to evaluate for possible gastrointestinal bleeding.

BENIGN DISORDERS

Prolapse

Disorders of pelvic floor support are common in older women. Risk factors include trauma from prior vaginal delivery, obesity, connective tissue abnormalities, and estrogen deficiency. The patient may complain of a pressure sensation or feeling of heaviness in the perineum or genitals. Back pain may be associated with prolapse caused by anterior tension on the uterosacral ligaments. Standardized terminology has been developed to describe various degrees of pelvic organ prolapse (Table 100-1).

A cystocele is a protrusion of the bladder through the anterior vaginal wall. This occurs because of weakness of the pubocervical fascia. Small cystoceles may be associated with urinary incontinence. Larger cystoceles tend to cause obstructive voiding symptoms because of associated hypermobility and angulation of the urethra. Some women may need to manually reduce the cystocele in order to initiate micturition or void to completion. A rectocele is a protrusion of the rectum through the posterior vaginal wall. This is caused by a weakness of the perirectal fascia. Patients may experience significant difficulty with defecation including constipation or a need to strain. An enterocele is a herniation of small bowel and peritoneum through the apical vagina or between the uterosacral ligaments and the rectovaginal space. It is the only true hernia among the various forms of prolapse. Enterocele is more common in women who have undergone hysterectomy as a result of a loss of support of the vaginal cuff. Uterine prolapse may result

Table 100-1   Grades of Pelvic Organ Prolapse

Grade	Characteristic
Grade I	Prolapse extends only into proximal half of the vagina
Grade II	Prolapse extends into the distal half of the vagina but does not protrude beyond introitus
Grade III	Prolapse protrudes beyond the vaginal introitus with standing or Valsalva
Grade IV	Prolapse protrudes beyond the vaginal introitus at rest

Table 100-2   Management Options for Pelvic Organ Prolapse

Biobehavioral therapy
   Pelvic floor muscle exercises (Kegel's)
   Biofeedback
   Electrical stimulation

Pessary

Topical estrogen replacement

Surgery
   Anterior colporrhaphy
   Posterior colporrhaphy
   Vaginal or abdominal sacrocolpopexy
   Hysterectomy
   Colpocleisis

from defects in support from the cardinal or uterosacral ligaments. Procidentia refers to an eversion of the entire vagina that may include a uterine prolapse.

Management of prolapse disorders may be surgical or nonsurgical (Table 100-2). Pelvic floor (Kegel's) exercises may be helpful to increase pelvic floor strength. These can be augmented with biofeedback therapy or electrical muscle stimulation. Pessaries may also be used to support the prolapse. They are particularly useful in women for whom surgery would be contraindicated. Pessaries come in a wide variety of shapes and sizes, and must be fit to the patient's specific anatomy. Topical estrogen and antibiotic creams are often used to help prevent infection or erosion of the vaginal epithelium. If the patient is unable to remove and replace the pessary herself, monitoring by a visiting nurse may be helpful. Periodic inspection is important to help prevent complications. Anecdotal reports of neglected pessary causing erosion or fistulae have been described.

Surgery may be indicated if the patient is an appropriate candidate based on her overall functional health and comorbidity status. Rectoceles are typically repaired with a transvaginal approach. Cystoceles and enteroceles may be repaired with either a transvaginal or transabdominal approach. Hysterectomy may be required for treatment of uterine prolapse. In patients who are no longer sexually active, a colpocleisis procedure which closes the vaginal introitus may be considered as definitive treatment for prolapse. A preoperative evaluation for stress urinary incontinence should also be performed so that concomitant surgery may be done if indicated. Surgical repair of pelvic organ prolapse may also help improve sexual function and satisfaction.

Vaginitis and Vulvovaginitis

Bacterial vaginosis may cause vaginal itching or discharge. Infection with coliform organisms may occur, particularly in women with fecal incontinence. Other infectious agents, including *Gardnerella vaginalis* and *Trichomonas vaginalis,* are also common. *Gardnerella* infections are characterized by a watery, foul-smelling discharge. The presence of "clue" cells on wet prep, or a positive "whiff" test that reveals a fish-like odor with addition of potassium hydroxide, confirm the diagnosis. Oral metronidazole, 500 mg bid for 1 week, is generally effective for treatment. Trichomonas infections typically present with intense pruritus and a frothy vaginal discharge. Inflammation with "strawberry spot" lesions may be visible on the cervix or vaginal mucosa. Oral metronidazole is the preferred treatment. Screening for sexually transmitted diseases may be indicated depending on the patient's sexual history and symptoms.

Candidal vulvovaginitis is the most common fungal infection of the female genital tract. Risk factors include obesity, diabetes, and immunosuppression. Topical antifungal medications are commonly used to treat the infection. If symptoms persist or in cases of severe infection, oral fluconazole or other systemic antifungal medications may be indicated.

Atrophic vaginitis is common in older women. Decreased estrogenization after menopause leads to a thinning of the vaginal mucosa. The tissue typically appears pale, although inflammation and telangiectatic changes may be present. Vaginal fluid becomes more alkaline and this leads to a loss of *Lactobacillus* which forms the normal vaginal flora. This can predispose women to an increased incidence of urinary tract infection. Sexually active women may also experience dyspareunia because of a lack of natural vaginal lubrication. Although oral hormone replacement therapy may lead to a partial improvement in symptoms, topical estrogen administration is generally the preferred method of administration to achieve adequate tissue levels. Topical estrogen replacement is usually provided with vaginal cream three times a week at bedtime. This helps to acidify the vaginal fluid and leads to regrowth of the normal flora. There is evidence that vaginal estrogen replacement therapy may help to prevent recurrent urinary tract infections in elderly women. Newer preparations of estrogen administered as either vaginal tablets or hormone infused rings may offer an effective and less cumbersome alternative to traditional estrogen creams.

Contact dermatitis may be caused by soaps or feminine hygiene sprays. Douching is generally discouraged because it washes away the normal vaginal flora and secretions which serve to lubricate the tissues and help prevent infection. Low-dose topical steroids may be indicated if contact dermatitis persists after elimination of the inciting agent.

Urethral Caruncle

A urethral caruncle is a prolapse of the urethral mucosa that may be associated with loss of support of the periurethral fascia. Urethral caruncles are typically asymptomatic although patients may experience pain or bleeding. Topical estrogen cream may help to alleviate symptoms. If symptoms persist, excision or cauterization may be performed.

Dermatologic Conditions

Lichen sclerosus is a chronic dermatosis that causes thinning of the vulvar epithelium and fibrosis of the underlying dermis. Symptoms include labial shrinkage and pruritus. Visual inspection reveals epithelial thinning with an overlying fine silver-white scale. Stenosis of the vaginal introitus may occur in severe cases. Biopsy should be performed to confirm the diagnosis. Treatment generally involves administration of topical steroids. Surgical correction of introital stenosis may be useful to treat dyspareunia and sexual dysfunction.

Squamous hyperplasia of the vulva typically presents with a thickened, raised white lesion that is often pruritic. Biopsy may be necessary to confirm the diagnosis and differentiate this benign lesion from vulvar carcinoma. Histologic analysis reveals hyperplastic keratinized squamous epithelium. There may be an associated contact dermatitis. Elimination of the inciting agent and treatment with topical steroids generally alleviates the symptoms.

Condyloma acuminata may occur at any age and are associated with exposure to human papillomavirus (HPV). Subtypes 16 and 18 are associated with an increased risk for cervical cancer. Treatment options include surgical excision, destruction of the lesions with carbon dioxide (CO_2) laser, or topical application of podophyllin.

Pigmented vulvar lesions raise the suspicion for melanoma. Excisional biopsy is typically indicated. Additional evaluation and management issues for vulvar melanoma are discussed in the section on gynecologic malignancies.

Sexual Dysfunction and Dyspareunia

To date, there has been little scientific research on the psychosocial or physiologic aspects of sexual dysfunction in older adult women. However, there is increased interest in this topic among both the scientific community and the lay public. The incidence of sexual dysfunction appears to increase with advancing age. However, the etiology of these changes is still poorly understood. Comorbid conditions such as cardiovascular disease, osteoarthritis, urinary incontinence, and stroke may negatively influence sexual function. Patients with complaints of decreased libido or sexual dysfunction should also be screened for other signs of depression. Although concerns about sexual health are common among women of all ages, elderly women may be reluctant to discuss these issues with their health care providers. An empathic clinician who raises the topic during the history and physical examination may be able to diagnose and treat these conditions and improve a patient's overall quality of life.

Dyspareunia, or pain with sexual activity, is a common complaint in older women. This may be caused by a lack of natural lubrication or stenosis of the vaginal introitus. Vaginismus is a muscular spasm of the vaginal wall that may cause severe pain. Vulvodynia and vulvovestibulitis are chronic conditions characterized by vulvar pain, itching, and dyspareunia. Although the exact etiologies are unknown, several theories have been proposed, including autoimmune changes and pelvic neuropathy with enhanced pain perception. Treatment is empiric, and the goal of therapy is to reduce the severity of symptoms. Dietary modification with elimination of caffeine, acidic foods and beverages, and alcohol may be beneficial. Low-dose tricyclic antidepressants may be helpful for reducing neuropathic pain. These medications should be used with caution in elderly women as a consequence of their significant potential anticholinergic side effects.

Fistulae

A fistula is a communication between two hollow organs or between a hollow organ and the skin surface. Vesicovaginal and ureterovaginal fistulae typically present with continuous urinary leakage. These may occur as the result of iatrogenic trauma during pelvic surgery such as hysterectomy. Other common causes include new or recurrent gynecologic malignancy or tissue erosion caused by pelvic radiation. Fistulae associated with radiation changes may not clinically manifest until years after the course of therapy is complete. Colovesical fistulae typically occur in patients with a history of colonic diverticulosis or diverticulitis. Patients may present with recurrent urinary tract infections with multiple coliform organisms. Pneumaturia (passage of gas in the urinary stream) may also occur.

Clinical evaluation for fistula is focused on finding the location and etiology of the fistula tract. This may require multiple imaging studies such as pelvic computerized tomography (CT), voiding cystourethrography (VCUG), or cystourethroscopy and vaginoscopy. Biopsies of the fistula tract should be obtained in women with a history of any gynecologic or other pelvic malignancy.

Surgical treatment is generally indicated for the management of fistulae. Depending on the size and location of the fistula, this may be performed through either a transvaginal or transabdominal approach. The goals of surgery include excision of the fistula tract and closure of the adjacent normal tissue. The repair must be done with no tissue tension in order to prevent recurrence. Interposition of omentum or other vascularized tissue such as a labial fat pad flap as part of a multilayer closure can help prevent breakdown of the repair.

Ovarian Cystic Disease

Ovarian cysts are a common clinical finding in both younger and older women. These may be simple benign cysts, or they may be more complex. On ultrasonographic and CT imaging, benign cysts are characterized by thin walls, lack of internal echoes or septations, and homogeneous fluid density. Evidence of complex cystic changes including septations, echogenicity, or variable density should raise suspicion for ovarian tumors. Serum levels of CA125, an ovarian tumor marker, should be checked, and are usually elevated in cases of malignancy. Hemorrhagic cysts may persist and can become calcified with time. Polycystic ovarian disease may be associated with other endocrinologic abnormalities including hirsutism and loss of libido. Laparoscopic excision may be beneficial for the evaluation of suspicious ovarian cystic lesions in elderly women.

Ovarian Torsion

Ovarian torsion is uncommon in elderly women, but should be included in the differential diagnosis of acute lower abdominal or pelvic pain. Physical examination typically reveals pelvic or adnexal tenderness, and a mass may be palpable. Ultrasonography is helpful to confirm the diagnosis. Diminished or absent arterial flow may be evident on Doppler flow analysis. Surgical excision is indicated, and laparoscopy may be particularly useful in this clinical setting.

Endometriosis

Symptomatic endometriosis is uncommon in elderly women. However, women who have suffered from endometriosis earlier in life may continue to have problems after menopause. Symptoms may include chronic pelvic pain, bloating, and episodic vaginal bleeding. Evaluation and management may include laparoscopy, surgical excision, or systemic hormonal manipulation.

GYNECOLOGIC MALIGNANCIES

Malignant disorders of the female genital tract represent a significant risk of morbidity and mortality for elderly women. All of the common gynecologic malignancies demonstrate an increase in age-specific incidence up to the ninth decade. Increased screening efforts with routine pelvic examination and Pap smear testing have helped to improve the rate of early detection and treatment, particularly for cervical cancer. However, screening is still underused in elderly women.

The development and implementation of routine screening tests for other gynecologic malignancies remains more controversial. In addition, the age at which screening may be safely stopped has not been adequately established. Clinicians should maintain a high index of suspicion for gynecologic cancers. Radical surgery may be warranted, and the overall complication rate is generally not significantly different from younger patients. Age alone should not be considered a risk factor for surgical complications. Overall survival from gynecologic malignancies differs significantly based on the type of tumor and is highly dependent on disease stage at the time of treatment (Table 100-3).

Postmenopausal Vaginal Bleeding

Dysfunctional vaginal bleeding should always be considered abnormal and a thorough clinical evaluation to identify the underlying etiology should be performed. A variety of both benign and malignant conditions are included in the differential diagnosis (Table 100-4). The greatest concern is for possible gynecologic cancer. Other causes include systemic estrogen or progesterone use or vaginal atrophy associated with decreased estrogen levels. Women with an intact uterus should receive progesterone in addition to estrogen replacement therapy to prevent the development of endometrial hyperplasia and endometrial cancer. Persistent bleeding may require adjustment or discontinuation of hormone replacement therapy.

Patients with complaints of dysfunctional bleeding should undergo careful history and pelvic examination. Additional diagnostic studies may be warranted. Pelvic

Table 100-3 Estimated Overall 5-year Cancer Survival Based on Disease Stage*

Cancer Type	Stage I	Stage II	Stage III	Stage IV
Endometrial†	54–88%	40–76%	22–57%	12–18%
Ovarian	80–90%	65–70%	30–59%	17%
Cervical	80–95%	74–77%	46–52%	20–29%
Vulvar	85%	69%	40%	22%
Vaginal	74%	50%	32%	0–18%

* Stage includes all substages.

† Ranges for endometrial cancer include both clinical and surgical stages.

The complete staging system for all gynecologic malignancies can be found in Greene FL et al (eds): *AJCC Cancer Staging Manual*, 6th ed. New York, Springer, 2002.

SOURCE: Data summarized from FIGO annual report. *J Epid Biostat* 6:1, 2001.

ultrasonography is a very useful test in the diagnosis of endometrial hyperplasia and cancer. These diagnoses are rare if the endometrial thickness is less than 5 mm. Endometrial thickening greater than 5 mm should raise the suspicion for malignancy and prompt additional evaluation with

Table 100-4 Differential Diagnosis of Postmenopausal Vaginal Bleeding

Cancer
  Endometrial
  Cervical
  Vaginal
  Vulvar
  Ovarian
  Metastatic spread from other sites
    to genitourinary system

Atrophy
  Atrophic vaginitis
  Atrophic cervicitis

Benign polyps
  Endometrial
  Cervical

Urethral caruncle

Endometrial hyperplasia

Estrogen stimulation of endometrium
  Exogenous estrogen replacement
  Endogenous estrogen production
    (functional ovarian tumor)

Systemic coagulopathy

Vaginal mucosal erosion or laceration
  Pessary
  Trauma
  Sexual abuse

Urinary tract infection

endometrial biopsy or formal dilation and curettage. Direct visualization with hysteroscopy can be also be performed during these procedures and may help to increase overall diagnostic accuracy.

Cancers

Endometrial Cancer

Endometrial cancer is the most common gynecologic malignancy in the United States. Approximately 36,000 new cases are diagnosed annually, and it is the fourth leading cancer among American women. Risk factors for endometrial cancer include nulliparity, prolonged exposure to unopposed estrogens, and obesity. Postmenopausal vaginal bleeding is the most common presenting symptom.

A Pap smear alone is not adequate for diagnosis or exclusion of endometrial cancer because only 35 to 50 percent of patients with endometrial cancer will have an abnormal finding on Pap smear cytology. Additional evaluation with pelvic ultrasonography and either endometrial biopsy or dilation and curettage is required.

Radical hysterectomy remains the mainstay of treatment for endometrial cancer. In women who cannot undergo surgery because of significant comorbid disease, radiation and chemotherapy may be used. Recent studies suggest a role for laparoscopy in early stage disease. Prognosis is dependent on the stage of disease (see Table 100-3). The overall 5-year survival for all stages is approximately 65 percent. Older women and those with more advanced tumor stage have a generally worse prognosis.

Ovarian Cancer

Ovarian cancer is the second most common gynecologic malignancy in elderly women. It is particularly dangerous because symptoms may be vague and they may not appear until late in the disease process. Current screening tests, including ultrasonography and tumor markers, are of somewhat limited value except in high-risk patients. Abdominal pain, distension, and gastrointestinal problems can occur from ovarian cancers. After menopause, the ovaries are typically atrophic and small. Therefore, any evidence of a palpable ovary on physical examination in elderly women should raise suspicion for a possible ovarian tumor.

The peak incidence of ovarian cancer occurs in the fifties and sixties. Identified risk factors for ovarian cancer include nulliparity, prolonged estrogen exposure, and mutations of the BRCA-I and BRCA-II genes. Complex ovarian cysts should be surgically explored to evaluate for malignancy. Laparoscopy may be helpful, and serum levels of the tumor marker CA125 should be obtained.

Surgical debulking is the primary form of therapy for ovarian cancer. Prognosis depends on the stage of disease at the time of diagnosis. Adjuvant platinum-based intravenous chemotherapy is often used and may improve overall survival. Intraperitoneal chemotherapy may also be used to treat metastatic ovarian cancer. Administration of chemotherapeutic agents directly into the peritoneal cavity offers the advantage of higher tissue concentrations compared to intravenous therapy. However, both routes of administration are associated with significant risks for chemotherapy related morbidity.

Because most ovarian tumors are diagnosed at a late stage, the overall prognosis is poor, and the 5-year survival rate for stage IV disease is generally less than 20 percent. Recent studies suggest a potential role for biologic response modifiers such as interferon and the interleukins in the treatment of ovarian cancer.

Cervical Cancer

Cervical cancer is the third most common gynecologic malignancy seen in the United States. It occurs in all age groups, but is most commonly diagnosed in patients in their forties and fifties. The risk of cervical cancer in women who have previously undergone a supracervical or partial hysterectomy is identical to that of women with an intact uterus.

Routine Pap smear screening has helped to improve rates of early detection and treatment of cervical cancer. It is now generally recommended that women older than age 50 years undergo pelvic examination with a Pap smear at least once every 3 years if all prior surveillance smears were normal. Examinations should be done annually in women with history of cytologic evidence of dysplasia. Colposcopy with additional biopsies or cervical conization may be necessary to establish the diagnosis. Women who are sexually active with multiple partners should also undergo annual Pap smear testing.

Exposure to HPV is felt to be a risk factor for development of cervical cancer. In particular, HPV subtypes 16 and 18 increase the risk and are found in more than 75 percent of all cervical tumors.

Symptoms are variable and depend on tumor stage. Some women may experience dysfunctional vaginal bleeding. Women who are sexually active may complain of postcoital bleeding or pain. Early tumors are often silent and are usually diagnosed by Pap smear screening.

Radical hysterectomy is the primary treatment for cervical cancer. Surgery is generally well-tolerated, and age has not been identified as a risk factor for perioperative complications. Adjuvant radiation or chemotherapy may be used to treat locally advanced disease or as palliation for metastases. Recent studies demonstrate that radiation may be administered safely in elderly women. Metastatic disease has an extremely poor prognosis.

Vulvar Cancer

Vulvar cancer is the fourth most common gynecologic cancer, accounting for approximately 3 percent of all malignancies of the female genital tract. The most common presenting symptoms are pruritus, pain, and a palpable vulvar lesion. Histology typically reveals squamous cell carcinoma. Surgical excision is indicated, and radical vulvectomy with inguinal lymphadenectomy may be required to treat late-stage tumors.

Prognosis depends on tumor stage (see Table 100-3). The overall 5-year survival for early stage lesions is 80 to 90 percent. If lymph node metastases are present, the overall survival drops significantly to 15 to 30 percent. Clinical performance status has been shown to be more important than patient age as a predictor of perioperative complications and survival. Adjuvant radiation and chemotherapy may be useful to treat local recurrences or to shrink tumors prior to surgical intervention.

Malignant melanoma of the vulva is relatively rare. However, melanoma should be considered in the differential diagnosis of pigmented vulvar lesions. This is particularly true if the lesion has irregular borders or has increased in size. Excisional biopsy is indicated, and radical vulvectomy with wide surgical margins of at least 1 cm may be necessary to adequately treat the tumor. The depth of invasion and tumor spread both affect overall prognosis. The number of positive lymph nodes is also a strong predictor of progression.

Vulvar intraepithelial neoplasia (VIN) is a term used to describe histologic findings of squamous dysplasia and squamous cell carcinoma in situ. It is generally considered a premalignant condition although there is some controversy on this point. Risk factors include cigarette smoking and HPV exposure. The most common symptom of VIN is pruritus. The overall incidence of VIN does not appear to increase with age after menopause. Multifocal lesions are common and treatment is accomplished with carbon dioxide laser ablation. Multiple treatment sessions may be required and close observation is critical. The presence of high-grade VIN near invasive vulvar carcinomas has been associated with poor prognosis.

Vaginal Cancer

Vaginal cancers are uncommon and account for approximately 1 percent of all female genital tract malignancies. Approximately 95 percent of these lesions are squamous cell carcinomas. The remaining tumor types include adenocarcinoma, clear cell carcinoma, and malignant melanoma. The most common presenting symptom is dysfunctional vaginal bleeding. Postcoital bleeding or pain may occur in sexually active women. Tumors that involve the anterior vaginal wall may invade into the urethra and cause symptoms of voiding dysfunction. Women who have had prior gynecologic cancers, particularly cervical cancer, are at increased relative risk for development of vaginal cancer.

Radiation therapy is the primary treatment choice for vaginal cancers, although adjuvant chemotherapy and surgery may also be used. Surgical therapy may be particularly useful for early stage tumors and those involving the proximal vagina. Prognosis depends on tumor type and stage. Overall 5-year survival estimates range from 25 to 48 percent.

Vaginal intraepithelial neoplasia (VAIN) refers to areas of vaginal dysplasia or carcinoma in situ. Three grades of VAIN are recognized, and most lesions are of moderate grade (grade 2). Multifocal lesions are common. Treatment is generally done with carbon dioxide (CO_2) laser ablation. This may be difficult if lesions are located in the vaginal angles. Multiple treatment sessions may be required, and close cytologic monitoring is necessary.

SUMMARY

Gynecologic disorders are common in elderly women. A wide variety of both benign and malignant conditions may occur. Clinicians need to ask patients about symptoms and be diligent about performing pelvic examination and screening tests such as Pap smears when indicated. Surgical treatment may be accomplished in most patients who do not have significant comorbid disease. Early diagnosis and treatment of gynecologic disorders can help to significantly improve both the length and quality of life for older adult women.

REFERENCES

American College of Obstetricians and Gynecologists: *Pelvic Organ Prolapse.* Technical Bulletin No. 214. Washington, DC, American College of Obstetricians and Gynecologists, 1995.

Beller U et al: Carcinoma of the vagina. FIGO annual report. *J Epid Biostat* 6:141, 2001.

Beller U et al: Carcinoma of the vulva. FIGO annual report. *J Epid Biostat* 6:153, 2001.

Benedet JL et al: Carcinoma of the cervix. FIGO annual report. *J Epid Biostat* 6:5, 2001.

Creasman W et al: Carcinoma of the corpus uteri. FIGO annual report. *J Epid Biostat* 6:45, 2001.

Geisler JP, Geisler HE: Radical hysterectomy in the elderly female: A comparison to patients age 50 or younger. *Gynecol Oncol* 80:258, 2001.

Griebling TL, Nygaard IE: The role of estrogen replacement therapy in the management of urinary incontinence and urinary tract infection in postmenopausal women. *Endocrinol Metab Clin North Am* 26:347, 1997.

Heintz APM et al: Carcinoma of the ovary. FIGO annual report. *J Epid Biostat* 6:107, 2001.

Hyde SE et al: The impact of performance status on survival in patients of 80 years and older with vulvar cancer. *Gynecol Oncol* 84:388, 2002.

Langkilde NC et al: Surgical repair of vesicovaginal fistulae: A ten-year retrospective study. *Scand J Urol Nephrol* 33:100, 1999.

Mandelblatt JS, Yabroff KR: Breast and cervical cancer screening for older women: Recommendations and challenges for the 21st century. *J Am Med Womens Assoc* 55:210, 2000.

Nusbaum MR et al: The high prevalence of sexual concerns among women seeking routine gynecologic care. *J Fam Pract* 49:299, 2000.

Benign Prostate Disorders

CATHERINE E. DUBEAU

DEFINITION

Benign prostatic hyperplasia (BPH) is the benign proliferation of stromal and/or epithelial prostate tissue. BPH first develops in the third decade, and prostate volume continues to increase with age until approximately the seventh decade, after which BPH volume shows an inconsistent or negative relationship with age. Histologic evidence of BPH is nearly universal in older men, yet prostate enlargement results in only about half of them. Voiding symptoms occur in approximately half of men with prostate enlargement. Consequently, the term *benign prostatic hyperplasia* should be reserved for the specific pathohistology, distinct from benign prostate enlargement (BPE) and bladder outlet obstruction (BOO). In this chapter, *benign prostate disease* indicates the total complex of BPH, BPE, and BOO. The symptoms usually associated with benign prostate disease—urgency, frequency, nocturia, slow stream, hesitancy, incomplete emptying, postvoiding dribbling, straining to void—have many etiologies, and therefore are best described as *lower urinary tract symptoms* (LUTS) and not *prostatism*. Besides prostate disease, LUTS may result from age-related physiologic lower urinary tract changes, comorbid conditions, or medications, and can occur in many older women.

EPIDEMIOLOGY

Epidemiologic studies for benign prostate disease are complicated by variable definitions of disease (LUTS, BPH, BPE, transurethral resection) and a mix of retrospective and prospective methods. LUTS are significantly associated with diabetes, hypertension, cardiovascular disease, diuretics, nocturnal polyuria (excess urine production), and the age-related decrease in urine flow rate (which is independent of BOO). Identified BPH risk factors include age, physical inactivity, high protein (meat) and fat intake (especially polyunsaturated fatty acids), diabetes, high insulin levels, obesity, and low high-density lipoprotein levels. Potential protective factors are micronutrients (zinc, selenium, vitamin E, lycopene, phytoestrogens, phytosterols), diet rich in vegetables, physical activity, and moderate alcohol consumption. Results regarding smoking are variable, and vasectomy is not a risk factor. Together, these factors suggest a role for sympathetic activity, androgen–estrogen balance, and smooth-muscle proliferation in the etiology of benign prostate disease.

BPH occurs in nearly 80 percent of men by age 80 years. Population-based studies indicate that 28 to 35 percent of older men without previous prostate surgery have moderate to severe LUTS. Mean prostate volume increases with age but is very variable; the strongest predictor of increased volume is prostate-specific antigen (PSA) level >1.4 to 2 ng/mL. On a population basis, LUTS increase linearly over time, with the fastest rate during the seventh decade. Among individual men, LUTS decrease in at least one-third without treatment. Nearly 25 percent of men older than age 80 years receive treatment for (presumed) BPH-related LUTS. Natural history studies and randomized intervention trials consistently demonstrate that symptomatic progression of benign prostate disease is not inevitable, and is independent of BOO. The rate of acute urinary retention is low: in a meta-analysis including 6100 moderately symptomatic men, the rate was 13.7 per 1000 patient-years overall and 34.7 per 1000 patient-years in men older than 70 years or on anticholinergic agents.

PATHOPHYSIOLOGY

Hyperplasia occurs when prostate cell proliferation exceeds programmed cell death (apoptosis), caused by either stimulation of cell growth, inhibition of apoptosis, or a combination. BPH occurs predominantly in the prostatic periurethral transitional zone. The characteristic combination of stromal and epithelial hyperplasia are androgen- and aging-dependent, and involve numerous paracrine and autocrine factors. BPH and prostate cancer are genetically distinct; for example, gene expression profiling reveals CAG repeat polymorphism in the androgen-receptor gene in prostate cancer but not BPH.

The dominant trophic androgen is dihydrotestosterone, produced by 5α reduction of testosterone within the prostate. Additional factors supporting prostate cell growth include inflammatory cytokines (e.g., interleukin-8), autocrine cytokine growth factors, and neuroendocrine cell products. Stromal–epithelial interactions regulating

Table 101-1   Lower Urinary Tract Factors Causing Divergence in Prevalence Between BPH, BPE, BOO, and LUTS

Factors	Impact
Ratio of stromal to epithelial hyperplasia: stromal proliferation occurs in 50%, glandular in 25%, and mixed in 25%	Stromal glands tend to be smaller, more symptomatic, have worse symptomatic response to prostatectomy.
Location of BPH nodules	Occur predominantly in central transitional and periurethral zones of the lateral prostate, thus predisposing to prostatic urethra compression. Enlarged median lobes may compress the bladder base without causing BOO.
Fibroelastic properties of prostate capsule	Altered compliance may decrease urethral patency in the absence of mechanical BOO.
α-Adrenergic innervation of prostate	Increased number of α-adrenergic receptors (primarily α_{1C}) mediating smooth-muscle contraction. Magnitude of contractile responsiveness increased in BPH.
Variability in detrusor muscle structure and function	Increased connective tissue infiltration; smooth-muscle hypertrophy and disintegration; decreased autonomic neuronal number; conversion from predominantly β-adrenergic (inhibitory) to α-adrenergic (stimulatory) responsiveness.
Detrusor overactivity	BOO associated with detrusor overactivity (DO), but causality unclear: DO occurs in normal asymptomatic older men and women. DO resolves in up to two-thirds of men after transurethral prostatectomy, yet tends to persist in the very elderly.
Atherosclerotic disease	May cause detrusor ischemia leading to impaired contractility.

BOO, bladder outlet obstruction; BPE, benign prostatic enlargement; BPH, benign prostatic hyperplasia; LUTS, lower urinary tract symptoms.

proliferation also involve interactions between androgens, estrogens, and stimulatory and inhibitory peptide growth factors (e.g., fibroblast growth factor-2, transforming growth factor-β).

The divergence in prevalence between BPH, BPE, BOO, and LUTS results from many lower urinary tract factors (Table 101-1). Of additional importance are the numerous medical conditions and medications that cause LUTS independent of any prostate disease (see Chap. 123).

CLINICAL PRESENTATION

Benign prostate disease may be asymptomatic, produce variable types and severity of LUTS, and, rarely, cause hematuria (from prostatic varices) and urinary retention (<5 percent). BPH, BPE, BOO, and LUTS do not always coexist: LUTS may be independent of prostate disease; BPH can cause LUTS without BPE or BOO; BOO can result from urethral strictures independent of BPE; and men with severe BOO and urinary retention may be asymptomatic.

EVALUATION

Lower Urinary Tract Symptoms

LUTS are the usual motivation for men to seek evaluation, especially when symptoms bother, worry, or embarrass them. The distinction between "irritative" and "obstructive" LUTS should be avoided because it does not increase specificity or correlate with symptom bother, severity, and urodynamic findings. "Irritative" symptoms can result from "obstructive" physiology (e.g., frequency from severe BOO with overflow), and "obstructive" symptoms from "irritative" causes (e.g., slowed urine stream from detrusor hyperactivity with impaired contractility). Older men especially should be evaluated for causes of LUTS independent of prostate disease. Nocturia is often the only and most bothersome symptom, and its many causes are often overlooked (Table 101-2).

The American Urological Association (AUA) symptom index (range, 0 to 35) (used worldwide as the International Prostate Symptom Score [IPSS]) is used to quantify symptom severity at baseline and over time. They should not be used for screening or diagnosis because LUTS are not specific for BPH. AUA score changes ±5 points have an 80 percent probability of indicating a true clinical change; any magnitude of change, however, can be caused by comorbid factors independent of benign prostate disease.

Quality of Life

The effect of LUTS on quality of life is central, because the need for treatment depends on symptom impact alone for the majority of men. Quality-of-life domains include

Table 101-2   Etiology of Nocturia

Category	Causes
Sleep disturbance	Insomnia Depression Medications Alcohol Obstructive sleep apnea
Increased nocturnal urine output	Congestive heart failure Pedal edema (venous insufficiency, NSAIDs, gabapentin, rosiglitazone) Obstructive sleep apnea Late-day diuretics (medications, caffeine, alcohol)
Lower urinary tract	Benign prostate disease Overflow incontinence Urinary tract infection

NSAIDs, nonsteroidal antiinflammatory drugs.

interference with daily activities, work, sleep, and sexual function; worry, embarrassment, and impaired self-esteem; and physical discomfort. The AUA symptom score include a quality-of-life question (not scored as part of symptom severity) that correlates well with the total symptom score. Perception of bother, however, often is independent of LUTS severity, and bother from an individual symptom may be more important than from total symptoms. Older men are bothered significantly more by nocturia, frequency, and urgency—independent of overall LUTS severity and BOO. Specifically asking men about their most bothersome symptom can help target treatment, especially given the many etiologies of LUTS in older men.

Comorbid Diseases and Factors

The evaluation of older men with LUTS closely parallels that of older persons with urinary incontinence (see Chap. 123). The first step in evaluation should be a full investigation of potential factors other than benign prostate disease that cause LUTS. The medical history and review of systems should include questions about: hematuria, dysuria, and pelvic pain (rare in benign prostate disease, more suggestive of infection, bladder stone, prostate and bladder cancers); previous episodes of urinary retention; cardiac symptoms (regarding possible congestive heart failure); bowel and sexual function (clues to potential sacral and pelvic neuropathies); type and amount of fluid intake (regarding frequency and nocturia); and sleep disturbance. All medications (including nonprescription drugs) must be reviewed, with a focus on drugs that decrease detrusor contractility (anticholinergics, calcium channel blockers), diuretics, agents associated with pedal edema (nifedipine, nonsteroidals, rosiglitazone, gabapentin), and α-adrenergic agents.

Physical Exam

Given the many medical causes of LUTS, a complete physical exam is necessary. Older men especially should have cognition, function, and mobility evaluated, as their deficits contribute to voiding difficulty. The neurologic exam should include the bulbocavernosus reflex, anal wink, and perineal sensation to assess sacral nerve integrity.

Digital rectal exam provides information about prostate nodularity, rectal tone, masses, and stool impaction. Digital rectal exam is inaccurate and poorly reproducible for prostate volume, even when performed by specialists. BPH adenomas can occur in the anterior prostate or median lobe, inaccessible to rectal palpation. Moreover, prostate volume—either by digital rectal exam, cystoscopy, ultrasound, or weight of tissue resected at transurethral prostatectomy—is not associated with BOO. Prostate volume is important only for choosing between transurethral and open surgical approaches (see Surgery below).

Testing

Bladder Diaries (Frequency–Volume Charts)

Bladder diaries recording time and volume of all voids (continent and incontinent) over several days can be very helpful in evaluating the role of urine output in frequency and nocturia. Several studies (albeit primarily in women) show that bladder diaries are reliable and valid. Quantifying symptoms in diaries provides a baseline severity measure, and an objective assessment of factors driving severity and bother. In a descriptive study of 160 men with LUTS, nocturia and daytime frequency (but neither 24-hour nor nocturnal output) were significantly associated with AUA score; daytime frequency and low voided volume were associated with quality of life. Bladder diaries can differentiate volume-related from lower urinary tract causes of frequency and nocturia (Table 101-3).

Table 101-3   Using Bladder Diary Information to Determine the Cause of Nocturia

	Mr. A	Mr. B
Nocturia	3 times/8 hour night	3 times/8 hour night
Nocturnal output	700 mL	400 mL
Functional bladder capacity (FBC)	250 mL	250 mL
Predicted nocturnal voids	3 voids	1.6 voids

Nocturnal output = total volume of all voids from bedtime to awakening (including first morning void); functional bladder capacity (FBC) = (total bladder capacity − post-voiding residual volume (PVR)) and is estimated by the modal voided volume; predicted nocturnal voids = (nocturnal output ÷ FBC).

In this example, Mr. A's actual nocturia is equal to the amount predicted by his output and FBC. His further evaluation and treatment should be directed at nonlower urinary tract causes of nocturnal diuresis. Mr. B has more nocturia than would be predicted by his nocturnal output. His nocturia is a result of either lower urinary tract disease or medical conditions causing sleep disturbance (but not associated with nocturnal diuresis).

Postvoiding Residual Volume

Expert opinion recommends postvoiding residual volume (PVR) testing for all men with LUTS, despite definitive supporting evidence. Certainly, a PVR should be done in men with coexistent neurologic disease, impaired renal function, who are taking bladder-suppressant medications, or who have failed empiric therapy. Especially in older men, elevated PVR is not specific for BOO, and may reflect detrusor underactivity (a result of either age, disease, and/or medication). Randomly selected community men have small PVRs (75th percentile, 35 mL). In a large randomized control trial of moderately symptomatic men, baseline mean PVR was approximately 110 ± 74 mL. PVR is not associated with age, AUA symptom score, quality of life indices, or maximum flow rate. PVR correlates modestly with prostate volume (rank correlation coefficient $[r_s] = 0.24$), and men with prostates over 30 g are 2.5 times more likely to have PVR >50 mL than are men with smaller glands. The latter is important because PVR >50 mL increases the risk of acute urinary retention nearly threefold over 3 to 4 years.

PVR can be done by urethral catheterization or ultrasound. Inability to pass an urethral catheter is usually a result of sphincter spasm and not BOO. Radiographic PVR estimates are only qualitative. Elderly persons tend to have a larger PVR in the morning, which can increase within-patient PVR variability. PVR, peak flow rate, and age can be combined in an algorithm to diagnose BOO (Fig. 101-1); its sensitivity is 90 percent (versus 55 percent for flow rate alone) and specificity 43 percent (63 percent in men older than age 75 years).

Laboratory Testing

Men with LUTS need urinalysis to exclude hematuria, glycosuria, pyuria, and bacteriuria, and blood urea nitrogen and creatinine to assess renal function. Those with frequency and nocturia additionally should be checked for hypercalcemia and diabetes. If the man is a candidate for and would desire curative treatment of localized prostate cancer, or if a prostate cancer diagnosis would modify his management, then screening with PSA should be considered (see Prostate Cancer).

Radiographic Tests

Voiding cystourethrography (VCUG) provides a dynamic evaluation of the urethral outlet during voiding, yet its sensitivity and specificity for BOO are unknown. Intravenous pyelography (IVP) and renal ultrasound are not required routinely because significant hydronephrosis occurs in only 3 to 10 percent of men with LUTS, and the association between elevated PVR and hydronephrosis in individual men is unclear. IVP is indicated with hematuria, recurrent urinary tract infections, previous lower urinary tract surgery, or bladder stones to evaluate upper and lower tracts. Although radiographic bladder base indentation and shadowing correlate with BOO, their detection is inconsistent. Bladder trabeculation correlates with detrusor overactivity but not BOO (hence its frequent observation in elderly women).

Specialized Testing

Urine Flow Rate Most expert groups consider flow rate testing optional. Peak flow rate measurement requires a flowmeter. Flows should be scanned for artifacts because flow rate is falsely elevated by straining. Low urine flow rates result from either impaired detrusor contractility, BOO, or a low bladder volume (alone or in combination). Independent of BOO, low flow rate is more prevalent in older men and women. Flow rate is very sensitive for BOO

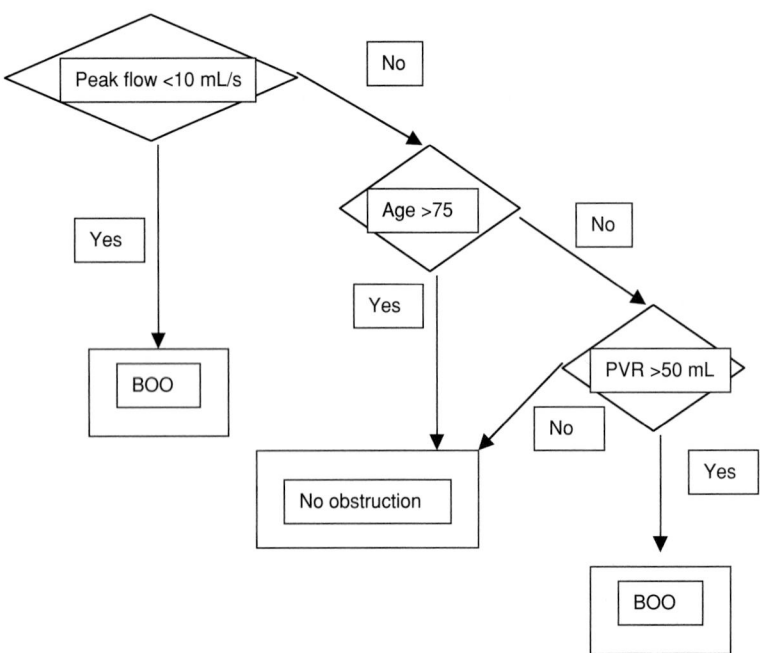

Figure 101-1 Algorithm for diagnosis of BOO in elderly men. BOO, bladder outlet obstruction; PVR, postvoiding residual volume. Reproduced with permission from DuBeau CE et al: Improving the utility of urine flow rate to exclude outlet obstruction in men with voiding symptoms. *J Am Geriatr Soc* 46:1118, 1998.

(peak flow >12 mL/s for voids ≥150 mL excludes BOO), but low flow rates are not specific.

Urodynamic Studies   Basic urodynamic tests for LUTS are cystometry and pressure-flow study. Cystometry measures bladder pressure during filling, detrusor stability (versus overactivity), contractility, and compliance. Pressure-flow study simultaneously measures flow rate versus bladder pressure during voiding; nomograms (e.g., Griffiths) are used to evaluate plots for BOO and detrusor contractility. Voiding profilometry (simultaneous measure of voiding detrusor and urethral pressures) is comparable to pressure-flow studies for BOO diagnosis, and may be easier to perform in frail patients.

The need for urodynamic studies in all men with LUTS remains controversial. The Agency for Health Care Policy and Research (AHCPR) BPH guideline designates urodynamic studies as "optional," its use to be based on physician judgment. In the United States, the majority of men undergoing transurethral prostatectomy (TURP) do not have preoperative urodynamic studies. Arguments for urodynamic studies include obstructed men have better TURP outcomes than do men without BOO; pressure flow is the criterion standard for BOO diagnosis; and the causes of LUTS in older men are diverse, often multiple, and may not be distinguishable without urodynamic studies. However, urodynamic studies are invasive, costly, and require specialized equipment and expertise. The improvement in TURP outcome for men with BOO is marginal, making definitive BOO diagnosis less pressing. Urodynamic studies should be considered when elderly men desire surgical treatment, to exclude conditions that do not require surgery (especially detrusor hyperactivity with impaired contractility); empiric treatment has failed; or when there is Parkinson's disease and spinal cord injury.

Cystoscopy   Cystoscopy should not be used diagnostically for BOO because it evaluates the prostate at rest and not during micturition, and can have false-positive results for BOO. In men already selected for surgery, or with hematuria or pelvic pain, cystoscopy provides needed information about prostate length, median lobe enlargement, and intravesical pathology (e.g., tumors, stones, marked trabeculation).

MANAGEMENT

Deciding on Treatment

Patient Preferences

Treatment decisions must be patient-centered because BPH, BPE, and BOO have small risks of morbidity and variable subjective impact. No treatment for benign prostate disease prolongs life or guarantees durable cure, and "watchful waiting" and lifestyle changes provide relief with little risk for many men. Considerations for discussion include: symptom severity and bother; preference for immediate versus delayed LUTS improvement; treatment outcomes and morbidity; short- and long-term costs; and ability to comply with long-term monitoring. Providers should

offer guidance in tailoring treatment so patients are supported in—and not burdened by—decision making. Video or print decision aids can help both patients and physicians weigh treatment risks and benefits.

Quality of life and symptom bother usually drive treatment decisions. These can be quantified by symptom indices, specific quality of life measures, and overall and specific symptom bother. The most bothersome symptom or most impacted quality of life domain should contribute to treatment choice. Nocturia, although often very bothersome, responds poorly to prostate-specific therapy; treatment should focus first on nonlower urinary tract causes. Men most bothered by worry may be relieved by evaluation and reassurance alone, while symptom relief should be the focus when LUTS interfere with daily activities.

Comorbidity

Multiple medical problems, frailty, and short life expectancy need not preclude treatment of benign prostate disease. The broad range of available therapies permits tailoring to desired immediacy of symptom relief, treatment invasiveness and morbidity, and patient comorbidity. These factors are discussed in the following sections on treatment.

Care Settings

Noninvasive treatments are possible in all care settings where clinical and compliance monitoring and medication adjustment are possible. Assisted-living residents will require either community or inpatient skilled nursing after surgical interventions. Across settings, surgery may not be desirable for men at high risk for in-hospital functional and cognitive decline.

Nonpharmacological Management

Lifestyle Changes

Many of the same voiding hygiene and behavioral approaches used for urinary incontinence reduce LUTS and their impact. Unhurried voiding without straining can improve bladder emptying. Addition of an afternoon diuretic may reduce nocturia in men with large nocturnal urine diuresis. Adjustment of lifestyle factors such as diet and physical activity may improve benign prostate disease (see "Prevention" later in this chapter).

Watchful Waiting

The natural history of BPH-related LUTS and the large placebo effects seen in randomized controlled BPH trials support the use of watchful waiting, the monitoring of men not given specific treatment. Men most appropriate for watchful waiting have mild to moderate LUTS, are comfortable with this approach, can be followed reliably, and have a normal or low PVR. They should be counseled to avoid medications that can cause urinary retention (e.g., over-the-counter "cold" tablets containing α-agonists and antihistamines), and monitored carefully if given anticholinergic or calcium channel-blocking drugs. Watchful waiting patients must be followed at least yearly to monitor symptoms, renal function, PVR, and (if appropriate) PSA.

In the largest randomized trial of watchful waiting versus TURP (556 men with moderate LUTS), TURP had significantly greater symptom improvement at 3 years (mean symptom score decrease was 66 percent), yet watchful waiting results were not trivial (−38 percent). One-third of watchful waiting men crossed-over to TURP, but absolute watchful waiting failure rates were low (urinary retention 2.9 percent, PVR >350 mL 5.8 percent, increased LUTS 4.3 percent). TURP decreased symptom bother and improved activities of daily living significantly more than watchful waiting; there were no significant differences in sexual performance, general well being, and social activities. LUTS improved less in those men least bothered at baseline, especially in the TURP group.

Medications

α-Adrenergic Blockers

α_1-Selective adrenergic blockers reduce BPH-related LUTS by several proposed mechanisms, including decreasing contractility of prostate capsule, tissue, and urethra; increasing tumor growth factor (TGF)-β and thus tissue apoptosis; and/or improving vascular flow to the detrusor. Overall, α blockers decrease mean IPSS scores over placebo by −3.9 points (95% CI −5.5, −3.3), with the largest decrease in men with severe LUTS. Time to onset of action is 2 to 4 weeks. Efficacy appears durable, although most long-term data come from open label trials. α Blockers have not been found to improve quality of life or prevent urinary retention. Symptom response is not related to the ratio of stromal to epithelial prostate tissue. Agents available in the United States are prazosin (1 to 2 mg twice a day), terazosin (2 to 10 mg daily), doxazosin (4 to 8 mg daily), and the α_{1A}-selective tamsulosin (0.4 mg daily). Randomized controlled trials show no significant differences between agents in symptom reduction.

Side effects include asthenia, headache, dizziness, lightheadedness, and orthostatic hypotension. Withdrawal rates in published trials are 10 to 15 percent, and are possibly higher in practice. For all agents, side effects increase with higher doses. Retrograde or delayed ejaculation occurs with tamsulosin (0 to 14 percent) but not other α blockers. Dizziness and withdrawal rates are significantly higher than placebo with terazosin and doxazosin, but not tamsulosin. Dizziness from terazosin (19 percent) is not related to age ($< / \geq 65$ years) or changes in blood pressure. Significant blood pressure drops and orthostatic hypotension are more likely in men with hypertension (whether treated or not). Slow titration from minimal starting doses and nighttime dosing mitigate first-dose hypotension. Men with diastolic dysfunction or taking other antihypertensives need to be carefully monitored. Although α blockers seem optimal for men with both LUTS and hypertension, they are not recommended as first-line hypertension agents. Also, the Antihypertensive and Lipid Lowering Treatment to Prevent Heart Attack Trial (ALLHAT) found that doxazosin increased the risk for congestive heart failure in men with cardiac risk factors.

Finasteride

Finasteride causes prostate involution by blocking the 5α reduction of testosterone to dihydrotestosterone in the prostate. Prostate volume decreases by at least one-third in 36 percent after a year. Treatment with 5 mg daily results in significant yet modest symptom improvement at 4 years (mean IPSS decrease −1.6 [95 percent CI −2.5, −0.7]). Because time to symptom decrease greater than placebo is 10 months, finasteride is not appropriate if quick improvement is desired or life expectancy is short.

Finasteride is less effective than terazosin in reducing LUTS. Two randomized controlled trials (RCTs) found that combining finasteride and α blockers did not increase efficacy. However, unlike α blockers, finasteride reduces the risk of urinary retention (1.1 percent versus 2.7 percent with placebo, number needed to treat (NNT)62) and TURP (4.2 percent versus 6.5 percent with placebo, NNT 44). Combined data from six RCTs indicate that prostate volume accounts for 80 percent of outcome variability. Overall results are best with prostates >40 g; large volume prostates (>60 g versus <20 g) have 55 percent greater decrease in IPSS score and decreased urinary retention and/or TURP (8.3 percent versus 19.9 percent, NNT 8). Because prostate volume correlates with PSA, high PSA levels (3.3 to 12 ng/mL) also are associated with better outcomes. Cost-effectiveness studies in men with moderate LUTS found finasteride less expensive with more quality-adjusted life years than watchful waiting (over ≤3 years) and TURP (over ≤14 years). Its high cost decreases the cost-effectiveness over time. Sustained drug effect requires lifetime use because prostate growth resumes when finasteride is stopped.

Finasteride decreases PSA levels by as much as 40 to 60 percent after 1 year in about one-third of men. One study found no difference in prostate cancer detection between finasteride and placebo, but heterogeneity in PSA response to finasteride may affect screening in individual patients. If PSA remains stable or increases in a compliant patient on finasteride, the patient should be evaluated with prostate biopsy. Despite maintained or increased testosterone levels, finasteride causes adverse sexual effects (decreased libido [6 percent], low ejaculate volume [4 percent], impotence [8 percent], gynecomastia [0.4 percent]). Although there are no long-term studies, finasteride appears to have little effect on serum lipids or bone density.

Phytotherapy

Plant-derived compounds are widely used to treat BPH-related LUTS, and systematic reviews support their efficacy. Compared with placebo, saw palmetto (from the dwarf palm tree *Serenoa repens*) improves LUTS (risk ratio 1.75; 95% CI 1.21, 2.54), decreases nocturia (weighted mean difference [WMD] −0.76 episodes; 95% CI −1.22, −0.32), and increases flow rate (WMD 1.93 mL/s; 95% CI 0.72, 3.14 mL/s). In two studies, symptomatic improvement was similar to finasteride. β-Sitosterols improve LUTS more than placebo (WMD for IPSS reduction −4.9 points [95% CI −6.3, −3.5]; WMD for flow rate 3.9 mL/s [95% CI 0.91, 6.9 mL/s]). Cernilton (pollen from the rye grass *Secale cereale*) also improves LUTS more than placebo (risk ratio 2.40, 95% CI 1.21, 4.75), but not flow rate. These agents have few to no reported side effects, but long-term data are lacking. Many studies suffer from short-term treatment (typically 4 to 24 weeks) and lack of standardized preparations.

Antiandrogens

Prostate involution can result from testosterone reduction by LHRH agonists or androgen receptor inhibitors. Small case series found that these agents facilitated indwelling catheter removal in frail older men. In one controlled trial, leuprolide caused significantly greater prostate reduction than placebo, but symptom relief was delayed until week 48. Side effects include impotence, weight gain, hot flashes, diarrhea, and gynecomastia; for frail men, most of these are tolerable. For most men, however, the high costs and morbidity make these agents undesirable. Prostate growth can resume when these agents are stopped.

Surgery

Transurethral Resection of Prostate

TURP remains the standard against which other treatments are compared because it has the highest rate of symptom improvement—generally 80 to 88 percent. The advent of new procedures and the low number of randomized trials has not diminished its central role.

The absolute indications for TURP are urodynamic evidence of high grade BOO, urinary retention (medical causes excluded), recurrent urinary infections, hydronephrosis, recurrent hematuria, and renal impairment. These indications account for nearly one-third of all TURPs, and for 50 to 60 percent of operations in men older than age 80 years.

TURP reduces LUTS significantly more than watchful waiting (90 percent versus 39 percent; IPSS difference at 7.5 months 10.4 [95% CI 8.5, 12.3]). Men with urodynamic BOO have better symptomatic outcomes. Quality of life, however, improves only in men with severe LUTS. At 5 years TURP has less treatment failure (increased LUTS, high PVR, retention, renal insufficiency, stones, death) (10 percent versus 21 percent, NNT 9), despite a 36 percent crossover from watchful waiting to TURP. Reoperation rate across trials is 1 percent per year. Efficacy declines over time; percent of surviving men with improved LUTS falls from 87 percent at 3 months to 75 percent at 7 years. Success rates tend to be lower in older men (<80 percent), often with a concomitant increase in morbidity (see below). Studies of TURP cost-effectiveness in the United States are complicated by marked geographic variability in operation rates, charges, and length of stay. Whether TURP prevents late detrusor compensation from BOO is unclear, and the true proportion of men at risk is unknown.

TURP morbidity includes retrograde ejaculation (74 percent); erectile dysfunction (14 percent, rate increases with age); immediate surgical complications (12 percent); urinary incontinence (5 percent); bleeding requiring transfusion (2 percent); failure to void; and infection. A single RCT found no significant difference between TURP and watchful waiting for erectile dysfunction and incontinence. Men older than age 80 years have higher rates of early complications (30 to 40 percent), late complications (13 to 22 percent), reoperation (4 percent per year), and perioperative mortality (2 to 3 percent versus 0.4 percent). Long-term survival rates are not different from age-matched controls. Many studies of TURP in elderly men, however, did not adjust for increased comorbidity with age.

Open Prostatectomy

Open prostatectomy by an abdominal or perineal approach is reserved for men with very large glands (>60 g) because the time required for transurethral resection would significantly increase perioperative complications. Open procedures account for only ≤5 percent of prostatectomies. Many surgeons prefer to perform an "incomplete" TURP to avoid the morbidity of abdominal or perineal surgery. In retrospective studies, open prostatectomy has lower reoperation rate and mortality than TURP, but these studies did not adequately control for increased age and comorbidity in TURP patients or the secular trend of decreasing TURP mortality in older men.

Prostate Incision

Men with small glands (<30 g) can be treated with transurethral incision of the prostate (TUIP or prostatotomy). TUIP is a technically simpler procedure than resection that can be done with local anesthesia and in a shorter operation time. RCTs comparing TUIP with TURP show similar symptomatic efficacy at 1 year. In a select case series with 2-year follow-up, only 8 percent of TUIP patients required later TURP. Additional advantages of TUIP include less bleeding complications and retrograde ejaculation. TUIP has the potential to be a safe and effective alternative for older men with high operative risk, BOO, and a small prostate in whom noninvasive treatment has failed.

Laser Prostatectomy

Despite the introduction over the last 10 years of a wide variety of laser systems to destroy prostate tissue, the long-term role of laser prostatectomy is unclear. Different laser systems yield results of variable definition, consistency and efficacy, making comparisons difficult. In RCTs, TURP is superior to noncontact lasers for symptom improvement, flow rate, and quality of life at 7 months; outcomes become equivalent at 1 year. The single 5-year study found higher reoperation rates with laser (38 percent), even with a TURP reoperation rate (16 percent) higher than in nearly all other studies. Despite its advantage as an outpatient procedure, laser prostatectomy requires longer post-operative catheterization and more infections and urethral irritation. Side effects vary by technique, and include impotence, retrograde ejaculation, increased urgency and frequency for several weeks, incontinence, and bladder neck stricture. Unlike TURP, laser procedures provide no tissue for prostate cancer detection. Given these considerations, laser prostatectomy (like balloon dilation before it) may fall from the therapeutic armamentarium.

Microwave Hyperthermia

Transurethral microwave thermotherapy is another outpatient procedure for destroying prostate tissue. Repeated treatments are usually required. Small, short-term trials show variable results compared with TURP, sham procedures, and terazosin; improvement in LUTS and flow rate are typically modest. The longest RCT (median follow-up 33 months) found TURP markedly superior in decreasing IPSS and complications. The future of this treatment also is uncertain.

Other Approaches

Transurethral needle ablation was less effective than TURP in a 1-year RCT (IPSS decrease 13.6 versus 16 points), although morbidity was less (retrograde ejaculation 0 percent versus 38 percent; bleeding 32 percent versus 100 percent). Prostatic urethral stents can restore spontaneous voiding in frail men with retention who are not surgical candidates or for whom long-term catheterization is undesirable. However, trials have been small, short-term, and nonrandomized, and these devices are complicated by immediate increased LUTS, stent encrustation or migration, infection, urinary incontinence, and retention.

PREVENTION

Prevention of benign prostate disease may be possible by several lifestyle factors. The data on risk and protective factors suggest that increased physical activity, a diet low in meat and fat and high in vegetables and micronutrients, and moderate alcohol consumption may prevent or slow the development of benign prostate disease. Weight loss in obesity, good glycemic control in diabetes, and treatment of high cholesterol also may be important. However, there are no intervention trials to support these suggestions. In men with LUTS, finasteride decreases the risk for TURP and urinary retention; avoidance of anticholinergic agents, calcium channel blockers, and α-adrenergic agonists may decrease the risk of urinary retention.

REFERENCES

Barry M, Roehrborn C: Benign prostatic hyperplasia. *Clin Evid* 775, 2002.

Barry MJ: Evaluation of symptoms and quality of life in men with benign prostatic hyperplasia. *Urology* 58:25, 2001.

Donovan JL et al: A randomized trial comparing transurethral resection of the prostate, laser therapy, and conservative management for lower urinary tract symptoms associated with benign prostatic enlargement: the ClasP study. *J Urol* 164:65, 2000.

Flanigan RC et al: 5-yr outcome of surgical resection and watchful waiting for men with moderately symptomatic BPH: VA cooperative study. *J Urol* 160:12, 1998.

Guthrie RM, Siegel RL. A multicenter, community-based study of doxazosin in the treatment of concomitant hypertension and symptomatic benign prostatic hyperplasia: the Hypertension and BPH Intervention Trial (HABIT). *Clin Ther* 21:1732, 1999.

McConnell JD et al. *Benign Prostatic Hyperplasia: Diagnosis and Treatment. Clinical Practice Guideline,* Number 8. AHCPR Publication No. 94-0582. Rockville, MD: Agency for Health Care Policy and Research, 1994.

McConnell JD et al: The effect of finasteride on the risk of acute urinary retention and the need for surgical treatment among men with benign prostatic hyperplasia. Finasteride Long-Term Efficacy and Safety Study Group. *N Engl J Med* 338:557, 1998.

Wilt T et al: Beta-sitosterols for benign prostatic hyperplasia. *Cochrane Database Syst Rev* 2:CD001043, 2000.

Wilt T et al: Cernilton for benign prostatic hyperplasia. *Cochrane Database Syst Rev* 3:CD001423, 2002.

Wilt TJ et al: Tamsulosin for treating lower urinary tract symptoms compatible with benign prostatic obstruction: a systematic review of efficacy and adverse effects. *J Urol* 167:177, 2002.

Wilt TJ et al: Saw palmetto extracts for treatment of benign prostatic hyperplasia: A systematic review. *JAMA* 280:1604, 1998.

Wilt TJ et al: Terazosin for treating symptomatic benign prostatic obstruction: A systematic review of efficacy and adverse effects. *BJU Int* 89:214, 2002.

Sexual Dysfunction in Older Persons

JOHN E. MORLEY • SYED H. TARIQ

Expressions of sexuality remain important throughout the life span. While, as Ann Landers has suggested, cuddling may be a sufficient expression of sexuality for some older persons, many others remain interested in having sexual intercourse throughout the life span (see Chap. 98). Over the last 20 years, there has been a dramatic increase in our knowledge concerning erectile dysfunction. This has led to the emergence of explicit sexuality in older males as typified by the television advertisements for sildenafil (Viagra), which use older men. In addition there has been an increased awareness of the role of testosterone decline in the aging male and the effects of testosterone replacement, not only in improving libido but also as a putative therapy for frailty. In comparison to the increased awareness of the role of sexual dysfunction in determining the quality of life in males, there has been a paucity of studies examining the prevalence, causes, and effects of sexual dysfunction in women. There is increasing interest in the effects of cognitive dysfunction on sexuality. In recent years increasing attention has been paid to the needs of the older homosexual. A small amount of literature is emerging suggesting that alternative sexual lifestyle practices still occur in older persons and create a variety of issues for consideration by the physician who cares for the elderly person. The importance of sexuality is liable to increase as the baby boomers, who are the products of the sexual revolution of the sixties, enter their retirement years.

The complete expression of sexuality represents a delicate balance of social, cultural, psychological, hormonal, and physical factors as outlined in Table 102-1. While this complexity applies at all ages, aging and old age introduce special considerations that are the focus of this chapter.

SEXUAL FUNCTION AND THE OLDER FEMALE

There is surprisingly little data on the physiologic changes related to sexuality in older women. Masters and Johnson in their pioneering studies on women investigated the effects of the aging process in 11 women older than age 60 years. Compared with younger women, preorgasm there would appear to be less vasocongestion in breast tissue and a reduction in vaginal lubrication. As the plateau phase is reached there is less vasocongestion of the vaginal wall, and less fullness of the clitoris and the fat pad over the mons. Transcervical, vaginal, and uterine tenting are minimized. Engorgement of the areolae and labia is less pronounced. Expansion of the vaginal inner wall still occurs. With the onset of orgasm there is a reduction in orgasmic platform contractions which in some cases may be associated with painful spastic contractions. Following orgasm, during the resolution phase, clitoral tumescence and retraction and the vasocongestion of the vagina is more rapidly lost. On the other hand, nipple erection returns more slowly to the basal state. Table 102-2 summarizes these changes.

A number of studies have determined the frequency of sexual intercourse in women older than 60 years of age. In women aged 60 to 70 years of age, sexual activity was present in from 30 to 78 percent depending on the study. Between 70 to 79 years of age, sexual activity declined to 11 to 74 percent, and beyond 80 years of age the frequency ranged from 8 to 43 percent. On the average, women older than 70 years of age who are sexually active have intercourse just under once a week. In the Sepulveda Veterans administration medical center study, 73 percent enjoyed sexual intercourse and 27 percent reported that they tolerated it. Masturbation has been reported to occur in 40 to 47 percent of older women. Just under 8 percent masturbate at least once a week.

Overall, females over 60 years of age believe that sexuality plays an important role in the maintenance of physical and mental health. Orgasm is an important part of the sexual experience for just under half of older females. Sexual variety, for example, oral sex, is considered an important part of the sexual experience. Masturbation is an acceptable sexual outlet for older females.

Sexual dysfunction is very common in women aged 40 to 60 years. Studies have found a prevalence from 30 to 63 percent. The major reported problems are lack of sexual

Table 102-1 Social and Psychological Factors that may Modulate Sexual Responsiveness in the Middle- and Late-Adult Life Persons

Middle Life (40–60 yrs)	Late Life (60+ yrs)
Adolescent children in house	Bereavement
Reentry into job market	Lack of socially approved partner
Career pressures	Adjusting to bereavement
Demands of aging parents	Coping with spousal illness
Social pressures	Dependency due to illness
Children leaving home (return to the couple)	Agist attitudes
Loss of self-esteem from being homemaker	Children's negative attitudes to sex
Melancholia of middle age	Adaptation to changing body image
Adaptation to changing body image	Previous sexual experiences
Previous sexual experiences	Institutionalization
Dysphoria	Dysphoria
	Cognitive impairment

desire, anorgasmia, vaginal dryness, dyspareunia, and incontinence during intercourse. Sexual activity and sexual interest decline over the menopausal transition as found in both cross-sectional and longitudinal studies. The decline in testosterone, rather than estrogen, levels is the best predictor of changes in sexual desire following the menopause. In many cases, the sexual dysfunction that occurs at midlife is associated with psychological difficulties, especially dysphoria.

In older women there is a paucity of studies on sexual dysfunction. Dyspareunia (pain on intercourse) occurs at some time in life in approximately 10 percent of women. Orgasms occur less often in older women. Approximately one-third of older women are unhappy with their sexual experiences most of the time. The lack of a male partner or erectile dysfunction in their partner represents a major barrier to sexual expression in many older women.

Sexual Dysfunction in Older Women

Ovarian failure is a physiologic event that is often associated with a group of symptoms and consequences that can be considered pathologic. Menopause is the era in the life of every middle-aged woman that reflects that failure and the consequences of associated decline in ovarian hormones.

It is the subject of a separate chapter devoted to this topic, which includes information on the role of estrogen deficiency and hormone replacement therapy on aspects of female genitourinary structure and libido that relate to sexual dysfunction in the postmenopausal woman. However, most information suggests that female sexual function is largely presumed (and possibly even enhanced) following the cessation of menses.

However, as in the premenopausal state, sexual dysfunction in individual older women is a relatively common and frequently underdiagnosed problem. The role of androgens in treatment has received special attention. Minimal data are available on the use of testosterone in older women. Testosterone has been used to improve libido. In addition, testosterone, when given with estrogens, further decreases hot flashes and improves general well being. Testosterone decreases estrogen side effects such as headaches and mastalgia. Testosterone increases bone mineral density and lean body mass in postmenopausal women. Testosterone deficiency is the leading candidate for the rapid decline in muscle mass that occurs in females following the menopause.

For women an oral form of testosterone (methyltestosterone) is available in combination with estrogen (Estratest). Methyltestosterone may increase liver enzymes. Testosterone patches have been developed for women. Testosterone gel can either be compounded by local pharmacists or obtained from AndroGel packets. Testosterone pellets can be implanted subcutaneously. Testosterone cream application locally can be used for treating atrophic vulvar dystrophy. It has been suggested that testosterone cream applied to the clitoris will increase orgasm in anorgasmic women. Tibolone is a unique agent that has mixed estrogenic-progestogenic-androgenic properties and as such appears to be an ideal replacement therapy. Side effects of testosterone therapy include hirsutism, deepening of the voice, and oily skin Dehydroepiandrosterone (DHEA) has mixed androgenic/estrogenic properties in postmenopausal women. It increases libido in women older than 70 years of age. Its use is not recommended because of the variable quality of DHEA products in the health food stores and its potentially carcinogenic effects on the postmenopausal breast. Urogenital also play has been associated with a variety of symptoms that can alter sexual function (Table 102-3).

The Older Lesbian

There is increasing awareness of the presence of a relatively large cohort of older lesbian women who have unique health needs. In this population, both better mental health and less suicidal ideation is associated with less loneliness, lower internalized homophobia, higher self-esteem, and a greater number of persons knowing about the lesbians' sexual identity. Disclosure of sexual identity to friends and family has been associated with greater levels of social support. Mary Adelman, in *In Long Time Passing: Lives of Older Lesbians* (Boston, Alyson Publications, 1986), has provided some important anecdotal insights into the problems that often face the older lesbian.

Table 102-2   Effects of Aging on the Sexual Response

Phase	Female	Male
Excitement (Arousal)	Decreased vaginal lubrication Decreased expansion of vagina Decreased breast vasocongestion Less flattening of labia majora Less vasocongestion labia minora	Delay in obtaining erection Diminished vasocongestion Decreased muscle tensing Decreased scrotal tensing
Plateau	Less areolar engorgement Labia does not change color Limited expansion of inner vagina Tenting of transcervical vagina decreased Uterine elevation less marked Decreased clitoral size Decreased fullness of mons	Decreased Cowper's gland secretion Diminished pre-ejaculation secretion Ejaculatory inevitability is lost
Orgasmic	Decreased contractions Painful, spastic contractions	Shorter duration Decreased ejaculatory force Spastic prostate contractions Less firm erections
Plateau	Clitoral tumescence and retraction more rapid Nipple erection returns to baseline more slowly	More rapid detumescence Longer refractory period

Specific issues that the geriatrician needs to be aware of in dealing with older lesbian women include (1) recognition of the partner who may become the caregiver for an older lesbian. In some cases, this can cause major conflict between the patient, the patient's family, and the patient's lifetime partner. (2) Care to see that adequate cervical cancer screening has been completed, as many lesbian women believe this is less necessary because of their sexual orientation. In contrast, lesbian women tend to be more likely to have breast cancer screening than the general population. (3) The presence of a greater alcohol and marijuana use than in the general population. While there is large variability in the populations' drug use, screening for excess alcohol use is important. (4) Awareness that sexually transmitted diseases may be present in women who only have other women as partners. (5) Awareness of the impact of homophobia on their health. (6) Specific retirement and leisure issues that can be unique to this population. (7) Increased awareness by the health care provider of "hidden" abuse that can occasionally occur in these relationships. (8) Encouraging a lesbian to fill out an appropriate health care directive to ensure that her health decisions are made by the person of her choice.

A number of social organizations have developed to provide support and services for older lesbians. These include Gays and Lesbians Older and Wiser (GLOW) in the Midwest and Gay and Lesbian Outreach to Elders (GLOE) in San Francisco. Health care workers need to be aware of these options in their community for older lesbians.

Good research into the social and health needs of older lesbians is lacking. Most available data is based on anecdotal reports or small-scale studies. This is an area where there is a need for more data to guide the health care professional.

The Effect of Specific Diseases on Sexuality, Especially in Older Women

Diseases can interfere with sexuality either by direct effects, for example, dyspnea, angina, pain or by altering body image. Physicians' office should have easily accessible brochures available for patients that discuss the effects of various diseases on sexuality. Table 102-4 is an example for counseling patients after a myocardial infarction. Such brochures should be gender neutral whenever possible.

Incontinence occurs during intercourse in approximately 25 percent of women at some time. Urinary

Table 102-3   Symptoms Associated with Urogenital Atrophy

Pruritus

Burning

Dryness

Dysuria

Dyspareunia

Bleeding

Infection

Frequent small volume urination

Incontinence

Postvoid dribbling

Table 102–4   Instructions for Patients and their Spouses after Myocardial Infarction

1. Sexual activity may be resumed as soon as you can bring your heart rate to 120 beats per minute without occasioning chest pain or shortness of breath, the equivalent of climbing two flights of stairs rapidly.
2. If chest pain develops during intercourse, take a nitroglycerine. If the pain does not subside within 15 minutes, consider this an emergency.
3. If chest pain regularly develops during sexual intercourse, take a nitroglycerine 10 minutes before attempting sex.
4. No sexual position is the best or is prohibited. Some patients may find one position preferable for their needs.
5. Altered desire after a heart attack is usually due to psychological factors, such as fear of another attack. Please discuss these problems with your physician.
6. Altered ability to obtain an erection after a heart attack may be due to medications or to vascular disease of the penis. These are both treatable. Please discuss this with your physician.
7. If the female has decreased vaginal lubrication or pain during intercourse, ask your physician to prescribe a lubricant or, in some cases, you may need estrogen replacement.
8. There is no time of day during which we know that sex is safer or more dangerous. Please be advised that sexual activity in a novel situation, for example, with a partner other than your spouse, appears to be associated with increased problems.
9. Discuss your sexual needs and concerns frankly with your spouse.
10. Any questions or concerns you have should be brought to the attention of your physician or nurse. It is best that both you and your spouse read these instructions. Feel free to have your spouse discuss his or her problems with the health professional team.

SOURCE: Developed by JE Morley for patient counseling.

incontinence is associated with decreased sexual intimacy in nearly 50 percent of women attending an incontinence clinic. Reasons for the reduction in sexual activity included bed wetting and associated need for separate beds, urine leaking during coitus, associated dyspareunia, and depression. Urge incontinence appears more likely to lead to major sexual dysfunction than does stress incontinence. Postcoital desire to urinate is common in older women. Atrophic changes result in dysuria and "honeymoon cystitis." Treatment consists of using an appropriately formulated lubricant, for example, Astroglide, and/or estrogen.

Hysterectomies are performed more commonly in the United States than in the rest of the world. Absence of a uterus can result in decreased vasocongestion, diminished ballooning of the vagina, and a loss of uterine contraction during orgasm. Vaginal scarring may lead to discomfort and/or dyspareunia. However, there is little evidence that hysterectomy alters sexual performance. Overall, changes in sexuality following hysterectomy are more often related to the woman's and her spouse's beliefs. Both the patient and her spouse need to be appropriately educated following hysterectomy to avoid becoming a victim of the many mythologies concerning the impact of hysterectomy on sexuality. When women are considering a hysterectomy, they need to be educated on alternatives such as myomectomy, endometrial resection of submucous fibroids, and conservative treatments for endometriosis. The potential effects of prophylactic removal of the ovaries need to be fully discussed. Decisions on whether or not to have a hysterectomy should involve a true collaboration between the woman and her gynecologist.

Stroke is associated with decreased libido (particularly left brain infarction), frequency of intercourse, and orgasm. Major reasons for these changes were attributed to decreased maneuverability and fear of another stroke. The physician needs to encourage the use of alternative sexual positions and pillows and to educate the spouse of a person with homonymous hemianopsia and hemineglect to make approaches from the visually intact side. Physicians need to control high blood pressure to allow reassurance that sexual intercourse is unlikely to precipitate another stroke. Depression, which can occur in up to one-third of women following a stroke, needs to be diagnosed and treated.

Hemodialysis is associated with decreased vaginal lubrication, anorgasmia, and a decline in frequency of intercourse. Depression commonly occurs in these patients and may be the cause of the decreased sexuality. Diabetes mellitus is associated with decreased vaginal lubrication and clitoral nerve degeneration. However, changes in libido and orgasmic frequency are more likely to be a result of failure to cope with the disease process and/or depression than the disease per se.

Ostomies result in a decrease in sexual activity and, in many cases, associated dyspareunia. Persons with ileostomies tend to do better than those with colostomies. Persons with chronic pain have nearly twice the prevalence of sexual difficulties as does the general population.

Osteoarthritis of the hip not only decreases sexual activity because of pain but also because of joint stiffness, creating difficulties in positioning for sexual intercourse. Rheumatoid arthritis is associated with a decreased libido and orgasm. Side-by-side or rear entry position, together with innovative use of pillows, often are necessary for intercourse to occur. Use of pain medication prior to intercourse may be necessary. Arthritis of the hands can prevent masturbation. In these cases a vibrator may be helpful. Sjögren's syndrome and xerostomia are associated with decreased salivary flow leading to a reduction in oral–genital contact. Sjögren's can also result in a dry, atrophic vagina, and dyspareunia.

Breasts and their stimulation play an important role in female sexuality. Breast cancer, therefore, represents a major factor in altering sexual adjustment. Mastectomy creates major changes in sexual activity. Women who receive breast-conserving therapy have better sexual outcomes than those who have a modified radical mastectomy. Following mastectomy nipple stimulation decreases. If there is discomfort from scar tissue on the side of the removed breasts, using a small pillow or female astride position might be useful alternatives. Presurgical counseling prior to mastectomy of both the patient and her partner improves sexual functioning following mastectomy. Partners need to be encouraged to communicate with one another, as the spouse often limits comments in fear of offending his wife. Two special issues exist for African American women following mastectomy: knowing where prostheses that are appropriate for the person's skin coloring are available and where to find support groups specifically for them.

Sexual Assault of Older Women

Older women can be the victims of rape, which is often associated with physical violence. Vaginal vault tears are not rare in the older women, with an atrophic vagina, who is sexually assaulted. Prophylaxis for venereal disease should be provided. Recognition of the fear and humiliation associated with sexual assault in an older woman is important, as is follow-up and support to prevent depression. Physicians in nursing homes need to be aware of the fact that sexual assault on residents by workers or other patients may occur. In these cases, completing the full rape investigation kit sample collection rapidly after the event is a key component in the physician's response.

Management Issues

It is important that physicians ask older females about problems associated with sexuality. Sexual therapy involves four stages:

- Permission giving, for example, permission to indulge in sexual fantasies or to assume new sexual positions.
- Provision of limited information, for example, provision of graded erotic exercises that are acceptable to the person's cultural background or how to stretch the vagina prior to resuming intercourse following a long period of celibacy.
- Specific suggestions, for example, use of vibrators, how to do paraclitoral stimulation or the use of lubricants such as Astroglide.
- Sex therapy, for example, dealing with deep seated issues or couples counseling.

There is no evidence that sildenafil improves sexuality in women. Depression or anxiety can be important inhibitors of sexual activity.

It is important to increase the awareness that, when desired, sexuality is an important component of mental health. Sex represents a key form of enjoyment for many older women. Sex is a natural body function. In older women, sexual dysfunction needs to be approached from the biopsychosocial paradigm. While for some women testosterone, antidepressants, or pain medication may alleviate problems; in the majority of women counseling, education, and support groups are the key to successful therapeutic outcomes.

SEXUALITY AND THE OLDER MALE

Three major issues exist as far as sexuality and the older male is concerned. These are libido concerns, erectile dysfunction, and couples conflict. Before any intervention is undertaken in an older male, it is essential that any conflicts between the male and his partner are explored. Enhancing a male's libido or improving his erectile dysfunction will often cause major conflicts if the partner is uninterested in these outcomes. For some males the ability to have an erection is equated to their immortality. We have provided a number of patients with vacuum tumescence devices, which are then stored in the garage, so that the male knows he has the ability to have an erection if he really needs it. Older males' sexual partners are not always the obvious or expected person. The physician needs to determine the sexual partner without others present.

Libido

Libido or the enthusiasm for sex is dependent on one's testosterone level, the learned responses of the individual, and their general health-related quality of life. Testosterone levels decline in the male older than age 30 years at the rate of approximately 1 percent per year. This has been demonstrated in both cross-sectional and longitudinal studies. The fall in testosterone is accompanied by both an increase in sex hormone-binding globulin (SHBG) and by an increase in the affinity of SHBG for testosterone. This results in the tissue-available testosterone being much lower than the total testosterone level in older men. For these reasons free testosterone or the calculated free testosterone index are inappropriate measurements of hypogonadism in older men. The assays recommended for measuring gonadal status in older men are the free testosterone by dialysis and the bioavailable testosterone (free and albumin-bound testosterone). The free testosterone by analog assay is an inappropriate measure of gonadal status. This assay is the one most commonly provided when a practitioner orders a "free testosterone" in the United States.

When bioavailable testosterone is used to determine whether or not men are hypogonadal, 2 to 5 percent of men in their forties and 35 to 70 percent of men in their seventies are found to be hypogonadal. This large range in different studies represents the lack of truly appropriate epidemiologic studies being undertaken. In the studies so far, the samples have been enriched either for excessively healthy males or for those with some degree of problems. It has been estimated that there are 4 to 5 million untreated men with hypogonadism in the United States.

The decline in testosterone secretion in aging males is predominantly caused by chaotic secretion of

Table 102-5 The Androgen Deficiency in Aging Male (ADAM) Questionnaire

			A positive answer represent yes to 1 or 7 or any 3 other questions.
(Circle one)			
Yes	No	1.	Do you have a decrease in libido (sex drive)?
Yes	No	2.	Do you have a lack of energy?
Yes	No	3.	Do you have a decrease in strength and/or endurance?
Yes	No	4.	Have you lost height?
Yes	No	5.	Have you noticed a decreased enjoyment of life?
Yes	No	6.	Are you sad and/or grumpy?
Yes	No	7.	Are your erections less strong?
Yes	No	8.	Have you noticed a recent deterioration in your ability to play sports?
Yes	No	9.	Are you falling asleep after dinner?
Yes	No	10.	Has there been a recent deterioration in your work performance?

gonadotrophin-releasing hormone, which results in a decline in luteinizing hormone (LH) secretion. This results in less LH to drive the failing testes with the result that testosterone secretion declines. In addition, the negative feedback of testosterone on the pituitary is more potent in older males.

Bioavailable testosterone levels have been correlated not only with libido but also with sleep erections and quality of erections. Testosterone treatment increases libido and nighttime erections. Testosterone therapy, while having only a small effect on true erectile dysfunction, clearly increases the "hardness" of the erection. This is because testosterone is essential for the activity of nitric oxide synthase. Nitric oxide increases the relaxation of the smooth muscle of the corpora cavernosa. In some patients who fail sildenafil, testosterone therapy will result in erections occurring after sildenafil.

Besides its effects on libido, testosterone therapy in older males has also increased lean body mass, decreased fat mass, increased strength, enhanced some aspects of cognition, increased bone mineral density (predominantly due to its aromatization to estrogen), decreased angina, decreased leptin and increased functional status. These effects may be a more important reason for testosterone replacement therapy in the older male than the effects of testosterone on libido and sexual function.

The Saint Louis University Androgenic Deficiency in Aging Males (ADAM) questionnaire is a simple 10-question forced yes-or-no-answer questionnaire that has good sensitivity and specificity for detecting males with hypogonadism (Table 102-5). Depression is a major cause of a false positive for this questionnaire. The questionnaire is widely used throughout the world and has been translated into a number of different languages. Persons who answer positively to the questionnaire should have a bioavailable or free testosterone measured on at least two occasions, a week apart (major week-to-week variation of testosterone levels has been demonstrated). Only when these values are

low should treatment be undertaken. It is important at this juncture to acknowledge that testosterone replacement in the absence of clear-cut hypogonadism is controversial, and no clear consensus has emerged regarding this case.

Testosterone replacement therapy can be either given by injections, transdermally (patch or gel), pellets, or orally (not at present in the United States). Injection therapy, although inexpensive, tends to give values of testosterone that exceed the physiologic range. The other therapies all produce values within the physiologic range. Patches tend to produce a relatively high degree of skin irritation (5 to 30 percent). Transscrotal patches are unacceptable to most men. The gel preparation has been very successful and has a low incidence of skin irritation. Testosterone undecenoate, an oral product, has been successfully used in the rest of the world for more than 20 years. Methyltestosterone is an oral product that is available in the United States. Its use is not recommended because of the potential liver toxicity of this formulation. Before treating males with testosterone, a normal prostate-specific antigen (PSA) and hematocrit needs to be documented. The PSA and the hematocrit need to be obtained every 6 months during therapy. Other side effects of testosterone therapy include gynecomastia and water retention. The effects of testosterone on patients with sleep apnea are variable. Where possible, sleep apnea should be treated before commencing testosterone replacement.

Erectile Function and the Older Male

As is the case with the female, a number of changes occur in the male sexual response with aging (see Table 102-2). With aging, it takes longer for an erection to develop and there is less scrotal vasocongestion. The final erection is less firm, but may remain tumescent longer before ejaculation. Orgasm is quicker and associated with a decreased volume and force of ejaculation. Detumescence is more rapid but it takes longer for the vasocongestion to resolve.

The period before the subsequent erection can be obtained is prolonged.

Erectile Dysfunction

Erectile dysfunction (impotence) is defined as the inability to obtain and sustain an erection adequate for intercourse on at least two-thirds of attempts. Erectile dysfunction (ED) is extremely common, accounting for 525,000 outpatient visits a year. Severe ED is present in 20 million males in the United States, and if males with some degree of ED are included, this number rises to 30 million. The Massachusetts Male Aging Study reported that the incidence of ED was 5 percent at 40 years of age and 15 percent at 70 years of age. Total ED occurred in 10 percent of these men. Of men older than age 40 years who visited a physician, 34 percent had ED. Despite this high prevalence, it is important to recognize that aging per se is not a cause of ED.

ED is a major factor resulting in a decline in health related quality of life. Up until the 1980s, ED was considered to be primarily caused by psychological factors. In the pioneering study of Slag and his colleagues published in *JAMA* in 1983, this myth was exploded when they could find only 14 percent of patients with ED in a large series to have a primary psychogenic cause. It is now accepted that most ED has an organic primary etiology, although in many males, there may also be an emotional component. When ED first starts, the male begins to become stressed at the time of intercourse. This results in norepinephrine release with a decrease in smooth muscle relaxation and, therefore, poorer erections. This condition is known as performance anxiety and is a component of most early organic ED.

An erection occurs when erotic stimuli (or the fantasizing about erotic events) results in a relaxation of the smooth muscle of the corpora cavernosa allowing blood to rush into the corporal sinusoids. This distension of the corporal sinusoids leads to obstruction of venous outflow by compressing the venous plexuses against the tunica albuginea. These events are mediated by neuronal messages from the central nervous system to the thoracolumbar spinal cord and then to the penis. Parasympathetic nerves that inhibit contraction of the smooth muscle of the corpora cavernosa come from the sacral spinal nerve (S2 to S4) to the penis via the nervi erigentes. Erections caused by penile stimulation are mediated through the sacral nerve center involving the pudendal nerve. This mechanism is also important in the maintenance of an erection during intercourse. Persons with pudendal nerve neuropathy lose their erection soon after penetration.

Relaxation of the smooth muscle of the corpora cavernosa is mediated by nonadrenergic noncholinergic neurotransmitters. These are under control of acetylcholine from the parasympathetic nerves and α-adrenergic receptors. The major mediator of smooth-muscle relaxation is nitric oxide (NO). NO is produced by nitric oxide synthase, an enzyme whose production is regulated by testosterone. NO activates guanylyl cyclase resulting in the production of cyclic guanosine monophosphate (cGMP). Relaxation of the cavernosal smooth muscles occurs because cGMP inhibits influx of calcium into these cells. cGMP is degraded by phosphodiesterase-5, and thus inhibitors of this enzyme, such as sildenafil, enhance erectile performance. Prostaglandin E_1 and vasoactive intestinal peptide also play a role in the smooth muscle relaxation associated with obtaining a penile erection. The penis is kept in the flaccid state by input from noradrenergic (α_2), nerves, as well as by the local release of endothelin. Another factor involved in the decline in erectile capacity with aging is the increase of collagen cross-linking within the corpora cavernosa, resulting in reduced compliance of type 3 collagen fibers. This is an important factor in the pathogenesis of ED in patients with diabetes mellitus.

There are numerous causes of ED. Table 102-6 compares the causes of erectile dysfunction as reported by a variety of different referral centers. The role of hypogonadism in ED is controversial. It is clearly necessary for the full elaboration of NO synthase. Certainly, extremely low levels can be associated with complete ED and in these cases testosterone can restore erectile function to normal. However, in most cases, testosterone therapy may improve erectile capacity slightly and only for a few months. In these cases, it is clearly not the major cause of ED.

While psychogenic causes of ED are relatively rare, they need to be excluded. Depression is a cause of ED that is readily treatable. Persons with anxiety will have increased circulating norepinephrine making obtaining an erection more difficult. The "widower's syndrome" is a unique cause of ED seen in older men. It occurs in a male who has been happily married for a long time and whose spouse dies. A female friend of the family who has also lost a partner may then start to take care of the male doing cooking and chores around the house. After a time, she then suggests that they should have intercourse. The male, not wanting to lose the domestic help, but at the same time not finding this female an appropriate sexual partner develops ED to protect himself from having to have intercourse. Marital discord and sexual phobias may also cause ED.

Atherosclerotic vascular disease is the most common cause of ED in older males. Not only does it cause blockage of the penile arteries, but it also causes venous leaks. Persons with ED caused by vascular disease are at extremely high risk of developing other vascular disease, that is, myocardial infarction or stroke, within 2 years of the diagnosis of ED. For this reason, all males with ED from a vascular cause should be provided with appropriate counseling and screening for the prevention of cardiovascular disease. Persons with hypertension can develop ED, which resolves when the blood pressure is controlled because of a decrease in penile vascular engorgement. However, treatment of hypertension can result in ED caused by the direct effects of the medications on the erectile process.

A variety of neurologic conditions can result in ED. The presenting feature for approximately half the males with multiple sclerosis is ED. It is particularly troublesome as the ED may be present for a time and then disappear, only to return at a later date during another multiple sclerosis flare. Strokes and temporal lobe epilepsy can also lead to ED. Spinal cord injury often is associated with ED. Following surgery for adenocarcinoma of the prostate, up to half of males may have ED.

Table 102-6 Causes of Erectile Dysfunction in Older Persons in Different Clinic Situations

Clinic	Referral base (Reference)				
	Endocrine (a)	Urology (b)	Sex Therapist (c)	FP (d)	Medical Outpatient (e)
Number of Patients	105	165	101	154	120
Mean age (range)	?	? (19–79)	40	50.3 (21–79)	59.4
Etiologic factor (percent)					
Endocrine	44	6	45	24	29
Hypogonadism	26	6	39	23	19
Thyroid	3	-	4	-	4
Hyperprolactinoma	8	-	2	-	6
Diabetes mellitus	7	19	2	20	9
Vascular	-	8	1	37	-
Neurogenic	-	4	2	5	7
Surgical/trauma	-	8	-	-	-
Urologic	-	8	-	49	6
Alcoholism	3	0.6	-	7	7
Systemic Disease	6	-	2	5	5
Medication	7	2	0	12	25
Psychiatric	14	-	-	-	-
Psychogenic	14	51	19	60	14
Unknown	19	0.6	-	0	7

Clinic	Referral base (Reference)			
	Outpatient Clinic (f)	Urology (g)*	Outpatient (h)	Outpatient (i)
Number of Patients	93	31	121	297
Mean age (range)	61(50–80)	53(32–76)	68(60–85)	66(27–98)
Etiologic factor (percent)				
Endocrine	35	-	-	54
Hypogonadism	9.6	19	2.6	43–81
Thyroid	2	-	-	-
Hyperprolactinoma	4	-	-	0.3
Diabetes mellitus	22	-	-	27–29
Vascular	37.6	68	21	39–55
Neurogenic	17	26	17¶/11**	3–10
Surgical/trauma	-	-	-	-
Urologic	19	3	1.3	7–12
Alcoholism	20	-	-	12–14
Systemic disease	-	-	-	-
Medication	67	-	4	58
Psychiatric	-	-	-	18–5
Psychogenic	15	19	9.2	9–3
Unknown	-	-	4	-

SOURCE: *All diabetic male patients
¶Diabetic-neuropathy/**non-diabetic-neuropathy
a. Spark et al. JAMA 263:750, 1980
b. Montague et al. Urology 14:545, 1979
c. Legros et al. Clin Psychoendocrinology 1:301, 1978
d. Collins et al. Can Med Assoc J. 128:1393, 1983.
e. Slag et al. JAMA 269:1736,1983
f. Davis et al. West J Med. 142:499, 1985.
g. Lehman & Jacobs. J Urology 129:2191, 1983.
h. Kaiser et al. J Am Geriat Soc. 36:511, 1988
i. Tariq et al. Unpublished series

A number of systemic disorders are commonly associated with ED. These include renal failure, chronic obstructive pulmonary disease (COPD), and diabetes mellitus. Persons with low PaO_2 have very low testosterone levels and a decrease in cavernosal nitric oxide. Oxygen therapy improves erectile capacity in men with COPD. Males with diabetes mellitus have lower testosterone levels than other males. However, the major cause of ED in diabetes appears to be the presence of atherosclerosis. Endocrine disorders such as hyperprolactinemia (prolactinomas), hyperthyroidism, and hypothyroidism are responsible for ED in 1 in 20 males. Peyronie's disease occurs because of plaque formation in the penis. It is associated with pain on erection, and often with a deformed erection.

Cigarette smoking is the major drug-induced cause of ED. Smoking causes ED both from the direct effects of nicotine causing smooth-muscle contraction in the corpora and from the long-term effects caused by accelerated atherosclerosis. Alcohol is known to provoke desire but to diminish performance. Opiate addiction is associated with low testosterone levels.

Numerous medications are associated with ED. Some medicines also interfere with desire and/or ejaculation. The major classes of medication producing ED include anticholinergic antidepressants (with the exception of trazodone), antihistamines, antihypertensives, antipsychotics, H_2-receptor antagonists, metoclopramide, barbiturates, anticonvulsants, and antiandrogens (megestrol acetate, spironolactone, digitalis, ketoconazole, gonadotropin-releasing hormone [GnRH] antagonists, and estrogens).

At this time, a complete sexual history and physical examination represents a key to developing an appropriate management plan for the male with ED. The International Index of Erectile Function is recommended as a good questionnaire to use to evaluate ED. Severe injuries to the penis when young and long-distance bicycle riding are both associated with ED. A careful history should also be obtained from the partner. This history should include the feelings about their partner's ability to obtain an erection. If psychological or couples problems exist, or if the patient is depressed, these conditions should be treated before pursuing the direct management of ED. Determination of nocturnal penile tumescence is no longer recommended in the work-up of ED. Work-up of vascular disease can be done. The easiest of these tests to perform is the Penile Brachial Pulse Index (PBPI). However, the large variability in results has led to it rarely being used. More complex tests used by urologists include pulsed Doppler ultrasonography for arterial function, dynamic infusion cavernosometry for vascular leaks, and penile arteriography to establish the potency of the arterial tree from the aortic bifurcation to the penis. In some cases, direct intracavernosal injection of prostaglandin E_1 may be useful to determine the patency of the arterial system and whether or not a venous leak exists.

Table 102-7 lists the various treatment options. Counseling should be part of the treatment of all patients with ED. This should include discussion of safe-sex options. The different options should be discussed with the patient and his partner. This should include a discussion of the cost of the agents, as well as their effectiveness and side effects. Counseling to stop smoking is a key component for long-term success. Medications should be reviewed and stopped or changed to ones less likely to result in ED, such as angiotensin-converting enzyme inhibitors.

At present most patients will choose sildenafil (Viagra), which is a phosphodiesterase-5 inhibitor. Before sildenafil became available, we used pentoxifylline, a nonspecific phosphodiesterase inhibitor, with some success. Two other phosphodiesterase-5 inhibitors are in clinical trials: IC351 and vardenafil. Sildenafil is effective in 50 to 70 percent of persons in whom it has been tried. It appears to be less effective in persons with diabetes mellitus and over 70 years of age men. It takes about an hour for its onset of action and requires tactile or erotic stimulation to produce its effect. It cannot be given to persons receiving nitrates because

Table 102-7   Treatment Options for Men with Erectile Dysfunction

MEDICATIONS:

- Phosphodiesterase inhibitors
  -sildenafil
  -vardenafil
  -IC351
  -pentoxifylline
- Apomorphine slow release
- Yohimbine
- Testosterone (usually as an adjunct in persons with low libido)
  -Oral[§]
  -Transdermal.
    -patch
    -gel
  -Injection
- Zinc (if zinc deficient)
- Intracavernosal agents
  -Prostaglandin E1
  -Phentolaine
  -Papavenne
- Transpenile[⊥]
  -Nitroglycerine
  -Minoxidil

VACUUM TUMESCENT DEVICES SURGICAL THERAPY

- Prosthesis
  -semirigid
  -inflatable
- Arterial surgery
- Venous surgery

PSYCHOLOGICAL THERAPY
- Treat Depression
- Couples Counseling

SOURCE: ⊥ not recommended, § not available in USA.

of the increased propensity of sudden death. The major side effects are dyspepsia, headache, dizziness, and visual changes. Its effect can last up to 24 hours.

Apomorphine slow release (Uprima) is another oral agent used to treat ED. It works through dopaminergic pathways and its mechanisms of action is completely different from sildenafil. The major side effect is nausea and vomiting. It is somewhat less effective than sildenafil in producing erections.

Intracavernosal injections of vasodilators such as prostaglandin E_1, papaverine, and/or phentolamine are more effective than oral agents at producing erections (70 to 100 percent effective). Prostaglandin E_1 (PGE_1)causes some local pain in approximately 20 percent of patients. Local bruising can be a problem. Priapism (prolonged erection) may require injection of norepinephrine directly into the penis. Repeated penile injections have a small risk of fibrosis. Occasionally, these injections can lead to systemic hypotension.

The medicated urethral system for erection (MUSE) involves inserting a pellet of PGE_1 into the urethra. Success rate is much lower than with intracavernosal injections. It is used with a constriction band (Actis) at the base of the penis in an attempt to reduce venous leakage. A number of penile creams, including nitroglycerin and minoxidil, have been used to increase erectile function. Their success rate has not been sufficient for them to be marketed in the United States.

Vacuum tumescence devices have been used for more than 100 hundred years. They consist of either a manual or battery-powered vacuum cylinder that is removed after the erection has been obtained and a constrictor band slipped over the base of the penis. They are somewhat cumbersome to use. Acceptance is low in most couples.

Yohimbine has been used for many years to promote erectile function. It is slightly better than placebo in patients with ED caused by psychogenic causes. It can produce hypertension and cause liver dysfunction. Its use will probably disappear with the availability of Uprima. Severe zinc deficiency can lead to low testosterone and ED. Diuretics, cirrhosis, diabetes mellitus, and renal failure can all result in zinc deficiency.

Penile prostheses remain the gold standard for outcomes in ED, although most men will choose another treatment, and many will accept ED rather than having surgery. Penile prostheses are highly acceptable, with more than 80 percent of men and partners being happy with the outcome. The major complications associated with penile prostheses are infection or insertion of the wrong size. There are two types of penile prostheses: the semirigid rods and the inflatable. Some older persons with arthritis cannot successfully inflate a prostheses. Inflatable prostheses have a failure rate at 5 years of approximately 30 percent. For most older persons, the semirigid prostheses would appear to be the prostheses of choice.

In the last 20 years, there have been major advances in the ability to treat ED. At this stage, the majority of older males with ED can be treated. Treatment of ED can result in dramatic improvements in health-related quality of life, not only for the male but also for his partner.

Complementary Medicine and Sexuality

A tricyclic triterpene alcohol, ambrein is obtained from Ambra grisea and increases LH and testosterone. Cantharidin ("Spanish fly") is a phosphodiesterase inhibitor obtained from blister beetles. It produces congestion of the corpora and inflammation. This agent can produce hematuria and other morbidity. Ginsenosides, derived from Panax ginseng, produce stimulation of NO synthase. At present, no clinical trials demonstrating convincing efficacy of these products are available.

Prostate Cancer and Sexual Quality of Life

Nearly one-half of men undergoing radical prostatectomy for adenocarcinoma of the prostate will have erectile dysfunction. Nerve sparing surgery can improve the outcomes during prostate surgery. An equally important factor in sexual quality of life in patients with prostate cancer is when they have an orchiectomy or receive GnRH analogs to reduce their testosterone levels. Males with orchiectomy may have psychological problems related to the loss of testes. Both groups develop decreased libido. Hot flashes and night sweats are not rare following these treatments. In addition, these males can suffer from fatigue, loss of muscle mass and strength, decreased bone mineral density, and a decreased hematocrit related to testosterone deficiency. In one study, orchiectomy patients had a better perception of their overall health and were more likely to consider themselves cured of prostate cancer than those receiving GnRH analogs. A separate issue is whether a patient who has had surgery for prostate cancer and then develops testosterone deficiency (andropause) may then be considered a candidate for testosterone therapy. This area is highly controversial. However, a consensus is emerging that if the male has had a PSA of 0 for 3 to 5 years, testosterone replacement into the low physiologic range may be appropriate. The PSA needs to be carefully monitored initially at 6 weeks and 3 months, and then every 4 months thereafter. The patient needs to be informed that long term outcomes of this approach are unknown.

Male Homosexuality

A number of older men are homosexual. The physician needs to be aware of the sexual orientation of patients. Unprotected sex occurs in approximately 10 percent of older homosexuals. The potential of an older male indulging in unprotected sex increases if they are lonely, and decreases if they are married. Acquired immunodeficiency syndrome (AIDS) is increasingly seen among older men (see Chap. 87). Education regarding safe-sex practices remains important in the older population. As with the older lesbian, the older male homosexual should be encouraged to have an advanced directive for health to allow decisions to be made by his partner. Caregiving issues need to be discussed. Family conflicts may lead to depression. If the older male is a member of the "leather" community, counseling concerning possible dangers associated with sadomasochistic behavior should be undertaken. This will also create difficulties for the physician in distinguishing between abuse and consensual sexual behavior. Awareness of appropriate support groups for older gays should exist. When orchiectomy is being carried out in an older gay male, the importance of testes in his sexual play needs to determine the need for the insertion of testicular prostheses. Older males with a history of anal sex should be regularly examined for anal cancer, as its prevalence is increased in persons who have had sexually transmitted infections. This appears to be a result of the presence of human papillomavirus-16. The physician needs to be aware of the benefits of testosterone (or other anabolic steroids) in the treatment of muscle wasting in males with AIDS.

SEXUALLY TRANSMITTED DISEASES

An article in *Age and Ageing* titled, "Age is no bar to sexually acquired infections." The geriatrician needs to have awareness that the incidence of sexually transmitted diseases in patients older than 65 years of age is significant in both males and females for newly acquired disease and the sequelae of disease obtained at a younger age. Sexually transmitted diseases seen in older persons include gonorrhea, syphilis, chlamydia, trichomonas, and human papillomavirus. Ten percent of all AIDS cases diagnosed in the United States are in persons older than 50 years of age. This represents nearly 20,000 persons. Education regarding safe sex remains a prerogative of health professionals throughout the patient's life span.

ALTERNATIVE SEXUALITY

Numerous alternative sexual practices (fetish behavior or paraphilias) are present in the younger population. Many persons who indulge in these behaviors continue them into late life, but they rarely come to the attention of physicians. A classic example is transvestism (cross-dressing), which would not be recognized unless the patient arrived in the doctor's office dressed in the clothes of the opposite sex. Infantilism (wearing diapers and needing to be treated as a baby) has been reported to occur in an 80-year-old male who had indulged in this behavior periodically throughout his life. Allopotemnophillia (a sexual preference for amputees) and autoapotemnophillia (a desire for amputation as an enhancement of one's sexuality) have likewise been seen in older men and women. Anal eroticism, including the insertion of a variety of objects into the rectum for sexual gratification, also occurs in older persons. The relationship of the common practice of demented persons to "digging out" feces and playing with feces to anal fetishism during their younger years is worthy of exploration.

Autoerotic deaths have been recognized to occur among older persons in the forensic literature. These range from a 77-year-old widower who died from a myocardial infarction while masturbating with a vacuum cleaner and a hair dryer to autoerotic asphyxial deaths. Accidental asphyxial deaths usually occur from hanging and can be associated with a variety of bondage techniques and cross-dressing.

Sadomasochism is the preferred sexual behavior of a small percentage of the population. For some, this can include severe whippings and/or cutting the skin with a knife (particularly in the genital area). Nipple torture can result in severe bruising of the breasts. Bondage can result in rope burns and mummification can lead to asphyxiation. Physicians need to be aware of these practices, both so that they can give advice on the potential dangers of these behaviors in older person (e.g., poor wound healing) and also to differentiate these consensual sexual practices from elder abuse, although obviously the line between elder abuse and consensual sadomasochism can be blurred in many cases. This becomes particularly true when one or the other partner becomes cognitively impaired.

Pedophilia is another important area for the physician to be aware of. Grandfather incest is not rare and inappropriate touching of young relatives is even more common. Pedophilia outside the family circle also continues to occur in older men. These men may seek treatment for hypogonadism. Clearly this creates a major ethical conundrum for the physician. Pedophilia can occur for the first time or activity can increase when an older person develops cognitive impairment.

As is the case with paraphilias in younger persons, the physician needs to be nonjudgmental and supportive where the paraphilia is not injurious to the patient or others. Where the behavior is harmful, the physician, nurses, and social workers need to be prepared to aggressively intervene, even to the extent of contacting law enforcement officials when appropriate. A separate series of issues exists when the alternative sexual behavior occurs in a person with dementia.

SEXUALITY AND DEMENTIA

Dementia can lead to the disinhibition of normal social restraints resulting in hypersexuality and/or paraphilic behavior. Besides dementia, other neurologic and psychiatric conditions can lead to unacceptable sexual behaviors. These include mania, frontal lobe epilepsy, brain tumors, septal injury and the Klüver-Bucy syndrome (decreased drive in general associated with increased sexuality and oral behaviors caused by bilateral medial temporal lobe lesions).

The most common disturbing behaviors in patients with dementia include making inappropriate sexual remarks, showing a marked sexual interest in other persons to the level of disturbing the spouse, exposure of genitals (exhibitionism), touching or rubbing against a nonconsenting adult (frotteurism) and sexual activity with other demented persons. As alluded to in previous situations, pedophilia and rape can also occur as the result of cognitive impairment.

In many cases, treatment can successfully be accomplished by behavior modification, such as careful avoidance of contact that may be considered sexual, not "flirting" with the patient, and firmly telling the person to stop the behavior; along with reassurance of the caregiver that these behaviors are caused by cognitive impairment.

In some cases, pharmacologic therapy may be appropriate, but in many cases, there is a tendency for health professionals to look for a drug solution before using behavioral options. No controlled trials exist on the efficacy of any of the drugs presently used to treat hypersexuality in demented persons and thus treatment recommendations are based on anecdotal case reports. Selective serotonin reuptake inhibitors (SSRIs) appear to decrease libido and may be effective in treating hypersexuality. Fluvoxamine may be the preferred agent because of its antiobsessional effects. Prostagestational agents (megestrol acetate and medroxyprogesterone acetate) lower testosterone and have been used to treat undesirable sexual behaviors. Unfortunately, these drugs then increase the likelihood of undesirable side effects caused by hypogonadism, that is, sarcopenia, osteoporosis, and decreased cognition and are associated with an increase in deep vein thrombosis. Cyproterone acetate is an antiandrogen that blocks testosterone effects at the receptor level. Estrogens are reported to decrease hypersexuality. Estrogens increase cardiovascular disease and thromboembolic disease in males. Gonadotrophin-releasing hormone analogs result in a decrease in pituitary production of LH and a decrease in testosterone. They have been used to treat a patient with the Klüver-Bucy syndrome and a patient with Huntington's disease who was an exhibitionist. Patients receiving this therapy have reported hot flashes and have developed the effects of hypogonadism. It is important for the geriatrician to recognize that, with the exception of the SSRIs, all of these drugs are likely to accelerate frailty in an older person because of the hypogonadism they induce. Thus, they should be used only as a last resort in the truly unmanageable patient.

SEXUALITY IN LONG-TERM CARE

A small number of studies in nursing homes have identified the major barriers to sexual expression in the nursing home as lack of privacy, lack of a partner, physical illness, erectile dysfunction, and dyspareunia. The majority of patients in nursing homes view themselves as sexually unattractive. Despite increased awareness of the sexual needs of persons living in nursing homes, the majority of staff have minimal understanding of the sexuality of residents in nursing homes. Education programs for nursing staff are a key to improving attitudes to sexuality in nursing homes. In particular, many staff find masturbatory behavior objectionable and will stop the resident rather than withdrawing quietly and allowing the resident privacy.

Providing residents privacy while spending time with their partner is a key to allowing full expression of sexuality in the nursing home. Providing privacy for sexual expression is an issue in nursing homes. While the provision of "quiet rooms" or the use of "do not disturb" signs provides a partial solution for conjugal visits, it can heighten embarrassment for the resident.

Another major issue is the development of romantic liaisons between two residents in the nursing home. When is a resident too cognitively impaired to consent to a romantic liaison with another resident? What should be the ethical approach when a resident who is still married forms a romantic liaison with another resident? What is the appropriate approach when children disapprove of a romantic liaison formed by their parent? Unfortunately, these and other issues have no simple solutions and the ethically appropriate answer requires a high degree of individualization, as well as education of family members.

To limit the problems of sexually inappropriate behaviors in nursing homes all staff should follow a series of simple rules:

- Do not allow residents to have sexually suggestive interactions with staff. Encouragement of these "cute" behaviors can often lead to misunderstanding of boundaries by the cognitively impaired resident.
- Reward appropriate behaviors and ignore sexually inappropriate behaviors.
- Redirect behavior wherever possible.
- State explicitly that certain behaviors are unacceptable whenever they occur.
- Isolate residents from persons whom they are interacting with inappropriately, and where necessary, use staff of the same sex to provide care.
- When residents masturbate publicly, take them to their room. Also consider clothing that is more difficult for the cognitively impaired person to remove.

CONCLUSION

Sexuality in its full expression represents an important component of quality of life. Sexuality in older persons is an area that has received minimal attention from health care professionals. The ability to fully express sexuality as one grows older involves biological (hypogonadism, erectile dysfunction, and disease), psychological (depression, attitudes to sexuality, perception of sexual attractiveness), and social (social interactions, partner availability, physical fitness, community education, and awareness of sexuality) aspects. The physician who cares for the elderly needs not only to have knowledge of the options available to the older persons experiencing problems with their sexuality but also needs to openly discuss the importance of sexuality with older patients. A sexual history remains a component of good holistic medical care regardless of the age of the patient.

REFERENCES

Al-Azzawi F: The menopause and its treatment in perspective [review]. *Postgrad Med J* 77(907):292, 2001.

Ambler N et al: Sexual difficulties of chronic pain patients. *Clin J Pain* 17(2):138, 2001.

Claes JA, Moore W: Issues confronting lesbian and gay elders: The challenge for health and human services providers. *J Health Hum Serv Admin* 23(2):181, 2000.

Cormier BM et al: Pedophilic episodes in middle age and senescence: An intergenerational encounter. *Can J Psychiatry* 40(3):125, 1995.

D'Augelli AR et al: Aspects of mental health among older lesbian, gay, and bisexual adults. *Aging Ment Health* 5(2):149, 2001.

Gelfand MM: Sexuality among older women [review]. *J Womens Health Gend Based Med* 9(Suppl 1):S15, 2000.

Goodwin J et al: Grandfather–granddaughter incest: A trigenerational view. *Child Abuse Negl* 7(2):163, 1983.

Kamel HK: Sexuality in aging: Focus on institutionalized elderly. *Ann Long-Term Care* 9:64, 2001.

Korenman SG: New insights into erectile dysfunction: A practical approach [review]. *Am J Med* 105:135, 1998.

McNagny SE: Prescribing hormone replacement therapy for menopausal symptoms [review]. *Ann Intern Med* 131(8):605, 1999.

Morales A et al: Andropause: A misnomer for a true clinical entity [review]. *J Urol* 163(3):705, 2000.

Morley JE: Androgens and aging. *Maturitas* 38(1):61, 2001.

Morley JE: Sexual function and the aging woman, in Morley JE, Korenman SG (eds): *Endocrinology and Metabolism in the Elderly*. Boston, Blackwell Scientific, 1992 p 307.

Morley JE, Perry HM: Androgen deficiency in aging men: Role of testosterone replacement therapy. *J Lab Clin Med* 135(5):370, 2000.

Rogstad KE, Bignell CJ: Age is no bar to sexually acquired infection. *Age Ageing* 20(5):377, 1991.

Rymer J, Morris EP: Menopausal symptoms [review]. *BMJ* 321(7275):1516, 2000.

Slag MF et al: Importance in medical clinic outpatients. *JAMA* 249:1736, 1983.

Vasconcelos C et al: Sexually transmitted diseases in the elderly. Review of 28 cases. *Eur J Dermatoll* 10(7):567, 2000.

Trophic Factors and Male Hormone Replacement

J. LISA TENOVER

There continues to be a growing interest in a number of hormones that decline in serum level with normal aging and that have anabolic, antiosteopenic, or other beneficial properties, at least when given to young adults with known deficiencies in these hormones. The decrease in the serum levels of these hormones seen with normal aging often parallels changes in the organs and physiologic functions on which they have an impact. These observations suggest that replacing them may prevent, stabilize, or even reverse some of the detrimental target-organ changes seen with aging, thereby prolonging life or improving the functional status of older persons. These agents are often referred to as trophic factors because they may promote cellular growth and metabolism at multiple sites.

Several hormones have been suggested to be trophic factor candidates, but the major ones currently being considered are growth hormone (GH) (or elements of the GH axis) and dehydroepiandrosterone (DHEA). In addition, gender-specific sex hormones, testosterone in the male and estrogen in the female, qualify in some respects as trophic factors. In the lay press, GH, DHEA, and, in some cases, testosterone have been espoused as potential "magic bullets," the "fountain of youth," "elements to stop the clock," and "antiaging hormones." However, many questions remain about their role, if any, in the prevention of age-related changes or in the treatment of aging syndromes such as frailty. Given the data indicating that dietary restriction in rodents, a model for prolonging life, often produces declines in the same hormone levels, it could be inferred that similar declines with age are not always maladaptive.

The emphasis of this chapter will be to review what is known about age-related changes in the levels and physiology of the GH axis, DHEA, and, in the male, testosterone and to review what is known about the beneficial and detrimental effects of hormone replacement therapy in older people. Estrogens and estrogen therapy are discussed in other chapters.

AGING-RELATED CHANGES TARGETED BY TROPHIC FACTOR ADMINISTRATION

The range of potential beneficial effects of trophic hormone replacement is quite extensive and can involve improvements in body composition, energy, sexual interest and performance, immune function, bone density, wound healing, mood, and cognitive function. Some of these potential benefits may be sought by middle-aged adults (e.g., increasing energy, improving mood, increasing libido or sexual performance), whereas others may have a more profound significance for elderly persons (e.g., improving osteopenia, sarcopenia, and muscle function). Table 103-1 lists some of the target-organ areas of interest, their changes with age, and the reported or hypothesized changes effected by trophic hormone replacement.

Body Composition and Strength

Advancing age is associated with significant alterations in body composition in both men and women. In one cross-sectional study assessing body composition in 18- to 85-year-old men and women, body fat was noted to increase from 18 percent to 36 percent in men and from 33 percent to 44 percent in women. With normal aging, there also is a decline in the amount of fat-free (lean body) mass, the principal component of which is muscle (Chapter 91). More important than muscle mass, from a functional point of view, is muscle strength. Multiple longitudinal and cross-sectional studies also have demonstrated a decrease in muscle strength with aging. Muscle strength is a complex phenomenon affected by many factors, but age-related general declines in muscle strength correlate with declines in muscle mass, although the former decreases more profoundly than the latter.

Significant declines in muscle mass and strength with age are strong predictors of functional problems. The

Table 103-1 Common Target-Organ or Functional Changes With Age Compared With Postulated Effects of Replacement Therapy With Growth Hormone, Testosterone, or Dehydroepiandrosterone in Older Persons

Target Organ and/or Function	Age Effect	Postulated Change With		
		GH/IGF	T	DHEA
Muscle mass	↓	↑	↑	↑
Muscle strength	↓	↑	↑	↑
Fat mass	↑	↓	↓	↓
Bone mass	↓	↑	↑	↑
Cellular immunity	↓	↑	NC	↑
Libido	↓	NC	↑	NC
Sense of well-being	NC/↓	↑	↑	↑

GH/IGF, growth hormone/insulin-like growth factor; T, testosterone; DHEA, Dehydroepiandrosterone; ↑, increase; ↓, decrease; NC, no change.

clinical correlates of sarcopenia, the age-related loss of skeletal muscle, include falls, fractures, loss of mobility, and loss of ability to perform the basic activities of daily living. With regard to body composition, to be a clinically useful trophic factor in older adults, a treatment should produce not only improvement in muscle mass but also improvement in or stabilization of muscle strength and overall function.

The metabolic consequences of alterations in body composition with age and the potential for improvement with the use of replacement therapy also need to be considered. For example, yet unproved consequences of sarcopenia include a lower basal metabolic rate, abnormal thermoregulation, impaired glucose metabolism, and worsening of osteopenia. Increases in body fat with age also may contribute to the decreased insulin sensitivity common in older individuals.

Bone Mass

The loss of bone mass and the decrease in bone density, with the concomitant increased risk for fracture, is well known in aging females (as discussed in other chapters). The loss of bone mass with age in males is less appreciated but is becoming a more important medical problem as men live longer (Figure 103-1). After age 60, hip fracture rates in men increase dramatically, doubling each decade. By age 80, proximal femur fracture rates in white men approach 1.3 percent per man-year. Similarly, vertebral wedge fracture deformities are not rare in men (occurring in up to 24% of community-dwelling men aged 53–75 years) and appear to be related to osteopenia. In both cross-sectional and longitudinal studies, healthy men were shown to lose bone mass with age. Typical bone loss rates for vertebral bone in men aged 30 to 80 years were 1.2 percent per year in cross-sectional studies and about 2 percent per year in longitudinal studies. Cortical bone was lost less rapidly, at a rate of 0.2 to 1 percent per year.

Immune Function

Immune function declines with age and may contribute to an increased incidence of infection and cancer. Age-related changes in immunity primarily involve T-cell function, such a decrease in the proliferative response to mitogens and diminished interleukin-2 (IL-2) production. Altered B-cell function also occurs with aging, leading to a decreased ability to generate antibodies in response to an antigenic stimulus.

Libido and Mood

Measures of libido such as sexual thoughts and sexual enjoyment generally decline with age in both men and women. Other aspects of psychological health, such as sense of well-being, ability to cope with stress, and general "energy" level, do not necessarily change with age but represent problematic areas for some elderly patients and

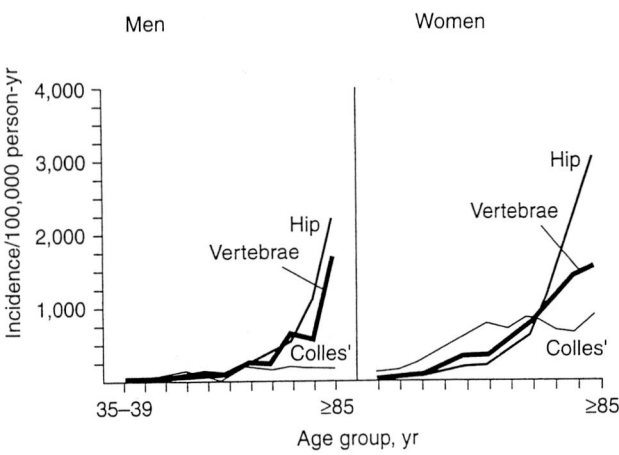

Figure 103-1 Age-specific rates of fracture in men and women from Rochester, Minnesota. Reprinted with permission from Melton LG, *Trends Endocrinol Metab* 3:224, 1993.

are evaluated as end points in several trophic factor replacement studies.

GROWTH HORMONE

Physiology and Changes with Aging

Growth hormone is secreted by the anterior pituitary gland under control of the hypothalamus (Chapter 65). GH secretion occurs predominantly after the onset of sleep, and the hormone degrades rapidly in serum, making single GH measurements difficult to interpret. GH stimulates the production of insulin-like growth factor 1 (IGF-1) in the liver and other tissues, and many of the actions of GH are mediated through IGF-1. In contrast to GH serum levels, those of IGF-1 show little diurnal variation, and so measurement of IGF-1 levels can provide a reasonable index of the status of the GH axis in an individual. Most studies have shown a decline in both 24-hour serum GH levels and serum IGF-1 levels with age.

Low GH levels that may accompany normal aging cannot be considered equivalent to low GH levels in GH-deficient adults with hypothalamic-pituitary disease. A comparison of age-matched and body mass index–matched persons older than 60 years who had low GH levels due to normal aging or were GH-deficient because of hypothalamic-pituitary disease demonstrated that 24-hour GH profiles, IGF-1 levels, and median arginine-stimulated peak GH levels were all markedly lower in the GH-deficient group. These observations could mean that physiologic changes brought about by GH replacement therapy in GH-deficient patients (those with hypothalamic-pituitary disease) may not translate directly into similar effects in the normal aging population. Also, although GH and IGF-1 levels both tend to decline with age, on an individual basis it is often possible to find normal GH levels and low IGF-1 levels, or visa versa, in older people, which suggests that responsiveness to intrinsic GH varies considerably in this group.

On the other hand, truly GH-deficient elderly individuals (those with low GH and low IGF-1 levels and with multiple pituitary hormone deficiencies) have been shown to respond to GH replacement therapy in a manner similar to that observed in younger GH-deficient adults.

A decline in sex steroid levels with age may contribute to a decrease in GH secretion, especially in postmenopausal women. The correlation of spontaneous and GH-releasing hormone (GHRH)-stimulated GH secretion with plasma estradiol levels and the enhancement of GH secretion by estrogen replacement therapy both suggest that the decline in GH secretion with age in women may be due in part to changes in estrogen-mediated effects on GHRH secretion. Although testosterone is known to enhance peak plasma GH secretion in peripubertal males, the contribution of testosterone to the decline in GH secretion in older men is unclear. Some studies involving young adult hypogonadal men treated with testosterone have shown an increase in 24-hour GH levels and serum IGF-1 levels, whereas others have not. Supraphysiologic amounts of testosterone given to young adult men, and in one study to older men, were shown to increase IGF-1 levels, but to date, short-term physiologic testosterone replacement and androgen withdrawal studies in older men have failed to show any significant effect on the GH axis.

Growth Hormone Therapy in Older Adults

Body Composition and Strength

Several cross-sectional studies have demonstrated a correlation between musculoskeletal frailty and serum IGF-1 levels, but the correlations were weak. When given to GH-deficient adults with hypothalamic-pituitary disease, GH was shown to result in a decline in fat mass and an increase in lean body mass. Similarly, beginning with the investigation by Rudman and coworkers in 1990, there have been several studies in which GH was administered to healthy older persons with somewhat low IGF-1 levels and body composition changes evaluated as outcome; nearly all these studies reported an increase in lean body mass and a decline in fat mass with therapy (Table 103-2). Most GH replacement studies involving older adults where body composition was evaluated have included only men. The few studies that have included women have reported variable effects of GH or GHRH on lean body mass and fat mass, with the magnitude of the effects, if they occurred at all, being generally less than that seen in men.

One study in which GH was administered to obese men demonstrated a decline in fat mass accompanied by a small increase in insulin sensitivity. There are no data indicating whether such metabolic benefits of GH replacement in men can be sustained or if they can translate into meaningful clinical benefits. Although increases in GH and IGF-1 levels in elderly men have been shown to lead to an increase in lean body mass, only one study has reported a change in strength accompanying these lean mass changes (Table 103-2), with the reported strength changes being very modest. These results might suggest that attaining "young" levels of IGF-1 alone cannot restore musculoskeletal function in elderly persons.

Resistance exercise elevates GH levels in healthy young adults, and cross-sectional analyses in older adults have shown that IGF-1 serum levels are higher in older adults who exercise compared with those who do not. However, several studies on resistance and endurance training in healthy older men and women have demonstrated that such exercise does not significantly increase serum IGF-1 levels and that the GH increase in response to exercise is much less than that in young adults. Studies in which GH and exercise together were evaluated in elderly men have shown that despite larger increases in lean body mass in the GH-plus-exercise group compared with the exercise-alone group, GH administration added nothing over exercise alone in terms of changes in strength.

Bone

The importance of GH for normal skeletal growth during childhood and adolescence is established, but much less is known about its effects on the adult skeleton. GH-deficient middle-aged adults have reduced bone mineral density

Table 103-2 Reported Effect of Growth Hormone, Growth Hormone–Releasing Hormone, or Growth Hormone–Releasing Hormone Analogs on Body Composition and Strength in Healthy Older Adults

Agent	N*	Sex	Length of Treatment (wk)	Changes in Body Composition With Therapy†		
				Lean Mass	Body Fat	Strength
GH	21	M	26	↑ (9%)	↓ (14%)	—
GH	26	M	52	↑ (6%)	↓ (15%)	—
GH	10	M	10	↑ (3%)	↓ (12%)	NC
GH	26	M	6	↑ (4%)	↓ (13%)	NC
GH	8	M	16	↑ (8%)	↓ (12%)	NC
GH	15	M	26	↑ (6%)	↓ (10%)	—
GHRH	9	M	6	NC	NC	↑
Analog	9	M	16	↑ (2%)	NC	—
GH	13	F	26	NC	↓ (9%)	—
GH	11	F	26	↑ (6%)	NC	—
Analog	10	F	16	NC	NC	—

GH, growth hormone; GHRH, growth hormone–releasing hormone; M, male; F, female; ↑, increase; ↓, decrease; NC, no change.
*Number of participants in study on active therapy.
† Body composition changes noted by direction of change, with percentage change in parentheses.

(BMD) when compared with healthy age- and gender-matched controls, and in most studies, GH replacement in middle-aged GH-deficient adults has resulted in a modest increase in BMD. However, studies comparing older (>60 years) persons with a GH deficiency (hypothalamic-pituitary disease) with healthy elderly persons matched by age, gender, and body mass index have not found a difference between the two groups in terms of BMD. These results might suggest that lower GH levels in late life may not have the same magnitude of effect on bone that they appear to have before and throughout middle age. In their original 1990 study in which they gave GH to older men for 6 months, Rudman and coworkers reported a 1.6 percent increase in spine BMD with therapy. One other study noted a 0.9 percent increase in BMD in older men after 6 months of GH therapy. However, all other studies to date using GH or GHRH therapy in elderly men or women have demonstrated no changes in BMD with these therapies alone, despite the fact that most GH replacement studies noted changes in the biochemical parameters of bone turnover.

Other Effects

The effects of GH administration on serum lipoprotein levels are uncertain. Some studies have reported a small decrease in serum total cholesterol and/or low-density-lipoprotein cholesterol levels with GH therapy, whereas other have noted no change in lipoprotein levels. A study involving men treated with GH and exercise showed that GH therapy had no effect on mood or on cognitive function test performance.

Growth Hormone Analogs and Other Related Agents

In addition to the lack of significant clinical findings noted thus far in replacement studies involving GH in elderly persons, there are some theoretical limitations to the use of GH as an anabolic agent. This hormone can impair glucose tolerance, and hepatic production of IGF-1 in response to GH can be greatly diminished in catabolic states. The use of IGF-1 alone also has limitations in that it can lead to hypoglycemia, and its administration can downregulate GH secretion even further. Also, IGF-1 administered alone leads to a decrease in levels of IGF-binding proteins, which results in more rapid IGF-1 degradation and decreased delivery to tissues. Some investigators have speculated that the coadministration of GH and IGF-1 may be more tolerable and beneficial than the administration of either agent alone.

Alternatively, the stimulation of endogenous GH, through the use of GHRH, GHRH analogs, or GH secretagogues, could offer some physiologic advantages. Among these would be the maintenance of counter-regulatory mechanisms and the pulsatile release of GH. In addition, many of these agents can be delivered either orally or intranasally rather than requiring injections. Results of short-term studies on GHRH or GHRH analogs administered to elderly persons have shown small or no changes in body composition, although serum IGF-1 levels were increased significantly (Table 103-2). A study involving elderly men and women, both treated for 16 weeks with either a GHRH analog or a placebo, reported an increase in both sense of well-being and libido in the men given GHRH compared with those given a placebo; for the women, there was no difference in these parameters between placebo and GHRH treatment. There have been no reports as yet of the effect of nonpeptidyl orally active GH secretagogues on the body composition of older persons, although their administration also leads to an increase in GH and IGF-1 serum levels.

In one study a GH secretagogue was given along with alendronate and the effects on BMD evaluated; the GH secretagogue did not substantially increase BMD over the values obtained with alendronate alone.

Growth Hormone and Sex Steroid Coadministration

Because levels of both GH and the major sex steroids (estradiol in women and testosterone in men) decline with age, it is possible that these changes may have concomitant effects on muscle, fat, and bone mass. Therefore, replacement therapy for older persons using both GH and the appropriate sex steroid has undergone limited evaluation. In one study generally healthy men and women older than 65 years of age were given GH, estradiol (women) or testosterone (men), both, or neither for 26 weeks, and the effects on body composition and bone were noted. In the women, GH did not augment the effect of hormone replacement therapy on BMD, and hormone replacement therapy did not augment the effect of GH on body composition. In men, the administration of both GH and testosterone led to a decrease in body fat and an increase in lean body mass, and for both these parameters the effect of the two treatments together was greater than that for either used alone.

Adverse Effects of Growth Hormone

A high incidence (up to 50%) of adverse effects have been reported in studies on healthy older adults receiving GH. Many studies used GH doses similar to those used for replacement therapy in GH-deficient adults. The incidence of side effects and the study dropout rate were proportional to the GH dose and the IGF-1 level obtained. Because adverse events seem to be dose-related, more recent GH trials have used lower doses for elderly participants, with somewhat fewer study dropouts and reported adverse effects. Table 103-3 lists the adverse effects that have occurred or have been postulated to occur with GH or IGF-1 therapy. Among the adverse events noted in published replacement studies involving men were gynecomastia, hyperglycemia, arthralgias, fluid retention, and the development of carpal tunnel syndrome. For studies that included women, arthralgias, joint swelling, fluid retention, and carpal tunnel syndrome were the predominant complaints. Studies involving IGF-1 replacement have noted problems with hypoglycemia, parotid tenderness, headaches, and orthostatic hypotension. The long-term effects of GH or IGF-1 replacement on the development or exacerbation of neoplasms are unknown but are of concern given that acromegaly is associated with an increased incidence of colon and breast cancer, IGF-1 has known mitogenic action on most cell types and protects against apoptosis, and IGF-1 receptors

Table 103-3 Potential or Reported Adverse Effects of Growth Hormone or Insulin-like Growth Factor 1 Replacement Therapy in Older Men and Women

With growth hormone
Hyperglycemia
Arthralgias/joint swelling
Carpal tunnel syndrome
Fluid retention
Gynecomastia (men)
With insulin-like growth factor 1
Hypoglycemia
Parotid tenderness
Headache
Orthostatic hypotension
With either
Development of exacerbation of neoplasms, especially colon and breast

are found in some human tumors. GH and IGF-1 must be administered by injection, and a year of replacement therapy with recombinant human GH can cost more than $10,000.

Growth Hormone in Catabolic States

Because of the effect of GH on nitrogen conservation and body composition, short-term GH administration has been used in several catabolic settings. In younger adults, GH adjunctive therapy has been evaluated for patients with severe burns, undergoing long-term treatment with glucocorticoids, in respiratory failure, and with acquired immunodeficiency syndrome (AIDS)-associated wasting. In most studies, short-term GH administration resulted in nitrogen conservation and in some functional benefits, including preservation of muscle strength, reduction in wound infections, acceleration of wound healing, and a shortened hospital stay. In older adults, short-term GH therapy has been evaluated in patients following abdominal surgery, in patients with severe burns, in underweight patients with chronic obstructive pulmonary disease (COPD), in patients who have experienced recent weight loss, and in chronically malnourished elderly persons. In most studies, nitrogen balance was improved, body weight increased, and for COPD patients, maximal inspiratory effort improved. These studies suggest that short-term GH therapy (along with nutritional support) may help improve the nitrogen balance and may attenuate the muscle loss seen in certain illnesses. On the other hand, a study on GH administered to critically ill patients in intensive care units following abdominal surgery, multiple trauma, or acute respiratory failure demonstrated that GH therapy doubled the in-hospital mortality rate compared to placebo treatment. It was felt that these patients may have been negatively affected by the hypermetabolic and proinflammatory effects of GH, as most died of a rapid onset of septic shock and multiple-organ failure. The anabolic effects of GH secretagogue or

IGF-1 administration for catabolic states in elderly patients have not been evaluated.

TESTOSTERONE IN OLDER MALES

Hormonal replacement therapy for postmenopausal women has been studied and discussed extensively for many years. However, hormonal replacement therapy for the aging male has been less thoroughly evaluated. Although data are limited, there is information suggesting that, at least in some older men, androgen replacement therapy may be beneficial.

Physiology and Changes with Aging

A further discussion of this topic appears in Chapter 65. Most (about 95%) of the serum testosterone in men is produced by the Leydig cells of the testes and released into the circulation in a pulsatile manner under stimulatory control by luteinizing hormone (LH). The remainder of the serum testosterone comes from conversion from adrenal androgens, largely androstenedione. Nearly all testosterone, which is the most plentiful androgen in the human male, circulates in blood bound to two proteins, albumin and sex hormone–binding globulin (SHBG); only about 1 percent to 2 percent of testosterone circulates totally free in plasma. Testosterone is tightly bound to SHBG, whereas its affinity for albumin is weak. Because of the strong affinity of testosterone for SHBG, the portion of plasma testosterone not bound to SHBG is often called bioavailable testosterone. Epidemiologic studies have shown that it is the amount of bioavailable testosterone that best correlates with parameters such as BMD and sexual function in older men and is predictive for the development of frailty in inner-city African-American males. It is not known, however, if non-SHBG (bioavailable) testosterone is the component of testosterone that is truly bioavailable to every androgen target organ; for example, data suggest that testosterone bound to SHBG may be available to the prostate.

Not all target-organ effects of testosterone are attributable to the steroid directly but may be the result of one of its metabolites. Testosterone can be converted to 17β-estradiol through the action of an aromatase enzyme. In men, the majority of estrogen presumably results from the action of an aromatase enzyme in adipose tissue rather than from direct production by the testes. Testosterone can also be converted, via a 5α-reductase, to dihydrotestosterone (DHT), which is the predominant androgen in some organs such as the prostate. Although some DHT is found in serum, most of the effects of DHT at the target-organ level are likely due to its formation from testosterone locally. Both testosterone and DHT affect target organs through their interaction with the same intracellular androgen receptor.

Serum levels of total testosterone, free testosterone, and bioavailable testosterone, but not DHT, decline with normal aging in many men. Cross-sectional studies, as well as at least three longitudinal studies, support this age-related change. Most data on testosterone levels and age come from studies involving predominantly white men of western European descent. Some smaller cross-sectional evaluations of men of African-American or Asian descent, however, suggest that these ethnic groups also may demonstrate this age-related testosterone decline. Figure 103-2 demonstrates the longitudinal effects of aging on total testosterone levels and the free testosterone index (total testosterone/SHBG) as determined in 890 men in the Baltimore Longitudinal Study of Aging (BLSA). These data indicate an average testosterone decline of 1.24 nmol/L per decade of age beginning at about 30 years of age.

The decline in serum testosterone level with normal aging is largely due to a decrease in production by the testes, which become less responsive to gonadotropin stimulation. The hypothalamus also seems to play a role because there is an age-related increase in sensitivity to sex steroid negative feedback. The peripheral conversion of testosterone to estrogens is higher in older men, probably because of the age-related increase in adipose mass. In addition, SHBG levels increase significantly with normal male aging, which results in a decline in bioavailable testosterone much more profound than the decline in total testosterone.

Although age alone has a strong predictive value for lower plasma testosterone levels, concomitant diseases such as diabetes mellitus, liver disease, and hemochromatosis can also contribute. Certain medications also have been associated with lower testosterone levels, including ketoconazole, cimetidine, and glucocorticoids. As they age, not all men develop testosterone levels low enough for them to become obviously hypogonadal. The prevalence of true hypogonadism in the older male population is uncertain, largely because there is no agreement on how to define testosterone deficiency in this age group. There is no target-organ change, physiologic finding, or symptom that readily provides a definition, and in general, measurements of serum LH levels are not helpful. Unlike the thyroid hormone axis, where serum thyroid-stimulating hormone levels can assist in the diagnosis of hypothyroidism, serum LH levels in most older men, even those with quite low testosterone levels, are usually within the normal range for young adult men. It also may be that no one serum level of testosterone can define all older men as hypogonadal; the desired level of testosterone that maximizes target-organ effects may vary according to the androgen target organ of interest as well as differ among individuals.

Currently, rather than defining the level of testosterone that makes the average older man testosterone-deficient, replacement studies have recruited older men with baseline testosterone levels at or below the lower limit of the normal range for young adult men and evaluated their androgen target-organ responses to testosterone therapy. This strategy allows testosterone to be raised to levels 100 to 200 percent above baseline but still be maintained within the normal physiologic young adult range. Table 103-4 presents some examples of the prevalence of various levels of testosterone deficiency as defined by some of these studies.

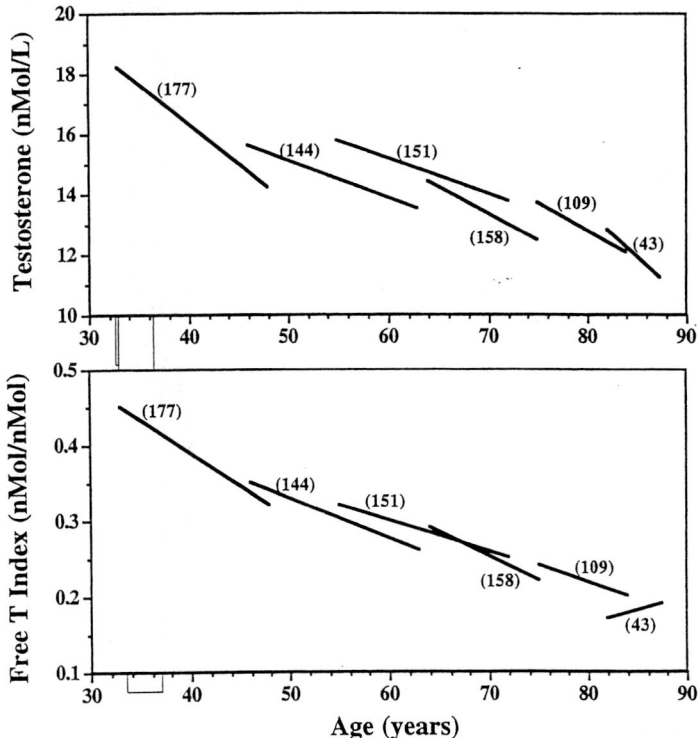

Figure 103-2   Longitudinal effects of age on plasma total testosterone levels and free testosterone index in men from the Baltimore Longitudinal Study of Aging. Reprinted with permission from Harman SM et al, *J Clin Endocrinol Metab* 86(2):724, 2001. Copyright © The Endocrine Society.

Testosterone Replacement in Older Men

Rigorous scientific investigation of the benefits and risks of androgen replacement therapy for older men is now only in about its second decade, and no large, multicenter controlled clinical trials of this therapy have been undertaken as yet. Clinical studies on androgen replacement therapy in older men have defined testosterone deficiency using a range of hormonal values, have been predominantly carried out in healthy men between the ages of 60 and 75 years, have involved small numbers of study participants, have evaluated therapy over relatively short periods (mostly 12 months or less), have not always been blinded to treatment or been placebo-controlled, and have utilized various modes of androgen therapy. Nonetheless, it is possible to evaluate the trends in the observed outcomes.

Table 103-4   Prevalence of Study-Defined Testosterone Deficiency in Older Men

Study*	Age (y)	N	Serum Total Testosterone level (ng/dL)	Percentage of Population
1	50–87	817	<300	11.4
2	20–100	300	<317	22 (60–80 y)
				36 (70–100 y)
3	60–83	379	<350	36
			<300	19
			<250	8
4	75–101	77	<245	33
5	60–91	685	<325	19 (60–69 y)
				28 (70–79 y)
				49 (80+ y)

*1, Lunglmayr (rural Austria); 2, Vermeulen and Kaufman (Belgium); 3, Tenover (Seattle, WA, and Atlanta, GA); 4, Morley et al (Albuquerque, NM); 5, Harman et al (Baltimore, MD; BLSA)

Table 103-5 Testosterone Supplementation Effects on Body Composition and Strength in Older Men

Length of Treatment (mo)	N	Change in Composition		Change in Strength	
		Fat Mass	Lean Mass	Grip	LE
1	6	—	—	—	↑
2	9	—	—	↑	—
3	7	—	NC	NC	NC
3	13	NC	↑ (3%)	NC	—
3	8	NC	—	↑	—
9	31	↓ (6%)	NC	—	—
12	17	NC	—	↑	—
18	29	↓ (14%)	↑ (5%)	—	—
36	54	↓ (14%)	↑ (4%)	NC	NC

LE, lower extremity strength; ↓, decrease; ↑, increase; NC, no change.
*Trend and mean percentage change.

Body Composition and Strength

There have been several published studies in which body composition and/or muscle strength has been evaluated in older men during androgen therapy. Table 103-5 summarizes the body composition and strength changes that have been observed in these trials. Changes in body composition with testosterone therapy have occurred consistently: a decline in body fat, an increase in lean body mass, or both. The magnitude of the fat mass changes in older men appears similar to that seen with testosterone replacement in young hypogonadal men, whereas the lean body mass changes produced are usually less dramatic. A small number of studies have suggested that insulin sensitivity may increase with testosterone therapy in the older population, but whether this is due to the therapy-related decline in fat mass is not known.

The strength changes observed with testosterone replacement therapy have been variable (Table 103-5). When strength was shown to improve with treatment, the magnitude of the change reported was not large, making the clinical relevance of these changes uncertain. Only two studies have evaluated the effect of testosterone therapy on some aspect of physical function, and only one showed an improvement with treatment.

Bone

Studies on androgen replacement therapy in older men evaluating the effects on bone have all utilized testosterone as the treatment androgen. This may be important because testosterone is converted to estradiol in vivo and older men receiving testosterone often show a substantial increase in plasma estradiol levels. Because bioavailable estradiol has been found to be a better predictor of BMD in older men than any component of testosterone, it is possible that the effects of testosterone replacement therapy on

bone in older men are mediated through its conversion to estradiol.

The published studies on testosterone replacement in older men have lasted from 3 to 36 months, with the shorter studies measuring biochemical parameters of bone turnover and the longer studies evaluating BMD. Some, but not all, of the studies enrolled older men who were osteoporotic at baseline, and one evaluated testosterone therapy in men taking chronic glucocorticoids. In general, the rate of bone degradation seemed to be slowed by testosterone replacement and BMD seemed to be increased. Table 103-6 summarizes the results from studies that measured BMD. Whether positive effects on BMD can be maintained over longer periods of time than have been studied and the optimal level of testosterone replacement required to achieve maximal benefit for bone are both unknown at this time. There are as yet no data on the effect of testosterone replacement therapy on fracture rates in older men.

Sexual Function, Mood, and Cognition

No clinical trials have evaluated the effect of testosterone therapy on aspects of sexual function in healthy older men with low or low-normal testosterone levels. However, some studies have evaluated the effects of raising serum testosterone levels in older men with various types of sexual dysfunction. In general, it appears that the majority of older men probably have androgen levels higher than the threshold required for behavioral activation, with libido usually being fully functional at relatively low levels of serum testosterone. On the other hand, there is some indication that the threshold for androgen activation of sexual function may increase with age, and some men with low libido and low-normal testosterone levels have shown an improvement in libido with testosterone supplementation. In general, studies do not support a role for testosterone

Table 103-6 Testosterone Therapy Effects on Bone Mineral Density in Older Men

Length of Treatment (mo)	N	Change in Bone Mineral Density	
		L-Spine	Other Site
12	4	↑	—
12	4	↑	↑
12	34	NC	↑
18	29	↑	—
36	8	Slowed ↓	
36	54	↑	—

↑, increase; ↓, decrease; NC, = no change.

"deficiency" in the pathogenesis of erectile dysfunction in older men.

Several blind, placebo-controlled testosterone replacement studies involving older men have evaluated its effects on sense of well-being and other aspects of mood. Although the study numbers are small, they generally have found that men taking testosterone report an improved or greater sense of well-being compared with men receiving a placebo.

There have been only a limited number of clinical trials on the effects of testosterone replacement on cognitive function. Small improvements in visual memory have been reported with this therapy, whereas several preliminary reports have noted improvement in trail-making, spatial, and verbal memory tests.

Cardiovascular System

Compared with premenopausal women, men have a higher incidence of cardiovascular disease and mortality. Whether this sexual dichotomy is due largely to a protective effect of estrogens in women or whether androgens have a detrimental impact on the cardiovascular system in men is not yet known. Epidemiologic studies have demonstrated that low, rather than high, serum testosterone levels are associated with an increased risk of cardiovascular disease in older men. Therefore, it is currently unknown whether testosterone replacement in older men would be beneficial, detrimental, or neutral with regard to the cardiovascular system. Factors associated with a risk for cardiovascular disease that might be affected by sex steroids include serum lipoprotein levels, vascular tone, platelet and red-blood-cell clotting parameters, and direct atherogenesis. There are no data as of yet on the effects of testosterone therapy in older men on most of these parameters. Several studies have suggested that testosterone therapy may decrease platelet aggregation or positively affect vasomotor tone, but these data need to be expanded. The effects of testosterone therapy on serum lipoprotein levels in older men have been more extensively investigated. In general, parenteral testosterone therapy has led to a decrease in total and low-density-lipoprotein cholesterol levels, a decrease

in lipoprotein(a) levels, and no change or a small decrease in high-density-lipoprotein cholesterol levels. These changes in serum cholesterol levels with testosterone therapy were generally modest, and the ultimate impact on cardiovascular disease is unknown.

Androgens in Catabolic States

Although parenteral testosterone has not been evaluated for its anabolic actions in older persons with catabolic states, several studies have investigated anabolic steroids, such as nandrolone, in such settings. Studies have involved ill surgical patients supported by intravenous nutrition, patients following severe burn injury, and frail elderly patients following hip fracture. Many of these studies have demonstrated a minor increase in nitrogen balance with anabolic steroid treatment but no significant changes in body composition, strength, or rehabilitation time; anabolic therapy has been reported to accelerate healing following severe burn injury. Complications such as water retention, edema, and lipoprotein abnormalities and, in women, unwanted virilizing effects, have been reported in these settings.

Adverse Effects of Testosterone

Table 103-7 lists potential or reported adverse effects of testosterone therapy in older men. Liver toxicity, although known to occur with oral methylated agents, has not been seen with parenteral forms of therapy. Fluid retention is possible, especially during the first few months of therapy, but is not as dramatic as in the case of oral anabolic steroids. No studies on testosterone replacement therapy in older men have reported problems with peripheral edema or exacerbation of hypertension or with congestive heart failure, but these studies have included only relatively healthy men. In chronically ill, frail, elderly men, fluid retention might pose a concern. Tender breasts or gynecomastia occurs in a small number of older men receiving testosterone therapy, perhaps because of the relatively greater increase in serum estradiol levels (as compared with serum testosterone

Table 103-7 Potential or Reported Adverse Effects of Testosterone Replacement Therapy in Older Men

Liver toxicity

Fluid retention
   Peripheral edema
   Exacerbation of hypertension
   Worsening of congestive heart failure

Breast tenderness or gynecomastia

Exacerbation of sleep apnea

Development of polycythemia

Exacerbation of benign or malignant prostate disease

Increase risk of cardiovascular disease
   Effects on clotting
   Effects on vasomotor tone
   Effects on rate of atherogenesis

levels) that occurs with the therapy. In several studies, testosterone supplementation has been shown to exacerbate sleep apnea, but this result has not been found uniformly.

Testosterone replacement therapy in older men can often cause a significant increase in red blood cell mass and hemoglobin levels. The increases reported are much larger than those usually observed when young hypogonadal men are given testosterone replacement. In some cases, where polycythemia has developed, it has been necessary to either terminate therapy or decrease the dose of testosterone used in the older men. While the coexistence of sleep apnea and elevated body mass index seems to contribute to the development of polycythemia in certain older men, this has not been the case for many of the men studied. The method of testosterone replacement may affect the magnitude of the change in red blood cell mass, with methods that give a more uniform level of testosterone within the physiologic range throughout the dosing period showing less of an effect.

Androgens have a role in promoting both benign prostatic hyperplasia (BPH) and prostate cancer, diseases common in older men. Androgen deprivation therapy has been used in the treatment of both these disorders, but the role of testosterone supplementation as a potential promoter of prostate disease in older men is not known. Several testosterone replacement studies involving men aged 40 to 89 years have evaluated serum levels of prostate-specific antigen (PSA), prostate size, or functional prostate parameters. The large majority of these studies have reported no significant change in PSA serum levels or other prostate parameters. However, because both prostate cancer and BPH are diseases with long natural histories, and the observation time for testosterone therapy in older men is limited to less than 1500 man-years, the long-term effects of testosterone supplementation on the prostates of older men is still of concern. As noted previously, the overall risk/benefit ratio for testosterone therapy in terms of the cardiovascular

system in older men is not known, and so this is also an area where potential adverse effects can occur.

In the United States three major types of delivery systems are currently available for testosterone replacement: long-acting injectable testosterone esters, such as testosterone enanthate or cypionate; patches, either scrotal or transdermal; and a transdermally applied gel. The disadvantages of injectable esters include the necessity for intramuscular injection, with possible discomfort at the injection site, and the nonphysiologic plasma testosterone profiles that result from these injections. The disadvantages of patches include local skin irritation, the need to shave the skin prior to application if the area is hirsute, and the occasional unreliable testosterone plasma levels that can result if the patches do not adhere correctly. The major disadvantage of testosterone gel at this point is its cost. The current cost of therapy with injectable testosterone esters ranges from $20 to $50 per month, including the cost of an office visit to receive the injection. Testosterone replacement by scrotal or transdermal patch currently costs between $80 and $115 per month, and testosterone gel costs about $130 to $145 per month.

Androstenedione

Androstenedione is a weak androgenic steroid produced by the adrenal glands. It is available as an over-the-counter dietary supplement and has been promoted as both an antiaging and an anabolic agent. Androstenedione is a precursor of testosterone but can also be converted to estrogens. In men and women, short-term usage may increase testosterone levels slightly, but the effect seems to be transient; plasma levels of estradiol and estrone also have been reported to increase with androstenedione use. Several studies have evaluated the effect of androstenedione on strength, alone or combined with exercise training. No improvements in body composition or strength were observed, and lipid profiles were adversely affected. Because androstenedione is a dietary supplement and is not regulated by the US Food and Drug Administration, the content and purity of the ingredients is controlled by the manufacturers.

DEHYDROEPIANDROSTERONE AND DEHYDROEPIANDROSTERONE SULFATE

Physiology and Changes With Aging

Dehydroepiandrosterone (DHEA) and its sulfate (DHEAS) are the most abundant steroids in humans. In women, DHEA is synthesized almost exclusively by the zona reticularis of the adrenal gland cortex, whereas in men, 5 percent to 30 percent comes from the testes. DHEA is released into the circulation in its water-soluble form, DHEAS, which is the most abundant hormone in human blood. DHEA and DHEAS (DHEA/S) are the progenitors of male and female sex steroids—testosterone, estradiol, and progesterone— and the glucocorticoid corticosterone.

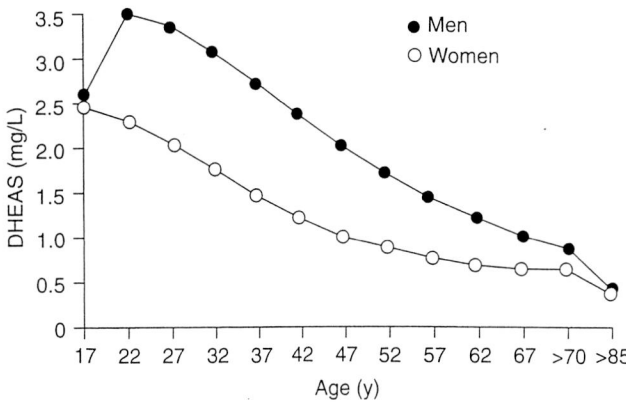

Figure 103-3 Age-related decline in dehydroepiandrosterone sulfate (DHEAS) blood levels in humans. Reprinted with permission from Watson et al, *Drugs Aging* 9(4):276, 1996.

Although DHEA/S was isolated in 1934, investigation of its role in endocrine physiology has been relatively recent. DHEA/S serum levels are high in the fetus, peak in young adulthood, and then decrease with age in both men and women; serum levels of DHEA/S decline more markedly with age than those of any other steroid. At age 65 years, both men and women have about 10 percent to 20 percent of the DHEA/S serum levels they did at age 20 years (Figure 103-3). Most studies have reported a 10 percent to 30 percent higher level of DHEA/S in men than in women, but this gender difference becomes less marked after age 50. There are also genetic differences, with Japanese men having significantly lower levels of DHEA/S than white men. The decline in serum levels with age is largely due to a decrease in DHEA/S production and meets several criteria for being a biomarker of aging, such as cross-sectional and longitudinal linear declines with age and stability of interindividual differences over time.

In most investigations of the effects of DHEA/S supplementation, rats, mice, or dogs have been used as the animal model system. In terms of their extrapolation to humans, the findings from such studies should be considered with caution because, unlike humans and other primates, which secrete large quantities of DHEA/S from their adrenals, rats, mice, and dogs normally secrete only a minute quantity of DHEA/S. Other aspects of endocrine physiology that make the role of DHEA/S difficult to explain include the lack of a dedicated feedback mechanism, such as governs plasma cortisol or testosterone, and the failure, as of yet, to identify specific receptors for DHEA/S. Nonetheless, the large DHEA/S concentrations available to act as a reservoir for substrate conversion, the dramatic change in serum DHEA/S levels with human aging, and the finding that caloric restriction in primates slows the postmaturational decline in serum DHEA/S levels have all made this hormone a target of investigation as a potential trophic factor. Currently, however, the essential biological effects and risks of this hormone are unknown and have not been tested in a long-term clinical trial. Human trials with DHEA/S are limited, involve only small numbers of participants, and vary widely in participant characteristics; thus

extrapolation of the data to the geriatric patient population is not always possible.

Dehydroepiandrosterone Sulfate Replacement in Older Adults

Immune Function

Based on rodent studies, some of which have shown that the administration of DHEA/S can result in an increase in the production of antibodies to vaccines, stimulation of T-cell proliferation and IL-2 production in response to mitogens, a decrease in mortality from a viral challenge, and quicker healing of burns, the possibility that human immune function can improve with DHEA/S supplementation has begun to be evaluated, although currently studies are limited.

Human studies that have demonstrated an effect of DHEA/S on immune function include (1) DHEA/S treatment of middle-aged women with systemic lupus erythematosus for 3 to 6 months, which resulted in a decline in proteinuria and the corticosteroid requirement; (2) DHEA/S given to a small number of older persons for 5 months, which caused an increase in various types of immune cells, enhancement of B- and T-mitogenic responses, and an increase in the in vitro mitogenic stimulation of IL-2 and IL-6 production; and (3) treatment of postmenopausal women for 3 weeks with DHEA/S, which resulted in increased natural killer cell cytotoxicity, a decreased number of CD4 (T-helper) cells, and an inhibited T-cell mitogenic response.

Conversely, several human studies have shown little or no effect of DHEA/S supplementation on the human immune system, including (1) evaluating megadoses given to younger symptomatic human immunodeficiency virus (HIV)-infected individuals and noting no improvement in immune parameters and (2) evaluating DHEA/S prior to influenza vaccination in elderly patients and observing no improvement in immune response. At this time, the improvements in immune action seen with DHEA/S supplementation in the rodent model have yet to be replicated in humans.

Cardiovascular System

Dehydroepiandrosterone sulfate has demonstrated anticlotting and antiatherosclerotic properties in animal studies. In human epidemiologic studies, the serum concentration of this agent has been found to be much lower in men with coronary artery disease compared with healthy age-matched men, even when stuudies were controlled for smoking or concomitant high cholesterol levels. Plasma levels of DHEA/S have been shown to be inversely proportional to the incidence of death from cardiovascular disease in older men, but directly proportional to the incidence of death from cardiovascular disease in older women. Prospective studies have failed to confirm an inverse association between serum DHEA/S levels and angiographically defined coronary atherosclerosis in men.

The effects of supplementation with DHEA/S on human platelet aggregation have been evaluated in a small number of young men, and results have shown a prolongation of time to platelet aggregation. In one study, DHEA/S was also found to decrease the concentrations of plasma plasminogen activator inhibitor type 1 (PAI-1) and tissue plasminogen activator (tPA) antigen, which may protect against heart disease. A study of healthy young men reported that suprapharmacologic doses of DHEA/S (1600 mg/d) given for 4 weeks resulted in a decline in levels of low-density-lipoprotein cholesterol and total cholesterol. However, these results were not confirmed by a subsequent similar study of young men. In most DHEA replacement studies involving older adults, plasma lipid and lipoprotein levels have not changed. A few studies have reported a small decrease in low-density-lipoprotein cholesterol in women, but not in men, with DHEA/S treatment. Overall, how these effects of DHEA/S might translate into any beneficial effect in protecting against cardiovascular disease in elderly people is unknown.

Body Composition

A few studies on humans have shown a decline in body fat and/or an increase in muscle mass with DHEA/S administration, but most investigations have failed to demonstrate any significant effects of DHEA/S on body composition. One study, in which men and women were given DHEA/S at a dose of 100 mg/d for 1 year, demonstrated an increase in lean body mass in both men and women and a decline in fat mass in men. In contrast, three other studies in which DHEA/S was given to older men in doses ranging from 100 to 1600 mg/d for 1 to 4 months found no change in total weight, body fat mass, or lean body mass. In several investigations, DHEA/S supplementation has been found to improve insulin sensitivity and reduce fasting glucose and oral glucose tolerance. Other investigations have not found such an effect, and one study involving postmenopausal women given high-dose DHEA/S reported an induction of insulin resistance with DHEA/S treatment. The variability of the doses of DHEA/S utilized and the types of patients evaluated (obese, middle-aged, older, diabetic, and nondiabetic) in the various studies have been great, making it difficult to make any general statements about the effects of DHEA/S on body composition and carbohydrate metabolism.

Other Effects

Clinical trials investigating DHEA/S effects on bone are limited. Daily administration of a 10 percent DHEA vaginal cream to 14 postmenopausal women for 12 months significantly increased BMD at the hip and improved the level of biochemical markers for bone turnover. On the other hand, no change in hip and vertebral BMD or biochemical bone turnover parameters was noted in 16 older men and women after 6 months of 100 mg/d DHEA given orally.

Early DHEA/S replacement trials lasting up to 12 months reported an increase in physical and psychological well-being compared to a placebo. However, at least six studies have failed to show any effect of DHEA/S therapy on various aspects of mood in either men or women. Two placebo-controlled, blind studies in which older men were given DHEA/S at 100 mg/d for 3 to 4 months reported no effect on aspects of sexual function. DHEA/S supplementation

Table 103-8 Potential or Reported Adverse Effects of Therapy With Dehydroepiandrosterone and Dehydroepiandrosterone Sulfate in Older Persons

Reported (in women)
Acne
Hirsutism
Hair loss
Deepening of voice
Hepatitis
Potential (men and women)
Acceleration of neoplasms
Prostate
Breast
Endometrium
Toxicity from impurities in various preparations

has failed to improve performance on cognitive tests of speed, attention, and episodic memory in the few studies where these tests have been administered.

Adverse Effects of Dehydroepiandrosterone Sulfate

No data are available on the long-term safety of DHEA/S given in replacement doses. Table 103-8 lists the potential or reported adverse effects of DHEA/S. In one study, increased liver enzyme levels and transient clinical hepatitis occurred in one of eight women after a single oral dose of a micronized DHEA preparation. However, in most studies to date, the adverse effects of DHEA administration have not been serious. Because DHEA/S can be converted to both active androgens and estrogens, it is possible that their use might accelerate the growth of prostate, breast, or endometrial cancer; therefore, their use in persons with these cancers should be avoided. Various androgenic effects, including acne, hirsutism, hair loss, and deepening of the voice, have been reported with the use of DHEA/S in women. Currently, these compounds are not regulated by the US Food and Drug Administration, and so the possible presence of potentially injurious impurities in the various preparations is of some concern. At this time, A 1-month supply of 100 mg/d DHEA/S currently costs about $35, with usual dosages being 25 to 150 mg/d in three to four divided doses.

REFERENCES

Bakhshi V et al: Testosterone improves rehabilitation outcomes in ill older men. *J Am Geriatr Soc* 48:550, 2000.

Broeder CE et al: The andro project: Physiological and hormonal influences of androstenedione supplementation in men 35 to 65 years old participating in a high-intensity resistance training program. *Arch Intern Med* 160:3093, 2000.

Christmas C et al: Growth hormone and sex steroid effects on bone metabolism and bone mineral density in healthy aged women and men. *J Gerontol Med Sci* 57A:M12, 2002.

Harman SM et al: Longitudinal effects of aging on serum total and free testosterone levels in healthy men. *J Clin Endocrinol Metab* 86:724, 2001.

Horani MH, Morley JE: The viability of the use of DHEA. *Clin Geriatr* 5:34, 1997.

Hornsby PJ: DHEA: A biologist's perspective. *J Am Geriatr Soc* 45:1395, 1997.

Matsumoto AM: Andropause: Clinical implications of the decline in serum testosterone levels with aging in men. *J Gerontol Med Sci* 57A:M76, 2002.

Melton LJ: Epidemiology of osteoporosis. *Trends Endocrinol Metab* 3:224, 1992.

Morales AJ et al: Effects of replacement doses of dehydroepiandrosterone in men and women of advancing age. *J Clin Endocrinol Metab* 78:1360, 1994.

Munzer T et al: Effects of GH and/or sex steroid administration on abdominal subcutaneous and visceral fat in healthy aged women and men. *J Clin Endocrinol Metab* 86:3604, 2001.

Nippoldt TB: Dehydroepiandrosterone supplements: Bringing sense to sensational claims. *Endocrine Pract* 4:106, 1998.

Papadakis MA et al: Growth hormone replacement in healthy older men improves body composition but not functional ability. *Ann Intern Med* 124:708, 1996.

Rosen CJ: Growth hormone and aging. *Endocrine* 12:197, 2000.

Rudman D et al: Effects of human growth hormone in men over 60 years old. *N Engl J Med* 323:1, 1990.

Snyder PJ et al: Effect of testosterone treatment on body composition and muscle strength in men over 65 years of age. *J Clin Endocrinol Metab* 84:2647,1999.

Sullivan DH et al: Side effects resulting from the use of growth hormone and insulin-like growth factor-I as combined therapy to frail elderly patients. *J Gerontol Med Sci* 53A:M183, 1998.

Tenover JL: Topical review: Testosterone replacement therapy in older adult men. *Int J Androl* 22:300, 1999.

Vermeulen A: Clinical review 24: Androgens in the aging male. *J Clin Endocrinol Metab* 73:221, 1991.

NEUROPSYCHIATRY

Cellular and Neurochemical Aspects of the Aging Human Brain

MARK P. MATTSON

Many cellular and molecular aspects of brain aging are shared with other organ systems, including increased oxidative damage to proteins, nucleic acids, and membrane lipids, impaired energy metabolism, and the accumulation of intracellular and extracellular protein aggregates. On the other hand, there are age-related changes that are unique to the nervous system, resulting from the unsurpassed molecular complexity of neural cells, which express approximately 50 to 100 times more genes than cells in other tissues. For example, complex cellular signal transduction pathways involving neurotransmitters, trophic factors, and cytokines that are involved in regulating neuronal excitability and plasticity are subject to modification by aging. This chapter describes cellular and molecular changes that occur in the brain during aging and how such changes may predispose neurons to degeneration in disorders such as Alzheimer's disease (AD), Parkinson's disease (PD), and Huntington's disease (HD).

STRUCTURAL CHANGES IN THE AGING BRAIN

Structural changes in both neurons and glial cells occur during aging. The changes include nerve cell death, dendritic retraction and expansion, synapse loss and remodeling, and glial cell reactivity. Such structural changes may result from alterations in cytoskeletal proteins and the deposition of insoluble proteins such as amyloid in the extracellular space. Alterations in cellular signaling pathways that control cell growth and motility may contribute to both adaptive and pathological structural changes in the aging brain.

Cytoskeletal and Synaptic Changes

The cell cytoskeleton consists of polymers of different sizes and protein compositions. The three major types of polymers are actin microfilaments (6 nm in diameter), microtubules (25 nm in diameter), which are comprised of tubulin, and intermediate filaments (10 to 15 nm in diameter), which are made of specific intermediate filament proteins that are different in different cell types (e.g., neurofilament proteins in neurons and glial fibrillary acidic protein in astrocytes). To regulate the processes of filament assembly and depolymerization, and to link the cytoskeleton to membranes and other cell structures, neurons and glial cells employ an array of cytoskeleton-associated proteins. For example, neurons express several microtubule-associated proteins (MAPs) that are differentially distributed within the complex architecture of the cells; MAP-2 is present in dendrites but not in the axon, whereas tau is present in axons but not in dendrites. While there are no major changes in the levels of the major cytoskeletal proteins with aging, there are changes in the cytoskeletal organization and in posttranslational modifications of cytoskeletal proteins. For example, increased levels of phosphorylation of tau occurs in some brain regions, particularly those involved in learning and memory (e.g., hippocampus and basal forebrain). In addition, there is evidence that calcium-mediated proteolysis of MAP-2 and spectrin (a protein that links actin filaments to membranes) is increased in some neurons during aging. Oxidation of certain cytoskeletal proteins is suggested by studies demonstrating their modification by glycation and covalent binding of the lipid peroxidation product 4-hydroxynonenal (see "Free Radicals and the Aging Brain" later in this chapter). A consistent feature of brain aging in humans and laboratory animals is an increase in levels of glial fibrillary acidic protein, which may represent a reaction to subtle neurodegenerative changes.

Synapses are dynamic structural specializations where neurotransmission and other intercellular signaling events occur. There is considerable evidence for synaptic "remodeling" in the brain as we age, which is likely related to

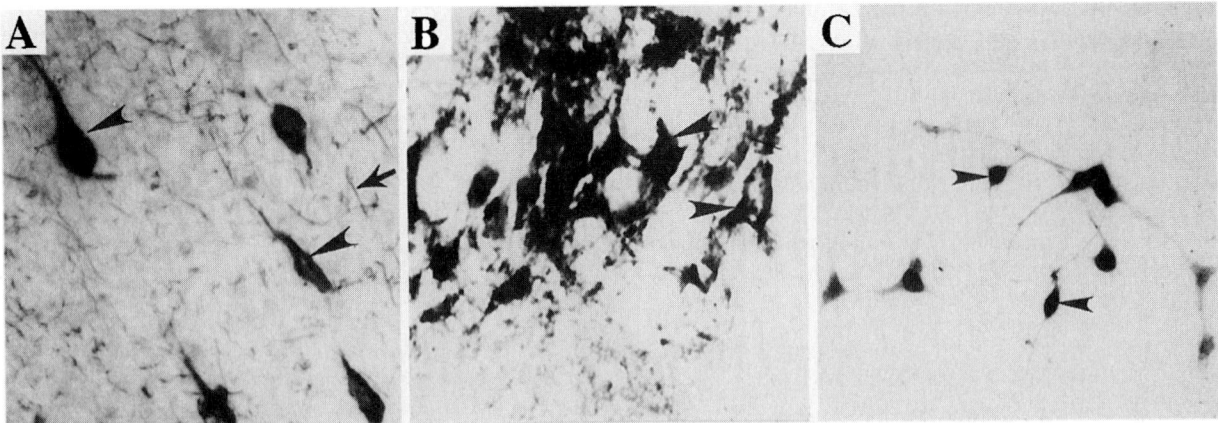

Figure 104-1   Neuronal cytoskeletal pathology in Alzheimer's disease is mimicked in experimental systems by insults that increase intracellular calcium levels and induce oxidative stress. *(A)* Section of hippocampal tissue from an AD patient immunostained with an antibody against the microtubule-associated protein tau. Note strong staining of degenerating "tangle-bearing" neuronal cell bodies *(arrowheads)*. *(B)* Section of hippocampus from an adult rat that had been administered the seizure-inducing excitotoxin kainate 6 hours previously. The section was immunostained with an antibody against the microtubule-associated protein tau. Note strong staining of degenerating neurons *(arrowheads)*. *(C)* Human embryonic cerebral cortical neurons in culture that were left untreated (control) or were exposed for 2 hours to a calcium ionophore. Cells were then stained with a antibody against ubiquitin, a stress-responsive protein present in degenerating neurons in AD.

changes in dendritic arbors and neuronal numbers. For example, there may be decreases in synaptic numbers in some brain regions, but these may be offset by increases in the size of the remaining synapses. In other brain regions, no loss of synapses can be discerned.

In contrast to usual, striking alterations in the neuronal cytoskeleton and synapses occur in neurodegenerative disorders such as AD, PD, and HD. Neurofibrillary tangles are filamentous accumulations of tau protein that form in the cytoplasm of degenerating neurons (Fig. 104-1). Neurons with tangles have a decreased number of microtubules, and often exhibit accumulations of MAP-2 and tau in the cell body. Tau is excessively phosphorylated in neurofibrillary tangles, which may result from reduced phosphatase activity as a consequence of oxidation or covalent modification by lipid peroxidation products. In PD, structures called Lewy bodies form in neurons, and are comprised of abnormal accumulations of neurofilaments, with associated MAPs (particularly MAP-1b) and actin-related proteins such as gelsolin. In amyotrophic lateral sclerosis, lower motor neurons are filled with massive accumulations of neurofilaments which concentrate in proximal regions of the axon. While the specific molecular events involved in formation of the cytoskeletal alterations in different neurodegenerative disorders have not been established, there is increasing evidence for major roles of aberrant elevation of intracellular calcium levels and increased oxidative stress. Conditions that elevate intracellular calcium levels (e.g., exposure to glutamate or calcium ionophores) and induce oxidative stress (e.g., exposure to Fe^{2+} and amyloid β-peptide [$A\beta$], or expression of mutant Cu/ZnSOD) can elicit changes in the cytoskeleton in experimental animal and cell culture models that are similar to those seen in the human disorders (Figs. 104-1 and 104-2).

Synapse loss occurs in neurodegenerative disorders and is strongly correlated with clinical symptoms. Accumulating data suggest that synaptic degeneration, resulting from excitotoxic events localized to synapses, may initiate the neuronal death process in AD, PD, HD, and stroke. Glutamate receptors are highly concentrated in postsynaptic dendritic spines, which represent sites of massive calcium influx during normal physiologic synaptic transmission. Age-related decreases in energy availability and increases in oxidative stress, and disease-specific alterations such as amyloid accumulation in AD and trinucleotide expansions of the huntingtin protein, may render synapses vulnerable to excitotoxic injury (see below).

Vascular Changes

As in other organ systems, vessels that supply blood to the brain are vulnerable to age-related atherosclerosis and arteriosclerosis, which render the vessels susceptible to occlusion or rupture (stroke), a major cause of disability and death in the elderly population. Reduced brain perfusion in the absence of overt stroke may play a role in age-related cognitive dysfunction. Decreased cerebral blood flow occurs with advancing age and is accompanied by declines in cerebral metabolic rate for oxygen and glucose use. Age-related changes in cerebral vasculature are generally similar to those that occur in vessels elsewhere in the body and are therefore likely to result from common cellular and molecular changes, including oxidative damage to vascular endothelial cells and an inflammatory response in which macrophages may penetrate the blood–brain barrier (Fig. 104-3). Age-dependent cerebral vascular changes are strongly linked to heart disease and hypertension. Interestingly, apolipoprotein E polymorphisms are linked to increased risk of both atherosclerosis and AD, with the apolipoprotein E4 increasing the risk. This association suggests that age-related vascular changes may make an important contribution to the neurodegenerative process in AD. Finally, important transport functions of cells (endothelial cells and astrocytes) that comprise the blood–brain barrier may also be impaired in the aging brain and more so in

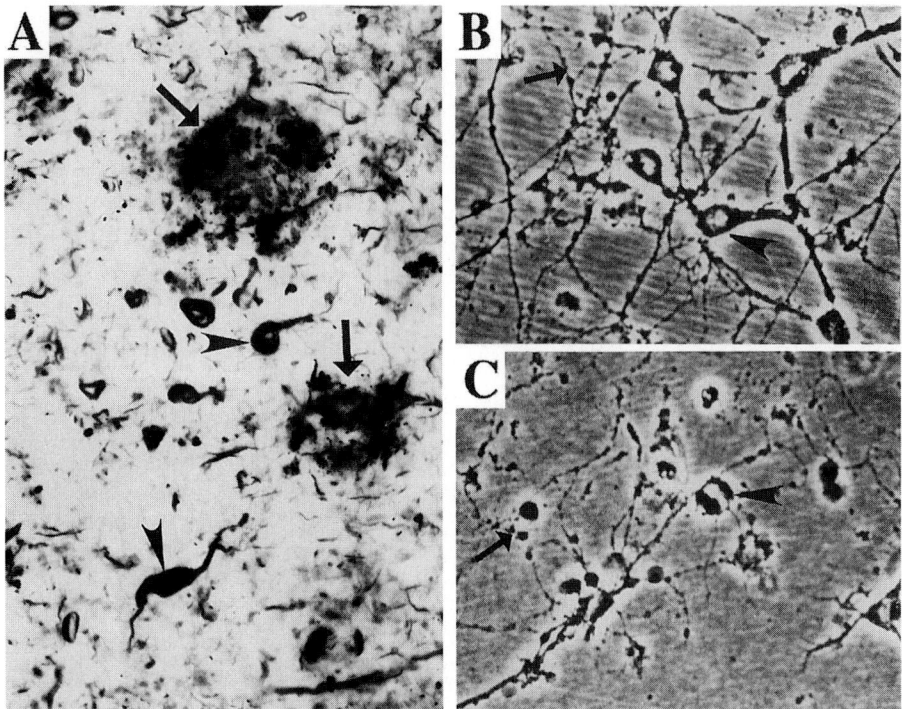

Figure 104-2 Histologic and experimental evidence that amyloid deposition plays a role in the neurodegenerative process in Alzheimer's disease. *(A)* Section of hippocampal tissue from an AD patient immunostained with an antibody against the microtubule-associated protein tau. Note strong staining of degenerating "tangle-bearing" neuronal cell bodies *(arrowheads)* and neurites associated with amyloid plaques *(arrow). (B and C)* Phase-contrast micrographs of cultured rat hippocampal neurons that had been exposed for 24 hours to amyloid β-peptide $(A\beta)$ alone *(B)* or in combination with corticosterone *(C)*. Note that neurites in the culture exposed to $A\beta$ alone are beginning to exhibit signs of damage *(arrow)*, while the neuronal cell bodies still appear undamaged *(arrowhead)*. Corticosterone exacerbated the damage to neurons exposed to $A\beta$. See Goodman et al: *J Neurochem.* 66:1836, 1996.

AD. Many of the same behavioral and dietary approaches now recognized to forestall cardiovascular disease may also forestall cerebrovascular disease; these include engaging in physical and mental activities, a low calorie intake, and a high antioxidant intake.

Amyloid Accumulation

$A\beta$ is a 40- to 42-amino-acid peptide that arises from a much larger membrane-spanning β-amyloid precursor protein (APP). During normal aging, and to a much greater extent in AD, $A\beta$ forms insoluble aggregates (plaques) in the brain parenchyma and vasculature (Fig. 104-4). Amyloid plaques accumulate most heavily in brain regions involved in learning and memory processes such as the hippocampus and entorhinal cortex. In AD, the accumulation of $A\beta$ in the brain is correlated with the amount of neuronal degeneration and with the severity of cognitive impairment. Although the cause(s) of the majority of cases of AD is unknown, some AD cases are caused by mutations in APP, presenilin-1, or presenilin-2; mutations in each of these proteins result in increased production of self-aggregating neurotoxic forms of $A\beta$. $A\beta$ can be neurotoxic, and can increase neuronal vulnerability to metabolic, excitotoxic, and oxidative insults. The sequence of events involved in $A\beta$-induced neuronal injury and death may involve induction of membrane lipid peroxidation, which

generates a toxic aldehyde called 4-hydroxynonenal that covalently modifies proteins involved in maintenance of cellular ion homeostasis and energy metabolism, including the plasma membrane Na^+/K^+ and Ca^{2+} ATPases (adenosine triphosphatases), glucose transporters, and glutamate transporters. This may lead to excessive elevation of intracellular calcium levels, mitochondrial dysfunction, and a form of cell death called apoptosis. In addition to its likely involvement in the neurodegenerative process, $A\beta$ may also disrupt neurotransmitter signaling pathways. For example, $A\beta$ impairs coupling of muscarinic acetylcholine receptors to their downstream GTP (guanosine triphosphate)-binding effector protein, an action that likely contributes to the well-established deficits in cholinergic signaling pathways in AD. Finally, $A\beta$ may also contribute to vascular damage and inflammatory processes in the aging brain.

FREE RADICALS AND THE AGING BRAIN

A free radical is any molecule with an unpaired electron in its outer orbital; in biological systems, oxygen-based molecules are the predominant free radical species (Fig. 104-5). A major oxyradical in cells is superoxide $(O_2^-\cdot)$ which is generated during the mitochondrial electron transport process; superoxide dismutases (MnSOD and Cu/ZnSOD) eliminate $O_2^-\cdot$ by converting it to hydrogen peroxide (H_2O_2). H_2O_2 can be converted to hydroxyl radical

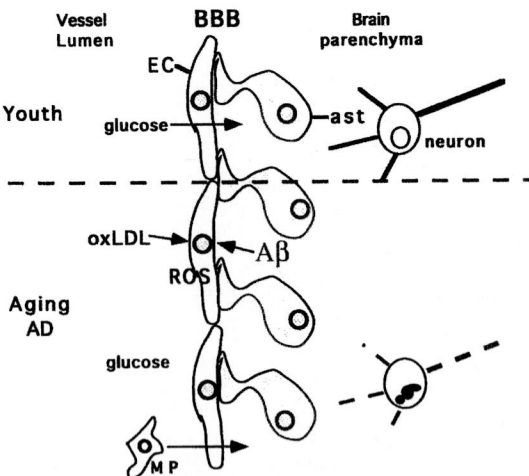

Figure 104-3 Adverse effects of aging and Alzheimer's disease on endothelial cells and the blood–brain barrier. Vascular endothelial cells (EC) and associated astrocyte (ast) processes form the blood–brain barrier (BBB), which plays important roles in transporting nutrients (e.g., glucose) into the brain, while at the same time preventing movement of toxic substances and blood cells such as macrophages (MP). With aging, and more so in AD, oxidative damage to endothelial cells results from exposure to oxidized LDL and amyloid β-peptide (Aβ). Oxidative stress impairs transport functions of the EC and promotes penetration of MP into the brain parenchyma. Such compromise of the vasculature results in reduced nutrient availability to neurons and inflammatory processes that promote degeneration of neurons.

(OH•) via the Fenton reaction which is catalyzed by Fe^{2+} and Cu^+. Peroxynitrite ($ONOO^-$) arises from the interaction of nitric oxide (NO) with O_2^-; calcium influx is a major stimulus for NO production. While OH• and $ONOO^-$ can cause direct damage to proteins and deoxyribonucleic acid (DNA), their major means of damaging cells is by attacking fatty acids in membranes and initiating a process called lipid peroxidation. Studies of aging have provided compelling evidence that there is an increase in production and accumulation of oxyradicals in essentially all tissues in the body during the aging process, including in the brain.

Lipid Peroxidation

Levels of lipid peroxidation products such as lipid peroxides and 4-hydroxnonenal are significantly elevated in the brain parenchyma and cerebrospinal fluid in AD (see Fig. 104-5). Immunohistochemical analyses of brain tissue from AD and PD patients, and spinal cord tissue from amyotrophic lateral sclerosis (ALS) patients, using antibodies directed against 4-hydroxynonenal adducts revealed increased levels of 4-hydroxynonenal in association with degenerating neurons and neuritic plaques suggesting a role for this aldehyde in the neurodegenerative process. Studies of cell culture and animal models of AD and ALS show that lipid peroxidation can impair the function of the plasma membrane glucose and glutamate transporters and render neurons vulnerable to excitotoxicity and apoptosis.

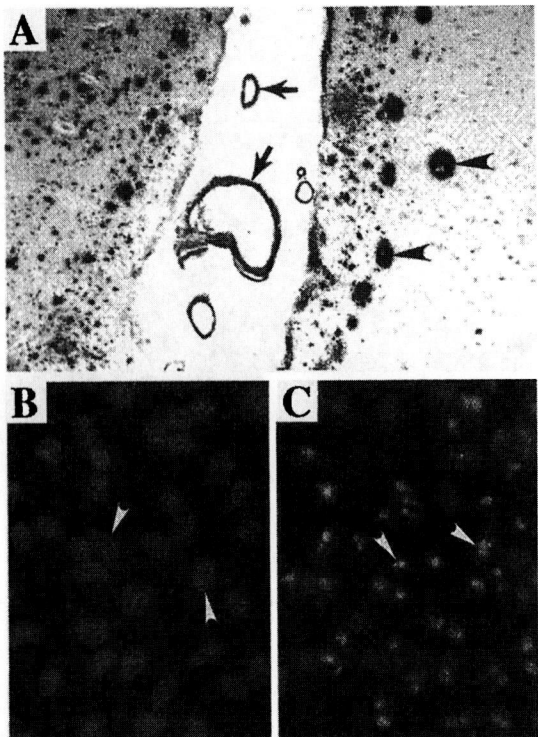

Figure 104-4 Amyloid deposits in the brain parenchyma and cerebral vessels: evidence that amyloid damages vascular endothelial cells. (A) Section of hippocampal tissue from an AD patient. The section was immunostained with an antibody against amyloid β-peptide (Aβ). Note numerous Aβ deposits of various sizes in the brain parenchyma (*arrowheads* point to large plaques) and cerebral blood vessels (*arrows*). (B and C) Cultured vascular endothelial cells were exposed for 24 hours to saline (B) or Aβ (C), and were then stained with the fluorescent deoxyribonucleic acid (DNA)-binding dye HOECHST 33342. The nuclear DNA in cells not exposed to Aβ exhibits the normal diffuse uniform distribution, while the chromatin in the cells exposed to Aβ exhibits condensation and fragmentation consistent with apoptotic death. Adapted from Blanc EM et al: Amyloid β-peptide disrupts barrier and transport functions and induces apoptosis in vascular endothelial cells. *J Neurochem* 68:1870, 1997.

Administration of antioxidants such as vitamin E to cultured cells and transgenic mice expressing mutations that cause AD or ALS can retard the neurodegenerative process, suggesting a causal role for lipid peroxidation in these diseases.

Protein Oxidation

Levels of protein oxidation, measured as protein carbonyls, are significantly elevated in the brains of aged rodents, and such age-associated protein oxidation can be prevented by administration of antioxidants. Studies of membrane structure have provided evidence for oxidation-related alterations in membrane protein conformation in old rodents. Studies of brain tissues of patients with AD and PD have revealed increased levels of protein oxidation in vulnerable

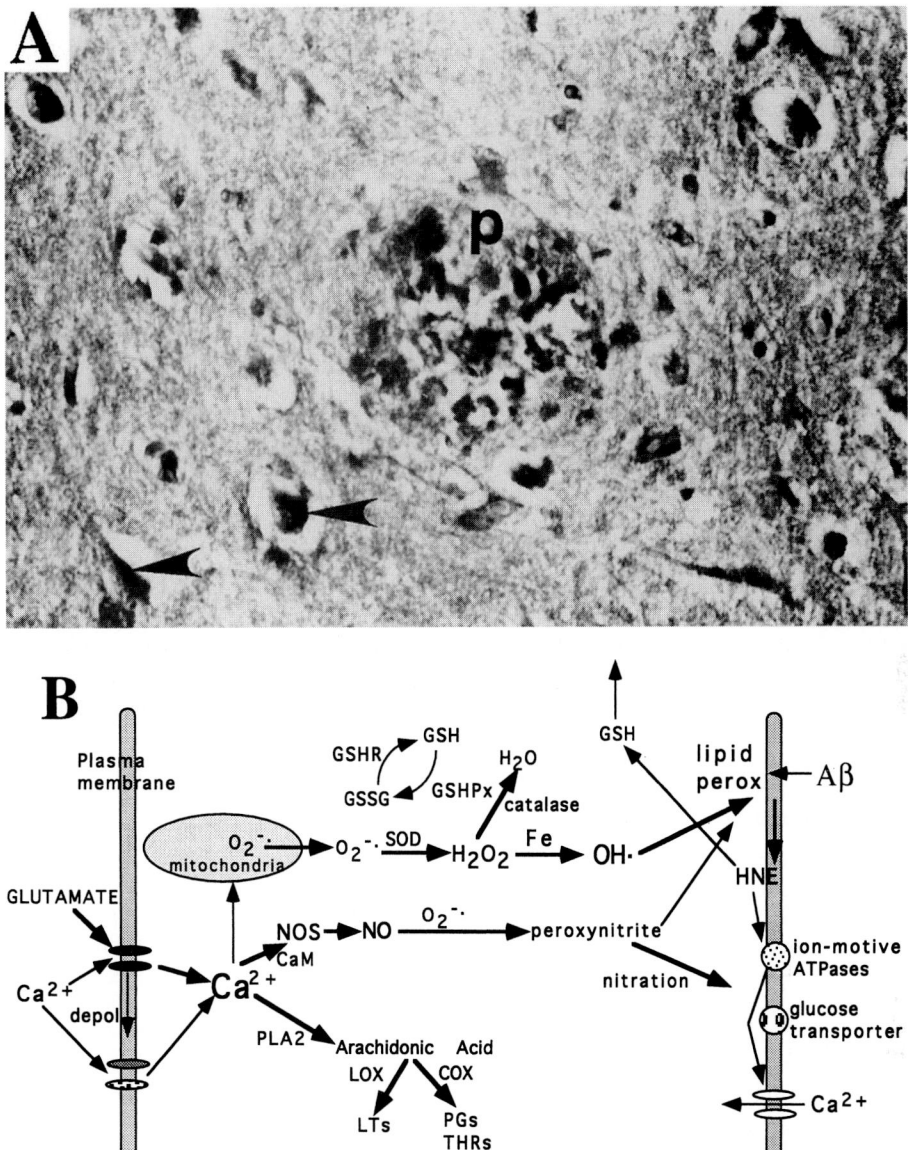

Figure 104-5 Possible sources of oxidative stress contributing to dysfunction and degeneration of neurons in aging and Alzheimer's disease. *(A)* Section of hippocampal tissue from an AD patient. The section was immunostained with an antibody that recognizes lipid peroxides which are by-products of membrane lipid peroxidation. Note immunoreactivity associated with neuritic plaques (p) and neurofibrillary tangles *(arrowheads)*. *(B)* The major cellular source of reactive oxygen species in neurons is mitochondria where O_2^-. is generated during the electron transport process. The superoxide dismutase enzymes (SOD) convert O_2^- to H_2O_2. Fe^{2+} catalyzes the production of OH• from H_2O_2, while glutathione peroxidase (GSHPx) and catalase detoxify H_2O_2. Peroxynitrite can be formed by the interaction of O_2^- with nitric oxide (NO). Both OH•, and peroxynitrite induce membrane lipid peroxidation (MLP), which may occur in the plasma membrane, mitochondrial membranes, and endoplasmic reticulum (ER) membranes. During aging and in age-related neurodegenerative disorders agents such as amyloid β-peptide (Aβ) can induce MLP. MLP liberates the aldehyde 4-hydroxynonenal (HNE) which impairs the function of membrane transporters (glucose and glutamate transporters, and ion-motive ATPases) and ion channels, and thereby alters their activities. Reduced glutathione (GSH) binds and detoxifies HNE, thereby serving an important neuroprotective role. The antiapoptotic gene product Bcl-2 may act, in part, by suppressing MLP in plasma, mitochondrial, and ER membranes. Elevation of intracellular calcium levels, as induced by glutamate, promotes oxyradical production and MLP by inducing NO and O_2^- production, and by activating phospholipases resulting in production of arachidonic acid, which is then acted upon by cyclooxygenases (COX) and lipoxygenases (LOX). Modified from Mattson MP, Trends Neurosci 1997; 20:395.

brain regions and, in particular, in degenerating neurons. Oxidation of proteins impairs their function and is therefore a likely contributor to age-related cellular dysfunction and neuronal degeneration. Progressive addition of sugar residues to many different proteins occurs during the aging process. This process, called glycation, may promote oxidative stress in cells. Two proteins that have been shown to be heavily glycated in AD are Aβ and tau, the major components of plaques and neurofibrillary tangles, respectively.

DNA Damage

Very little nuclear DNA damage occurs in the nervous system during usual aging, but DNA damage may contribute to the pathogenesis of neurodegenerative disorders. Damage to nuclear DNA in striatum of HD patients, and in hippocampus and vulnerable cortical regions of AD patients, has been documented. Specifically, levels of 8-hydroxyguanosine are increased. This DNA damage may be caused by oxyradicals, with hydroxyl radical and peroxynitrite being the major culprits. Progressive oxidative damage to mitochondrial DNA occurs during aging, and may be exacerbated in neurodegenerative disorders. Mitochondrial DNA is particularly prone to damage because this organelle is the site where the vast majority of free radicals are generated and because cells do not possess effective systems for repair of damaged mitochondrial DNA. Damage to mitochondrial DNA can lead to failure of electron transport and reduced adenosine triphosphate (ATP) production. Moreover, the important calcium sequestering function of mitochondria may be compromised as the result of age-related DNA damage which may increase neuronal vulnerability to excitotoxicity and apoptosis.

Mechanisms that Promote Oxidative Stress in Aging and Neurodegenerative Disorders

Mitochondria-derived oxyradicals are likely to play a central role in the cumulative oxidative damage to various cellular constituents that accrues with aging. Age-related impairments in energy availability and metabolism may contribute to an acceleration of oxyradical production with aging. The importance of mitochondrial oxyradical production in aging, in general, is underscored by recent studies of the mechanism whereby caloric restriction extends life span in rodents and nonhuman primates. Levels of cellular oxidative stress (as indicated by oxidation of proteins, lipids, and DNA) are decreased in many different nonneural tissues of rats and mice maintained on a calorie-restricted diet (30 to 40 percent reduction in calories). Recent studies suggest that levels of oxidative stress are also reduced in the brains of calorie-restricted rodents. The current dogma for the underlying mechanism is that reduced mitochondrial metabolism because of reduced energy availability results in a net decrease in mitochondrial ROS production over time, and hence less radical-mediated cellular damage. Thus, one factor contributing to brain aging is simply the constant production of oxyradicals and resultant progressive damage to cellular components.

In addition to the oxyradical damage that accrues with usual aging, there are specific initiators of oxidative stress that appear to play key roles in different age-related neurodegenerative disorders. For example, in AD the increased generation and accumulation of Aβ may be a pivotal event that enhances oxidative stress in neurons. There is evidence that increased levels of Fe^{2+} in the substantia nigra plays a role in the degeneration of dopaminergic neurons in PD. The damage to neurons in the brain of stroke victims is the result of a combination of factors including excessive calcium influx and the presence of blood components such as Fe^{2+} and thrombin. In HD, the presence of trinucleotide repeats in the Huntingtin protein may induce oxidative stress in striatal neurons by a yet-to-be-determined mechanism.

ALTERATIONS IN ENERGY METABOLISM AND MITOCHONDRIAL FUNCTION IN THE AGING BRAIN

During the aging process, changes that occur in cerebral blood vessels, as well as in the neural cells themselves, appear to result in reduced energy availability to neurons. These age-related changes may be accelerated in several different neurodegenerative disorders including AD and PD.

Cerebral Metabolism

Reduced glucose use, and changes in enzymes involved in energy metabolism, may occur during normal aging, but are not dramatic. Studies of aging rodents document decreases in glucose and ketone body oxidation, oxygen consumption, local cerebral glucose use, and glycolytic compounds (e.g., fructose-1,6-diphosphate). Additional studies show that brain cells in older animals exhibit increased vulnerability to metabolic stresses. Incorporation of glucose into amino acids declines in the brains of aging mice, and older people are much more vulnerable to metabolic encephalopathy than are young people. In contrast to normal aging, activities of several enzymes involved in energy metabolism are severely reduced in AD brain tissues. Three such enzymes, which are involved in mitochondrial oxidative metabolism, are the pyruvate dehydrogenase complex, the α-ketoglutarate dehydrogenase complex, and cytochrome c oxidase. These defects may result from age-associated oxidative damage to the DNA encoding these enzyme systems and/or reduced activity of the proteins in these systems.

Another factor that may contribute to reduced neuronal energy metabolism is impairment of the function of glucose transporter proteins in neuronal membranes. Studies of postmortem brain tissues of AD patients document reduced levels of glucose transporters, and experimental studies of cultured hippocampal neurons and synaptosomes show that insults relevant to the pathogenesis of AD (exposure to Aβ and oxyradical-generating agents) can impair glucose transport (Fig. 104-6). Impairment of glucose transport and mitochondrial dysfunction would be expected to lead to ATP depletion and render neurons vulnerable to excitotoxicity.

Mitochondrial Function

Age-related structural changes in synaptic mitochondria have been reported and include a decrease in numbers and increase in size. During normal aging levels of

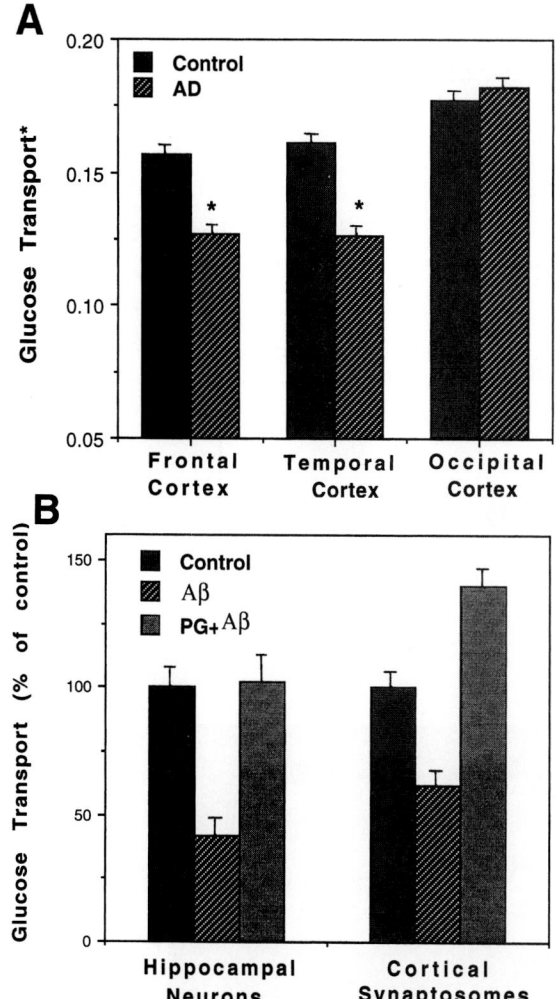

A

B

Figure 104-6 Evidence for reduced glucose transport in Alzheimer's disease. *(A)* Levels of glucose uptake into different brain regions of Alzheimer's patients and age-matched control subjects were quantified by dynamic positron emission tomography using [^{18}F]-fluorodeoxyglucose. Values are the rate constant K_1 expressed in mL/g/min and reflect glucose transport across the blood–brain barrier and into brain cells. *p <0.05 compared to corresponding value for control subjects. Adapted from Jagust et al: *J Cereb Blood Flow Metab* 11: 323, 1991. *(B)* Cultured embryonic rat hippocampal neurons, or cortical synaptosomes from adult rats, were pretreated with vehicle or the antioxidant propyl gallate (PG), and were then exposed for 2 hours to saline (control) or Aβ. Glucose transport was quantified. Note that Aβ caused a decrease in glucose transport, and that PG blocked the effect of Aβ. Adapted from Mark et al. *J Neurosci* 17:1046, 1997, and Keller et al: *J Neurochem* 69:273, 1997.

mitochondrial protein synthesis are unchanged. However, decreases in synthesis of specific mitochondrial proteins that are components of the electron transport chain occur in aging rodents. Damage to mitochondrial DNA progressively increases in somatic cells during the aging process, with the most pronounced damage occurring in postmitotic cells such as neurons. Mitochondrial dysfunction has been linked to several neurodegenerative disorders (Fig. 104-7). In PD there are marked decreases in complex I

and α-ketoglutarate dehydrogenase activities. Exposure of cultured dopaminergic neurons to insults relevant to the pathogenesis of PD (e.g., MPTP and Fe^{2+}) cause mitochondrial dysfunction. In AD, cytochrome c oxidase and α-ketoglutarate dehydrogenase activity levels are markedly reduced in vulnerable brain regions. Interestingly, mitochondrial deficits are also observed in nonneuronal cells, including platelets and fibroblasts, of AD patients. When mitochondria from platelets of AD patients are introduced into cultured neuroblastoma cells, levels of oxidative stress are increased suggesting an important contribution of mitochondrial alterations to the increased oxidative stress present in neurons in AD brain. Mitochondrial alterations in neurons have been documented in studies of mouse models of AD (APP and presenilin mutant mice), PD (α-synuclein mutant mice), HD (huntingtin mutant mice), and stroke (middle cerebral artery occlusion).

NEURONAL ION HOMEOSTASIS IN THE AGING BRAIN

Among the properties of neurons that set them apart from many other cell types is their excitability, which is regulated by a complex array of neurotransmitters and ion channels. Neurons express voltage-dependent sodium channels, as well as multiple types of calcium and potassium channels that are differentially expressed among neuronal populations, and are segregated in different cellular compartments (e.g., L-type calcium channels in the cell body, N-type calcium channels in the dendrites, and T-type calcium channels in presynaptic terminals). In addition, neurons possess ion-motive ATPases that play critical roles in reestablishing ion gradients following neuronal stimulation. A variety of age-related alterations in electrophysiologic parameters of neurons have been described in rodents and, in some cases, in humans, including increased thresholds for induction of action potentials in cranial nerves, increased after hyperpolarizations in hippocampal neurons, and impaired long-term potentiation of synaptic transmission in the hippocampus. Moreover, a generalized decrease in neuronal inhibition appears to occur during the aging process.

The calcium ion plays fundamental roles in regulating neuronal survival and plasticity in both the developing and adult nervous system. Calcium mediates the effects of neurotransmitters and neurotrophic factors on neurite outgrowth, synaptogenesis, and cell survival in many different regions of the developing nervous system, and in the adult nervous system, calcium regulates neurotransmitter release from presynaptic terminals and postsynaptic changes associated with learning and memory processes. Aging may result in decreases in the activity of the plasma membrane calcium ATPase and in levels of calcium-binding proteins, while increasing calcium influx through voltage-dependent channels and increasing the activation of calcium-dependent proteases. The factors that promote impaired calcium homeostasis in neurons in aging and age-related neurodegenerative disorders likely include increased levels of oxidative stress and metabolic compromise (see above).

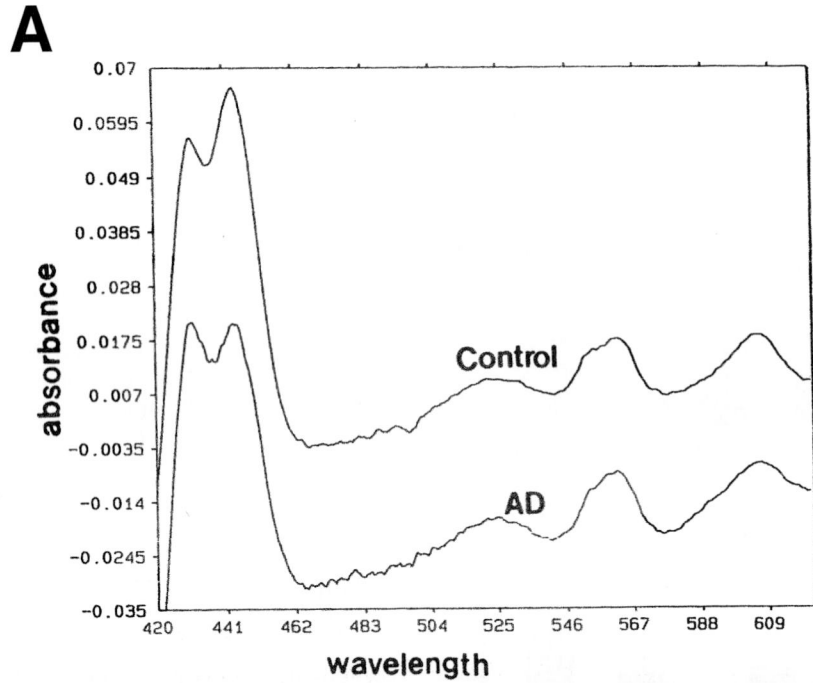

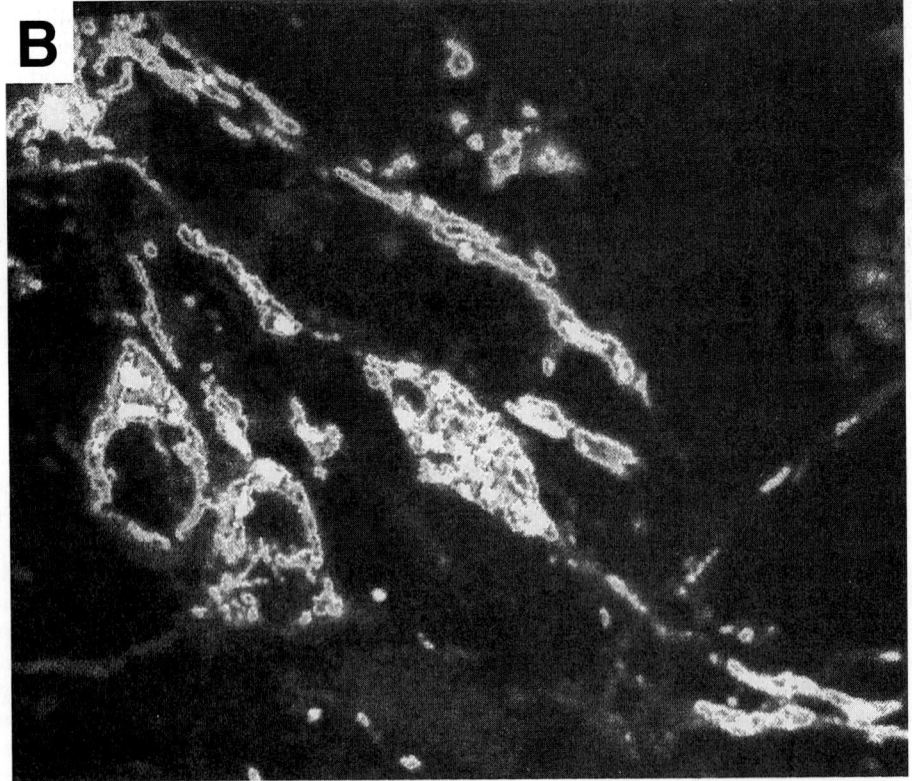

Figure 104-7   Evidence for mitochondrial dysfunction neurodegenerative disorders. *(A)* Reduced-oxidized difference spectra in isolated brain mitochondria from control and Alzheimer's disease (AD) patients. The spectra reflect levels of electron transport function in the mitochondria. Note reduced levels of cytochromes b, c_1, and aa_3 in mitochondria from the AD patients. Adapted from Parker et al: *Neurology* 44:1090, 1994. *(B)* Confocal laser scanning microscope image of mitochondrial reactive oxygen species levels (dihydrorhodamine 123 fluorescence) in cultured rat hippocampal neuron that had been exposed to amyloid β-peptide for 4 hours. Note high levels of fluorescence in mitochondria indicating the presence of extensive mitochondrial oxidative stress. Adapted from Mark et al: *Brain Res* 756:205, 1997.

NEUROTRANSMITTER SIGNALING IN THE AGING BRAIN

A number of alterations in different neurotransmitter systems have been documented in studies of aging rodents, and in analyses of brain tissues from humans with age-related neurodegenerative disorders. While some of these alterations likely result from neuronal degeneration, others appear to occur in the absence of cell injury.

Cholinergic Systems

Acetylcholine is employed as a neurotransmitter in select populations of neurons in the brain, prominent among which are basal forebrain neurons that innervate widespread regions of neocortex and to the hippocampus; these cholinergic neurons are known to play key roles in learning and memory processes in humans and rodents. Deficits in one or more aspects of cholinergic signal transduction may occur with aging including choline transport, acetylcholine synthesis, acetylcholine release, and coupling of muscarinic receptors to their GTP-binding effector proteins. Cholinergic deficits are much more severe in AD patients and also differ qualitatively from the changes observed during normal aging. Particularly striking is a reduced ability of muscarinic agonists to activate GTP-binding proteins in cortical neurons (Fig. 104-8). Increased levels of membrane lipid peroxidation in neurons may contribute to impaired cholinergic signaling; for example, $A\beta$, Fe^{2+} and the lipid peroxidation product 4-hydroxynonenal can impair coupling of muscarinic receptors to the GTP-binding protein G_{q11} (Fig. 104-8).

Dopaminergic Systems

Very prominent reductions in both pre- and postsynaptic aspects of dopaminergic neurotransmission occur during brain aging. Decreases in dopamine levels and dopamine transporter levels in the striatum occur with advancing age, and there is an age-related decrease in levels of D_2 receptor-binding sites in striatum. As with cholinergic signal transduction, there also appears to be an age-related impairment of coupling of dopamine receptors to their GTP-binding effector proteins. The contribution of oxidative stress to changes in dopaminergic signaling has not been established, although the prominent role of oxyradicals in the pathogenesis of PD argue that similar oxidative processes contribute to dopaminergic dysfunction during normal aging. These changes in dopaminergic signaling likely play a role in age-related deficits in motor control and may explain the fact that the elderly are susceptible to extrapyramidal effects of dopamine receptor antagonist drugs.

Monoaminergic Systems

Norepinephrine and serotonin are the major monoamine neurotransmitters in the brain. Noradrenergic neurons are located primarily in the locus caeruleus and serotonergic

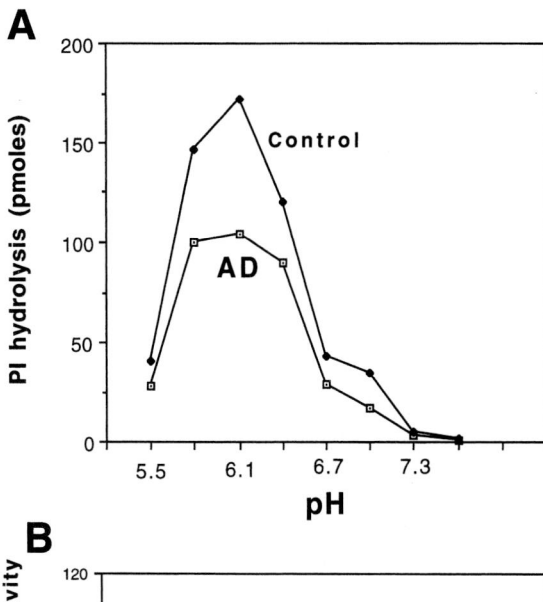

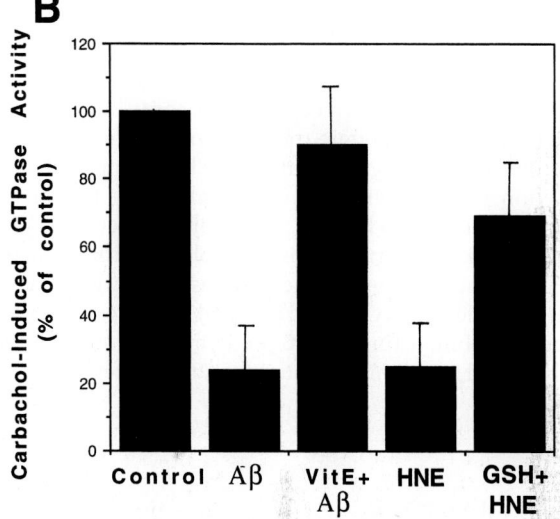

Figure 104-8 Impact of oxidative stress and Alzheimer's disease on muscarinic cholinergic signal transduction. *(A)* Levels of [³H]-PI hydrolysis induced by GTPγS plus carbachol (muscarinic acetylcholine receptor agonist) in membranes from brains of AD patients and age-matched controls. Note reduced levels of ligand-induced PI hydrolysis in the membranes from the AD patients. Adapted from Jope et al: *Neurobiol Aging* 15:221, 1997. *(B)* $A\beta$ and membrane lipid peroxidation impair coupling of muscarinic receptors to the GTP-binding protein G_{q11} in cultured cerebral cortical neurons. Cultured rat cortical neurons were exposed for 3 to 4 hours to vehicle (control), $A\beta$, vitamin E (VitE) plus $A\beta$, 4-hydroxynonenal (HNE), or glutathione ethyl ester (GSH) plus HNE. Membranes were then isolated and levels of carbachol-induced GTPase activity were quantified. Note that $A\beta$ and HNE impaired coupling of the muscarinic receptors to the GTP-binding protein, and that the antioxidants vitamin E and GSH attenuated the impairments. Adapted from Kelly et al: *Proc Natl Acad Sci U S A* 93:6753, 1996, and Blanc EM et al: Amyloid β-peptide disrupts barrier and transport functions and induces apoptosis in vascular endothelial cells. *J Neurochem* 68:1870, 1997.

neurons in the raphe nucleus; both types of neurons project to widespread regions of cerebral cortex. There are several subtypes of receptors for norepinephrine which each couple to GTP-binding proteins. There are also several subtypes of serotonin receptors, some of which couple to

GTP-binding proteins and others of which are ligand-gated ion channels. There appear to be increased levels of norepinephrine with aging in some brain regions, while levels of α_2-adrenergic receptors may decrease in cerebral cortex with advancing age. Levels of serotonin may decrease in the striatum, hippocampus, and cerebral cortex. Age-related decreases in levels of evoked serotonin release and of serotonin binding sites have been reported, and may contribute to affective disorders such as depression.

Amino Acid Transmitter Systems

The amino acid glutamate is the major excitatory neurotransmitter in the human brain. Glutamate stimulates inotropic receptors that flux calcium and sodium; excessive activation of inotropic glutamate receptors may play a role in the degeneration of neurons in several age-related disorders including stroke, AD, PD, and HD. Levels of inotropic glutamate receptors were reported to decrease with aging, but these decreases may be the result of degeneration of the neurons expressing the receptors. The contribution of dysfunction of glutamatergic transmission, in the absence of neuronal death, to age- and disease-related deficits in brain function is unknown. The major inhibitory neurotransmitter in the human brain is γ-aminobutyric acid (GABA). Relatively little information is available concerning the impact of aging on GABAergic systems, although levels of glutamate decarboxylase and GABA-A binding sites may be decreased. Interestingly, GABAergic interneurons are typically spared in various neurodegenerative disorders including AD.

NEUROENDOCRINE CHANGES IN THE AGING BRAIN

A variety of age-related alterations in neuroendocrine systems have been documented. Of particular importance for human brain aging and neurodegenerative disorders are changes in levels of steroid hormones, particularly glucocorticoids and estrogens. There is considerable evidence for age-related alterations in the diurnal regulation of circulating glucocorticoid levels, and an increase in the mean level. Moreover, regulation of the hypothalamic–pituitary–adrenal axis is altered in AD patients, such that plasma levels of glucocorticoids are increased. Increased levels of glucocorticoids, including those induced by physiologic or psychological stress, can increase the vulnerability of hippocampal neurons to injury and death induced by ischemic and excitotoxic insults, suggesting that glucocorticoids may have a negative impact on the outcome of both acute (e.g., stroke) and chronic (e.g., AD) age-related neurologic disorders. Estrogen (17β-estradiol) may have a beneficial effect on brain aging. Epidemiologic studies suggest a reduced risk of AD in postmenopausal women who take estrogen replacement therapy (Fig. 104-9), and elderly women who take estrogens perform better on cognitive tasks. Animal and cell culture studies have shown

that 17β-estradiol can protect neurons from being damaged and killed by insults relevant to ischemia and AD including glucose deprivation, exposure to Aβ, and expression of AD-linked presenilin mutations (Fig. 104-9).

IMMUNOLOGIC FACTORS IN BRAIN AGING

While the blood–brain barrier limits access of circulating lymphocytes to neurons in the brain, it is becoming increasingly evident that the brain is by no means devoid of immune responses. The brain possesses resident immune effector cells called microglia that may respond to age- and disease-related neurodegenerative processes. Some data suggest that a decline in peripheral immune function during aging may lead to an autoimmune-like phenomenon in the brain wherein microglia are activated. Inflammatory processes are associated with, and contribute to, the neurodegenerative process in AD and other age-related neurodegenerative disorders; these include activation of microglia in the affected brain regions, increased local cytokine production in association with the neuropathologic changes, and activation of components of the complement cascade system. Moreover, epidemiologic and clinical data suggest that antiinflammatory agents may suppress the development of AD. Collectively, the emerging data suggest a role for chronic inflammatory reactions in the pathogenesis of at least some neurodegenerative disorders.

NEUROTROPHIC FACTORS IN THE AGING BRAIN

Neurotrophic Factors Counteract Age- and Disease-Related Neurodegeneration

Cells in the nervous system produce a variety of proteins which serve the function of promoting neuronal survival and growth, and protecting the neurons against injury and death. Examples of such "neurotrophic factors" include nerve growth factor (NGF), basic fibroblast growth factor (bFGF), brain-derived neurotrophic factor (BDNF), and insulin-like growth factor (IGF). Neurotrophic factors are remarkable in that they can protect neurons against a variety of insults relevant to the pathogenesis of age-related neurodegenerative conditions. For example, bFGF can protect hippocampal and cortical neurons against metabolic, oxidative, and excitotoxic insults, and can greatly reduce brain damage in rodent models of stroke. One or more neurotrophic factors have also been shown to protect particular neuronal populations against neurodegenerative disorder-specific insults. Thus, BDNF protects dopaminergic neurons against MPTP toxicity (PD model), while bFGF and sAPP (secretory domain of the β-amyloid precursor protein) protect hippocampal neurons against Aβ toxicity (AD model). There appear to be two general mechanisms whereby neurotrophic factors prevent neuronal degeneration; they increase cellular resistance to oxidative stress and they stabilize cellular calcium homeostasis. These actions

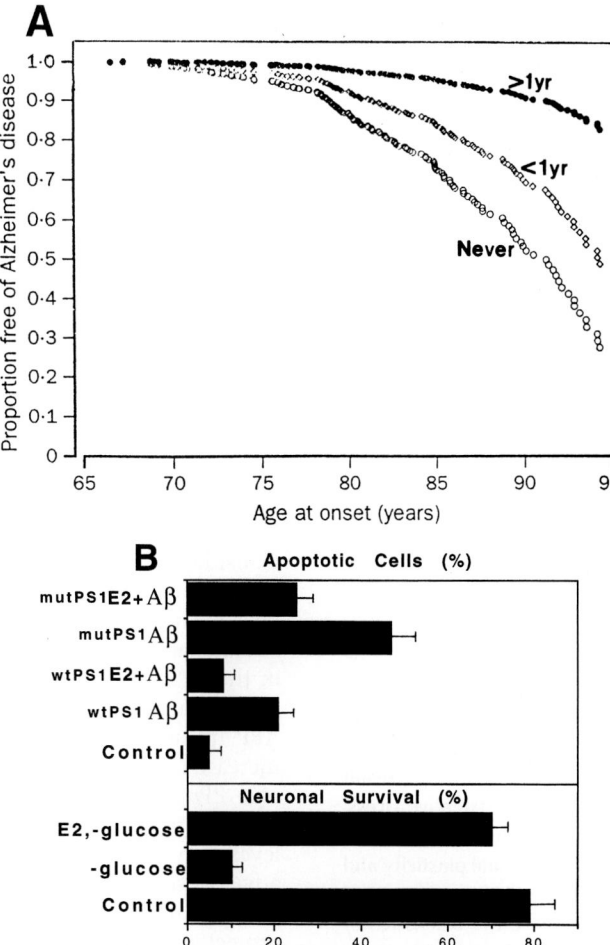

Figure 104-9 Estrogen protects women against Alzheimer's disease, and protects cultured neurons against genetic and environmental factors linked to Alzheimer's disease. *(A)* Plot of proportion of the study group free of Alzheimer's disease as a function of age in postmenopausal women receiving estrogen replacement therapy more than 1 year, less than 1 year, or not at all. Adapted from Tang et al: *Lancet* 348:429, 1996. *(B)* The lower portion of the graph shows data from cultured rat hippocampal neurons that were deprived of glucose (–glucose) for 24 hours in the absence or presence of 17β-estradiol (E2); control cultures were not deprived of glucose. The percentage of neurons surviving was quantified. Note that 17β-estradiol largely prevented neuronal death. The upper portion of the graph shows data from cultured PC12 cells overexpressing either wild-type presenilin-1 (wtPS1) or mutant presenilin-1 (mutPS1). Cultures were exposed to either Aβ alone or in combination with 17β-estradiol (E2); control cultures were not exposed to Aβ. The percentage of cells undergoing apoptotic cell death was quantified. Note that apoptosis was enhanced in cells expressing mutant PS-1, and that 17β-estradiol largely prevented the apoptosis. Adapted from Goodman et al: *J Neurochem* 66:1836, 1996, and Mattson et al: *Neuroreport* 8:3817, 1997.

of neurotrophic factors appear to result from induction of the expression of antioxidant enzymes (e.g., superoxide dismutases and glutathione peroxidase) and calcium-regulating proteins (e.g., the calcium-binding protein calbindin). In addition to preserving existing neurons, neurotrophic factors may stimulate the production of new neurons from so-called stem cells. Such neural stem cells may be able to replace lost or damaged neurons, and are therefore receiving considerable attention for their potential use in the treatment of neurodegenerative disorders.

"Use it or Lose it"

An intriguing feature of neurotrophic factors is that their expression is increased by activity in neuronal circuits.

Experimental studies in cell culture and in vivo show that such activity-dependent production of neurotrophic factors plays a major role in promoting neuronal survival and neurite outgrowth. Rearing of rodents in an "intellectually enriched" environment results in expansion of dendritic arbors and increased numbers of synapses in hippocampus and certain regions of cerebral cortex. Moreover, epidemiologic data suggest that humans with "active" minds have a reduced risk for developing AD as they age. When taken together with data showing that neurotrophic factors can protect brain neurons against insults relevant to usual brain aging and neurodegenerative disorders (oxidative, metabolic, and excitotoxic insults), these findings suggest a "use it or lose it" scenario of brain aging in which brain activity induces expression of neurotrophic factors which, in turn, promote neuronal growth and plasticity (Fig. 104-10).

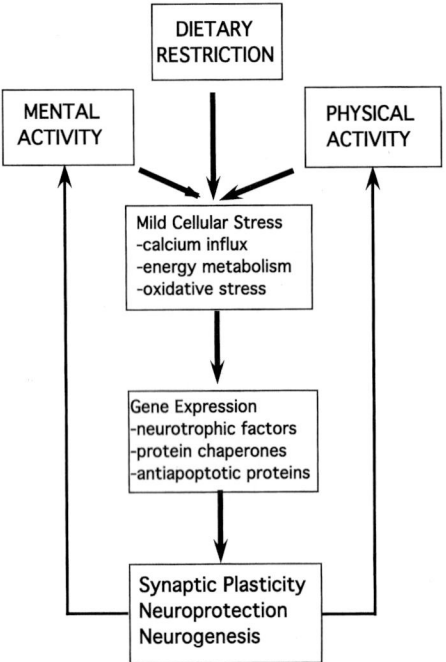

Figure 104-10 Mechanisms whereby dietary restriction, and mental and physical activities, promote successful brain aging. Dietary restriction, and stimulation of activity in neuronal circuits by mental and physical activities, induce mild stress in neurons as the result of reduced energy availability, calcium influx, and oxidative stress. The neurons respond to the stress by upregulating the expression of genes that encode proteins that promote neuronal plasticity and survival including neurotrophic factors, heat shock proteins, and antiapoptotic proteins. These changes increase the resistance of neurons to age-related diseases by promoting synaptic plasticity, cell survival, and neurogenesis.

GENETIC FACTORS IN BRAIN AGING AND NEURODEGENERATIVE DISORDERS

Longevity Genes

Individuals inherit two apolipoprotein E alleles, of which there are three isoforms (E2, E3, and E4). The E2 allele has been linked to increased life span and reduced incidence of AD; this "longevity gene" may act, in part, by reducing atherosclerotic processes in the vasculature. Another possible longevity gene is that encoding an isoform of angiotensin-converting enzyme, although its mechanistic links to aging are unclear. Finally, the multigene major histocompatability system appears to influence life span, and may act by sustaining functions of the immune system.

Disorder-Specific Genes

Considerable progress has been made in identifying genetic factors that play roles in AD. Three different genes have been identified in which mutations cause early-onset autosomal dominant familial AD (Fig. 104-11). Mutations in the APP gene on chromosome 21 are located immediately adjacent to the $A\beta$ sequence. Expression of mutant APP in cultured cells and transgenic mice results in an increase in production of $A\beta$ and a decrease in production of sAPPα. The increase in $A\beta$ may promote plaque formation and associated neurotoxicity. The decrease in sAPPα levels may also play an important role in the neurodegenerative consequences of APP mutations, because sAPPα normally promotes neuronal survival and plasticity and can protect neurons against excitotoxic and oxidative injury. The two other genes causally linked to early onset familial

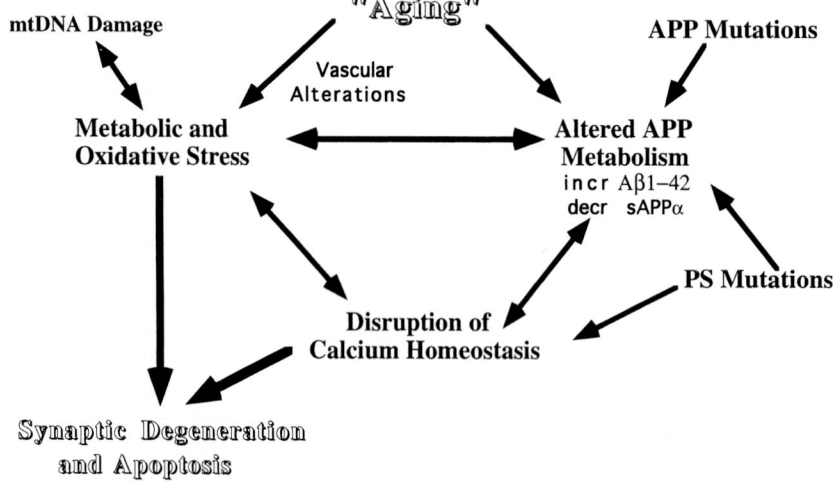

Figure 104-11 Interactions of aging and genetic factors in the pathogenesis of neurodegenerative disorders: Alzheimer's disease as an example. The aging process is associated with increases in cellular oxidative stress and metabolic impairment. Metabolic and oxidative stress disrupt neuronal calcium homeostasis and promote excitotoxic synaptic degeneration and apoptotic cell death. Mutations in the β-amyloid precursor protein (APP) and presenilins (PS) result in altered proteolytic processing of APP, increased production of amyloid β-peptide (Aβ1-42) and decreased sAPPα production. The result of these mutations is impaired calcium homeostasis and increased age-related oxidative stress. Vascular alterations contribute to reduced energy availability to neurons and increased oxidative stress. Adapted from Mattson Mol Cell Biol 1:120, 2000.

AD are called presenilin-1 (PS-1) and presenilin-2 (PS-2). PS-1 is located in chromosome 14 and PS-2 is located in chromosome 1. PS-1 and PS-2 are integral membrane proteins localized in the endoplasmic reticulum of neurons throughout the brain. Studies of cultured cells and transgenic mice expressing PS-1 mutations have shown that the mutations increase $A\beta$ production and sensitize neurons to death induced by metabolic and oxidative insults. The pathogenic action of presenilin mutations may involve perturbed regulation of endoplasmic reticulum calcium.

Several age-related inherited neurodegenerative conditions are caused by trinucleotide repeats in specific genes. The best known such disorder is HD in which polyglutamine repeats in the huntingtin gene promote degeneration of neurons in the caudate/putamen and cerebral cortex. Other examples include spinal and bulbar muscular atrophy, fragile X syndrome, spinocerebellar ataxia type 1, and Machado–Joseph disease. Trinucleotide repeat mutations do not follow strict rules of mendelian inheritance, as they are unstable and change size in successive generations. The mechanism(s) whereby expansions of trinucleotide repeats cause neuronal degeneration have not been established, but recent findings suggest roles for protein aggregation and oxidative stress. ALS is a disorder in which lower motor neurons in the spinal cord, and to a lesser extent neurons in the motor cortex, degenerate resulting in progressive paralysis. A small percentage of cases of ALS are caused by mutations in the gene encoding the antioxidant enzyme Cu/ZnSOD, which appear to alter the properties of the enzyme so that it produces hydroxyl radical and peroxynitrite. Finally, several "predisposition" genes have been identified in which polymorphisms or mutations increase the risk for developing one or more age-related neurodegenerative disorders. For example, inheritance of the E4 allele or mutations in the mitochondrial DNA encoding cytochrome C oxidase increase the risk for AD.

DIETARY FACTORS IN BRAIN AGING AND NEURODEGENERATIVE DISORDERS

It recently became evident that diet can affect one's risk of age-related neurodegenerative disorders. In particular, emerging findings indicate that several dietary risk factors for prominent age-related diseases including cardiovascular disease, cancer, and diabetes are also risk factors for AD, PD, and stroke.

Calorie Intake

The only known means of increasing the life span of rodents and nonhuman primates is by decreasing their calorie intake; both maximum and mean life span can be increased by up to 40 percent. The average life span of humans is certainly decreased by overeating, although it remains to be determined whether maximum life span can be increased. Epidemiologic data suggest that individuals with a low calorie intake are at a reduced risk for AD and PD. Biochemical markers of aging, and deficits in learning and memory and motor function, are retarded in rodents maintained on dietary restriction. Recent studies show that neurons in the brains of rats and mice maintained on dietary restriction are more resistant to dysfunction and death in experimental models of AD, PD, HD, and stroke. The mechanism whereby caloric restriction increases the resistance of neurons to the adverse effects of aging is by stimulating the expression of genes that promote neuronal plasticity and survival (see Fig. 104-10). These genes include those that encode neurotrophic factors such as BDNF and NGF, and protein chaperones such as heat shock protein-70 and glucose-regulated protein-78. Thus, the benefits of dietary restriction may result from a hormesis mechanism akin to the beneficial effects of physical exercise on skeletal muscle and blood vessels.

Folic Acid (Homocysteine)

It was recognized long ago that folic acid deficiency can cause abnormalities in the developing nervous system. Subsequently, it was shown that people with low levels of folic acid tend to have elevated levels of homocysteine and that this condition is associated with increased risk of cardiovascular disease and stroke. Homocysteine is produced during metabolism of methionine, and folic acid plays an important role in removing homocysteine via remethylation. Epidemiologic findings suggest that people with elevated homocysteine levels may be at increased risk of AD and PD. Animal studies support a cause–effect relationship between elevated homocysteine levels and neuronal vulnerability to neurodegenerative disorders. For example, hippocampal neurons of APP mutant mice (AD model), and substantia nigra dopaminergic neurons in mice given MPTP (PD model), exhibit increased vulnerability to degeneration when maintained on a folic acid-deficient diet. By increasing homocysteine levels, folic acid deficiency may promote accumulation of DNA damage by inhibiting DNA repair. In neurons, the increased DNA damage can trigger apoptosis, particularly under conditions of increased oxidative or metabolic stress, as occur during aging.

Antioxidants

Neurons are clearly subjected to increased levels of oxidative stress during normal aging, and more so in neurodegenerative disorders. It is therefore reasonable to consider the possibility that dietary antioxidants might promote successful brain aging. Epidemiologic findings support a protective effect of antioxidants in fruits and vegetables against stroke, and possibly AD. Studies of animal models of AD, PD, HD, stroke, and ALS have documented beneficial effects of some antioxidants. Positive effects have been reported for several commonly used dietary supplements, including vitamin E, creatine, and ginkgo biloba. However, the effects of such antioxidants are relatively subtle compared to the quite striking neuroprotective effects of dietary restriction.

CONCLUSION

Structural changes occur in the brain during aging and appear to be compensatory responses to adverse changes in cellular metabolism that occur during the aging process. There are several biochemical processes that may predispose neurons to dysfunction and death in aging and neurodegenerative disorders. At the cellular and molecular levels these changes include, increased levels of oxidative stress, impaired mitochondrial function, and energy metabolism, and dysregulation of neuronal calcium homeostasis. Disease-specific initiators of neuronal degeneration are being identified and include increased production of Aβ and reduced production of sAPPα in AD; trinucleotide repeat expansions in HD and related disorders; and dopamine- and Fe^{2+}-mediated free radical production in PD. As in many other organ systems, untoward changes in blood vessels may contribute greatly to age-related declines in cell function and tissue damage in the brain. A role for chronic inflammatory processes involving microglial activation is implicated in the pathogenesis of some neurodegenerative disorders. Neurodegenerative cascades may be countered by neurotrophic signaling pathways that promote neuronal survival and adaptation; these pathways are stimulated by brain activity, such that individuals with a high level of "intellectual" activity have a reduced risk for AD. Genetic causal and risk factors for neurodegenerative disorders are being identified and characterized, leading to new insights into disease pathogenesis. Successful brain aging may be promoted through dietary manipulations with dietary restriction and supplementation with folic acid and antioxidants being the most notable.

REFERENCES

Bertoni-Freddari C et al: Synaptic structural dynamics and aging. *Gerontology* 42:170, 1996.

Blanc EM et al: Amyloid β-peptide disrupts barrier and transport functions and induces apoptosis in vascular endothelial cells. *J Neurochem* 68:1870, 1997.

Blass JP: Metabolic alterations common to neural and non-neural cells in Alzheimer's disease. *Hippocampus* 3:45, 1993.

Bowling AC, Beal MF: Bioenergetic and oxidative stress in neurodegenerative diseases. *Life Sci* 56:1151, 1995.

de la Torre JC: Cerebromicrovascular pathology in Alzheimer's disease compared to normal aging. *Gerontology* 43:26, 1997.

Disterhoft JF et al. (eds): Calcium hypothesis of aging and dementia. *Ann N Y Acad Sci* 747:1, 1994.

Dustman RE et al: Life span changes in electrophysiological measures of inhibition. *Brain Cogn* 30:109–126, 1996.

Evans DA et al: Somatic mutations in the brain: Relationship to aging? *Mutat Res* 338:173, 1995.

Finch CE, Cohen DM: Aging, metabolism, and Alzheimer disease: Review and hypotheses. *Exp Neurol* 143:82, 1997.

Jucker M, Ingram DK: Murine models of brain aging and age-related neurodegenerative diseases. *Behav Brain Res* 85:1, 1997.

Kalaria RN et al: Molecular aspects of inflammatory and immune responses in Alzheimer's disease. *Neurobiol Aging* 17:687, 1996.

Landfield PW: The role of glucocorticoids in brain aging and Alzheimer's disease: An integrative physiological hypothesis. *Exp Gerontol* 29:3, 1994.

Markesbery WR: Oxidative stress hypothesis in Alzheimer's disease. *Free Radic Biol Med* 23:134, 1997.

Mattson MP: Apoptosis in neurodegenerative disorders. *Nat Rev Mol Cell Biol* 1:120, 2000.

Mattson MP: Cellular actions of β-amyloid precursor protein, and its soluble and fibrillogenic peptide derivatives. *Physiol Rev* 77:1081, 1997.

Mattson MP et al: Suppression of brain aging and neurodegenerative disorders by dietary restriction and environmental enrichment: molecular mechanisms. *Mech Aging Dev* 122:757-, 2001.

Mattson MP, Geddes JW (eds): The aging brain. *Adv Cell Aging Gerontol* 2:1, 1997.

Morrison JH, Hoff PR: Life and death of neurons in the aging brain. *Science* 278:412, 1997.

McEwen BS et al: Oestrogens and the structural and functional plasticity of neurons: Implications for memory, ageing and neurodegenerative processes. *Ciba Found Symp* 191:52, 1995.

Rao MS, Mattson MP: Stem cells and aging: Expanding the possibilities. *Mech Aging Dev* 122:713, 2001.

Riedel WJ, Jolles J: Cognition enhancers in age-related cognitive decline. *Drugs Aging* 8:245, 1996.

Sohal RS, Weindruch R: Oxidative stress, caloric restriction, and aging. *Science* 273:59, 1996.

Wisniewski T, Frangione B: Molecular biology of brain aging and neurodegenerative disorders. *Acta Neurobiol Exp (Warsz)* 56:267, 1996.

Zielasek J, Hartung HP: Molecular mechanisms of microglial activation. *Adv Neuroimmunol* 6:191, 1996.

Aging and Cognition: What is Normal?

SUZANNE CRAFT • BRENNA CHOLERTON • MARK REGER

"Age does not depend upon years, but upon temperament and health. Some men are born old, and some never grow so."

Tyron Edwards

"A man is as old as his arteries."

Thomas Sydenham

The dogma that aging brings inevitable cognitive decline is being challenged by studies of the rapidly expanding oldest segment of our society, adults older than 60 years of age. Although some aspects of cognition are affected by aging, many changes in cognition previously considered the unavoidable consequence of brain senescence may instead result from incremental insults on brain function associated with aging-related medical conditions. The detection of such changes, which may stabilize or even reverse with appropriate intervention, and their differentiation from the cognitive changes associated with neurodegenerative disease or other neurologic disorders is a critical task. This chapter describes changes in various cognitive abilities that occur with normal aging and with common age-related medical and neurologic conditions.

THE EFFECTS OF NORMAL AGING ON COGNITIVE FUNCTION

General Intellectual Functioning

Intelligence is generally measured by summing the scores on a variety of verbal and performance subtests. Studies of aging consistently show that subtests measuring verbal abilities remain stable with normal aging. In contrast, subtests that require nonverbal creative thinking and new problem-solving strategies show a slow decline with age. Horn and Cattell suggest that with aging, crystallized abilities (information and skills gained from experience) remain relatively intact, while fluid intelligence, which involves flexible reasoning and problem solving approaches, declines. Numerous studies document this general pattern

in both cross-sectional and longitudinal research designs. Below, we review the literature on the effects of normal aging on specific cognitive functions (Table 105-1).

Attention

Attention involves the ability to focus on one or more pieces of information (auditory or visual) long enough to register and make meaningful use of the data. Attention requires both simple and complex immediate processing and provides a foundation for working memory and other cognitive functions. Sustained attention, or vigilance, entails attending to one type of information over a period of time. After controlling for reaction time and sensory changes, sustained attention and strategies for maintaining vigilance do not appear to change significantly with age. Divided attention, or the ability to concentrate on more than one piece of information at a time, may worsen with age although research in this area has produced mixed results. Increased distractibility (difficulty blocking out irrelevant or salient stimuli), decreased use of effective strategies, and reduced processing speed may be responsible for some of the noted declines in divided attention. Pronounced impairment of attention is not typical of normal aging, however, and a complete evaluation of medical and psychosocial issues is warranted in individuals who demonstrate such changes. Attention may be negatively impacted by perceptual or sensory changes, illness, chronic pain, certain medications, and psychological disturbance (in particular, depression and anxiety), all of which are common in an older population. As the ability to effectively attend is a requisite for nearly all other cognitive functions, it is important to identify the cause of attentional impairment whenever possible and to implement any changes in medications or treatment that may help to resolve these problems.

Executive Functions

Executive functions include the ability to control and direct behavior, make meaningful inferences and appropriate

Table 105-1 Cognitive Effects of Normal Aging

	Preserved Cognitive Functions	Cognitive Functions Showing Decline
General intellectual functioning	Crystallized, verbal intelligence	Fluid, nonverbal intelligence, speed of information processing
Attention	Sustained attention, primary attention span	Divided attention (possibly)
Executive function	"Real world" executive tasks	Novel executive tasks
Memory	Remote memory, procedural memory, semantic recall	Learning and recall of new information
Language	Comprehension, vocabulary, syntactic abilities	Spontaneous word finding, verbal fluency
Visuospatial skills	Construction, simple copy	Mental rotation, complex copy, mental assembly
Psychomotor functions		Reaction time

judgments, plan and carry out tasks, manipulate multiple pieces of information at one time (working memory), complete complex motor sequences, and solve abstract and complex problems. Neuropsychological test performance on executive tasks declines slightly with age, and several current theories posit that deficits in working memory and executive function underlie many age-related changes in cognition. Neurocognitive tasks that require response inhibition, such as the Wisconsin Card Sort Test, Stroop Color-Word Test, and Brown–Peterson Distractor Test may be affected. However, many researchers suggest that a reduction in cognitive processing speed rather than executive function per se may be partly responsible for decreased performance on executive tasks. It should be noted that changes in the executive system that occur with normal aging are much less severe than the deficits associated with dysexecutive syndromes, including those caused by stroke, heavy and prolonged alcohol use, head injury, and some neurodegenerative diseases. In fact, successful aging appears to produce little impact on "real world" executive functions requiring planning and executing multiple tasks. Thus, it is important to assess an individual's actual functional abilities in addition to performance on neuropsychological tests of executive function.

Memory

Memory changes are perhaps the most common cognitive complaints reported by older adults. Patients often wonder if their subjective concerns reflect normal age-related changes, or some pathologic condition. For patients with a family history of Alzheimer's disease or other dementia, even minor memory failings can cause significant anxiety. One difficulty in answering such questions lies in the complex nature of the memory process. Different forms of memory are invoked when learning new information (declarative memory), recalling prior life events (remote memory), recalling general knowledge not tied to a specific

event (semantic memory), and remembering procedures for performing tasks such as riding a bicycle (procedural memory). Some conditions result in modality-specific deficits, differentially affecting verbal or visual memory. A number of models describe the different stages or processes involved in forming and recalling memories. The modal model includes sensory, short-term (working), and long-term memory. A patient must first sense and attend to a given stimulus. A large amount of information is briefly held in sensory memory. Information is then rehearsed or manipulated in short-term or working memory. Although many factors are involved in determining what information is transferred to long-term storage, sufficient rehearsal is a common requirement for successful transfer. From this brief review of the memory process, it is clear that when a patient complains of memory changes, additional information is required to make sense of the problem.

Although it is true that some older adults continue to demonstrate memory performances comparable to young adults, on average, even healthy aging patients do show changes in some aspects of memory. For example, when a large group of healthy, nondemented elderly subjects were followed over a 7-year period, a general memory factor showed significant decline. Other studies have attempted to describe which aspects of memory change with healthy aging. In general, elderly subjects without significant illness demonstrate increased difficulty learning new information with aging. When older adults are given repeated chances to practice learning new information, they continue to remember significant portions as they age, but they demonstrate a slower learning curve and a lower total amount learned.

Although healthy older adults may retain slightly less information after a delay than do younger adults, this effect is less pronounced than the slowed learning rate. For delayed memory tests, patients are generally asked to recall information 15 to 60 minutes after the initial exposure. Although patients recall less at the delay with age, they generally retain a stable proportion of the information that they initially learned. On a commonly used story recall measure, Malec et al. found that among their oldest subjects (age 85 years and older), 90 percent of them retained at least 50 percent what they initially learned about the story. This is especially impressive because their sample included patients with minor medical problems. Although the strength of this effect may be test-specific, in general longitudinal studies of aging show small, but statistically significant, declines in delayed memory with age, particularly on tests of visual memory. Some older adults also appear less likely to use cognitive strategies to aid memory than younger subjects. This may be a result of generational differences in learning style. However, it may be significant because the use of memory strategies (i.e., grouping vegetables and clothing items for easier recall) reduces the age effect observed on free recall tests.

A number of memory processes do not appear to change with successful aging. Remote memory, that is recall of events that occurred in the distant past, remains relatively intact, as does sensory memory. In addition, while elderly patients often have medical problems that limit physical movement, procedural memory appears to be unaffected by healthy aging. Lastly, semantic memory, such as vocabulary and general information about the world, remains largely unchanged until very old age.

Longitudinal studies consistently show that as groups age, the variability in cognitive performance increases. Overall, studies of healthy aging suggest that there are some statistically significant declines in memory in late life. However, the memory functions of patients who age successfully are typically adequate for the demands of independent living.

Language

Language abilities incorporate multiple levels of processing, and general language functions tend to remain relatively stable with increasing age. Some linguistic abilities, however, particularly those involving language output, show reliable decline beginning in the later years. As with other cognitive functions, there are multiple potential intervening factors, including trauma, illness, and sensory disruption, that may lead to more severe changes in the language functions.

Language Comprehension

Language comprehension involves discerning the simple and complex rules of language and incorporating both visual and auditory information into a meaningful concept, and is generally associated with few age-related impairments. The ability to recognize basic word structure and word representation is typically measured using "lexical-decision" tasks (in which letters are rapidly presented and the person is asked to identify whether or not it is a word), and simple word reading tasks. While some studies suggest an inverse relationship between performance on these tasks and age, it is generally believed that such changes are the result of decreased reaction time and processing speed rather than the ability to comprehend word structure

and meaning. In addition, there is some indication that the level of lexical processing changes slightly with age, in that older adults tend to rely more on word recognition than do younger adults, while ignoring other factors such as word length. Phonologic understanding of language does not appear to change significantly with age, although hearing loss may appear to reduce auditory comprehension. Overall, it is generally accepted that language comprehension remains relatively intact throughout the life span.

Language Production

Basic syntactic abilities do not appear to change significantly with advancing age, although minor repetitions, longer pauses, and an increased use of pronouns and other vague words while speaking have been noted. Additionally, a recent longitudinal study suggests a decline in spoken grammatical complexity during the eighth decade of life. The authors note, however, that Kemper et al. demonstrated a high individual variability throughout the life span in terms of syntactic aptitude.

Semantic abilities involve aptitude with naming and retrieving long-stored information. There is a steady increase in vocabulary knowledge throughout middle adulthood, and such knowledge typically remains stable in the later years. A frequent complaint from older adults, however, involves the "tip-of-the-tongue" phenomenon, in which there is a notable struggle with spontaneous word finding. In contrast to the dysnomia that often accompanies dementia, however, such changes appear to result primarily from difficulties accessing rather than storing information, and thus there is usually a marked improvement when cues are given. Verbal fluency, the rate at which a person can spontaneously produce words belonging to a single phonemic or semantic category, also appears to change somewhat with age. Multiple research findings support a decrease in semantic fluency ("name all the animals you can"), while phonemic fluency ("tell me as many words as you can that begin with the letter F") generally remains stable. In terms of strategy, Troyer et al. suggest that younger adults tend to produce more words and to change categories more frequently than do older adults on semantic fluency tasks, while older subjects generate the same amount of words but more "clusters" on tasks of phonemic fluency. Thus, older subjects rely more on structural word knowledge than on word meaning.

Visuospatial Skills

Visuospatial skills are commonly tested by constructional tasks in which patients are asked to draw figures or assemble objects. In general, as patients age, they become slower at completing visuospatial tasks. However, as noted, one of the more consistent findings in the field is that normal aging is associated with general slowing of psychomotor and cognitive speed. Therefore, performance on tests of visuospatial functioning is often confounded by slowing. Some studies have attempted to separate the effects of the two domains. For instance, when the commonly used Wechsler Block Design test is scored without regard to time, no

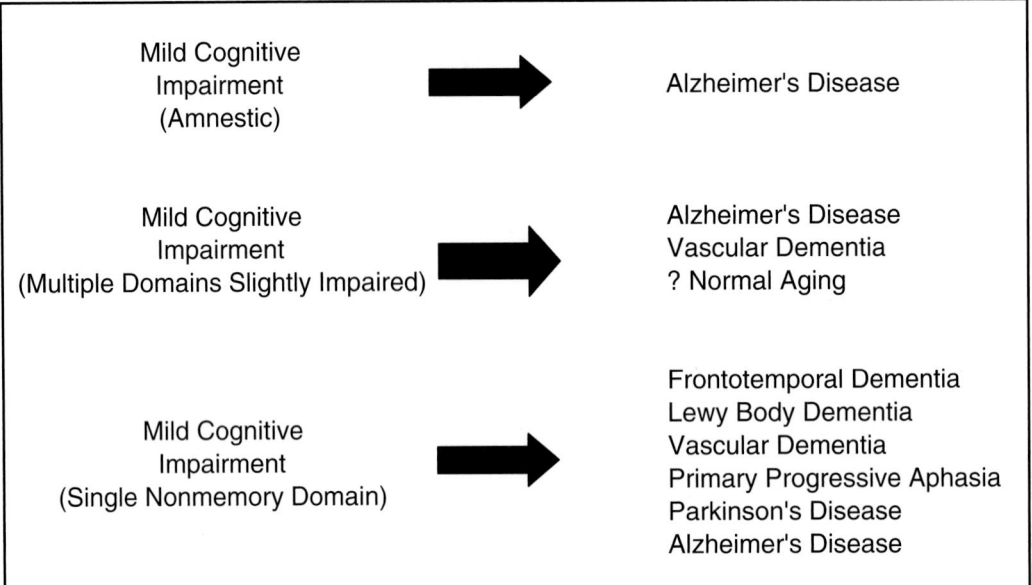

Figure 105-1   Heterogeneity of the term *mild cognitive impairment* Figure reproduced by permission: Petersen, et al., *Archives of Neurology* 2001 58;1987. Copyrighted 2001 American Medical Association.

decline with aging is often observed. Similarly, an 11-year follow-up of elderly subjects by Laursen analyzed both speed and quality of performance (errors) on a parallelogram test. As expected, speed declined with age, but the quality of the performance actually improved significantly. This body of literature suggests that declining speed contributes to some of the findings that report visuospatial processing deficits in normal aging.

Speed does not appear to account for all of the visuospatial changes observed in healthy aging, however. Mental rotations of objects or spatial coordinates, accurate copy of complex geometric designs, and mental assembly of objects typically worsen with age even when unlimited time is allowed to perform such tasks. Furthermore, when speed is included in scoring, some studies have reported disproportionate slowing on visuospatial tasks compared to verbal tasks. Overall, some studies may exaggerate the visuospatial decline observed in normal aging because of the role speed plays in many tasks used to assess visuospatial function. However, abstract spatial abilities may decline with age, even when speed is controlled.

Psychomotor Functions

A consistent finding among aging populations is significantly increased reaction time related to both a general reduction in the speed of cognitive processing and to changes in peripheral motor skills. Age-related declines in brain dopamine activity and periventricular white matter changes may be associated with reduced cognitive speed and basic motor functions. As a result, performance on tests requiring speed and quick reaction to stimuli are likely to decline. As previously noted, increased psychomotor speed and reaction time are believed to underlie many of the age-related changes noted on neurocognitive testing, particularly tasks involving perceptual speed, attention, and working memory. In addition, changes in psychomotor

functions can be associated with changes in real world tasks, such as driving. As a result, it is important to monitor the manner in which physical changes are impacting an individual's level of safety in performing daily activities. Reaction time training can be effective in healthy older populations, and safe driving courses have been found to decrease overall accident rates.

COGNITIVE EFFECTS OF COMMON AGE-RELATED MEDICAL CONDITIONS

The following section reviews cognitive symptoms associated with common disease affecting older adults. Table 105-2 summarizes these symptoms.

Cardiovascular Disease

In addition to increasing the risk for developing stroke and/ or vascular dementia, cardiovascular disease potentially jeopardizes cognitive function via multiple mechanisms.

Coronary Artery Bypass Graft Surgery

Cognitive impairment subsequent to coronary artery bypass graft (CABG) surgery has been reported in up to 80 percent of patients, and older age significantly increases the risk for development of such complications. A wide range of cognitive deficits, including problems with attention and concentration, processing speed, memory, and visuospatial function, have been noted in patients immediately following surgery. Initial reports suggested that postoperative cognitive function stabilizes or even improves after a period of approximately 12 months in those patients who demonstrate initial decline. However, recent longitudinal data provide evidence that such patients are at high risk for continued cognitive deterioration 5 years postsurgery. For example, one study by Newman et al. found that 42 percent of patients showed a significant decline in one or more areas of cognitive function 5 years postsurgery, including verbal and visual memory, attention and concentration, and general cognition. Notably, post-CABG neurocognitive status is related to overall quality of life, and current recommendations underscore the importance of closely monitoring cognitive status in the years following cardiac surgery.

Hypertension

Essential hypertension is associated with cognitive impairment independent of secondary disease or organ damage, particularly in older patients. Potential cognitive effects of primary hypertension include reductions in mental status, slowed reaction time, reduced attention and vigilance, weakened executive function, poor verbal fluency, and impaired visual organization and construction. Memory functions, including spatial recall, verbal recall, and word recognition, may also be affected in some hypertensive patients. In addition, secondary effects of hypertension may lead to an increased risk for cognitive decline in older age. For example, uncontrolled hypertension potentiates the development of subcortical white matter lesions. While there is currently debate concerning the extent to which hypertension and related subcortical effects overtly impact cognition, recent findings suggest that hypertension is a significant risk factor for dementia and that treating hypertension reduces this risk.

Nutritional Deficiency

Older adults are at considerable risk for nutritional deficiencies as a consequence of poor diet and malabsorption syndromes. Growing evidence suggests that deficiencies of micronutrients such as the B vitamins folate, B_{12}, and B_6 may be associated with impairments of attention, memory, and abstract thinking. Some studies suggest that supplementation may improve cognitive performance in deficient individuals.

The amino acid homocysteine is an independent risk factor for cerebrovascular and cardiovascular disease. In patients with both Alzheimer's disease (AD) and vascular dementia (VaD), elevated plasma homocysteine levels have been reported, and recent studies suggest that homocysteine levels are related to cognitive function in normal aging. Reduced performance on tests of mental status, nonverbal pattern abstraction, construction, and processing speed are reported in patients with high plasma homocysteine. Given that plasma homocysteine and folate levels are inversely related, it is conceivable that such cognitive deficits are related to reduced folate rather than to increased homocysteine per se. Recent data suggest, however, that homocysteine increases the risk for cognitive decline independent of both folate levels and other vascular risk factors.

Type 2 Diabetes Mellitus

Much attention has been given to the rampant epidemic of type 2 diabetes mellitus in older adults, a trend thought to be largely attributable to obesity and physical inactivity.

Current prevalence estimates suggest that 20 percent of adults older than 65 years of age are afflicted with type 2 diabetes mellitus. The negative impact of type 2 diabetes mellitus on multiple medical systems is well known. The clear impact of type 2 diabetes mellitus on cognitive function in older adults is less-widely known. These patients show pronounced impairment in attention and verbal memory when compared to healthy age-matched adults. Complex attentional impairment is most common, involving the inability to handle multiple streams of information or attend to information in the face of competing stimuli. Verbal memory deficits typically affect the ability to encode new verbal information. The magnitude of such impairment may vary from subtle subjective complaints to pronounced impairment that interferes with daily activities and may interfere with the patient's ability to adhere to complex treatment regimens. The mechanisms causing attentional and memory impairments are likely multifactorial and include vascular factors, in addition to the potential negative effects of hyperglycemia and glucose toxicity thought to cause oxidative injury. Recent work also suggest that insulin resistance, independent of hyperglycemia, may have negative consequences on brain systems mediating memory and attention. This intriguing possibility has implications for therapeutic approaches to treating type 2 diabetes mellitus, suggesting that strategies focused on improving insulin sensitivity may be preferable to those focused on augmenting insulin levels. Successful treatment of type 2 diabetes mellitus has been shown to improve cognitive function. The importance of treating and preferably preventing type 2 diabetes mellitus has been underscored by recent findings that it is a risk factor for various forms of neurodegenerative disease, including Alzheimer's disease, vascular dementia, and Parkinson's disease.

Oxygen Deprivation

Chronic Obstructive Pulmonary Disease

Emphysema and chronic bronchitis obstruct airflow, resulting in hypoxemia and hypercapnia. Cognitive dysfunction is commonly observed in chronic obstructive pulmonary disease (COPD), although the specific skills affected appear to be broad and diffuse. Deficits in verbal and visual memory, attention, abstraction, psychomotor speed, information processing speed, and general intelligence have all been reported. These changes in cognition appear to be caused by hypoxemia. The decrease in arterial oxygen partial pressure correlates with neuropsychological impairments, and most studies indicate that oxygen therapy results in modest improvements in cognition. Depression is also common in COPD and must be considered as another cognitive risk factor.

Obstructive Sleep Apnea

The prevalence of obstructive sleep apnea increases in geriatric populations. Many patients remain unaware of the disorder and report associated symptoms only when specifically queried. Cognitive changes in obstructive sleep apnea

Table 105–2 Possible Cognitive Effects of Common Age-Related Medical Conditions

	Symptom Course	Increased risk for Developing Dementia?	Memory	Attention	Executive Functions	Language	Visuospatial Function	Psychomotor Function	Behavior
Cardiac surgery	Symptom onset immediate after surgery, improvement noted in first year, then further decline possible in some patients	AD, VaD	Verbal and visual memory deficits possible several years after surgery	Reduced attention	Variable	No significant changes noted	May lead to impaired visual organization and construction	Reduced reaction time, general slowing	Depression common after surgery
Hypertension	May improve with antihypertensive treatment	AD, VaD	Verbal and visual recall and recognition deficits in some patients	Reduced attention and vigilance	Impairment in working memory and other executive function	Reduced verbal fluency	May lead to impaired visual organization and construction; more likely with comorbid diabetes	Reduced reaction time, general slowing	Variable
Diabetes	May improve with insulin or insulin-sensitizing agents	AD, VaD, PD	Verbal memory impairment related to deficits in encoding new information	Reduced complex attention, simple attention variable	Impairments in abstract reasoning and concept formation	No significant changes noted	Variable, more likely with comorbid hypertension	No significant changes noted	Variable
COPD	May improve with oxygen therapy	Unkown	Verbal and visual memory deficits	Reduced attention	Impairment in abstract thinking	No significant changes noted	No significant changes noted	Reduced reaction time, general slowing	Depression common
Sleep Apnea	May improve with CPAP treatment	Unkown	Verbal and visual memory deficits	Reduced attention	Impairment in general executive function; esp. working memory	No significant changes noted	No significant changes noted	Reduced reaction time, general slowing	Depression and irritability related to sleep disruption
Nutritional deficiency	May improve with supplementation, although some effects of low vitamin B₁₂ may persist	Wernicke-Korsakoff syndrome	Recall deficits	Reduced attention	Impairment in abstract thinking	No significant changes noted	Nonverbal pattern abstraction, construction impaired in high homocysterine	Reduced processing speed in patients with high homocysterine	Variable
Hypothyroidism	May improve with thyroid treatment, although some patients do not return to baseline	AD	Recall deficits, intact recognition	Variable	Variable	No significant changes noted	Reduced visuospatial function	Reduced reaction time, general slowing	Depression

AD, Alzheimer's disease; COPD, chronic obstructive pulmonary disease; PD, parkinsonian dementia; VaD, vascular dementia can be diverse, but generally include attention, concentration, executive functioning, verbal and visual learning, and working memory. Tests of global functioning have also revealed differences compared to healthy elderly patients without obstructive sleep apnea. There is debate regarding whether the cognitive deficits are caused by hypoxia, hypersomnolence, or both. However, severity of hypoxemia appears to relate to cognitive functioning, and continuous positive airway pressure treatment improves cognitive functioning in many patients.

Thyroid Dysfunction

There are a number of thyroid disorders that result in hypo- or hyperthyroidism. Hypothyroidism, even at subclinical levels, appears to be associated with cognitive changes. Deficits may be observed in visuospatial skills, psychomotor speed, and memory. There is some evidence that the memory deficits are related to retrieval rather than to immediate recall or learning; thus, disproportionately better performance may be observed on tests of cued or recognition memory than on free recall tests. Thyroid replacement therapy frequently improves cognitive functioning, although skills may not return to baseline levels in some patients. Hyperthyroid episodes may result in cognitive changes that last for many years. Symptoms may include attention and executive functioning deficits, and memory impairment. Hyperthyroid dementia is less common than in hypothyroidism, and is also generally less severe. Thyroid hormone abnormalities occur in a large proportion of patients with dementia. Therefore, levels should be routinely monitored as a treatable contributor to cognitive decline.

Depression

Depression is an increasingly common problem in older adults. Multiple situational risk factors for depression in older age include the loss of social support, death of family members and close friends, changing social roles, and physical limitations. Depressive symptoms, including lack of initiation, poor attention and concentration, and mild memory impairment can mimic early signs of dementia and may potentially lead to misdiagnosis and/or lack of appropriate medical intervention. As depression is a potentially reversible cause of cognitive impairment, the differential diagnosis between depression and dementia is vital when evaluating elderly patients. Factors that are useful in discriminating between depression and dementia include the clinical course of symptoms, relationship to a specific crisis or stressful event, history of previous psychiatric problems, quality of effort, and level of impaired processing on cognitive evaluation (Table 105-3).

Recent findings suggest that late-onset depression is an independent risk factor for the development of neurodegenerative diseases, such as AD and vascular dementia, and some hypothesize that depression may actually represent a preclinical phase of progressive dementia. In patients with early cognitive loss, depressive symptoms may represent realistic self-evaluation of such decline and/or

may coincide with actual changes in neuroendocrinologic status. In the absence of predisposing situational factors, late-onset affective disorders are quite rare. For such cases, cognitive ability and independent functional status must be carefully evaluated, and an in-depth qualitative analysis of depressive symptoms may be useful. Major depressive disorder is associated with a range of affective, cognitive, and vegetative symptoms, while depressive symptoms in early dementia are more likely to include cognitive and motivational symptoms (e.g., poor concentration, lack of initiation) in the relative absence of central affective disturbance. Continued monitoring of the cognitive status of depressed elderly patients is essential in order to rule out progressive cognitive decline.

Medications

A number of medications have the potential to cause both subtle cognitive changes and alterations in overall mental status, particularly in the elderly population. Medications known to adversely affect cognitive status include opiates and opioid-like analgesics, benzodiazepines, anticonvulsants, antipsychotic and antidepressant medications, antiparkinsonian agents, central nervous system stimulants, antihistamines and decongestants, and certain cardiovascular medications. A variety of other medications, particularly those that readily cross the blood–brain barrier, may impact cognitive function in certain individuals. In addition, drug interactions in older adults can lead to more serious physiologic and cognitive consequences than those observed in younger adults, and adverse medication interactions are more likely to occur in an older population. As a result, changes in cognitive status must be carefully evaluated in light of a patient's current medication profile.

Certain medications may, in fact, enhance cognitive function in older adults and aid in the prevention of cognitive decline. The cholinesterase inhibitors donepezil, rivastigmine, galantamine, and tacrine stabilize and even improve general cognitive function in some patients with Alzheimer's disease. Medications currently being evaluated for potential reduction of risk for cognitive decline in both healthy aging and dementia include statins, nonsteroidal antiinflammatory drugs (NSAIDs), antioxidant vitamin supplements, and estrogen replacement therapy.

Delirium

Older adults are at a significantly increased risk for developing delirium, particularly following surgery or in response to medication changes or interactions. Delirium is a reversible condition that can be distinguished from most neurodegenerative diseases by a rapid onset of symptoms that include significant disorientation and disturbance in consciousness, reduced awareness of the environment, and attention deficits. While recent memory is generally impaired, altered consciousness is the primary indicator of delirium. Hallucinations, delusional thinking, and other disturbed thought processes may also be present. Delirium usually resolves quickly, but may persist for several weeks. It should also be noted that postoperative delirium may

Table 105-3 Depression versus Alzheimer's Disease

	Depression	Alzheimer's Disease
Symptom history		
Onset	Distinct, often related to a specific traumatic event or loss	Insidious onset
Progression	Rapid	Slow
Patient's description of symptoms	Detailed	Few details
Psychiatric symptoms/history		
Depressive symptoms	Affective, vegetative, cognitive	Cognitive, some vegetative
Psychiatric history	History of one or more depressive episodes usual	May or may not have a history of depression
Cognition		
Effort on testing	Often poor	Usually effortful
Memory		
Recent	Recall improves with cuing/recognition	Impaired, recall does not improve with cuing/recognition
Remote	May be impaired, may have memory "gaps"	Not impaired until late in disease
Procedural	May be impaired	Not impaired
Attention/concentration	Impaired	Impaired
Language	Assisted by semantic strategies	Unable to use semantic strategies

signify the presence of a beginning dementia. A primary concern is to identify and treat the underlying cause while providing a supportive and nonthreatening environment for the patient.

NEURODEGENERATIVE DISEASE

The following section reviews the cognitive and behavioral profiles associated with common neurodegenerative disorders (Table 105-4). Early identification of such disorders, many of which are diagnosed solely on these parameters, has become increasingly important because of potential therapies that may delay disease progression.

Alzheimer's Disease

Alzheimer's disease (AD), the most prevalent of the primary neurodegenerative disorders, causes profound progressive cognitive and functional impairments. While confirmatory diagnostic procedures require histopathologic evaluation at autopsy, probable AD may be diagnosed on the basis of a thorough clinical assessment. The most widely accepted diagnostic standards for probable AD are the National Institute of Neurological and Communicative Disorders and Stroke (NINCDS) and the Alzheimer's Disease and Related Disorders Association (ADRDA) criteria, and include the following: (1) dementia as noted on clinical examination and established by neuropsychological testing; (2) significant impairment in two or more areas of cognition; (3) progressive memory decline; and (4) absence of other medical or psychiatric conditions, including delirium, as the cause for memory impairment. Current debate surrounds the value of an almost purely exclusionary diagnosis, and as a result potential cerebrospinal fluid markers (elevated β-amyloid or tau proteins), structural and functional changes on brain scan, and genetic factors are under close scrutiny for their potential diagnostic utility. In the absence of such tools, however, the current conventional diagnostic criteria are considered to be reasonably accurate, particularly when the evaluation is comprehensive and includes a complete medical and psychosocial history, medical evaluation, and neurocognitive testing.

Patient History

A complete medical and psychosocial history is a vital component of any dementia assessment. Such a history should be obtained both from the patient and a reliable informant, preferably someone who has regular contact with the patient and who has an adequate opportunity to observe their daily functional abilities. Typically, a patient in the earliest stages of AD will not exhibit deficits in basic self-care. However, more complex daily tasks, including driving, finances, shopping, and other chores and activities, are likely to be affected. A gradually progressive course and insidious onset of cognitive symptoms is a hallmark of AD, thus a careful history regarding the nature and timing of symptom onset and progression must be obtained. An inventory of all current medical concerns, past major medical problems, and medications must be evaluated in order to rule out conditions that may be either causing cognitive problems or influencing their expression.

Table 105-4 Early cognitive symptoms associated with different dementia types

| | Symptom Onset | Progession, rate | Memory | | | | Attention | Executive Functions | Language | Visuospatial Function | Psychomotor Function | Behavior |
			Recent	Recognition intact?	Remote intact?	Procedural intact?						
Alzheimer's disease (AD)	Insidious	Steady, gradual	Significantly impaired declarative recall	N	Y	Y	Intact primary span; impaired selective/divided attention	Mildly impaired working memory, response inhibition, general problem-solving	Semantic organizational abilities significantly impaired, mild anomia	Simple construction intact, complex visual reasoning impaired	If present, symptoms are mild	Depression common
Vascular dementia (VaD)	May be insidious or acute	Stepwise, varied	Possible deficits	Y	Y	Y	Intact primary span; impaired selective/divided attention	Significantly more impaired than AD and relative to performance on verbal memory tasks	Verbal fluency impaired	Relatively preserved, although may be affected by executive impairments	Slowing, possible discrete motor problems depending on distrbution of vascular changes	Depression common
Frontotemporal dementia (FTD)	Insidious	Steady, rapid	Relatively preserved	Y	Y	Y	Intact primary span; impaired selective/divided attention	Impaired across a range of executive functions	Verbal fluency impaired	Relatively preserved, although may be affected by executive impairments	May exhibit ideational apraxia	Significant behavioral changes: apathy/ blunting, disinhibition, lack of insight, etc.
Primary progressive aphasia (PPA)	Insidious	Steady, varied	Preserved recall, may score poorly on verbal memory tests	Y	Y	Y	Preserved	Preserved	*Nonfluent PPA:* Anomic aphasia, poor articulation, dysarthria, relatively preserved comprehension; *Fluent PPA:* Impaired comprehension, anomia, intact speech rate & prosody	In semantic dementia, may have visual agnosia	*Nonfluent PPA:* Buccofacial apraxia	Changes unlikely

(Continued)

Table 105-4 (*Continued*)

	Symptom Onset	Progression, rate	Memory: Recent	Memory: Recognition intact?	Memory: Remote intact?	Procedural intact?	Attention	Executive Functions	Language	Visuospatial Function	Psychomotor Function	Behavior
Parkinson's disease (PD)	Insidious	Varied	Possible deficits	Y	Y	N - possible impairments	Intact primary attention span, impaired selective/divided attention	Difficulty planning/ shifting set	Verbal fluency, mechanical aspects of speech impaired	May be impaired	Resting tremor, bradykinesia, rigidity, postural instability, shuffling gait	Depression common, may exhibit hallucinations/ delusions, less common that DLB
Dementia with Lewy Bodies (LDB)	Insidious	Steady, gradual	Mild impairment, less than AD	Variable	Y	Y	Significant fluctuations in attention	Variable	Variable; fluency may be impaired	Impaired construction, copy, visuospatial planning and problem-solving	May exhibit a range of Parkinsonian symptoms	Hallucinations, delusions, depression
Progressive supranuclear palsy (PSP)	Insidious	Steady, gradual	Mild impairment, less than AD	Variable	Y	Y	Impaired selective/divided attention	Impaired across a range of executive functions	Verbal fluency impaired	May be impaired	vertical supranuclear gaze palsy; postural instability	Apathy, disinhibition
Persistent alcohol dementia	Deficits persist after *d/c* alcohol use	May worsen over time	Impairment on recall, not more than other functions	Variable	Y	Y	Impaired sustained attention	Abstraction, mental flexibility, perseveration, confabulation, impaired judgment, reduced ability to care for self	Preserved	Visual scanning, visuospatial organization impaired	May exhibit cerebellar tremor, impaired gait	Apathy, depression

Condition												
Wernicke-Korsakoff's syndrome	Acute (initial phase)	Steady, gradual (chronic phase)	Significant impairment on declarative recall relative to other deficits (semantic memory spared)	N	N	Variable	Impaired across all attentional functions	Similar profile to persistent alcohol dementia	Presevered	Visual scanning, visuospatial organization impaired	Impaired gait, abnormal reflexes, other movement abnormalities	Personality change prominent feature, inappropriate behavior
Prion disease	Insidious	Steady, rapid	Nonspecific impairments reported	Y	Y	Y	Nonspecific impairments reported	Reduced problem solving ability	Generally preserved	Generally intact	May exhibit impaired reflexes and coordination	Apathy, emotional lability, impaired sleep, appetite loss
Normal pressure hydrocephalus (NPH)	Insidious	Varied, potentially reversible	Not prominently impaired	Y	Y	Y	Primary deficits in attention	Nonspecific impairments in executive function reported	Generally preserved	Generally intact	wide-based gait or other balance disturbance, urinary incontinence	May present with a confusional state
Human immunodeficiency virus (HIV)	Usually later in the disease course	Varied	Variable	Variable	Y	Y	Nonspecific impairments reported	Nonspecific impairments in executive function reported	Generally preserved	Generally intact	Generally intact	Depression common
Neurosyphilis	Many years after initial infection	Varied, potentially reversible	Variable	Variable	Y	Y	Variable	Variable	Generally preserved	Generally intact	May be ataxic	Hallucinations, delusions, personality change, mood disturbance

Medical Examination

An important goal of the medical evaluation is to exclude the presence of medical conditions that may be responsible for the observed cognitive deficits. It is critical to investigate potentially reversible causes of dementia such as uncontrolled liver or kidney disease, adverse reactions to medications, and delirium. Laboratory blood tests can aid in ruling out systemic illnesses or organ malfunction. Structural brain scans are used to evaluate major cerebrovascular events, tumors, normal pressure hydrocephalus, and other neurologic conditions, while functional brain scans identify patterns of activity that may be useful in classifying dementia type.

Neuropsychological Assessment

Neuropsychological assessment of cognitive function not only provides confirmatory evidence for cognitive impairment, but may also aid in clarification of dementia type. Given the extensive variation in rate of AD progression between patients, regular neuropsychological examinations can also provide information regarding an individual's rate of progression and remaining cognitive strengths. Perhaps one of the most valuable assets of neuropsychological evaluation is the sensitivity of the tests to early cognitive decline. Although there is debate regarding the usefulness of providing an early AD diagnosis, it is generally accepted that such a diagnosis allows patients to avail themselves of current and emerging therapies, as well as to make decisions regarding health care, finances, and legal issues while still competent. In a typical neuropsychological evaluation, patients are given tests that sample a variety of domains of cognitive function. Results are compared to normative data based on age, and also to an individual's estimated premorbid abilities (based on educational and occupational background and performance on tests that tend to remain stable over time). Pattern analysis of test results, in combination with data from the patient history and medical evaluation, is then used to generate diagnostic possibilities. The following sections discuss cognitive impairment patterns typical in patients with Alzheimer's disease.

Memory   The hallmark of Alzheimer's disease, and most often the first cognitive symptom of the disorder, is anterograde amnesia, evidenced by difficulty with learning new information. Deficits are noted in declarative memory as a result of prominent impairment in information encoding, retrieval, and, in particular, storage of new material. Patients are likely to exhibit deficits in recent episodic recall, and they or their caregivers often report misplacing items, forgetting recent events or conversations, and frequently repeating questions or statements. In contrast to impaired episodic recall and difficulty learning new information, procedural memory is rarely impaired, and remote memory remains relatively intact until later stages of the disease.

To adequately evaluate short-term memory loss and to establish a pattern of impaired retrieval, neuropsychological evaluations include tests of both immediate and delayed verbal and visual recall. Tests such as the Folstein

Mini-Mental Status Examination (MMSE) and other diagnostic screening instruments assess general mental status and orientation, but are not adequate for a comprehensive understanding of memory impairment. To satisfactorily assess a person's true memory ability, Zec recommends using tasks that are high in cognitive demand, that exceed the primary memory span (such as story recall and list-learning tasks that include at least 10 items), and that have a recognition component. On neuropsychological examination, verbal and visual free immediate and delayed recall and recognition are significantly impaired in AD patients relative to same-age peers, and patients typically exhibit a high number of intrusion errors and repetitions. Semantic recall is generally the most predominantly impaired, and thus verbal recall tasks are often the most sensitive to early memory loss.

Attention and Executive Function   Certain aspects of attention and concentration are often impaired early in the disease process, and recent research has supported that it may in fact be one of the earliest abilities affected in AD. While patients with AD are likely to have relatively intact simple attention (e.g., primary memory span), tests requiring selective and divided attention are likely to be impaired, particularly as task demands increase. This pattern of performance strongly supports the presence of a deficit in working memory (the ability to simultaneously attend, process, and respond to multiple pieces of information) early in the disease process, and a converging body of evidence supports a primary executive component in AD.

In addition to problems on tasks of complex attention and working memory, patients are likely to exhibit mild deficits in response inhibition, evidenced by intrusion errors and perseverative responses, on neuropsychological testing. Deficits in abstract reasoning, general problem solving ability, and making appropriate judgments are also commonly noted. In assessing for judgment and abstraction, patients may be asked the meaning of proverbs (e.g., "you can lead a horse to water but you can't make it drink"), and are often given hypothetical situations in which they must decide an appropriate course of action (e.g., "What would you do if you were in a crowded shopping mall and saw smoke and fire?"). On these tasks, even early AD patients may provide incorrect or inappropriate responses.

Language   Semantic processing is considered the primary language deficit in AD, and is present in more than half of all AD patients at the time of diagnosis. Word-finding problems are commonly reported in both AD and normal aging, but patients with AD have more severe deficits and are more likely to produce a significantly higher number of semantic paraphasias and circumlocutions. Patients are generally impaired on tasks of confrontational naming, and, unlike changes that occur with normal aging, are not likely to be assisted by cues. Syntactic processing, in contrast to semantic processing, is typically unaffected in mild AD. For example, patients with early AD can typically process even complex sentences at the same level as their healthy counterparts, and generally remain unimpaired on repetition and fluent speech. Verbal fluency tasks are particularly useful in evaluating both semantic and syntactic processing.

Semantic, or category fluency (e.g., "tell me as many animals as you can") is generally impaired disproportionately to syntactic, or phonemic fluency (e.g., "tell me as many words that begin with the letter __") in AD. While decreased information processing and working memory may impair an AD patient's responses on certain syntactic processing tasks, and comprehension and intelligible speech are likely to decline slowly as the disease advances, patients who present first with nonfluent aphasia or impaired comprehension should be carefully evaluated for other conditions.

Visuospatial Function Deficits in visuospatial abilities are frequently seen in AD patients, although they generally appear later than memory and language deficits. Patients may become lost in familiar places (e.g., grocery store) or while driving. Eventually, disorientation may lead to confusion in one's own home and subsequent wandering behavior. Early deficits however, are more likely to involve visuospatial problem solving. Neuropsychological tests commonly used involve comparing simple construction or copying, typically not impaired early in the disease, to complex visual reasoning. The presence of constructional apraxia early in the disease may indicate greater pathology in visual processing areas of the brain and has been associated with more rapid symptom progression. In general, more complex drawing tasks, such as three-dimensional figure copy, may be more precise measures of the most common early visual spatial deficits in AD than simple copying tasks.

Motor Function While motor dysfunction has not been typically considered to be a defining symptom of AD, recent research suggests that AD patients may display impairments in gait, motor speed, and general level of activity even in the mild stages of the disease. In addition, converging evidence provides support for greater overlap between AD and Lewy body dementia, making motor changes such as tremor or gait disturbance more likely in these patients. Importantly, there have been reports of gait disturbance in patients taking cholinesterase inhibitors, a factor that should be carefully monitored when prescribing these medications.

AD patients may also exhibit mild ideomotor and ideational apraxia (deficits in skilled movements) as a result of concrete responses, lack of sufficient external cues, or a disruption in conceptualization ability. However, moderate to severe apraxia is not generally present until later stages of the disease. Incorporating an apraxia assessment into a dementia evaluation is useful, however, particularly for excluding other disorders that may initially present with more severe skilled movement disorders.

Behavioral Changes

As mentioned previously, depression is common in patients with AD, and may manifest as apathy, indifference, poor initiation, or emotional lability. Irritability, agitation, and paranoid ideation are also common in AD, and may worsen with disease progression, prompting wandering behavior and aggressive outbursts. Repetitive and aimless behavior may also increase as the disease progresses. More severe psychotic symptoms, such as hallucinations and severe delusions, have been reported in some patients with early AD, but are typically rare in the absence of coexisting disorders. Given the wide range of behaviors that may be exhibited in an AD patient, it is imperative that the patient's family be provided with ample dementia education, that they have access to social support, and that they possess the coping skills necessary to provide adequate care.

Awareness of Deficits

Patients in the early stages of AD typically vary in their level of deficit awareness. Whatever the starting point, deficit awareness declines with disease progression. Even when patients do acknowledge their cognitive decline, however, such awareness may not be "complete" as a result of deficits in executive function. For example, patients may be unable to translate cognitive problems into functional problems, and as a result may not understand how their deficits affect certain activities, such as driving, cooking, and finances. Again, providing the patient's caregivers with access to education can increase the likelihood that patients will comply with physician recommendations to limit certain unsafe behaviors.

Variant AD Presentations

While the primary early deficit in AD most often involves recent memory, there are several reported cases of variant forms of AD that involve primary deficits in language, visuospatial function, or central executive function. In such cases, differential diagnoses, including frontotemporal dementia, primary progressive aphasia, Lewy body dementia, and others must be carefully considered prior to assigning a diagnosis of AD.

Mild Cognitive Impairment

The term "mild cognitive impairment" has been used to describe cognitive impairment in aging that does not meet the criteria for dementia and that is not the result of a known medical condition. Petersen and colleagues proposed a set of criteria for diagnosing mild cognitive impairment that includes (1) subjective memory concerns, (2) objective impairment in memory on neuropsychological testing, (3) absence of dementia, and (4) absence of functional complaints. Longitudinal research suggests that 80 percent of those diagnosed with mild cognitive impairment will go on to develop Alzheimer's disease within 5 to 8 years, and will convert at a rate of approximately 10 to 15 percent per year as compared to general population conversion rates of 1 to 2 percent. The term "amnestic" mild cognitive impairment is currently used to differentiate between isolated impairment in memory versus impairments in other cognitive functions. Given the above-noted conversion rates, it is proposed that amnestic mild cognitive impairment may actually be a preclinical stage of AD, while nonamnestic mild cognitive impairment may represent early onset of other forms of dementia, including frontotemporal, Lewy body, and vascular dementias. Neuropsychological assessment can be particularly useful in distinguishing between normal age-related changes and mild cognitive impairment.

Vascular Dementia

VaD is a controversial and heterogenous nosologic construct. This heterogeneity complicates efforts to identify characteristic cognitive profiles. According to NINDS-AIREN criteria, six vascular "subtypes" ascribe dementia to multiple large infarcts, strategic single infarcts, small vessel disease, hypoperfusion, hemorrhage, or miscellaneous vascular insult. It is likely that dementia caused by small-vessel disease is the most common form of vascular dementia and provides the most uniform pattern of cognitive impairment. Cognitive profiles of these patients at early stages typically reveal executive function deficits, reduced verbal fluency, and slowing, with preservation of cued memory and an absence of intrusions. Depression, irritability and lack of initiative are also common. Looi and Sachdev noted the difficulty in differentiating vascular dementia from Alzheimer's disease, because current criteria for dementia require memory impairment, and impairment in one additional cognitive domain. For adults with vascular dementia, memory impairment may not occur until later in the disease process; thus these patients have more progressed dementia and greater cognitive impairment at the time of diagnosis. A review of studies differentiating between early stage Alzheimer's disease and vascular dementia found that the latter group had more pronounced deficits in executive function on tests such as the Wisconsin Card Sorting tests and the executive function scale of the Mattis Dementia Rating Scale than did adults with AD. Interestingly, performance between the two groups was similar on tests of selective attention and working memory such as the Trail-Making Test and Stroop Color-Word Interference test. In contrast, VaD patients had better performance than AD patients on tests of verbal learning and story recall, such as the California Verbal Learning Test and the Logical Memory subtest of the Wechsler Memory Scale-III (WMS-III), with fewer intrusions. It is important to note that as both VaD and AD progress, the cognitive profiles become more similar, so that differentiating midstage disease is very difficult. In addition, recent neuropathologic studies show that many patients previously diagnosed with vascular dementia because of the presence of vascular risk factors such as diabetes, hypertension, and radiologic evidence of ischemia, have prominent AD pathology as well. Prevalence estimates of the co-occurrence of AD and vascular dementia range from 20 to 40 percent of patients with dementia. Few studies have attempted to differentiate between mixed AD/VaD and either form of dementia on a neuropsychological basis, although Bowler et al. suggest that mixed dementia most closely resembles VaD from a cognitive perspective. Results from the Nun Study demonstrate that vascular pathology increases the likelihood that patients with neuropathologic AD will show significant cognitive impairment. Finally, cognitive profiles for other forms of VaD, such as multiple large-vessel or single-strategic infarcts, are highly idiosyncratic, depending on lesion location and volume.

Frontotemporal Dementia

Frontotemporal dementia (FTD) is a diagnostic category used to describe a number of conditions, including Pick's disease, progressive aphasia, semantic dementia, behavioral disorder and dysexecutive syndrome, familial chromosome 17-linked frontal lobe dementia, FTD of the non-Alzheimer's type, and other histopathologic classifications. FTD is estimated to account for 3 to 20 percent of dementia cases. Prototypical symptoms of FTD include personality change and slowly progressive executive dysfunction. Patients often present with behavioral disturbance that includes disinhibition, a lack of conformity to social norms, perseveration, emotional blunting, and a lack of insight. Neuropsychological testing generally reveals impaired selective and divided attention, difficulty shifting mental set, poor abstraction, and impaired verbal fluency. Perseverative errors are common. Spatial skills are relatively preserved, except when organizational skills are required for completion of the task. Unfortunately, the MMSE is not very helpful in diagnosing early FTD because many patients score within normal limits.

Both the personality changes and cognitive dysfunction observed at early stages of FTD exceed those seen in normal aging. The most difficult differential diagnosis is between FTD and AD. Age of onset for FTD is typically in the late fifties or early sixties, although exceptions are observed. Therefore, on average, FTD patients show symptoms about a decade earlier than AD patients. As with AD, FTD patients show insidious onset of symptoms with a gradual progression. Although comparisons of AD and FTD groups do not always reveal significantly different cognitive profiles, in general, FTD patients show relatively spared memory performance in comparison to their executive and language functioning, especially when memory cues are provided. Apraxia is also more common than in AD. Often a multidisciplinary approach may be most helpful in the differential diagnosis since studies indicate that up to 75 percent of pathologically confirmed FTD patients also appear to meet clinical criteria for probable AD.

Primary Progressive Aphasia

Primary progressive aphasia (PPA) has been described as the fifth most common cause of dementia. The diagnosis of PPA requires isolated language dysfunction for 2 years, with all other areas of cognition remaining largely intact, and the absence of radiologic evidence of cerebrovascular or other neurologic injury that would account for the aphasia. In the initial stages of PPA, anomia is inevitably present consisting of impaired object naming, more generally impaired word finding, or both. Two broad categories of PPA are defined by the presence of additional language impairment. Nonfluent PPA is characterized by labored articulation, occasional dysarthria, dyscalculia, and buccofacial apraxia, with preserved comprehension except for complex sentences with embedded clauses. In fluent PPA (also called PPA with verbal semantic comprehension deficits), word-finding pauses may still be evident, although speech rate and prosody are largely preserved. Comprehension is impaired, and patients may have difficulty both with naming objects and with pointing to objects when given their names. They are still able to demonstrate the use of such objects appropriately, however, reflecting intact knowledge of object meaning. As the disease progresses, speech becomes empty and paraphasic. A related condition, semantic dementia, is diagnosed when fluent PPA is accompanied by impairment in visual recognition of objects, and the semantic meaning of both words and objects is lost. Patients with semantic dementia display prominent visual agnosias and can no longer demonstrate object use accurately.

Because anomia and other language deficits may occur in a number of neurodegenerative conditions, the differential diagnosis of PPA rests on the clear demonstration that nonlinguistic cognitive and behavioral functions are intact for the first 2 years of the disease. The examiner must carefully determine whether poor performance on memory and other nonlanguage tests is a result of language deficits such as impaired comprehension of instructions. The onset of PPA is typically in the fifth or sixth decade of life, and its rate of progression varies greatly. As the disease progresses, however, other cognitive functions become impaired, as does the patient's ability to carry out functional activities. Thus, making a diagnosis of midstage PPA is difficult at best. Differential diagnosis is also complicated by the heterogenous etiologies of PPA. The majority of patients have nonspecific focal atrophy of perisylvian language areas. A subgroup have AD-like pathology although not in brain regions typically associated with AD. Another sub-group have Pick's pathology, although not the flagrant behavioral and executive function deficits of typical Pick's disease.

Lewy Body Disease

Although the following diseases have a number of different neuropathologic features, a common shared characteristic is the presence of Lewy bodies, abnormal intracytoplasmic inclusion deposits, on neuropathologic exam.

Parkinson's Disease

At its early stages, Parkinson's disease (PD) can be difficult to differentiate from normal aging. Most patients initially present with a resting tremor. Other cardinal symptoms include bradykinesia, rigidity, and postural instability. Patients may also present with a shuffling gait, masked facies, and depression. Although there has been significant variability across estimates of the frequency of dementia in PD, it appears that approximately a third of these patients develop dementia. Relatively healthy elderly patients can present with a number of these symptoms for unrelated problems. For instance, essential tremors are not uncommon and patients with arthritis often show slowed motor movements.

Typically, even nondemented PD patients show slight cognitive deficits across a range of cognitive domains that are often conceptualized as executive dysfunction. PD with dementia is usually characterized by visuospatial deficits, attentional impairment, difficulty planning or shifting to a new stimulus, slowed information processing speed, and mildly impaired memory recall. Memory impairment is most frequently attributable to a retrieval deficit since recognition is generally intact. Procedural learning may be impaired, a pattern atypical in normal aging or in AD. Some language skills are intact, such as vocabulary, while others that tap additional cognitive domains, such as verbal fluency, are impaired. Mechanical aspects of speech are often impaired as well. Although PD has been characterized as a subcortical dementia to distinguish it from cortical dementias such as AD, this characterization has been criticized more recently and may serve simply as a gross depiction of the cognitive profile.

Dementia with Lewy Bodies

According to consensus criteria for probable dementia with Lewy bodies (DLB), cognition must be carefully assessed. A progressive cognitive decline, usually over the course of a number of years, must be observed to a degree that it disables the patient. In addition the patient must show some combination of fluctuations in attention, recurrent visual hallucinations, or spontaneous parkinsonism. Many patients may also present with other psychotic symptoms, neuroleptic sensitivity, and a history of falls and syncopal attacks. Based on these criteria, the differential diagnosis between DLB and Parkinson's disease is obviously difficult. At this time, the differential diagnosis is based purely on the timing of the onset of the cognitive symptoms. A Parkinson's patient who develops cognitive symptoms after one year of motor symptoms is classified as "Parkinson's disease with dementia." Earlier cognitive symptoms indicate DLB.

The differential diagnosis between DLB and AD can also be difficult. Ballard and colleagues reported that the presence of hallucinations in patients with MMSE scores greater than 20 was highly suggestive of DLB in prospectively studied cases. Neuropsychological studies have identified typical cognitive profiles that may aid in diagnosis. In DLB, patients have more difficulty than AD patients in copying complex designs, assembling pieces of an object, or completing other tasks requiring visuospatial skills. In contrast, AD subjects generally show significantly more impairment on delayed recall tasks than patients with DLB. DLB patients have attentional skills that are generally equivalent to those of AD patients; however, patients with DLB exhibit significant attentional fluctuations. As a result, evaluating attention over time is more helpful than the overall severity of attention problems in the differential diagnosis. The clinical overlap of the two diseases may be related, in part, to the pathological overlap of the diseases. Neuropathologic studies indicate that the majority of DLB cases have Alzheimer pathology (especially plaques) and that Lewy bodies are common in AD patients. Finally, these cognitive profiles are most evident early in the course of the diseases. As the diseases progress, all cognitive functions become impaired and neuropsychological testing is less helpful for diagnosis.

Progressive Supranuclear Palsy

Progressive supranuclear palsy (PSP) is less common than PD. Although Lewy bodies are found in only the minority of PSP cases, PSP is frequently misdiagnosed as PD. A core feature of the disorder is vertical supranuclear gaze palsy, although this symptom may not present early in the course of the disease. Patients also present with postural instability, and falls are often seen shortly after onset. Cognition is characterized by mental slowing and executive dysfunction. Memory impairments are observed, but they are not as severe as in AD. Language functions resemble those seen in PD. Visual spatial deficits and increased apathy are also observed.

Alcohol-Related Dementia

Recent epidemiologic analyses suggest that mild to moderate alcohol use reduces the risk for developing certain dementias, including Alzheimer's disease and vascular dementia. Chronic and profound alcohol use, however, can have a negative effect on cognition and may exacerbate the cognitive symptoms of other dementias and brain injuries. Poor nutrition (thiamine deficiency in particular) resulting from alcohol abuse is a primary contributor to the onset of cognitive problems. In addition, liver disease itself can interfere with thiamine regulation in the brain and may be a factor in the multiple cognitive and motor impairments associated with long-term alcohol use. Chronic alcoholics are often impaired on neurocognitive tests even following a period of abstinence, and many continue to show cognitive deficits indefinitely.

Persistent Alcohol Dementia

Alcohol dementia involves impairment in more than one area of cognitive function that persists after the patient stops drinking for a period of time. Visuospatial problem solving deficits and executive problems, including apathy, decreased judgment, and reduced interest in self-care, are prominent in these patients. Memory problems, particularly anterograde amnesia, are also common, but are generally not more impaired than other cognitive domains, and recognition is often intact. Typical neuropsychological sequelae include impairments on tasks requiring visual scanning, visuospatial organization, perceptual–motor speed, sustained attention, abstraction, and mental flexibility, while language functions are generally preserved. Perseveration and confabulation are common indicators of impaired executive function in the responses of patients with chronic alcohol use.

Wernicke–Korsakoff Syndrome

The most severe neurologic outcome of heavy and prolonged alcohol use, and the result of critical malnutrition, is Wernicke–Korsakoff syndrome. In contrast to patients with persistent alcohol dementia, Wernicke–Korsakoff patients exhibit an acute symptom onset, often beginning with a grave confusional state, nystagmus, and significant ataxia. During this phase, symptoms progressively and rapidly worsen if treatment (immediate thiamine replacement) is not applied. This phase is almost always followed by a chronic and progressive stage that is associated primarily with impaired frontal and cerebellar functions. Unlike persistent alcohol dementia, Wernicke–Korsakoff patients

have significant impairments in memory relative to other cognitive effects, and memory impairment includes both retrograde and anterograde amnesia for episodic events, frequently with prominent confabulation. In contrast to Alzheimer's disease, semantic memory is relatively spared in the Wernicke–Korsakoff patient. Patients show a characteristic gradient of remote memory impairment, with better recall for remote events and progressively reduced recall of recent events. As with persistent alcohol dementia, executive dysfunction and visuospatial impairments are also significant symptoms of the syndrome. Cerebellar atrophy and peripheral nerve damage lead to impaired gait, decreased or abnormal reflexes, and other movement abnormalities in these patients.

Prion Diseases

The prion diseases are a group of rare fatal spongiform encephalopathies that result from mutations and polymorphisms in the prion protein gene (PrP), causing rapid neurodegeneration. These diseases, of which Creutzfeldt–Jakob is the most well known, produce a profound and quickly progressive dementia, and may be sporadic, familial, or infectious. Sporadic cases are the most common, and are generally diagnosed in people in their sixties, with a typical age range between 40 and 80 years. Early cognitive signs of the prion diseases are usually vague and nonspecific, such as poor memory, concentration, and problem solving. Initially, there are also often psychiatric symptoms, including apathy, emotional lability, impaired sleep, and appetite loss. Early frank neurologic symptoms are not common, but as the disease progresses, hyperreflexia, impaired coordination, changes in saccadic eye movements, and incontinence may occur. Given the early vague symptoms and dearth of neurologic symptoms, patients are not likely to present for evaluation until they are in the more moderate to advanced stages, which can occur in a matter of months. Diagnosis typically involves measuring electroencephalographic changes, hyperintensities on magnetic resonance imaging, and abnormal 14-3-3 protein deposits in the cerebrospinal fluid. The most common differential diagnoses include depression, AD, and LBD.

Normal Pressure Hydrocephalus

Normal pressure hydrocephalus (NPH) is a potentially reversible progressive dementia that makes up approximately 6 percent of the dementia cases. Abnormalities in the production, absorption, or flow of cerebrospinal fluid (CSF) results in ventricular dilatation. Patients may present with a triad of clinical symptoms that include gait or balance disturbance, urinary incontinence, and cognitive deficits. Unlike most other dementias, cognitive symptoms often present later in the course. This can make early clinical diagnosis difficult because gait abnormalities and incontinence have a variety of etiologies in geriatric populations. Radiographic evidence and intraventricular pressure measurement aid in the diagnosis. When cognitive deficits are present, they most frequently fall in executive functioning. Although many subjects may have subjective memory complaints, memory deficits are not a prominent early symptom, and some memory declines are attributable to attention problems, which are more common.

When treated, a ventriculoperitoneal shunt is usually used to divert CSF for better absorption. However, surgery in geriatric populations always involves added risks, and the benefits of shunt surgery remain unclear. A wide variety of success rates have been reported. Patients with the full triad of symptoms appear to respond best to shunt surgery. Gait problems show the most frequent improvement, while cognitive function improves in the fewest patients. Savolainen and colleagues recently reported findings from a 5-year follow-up of NPH patients with and without shunt surgery. One year after surgery, 72 percent of shunted cases showed improvement in activities of daily living, as compared to 27 percent of those who did not undergo shunt procedures. However, there were no postoperative neuropsychological improvements. Improvements in gait and incontinence were observed after 1 year in 69 percent and 64 percent of subjects, respectively. These rates declined at the 5-year follow-up (47 percent and 29 percent remained "better," respectively). Consistent with other findings, neuropsychological testing was not useful for predicting response to surgery.

Human Immunodeficiency Virus

Although there is often the perception that geriatric patients are not at risk for human immunodeficiency virus (HIV) infection, the Centers for Disease Control; reported that 10 percent of all HIV cases in the United States are in patients 50 years of age or older. In addition, 10 percent of people older than age 50 years have at least one risk factor for contraction of the disease. The earliest cognitive areas affected are usually speed of information processing, attention, and motor speed. A subgroup of patients progress to HIV-associated dementia which is usually characterized by impairments in executive functioning, psychomotor speed, and memory.

Neurosyphilis

Neurosyphilis is an advanced syphilitic infection that may present with hallucinations, delusions, mood disturbance, personality change, strokes, ataxia, or cognitive decline. Deficits are observed in short-term memory and mental status with progressive cognitive decline in all areas of functioning. Although neurosyphilis is often classified as a reversible dementia, there is only limited evidence to support cognitive benefits with treatment. The onset of dementia in neurosyphilis often occurs several decades after contraction of the disease. Therefore, neurosyphilis should be considered in a differential diagnosis of dementia of unclear etiology in geriatric patients.

CONCLUSIONS

We have greatly furthered our understanding that age-related medical conditions not considered classically neurologic in nature can nevertheless impact the central nervous system and thereby affect cognition. This knowledge has led to the realization that many of the changes in cognition previously thought to be unavoidable concomitants of normal aging are in fact preventable, and in some cases, even reversible. The deleterious consequences of not treating such disorders has become evident, given that many common diseases such as type 2 diabetes and hypertension appear to be risk factors for dementia. In turn, early identification of dementia or the prodromal condition mild cognitive impairment will become critical as therapeutic options for delaying disease progression proliferate. Careful characterization of cognitive status through neuropsychological assessment can provide the clinician with essential information to determine whether the patient is experiencing symptoms that warrant concern or further treatment. As the field of geriatrics approaches the goal of controlling or even preventing endemic late-life chronic diseases, it will become increasingly clear that the cognitive changes that occur with healthy aging are fewer than we thought, that they are more subtle in nature, and that they should not affect our ability to have rich, active lives into our eighties and beyond.

REFERENCES

Anstey K, Christensen H: Education, activity, health, blood pressure, and apolipoprotein E as predictors of cognitive change in old age: A review. *Gerontology* 46:163, 2000.

Ballard C et al: Psychiatric morbidity in dementia with Lewy bodies: A prospective clinical and neuropathological comparative study with Alzheimer's disease. *Am J Psychiatry* 156:1039, 1999.

Berger A et al: The occurrence of depressive symptoms in the preclinical phase of AD. *Neurology* 53:1998, 1999.

Bowler J et al: Conceptual background to vascular cognitive impairment. *Alzheimer Dis Assoc Disord* 13(Suppl 3):S30, 1999.

Burke D, MacKay D: Memory, language, and ageing. *Phil Trans R Soc Lond* 352:1845, 1997.

Butterworth, R: Cerebral dysfunction in chronic alcoholism: Role of alcoholic liver disease-review. *Alcohol Alcohol Suppl* 2:259, 1994.

Calvaresi E, Bryan J: B vitamins, cognition, and aging: A review. *J Gerontol B Psychol Sci Soc Sci* 56:P327, 2001.

Christensen H: What cognitive changes can be expected with normal ageing? *Aust N Z J Psychiatry* 35:768, 2001.

Collinge J: Prion diseases of humans and animals: their causes and molecular basis. *Annu Rev Neurosci* 24:519, 2001.

Crawford S, Channon S: Dissociation between performance on abstract tests of executive function and problem solving in real-life-type situations in normal aging. *Aging Ment Health* 6:12–21, 2002.

Duke L, Seltzer B, Seltzer J, et al: Cognitive components of deficit awareness in Alzheimer's disease. *Neuropsychology* 16:359, 2002.

Duthie S et al: Homocysteine, B vitamin status, and cognitive function in the elderly. *Am J Clin Nutr* 75:908, 2002.

Elias P et al: NIDDM and blood pressure as risk factors for poor cognitive performance: The Framingham study. *Diabetes Care* 20:1388, 1997.

Eustache F et al: Healthy aging, memory subsystems and regional cerebral oxygen consumption. *Neuropsychologia* 33:867, 1995.

Grossman M: Frontotemporal dementia: A review. *J Int Neuropsychol Soc* 8:566, 2002.

Horn J, Cattell R: Age differences in fluid and crystallized intelligence. *J Educat Psychol* 57:253, 1967.

Kemper S et al: Longitudinal change in language production: Effects of aging and dementia on grammatical complexity and propositional content. *Psychol Aging* 16:600, 2001.

Laursen P: The impact of aging on cognitive function. An 11-year follow-up study of four age cohorts. *Acta Neurol Scand* S172:7, 1997.

Looi J, Sachdev P: Differentiation of vascular dementia from AD on neuropsychological tests. *Neurology* 53:670, 1999.

Luszcz M, Bryan J: Toward understanding age-related memory loss in adulthood. *Gerontology* 45:2, 1999.

Malec J et al: Neuropsychology and normal aging: The clinician's perspective, in Parks RW et al. (eds): *Neuropsychology of Alzheimer's Disease and Related Disorders.* New York, Oxford University Press, 1993.

Mayeux R et al: Memory performance in healthy elderly without Alzheimer's disease: Effects of time and apolipoprotein-E. *Neurobiol Aging* 22:683, 2001.

McKhann G et al: Clinical diagnosis of Alzheimer's disease: Report of the NINCDS-ADRDA work group under the auspices of Department of Health and Human Services Task Force on Alzheimer's Disease. *Neurology* 34:939, 1984.

Mesulam M: Primary progressive aphasia. *Ann Neurol* 49:425, 2001.

Miller J: Homocysteine, Alzheimer's disease, and cognitive function. *Nutrition* 16:675, 2000.

Newman M et al: Longitudinal assessment of neurocognitive function after coronary-artery bypass surgery. *N Engl J Med* 344:2874, 2001.

Newman M et al: Report of the substudy assessing the impact of neurocognitive function on quality of life 5 years after cardiac surgery. *Stroke* 32:2874, 2001.

Pasquier F: Early diagnosis of dementia: Neuropsychology. *J Neurol* 246:6, 1999.

Petersen R et al: Current concepts in mild cognitive impairment. *Arch Neurol* 58:1985, 2001.

Reaven G et al: Relationship between hyperglycemia and cognitive function in older NIDDM patients. *Diabetes Care* 13:16, 1990.

Salmon D et al: Alcoholic dementia and related disorders, in Parks RW et al. (eds): *Neuropsychology of Alzheimer's Disease and Related Disorders.* New York, Oxford University Press, 1993 p 186.

Savolainen S et al: Five-year outcome of normal pressure hydrocephalus with or without a shunt: Predictive value of clinical signs, neuropsychological evaluation, and infusion test. *Acta Neurochir* 144:512, 2002.

Saxton J et al: Alcohol, dementia, and Alzheimer's disease: comparison of neuropsychological profiles. *J Geriatr Psychiatry Neurol* 13:141, 2000.

Smith M et al: Constructional apraxia in Alzheimer's disease: Association with occipital lobe pathology and accelerated cognitive decline. *Dementia* 12:281, 2001.

Snowdon D et al: Brain infarction and the clinical expression of Alzheimer disease. The Nun Study. *JAMA* 277:813, 1997.

Spieler D, Balota D: Factors influencing word naming in younger and older adults. *Psychol Aging* 15:225, 2000.

Storey E et al: Patterns of cognitive impairment in Alzheimer's disease: Assessment and differential diagnosis. *Front Biosci* 7:e155, 2002.

Troyer A et al: Clustering and switching as tow components of verbal fluency: Evidence from younger and older healthy adults. *Neuropsychology* 11:138, 1997.

Zec R: Neuropsychological functioning in Alzheimer's disease, in Parks RW et al. (eds): *Neuropsychology of Alzheimer's Disease and Related Disorders.* New York, Oxford University Press, 1993 p 3.

Zekry D et al: Mixed dementia: epidemiology, diagnosis, and treatment. *J Am Geriatr Soc* 50:1431, 2002.

Cerebrovascular Disease

J. PHILLIP KISTLER • M.A. TOPÇUOGLU • FERDINANDO S. BUONANNO

Although cerebral vascular disease is the third leading cause of death in the United States after heart disease and cancer, it remains the single most important cause of disability. One of several pathologic processes that either lead to occlusion or rupture of an extra- or intracranial artery or vein produces the clinical manifestation of cerebral vascular disease in terms of primary ischemic stroke, transient ischemic attacks (TIAs) and/or primary hemorrhagic stroke. With either TIA or primary ischemic or hemorrhagic stroke, the prelude to acute, chronic, or preventive therapy is precise diagnosis. The diagnostic formulation must not only establish that the clinical entity is an ischemic stroke or TIA, or a hemorrhagic stroke, but also must localize and characterize the precise arterial or venous pathologic process causing the stroke, as well as elucidate the nature of the spared collateral circulation (Figs. 106-1 and 106-2). This chapter focuses on identifying this pathologic process as the pivot on which hinge rational medical and/or surgical treatments or preventive strategies. For both primary ischemic and/or primary hemorrhagic stroke, as for TIAs, the precise pathophysiologic process divides logically into specific stroke or TIA subtypes.

ISCHEMIC STROKE OR TIA SUBTYPE

Pathophysiology and Clinical Presentation

It is important to recognize that ischemic stroke and/or TIAs share the same pathophysiologic causation in terms of the underlying arterial pathology. The terms "stroke" and "TIA" are no more a diagnosis that dictates a specific therapeutic strategy than are the terms "fever" and "abdominal pain." Just as the primary care physician would treat the pneumococcal pneumonia giving rise to the fever, or the pancreatitis giving rise to abdominal pain, so should the underlying arterial pathophysiology of the ischemic stroke or TIA be the focus of a treatment strategy. The term "cerebral vascular accident (CVA)" should be discarded and the terms "TIA" and "ischemic stroke" should be complemented by terms defining their pathophysiologic subtype. Primary ischemic stroke and transient cerebral ischemia (TIA) conveniently divide into four ischemic or TIA subtypes: (1) large artery atherothrombotic (15 percent);

(2) embolic (57 percent—cardiac, ascending aorta, or unknown source); (3) small vessel lacunar (25 percent); and (4) other (3 percent), such as arterial dissection, venous sinus occlusion, and arteritis. The percentages of the various ischemic stroke or TIA subtypes or pathophysiologic cause identified in the National Institutes of Health Stroke Databank vary with different ethnic population groups.

When transient or sustained focal neurologic symptoms or signs develop in a patient, the history, physical examination, and neurologic examination suggest that it is a stroke, and may even suggest the pathophysiologic subtype. This presumed pathophysiologic TIA or stroke subtype diagnosis requires immediate noninvasive assessment of the extra- and intracranial arterial system, focusing on the arteries supplying the suspected symptomatic arterial territory. This includes the large arteries from the aortic arch to the locus of ischemia or infarct. The "parent" artery pathology—or lack thereof—then confirms the subtype, namely, large artery atherothrombotic, embolic, small vessel disease, or other. Often an embolus has fragmented and migrated, leaving the parent vessel patent, or it may have entered a branch of the parent vessel not shown in the scheme outlined in Figure 106-2. In that case, embolism is suggested only by the specific territory of the infarction. When a small infarction occurs in the territory of a single penetrating vessel deep in the brain (as might arise from the basilar artery, the middle cerebral artery stem, or the arteries of the circle of Willis), a small vessel lacunar stroke is diagnosed. To confirm the clinically suspected presumed pathophysiologic diagnosis, computed tomography (CT) scanning alone in the acute or subacute phase is inadequate. CT usually identifies an intracranial hemorrhage, but may miss a subarachnoid hemorrhage. Ischemic infarction may not be demonstrable by noncontrast CT for 12 to 14 hours after symptom onset; additionally, infarction involving only the cortical surface supratentorially, or infarction in the posterior fossa, can often be obscured by bone artifact. Therefore, contrast CT angiography, magnetic resonance imaging (MRI) with MR angiography, and/or carotid duplex Doppler and transcranial Doppler, should be obtained to outline the parent vessels (see Fig. 106-2), before specific treatment based on the pathologic process can be devised. Only with precise knowledge of the parent vessel pathology, or its absence, can therapy be properly addressed—whether it be thrombolytic, antithrombotic, or antiplatelet, interventional intraarterial, or surgical. The following sections outline each of the four ischemic stroke and TIA subtypes in terms of their pathophysiologic process and clinical presentation. A discussion of a focused diagnostic approach to confirm that clinically presumed diagnosis follows. Based on the particular TIA or stroke subtype and its causative pathologic process, acute, subacute, and preventive management strategies, can then be addressed.

Large Vessel, Atherothrombotic Stroke/TIA

Atherothrombotic cerebral vascular disease accounts for only 15 percent of all ischemic infarcts in the National Institutes of Health (NIH) Stroke Databank. As occurs in the heart, the atheromatous process occurs in strategically focal locations with predilection for four extra- and intracranial arterial locations (see Fig. 106-2): (1) the internal carotid artery origin, (2) or its siphon portion, (3) the middle cerebral stem, and (4) the vertebrobasilar junction. Although the origin of the common carotid artery and the vertebral arteries also are sites of atheromatous disease, they are less-often implicated in stroke or TIA. At each of the sites of predilection, two mechanisms are responsible for causing the stroke or TIA: (1) atherothrombotic plaque with clot formation that either occludes the vessel and gives rise to an embolic fragment that occludes a more distal vessel, that is, artery-to-artery embolus or thrombus that propagates into a distal vessel; or (2) the atherothrombotic process might occlude or narrow the vessel to such a degree that distal flow is diminished and not compensated via the circle of Willis, that is, low-flow stroke or TIA. Generally, both artery-to-artery embolism and low-flow stroke occur when the vessel is narrowed by the atheromatous process to a degree that decreases pressure across the arterial segment, that is, producing 70 percent or greater diameter stenosis, or frank occlusion. A TIA is said to occur if symptoms clear within an arbitrarily set time of 24 hours. In artery-to-artery embolic events, symptoms may last for shorter periods of time and in low-flow transient ischemic events they may last only minutes to as long as an hour or more. Often, artery-to-artery or low-flow transient ischemic events may be associated with an MRI-proven area of infarction, notwithstanding resolution of the symptoms. When symptomatic stroke ensues in this setting, it is because the artery-to-artery embolic fragment lodges in an intracranial vessel unable to be adequately collateralized via the circle of Willis, or the clot propagates and occludes the vessel. The latter case occurs most prominently with internal carotid artery origin occlusion and propagation of the clot distally into the middle cerebral stem (see Figs. 106-1 and 106-2).

Low-flow stroke or TIA occurs less often from a cervical lesion because the circle of Willis distally provides collateral circulation. However, low-flow stroke or TIA occurs more often with atheromatous disease in the distal vertebral or in the basilar arteries. Similarly, the frequency of low-flow stroke or TIA increases when the atheromatous process is in the middle cerebral stem and compromises the ability of the circle of Willis to provide sufficient collateral flow. In more than 50 percent of the population, the circle of

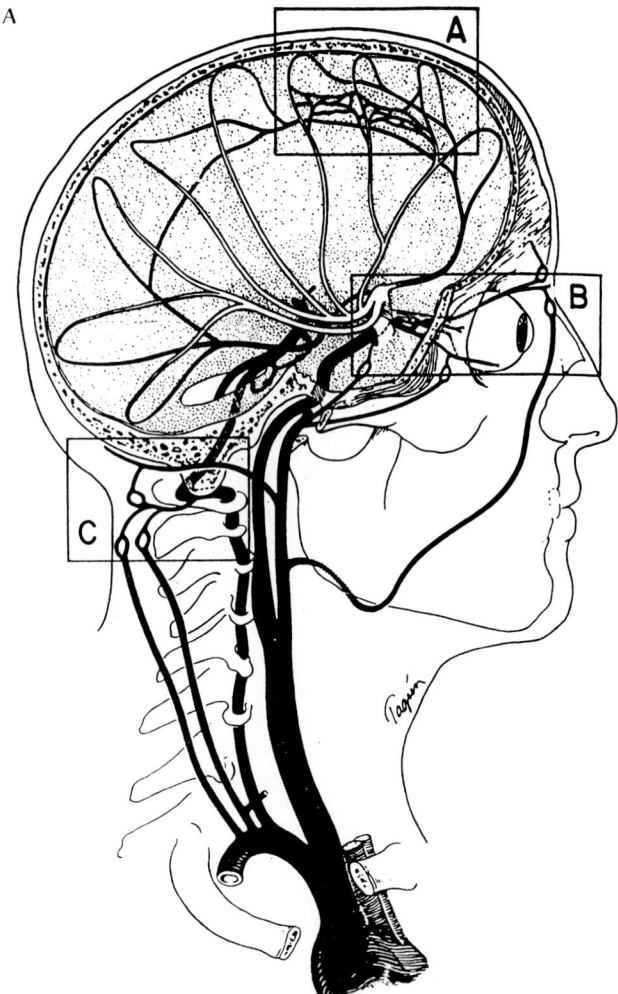

Figure 106-1 (*A*) Arrangement of the major arteries of the right side carrying blood from the heart to the brain. Also shown are vessels of collateral circulation that may modify the effects of cerebral ischemia (A, B, and C). Not shown is the circle of Willis, which also provides a source for collateral circulation. *A.* The anastomotic channels between the distal branches of the anterior and middle cerebral artery, termed borderzone or watershed anastomotic channels. Note that they also occur between the posterior and middle cerebral arteries and the anterior and posterior cerebral arteries. *B.* Anastomotic channels occurring through the orbit between branches of the external carotid artery and ophthalmic branch of the internal carotid artery. *C.* Wholly extracranial anastomotic channels between the muscular branches of the ascending cervical arteries and muscular branches of the occipital artery that anastomose with the distal vertebral artery. Note that the occipital artery arises from the external carotid artery, thereby allowing reconstitution of flow in the vertebral from the carotid circulation. Courtesy of C. M. Fisher, MD.

Willis is incompetent, with one or more of the connecting arteries atretic or functionally inadequate (see Fig. 106-2); in this circumstance, low-flow TIA or stroke may arise from atherothrombosis at the internal carotid artery origin or in its petrous or siphon portions.

Because of the advent of thrombolytic therapy, acute stroke diagnosis and management strategies differ

B

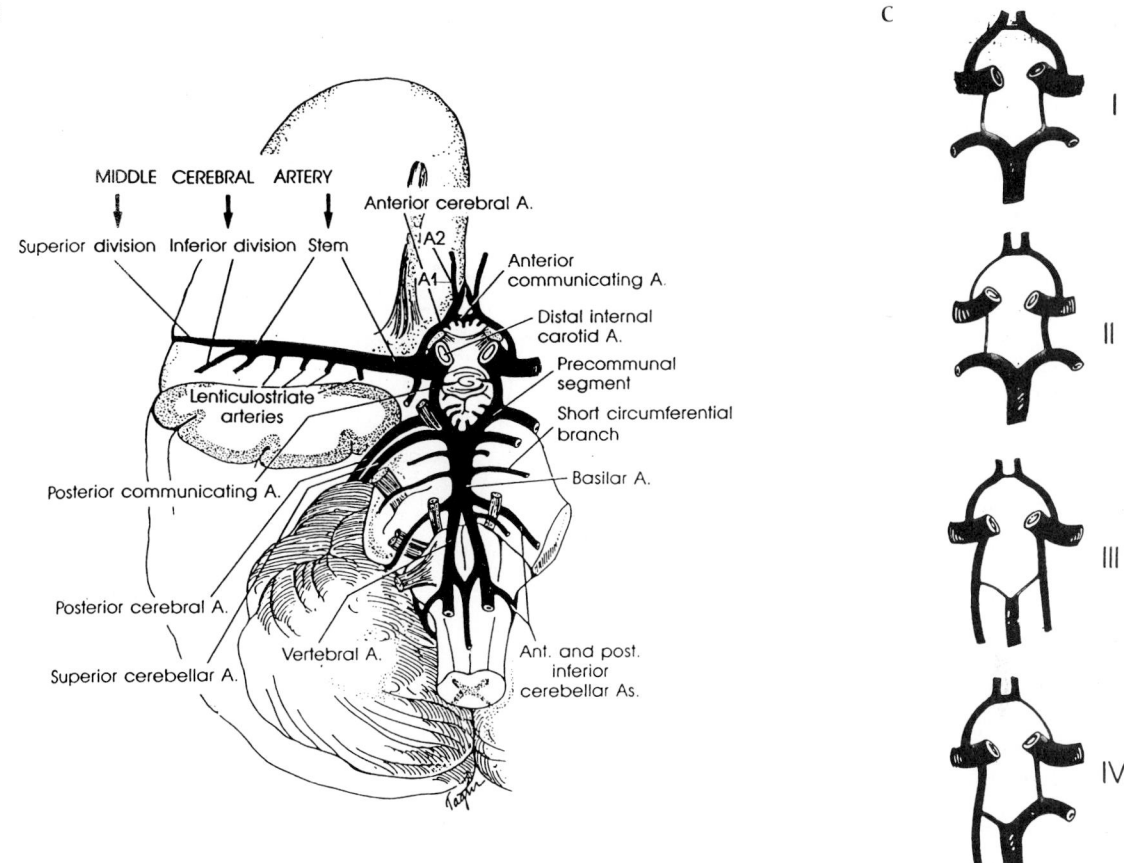

Figure 106-1 (*Continued*) (*B*) Diagram of the brainstem, cerebellum, inferior right frontal lobe, and temporal lobe transected. Principal branches of the vertebral basilar arterial system are pictured. Small branches of the vertebral and basilar artery that penetrate the medulla and pons are not pictured. The stem of the middle cerebral artery with its small, deep-penetrating lenticulostriate arteries and the circle of Willis with its small, deep-penetrating branches, are shown. Roman numerals I, II, III, and IV represent some of the possible variations of the circle of Willis caused by atresia of one or more of its arterial components.

significantly from those for subacute stroke or TIA. Acute treatment strategies for all subtypes of stroke are discussed at the end of the ischemic section. In subacute stroke or TIA, the evaluation and management is best directed in relation to the specific pathophysiologic subtype, as outlined in the sections that follow.

Atherothrombotic disease of the anterior cerebral circulation (origin of the internal carotid artery, its major branches, and the common carotid artery) In this arterial territory, atheroma occurs most often at the bifurcation of the common carotid artery, and usually begins on the posterior wall of the internal carotid artery origin. Most often, such atheroma becomes symptomatic after it has narrowed the lumen by 70 percent, leaving a residual lumen diameter of 1.5 mm—the point where the pressure begins to drop across the stenosis, allowing both embolic or low-flow ischemic TIA and stroke to occur. Embolism from thrombus forming in an ulcerated crater may occur at 50 to 70 percent stenosis, but it is much less common, and very rarely occurs with lesser degrees of stenosis. Embolism can also occur if the atheromatous process occludes the internal carotid artery origin forming a thrombus at the site. At times, the occluding thrombus may also propagate without

embolizing, reaching the ophthalmic artery origin and producing monocular blindness, or extending even more distally to the middle cerebral artery origin and producing a devastating, total, middle cerebral territory stroke.

Low-flow symptoms caused by internal carotid artery origin stenosis occur only if two conditions exist: (1) the lesion has to be hemodynamically significant, that is, severe enough to provoke a drop in pressure across the lesion, which is a situation supervening at a residual lumen diameter ≤1.5 mm; and (2) collateral flow distally through the circle of Willis or external carotid artery ophthalmic routes is inadequate, leading to a low pressure state either in the middle cerebral artery or in one or both of the anterior cerebral arteries. The posterior cerebral artery (PCA) territory may also be vulnerable to low flow when this artery arises directly from the internal carotid artery, that is, a "fetal PCA."

Atheromatous disease in the internal carotid artery siphon occurs less often, but shares the same type of physiologic mechanisms for TIA and stroke. By contrast, middle cerebral stem atheromatous lesions mainly cause low-flow TIA or stroke. Emboli to the middle cerebral artery branches from that source occur less frequently and tend to be small. Common carotid origin stenosis rarely causes

A

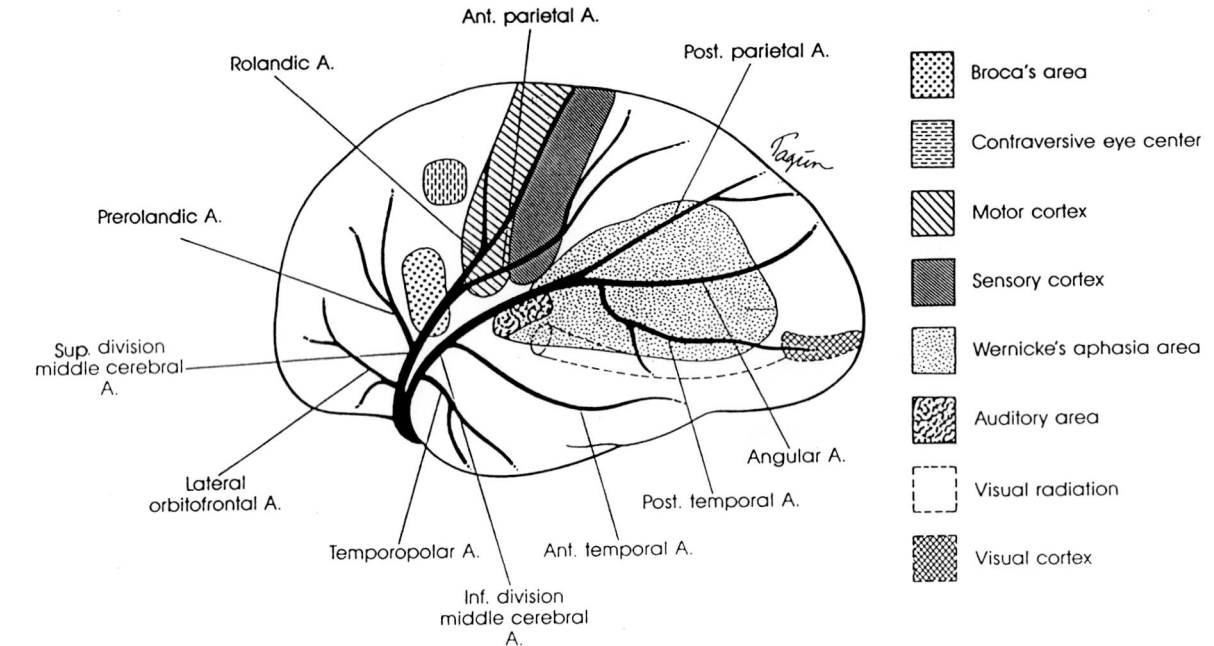

B

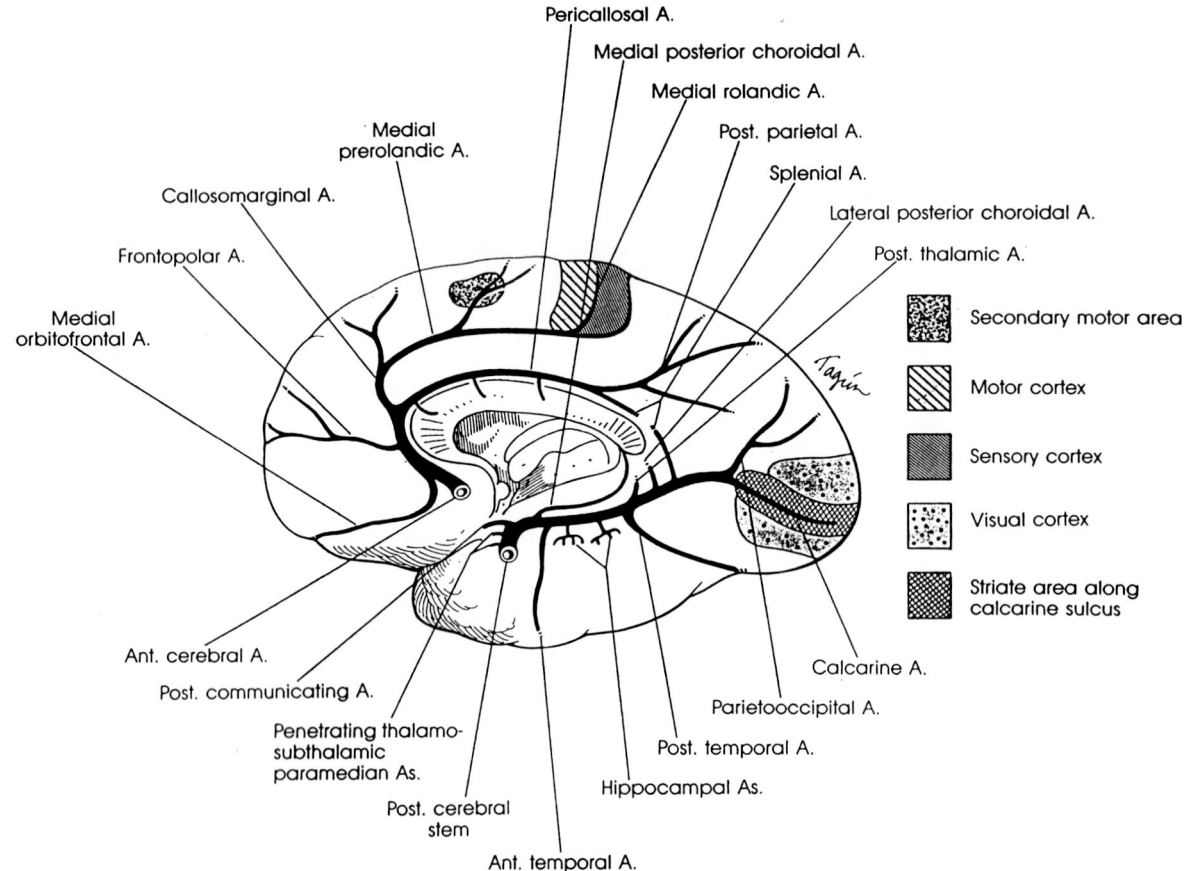

Figure 106-2 (*A*) Diagram of a cerebral hemisphere, lateral aspect, showing the branches and distribution of the middle cerebral artery and the principal regions of cerebral localization. Note the bifurcation of the middle cerebral artery into a superior and inferior division. Courtesy of C. M. Fisher, MD. (*B*) Diagram of a cerebral hemisphere, medial aspect, showing the branches and distribution of the anterior cerebral artery and the principal regions of cerebral localization. Courtesy of C. M. Fisher, MD.

symptoms, but when they occur, they are most commonly caused by embolism to a distal intracranial artery.

The clinical manifestations emanating from each of these atherothrombotic sites depend on the precise location of the ischemia, whether in the territory of the ophthalmic artery, the middle cerebral artery, or the anterior choroidal artery. Transient monocular blurring or blindness, often with a shade lowering or telescopic effect, points to the *ophthalmic artery* territory as the one ischemic.

Middle cerebral artery territory symptoms may conveniently be divided into those involving the stem territory (M1 segment, Fig. 106-2) and those symptoms resulting from ischemia in the superior or inferior territory division or one of their cortical surface branches (see Figs. 106-1 and 106-2). When the stem of the middle cerebral artery is occluded, a complete middle cerebral artery syndrome occurs. It produces a complete hemiplegia equally involving the face, arm, hand, leg, and foot because of the ischemia in the small penetrating (lenticulostriate) arteries that arise from the middle cerebral stems supplying the basal ganglia and internal capsule. Eye deviation toward the ischemic hemisphere occurs when either hemisphere is affected. In addition, ischemia in the upper and lower division cortical surface branches of the middle cerebral artery gives rise to global or partial aphasia (dominant hemisphere) and to neglect and apractognosia (nondominant hemisphere). Partial syndromes occur when emboli occlude the superior or inferior division itself, or one of their branches. Which cortical surface structures are involved depends on the level of occlusion and degree of cortical surface collateral flow (see Fig. 106-1).

Low-flow syndromes occur when the internal carotid artery occlusion is not supported by adequate collateralization distally. They include recurrent transient brief episodes of hip and shoulder weakness, arm and leg weakness, speech trouble, and face or tongue numbness or weakness, many of which are similar, that is, stereotyped. Cortical surface infarcts secondary to low flow tend to occur in the distal field of the middle cerebral artery branches, before they anastomose with the anterior or posterior cerebral artery cortical surface branches, or in the distal field of the lenticulostriate penetrating artery, affecting the deep white matter of the corona radiata. Smaller emboli cause single superior or inferior branch of the middle cerebral artery syndromes, or partial branch syndromes. In the superior division, these might result in unilateral hand, hand and arm, or hand, arm, and shoulder weakness, unilateral face weakness, or difficulty getting words out. Inferior division branch embolic syndromes include difficulty with reading, writing, auditory comprehension of language, or garbled speech with normal motor ability. Paraphasic errors abound in both inferior and superior division syndromes. Visual neglect occurs most noticeably on the left in nondominant syndromes, but may also occur on the right with dominant syndromes.

Anterior cerebral artery   Anterior cerebral arteries divide into two segments: part of the circle of Willis (A1 or stem) and the postcommunal (A2) segment distal to the anterior communicating artery (see Fig. 106-1). The A1 segment gives rise to several deep penetrating arteries that supply the anterior limb of the internal capsule, the anterior

perforate substance, medullar anterior hypothalamus, and posterior part of the head of the caudate nucleus. Infarction in these territories are most often caused by an embolus. If the A2 segments of both right and left anterior cerebral arteries arise from a single anterior cerebral artery A1 segment, symptoms occur in both hemispheres and include bilateral leg weakness. The most common symptoms of A2 segment occlusion are foot and leg weakness, incontinence, and—occasionally, when both A2 segments are affected—abulia; gait apraxia and forced grasping may also occur.

Anterior choroidal artery   This artery arises from the internal carotid artery and supplies the posterior limb of the internal capsule and its posterolateral white matter, through which pass some of the geniculocalcarine fibers. The complete clinical syndrome consists of contralateral hemiparesis, hemianesthesia, and a visual field cut. However, because this territory is also supplied by penetrating vessels of the middle cerebral artery stem and the posterior communicating and posterior choroidal arteries, syndromes with minimal deficits occur and patients frequently recover.

Internal carotid artery   The clinical picture of internal carotid occlusion varies depending on whether the cause of the ischemia is propagated thrombus, embolism, or low flow to the distal intracranial arteries. The middle cerebral artery territory is the most often affected. With a competent circle of Willis, occlusion of the internal carotid artery can be asymptomatic if it does not have an associated embolic or propagated thrombotic component. The symptoms can vary, but are similar to those of the middle or anterior cerebral artery described above. A complete middle cerebral syndrome occurs when it is occluded by thrombus or embolism. Embolic or low-flow TIAs or minor strokes occur with the same symptoms as those mentioned for the middle cerebral artery. Transient monocular blindness as a consequence of ischemia of the ophthalmic territory is also prominent.

Common carotid artery   All of the neurologic symptoms of internal carotid artery stenosis or occlusion can occur with common carotid artery thrombosis or an atherothrombotic lesion occurring at its origin. But the occurrence of transient ischemia or ischemia stroke arising from disease in the common carotid artery is far less than that of the internal carotid artery. Bilateral common carotid occlusions can cause faintness on arising, recurrent loss of consciousness, bilateral dim vision, headache, atrophy of the iris, pericapillary arteriovenous malformations, rubeosis iridis, optic atrophy, and claudication of the jaw muscles. They are associated with an incomplete aortic arch syndrome and have been associated with various combinations of carotid, subclavian, and innominate stenosis or occlusion.

Atherothrombotic disease of the posterior cerebral circulation: vertebrobasilar and posterior cerebral arteries and their branches   As it does in the carotid artery, atherosclerosis has a predilection for certain parts of the posterior circulation–most frequently, the distal vertebral artery and the lower to midbasilar artery (see Fig. 106-1).

Vertebral and posterior inferior cerebellar artery An occlusion of the distal vertebral or its major branch, the posterior inferior cerebellar artery (PICA), is frequently caused by atherothrombosis, but on many occasions, it is caused by an embolus. An occlusion of either artery produces infarction in the lateral medulla, which often causes a TIA or minor stroke before the larger, completed stroke. The symptoms and signs vary, but the most frequent include vertigo, nausea and vomiting, hoarseness, dysphagia, ipsilateral facial numbness associated with impaired sensation of pain and heat over the ipsilateral face and contralateral arm and leg, ipsilateral Horner's syndrome, and ipsilateral limb ataxia. The posterior inferior cerebellar artery also supplies the posterior inferior cerebellum that may become infarcted if collateral circulation from the superior cerebellar artery is inadequate. The infarct resulting from vertebral occlusion does not differ anatomically from that produced by PICA occlusion, except for a greater involvement of the restiform body in the latter. Nevertheless, involvement of the cerebellum does not appreciably alter the clinical picture, except for edema formation which may increase the pressure in the posterior fossa enough to result in progressive obtundation and death; although cerebellar edema can be treated with osmotic agents, that is, mannitol, surgical decompression may be necessary.

Basilar artery TIA usually heralds atherothrombotic basilar artery occlusion and the consequent accompanying devastating brainstem infarction. The symptoms of a TIA in the territory of the distal vertebral and the basilar artery are more varied than in the carotid-middle cerebral territory because of the many different neuronal structures involved. Moreover, brainstem TIAs may be caused by disease either of the small penetrating branches of the basilar or vertebral artery or of the basilar or vertebral arteries themselves. The disease process may be atherothrombotic, involving the proximal origins of these small branch vessels, or lipohyalinotic, involving the small vessels deeper in the brainstem (see "Lacunar or Small Vessel Disease" later in this chapter). In general, small vessel disease is less threatening than disease of the basilar trunk. Therefore, when brainstem TIA or acute stroke occurs, it is extremely important to determine whether the problem lies in the basilar artery or in one of its smaller branches. Disease of a basilar branch usually produces unilateral symptoms of infarction, whereas disease of the basilar artery itself produces bilateral symptoms. Transient dizziness associated with diplopia, dysarthria and numbness around the mouth strongly indicate the presence of basilar insufficiency. Other important symptoms occurring less often include a general profound feeling of weakness of the entire body, staggering and/or a feeling of propulsion. Bilateral signs such as gaze paresis or internuclear ophthalmoplegia associated with ipsilateral sensory loss or weakness signifies ischemic infarction in both sides of the pons—a situation that occlusive disease of a penetrating-artery branch cannot produce. On the other hand, basilar branch disease produces symptoms that refer to only one side of the brainstem. Many such basilar branch syndromes have been described; others await clinical correlation. In both instances, that is, basilar artery proper or its branches, the neurologic deficit may fluctuate, and usually is of low-flow type; artery-to-artery embolic TIA occur, but much less often, usually from embolism to the small basilar branches from a proximal or distal vertebral atheromatous lesion. In the case of an artery-to-artery embolic TIA or minor stroke, the events are single and tend not to fluctuate.

Major basilar branches: anterior inferior cerebellar artery, superior cerebellar artery, posterior cerebral artery These major artery branches of the basilar artery produce their own distinct pathophysiologic syndromes. They are most often caused by artery-to-artery embolism from an atherothrombotic source, that is, the proximal basilar artery or the proximal or distal vertebral artery. Less often, an aortic or cardiogenic source is found. Rarely, primary atherothrombotic occlusion at their origins is the cause of the stroke or TIA.

Superior cerebellar artery Occlusion of the superior cerebellar artery results in one or more of the following symptoms: ipsilateral cerebellar ataxia (middle and/or upper cerebellar peduncle, or dentate nucleus), nausea and vomiting, dysarthria and contralateral loss of pain and temperature sensation over the extremities, body and face (spinal and trigeminal thalamic tract), and ataxic tremor of the ipsilateral upper extremity. Horner's syndrome, partial deafness, and palatal myoclonus may occur rarely. Partial syndromes occur frequently.

Anterior inferior cerebellar artery Occlusion of the anterior inferior cerebellar artery produces variable degrees of infarction because the size of this artery varies inversely with that of the posterior inferior cerebellar artery. The territory it supplies usually includes the lateral midpons, middle cerebellar peduncle, and cerebellum. The principal symptoms include ipsilateral deafness, facial weakness, vertigo (whirling dizziness), nausea, vomiting, nystagmus, tinnitus, cerebellar ataxia, Horner's syndrome, and paresis of conjugate lateral gaze. The opposite side of the body loses pain and temperature sensation. An occlusion close to the origin of the artery may cause cortical spinal tract signs.

Paramedian and short circumferential branches Occlusion of one of the 5 to 7 short circumferential branches of the basilar artery effects the lateral two-thirds of the pons and/or middle or superior cerebellar peduncle, whereas occlusion of one of the 7 to 10 paramedian branches of the basilar artery effects a wedge-shaped area on either side of the medial pons. Many brainstem syndromes with cranial nerve abnormalities and crossed hemiplegia have been given eponyms; others await description.

Posterior cerebral artery Arising from the bifurcation of the top of the basilar artery, each posterior cerebral artery divides into two segments, each with its distinct clinical pathophysiologic syndrome. (1) The proximal precommunal segment beginning at the top of the basilar artery and going to the posterior communicating artery takeoff gives penetrating branches to the subthalamus, thalamus, and midbrain. (2) The postcommunal segment supplies the medial inferior temporal lobe and the medial occipital lobe distally. Twenty percent of the time, one or both of the right or left posterior cerebral artery precommunal (P1) segments are atretic. The postcommunal (P2) segment is then supplied by the internal carotid artery via the posterior communicating artery. The majority of ischemic syndromes, TIA, or stroke, result from embolism (artery-to-artery, cardioaortic, or unknown source) to the pre- and postcommunal segments and/or one of their branches. Primary atherothrombotic disease of the posterior cerebral artery is much less common.

Precommunal posterior cerebral artery syndromes include midbrain, subthalamic, and thalamic signs that vary depending on whether the embolus occludes the top of the basilar area, the right or left posterior cerebral artery precommunal segment, that is, the stem, or the penetrating artery branch of the precommunal segment. Coma and quadriplegia result from a top of the basilar occlusion that is devastating. But branch syndromes abound otherwise, usually with third nerve and contralateral motor or sensory findings. At the very top of the basilar artery, a single large medial mesencephalic artery, the artery of Percheron, penetrates upward to supply both sides of the subthalamus as well as part of the midbrain. The resulting syndrome is one of bilateral ptosis, paralysis of upgaze, and sleepiness caused by involvement of the periaqueductal gray and the mesencephalic reticular formation. When only a single penetrating precommunal artery territory is involved, small vessel lacunar disease results (see "Lacunar or Small Vessel Disease" later in this chapter).

Postcommunal posterior cerebral artery syndromes include cortical branches to the medial inferior temporal lobe, giving rise to memory loss and delirium, and branches to the medial occipital lobe, giving rise to homonymous visual field defects. Distal field border zone ischemia of the posterior cerebral and middle cerebral arteries give rise to visual impairment syndromes that include inability to recognize faces or pictures or to put items in a picture together to form an object (Balint's syndrome).

Lacunar or Small Vessel Disease

As defined by C. Miller Fisher through fastidious brainstem serial section, lacunar infarct results from an occlusion of a small single penetrating artery arising from the circle of Willis, the middle cerebral stem, the basilar artery or either distal vertebral arteries. It is caused by a lipohyalinotic narrowing or occlusion in the mid-distal part of the artery, or by an atherothrombotic lesion at its origin; embolism is rarely the cause. So-called lacunar strokes account for 25 percent of all strokes in the National Institutes of Health Stroke Data Bank. These penetrating arteries vary in size from 100 to 400 microns in diameter, rendering the infarct size finite from 0.5 cm to 1.5 cm in diameter, and usually no more than 3 cm long. These infarcts cause recognizable clinical syndromes that evolve over hours to days, and may be preceded by transient symptoms (lacunar TIAs). The location of the ischemia determines the nature and severity of the symptoms. Recovery occurs often within days, but in some with especially strategically placed infarcts, significant disability is persistent.

The most common lacunar syndromes are the following:

- *Pure motor hemiparesis* from an infarct in the posterior limb of the internal capsule or basis pontis. The face, arm, leg, foot, and toes are equally paretic or plegic, but with no sensory deficit. The weakness may be intermittent (TIA), progress in a stepwise manner, or appear abruptly. The progression may result in a complete hemiplegia. Improvement almost to normal occurs in many cases.
- *Pure sensory stroke* from an infarct in the ventrolateral thalamus. This type of infarct produces face, arm, and leg sensory involvement with numbness, tingling, and loss of pain and temperature. The patient generally recovers but often is left with a sensory sensation that is abnormal. On rare occasions, an intolerable pain syndrome with dysesthesia occurs in the involved extremities some months afterwards (Dejerine–Roussy syndrome).
- *Ataxic hemiparesis* from an infarct in the basis pontis or dysarthria and *clumsy hand/arm syndrome* caused by an infarct in the basis pontis or corona radiata near the genu of the internal capsule.
- *Pure motor hemiparesis with aphemia* caused by lacunar infarctions of the genu and anterior limb of the internal capsule and adjacent corona radiata white matter. (Aphemia is loss of the ability to recognize what one is saying.)

Before antihypertensive therapy, multiple lacunar infarctions often occurred in a single patient, producing bilateral pyramidal and corticobulbar motor system signs, dysarthria, and a slowed abulic mental state with emotional lability, that is, pseudobulbar palsy.

Careful attention to antihypertensive, diabetic, and dyslipidemic therapies offer the best form of prevention. In all lacunar stroke or TIA, it is essential to ascertain that the large arteries at the base of the brain giving rise to the penetrating small arteries, that is, the basilar artery, the middle cerebral artery stem, or the posterior cerebral artery stem, are not, in themselves, harboring a thrombus threatening their occlusion and causing the lacunar syndrome (see Evaluation and Therapeutic Strategies below).

Embolic Stroke/TIA Subtype

In this pathophysiologic stroke subtype, the embolic fragment occluding the intracranial vessel leading to the ischemia or infarction did not arise from an extra- or intracranial atherothrombotic arterial source or dissection, but rather derived from the aortic arch, the heart, or an unknown source (cryptogenic stroke).

Embolic strokes are diagnosed when a sudden or stuttering neurologic deficit appears in the territory of a large intracranial artery at the base of the brain or in one of its major branches, and the extra- or intracranial arterial supply to the ischemic zone does not have a detectable thick stenotic or thrombotic occlusive lesion as detected by ultrasonography, MRI, or CT angiographic imaging. While an embolic fragment may be seen to occlude the vessel or a distal branch, often the suspected embolic material lyses and migrates before it can be detected within the vessel. When this definition is used, embolic stroke accounts for fully 60 percent of all strokes in the NIH Stroke Databank. It is most convenient to divide these types of emboli into treatment categories. First, those commonly accepted cardiac source emboli where antithrombotic therapy is standard of practice. Second, commonly accepted cardiac source emboli where antithrombotic therapy is contraindicated, as in bacterial endocarditis. Third, those possible cardioaortic sources that can only be diagnosed by transthoracic echocardiogram or transesophageal echocardiogram, in which debate exists as to the best therapy, be it antithrombotic, antiplatelet, or cardio-interventional. Fourth, those truly cryptogenic strokes in which a possible or definite cardiac and aortic source is excluded (Table 106-1). With all of the source categories above, the level of activity of the hemostatic system may be a significant determinant in the incidence of local thrombus formation and embolism. Therefore, in addition to careful evaluation of the heart, evaluation of the hemostatic system and exclusion of a primary arterial source of embolism is essential in order to plan appropriate pathophysiologic-based treatment.

The clinical presentation of embolism in the anterior and posterior cerebral circulation is similar to that of artery-to-artery embolism where a primary extra- or intracranial arterial source is detected as the cause. The nature and severity of the symptoms depends entirely on the location of the embolic fragment occluding the artery and the spared collateral circulation to its cerebral territory. The artery occluded, in turn, depends on the size of the embolic fragment and the extracranial artery it enters. In the case of an embolic fragment ending in the vertebral artery, it may migrate, stop, and then migrate again, leaving a trail of infarcted tissue from the cerebellum and lower brainstem to the upper brainstem, thalamus, and temporal and occipital lobes. Embolic fragments that enter the middle cerebral stem often disperse to branches of the superior and inferior division of the middle cerebral artery, giving rise to a patchy infarct in the deep or basal lenticulostriate arterial territory, and in the cortical surface branch territories.

In every case of embolic stroke, embolism from an infected heart valve should be considered because of the devastating consequences if not detected. Subacute bacterial endocarditis may have a very subtle presentation. A normal erythrocyte sedimentation rate at the time of the initial evaluation is a quick means of excluding it.

Other Causes of Cerebral Infarction

Although other causes of cerebral infarction account for only 3 percent of all stroke in the NIH Stroke Databank, they are extremely important because their precise pathophysiologic diagnosis can lead to effective treatment.

Dissection of the cervical cerebral arteries is, by far, the most common cause of stroke in this category subtype.

Table 106-1 Embolic Stroke Classification

I. **Cardiac source is definite**: antithrombotic therapy generally considered standard of practice.
  1. Left ventricular thrombi
  2. Left atrial thrombi
  3. Rheumatic valvular disease
  4. Mechanical prosthetic valves
  5. Bioprosthetic heart valves
  6. Atrial fibrillation*
  7. Nonbacterial thrombotic endocarditis

II. **Cardiac source is definite**: anticoagulation considered hazardous.
  1. Bacterial endocarditis
  2. Atrial myxoma

III. **Cardiac source is possible**: synonyms in the literature include "unknown source," "cryptogenic stroke"—these diagnoses are made by transthoracic or transesophageal echocardiogram. The efficacy of antiplatelet versus antithrombotic therapy is unknown.
  1. Mitral annular calcification
  2. Left ventricular dysfunction and dilated cardiomyopathy
  3. Status postmyocardial infarction with and without left ventricular aneurysm or thrombi
  4. Left atrial spontaneous echo contrast
  5. Patent foramen ovale
  6. Atrioseptal aneurysm
  7. Valvular strands

IV. **Ascending aortic atheromatous disease**: mobile plaque 4 mm or greater.

V. **Truly unknown source embolic stroke.**

*Antithrombotic therapy efficacy proven by randomized trial.

Generally, dissection begins at the point where the internal carotid artery enters the petrous bone, or in the vertebral artery, as it transverses the foramen transversarium. The dissections divide the media or the media and intima, and clot forms in the division. The lumen may be compromised or occluded and thrombus may form in it if the dissection ruptures into the lumen or if it occludes. Trauma, either severe or trivial, is often the cause, but Valsalva maneuvers with coughing and vomiting, and weight-lifting or chiropractic manipulations are other associations. Spontaneous dissections are not uncommon. Dissections occur at all ages, but are a frequent cause of stroke in school-age children or young adults. The clinical hallmark of carotid dissection is a Horner's syndrome, which occurs in 50 percent of instances. Cervical pain, or pain behind the eye, occurs frequently. Carotid artery-to-artery embolism or low-flow infarction syndromes occur, just as they do for atherothrombotic disease of the internal carotid artery. Similar pathophysiologic circumstances exist for vertebral artery dissections; with them, cervical spine pain is the suggestive symptom. The most common site of infarction in vertebral dissection is the lateral medulla, with or without concomitant involvement of a posterior cerebral artery territory. Dizziness, ataxia of gait, nausea and vomiting with a unilateral Horner's syndrome, and ipsilateral face numbness with contralateral body numbness are the hallmark symptoms. Occasionally, diplopia and a hoarse voice are evident. Artery-to-artery emboli arising from a thrombus at the site of dissection in the vertebral artery may migrate to distal branches of the basilar artery, producing brainstem, cerebellar, or thalamic infarction. Although not proven by randomized clinical trial, our experience suggests intravenous heparin acutely, followed by 4 to 6 months of antithrombotic therapy (warfarin, international normalized ratio [INR] 2 to 3), is helpful in preventing recurrent or worsening stroke.

Fibromuscular dysplasia occurs in the extracranial carotid artery. On angiography, it looks like a ruffled sock. It is rarely symptomatic unless it becomes hemodynamically significant; then, both embolic or low-flow TIA or stroke can occur. Generally, antiplatelet therapy is used for prevention, but no clinical trial evidence exists in its support. Antithrombotic therapy and interventional arterial therapy are possible options after symptoms have occurred.

Arteritis caused by bacterial or syphilitic infection is no longer a common cause of cerebral thrombosis. Other arteritides are rare, but can cause cerebral thrombosis. Necrotizing granulomatous arteritis, occurring alone or in association with polyarteritis nodosa or Wegener's granulomatosis, involves the distal small branches (less than 2 mm diameter) of the main intracranial arteries and produces small ischemic infarcts in the brain, optic nerve, and spinal cord. The disease, although rare, is relentlessly progressive. Often, there is cerebrospinal fluid pleocytosis. In some cases, glucocorticoid therapy (prednisone, 40 to 60 mg/d) has been helpful, as has immunosuppressive therapy (e.g., cyclophosphamide). Idiopathic giant cell arteritis involving the great vessels arising from the aortic arch (Takayasu's syndrome) may, on occasion, cause carotid or vertebral thrombosis; nevertheless, it is an infrequent cause of the aortic arch syndrome in the western hemisphere.

Temporal arteritis (cranial arteritis)   This is a relatively common affliction of elderly persons, in which the external carotid system—particularly the temporal arteries—is the site of a subacute granulomatous infiltration with an exudate of lymphocytes, monocytes, neutrophilic leukocytes, and giant cells. Usually, the most severely affected parts of the artery become thrombosed. Headache or facial pain is the chief complaint. The inflammatory nature of the illness is indicated by one or more of the following: fever, slight leukocytosis, increased erythrocyte sedimentation rate, and anemia. Systemic manifestations include anorexia, loss of weight, malaise and polymyalgia rheumatica. Occlusion of the branches of the ophthalmic artery results in blindness of one or both eyes. Occasionally an ophthalmoplegia caused by involvement of extrinsic ocular muscles occurs. In some cases, an arteritis of the aorta and its major branches, including the carotids, subclavian, coronary, and femoral arteries, has been found at postmortem examination. Significant inflammatory involvement of the intracranial arteries is rare, but strokes occur occasionally on the basis of occlusion of the internal carotid, middle cerebral, or vertebral arteries. The diagnosis depends on the finding of a tender thrombosed or thickened cranial artery and demonstration of the lesion in a biopsy specimen. The hallmark symptom is transient blindness. When that occurs in patients older than age 50 years, a sedimentation rate with a fibrinogen level and complete blood count should be done urgently. Corticosteroids may bring striking relief and prevent blindness. Prednisone is most often used, beginning with large daily doses of 80 to 100 mg/d and then tapering over 2 to 4 weeks using the sedimentation rate as a guide.

Moyamoya disease   Moyamoya disease is a poorly understood occlusive disorder involving large intracranial arteries, especially the distal internal carotid artery, and the stem of the middle cerebral artery, as well as the anterior cerebral artery. The lenticulostriate arteries develop a rich collateral network around the middle cerebral occlusive lesion giving the impression of a puff of smoke on cerebral angiography. Other collaterals include transdural anastomoses between the cortical surface branches of the middle cerebral artery and the scalp arteries. The disease mainly occurs in the Oriental population, but should be suspected when TIAs or stroke occur in children or young adults. Its etiology is unknown. There have been few pathologic studies; they suggest that hyalinotic fibrous type material is associated with the arterial narrowing and microaneurysm formation. The best treatment is not known. Although no formal study has been performed to determine the optimal treatment of patients with symptoms of ischemia or infarction, steroids, aspirin, or ticlopidine, and, occasionally, vasodilators, have been used because of the occurrence of hemorrhage (both intraparenchymal and subarachnoid) from rupture of the small, fragile anastomotic channels, or from rupture of the microaneurysms occurring in the perforating arteries from the circle of Willis. Anticoagulation is not recommended in all symptomatic cases, but rather on a case-by-case basis. In the case of hemorrhage, of course, hematoma evacuation and ventricular drainage are indicated. A variety of surgical revascularization procedures have been proposed: cervical sympathectomy, omentum transplantation, superficial temporal artery–middle cerebral artery bypass, or encephaloduroarteriosynangiosis (EDAS), but the efficacy of these treatments has not been established.

Reversible cerebral segmental vasoconstriction Reversible, widespread segmental vasoconstriction has been noted in patients with severe headache and fluctuating neurologic symptoms and signs. Occasionally, cerebral infarction has ensued. The etiology is unknown. Eclampsia, the postpartum period, head injury, migraine, and sympathomimetic intoxication are all associated with this entity. Conventional contrast angiography is the only definitive means of establishing the diagnosis. Cerebrospinal fluid is normal in most cases, but an elevated protein and a slight lymphocytic pleocytosis has been found in some cases. No effective therapy is known. Maintenance of normal systemic arterial pressure or even increasing it modestly with adequate hydration seems important on empirical grounds. Glucocorticoids and vasodilators such as a calcium channel blocking agent or intravenous nitroglycerin might be considered.

Cerebral autosomal dominant arteriopathy with subcortical infarcts and leukoencephalopathy syndrome Cerebral autosomal dominant arteriopathy with subcortical infarcts and leukoencephalopathy (CADASIL) is a rare primary arteriolopathy affecting cerebral white matter medullary vessels. The typical clinical symptom complex includes late-onset migraine with aura, recurrent stroke and/or TIAs, neuropsychiatric problems such as depression, bipolar disease, or subcortical dementia with pseudobulbar features occurring in persons between 40 and 50 years of age. Cerebrospinal fluid examination and cerebral angiography are normal. There is no specific treatment to date. Cerebral, leptomeningeal, or skin biopsy with electromicroscopic demonstration of typical osmophilic granular deposits in or around the vascular smooth muscle cells of the tunica media and basal lamina matrix are diagnostic. Recently, a specific genetic defect was identified in the Notch-3 gene in chromosome 19q.13.1; it may be possible in the near future to screen family members at risk.

Binswanger's subcortical leukoencephalopathy An unusual disorder related to small-vessel hypertensive disease, chronically progressive, and associated with a particular type of demyelination, Binswanger's disease usually produces diffuse vascular lesions in the subcortical layers of the cerebral hemispheres. Usually affecting individuals around 50 years of age, it is characterized by fluctuations in mood and consciousness, perhaps even seizures; a dementia may be an early and prominent symptom preceded or accompanied by symptoms and signs of one or more small vessel infarctions. Confusional states, memory difficulties, and abulia are prominent, and sometimes accompanied by focal cortical–subcortical deficits such as aphasia, apraxia, or neglect. Focal neurologic deficits, or uni- or bilateral limb signs may lead to a pseudobulbar state; gait difficulties are prominent. There is often evidence of vascular compromise in other body districts.

Binswanger's disease must be differentiated from disorders with prominent subcortical white matter involvement on CT or MRI; these include hypertensive encephalopathy, cerebral amyloid (congophilic) angiopathy, CADASIL, normal pressure hydrocephalus, and Alzheimer's disease.

Evaluation

The initial history and physical is the hallmark of the evaluation to obtain a presumed pathophysiologic stroke or TIA subtype diagnosis. The initial electrocardiogram and blood work should include a sedimentation rate and C-reactive protein as a screen for subacute bacterial endocarditis. In addition, the standard complete blood count, platelet count, and general chemistry examination is essential. None of those laboratory assessments should interfere with the urgent timing of neuroimaging and ultrasound studies. The history and physical examination suggesting the presumed pathophysiologic diagnosis that includes the presumed arterial cause, that is, the status of the parent vessel supplying the ischemic territory, should be urgently confirmed. Special clotting studies are not essential urgently, but are often helpful prior to any therapeutic intervention. They are extremely helpful in patients with suspected embolic stroke. They include not only the standard partial thromboplastin time, prothrombin time, INR and platelet count, but also protein C, protein S, and antithrombin 3. In addition, detection of antiphospholipid antibodies, factor V Leiden mutation, and prothrombin gene polymorphism, are of probable importance. The screen of thyroid function with a thyroid stimulating hormone has helped us in identifying a clinically inapparent hyperthyroidism, a condition that may be associated with atrial fibrillation and embolism. In the initial blood evaluation, cardiac enzymes are also essential to rule out an associated myocardial infarction.

Urgent confirmation of the arterial pathology is essential but, in many smaller hospitals, neither CT angiography nor carotid or transcranial Doppler carotid ultrasonography are readily available. In that situation, a plain brain CT scan is essential to rule out hemorrhage prior to the institution of thrombolytic, antithrombotic and/or antiplatelet therapy.

In those institutions where it is possible to evaluate the parent vessel arterial supply to the ischemic zone, the following neuroimaging and neurosonology studies are considered.

CT or CT angiography is an extremely rapid, accurate way of identifying the pathology in the parent vessel from the origin of the aortic arch to the ischemic zone distal to the great vessels at the base of the brain (vessels shown in Fig. 106-1B). The perfusion time of dye injected to obtain a CT angiogram can give clues as to the size of the ischemic zone. The CT scan alone has difficulty in identifying acute infarction prior to the first 12 hours. In addition, CT scanning may miss a small cortical surface embolic infarct or one in the cerebellum or brainstem because of the approximation of the bones of the skull. Such infarcts may be identifiable only by MRI imaging.

MRI or MRA (magnetic resonance angiography) is the best way of identifying infarcts accurately in terms of their extent and location. Susceptibility sequences identify subacute hemorrhagic infarcts and areas of hemorrhage that might be associated with amyloid angiopathy not otherwise identifiable. Areas of ischemia without infarction, especially supratentorially, may be identified with the use of gadolinium and the proper MRI pulse sequences. MRA, especially when enhanced with gadolinium, can outline the parent vessel pathology from the arch all the way through to the branches of the major vessels at the base of the brain. The disadvantage of MRI imaging is the time it takes for the scan to be obtained. In addition, because of the small head diameter of the imaging system, there is a significant claustrophobic effect in approximately 10 percent of patients. These disadvantages decrease its efficacy in hyperacute stroke state, where the most urgent issue is elucidating the nature of the arterial pathology of the parent vessel leading to the ischemic infarct and the exclusion of hemorrhages, tasks CT and CT angiogram perform admirably.

Neurosonology tests include *carotid duplex Doppler* and *transcranial Doppler* assessment of the extra- and intracranial arterial system. *Carotid duplex Doppler* allows assessment of flow at the bifurcation of the common carotid artery, including flow in the proximal internal carotid artery; in addition, flow in the middle portion of the vertebral artery can be assessed to identify more proximal or distal obstructive lesions. *Transcranial Doppler* allows assessment of flow of the intracranial carotid artery and flow in the ophthalmic artery through the transorbital approach. The transtemporal approach permits assessment of flow in the middle, anterior, and posterior cerebral artery stems. The occipital foramen magnum approach easily and reliably allows determination flow in the distal vertebral artery and in the basilar artery. These ultrasound studies allow for immediate evaluation of the stroke or TIA presumed subtype and are important in all four stroke subtypes. They can identify the presence and severity of an obstructive lesion in the parent vessel as well as identify the presence of collateral flow to the ischemic zone. Their disadvantage is that, on some occasions, the parent vessel of interest escapes examination. Nevertheless, in atherothrombotic stroke, often the severity and location of the atherothrombotic parent vessel lesion and the nature of the spared collateral flow can be identified. In addition, in an embolic stroke, migration and lysis of an embolism in a parent vessel can be noted by detecting normal flow in that vessel. In lacunar small-vessel stroke, the diagnosis can be supported by the identification of normal flow in the parent vessel to the penetrating artery that is suspected of being occluded. In dissection of the carotid or vertebral artery extracranially, obstruction of flow proximally in the vessel can be identified if the dissection is severe enough to affect flow distally. In cases of temporal arteritis, the pathology can be suspected by duplex ultrasound of the temporal area. These neurosonology tests allow for ease in following these arterial lesions in terms of their progression or resolution. These tests have the advantage of being simple, can be used by the physician similar to the cardiologist's stethoscope examination, and are highly portable. We use these tests to identify acutely the suspected problem, but always confirm with neuroimaging studies. We then use these tests to follow the progression of the arterial pathology subacutely and chronically. The quantification of carotid artery atheromatous disease and its progression is an especially important use of carotid duplex Doppler combined with transcranial Doppler.

Cardiac Evaluation

Cardiac evaluation, in addition to an electrocardiogram, cardiac enzymes, and sedimentation rate acutely obtained, should include, on a subacute basis, cardiac ultrasonography and cardiac monitoring when an embolic stroke is considered in the differential diagnosis. That would, therefore, include lacunar strokes in addition to embolic strokes. Echocardiography generally starts with transthoracic echocardiogram but, in cases where the diagnosis is not obvious, transesophageal echocardiogram is considered, especially when the obvious diagnostic source is important in deciding a precise preventive treatment. Contrast echocardiography or contrast transcranial Doppler ultrasonography can easily identify patients who have a patent foramen ovale. Cardiac monitoring on a portable basis is very helpful if atrial fibrillation or other cardiogenic arrhythmias are to be considered. Only then can precise therapeutic preventive strategies be planned.

Therapeutic Strategies

With the acute onset of neurologic deficits suggesting ischemia, the essential therapeutic goal is to prevent worsening and to try to facilitate or reestablish blood flow to the ischemic zone. The therapeutic strategy should always be guided by pathophysiology, whether presumed (history and physical) or confirmed (history, physical, and positive neuroimaging or neurosonology confirmatory diagnostic study). The diagnosis should include not only one of the four stroke or TIA subtypes noted earlier, but also the presence or absence of pathology in the parent vessel supplying the ischemic zone and the extent of the spared collateral flow to it. The time of onset to treatment determines the therapeutic options. Three phases exist: (1) the hyperacute (1 to 3 hours)–acute (3 to 12 hours) phase; (2) the subacute phase; and (3) the preventive phase.

Hyperacute/Acute

In this hyperacute/acute phase, the goal is to open the occluded parent artery. Obviously, knowledge as to whether or not it is occluded and where the occlusion lies, is essential before proceeding. But, in many hospital situations, this is not possible in the first 3 hours. In that setting, intravenous thrombolysis with recombinant tissue-type plasminogen activator (rt-PA) is acceptable practice, but only if CT scanning excludes hemorrhage at the time of the onset of the deficit. This approach meets the criteria set up by the NIH-sponsored tissue plasminogen activator (t-PA) trial. Intravenous t-PA has not been approved for suspected stroke that is more than 3 hours old or if the stroke is noted on the CT scan as an infarct. Occasionally in this setting, if a basilar or middle cerebral stem clot is suspected, intravenous t-PA is given and the patient is rapidly transported to a facility in which intraarterial thrombolysis is considered. This therapy is not proven effective by randomized trial design, although both the PROACT (Prolyse in Acute Cerebral Thromboembolism) and the EMS (Emergency Management of Stroke) bridging trials demonstrated better angiographic recanalization in the treatment groups. Thus, intraarterial thrombolysis applied with alacrity in the first 3 hours (for the middle cerebral stem) or 12 hours (in the case of a basilar clot) benefits some patients, sparing them from what would have been a devastating, major middle cerebral or basilar territory stroke. In all instances where thrombolytic therapy is considered, whether it be intravenous or intraarterial, severe hemorrhagic complications are a possible outcome. Therefore, the stroke severity and the therapeutic gain anticipated by the physician should be sufficient to warrant the treatment risks.

Intraarterial thrombolysis is occasionally considered for patients with a basilar thrombus up to 12 hours because in the posterior circulation, particularly the brainstem and cerebellum, a rich collateralization can sustain the ischemic brain without infarcting, for longer periods of time. Intraarterial or intravenous thrombolysis supratentorially in the anterior circulation from 3 to 6 hours after symptom onset is also occasionally attempted, but its efficacy remains to be established.

Intravenous heparin is also associated with hemorrhagic complications, but it may be safer. Theoretically, it is meant to stop clot propagation, but not lyse it. Its efficacy has not been proven by randomized trial. Heparin is generally considered after the decision has been made whether or not to use IV t-PA. The rationale for giving it is to stop clot propagation in the parent vessel, that is, the occluded vessel causing the ischemia. It is also given to prevent further artery-to-artery embolization or cardiac embolization. Four therapeutic settings apply regarding intravenous heparin. First, large-vessel atherothrombotic disease to prevent clot propagation from the atherothrombotic locus, or to prevent further embolization from the atherothrombotic site. Second, embolic stroke from a cardiac or aortic source where the embolus remains in the stem of the middle cerebral artery, the internal carotid artery or the basilar artery, that is, one of the parent vessels, and the deficit is submaximal, that is, the deficit could worsen if the embolus propagates as a thrombus. Third, in lacunar stroke, it is occasionally given when the motor weakness is relentlessly progressive. Its efficacy has not been very high in this setting in our hands. Fourth, it is of benefit in patients who have dissections or sinovenous thrombosis; only in the latter setting has the efficacy of heparin been proven in a randomized trial.

Subacute

The subacute phase signifies that intravenous or intraarterial thrombolysis is no longer an option. Heparin is the therapeutic option, for the reasons outlined above. But heparin's therapeutic efficacy has not been established by randomized trial design as has rt-PA. We use it for the indications stated above, but the individual physician must decide on a case by case basis. We avoid heparin use if the infarction is deep in the basal ganglia, that is, the territory of the lenticulostriate arteries, because of the higher rate

of hemorrhagic complications when the infarct is in this location.

Surgical therapeutic options can be considered in this subacute phase. Urgent carotid endarterectomy may be considered if the patient has a severe carotid stenosis with an inadequate collateral supply through the circle of Willis or the external carotid artery ophthalmic system. In this setting, the resultant low-flow stroke can be devastating, while emergency endarterectomy can be highly effective. Carotid endarterectomy for mild to moderate stroke or TIA in the territory of the internal carotid artery has also been proven effective, this by randomized trial design (the North American Symptomatic Carotid Endarterectomy Trial [NASCET] study). But severe stroke in the middle cerebral artery territory in which further worsening would only be minimal, that is, the deficit is almost maximal, is not appropriate for endarterectomy in the subacute phase. If the patient improves in rehabilitation to the point where worsening of the deficit would be problematic, then endarterectomy can be reconsidered. If low-flow stroke is not the issue, surgery can be planned in patients with mild to moderate deficits on an elective basis after careful consideration of the cardiomedical status. The surgical morbidity should be no greater than 2 percent for surgery to be considered efficacious.

The only other surgical therapeutic option in this subacute phase is that of hemicraniectomy. That is considered in the nondominant hemisphere when cerebral edema progresses to the point where it will worsen the deficit and/or lead to death. The patient is generally young enough to make a reasonable recovery that would allow the dominant hemisphere to function well and the patient to have good language-dependent behavior.

Preventive

There are two important aspects of preventive therapy. First, the control and prevention strategies related to the primary risk factors for all stroke subtypes and, second, preventive strategies directed toward the specific stroke or TIA subtype in the particular patient.

Preventive strategies for controlling primary risk factors
Treatment of hypertension is, by far, the most important aspect of risk factor control. Angiotensin-converting enzyme (ACE) inhibitors are especially helpful in this regard because of their association with myocardial infarction (MI) and stroke prevention in large trials. Control of lipids are also important. Following the Third Report of the National Cholesterol Education Program Expert Panel on Detection, Evaluation, and Treatment of High Blood Cholesterol in Adults (ATPIII) guidelines for prevention of MI, the primary goal is lowering the LDL. Risk factor adjustment including diet, exercise, weight reduction, cessation of smoking, and diabetes management are all important first steps. Hydroxymethylglutaryl coenzyme A (HMG-CoA) reductase inhibitors ("statins") are also associated with MI reduction, as well as with stroke-risk reduction. Attention to homocysteine metabolism and B-vitamin metabolism is helpful in the prevention of early atherothrombosis, and may possibly be helpful in the prevention of embolism. Homocysteine levels and folic acid levels should be checked

on a fasting basis and the proper B-vitamins given. Antioxidants, in particular vitamin E, may not be helpful, and could interfere with the beneficial effects of LDL reduction on HDL metabolism.

Preventive therapy directed toward the specific stroke/TIA subtype Therapy directed toward preventing the specific stroke subtypes consists of two aspects: (1) antiplatelet versus antithrombotic therapy and (2) surgical strategies.

Antithrombotic versus antiplatelet therapy Antithrombotic therapy is accepted as standard of practice in the cardiac conditions outlined in Table 106-1; but only in the case of atrial fibrillation has this treatment been proven by randomized clinical trial. The INR goal is 2 to 3, except in certain prosthetic valvular conditions, where an INR of 2.5 to 3.5 is recommended. Warfarin anticoagulation is contraindicated in infective endocarditis and in left atrial myxomatous syndromes because of associated cortical surface mycotic and myxomatous aneurysm with the risk of hemorrhage. In all other possible causes of cardioaortic embolism, as in cases of cryptogenic embolism, debate exists as to the efficacy of antithrombotic therapy. Aspirin or other antiplatelet agents have been prescribed in lieu of antithrombotic therapy; but their efficacy also has not been proven by randomized clinical trials. Stroke and TIA subtypes were not identified in those studies in which aspirin was compared to placebo or to another antiplatelet agent (Plavix or Anturane) for the secondary prevention of recurrent stroke or TIA after a previous minor primary stroke or TIA. One study in which the primary and secondary stroke subtypes were accurately identified was the Warfarin Aspirin Recurrent Stroke Study (WARSS), which compared the efficacy of warfarin to aspirin in secondary stroke prevention. When all of the stroke primary and secondary subtypes were lumped together in the randomization process and in the secondary stroke end point diagnoses, the data was inconclusive. When the data for primary individual stroke subtype was analyzed in terms of secondary stroke prevention, there was a trend in favor of antithrombotic therapy. This category of embolism is generally treated with warfarin for 6 months, followed by aspirin or another form of antithrombotic therapy. We also use warfarin to manage patients with symptomatic atherothrombotic middle cerebral stem or basilar artery disease. In addition, we manage carotid or vertebral dissection with warfarin. The INR goal in all of these conditions is 2 to 3. Generally, for dissection, we continue the warfarin for 6 months; then if ultrasonographic evidence or noninvasive neuroimaging evidence suggests the arteries are open and symptom-free, we switch to aspirin. In some cases, we switch to aspirin even though the artery is still narrowed at the point of dissection or even occluded.

Surgical therapy Carotid endarterectomy is the only widespread surgical therapy available in ischemic stroke. Two clinical settings apply, with different criteria: (1) symptomatic disease and (2) asymptomatic disease. The efficacy of carotid endarterectomy for symptomatic disease when it presents with a mild to moderate stroke or transient cerebral ischemic attack has been proven by randomized trial design for patients with a 70 percent stenosis or greater. The efficacy of carotid endarterectomy when a patient has 50 to 70 percent stenosis in this setting has also been demonstrated, but at a less robust power. The NASCET established this efficacy only if the surgical morbidity was <5 percent. It is, therefore, recommended in most centers to have a surgical morbidity of 2 percent or less. Carotid disease is a marker of cardiac disease. Careful consideration of patients' cardiac status prior to endarterectomy is essential. Precise assessment of the degree of severity of the stenosis and its effect intracranially is extremely helpful. In addition, an image through CT angiography or MRI angiography is also helpful in identifying the pathology not only in the internal carotid artery origin, but also in the arteries distally and in the arteries providing collateral flow. Neither CT angiography or MRI angiography can quantify the degree of stenosis when it becomes hemodynamically significant as well as can carotid duplex Doppler and transcranial Doppler. There now exist 100 percent specific criteria noted by transcranial duplex Doppler for identifying such a lesion.

Asymptomatic carotid stenosis Natural history studies and the modern endarterectomy trials point out that symptoms (low-flow transient ischemia or embolic ischemia, transient or permanent) most often occur as a result of internal carotid artery origin stenosis that is severe enough to produce a pressure drop across it. This occurs between 70 percent and 75 percent residual lumen diameter reduction or 1.5 mm actual residual lumen diameter. Duplex Doppler assessment of flow at the bifurcation of the common carotid artery and transcranial Doppler assessment of distal internal carotid artery, ophthalmic artery, and middle, anterior, and posterior cerebral artery stem flow can accurately identify such lesions. Confirmation by CT angiography and/or MR angiography virtually eliminates the need for conventional intraarterial angiography and its risks. To date, the one endarterectomy trial allowed to come to completion used 50 percent stenosis as a guideline for randomization to surgery versus medical therapy. Naturally, the event rate in that trial was extremely low. That is the reason why the benefit of surgery was only suggested after 5 years, but not before. Well over 80 percent of the patients in that trial had <80 percent stenosis. The number of events did not allow for correlation between the degree of stenosis and the efficacy of surgery as occurred positively with the NASCET study.

The NASCET investigators, therefore, suggest that endarterectomy should only be considered in symptomatic cases and only after carotid angiography. We have argued that the decision whether or not to operate in an asymptomatic patient should be based on available data on the risk associated with the degree of stenosis and the activity of the atheromatous carotid lesion, in addition to issues of medical and surgical morbidity.

Our neurology service continues to take this approach for three reasons. First, natural history studies show a high rate of stroke in patients with asymptomatic carotid stenosis of 75 percent or more. Second, NASCET demonstrated that the majority of carotid atherothrombotic strokes (80 percent) occur without warning symptoms. Third, in patients in NASCET with stenosis of 70 percent or more, increasing degrees of stenosis were associated with higher rates of stroke and greater benefit from endarterectomy.

Our data from transcranial Doppler and duplex ultrasound studies suggest that a stenosis with a residual luminal diameter of 1.5 mm (i.e., 70 to 75 percent stenosis) represents the point at which a pressure drop across the stenosis occurs in most patients; that is, the point at which the stenotic lesion at the origin of the internal carotid artery becomes hemodynamically important. When the stenosis has hemodynamic consequences, the collateral flow through the ophthalmic artery or through the circle of Willis is called into play. If collateral flow is not adequate, low-flow transient ischemic attacks and infarcts develop. If collateral flow is adequate, patients should remain free of low flow symptoms (transient ischemic attack or stroke).

Our concern is that reduced flow in the internal carotid artery, supplemented by good collateral flow distally, may promote the formation of thrombi at the origin of the internal carotid artery; such thrombi may embolize or propagate distally to cause sudden stroke. We, therefore, recommend surgery for asymptomatic patients whose lesions have progressed to this point, that is, those with stenosis of 70 to 75 percent or more. To reduce the morbidity associated with surgery, we avoid transfemoral angiography. Instead, we identify hemodynamically important lesions on the basis of our 100 percent-specific criteria for hemodynamic importance, based on duplex and transcranial Doppler ultrasonography, combined with MRA or CT angiography. In the experience of our surgical team, morbidity is no greater than that in the Asymptomatic Carotid Atherosclerosis Study (2.3 percent) for patients deemed to have a low risk of cardiac complications.

We further suggest that patients with hemodynamically important, asymptomatic carotid artery stenosis identified on ultrasonography form the basis of a definitive surgical trial that will carefully define subtypes of strokes (i.e., the end point) on the basis of state-of-the-art technology. Ongoing trials comparing surgery with angioplasty might incorporate these hemodynamic issues into their design as well. Until such a trial is completed, we believe the decision whether to operate should be based on the hemodynamic importance of the carotid lesion and the risk to the individual patient, rather than on a uniform policy of using medical treatment in all patients with asymptomatic carotid artery stenosis.

INTRACRANIAL HEMORRHAGE

Of the many causes of nontraumatic intracranial hemorrhage, four are particularly common: (1) deep hypertensive intracerebral hemorrhage; (2) lobar hemorrhage; (3) ruptured saccular aneurysm; and (4) ruptured arteriovenous malformation or cavernous angioma.

Deep Hypertensive Intracerebral Hemorrhage

Hypertensive hemorrhages typically occur in one of four sites: (1) the putamen and adjacent internal capsule; (2) the

thalamus; (3) the pons; and (4) the cerebellum. They rarely originate in the central white matter of the hemispheres. A penetrating artery arising from the middle cerebral stem, basilar artery, or circle of Willis is generally the source of the hemorrhage, the same vessels that form lipohyalinosis and occlude, giving rise to a lacune as a result of hypertension. Each of the four sites of intracerebral hemorrhage produces a characteristic clinical syndrome. For *putaminal hemorrhage*, the eyes are deviated conjugately to the side of the hemorrhage and there is a contralateral hemiplegia. Stupor is evident at the onset in most cases. *Thalamic hemorrhage* has a similar clinical state unless the mass effect is directed downward; in that case, the eyes deviate downward and inward. Unequal pupils and skewed deviation with the eye on the side opposite the hemorrhage being displaced down and medially is also seen. *Pontine hemorrhage* produces deep coma, quadriplegia, decerebrate rigidity, and impairment of horizontal eye movements with pinpoint pupils. *Cerebellar* hemorrhage presents with vomiting and instability of gait; these may be the only signs. However, forced deviation of the eyes to the opposite side or an ipsilateral sixth nerve palsy may be noted. Less-frequent ocular signs include blepharospasm, involuntary closure of one eye, and skew deviation. Dysarthria may also occur. Babinski signs and bifacial weakness occur late. Hemiparesis or hemiplegia is not part of the clinical picture until coma has set in from pressure in the posterior fossa. Laboratory evaluation includes CT scan, which well delineates the hemorrhage. Even in cases of hypertensive hemorrhage in younger people, it is suggested that an MR angiography, a CT angiogram, or conventional angiogram be done when the hemorrhage absorbs in order not to miss an arteriovenous malformation. Lumbar puncture carries considerable risk.

The size and location of the hematoma determine the treatment and prognosis. Supratentorial hematomas >5 cm in diameter have a poor prognosis. Infratentorial hematomas >3 cm in size are generally fatal if they are in the pons. Edema in the week following the hemorrhage worsens the prognosis in all cases. Surgical removal of the supratentorial hemorrhage is controversial. If the hemorrhage is large enough to produce coma and it is in the nondominant hemisphere, surgical evacuation can be considered. By contrast, surgical removal of a cerebellar hemorrhage can be life-saving and result in a good recovery. It should be considered in all cases of cerebellar hemorrhage. If the hemorrhage is small and the patient is fully alert without dysarthria, upgoing toes, or facial weakness, the patient may be observed carefully. In instances where there is stupor and the hemorrhage is >2 cm in size, surgery should be performed. Osmotic agents including mannitol can be used in cases of intracerebral hemorrhage, but are generally considered temporizing therapy, gaining time while preparing for surgery.

Lobar Hemorrhage

Lobar hemorrhages occur spontaneously in the supratentorial white matter of all lobes of the brain. They have a slower onset than hypertensive hemorrhage, often evolving over hours and usually produce milder deficits. Frontal hemorrhage causes frontal headache and severe contralateral arm weakness, with little or no facial or crural weakness. Parietal hemorrhage produces a headache localized to anterior temporal regions, and a hemisensory deficit. Left temporal hemorrhage causes pain around the ear, fluent aphasia with poor comprehension, but retained repetition. Occipital hemorrhage presents with severe pain around the homolateral orbit and with a dense hemianopsia. A precise cause is found in a significant number of cases: amyloid angiopathy and vascular malformations are the most common; metastatic disease is less frequent, but well known. The location of the hemorrhage often suggests the etiology: frontal hemorrhages from aneurysms; trigone and parieto-occipital hemorrhages as complications of anticoagulation; basal ganglia and posterior fossa hemorrhages in hypertension. Most lobar hematomas, although more readily approachable surgically than centrencephalic hypertensive hemorrhages, carry a better prognosis and often do not require surgery, unless a result of aneurysm or arteriovenous malformation.

Amyloid Angiopathy

A cause of both single and recurrent hemorrhages in the elderly population, amyloid angiopathy is diagnosed conclusively only by postmortem demonstration of congo red or β-amyloid staining of amyloid in the media of cortical and leptomeningeal arterioles. But the clinical history of repeated supratentorial lobar hemorrhages and the demonstration of silent, small, 1- to 2-mm areas of subcortical white matter old hemorrhages by MRI (susceptibility pulse sequences), strongly suggest the diagnosis. These small, silent hemorrhages may be the cause of recurrent focal symptoms often seen in these patients. Other than avoidance of anticoagulants, treatment options remain elusive. Some suspected cases have had an angiitis associated with them that may respond to steroids; brain biopsy is suggested if angiitis is suspected prior to initiation of therapy.

Lobar Hemorrhages Caused by Metastatic Disease

Cerebral metastases, particularly malignant melanoma, may give rise to hemorrhage. Usually the metastases are multiple and can easily be demonstrated by MRI or CT scanning, both with contrast.

Vascular Malformations

Increasingly recognized with advances in neuroimaging techniques, vascular malformations are classified into four types: venous malformations, capillary telangiectasias, arteriovenous malformations, and cavernous malformations or angioma.

Venous malformations consist of anomalous veins that, while not associated with arterial feeders, nevertheless provide functional venous drainage, and are usually asymptomatic.

Capillary telangiectasias are small, often punctate, lesions composed of small clusters of dilated capillaries with normal intervening parenchyma. Small capillary telangiectasias in basal ganglia areas or in the brainstem are usually asymptomatic (i.e., discovered at autopsy), but occasionally rupture and produce a devastating hematoma.

Arteriovenous malformations and *cavernous malformations* are clinically significant because of their potential for producing hemorrhage and neurologic deficits.

Arteriovenous malformations consist of a tangle of abnormal vessels forming an abnormal communication between the arterial and venous systems. Most are developmental arteriovenous fistulas in which the constituent blood vessels enlarge and grow with the passage of time. They vary in size from a small blemish a few millimeters in diameter to a huge mass of tortuous channels composing an arteriovenous shunt of sufficient magnitude to raise the cardiac output. Hypertrophic dilated arterial "feeders" approach the main lesion and then disappear into a network of thin-walled blood vessels, which are the source of rupture, although some (perhaps 10 percent) may harbor berry aneurysms. Arteriovenous malformations occur in all parts of the brain, brainstem, and spinal cord, but larger ones are most frequently located in the hemispheres.

The chief clinical symptoms and signs are headache, seizures, and findings associated with rupture. When headache occurs (without bleeding), it may be hemicranial and throbbing, like migraine, or diffuse. A hemiplegia may accompany a headache, resembling the syndrome of hemiplegic migraine. Focal seizures that become generalized occur in approximately 30 percent of cases and are sometimes difficult to control with antiepileptic drugs. In half of the cases, arteriovenous malformations manifest with an intracerebral hemorrhage. In most of these cases, the hemorrhage is mainly intraparenchymal with a small amount of spillage into the subarachnoid space. Blood is usually not deposited in the basal cisterns, thus symptomatic vasospasm is rare. When the hemorrhage occurs, it may be large leading to death or small, giving rise to focal symptoms. Large supratentorial arteriovenous malformations may be associated with an audible bruit, sometimes even self-audible. Headache at the onset of the rupture is common and it may be difficult to distinguish it from the headache present in nonruptured arteriovenous malformations.

Cavernous malformations represent approximately 10 percent of all intracranial vascular malformations. Located within the brain parenchyma, without site of predilection, they are composed of thin-walled, dilated vessels, like a mulberry, devoid of intervening normal brain, and often surrounded by a ring of hemosiderin, a residuum of prior hemorrhage(s). Cavernous malformations may be multiple in as many as 3.6 percent of patients; in some families, multiple cavernous malformations appear to be inherited as an autosomal dominant trait, with the gene recently identified on chromosome 7.

As for arteriovenous malformations, symptoms of cavernous malformations are seizures, headaches, or neurologic deficits associated with rupture. Hemorrhages are usually small and circumscribed, but on occasion can be quite large, or clinically devastating because of their critical location, for example, in the pons. The risk of hemorrhage may be as high as 20 percent; repeated hemorrhages are often associated with progressive neurological disability.

The management of patients with arteriovenous malformations is best accomplished by an experienced team approach consisting of neurosurgeons and physicians who can consider surgical versus intraarterial obliteration of the malformation or aneurysm. Radiosurgical obliteration may also be an option in some cases (i.e., deep, inaccessible lesions associated with repeated hemorrhages or progressive neurologic deficits). Each case requires a unique approach that takes into account the extent and location of the arteriovenous malformation, the feasibility and safety of the various therapeutic approaches, and the assumption of a 3 percent per year rate of initial hemorrhage for arteriovenous malformations. In cavernous malformations, the risk of rehemorrhage may be substantially higher, perhaps 20 percent per year.

Subarachnoid Hemorrhage

Although sometimes a result of other causes (such as blood dyscrasia or leukemia, trauma, tumors such as ependymoma or meningioma, glioblastoma, renal cell, or metastasis, or, rarely, venous sinus disease or meningitis), by far the most common cause of subarachnoid hemorrhage is rupture of a berry aneurysm.

Ruptured saccular "berry" aneurysms at the branch points of the arteries at the base of the brain give rise to subarachnoid hemorrhage, or sometimes intracerebral hemorrhage. The internal elastic lamina is interrupted, giving aneurysmal outpouching that appears like a berry. Although they are usually single, they can be multiple in 15 to 20 percent of cases. The most common sites are the anterior communicating artery, the junction of the posterior communicating artery with the internal carotid artery, the middle cerebral stem bifurcation, the top of the basilar artery bifurcation, the origin of the major branches of the basilar artery and at the origin of the posterior inferior cerebellar artery. Intracranial aneurysms can be associated with coarctation of the aorta or with polycystic kidneys.

Prodromal symptoms and signs prior to rupture occur in as many as a third of cases. These symptoms may include headache, diplopia, or blurred vision. Pinpoint pain behind the eye with or without a third nerve palsy is the most common and indicates the presence of an aneurysm at the posterior communicating artery–internal carotid artery junction. It represents a medical emergency. Juxtaclinoid aneurysms compress the optic nerve, leading to amblyopia. Supraclinoid aneurysms can be confused with suprasellar tumors, perhaps producing a hypothalamic syndrome. Aneurysms in the vertebrobasilar system can produce occipital headaches and cerebellar or long-tract signs as well as cranial nerve deficits.

Once rupture occurs, the clinical syndromes are best divided into the *hemorrhage onset syndrome* and the *delayed onset syndrome*. The *hemorrhage onset syndrome* consists of a sudden, severe headache with or without loss of consciousness. Nausea and vomiting invariably occur on awakening.

If the hemorrhage ruptures into the brain substance, stupor and focal signs appear which relate to the site of the rupture. Anterior communicating artery aneurysmal rupture produces a quiet, slowed or retarded abulic state with a crural paresis, or hemiplegia predominating in the leg, while middle cerebral bifurcation aneurysms rupture into the brain substance and often produce a faciobrachial hemiparesis, with aphasia if the dominant hemisphere is involved. *Delayed clinical syndromes* mainly consist of rerupture syndromes, hydrocephalus, and the syndromes resulting from cerebral vasospasm. *Rerupture* is most frequent during the first 72 hours after the initial rupture. Early surgical intervention or intraarterial obliteration now precludes many reruptures (low grade). *Fever* ($\geq 38°C$) in the absence of a discernible infective etiology, is common in subarachnoid hemorrhage, and in some instances, may be confused with a florid meningitis. *Hydrocephalus* may be acute in the first day or two after the subarachnoid hemorrhage and might require ventricular drainage. Delayed hydrocephalus presents several days to weeks after the subarachnoid hemorrhage and may require ventriculoperitoneal shunting. Worsening stupor is a sign of both early and delayed hydrocephalus. *Cerebral vasospasm* usually develops between days 4 and 14 following the subarachnoid hemorrhage. Its location and severity has been related to the extent and location of the subarachnoid blood, especially presence of thick clot around the artery developing spasm. In 30 percent of cases, the spasm is severe enough to give rise to ischemic symptoms; infarction may ensue. In middle cerebral stem spasm, the resulting infarction may cause devastating edema. Volume expansion and blood pressure elevation together with calcium channel blockers are often used, but may not be successful; regional, intraarterial nicardipine infusions, or angioplasty of the artery in spasm, may be required.

Because of the above complications and the highly technical neurosurgical and interventional arterial approaches that are available to obliterating the aneurysm, as well as the specialized neurointensive care required, the patient should be managed in a center capable of carrying out these maneuvers.

REFERENCES

Adelson PD, Scott RM: Pial synangiosis for moyamoya syndrome in children. *Pediatr Neurosurg* 23:26, 1995.

Atrial Fibrillation Investigators: Risk factors for stroke and efficacy of antithrombotic therapy in atrial fibrillation: Analysis of pooled data from five randomized controlled trials. *Arch Intern Med* 154:1449, 1994.

Ay H et al: Diffusion-weighted imaging identifies a subset of lacunar infarction associated with embolic source. *Stroke* 30:2644, 1999.

Barnett HJM et al: Causes and severity of ischemic stroke in patients with internal carotid artery stenosis. *JAMA* 283:1429, 2000.

Barnett HJM et al: Benefit of carotid endarterectomy in patients with symptomatic moderate or severe stenosis. *N Engl J Med* 339:1415, 1998.

Brott T, Bogousslavsky J: Treatment of acute ischemic stroke. *N Engl J Med* 343:710, 2000.

Can U et al: Transcranial Doppler ultrasound criteria for hemodynamically significant internal carotid artery stenosis based on residual lumen diameter calculated from en bloc endarterectomy specimens. *Stroke* 28:1966, 1997.

Caplan LR et al: Should thrombolytic therapy be the first-line treatment for acute ischemic stroke? Thrombolysis—not a panacea for ischemic stroke. (Invited clinical debate.) *N Engl J Med* 337:1309, 1997.

Chambers BR, Norris JW: Outcome in patients with asymptomatic neck bruits. *N Engl J Med* 315:860, 1986.

Einhaupl KM et al: Heparin treatment of sinus venous thrombosis. *Lancet* 338:597, 1991.

Executive Committee for the Asymptomatic Carotid Atherosclerosis Study: Endarterectomy for asymptomatic carotid artery stenosis. *JAMA* 273:1421, 1995.

Fisher M: Occlusion of the internal carotid artery. *Arch Neurol Psychiatry* 65:346, 1951.

Fleisher LA, Eagle KA: Lowering cardiac risk in noncardiac surgery. *N Engl J Med* 345:1677, 2001.

Furlan A et al: Intra-arterial prourokinase for acute ischemic stroke. The PROACT II study: A randomized controlled trial. Prolyse in acute cerebral thromboembolism. *JAMA* 282:2003, 1999.

Gilon D et al: Lack of evidence of an association between mitral-valve prolapse and stroke in young patients. *N Engl J Med* 341:8, 1999.

Greenberg SM: Cerebral amyloid angiopathy. Prospects for clinical diagnosis and treatment. *Neurology* 51:690, 1998.

Hunter GJ et al: Assessment of cerebral perfusion and arterial anatomy in hyperacute stroke with three-dimensional functional CT: Early clinical results. *AJNR Am J Neuroradiol* 19:29, 1998.

Kistler JP: Cerebral embolism. *Comprehen Ther* 22:515, 1996.

Kistler JP et al: Cerebrovascular diseases, in Isselbacher KJ et al. (eds): *Harrison's Principles of Internal Medicine,* 13th ed. New York, McGraw-Hill, 1994, p 2233.

Kistler JP et al: Effects of low-intensity warfarin anticoagulation on level of activity of the hemostatic system in patients with atrial fibrillation. *Stroke* 24:1360, 1993.

Kistler JP et al: Carotid endarterectomy—Specific therapy based on pathophysiology. *N Engl J Med* 325:505, 1991.

Kistler JP, Furie KL: Carotid endarterectomy revisited [editorial]. *N Engl J Med* 342:1743, 2000.

Kistler JP, Furie KL: Patent foramen ovale diameter vs. embolic stroke: A part of the puzzle [editorial]? *Am J Med* 109:506, 2000.

Kistler JP, Furie KL: Strategic location of large-vessel atherothrombotic cerebral vascular disease. *Arch Neurol* 56:1329, 1999.

Lewandowski CA et al: Combined intravenous and intra-arterial r-TPA versus intra-arterial therapy of acute ischemic stroke. Emergency management of stroke (EMS) bridging trial. *Stroke* 30:2598, 1999.

Maraire JN, Awad IA: Intracranial cavernous malformations: Lesion behavior and management strategies. *Neurosurgery* 37:591, 1995.

Mas J-L et al: Recurrent cerebrovascular events associated with patent foramen ovale, atrial septal aneurysm, or both. *N Engl J Med* 345:1740, 2001.

Matsushima T et al: Surgical treatment for pediatric patients with moyamoya disease by indirect revascularization procedures (EDAS, EMS, EMAS). *Acta Neurochir (Wien)* 98:135, 1989.

Michelsen WJ: Natural history and pathophysiology of arteriovenous malformations. *Clin Neurosurg* 26:307, 1979.

Mohr JP et al: A comparison of warfarin and aspirin for the prevention of recurrent ischemic stroke. *N Engl J Med* 345:1444, 2001.

North American Symptomatic Carotid Endarterectomy Trial Collaborators: Beneficial effects of carotid endarterectomy in symptomatic patients with high-grade carotid stenosis. *N Engl J Med* 325:445, 1991.

Oliveira-Filho J et al: Diffusion-weighted magnetic resonance imaging identifies the "clinically relevant" small-penetrator infarcts. *Arch Neurol* 57:1009, 2000.

Oliveira-Filho J, Koroshetz WJ: Acute evaluation and management of ischemic stroke, in Rose BD (ed): *UpToDate.* Wellesley, MA, UpToDate Inc, 2001.

Ropper AH, Davis KR: Lobar cerebral hemorrhages: Acute clinical syndromes in 26 cases. *Ann Neurol* 8:141, 1980.

Rosenberg RD, Aird WC: Vascular-bed-specific hemostasis and hypercoagulable states. *N Engl J Med* 340:1555, 1999.

Sacco RL et al: Infarcts of undetermined cause: The NINCDS Stroke Data Bank. *Ann Neurol* 25:382, 1989.

Singhal AB et al: Cerebral vasoconstriction and stroke after use of serotonergic drugs. *Neurology* 58:130, 2002.

Sorensen AG et al: Hyperacute stroke: Simultaneous measurement of relative cerebral blood volume, relative cerebral blood flow, and mean tissue transit time. *Radiology* 210:519, 1999.

Suwanwela N et al: Carotid Doppler ultrasound criteria for internal carotid artery stenosis based on residual lumen diameter calculated from en bloc carotid endarterectomy specimens. *Stroke* 27:1965, 1996.

The Boston Area Anticoagulation Trial for Atrial Fibrillation Investigators: The effect of low-dose warfarin on the risk of stroke in patients with nonrheumatic atrial fibrillation. *N Engl J Med* 323:1505, 1990.

The National Institute of Neurological Disorders and Stroke rt-PA Stroke Study Group: Tissue plasminogen activator for acute ischemic stroke. *N Engl J Med* 333:1581, 1995.

van Swieten JC, Caplan LR: Binswanger's disease. *Adv Neurol.* 62:193, 1993.

Wolf PA et al: Atrial fibrillation: A major contributor to stroke in the elderly. *Arch Intern Med* 147:1561, 1987.

Wu O et al: Predicting tissue outcome ion acute human cerebral ischemia using combined diffusion- and perfusion-weighted MR imaging. *Stroke* 32:933, 2001.

Dementias Including Alzheimer's Disease

JOHN P. BLASS

DEFINITIONS

Dementia is a syndrome, not a disease. The exact number of disorders that can can cause dementia depends on how finely one wants to split diagnostic categories. The neuropathologic changes characteristic of Alzheimer's disease (AD) are found in the brains of 85 percent or more of people older than age 65 who die with dementia and are autopsied. Often concomitant changes of vascular disease or other conditions that can themselves cause dementia are found in their brains as well. In the past, the terms "senility" and "senile dementia" were used as synonyms for AD.

Dementia is currently defined as global cognitive impairment that is irreversible and occurs in a clear sensorium. "Global cognitive impairment" requires impairment in memory and in at least two other cognitive domains. "Irreversible" distinguishes permanent dementia from transient delirium. "A clear sensorium" is required because obtundation or stupor suggests delirium rather than dementia.

A clear distinction between transient delirium and permanent dementia is conventional in internal medicine at this time (see Chapter 117). However, dementia—even subclinical dementia—predisposes to the development of delirium, and conditions that can cause transient delirium can often cause permanent dementia if they are severe enough and last long enough (e.g., hypoxia or hypoglycemia). Delirium and dementia have been described as two poles of a spectrum of "brain failure," delirium being functional and dementia anatomic. Often patients have both, simultaneously.

HISTORICAL ASPECTS

Most if not all societies have recognized that feebleness of mind as well as of body often accompanies aging; for example, Shakespeare referred to the "seventh age of man."

In 1907 Alois Alzheimer described a patient with pathologic jealousy who subsequently developed dementia. At autopsy she was found to have lesions in her brain similar to those he frequently found in the brains of old people. He described her condition as a form of "premature aging." He and his coworkers were not clear on the extent to which the clinical syndrome was the result of the lesions he saw on silver staining or the result of cerebrovascular disease. Despite enormous increases in knowledge about this condition, occurring particularly over the last 20 years, the definition of the disorder remains the same. All dementia with Alzheimer's lesions is now classified as a single illness, whether of earlier or later onset. The term "senile dementia" has largely disappeared.

In this chapter, AD is discussed in some detail. Other causes of dementia are considered in the context of a differential diagnosis, as is delirium. For more extensive discussions of the other conditions, see Chapters 105, 109, and 117.

ALZHEIMER'S DISEASE AND ALZHEIMER'S DEMENTIA

Definition

Alzheimer's disease is conventionally defined by a clinical-pathologic correlation even though it is now clear that the clinical syndrome can occur without the pathologic findings, and the neuropathology without clinically significant disability. A dementia syndrome clinically indistinguishable from Alzheimer's dementia can be caused by a number of other diseases. When the neuropathology has been examined in prospective population-based studies, perhaps a third to a half of people who died with the full panoply of Alzheimer's neuropathology were not considered clinically demented while they were alive. Pathology without symptoms was even found in a nun who showed normal responses on detailed neuropsychological testing shortly before she died at age 101.

To avoid ambiguity, this chapter makes a distinction between Alzheimer's disease and Alzheimer's dementia.

Alzheimer's disease refers to the human *neuropathologic* condition with its attendant neurobiological abnormalities. Alzheimer's dementia refers to *clinically* significant dementia in a person who has Alzheimer's disease. This usage depends on direct, quantifiable observations of brain tissue at autopsy and of behavior during life. It avoids implicit assumptions about the relationship of the neuropathology to the behavior.

Incidence and Prevalence

Knowing the frequency with which Alzheimer's disease occurs requires population-based, autopsy-controlled studies. There are relatively few of these compared to clinical epidemiologic studies. Available data suggest that in western societies perhaps 30 percent or more of people who die after the age of 65 have lesions in their brain that meet consensus criteria for a neuropathologic diagnosis of Alzheimer's disease. Careful clinical studies involving African and East Asian populations suggest that the age-adjusted frequency of Alzheimer's disease is of the same order in these populations. Age is the most important risk factor for Alzheimer's disease, and so people must live long enough to develop it.

Alzheimer's dementia appears to be less common than AD (Table 107-1). In an epidemiologically valid, autopsy-controlled study in Finland involving sibjects 85 years and older, the incidence of AD based on neuropathology was 33 percent, but that of clinical dementia was only 16 percent. Presumably all the subjects with dementia did not have AD. This study therefore suggests that in this population less than half of the people who had the neuropathology of AD also had full blown, clinically disabling Alzheimer's dementia clinically significant enough for them to come to the attention of the nationalized health care service in this highly developed northern European country. When milder degrees of cognitive impairment are included, the incidence of abnormalities associated with Alzheimer's neuropathology is higher. An example is provided by an autopsy-controlled study of a religious community in the United States. Detailed neuropsychological evaluations documented the frequent existence of varying degrees of milder cognitive impairment in most people who had definite Alzheimer's neuropathology without dementia (Table 107-1).

Full-blown dementia of all types has been reported to occur in about 5 percent to 25 percent of the elderly population. When less severe degrees of cognitive impairment are included, the reported incidence has been as high as 50 percent. The incidence doubles every decade between the seventh and the ninth. Socioeconomic factors—and therefore race and ethnicity—can influence how much care is given to people who can no longer care for themselves and therefore influence how long people with dementia survive.

Etiology

Risk factors for AD include aging, genes, and the environment. Aging is the most important risk factor for AD. Except for rare familial forms, Alzheimer's disease is essentially a disease of those older than 65 years of age. Whether the incidence of AD and Alzheimer's dementia peaks in the ninth decade or continues to rise even in people in their nineties and older continues to be debated. Difficulties in resolving this issue include the relatively smaller numbers of people who reach these advanced ages and their relatively high burden of other illnesses. If the incidence of AD peaks and then falls, it is a disease that tends to occur in a particular age range rather than a disorder that is a result of progression of "the aging process itself." A currently popular hypothesis is that free radicals are important in mediating the effects of aging. The role of free radicals in AD is discussed below.

Genes for AD include 4 that are well established and perhaps 50 others that have been postulated on the basis of more limited and contradictory studies (Table 107-2). Genes in which mutations are established that lead to early-onset AD in susceptible families include those for the amyloid precursor protein (APP) and for presenilin 2 (PS2) and presenilin 1 (PS1). Mutations in the *APP* gene are rare, and in *PS2* are even rarer. Mutations in *PS1* are the most common known cause of early-onset familial AD although they appear in only a minority of the affected

Table 107-1 Relation of Memory Impairment to Alzheimer Neuropathology

Pathology	Memory* Intact	Impaired, Without Dementia	Dementia
None	10	0	0
Mild	30	11	11
Moderate	9	7	12
Severe	3	9	28

*Numbers refer to number of patients out of a total of 130. Of patients with neuropathologic stigmata of Alzheimer's disease, 53 percent did not meet the neuropsychologic criteria for dementia. Of patients with moderate or severe neuropathology, 41 percent did not meet the criteria for clinical dementia.

SOURCE: Data from Riley KP, Snowden DA et al: Alzheimer's neurofbrillary pathology and the spectrum of cognitive function: Findings from the Nun study. *Ann Neurol* 51:567, 2002.

Table 107-2 Genes for Alzheimer's Disease*

Gene	Chromosome	Frequency
Familial, early-onset type		
PS1	14	Common in early-onset familial disease, not in the more usual later-onset disease.
APP	21	Rare even in early-onset familial disease, normal in other patients.
PS2	1	Very rare even in early-onset familial disease.
Later-onset type		
APOE	19	The ε4 allele increases the risk of Alzheimer's dementia, the ε2 allele appears to protect, and the ε3 allele appears to be neutral.

*Many other genes have been proposed to be involved but have not been robustly confirmed (e.g., abnormalities in mitochondrial DNA). See htpp://www.alzforum.org for a continually updated internet listing of genes proposed to be biological risk factors for Alzheimer's dementia.

families. Presenilins may be involved in the metabolism of APP, specifically as γ-secretases contributing to formation of the characteristic Alzheimer's amyloid. Presenilins have other important actions as well—for instance on Notch, a key molecule in the control of differentiation.

The ε4 allele of the APOE gene (APOE4) is the only gene known to be a risk factor for later-onset AD. The ε3 allele is believed to be relatively neutral, and the ε2 assay to be relatively protective. The APOE gene encodes apolipoprotein E, which participates in cholesterol metabolism, and the metabolism of cholesterol in the Alzheimer's brain has recently become a subject of intense interest. It should be noted, however, that APOE4 predisposes to a number of diseases including cardiovascular disease. APOE can also be thought of as an "aging" gene, because with age the proportion of the population possessing the ε4 allele diminishes, whereas the proportion with the ε2 allele increases.

A discussion of genes less well established to be linked with AD is beyond the scope of this chapter. Being female is associated with a higher risk of developing Alzheimer's dementia. Whether this is because more women live to the age of risk or because they have two X chromosomes is still being debated.

An environmental factor that has been clearly linked to AD is head injury; an environmental factor robustly associated with Alzheimer's dementia is a low level of education. Head injury even in early life has been shown to predispose to the development of AD. The effect may be more marked in patients possessing the APOE4 gene. A head injury by itself can cause brain damage, accumulation of APP, and dementia.

Having only a very limited education predisposes to the clinical expression of Alzheimer's dementia. The education effect is most noticeable in the illiterate; university graduates have little or no advantage in this regard compared to those who finish the equivalent of junior high school. The education effect may simply be a matter of patients with minimal literacy performing more poorly on standardized tests. It has been proposed but not documented biologically that this effect is mediated by an "increased synaptic reserve." Nuns who had fewer verbal skills in adolescence were found to be more likely to develop dementia when they were older.

Other environmental risk factors for AD have been proposed, such as exposure to aluminum. None has as yet been established.

Pathology of Alzheimer's Disease

Three phases have marked the investigation of the neuropathology of AD. The first phase (ca. 1907–1950) was dominated by tissue staining, including the silver staining procedures used by Alzheimer. This research led to a description of the neuritic plaques and neurofibrillary tangles (NFTs) that are the hallmarks of the disease. The second phase (the 1950s and 1960s) utilized electron microscopy to characterize the ultrastructure of the lesions. These studies led to recognition that the classic neuritic plaque consists of a central core of "dense" amyloid surrounded by degenerating nerve endings and that NFTs consist of characteristic paired helical filaments (PHFs) with a distinctive periodicity. The third phase (the late 1970s to the present) has utilized modern immunologic, cell biological, biochemical, and molecular techniques.

Careful immunohistochemistry studies allowed the staining of specific molecules and specific epitopes within these molecules. Among the many antibodies now used to characterize AD pathologically are monoclonal antibodies to specific epitopes of APP, of its Aβ derivative (which accumulates in the distinctive Alzheimer plaques), and of the tau proteins in PHFs that are a major constituent of the characteristic NFTs. These techniques allow staining of early plaques, differentiation of different forms of the Aβ peptide that accumulate in plaques, and detection of the form of the tau protein that accumulates in NFTs.

Biochemical and molecular analyses of disrupted Alzheimer's brain and of cells in tissue culture have detected a large number of abnormalities associated with AD. More recently these investigations have involved molecular genetics. Biochemical and molecular analyses interrelate positively with the use of specific antibodies because antibodies can be used to localize molecular and chemical abnormalities that have been demonstrated by direct analyses.

The pathology of AD is now believed to proceed from "diffuse plaques" to "burned-out" plaques. According to this scheme, the first neuropathologic manifestation is the extracellular accumulation of diffuse plaques consisting largely of APP. These are reversible and develop as a rather nonspecific response to various kinds of injuries including hypoxia-ischemia and head trauma. The metabolism of APP through a quantitatively minor pathway, which utilizes β- and γ-secretases instead of α-secretase, leads to formation of the amyloidogenic Aβ peptide. The form of Aβ that contains 42 amino acids (Aβ_{42}) appears to be a much more effective nidus for amyloid deposition than the shorter forms (Aβ_{40} and Aβ_{38}). "Classic" plaques contain a center of amorphous material containing predominantly Aβ_{40}. Enough of the material is in a β-pleated sheet formation to stain metachromatically with Congo red dye and therefore be classified as amyloid. Materials other than Aβ are also present in Alzheimer's plaques but have been less investigated. The amyloid core is surrounded by degenerating nerve endings of various types often including cholinergic nerve endings. In a burned-out plaque, the nerve endings have largely disappeared. In most clinical-pathologic correlations, plaque density accounts for less than 10 percent of the clinical variability.

The other characteristic lesions in AD are NFTs. They are made up of PHFs, which are themselves made up of highly phosphorylated tau proteins. The high degree of phosphorylation of tau proteins in NFT is probably due to a failure of dephosphorylation postmortem. NFTs normally occur intracellularly, but when neurons die, they can be left behind as extracellular "ghost tangles." NFTs, like diffuse plaques, are found in a variety of brain diseases. The density of NFTs correlates with clinical disability only a little better than plaque density does.

Other lesions typically found in neuropathologic studies on Alzheimer's brain include Hirano bodies and granulovacuolar degeneration.

Neurons, particularly large ones, diminish in number in AD. The extent to which there is true loss rather than just shrinkage remains unclear. Immunohistochemistry studies demonstrate a clear loss of synaptic marker proteins, and the loss of synapses correlates better with the extent of clinical disability than either plaque density or number of NFTs does. Gliosis does occur. Beyond age 70, the overlap in mass between the brains of AD victims and those of cognitively intact people is so great as to make this effect of little diagnostic use.

The pathology of AD has been extensively reviewed, and consensus criteria for the diagnosis have been set. With increasing age, these criteria require more plaques and tangles to be present to make the diagnosis. In general, like other tissues, the brain is believed to become more sensitive to insults with increasing old age. The consensus criteria therefore imply that the plaques and tangles themselves may not be the direct *proximate* cause of clinical disabilities.

Bilateral hippocampal damage is a characteristic finding in AD and probably contributes to clinical disability. Bilateral hippocampal damage from any cause impairs memory, often severely. Imaging studies suggest that hippocampal damage correlates well with the degree of cognitive impairment in living patients.

More detailed discussions of the pathology of AD are available in earlier editions of this book, including pictures of typical plaques and tangles.

Pathophysiology of Alzheimer's Disease

A number of competing theories emphasize different aspects of the pathophysiology of AD, but these theories are not mutually exclusive.

The amyloid cascade hypothesis is by far the most widely held of these proposals. This hypothesis states that the pivotal event in AD is abnormal metabolism of APP, with the accumulation of Aβ amyloid. The arguments in favor of this view have recently been summarized elegantly and in detail by Selkoe. In brief, amyloid plaques are found more frequently in the brains of old people with dementia than in the brains of cognitively intact old people. Mutations in the gene for APP are associated with early-onset dementia in several well-characterized families, although the amyloid gene is normal in patients with the common, later-onset form of the disorder. Many, although by no means all, preparations of Aβ peptides damage cells in tissue culture and brain in vivo. The damage caused by injecting Aβ peptides into the brain can interfere with aspects of learning such as long-term potentiation.

Difficulties with the amyloid cascade hypothesis have been reviewed recently by Robinson and Bishop. One problem is that in most studies variations in the amyloid load account relatively poorly for the variance in cognitive function in patients with AD (Table 107-1).

A second problem is that amyloid production is increased in response to many injuries, including hypoxia-ischemia and brain trauma. Intuitively, it seems more likely that this response has evolved to protect the brain rather than to harm it. APP appears to be able to act as a free-radical scavenger. It can also act as a bioflocculant, that is, as a chaperone protein and an agent that complexes potentially toxic metals. APP production may start out as a protective mechanism but then go too far and become damaging. (Analogously, inflammation often starts out as a protective mechanism but then itself becomes a treatable source of tissue damage.) Abundant evidence indicates that Aβ peptides damage tissues by mechanisms involving free radicals. The oxidized form of a free-radical scavenger is inherently a potentially damaging prooxidant. APP and Aβ peptides may start out as antioxidants but become sources of free-radical damage once they accumulate in oxidized form.

Some of the data cited in favor of the amyloid cascade hypothesis allow alternate interpretations. For instance, learning disabilities in transgenic amyloid mice have been proposed to be proof of the primacy of amyloid in this disorder. However, only a minority of amyloid-bearing transgenic mice show learning deficits, and these deficits tend to be subtle. Even double mutants with enormous amyloid loads in their brains, exceeding anything seen in humans, do not show major learning disabilities compared to nontransgenic members of the same mouse strain. The data from transgenic amyloid mice could be used to argue that amyloid is not all that toxic.

In theory, therapeutic attempts to reduce the amount of amyloid in an Alzheimer's brain could provide a rigorous test of this widely held hypothesis. Human trials of a vaccine designed to remove amyloid have been stopped because of complications (see below).

Neurofibrillary tangles have also been proposed to damage the brain in AD. Mutations of the gene for tau proteins that accumulate in NFTs lead to frontotemporal dementias that are pathologically and clinically different from Alzheimer's dementia. Because tau proteins are involved in cytoskeletal functions, many investigators have assumed that NFTs impair cytoskeletal functions including intracellular transport.

Inflammation characteristically occurs in the Alzheimer's brain. It is complement-mediated and non-exudative. By analogy with disease in other tissues, this inflammation is widely thought to begin as a protective response and then progress to the point where it becomes damaging. Relatively small retrospective studies have indicated that people taking nonsteroidal anti-inflammatory drugs (NSAIDs) are at less risk of developing Alzheimer's dementia. Although prednisone is known to be an effective treatment for many kinds of inflammatory diseases of the brain, it had no effect on the progression of Alzheimer's dementia in a meticulous, large, prospective trial. The results of that trial argue against inflammation being a major source of continuing brain damage in AD.

Oxidative stress is also present in the Alzheimer's brain. There is evidence of oxidative damage to nucleic acids, lipids, and proteins. Often, however, the quantitative level of damage is so low as to raise questions about its physiologic significance. Free radicals—for instance, NO—are necessary for normal physiologic functions. The extent to which oxygen free radicals in AD are an appropriate response to damage rather than a source of brain damage requires further study.

Impaired brain metabolism is an essentially invariant finding in AD and includes impairments in key components of mitochondrial metabolism as well as overall reductions in glucose oxidation in patients with concomitant Alzheimer's dementia.

Multiple causes and mechanisms probably contribute to AD. In biology the concept of a "cause" is complex, as pointed out by Aristotle, among others,. The *ultimate* cause of AD appears to be a combination of genes, environment, and aging (see "Etiology" earlier in this chapter). The *material* cause of AD appears to be the panoply of neurobiological abnormalities characteristic of AD. Toxic fragments of APP are widely thought to have a pivotal role. The abnormality that fulfills the requirements for the *proximate* cause of the clinical disability of Alzheimer's dementia is cerebrometabolic deficiency. It occurs whenever dementia occurs. Significant metabolic insufficiency from any cause essentially always causes cognitive disability in humans and experimental animals (e.g., hypoxia, hypoglycemia). Treatments designed to ameliorate the deficits in brain metabolism have been reported to improve cognition in patients with AD (see below).

Impairment of cerebral metabolism leads directly to the changes in cholinergic and other neurotransmitter functions and to changes in intracellular second messengers comparable to those that occur in AD. These deficiencies in the brain's capacity for inter- and intracellular signaling appear to be the *immediate* cause of the clinical disabilities in Alzheimer's dementia. They can be described as defects in the brain's information-processing apparatus. The direct importance of defects in intercellular signaling agrees with the efficacy of neurotransmitter therapy discussed below and the evidence of loss of synaptic markers discussed above.

OTHER DEMENTIA DISORDERS

Vascular Disease

The role of vascular disease in dementia disorders of the elderly is important, complex, and unsettled. For the first three-quarters of the twentieth century, "cerebral arteriosclerosis" was the most widely accepted cause of dementia in the elderly population (then called senile dementia or senility). Plaques and tangles were thought to be important in earlier-onset dementia of the Alzheimer's type (then called Alzheimer's disease). In the middle of the 1970s, the pendulum swung in the opposite direction. The view became widespread that dementia due to cerebrovascular disease was the result of multiple infarcts requiring the loss of approximately 100 mL of brain to become clinically significant. This condition was named multi-infarct dementia, a category still used in several major classifications of disease. The frequent coexistence of cerebrovascular disease and AD was called mixed dementia.

More recent epidemiologic studies have documented convincingly that vascular disease is an independent risk factor for the development of dementia with Alzheimer's neuropathology. Risk factors for vascular disease are turning out to be independent risk factors for AD, including hypertension during middle life, pathologic levels of blood cholesterol and other lipids, and homocysteinemia. NSAIDs may protect against Alzheimer's dementia by protecting against vascular disease. In 1986 Brun and Englund examined Weigert-stained serial vertical sections of brains of patients with well-documented Alzheimer's dementia. More than 90 percent had white-matter lesions of the Binswanger type to an extent adequate to account for their dementia. This technically demanding study has not, to my knowledge, been independently repeated. A conservative view is that when it occurs—as it so often does—vascular disease including microvascular disease contributes to AD and dementia, but vascular disease by itself is an unusual cause of the dementia syndrome.

Patients with cerebrovascular disorders without degenerative disease are rarely seen in memory disorder clinics in the United States and most European countries. Even patients who have had multiple strokes and have obvious cognitive disabilities are typically seen instead in cerebrovascular and/ or stroke clinics. This triage reflects in part the organization of the health care system. However, as noted above, the typical neuropsychological abnormalities of dementia involve bilateral hippocampal damage. The organization of the human cerebrovascular system is such that bilateral hippocampal damage is unlikely to result from a stroke alone. This type of damage can of course result from global cerebral ischemia like that accompanying cardiac arrest and resuscitation.

Dementia With Parkinsonian Features

The clinical entities in dementia with parkinsonian features are defined by specific patterns of clinical-pathologic correlations (Chapters 108 and 109). Intermediate forms that do not fit easily into any of the standard categories are also seen. In these conditions, motor manifestations of parkinsonism accompany progressive dementia. Prominent manifestations of psychiatric disease are often present even early in the course of the disease. These disorders include Lewy body dementia (LBD), progressive supranuclear palsy (PSP), and several others. In LBD, the Lewy bodies characteristically found in the pars compacta of the substantia nigra in Parkinson disease (PD) are found in the cerebral cortex as well. About half of patients with autopsy-proven LBD also have enough characteristic neuropathologic lesions of AD for that diagnosis to be made as well. Diffuse Lewy body dementia has been recognized only relatively recently. It is tempting to speculate that it may be responsible for the old observation that dementia is a common complication of PD.

Frontotemporal Dementias

Frontotemporal dementias includes Pick's disease as well as a number of related disorders in which the characteristic Pick's bodies are not found (Chapter 109). Psychiatric manifestations and more variably aphasia are described as being prominent even early in the course of the disease. The age of onset is typically younger than for Alzheimer's dementia or LBD. Mutations in the genes encoding tau proteins have been found in a number of families with these disorders.

Normal Pressure Hydrocephalus

Impairment of the drainage of cerebrospinal fluid can be an important consequence of head trauma, with resulting pressure on the brain and loss of mental ability. A similar syndrome, normal pressure hydrocephalus (NPH), can occur in people with no known history of brain trauma. The characteristic clinical triad is dementia, gait disturbance, and incontinence—particularly urinary incontinence. The syndrome is said to respond well to shunting. Expert reading of computed tomography (CT) or magnetic resonance imaging (MRI) scans and careful clinical correlation by a specialist are needed to avoid inappropriate surgery.

Other Neurologic Diseases

Intellectual functions are widely represented in the brain, with the result that many types of brain damage can more or less impair higher intellectual functions. Whether the intellectual impairment is clinically significant or not can depend on what the patient is asked to do, including performing on neuropsychological tests. Referral to a specialist is in order when such a condition is suspected.

Psychiatric Diseases

Dementia can result from brain diseases that are now classified as psychiatric. Furthermore, in most patients with dementia, psychiatric complications typically occur sometime in the course of the disease.

Depression

Depression can complicate dementia, be the presenting sign of a dementing illness, and mimic dementia. Depression in older people can be a continuing manifestation of a life-long illness. Depression with an onset late in life is often a presenting manifestation of a brain disease, cerebrovascular or degenerative or both. Depression can be the only obvious clinical consequence of an otherwise silent stroke. If patients with late-onset depression live long enough, most of them end up with an obvious dementing illness. As a generalization, patients with depression can be distinguished from those with dementia because the former do relatively well in nonthreatening testing without sharp time constraints by a neuropsychologist who is a skilled clinician.

Psychoses

Progressive diseases of the brain can present with primarily psychiatric manifestations and then go on to cause dementias as well. The original Latin name for schizophrenia was *dementia praecox*. Generally, the diagnosis of Alzheimer's dementia is not made confidently in a patient with a previous history of severe psychiatric disease, except at autopsy.

CLINICAL EVALUATION OF PATIENTS WITH DEMENTIA

Confusion in an elderly patient can be a nonspecific manifestation of disease. Infections, heart attacks, and a variety of other common diseases can present clinically as loss of mental ability in older people, particularly in those who have subclinical AD or another brain disorder. Working out the cause(s) of the confusion and finding a way to help the patient and the caregivers is a classic challenge for geriatricians.

History

By definition, confused patients are poor historians. Their history must come from an informant. Even practicing physicians who know their patients well need to be wary of the development of a new disease that contributes to the loss of mental function. A much more extensive workup is needed for a confused patient without a reliable history—for instance, a patient seen first in an emergency department.

Distinguishing dementia from delirium requires a valid clinical history. Patients with dementia are said to be attentive, whereas delirious patients are not, but making clinical judgments about attentiveness can be difficult, and patients can have a delirium superimposed on a dementia. Probably it is not safe to diagnose dementia unless a reliable history of cognitive difficulties goes back at least 6 months and preferably more.

The onset of Alzheimer's dementia is characteristically insidious. Patients with Alzheimer's dementia or other degenerative dementias can, however, also have strokes or other acute events that lead to clinical deterioration. A family can describe the onset of dementia as occurring suddenly after the death of a spouse or other caregiver who had been concealing the patient's long-standing progressive disability.

A family history of dementia supports a diagnosis of Alzheimer's dementia. The lack of such a history does not disprove the diagnosis but should raise the index of suspicion of other disorders, assuming the family history has not been truncated. Often when a detailed family tree is diagrammed, relatives who deny a family history of dementia can recall a relative who became forgetful in old age.

Recognizing depression or another psychiatric disability is important. Depression is not only unpleasant for the patient but also appears to be associated with decreased survival even in the absence of suicide. The results of treatment can be very gratifying, even if the patient suffers from concomitant AD or another neurodegenerative disorder. Psychotic manifestations are very common in the course of a dementing illness.

A comprehensive medical history also provides information about other neurologic or medical disorders that can contribute to cognitive problems. Obtaining a list of the medications the patient is actually taking is critical; all nonprescription medications should be listed including, but not limited to, over-the-counter antihistaminics. A 73-year-old patient of mine appeared to have Alzheimer's dementia until her daughter found and took away the Quaalude her mother had been secretly abusing.

Epidemiologic investigations have disproved some of what were previously thought to be characteristics of Alzheimer's dementia. To state that it is a steadily progressive disease without improvement is to oversimplify. Recent large studies indicate that about a third of patients do not progress over a year, even without treatment. A few actually appear to improve clinically. The length of survival depends on intercurrent disease and on the care these patients receive, because they lose the ability to care for themselves. In a socioeconomically favored population studied before therapy became available, mean survival was 8 years. Shorter survivals have also been reported, as well as survivals for two decades or more after the diagnosis. Like many diseases of the brain, Alzheimer's dementia often develops asymmetrically. In the earlier stages and midstages, patients can have more problems with language than with spatial orientation, or vice versa. They can have more prominent psychiatric abnormalities than problems with cognition, as did Alzheimer's original patient. Eventually, as the dementia progresses, more faculties tend to be lost until the patient ends up in a chronic vegetative state.

The diagnosis of Alzheimer's dementia during life is clinical. In prospective series, about 85 percent or even more of patients older than 65 years who come to a clinic with memory problems turn out at autopsy to have enough plaques and tangles to make a diagnosis of AD. In many of the remaining 15 percent, the diagnoses are often obvious on clinical examination—not only diagnoses of other brain diseases such as parkinsonism or long-standing schizophrenia but also medical diagnoses such as hypothyroidism and pernicious anemia. Diagnostic accuracy as determined by pathology studies can be close to 100 percent with appropriate, careful workups and a willingness not to make a hasty diagnosis.

Physical and Neurologic Examinations

On physical examination the classic physical findings of Alzheimer's dementia are only the cognitive and behavioral abnormalities. Patients with Alzheimer's dementia can be strikingly physically healthy early in the course of their disease. A proverbial example is the lady who is still a superb tennis player although she can no longer keep score. On the other hand, AD and other dementia disorders do not protect against other illnesses that can themselves impair cognitive performance. Chronic delirium due to a chronic medical illness or inappropriate medications (including over-the-counter medications such as antihistamines) can lead to a mistaken diagnosis of dementia. The presence of clear-cut neurologic signs such as signs of parkinsonism in a patient with dementia generally calls for referral to a specialist.

Neuropsychological Evaluation

Neuropsychological studies are perhaps the single most important part of the evaluation of a patient with a cognitive disability. They examine the patient's presenting complaint directly, systematically, and in detail (Chapter 105). Caring for a patient with dementia without performing a neuropsychological examination is like caring for a cardiac patient without obtaining an electrocardiogram or measuring blood cholesterol levels—possible, but hardly modern medicine. Neuropsychologists, like consulting physicians, should include in their reports a brief summary of diagnostic conclusions written in language meaningful to a typical physician or nurse.

Probably the most widely used single test for evaluating mental status in the elderly is the Mini-Mental State Examination (MMSE) originally developed by Folstein, Folstein, and McHugh. This neuropsychological instrument has been widely translated. It has clear floor-and-ceiling effects and education effects and is now most often used as a screening test. Sophisticated, well-validated neuropsychological instruments have been developed to measure both cognition and ability in activities of daily living in patients with cognitive impairments. Their advantages and disadvantages are discussed in Chapter 105.

Neuroimaging

At this time, complete evaluation of a patient with dementia in the United States conventionally includes a neuroimaging study, either CT imaging or MRI. The yield of clinically significant abnormalities discovered by imaging is low in patients with dementias unless they have other abnormalities that call for obtaining a brain scan.

Several newer radiologic techniques are still in the research stage. Perhaps the most promising is examination of the hippocampus and related structures by MRI. In the future, a diagnostic role for these expensive techniques may be defined in cases where the differential diagnosis of dementia is difficult. It may also become possible to measure the burden of amyloid plaques cost-effectively by brain imaging. Such a technique would provide a definitive diagnosis because it would measure the biological abnormality that defines AD and distinguishes it from other forms of dementia.

Clinical Laboratory Studies

A conventional clinical laboratory evaluation of a patient with dementia consists of a complete blood count, urinalysis, and chemistry studies including measures of thyroid function (including thyrotropin). Levels of vitamin B_{12} and folate are usually measured although the yield of useful information obtained from these studies is very low. Tests for syphilis are not now recommended by most experts, although we have found them valuable in our catchment area. A test for Lyme disease is often performed in areas where this disease is endemic. Other tests are used for more specific indications. A laboratory evaluation for "confusion" in a patient presenting without a useful history is of course more extensive and includes screening for drugs and other toxins.

TREATMENT OF DEMENTIAS

Dementias including Alzheimer's dementia are now, in general, treatable although not curable diseases—in the sense that chronic heart failure and chronic obstructive pulmonary disease are treatable even when not curable. Research over the last three decades has made therapeutic nihilism in this area out of date.

Treatment of Behavior

Behavioral "psychiatric" symptoms develop in a high proportion of patients with dementias including Alzheimer's dementia. Recent estimates are as high as 90 percent. The form the psychiatric manifestations take (including "manifest content") is influenced by cultural, family, and personal variables as well as the neurobiology. Behavioral abnormalities often bother families and other caregivers more than a simple "loss of memory" or other aspects of impaired cognition, particularly as the disease progresses and the behavioral abnormalities become more socially unacceptable. Treatment directed at behavior is a mainstay of the clinical treatment of patients with AD. It typically involves both behavioral interventions and medication.

There is a large, continuously growing literature on behavioral interventions for Alzheimer's dementia. The basic principle is to adjust the circumstances of each patient's life

to that patient's remaining abilities. Because the disease is typically progressive, adjusting the environment is usually a continual process. When a patient should be placed in a nursing home or other institutional setting is an individual decision to be made by each family unit. Ethnic and other social differences play a major role, as does the personality of the caregiver(s) and the closeness of the relationship between caregiver and patient. A strong indication for placement is that the major caregiver is breaking down—physically or psychologically—under the burden of care. If a devoted spouse or other caretaker needs to be hospitalized or dies, the patient will likely require emergency placement, with all the compromises that this implies. Another indication for placement is that the patient no longer recognizes the caregiver. At this point, the caregiver might just as well be someone working an 8-hour shift. A person who has no family or other caregiver may require nursing home placement at an earlier stage of dementia than a person with a strong support system.

Medications are used to modify target symptoms in dementias as in other psychiatric disorders. The drugs now favored for the treatment of depression are selective serotonin reuptake inhibitors (SSRIs), with the use of newer medications or tricyclics when needed. Risperdal and olanzapine are currently the favored medications for treating psychosis, agitation, and aggression, although Risperdal carries the risk of parkinsonian side effects. Before deciding how vigorously hallucinations and delusions should be treated, it is important to find out who, if anyone, is bothered by them. For anxiety, short-acting benzodiazepines are often used. For unclear reasons, some patients respond well to one medication but not to several others in the same class. Optimal clinical practice requires empiricism as well as the use of guidelines. In choosing doses, the general rule is to "start low, go slow, but give enough." In other words, individualize doses. Behavioral tensions can often be eased by surprisingly low doses of Risperdal—as little as a few hundred micrograms in solution. Whether the clinical benefit of these low doses comes from empowering the caregiver or from modifying the patient's behavior is unclear but is also relatively unimportant in clinical management.

Neurotransmitter Therapy

The mainstay of neurotransmitter therapy for Alzheimer's dementia is cholinesterase inhibition. The most widely used medication is donepezil (Aricept). Recent, rigorous, yearlong, multicenter studies in both Europe and the United States have shown the unequivocal benefits of treatment with donepezil and that it is possibly effective in slowing the progression of the illness (Figure 107-1). Other cholinesterase inhibitors are now also on the market in the United States, including rivastigmine (exelon) and galanthamine (Reminyl). Unlike donepezil, they require bid dosing and need to be carefully titrated upward to avoid gastrointestinal side effects. They appear to have similar clinical benefits when used properly. Tetrahydroaminoacridine (THA, Cognex) is now used less frequently because liver toxicity must be monitored. Cholinesterase inhibitors have also been reported to benefit patients with LBD, but research has been less extensive.

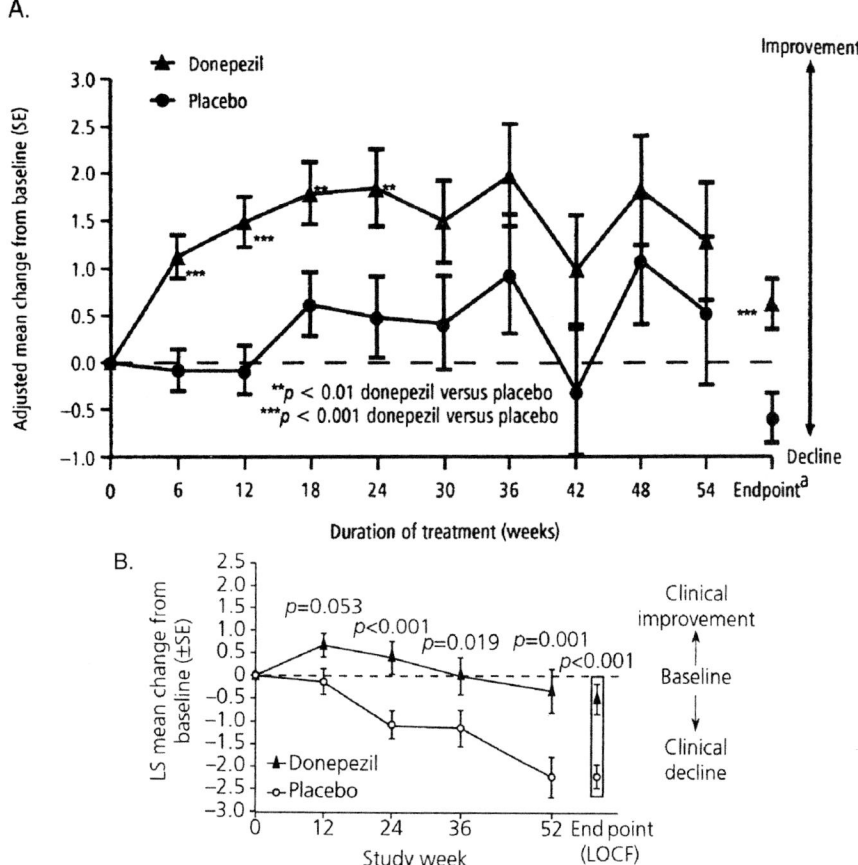

Figure 107-1 The effects of donepezil (Aricept) on Alzheimer's dementia. The graphs compare the change in performance on a robust neuropsychological test, the Mini-Mental Status Examination, in patients with Alzheimer's disease treated with donepezil and patients with Alzheimer's disease given a placebo. Both studies were prospective, double-blind, multicenter investigations. (A) A study in the United States, (B) a study in northern Europe.

A wide variety of other neurotransmitter agonists were tested in patients with Alzheimer's disease during the 1980s. These studies essentially found that antidepressants with serotonergic action appear to improve the depressive symptoms in patients with AD and any cognitive manifestations secondary to the depression. Ritalin can transiently "energize" some patients. Other neurotransmitter agents have not proven useful.

Treatments for Slowing Disease Progression

A major aim of research on the treatment of dementias, including Alzheimer's dementia, is to slow—or hopefully even stop or reverse—the damage to and loss of neurons characteristic of these diseases. Research in this area is very active. However, the great variability in the course of Alzheimer's dementia makes such studies difficult and expensive. For instance, compare the rate of progression of the placebo-treated groups in the two studies shown in Figure 107-1. A compelling demonstration that disease progression is slowed will require large, long, expensive studies.

Therapy with certain nonsteroidal anti-inflammatory medications appeared to reduce the incidence and prevalence of Alzheimer's dementia in retrospective epidemiologic studies. Direct evidence for (or against) a beneficial

effect in patients with established disease is not, however, yet available. As noted above, prednisone has not proven useful.

Antioxidants have been proposed to be of benefit in Alzheimer's dementia and perhaps other dementias. A lower than expected incidence of Alzheimer's dementia has been reported in people who regularly ingest vitamin C and vitamin E in a prospective study of a large population. Vitamin E was reported to delay progress in patients with established Alzheimer's dementia, but the statistical analysis of the study has been questioned. Other antioxidants are currently undergoing active investigation.

Postmenopausal hormone replacement, notably with estrogens, has been associated with a reduced incidence of Alzheimer's dementia in epidemiologic studies. However, the small proportion of American women who receive postmenopausal hormone replacement therapy represents a highly self-selected subset. Hormone replacement was ineffective in a large study. However, a subsequent small study using high doses of estrogen claimed to be beneficial. A rigorous prospective trial to determine whether or not estrogen replacement reduces the incidence of Alzheimer's dementia is now underway.

Attempts to prevent or treat Alzheimer's dementia by inhibiting the formation of amyloid or removing it once it has formed continue to be one of the goals of current research. Vaccination against $A\beta$ peptide has been associated with deterioration in function in a significant number of patients, reportedly a result of encephalitis.

Predicting the future is always dangerous, but current trends suggest that future reviews on AD and other dementing disorders will be able to describe treatments that are much more effective than those now available.

REFERENCES

Blass JP: Alzheimer's disease and Alzheimer's dementia: Distinct but overlapping entities. *Neurobiol Aging* 2002; in press.

Blass JP. The Mitochondrial Spiral: An adequate cause of dementia in the Alzheimer syndrome. *Ann NY Acad Sci* 2000; 924: 170.

Brun A, Englund E. A white matter disorder in dementia of the Alzheimer type: A pathoanatomical study. *Ann Neurol* 1986; 19: 253.

Dickson DW. Neuropathology of Alzheimer's disease and other dementias. *Clin Geriatr Med* 2001; 17: 209.

Jellinger K. Pure hippocampal sclerosis: a rare cause of dementia mimicking Alzheimer's disease. *Neurology* 2000; 55: 739.

Mohs RC, Doody RS et al. A placebo-controlled study of donepezil in patients with mild to moderate AD. *Neurology* 2001; 57: 489.

Polvikoski T, Sulkava R et al: Prevalence of Alzheimer's disease in very elderly people: a prospective neuropathological study. *Neurology* 2001; 56: 1690.

Riley KP, Snowdon DA, Markesbery WR. Alzheimer's neurofibrillary pathology and the spectrum of cognitive function: Findings from the Nun Study. *Ann Neurol* 2002; 51: 567.

Robinson SR, Bishop GM. Aβ as a bioflocculant: Implications for the amyloid hypothesis of Alzheimer's disease. *Neurobiol Aging* 2002; 23: 1052–1072.

Selkoe DJ. Alzheimer's disease: genes, proteins, and therapy. *Physiol Rev* 2001; 81:741.

Snowdon DA. Aging and Alzheimer's disease: Lessons from the nun study. *Gerontologist* 1997; 37: 150.

Winblad B, Engedal K et al: A 1-year, randomized placebo-controlled study of donepezil in patients with mild to moderate AD patients. *Neurology* 2001; 57: 481.

Parkinson's Disease and Related Disorders

STANLEY FAHN

DISTINGUISHING BETWEEN PARKINSON'S DISEASE AND PARKINSONISM

The syndrome of parkinsonism must be understood before you can understand what Parkinson's disease (PD) is. Parkinsonism is defined by any combination of six specific motoric features: tremor at rest, bradykinesia, rigidity, loss of postural reflexes, flexed posture, and the freezing phenomenon (where the feet are transiently "glued" to the ground). Not all six of these cardinal features need be present, but at least two should be before the diagnosis of parkinsonism is made, with at least one of them being tremor at rest or bradykinesia. Parkinsonism is divided into four categories (Table 108-1). PD or primary parkinsonism is the principal focus of this chapter; not only is it the one that is most commonly encountered by the general clinician, it is also the one on which much research has been expended and the one we know the most about. The great majority of cases of primary parkinsonism are sporadic, but in the last few years several gene mutations have been discovered to cause PD (Table 108-2). Whether genetic or idiopathic in etiology, the common denominator is that this group of primary parkinsonism is not caused by known insults to the brain (the main feature of secondary parkinsonism) and is not associated with other motor neurologic features (the main feature of Parkinson-plus syndromes). The uncovering of genetic causes of primary parkinsonism has shed light on probable pathogenetic mechanisms that may be a factor in even the more common idiopathic cases of PD. It may even turn out that many of the idiopathic cases will be linked to gene mutations, discoveries yet to be made. Although the term "idiopathic PD" has been applied to primary parkinsonism, the fact that there are known genetic causes should encourage us to adopt the term "primary parkinsonism" rather than "idiopathic parkinsonism."

Three of the most helpful clues that one is likely dealing with a category of parkinsonism other than PD are (1) a symmetric onset of symptoms (PD often begins on one side of the body), (2) a lack of a substantial clinical response to adequate levodopa therapy, and (3) the absence of rest tremor. The presence of any of these features does not necessarily exclude a diagnosis of PD, but the likelihood that the cause belongs in another category of parkinsonism is high. Table 108-3 lists the clinical features suggesting a diagnosis favoring the other parkinsonian disorders and not PD. One common misdiagnosis is caused by essential tremor, which can even be unilateral, although it is more commonly bilateral. Helpful in the diagnosis is the tremor caused by PD is a rest tremor, whereas essential tremor is not present at rest, but appears with holding the arms in front of the body and increases in amplitude with intention activity of the arm, such as with handwriting or performing the finger-to-nose maneuver.

PD begins insidiously and gradually worsens. Symptoms, such as rest tremor, can be intermittent in the beginning, becoming present only in stressful situations. Patients with PD can live 20 or more years, depending on the age at onset; the mortality rate is about 1.5 times that of normal individuals the same age. Death in PD is usually a result of some concurrent unrelated illness or a result of the effects of decreased mobility, aspiration, or increased falling with subsequent physical injury. The Parkinson-plus syndromes typically progress at a faster rate and often cause death within 9 years. Thus, the diagnosis of PD is of prognostic importance, as well as of therapeutic significance, because it almost always responds to at least a moderate degree to levodopa therapy, whereas the Parkinsonplus disorders do not. While it may be difficult to distinguish between PD and Parkinson-plus syndromes in the early stages of the illness, with disease progression over time, the clinical distinctions of the Parkinsonplus disorders become more apparent with the development of other neurologic findings, such as cerebellar ataxia, loss of downward ocular movements, and autonomic dysfunction (e.g., postural hypotension, loss of bladder control, and impotence).

There are no practical diagnostic laboratory tests for PD, and the diagnosis rests on the clinical features or by excluding some of the other causes of parkinsonism. The research tool of fluorodopa positron emission tomography (PET) measures levodopa uptake into dopamine nerve terminals,

Table 108-1   Classification of the Parkinsonian States

I. Primary Parkinsonism (Parkinson's disease)

  A. Sporadic
  B. Known genetic etiology (see Table 108-2)

II. Secondary Parkinsonism (environmental etiology)

  A. Drugs
    1. Dopamine receptor blockers (most commonly antipsychotic medications)
    2. Dopamine storage depletors (reserpine)
  B. Postencephalitic
  C. Toxins: Mn, CO, MPTP, cyanide
  D. Vascular
  E. Brain tumors
  F. Head trauma
  G. Normal pressure hydrocephalus

III. Parkinsonism-plus syndromes

  A. Progressive supranuclear palsy
  B. Multiple system atrophy
  C. Cortical–basal ganglionic degeneration
  D. Parkinson–dementia–ALS complex of Guam
  E. Progressive pallidal atrophy
  F. Diffuse Lewy body disease (DLBD)

IV. Heredodegenerative disorders

  A. Alzheimer's disease
  B. Wilson's disease
  C. Huntington's disease
  D. Frontotemporal dementia on chromosome 17q2l
  E. X-linked dystonia-parkinsonism (in Filipino men; known as lubag)

NOTE: ALS, amyotrophic lateral sclerosis; CO, carbon monoxide; Mn, manganese; MPTP, 1-methyl-4-phenyl-1,2,3,6-tetrahydropyridine.

and this shows a decline of approximately 5 percent per year of the striatal uptake. A similar result is seen using ligands for the dopamine transporter, either by PET or by single-photon emission computed tomography (SPECT); these ligands also label the dopamine nerve terminals. All these neuroimaging techniques reveal decreased dopaminergic nerve terminals in the striatum in both PD and the Parkinson-plus syndromes, and do not distinguish between them. A substantial response to levodopa is most helpful in the differential diagnosis, indicating presynaptic dopamine deficiency with intact postsynaptic dopamine receptors, features typical for PD.

The development of dementia in a patient with parkinsonism remains a difficult differential diagnosis. If the patient's parkinsonian features did not respond to levodopa, the diagnosis is likely to be Alzheimer's disease, which can occasionally present with parkinsonism. If the presenting parkinsonism responded to levodopa, and the patient developed dementia over time, the diagnosis could be either PD or diffuse Lewy body disease (DLBD). If hallucinations

occur with or without levodopa therapy, DLBD is the most likely diagnosis. DLBD is a condition where Lewy bodies are present in the cerebral cortex as well as in the brainstem nuclei. The heredodegenerative disease, known as frontotemporal dementia, is an autosomal dominant disorder caused by mutations of the tau gene on chromosome 17; the full syndrome presents with dementia, loss of inhibition, and parkinsonism, and sometimes muscle wasting.

Some adults may develop a more benign form of PD, in which the symptoms respond to very-low-dosage levodopa, and the disease does not worsen severely with time. This form is usually caused by the autosomal dominant disorder known as dopa-responsive dystonia, which typically begins in childhood as a dystonia. But when it starts in adult life, it can present with parkinsonism. There is no neuronal degeneration. The pathogenesis is a result of a biochemical deficiency involving dopamine synthesis. The gene defect is for an enzyme (guanosine triphosphate [GTP] cyclohydrolase I) required to synthesize the cofactor for tyrosine hydroxylase activity, the crucial rate-limiting first step in the synthesis of dopamine and norepinephrine. Infantile parkinsonism is a result of the autosomal recessive deficiency of tyrosine hydroxylase, another cause of a biochemical dopamine deficiency disorder.

Table 108-2   Genetic Forms of Primary Parkinsonism

Name of Gene	Protein	Chromosome
Autosomal dominant tranmission		
PARKI	α-Synuclein	4q2l–q22
PARK3	?	2p13
PARK4	Iowa pedigree: PD/ET	4p15
PARK5	Ubiquitin C-terminal Hydrolase-Ll (UCH-LI)	4p14
PARK8	?	12p11.2–ql3.1
Dopa-responsive dystonia		14q22.1–q22.2
Autosomal recessive tranmission		
PARK2	Parkin (ubiquitin ligase)	6q25.2–q27
PARK6	?	1p35–p36
PARK7	?	1p36
PARK9	?	1p32
Tyrosine hydroxylase deficiency		11p11.5

Table 108-3 Criteria to Exclude the Diagnosis of Parkinson's Disease in Favor of Another Cause of Parkinsonism

Criteria	Likely Diagnosis
1. History of:	
Encephalitis	Postencephalitic
Exposure to carbon monoxide, manganese, or other toxins	Toxin-induced
Recent exposure to neuroleptic medication	Drug-induced
2. Onset of parkinsonian symptoms following:	
Head trauma	Posttraumatic
Stroke	Vascular
3. Presence on examination of:	
Cerebellar ataxia	OPCA, MSA
Loss of downward ocular movements	PSP
Pronounced postural hypotension not caused by concurrent medication	MSA
Pronounced unilateral rigidity with or without dystonia, apraxia, cortical sensory loss, alien limb	CBGD
Myoclonus	CBGD, MSA
Falling or freezing of gait early in the course of the disease	PSP
Autonomic dysfunction not caused by medications	MSA
Excessive drooling of saliva	MSA
Early dementia or hallucinations from medications	DLBD
Dystonia induced with low dose levodopa	MSA
4. Neuroimaging (MRI or CT scan) revealing:	
Lacunar infarcts	Vascular
Sapacious cerebral ventricles	NPH
Cerebellar atrophy	OPCA, MSA
Atrophy of the midbrain or other parts of the brainstem	PSP, MSA
5. Effect of medication:	
Poor response to levodopa	PSP, MSA, CBGD, Vascular, NPH
No dyskinesias despite high-dosage levodopa	Same as above

NOTE: CBGD, cortical–basal ganglionic degeneration; DLBD, diffuse Lewy body disease, also called dementia with Lewy bodies; MSA, multiple system atrophy; NPH, normal pressure hydrocephalus; OPCA, olivo-ponto-cerebellar atrophy which can be one form of MSA; PSP, progressive supranuclear palsy.

PATHOLOGY OF PARKINSONS DISEASE AND PARKINSON-PLUS SYNDROMES

PD and the Parkinson-plus syndromes have in common a degeneration of substantia nigra pars compacta dopaminergic neurons, with a resulting deficiency of striatal dopamine caused by loss of the nigrostriatal neurons. Accompanying this neuronal loss is an increase in glial cells in the nigra and a loss of the neuromelanin normally contained in the dopaminergic neurons. In PD, intracytoplasmic inclusions, called Lewy bodies, are usually present in many of the surviving neurons. It is recognized today that not all patients with PD have Lewy bodies, for those with a homozygous mutation in the PARK2 gene, mainly young-onset PD patients, have nigral neuronal degeneration without Lewy bodies. Lewy bodies contain many proteins, including the fibrillar form of α-synuclein, discovered because PARK1's mutations involve the gene for this protein. There are no Lewy bodies in the Parkinson-plus syndromes.

A pathologic feature of multiple system atrophy (MSA) is the presence of inclusions in oligodendroglia; these inclusions also contain α-synuclein. Progressive supranuclear palsy (PSP) and cortical–basal ganglionic degeneration (CBGD) contain tau filaments, and these two diseases share similar clinical features, especially in the late stages of these diseases. PSP, though, shows neurofibrillary tangles in the substantia nigra and other nuclei, while CBGD shows ballooned neurons, especially in areas of the cerebral cortex.

CAUSE AND PATHOGENESIS OF PD AND PARKINSON-PLUS SYNDROMES

Other than known genetic causes of PD (see Table 108-2), the etiology of these disorders remains unknown. Alterations in the tau gene have been implicated for PSP and CBGD. The three identified genes causing PD all point to an impairment of protein degradation with a build up of toxic proteins that cannot be degraded via the ubiquitin–proteasomal pathway. This has led to the concept that perhaps most, if not all, cases of sporadic PD have an impairment of protein degradation. A current hypothesis is that oxidative stress with the formation of oxyradicals, such as dopamine quinone, can lead to reactions with α-synuclein to form oligomers of α-synuclein (so-called protofibrils), which accumulate because they cannot be degraded by the ubiquitin–proteasomal pathway, leading, finally, to cell death. Other pathogenetic mechanisms being considered are (1) other effects from oxidative stress, such as the reaction of oxyradicals with nitric oxide to form the highly reactive peroxynitrite radical, (2) impaired mitochondria leading to both reduced adenosine triphosphate (ATP) production and accumulation of electrons that aggravate oxidative stress, with the final outcome being apoptosis and cell death, and (3) inflammatory changes in the nigra, producing cytokines that augment apoptosis. These concepts on pathogenesis are leading researchers to test agents that affect these potential mechanisms in an attempt to reduce the rate of neurodegeneration in PD.

EPIDEMIOLOGY AND CLINICAL FEATURES OF PD

Although PD can develop at any age, it is most common in older adults, with a peak age at onset around 60 years. The likelihood of developing it increases with age, with a lifetime risk of approximately 2 percent. A positive family history doubles the risk of developing PD to 4 percent. Twin studies indicate that PD with an onset younger than age 50 years is more likely to have a genetic relationship than for patients older than age 50 years at onset.

The early symptoms and signs of PD are rest tremor, bradykinesia, and rigidity; these are related to progressive loss of nigrostriatal dopamine. These signs and symptoms result from dopamine deficiency and are usually correctable by levodopa and dopamine agonists. As PD progresses over time, non–dopamine-related symptoms develop, such as flexed posture, the freezing phenomenon and loss of postural reflexes; these do not respond well to levodopa therapy. Moreover, increasing bradykinesia that is not responsive to levodopa can appear as the disease worsens. These intractable symptoms lead to disability.

While the motor symptoms of PD dominate the clinical picture—and even define the parkinsonian syndrome—many patients with PD have other complaints that have been classified as *nonmotor*. These include fatigue, depression, anxiety, sleep disturbances, constipation, bladder and other autonomic disturbances (sexual, gastrointestinal), and sensory complaints. Sensory symptoms that include pain, numbness, tingling, and burning in the affected limbs occur in approximately 40 percent of patients. Behavioral and mental alterations include changes in mood, decreased motivation and apathy, slowness in thinking (bradyphrenia), and a declining cognitive capacity.

PRINCIPLES OF THERAPY

Parkinson-plus syndromes respond poorly to medications, so the emphasis here is on the treatment of PD. Certain principles serve as guidelines.

Neuroprotective therapy. So far no drug or surgical approach unequivocally slows the rate of progression of PD, but if any drug could be proven to delay the progression of the disease process, it should be incorporated early.

Encourage exercise to keep the patient mobile. An active exercise program encourages the patient to participate in his or her own care, allows muscle stretching and full range of joint mobility, and enhances a better mental attitude toward fighting the disease. One of the nonmotor symptoms of PD is the tendency to be passive with decreased motivation. Encouraging activity helps fight these symptoms.

Individualize therapy. No two patients are identical; each presents with a unique set of symptoms, signs, response to medications, and a host of social, occupational, and emotional problems that need to be addressed. The treatment of PD, therefore, needs to be individualized. One takes into account the severity of the patient's symptoms, the degree of functional impairment, the expected benefits and risks of available therapeutic agents, and the age of the patient. Younger patients are more likely to develop motor fluctuations and dyskinesias from anti-PD medication; while older patients are more likely to develop confusion, sleep–wake alterations, dementia, and psychosis.

MEDICAL THERAPY OF PD

Treatment of patients with PD can be divided into three major categories: physical (and mental health) therapy, medications, and surgery. Physical exercise was mentioned above, and should be implemented as soon as the diagnosis is made, but it is useful in all stages of disease. In the early stages of the disease, the joints should be fully stretched to compensate for the tendency of the patient to have a reduced range of motion. In advanced stages of PD, formal physical therapy is more valuable by keeping the joints from becoming frozen, and by providing guidance how best to remain independent in mobility, particularly with gait training. Medications are the mainstay of therapy, but new surgical procedures are becoming appropriate for patients with advanced PD, who are no longer adequately controlled by medications.

Dopamine replacement therapy is the major medical approach to treating PD, and a variety of dopaminergic agents are available (Table 108-4). The most powerful drug is levodopa. It is usually administered with a peripheral decarboxylase inhibitor to prevent formation of dopamine in the peripheral tissues. Such combination drugs are available in standard and slowrelease formulations. The former allows a more rapid and predictable "on," and the latter allows for a slightly longer plasma half-life, but with a slower and less predictable "on." Besides being metabolized by aromatic amino acid decarboxylase, levodopa is also metabolized by catechol-O-methyltransferase (COMT) to form 3-O-methyldopa. Two COMT inhibitors are available: entacapone and tolcapone. These agents extend the plasma half-life of levodopa without increasing its peak plasma concentration, and can thereby prolong the duration of action of each dose of levodopa. Although levodopa is the most effective drug to treat the symptoms of PD, approximately 60 percent of patients develop troublesome complications

Table 108-4 Dopaminergic Agents

Dopamine precursor: levodopa

Peripheral decarboxylase inhibitors: carbidopa, benserazide

Dopamine agonists: bromocriptine, pergolide, pramipexole, ropinirole, apomorphine, and cabergoline

Catechol-*O*-methyltransferase inhibitors: tolcapone, entacapone

Dopamine releaser: amantadine

Peripheral dopamine-receptor blocker: domperidone

Monamine oxidase type B inhibitor: selegiline, lazabemide, rasagiline

of disabling response fluctuations ("wearing-off" effect) and dyskinesias after 5 years of levodopa therapy, and younger patients (younger than 60 years of age) are particularly prone to develop these problems even sooner.

It should be pointed out that it is not safe to discontinue levodopa suddenly, for such action can induce the neuroleptic-like malignant syndrome of fever, sweating, rigidity, and mental confusion and obtundation.

The next most powerful drugs in treating PD symptoms are the dopamine agonists. Several of these are available. Apomorphine may be the most powerful, but it needs to be injected or taken sublingually. The others agonists are effective orally. Pergolide, pramipexole and ropinirole appear to be equally effective, and all are more powerful than bromocriptine. Cabergoline and lisuride are not available in the United States. Cabergoline has the longest halflife and therefore may prove ultimately to be most useful. Dopamine agonists are more likely to cause hallucinations, confusion and psychosis, especially in the elderly person. Thus, it is safer to use levodopa in patients older than age of 70 years. Controlled clinical trials reveal that dopamine agonist therapy is less likely to produce dyskinesias and the wearing-off phenomena than levodopa. But these trials also showed that levodopa provides greater symptomatic benefit that do dopamine agonists. The neuroimaging component of these studies reveals that striatal dopamine nerve terminals disappear at a faster rate with levodopa treatment than with the agonists. There is uncertainty how to apply the information gleaned from these studies to the patient, and a frank discussion between physician and patient should lead to the appropriate treatment for that individual.

Amantadine has several actions; it has antimuscarinic effects, but more importantly, it can activate release of dopamine from nerve terminals, block dopamine uptake into the nerve terminals, and block glutamate receptors. Its dopaminergic actions make it a useful drug to relieve symptoms in approximately two thirds of patients, but it can induce livedo reticularis, ankle edema, visual hallucinations, and confusion. Its antiglutamatergic action is useful in reducing the severity of levodopa-induced dyskinesias.

Elderly persons do not tolerate amantadine well because of the mental adverse effects. Domperidone is a peripherally active dopamine receptor blocker and is useful in preventing gastrointestinal upset from levodopa and the dopamine agonists. It is not available in the United States, but can be obtained from other countries. Monoamine oxidase type B (MAO-B) inhibitors (e.g., selegiline) offer mildly effective symptomatic benefit and are without the hypertensive "cheese effect" seen with MAO-A inhibitors, and therefore can be used in the presence of levodopa therapy. Although there has been considerable debate about possible protective benefit with selegiline, recent studies evaluating its longterm use indicate that selegiline is associated with less freezing of gait and with a slower rate of clinical worsening when compared to placebo-treated subjects. These benefits appear to be separate from its mild symptomatic effects because all subjects were receiving symptomatic benefit from concurrent levodopa therapy.

Nondopaminergic agents (Table 108-5) are also useful to treat many PD symptoms. Antimuscarinic drugs have been widely used since the 1950s, but these are much less effective than the dopaminergic agents, including amantadine. Because of sensitivity to memory impairment and hallucinations in the elderly population, antimuscarinics should be avoided in patients older than age 70 years. Antihistaminics have mild anticholinergic properties and can serve as alternatives to antimuscarinic drugs in the elderly population. Another alternative agent is amitriptyline because it also has anticholinergic properties. Because depression is common in patients with PD, this symptom needs to be addressed; the tricyclics and selective serotonin reuptake inhibitors are useful antidepressants. It is not certain if one type of antidepressant class of compounds is superior to the other in treating the depression accompanying PD. If insomnia is a problem for the patient, using an antidepressant that is also a soporific can be doubly advantageous, such as amitriptyline given at bedtime.

Psychosis induced by levodopa and the dopamine agonists can usually be controlled by quetiapine and clozapine

Table 108-5 Nondopaminergic Agents

Antimuscarinics: trihexyphenidyl, benztropine, ethopropazine, etc.

Antihistaminics: diphenhydramine, orphenadrine

Antiglutamatergics: amantadine, dextromethorphan

Antidepressants: selective serotonin reuptake inhibitors, tricyclics

Antipsychotics: clozapine, quetiapine, olanzapine

Antistress: benzodiazepines: diazepam, lorazepam, alprazolam

Antiorthostasis: fluodrocortisone, midodrine (ProAmatine)

Muscle relaxants: cyclobenzaprine, diazepam, baclofen

without worsening the parkinsonism. Other antipsychotic agents are more likely to worsen the parkinsonism, therefore they should be avoided. Clozapine appears to be more effective than quetiapine, but because clozapine treatment requires weekly white blood cell counts, quetiapine should be tried first. Another useful class of drugs is the benzodiazepines to reduce anxiety, which can decrease parkinsonian tremor that is exacerbated by stress. Diazepam is usually well tolerated and does not exacerbate parkinsonian symptoms. Lorazepam and alprazolam are other agents in this class of drugs. Muscle relaxants might help overcome "off" dystonia and peakdose dystonia that patients on levodopa therapy sometimes develop. Coenzyme Q10 is currently being tested in a controlled clinical trial to determine whether it has protective effects.

MOTOR COMPLICATIONS OF LEVODOPA THERAPY

Many patients on levodopa therapy develop motor complications (Table 108-6). Response fluctuations usually begin as mild wearingoff, which can be defined as when an adequate dosage of levodopa does not last at least 4 hours. Typically, in the first couple of years of treatment, there is a long duration response so that the timing of doses of levodopa is not important. Over time, the long duration response becomes lost, and only a short duration response occurs; patients then develop the wearing off phenomenon. The "offs" tend to be mild at first, but over time become

Table 108-6 Pattern of Development of Response Fluctuations, Dyskinesias, and Other Complications

Dyskinesias (chorea and dystonia)
Peak-dose dyskinesias
Diphasic dyskinesias
Fluctuations
Wearing-off
Delayed "ons"
Dose failures
Sudden, unpredictable "offs" (on–offs)
Early morning "off" dystonia
"Off" dystonia during day
Alertness
Drowsy from a dose of levodopa
Reverse sleep–wake cycle
Behavioral and cognitive
Vivid dreams
Benign hallucinations
Malignant hallucinations
Delusions
Paranoia
Confusion
Dementia

deeper with more severe parkinsonism; simultaneously, the duration of the "on" response becomes shorter. Eventually, some patients develop random, sudden "offs" in which the deep state of parkinsonism develops over minutes rather than tens of minutes, and they are less predictable in terms of timing with the dosings of levodopa. Many patients who develop response fluctuations also develop abnormal involuntary movements, that is, dyskinesias.

Treatment of the "Wearing-off" Phenomenon

The wearing off phenomenon, when mild, may be ameliorated slightly with the addition of selegiline (introduced as 5 mg daily, and increasing to 5 mg twice daily, as necessary). Selegiline potentiates the action of levodopa, and its introduction can induce confusion and psychosis, particularly in the elderly person. A lower dose of levodopa may be necessary. Sinemet CR (continuous-release carbidopa/levodopa) can also be effective in patients with mild wearingoff, and one can gradually switch from standard carbidopa/levodopa to Sinemet CR. Because it takes more than an hour for a dose of continuous-release medication to become effective, most patients also require supplemental standard carbidopa/levodopa to obtain an adequate response. One can attempt to use standard carbidopa/levodopa alone, giving the doses closer together, but ultimately, most patients develop progressively shorter durations of effectiveness from these doses, so patients could require as many as six or more doses per day. Eventually, dose failures as a consequence of poor gastric emptying often develop.

Dopamine agonists, which have a longer biological half-life than levodopa, can also be used in combination with standard Sinemet or Sinemet CR. The addition of a dopamine agonist tends to make the "off" state less severe when used in combination with carbidopa/levodopa. The addition of a dopamine agonist, however, will likely increase dyskinesias; in this situation the dosage of levodopa would need to be reduced.

COMT inhibitors are useful for treating wearingoff. COMT is the enzyme that catalyzes the conversion of dopa and dopamine to their methylated derivatives, so COMT inhibitors extend the duration of levodopa's effect without increase in the peak plasma concentration. Two COMT inhibitors are available: entacapone and tolcapone. Entacapone has a short half-life and is given at 200 mg with each dose of carbidopa/levodopa. For the many patients who have "offs" at a specific time of day, entacapone can be strategically given just with the dosage of carbidopa/levodopa that Precedes this "off" period. Tolcapone, with a longer half-life, is taken three times daily. Diarrhea and hepatic enzyme changes are sometimes adverse effects from tolcapone; hepatotoxicity has led to four deaths, so a patient's liver enzymes must be monitored biweekly, and it should be used only if entacapone is unsuccessful. The patient needs to sign a consent form to take tolcapone. A typical dose of tolcapone is 100 mg tid, with an increase to 200 mg tid possible, should the need arise. The COMT inhibitors are effective immediately; stopping them eliminates their benefit immediately.

Treatment of Dyskinesias

Levodopa-induced dyskinesias are involuntary movements and occur in two major forms: chorea and dystonia. Choreic movements are irregular, purposeless, nonrhythmic, abrupt, rapid, unsustained movements that seem to flow from one body part to another. Dystonic movements are more sustained, twisting contractions. Many patients probably have a combination of chorea and dystonia. Dystonia is a more serious problem than chorea because it is usually more disabling.

Peak dose dyskinesias occur when the plasma concentration of levodopa is at its peak, and the brain concentration of levodopa and dopamine is too high. Reducing the individual dose can resolve this problem. But the patient may need to take more frequent doses at this lower amount because reducing the amount of an individual dose also reduces the duration of benefit. More frequent dosings of levodopa tends to lead to delayed "ons" and, eventually, to dose failures. A simple approach is to add amantadine. Possibly because of its antiglutamatergic action, amantadine can suppress the severity of dyskinesias. Start with a dose of 100 mg bid and increase up to 200 mg bid, if necessary. Another approach is to substitute higher doses of a dopamine agonist while lowering the dose of carbidopa/levodopa. Dopamine agonists are less likely to cause dyskinesias, and therefore can usually be used in this situation quite safely. If lowering the dose of levodopa results in more severe "off" states, then the agonists become more important. Sinemet CR is not helpful because there is the danger of increased dyskinesias at the end of the day as the blood levels become sustained from frequent dosings. Once dyskinesias appear with Sinemet CR, they last for a considerable duration of time because of the slow decay in the plasma levels. In some patients peakdose chorea and dystonia occur at sub-therapeutic doses of levodopa, and lowering the dosage will render a patient even more parkinsonian. Such patients are candidates for deep brain stimulation (see below under surgical treatment).

Diphasic dyskinesias are dyskinesias that occur at the beginning and end of dose, not during the time of peak plasma and brain levels of levodopa. They tend to affect particularly the legs with a mixture of chorea and dystonia. Because the mechanism is unclear, treatment of diphasic dyskinesias is difficult. In this situation, one should use a dopamine agonist as the major pharmacologic agent with supplementary levodopa.

"Off" dystonia and painful "off" cramps could be listed in both dyskinesias and fluctuations, because these dystonias occur when the patient is "off." Dystonic spasms, therefore, can be either a sign of levodopa overdosage, as in peakdose dyskinesias, or occur when the plasma level of levodopa is low, such as in early morning before the first dose of levodopa. "Off" dystonia can occur anytime when the patient is "off." Preventing "offs" is the best way to control them. An effective treatment is to use a dopamine agonist as the major pharmacologic agent with supplementary levodopa. Baclofen has also been report to benefit some patients. Bedtime Sinemet CR may be useful to prevent early morning dystonia, but some patients need to set the alarm early to take a dose of carbidopa/levodopa and then fall back to sleep and awaken at their usual time.

TREATMENT OF NONMOTOR FEATURES

Nonmotor symptoms can also occur as complications from dopaminergic therapy of PD. *Mental changes of psychosis, confusion, agitation, hallucinations, paranoid delusions, and excessive sleeping* are probably related to activation of dopamine receptors in nonstriatal regions, particularly the cortical and limbic structures. Elderly patients and patients with concomitant dementia are extremely sensitive to small doses of levodopa. But all patients with PD, regardless of age, can develop psychosis if they take excess amounts of levodopa as a means to overcome "off" periods. Psychosis and hallucinations can often be eliminated by reducing the antiparkinsonian drugs. All antiparkinson drugs have the potential to induce psychosis, so the less-efficacious drugs should be withdrawn first. Accordingly, selegiline, amantadine, anticholinergics, and dopamine agonists should be withdrawn in that order, reserving levodopa as the most effective agent. If psychosis persists, atypical antipsychotics need to be used. These "atypicals" antipsychotics are so-called because they usually do not induce or worsen parkinsonism, and therefore can be used in patients with PD. The two most atypical antipsychotics are quetiapine and clozapine. Clozapine is more effective than quetiapine, but, unfortunately, clozapine induces agranulocytosis in approximately 1 to 2 percent of patients. Patients must have their blood counts monitored weekly for this potential complication, and then discontinue the drug if leukopenia develops. This inconvenience can be avoided if quetiapine is effective, so one should start treatment with quetiapine. Both quetiapine and clozapine often cause drowsiness, so bedtime dosing is recommended. Quetiapine can cause falling, and clozapine can cause seizures with high doses. For quetiapine, start with a 25-mg tablet hs, and increase as needed until benefit or adverse effects are encountered. For clozapine start with half of the 25-mg strength tablet at bedtime, and increase the dose as needed.

An altered sleep–wake cycle of drowsiness during the daytime, particularly after a dose of levodopa, and insomnia at night are fairly common in elderly patients and often accompany confusion. If a patient becomes drowsy after each dose of medication, reducing the dose may correct this problem. If the patient is generally drowsy during the daytime and remains awake at night, this makes it difficult for the care provider. It is important to get the patient onto a sleep–wake schedule that fits with the rest of the household. Efforts must be made to stimulate the patient physically and mentally during the daytime and force the patient to remain awake; otherwise, the patient will not be able to sleep at night. At night, the patient should then be drowsy enough to be able to sleep. If this fails, it may be necessary to use stimulants in the morning and sedatives at night in order to reverse the altered state. This should be done in addition to prodding the patient to remain awake during the day. Drugs such as methylphenidate and amphetamine are usually well tolerated by patients with PD. A 10-mg dose of either of these two drugs, repeated once if necessary, may be helpful. To encourage sleep at night, a hypnotic may be necessary in addition to using daytime stimulants. It should be noted that strong sedatives, such as barbiturates, are poorly tolerated by patients with PD.

Milder hypnotics, such as benzodiazepines and zolpidem, are usually taken without difficulty.

Orthostatic hypotension can be caused by levodopa, dopamine agonists, and other drugs taken by the patient, such as tricyclic antidepressants. These other drugs should be discontinued. If orthostatic hypotension remains, it can sometimes be managed by using support stockings, NaCl, midodrine (ProAmatine) and fludrocortisone (Florinef), but often the dosage of levodopa needs to be reduced.

Constipation is common in PD. It may be further aggravated by anticholinergics. Besides changing dietary habits by increasing intake of more fiber and dried fruits, polypropylene glycol (Mira-Lax) can be effective. For those who have bloating because of suppression of peristalsis when they are "off," keeping them "on" with levodopa is beneficial.

Depression is a common nonmotor symptom in PD, probably related to the reduction of all brain monoamines in this disease. Depression must be treated, not only for its own sake, but because its presence interferes with a good response to antiparkinson drugs. It often responds to tricyclic antidepressants, such as amitriptyline, nortriptyline, and protriptyline. Because of its anticholinergic and soporific effects, amitriptyline can be useful for these properties as well as for its antidepressant effect. Protriptyline, on the other hand, has no anticholinergic effect and can be useful when this property is not needed. Selective serotonin reuptake inhibitors, such as fluoxetine, sertraline, and paroxetine are also effective agents for treating depression in PD, but may aggravate parkinsonism if antiparkinsonian drugs are not being used concurrently. The newer agents nefazodone and venlafaxine with a combination of serotonin and norepinephrine reuptake inhibition are also effective. Electroconvulsive therapy (ECT) can be effective in patients with severe, intractable depression, and it can sometimes transiently improve the motor symptoms of PD as well.

SURGICAL THERAPY

Surgery for PD is becoming increasingly available as new techniques of electrical stimulation have been developed, while a better understanding of basal ganglia physiology has occurred. Stereotaxic deep brain stimulation (DBS) is fast becoming the treatment of choice because ablative lesioning is more risky for inducing neurologic deficits. With stimulating electrodes, the stimulation can be adjusted, and the electrodes could be removed if required. However, DBS is more costly, and frequent adjustments of the stimulator are usually needed. The location of the stereotaxic target is the other major factor that needs to be individualized for each patient. The thalamus, particularly the ventral intermediate nucleus, appears to be the most successful target for controlling tremor, but this target does not eliminate bradykinesia so stereotaxic thalamotomy or thalamic DBS is not a preferred choice today. The globus pallidus interna is a more satisfactory target for controlling choreic and dystonic dyskinesias. But the subthalamic nucleus appears to be best target for controlling bradykinesia. DBS of the subthalamic nucleus, by reducing bradykinesia, allows for a reduction of levodopa dosage, thus reducing the severity of dyskinesias as well. This surgical approach seems the most promising. Surgical procedures for patients with PD are best performed at specialty centers with an experienced team of a neurosurgeon, neurophysiologist to monitor the target during the operative procedure, and neurologist to program the stimulators. The patient needs close follow-up to adjust the stimulator settings to their optimum.

REFERENCES

Lansbury PT Jr, Brice A: Genetics of Parkinson's disease and biochemical studies of implicated gene products. *Curr Opin Genet Develop* 12:299, 2002.

Marek K et al: Dopamine transporter brain imaging to assess the effects of pramipexole vs levodopa on Parkinson disease progression. *JAMA* 287:1653, 2002.

Shoulson I et al: Impact of sustained deprenyl (Selegiline) in levodopa-treated Parkinson's disease: A randomized placebo controlled extension of the deprenyl and tocopherol antioxidative therapy of parkinsonism trial. *Ann Neurol* 51:604, 2002.

Tanner CM et al: Parkinson disease in twins—An etiologic study. *JAMA* 281:341, 1999.

Other Neurodegenerative Disorders

JAMES R. BURKE

Neurodegenerative diseases are characterized by selective neuronal loss and increasing frequency with age. Symptoms begin after normal development and decades of normal function. This chapter describes some of the less-common neurodegenerative diseases, including motor neuron disease, focal cortical atrophies, cerebellar degeneration, Lewy body dementia, and Parkinson-plus syndromes.

MOTOR NEURON DISEASE

Motor neuron diseases are characterized by selective loss of upper and/or lower motor neurons (UMN and LMN). The specific pattern of UMN and LMN loss determines the clinical presentation. UMN degeneration causes spasticity, hyperreflexia, and extensor plantar responses (Babinski's sign), while LMN loss results in muscle weakness, atrophy, cramps, and fasciculations. Bilateral UMN degeneration results in pseudobulbar palsy, which is the combination of dysarthria, dysphagia, and emotional lability. Neuronal loss in the lower brainstem (bulbar) causes dysarthria and dysphagia.

Amyotrophic lateral sclerosis (ALS; also known as Lou Gehrig's disease), the most common form of motor neuron disease (65 percent of motor neuron disease), affects both upper and lower motor neurons. Less-common forms of motor neuron disease include pure lower motor neuron degeneration (progressive muscular atrophy or progressive bulbar palsy) and pure upper motor neuron loss (primary lateral sclerosis or progressive pseudobulbar palsy). Patients may present with selective upper or lower motor neuron degeneration, but over time, the other type of motor neuron may begin to degenerate and the disease is then classified as ALS.

Two-thirds of ALS patients present with symptoms in the limbs, and 25 percent begin with bulbar symptoms. Bulbar symptoms are common in older individuals and are the presenting sign in 50 percent of patients older than age 70 years. Patients with ALS often report muscle cramps and examination may show muscle atrophy and fasciculations. ALS does not affect sensory, cerebellar or extraocular muscle function. Surprisingly, motor neuron disease can be associated with dementia. Frontal lobe dementia occurs in approximately 5 percent of motor-neuron-disease patients (see "Frontal Lobe Degeneration" later in this chapter).

The incidence of ALS is approximately 1 per 100,000 population with a prevalence of 5 per 100,000 population. Prevalence is similar in all races, but men are more commonly affected than women. ALS rarely occurs before 40 years of age and most cases occur between 40 and 70 years. The average age of onset is 60 years. ALS progresses rapidly and 50 percent of patients die within 26 to 38 months of symptom onset. Long-term survival does occur—25 percent of patients remain alive at 5 years after diagnosis and 8 to 15 percent at are alive at 10 years. Rapidly fatal disease is associated with increased age and bulbar-onset, but predictors of long-term survival remain elusive. Figure 109-1 shows the relation between age at symptom onset in ALS and duration of survival.

The diagnosis of motor neuron disease is based on history and examination with electrophysiologic, blood, and imaging studies used to confirm the diagnosis and exclude other etiologies. The electromyogram (EMG) in ALS demonstrates muscle denervation with preserved nerve conduction velocities. Rarely, ALS-like clinical presentations may occur with vitamin B_{12} deficiency, thyroid dysfunction, heavy metal toxicity, human immunodeficiency virus (HIV) infection, vasculitis, and dysproteinemia. Antibodies to gangliosides and other neuronal antigens are commonly reported, but their clinical significance is unclear. Magnetic resonance imaging (MRI) of the brain and spinal cord is used to rule out compressive myelopathy and masses in the region of the foramen magnum.

Treatment of motor neuron disease is primarily supportive with attention focused on emotional support and frank discussion of end-of-life issues and choices. Riluzole is the one medication currently approved for treatment of patients with ALS (Rilutek; Rhone-Poulenc Rorer). A

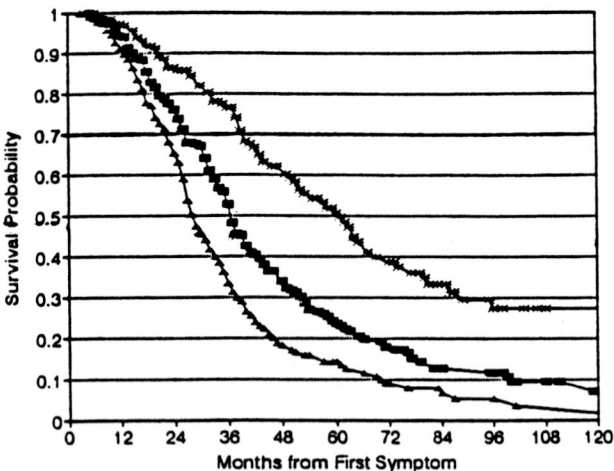

Figure 109-1 Kaplan-Meier plots of survival probabilities in amyotrophic lateral sclerosis patients as a function of age at onset of symptoms. Patients younger than age 45 years (*asterisks*); aged 45 to 65 years (*filled squares*); and older than age 65 years (*filled triangles*) at age of first symptoms. Reproduced with permission of Oxford University Press from Haverkamp L et al: Natural history of amyotrophic lateral sclerosis in a database population. Validation of a scoring system and a model for survival prediction. *Brain* 118:707, 1995.

Cochrane Library meta-analysis of the use of riluzole in ALS examined two studies containing a total of 794 patients treated with riluzole and 320 patients on placebo. The 100-mg dose of riluzole decreased death in the treated group at 12 months (odds ratio 0.57 [95% CI, 0.41 to 0.80]), but there was no beneficial effect on bulbar function or muscle strength. Riluzole's mechanism of action is unproven, but its pharmacologic properties include inhibition of release of the neurotransmitter glutamate and inactivation of voltage-dependent sodium channels, which may decrease excitotoxicity.

Symptomatic therapy of ALS includes treatment of muscle cramps, joint pain, and spasticity. Muscle cramps can be minimized by daily, repeated stretching of affected muscles. Joint pain commonly occurs as a result of disuse and loss of muscle support. Regular use of nonsteroidal antiinflammatory drugs may be helpful in reducing arthralgia. Spasticity responds to treatment with baclofen (Lioresal; Geigy Pharmaceuticals), tizanidine (Zanaflex; Athena Neurosciences), or botulinum toxin injections. Benzodiazepines can be useful for decreasing spasticity, but sedation limits effectiveness.

Pathologic examination of the spinal cord in ALS demonstrates a dramatic decrease in the population of large cervical and lumbar motor neurons. Brainstem motor nuclei also show significant neurodegeneration, but cranial nerve nuclei innervating the extraocular muscles are spared. Brains from patients with prominent UMN signs show marked loss of large pyramidal neurons in motor cortex. Atrophy of cortical neurons in the frontal lobe is common in patients with ALS-associated dementia. Degenerating neurons may contain inclusions of neurofilament, lipofuscin, Bunina bodies (dense granular eosinophilic inclusions) or Hirano bodies (rod-shaped inclusions).

ALS is primarily a sporadic disease, but 10 percent of patients have a positive family history. Most inherited ALS is transmitted as an autosomal dominant disorder, but early onset of autosomal recessive disease has been reported. Twenty percent of patients with autosomal dominant ALS have mutations in the superoxide dismutase 1 gene (SOD1). More than 70 different mutations in SOD1 have been identified in familial ALS, but mutations in SOD1 are not present in the sporadic form of the disease.

SOD1 provides a cellular defense against oxygen free radicals, but how mutations in this enzyme lead to disease is unknown. Pathogenesis is not simply related to a decrease in dismutase activity. Transgenic mice that express a human SOD protein containing an ALS causing mutation plus normal levels of mouse SOD still develop symptoms and signs of ALS. Additionally, supplementation of antioxidant defenses with Vitamin E is not successful in slowing progression of ALS in humans. Interestingly, Vitamin E delayed symptom onset in transgenic mice carrying mutant SOD1, but was ineffective in prolonging survival after symptom onset. In contrast, riluzole treatment of SOD1 transgenic mice did not delay symptom onset, but prolonged life after symptoms developed. These findings suggest separate mechanisms may be responsible for disease onset and progression.

The cause of sporadic ALS is unknown, but multiple etiologies have been proposed. Elevated concentrations of the excitatory amino acid neurotransmitters, glutamate and aspartate, can kill neurons by a process called excitotoxicity. Cerebrospinal fluid (CSF) from patients with ALS has threefold higher concentrations of excitatory amino acids than control CSF, a finding that is consistent with a role for excitotoxicity in pathogenesis. The cause for increased concentrations of aspartate and glutamate is unknown, but dysfunctional transport may cause a persistent elevation in the concentration of excitatory amino acids in the region of susceptible neurons. Glutamate transporters are responsible for removing excitatory amino acids from the extracellular space and impaired transport is found in effected regions of ALS brain and spinal cord. More than half of the patients with sporadic ALS have a 30 to 95 percent reduction in excitatory amino acid transporter 2. Defects in glutamate transport in sporadic ALS may be related to errors in ribonucleic acid (RNA) processing of the excitatory amino acid transporter messenger RNA.

Other candidates for pathogenesis in ALS include increased oxidative stress, autoimmune mechanisms and cytoskeletal abnormalities, but direct proof is lacking. Autoantibodies to calcium channel and other antigens are commonly found in ALS, but it is unclear whether they are an epiphenomenon or play a role in disease propagation. Aggregates of the cytoskeletal protein neurofilament accumulate in degenerating ALS motor neurons and may be important in pathogenesis. Transgenic mice expressing mutant neurofilament develop clinical and pathologic features of motor neuron disease. Mutations in a neurofilament gene have been detected in a small number of patients with sporadic ALS, but the clinical relevance of these mutations is unknown. It is likely that the etiology of ALS is multifactorial with numerous factors contributing to pathogenesis.

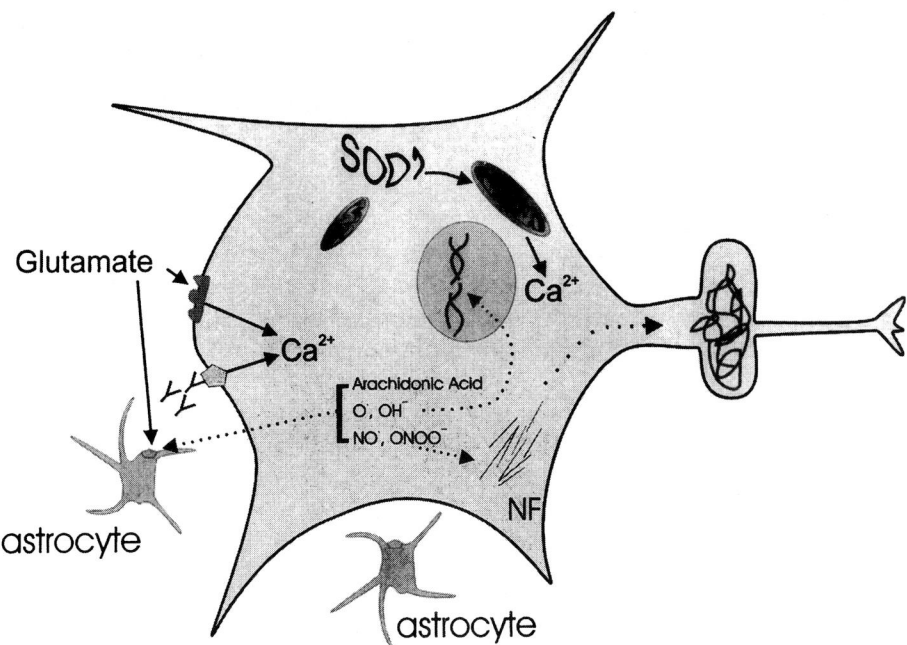

Figure 109-2   Mechanisms of motor neuron degeneration. Motor neurons are subject to various cellular insults that may intersect, leading individually or in concert to selective degeneration. For example, either excess glutamate or calcium channel antibodies may lead to increased intracellular calcium. Increased production of radical species may directly damage neurofilaments, leading to their accumulation, or damage to glutamate transporters, leading to excess glutamate, excitotoxicity, and additional oxidative stress. NF, neurofilament. Reproduced with permission of Lippincott Raven from Rothstein JD: Excitotoxicity hypothesis. *Neurology* 47:S19, 1996.

Figure 109-2 is a schematic of mechanisms of motor neuron degeneration.

FOCAL ATROPHIES

The focal atrophies are a group of disorders named for the presence of well-circumscribed areas of cortical degeneration surrounded by normal appearing cortex. Focal atrophy can be the result of many different pathologies. Regardless of the pathologic etiology, the clinical symptoms and signs are determined solely by the location of neuronal degeneration. Genetic studies show that more than one type of focal atrophy can occur within a single family, suggesting a common genetic factor can cause degeneration of different neuronal populations.

Frontal Lobe Degeneration

Degeneration of neurons in the frontal lobe leads to dementia, which is characterized by personality change with lack of insight, impaired judgment, and disinhibition. Individuals with frontal lobe degeneration may present with anxiety, depression, or emotional indifference. Social interactions and neglect of personal hygiene are common. Many of the problems in frontal lobe dementia can be attributed to marked deficits in attention and concentration.

In contrast to Alzheimer's disease where memory loss is a prominent early feature, frontal lobe dementia is primarily a disorder with behavioral disturbance and disordered thinking with relatively preserved memory. A useful way to distinguish between behavioral changes associated with Alzheimer's disease and frontal lobe dementia is to note whether memory problems precede personality change. If memory problems are the presenting problem, then the patient is more likely to have Alzheimer's disease. But if personality change is the presenting symptom, then frontal lobe degeneration is more likely. Later stages of frontal lobe degeneration show progressive impairment in language with deficits in expressive and receptive speech. The motor system remains uninvolved until late in the course when extrapyramidal signs may develop (except in families with frontal lobe dementia associated with parkinsonism [see in the section on Frontal Lobe Degeneration]). Progression to profound dementia is insidious and therapy is limited to attempts at behavioral control.

Frontal lobe dementia accounts for 5 to 10 percent of all cases of dementia and is more common in clinics where younger individuals are evaluated (the typical age of onset is between 45 and 65 years). Patients with frontal lobe dementia are frequently first evaluated by psychiatrists because of the prominence of behavioral symptoms. A positive family history is present in approximately half the patients. The average duration of illness is 8 years, but survival for 10 to 15 years is not unusual.

Laboratory testing including CSF examination is unrevealing, but electroencephalogram (EEG) may show focal slowing, especially in advanced cases. Neuropsychological testing can be helpful in quantifying deficits and identifying the characteristic features of frontal lobe dysfunction. Imaging studies may demonstrate frontal and/or temporal lobe atrophy, especially later in the illness. Positron emission tomography (PET) and single-photon

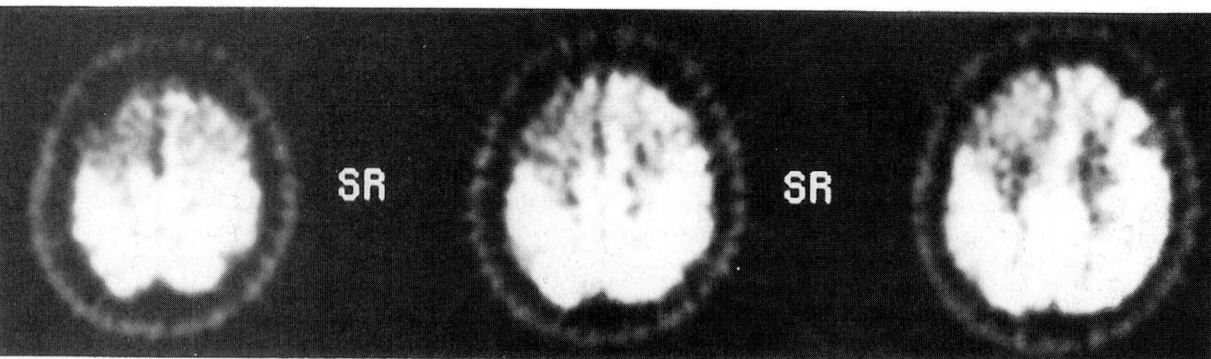

Figure 109-3   Fluorodeoxyglucose positron emission tomograph showing frontal lobe hypometabolism in patient with frontal lobe dementia. Courtesy of Sharon Hamblen and A. Al-Sugair, MD, Department of Radiology, Duke University Medical Center.

emission computed tomography (SPECT) frequently show bilateral frontal lobe hypometabolism or hypoperfusion. Figure 109-3 is an example of a fluorodeoxyglucose PET scan from a patient with severe frontal lobe dementia showing characteristic bilateral frontal lobe hypoperfusion.

Examination of the brain from patients with frontal lobe dementia demonstrates focal atrophy of the frontal and/or anterior temporal lobes. Several pathologic entities can cause this clinical syndrome including frontal lobe degeneration of the non-Alzheimer's type (which is also called "dementia lacking distinctive histologic features"), Pick's disease, and progressive subcortical gliosis. Frontal lobe degeneration of the non-Alzheimer's type is the most common pathology associated with frontal lobe dementia. The pathologic findings include spongy vacuolation and focal neuronal degeneration in layer II of frontal and temporal cortex. Intraneuronal and glial aggregates of hyperphosphorylated tau are frequently seen, but the classic inclusions of Pick's, Parkinson's, or Alzheimer's disease are absent. This nonspecific frontal lobe pathology is also called frontotemporal dementia. The common occurrence of abnormal accumulations of tau in sporadic and inherited forms of frontal lobe dementia and other forms of focal cortical atrophy have led some to characterize these disorders as "tauopathies." Pick's disease has spongiform changes and ballooned neurons some of which contain argyrophilic deposits known as Pick bodies. Pick bodies are composed of the cytoskeletal proteins neurofilament, tubulin and tau. Other causes of frontal lobe degeneration include bilateral infarction of the frontal lobe white matter, Creutzfeldt–Jakob disease, progressive subcortical gliosis, bilateral thalamic infarct, and, most commonly, a frontal lobe variant of Alzheimer's disease. Frontal lobe dementia can also occur with motor neuron disease.

Autosomal dominant frontal lobe dementia is associated with pathologic features of frontal lobe degeneration of the non-Alzheimer's type. Some inherited forms of frontal lobe dementia are caused by mutations in the tau gene on chromosome 17q21, and more than 20 disease-associated mutations have been identified.

As mentioned previously, neurodegenerative diseases can display marked heterogeneity, and this is well described in families with frontotemporal dementia. Individuals in a single family can present with typical frontal lobe dementia, parkinsonism, other focal cortical atrophy syndrome

or even motor neuron disease. This phenotypic variability within families inheriting a common mutation suggests that the same pathogenesis can cause degeneration of several different susceptible neuronal populations.

Primary Progressive Aphasia

Primary progressive aphasia (PPA) is a syndrome in which patients slowly develop a nonfluent, anomic aphasia. Speech is effortful, telegraphic and hesitant with frequent semantic (word choice) and phonemic (sound-based) errors. Repetition, reading, and writing are impaired, but comprehension is initially preserved. The disease progresses slowly and initially does not affect other faculties, such as memory, nonlanguage cognitive skills, and insight. As the disease progresses, impaired comprehension occurs, and ultimately patients become mute. Although some patients continue to have only language impairment, at least 75 percent of patients who present with PPA ultimately develop nonlanguage deficits. Less commonly, the first sign of PPA is a fluent, Wernicke's-like aphasia with impaired comprehension. Limited evidence suggests that aggressive speech therapy early in the course of the disease may transiently improve language function.

The average age of onset of PPA is 60 years and duration of isolated language problems ranges from 1 to 15 years (median 4.5 years). Diagnosis of PPA is based on history and physical examination. Laboratory testing is uninformative, but EEG may show left hemisphere slowing (25 percent) or, less commonly, bilateral or diffuse abnormalities. Computed tomography (CT) and MRI typically show left temporal lobe atrophy, but up to one-half of imaging studies are normal especially early in the course of the disease. Functional neuroimaging, PET, and SPECT may demonstrate left temporal hypometabolism.

The differential diagnosis of PPA includes stroke, mass lesion, and Alzheimer's disease. Dominant hemisphere stroke involving the language centers produces aphasia, which is similar, or identical, to the language deficit in PPA. The aphasia in stroke, however, occurs acutely making confusion with the slowly progressive symptoms of PPA unlikely. A slow growing mass in the language center could produce aphasia and mimic PPA, so to exclude this possibility an imaging study is necessary. Aphasia is common in Alzheimer's disease, but is almost invariably associated with early memory loss or other cognitive impairment.

The characteristic gross pathologic lesion in PPA is focal atrophy of the left anterior temporal region. Pathologic involvement of other areas depends on the patient's clinical state at the time of death. Microscopic findings in PPA include focal spongiform changes, focal neuronal degeneration, and accumulations of tau protein (resembling the pathologic findings in frontal lobe degeneration of the non-Alzheimer's type). Identical clinical presentations can be caused by Pick's disease, Alzheimer's disease, and Creutzfeldt–Jakob disease.

PPA is primarily a sporadic disorder, but can be inherited as an autosomal dominant disease. Families containing individuals with PPA and/or frontal lobe dementia have been described and linked to mutations in the tau gene on chromosome 17.

Corticobasal Degeneration

Focal atrophy of the parietal lobe and basal ganglia dysfunction leads to corticobasal degeneration (CBD). The clinical presentation of CBD is variable, but common features include asymmetric apraxia, the loss of ability to perform a skilled movement, and parkinsonism. The apraxia in CBD is striking; patients are virtually unable to use the affected extremity despite good comprehension of verbal commands and normal strength. In addition to apraxia, patients demonstrate cortical sensory loss (impaired stereognosis, graphesthesia, two-point discrimination, and double simultaneous stimulation) and action tremor. Dystonic posturing develops later and, finally, the limb is useless. Symptom progression is highly variable with no fixed order of development. CBD differs from Alzheimer's disease, which is also associated with apraxia, because in CBD other cognitive functions are preserved. A diagnosis of CBD should be considered in individuals who present with an early history of severe apraxia and then develop cognitive impairment.

More than 50 percent of patients with CBD develop alien limb phenomenon. Alien limb is limb movement without patient awareness. The movements can be purposeful (e.g., touching the face), antagonistic, (e.g., preventing the other hand from performing a task or inappropriate touching of others), or random (e.g., simple limb elevation). Reflex myoclonus is common and can be induced by light touch, pin prick, or attempted movement. Occasionally patients with CBD may present with apraxia of gait or speech.

Basal ganglia features of CBD include bradykinesia and rigidity mimicking Parkinson's disease. Other neurologic signs in patients with CBD include postural instability, supranuclear gaze palsy, aphasia (similar to primary progressive aphasia) and behavioral abnormalities (similar to those seen in frontal lobe dementia). The common finding of apraxia, aphasia, and behavioral problems in some patients has led to the hypothesis that CBD, PPA, and frontal lobe dementia are all subtypes of a single disorder, perhaps with tau abnormalities as a common factor (see below).

CBD is a rare disorder that typically begins in the sixth decade or later. It is slowly progressive with death occurring on average 5 or 10 years after onset of apraxia. Apraxia may remain restricted to a single limb for several years before spread inevitably occurs. In the latter stages of illness, dysphagia develops and aspiration becomes a significant risk. Management of patients with CBD is supportive. Dopamine replacement therapy does not produce any significant improvement in the basal ganglia symptoms or signs, but clonazepam can be helpful in controlling myoclonus. Occurrence of CBD is not associated with any environmental or genetic risk factors.

Diagnosis of CBD is based on history and physical examination. There are no diagnostic laboratory tests. EEG may be normal or show focal slowing. Neuroimaging and PET scans can support the diagnosis but are not sufficiently unique to exclude other diagnostic possibilities. MRI of patients with CBD frequently shows asymmetric atrophy involving the frontoparietal region. PET scans demonstrate decreased glucose metabolism in the frontoparietal region, contralateral to the most severely affected side.

The diagnosis of CBD is not difficult if the clinical picture is fully expressed. Early in the course, however, other etiologies can have similar presentations, including focal parietal lobe lesions such as infarcts, vascular malformations, or tumors. Imaging studies should exclude these possibilities. If basal ganglia symptoms predominate early in the course of the disease, misdiagnosis of Parkinson's disease or progressive supranuclear palsy is common. Parkinson and Parkinson-like syndromes can have similar clinical presentations, but the presence of asymmetric parietal cortex sensory loss and apraxia strongly suggests CBD. Similar clinical features may also occasionally occur with Alzheimer's disease, Pick's disease, Creutzfeldt–Jakob disease, and dementia with Lewy bodies.

The major pathologic features of CBD include tau-positive neuropil threads and grains, swollen neurons, neurofibrillary tangles, and glial inclusions. Gross examination of the brain reveals focal atrophy with asymmetric enlargement of sulci in the parietal lobe. Neuronal loss and gliosis are found in the cortex and pars compacta of the substantia nigra. Cortical neurons are pale, or achromatic, and swollen, but Pick bodies are absent. Substantia nigra neurons have intracytoplasmic inclusions, but the inclusions differ from the Lewy bodies seen in Parkinson's disease. CBD is a sporadic disorder, but patients have an overrepresentation of a specific tau gene haplotype compared to control individuals.

Cerebellar Degeneration

Cerebellar degenerations are a heterogeneous group of disorders linked by prominent ataxia. In this chapter, discussion is restricted to cerebellar degeneration with onset in adulthood. Most of the degenerative cerebellar disorders that meet this criterion are sporadic and idiopathic, but one-third are inherited. Few patients have pure cerebellar dysfunction and the presence of other neurologic findings has led to a complex nosology. It is not necessary for the nonspecialist to remember the clinical features of each disorder, but it is useful to have a framework so that one can approach a patient with ataxia in a logical and efficient manner.

Clinical features of ataxia include disturbed gait, limb incoordination, tremor, dysarthria, and abnormal eye movements. An ataxic gait is wide-based and is frequently compared to that of an intoxicated individual. Subtle gait ataxia can be demonstrated by having patients walk heel-to-toe (tandem gait). Ataxic limb movements can be divided into two components: dysmetria, erratic jerky course during purposeful movement, and dysdiadochokinesis, impaired fine or alternating repetitive movements. Both abnormalities are commonly present in ataxic patients. The earliest symptom of limb ataxia is impairment of fine movements. Patients will typically describe limb ataxia as clumsiness. Caution must be exercised in interpreting cerebellar dysfunction in the presence of sensory loss or weakness because fine movements in weak or anesthetic limbs can appear ataxic. Cerebellar tremor is most apparent during purposeful movements. Speech abnormalities in cerebellar disease are described as scanning and explosive. Scanning refers to slow, slurred speech with increased separation between syllables. Explosive speech is caused by impaired coordination of breathing and speech so that volume regulation is irregular. Often cerebellar speech is only slurred and can be difficult to distinguish from spastic dysarthria. Common eye movement abnormalities in patients with cerebellar degeneration are jerkiness of smooth pursuit, ocular dysmetria (overshoot when approaching a target) and slow saccades.

There are three major clinical presentations of sporadic cerebellar degeneration. Patients with onset after 55 years of age frequently have prominent midline cerebellar dysfunction that leads to gait ataxia with mild limb dysfunction. Cerebellar speech may be present, but is frequently mild. A second group of patients develops symptoms between 35 and 55 years of age with cerebellar deficits combined with dementia and peripheral neuropathy. This group is also at increased risk for developing symptoms and signs of multiple system atrophy (see "Multiple System Atrophy" later in this chapter). The third group has cerebellar ataxia beginning in the fifth or sixth decade with prominent resting and intention tremor. Late-onset, sporadic cerebellar ataxia is a slowly progressive disorder with loss of independent ambulation developing 5 to 20 years after symptom onset. Poor prognostic signs include development of multiple system atrophy or evidence of brainstem atrophy on MRI.

Pharmacologic treatments for ataxia are generally unsuccessful. Small studies suggest modest efficacy of buspirone, acetazolamide, amantadine, and transdermal physostigmine for treatment of varying types of ataxia, but double-blinded, placebo-controlled trials are lacking. Occupational therapy is useful in educating patient's and families about coping strategies for ataxia and to provide prosthetics to minimize the amplitude of ataxic movements.

One-third of adult-onset ataxia is inherited, and most is transmitted in an autosomal dominant pattern. More than 10 forms of autosomal dominant cerebellar degeneration have been described with varying associated findings including: optic atrophy, pigmentary retinopathy, ophthalmoplegia, dementia, pyramidal and extrapyramidal dysfunction and peripheral neuropathy (see Table 109-1 for information on chromosomal localization and clinical phenotype of some of the ataxia mutations). Age of onset

Table 109-1   Genotype Classification of the Spinocerebellar Ataxias

Name	Locus	Phenotype
SCA type 1 (autosomal dominant type 1)	6p22-p23 with CAG repeats	Ataxia with ophthalmoparesis, pyramidal and extrapyramidal findings
SCA type 2 (autosomal dominant type 2)	12q23-24.1	Ataxia with slow saccades and minimal pyramidal and extrapyramidal findings
SCA type 3 (autosomal dominant type 3)	14q24.3-qter: allelic at the Machado–Joseph disease locus	Ataxia with ophthalmoparesis and variable pyramidal and extrapyramidal findings
SCA type 4 (autosomal dominant type 4)	16q22.1	Ataxia with normal eye movements, sensory axonal neuropathy, and pyramidal signs
SCA type 5 (autosomal dominant type 5)	Centromeric region of chromosome 11	Ataxia and dysarthria
Machado–Joseph disease	14q24.3-q32 with CAC repeats	Ataxia with ophthalmoparesis and variable pyramidal–extrapyramidal and amyotrophic features
Dentatorubropallidouysian atrophy (autosomal dominant)	12p12-ter with CAG repeats	Ataxia, choreoathetosis, dystonia, seizures, myoclonus, and dementia

NOTE: Table includes only the autosomal dominant forms of the ataxias with chromosomal localization and summary of clinical phenotype.
SOURCE: Reproduced with permission of Wiley-Liss, Inc. from Rosenberg RN: The genetic basis of ataxia. *Clin Neurosci* 8:1, 1995.

differs in the various forms of inherited autosomal dominant ataxia, but in general early onset (age 40 years or younger) is associated with more aggressive disease. Specific diagnosis at the bedside is difficult because associated clinical features can vary even among individuals in a single family, but genetic testing is becoming increasingly common. Good, current descriptions of the inherited cerebellar degenerations, and other genetic disorders, can be found in Online Mendelian Inheritance in Man (OMIM) on the World Wide Web at http://www.ncbi.nlm.nih.gov/omim.

Several genes causing late-onset cerebellar ataxias are known. Each contains an expanded trinucleotide repeat in the coding region of the disease gene. The trinucleotide repeat is identical in each CAG, and codes for the amino acid glutamine. Unaffected individuals generally have fewer than 30 CAG repeats, while affected persons have more than 40. The length of the polyglutamine repeat is the major determinant of age of onset. Individuals with longer repeats develop early onset of symptoms. Figure 109-4 shows the relationship between repeat length and age of symptom-onset in patients with spinocerebellar ataxia type I. SCA6 is an exception to the rule that disease is only associated with CAG repeat lengths greater than 40. Individuals with SCA6 commonly have 20–30 CAG repeats. The polyglutamine expansion in SCA6 gene is contained in a calcium channel gene and may have a different pathogenetic mechanism than the other CAG repeat diseases. Expanded CAG repeats also cause Huntington's disease and spinobulbar muscular atrophy (Kennedy's disease).

Polyglutamine repeat length varies from generation to generation and pathologic-length repeats are more likely to expand than contract, especially when the disease gene is inherited paternally. The increased likelihood that long repeats will expand is the molecular explanation for the clinical observation that disease onset within a family occurs at younger ages in succeeding generations (i.e., anticipation).

The function of the ataxia disease genes and the effect of having >40 consecutive glutamines, is unknown. It is believed that these mutations cause disease by a gain-of-function mechanism rather than by loss of normal function. Polyglutamine domains can mediate protein–protein interactions, so pathogenesis may be caused by quantitative or qualitative changes in these interactions. Cytoplasmic and nuclear intraneuronal protein aggregates are common in polyglutamine repeat diseases and may be important in pathogenesis. Sequestration of transcription factors and other essential factors by polyglutamine proteins has been suggested to be the critical event leading to selected neuronal loss.

Laboratory testing is available to detect the trinucleotide repeat expansion in known disease genes, but more ataxia genes remain to be discovered. At present, a patient with a clear family history of autosomal dominant cerebellar ataxia has approximately a 50 percent chance of having a mutation in a known disease gene. It is becoming increasingly common to find patients with no family history of ataxia, but who possess a mutation in one of the ataxia genes. The discovery of new mutations has important implications for patient counseling. Some "sporadic" cerebellar ataxias are actually the result of new mutations (i.e., expansion of the CAG repeat from normal to pathologic length) and will be transmitted to subsequent generations. Patients should not be assured that their ataxia is not caused by an inherited disease simply because there are no other affected family members.

The evaluation of adult-onset ataxia includes a careful history, especially the nature of onset (acute versus subacute versus chronic), presence of other neurologic or medical complaints, and family history. Acute onset ataxia is rarely confused with degenerative disorders and can be caused by stroke, hemorrhage, infection, or intoxication (alcohol, solvents; thallium, lead, and drugs, especially anticonvulsants). Subacute development of ataxia may be a sign of hydrocephalus caused by posterior fossa mass, abscess or chronic infection. Subacute ataxia can also occur as a result of HIV infection or a paraneoplastic syndrome, most commonly associated with small-cell lung, ovarian cancer or Hodgkin's disease. Laboratory conformation of paraneoplastic cerebellar degeneration can be made by detection of the antineuronal antibody anti-Yo. Paraneoplastic syndromes can predate the diagnosis of cancer by years, so occurrence of subacute cerebellar degeneration in a patient without a diagnosis of cancer should still lead to a thorough search for occult neoplasm. Paraneoplastic cerebellar degeneration can occasionally present with an indolent course suggesting degenerative disease. Chronic development of ataxia commonly is due to alcoholism, but other causes include idiopathic or inherited degenerative disease, Creutzfeldt–Jakob disease, vitamin E deficiency, hypothyroidism and, rarely, multiple sclerosis. Laboratory evaluation for individuals with chronic ataxia should include thyroid studies, Vitamin E levels, heavy metal screen, and MRI.

Pathologic features of the cerebellar degenerations vary depending on the associated neurologic features. In general

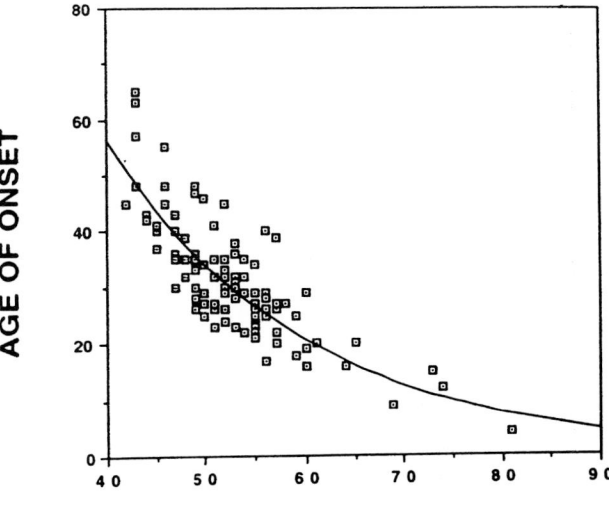

Figure 109-4 Relationship between the age at onset and the repeat length of the expanded allele in 113 patients affected with SCA1. Reproduced with permission of the University of Chicago Press from Ranum LPW et al: Molecular and clinical correlations in spinocerebellar ataxia type 1: evidence for familial effects on the age at onset. *Am J Hum Gene.* 55:244, 1994.

the cerebellum is atrophic with loss of Purkinje cells and proliferation of Bergmann glia. Surviving Purkinje cells may contain axonal swellings called torpedoes, which are composed of neurofilament. There are no pathognomonic pathologic features found in all forms of disease.

NEURODEGENERATIVE DISEASES PRESENTING AS PARKINSONISM

Parkinson's disease was described in 1817 by the English physician James Parkinson. The clinical features he noted remain the pillars of diagnosis and include bradykinesia, rigidity, rest tremor, and postural instability. Unfortunately, there are a significant number of diseases that mimic Parkinson's disease and a diagnostic error rate of 25 percent for Parkinson's disease is common. Idiopathic Parkinson's disease is not discussed in this chapter.

Parkinsonism is common in dementia. At least one-third of Alzheimer's disease patients display bradykinesia, rigidity, and shuffling gait at some point in the illness. This section describes some of the neurodegenerative disease mimics of Parkinson's disease and how they can be distinguished from idiopathic Parkinson's disease.

Progressive Supranuclear Palsy

Progressive supranuclear palsy (PSP) is a common neurodegenerative mimic of Parkinson's disease. It usually begins between the ages of 50 and 75 years (median age 63 years) with symptoms and signs resembling Parkinson's disease, but there are several differences. The most distinctive clinical feature of PSP is vertical gaze paresis. Patients with PSP initially lose voluntary downgaze. Subsequently upgaze is impaired and finally horizontal eye movements leave the eyes immobile to voluntary command. The eyes will, however, move in response to head turning. Eye movement in response to passive head turning indicates the pathologic lesion is supranuclear to the nerves innervating the extraocular muscles. Supranuclear gaze palsy causes patients to have significant problems descending stairs and searching for objects directly in front of them. Supranuclear gaze palsy is uncommon in idiopathic Parkinson's disease.

There are a number of distinguishing features between PSP and Parkinson's disease. Individuals with PSP and Parkinson's disease have abnormal tone, but rigidity in PSP is mainly axial, while in Parkinson's it primarily affects the limbs. The onset of rigidity also differs. In PSP rigidity develops symmetrically, but rigidity in Parkinson's disease has an asymmetric onset. Tremor and posture are other areas of divergence. Patients with PSP have minimal rest tremor and posture is extended, while individuals with Parkinson's disease have prominent tremor and stooped posture. Another characteristic difference is the minimal or absent response to dopamine therapy in PSP.

Dementia occurs in both PSP and Parkinson's disease but is much more common in PSP. The clinical features of dementia in PSP are similar to frontal lobe dementia with prominent inattention and apathy. Patients with PSP display a characteristic wide-eyed, expressionless stare giving a look of persistent surprise. They also commonly have problems with dysequilibrium leading to frequent falls (especially backwards).

Diagnosis of PSP is based on history and physical examination. Laboratory testing is of limited utility. MRI of patients with PSP is often normal, especially early in the course of the disease, but in more advanced cases MRI may show midbrain atrophy. PSP is frequently misdiagnosed as Parkinson's disease or multiple systems atrophy especially if eye movement abnormalities are not prominent. It must be cautioned that overreliance on supranuclear gaze palsy can also lead to misdiagnosis. This eye movement abnormality can be seen in cortical-basal degeneration, olivopontocerebellar atrophy (OPCA) form of multiple system atrophy, diffuse Lewy body disease, Creutzfeldt–Jakob disease, Whipple's disease, and Niemann Pick type C, or as a result of strokes.

The prevalence of PSP is approximately 1.4 cases per 100,000 population and men account for two-thirds of patients. PSP is responsible for approximately 5 percent of cases of parkinsonism. There are no known genetic or environmental risk factors. There is a report of a single family with two affected individuals. The median survival from symptom onset to death is 6 years, with a range from 6 months to 9 years. The usual cause of death is aspiration pneumonia.

Pathologic examination of the brain in PSP shows midbrain atrophy with relatively well-preserved cerebral cortex. The main histopathologic features of PSP are neuronal loss, frequent neurofibrillary tangles and gliosis. Neuronal loss is seen in the globus pallidus, substantia nigra pars compacta, locus coeruleus, subthalamic nucleus, and the superior colliculi. The neurofibrillary tangles in PSP are ultrastructurally different from the 20- to 24-nm twisted filaments seen in Alzheimer's disease, but both are composed of the cytoskeletal protein tau. PSP tangles are straight 15-nm filaments. Aggregates of tau are found in the processes of glial cells and neuropil threads are common. Determination of tau genotypes in PSP show overrepresentation of the same specific tau haplotypes found in CBD suggesting that this form of tau predisposes to neurodegenerative disease, but other genetic or environmental factors determine which groups of neurons degenerate.

Multiple System Atrophy

Multiple system atrophy (MSA) is, as the name implies, a diverse group of disorders involving degeneration of different neuronal populations. Clinical features of MSA include a combination of parkinsonism, autonomic failure, cerebellar degeneration, and/or pyramidal tract dysfunction. In a large study of patients with MSA, approximately half the patients presented with parkinsonian features and half with autonomic failure. Later in the disease course, however, both findings were present in almost all patients. MSA can also present with cerebellar or corticospinal tract findings. Ultimately half of all patients develop cerebellar and/or pyramidal tract dysfunction. Despite the clinical variability, there are characteristic pathologic features that suggest a common pathogenetic mechanism and provide a rationale for classifying these patients as a single group.

Differentiation of MSA from idiopathic Parkinson's disease is difficult early in the disease course, but several predictive factors are suggested. Distinguishing features of MSA include symmetric onset of parkinsonism, absence of early rest tremor, rapid clinical deterioration, absent or transient responsiveness to dopamine replacement and impaired autonomic function. Autonomic features include orthostatic hypotension, urinary retention or incontinence, and/or impotence. Similarly, cerebellar dysfunction in MSA may be difficult to distinguish from other forms of cerebellar degeneration unless other clinical features are present, such as parkinsonism or autonomic failure. Corticospinal tract signs include spasticity, increased reflexes, Babinski signs, and pseudobulbar palsy.

When parkinsonian features predominate, MSA is often called striatonigral degeneration. If autonomic features predominate, it is called Shy–Drager syndrome, and when cerebellar features are prominent it is called OPCA.

MSA is a sporadic disorder of unknown cause. The prevalence of MSA is unknown, but autopsy studies show that 7 to 20 percent of patients diagnosed with Parkinson's disease have pathologic evidence of MSA. The median age of onset is 60 years. Survival is variable and ranges from 2 to 20 years. Median survival from onset of motor symptoms in MSA is 7.5 years, and half of patients are wheelchair bound within 5 years of onset of motor disturbance. The predominant symptom at initial clinical presentation does not have a major effect on survival.

Diagnosis of MSA is by history and physical examination. Misdiagnosis is common, especially early in the course before all symptoms and signs have developed. MRI may be helpful in diagnosis of striatonigral degeneration-type MSA if low signal intensity in the putamen on T2-weighted images is seen, or in OPCA, if cerebellar and brainstem atrophy is present. Unfortunately, atrophy is marked only late in the course of OPCA.

Disorders commonly misdiagnosed as MSA include Parkinson's disease, PSP, Lewy body dementia, primary autonomic failure, and cerebellar degeneration. Autonomic dysfunction can occur late in the course of idiopathic Parkinson's disease, but the late onset and previous long-term response to dopamine replacement makes confusion with MSA unlikely. The mechanism underlying late onset autonomic failure in Parkinson's disease is unknown. Dementia with Lewy bodies is discussed in detail in the section on that disorder, below. Primary autonomic failure is autonomic failure without associated basal ganglia, cerebellar, or pyramidal deficits.

Treatment of MSA varies depending on the symptom to be treated. Bradykinesia and rigidity are treated with dopamine replacement. Some MSA patients with parkinsonism have a good, if transient, response to dopamine supplementation so a therapeutic trial is worthwhile. Cerebellar symptoms are refractory to treatment and no drugs are currently approved for this indication.

Management of autonomic dysfunction is complex and many therapeutic options are available. Individuals with orthostatic hypotension should be educated about increasing salt intake, avoiding rapid changes in position, carbohydrate-induced postprandial hypotension, exacerbation of symptoms by alcohol consumption and straining during micturition or defecation. Supine hypertension is a significant problem. Raising the head of the patient's bed by 20 degrees treats supine hypertension and may minimize postural hypotension by reducing nocturnal diuresis and sodium loss. If these simple measures are insufficient, the next step in managing symptoms is use of devices that prevent venous pooling upon standing. These devices include elastic stockings (Jobst stockings). Positive-pressure anti-gravity suits can be effective, but difficult to use in daily life. Some experts do not recommend use of elastic stockings because most pooling of blood occurs in the splanchnic circulation, not in the legs.

Most patients ultimately require pharmacologic management to reduce postural hypotension. The first-line agent for treatment of orthostatic hypotension is a mineralocorticoid such as fludrocortisone (Florinef; Apothecon). Mineralocorticoids increase fluid retention, which raises blood pressure, but this may exacerbate or cause supine hypertension. Sympathomimetics, such as ephedrine, can be used to raise blood pressure, but they are often associated with tachycardia and tremor. Midodrine (ProAmatine; Roberts Pharmaceuticals) can be useful to control hypotension. It is a prodrug that is metabolized to form an α_1 agonist that raises blood pressure by increasing arteriolar and venous vascular tone. The advantages of midodrine include brief duration of action (approximately 3 hours), absence of tachycardia and no effect on circulating blood volume. Patients must be cautioned about supine hypertension and avoiding other sympathomimetics including pseudoephedrine in over-the-counter medications. Nocturnal polyuria can be reduced by use of intranasal administration of vasopressin, but monitoring to prevent hyponatremia is required. Caffeine may be of benefit in postprandial hypotension, but the effect is modest. Constipation should be treated with high-fiber diets, stool softeners, and laxatives. Urinary retention may require intermittent catheterization. Impotence can be treated with transurethral alprostadil, a synthetic prostaglandin E_1, or intracavernous injections of Regitine, a combination of papaverine with phentolamine, an α-adrenergic blocker, which causes erection by relaxation of smooth muscle and vasodilatation. Caution should be exercised before prescribing sildenafil citrate (Viagra) because it may worsen hypotension.

Pathologic findings in MSA vary depending upon the clinical features. In patients with prominent ataxia (OPCA type), there is significant atrophy of the cerebellum and brainstem. If parkinsonian symptoms predominate (striatonigral degeneration type), then atrophy and a characteristic gray-green discoloration of the putamen is seen. Gross atrophy of the spinal cord is not seen even in patients with severe autonomic failure (Shy–Drager type). The characteristic cellular pathology in all forms of MSA is glial cytoplasmic inclusions. The inclusions are not detected by hematoxylin and eosin, but are easily seen with silver stains. The inclusions are most prominent in the motor and premotor cortex, putamen, globus pallidus, subthalamus, brainstem motor nuclei, and in the intermediolateral column of the spinal cord. On electron microscopy the glial inclusions are seen as 10- to 20-nm filaments with variable immunoreactivity for ubiquitin and tau. Neuronal cytoplasmic inclusions are also found in the putamen and pons. The neuronal inclusions possess similar ultrastructure and staining characteristics to the filamentous glial inclusions.

Dementia with Lewy Bodies

Lewy bodies are intraneuronal cytoplasmic inclusions that are found in the substantia nigra of patients with Parkinson's disease. Over the past 20 years, however, it has been increasingly recognized that Lewy bodies are also found in the cortex of individuals with dementia who do not have Parkinson's disease. The relationship between cortical Lewy bodies and dementia is not simple because cortical Lewy bodies commonly coexist with pathologic changes associated with Alzheimer's or Parkinson's disease. A recent pathologic study demonstrated that Lewy bodies are found in the amygdala of 60 percent of patients with sporadic Alzheimer's disease. The presence of cortical Lewy bodies is significant because they modify the clinical presentation of dementia and may reflect a different pathogenetic mechanism from Alzheimer's or Parkinson's disease. This coexistence of pathologic lesions has led to significant diagnostic confusion about whether Lewy body dementia is a variant of Alzheimer's or Parkinson's disease. Lewy bodies without any other pathology can also cause dementia. Dementia with Lewy bodies (DLB), therefore, is a heterogeneous disorder whose clinical features vary depending on associated pathologic findings.

The following description of the clinical presentation of Lewy body dementia includes patients with some pathologic features of Alzheimer's disease. The earliest symptom of dementia with Lewy bodies is parkinsonism, but cognitive changes typically develop within 1 year of the motor symptoms. Patients with DLB are more likely to experience bradykinesia, rigidity and postural changes than rest tremor. Cognitive impairment in DLB is characterized by slowed thought processes and difficulty with sequencing and planning, but memory is also impaired.

The most notable clinical feature of DLB is marked day-to-day fluctuation in performance. The fluctuations are much more dramatic than the "good days–bad days" commonly reported with Alzheimer's disease and these transient confusional episodes may mimic delirium. Early in the course of DLB, visual and/or auditory hallucinations are common but unusual in Alzheimer's disease. Many patients with DLB have episodic loss of consciousness and unexplained falls. Neuroleptics should be used with caution in individuals with Lewy body dementia because patients with DLB are more sensitive to the extrapyramidal side effects of these medications than patients with Alzheimer's disease. Cholinesterase inhibitors can be useful in improving attention and concentration similar to their effect in Alzheimer's disease.

The Consortium on DLB has proposed clinical criteria for the diagnosis of DLB, including early findings of dementia, hallucinations, and parkinsonism. In an autopsy series, the sensitivity and specificity of these criteria were 53 percent and 83 percent, respectively, at the patient's initial visit, and 90 percent and 68 percent using data from all visits.

The prevalence of DLB as a cause of dementia is unclear because of the common occurrence of Lewy bodies and other pathology makes determining which pathology is primary difficult. Despite this caveat diffuse Lewy bodies are found in the brains of at least 10 percent of all demented patients. The mean age of onset of DLB is 67 years with a male:female ratio of 1.7:1. There are no diagnostic tests for dementia with Lewy bodies and MRI findings are nonspecific. Fluorodeoxyglucose PET scans of patients with probable DLB demonstrate greater glucose hypometabolism in the visual association cortex compared to patients with Alzheimer's disease, which may explain the frequent occurrence of visual hallucinations in DLB. SPECT scanning shows a similar decrease in occipital perfusion. It is unclear whether the abnormal findings on PET or SPECT scans will be a useful adjunct to accurately diagnose DLB in the clinic. EEG may show diffuse slowing early in the course. Average life expectancy following symptom onset in DLB is 6 to 12 years.

Treatment of dementia with Lewy bodies is primarily supportive. Dopamine replacement can be attempted to decrease parkinsonism, but frequently worsens hallucinations and confusion. Hallucinations can be treated with dopamine blocking agents, but will likely worsen extrapyramidal symptoms. If treatment of hallucinations is necessary, use a neuroleptic with few extrapyramidal side effects such as clozapine, risperidone, quetiapine, ziprasidone, or olanzapine.

Dementia with Lewy bodies is frequently misdiagnosed as Alzheimer's disease, Parkinson's disease, or one of the other Parkinson's disease mimics discussed above. In advanced dementia, DLB is difficult to distinguish from

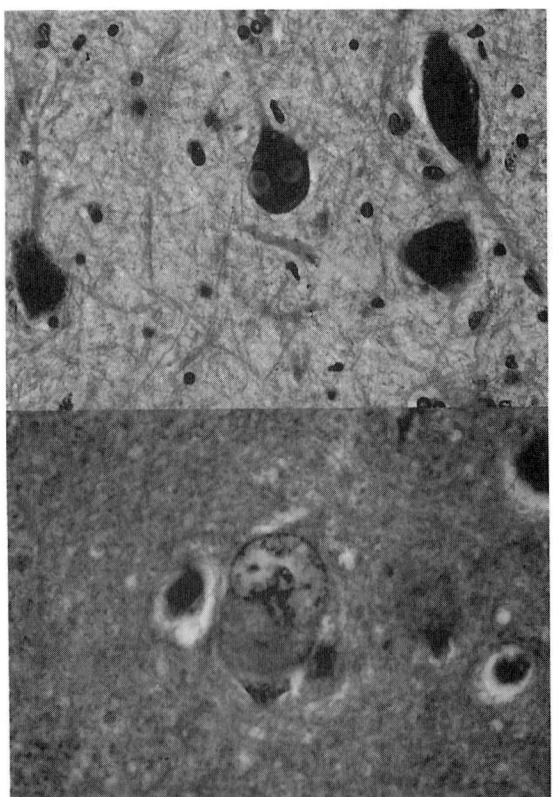

Figure 109-5 *Top,* Neuron containing classic Lewy body. Center neuron contains two large Lewy bodies. *Bottom,* Neuron containing diffuse or cortical Lewy body. Center cell with expanded, homogeneous, pale pink cytoplasm. Hematoxylin and eosin staining. Courtesy of Christine Hulette, MD, Department of Pathology, Duke University Medical Center.

Alzheimer's disease because parkinsonism occurs in both disorders. Similarly, early confusion about diagnosis may occur with Parkinson's disease, if parkinsonian symptoms and signs predominate and dementia is mild. Notably parkinsonism in DLB is not responsive to dopamine replacement.

The pathologic hallmark of dementia with Lewy bodies is numerous diffuse Lewy bodies in cortical neurons. They are most frequently located in small and medium size pyramidal neurons in deeper layers of cortex. Diffuse Lewy bodies differ from classic Lewy bodies in two ways: location and appearance. Classic Lewy bodies are found in the substantia nigra and locus coeruleus in Parkinson's disease, whereas diffuse Lewy bodies are primarily located in cortex. Classic Lewy bodies are eosinophilic, cytoplasmic, neuronal inclusions with a hyaline core, a pale peripheral halo. They are easily seen with routine hematoxylin and eosin (H&E) staining. Diffuse Lewy bodies have a less-prominent central core and halo, and are poorly stained with H&E. Figure 109-5 shows appearance of classic and diffuse Lewy bodies. Lewy bodies are a complex protein aggregate with the major components α-synuclein, neurofilament, and ubiquitin.

SUMMARY

Clinical and pathologic heterogeneity are common in neurodegenerative disorders even when the disorder is the result of mutation in a single gene. This heterogeneity demonstrates that a common pathogenetic event can cause neurodegeneration in different neuronal populations. The identity of the susceptible neuronal population determines the specific clinical and pathologic features, but the basis of selective neuronal death is unknown. The goal of future therapy is to identify mechanisms responsible for neurodegeneration and to develop ways to block cell death.

REFERENCES

Ballard C et al: Attention and fluctuating attention in patients with dementia with lewy bodies and Alzheimer disease. *Arch Neurol* 58:977, 2001.

Ben Shlomo Y et al: Survival of patients with pathologically proven multiple system atrophy: A meta-analysis. *Neurology* 48:384, 1997.

Borasio GD et al: Clinical characteristics and management of ALS. *Semin Neurol* 21:155, 2001.

Center for Medical Genetics, Johns Hopkins University (Baltimore) and National Center for Biotechnology Information, National Library of Medicine (Bethesda): Online Mendelian Inheritance in Man, OMIM, 1996 at: http://www.ncbi.nlm.nih.gov/Omim/.

Chaudhuri KR: Autonomic dysfunction in movement disorders. *Curr Opin Neurol* 14: 505, 2001.

Gomez-Tortosa E et al: Clinical and quantitative pathologic correlates of dementia with Lewy bodies. *Neurology* 53: 1284, 1999.

Kertesz A et al: The corticobasal degeneration syndrome overlaps progressive aphasia and frontotemporal dementia. *Neurology* 55: 1368, 2000.

Knopman DS: An overview of common non-Alzheimer dementias. *Clinics Geriatr Med* 17:281, 2001.

Litvan I: Therapy and management of frontal lobe dementia patients. *Neurology* 56: S41, 2001.

Mark MH: Lumping and splitting the Parkinson plus syndromes: Dementia with Lewy bodies, multiple system atrophy, progressive supranuclear palsy, and cortical-basal ganglionic degeneration. *Neurol Clin* 19:607, 2001.

McKeith IG et al: Prospective validation of consensus criteria for the diagnosis of dementia with Lewy bodies. *Neurology* 54:1050, 2000.

Mesulam MM: Primary progressive aphasia. *Ann Neurol* 49:425, 2001.

Miller RG et al: Riluzole for amyotrophic lateral sclerosis (ALS)/motor neuron disease (MND). *Cochrane Database Syst Rev* CD001447, 2001.

Nestor P et al: Non-Alzheimer dementias. *Semin Neurol* 20:439, 2000.

Paulson H et al: Ataxia and hereditary disorders. *Neurol Clin* 19:759, 2001.

Snowden JS: Frontotemporal dementia. *Br J Psychiatry* 180:140, 2002.

Wenning GK et al: Multiple system atrophy. *Semin Neurol* 21:33, 2001.

Traumatic Brain Injury In Elderly Patients

EUGENIO R. ROCKSMITH • BARRY D. JORDAN

During the last decade the number of Americans beyond the age of 60 has increased dramatically, with the sharpest increase in those 80 years of age and greater. This trend is predicted to continue into the future along with a proportional rise in the number of elderly patients with traumatic brain injury (TBI). Regardless of mechanism of injury, the pathophysiological response of the elderly to TBI has been hypothesized to differ from the response in younger adults and children. This chapter will first review a general classification of brain injury and will focus on TBI in the elderly, specifically discussing consequences, clinical evaluation, management, and outcome.

EPIDEMIOLOGY

Depending on geographical location and various socioeconomic factors the annual incidence of TBI in the United States varies between 160 and 375 per 100,000 persons per year. Based upon national data in the U.S. in 1998 it was estimated that 67,500 deaths and 417,200 nonfatal hospital admissions attributed to TBI occur annually. This number increases substantially when 1,637,000 self-reported but non-hospitalized cases are considered. Age-specific brain injury incidence rates tend to have a bimodal distribution with the highest incidences among persons aged 15 to 24 and 75 years or older. There is a third, smaller peak in incidence in children 5 years of age or younger.

Risk factors include ethnicity (a higher incidence of brain injury in under-represented groups), socioeconomic status (a higher incidence in lower socioeconomic groups), gender (a higher incidence in men), and alcohol usage. Increasing age has been reported to be a risk factor for an individual having an abnormal computed tomography (CT) scan after TBI. Athletes participating in contact sports (e.g. boxing, football, hockey, soccer) also have an increased risk of sustaining TBI. In today's society motor vehicle accidents (MVA) are the most frequent cause of TBI. However, in the elderly population, falls tend to be a common cause of acute TBI.

CLASSIFICATION OF HEAD INJURY

TBI can be classified into four major categories: skull fractures, diffuse brain injury, focal brain injury, and penetrating brain injury. Diffuse injuries include cerebral concussion and diffuse axonal injury. Focal injuries include epidural hematoma, subdural hematoma, cerebral contusion and intracerebral hemorrhage. Penetrating injuries are those injuries where foreign objects or missiles penetrate the calvarium and brain (e.g. bullet).

Skull Fractures

Skull fractures can be classified into linear, depressed or basilar. In general, severe TBI may be associated with a higher incidence of skull fractures. However a severe TBI does not require the presence of skull fracture, nor does a skull fracture necessarily imply a severe brain injury. The presence of a skull fracture does imply a high energy impact. Linear skull fractures involving the vault may occur in 62 percent of patients with severe TBI. A linear skull fracture increases the risk of an intracranial hematoma and contusion. A linear skull fracture of the vault typically does not require any further treatment unless it crosses a sinus or venous structure. Depressed skull fractures are those fractures where the outer table of a fractured skull segment lies below the inner table of surrounding intact skull. This usually occurs when the skull is struck forcibly with objects such as a club or baseball bat that transmit a large amount of energy over a small area. Depressed skull fracures have an increased risk of posttraumatic seizures. Depressed skull fractures can be further categorized as closed (i.e. not associated with a scalp laceration) or compound (i.e. associated with a scalp laceration). Compound depressed skull fractures are more likely to be associated with risk of central nervous system (CNS) infection. Fragments depressed more than the thickness of the skull typically require elevation. Basilar skull fractures can involve the cribiform plate of the ethmoid bone, the orbital plate of the frontal bone, the sphenoid bone, the petrous and squamous portions of the temporal bone, and the occipital bone. Basilar skull fractures may be complicated by CNS infection secondary to direct contact with sinuses or middle ear. Patients with basilar skull fractures may present with rhinorrhea, otorrhea, facial nerve palsy, postauriclar hematoma (Battle's sign), periorbital ecchymosis (raccoon's eye), hemotympanum or eight nerve dysfunction.

Diffuse Brain Injury

Diffuse brain injuries can be classified according to a spectrum ranging from mild concussion to severe diffuse axonal injury. Diffuse brain injuries result from the sudden acceleration, deceleration, and/or rotation of the brain following a blunt impact.

Concussion: Concussion is defined as an immediate and reversible impairment of neurological function secondary to mechanical forces to the head that does not result in gross structural damage to the brain. In mild concussion the patient may experience cognitive dysfunction (e.g. disorientation, posttraumatic amnesia), behavioral disturbance (e.g. agitation, irritability), and/or neurophysical impairment (e.g. dizziness, motor incoordination, disequilibrium) without loss of consciousness (LOC). In more severe cases of concussion the patient experiences transient LOC (less than 6 hours) along with cognitive, behavioral, and/or neurophysical impairments. The signs and symptoms of concussion are primarily secondary to a neurophysiological disruption because gross structural damage typically does not occur and brain imaging is normal. However, microscopic or subcellular neuropathological changes can not be ruled out.

Patients with persistent neurological symptoms after a concussion are experiencing a post-concussion syndrome (PCS). Patients with this syndrome complain of headache, dizziness, vertigo, irritability, poor concentration, memory impairment and fatigue. The neurological examination and neuroimaging are usually normal but detailed neuropsychological testing may reveal subtle cognitive impairment. The duration of the PCS is highly variable. Typically symptoms tend to resolve in 1 month but symptoms can last up to 3 months.

Diffuse Axonal Injury (DAI): DAI is characterized by posttraumatic coma lasting 6 hours or longer in the absence of focal lesions on brain imaging. Patients experiencing DAI may remain in coma from days to weeks. Severe cases of DAI may be associated with decorticate or decerebrate posturing. Shearing injury to the white matter tracts more typically occur in the midbrain-diencephalon, cerebral hemispheres, corpus callosum, and the cerebellar peduncles causing punctate hemorrhages and edema. The most common cause of DAI is a high velocity acceleration-deceleration injury of the head associated with a vehicular accident. Compared to the elderly, young adutls more often sustain diffuse axonal injury without extra-axial hemorrhaging.

Focal Brain Injury

Focal brain injuries include cerebral contusions and intracranial hematomas. The older the patient the greater the risk of hematoma formation and its sequelae. In part this may be due to the decreased compliance of the older brain and it's vasculature.

Epidural Hematoma (EDH): Rupture of a meningeal artery as a consequence of direct skull trauma (usually a fracture) results in the formation of an EDH. In an EDH, blood accumulates in the epidural space causing compression of the brain parenchyma. The most common source for an EDH is the rupture of the middle menningeal artery associated with a temporal bone fracture. The pathognomic finding in CT imaging of the brain is a lenticular shaped extraparenchymal accumulation of blood adjacent to the skull and above dura. The classic clinical presentation of an acute EDH is an immediate loss of consciousness followed by a lucid interval. Subsequently, the patient develops neurological symptoms such as headache, nausea, vomiting, and drowsiness, which can progress to confusion and ultimately coma if appropriate medical care is not instituted. Mortality from EDH is primarily due to herniation of brain parenchyma. Life threatening herniation may occur less frequently in the elderly due to the presence of atrophy.

Subdural Hematoma (SDH): SDHs occur when the bridging veins between the brain and the dural sinuses are ruptured. SDHs are classified as acute, subacute, or chronic, depending upon the time between the onset of hemorrhage and presentation. Acute SDHs are rapidly evolving and typically present immediately or within 3 days of onset. Subacute SDH present anywhere from 3 to 21 days after onset. Chronic SDHs are more slowly evolving and insidious in their presentation. Chronic SDHs present at least 3 weeks after the initial onset of bleeding. Typically patients with chronic SDHs present with a gradual deterioration of intellectual functioning and consciousness with few or subtle lateralizing signs. In the elderly, a chronic SDH is in the differential diagnosis of dementia.

Cerebral Contusion (CC): CCs are heterogenous areas of necrosis, infarction, hemorrhage or edema within the brain parenchyma. CT or magnetic resonance imaging (MRI) often reveal both coup and contre-coup lesions caused by acceleration and decleration forces upon the brain. A coup lesion occurs as a direct result of injury to the parenchyma underlying the point of impact on the skull. A contre-coup lesion occurs when the parenchyma on the side opposite the site of impact is contused as it strikes the bony calvarium. These types of lesions occur most commonly in the fronto-temporal regions.

Intracerebral Hemorrhage (ICH): Traumatic ICH are well defined homogeneous collections of blood within the brain parenchyma. Although they can occur in many locations, they are most commonly observed in the frontal and temporal lobes. The signs and symptoms exhibited by the patient are related to the size and location of the hematoma and amount of ensuing edema. ICH can result from depressed skull fractures, penetrating brain injuries, or acceleration-deceleration injuries.

Penetrating Brain Injury

In a penetrating brain injury the projectile (e.g. bullet) penetrates the calvarium and enters the brain parenchyma resulting in damage along the path of the projectile. If the projectile enters the skull and exits at another location it is considered a perforating injury. Penetrating brain injuries are commonly complicated by associated injuries such as scalp lacerations, skull fractures, cerebral contusions, and intracranial hemmorrhage. Patients exhibiting penetrating brain injuries are at a high risk or seizures and CNS infection. Associated scalp injuries may be the source of significant blood loss. Skull fractures distant to the entry/exit sites can also occur. Contusions can occur at the entry site, contracoup to the entry site, and in the subfrontal region. Subfrontal contusions can occur from forceful craniocaudal displacement at the time of injury.

NEUROLOGICAL CONSEQUENCES OF TBI

A variety of neurological consequences can be encountered as the result of a TBI. These neurological sequelae can be grouped into neurophysical, cognitive, and behavioral complications (see Table 110-1). However, certain neurological conditions (e.g. postconcussion syndrome) may encompass selected aspects of the neurophysical, cognitive, and behavioral complications of TBI (see above discussion of postconcussion syndrome). Although medical complications of TBI such as cardiopulmonary dysfunction, deep venous thrombosis, disseminated intravascular coagulation,

Table 110-1 Neurologic Consequences of Traumatic Brain Injury

Neurophysical	Cognitive	Behavioral
Posttraumatic headache	Attention/ concentration	Agitation/ aggression
Posttraumatic vertigo	Memory	Anxiety
Posttraumatic seizures	Executive	Depression
Posttraumatic hydrocephalus	Language	Apathy/abulia
Cranial neuropathies	Visuospatial	Hallucinations/ delusions
Arachnoid cyst		Mania/euphoria
Movement disorders		Irritability
CSF fistulas		Disinhibition/ impulsivity
Intracranial vascular anomalies		
Subdural hygromas		
Posttraumatic CNS infections		
Motor impairment		

and electolyte imbalance can occur, a detailed discussion of these issues are beyond the scope of this chapter.

Neurophysical

Posttraumatic Headache: A variety of headache types can be encountered after TBI. These include tension, migraine, mixed tension-migraine, cluster, and posttraumatic dysautonomic cephalgia. Although a detailed discussion of the diagnosis and management is beyond the scope of this chapter, any individual that has experienced a TBI and has a significant headache should have CT or MRI performed to rule out a space occupying lesion.

Posttraumatic Vertigo: Posttraumatic vertigo can be an immediate or delayed complication of TBI. Acute posttraumatic vertigo results from sudden trauma to the labyrinthine (labyrinthine concussion) that may or may not be associated with a fracture of the temporal bone. Positional vertigo can occur days to weeks after TBI and is characterized by sudden attacks of vertigo with changes in head position. Rupture of the oval or round window can result in a perilymphatic fistula. These patients will present with intermittent vertigo and/or sensorineural hearing loss and may be confused with Meniere's disease. Most cases of posttraumatic vertigo will subside within a few months. Perilymphatic fistulas can heal spontaneously but surgical repair may be considered in refractory cases. Vertigo can also be secondary to direct trauma to the brainstem, cerebellum, or eighth cranial nerve.

Post-traumatic Seizures (PTS): PTS are classified as early and late. Early PTS occur within 7 days of head injury. The risk is increased with prolonged unconsciousness and with patients who have sustained skull fractures, SDH, intracerebral hemorrhages, cerebral contusions, and focal neurologic findings. Late PTS occur greater than 7 days after head injury. The risk is increased with unconsciousness greater than 24 hours, depressed skull fractures, intracranial hematomas, early seizures, and age 65 years or older (Table 110-2). There is no consistent correlation between EEG abnormalities in the first year after TBI and the development of late epilepsy. The 30 year cumulative incidence of unprovoked seizures in patients with moderate and severe TBI is 4.2 percent and 16.7 percent, respectively. The mangement of PTS in the elderly is similar to that in

Table 110-2 Risk Factors for Posttraumatic Seizures

Glasgow Coma Scale (GCS) score <10
Cortical contusion
Depressed skull fracture
Subdural hematoma
Epidural hematoma
Intracerebral hematoma
Penetrating head wound
Seizure within 24 hours of injury

other populations. Seizure prophlaxis after TBI using either phenytoin, carbamazepine or valproate is only recommended for 7 days after injury if no seizures have occurred.

Posttraumatic Hydrocephalus (PTH): Obstructive or communicating hydrocephalus can complicate TBI. The pathophysiological mechanism of acute obstructive hydrocephalus is a midventricular shift with occlusion to the CSF outflow, while delayed communicating hydrocephalus is due to defective CSF absorption by clogged arachnoid villi secondary to blood products. PTH may be responsible for slow or failed recovery in the rehabilitation setting. Risk factors for PTH include intraventricular or subarachnoid hemorrhages and meningitis. Initial signs and symptoms of acute hydrocephalus may include intermittent headache, nausea, vomiting, confusion, and drowsiness later followed by intellectual detioration, psychomotor retardation, gait abnormality, and urinary incontinence.

Cranial Neuropathies (CN): The most commonly injured cranial nerves in the setting of TBI are the olfactory nerve (CN I), the facial nerve (CN VII), vestibulocochlear nerve (CN VIII) and the cranial nerves subserving oculomotor function. Anosmia is a common symptom secondary to TBI and is secondary to damage of CN I fibers as they traverse the cribiform plate. Damage to CN VII and CN VIII resulting from TBI may occur individually or simultaneously and are usually due to a fracture of the temporal bone. Diplopia secondary to injury to CN III, IV, and/or VI is another common symptom resulting from TBI. Another common cause of oculomotor dysfunction is extraocular muscle entrapment resulting from orbital or facial fractures.

Arachnoid Cyst: Arachnoid cyst formation can occur as a result of TBI and has also been known to rupture as a consequence of TBI. Arachnoid cysts can occur from head trauma in infancy and may not manifest symptoms for years later. Arachnoid cysts are most often located in the middle cranial fossa and may rupture secondary to TBI. Rupture of the cyst can result in formation of a subdural hematoma or hygroma and contribute to elevation of intracranial pressure (ICP).

Movement Disorders: Tremors of low or high frequency, dystonia, myoclonus, parkinsonism, tics, and ballismus may occur as a sequelae of TBI. Posttraumatic movement disorders are more commonly associated with severe TBI. Movement disorders associated with mild to moderate TBI tend to be transient and less disabling. The onset of the movement disorder can be delayed for several months and it can be transient or persistent. A focal lesion in the basal ganglia or disruption of the cortico-basal ganglionic connections is often implicated; however, CT or MRI evidence may be lacking. Poor responsiveness to pharmacotherapy is frequently encountered.

Cerebrospinal Fluid (CSF) Fistulae: Leakage of CSF resulting from a dural tear may occur in patients who have sustained a basal skull fracture and/or a TBI with damage to the ethmoid bone. The most common symptom is otorhinorhea and most of the fistulae close spontaneously within several days. Persistent otorhinorhea can increase the risk of meningitis.

Intracranial Vascular Anomalies: Traumatic arteriovenous fistulas (AVF) and traumatic aneurysms are rare but serious complications of TBI. Although more common in younger men, a traumatic AVF can form secondary to a depressed skull fracture or penetrating trauma in any age group. It occurs most frequently between the carotid artery and cavernous sinus and presents as headache, proptosis, hyperlacrimation and opthalmoplegia. Rupture of the fistula can be fatal. Traumatic aneurysms are very rare and are typically caused by penetrating trauma. Most are false aneurysms caused by a disruption of the vessel wall followed by thrombosis and the formation of a pseudoaneurysm wall. SAH may follow several days to weeks after the trauma and may impede clinical recovery.

Subdural Hygroma (SH): A collection of CSF mixed with blood products that forms in the subdural space is called a subdural hygroma (SH). Although the pathophysiology is not clear, it has been postulated that a tear in the arachnoid secondary to trauma allows CSF to flow into the subdural space, where it is trapped by the torn arachnoid functioning as one way valve. If CSF continues to escape into the subdural space it can expand and cause a subdural mass capable of producing clinical signs and symptoms. Similiar to the SDH, the SH can be associated with parenchymal brain damage after TBI. Clinically a SH presents as a SDH several days to weeks after the trauma, and the diagnosis must be made by CT or MR brain imaging.

Posttraumatic CNS Infections: Posttraumatic infections of the CNS can include meningitis, brain abscess, infection of CNS prosthetic devices, subdural empyema and epidural abscess. Infections of the CNS following trauma occur from hematogenous spread from a distant extracranial foci or from direct contact with a contiguous site such as a sinus cavity or bone. Meningitis represents the most common posttraumatic infection of the CNS and can be associated with CSF leak. Brain abscess are infrequent posttraumatic infections and tend to be associated with depressed skull fractures, gunshot wounds, retained bone fragments, postsurgical hematomas, fluid collections, wound infections, CSF fistula and concomitant injury to the paranasal sinuses. Ventriculoperitoneal shunts, ventriculostomies, ICP monitors, and indwelling reservoirs are prosthetic devices that can become infected following TBI. Subdural empyema is a purulent collection between the arachnoid and dura and is an infrequent complication of TBI. Epidural abscesses more commonly involve the spinal cord but on occasion may invole the cranium.

Motor Impairment: Motor impairment due to TBI is characteristically described by upper motor neuron signs including weakness, hypertonicity, and hyperreflexia. Motor impairment can result in significant difficulty with gait and ambulation. In addition one may also encounter decreased motor speed and decreased coordination. Movement disorders can also complicate TBI and are discussed above. In addition to focal weakness or hemiparesis, the risk of spasticity and contractures of the extremities are also of concern. The management of spasticity will often require the administration of antispasmodics such lioresal, diazepam, or tizanidine, however these medications tend to be more effective in the treatment of spasticity of spinal orign. Furthermore, achieving appropriate drug levels may be associated with increased somnolence and lethargy, especially in the elderly. Accordingly, the management of spasticity may require botulinum toxin injections, serial casting, or intrathecal administration of lioresal. Hetero-topic ossification (formation of new bone in an abnormal location) involving skeletal muscle after TBI can also impede motor function.

Cognitive Impairment

Cognitive dysfunction represents a common and profound complication of TBI especially in older individuals. Since the frontal and temporal lobes are susceptible to the effects of trauma, cognitive function and speed of information processing can be affected. In the elderly, the cognitive outcome of TBI patients is influenced by premorbid functioning. Ageing in the average adult is often associated with cognitive decline, especially in the areas of memory and information processing speed. This decline may affect cognitive outcome following TBI.

Attention: Deficits in attention and concentration (the capacity to maintian attention on a fixed stimulus for a period of time) are often profound and can be associated with any type of mild to severe TBI. Once a patient has awakened from coma and exhibits a normal level of arousal and alertness, deficits in attention can impact upon overall cognitive function, speed of information processing, and behavior. Individuals with difficulties in basic attention are unable to effectively perceive internal or external cues and interact appropiately with their environment. In addition to impairment in basic or simple attention, deficits in sustained attention or vigilance as well as divided attention may also be encountered.

Memory: Memory is a commonly affected cognitive domain after TBI and can be a transient or permanent deficit. Memory dysfunction can present as anterograde (posttraumatic) amnesia, retrograde (pretraumatic) amnesia, or posttraumatic memory impairment. The duration of anterograde or posttraumatic amnesia (PTA) is considered a prognostic indicator of the severity of the TBI and can be assessed by the Galveston Orientation and Amnesia Test. Retrograde amnesia, defined as loss of the ability to remember information stored prior to the injury, usually recovers much more quickly and completely depending on the patient's mental status. After the resolution of PTA and the restoration of orientation, patients may exhibit more persistant problems with memory function. This posttraumatic memory impairment (PTMI) may be transient or permanent. More persistant or permanent PTMI is associated with more moderate to severe memory impairment and probable disruption of the structures subserving memory function (e.g. hippocampus, thalamus, frontal lobes).

Executive Function: Like memory, executive function is very susceptible to the effects of TBI because of its neuroanatomic location in relation to the bony calvarium. The executive system is located in the bilateral frontal lobes and controls such functions as planning, organization, problem solving, initiation, execution, and regulation of behavior. Essentially this system enables the human organism to function in every-day life and adapt to unexpected changes. Subtle deficits in executive function may not be obvious to the causual observer, but can be detected with detailed neuropsychological testing.

Language: Primary aphasia or language dysfunction not attributable to cognitive impairment is less frequently encountered after TBI unless there is focal involvement of the language dominant (usually left) cerebral hemisphere. The most common disturbance of language noted after brain injury is anomia or word finding difficulty. Typically, after a TBI, speech is fluent with circumlocution and paraphasic errors and relative sparing of comprehension and repetition. Pragmatic language deficits after TBI can also occur and include impaired prosody, ungrammatical syntax, perseveration, frequent interruptions of others, abrupt shift of topics, decreased initiation, limited listening, decreased intelligibility, and a constricted operational vocabulary.

Visuospatial and Visuoconstructive Skills: In a majority of patients experiencing TBI, visuospatial and visuoconstrutional skills are relatively preserved unless there is focal brain injury affecting the posterior aspects of the non-language dominant (usually right) cerebral hemisphere. Injury to the anterior non-dominant cerebral hemisphere can result in constructional difficulties but this may represent more of an impairment of executive function and attention. The characteristic rostrocaudal gradient of tissue destruction and the smooth, convex skull surface overlying the posterior cortices usually affords the visuospatial processing system protection, even in the setting of a severe TBI.

Behavioral Complications

The spectrum of neuropsychiatric symptoms after TBI is diverse and depends on the severity, type, and location of the brain injury. Other factors that may influence behavioral outcome following TBI include premorbid personality, litagation, environmental factors, posttraumatic seizures, and response to cognitive limitations. Although increasing age has a negative influence on cognitive function, the impact of old age on the behavioral outcome from TBI needs to be further ellucidated.

Agitation/Aggression: Patients emerging from coma are initially very agitated and delirious. Though some studies have found post-injury agitation to be a good prognostic sign, if not well managed it can be detrimental to the patient's recovery. Agitated patients are typically confused and benefit from a limited amount of external stimulation. Often the agitation is more significant in the evening and at night. In addition to behavioral modification strategies, clinicians have at their disposal several categories of pharmacologic intervention. However, in the elderly TBI population one must use extreme caution as the pharmacokinetics of most drugs vary in older individuals. The clinician must also consider the observation that the traumatized brain often exhibits greater sensitivity to centrally acting medication. The pharmacological management of the agitated patient is dependent upon the symptoms associated with the agitation. Potential medications include antidepressants, atypical antipsychotics, and mood stabilizers (e.g. carbamezapine, valproate, neurontin). In agitated elderly patients it is best to start out with low dosages and avoid the use of high potency neuroleptics (i.e. haloperidol). Low dosages of risperidone or olanzapine may be beneficial without causing significant extrapyramidal symptoms, confusion, or other anti-cholinergic side effects.

Anxiety: A variety of anxiety disorders may be encountered after a TBI. These include generalized anxiety, obsessive-compulsive disorders, panic disorder, phobias, and posttraumatic stress. Anxiety experienced by TBI patients usually tends to be generalized and characterized by tension, worry, and fearfulness. Not infrequently, a generalized anxiety disorder may be noted in the setting of depression and may be associated with a right hemispheric lesion. Although relatively uncommon, obsessive-compulsive disorders (OCDs) may also be observed after mild to severe TBI and is most likely secondary to dysfunction of the frontal-subcortical cicuits. Patients with OCD may respond to selective serotonin uptake inhibitors (SSRI). Catastrophic panic and agitation following TBI may be associated with the realization of neurological and physical impairment. Phobic symptoms following TBI may result from avoidance of the situation that caused the injury. Social phobias may be related to low self-esteem and impaired social judgement. Post-traumatic stress disorder (PTSD) can be an immediate or delayed consequence of TBI and often presents with hyperalertness (exaggerated startle response), sleep disturbance, guilt, difficulty concentrating, memory impairment, avoidance of activities that precipitate recollection of the event, and/or increased symptoms when exposed to events that resemble the traumatic event.

Depression: Another common behavioral problem seen in the setting of TBI is depression. Depression can occur as a direct neurobiological disturbance (e.g., neurochemical imbalances in the brain) secondary to the TBI or can be a reactive psychological response to neurological and physical impairment. Patients in the delirious and disoriented stages post-TBI do not have enough insight to appreciate their conditions. However, once the patients become more aware there is an increased risk of depression. Depression in the elderly TBI patient should be managed similarly to any other type of geriatric depression. Strongly anticholinergic antidepressants should be avoided because of potential cognitive side effects. SSRI are typically the drug of choice for the management of depression, however patients exhibiting agitation as part of their depressive symptoms may be treated with low dose Trazodone.

Apathy and Abulia: Apathy, abulia, or indifference can be seen with injury to the frontal lobes, in particular the medial frontal lobe. Apathy can occur with or without depression. A clear distinction between apathy and depression should be acknowledged because the treatment for apathy is different than for depression. Patients exhibiting apathy or abulia may benefit from the use of pschostimulants or a dopamine agonist, such as bromocriptine.

Hallucinations and Delusions: Signs of psychosis (i.e. hallucinations and delusions) are relatively infrequent neurobehavioral complications of TBI and may be encountered in the setting of agitation or associated with posttraumatic epilepsy. Psychosis can be a an early or late manifestation of TBI. The use of potent neuroleptics (e.g. haloperidol) should, when possible, be avoided in the elderly. Their anti-cholinergic effects can worsen intellectual function and memory impairment. In addition they may delay recovery. The newer generation anti-psychotics (e.g. risperidone) have fewer cognitive side effects.

Mania and euphoria: Secondary mania can be a consequence of TBI and may be more frequently associated with lesions involving the right hemisphere, thalamus, basal ganglia, and limbic related areas such as the orbitofrontal and basotemporal cortices. Aggressive behavior may be more frequently encountered in patients with mania and an association between posttraumatic seizures and mania has also been observed. Anticonvulsants with mood stabilizing properties such carbamezapine, valproate, or neurotin may be effective in the pharmacological management of mania. Lithium may also be of benefit but may be associated with significant side-effects especially in the elderly.

Irritability: Irritability represents a relatively common behavioral disturbance following TBI and can occur with or without agitation/aggression. Irritability can be an immediate or delayed complication of TBI. Irritability can be a direct result of the TBI or consequence of perceived deficits following a TBI. Characteristically, irritability can be exemplified by mood swings, anger, impatience, difficulting coping, and increased arguing. The acute onset of irritability may be associated with a higher frequency of left cortical lesions. Delayed onset irritability tends to be associated with poor social functioning and more impairment with activities of daily living. Extreme irritation can result in aggressive behavior.

Disinhibition/Impulsivity: Impulsivity can be defined as the failure to resist an impulse, drive, or temptation that is harmful to oneself of others. These symptoms result from frontal lobe dysfunction and can be manifested by utterances of profanity, immature behavior, capriciousness, hypersexuality and poor safety awareness. Often they persist for several weeks to months. Lack of insight into their deficits often results in these patients sustaining additional injury in the post-acute setting.

MANAGEMENT OF TRAUMATIC BRAIN INJURY

The principles of management of TBI in the elderly depends upon the type and severity of the injury (Table 110-3). The initial management requires the assessment of ventilatory and circulatory function. Once cardiovascular and pulmonary function has been stablized, a general physical exam establishes the extent of multisystem trauma and the neurological exam determines the severity of the brain injury. The Glasgow Coma Scale (GCS) (see Table 110-4) is the most widely used assessment scale to determine the

Table 110-3 Principles of Management of Traumatic Brain Injury in the Elderly Patient

Maintain circulatory and ventilatory function

Expeditious surgical intervention

Control intracranial pressure

Maintain cerebral blood flow

Maintain normal physiologic functions

Table 110-4 Glasgow Coma Scale

Response		Score
Verbal:	None	1
	Incomprehensible sounds	2
	Inappropriate words	3
	Confused	4
	Oriented	5
Eye opening:	None	1
	To pain	2
	To speech	3
	Spontaneously	4
Motor:	None	1
	Abnormal extension	2
	Abnormal flexion	3
	Withdraws	4
	Localizes	5
	Obeys	6

severity of a brain injury. It measures best eye opening, best verbal response, and best motor response; the combined score ranges from 3 to 15. The management of TBI is also determined by the relative risk of significant intracranial injury (Table 110-5).

Mild TBI (GCS = 13−15) is often synonymous with the term concussion in the clinical literature and represents the most frequent type of TBI. The management of mild TBI is primarily observational since most concussions tend to be self limited. However, the postconcussion syndrome may be encountered and may require symptomatic treatment of headache, dizziness, cognitive impairment or behavioral disturbance. Complicated mild TBI (i.e. patients that present clinically as mild TBI but exhibit an abnormal CT or MRI) may require more definitive treatment depending upon the lesion noted. Considering the increased risk of hematoma formation in elderly TBI patients, there should be a lower threshold for obtaining a head CT in all patients of age 65 and greater, especially if they have experienenced LOC, amnesia, or headaches.

Approximately 10 percent of all TBI will be of moderate severity (GCS = 9−12). These patients tend to be confused or somnolent and exhibit focal neurological deficits such as hemiparesis. Any individual that experiences a moderate TBI should have an immediate CT scan of the head to rule out an intracranial hematoma, brain edema, and/or mass effect. A reasonable percentage of patients may require neurosurgical intervention. Ten to twenty percent of moderate TBI will deteriorate and should be managed as a severe TBI.

Patients with severe TBI exhibit a GCS of 3−8 and are technically in coma. The management of severe TBI requires the resuscitation of blood pressure and oxygenation, intracranial pressure monitoring, the maintenance of cerebral perfusion pressure, and the management of intracranial pressure. Cerebral edema and elevated ICP develop in 40 percent of patients with severe TBI. Emergent treatment to reduce ICP should be initiated at a threshold of 20–25 mm Hg. Hyperventilation results in cerebrovascular vasoconstriction, thus lowering intracranial blood volume and ICP. Osmotic diuretics (i.e. mannitol) cause a rapid shift of fluid from the surrounding brain into the intravascular space. Barbiturates exert their effects through the reduction of cerebral metabolic demands and the corresponding reduction in blood flow. Definitive treatment of elevated ICP involves the surgical placement of a ventriculostomy drain. Intracranial mass lesions (EDH, SDH) causing greater than 5 mm of midventricular shift should be evacuated immediately. If the shift is less than 5 mm, the patient should be observed closely with ICP monitoring. If neurologic deterioration is noted or if ICP exceeds 25 mm Hg, emergent hematoma evacuation should be performed.

OUTCOME

In the general TBI population, several factors are associated with poorer outcome. These include anemia (hematocrit <30 percent), arterial hypercarbia ($p_{CO_2} > 45$ mm Hg), arterial hypoxemia (PO2 < 60 mm Hg) and arterial hypotension (systolic blood pressure < 90 mm Hg) (Table 110-6). In addition a lower GCS score, longer duration of posttraumatic amnesia, increased duration of LOC, and

Table 110-5 Relative Risk of Significant Intracranial Injury After Closed Head Injury

Low Risk	Moderate Risk	High Risk
Asymptomatic	Mental status alterations	Lethargy, depressed consciousness
Mild headache/dizziness	Severe progressive headache	Focal neurologic finding
Scalp injury	Alcohol, drug intoxication	Decreasing consciousness
No moderate or high-risk factors	Posttraumatic seizures	
	Protracted vomiting	
	Younger than age 2 years	
	Multiple trauma	
	Facial fractures	

Table 110-6   Percentage of Poor Outcomes Associated with Systemic Insults in Head Trauma

Systemic Insults	Poor Outcome*
Arterial hypoxemia (PO$_2$ <60 mmHg)	59%
Arterial hypotension (SBP <90 mmHg)	65%
Anemia (hematocrit <30%)	62%
Arterial hypercarbia (P$_{CO2}$ >45 mmHg)	78%
No systemic insults	35%

SBP, systolic blood pressure.

*Includes severe disability, vegetative state, and death.

brainstem abnormalites (e.g., pupillary nonreactivity, loss of oculocephalic reflexes) are associated with poor outcomes following TBI. In the elderly, outcome from TBI is less favorable than in young adults secondary to a limited neuronal reserve, more associated comorbidity, and a reduced capacity for recovery.

A preponderence of clinical and epidemiological data supports the theory that older TBI patients fare worse than younger patients. Clinically, age has been noted to be significantly associated with an abnormal CT scan after TBI and correlated with increased morbidity and mortality. These findings have been corroborated by many studies. A study comparing 1571 patients under age 65 with 449 patients aged 65 years or over, found that in the elderly, intracranial hematomas were more common and mortality rates were higher. In addition, the length of hospital stay was also longer among the elderly. Another study compared mortality rates and Glasgow Outcome Scale (GOS) scores in 90 patients aged 60 years or older with 79 patients aged 20 to 40 years, all with GCS scores of 5 or less. Their conclusions were that in comparison to younger patients the elderly had a higher mortality, had worse functional recovery and consumed more resources per favorable outcome. In a recent study it has been noted that mortality from TBI is higher in those age 65 and older, at all levels of head injury. In addition, the functional outcome of these patients was worse at the time of hospital discharge.

Several hypotheses based on scientific animal observations have been proposed to explain the differential outcomes among elderly TBI patients compared to younger TBI patients. At a cellular level, older patients may exhibit a greater sensitivity to glutamate toxicity. In addition, early glial response that occurs post-trauma may differ according to age. Younger rats tend to form less scar tissue in response to a given lesion compared to older rats. It has been postulated that the increased scar formation in older rats may inhibit or limit a regenerative response of the recovering brain. A third experimental observation is that the aging brain may exhibit reduced neuronal plasticity. Infant monkeys with unilateral lesions of the motor cortices exhibited less motor impairment than adult monkeys with similar lesions. This was attributed to a greater capacity for neural plasticity in the immature central nervous system.

In addition to the elderly experiencing poorer outcomes after TBI, epidemiological and clinicopathological evidence suggests that premorbid head trauma may play an etiologic role in the development of Alzheimer's disease (AD) in later life. Several case control studies have noted an increased risk of AD in patients that experienced a previous TBI that was associated with LOC. The risk of AD secondary to TBI may be particularly increased in those individuals that also possess the apoliprotien ε4 allele. The biological plausibility of TBI predisposing to the development of AD is supported by the neuropathological observations of boxers that exhibit dementia pugilistica (DP). Brains of boxers with DP demonstrate the presence of neurofibrillary tangles, diffuse amyloid deposition, and a central cholinergic deficiency.

CONCLUSION

In general, the outcome following TBI in the elderly is less favorable than that of younger adults and adolescents. Although the exact mechanism for this phenomenon has not been disclosed, it has been hypothesized that the brain's physiological response to trauma in the elderly may be different and that there is less functional reserve of the brain secondary to the aging process.

REFERENCES

Alberico AM et al: Outcome after severe head injury: Relationship to mass lesions, diffuse injury, and ICP course in pediatric and adult patients. *J Neurosurg* 67:648, 1987.

Annegers JF et al: Seizures after head trauma: A population study. *Neurology* 30: 683, 1980.

Annegers JF et al: A population based study of seizures after traumatic brain injuries. *N Engl J Med* 338:20, 1998.

Annegers JF et al: Risk of recurrences after an initial unprovoked seizure. *Epilipsia* 27:43, 1986.

Bowers AS, Marshall LF: Outcome in 200 consecutive cases of severe head injury treated in San Diego county: A prospective study. *Neurosurgery* 6:237, 1980.

Braakman R et al: Interobserver agreement in Assessment of motor response of Glasgow Coma Scale. *CI Neurol Neurosurg* 80:100, 1977.

Chestnut RM et al: The role of secondary brain injury in determining outcome from severe head injury. *J Trauma* 34:216, 1993.

Choi JU, Kim DS: Pathogenesis of arachnoid cyst: congenital or traumatic. *Pediatr Neurosurg* 29:260, 1998.

Donaldson JW et al: Arachnoid cyst rupture with concurrent subdural hygroma. *Pediatr Neurosurg* 32:137, 2000.

Fielding K, Rowley G: Reliability of assessment by skilled observers using Glasgow Coma Scale. *Aust J Adv Nursing* 7:13, 1990.

Gaufin L et al: Release of anti-diuretic hormone during mass-induced elevation of intracranial pressure. *J Neurosurg* 46:627, 1977.

Gronwall D: Advances in the assessment of attention and information processing after head injury. In Levin HS, Grafman J, Eisenberg HM, (eds): Neurobehavioral Recovery from Head Injury. New York, Oxford University Press, 1987.

Gudeman SK et al: Indications for operative treatment And operative technique in closed head injury. In: Becker DP, Gudeman SK, Eds. Textbook of Head injury. Philadelphia: WB Saunders, 1989, 128.

Hoff J et al: Traumatic subdural hygroma. *J Trauma* 13:870, 1973.

Jennett B: Epilepsy After Non-missile Injuries, ed 2. Chicago, Year Book Medical Publishers, 1975.

Jongkees LBW: On peripheral facial nerve paralysis. *Arch Otolaryngol* 95: 317, 1972.

Jorge RE et al: Depression and anxiety following traumatic brain injury. *J Neuropsychiatry Clin Neurosci* 5: 369, 1993.

Jorge RE et al: Secondary mania following traumatic brain injury. *Am J Psychiatry* 150:916, 1993.

Kennard MA: Age and other factors in motor recovery from precentral lesions in monkeys. *American Journal of Physiology,* 115:138, 1936.

Krauss JK et al: Post-traumatic movement disorders in survivors of severe head injury. *Neurology* 1996:47; 1488.

Leramo OB, Rao AB: Diplopia and diabetes insipidus secondary to type II fracture of the sella turcica: case report. *Can J Surg* 30:53, 1987.

Levin HS et al: Disproportionately severe memory deficit in relation to normal intellectual functioning after closed head injury. *J Neurol Neurosurg Psychiatry* 51:1294, 1988.

Levin HS et al: Longterm neuropsychological outcome of closed head injury. *J Neurosurg* 50:412, 1979.

Levin HS et al: The Galveston Orientation and Amnesia Test: a practical scale to assess cognition after head injury. *J Merv Ment Dis* 1979;167:675.

Licata C et al: Post-traumatic Hydrocephalus. *J Neurosurg Sci* 45:141, 2001.

Marshall LF et al: The outcome of severe closed head injury. *J Neurosurg* 75:S28, 1991.

Marmarou A et al: Significance of intracranial hypertension in severe head injury. *J Neurosurg* 47:503, 1977.

Mosenthal AC et al: Isolated traumatic brain injury: age is an independent predictor of mortality and early outcome. *J Trauma* 52:907, 2002.

Nabil B et al: Post-Traumatic Tremor. *Neurology* 1989;39:103.

Neatherlin JS: Head trauma in the older adult population. *Crit Care Nurs Q* 23:49, 2000.

Oddy M et al: Social adjustment after closed head Injury: A further follow-up seven years after injury. *J Neurol Neurosurg Psychiatry* 48:564, 1985.

Olney JW: Excitotoxin-mediated neuronal death in youth and old age. *Prog Brain Res* 1990; 86:37.

Pennings JL et al: Survival after severe brain injury in the aged. *Arch Surg* 128:787, 1993.

Pentland B et al: Head injury in the elderly. *Age Ageing* 15:193, 1986.

Reyes RL et al: Traumatic Head Injury: Restlessness and agitation as prognosticators of physical and psychological improvement in patients. *Arch of Phys Med Rehab* 62:20, 1981.

Russel WR, Nathan PW: Traumatic amnesia. *Brain* 69:183, 1946.

Samie MR et al: Post-traumatic midbrain tremors. *Neurology* 1990;40:62.

Teasdale G, Jennett B: Assessment of coma and impaired consciousness: a practical scale. *Lancet* 1974;1:81.

Epilepsy in the Elderly

JAMES A. FERRENDELLI • HOWARD L. KIM

Many neurologic disorders become more frequent with advancing age, and elderly people are particularly susceptible to seizures and epilepsy. Therefore it is important that physicians have a basic clinical understanding of seizure disorders. The majority of elderly patients who have epileptic seizures readily respond to treatment. However, older patients are frailer and have significant age-related physiologic changes and comorbid conditions that present unique challenges and constraints for physicians.

Seizure disorders encompass a broad range of seizures and epilepsies. The term "seizure" itself is nonspecific and refers to a sudden transient change in brain function that can be caused by a wide variety of medical conditions. In contrast, the term "epilepsy" refers to any central nervous system (CNS) disorder that predisposes an individual to having recurrent seizures. An epileptic seizure is specifically defined by changes in perception and/or behavior caused by excessive, uncontrolled, hypersynchronized electrical discharges from the cerebral cortex. Almost any neurologic or systemic process that causes a sufficient perturbation of cerebral function can provoke an epileptic seizure. These causative factors may be acute or chronic. The term "ictal" refers to the occurrence of the epileptic seizure, and the terms "interictal" and "postictal" refer to the time period between seizures and immediately following the seizure, respectively. The postictal period may be marked by transient focal and/or generalized neurologic impairments. The electrical and clinical changes of an epileptic seizure are usually tightly linked, but they can become disassociated in certain conditions. A person who has a single seizure does not have epilepsy.

A diagnosis of epilepsy also implies a persistent chronic abnormality, and so reversible processes that acutely provoke seizures, such as drug intoxication and/or withdrawal and hypoglycemia do not constitute epilepsy. It is important to remember that seizures and epilepsies are not diseases but neurologic disorders (symptoms and signs) of an underlying disease process. The key to diagnosing and treating seizure disorders is to recognize the relevant symptoms, organize them into a meaningful syndrome that helps define a specific etiology, and provide effective treatment and an accurate prognosis.

CLASSIFICATION

In 1981 and 1989 the International League Against Epilepsy (ILAE) established classification schemes for epileptic seizures and epilepsy syndromes, respectively, that segregate different entities by their specific clinical and electroencephalographic (EEG) features. Basically, epileptic seizures can be divided into two broad categories: partial (focal) and generalized. Conceptually, the electrical component of a partial seizure starts in a discrete focal cortical region and may spread to involve other brain regions during the ictus. The associated clinical changes presumably reflect the specific function of the affected brain region, such as tingling or numbness with somatosensory (parietal) cortical involvement. Partial seizures are further divided into two groups: simple and complex. The term "simple" denotes that the patient's awareness is completely intact during the ictus, whereas the term "complex" means that awareness is impaired or lost. It is important to note that although patients may appear awake during a complex partial seizure, they are actually unaware. Complex partial seizures were formerly known as psychomotor seizures. Simple partial seizures are subdivided into motor, sensory, autonomic, and psychic groups based on the specific type of ictal symptom(s). Interictal EEG recordings for patients with partial seizures may reveal specific focal or multifocal epileptiform abnormalities, namely, spikes or sharp waves (Figure 111-1).

In contrast, generalized seizures simultaneously start with a widespread distribution involving both cerebral hemispheres, presumably synchronized via subcortical mechanisms. There are several basic types of generalized seizures including absence, tonic, atonic, myoclonic, and tonic-clonic. Absence seizures and generalized tonic-clonic (GTC) seizures were formerly known as petit mal and grand mal seizures, respectively. Even though GTC seizures represent a type of generalized seizure, partial seizures can propagate extensively throughout the brain and, in a process known as secondary generalization, eventually progress to GTC seizures. Interictal EEG recordings for patients with generalized seizures often display widespread synchronous epileptiform abnormalities,

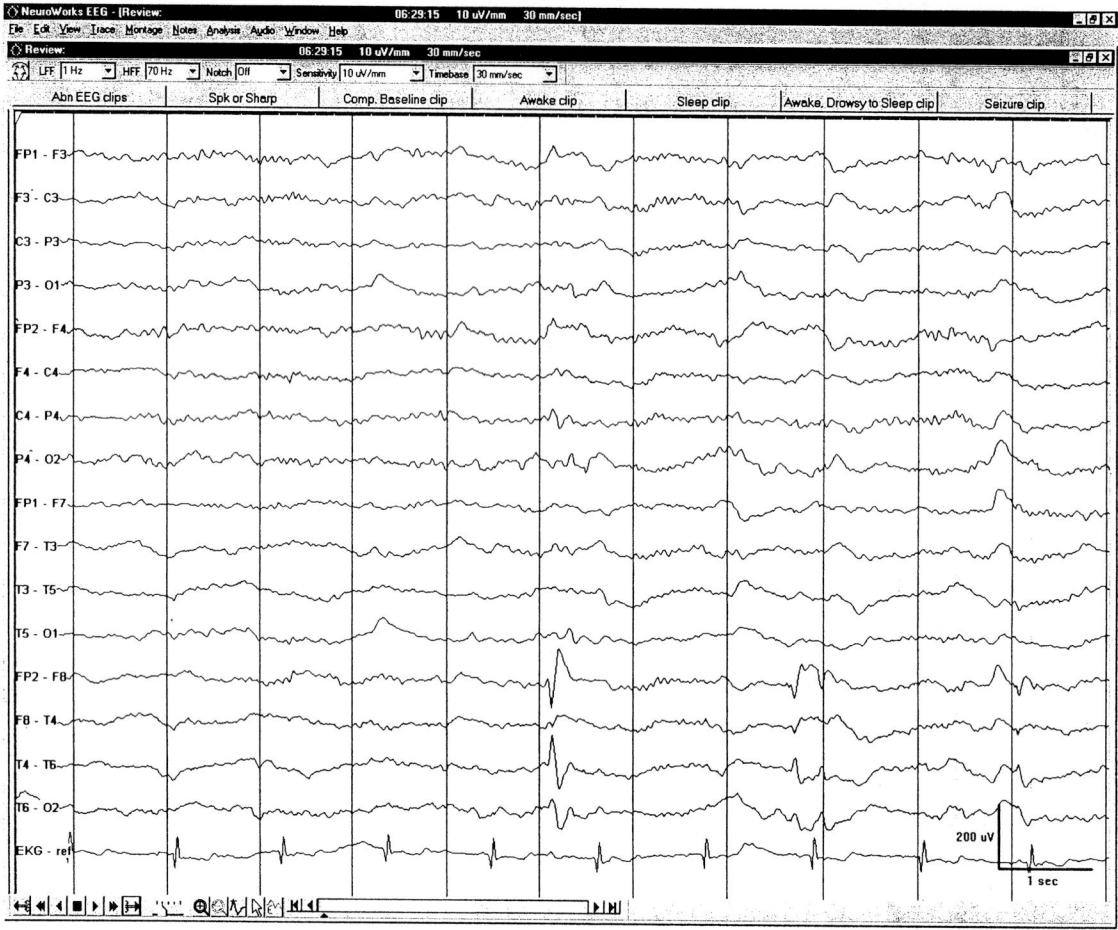

Figure 111-1   Focal sharp waves in the right temporal region.

namely, generalized spike– and polyspike–wave complexes (Figure 111-2).

Similarly, epilepsy syndromes can be divided into two categories: localization-related (focal) and generalized. Each of these categories is subdivided into idiopathic, cryptogenic, and symptomatic groups. Idiopathic epilepsies largely comprise the age-related epilepsy syndromes arising during the first two decades of life and often have a genetic component. Cryptogenic and symptomatic epilepsies represent epilepsy syndromes associated with acquired neurologic abnormalities and/or established etiologies such as head trauma, hippocampal sclerosis, low-grade tumors, vascular malformations, cortical malformations, and inborn errors of metabolism. The combination of specific clinical features (age of onset, clinical course, family history), seizure type(s), and neurodiagnostic study findings (EEG, head magnetic resonance imaging [MRI]) define the individual epilepsy syndromes within these groups. Cryptogenic and symptomatic focal epilepsies are further segregated by the putative brain location of seizure origin (e.g., temporal lobe epilepsy).

Status epilepticus (SE) deserves special consideration because it is often an emergent life-threatening condition, and it is categorized separately in an addendum to the 1981 ILAE classification. The Epilepsy Foundation of America Working Group defines SE as more than 30 minutes of either continuous epileptic seizure activity or two or more sequential seizures without full recovery of consciousness between seizures. SE can be further subdivided into two broad descriptive categories: generalized convulsive and nonconvulsive. Generalized convulsive status epilepticus (GCSE) is a neurologic emergency consisting of uncontrolled GTC seizures, and it is associated with significant morbidity and mortality. Nonconvulsive status epilepticus (NCSE) may consist of uncontrolled absence, simple or complex partial, or subtle myoclonic seizures. It also requires emergent evaluation and treatment although the ictus itself is not considered imminently lethal as in GCSE.

CLINICAL CHARACTERISTICS OF EPILEPTIC SEIZURES

Epileptic seizures usually manifest five cardinal traits. They are (1) spontaneous, (2) recurrent, (3) paroxysmal, (4) stereotypical, and (5) brief. Virtually any episodic alteration of perception and/or behavior exhibiting these traits should be considered suggestive of epileptic seizures. The precise clinical characteristics of an epileptic seizure mainly depend on whether it is generalized or partial (simple or complex).

Partial seizures are quite protean, although there are some consistent themes. Simple partial sensory seizures can cause alterations or hallucinations of a somatosensory,

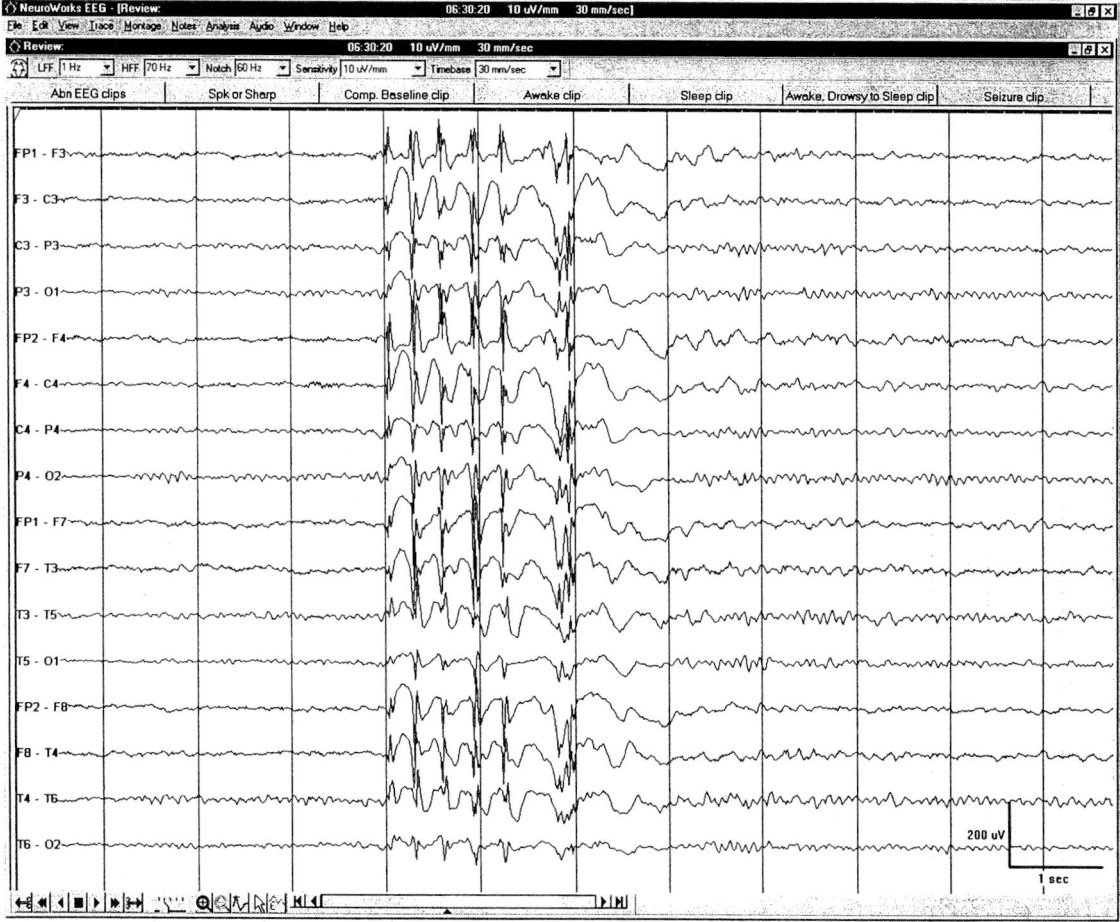

Figure 111-2 Generalized spike-wave complexes.

visual, auditory, olfactory, gustatory, or vestibular nature. Examples include tingling, numbness, flashing lights, sounds, voices, unusual odors or taste (usually unpleasant), and vertigo (rare). Simple partial motor seizures consist of either tonic stiffening or repetitive clonic jerks of one or more limbs, the face, the head, or the body. These motor manifestations are usually unilateral. Some simple partial motor seizures start in one part of the body and then migrate over a brief period of time to involve other parts (the "Jacksonian march"). Simple partial autonomic seizures are characterized by a variety of visceral manifestations such as nausea, emesis, and epigastric sensations (fullness or "butterflies"), as well as by pallor, flushing, mydriasis, and piloerection. Simple partial psychic seizures can cause different emotional or cognitive symptoms such as fear, euphoria, *déjà vu*, *jamais vu*, distortions of time, aphasia, and forced memories or thoughts.

The brief symptom(s) of simple partial sensory, autonomic, or psychic seizures, that is, an aura, may herald progression to a complex partial seizure. These seizures consist principally of an impairment of awareness associated with blank staring, diminished responsiveness, speech and behavioral arrest, and automatisms lasting up to a few minutes. The degree of impaired awareness is variable. It can range from a dazed, dreamlike state to a frank loss of awareness even though patients appear to be awake.

Some complex partial seizures manifest ictal automatisms. Rudimentary ones include hand-fidgeting, lip smacking, chewing, or swallowing movements. More elaborate automatisms include wild flailing of the limbs, pelvic thrusting, vocalizations, and detailed polyarticular movements or postures (writing movements, bicycling movements of the legs, driving motions of the arms). Automatisms usually occur when the patient experiences an impairment of awareness during the seizure, although there are some rare exceptions. During the immediate postictal period following some seizures, patients may experience transient neurologic deficits such as confusion, dysmnesia, aphasia, numbness, or hemiparesis (also known as Todd's paralysis). However, this mild postictal phase may be preempted if the simple or complex partial seizure secondarily generalizes into a GTC seizure. Secondary generalization may be briefly heralded by forced deviation of the head and eyes to the side contralateral to the source of the seizure. Complex partial seizures arising from the medial temporal lobe characteristically start with an aura of *déjà vu*, fear, or an olfactory hallucination, followed by a bland period of staring, speech and behavioral arrest, impaired responsiveness, lip smacking or swallowing, and fidgeting automatisms of the hands that may resemble absence seizures. Postictally, patients are usually confused and dysmnesic. These seizures usually can be easily distinguished from absence seizures because the latter are briefer and almost never associated with auras or postictal states. In contrast, complex partial seizures arising from the frontal lobes are often not associated with an aura and may be characterized by milder impairments in consciousness, a briefer duration, vigorous or bizarre automatisms, and inconspicuous postictal states. Partial seizures arising from the frontal lobes also tend to secondarily generalize more frequently than those arising from the medial temporal lobes.

There is a tendency for elderly patients who develop partial seizures to demonstrate more prominent sensory and/or motor features, presumably because of the higher incidence of etiologic strokes. Focal epilepsy and complex partial seizures may manifest some clinical changes over time in a significant proportion of elderly patients. In most, complex partial seizures become less conspicuous, with a reduction in gestural and other behavioral automatisms. The seizure may appear just as brief unresponsiveness or mild confusion. Secondarily GTC seizures often remit with advancing age. However, a minority of patients may experience worsening epilepsy with the appearance of violent motor activity or a higher frequency of GTC seizures. Elderly people also tend to have longer, more robust postictal symptoms, such as Todd's paralysis or confusion. In young patients, these symptoms usually resolve within 30 minutes, whereas in elderly patients they may last as long as 4 to 8 days. However, a physician must be careful not to miss a new pathologic process with a longer, atypical presentation. Rarely, a deceptive initial presentation of NCSE (complex partial or absence seizures) appearing as prolonged confusion, stupor, catatonia, or a "pseudodementia" is observed in elderly individuals with new-onset epileptic seizures. This condition may occur in the setting of various psychotropic and nonpsychotropic drug treatments, benzodiazepine withdrawal, metabolic aberrations, or chronic alcoholism.

Absence seizures are characterized by an abrupt impairment of consciousness associated with blank staring, unresponsiveness, and rudimentary automatisms lasting 10 to 20 seconds. Witnesses may mistakenly believe that patients are inattentive or daydreaming rather than seizing. Myoclonic seizures consist of bilateral, lightning-like jerks of the limbs and body. They can vary in severity from a subtle twitch to a violent motion that causes the patient to drop items or fall. They occur either singly or in irregular clusters that may resemble coarse tremors. Generalized tonic and atonic seizures (sometimes described as "drop attacks") consist of either a sudden increase or decrease in whole-body tone, respectively. They usually last no more than 20 to 30 seconds. Despite their brevity, they can cause significant injury to ambulatory patients as a result of unprotected falls. Consciousness is impaired during these seizures. GTC seizures start with a sudden increase in muscle tone involving the whole body and all the limbs (causing falls), which is associated with a loss of consciousness, hoarse vocalizations, and apnea, quickly followed by vigorous repetitive clonic jerking of all the limbs. These seizures are also accompanied by hypoxemia and autonomic hyperactivity, along with tachycardia, hypertension, and sometimes emesis or bladder or bowel incontinence. These systemic alterations can compromise elderly individuals with preexisting cardiopulmonary problems. Postictally, patients are lethargic or stuporous and thus at significant risk for aspiration. Most GTC seizures do not exceed 2 minutes.

EPIDEMIOLOGY

Epilepsy is one of the most common neurologic disorders and has its highest incidence in the elderly population. An extensive population-based study by Hauser et al. in Rochester, Minnesota, revealed that the age-adjusted incidences of initial unprovoked seizures and epilepsy were 61 per 100,000 and 44 per 100,000, respectively. The cumulative incidences of initial unprovoked seizures and epilepsy through age 74 were 3 percent and 4.1 percent, respectively. These figures displayed similar bimodal distributions across the extremes of age, with the highest incidence in persons aged 75 years and older (100+ per 100,000) following an early peak during the first year of life. Notably, the incidence of epilepsy in the elderly population almost doubled (although it fell in children) over the 50-year duration of this study. Similar age-specific prevalence and incidence trends have been observed in Europe. Epilepsy tends to be more common in males, and this gender specificity is highlighted in the elderly population. Focal epilepsies (57 percent) constitute the majority of epilepsy cases in the general population, followed by generalized epilepsies (39 percent). In particular, focal epilepsies with complex partial seizures (37 percent) are more common than generalized epilepsies with GTC seizures (23 percent). This finding is in contradistinction to the widespread notion that GTC seizures are the most common manifestation of epilepsy. The incidence of focal epilepsies predominates with advancing age, peaking at ages 65 years and older, whereas generalized epilepsies peak during the first 5 years of life (Figure 111-3). Generalized epilepsies in elderly people usually represent the persistence of childhood or juvenile-onset epilepsy or myoclonic seizures in the setting of a diffuse anoxic brain injury.

In another study involving the Rochester, Minnesota, population made by Hesdorffer et al., the age-adjusted incidence of SE was 18.3 per 100,000 with a cumulative incidence through age 74 years of 0.4 percent. The majority (54 percent) of SE cases were not associated with a preexisting diagnosis of epilepsy. The age- and gender-specific distributions of SE mirrored the findings for other epileptic disorders: SE occurs in a bimodal distribution, peaking at less than 1 year old and more than 60 years old, with the highest incidence in the latter group, particularly in males. The majority of nonfebrile SE cases were GCSE (45 percent, including both primary and secondarily generalized cases). NCSE with simple or complex partial seizures constituted another large proportion (41 percent) of cases, whereas SE with absence or myoclonic seizures accounted for the remaining 14 percent. In contrast, NCSE with partial seizures was more than two times more common in elderly people than any other type of SE, except that GCSE predominated in SE in elderly persons exceeding 24 hours. The duration of SE was longer in elderly patients (and in children less than 1 year old) compared to other age groups, often lasting at least 2 hours.

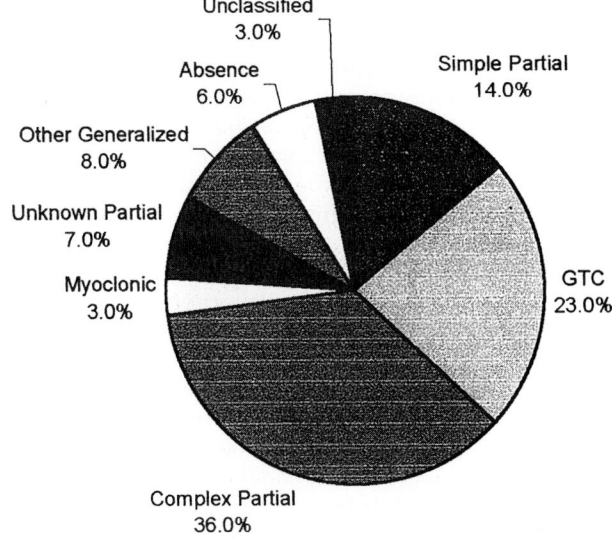

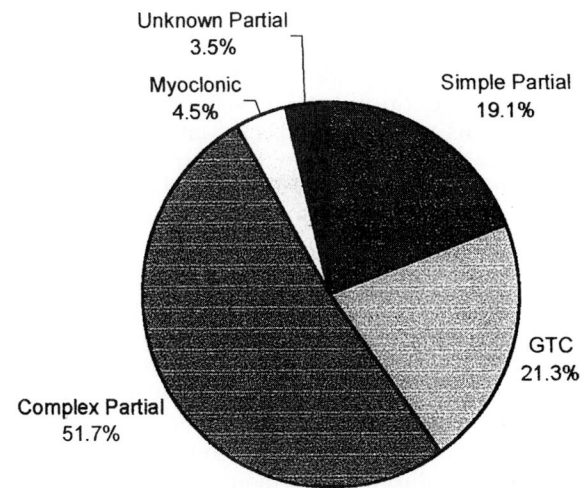

Figure 111-3 Proportion of different epilepsies by seizure type. Top chart: General population. Bottom chart: Elderly population. GTC: Generalized tonic-clonic. Top chart adapted from WA Hauser et al: Epilepsia 34(3):453, 1993. Bottom chart adapted from WA Hauser, Epilepsy in the Elderly, AES CME monograph.

CAUSES OF SEIZURES IN ELDERLY PATIENTS

The majority of seizure disorders arising in old age are due to symptomatic causes that are often age-dependent. Acute symptomatic causes of seizures are manifold, including drug intoxication or withdrawal, CNS infections, head trauma, acute stroke (hemorrhagic and nonhemorrhagic), electrolyte disorders, hypoglycemia, nonketotic hyperglycemia, hepatic failure, uremia, and endocrinologic disorders. In adults, alcohol withdrawal, strokes, and electrolyte disorders were the three most common identified causes of acute symptomatic seizures in a Swedish population-based study. Elderly patients may be at particular risk for drug-induced seizures given the ubiquity of polypharmacy in this patient population. Drug-induced seizures accounted for 1.7 percent of all seizures in a

hospital-based study. The majority (96 percent) of the patients had GTC seizures, although a minority of these seizures were partial with secondary generalization. Isoniazid and psychotropic medications were the most common provocative medications; isoniazid, bronchodilators, lidocaine, and insulin tended to cause multiple seizures.

Cerebrovascular disease is the most frequent cause of seizures in elderly people, and about 10 percent of individuals who have had a stroke have epileptic seizures. Seizures are more common sequelae of hemorrhagic strokes than nonhemorrhagic ones. The majority of early seizures (<2 weeks) occur within the first 24 to 48 hours of a stroke, and only a minority of these patients develop epilepsy. The majority of patients with a late occurrence (>2 weeks) of seizures develop epilepsy. Clinically silent strokes also have been implicated as a cause of late-onset epilepsy.

Other symptomatic causes of epilepsy in elderly persons may be static or progressive. In addition to stroke, other frequent etiologies are cerebral tumors and dementias. Epileptic seizures may herald the presence of different types of primary and metastatic cerebral tumors. Patients who have epilepsy as the initial symptom tend to have low-grade tumors and better prospects for survival. Patients with Alzheimer's disease and other types of dementia have six and eight times higher age-adjusted risks of developing epilepsy, respectively, with partial or generalized-onset seizures. Interestingly, epilepsy in patients with dementia is not exclusively limited to advanced cases but can occur within 3 to 4 years of dementia onset. Closed head trauma is another important etiology for epilepsy in elderly individuals. Most seizures start within the first 1 to 2 years following the injury.

DIFFERENTIAL DIAGNOSIS

Many episodic symptoms and disorders can mimic seizures in elderly people. Older individuals are particularly prone to syncope, given their prevalence of cardiac disease, dysautonomia, and predisposing medications. Patients with syncope may have some premonitory aura-like symptoms, such as light-headedness, nausea, and clamminess. In addition, they may manifest brief tonic body stiffening and/or fragmentary myoclonic jerks during syncope (also known as convulsive syncope) that sometimes can be difficult to distinguish from epileptic seizures. However, unconsciousness caused by syncope is usually much briefer than that associated with epileptic seizures and is not followed by prominent postictal confusion, dysamnesia, or focal neurologic symptoms. Patients experiencing a complex partial or GTC seizure usually claim to have had a longer subjective period of unconsciousness (lasting minutes to hours) compared to the period observed by witnesses. Transient confusion, delirium, amnesia, or unresponsiveness caused by sedating medications, metabolic dysfunction, or fluctuations in dementia may be mistaken for complex partial seizures or NCSE. Transient ischemic attacks (TIAs) occasionally may be mistaken for epileptic seizures or postictal Todd's paralysis. Rarely, some TIAs cause limb-shaking movements. Transient global amnesia (TGA) may cause a prolonged subjective loss of consciousness, but patient responsiveness and behavior remain relatively intact during the episode. TGA typically lasts much longer than most complex partial and absence seizures, and it occurs as a single episode in most people. Movement disorders manifesting variable tremors or dystonia may resemble simple partial motor or myoclonic seizures. Tremors typically display faster frequencies and greater rhythmicity and duration than these types of epileptic seizures. Also, most movement disorders remit during sleep, whereas epileptic seizures still occur (or may even be predominant) during sleep. Migrainous auras rarely are mistaken for epileptic seizures. Migraines last longer than most epileptic seizures. Headaches are not a common ictal feature of epileptic seizures although many patients may have a headache postictally. Older patients are more likely to develop a variety of sleep disorders that may resemble a variety of nocturnal epileptic seizures. These disorders include obstructive sleep apnea (OSA), periodic limb movement disorder of sleep (PLMD), and random eye movement (REM) sleep behavior disorder. Patients with excessive daytime sleepiness caused by OSA or PLMD may experience "micro sleeps" with automatic behaviors, perceived as episodic amnesia or impairment of consciousness. PLMD may also be mistaken for myoclonic or GTC seizures. The hyperkinetic oneiric motor activity of REM sleep behavior disorder may be mistaken for complex partial seizures although REM episodes usually are not as stereotypical as the latter. All-night polysomnography can identify these sleep disorders. Finally, pseudoseizures due to underlying psychological problems are frequently mistaken for epilepsy, particularly in younger patients. Pseudoseizures are uncommon in elderly individuals, but they do occur. The identification of pseudoseizures is an important indication for video-EEG monitoring.

EVALUATION

A thorough evaluation of patients with epilepsy begins with a good medical history. Because a patient is unlikely to manifest a seizure during an office visit, it is imperative for a physician to obtain an adequate description of the patient's seizures to determine their characteristics. Patients may not be aware of their seizures or may downplay their significance. Elderly patients may effusively fixate on multiple extraneous symptoms or may have cognitive problems that impede their ability to communicate reliable information. Hence, the physician needs persistence in obtaining a second-hand medical history from family members, friends, or caregivers. A complete physical and neurologic examination is required for all patients.

Once the physician determines that the patient's seizure are probably epileptic, reviewing the history and performing the physical examination must be focused on finding the underlying cause or at least the pathophysiologic process. Late-onset partial seizures are almost always caused by acquired processes. If the seizures started recently, an acute etiology should be ruled out, particularly an imminently life-threatening or reversible one. The history and physical examination clearly indicate which serum and urine laboratory studies should be ordered, but conventional studies include a multichemistry panel, liver function tests,

a complete blood count (CBC) with a differential and a platelet count, and urinalysis. A lumbar puncture for cerebrospinal fluid (CSF) collection and a CSF analysis are necessary for some patients, especially those with suspected CNS infection or inflammation or with carcinomatous meningitis. A computed tomography (CT) scan of the head should be obtained prior to a lumbar puncture to determine that the procedure can be performed safely.

If a patient clearly experiences recurrent epileptic seizures as part of long-standing epilepsy, the physician must determine the patient's epilepsy syndrome because certain syndromes are associated with specific etiologies, treatments, and prognoses. Generalized epilepsies in elderly patients may represent the persistence of an earlier childhood or juvenile-onset epilepsy syndrome. Because late-onset epilepsy is usually a cryptogenic or symptomatic focal epilepsy, the evaluation should focus on finding an underlying structural abnormality. MRI studies of the head are a crucial part of the evaluation because they are vastly superior to CT studies in detecting a wide variety of CNS pathologies. Thin-section coronal MRI views of the temporal lobes allow adequate visualization of deep hippocampal structures, which are commonly involved in temporal lobe epilepsy.

Electroencephalography deserves special consideration because it is a critical tool in evaluating epileptic disorders. Patients may display specific interictal EEG abnormalities characterized by spikes, sharp waves, or spike–wave complexes. Their morphology and distribution help identify different types of focal and generalized epilepsies. In particular, elderly patients with epilepsy tend to have focal epileptiform abnormalities located in the temporal lobes. EEG recording is also the only definitive modality for confirming the presence of ongoing epileptic seizures such as NCSE. An EEG must be interpreted with caution. A normal EEG study does not exclude the diagnosis of epileptic seizures or epilepsy. Like clinical seizures, interictal epileptiform abnormalities also occur randomly and may be missed during one or more EEG recordings. In detecting interictal epileptiform abnormalities, the yield can be increased by using outpatient ambulatory EEG monitoring. Currently, the most reliable procedure for diagnosing epileptic seizures is video-EEG monitoring. With this procedure, a patient's EEG is continuously recorded along with audio and video recordings of physiologic functions in a time-synchronized fashion so that the seizures can be studied and precisely identified. Video-EEG monitoring studies are usually performed in specially designed hospital telemetry monitoring rooms. This type of monitoring is indicated for patients who do not respond to medical therapy, have atypical seizure-like attacks of an uncertain nature, or need evaluation for epilepsy surgery. Unfortunately, this valuable type of study is underutilized in elderly patients despite its established diagnostic value in this age group.

TREATMENT

The main strategy in treating epileptic seizures is to treat the underlying cause if possible. For example, if a patient has hypoglycemia-induced GTC seizures, the best treatment is

Table 111-1   Use of Old and New Antiepileptic Drugs in Elderly Patients

Generation	Antiepileptic Drug	Starting Dose (mg)	Proposed Dose Titration (total mg/d)	Titration Interval (weeks)	Proposed Maintenance Dose (total mg/d)
First	Carbamazepine	50–100 bid	100–200	1–2	100–400 divided bid-tid
	Clonazepam	0.25–0.5 qd	0.25–0.5	1	0.5–1.0 divided bid-tid
	Ethosuximide	250 qd	250	2	500–1000 divided bid-tid
	Phenobarbital	15–30 qd	15–30	2	30–120 divided qhs-bid
	Phenytoin	100–200 qd	50	1–2	100–300 divided qd-bid
	Primidone	125 qd-bid	125	2	250–750 divided bid-tid
Second	Felbamate*	200 bid	200–400	2	800–2400 divided tid-qid
	Gabapentin	100 tid	300	1	900–3600 divided tid-qid
	Lamotrigine†	25–50	25–50	2	100–400 divided bid
	Levetiracetam	250–500 bid	500–1000	2	1000–3000 divided bid-tid
	Oxcarbazepine	150 bid	150–300	2	300–1200 divided bid
	Tiagabine	2 qd-bid	2–4	1–2	24–48 divided bid
	Topiramate	25 bid	25–50	2	200–400 divided bid
	Valproate	125–250 bid	250–500	1–2	750–1500 divided tid
	Zonisamide	100 qd	100	2	200–600 divided bid

*Avoid using in the elderly; may cause acute fulminant hepatic failure or aplastic anemia; some cases are fatal.

†May cause a dose-dependent rash; dosing depends on whether the patient is concurrently taking an inducer or inhibitor of hepatic cytochrome P450 enzymes.

an intravenous glucose infusion. If the patient's seizures have consistent provoking factors, such as sleep deprivation, these situations need to be assiduously avoided. The underlying cause of epilepsy is not readily identifiable or treatable in many patients. Therefore epileptic disorders must be treated symptomatically using antiepileptic drugs (AEDs) (Table 111-1). The selection of an AED should balance efficacy with safety and tolerability. AEDs must be prescribed judiciously in elderly patients in light of their age-related pharmacokinetic and pharmacodynamic changes, comorbid medical problems, and concurrent use of medications. Unfortunately, pivotal AED trials often exclude elderly patients, and the resulting treatment recommendations may not be ideally suited for them. Treatment using one AED (monotherapy) should be the primary

goal because polytherapy increases the risk of problematic side effects or drug interactions. The AED dose should be titrated primarily to clinical effect, that is, the remission of seizures and the absence of intolerable side effects.

Age-related pharmacokinetic and pharmacodynamic changes are important considerations when AEDs are used to treat elderly patients with epilepsy. An AED pharmacokinetic profile involves four main components: absorption, distribution, metabolism, and excretion. Elderly patients may take concurrent medications that reduce the absorption of certain AEDs, thus decreasing their bioavailability. AED distribution in elderly persons is affected by reductions in serum protein binding and volume of distribution. Elderly individuals have lower concentrations of circulating plasma proteins (i.e., albumin). This reduction increases the free fraction of circulating AEDs that normally have high protein-binding affinities. This free fraction of AED is the biologically active component that is poorly reflected in routine measurements of the total AED level. Total AED levels are more reliable in detecting the concentrations of drugs that are not highly protein-bound (<70%) or have a constant ratio of bound to free drug over a wide range of serum concentrations. Hence, in elderly persons it is often more beneficial to measure free AED levels than routine total AED levels. Older patients also have lower amounts of total body water, which reduces the volume of distribution, potentially increasing the AED concentration for a given dose. The ratio between fat and lean muscle is also greater, which increases the volume of distribution for fat-soluble AEDs. This shift prolongs the AED elimination half-life if it is not compensated by increased AED clearance. Hepatic metabolism is slowed by reductions in hepatic mass, blood flow, and hepatic enzyme activity (especially the cytochrome P450 system), which raise the serum half-lives of AED metabolized by this system. Many conventional AEDs, such as phenytoin, phenobarbital, carbamazepine, and sodium valproate, are extensively metabolized by the liver. Renal clearance is reduced because of decreased renal mass, blood flow, and glomerular filtration. This may be a particular problem for some newer-generation AEDs such as gabapentin and topiramate, which primarily undergo renal excretion. In addition to problems caused by pharmacokinetic properties, older patients may have different pharmacodynamic responses than younger patients. Elderly patients are often more sensitive to the therapeutic and toxic side effects of many neurotropic medications independent of their pharmacokinetic effects. These issues are compounded by the other age-related problems of comorbidities (e.g., dementia) and polypharmacy, which cause a wide variety of potential drug interactions. These observations support the "low-and-slow" rule for AED therapy in elderly people: Doses should be started at lower amounts and titrated slowly.

The effectiveness of an AED depends on the targeted epileptic seizure(s). Certain AEDs are more effective for generalized versus partial seizures (Table 111-2) although there is a significant overlap. In the United States, first-generation AEDs, particularly phenytoin, carbamazepine, and phenobarbital, are the most commonly prescribed treatments for epileptic seizures in elderly individuals. The comparative efficacy and tolerability of these AEDs, as well as primidone and valproate, have been rigorously studied in focal epilepsy. All these AEDs can control partial and secondarily generalized seizures, although primidone and phenobarbital are not tolerated as well as the others because of acute dose-related side effects such as nausea, sedation, dizziness, and ataxia. Phenytoin has an advantageous serum half-life of approximately 24 hours and a widely available sustained-release capsule formulation that allows once-a-day dosing in most patients. It is also available in oral suspension and intravenous formulations. Parenteral administration of phenytoin should be avoided. When given by intramuscular injection, it is erratically absorbed and causes muscle necrosis; intravenous infusion may cause serious side effects, namely, hypotension and cardiac arrhythmias. A safer derivative

of phenytoin, fosphenytoin, can be given intramuscularly or intravenously and should be used instead if parenteral administration is required. Carbamazepine and valproate have relative short serum half-lives of approximately 8 to 10 hours that require tid or qid dosing and may cause significant fluctuations in serum concentrations. However, two sustained-release formulations are available for carbamazepine (Carbatrol, Tegretol XR) that require only bid dosing. Valproate tablets (Depakote) provide a delayed release, although the sprinkle formulation has a sustained-release delivery. Valproate is also available in an intravenous formulation (Depacon). Phenobarbital has a long serum half-life of 36 to 72 hours, particularly in older patients. It can be dosed once a day, specifically at bedtime because its causes sedation. Phenytoin, carbamazepine, and valproate are highly protein-bound. All these AEDs are extensively metabolized by the liver and can cause numerous drug interactions. Phenytoin and carbamazepine are potent inducers of cytochrome P450 enzymes; valproate is an inhibitor. The acute dose-related side effects of all these medications are similar, namely, nausea, emesis, dizziness, blurry vision, nystagmus, ataxia, and sedation. These side effects are more problematic in elderly patients who may already be at a significant risk of falling. Phenobarbital may cause more sedation and cognitive deficits compared to other AEDs. Depakote causes an action tremor of the hands and weight gain. These common AEDs can also cause rare idiosyncratic reactions such as a rash (including Stevens–Johnson syndrome and toxic epidermal necrolysis), fever, hepatitis, and various blood dyscrasias. Additionally, sodium valproate and carbamazepine can cause pancreatitis and hyponatremia, respectively. Phenytoin and phenobarbital may produce noticeable integumentary changes, namely, gingival hyperplasia and Dupuytren's contractures, respectively. All these AEDs can increase bone demineralization that may aggravate osteoporosis in elderly people.

Newer (second-generation) AEDs also control a variety of partial and generalized seizures. So far, there have been no published randomized double-blind trials comparing these AEDs. Meta-analysis of their add-on trials does not indicate outstanding differences in efficacy among these medications. There is little evidence suggesting that the newer AEDs are significantly better than the first-generation AEDs in controlling seizures, but they do appear to be better tolerated. Most new AEDs are not significantly protein-bound. Many are not extensively metabolized by the liver and primarily rely on renal clearance. These properties reduce the risk of problematic drug interactions. However, these newer AEDs will need further study to define their advantages in terms of efficacy and tolerability in different epilepsy populations such as older patients.

It is important to consider several nonmedical factors that may hamper pharmacologic therapy in older individuals. Elderly patients often have poor vision, which makes it difficult to read fine-print drug instructions or increases the risk of taking the wrong medication. Hearing and cognitive problems may impair their ability to understand and follow complex verbal instructions. Physical handicaps also may prevent them from self-administering medications or cutting pills. The rising cost of AEDs is another important consideration. Despite the benefits espoused by

Table 111-2 Spectrum of Efficacy of Antiepileptic Drugs in Adults

Antiepileptic Drug	Partial Seizures	Generalized Tonic-Clonic Seizures	Absence Seizures	Myoclonic Seizures	Tonic/Atonic Seizures
Carbamazepine	++	++	−	−	−
Clonazepam	++	++	+/−	++	+/−
Ethosuximide	−	−	++	−	−
Phenobarbital	++	++	+	+	+
Phenytoin	++	++	−	−	+
Primidone	++	++	+	+	+
Felbamate*	++	++	++	++	++
Gabapentin	++	++	−	−	−
Lamotrigine	++	++	++	++	++
Levetiracetam	++	++	+	+	+
Oxcarbazepine	++	++	−	−	−
Tiagabine	++	++	−	−	−
Topiramate	++	++	+	++	++
Valproate	++	++	++	++	++
Zonisamide	++	++	+	+	+

++, beneficial effect; +, may have beneficial effect; +/−, may have either beneficial or detrimental effect; −, no effect or detrimental effect.

*Avoid using in the elderly; may cause Salminant heptic Saileve or aplastic anemia; some cases are fatal.

a pharmaceutical company, it does no good to prescribe a medication if it will cause excessive financial hardship for the patient. Patients may try to skip doses in an effort to extend prescription refill intervals. Extra time, consideration, and effort on the part of the physician are required to ameliorate these problems so that AED treatments are tailored to an individual patient's specific needs. Monotherapy using the simplest dosing schedule is the goal, preferably never exceeding bid dosing. Multiple drug doses and pill splitting should to be avoided if possible.

Generalized convulsive status epilepticus is a neurologic emergency that requires special treatment. The Epilepsy Foundation of America has published treatment guidelines for this condition. Once GCSE is recognized, the patient's airway should be secured and oxygenation maintained. Monitoring of vital signs, an electrocardiogram (ECG), and pulse oximetry should be initiated. Intravenous access should be established and blood samples drawn for glucose level determination, serum chemistry analysis, a CBC, toxicology screens, and measurement of AED levels (if applicable). If the patient is hypoglycemic, 100 mg of thiamine should be given followed by 50 mL of 50 percent glucose intravenously. Lorazepam (0.1 mg/kg) should be administered intravenously at 2 mg/min. If it is unavailable, 0.2 mg/kg of diazepam can be given instead at 5 mg/min. The patient should be monitored closely for respiratory compromise or hypotension. If GCSE still continues after

5 minutes, intravenous fosphenytoin in a dose of 15 to 20 mg phenytoin equivalents (PE)/kg should be administered at 100 to 150 mg PE/min. Note that fosphenytoin is dosed as sodium phenytoin equivalents because fosphenytoin is equivalent to sodium phenytoin in a 3:2 ratio. If GCSE persists after the administration of 20 mg PE/kg of fosphenytoin, additional doses of 5 mg PE/kg can be given to a maximum dose of 30 mg PE/kg. Even though fosphenytoin causes hypotension less commonly than phenytoin, the patient's ECG and blood pressure readings should still be closely monitored during infusion. If GCSE continues, 20 mg/kg of intravenous phenobarbital should be administered. At this point, the patient will almost certainly need intubation and mechanical ventilation if such support has not already been provided. Intravenous fluid boluses or vasopressors may be needed to control hypotension. If GCSE continues even after all these measures, the patient will need to be anesthetized. Pentobarbital is a common choice despite its significant cardiovascular side effects. In addition, the patient should undergo EEG monitoring to detect any persistent electrographic (nonconvulsive) seizure activity. Most patients with GCSE should be evaluated and treated by a specialist.

A minority of patients have epilepsy that remains intractable to multiple AEDs. In younger patients, different epilepsy surgery procedures may produce complete remission or significant palliation of their disease. Vagal nerve stimulation is a palliative nonneurosurgical treatment option using an implanted device similar to a cardiac pacemaker. Although these riskier procedures are usually avoided in elderly patients, some case series indicate a potential role for such therapy in some older patients, particularly the use of vagal nerve stimulation. These treatment options merit some consideration in select elderly patients with problematic intractable epilepsy, and these cases should be evaluated at an experienced epilepsy center. However, these interventional procedures require further study to fully define the safety and tolerability envelope for elderly individuals.

Prognosis

The prognosis for epilepsy encompasses treatment response, mortality, and quality of life (QOL). The overall prognosis for seizure control is good in the majority of epileptic patients, and elderly patients are no exception. At least 60 percent of older individuals (aged 60 years and older) experience a sustained remission of their seizures. Lower seizure remission rates are associated with remote symptomatic and cryptogenic etiologies, partial seizures, and frequent seizures prior to AED treatment. If a patient's seizures are not controlled by the first appropriate AED, the odds for remission decrease sharply with each subsequent AED trial, becoming negligible after the third AED. However, the odds of remission after failure of the first AED are better if the failure was due to intolerable side effects rather than inefficacy. Judicious reconsideration of the diagnosis and treatment is required if a patient's epilepsy remains intractable after two or three adequate AED trials. The physician should ask the following questions: Is the diagnosis of epilepsy correct? Has the underlying etiology been adequately treated or is there a new exacerbating factor? Is the selected AED appropriate for the patient's type of epileptic seizure(s)? Are sufficient doses of the AED being used? Is the patient complying with the prescribed treatment? Are there confounding drug interactions? If the diagnosis of epilepsy is uncertain, video-EEG monitoring should be considered to confirm the diagnosis. The determination of serum AED levels (total and free) may be helpful in assessing the adequacy of AED dosing, drug interactions, and noncompliance.

Mortality in elderly patients with epilepsy (aged 60 years and older) is up to three times greater than in the nonepileptic elderly population. The standardized mortality rates in the former group tend to be lower than in the younger adult epilepsy population only because the expected death rate in the older age bands is relatively high. Although elderly patients may be injured during an epileptic seizure, it is unusual for them to die during a seizure, even during SE. Most mortality appears to be related to the underlying cause of epilepsy. Not surprisingly, mortality rates tend to be higher in patients with symptomatic etiologies of epilepsy and during the first few years following diagnosis. Most deaths in older epileptic patients are caused by ischemic heart disease, cerebrovascular disease, and pneumonia. Surprisingly, older age has not been demonstrated as an independent risk factor for sudden, unexpected death

in epilepsy. Older age is a significant risk factor for short-term mortality in SE, with an 18-fold higher relative risk than for patients younger than 20 years old.

There is a paucity of systematic QOL studies involving elderly persons with epilepsy. One would expect older patients with epilepsy to experience a reduction in QOL satisfaction just like younger ones, although specific domains may be differentially affected. Elderly individuals may be expected to express even greater dissatisfaction given the increased occurrence of comorbid illnesses and psychiatric problems with advancing age. However, current data indicate that QOL differences depend on the age of epilepsy onset rather than just the presence of epilepsy. Older patients with epilepsy that occurs later in life tend to be more anxious and depressed and have a poorer QOL than those with epilepsy that occurs earlier in life. However, older patients often feel less stigmatized by their condition than younger patients.

CONCLUSION

Epilepsy in elderly individuals presents a variety of diagnostic and treatment challenges. In the coming years, physicians will need a comprehensive understanding of epilepsy to treat the expanding number of elderly patients. When an elderly person with seizures is evaluated, the precise nature of the disturbance should be identified first. If it is epilepsy, the type of epileptic seizure and the probable epilepsy syndrome should then be determined. Any acute symptomatic etiologies must be promptly identified and treated. If the underlying etiology is idiopathic, cryptogenic, or chronic, AEDs are the primary treatment for the epilepsy. AED treatment in older individuals requires careful selection and substantial knowledge in light of the problematic pharmacokinetic and pharmacodynamic features of this patient population. Adequate trials of monotherapy should take precedence over any polytherapy. The overall prognosis for seizure control in elderly patients is good, although mortality is largely dependent on etiologic or comorbid disease. Although complete remission of epileptic seizures is a desired goal, the treatment should not significantly compromise the patient's QOL. Enhancing other domains of QOL is especially important in elderly patients with intractable epilepsy because many are ineligible for aggressive interventional treatments. Future clinical epilepsy research needs to focus on elderly individuals to define optimal treatments, management strategies, and QOL issues in this unique patient population.

REFERENCES

Baker GA et al: The quality of life of older people with epilepsy: Findings from a UK community study. *Seizure* 10:92, 2001.

Cockerell OC et al: Prognosis of epilepsy: A review and further analysis of the first nine years of the British National General Practice Study of Epilepsy, a prospective population-based study. *Epilepsia* 38(1):31, 1997.

Commission on Classification and Terminology of the ILAE. Proposal for revised clinical and electroencephalographic classification of epileptic seizures. *Epilepsia* 22:489, 1981.

Commission on Classification and Terminology of the ILAE. Proposal for revised classification of epilepsies and epileptic syndromes. *Epilepsia* 30(4):389, 1989.

DeToledo J. Changing presentation of seizures with aging: Clinical and etiological factors. *Gerontology* 45:329, 1999.

Drury I, Beydoun A. Interictal epileptiform activity in elderly patients with epilepsy. *Electroencephalogr Clin Neurophysiol* 106:369, 1998.

Forsgren L et al: Incidence and clinical characterization of unprovoked seizures in adults: A prospective population-based study. *Epilepsia* 37(3):224, 1996.

Godfrey JW et al: Epileptic seizures in the elderly: II. Diagnostic problems. *Age Aging* 11(1):29, 1982.

Greenblat DJ et al: Implications of altered drug disposition in the elderly: Studies of benzodiazepines. *J Clin Pharmacol* 29:866, 1989.

Hauser WA et al: Incidence of epilepsy and unprovoked seizures in Rochester, Minnesota, 1935–1984. *Epilepsia* 34(3):453, 1993.

Hesdorffer DC et al: Dementia and adult-onset unprovoked seizures. *Neurology* 46:727, 1996.

Hesdorffer DC et al: Incidence of status epilepticus in Rochester, Minnesota, 1965–1984. *Neurology* 50(3):735, 1998.

Kwan PK, Brodie MJ. Early identification of refractory epilepsy. *N Engl J Med* 342:314, 2000.

Lancman M et al: Usefulness of prolonged video-EEG monitoring in the elderly. *J Neurol Sci* 142:54, 1996.

Lhatoo SD et al: Mortality in epilepsy in the first 11 to 14 years after diagnosis: Multivariate analysis of a long-term, prospective, population-based cohort. *Ann Neurol* 49:336, 2001.

Logroscino G et al: Short-term mortality after a first episode of status epilepticus. *Epilepsia* 38(12):1344, 1997.

Marson AG et al: Levetiracetam, oxcarbazepine, remacemide, and zonisamide for drug resistant localization-related epilepsy: A systematic review. *Epilepsy Res* 46:259, 2001.

Marson AG et al: New antiepileptic drugs: A systematic review of their efficacy and tolerability. *BMJ* 313:1169, 1996.

Mattson RH et al: Department of Veterans Affairs Epilepsy Cooperative Study No. 264 Group: A comparison of valproate with carbamazepine for the treatment of complex partial seizures and secondarily generalized tonic-clonic seizures in adults. *N Engl J Med* 327:767, 1992.

Mattson RH et al: Comparison of carbamazepine, phenobarbital, phenytoin, and primidone in partial and secondarily generalized tonic-clonic seizures. *N Engl J Med* 313:145, 1985.

Messing RO, Closson RG: Drug-induced seizures: A 10-year experience. *Neurology* 34:1582, 1984.

Roberts RC et al: Clinically unsuspected cerebral infarction revealed by computed tomography scanning in late onset epilepsy. *Epilepsia* 29(2):190, 1988.

Sander JWAS, Shorvon SD. Epidemiology of the epilepsies. *J Neurol Neurosurg Psychiatry* 61:433, 1996.

Silverman IE et al: Poststroke seizures. *Arch Neurol* 59:195, 2002.

Sirven JI et al: Temporal lobectomy outcome in older versus younger adults. *Neurology* 54:2166, 2000.

Sirven JI et al: Vagus nerve stimulation for epilepsy in older adults. *Neurology* 54:1179, 2000.

Smith DF et al: The prognosis of primary intracerebral tumors presenting with epilepsy: The outcome of medical and surgical management. *J Neurol Neurosurg Psychiatry* 54:915, 1991.

Stephen LJ et al: Bone density and antiepileptic drugs: A case-controlled study. *Seizure* 8:339, 1999.

Tatum WO et al: Epileptic pseudodementia. *Neurology* 50:1472, 1998.

Thomas P et al: "De novo" absence status of late onset: Report of 11 cases. *Neurology* 42:104, 1992.

Tinuper P et al: Partial epilepsy of long duration: Changing semiology with age. *Epilepsia* 37(2):162, 1996.

Walczak TS et al: Incidence and risk factors in sudden unexpected death in epilepsy. *Neurology* 56:519, 2001.

Willmore LJ. The effect of age on pharmacokinetics of antiepileptic drugs. *Epilepsia* 36(suppl 5):S14, 1995.

Working Group on Status Epilepticus. Treatment of convulsive status epilepticus: Recommendations of the Epilepsy Foundation of America's Working Group on status epilepticus. *JAMA* 270(7):854, 1993.

Late-Life Mood Disorders

WILLIAM J. APFELDORF • GEORGE S. ALEXOPOULOS

Depression, anhedonia, anxiety, fearfulness, and suspiciousness are not normal consequences of aging. Depression in older adults causes distress and suffering, and also leads to impairments in physical, mental, and social functioning. In the United States, mental disorders collectively account for more than 15 percent of the overall burden of disease from all causes and slightly more than the burden associated with all forms of cancer. Major depression alone ranked second only to ischemic cardiac disease in magnitude of disease burden. Pharmacologic and nonpharmacologic treatments are available that may provide symptom reduction and easing of disability when targeted to specific symptoms and syndromes. Despite being associated with morbidity and mortality, and despite the availability of treatment, depression often goes undiagnosed and untreated. The startling reality is that a substantial proportion of older patients receive no treatment or inadequate treatment for their depression. Part of the problem is that depression in older adults is hard to disentangle from the many other disorders that affect older people, and that its symptom profile is somewhat different from that in younger adults. Depressive symptoms are far more common than full-criteria major depression. However, several depressive symptoms represent conditions that can be as disabling as major depression. Additionally, mental health and mental illness are not polar opposites, but are points on a continuum. Mental health is a state of successful performance of mental functioning, resulting in productive activities, fulfilling relationships with other people, and the ability to adapt to change and to cope with adversity. Mental health is indispensable to personal well-being, family and interpersonal relationships, and contribution to community or society. Mental illnesses are health conditions characterized by alterations in thinking, mood, and/or behavior associated with distress and impaired functioning. Therefore, neglecting to identify and treat depressive disorders may be devastating not just to the elderly individual, but also to the family and the community.

DIAGNOSING GERIATRIC DEPRESSIVE DISORDERS

Several syndromes of geriatric depression have been identified and are included in the current *Diagnostic and Statistical Manual for Mental Disorders, Fourth Edition–Transitional* (DSM-IV-TR) classification system (Table 112-1). However, the diagnosis of psychiatric disorders in elderly patients is complicated by several factors. The presence of multiple comorbid conditions is the rule, rather than the exception, in geriatric patients. The signs and symptoms of psychiatric disorders may overlap with signs and symptoms of many medical illnesses, complicating diagnostic assessment. Medical and neurologic disorders may result in persistent psychiatric syndromes that will remit only when the underlying medical disorders are addressed. Older patients are likely to be taking a large number of medications, some of which (e.g., steroids, reserpine, alpha-methyldopa) can cause or contribute to depression. Psychiatric disorders may have late onset, so the clinician cannot be guided by previous history. Elderly patients may underreport psychological symptoms or ascribe symptoms to other somatic concerns. Finally, there are currently no biologic gold standard tests that can confirm specific geriatric psychiatric disorders. To overcome these factors, clinicians may use the reports of family informants or caregivers to supplement information provided by the patient. In addition, the adoption of an all-inclusive approach enables treatment of psychiatric disorders as a search for a medical or neurologic disorder is conducted.

Major Depression

The diagnosis of major depression requires five of the following nine symptoms for at least 2 weeks: depressed mood; diminished interest or pleasure in all or almost all activities; weight loss or gain (more than 5 percent of body weight); insomnia or hypersomnia; psychomotor agitation or retardation; fatigue; feelings of worthlessness or inappropriate guilt; reduced ability to concentrate; recurrent thoughts of death or suicide. Depressed mood or loss of interest or pleasure is necessary to meet criteria for major depression, and either must be one of the five required symptoms.

Although not part of the diagnostic criteria, nondemented elderly individuals often have cognitive impairment when they develop depression, including disturbances in attention, speed of mental processing, and executive

Table 112-1 Definitions of DSM-IV-TR Mood Disorders

Mild episode of major depression
　Few, if any, symptoms in excess of those required to make the diagnoses and symptoms result in only minor impairment in overall functioning or in social activities or relationships with others.

Severe episode of major depression
　Several symptoms in excess of those required to make the diagnosis and symptoms markedly interfere with overall functioning or with social activities or relationships with others.

Severe episode of major depression with psychotic features
　Several symptoms in excess of those required to make the diagnosis and symptoms markedly interfere with overall functioning or with social activities or relationship with others. Delusions or hallucinations are present.

Minor depressive disorder (subsyndromal depression)
　One or more periods of depressive symptoms that are identical to those present in major depressive episodes in duration, but which involve fewer (two or three) symptoms and less impairment.

Dysthymia
　Chronic symptoms of depression (depressed mood plus at least two more symptoms) that occur for most of the day, more days than not, for at least 2 years. It is distinguished from major depressive disorder by the presence of chronic, less-severe depressive symptoms that have been present for many years, as opposed to one or more discrete major depressive episodes.

Bipolar depression
　Major depression occurring in person with history of manic or hypomanic episodes.

function, even when they are not demented. Processing speed and working memory deficits persist after remission of geriatric depression and may be a trait marker of this disorder.

Dysthymia

Dysthymia is defined as a chronic depression (more than 2 years) of mild or moderate severity. Depressed mood is the cardinal symptom of dysthymia and should not be absent for longer than two months. The DSM-IV-TR criteria require that at least two of the following symptoms be present: poor appetite or overeating; insomnia or hypersomnia; fatigue; low self-esteem; poor concentration or difficulty in making decisions; and hopelessness. In elderly patients, major depression, dysthymia, and even clinically significant depressive symptomatology that does not meet criteria for a distinct depressive syndrome occur frequently in the context of neurologic and medical disorders and pose diagnostic difficulties.

Psychotic Depression

Patients with psychotic depression, as a rule, have delusions, while hallucinations are less frequent. The usual themes of depressive delusions are guilt, hypochondriasis, nihilism, persecution, and sometimes jealousy. Depressive delusions can be distinguished from delusions of demented patients in that the latter are less systematized and less congruent to the affective disturbance. Psychotic depression occurs in 20 to 45 percent of hospitalized elderly depressives and in 3.6 percent of elderly depressives living in the community.

Bipolar Disorder

The diagnosis of bipolar disorder is categorized by course and family history. Type I consists of patients who are hospitalized at least once for a manic episode and who also have a history of major depressive episodes. Type II includes patients with mild manic (hypomania) and depressive episodes. Type III patients have cyclothymic mood fluctuations without major depression or mania. Type IV patients have manic states resulting from medical illness or drugs; mania emerging during antidepressant treatment is not considered organic mood disorder. Type V patients have histories of major depression only with a family history of bipolar disorder. Mania or hypomania constitutes 5 to 10 percent of the diagnoses of elderly patients. However, limited information is available concerning the prevalence of bipolar disorders in the elderly community. In a sample of 923 elderly persons studied in the Epidemiologic Catchment Area Study, no manic cases were identified. Most patients with manic syndromes have bipolar mood disorder. Some cases of mania may be etiologically related to medical diseases and drugs. Manic symptoms and signs may be part of schizoaffective disorder, a condition related to bipolar disorder. Schizoaffective disorder is infrequently diagnosed in geriatric patients.

It has been suggested that mania associated with medical disorders or drug treatment as a rule has onset after 40 years of age. Mania with onset during senescence is associated with coarse brain disease. Cerebrovascular disease, especially right-sided lesions, is implicated in late-onset mania. The course and outcome of manic states in geriatric patients are unclear. As manic states in this age group probably represent various disorders with multiple biological determinants, no single characterization of "mania" can be considered to be prototypic. Disorientation, delirium, and reversible cognitive dysfunction have been described in mania patients. It is unclear whether reversible cognitive dysfunction in mania leads to persistent cognitive dysfunction and dementia at follow-up, as it does in depression. Older age appears to be associated with chronic mania, and there is a suggestion of an association between later age at onset and greater duration of episode, as well as shorter intervals between episodes.

Adjustment Disorder with Depressed Mood

Negative life events are associated with increased depressive symptoms in the elderly person. Financial problems, socioeconomic deprivation, poor physical health, disability, and social isolation are significant contributors to depressive symptomatology in late life. Other causes of adjustment disorders in the elderly person are relocation to a long-term care facility and bereavement because of loss of a spouse. Marked increases in the risk for medical morbidity and mortality occur following involuntary relocation. However, when elderly persons have control over such decisions, and when they move to a high-quality institution, relocation may have a neutral or even a beneficial effect.

Complicated Bereavement

Approximately 10 to 20 percent of persons who lose their spouse develop clinically significant depressive symptoms in the first year of bereavement. If left untreated, the depression persists. Older persons appear to be at lower risk for developing depressive symptoms or syndromes than younger adults during the first months of widowhood. However, by the end of the second year, older and younger individuals have same rates of major depression. In fact, the prevalence of major depression continues to increase during the second year of bereavement. At the end of the second year after loss, 14 percent of the bereaved individuals have major depression, a percentage much higher than the prevalence of major depression in the elderly community population (1 percent). Bereaved elderly individuals who do not meet criteria for major depression often have significant depressive symptomatology that can contribute to compromised function, disability, and impaired quality of life.

OTHER SYNDROMES OF LATE-LIFE DEPRESSION

Several syndromes of geriatric depression have been described. Research on these syndromes has facilitated the development of pathogenetic hypotheses and stimulated research on brain mechanisms in geriatric depression. While some clinically useful information was derived from the description of these syndromes, their main contribution to the field has been heuristic.

Late-Onset Depression

It has been suggested that depression with onset of first episode in late life includes a large subgroup of patients with neurologic brain disorders that may or may not be evident when the depression first appears. Compared to early onset geriatric depressives, patients with late-onset depression appear to have less-frequent family history of mood disorders, higher prevalence of dementing disorders, more impairment in neuropsychological tests, higher rate of dementia development on follow-up, more neurosensory hearing impairment, greater enlargement in lateral brain ventricles, and more white matter hyperintensities.

The late-onset syndrome has served as the basis of pathogenetic hypotheses linking neurologic brain abnormalities to development of late-life depression and stimulated research on specific brain abnormalities underlying geriatric depressive disorders. However, there have been significant limitations in using age of onset as a distinguishing clinical characteristic. On a clinical level, onset of depression is difficult to identify, especially in patients whose early episodes are of mild severity. On a theoretical level, an episode occurring in late life may be contributed to by neurologic brain changes regardless of whether the patient had or had no other depressive episodes in early life.

Depression with Reversible Dementia

Some elderly depressed patients develop a reversible dementia syndrome that improves or completely subsides after remission of depression. This syndrome has been termed "pseudodementia," "depression with reversible dementia," and "dementia of depression," and mainly occurs in patients with late-onset depression. Depressed elderly patients who remain with some cognitive impairment even after improvement of depression usually have an early state dementing disorder whose cognitive manifestations are exaggerated when the depressive syndrome is superimposed. It appears that even patients with more or less complete cognitive recovery have high rates of irreversible dementia (approximately 40 percent within 3 years) on follow-up. Most of these patients do not meet criteria for dementia for 1 to 2 years after the initial episode of depression with reversible dementia. Therefore, identification of a "reversible dementia" syndrome in elderly depressives constitutes an indication for thorough diagnostic work-up aimed at the identification of treatable dementing disorders and frequent follow-up.

Vascular Depression

It has been proposed that cerebrovascular disease may predispose, precipitate, or perpetuate some geriatric depressive syndromes. The comorbidity of depression and vascular disease and risk factors and the association of ischemic lesions to distinctive behavioral symptomatology support the vascular depression hypothesis. Elderly patients with vascular depression have greater overall cognitive impairment and disability than do the nonvascular depression group. Fluency and naming are most impaired in vascular depression. Patients with vascular depression have more apathy and retardation and less agitation, as well as less guilt and greater lack of insight. Disruption of prefrontal systems or their modulating pathways by single lesions or by an accumulation of lesions exceeding a threshold have been hypothesized to be central mechanisms in vascular depression.

Depression–Executive Dysfunction Syndrome

Clinical, structural, and functional neuroimaging and neuropathology studies suggest that frontostriatal dysfunction contributes to the pathogenesis of at least some late-life depressive syndromes. Based on these findings, the "depression–executive dysfunction syndrome" has been described and conceptualized as an entity with pronounced frontostriatal dysfunction. On a clinical level, the syndrome is characterized by psychomotor retardation, reduced interest in activities, suspiciousness, impaired instrumental activities of daily living, and limited vegetative symptoms. The clinical significance of identifying the "depression–executive dysfunction syndrome" of late life is that emerging evidence suggests that the syndrome has poor or slow and unstable response to classical antidepressants.

Depression of Alzheimer's Disease

Depressive symptoms and syndromes are common in Alzheimer's patients. Recently, the National Institute of Mental Health's provisional diagnostic criteria for depression in Alzheimer's disease were developed to assist clinicians in making the diagnosis and to promote research on the mechanisms and treatment of these disorder. The criteria require (1) establishing the diagnosis of dementia of the Alzheimer's type and (2) identifying clinically significant depressive symptoms. Clinical assessment should focus on the temporal associations between the onset and course of the depression and the dementia in order to establish that the depression is not better accounted for by an idiopathic depression, other mental disorders, other medical conditions, or adverse effects of medication.

The criteria require that three (or more) depressive symptoms be present during the same 2-week period and represent a change from previous functioning; at least one of the symptoms must be either depressed mood or decreased positive affect or pleasure. Depressive symptoms, part of the criteria are (1) clinically significant depressed mood (e.g., depressed, sad, hopeless, discouraged, tearful); (2) decreased positive affect or pleasure in response to social contacts and usual activities; (3) social isolation or withdrawal; (4) disruption in appetite; (5) disruption in sleep; (6) psychomotor changes (e.g., agitation or retardation); (7) irritability; (8) fatigue or loss of energy; (9) feelings of worthlessness, hopelessness, or excessive or inappropriate guilt; (10) recurrent thoughts of death, suicidal ideation, plan, or attempt. Symptoms that, in the clinician's judgment, are clearly caused by a medical condition other than Alzheimer's disease, or that are a direct result of nonmood-related dementia symptoms (e.g., loss of weight because of difficulties with food intake) should not be used in making the diagnosis of depression of Alzheimer's disease.

Caregivers' Depression

Individuals caring for disabled family members often develop depressive symptoms or syndromes. Depressive symptoms are twice as common among caregivers than among noncaregivers. Depression is most likely to occur during long-term caregiving. Behavioral problems by the care recipient and limited help from family and friends contribute significantly to caregiver burden and predispose to symptoms of depression. Approximately 25 percent of caregivers develop significant symptoms of depression following nursing home placement of the care recipient. Male caregivers underreport depression, as compared to female caregivers. Similarly, African American caregivers report less depression and role strain than their white counterparts, although there was no interaction between race and caregiver distress. Once identified, depression remains relatively unchanged over time in female caregivers but worsens in male caregivers.

EPIDEMIOLOGY

Epidemiologic studies show that major depression occurs in 1 percent of the general elderly population while 3 percent of community residing elderly individuals suffer from dysthymia and 8 to 15 percent have clinically significant depressive symptomatology. Several studies have shown that the prevalence of geriatric depression is much higher in medical settings than in the community. In mixed-age patients treated in primary care settings, clinically significant depressive symptoms and signs were identified in 17 to 37 percent of patients. Approximately 30 percent of these patients have major depression, while the remainder have a variety of depressive syndromes that could benefit from medical attention. In medically hospitalized patients, major depression occurs in 11 percent and less severe, yet clinically significant depressive symptomatology, is identified in 25 percent of the population.

Elderly persons who reside in long-term care settings suffer higher rates of depression than do those living in the community, and half of those relocated to nursing homes are at increased risk for depression. Depression estimates in nursing home residents range from 12 to 22.4 percent for major depression and an additional 17 to 30 percent for minor depression. Approximately 13 percent of residents develop new episodes of major depression in a 1-year period, and another 18 percent develop new depressive symptoms.

Patients with dementia develop depression at a higher rate than the general population. Depressive symptoms of varying severity were found in approximately half of patients with dementia, and major depression disorder was diagnosed in 17 to 31 percent of demented patients. In Alzheimer's patients, major depression occurs in approximately 15 percent of patients, and less severe symptoms in 30 to 40 percent of the demented population. Depression occurs in approximately 25 percent of patients with cerebrovascular disease: 30 to 60 percent of stroke patients experience depression within 24 months of having a stroke. Patients with parkinsonism also have a high prevalence of depression, up to 40 percent.

COURSE

Depression is a chronic illness with relapses and recurrences; "relapse" denotes the reappearance of full syndromal depression within 6 months of remission of the index episode; and "recurrence" denotes the reappearance of depression beyond 6 months from the end of the index episode. In a large observational study of depressed patients, a cumulative recurrence rate of 85 percent was noted, with the majority of patients suffering a recurrence within 5 years. While most studies of recurrence risk have been conducted in mid-life patients, available data in the elderly population suggest that elderly patients have similar rates of recurrence; however, the time between episodes is shorter, with most relapses and recurrences occurring within 2 years. These observations highlight the importance of keeping patients well following the acute treatment of a depressive episode, via continuation and maintenance therapy. The primary goal of continuation therapy is to prevent relapse; and the primary goal of maintenance therapy is to prevent recurrence and to prolong recovery.

Within the clinical context of old-age depression are vulnerabilities to relapse, recurrence, and chronicity. In particular, the coexistence of depression in later life with chronic medical illnesses may represent a vulnerability to relapse and chronicity. The disability of chronic medical illnesses sets the stage for demoralization and depression; conversely, depression itself can and does amplify the disability of coexisting medical illnesses. Advanced age, female gender, medical burden, severity of depression, and cognitive dysfunction predict disability. Furthermore, the cooccurrence of depression in older adults with multiple personal losses and bereavement with chronic insomnia, with risk factors to cerebrovascular disease and to neurodegenerative disorders such as Alzheimer's disease and Parkinson's disease, with progressive depletion of psychosocial resources, and with limited access to adequate treatment may contribute to a relapsing, chronic illness course.

CONSEQUENCES OF LATE LIFE DEPRESSION

Medical Burden

Geriatric depression, as a rule, occurs in the context of multiple medical illnesses. A recent study showed that patients with any medical diagnosis were twice as likely to develop depression than were patients without a medical diagnosis. The total mean number of medical diagnoses in depressed patients was 7.9, as compared to 3.0 medical diagnoses in nondepressed patients. These differences persisted when the elderly group was examined separately.

There is evidence that depression increases mortality in hospitalized patients even when the severity of medical illnesses and disability is controlled. Depression is associated with increased mortality in residents of nursing homes and congregate apartments. It has been reported that presence of major depression on admission to a nursing home increases the likelihood of death by 59 percent 1 year later. The effect of depression on mortality was independent of other medical health parameters.

Depression may increase medical morbidity. Depressive symptoms, especially chronic symptoms, are associated with more medical morbidity than other psychiatric disorders of late life. In older community residents, long-term, but not short-term, depressive symptoms had an adverse impact on health. In contrast, medical burden contributed only to short-lived depressive symptoms. In elderly medical inpatients, those with six depressive symptoms had greater comorbid illness, cognitive impairment, and functional impairment. Depression may adversely affect the prognosis of comorbid disease, as suggested by evidence of prolonged recovery from illness, long hospital stays, increased medical complications and earlier mortality in depressed patients. Increased mortality risk has been reported in depressed, as compared to nondepressed, medical and psychiatric patients.

Depression worsens the outcomes of medical disorders. Depression after surgery is associated with poorer recovery in both functional and psychosocial status. Among patients hospitalized after hip fractures, those with chronic or acute cognitive and depressive symptoms had poorer functional recovery 1 year after discharge than did those patients who did not. Similarly, patients who had more contact with family and friends after leaving the hospital had better recovery than did those patients who had less contact. Depressed medical patients stay in bed more days, as compared to patients with chronic diseases such as chronic lung disease, diabetes, arthritis, and hypertension. Depression increases the perception of poor health and use of medical services. Depressed primary care patients had almost twice the number of appointments per year, as compared to nondepressed patients. Depressed patients had more than twice the number of hospital days over the expected length of stay, as compared to nondepressed patients. Finally, 65 percent of depressed patients received more than five medications, as compared to 35.6 percent of nondepressed patients.

Depression increases the perception of poor health and use of medical services. In primary care clinic populations, 75 percent of distressed overusers were found to have clinically significant depressive symptomatology. Depressed primary care patients had almost twice the number of appointments per year, as compared to nondepressed patients (5.3 versus 2.9). Depressed patients had more than twice the number of hospital days over the expected length of stay, as compared to nondepressed patients. Finally, 65 percent of depressed patients received more than five medications, as compared to 35.6 percent of nondepressed patients.

Depression increases the economic burden on the health care system. Data from a large health maintenance organization population suggest that the health care cost of depressed medical patients is twice that of nondepressed patients with similar levels of medical morbidity.

Dementing Disorders

Depressive symptoms of varying intensity occur in approximately 50 percent of demented patients. The point prevalence of major depression or clinically significant depressive symptomatology is approximately 17 percent in Alzheimer's patients. There is some evidence that family history of mood disorder predisposes Alzheimer's patients to develop depression. Subcortical dementias (vascular dementia, Parkinson's disease, and Huntington's disease) are more likely to be complicated by depression than cortical dementias (Alzheimer's disease).

Depression is often a prodrome to dementing disorders. Individuals with late-life depression and dementia that subsides after remission of depression ("pseudodementia") frequently develop dementia within a few years after the onset of depression. History of depression is associated with increased incidence of Alzheimer's disease. Depressive symptoms were associated with poorer cognitive function at baseline and with cognitive decline during follow-up. Depressive symptoms are common in elderly individuals who later develop dementia. Among elderly individuals with subclinical cognitive dysfunction, those who developed dementia 3 years later had more depressive symptoms. As subjects were progressing to dementia, they exhibited fewer affective symptoms and more agitation and psychomotor slowing. These changes paralleled reduction of cerebral blood flow in the left temporal region.

Depression may be a risk factor for development of dementing disorders in late life. Lifetime history of depression may increase the risk of Alzheimer's disease, regardless of presence or absence of family history of dementing disorders. In elderly twins, depression was one of risk factors for development of dementia regardless of the presence or absence of an ApoE4 allele. Depressive symptoms and diagnoses were found to be associated with cognitive decline and high risk for Alzheimer's disease. In a meta-analytic study, history of depression was associated with onset of Alzheimer's disease after the age of 70 years only when depressive symptoms had appeared within 10 years before the onset of dementia. However, depression with onset more than 10 years before the diagnosis of dementia was associated with onset of Alzheimer's disease at any age, suggesting that previous depression can sometimes represent a risk factor in some patients and a prodromal expression of dementing illness in others.

Disability

Disability consists of problems with self-care, household activities, getting around, understanding and communicating, getting along with others, and participating in society.

Disability compromises quality of life and has various negative outcomes such as high rate of hospital admissions, nursing home placement, mortality, and even morbidity for specific medical conditions. While disability has a reciprocal relationship with psychiatric and medical disorders, it constitutes a distinct functional dimension of health status.

Depression is the second leading cause of disability in the United States. Depression may lead to disability in medically healthy elderly individuals directly, and by contributing to and increasing the impact of medical burden. Moreover, disability resulting from medical or neurologic illnesses is a risk factor for depressive disorders in late life. Therefore, depression and disability interact with each other in a variety of ways with potentially detrimental consequences.

The course of disability parallels the course of depression. In community-residing individuals, residual depressive symptoms covary with disability over time. Reduction in the levels of depression was shown to result in approximately 50 percent reduction in disability days 1 year later. In patients with chronic obstructive pulmonary disease, nortriptyline was superior to placebo in improving both depression and day-to-day function, although it did not influence the physiologic measures of pulmonary insufficiency.

In elderly populations, disability often has been classified as impairment in self-maintenance functions (ability to eat, dress, groom, bathe, use the toilet and ambulate) and impairment in instrumental activities of daily living (IADL), including the ability to go to places out of walking distance, shop for groceries, prepare meals, do housework, launder clothes, use the telephone, take medications, and manage money. Clinical findings ascertained during a comprehensive clinical examination of depressed elderly patients (that is, severity of depression, cognitive impairment, medical burden) and appear to predict approximately 40 percent of the variance in instrumental activities of daily living. Self-maintenance is predicted by different demographic and clinical factors than IADL in depressed elderly patients. Among older depressed adults, impairment in self-maintenance competence is associated with increasing age, more severe chronic medical illness, psychomotor retardation, and lower subjective social support, while depressed mood had a lower impact. Unlike self-maintenance skills, IADL are significantly influenced by depressive symptoms and signs. Specific depressive symptoms can uniquely contribute to IADL impairment. In depressed elderly psychiatric patients, IADL impairment was found to be associated with high severity of depression, and more specifically with anxiety, depressive ideation, apathy, psychomotor retardation, and weight loss, but with less pathologic guilt. Similar findings have been reported in community-residing elderly individuals, in whom IADL impairment was associated with dysphoria, sleep disturbance, appetite disturbance, feelings of guilt, death wishes and suicidal thoughts, loss of interest, concentration difficulties, psychomotor change, and loss of energy.

Executive dysfunction (initiation–perseveration) seems to have a stronger relationship to IADL impairment than to other cognitive impairments in depressed elderly patients. A similar association between executive dysfunction and disability was reported in nondepressed patients with Alzheimer's disease of mild to moderate severity. Because both geriatric depression and executive dysfunction often occur in patients with frontostriatal impairment, these observations raise the question of whether disability is an early indicator of impairment of the frontal and prefrontal areas.

Suicide

Suicide is more frequent in elderly individuals than in any other population. In 1989, the suicide rate in the United States was 12.2 per 100,000 population. Americans older than 65 years of age had a suicide rate of 20.1 per 100,000, almost twice that of the general population. Suicide rates consistently increase in males and reach their highest level in the oldest age group. In contrast, female suicide rates increase slightly with age, peak in middle adulthood, and decline in late life. In 1989, the suicide rate for men older than 65 years was 40.7 per 100,000, while the suicide rate for women of similar age was 5.9 per 100,000. White men older than age 65 years had the highest suicide rate (43.5 per 100,000), followed by nonwhite men (15.7 per 100,000), white women (6.3 per 100,000), and nonwhite women (2.8 per 100,000). Although suicide is more frequent in elderly patients than in younger patients, the rate of suicide for elderly individuals steadily decreased from the 1930s to 1980. However, the suicide rate began to rise again in the 1980s. Demographic differences between persons who contemplate or attempt suicide and those who commit suicide suggest that these populations are dissimilar. Approximately 60 percent of suicide victims are men, but 75 percent of those who attempt suicide are women. Suicide victims as a rule use guns or hang themselves, whereas 70 percent of suicide attempters take a drug overdose, and 22 percent cut or slash themselves.

Depression is the most common psychiatric diagnosis in elderly suicide victims, unlike younger adults in whom substance abuse alone or with comorbid mood disorders is the most frequent diagnosis. Major depression was identified in 80 percent of suicide victims older than 74 years of age, while its frequency ranged from 3.1 to 29.4 percent in younger victims. These findings indicate that depression is the psychiatric disorder most likely to increase risk of successful suicide in the elderly.

Suicidal ideation is a risk factor for suicide in both young and elderly patients. In younger psychiatric outpatients, suicidal ideation appears to predict completed suicide with 53 percent sensitivity, 83 percent specificity, and 4.2 percent predictive value. The sensitivity (80 percent) and predictive value (5.6 percent) of suicidal ideation is even higher in geriatric psychiatric outpatients. Despite the high frequency of suicide in late life, suicidal attempts and suicidal ideation decrease with aging. Older adults commit more carefully planned and lethal self-destructive acts, and give fewer indications of suicidal intent. Therefore, while suicide attempts are rarer in old age than in young age, their lethality is increased.

The clinical profile of depressed elderly suicide victims suggests that, with treatment, their prognosis would be favorable. Most elderly suicide victims have a mild to moderately severe depression, no previous depressive episodes, and no comorbid substance abuse or personality disorders. These characteristics predict good response to treatment. One-third of elderly persons report loneliness as the principal reason for considering suicide. Approximately 10 percent of elderly individuals with suicidal ideation report financial problems, poor medical health, or depression as reasons for suicidal thoughts. Psychological autopsy studies suggest that most elderly persons who commit suicide have had a psychiatric disorder, most commonly depression. However, often the psychiatric disorders of suicide victims do not receive medical or psychiatric attention. More elderly suicide victims are widowed and fewer are single, separated, or divorced, than younger adult victims. Violent methods of suicide are more common in the elderly, but alcohol use and psychiatric histories appear to be less frequent. Most elderly persons who commit suicide communicate their suicidal thoughts to family or friends prior to the act of suicide.

ETIOLOGIC CONTRIBUTORS TO DEPRESSION AND DYSFUNCTION

Despite major advances, the etiology of depression is not fully understood. Both biological and psychosocial factors clearly play important roles. In late-onset depression, several risk factors have been identified. Persistent insomnia, occurring in 5 to 10 percent of older adults, is a known risk factor for the subsequent onset of depression. Grief following the death of a loved one is an important risk factor for both major and minor depression.

Frontostriatal dysfunction contributes to the pathogenesis of at least some late-life depressive syndromes. The frontal lobe is connected to the basal ganglia through five contiguous, nonoverlapping parallel zones (cortico-striato-pallido-cortical pathways). Three cortico-striato-pallido-cortical pathways may be relevant to depression as damage of these pathways leads to behavioral abnormalities that resemble in part the depressive syndrome. Damage of the orbitofrontal circuit may lead to disinhibition, irritability, and diminished sensitivity to social cues. Damage of the anterior cingulate may result in apathy and reduced initiative. Damage of the dorsolateral circuit may result in difficulties in set shifting, learning, and word list generation.

Clinical studies demonstrate that patients with disorders of subcortical structures often develop depression. Moreover, the executive abnormalities of depressed elderly patients are similar to those of patients with basal ganglia disorders. Structural neuroimaging studies of depressed elderly patients have revealed abnormalities consistent with frontostriatal impairment. Volume reduction in the subgenual anterior cingulate has been reported in familial major depression. Bilateral white matter hyperintensities (WMH) are prevalent in geriatric depression and mainly occur in subcortical structures and their frontal projections. Lesions localized in the basal ganglia and their frontal projections are associated with a high incidence of depression. Neuropathologic studies identified abnormalities in frontal structures. Reduction in glia of the subgenual prelimbic anterior cingulate gyrus has been demonstrated in unipolar depressed patients. Abnormalities in neurons of the dorsolateral prefrontal cortex have also been documented in unipolar disorder. Functional neuroimaging studies suggest that depression is associated with abnormal metabolism (mostly increased) in limbic regions, including the amygdala, the pregenual and subgenual anterior cingulate and the posterior orbital cortex, as well as the posterior cingulate and the medial cerebellum. In contrast, the lateral and dorsolateral prefrontal cortex, the dorsal anterior cingulate (located posterior to the pregenual cingulate), and the caudate have reduced blood flow during depression. Bilateral activation of the dorsal anterior cingulate and the hippocampus has been reported in severely depressed, nondemented elderly patients performing a word activation task (Fig. 112-1). Similarly, younger patients with mood disorders, when challenged with the Stroop response interference task, demonstrated blunted activation of the left anterior cingulate and minimal activation of the right anterior cingulate gyrus, as compared to normal controls. Instead, patients with mood disorders showed increased activity in the left dorsolateral prefrontal and visual cortex. Taken together, these findings underscore the importance of subcortical neural systems in mediating development of depression.

Clinical and electrophysiologic indices of frontostriatal dysfunction appear to influence the course of geriatric depression. Executive impairment, the neuropsychological expression of frontostriatal dysfunction, was reported to predict poor or delayed antidepressant response of geriatric major depression, while memory impairment did not influence the response to antidepressants. Poor or slow antidepressant response was associated with psychomotor retardation, a behavioral disturbance that may result from frontostriatal dysfunction. In addition to chronicity, executive dysfunction is associated with relapse and recurrence of geriatric major depression and with residual depressive symptomatology.

The causes of brain abnormalities in geriatric depression are multifactorial. It has been proposed that hypercortisolemia occurring during depressive episodes leads to atrophy of the hippocampus. Apolipoprotein E (apoE) is associated with late-life depression, as well as with hippocampal volume loss. Among nondemented elderly individuals, the rate of volumetric loss was significantly greater among those with an apoE4 allele compared to individuals without apoE4 alleles. Depression is common in individuals with vascular diseases or vascular risk factors. Moreover, late-life depression is a frequent complication of stroke. Lacunar infarct in the basal ganglia has the highest comorbidity with depression. Left hemisphere lesions, especially close to the frontal pole, are most frequently associated with poststroke depression, while subcortical atrophy appears to be a predisposing factor. These observations suggest that degenerative and vascular processes contribute to the brain abnormalities identified in late-life depression.

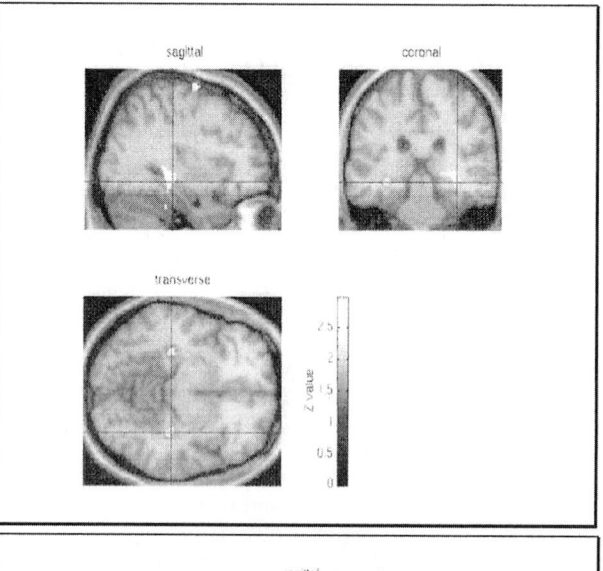

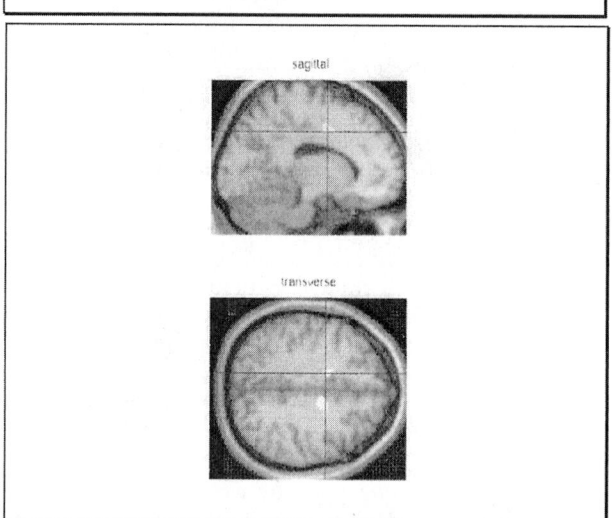

Figure 112-1 Positron emission tomography scans of elderly depressed subjects versus normal elderly subjects during paced word generation task. Comparing elderly depressed patient and healthy comparison subjects undergoing [^{15}O]H$_2$O positron emission tomography scans during a paced word generation task and resting condition reveal bilateral activation deficits in the dorsal anterior cingulate gyrus and hippocampus of the depressed subjects. Courtesy of de Asis JM et al: Hippocampal and anterior cingulate activation deficits in patients with geriatric depression. *Am J Psychiatry* 158:1321, 2001.

ASSESSMENT

Initial Evaluation

The most important symptoms in diagnosing depression in an older patient include sad, downcast mood, frequent tearfulness, and recurrent thoughts of death and suicide (Table 112-2). Other symptoms include diminished interest in pleasurable activities; feelings of hopelessness or helplessness; feelings of worthlessness, guilt, or self-reproach; avoidance of social interactions or going out; psychomotor agitation or retardation; difficulty making decisions; and difficulty in planning daily activities. Underreporting of depressive symptoms often complicates the

Table 112-2 Symptoms to Assess in Diagnosing Depression in an Older Patient

Most important symptoms

- Sad, downcast mood; poor spirits (blue); frequently feels like crying
- Recurrent thoughts of death or suicide

Other important symptoms

- Diminished interest in pleasurable activities and hobbies
- Feelings of hopelessness or worthlessness
- Feeling that life is empty
- Feelings of guilt
- Avoiding social interactions or going out
- Feeling of helplessness
- Psychomotor agitation (restlessness, fidgeting) or retardation
- Difficulty making decisions
- Difficulty initiating new projects

Symptoms that are sometimes helpful

- Family history of mood disorders
- Appetite change or weight loss'
- Feeling worse in the morning
- Loss of energy/fatigue
- Insomnia or hypersomnia
- Fear that something bad is going to happen
- Difficulty with memory or problems concentrating
- Preoccupation with poor health or physical limitations

diagnosis of late-life depression. The current cohort of elderly patients is most likely to report physical symptoms such as lack of sleep, energy, appetite, and weight loss, rather than sadness, feelings of guilt, suicidal ideation, hopelessness, and worthlessness. Depressed elderly patients often have anhedonia rather than sadness. As these symptoms may originate from medical disorders, depression may be overlooked.

As part of the initial evaluation of depression in an older person, a focused psychiatric history and examination and a clinical examination of cognitive functions are crucial. Also recommended are medical history, physical and neurological examinations, and laboratory tests, including thyroid stimulating hormone levels, chemistry screen, complete blood count, and medication levels if needed. Often, an electrocardiogram, serum B_{12} and folate levels, and urinalysis are also obtained. These recommendations reflect the need to diagnose coexisting medical conditions that may be contributing to the depression or that might complicate its treatment.

As part of the evaluation, it is important to assess for current alcohol or substance use problems, for medications that can cause depression, and for dementing disorders. Alcohol or substance abuse may lead to withdrawal

syndromes. A patient who continues to use alcohol or substances of abuse, or a medication known to cause depression, frequently will not have a robust treatment response. Complicated medication regimens may lead to the accidental misuse of medications. Comorbid dementia not only complicates the assessment of depression but also requires planning for the long-term care of these patients. The elderly may also be subjected to physical, verbal, or emotional abuse by caregivers or relatives. In addition, it is important to evaluate the patient's level of functioning, environmental problems, recent loss, and new functions the person has had to assume.

Suicide Risk

The majority of elderly suicide victims see their physicians within a few months of their death and more than a third see their physicians within the week of their suicide. Therefore, reliable assessment of suicide risk is critical because protective measures may avert suicide (Table 112-3). Several clinical characteristics can be used to assess the risk for suicidal ideation in depressed elderly patients. During episodes of depression, suicidal ideation is associated with severity of depression, poor social support, and history of serious suicide attempts. Patients with severe depression and IADL impairment were more likely to have history of suicide attempts. Poor social support and history of serious suicide attempts are associated with suicidal ideation even in the context of mild depression.

Some clinical characteristics predict the course of suicidal ideation. At the initial evaluation, suicidal ideation and history of serious suicide attempts are strong predictors of the evolution of suicidal ideation over time. During follow-up examinations, severity of depression, medical burden, disability, and social support predict the longitudinal course of suicidal ideation. However, severity of concurrent depression is the main determinant of fluctuations in suicidal ideation over time. The relationship of geriatric depression to suicidal ideation suggests that identification and appropriate treatment of depression can improve suicidal ideation and ultimately lower the risk of suicide.

Older patients with major medical illnesses or a recent loss should be evaluated for depressive symptomatology

Table 112-3 Suicide Risk

Patients at highest risk for suicide
  Highest risk: white males older than 80 years of age
  High risk: white males 65 to 80 years of age

Most important risk factors for suicide

- Severity of depression
- Psychotic depression
- Alcoholism
- Recent loss or bereavement
- Abuse of sedatives/hypnotics
- Development of disability
- Abuse of pain killers

and suicidal ideation and plans. Thoughts and fantasies about the meaning of suicide and life after death may reveal information that the patient is unable to share directly. There should be no reluctance to question patients about suicide because such questions do not increase the likelihood of suicidal behavior.

Depressive Syndromes not Meeting Diagnostic Criteria

The majority of depressed elderly patients treated in primary care do not meet diagnostic criteria for depressive disorders. Six to 8 percent of primary care patients meet criteria for major depression and major depression occurs in 9 percent of elderly primary care patients. The remainder have clinically significant depressive symptomatology. In medical populations, 25 percent of minor depressions evolve into major depression within a 2-year period. Minor depression is often the diagnosis of elderly suicide victims. These observations underscore the need for close follow-up and for use of antidepressants and/or psychotherapy if depressive symptoms persist or worsen.

Dementing Disorders

The similarity of depressive manifestations with symptoms and signs of dementing disorders often poses diagnostic problems. Early stage Alzheimer's patients show loss of interest, decreased energy, difficulty in concentration, and agitation or retardation. Apathy, a characteristic of frontal lobe syndrome, may be misidentified as retarded depression. Sad, downcast mood, and psychic rather than vegetative features are useful in distinguishing depressed-demented patients from patients with dementia alone. It remains unclear whether depression is associated with the degree of cognitive impairment in demented patients. Demented patients may be unable to identify and express dysphoric feelings. For this reason, examination should rely on caregiver reports as well as examination of the patient. Identification of depression in demented patients is important since they may respond to drug therapy or electroconvulsive therapy (ECT).

TREATMENT

Acute Treatments

Pharmacotherapy

Antidepressants, regardless of class, lead to improvement of depressive symptomatology in approximately 60 percent of elderly patients, while the placebo response rate is 30 to 40 percent. Even among responders, a significant number of elderly patients continue to have significant residual symptomatology.

Older patients can benefit from the same psychopharmacologic agents as younger patients. However, the clinician must be aware that aging and medical conditions associated with aging have an impact on pharmacokinetics and increase the sensitivity to side effects even at low plasma concentrations of antidepressants.

Four families of antidepressants are available for the treatment of geriatric depression: selective serotonin reuptake inhibitors (SSRIs), tricyclics, monoamine oxidase inhibitors (MAOIs), and atypical antidepressants. It is crucial that antidepressant drugs are given to achieve adequate plasma levels and at adequate dosages for a sufficient length of time.

An adequate antidepressant trial in the elderly is longer than that of younger adults. A complete response often occurs after 6 to 12 weeks of treatment. However, if there are no signs of improvement by the fourth week of treatment, most clinicians consider the antidepressant trial a failure.

Selective Serotonin Reuptake Inhibitors

Several studies show that fluoxetine, sertraline, paroxetine, and citalopram are more effective than placebo in depressed elderly outpatients. The dosages of SSRIs should be increased gradually. Recommended starting daily dosages are fluoxetine 10 mg, paroxetine 10 to 20 mg, sertraline 25 to 50 mg, and citalopram 10 to 20 mg. For most patients, daily dosages of fluoxetine 20 mg, paroxetine 20 to 30 mg, sertraline 75 to 100 mg, and citalopram 20 to 30 mg are sufficient, although higher dosages are required by some. The SSRI fluvoxamine may be effective in the treatment of geriatric depression, although research data are sparse.

The main advantage of SSRIs is their safety. With the exception of allergy, they have few, if any, dangerous side effects. Even when these drugs are not tolerated, the side effects consist of subjective discomfort rather than risk to the patient. Nausea, restlessness, insomnia, headache, diarrhea, and sexual dysfunction are the most frequent side effects in the elderly. Inappropriate secretion of antidiuretic hormone may lead to hyponatremia, confusion, and falls in the elderly, but it is rare.

SSRIs interact with drugs frequently used in the depressed elderly. Fluoxetine, sertraline, and paroxetine inhibit the cytochrome P450 2D6 liver cytochrome isoenzyme. This pathway is essential for the hydroxylation of nortriptyline and desipramine and the metabolism of antipsychotics and type 1A antiarrhythmic drugs (encainide, flecainide), beta-blockers, and verapamil whose plasma levels may be raised in SSRI-treated patients. Therefore, reduction of dosages and monitoring of plasma levels of tricyclic antidepressants and of antipsychotic and antiarrhythmic drugs are required in patients treated with fluoxetine, sertraline, or paroxetine. Norfluoxetine, the metabolite of fluoxetine, inhibits the P450 3A4 isoenzyme, which is responsible for the metabolism of alprazolam, triazolam, carbamazepine, quinidine, erythromycin, terfenazine, and astemizole, and may lead to an increase in the plasma level of these agents. For these reason, when fluoxetine is prescribed, reduction and monitoring of dosages of drugs metabolized by the 2D6 and the 3A4 isoenzymes is required. Fluvoxamine inhibits the P450 3A4 and the 1A2 cytochrome isoenzymes but does not significantly inhibit the 2D6 isoenzyme. Drugs metabolized by the 3A4 and the 1A2 isoenzymes should be cautiously prescribed in fluvoxamine-treated patients. Fluvoxamine may produce a threefold decrease in theophylline clearance by inhibiting the 1A2 isoenzyme, which is responsible for its metabolism.

Tricyclic Antidepressants

The most commonly used tricyclic antidepressants are nortriptyline and desipramine because they have lower potential for sedation and weaker anticholinergic action than other tricyclics. Nortriptyline rarely produces orthostatic hypotension and may be favored over other tricyclics for this reason. Antidepressant response to tricyclics depends on their plasma levels and the duration of acute treatment. Elderly patients require plasma levels similar to those of younger adults in order to respond to treatment with tricyclic antidepressants: 50 to 150 ng/mL for nortriptyline and >115 ng/mL for desipramine. However, such plasma levels may be achieved with lower dosages in the elderly (nortriptyline 1 to 1.2 mg/kg and desipramine 1.5 to 2 mg/kg).

Tricyclics are contraindicated in patients with cardiac conduction defects. Nortriptyline and desipramine have properties similar to those of type 1A antiarrhythmic drugs (quinidine-like drugs). When administered to patients with right- or left-bundle-branch block, tricyclics may cause second-degree block in approximately 10 percent of cases. For this reason, an electrocardiogram (ECG) should always precede the use of tricyclics. The type 1A properties of tricyclics necessitate cautious use of these drugs in patients with ischemic heart disease. The multicenter Cardiac Arrhythmia Suppression Trial demonstrated that type 1A antiarrhythmics increase cardiac mortality in postmyocardial infarction patients. Although tricyclic antidepressants were not used in this study, the type 1A antiarrhythmic properties of tricyclic antidepressants suggest cautious use in depressed patients with ischemic heart disease.

Tricyclic antidepressants have anticholinergic properties. For this reason, these drugs should be avoided in patients with prostatic hypertrophy or narrow angle glaucoma. High intellectual functions, orthostatic blood pressure, the ECG, and the ability to urinate should be monitored frequently in depressed elderly patients receiving nortriptyline or desipramine. There is little justification for using the cyclic agents amitriptyline, imipramine, doxepin, maprotiline, or amoxapine as antidepressants in the elderly, because they have stronger sedating and anticholinergic properties than do the secondary amines.

Monoamine Oxidase Inhibitors

The MAOI phenelzine may be effective in the treatment of major depression of patients in their mid-sixties. However, there is limited research experience on MAOIs in depressed patients. When MAOIs are used in this population, low dosages should be prescribed, for example, phenelzine 30 to 45 mg daily or tranylcypromine 20 to 30 mg daily. Orthostatic hypotension is the most frequent side effect of MAO inhibitors. This side effect is of concern in the elderly

patient because it may lead to falls and fractures, especially of the hip or the humerus. Other side effects include weight gain, insomnia, lack of energy, and daytime somnolence in phenelzine-treated patients, and nervousness, insomnia, and excessive perspiration in tranylcypromine-treated patients. Peripheral neuropathy occurs in a small percentage of patients on MAOIs; it responds to pyridoxine, which may be prescribed prophylactically. Sympathomimetic amines, monoamine precursors, tricyclic antidepressants, SSRIs, venlafaxine, concomitant administration of two MAOIs, and tyramine-rich food may cause a hypertensive crisis and should be avoided in patients on MAOIs. Drug interactions and diet restrictions often prevent the use of MAOIs in the elderly. Moclobemide, a reversible inhibitor of type A MAO has a mild interaction with tyramine-rich food because of its short elimination half-life and its reversible inhibition of MAO. For this reason, moclobemide is regarded as safer than the classical MAOIs. Moclobemide appears to have neuroprotective properties through its antioxidant action. Studies are underway to examine the efficacy of moclobemide in patients with cerebrovascular and degenerative brain disorders. However, moclobemide is not available in the United States.

Other Antidepressants

Studies of younger adults suggest that bupropion is of comparable efficacy to tricyclics and SSRIs, but limited research experience exists in depressed geriatric patients. Bupropion has does not appear to influence cognitive function and heart rate or rhythm. It was found to be safe in a sample of patients with a variety of heart disorders. Bupropion has few drug interactions, but it should not be prescribed in patients receiving MAOIs. Bupropion may exacerbate preexisting hypertension. For this reason, monitoring of blood pressure is required. Seizures have been reported in 0.4 percent of patients treated with bupropion. The risk of seizures can be minimized by use of a slow-release preparation, slow introduction of bupropion (100 mg daily), use of twice-a-day dosages, and restriction of the total daily dosage to 450 mg. Most elderly patients require 150 mg of bupropion twice daily, but higher dosages (e.g., 400 mg daily) may be used.

Venlafaxine, a reuptake inhibitor of serotonin and norepinephrine, was found effective in the treatment of younger adults with major depression resistant to drugs or ECT. A significant advantage of venlafaxine is its few drug–drug interactions; no clinically significant interactions have been reported, except a life-threatening serotonin syndrome following coadministration with MAOIs. Frequent side effects include nausea, insomnia, sweating, and mild increases in blood pressure requiring monitoring. Elderly patients appear to require dosages comparable to those of younger adults. Daily dosages of 75 to 200 mg are adequate for the majority of elderly patients. Nausea, a rather frequent side effect of venlafaxine, can be minimized by a slow increase of the daily dosage. Blood pressure should be monitored, especially in patients receiving dosages above 225 mg daily, because venlafaxine can increase blood pressure. Extended release preparations of venlafaxine should be favored because they can be administered once a day and lead to better compliance.

Nefazodone promotes sleep and has anxiolytic effects. Nefazodone is well tolerated and safe in overdose, does not influence sleep architecture and does not cause sexual dysfunction. However, sedation and need for two daily dosages may be a problem for some elderly patients. A total daily dosage of 150 to 300 mg is usually sufficient, but higher dosages (up to 500 mg) may be required. Cognitive function examination should be done in patients treated with nefazodone, because this drug may lead to dose-related cognitive side effects. Nefazodone inhibits the P450 3A4 isoenzyme of the liver. The 3A4 is responsible for the metabolism of alprazolam and triazolam. These drugs should be cautiously prescribed and preferably avoided in patients receiving nefazodone.

Dextroamphetamine and methylphenidate are relatively ineffective in elderly patients with primary major depression. However, psychostimulants appear to improve apathy and anergy in medical patients or cognitively impaired patients. Dextroamphetamine or methylphenidate at dosages 5 to 10 mg in the morning and at noon is sufficient. In the elderly patient, psychostimulants have rapid onset of action, minimal side effects, limited potential for tolerance, and low risk for addiction.

Electroconvulsive Therapy

ECT is equally effective as an acute treatment of severe depression and mania. ECT should be favored in patients with severe mood syndromes who may be unable to tolerate the long waiting imposed by the gradual introduction of antidepressants or mood stabilizers and the slow onset of drug action. ECT can also be prescribed in patients with cardiac conduction deficits, prostatic hypertrophy, or glaucoma, conditions that increase the risk of treatment with tricyclics. The average number of ECTs required for the treatment of major depression is nine. Administration of three ECTs weekly appears to produce a more rapid recovery than ECT given once a week. Less-frequent ECT is associated with less cognitive impairment, but no differences were found 1 month after ECT completion between the group that had ECT three times weekly and the group that had it twice weekly.

ECT is a safe treatment with a mortality rate of 0.01 percent. The majority of deaths (67 percent) related to ECT is a result of cardiac complications and occur immediately after ECT or within a few hours after treatment. With adequate medical evaluation, monitoring during and after ECT, and appropriate intervention, most cardiovascular events related to ECT have a benign outcome. Geriatric patients sometimes develop prolonged confusion after ECT and may be prone to falls.

Dementing disorders are not a contraindication to ECT. Demented patients are more prone to delirium and prolonged memory impairment than are nondemented patients. However, administration of ECT once or twice a week may reduce the occurrence of these complications. There is no evidence that ECT accelerates the course of dementing disorders.

ECT is contraindicated in patients with recent myocardial infarction because that increases the risk of arrhythmias. ECT should not be administered in patients with intracranial tumors because it may lead to delirium, herniation or death. ECT appears to be reasonably safe 1 month after a cerebrovascular accident.

Antipsychotics

Hallucinations or delusions may be part of the presentation of psychotic depression, but may also be related to certain medical disorders including encephalopathies such as heavy metal poisoning, endocrinopathies, vitamin deficiencies, and autoimmune and metabolic disorders. Neurologic disorders associated with psychotic symptoms include dementias, epilepsies, hydrocephalus, multiple sclerosis, tumors, encephalitis, neurosyphilis, and intoxication/withdrawal from alcohol and other substances with central nervous system actions. The same neuroleptic drugs used to treat psychosis in younger adults are used in the elderly patient. Use of neuroleptics will produce a positive response in 60 to 70 percent of elderly psychotic patients, most likely through dopamine receptor blockade. Tardive dyskinesia occurs in approximately 40 percent of elderly patients who receive continuous treatment with classical neuroleptics. Typical high potency neuroleptic agents, such as haloperidol and perphenazine, are less sedating than lower-potency neuroleptics, but carry the risk of dystonia, akathisia, and parkinsonism. Neuroleptic malignant syndrome, malignant hypertension, and agranulocytosis are rare but potentially lethal complications of treatment. Risperidone, olanzapine, quetiapine, and ziprasidone are newer atypical antipsychotic agents with potential benefit for the elderly, but results of long-term use are sparse.

The lowest possible dosages should be used and increased gradually (Table 112-4). The clinician must monitor response carefully and inform the patient, close family, and caregivers about potential side effects. Attempts should be made periodically to reduce the dosage or to discontinue neuroleptics with monitoring of symptomatology for exacerbation, which may not occur until several weeks following dosage reduction. The Omnibus Budget Reconciliation Act of 1987 (OBRA) requires ongoing monitoring of neuroleptics administered to nursing home residents. Monitoring includes early examination for tardive dyskinesia, documentation of dose reduction trials to see whether symptom presentations change, and ongoing documentation justifying continued need for neuroleptics.

Psychotherapy

Interpersonal therapy (IPT), cognitive–behavioral therapy (CBT), problem-solving therapy (PST), and perhaps psychodynamic psychotherapies are as effective as antidepressant drugs in the acute treatment of depressed elderly outpatients. IPT is a brief focused psychotherapy; it addresses four factors that often are part of the interpersonal context of depressed patients: grief, role transitions, role disputes,

Table 112-4 Adequate Dose of Pharmacotherapy

Antidepressants	Average Starting Dose (mg/d)	Average Target Dose After 6 Weeks of Treatment (mg/d)	Usual Highest Final Acute Dose (mg/d)
Buproprion SR	100	150–300	300–400
Citalopram	10–20	20–30	30–40
Desipramine*	10–40	50–100	100–150
Fluoxetine	10	20	20–40
Fluvoxamine	25–50	50–200	100–300
Mirtazapine	7.5–15	15–30	30–45
Nefazodone	50–100	150–300	300–500
Nortriptyline*	10–30	40–100	75–125
Paroxetine	10–20	20–30	30–40
Phenelzine	15	30–45	30–75
Sertraline	25–50	50–100	100–120
Venlafazine XR	37.5	75–225	150–225

Antipsychotics	Average Starting Dose (mg/d)	Average Target Dose Range (mg/d)	Usual Highest Final Acute Dose (mg/d)
Haloperidol	0.5	0.5–5.0	2.0–7.0
Olanzapine	2.5	2.5–10	7.5–15
Perphenazine	2–4	4–10	8–24
Quetiapine	25–50	50–300	100–400
Risperidone	0.25–0.5	0.5–4.0	1–5
Ziprasidone†	—	—	—

*Monitoring plasma levels is recommended for this medication. Recommended target blood levels: desipramine, 115–200 ng/mL; nortriptyline, 50–150 ng/mL.

†Ziprasidone is an atypical antipsychotic newly approved for use in the United States. Experience to date is too limited to provide dose ranges.

and interpersonal deficits. Beyond its efficacy in the acute treatment of depression, antidepressant medication combined with monthly IPT sessions was superior to either treatment alone in preventing recurrence and prolonging recovery in elderly patients with recurrent unipolar depression. The superiority of combined treatment was especially evident in subjects aged 70 years and older. CBT is based on the theory that cognitive and behavioral symptoms initiate and maintain the depressive syndrome. CBT uses a variety of learning theory-based approaches that seek to reduce pathological ideas and behaviors associated with depression. CBT alone (16 to 20 sessions), desipramine alone, and CBT combined with desipramine were all found effective in the treatment of geriatric depression of mild to moderate severity. CBT combined with desipramine was more effective than desipramine alone. PST targets depression by teaching patients skills for improving their ability

to deal with everyday problems as well as major life events: this goal is accomplished by providing patients structure for approaching problems and negotiating their daily lives by teaching problem solving skills explicitly. The relative benefit of PST alone or combined with pharmacotherapy has not yet been established. Despite their efficacy and the lack of side effects, psychotherapies remain underutilized in geriatric depression.

Family interventions are useful in the treatment of geriatric mood disorders. Caregivers of elderly patients, and especially caregivers of demented patients, often develop depression themselves that can be effectively addressed by psychotherapeutic or family interventions. Since most elderly depressed patients depend on family members for emotional support and for their day-to-day functioning, treatment approaches that include selected family members may be particularly effective.

Treatment Efficacy, Medical Burden, and Cognitive Impairment

There is evidence that medical burden does not significantly interfere with antidepressant response. In a large multicenter study, fluoxetine was well tolerated (discontinuation rate 11.6 percent) but its efficacy was somewhat lower than that reported in younger adults (remission: 31.6 percent, response: 43.9 percent). History of medical illness (number of chronic medical conditions), but not current medical burden, was associated with greater response to fluoxetine and with lower placebo response. Antidepressant treatment can improve mood, physical symptoms, and function in depressed patients with emphysema. Similarly, a variety of psychotherapies have been found effective both in the acute treatment of depressed elderly patients as well in prevention of relapse and recurrence. Therefore, both antidepressants and psychotherapy have the potential to reduce depressive symptoms and disability.

While limited information from systematic studies exists, most clinicians believe that depressed-demented patients respond favorably to antidepressant drugs. Most depressed-demented patients require dosages of antidepressants comparable to those of nondemented elderly depressed patients. Treatment of depression in dementia has important implications. Effective treatment can reduce the suffering of depressed-demented patients and improve the quality of life of their families. Improvement of depression can reduce "excess disability" in demented patients and allow them to remain in the community. Finally, reduction of depressive symptoms can ameliorate the cognitive dysfunction contributed by depression and permit clinicians to determine the stage of dementia and advise patients and families about future treatment needs.

Continuation and Maintenance Treatments

Depression is a recurrent disorder. Once recovery is achieved, continuation treatment should be administered for at least 6 months with the same dosages of the antidepressant that was used during acute treatment. Failure to provide continuation treatment results in relapse in 30 to 35 percent of cases (reemergence of the index episode).

After being well for 6 months, patients are at risk for a new episode of depression. History of three or more episodes is the strongest predictor of recurrence. Other predictors are high severity of the initial episode, persisting anxiety, and advanced age. Patients at high risk for recurrence should have maintenance treatment for at least 1 to 2 years.

It is estimated that 70 percent of patients fail to take 25 to 50 percent of the dosages of their medications. Older patients and their families may not understand the importance of taking medications as prescribed. Concurrent medical illnesses can interfere with antidepressant response or attainment of adequate dosages. Alcoholism and other substance abuse may undercut pharmacotherapy. Difficulties accessing health care may hinder the ability of elderly, especially functionally impaired elderly, to obtain adequate treatment.

Treatment of Geriatric Mania

Lithium is an effective treatment for elderly mania patients. However, lithium may be less effective in mania complicated by neurologic and medical disorders than in uncomplicated mania. Elderly patients tend to show high lithium plasma levels at relatively low dosages because of an age-associated reduction in renal clearance. About one-half to two-thirds of the dosage required for young adults is usually sufficient for elderly individuals. The half-life of lithium is approximately 24 hours in the seventh decade of life. Therefore, steady-state pharmacokinetics is anticipated 5 or more days after the stabilization of the daily dosage. Elderly persons have a high increase of pharmacodynamic sensitivity to lithium and tend to have a fine tremor and even myoclonus at plasma levels considered to be therapeutic for young adults. It has been suggested that lithium plasma levels of 0.3 to 0.6 mEq/L are clinically effective in elderly individuals. However, controlled studies are lacking. The onset of action of lithium is slow and may require several days or weeks.

A large number of elderly patients develop intolerable side effects when treated with lithium, and therefore it should be avoided or discontinued in these patients. Elderly patients develop lithium-induced tremor more frequently than younger patients. Lithium may induce or worsen cognitive impairment, and this side effect is more prominent in dementia patients. In elderly mania patients, delirium can develop at lithium levels at or even below the therapeutic lithium plasma level range. Patients with Parkinson's disease and patients receiving neuroleptics are prone to lithium-induced delirium. Delirium and cerebellar dysfunction may last for weeks after lithium discontinuation. Lithium can worsen rigidity and tremor in patients with Parkinson's disease or produce parkinsonism in neurologically intact patients. Sinoatrial block can be caused by lithium. Cardiac drugs, including digitalis and beta-blockers, increase the risk for sinoatrial block. Salt depletion caused by vomiting or diarrhea, thiazide diuretics, nonsteroidal antiinflammatory drugs, and angiotensin-converting enzyme inhibitors may raise lithium plasma levels and lead to toxicity.

Anticonvulsant drugs such as carbamazepine and sodium valproate appear to have antimanic action in younger adults. Anecdotal evidence suggests that carbamazepine and sodium valproate are effective in elderly mania patients. A retrospective study of hospitalized manic elderly patients suggests that subjects receiving valproate (plasma levels 65 to 90 ng/mL) had a similar response rate (75 percent versus 82 percent) to those treated with lithium (plasma levels above 0.79 mEq/L). History of poor response to lithium does not preclude response to anticonvulsants. Some evidence exists that carbamazepine and valproate are more effective than lithium in rapidly cycling patients with dysphoric mania. Patients with neurologic brain diseases may be responsive to sodium valproate. Complete blood count and liver function tests should be obtained before treatment with carbamazepine and valproate. Elderly mania patients tend to develop a higher valproate plasma free fraction of valproate than younger patients, but the clinical significance of a high valproate free fraction in unclear.

Carbamazepine may cause sedation, confusion, and ataxia in a dose-dependent fashion. Carbamazepine-treated patients should have frequent complete blood counts because carbamazepine can cause leukopenia (white blood cells below 4,000/mm^3) in approximately 2 percent of cases. Approximately one-half of the patients who develop carbamazepine-induced leukopenia have a drop in white blood cell count within the first 16 days of treatment. Valproate causes leukopenia in 0.4 percent of patients, a percentage comparable to that of tricyclic antidepressants.

Lithium and mood stabilizers have a delayed onset of action. For this reason, lorazepam or low dosages of atypical antipsychotics may be used in the early treatment of acutely agitated elderly manic patients. Haloperidol may be used in patients who are unable to take oral medications.

ECT is highly effective as an acute treatment of mania. Approximately 80 percent of ECT-treated mania patients achieve remission or marked clinical improvement. ECT is effective even in mania patients who are resistant to drug therapy. Clinical improvement after ECT is a primary therapeutic effect rather than a result of an ECT-induced organic brain syndrome. The number of ECT treatments required to treat mania is comparable to that for treating depression. Mania patients often have a lower seizure threshold than depressed patients. Because it is well-tolerated by most geriatric patients, ECT is the treatment of choice for elderly manic patients who are unable to tolerate drug therapy or have a severe behavioral disturbance that needs to be brought under control.

Treatment of Bereavement

The treatment of a bereaved elderly person depends on the severity of symptomatology. If major depression develops during the bereavement period, antidepressant treatment should be administered. Best outcomes for major depression associated with bereavement are achieved when psychotherapy is combined with a psychosocial intervention such as interpersonal therapy.

Bereaved persons with depressive symptomatology that does not meet criteria for major depression may benefit by brief focused psychotherapy. Interpersonal therapy lends itself well for this purpose because it addresses issues related to loss, depression, and change of roles.

Most elderly bereaved individuals do not develop depressive syndromes or clinically significant depressive symptoms. Therefore, prophylactic treatment is not recommended for the whole elderly bereaved population. However, self-help groups, counseling, group therapy, and individual dynamic psychotherapy may be helpful and they should be considered for individuals with an intense reaction to loss or history of depression.

SELECTED RECOMMENDATIONS FROM THE EXPERT CONSENSUS STUDY

Clinical research, as well as meta-analytic studies, provides reliable data for characterizing the clinical presentation of psychiatric syndromes and for testing the efficacy and safety of specific treatments. However, the clinical complexity of late life depression and the number of possible combinations and sequences of available treatments make it difficult to provide clear recommendations based entirely on clinical trial data. The survey was sent to 50 national experts on geriatric depression. Consensus on each option was defined as a nonrandom distribution of scores by chi-square "goodness-of-fit" test. What follows are selected conclusions adapted from the *Expert Consensus Guideline Series: Pharmacotherapy of Depressive Disorders in Older Patients* (see Alexopoulos et al.).

1. Consider the presence of a psychiatric disorder when there is a change in usual behavior, thought pattern, or attitude. Families and caregivers may provide important information on history and present state to aid in defining the current symptoms and impairments.

2. Biological, psychologic, and social factors contribute to late-life depression, and it has biological, psychological, and social consequences. Late-life depression occurs in the context of medical and neurologic illnesses, disability, and psychosocial stress, and is best evaluated by assessing all these areas. Untreated geriatric depression carries significant medical morbidity, mortality, and disability, and can adversely impact families and caregivers. The goals of treatment extend beyond reduction of depressive symptoms and suicidal ideation, and include prevention of relapse and recurrence, improvement of cognitive and functional status, and development of skills needed for coping with handicaps and psychosocial stressors.

3. Primary care physicians treat most depressed elderly patients. Workup should include efforts to identify medical, neurologic, or drug-related disorders that may contribute to current problems. Comorbidity is common, but does not obviate the need to actively address and treat the depressive disorder. Correction of underlying medical abnormalities is a necessary, but often not a sufficient, intervention. Patients with psychotic depression, bipolar depression, or suicidal ideation benefit from early referral for specialized psychiatric care.

4. The elderly are at high risk for successful suicide, and older white men present the highest risk. The risk markedly increases after the age of 80 years. Severity of depression, psychotic symptoms, alcoholism or abuse of sedatives, recent loss or bereavement, and recent development of disability are important risk factors for suicide in depressed elderly patients. Suicide risk needs to be assessed and addressed in elderly depressed individuals.

5. Be prepared to offer treatment for patients with geriatric depression. In nonpsychotic geriatric depression, combination of antidepressants and psychotherapy is the preferred treatment for both severe and mild cases. Drug treatment alone or psychotherapy alone is an alternative choice in mild geriatric depression. Drug treatment and ECT are the alternative choices in severe geriatric depression. ECT should be considered in patients who failed adequate antidepressant trials, or

have severe depression with high suicide risk. Sequential, not overlapping, treatment trials targeting specific syndromes avoids the dangers of polypharmacy. Failure to respond to one agent does not preclude response to an alternate agent. Psychotic depression is the exception to this guideline, and treatment should include both antidepressant and antipsychotic medications. Difficulties with compliance must be addressed to ensure that adequate treatment is delivered and overdosing is prevented.

6. Many effective agents are available for the treatment of geriatric depression. For pharmacological treatment of geriatric nonpsychotic depression, SSRIs (such as citalopram or sertraline) followed by venlafaxine-XR are current recommended treatments. Alternate medications include bupropion-SR, and mirtazapine. Tricyclic antidepressants (nortriptyline or desipramine) are a reasonable alternative treatment in severe geriatric depression. Because of dose-related changes in physiology and pharmacokinetics, doses should be increased slowly in elderly patients and potential side effects and medication interactions need to be monitored. The minimal length of antidepressant trial should be 3 to 4 weeks and the maximum length should be 6 to 7 weeks before switch to another antidepressant or an augmentation agent is used.

7. Interpersonal therapy, cognitive-behavioral therapy, supportive psychotherapy, and problem-solving therapy are beneficial psychotherapeutic approaches for older depressed patients. The choice of psychosocial interventions will depend of the patient's specific needs and the availability of such services in the community.

8. For continuation and maintenance treatment, the dosages should be used that were found effective during acute treatment, for at least 1 year. The length of maintenance treatment should be increased in patients with multiple prior episodes. In a patient with psychotic depression who achieves remission following treatment with an antidepressant and an antipsychotic, the antipsychotic drug should be continued for at least 6 months. For a depressed patient who failed antidepressants but responded to ECT, antidepressants (other than the one to which the patient previously failed to respond) should be used for continuation/maintenance treatment. Continuation/maintenance ECT is another option.

9. Inform patients and families of the benefits and risks of treatment. Psychoeducational interventions are important in helping patients and their families facilitate rational decisions, avoid undertreatment, and improve adherence.

REFERENCES

Alexopoulos GS: New concepts for prevention and treatment of late-life depression. *Am J Psychiatry* 158:835, 2001.

Alexopoulos GS et al: The expert consensus guideline series: Pharmacotherapy of depressive disorders in older patients. *Postgrad Med.* October 2001 (Spec No): 1–86.

American Psychiatric Association: *Diagnostic and Statistical Manual of Mental Disorders, 4th Edition–Transitional.* Washington DC, American Psychiatric Press, 2000.

Bassuk SS et al: Depressive symptomatology and incident cognitive decline in an elderly community sample. *Arch Gen Psychiatry* 55:1073, 1998.

Conwell Y et al: Age differences in behaviors leading to completed suicide. *Am J Geriatr Psychiatry* 6:122, 1998.

Dennis MS, Lindesay J: Suicide in the elderly: The United Kingdom perspective. *Int Psychogeriatr* 7:263, 1995.

Drevets WC: Neuroimaging studies of mood disorders. *Biol Psychiatry* 48:813, 2000.

Farran CJ et al: Race, finding meaning, and caregiver distress. *J Aging Health* 9:316, 1997.

Hays JC et al: Social correlates of the dimensions of depression in the elderly. *J Gerontol B Psychol Sci Soc Sci* 53:P31, 1998.

Katz IR et al: Depression in older patients in residential care: Significance of dysphoria and dimensional assessment. *Am J Geriatr Psychiatry* 3:161, 1995.

Krishnan KRR et al: MRI-defined vascular depression. *Am J Psychiatry* 154:497, 1997.

Kumar A et al: Atrophy and high-intensity lesions: Complementary neurobiological mechanisms in late-life depression. *Neuropsychopharmacol* 22:264, 2000.

Lesser I et al: Cognition and white matter hyperintensities in older depressed adults. *Am J Psychiatry* 153:1280, 1996.

Meeks S et al: Longitudinal relationships between depressive symptoms and health in normal older and middle-aged adults. *Psychol Aging* 15:100, 2000.

Mental Health: A Report of the Surgeon General. Chap. 5. 1999. U.S. Department of Health & Human Services. U.S. Department of Health & Human Services, Substance Abuse & Mental Health Services Admin, Center for Mental Health Services, NIH, NIMH, Rockville, MD pp 331–401.

Reynolds CF et al: Nortriptyline and interpersonal psychotherapy as maintenance therapies for recurrent major depression: A randomized controlled trial in patients older than 59 years. *JAMA* 281(1):39, 1999.

Riley KP et al: Cognitive function and apolipoprotein E in very old adults: Findings from the Nun study. *J Gerontol B Psychol Sci Soc Sci* 55:S69, 2000.

Ritchie K et al: Depressive illness, depressive symptomatology, and regional cerebral blood flow in elderly people with subclinical cognitive impairment. *Age Ageing* 28:385, 1999.

Steffens DC et al: Disability in geriatric depression. *Am J Geriatr Psychiatry* 7:34, 1999.

Unutzer J et al: Patterns of care for depressed older adults in a large-staff model HMO. *Am J Geriatr Psychiatry* 7(3):235, 1999.

Schizophrenia

NADEEM MIRZA • PETER V. RABINS • TREY SUNDERLAND

Schizophrenia affects approximately 1 percent of the population; 10 percent of the schizophrenic population has onset after age 45 years. This relatively low incidence of schizophrenia is offset by a chronic debilitating course of the illness resulting in direct care expenditures estimated to approach 50 billion dollars annually.

DEFINING SCHIZOPHRENIA

Schizophrenia is difficult to define in part because its characteristic signs and symptoms lay beyond the realm of what most of us experience as normal. In the broadest terms, schizophrenia is a syndrome of disordered mental processes. Essential abnormalities include (1) firmly held, false beliefs known as delusions; (2) sensory perceptions without external stimulation dubbed hallucinations; and (3) aberrant organization or form of thought processes (thought disorder). An exclusionary criterion, (4) no evidence of a mood (affective) or medical disorder that could account for the presentation, rules out other potential diagnoses.

PATHOGENESIS

Despite substantial advances in schizophrenia research, its underlying pathophysiology is unknown. Principal hypotheses regarding causation include altered expression of genes, neuroimmunovirology, and hypoxic damage during gestation and birth. In addition, several neuropeptide abnormalities have been hypothesized (the most strongly implicated peptide being neurotensin) along with neuroanatomic theories emphasizing the role of limbic system, frontal cortex, and basal ganglia abnormalities.

Indirect support for frontal lobe involvement in schizophrenia comes from observation of inconsistent features such as abnormal eye movements, neurophysiologic deficits, decreased blood flow to the frontal lobes and "negative" symptoms.

Increased temporal lobe activity may relate to the positive symptoms (particularly hallucinations) of schizophrenia. Auditory hallucinations are related to morphologic characteristics of the superior temporal gyrus, and functional brain imaging has found a relationship between changes in blood flow and auditory hallucinations in Broca's area in the left temporal lobe. Neuronal circuits involving cortical and limbic areas are also implicated in auditory hallucinations. Conceptual disorganization is related to morphologic abnormalities in Wernicke's area, which is not surprising because this area is involved in conceptualization and organization of speech.

Biochemical theories of schizophrenia implicate dopamine, serotonin, norepinephrine, glutamine, glycine, and γ-aminobutyric acid (GABA) neurotransmitter systems. It is likely there is primary and secondary involvement of multiple systems.

Dopamine (DA) is thought to play a central, but complex, role in schizophrenia. Dopamine exerts its effects through at least five receptor subtypes and also interacts with other neurotransmitter systems. The positive symptoms of schizophrenia are thought to involve increased subcortical dopamine activity and blockade of DA type 2 (D2) receptors. Additional blockade of D2 receptors is likely the mechanism by which older, typical antipsychotic agents show efficacy for reducing positive symptoms. However, evidence suggests that negative symptoms may relate to decreased cortical dopamine activity with typical antipsychotic agents showing no benefit.

Serotonin (5-HT) projections arise from two midbrain nuclei. The dorsal raphe nucleus projects to the cortex and to striatal regions. The medial raphe nucleus projects to limbic regions. Serotonin projections inhibit dopamine functions at two levels. At midbrain levels, they inhibit firing of dopamine cells from the substantia nigra. In the striatum and cortex, they inhibit the synaptic release of dopamine. This may explain why 5-HT agonists induce extrapyramidal symptoms, while blockade of 5-HT receptors diminishes the extrapyramidal side effects of dopamine antagonism. There are three families of 5-HT receptors: 5-HT1 activates G protein-mediated signal transduction; 5-HT2 receptors activate phosphoinositol-mediated signal transduction; and 5-HT3 receptors modulate the function of ion-gated channels. Negative symptoms are thought to involve decreased dopamine transmission in the prefrontal cortex. Thus, drugs that inhibit serotonergic transmission and increase prefrontal dopamine transmission appear more likely to improve negative symptoms.

Table 113-1 DSM-IV-TR Criteria for Schizophrenia

Criterion A. Characteristic symptoms:
Delusions
Hallucinations
Disorganized speech
Grossly disorganized or catatonic behavior
Negative symptoms—affective flattening, poverty of speech, avolition, anergia

- Two or more symptoms present for at least 1 month (less if successfully treated)
- Only one symptom required if delusions are bizarre, or if hallucinations consist of multiple voices conversing, or a voice keeping a running commentary

Criterion B. Social/occupational dysfunction:
Self-care
Work
Interpersonal relations

- Level of functioning in one or more of these areas has fallen below the level achieved prior to onset

Criterion C. Duration:
Continuous signs, including prodromal, active, and residual phases of illness, persist for at least 6 months. These signs may include attenuated forms of delusions or hallucinations (odd beliefs or unusual perceptual experiences), or may be manifested by negative symptoms only.

Criterion D. Schizoaffective and mood disorder exclusion:
Mood episodes occurring during the active phase must be relatively brief in comparison to the duration of the active and residual phases.
Otherwise, no concurrent major depressive, manic, or mixed episodes have occurred during the active phase of the illness.

Criterion E. Substance/general medical condition exclusion:
The episode is not a direct result of physiologic effects of a medication, drug of abuse, or a general medical condition.

Criterion F. Relationship to a pervasive developmental disorder:
In the setting of a preexisting diagnosis of autism or other pervasive developmental disorder, the diagnosis of schizophrenia is made only if prominent delusions or hallucinations are present for at least 1 month, or less, if successfully treated.

Norepinephrine (NE) plays a significant role in the body's response to stress and is involved in modulating dopaminergic systems. Elevations in NE levels have been reported in cerebrospinal fluid (CSF), plasma, and brain tissue from patients with paranoid schizophrenia. Explanations for these observations remain unclear; however, research suggests alterations in NE metabolism or in response to stress in some schizophrenic patients.

Glutamate is an excitatory and glycine an inhibitory neurotransmitter. Both glutamate and glycine are involved in the regulation of the N-methyl-D-aspartate (NMDA) receptor. Ketamine, a glutamate/NMDA antagonist, produces an acute schizophrenic-like state in healthy individuals that includes concept disorganization, perceptual alterations, cognitive deficits, and negative symptoms. There is evidence that prefrontal glutaminergic systems are involved in mediating conceptual disorganization further implicating a role for this neurotransmitter in schizophrenia.

GABA is an inhibitory neurotransmitter. Evidence suggests that individuals with schizophrenia have low levels of this neurotransmitter, which may lead to inadequate inhibition of the frontal cortex, thus explaining the loss of selective attention seen in some individuals with schizophrenia.

DIAGNOSIS

The diagnostic criteria for schizophrenia are listed in the *Diagnostic and Statistical Manual of Mental Disorders, Fourth Edition, Text Revision* (DSM-IV-TR). Six criteria, designated A to F, must be met before a diagnosis of schizophrenia is made. Criterion A outlines the characteristic symptoms of the active phase of schizophrenia, which includes the presence of at least two of the following for a minimum of 1 month, or less, if successfully treated: delusions, hallucinations, disorganized speech, grossly disorganized or catatonic behavior, and negative symptoms. Only one symptom, delusions or hallucinations, is necessary if the delusions are bizarre or if the hallucinations involve voices keeping a running commentary of the patient's behavior. Criterion B requires significant deterioration in an individual's level of social and occupational functioning (self-care, employment, or interpersonal relations) since the onset of the disturbance. Criterion C lists duration requirements of a minimum of 6 months of prodromal, active, and residual phase symptoms. Criterion D excludes patients who meet diagnostic criteria for other psychiatric disorders such as schizoaffective disorder, or other disorders involving a preponderance of mood related symptoms. Criterion E excludes patients in whom symptoms are related to the use of a substance of abuse, a medication, or a general medical condition. Criterion F establishes symptom (delusions or hallucinations) and duration (minimum of 1 month, or less, if successfully treated) requirements before the diagnosis of schizophrenia is made in a person who is known to suffer from a pervasive developmental disorder (mental retardation, autism, Rett's disorder, Asperger's disorder). Table 113–1 highlights the DSM-IV-TR criteria for schizophrenia.

LATE-ONSET AND VERY-LATE-ONSET SCHIZOPHRENIA

Given the propensity for schizophrenia to begin during youth, the onset of symptoms during late adulthood suggests a degenerative or other structural brain disease. However, in the absence of organic illness and major depression, evidence supports the presentation of schizophrenia throughout the life span, including old age.

DIFFERENTIAL DIAGNOSIS

Other conditions that present with delusions, hallucinations, and other criterion A symptoms need to be differentiated from schizophrenia.

Brief psychotic disorder patients manifest at least one criterion A symptom of delusions, hallucinations, disorganized speech, or grossly disorganized or catatonic behavior. Formerly known as brief reactive psychosis, the diagnosis of brief psychotic disorder no longer requires appearance of symptoms temporally related to a significant life stressor. Duration of symptoms last a minimum of 1 day but less than 1 month, with a full return to baseline level of functioning.

Schizophreniform disorder applies to those patients fulfilling diagnostic criteria for schizophrenia save for disturbance of social or occupational dysfunction and for duration of symptoms. Therefore, two criterion A symptoms (delusions, hallucinations, disorganized speech, grossly disorganized or catatonic behavior, or negative symptoms), or the sole symptom of bizarre delusions or hallucinations of a voice keeping a running commentary of the person's behavior or voices conversing must be present for at least 1 month. Social or occupational dysfunction will likely be seen but is not a diagnostic criterion. Duration of psychotic, prodromal, and residual symptoms last a minimum of one but no more than 6 months.

Schizoaffective disordered patients meet criterion A for schizophrenia as well as criteria for a major depressive, a manic, or a mixed (major depressive and manic) episode at some time during the course of the illness. Thus, two criterion A symptoms (delusions, hallucinations, disorganized speech, grossly disorganized or catatonic behavior, or negative symptoms—affective flattening, alogia, or avolition), or the sole symptom of bizarre delusions or hallucinations of a voice keeping a running commentary of

the person's behavior or voices conversing must be present for at least 2 weeks. The exception here is the existence of delusions or hallucinations for at least 2 weeks without prominent mood symptoms. This criterion serves to rule out psychoses solely caused by a major depressive, bipolar, or mixed disorder. However, the symptoms of mood disturbance will ultimately be present for a substantial part of the total duration of the illness.

Delusional disorder is characterized by nonbizarre delusions and the patient never having met criteria for schizophrenia. In contrast to bizarre delusions that are regarded by the person's culture as clearly implausible (having one's thoughts read by others), nonbizarre delusions are within the realm of possibility in real life (being infected or followed) but without factual basis. Common delusions include jealousy (e.g., a sexual partner is unfaithful), erotomania (e.g., a person of power is in love with them), grandiosity (remarkable power or knowledge), being controlled (unusual feelings or impulses of being controlled by outside forces), and delusions of reference wherein objects or people in the individual's environment have unusual significance.

Major depressive disorder frequently can cause delusions and hallucinations. These patients meet diagnostic criteria for a major depressive disorder, although the depressive symptoms may be obscured by the delusions or hallucinations. To identify major depressive disorder with psychotic features, one looks to characterize the timing and duration of the delusions and hallucinations. Generally, the psychiatric history reveals the development of persistent depression with melancholic features first, and later, emergence of psychotic symptoms.

Bipolar disorder, depressed, manic, or mixed episode may include delusions and hallucinations but in the setting of prominent mood symptoms. Like major depressive disorder with psychotic features, this diagnosis may be confused with schizophrenia when the current presentation is one of overt psychoses. A thorough psychiatric history will often reveal an uninterrupted mood (depressed, manic, or mixed) pattern with delusions or hallucinations that are mood congruent, that is, can be related to a change in the person's self-attitude, e.g. "I'm a horrible person" in depression and "I'm all powerful" in mania.

Substance and medication use or withdrawal can lead to the production of psychotic symptoms. Given the often prominent nature of delusions and hallucinations, difficulty establishing the timing of substance use or withdrawal and presentation of psychotic symptoms, and the high comorbidity of schizophrenia with substance abuse and addiction, this diagnosis can be difficult to make and is frequently confused with schizophrenia. Ultimately, evidence from the history, physical, or laboratory exam suggests the onset of symptoms within 1 month of substance or medication use, intoxication, or withdrawal, and a diagnosis of substance-induced psychotic disorder can be established.

Psychotic disorder, not otherwise specified, is used when symptoms of delusions, hallucinations, disorganized speech, grossly disorganized or catatonic behavior are present, but evidence favoring a more specific diagnosis is inadequate at the time of evaluation. As further information

Table 113-2 Psychiatric Illnesses with Schizophrenic-like Symptoms

Brief Psychotic Disorder
Core symptoms: delusions, hallucinations, disorganized speech, grossly disorganized or catatonic behavior

- At least one symptom must be present
- Duration of symptoms between 1 day and 1 month

Schizophreniform Disorder
Core symptoms: delusions, hallucinations, disorganized speech, grossly disorganized or catatonic behavior, negative symptoms—affective flattening, poverty of speech, avolition, anergia

- Criteria same as schizophrenia
- Duration of symptoms greater than 1 month but less than 6 months

Schizoaffective Disorder
Core symptoms: delusions, hallucinations, disorganized speech, grossly disorganized or catatonic behavior, negative symptoms—affective flattening, poverty of speech, avolition, anergia

- Criteria same as schizophrenia
- Two-week period of depressed mood plus four or more depressive symptoms: decreased interest or pleasure; significant weight loss or gain; insomnia or hypersomnia; motor slowing or restlessness; loss of energy; guilt; inability to concentrate; thoughts of death/wanting to die
- Delusions and hallucinations must exist for 2 weeks in the absence of significant mood symptoms

Delusional Disorder
Core symptoms: nonbizarre delusions (situations that could occur in real life such as being followed, poisoned, deceived, infected)

- Has never met criteria for schizophrenia
- Functioning is not severely impaired

Major Depressive Disorder, Severe with Psychotic Features
Core symptoms: delusions, hallucinations

- Criteria are met for major depressive disorder
- Delusions or hallucinations are present

Bipolar 1 Disorder, Manic, Depressed, or Mixed, Severe with Psychotic Features
Core symptoms: delusions, hallucinations

- Criteria are met for bipolar disorder (manic, depressed, or mixed episode)
- Delusions or hallucinations are present

Substance-induced Psychotic Disorder
Core symptoms: delusions, hallucinations

- Evidence from history, physical, or laboratory exam of onset of symptoms during or within 1 month of substance intoxication or withdrawl
- Evidence that substance use is related to the disturbance

Psychotic Disorder, Not Otherwise Specified
Core symptoms: delusions, hallucinations, disorganized speech, grossly disorganized or catatonic behavior

- Available information is inadequate to make a specific diagnosis
- The clinician is unable to determine whether the symptoms are primary, caused by a general medical condition, or substance induced

Hallucinations of Grief
Core symptoms: illusions (false perceptions or misinterpretations), isolated hallucinations (frequently auditory or visual)

- Common phenomenon
- Maintains awareness that the experience was not real
- The experience is generally brief and variable (not the same each time)

Table 113-3 Drugs of Abuse and Medical Conditions Associated with Delusions or Hallucinations

Intoxication/Withdrawl	Neurologic/Medical	Endocrine
Alcohol	Adrenoleukodystrophy	Addison's disease
Amphetamines	Alzheimer's disease	Cushing's disease
Cannabis	Cerebrovascular accident	Hypothyroidism
Cocaine	Delirium	Hyperthyroidism
Hallucinogens	Friedreich's ataxia	Hypoparathyroidism
Inhalants	Huntington's disease	Hyperparathyroidism
Opioids	Metachromatic leukodystrophy	
Sedative–hypnotics	Phenylketonuria	**Infectious**
	Porphyria, acute intermittent	Brain abscess
Developmental	Seizures, complex partial	Meningitis
Asperger's syndrome	Systemic lupus erythematosus	Encephalitis
Autism	Traumatic brain injury	
Mental retardation	Tumors	**Additional syndromes**
Rett's syndrome		Heavy metal intoxication

becomes available, a more specific diagnosis may be applicable.

Hallucinations of grief are a common, normal phenomenon associated with loss of a loved one. They generally involve the experience of seeing or hearing the deceased person; however, the patient will recognize this as not real. Table 113–2 summarizes psychiatric illnesses involving schizophrenic-like symptoms.

Differential Diagnosis of Delusions and Hallucinations

A large number of neuropsychiatric and medical illnesses can cause delusions or hallucinations. Elderly persons are at increased risk because of a high prevalence of medical conditions and widespread use of multiple medications. Many medications lead to delirium and this risk is exaggerated by the frequency of drug–drug interactions. Table 113–3 is a list of the more common causes of schizophrenic-like symptoms.

PHARMACOLOGIC TREATMENTS

Antipsychotic medication guidelines established by the Health Care Financing Administration (HCFA) state that antipsychotic agents should be restricted to use for primary psychotic disorders or for specific nonpsychotic behavior. For nonpsychotic behavior, antipsychotic drugs should be used only when behavior is associated with an organic mental syndrome, such as delirium, dementia or amnesia, along with other psychotic and/or agitated behaviors when such behaviors present a danger to the patient or to others. Antipsychotic medications are often divided into two broad, generalized categories—typical and atypical. This classification is based largely upon theoretical mechanisms of action and side-effect profiles. Typical antipsychotics (e.g., haloperidol, perphenazine, molindone) primarily target the dopamine system while atypical

agents (e.g., risperidone, olanzapine, quetiapine) modulate dopamine and serotonin systems. Until recently, the most commonly used medications to treat late-life psychosis were typical antipsychotics. Although therapeutically effective they also were associated with significant side effects.

Typical antipsychotic medications primarily target the dopamine system and are effective in treating positive symptoms, but they show little efficacy in the treatment of negative symptoms. Atypical antipsychotics have comparable efficacy to typical agents in treating positive symptoms but are superior to typical agents in the management of negative symptoms. Relative to typical antipsychotics, atypical agents have a more favorable side-effect profile especially in the treatment of elderly populations. Current prescribing practices now favor the use of atypical neuroleptics as the first-choice treatment for late-life psychosis. Dosing strategies in the elderly patient should consider issues relevant to metabolism and adherence. Elderly populations in general are extremely sensitive to the neurotoxic effects of all neuroleptics and are especially prone to developing extrapyramidal symptoms (EPS). In settings such as nursing homes, neuroleptics may be prescribed for inappropriate reasons (control of nonpsychotic, annoying behaviors) or, conversely, not prescribed in appropriate situations because of fears of side effects. Educational programs for patients and care providers directed towards improving the understanding of complex behaviors, the risks and benefits of antipsychotic medication use, and the nonpharmacologic strategies for managing behaviors will contribute to improved safety, care, and adherence to prescribed therapeutic regimes.

The following is a brief description of the currently available, FDA-approved, atypical antipsychotic agents.

Clozapine (Clozaril) was the first atypical agent approved by the FDA. Clozapine is an antagonist of serotonergic (5-HT2A) and D2 receptors but also effects muscarinic, cholinergic, adrenergic and histaminergic receptors. More common side effects include hypotension, weight gain, sedation, constipation or diarrhea, sialorrhea, and

Table 113-4 FDA-approved Atypical Antipsychotic Medications

General Name	Trade Name	Starting Dose (mg/d)	Dose Range (mg/d)	Side Effects
Clozapine	Clozaril	6.25–12.5 bid	75–450	Agraulocytosis, sedation, tachycardia
Risperidone	Risperdal	0.25–0.5	0.25–2	Hypotension, sedation
Olanzapine	Zyprexa	2.5–5	2.5–15	Sedation, weight gain
Quetiapine	Seroquel	12.5–25 bid	100–400	Sedation, postural hypotension
Ziprasidone	Geodon	20 bid	40–80	QTc prolongation

tachycardia. Baseline and weekly white blood cell (WBC) studies must be conducted during the first 6 months of therapy because of the possible occurrence of serious alterations in granulocytes, monocytes, platelets, and eosinophils. Increasing age is a significant risk factor for clozapine-induced agranulocytosis. While clozapine has proven efficacy in patients with schizophrenia, its use is limited to patients who are unresponsive to other antipsychotic medications because of its potentially serious side-effects. The recommended starting dose is 6.25 to 12.5 mg daily, with maintenance at the lowest effective dose.

Risperidone (Risperdal) was the second atypical agent approved by the FDA. It is an antagonist of 5-HT2A, D2, and noradrenergic receptors, but it appears to have little involvement with cholinergic receptors. More common side effects are hypotension and EPS. Conservative starting doses for the elderly are 0.25 to 0.5 mg daily, with maintenance doses seldom exceeding 2 mg/d. Risperidone is available in tablet, liquid, and depot forms.

Olanzapine (Zyprexa) has a pharmacologic profile resembling that of clozapine. It displays greater antagonistic activity at 5-HT2A than at D2 receptors, while also antagonizing muscarinic, cholinergic, adrenergic, and histaminergic receptors. More common side effects include weight gain, dizziness, sedation, and orthostasis. Starting doses of 2.5 to 5 mg are advised in the elderly patient, with maintenance doses ranging from 5 to 15 mg. Olanzapine tablets start at 2.5 mg with an orally disintegrating (Zydis) form available in 5 mg doses.

Quetiapine (Seroquel) also displays antagonist effects at 5-HT2A and D2 receptors. The more common side effects of this medication include somnolence, hypotension and a low occurrence of EPS. An association with cataract formation was documented in animal testing, resulting in recommendations for baseline and biannual eye examinations. Initial doses should begin at 12.5 to 25 mg twice daily, with maintenance doses of approximately 100 to 400 mg.

Ziprasidone (Geodon) has a high affinity for 5-HT2A receptors and moderate affinity for D2 and D3 receptors. More common side effects include nausea, dyspepsia, insomnia, and QTc prolongation, and a low incidence of orthostatic, sedative, and anticholinergic effects. Because of its capsular form, dosing begins at 20 mg twice each day, with adjustments to the lowest effective dose, ranging from 20 to 40 mg twice per day. Table 113–4 is a list of currently available atypical antipsychotic medications.

The side effects of antipsychotic medications can be divided into neurologic and nonneurologic. Neurologic side effects are typified by production of EPS (akathisia, dystonia, and parkinsonism). These symptoms are thought to occur when striatal D2 receptor occupancy exceeds approximately 80 percent and, given their high affinity for D2 receptors, EPS is more frequently experienced when typical antipsychotic agents are used. Akathisia is characterized by mental and physical restlessness and agitation and may present at any time during the course of treatment. Acute dystonia generally presents early in treatment and is characterized by muscular spasms, potentially involving any muscle group. Muscular spasms are most commonly observed to involve the neck, face, tongue, and eyes. Drug-induced parkinsonism is generally observed after the initial weeks or months of treatment. Management of acute EPS is generally accomplished by using anticholinergic medications such as diphenhydramine or benztropine. Tardive dyskinesia (TD) is a chronic movement disorder associated with long-term use of antipsychotic medications, and elderly populations are at significantly increased risk for developing TD. Prevention of TD includes careful monitoring for the earliest signs of development, using the lowest effective doses, and periodic assessment for need to continue antipsychotic medications. Neuroleptic malignant syndrome (NMS) is a relatively uncommon, but potentially lethal condition that is associated with the use of antipsychotic medications. Muscle rigidity, high temperature, increases in muscle enzymes and leukocytosis are objective signs of NMS. In the face of NMS, early diagnosis and withdrawal of medications is key. Nonneurologic side effects of antipsychotic medications include liver dysfunction, hypotension, blood dyscrasias, and hormonal alterations such as hyperprolactinemia. Management includes early recognition, dose reductions, medication discontinuation, and alternative medication trials, if warranted.

REFERENCES

American Psychiatric Association: *Diagnostic and Statistical Manual of Mental Disorders, Fourth Edition, Text Revision.* Washington, DC, American Psychiatric Association, 2000.

Charney DS, Nestler EJ, Bunney BS (eds): *Neurobiology of Mental Illness.* New York, Oxford University Press, 1999.

General Topics in Geriatric Psychiatry

ANAND KUMAR

PERSONALITY DISORDERS IN THE ELDERLY POPULATION

A personality disorder (PD) can be defined as an enduring maladaptive pattern of behavior that is pervasive and seen across a broad range of personal and social circumstances. The behavior interferes with the individual's psychological, occupational, and social well-being and is always at marked variance with societal and cultural norms of appropriate behavior. The pattern is also long-standing, and its onset can be traced to late adolescence or early adulthood. Further, the behavior is not accounted for by another mental disorder, the direct physiologic effects of a substance, or a general medical disorder.

The diagnosis of a PD requires a comprehensive assessment of the individual's long-term pattern of functioning. Often a single interview, including a comprehensive mental status examination, is inadequate for making a proper diagnosis of a PD. Observing the individual's behavior in diverse social situations across time and integrating collateral information from reliable informants are necessary before a diagnosis of PD can be made with clinical certainty.

Classification of Personality Disorders

The *Diagnostic and Statistical Manual* (DSM) of the American Psychiatric Association lists several PDs based on primary behavioral characteristics that dominate the clinical picture. The DSM also provides operational clinical criteria for the diagnosis of individual disorders and groups PDs into the clusters listed below based on certain broad similarities in manifest behavior. This approach treats these disorders as independent categories largely distinct from one another. Clinically, patients often present with a combination of features and share characteristics with patients from other categories. Overlap is more likely to occur within a specific cluster.

1. Cluster A comprises personalities manifested by behavior that can be described as eccentric or odd. This subgroup is broadly associated with behavioral characteristics such as magical thinking, strange or bizarre ideas, and hypervigilant behaviors. It includes schizotypal, paranoid, and schizoid PDs. Overt features of psychosis such as hallucinations and delusional thinking are not typically part of the clinical picture. However, there is a certain strangeness in the thought content and overall pattern of interactions exhibited by patients with Cluster A disorders.

2. Cluster B includes volatile and erratic personalities often manifested by explosive and other unpredictable behaviors. Patients with Cluster B disorders typically have difficulty regulating and modulating emotion and affect. Difficult interpersonal relationships, promiscuity, increased sensitivity to rejection together with an inflated sense of self-worth, and substance abuse are often encountered in patients with diagnoses in this group of disorders. Antisocial, borderline, narcissistic, and histrionic PDs are included in Cluster B.

3. Cluster C consists largely of personalities characterized by fearfulness and withdrawal and includes subtypes such as dependent, obsessive-compulsive, and avoidant PDs. Some patients with these types of disorders are somewhat reclusive and have difficulty expressing emotions appropriately. They can be thought of as "underexpressing" emotions and provide an interesting contrast to patients with Cluster B disorders.

Personality Traits

Personality traits are enduring patterns of perceiving, thinking about, and relating to the environment across a range of personal and social situations. They can be considered innate characteristics that help define an individual in the larger social milieu in which they operate. Traits can be either adaptive or maladaptive, depending both on the trait (the quality) and the circumstances. Traits that are adaptive and/or helpful under one set of conditions may prove maladaptive under a different set of circumstances.

For example, under stress, traits that may appear neutral under normal circumstances may result in clinical decompensation and dysfunctional behaviors. Traits are widely considered to have genetic and biological underpinnings. However, environmental influences are likely to attenuate individual traits and play an important role in their evolution, especially in the early years of development. Personality traits commonly observed and studied include introversion, extroversion, neuroticism, and openness to new experience (i.e., novelty-seeking behavior).

Patients who are clinically impaired but do not meet standard criteria for the diagnosis of a PD may be thought of as having trait disturbances or subsyndromal PDs. The differences between subsyndromal PDs and disorders that meet standard diagnostic criteria for PDs are not qualitative but are more typically differences in degree of impairment. However, it is important both conceptually and clinically to distinguish between individuals who display abnormal behaviors only under conditions of extreme stress from those with a persistent pattern of dysfunctional behaviors.

Changes in Personality Traits With Aging

Most personality traits remain constant throughout the life span. Longitudinal studies using personality inventories demonstrate that personality traits and patterns generally remain consistent over the entire life span although they may be attenuated by increasing life experience and social maturation. Neurobiological changes with aging may also contribute to changes in overt behavior with aging. Characteristics such as extroversion and openness to new experiences have been reported to decrease with increasing age. This decrease in extroversion with age is one of the more consistent findings in trait and personality studies that focus on changes across the life span. Older individuals have been demonstrated to be more orderly, stable, and less active than younger individuals. Impulsiveness and novelty-seeking behaviors may also occur to a lesser degree in elderly subjects.

Although changes in personality with increasing age and maturation are somewhat subtle, more dramatic changes have been observed under special circumstances such as injury to the brain and/or major changes in the environment. The classic case of Phineas Gage, who received a piercing wound to the orbitofrontal cortex and subsequently developed new personality traits including irritability, indifference to appearance, and a lack of concern for "the feelings of others," exemplifies how striking changes in personality can occur in the absence of major neurologic sequelae. Personality changes have also been reported following strokes and the onset of degenerative disorders such as Alzheimer's disease. In some instances the change is an exacerbation of a previous personality characteristic. Major environmental changes, including placement in a nursing home or in a position of dependency created by a chronic illness and/or disability, can also result in fundamental changes in attitudes and behavior often described as personality changes. The term "personality" is used loosely in these instances and often denotes changes in behavior and interests secondary to injury to the central nervous system (CNS) and/or environmental changes.

The Prevalence of Personality Disorders in the Elderly

In a meta-analysis of published studies on PDs in patients aged 50 and older, Abrams and colleagues reported that about 10 percent of subjects older than age 50 met DSM criteria for having a PD. The 11 studies used in this meta-analysis showed a wide range in the estimated prevalence of PDs in the study samples ranging from 6 percent to 30 percent. The meta-analysis also revealed that the most common PD in older adults was obsessive-compulsive PD (35%) followed by dependent PD (2%) and PDs not otherwise specified (clinically significant disorders not meeting criteria exclusively for any specific category) (2%). The rate of occurrence of each of the other PDs in this age group was 1 percent or less. There were no noticeable gender differences in elderly people with PDs. This pattern differs from the prevalence and distribution of PDs in individuals younger than age 50. In younger adults the distribution is dependent (6%), antisocial (3%), obsessive-compulsive (3%), and histrionic PD (2%).

Several factors influence the estimated prevalence of PDs. The method used to make a diagnosis affects the accuracy of the diagnosis. These factors include differences in structured interviews versus subjective reports versus retrospective chart reviews. The diagnosis also varies with the setting in which patients are identified, namely, inpatient care versus ambulatory care versus long-term care. The availability, or lack thereof, of reliable collateral sources of information additionally influences the diagnostic precision in studies on PDs. These methodologic factors should be considered when comparing different estimates of the prevalence of PDs.

Changes in Personality Disorders With Age

Longitudinal studies indicate that there are differences in the natural progression of the various PDs with age. In general, it has been demonstrated that patients with diagnoses of PDs in Cluster B, characterized by a compromise in the regulation and modulation of affect, improve as they grow older. Patients with diagnoses of these disorders demonstrate less impulsivity and aggression with age. More specifically, studies indicate that in antisocial PD, there is a trend toward improvement or remittance in symptoms in the majority of individuals who survive to late life. Follow-up studies also demonstrate that patients with diagnoses of borderline PDs, typically characterized by a marked lack of emotional control, also improve symptomatically in middle age and late life. PDs in Cluster A, such as paranoid and schizotypal PDs, and those characterized by overcontrol of emotions and affect, such as obsessive-compulsive PDs, remain largely unchanged with age. The specific neurobiological and psychosocial changes responsible for some of the observed changes in behavior and interpersonal style remain unclear.

The accurate diagnosis of PDs in elderly people faces several challenges. By definition, this diagnosis is based on a lifelong, maladaptive pattern of behavior. Several limitations, including difficulty in obtaining an accurate history of earlier behavioral patterns, failure of patients to acknowledge a history of interpersonal difficulties, and difficulty in obtaining access to medical and psychiatric records compromise the ability to establish a lifelong pattern of dysfunction. In addition, some of the behavioral characteristics of humans change with age, and consequently the clinical presentation of PDs in older adults may differ from that in younger adults. Diagnostic criteria for PDs, largely based on experience with younger patients, may not be optimal for older individuals. Additional factors that complicate a diagnosis of PD in elderly people include the coexistence of medical and neurologic disorders such as parkinsonism and Alzheimer's disease. These disorders modify behavior and cognition, thereby complicating the diagnosis of PDs in elderly patients. If one adheres to convention, the diagnosis of a late-onset PD cannot be made because a lifelong pattern of maladaptive behavior is required. Although this nosologic barrier might preclude a diagnosis of late-onset PD, it is not unusual to observe changes in the personality of individuals with degenerative, vascular, and other CNS insults, especially when the frontal lobes and circuits are involved. Whether one considers these late-onset behavioral changes PDs, personality changes, or simply pervasive behavioral changes, the nosologic arguments should not obscure the need for ongoing behavioral treatment of the patient.

Comorbidity

Personality disorders often coexist in elderly patients with other psychiatric disorders such as major depression. Older individuals with clinically significant mood disorders are more likely to receive a diagnosis of a Cluster C than a Cluster B disorder. Certain subtypes like dependent, avoidant, and obsessive-compulsive PDs are more frequently diagnosed in elderly patients during an episode of clinical depression. In contrast, younger adults more commonly receive diagnoses of disorders belonging to both Cluster B and C categories. These results are consistent with other longitudinal studies suggesting that certain PDs in Cluster B appear to be less prevalent in elderly than in younger populations. It has also been demonstrated that patients with late-onset mood disorders receive diagnoses of PDs less frequently than patients with early-onset disorders.

The diagnosis of a PD cannot be made with any degree of certainty during an episode of clinical depression or other major psychiatric disturbance. A resolution of symptoms is needed before such a diagnosis can be made, as normal interepisodic functioning precludes the diagnosis of a PD. There are also preliminary indications that PDs complicate the treatment of depression in terms of both short-term response and more long-term outcomes. Individuals with a PD respond poorly to pharmacologic treatment of depression. A PD can also contribute to residual symptoms of depression that persist following pharmacologic intervention. Further, a PD can also interfere with short-term psychotherapy in elderly patients with major depression. The effect of a PD on the treatment of concurrent psychiatric disorders is clearly deleterious and should be considered in the treatment of older patients.

Etiology of Personality Disorders

Historically, the study of PDs in psychiatry was dominated by psychodynamic theories and related psychosocial models. It was widely believed that most PDs resulted from poor parenting and/or dysfunctional domestic and social environments and interactions. Treatment of these disorders was therefore largely psychosocial in nature. A widely held view was that unlike axis 1 disorders, such as schizophrenia and manic depression, PDs had minimal biological substrates. Although this may still represent a minority opinion, the biological basis of temperament, personality traits, and PDs is receiving increasing attention in psychiatry and behavioral neuroscience.

Studies on twins with PDs suggest a strong genetic component in many PDs, including disorders belonging to Clusters A, B, and C. There is a large variability in the heritability of the different PDs, with schizoid, paranoid, and avoidant PDs showing less heritability than some of the other disorders in one study. Some PDs like schizotypal PD may be biologically and/or genetically linked to schizophrenia. Although evidence supporting an important role for heritability in PDs is increasing, the question of precisely what is being inherited is an intriguing and important one. There are preliminary suggestions that personality traits and temperaments are genetically determined, at least in part. The precise combination of traits inherited and the interaction between these traits and the environment may well determine the overall clinical picture. At their core, PDs represent a collection of behavioral features that are socially maladaptive. Behavioral elements such as aggression, affective lability, impulsivity, and cognition may be differentially influenced and controlled by genes. The interplay between biological mechanisms and experience mediated by environmental interactions may be influential in the pathophysiology of PDs. The cultural context, together with the conceptual framework and diagnostic system used, undoubtedly influence the final diagnosis a patient receives. Despite the paucity of studies and the methodologic challenges, the biological basis of PDs is an exciting area that is likely to receive increasing scientific attention in the future.

Treatment, Management, and Implications

In general, patients with PDs are difficult to care for and treat in both medical and psychiatric settings. They often do not conform to traditional expectations of patient behavior in nearly all medical settings. Several aspects of their behavior appear self-defeating, and they have come to typify the "high-maintenance" patient encountered in most clinical settings. Patients with PDs have limited insight into their situation and behavior, which clearly creates a barrier to their ongoing care and treatment. Treatment resistance and noncompliance with pharmacologic and other regimens are not uncommon in these individuals. Behavioral treatment often involves interventions with antidepressants, antianxiety agents, and tranquilizers at different times depending on the most disabling symptoms clinically apparent during that phase. Once a diagnosis of PD is made or suspected, consultation with psychiatrists and psychologists experienced in dealing with the behavioral challenges posed by these patients may be clinically useful. Patients with a diagnosis of such disorders are often better treated by teams that can readily provide pharmacologic and psychological expertise. A professional interest in and a commitment to the treatment of patients with chronic behavioral disorders is often necessary to implement and sustain the long-term interventions necessary to achieve clinically significant improvement in such patients.

SUBSTANCE ABUSE IN THE ELDERLY POPULATION

Alcohol Abuse

Alcohol abuse in the elderly population is a significant medical and public health problem, although it has received scant attention in medical and health policy circles. The terms "substance dependence" and "substance abuse" both allude to maladaptive patterns of psychoactive substance use. The symptoms of the dependence syndrome often include physiologic symptoms of tolerance and withdrawal, whereas the term "abuse" refers to patterns of use that do not meet the threshold for a diagnosis of drug dependence. Although distinctions between alcohol dependence and alcohol abuse are often drawn in the literature, these terms are used interchangeably in this chapter as there are several overlapping features that permit them to be conceptually treated as components of the same disorder. Epidemiologic studies indicate that the 1-year prevalence of alcohol use disorders among community-dwelling elderly people aged 65 and older is approximately 3 percent in men and 0.46 percent in women. These figures are lower than estimates of alcohol abuse in middle-aged populations (aged 45 to 64 years old), which are about 7.85 percent in men and 1.0 percent in women. The prevalence of alcoholism is higher in clinical than in community studies and has been estimated to be greater than 10 percent among patients admitted to medical units. Heavy drinking can be defined as having more than two drinks per day. With this definition, approximately 6 percent of older adults are considered heavy users of alcohol.

The overall consumption of alcohol is lower in the elderly population when compared with nongeriatric adult populations. Attrition from alcohol-related deaths may be a factor in the lower prevalence of alcohol abuse by elderly people. The increased physiologic effects of small amounts of alcohol, together with medical problems and fewer social events, which reduce access to drinking, are additional factors that contribute to the reduced alcohol intake observed in elderly people. What is less clear is whether this finding represents a real decrease in the consumption of alcohol with age or more accurately reflects cohort differences in the alcohol consumption patterns between older and younger individuals studied cross-sectionally. Longitudinal studies indicate that there is little change in alcohol consumption in people as they age.

Special Characteristics of Elderly People

Elderly people represent the fastest growing segment of the population, and most psychiatric and behavioral disorders are detected and treated in primary care and general medical settings. It is therefore important that physicians working in these settings familiarize themselves with the fundamentals of substance and alcohol abuse in the elderly population, including knowledge of its impact, appropriate methods of diagnosis, and adequate referral patterns. About two-thirds of elderly alcoholic patients have a long history of alcohol abuse. The other third have a history consistent with late-onset abuse. A family history of alcoholism is more often obtained in the early-onset cases. It has been suggested that stressors such as bereavement and retirement may contribute to late-onset drinking, although retirement per se is not a strong predictor of patterns of alcohol abuse for most individuals. Despite the significant clinical impact of alcohol use in the elderly population, alcohol problems are often undetected and untreated in older persons. The factors that contribute to this underrecognition are physician unawareness of alcohol abuse and its potential medical and psychosocial impact and the reluctance of the patient to volunteer information or acknowledge alcohol consumption. Other factors such as limited access to collateral sources of information and attributing the symptoms and signs of alcohol abuse to medical problems also limit the diagnosis of alcohol abuse in elderly people.

Biological Changes With Aging

Biological changes with aging render older individuals more vulnerable to the effects of alcohol. Changes in the volume of distribution produced by a decrease in lean body mass result in higher peak levels for a given dose of alcohol. Older people frequently ingest prescription medications for multiple comorbid medical disorders, and therefore the potential for drug–alcohol interactions is high. Drug absorption is affected by delayed gastric emptying and increased small bowel transit time related to alcohol use. Blood flow through the liver and metabolic capacity decrease with age. While acute alcohol use may impair liver function, more chronic use of alcohol results in the induction of hepatic microsomal enzymes that may enhance drug metabolism. In addition, heavy drinkers who are malnourished may have hypoalbuminemia and altered protein-binding ability. These physiologic factors complicate the pharmacodynamics and pharmacokinetics of alcohol use in older people and contribute to some of the unique presentations of alcohol use in this age group.

Clinical Presentations of Alcohol Abuse in Elderly People

Alcohol-related disorders often do not manifest clinically in elderly adults as they do in younger adults. The stereotypic image of skid row and its social and clinical presentations is infrequently, if at all, seen in the elderly population. Medical and psychosocial factors influence the clinical presentation of alcohol-related disorders in older people, and their presentation often differs from that observed in younger adults. Several psychological and medical factors affect the presentation of alcohol-related problems in elderly patients.

Clinical Presentations

Several unique features of the presentation of an elderly patient with an alcohol problem should be considered.

1. Patients with alcohol problems may present with symptoms and signs that resemble those of other psychiatric conditions such as a mood disorder or a dementia. Anxiety disorders and sleep disturbances may also be the main presenting complaint of an individual with an alcohol problem. Symptoms and signs of depression may sometimes be a consequence of heavy drinking, and at other times alcohol abuse may reflect attempts at self-medication in a depressed or very anxious patient. Problems with memory, concentration, abstraction, and other cognitive skills may be the main presenting complaint in an elderly patient with an alcohol problem. They may be associated with an impairment in driving skills and a history of recent driving difficulties and/or infractions. Further, the cognitive impairment may not meet criteria for dementia and may resolve over a period of months if alcohol intake is stopped.
2. Alcohol abuse may present as medical and/or neurologic problems requiring medical attention. Medically complex patients with alcohol problems may make frequent trips to the emergency department or to primary care settings to seek treatment for medical disorders without discussing their alcohol problem. Presenting features include delirium, dehydration, malnutrition, gait disturbances, head trauma, and recurring falls. The impact of alcohol on gait, superimposed on osteoporosis, places these patients at high risk for hip fractures. Liver disease, late-onset seizure disorders, neuropathy, and myopathy are some of the other medical disorders found in elderly patients with alcohol problems. Chronic pain is sometimes associated with long-standing medical disorders, and self-medication with alcohol may result from this combination. Alcohol use can also exacerbate chronic medical problems such as diabetes, hypertension, gastritis, and parkinsonism. Frequent visits to the emergency department or the physician's office with an array of seemingly unrelated medical problems should alert the clinician to the possibility of alcohol abuse in these patients.
3. Finally, there are mildly dependent patients, so-called quiet drinkers without a specific complaint who may have developed tolerance to alcohol over the years. Although these types of patients may not present with an immediate problem, the identification of problem drinking in this subgroup of individuals facilitates preventive intervention to reduce the future occurrence of medical, neurologic, and psychiatric problems.

The Diagnosis of Alcoholism in Elderly Patients

A comprehensive history, including a history of problem drinking and related medical and social consequences, is central to the diagnosis of alcohol abuse in elderly individuals. A detailed, systematic description of drinking practices provided by patients and reliable collateral sources remains the primary clinical method of making a diagnosis of alcohol abuse. Any mention of driving infractions and "hangovers," while not typical in elderly people, should be probed when obtaining the history. Screening instruments such as the CAGE measure (Table 114-1) and the geriatric version of the Michigan Alcoholism Screening Test (MAST-G) can be useful adjuncts in making a diagnosis of alcohol problems in older adults. Questionnaires alone are insufficient to identify problem drinkers. Specific questions referring to the amount of alcohol consumed and the frequency of drinking, together with the use of instruments such as the CAGE screen, can help identify an increasing number of problem drinkers. A denial of alcohol problems, defensiveness, and frank irritability are often observed in clinical practice. Building a careful rapport with patients, interfacing with relatives, caregivers, and those within the patient's social network, and reviewing medical records are important steps in building a comprehensive information base.

In addition, a detailed physical and laboratory examination can also provide clues to excessive alcohol intake. These include signs of chronic liver disease, peripheral neuropathy, and cerebellar ataxia. Their presence should increase the suspicion of an underlying alcohol-related

Table 114-1   Ewing's CAGE Screening Measure*

1. Have you ever felt you ought to Cut down on your drinking?
2. Have people Annoyed you by criticizing your drinking?
3. Have you ever felt bad or Guilty about your drinking?
4. Have you ever had a drink first thing in the morning to steady your nerves or get rid of a hangover ("Eye opener")?

*Positive answers to two or more questions suggest an alcohol problem at some time, although the problem may not currently be active.

Source: Reprinted with permission from Ewing JA: Detecting alcoholism: The CAGE questionnaire. *JAMA* 252: 1905, 1984.

problem. Laboratory testing may also be useful in certain instances, and findings such as higher mean corpuscular volume, anemia, and elevated liver enzyme levels should heighten the suspicion of recurrent alcohol abuse.

The Genetic Basis of Alcoholism

Converging lines of evidence indicate that alcoholism has a strong genetic component. Family studies demonstrate a three- to fivefold increased risk for alcoholism in siblings and first-degree relatives of affected individuals. The risk of alcoholism is increased in children of alcoholics who have been adopted and raised away from their biological parents. Studies involving twins also suggest a strong genetic component with heritability in the 50 percent to 60 percent range.

As in the case of other complex genetic diseases, it is likely that multiple interacting genes contribute to alcoholism. The initial thrust of studies aimed at determing the genetic basis of alcoholism focused on identifying candidate genes. This approach has been successful in describing the contributions made by genes responsible for alcohol metabolism. The only finding that has been consistently replicated in genetic studies on alcoholism has been identification of the protective effects of certain functional polymorphisms of the enzyme alcohol dehydrogenase (ADH) and the mitochondrial enzyme aldehyde dehydrogenase (ALDH2). Most ingested alcohol is metabolized to acetaldehyde by ADH and the microsomal cytochrome P450 system in the liver. *ALDH2* is present as a polygene family on chromosome 4 consisting of seven genes, two of which, *ADH2* and *ADH3,* are functionally polymorphic. ALDH is present in the cytoplasm and the mitochondria of liver cells. Studies consistently show that in specific populations (subgroups of Asians) functional polymorphisms in the ADH and ALDH2 enzymes result in a lower risk for alcoholism. Individuals with a functional variant of the enzyme ALDH2, coded for by the *ALDH2*2* allele, have elevated levels of acetaldehyde even after drinking small amounts of alcohol. This results in flushing and other unpleasant effects that serve as natural aversive conditioning similar to that observed with the alcohol–disulfiram reaction. Alcohol intake and abuse are consequently lower in ethnic groups with these polymorphisms.

Several candidate genes, including the dopamine-2 receptor gene (*DRD2*) on chromosome 11 and the serotonin transporter gene (*HTT*), have been implicated in the etiopathogenesis of alcoholism. However, failure to replicate preliminary findings in larger study samples has characterized much of the effort to identify genetic loci underlying a predisposition to alcoholism in humans. Differences in clinical definition of the disease state and phenotypic and genetic variability among populations have contributed to the inconsistency in results. The Collaborative Study on the Genetics of Alcoholism (COGA) is a multicenter study designed to standardize clinical assessment and related methodologic considerations to facilitate the identification of loci contributing to a predisposition to alcoholism. "Hot spots"—areas that harbor genes that may be associated with this disorder—have been identified on chromosomes 1, 2,

and 7. However, even within the COGA study (primarily focused on whites and African Americans), differences in definitions of disease can result in different findings. In another study focused on a American Indian population in the Southwest, linkages were reported to chromosomes 4 and 11. These disparate observations perhaps more accurately reflect overlapping subsets of loci that contribute to the disease rather than spurious findings. Additional methodologic refinements, together with the use of large study samples comprising affected individuals and their families, will be needed to more precisely determine the genes that confer a vulnerability to alcoholism. Most of these studies focused on adults with the disease phenotype. The study of the genetic and biological basis of alcohol abuse in elderly adults remains obscure, although the principles underlying alcohol abuse in younger adults may be relevant to this disorder in older adults. More focused studies in the elderly population are needed to better characterize the underlying substrates in this age group.

Treatment of Patients With Alcohol Problems

The treatment of patients with alcohol problems can be conceptualized and divided into three phases:

1. Proper diagnosis of alcohol abuse and coexisting medical and psychiatric problems
2. Short-term management of alcohol withdrawal when necessary and concurrent management of medical and psychiatric comorbidities
3. Long-term management of alcohol abuse in order to prevent a further relapse.

Short-Term Management of Alcohol Abuse

The treatment of acute alcohol withdrawal is often best undertaken in an inpatient medical or psychiatric setting. Short-term medical treatment typically consists of the administration of intravenous fluids and nutritional supplements and the appropriate use of benzodiazepines to treat the psychological as well as the physiologic correlates. If the patient is withdrawing from alcohol, the diagnosis of an anxiety disorder or depression should be deferred until they are past the acute withdrawal phase. This practice facilitates a more reliable diagnosis of depression and anxiety, which can then be treated. Concurrent medical problems must also be attended to during the acute phase of alcohol withdrawal.

Long-Term Treatment of Alcohol Abuse

The combination of pharmacologic and psychosocial approaches has proved to be more effective than either approach in isolation. Psychosocial treatment includes supportive psychotherapy for the patient and the family and attendance at meetings sponsored by Alcoholics Anonymous or a similar organization. Involving a family member or caregiver who is closely associated with the patient often improves the chances of compliance with psychological treatment. Elderly patients are also more likely to engage successfully in group settings that are more age-appropriate and where younger, boisterous alcoholic patients are less likely to be present. Cognitive-behavioral therapy and addressing issues such as self-esteem may also improve the chances of long-term sobriety in these patients.

Pharmacologic Treatment

Alcohol craving has long been identified as a cause of chronic abuse and relapse in patients with alcohol problems. In this context, craving can be conceptualized as a neuronal state resulting from years of alcohol use that undermines free will and causes the individual to consume alcohol in spite of cognitive appreciation of its deleterious effects. Recently, craving has emerged as a target for the development and use of pharmacologic compounds that could help minimize relapse in patients being treated for alcohol abuse. Craving is believed to have a biological basis, and the opioid γ-aminobutyric acid (GABA) and the dopaminergic and glutamate systems have been implicated in this disorder.

Preclinical work suggests that the opiate system may play a role in cravings. The opiate antagonist naltrexone reduces both free alcohol consumption and consumption secondary to reinforced behavior (pressing a bar) in rats, mice, and monkeys. Based on these observations, human studies were initiated to examine the effects of this agent in reducing relapse in alcohol-dependent individuals. Evidence now indicates that naltrexone reduces the risk of relapse and also promotes abstinence. Preliminary observations also suggest that its effects are mediated by reducing craving, although more work is needed to confirm the precise mechanism of action. The main side effects of naltrexone are nausea, abdominal pain, and headache. The standard starting dose is 25 to 50 mg/d, which can be gradually increased up to 300 mg/d. Although most of the published studies have examined the short-term effects (after 12 weeks of treatment) of naltrexone in humans, the optimal duration of treatment has not been determined.

Acamprosate

Acamprosate (calcium homotaurinate) is a derivative of the naturally occurring amino acid taurine and blocks alcohol consumption in animals. Acamprosate appears to modulate glutaminergic transmission, which is believed to be involved in mediating the chronic effects of alcohol and substance abuse sensitization. Acamprosate also reduced free alcohol consumption and alcohol relapse in rodent models. Clinical studies demonstrate that it reduces time to first drink and number of days of abstinence in humans when compared with a placebo. The reduction of craving has been suggested as the likely mechanism of action, although this remains unconfirmed. The relative efficacy of acamprosate in structured psychosocial interventions such as cognitive-behavioral therapy is unknown. Although most trials indicate that the impact of acamprosate on time to first drink is evident in the first 3 months of the trial, the optimal duration of treatment in general clinical settings is yet to be established.

Disulfiram

Disulfiram has been used in the management of alcoholism for several decades. It is based on the principle of aversive conditioning and blocks the enzyme ADH, thereby leading to the accumulation of acetaldehyde following alcohol ingestion. This leads to flushing, nausea, vomiting, and autonomic changes that are relatively unpleasant to the drinker. It does not reduce craving and requires a high degree of motivation. An acamprosate-disulfiram combination has been shown to be more effective in reducing relapse than either drug alone.

Advantages of Moderate Social Drinking

The use of a small amount of alcohol has been advocated as a safe and sometimes desirable social adjuvant in elderly individuals. This assumption forms the basis of the "happy hour," which has become commonplace in some elderly residential settings. Alcohol is often thought of as an appetite stimulant and is sometimes inappropriately used to facilitate sleep in elderly patients. Reports from France and elsewhere suggest that moderate amounts of wine drinking may increase cognitive performance in individuals who abstain from alcohol. There have also been reports suggesting that moderate alcohol use may be associated with lower mortality and morbidity from coronary artery disease when abstainers are compared with heavy alcohol users. It has been suggested that alcohol elevates the level of high-density-lipoprotein (HDL) cholesterol, including a subfraction HDL3 with antiatherogenic activity, although apparently it does not work on the most elevated antiatherogenic subfraction HDL2. Alcohol may also reduce platelet aggregation and could potentially have other anticoagulant effects that may explain the epidemiologic findings. However, the potential benefits of mild to moderate alcohol use should be carefully weighed against the other negative effects of alcohol.

Benzodiazepine Abuse in the Elderly Population

Benzodiazepines are among the most widely prescribed drugs in the United States, and elderly adults are given a disproportionate number of drug prescriptions by general internists, primary care providers, and other specialists. Older people rarely abuse benzodiazepines for their psychoactive effects, and the illicit use of these drugs is seldom seen in the elderly population. Patterns of dependence secondary to prolonged prescription drug use are more commonly encountered in this group. Benzodiazepines are often prescribed for older people for treatment of insomnia and anxiety, although a scientific basis has not been established for their long-term use in treating generalized anxiety disorder. The other primary indication for the use of benzodiazepines is panic disorder, which occurs relatively infrequently in elderly people. Complaints of insomnia increase with age, and benzodiazepines are a partial solution, at best, to the problems of compromised sleep in elderly individuals. The primary limitation of benzodiazepine use in the management of sleep disturbances in older people is that their efficacy diminishes after several weeks of treatment. Many patients continue to experience chronic anxiety and depression despite taking benzodiazepines, and few seek assistance from mental health professionals. Most elderly benzodiazepine abusers obtain drugs from their primary care physicians. Benzodiazepine abuse is also high in caregivers of patients with dementia.

Compared with nonelderly adults, elderly individuals clear benzodiazepines more slowly, and repeated doses produce higher steady-state concentrations. Psychomotor slowing and sedation occur with lower doses, and comparable doses result in higher plasma levels in elderly patients than in younger ones. Adverse effects are common in patients who take high doses of agents with a long half-life, although they are also observed in patients who use agents with short half-lives. Elderly people are particularly vulnerable to the negative effects of benzodiazepines, such as impairments in cognition, coordination, balance, and driving skills. Older people are also at risk for falls, and benzodiazepine use increases this risk.

After long-term therapeutic use of benzodiazepines, sudden discontinution of their use leads to unpleasant withdrawal effects. Abrupt discontinuation often results in rebound insomnia together with other effects such as anxiety, fatigue, tremulousness, concentration difficulties, and restlessness. Withdrawal symptoms are more likely following 12 months of benzodiazepine use. It is estimated that a high percentage (90 percent to 100 percent) of mixed-age and elderly patients who discontinue long-term benzodiazepine use experience some rebound symptoms. This effect is enhanced by abrupt withdrawal, dependence on high doses, the use of agents with short half-lives, and concurrent alcohol use. In elderly patients the effects of benzodiazepine withdrawal are sometimes overlooked and prematurely attributed to comorbid medical disorders. Although age per se does not increase the risk for withdrawal symptoms, older adults have more difficulty remaining abstinent following discontinuation of the use of benzodiazepines. Recommended strategies include a slow, gradual taper over several weeks, which may extend up to a month. Replacing a short-acting agent with one with a longer half-life to facilitate the taper and the concurrent use of other agents to minimize discomfort should also need be considered.

Use of Narcotic Analgesics and Nonprescription Drugs

The abusive use of prescription narcotics in the elderly population is not common but may be encountered clinically. Narcotics may be prescribed for a variety of painful nonmalignant conditions such as neuropathy and arthritis. Tolerance and dependence can occur without abuse, and these risks should be carefully considered when prescribing narcotics for elderly patients. These individuals are the most

frequent users of nonprescription drugs for the treatment of mild illnesses, and although expectations about the clinical efficacy of these drugs are modest, their use remains high among well-educated people with high incomes. Individuals who believe in the "naturalistic" treatment of medical disorders are more likely to seek nonprescription remedies for minor medical ailments. It is an estimated that 19 percent of elderly patients have had at least one adverse drug reaction and that the likelihood of an adverse reaction increases with the number of disorders and the number of drugs used to treat them. The additive effects of multiple prescription and nonprescription drugs render elderly patients especially vulnerable to adverse drug reactions. Further, users of nonprescription drugs often fail to read the directions and adverse warnings that accompany these medications.

Nonprescription drugs are primarily used as hypnotics and stimulants. Over-the-counter hypnotics are predominantly agents with antihistaminic and anticholinergic properties used to facilitate sleep. The use of drugs with anticholinergic properties may result in drug-induced delirium and mild cognitive signs and symptoms, and these agents may interact with other drugs with anticholinergic properties. Consequently, complaints such as urinary retention and constipation are commonly encountered in elderly patients. Sympathomimetics are often components of antihistamine compounds found in cold remedies and also pose some risk to older persons. The use of laxatives and antacids is frequent in older adults and, like vitamins and minerals, these substances are sometimes used in amounts greatly exceeding the recommended dose. In general, physicians should routinely inquire about the use of over-the-counter medications by their patients, as many elderly patients may not consider these "active medicines" with a potential for drug–drug interactions.

SUICIDE

Suicide is among the leading causes of death in the United States and accounts for approximately 30,000 deaths per year or 1.4 percent of all deaths. Elderly individuals account for a disproportionate number of suicide deaths (Fig. 114-1). Further, mood disorders are more prevalent in women than in men across the age spectrum, although successful suicide is disproportionately higher in men, especially elderly men.

Risk Factors

The biological and psychological underpinnings of suicide are complex, and it is prudent to consider the totality of the clinical circumstances associated with suicide while conceptualizing its etiologic basis and effective management strategies. Clinical and epidemiologic studies have consistently identified certain risk factors that are associated with and increase the likelihood of suicide. These include a major psychiatric disorder, increasing age, being male, loneliness, and a past history of suicide attempts. Additional correlates include substance abuse, a PD, and widowhood.

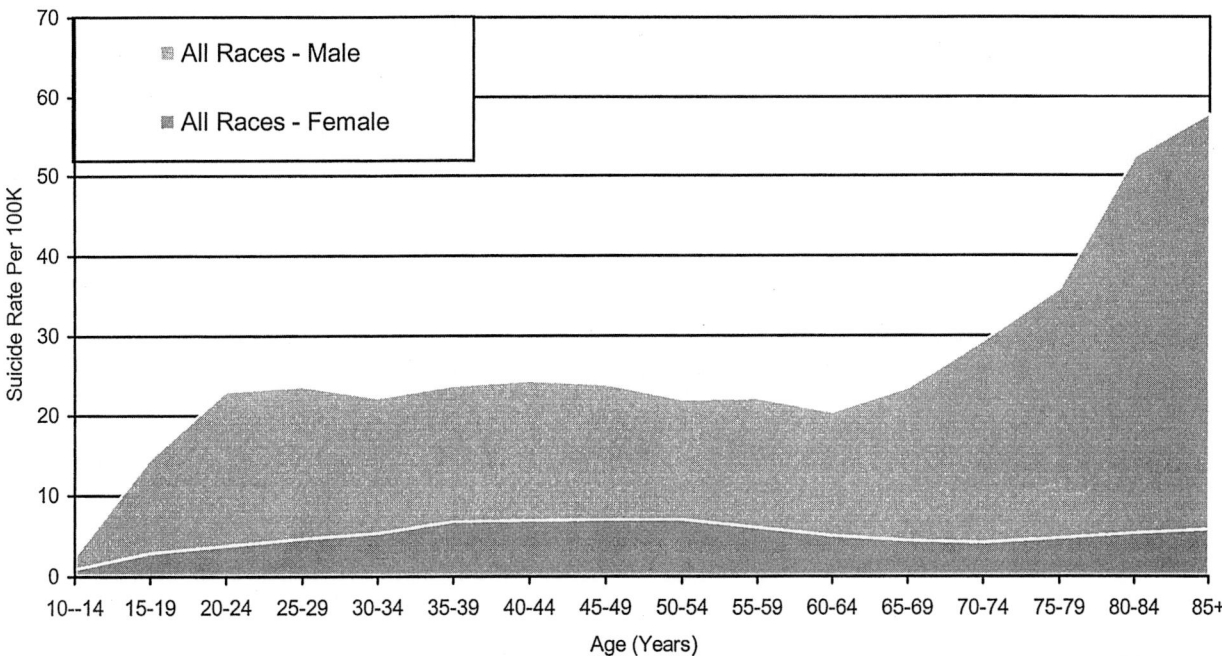

Figure 114-1   U.S. suicide rates by age and gender-1998.
Source: National Centers for Health Statistics.

The risk factors for suicide in elderly people are listed in Table 114-2.

Psychological Autopsy

The term "psychological autopsy" is applied to a series of interviews primarily designed to reconstruct the social and psychological circumstances surrounding the suicide death of a patient. This technique was originally developed in the Los Angeles medical examiner's office to augment the coroner's investigation of equivocal deaths. Since then, the psychological autopsy approach has been utilized by several research groups in order to better characterize and study the clinical correlates of patients who complete suicide. This approach has been used to examine adolescent, adult, and elderly cases of suicide. Much of the current understanding of the risk factors and psychiatric diagnoses associated with suicide has come from systematic psychological autopsy studies. Although prospective studies for identifying risk factors are optimal in most clinical situations, they

Table 114-2   Risk Factor for Suicide in Elderly People

Major depressive disorder
Male
Physical and/or somatic complaints
Social isolation
Alcohol abuse
Personality disorder

are highly inefficient in the study of rare disorders and disorders with poorly delineated risk factors, such as suicide. Consequently, we rely on retrospective gathering of information in order to describe and better appreciate the circumstances surrounding suicide.

An approach commonly used in psychological autopsies is to contact the spouse, a first-degree relative, or the caregiver of a suicide victim within days or weeks following the suicide. The initial contact via letter and/or telephone is followed by a detailed psychological and/or psychosocial interview using validated instruments and established diagnostic criteria. Often, a consensus diagnosis is obtained after family members are interviewed by trained clinical personnel. Data from medical charts and physician interviews is often used to supplement that obtained from caregivers. Information from these diverse sources is then integrated in order to obtain a holistic picture of the patient's psychological and medical status around the time of suicide. The psychological autopsy approach has a few intrinsic methodologic limitations such as the retrospective nature of the data gathering, errors in recall, and concern about telescoping information (attributing remote events and circumstances to more recent time frames). Despite these limitations, this approach remains a fairly reliable, widely used method in suicide research.

Limitations of Official Suicide Statistics

The diagnosis of suicide is typically based on the final verdict of suicide issued by the office of the medical examiner or coroner. This verdict is generally returned only if there is unambiguous evidence that the death was self-inflicted and that the deceased intended to end their life. In most instances, the standard of proof remains relatively high before a verdict or diagnosis of suicide is issued. This leaves open the possibility that a case with an "open verdict," where the death is considered to be of undetermined origin, is actually a case of suicide where the evidence did not meet the standard required for the verdict. Studies have also found marked variability in the coroner's report on suicide even in cases where the clinical circumstances are comparable and equally suggestive. The courts and coroners' offices also exhibit a gender bias in suicide verdicts. Collectively, these observations suggest that official suicide statistics often tend to be underestimates of the true figures.

Mental Disorders in Suicide

Psychological autopsy studies, both in the United States and in Europe, indicate that about 90 percent of patients who commit suicide have received a major psychiatric diagnosis. In the elderly population, the most common diagnosis associated with suicide is unipolar major depressive disorder (MDD). In samples from the nongeriatric adult population, the combination of a mood disorder and substance abuse is commonly found in suicide victims. In adolescents and young adults, major psychotic disorders, substance abuse, and mood disorders are the three most common psychiatric disorders associated with patients who commit suicide. Reports from both the United States and Europe suggest that approximately 50 percent of patients who commit suicide have had some contact with health service personnel in the month preceding the suicide. In most cases, contact was made with an internist or a general practitioner or family doctor. Very often, elderly patients do not express any suicidal ideation to the contact in the health care network and are often seen for somatic complaints associated with medical problems. It has been consistently noted that a referral to specialized psychiatric or geropsychiatric services is relatively uncommon in these individuals. A high percentage of patients seen in these settings do not receive a psychiatric diagnosis and consequently do not obtain treatment. A subgroup of patients who receive treatment are often inadequately treated for depression.

Pain and prior suicide attempts are also more common in individuals who commit suicide. Poor physical health, that is, medical comorbidity and depression, are closely linked in elderly individuals. It is therefore not surprising that in the elderly population many suicides are associated with comorbid medical disorders. A striking association between cancer and suicide has been found in certain studies. It is noteworthy that a clinically significant mood disturbance may be the first presenting sign of an occult malignancy such as cancer of the pancreas.

Studies on attempted suicide have helped to clarify some of the salient clinical features associated with an increased risk for suicide. Suicide attempts are more lethal in the elderly population. The ratio of attempted to successful suicide in this group is 4:1 compared with ratios between 8:1 and 20:1 in the general population. Studies on suicide attempts in elderly psychiatric inpatients further corroborate the observation that unipolar MDD is a common correlate of suicide in older people. Social isolation, being

unmarried, and impaired physical health are some of the other correlates of attempted suicide in elderly persons. In this group, drug overdose is the method most frequently used in suicide attempts. Prescription drugs, benzodiazepines, analgesics, and antidepressants are commonly used. More violent attempts at suicide such as wrist and throat slashing and the use of firearms have also been reported. The similarities between the risk factors for successful and unsuccessful suicide make the study of those who attempt suicide useful in obtaining a better understanding of the clinical and biological basis of suicide. These investigations support the observation that completed suicides are often associated with more depressive illness, physical burdens, and functional limitations.

Biological Correlates of Suicide

Several studies have tried to ascertain the biological correlates and basis of suicide across age groups. Most postmortem studies are restricted to younger and middle-aged patients who commit suicide, and there is minimal information on the biological correlates of suicide in elderly people. The serotonin system has been consistently implicated in suicide, and serotonin may have a role in suicide that is relatively independent of its role in the pathophysiology of depression. Serotonin levels are also reduced in suicides of patients with a diagnosis of schizophrenia. A low level of cerebrospinal fluid hydroxyindoleacetic acid (HIAA), a metabolite of serotonin, is strongly associated with suicidal behavior, and the degree of metabolite reduction correlates with the lethality of the suicide attempt; patients who make the most lethal attempts have the lowest concentrations of HIAA in the cerebrospinal fluid. Observation of a reduced concentration of presynaptic serotonin receptor markers in the prefrontal cortex in people who successfully commit suicide further corroborates the relationship between serotonin function and suicide. The changes detected included a decrease in presynaptic serotonin transporter sites and the presence of a related serotonin nontransporter-binding site. These changes appear to be more obvious in the ventral prefrontal cortex than in the dorsolateral prefrontal region. However, an alteration in the level of serotonergic markers is not associated with a reduction in the number of neurons in the dorsal raphe nuclei, which are a principal source of serotonergic afferents to the neocortex. A preliminary report suggests that there may be more serotonergic neurons in the dorsal raphe nucleus in the brains of suicide victims when compared with those of controls. Also, postsynaptic receptors such as the serotonin receptors $5HT_{1A}$ and $5HT_{2a}$ appear to be increased in number in the prefrontal cortex of suicide victims. This may reflect a compensatory upregulation in response to reduced serotonergic activity. Levels of molecular markers for serotonin function may also be lower in the brains of suicide victims when compared with those of controls. Collectively, these data suggest that reduced serotonergic input, especially to the ventral prefrontal cortex, may be an important element in vulnerability to suicide.

Changes in noradrenergic measures have also been identified in brain tissue from suicide victims, albeit less consistently. Levels of norepinephrine appear to be lower in the brainstems of these individuals, and levels of alpha$_2$-adrenergic autoreceptors appear to be increased. This is associated with an increase in the levels of tyrosine hydroxylase, which is the rate-limiting enzyme in the biosynthesis of norepinephrine. There may also be fewer neurons in the locus ceruleus in suicide victims when compared with those in controls. These findings suggest that noradrenergic activity may be increased in these individuals. These observations are consistent with increased stress preceding a suicidal event.

Gross neuropathologic studies on brain tissue of patients who committed suicide reveal nonspecific features such as dilated ventricles and cerebral atrophy. These observations are consistent with in vivo neuroanatomic studies on patients diagnosed with mood disorders. The evidence of a stroke has been demonstrated in some postmortem studies. In a case-control study of the brain tissue of elderly patients who committed suicide, Alzheimer's disease pathology was more frequently seen in the brains of suicide victims than in those of controls. Alternative explanations such as decreased plasticity and synaptic repair and more selective regeneration of neurotransmitters have been offered as the biological basis of suicide. However, more focused morphometric and molecular studies using brain tissue from patients who have been well characterized clinically are needed to better appreciate the neurobiological basis of suicide. A combination of other biological and psychological factors such as the presence of clinical depression, hopelessness, and social isolation may determine the final outcome for such patients. Correlative studies comparing psychological autopsy findings and neurobiological findings in the same patients will further enhance our understanding of the biological basis of suicide.

Treatment

Psychological autopsies and other descriptive studies have helped to identify risk factors for suicide that have major implications for the proper identification and treatment of patients in medical and psychiatric settings. The vast majority of elderly patients with clinical depression are seen and treated by internists and primary care physicians. Therefore physician education is central to the diagnosis and treatment of patients at risk for suicide. Important risk factors occurring either in isolation or in combination should alert physicians to the possibility of or risk for suicide in these patients, which should lead to a more thorough mental status examination and an inquiry into the symptoms and signs of depression, including suicidal ideation. Case identification should be followed by a referral to appropriate experts in the field of psychiatry and geriatric psychiatry. Adequate monitoring throughout the system, together with the implementation of appropriate treatment with pharmacologic and psychotherapeutic interventions over the long term, are necessary steps in patient treatment. The Prevention of Suicide in Primary Care Elderly Collaborative Trial (PROSPECT) funded by the National Institute of Mental Health is an ongoing multicenter study designed to examine the impact of behavioral intervention

(psychotherapeutic) and pharmacological approaches to reducing suicidal ideation in primary and general medical settings. Although several high-risk indices have been consistently identified in numerous psychological autopsies of suicide, they should be conceptualized as providing a foundation on which more focused prospective studies integrating neurobiological and psychological factors can be developed. In the future, a combination of clinical and biological markers may help in the early identification of patients at increased risk for suicide. This will facilitate the implementation of effective management strategies aimed at reducing suicide in all age groups including the elderly.

SUBSYNDROMAL DEPRESSION

Depression in later life has serious health consequences, including increased mortality related to suicide and medical illness and amplification of disability associated with medical and cognitive disorders, often resulting in increased health care costs. Although major depression is the most studied, most well-defined depressive syndrome, other syndromes and subsyndromal disorders are also associated with significant functional impairment and disability. These include increased visits to physicians' offices and emergency departments, increased use of tranquilizers, suicide attempts and loss of productivity, and absenteeism. Despite their clinical importance, these clinical categories have received only scant attention in the psychiatric literature.

Current nosologic approaches in psychiatry classify mood disturbances that do not meet the threshold for MDD into several categories with subtle distinctions among them. They include dysthymic disorder (chronic minor depression), mood disorder due to a general medical condition, substance-induced mood disorder, adjustment disorder, and depressive disorder not otherwise specified. Other terms such as "subthreshold depression" and "minor depression" have also been used to characterize subgroups of patients with nonmajor depression. This exhaustive list of mood disorders does not, however, cover all categories of clinically significant depression.

The relationship of these clinically significant categories to MDD is dynamic and tends to change over time. Prospective longitudinal data from studies involving young adult patients reveal that subthreshold depression, and other forms, may be both an antecedent to and a sequela of MDD, thereby providing evidence for the validity of the spectrum concept of depression. About 20 percent of patients with a diagnosis of minor depression have a lifetime diagnosis of major depression. As many as one-third to one-half of patients with major depression do not fully recover and have residual symptoms consistent with minor depressive syndrome. Several nosologic entities can be subsumed under the rubric of nonmajor clinically significant depression, thereby complicating the overall picture both conceptually and clinically. Despite its broad impact and clinical relevance, information on the natural course, neurobiological correlates, and treatment response of nonmajor depression is fragmentary at present. Studies consistently report the undertreatment of depressed elderly patients in primary care and nursing home settings, underscoring the importance of recognizing nonmajor depression.

Prevalence

The existing clinical and semantic overlap makes any assumptions about the true prevalence of nonmajor depression difficult to ascertain precisely. In older individuals, minor and other nonmajor forms of clinical depression are more prevalent than MDD. The prevalence of clinically significant nonmajor depression in community-dwelling older people is in the 5 percent to 15 percent range, whereas MDD occurs in 1 percent to 3 percent of elderly individuals. Despite methodologic differences, there is an emerging consensus that the prevalence of minor depression changes with age: There is an increase in the third decade, a decrease in middle age, a steady increase in old age, and a very steep increase in the eighth decade. This phenomenon appears to be unrelated to the increased mortality, somatization, or increased institutionalization in depressed elderly individuals. For example, clinically significant depression affects about 10 percent to 15 percent of residents of long-term care facilities and a comparable number of patients treated in a primary care setting. In all settings, the prevalence of nonmajor depression and depression symptoms is two- to fourfold higher than that of major depression. It is estimated that 3 percent to 16 percent of medical outpatients suffer from minor depression and mood disorders that adversely impact compliance and the outcome of medical illnesses. Both major and less severe forms of depression also occur when there is vascular, degenerative insult to the brain. Although estimates vary, the prevalence of MDD and less severe forms of depression is estimated to be in the 10 percent to 40 percent range in patients with Alzheimer's disease or parkinsonism or who have suffered a stroke. About half of such patients have a subsyndromal form of depression.

Distinctive Clinical Features in Elderly Patients

The presentation of mood disorders in elderly patients differs in some important respects from that in younger patients. Elderly patients are less likely to acknowledge sadness and mood symptoms than younger patients are. They often present with somatic complaints such as fatigue, loss of energy, and other nonspecific cardiorespiratory and gastrointestinal symptoms. Persistent complaints about sleep should also alert clinicians to the possibility of depression. In addition, it is not uncommon for elderly patients to report cognitive complaints like memory impairment and poor concentration and to minimize mood symptoms, especially during the initial phase of assessment. Significant losses, such as the death of a spouse, contribute to the increased social isolation experienced by elderly people. The totality of the clinical picture should be carefully considered, as these symptoms are often attributed exclusively to medical disorders and/or to life circumstances, frequently resulting in the underrecognition of depression in late life.

Neurobiological Correlates

The neurobiological correlates of subsyndromal mood disorders have been examined using neuroimaging and cognitive probes of brain structure and/or function. Further, genetic studies also have the potential to clarify the biological status of subsyndromal disorders. Neuroimaging studies in mood disorders are largely restricted to patients with MDD. Magnetic resonance imaging (MRI) studies demonstrate that patients with late-life MDD have smaller focal brain volumes and larger high-intensity lesion volumes in the neocortical and subcortical regions when compared with controls. Focal reductions in brain volume have been identified in the prefrontal region, hippocampus, and caudate nucleus. The physiologic correlates of MDD in late life include widespread reductions in glucose metabolism and cerebral blood flow on positron emission tomography, xenon-133 inhalation, and single-photon-emission computed tomography. In MDD, glucose hypometabolism took place in the neocortical and subcortical regions. Cerebral blood flow and metabolism were reduced in the prefrontal cortical, superior temporal, and anterior parietal areas.

Our recent study demonstrated that patients with late-onset minor depression had smaller prefrontal lobe volumes when compared with age-matched nondepressed controls (Fig. 114-2). Our findings indicate that patients with minor depression present with specific neuroanatomic abnormalities comparable to those observed in patients in the major depression group but significantly different from

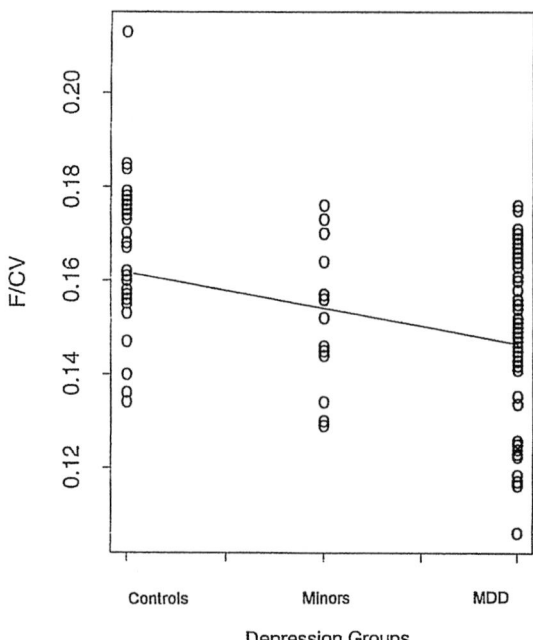

R-squared=0.23, p-val for group=0.0003

Adjusted for Age, Gender, Age*Gender
Evaluated at Age=70 for Females

Figure 114-2 A regression plot for normalized prefrontal volume in all of the three groups after age and gender corrections. F/CV, prefrontal volume/cranial volume.

those seen in the controls. Normalized prefrontal lobe volumes showed a significant linear trend with severity of depression, with volumes decreasing with illness severity. Whole-brain volumes did not differ significantly among the groups. These findings suggest common neurobiological substrates for all clinically significant forms of depression with a late onset and support the spectrum hypothesis of depression. Neuroanatomic abnormalities may represent one aspect of a broader neurobiological tendency toward mood disorders in late life.

Preliminary unpublished observations from our laboratory suggest that patients with minor depression have neuropsychological impairments between those of patients with MDD and those of controls. In a study involving patients with late-onset major and minor depression and controls, we investigated whether cognitive abilities decreased with increasing severity of depression. Our results indicate that in domains such as verbal recall, executive functioning, processing speed, maintenance of set, and working memory, patients with minor depression (operationally defined using modified DSM IV criteria) had scores between those of the MDD and control groups. This decline in cognitive performance parallels a similar trend in brain volumes demonstrated on MRI.

Polysomnographic findings in adult patients with subthreshold depression revealed shortened random eye movement (REM) latency, increased REM sleep, redistribution of REM to the first part of the night, classic diurnality, a high rate of family history of mood disorders, and a positive response to antidepressant medication and sleep deprivation. Rather than being incidental, the REM disturbances in the foregoing studies appeared consistently in the subthreshold affective group, which suggests a common neurophysiological substrate for subthreshold and melancholic depression.

One study examined first-degree relatives of probands with a diagnosis of minor depression, major depression, dysthymia, and "double depression" in adults. When morbidity risks were calculated for the first-degree relatives using the maximum likelihood approach, they showed comparable risks for depression in first-degree relatives of probands with MDD, minor depression, and dysthymia. It was concluded that from a genetic perspective major depression, recurrent depression, minor depression, and double depression are closely linked. Some of the studies elucidating the biological basis of subsyndromal depression involved nonelderly study samples, and collectively they appear somewhat fragmentary. However, despite their preliminary nature, they suggest that there may be a biological basis for most, if not all, clinically significant nonmajor disorders of mood in adult and elderly populations.

Management

Both pharmacotherapy and structured psychotherapy have been used to treat subsyndromal depression. Several ongoing collaborative trials are addressing the effectiveness of pharmacologic and nonpharmacologic treatment of depression in primary care settings. Two current collaborative trials include PROSPECT, supported by the NIMH, and the

Improving Mood: Promoting Access to Collaborative Treatment for Late Life Depression (IMPACT) study supported by the Hartford Foundation, both of which are evaluating the effectiveness of models in the practices of nurse health specialists. The PROSPECT study was designed to evaluate the extent to which intervention targeting depression in older primary care patients could reduce risk factors for suicide, including suicidal ideation, hopelessness, and depression.

Preliminary studies indicate that both antidepressants and structured psychotherapy may be effective in elderly patients with minor depression. The selective serotonin reuptake inhibitor Paroxetine has been shown to be more expeditious than therapy in the treatment of subsyndromal depression in the elderly population. As the multicenter treatment trials are completed, more definitive data will become available on the relative efficacy of the various therapies for nonmajor depression in elderly patients.

In summary, the collective evidence indicates that subsyndromal forms of depression in adults and elderly persons have striking clinical correlates and sequelae. They overlap clinically with and are phenomenologically related to MDD. The emerging evidence also suggests that major and subsyndromal forms of depression may have a common biological basis. Additional research will further clarify the precise neurobiological links between these groups of disorders. Management strategies must be tailored to assist in the early identification of and ongoing treatment of patients with these disorders.

REFERENCES

Abrams RC et al: Personality disorder correlates of late and early onset depression. *J Am Geriatr Soc* 42:727, 1994.

Abrams RC, Horowitz SV: Personality disorders after age 50: A meta-analysis. *J Personal Disord* 10:271, 1996.

Adams WL et al: Alcohol abuse in elderly emergency department patients. *J Am Geriatr Soc* 40:1236, 1992.

Adams WL et al: Alcohol intake in the healthy elderly: Changes with age in a cross-sectional and longitudinal study. *J Am Geriatr Soc* 38:211, 1990.

Adams WL et al: Alcohol-related hospitalizations of elderly people: Prevalence and geographic variation in the United States. *JAMA* 270:1222, 1993. [See erratum in *JAMA* 270(17):2055, 1993.]

American Psychiatric Association: *Diagnostic and Statistical Manual of Mental Disorders*, 4th ed. Washington DC, American Psychiatric Association, 1994.

Anton RF: Pharmacologic approaches to the management of alcoholism. *J Clin Psychiatry* 62(suppl 20):11, 2001.

Atkinson RM: Aging and alcohol use disorders: Diagnostic issues in the elderly. *Int Psychogeriatr* 2:55, 1990.

Atkinson RM: Alcoholism in the elderly population. *Mayo Clin Proc* 63:825, 1988.

Beekman AT et al: Consequences of major and minor depression in later life: A study of disability, well-being, and service utilization. *Psychol Med* 27:1397, 1997.

Blazer D, Williams CD: Epidemiology of dysphoria and depression in an elderly population. *Am J Psychiatry* 137:439, 1980.

Blow FC et al: Age-related psychiatric comorbidities and level of functioning in alcoholic veterans seeking outpatient treatment. *Hosp Community Psychiatry* 43:990, 1992.

Brent DA: The psychological autopsy: Methodological considerations for the study of adolescent suicide. *Suicide Life Threat Behav* 19:43, 1989.

Bruce ML, Pearson JL: Designing an intervention to prevent suicide: PROSPECT (Prevention of Suicide in Primary Care Elderly Collaborative Trial). *Dialog Clin Neurosci* 1:100, 1999.

Cattell H, Jolley DJ: One hundred cases of suicide in elderly people. *Br J Psychiatry* 166:451, 1995.

Comings DE et al: A multivariate analysis of 59 candidate genes in personality traits: The temperament and character inventory. *Clin Genet* 58:375, 2000.

Conwell Y et al: Completed suicide among older patients in primary care practices: A controlled study. *J Am Geriatr Soc* 48:23, 2000.

Conwell Y et al: Relationships of age and axis I diagnoses in victims of completed suicide: A psychological autopsy study. *Am J Psychiatry* 153:1001, 1996.

Davidson DM: Cardiovascular effects of alcohol. *West J Med* 151:430, 1989.

Davidson RJ: Toward a biology of personality and emotion. *Ann NY Acad Sci* 935:191, 2001.

Delafuente JC et al: Drug use among functionally active, aged, ambulatory people. *Ann Pharmacother* 26:179, 1992.

Draper B: Attempted suicide in old age. *Int J Geriatr Psychiatry* 11:577, 1996.

Ekelund J et al: Association between novelty seeking and the type 4 dopamine receptor gene in a large Finnish cohort sample. *Am J Psychiatry* 156:1453, 1999.

Ewing JA: Detecting alcoholism. The CAGE questionnaire. *JAMA* 252:1905, 1984.

Fava M et al: Patterns of personality disorder comorbidity in early-onset versus late-onset major depression. *Am J Psychiatry* 153:1308, 1996.

Fawcett J et al: Assessing and treating the patient at risk for suicide. *Psychiatric Ann* 23:244, 1993.

Fink A et al: Alcohol-related problems in older persons: Determinants, consequences, and screening. *Arch Intern Med* 156:1150, 1996.

Fogel BS, Sadavoy J: Somatoform and personality disorders, in Sadavoy J et al (eds): *Comprehensive Review of Geriatric Psychiatry—II,* 2nd ed. Washington, DC, American Psychiatric Press, 1996, p 637.

Foroud T, Li TK: Genetics of alcoholism: A review of recent studies in human and animal models. *Am J Addict* 8:261, 1999.

Ganzini L, Atkinson RM: Substance abuse, in Sadavoy J et al (eds): *Comprehensive Review Of Geriatric Psychiatry—II,* 2nd ed. Washington, DC, American Psychiatric Press, 1996.

Harwood DM et al : Suicide in older people: Mode of death, demographic factors, and medical contact before death. *Int J Geriatr Psychiatry* 15:736, 2000.

Heath AC et al: Genetic and environmental contributions to alcohol dependence risk in a national twin sample: Consistency of findings in women and men. *Psychol Med* 27:1381, 1997.

Heikkinen ME, Lonnqvist JK: Recent life events in elderly suicide: A nationwide study in Finland. *Int Psychogeriatr* 7:287, 1995.

Henriksson MM et al: Mental disorders in elderly suicide. *Int Psychogeriatr* 7:275, 1995.

Higgins JP et al: Alcohol, the elderly, and motor vehicle crashes. *Am J Emerg Med* 14:265, 1996.

Judd LL et al: A prospective 12-year study of subsyndromal and syndromal depressive symptoms in unipolar major depressive disorder. *Arch Gen Psychiatry* 55:694, 1998.

Kales A et al: Rebound insomnia: A potential hazard following withdrawal of certain benzodiazepines. *JAMA* 241:1692, 1979.

Koob GF et al: Neurocircuitry targets in ethanol reward and dependence. *Alcohol Clin Exp Res* 22:3, 1998.

Kumar A et al: Late-onset minor and major depression: Early evidence for common neuroanatomical substrates detected by using MRI. *Proc Natl Acad Sci USA* 95:7654, 1998.

Kumar A et al: Regional cerebral glucose metabolism in late-life depression and Alzheimer disease: A preliminary positron emission tomography study. *Proc Natl Acad Sci USA* 90:7019, 1993.

Kumar A, Cummings J: Depression in neurodegenerative disorders and related conditions, in Gotheir S, Cummings J (eds): *Alzheimer's Disease and Related Conditions.* London, Martin Dunitz, 2001.

Kunik ME et al: Personality disorders in elderly inpatients with major depression. *Am J of Geriatr Psychiatry* 1:38, 1993.

Lavretsky H, Kumar A: Nonmajor clinically significant depression: Old concepts, new insights. *Psychiatr Serv* 54:297, 2003.

Mann JJ: The neurobiology of suicide. *Nat Med* 4:25, 1998.

O'Donnell I, Farmer R: The limitations of official suicide statistics. *Br J Psychiatry* 166:458, 1995.

O'Malley SS et al: Naltrexone and coping skills therapy for alcohol dependence: A controlled study. *Arch Gen Psychiatry* 49:881, 1992.

Ozdemir V et al: Pharmacokinetic changes in the elderly: Do they contribute to drug abuse and dependence? *Clin Pharmacokinet* 31:372, 1996.

Prigerson HG et al: Older adult patients with both psychiatric and substance abuse disorders: Prevalence and health service use. *Psychiatr Q* 72:1, 2001.

Ray WA et al: Benzodiazepines of long and short elimination half-life and the risk of hip fracture. *JAMA* 262:3303, 1989.

Reich T et al: Genome-wide search for genes affecting the risk for alcohol dependence. *Am J Med Genet* 81:207, 1998.

Rickels K et al: Long-term benzodiazepine users 3 years after participation in a discontinuation program. *Am J Psychiatry* 148:757, 1991.

Rickels K et al: Long-term therapeutic use of benzodiazepines. I. Effects of abrupt discontinuation. *Arch Gen Psychiatry* 47:899, 1990. [See erratum in *Arch Gen Psychiatry* 48(1):51, 1991.]

Rubio A et al: Suicide and Alzheimer's pathology in the elderly: A case-control study. *Biol Psychiatry* 49:137, 2001.

Schneider LS et al: Personality in recovered depressed elderly. *Int Psychogeriatr* 4:177, 1992.

Silk KR: Borderline personality disorder: Overview of biologic factors. *Psychiatr Clin North Am* 23:61, 2000.

Torgersen S et al: A twin study of personality disorders. *Comp Psychiatry* 41:416, 2000.

Tune L et al: Anticholinergic effects of drugs commonly prescribed for the elderly: Potential means for assessing risk of delirium. *Am J Psychiatry* 149:1393, 1992.

Underwood MD et al: Morphometry of the dorsal raphe nucleus serotonergic neurons in suicide victims. *Biol Psychiatry* 46:473, 1999.

Volpicelli JR et al: Naltrexone and alcohol dependence: Role of subject compliance. *Arch Gen Psychiatry* 54:737, 1997.

Management of Agitation in Dementia

BALU KALAYAM

"The first noticeable symptom of illness was suspiciousness of her husband ... believing that people were out to murder her ... she screams that her doctor wants to cut her open; at times, she seems to have auditory hallucinations."

Alois Alzheimer (1907)

Those were descriptions recorded, in 1907, of behavior of a patient with Alzheimer's disease by Dr. Alois Alzheimer. Behavioral changes are common in patients with dementia and often present as emotional distress, and as anxiety and agitation. The consensus statement of The International Psychogeriatric Association meeting of 1996 notes that although cognitive disturbance is the hallmark feature of dementia, a constellation of symptoms commonly called behavioral symptoms are important features of the illness. They note that symptoms of disturbed perception, thought content, mood, and behavior are frequent occurrences in patients with dementia. Clinically, this may present in a range of behavior from nervousness; motor restlessness; frequent verbalizations that are often disruptive; physical restlessness, including kicking, biting, scratching, and hitting that occur during cares or otherwise; and wandering; to irrational beliefs and misperceptions. Commonly, and sometimes collectively, this behavior is often referred to as agitation. The agitation may be short-lived, repetitious, or protracted. When very mild, the agitation is sometimes viewed by the patient's family or caregivers as a change in their personality. The person may act in ways that are uncharacteristic or inappropriate for him or her, such as fidgeting, stubbornness, hostility, impatience, or poor tolerance. When more severe, the agitation is often disruptive or even dangerous and may force the caregiver to supervise or reassure the patient constantly.

PREVALENCE

Agitation requiring professional intervention is uncommon in older adults free of psychiatric or neurologic disease. Agitation and physical aggression are noted in approximately one-fourth of all patients with dementia, as reported by Lyketsos et al. An increase in prevalence of these symptoms is also noted with increase in the severity of dementia. In a study of the elderly population living in the community, agitation and physical aggression were noted 8.5 times more often in demented than in nondemented elderly residents; additionally, delusions were noted 8 times more often and hallucinations were noted 23 times more often in demented than in nondemented elderly residents. Of the 329 patients subjects diagnosed with dementia in the study, agitation and physical aggression was noted in up to 24 percent, delusions in 19 percent, and hallucinations in 14 percent. Agitation was noted in 13 percent of patients with mild dementia, as compared to 24 percent of patients with moderate dementia, and to 29 percent of patients with severe dementia. The categories of dementia seen in the subjects included Alzheimer's disease, vascular dementia, and combined vascular and degenerative dementia. Differences were observed in the frequency of behavioral disturbances at different stages of illness. Significant differences occurred in the incidence of agitation/aggression (13 percent, mild dementia; 24 percent, moderate dementia; 29 percent, severe dementia) and in the incidence of aberrant motor behavior (3 percent, mild dementia; 7 percent, moderate dementia; 19 percent, severe dementia).

In an earlier analysis of 100 patients with autopsy-confirmed diagnosis of Alzheimer's disease, Jost and Grossberg noted in a retrospective analysis that symptoms of agitation including irritability, restlessness, and aggression were the most prevalent behavioral disturbance in their patients. Symptoms of agitation were noted in 81 percent of their cases, whereas 45 percent of patients exhibited psychotic symptoms, including hallucinations, paranoia, accusatory behavior, and delusions. Depressive mood change, social withdrawal, and suicidal ideation were seen in 72 percent of the patients. While the authors note psychotic symptoms both before and following clinical diagnosis of Alzheimer's disease in their sample, agitation usually followed clinical diagnosis of the disease. Depression and social withdrawal were usually observed prior to clinical diagnosis, and were often the earliest identifiable behavioral symptom, seen as early as 2.5 to 3 years prior to the diagnosis of Alzheimer's disease.

Severe agitation is frequently a reason families decide to seek hospitalization or institution-based care, and the cost of institutionalization is the largest component of expense in the care of the elderly demented patient. Behavioral symptoms that commonly trigger admission to a nursing home are seen in a large proportion of nursing home admissions. A prospective study by Rovner and colleagues found 79 of 459 consecutive admissions to nursing homes had dementia that was complicated by behavioral symptoms, including agitation, physical aggression, delusions, or depression. Agitation and psychosis in demented patients can lead to premature institutionalization. Changes in behavior are a stronger predictor of institutionalization in these patients than decline in cognitive status.

CLINICAL MANAGEMENT

General Principles

A thorough assessment of the agitated patient is essential, because these patients often have general medical and/or neuropsychiatric syndromes that may be responsible for, or in part contribute to, the agitation (Table 115-1). The correction of these factors can be associated with decrease in caregiver burden, preservation of the patient's quality of life, and reduced likelihood for relocation or premature institutionalization. It is therefore crucial to develop a systematic approach to differential diagnosis that focuses on the causes of agitation in individual patients. A host of conditions is associated with agitation (Table 115-1). Agitation often accompanies delirium, and may be secondary to acute pain or other chronic pain syndromes, or from the distress that accompanies the onset or exacerbation of a physical illness. The clinician should be particularly alert to potential drug interactions or over-the-counter medications used by the patient that may result in confusion, restlessness, or agitation. Although agitation and aggression are often the direct result of dementia, the differential diagnosis to pursue potential medical contributions should be meticulous. Attention should specifically be directed to ruling out misuse or accidental use of medications; central nervous system (CNS) toxic reactions from medications; systemic reactions from drugs, for example, electrolyte imbalance; concurrent urinary tract or upper respiratory infection; recent stroke; poor nutritional state, including dehydration; occult head trauma; and severe constipation or fecal impaction. Other possible causes to consider are thyroid dysfunction; congestive heart failure; poorly controlled diabetes; orthostatic hypotension; alcohol- or substance-induced disorder; occult long-bone fracture associated with any recent fall; the presence of common neuropsychiatric syndromes, including psychosis; mood and anxiety disorders; "sundowning"; and agitation that results from change in caregivers and routines, noise, move to new or unfamiliar surroundings, and social isolation that is especially associated with sensory deprivation resulting from poor hearing and vision.

Table 115-1 Differential Diagnosis of Agitation

Secondary to delirium
 Urinary tract infection
 Lung and respiratory tract infections
 Poorly controlled diabetes
 Congestive heart failure
 Hypoxia and chronic obstructive pulmonary disease
 Recent surgery
 Occult head trauma
 Renal insufficiency
 Anemia
 Hypoperfusion states
 Sensory impairment
 Cerebrovascular disease
 Thyroid disease

Iatrogenic states
 Drug interactions
 Anticholinergic and other drug toxicities
 Drug withdrawal states

Other physical causes
 Fecal impaction
 Urinary retention
 Pain syndromes
 Immobilization

Environmental triggers
 Relocation
 Interpersonal changes/difficulties
 Ambient noise and inadequate lighting

Psychiatric disorders
 Dementia
 Depression
 Pscychosis
 Mania
 Anxiety state
 "Sundowner's syndrome"

Patient Examination

Assessment of the agitated patient begins with proper bedside examination that consists of obtaining a focused history and examining the patient's psychiatric, cognitive, neurologic, and medical status. Most applicable to the history are recognizing changes in the patient's behavior and physical health; recent trauma, including falls; change in medications, including their doses; the addition of a new drug; change in the characteristics of physical care delivery, including location and personnel; and change in nutritional status.

Careful consideration should be given to uncover toxic effects of drugs and potential for any drug interaction that may exist in the older adult. This population is often on multiple medications that are metabolized much more slowly than in younger adults. Elderly persons are often frail. They are particularly sensitive to adverse consequences of a drug interaction that can be mistakenly identified as a new symptom or exacerbation of an underlying illness.

Laboratory assessments, including urinalysis, a complete metabolic panel, thyroid function test, vitamin B_{12} assay, urine culture, chest x-ray, electrocardiogram, and urine toxicology, can clinch the diagnoses in trying to rule out systemic diseases and metabolic changes. Other tests that are helpful include brain imaging, when applicable, and assessment of serum drug levels, particularly for patients receiving digoxin, anticonvulsants, tricyclic antidepressants, and theophylline.

Several clinically meaningful instruments are available to rate the severity of behavioral symptoms in agitated patients. Although these instruments are not homogenous in their characteristics, they can be a valuable resource to track the effects of interventions and their clinical course during progression of a disease. The commonly used instruments differ in their psychometric properties, their characterization of the patient's behavior, the stage of a dementing illness that was studied, characteristics of patient sample used during the design of the instrument, and the time frame over which behavior is examined. Other features that differentiate the instruments are the organization of behavior in domains in some instruments (e.g., psychosis, agitation), the generation of data by patient observation versus caregiver reports, and whether the behavior is recorded by its frequency of occurrence or by its severity. The more commonly used instruments include the Brief Psychiatric Rating Scale (BPRS), the Behavior Pathology in Alzheimer's Disease (BEHAVE-AD) scale, the Cohen–Mansfield Agitation Inventory (CMAI), ADAS-Noncognitive Subscale, the Behavior Rating Scale for Dementia of the Consortium to Establish a Registry for Alzheimer's Disease (CERAD-BRSD), and the Neuropsychiatric Inventory (NPI). Table 115-2 summarizes the features of these scales.

The BPRS, which was initially designed to provide a resourceful tool for rapid assessment in psychopharmacologic studies, consists of 18 items rated on a 7-point severity scale. The ratings are derived based on the clinical experience of the examiner in recognizing the different levels of symptoms. It also provides a measure of overall level of psychopathology among five factors, including depression, agitation, cognitive dysfunction, psychotic distortion, and hostility/suspiciousness. The tool is intended for use as a present-state interview.

Other instruments are also available. The BEHAVE-AD scale assesses 25 behaviors in 7 areas, namely, paranoid and delusional symptoms, hallucinations, activity disturbances, aggressiveness, diurnal rhythm disturbances, affect or mood state, anxieties and phobias. The CMAI is a nurse's rating questionnaire that can be easily used with a nurse's aide at the patient's residence or in a community facility. It consists of 29 "agitated behaviors" clustered in four factors: aggressive behavior, physically nonaggressive behavior, verbally agitated behavior, and hiding/hoarding behavior. The instrument uses a 7-point rating scale from 1 (never) to 7 (several) times per hour. The ADAS-Noncognitive Subscale assesses behavior in the areas of tearfulness, depression, concentration, uncooperativeness, delusions,

Table 115-2 Rating Scales in the Behavioral Assessment of Dementia

Brief Psychiatric Rating Scale (BPRS)
  Eighteen items are rated by an experienced clinician using a seven-point severity scale. Has been used extensively in assessment of psychopathology in treatment studies.

Behavioral Pathology in Alzheimer's Disease Scale (BEHAVE-AD)
  Twenty-five well defined behaviors are assessed in seven areas: paranoid and delusional thinking; hallucinations; activity disturbances; aggression; diurnal rhythm disturbances; affective disturbances; and anxieties and phobias.

Behavioral Rating Scale for Dementia of the Consortium to Establish a Registry for Alzheimer's disease (CERAD-BRSD)
  Administered to caregivers in the form of a standardized semistructured clinical interview to elicit information on frequency of behaviors in relevant clinical domains encompassing features of depression, psychosis, defective self-regulation, agitation/irritability, vegetative functions, apathy, aggression, and affective lability.

Cohen–Mansfield Agitation Inventory (CMAI)
  A nursing questionnaire rating 29 "agitated behaviours" that uses a 7-point frequency scale ranging from 1 (never) to 7 (several times per hour). The items are organized in four factors (aggressive behavior, physically nonaggressive behavior, verbally agitated behavior, and hiding/hoarding behavior).

ADAS Noncognitive Subscale
  Behaviors of tearfulness, depression, poor concentration, uncooperativeness, delusions, hallucinations, pacing, motor activity, tremors, and appetite are assessed on a 0 to 5 severity scale.

Neuropsychiatric Inventory (NPI)
  Assesses neuropsychiatric disturbances common in dementia, namely, delusions, hallucinations, agitation, dysphoria, anxiety, apathy, irritability, euphoria, disinhibition, aberrant motor behavior, nighttime behavior disturbances, and eating disturbances.

hallucinations, pacing, motor activity, tremors, and appetite on a 6-point severity scale. The CERAD-BRSD is an instrument that uses a semistructured interview that is administered to caregivers to elicit information on the frequency of behaviors. In its revised form the scale has 48 items that rate behavior in 8 clinically relevant domains in Alzheimer's disease: depressive features, psychotic features, defective self-regulation, irritability/agitation, vegetative features, apathy, aggression, and affective lability. The NPI addresses all of these domains plus euphoria and disinhibition. The instrument assesses behavior on the basis of frequency as well as severity.

Both pharmacologic and environmental interventions are important in managing agitation that persists following treatment of pertinent physical illnesses. Environmental intervention may alone suffice in managing cases with mild or intermittent agitation where the behavior poses minimal risks or danger for damage to property or injury to the patient or others. However, pharmacologic interventions become necessary if environmental changes are not effective, or if the agitation is severe and presents increased risks of injury to the patient or others, or damage to property.

Environmental Interventions

Environmental interventions that are recommended and proven to be useful range from patient and family education, to appropriate structural changes, and to provision of continuous supervision by a family member or aide. Family education in the management of the agitated demented patient is critical and can be offered both as direct education by the physician and other clinicians involved in the patient's care or through support groups. A predictable routine of daily cares should be established for each patient. Interventions should be implemented to (1) identify specific precipitants for agitation and develop a patient management plan; (2) reduce isolation; (3) provide orienting stimuli (clocks, radios, pictures of other family, newspapers); (4) separate noisy disruptive patients in institutional settings from quieter peers; (5) make/leave way for pacing and wandering without increasing the risk of elopement; (6) control access to doorways; (7) maintain adequate and appropriate lighting at all times; (8) provide pleasant experiences (e.g., recreational activities, ethnic foods and other culturally oriented activities, pets, stuffed animals); and (9) maintain flexibility and experiment with targeted changes of daily activities and schedule. In rare instances, physical restraints (such as Posey, Geri-chair) may be necessary, and when implemented, should be done with sensitivity, monitored carefully, and not kept in place any longer than necessary.

Pharmacologic Interventions

Severe agitation when associated with delirium may require medication, especially when the behavior disrupts medical care and poses risks to the patient and others. The treatment of agitation associated with the onset of delirium is often brief, and drugs may be tapered when the medical condition becomes stable and the behavior is improved. Conventional high-potency antipsychotic medications such as haloperidol and fluphenazine are still the drugs of choice, although newer agents, including risperidone and olanzapine, may be considered. If the agitation is associated with alcohol or benzodiazepine withdrawal, a short-acting benzodiazepine that is easily metabolized may be favored in divided doses rather than an agent with a long half-life (e.g., diazepam).

Agitation may be secondary to or associated with psychotic symptoms in demented patients. Psychotic symptoms in such instances may manifest as hallucinations or as paranoid delusions (e.g., patient accusing others of stealing their personal possessions, convictions of spousal infidelity, or believing that family members are impostors). Hallucinations are infrequent symptoms of dementia and as such should be differentiated from pseudohallucinations (e.g., the Charles Bonnet syndrome where the patient's understanding of the hallucinatory behavior is commonly preserved in conditions with visual pathology) and confabulated delusions (e.g., reports of having seen nonexistent visitors at night). In prescribing antipsychotic agents for treatment of agitation with psychosis, conventional agents are preferred for intramuscular administration and for use of an antipsychotic agent in the short-term. However, atypical antipsychotic agents (risperidone, olanzapine, quetiapine) are favored over conventional agents (e.g., haloperidol, fluphenazine) especially when used over long periods. Atypical antipsychotics have a significantly lower risk for inducing tardive dyskinesia, as well as several anticholinergic side effects, as compared to conventional neuroleptic agents. In a prospective study by Jeste et al. of elderly patients treated with risperidone versus haloperidol, tardive dyskinesia at the end of 9 months of treatment was noted to develop in 4 percent of the patients treated with risperidone, as compared to 30 percent of patients treated with haloperidol.

Depressive disorders in the elderly patient with dementia may manifest with agitation. The depressive disorder may be missed or difficult to detect because symptoms of depression often resemble those of general medical illnesses (apathy, anorexia, weight loss) or of dementia (anhedonia, flat affect). The presence of a depressed mood is often what facilitates the diagnosis, although mood may fluctuate widely over the course of a day. Proper diagnosis is facilitated when the clinician is alert to the presence of a depressed mood with associated vegetative symptoms (sleep and appetite disturbance), nonverbal cues (sad affect, irritability, frequent crying), and verbally expressed feelings of guilt, hopelessness, wishes for life to end, or passive or active suicidal thoughts. The treatment of depressive states in the elderly demented patient varies both with the severity of mood disturbance, its effect on comorbid medical illnesses, and the presence of psychotic symptoms and of suicidal preoccupation. Mild to moderate depressive symptoms are treated with antidepressant medications alone. For severe depression without psychosis the treatment of choice is an antidepressant medication, although electroconvulsive therapy may need to be considered. For more severe major depression with psychosis the treatment of choice is an antidepressant medication in combination with an antipsychotic agent, although electroconvulsive therapy may also be indicated.

"Sundowning" is a syndrome of disorientation, confusion, and agitation that often starts in the middle to late afternoon and progressively worsens through the evening into the night. Numerous explanations have been proposed to explain this syndrome including the lack of visual cues in the dark, difficulty with sensory integration, and instability of circadian rhythm. The syndrome can result in particularly dangerous behavior, such as falls while climbing out of bed and risks associated with elopement. Orienting environmental manipulations (e.g., providing familiar objects, adequate lighting, and access to radios and televisions) can be helpful. However, with more severe behavioral disturbance pharmacologic interventions are required. Medications that have potential benefit include drugs that promote sleep at night (e.g., trazodone) and those that diminish confusion (e.g., risperidone, olanzapine, and some of the high-potency antipsychotic agents such as haloperidol).

Insomnia can be a particularly distressing symptom in the elderly person that may be associated with agitation, particularly in demented patients. Although insomnia may be in part an expected consequence of aging, identifiable causes, such as distress associated with underlying medical conditions and pain, should be recognized and treated appropriately. Administration of a hypnotic medication (e.g., zolpidem, zaleplon, or lorazepam) may be helpful in the short-term, and trazodone or nefazodone may be useful in the long-term. It is best to avoid the use of benzodiazepine agents, as sleep medications especially those with a longer half-life (e.g., flurazepam), because of the increased risks of falls, confusion, and sometimes paradoxical agitation that is associated with their use.

Agitation may be a concomitant feature of an anxiety syndrome in some demented patients. The demented patient with anxiety and agitation may seek frequent reassurance and complain of feeling tense and anxious. These complaints are sometimes accompanied by somatic symptoms, including palpitation, hyperventilation, gastrointestinal distress, and increased urinary frequency and urgency. Psychological manifestations of anxiety may present as fears for the safety of loved ones, distress over making and keeping scheduled appointments and plans, discomfort with medical procedures and blood work, and the like. Treatment should include reassurance and support, and frequent attempts to educate the patient. Pharmacologic agents for *short-term* treatment may include low-dose benzodiazepine or trazodone (e.g., lorazepam used before a procedure). Both trazodone and the serotonergic reuptake inhibitors have been used for longer-term management of more persistent and severe anxiety and agitation.

Musculoskeletal pain is a common problem of the elderly person. In some patients, the pain may persist, leading to agitation despite the use of comfortable positioning and general approaches of pain management. Treatment with a selective serotonergic inhibitor agent is recommended when commonly used analgesic medications and nonsteroidal antiinflammatory agents do not relieve the pain.

A frequent behavioral complication of dementia is the expression of anger or aggression that is unprovoked and not explained by any other syndrome such as a psychosis, underlying mood disturbance, anxiety state, or physical or metabolic changes. The aggression may be mild and limited to specific situations (such as presence of a noisy roommate, or during bathing or toileting) or may be persistent. Severe aggression may be persistent or show a recurrent pattern, and can be a source of physical injury to peers and caregivers. Divalproex, serotonergic reuptake inhibitor agents, carbamazepine, risperidone, and other commonly used neuroleptics have been tried in the management of unexplained agitation and aggression with varying degrees of success. The high-potency neuroleptics, risperidone and olanzapine, are favored in the management of an acute situation.

Finally, several of the currently available cholinomimetic agents (e.g., donepezil, rivastigmine, galantamine) and newer agents such as memantine are potential resources for the management of behavioral symptoms of dementia. Extensive clinical trials using these agents show a decrease in the incidence of behavioral symptoms, as compared to placebo, in the course of course of treatment of patients with Alzheimer's disease and vascular dementia.

Several challenging situations arise during the clinical management of the agitated demented patient and several of those remain unanswered. These situations include the selection of appropriate agents as first-line treatment, managing patients who show insufficient response to treatment, deciding when to switch to a different pharmacologic agent or to combine psychotropic drugs, and how long to continue treatment or when to taper a medication when the patient is showing response. Other issues include the doses of the different medications used, their side effects, potential long-term consequences, and drug interactions. Even though these issues are not sufficiently addressed in systematic clinical studies, the author wishes to direct the reader to answers that can be found for at least some of these questions in consensus statements of researchers and clinicians involved in the care of the demented elderly patient.

REFERENCES

Alexopoulos GS et al: Pharmacotherapy of depressive disorders in older adults—A summary of the expert consensus guidelines. *J Psychiatr Pract* 7:361, 2001.

Alexopoulos GS et al: Treatment of agitation in older persons with dementia. Expert consensus guideline series. *Postgrad Med* 1998.

Alzheimer A: Uber eine eigenartige Erkraukung der Hirnrinde. *Allegmeine Zeitschrift für Psychiatrie* 64:146, 1907.

Finkel SI et al: Behavioral and psychological symptoms of dementia: A consensus statement on current knowledge and implications for research and treatment. *Am J Geriatr Psychiatry* 6:97, 1998.

Jeste DV et al: Conventional vs. newer antipsychotics in elderly patients. *Am J Geriatr Psychiatry* 7:70, 1999.

Jost BC, Grossberg GT: The evolution of psychiatric symptoms in Alzheimer's disease: A natural history. *J Am Geriatr Soc* 44:1078, 1996.

Lyketsos CG et al: Mental and behavioral disturbances in dementia: Findings from the Cache County Study on Memory in Aging. *Am J Psychiatry* 157:708, 2000.

Rovner BW et al: Psychiatric diagnosis and uncooperative behavior in nursing homes. *J Geriatr Psychiatry Neurol* 5:102, 1992.

Tariot PN, Schneider LS: Nonneuroleptic treatment of complications of dementia: Applying clinical research to practice, in Nelson JC (ed): *Geriatric Psychopharmacology.* New York, Marcel Dekker, 1998.

Winblad B et al: Severe dementia: A common condition entailing high costs at individual and societal levels. *Int J Geriatr Psychiatry* 14:911, 1999.

GERIATRIC SYNDROMES

Frailty and Failure to Thrive

LINDA P. FRIED • JEREMY WALSTON

The identification, evaluation, and treatment of frail older adults is a cornerstone of the practice of geriatric medicine. This is the case for several reasons. First, the frail elderly are generally the older adults most in need of health care, community and informal support services, and long-term care. Second, given the increasing numbers and proportion of older adults in the population, our obligation to provide care for a commensurately increasing subgroup of frail individuals is a critical clinical and public health concern. It is thought that between 10 and 25 percent of persons aged 65 years and older are "frail," with the proportions increasing dramatically with increasing age. According to the AMA *White Paper on Elderly Health* (1990), "after the age of 85, 46 percent of those living in the community fall into this group of frail elderly." Finally, and centrally, much of geriatric medicine is directed toward the care of the frail older adult because of the health risks and needs associated with being frail. Many geriatric interventions, such as geriatric assessment, are thought to be most cost-effectively targeted to the frail elderly population. This is the subset most likely to benefit from such comprehensive evaluation and preventive interventions and team-based care.

Geriatricians often state that the clinical expert can readily distinguish a frail from a nonfrail older person. Frail individuals are perceived to constitute those older adults at highest risk for a number of adverse health outcomes, including dependency, institutionalization, falls, injuries, acute illness, hospitalization, slow or blocked recovery from illness, and mortality (Fig. 116-1). Thus, a clinical "sense" of frailty exists. There is still no explicitly agreed-upon, standard clinical definition of frailty or of failure to thrive that would assist identification of this high-risk subset of the population *prior to* the onset of these adverse outcomes. However, there is a building consensus as to the clinical markers of frailty, suggesting standardized definitions. Such definitions are needed to teach geriatric medicine, to develop useful screening tools to identify the people at high risk for poor outcomes and those most likely to benefit from geriatric care, to target interventions effectively, and to further guide clinical and molecular research in the field of geriatric medicine to define underlying etiology.

This chapter considers the currently used definitions of frailty and failure to thrive, proposes a definition and framework that could organize our understanding of the physiologic characteristics of these syndromes and their possible etiologies, and reviews potential treatments and preventive strategies.

DEFINITION OF FRAILTY AND FAILURE TO THRIVE

Frailty

We suggest that frailty and failure to thrive represent a continuum of a clinical syndrome, with failure to thrive being the most extreme manifestation that is associated with a low rate of recovery and presages death. The manifestations of frailty that are most widely agreed upon in the literature are a constellation of symptoms including weight loss, weakness, fatigue, inactivity, and decreased food intake (see Fig. 116-1). In addition, signs of frailty are frequently cited as components of the syndrome; these include sarcopenia (decreased muscle mass), balance and gait abnormalities, deconditioning, and decreased bone mass (osteopenia). Each of these clinical characteristics is highly predictive of a range of adverse outcomes clinically associated with frailty, including decline in function, institutionalization, and mortality. Consistent with the definition of a syndrome, the phenotype of frailty may vary across this constellation of possible manifestations, with multiple components present, but not always the same ones from individual to individual.

Disability and Comorbidity: Are They Indicators of Frailty?

The literature has, historically, also used the term frailty as synonymous, variously, with one or more of the following characteristics: extreme old age, disability, and the presence of multiple chronic diseases (comorbidity) and/or geriatric syndromes. Each of these characteristics has been used as a measure of frailty itself. Reviewed here are the bases for such use and their limitations. First, in terms of disability, measures that have been used as indicating frailty include

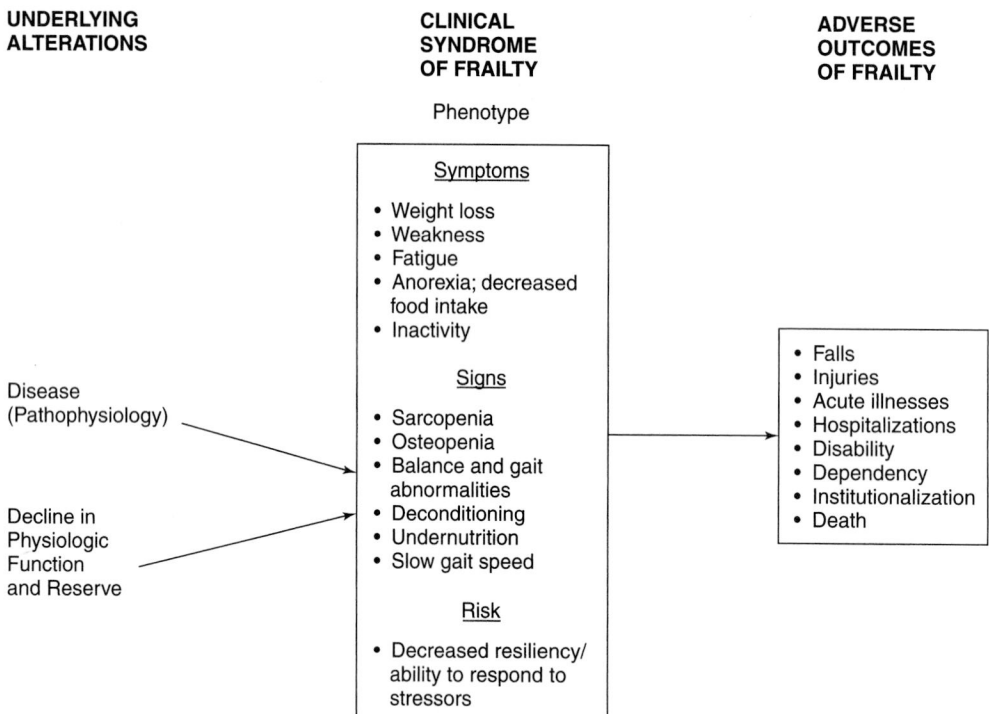

Figure 116-1 Modal pathway of frailty. The clinical phenotype of frailty which is associated with causing adverse health outcomes, and appears to result from declines in physiologic function and reserve, as well as disease precipitants.

chronic limitations or dependency in mobility and/or activities of daily living (ADLs) or instrumental activities of daily living (IADL). Such disability is highly prevalent in the older population, particularly those older than age 75 years, and it is associated with fair or poor health or declines in health, as reported by the individual. Disability is also a predictor of future risk; for example, it is associated with increased use of physician services, hospitalizations, and mortality. Thus, older adults with physical disability are a group at high risk for other adverse outcomes. A clinician is more likely to consider a patient with problems ambulating as being frail than another patient who has no such difficulty. Use of disability as an indicator of frailty can assist in the identification of those with special medical and service needs and in planning for service provision at an organizational level. However, clinical experience suggests that, while many (but not all) frail individuals are disabled, not all disabled individuals are frail. This was supported in a survey of geriatricians, in which 98 percent of respondents thought that frailty and disability were not the same. Recent evidence from a population-based study proposing a phenotype of frailty, as indicated in Figure 116-1, found that there is, in fact, overlap between those who are frail and those who are disabled; however, they are not identical (Fig. 116-2). Disability is likely an outcome of frailty or even a contributor to frailty, rather than the essence of frailty itself. Disability does not appear to be synonymous with frailty.

The presence of multiple chronic diseases (comorbidity) is often used as another marker of frailty. Not surprisingly, comorbidity is associated with increased risk of adverse outcomes, as evidenced by higher short- and long-term mortality rates and significantly increased physical

disability, compared to those without diseases. However, the presence of two or more diseases may not, in itself, identify the highest-risk groups or those most frail. For example, analysis of longitudinal follow-up of persons age 70 years and older, surveyed in the Health Interview Survey Supplement on Aging, showed rates of new confinement to bed or chair for those with two or more chronic diseases (considering arthritis, heart disease, stroke, diabetes, cancer, cataracts, and broken hip) only slightly higher than those for all persons age 70 years and older—24 versus 17 percent, respectively—were newly confined after 2 years. In contrast, 36 percent of those with physical disability as well as two or more chronic diseases were newly confined to a bed or chair after 2 years, as were 42 percent of those age 80 years and older who also had the other characteristics of disability and comorbidity. Thus, comorbidity alone does not appear to capture the group at highest risk of adverse outcomes, which is theoretically the group that would be frail. This may be because just identifying the presence of a chronic disease does not specify those with severe disease. Alternatively, other factors are contributors to frailty, beyond disease itself. Overall, the presence of comorbidity alone may also not be synonymous with frailty (see Fig. 116-2).

These population-based data are supported by conclusions from a consensus conference of geriatricians and gerontologists. This group concurred that the presence of chronic disease, in itself, is generally not sufficient to define the older adult who is frail. Rather, it was thought that other physiologic processes may be more central to the development of frailty. It is hypothesized that diseases, acute or chronic, may worsen the health and functional status of an individual who is highly vulnerable because of an

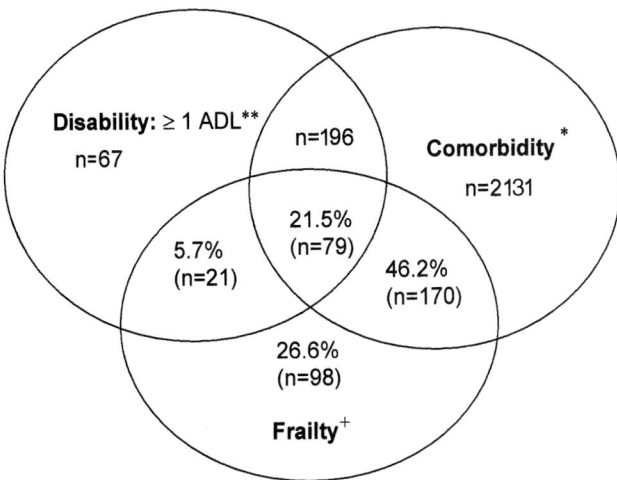

Figure 116-2 Venn diagram displaying extent of overlap of frailty with ADL disability and comorbidity (two or more diseases). Total represented: 2762 subjects who had comorbidity and/or disability and/or frailty. Number of each subgroup indicated in parentheses. + Frailty: overall, n = 368 frail subjects (both cohorts). *Comorbidity: overall, n = 2576 with 2 or more of the following 9 diseases: myocardial infarction, angina, congestive heart failure, claudication, arthritis, cancer, diabetes, hypertension, chronic obstructive pulmonary diseased. Of these, 249 were also frail. ** Disabled: overall, n = 363 with an ADL disability; of these, 100 were frail. Reprinted with permission from Fried LP et al: Frailty in older adults: Evidence for a phenotype. *J Gerontol A Biol Sci Med Sci* 56A:M146, 2001.

already-existing physiologic state of frailty. Alternatively, specific end-stage diseases may initiate a physiologic cycle of frailty in vulnerable older adults.

Proposed Definition of Frailty

The most widely agreed upon definition of frailty is that it represents a state of age-related physiologic vulnerability, resulting from impaired homeostatic reserve and a reduced capacity of the organism to withstand stress. It has been suggested that this decline in reserve occurs across multiple physiologic systems. Those central to the syndrome of

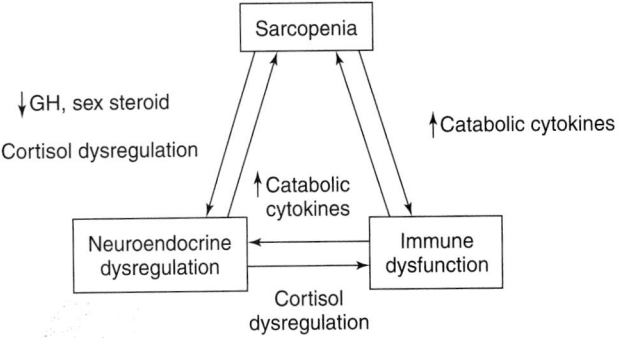

Figure 116-3 Age-related physiologic changes that are proposed as central to the syndrome of frailty. These changes underlie much of the poor response to stressors and the vulnerable state exhibited by frail individuals.

frailty appear to be neuromuscular changes resulting in sarcopenia, neuroendocrine dysregulation and immunologic dysfunction (Fig. 116-3 and Table 116-1). Declines in each of these physiologic realms or aggregate declines in multiple systems can leave the frail older adult vulnerable to many types of stressors. The nature of declines in each of these systems is discussed further in the following sections.

Age-Related Physiologic Declines

Age-related declines have been described in a number of physiologic characteristics, including creatinine clearance, forced expiratory volume, nerve conduction velocity, insulin sensitivity, muscle mass, strength, and VO_2max (maximum oxygen uptake). Such age-related declines in VO_2max are exemplified in Figure 116-4, in which data are summarized that show a progressive decline beginning in the fourth decade and then accelerating around age 70 years.

It has been suggested that within each system that declines in function with age, frailty may emerge from a particular severity of these decrements in physiologic reserve. For example, with VO_2max, it appears that declines to a threshold level may be necessary for the individual to be compromised in terms of functioning or inability to tolerate

Table 116-1 Clinical Signs and Symptoms of Age-Related Physiologic System Declines Central to the Syndrome of Frailty

Sarcopenia	Immune Dysfunction	Dysregulation Neuroendocrine
↓ Skeletal muscle mass	↑ Memory cells	↓ Growth hormone
↓ VO_2max	↓ Naïve cells	↓ Estrogen
↓ Strength and exercise tolerance	↓ IL-2	↓ Testosterone
↓ Thermoregulation	↓ IgG, IgA	Cortisol dysregulation
↓ Energy expenditure	↑ IL-6, IL-1B	↑ Sympathetic tone
↑ Insulin resistance	↓ Mitogen response	

Ig, immunoglobulin; IL, interleukin; VO_2max, maximum oxygen update.

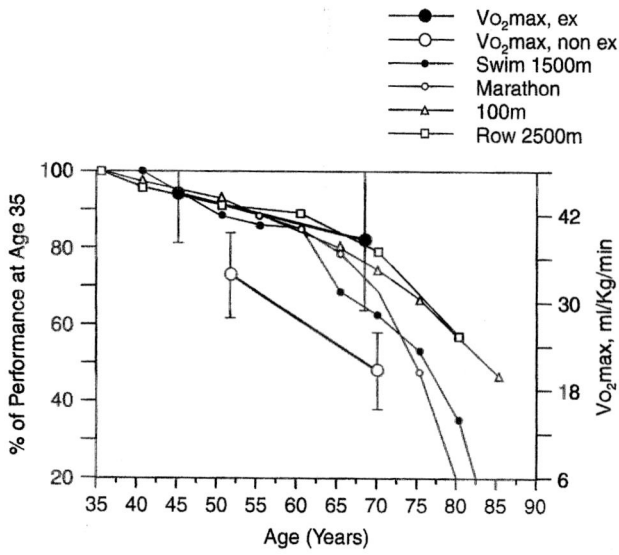

Figure 116-4   Change in exercise performance and VO₂max over time, as reported in six studies. Reprinted with permission from Bortz WM: The physics of frailty. *J Am Geriatr Soc* 41:1004, 1993.

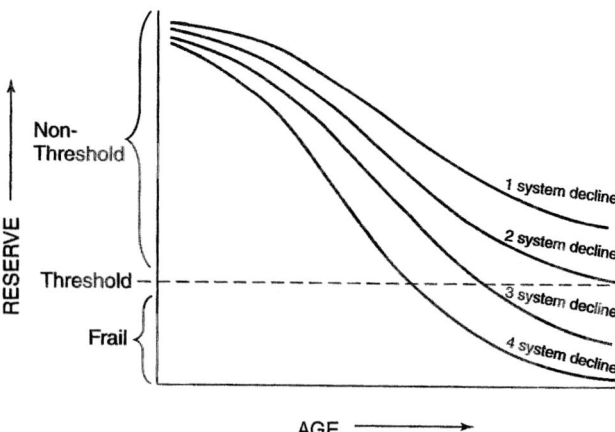

Figure 116-5 Theoretical figure showing the aggregate effect of declines in function across multiple organ systems, especially muscular, neuroendocrine and immunologic. A multiplicity of systems affected is likely to increase risk through cumulatively decreasing ability to respond to stressors and maintain homeostasis.

an acute exercise stress. These changes in different systems may occur at different rates as people age, but may result in an aggregate decreasing physiologic reserve with which the organism can respond to stressors.

The cumulative impact of declines in multiple systems may underlie what is frequently considered a hallmark of frailty: vulnerability to stressors and compromised ability to maintain homeostasis. Frailty appears, especially to become apparent in terms of physiologic ability to respond appropriately in dynamic situations, that is to stressors such as exercise, temperature extremes or acute illness, more than to declines noted in a resting state. Underlying this could be a decreased range and complexity of responsiveness that the organism is capable of. Lipsitz and Goldberger suggested that a progressive loss of complexity

in physiologic systems with aging can be demonstrated, for example, in decline in heart rate variability with aging or in the regulation of anterior pituitary hormone secretion in older adults (Table 116-2). The result of such decline in complexity may be a narrowing of regulatory control, and thus decreased effectiveness of compensatory responses under stress. Overall, the aggregate loss of reserve across systems may lead to an overall decline in the ability of the whole organism to tolerate stressors, and, thus, to the risk of adverse health outcomes associated with being frail (Fig. 116-5).

The Cycle—and Spiral—of Frailty

While these declines in reserve in multiple systems may explain the high risk for adverse outcomes that clinicians associate with frailty, it does not necessarily explain the

Table 116-2   Examples of Decreased Structural (Anatomic) and Functional (Physiologic) "Complexity" in Advanced Age

	Measure of Complexity	Age Effect
Anatomic structures	Branching arbor	Dendrite loss and reduced branching
Neuronal dendrites		
Bone trabeculae	Meshwork	Trabecular loss, disconnection
Physiologic systems	Dimension, entropy	Decrease
Heart rate variability		
Blood pressure variability	Dimension, entropy	Decrease
Pulsatile thyrotropin release	SD of interpulse interval	Decrease
Electroencephalographic evoked potentials	Range of frequencies evoked	Decrease
Auditory	Range of audible frequencies	High-frequency loss

SD, standard deviation.

SOURCE: Adapted from Lipsitz LA and Goldberger AL (1992).

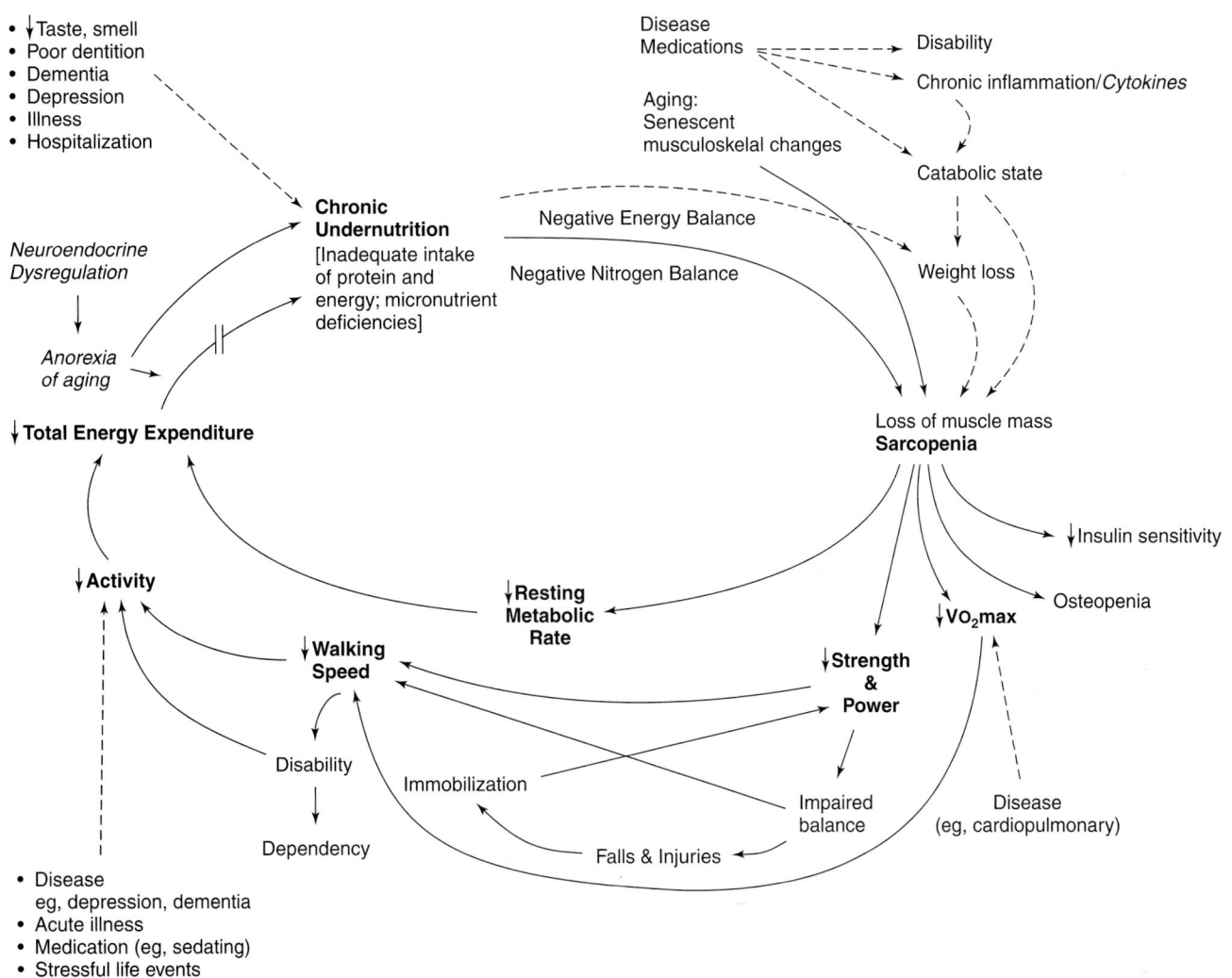

- ↓Taste, smell
- Poor dentition
- Dementia
- Depression
- Illness
- Hospitalization

Neuroendocrine
Dysregulation

Anorexia
of aging

↓ **Total Energy Expenditure**

Disease
Medications ⤏ Disability

⤏ Chronic inflammation/*Cytokines*

Aging:
Senescent
musculoskelal changes

Catabolic state

Chronic
Undernutrition
[Inadequate intake
of protein and
energy; micronutrient
deficiencies]

Negative Energy Balance

Negative Nitrogen Balance

Weight loss

Loss of muscle mass
Sarcopenia

↓Insulin sensitivity

Osteopenia

↓**Activity**

↓**Resting**
Metabolic
Rate

↓**Walking**
Speed

↓VO₂max

Disability

Immobilization

↓**Strength**
&
Power

Impaired
balance

Disease
(eg, cardiopulmonary)

Dependency

Falls & Injuries

- Disease
  eg, depression, dementia
- Acute illness
- Medication (eg, sedating)
- Stressful life events
- Falls

Figure 116-6   The cycle of frailty. Key components of frailty that appear to underlie its phenotypic manifestations in a negative cycle are chronic undernutrition; sarcopenia; declines in strength, power, and exercise tolerance; and declines in activity and total energy expenditure. Factors that could precipitate or exacerbate this core cycle are indicated with dashed lines. Factors in which a relationship is hypothesized are indicated in italics.

syndrome of weakness, weight loss, and decreased activity, as well as balance and gait abnormalities, that is also associated with frailty (see Fig. 116-1). Recent research on aging provides a basis for proposing an integration of these clinical presenting symptoms and signs as manifestations of a downward cycle of energetics that may occur as a second stage of frailty, when aggregate reserve has declined to a threshold level and, particularly, occurring in relation to sarcopenia. We suggest that underlying this clinical syndrome of frailty may be a cycle of undernutrition relative to activity level, with resulting negative nitrogen and energy balance, loss of muscle mass (sarcopenia) and bone mass (osteopenia), and further declines in strength, exercise tolerance and activity level.

Figure 116-6 portrays this vicious cycle—or spiral—of the syndrome of frailty, based on current evidence. This cycle may begin at any point shown. For example, let us start with nutritional intake. There is reasonable evidence that aging is associated with decreased ability to appropriately

modulate food intake to match with total energy expenditure, with increased likelihood of inadequate dietary intake. This anorexia of aging can be compounded by many factors that can decrease food intake, including decreased taste and smell, poor dentition, depression, dementia and illness. Energy intake lower than caloric needs because of energy expenditure can lead to a state of chronic protein–energy undernutrition or malnutrition, loss of body protein, and a negative nitrogen balance. This chronic state contributes to loss of lean body mass alone, or, with malnutrition, fat loss as well. The major component of lean body mass is skeletal muscle, and loss of muscle mass results in sarcopenia. The latter can also result from senescent changes in muscle, perhaps genetically controlled. Sarcopenia, or decreased muscle mass, then contributes to loss of strength and decline in maximal exercise tolerance (VO₂-max). The latter two changes are known to then contribute to slowed walking speed. Past a certain level of severity, they are also likely to contribute to disability in tasks requiring strength and/or exercise tolerance. Finally, sarcopenia also leads to a decrease in resting metabolic rate which, together with further declines in activity resulting from decreased strength, exercise tolerance and disability, causes a further decline in total energy expenditure. Entry at a number of other points shown in Figure 116-6 could also precipitate the cycle. Thus, a core cycle of negative energy balance is consistent with the clinical phenotype of frailty, and is suggestive of a wasting syndrome.

This negative energetics cycle can help explain the phenotype of frailty (see Fig. 116-1), unifying the relationship of weakness, weight loss, inactivity, and decreased food intake. In fact, there are scientifically well-established relationships for each sequential pair in this cycle, with the exception of the mismatch between energy expenditure and intake, for which there is supportive but not definitive data. This hypothesis requires verification. It provides an explanation as to the co-occurrence of these components of the phenotype that are cited by clinicians. It also supports findings from a recent survey of one group of geriatricians, 100 percent of who thought that frailty was most likely to be found in individuals with more than one defining characteristic.

Triggering the Cycle

Much of this cycle of frailty can be explained through intrinsic age-related changes at each point in the core cycle, leading to a number of potential initiation points (see Fig. 116-6). One major point of initiation is sarcopenia itself. It is known that fat-free mass declines by approximately 15 percent between the third and eighth decades and leads, in itself, to declines in basal metabolic rate. One study has reported declines in strength of 24 to 36 percent in men between ages 50 and 70 years, primarily as a result of selective atrophy of type II muscle fibers. Others report declines in muscle strength of 15 percent per decade in the sixth and seventh decades, and 30 percent thereafter, again especially related to declines in the number of type II muscle fibers. There is a related loss of total body potassium with age, in men occurring from ages 41 to 60 years, and in women after age 60 years.

Maximal exercise tolerance, or VO_2-max, also declines with age. The amount attributed to age per se is a decline of 0.5 percent per year from ages 25 to 65 years (see Fig. 116-3). This may accelerate thereafter, although the latter may be a result of superimposed declines in activity. Each of these changes with age, along with basal metabolic rate and the anorexia of aging, could be an initiating point in the cycle of frailty. The core components of this cycle of frailty appear related to aging and not necessarily because of disease.

The Importance of Trigger Events in Frailty and Failure to Thrive

Several authors have proposed that frailty and failure to thrive become manifest when a trigger event occurs. This event or events, such as acute illness, injury, or an adverse life event, can precipitate decline. In the presence

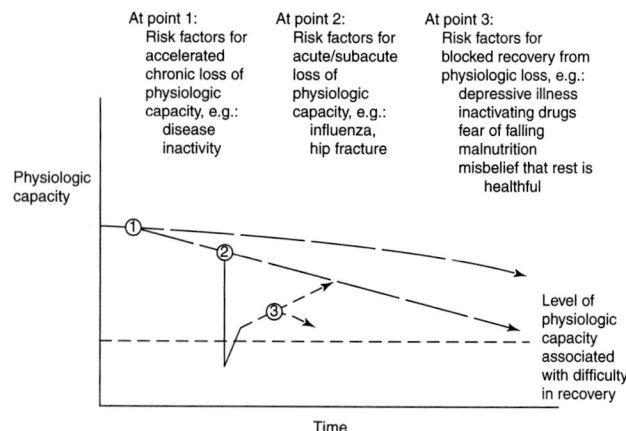

Figure 116-7 Importance of trigger events in frailty and failure to thrive: conceptual model of how risk factors precipitate frailty and of incomplete, blocked recovery after event. Reprinted with permission from Buchner DM, Wagner EH. Preventing frail health. *Clin Geriatr Med* 8:1, 1992.

of underlying loss of reserves, declines in activity level and energy or micronutrient intake because of the trigger event may precipitate the syndrome of frailty, and the individual may not be able to fully recover. Episodic negative energy balance and incomplete recovery from each trigger event may be an important pattern for progression toward frailty (Fig. 116-7) and initiation of the frailty cycle (see Fig. 116-6). There may be profound obstacles to recovery from these events, particularly related to correcting the negative energetics cycle.

Frailty, Disability, Falls, and Disease

This cycle also provides a framework for understanding the relationship between frailty and disability. It suggests a cause–effect relationship between the two, with frailty likely causing a particular aspect of disability, which results when a threshold severity of weakness and decreased exercise tolerance is crossed. These effects of frailty on physical function are, thus, largely to be found in difficulty ambulating and with other tasks requiring exercise tolerance and strength (from stair climbing and heavy housework to transferring from a bed, chair or toilet), and affected by the declines in balance and slowed walking speed associated with the frailty cycle. Thus, in this conceptual framework, physical disability is an outcome of being frail, and frailty leads to limitations in performing tasks dependent on strength and energy. This definition of frailty refers, thus, to a physiologic state that increases the risk of disability, likely occurring when a certain level of severity of frailty is reached. There are many other pathways to disability through specific diseases, which may impact on other aspects of physical function and not include the syndrome of frailty in the causal pathway.

Thus, while some types of disability can be an outcome of frailty, disability does not appear to be an integral, causal part of the cycle. Other characteristics that clinicians often associate with frailty may also be an outcome of frailty, but they are not solely a result of being frail. Falls are one example. As shown in Figure 116-6, falling is known to result from declines in strength and postural stability, and could thus result from the cycle of frailty. Speechley and Tinetti showed that falls occur in both frail and nonfrail, or vigorous, older individuals. They developed and applied a definition of frail individuals as having four or more of the following characteristics: age older than 80 years, balance and gait abnormalities, infrequent walking for exercise, decreased strength in shoulder and/or knees, lower extremity disability, depression, sedative use, and near vision loss. The "frail" group fell three times more frequently than the vigorous group (52 versus 17 percent), but falls were still common among the vigorous group. However, the percentage of falls resulting in serious injury was much higher in the vigorous group than the "frail" group (22 versus 6 percent). The circumstances of falling also differed between the two groups: the "frail" group were most likely to fall at home, while the vigorous group primarily fell in more active endeavors—away from home or on stairs. Thus, while the fact of falling may not differentiate frail from nonfrail individuals, the situations and injuries associated with falling may be important in providing insight into who is and is not frail.

Figure 116-6 suggests that frailty can result exclusively from changes of aging, and unrelated to disease. However, diseases can, potentially, impact on every point in the cycle. In some cases, they may actually initiate the aging-related cycle. One example of this could be depression leading to declines in activity and/or energy intake, which then precipitates the cycle of frailty. Some diseases could also, potentially, precipitate frailty as part of their end-stage pathophysiology. In this scenario, catabolic states, resulting, for example, from chronic inflammation or endstage congestive heart failure, could lead to sarcopenia and then precipitate the resulting cycle (see Fig. 116-6).

This cycle of negative energy balance, sarcopenia, and decreasing activity may identify many who are frail. However, these factors are not always present or clinically evident in persons clinically thought to be frail, or who, post hoc, demonstrate an inability to tolerate even minor stressors. Clinical observation suggests that some older individuals may not display this phenotype, may be active and functioning well, and yet, in the face of a stressor such as a hip fracture, display little reserve and manifest unexpected but catastrophic decline. These individuals may be in an earlier stage of the frailty cycle that is not yet clinically apparent. Those with one or two of the phenotypic characteristics are at 2.5-fold increased risk of progression to frailty (defined as three or more characteristics over 3 years) than are those with none of the characteristics, supporting the hypothesis of a subclinical stage of frailty. However, it is likely that this cycle is not entirely explanatory of frailty.

In fact, while this cycle of negative energy balance matches the clinical phenotype of frailty, it does not fully explain the vulnerability to stressors and decreased reserve that is central to the definition of frailty. Frailty is likely more complex than this cycle alone. A more complete explanation would exist if the phenotype of frailty that results from this cycle were superimposed on the less readily apparent processes that contribute to vulnerability and risk via decreases in physiologic reserve. It may even be that the declines in reserve (see Fig. 116-5) precede the development of the clinical syndrome of frailty displayed in Figures 116-1 and 116-6.

This combined process of decreased reserve and a negative energetics cycle may well, in some individuals, progress to become a downward spiral of frailty. Outcomes of this spiral could include falls and disability, which in themselves could exacerbate declines in activity and worsen the downward spiral. The literature to date also suggests that an end stage of this spiral may be manifested as "failure to thrive."

Failure to Thrive

Frailty and failure to thrive are sometimes used interchangeably. *Failure to thrive*, however, is generally thought to indicate something beyond the vulnerability for *future* events associated with frailty. It is more often used in the context of the end stage of decline, often *after* these events have occurred and when the decline may be irreversible. In addition, failure to thrive may well be a final, common end stage process of both frailty and severe chronic diseases (such as congestive heart failure, malignancy, human immunodeficiency virus [HIV], and dementia).

The term failure to thrive is drawn from pediatrics. It was initially applied to elderly nursing home residents who gradually lost weight, declined in physical and cognitive function, withdrew from social activity, and had a poor appetite. Depression is often seen as a component, as is impaired cognition. While the term is used as a clinical diagnosis, there is controversy about doing so because of concern that it reinforces pejorative and fatalistic images of aging.

The hallmark of failure to thrive is unexplained weight loss, possibly caused by malnutrition and resulting loss of fat, as well as muscle mass. Dysregulated physiologic systems, such as chronic inflammation, may also contribute (see Fig. 116-3). Thus, failure to thrive can be associated with sarcopenia and many of the resulting complications associated with frailty. It is hypothesized that failure to thrive may be a manifestation of loss of physiologic reserve. It is also reported to be a syndrome presenting with metabolic abnormalities, including hypoalbuminemia, low creatinine, acquired hypocholesterolemia and anemia of chronic disease, and pressure ulcers, along with the weight loss and sarcopenia.

The individual components associated with failure to thrive are, in themselves, predictive of mortality. For example, among people ages 45 to 74 years who participated in the First National Health and Nutrition Examination Survey (1971–1975) and who survived the next 5 years, mortality through 1987 was twice as likely in subjects who lost 15 percent or more of their maximum weight, compared to those who lost less than 5 percent. Additionally, hypoalbuminemia is associated with a two- to fourfold increased mortality risk, as compared to those with normal albumin, among adults age 71 years and older. Similarly, hypocholesterolemia is associated with increased risk of mortality.

Several reports describe series of patients with unexplained weight loss or with diagnoses of failure to thrive.

In one series of older outpatients, the incidence of unexplained weight loss was 13 percent (Wallace, 1995). However, of 15 people in this sample who subsequently died, 6 died of heart disease, 6 died of cancer, and 3 died of infection, suggesting that the unexplained weight loss may have been a result of occult disease. In a second series of inpatients admitted with a diagnosis of failure to thrive, the most common etiologies were found to be dementia, depression, delirium, drug reactions and chronic diseases (Palmer, 1990). A third study on people age 65 years and older in an intermediate-care facility who became bed bound during a 1-year period showed an incidence of 13 per 1000 (Clark et al., 1990). Forty-two percent had lost at least 5 pounds in the prior 6 months. Medical diagnoses were identified in all, and almost half died within 6 months. A fourth study looking at all patients older than age 65 years admitted with a diagnosis of failure to thrive to one hospital in a 1-year period described the presenting symptoms and signs as poor appetite (55 percent), pain control needs (43 percent), malnutrition (40 percent), falling (36 percent), and memory impairment (40 percent) (Berkman et al., 1989). The mean number of diagnoses was 6, and 21 percent had 9 or more. In this sample, 55 percent were limited in their ability to undertake rehabilitation and 57 percent in their ability to follow medical recommendations. Discharge diagnoses included cancer (20 percent), nervous and mental disorders (13 percent), respiratory disorders (9 percent), digestive disorders (6 percent), circulatory problems (5 percent) and pancreatic disease (5 percent), as well as nutritional disorders (12 percent). Sixteen percent of this group died during hospitalization. It was concluded by the authors that the diagnosis of failure to thrive "seems to be used when the elderly patient's ability to live with multisystem disease, cope with the ensuing problems, and manage his/her care are remarkably diminished and no longer responsive to medical and nonmedical interventions." Thus, clinically, the term failure to thrive is often used to represent end-stage disease(s). It may also represent the more irreversible end of the natural history of the syndrome of frailty.

A UNIFYING PHYSIOLOGIC FRAMEWORK TO UNDERSTAND THE CLINICAL SYNDROME OF FRAILTY

We suggest that the clinical presenting symptoms and signs of frailty are manifestations of an underlying, cardinal physiologic decline in reserve of multiple physiologic systems, plus a downward spiral related to energetics, and that both of these integrated processes are highly associated with aging and are not disease-specific. Three physiologic systems appear to be integral components of frailty and key to understanding the causes of the vulnerability to stressors associated with the syndrome. They are sarcopenia, or loss of lean body mass, immune dysfunction, and neuroendocrine dysregulation (see Fig. 116-3). We propose that age-related changes in these three systems are all major contributors to the syndrome of frailty. Their impact is, in part, a result of their direct effects, and in part because each influences the other two physiologic systems. In addition, decline

Table 116-3 Proposed Provocations That May Trigger or Accelerate the Syndrome of Frailty

Chronic or acute psychological stress

Disuse, low activity

Injury causing physical disability and low activity

Dietary factors including decreased micronutrients and protein calorie malnutrition

across the three systems likely has a summary physiologic effect that explains a frail individual's aggregate vulnerability to stressors and to poor clinical outcomes. In each of these physiologic realms, there are important component declines or dysregulations that leave the frail older adult vulnerable to many types of stressful events, including exertion, temperature extremes, emotion, infection, medications, and medical illnesses (Table 116-3). We first review the changes in each individual component system, and then propose an integrating framework that may be explanatory of the clinical syndrome.

Component Systems of Frailty

Sarcopenia

It is well established that sarcopenia, or the decline in muscle mass associated with aging, advances steadily starting at approximately age 35 years. This process may progress to the point where up to 50 percent of lean body mass (mostly skeletal muscle) is lost and replaced with fibrotic and/or adipose tissue. This cumulative loss of muscle mass has a profound impact on functional abilities of individuals in the oldest age groups via resulting decreased strength and exercise tolerance, weakness and fatigue, and diminished ability to perform many activities of daily living. Declines in strength are, further, risk factors for poor balance, slowed gait, and falling. It is well known that a decline in VO_2max of 0.5 to 1 percent per year starts around age 35 years (see Fig. 116-4). Part of this loss is a result of declines in physical activity with age, but much of it correlates with the loss in lean body mass seen with age. Age-related sarcopenia is, therefore, the major component in the marked decrease in exercise tolerance seen in older, frail individuals.

The loss of skeletal muscle has substantial metabolic consequences beyond the loss of strength. Skeletal muscle is a major component in energy expenditure, and loss of skeletal muscle declines results in resting metabolic rate seen with aging. The direct metabolic consequences of this lower metabolic rate are unclear. However, thermoregulation appears to be a critical component in this axis, and much of the cold and heat intolerance seen in older individuals is related to this phenomena. Finally, the gradual replacement of lean tissue with fat (and fibrous tissue) is partly responsible for the increasing insulin resistance and glucose intolerance seen in middle-age and older-age groups. As insulin is one of the major anabolic hormones, decreasing levels of insulin effectiveness at a tissue level may contribute to the generalized catabolic state that characterizes frail individuals.

The extent of sarcopenia varies between older individuals. Muscle mass maintenance is dependent on a number of regulatory and environmental factors, including exercise, medications, acute or chronic illnesses, growth hormone, other neuroendocrine factors, and genetics. Whatever the contributors to sarcopenia in a given individual, people with the greatest lean tissue loss are among the most vulnerable to falls and injuries.

Immune Dysfunction

The immune system is composed of a complex and interactive group of organs, tissues, and cells that act, in sum, to defend the host organism against pathogens and malignancies. The system must respond and adapt quickly and appropriately in order to protect the individual, while at the same time preserving normal host tissue. A large body of literature offers supportive, but sometimes conflicting, evidence that marked age-related changes occur in immune function. These changes have been observed at an organ level, a cellular level, and a molecular genetic level. It appears that the sum of these complex age-related changes make the host more vulnerable to infection. At the same time, emerging evidence supports the concept that elderly individuals, especially very old individuals, have abnormally elevated levels of catabolic cytokines that contribute to a chronic inflammatory state. This age-related immune system dysfunction appears to be most exaggerated in the frailest elderly individuals, with vulnerability to infections and a generalized inflammatory state potentially contributing to the physiologic declines of sarcopenia and neuroendocrine dysregulation and a downward spiral of frailty. A summary of the changes that may contribute to the immune dysfunction associated with frailty follows.

Increased Vulnerability to Infection: Cellular Immunity
T cells are the cornerstone of cellular immunity and provide critical sensing, processing, and messenger roles in mounting an immune response. Many subsets of T cells, characterized by surface receptors and functional roles, have been identified. Several component changes in T-cell function contribute to age-related immune dysfunction. The overall number of T cells declines in aging organisms, and the ratios of T-cell subsets change. The latter is partly a result of the proportionally greater loss of naïve T cells, the subset of cells that have not been exposed to antigens in the past. A concomitant proportional increase in T-memory cells has also been observed, and this may also influence the decreased response to newer antigens. Although there is a proportional increase in the pool of these memory cells, they appear to be less effective than memory cells of younger individuals. This likely results in the shorter duration of effectiveness of immunizations in older, as compared to younger, individuals. Animal and human studies show an age-related decrease in ability to mount T-cell proliferation in response to antigenic stimulation. A potential reason for loss of immune system responsiveness is the decline in ability of T cells to secrete interleukin-2 (IL-2), a cytokine critical in mounting hypersensitivity

responses, generation of cytotoxic cells, and stimulation of B-cell proliferation and, hence, humoral immunity.

Humoral Immunity   Humoral immunity is the component of the immune system responsible for generating specific antibodies that act to isolate and render pathogens ineffectual. The B cell is the major component of this system. It is well known that the production of antibodies declines with age. As these antibodies act as first-line defense against antigens of all kinds, lower levels of these would be expected to make the older, frail individual more vulnerable to attack and to the spread of infection. It is unclear whether these changes are caused by age-related changes in B-cell responsiveness or to decline in total number. Both of these changes may be a result of the T-cell changes characterized above and hence the lack of appropriate stimulation of humoral immunity.

The combined result of these age-related changes in humoral and cellular immunity alters the organisms' ability to respond to infectious challenge. Like most physiologic changes associated with aging, there is a large amount of individual variability that makes some more vulnerable to infection than others. We suggest that those with the syndrome of frailty would include the subset of older individuals with the most immune vulnerability. Support for this comes from a Swedish study that evaluated immune function in an ambulatory, healthy cohort ages 86 to 92 years. Three groups were identified based on T-cell proliferation capacity, T-helper–to–T-suppressor cell ratio, and total B-cell numbers. After 2 years, the group with the lowest T-cell proliferation capacity, lowest T-helper–to–T-suppressor ratio, and lowest total B-cell number had the highest mortality (Fig. 116-8).

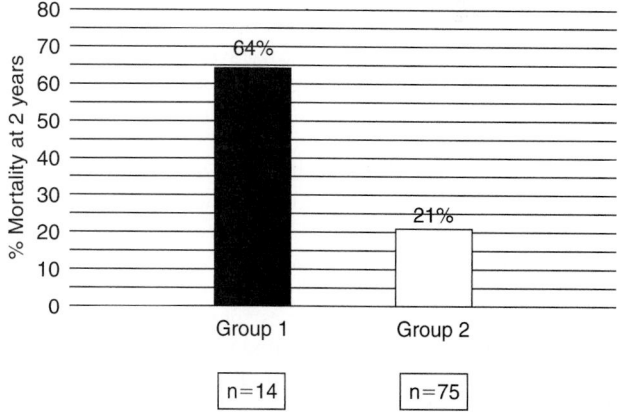

Immune Function and Mortality

Figure 116-8   Identification of most vulnerable group by immune function status: 2-year mortality data from apparently healthy Swedish individuals ages 86 to 92 years, grouped according to immune function status. Group one had significantly lower T-cell proliferation in response to antigen exposure, lower total CD4 counts, CD4/CD8 ratio, and lower CD19 (B-cells) as compared to group 2. Mortality reached 64 percent at 2 years in group 1 and 12 percent in group 2 (p = 0.0008). Adapted with permission from Ferguson F et al: Immune parameters in a longitudinal study of a very old population of Swedish people. *J Gerontol A Biol Sci Med Sci 50:B378, 1995.*

Generalized Inflammation   A number of authors have reported generalized immune system activation related to age. This may contribute to the development of the syndrome (and cycle) of frailty through pathologic influences on other physiologic systems. Specifically, the level of autoantibodies not related to identifiable autoimmune diseases increases with age. However, generalized autoimmune tissue damage that would contribute to age-related functional decline has never been identified, although studies of specific autoantibodies and their potential role in immune dysfunction continue.

A number of mediators of inflammation are elevated in older adults, and in some cases are associated with physical disability not related to specific disease states. Age-related increases in the inflammatory cytokines IL-6, IL-1B, and tumor necrosis factor (TNF)-α have been identified. Elevated IL-6 in particular correlates with a number of poor outcomes in older adults, including the development of disability and early mortality. In fact, one study has demonstrated a correlation between elevated IL-6 and a phenotype of frailty. These increased levels likely stem from declining regulatory mechanisms that allow an activated cell to continue the secretion of these potent catabolic agents well after the stimulus is over. Long-term exposure to higher levels of these agents may contribute to the cycle of frailty via catabolic influences on skeletal muscle (increased sarcopenia), and worsening neuroendocrine dysregulation via increased stimulation of the adrenocortical axis (see Fig. 116-3). We suggest that the sum of increased vulnerability to infection along with the increased inflammatory state leads to a subset of individuals with more phenotypic wasting and especially vulnerable to stressors, thus potentially contributing to the development of frailty.

Neuroendocrine Dysregulation

The neuroendocrine system in its normal state is a highly integrated and complex regulatory system that monitors environmental and other sensory input and maintains homeostatic balance via nerve and endocrine signaling to end-organ systems. This balance is critical in maintaining homeostasis for basal functioning, as well as in providing much of the dynamic signaling that allows appropriate hormonal and neuronal response to environmental changes or other stressors. It is apparent that many components of this intricate system change with age. The best known example of this change is the loss of estrogen in women at the time of menopause. This age-related phenomenon leads to alteration in several metabolic functions, including maintenance of bone and lean tissue mass. Declines in the latter lead to declining metabolic rate. Other examples of these changes with age include declines in growth hormone level, increase in sympathetic nervous system tone, and altered cortisol secretory patterns, among others (see Table 116-1).

Many of the observed neuroendocrine changes are related to a loss of the coordinating mechanisms and fine regulation of the component systems. Some investigators have related a loss of complexity with aging to the chaos theory, and have identified several physiologic systems, including neuroendocrine systems, that demonstrate this "chaos" or loss of complexity with age (see Table 116-2). There is

intriguing evidence that there is an associated loss of physiologic complexity in a number of systems with age, which may contribute to a different kind of loss of reserve, the range and accuracy of responsiveness of the system. In the neuroendocrine systems, normal responses are often pulsatile and quickly turned "on" and "off." However, the complex network of control begins to function less sensitively with advanced age, leaving neuroendocrine systems with lagging or slowed responses to normal stimuli and slow or sluggish negative feedback mechanisms. The latter can lead to slowed turning off of responses to stressors, as well as delay in initiating them in the first place. As many of the neuroendocrine pathways are complex and interrelated, the loss of complexity and decline of one system likely impacts on many others, leading to a cumulative loss of regulation across multiple systems. Given that these changes are most apparent in the oldest individuals and that the systems affected are critical in the response to stressors of all kinds, we hypothesize that this dysregulation is central to the syndrome of frailty.

Stress Response Hormones   Part of the definition of frailty involves excess vulnerability to stressors. The most important neuroendocrine responses to stress in humans are the activation of the sympathetic nervous system, with its concomitant release of epinephrine and norepinephrine and the elevation of plasma glucocorticoid levels. These comprise key physiologic responses to stressors of all kinds, including physical danger (exertion, temperature extremes, infection, inflammation), psychological distress (anxiety, depression, fear, social isolation), and pain. The events that follow the secretion of these stress hormones are many, including the well known physiologic responses of tachycardia, dilation of the airways, hyperalertness, and a short-term increase in muscular strength, all related to immediate effects of β-adrenergic receptor stimulation. The immediate effects of the glucocorticoids are less-well studied, but these include short-term elevation of glucose and lipid levels. This pathway may be a major source of energy liberation during the stress response. In a well-regulated system, these pathways are very finely tuned and function to minimize the impacts of dangerous situations and stressful encounters. However, the long-term effects of chronically or repeatedly activated stress response systems may well be deleterious, especially if the responses are prolonged.

Many studies show that baseline activity of these stress-response systems are elevated with age, that is, higher baseline sympathetic nervous system activity and tone and elevated cortisol levels. There is evidence that these responses, while beneficial in the short-term, can, in the long-term, lead to pathologic changes in this and other systems. From rodent studies, it is known that long-term exposure to cortisol leads to the loss of important regulatory elements on the hippocampus, with the loss of negative feedback and, hence, inhibition of this stress response. This, in turn, leads to higher and more active cortisol systems. The potential long-term clinical outcome of chronic overproduction of cortisol in response to stress includes suppressed immune function, increased insulin resistance and adipose tissue, and loss of lean and bone mass.

The elevation of sympathetic nervous system output with aging is well known, as demonstrated in most studies in humans and in mammals. The exact mechanism of the decline of tight regulation in this system is unknown. The end-organ response to this system also declines with age, so that the responses to the chronically elevated levels of norepinephrine and epinephrine are not as vigorous. However, there is evidence that the increased activity of the locus ceruleus (brain center for sympathetic nervous system activity) elevates corticotropin-releasing factors (CRF), which, in turn, causes an increasing level of cortisol secretion, leading to further dysregulation of the stress response. Other effects of long-term elevated sympathetic tone are less-well studied.

Growth Hormone   Growth hormone (GH) and its major messenger molecule, insulin-like growth factor-1 (IGF-1), play a critical role in the growth and development of immature organisms, and remains an important component of development and maintenance of lean body mass well into adulthood and older age. This hormone is generally released from the pituitary gland in a pulsatile fashion, and a gradual loss in this pulsatile secretion occurs with aging. Many studies have demonstrated that the loss of normal GH secretion has an impact on the maintenance of both lean body mass and bone mass, which are both components of the frailty phenotype. Supplementation of growth hormone in older men with low IGF-1 levels can result in a small (4 percent) increase in lean body mass. This does not, however, result in increases in strength or endurance over 6 months.

Estrogen and Testosterone   The finely regulated female reproductive neuroendocrine pathway changes markedly at the onset of menopause. This sudden, age-related loss of estrogen from ovarian failure and the hypothalamic dysregulation of gonadotropins has a profound effect on women, with rapid decline in bone mineral density, loss of lean body mass and increased fat mass, and increased cardiovascular risk accompanying this change. The male reproductive neuroendocrine system also undergoes age-related changes that include a gradual loss in testosterone levels and an increasing sensitivity to the negative feedback effects of testosterone on the hypothalamus. These decreased levels of sex hormones may have an effect on frailty via a direct contribution to decline in lean tissue (sarcopenia).

Dehydroepiandrosterone   The adrenal cortex secretes dehydroepiandrosterone (DHEA) at low levels until age 5 years, when it increases markedly and peaks at age 20 years. Secretion then gradually falls to low levels in old age. There are a number of suggestive, but conflicting, studies that may support a role for this hormone in the maintenance of lean body mass and appropriate immune function. In fact, a number of human and rodent trials suggest a role for this steroid in the suppression of catabolic or inflammatory cytokines (IL-6, IL-1B) and the induction of the immune stimulatory cytokine IL-2. Hence, a low level of this steroid, as part of the neuroendocrine dysregulation of old age, may contribute to the primary physiologic characteristics of frailty.

Other Metabolic Pathways   The neuroendocrine system is also the major force in the regulation of several critical homeostatic functions, including maintenance of body weight, appetite regulation, thirst centers, and thermoregulation. Recently elucidated hormones and ligands include leptin and the leptin receptor, neuropeptide Y and the neuropeptide Y5 receptor subtype in the hypothalamus. In addition, important connections between the sympathetic nervous system and these pathways have helped to define the centrality of these pathways in appetite control, body composition, and energy expenditure. To date, there has been little study of age-related changes in these pathways. However, given other neuroendocrine dysregulations, this pathway may be found to play a contributory role in the underlying physiologic changes in body composition related to frailty.

Interactions Between the Physiologic Components

The aggregate effect of these age-related changes of sarcopenia, immune dysfunction, and neuroendocrine dysregulation is likely to increase the vulnerability of the organism to stressors of all kinds, with decreased ability to adapt, compensate, or modulate (see Fig. 116-3). Each of these physiologic components of frailty has significant effects on the others, leading to or accelerating declines in other regulatory mechanisms that, in turn, may contribute to a clinical outcome of frailty that is independent of any specific disease process. For example, age-related loss of testosterone, estrogen, and dehydroepiandrosterone sulfate (DHEAS) leads to increased production of serum IL-6. Chronic elevation of IL-6 accelerates the loss of muscle mass as well as contributing to the decline in growth hormone and IGF-1. This further accelerates the loss of muscle mass. This underlying physiology can be acutely worsened by many triggering events such as disease, medication, injury, or depression, as described above.

A complex and interactive network that is only partially understood connects each of the three primary physiologic components of frailty. Several examples were listed in the discussion above of components of the physiologic system declines. In sum, these interrelated physiologic alterations contribute and accelerate the other physiologic components, thus accelerating the cycle of frailty.

Disease and the Physiology of Frailty

No discussion of frailty in older adults would be complete without addressing the interaction between physiologic alterations found in frailty and disease. Evidence that there are physiologic correlates of frailty such as elevated IL-6, increased C-reactive protein (CRP), and increased clotting factors raises the possibility that the underlying physiology of frailty is partly responsible for the exacerbation of disease states and of poor clinical outcomes experienced by many frail, older adults. For example, there is a correlation between frailty and CRP, a marker of inflammation that is driven by elevated serum IL-6. CRP is, in turn, associated with myocardial infarction, perhaps because of its role in amplifying inflammation. In addition, frailty is associated with increases in several clotting factors likely driven by

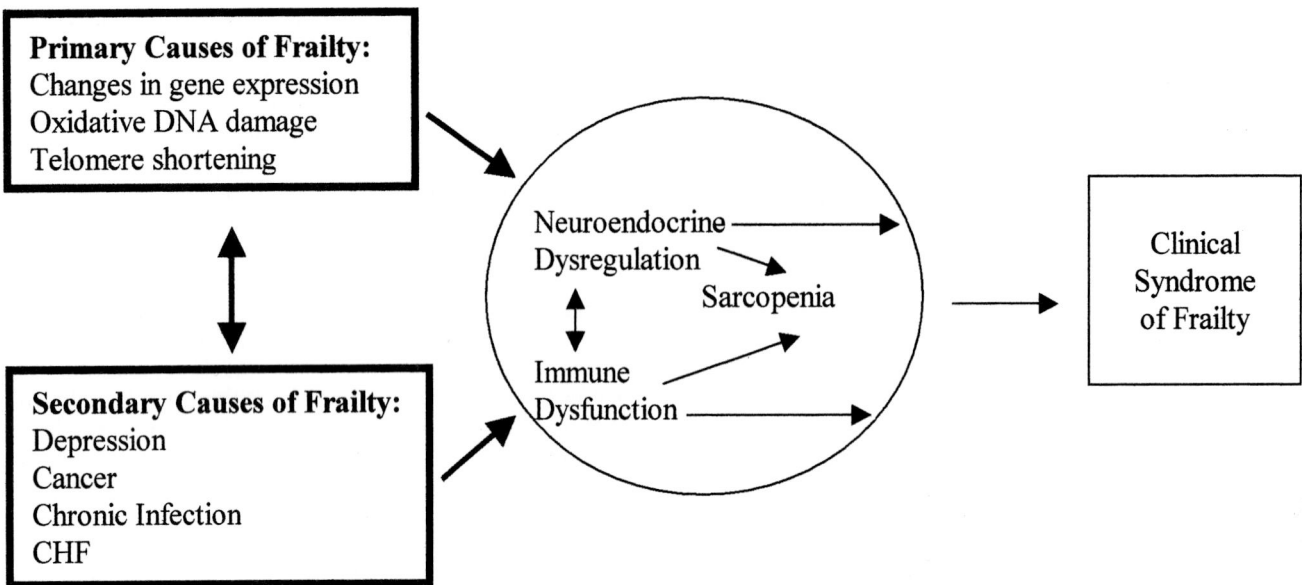

Figure 116-9 Hypothetical causal pathway of frailty focused on primary, age-related mechanisms, and secondary disease-related mechanisms. We hypothesize that both mechanisms can trigger the physiology of frailty, and that there is substantial interaction between primary and secondary mechanisms.

inflammation which, in turn, are part driven by increased CRP and IL-6. An altered clotting state may drive some disease states, such as cardiovascular and cerebrovascular disease, and may partly explain subsequent adverse clinical outcomes observed in frail, older adults.

Although evidence is emerging that the physiology of frailty may lead to many clinical consequences, it is also apparent that many specific disease states can trigger alterations in the immune system, the neuroendocrine system, and in skeletal muscle similar to those found in frailty. For example, many of the wasting symptoms observed in malignancy, congestive heart failure, depression and rheumatoid arthritis result, in part, from inflammatory cytokines and altered neuroendocrine axes. In fact, Newman et al. recently identified subclinical cardiovascular disease, as measured by arterial plaque burden, as an important correlate of frailty, suggesting a disease-based physiologic trigger for frailty in a subset of older adults. Future studies of the interaction between disease states and the physiologic changes associated with frailty will be necessary to help unravel etiologies and to develop more effective treatments for both frailty and wasting symptoms of specific disease states. Figure 116-9 displays a causal pathway for frailty that depicts two potential etiologies for frailty. The first, primary frailty, results from age-related changes described in detail below. Secondary frailty results from specific disease states. It is likely that both changes contribute to the development of frailty, likely through the same physiologic pathway described above.

Potential Molecular Mechanisms that Might Predispose to Frailty

The presence of a cycle of frailty, a spiral of decline, and underlying physiologic vulnerability caused by dysregulation and multiple systems that appears to be independent of disease and related to age, suggests that basic underlying mechanisms related to the aging process itself may be responsible for the development of this vulnerability. Despite the tremendous complexity of the study of human aging, great progress has been made over the past several years in the understanding of several molecular processes that lead to functional decline in cellular pathways. Some of these molecular processes, including oxidative genomic and mitochondrial deoxyribonucleic acid (DNA) damage, oxidative and glycation protein changes, and finite cellular reproductive capacity and cell senescence, may play a role in increasing vulnerability. Although none of these processes has been directly linked to any of the physiologic states proposed to underlie frailty, it is likely that many of these mechanisms contribute in meaningful ways to the complex molecular changes of aging and the accompanying functional decline seen in frailty. Because the underlying molecular etiology of the syndrome of frailty, much like the phenotype and physiology, is likely to be highly complex, studies to evaluate these potential mechanisms and their complex interactions will be crucial in the identification of preventive and treatment modalities for the syndrome of frailty. A summary of molecular factors that may contribute to the syndrome of frailty follows (see also Table 116-4).

Oxidative DNA Damage and Repair The generation of free radicals from oxidative phosphorylation and other cellular metabolic processes is well known to damage both genomic and mitochondrial DNA. This is especially true in the most metabolically active tissues, where the highest number of free radical products are generated. In genomic DNA, a number of cellular mechanisms normally repair the damage and allow transcriptional and cellular reproductive processes to continue unaltered. However, there is evidence that the functionality of these repair mechanisms

Table 116-4 Age-Related Molecular/Cellular Processes That May Contribute to Frailty

Cumulative oxidative damage to DNA
   Decline in repair capabilities
   Transcription abnormalities
   Unstable RNA transcripts

Mitochondrial DNA deletions/mutations
   Decline in bioenergetic molecules

Replicative senescence
   Telomere shortening

Protein alterations
   Glycation
   Oxidation

change with age, leading to a decline in mutagenesis in DNA, and hence the potential for functional decline in a number of systems.

Support for these age-related changes in DNA repair and the cumulative functional decline related to this comes from evidence as to mechanisms of several progeroid syndromes. Werner's syndrome is an autosomal recessive disorder that has been linked to the helicase gene located on chromosome 8. Individuals homozygous for a mutation in this gene develop an accelerated aging phenotype that is characterized by skin and hair changes in the teens and 'twenties, glucose intolerance, osteoporosis, cataract development, and hypogonadism in the 'twenties and 'thirties, and premature death in the 'forties. Helicase is an enzyme critical for unwinding the double-helix structure of DNA which, in turn, allows DNA reproduction and transcription. Without this enzyme, cellular reproductive processes and normal transcription cannot take place, leading to abnormalities in a wide variety of systems and early functional decline. The phenotype of individuals with Werner's syndrome is similar to that of frail individuals, suggesting some mechanistic overlap. However, some differences in clinical outcomes, such as the common development of sarcomas and development of osteoporosis in the cortical,

rather than trabecular, bones, makes it clear that this is not the only mechanism that may impact on the development of the frailty phenotype.

Additional support for cumulative DNA damage contributing to frailty comes from studies of the enzyme poly(ADP-ribose)polymerase. This enzyme is activated when DNA strands are broken. Overproduction of this enzyme leads to consumption of nicotinamide adenine dinucleotide-positive (NAD+) for replenishment of the enzyme. This, in turn, leads to depletion of adenosine triphosphate (ATP), the other major energy-supplying molecule of the cell. The large-scale activation of this enzyme in acute ischemic events has been shown to lead to the irreversible decline in the steady-state cellular levels of ATP and NAD and to cell death. However, it is not yet known whether this mechanism can cause cell death or a significant slowdown in metabolic processes on a more chronic basis. If so, this could prove to be a key pathway in the gradual breakdown of metabolic integrity, and the physiologic disarray and dysregulation seen in frailty (Fig. 116-10).

Age-Related Mitochondrial DNA Damage Mitochondrial DNA is especially vulnerable to cumulative oxidative damage generated by free radicals from oxidative phosphorylation. There are a number of reasons for this. First, the mitochondrial genome does not have mechanisms for DNA repair. Second, mitochondrial DNA is especially vulnerable to oxidative damage because mitochondria are the major source of oxidative phosphorylation and, hence, free radical production. The mitochondrial genome encodes for enzymes critical in the process of transforming glucose into a usable form of energy (ATP), which is then used in many cellular processes that maintain homeostasis. Many studies show large areas of mitochondrial DNA deletion and a number of mutations that accumulate with age. This damage could potentially affect the energy production pathways that are critical for the maintenance of most cellular and metabolic integrity. Given the marked fatigue and lack of energy that many frail individuals exhibit, and the reduced ability to respond to a variety of stimuli, this molecular pathway critical for the generation of usable energy may well play a crucial role in the development of frailty.

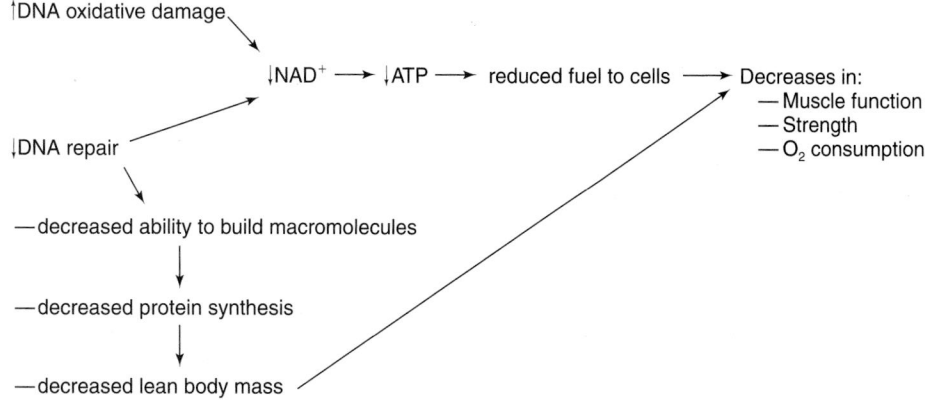

Figure 116-10 Hypothetical pathway for low energy state of frailty related to DNA repair defects and loss of bioenergetic molecules. (Adapted with permission from Grossman L: The role of DNA damage and its repair in the aging process. *Aging* (Milano) 4:252, 1992.)

Replicative Senescence Hayflick and other investigators in the 1960's found that cells in culture have a finite number of reproductive cycles and that the number of senescent cells rise exponentially with the age of the culture. In addition, it was noted that short-lived species have the lowest number of cellular reproductive cycles. Although most of these findings have been demonstrated in cell culture, one could hypothesize that, in vivo, cells critical to metabolic or homeostatic processes would eventually arrive at the senescent state. This mechanism would be consistent with the phenotype of frailty and, especially, failure to thrive, given that frail, older individuals have lost much responsive capacity and this could result from such cellular senescence.

One potential mechanism for this finite number of cell divisions and the development of cellular senescence is the loss of the telomere region of chromosomes. Telomeres are repeating DNA base pairs that are located at the ends of chromosomes which act as protective caps for the critical coding sequences further inside the chromosome. With each cellular division, chromosomal unwinding must take place and new DNA strands must be synthesized. With each unwinding, some of the telomeric DNA is lost from the most distal ends of the chromosome. Normally, the enzyme telomerase replaces these bases, effectively capping and protecting the gene coding regions located further inside the chromosomes. Telomerase is gradually lost with age and, therefore, the protective segments of DNA are gradually lost over time, exposing the coding regions of the chromosome to base pair loss. This, in turn, may lead to the loss over time of the expression of a variety of genes that may be critical in the maintenance of homeostatic processes.

Protein Modifications Proteins are vulnerable to both pre- and posttranslational modification that may affect long-term function. Free oxygen radicals and derivative molecules are known to alter amino acids in a variety of ways, many of which have functional consequences. Intracellular repair mechanisms normally correct many of these changes. However, over time, the accumulation of modified proteins may be expected to have functional consequences. For example, metal-catalyzed oxidation byproducts have been demonstrated to cause cumulative damage in critical enzyme pathways such as cytochrome P450, and nicotinamide adenine dinucleotide (reduced form) (NADH) and nicotinamide adenine dinucleotide phosphate (NADPH) oxidases. Age-related accumulations of these altered, and hence less effective, proteins may well contribute to the phenotype of frailty. Another well-studied pathway of protein alteration is glycation leading to advanced glycation end-products (AGEs). These products accumulate with age, potentially changing structure and function of critical proteins in regulatory pathways.

In summary, a number of age-related molecular processes, including cumulative oxidative genomic and mitochondrial DNA damage, oxidative and glycation protein changes, finite cellular reproductive capacity, and cell senescence may all play a role in increasing vulnerability to physiologic stressors. Most of these mechanisms have not been directly linked to changes seen in vivo. However,

changes in bioavailable energy, altered cellular reproduction and altered protein constitution may all contribute to the underlying alterations in normal physiology seen in frailty.

DIAGNOSIS AND TREATMENT

Diagnosis and therapeutic approaches can be based on our growing understanding of frailty. The first premise of evaluation is to seek to identify vulnerable, frail individuals before the occurrence of the adverse outcomes for which they are at risk. Such a clinical approach should include careful attention to identification of secondary frailty because of latent or undertreated disease that could be causing weight loss or decreased nutritional intake. A number of diseases which are responsive to therapy can cause wasting, including congestive heart failure, diabetes, thyroid diseases, tuberculosis and other chronic infections, undiagnosed cancer, and inflammatory conditions such as temporal arteritis. Psychological conditions such as depression, psychosis and grief—as well as dementia—can also present in this manner. Whether or not frailty is a result of underlying disease, focus should also be placed on prevention of related adverse outcomes, including falls and disability. Evaluation should also include screening for factors that may exacerbate vulnerability for these outcomes, such as medications, with intervention as indicated. Outpatient Comprehensive Geriatric assessment with patient-centered goal setting, family involvement, and regular follow-up by a trained health care provider helps facilitate the identification of problems in need of intervention and also ensure follow-up. It has been demonstrated to slow functional decline and reduce symptoms in frail older adults.

If other diseases are ruled out as the cause of frailty or failure to thrive, that is if it appears to be primary, a goal should be to institute supportive interventions early. These include targeting the environmental provocations that can trigger or accelerate the manifestations of frailty, especially low activity, inadequate nutrition and catabolic medications. The goal of this intervention would be prevention of loss of muscle mass and improvement in strength and energy.

Attention to maintaining strength and nutritional intake may include prescription of regular exercise, as well as nutritional supplementation if indicated. In addition, screening of frail individuals should evaluate factors such as depression that may contribute to decreased activity or food intake. There is now good evidence indicating that resistance exercise to increase strength of a frail older adult has potential from both a preventive and therapeutic point of view. In very frail nursing home patients, ages 72 to 98 years, progressive resistance exercise training over a 10-week period was shown to improve strength, gait velocity, stair-climbing power and spontaneous physical activity (Fiatarone et al., 1994). Greatest benefit from this weight-lifting exercise was seen in those who were initially weakest but did not have severe muscle atrophy. This suggests a group with more recent onset of weakness. These findings indicate benefit from exercise for even the most frail, while suggesting that improvement is greatest if declines in strength are caught earlier, rather than later. At the other end of the spectrum, primary prevention of frailty through regular strength training also has good potential. In one study of 40 postmenopausal women ages 50 to 70 years, high-intensity strength training exercises 2 days per week led to increased bone mineral density in the femoral neck and lumbar spine, plus significantly improved muscle mass, muscle strength and dynamic balance in those receiving training, compared to controls. In addition, as with the nursing home patients engaging in resistance exercise (above) the exercise group increased their energy expenditure 27 percent in activities outside of the intervention itself, compared with the controls who decreased their energy expenditure by 25 percent. Thus, resistance training appeared to improve a number of risk factors for frailty, as well as for osteoporotic fractures. Evans has also reported that high-intensity strength training appears to have highly anabolic effects in the elderly population. He reported a 10 to 15 percent decrease in nitrogen excretion at the initiation of such training, which persisted for 12 weeks. That is, progressive resistance training improved nitrogen balance. As a result, older patients performing resistance training had a lower mean protein intake requirement than did sedentary subjects. In contrast, aerobic exercise causes an increase in protein requirements. Overall, it is notable that increases in strength from high intensity strength training are substantially greater than those seen with growth hormone.

Preservation of fat-free mass and prevention of sarcopenia should help prevent the decrease in metabolic rate described in association with frailty. Maintenance of strength should facilitate maintenance of exercise tolerance, both directly and because those with improved strength appear to engage more spontaneously in other activities. In prevention of frailty, this appears to be a critical stage, both to prevent the downward cycle towards failure to thrive and to prevent disability. Otherwise, with declining exercise tolerance, activities of daily living start to take up larger proportions of VO_2max, with highly sedentary older adults requiring as much as 90 percent of their VO_2max to carry out basic self-care tasks.

The role of nutritional supplementation in treating frailty is less-well defined. In a trial of resistance exercise and nutritional supplementation in frail nursing home patients, total energy intake did not increase in those exercising (without nutritional supplementation) or in those receiving nutritional supplementation but no exercise, as compared to controls. This was the case even though this population had a marginal nutritional intake at baseline. Only with both exercise and nutritional supplement did energy intake increase; these people gained weight but not fat free mass. Additionally, Poehlman's research indicates that older men and women have to increase energy expenditure by 1000 kcal/wk to get compensatory increases in energy intake (food) and increases in resting metabolic rate.

Hormonal Therapy

A number of endocrine system changes have been noted with age. These include falling levels of estrogen, testosterone, growth hormone, and DHEA. While several of these changes are measurable, there is no clear evidence that these changes in and of themselves are diagnostic of the syndrome of frailty. However, in combination with other physiologic changes, the endocrine changes may well contribute to the syndrome of frailty. These hormones are important in the maintenance of lean body mass and bone mineral density. Several studies have looked at replacement therapies for the prevention or treatment of hormonal declines and in some cases of lean body mass decline.

The best known and accepted hormonal therapy is estrogen replacement. There is little evidence to show that it prolongs survival or increases lean body mass, but it does help maintain bone mineral density and may play a role in the prevention of cardiovascular disease and in dementia. Testosterone levels do not decline as precipitously in men as estrogen does in women at the menopause, and there appears to be a large amount of variability in levels between elderly men. While it is clear that testosterone replacement therapy in hypogonadal younger men leads to increased muscle mass, it is not clear that muscle mass increases in older men who are hypogonadal and are treated with physiologic replacement doses. In addition, supplementation is associated with increased risk for benign prostatic hypertrophy and potential stimulatory effects of the hormone on preexisting prostate cancer.

Growth hormone levels decline in older age groups. Replacement protocols have shown some efficacy in increasing lean body mass, in decreasing fat mass, and in slowing the catabolic effects of acute and chronic diseases or injuries such as hip fracture and infections. However, it is not clear that such changes due to growth hormone replacement can be sustained, and there is no evidence that supplementation improves functional status in growth hormone deficient men. In addition, the long-term risks of growth hormone replacement on tumor development remain unclear. Therefore, there is currently no clear indication for growth hormone use in relation to lean body mass loss with age.

In recent years, attention has focused on the adrenal hormone DHEA and its effects on immune function, lean body mass, fat mass, and cardiovascular disease. It is clear that DHEA falls to very low levels in old age, and those with the lowest levels appear to have the lowest level of functionality as measured by activities of daily living. Replacement trials have shown some improvement in lean body mass and decreasing fat mass, but little or no improvement in strength in younger individuals. Given the conflicting data and limited safety information on long term use of the hormone replacement, it does not appear that DHEA has a place in the treatment of frailty at the present time.

SUMMARY

Frailty and failure to thrive appear to comprise a continuum of decline in reserve and ability to respond effectively to stressors. Clinical signs and symptoms include weight loss, loss of muscle mass and declines in energy and activity level. Secondary frailty could be initiated by chronic disease, but there may well be a primary form of frailty which is age, and not disease related. A number of events can serve as triggers or contribute to the cycle of frailty, including acute illness, psychological stressors, depression, malnutrition, or injury-causing disability. There is potential for this syndrome to become a self-perpetuating cycle, or downward spiral. Presence of frailty is an independent predictor of mortality, disability, falls, and hospitalization.

The physiologic systems involved in the development of this vulnerability include sarcopenia, neuroendocrine dysregulation, and immune dysfunction. A number of alterations within each system influence the development and progression of frailty. Disease states clearly influence frailty, and the physiology of frailty likely influences disease states. Molecular changes likely underlie the changed physiology, including cumulative oxidative damage to genomic and mitochondrial DNA, replicative senescence and protein alterations.

Clues to the diagnosis of frailty are mostly related to weight loss, weakness, slowed performance, and vulnerability. Exercise, especially resistance exercise, appears to be a particularly important mode of prevention and treatment of frailty. More research into the underlying physiologic basis of frailty may reveal more specific diagnostic and treatment protocols. The construct of frailty presented here represents a framework from which new research into this important area can evolve.

REFERENCES

Berkman B et al: Failure to thrive: Paradigm for the frail elderly. *Gerontologist* 2:654, 1989.
Bortz WM IV, Bortz WM II: How fast do we age? Exercise performance over time as a biomarker. *J Gerontol A Biol Sci Med Sci* 51A:M223, 1996.
Bortz WM II: The Physics of frailty. *J Am Geriatr Soc* 41:1004, 1993.

Buchner DM, Wagner EH: Preventing frail health. *Clin Geriatr Med* 8:1, 1992.
Clark LP et al: Taking to bed. Rapid functional decline in an independently mobile older population living in an intermediate-care facility. *J Am Geriatr Soc* 38:967, 1990.
Evans WJ: What is sarcopenia? *J Gerontol* 50A:5, 1995.
Evans WJ: Exercise, nutrition and aging. *Clin Geriatr Med* 11:725, 1995.
Fiatarone MA, Evans WJ: The etiology and reversibility of muscle dysfunction in the aged. *J Gerontol* 48:77, 1993.
Fiatarone MA et al: Exercise training and nutritional supplementation for physical frailty in very elderly people. *N Engl J Med* 330:1769, 1994.
Fried LP et al: Conference on the physiologic basis of frailty. *Aging Clin Exp Res* 4:251, 1992.
Fried LP et al: Frailty in older adults: Evidence for a phenotype. *J Gerontol A Biol Sci Med Sci* 56:M146, 2001.
Lipsitz LA, Goldberger AL: Loss of "complexity" and aging. Potential applications of fractals and chaos theory to senescence. *JAMA* 267:1806, 1992.
Nelson ME et al: Effects of high-intensity strength training on multiple risk factors for osteoporotic fractures. *JAMA* 272:1909, 1994.
Newman AB et al: Associations of subclinical cardiovascular disease with Frailty. *J Gerontol A Biol Sci Med Sci* 56:M1158, 2001.
Palmer RM: A "Failure to thrive" in the elderly: Diagnosis and management. *Geriatrics* 45:47-50,53, 1990.
Poehlman ET et al: Sarcopenia in aging humans: The impact of menopause and disease. *J Gerontol* 50A:73, 1995.
Roberts SB: Effects of aging on energy requirements and the control of food intake in men. *J Gerontol* 50A:101, 1995.
Roubenoff R, Rall LC: Humoral mediation of changing body composition during aging and chronic inflammation. *Nutr Rev* 51:1, 1993.
Speechley M, Tinetti M: Falls and injuries in frail and vigorous community elderly persons. *J Am Geriatr Soc* 39:46, 1991.
Verdery RB: Failure to thrive in older people. *J Am Geriatr Soc* 44:465, 1996.
Wallace JL et al: Involuntary weight loss in older outpatients: Incidence and clinical significance. *J Am Geriatr Soc* 43:329, 1995.
Walston J et al: Frailty is associated with activation of the inflammation and coagulation systems, and with glucose intolerance, independent of clinical comorbidities: Results from the Cardiovascular Health Study. *Arch Intern Med* 162:2333–2341, 2002.

Delirium

JOSEPH V. AGOSTINI   •   SHARON K. INOUYE

Delirium, defined as an acute disorder of attention and global cognitive function, is a common, serious, and potentially preventable source of morbidity and mortality for hospitalized older persons. It occurs in 14 to 56 percent of such persons, and represents the most frequent complication of hospitalization for this group. With the aging of the US population, delirium has assumed heightened importance because persons aged 65 years and older presently account for more than 48 percent of all days of hospital care. Based on current US national vital health statistics, each year delirium complicates hospitalization for more than 2.3 million older patients, involving more than 17.5 million inpatient days, and accounting for more than $4 billion (1994 dollars) of Medicare expenditures per year. Importantly, substantial additional costs linked to delirium accrue after hospital discharge because of the increased need for institutionalization, rehabilitation services, closer medical follow-up, and home health care. Delirium often initiates a cascade of events in older persons, leading to a downward spiral of functional decline, loss of independence, institutionalization, and, ultimately, death. These statistics highlight the importance of delirium from both clinical and health policy perspectives. In fact, a recent consensus panel identified delirium as among the top three target conditions for quality-of-care improvement for vulnerable older adults. With its common occurrence, its frequently iatrogenic nature, and its close linkage to the processes of care, incident delirium can serve as a marker for the quality of hospital care and provides an opportunity for quality improvement.

DEFINITION

The definition of and diagnostic criteria for delirium continue to evolve (Table 117-1). The standardized criteria for delirium that appear in the American Psychiatric Association's *Diagnostic and Statistical Manual of Mental Disorders, Fourth Edition* (DSM-IV) remain the current diagnostic standard. Expert consensus was used to develop these criteria, however, and performance characteristics such as diagnostic sensitivity and specificity have not been reported for DSM-IV criteria. An empirically designed tool, the Confusion Assessment Method (CAM), provides a brief, validated diagnostic algorithm that is currently in widespread use for identification of delirium. The CAM algorithm relies on the presence of acute onset and fluctuating course, inattention, and either disorganized speech or altered level of consciousness. The algorithm has a sensitivity of 94 to 100 percent, specificity of 90 to 95 percent, and high interrater reliability. Given the uncertainty of diagnostic criteria for delirium, a critical area for future investigation is to establish more definitive criteria, including epidemiologic and phenomenologic evaluations assisted by advances in functional neuroimaging and other potential diagnostic marker tests.

EPIDEMIOLOGY

Occurrence Rates

Most of the epidemiologic studies of delirium involved hospitalized older patients, in whom the highest rates of delirium occur. Reported rates vary based upon the subgroup of patients studied and the setting of care (e.g., rehabilitative, intensive care, surgical). Previous studies estimated the prevalence of delirium—present at the time of hospital admission—at 14 to 24 percent, and the incidence of delirium—new cases arising during hospitalization—at 6 to 56 percent. The rates of delirium in high-risk hospital venues, such as the intensive care unit and posthip fracture settings, range from 60 to 80 percent and 15 to 53 percent, respectively. While not well-studied, delirium rates in the nursing home setting in two studies were 14 percent and 41 percent. The rates of delirium in all older persons presenting to the emergency department in several studies have ranged from 10 to 30 percent. While less frequent in the community setting, delirium is an important presenting symptom to emergency departments and community physicians, and often heralds serious underlying disease. Delirium is often unrecognized; previous studies have documented that clinicians fail to detect up to 70 percent of affected patients across all of these settings. Furthermore, the presence of delirium portends a potentially poor prognosis; hospital mortality rates in patients with delirium range from 25 to 33 percent, as high as mortality rates associated with acute myocardial infarction or sepsis.

Table 117-1 Diagnostic Criteria for Delirium

Diagnostic and Statistical Manual (DSM-IV) Diagnostic Criteria

A. A disturbance of consciousness (i.e., reduced awareness of the external environment) with reduced ability to focus, sustain, or shift attention.

B. A change in cognition (such as memory deficit, disorientation, language disturbance) or the development of a perceptual disturbance that is not better accounted for by a preexisting dementia.

C. The disturbance develops over a short period of time (usually hours to days) and tends to fluctuate over the course of a 24-hour period.

D. Evidence from the history, physical examination, or laboratory findings that the disturbance is caused by an underlying organic condition or is the direct physiologic consequences of a general medical condition or its treatment.

The Confusion Assessment Method (CAM) Diagnostic Algorithm*

Feature 1. Acute onset and fluctuating course
    This feature is usually obtained from a reliable reporter, such as a family member, caregiver, or nurse, and is shown by positive responses to these questions: Is there evidence of an acute change in mental status from the patient's baseline? Did the (abnormal) behavior fluctuate during the day, that is, tend to come and go, or did it increase and decrease in severity?

Feature 2. Inattention
    This feature is shown by a positive response to this question: Did the patient have difficulty focusing attention, for example, being easily distractible, or have difficulty keeping track of what was being said?

Feature 3. Disorganized thinking
    This feature is shown by a positive response to this question: Was the patient's thinking disorganized or incoherent, such as rambling or irrelevant conversation, unclear or illogical flow of ideas, or unpredictable switching from subject to subject?

Feature 4. Altered level of consciousness
    This feature is shown by any answer other than "alert" to this question: Overall, how would you rate this patient's level of consciousness (alert [normal], vigilant [hyperalert], lethargic [drowsy, easily aroused], stupor [difficult to arouse], or coma [unarousable])?

*The ratings for the CAM should be completed following brief cognitive assessment of the patient, for example, with the Mini-Mental State Examination. The diagnosis of delirium by CAM requires the presence of features 1 and 2 and of either 3 or 4.
SOURCE: American Psychiatric Association (1994) and Inouye SK et al (1990).

Multifactorial Etiology

The etiology of delirium is usually multifactorial, like many other common geriatric syndromes, such as falls, incontinence, and pressure sores. Although there may be a single cause of delirium, more commonly, delirium results from the interrelationship between patient vulnerability at the time of admission (i.e., predisposing factors) and the occurrence of noxious insults during hospitalization (i.e., precipitating factors). For example, patients who are highly vulnerable to delirium at baseline (e.g., such as patients with dementia or serious illness) can experience acute delirium after exposure to otherwise mild insults, such as a single dose of a sedative medication for sleep. On the other hand, older patients with few predisposing factors (low baseline vulnerability) would be relatively resistant, with precipitation of delirium only after exposure to multiple potentially detrimental insults, such as general anesthesia, major surgery, multiple psychoactive medications, immobilization, and infection (Fig. 117-1). Moreover, based on predictive models of delirium, the effects of multiple risk factors appear to be cumulative. Clinically, the overall importance of the multifactorial nature of delirium is that removal or treatment of one risk factor alone often fails

to resolve delirium. Instead, addressing many or all of the predisposing and precipitating factors for delirium is often required before the delirium improves.

Predisposing Factors

Predisposing factors for delirium include preexisting cognitive impairment or dementia, advanced age, severe underlying illness and comorbidity, functional impairment, male gender, depression, chronic renal insufficiency, dehydration, malnutrition, alcohol abuse, and sensory impairments (vision or hearing) (Table 117-2). Preexisting cognitive impairment, or dementia, is a powerful and consistent risk factor for delirium demonstrated across multiple studies, and patients with dementia have a two- to fivefold increased risk for delirium. Moreover, up to half of delirious patients have an underlying dementia. Nearly any chronic medical condition can predispose to delirium, ranging from diseases involving the central nervous system (e.g. Parkinson's disease, cerebrovascular disease, mass lesions, trauma, infection, collagen vascular disease), to diseases outside the central nervous system, including infectious, metabolic, cardiac, pulmonary, endocrine, or neoplastic

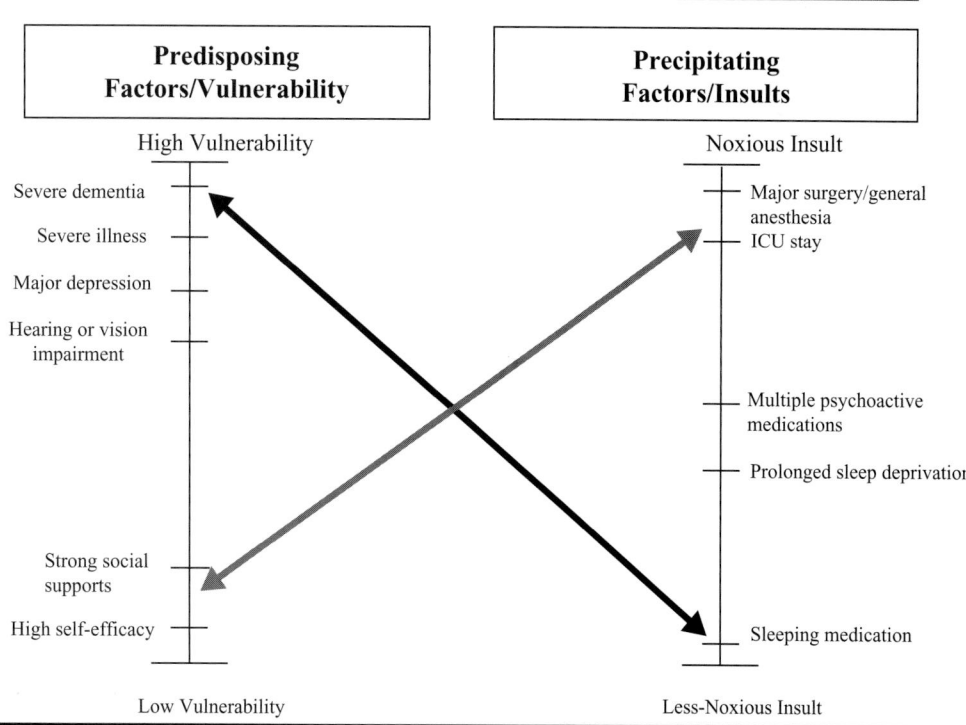

Figure 117-1 Multifactorial model for delirium. The etiology of delirium involves a complex interrelationship between the patient's underlying vulnerability or predisposing factors (*left axis*) and precipitating factors or noxious insults during hospitalization (*right axis*). For example, a patient with high vulnerability, such as with severe dementia, underlying severe illness, hearing or vision impairment, might develop delirium with exposure to only one dose of a sleeping medication. Conversely, a patient with low vulnerability would develop delirium only with exposure to many noxious insults, such as general anesthesia and major surgery, ICU stay, multiple psychoactive medications, and prolonged sleep deprivation.
SOURCE: Adapted from Inouye SK: Delirium in hospitalized older patients, in Palmer RM (ed): *Clinics in Geriatric Medicine* 1998; P 745.

etiologies. Independent predisposing risk factors for delirium at the time of hospital admission validated in a predictive model include severe underlying illness, vision impairment, baseline cognitive impairment, and high blood urea nitrogen (BUN): creatinine ratio (used as an index of dehydration). Similar predictive models that identify predisposing factors in other patient populations, for example in surgical patients and long-term care residents, are needed to better understand the contribution of baseline patient characteristics to delirium risk.

Precipitating Factors

Major precipitating factors identified in previous studies include medication use (see section on Drug Use and Delirium), immobilization, use of indwelling bladder catheters, use of physical restraints, dehydration, malnutrition, iatrogenic events, medical illnesses, infections, metabolic derangement, alcohol or drug intoxication or withdrawal, environmental influences, and psychosocial factors (see Table 117-2). Decreased mobility is strongly associated with delirium and concomitant functional decline. The use of medical equipment and devices (e.g., indwelling bladder catheters and physical restraints) may further contribute to immobilization. Major iatrogenic events occur in 29 to 38 percent of older hospitalized adults (three to five

times the risk when compared with adults younger than 65 years old). Examples include complications related to diagnostic or therapeutic procedures, allergic reactions, and bleeding caused by overanticoagulation. Many of these events potentially are preventable. Disorders of any major organ system, particularly renal or hepatic failure, can precipitate delirium. Occult respiratory failure has emerged as an increasing problem in elderly patients, who often lack the typical signs and symptoms of dyspnea and tachypnea. In older adults, acute myocardial infarction and congestive heart failure may present with delirium or "failure to thrive" as the cardinal feature, and minimal or none of the usual symptoms of angina or dyspnea. Occult infection, due to pneumonia, urinary tract infection, endocarditis, abdominal abscess, or infected joint, is a particularly noteworthy cause of delirium because older patients may not present with leukocytosis or a typical febrile response. Metabolic and endocrinologic disorders, such as hyper- or hyponatremia, hypercalcemia, acid–base disorders, hypo- and hyperglycemia, and thyroid or adrenal disorders, may also contribute to delirium. The precipitating factors for delirium in hospitalized older patients that have been validated in a predictive model include use of physical restraints, malnutrition, more than three medications added during the previous day (more than 70 percent of these were psychoactive drugs), indwelling bladder catheter, and any iatrogenic event. The presence of these independent

Table 117-2 Predisposing and Precipitating Factors for Delirium

Predisposing factors

- Dementia or underlying cognitive impairment
- Severe illness
- Comorbidity
- Depression
- Vision and/or hearing impairment
- Functional impairment, inactivity
- Volume depletion
- Chronic renal insufficiency

- Structural brain abnormality or previous stroke
- History of alcohol abuse
- History of delirium
- History of falls
- Advanced age
- Baseline use of psychoactive drugs
- Male gender
- Malnutrition

Precipitating factors

- Psychoactive drugs
- Immobilization
- Indwelling bladder catheters
- Physical restraints
- Dehydration
- Poor nutritional status
- Iatrogenic complications
- Intercurrent medical illnesses
- Major surgical procedure

- Metabolic derangements (electrolytes, glucose, acid–base)
- Infections
- Hypoxia
- Alcohol or drug intoxication or withdrawal
- Sensory deprivation
- Sensory overload
- Pain
- Emotional stress, bereavement
- Prolonged sleep deprivation

factors contributes to delirium risk in a predictable and cumulative manner, yet each risk factor is potentially modifiable.

Drug Use and Delirium

In 40 percent or more of delirium cases, use of one or more specific medication contributes to its development. While medications often incite delirium, they are also the most common remediable cause of delirium. A broad array of medications and their metabolites can lead to delirium; the most common are those with known psychoactive effects, such as sedative-hypnotics, anxiolytics, narcotics, H_2-blockers, and medications with anticholinergic activity (Table 117-3). In previous studies, use of any psychoactive medication was associated with a fourfold increased risk of delirium, while use of two or more psychoactive medications was associated with a fivefold increased risk. Sedative–hypnotic drugs are associated with a 3- to 12-fold increased risk of delirium; narcotics with a 3-fold risk; and anticholinergic drugs with a 5- to 12-fold risk. The incidence of delirium, similar to other adverse drug events, increases in direct proportion to the number of medications prescribed, because of the effects of the medications themselves, as well as to the increased risk of drug–drug and drug–disease interactions. Recent studies provide compelling evidence that suboptimal medication management, ranging from inappropriate use to overuse of psychoactive medications, occurs commonly in older adults in the hospital and in community settings, and suggests that many cases of delirium and other related adverse drug events may be preventable. As the number of prescription and over-the-counter drugs consumed by the older population increases, review of potentially problematic medications

will remain an important step in the search for predisposing factors in the patient with delirium.

PATHOPHYSIOLOGY

The fundamental pathophysiologic mechanisms of delirium remain unclear. Delirium is thought to represent a functional rather than structural lesion, with characteristic electroencephalographic (EEG) findings demonstrating global functional derangements and generalized slowing of cortical background (alpha) activity. The leading current hypotheses view delirium as the final common pathway of many different pathogenic mechanisms, resulting from dysfunction of multiple brain regions and neurotransmitter systems. Evidence from EEG, evoked-potential studies, and neuroimaging studies suggest predominantly right-sided abnormalities in delirium localized to the prefrontal cortex, thalamus, basal ganglia, temporoparietal cortex, fusiform, and lingual gyri. Associated neurotransmitter abnormalities involve elevated brain dopaminergic function, reduced cholinergic function, or a relative imbalance of these systems. Serotonergic activity may interact to regulate or alter activity of these other two systems, and serotonin levels may be either increased or decreased. The stress response associated with severe medical illness or surgery involves sympathetic and immune system activation, including increased activity of the hypothalamic–pituitary–adrenal axis with hypercortisolism, release of cerebral cytokines that alter neurotransmitter systems, alterations in the thyroid axis, and modification of blood–brain barrier permeability. Age-related changes in central neurotransmission, stress management, hormonal regulation, and immune response may contribute to the increased vulnerability of older persons to delirium. The description of delirium as "acute

Table 117-3   Drugs Associated with Delirium

Sedatives/hypnotics
  Benzodiazepines (especially flurazepam, diazepam)
  Barbiturates
  Sleeping medications (diphenhydramine, chloral
  hydrate)

Narcotics (especially meperidine)

Anticholinergics
  Antihistamines (diphenhydramine, hydroxyzine)
  Antispasmodics (belladonna, Lomotil)
  Heterocyclic antidepressants (amitriptyline,
  imipramine, doxepin)
  Neuroleptics (chlorpromazine, haloperidol,
  thioridazine)

Incontinence (oxybutynin, hyoscyamine)
  Atropine/scopolamine

Cardiac
  Digitalis glycosides
  Antiarrhythmics (quinidine, procainamide, lidocaine)
  Antihypertensives (beta-blockers, methyldopa)

Gastrointestinal
  H$_2$-antagonists (cimetidine, ranitidine, famotidine,
  nizatidine)
  Proton pump inhibitors
  Metoclopramide (Reglan)
  Herbal remedies (valerian root, St. John's wort,
  kava kava)

brain failure"—involving multiple neural circuits, neurotransmitters, and brain regions—suggests that understanding delirium may help to elucidate the essential underlying mechanisms of brain functioning.

PRESENTATION

Cardinal Features

Acute onset and inattention are the central features of delirium. Determining the acuity of onset requires accurate knowledge of the patient's prior cognitive status. Pinpointing the origin and time course of changes in mental status often entails obtaining historical information from another close observer, such as a family member, caregiver, or nurse. Typically with delirium, the mental status changes occur over hours to days, in contrast to the changes that occur with dementia, which present insidiously over weeks to months. Another key feature is the fluctuating course of delirium, with symptoms tending to wax and wane in severity over a 24-hour period. Lucid intervals are characteristic, and the reversibility of symptoms within a short time can deceive even an experienced clinician. Inattention is manifested as difficulty focusing, maintaining, and

shifting attention or concentration. With simple cognitive assessment, patients may display difficulty with straightforward repetition tasks, digit spans, or recitation of the months of the year backward. Delirious patients appear easily distracted, experience difficulty with multistep commands, cannot follow the flow of a conversation, and often perseverate with an answer to a previous question. Additional major features include a disorganization of thought and altered level of consciousness. Disorganized thoughts are a manifestation of underlying cognitive or perceptual disturbances, and can be recognized by disjointed and incoherent speech, or an unclear or illogical progression of ideas. Clouding of consciousness is typically manifested by lethargy, with a reduced awareness of the environment that may show diurnal variation. Although not cardinal elements, other frequently associated features include disorientation (more commonly to time and place than to self), cognitive impairments (e.g., memory and problem-solving deficits, dysnomia), psychomotor agitation or retardation, perceptual disturbances (e.g., hallucinations, misperceptions, illusions), paranoid delusions, emotional lability, and sleep–wake cycle disruption.

Tools for Evaluation of Delirium

Table 117-4 describes the most widely-used instruments for identification of delirium, along with their performance characteristics. These include CAM, the Delirium Rating Scale (DRS), the Delirium Symptom Interview (DSI), and the Memorial Delirium Assessment Scale (MDAS). Each instrument has strengths and limitations, and the choice among them depends on the goals for use. Notably, the evaluation for the CAM has been adapted recently as the CAM-ICU for nonverbal or intubated patients. In addition, the DRS–Revised-98 version allows more refined measurements of delirium severity over a broad range of symptoms.

Forms of Delirium

The clinical presentation of delirium can take two main forms, either hypoactive or hyperactive. The hypoactive form of delirium is characterized by lethargy and reduced psychomotor functioning, and is the more common form in older patients. Hypoactive delirium often goes unrecognized and carries an overall poorer prognosis. By contrast, the hyperactive form of delirium presents with symptoms of agitation, increased vigilance, and often concomitant hallucinations; its presentation rarely remains unnoticed by caregivers or clinicians. Importantly, patients can fluctuate between the hypoactive and hyperactive forms—the mixed type of delirium—presenting a challenge in distinguishing the presentation from other psychotic or mood disorders. Moreover, recent recognition of partial or incomplete forms of delirium has brought attention to the persistence of symptoms among older patients, particularly during the resolution stages of delirium, when manifestation of the full syndrome may not be apparent. Partial forms of delirium also adversely influence long-term clinical outcomes.

Table 117-4   Sample Instruments Used to Evaluate Delirium

Description	Domains	Validation	Reference Standard	Reliability	Feasibility
Confusion Assessment Method (CAM)					
Nine operationalized delirium criteria scored according to CAM algorithm. Shortened version uses four criteria. Based on observations made during interview with MMSE, by trained lay or clinical interviewer.	Onset/course Attention Organization of thought Level of consciousness Orientation Memory Perceptual problems Psychomotor behavior Sleep—wake cycle	Sensitivity = 0.94–1.0 (n = 26 delirious patients) Specificity = 0.90–0.95 (n = 30 controls without delirium) Convergent agreement with four other cognitive measures Ability to distinguish delirium and dementia verified	Gero-psychiatrists' diagnoses based on clinical judgment and DSM-III-R criteria	Interrater: K = 1.0 overall	Observer-rated: 10–15 minutes for cognitive testing and completion of rating
CAM–ICU					
Uses four CAM criteria. Cognitive assessment adapted for use in nonverbal or ventilated patients.	Onset/course Attention Organization of thought Level of consciousness	Sensitivity = 0.93–1.0 Specificity = 0.98–1.0 (n = 91 patients)	Delirium expert clinicians' ratings based on DSM-IV criteria	Interrater: K = 0.96 overall	Observer-rated: <5 minutes for cognitive assessment and completion of rating
Delirium Rating Scale (DRS)					
Ten-item rating, with additive score 0 to 32, designed to be completed by a psychiatrist after complete psychiatric assessment. Useful to rate severity.	Onset/course Cognitive status Perceptual problems Delusions Psychomotor behavior Emotional lability Sleep–wake cycle Physical disorder	No overlap in scores between delirious group (n = 20) and three control groups: demented (n = 9), schizophrenic (n = 9), and normal (n = 9) Convergent agreement with two other cognitive measures Ability to distinguish delirium and dementia verified	Consult-liaison psychiatrist's diagnosis based on DSM-III criteria	Interrater: intraclass correlation coefficient = 0.97	Observer-rated: based on lengthy interview and detailed assessment (time not specified)
Delirium Symptom Interview (DSI)					
Includes interview with brief cognitive assessment and rating scale for 7 symptom domains of delirium, by trained lay or clinical interviewer.	Course Organization of thought Level of consciousness Orientation Perceptual problems Psychomotor behavior Sleep–wake cycle	Sensitivity = 0.90 Specificity = 0.80 (n = 30 "cases", 15 non-cases, 3 borderline, 2 disagreements by psychiatrist and neurologist). Ability to distinguish delirium and dementia not tested	Psychiatrist's and neurologist's assessments based on presence of any 1 of 3 "critical symptoms" (disorientation, disturbance of consciousness, or perceptual disturbance)	Interrater: K = 0.90 overall	Observer-rated part; 15+ minutes for interview, plus additional time for completion or rating (not specified)

(Continued)

Table 117-4 (*Continued*) Sample Instruments Used to Evaluate Delirium

Description	Domains	Validation	Reference Standard	Reliability	Feasibility
Memorial Delirium Assessment Scale (MDAS)					
Ten-item scale, with additive score 0 to 30 using cognitive testing and behavioral observations, by experienced mental health professionals. Designed to rate delirium severity, not for screening or diagnosis.	Level of consciousness Orientation Memory Digit span Attention Organization of thought Perceptual problems Delusions Psychomotor behavior Sleep–wake cycle	Sensitivity = 0.82 Specificity = 0.75 (with score = 10; n = 33: 17 delirium, 8 dementia, 8 other psychiatric)	Consult-liaison psychiatrist's diagnosis using DRS, MMSE, and Clinician's Global Rating of delirium severity	Interrater: intraclass correlation coefficient = 0.92 overall	Observer-rated in part; 10+ minutes for administration

Abbreviations: DSM-III = *Diagnostic and Statistical Manual of Mental Disorders*, 3rd ed.; DSM-III-R = *Diagnostic and Statistical Manual of Mental Disorders*, 3rd ed. rev.; DSM-IV = *Diagnostic and Statistical Manual of Mental Disorders*, 4th ed.; K = Kappa coefficient; MMSE = Mini-Mental State Examination; n = number of subjects.

SOURCE: Inouye SK et al (1990); Ely EW et al; Trzepacz P et al: A symptom rating scale for delirium. *Psychiatry Res* 23:89, 1988; Albert M et al; and Breibart W et al (1997).

PROGNOSIS

Delirium is an important independent determinant of prolonged length of hospital stay, increased mortality, increased rates of nursing home placement, and functional and cognitive decline—even after controlling for age, gender, dementia, illness severity, and baseline functional status.

Delirium has long been thought to be a reversible, transient condition. Recent research on the duration of delirium symptoms, however, provides evidence that delirium may persist for much longer than previously recognized. In fact, delirium symptoms generally persist for a month or more, and as few as 20 percent of patients attain complete symptom resolution at 6-month follow-up. In addition, those patients with extant cognitive impairment may experience greater deleterious effects than comparable non-dementia patients. The chronic detrimental effects are likely related to the duration, severity, and underlying cause(s) of the delirium, in addition to the baseline vulnerability of the patient. The contribution of delirium itself to permanent cognitive impairment or dementia remains controversial; however, previous studies document that at least some patients post-delirium never recover their baseline level of cognitive function. Thus, delirium and dementia may represent two ends along a spectrum of cognitive impairment with "chronic delirium" and "reversible dementia" falling along this continuum.

EVALUATION

The acute evaluation of delirium centers on three main tasks that occur simultaneously: (1) establishing the diagnosis of delirium; (2) determining the potential cause(s) and ruling out life-threatening contributors; and (3) managing the symptoms. Delirium is a clinical diagnosis, relying on astute observation at the bedside, careful cognitive assessment, and history taking from a knowledgeable informant to establish a change from the patient's baseline functioning. Identifying the potentially multifactorial contributors to the delirium is of paramount importance, because many of these factors are treatable, and if left untreated, may result in substantial morbidity and mortality. Because the potential contributors are myriad, the search requires clinical judgment combined with a thorough medical evaluation. The challenge is enhanced by the frequently nonspecific or atypical presentation of the underlying illness in older persons. In fact, delirium is often the *only* sign of life-threatening illness, such as sepsis, pneumonia, or myocardial infarction in older persons.

A thorough history and physical examination constitute the foundation of the medical evaluation of suspected delirium. The first step in evaluation should be to establish the diagnosis of delirium through careful cognitive assessment and to determine the acuity of change from the patient's baseline cognitive state. Because cognitive impairment may easily be missed during routine conversation, brief cognitive screening tests, such as the Mini-Mental Status Examination and the CAM, should be used. The degree of attention should be further assessed with simple tests such as a forward digit span (inattention indicated by an inability to repeat five digits forward) or recitation of the months of the year backward. Of note, a delirium tool to assess nonverbal (e.g., mechanically ventilated) patients, the CAM-ICU, has recently been developed and validated for use in critically ill older persons. A targeted history, focusing on baseline cognitive status and chronology of recent mental status changes, should be elicited from a reliable informant. In addition, such historical data as intercurrent illnesses, recent adjustments in medication regimen, the possibility of alcohol withdrawal, and pertinent environmental changes may point to potential precipitating factors of delirium.

The physical examination should include a detailed review that focuses on potential etiologic clues to an underlying or inciting disease process. Vital sign assessment is important to identify fever, tachycardia, or decreased oxygen saturation, each of which may point to specific disease processes. Ausculatory examination may suggest pneumonia or pulmonary effusion. A new cardiac murmur or dysrhythmia may suggest ischemia or congestive heart failure. Gastrointestinal examination should focus on evidence of an acute abdominal process, such as occult bleeding, perforated viscus, or infection. Patients with delirium may also demonstrate nonspecific focal findings on neurologic examination, such as asterixis or tremor, although the presence of any new neurologic deficit should raise suspicion of an acute cerebrovascular event. As previously mentioned, in many older patients and in those with cognitive impairment, delirium may be the initial manifestation of a serious new disease process. Therefore, attention to early localizing signs on serial physical examinations is important.

A complete medication review, including over-the-counter medications, is critical, and any medications with known psychoactive effects should be discontinued or minimized whenever possible. Because of pharmacodynamic and pharmacokinetic changes in aging adults, these medications may cause deleterious psychoactive effects even when prescribed at customary doses and with serum drug levels that are within the "therapeutic range."

Notwithstanding the growing recognition of geriatric syndromes such as delirium, there is little evidence-based research that assesses the predictive value of laboratory and other diagnostic testing in the evaluation of delirium. Consequently, laboratory evaluation should be guided by clinical judgment, taking into account specific patient characteristics and historical data. An astute history and physical examination, medication review, focused laboratory testing (e.g., complete blood count, chemistries, glucose, renal and liver function tests, urinalysis, oxygen saturation), and search for occult infection should help to identify the majority of potential contributors to the delirium. Obtaining additional laboratory testing such as thyroid function tests, B_{12} level, cortisol level, drug levels or toxicology screen, syphilis serologies, and ammonia level should be based on a patient's distinct clinical presentation. Further diagnostic work-up with an electrocardiogram, chest radiograph, and/or arterial blood gas determination may be

Table 117-5 Differential Diagnosis of Altered Mental Status

Characteristic	Delirium	Dementia	Depression	Acute Psychosis
Onset	Acute (hours to days)	Progressive, insidious (weeks to months)	Either acute or insidious	Acute
Course over time	Waxing and waning	Unrelenting	Variable	Episodic
Attention	Impaired, a hallmark of delirium	Usually intact, until end-stage disease	Decreased concentration and attention to detail	Variable
Level of consciousness	Altered, from lethargic to hyperalert	Normal, until end-stage disease	Normal	Normal
Memory	Impaired commonly	Prominent short- and/or long-term memory impairment	Normal, some short-term forgetfulness	Usually normal
Orientation	Disoriented	Normal, until end-stage disease	Usually normal	Usually normal
Speech	Disorganized, incoherent, illogical	Notable for parsimony, aphasia, anomia	Normal, but often slowing of speech (psychomotor retardation)	Variable, often disorganized
Delusions	Common	Common	Uncommon	Common, often complex
Hallucinations	Usually visual	Sometimes	Rare	Usually auditory and more complex
Organic etiology	Yes	Yes	No	No

appropriate for patients with pulmonary or cardiac conditions. The indications for cerebrospinal fluid examination, brain imaging, or electroencephalography remain controversial. Their overall diagnostic yield is low, and these procedures are probably indicated in less than 5 to 10 percent of delirium cases. Lumbar puncture with cerebrospinal fluid examination is indicated for the febrile delirious patient when meningitis or encephalitis is suspected. Brain imaging (such as computed tomography or magnetic resonance imaging) should be reserved for cases with new focal neurologic signs, with history or signs of head trauma, or without another identifiable cause of the delirium. Of note, some neurologic symptoms are associated with delirium, including tremor and asterixis. Electroencephalography, which has a false-negative rate of 17 percent and a false-positive rate of 22 percent for distinguishing between delirious and nondelirious patients, plays a limited role and is most commonly employed to detect subclinical seizure disorders and to differentiate delirium from nonorganic psychiatric conditions.

Distinguishing a long-standing confusional state (dementia) from delirium alone, or from delirium superimposed on dementia, is an important, but often difficult, diagnostic step. These two conditions can be differentiated by the acute onset of symptoms in delirium, with dementia presenting much more insidiously, and by the impaired attention and altered level of consciousness associated with delirium. The differential diagnosis of delirium can be extensive and includes other psychiatric conditions such as depression and nonorganic psychotic disorders (Table 117-5). Although perceptual disturbances, such as illusions and hallucinations, can occur with delirium, recognition of the key features of acute onset, inattention, altered level of consciousness, and global cognitive impairment will enhance the identification of delirium. Differentiating among diagnoses is critical because delirium carries a more serious prognosis without proper evaluation and management, and treatment for certain conditions such as depression or affective disorders may involve use of drugs with anticholinergic activity, for example, which could exacerbate an unrecognized case of delirium. At times, working through the differential diagnosis can be quite challenging, particularly with an uncooperative patient or when an accurate history is unavailable, and the diagnosis of delirium may remain uncertain. Because of the potentially life-threatening nature of delirium, however, it is prudent to manage the patient as having delirium and search for underlying precipitants (e.g., intercurrent illness, metabolic abnormalities, adverse medication effects) until further information can be obtained.

Figure 117-2 presents an algorithm for the evaluation of altered mental status in the older patient. The initial steps center on establishing the patient's baseline cognitive functioning and the onset and timing of any cognitive changes. Chronic impairments, representing changes that occur over months to years, are most likely attributable to

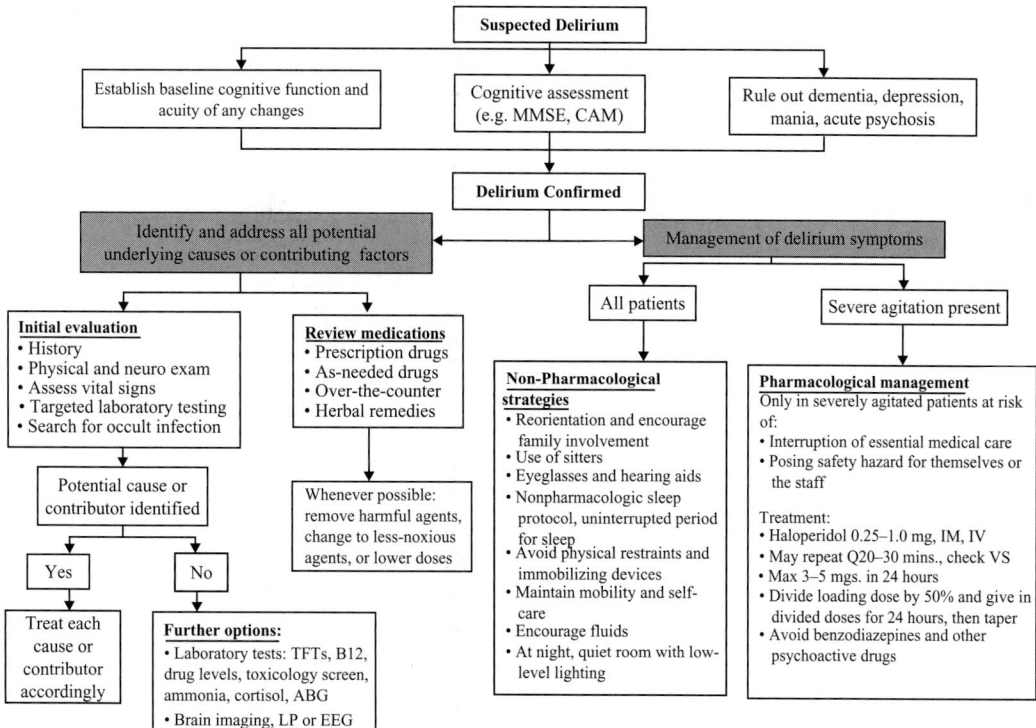

Figure 117-2   Flowchart for evaluation of suspected delirium in an older person. ABG = arterial blood gas; B12 = cyanocobalamin for vitamin B$_{12}$ level; CAM = Confusion Assessment Method; EEG = electroencephalography; LP = lumbar puncture; MMSE = Mini-Mental State Examination; neuro exam = neurologic examination; TFTs = thyroid function tests (e.g., T4, thyroid index, thyroid-stimulating hormone); VS = vital signs.

Source: Adapted from Inouye SK: Delirium and other mental status problems in the older patient, in Goldman L, Bennett JC (eds): *Cecil Textbook of Medicine,* 21st edition. Philadelphia, WB Saunders company, 1999, 18.

a dementia, which should be evaluated accordingly (see Chap. 106). Acute alterations, representing abrupt deteriorations in mental status, occur over hours to weeks, although they may be superimposed on an underlying dementia. They should be further evaluated with cognitive testing to establish the presence of delirium. In the absence of notable delirium features (see "Presentation" earlier in this chapter), subsequent evaluation should focus on the possibility of major depression, acute psychotic disorder, or other psychiatric disorders (see Chaps. 112, and 113).

PREVENTION

Primary prevention, that is, preventing delirium before it develops, is the most effective strategy for reducing delirium and its associated adverse outcomes, which range from functional disability to longer lengths of hospital stay and institutionalization. Table 117-6 describes well-documented delirium risk factors and tested preventive interventions to address each risk factor. A controlled clinical trial demonstrated the effectiveness of a delirium prevention strategy targeted towards these risk factors. The selection of risk factors was based upon their clinical relevance and the degree to which they could be modified by employing practical and feasible interventions. Compared with standard care, implementation of these preventive interventions resulted in a 40 percent risk reduction for delirium in hospitalized older patients.

The Hospital Elder Life Program (HELP) represents an innovative strategy of hospital care for older patients, designed to incorporate the tested delirium prevention strategies and to improve overall quality of hospital care. Hospital-wide programs such as HELP underscore the importance of an interdisciplinary team's contributions to the prevention of delirium. For example, trained volunteers and family members can play roles in daily orientation, therapeutic recreation activities, and feeding assistance. Physical rehabilitation experts and nurses can assist with mobilization and the incorporation of daily exercises to prevent functional decline. Dietitians can help to maximize appropriate caloric intake and oral hydration in acutely ill patients. Consultant pharmacists, chaplains, and social workers also may provide specialized expertise to address patient care issues pertinent to individuals at risk for delirium.

Proactive geriatric consultation has been demonstrated to reduce the risk of delirium posthip fracture by 40 percent in a randomized controlled trial. The targeted multicomponent consultation strategy focused on 10 domains, namely adequate brain oxygen delivery, fluid/electrolyte balance, pain management, reduction in psychoactive medications, bowel/bladder function, nutrition, early mobilization, prevention of postoperative complications, appropriate environmental stimuli, and treatment of delirium (Table 117-7). The recommendations were carried out with good adherence (77 percent), and provided a feasible and effective approach to address a leading complication of hip fracture surgery. Although not yet tested, this multicomponent approach is likely to be effective at reducing the risk of delirium in high-risk patients other than those with posthip fracture repair.

On a larger scale, preventive efforts for delirium will require system-wide changes and large-scale shifts in local and national policies and approaches to care. Recommended changes include routine cognitive and functional assessment on admission of all older patients; monitoring mental status as a "vital sign"; education of physicians and nurses to improve recognition and heighten awareness of the clinical implications; enhanced geriatric physician

Table 117-6 Delirium Risk Factors and Tested Interventions

Risk Factor	Intervention Protocol
Cognitive impairment	• Orienting communication, including orientation board • Therapeutic activities program
Immobilization	• Early mobilization (e.g., ambulation or bedside exercises) • Minimizing immobilizing equipment (e.g., restraints, bladder catheters)
Psychoactive medications	• Restricted use of PRN sleep and psychoactive medications (e.g., sedative–hypnotics, narcotics, anticholinergic drugs) • Nonpharmacologic protocols for management of sleep and anxiety
Sleep deprivation	• Noise-reduction strategies • Scheduling of nighttime medications, procedures, and nursing activities to allow uninterrupted period of sleep.
Vision impairment	• Provision of vision aids (e.g., magnifiers, special lighting) • Provision of adaptive equipment (e.g., illuminated phone dials, large-print books)
Hearing impairment	• Provision of amplifying devices; repair hearing aids • Instruct staff in communication methods
Dehydration	• Early recognition and volume repletion

Source: Inouye SK et al (1999).

Table 117-7   Preventive Interventions after Hip Fracture

Risk Factor	Intervention
Hypoxia	• Supplemental oxygen • Raise systolic blood pressure • Transfusion to Hct >30%
Fluid/electrolyte imbalance	• Restore serum sodium, potassium, glucose • Treat fluid overload or dehydration
Pain	• Around-the-clock acetaminophen • Low-dose morphine, oxycodone for break-through pain
Psychoactive medications	• Minimize benzodiazepines, anticholinergics, antihistamines • Eliminate drug interactions and redundancies
Bowel/bladder dysfunction	• Treat constipation • Discontinue urinary catheter by postoperative day 2, screen for retention or incontinence
Poor nutrition	• Provide dentures, assistance • Supplements or enteral nutrition
Immobilization	• Early mobilization (out of bed postoperative day 1) • Physical therapy

Postoperative complications	• Monitor and treat for:
	    Myocardial ischemia
	    Atrial arrhythmias
	    Pneumonia
	    Pulmonary embolus
	    Urinary tract infection

Sensory deprivation	• Use glasses and hearing aids • Provide clock and calendar • Provide radio and soft lighting
Treatment of agitation	• Diagnostic work-up • Reassurance, family presence, sitter • If pharmacologic management necessary, use haloperidol

SOURCE: Marcantonio ER et al.

and nursing expertise at the bedside; incentives to change practice patterns that lead to delirium (e.g., immobilization, use of sleep medications, bladder catheters, and physical restraints); and creation of systems that enhance high-quality geriatric care (e.g., geriatric expertise, case management, clinical pathways, and quality monitoring for delirium). Implementing these changes will impact not only on delirium, but will result in high-quality hospital care more generally.

MANAGEMENT

Pharmacologic Management

The recommended management approach for all delirious patients begins with nonpharmacologic strategies (see "Nonpharmacologic Management" and "Nonpharmacologic Sleep Protocol" later in this chapter), which usually result in successful symptom amelioration. In selected cases, such strategies must be supplemented with a pharmacologic approach, usually reserved for patients in whom delirium symptoms would result in interruption of needed medical therapies (e.g., mechanical ventilation, central lines) or may endanger the safety of the patient or other persons. However, prescribing any drug requires balancing the benefits of delirium management against the potential for adverse medication effects, because no drug is ideal for the treatment of delirium symptoms. Sometimes the decision to prescribe may be influenced by other members of the clinical team, the family, or caregivers. All interested parties should understand that the choice of almost any medication may further cloud the patient's mental status and obscure efforts to monitor the course of the mental status change. Consequently, any drug chosen should be initiated at the lowest starting dose for the shortest time possible. In general, neuroleptics are the preferred agents of treatment, with haloperidol being the agent in most widespread use, whose effectiveness has been established in a randomized clinical trial. Haloperidol is available in parenteral form and is associated with less postural blood pressure changes and fewer anticholinergic side effects compared with thioridazine; however, high-potency antipsychotics such as haloperidol are associated with a higher rate of extrapyramidal side effects and acute dystonias. The intravenous route can be used when parenteral administration is required, which results in a rapid onset of action and a short duration of effect, whereas oral or intramuscular use is associated with a more optimal duration of action. The recommended starting dose is 0.5 to 1.0 mg haloperidol orally or parenterally. The dose may be repeated every 30 minutes after the vital signs have been rechecked and until sedation has been reached. The clinical end point should be an awake but manageable patient, a goal that can be achieved by following the general geriatric prescribing principle, "start low and go slow." Most older patients naïve to prior treatment with a neuroleptic should require a total loading dose of no more than 3 to 5 mg of haloperidol. A subsequent maintenance dose consisting of one-half of the loading dose should be administered in divided doses over the next 24 hours, with doses tapered over the ensuing several days as the agitation resolves.

Other Pharmacologic Approaches

Benzodiazepines (e.g., lorazepam) are not recommended as first-line agents in the treatment of delirium because of their increased propensity to cause oversedation and to exacerbate acute mental status changes. However, they remain the treatment of choice for delirium caused by seizures and alcohol- and medication-related withdrawal syndromes. While other drugs have been advocated for use in treatment of delirium, their use has been evaluated only in case series or uncontrolled studies and is not recommended. These drugs include the newer atypical antipsychotic agents, procholinergic agents (such as donepezil), and serotonin receptor antagonists (such as trazodone). While the newer antipsychotic drugs (such as risperidone, olanzapine, and quetiapine) have the potential for fewer sedative and extrapyramidal effects, they have not yet been evaluated in randomized clinical trials.

Nonpharmacologic Management

Nonpharmacologic approaches are the mainstays of treatment for every delirious patient. These approaches include strategies for reorientation and behavioral intervention, such as ensuring the presence of family members, use of sitters, and transferring a disruptive patient to a private room or closer to the nurse's station for increased supervision. Orienting influences such as calendars, clocks, and the day's schedule should be prominently displayed, along with familiar personal objects from the patient's home environment (e.g., photographs and religious artifacts). Personal contact and communication are critical to reinforce patient awareness and encourage patient participation as much as possible. Communication should incorporate repeated reorientation strategies, clear instructions, and frequent eye contact. Correction of sensory impairments (i.e., vision and hearing) should be maximized as applicable for individual patients by encouraging the use of eyeglasses and hearing aids during the hospital stay. Mobility and independence should be promoted; physical restraints should be avoided because they lead to decreased mobility, increased agitation, and greater risk of injury. Patient involvement in self-care and decision-making should also be encouraged. Other environmental interventions include limiting room and staff changes and providing a quiet patient care setting with low-level lighting at night. An environment with decreased noise allowing for an uninterrupted period for sleep at night is of crucial importance in the management of delirium. This may require unit-wide changes in the coordination and scheduling of nursing and medical procedures, including medication dispensing, vital sign recording, and administration of intravenous medications and other treatments. Hospital-wide changes may be needed to ensure a low level of noise at night, including minimizing hallway noise, overhead paging, and staff conversations.

Nonpharmacologic Sleep Protocol

Nonpharmacologic approaches for relaxation and sleep can be effective for management of agitation in delirious patients and for prevention of delirium through minimization of psychoactive medications. The nonpharmacologic sleep protocol includes three components: (1) a glass of warm milk or herbal tea; (2) relaxation music or tapes; and (3) back massage. This protocol was demonstrated to be feasible and effective. Use of the protocol reduced the use of sleeping medications from 54 percent to 31 percent ($P < .002$) in a hospital environment.

SPECIAL ISSUES

Long-Term Care Setting

While the vulnerable, frail nursing home population represents a potentially high-risk group, delirium has been relatively neglected as an area of clinical investigation in this setting. Many episodes of agitation and behavioral changes in this environment may potentially be due to delirium. Few studies have examined occurrence rates or risk factors. Moreover, the validity of the Minimum Data Set for identification of delirium has not been systematically examined.

Palliative Care Setting

Management of delirium at the end of life poses particular challenges. Because delirium occurs in more than 80 percent of patients at the end of life, it is considered nearly inevitable in the terminal stages by most hospice care providers, and may serve as a predictor of approaching death. Establishing the goals of care with the patient and family is a crucial step, including discussions about the potential causes of the delirium, intensity of medical evaluations considered appropriate, and the need for titration between alertness and adequate control of pain and agitation. For example, some patients may wish to preserve their ability to communicate as long as possible, while others may focus on comfort perhaps at the expense of alertness. Physicians must be cognizant that even in the terminal phase, many causes of delirium are potentially reversible and may be amenable to interventions (e.g., medication adjustments, treatment of dehydration, hypoglycemia, or hypoxia) that may improve comfort and quality of life. However, the burdens of evaluation (e.g., invasive testing) or treatment (e.g., reduction in narcotic dose) may not be consistent with the goals for care. In all cases, symptom management should begin immediately, while evaluation is underway. Nonpharmacologic approaches should be instituted in all patients, with pharmacologic approaches for selected cases. Haloperidol remains the first-line therapy for delirium in terminally ill patients. In end-of-life care, there is a lower threshold for the use of sedative agents. Sedation may be indicated as an additional therapy for management of severe agitated delirium in the terminally ill patient, which can cause considerable distress for the patient and family. Because sedation poses the risks of decreased meaningful interaction with family, increased confusion, and respiratory depression, this choice should be made in conjunction with the family according to the goals for care. If sedation is indicated, an agent that is short-acting and easily titrated to effect is recommended. Lorazepam (starting dose 0.5 to 1.0 mg po, IV, or SQ) is the recommended agent of choice.

Ethical Issues

In a condition characterized by acute fluctuations in attention and decision-making capacity, delirium presents formidable challenges to the ethical care of afflicted patients (see Chaps. 10 and 29). Recent research has highlighted the importance of determining and appropriately documenting cognitive impairment prior to initiating nonemergent treatments. Cognitive assessments in patients with suspected delirium help to ensure that appropriate surrogate decision makers (e.g., family members or caregivers) are involved in representing a patient's wishes, and understanding the risks and benefits of procedures and treatments. Because the patient may exhibit periods of lucidity in delirium, there may be times during which the informed consent process can and should involve the patient. Following resolution of an acute delirium episode, the clinician should

be cognizant of ongoing subclinical manifestations of delirium, or partial forms of delirium, that may be important for considerations of both the long-term management and decision-making capacity of the patient.

REFERENCES

Agostini JV et al: Cognitive and other anticholinergic effects of diphenhydramine in hospitalized older patients. *Arch Intern Med* 161:2091, 2001.

Albert M et al: The delirium symptom interview. *J Geriatr Psychiatry Neurol* 5:14, 1992.

American Psychiatric Association: *Diagnostic and Statistical Manual of Mental Disorders (DSM-IV)*, 4th ed. Washington, DC, American Psychiatric Association, 1994.

American Psychiatric Association: Practice guideline for the treatment of patients with delirium. *Am J Psychiatry* 156(5 Suppl):1, 1999.

Breitbart W et al: A double-blind trial of haloperidol, chlorpromazine, and lorazepam in the treatment of delirium in hospitalized AIDS patients. *Am J Psychiatry* 153:231, 1996.

Breitbart W et al: The Memorial Delirium Assessment Scale. *J Pain Symptom Manage* 13:128, 1997.

Creditor MC: Hazards of hospitalization of the elderly. *Ann Intern Med* 118:219, 1993.

Elie M et al: Delirium risk factors in elderly hospitalized patients. *J Gen Intern Med* 13:204, 1998.

Ely EW et al: Delirium in mechanically ventilated patients: Validity and reliability of the confusion assessment method for the intensive care unit (CAM-ICU). *JAMA* 286:2703, 2001.

Inouye SK et al: Clarifying confusion: The confusion assessment method. A new method for detection of delirium. *Ann Intern Med* 113:941, 1990.

Inouye SK et al: A predictive model for delirium among hospitalized elderly persons based on admission characteristics. *Ann Intern Med* 119:474, 1993.

Inouye SK, Charpentier PA: Precipitating factors for delirium in hospitalized elderly persons: Predictive model and inter-relationship with baseline vulnerability. *JAMA* 275:852, 1996.

Inouye SK et al: A clinical trial of a multicomponent intervention to prevent delirium in hospitalized older patients. *N Engl J Med* 340:669, 1999.

Inouye SK et al: Delirium: A symptom of how hospital care is failing older persons and a window to improve quality of hospital care. *Am J Med* 106:565, 1999.

Marcantonio ER et al: Reducing delirium after hip fracture: A randomized trial. *J Am Geriatr Soc* 49:516, 2001.

Meagher DJ: Delirium: Optimizing management. *BMJ* 322:144, 2001.

Rothschild JM et al: Preventable medical injuries in older patients. *Arch Intern Med* 160:2717, 2000.

Trzepacz PT: The neuropathogenesis of delirium: A need to focus our research. *Psychosomatics* 35:374, 1994.

Trzepacz PT et al: Validation of the Delirium Rating Scale–Revised-98: Comparison with the Delirium Rating Scale and Cognitive Test for Delirium. *J Neuropsychiatry Clin Neurosci* 13:229, 2001.

Falls

MARY B. KING

DEFINITION

Falls are common in older persons. A fall injury is costly in terms of morbidity, loss of physical function and independence, and mortality, as well as health care dollars. Falls have not always been recognized as a serious health problem; prior to the 1940s, a fall was considered an unpredictable event that could not be prevented. In the past 20 years, however, research studies have shown the incidence and consequences of falls, revealed their multifactorial etiology, and demonstrated that they can be prevented by treating the factors that increase an older person's risk of falling. Effective treatment requires a multidisciplinary approach. Perhaps because of this, fall prevention is not widely practiced in clinical settings outside of specialized geriatric assessment clinics; thus, falls remain an undertreated public health issue.

This chapter addresses nonsyncopal falls—unintentional events in which a person comes to rest on the floor or ground that are not caused by loss of consciousness, stroke, seizure, or overwhelming force. Falls in three different settings—the community, skilled nursing facilities, and hospitals—are discussed, as reasons for falling and, therefore, interventions differ by site.

INCIDENCE AND CONSEQUENCES OF FALLS

Incidence

Approximately 35 to 40 percent of persons age 65 years and over fall in a given year; half of persons who fall do so more than once. The incidence increases steadily after age 60 years; approximately 50 percent of persons age 80 years and older fall in a year. Women are more likely to fall than men. More than half of all falls in the community happen in the home. The rates for falls in skilled nursing facilities and hospitals are almost three times that for community-dwelling elders, and are estimated at 1.5 falls per bed per year.

Fall Injuries

Incidence

Although young children and athletes also have a high incidence of falls, older persons are at high risk of injury with a fall because of age-related changes such as slow reaction time, impaired protective responses, and comorbid diseases such as osteoporosis. As a result, serious fall injuries, including fractures, lacerations, serious soft-tissue injuries, and head trauma, occur in 5 to 15 percent of falls in the community. Injury rates are higher, from 10 to 25 percent of falls, in institutional settings. Approximately 8 percent of persons age 65 years and older visit an emergency department because of a fall-related injury each year; almost half of these persons are admitted to the hospital for treatment. Older persons are often unable to get up from the ground or floor after a fall, resulting in long lies with the risk of pneumonia, dehydration, and rhabdomyolysis. Fractures, most commonly of the hip, pelvis, femur, vertebrae, humerus, hand, forearm, leg, and ankle, occur in approximately 3 percent of falls. Conversely, falls account for 87 percent of all fractures and for more than 95 percent of hip fractures in this group. Falls are the second leading cause of brain and spinal cord injury in older adults.

Hip Fractures

Hip fractures are probably the most dreaded fall-related injury, as approximately half of older persons who sustain a hip fracture cannot return home or live independently after the fracture. The incidence of hip fracture has risen for both men and women in recent years; women sustain about three times as many hip fractures as men (Fig. 118-1). In 1998, there were almost 332,000 hip fractures in the United States. The hospital admission rates for hip fractures increased by 18 percent in men and 30 percent in women between 1988 and 1999.

Death

In the United States, unintentional injury is the fifth leading cause of death in persons age 65 years and older; falls

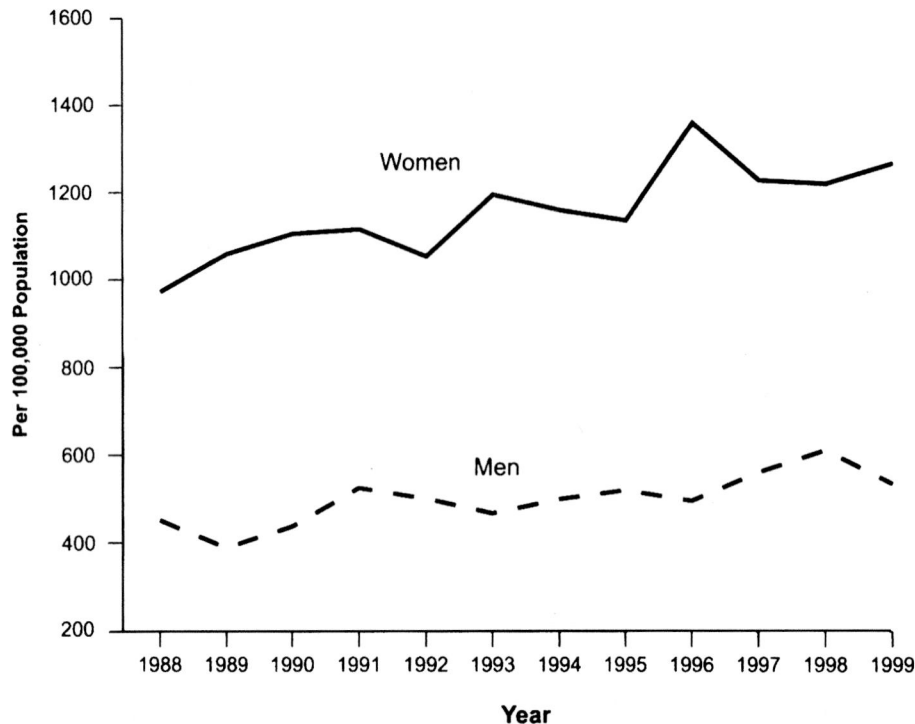

Figure 118-1   Rates of hospital admission for hip fractures for men and women ages 65 years and older in the United States, 1988–1999. Rates are per 100,000 population. Adapted from National Center for Health Statistics (NCHS), National Hospital Discharge Surveys. National Center for Injury Prevention and Control, with permission, Centers for Disease Control and Prevention (CDC) website at: http://www.cdc.gov/ncipc/.

are the cause of two-thirds of the deaths resulting from injuries in this age group. In 1998, approximately 9600 older persons died as the result of a fall. The death rate from falls for men in this age group is approximately 20 percent higher than that for women; deaths as a consequence of falls increased in both men and women from 1988 to 1998 (Fig. 118-2).

Other Consequences of Falling

Falls are costly for older persons, both in terms of health care dollars and in loss of physical function and independence. Fall-related injuries account for approximately 6 percent of all health care expenses for persons age 65 years and older in the United States. The cost of a hip fracture was recently estimated at $16,300 to $18,700 for care during the first year following injury. Falls also take a toll on an older person's independence and quality of life. Falls account for approximately 20 percent of restricted activity days in older people—more than for any other health condition. In addition to immediate curtailment of activity, older persons who have a fall injury may restrict activity for several months or longer after the injury because of residual physical impairment or because of fear of falling again. Fear of falling occurs in at least 50 percent of those who fall, and leads to restriction of activities in 10 to 25 percent. Finally, falls and fall injuries are a major determinant of nursing home placement.

ETIOLOGY OF FALLS AND FALL INJURIES

A fall occurs when a person's center of gravity moves over or outside of his or her base of support and insufficient, ineffective, or no effort is made to restore balance. Classification schemes have been developed to explain how falls occur. One such scheme classified falls according to cause, namely extrinsic, or as a consequence of slips, trips, and other environmental factors that perturbed balance; intrinsic, or as a consequence of deficits in balance, mobility, cognitive or sensory function; nonbipedal falls, such as falling out of bed; or nonclassifiable falls. Falls have also been classified by most likely immediate cause, including environmental factors, balance or gait disorder, drop attack, dizziness, or postural hypotension. However, while observation may suggest that one factor predominates, more often it is the interaction of multiple factors that results in a fall (Fig. 118-3). Intrinsic, personal characteristics, in conjunction with pharmacologic and behavioral factors, can alter resting balance or affect an older person's postural responses to challenges posed by the environment, or posed simply by movements such as transfers or walking.

Risk Factors for Falling
Age-Associated Changes and Chronic Disease

Prospective and retrospective community- and nursing home-based studies in the past 15 years have identified a number of factors that increase an older person's risk of

reducing falls. There have been no trials of interventions to improve vision, postural hypotension, or footwear as single factor interventions. Educational programs for older persons about fall risk factor modification have not been effective by themselves in preventing falls.

Multifactorial Interventions

Several studies employing a multidisciplinary, multifactorial approach to risk factor reduction in community-dwelling older persons have been published, and more are being completed. Effective components of these studies include exercise programs, reduction in the number and dosage of medications, treatment of postural hypotension and other cardiovascular disorders, and treatment of visual impairment. One strategy that has been successful has been a combination of assessment and treatment in the home by a nurse, and/or a physical or occupational therapist, and medical risk factor assessment and treatment in an outpatient office setting. Modifications of the home environment to improve home safety as part of a multifactorial intervention have been of equivocal or no efficacy. None of the intervention studies has had enough participants to show a reduction in fall injuries.

Strategy for Decreasing Falls and Fall Injuries

The most effective fall-prevention programs require coordination of efforts by several health care disciplines to treat the older person who is at risk for falls. The strategy is first to screen for fall risk, and then to perform a thorough assessment and create a treatment plan for those who are likely to fall in the future.

Screen for Fall Risk

All older persons seen for routine medical care should be screened for fall risk by asking, at least once a year, if they have fallen. They should be observed getting up from a chair and walking across a room for difficulty with the activity, unsteadiness, or use of an assistive device. If there is no history of falls and no problem with balance, mobility, or gait, then no specific fall risk assessment is necessary (Fig. 118-5). However, in all healthy older adults, routine vision and hearing screening, regular review and reduction, when possible, of medications, screening for and treatment of osteoporosis, exercise prescription, and discussion of home safety, can aid fall prevention.

Multifactorial Assessment

If there is a history of one or more falls, or if the person has problems with mobility or gait, then a more detailed fall risk assessment is warranted (see Fig. 118-5). Other potentially high-risk times are during acute illness, after hospital or emergency department discharge, or after introduction of new medications. Determination of risk factors for falls is within the capability of the primary care provider; it requires a systematic approach and a plan of treatment that often requires coordination among several different specialties and disciplines. Referral to a geriatric specialist with resources to coordinate multidisciplinary care may be the most effective way to accomplish fall risk assessment and treatment. The assessment should include history taking and medication review, physical examination, including physical performance testing, and, when indicated, assessment of the home environment. It is important to look for all possible contributing factors, as the concept of risk reduction is to treat as many factors as possible to lessen the likelihood of a fall.

The medical history should focus on information about physical function, mobility, use of an assistive device such as a cane or walker, performance of activities of daily living, previous falls and fractures, and acute or chronic medical problems. If the person has fallen, details of fall circumstances, including setting and activity at the time of the fall, can help determine specific risk factors for future falls. A list should be made of the dose and frequency of all medications that the older person actually takes, including over-the-counter medications. This can be done by "brown bag" review of medications in the office, or, if the older person is eligible for visiting nurse services, by a nurse in the home.

Aspects of the physical examination that pertain to fall risk are checking blood pressure lying and standing after 3 minutes, pulse (looking for cardiac arrhythmias and appropriate response to positional change), hearing and visual acuity screening, examination of joints for range of motion and evidence of arthritis, and of the feet for deformity and painful lesions. A neurologic examination should be done, including mental status testing, cranial and peripheral nerve function, reflexes, muscle strength, and cerebellar and sensory function. Tests of functional gait and balance maneuvers during usual activities should be part of a fall risk assessment (Table 118-3). The Timed Up and Go Test can be done in less than 1 minute in an office setting, and has high sensitivity and specificity in predicting fall risk. Other measures, such as the Performance-Oriented Mobility Assessment, give more specific information about balance, gait, and mobility impairment, but take longer to perform and are best used for assessment prior to a rehabilitative program. Laboratory testing is determined by the history and physical examination, and may include a complete blood count, fasting blood glucose, electrolytes, blood urea nitrogen (BUN) and creatinine, thyroid-stimulating hormone (TSH), B_{12} level, and levels of medications such as digoxin and anticonvulsants. Testing for osteoporosis will determine the need for medication to improve bone density and therefore reduce risk of fracture. Radiographs, such as cervical spine films, and computed tomography or magnetic resonance imaging of the brain, are only indicated if diseases that would be diagnosed by these tests are suspected.

Multidisciplinary Treatment

Once the older person's risk factors for falls have been determined, an individually tailored, multidisciplinary treatment plan can be put in place. The key components of such a plan include one or more of the following: (1) exercise to improve deficits in balance, mobility, and strength;

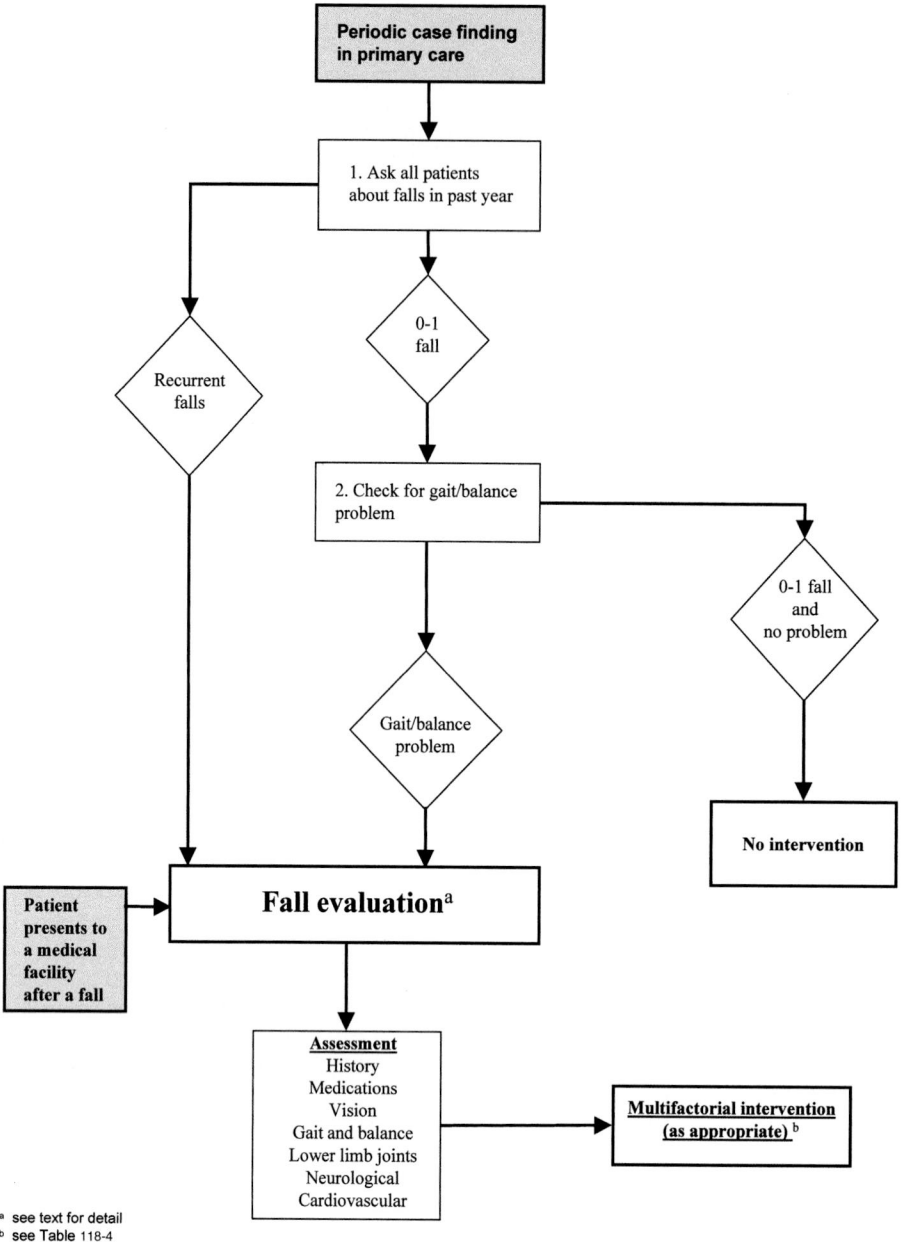

Figure 118-5 Algorithm summarizing screening, assessment, and management of falls. Modified with permission from Anonymous: Guideline for the prevention of falls in older persons. American Geriatrics Society, British Geriatrics Society, and American Academy of Orthopaedic Surgeons Panel on Falls Prevention. *J Am Geriatr Soc* 49:664, 2001.

(2) correction of sensory deficits (vision, hearing, vestibular and proprioceptive function); (3) evaluation and treatment of postural hypotension; (4) review and reduction of medications; (5) treatment of foot problems; and (6) environmental modification and use of adaptive equipment, if indicated. Table 118-4 summarizes possible interventions for factors that contribute to falling.

Physical therapy, with instruction in exercises to improve balance and mobility, is an important part of the fall-prevention strategy. Progressive exercises under the guidance of a physical therapist can help the older person improve confidence and reduce fear of falling. Older persons can also be taught how to get up from the floor in order to prevent a long lie as a result of a fall.

Other strategies for older persons with limited mobility include wearing an emergency call device in order to summon help or to have a telephone within reach in case of a fall. Treatment of osteoporosis can reduce the likelihood of a fracture with a fall. The use of hip protectors by persons with osteoporosis who are at risk for falls has been shown to dramatically reduce the incidence of hip fractures when they are worn (see "Hip Protectors" later in this chapter).

FALLS IN SKILLED NURSING FACILITIES

The general approach to fall-risk evaluation and treatment in nursing home residents is the same as with older people

Table 118-3 Observation of Position Changes, Balance Maneuvers, and Gait Components Used in Daily Activities that Indicate Fall Risk if Not Performed Adequately

Maneuver	Measure(s) in Which It Is a Component	Observation: Abnormality in Performance that Indicates Fall Risk
		Position Change or Balance Maneuver
Getting up from a chair*	A,B	Does not get up with single movement; pushes up with arms or moves forward in chair first; unsteady on first standing
Sitting down in a chair*	A,B	Plops in chair; does not land in center of chair
Withstanding pull back at waist	A	Moves feet; begins to fall backward; grabs object for support
Side-by-side standing with eyes open	A	Feet not touching side by side; moves feet; begins to lose balance or grabs object for support
Semitandem, tandem standing	C	Cannot maintain stances for 10 seconds (same as above)
Standing on one leg	A	Cannot maintain stance for 5 seconds (same as above)
Bending over	A	Unable to bend over to pick up small object (e.g., pen) from floor; grabs object to pull up on; requires multiple attempts to arise
Neck turning	C	Moves feet; grabs object for support; complains of vertigo, dizziness, or unsteadiness
		Gait Component or Maneuver
Gait initiation	A,B	Hesitates; stumbles; grabs object for support
Step height (raising feet with stepping)	A,B	Does not clear floor consistently (scrapes or shuffles); raises foot too high (more than 2 inches)
Step continuity	A,B	After first few steps, does not consistently begin raising one foot as other foot touches floor
Step symmetry	A,B	Step length not equal (pathologic side usually has longer step length—problem may be in hip, knee, ankle, or surrounding muscles)
Path deviation	A,B	Does not walk in straight line; weaves side-to-side
Turning	A,B	Stops before initiating turn, staggers; sways; grabs object for support
Stepping over obstacles	A	Unable to step over obstacles or loses balance
Gait speed	A	Unable to increase walking speed without losing balance
	B	Takes longer than 10 seconds to stand up from chair, walk 3 m, turn, walk back to chair and sit

Maneuvers that are components of physical performance tests are indicated as follows: A, Performance-Oriented Mobility Assessment; B, Timed Up and Go Test; C, other maneuvers.
*Use hard, armless chair.
SOURCE: Modified with permission from Tinetti ME and Ginter SF: Identifying mobility dysfunctions in elderly patients. *JAMA* 259:1190, 1988.

living in the community, although the relative importance of individual risk factors for falls in each setting differs. While most community-dwelling elderly persons have as their goal to increase function and maintain independence, nursing home residents and their family members and caregivers must weigh the risk of decreased safety that may accompany independent mobility, particularly as frailty increases. The focus of fall risk assessment and treatment

in skilled nursing facilities is to find the least-restrictive means by which the resident can move safely. Because it is less likely that personal risk factors due to age and chronic disease can be modified sufficiently to prevent falls, and because the opportunity for observation and supervision is greater in the nursing home setting, more emphasis should be placed on improving individual patient safety within the environment.

Table 118–4 Multidisciplinary Treatment of Factors Contributing to Fall Risk

Factor Contributing to Fall Risk	Treatment*
Age-Associated or Caused by Chronic Disease	
Impaired balance, gait, mobility	
Neurologic disease, with impaired strength, sensation, balance, gait, tone, and/or coordination	M: Diagnose and treat specific disease (e.g., Parkinson's disease, stroke, normal pressure hydrocephalus)
	R: Physical therapy; balance and gait training; correct walking aid
	E: Home safety assessment; appropriate adaptations (e.g., high, firm chairs, raised toilet seats, grab bars in bathroom)
Dementia, with impaired gait, apraxia	M: Diagnose and treat specific disease; minimize centrally acting medications
	R: Supervised exercise and walking
	S: Evaluate home safety; need for supervision
Musculoskeletal disease	M: Diagnose and treat specific diseases; referral to podiatry, if indicated, for foot care
Muscle weakness	
Arthritides with back/joint deformity causing postural instability	R: Physical therapy with muscle strengthening exercises, balance, and gait training; correct walking aid; correct footwear
Feet: pain, deformity	E: Home safety assessment; appropriate adaptations
Sensory impairment	
Vision: acuity, accommodation, contrast sensitivity	M: Referral for refraction; cataract extraction
	R: Balance and gait training
	E: Home safety assessment with attention to good lighting
Hearing: spatial disorientation, balance impairment, distorted environmental signals caused by decreased auditory input	M: Cerumen removal; audiologic evaluation with hearing aid if appropriate
Vestibular dysfunction: spatial disorientation at rest; balance impairment especially with head or body turning	M: Avoid vestibulotoxic drugs; surgical ablation
	R: Habituation exercises
	E: Good lighting (increased reliance on visual input); home safety assessment
Proprioceptive: cervical disorders; peripheral neuropathy; spatial disorientation during position changes or while walking on uneven surfaces or in dark	M: Diagnose and treat specific disease (e.g., spondylosis, B_{12} deficiency, diabetes mellitus)
	R: Physical therapy; balance and gait training; correct walking aid
	E: Good lighting (increased reliance on visual input); appropriate footwear; home safety assessment
Impaired perception or concentration	
Dementia: impaired judgment, problem solving	See "Dementia" above
Depression: poor concentration or awareness?	M: Watch for adverse medication effects
	E: Home safety assessment
Postural hypotension	
Impaired cerebral blood flow leading to fatigue, weakness, postural instability; syncope if severe	M: Diagnose and treat specific diseases; review medications and reduce/eliminate offending ones; adequate salt and water intake
	R: Graded pressure stockings; dorsiflexion and hand flexion exercises prior to arising

(Continued)

Table 118-4 (*Continued*) Multidisciplinary Treatment of Factors Contributing to Fall Risk

Factor Contributing to Fall Risk	Treatment*
Pharmacologic	
Total number and dose of medications Taking ≥4 medications	M: Regular review and reduction, when possible, of number and dose of medications, including nonprescription medications; consider nonpharmacologic treatments; start medications low and increase slowly
Specific medications Sedatives, antidepressants, neuroleptics, diuretics, antihypertensives, antiarrhythmics, anticholinergic medications	
Other Change in dose; new medications	
Situational and Environmental Factors	
Onset of acute illness	M: Diagnose and treat specific diseases; close supervision of mobility
Hospital or emergency department discharge	M: Review medications and doses; look for adverse effects of new medications; evaluate balance, mobility R: Physical therapy if indicated E: Home safety assessment S : Assess need for increased supervision
Risk-taking behavior	S: Assess need for increased supervision or community services R: Recommend avoiding only clearly hazardous and unnecessary activities (e.g., climbing on chairs); balance and gait training E: Home safety assessment
Environmental hazards	E: Home safety assessment

*E, environmental; M, medical; R, rehabilitative; S, social services/case management.

Evaluation

A careful assessment of risk factors for falls is important for all residents on admission, at yearly examinations, with a significant change in condition, or after a fall. The history may be difficult to obtain due to cognitive impairment, and may require input from family members or caregivers. Specific symptoms such as dizziness, foot or joint pain, weakness, or decreased sensation, if elicited, may indicate acute or chronic diseases that contribute to fall risk. As in community-dwelling older adults, the physical examination should include checking for postural changes in blood pressure, screening for cognitive, vision, and hearing impairment, examination of cardiovascular, musculoskeletal, and neurological systems, and examination of the feet. Tests of balance, transfers, and gait, and observation for proper use of assistive devices are also part of the evaluation. Laboratory testing may be of help in diagnosing or evaluating specific chronic diseases.

Pharmacologic and situational factors play a key role in fall risk in the nursing home. Risk assessment should include regular medication review and reduction, if possible. Medication use, particularly of psychotropic medications,

is an important contributor to fall risk in this setting, as this is a factor that potentially can be modified. Because of the prevalence of chronic disease, nursing home residents are likely to be on more than four medications, and may be less able to identify symptoms of adverse reactions to drugs, such as fatigue and dizziness, that increase risk of falling. Early recognition of acute illnesses, such as urinary tract infection or pneumonia which are likely to begin with symptoms of impaired cognition or mobility, can lead to treatment and preventive measures to keep the older person from falling.

After a fall, there may be greater opportunity to get accurate information about fall circumstances and to evaluate the resident because of closer supervision by health care professionals in this setting as compared to the community. Symptoms of dizziness may suggest postural hypotension or medication effect; symptoms or signs of acute infection, myocardial infarction, heart failure, or stroke may be elicited. The time and location of the fall may give clues as to the most effective intervention. A fall in the hallway after lunch may indicate postprandial hypotension; a fall in the bathroom near bedtime when nursing staff are helping other residents may indicate the need for scheduled toileting or greater supervision at that time. Examination of footwear and condition of assistive devices may also lead to interventions to prevent future falls.

Treatment

Multifactorial Approach

As in community fall prevention and risk reduction, a multifactorial approach is most effective in the nursing home setting; however, the risk factors targeted may be different. Because poor balance and decreased mobility are such important predictors of falls, interventions have been designed specifically to address these impairments. However, while studies have shown that it is possible to improve balance and strength with exercise in nursing home residents, these improvements have not resulted in fewer falls. Studies of other interventions to address single risk factors, such as psychotropic medication reduction, have not been done.

To date, there have been two randomized controlled trials of multifactorial risk reduction interventions. One demonstrated a significant reduction in the number of residents with recurrent falls and a trend toward fewer injurious falls, and the other a reduction in number of falls and hip fractures and an increase in time to first fall. The multidisciplinary interventions included education of patient care staff, ensuring environmental safety, fitting and repair of assistive devices, reduction of psychotropic medications, instruction in safe transfers and walking, exercise classes, and the use of hip protectors.

Maintaining a safe environment is of great importance in the nursing home setting, as environmental factors play a larger role in fall risk for patients with impaired mobility and cognition. Attention should be paid to floors, removing clutter and unstable furniture such as rolling tray tables, and lighting. Beds should be low enough so that the resident can sit with knees bent to 90 degrees and feet on the floor. Use of half-rails can improve safety and aid in transfers in and out of bed. Chairs should be firm, with arms. Bathrooms should be equipped with rails and, if appropriate, raised toilet seats.

Alternatives to Restraints

In the past decade, there have been widespread efforts to reduce the use of physical and chemical restraints and to find alternatives to prevent falls in nursing home residents. The use of restraints has not been shown to decrease the incidence of fall injuries. Bed and chair alarms to alert caregivers that residents are getting up are alternatives to restraints for fall prevention. Low beds and mats placed on the floor next to the bed reduce the risk of injury with a fall. Additional alternatives to restraint use to reduce fall risk include structured group activities to increase supervision of at-risk residents, scheduled toileting, particularly before and after meals, and attention to the safe use of assistive devices.

Hip Protectors

In the setting of a skilled nursing facility, ambulatory older persons at risk for falls also are likely to have osteoporosis. Treatment of risk factors for falls and osteoporosis are not sufficient to prevent all falls and fractures, particularly in residents who have low bone density. One option for treatment is the use of hip protectors, which attenuate the force of a fall on the hip. Those studied most extensively consist of foam or plastic pads placed inside pockets on a stretchy undergarment so that the protectors lie over the greater trochanter of each hip. The undergarment is designed to be fairly easy to wear without affecting walking or sitting. In a subgroup of three randomized controlled trials of hip protectors, the incidence of hip fractures was reduced by 76 percent in older persons in the intervention group, compared with controls. The use of hip protectors may also improve confidence and reduce fear of falling. However, compliance with hip protectors is problematic because of difficulty pulling the undergarment up or down for toileting, discomfort, poor fit, skin irritation, or lack of perceived risk for hip fracture.

HOSPITAL FALLS

Risk Factors

Patients at risk for falls in the hospital are those with chronic or acute cognitive impairment; weakness and difficulty with balance, transfers, or gait; need for frequent toileting because of urinary frequency, incontinence, or diarrhea; medication use; history of a previous fall at home or, more significantly, in the hospital; and age 65 years and older. Various assessment tools have been created to identify patients at risk for falls; however, these tools have not been demonstrated to be more accurate than clinical judgment in predicting falls.

Preventive Measures

There have been no randomized, controlled trials of interventions to reduce falls in the hospital, yet fall prevention has been a focus of hospitals and hospital regulatory agencies. Although there are no studies to support it, a multifactorial approach has been employed most commonly to reduce the risk for falls. Risk-reduction programs include education of staff, patients, and relatives about the risk of falling during hospitalization. Many include fall risk assessment and identification of persons at risk by some type of marker in the chart, on the patient's wristband, and/or in the patient's room. Strategies to address specific risk factors are used, such as physical therapy to improve gait and balance; scheduled toileting for those with elimination issues; use of low beds, half-rails on the bed, and nonskid footwear for patients with mobility problems; and increased supervision for patients with cognitive impairment. The use of physical restraints in acute care settings is

Table 118-5 Questions for Future Research on Fall Prevention

1. What is the cost-effectiveness of recommended strategies?
2. Can fall-prone individuals be risk stratified in terms of who will most benefit from assessment and interventions?
3. What are the effective elements for fall prevention among hospital inpatients?
4. How can falls best be prevented in patients with cognitive impairment and dementia?
5. What are the effective elements of exercise programs (such as type, duration, intensity, and frequency)?
6. What are the effective elements of cardiovascular programs for fall prevention?
7. For whom and when is home assessment by an occupational therapist or other home care specialist effective?
8. What is the effectiveness of assistive devices (e.g., canes and walkers/Zimmer frames) used alone as a strategy for preventing falls?
9. What is the effect of restraint removal, coupled with other specific interventions, on falls and serious injuries?
10. Does treatment of visual problems prevent falls?
11. What is the safest footwear for people who have fallen or are at risk of falling?
12. What is the role of hip protectors in persons who have fallen or are at risk of falling and what are the most effective designs?

SOURCE: Reproduced with permission from Anonymous: Guideline for the prevention of falls in older persons. American Geriatrics Society, British Geriatrics Society, and American Academy of Orthopaedic Surgeons Panel on Falls Prevention. *J Am Geriatr Soc* 49:664, 2001.

controversial. There is no evidence showing that restraints prevent falls in these patients.

AREAS FOR FUTURE RESEARCH

Although much is now known about falls and their consequences, there are still questions about what the best, most cost-effective interventions are to prevent falls and fall injuries. The recently-published "Guideline for the Prevention of Falls in Older Persons" listed 12 questions for future research (Table 118-5). Within the current US health care system, care is not coordinated among different providers and disciplines and is aimed more at treatment rather than prevention of disease. Given these constraints, studies need to be done of fall prevention in community practice settings. Research studies of interventions that have been successful generally have targeted older persons at risk for falling; yet more needs to be learned about who will benefit most from fall prevention efforts, particularly in nursing home and hospital settings. The most effective treatment of specific impairments, such as visual problems, dementia, and cardiovascular disease, to reduce falls remains untested. The role of assistive devices and the best design for footwear and hip protectors need to be determined.

CONCLUSION

Falls are common in older persons, and are costly in terms of injury, loss of function, and health care dollars. There is now evidence that multidisciplinary programs aimed at reducing multiple risks for falls are effective in preventing falls in a community research setting. The evidence is less compelling for nursing home and hospital falls. Screening for fall risk, careful assessment of older persons who have fallen or have mobility impairment, and oversight of an individualized, multidisciplinary risk reduction plan are important components of the care of geriatric patients.

REFERENCES

Anonymous: Guideline for the prevention of falls in older persons. American Geriatrics Society, British Geriatrics Society, and American Academy of Orthopaedic Surgeons Panel on Falls Prevention. *J Am Geriatr Soc* 49:664, 2001.

Gillespie LD et al: Interventions for preventing falls in elderly people (Cochrane Review). *The Cochrane Library,* Issue 4, 2001. Oxford: Update Software.

Jensen J et al: Fall and injury prevention in older people living in residential care facilities: A cluster randomized trial. *Ann Intern Med* 136:733, 2002.

Leipzig RM et al: Drugs and falls in older people: A systematic review and meta-analysis: I. Psychotropic drugs. *J Am Geriatr Soc* 47:30, 1999.

Leipzig RM et al: Drugs and falls in older people: A systematic review and meta-analysis: II. Cardiac and analgesic drugs. *J Am Geriatr Soc* 47:40, 1999.

Mahoney J et al: Risk of falls after hospital discharge. *J Am Geriatr Soc* 42:269, 1994.

National Center for Injury Prevention and Control, Centers for Disease Control and Prevention (CDC) web site at: http//www.cdc.gov/ncipc/.

National Safety Council web site at: http://www.nsc.org/issues/fallstop.htm.

Nevitt MC et al: Risk factors for recurrent nonsyncopal falls. A prospective study. *JAMA* 261:2663, 1989.

Oliver D et al: Do hospital fall prevention programs work? A systematic review. *J Am Geriatr Soc* 48:1679, 2000.

Parker MJ et al: Hip protectors for preventing hip fractures in the elderly (Cochrane Review). *The Cochrane Library,* Issue 4, 2001. Oxford: Update Software.

Perell KL et al: Fall risk assessment measures: An analytic review. *J Gerontol Med Sci* 56A:M761, 2001.

Podsiado D, Richardson S: The timed "Up & Go": A test of basic functional mobility for frail elderly persons. *J Am Geriatr Soc* 39:142, 1991.

Ray WA et al: A randomized trial of a consultation service to reduce falls in nursing homes. *JAMA* 278:557, 1997.

Rubenstein LZ et al: Falls in the nursing home. *Ann Intern Med* 121:442, 1994.

Tinetti ME et al: Risk factors for falls among elderly persons living in the community. *N Engl J Med* 319:1701, 1988.

Tinetti ME, Ginter SF: Identifying mobility dysfunctions in elderly patients. *JAMA* 259:1190, 1988.

Sleep Disorders

MAIRAV COHEN-ZION • SONIA ANCOLI-ISRAEL

Recent research has led to many new developments and a better understanding of healthy and abnormal sleep in the geriatric population. This chapter reviews normal age-related changes in sleep and common sleep disturbances that affect older adults. Each section reviews a sleep disorder and includes information on presentation, etiology, pathophysiology, evaluation, and management.

CHANGES IN SLEEP WITH AGING

Approximately 50 percent of community-dwelling elderly persons complain of some form of sleep difficulty. Subjective and objective reports show that when compared to their younger counterparts, older adults take longer to fall asleep, have lower sleep efficiency (defined as the amount of sleep given the amount of time in bed), have more nighttime awakenings, wake up earlier than they would like in the morning, and require more daytime naps (Table 119-1). Polysomnographic sleep recordings have confirmed that there is a significant reduction in slow wave sleep and rapid eye-movement (REM) sleep with older age. Multiple sleep latency tests (MSLTs), which are objective measures that assess daytime sleepiness, indicate that older adults are significantly sleepier throughout the day than are younger adults.

One central question raised by researchers in the field is whether these age-related changes represent a decrease in the need for sleep or a decrease in the ability to sleep. Although this question is still being debated and there is no clear consensus on whether there is a reduced need for sleep, there is clearly a reduced ability to sleep in this population. As discussed in this chapter, sleep difficulties in this population are associated with several factors, including specific sleep disorders, changes in the endogenous circadian clock, medical and psychiatric illness, and medication intake (Table 119-2). Recent developments in sleep research have identified several effective treatments for many of these sleep difficulties. Given the high prevalence of sleep complaints and sleep disorders in this population, there is a clear need for increased awareness, assessment, and treatment of these sleep disturbances.

SLEEP-DISORDERED BREATHING

Definition

Sleep-disordered breathing (SDB) is characterized by respiratory events, including hypopneas (partial respiration) and/or apneas (complete cessation of respiration), during sleep. These respiratory events occur repeatedly over the course of the night with each respiratory event lasting a minimum of 10 seconds. The number of apneas per hour of sleep is called the apnea index (AI), the number of hypopneas per hour of sleep is called the hypopnea index (HI), and the number of apneas and hypopneas per hour of sleep is called the respiratory disturbance index (RDI). Clinical diagnosis of SDB is traditionally given when a patient has an RDI of 10 to 15.

The cessations in breathing in SDB lead to repeated arousals from sleep, as well as to reductions in blood oxygen levels over the course of the night, which result in nighttime hypoxemia.

Epidemiology

SDB is more common in older than younger adults. Table 119-3 summarizes several potential age-dependent risk factors in the development of SDB. The prevalence of SDB is approximately 4 to 9 percent in middle-aged men and women (age 30 to 60 years), compared to 45 to 62 percent in older adults (age 60+ years). In addition, within the older population, SDB is more common in men than in women and in patients with hypertension. Some research suggests that SDB is more severe in older African Americans than in older whites.

Pathophysiology

There are three types of apneic events: central, obstructive, and mixed. Central events are a result of a dysfunction of the respiratory neurons. Obstructive events are caused by anatomic obstruction of the upper airways despite

Table 119-1 Subjective and Objective Complaints of Older Adults

Subjective	Objective
Spend too much time in bed	Decrease in delta (stages 3 and 4) sleep
Spend less time asleep	Decrease in rapid eye-movement sleep
Increase in number of awakenings	Significant increase in awakenings
Increase in time to fall asleep	Increase in frequency of sleep disorders/problems
Less satisfied with sleep	Reduced sleep efficiency
More tired during the day	Significant increase in daytime sleepiness
Napping more often and longer	Increase in number of naps

respiratory effort. Mixed events are a combination of central and obstructive components.

Presentation

The cardinal symptoms of SDB are snoring and excessive daytime sleepiness. It is often one or both of these two symptoms that brings the patient to seek evaluation and treatment of this sleep disorder.

The snoring is reflective of the airway collapse and is a component of the breathing cessation during an apneic event. It may be extremely loud, being heard all over the house. Often bed partners have moved into separate bedrooms. While not all snoring is associated with sleep apnea, snoring alone is associated with increased risk of ischemic heart disease and stroke.

The excessive daytime sleepiness in SDB is associated with both repeated nighttime awakenings, which

Table 119-2 Causes of Sleep Disturbances in Older Adults

Circadian rhythm changes
Primary sleep disturbances (e.g., SDB, PLMS, RBD)
Medical illness (e.g., hyperthyroidism, arthritis)
Psychiatric illness (e.g., depression, anxiety disorders)
Multiple medications, alcohol, caffeine
Dementia
Poor sleep hygiene habits

PLMS, periodic leg movements in sleep; REM, rapid eye-movement behavior disorder; SDB, sleep-disordered breathing.

Table 119-3 Potential Age-Dependent Risk Factors in SDB

Increased body mass index (central obesity)
Decreased muscle tension
Changes in airway anatomy
Increased airway collapsibility
Decreased thyroid function
Decreased lung volume

frequently follow the apneic events, and with the hypoxia. Daytime sleepiness may manifest as being unable to stay awake during the day or falling asleep at inappropriate times during the day. Patients with excessive daytime sleepiness secondary to SDB may fall asleep while reading, watching television, or at the movies, while in conversation with a group of friends, or while driving. Daytime sleepiness can be a very debilitating symptom, causing social and occupational difficulties, reduced vigilance, and cognitive deficits, including decreased concentration, slowed response time, and memory and attention difficulties. These symptoms may be particularly relevant to older adults who are at an increased risk of developing such symptoms with aging. SDB may unnecessarily further exacerbate these cognitive deficits.

SDB is often associated with other serious health problems, including hypertension and cardiac and pulmonary problems, which can then lead to increased risk of mortality. While cause and effect has not yet been determined, treating the SDB reduces the severity of the hypertension and heart disease, and reduces the risk of shorter survival. Recent research indicates that even those patients with only five events per hour of sleep are at greater risk for developing hypertension.

Patients with SDB are often overweight. While obesity may be less of an issue in the older population, body mass index (the ratio of weight to height) is the best predictor of the presence or absence of SDB. Nevertheless, the presence of SDB should not be overlooked in the older patient of normal or even slender weight.

Upon initial evaluation, sleep complaints such as snoring and/or gasping and excessive daytime sleepiness may be suggestive of SDB. The assessment should begin with a thorough sleep history from the patient, including information on daytime behavior. Because the patient is often unaware (or not disturbed) by the loud snoring or cessations in breathing during the night, it is helpful to have the patient's bed partner present at the assessment interview. The clinician should examine the patient's airway and throat to check for obstruction of the airway. It is important that the medical history include information on history of hypertension and any cardiac or pulmonary problems. The clinician should also collect information on recent weight gain or obesity (excess fatty tissue may contribute to airway obstruction), smoking history (may irritate oropharynx and/or nicotine may affect central nervous system), alcohol intake, and intake of any sedating medications (may result in airway relaxation thus facilitating obstruction).

If the clinician suspects SDB, the patient should be referred for an overnight polysomnographic (PSG) recording in a sleep disorders clinic, or for ambulatory monitoring in the patient's home. Based on the results of the objective recording, recommendations for treatment can be suggested.

Management

Most pharmacologic treatments for SDB are ineffective; however, there are several effective nonpharmacologic treatments that have become first-line treatment of SDB.

Positive Airway Pressure

The most common treatment for SDB is positive airway pressure. The are several types of devices that provide positive airway pressure, including continuous positive airway pressure (CPAP), bilevel positive airway pressure (BiPAP), and auto-CPAP. CPAP is composed of a nose mask, which is connected via a hose to a machine that provides continuous air pressure . The air pressure acts as a splint to maintain the opening of the upper airway, thereby preventing the obstruction or collapse of the airway. The degree of air pressure (traditionally, 5 to 20 cm H_2O) is set individually for each patient at the sleep laboratory and is dependent on the patient's RDI or the severity of the patient's SDB. CPAP alleviates all snoring and most of the apneic events, repeated awakenings, and nighttime hypoxemia in these patients. This intervention is also very effective in the reduction of daytime sleepiness.

BiPAP was designed to allow for the variation in positive airway pressure during expiration and inspiration. The device looks and acts similarly to CPAP but rather than providing continuous airway pressure, the BiPAP device has reduced expiratory positive airway pressure (EPAP) when compared to the inspiratory positive airway pressure (IPAP). The BiPAP prevents the obstruction of the airway by using lower EPAP levels when compared to CPAP. At this time, there are no data to suggest that BiPAP is more effective than CPAP, however some reports suggest better compliance with BiPAP when compared to CPAP.

The auto-CPAP was designed to allow for the overnight variability in airway pressure, which is adjusted automatically depending on the extent of airway obstruction. In contrast to the constant airway pressure in traditional CPAP, this device adjusts for periods of reduced obstruction by providing lower airway pressure, while providing greater airway pressure with increases in obstruction. To date, no studies suggest increases in compliance with the auto-CPAP when compared to other positive airway pressure devices.

Clinicians should be aware of possible poor patient compliance, however, as these devices are recommended for nightly use and are a long-term management approach. The addition of a humidifier to some units reduces the discomfort and possible nasal irritation sometimes associated with the use of these devices.

Surgical Interventions

There are several different surgical approaches for the treatment of SDB, including (1) nasal reconstruction which corrects nasal valve collapse, septal deviations, and turbinate hypertrophy; (2) uvulopharynpalatoplasty (UPPP) which corrects pharyngeal obstruction by removal of pharyngeal tissue, including soft palate, uvula, tonsillar pillars, and tonsillar tissue; (3) laser-assisted uvulopharynpalatoplasty (LAUP), which has the same standard procedure as UPPP, but uses a laser to remove the pharyngeal tissue; (4) genioglossus advancement, which corrects by the forward advancement of the insertion of the tongue (usually in conjunction with UPPP or LAUP); and (5) hyoid myotomy, which corrects hypopharyngeal obstruction by suspending the hyoid bone to the superior edge of the larynx (usually in conjunction with UPPP or LAUP).

The surgical approach or combination of approaches (including nonsurgical) chosen for an individual patient is decided on a case-by-case basis and is dependent on the location and the type of obstruction present. Depending on the choice of surgical approach, the effectiveness of the intervention in reducing RDI varies from 48 to 72 percent and depends on the severity of the SDB and the obstruction.

Oral Appliances

Oral devices are appropriate for the management of milder forms of obstructive sleep apnea and snoring. The two most common oral devices are the tongue retaining device (TRD) and the mandibular advancement device (MAD). These oral appliances are anchored on the patient's teeth or gums and work by moving the tongue or the mandibular forward, thereby preventing obstruction at the hypopharyngeal level. Depending on the type of device used, the effectiveness of this approach in decreasing RDI and increasing blood oxygen saturation levels varies from 40 to 81 percent. Clinicians need to be aware of possible side effects, including pain or discomfort in the temporomandibular joint or short-term occlusion abnormalities when removing the appliance, which occurs in an estimated 30 percent of patients. Newer devices can be used with dentures, which makes them particularly appropriate for use in the older patient.

Diet and Lifestyle

There are several dietary and lifestyle factors that can exacerbate SDB, such as obesity, alcohol intake, and smoking. Obesity is a common problem in patients with obstructive sleep apnea, as the additional fatty tissue often results in the obstruction of the upper airways. These patients will benefit significantly from weight loss, which sometimes dramatically reduces or even eliminates apneic events.

Alcohol and certain medications, such as sedative-hypnotics, narcotics, and barbiturates, have a depressant effect on the upper airway musculature and may exacerbate SDB. Furthermore, given the usually high number of prescriptions taken by older patients, clinicians should be diligent when prescribing sedating medications, particularly to those older patients who are at higher risk for SDB.

Smoking is also associated with exacerbation of SDB. Although the mechanism is not fully understood at this time, several theories have been suggested, including irritation of oropharynx by cigarette smoke and the possible effect of nicotine on the central nervous system.

Finally, for patients with mild SDB, positional SDB, or positional snoring, body position during sleep may account for many of the respiratory events in these cases. The supine position is associated with the majority of the positional apneic events, which are likely a result of the relaxation of the anterior neck and oropharyngeal structures while in this position. A simple behavioral technique for dealing with positional apnea is to place a tennis ball in a pocket sewn to the back of a night shirt, thereby deterring the patient from sleeping on his or her back and preventing positional respiratory events.

PERIODIC LIMB MOVEMENTS IN SLEEP

Definition

Periodic limb movements in sleep (PLMS) is characterized by clusters of repeated leg (or sometimes arm) jerks that occur approximately every 20 to 40 seconds over the course of the night. These clusters of movements last on average 0.5 to 5 seconds and cause repeated brief awakenings. The number of limb movements followed by arousals per hour of sleep is called the periodic limb movement index (PLMI). Clinical diagnosis of PLMS is typically given when a patient has a PLMI >5.

Another disorder, often comorbid with PLMS, is restless leg syndrome (RLS). RLS is characterized by dysesthesia in the legs, usually described by patients as "a creeping crawling sensation" or as "pins and needles," which can only be relieved with vigorous movement. These sensations often occur in the evening or whenever the patient is in a restful, relaxed state.

Epidemiology

The prevalence of PLMS increases significantly with age. The prevalence of PLMS in older adults is estimated at 45 percent, compared to 5 to 6 percent in younger adults. There is no gender difference. Most patients with RLS also suffer from PLMS. In addition, PLMS may be comorbid with SDB.

Pathophysiology

The exact mechanisms underlying PLMS are not fully understood; however, current hypotheses suggest possible dysfunction of the dopamine and/or the opiate system. These theories are derived from the therapeutic effects of dopamine agonists and opiates in RLS and PLMS.

Presentation

The most common complaints of patients with PLMS are sleep initiation insomnia, sleep maintenance insomnia, and excessive daytime sleepiness. Patients may or may not be aware of leg kicks or jerks. Some may complain simply of having difficulty falling asleep or staying asleep with no knowledge that they kick. Often, bed partners may be aware of the leg movements and may have moved into separate beds.

As many patients with PLMS also suffer from RLS, patients may also complain of discomforting sensations in their legs during the day. Clinicians should assess patients with symptoms of RLS for anemia, uremia, and peripheral neuropathy prior to treatment.

Evaluation

Patients are often unaware of the multiple nighttime awakenings and the associated sleep loss, therefore is it often helpful to have the patient's bed partner present at the assessment interview. An accurate diagnosis of PLMS can only be made with a very clear report of leg movements or by recording limb movements and associated arousals. This can be accomplished via an overnight polysomnographic recording in the sleep disorders laboratory, or in the home with unattended monitoring. Additionally, several actigraph devices, placed on the ankle, have been validated against PSG for measurement of PLMS.

Management

Several pharmacologic treatments for PLMS target the leg movements and/or the associated arousals (Table 119-4). Benzodiazepines (e.g., clonazepam, temazepam) work by decreasing the number of arousals, but do not significantly reduce the number of limb movements. Benzodiazepines are contraindicated in patients with SDB; as PLMS is often comorbid with SDB, clinicians should be cautious when prescribing benzodiazepines. Clinicians should also be aware of possible daytime sedation resulting from these longer-acting medications. In contrast, opiate agents (e.g., codeine, propoxyphene hydrochloride) inhibit most leg jerks but do not eliminate all arousals. These agents may also have a beneficial effect on the dysesthesia in RLS. Carbidopa/levodopa (a dopaminergic agent) is effective in reducing both the limb jerks and the associated arousals. However, shifting of limb movements from the nighttime to the daytime may occur.

Currently, the first-line treatment for PLMS is either pergolide or pramipexole, as they both reduce or eliminate both the limb jerks and the associated arousals without shifting the rhythm of the leg movements.

CIRCADIAN RHYTHMS SLEEP DISORDERS

Definition

Circadian rhythms refer to 24-hour biological rhythms that control many physiologic functions, such as endogenous hormone secretions, core body temperature, and the sleep–wake cycle. These rhythms originate in the suprachiasmatic nucleus (SCN) in the anterior hypothalamus, which houses

Table 119-4 Pharmacologic Treatments of Periodic Leg Movements in Sleep

Class	Generic	Brand	Dose	Intake (Before Bedtime)
Benzodiazepines	Clonazepam	Klonopin	0.25–2 mg	30–60 minutes
	Tempazepam	Restoril	15–30 mg	30–60 minutes
Opiate agents	Codeine	Tylenol #3/#4	30–60 mg (codeine)	30–60 minutes
	Propoxyphene hydrochloride	Darvon	65–135 mg	30–60 minutes
Dopaminergic agents	Carbidopa/levodopa	Sinemet	25/100–25/250 mg	30–60 minutes
	Pergolide	Permax	0.05–0.25 mg	30–60 minutes
	Pramipexole	Mirapex	0.25–0.75 mg	30–60 minutes

the internal circadian pacemaker. Circadian rhythms are synchronized to the 24-hour day by other internal rhythms, as well as by external zeitgebers (literally time-givers or cues) such as light. The sleep–wake cycle is primarily synchronized by internal rhythms, such as core body temperature and the endogenous melatonin cycle, and the external light/dark rhythm, which asserts its effect on the sleep–wake cycle via the retinohypothalamic visual pathway. For example, as core body temperature drops, individuals get sleepy; as core body temperature rises, individuals wake up.

As people age, the sleep–wake circadian rhythm becomes less synchronized to external cues; that is, the rhythms may no longer have the same response to the external cues. In addition, with age, the sleep–wake circadian rhythm becomes much weaker (less robust), thus the periods of sleep–wake are less consistent across the 24-hour day.

Another circadian rhythm change in older age is the shifting, or advancing, of the sleep/wake cycle. This circadian rhythm disorder is called advanced sleep phase syndrome (ASPS), a condition in which the sleep–wake rhythm and the core body temperature rhythm are advanced, as compared to those of younger adults. Older adults with ASPS get sleepy in the early evening and wake up in the early morning hours, in part because the core body temperature is dropping earlier in the evening (perhaps at about 7:00 P.M. or 8:00 P.M.) and rising about eight hours later, at about 3:00 A.M. or 4:00 A.M.

Epidemiology

Prevalence of ASPS is approximately 1 percent in middle-aged adults. Although the prevalence in older adults is known to increase, the exact percentage has not been established. This may be partly because these patients have learned to function with the changes in their circadian clocks, and therefore do not present for treatment.

Pathophysiology

Changes in the sleep–wake cycle are likely caused by changes in the core body temperature cycle, in decreased light exposure, and to environmental factors. More recent research suggests there may also be a genetic component.

Presentation

The most common complaints of patients with ASPS are being sleepy early in the evening and waking up too early in the morning. If patients with ASPS went to bed as their core body temperature was dropping, for example, around 7:00 P.M. or 8:00 P.M., they would have little difficulty falling asleep and would sleep for a full night, about 8 hours. As explained above, that would result in their waking up somewhere between 3:00 A.M. and 4:00 A.M. An additional problem results when these patients, although sleepy, do not go to bed until later in the evening, but continue to awaken early in the morning, thus not being in bed long enough to get a full night's sleep. This significant sleep loss can result in daytime sleepiness, often resulting in daytime naps.

The weakening of the circadian rhythm in older age may also result in increased awakenings during the night.

Evaluation

As symptoms of ASPS are very similar to symptoms of sleep-maintenance insomnia, clinicians may have difficulty distinguishing between the two disorders. To implement the correct treatment, appropriate evaluation is imperative. When assessing for ASPS, the clinician should obtain an extensive sleep history (Table 119-5) and at least 1 to 2 weeks of sleep diaries, which can be sent to the patient several weeks prior to their treatment. If possible, the patient should also wear a wrist actigraph from several days to 1 week, allowing for the objective examination of the shifting of the sleep–wake cycle. If these assessments suggest early evening sleepiness and early evening bedtimes along with early morning awakenings, the clinician should suspect ASPS.

Management

As shifting of the circadian rhythm is a common and expected development in older age, patients should be educated that ASPS is not a medical disorder and does not necessarily need to be treated. Treatment is dependent on the extent of the discomfort the ASPS has on the day-to-day life of the patient. Patients often complain that their waking hours are no longer consistent with societal norms,

Table 119-5 Sample Sleep Diary

Name: _____					Date: _____ to _____		
	Monday	Tuesday	Wednesday	Thursday	Friday	Saturday	Sunday
1. Bed time							
2. Time taken to fall asleep (after lights off)							
3. Number of nighttime awakenings							
4. Wake-up time							
5. Time out of bed (morning)							
6. Total sleep time (night only)							
7. Total wake time (night only)							
8. Nap time (if any)							
9. Medication (time/dosage)							
10. Alcohol (time/dosage)							
11. How was your sleep last night?*							
12. How tired were you in the morning?**							

*1 = excellent to 5 = very poor; **1 = not tired to 5 = very tired.

causing them to be awake (or asleep) when those around them are not.

Nonpharmacologic therapies are the treatment of choice in patients with ASPS, particularly bright-light therapy.

Bright-Light Therapy

As bright light is the most influential external zeitgeber on the sleep–wake circadian rhythm, it is not surprising that it is also the most appropriate and effective treatment for circadian rhythm disturbances. By increasing light exposure during specific times of the day, it is possible to advance or delay the sleep–wake circadian rhythm. Specifically, exposure to bright light in the early morning will advance the rhythm (i.e., patient will become sleepier earlier), whereas exposure to bright light in the late afternoon or early evening will delay the rhythm (i.e., patient will become sleepier later in the day allowing them to stay alert longer). Exposure to bright light will not only shift the sleep–wake circadian rhythm but will also shift related rhythms such as core body temperature and endogenous melatonin.

Older persons are exposed to significantly less bright light than their younger counterparts. Reports show that healthy older adults receive on average only 60 minutes of bright light a day (>2000 lux), whereas elderly demented patients living in the community receive on average 30 minutes of bright light a day (>2000 lux), and demented nursing home patients receive on average no light >2000 lux and only 10 minutes of bright light a day >1000 lux.

To delay the advanced sleep–wake rhythm, patients with ASPS should be exposed to bright light (minimum >2500 lux) for approximately 2 hours a day during the late afternoon to early evening. The best source of bright light is sunlight, therefore patients should attempt to spend time outdoors in the late afternoon. Because the mechanism of the light is primarily through the eyes, sunglasses should not be worn. However, sunglasses should be worn in the morning hours to avoid having rhythms advance even more. Normal room light is not generally bright enough to shift rhythms. Therefore, if the patient is unable to spend 2 hours a day outdoors, another option is a special commercially available "light box," which provides a minimum of 2500 lux light exposure.

Melatonin

Melatonin is an endogenous hormone secreted primarily at night by the pineal gland. The secretion of melatonin is in part stimulated by darkness and inhibited by light, and is thus synchronized with the sleep–wake circadian rhythm.

Melatonin secretion decreases gradually with age, which may be an important element in the development of disturbed sleep and shifted rhythms in this population. Melatonin has been shown to appropriately synchronize the sleep–wake circadian rhythms as well as promote good quality sleep in several populations suffering from inappropriately synchronized rhythms, such as blind persons and persons suffering from jet lag. Currently, melatonin replacement therapy is being explored as a treatment for ASPS. Clinicians should be cautious when recommending melatonin for use on a regular basis. Although there are no reports to date of any significant long-term side effects of melatonin, longitudinal studies remain too brief to make any definite conclusions at this time. Moreover, melatonin is considered an nutritional supplement and is not regulated by the Food and Drug Administration. Therefore, there are no clear guidelines for correct timing and dosage of melatonin, and no management of the exact composition, purity, or dosage of melatonin sold over-the-counter.

REM SLEEP BEHAVIOR DISORDER

Definition

REM behavior disorder (RBD) is characterized by a dissociated state during which complex motoric behaviors occur, most likely resulting from an intermittent lack of skeletal muscle atonia that is typically present during REM sleep. RBD usually occurs during the second half of the night, when REM is more prevalent. Nighttime behaviors in RBD include vigorous and complex body movements and actions, such as walking, talking, and eating.

Epidemiology

The prevalence of RBD is unknown. However, recent reports suggest elderly men may be at higher risk for developing RBD.

Pathophysiology

To date the etiology of RBD remains unknown. Some reports suggest that acute RBD is associated with the intake of tricyclic antidepressants, fluoxetine, and monoamine oxidase inhibitors, and withdrawal from alcohol or sedatives. In contrast, chronic RBD has been associated with narcolepsy, and other idiopathic neurodegenerative disorders, such as dementia and Parkinson's disease.

Presentation

Patients engage in complex motoric behaviors over the course of the night and may be unable to recollect these actions in the morning. Patients' recollections of their dreams suggest these nighttime activities and movements may be the acting out of patient dreams, made possible by the lack of muscle atonia during REM sleep. Movements may be violent and may harm the patient and/or the patient's bed partner.

Evaluation

Assessment of RBD should include a complete sleep history. Because patients may be unaware of their behaviors over the course of the night, bed partners should also be interviewed. Clinicians should acquire a simultaneous overnight PSG and video recording of nighttime behavior in order to examine whether there is a link between REM sleep and the complex behaviors exhibited by the patients. When examining the PSG, clinicians should be attentive to any marked elevations in muscle tone and/or limb movements in the electromyogram (EMG) recording, specifically during REM sleep, when such features are normally rare.

Management

Pharmacologic Interventions

To date there have been only a few reports of pharmacologic treatments for RBD, with promising initial results. Currently, clonazepam is the most prescribed pharmacologic treatment for RBD. Clonazepam acts by inhibiting nighttime motoric movements, without directly affecting muscle tone. It has been shown to result in cessation (partial or complete) of abnormal body movements during the night in 90 percent of RBD patients. If the medication is stopped, all symptoms return. Patients may complain of excessive daytime sleepiness because of this drug's long half-life. If clonazepam is contraindicated, several alternative drugs have shown some positive effects in RBD, including tricyclic antidepressants and dopaminergic agents.

Lifestyle

Clinicians should educate RBD patients and their bed partners on making changes in bedtime/sleeping routines and environment, in order to make the bedroom safer and to decrease the potential for injurious behavior during the night. For example, heavy curtains should be placed on bedroom windows, and doors and windows should be locked at night if there is risk of the patient wandering out of bed during the night and engaging in complex behaviors. If the patient is extremely active or violent during the night, heavy or breakable objects should be removed or from the vicinity of the bed, and if needed, patients may want to sleep on a mattress placed on the floor to avoid falling off the bed and/or hurting themselves or their bed partners.

INSOMNIA

Definition

Insomnia is a complaint of low quantity and/or poor quality sleep, resulting in a sense of nonrestorative sleep. There are several different types of insomnia, including sleep onset insomnia (an inability to initiate sleep), sleep maintenance insomnia (an inability to maintain sleep throughout the night), early morning insomnia (awakening early in the morning with an inability to return to sleep), and pathophysiologic insomnia (behaviorally conditioned insomnia associated with maladaptive cognitions and/or behaviors). Although older adults can suffer from any of the types of insomnia, the most common complaints in the elderly are of sleep maintenance insomnia and early morning insomnia.

Insomnia is also classified based on the length of time the complaint has persisted, with transient insomnia lasting only a few days prior to or during a brief stressful experience, short-term insomnia lasting a few weeks during an extended period of stress and adjustment, and chronic insomnia last several months to years, which may have begun following a discrete event, but lasted even after the antecedent event is no longer relevant. In many cases of chronic insomnia, the inability to sleep may have become a conditioned response and may be associated with poor sleep hygiene.

Epidemiology

The prevalence of insomnia is greater in older than younger adults. Approximately 40 to 50 percent of older adults complain of chronic sleep onset or sleep maintenance insomnia, with women reporting more insomnia than men.

Pathophysiology

There are multiple factors that may play a causal role in the development of insomnia. Insomnia is often secondary to medical, psychiatric, or psychosocial conditions, and/or to the treatment of these conditions. Medical illnesses common in the elderly population, such as arthritis, cardiovascular disease, pulmonary disease, chronic pain disorders, and other illnesses associated with physical discomforts, are often antecedents for insomnia. Major life changes, such as retirement and death of loved ones, can also lead to insomnia. These psychosocial and environmental factors may cause or exacerbate psychiatric and/or sleep difficulties. Depression and anxiety disorders are therefore some of the most common causes for sleep disturbances in the elderly person.

Pharmacologic treatments for such conditions often exert either a sedating or alerting effect (Table 119-6). These alerting or stimulating drugs, when taken late in the day, may cause difficulty falling asleep at night. On the other hand, sedating drugs taken early in the day may lead to excessive daytime sleepiness and daytime napping behavior, which may contribute to sleep onset insomnia or may further exacerbate and maintain the existing insomnia.

Presentation

Complaints of insomnia may vary significantly from patient to patient. Apart from the inability to sleep at various periods of the night (early, middle, or late), patients often complain of excessive daytime sleepiness leading to daytime napping and decreased mental functioning.

Table 119-6 Effect of Common Drugs Taken by Older Adults

Sedating	Alerting
Hypnotics	Alcohol
	Nicotine
Antihypertensives	Central nervous system stimulants
Antihistamines	Thyroid hormone
Tranquilizers	Bronchodilators
Antidepressants	Corticosteroids
	Beta-blockers
	Calcium channel blockers

Evaluation

As detailed above, insomnia is usually a symptom of another underlying problem, such as medical, psychiatric, or psychosocial, but is usually not a sleep disorder in itself. The best approach to the treatment of insomnia is to first assess the cause of the complaint. Evaluation of insomnia should begin with a thorough medical, psychiatric, and sleep assessment, and a review of recent medication intake (including time of medication ingestion). The clinician should also request 1 to 2 weeks of sleep diaries in order to obtain an exact description of the nature of the insomnia. In addition, the clinician needs to collect information on the characteristics, onset, duration, and severity of the insomnia, as well as on any factors that may contribute to the sleep condition, such as sleep hygiene practices, diet, alcohol intake, and smoking history.

Management

If the insomnia is clearly caused in response to another primary condition, that condition should be treated first to see if the insomnia subsides following treatment. If no primary condition can be identified, or if there is no change in the insomnia following the treatment of the primary condition, there are several behavioral and pharmacologic interventions and lifestyle changes that may aid in the management of the insomnia. Overall, given the high prevalence of medication prescribed for this population, clinicians should attempt to implement behavioral treatments prior to attempting pharmacologic interventions.

Nonpharmacologic Interventions

Nonpharmacologic treatments include behavioral, cognitive, and educational approaches. These treatments attempt to change the inappropriate or maladaptive behaviors or cognitions associated with sleep. These treatments are particularly effective in cases of psychophysiologic insomnia where the initial cause of the insomnia may no longer be present. Even in cases where a medical or psychiatric illness is at the core of the insomnia, nonpharmacologic

Table 119-7 Sleep Hygiene Rules for Older Adults

Check effect of medication on sleep and wakefulness

Avoid caffeine, alcohol, and cigarettes after lunch

Limit liquids in the evening

Keep a regular bedtime–waketime schedule

Avoid naps or limit to 1 nap a day, no longer than 30 minutes

Spend time outdoors (without sunglasses), particularly in the late afternoon or early evening

Exercise

Table 119-8 Instructions for Stimulus-Control Therapy for Older Adults

Patient should only go to bed when tired or sleepy.

If unable to fall asleep within 20 minutes, patient should get out of bed (and bedroom if possible). While out of bed, do something quiet and relaxing.

Patient should only return to bed when sleepy.

If unable to fall asleep within 20 minutes, patient should again get out of bed.

Behavior is repeated until patient can fall asleep within a few minutes.

Patient should get up at the same time each morning (even if only after a few hours of sleep).

Naps should be avoided.

interventions can be a complement to the treatment of the primary condition.

Many nonpharmacologic interventions are effective in producing short-term and long-term positive changes in sleep habits, as well as the subjective perception of better sleep. Below are examples of the most common nonpharmacologic interventions.

Sleep Hygiene Sleep hygiene is an educational approach designed to give insomniacs, as well as the general population, a list of guidelines on how to maintain healthy sleep–wake routines. Poor sleep habits are associated with a reduction in nighttime sleep quality and difficulties with alertness during the day. When the clinician is collecting the patient's sleep history, information should also be collected on any disruptive nighttime or daytime behaviors that may be affecting the patient's sleep. Table 119-7 summarizes sleep hygiene rules specifically adapted for older adults. Sleep hygiene rules can also be incorporated with other treatments for sleep difficulties in this chapter.

Stimulus-Control Therapy Stimulus-control therapy was developed for the management of psychophysiologic insomnia. Patients often have negative associations with the bedroom environment leading to arousal. These associations can be redefined for the patient by associating the sleep environment with positive and calming cues thereby promoting sleep.

Stimulus-control therapy requires that patients only go to bed when they feel tired enough to fall asleep. Patients should avoid any stimulating or arousing activities prior to bedtime, such as watching television, reading exciting books, or watching the alarm clock. If the patient cannot fall asleep within 20 minutes, the patient should get out of bed and return to bed only when the patient feels tired enough to be able to fall asleep. For a regular sleep period to develop, the patient should wake up and get out of bed at the same time everyday (including weekends). Napping behavior should be avoided, so that the need for sleep can accumulate. However, some modification is possible in the case of older adults who may be allowed to nap during the day (if absolutely necessary), but for no longer than 30 minutes, so as not to interfere with sleep onset. These rules should be followed at sleep onset for sleep

onset insomnia or upon each awakening for patients with sleep maintenance insomnia. Table 119-8 summarizes the instructions for stimulus-control therapy. The patient may initially resist this method because it may require significant effort on the part of the patient and may initially reduce the sleep period and increase daytime sleepiness. Therefore, to increase compliance when recommending this method to the patient, the clinician should explain the underlying theory behind this approach.

Sleep-Restriction Therapy Sleep-restriction therapy was developed in response to the clinical observation that patients with sleep difficulties often spend a significant amount of time in bed unsuccessfully attempting to fall asleep. This inability to fall asleep in an appropriate amount of time results in anxiety and frustration, which, over time, can lead to the development of psychophysiologic insomnia. In addition, spending too much time in bed can lead to fragmented sleep. This method is designed to reduce the amount of time the patient spends awake in bed, thus increasing sleep efficiency. As described above, sleep efficiency is defined as the amount of time asleep given the amount of time in bed. Ideally, an individuals sleep efficiency will be 90 percent or greater.

Sleep-restriction therapy requires the patient to fill out sleep logs for 1 to 2 weeks. Based on these sleep logs, the average amount of time the patient sleeps a night is calculated. The patient is only allowed to spend this amount of time, plus 15 minutes, in bed each night for the following week. For example, if the patient reports sleeping an average of only 5 hours a night, the patient is only allowed to be in bed 5 hours and 15 minutes. Although this reduction in time in bed causes an initial reduction in time spent asleep and possible sleep deprivation, it is likely to lead to shorter sleep onset and sleep consolidation in the long run. Patients should also wake up at the same time each day and avoid daytime napping. In our example, if the patient's normal time to awaken is 6:00 A.M. and they estimate they sleep for only 5 hours, they would not be allowed to go to bed until 12:45 A.M. Once sleep efficiency

Table 119-9   Instructions for Sleep-Restriction Therapy for Older Adults

Calculate the average amount of time in bed per night reported by patient.
Patient is only allowed to stay in bed for this amount of time plus 15 minutes.
Patient must get up at the same time each day.
Daytime napping should be strictly avoided.
When sleep efficiency has reached 80 to 85%, patient can go to bed 15 minutes earlier.
This procedure should be repeated until patient can sleep for 8 hours (or period needed for a good night's sleep).

has reached 80 to 85 percent, the time allowed to spend in bed at night is increased by 15 minutes at the start of the night, so that now the patient would go to bed at 12:30 A.M. This pattern is repeated until the patient is in bed, able to sleep 8 hours or the number of hours that affords the patient a good night's sleep.

To increase compliancy, clinicians should help the patient understand the underlying theory behind this method and educate them on some initial difficulties they should expect, such as initial sleep loss and daytime sleepiness. Table 119-9 summarizes the instructions for sleep-restriction therapy.

Pharmacologic Interventions

Medications, such as antidepressants and hypnotics, are often the most commonly used therapy for insomnia. Clinics should exercise caution when prescribing longer-acting hypnotics to this population, as these medications have several side effects that may be particularly pronounced in the elderly person. Side effects of longer-acting hypnotics include changes in sleep architecture, specifically reduction in delta or deep sleep, morning hangover leading to excessive daytime sleepiness, poor motor coordination, and visuospatial problems that increase the risk for injury in the population. Patients' sleep should be evaluated regularly, especially prior to renewing the prescription of the longer-acting hypnotic, as tolerance is common with this class of drugs and thus insomnia symptoms may return regularly.

Finally, when the time has come to terminate treatment, withdrawal should be very gradual to reduce the likelihood for rebound insomnia.

If after careful consideration, the best course of treatment is sleep medication, the approach to consider would be the shorter-acting, nonbenzodiazepine hypnotics such as zolpidem or zaleplon. The short-acting hypnotics are absorbed quickly and because of the shorter half-life, reduce both sleep onset latency and the risk for daytime sleepiness the following day. Because of zaleplon's 1-hour half-life, it can also be taken following awakenings in the middle of the night. Table 119-10 summarizes common pharmacologic treatments of insomnia.

SPECIAL ISSUES

Sleep in Institutionalized Elderly Patients and Neurodegenerative Disorders

The sleep of older adults living in nursing homes is known to be extremely disturbed. Nursing home patients suffer from severely fragmented sleep, often to the extent that there is not a single hour in a 24-hour day that is spent fully awake or asleep. A common reason for the institutionalization of an elderly person is frequent nocturnal awakenings with wandering and confusion.

Environmental factors in the nursing home may also contribute to the reduction in the quality of sleep. In the nursing home, noise and light exposure occurs intermittently throughout the night and contributes to the disruption of sleep for the patients. Patients in the nursing home spend a significant amount of the 24-hour day in bed, leading the patients to rapidly cycle between sleep and wake during this time. Changes in sleep hygiene and the sleep environment of nursing home patients, may greatly improve the sleep quality in this population. Table 119-11 summarizes a list of strategies for dealing with sleep–wake disturbances in the institutionalized elderly patient. The purpose of these strategies is to help both patients and nursing home staff reduce the nighttime disturbances in the sleeping environment, while promoting stronger and more defined sleep–wake cycles.

Many nursing home patients suffer from neurodegenerative disorders such as Alzheimer's disease, Parkinson's disease, Huntington's disease, and some forms of dementia. These disorders are associated with a high prevalence of sleep disorders. Sleep disturbances affect elderly persons

Table 119-10   Sample of Hypnotic Treatments of Insomnia

Generic	Brand	Dose (mg)	Rate of Action (Minutes)	Half-life (Hours)
Temazepam	Restoril	7.5–30	45–60	10–20
Triazolam	Halcion	0.125–0.5	15–30	1.5–5.5
Zolpidem	Ambien	5–10	15–30	2.5–3.0
Zaleplon	Sonata	5–10	15–30	1

Table 119-11 Sleep Hygiene Rules for Nursing Homes Patients

Limited the amount of time in bed, particularly during the day.

Limited naps to 1 hour once a day, early in the afternoon.

Keep regular sleep–wake schedule (if possible similar to prior home routine).

Keep regular meal schedule (if possible patients should not eat in bed).

Avoid caffeinated beverages and food.

Limit nighttime noise.

Ensure that patient rooms are as dark as possible during the night.

Ensure that patient environment is brightly lit during the day.

Encourage exercise appropriate for each patient.

Match roommates on sleep–wake behavior.

Assess patients for possible sleep problems and initiate specific treatment.

Check medications for sedating/alerting effects.

with neurodegenerative disorders differently than they affect "healthy" older adults. For example, Alzheimer's disease patients suffer from progressive increases in the duration and frequency of nocturnal awakenings, increases in daytime napping, and decreases in slow-wave sleep and REM sleep, when compared to healthy older adults. Many of the coping strategies summarized in Table 119-11 are also relevant to patients suffering from neurodegenerative disorders, particularly the need for significant light exposure during the day, increasing daytime activity and exercise, and decreasing the need for daytime napping.

It was previously mentioned that older adults have higher rates of sleep-disordered breathing than do younger adults. Research also shows that patients suffering from neurodegenerative disorders and patients living in nursing homes suffer from an even higher prevalence of sleep-disordered breathing. Recent reports also suggest a possible relationship between sleep-disordered breathing and exacerbation of cognitive impairments. Consequently, clinicians should be even more attentive to symptoms of sleep-disordered breathing in this population.

REFERENCES

Ancoli-Israel S: Insomnia in the elderly. A review for the primary care practitioner. *Sleep* 23(Suppl 1):S23, 2000.

Ancoli-Israel S: Sleep problems in older adults: Putting myths to bed. *Geriatrics* 52(1):20, 1997.

Ancoli-Israel S et al: Identification and treatment of sleep problems in the elderly. *Sleep Med Rev* 1(1):3, 1997.

Bliwise DL: Dementia, in Kryger MH et al. (eds): *Principles and Practice of Sleep Medicine,* 3d ed. Philadelphia, WB Saunders, 2000, p 1058.

Bootzin RR, Epstein D: Stimulus control, in: Lichstein KL, Morin CM (eds): *Treatment of Late-life Insomnia.* Thousand Oaks, CA, Sage Publications, 2000, p 167.

Foley DJ et al: Incidence and remission of insomnia among elderly adults: An epidemiologic study of 6800 persons over three years. *Sleep* 22 (Suppl 2):S366, 1999.

McCurry SM et al: Treatment of sleep disturbances in Alzheimer's disease. *Sleep Med Rev* 4(6):603, 2000.

Morin CM et al: Behavioral and pharmacological therapies for late-life insomnia. *JAMA* 281(11):991, 1999.

Phillips B, Ancoli-Israel S: Sleep disorders in the elderly. *Sleep Med* 2(2):99, 2000.

Shochat T et al: Sleep disorders in the elderly. *Curr Treat Options Neurol* 3(1):19, 2001.

Vitiello MV: Sleep disorders and aging: Understanding the causes. *J Gerontol* 52A(4):M189, 1997.

Dizziness

AMAN NANDA • RICHARD W. BESDINE

DEFINITION

Dizziness is used to describe an abnormal sensation of unsteadiness or motion in space. Dizziness has been arbitrarily defined on the basis of duration as acute (present for less than 1 or 2 months) or chronic (present for more than 1 or 2 months). The differential diagnosis of acute dizziness is similar in younger and older persons and management of acute dizziness is not different in older persons as compared to younger adults, except that recovery may be more prolonged. This chapter focuses on chronic dizziness.

EPIDEMIOLOGY

The prevalence of dizziness ranges from 4 to 30 percent in persons age 65 years or older, and more commonly is reported by women than men. In one study of persons age 65 years and older, the likelihood of reporting dizziness increased by 10 percent for every 5 years of increasing age.

Chronic dizziness is associated with a number of comorbid conditions, including falls, functional disability, orthostatic hypotension, syncope, and strokes. In one prospective study of older persons with dizziness, after 2 years of follow-up, dizzy older persons were more likely to become disabled than were those who were not, although mortality was no different. Dizziness has a negative effect on the quality of life among older persons. Chronic dizziness is also associated with fear of falling, worsening depressive symptoms and self-rated health, and decreased participation in social activities.

PATHOPHYSIOLOGY

Dizziness is a sensation of postural instability or imbalance. Maintenance of balance and equilibrium is complex, achieved by integration of sensory information obtained from vestibular, proprioceptive, visual, and auditory systems by the cerebral cortex and cerebellum, leading to appropriate balance maintaining responses. Abnormal function in any one or a combination of these systems may result in imbalance and the sensation of dizziness.

The vestibular system maintains spatial orientation at rest and during acceleration. Elements of the vestibular system and its connecting pathways include the semicircular canals, utricle, saccule, vestibular nerve, vestibular nuclei, vestibulospinal tracts, and vestibulocerebellar pathways. Diseases affecting this system and producing dizziness include Ménière's disease, benign paroxysmal positional vertigo, recurrent vestibulopathy, labyrinthitis/vestibular neuronitis, acoustic neuroma, and drug toxicity (especially aminoglycosides). Age-related changes have also been reported in the sensory (hair) cells in the semicircular canals, saccule, and utricle.

The proprioceptive system consists of mechanoreceptors in the joints, peripheral nerves, and posterior columns, and multiple central nervous system (CNS) connections. Proprioception contributes to equilibrium by providing information about changes in body position, and helping mediate the body's response to position change. Common disorders include peripheral neuropathy associated with diseases such as diabetes or vitamin B_{12} deficiency and cervical degenerative disorders. There are few data on age-related changes in proprioception. One study reported a substantial decline in joint position sense with aging, while another found no major changes.

Vision provides important information about spatial orientation, and is relied upon particularly when vestibular and/or proprioceptive function is impaired. Common ocular diseases include cataracts, macular degeneration, and glaucoma. Age-related visual changes include decrease in each of visual acuity, dark adaptation, contrast sensitivity, and accommodation. Hearing also provides spatial clues, but to a lesser extent than vision. Impairment in hearing, common in older persons, may be secondary to age-related changes, or to disease processes.

The cerebral cortex and cerebellum, along with their synaptic networks, integrate information and supply the musculoskeletal system with information for appropriate responses. Because of multiple and complex connections, essentially any central nervous system disorder can lead to imbalance which may manifest as dizziness.

CLASSIFICATION

Dizziness is described using many names, including vertigo, lightheadedness, dysequilibrium, giddiness, wooziness, and spinning. The sensation of dizziness is commonly categorized as vertigo, dysequilibrium, presyncope, and other. In addition to these four types, another category, mixed dizziness, is a combination of two or more of the above types. Mixed dizziness is the most common type of dizziness reported by older persons.

Vertigo, a sensation of spinning, in which the individual perceives movements of the environment in relation to the body (objective vertigo) or vice versa (subjective vertigo). Vertigo is often assumed to result from disorders of the vestibular system and its connecting pathways although other causes of dizziness such as cervical disorders may present as vertigo as well.

Dysequilibrium refers to feelings of unsteadiness or imbalance primarily involving the lower extremities or trunk rather than the head. The person often expresses the feeling that he/she is about to fall. Dysequilibrium results mostly from disorders of the proprioceptive system, musculoskeletal weakness, or cerebellar disease.

Presyncope is a feeling of lightheadedness or impending faintness or the sensation that one is about to pass out. Presyncope usually results from hypoperfusion of the brain; cardiovascular causes (including vasovagal disorders) are common causes in older persons.

Often the sensation does not fit any of the above three types. The patient may describe "whirling," "tilting," "floating," and other nonspecific sensations. Furthermore, the correlation between sensations and organ systems is not as consistent among older persons as younger persons. Thus, the sensation reported does not have diagnostic specificity in older patients.

In addition, although dizziness may be a symptom of one or more discrete diseases, multifactorial etiologies of dizziness are common in older persons. Chronic dizziness is associated with risk factors such as angina, myocardial infarction, arthritis, diabetes, stroke, syncope, anxiety, depressive symptoms, impaired hearing, and polypharmacy. In a recent population-based study of community-dwelling older persons, the factors that were independently associated with dizziness included anxiety, depressive symptoms, impaired hearing, the use of five or more medications, postural hypotension, impaired balance, and a past history of myocardial infarction. Almost 70 percent of patients with five or more of the above risk factors reported dizziness, whereas only 10 percent of patients with none of these factors reported dizziness. These findings suggest that dizziness, in a subset of older persons, may be a geriatric syndrome that is the result of the accumulated effect of multiple coexisting risk factors and diseases.

Thus, as presented in the following section, dizziness may be the presenting complaint of a discrete disease or the results of contributing multiple factors.

Discrete Diseases Causing Dizziness

Vestibular Disorders

Vestibular diseases have been reported in anywhere from 4 to 71 percent of older persons with dizziness. The most common vestibular disorders causing chronic dizziness in older persons are Ménière's disease, benign paroxysmal positional vertigo, recurrent vestibulopathy, the effects of ototoxic medications, and acoustic neuroma.

Ménière's disease　Ménière's disease, also called endolymphatic hydrops, is reported in 2 to 8 percent of older patients with dizziness. It is a debilitating disorder of the inner ear, consisting of a triad of recurrent episodic vertigo, tinnitus, and fluctuating sensorineural hearing loss. A sensation of fullness in the inner ear is common. Episodes of true vertigo usually last for 1 to 24 hours. The patient may complain of nausea, vomiting, and headaches during the episodes. The exact cause is unknown, but the pathology is characterized by excess endolymph within the cochlea and vestibular labyrinth. The disease is unilateral in a majority of patients; men and women are affected equally. In a 14-year follow-up study, the episodes of vertigo disappeared in 50 percent of patients and improved in 28 percent, while hearing in the affected side was absent in 48 percent and impaired in 21 percent of the patients.

Benign paroxysmal positional vertigo　Benign paroxysmal positional vertigo (BPPV) has been reported to be the cause of dizziness in 4 to 34 percent of cases. In this condition, patients report sudden-onset, episodic vertigo, often associated with nausea and/or vomiting, precipitated by changes in the position of the head, such as rolling over in bed, getting in and out of bed, or bending forward to pick something up. It is classically accompanied by rotational nystagmus. In most cases, the etiology is unknown, although some patients have a history of head injury or viral neurolabyrinthitis. Benign paroxysmal positional vertigo results from freely moving particulate matter within the posterior semicircular canal. These particles most likely are dislodged otoconia, which are tiny calciferous granules that make up part of the receptor mechanism in the otolithic apparatus. It is postulated that movement of these free-floating particles cause alteration in the endolymphatic pressure, resulting in episodes of vertigo and nystagmus. In one study, researchers reported that otoconia undergo degenerative changes, which may lead to their dislodgment from the utriculus. A definitive diagnosis of BPPV can be made by the Dix–Hallpike test described under "Evaluation" later in this chapter.

Recurrent vestibulopathy　Recurrent vestibulopathy is an idiopathic disorder characterized by recurrent episodes of vertigo without auditory or neurologic symptoms or signs. The vertigo usually lasts from 5 minutes to 24 hours. It is differentiated from Ménière's disease by the absence of auditory symptoms. Over 8.5 years of follow-up, spontaneous recovery was reported in 62 percent patients. The diagnosis was changed to Ménière's disease or benign positional vertigo in 14 percent and 8 percent of patients, respectively.

Acoustic neuroma　Acoustic neuroma, also known as cerebellopontine angle tumor, is a benign tumor of the eighth cranial nerve, and is reported in 1 to 3 percent of older persons with dizziness. Clinical features include tinnitus and progressive unilateral sensorineural hearing loss, particularly for the higher frequencies. Patients complain more often of a feeling of unsteadiness rather than of true vertigo. Patients with large tumors may also complain of occipital headache, diplopia, paresthesias in trigeminal or facial nerve distribution, and/or ataxic gait.

Central Nervous System Disorders

The frequency of cerebrovascular disease ranges from 4 percent to 70 percent among older persons with dizziness. Patients with transient ischemic attack (TIA) or stroke involving vertebrobasilar distribution commonly present with dizziness, along with diplopia, or dysarthria, numbness, or weakness. Dizziness rarely is a presenting symptom in patients with anterior or posterior cerebral artery ischemia or with internal carotid artery disease. The patient may complain of either a rotatory or nonrotatory dizziness along with other neurologic symptoms and signs. A number of specific stroke syndromes present with dizziness, including cerebellar infarction and posterior lateral medullary artery infarction, also known as Wallenberg's syndrome.

Other central nervous disorder causes of dizziness include Parkinson's disease and basilar artery migraine. The latter is rare in older persons.

Psychiatric Causes

Anxiety, depression, obsessive-compulsive disorder, panic disorder, and other psychiatric conditions are among the most common causes of chronic dizziness in young adults. In older persons as well, psychiatric conditions are often associated with dizziness. Common psychiatric conditions causing or contributing to dizziness in older persons include depressive and anxiety disorders. Recent studies show that depressive symptoms are associated with symptoms of dizziness, while, conversely, persons who have chronic dizziness are at increased risk of depression, suggesting a reciprocal relationship between dizziness and depressive symptoms among older persons.

Systemic Causes

Hypothyroidism, anemia, electrolyte imbalance, hypertension, coronary artery disease, congestive heart failure, and diabetes mellitus are commonly found in patients with dizziness, although the frequency of dizziness as a symptom of each is low. Studies have found an independent association between dizziness and a history of hypertension, angina, myocardial infarction, and diabetes mellitus. Systemic disorders may contribute to instability or dizziness by affecting the sensory, central, or effector components. These systemic disorders may also cause decreased cerebral perfusion or oxygen delivery, fatigue, or confusion, each of which may subsequently lead to a sensation of instability or dizziness.

Orthostatic Hypotension

Orthostatic hypotension is a primary or contributing cause in 2 to 15 percent of older persons with dizziness. There is a long list of causes of orthostatic hypotension (see Chap. 124). Although there is no consensus on the definition of orthostatic hypotension in older adults, commonly noted criteria include a 20 mmHg drop in systolic blood pressure, a 10 mmHg drop in diastolic blood pressure, or typical symptoms associated with any drop in blood pressure after standing from a supine position. Another entity reported in literature is postural dizziness, in which patients complain of dizziness on standing from a supine position but have no drop in blood pressure. In these studies, a subset of patients who have orthostatic blood pressure changes do not complain of dizziness, suggesting that orthostatic changes in blood pressure may be asymptomatic, while, conversely, all dizziness with postural changes may not be caused by a drop in blood pressure. Vestibular dysfunction is thought to account for the postural dizziness not accompanied by postural blood pressure drops.

Postprandial Hypotension

Another important entity to consider in older persons is postprandial hypotension. Postprandial hypotension is defined as a decrease in systolic blood pressure of 20 mmHg or more in a sitting or standing posture within 1 to 2 hours of eating a meal; dizziness often is a symptom. In a recent study, the effects of postprandial hypotension and orthostatic hypotension were found to be additive but not synergistic, suggesting that the two entities have different pathophysiologic mechanisms. Chapter 121 discusses cardiovascular disorders that can cause dizziness as well as syncope.

Medications

Many classes of drugs can cause or contribute to dizziness, such as antihypertensives, antiarrhythmic agents, anticonvulsants, antidepressants, anxiolytics, antibiotics (aminoglycosides, macrolides, and vancomycin analogs), antihistamines, nonsteroidal antiinflammatory agents, and over-the-counter cold and sleep preparations. These agents cause dizziness through different mechanisms. Antihypertensive agents can cause dizziness simply by lowering blood pressure to a level at which the postural drop in pressure becomes symptomatic. Calcium channel blockers, nitrates, and hydralazine are common offenders. Loop diuretics such as furosemide can cause dizziness by ototoxicity or volume depletion. Antiarrhythmics, anticonvulsants, and anxiolytics are responsible for dizziness because of their effects on the central nervous system. Tricyclic antidepressants, antihistamines, and cold preparations cause dizziness through their anticholinergic properties. Antibiotics (e.g., aminoglycosides, macrolides, and vancomycin analogs), nonsteroidal antiinflammatory agents, and loop diuretics cause dizziness through ototoxicity, especially in the presence of impaired renal function, which decreases their clearance. The aminoglycosides are especially hazardous because of their toxicity to both the kidney and vestibule.

Apart from risks conferred by specific toxicity of drugs, studies have also reported an association between dizziness and the number of medications taken, independent of the effect of comorbid diseases.

Cervical Causes

Disorders of the cervical spine as a cause of dizziness in older persons have been reported in the range of 0 to 57 percent. Patients with cervical dizziness usually present with vague lightheadedness or vertigo associated with turning of the head. Both vascular and proprioceptive mechanisms have been proposed to explain cervical dizziness.

Obstruction of the vertebral arteries is thought to be the most common vascular mechanism of cervical dizziness. One hypothesis suggests that in the presence of atheromatous narrowing of one vertebral artery, rotation of the head may cause sufficient obstruction of the contralateral vertebral artery to produce ischemia of the brainstem. Another hypothesis suggests that turning the head or neck results in compression of adjacent vertebral artery by a strategic osteoarthritic spur, causing a transient disruption of the blood flow.

Degenerative changes in the cervical spine may cause dizziness because of impairment of the cervical proprioceptive mechanoreceptors. These receptors provide information for postural control via the vestibulospinal tract. The patient may present with decreased range of motion and radicular pain in the neck upon movement, as well as dizziness.

EVALUATION

Evaluation of dizziness can be a complex and challenging task for clinicians. The differential diagnosis is broad and the literature offers no evidence-based clinical practice guidelines. Optimal care requires the identification and treatment of the discrete diseases causing dizziness when possible. If a discrete treatable disease cannot be found, then the objective becomes maximum symptomatic improvement of dizziness. Based on these objectives and on the available evidence, a stepwise approach is recommended for the evaluation of chronic dizziness, proceeding from careful history and physical examination to screening laboratory tests. A targeted battery of more elaborate and expensive tests is indicated only when routine evaluation suggests a specific disease entity and the results of these tests are likely to influence the management. For the majority of older persons in whom a routine evaluation does not suggest a single discrete cause, the clinician should try to focus on identifying various factors (Table 120-1) that might be contributing to dizziness, some of which are likely to be modifiable. When etiology is multifactorial, identifying and treating one or more contributing factors may improve, if not eliminate, the dizziness.

History

Patients should be asked to describe the feelings of dizziness in their own words, supplemented by directed questions. Narrowing the differential diagnosis can occur following a careful history, but older patients often describe a vague sensation such as "whirling," or "giddiness," or a combination of sensations. Determining whether the attacks are episodic or continuous may help in identifying a specific disease. For example, patients with Ménière's disease or BPPV will usually have episodic dizziness, while psychogenic dizziness is usually continuous. Frequency and duration of dizziness also should be determined. Episodic dizziness lasting less than 1 minute suggests BPPV, 5 to 120 minutes suggest TIA or migraine, while episodes longer than 120 minutes suggest Ménière's disease or recurrent vestibulopathy. One should also ask about any precipitating factors of dizziness, such as missing a meal, drinking alcohol, taking a medication, standing from a lying position, rolling over in bed, changing the position of the head or neck such as looking up or from side to side, bending forward to pick something up, micturition, or defecation. Any relationship between the onset of dizziness and meals should be sought, because postprandial hypotension is common, especially in frail older persons. The patient should also be asked about any symptoms associated with dizziness. For example, patients with Ménière's disease often will complain of tinnitus, fullness in ear, and fluctuating hearing loss. Patients with vertebrobasilar involvement may complain of double vision, dysarthria, or sudden blackouts. Patients with cervical arthritis may also complain of associated pain in the neck on movement. The clinician should also ask about comorbid conditions such as anemia, cardiac diseases, or diabetes which may contribute to dizziness. One should look for any symptoms of depression or anxiety disorders; use of screening instruments can be helpful (see Chap. 112). Finally, all medications, including over-the-counter medications, should be reviewed as potential contributors to dizziness.

Physical Examination

The clinician should do a focused physical examination, keeping in mind the complex pathophysiology and broad differential diagnosis of dizziness. The examiner should look for spontaneous nystagmus on cranial nerve testing. The nystagmus is vertical in central lesions and horizontal or rotatory in peripheral lesions. The nystagmus of central lesions is not suppressed by visual fixation; in peripheral lesions nystagmus can be suppressed by visual fixation. One should also test for near and distant vision. The ear examination should include both a hearing test (whisper test or audioscope) and an otoscopic examination to rule out cerumen impaction or any structural abnormalities. Blood pressure should be tested both in supine and standing positions to rule out orthostatic hypotension after at least 5 minutes of quiet lying. One should examine the neck for local tenderness and restrictions in the range of movement which can result from cervical arthritis. One should also consider that the patient might voluntarily restrict the range of neck movement in order to minimize dizziness secondary to vestibular dysfunction; such patients may respond well to vestibular rehabilitation.

A neurologic examination should include cranial nerves, the motor and sensory systems, and gait and balance. In the cranial nerve examination, one should look for diplopia, dysarthria, or facial paresthesia to rule out vertebrobasilar involvement. An absence of corneal reflex may suggest acoustic neuroma, especially if accompanied with unilateral hearing loss, tinnitus, and cerebellar

Table 120-1 Possible Contributors to Chronic Dizziness

Contributor	History	Examination	Possible Causes	Potential Interventions
Vision	Use of bifocals or trifocals	Abnormalities in near/distant acuity; contrast sensitivity; depth perception	Cataract; glaucoma; macular degeneration; perceptual difficulties with glasses	Appropriate refraction; consider avoiding bifocals or trifocals; drugs for glaucoma; surgery; good lighting without glare
Hearing	Deafness in one or both ears; difficulty hearing in social situations	Abnormal findings with Rinne's test, Weber's test, whisper test, or audiometry	Presbycusis; otosclerosis	Hearing aid; surgery (for otosclerosis); hearing rehabilitation; listening devices
Vestibulocochlear system	True vertigo, worse in dark or with specific head positions; tinnitus; history of aminoglycosides, furosemide, aspirin use; ear surgery; ear or mastoid infections	Nystagmus (horizontal or rotary nystagmus suggests a peripheral vestibular disorder; vertical nystagmus suggests a central disorder); decreased neck range of motion; decreased hearing; abnormal Hallpike maneuver; abnormal vestibular testing	Drug toxicity; previous infections, tumor (e.g. acoustic neuroma); previous surgery; vascular (e.g. brain stem infarct); benign positional vertigo; Ménière's disease	Avoid toxic drugs and long-term vestibular suppressants; remove earwax; vestibular rehabilitation; surgery
Peripheral nerves	Worse in dark or on uneven surfaces or inclines	Decreased neck range of motion; signs of radiculopathy or myelopathy; clumsiness with fine motor tasks; mild spastic gait; increased tone	Spondylosis; degenerative or inflammatory arthritis	Treatment of underlying disease; cervical or balance exercises; consider surgery
Cerebral hypoperfusion	Presyncope; near fainting	Postural hypotension; signs of underlying disease	See causes for syncope in Chap. 121; cardiovascular and pulmonary diseases; anemia	Treatment of underlying disease
Hypotension				
Postprandial	Symptoms within 1 hour of eating	Hypotension after meals	Postprandial hypotension	Small meals; avoid exertion after meals; avoid hypotensive drugs near meals; have caffeine with meals
Postural	Near fainting—worse when getting up, walking, exercising; complaints consistent with predisposing diseases; may be asymptomatic; history of predisposing drugs	Blood pressure and heart rate; signs of predisposing diseases	Drugs, volume/salt depletion; deconditioning; Parkinson's syndrome; diabetes; autonomic dysfunction; vasovagal attack	Treatment of salt and water repletion; reconditioning exercises; ankle pumps or hand clenching; slow rising; elevate head of bed; graduated stockings; lowest effective dosage of essential contributing drugs

(Continued)

Table 120-1   (*Continued*) **Possible Contributors to Chronic Dizziness**

Contributor	History	Examination	Possible Causes	Potential Interventions
Cardiac dysfunction	Variable, depending on specific etiology	Cardiac auscultation, ECG, echocardiography	Cardiac arrhythmias, valvular lesions, myocardial ischemia, myxoma, hypertrophic cardiomyopathy	Variable, depending on specific etiology
Brainstem	Any sensation (e.g., vertigo, near fainting, wooziness); transient neurologic symptoms (e.g., slurred speech, visual change, one-sided weakness); symptoms on looking up	Findings may be transient or fixed; ataxia	Transient ischemic attack; brainstem infarct; vertebrobasilar insufficiency	Low-dose aspirin; assistive device if ataxic
Metabolic diseases	Symptoms of underlying disease	Signs of underlying disease	Any metabolic disease, (e.g., thyroid disorders, diabetes)	Treatment of underlying disease
Medications				
Past	Vestibulocochlear symptoms (see above)	See above under vestibulocochlear system	See above under vestibulocochlear system	See above under vestibulocochlear system
Current	Confusion; fatigue; weakness; dizziness often vague, may be constant	May have postural hypotension	Specific: Nitrates, beta-blockers, antidepressants, antipsychotics, anticholinergics; vestibular depressants, benzodiazepines, others General: total number and dose of all drugs	Eliminate, substitute, or reduce specific offending drugs if possible; reduce all other drugs to lowest effective dose possible; remember over-the-counter drugs
Depression, anxiety	Constant dizziness; multiple somatic complaints; poor concentration; positive results on anxiety or depression screening; vegetative complaints (sleep, appetite)	See Chap. 112	Depression, anxiety	Thorough consideration of risks and benefits of antidepressant drug; counseling

SOURCE: Adapted from Beers MH et al: The Merck Manual of Geriatrics. Third Edition. Whitehouse Station, NJ, Merck Research Laboratories, 2000, p. 181.

signs. The presence of cogwheel rigidity and bradykinesia is suggestive of parkinsonism. Although most of the abnormalities detected in the balance examination are not specific, the presence of a positive Romberg's sign with the eyes closed is suggestive of an abnormality of proprioception and/or the vestibular system. A wide-based stance, a worsening of the gait with the eyes closed, and an improvement in gait with minimal hand-held assistance of the examiner, in combination, suggest a proprioceptive deficit.

In addition to the history and physical examination, clinicians can also perform certain provocative tests at the bedside or in the office which may help in detecting abnormalities of the vestibular system.

Provocative Tests

These tests include the Dix–Hallpike, head-thrust, post-headshake, and stepping tests. The Dix–Hallpike test establishes the diagnosis of BPPV (Fig. 120-1)(Color Plate 31).

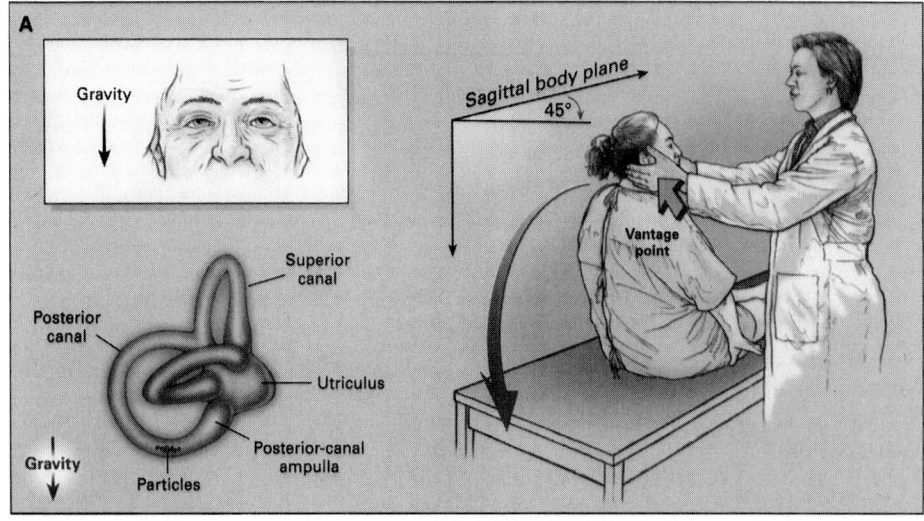

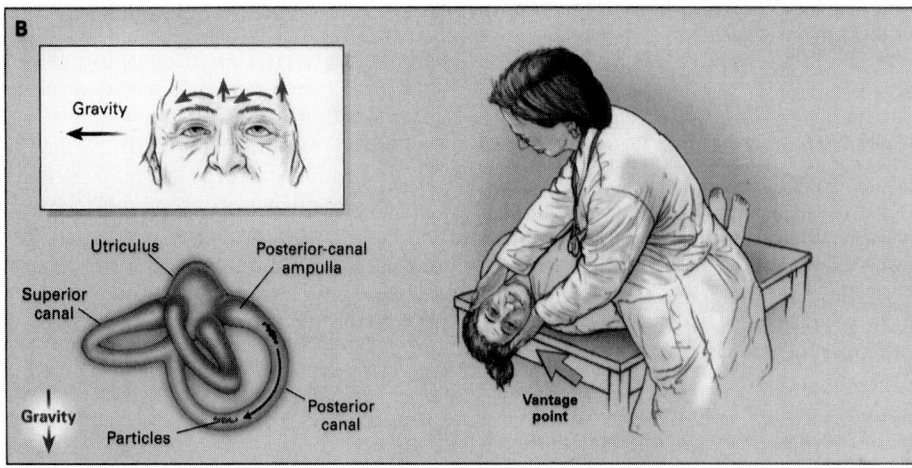

Figure 120-1 Dix-Hallpike test. SOURCE: Furman JM, Cass SP: Benign Paroxysmal Positional Vertigo. *N Engl J Med* 341:1590, 1999. Copyright © 1999 Massachusetts Medical Society. All rights reserved.

In this test, the patient is asked to sit on an examination table with the head rotated 45 degrees to one side. The patient is then asked to fix his/her vision upon the examiner's forehead. The examiner, while holding the patient's head firmly in the same position, moves the patient from a seated to a supine position with the head hanging below the edge of the table. If the ipsilateral ear is affected then this maneuver will result in vertigo and nystagmus. If present, the direction, latency, and duration of nystagmus, and duration of vertigo should be noted. The diagnostic criteria for BPPV are (1) vertigo accompanied by a rotatory nystagmus; (2) a latency of 1 to 5 seconds between the completion of the maneuver and the onset of vertigo and nystagmus; (3) paroxysmal nature of the vertigo and nystagmus (lasting for 10 to 20 seconds); and (4) fatigability, that is, a decrease in the intensity of the vertigo and nystagmus with repeated testing.

The head-thrust and postheadshake tests can help in determining if the vestibuloocular reflex (VOR) is intact. The VOR helps maintain visual stability during head movement. It functions according to the information relayed by the vestibular nucleus to the sixth cranial nerve nucleus in the pons, as well as to the third and fourth cranial nerve nuclei in the midbrain through the median longitudinal fasciculus.

The head-thrust test requires the patient to fix the vision on the examiner's nose, while the head is quickly turned approximately 10 degrees to the left or right. If the VOR is intact, the eyes will stay fixed to the target. But in patients with a vestibular defect, the eyes move with the head away from the target before a corrective saccade back to it. For instance, head thrusts to the left in patients with left-sided vestibular lesions will cause a slipping away of the pupils from the target followed by a corrective movement, whereas head thrusts to the right will produce a normal visual response.

Using Frenzel lenses to eliminate fixation of vision, the postheadshake test calls for the head to be rotated for approximately 10 seconds, either passively by the examiner or actively by the patient at a frequency of approximately 2 Hz in the horizontal plane, after which the examiner checks for nystagmus. If there is a unilateral peripheral vestibular lesion, a horizontal nystagmus will result; the fast phase will usually beat away from the side of the lesion. With central lesions, the nystagmus may be vertical.

Unterberger originally introduced the stepping test, later modified by Fukuda. A positive stepping test suggests a lesion in the vestibular or vestibulospinal system. In this test, the patient stands at the center of a circle which is divided into sections with lines intersecting at 30-degree angles. Blindfolded, the patient is asked to stretch out both arms at 90 degrees to the body and then to flex and raise high one knee and then the other, and to continue stepping in place at a normal walking speed for a total of 50 or 100 steps. The blindfolded patient marches and the examiner watches for deviation from the straight line. If there is a unilateral vestibular lesion or acoustic neuroma, a gradual rotation of the body (more than 30 degrees) toward the affected side will occur.

These tests are more useful in detecting unilateral than bilateral vestibular dysfunction. Upon finding any abnormalities, one can proceed with specialized vestibular function tests such as electronystagmography and rotational chair test described under "Laboratory Tests". Clinicians must be aware that compensatory mechanisms may mask a vestibular deficit when these tests are used in patients with longstanding vestibular loss. There are no data addressing the specificity or sensitivity of these tests in older persons.

Laboratory Tests

There is no standardized approach for laboratory testing for patients with chronic dizziness. However, a modest baseline battery of tests should be done in all elderly persons with chronic dizziness to rule out common modifiable contributors to dizziness. Thus, a hematocrit, basic metabolic panel, thyroid function tests, and vitamin B_{12} levels should be done in all patients to rule out anemia, diabetes, azotemia, hypothyroidism, and vitamin B_{12} deficiency.

Further testing should be tailored to the situation. Audiometry should be done in patients with a history of fluctuating or gradual hearing loss. An audiogram will reveal sensorineural loss in both Ménière's disease and acoustic neuroma; the hearing loss will be greater in lower frequencies in Ménière's disease and in higher frequencies in acoustic neuroma. An electrocardiogram is indicated if there is a suspicion of myocardial infarction or cardiac arrhythmia. Holter or event monitoring, or tilt table testing is indicated only in selected patients with unexplained syncope.

In patients with a suspicion of cervical osteoarthritis, radioimaging of the cervical spine can be considered, but the frequency of false-positives is great. Neuroimaging is needed when a stroke or cerebellopontine tumor is suspected. Magnetic resonance imaging is preferred over computed tomography scans because of its greater sensitivity, particularly for lesions in the brainstem. Doppler studies or a magnetic resonance angiogram may be needed to detect vertebrobasilar insufficiency.

Abnormalities of the peripheral vestibular system can be evaluated by performing special tests, such as electronystagmography (ENG) including caloric testing, a rotational chair test, and computerized posturography. These tests can provide data that help confirm history and physical examination data; however, abnormalities are common in older persons without dizziness, so a positive test is often nonspecific and nondiagnostic.

In ENG, movements of the eyes (nystagmus) are recorded in the form of tracings with the help of electrodes placed around the eyes. These electrodes record changes in scalp potential produced by the corneal-retinal potential in response to visual and vestibular stimuli, which can be either spontaneous or provoked by caloric stimuli of warm and cold water in the external ear canal. In caloric testing, each ear is stimulated first with warm (111°F [44°C]) and then with cold water (86°F [30°C]), each instilled over 30 seconds. When vestibular function is normal, the temperature change will result in nystagmus, but there will be decreased or no response in an ear on the side of peripheral vestibular disorder. The caloric test assesses the symmetry of vestibular function, and is useful in detecting unilateral vestibular lesions. However, patients with bilateral vestibular loss or patients in whom caloric testing can not be performed should undergo rotational chair testing.

A rotational chair test, in addition to quantifying the extent of lesions in patients with bilateral peripheral vestibular loss, also helps reveal the degree of peripheral or central vestibular dysfunction. In this test, the patient is seated on a chair in a dark room, and eye movements are recorded when the chair is rotated at different frequencies.

Computerized posturography evaluates the ability of the patient to maintain balance in response to individual or combinations of visual, vestibular, or proprioceptive stimuli while standing on a platform that can be perturbed in three dimensions. This test may be helpful in providing additional confirmatory data when there is a suspicion of peripheral vestibular pathology, but ENG or rotational chair testing are equivocal. In addition, computerized posturography may be the only positive test in the case of central vestibular and extravestibular CNS pathology. Posturography also may be helpful in determining which patients with dizziness are likely to benefit from physical rehabilitation.

MANAGEMENT

Clinicians often feel frustrated in managing patients with dizziness. As discussed in the previous section, the goal should be to identify and treat the causes of dizziness. However, in many patients with chronic dizziness, a single specific diagnosis may be elusive in the presence of multiple factors contributing to dizziness. In these patients, instead of focusing on a single diagnosis-oriented approach, one should try to identify and treat as many of these contributing or causative factors as possible, recognizing that some may not be modifiable. The result of such an approach usually is a decrease in the disability associated with dizziness.

Systemic disorders such as anemia, metabolic derangements, vitamin B_{12} deficiency, and thyroid abnormalities should be corrected. Correction of vision and hearing deficits is very important. Anxiety and depression should be treated. Medications potentially contributing to dizziness, including over-the-counter medicines, should be identified and either be withdrawn or reduced. The ideal approach should be to stop a potentially offending medication rather than adding new ones.

Pharmacologic Therapy

Drugs commonly used as vestibular suppressants include antihistamines (e.g., meclizine), anticholinergic agents (e.g., scopolamine), and benzodiazepines (e.g., diazepam). Vestibular suppressants are more effective when used for acute episodes of dizziness than for chronic dizziness. Many vestibular suppressants themselves may cause dizziness. Scopolamine should not be used in elderly persons because of its anticholinergic side effects. Meclizine, a weak antihistaminic agent, is usually given in doses of 12.5 to 25 mg three times daily as needed. These medications should be used only temporarily as their prolonged use may compromise central and peripheral adaptation and thus, paradoxically, prolong the dizziness. Benzodiazepines may at times, however, be indicated as a long-term vestibular suppressant in persons with severe unilateral lesions who are not surgical candidates.

Vestibular Rehabilitation

Vestibular rehabilitation plays an important role in managing patients with peripheral or central vestibular causes of dizziness by enhancing the adaptation of the vestibular system. Vestibular rehabilitation consists of exercises combining movements of eyes, head, and body designed to stimulate the vestibular system. At first these exercises may worsen the dizziness, but with continued practice and gradual increase in the frequency, these exercises improve dizziness, probably through central adaptation and habituation. These exercises also may help patients alleviate anxiety and fears in performing various activities. Improvement is usually seen after 6 to 8 weeks of vestibular rehabilitation. Patients should perform these exercises initially under the supervision of a trained specialist such as a physical therapist, and later independently at home.

In patients with cervical dizziness, physical therapy can substantially decrease the frequency and severity of dizziness and neck pain, and can improve postural stability. Some patients may benefit from cervical collars or cervical traction.

Patients suffering from BPPV can be treated by performing one of two bedside maneuvers, Epley's canalith repositioning procedure or Brandt's and Daroff's exercises. Epley's canalith repositioning procedure (Fig. 120-2) (Color Plate 32) is performed to move free-floating particles from the posterior semicircular canal into the utricle of the labyrinth by the effects of gravity, thereby eliminating fluctuation of the endolymphatic pressure in the semicircular canals. In this five-position procedure, the patient is asked to sit on a table and a vibrator is applied to the ipsilateral mastoid process. Next, the patient is made to lie down supine on the examining table with the head rotated 45 degrees toward the affected ear and hanging below the edge of the table, similar to the Dix–Hallpike test. This position will induce vertigo. Once the vertigo subsides, the head is rotated 45 degrees to the opposite side, which may induce vertigo again. Then the head and body are rotated further in the same direction until the head is facing downward. Subsequently, while holding the head in the same position, the patient sits up. Finally, the head is turned forward with the chin down by about 20 degrees. The examiner holds the head in each of these positions for approximately 10 to 15 seconds or until the vertigo subsides. The patient should be told not to lie flat for the next 24 to 48 hours.

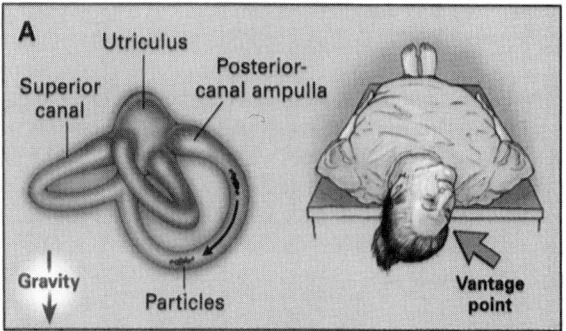
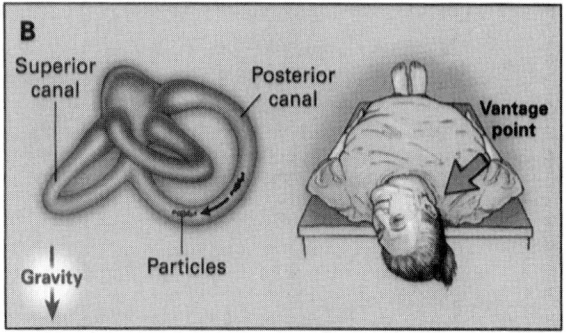
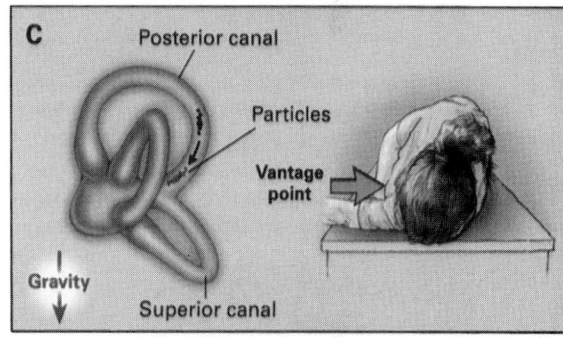
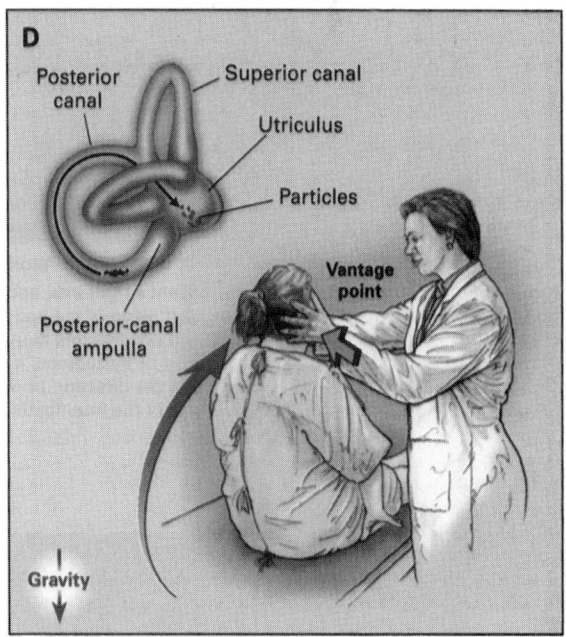

Figure 120-2 Epley's canalith repositioning procedure. SOURCE: Furman JM, Cass SP: Benign Paroxysmal Positional Vertigo. *N Engl J Med* 341:1590, 1999. Copyright © 1999 Massachusetts Medical Society. All rights reserved.

Alternatively, a cervical collar can be used to prevent loose particles from sliding back to the posterior semicircular canals. There are no data to support these recommendations. These maneuvers can be performed without using the vibrator although the results are said to be not as good. This maneuver can be repeated at weekly intervals until vertigo ceases and the Dix–Hallpike test is negative.

Brandt's and Daroff's exercises can be used in patients who cannot keep their heads upright for 24 to 48 hours as recommended in Epley's maneuver. The patient can do the exercises at home without the presence of a physician or therapist. These exercises probably work by habituation. The patient is asked to sit on the edge of the bed with eyes closed and to rotate the head horizontally by approximately 45 degrees. The patient then lies down on the side opposite to the direction of head rotation and waits for at least 30 seconds or until the vertigo has resolved. The movement is then repeated in the opposite direction. Patients can repeat these exercises every 3 hours and can stop them 2 to 3 days after becoming symptom-free. Improvement usually occurs after 1 to 2 weeks of exercises.

Surgery

Surgery is reserved for a small group of patients who fail pharmacologic treatment or vestibular rehabilitation, or who have cerebellopontine angle tumors. Patients with uncontrolled Ménière's disease can have a transmastoid labyrinthectomy, or partial vestibular neurectomy, or endolymphatic sac decompression. Very rarely, patients with benign paroxysmal positional vertigo who do not respond to repeated canalith repositioning procedures may benefit from disabling of the semicircular canal either by singular neurectomy or by occluding the posterior semicircular canal.

PATIENT EDUCATION

Patient education plays a very important role in the management of chronic dizziness. Understanding the basic pathophysiology of dizziness often alleviates associated anxiety. Education also helps patients to modify activities appropriately, thus encouraging patients to cope actively with their dizziness. While most patients need to be advised to be more active, some should be told to avoid looking up or bending down, when these motions clearly precipitate cervical dizziness attacks. Home modifications to reduce neck extension can include storing commonly used items on lower shelves. When orthostatic hypotension is present, patients should be instructed to rise slowly from a supine or sitting position. They should also flex their hands and feet a few times before standing and should never try to walk while feeling dizzy. They should avoid over-the-counter medications such as sleeping pills and cold and allergy medicine, and should ingest a sufficient amount of water.

ACKNOWLEDGMENT

The authors wish to thank Philip D. Sloane, MD, MPH for his valuable comments.

REFERENCES

Boult C et al: The relation of dizziness to functional decline. *J Am Geriatr Soc* 39:858, 1991.

Colledge NR et al: Evaluation of investigations to diagnose the cause of dizziness in elderly people: A community-based controlled study. *BMJ* 313:788, 1996.

Colledge NR et al: The prevalence and characteristics of dizziness in an elderly community. *Age Ageing* 23:117, 1994.

Davis LE: Dizziness in elderly men. *J Am Geriatr Soc* 42:1184, 1994.

Drachman DA, Hart CW: An approach to the dizzy patient. *Neurology* 22:323, 1972.

Ensrud KE et al: Postural hypotension and postural dizziness in elderly women. *Arch Intern Med* 152:1058, 1992.

Grimby A, Rosenhall U: Health-related quality of life and dizziness in old age. *Gerontology* 41:286, 1995.

Kao A et al: Validation of dizziness as a possible geriatric syndrome. *J Am Geriatr Soc* 49:72, 2001.

Katsarkas A: Dizziness in aging. A retrospective study of 1194 cases. *Otolaryngol Head Neck Surg* 110:296, 1994.

Lawson J et al: Diagnosis of geriatric patients with severe dizziness. *J Am Geriatr Soc* 47:12, 1999.

Norre ME, Beckers A: Benign paroxysmal positional vertigo in the elderly. Treatment by habituation exercises. *J Am Geriatr Soc* 36:425, 1988.

Sloane PD, Baloh RW: Persistent dizziness in geriatric patients. *J Am Geriatr Soc* 37:1031, 1989.

Sloane PD et al: The vestibular system in the elderly: Clinical implications. *Am J Otolaryngol* 10:422, 1989.

Sloane P et al: Dizziness in a community elderly population. *J Am Geriatr Soc* 37:101, 1989.

Sloane PD et al: Psychological factors associated with chronic dizziness in patients' aged 60 and older. *J Am Geriatr Soc* 42:847, 1994.

Sloane PD et al: Dizziness: State of the science. *Ann Intern Med* 134:823, 2001.

Tinetti ME et al: Health, functional, and psychological outcomes among older persons with chronic dizziness. *J Am Geriatr Soc* 48:417, 2000.

Tinetti ME et al: Dizziness among older adults: A possible geriatric syndrome. *Ann Intern Med* 132:337, 2000.

Walker MF, Zee DS: Bedside vestibular examination. *Otolaryngol Clin North Am* 33(3):495, 2000.

Yardley L et al: A randomized controlled trial of exercise therapy for dizziness and vertigo in primary care. *Br J Gen Pract* 48:1136, 1998.

Syncope

ROSE ANNE KENNY

DEFINITION

Syncope (derived from the Greek words, "syn" meaning "with" and the verb "koptein" meaning "to cut," or more appropriately in this case, "to interrupt") is a symptom, defined as a transient, self-limited loss of consciousness, usually leading to falling. The onset of syncope is relatively rapid, and the subsequent recovery is spontaneous, complete, and usually prompt.

EPIDEMIOLOGY

Syncope is a common symptom experienced by up to 30 percent of healthy adults at least once in their lifetime. Syncope accounts for 3 percent of emergency department visits and 1 percent of medical admissions to a general hospital. Syncope is the seventh most common reason for emergency admission of patients older than age 65 years. The prevalence of syncope in a chronic care facility is close to 23 percent over a 10-year period, with an annual incidence of 6 percent, and recurrence rate of 30 percent over 2 years.

Syncope from a cardiac cause is associated with higher mortality rates irrespective of age. In patients with a noncardiac or unknown cause of syncope, older age, a history of congestive cardiac failure, and male sex are important prognostic factors of mortality. It remains undetermined whether syncope directly is associated with mortality or is merely a marker of more severe underlying disease.

PATHOPHYSIOLOGY

The temporary cessation of cerebral function that causes syncope results from transient and sudden reduction of blood flow to parts of the brain (brainstem reticular activating system) responsible for consciousness.

Regardless of the etiology, the underlying mechanism responsible for syncope is a drop in cerebral oxygen delivery below the threshold for consciousness. Cerebral oxygen delivery, in turn, depends on both cerebral blood flow and oxygen content. Any combination of chronic or acute processes that lowers cerebral oxygen delivery below the "consciousness" threshold may cause syncope. Age-related physiologic impairments in heart rate, blood pressure, cerebral blood flow, in combination with comorbid conditions and concurrent medications account for the increased prevalence of syncope in the older person. The blunted baroreflex sensitivity with aging is manifested as a reduction in the heart rate response to hypotensive stimuli. Older people are prone to reduced blood volume due to excessive salt wasting by the kidneys as a result of a decline in plasma renin and aldosterone, a rise in atrial natriuretic peptide, and concurrent diuretic therapy. Low blood volume together with age-related diastolic dysfunction can lead to a low cardiac output, which increases susceptibility to orthostatic hypotension and vasovagal syncope. Cerebral autoregulation, which maintains a constant cerebral circulation over a wide range of blood pressure changes, is altered in the presence of hypertension and possibly by aging; the latter is still controversial. In general, it is agreed that sudden mild to moderate declines in blood pressure can affect cerebral blood flow markedly and render an older person particularly vulnerable to presyncope and syncope. Syncope may thus result either from a single process that markedly and abruptly decreases cerebral oxygen delivery or from the accumulated effect of multiple processes, each of which contributes to the reduced oxygen delivery (see Table 121-1).

Multifactorial Etiology

Up to 40 percent of patients with recurrent syncope will remain undiagnosed despite extensive investigations, particularly older patients who have marginal cognitive impairment and for whom a witnessed account of events is often unavailable. The high frequency of unidentified causes in clinical studies may occur because patients failed to recall important diagnostic details, because of the stringent diagnostic criteria used in clinical studies, or because the syncopal episode resulted from a combination of chronic and acute factors rather than from a single obvious disease process. Indeed, a multifactorial etiology likely explains many cases of syncope in older persons who are predisposed because of multiple chronic diseases and medication effects superimposed on the age-related physiologic

Table 121-1 Causes of Syncope

Neurally mediated reflex syncopal syndromes
- Vasovagal faint (common faint)
- Carotid sinus syncope
- Situational faint

    Acute hemorrhage

    Cough, sneeze

    Gastrointestinal stimulation (swallow, defecation, visceral pain)

    Micturition (postmicturition)

    Postexercise

    Pain, anxiety
- Glossopharyngeal and trigeminal neuralgia

Orthostatic
- Aging
- Hypertension and antihypertensives
- Autonomic failure

    Primary autonomic failure syndromes (e.g., pure autonomic failure, multiple system atrophy, Parkinson's disease with autonomic failure)

    Secondary autonomic failure syndromes (e.g., diabetic neuropathy, amyloid neuropathy)
- Medications (see table 121-2)
- Volume depletion

    Hemorrhage, diarrhea, Addison's disease, diuretics, febrile illness, hot weather

Cardiac Arrhythmias
- Sinus node dysfunction (including bradycardia/ tachycardia syndrome)
- Atrioventricular conduction system disease
- Paroxymal supraventricular and ventricular tachycardias
- Implanted device (pacemaker, internal cardioverter-defibrillator) malfunction
- Drug-induced proarrhythmias

Structural cardiac or cardiopulmonary disease
- Cardiac valvular disease
- Acute myocardial infarction/ischemia
- Obstructive cardiomyopathy
- Atrial myxoma
- Acute aortic dissection
- Pericardial disease/tamponade
- Pulmonary embolus/pulmonary hypertension

Cerebrovascular
- Vascular steal syndromes

Multifactorial

Table 121-2 Some Drugs that can Cause or Contribute to Syncope

Drug	Mechanism
Diuretics	Volume depletion
Vasodilators Angiotensin-converting enzyme inhibitors Calcium channel blockers Hydralazine Nitrates α-Adrenergic blockers Prazosin	Reduction in systemic vascular resistance and venodilation
Other antihypertensive drugs α-Methyldopa Clonidine Guanethidine Hexamethonium Labetalol Mecamylamine Phenoxybenzamine	Centrally acting antihypertensives
Drugs associated with torsade de pointes Amiodarone Disopyramide Encainide Flecainide Quinidine Procainamide Solatol	Ventricular tachycardia associated with a prolonged QT interval
Digoxin	Cardiac arrhythmias
Psychoactive drugs Tricyclic antidepressants Phenothiazines Monamine oxidase inhibitors Barbiturates	Central nervous system effects causing hypotension; cardiac arrhythmias
Alcohol	Central nervous system effects causing hypotension; cardiac arrhythmias

changes described above. Common factors that, in combination, may predispose to, or precipitate, syncope include anemia, chronic lung disease, congestive heart failure, and dehydration. Table 121-2 lists medications that may contribute to, or cause, syncope.

Individual Causes of Syncope

Table 121-1 lists individual common causes of syncope. Strict diagnostic criteria are essential for accurate diagnosis and management. The most frequent individual causes of syncope in older patients are neurally mediated syndromes, including carotid sinus syndrome, orthostatic hypotension, vasovagal syndromes, and postprandial hypotension, as well as arrhythmias, including both tachyarrhythmias and

Table 121-3 Disorders Commonly Misdiagnosed as Syncope

- Transient ischemic attacks (TIA) of carotid or vertebrobasilar origin
- Hypoglycemia and other metabolic disorders
- Some forms of epilepsy
- Alcohol and other intoxicats
- Hyperventilation with hypocapnia

bradyarrhythmias. These disease processes are described in the next section. Table 121-3 lists disorders that may be confused with syncope and which may, or may not, be associated with loss of consciousness.

PRESENTATION

As noted, the underlying mechanism of syncope is a transient cerebral hypoperfusion. In some forms of syncope, there may be a premonitory period in which various symptoms (e.g., light-headedness, nausea, sweating, weakness, and visual disturbances) offer warning of an impending syncopal event. Often, however, loss of consciousness occurs without warning. Recovery from syncope is usually accompanied by almost immediate restoration of appropriate behavior and orientation. Amnesia for loss of consciousness occurs in many older individuals and in those with cognitive impairment. The postrecovery period may be associated with fatigue.

Syncope and falls are often considered two separate entities with different etiologies. Recent evidence suggests, however, that these conditions may not be distinctly separate. In older adults, determining whether patients who have fallen have had a syncopal event can be difficult. Half of syncopal episodes are unwitnessed, and older patients may have amnesia for loss of consciousness. Amnesia for loss of consciousness has been observed in half of patients with carotid sinus syndrome who present with falls, and in a quarter of all patients with carotid sinus syndrome, irrespective of presentation. More recent reports confirm a high incidence of falls in addition to traditional syncopal symptoms in older patients with sick sinus syndrome and atrioventricular conduction disorders. Thus, syncope and falls are often indistinguishable and may, in some cases, be manifestations of similar pathophysiologic processes. The presentation of specific causes of syncope are presented in the following sections.

EVALUATION

The initial step in the evaluation of syncope is considering whether there is a specific cardiac or neurologic etiology or whether the etiology is likely multifactorial. The starting point for the evaluation of syncope is a careful history and physical examination. A witness account of events is important to ascertain when possible. Three key questions should be addressed during the initial evaluation: (1) Is

loss of consciousness attributable to syncope or not? (2) Is heart disease present or absent? (3) Are there important clinical features in the history and physical examination that suggest the etiology?

Differentiating true syncope from other "nonsyncopal" conditions associated with real or apparent loss of consciousness is generally the first diagnostic challenge and influences the subsequent diagnostic strategy. Heart disease is an independent predictor of a cardiac cause of syncope, with a sensitivity of 95 percent and a specificity of 45 percent.

Patients frequently complain of dizziness alone or as a prodrome to syncope and unexplained falls. The clinical features of dizziness might guide the diagnosis. Four categories of symptoms—vertigo, dysequilibrium, light-headedness, and others—have been recognized (see Chap. 120). Light-headedness often is associated with an underlying cardiovascular cause of symptoms, although the category of sensation has neither the sensitivity nor specificity in older, as in younger, patients. Dizziness is more likely to be attributable to a cardiovascular diagnosis if associated with pallor, syncope, prolonged standing, or the need to lie down or sit down when symptoms occur.

Initial evaluation may lead to a diagnosis based on symptoms, signs or electrocardiogram (ECG) findings. Under such circumstances, no further evaluation is needed, and treatment, if any, can be planned. More commonly, the initial evaluation leads to a suspected diagnosis (see Table 121-1), which needs to be confirmed by directed testing. If a diagnosis is confirmed by specific testing, treatment may be initiated. On the other hand, if the diagnosis is not confirmed, then patients are considered to have unexplained syncope and should be evaluated following a strategy such as that outlined in Fig. 121-1. It is important to attribute a diagnosis, if possible, rather than assume that an abnormality known to produce syncope or hypotensive symptoms is the cause. To attribute a diagnosis, patients should have symptom reproduction during investigation and, preferably, alleviation of symptoms with specific intervention. It is not uncommon however, for more than one predisposing disorder to coexist in older patients, rendering a precise diagnosis difficult.

The most important issue in patients with unexplained syncope is the presence of structural heart disease or an abnormal ECG. These findings are associated with a higher risk of arrhythmias and a higher mortality at 1 year. In these patients, cardiac evaluation consisting of echocardiography, stress testing, and tests for arrhythmia detection, such as prolonged electrocardiographic and loop monitoring or electrophysiologic study, are recommended. The most alarming ECG sign in a patient with syncope is probably alternating complete left and right bundle-branch block, or alternating right bundle-branch block with left anterior or posterior fascicular block, suggesting trifascicular conduction system disease and intermittent or impending high-degree arteriovenous (AV) block. Patients with bifascicular block (right bundle-branch block plus left anterior or left posterior fascicular block, or left bundle-branch block) are at higher risk of developing high-degree AV block. A significant problem in the evaluation of syncope and bifascicular block is the transient nature of high-degree

Syncope

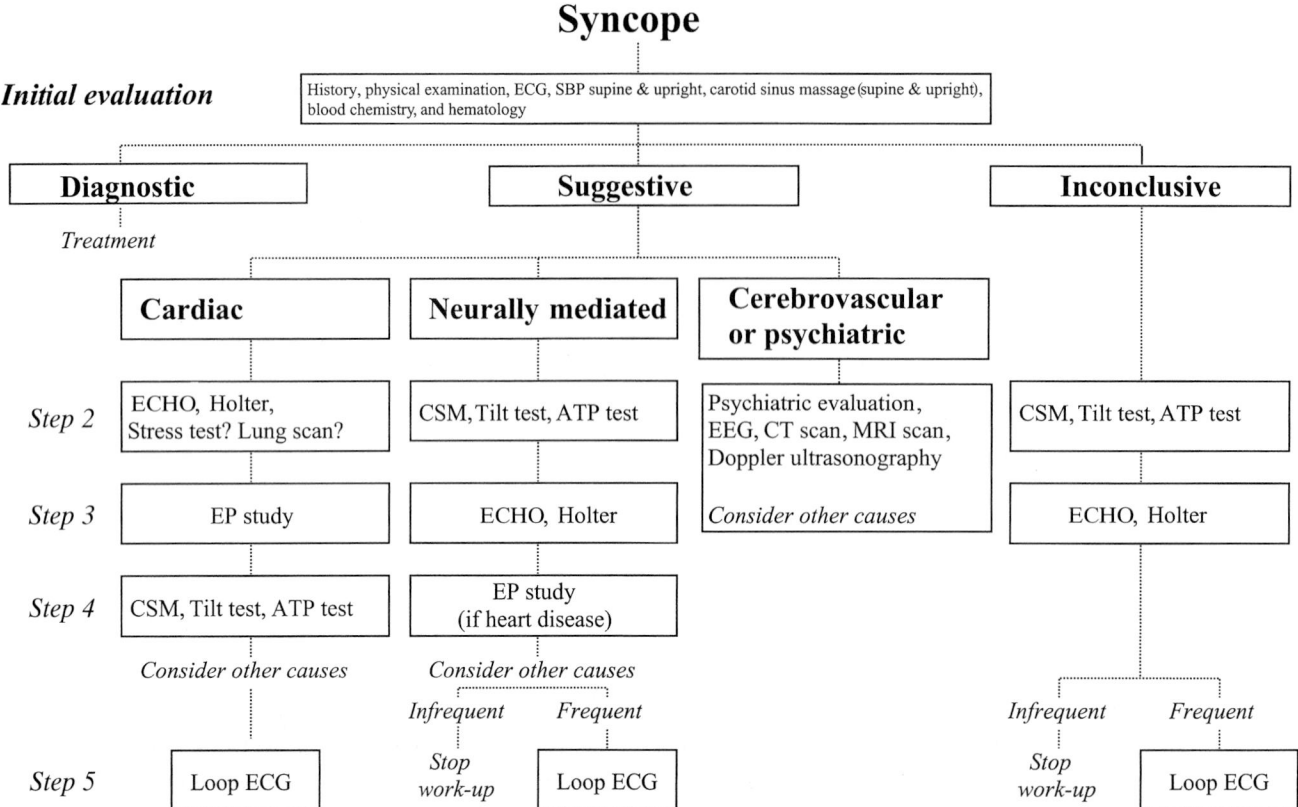

Figure 121-1 A flowchart approach to the evaluation of syncope for all age groups based on the recommendations from the European Society Task Force on Syncope. ATP test, adenosine provocation test; CSM, carotid sinus massage; ECHO, echocardiogram; EEG, electroencephalogram; EP study, electrophysiologic study; ECG, electrocardiogram.

AV block and, therefore, the long periods required to document it by ECG.

In patients without structural heart disease and a normal ECG, evaluation for neurally mediated syncope should be considered. The tests for neurally mediated syncope consist of tilt testing and carotid sinus massage.

The majority of older patients with single or rare episodes of syncope likely have a multifactorial etiology, and thus both predisposing and precipitating causes should be sought in the history, examination, and laboratory evaluation.

The presentation, evaluation, and management of individual causes of syncope are presented in the following sections.

CAROTID SINUS SYNDROME AND CAROTID SINUS HYPERSENSITIVITY

Pathophysiology

Carotid sinus syndrome is an important but frequently overlooked cause of syncope and presyncope in older persons. Episodic bradycardia and/or hypotension resulting from exaggerated baroreceptor mediated reflexes or carotid sinus hypersensitivity characterize the syndrome. The syndrome is diagnosed in persons with otherwise unexplained recurrent syncope who have carotid sinus hypersensitivity.

The latter is considered present if carotid sinus massage produces asystole exceeding 3 seconds (cardioinhibitory), or a fall in systolic blood pressure exceeding 50 mmHg in the absence of cardioinhibition (vasodepressor) or a combination of the two (mixed).

Epidemiology

Up to 10 percent of the healthy aged population have carotid sinus hypersensitivity. The prevalence is higher in the presence of coronary artery disease or hypertension. Abnormal responses to carotid sinus massage are more likely to be observed in individuals with coronary artery disease and in those on vasoactive drugs known to influence carotid sinus reflex sensitivity such as digoxin, beta-blockers and α-methyldopa. Other hypotensive disorders, such as vasovagal syncope and orthostatic hypotension, coexist in one-third of patients with carotid sinus hypersensitivity. In centers that routinely perform carotid sinus massage in all older patients with syncope, carotid sinus syndrome is found in 20 to 45 percent. This frequency needs to be interpreted within the context that these centers evaluate a preselected group of patients who have a higher likelihood of carotid sinus syndrome than the general population of older persons with syncope.

Carotid sinus syndrome is virtually unknown before the age of 50 years; its incidence increases with age thereafter.

Males are more commonly affected than females. Carotid sinus syndrome is associated with appreciable morbidity. Approximately half of patients sustain an injury, including a fracture, during symptomatic episodes. In a prospective study of falls in nursing home residents, a threefold increase in the fracture rate in those with carotid sinus hypersensitivity was observed. Indeed, carotid sinus hypersensitivity can be considered as a modifiable risk factor for fractures of the femoral neck. Carotid sinus syndrome is not associated with an increased risk of death. The mortality rate in patients with the syndrome is similar to that of patients with unexplained syncope and the general population matched for age and sex. Mortality rates are similar for the three subtypes of the syndrome.

The natural history of carotid sinus hypersensitivity has not been well investigated. In one study, the majority (90 percent) of persons with abnormal hemodynamic responses but without syncopal symptoms, remained symptom free during a follow-up over 19 ± 16 months, while half of those who presented with syncope had symptom recurrence.

Presentation

The syncopal symptoms are usually precipitated by mechanical stimulation of the carotid sinus such as head turning, tight neckwear, neck pathology and by vagal stimuli such as prolonged standing. Other recognized triggers for symptoms are the postprandial state, straining, looking or stretching upwards, exertion, defecation, and micturition. In a significant number of patients, no triggering event can be identified. Abnormal response to carotid sinus massage (see section on Carotid Sinus Massage) may not always be reproducible necessitating repetition of the procedure if the diagnosis is strongly suspected.

Evaluation

Carotid Sinus Massage

Carotid sinus reflex sensitivity is assessed by measuring heart rate and blood pressure responses to carotid sinus massage (Fig. 121-2). Cardioinhibition and vasodepression are more common on the right side. In patients with cardioinhibitory carotid sinus syndrome, more than 70 percent have a positive response to right-sided carotid sinus massage, either alone or in combination with left-sided carotid sinus massage. There is no fixed relationship between the rate of heart rate slowing and the degree of fall in blood pressure.

Carotid sinus massage is a crude and unquantifiable technique, and is prone to both intra- and interobserver variation. More scientific diagnostic methods using neck chamber suction or drug-induced changes in blood pressure can be used for carotid baroreceptor activation, but are not suitable for routine clinical use. The recommended duration of carotid sinus massage is from 5 to 10 seconds. The maximum fall in heart rate usually occurs within 5 seconds of the onset of massage (Fig. 121-3).

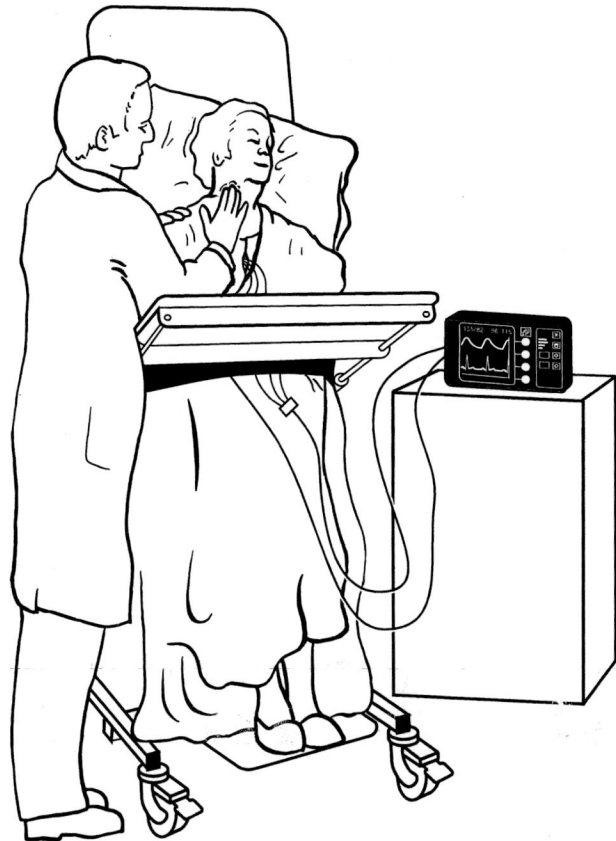

Figure 121-2 Procedure for carotid sinus massage while upright.

Complications resulting from carotid sinus massage include cardiac arrhythmias and neurologic sequelae. Fatal arrhythmias, including both asystolic and ventricular, are extremely uncommon and have generally only occurred in patients with underlying heart disease undergoing therapeutic, rather than diagnostic, massage. Digoxin toxicity has been implicated in most cases of ventricular fibrillation. Neurologic complications result from either occlusion of, or embolization from, the carotid artery. Several authors report cases of hemiplegia following carotid sinus stimulation, often in the absence of hemodynamic changes. Complications from carotid sinus massage, however, are uncommon. In a prospective series of 1000 consecutive cases, no patient had cardiac complications and 1 percent had transient neurologic symptoms that resolved. Persistent neurologic complications were uncommon, occurring in 0.04 percent. Carotid sinus massage should not be performed in patients who have had a recent cerebrovascular event or myocardial infarction.

Symptom reproduction during carotid sinus massage was regarded by early investigators as essential in the diagnosis of carotid sinus syndrome. Older patients, however, may manifest reproducibly abnormal hemodynamic responses without symptoms. Spontaneous symptoms usually occur in the upright position. It may thus be worth repeating the procedure, with the patient upright on a tilt table, even after demonstrating a positive response when supine. This reproduction of symptoms aids in attributing the episodes to carotid sinus hypersensitivity especially in

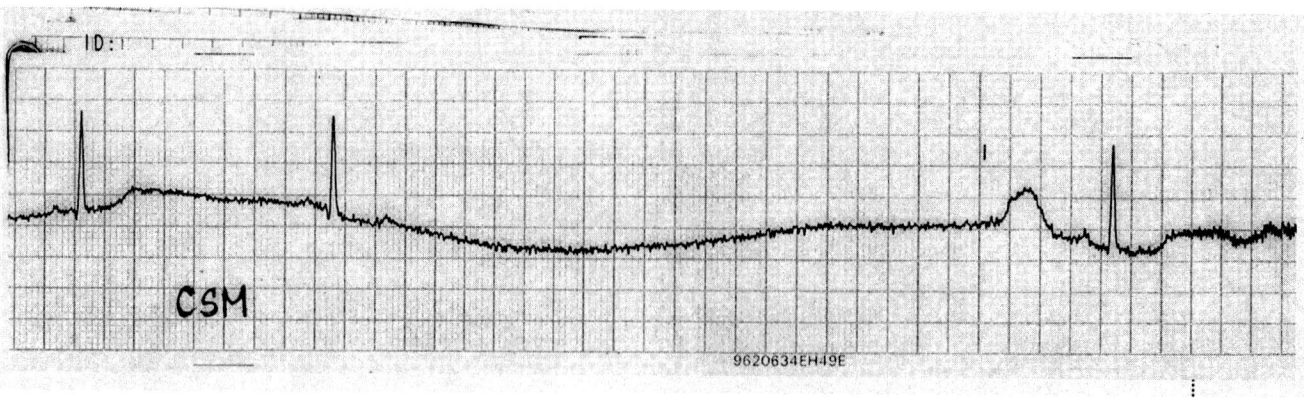

Figure 121-3 Cardioinhibitory carotid sinus response asystole of 5.2 seconds.

patients with unexplained falls who deny loss of consciousness. In one-third of patients a diagnostic response is only achieved during upright carotid sinus massage.

Management

No treatment is necessary in persons with asymptomatic carotid sinus hypersensitivity. There is no consensus, however, on the timing of therapeutic intervention in the presence of symptoms or syncopal episodes. Considering the high rate of injury in symptomatic episodes as well as the low recurrence rate of symptoms, it is prudent to treat all patients with a history of two or more symptomatic episodes. The need for intervention in those individuals with a solitary event should be assessed on an individual basis, taking into consideration the severity of the event and the patient's comorbidity.

Treatment strategies in the past included carotid sinus denervation achieved either surgically or by radioablation. Success rates with radioablation were variable and the procedure has largely been abandoned. Surgical denervation has been reported to relieve symptoms in approximately two-thirds of patients, but is not without risk of postoperative orthostatic hypotension and hypertensive crises. Denervation surgery is still occasionally considered in patients with coexisting neck pathology or with vasodepression resistant to drug therapy.

Atrioventricular sequential pacing, chamber cardiac pacing, is the treatment of choice in patients with symptomatic cardioinhibitory carotid sinus syndrome. Atrial pacing is contraindicated in view of the high prevalence of both sinoatrial and atrioventricular block in patients with carotid sinus hypersensitivity. Ventricular pacing abolishes cardioinhibition but fails to alleviate symptoms in a significant number of patients. Such symptoms result from either aggravation of a coexisting vasodepressor response or the development of pacemaker-induced hypotension, referred to as pacemaker syndrome. The latter occurs when ventriculoatrial conduction is intact, as is the case for up to 80 percent of patients with the syndrome. Dual-chamber pacing results in significantly less vasodepression than ventricular pacing during both supine and upright carotid sinus massage. Moreover, with maintenance of atrioventricular synchrony, there is no risk of pacemaker syndrome. With appropriate pacing, syncope

is abolished in 85 to 90 percent of patients with cardioinhibition.

In a recent report of cardiac pacing in older fallers with a mean age of 74 years who had cardioinhibitory carotid sinus hypersensitivity, falls during 1 year of follow up were reduced by two-thirds in patients who received dual-chamber systems; syncopal episodes were reduced by half. More than 50 percent of the patients in the aforementioned series had gait abnormalities and 75 percent had balance abnormalities that would render individuals more susceptible to falls under hemodynamic circumstances, thus further suggesting the multifactorial nature of many falls and syncopal episodes.

Treatment of vasodepressor carotid sinus syndrome is less successful because of poor understanding of its pathophysiology. Ephedrine has been reported to be useful, but long-term use is limited by side effects. Dihydroergotamine is effective but poorly tolerated. Fludrocortisone, a mineralocorticoid widely used in the treatment of orthostatic hypotension, is used in the treatment of vasodepressor carotid sinus syndrome with good results, but its use is limited in the longer term by adverse effects. The medical treatment of vasodepressor carotid sinus syndrome remains unsatisfactory.

ORTHOSTATIC HYPOTENSION

Pathophysiology

Orthostatic or postural hypotension is arbitrarily defined as either a 20 mmHg fall in systolic blood pressure or a 10 mmHg fall in diastolic blood pressure on assuming an upright posture from a supine position. Orthostatic hypotension implies abnormal blood pressure homeostasis and is a frequent observation with advancing age. Prevalence of postural hypotension varies between 4 percent and 33 percent among community-living older persons, depending on the methodology used. Higher prevalence and larger falls in systolic blood pressure have been reported with increasing age and often signifies general physical frailty. Orthostatic hypotension is an important cause of syncope, accounting for 14 percent of all diagnosed cases in a large series on syncope. In a tertiary referral clinic dealing with unexplained syncope, dizziness, and falls,

32 percent of patients older than age 65 years had orthostatic hypotension.

Aging

The heart rate and blood pressure responses to orthostasis occur in three phases: (1) an initial heart rate and blood pressure response, (2) an early phase of stabilization, and (3) a phase of prolonged standing; all are influenced by aging. The maximum rise in heart rate and the ratio between the maximum and the minimum heart rate in the initial phase decline with age, implying a relatively fixed heart rate irrespective of posture. Despite a blunted heart rate response, blood pressure and cardiac output are adequately maintained on standing in active, healthy, well-hydrated, and normotensive older persons. The underlying mechanism involves decreased vasodilatation and reduced venous pooling during the initial phases, and increased peripheral vascular resistance after prolonged standing. However, in older persons with hypertension and cardiovascular disease receiving vasoactive drugs, these circulatory adjustments to orthostatic stress are disturbed, rendering them vulnerable to postural hypotension.

Hypertension

Hypertension further increases the risk of hypotension by impairing baroreflex sensitivity and reducing ventricular compliance. A strong relationship between supine hypertension and orthostatic hypotension has been reported among unmedicated institutionalized older persons. Hypertension increases the risk of cerebral ischemia from sudden declines in blood pressure. Older persons with hypertension are more vulnerable to cerebral ischemic symptoms even with modest and short-term postural hypotension, because the threshold for cerebral autoregulation is altered by prolonged elevation of blood pressure. In addition, antihypertensive agents impair cardiovascular reflexes and further increase the risk of orthostatic hypotension.

Medications

Drugs (see Table 121-2) are important causes of orthostatic hypotension. Ideally, establishing a causal relationship between a drug and orthostatic hypotension requires identification of the culprit medicine, abolition of symptoms by withdrawal of the drug, and rechallenge of the drug to reproduce symptoms. Rechallenge is often omitted in clinical practice in view of the potential serious consequences. In the presence of polypharmacy, which is common in the older person, it becomes difficult to identify a single culprit drug because of the synergistic effect of different drugs and drug interactions. Thus, all drugs should be considered as possible contributors to orthostasis.

Other Conditions

A number of nonneurogenic conditions are also associated with postural hypotension. These conditions include myocarditis; atrial myxoma; aortic stenosis; constrictive pericarditis; hemorrhage; diarrhea; vomiting; ileostomy; burns; hemodialysis; salt-losing nephropathy; diabetes insipidus; adrenal insufficiency; fever; and extensive varicose veins. Volume depletion for any reason is a common sole, or contributing, cause of postural hypotension, and, in turn, of syncope.

Primary Autonomic Failure Syndromes (see also Chap. 124)

Three distinct clinical entities, namely pure autonomic failure (PAF), multiple system atrophy (MSA) or Shy–Drager syndrome (SDS), and autonomic failure associated with idiopathic Parkinson's disease (IPD) are associated with orthostasis. PAF, the least common and a relatively benign entity, was previously known as idiopathic orthostatic hypotension. This condition presents with orthostatic hypotension, defective sweating, impotence, and bowel disturbances. No other neurologic deficits are found and resting plasma noradrenaline levels are low. MSA is the most common and has the poorest prognosis. Clinical manifestations include features of dysautonomia and motor disturbances as a result of striatonigral degeneration, cerebellar atrophy, or pyramidal lesions. Additional neurologic deficits include muscle atrophy; distal sensorimotor neuropathy; pupillary abnormalities; restriction of ocular movements; disturbances in rhythm and control of breathing; life-threatening laryngeal stridor; and bladder disturbances. Psychiatric manifestations and cognitive defects are usually absent. Resting plasma noradrenaline levels are usually within the normal range, but fail to rise on standing or tilting. The prevalence of autonomic failure in Parkinson's disease is not precisely known. Cerebellar and pyramidal signs are not seen. Orthostatic hypotension in Parkinson's disease can be a result of factors other than dysautonomia, such as side effects of antiparkinsonian drugs.

Secondary Autonomic Dysfunction

Autonomic nervous system involvement is seen in several systemic diseases. A large number of neurologic disorders are also complicated by autonomic dysfunction that may involve several organs leading to a variety of symptoms in addition to orthostatic hypotension including anhidrosis, constipation, diarrhea, impotence, retention of urine, urinary incontinence, stridor, apneic episodes, and Horner's syndrome. Among the most serious and prevalent conditions associated with orthostatic hypotension caused by autonomic dysfunction are diabetes; multiple sclerosis; brainstem lesions; compressive and noncompressive spinal cord lesions; demyelinating polyneuropathies (Guillain Barré's syndrome); chronic renal failure; chronic liver disease; and connective-tissue disorders.

Presentation

The clinical manifestations of orthostatic hypotension are caused by hypoperfusion of the brain and other organs. Depending on the degree of fall in blood pressure and cerebral hypoperfusion, symptoms can vary from dizziness to syncope associated with a variety of visual defects, from blurred vision to blackout. Other reported ischemic symptoms of orthostatic hypotension are nonspecific and include lethargy and weakness, suboccipital and paravertebral muscle pain, low back ache, calf claudication, and angina. Several precipitating factors for orthostatic hypotension have been identified, including speed of positional change, prolonged recumbency, warm environment, raised intrathoracic pressure (coughing, defecation, micturition) physical exertion and vasoactive drugs.

Evaluation

The diagnosis of orthostatic hypotension involves a demonstration of a postural fall in blood pressure after active standing. Reproducibility of orthostatic hypotension depends on the time of measurement and on autonomic function. The diagnosis may be missed on casual measurement during the afternoon. The procedure should be repeated during the morning after maintaining supine posture for at least 10 minutes. Sphygmomanometer measurement is as sensitive as sophisticated phasic blood pressure measurements and active standing is as diagnostic as head up tilting. Once a diagnosis of postural hypotension is made, the evaluation involves identifying the cause or causes of orthostasis mentioned above.

Management (Table 121–4)

The goal of therapy for symptomatic orthostatic hypotension is to improve cerebral perfusion. There are several nonpharmacologic interventions for orthostatic hypotension, including avoidance of precipitating factors for low blood pressure, elevation of the head of the bed at night, and application of graduated pressure from an abdominal support garment or from stockings. Medications known to contribute to postural hypotension should be eliminated or reduced. There are reports to suggest benefit from implantation of cardiac pacemakers, in a small number of patients, by increasing heart rate during postural change. However, the effects of tachypacing on improving cardiac output in patients with maximal vasodilatation remains conjectural. A large number of drugs have been used to raise blood pressure in orthostatic hypotension, including fludrocortisone, midodrine, ephedrine, desmopressin (DDAVP), octreotide, erythropoietin, and nonsteroidal antiinflammatory agents. Fludrocortisone (9-α-fluohydrocortisone), in a dose of 0.1 to 0.2 mg, causes volume expansion, reduces natriuresis and sensitizes α-adrenoceptors to noradrenaline. In older people, the drug is poorly tolerated in larger doses and for long periods. Reported adverse effects in the older person include hypertension, cardiac failure, depression, edema, and hypokalemia. Midodrine is a directly acting sympathomimetic vasoconstrictor of resistance vessels. Treatment is started at a dose of 2.5 mg three times daily and requires gradual titration to a maximum dose of 45 mg/d. The adverse effects include pilomotor erection, gastrointestinal symptoms, and cardiovascular and central nervous system toxicity. Side effects are usually controlled by dose reduction. Midodrine is comparable in its efficacy with other sympathomimetic agents but is better tolerated. Midodrine is an effective and well-tolerated treatment for moderate

Table 121–4 Management of Orthostatic Hypotension in Older Persons

Identify and treat correctable causes

Reduce or eliminate drugs causing orthostatic hypotension
(see Table 121-2)

Avoid situations that may exacerbate orthostatic hypotension
    Standing motionless
    Prolonged recumbency
    Large meals
    Hot weather
    Hot showers
    Straining at stool or with voiding
    Isometric exercise
    Ingesting alcohol
    Hyperventilation
    Dehydration

Raise the head of the bed to 5- to 20-degree angle

Wear waist-high custom-fitted elastic stockings and an abdominal binder

Participate in physical conditioning exercises

Controlled postural exercises using the tilt table

Avoid diuretics and drink salt-containing fluids (unless congestive heart failure is present)

Drug therapy
    Caffeine
    Fludrocortisone
    Midodrine
    Desmopressin

to severe orthostatic hypotension. It significantly increases standing blood pressure and improves symptoms of orthostatic hypotension. Reported side effects have been mostly mild and only 7 percent of patients discontinue treatment because of supine hypertension. DDAVP has potent antidiuretic and mild pressor effects. Intranasal doses of 5 to 40 microgram at bed time are useful. The main side effect is water retention. This agent can be combined with fludrocortisone with synergistic effect. The drug treatment for orthostatic hypotension requires frequent monitoring for supine hypertension, electrolyte imbalance and congestive heart failure.

VASOVAGAL SYNCOPE

Pathophysiology

The normal physiologic responses to orthostasis are an increase in heart rate, rise in peripheral vascular resistance (increase in diastolic blood pressure), and minimal decline in systolic blood pressure, to maintain an adequate cardiac output. In patients with vasovagal syncope, these responses to prolonged orthostasis are paradoxical. The precise sequence of events leading to vasovagal syncope are not fully understood. The possible mechanism involves a sudden fall in venous return to heart, rapid fall in ventricular volume and virtual collapse of the ventricle because of vigorous ventricular contraction. The net result of these events is stimulation of ventricular mechanoreceptors and activation of Bezold–Jarisch reflex leading to peripheral vasodilatation (hypotension) and bradycardia. Negative inotropic agents (beta-blockers) can reportedly avert or diminish these responses in spontaneous or head-up tilt-induced vasovagal syncope. Several neurotransmitters, including serotonin, endorphins, and arginine vasopressin, play an important role in the pathogenesis of vasovagal syncope, possibly by central sympathetic inhibition, although their exact role is not yet well understood.

Healthy older persons are not as prone to vasovagal syncope as younger adults. Because of an age-related decline in baroreceptor sensitivity, the paradoxical responses to orthostasis (as in vasovagal syncope) are possibly less marked in older persons. Thus situational syncope is less common in older age. However, in the presence of hypertension and atherosclerotic cerebrovascular disease, excessive loss of baroreflex sensitivity leads to dysautonomic responses during prolonged orthostasis (in which blood pressure and heart decline steadily over time) and patients become susceptible to vasovagal syncope. Diuretic or age-related contraction of blood volume further increases the risk of syncope.

Presentation

The hallmark of vasovagal syncope is hypotension and/or bradycardia sufficiently profound to produce cerebral ischemia and loss of neural function. Vasovagal syncope has been classified into cardioinhibitory (bradycardia), vasodepressor (hypotension), and mixed (both) subtypes, depending on the blood pressure and heart rate response. In most patients, the manifestations occur in three distinct phases: a prodrome or aura, loss of consciousness, and postsyncopal phase. A precipitating factor or situation is identifiable in most patients. Common precipitating factors include extreme emotional stress, anxiety, mental anguish, trauma, physical pain or anticipation of physical pain (e.g., anticipation of venesection), warm environment, air travel, and prolonged standing. The commonest triggers in older individuals are prolonged standing and vasodilator medication. Some patients experience symptoms in specific situations such as micturition, defecation, and coughing. Prodromal symptoms include extreme fatigue; weakness; diaphoresis; nausea; visual defects; visual and auditory hallucinations; dizziness; vertigo; headache; abdominal discomfort; dysarthria; and paresthesias. The duration of prodrome varies greatly from seconds to several minutes, during which some patients take actions such as lying down to avoid an episode. The syncopal period is usually brief during which some patients develop involuntary movements usually myoclonic jerks but tonic clonic movements also occur. Vasovagal syncope may masquerade as epilepsy. Recovery is usually rapid, but some patients can experience protracted symptoms such as confusion, disorientation, nausea, headache, dizziness, and a general sense of ill health.

Evaluation

Several methods have evolved to determine an individual's susceptibility to vasovagal syncope such as Valsalva maneuvers, hyperventilation, ocular compression, and immersion of the face in cold water. However these methods are poorly reproducible and lack correlation with clinical events. Using the strong orthostatic stimulus of head-upright tilting and maximal venous pooling, vasovagal syncope can be reproduced in a susceptible individual. Head-up tilting as a diagnostic tool was first reported in 1986; the validity of this technique in identifying susceptibility to neurocardiogenic syncope has been established. Subjects are tilted head up for 40 minutes at 70 degrees. Heart rate and blood pressure are measured continuously throughout the test. A test is diagnostic or positive if symptoms are reproduced with a decline in blood pressure of greater than 50 mmHg or to less than 90 mmHg. This may be in addition to significant heart rate slowing. As with carotid sinus syndrome, the hemodynamic responses are classified as vasodepressor, cardioinhibitory, or mixed. The cardioinhibitory response is defined as asystole in excess of 3 seconds or heart rate slowing to less than 40 bpm for a minimum of 10 seconds.

The sensitivity of head-up-tilting can be further improved by provocative agents that accentuate the physiologic events leading to vasovagal syncope. The most widely used agent is intravenous isoprenaline, which enhances myocardial contractility by stimulating β-adrenoreceptors. Isoprenaline is infused, prior to head-up tilting, at a dose of 1 μg per minute and gradually increased to a maximum dose of 3 μg per minute to achieve a heart rate increase of 25 percent. Although the sensitivity of head-up tilt testing improves by approximately 15 percent, the specificity is reduced. In addition, as a result of the decline in β receptor sensitivity with age, isoprenaline may be less useful as a provocative agent in elderly patients with a higher incidence adverse effects. The other agent that can be used as a provocative agent is sublingual nitroglycerin, which, by reducing venous return as a consequence of vasodilatation, can enhance the vasovagal reaction in susceptible individuals. Nitroglycerin provocation during head-up tilt testing is preferable to other provocative tests in older patients. The duration of testing is less, and the sensitivity and specificity are better than for isoprenaline. Adenosine (ATP) has recently been described as a further diagnostic test (Figure 121-1).

Management

Avoidance of precipitating factors, including vasodilating drugs, and evasive actions such as lying down during prodromal symptoms, have great value in reducing episodes of vasovagal syncope. However, many patients experience symptoms without warning, necessitating drug therapy. A number of drugs are reported to be useful in alleviating symptoms. Beta-blockers (e.g., atenolol 50 mg/d), by their negative inotropic actions, decrease the force of ventricular contraction, and thereby reduce the degree of mechanoreceptor discharge; they are useful in vasovagal syncope. Because of its negative inotropic and anticholinergic effects, disopyramide (200 mg twice daily) has been recommended, but its efficacy is dubious. Fludrocortisone (100 to 200 μg/d) works by its volume-expanding effect. Recent reports suggest that serotonin antagonists such as fluoxetine (20 mg/d) and sertraline hydrochloride (25 mg/d) are effective in symptom relief. The efficacy of midodrine in the management of vasovagal syncope was recently observed in a double-blind randomized controlled trial. More than 50 percent of patients experienced significant symptomatic improvement, delayed response to head-up tilting, and improvement in quality of life. Midodrine acts by reducing peripheral venous pooling and thereby improving cardiac output. Elastic support hose, relaxation techniques (biofeedback), conditioning using repeated head-up tilt as therapy, and muscle contraction maneuvers are useful adjuvant therapies. Permanent cardiac pacing is beneficial in some patients who have recurrent syncope and cardioinhibitory responses. Dual-chamber pacing is the preferred mode of pacing.

POSTPRANDIAL HYPOTENSION

The effect of meals on the cardiovascular system was appreciated from postprandial exaggeration of angina, which was demonstrated objectively by deterioration of exercise tolerance following food. Postprandial reductions in blood pressure manifesting as syncope and dizziness were subsequently reported leading to extensive investigation of this phenomenon. In healthy older subjects, systolic blood pressure falls by 11 to 16 mmHg, and heart rate rises by 5 to 7 beats per minute 60 minutes after meals of varying compositions and energy content. However the change in diastolic blood pressure is not as consistent. In older persons with hypertension, orthostatic hypotension, and autonomic failure, the postprandial blood pressure fall is much greater with no corresponding rise in heart rate. These responses are marked if the energy and simple carbohydrate content of the meal is high. However in the majority of fit, as well as frail, older persons, most of these hypotensive episodes go unnoticed.

Postprandial physiologic changes include increased splanchnic and superior mesenteric artery blood flow at the expense of peripheral circulation and a rise in plasma insulin levels without corresponding rises in sympathetic nervous system activity. Vasodilator effects of insulin and other gut peptides, including neurotensin and vasoactive intestinal polypeptide, are thought to be responsible for postprandial hypotension, although the precise mechanism remains uncertain. The clinical significance of a fall in blood pressure after meals is difficult to quantitate. However, postprandial hypotension is causally related to recurrent syncope and falls in older persons. In the author's experience, postprandial symptoms occur in, at best, 20 percent of patients with symptomatic orthostatic hypotension. A reduction in simple carbohydrate content of food, its replacement with complex carbohydrates or high protein,

high fat, and frequent small meals are effective interventions for postprandial hypotension. Drugs useful in the treatment of postprandial hypotension are fludrocortisone and indomethacin, octreotide, and caffeine. Given orally along with food, caffeine prevents hypotensive symptoms in fit as well as in frail older persons, but should preferably be given in the mornings, as tolerance develops if it is taken throughout the day.

SUMMARY

Syncope is a common symptom in older adults due to age-related neurohumoral and physiologic changes plus chronic diseases and medications that reduce cerebral oxygen delivery through multiple mechanisms. Common individual causes of syncope encountered by the geriatrician are carotid sinus syndrome, orthostatic hypotension, vasovagal syncope, postprandial syncope, sinus node disease, and atrioventricular block. Algorithms for the assessment of syncope are similar to those for young adults, but the prevalence of carotid sinus syndrome and cardiac conduction disease is higher in older adults and the etiology is more often multifactorial. A systematic approach to syncope is needed with the goal being to identify either a single likely cause or multiple treatable contributing factors. Management is then based on removing or reducing the predisposing or precipitating factors through various combinations of medication adjustments, behavioral strategies, and more invasive interventions, such as cardiac pacing in select cases.

REFERENCES

Alboni P et al: The diagnostic value of history in patients with syncope with or without heart disease. *J Am Coll Cardiol* 37:1921, 2001.

Allcock LM, O'Shea D: Diagnostic yield and development of a neuro-cardiovascular investigation unit for older adults in a district general hospital. *J Gerontol A Biol Sci Med Sci* 55(8):M458, 2000.

Brignole M et al: Guidelines on management (diagnosis and treatment) of syncope. *Eur Heart J* 22(15):1256, 2001.

Guideline for the prevention of falls in older persons. American Geriatrics Society, British Geriatrics Society, and American Academy of Orthopaedic Surgeons Panel on Falls Prevention. *J Am Geriatr Soc* 49:664, 2001.

Kenny RA (ed): Falls and syncope in elderly patients. Clin Geriatr Med 18(2): 141–366, 2002.

Kenny RA et al: Carotid sinus syndrome: Modifiable risk factors for non-accidental falls in older adults. *J Am Coll Cardiol* 38(5):1491, 2001.

Kenny RA et al: The Newcastle protocols for head-up tilt-table testing in the diagnosis of vasovagal syncope, carotid sinus hypersensitivity, and related disorders. *Heart* 83(5):564, 2000.

Lipsitz LA et al: Postprandial reduction in blood pressure in the elderly. *N Engl J Med* 309:81, 1983.

Lipsitz LA et al: Intra-individual variability in postural blood pressure in the elderly. *Clinical Science* 69:337, 1985.

McIntosh SJ et al: Outcome of an integrated approach to the investigation of dizziness, falls, and syncope in elderly patients referred to a syncope clinic. *Age Ageing* 22:53, 1993.

Pressure Ulcers

RICHARD M. ALLMAN

DEFINITION

A pressure ulcer is any lesion caused by unrelieved pressure resulting in damage of underlying tissue. Synonymous terms include pressure ulcers, decubitus ulcers, and bedsores, but because pressure is the primary pathophysiologic factor in the development of these lesions, pressure ulcer is the preferred term. The terms decubitus ulcer and bedsore imply that the lesions occur only when lying down, but some of the most severe pressure-induced cutaneous injuries may occur as a result of prolonged sitting.

Pressure ulcers may present as nonblanchable erythema over a bony prominence or as areas of epithelial loss, skin breakdown, blisters, or skin necrosis manifested by eschar formation. Stage I lesions present as nonblanchable erythema of intact skin. Discoloration of skin, warmth, edema, or induration also may be indications of stage I lesions in persons with darker skin. These stage I lesions are associated with a 10-fold increased risk of subsequent development of higher-stage ulcers. Partial-thickness skin loss involving the epidermis and/or the dermis is defined as stage II. Stage III ulcers extend into the subcutaneous tissues to the deep fascia and typically show undermining. Stage IV lesions involve muscle and/or bone. Full-thickness injury, manifested by eschar, frequently involves muscle and bone but cannot be staged until the eschar is removed. Pressure-induced subepidermal blisters typically occur on the heels. Their depth cannot be determined by clinical examination.

EPIDEMIOLOGY

The prevalence of stage II and greater pressure ulcers among patients in acute-care hospitals ranges from 3 to 11 percent, and the incidence during hospitalization is between 1 and 3 percent. Among patients expected to be confined to bed or chair for at least 1 week, the prevalence of stage II and greater pressure ulcers is as high as 28 percent, and the incidence during hospitalization ranges between 8 and 30 percent. Pressure ulcers generally occur within the first 2 weeks of hospitalization, and of those patients with an ulcer, 54 percent develop them after admission. More than 50 percent of pressure ulcers occur in persons older than age 70 years.

The prevalence of pressure ulcers in nursing homes is very similar to that reported in acute-care hospitals. As many as 20 to 33 percent of patients admitted to nursing homes have a stage II or greater pressure ulcer. The incidence of pressure ulcers among newly admitted residents without ulcers and who remain in a nursing home for 4 weeks is between 11 and 14 percent.

Sepsis is the most serious complication of pressure ulcers. There are 3.5 episodes of pressure ulcer-associated bacteremia per 10,000 discharges. Of these episodes of pressure ulcer-associated bacteremia, the pressure ulcer is the probable source in nearly half the cases. When the pressure ulcer is the source of bacteremia, the in-hospital mortality is nearly 60 percent. Clinicians should be aware that transient bacteremia occurs after débridement of pressure ulcers in as many as 50 percent of patients.

Other infectious complications of pressure ulcers include local infection, cellulitis, and osteomyelitis. Infected pressure ulcers are the most common infection found in skilled nursing facilities and are reported in 6 percent of residents. Among patients with nonhealing pressure ulcers, 26 percent of ulcers have underlying bone pathology consistent with osteomyelitis. Infected pressure ulcers may be deeply undermined and lead to pyarthrosis or penetrate into the abdominal cavity. Secondary amyloidosis also can be a complication of chronic suppurative pressure ulcers. Infected pressure ulcers also can serve as reservoirs for nosocomial infections with antibiotic-resistant bacteria.

Pressure ulcers are associated with prolonged and expensive hospitalizations. Even after adjusting for other factors associated with increased length of stay, the association remains significant. The in-hospital development of pressure ulcers is associated with increased Medicare payments up to 1 year after discharge from the hospital. Eighty-four percent of the total cost of pressure ulcer treatment for nursing home residents is attributed to those residents who require hospitalization for an ulcer.

Many people with pressure ulcers have pain. Although as many as one-half of hospitalized patients with pressure ulcers cannot describe the pain, 59 to 85 percent of those who can provide such a description report at least some pain. Of these, 45 percent describe the ulcer-associated pain as distressing or horrible. Only 2 percent of patients receive analgesic medication within 4 hours of reporting such pain.

Increased death rates are consistently observed in elderly individuals who develop pressure ulcers. In addition, failure of an ulcer to heal or improve has been associated with a higher rate of death in nursing home residents. The death rate among bed- and chair-bound patients who develop a pressure ulcer during hospitalization is 60 percent 1 year after discharge, whereas the death rate for patients who do not develop a pressure ulcer is 38 percent.

PATHOPHYSIOLOGY

Four factors are implicated in the pathogenesis of pressure ulcers: pressure, shearing forces, friction, and moisture. Animal studies show repeatedly that muscle and subcutaneous tissues are more sensitive to pressure-induced injury than the epidermis. Contact pressures of 60 to 70 mmHg for 1 to 2 hours lead to degeneration of muscle fibers. In the dog, skin ulceration occurred over the greater trochanter after exposure to contact pressures of 150 mmHg for 9 to 12 hours or pressures of 500 mmHg for 2 to 6 hours. Because dogs do not have a layer of subcutaneous tissue comparable with that of humans, investigators have studied the effect of pressure over the trochanter of pigs. Pigs have tissue layers more comparable with human skin. In these latter experiments, full-thickness injury required exposure to higher pressures: 600 mmHg for 11 hours or 200 mmHg for 16 hours.

Depending on the methodology used, pressures measured under bony prominences such as the sacrum and greater trochanter can be as high as 100 to 150 mmHg when humans are lying on a regular hospital mattress. The pressures obtained are sufficient to decrease the transcutaneous oxygen tension to nearly zero. In seated persons, the pressures measured under the ischial tuberosities may easily reach 300 mmHg. Although the magnitude of these pressures may not be sufficient to cause full-thickness tissue injury without prolonged exposure to pressure, other factors can lower the pressure or time required to cause the full-thickness injury observed clinically. Repeated exposures to pressure will cause skin necrosis at lower pressures. Other data suggest that loss of subcutaneous tissue also can lower the threshold for skin breakdown as a consequence of pressure.

Shearing forces lower the amount of pressure required to cause damage to the epidermis. Shearing forces are tangential forces that are exerted when a person is seated or the head of the bed is elevated and the person slides toward the floor or the foot of the bed. The sacral skin is held in place by friction while the gluteal vessels are angulated and elongated. Such forces decrease the amount of pressure required to occlude blood vessels and are likely important in the development of deep tissue injury. One study found that the shearing forces of seated elderly and paraplegic patients are threefold greater and blood flow is about one-third that of healthy young adults, although the contact pressures are similar.

In experimental studies, friction causes intraepidermal blisters. When unroofed, these lesions result in superficial erosions. This kind of injury can occur when a patient is pulled across a sheet or the patient has repetitive movements that expose a bony prominence to such frictional forces. Intermediate degrees of moisture increase the amount of friction produced at the rubbing interface, whereas extremes of moisture or dryness decrease the frictional forces between two surfaces rubbing against each other. In addition to its impact on frictional forces, skin moisture may directly lead to maceration and epidermal injury.

The effects of pressure on tissues overlying bony prominences are likely caused by ischemia and the accumulation of cellular toxins associated with the occlusion of blood and lymphatic vessels rather than mechanical injury. Injury caused by pressure alone typically will begin in deeper tissues and spread toward the skin surface. If relieved, the normal response to pressure is hyperemia, but if persistent, pressure-induced ischemia leads to endothelial swelling and vessel leak. As plasma leaks into the interstitium, diffusing distances between the cellular elements of skin and blood vessels increase. Ultimately, hemorrhage occurs and leads to nonblanchable erythema of the skin, a stage I pressure ulcer. In bacteremic experimental animals, bacteria will be deposited at sites of pressure-induced injury and set up a deep suppurative process. This may explain the occurrence of deep pressure ulcers with apparently normal overlying skin or simply a draining sinus. The accumulation of edema fluid, blood, inflammatory cells, toxic wastes, and possibly bacteria ultimately and progressively leads to the death of muscle, subcutaneous tissue, and finally, epidermal tissue. The damage caused by shearing forces probably is mediated by pressure-induced ischemia in deep tissues as well as direct mechanical injury to subcutaneous tissue. Friction and moisture are most important in the development of superficial lesions, but their effects are likely to be greatest when excessive pressures are also present.

PRESENTATION

Any disease process leading to immobility and limited activity levels, whether a spinal cord injury, dementia, Parkinson's disease, severe congestive heart failure, or lung disease, increases the risk of pressure ulcers. In one study of geriatric patients, spontaneous nocturnal movements were counted using a device attached to the patient's mattresses. No patients with 51 or more spontaneous movements during the night developed a pressure ulcer, but 90 percent of patients with 20 or fewer spontaneous movements developed an ulcer.

Risk factors for stage II and greater pressure ulcers consistently identified by prospective studies other than limitations in mobility and activity levels include incontinence, nutritional factors, and altered level of consciousness. When examined separately, prospective studies have suggested that fecal incontinence, but not urinary incontinence, is a risk factor among patients in the acute-care hospital. Nutritional factors found to be associated significantly with pressure ulcer development include a decreased lymphocyte count, hypoalbuminemia, inadequate dietary intake, decreased body weight, and a depleted triceps skin fold.

Other factors associated with a higher incidence of stage II or greater pressure ulcers in one or more prospective studies include dry skin, increased body temperature, decreased blood pressure, and increased age. The functional impairment associated with the age-related increase in disease prevalence may explain the association of age with increased risk of pressure ulcers in part, but age-related changes in the skin may predispose the elderly patient to pressure-induced cutaneous injury independent of immobility.

Among bed- and chair-bound hospitalized patients, no pressure ulcer developed after 3 weeks of follow-up in the absence of any of these factors: inability to reposition (immobility), dry skin, nonblanchable erythema of intact skin (a stage I pressure ulcer), lymphopenia, or body weight under 58 kg. In contrast, the 3-week incidence for patients with one, two, or three or more of these factors was 11.4, 39.6, and 67.9 percent, respectively.

ASSESSMENT

The appropriate management of patients with pressure ulcers requires assessment and treatment of underlying diseases and conditions that have put the person at risk for development of a pressure ulcer and may prevent the lesion from healing. Nutritional assessment is particularly important. The location, stage, size, and wound characteristics of all pressure ulcers should be recorded. This includes assessment for sinus tracts, undermining, tunneling, exudate, necrotic tissue, granulation tissue, and epithelialization. The clinician also should document the status of the skin surrounding the ulcer.

Follow-up assessments should be repeated at least weekly to determine whether an ulcer is improving or not. These follow-up assessments may be limited to an estimation of an ulcer's surface area by multiplying its perpendicular length and width, assessing the amount of exudate present (none, light, moderate, or heavy), and determining the type of tissue present (necrotic, slough, granulation, or epithelial tissue). These assessment components can be used to determine a Pressure Ulcer Scale for Healing (PUSH) wound status score. Within 2 to 4 weeks, a pressure ulcer should show improvement based on these assessments. Reductions in ulcer size over a 2-week period predict subsequent complete healing. Therefore, if there is no evidence of ulcer improvement based on the parameters in the PUSH tool, then changes in management strategy should be considered.

Surrounding erythema may represent cellulitis, whereas purulent drainage suggests local wound infection. The presence of necrotic tissue or a darkly pigmented eschar identifies a wound unlikely to heal without débridement. Sinograms may be required to delineate the extent of pressure ulcers associated with a sinus tract.

Bacterial counts of greater than 100,000 colonies per gram of tissue in pressure ulcers correlate well with poor wound healing and wound graft failure. In particular, *Pseudomonas aeruginosa*, *Providencia*, and *Proteus* species, and anaerobic bacteria reportedly are associated with poorly healing ulcers. Despite this, because all stages II, III, and

IV ulcers are colonized with bacteria, swab cultures have no diagnostic value and should not be used. When signs of advancing cellulitis or systemic infection accompany a pressure ulcer, a culture of fluid obtained by needle aspiration or of tissue obtained by ulcer biopsy may be helpful. If an ulcer does not show improvement or evidence of local infection persists after ulcer care measures have been in place for 4 or more weeks, then quantitative bacterial cultures of the ulcer base and bone biopsy for culture and histology should be considered.

The diagnosis of osteomyelitis beneath a pressure ulcer can be difficult because there may be radiographic changes in the underlying bone due to pressure that may mimic changes seen in osteomyelitis. However, among patients with a nonhealing ulcer, the presence of an abnormal plain bone radiograph, a leukocyte count of more than 15.0×10^9 per liter, or an erythrocyte sedimentation rate of 120 mm/h suggests that the probability of underlying osteomyelitis is nearly 70 percent. On the other hand, if all three tests are normal, the probability of osteomyelitis is less than 5 percent. Thus, any of these abnormalities in an individual with a nonhealing pressure ulcer should prompt consideration of a bone biopsy and culture to confirm the diagnosis and to guide therapy.

When performed, bacteriologic studies of infected pressure ulcers often identify multiple organisms. The most common isolates include gram-negative aerobic rods. These account for 45 percent of isolates from patients with sepsis caused by pressure ulcers. Gram-positive aerobic cocci also are frequent and account for 39 percent of isolates. Bacteroides species are the most common anaerobic isolates, accounting for 16 percent of the total. The frequency of polymicrobial sepsis in patients with bacteremia due to a pressure ulcer ranges from 20 to 38 percent. Foul-smelling lesions are very likely to be infected with anaerobic organisms, but the absence of odor does not exclude infection with anaerobes. Stages III and IV lesions are also more likely to be infected with anaerobes.

MANAGEMENT

Drugs

Nutritional factors seem to be particularly important in the management of patients with pressure ulcers. A daily high-potency vitamin and mineral supplement is recommended for all patients suspected of vitamin deficiencies.

Systemic antibiotics are indicated for patients with sepsis, cellulitis, or osteomyelitis or for the prevention of bacterial endocarditis in persons with valvular heart disease and who require débridement of a pressure ulcer. Because of the high mortality of sepsis associated with pressure ulcers despite appropriate antibiotics, broad-spectrum coverage for aerobic gram-negative rods, gram-positive cocci, and anaerobes is indicated pending culture results in patients with suspected bacteremia. Ampicillin sulbactam, imipenem, meropenem, ticarcillin clavulanate, piperacillin tazobactam, and a combination of clindamycin or metronidazole with ciprofloxacin, levofloxacin, or an aminoglycoside are appropriate choices for initial antibiotic therapy.

Vancomycin may be required for methicillin-resistant *Staphylococcus aureus* (MRSA). In septic patients, urgent surgical débridement of necrotic tissue is necessary to remove the source of the bacteremia.

Stage I and II ulcers infrequently require the use of any specific topical therapy, but data are available to suggest that deeper ulcers, particularly when there is evidence of local infection, may benefit from topical antibiotics. A 2-week trial of a topical antibiotic, such as silver sulfadiazine, can be considered for clean pressure ulcers that are not healing or are continuing to produce exudate after 2 to 4 weeks of optimal management. On the other hand, clinicians should not use povidone-iodine, iodophor, sodium hypochlorite, hydrogen peroxide, or acetic acid as topical therapies. These antiseptic agents have been shown to be toxic to fibroblasts and to impair wound healing.

Nonpharmacologic

Protein intake is one of the most important predictors of pressure ulcer improvement. Adequate dietary intake should be provided to prevent malnutrition, and nutritional deficiencies should be corrected in a way consistent with the overall goals of therapy. For malnourished patients with pressure ulcers, nutritional support providing 30 to 35 cal/kg per day and 1.25 to 1.5 g protein per kilogram per day may be needed to achieve a positive nitrogen balance.

Treatment of pressure ulcers necessitates the use of all the preventive measures needed for individuals at risk for pressure ulcers described below, including the use of a pressure-reducing device. Some of the air or foam products used for prevention probably are adequate for many patients with pressure ulcers, but some patients may require the use of one of the more expensive, specialized beds available.

One such specialized device is the air-fluidized bed. Air-fluidized beds contain microspheres of ceramic glass, and warm, pressurized air is forced up through the beads so that they take on the characteristics of a fluid. The beads are covered by a filter sheet that allows air to escape but not the beads. Patients then float on the beads, with pressures reduced under prominences.

Hospitalized patients provided with air-fluidized bed therapy show a significant decrease in pressure ulcer surface area on air-fluidized therapy, whereas pressure ulcers treated conventionally show an increase in size. After adjusting for other factors associated with improvement, air-fluidized therapy is associated with a greater than fivefold increase in the odds of pressure ulcer improvement compared with conventional therapy. Although air-fluidized therapy increased the odds of improvement, only 12 percent of hospitalized patients achieved healing of the largest pressure ulcer.

Other specialized beds are available for treatment of patients with pressure ulcers. Low-air-loss beds consist of large fabric cushions that are constantly inflated with air. In contrast to air-fluidized beds, the cushions of low-air-loss beds are fitted on a regular hospital bed frame. This allows the head of these beds and the beds themselves to be raised or lowered. These features facilitate patient transfers and eliminate the difficulties associated with trying to keep a patient's head elevated when he or she is on an air-fluidized bed. Randomized, controlled trial data from nursing home residents suggest that pressure ulcer areas decrease three times faster when low-air-loss beds are used as compared with conventional care.

The clinical effectiveness of low-air-loss beds has not been compared with that of air-fluidized beds. Air-fluidized beds may be better able to reduce damage due to pressure, shear, and friction, and the warm environment of air-fluidized beds may reduce catabolism. On the other hand, air-fluidized beds are more expensive than low-air-loss beds and have a drying effect on tissues that may or may not be desired in certain clinical situations. The use of air-fluidized beds, low-air-loss beds, or similar dynamic support surfaces should be considered when there are large, multiple, or full-thickness (stages III or IV) pressure ulcers; when an individual has fewer than two turning surfaces free of pressure ulcers; after reconstructive surgery for pressure ulcers; or when an individual has experienced recurrent ulceration and an inability to heal on a static pressure-reducing device.

Other specialized beds have been developed that automatically reposition immobilized subjects. A low-air-loss bed with this capability is available, whereas other devices automatically turn patients from side to side on a more traditional support surface. These beds are generally more expensive than both the air-fluidized and regular low-air-loss beds. Without more data to suggest that these beds with automatic repositioning capability improve clinical outcome, there appears little justification to use them for treatment or prevention of pressure-induced cutaneous injury. On the other hand, they may be useful in preventing the pulmonary complications of immobility, particularly in spinal cord injury patients.

When necrotic tissue is present, an appropriate approach to débridement should be selected. This can include sharp débridement using a scalpel or scissors; mechanical approaches such as wet-to-dry dressings, hydrotherapy, irrigation, or dextranomers; enzymatic approaches (collagenase); or autolytic techniques using a synthetic dressing cover and permitting wound fluids to destroy necrotic tissues. Autolytic approaches are contraindicated in infected ulcers. A 19-gauge 35-mL syringe is recommended when wound irrigation is used to facilitate wound cleansing. Dry heel eschar may be left in place if there is no evidence of underlying infection.

Once an ulcer is clean and granulation or epithelialization begins to occur, then a moist wound environment should be maintained without disturbing the healing tissue. Superficial lesions heal by migration of epithelial cells from the borders of an ulcer, whereas deep lesions heal as granulation tissue fills the base of the wound. Controlled trials suggest that the use of occlusive dressings such as transparent films and hydrocolloid dressings improves healing of stage II pressure ulcers. These dressings may remain in place for several days and allow a layer of serous exudate to form underneath the dressing, facilitating epithelial migration. Such occlusive dressings have not proven to be more effective in healing stage III and IV ulcers but reduce the nursing time required for their treatment.

Alternatively, gauze dressings kept moistened with normal saline can be used for clean stages III and IV pressure ulcers. Moist dressings should be kept off surrounding intact skin to avoid macerating normal tissues.

When pain is present, adequate analgesia should be provided to patients, especially when sharp débridement is performed. Electrotherapy may be considered for clean stages III and IV ulcers when no improvement is noted after 4 weeks of otherwise optimal therapy.

A multitude of surgical procedures is available for the treatment of pressure ulcers. These include primary closure, skin grafts and myocutaneous flaps, and removal of underlying bony prominences. Radical procedures, such as amputation and hemicorporectomy, are sometimes required in complicated and extensive, infected pressure ulcers. Removal of ischial tuberosities can be complicated by urethral fistula formation and should not be done.

The outcomes of flap surgery for pressure ulcer closure among traumatic paraplegics (mean age 32 years) and non-traumatic, nonparaplegics with immobility caused by cerebral dysfunction and chronic illness (mean age 73 years) have been compared. The operative complication rate in both groups is greater than 30 percent. Complications include dehiscence, flap infection, necrosis, and hematoma. More than 70 percent of the ulcers heal by the time of hospital discharge in both groups, but the mean length of stay is shorter for younger patients.

After a mean follow-up of 11 months, the traumatic paraplegic group has a 79 percent ulcer recurrence rate, as compared with 40 percent in the older group after a mean follow-up of 8 months. On the other hand, none of the younger patients develop new ulcers, while 29 percent of the older patients do. Mortality is less than 5 percent for the younger group, but reaches 50 percent in the older group. These data raise serious questions about the benefits of surgical closure for pressure ulcers. Randomized, controlled trials are needed to define the appropriate use of such procedures in geriatric patients.

Multitudes of treatments have been advocated for the treatment of pressure ulcers without sufficient data to support their use. Such treatments include the use of hyperbaric oxygen. A number of topical agents and growth factors are being developed that may stimulate wound healing. Preliminary trial data suggest that recombinant platelet derived growth factor may improve healing of stage III pressure ulcers. Definitive trials have not confirmed these preliminary findings.

PREVENTION

Bed- and chair-bound individuals or those with impaired ability to reposition should be assessed for additional risk factors that increase risk for developing pressure ulcers on admission to acute-care and rehabilitation hospitals, nursing homes, home care programs, and other health care facilities. A systematic risk assessment can be accomplished by using a validated risk-assessment tool such as the Braden Scale or Norton Scale. Pressure ulcer risk should be reassessed when there is a change in activity or mobility levels.

Table 122-1   Skin Care and Early Treatment Recommendations

1. Systemically inspect skin daily.

2. Clean skin with a mild cleansing agent at the time of soiling and at routine intervals, avoiding hot water and minimizing force and friction applied to the skin.

3. Minimize skin drying caused by low humidity and exposure to cold, and use moisturizers for dry skin.

4. Minimize skin exposure to moisture caused by incontinence, perspiration, or wound drainage. If incontinence cannot be controlled, after appropriate assessment and treatment, use an absorptive brief or underpad. Topical agents that act as barriers to moisture also can be used.

5. Minimize skin injury caused by friction and shear by using proper positioning, transferring, and turning techniques; lubricants such as corn starch and creams; and protective films, dressings, and pads over bony prominences.

6. Ensure adequate dietary intake and correct nutritional deficiencies in a way consistent with overall goals of therapy.

7. Institute rehabilitation efforts if consistent with overall goals of therapy.

8. Document all interventions and outcomes.

Appropriate skin care may reduce the risk of pressure ulcer development. A number of skin care recommendations are outlined in Table 122–1. Massage over bony prominences should be avoided because it may decrease blood flow and result in deep tissue injury.

Historically, frequent repositioning has been the primary method of preventing pressure ulcers. One study demonstrated that the incidence of pressure ulcers was one-third that observed in historical controls when elderly at-risk patients were repositioned on a regular schedule. Patients at highest risk were repositioned every 2 to 3 hours, whereas lower-risk patients were repositioned two to four times per day. The nurse-to-patient ratio was higher and greater attention was paid to the problem of incontinence in the study group than in the control patients. In addition to a lower incidence, the ulcers that developed in the study group were less severe than those observed in the group not repositioned on a regular schedule. These beneficial effects were noted, although the patients who were repositioned generally were at higher risk than the historical controls. Although the study group did not have a concurrent control group, and the independent role of repositioning on patient outcome is uncertain, these data support the recommendation that at-risk patients should be repositioned every 2 hours if consistent with overall patient goals. Pressure-reducing support surfaces may reduce the frequency of repositioning required in some patients. Controlled trials are required to define the optimal repositioning schedules for patients on such surfaces.

Repositioning should be performed so that a person at risk is positioned without pressure on vulnerable bony prominences. Most of these sites are avoided by positioning patients with the back at a 30-degree angle to the support surface, alternatively from the right to left sides and the supine position. At-risk patients should never be repositioned with the back at a 90-degree angle to the support surface because such a position exposes the greater trochanter and lateral malleolus to excessive pressure. The use of pillows between the legs, behind the back, and supporting the arms will aid in maintaining optimal positioning. If a person with limited ability to change position needs to sit in a chair or to have the head of the bed elevated, he or she should not remain in the chair for more than 1 hour at a time. When possible, individuals should be taught to shift weight every 15 minutes while seated. The head of the bed should be maintained at the lowest degree of elevation consistent with medical conditions and other restrictions, and the amount of time the head of the bed is elevated also should be limited. This will decrease exposure of the sacral area to shearing forces that may predispose to deep-tissue injury.

Frequently despite nurses' best efforts, the use of proper positioning techniques is not sufficient or possible, and pressure ulcers occur. While one should not rely on a pressure-reducing device to substitute for good nursing care, such a mattress or support surface is indicated for persons at high risk for pressure ulcers. One randomized, controlled trial in Europe showed that the use of water mattresses or alternating air mattresses decreased the incidence of pressure ulcers by one-half compared with the use of conventional hospital mattresses. The comparability of these devices to those used in the United States is uncertain.

A number of products and devices are marketed for the prevention and treatment of pressure ulcers in the United States. Sheepskins and 2-inch convoluted foam pad products are very popular and relatively inexpensive. Unfortunately, they do not have the capability to decrease pressure enough to eliminate risk of cutaneous injury. Alternating air mattresses consist of interconnecting air cells that are alternately inflated and deflated with a bedside pump. The alternating air mattresses intermittently relieve pressures at sites of bony prominences and may provide protection against tissue injury by this mechanism.

Some air mattresses have interconnecting air cells that may deflate or inflate when a person changes position on them and do not require a bedside pump. These air mattresses and some thicker foam products with different configurations or densities than the typical "egg crate" foam mattress are reportedly capable of decreasing skin pressures to below capillary filling pressure under most bony prominences.

Water mattresses are heavy, they can leak, and they theoretically increase the risk of maceration because they are made of impermeable materials. Moreover, nursing tasks are made more difficult using a water mattress. On the other hand, randomized trial data suggest that water

mattresses can be useful for preventing pressure ulcers. Water mattresses may be most appropriate for non-acute-care settings.

The use of foam-padded chairs, stretchers, and wheelchairs also may be helpful in lowering the incidence of pressure ulcers. Pillows under the length of the lower leg can totally relieve pressure on the heels of immobile individuals. Donut cushions should not be used because they decrease blood flow to the skin in the center of the cushion .

In summary, a pressure-reducing foam, static air, alternating air, gel, or water mattress is indicated for any individual found to be at risk for developing pressure ulcers. Lifting devices such as a trapeze or bed linen to move (rather than drag) can minimize friction- and shear-induced injuries during transfers and position changes. Specialty beds such as the air-fluidized and low-air-loss beds described above are most commonly used for the treatment of pressure ulcers rather than for prevention.

Several studies show a significant decrease in pressure ulcer incidence after an educational program and a multidisciplinary team approach to the problem of pressure ulcers are implemented. Such educational programs should be directed at all levels of health care providers, patients, and family or caregivers.

SPECIAL ISSUES

Despite the potential for future treatments, currently available data suggest that pressure ulcers require long periods of treatment, and many pressure ulcers never heal. Only 12 percent of patients show healing of their largest pressure ulcer in acute care settings. Among nursing home residents, healing rates for stage II ulcers range from 25 to 42 percent after 4 weeks of treatment. For stages III and IV ulcers, no ulcers achieve healing after 4 weeks. The best healing rate reported even after 6 months of treatment is 59 percent. These data highlight the importance of identifying those persons who are at risk for pressure ulcers and implementing the preventive strategies described in this chapter.

Decisions about implementing preventive interventions such as frequent repositioning or the use of tube feeding to optimize nutritional status in persons with pressure ulcers must take into account goals of treatment and the person's treatment preferences. Some persons may have underlying comorbidity, such as arthritis or metastatic cancer, making frequent repositioning painful and burdensome. In such cases, comfort measures may be the primary management goal, rather than pressure ulcer prevention or cure.

REFERENCES

Allman RM: Outcomes in prospective studies and clinical trials. *Adv Wound Care* 8(Suppl):61, 1995.

Allman RM: Pressure ulcer prevalence, incidence, risk factors, and impact. *Clin Geriatric Med* 13:421, 1997.

Allman RM et al: Pressure ulcer risk factors among hospitalized patients with activity limitation. *JAMA* 273:865, 1995.

Bergstrom NI. Strategies for preventing pressure ulcers. *Clin Geriatr Med* 13:437, 1997.

Frantz RA: Adjuvant therapy for ulcer care. *Clin Geriatr Med* 13:553, 1997.

Goode PS, Thomas DR: Pressure ulcers: local wound care. *Clin Geriatr Med* 13:543, 1997.

Mustoe TA et al: A Phase II study to evaluate recombinant PDGF-BB in the treatment of stage III/IV pressure ulcers. *Arch Surg* 129:213, 1994.

Niazi ZBM, Salzberg CA: Operative repair of pressure ulcers. *Clin Geriatr Med* 13:587, 1997.

Remsburg RE, Bennett RG: Pressure-relieving strategies for preventing and treating pressure sores. *Clin Geriatr Med* 13:513, 1997.

Stotts NA et al: An instrument to measure healing in pressure ulcers: Development and validation of the Pressure Ulcer Scale for Healing (PUSH). *J Gerontol Med Sci* 56A:M795, 2001.

Thomas DR et al: Hospital-acquired pressure ulcers and risk of death. *J Am Geriatr Soc* 44:1435, 1996.

Incontinence

JOSEPH G. OUSLANDER • THEODORE M. JOHNSON II

DEFINITION AND EPIDEMIOLOGY

Defined as the involuntary loss of urine in sufficient amount or frequency to be a social and/or health problem, urinary incontinence is a common and bothersome condition in elderly persons. The prevalence of incontinence increases with age and is higher in women than men. Among community-dwelling older women, the prevalence of any urinary incontinence is approximately 30 percent; among older men, it is approximately 15 percent. The prevalence in older community-dwelling persons of urinary incontinence with multiple episodes per week and/or the use of pads is close to 10 percent. The prevalence approaches 60 percent among nursing home residents. Incontinence ranges in severity from occasional episodes of dribbling small amounts of urine to continuous urine leakage with concomitant fecal incontinence. In addition, many older people who do not have "loss of urine" have bothersome lower urinary tract symptoms such as urgency, frequency, and nocturia that require changes in lifestyle and/or the use of pads.

Physical health, psychological well-being, social status, and the costs of health care can all be adversely affected by incontinence. Urinary incontinence can be cured especially in those who have adequate mobility and mental functioning. Even when not curable, incontinence can always be managed in a manner that will keep patients comfortable, make life easier for caregivers, and minimize costs of caring for the condition. Because many elderly patients are embarrassed to discuss their incontinence and may not be aware that treatment is available, it is essential for specific questions about incontinence to be included in periodic assessments and for incontinence to be noted as a problem (Table 123-1). This chapter briefly reviews the pathophysiology of incontinence in older persons and provides detailed information on the evaluation and management of this condition.

PATHOPHYSIOLOGY AND CLASSIFICATION

Continence requires effective functioning of the lower urinary tract, adequate cognitive and physical functioning, motivation, and an appropriate environment (Table 123-2).

Anatomic and physiologic aspects of the lower urinary tract, as well as functional, psychological, and environmental factors, contribute to the pathophysiology of incontinence in older people. Normal urination is a complex process; the neurophysiology of urination remains incompletely understood. Proper bladder filling and emptying are influenced by higher centers in the brainstem, cerebral cortex, and cerebellum. The cerebral cortex exerts a predominantly inhibitory influence and the brainstem facilitates urination. Consequently, loss of the central cortical inhibiting influences over the sacral micturition center from diseases such as stroke and parkinsonism can produce incontinence in older patients. Disorders of the brainstem and suprasacral spinal cord can interfere with the coordination of bladder contraction and urethral relaxation, and interruptions of the sacral innervation can cause impaired bladder contraction and problems with continence.

At the most basic level, urination is governed by a reflex centered in the sacral micturition center. During normal bladder filling, afferent pathways (via somatic and autonomic nerves) carry information on bladder volume to the spinal cord. Motor output is adjusted accordingly (Fig. 123-1). Sympathetic tone closes the bladder neck and inhibits parasympathetic tone (thus relaxing the dome of the bladder); somatic innervation maintains tone in the pelvic floor musculature (including striated muscle around the urethra). Voluntary pelvic floor muscle contracture also leads to inhibitions of parasympathetic tone. For bladder emptying, sympathetic and somatic tone diminish, and parasympathetic cholinergically mediated impulses cause the bladder to contract. Normal urination is a dynamic process, requiring the coordination of several physiologic processes. Under normal circumstances, as the bladder fills, bladder pressure remains low (<15 cm H_2O). The bladder volume at first urge to void is variable but generally occurs at between 150 and 350 mL; normal bladder capacity is 300 to 600 mL. When normal urination is initiated, the detrusor contracts and detrusor pressure increases until it exceeds urethral resistance (which lowers when the bladder contracts) and urine flow occurs. If at any time during bladder filling total bladder pressure exceeds outlet resistance, urinary leakage occurs. Transmitted intraabdominal pressure alone by coughing or sneezing may cause leakage in someone with low outlet resistance

Table 123-1   Asking about Urinary Incontinence

Questions about incontinence should be open-ended and phrased in language easily understood by the patient:

"Tell me about any problems you are having with your bladder?"

"Tell me about any trouble you are having holding your urine (water)?"

If the responses to the above questions are negative, following up with questions may be helpful:

"How often do you lose urine when you don't want to?"

"How often do you wear a pad or other protective device to prevent urinary accidents?"

Source: Fantl JA et al. Urinary Incontinence in Adults: Acute and Chronic Management. Clinical Practice Guideline No. 2, 1996 Update. Rockville, MD: U.S. Department of Health and Human Services, Public Health Service, Agency for Health Care Policy and Research. AHCPR Publication No. 96-0682, 1996.

pressure or urethral sphincter weakness. Alternatively, the bladder can contract involuntarily and cause urinary leakage.

Basic Causes

Urologic, neurologic, psychological, and functional factors may contribute to incontinence. As is the case for a number of other common geriatric problems, multiple disorders often interact to cause urinary incontinence. Determining the cause or causes facilitates proper management. Several age-related changes can contribute to the development of urinary incontinence. In general, bladder capacity declines with age and residual urine following voiding increases. The prevalence of involuntary bladder contractions also increases with age. These contractions are found in 40 to 75 percent of elderly incontinent patients. They are, however, also found in 5 to 10 percent of elderly continent women and in up to one-third of elderly men with no or minimal urinary symptoms. While involuntary bladder

contractions do not always result in urinary incontinence, when combined with impaired mobility, these contractions likely account for a substantial proportion of incontinence in elderly functionally disabled patients. Aging is also associated with a decline in bladder outlet and urethral resistance pressure in women. While this is understood to be related to laxity of pelvic structures associated with prior childbirths, the association between parity and incontinence is weak in women older than 65 years of age. Obesity, deconditioned muscles, and hysterectomy also predispose women to the development of stress incontinence. White women appear to be more likely to have stress urinary incontinence than do African American women. In men, prostatic enlargement is associated with nocturia, decreased urine flow rates, and detrusor motor instability and can lead to urge and/or overflow types of incontinence. Many older individuals of both sexes have impaired bladder contractility, often in combination with detrusor hyperactivity (a condition termed *detrusor hyperactivity with impaired*

Table 123-2   Requirements for Continence

Effective lower urinary tract function

Storage

Accommodation by bladder of increasing volumes of urine under low pressure

Closed bladder outlet

Appropriate sensation of bladder fullness

Absence of involuntary bladder contractions

Emptying

Bladder capable of contraction

Lack of anatomic obstruction to urine flow

Coordinated lowering of outlet resistance with bladder contractions

Adequate mobility and dexterity to use toilet

Adequate cognitive function to recognize toileting needs

Motivation to be continent

Absence of environmental and iatrogenic barriers

Source: Adapted from Kane RL et al.

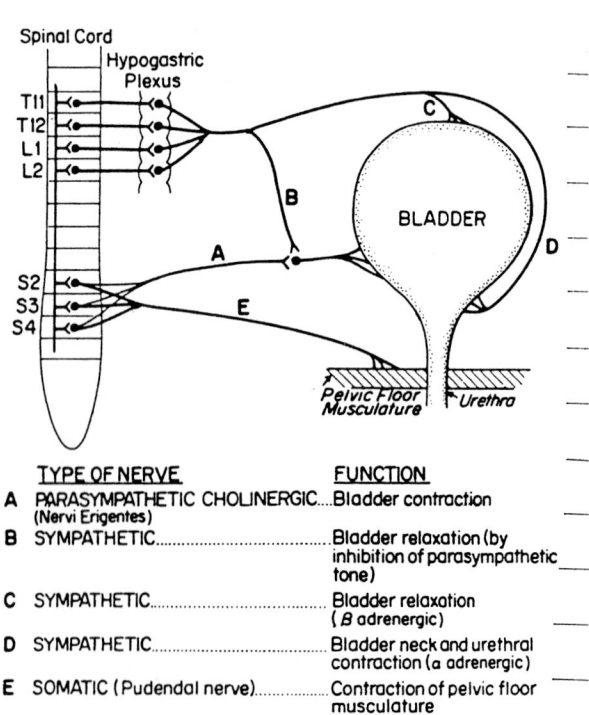

TYPE OF NERVE	FUNCTION
A PARASYMPATHETIC CHOLINERGIC (Nervi Erigentes)	Bladder contraction
B SYMPATHETIC	Bladder relaxation (by inhibition of parasympathetic tone)
C SYMPATHETIC	Bladder relaxation (β adrenergic)
D SYMPATHETIC	Bladder neck and urethral contraction (α adrenergic)
E SOMATIC (Pudendal nerve)	Contraction of pelvic floor musculature

Figure 123-1 Peripheral nerves involved in micturition. Reprinted with permission from Kane et al.

Table 123-3 Reversible Conditions that Cause or Contribute to Urinary Incontinence in Older Persons

Condition	Management
Conditions affecting the lower urinary tract	
Urinary tract infection (symptomatic with frequency, urgency, dysuria, etc.)	Antimicrobial therapy
Atrophic vaginitis/urethritis	Topical estrogen
Postprostatectomy	Behavioral interventions
	Avoid further surgical therapy until it is clear condition will not resolve
Stool impaction	Disimpaction; appropriate use of stool softeners, bulk-forming agents, and laxatives if necessary; implement high fiber intake, adequate mobility and fluid intake
Drug side effects (see Table 123-4)	
	Discontinue or change therapy if clinically appropriate. Dosage reduction or modification (e.g., flexible scheduling of rapid-acting diuretics) may also help
Increased urine production	
Metabolic (hyperglycemia, hypercalcemia)	Better control of diabetes mellitus; therapy for hypercalcemia depends on underlying cause
Excess fluid intake	Reduction in intake of diuretic fluids (e.g., caffeinated beverages)
Volume overload	
Venous insufficiency with edema	Support stocking
	Leg elevation
	Sodium restriction
	Diuretic therapy
Congestive heart failure	Medical therapy
Impaired ability or willingness to reach a toilet	
Delirium	Diagnosis and treatment of underlying cause(s) of acute confusional state
Chronic illness, injury, or restraint that interferes with mobility	Regular toileting
	Use of toilet substitutes
	Environmental alterations (e.g., bedside commode, urinal)
Psychological	Remove restraints if possible
	Appropriate pharmacologic and/or nonpharmacologic treatment

SOURCE: Fantl JA et al. Urinary Incontinence in Adults: Acute and Chronic Management. Clinical Practice Guideline No. 2, 1996 Update. Rockville, MD: U.S. Department of Health and Human Services. Public Health Service, Agency for Health Care Policy and Research. AHCPR Publication No. 96-0682,1996.

contractility, or DHIC). These individuals have evidence of widespread muscle degeneration on detrusor muscle biopsy.

Acute and Reversible Causes

The distinction between acute (or reversible) forms of incontinence and persistent (or established) incontinence is clinically important. *Acute incontinence* refers to those situations in which the incontinence is of sudden onset, usually related to an acute illness or an iatrogenic problem, and subsides once the illness or medication problem has been resolved. *Persistent incontinence* refers to incontinence that is unrelated to an acute illness and persists over time.

Several of the reversible factors discussed below also can contribute to persistent forms of incontinence.

The potentially reversible causes of urinary incontinence are outlined in Table 123-3. These causes include impaired ability (or willingness) to reach a toilet, conditions that affect the lower urinary tract, conditions that cause or contribute to polyuria, and iatrogenic factors. Because of urinary frequency and urgency, many older persons, especially those limited in mobility, carefully arrange their schedules (and may even limit social activities) in order to be close to a toilet. Thus, an acute illness can precipitate incontinence by disrupting this delicate balance. Hospitalization, with its attendant environmental barriers (such as bed rails), and the delirium and immobility that often accompany acute illnesses in older patients can contribute

Table 123-4 Medications that Can Potentially Affect Continence

Type of Medication	Potential Effects on Continence
Diuretics	Polyuria, frequency, urgency
Anticholinergics	Urinary retention, overflow incontinence, stool impaction
Psychotropics	
Antidepressants	Anticholinergic actions, sedation
Antipsychotics	Anticholinergic actions, sedation, immobility
Sedative–hypnotics	Sedation, delirium, immobility, urethral muscle relaxation
Narcotic analgesics	Urinary retention, fecal impaction, sedation, delirium
α-Adrenergic blockers	Urethral relaxation
α-Adrenergic agonists	Urinary retention
Angiotensin-converting enzyme inhibitors	Cough precipitating stress incontinence
β-Adrenergic agonists	May contribute to urinary retention
Calcium channel blockers	May contribute to urinary retention
Alcohol	Polyuria, frequency, urgency, sedation, delirium, immobility
Caffeine	Polyuria, bladder irritation

SOURCE: Adapted from Kane RL et al.

to acute incontinence. Acute incontinence in these situations is likely to resolve with resolution of the underlying acute illness. In a substantial proportion of patients, incontinence may persist for several weeks after hospitalization and should be further evaluated.

Fecal impaction is a common problem in both acutely and chronically ill elderly patients. Impaction may cause mechanical obstruction of the bladder outlet with overflow-type incontinence and reflex bladder contractions induced by rectal distension. Relief of a fecal impaction can lead to resolution of urinary, as well as fecal, incontinence. Urinary retention with overflow incontinence should be considered in any patient who suddenly develops urinary incontinence. Immobility; anticholinergic, narcotic, calcium channel blocking, and beta-adrenergic medications; and fecal impaction can all precipitate overflow incontinence in an older patient. In addition, urinary retention may be an acute manifestation of an underlying process causing spinal cord compression.

Inflammation of the lower urinary tract may precipitate or exacerbate incontinence. Atrophic vaginitis and urethritis are common among older women and can cause dysuria, urgency, and frequency that can contribute to incontinence. Physical signs include patchy erythema and increased vascularity of the labia minora and vaginal epithelium, petechiae and friability, and urethral erythema often with an inflamed caruncle (dark or bright red epithelium usually at the inferior aspect of the urethra). Topical estrogen therapy, as discussed under "Drug Treatment" later in this chapter, may be helpful. Acute urinary tract infection also can precipitate or exacerbate incontinence. However, urine loss among older patients with *chronic* incontinence, especially

frail nursing home residents, with otherwise asymptomatic bacteriuria (with or without pyuria) does not appear to improve when the bacteriuria is eradicated. These patients therefore should not be treated with antibiotics because of the costs and risks unless the incontinence is new or acutely worsened.

Diuretics (especially the rapid-acting loop diuretics) and conditions that cause polyuria, including hyperglycemia and hypercalcemia, can precipitate acute incontinence. Patients with volume-expanded states, such as those with congestive heart failure and lower extremity venous insufficiency, may have polyuria at night, which can contribute to nocturia and nocturnal incontinence. As is the case in many other conditions in geriatric patients, a wide variety of medications can play a role in the development of incontinence in elderly patients (Table 123-4). Whether the incontinence is acute or persistent, the potential role of these medications in causing or contributing to a patient's incontinence should be considered. When feasible, stopping the medication, switching to an alternative, or modifying the dosage schedule can be an important component (and possibly the only one necessary) of the treatment for incontinence.

Persistent Incontinence

Table 123-5 lists the clinical definitions and common causes of persistent urinary incontinence. These types can overlap with each other, and an individual patient may have more than one type simultaneously. Three of these types of incontinence—stress, urge, and overflow—result from one

Table 123-5 Basic Types and Causes of Persistent Urinary Incontinence

Type	Definition	Common Causes
Stress	Involuntary loss of urine (usually small amounts) with increases in intraabdominal pressure (e.g., cough, laugh, exercise)	Weakness of pelvic floor musculature and urethral hypermobility Bladder outlet or urethral sphincter weakness Postprostactectomy sphincter weakness
Urge	Leakage of urine (variable but often larger volumes) because of inability to delay voiding after sensation of bladder fullness is perceived	Detrusor hyperactivity, isolated or associated with one or more of the following: Local genitourinary condition such as tumors, stones, diverticuli, or outflow obstruction CNS disorders such as stroke, dementia, parkinsonism, spinal cord injury
Overflow	Leakage of urine (usually small amounts) resulting from mechanical forces on an overdistended bladder or from other effects of urinary retention on bladder and sphincter function	Anatomic obstruction by prostate, stricture, cystocele Acontractile bladder associated with diabetes mellitus or spinal cord injury Neurogenic (detrusor–sphincter dyssynergy), associated with multiple sclerosis and other suprasacral spinal cord lesions Medication effect (see Table 123-4)
Functional	Urinary accidents associated with inability to toilet because of impairment of cognitive and/or physical functioning, psychological unwillingness, or environmental barriers	Severe dementia and other neurological disorders Psychological factors such as depression and hostility

SOURCE: Adapted from Kane RL et al.

or a combination of two basic abnormalities in lower genitourinary tract function:

1. Failure to store urine, caused by a hyperactive or poorly compliant bladder or by diminished outflow resistance; and/or
2. Failure to fully empty the bladder, caused by a poorly contractile bladder or by increased outflow resistance.

Stress incontinence is common in elderly women, especially in ambulatory clinic settings. The symptoms of stress incontinence are very specific: leakage coincident with increases in intraabdominal pressure caused by coughing, sneezing, laughing, or exercising. Stress incontinence may be infrequent and involve very small amounts of urine. It may need no specific treatment in women who are not bothered by it. On the other hand, it may be so severe and/or bothersome that it has rendered the person housebound. Among women it is most often associated with weakened supporting tissues resulting in hypermobility of the bladder outlet and urethra and caused by lack of estrogen, obesity, previous vaginal deliveries, and/or surgery. Some women, generally those who have had previous lower urinary tract surgery, have intrinsic urethral weakness with failure of the urethra to coapt and prevent urine loss. These patients tend to have severe incontinence and sometimes constant wetting. Stress incontinence is unusual in men, but it can

occur after transurethral surgery and/or radiation therapy for lower urinary tract malignancy when the anatomic sphincters are damaged.

Urge incontinence can be caused by a variety of lower genitourinary and neurologic disorders (see Table 123-5). This type of incontinence is characterized by a sudden strong desire to void, accompanied by a fear of leakage, and followed by urine loss. The amount of urine lost is variable and largely dependent on sphincter function and the ability of the patient to abort a bladder contraction. Urge incontinence often occurs as a component of the "overactive bladder" syndrome, which includes daytime urinary frequency and nocturia. Urge incontinence is most often, but not always, associated with involuntary bladder contractions. Some patients have a poorly compliant bladder without involuntary contractions (e.g., interstitial cystitis or following irradiation). A subgroup of elderly incontinent patients with detrusor hyperactivity also has impaired bladder contractility, emptying less than one-third of their bladder volume with involuntary contractions on urodynamic testing. These patients may be predisposed to significant urinary retention and may require training to learn to completely empty their bladder with voiding.

Urinary retention with *overflow incontinence* can result from anatomic or neurogenic outflow obstruction, a hypotonic or acontractile bladder, or both. Symptoms of overflow incontinence are nonspecific; they may be similar to urge or stress symptoms or may be leakage without warning. The most common causes include prostatic enlargement, diabetic neuropathic bladder, and urethral stricture. Low spinal cord injury and anatomic obstruction in women (caused by pelvic prolapse and urethral distortion) are less common causes of overflow incontinence in older patients. Several types of drugs also can contribute to this type of persistent incontinence (see Table 123-4). Some patients with suprasacral spinal cord lesions (e.g., multiple sclerosis) develop detrusor–sphincter dyssynergy and consequent urinary retention, which must be treated similarly to overflow incontinence; in some instances, a sphincterotomy is necessary.

Functional incontinence results when an elderly person is unable or unwilling to reach a toilet on time. Recognizing and removing these barriers to continence are critical to appropriate management. Factors that cause functional incontinence (such as inaccessible toilets and psychological disorders) also can exacerbate other types of persistent incontinence. Patients with incontinence that appears to be predominantly related to functional factors also may have abnormalities of the lower genitourinary tract, most commonly detrusor hyperactivity. In some patients, it can be very difficult to determine whether the functional factors or the genitourinary factors predominate without a trial of specific types of treatment.

Many older patients have "mixed" types of incontinence. Most common are combinations of urge and stress incontinence among older women and a combination of urge and functional incontinence among nursing home residents.

EVALUATION

Federal clinical practice guidelines from the Agency for Health Care Policy and Research (AHCPR, now Agency for Healthcare Research and Quality [AHRQ]) and the Resident Assessment Instrument for nursing homes (which includes a section on continence in the Minimum Data Set and a Resident Assessment Protocol on continence and catheter management) recommend a basic diagnostic evaluation. This evaluation includes a history (which can be enhanced by a bladder record), a physical examination, a urinalysis, and a postvoid residual determination. A number of other diagnostic studies are indicated in selected patients (Table 123-6). Figure 123-2 summarizes the recommended diagnostic evaluation of incontinent older patients.

The objectives of the basic evaluation are threefold:

1. To identify potentially reversible conditions that might be contributing to the incontinence (see Table 123-3);
2. To identify conditions that require further diagnostic tests and/or referral for gynecologic or urologic evaluation; and
3. To develop a management plan, which may include referral for further evaluation or a therapeutic trial of behavioral and/or pharmacologic therapy.

In patients with the sudden onset of incontinence (especially when associated with an acute medical condition and hospitalization), the potentially reversible causes of acute

Table 123-6 Components of the Diagnostic Evaluation of Persistent Urinary Incontinence*

All Patients
  History (a bladder record may be helpful)
  Physical examination
  Urinalysis
  Postvoid residual determination

Selected Patients
  Laboratory studies
    Urine culture
    Urine cytology
    Blood glucose, calcium
    Renal function tests
    Renal ultrasound
  Gynecologic evaluation
  Urologic evaluation
  Cystourethroscopy
  Urodynamic tests
    Simple
      Observation of voiding
      Cough test for stress incontinence
      Simple (single channel) cystometry
      Urine flowmetry (for men)
    Complex
      Multichannel cystometrogram
      Pressure-flow study
      Leak point pressure
      Urethral pressure profilometry
      Sphincter electromyography
      Videourodynamics

*NOTE: See Table 123-7.
SOURCE: Adapted from Kane RL et al.

incontinence (see Table 123-3) can be ruled out by a brief history, a physical examination, and basic laboratory studies including urinalysis, culture, and tests for serum glucose or calcium, if indicated.

The history should focus on the characteristics of the incontinence, on current medical problems and medications, and on the impact of the incontinence on the patient and caregivers. The incontinence should be characterized in terms of frequency, timing, and amount of leakage; and symptoms of voiding difficulty including hesitancy, intermittent stream, and straining to void. Symptoms of urge versus stress incontinence should be sought, recognizing that symptom history does not perfectly predict subtype of urinary incontinence. Bladder records such as the one shown in Fig. 123-3 can be helpful in characterizing symptoms, as well as in following the response to treatment. The physical examination includes abdominal, rectal, and genital examinations, as well as an evaluation of lumbosacral innervation. The pelvic examination in women includes inspection for significant prolapse, signs of inflammation suggestive of atrophic vaginitis, and a cough test to detect stress incontinence. The latter is best done in the standing

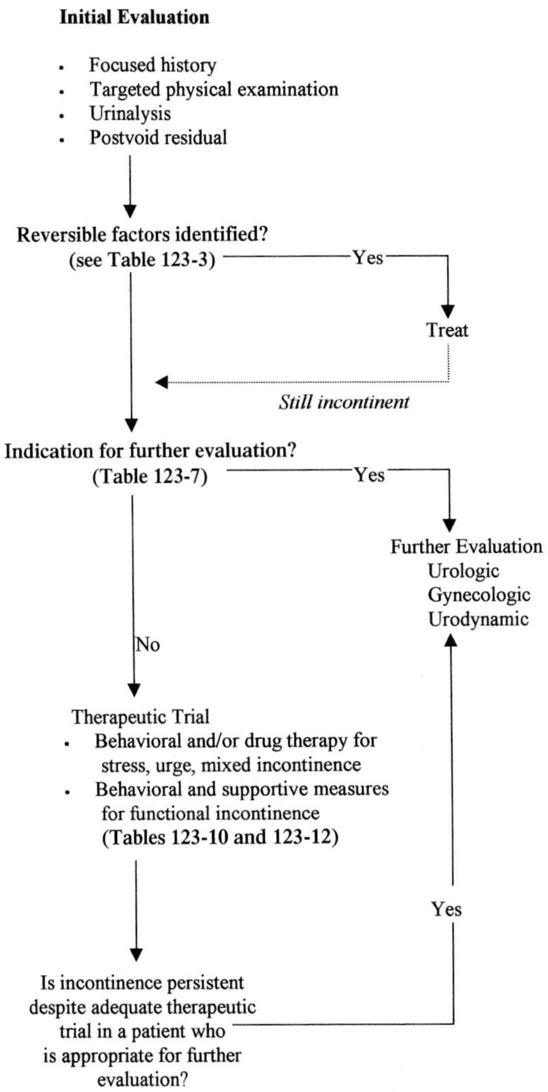

Initial Evaluation

- Focused history
- Targeted physical examination
- Urinalysis
- Postvoid residual

↓

Reversible factors identified?
(see Table 123-3) ———————— Yes ————

↓   ↓

                                          Treat

                              Still incontinent

↓

Indication for further evaluation?
(Table 123-7) ———————— Yes ————

                                           ↓

                              Further Evaluation
                              Urologic
                              Gynecologic
                              Urodynamic

No

↓

Therapeutic Trial
- Behavioral and/or drug therapy for
  stress, urge, mixed incontinence
- Behavioral and supportive measures
  for functional incontinence
  (Tables 123-10 and 123-12)

                                          Yes

↓

Is incontinence persistent
despite adequate therapeutic
trial in a patient who
is appropriate for further
evaluation?

Figure 123-2 Summary of assessment of geriatric urinary incontinence (see referenced tables and text for details).

position while the patient has a comfortably full bladder, but not a strong sense of urgency. The patient should be positioned over a pad or towel next to a commode and then should be asked to cough forcefully. Leakage simultaneously with coughing documents stress incontinence; delayed leakage (e.g. after 3 seconds) or the initiation of voiding generally indicates a cough-induced bladder contraction. Special attention should be given to mobility and mental status, because impairments may be either causing the incontinence or interacting with urologic and neurologic disorders to worsen the condition. Patients with nocturia and nocturnal incontinence should be examined for signs of congestive heart failure or venous insufficiency with edema.

Urinalysis should be performed to look for hematuria and glucosuria. Clean urine specimens are often difficult to obtain from frail incontinent patients but can be performed reliably without first resorting to in-and-out catheterization. For men who cannot void spontaneously, a condom-type catheter can be used after cleaning the penis

to collect a specimen that accurately reflects bladder urine. While there is a clear relationship between acute symptomatic urinary tract infection and incontinence, the relationship between asymptomatic bacteriuria and incontinence is controversial. In nursing home populations, there is no benefit to treating bacteriuria in patients with chronic, stable incontinence. For patients in other settings, it is difficult to make clear recommendations. For the initial evaluation of incontinence among noninstitutionalized incontinent patients, it is reasonable to eradicate the bacteriuria once and observe the effect on the incontinence.

A postvoid residual volume (PVR) determination should be performed to exclude significant urinary retention. Neither the history nor the physical examination is sensitive or specific enough for this purpose in geriatric patients. The PVR determination can be done by portable ultrasonography if equipment is available. To be accurate, the PVR determination should be done within a few minutes of a spontaneous continent or incontinent void. PVR values of less than 100 mL in the absence of straining to void generally reflect adequate bladder emptying in geriatric patients, whereas PVR values greater than 200 mL are abnormal; values in between must be interpreted in light of other patient symptoms and the representativeness of the void.

Clinical practice guidelines do not recommend that all incontinent elderly patients undergo a urologic, gynecologic, or complex urodynamic evaluation. Many patients can be treated with a trial of behavioral and/or drug therapy after the initial evaluation is completed and potentially reversible factors are addressed. Table 123-7 lists examples of criteria for referring incontinent geriatric patients for further urologic, gynecologic, and/or urodynamic evaluations.

MANAGEMENT

Several therapeutic modalities are used in managing incontinent patients (Table 123-8).

Special attention should be paid to the management of acute incontinence, which is most common in elderly patients in acute care hospitals. A common approach to elderly incontinent patients in acute hospitals is indwelling catheterization. In some instances, this practice is justified by the need for accurate measurement of urine output during the acute phase of an illness. In many instances, however, it is unnecessary and poses a substantial and unwarranted risk of catheter-induced infection and may prolong immobilization. Although other procedures may be more difficult and time-consuming, making toilets and toilet substitutes accessible and combining this accessibility with some form of scheduled toileting are probably a more appropriate approach. Using launderable or disposable and highly absorbent bed pads and undergarments may be more costly than catheters, but probably will result in less morbidity in the long run. All the factors that can cause or contribute to a reversible form of incontinence (see Table 123-3) should be attended to in order to maximize the potential for regaining continence.

Supportive measures are critical in managing all forms of incontinence and should be used in conjunction with

BLADDER RECORD

Day:_____   Date:_____/_____.

                                                  month   day

INSTRUCTIONS:

1) In the 1st column make a mark every time during the 2-hour period you urinate into the toilet

2) Use the 2nd column to record the amount you urinate (if you are measuring amounts)

3) In the 3rd or 4th column, make a mark every time you accidentally leak urine

Time Interval	Urinated in Toilet	Amount	Leaking Accident	or	Large Accident	Reason for Accident *
6-8 am						
8-10 am						
2-4 pm						
4-6 pm						
6-8 pm						
8-10 pm						
10-12 pm						
Overnight						

Number of pads used today: _____

* For example, if you coughed and have a leaking accident, write "cough".
If you had a large accident after a strong urge to urinate, write "urge".

Figure 123-3 Example of a bladder record for ambulatory care settings. Reprinted with permission from Kane et al.

other, more specific treatment modalities. Education, environmental manipulations, appropriate use of toilet substitutes, avoidance of iatrogenic contributions to incontinence, modifications of diuretic and fluid intake patterns, caffeine, and good skin care are all important.

Specially designed incontinence undergarments and pads can be very helpful in many patients, but they must be used appropriately. Although they can be effective, several caveats should be raised:

1. Garments and pads are a nonspecific treatment;
2. Many patients are curable if treated with specific therapies, and some have potentially serious factors underlying their incontinence that must be diagnosed and treated;
3. Patients often prefer more specific incontinence therapy designed to restore a normal pattern of voiding and continence; and
4. Incontinence garments and pads generally are not covered by third-party payers and can be expensive.

To a large extent, the optimal treatment of persistent incontinence depends on identifying the type or types.

Table 123-9 outlines the primary treatments for the basic types of persistent incontinence in the geriatric population. Each treatment modality is briefly discussed below.

Behavioral Interventions

Many types of behavioral interventions have been described for the management of urinary incontinence. These are either patient dependent (i.e., require adequate function and motivation of the patient), in which the goal is to restore a normal pattern of voiding and continence, or caregiver dependent, which can be used for functionally disabled patients, in which the goal is to keep the patient and the environment dry. Table 123-10 summarizes these interventions. The patient-dependent interventions generally involve the patient's continuous, self-monitoring use of a record such as the one depicted in Fig. 123-3.

To be successful, patient-dependent interventions require a functional, motivated patient capable of learning and practice, and a skilled, enthusiastic trainer. These are structured intervention programs that have education, counseling, and frequent patient contact. Pelvic muscle

Table 123-7   Examples of Criteria for Referral of Incontinent Geriatric Patients for Further Urologic, Gynecologic, or Urodynamic Evaluation

Criteria	Definition	Rationale
History		
Recent history of lower urinary tract or pelvic surgery or irradiation.	Surgery or irradiation involving the pelvic area or lower urinary tract within the past 6 months.	A structural abnormality relating to the recent procedure should be sought.
Recurrent symptomatic urinary tract infections.	Three or more symptomatic episodes in a 12-month period.	A structural abnormality or pathologic condition in the urinary tract predisposing to infection should be excluded.
Physical examination		
Marked pelvic prolapse	A prominent cystocele that descends the entire height of the vaginal vault with coughing during speculum examination.	Anatomic abnormality may underlie the pathophysiology of the incontinence, and selected patients may benefit from surgical repair.
Marked prostatic enlargement and/or suspicion of cancer.	Gross enlargement of the prostate on digital exam; prominent induration or asymmetry of the lobes.	An evaluation to exclude prostate cancer may be appropriate.
Postvoid residual		
Difficulty passing a 14-French straight catheter.	Impossible catheter passage, or passage requiring considerable force, or a larger, more rigid catheter.	Anatomic blockage of the urethra or bladder neck may be present.
Postvoid residual volume >200 mL.	Volume of urine remaining in the bladder within a few minutes after the patient voids spontaneously in as normal a fashion as possible.	Anatomic or neurogenic obstruction or poor bladder contractility may be present.
Urinalysis		
Hematuria.	Greater than 5 red blood cells per high-power field on microscopic exam in the absence of infection.	A pathologic condition in the urinary tract should be excluded.
Therapeutic trial		
Failure to respond.	Persistent symptoms that are bothersome to the patient after adequate trials of behavioral and/or drug therapy.	Urodynamic evaluation may help guide specific therapy.

SOURCE: Adapted from Kane RL et al.

(Kegel) exercises are effective for urge, stress, and mixed stress–urge incontinence. These exercises consist of repetitive contractions of the pelvic floor muscles. This procedure can be taught by brief verbal or written instruction. Instruction can be provided by having a patient squeeze the examiner's inserted finger during a vaginal or rectal examination (without doing a Valsalva maneuver, which is opposite of the intended effect). Once learned, the exercises should be practiced many times throughout the day (e.g., 3 to 5 sets of 10 contractions building up from 3 seconds to 10 seconds in duration). Biofeedback can be especially helpful for teaching patients who bear down (increasing intraabdominal pressure) when attempting to contract pelvic floor muscles. Biofeedback involves the use of bladder, rectal, or vaginal pressure or electrical activity recordings to train patients to contract pelvic floor muscles while leaving the abdominal muscles relaxed. The use of biofeedback may be limited by the requirement for equipment, software, and trained personnel; in addition, some of these techniques are relatively invasive and require the use of vaginal or rectal sensors. Electrical stimulation, introduced either vaginally or rectally, also has been used to help identify and train muscles in the management of stress incontinence and inhibit involuntary bladder contractions in patients with urge incontinence. However, this technique is not acceptable to many older patients and has not been well studied or used to any great degree in the elderly population in the United States.

Other forms of patient-dependent interventions include bladder training and bladder retraining. Bladder training involves the educational components taught during biofeedback, without the use of biofeedback equipment.

PART VI GERIATRIC SYNDROMES

Table 123-8 Treatment Options for Geriatric Urinary Incontinence

---

Behavioral interventions (see Table 123-10)

    Patient-dependent
        Pelvic muscle exercises
        Bladder training
        Bladder retraining
        Adjunctive techniques
            Biofeedback
            Electrical stimulation
            Vaginal cones
    Caregiver dependent
        Scheduled toileting
        Habit training
        Prompted voiding

Drugs (see Table 123-12)

    Bladder Relaxants
    α Agonists
    α Antagonists
    Estrogen

Periurethral injections

Surgery

    Bladder neck suspension
    Removal of obstruction or pathologic lesion

Mechanical devices

    Urethral Plugs
    Artificial sphincters

Nonspecific Supportive Measures

    Education
    Modifications of medication intake
    Avoid caffeine
    Use of toilet substitutes
    Environmental manipulations
    Garments and pads

Catheters

    External
    Intermittent
    Indwelling

SOURCE: Adapted from Kane RL et al.

Table 123-9 Primary Treatments for Different Types of Geriatric Urinary Incontinence

Type of Incontinence	Primary Treatments
Stress	Pelvic muscle (Kegel) exercises Other behavioral interventions α-Adrenergic agonists Periurethral injections Surgical bladder neck suspension
Urge	Bladder training Bladder relaxants
Overflow	Surgical removal of obstruction Intermittent catheterization (if practical) Indwelling catheterization

Functional	Behavioral interventions
	   (caregiver dependent)
	Environmental manipulations
	Incontinence undergarments
	   and pads

SOURCE: Adapted from Kane RL et al.

Patients are taught pelvic muscle exercises and strategies to manage urgency and are taught to use bladder records regularly. There is some evidence that these techniques are as effective as biofeedback in a selected group of cognitively intact, motivated elderly patients. Bladder retraining as described here is used primarily after a period of temporary bladder catheterization. Table 123-11 is an example of a bladder-retraining protocol. This protocol is applicable to patients who have had an indwelling catheter for monitoring of urinary output during a period of acute illness or for treatment of urinary retention with overflow incontinence. Such catheters always should be removed as soon as possible, and this type of bladder-retraining protocol should enable most indwelling catheters to be removed from patients in acute care hospitals as well as some residents in long-term care settings. A patient who continues to have difficulty voiding after 1 to 2 weeks of such a bladder-retraining protocol should be examined for other potentially reversible causes of voiding difficulties. When difficulties persist, a urologic referral should be considered to rule out correctable lower genitourinary pathologic conditions.

The goal of caregiver-dependent intervention such as scheduled toileting, habit training, and prompted voiding is to prevent incontinence episodes rather than to restore a normal pattern of voiding and complete continence. Highly motivated caregivers are essential for these interventions to be successful on an ongoing basis. Scheduled toileting involves putting the patient on the toilet at regular intervals, usually every 2 hours during the day and every 4 hours during the evening and night regardless of the presence or absence of the patient's expressed desire to void. Habit training involves a schedule of toileting that is individually modified according to the patient's pattern of continent voids and incontinence episodes. *Prompted voiding* is a behavioral protocol that involves focusing the patient's attention on his or her bladder by asking if the patient is wet or dry, asking (prompting) the patient to attempt to void (up to three times) every 2 hours during the day, toileting the patient if he or she responds positively, giving personal interaction as a social reward for attempting to toilet and maintaining continence, and offering fluids routinely.

Table 123-10 Examples of Behavioral Interventions for Urinary Incontinence

Procedure	Definition	Types of Incontinence	Comments
Patient dependent			
Pelvic muscle (Kegel) exercises	Repetitive contraction and relaxation of pelvic floor muscles with use in everyday situations that precipitate leakage	Stress and urge	Requires adequate function and motivation; biofeedback often helpful for teaching
Bladder training	Use of education, bladder records, pelvic muscle, and other behavioral techniques	Stress and urge	Requires trained therapist, adequate cognitive and physical functioning, and motivation
Bladder retraining	Progressive lengthening or shortening of intervoiding interval, with intermittent catheterization used in patients recovering from overdistension injuries with persistent retention	Acute (e.g., postcatheterization with urge or overflow, poststroke)	Goal is to restore normal pattern of voiding and continence; requires adequate cognitive and physical function and motivation
Caregiver dependent			
Scheduled toileting	Routine toileting at regular intervals (scheduled toileting)	Urge and functional	Goal is to prevent wetting episodes; can be used in patients with impaired cognitive or physical functioning; requires staff or caregiver availability and motivation
Habit training	Variable toileting schedule based on patient's voiding patterns	Urge and functional	Goal is to prevent wetting episodes; can be used in patients with impaired cognitive or physical functioning; requires staff or caregiver availability and motivation
Prompted voiding	Offer opportunity to toilet every 2 hours during the day; toilet only on request; social reinforcement; routine offering of fluids	Urge, stress, mixed, functional	Same as above; 25–40% of nursing home residents respond well during the day, and can be identified during a 3-day trial

SOURCE: Adapted from Kane RL et al.

Between 25 and 40 percent of nursing home residents respond very well to daytime prompted voiding, and these responders can be identified by carrying out a 3-day trial of the intervention. Care for incontinence at night should be individualized. Routine incontinence care can be very disruptive to sleep. Because older people tend to awaken frequently at night, one way to individualize toileting is to check on the patient every hour or two, and only prompt to toilet when he/she is found awake.

Drug Treatment

Table 123-12 lists the drugs used to treat incontinence. Although most efficacy trials of drug treatment have been in younger populations, better data for older patients are now available for some drugs. Drug treatment should

be prescribed in conjunction with one or more behavioral interventions. For urge incontinence, drugs with anticholinergic and bladder smooth-muscle relaxant properties are used. Most studies suggest a reduction of 60 to 70 percent in the frequency of incontinence episodes with drug therapy in selected older adults. These drugs may have bothersome systemic anticholinergic side effects, especially dry mouth and constipation. Anticholinergic agents may precipitate urinary retention in some patients; men with some degree of outflow obstruction, diabetic patients, and patients with impaired bladder contractility are at the highest risk and should be followed carefully. Patients with Alzheimer's disease must be followed for the development of drug-induced delirium, although it is unusual. Several studies suggest that cognitive and physical functional impairments are associated with poor responses to bladder relaxant drug therapy. The results of these studies should

Table 123-11   Example of a Bladder Retraining Protocol

Objective: To restore a normal pattern of voiding and continence after the removal of an indwelling catheter.

1. Remove the indwelling catheter (clamping the catheter before removal is not necessary).
2. Treat urinary tract infection if present.
3. Initiate a toileting schedule. Begin by toileting the patient:

    a. Upon awakening
    b. Every 2 hours during the day and evening
    c. Before getting into bed
    d. Every 4 hours at night

4. Monitor the patient's voiding and continence pattern with a record that allows for the recording of:

    a. Frequency, timing, and amount of continent voids
    b. Frequency, timing, and amount of incontinence episodes
    c. Fluid intake pattern
    d. Postvoid catheter volume

5. If the patient is having difficulty voiding (complete urinary retention or very low urine outputs, e.g., <240 mL in an 8-hour period while fluid intake is adequate):

    a. Perform bladder ultrasonography or in-and-out catheterization, recording volume obtained, every 6 to 8 hours until residual values are <200 mL
    b. Instruct the patient on techniques to trigger voiding (e.g., running water, stroking inner thigh, suprapubic tapping) and to help completely empty bladder (e.g., bending forward, suprapubic pressure, double voiding)
    c. If the patient continues to have high residual volumes after 3 to 4 weeks, consider urodynamic evaluation

6. If the patient is voiding frequently (i.e., more often than every 2 hours):

    a. Perform postvoid residual determination to ensure the patient is completely emptying the bladder
    b. Encourage the patient to delay voiding as long as possible and instruct the patient to use techniques to help completely empty bladder
    c. If the patient continues to have frequency and nocturia, with or without urgency and incontinence:

        (1) Rule out other reversible causes (e.g., urinary tract infection medication effects, hyperglycemia, and congestive heart failure)
        (2) Consider trial of bladder relaxant if postvoid residuals are low

SOURCE: Adapted from Kane RL et al.

not, however, preclude a treatment trial in this patient population when they make frequent attempts to toilet yet remain incontinent. Newer long-acting anticholinergic drugs for urge incontinence are as effective as immediate release preparations, but with a lower incidence of bothersome side effects.

For stress incontinence, drug treatment involves a combination of an α-agonist and estrogen. Phenylpropanolamine was the most studied agent used for stress incontinence, but is no longer available because of the increased risk of intracranial hemorrhage in women (who were using the drug as a dietary supplement not as an incontinence treatment). Pseudoephedrine is now the most commonly used agent for stress incontinence. Drug treatment is appropriate for motivated patients who (1) have mild to moderate degrees of stress incontinence, (2) do not have a major anatomic abnormality such as a large cystocele, and (3) do not have a contraindication to these drugs such as poorly controlled hypertension in the case

of α-agonists. These patients also may respond to behavioral interventions. Studies suggest that the two treatment modalities are roughly equivalent, with about three-fourths of patients reporting improvement. A combination is also a reasonable approach for some patients. Oral estrogen, in studies using hormonal replacement dosages, has shown no effect on stress incontinence episodes in hypoestrogenemic incontinent women. Estrogen is likely effective, however, in combination with an α-agonist for stress incontinence (see Chap. 75 for further discussion of oral estrogen use). Topical estrogen is also used, either chronically or on an intermittent basis (i.e., 1- to 2-month courses), for the treatment of irritative voiding symptoms and urge incontinence in women with atrophic vaginitis and urethritis. Although no specific topical treatment regimen has been shown to be more effective than others, therapy usually involves 0.5 to 1 g of vaginal cream nightly for 1 to 2 months and then a maintenance dose two or three times per week. Several months of therapy is often necessary to observe

Table 123-12 Drugs Used to Treat Urinary Incontinence

Drugs	Dosages	Mechanisms of Action	Type of Incontinence	Potential Adverse Effects
Anticholinergic and antispasmodic agents				
Oxybutynin (Ditropan, immediate release)	2.5–5.0 mg tid	Increase bladder capacity; diminish involuntary bladder contractions	Urge or mixed with urge predominant	Anticholinergic (dry mouth, blurry vision, elevated intraocular pressure, delirium, constipation)
Oxybutynin (extended release; Ditropan (XL)	5–30 mg qd (most often 10 mg qd)			Above, but with less dry mouth
Tolterodine (Detrol LA)	4 mg qd			Above, but with less dry mouth
Hyoscamine (Levsin)	0.125 mg tid			Anticholinergic
Propantheline (Pro-Banthine)	15–30 mg tid			Anticholinergic
Dicyclomine (Bentyl)	10–20 mg tid			Anticholinergic
Imipramine (Tofranil)	25–50 mg tid			Above effects plus postural hypotension, cardiac conduction disturbances
α-Adrenergic agonists				
Pseudoephedrine (Sudafed)	30–60 mg tid	Increase urethral smooth-muscle contraction		Headache, tachycardia, elevation of blood pressure
Imipramine (Tofranil)	25–50 mg tid			As listed above
Conjugated estrogens				
Topical	0.5–1.0 g per application	Strengthen periurethral tissues	Urge associated with atrophic vaginitis	
Vaginal ring (Estring)	One ring every 3 months			
Cholinergic agonists				
Bethanechol (Urecholine)	10–30 mg tid	Stimulate bladder contraction	Overflow incontinence with atonic bladder	Bradycardia, hypotension, bronchoconstriction, gastric acid secretion
α-Adrenergic antagonist				
Terazosin (Hytrin)	1–10 mg qhs	Relax smooth muscle of urethra and prostatic capsule	Urge incontinence associated with prostatic enlargement	Postural hypotension
Doxazosin (Cardura)	1–8 mg qhs			
Prazosin (Minipress)	1–2 mg tid			
Tamsulosin (Flomax)	0.4–0.8 mg qd			

SOURCE: Adapted from Kane RL et al.

therapeutic benefit. A small vaginal ring that slowly releases estrogen and vaginal tablets are now available in the United States.

Many elderly women have symptomatically and urodynamically a combination of both urge and stress incontinence. A combination of estrogen and imipramine would, at least in theory, be appropriate for these patients because imipramine has both anticholinergic and α-adrenergic effects. However, imipramine poses a risk of postural hypotension in addition to its marked anticholinergic effects. If urge incontinence is the predominant symptom, a combination of estrogen and bladder relaxant would be appropriate. Behavioral interventions are also an effective approach for women with mixed incontinence.

Drug treatment for chronic overflow incontinence using a cholinergic agonist or an α-adrenergic antagonist is usually not efficacious. Bethanechol may be helpful when given subcutaneously for a brief period in patients with persistent bladder contractility problems after an overdistension injury, but the drug is generally not effective as a long-term oral therapy. Although α-adrenergic blockers are beneficial in relieving symptoms of benign prostatic hyperplasia, they are probably not efficacious for long-term treatment of elderly patients with overflow incontinence and a significant degree of urinary retention (i.e., residuals consistently greater than 200 to 300 mL).

Surgery and Periurethral Injection

Surgery should be considered for elderly women with stress incontinence unresponsive to nonsurgical treatment and for women with a significant degree of pelvic prolapse. As with many other surgical procedures, patient selection and the experience of the surgeon are critical to success. Any woman being considered for surgical therapy should have a thorough evaluation, including urodynamic tests, before undergoing the procedure. Newly modified techniques of bladder neck suspension and the use of periurethral collagen injections can be done with minimal risks. However, many elderly women with severe incontinence associated with intrinsic urethral weakness require a sling procedure rather than a simple bladder neck suspension. Urinary retention can occur after surgery, but it is usually transient and can be managed by intermittent catheter drainage. Periurethral injections appear to be most appropriate for women with intrinsic urethral weakness. Repeated injections are usually necessary to maintain effectiveness.

Surgery may be indicated in men in whom incontinence is associated with outflow obstruction. Men who have had complete urinary retention are likely to have another episode within a short period of time and should have a prostatic resection, as should men with incontinence associated with enough residual urine to be causing recurrent symptomatic infections or hydronephrosis. In men who do not meet these criteria the decision should be based on weighing carefully the degree to which the symptoms bother the patient, the potential benefits of surgery (obstructive symptoms often respond better than irritative symptoms), and the risks of surgery (which may be minimal with newer prostate resection techniques).

CATHETERS AND CATHETER CARE

Three basic types of catheters and catheterization procedures are used for the management of urinary incontinence: external catheters, intermittent straight ("in-and-out") catheterization, and chronic indwelling catheterization. External catheters generally consist of some type of condom connected to a drainage system. Improvements in design and observance of proper procedure and skin care when applying the catheter decrease the risk of skin irritation, as well as the frequency with which the catheter falls off. Studies of complications associated with the use of these devices have been limited. Existing data suggest that patients with external catheters are at increased risk of developing symptomatic infection. External catheters should be used only to manage intractable incontinence in male patients who do not have urinary retention and who are extremely physically dependent. An external catheter for use in female patients is available commercially, but its safety and effectiveness have not been well documented in the elderly population.

Intermittent catheterization can help in the management of patients with urinary retention and overflow incontinence. The procedure can be carried out by either the patient or a caregiver and involves straight catheterization two to four or more times daily, depending on residual urine volumes. The goal is to keep residual urine volume generally less than approximately 300 mL. In the home setting, the catheter should be kept clean (but not necessarily sterile). Studies conducted largely among younger paraplegic patients show that this technique is practical and reduces the risk of symptomatic infection compared with the risk associated with chronic catheterization. Self-intermittent catheterization is also feasible for elderly female outpatients who are functional and willing and able to catheterize themselves. The technique may be especially useful following removal of an indwelling catheter in a bladder-retraining protocol (see Table 123-11). However, elderly nursing home residents, especially men, may be difficult to catheterize. Anatomic abnormalities commonly found in the lower urinary tracts of elderly patients may

Table 123-13 Indications for Chronic Indwelling Catheter Use

Urinary retention that
  Is causing persistent overflow incontinence, symptomatic infections, or renal dysfunction
  Cannot be corrected surgically or medically
  Cannot be managed practically with intermittent catheterization

Skin wounds, pressure sores, or irritations that are being contaminated by incontinent urine

Care of terminally ill or severely impaired for whom bed and clothing changes are uncomfortable or disruptive

Patient preference

SOURCE: Adapted from Kane RL et al.

Table 123-14 Key Principles of Chronic Indwelling Catheter Care

1. Maintain sterile, closed, gravity drainage system.
2. Avoid breaking the closed system.
3. Use clean techniques in emptying and changing the drainage system; wash hands between patients in institutionalized setting.
4. Secure the catheter to the upper thigh or lower abdomen to avoid perineal contamination and urethral irritation caused by movement of the catheter.
5. Avoid frequent and vigorous cleaning of the catheter entry site; washing with soapy water once per day is sufficient.
6. Do not routinely irrigate.
7. If bypassing occurs in the absence of obstruction, consider the possibility of a bladder spasm, which can be treated with a bladder relaxant.
8. If catheter obstruction occurs frequently, increase the patient's fluid intake and acidify the urine by dilute acidic irrigations.
9. Do not routinely use prophylactic or suppressive urinary antiseptics or antimicrobials.
10. Do not do routine surveillance cultures to guide management of individual patients because all chronically catheterized patients have bacteriuria (which is often polymicrobial) and the organisms change frequently.
11. Do not treat infection unless the patient develops symptoms; symptoms may be nonspecific, and other possible sources of infection should be carefully excluded before attributing symptoms to the urinary tract.
12. If a patient develops frequent symptomatic urinary tract infections, a genitourinary evaluation should be considered to rule out pathologic lesions such as stones, periurethral or prostatic abscesses, or chronic pyelonephritis.

SOURCE: Adapted from Kane RL et al.

increase the risk of infection because of repeated straight catheterizations. In addition, using this technique in an institutional setting, which may have an abundance of organisms relatively resistant to many commonly used antimicrobial agents, may yield an unacceptable risk of nosocomial infections. Using sterile catheter trays for these procedures would be very expensive. Thus, it may be extremely difficult to implement such a program in a typical nursing home setting.

Chronic indwelling catheterization, when used for periods of months to years, has been shown to increase the incidence of a number of complications, including chronic bacteriuria, bladder stones, periurethral abscesses, and even bladder cancer. Elderly nursing home residents managed by this technique, especially men, are at relatively high risk of developing symptomatic infections. Given these risks, it seems appropriate to recommend that the use of chronic indwelling catheters be limited to certain specific situations (Table 123-13). When indwelling catheterization is used, certain principles of catheter care should be observed in an attempt to minimize complications (Table 123-14).

FECAL INCONTINENCE

Fecal incontinence is less common than urinary incontinence. Its occurrence is relatively unusual in elderly patients who are continent of urine. Thirty to 50 percent of elderly patients in institutional settings with frequent urinary incontinence, however, also have episodes of fecal incontinence. This coexistence suggests common pathophysiologic mechanisms.

Defecation, like urination, is a physiologic process that involves smooth and striated muscles, central and peripheral innervation, coordination of reflex responses, mental awareness, and physical ability to get to a toilet. Disruption of any of these factors can lead to fecal incontinence.

The most common causes of fecal incontinence are problems with constipation and laxative use, neurologic disorders, and colorectal disorders (Table 123-15). In patients who are fed by enteral tubes, hyperosmotic feedings can precipitate diarrhea and fecal incontinence. Diluting the feedings or using slow continuous infusion is sometimes helpful. Constipation is extremely common in elderly persons and, when chronic, can lead to fecal impaction and incontinence. The hard stool (or scybalum) of fecal impaction irritates the rectum and results in the production of mucus and fluid. This fluid leaks around the mass of

Table 123-15 Causes of Fecal Incontinence

Fecal impaction

Constipation

Laxative overuse or abuse

Hyperosmotic enteral feedings

Neurologic disorders
  Dementia
  Stroke
  Spinal cord disease

Colorectal disorders
  Diarrheal illnesses
  Diabetic autonomic neuropathy
  Rectal sphincter damage

impacted stool and precipitates incontinence. Constipation is difficult to define; technically, it indicates fewer than three bowel movements per week, although many patients use the term to describe difficult passage of hard stools or a feeling of incomplete evacuation. Poor dietary and toilet habits, immobility, and chronic laxative abuse are the most common causes of constipation in elderly persons. Appropriate management of constipation prevents fecal impaction and resulting fecal incontinence. The management of constipation is discussed thoroughly in Chapter 52.

Fecal incontinence is sometimes amenable to biofeedback therapy, although many elderly demented patients are unable to cooperate. For those patients with end-stage dementia, a program of alternating constipating agents (if necessary) and laxatives in a routine schedule (such as giving laxatives and enemas three times a week) is effective in controlling defecation in many patients with fecal incontinence. Functionally dependent patients should be toileted regularly after a meal to take advantage of, or possibly regain, the gastrocolic reflex. Experience suggests that these measures should permit management of even severely cognitively impaired patients. As a last resort, specially designed incontinence undergarments are sometimes helpful in managing fecal incontinence and preventing skin irritation and other complications.

REFERENCES

Abrams P, Klevmark B: Frequency volume charts: An indispensable part of lower urinary tract assessment. *Scand J Urol Nephrol Suppl* 179:47, 1996.

Brown JS et al: Urinary incontinence in older women: Who is at risk? Study of Osteoporotic Fractures Research Group. *Obstet Gynecol* 87(5 Pt 1):715, 1996.

Brown JS et al: Urinary incontinence: Does it increase risk for falls and fractures? Study of Osteoporotic Fractures Research Group. *J Am Geriatr Soc* 48(7):721, 2000.

Burgio KL et al: Behavioral vs. drug treatment for urge urinary incontinence in older women: A randomized controlled trial. *JAMA* 280(23):1995, 1998.

DuBeau CE et al: The impact of urge urinary incontinence on quality of life: Importance of patients' perspective and explanatory style. *J Am Geriatr Soc* 46(6):683, 1998.

Fantl JA et al: Efficacy of estrogen supplementation in the treatment of urinary incontinence. The Continence Program for Women Research Group. *Obstet Gynecol* 88(5):745, 1996.

Johnson TM 2nd et al: Self-care practices used by older men and women to manage urinary incontinence: Results from the national follow-up survey on self-care and aging. *J Am Geriatr Soc* 48(8):894, 2000.

Kane RL et al: *Essentials of Clinical Geriatrics,* 4th ed. New York, McGraw-Hill, 1999.

Malone-Lee JG et al: Tolterodine: A safe and effective treatment for older patients with overactive bladder. *J Am Geriatr Soc* 49(6):700, 2001.

Ouslander JG et al: Prompted voiding for nighttime incontinence in nursing homes: Is it effective? *J Am Geriatr Soc* 49(6):706, 2001.

Resnick NM: Geriatric incontinence. *Urol Clin North Am* 23(1):55, 1996.

Smoger SH et al: Urinary incontinence among male veterans receiving care in primary care clinics. *Ann Intern Med* 132(7):547, 2000.

Thom DH et al: Medically recognized urinary incontinence and risks of hospitalization, nursing home admission, and mortality. *Age Aging* 26:367, 1997.

Wagner TH, Hu TW: Economic costs of urinary incontinence in 1995. *Urology* 51(3):355, 1998.

Disorders of Temperature Regulation

ITAMAR B. ABRASS

Temperature dysregulation in the elderly is an example of the declining regulation of homeostatic mechanisms that occurs with advancing age. Elderly persons are less able to adjust to extremes of environmental temperatures. Hypothermic and hyperthermic states are predominantly disorders of the elderly population. Despite underreporting of these disorders, there is evidence that morbidity and mortality increase during particularly hot or cold periods, especially among ill elderly persons. Much of this illness is caused by an increased incidence of cardiovascular disorders (myocardial infarction and stroke) and infectious diseases (pneumonia) during periods of temperature extremes.

HYPOTHERMIA

Epidemiology

Studies in the United Kingdom reveal that hypothermia is a common finding among elderly people during the winter, when homes are usually heated to less than 21°C (70°F). As might be expected, there is a similar seasonal occurrence in the United States and Canada. In Great Britain, as many as 3.6 percent of all patients older than 65 years admitted to the hospital are hypothermic. In a population study, 10 percent of elderly people living at home were found to be on the borderline of hypothermia, with a deep-body temperature of less than 35.5°C (96°F).

Pathophysiology

Hypothermia is defined as a core temperature (rectal, esophageal, tympanic) of less than 35°C (95°F). The susceptibility of elderly persons to hypothermia is related to both disease and physiologic change. The thermoregulatory center maintains body temperature through control of sweating, vasoconstriction and vasodilation, chemical thermogenesis, and shivering. A diminished sensation of cold and impaired sensitivity to changes in temperature are associated with poor thermoregulation in elderly individuals and can lead to maladaptive behavior in cold environments. In older adults, shivering is often observed to be less intense, despite a greater loss of core temperature. Because maximal shivering increases heat production threefold to fivefold greater than at the resting level, elderly persons with less efficient or reduced shivering processes are at increased risk for hypothermia.

The mechanisms by which adrenergic deficits contribute to hypothermia in the elderly population have not been defined. However, an abnormal autonomic vasoconstrictor response to cold is a key factor in the temperature dysregulation associated with aging. This autonomic dysregulation is also manifested in a higher incidence of orthostatic hypotension in people at risk for hypothermia. Diminished thermogenesis is another key factor in temperature dysregulation in elderly individuals. Aging is associated with diminished beta-adrenergically mediated thermogenesis. The metabolic rate is also lower in older people owing to a decrease in lean body mass, thus contributing to the risk of hypothermia in these individuals. The thermic effect of feeding may also be diminished in elderly persons. Because body fat contributes to insulation against heat loss, thin elderly persons with a decreased fat mass are also at increased risk for hypothermia.

Besides actual exposure to cold, there are a host of factors predisposing to hypothermia. Disorders associated with decreased heat production include hypothyroidism, hypoglycemia, starvation, and malnutrition. The most common endocrinopathy associated with hypothermia is hypothyroidism, a condition in which as many as 80 percent of patients have a low body temperature as a result of the associated depression of metabolic rate and calorigenesis. Hypoglycemia also reduces shivering, probably by a central effect. Hypothermia may occur in 50 percent or more of patients with hypoglycemia. Starvation and malnutrition may contribute to the risk of hypothermia because of the decrease in lean body mass and energy stores for calorigenesis as well as the loss of body fat with its insulating effect. Immobility and decreased activity due to such disorders as stroke, arthritis, and parkinsonism also may lead to decreased heat production. In patients with parkinsonism, autonomic dysfunction may also contribute to temperature dysregulation.

Thermoregulatory impairment may occur as a result of hypothalamic and central nervous system dysfunction or may be drug-induced. Trauma, hypoxia, tumor, or cerebrovascular disease may impair the central regulation of temperature. The drugs most commonly associated with hypothermia are ethanol, barbiturates, phenothiazines, benzodiazepines, anesthetic agents, and opioids. Ethanol predisposes to hypothermia in acting as a vasodilator, a central nervous system depressant, an anesthetic, a cause of hypoglycemia, and a risk factor for trauma and environmental exposure. Phenothiazines inhibit shivering by exerting a peripheral curarizing effect.

In sepsis, hypothermia reflects an alteration in the hypothalamic set point and a diminished and often paradoxical host response to pyrogenes in the setting of overwhelmed host defenses. In cardiovascular disease, the circulatory system may not be able to respond to the stress of changes in body temperature or to the demands of such counterregulatory mechanisms as shivering.

Particularly in elderly individuals, living alone or being alone, lack of central heating, failure to use heating (whatever the type), and dementia or confusion are associated with an increased risk for hypothermia. In one survey of elderly people, only 1 in 10 was aware of the dangers of accidental hypothermia.

Clinical Presentation

As stated previously, hypothermia is defined as a core temperature of less than 35°C (95°F). Essential to the diagnosis is early recognition with a low-recording thermometer. Ordinary thermometers do not register low temperatures. Because early signs are nonspecific and subtle, a high index of suspicion must exist to allow an early diagnosis. A history of known or potential exposure is helpful, but elderly patients can become hypothermic even at modest temperatures. Early signs that occur at core temperatures of 32° to 35°C (90° to 95°F) include fatigue, weakness, slowness of gait, apathy, slurred speech, confusion, and cool skin. Patients may complain of a sensation of being cold and may be shivering. As hypothermia progresses (28°–30°C [82°–86°F]), the skin becomes cold. Hypopnea and cyanosis are present, at first because of decreased metabolic demands and later owing to depression of the central respiratory drive. Bradycardia, atrial and ventricular arrhythmias, and hypotension also occur. Semicoma or coma and muscular rigidity are present. Consciousness is commonly lost at a brain temperature between 32° and 30°C (90° and 86°F). Reflexes are slowed, and pupils are poorly reactive. Generalized edema and polyuria or oliguria may be present. Cold exposure is associated with both water and solute diuresis. Volume contraction occurs because of diuresis and also because of some degree of extracellular and intracellular water shift.

As the core temperature falls to less than 28°C (82°F), the skin becomes very cold; individuals become unresponsive, rigid, and areflexive and have fixed, dilated pupils. Apnea and ventricular fibrillation are frequently present. Patients may sometimes be mistaken for dead. Case reports describe patients who have survived after being discovered without respiration or pulse.

The most significant early complications of severe hypothermia are arrhythmias and cardiorespiratory arrest. Later complications include bronchopneumonia and aspiration pneumonia. The cough reflex is depressed by hypothermia, and the cold results in the production of large quantities of thick, tenacious bronchial secretions, predisposing the patient to the previously mentioned complications. Pulmonary edema may occur, especially in individuals with prior cardiovascular disease. Pancreatitis and gastrointestinal tract bleeding are frequent complications, although massive hemorrhage is unusual. Acute renal failure may occur. Intravascular thrombosis is a complication of hemoconcentration and the temperature-induced changes in viscosity.

Electrocardiogram (ECG) abnormalities are common. The most specific ECG finding is a J wave (Osborne wave) following the QRS complex. This abnormality disappears as the temperature returns to normal. Other common abnormalities include bradycardia and a prolonged P-R interval, QRS complex, and QT segment, as well as atrial fibrillation, premature ventricular contractions, and ventricular fibrillation. ECG changes may simulate those of acute myocardial ischemia or infarction.

Frequently, the most difficult differential diagnosis in hypothermia is hypothyroidism, a common cause of hypothermia. A previous history of thyroid disease, a neck scar from previous thyroid surgery, and a delay in the relaxation phase of deep tendon reflexes may assist in the diagnosis of hypothyroidism.

Treatment

Emergency Care

In the field, a hypothermic person should immediately be removed from the cold environment, windy areas, and contact with cold objects. Wet clothing should be removed to prevent further heat loss. Top and bottom blankets should be used (covers may need to be preheated to avoid a drain of heat from the patient's body). The patient should be moved carefully, as a cold, bradycardic heart is extremely irritable and even minor stimuli can precipitate ventricular fibrillation or asystole. Cardiac monitoring should be started as soon as possible. Patients with a detectable heartbeat who are breathing spontaneously, no matter how slowly, should not be subjected to unnecessary procedures such as chest compression or the placement of a pacemaker. Patients in asystole or ventricular fibrillation should be resuscitated, but a cold heart may be relatively unresponsive to drugs or electrical stimulation. Intravenous fluids, preferably 5 percent dextrose normal saline without potassium, should be warmed before being used.

General Support

At the hospital, general supportive therapy for severe hypothermia consists of intensive care management of complicated multisystem dysfunctions. Mortality is usually greater than 50 percent for severe hypothermia. It increases with age and is particularly related to underlying disease. Every attempt should be made to assess and treat any contributing medical disorder (e.g., infection, hypothyroidism, or hypoglycemia). Underlying infections are common. Hypothermia in elderly patients should be promptly treated as sepsis unless proved otherwise. If hypothyroidism is suspected, the patient should be treated with 0.5 mg levothyroxine intravenously and corticosteroids. Although patients should undergo continuous ECG monitoring, central lines should be avoided if possible because of myocardial irritability.

Because metabolism is delayed, most drugs have little effect in a severely hypothermic patient, but they may cause problems once the patient is rewarmed. Arrhythmias are resistant to cardioversion and drug therapy. Insulin is ineffective at temperatures of less than 30°C (86°F) and should be avoided in a hyperglycemic hypothermic patient. If given during hypothermia, insulin may cause hypoglycemia as the patient is rewarmed. Insulin resistance improves spontaneously as the core body temperature rises. In chronic hypothermia (lasting longer than 12 hours), volume depletion may be severe, and volume repletion may be needed as rewarming occurs. Blood gases should be observed to assess respiratory function. Oxygen therapy, suctioning, and endotracheal intubation may be required. Serious arrhythmias, acidosis, and fluid and electrolyte disorders usually respond to therapy only after rewarming has been accomplished. It is preferable to stabilize the patient and immediately undertake specific rewarming techniques.

Rewarming

Passive rewarming with insulating material and placement of the patient in a warm environment (>70°F [>21°C]) is generally adequate for those with mild (>32°C [>90°F]) hypothermia. Active external rewarming (electric blankets, warm mattresses and hot-water bottles, submersion in a warm water bath) is a more rapid technique of rewarming than passive procedures. However, active external rewarming has been associated with increased morbidity and mortality. Cold blood may suddenly be shunted to the core, further decreasing the core temperature. Peripheral vasodilation resulting from external rewarming can precipitate hypovolemic shock by decreasing the circulatory blood volume.

For more severe hypothermia (<32°C [<90°F]), core rewarming is necessary. Several techniques for core rewarming have been used, but positive results have been reported only from small, uncontrolled studies. Mediastinal lavage is effective, but it is a major surgical procedure. Extracorporeal circulation is a rapid method for rewarming but requires a special hospital unit; also, there is a risk of hypotension and of bleeding with the use of heparin. Continuous arteriovenous rewarming (CAVR) has been used

to treat hypothermia in critically ill patients. In this procedure, percutaneously placed femoral arterial and venous catheters are connected to the inflow and outflow side of a countercurrent fluid warmer to create a fistula through the heating mechanism. In a study comparing CAVR with standard rewarming techniques, CAVR was associated with improved survival after moderately severe injury and a significant reduction in blood and fluid requirements, organ failure, and length of stay in the intensive care unit. Another approach is to use gastric lavage, in which balloons are placed in the stomach and filled with water. With this method, a smaller area is rewarmed than in peritoneal dialysis, and local pharyngeal irritation may precipitate an arrhythmia.

Peritoneal dialysis and inhalation rewarming may be the most practical techniques in most institutions. However, inhalation therapy may not be as effective in moderate to severe hypothermia as it is in mild hypothermia. Peritoneal dialysis (40°C [104°F]) carries little risk for the patient, is easy to perform, requires simple equipment, and can be performed in any hospital. Dialysis with 2 L of a potassium-free solution and rapid instillation and immediate removal are preferred. Normothermia is usually accomplished within six to eight exchanges. Enemas are infrequently used but can be employed in conjunction with dialysis.

HYPERTHERMIA

Epidemiology

In the United States, approximately 5000 deaths occur annually as a direct result of heatstroke, and two-thirds of the victims are older than 60 years. Hyperthermia can contribute to increased morbidity and mortality from various cardiovascular diseases in elderly persons. In the past, a significant number of deaths during heat waves occurred in nursing home residents. Increased awareness of the problem has probably benefited this group of elderly patients. During the 1984 New York City heat wave, the death rate for those older than 75 years increased by almost 50 percent, but the increase was limited almost exclusively to noninstitutionalized elderly persons.

Women appear to be more susceptible to the lethal effects of heatstroke. In the 1984 New York City heat wave mortality increased by 66 percent for women, compared with 39 percent for men. A similar sex distribution was seen in the St. Louis and Georgia heat waves of 1983, when 77 percent of excess deaths occurred in women.

Pathophysiology

Heatstroke is defined as an acute failure to maintain normal body temperature in the setting of a warm environment. Elderly people usually present with nonexertional heatstroke due to impaired heat loss and a failure of homeostatic mechanisms. As with hypothermia, the susceptibility of elderly people to heatstroke is related to both disease and physiologic changes.

Impairment of the thermoregulatory system by diminished or absent sweating is an important cause of heat exhaustion and heatstroke in a hot environment. Deaths of elderly persons during a heat wave can usually be ascribed to heart or other cardiovascular disease exacerbated by heat stress. However, some morbidity is directly related to primary thermoregulatory failure. The sweating response to thermal and neurochemical stimulation has been found to be reduced in elderly people compared with that in younger adults. There is also a higher core temperature threshold at which sweating can be initiated. A delayed development of skin vasculature dilation and diminished cardiac output and splanchnic circulation redistribution with heating also interfere with heat loss in elderly people. Some of these changes in sweat rate and blood flow may, however, be related more to deconditioning than to aging per se. When the maximum oxygen uptake is matched between younger and older men, there is no significant difference in the sweat rate or forearm blood flow during exercise. However, when young men are compared with sedentary older men, there is a decreased response in these parameters with age. Impaired sensitivity to changes in temperature may lead to maladaptive behavior in warm environments. Acclimatization to heat may be less likely to occur in elderly compared with young people and may thus contribute to the physiologic deficits.

Inability to take appropriate measures such as removing heavy clothing, moving to a cooler environment, and increasing fluid intake increases the risk for heatstroke in elderly individuals with limited mobility. Living alone and confusion add to this risk. Elderly individuals with cardiovascular disease may not be able to increase their cardiac output adequately in response to heat stress. Congestive heart failure, diabetes mellitus, obesity, and obstructive lung disease have been associated with an increased risk of death in heatstroke victims. Other risk factors for death from heatstroke are alcoholism, the use of tranquilizers and anticholinergics, and a reduction in physical activity. Elderly people are more likely to be taking multiple drugs, some of which may impair the response to a warm environment. Anticholinergics, phenothiazines, and antidepressants lead to hypohidrosis. Diuretics may be associated with hypovolemia and hypokalemia, and beta-blockers may depress myocardial function.

Clinical Presentation

Heatstroke is characterized by a core temperature of greater than 40.6°C (105°F), severe central nervous system dysfunction (psychosis, delirium, coma), and anhidrosis (hot, dry skin). Earlier manifestations, termed heat exhaustion, are nonspecific and include dizziness, weakness, a sensation of warmth, anorexia, nausea, vomiting, headache, and dyspnea.

Complications of heatstroke include congestive heart failure and a host of cardiac arrhythmias, cerebral edema with seizures and diffuse and focal neurologic deficits, hepatocellular necrosis with jaundice and liver failure, hypokalemia, respiratory alkalosis and metabolic acidosis, and hypovolemia and shock. Rhabdomyolysis, disseminated intravascular coagulation, and acute renal failure are less frequent in elderly than in younger patients with exertional heatstroke. The ultimate complication, death, occurs in as many as 80 percent of patients once the full syndrome of heatstroke is manifest.

Treatment

The key to treating hyperthermia is rapid cooling. It should be started immediately in the field, and the core body temperature should be brought to 39°C (102°F) within the first hour. The duration of hyperthermia is the major determinant of the ultimate outcome. Ice packs and ice-water immersion are superior to convection cooling with alcohol sponge baths or electric fans. Complications require intensive multisystem care.

CONCLUSIONS

Prevention appears to be the most appropriate approach to the management of temperature dysregulation in the elderly. Educating older adults about their susceptibility to hypothermia and hyperthermia in environmental temperature extremes, educating them about appropriate behavior under such conditions, and close monitoring of the most vulnerable elderly individuals should help reduce the morbidity and mortality from these disorders.

REFERENCES

Anderson RK, Kenney WL: Effect of age on heat-activated sweat gland density and flow during exercise in dry heat. *J Appl Physiol* 63:1089, 1987.

Avery CE, Pestle RE: Hypothermia and the elderly: Perceptions and behaviors. *Gerontologist* 27:523, 1987.

Barnard CN: Hypothermia: A method of intragastric cooling. *Br J Surg* 44:269, 1956.

Bristow G: Treatment of accidental hypothermia with peritoneal dialysis. *Can Med Assoc J* 118:764, 1978.

Collins KJ et al: Accidental hypothermia and impaired temperature homeostatis in the elderly. *BMJ* 1:353, 1977.

Collins KJ et al: Shivering thermogenesis and vasomotor responses with convective cooling in the elderly. *J Physiol* 320:76, 1981.

Collins KJ, Exton-Smith AN: Thermal homeostasis in old age. *J Am Geriatr Soc* 31:519, 1983.

Curley FJ, Irwin RS: Disorders of temperature control: I. Hyperthermia. *J Intensive Care* 1:5, 1986.

Danzl DF et al: Multicenter hypothermia survey. *Ann Emerg Med* 16:1042, 1987.

Danzl DF, Pozos PS: Accidental hypothermia. *N Engl J Med* 331:1756, 1994.

Darowski A et al: Hypothermia and infection in elderly patients admitted to hospital. *Age Ageing* 20:100, 1991.

Elia M et al: Total energy expenditure in the elderly. *Eur J Clin Nutr* 54(suppl 3):S92, 2000.

Fox RH et al: Body temperature in the elderly: A national study of physiological, social, and environmental conditions. *BMJ* 1:200, 1963.

Frank SM et al: Age-related thermoregulatory differences during core cooling in humans. *Am J Physiol Regul Integr Comp Physiol* 279:R349, 2000.

Gentilello LM et al: Continuous arteriovenous rewarming: Rapid reversal of hypothermia in critically ill patients. *J Trauma* 32:316, 1992.

Granberg PO: Human physiology under cold exposure. *Arctic Med Res* 50(suppl 6):23, 1991.

Gregory RT, Doolittle WH: Accidental hypothermia: II. Clinical implications of experimental studies. *Alaska Med* 15:48, 1973.

Halle A, Repasy A: Classic heatstroke: A serious challenge for the elderly. *Hosp Pract* 22:26, 1987.

Heat -associated mortality —New York City. *MMWR Morb Mortal Wkly Rep.* 33:430, 1984.

Hudson LD, Conn RD: Accidental hypothermia: Associated diagnoses and prognosis in a common problem. *JAMA* 227:37, 1974.

Inoue Y et al: Relationship between skin blood flow and sweating rate, and age related regional differences. *Eur J Appl Physiol Occup Physiol* 79:17, 1998.

Kerckhoffs DA et al: Effect of aging on beta-adrenergically mediated thermogenesis in men. *Am J Physiol* 274:E1075, 1998.

Kilbourne EM et al: Risk factors for heat stroke: A case-control study. *JAMA* 247:3332, 1982.

Maresca L, Vasko JS: Treatment of hypothermia by extracorporeal circulation and internal rewarming. *J Trauma* 27:89, 1987.

Mattu A et al: Electrographic manifestations of hypothermia. *Am J Emerg Med* 20:314, 2002.

Matz R: Hypothermia: Mechanisms and countermeasures. *Hosp Pract* 21:45, 1986.

Medical Letter Advisory Panel: Treatment of hypothermia. *Med Lett* 36:116, 1994.

Miescher E, Fortney SM: Responses to dehydration and rehydration during heat exposure in young and older men. *Am J Physiol* 257:R1050, 1989.

Minson CT et al: Age alters the cardiovascular response to direct passive heating. *J Appl Physiol* 84:1323, 1998.

Natsume K et al: Preferred ambient temperature for old and young men in summer and winter. *Int J Biometeorol* 36:1, 1992.

Nielsen HK et al: Hypothermic patients admitted to an intensive care unit: A fifteen year survey. *Danish Med Bull* 39:190, 1992.

Poehlman ET, Horton ES: Regulation of energy expenditure in aging humans. *Annu Rev Nutr* 10:255, 1990.

Reuler JB: Hypothermia: Pathophysiology, clinical settings, and management. *Ann Intern Med* 89:519, 1978.

Richardson D et al: Attenuation of the cutaneous vasoconstrictor response to cold in elderly men. *J Gerontol Med Sci* 47:M211, 1992.

Semenza JC et al: Heat-related deaths during the July 1995 heat wave in Chicago. *N Engl J Med* 335:84, 1996.

Simon HB: Hyperthermia. *N Engl J Med* 329:483, 1993.

Tankersley CG et al: Sweating and skin blood flow during exercise: Effects of age and maximal oxygen uptake. *J Appl Physiol* 71:236, 1991.

Vans E et al: Thermally-induced cutaneous vasodilation in aging. *J Gerontol Med Sci* 48:M53, 1993.

White JD et al: Controlled comparison of radio wave regional hyperthermia and peritoneal lavage rewarming after immersion hypothermia. *J Trauma* 25:989, 1985.

White JD et al: Rewarming in accidental hypothermia: Radio wave versus inhalation therapy. *Ann Emerg Med* 16:50, 1987.

Wongsurawat N et al: Thermoregulatory failure in the elderly. *J Am Geriatr Soc* 38:899, 1990.

Elder Mistreatment

MARK LACHS

DEFINITIONS

In the broadest context, *elder mistreatment* subsumes a variety of activities perpetrated upon an older person by others. Some proposed strategies for defining or classifying elder mistreatment have been based on abuse type (e.g., physical versus verbal abuse), motive (e.g., intentional versus unintentional neglect), perpetrator relationship (e.g., family versus paid caregiver), and setting (e.g., community versus nursing home). There is as yet no universally agreed definition or classification of elder mistreatment. Nonetheless, the clinician attempting to care for a victimized older person or understand the spectrum of elder mistreatment will encounter several thematically similar definitions. For example, the older Americans Act of 1975 defines elder abuse as "the willful infliction of pain, injury, or mental anguish." This definition has been adopted, and/or modified, by many state protective service agencies that investigate cases of abuse. Table 125-1 lists other representative definitions and examples of elder mistreatment. An important feature of elder mistreatment, and other forms of family violence, is that multiple types of mistreatment, such as physical and verbal abuse, neglect, and financial exploitation frequently coexist in the same abuser–victim dyad.

Virtually all experts, clinicians, and reasonable lay persons will agree that egregious instances of physical violence such as punching, hitting, slapping, or assaulting an older person with a gun or other weapon is elder abuse. The most contentious definitional (and clinical) area relates to elder neglect, because the term neglect immediately implies that a caregiving obligation—such as providing food, medicines, or care—has not been met. This, in turn, raises difficult questions that must, with clinical judgment and experience, be considered in the context of the older adult's environment. For example, what are reasonable community standards for the frequency of bathing an assaultive spouse with Alzheimers disease? Does that standard change if the designated caregiver also suffers from chronic diseases that precludes perfect hygiene for their impaired family member? What if this inadequate care enables the "victim" to live at home long after other families would have considered nursing home placement? Who exactly is the responsible caretaker, especially when multiple adult children are available to assume that role, but only one has "stepped up" because of birth order or some other arbitrary circumstance? And is it fair to label that adult child an "elder neglector" when caregiving becomes physically impossible without the assistance of siblings?

These difficult questions also highlight the fact that clinicians caring for elder abuse victims often find themselves working closely with alleged perpetrators of abuse and neglect, as these individuals are often the primary caregivers.

EPIDEMIOLOGY

However it is defined, elder mistreatment is common. Over the past 15 years, several prevalence studies have been conducted in different countries. These studies have used primarily self-report for case finding and validated family violence scales for case definition. Pillemer and Finkelhor conducted the most commonly cited study in the United States. Surveying residents of metropolitan Boston by telephone, the investigators calculated a prevalence of 32 per 1000 population (i.e., 3.2 percent of the 2010 individuals surveyed reported having been victims of elder mistreatment at least once since turning age 65 years). In this study, cases of abuse exceeded cases of neglect. This estimate is consistent with that calculated in a number of similar studies throughout the world, with prevalences generally in the 2 to 5 percent range.

A less-consistent epidemiologic picture emerges when one attempts to discern risk factors for elder mistreatment from the literature (Table 125-2). The most consistent findings relate to the relationship of the abuser to victim; most studies report that spouses and adult children are the most common perpetrators. Studies also show that when adult children are the abusers, sons and daughters are often equally implicated, and at least one study has found daughters to be the more common abuser. These findings must be viewed cautiously in that women are far more likely to be the de facto or designated care providers to frail older adults and are, therefore, more "at risk" for being accused of mistreatment should caregiving fall short of any arbitrary standard.

The most discordant literature is in the area of victim risk factors. Here the literature has produced inconsistent

Table 125-1 Some Representative Definitions of Elder Mistreatment

Mistreatment Category	Definition	Examples
Physical abuse	Acts of violence that may result in pain, injury, impairment, or disease	• Pushing, striking, slapping, force-feeding • Incorrect positioning • Improper use of restraints or medications • Sexual coercion or assault
Neglect	The failure to provide the goods or services necessary for optimal functioning or to avoid harm	• Withholding of health maintenance care • Failure to provide physical aids such as eyeglasses, hearing aids, false teeth • Failure to provide safety precautions
Financial or material abuse	The misuse of the elderly person's income or resources for the financial or personal gain of a caretaker or advisor	• Denying the older person a home • Stealing money or possessions • Coercing the older person into signing contracts
Psychological or verbal abuse	Conduct that causes mental anguish	• Verbal berating, harassment, or intimidation • Threats of punishment or deprivation • Treating the older person like an infant • Isolating the older person from others

SOURCE: Adapted from American Medical Association Diagnostic and Treatment Guidelines on Elder Abuse and Neglect.

findings with respect to gender, functional disability, cognitive impairment, social network, and a variety of other factors proffered by elder abuse theorists. A particularly contentious area has been spawned by the "dependency theory" of mistreatment which holds that mistreatment occurs when the victim becomes inordinately dependent upon the caregiver for a variety of medical and nonmedical needs. Again, studies show an inconsistent relationship between functional disability and elder mistreatment. In fact, a more consistent finding in the literature is the converse; the perpetrators are often dependent upon the victims for financial support and housing.

The disparate findings probably derive from two major factors. The first is the methodologic quality of the studies, which have been highly variable and rife with susceptibility and other biases. The second relates to the heterogeneous nature of elder abuse cases. Elderly protective services workers and clinicians experienced in elder mistreatment know that the term elder mistreatment subsumes many situations—abusive spousal relationships that have "aged," caregivers to dementia patients who lash out in frustration, and physically abusive adult children with poorly managed mental health or substance abuse problems, are but a few examples. Epidemiologic studies that attempt to discern risk factors without acknowledging this reality probably are measuring an "average" effect.

Whatever risk factors are identified in previous and future research, it should not foster a complacency wherein an absence or paucity of such factors causes the clinician to lower his or her guard. Elder mistreatment crosses all ethnic and socioeconomic boundaries, and a high index of clinical suspicion is paramount for identification.

PATHOPHYSIOLOGY

Theories of elder mistreatment abound; three deserve detailed treatment here, because they may have clinical relevance with regard to the types of interventions contemplated in confirmed cases of mistreatment. The most commonly cited theory contends that family violence is a learned behavior, and that abused children grow up to potentially abuse not only their children, but also perhaps spouses and their parents. This is sometimes referred to as the transgenerational violence theory of mistreatment.

The dependency theory of mistreatment holds that abuse is fostered by situations in which victims have a degree of functional and/or cognitive disability that results in activities of daily living (ADL) impairment and overwhelming care needs. Closely associated with this paradigm is another theory—that of the "stressed caregiver."

The psychopathology of the abuser theory shifts focus away from the victim and argues that elder mistreatment is firmly rooted in mental health problems of the abuser. Examples include personality disorders, poorly or undertreated schizophrenia, alcoholism, and other substance abuse problems.

Discerning the underlying causes of elder mistreatment is essential in fashioning an intervention plan (see "Treatment" later in this chapter).

PRESENTATION

For a variety of reasons, the identification of elder mistreatment is one of the most difficult clinical challenges in geriatric medicine. First, many chronic diseases whose

Table 125-2 Possible Risk Factors for Elder Mistreatment

Factor	Mechanism
Victim poor health and functional impairment	Disability reduces elder's ability to seek help and/or defend self.
Cognitive impairment	Aggression toward caregiver and disruptive behaviors resulting from dementia precipitate abuse. Higher rates of abuse have been found among dementia patients.
Abuser deviance	Abusers likely to abuse alcohol or drugs and to have serious mental illness, which, in turn, leads to abusive behavior.
Abuser dependency	Abusers are very likely to depend on the victim financially, for housing, and in other areas. Abuse results from relative's (especially adult children's) attempts to obtain resources from the elder.
Living arrangement	Abuse much less likely among elders living alone. A shared living situation provides greater opportunities for tension and conflict that generally precede abusive incidents.
External stress	Stressful life events and chronic financial strain decrease the family's resistance and increase likelihood of abuse.
Social isolation	Elders with fewer social contacts more likely to be victims. Isolation reduces the likelihood that abuse will be detected and stopped. In addition, social support can buffer against the impact of stress.
History of violence	Particularly among spouses, prior history of violence in the relationship may be predictive of elder abuse in later life.

SOURCE: Reprinted with permission from Lachs MS, Pillemer K: Current concepts: Abuse and neglect of elderly persons. *N Engl J Med* 332:437, 1995.

prevalence is high in older adults may have clinical manifestations that mimic abuse. If elder abuse is present, the clinician may ascribe those findings to chronic disease rather than family violence. If elder abuse is absent, the clinician may erroneously attribute findings from another disease to elder mistreatment. Second, the setting in which an elder mistreatment evaluation occurs is often quite challenging . The environment may be hurried (e.g., the emergency department), and the presence of the suspected abuser only adds pressure to what is already likely to be a stressful encounter. Lastly, the competent identification and management of mistreatment propels the clinician into a world that he or she is likely to be unfamiliar with—a world that includes mandatory reporting statutes, adult protective service workers, and a criminal justice system with a vocabulary that is foreign to many medical professionals. Given these educational, emotional, and systematic obstacles, it is not surprising that elder mistreatment often is missed or unreported in the context of "customary care."

Thus, clinicians need to consider elder mistreatment in the differential diagnosis of many or most of the clinical presentations they encounter. Fractures may result from osteoporosis or force or both. Depression may be related to neurotransmitter imbalances or a hopeless abusive environment. Malnutrition may be the result of any number of chronic illnesses inexorably worsening, or from the withholding of sustenance.

Dramatic injuries or neglect pose no particular diagnostic challenge. Fractures, burns, contusions, and lacerations, particularly when a credible history accompanies,

immediately lead to the diagnosis. On the other extreme, subtle presentations that mimic chronic disease are highly challenging. Examples include chronic diseases that frequently decompensate despite a care plan and adequate resources (e.g., repeated emergency room visits for congestive heart failure or chronic obstructive pulmonary disease [COPD] exacerbation). Indeed, because elder mistreatment can be defined so broadly, there are very few presenting signs or symptoms in the geriatric patient for which elder mistreatment is not in the differential diagnosis.

Many instruments have been devised for the screening or evaluation of elder mistreatment, but they are not applicable to all settings and have not been validated against some external standard, because this would be difficult to create. Rather, they can serve as useful "checklists" for a thorough evaluation. Table 125-3 suggests a system-by-system approach. The importance of heightened awareness cannot be overemphasized in considering the diagnosis. Not infrequently, clues about potential mistreatment come from ancillary staff who observe the abuser–victim dyad away from the physician (e.g., office reception staff, visiting nurses). A general sense that something is amiss in the patient's environment (such as caustic interaction between parties, poor hygiene or dress, frequently missed medical appointments, or failure to adhere with a clearly designated treatment strategy) can all be important clues.

Patient and alleged perpetrator should be interviewed separately and alone. Although there is an emerging consensus that patients of all ages should be routinely screened for family violence, an optimal strategy or instrument has

Table 125-3　Potential Clinical Manifestations of Mistreatment and Assessment

Target	Assessment
History from elder	Interview patient alone; direct inquiries regarding physical violence, restraints, or neglect; precise details about nature, frequency and severity of events Functional status (independence with activities of daily living [ADL]) Who is designated caregiver if ADL impairment is present?
History from abuser	Should also be interviewed alone; best left to professionals with experience in this area; avoid confrontation in the information gathering phase. Interview other sources if possible Recent psychosocial factors (bereavement, financial stresses) Caregiver understanding of patient's illness (care needs, prognosis, etc.) Caregiver explanations for injuries or physical findings
Behavioral observation	Withdrawal Infantalizing of patient by caregiver Caregiver who insists on providing the history
General appearance	Hygiene Cleanliness and appropriateness of dress
Skin/mucous membranes	Skin turgor, other signs of dehydration; multiple skin lesions in various stages of evolution Bruises, decubiti; how established skin lesions have been cared for
Head and neck	Traumatic alopecia (distinguishable from male pattern alopecia on a basis of distribution) Scalp hematomas Lacerations, abrasions
Trunk	Bruises, welts; shape may suggest implement (e.g., iron/belt)
Genitourinary	Rectal bleeding Vaginal bleeding Decubiti, infestations
Extremities	Wrists or ankle lesions suggest restraint use or immersion burn (stocking/glove distribution)
Musculoskeletal	Examine for occult fracture, pain; observe gait
Neurologic/psychiatric	Thorough evaluation to assess focality Depressive symptoms, anxiety
Mental status	Formal mental status testing (e.g., Mini-Mental State Examination); cognitive impairment suggests delirium or dementia and plays a role in assessing decision-making capacity Psychiatric symptoms including delusions and hallucinations
Imaging	As indicated from the clinical evaluation
Laboratory	As indicated from the clinical evaluation (drug levels) Albumin, blood urea nitrogen, and creatinine toxicology
Social and financial resources	Other members of social network available to assist the elder; financial resources Crucial in considering interventions that include alternate-living arrangements and home services

SOURCE: Reprinted with permission from Lachs MS, Pillemer K: Current concepts: Abuse and neglect of elderly persons. *N Engl J Med* 332:437, 1995.

not emerged. Patients should be asked candidly and calmly about the etiology of any unexplained injuries or other findings. Often patients are at first unwilling to speak candidly about being an elder abuse victim for reasons of embarrassment, shame, or fear of retribution from the perpetrator who is not infrequently a caregiver.

Interview of the suspected abuser is a tricky and potentially dangerous undertaking. On the one extreme, elder abusers who are presented with an empathetic, nonjudgmental ear to describe their stresses and actions will sometimes describe their situations at great length and in great detail. On the other hand, all forms of domestic abuse share

Table 125-4   Safety Plan for Victims of Elder Mistreatment or Other Victims of Family Violence with Capacity Who Insist on Remaining in an Abusive Environment

Time Frame	Activity
Prior to violent or abusive episode	Recognize patterns that lead to abusive behavior (e.g., abuser alcohol use).
	Determine who in the social network is available to assist when such an episode occurs through explicit conversations with neighbors, friends, other relatives.
	Be aware of elder domestic violence programs, shelters, and other resources in the local community available to assist; know their contact numbers.
	Have essential resources readily available if the patient needs to leave quickly (e.g., money, ATM cards, credit cards, drivers license, keys, identification, social security card, other important documents).
	Practice implementing safety plan (e.g., mock 911 call). Consider creating a "code" with a friend or neighbor so that the patient can communicate danger in the presence of the abuser.
During violent or abusive episode	Implement safety plan quickly and with discretion.
	Consider appeasing abuser briefly (if this does not cause a danger) so that safety plan may be implemented.
	Use of self-protective behaviors such as a weapon should be considered with the utmost caution.
After violent or abusive episode	Recognize that family violence is a chronic problem that usually recurs and escalates.
	Change locks as soon as possible.
	Strongly consider order of protection.
	Let neighbors and landlord know that abusive individual no longer lives in the home.

a pattern wherein abusers gain and control access to their victims. An elder abuser graphically confronted with allegations of mistreatment may move to sequester a frail victim in such a way that a frail isolated older adult loses access to critically needed medical and social services. Whenever possible, assistance from providers skilled in elder abuse evaluation and management should be enlisted to assist in such undertakings.

Treatment/Management

There are no randomized intervention studies of reasonable quality on elder mistreatment, and the clinician confronted with a confirmed case is best served by a resourceful approach that combines experience, clinical judgment, and local resources. A dogmatic or algorithmic approach to all elder mistreatment cases ignores the enormous heterogeneity of the entity, including the type(s) of mistreatment being concurrently perpetrated, the underlying mechanisms, patient comorbidities, caregiver burden issues, and the available resources (both familial and community) that can be brought to bear on the issue. A more sensible approach may be the multipronged strategy increasingly used to treat other geriatric syndromes that have multifactorial etiologies. The paradigm may be a useful one in that elder mistreatment can be likened to geriatric syndromes. That is, there may be multiple "host" and environmental contributors, decompensation may be accelerated by other medical and social problems, and some of the contributors may be more remediable than others. The physical elder abuse

victim with severe COPD and an abusive schizophrenic child-caregiver will need an entirely different series of interventions than the dementing spouse who has suffered life-long domestic violence that is now worsening.

The first step in confronting any confirmed case of family violence is insuring the safety of the victim. First, the immediate threat of danger to the victim should be ascertained. Even if there is no immediate threat, a *safety plan* is critical in the management of all forms of family violence (Table 125-4). What are the specific steps the victim should take if the perpetrator of mistreatment becomes acutely violent? Options include calling the local police department, accessing shelters, emergency department use/hospital admission, or respite care in some evolved systems of long-term care. Additionally, in most states, cases of elder abuse must be reported to adult protective services agencies. This typically results in a home visit to adjudicate the veracity of such a report. State protective service agencies vary widely with respect to their caseloads and available resources; ideally a coordinated approach that brings to bear their expertise and resources in collaboration with the physician and multidisciplinary team produces the best response.

However, the safety plan paradigm will have limited utility in many cases of elder mistreatment because of victim frailty and/or cognitive impairment that limits the use of self-protective behaviors. Frequently, physicians find themselves in the predicament of caring for an elder mistreatment victim who lacks capacity. Here the likely intervention will involve the appointment of a guardian in collaboration with adult protective service agencies or other elder social service programs in the community that serve such functions. In such a proceeding, the physician's role is to provide objective evidence that documents the lack of decision-making capacity. The physician may also have a role in ensuring the alleged perpetrator of mistreatment does not become the guardian.

One of the most frustrating situations for professionals working with victims of family violence is the individual who retains decision-making capacity but insists on remaining in an abusive environment. Here the physician's role is to educate the patient about the tendency of family violence to escalate and to review the safety plan created. The physician should also explain to the patient that even if services are refused, the doctor remains an important and available resource, should the situation change.

Special Situations

Elder mistreatment may also occur in institutional settings, and the physician has a role in detecting these cases as well. Substantial regulatory safeguards have been progressively enacted since the 1970s to protect residents of long-term care facilities; these include mandatory criminal background checks of all employees, ombudsman programs to adjudicate complaints of mistreatment, and components of the omnibus budget reconciliation act of 1987, which includes residents rights provisions (e.g., minimization of restraints). In some contexts, the failure to create or follow a reasonable plan of care for the long-term care residents may be viewed as abusive or neglectful. One recent area of interest has been abuse and neglect that occurs in nonnursing home long-term care environments (e.g. assisted-living and board and care environments), because these facilities generally are under considerably less regulation.

Physicians have an important role in the detection of these institutional cases, as they may see potential manifestations of nursing home elder mistreatment in facilities or emergency departments as part of providing customary care.

SUMMARY

Elder mistreatment is a prevalent problem with many potential manifestations. The epidemiology of injuries and other clinical findings are not completely understood, but this does not preclude the clinician from taking an active role in its detection and management. Studies show elder mistreatment victims to be at substantial independent risk of death and quality-of-life decline, and the syndrome should be afforded the same vigilance that physicians devote to other "traditional" medical problems in geriatrics.

REFERENCES

American Medical Association Diagnostic and Treatment Guidelines on Elder Abuse and Neglect. Chicago, 1992.

Johnson T: *Elder Mistreatment: Deciding Who is at Risk.* Westport CT, Greenwood Press, 1991.

Lachs MS et al: Risk factors for reported elder abuse and neglect: A nine-year observational study. *Gerontologist* 37(4):469, 1997.

Lachs MS et al: The mortality of elder mistreatment. *JAMA* 280:428, 1988.

Pillemer K, Finkelhor D: The prevalence of elder abuse: A random sample survey. *Gerontologist* 28:51, 1988.

I N D E X

Parkinsonism from, 221
policy issues in, 228
prescribing in, approach to, 228–230,
229t
current therapies in, 228–229, 229t
discontinuation of potentially
unnecessary therapy in, 229
dose reduction in, 230
nonpharmacologic approaches in,
229–230
prescription
misuse of, 87
prescribing of, 98
cascades of, 221–223, 223f
in nursing homes, 207
quality of, 220–221, 222t
on sexuality, 1280
underuse of beneficial therapy in,
223–225
with beta-blocker therapy post MI,
224
with hypertension, 223–224
opioid analgesia and cancer pain in,
224
for osteoporosis, 224
warfarin in atrial fibrillation and,
224–225
use of (See Drug therapy)
Dual-energy x-ray absorptiometry, for
bone mineral density, validity
of, 133
Ductal carcinoma in situ, 688–689
"Dumping syndrome," 638
Duodenal disorders
H. pylori infection, 628–630, 629t
peptic ulcer disease, 630–633 (See also
Peptic ulcer disease)
Duodenitis, acute erosive, 633
Durable power of attorney, 354–355
Dying patient, 323–334
depression in, 328, 330t–331t
end-of-life decision making in,
facilitating, 325–326, 326t
hospice for, 332–334, 333f
management of specific symptoms in,
326–332, 328t
anorexia and weight loss, 329
constipation, 329
depression, 328, 330t–331t
dyspnea, 329
general principles, 326, 327t
nausea and vomiting, 329
other, 329, 332
pain, 326–328, 328t
palliative care for, 323–325, 332–334,
333t
approach to, 323–325, 324f, 325t
definition of, 323
history of, 323, 324t
Dysequilibrium, 1544
Dyskinesias, levodopa-induced, 1407
Dyslipidemia. See Dyslipoproteinemia
Dyslipoproteinemia, 875–890
in diabetes mellitus, 428
epidemiology of, 876, 878–879,
879f
exercise on, 940–941

hyperlipoproteinemia
classification of, 876, 879t
elevated LDL-C, 882, 882f
elevated total, 882, 882f
epidemiology of, 876, 878–879, 879f
mechanisms of, 879–881, 880f
subclasses of, 876, 879t
hypocholesterolemia, 881
intervention trials on, 884–887
cholesterol management in, 887,
889t
hormone replacement therapy in,
886–887
lifestyle in, 884–885, 885t
pharmacologic, 886
lipoprotein risk factors for CHD and,
881–884
apolipoprotein E4 allele, 883–884
atherogenic LDL pattern B
phenotype, 883
elevated total, 882, 882f
homocysteine, elevated, 884
LDL-C
elevated, 882, 882f
reduced, 882–883
Lp(a), elevated, 884
mechanisms of, 879–881, 880f
diet change in, 880
lipid metabolism changes in, 881
physical fitness declines in, 880–881
total and central adiposity increases
in, 880
screening and treatment of, 887–890,
887f–890t
Cholesterol Education Program
Adult Treatment Panel III report
in, 887–889, 888t
Framingham Risk Score for,
887–889, 888t
hypertriglyceridemia in, 889–890
with no risk factors, 889
Dyspareunia, 1297–1298
Dysphagia, 613–622. See also Swallowing
algorithm for, 613, 614f
assessment tools for, 1194–1195, 1194t
definition of, 1193
differential considerations for,
1202–1206
etiologies in, 1202–1205
conditions in, 1202–1203
disease in, 1203–1205, 1203t,
1204t
medications in, 1204, 1204t
warning signs in, 1203, 1204t
symptoms in, 1205–1206, 1205t
esophageal, 593–594, 617–622
achalasia in, 617–619, 618f
causes of, 617, 617t
dysphagia aortica in, 621
esophageal cancer in, 620
infections of esophagus in, 621
medication-induced, 620–621
peptic stricture in, 620, 620f
rings and webs in, 620–621
scleroderma in, 620
spastic esophageal motor disorders
in, 619–620, 619f

impact of, 1193–1195
interventions for, 1209–1211
compensatory, 1209–1210
rehabilitative, 1210–1211
medical management of, in subacute
care, 189–190, 190t
oropharyngeal, 593–594, 613–617
causes of, 613–616, 615t
central nervous system, 613–615,
615t
local structural lesions, 615, 615t
other neuromuscular, 615, 615t
sphincter dysfunction, 615–616
Zenker diverticulum, 616, 616t
diagnosis of, 613, 614f
evaluation of, 616
treatment of, 616–617
prevention of, 1211–1212
mealtime atmosphere in, 1211
medications in, 1211
oral hygiene in, 1211
oral vs. nonoral intake in, 1211–1212
screening for, 1206
senescent swallowing in, 1199–1202
changes in, 1199–1201,
1200f–1201f, 1202t
neurophysiologic correlates of, 1202
team approach to, 1206–1209
instrumental examination in,
1207–1208
screening form for, 1206, 1207t
swallowing assessment in
fiberoptic endoscopic evaluation,
1209
focused, 1206
noninstrumental, 1206–1207,
1208t
oropharyngeal videofluoroscopic,
1208–1209
summary of, 1209
Dysphagia aortica, 621
Dysplastic nevi, 758, 758f, 759f
Dyspnea. See also Breathing
in dying patient, 329
Dysthymia, 1444, 1444t
Dystrophies
facioscapulohumeral, 1007
late-onset limb girdle, 1007
oculopharyngeal, 1007

E
Ear. See also Auditory changes
anatomy and physiology of,
1241–1243, 1242f–1243f
Early diastolic filling, 413
Early-onset aging, and familial
Alzheimer's disease, 24
Economic assessment, 104
Ectopy
atrial, epidemiology of, 475–476
ventricular, 478f, 481
epidemiology of, 475–476
management of, 478f, 481
EGb 761, for dementia, 235
Elder mistreatment. See Mistreatment,
elder
Elderly ratio, 57–59, 57f

COLLEGE OF OSTEOPATHIC MEDICINE
LEARNING CENTER

ISBN 0-07-140216-0

90000

9 780071 402163

Principles of Geriatric Medicine & Gerontology